TEXTBOOK OF
Gastroenterology

VOLUME ONE

EDITOR
TADATAKA YAMADA, MD

*John G. Searle Professor and Chairman, Department of
Internal Medicine, Professor of Physiology, Physician-in-Chief,
University of Michigan Medical Center, Ann Arbor, Michigan*

ASSOCIATE EDITORS
DAVID H. ALPERS, MD

*Professor of Medicine, Chief, Gastroenterology Division, Washington University
School of Medicine, St. Louis, Missouri*

CHUNG OWYANG, MD

*Professor of Internal Medicine, Division Chief of Gastroenterology, University
of Michigan Medical Center, Ann Arbor, Michigan*

DON W. POWELL, MD

*The Edward Randall and Edward Randall, Jr. Chair in Internal Medicine,
Professor and Chairman of Internal Medicine, Professor of Physiology and
Biophysics, The University of Texas Medical Branch Hospitals at Galveston,
Galveston, Texas*

FRED E. SILVERSTEIN, MD

*Professor of Medicine, University of Washington School of Medicine,
Seattle, Washington*

J.B. LIPPINCOTT COMPANY
Philadelphia

New York   London   Hagerstown

Acquisitions Editor: Dean Manke
Developmental Editor: Richard Winters
Project Editors: Marian A. Bellus and Melissa McElroy
Indexer: Maria Coughlin
Designer: Susan Hess Blaker
Design Coordinator: Doug Smock
Production Manager: Caren Erlichman
Production Coordinator: Kevin P. Johnson
Compositor: TAPSCO, Inc.
Printer/Binder: The Courier Book Co./Westford

6 5 4 3 2

Library of Congress Cataloging-in-Publication Data

Textbook of gastroenterology/editor, Tadataka Yamada; associate
  editors, David H. Alpers . . . [et al.].
      p.   cm.
    Includes bibliographical references.
    Includes index.
    ISBN 0-397-51227-9 (vol 1).—ISBN 0-397-50978-2 (2 vol set)
    1. Gastroenterology.   2. Gastrointestinal system—Diseases.
  I. Yamada, Tadataka.   II. Alpers, David H.
    [DNLM: 1. Gastrointestinal Diseases.   WI 100 T3551]
  RC801.T48   1991
  616.3'3—dc20
  DNLM/DLC
  for Library of Congress   90-6386
                                                                CIP

The authors and publisher have exerted every effort to ensure that drug selection and dosage set forth in this text are in accord with current recommendations and practice at the time of publication. However, in view of ongoing research, changes in government regulations, and the constant flow of information relating to drug therapy and drug reactions, the reader is urged to check the package insert for each drug for any change in indications and dosage and for added warnings and precautions. This is particularly important when the recommended agent is a new or infrequently employed drug.

CONTRIBUTORS

ANTOINE ADENIS, MD

Assistant, Department of Medical Oncology, Centre Oscar
Lambret, Lille Cedex, France

DAVID A. AHLQUIST, MD

Associate Professor, Mayo Medical School, Consultant in
Gastroenterology, Mayo Clinic, Rochester, Minnesota

DENNIS J. AHNEN, MD

Associate Professor of Medicine, University of Colorado
School of Medicine, Staff Physician and Chief, Section of
Gastroenterology, Denver Veterans Affairs Medical Center,
Denver, Colorado

NAOMI P. ALAZRAKI, MD

Professor of Radiology, Emory University School of
Medicine, Co-Director of Nuclear Medicine, Emory
University Hospital, Chief, Nuclear Medicine, Veterans
Affairs Hospital, Atlanta, Georgia

MICHAEL B. ALBERT, MD

Assistant Professor of Medicine, George Washington
University Medical Center, Washington, DC

DAVID H. ALPERS, MD

Professor of Medicine, Chief, Gastroenterology Division,
Washington University School of Medicine, St. Louis,
Missouri

SINN ANURAS, MD, PE

Professor of Medicine, Director, Division of
Gastroenterology, Texas Tech University Health Sciences
Center, Vice-President, University Medical Center,
Lubbock, Texas

DAVID C. AUTH, PhD

Professor of Bioengineering, University of Washington
School of Medicine, Seattle, Washington, Chairman, Heart
Technology, Inc., Bellevue, Washington

MARK W. BABYATSKY, MD

Research Fellow, Harvard Medical School, Massachusetts
General Hospital, Boston, Massachusetts

DENNIS M. BALFE, MD

Associate Professor of Radiology, Chief, Gastrointestinal
Radiology, Washington University School of Medicine,
Barnes Hospital, St. Louis, Missouri

JEFFREY L. BARNETT, MD

Assistant Professor of Internal Medicine, Division of
Gastroenterology, University of Michigan Medical School,
Ann Arbor, Michigan

RICHARD L. BARON, MD

Professor of Radiology, University of Pittsburgh School of
Medicine, Director of Body CT/MR, Presbyterian
University Hospital, Pittsburgh, Pennsylvania

KIM E. BARRETT, PhD

Assistant Professor of Medicine in Residence, University of
California, San Diego, School of Medicine, San Diego,
California

JOSE BEHAR, MD

Professor of Medicine, Division of Biomedical Sciences,
Brown University, Associate Director, Division of
Gastroenterology, Rhode Island Hospital, Providence,
Rhode Island

STANLEY BERNARD BENJAMIN, MD

Professor of Medicine, Chief, Division of Gastroenterology,
Georgetown University Hospital, Washington, DC

PIERO BIANCANI, PhD

Professor of Medicine, Brown University, Rhode Island
Hospital, Providence, Rhode Island

EDGAR C. BOEDEKER, MD

Associate Professor of Medicine, Uniformed Service,
University of the Health Sciences, Chief, Gastroenterology
Division, Walter Reed Army Institute of Research, Walter
Reed Army Medical Center, Washington, DC

C. RICHARD BOLAND, MD

Associate Professor of Internal Medicine, Division of Gastroenterology, University of Michigan Medical School, Chief, Gastroenterology Section, Veterans Affairs Medical Center, Ann Arbor, Michigan

JOEL C. BORNSTEIN, PhD

NH and MRC, Research Fellow and Senior Lecturer, Physiology Department, Flinders University School of Medicine, Bedford Park, Australia

GREGORY A. BOYCE, MD

Assistant Professor of Medicine, Division of Digestive Diseases and Nutrition, University of South Florida College of Medicine, Tampa, Florida

H. WORTH BOYCE, JR., MD

Professor of Medicine, Director, The Center for Swallowing Disorders, Department of Internal Medicine, Division of Digestive Diseases and Nutrition, University of South Florida College of Medicine, Tampa, Florida

EUGENE M. BOZYMSKI, MD

Professor of Medicine, Co-Chief, Division of Digestive Diseases and Nutrition, University of North Carolina at Chapel Hill School of Medicine, Attending Physician, University of North Carolina Hospitals, Chapel Hill, North Carolina

THOMAS A. BRASITUS, MD

Walter Lincoln Palmer Distinguished Service Professor of Medicine, University of Chicago, Director, Section of Gastroenterology/Nutrition, University of Chicago Hospitals and Clinics, Chicago, Illinois

JEFFREY J. BROWN, MD

Assistant Professor of Radiology, Mallinckrodt Institute of Radiology, Washington University School of Medicine, St. Louis, Missouri

JEAN MARC BRUNETEAUD, MD

Associate Professor of Medicine, Lille School of Medicine, Hospital Claudia Hureiez, La Madeleine, France

GREGORY B. BULKLEY, MD

Mark W. Ravitch Professor of Surgery, Associate Professor, Department of Surgery, Johns Hopkins University School of Medicine, Baltimore, Maryland

RANDALL W. BURT, MD

Associate Professor of Medicine, University of Utah School of Medicine, Salt Lake City, Utah

RICARD CALABUIG, MD

Postdoctoral Fellow, Servei de Crrurdia General Hospital de la Santa Creui Sant Pau, Universitat Autonoma de Barcelona, Barcelona, Spain

DONALD O. CASTELL, MD

Rorer Professor of Medicine, Director, Division of Gastroenterology and Hepatology, Jefferson Medical College, Philadelphia, Pennsylvania

KYUNG J. CHO, MD

Professor of Radiology, Director, Division of Cardiovascular Radiology, University of Michigan Medical School, Ann Arbor, Michigan

SITA CHOKHAVATIA, MD

Assistant Professor, Department of Internal Medicine, Division of Gastroenterology, Texas Tech University Health Sciences Center, Lubbock, Texas

JAMES CHRISTENSEN, MD

Professor of Internal Medicine, University of Iowa College of Medicine, University of Iowa Hospitals and Clinics, Iowa City, Iowa

PAUL E. CHRISTIAN, CNMT

University of Utah, Salt Lake City, Utah

RAY E. CLOUSE, MD

Associate Professor of Medicine, Washington University School of Medicine, Associate Physician, Barnes Hospital, St. Louis, Missouri

THOMAS J. COLTURI, MD

Assistant Professor of Internal Medicine, Section of Gastroenterology, Medical College of Ohio, Member, Gastroenterology Consultants of Northwest Ohio, Toledo, Ohio

DAVID H. B. CORT, MD

Consultant in Gastroenterology, St. Luke's Hospital, St. Louis, Missouri

DAVID W. CRABB, MD

Associate Professor of Medicine and Biochemistry, Indiana University School of Medicine, Indianapolis, Indiana

KAREN D. CRISSINGER, MD, PhD

Assistant Professor of Pediatrics and Physiology, Division of Pediatric Gastroenterology and Nutrition, Louisiana State University Medical Center, Shreveport, Louisiana

DARYL F. DAUGHERTY, MD

Assistant Professor of Internal Medicine, Division of Gastroenterology, University of Michigan Medical School, Ann Arbor, Michigan

NICHOLAS O. DAVIDSON, MD

Associate Professor of Medicine, University of Chicago Hospitals and Clinics, Chicago, Illinois

HAILE T. DEBAS, MD, FRCS(C)

Professor and Chairman, Chief of Surgery, Department of General Surgery, University of California San Francisco School of Medicine, San Francisco, California

JOHN DEL VALLE, MD

Assistant Professor of Internal Medicine, Division of
Gastroenterology, University of Michigan Medical Center,
Ann Arbor, Michigan

KIERTISIN DHARMSATHAPHORN, MD

Associate Professor of Medicine, University of California,
San Diego Attending Physician, University of California,
San Diego Medical Center, San Diego, California

CHARLES D. DIETZEN, MD

Assistant Professor of Surgery, Louisiana State University
School of Medicine, New Orleans, Louisiana

EUGENE P. DIMAGNO, MD

Professor of Medicine, Mayo Medical School, Consultant in
Gastroenterology, Mayo Clinic and Foundation, Rochester,
Minnesota

WILLIAM O. DOBBINS, III, MD

Professor of Internal Medicine, University of Michigan
Medical School, Gastroenterologist, Veterans Affairs
Medical Center, Ann Arbor, Michigan

DOUGLAS A. DROSSMAN, MD

Professor of Medicine and Psychiatry, Division of Digestive
Diseases and Nutrition, University of North Carolina at
Chapel Hill, Attending Physician, University of North
Carolina Hospitals, Chapel Hill, North Carolina

QUAN-YANG DUH, MD

Assistant Professor of Surgery, University of California San
Francisco School of Medicine, Veterans Administration
Medical Center, San Francisco, California

HERBERT L. DUPONT, MD

Mary W. Kelsey Professor and Director, Center for
Infectious Diseases, The University of Texas Health Science
Center at Houston, Medical School and School of Public
Health, Attending Physician, Internal Medicine, Hermann
Hospital, Houston, Texas

GREGORY L. EASTWOOD, MD

Professor of Medicine, Dean, School of Medicine, Medical
College of Georgia, Augusta, Georgia

GRACE H. ELTA, MD

Associate Professor of Internal Medicine, Division of
Gastroenterology, University of Michigan Medical School,
Ann Arbor, Michigan

WENDY R. EWART, MD

Senior Lecturer in Physiology, The London Hospital
Medical College, Associate Director, Gastrointestinal
Science Research Unit, The London Hospital, London,
England

WILLIAM A. FAJMAN, MD

Associate Professor of Radiology, Emory University School
of Medicine, Atlanta, Georgia

ANDREW P. FEINBERG, MD, MPH

Associate Professor, Department of Internal Medicine and
Human Genetics, University of Michigan Medical School,
Attending Physician, University of Michigan Hospital, Ann
Arbor, Michigan

JAMES W. FRESTON, MD, PhD

Professor and Chairman, Department of Medicine,
University of Connecticut School of Medicine, John
Dempsey Hospital, University of Connecticut Health
Center, Farmington, Connecticut

HANS FROMM, MD

Professor of Medicine, Director, Division of
Gastroenterology and Nutrition, George Washington
University Medical Center, Washington, DC

JOHN B. FURNESS, PhD

Professor, Chief Hospital Scientist, Flinders Medical Center,
Bedford Park, Australia

J. E. GEENEN, MD

Clinical Professor of Medicine, Division of
Gastroenterology, Medical College of Wisconsin,
Milwaukee, Wisconsin, Director, Digestive Disease Center,
St. Luke's Hospital, Racine, Wisconsin

MARTIN L. GOLDMAN, MD

Professor of Radiology, University of Washington School of
Medicine, Chief of Vascular and Interventional Radiology,
University of Washington Medical Center, Seattle,
Washington

D. NEIL GRANGER, PhD

Professor and Head of Physiology, Louisiana State
University Medical Center, Shreveport, Louisiana

PETER B. GREGORY, MD

Professor of Medicine (Clinical), Associate Dean—Clinical
Affairs, Medical Director Faculty Practice Program,
Stanford University Medical Center and Clinic, Stanford,
California

RICHARD L. GUERRANT, MD

Professor of Medicine, Head, Division of Geographic
Medicine, University of Virginia School of Medicine,
Attending Physician, University of Virginia Health Science
Center, Charlottesville, Virginia

JORGE J. GUMUCIO, MD

Associate Professor of Internal Medicine, Division of
Gastroenterology, University of Michigan Medical School,
Veterans Affairs Medical Center, Ann Arbor, Michigan

RODGER C. HAGGITT, MD

Professor of Pathology, Adjunct Professor of Medicine,
University of Washington School of Medicine, Director
Hospital Pathology, University of Washington Medical
Center, Seattle, Washington

WILLIAM L. HASLER, MD

Instructor of Internal Medicine, Division of Gastroenterology, University of Michigan Medical School, University of Michigan Medical Center, Ann Arbor, Michigan

WILLIAM D. HEIZER, MD

Professor of Medicine, University of North Carolina at Chapel Hill, Division of Digestive Diseases and Nutrition, School of Medicine, Co-Director, Nutrition Support Service, University of North Carolina Hospitals, Chapel Hill, North Carolina

HANS HERLINGER, MD

Professor of Radiology (Emeritus), Hospital of the University of Pennsylvania, Philadelphia, Pennsylvania

DAVID R. HILL, MD

Assistant Professor of Medicine, Director of International Travelers Medical Service, University of Connecticut School of Medicine, Farmington, Connecticut

BEVERLY HOLCOMBE, PharmD

Clinical Specialist, Nutrition Support Service, Department of Pharmacy, University of North Carolina Hospitals, Clinical Assistant Professor, Division of Pharmacy Practice, School of Pharmacy, University of North Carolina, Chapel Hill, North Carolina

PETER R. HOLT, MD

Professor of Medicine, Columbia University College of Physicians and Surgeons, Chief, Division of Gastroenterology, St. Luke's Hospital Center, New York, New York

K. HUIBREGTSE, MD

Associate Professor of Medicine, University of Amsterdam, Academic Medical Centre, Meiberdreef, The Netherlands

JON I. ISENBERG, MD

Professor of Medicine, University of California, San Diego, School of Medicine, Head, Division of Gastroenterology, University of California San Diego Medical Center, La Jolla, California

DENNIS M. JENSEN, MD

Professor of Medicine, University of California, Los Angeles, School of Medicine, Division of Gastroenterology, UCLA Center for the Health Sciences, Veterans Affairs Medical Center, Los Angeles, California

ROBERT T. JENSEN, MD

Chief, Cell Biology Section, Digestive Diseases Branch, National Institutes of Health, Bethesda, Maryland

GEOFFREY C. JIRANEK, MD

Clinical Assistant Professor of Medicine, Division of Gastroenterology, Department of Medicine, University of Washington, Staff Physician, Virginia Mason Medical Center, Seattle, Washington

JOSEPH L. JORIZZO, MD

Professor and Chairman of Dermatology, Bowman Gray School of Medicine of Wake Forest University, North Carolina Baptist Hospital, Winston-Salem, North Carolina

MARTIN F. KAGNOFF, MD

Professor of Medicine, University of California San Diego School of Medicine, Attending Physician, University of California, San Diego Medical Center, La Jolla, California

NEIL KAPLOWITZ, MD

Professor of Medicine, University of Southern California, School of Medicine, Chief, Division of Gastrointestinal and Liver Diseases, University of Southern California, Los Angeles County Medical Center, Los Angeles, California

KEIICHI KAWAI, MD

Professor of Preventive Medicine, Kyoto Prefectural University of Medicine, Kawaramachi-Hirokoji, Kamigyo-ku, Kyoto, Japan

KEITH A. KELLY, MD

Professor and Chairman of Surgery, Mayo Clinic and Foundation, Mayo Medical School, Consultant in Surgery, Rochester Methodist Hospital, Saint Mary's Hospital, Rochester, Minnesota

PATRICK W. KELLEY, MD

Chief, Department of Advanced Preventive Medicine Studies, Department of Army, Walter Reed Army Institute for Research, Washington, DC

MICHAEL B. KIMMEY, MD

Assistant Professor of Medicine, Division of Gastroenterology, Department of Medicine, Director of Therapeutic Endoscopy, University of Washington Medical Center, Seattle, Washington

NANCY B. KIVIAT, MD

Associate Professor of Pathology, University of Washington School of Medicine, Director of Cytology, Harborview Medical Center, Seattle, Washington

KENNETH B. KLEIN, MD

Research Associate Professor of Medicine, Division of Digestive Diseases and Nutrition, University of North Carolina at Chapel Hill, School of Medicine, Attending Physician, University of North Carolina Memorial Hospitals, Chapel Hill, North Carolina

FREDERICK A. KLIPSTEIN, MD

Professor of Medicine and Microbiology, University of Rochester School of Medicine, Attending Physician, Strong Memorial Hospital, Rochester, New York

DONALD P. KOTLER, MD

Associate Professor of Clinical Medicine, Columbia University, College of Physicians and Surgeons, Associate Attending Physician, St. Luke's-Roosevelt Hospital Center, New York, New York

RICHARD A. KOZAREK, MD

Associate Clinical Professor of Medicine, University of Washington School of Medicine, Chief of Gastroenterology, Virginia Mason Clinic, Seattle, Washington

LOREN LAINE, MD

Assistant Professor of Medicine, University of Southern California School of Medicine, Physician Specialist, Los Angeles County—University of Southern California Medical Center, Los Angeles, California

J. THOMAS LAMONT, MD

Professor of Medicine, Boston University School of Medicine, Chief, Section of Gastroenterology, University Hospital, Boston, Massachusetts

PETER LANCE, MA, MB, MRCP(UK)

Assistant Professor of Medicine, State University of New York at Buffalo, Director, Gastrointestinal Section, Veterans Administration Medical Center, Buffalo, New York

ERIC B. LARSON, MD, MPH

Professor of Medicine, University of Washington Medical School, Medical Director, University of Washington Medical Center, Seattle, Washington

IGOR LAUFER, MD

Professor of Radiology, Chief, Gastrointestinal Radiology, Hospital of the University of Pennsylvania, Philadelphia, Pennsylvania

EMANUEL LEBENTHAL, MD

Professor and Chairman, Department of Pediatrics, Hahnemann University, Philadelphia, Pennsylvania

SUM PING LEE, MD, PhD

Professor of Medicine, University of Washington School of Medicine, Staff Physician, Veterans Administration Medical Center, Seattle, Washington

AARON LERNER, MD

Senior Lecturer in Pediatrics, Faculty of Medicine, Technion Israel Institute of Technology, Haifa, Israel

DOUGLAS S. LEVINE, MD

Assistant Professor of Medicine, Division of Gastroenterology, Department of Medicine, University of Washington, Seattle, Washington

MARC S. LEVINE, MD

Professor of Radiology, Hospital of the University of Pennsylvania, Philadelphia, Pennsylvania

MICHAEL D. LEVITT, MD

Professor of Medicine, University of Minnesota, Associate Chief of Staff for Research, Veterans Administration Medical Center, Minneapolis, Minnesota

ELLEN LI, MD, PhD

Assistant Professor, Division of Gastroenterology, Department of Medicine, Assistant Physician, Barnes Hospital, St. Louis, Missouri

YONG F. LI, MD

Research Scientist, Department of Surgery, The University of Texas Medical School at Houston, Houston, Texas

RODGER A. LIDDLE, MD

Associate Professor of Medicine, Duke University School of Medicine, Chief, Gastroenterology Section, Veterans Administration Medical Center, Durham, North Carolina

CHARLES LIEBOW, DMD, PhD

Professor, Director of Research, Department of Oral and Maxillofacial Surgery, School of Dental Medicine, State University of New York at Buffalo, Buffalo General Hospital, Buffalo, New York

HENRY C. LIN, MD

Assistant Professor of Medicine, University of California Los Angeles, UCLA School of Medicine, Director, Section of Nutrition, Cedars-Sinai Medical Center, Los Angeles, California

MARK L. LLOYD, MD

Assistant Professor of Medicine, University of Wisconsin-Madison School of Medicine, Section of Gastroenterology, University of Wisconsin Hospital and Clinics, Madison, Wisconsin

JERRY F. LONDON, MD

Clinical Instructor of Medicine, Division of Digestive Diseases and Nutrition, University of North Carolina at Chapel Hill, School of Medicine, Attending Physician, University of North Carolina Hospital, Chapel Hill, North Carolina

CHARLES H. LU, MD

Associate Professor of Radiology, University of Iowa College of Medicine, Department of Radiology, University of Iowa Hospitals and Clinics, Iowa City, Iowa

SHELLY C. LU, MD

Assistant Professor of Medicine, University of Southern California School of Medicine, Physician Specialist, Los Angeles County—University of Southern California Medical Center, Los Angeles, California

MICHAEL R. LUCEY, MD, FRCP

Assistant Professor of Internal Medicine, Division of Gastroenterology, University of Michigan School of Medicine, University of Michigan Medical Center, Ann Arbor, Michigan

GORDON D. LUK, MD, PhD

Professor of Medicine and Molecular Biology and Genetics, Wayne State University School of Medicine, Director, Division of Gastroenterology, Harper Hospital/Detroit Medical Center, Detroit, Michigan

RICHARD P. MACDERMOTT, MD

T. Grier Miller Professor of Medicine, Chief, Gastrointestinal Section, Hospital of the University of Pennsylvania, Philadelphia, Pennsylvania

JAMES L. MADARA, MD

Associate Professor of Pathology, Harvard Medical School, Director of Gastrointestinal Pathology, Brigham and Womens Hospital, Boston, Massachusetts

ARTHUR M. MAGUN, MD

Assistant Professor of Medicine, Columbia University, College of Physicians and Surgeons, Associate Attending Presbyterian Hospital, New York, New York

GABRIEL M. MAKHLOUF, MD, PhD, FRCP

Professor of Medicine, Director of Gastroenterology Research, Medical College of Virginia, Virginia Commonwealth University, Richmond, Virginia

PETER MANNON, MD

Associate in Medicine, Duke University Medical Center, Durham, North Carolina

VINCENT MAUNOURY, MD

Centre Multidisciplinaire de Traitement, par Laser, Hopital Huriez, Lille, France

SUZANNE M. MATSUI, MD

Postdoctoral Fellow in Gastroenterology, Stanford University School of Medicine, Stanford, California

GEORGE B. MCDONALD, MD

Gastroenterology/Hepatology Section, Fred Hutchinson Cancer Research Center, University of Washington School of Medicine, Seattle, Washington

DAVID W. MCFADDEN, MD

Assistant Professor of Surgery, University of Cincinnati College of Medicine, University of Cincinnati Medical Center, Cincinnati, Ohio

KENNETH R. MCQUAID, MD

Assistant Clinical Professor of Medicine, Department of Internal Medicine, Division of Gastroenterology, University of California, San Diego School of Medicine, University of California, San Diego Medical Center, La Jolla, California

SHERMAN M. MELLINKOFF, MD

Emeritus Professor and Dean, University of California, Los Angeles, School of Medicine, Los Angeles, California

DMITRI S. MERINE, MD

Assistant Professor of Interventional Radiology, Department of Radiology, The Johns Hopkins Medical Institutions, Baltimore, Maryland

JAMES H. MEYER, MD

Gastrointestinal Section, Veterans Affairs Medical Center, Sepulveda, California

ABRAHAM G. MIRANDA, MD

Instructor of Clinical Medicine, Division of Infectious Diseases, The Hermann Hospital, Houston, Texas

CAROL A. MITTELSTAEDT, MD

Professor of Radiology and Obstetrics and Gynecology, University of North Carolina, School of Medicine, University of North Carolina at Chapel Hill, Director, Ultrasound Section, University of North Carolina Hospitals, Chapel Hill, North Carolina

FRANK G. MOODY, MD

Denton A. Cooley Professor, Chairman, Department of Surgery, The University of Texas Medical School at Houston, Chief of Surgery, The Hermann Hospital, Houston, Texas

JAMES R. MOORE, MD

Assistant Professor of Medicine, University of Connecticut School of Medicine, Farmington, Connecticut, Chief of Gastroenterology, Newington Veterans Administration Medical Center, Newington, Connecticut

A. R. MOOSSA, MD, FRCS

Professor and Chairman of Surgery, University of California, San Diego School of Medicine, Surgeon-in-Chief, University of California, San Diego Medical Center, La Jolla, California

SERGE MORDON, PhD

Research Physicist, Inserm, Institut National de la Saute et de la Recherche Medicale, Lille Cedex, France

RICHARD H. MOSELEY, MD

Assistant Professor of Medicine, Division of Gastroenterology, University of Michigan Medical School, Veterans Affairs Medical Center, Ann Arbor, Michigan

MICHAEL W. MULHOLLAND, MD

Assistant Professor of Surgery, University of Michigan Medical School, Attending Surgeon, University of Michigan Hospital, Ann Arbor, Michigan

GARRY A. NEIL, MD

Assistant Professor, Division of Gastroenterology-Hepatology, Department of Internal Medicine, University of Iowa College of Medicine, Staff Gastroenterologist, University of Iowa Hospitals and Clinics, Iowa City, Iowa

H. JUERGEN NORD, MD

Professor of Medicine, Director of Division of Digestive Diseases and Nutrition, Department of Internal Medicine, University of South Florida College of Medicine, Tampa, Florida

CAROL S. NORTH, MD

Assistant Professor of Psychiatry, Washington University School of Medicine, Barnes Hospital, St. Louis, Missouri

JEFFREY A. NORTON, MD

Head, Surgical Metabolism Section, Surgery Branch, National Cancer Institute, National Institutes of Health, Bethesda, Maryland

TIMOTHY T. NOSTRANT, MD

Associate Professor of Internal Medicine, University of Michigan Medical School, Associate Chief of Inpatient Services and Education, Division of Gastroenterology, University of Michigan Hospitals, Ann Arbor, Michigan

WARD A. OLSEN, MD

Professor of Medicine, University of Wisconsin–Madison, Head, Gastroenterology Section, Department of Medicine, University of Wisconsin Hospitals and Clinics, Chief of Gastroenterology, William S. Middleton Veterans Hospital, Madison, Wisconsin

FREDERICK H. OPPER, MD

Clinical Instructor in Medicine, Division of Digestive Diseases and Nutrition, University of North Carolina at Chapel Hill, School of Medicine, Chapel Hill, North Carolina

ROY C. ORLANDO, MD

Professor of Medicine, Division of Digestive Diseases and Nutrition, University of North Carolina at Chapel Hill School of Medicine, Attending Physician, University of North Carolina Hospitals, Chapel Hill, North Carolina

SUSAN L. ORLOFF, MD

General Surgery Resident, Department of Surgery, University of California, San Francisco, School of Medicine, San Francisco, California

JOSE M. ORTEGA, MD

Research Fellow, Department of Surgery, University of Texas Medical School at Houston, Houston, Texas

ANN OUYANG, MB, BS

Assistant Professor of Medicine, University of Pennsylvania School of Medicine, Hospital of the University of Pennsylvania, Philadelphia, Pennsylvania

CHUNG OWYANG, MD

Professor of Internal Medicine, Chief, Division of Gastroenterology, University of Michigan Medical Center, Ann Arbor, Michigan

RICHARD D. PEARSON, MD

Professor of Medicine and Pathology, University of Virginia School of Medicine, University of Virginia Health Sciences Center, Charlottesville, Virginia

CARLOS A. PELLEGRINI, MD

Department of Surgery, University of California San - Francisco School of Medicine, San Francisco, California

JOHN H. PEMBERTON, MD

Associate Professor of Surgery, Mayo Medical School, Mayo Clinic, Rochester, Minnesota

JAY A. PERMAN, MD

Associate Professor of Pediatrics, Director, Pediatric Gastroenterology and Nutrition, Johns Hopkins University School of Medicine, University of Maryland School of Medicine, Baltimore, Maryland

JEFFREY H. PETERS, MD

Clinical Assistant Professor, Ohio State University, Attending Surgeon, Ohio Digestive Diseases Institute, Columbus, Ohio

WILLIAM A. PETRI, JR., MD, PhD

Lucille P. Markey Scholar, Assistant Professor of Medicine and Microbiology, Division of Infectious Diseases and Geographic Medicine, University of Virginia Health Sciences Center, University Hospital, Charlottesville, Virginia

DANIEL K. PODOLSKY, MD

Associate Professor of Medicine, Harvard Medical School, Associate Physician, Chief, Gastrointestinal Unit, Massachusetts General Hospital, Boston, Massachusetts

JEFFREY L. PONSKY, MD

Associate Professor of Surgery, Case Western Reserve University School of Medicine, Director, Department of Surgery, Mount Sinai Medical Center in Cleveland, Cleveland, Ohio

DON W. POWELL, MD

The Edward Randall and Edward Randall, Jr. Chair in Internal Medicine, Professor and Chairman of Internal Medicine, Professor of Physiology and Biophysics, The University of Texas Medical Branch Hospitals at Galveston, Galveston, Texas

LINDA RANDOLPH, MD

Clinical Geneticist, Alfigen/The Genetics Institute, Medical Center, Pasadena, California

STEVEN E. RAPER, MD

Assistant Professor of Surgery, University of Michigan Medical School, Ann Arbor, Michigan

JEAN-PIERRE RAUFMAN, MD

Associate Professor of Medicine, State University of New York, Health Science Center at Brooklyn, Attending Physician, Division of Gastroenterology, Kings County Hospital Medical Center, Brooklyn, New York

GEORGIA M. REES, MD

Senior Fellow, Gastroenterology/Hepatology Section Fred Hutchinson Cancer Research Center, University of Washington School of Medicine, Seattle, Washington

BRIAN J. REID, MD

Assistant Professor of Medicine, Division of Gastroenterology, Department of Medicine, University of Washington, Seattle, Washington

PATRICK M. REILLY, MD

Research Fellow, Department of Surgery, Johns Hopkins University School of Medicine, Baltimore, Maryland, Resident, Department of Surgery, Medical Center of Delaware, Newark, Delaware

JAMES C. REYNOLDS, MD

Professor of Medicine and Physiology, Chief, Division of Gastroenterology and Hepatology, University of Pittsburgh School of Medicine, Pittsburgh, Pennsylvania

TELFER B. REYNOLDS, MD

Clayton G. Loosli Professor of Medicine, University of Southern California School of Medicine, Los Angeles, California

JOEL E. RICHTER, MD

Professor of Medicine, Director of Clinical Research, Division of Gastroenterology, The University of Alabama, School of Medicine, Birmingham, Alabama

CHARLES A. ROHRMANN, JR, MD

Professor and Vice Chairman of Radiology, University of Washington School of Medicine, Director of Gastrointestinal Radiology, University of Washington Hospitals, Seattle, Washington

MARC A. ROSENTHAL, DDS

Research Associate, Department of Oral and Maxillofacial Surgery, State University of New York at Buffalo, School of Dental Medicine, Research Faculty, Buffalo General Hospital, Buffalo, New York

JEROME I. ROTTER, MD

Director, Division of Medical Genetics, Cedars-Sinai Medical Center, Professor of Medicine and Pediatrics, UCLA School of Medicine, Cedars-Sinai Board of Governors', Chair in Medical Genetics, Los Angeles, California

STEPHEN E. RUBESIN, MD

Associate Professor of Radiology, Radiologist, Hospital of the University of Pennsylvania, Philadelphia, Pennsylvania

CYRUS E. RUBIN, MD

Professor of Medicine, Adjunct Professor of Pathology, Division of Gastroenterology, Department of Medicine, University of Washington, Seattle, Washington

WALTER RUBIN, MD

Professor of Medicine and Anatomy, Chief, Division of Gastroenterology, Vice-Chairman, Department of Medicine, Medical College of Pennsylvania, Attending Physician, Hospital of the Medical College of Pennsylvania, Philadelphia, Pennsylvania

NORBERT S. RUNKEL, MD

Chief Surgical Resident, Chirurgische Universitätsklinik Heidelberg, Germany

BRUCE A. RUNYON, MD

Associate Professor of Internal Medicine, Division of Gastroenterology/Hepatology, Department of Medicine, University of Iowa College of Medicine, Iowa City, Iowa

WILLIAM A. RUTALA, PhD, MPH

Research Associate Professor, Division of Infectious Diseases, Department of Medicine, University of North Carolina School of Medicine, Administrative Director, Department of Hospital Epidemiology, University of North Carolina Hospital, Chapel Hill, North Carolina

JAMES P. RYAN, PhD

Professor and Deputy Chairman of Physiology, Temple University School of Medicine, Philadelphia, Pennsylvania

SANJAY SAINI, MD

Assistant Professor of Radiology, Harvard Medical School, Assistant Radiologist, Massachusetts General Hospital, Boston, Massachusetts

DAVID M. SALTZBERG, MD

Assistant Professor of Medicine, Division of Gastroenterology, Department of Medicine, University of Maryland School of Medicine, Baltimore, Maryland

ROBERT S. SANDLER, MD, MPH

Associate Professor of Medicine, Division of Digestive Diseases and Nutrition, University of North Carolina at Chapel Hill, School of Medicine, Attending Physician, University of North Carolina Hospitals, Chapel Hill, North Carolina

JAMES M. SCHEIMAN, MD

Instructor in Internal Medicine, Division of Gastroenterology, University of Michigan School of Medicine, Staff Physician, University of Michigan Hospital, Director of Endoscopy Unit, Veterans Affairs Medical Center, Ann Arbor, Michigan

CHARLES M. SCHRON, MD

Associate Professor of Medicine, University of Cincinnati College of Medicine, Attending Physician, University of Cincinnati Medical Center, Cincinnati, Ohio

MARKUS SCHWAIGER, MD

Associate Professor of Internal Medicine, Division of Nuclear Medicine, University of Michigan Medical School, Director, Cardiovascular Nuclear Medicine, University of Michigan Medical Center, Ann Arbor, Michigan

JOHN SEKIJIMA, MD

Clinical Instructor in Gastroenterology, University of Washington School of Medicine, Staff Physician, Seattle Veterans Affairs Medical Center, Seattle, Washington

FERGUS SHANAHAN, MD, FRCPI, FRCP(C)

Assistant Professor of Medicine, University of California Los Angeles, UCLA School of Medicine, Los Angeles, California

ELIZABETH F. SHERERTZ, MD

Associate Professor of Dermatology, Bowman Gray School of Medicine, Wake Forest University, Winston-Salem, North Carolina

PHILIP M. SHERMAN, MD, FRCP(C)

Associate Professor of Pediatrics and Microbiology, University of Toronto Faculty of Medicine, Staff Gastroenterologist, The Hospital for Sick Children, Toronto, Ontario, Canada

FRED E. SILVERSTEIN, MD

Professor of Medicine, Division of Gastroenterology, Department of Medicine, University of Washington, Seattle, Washington

MICHAEL D. SITRIN, MD

Associate Professor of Medicine, Director, Clinical Nutrition Research Unit, University of Chicago/Pritzker School of Medicine, Chicago, Illinois

DAVID D. STARK, MD

Associate Professor of Radiology, Harvard Medical School, Boston, Massachusetts

MICHAEL L. STEER, MD

Professor of Surgery, Harvard Medical School, Associate Surgeon-in-Chief, Beth Israel Hospital, Boston, Massachusetts

WILLIAM F. STENSON, MD

Associate Professor of Medicine, Washington University School of Medicine, Chief, Division of Gastroenterology, Jewish Hospital of St. Louis, St. Louis, Missouri

ROBERT W. SUMMERS, MD

Professor of Internal Medicine, Division of Gastroenterology/Hepatology, University of Iowa College of Medicine, University of Iowa Hospitals and Clinics, Veterans Affairs Medical Center, Iowa City, Iowa

CHRISTINA M. SURAWICZ, MD

Associate Professor of Medicine, University of Washington School of Medicine, Director, Gastrointestinal Endoscopy, Harborview Medical Center, Seattle, Washington

NORMAN L. SUSSMAN, MD

Assistant Professor of Medicine, Baylor College of Medicine, Assistant Attending Physician, Medical Service, Harris County Hospital, Staff Physician, The Methodist Hospital, Veterans Administration Medical Center, Houston, Texas

FRED M. SUTTON, JR., MD

Assistant Professor of Medicine, Baylor College of Medicine, Chief of Gastroenterology, Ben Taub General Hospital, Houston, Texas

STEPHAN R. TARGAN, MD

Professor of Medicine, University of California, Los Angeles, UCLA School of Medicine, Los Angeles, California

PHILLIP I. TARR, MD

Assistant Professor of Pediatrics, Assistant Professor, Division of Gastroenterology and Infectious Diseases, University of Washington School of Medicine, Attending Physician, Children's Hospital and Medical Center, Seattle, Washington

IAN L. TAYLOR, MB, ChB (Hons), PhD

Professor of Medicine, Chief of Gastroenterology, Duke University Medical Center, Durham, North Carolina

DAVID A. THOMPSON, MD

Fellow, Colon and Rectal Surgery, University of Texas Medical School at Houston and The Hermann Hospital, Houston, Texas

COURTNEY M. TOWNSEND, JR, MD

Robertson-Poth Professor of Surgery, University of Texas Medical Branch, Galveston, Texas

PETER G. TRABER, MD

Assistant Professor of Internal Medicine, Division of Gastroenterology, University of Michigan Medical School, Ann Arbor, Michigan

GUIDO TYTGAT, MD, PhD

Professor of Medicine/Gastroenterology, University of Amsterdam Faculty of Medicine, Chief, Department of Gastroenterology/Hepatology, Academic Medical Centre, Amsterdam, The Netherlands

RAMA P. VENU, MD

Associate Clinical Professor of Medicine, Medical College of Wisconsin, Milwaukee, Wisconsin

ARNOLD WALD, MD

Associate Professor of Medicine, University of Pittsburgh, School of Medicine, Head, Gastroenterology Unit, Montefiore Hospital, Pittsburgh, Pennsylvania

PAUL B. WATKINS, MD

Assistant Professor of Internal Medicine, Division of Gastroenterology, University of Michigan Medical School, Ann Arbor, Michigan

JEROME D. WAYE, MD

Clinical Professor of Medicine, Mount Sinai School of Medicine (CUNY), Chief, Gastrointestinal Endoscopy Unit, Mount Sinai Hospital, Lenox Hill Hospital, New York, New York

DAVID J. WEBER, MD, MPH

Assistant Professor of Medicine, Department of Medicine and Epidemiology, University of North Carolina at Chapel Hill, School of Medicine and Public Health, Chapel Hill, North Carolina

JOEL V. WEINSTOCK, MD

Associate Professor of Medicine, Director of Gastroenterology/Hepatology, University of Iowa College of Medicine, University of Iowa Hospitals and Clinics, Iowa City, Iowa

JOHN W. WILEY, MD

Assistant Professor of Internal Medicine, Division of Gastroenterology, University of Michigan, Ann Arbor, Michigan

CHRISTOPHER B. WILLIAMS, BM, FRCP

Consultant Physician in Gastrointestinal Endoscopy, St. Mark's, St. Bartholomew's Hospitals, London, England

DAVID M. WILLIAMS, MD

Associate Professor of Radiology, University of Michigan Medical Center, Ann Arbor, Michigan

JOHN A. WILLIAMS, MD, PhD

Professor and Chairman, Department of Physiology, Professor, Department of Internal Medicine, University of Michigan Medical Center, Ann Arbor, Michigan

KENNETH H. WILSON, MD

Associate Professor of Medicine, Duke University School of Medicine, Duke University Medical Center, Veterans Affairs Medical Center, Durham, North Carolina

DAVID L. WINGATE, MD

Professor of Gastrointestinal Science, University of London, London Hospital Medical College, Consultant Gastroenterologist, London Hospital, London, England

TADATAKA YAMADA, MD

John G. Searle Professor and Chairman, Department of Internal Medicine, Professor of Physiology, Physician-in-Chief, University of Michigan Medical Center, Ann Arbor, Michigan

KENJIRO YASUDA, MD

Associate Chief, Department of Gastroenterology, Kyoto Second Red Cross Hospital, Kamigyo-Ku, Kyota, Japan

HARVEY S. YOUNG, MD

Assistant Professor of Medicine, Chief, Gastrointestinal Endoscopy, Stanford University School of Medicine, Stanford University Medical Center, Stanford, California

MICHAEL J. ZINNER, MD

Professor and Chairman of Surgery, University of California Los Angeles, UCLA School of Medicine, Los Angeles, California

PREFACE

The practice of gastroenterology has changed dramatically during the past 20 years. We have witnessed a logarithmic growth in the volume of information concerning the basic biology and biochemistry of the gut. This wealth of new knowledge not only has provided fresh insight into the pathogenesis of gastrointestinal diseases but also has identified the critical role of the gut in the physiology and pathology of other organ systems. There is every reason to expect that the pace of our scientific growth will continue in the years ahead.

In many instances, advances in the science of gastroenterology have been incorporated directly into clinical practice. This has led to the evolution of a large and ever-expanding armamentarium of diagnostic and therapeutic modalities for management of patients with gastrointestinal diseases. The ability to see the organ of pathology and to treat lesions directly without invasive surgical procedures is an advantage almost unique to gastroenterology. As a result, today's clinicians must think in ways not even imagined by their predecessors. Although the textbooks of the past have served us well, modern gastroenterology dictates a more integrated approach to science, technology, and clinical practice. In the *Textbook of Gastroenterology* the Editors address this need.

The *Textbook* begins with a section of chapters describing the basic mechanisms of normal and abnormal gastrointestinal function. This section of the *Textbook* is written so that fundamental scientific concepts can be understood by a reader who is not scientifically oriented. We hope to present the scientific basis of gastroenterology in such a fashion that it will provide insight into common clinical problems. The section is intended to serve both as a guide for clinicians who need to understand the pathophysiology of their patients' disorders and as a resource for serious students of gastroenterology.

A major shortcoming of textbooks that consist solely of descriptions of diseases is the lack of guidance for the reader in applying the information to the management of patients who present with symptoms or signs rather than diagnoses. Therefore, a major section of the *Textbook* consists of detailed chapters on the clinician's approach to patients presenting with common gastrointestinal problems.

As a fully comprehensive textbook, the *Textbook of Gastroenterology* has at its core an encyclopedic discussion of virtually all of the disease states encountered in practice. These chapters, comprising the bulk of the *Textbook,* have a classical structure that ensures the uniform coverage of all important points.

After the initial evaluation, physicians must choose from a battery of diagnostic and therapeutic modalities as they proceed with patient management. A full section describing all of the major technologies, both the longstanding and the very recent, available to clinicians today comprises the last section of the *Textbook.* This section discusses not only the theory and practical uses of these procedures but also the contraindictions and potential complications, the evaluation and assessment of the data obtained, and the future directions of the modality.

The purposes of the *Textbook of Gastroenterology,* then, are multiple: to teach the scientific basis of gastroenterology, to provide practical approaches to common gastrointestinal problems, to serve as an encyclopedic reference for gastrointestinal diseases, and to indicate the current applications and future directions of the technology of gastroenterology. Above all, the *Textbook* is planned to integrate the various demands of science, technology, expanding information, good judgment, and common sense in the diagnosis and management of gastrointestinal patients. The Editors intend the book to be as useful at the bedside as on an office shelf or a student desk. Because gastrointestinal complaints are among the most commonly encountered in clinical practice, we want our readers to include surgeons, primary care physicians, and nurses as well as gastroenterologists and other internists.

To achieve these goals, the finest experts in the field of gastroenterology have written this *Textbook.* Each chapter is prepared by an authority who is actively engaged in advancing our knowledge of the subject matter of the chapter. We believe that the expertise of this group of physicians and scientists has ensured that the *Textbook* will achieve its aims.

ACKNOWLEDGMENTS

The work of the editors was greatly facilitated by the expert assistance of Lori Ennis and Fran Frueh who collaborated as a team to complement editorial talents with interpersonal skills to maintain the high quality of the text and deliver the manuscript in a timely fashion. The editors also are indebted to the critical roles served by their administrative and secretarial assistants, Gail Evans, Pam Evans, Sandy Forest, Elsa Forero, Donna Hall, Mary Hill, Marie Jost, Don May, and Terry L. Reeves. In addition, the faculty and fellows of the Gastroenterology Divisions at the University of Michigan, Washington University in St. Louis, the University of North Carolina, and the University of Washington provided invaluable assistance in reviewing and critiquing all of the chapters in the *Textbook*.

The editors wish to express their gratitude to their superlative colleagues at J.B. Lippincott Company who gave birth to this project, nurtured it, and demonstrated throughout the entire 40 months of the project their commitment to quality, integrity, and excellence. Of the many people at Lippincott who have made this book possible, two deserve special recognition: Dean Manke and Richard Winters. The book would not have been possible without their exceptional talents.

In pursuance of this project, the editors benefited greatly from the patience and support of their families. It is with considerable pride that Leslie, Sanae, and Takao Yamada; Melanie Alpers; Jeannette Owyang; Ellie, Laura, and Mark Silverstein; and Curt and Chris Gerston are acknowledged for their contributions to this effort.

Finally, the editors wish to acknowledge the influence that the late Morton I. Grossman had on the progress of Gastroenterology as a science. It is the editors' fondest hope that this book will live up to his exacting standards and represent well the clinical discipline that he was so instrumental in establishing.

Tadataka Yamada, M.D.

CONTENTS

B. Motility   119

    TRACT   475
    Mark W. Babyatsky, Daniel K. Podolsky

    Embryology and Histogenesis   475
    Functional Maturation   479
    Growth and Differentiation in the Mature GI Tract   486

24. NEOPLASIA OF THE GASTROINTESTINAL TRACT   501
    C. Richard Boland, Andrew P. Feinberg

    The Cellular Biology of Tumor Development Carcinogenesis:
      An Introduction   501
    The Molecular Genetics of Tumor Development   511

25. PHARMACOLOGY OF THE GASTROINTESTINAL TRACT   518
    Paul B. Watkins

    Functional Anatomy of the Gastrointestinal Barrier   519
    The Metabolic Barrier of the GI Tract   523
    Secretion of Drugs by the Gut   528
    Alternate Routes for Drug Administration   529
    Summary   529

26. THE GASTROINTESTINAL MICROFLORA   532
    Kenneth H. Wilson

    Composition of the Flora   532
    Metabolism   536
    Suppression of Pathogens   537
    Effects of Antibiotics on the Flora   539
    Overall Interaction of the Microflora with the Host   540

II. APPROACHES TO COMMON GASTROINTESTINAL
    PROBLEMS   545

27. PSYCHOSOCIAL FACTORS IN THE CARE OF PATIENTS WITH
    GASTROINTESTINAL DISEASE   546
    Douglas A. Drossman

    Relationship of Biological and Psychosocial Factors
      in Gastrointestinal Illness   547
    Obtaining Psychosocial Data: The Interview   548
    Understanding the Data   550
    Psychosocial Treatment   556

28. APPROACH TO THE PATIENT WITH DYSPHAGIA   562
    Donald O. Castell

    Introduction   562
    Globus   562
    Classification   562
    Pathophysiologic Considerations   563
    History and Physical Examination   564
    Clinical Presentation   566
    Assessment   570
    Therapeutic Considerations   570

29. APPROACH TO THE PATIENT WITH CHEST PAIN   573
    Timothy T. Nostrant

    Introduction   573
    Causes of Chest Pain   573
    History   580
    Physical Examination   581
    Diagnostic Strategies   582
    Therapeutic Considerations   585

A. Esophagus   1066

53. **ESOPHAGUS: ANATOMY AND STRUCTURAL ANOMALIES**   1066
    Gregory A. Boyce, H. Worth Boyce, Jr.

    Embryology   1066
    Adult Anatomy   1066
    Histology   1069
    Developmental Anomalies   1071
    Mucosal Rings and Webs   1075
    Esophageal Diverticula   1076
    Esophageal Hiatal Hernia   1078

54. **MOTILITY DISORDERS OF THE ESOPHAGUS**   1083
    Joel E. Richter

    Introduction   1083
    Disorders of the Hypopharynx, Upper Esophageal Sphincter, and Cervical Esophagus   1083
    Achalasia   1090
    Spastic Motility Disorders of the Distal Esophagus   1104
    Esophageal Motility Disorders Associated with Systemic Diseases   1113

55. **REFLUX ESOPHAGITIS**   1123
    Roy C. Orlando

    Epidemiology   1123
    Etiology   1123
    Clinical Manifestations   1129
    Differential Diagnosis and Diagnostic Studies   1130
    Clinical Course and Complications   1134
    Therapy   1137
    Gastroesophageal Reflux in Children   1141
    Alkaline Reflux Esophagitis   1142

56. **ESOPHAGEAL INFECTIONS**   1148
    Jean-Pierre Raufman

    Epidemiology   1148
    Specific Infections   1149
    Esophageal Infection in AIDS   1157

57. **ESOPHAGEAL TUMORS**   1159
    Brian J. Reid

    Squamous Cell Carcinoma   1159
    Esophageal Adenocarcinoma   1165
    Clinical Course and Complications   1167
    Other Epithelial Tumors   1169
    Nonepithelial Tumors   1170

58. **MISCELLANEOUS DISEASES OF THE ESOPHAGUS**   1178
    Eugene M. Bozymski, Jerry F. London

    Caustic Injury to the Esophagus   1178
    Medication-Induced Esophageal Injury   1183
    Radiation Esophagitis   1184
    Foreign Bodies in the Esophagus   1185
    Systemic Diseases Affecting Esophagus   1186
    Dermatologic Diseases Affecting Esophagus   1187
    Esophageal Intramural Hematomas   1191
    Esophageal Injury and Rupture   1192

B. Stomach   1198

H. Miscellaneous 2086

IV. DIAGNOSTIC AND THERAPEUTIC MODALITIES IN GASTROENTEROLOGY   2219

TEXTBOOK OF
Gastroenterology

COLOR FIGURES

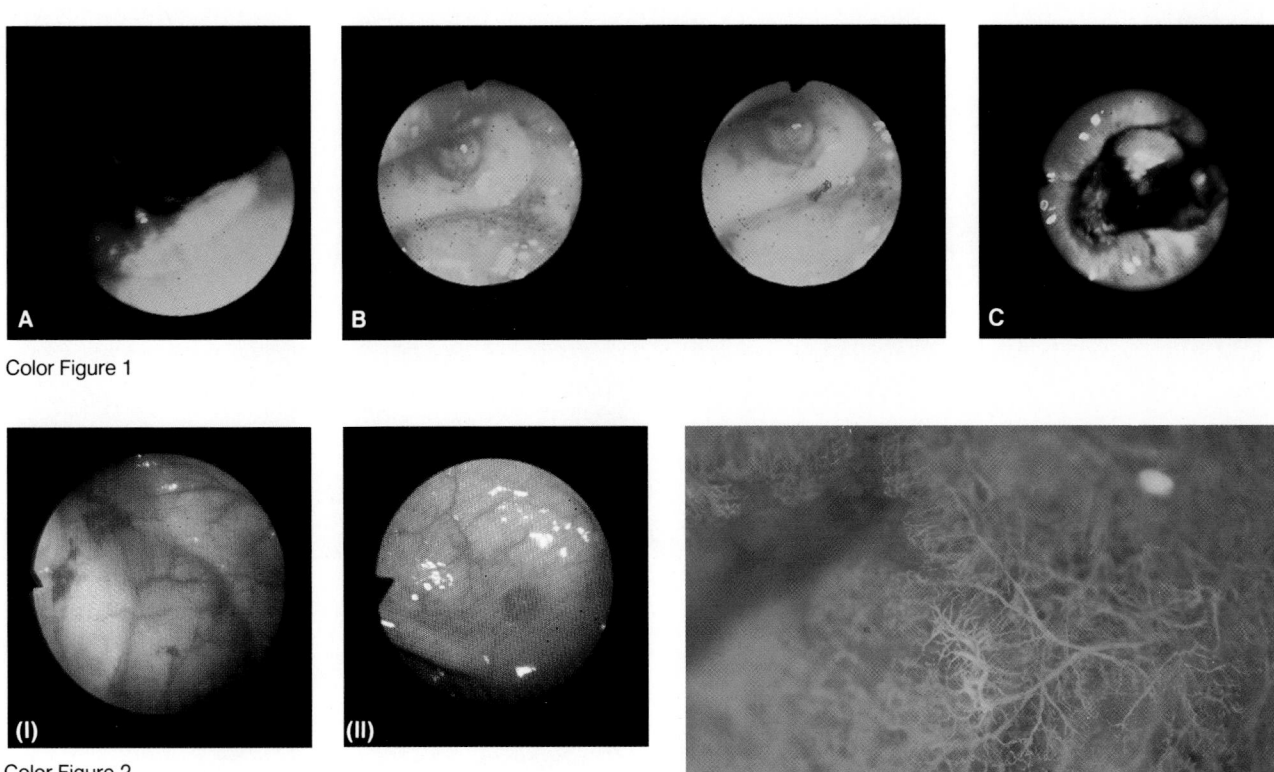

Color Figure 1

Color Figure 2

Color Figure 3

COLOR FIGURE 1. Three endoscopic pictures of stigmata of hemorrhage. **A,** Arterial spurting from a gastric ulcer crater. **B,** Visible vessel in a duodenal alcer that is not actively bleeding. **C,** Adherent blood clot obscuring most of this duodenal ulcer base.

COLOR FIGURE 2. Two endoscopic pictures of angiodysplastic lesions in the right colon.

COLOR FIGURE 3. Acrylic cast of a surgical colonic specimen showing the tuft of dilated vessels in angiodysplasia.

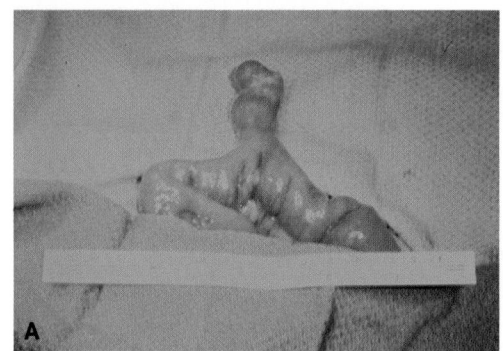

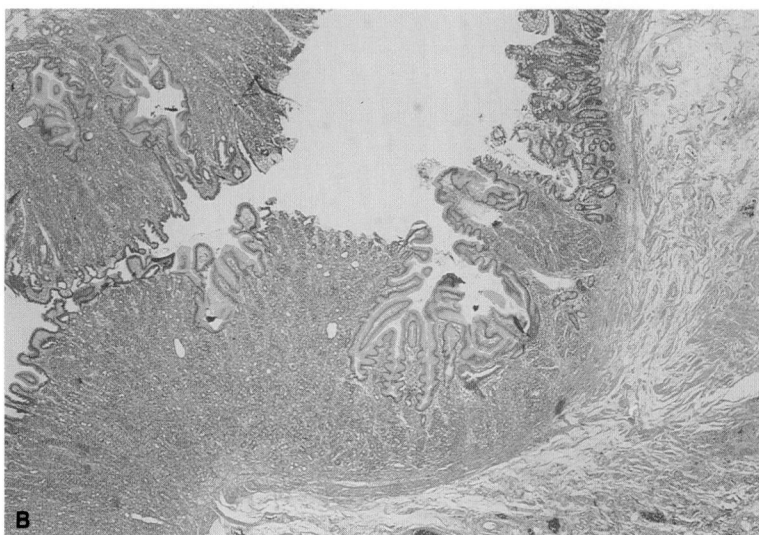

Color Figure 4

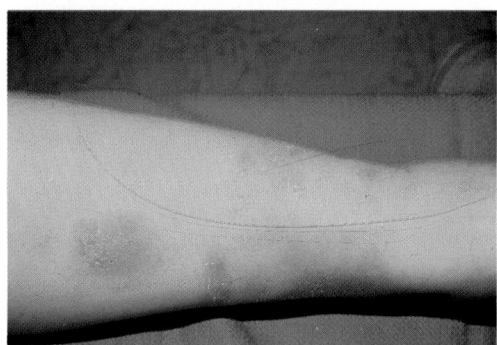

Color Figure 5

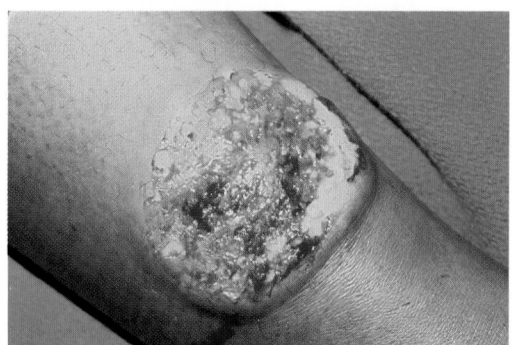

Color Figure 6

COLOR FIGURE 4. A, Operative picture of a gross specimen of a Meckel's diverticulum. **B,** Histologic slide from the same specimen showing gastric mucosa adjacent to ileal mucosa.

COLOR FIGURE 5. Erythema nodosum. These tender nodules occurred in association with ulcerative colitis.

COLOR FIGURE 6. Pyodema gangrenosum in a patient with Crohn's disease.

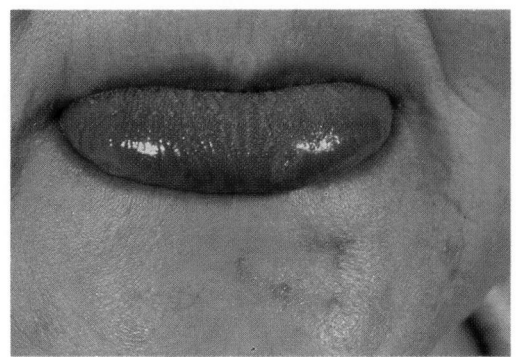

Color Figure 7

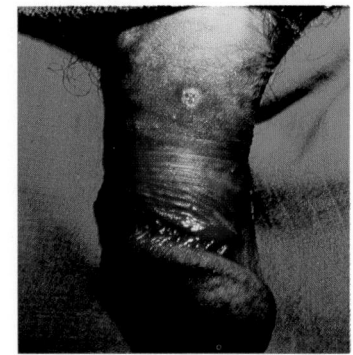

Color Figure 8

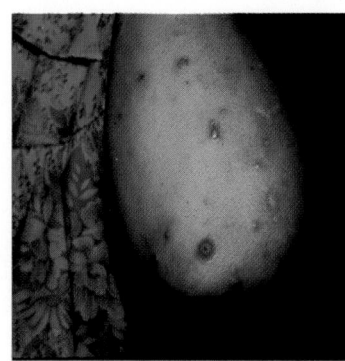

Color Figure 9

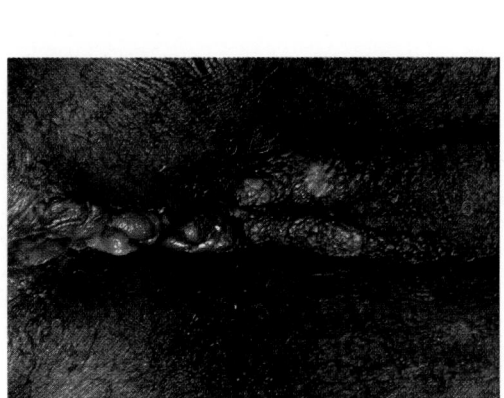

Color Figure 10

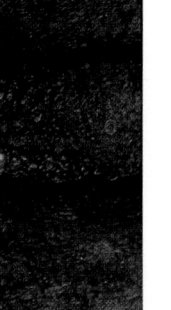

Color Figure 11

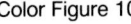

COLOR FIGURE 7. Aphthous ulcer involving the tongue in a patient with Behçet's disease.

COLOR FIGURE 8. Behcet's disease. Note the early genital aphtha showing features of pustular vasculitis.

COLOR FIGURE 9. Bowel-associated dermatosis-arthritis syndrome. Pustular vasculitis lesions in a patient with a blind loop after Billroth II surgery.

COLOR FIGURE 10. Amyloidosis. Note the perirectal amyloid nodules in this patient with multiple myeloma.

COLOR FIGURE 11. Typical telangiectasia of Osler-Weber-Rendu disease.

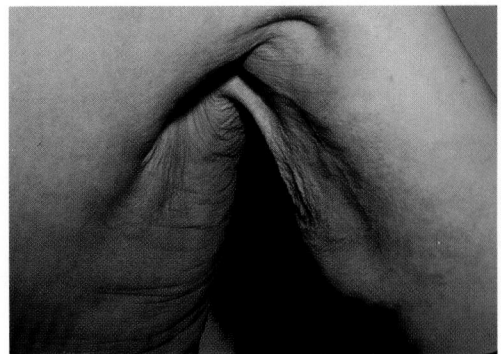

Color Figure 12

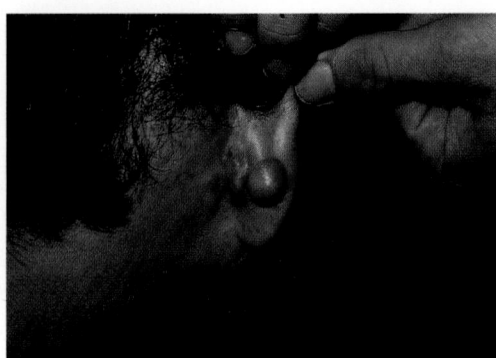

Color Figure 13

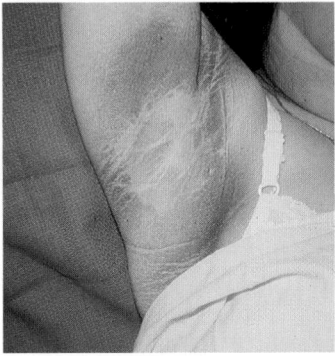

Color Figure 14

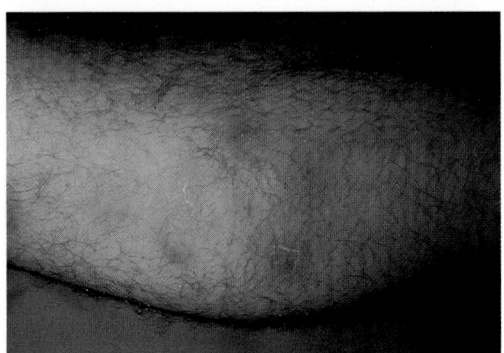

Color Figure 15

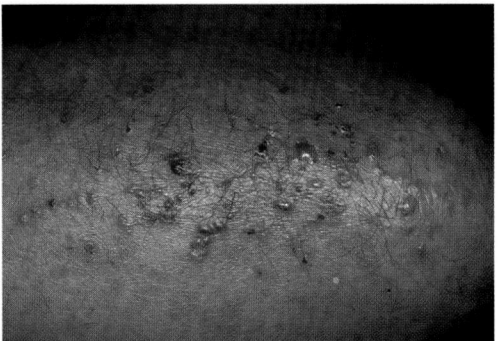

Color Figure 16

COLOR FIGURE 12. Pseudoxanthoma elasticum. Note the "chicken skin" appearance of the axillary skin.

COLOR FIGURE 13. Gardner's syndrome. Note the typical epidermal inclusion cyst. This patient had multiple other cystic nodules, particularly on the scalp.

COLOR FIGURE 14. Acanthosis nigricans in a nonobese adult patient.

COLOR FIGURE 15. Panniculitis presenting as tender erythematous nodules in a patient with pancreatitis.

COLOR FIGURE 16. Dermatitis herpetiformis. Both elbows were involved. Note intact vesicles and multiple crusted (excoriated) lesions.

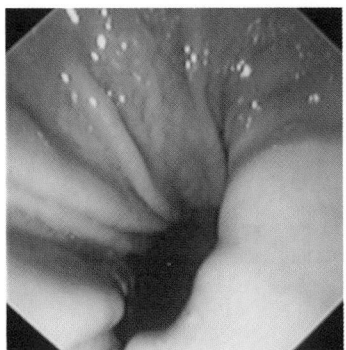

Color Figure 17

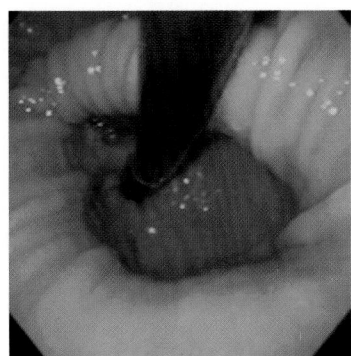

Color Figure 18

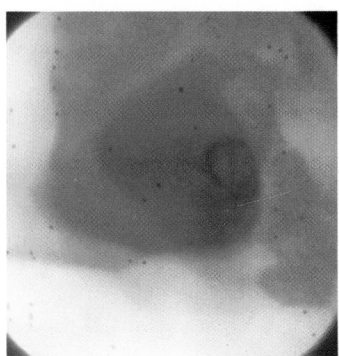

Color Figure 19

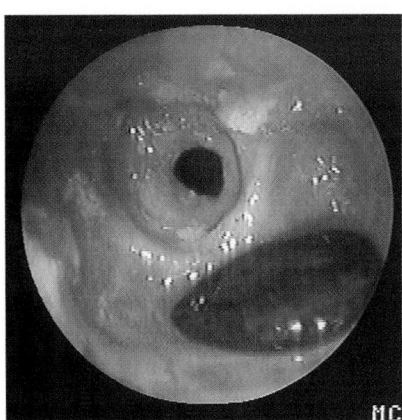

Color Figure 20

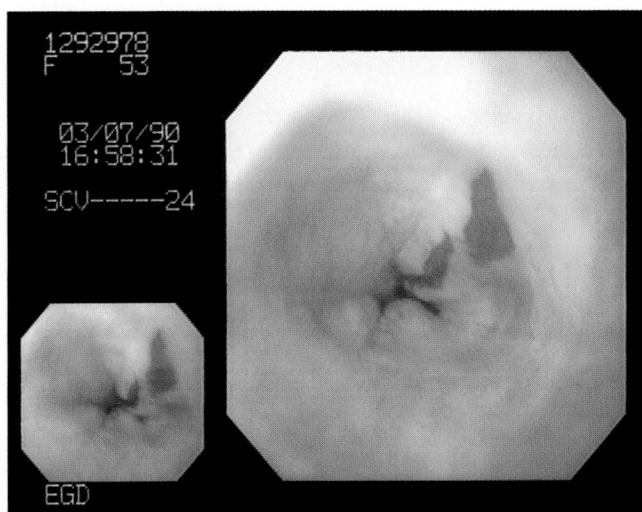

Color Figure 21

COLOR FIGURE 17. Antegrade endoscopic view into a hiatal hernia proximal to a patulous diaphragmatic hiatus. Note the gastric mucosal folds in the hernia pouch extending over the hiatal margin. The upper ends of the gastric mucosal folds are located about 1 cm distal to the squamocolumnar junction and coincide with the level of the true esophagogastric or muscular junction.

COLOR FIGURE 18. Retrograde view from the stomach into the hernia pouch through the patulous hiatus. Note the gastric folds coursing over the margin of the hiatal circumference.

COLOR FIGURE 19. Endoscopic appearance of the distal esophagus in a patient with circumferential-type Barrett's esophagus. Note that the red columnar epithelium completely lines the lower esophagus but merges proximally with the lighter stratified squamous epithelium of the mid-esophagus. (From Herlihy KJ, Orlando RC, Bryson JC, et al. Barrett's esophagus: Clinical, endoscopic, histologic, manometric and electrical potential difference characteristics. Gastroenterology 1984;86:436.)

COLOR FIGURE 20. "Watermelon esophagus." A watermelon seed lodged in a pseudodiverticulum above a very narrow esophageal stricture.

COLOR FIGURE 21. Nonpenetrating mucosal laceration following retching in a 53-year-old woman.

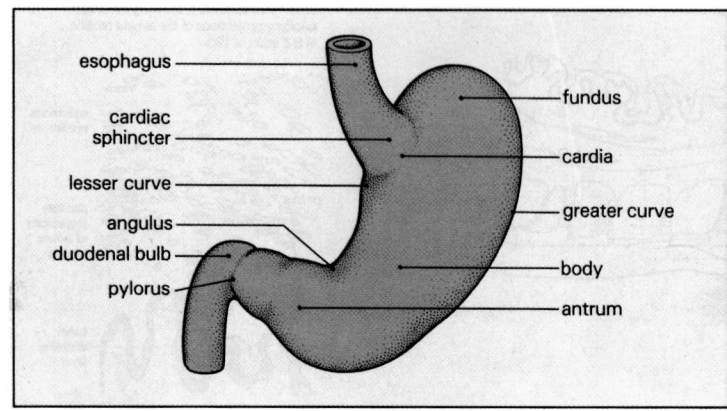

Color Figure 22

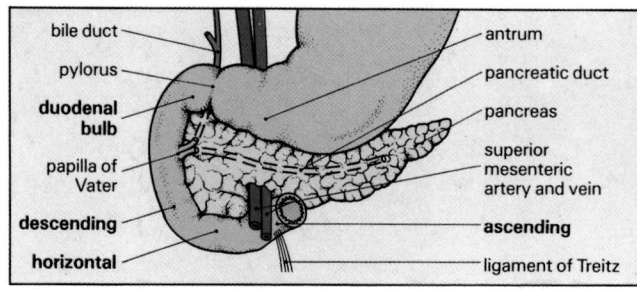

Color Figure 23

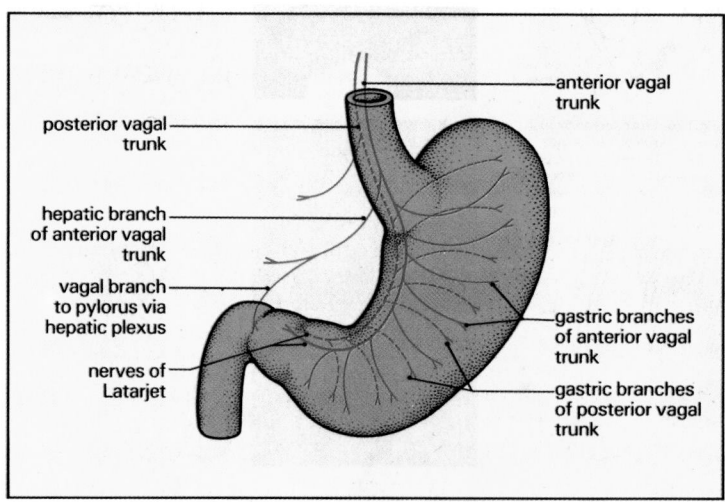

Color Figure 24

COLOR FIGURE 22. Diagram of the lower esophagus, stomach, and proximal duodenum. (From Misiewicz JJ, Bartram Cl, Cotton PB, Mee AS, Price AB, Thompson RPH. Atlas of Clinical Gastroenterology. London: Gower Medical Publishing, 1987:1.6.)

COLOR FIGURE 23. Diagram showing the anatomic relationships of the duodenum. (From Misiewicz JJ, Bartram Cl, Cotton PB, Mee AS, Price AB, Thompson RPH. Atlas of Clinical Gastroenterology. London: Gower Medical Publishing, 1987:4.2.)

COLOR FIGURE 24. Diagram showing the anatomic arrangement of the vagus nerves. (From Misiewicz JJ, Bartram Cl, Cotton PB, Mee AS, Price AB, Thompson RPH. Atlas of Clinical Gastroenterology. London: Gower Medical Publishing, 1987:1.7.)

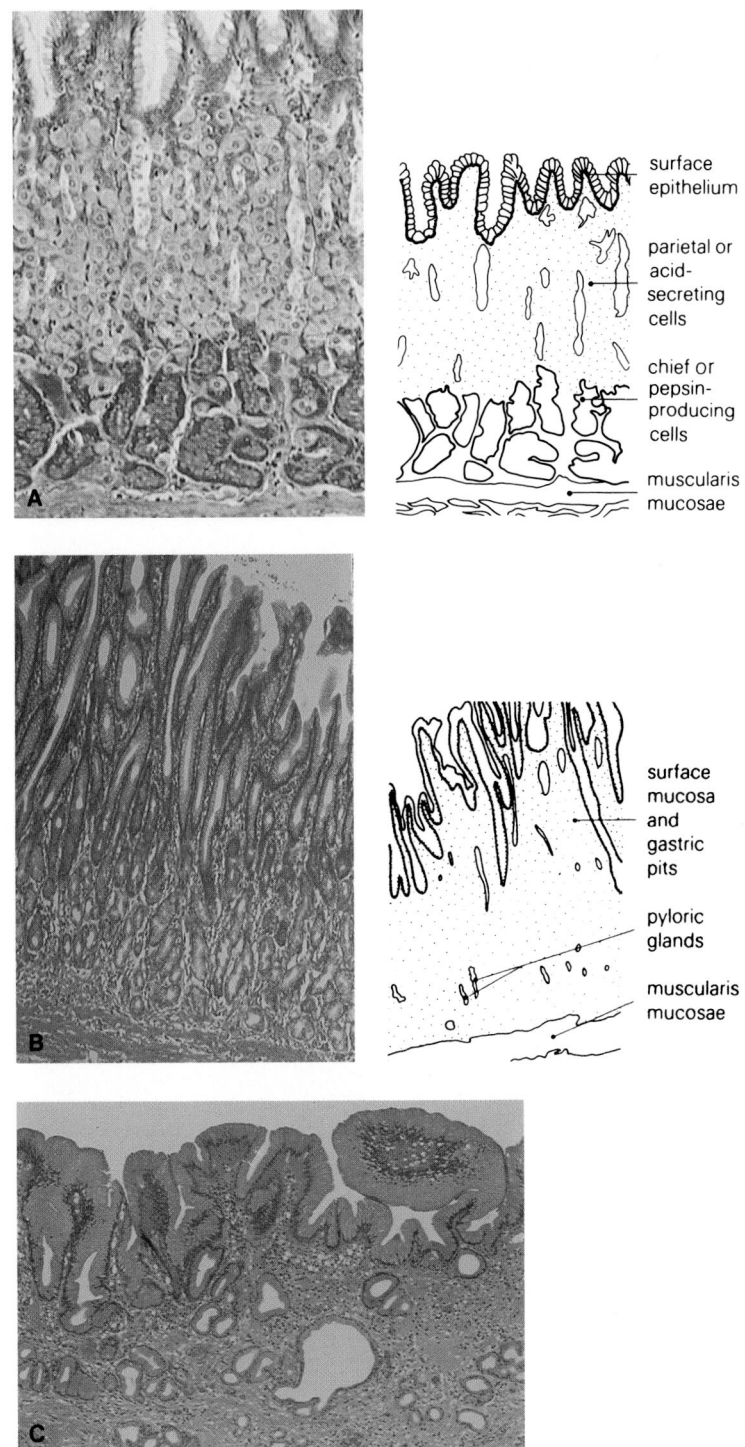

surface
epithelium

parietal or
acid-
secreting
cells

chief or
pepsin-
producing
cells

muscularis
mucosae

surface
mucosa
and
gastric
pits

pyloric
glands

muscularis
mucosae

COLOR FIGURE 25. **A,** Light photomicrograph of fundic-type gastric mucosa. Columnar mucus-secreting cells line the surface and pits, acid-secreting parietal cells (light staining cuboidal cells) predominate in the midportion of the mucosa, and pepsinogen-secreting chief cells (darker staining) are located deeper in the mucosa. (Hematoxylin and eosin, courtesy of Dr. P. Wheater.) (From Misiewicz JJ, Bartram CI, Cotton PB, Mee AS, Price AB, Thompson RPH. Atlas of Clinical Gastroenterology. London: Gower Medical Publishing, 1987:1.8.) **B,** Light photomicrograph of antral-type gastric mucosa. The gastric pits are deeper than in fundic mucosa. Mucus-secreting glands are deep in the mucosa and empty into the pits. (Hematoxylin and eosin.) (From Misiewicz JJ, Bartram CI, Cotton PB, Mee AS, Price AB, Thompson RPH. Atlas of Clinical Gastroenterology. London: Gower Medical Publishing, 1987:1.8.) **C,** Light photomicrograph of junctional gastric mucosa. Although the architecture is similar to fundic mucosa, the mucosa is thinner and the loosely arranged glands are devoid of parietal and chief cells. Hematoxylin and eosin. (From Mitros FA. Atlas of Gastrointestinal Pathology. London: Gower Medical Publishing, 1988:3.3.)

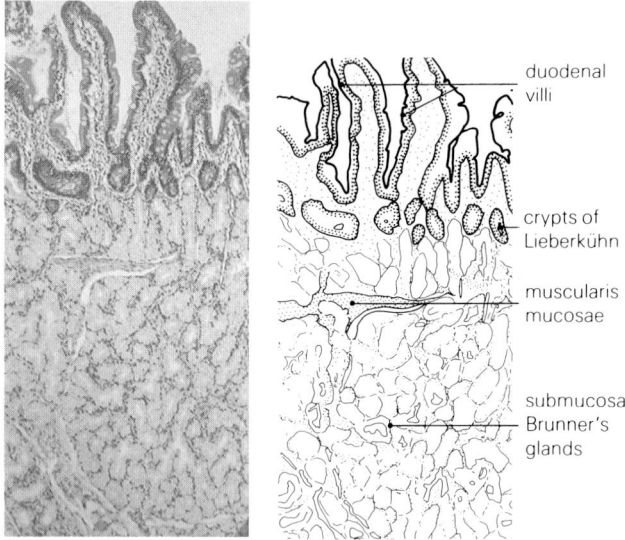

duodenal
villi

crypts of
Lieberkühn

muscularis
mucosae

submucosal
Brunner's
glands

Color Figure 26

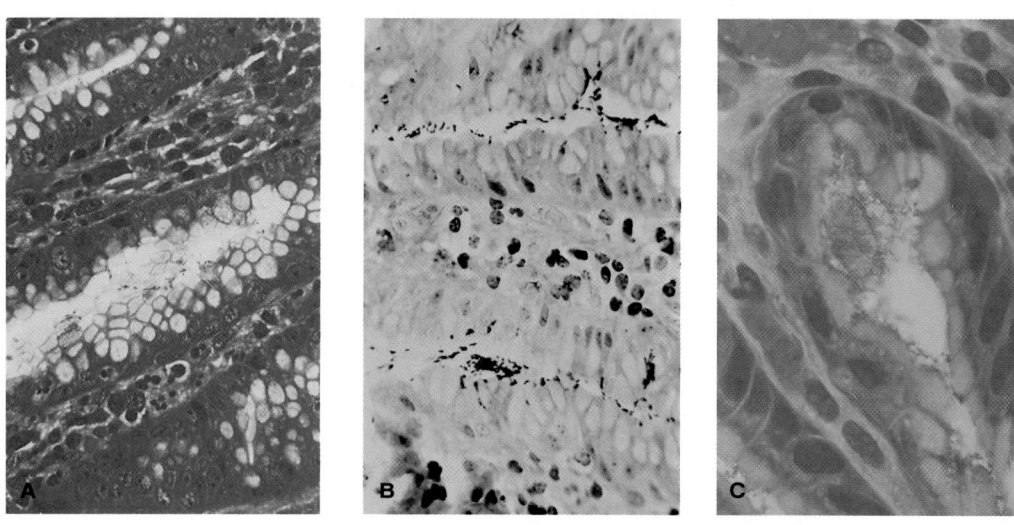

Color Figure 27

COLOR FIGURE 26.   Light photomicrograph of duodenal mucosa. Villi protrude from the mucosal surface. Columnar absorptive cells and goblet (mucous) cells cover the villi and line the crypts at the base of the villi. Clusters of clear-staining cells that secrete an alkaline mucus, called Brunner's glands, are found above and below the muscularis mucosae and empty into the base of the crypts (Hematoxylin and eosin). (From Misiewicz JJ, Bartram CI, Cotton PB, Mee AS, Price AB, Thompson RPH. Atlas of Clinical Gastroenterology. London: Gower Medical Publishing, 1987:4.3.)

COLOR FIGURE 27.   Gastric mucosal biopsy specimens positive for *Helicobacter pylori* with (**A**) Giemsa, (**B**) Warthin-Starry silver, and (**C**) hematoxylin and eosin stains. (Figure reproduced courtesy of Henry D. Appelman, University of Michigan Medical Center.)

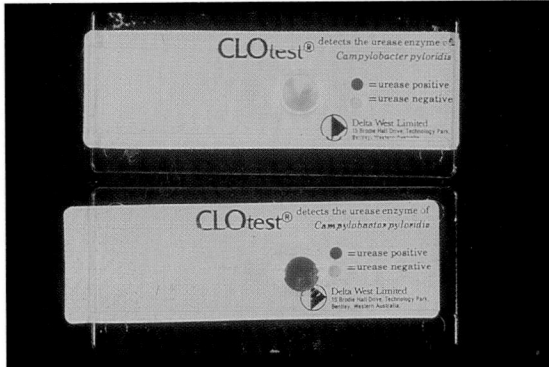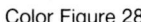

Color Figure 28

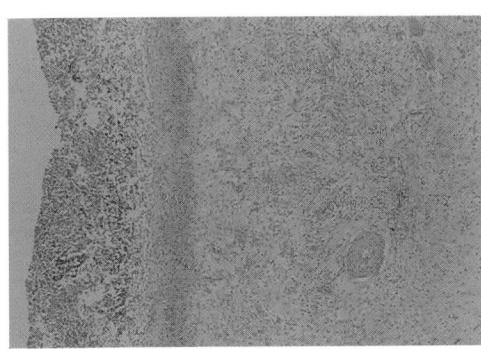

Color Figure 29

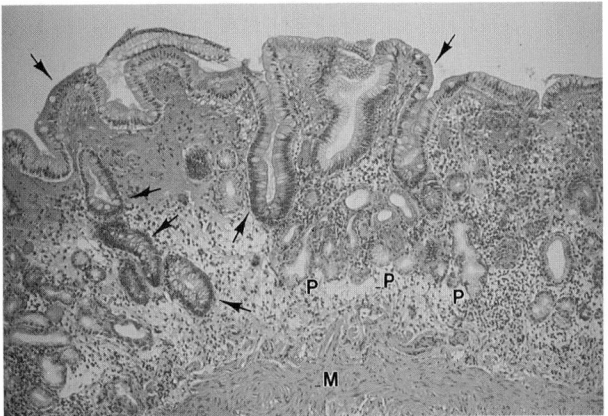

Color Figure 30

COLOR FIGURE 28. CLOtest—presence of Helicobacter pylori is indicated by pink color.

COLOR FIGURE 29. The pathology of peptic ulcer. This ulcer crater shows the four classic zones of activity: fibrinopurulent debris, active cellular infiltrate with neutrophils, granulation tissue, and collagenous scar (Approximately 2.5×). (From Mitros FA. Atlas of gastrointestinal pathology. Philadelphia and London: JB Lippincott and Gower.)

COLOR FIGURE 30. Pernicious anemia with severe atrophic gastritis (type A). A biopsy from the body of the stomach shows that the area occupied by gastric glands is reduced, and the lamina propria is reciprocally expanded and infiltrated predominantly by chronic inflammatory cells. Parietal and chief cells—normal constituents of gastric glands—cannot be seen and are replaced by mucous cells normally observed in pyloric glands (pseudopyloric metaplasia) and by intestinal-type cells (intestinal metaplasia). P denotes glands with pseudopyloric metaplasia; the arrows denote some areas of intestinal metaplasia; and M denotes the muscularis mucosae. Approximately 100×.

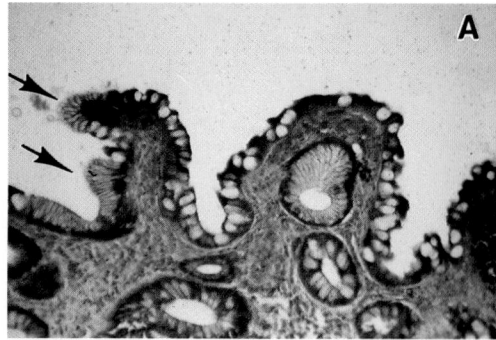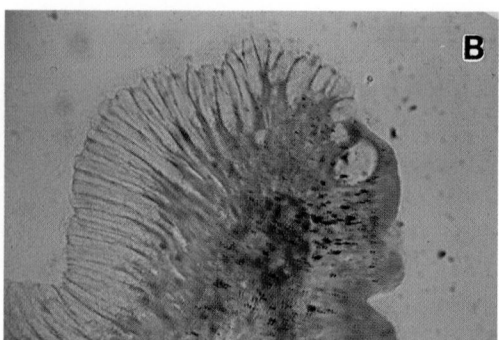

Color Figure 31

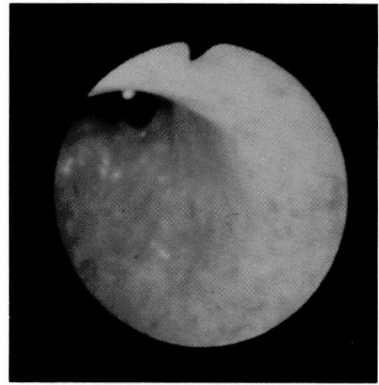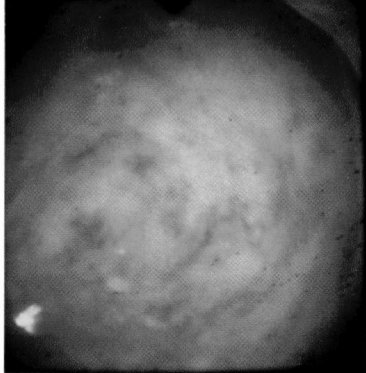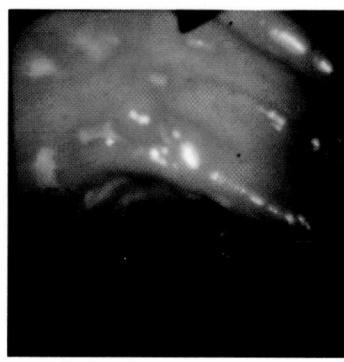

Color Figure 32   Color Figure 33   Color Figure 34

COLOR FIGURE 31A and B. As intestinal-type cells in complete intestinal metaplasia differentiate morphologically and biochemically from undifferentiated "crypt" cells, as illustrated in figure 61-32, they also develop the ability to function as differentiated intestinal villous cells (enterocytes). These two photomicrographs illustrate their ability to absorb lipid. Gastric specimens were frozen, and frozen sections stained with oil red O to demonstrate lipid. The specimen in Color Figure 31A was from a fasting patient with pernicious anemia. Lipid (in red) is observed in the lamina propria just below metaplastic surface intestinal cells, especially at or near the tips of short villi, which have formed on the gastric surface. The arrows indicate small patches of gastric-type mucous cells; the remainder of the surface epithelial cells are intestinal-type. Little lipid is observed beneath the surface epithelium of the normal stomach or beneath gastric-type surface cells in atrophic stomachs. The specimen illustrated in Color Figure 31B was obtained from the same patient 2 hours after a micellar solution of fatty acid and monoglyceride was infused into his stomach. The metaplastic intestinal cells on the right absorb the lipid, whereas the gastric-type surface mucous cells on the left do not. When studied by light and electron microscopy of serial biopsies, the differentiated villous cells of complete intestinal metaplasia appear identical to normal small intestinal enterocytes as they absorb lipid.[150] Thus, the presence of complete intestinal metaplasia seems to change the stomach from a primarily secretory organ to one that is more absorptive in nature.[115] (Figure A, approximately 105×. Figure B, approximately 500×.) (From Rubin W, Ross LL, Jeffries GH, Steinenger MH. Some physiologic properties of heterotopic intestinal epithelium. Its role in transporting lipid into the gastric mucosa. Lab Invest 1967;16:813.)

COLOR FIGURE 32. Mild ulcerative colitis with mucosal edema and some granularity.

COLOR FIGURE 33. Severe ulcerative colitis with total loss of mucosal detail, marked edema, granularity, and erythema. (Courtesy of Dr. Gary Zuckerman, Washington University, St. Louis, MO.)

COLOR FIGURE 34. Crohn's colitis with discrete small round ulcers separated by normal mucosa. (Courtesy of Dr. Gary Zuckerman, Washington University, St. Louis, MO.)

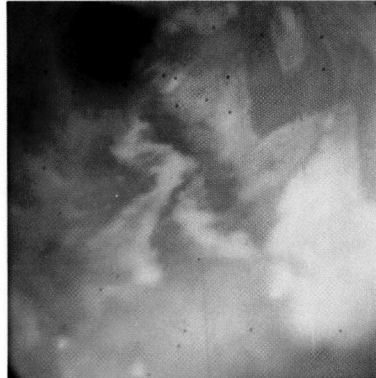

Color Figure 35

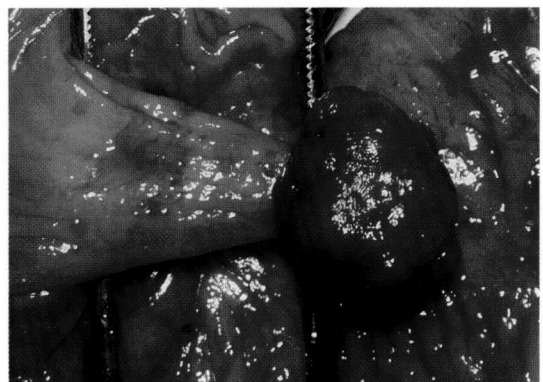

Color Figure 36

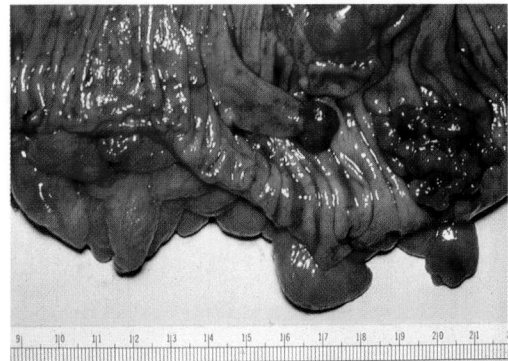

Color Figure 37

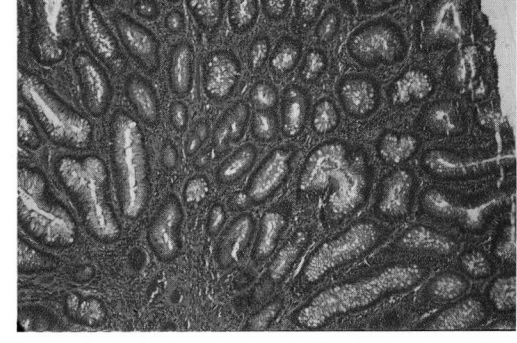

Color Figure 38

COLOR FIGURE 35. Crohn's colitis with long serpiginous ulcers. (Courtesy of Dr. Gary Zuckerman, Washington University, St. Louis, MO.)

COLOR FIGURE 36. Macroscopic appearance of a pedunculated tubular adenoma. The stalk is demonstrated by the forceps marking the base and the neck.

COLOR FIGURE 37. A synchronous pedunculated tubular adenoma adjacent to a sessile tubulovillous adenoma. Synchronous adenomas (not infrequently are found adjacent to each other. In this instance, a 1-cm pedunculated tubular adenoma is found about 5 cm away from a 3 cm sessile tubulovillous adenoma. Note the smooth surface of the tubular adenoma and the smooth lobulated surface of the tubulovillous (primarily tubular) adenoma.

COLOR FIGURE 38. Histologic appearance of a tubular adenoma with minimal dysplasia. Note the architectural features of closely packed epithelial tubules, with hyperchromatic elongated nuclei, but still with a predominant basal orientation, and a normal nuclear:cytoplasmic ratio.

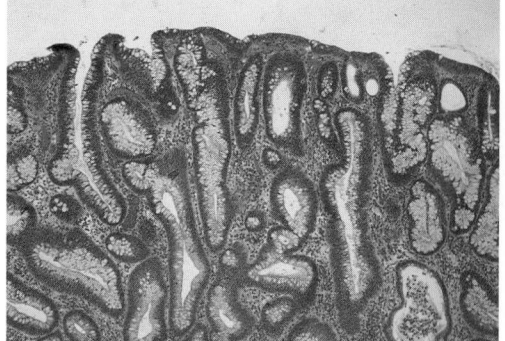

Color Figure 39

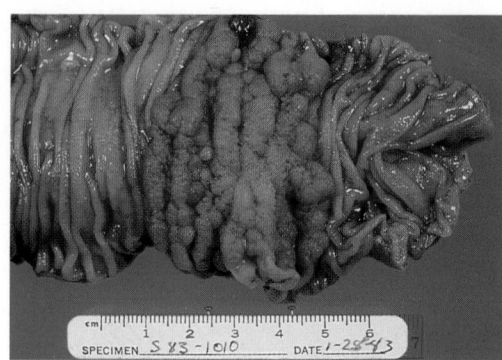

Color Figure 40

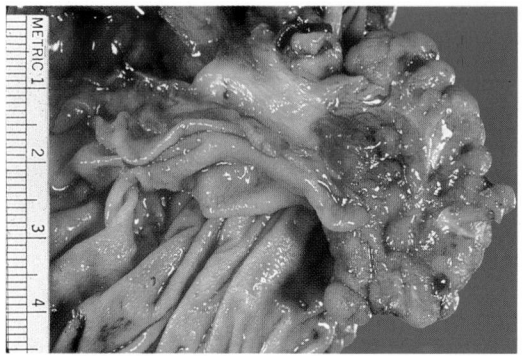

Color Figure 41

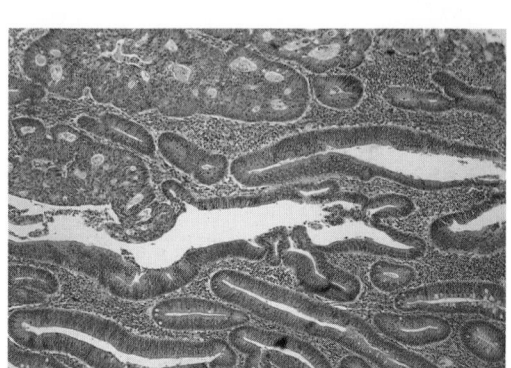

Color Figure 42

COLOR FIGURE 39. Histologic appearance of a tubular adenoma with moderate dysplasia. Note increased cellular crowding, pleomorphic hyperchromatic nuclei, with some loss of basal polarity and increased nuclear: cytoplasmic ratio.

COLOR FIGURE 40. Cecal villous adenoma that is virtually circumferential, with submucosal carcinomatous invasion. Note the sessile nature, cauliflower appearance with a shaggy, frondlike, friable surface. This is in contrast with the smoother lobulated surface seen in Figure 36.

COLOR FIGURE 41. Sectioned surface of a tubulovillous adenoma with early carcinoma extending into the neck of the stalk. Note the large size (4 cm) of the adenoma and the extent of carcinomatous tissue extending from the head of the adenoma into the stalk, obliterating the muscularis propria layers.

COLOR FIGURE 42. Histologic appearance of a tubulovillous adenoma with severe dysplasia and contiguous carcinoma. Note the hyperchromatic elongated nuclei with loss of basal polarity and the increased nuclear: cytoplasmic ratio. There is a sharp and drastic transition from these adenomatous features to carcinoma.

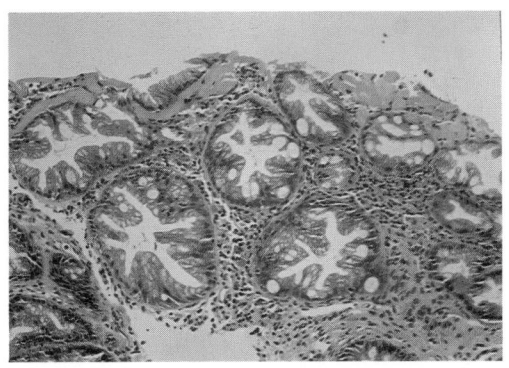

Color Figure 43

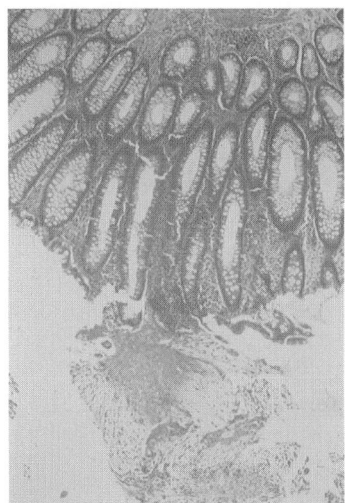

Color Figure 44

Color Figure 45

Color Figure 46

COLOR FIGURE 43. Histologic appearance of a hyperplastic polyp. Note the typical elongated glands with papillary infolding and increased mucus, which contribute towards a serrated surface appearance. The epithelial cells are well differentiated with abundant cytoplasm, normal nuclear: cytoplasmic ratio, and abundant secreted mucus. The nuclei are not hyperchromatic, retain their basal polarity, and show no dysplasia. Note also the characteristic "starfish" appearance of the hyperplastic crypts seen in cross section.

COLOR FIGURE 44. Histologic appearance of adenomatous epithelium in a predominantly hyperplastic polyp. This polyp should be managed as an adenoma, as the adenomatous areas are presumed to be premalignant.

COLOR FIGURE 45. Colonoscopic appearance of pseudomembranous colitis.

COLOR FIGURE 46. Biopsy of a pseudomembrane showing the typical summit lesion.

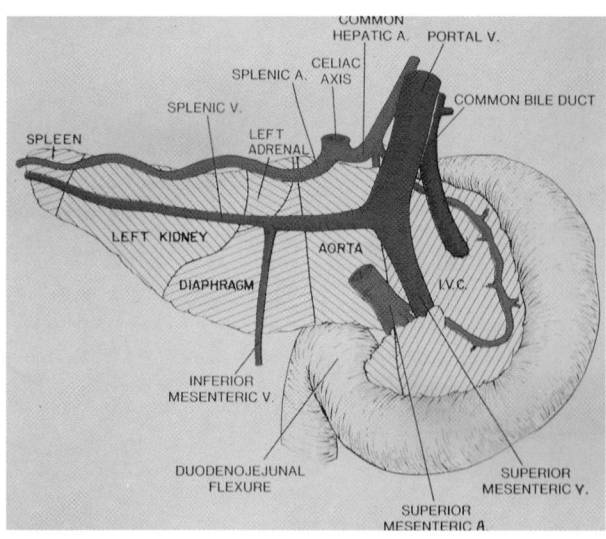

Color Figure 47

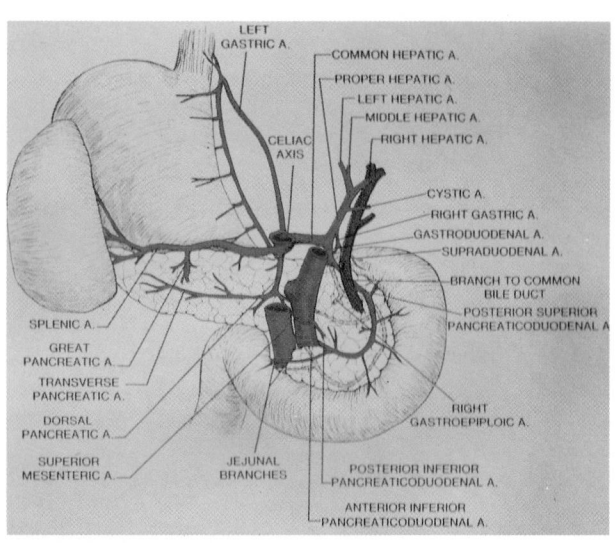

Color Figure 48

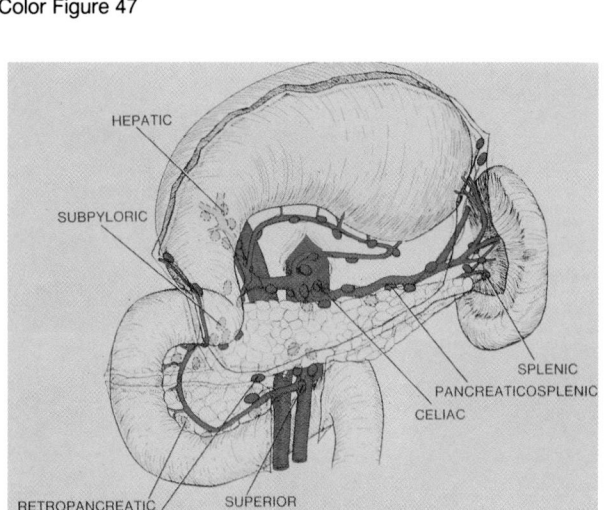

Color Figure 49

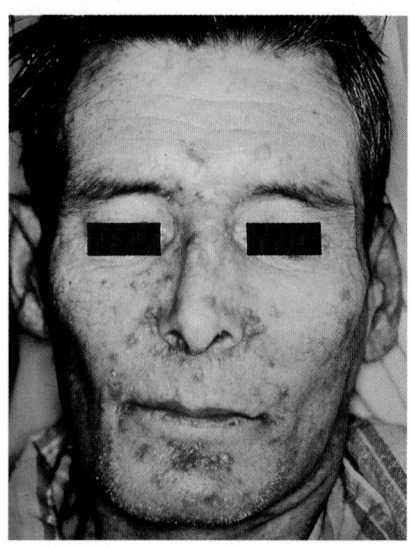

Color Figure 50

COLOR FIGURE 47.   The pancreas and duodenum viewed from their posterior aspect. The major posterior relations of the pancreas are indicated.

COLOR FIGURE 48.   Blood supply of the pancreas. The pancreas, duodenum, stomach, and spleen are viewed from their posterior aspects.

COLOR FIGURE 49.   Lymphatic drainage of the pancreas. The pancreas is viewed from its anterior aspect. The gastrocolic ligament has been divided along the greater curvature of the stomach, which has been retracted anterosuperiorly. The transverse mesocolon has been detached from the peritoneum of the posterior abdominal wall. Labels indicate representative lymph nodes in the major regional nodal groups.

COLOR FIGURE 50.   Migratory necrolytic erythema involving the face in a patient with metastatic glucagonoma. The typical skin lesions, which usually start on the extremities, intertriginous, or periorifical sites, are seen on this patient's face. The lesions initially are erythematous and scaly, later become raised and bullous, and finally crusty, as is evident here. The healing results in the hyperpigmentation. Angular cheilitis, which is a common feature in patients with glucagonoma, is also present in a mild form in this patient. The patient also shows loss of the buccal fat pad and temporal muscle wasting, indicative of the generalized wasting these patients characteristically develop.

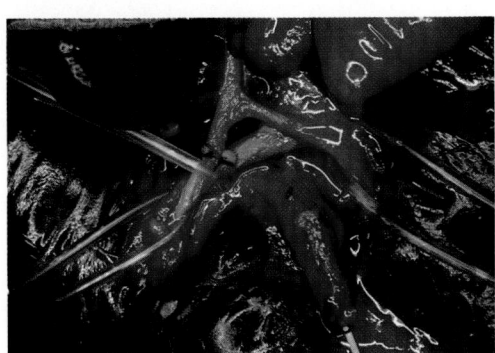 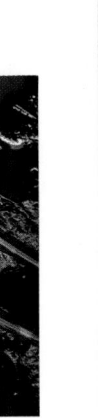

Color Figure 51   Color Figure 52

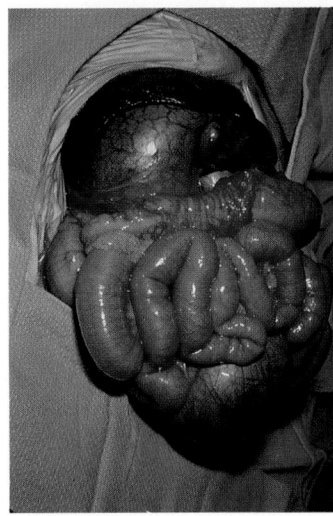 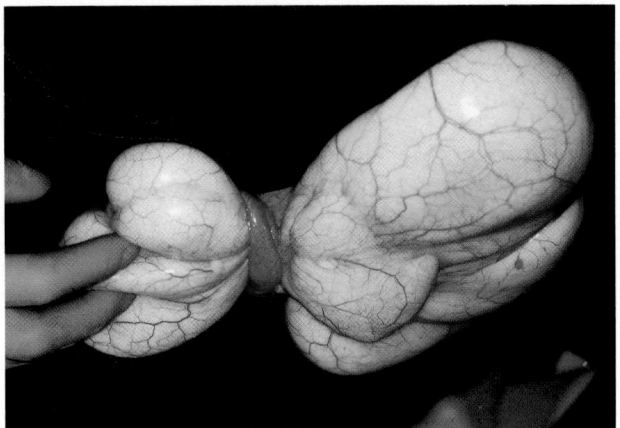

Color Figure 53   Color Figure 54

COLOR FIGURE 51. Photograph of the liver hilum in a patient with biliary atresia. The common hepatic artery is surrounded by a tape. The right and left hepatic arteries are well dissected at the hilum of the liver. The portal vein, surrounded by a tape, has been dissected and is visible behind the artery. The dissection has been completed and there is no extrahepatic biliary tract. (Courtesy of Dr. Michael Harrison.)

COLOR FIGURE 52. Photograph of a giant choledochal cyst. The large cyst is outside the abdomen; the gallbladder and cystic duct (normal) are attached to its top portion. (Courtesy of Dr. Michael Harrison.)

COLOR FIGURE 53. Choledochal cyst. The liver is visible above it and the intestine below. (Courtesy of Dr. Michael Harrison.)

COLOR FIGURE 54. Mesenteric cyst in an infant, as seen at the operating table.

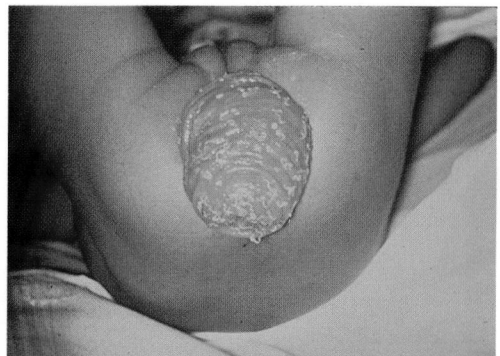

Color Figure 55

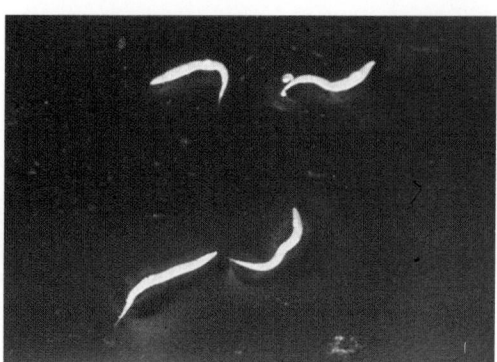

Color Figure 56

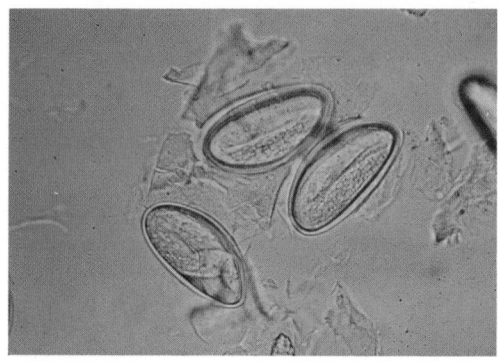

Color Figure 57

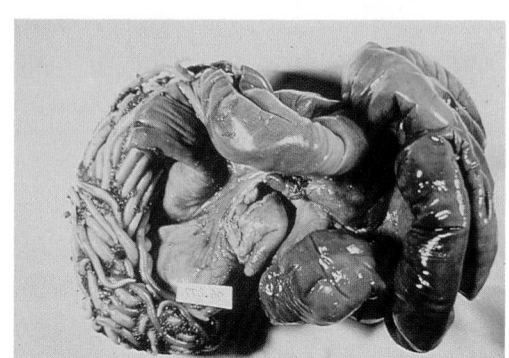

Color Figure 58

COLOR FIGURE 55. *Trichuris trichiura* associated with rectal prolapse in a child. Adult *T. trichiura* are seen as white threads on the mucosal surface. (Reproduced, by permission from JW Smith, et al., *INTESTINAL HELMINTHS*—revised reprint from the Atlas of Diagnostic Medical Parasitology Series. © 1976—revised 1984 by the American Society of Clinical Pathologists, Chicago)

COLOR FIGURE 56. Adult female *Enterobius vermicularis* (pinworm). Adult female pinworms may be found on the perianal skin or occasionally on the surface of stools. Adult females are 8 to 13 mm in length and 0.3 to 0.5 mm wide. The scale is in millimeters. (Reproduced, by permission from JW Smith, et al., *INTESTINAL HELMINTHS*—revised reprint from the Atlas of Diagnostic Medical Parasitology Series. © 1976—revised 1984 by the American Society of Clinical Pathologists, Chicago)

COLOR FIGURE 57. Embryonated eggs of *Enterobius vermicularis*. A cluster of typical eggs is seen in a cellulose tape preparation. Each ova contains an infective larva. Ova are 56 to 58 μm by 27 to 29 μm. (Reproduced, by permission from JW Smith, et al., *INTESTINAL HELMINTHS*—revised reprint from the Atlas of Diagnostic Medical Parasitology Series. © 1976—revised 1984 by the American Society of Clinical Pathologists, Chicago)

COLOR FIGURE 58. *Ascaris lumbricoides* in the intestine. Intestinal obstruction due to a mass of adult *A. lumbricoides* is seen in this autopsy specimen. Intestinal obstruction is an unusual complication of heavy *Ascaris* infection. (Reproduced, by permission from JW Smith, et al., *INTESTINAL HELMINTHS*—revised reprint from the Atlas of Diagnostic Medical Parasitology Series. © 1976—revised 1984 by the American Society of Clinical Pathologists, Chicago)

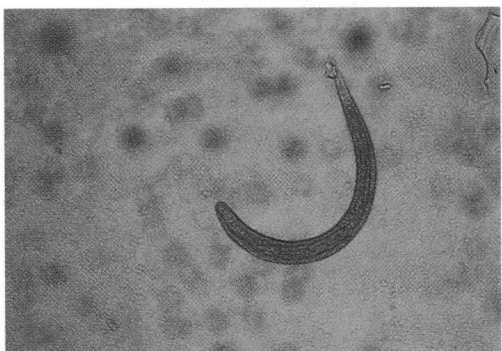

Color Figure 59

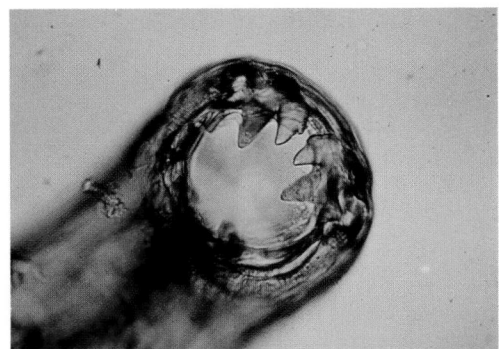

Color Figure 60

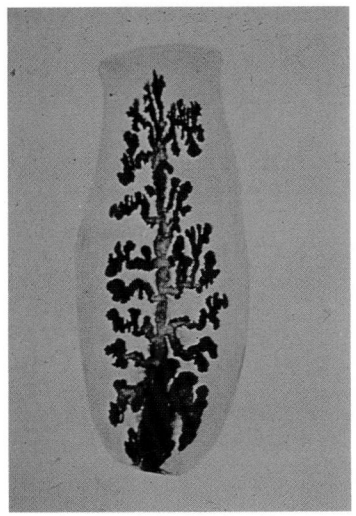

Color Figure 61

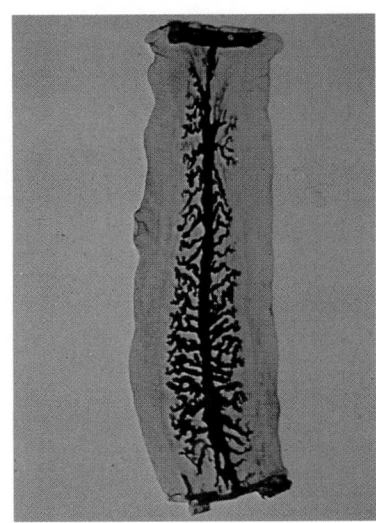

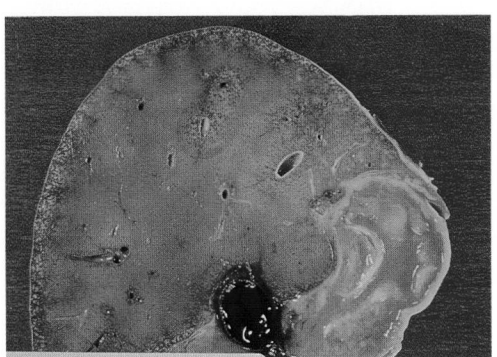

Color Figure 62

COLOR FIGURE 59. *Strongyloides stercoralis* rhabditiform larva (225 × 16 mm) in the stool of a patient with epigastic pain and eosinophilia. (Photomicrograph kindly provided by Richard L. Guerrant, MD, University of Virginia School of Medicine, Charlottesville, Virginia)

COLOR FIGURE 60. *Taenia saginata.* The scolex (brown) with its four suckers is seen at the lower left. Mature proglottids are found at the distal end of the worm. (Reproduced, by permission from JW Smith, et al., *INTESTINAL HELMINTHS*—revised reprint from the Atlas of Diagnostic Medical Parasitology Series. © 1976—revised 1984 by the American Society of Clinical Pathologists, Chicago)

COLOR FIGURE 61. Proglottids of *Taenia saginata* (right) and *T. solium* (left). Proglottids of *T. saginata* have uterine branches more lateral than those of *T. solium,* as illustrated in these India ink-injected proglottids. (Reproduced, by permission from JW Smith, et al., *INTESTINAL HELMINTHS*—revised reprint from the Atlas of Diagnostic Medical Parasitology Series. © 1976—revised 1984 by the American Society of Clinical Pathologists, Chicago)

COLOR FIGURE 62. *Echinococcus granulosus* (hydatid) liver cyst. Hydatid liver cysts have well-defined capsules with an irregular lining. They contain a semiopaque, tan liquid with hydatid "sand" composed of *protoscolicies,* each of which can mature to one adult worm. (Reproduced, by permission from JW Smith, et al., *INTESTINAL HELMINTHS*—revised reprint from the Atlas of Diagnostic Medical Parasitology Series. © 1976—revised 1984 by the American Society of Clinical Pathologists, Chicago)

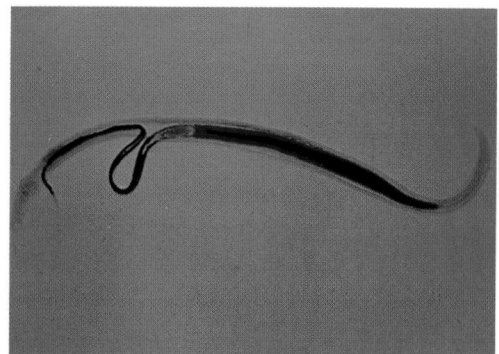

Color Figure 63

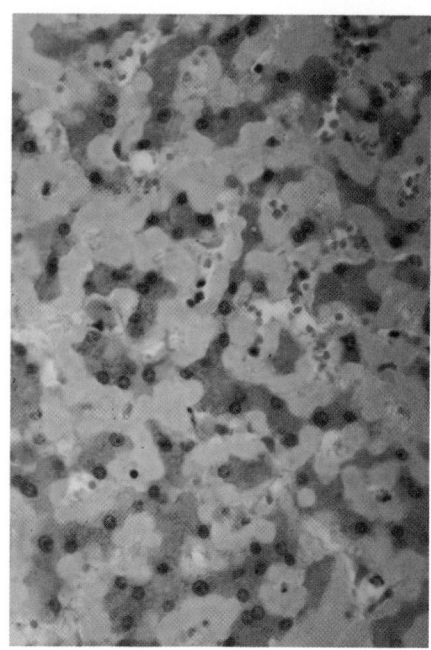

Color Figure 64

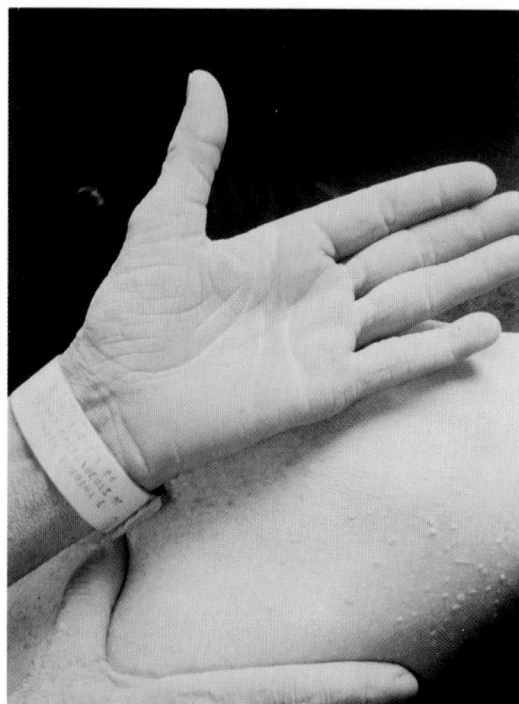

Color Figure 65

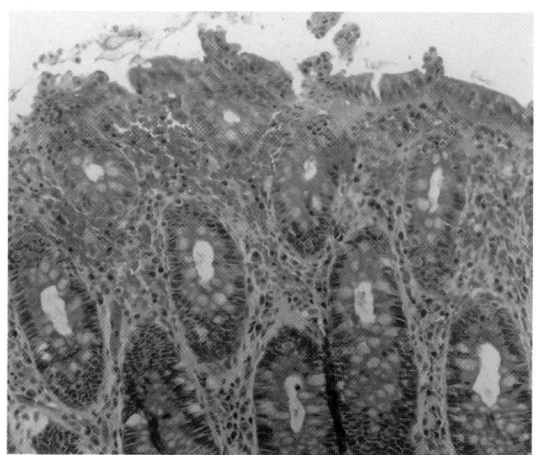

Color Figure 66

COLOR FIGURE 63. *Schistosoma mansoni,* adult worm pair (carmine stain). The long, slender female can be seen protruding from the gynecophoral canal of the larger male worm. *S. mansoni* pairs, such as these, usually reside in the mesenteric plexus in the distribution of the superior mesenteric vein. (Reproduced, by permission from JW Smith, et al., *INTESTINAL HELMINTHS*—revised reprint from the Atlas of Diagnostic Medical Parasitology Series. © 1976—revised 1984 by the American Society of Clinical Pathologists, Chicago)

COLOR FIGURE 64. Hepatic congestion and cirrhosis secondary to congestive heart failure (hematoxylin-eosin, ×100).

COLOR FIGURE 65. Hyperkeratosis of the palm and leg indicative of tylosis.

COLOR FIGURE 66. Colonic biopsy specimen of patient with hemolytic uremic syndrome showing intra-vascular coagulation and thrombotic microangiopathy (hematoxylin-eosin, ×16).

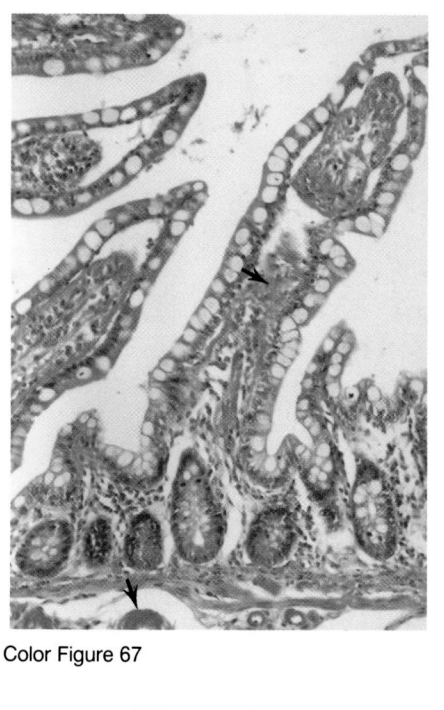
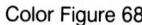

Color Figure 67

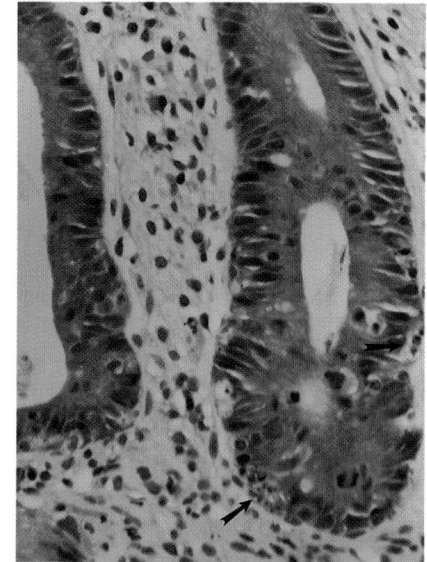

Color Figure 68

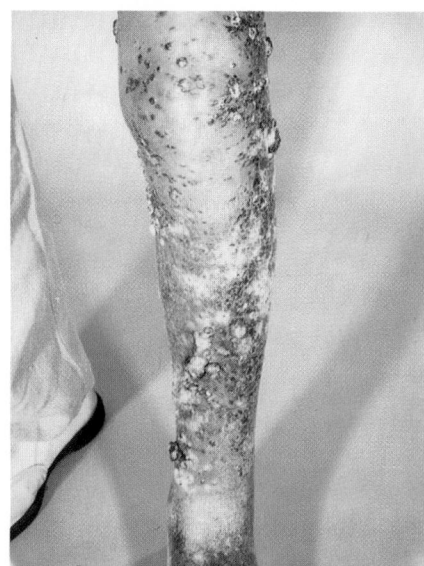
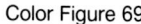

Color Figure 69

Color Figure 70

COLOR FIGURE 67. Amyloid infiltration of the small intestine (arrows) (Congo red, ×200).

COLOR FIGURE 68. Hodgkin's disease infiltrating liver (hematoxylin-eosin, ×25). Reed-Sternberg cells are indicated by arrows.

COLOR FIGURE 69. Kaposi's sarcoma of the lower extremities.

COLOR FIGURE 70. Rectal biopsy specimen from a patient showing crypt cell degeneration, which is the characteristic lesion of graft versus host disease (hematoxylin–eosin, ×100).

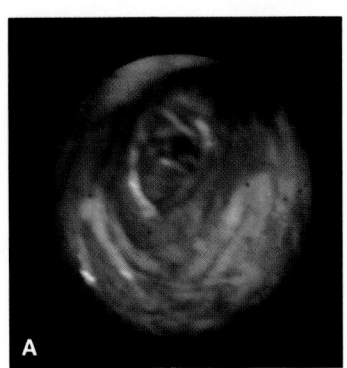

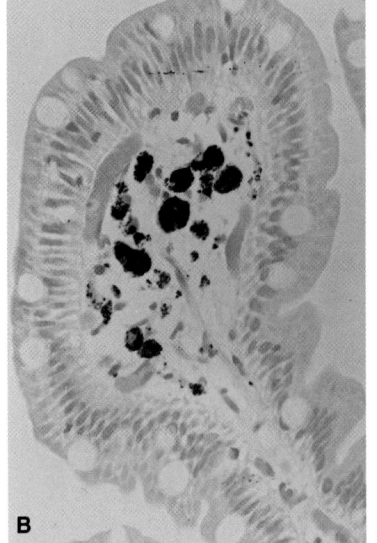

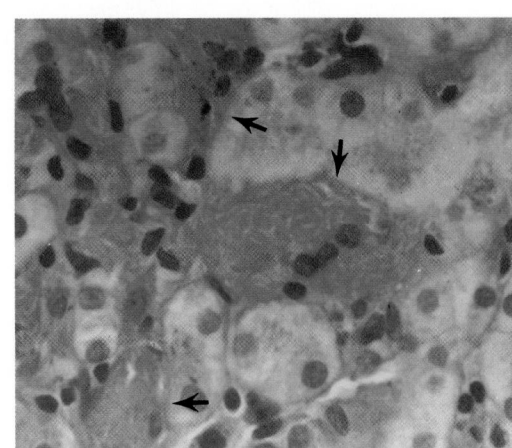

Color Figure 71

Color Figure 72

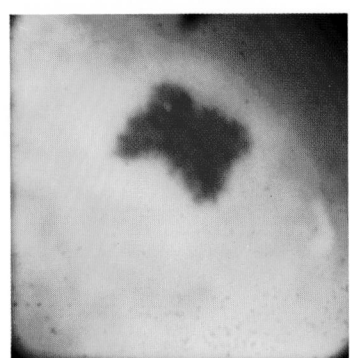

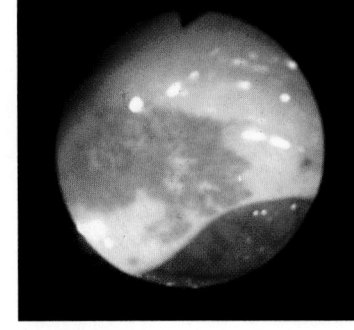

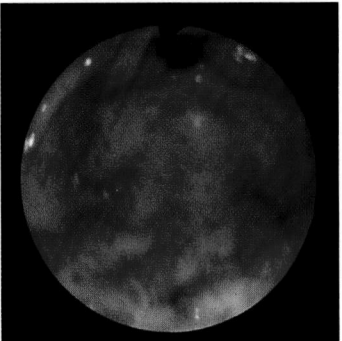

Color Figure 73

Color Figure 74

Color Figure 75

COLOR FIGURE 71. A, Endoscopic appearance of pseudomelanosis duodeni. **B,** Duodenal biopsy specimen from a patient with pseudomelanosis duodeni showing the deposition of pigment within lamina propria macrophages.

COLOR FIGURE 72. Gaucher disease of the liver. Arrows indicate multinucleated Gaucher cells (hematoxylin–eosin, ×400).

COLOR FIGURE 73. A well-demarcated, 3-mm, duodenal angiodysplastic lesion with fernlike margins. A pale ''halo'' is noted around this lesion (*arrow*).

COLOR FIGURE 74. Cecal angiodysplasia 1.5 cm in diameter detected during colonoscopic evaluation for chronic gastrointestinal bleeding. Frondlike margins are present for part of the lesion.

COLOR FIGURE 75. Gastric antral vascular ectasia detected in a 71-year-old male with chronic iron deficiency anemia and occult fecal blood. The intensely red stripes alternate with areas of more normal mucosa, providing the ''watermelon'' appearance.

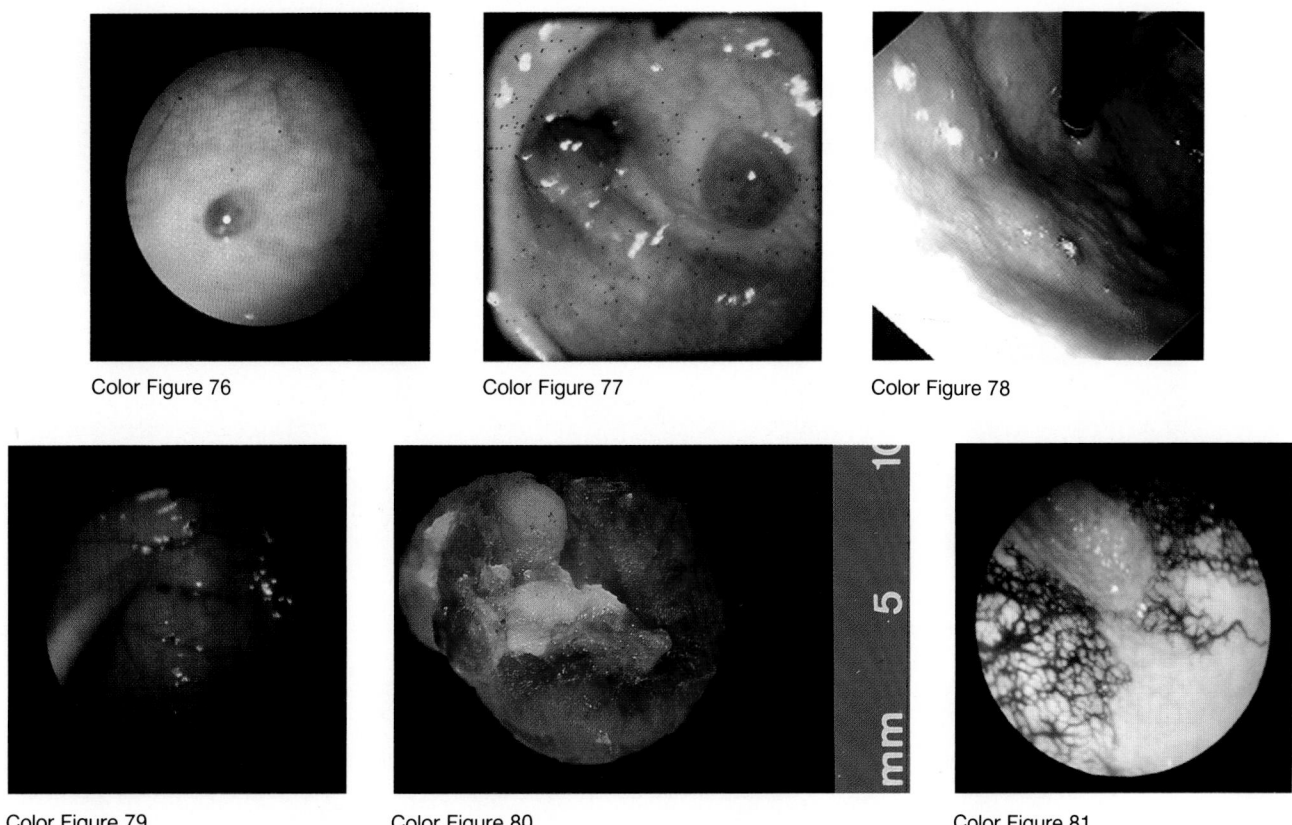

Color Figure 76   Color Figure 77   Color Figure 78

Color Figure 79   Color Figure 80   Color Figure 81

COLOR FIGURE 76. A 3–4 mm, capillary hemangioma with a smooth, round appearance detected at colonoscopy.

COLOR FIGURE 77. Well-circumscribed polypoid lesions of blue rubber bleb nevus syndrome in a 28-year-old man. These blue-red lesions of 1–2 cm in size were present in the colon (shown), stomach, and small intestine.

COLOR FIGURE 78. Protruding fibrin plug from a Dieulafoy's lesion on the lesser curvature of the proximal stomach. The endoscope is seen in retroflexion at the esophagogastric junction.

COLOR FIGURE 79. Small venous varicosities consistent with the diagnosis of multiple phlebectasia in the colon. The lesions in this case were 4–10 mm in size with a bluish discoloration.

COLOR FIGURE 80. Big particle biopsy of a large gastric erosion, removed with an electrosurgical snare.

COLOR FIGURE 81. Methylene blue scattering in villus atrophy due to gluten enteropathy.

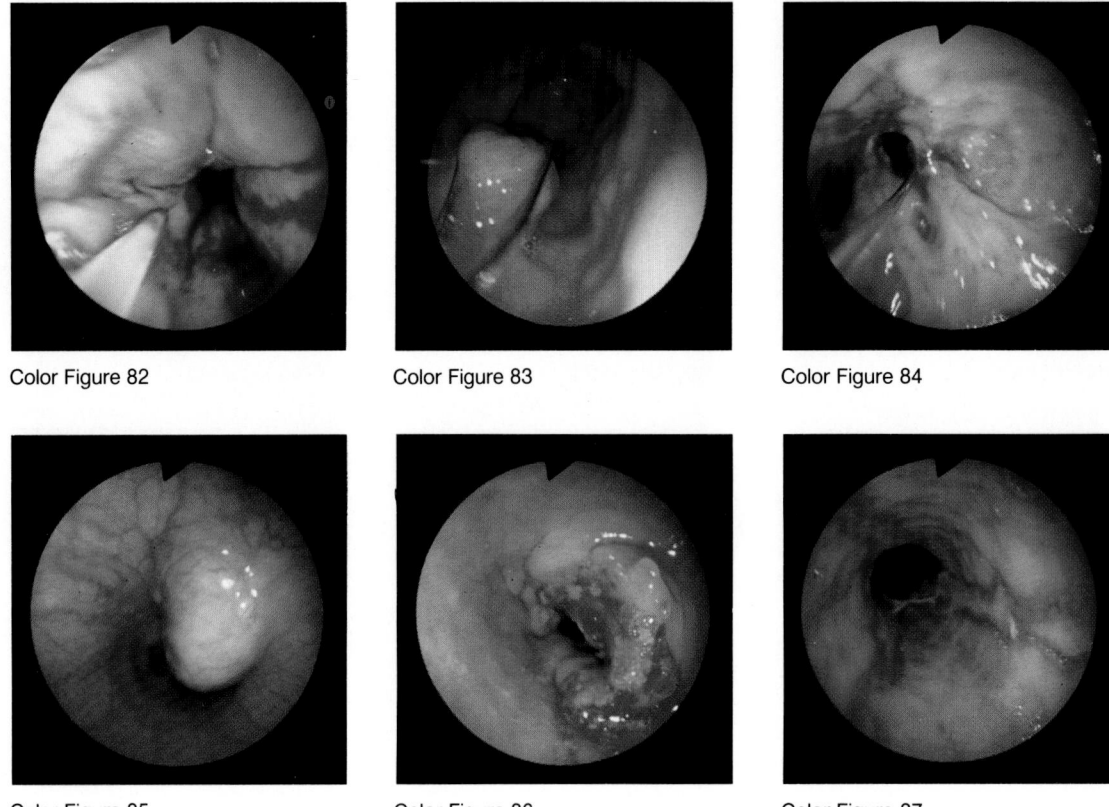

Color Figure 82 Color Figure 83 Color Figure 84

Color Figure 85 Color Figure 86 Color Figure 87

COLOR FIGURE 82. Technique of endoscopic sclerotherapy. The sclerotherapy needle is inserted in the variceal structure.

COLOR FIGURE 83. Polypectomy of gastric polyp; the snare loop is positioned around the sessile adenomatous polyp.

COLOR FIGURE 84. Eccentric reflux-induced stricture, through which a guidewire has been passed.

COLOR FIGURE 85. Esophageal leiomyoma.

COLOR FIGURE 86. Esophageal carcinoma obstructing the esophagus.

COLOR FIGURE 87. Example of reflux esophagitis grade II with confluent but noncircumferential erosions.

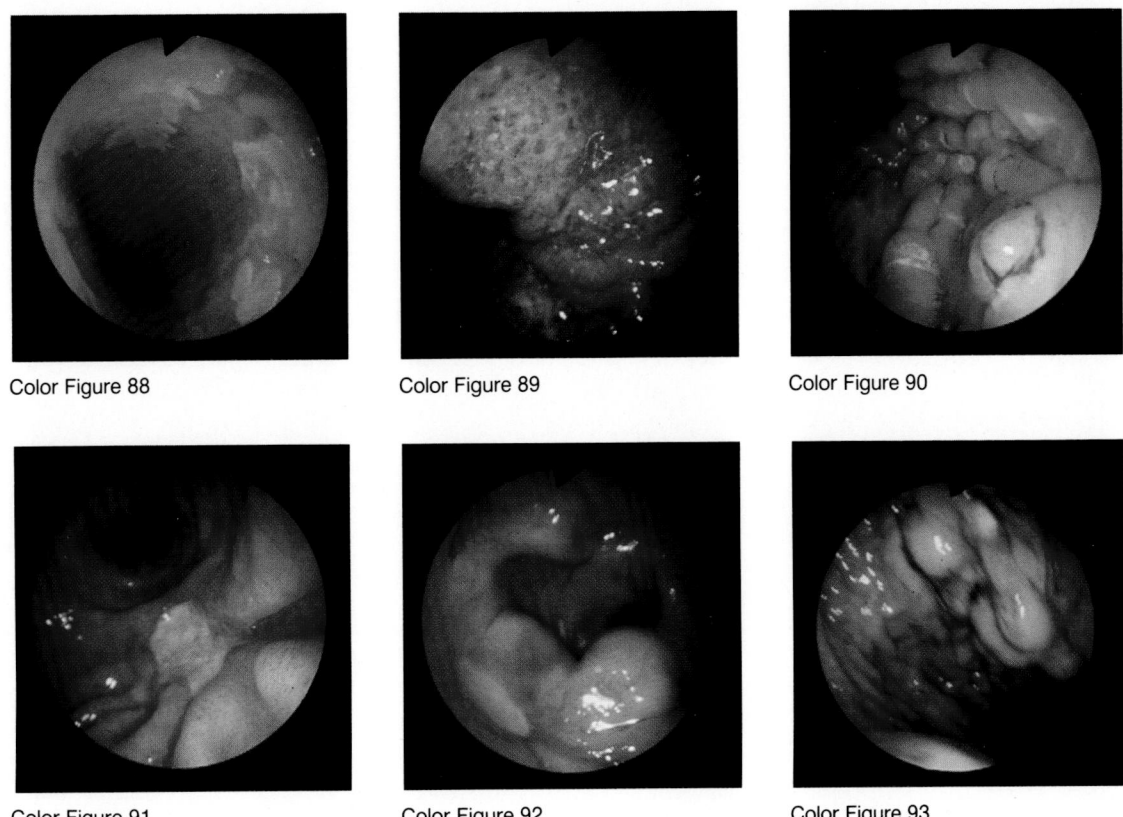

Color Figure 88

Color Figure 89

Color Figure 90

Color Figure 91

Color Figure 92

Color Figure 93

COLOR FIGURE 88. Example of a columnar-lined esophagus or Barrett's esophagus.

COLOR FIGURE 89. Endoscopic example of gastritis with punctate erythema and swelling.

COLOR FIGURE 90. Endoscopic example of erosive gastritis.

COLOR FIGURE 91. Atypical gastric ulceration, along the greater curvature, presumably NSAID-induced.

COLOR FIGURE 92. Deformed bulb due to scarring after prior ulceration and recurrent duodenal ulcer.

COLOR FIGURE 93. Gastric fundus varices.

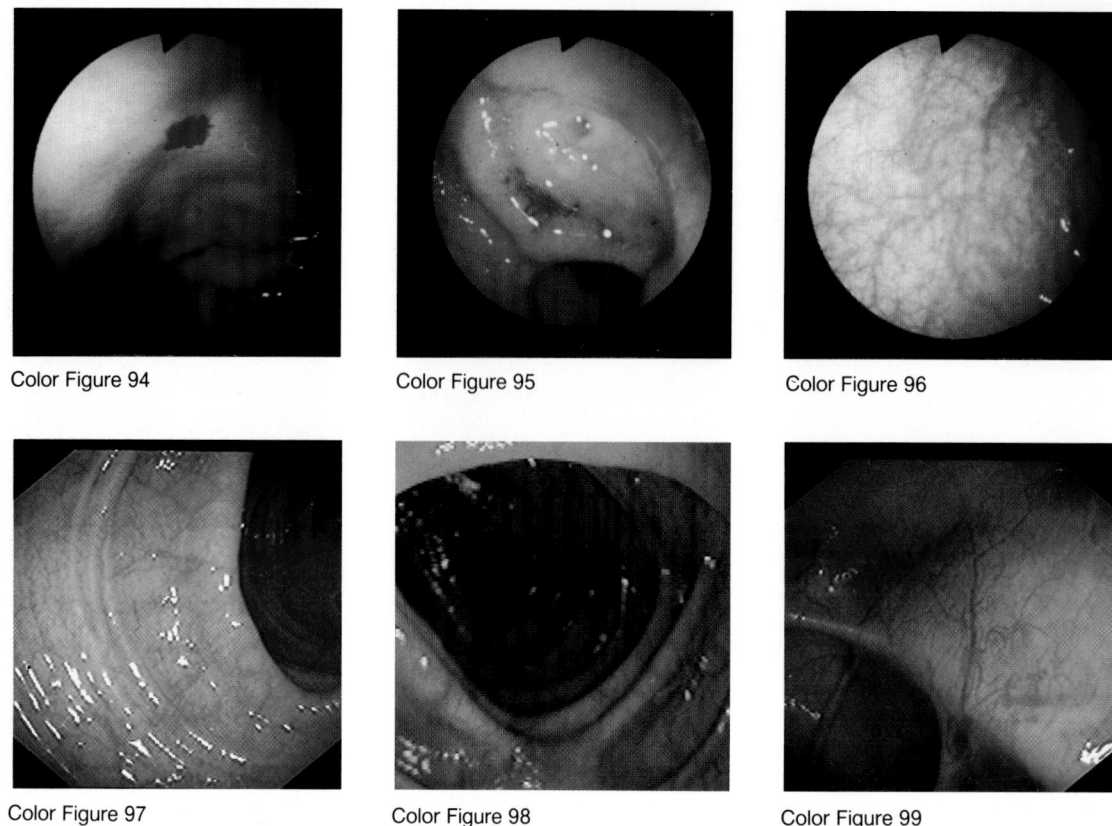

Color Figure 94

Color Figure 95

Color Figure 96

Color Figure 97

Color Figure 98

Color Figure 99

COLOR FIGURE 94. Gastric mucosal vascular anomaly.

COLOR FIGURE 95. Duodenal ulcer with visible vessel in the base of the ulcer.

COLOR FIGURE 96. Atrophic gastritis.

COLOR FIGURE 97. Sigmoid colon, circular outline with the "light reflex" over arcs of circular musculature, clearly indicating the center of the lumen for close-up steering purposes.

COLOR FIGURE 98. Transverse colon, showing the characteristic triangular outline resulting from the relative thickness of the three longitudinal teniae coli, compared to the thinner circular muscle.

COLOR FIGURE 99. Hepatic flexure showing the blue-gray impression of the liver; similar discoloration can be caused by other extracolonic viscera at the splenic flexure or in the distal colon. Note the longitudinal impression of a tenia as well as the transverse haustral folds.

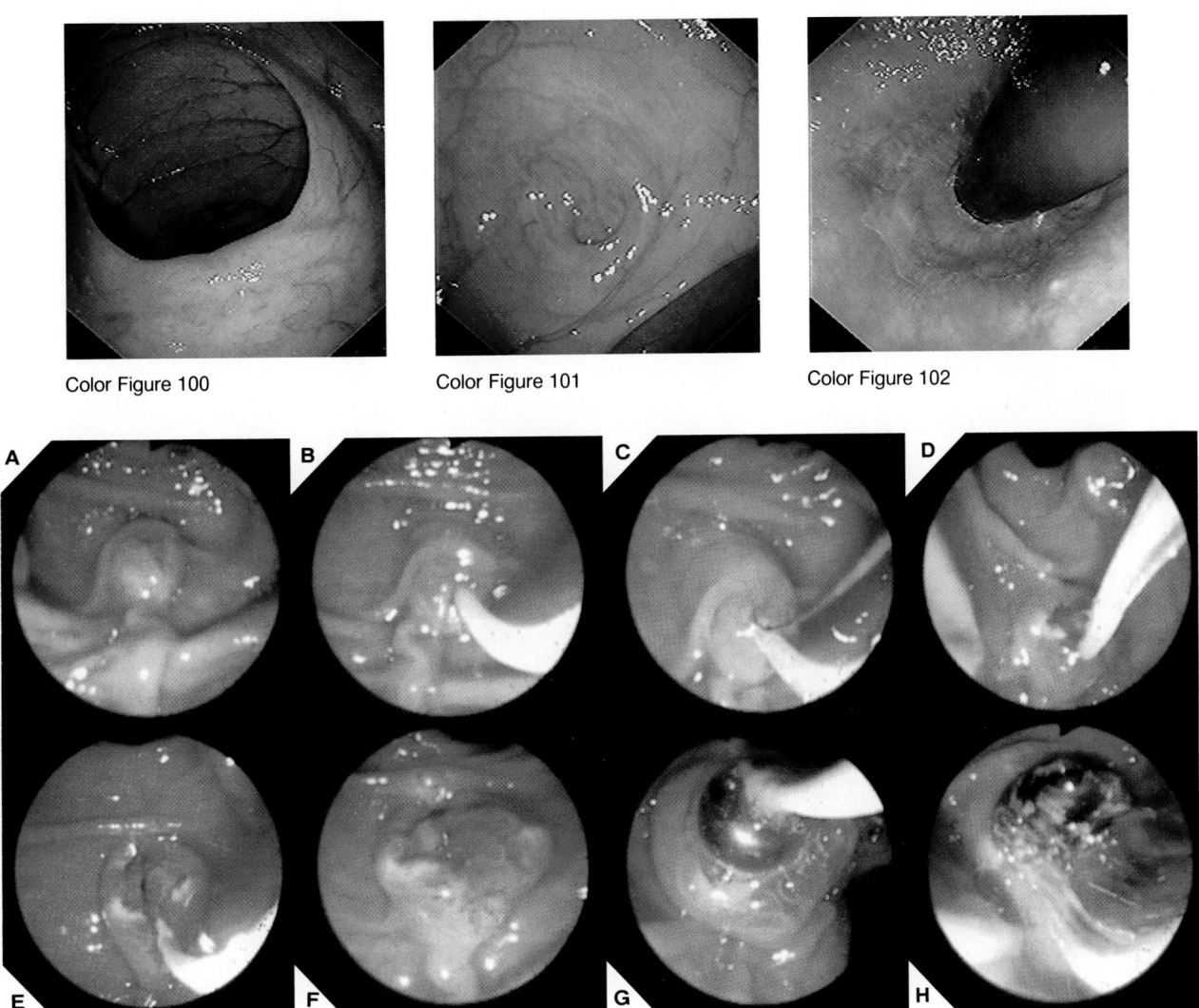

Color Figure 100   Color Figure 101   Color Figure 102

Color Figure 103

COLOR FIGURE 100. Ileocecal fold, showing the characteristic "notch" on a flattened fold. The notch denotes the superior labia of the ileocecal valve. The opening is just below the notch and cannot be seen without marked angulation of the instrument tip.

COLOR FIGURE 101. Appendix orifice, variable in configuration. Here, the orifice is round, but it may be a crescent slit. It is usually rather insignificant in appearance. The internal aspect remains the same after appendectomy.

COLOR FIGURE 102. Retroversion of the endoscope in the rectum is a useful maneuver to find or remove small polyps in the distal part of the rectal ampulla. The dentate (pectinate) line is seen to be serpiginous, at the junction of the squamous mucosa of the rectal canal (purple) and the columnar rectal mucosa.

COLOR FIGURE 103. The sequence of endoscopic sphincterotomy and stone extraction is demonstrated. A normal appearing papilla (**A**) is first cannulated with a diagnostic catheter (**B**). The papillotome is introduced into the papilla (**C**) and an incision is made using electrocautery (**D** and **E**) leaving a completed sphincterotomy (**F**). A balloon catheter is then used to calibrate the size of the sphincterotomy (**G**), followed by pulling the stone into the duodenum (**H**). (From Silverstein, Tytgat. Atlas of gastrointestinal endoscopy.)

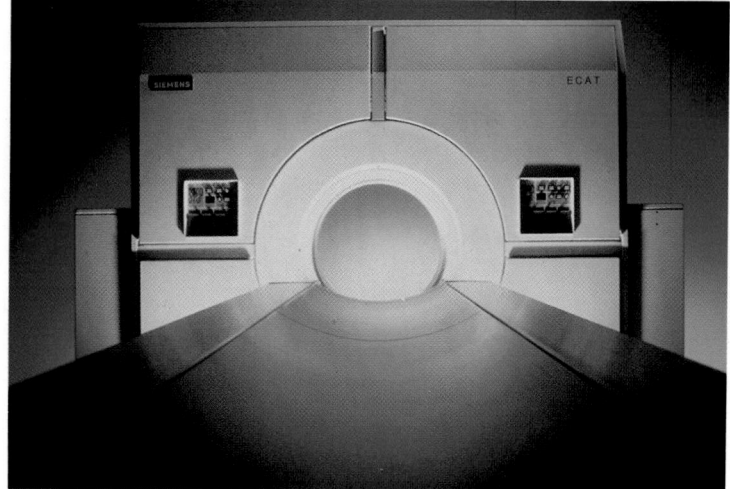

Color Figure 104

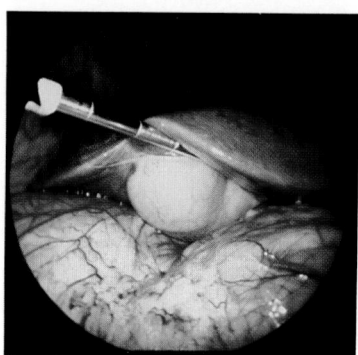

Color Figure 105

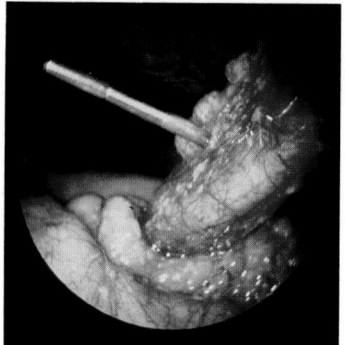

Color Figure 106

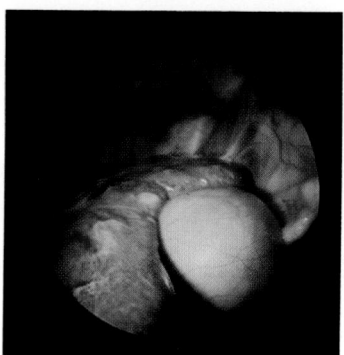

Color Figure 107

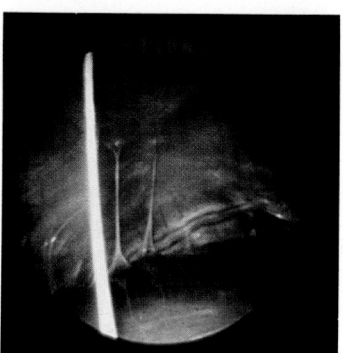

Color Figure 108

COLOR FIGURE 104. State-of-the-art positron emission tomography (PET) camera (Siemens/CTI 931) used for whole-body imaging. This instrument consists of 8 detector rings (512 detectors each), allowing simultaneous imaging of 15 planes (6.75 mm thick).

COLOR FIGURE 105. View of normal right upper quadrant showing liver margin elevated by a palpating probe passed by way of a 4-mm second puncture trocar. Elevation of the liver margin gives a clear view of the gallbladder and permits inspection for hidden focal lesions such as metastases. The omentum is in the lower left, and the gastric antrum is in lower right.

COLOR FIGURE 106. View of round and falciform ligaments and medial right hepatic lobe surfaces covered with many small metastases from carcinoma of the stomach. Metastases on the anterior gastric wall is shown just below the round ligament in lower center. All staging studies before laparoscopy, including computed tomography, indicated disease limited to the stomach. This laparoscopic diagnosis saved the patient a needless laparotomy.

COLOR FIGURE 107. The right hepatic lobe has a dark green lobular pattern indicative of severe cholestasis. The distended, tense gallbladder is due to common bile duct obstruction (Courvoisier sign). Along the medial margin of the right hepatic lobe are multiple 2- to 3-mm diameter metastases from carcinoma of the pancreas not detected by imaging studies before laparoscopy. Laparotomy was avoided, and an endoscopically placed biliary stent provided relief of bile duct obstruction.

COLOR FIGURE 108. This view of the right hepatic lobe reveals several ''violin string'' adhesions between liver and peritoneum caused by gonococcal perihepatitis. This young woman presented with recurrent, focal, perihepatic pain typical of the Curtis-Fitz-Hugh syndrome after developing gonococcal salpingitis.

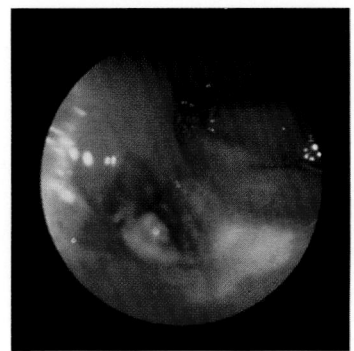

Color Figure 109

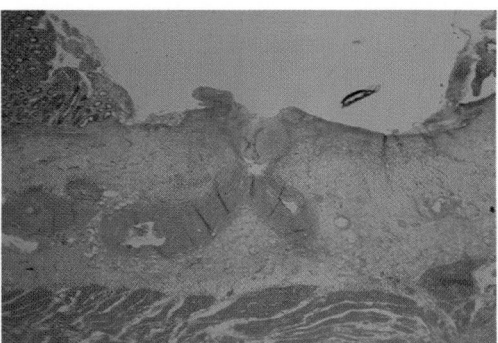

Color Figure 110

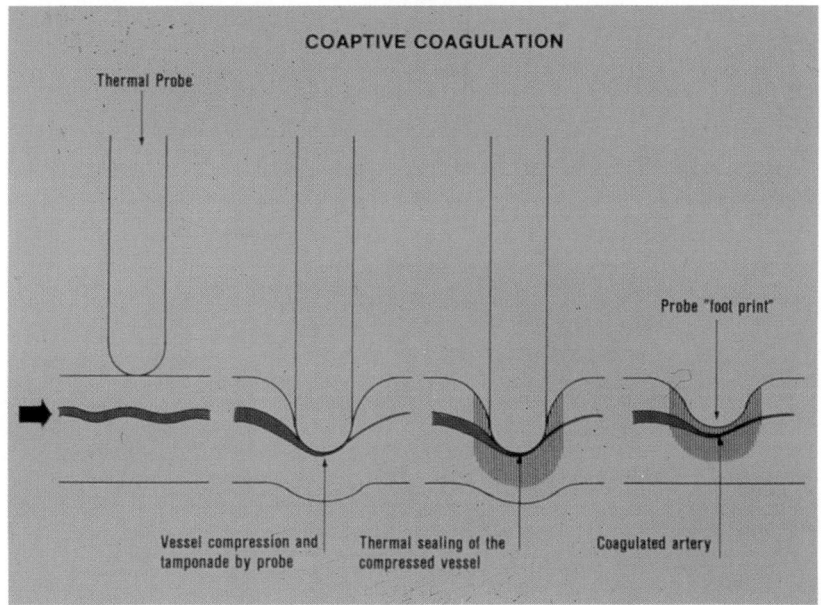

Color Figure 111

COLOR FIGURE 109. Nonbleeding visible vessel in a benign ulcer crater.

COLOR FIGURE 110. Histopathology of a nonbleeding visible vessel in a resected chronic gastric ulcer. Note there is a side hole in the artery, and an organizing clot protrudes into the ulcer crater from this. The artery is nearest to the ulcer base at the visible vessel site. (Courtesy of C. Paul Swain, M.D.)

COLOR FIGURE 111. Tamponade of coaptation, and effective coagulation of a submucosal artery by a contact probe. *Left,* patent artery. *Middle,* vessel compression by tamponade. *Right,* coagulated vessel and probe imprint. (From Johnston JH, Jensen DM, Auth D. Experimental comparison of endoscopic yttrium-aluminum-garnet laser, electrosurgery, and heater probe for canine gut arterial coagulation: The importance of vessel compression and avoidance of tissue erosion. Gastroenterology 1987;92:1101.)

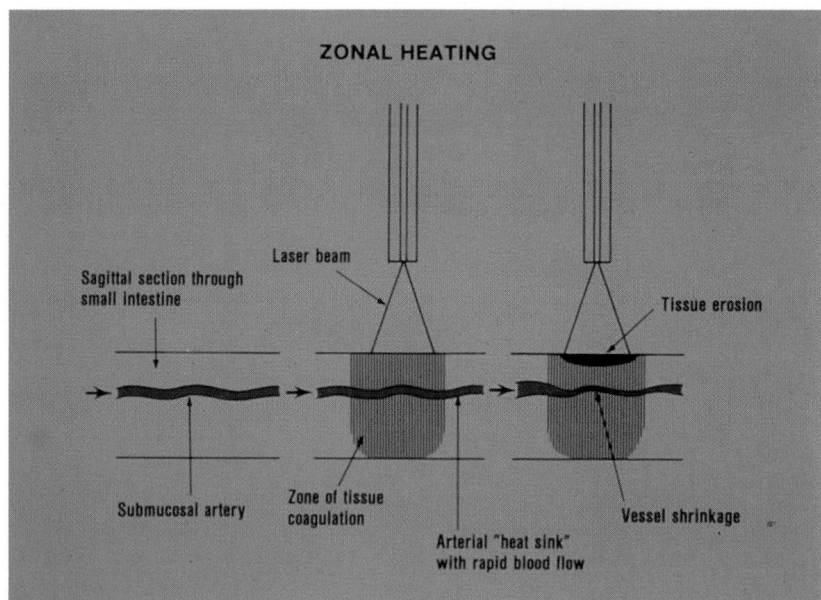

Color Figure 112

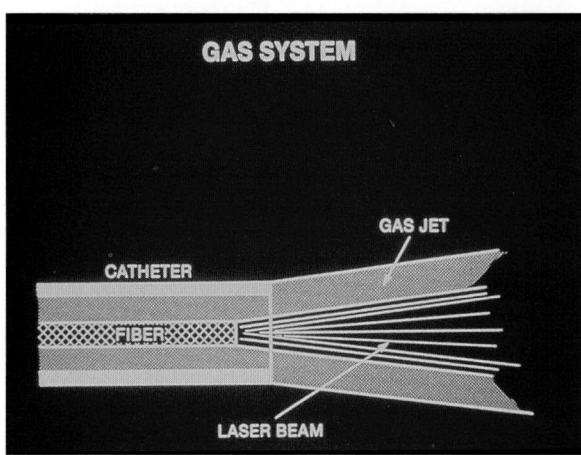

Color Figure 113

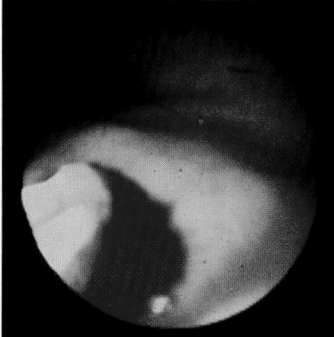

Color Figure 114

COLOR FIGURE 112. Zonal heating and coagulation with laser. *Left,* patent artery. *Middle,* en face coagulation of tissue transmurally without artery coagulation. *Right,* vessel shrinkage, tissue coagulation, and tissue erosion. (From Johnston JH, Jensen DM, Auth D. Experimental comparison of endoscopic yttrium-aluminum-garnet laser, electrosurgery, and heater probe for canine gut arterial coagulation: The importance of vessel compression and avoidance of tissue erosion. Gastroenterology 1987;92:1101.)

COLOR FIGURE 113. Laser catheter with coaxial CO_2 gas around central quartz lightguide. (Courtesy of Charles Enderby, Ph.D)

COLOR FIGURE 114. BICAP treatment of a bleeding ulcer. Tamponade of the ulcer with the large probe in a tangential approach.

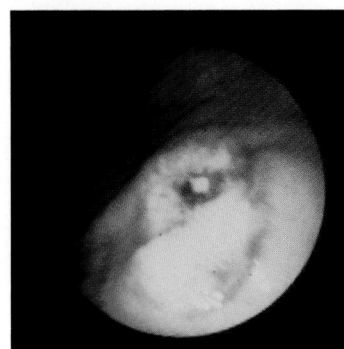

Color Figure 115

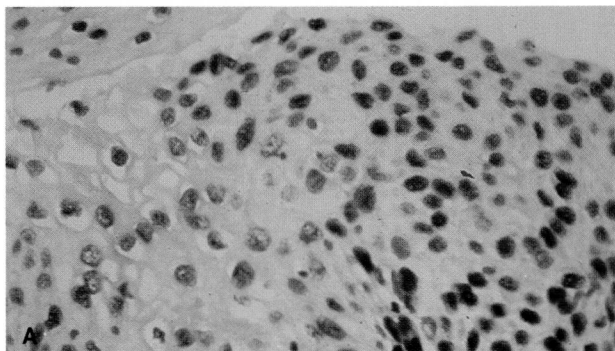

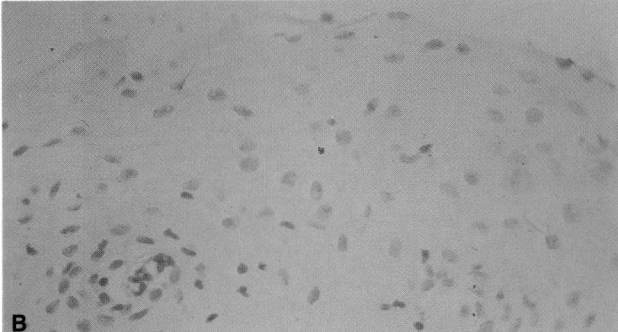

Color Figure 116

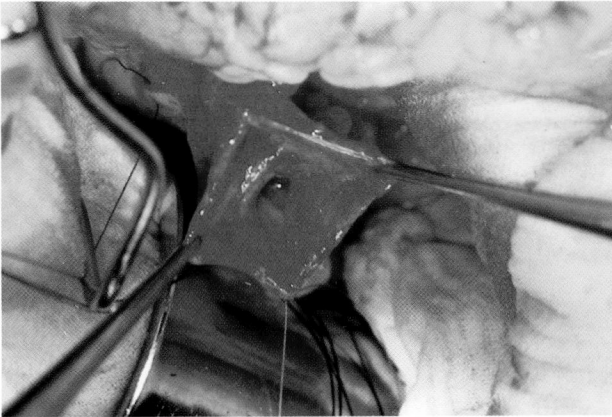

Color Figure 117

COLOR FIGURE 115. After BICAP coagulation of the actively bleeding ulcer, (see color Fig 114). Note the coagulated vessel in the ulcer crater.

COLOR FIGURE 116. In situ hybridization. Tissue sample positive for human papilloma viruses (HPV) by in situ hybridization. Three on one shows positive **A,** and negative **B,** controls, positive specimen **C,** for HPV 16 + 18 probes. (With permission, courtesy of Life Technology.)

COLOR FIGURE 117. Operative view of a sigmoid perforation that occurred during diagnostic colonscopy. The antimesenteric portion of the sigmoid colon has been torn open over a 15-cm segment.

I

Basic Mechanisms of Normal and Abnormal Gastrointestinal Function

A. COMPONENTS

1

The Enteric Nervous System and Its Extrinsic Connections

JOHN B. FURNESS
JOEL C. BORNSTEIN

The gastrointestinal tract is unique among mammalian organ systems in having a nervous system, the enteric nervous system, intrinsic to the organ. The enteric nervous system contains reflex pathways that are capable of functioning independently of central control, although in normal life the central nervous system continuously or intermittently modifies activity within the enteric nervous system. The enteric nervous system has essential roles in the control of motility, blood flow, and water and electrolyte transport.

In this chapter we have provided an overview of the major structural and functional features of the enteric nervous system. We have also discussed the connections between the intestine and the prevertebral ganglia in detail, because these ganglia are involved in enteroenteric reflexes acting via pathways that are external to the gastrointestinal tract and yet bypass the central nervous system. The organization and physiology of centers within the central nervous system from which the digestive system is influenced are covered in Chapter 3. In the present chapter we only deal with the ways in which pathways from the central nervous system make connections with enteric neurons.

STRUCTURAL ORGANIZATION OF THE ENTERIC NERVOUS SYSTEM

The enteric nervous system consists of a vast number of nerve cell bodies and their processes embedded in the wall of the gut. The number of enteric neurons in humans is estimated to be 10 to 100 million, which is about the same number of neurons as are in the spinal cord.[1] The nerve cell bodies are grouped in small aggregates, the enteric ganglia, which are connected by bundles of nerve cell processes to form two major ganglionated plexuses, the myenteric, or Auerbach's, plexus and the submucous plexus, which is often referred to as Meissner's plexus.

Location of Enteric Ganglia

The myenteric plexus lies between the longitudinal and circular layers of the muscularis externa and forms a continuous network around the circumference of the tubular digestive tract from the upper esophagus to the internal anal sphincter (Fig 1-1). Myenteric ganglia of similar size are found in the striated and smooth muscle parts of the human esophagus.[2] In those parts of the large intestine where the longitudinal muscle is gathered into taeniae, the myenteric plexus is prominent underneath the taeniae and is sparser over the rest of the colonic surface.

The submucous plexus of ganglia, which is located in the submucous layer, is only significant in the small and large intestines; extensive networks of interlinked ganglia are not found in the submucosa of the esophagus and stomach, although rare ganglia are sometimes encountered in these regions. Ganglia are occasionally found in the mucosa, usually in the connective tissue close to the muscularis mucosae.[3] Small ganglia are also found along the extrinsic nerves (the vagus, the pelvic, and the mesenteric nerves) as they enter the gut. Some of the ganglia associated with the extrinsic nerves are on the surface of the gut, particularly in the stomach and rectum; these are referred to as subserous ganglia. It should be emphasized, however, that the great majority of enteric neurons have their cell bodies in the ganglia of the myenteric or submucous plexuses. Enteric ganglia are also found in the biliary system and pancreas.

Nonganglionated Plexuses

A series of nonganglionated plexuses supply the layers of the tubular digestive tract (Fig 1-2).[3] These are the longitudinal muscle plexus, the circular muscle plexus, the plexus of the muscularis mucosae, and the mucosal plexus. A perivascular plexus is also found around arteries and arterioles in the gut wall.

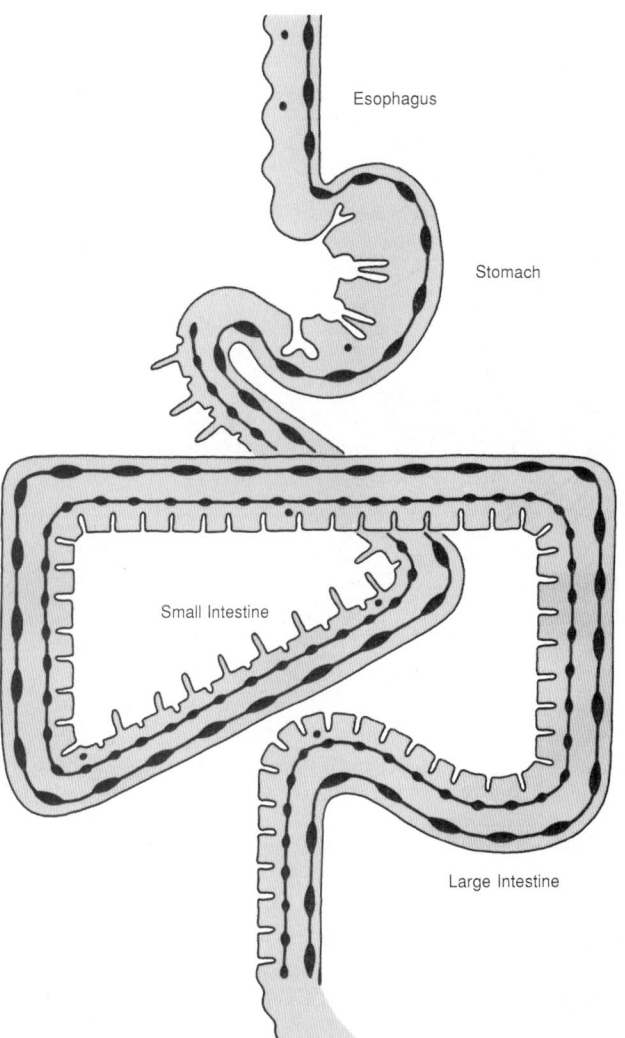

FIGURE 1–1. Distribution of enteric ganglia in the tubular digestive tract. The gastrointestinal tract is depicted in longitudinal section, to reveal the myenteric ganglia, which form a continuous plexus from the upper esophagus to the internal anal sphincter; the submucous plexus, which is prominent in the small and large intestines; and isolated ganglia in the gastric and esophageal submucosa and in the mucosa of the digestive tract.

The pattern of innervation of the longitudinal muscle differs according to the thickness of the muscle. In the human (and other species in which the longitudinal muscle is thick throughout the intestine) nerve fiber bundles that run parallel to the muscle are found throughout its thickness. These make up the longitudinal muscle plexus. In some species the longitudinal muscle of the small intestine is less than about 10 muscle cells thick. In these species (e.g., rabbit and guinea pig), nerve fiber bundles do not form a plexus within the longitudinal muscle. There is instead a tertiary plexus, which is a component of the myenteric plexus that lies against the inner surface of the longitudinal muscle (see Fig 1-4).[3,4] In the taeniae, which are formed from the longitudinal muscle of parts of the large intestine in humans and some other species, nerve fibers that innervate the muscle run parallel to the muscle through its thickness.

The circular muscle plexus is formed by parallel bundles of nerve fibers throughout this muscle layer. In addition, in some regions of the gastrointestinal tract the innervation of the circular muscle includes a dense layer of nerve fiber bundles. The presence of this plexus of nerve fibers and its position in relation to the circular muscle differs between species. In the small intestine of most mammals, including humans, the circular muscle has a thick outer layer and a thin inner layer of specialized muscle cells.[5,6] The dense plexus of nerve fibers that occurs between these two muscle layers in the small intestine is called the deep muscular plexus. The terminology was introduced by Cajal,[7] although he does not seem to have realized that a thin layer of muscle separates the deep muscular plexus from the submucous layer.

In the colon of most species, no inner specialized layer of the circular muscle is present and a dense layer of nerve fibers, similar to the deep muscular plexus, lies close against the inner surface of the circular muscle, adjacent to connective tissue of the submucosa. The plexus has been called the plexus entericus extremus by Stach.[8] This name does not describe its position very well, and it might be preferable to use a term introduced by Cajal,[7] the *submuscular plexus (plexus sous-musculeux)*, as suggested by Thuneberg[9] and Furness and colleagues.[10] An inner specialized muscle layer has been found in the human and the mouse colon.[11,12] In human colon, a deep muscular plexus is found between the two circular muscle layers.

Thuneberg[9] states that the circular layer of the stomach lacks an inner layer of specialized smooth muscle. In the stomach of dog and guinea pig, no dense plexus of nerve fibers near the inner surface of the circular muscle is readily discerned. In contrast, Faussone-Pellegrini and Cortesini[13] have reported a submuscular plexus in the human stomach. There are no reports of a dense inner plexus in the esophagus.

The circular muscle plexus continues into the circular muscle of the smooth muscle sphincters of the digestive tract, without any apparent change in form. The myenteric plexus also continues into the sphincter regions.

The muscularis mucosae consists of outer longitudinal and inner circular layers that are both innervated by nerve fibers running parallel to the muscle bundles. In the small intestine of small animals such as mice and rats, the muscularis mucosae is quite thin and is barely discernable in histologic sections.

The mucosal plexus is a network of fine nerve fiber bundles that lies beneath the mucosal epithelium. It is sparse in the esophagus but prominent in the stomach, small intestine, colon, and gallbladder. In the small intestine it is sometimes divided, for descriptive purposes, into subglandular, periglandular, and villous components, although these components are continuous with each other.

Myenteric Plexus

The arrangement of an area of the myenteric plexus of the human small intestine is shown in Figure 1-3, and part of the plexus from the guinea pig small intestine is shown in Figure 1-4 for comparison. The ganglia are flattened in the plane of the plexus. They are usually from one to three or four nerve cells thick, depending on the state of contraction and the size of the intestine, which varies considerably between species.[14] In any region, the sizes of ganglia vary over a large range. For example, in the small intestine of the guinea pig they vary from single cells to ganglia containing

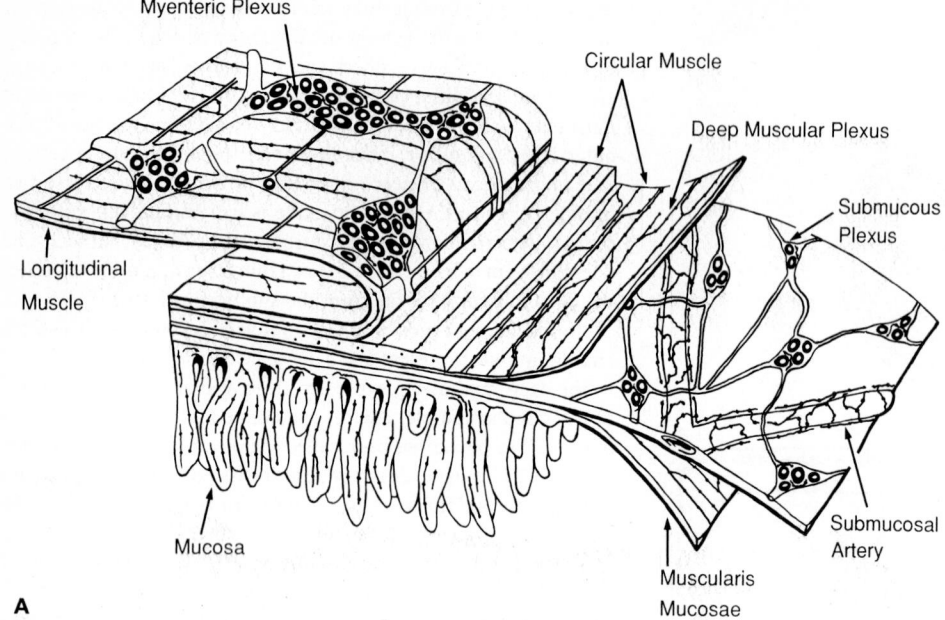

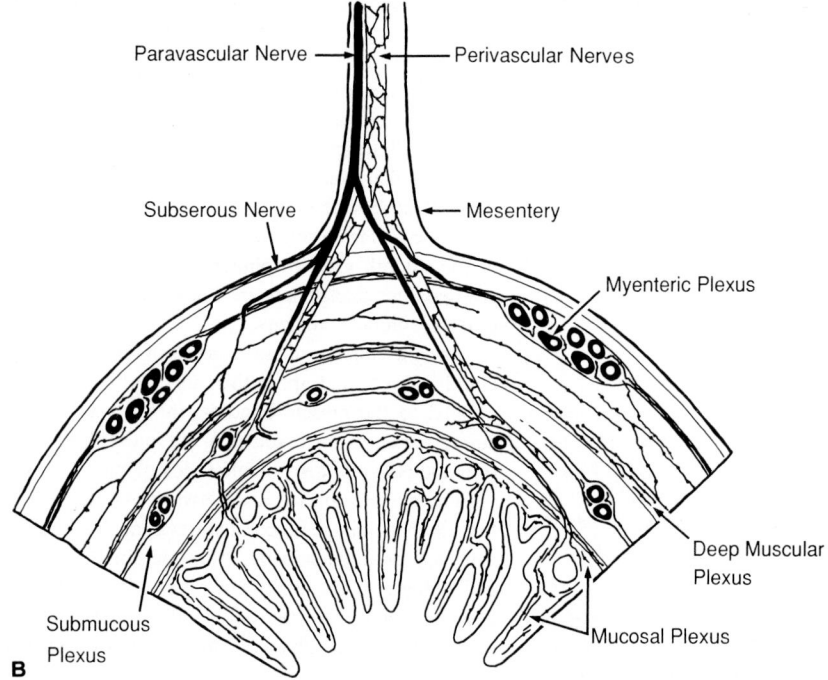

FIGURE 1–2. Diagrammatic representation of the enteric plexuses as they are seen in whole mounts of intestine, **A,** and in transverse section, **B.** (Modified from Furness JB, Costa M. Types of nerves in the enteric nervous system. Neuroscience 1980;5:1–20.)

about 160 nerve cell bodies. The pattern of ganglia, determined by their shapes and orientation, is quite different between regions and species, and is often readily identifiable as belonging to a particular part of intestine.[15] The ganglia are connected to each other by small bands of nerve fibers known as internodal strands (see Figs 1-3 and 1-4). The meshwork formed by the ganglia and the internodal strands is called the primary component of the myenteric plexus. Nerve strands that join with the primary plexus and run circumferentially constitute the secondary component of the plexus (see Figs 1-3 and 1-4).[4,16] Branches from the secondary strands run into the circular muscle to supply the innervation of that layer.[17] Nerve fiber bundles also run through the circular

muscle to connect the myenteric plexus with the submucosal and mucosal plexuses. These penetrating fiber bundles arise from the ganglia, from strands of the primary plexus, or from secondary strands and run almost directly through the circular layer.[18] A tertiary component of the myenteric plexus (see Fig 1-4) is found in some species in regions of the intestine where the longitudinal muscle layer is thin.

There are numerous targets for nerve cells in the myenteric plexus. The major targets are the muscularis externa, which receives most of its innervation from this source, the submucous ganglia, and other myenteric nerve cells. Myenteric nerve cells also provide nerve fibers to the mucosa, many of which are probably

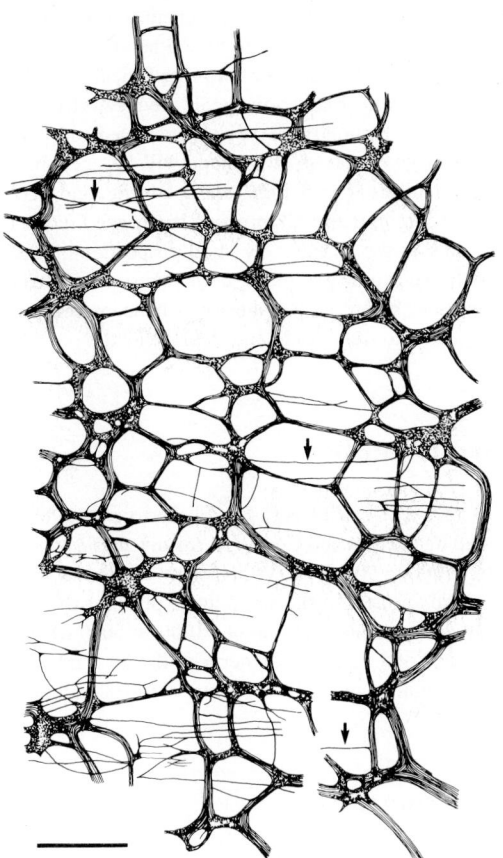

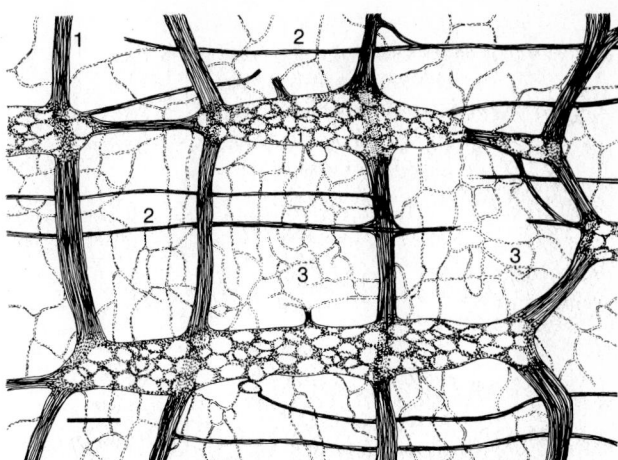

FIGURE 1-4. The three components of the myenteric plexus found in small animals are shown in a drawing of a whole mount from the guinea pig small intestine. Common to all species is the primary component of the plexus (*1*), consisting of the ganglia and internodal strands, and the secondary component (*2*), consisting of nerve strands lying parallel to the circular muscle. The tertiary plexus (*3*) is found only where the longitudinal muscle is thin and there is no longitudinal muscle plexus within the longitudinal layer. Calibration: 100 μm. (Modified from Furness JB, Costa M. The enteric nervous system. New York: Churchill Livingstone, 1987.)

FIGURE 1-3. Drawing of a whole mount of the myenteric plexus of the human small intestine, prepared by Auerbach and published in Henle's *Textbook of Histology* in 1871. Myenteric ganglia, internodal strands, and the small nerve trunks of the secondary component of the myenteric plexus (*arrows*) can be clearly seen. Calibration: 1 mm.

sensory nerve endings and nerve fibers that project to prevertebral ganglia.

Submucous Plexus

A continuous network, containing numerous small ganglia, is found in the submucosa throughout the small and large intestine. In many species two layers of ganglia are found, but in some regions there is only one layer.[19] Stach[20] has suggested that the outer plexus, which lies close to the circular muscle, be called Schabadasch's plexus and that the inner plexus be called Meissner's plexus, although there has been uncertainty over who should be credited with discovering each plexus. The validity of separately designating these plexuses is based on their containing different populations of neurons defined by their morphologic and histochemical characteristics.[21] Functional distinctions between the outer and inner submucous plexuses have yet to be demonstrated. Submucous ganglia are smaller and less regularly arranged than are myenteric ganglia.[22]

A major target of cell bodies in the submucosa is the intestinal mucosa, and the majority of secretomotor neurons have their cell bodies in this plexus.[23] Some neurons project from the submucosa to the myenteric plexus.[24] Others probably supply the muscularis mucosae of the small and large intestines, although this has only been shown directly for the dog.[10] Submucous neurons supply a few fibers to the inner circular muscle in some species.[10,25,26]

In the stomach, which almost entirely lacks submucous ganglia, the intrinsic innervation of the mucosa and muscularis mucosae comes from the myenteric plexus.

Ganglia of Biliary System and Pancreas

The biliary system and the pancreas develop from diverticula of the small intestine, and from this point of view the ganglia in their walls can be considered part of the enteric nervous system. A plexus of ganglia, similar to the enteric plexuses of the small intestine, but differing between species in its relation to tissue layers, is found in the gallbladder, cystic duct, and common bile duct.[3] Numerous nerve fibers are found in the muscle, around blood vessels, and in the mucosa of the biliary tract. Ganglia, connected to each other by small nerve trunks, are scattered through the pancreas to form a three-dimensional plexus in this solid organ. Nerve fibers are around the acini, around blood vessels, and in the islets.

MICROSCOPIC STRUCTURE OF THE ENTERIC NERVOUS SYSTEM

Neuron Shape

The nerve cells of the enteric ganglia can be classified into subgroups by their shapes (Fig 1-5). Classification has usually

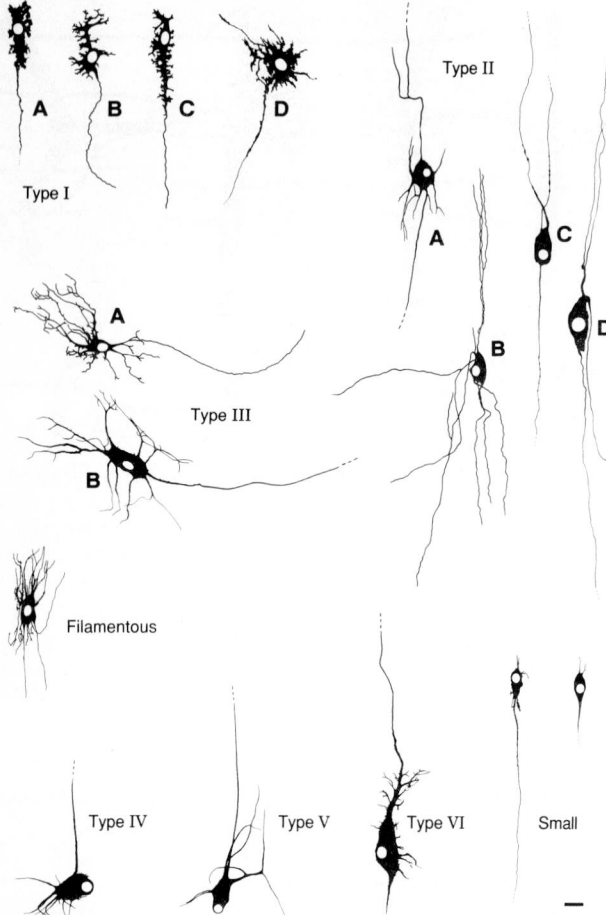

FIGURE 1–5. Shapes of myenteric neurons. These drawings are taken from whole mount preparations of the small intestine (except for type III, cell *a*). Dogiel type I neurons: *a* and *d* are from the guinea pig[28]; *b* and *c* are from human and guinea pig[27]. Dogiel type II neurons: *a* is a dendritic type II cell from pig[21]; *b* is from human[27]; *c* and *d* are from guinea pig[28]. Dogiel type III neurons: *a* is from the guinea pig large intestine[27]; *b* is from pig[21]. Filamentous neuron from the guinea pig[28]. Examples of types IV, V, and VI drawn by Stach from studies in the pig[21]. Small, simple neurons from the guinea pig[28]. Calibration: approximately 20 μm.

been based on the work of Dogiel,[27] who proposed that the shapes of nerve cells are related to their functions. Dogiel defined three cell shapes: type I, type II, and type III. The first two are readily recognized in different species and with various staining techniques. Type I neurons are generally flattened in the plane of the ganglia; they have oval cell bodies, prominent flattened (lamellar) dendrites, and a single long axon that often has spiny protuberances close to the cell body. Type II neurons have a spheroidal shape and give rise to several axons, usually 3 to 10, although some type II neurons are pseudounipolar.[28] A minority of type II neurons have tapering dendrites in addition to several long axon-like processes and are referred to as dendritic type II cells.[21] The majority of neurons seem to be type I or type II, but a variety of other shapes can be found. Stach[21] has classified these as types III to VI, based primarily on work in the pig. In the guinea pig small intestine, Furness and colleagues.[28] have described filamentous and small simple neurons (see Fig 1-5). The correlation between

shapes of nerve cells and their neurochemistry, electrophysiologic properties, and functions are discussed below.

Neurons of all classes, other than type II neurons, are effectively uniaxonal. By "effectively uniaxonal" we mean that if many neurons of a particular uniaxonal type are examined, only an occasional neuron that gives rise to two axons will be encountered.[28] For example, neurons with gamma-aminobutyric acid (GABA) immunoreactivity in the small intestine have type I morphology and project only to the muscle.[29] A small proportion of GABA nerve cells with two axons was found; both axons of such neurons went to the muscle, whereas the majority of neurons had a single axon that projected to the muscle and then divided.

Neuron Numbers

Counts of nerve cell densities published up to 1985 have been tabulated by Furness and Costa.[3] In the myenteric plexus, densities of about 2000 to 20,000 nerve cells/cm^2 are found in a variety of regions and species. In the submucous plexuses of the small and large intestines, densities of about 1000 to 5000 nerve cells/cm^2 are found. Total numbers of nerve cells are estimated to range from 3 to 4 million in small rodents to 10 to 100 million in humans.

Ultrastructure

The ultrastructures of enteric neurons and glia have been reviewed in detail elsewhere[3,30]; only a short summary is given here. The ganglia consist of compactly arranged nerve cell bodies, nerve fiber terminals, bundles of nerve fibers, and glial cells and their processes. Unlike other autonomic ganglia, they do not contain blood vessels or connective tissue cells, although septa of connective tissue sometimes separate parts of ganglia in large species, including humans. The supply of nutrients to the ganglia is therefore through the surrounding interstitial fluid. Hormones or drugs that act on the enteric ganglia must do so via this route. Therefore, it is perhaps significant that the cell bodies of many enteric neurons present large surface areas, that are not covered by glia, to the extracellular space.[30]

Nerve cell bodies in the myenteric ganglia of the guinea pig small intestine have been classified into eight types on the basis of their ultrastructure.[31]. No comparable study has been made in other species or regions, although from light microscopy it would be anticipated that similar diversity could be found. The type 6 neurons distinguished by Cook and Burnstock[31] have been shown, in the guinea pig small intestine, to have Dogiel type II morphology and to be AH neurons electrophysiologically.[32] As yet, other ultrastructurally defined types have not been characterized by light microscopy or electrophysiology. However, given the diverse shapes, chemistries, and roles of the enteric neurons, it seems likely that such correlations will be found.

Nerve fibers in the enteric ganglia are of two types, fibers of relatively uniform diameter (0.2 to 0.5 μm) and fibers that consist of varicosities, usually 1 to 2 μm in diameter, connected by short intervaricose segments, 0.2 to 0.5 μm thick.[30] It is generally considered that nonterminal parts of axons (i.e., parts that do not release transmitters) are nonvaricose, whereas the varicosities are points of transmitter release. Some neurons also have long fine dendrites that cannot be distinguished from axons if their full extents are not determined. The varicose parts of enteric axons, both those within ganglia and those associated with muscle or mucosal epithelium, are often hundreds of microns or millimeters long. In the ganglia this means that a single axon can contact many nerve cell bodies. Close contacts with nerve cells and their dendrites are of two types: those that have synaptic specializations, consisting of presynaptic accumulations of vesicles and postsynaptic densities, and those in which varicosities containing numerous synaptic vesicles come close to the cell, with no intervening glial cell, but in which no synaptic density is seen. The latter type of nonspecialized relationship is the most common. The majority of enteric neurons receive both specialized and nonspecialized contacts.[33-35] Particular types of contact do not seem to be associated selectively with the soma, dendrites, or axon.

Enteric varicosities contain various mixtures of vesicles, and a number of attempts have been made to classify nerve fibers in terms of their vesicular content.[30,36] No general agreement has yet emerged on the way that the vesiculated nerve endings can be classified. It certainly seems that no straightforward correlation is possible between vesicular content and the many types of nerve endings that can be recognized histochemically or are deduced to be present from physiologic experiments. Moreover, the vesicular content of a single axon can vary dramatically from one region to another.[31,34,37] Noradrenergic axons are the only type of axon in the enteric nervous system with a distinctive ultrastructure not shared by axons of other neuron types.[38] In the human myenteric plexus, noradrenergic axons contain numerous flattened vesicles.[39] Adequate distinctions between different nerve fibers can be made only with immunocytochemical methods.

Nerve fibers that innervate the muscle are arranged in bundles in which the individual fibers are partly surrounded by enteric glial cells.[30] No postjunctional specializations are apparent where vesicle containing fibers come close to the muscle cells, and close contacts by single nerve fibers are rare. Similarly, there are no specializations where nerve fiber bundles approach the mucosal epithelium.

ENTERIC NEUROTRANSMITTERS AND THE CHEMISTRY OF ENTERIC NEURONS

It has been known for many years that acetylcholine is the major transmitter for excitation at neuroneuronal synapses in the enteric nervous system. It is also a transmitter from excitatory motor neurons to intestinal muscle and from secretomotor neurons. The other principal autonomic transmitter, norepinephrine, is in sympathetic nerve fibers that supply the gastrointestinal tract from extrinsic ganglia. Physiologic and pharmacologic data indicate that additional transmitter substances exist within the enteric nervous system, and a large number of compounds with the potential to serve transmitter roles have been identified in enteric neurons (Table 1-1).[38] Some of these are discussed later in relation to specific functional classes of enteric neurons.

Evidence in the enteric nervous system and elsewhere indicates that many neurons contain several possible neurotransmitters.[40,41] However, it is clear that these co-localized substances do not have equal status as transmitters, because when several neurotransmitter substances are released together from a neuron they make different contributions to the transmission process. It seems to be common that one substance has the principal role in transmission. For example, vasoconstrictor neurons in many species contain both norepinephrine and neuropeptide Y. Transmission seems to depend on norepinephrine, and neuropeptide Y seems to have a subsidiary, or modifying, role. The chemistry of the subsidiary transmitters differs between species; for example, the noradrenergic neurons that cause inhibition of intestinal water and electrolyte secretion contain somatostatin in the guinea pig but not in other species, whereas the noradrenergic neurons that inhibit motility contain neuropeptide Y in the rat but not in the guinea pig. A broad range of experiments suggest that principal transmitters are constant between species; thus many of the species differences in neuronal chemistry that are observed are probably differences in the subsidiary transmitters. In this chapter we do not discuss all the substances that may participate in enteric neurotransmission in different species; much of this information has been the subject of recent reviews.[3,42,43]

The immunohistochemical localization of specific combinations of compounds in neurons provides a valuable investigative probe that allows the projections of individual neurons to be determined and their functions to be deduced, even when the role of the chemicals that are detected are not known. For example, neuropeptide Y immunoreactivity has been used as a marker of cholinergic secretomotor neurons in the small intestine of the guinea pig.[44]

FUNCTIONALLY DEFINED ENTERIC NEURONS

The following paragraphs provide a summary of the major classes of functionally defined enteric neurons and the substances that are deduced to act as their neurotransmitters. This is based largely on a recent review.[45]

Motor Neurons

Excitatory Muscle Motor Neurons. Excitatory neurons innervate the longitudinal and circular muscle and the muscularis mucosae throughout the digestive tract. The principal transmitter of these neurons is acetylcholine, which acts on the muscle via muscarinic receptors. In all or most mammals, probably including humans, the tachykinins, substance P and neurokinin A, are also released from excitatory motor neurons and contribute to excitation of both the longitudinal and circular muscle. The involvement of tachykinins is revealed after pharmacologic block of muscarinic receptors and appears to be more prominent at high rates of firing of the neurons.[46] Several drugs that are antagonists at tachykinin receptors on intestinal muscle have been developed; these have allowed the involvement of tachykinins in excitatory transmission to be clearly demonstrated.[45] An electron microscopic examination of the innervation of the circular muscle in the small intestine of the guinea pig indicates that acetylcholine and the tachykinins are likely to be contained in the same axons and released as co-transmitters.[47]

TABLE 1–1

Pharmacologically Active Substances, Possibly Neurotransmitters, in Enteric Neurons and Their Extrinsic Connections

Established Neurotransmitters

Acetylcholine (ACh): In interneurons, several classes of enteric motor neuron (see text), and vagal input neurons

Gastrin releasing peptide (GRP): In motor neurons to gastrin cells

Norepinephrine (NE): In sympathetic postganglionic neurons supplying the gastrointestinal tract

Substance P (SP) and gene-related products: In enteric excitatory motor neurons to muscle, possibly as a co-transmitter with acetylcholine

Vasoactive intestinal peptide (VIP) and gene-related products (PHI & PHM): In enteric inhibitory motor neurons to muscle, noncholinergic secretomotor neurons, and enteric vasodilator neurons

Presence in Neurons Demonstrated

Calcitonin gene-related peptide (CGRP): In enteric neurons and some extrinsic sensory neurons

Cholecystokinin (CCK): Probably present primarily as the octapeptide (CCK-8)

Dynorphin (DYN) and related gene products

Enkephalin (ENK) and related gene products

Galanin (GAL)

Gastrin releasing peptide (GRP): This peptide is in enteric neurons throughout the gut. Only in the gastric antral mucosa is its transmitter role established. GRP is also referred to as mammalian bombesin.

γ-Aminobutyric acid (GABA)

5-Hydroxytryptamine (5-HT or serotonin): Although this substance is almost certainly a neurotransmitter, its role is not known

Neuromedin U (NMU)

Neuropeptide Y (NPY): Co-localized with norepinephrine in sympathetic vasoconstrictor neurons and also present in enteric neurons

Neurotensin (NT) or a neurotensin-like peptide

Somatostatin (SOM)

Substance P (SP) and gene-related products (known collectively as tachykinins): These substances are in many enteric neurons in addition to the excitatory muscle motor neurons referred to above

Thyrotropin releasing hormone (TRH)

Vasoactive intestinal peptide (VIP) and related gene products: Although these are transmitters in some motor neurons (see above), they are also in neurons where their roles are not known.

Other Possible Neurotransmitters

Adenosine triphosphate (ATP) and/or related nucleotides

Endorphins

Histamine

Inhibitory Muscle Motor Neurons. Considerable controversy has surrounded the identification of the transmitter of these neurons, which are also referred to as enteric inhibitory neurons. The two substances that have been suggested as transmitters are adenosine triphosphate (ATP)[48] and vasoactive intestinal peptide (VIP).[49,50] While a role for ATP remains to be clearly proven, there is now little doubt that VIP does contribute to transmission from the neurons. The closely related peptide, PHI (PHM in humans) should be included with VIP. This peptide comes from the same precursor as VIP, it has a similar structure, and it acts similarly on intestinal muscle. In summary, the main evidence for VIP is as follows:(1) VIP-like immunoreactivity is in nerve fibers supplying the muscle of the intestine in all species studied (see tabulation in Furness and colleagues[38]; (2) VIP-like material is released when enteric inhibitory neurons are stimulated[45]; (3) VIP relaxes intestinal muscle[50]; and (4) when the effectiveness of VIP on intestinal muscle is reduced by antagonists or by immunoneutralization, transmission from enteric inhibitory neurons is antagonized.[50] Several studies suggest that more than one substance contributes to transmission from the enteric inhibitory neu-

rons.[51-53] Thus, present evidence suggests that the transmitters of these neurons are VIP/PHI(M) plus one or more unidentified substances.

Secretomotor Neurons (Water and Electrolyte Secretion). The mucosa of the small and large intestines is supplied by both cholinergic and noncholinergic secretomotor neurons.[54,55] Acetylcholine released from the cholinergic neurons acts on muscarinic receptors on the mucosal epithelium. The principal transmitter of the noncholinergic secretomotor neurons is likely to be VIP.[55,56]

Secretomotor Neurons (Gastric Acid Secretion). Secretomotor neurons are cholinergic and act on the parietal cells via muscarinic receptors. There is not space in this chapter to describe the roles of these neurons and their relation to hormonal control of gastric acid secretion. The reader is referred instead to the work of Furness and Costa[3] and to Chapter 13.

Enteric Vasodilator Neurons. Enteric vasodilator neurons have been most studied in the small and large intestines, although some evidence suggests that they also exist in the stomach.[57]

Local vasodilator reflexes can be elicited in the intestines by mechanical or chemical irritation of the mucosa; substantial evidence indicates that the vasodilator neurons are intrinsic to the intestine and are noncholinergic.[57] Recent experiments have provided direct evidence for vasodilator neurons with their cell bodies in the submucous plexus.[58] It is probable that the principal transmitter is VIP.[3,57]

When the vagus nerve is stimulated, both acid secretion and blood flow are enhanced; both effects are reduced by muscarinic antagonists. In almost all experiments to date, it is not possible to determine whether there is dilatation due to a direct vascular action of cholinergic neurons in addition to a functional hyperemia consequent on the secretomotor effect of vagal cholinergic pathways.[57] However, in a recent study in the rat, Thiefen and associates[59] have shown that centrally administered thyrotropin releasing hormone (TRH) stimulates a vagal pathway that causes gastric vasodilation after acid secretion is blocked by omeprazole. The secretion-independent flow increase was antagonized by atropine. There is also evidence for noncholinergic gastric vasodilator neurons that use VIP as a transmitter.[60]

Motor Neurons to Enteric Endocrine Cells. There are a wide variety of endocrine cells in the mucosa of the gastrointestinal tract and, because the mucosa is densely innervated, the majority of these cells have nerve fibers in close proximity. Despite this association, there is little information on the neuronal control of enteric endocrine cells, with the notable exception of the gastrin cells.

The secretion of gastrin is under the control of vagal and of intrinsic gastric pathways. The final neurons in both paths are in the stomach wall. Transmission from the neurons is mediated by a peptide, gastrin releasing peptide (GRP).[50]

Enteric Interneurons

Both structural and physiologic evidence point to the existence of interneurons in enteric reflex pathways. Although it is difficult to study the interneurons specifically (i.e., in isolation from the rest of a pathway) there is evidence that some of the neurons are cholinergic both in motility and in secretion controlling pathways. Structural and pharmacologic evidence also implicates 5-hydroxytryptamine (5-HT) as a transmitter in interneurons of descending pathways in the small intestine.[61-63]

Intrinsic Enteric Sensory Neurons

The intrinsic reflex pathways that are involved in the control of movement, blood flow, and secretion are activated via neurons that are sensitive to a number of stimuli, such as distention, luminal chemistry, and mechanical stimulation of the mucosa. These sensory neurons have their nerve cell bodies in the myenteric and submucous plexuses. It is not known what transmitters the sensory neurons with cell bodies in the myenteric plexus use. Those in the submucosa of the small intestine of the guinea pig are probably cholinergic.[64] The gastrointestinal tract is also supplied by numerous extrinsic sensory neurons with their cell bodies in dorsal root ganglia or in the sensory ganglia of the vagus nerve.[65]

Sympathetic Neurons

Norepinephrine is the principal transmitter of the sympathetic postganglionic neurons that supply the gastrointestinal tract.[3,66] These neurons are discussed in detail below.

Neurons of Vagal and Pelvic Motor Pathways

The vagus nerves contain the axons of neurons whose cell bodies lie within the brain stem. It is through these neurons that a variety of central effects on the upper gastrointestinal tract are mediated, for example, relaxation of the proximal stomach, enhancement of gastric peristalsis, secretion of acid, and promotion of gastrin secretion. In each case the vagal neuron does not act directly; the vagal neurons form synaptic connections with enteric neurons whose cell bodies are in the intrinsic ganglia of the gastrointestinal tract. By the convention used for other cranial autonomic pathways, the vagal neurons of these motor pathways are called parasympathetic preganglionic, or vagal preganglionic neurons. While this is a logical terminology, it has led some researchers to consider enteric neurons to be equivalent to parasympathetic postganglionic neurons. Reference to vagal input neurons as preganglionic wrongly implies that enteric neurons are really neurons in parasympathetic pathways, whereas they are neurons in complex circuits in which enteric reflexes of several types are integrated with signals from the central nervous system and from other parts of the gastrointestinal tract. In fact, the majority of enteric neurons do not receive direct vagal connections. Thus, it is misleading to use the term *parasympathetic neurons* for enteric neurons or the term *parasympathetic ganglia* for enteric ganglia. This distinction is in accord with the early definition of the autonomic nervous system by Langley[67] and with modern concepts of the enteric nervous system.[68,69]

Transmission from vagal input neurons to enteric neurons is mediated principally by acetylcholine acting on nicotinic receptors. All the effects of stimulating vagal motor pathways are blocked or substantially attenuated by drugs that block nicotinic receptors.

The primary effects of the pelvic nerves, so far as the gastrointestinal tract is concerned, are on movement, secretion, and blood flow in the distal colon and rectum. The pathways are analogous to those of the vagus nerve; pelvic input neurons with cell bodies in the sacral spinal cord form synapses on enteric neurons at which acetylcholine is an excitatory transmitter acting through nicotinic receptors.

PHYSIOLOGIC CHARACTERISTICS OF ENTERIC NEURONS

As has already been indicated, enteric neurons have a variety of characteristic shapes and neurochemistries. Relating these properties to their functions has been difficult because the morphologically distinct classes of enteric neurons are not segregated from each other within the enteric plexuses but are distributed apparently randomly among the ganglia. Thus, it has been difficult to record selectively the activity of functionally distinct neurons. This contrasts to other parts of the nervous system in which functionally distinct neurons are often grouped in separate nuclei; for example, somatic sensory neurons are located in the dorsal root ganglia, while the motor neurons they supply are in the ventral horn of the spinal cord.

Correlations of Physiology and Cell Body Shape

In recent years, the problem of correlating neuronal morphology and function has been addressed in a series of studies in the small intestine of the guinea pig.[44,62,64,70-73] Each of these studies used microelectrodes to identify the electrophysiologic properties of enteric neurons. The identified neurons were then injected with a dye (typically the fluorescent dye Lucifer yellow), and their shapes were determined. In both the myenteric plexus and the submucous plexus, the large multiaxonal, Dogiel type II neurons (see Fig 1-5) were found to have electrophysiologic characteristics that differed markedly from those of the other, uniaxonal classes of neurons. The clearest examples of these differences are seen in the synaptic inputs to the neurons and in their action potentials. The uniaxonal enteric neurons exhibit prominent fast excitatory synaptic potentials (ESPs) in response to electrical stimulation of

internodal strands in either the myenteric plexus or the submucous plexus (Fig 1-6). These fast ESPs appear to be mediated by acetylcholine acting through nicotinic receptors as they are blocked or markedly reduced by hexamethonium and tubocurarine (although the concentrations needed for this blockade are considerably higher than those needed to block similar responses in sympathetic ganglia). In contrast, the Dogiel type II neurons usually do not exhibit fast ESPs in response to electrical stimulation and when such responses are observed in neurons with this shape the fast ESPs are normally very small (Fig 1-7). The action potentials in the Dogiel type II neurons are large (Table 1-2), 75 to 110 mV in amplitude, and are normally followed by two separate phases of hyperpolarization (Fig 1-8). The first hyperpolarization lasts 20 to 100 ms and is similar to the undershoot seen in nearly all neurons following an action potential; it appears to be due to activation of a voltage-sensitive potassium channel.[74-76] The second hyperpolarization is characteristic of the Dogiel type II neurons and lasts 5 to 25 seconds; it is due to the opening of a calcium-sensitive potassium channel.[75] The calcium needed to open this potassium channel enters the Dogiel type II neuron during the action potential in the soma. These neurons can generate a soma action potential (in which the inward current is carried entirely by calcium ions) and slow hyperpolarization even when all the voltage sensitive sodium channels are blocked by tetrodotoxin. In contrast, the uniaxonal enteric neurons have action potentials that are completely blocked by tetrodotoxin; these action potentials are smaller and are followed only by the rapid hyperpolarization and not by the slow, calcium-dependent hyperpolarization (see Fig 1-8).

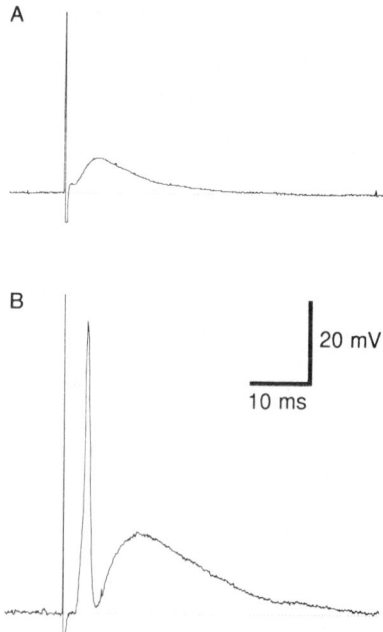

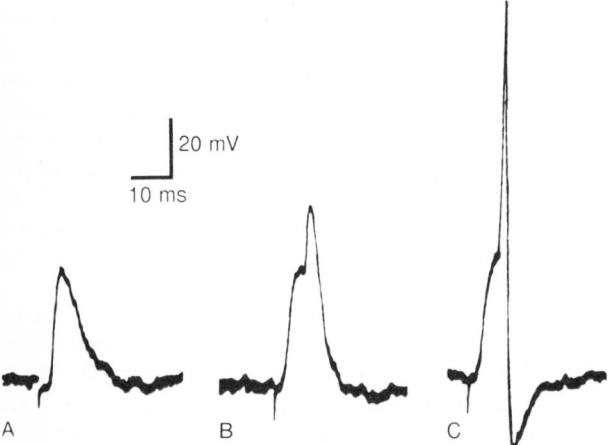

FIGURE 1-6. Cholinergic fast excitatory synaptic potentials (fast ESPs) recorded from enteric S neurons with intracellular microelectrodes. Brief stimulus artifacts precede each response. In **A,** only the ESP is seen; in **B,** the ESP has triggered a local response; and in **C,** the ESP has elicited an action potential. (From Nishi S, North RA. Intracellular recording from the myenteric plexus of the guinea pig ileum. J Physiol [London] 1973;231: 474–494.)

FIGURE 1-7. Fast ESPs recorded from an AH neuron, **A,** and from an S neuron, **B,** of the submucous plexus. The response in the AH neuron was the maximum that could be obtained; three fibers contributed to the response that failed to elicit an action potential. The response in the S cell from a single fiber elicited an action potential. (From Bornstein JC, Furness JB, Costa M. An electrophysiological comparison of substance P immunoreactive neurons with other neurons in the guinea pig submucous plexus. J Auton Nerv Syst 1989;26:113–120.)

TABLE 1–2

Resting Membrane Potentials (RMPs) and Amplitudes and 1/2-Widths* of Action Potentials Recorded in AH/Dogiel Type II Neurons and S/Uniaxonal Neurons†

CELL TYPE	RMP (mV)	AMPLITUDE (mV)	1/2-WIDTH (ms)	REFERENCES
AH/Dogiel type II	59.2 ± 1.3	83 ± 1	2.5 ± 0.1	70, 73
		87 ± 2	2.1 ± 0.1	74
S/uniaxonal	54.0 ± 2.9	68 ± 1	1.4 ± 0.1	70, 73

* 1/2-width is a standard measure of the duration of a response and is measured from half the maximum amplitude on the rising phase to half the maximum amplitude on the falling phase.
† All values given as mean ± standard error.

Thus, the multiaxonal Dogiel type II neurons are an electrophysiologically distinct class of enteric neuron with properties identical to the neurons first defined as AH (for afterhyperpolarizing) by Hirst and co-workers.[77] The uniaxonal enteric neurons have properties similar to those of sympathetic neurons and appear to be identical to the enteric neurons defined by these authors as S-neurons.[77]

Other classification schemes for enteric neurons have been based on a somewhat different array of electrophysiologic parameters, including input resistance (the electrical resistance of the whole cell body to passage of current), membrane potential, and the ability of neurons to fire action potentials during prolonged depolarizations.[63,78] However, because estimates of input resistance and membrane potential vary widely between authors (Table 1-3) the use of these parameters as distinguishing criteria may lead to confusion. Furthermore, the ability of a neuron to generate action potentials during a depolarization depends on its input resistance and membrane potential so that this feature may also harbor ambiguity.

Although there are clear biophysical differences between the AH/Dogiel type II neurons and the S/uniaxonal neurons, the question of whether the different classes of uniaxonal neurons can be separated on the basis of their electrophysiologic properties remains open. At least three different shapes of uniaxonal myenteric neurons have been identified in the small intestine of the guinea pig,[28] but the results available to date do not allow them to be distinguished electrophysiologically. In the submucous plexus, uniaxonal neurons can be distinguished on the basis of their neurochemistry and their synaptic inputs. However, unlike the uniaxonal neurons of the myenteric plexus, these neurons all have similar shapes.[44]

The results described here have been obtained from neurons of the small intestine of the guinea pig. There have been relatively few studies of the electrophysiologic properties of neurons from other parts of the intestine or from other species. Wood and his colleagues have described the properties of enteric neurons in the stomach,[79,80] colon,[81,82] and rectum[83] of the guinea pig. There have also been studies of myenteric neurons from the rat duodenum,[84] mouse colon,[85] and human colon.[86] However, the relationships between cell shape and electrophysiology have not yet been analyzed in these preparations. Nevertheless, it is clear from these papers that neurons analogous to AH- and S-neurons can be found elsewhere in the gastrointestinal tract and in other species.

Neurons are found in small ganglia associated with branches of the parasympathetic input nerves, the vagus and pelvic nerves, where they enter the stomach and large intestine. Properties of these neurons have been studied in the opossum stomach, and they appear to be similar to the S-neurons of the small intestine

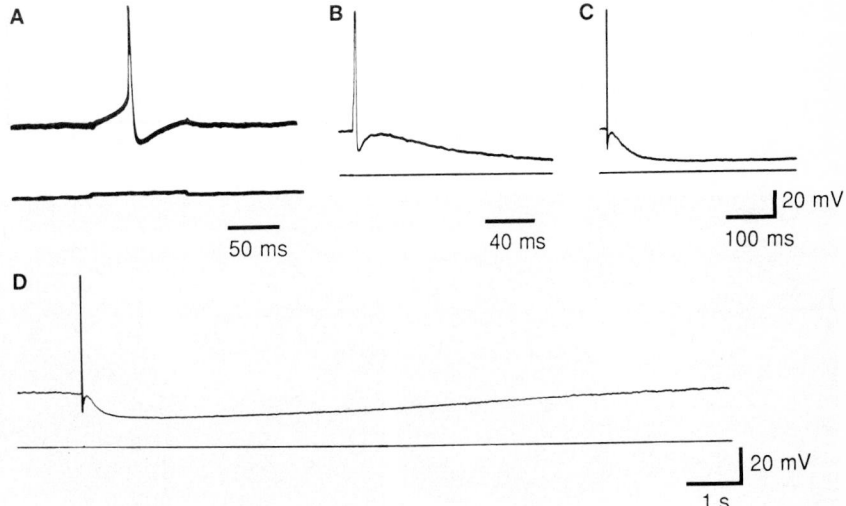

FIGURE 1–8. Action potentials elicited in an S neuron, **A**, and in AH neurons, **B,C**, and **D**, by intracellular current pulses. The action potential in the S neuron is followed by a brief period of hyperpolarization; the action potentials in AH neurons are followed by two phases of hyperpolarization, one brief, **B**, and the other prolonged, **C** and **D**. Note the differences in time scale. (From Hirst GDS, Holman ME, Spence I. Two types of neurons in the myenteric plexus of duodenum in the guinea pig. J Physiol [London] 1974;236:303–326.)

TABLE 1–3
Estimates of Input Resistances of Myenteric Neurons of the Guinea Pig Small Intestine*

NEURON TYPE	INPUT RESISTANCE (MΩ)	SOURCE
AH/Dogiel type II	190 ± 20	Iyer et al[73]
S/unixonal	270 ± 30	Iyer et al[73]
AH/Dogiel type II	125 ± 7	Hirst et al[74]
all neurons	125–250	Hirst et al[77]
AH/Dogiel type II	150 ± 19	Hodgkiss & Lees[70]
S/uniaxonal	153 ± 32	Hodgkiss & Lees[70]
Type 1†	58 ± 5	Nishi & North[78]
Type 2†	21 ± 2	Nishi & North[78]
All neurons	10–185	Wood[63]

* Values are given either as mean (± standard error) values for different electrophysiologically characterized classes of neurons or as a range including all classes of myenteric neurons.
† Electrophysiologically defined classes of myenteric neurons characterized on the basis of input resistance and action potential firing properties during prolonged depolarizing current pulses.

of the guinea pig; no neurons similar to AH-neurons were identified.[87]

Correlation of Physiology and Immunohistochemistry

The use of intracellular dyes to determine the shapes of electrophysiologically identified neurons has also facilitated studies in which the properties of these neurons have been correlated with their neurochemistry. In essence these experiments involve injecting an impaled neuron with the dye and then fixing the tissue and processing the preparation for immunohistochemical localization of one or more neurochemical markers, usually peptides. The dye is used to re-identify the impaled neuron, and whether it contains the chosen marker can then be determined (Fig 1-9). Studies of this type have allowed the electrophysiologic characteristics of the four functionally distinct classes of neurons in the submucous plexus of the small intestine of the guinea pig to be identified. Each of these classes of neurons is uniquely identified by the presence of a single neurochemical marker: the cholinergic secretomotor neurons contain neuropeptide Y as well as the enzyme choline acetyltransferase (ChAT), the noncholinergic secretomotor neurons contain VIP, the sensory neurons contain SP (substance P) together with ChAT, and the interneurons contain ChAT but no VIP, neuropeptide Y, or SP.[56,88] The neurons can also be distinguished on the basis of their electrophysiologic properties. For example, the sensory neurons appear to be AH/Dogiel type II neurons, while the secretomotor neurons are S/uniaxonal neurons, which can be distinguished from each other by their synaptic inputs. Both types of secretomotor neurons have fast ESPs, but the noncholinergic neurons also have inhibitory and slow excitatory inputs as described below.

Considerably more data will be necessary before clear conclusions about the functions and electrophysiology of neurochemically distinct classes of myenteric neurons are possible. This is because neurons in the myenteric plexus are rarely uniquely identified by a single neurochemical marker and the correlation studies to date have not allowed identification of more than one marker in a single impaled neuron. Nevertheless, some conclusions are possible for myenteric neurons from the small intestine of the guinea pig. All myenteric neurons immunoreactive for enkephalin, dynorphin, or VIP are S/uniaxonal neurons.[71,72,89] In contrast, 80% to 90% of

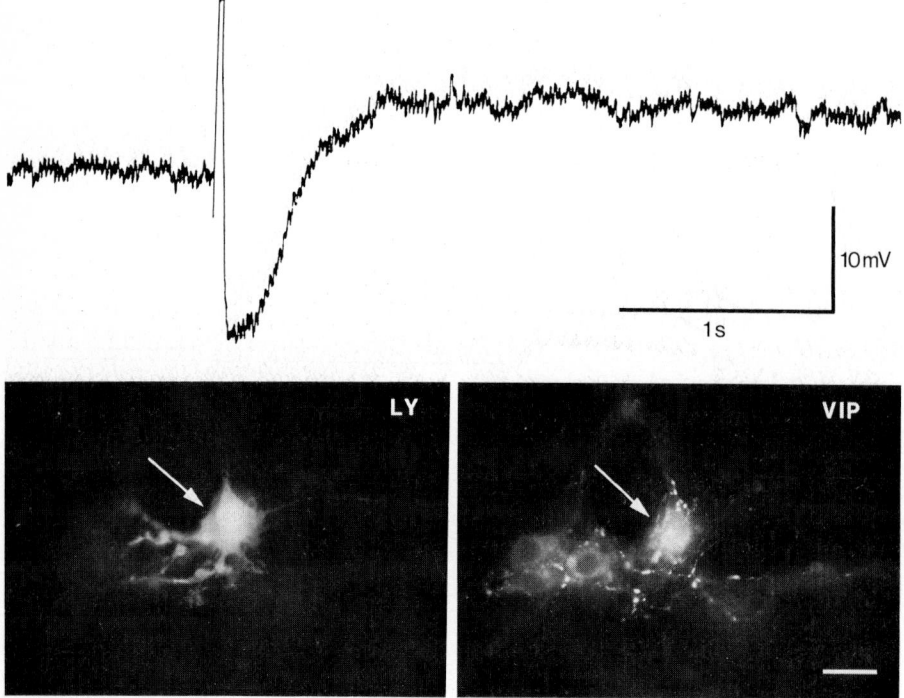

FIGURE 1–9. Recording of an inhibitory synaptic potential (ISP) in a secretomotor neuron of the submucous plexus of the guinea pig small intestine. The trace is of the intracellularly recorded membrane potential of the neuron. Electrical stimulation of a connecting strand gave rise to a fast ESP followed by an ISP. This preparation had been extrinsically denervated, so the inhibitory inputs came from intrinsic neurons. The recording electrode was used to fill the neuron with Lucifer yellow (LY). The tissue was then fixed and stained for VIP localization. The neuron was reactive for VIP (see micrograph), which indicates it to be a secretomotor neuron. Calibration: 20 μm. (From Bornstein JC, Costa M, Furness JB. Intrinsic and extrinsic inhibitory synaptic inputs to submucous neurons of the guinea pig small intestine. J Physiol [London] 1988;398:371–390.)

AH/Dogiel type II neurons are immunoreactive for the protein calbindin, but no S/uniaxonal neurons are reactive for this protein.[73]

Synaptic Inputs to Enteric Neurons

As already stated, neurons in both the myenteric plexus and the submucous plexus receive cholinergic fast excitatory inputs. This appears to be the major form of synaptic transmission in the enteric nervous system. Roughly 70% of all myenteric neurons and 90% of all submucous neurons receive such input, and in nearly all cases the input is sufficient to excite the receiving neurons to fire an action potential (see Fig 1-6). Furthermore, as described in more detail below, the synaptic responses evoked in neurons by physiologic stimuli consist primarily of bursts of fast ESPs. The other types of synaptic events, slow ESPs and inhibitory synaptic potentials (ISPs), are described separately for the myenteric and submucous ganglia.

Responses in Myenteric Neurons.
Whereas fast ESPs are largely confined to the S/uniaxonal neurons in the small intestine of the guinea pig, slow excitatory potentials (slow ESPs) can be evoked both in these neurons and in the AH/Dogiel type II neurons by electrical stimulation of the internodal strands. Slow ESPs can last between 15 and 120s (Fig 1-10)[90,91] and are seen in at least 75% of S/uniaxonal neurons and 40% of AH/Dogiel type II neurons.[92] The exact proportions of neurons exhibiting such responses depend on the stimulus conditions.[93]

Analysis of the slow ESPs suggests that they may actually be the net result of a number of different, superimposed responses, each producing superficially similar synaptic potentials.[93] A single electrical stimulus often evokes a slow ESP in an S/uniaxonal neuron, and much of this response (but not all of it) is blocked by muscarinic antagonists.[94]. Repetitive stimulation evokes slow ESPs in these neurons even in the presence of muscarinic antagonists. Thus, the slow ESPs in many S/uniaxonal neurons are the result of the action of at least two transmitters, acetylcholine acting through muscarinic receptors and one or more as yet unidentified transmitters. A small number of AH/Dogiel type II neurons also exhibit muscarinic slow ESPs in addition to a more prominent noncholinergic slow ESP that typically requires several stimuli to evoke it. Other AH/Dogiel type II neurons only have noncholinergic slow ESPs.

The nature of the transmitter responsible for the noncholinergic slow ESPs has been the subject of extensive speculation since these responses were first described by Wood and Mayer.[90] Several substances found within enteric nerve terminals, including 5-HT, substance P, VIP, and somatostatin, mimic the slow ESPs in myenteric neurons from the small intestine of the guinea pig.[63] Progress has been hindered substantially by the absence of appropriate antagonists for these substances.

In the guinea pig, many of the potential mediators of the slow ESPs are contained in nerve fibers that run for some distance along the intestine before contacting other myenteric neurons.[3] Circumferential lesions through the myenteric plexus leave an area from which all nerve terminals containing 5-HT or VIP have degenerated, but terminals containing substance P remain intact. Loss of 5-HT and VIP terminals has no effect on the slow ESPs recorded in S/uniaxonal neurons.[92] Thus, neither VIP nor 5-HT is necessary to evoke slow ESPs in S/uniaxonal neurons, whereas substance P, or another tachykinin, may mediate the slow ESPs in these neurons. The picture is somewhat more complicated for AH/Dogiel type II neurons. The lesions cause only a very slight reduction in the slow ESPs in these neurons, indicating that the major part of the response could be due to a tachykinin.[92] Nevertheless, there is compelling evidence that 5-HT may play a role in mediating slow ESPs in some of these neurons.[62] It is likely that the slow ESPs evoked by electrical stimulation of inputs to AH/Dogiel type II neurons may be produced by the interaction of several different neurotransmitters.

The reason why these different slow responses appear similar is that they are all mediated by a reduction in the potassium permeability of the neuronal membrane. Thus, discriminating between the different slow ESPs using electrophysiologic methods has been very difficult. The problem is compounded by the finding that there are several different types of potassium channels in the membranes of enteric neurons; AH/Dogiel type II neurons have at least five.[75,76] These include a voltage-sensitive channel opened during action potentials, the calcium-dependent channel described previously, a resting or background channel, and two channels that are only opened when the membrane potential is hyperpolarized. The calcium-dependent channel and the background channel are both partially open under resting conditions, and thus each may be closed during a slow ESP. Muscarinic agonists close both of these channels in AH/Dogiel type II neurons but have little effect on the other channels.[76] S/uniaxonal neurons do not have calcium-dependent channels that are open at rest; in these neurons only the background channel is altered by muscarinic agonists.[76] The channels involved in the noncholinergic slow ESPs have not yet been identified, but they will probably also prove to be the calcium-dependent and background potassium channels. It

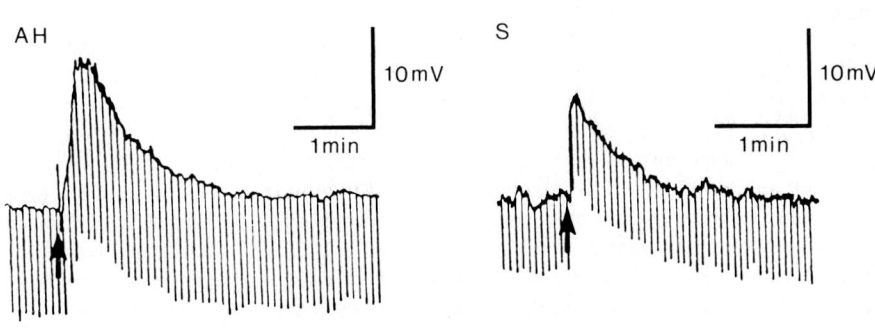

FIGURE 1–10. Examples of slow excitatory synaptic potentials (slow ESPs) in an AH and an S neuron of the myenteric plexus, in each case evoked by stimulating a connecting nerve strand at 10 Hz for three pulses. The amplitudes of the downward deflections are proportional to cell input resistance, which increases during the slow ESPs. (From Bornstein JC, North RA, Costa M, Furness JB. Excitatory synaptic potentials due to activation of neurons with short projections in the myenteric plexus. Neuroscience 1984; 11:723–731.)

has been shown that several agonists can each act through a different receptor in the membrane of either myenteric or submucous neurons to modulate a single potassium channel.[95,96]

Reducing the potassium permeability of the membrane increases the neuronal excitability in two ways. First, it depolarizes the cell membrane, bringing it closer to the threshold potential needed to trigger an action potential. Second, by increasing the input resistance of the cell it enhances the effect on the membrane potential of an applied current, thus making synaptic inputs and other small depolarizations more effective. Many slow ESPs in AH/Dogiel type II neurons also have a third effect on neuronal excitability by reducing or abolishing their characteristic slow afterhyperpolarizations, presumably by closing the calcium-sensitive potassium channels. This has the effect of making the neuron more able to fire prolonged, high-frequency trains of action potentials. The functional significance of this is discussed below.

The fast cholinergic ESPs and the slow ESPs are by far the most frequently observed synaptic potentials in myenteric neurons. The ISPs have been reported only very rarely and then only in a small proportion of neurons in the small intestine of the guinea pig.[90,91] It is possible that the methods of stimulation used (electrical stimulation of internodal strands with one or more pulses) may nonselectively stimulate both excitatory and inhibitory fibers. The dominant excitatory responses would tend to obscure any ISPs that may be evoked at the same time. Studies in which enteric reflex pathways are activated by physiologic stimuli have, however, also failed to evoke ISPs in myenteric neurons.[97,98] This suggests that any physiologic role for this type of synaptic potential may be confined to a very restricted group of myenteric neurons.

Synaptic Responses in the Submucous Plexus.

Electrophysiologic studies of submucous neurons have been confined to preparations from the small intestine and the cecum of the guinea pig.[44,99-102] About 90% of all submucous neurons exhibit fast ESPs and a large proportion of these also exhibit slow ESPs. The properties of these responses are similar to those observed in myenteric neurons. The fast ESPs are blocked by hexamethonium and are presumably mediated by acetylcholine acting through nicotinic receptors. The slow ESPs appear to be due to a reduction in potassium permeability.

Although several substances found within nerve terminals in the submucous plexus can mimic the slow ESPs, none can be shown unequivocally to be a transmitter. For example, lesions that cause a complete loss of substance P–containing nerve terminals in the submucous plexus reduce the number of neurons with slow ESPs but some remain.[103] It seems likely that the slow ESPs in this plexus are also the result of the actions of several different neurotransmitters including acetylcholine (acting through muscarinic receptors), substance P (and/or another tachykinin), 5-HT, and, possibly, VIP.

In contrast to myenteric neurons, ISPs are commonly observed in submucous neurons. Stimulation of the internodal strands evokes a substantial ISP in about 50% of neurons in the small intestine[44,99,100] and in up to 90% in the cecum.[102] Nearly all neurons with ISPs also exhibit slow ESPs, and all have fast ESPs. In the small intestine, these neurons all contain VIP and are probably noncholinergic secretomotor neurons (see Fig 1-10).[44,56,103] The ISP is due to a substantial increase in the potassium permeability of the membrane that leads to a hyperpolarization of up to 30 mV. Two separate ISPs have been identified. Short trains of stimuli

(one to five pulses at 10 to 30 Hz) evoke an ISP lasting up to 2 seconds; this is substantially depressed by α_2-receptor antagonists or by guanethidine. Longer trains evoke a much slower ISP that is resistant to blockade of norepinephrine receptors or release. Lesion studies, in which sources of nerve terminals extrinsic to the submucosa are caused to degenerate before the electrophysiologic analyses, confirm that there are two types of ISP in submucous neurons. One is mediated by norepinephrine released from sympathetic nerve terminals, and the other is mediated by a still unidentified transmitter released from the terminals of myenteric neurons projecting to the submucosa.[103]

Similar lesion studies have also partially revealed the sources of the excitatory synaptic inputs to the submucous neurons. Most submucous neurons receive fast cholinergic input both from neurons in the myenteric plexus and from neurons in the submucous plexus.[104] The slow ESPs in many of the submucous neurons appear to come from myenteric neurons, but some may come from submucous neurons.[103,104]

Presynaptic Inhibition.

Several studies have indicated that presynaptic inhibition may have an important role in the enteric nervous system. Sympathetic nerve stimulation reduces the amplitudes of fast ESPs in both myenteric and submucous neurons, probably by decreasing the amount of acetylcholine released.[105,106] Indeed, it appears that the presynaptic inhibitory effects of the sympathetic nerves are the primary mechanism by which they diminish the contractile activity of the gut.[3] This inhibition is mediated via α-receptors. Acetylcholine released from enteric nerve terminals can act presynaptically to regulate subsequent release of acetylcholine and possibly the transmitters mediating slow ESPs.[107] In the myenteric plexus, the amplitudes of fast ESPs decline markedly when the internodal strands are stimulated more frequently than about 0.05 Hz; this decline is, however, much reduced in the presence of muscarinic antagonists. Thus, both intrinsic and extrinsic pathways can produce presynaptic inhibition. Several other putative transmitters contained within enteric nerve terminals (e.g., dynorphin, enkephalin, GABA, and 5-HT) have been found in pharmacologic experiments to reduce transmitter release in the gastrointestinal tract. As yet no physiologic role has been established for any of these substances.

ENTERIC PATHWAYS FOR MOTILITY CONTROL

Details of the patterns of motility and their control in the different parts of the gastrointestinal system are given in Chapters 7 through 11. Although the organization of the enteric reflex pathways concerned with control of motility is being actively studied, no satisfactory model that links enteric neural circuitry to the complex patterns of movement that are described in later chapters has yet emerged. At the moment we are only able to provide a circuit analysis that deals with very simple stereotyped reflexes in the small intestine. These reflexes may provide the building blocks for the complex movements of the intestine, with the observed movements representing the superimposition and interaction of many simple reflexes. We will confine most of our discussion of the circuitry to the small intestine. It should be pointed out that many features are shared by the entire smooth muscle part of the gastrointestinal tract. In all regions, similar excitatory and inhibitory motor neurons supply the muscle and there are intrinsic reflexes that respond to the bulk and chemical nature of the luminal contents.

The general patterns of motility of the small intestine are similar in all mammals. The intestine exhibits cyclic changes of activity, collectively termed *migrating myoelectric complexes*, that pass along the intestine from the stomach to the terminal ileum. In humans, these cycles last about 90 minutes and are seen when the intestine is between digestive periods. The myoelectric complex is generated by the enteric nervous system. During digestion, irregular contractions are observed. This irregular activity consists of mixing and propulsive movements that are triggered by the contents of the intestine in three ways: by distension, by chemical stimulation of the mucosa, and by mechanical stimulation of the mucosa. Numerous studies, beginning during the past century and continuing to the present, show that reflex circuits for motility control are in the enteric nervous system and that they can operate entirely independent of central nervous system control (see Furness and Costa[3] for review).

The movements of the intestine are a result of the contractions and relaxations of the external longitudinal and external circular muscles and of the muscularis mucosae. However, the major role in determining the pattern of mixing and propulsive movements appears to be taken by the circular layer of the external muscle. Thus, we will concentrate on this layer. The analysis that follows comes primarily from work on the small intestine of the guinea pig.

Most investigators who have attempted to analyze enteric muscle motor reflexes have used isolated segments of intestine so that the influence of the central nervous system and of circulating hormones could be eliminated. This also simplifies recording from the muscle and enteric neurons. In such preparations, distension, or mechanical stimulation of the mucosa (by bending the villi with a small brush) elicits reflexes whose effects on the circular muscle can be recorded with intracellular microelectrodes (Fig.

1-11).[97,98,108,109] The major responses are depolarizing potentials (excitation) oral to the stimulus and hyperpolarizing potentials (inhibition) on the caudal side. This polarization of electrical responses is analogous to that of the mechanical events that are seen when the intestine is distended.[110] The responses to mucosal stimulation were not observed if the mucosa was removed, indicating that the sensory nerve endings are in the mucosa. The reflexes do not pass along the gut if the myenteric plexus is cut, whereas they are unaffected by interruption of the submucous plexus. Thus the reflex pathways must pass locally from the mucosa to the myenteric plexus and then along the intestine in this plexus. It is commonly observed that the intestine undergoes annular contractions or relaxations; that is, it does not contract or relax eccentrically. This is consistent with structural and electrophysiologic studies that show that motor neurons extend their processes circumferentially. In Figure 1-12, the shapes of the sensory neurons, interneurons, and motor neurons that are deduced from combined physiologic and structural studies in the small intestine of the guinea pig are illustrated.

In trying to unravel the reflex pathways, one of the problems has been to identify the primary sensory neurons. The only place for which there is reasonable progress is the small intestine of the guinea pig, where we propose that the AH/Dogiel type II neurons are sensory. It is interesting that, in 1899, Dogiel[27] recognized that these cells had a suitable morphology and therefore proposed them to be sensory. The electrophysiologic and morphologic properties of these neurons are discussed above (see also Fig 1-12). The sensory neurons that respond to mucosal stimulation should have nerve endings in the mucosa and provide outputs to other myenteric neurons. The only multiaxonal neurons in the myenteric plexus, and thus the only neurons likely to fulfill this criterion in the myenteric plexus, are the Dogiel type II neurons, many of which extend processes to the mucosa. Recent electrophysiologic evidence that the long axon-like processes of the type II neurons all conduct action potentials indicates that they could indeed receive sensory information via one process and relay it

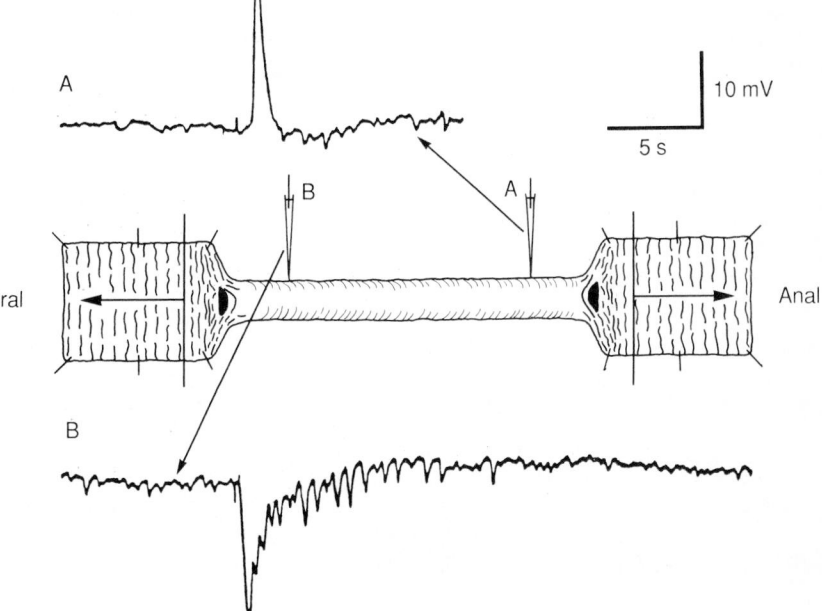

FIGURE 1–11. Mucosa-to-muscle reflexes in the small intestine. The villi of the opened ends of segments were distorted by brushing (*center panel*). This caused an ascending excitatory reflex, which gave rise to depolarizing potentials in the circular muscle oral to stimuli, **A**, and a descending inhibitory reflex, which gave rise to hyperpolarizing potentials anally, **B**. (From Smith TK, Furness JB. Reflex changes in circular muscle activity elicited by stroking the mucosa: An electrophysiological analysis in the isolated guinea pig ileum. J Auton Nerv Syst 1988;25: 205–218.)

via other processes to further neurons in a reflex pathway.[111] The other neurons in the myenteric plexus are uniaxonal and are thus unlikely to be sensory neurons, particularly because ultrastructural studies provide no evidence of there being outputs from these neurons other than via the axon. About 85% of AH/Dogiel type II neurons, and only Dogiel type II neurons in the small intestine of the guinea pig, contain calbindin-like immunoreactivity.[73,112] Examination of the projections and synaptic relations of the calbindin neurons shows that the major projections of these neurons within the myenteric plexus are circumferential, that they make synapses with the majority of other neurons, and that they also send processes to the mucosa.[18,113] The shapes and projections of Dogiel type II neurons have been examined after intracellular injection of dye (see Fig 1-12), and this confirms the morphologic deductions made for the subgroup containing calbindin.

Sensory neurons in the submucous plexus may also play a role in mediating the contractile reflexes evoked by stimulating the mucosa. A population of AH/Dogiel type II neurons has been identified in the submucous plexus and these have been found to be immunoreactive for both substance P and ChAT.[64] Distension-sensitive sensory neurons are located in the myenteric plexus[109,114,115] and may also be AH/Dogiel type II neurons. As yet, no direct evidence is available to support this supposition.

The projections of motor neurons to the circular muscle have been determined by mapping responses in the muscle to transmural nerve stimulation in normal pieces of intestine and in pieces in which nerve paths had been lesioned and allowed to degenerate.[116,117] The majority of excitatory and inhibitory motor neurons extend very little distance along the intestine, 1 to 2 mm, but they run up to half the distance around its circumference, 6 to 8 mm in the small intestine of the guinea pig (see Fig 1-12). A small proportion of motor neurons run along the intestine for 20 to 30 mm; long excitatory motor neurons run orally, and long inhibitory motor neurons run anally.

Enteric reflexes extend for several centimeters along the intestine from a single point of stimulus, in contrast to the sensory neurons and the majority of motor neurons, which implies that there are interneurons in the reflex pathways. Immunohistochemical studies, for example, those that examined serotonin and VIP pathways (see Furness and Costa[3]), provided structural evidence for myenteric interneurons. We also have evidence of these neurons from dye-filling experiments, which indicate that the interneurons run almost directly along the intestine (i.e. they do not run for more than about 1 mm circumferentially while they run along the intestine for 5 to 10 mm, in the small intestine of a guinea pig). These experiments also showed that the interneurons gave off small side branches along their course (see Fig 1-12), as had been previously found for serotonin neurons.[61]

Intracellular recordings have been made from enteric neurons during distention-evoked reflexes at sites anal to stimuli[97,98] and at both oral and anal sites during reflexes elicited by mucosal distortion (Fig 1-13). Fast ESPs are seen in neurons at distances from 0.5 to 2.5 cm from the stimuli. Because it appears that the primary sensory neurons extend only a few millimeters in the lengthwise direction of the intestine, the fast ESPs recorded at greater distances must be due to transmission from interneurons that project orally and anally along the intestine. This implies that the interneurons are cholinergic.

By combining the physiologic and morphologic studies, it is possible to draw a generalized pattern of the circuit for the reflexes initiated from the mucosa (Fig 1-14). When a small area of mucosa is stimulated, a band of myenteric plexus is activated via the circumferentially directed axons of the primary sensory neurons. Excitation is conducted from this region along ascending and descending pathways. There are a huge number of primary sensory neurons (in guinea pig about 500 per millimeter of intestine and about 3 to 4 per villus); thus considerable summation of sensory input can be expected in an area such as that drawn in Figure

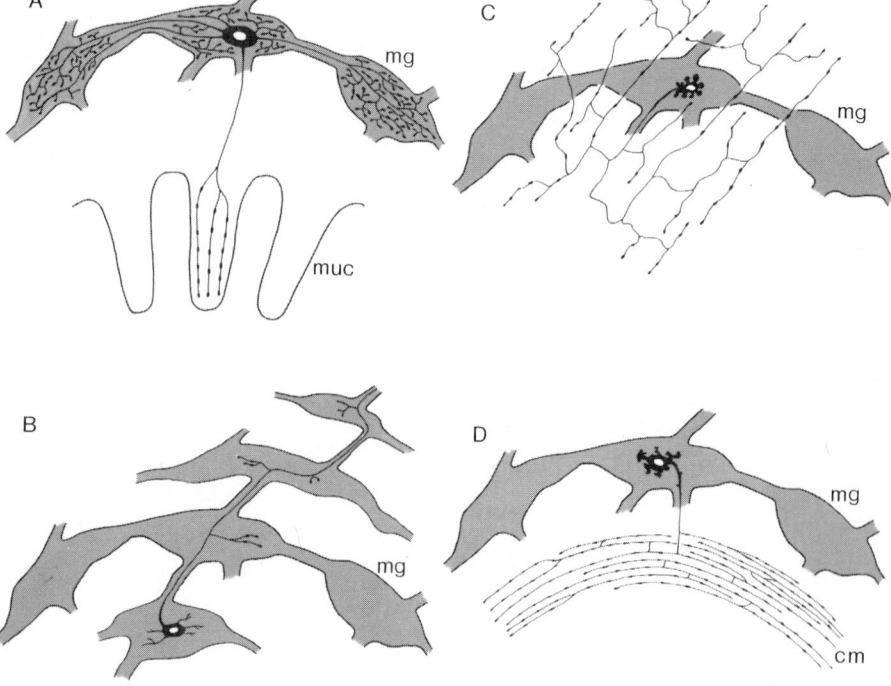

FIGURE 1–12. Drawings of enteric primary sensory neurons, **A;** interneurons, **B;** and motor neurons to the longitudinal muscle, **C;** and circular muscle, **D.** These drawings are derived from studies in the guinea pig small intestine. The morphologies of the sensory neuron, the interneuron, and the motor neuron to the longitudinal muscle are based primarily on filling neurons with the intracellular marker, biocytin. The morphology of the motor neuron to the circular muscle is based on a combination of results from histochemical and lesion studies.

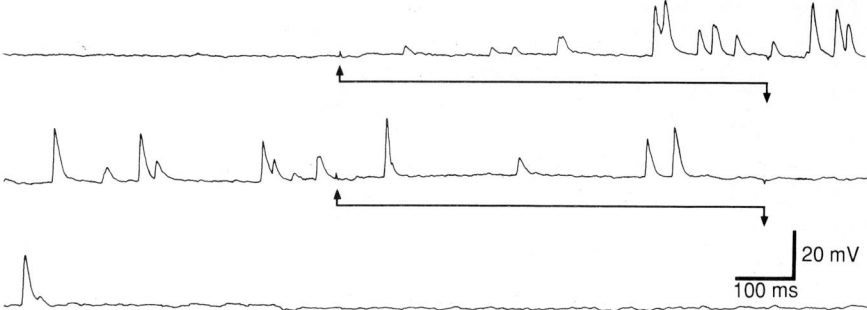

FIGURE 1–13. Continuous intracellular recording taken from a myenteric neuron of the guinea pig small intestine, showing responses recorded in an S/uniaxonal neuron 5 mm oral to a region of stimulation of the mucosa by villous distortion. This stimulus, applied for the periods indicated, elicited a series of fast ESPs in the neuron. This is the typical response of neurons when ascending excitatory reflexes are evoked.

1-14. The interneurons that lead out from an area of sensory activation probably do not provide significant circumferential divergence, because those interneurons that we have filled with dye all run almost directly along the intestine. However, the motor neurons do run circumferentially and so the response to reflex activation is spread around the intestine. Once more this is likely to involve a summed response to transmission from many neurons; Bornstein and co-workers[116] estimated that each smooth muscle cell is influenced by approximately 25 inhibitory motor neurons, and a similar convergence of excitatory influence can be expected.[117] Local averaging of the responses is probably contributed by the electrical communication between smooth muscle cells.

The sensory, AH/Dogiel type II, neurons are probably modulated by inputs from other neurons. AH neurons have prominent afterhyperpolarizations that are caused by prolonged increases in calcium-activated potassium conductance and that limit the firing rates of the neurons. Thus, action potentials that may arrive at high frequency from one axon can be gated at the cell body and output processes may fire at a significantly lower frequency (Fig 1-15). This gating effect of the cell body will be diminished if slow synaptic inputs that reduce potassium currents are active (see above and Fig 1-15). The slow synaptic inputs to AH neurons provide a mechanism through which enteric reflexes could be augmented. This could occur between regions (e.g., the gastrocolic reflex) or between mucosal and distention reflexes.

A NOTE ON THE UNDERLYING MUSCLE RHYTHMS

The smooth muscle of the gastrointestinal tract exhibits an endogenous rhythmic activity (see ch 4; Sanders and Publicover[118]), which takes the form of regular oscillations in membrane potential called slow waves that occur at frequencies of 3 to 12 per minute in humans. To cause contractions of the muscle, the slow wave amplitude needs to exceed a threshold. This is the electrical threshold for eliciting mechanical activity and is referred to as the "mechanical threshold." Once the mechanical threshold is reached, the relation between depolarization and contraction is quite steep.[118] Thus the reflexes that have been discussed act on this underlying rhythm. Activity of the neurons can move the membrane potential of the muscle below or further above the mechanical threshold, thus causing the rhythmic contractions of the gut to be stronger, weaker, or absent. The neurons can also influence the frequency of the contractions.[119]

INTERSTITIAL CELLS OF CAJAL

Cajal[7] proposed that the interstitial cells are a type of neuron that is intercalated between nerve fibers and the muscle. The cells have created considerable controversy. For some years it was uncertain which cells should receive this title, partly because Cajal's descriptions seem ambiguous. Now, thanks mainly to the investigations of Thuneberg, a consensus about the identification of the cells appears to have been reached.[9,120]

Two groups of interstitial cells are of greatest interest: those at the interface of the longitudinal and circular muscle coats and those near the inner surface of the circular muscle. These cells have a cell body region containing a single nucleus with a thin surround of cytoplasm and give rise to a number of long tapering processes, some of which branch (Fig 1-16). A number of light microscope studies indicated that the cells do not have morphologies and staining characteristics unequivocally typical of nerve cells,[121,122] and later electron microscopic studies made it quite clear that the cells are not neurons.[33,123-126] Most recent consid-

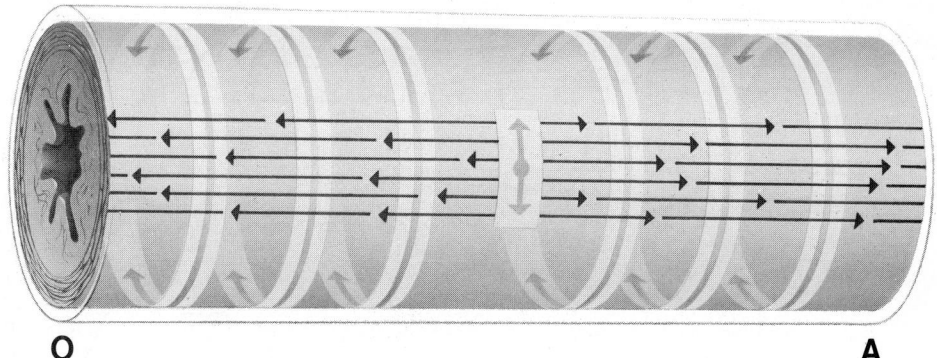

FIGURE 1–14. Schematic representation of the arrangement and connections of neurons of peristaltic reflexes to the circular muscle. Groups of sensory neurons provide inputs to myenteric neurons in circumferentially aligned bands (*green*). Interneurons run along the intestine with little divergence (*black arrows*). Motor neurons run circumferentially (*blue*) to excite or inhibit rings of intestine. See text for further details.

O   A

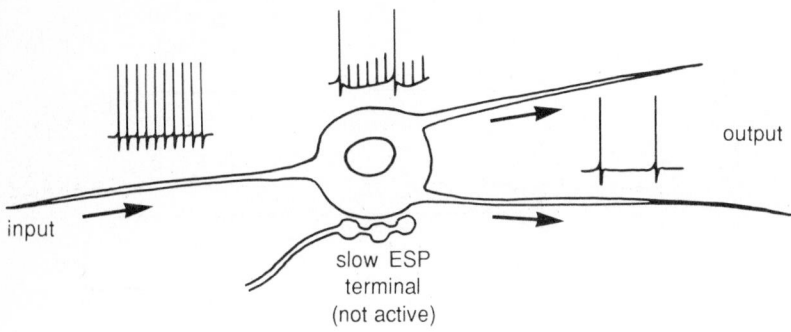

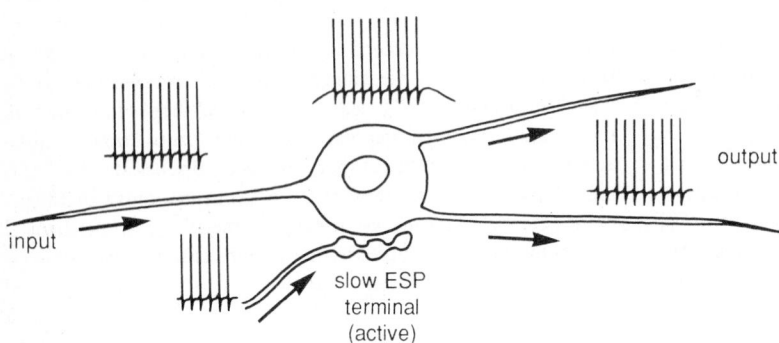

FIGURE 1–15. Illustration of the mechanism by which the passage of action potentials across the cell bodies of AH neurons is gated. If the AH neuron is not excited, **A,** an action potential that invades the cell body is followed by a prolonged hyperpolarization that prevents the active propagation of subsequent action potentials across the cell body for several seconds. If synaptic inputs causing slow ESPs are activated, **B,** the prolonged hyperpolarization is attenuated and the action potentials follow at a higher frequency. See text for further explanation. (From Furness JB, Costa M. The enteric nervous system. New York: Churchill Livingstone, 1987.)

erations have focused on two possibilities: either that they are a type of connective tissue cell or that they are cells responsible for the generation of spontaneous electrical activity that drives or controls the rhythmic oscillations in membrane potential (slow waves) seen in intestinal smooth muscle.

Ultrastructure of Interstitial Cells of Cajal

Literature on the ultrastructure of the interstitial cells does not present a consistent picture of these cells, possibly because there are genuine differences between the cells in different species or regions or because of the difficulty of being certain that cells examined in the electron microscope are the same as those identified by light microscopy. Those features that seem to be typical of the interstitial cells of Cajal have been summarized by Thuneberg.[9] The most pertinent are the following: 1) the presence of numerous mitochondria, suggesting a metabolically active cell; 2) large bun-

dles of intermediate filaments, especially in the processes, which distinguishes these cells from many others of the interstitium; 3) abundant surface caveolae and prominent smooth endoplasmic reticulum, consistent with the cell needing to sequester ions, as might be expected if it is acting as an electrical oscillator. Furthermore, the cells have few cisternae of rough endoplasmic reticulum, a feature that distinguishes them from fibroblasts, and they do not have any accumulations of synaptic vesicles, confirming that they are not neurons.

Relations to Other Cells

The strongest clues to their roles are perhaps the relations that they form with other cells. Interstitial cells of Cajal, especially those in the inner layers of the circular muscle, form close relations with smooth muscle cells.[9,33] These associations consist of numerous points where the adjacent cell membranes come within 10 nm over distances of 0.5 to 1 μm and form nexus junctions, sim-

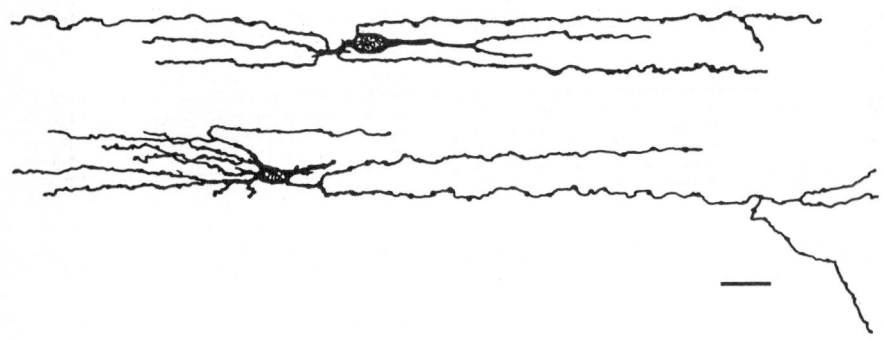

FIGURE 1–16. Interstitial cells of Cajal. These cells are from the region of the deep muscular plexus. Calibration: approximately 20 μm. (From Cajal SRy. Histologie du système nerveux de l'homme et des vertébrés. Paris: Maloine, 1911.)

ilar to those between individual cardiac or smooth muscle cells.[124,126-128] In some places (e.g., between the longitudinal and circular muscle layers of the small intestine), processes of each interstitial cell make close contacts with those of other interstitial cells. Thus, as Cajal originally described, the interstitial cells form a network that can be readily appreciated when the cells are stained in whole mount preparations.[9] Although close approaches occur between nerve fibers and interstitial cells, these could be expected because the cells are located where there are rich plexuses of nerve fiber bundles whose true targets could be the smooth muscle. There are no morphologic specializations that define autonomic neuroeffector junctions and, in the absence of direct physiologic evidence for the innervation of interstitial cells, the significance of close nerve fiber approaches is uncertain.

Physiologic Evidence for a Role of Interstitial Cells of Cajal

The supposition that the interstitial cells of Cajal generate or control the pacemaker activity of intestinal muscle was based on the location of the cells close to the site of generation of the pacemaker activity and their relation with smooth muscle and with each other.[9] To prove that they act as pacemakers requires a demonstration that the interstitial cells exhibit rhythmic changes in membrane potential, that these changes are effectively communicated to the muscle, and that without the interstitial cells the normal smooth muscle activity is not generated. Suzuki and associates[129] prepared strips of smooth muscle from the small intestine of the cat with and without the layer of interstitial cells and found that slow waves only occurred in the muscle when the interstitial cells were present. Interstitial cells isolated from the canine colon show rhythmic oscillations in membrane potential.[130] Thus there is both morphologic and physiologic evidence that is consistent with the interstitial cells of Cajal being involved in the generation of slow waves in the intestinal muscle, but direct evidence that rhythmic activity of interstitial cells drives rhythmic activity in the muscle is yet to be obtained.

ENTERIC PATHWAYS FOR SECRETOMOTOR CONTROL

Despite the fact that a dense innervation of the intestinal mucosa was demonstrated in the past century, and it was suggested more than a century ago that enteric neurons of the submucous plexus control water and electrolyte exchange,[131] this information is mentioned in almost no textbook. However, knowledge of the physiology of enteric control of water and electrolyte transport has advanced remarkably in recent years and similar diagrams of the underlying circuits have been deduced by investigators in different laboratories (Fig 1-17).[56,132] The circuits consist of sensory neurons with their endings in the mucosa and an integrating circuitry in the myenteric plexus that feeds back to secretomotor neurons with cell bodies in the submucous ganglia. There are two types of secretomotor neurons: cholinergic and noncholinergic. The noncholinergic neurons appear to mediate most of the local reflex response.

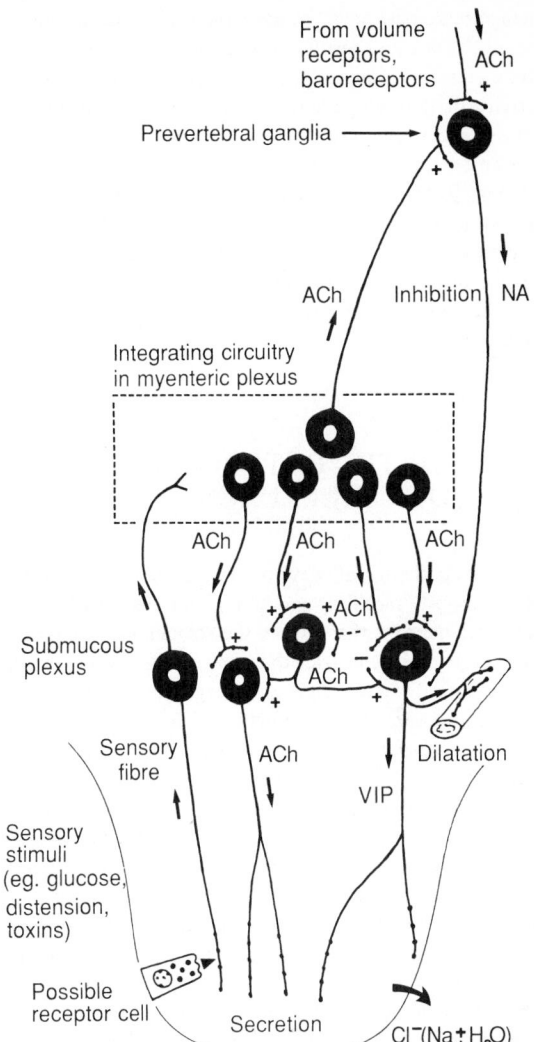

FIGURE 1–17. Diagram of enteric neural circuitry for control of water and electrolyte secretion, which combines knowledge of neural projections and of neuroneural transmission primarily from the guinea pig, information about the actions of secretomotor neurons from a variety of species, and data on the physiologic stimuli that can activate or inhibit secretomotor reflexes from experiments primarily on cats and rats.

Secretomotor reflexes can be initiated in a number of ways, physiologically by chemical or mechanical interaction of luminal contents with the mucosa or pathologically by toxins, such as cholera toxin or enterotoxins, in the lumen. In the small intestine an important physiologic stimulus appears to be the presence, or active uptake, of nutrients (it is not certain which of these is the stimulus). Nutrients such as glucose that are absorbed by a sodium co-transporter draw in sodium ions along with counter ions, mostly chloride ions, and water. At the same time, glucose, or its uptake, stimulates the enteric secretomotor reflex.[133] The secretomotor neurons stimulate the epithelial cells to pump chloride ions into the lumen, which will take with it counter ions, mostly sodium ions, and water. The gain on this reflex is not known, but it is likely to be greater than unity, that is, more water is secreted than is absorbed if the reflex is not controlled. Inhibitory control over the reflex is exerted by sympathetic neurons that are tonically active. Cutting the sympathetic pathways "releases the brake" on the enteric secretomotor reflex and results in what Bernard,[134] in 1859, called paralytic secretion. Logically, it might be expected that the level of activity of the sympathetic secretomotor inhibitory neurons would respond to measures of whole body water and electrolyte status. This is in fact so; they increase activity and thus reduce water and electrolyte secretion in response to hemorrhagic hypotension, unloading of the baroreceptors, or reduction in right atrial pressure.[135-138] Histochemical studies suggest that secretomotor neurons might cause a physiologically appropriate vasodilation, concomitant with secretion, via collaterals to submucous arterioles.[56]

SYMPATHETIC ENTEROENTERIC INHIBITORY REFLEXES

Separate sympathetic pathways to the gastrointestinal tract affect its blood supply, motility, and water and electrolyte secretion. Sympathetic neurons that supply the splanchnic vasculature are noradrenergic; they constrict the arterioles and arteries and the major mesenteric veins. Their physiologic roles, which primarily involve adjustments of the proportion of the cardiac output going to digestive organs, have been reviewed.[57] The influence of sympathetic pathways on electrolyte exchange has been discussed previously. Sympathetic neurons that inhibit motility do this in two ways, by constricting the sphincters and by inhibiting the contractile activity of the nonsphincter parts of the gastrointestinal tract. Sympathetic pathways may inhibit the muscle of the nonsphincter parts of the gastrointestinal tract both by presynaptic inhibition in the myenteric plexus and by direct inhibitory actions on the muscle.

The sympathetic enteroenteric inhibitory reflexes decrease motility. They are initiated in one part of the gastrointestinal tract and pass to other regions and back to the same region via prevertbral ganglia.[139] The existence of such reflexes whose pathways travel to the central nervous system and then back to the intestine via sympathetic ganglia was shown early this century. It was thus surprising when, in the 1940s, Kuntz and his colleagues showed convincingly that reflexes could be conducted from one part of the gastrointestinal tract to another via sympathetic prevertebral ganglia, even when these ganglia were completely isolated from central nervous connections (see review by Szurszewski and King[139]). It is now clear that there are two reflexes, a reflex via the spinal cord and a peripheral reflex.[3] The peripheral reflex can only be studied after the central pathways have been selectively inactivated. Under these circumstances the peripheral reflexes exhibit a higher threshold than the central reflexes. Szurszewski and King[139] suggest that the higher threshold may be a consequence of the loss of background synaptic input activity, which would normally increase the effectiveness of the peripheral reflexes.

A diagram of the peripheral enteroenteric reflex pathways and their relation to other sympathetic pathways is shown in Figure 1-18. It is not possible to survey all the evidence for the diagram in this chapter, so only major points are dealt with. Intestinofugal neurons that synapse in prevertebral ganglia were demonstrated by recording intracellularly from the ganglia in preparations consisting only of a segment of intestine connected to the ganglion that were completely removed from the body.[140] Activation of intestinal tension receptors evoked fast ESPs in a majority of nerve cells in the prevertebral ganglia.[140-142] The ESPs were blocked by nicotinic antagonists applied to the ganglia. Crowcroft and colleagues[140] suggested that the intestinofugal neurons were second order neurons in the sensory pathways, because they found that the responses in the ganglia were diminished by nicotinic blockers applied to the intestine. Structural studies have confirmed the presence of neurons with cell bodies in the intestine that send processes to prevertebral ganglia where they form synapses.[139] The cell bodies of the intestinofugal neurons were shown to be in the myenteric ganglia by injection of retrogradely transported dye into prevertebral ganglia.[143] A variety of neuropeptides are found in intestinofugal neurons; their possible significance has been discussed by Szurszewski and King.[139]

Considerable evidence suggests that sympathetic motility inhibiting neurons have little or no activity in undisturbed humans or animals,[3] although evidence for some ongoing activity has been summarized by Szurszewski and King.[139] Enteroenteric inhibitory reflexes affecting other parts of the intestine can be initiated by distention of any region. Most studies have dealt with reflexes affecting the stomach and intestine, but similar reflex pathways

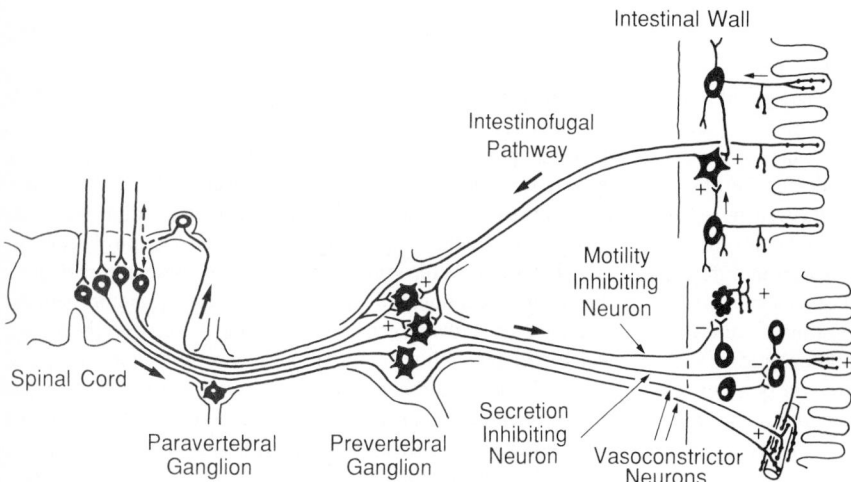

FIGURE 1-18. Connections of sympathetic pathways that affect intestinal motility, fluid exchange, and blood flow.

also affect the biliary system.[144] Inhibition of the stomach can also be caused by acidity or hypertonicity in the lumen of the upper small intestine; such reflexes are referred to as enterogastric reflexes. The enteroenteric inhibitory reflexes appear to have a protective role for the gastrointestinal tract.[3] In the case of enterogastric reflexes, the slowing of gastric emptying protects the duodenal mucosa from acid and osmotic stress.

SUMMARY

The enteric nervous system is the basis for intrinsic control of motility, epithelial water and electrolyte transport, and blood flow in the digestive tract. It is the medium through which extrinsic neurons control the gastrointestinal system.

> The reader is directed to Chapter 2, Gastrointestinal Hormones; Chapter 3, The Brain-Gut Axis; Chapter 4, Smooth Muscle of the Gut; Chapter 7, Esophageal Motor Function; Chapter 8, The Physiology of Gastric Motility and Gastric Emptying; Chapter 9, Motility of the Small Intestine; Chapter 10, The Motor Function of the Colon; Chapter 11, Motility of the Biliary Tree; Chapter 54, Motility Disorders of the Esophagus; Chapter 60, Disorders of Gastric Emptying; Chapter 67, Dysmotility of the Small Intestine; Chapter 80, Irritable Bowel Syndrome; Chapter 81, Motility Disorders of the Colon; Chapter 97, Postcholecystectomy Syndrome; Chapter 128, Evaluation of Gastrointestinal Motility: Methodological Considerations.

REFERENCES

1. Furness JB, Costa M. Types of nerves in the enteric nervous system. Neuroscience 1980;5:1.
2. Wattchow DA, Furness JB, Costa M, et al. Distributions of neuropeptides in the human esophagus. Gastroenterology 1987;93:1363.
3. Furness JB, Costa M. The enteric nervous system. Edinburgh: Churchill Livingstone, 1987:1
4. Stöhr P. Mikroskopische Studien zur Innervation des Magen-Darmkanales. Z Zellforsch Mikroskop Anat 1930;12:66.
5. Li P-L. Neue Beobachtungen über die Struktur des Zirculärmuskels im Dunndarm bei Wirbeltieren. Z Anat Entw-Gesch 1937;107:212.
6. Gabella G. Special muscle cells and their innervation in the mammalian small intestine. Cell Tissue Res 1974;153:63.
7. Cajal SRY. Histologie du système nerveux de l'homme et des vertébrés. Paris: Maloine, 1911
8. Stach W. Der Plexus entericus extremus des Dickdarmes und seine Beziehungen zu den interstitiellen Zellen (Cajal). Z Mikrosk Anat Forsch 1972;85:245.
9. Thuneberg L. Interstitial cells of Cajal. In: Wood JD, ed. Handbook of physiology, section 6: the gastrointestinal system, vol I. Washington, DC: American Physiological Society, 1989:349.
10. Furness JB, Lloyd KCK, Sternini C, Walsh JH. Projections of substance P, vasoactive intestinal peptide and tyrosine hydroxylase immunoreactive nerve fibres in the canine bowel, with special reference to the innervation of the circular muscle. Arch Histol Cytol 1990;53:129.
11. Faussone-Pellegrini M-S, Cortesini C. Ultrastructural peculiarities of the inner portion of the circular layer of colon: I. Research in the human. Acta Anat 1984;120:185.
12. Faussone-Pellegrini M-S. Ultrastructural peculiarities of the inner portion of the circular layer of the colon: II. Research on the mouse. Acta Anat 1985;122:187.
13. Faussone-Pellegrini M-S, Pantalone D, Cortesini C. An ultrastructural study of the interstitial cells of Cajal of the human stomach. J Submicrosc Cytol Pathol 1989;21:439.
14. Gabella G, Trigg P. Size of neurons and glial cells in the enteric ganglia of mice, guinea pigs, rabbits and sheep. J Neurocytol 1984;13:49.
15. Irwin DA. The anatomy of Auerbach's plexus. Am J Anat 1931;49:141.
16. Auerbach L. Fernere vorlaufige Mitteilung über den Nervenapparat des Darmes. Arch Pathol Anat Physiol 1864;30:457.
17. Wilson AJ, Llewellyn-Smith IJ, Furness JB, Costa M. The source of the nerve fibres innervating the circular muscle and forming the deep muscular plexus in the guinea-pig small intestine. Cell Tissue Res 1987;247:497.
18. Furness JB, Trussell DC, Pompolo S, et al. Calbindin neurons of the guinea-pig small intestine: quantitative analysis of their numbers and projections. Cell Tissue Res 1990;260:261.
19. Scheuermann DW, Stach W, Timmermans J-P, et al. Neuronspecific enolase and S-100 protein immunohistochemistry for defining the structure and topographical relationship of the different enteric nerve plexuses in the small intestine of the pig. Cell Tissue Res 1989;256:65.
20. Stach W. Der Plexus submucosus externus (Schabadasch) im Dünndarm des Schweins: I. Form, Struktur und Verbindungen der Ganglien und Nervenzellen. Z Mikroskop Anat Forsch 1977;91:737.
21. Stach W. A revised morphological classification of neurons in the enteric nervous system. In: Singer MV, Goebell H, eds. Nerves and the gastrointestinal tract. Lancaster, U.K.: Kluwer Academic Publishers, 1989:29.
22. Christensen J, Rick GA. Nerve cell density in submucous plexus throughout the gut of cat and opossum. Gastroenterology 1985;89:1064.
23. Keast JR, Furness JB, Costa M. Distribution of certain peptide-containing nerves and endocrine cells in the gastrointestinal mucosa in five mammalian species. J Comp Neurol 1985;236:403.
24. Kirchgessner AL, Gershon MD. Projections of submucosal neurons to the myenteric plexus of the guinea pig intestine: in vitro tracing of microcircuits by retrograde and anterograde transport. J Comp Neurol 1988;277:487.
25. Ekblad E, Winther C, Ekman R, Håkanson R. Projections of peptide-containing neurons in rat small intestine. Neuroscience 1987;20:169.
26. Ekblad E, Ekman R, Håkanson R, Sundler F. Projections of peptide-containing neurons in rat large intestine. Neuroscience 1988;27:655.
27. Dogiel AS. Ueber den Bau der Ganglien in den Geflechten des Darmes und der Gallenblase des Menschen und der Säugetiere. Arch Anat Physiol Leipzig 1899; Anat Abt Jg 1899:130.
28. Furness JB, Bornstein JC, Trussell DC. Shapes of nerve cells in the myenteric plexus of the guinea-pig small intestine revealed by the intracellular injection of dye. Cell Tissue Res 1988;254:561-571.
29. Furness JB, Trussell DC, Pompolo S, et al. Shapes and projections of neurons with immunoreactivity for gamma-aminobutyric acid in the guinea-pig small intestine. Cell Tissue Res 1989;256:293-301.
30. Gabella G. Structure of muscles and nerves in the gastrointestinal tract. In: Johnson LR, ed. Physiology of the gastrointestinal tract. New York: Raven Press, 1987:335.
31. Cook RD, Burnstock G. The ultrastructure of Auerbach's plexus in the guinea pig: I. Neuronal elements. J Neurocytol 1976;5:171.
32. Pompolo S, Furness JB, Bornstein JC, et al. Dogiel type II neurons in the guinea-pig small intestine: ultrastructure in relation to other characteristics. In: Singer MV, Goebell H, eds. Nerves in the gastrointestinal tract. Lancaster, U.K.: Kluwer Academic Publishers, 1989:57.
33. Gabella G. Fine structure of the myenteric plexus in the guinea-pig ileum. J Anat 1972;111:69.
34. Wilson AJ, Furness JB, Costa M. The fine structure of the submucous plexus of the guinea-pig ileum: I. The ganglia, neurons, Schwann cells and neuropil. J Neurocytol 1981;10:759.
35. Llewellyn-Smith IJ, Furness JB, Costa M. Ultrastructural analysis of substance P immunoreactive nerve fibers in myenteric ganglia of guinea-pig small intestine. J Neurosci 1989;2:167.

36. Costa M, Furness JB, Llewellyn-Smith IJ. Histochemistry of the enteric nervous system. In: Johnson LR, ed. Physiology of the gastrointestinal tract. New York: Raven Press, 1987:1.

37. Hoyes AD, Barber P. Axonal terminal ultrastructure in the myenteric ganglia of the guinea-pig stomach. Cell Tissue Res 1980;209:329.

38. Furness JB, Llewellyn-Smith IJ, Bornstein JC, Costa M. Chemical neuroanatomy and the analysis of neuronal circuitry in the enteric nervous system. In: Björklund A, Hökfelt T, Owman C, eds. Handbook of chemical neuroanatomy, vol 6, The peripheral nervous system. Amsterdam: Elsevier, 1988.

39. Llewellyn-Smith IJ, Furness JB, O'Brien PE, Costa M. Noradrenergic nerves in human small intestine: distribution and ultrastructure. Gastroenterology 1984;87:513.

40. Hökfelt T, Fuxe K, Pernow B. Progress in brain research, Vol 68, Coexistence of neuronal messengers: a new principle in chemical transmission. Amsterdam: Elsevier, 1986.

41. Furness JB, Morris JL, Gibbins IL, Costa M. Chemical coding of neurons and plurichemical transmission. Ann Rev Pharmacol Toxicol 1989;29:289.

42. Furness JB, Costa M. Identification of gastrointestinal neurotransmitters. In: Handbook of experimental pharmacology, Heidelberg and New York: Springer, vol 59, 1982:383.

43. Dockray GJ. Physiology of enteric neuropeptides. In: Johnson LR, ed. Physiology of the Gastrointestinal Tract. New York: Raven Press, 1987:41.

44. Bornstein JC, Costa M, Furness JB. Synaptic inputs to immunohistochemically identified neurones in the submucous plexus of the guinea-pig small intestine. J Physiol (Lond) 1986;381:465.

45. Furness JB, Costa M. Identification of transmitters of functionally defined enteric neurons. In: Wood JD, ed. Handbook of physiology, section 6: gastrointestinal system, vol I. Washington, DC: American Physiological Society, 1989:387.

46. Barthó L, Holzer P. Search for a physiological role of substance P in gastrointestinal motility. Neuroscience 1985;16:1.

47. Llewellyn-Smith IJ, Furness JB, Gibbins IL, Costa M. Quantitative ultrastructural analysis of enkephalin-, substance P-, and VIP-immunoreactive nerve fibers in the circular muscle of the guinea-pig small intestine. J Comp Neurol 1989;272:139.

48. Burnstock G. Neurotransmitters and trophic factors in the autonomic nervous system. J Physiol (Lond) 1981;313:1.

49. Fahrenkrug J. Vasoactive intestinal polypeptide: Measurement, distribution and putative neurotransmitter function. Digestion 1979;19:149.

50. Makhlouf GM, Grider JR, Schubert ML. Identification of physiological function of gut peptides. In: Makhlouf GM, ed. Handbook of physiology, section 6: the gastrointestinal system, vol II. Washington, DC: American Physiological Society, 1989:123.

51. Niel JP, Bywater RAR, Taylor GS. Apamin-resistant post-stimulus hyperpolarization in the circular muscle of the guinea-pig ileum. J Auton Nerv Syst 1983;9:565.

52. Costa M, Furness JB, Humphreys CMS. Apamin distinguishes two types of relaxation mediated by enteric nerves in the guinea-pig gastrointestinal tract. Naunyn-Schmiedeberg's Arch Pharmacol 1986;332:79.

53. Manzini S, Maggi CA, Meli A. Pharmacological evidence that at least two different non-adrenergic non-cholinergic inhibitory systems are present in the rat small intestine. Eur J Pharmacol 1986;123:229.

54. Cook HJ. Neural and humoral regulation of small intestinal electrolyte transport. In: Johnson LR, ed. Physiology of the gastrointestinal tract. New York: Raven Press, 1989:1307.

55. Keast JR. Mucosal innervation and control of water and ion transport in the intestine. Rev Physiol Biochem Pharmacol 1987;109:1.

56. Bornstein JC, Furness JB. Correlated electrophysiological and histochemical studies of submucous neurons and their contribution to understanding enteric neural circuits. J Auton Nerv Syst 1988;25:1.

57. Jodal M, Lundgren O. Neurohormonal control of gastrointestinal blood flow. In: Wood JD, ed. Handbook of physiology, section 6: the gastrointestinal system, vol I. Washington, DC: American Physiological Society, 1989:1667.

58. Neild TO, Surprenant A, Shen K-Z, Galligan JJ. Vasodilator nerves supplying arterioles of the small intestine. Neurosci Lett 1989;suppl 34:S128.

59. Thiefin G, Tache Y, Leung FW, Guth PH. Central nervous system action of thyrotropin-releasing hormone to increase gastric mucosal blood flow in the rat. Gastroenterology 1989;97:405.

60. Ito S, Ohga A, Ohta T. Gastric vasodilation and vasoactive intestinal peptide output in response to vagal stimulation in the dog. J Physiol (Lond) 1988;404:669.

61. Furness JB, Costa M. Neurons with 5-hydroxytryptamine–like immunoreactivity in the enteric nervous system: their projections in the guinea-pig small intestine. Neuroscience 1982;7:341.

62. Erde SM, Sherman D, Gershon MD. Morphology and serotonergic innervation of physiologically identified submucous neurons of guinea-pig's myenteric plexus. J Neurosci 1985;5:617.

63. Wood JD. Physiology of the enteric nervous system. In: Johnson LR, ed. Physiology of the gastrointestinal tract. New York: Raven Press, 1987:67.

64. Bornstein JC, Furness JB, Costa M. An electrophysiological comparison of substance P–immunoreactive neurons with other neurons in the guinea-pig submucous plexus. J Auton Nerv Syst 1989;26:113.

65. Grundy D, Scratcherd T. Sensory afferents from the gastrointestinal tract. In: Wood JD, ed. Handbook of physiology, section 6: the gastrointestinal system, vol I. Washington, DC: American Physiological Society, 1989:593.

66. Furness JB, Costa M. The adrenergic innervation of the gastrointestinal tract. Ergeb Physiol 1974;69:1.

67. Langley JN. The autonomic nervous system, part 1. Cambridge: Heffer, 1921.

68. Gershon MD. The enteric nervous system. Ann Rev Neurosci 1981;4:227.

69. Gershon MD. Colonization of the bowel and development of the enteric nervous system by precursors from the neural crest. In: Singer MV, Goebell H, eds. Nerves and the gastrointestinal tract. Lancaster, UK: Kluwer Academic Publishers, 1989:117.

70. Hodgkiss JP, Lees GM. Morphological studies of electrophysiologically-identified myenteric plexus neurons of the guinea-pig ileum. Neuroscience 1983;8:593.

71. Bornstein JC, Costa M, Furness JB, Lees GM. Electrophysiology and enkephalin immunoreactivity of identified myenteric plexus neurones in the guinea-pig small intestine. J Physiol (Lond) 1984;351:313.

72. Katayama Y, Lees GM, Pearson GT. Electrophysiological and morphological characteristics of vasoactive intestinal peptide (VIP)–immunoreactive neurones in the guinea-pig myenteric plexus. J Physiol (Lond) 1986;378:1.

73. Iyer V, Bornstein JC, Costa M, et al. Electrophysiology of guinea-pig myenteric neurons correlated with immunoreactivity for calcium binding proteins. J Auton Nerv Syst 1988;22:141.

74. Hirst GDS, Johnson SM, van Helden DF. The calcium current in a myenteric neurone of the guinea-pig ileum. J Physiol (Lond) 1985;361:297.

75. Hirst GDS, Johnson SM, van Helden DF. The slow calcium-dependent potassium current in a myenteric neurone of the guinea-pig ileum. J Physiol (Lond) 1985;361:315.

76. Galligan JJ, North RA, Tokimasa T. Muscarinic agonists and potassium currents in guinea-pig myenteric neurones. Br J Pharmacol 1989;96:193.

77. Hirst GDS, Holman ME, Spence I. Two types of neurones in the myenteric plexus of duodenum in the guinea pig. J Physiol (Lond) 1974;236:303-326.

78. Nishi S, North RA. Intracellular recording from the myenteric plexus of the guinea-pig ileum. J Physiol (Lond) 1973;231:474.

79. Schemann M, Wood JD. Electrical behaviour of myenteric neurones in the gastric corpus of the guinea pig. J Physiol (Lond) 1989;417:501.

80. Schemann M, Wood JD. Synaptic behaviour of myenteric neurones in the gastric corpus of the guinea pig. J Physiol (Lond) 1989;417: 519.

81. Wade PR, Wood JD. Electrical behavior of myenteric neurones in guinea-pig distal colon. Am J Physiol 1988;254:G522.

82. Wade PR, Wood JD. Synaptic behaviour of myenteric neurones in guinea-pig distal colon. Am J Physiol 1988;255:G184.

83. Tamura K, Wood JD. Electrical and synaptic properties of myenteric plexus neurones in the terminal large intestine of the guinea pig. J Physiol (Lond) 1989;415:275.

84. Brookes SJH, Ewart WR, Wingate DL. Intracellular recordings from cells in the myenteric plexus of the rat duodenum. Neuroscience 1988;24:297.

85. Furukawa K, Taylor GS, Bywater RAR. An intracellular study of myenteric neurons in the mouse colon. J Neurophysiol 1986;55: 1395.

86. Brookes SJH, Ewart WR, Wingate DL. Intracellular recordings from myenteric neurones in the human colon. J Physiol (Lond) 1987;390: 305.

87. King BF, Szurszewski JH. Intracellular recordings from vagally innervated intramural neurons in opossum stomach. Am J Physiol 1984;246:G209.

88. Furness JB, Costa M, Keast JR. Choline acetyltransferase and peptide immunoreactitivity of submucous neurons in the small intestine of the guinea pig. Cell Tissue Res 1984;237:329.

89. Lees GM, Leishman DJ, Pearson GT. Electrophysiological characteristics of guinea-pig myenteric plexus neurons immunoreactive for dynorphin A(1-8). In: Singer MV, Goebell H, eds. Nerves and the gastrointestinal tract. Lancaster, UK: Kluwer Academic Publishers, 1989;79.

90. Wood JD, Mayer CJ. Intracellular study of electrical activity of Auerbach's plexus in guinea-pig small intestine. Pflügers Arch 1978;374:265.

91. Johnson SM, Katayama Y, North RA. Slow synaptic potentials in the neurones of the myenteric plexus. J Physiol (Lond) 1980;301: 505.

92. Bornstein JC, North RA, Costa M, Furness JB. Excitatory synaptic potentials due to activation of neurons with short projections in the myenteric plexus. Neuroscience 1984;11:723.

93. Morita K, North RA. Significance of slow synaptic potentials for transmission of excitation in guinea-pig myenteric plexus. Neuroscience 1985;14:661.

94. North RA, Tokimasa T. Muscarinic synaptic potentials in guinea-pig myenteric plexus neurones. J Physiol (Lond) 1982;333:151.

95. Mihara S, North RA, Surprenant A. Somatostatin increases an inwardly rectifying potassium conductance in guinea-pig submucous plexus neurones. J Physiol (Lond) 1987;390:335.

96. Palmer JM, Wood JD, Zafirov DH. Transduction of aminergic and peptidergic signals in enteric neurones of the guinea pig. J Physiol (Lond) 1987;387:371.

97. Hirst GDS, McKirdy HC. A nervous mechanism for descending inhibition in guinea-pig small intestine. J Physiol (Lond) 1974;238: 129.

98. Hirst GDS, Holman ME, McKirdy HC. Two descending nerve pathways activated by distension of guinea-pig small intestine. J Physiol (Lond) 1975;244:117.

99. Hirst GDS, McKirdy HC. Synaptic potentials recorded from neurones of the submucous plexus of guinea-pig small intestine. J Physiol (Lond) 1975;249:369.

100. Surprenant A. Slow excitatory synaptic potentials recorded from neurones of guinea-pig submucous plexus. J Physiol (Lond) 1984;351:343.

101. Surprenant A. Two types of neurones lacking synaptic input in the submucous plexus of guinea-pig small intestine. J Physiol (Lond) 1984;351:363.

102. Mihara S, Katayama Y, Nishi S. Slow postsynaptic potentials on neurones of submucous plexus of guinea-pig caecum and their mimicry by noradrenaline and various peptides. Neuroscience 1985;16: 1057.

103. Bornstein JC, Costa M, Furness JB. Intrinsic and extrinsic inhibitory synaptic inputs to submucous neurones of the guinea-pig small intestine. J Physiol (Lond) 1988;398:371.

104. Bornstein JC, Furness JB, Costa M. Sources of excitatory synaptic inputs to neurochemically identified submucous neurons of the guinea-pig small intestine. J Auton Nerv Syst 1987;18:83.

105. Hirst GDS, McKirdy HC. Presynaptic inhibition at a mammalian peripheral synapse? Nature 1974;250:430.

106. Edwards FR, Hirst GDS, Silinsky EM. Interaction between inhibitory and excitatory synaptic potentials at a peripheral neurone. J Physiol (Lond) 1976;259:647.

107. Morita K, North RA, Tokimasa T. Muscarinic presynaptic inhibition of synaptic transmission in myenteric plexus of guinea-pig ileum. J Physiol (Lond) 1982;333:141.

108. Smith TK, Furness JB. Reflex changes in circular muscle activity elicited by stroking the mucosa: an electrophysiological analysis in the isolated guinea pig ileum. J Auton Nerv Syst 1988;25:205.

109. Smith TK, Bornstein JC, Furness JB. Distension-evoked ascending and descending reflexes in the circular muscle of the guinea-pig ileum: an intracellular study. J Auton Nerv Syst 1990;29:203.

110. Bayliss WM, Starling EH. The movements and innervation of the small intestine. J Physiol (Lond) 1899;4:100.

111. Hendriks R, Bornstein JC, Furness JB. An electrophysiological study of the projections of putative sensory neurons within the myenteric plexus of the guinea-pig ileum. Neurosci Lett 1990;110:286.

112. Furness JB, Keast JR, Pompolo S, et al. Immunohistochemical evidence for the presence of calcium binding protein in enteric neurons. Cell Tissue Res 1988;252:79.

113. Pompolo S, Furness JB. Ultrastructure and synaptic relationships of calbindin-reactive, Dogiel type II neurons in myenteric ganglia of guinea-pig small intestine. J Neurocytol 1988;17:771.

114. Hukuhara T, Miyake T. The intrinsic reflexes in the colon. Jpn J Physiol 1959;9:49.

115. Costa M, Furness JB. The peristaltic reflex: an analysis of nerve pathways and their pharmacology. Naunyn-Schmiedeberg's Arch Pharmacol 1976;294:47.

116. Bornstein JC, Costa M, Furness JB, Lang RJ. Electrophysiological analysis of projections of enteric inhibitory motor neurones in the guinea-pig small intestine. J Physiol (Lond) 1986;370:61.

117. Smith TK, Furness JB, Costa M, Bornstein JC. An electrophysiological study of the projections of motor neurones that mediate noncholinergic excitation in the circular muscle of the guinea-pig small intestine. J Auton Nerv Syst 1988;22:115.

118. Sanders KM, Publicover NG. Electrophysiology of the gastric musculature. In: Wood JD, ed. Handbook of physiology, section 6: the gastrointestinal system, vol I. Washington, DC: American Physiological Society, 1989;187.

119. Sanders KM, Smith TK. Electrophysiology of colonic smooth muscle. In: Wood JD, ed. Handbook of physiology, section 6: the gastrointestinal system, vol I. Washington, DC: American Physiological Society, 1989;251-271.

120. Kobayashi S, Furness JB, Smith TK, Pompolo S. Histological identification of the interstitial cells of Cajal in the guinea-pig small intestine. Arch Hist Cyt 1989;52:277.

121. Taxi J. Contribution a l'étude des connexions des neurones moteurs du système nerveux autonome. Ann Sci Nat Zool Biol Anim 1965;12: 413.

122. Botar J. The autonomic nervous system: an introduction to its physiological and pathological histology. Budapest: Akademiai Kiado, 1966.

123. Rogers DC, Burnstock G. The interstitial cell and its place in the concept of the autonomic ground plexus. J Comp Neurol 1966;126: 255.

124. Rumessen JJ, Thuneberg L, Mikkelsen HB. Plexus muscularis profundus and associated interstitial cells: II. Ultrastructural studies of mouse small intestine. Anat Rec 1982;203:129.

125. Faussone-Pellegrini M-S. Cytodifferentiation of the interstitial cells of Cajal related to the myenteric plexus of mouse intestinal muscle coat. Anat Embryol 1985;171:163.

126. Berezin I, Huizinga JD, Daniel EE. Interstitial cells of Cajal in the canine colon: a special communication network at the inner border of the circular muscle. J Comp Neurol 1988;273:42.

127. Komuro T. The interstitial cells in the colon of the rabbit. Cell Tissue Res 1982;222:41.

128. Faussone-Pellegrini M-S. Comparative study of interstitial cells of Cajal. Acta Anat 1987;130:109.

129. Suzuki N, Ladd Prosser C, Dahms V. Boundary cells between lon-

gitudinal and circular layers: essential for electrical slow waves in cat intestine. Am J Physiol 1986;250:G287.

130. Langton P, Ward SM, Carl A, et al. Spontaneous electrical activity of interstitial cells of Cajal isolated from canine proximal colon. Proc Natl Acad Sci USA 1989;86:7280-7284.

131. Pye-Smith PH, Brunton TL, West SH. Report of the committee appointed for the purpose of investigating the nature of intestinal secretion. In: British Association for the Advancement of Science (44th meeting). London: John Murray, 1874:54.

132. Lundgren O, Svanvik J, Jivegard L. Enteric nervous system: I. Physiology and pathophysiology of the intestinal tract. Dig Dis Sci 1989;34:264.

133. Sjövall H, Jodal M, Lundgren O. Further evidence for a glucose-activated secretory mechanism in the jejunum of the cat. Acta Physiol Scand 1984;120:437.

134. Bernard C. Leçons sur les liquides de l'organisme. Paris: Balliere, 1859.

135. Sjövall H, Jodal M, Redfors S, Lundgren O. The effect of carotid occlusion on the rate of net fluid absorption in the small intestine of rats and cats. Acta Physiol Scand 1982;115:447.

136. Sjövall H, Redfors S, Biber B, et al. Evidence for cardiac volume-receptor regulation of feline jejunal blood flow and fluid transport. Am J Physiol 1984;246:G401.

137. Sjövall H, Butcher P, Biber B, Martner J. Carotid sinus baroreceptor modulation of fluid transport and blood flow in the feline jejunum. Am J Physiol 1986;250:G736.

138. Redfors S, Hallbäck D-A, Sjövall H, et al. Affects of hemorrhage on intramural blood flow distribution, villous tissue osmolality and fluid and electrolyte transport in the cat small intestine. Acta Physiol Scand 1984;121:211.

139. Szurszewski JH, King BF. Physiology of prevertebral ganglia in mammals with special reference to inferior mesenteric ganglion. In: Wood JD, ed. Handbook of physiology, section 6: gastrointestinal system, vol I. Washington, DC: American Physiological Society, 1989:519.

140. Crowcroft PJ, Holman ME, Szurszewski JH. Excitatory input from the distal colon to the inferior mesenteric ganglion in the guinea pig. J Physiol (Lond) 1971;219:443.

141. Szurszewski JH, Weems WA. A study of peripheral input to and its control by postganglionic neurones of the inferior mesenteric ganglion. J Physiol (Lond) 1976;256:541.

142. Kreulen DL, Szurszewski JH. Reflex pathways in abdominal pre-vertebral ganglia: evidence for a colo-colonic inhibitory reflex. J Physiol (Lond) 1979;295:21.

143. Kuramoto H, Furness JB. Distribution of nerve cells that project from the small intestine to the coeliac ganglion in the guinea pig. J Auton Nerv Syst 1989;27:241.

144. Kuntz A, Buskirk Cvan. Reflex inhibition of bile flow and intestinal motility mediated through decentralized celiac plexus. Proc Soc Exp Biol 1941;46:519.

2

Gastrointestinal Hormones

IAN L. TAYLOR
PETER MANNON

History of Gut Endocrinology

The first hormone described was a gastrointestinal (GI) hormone, and this discovery, which was made in 1902, established endocrinology as a science.[1] Bayliss and Starling demonstrated that an extract made from canine duodenal mucosa stimulated the flow of pancreatic juice when infused intravenously into dogs. They also observed that perfusion of acid into the intestine stimulated pancreatic exocrine secretion even when all neural connections between the pancreas and intestine had been severed. They proposed that acid bathing the duodenal mucosa stimulated the release of a chemical messenger that was carried in the circulation to the pancreas. They called this substance "secretin" and invented the word "hormone" to describe a chemical messenger released into the circulation from one location to have effects on a distant target organ. The word "hormone" is derived from the Greek word meaning "to arouse to activity." Shortly thereafter, Edkins,[2] using an extraction technique similar to that described by Bayliss and Starling,[1] established that the antral mucosa contained a hormone (gastrin) that stimulated the stomach to secrete acid. The next gastrointestinal hormone was discovered in the small intestine over two decades later and was named cholecystokinin based on the fact that it caused contraction of the gallbladder.[3] The name "pancreozymin" was given to a hormone discovered in the mucosa of the jejunum that stimulated secretion of pancreatic enzymes.[4] The discovery of these and other blood-borne chemical messengers contradicted the prior dogma that held that all bodily functions were controlled by neural reflexes. It is only within the last decade that we have come to think of hormonal and neural control of gut function as a continuum so intimately interconnected as to be indivisible.

Major advances in peptide chemistry[3] during the middle of this century allowed elucidation of the structure of many of the gastrointestinal hormones that had been identified previously based on biologic activity.[5] Gastrin was the first peptide to be purified sufficiently[6] so that its amino acid sequence could be determined (Tables 2-1 and 2-2); the structures of secretin[7] and cholecystokinin[8] soon followed. Purification and analysis of the amino acid composition of pancreozymin and cholecystokinin revealed that they were one and the same hormone.[8] These structural studies established gastrointestinal hormones as peptides (i.e., compounds of relatively low molecular weight [MW] that, on hydrolysis, yielded two or more amino acids). Today, the term gastrointestinal *peptide* is often used instead of *hormone* if a definitive physiologic action has not been established.

Molecular Biology

The recent application of recombinant-DNA technology to the field of gastrointestinal endocrinology has allowed the determination of the structure of the DNA that encodes many of these peptides (Fig 2-1). Use of the genetic code to translate the DNA structure yields the amino acid structure of the peptide encoded. The molecular biology era was heralded by a number of apparently unconnected discoveries (for review, see reference 9). Important amongst these was the discovery of a number of enzyme families—restriction endonucleases, polymerases, and ligases. Polymerases allow the synthesis of complementary copies of DNA from RNA and DNA templates. Ligases cleave DNA at specific sites, leaving sticky ends that allow insertion (splicing) of foreign DNA into the spliced region. The discovery of a series of expression vectors now makes it possible to incorporate foreign DNA into heterologous cells that can translate and express the message encoded within it. Vectors, such as bacterial plasmids and viruses, with foreign DNA inserted in them can be introduced into bacterial hosts where they replicate their DNA at very high efficiency. Replication of these vectors within their bacterial host greatly amplifies the "recombinant DNA," allowing production of large amounts of both the DNA and the peptide it encodes.

TABLE 2–1
Amino Acid Sequences of Brain–Gut Peptides From Various Species

PEPTIDE	SPECIES	STRUCTURE
Cholecystokinin (58)	Human	VSQRTDGESRAHLGALLARYIQQARKAPSGRMSIVKNLQNLDPSHRISDRDYMGWMDF#
CCK 39		Y-------------------------------------#
CCK 33		K----------------------------#
CCK 22		Q------------------#
CCK 8		D-------#
CCK 5		G----#
Gastrin 34	Human	pQLGPQGPPHLVADPSKKQGPWLEEEEEAYGWMDF#
Gastrin 17		Q_____#
Gastrin 14		W-------------#
Secretin	Human	HSDGTFTSELSRLREGARLQRLLQGLL #
Glicentin	Pig	RSLQNTEEKSRSFPAPQTDPLDDPDQMTEDKRHSQGTFTSDYSKYLDSRRAQDFVQWLMNTKRNKNNIA
Glucagon		HSQGTFTSDYSKYLDSRRAQDFVQWLMNT#
VIP	Human	HSDAVFTDNYTRLRKQMAVKKYLNSILN #
PHI	Pig	HADGVFTSDFSRLLGQLSAKKYLESLI #
PHM	Human	KM #
GIP	Pig	YAEGTFISDYSIAMDKIRQQDFVNWLLAQKGKKSDWKHNITQ
Pancreatic	Human	APLEPVYPGDQATPEQMAQYAAELRRYINMLTRPRY #
polypeptide	Pig	YPAKPEAPGEDASPEELSRYYASLRHYLNLVTRQRY #
Peptide YY	Human	YPSKPDNPGEDAPAEDMARYYSALRHYINLITRQRY #
Neuropeptide Y		
Somatostatin 28	Human	SANSNPAMAPRERKAGCKNFFWKTFTSC
Somatostatin 14	Human	A-----------C
Motilin	Pig	FVPIFTYGELQRMQEKERNKGQ
Neurotensin	Human	PQLYENKPRRPYIL
Substance P	Pig	RPKPQQFFGLM#
Gastrin-releasing peptide (GRP 27)	Human	VPLPAGGGTVLTKMYPRGNHWAVGHLM #
Galanin	Pig	GWTLNSAGYLLGPHAIDNHRSFHDKYGLA #

pQ, pyroglutamyl; #, amide; y: tyrosine sulfate.
(Modified from Walsh JH. Gastrointestinal hormones. In: Johnson LR, ed. Physiology of the gastrointestinal tract. New York: Raven Press, 1989:183.)

TABLE 2–2
Single-Letter and Three-Letter Abbreviations
for Individual Amino Acids

AMINO ACID	ABBREVIATION	
	3-Letter	1-Letter
Alanine	Ala	A
Arginine	Arg	R
Asparagine	Asn	N
Aspartic acid	Asp	D
Asn or Asp	Asx	B
Cysteine	Cys	C
Glutamine	Gln	Q
Glutamic acid	Glu	E
Gln or Glu	Glx	Z
Pyroglutamyl	pGlu	pQ
Glycine	Gly	G
Histidine	His	H
Isoleucine	Ile	I
Leucine	Leu	L
Lysine	Lys	K
Methionine	Met	M
Phenylalanine	Phe	F
Proline	Pro	P
Serine	Ser	S
Threonine	Thr	T
Tryptophan	Trp	W
Tyrosine	Tyr	Y
Valine	Val	V

In the first application of this technology to the gastrointestinal field, analysis of the structure of the DNA encoding the antral hormone gastrin[10,11] confirmed the amino acid sequence of gastrin. These studies also revealed that gastrin was synthesized within a large precursor molecule from which the biologically active peptide was liberated by enzymatic activity within the G cell. The structure of many of the genes for brain–gut peptides has now been determined by use of similar methods.[9–11] In brief, single-stranded DNA complementary to a purified messenger RNA (mRNA) for a particular peptide can be cloned by use of an enzyme called reverse transcriptase. This can then be converted to double-stranded DNA by use of another enzyme, DNA polymerase. Once the complementary DNA (cDNA) copy has been synthesized, it can be inserted into the circular DNA of a plasmid. This involves cleaving the DNA with ligases and allowing the "sticky ends" of the plasmid DNA and the DNA insert to couple. The foreign DNA, once inserted into the plasmid, can be expressed and the synthetic product isolated in large amounts and in a much purer form relative to that obtained from crude tissue extracts.

The ability to clone genomic DNA necessitated the insertion of much longer DNA sequences into expression vectors. Derivatives of bacteriophage lambda were found to accommodate DNA fragments from 10 to 20 kilobase pairs. The construction of cosmids (hybrids of bacteria phages and plasmids) permitted insertion of DNA up to 40 to 50 kilobase pairs in length, which allowed the huge amount of genetic information encoded in genomic DNA to be stored in "libraries" from which information about a single peptide could be retrieved readily.[9]

Another technologic advance arose out of the use of synthetic fragments of DNA and RNA "hybridization probes" to bind and identify complementary RNA or DNA by use of the techniques[9] of Northern transfer (RNA) and Southern transfer (DNA). In these two techniques, either cellular RNA or a restriction endonuclease digest of genomic DNA is separated by agarose gel electrophoresis, and the polynucleotide fragments are transferred to nitrocellulose filters. The fragments can be identified by hybridization with ^{32}P-labeled cDNA or RNA probes. The development of automated instruments for the production of synthetic oligonucleotides allows construction of large probes, 80 to 100 bases in length, which can be used to identify recombinant and genomic DNA. They can be used to probe tissues at the microscopic level with enhanced specificity to determine which particular cell types are expressing a specific messenger RNA. These techniques have become so sensitive that gene mapping is possible, allowing identification of the actual arms of a chromosome upon which a particular gene is localized by hybridization of mitotic chromosome preparations with a tritium-labeled probe.

The ability to synthesize fragments of DNA and RNA as hybridization probes has led to the development of assay techniques that allow quantitation of messenger RNA levels in tissue extracts.[9] Cellular RNA can be isolated and separated by agarose gel electrophoresis, and polynucleotide species can be transferred to nitrocellulose filters. Extraction techniques for mRNA have been developed based on the presence of a "polyadenylated" tail, which is a structural characteristic of mRNA. Specific mRNA subtypes can be identified on nitrocellulose filters by hybridization with ^{32}P-labeled cDNA probes, and the amount of radioactivity hybridized to the filter gives a measure of the tissue content of the specific mRNA in question.

The information currently available about the structure, organization, and expression of genes is too great to summarize in a chapter such as this. However, it is worth commenting on some of these developments. For example, it is now known that the coding regions (called exons) of most genes are separated by intervening DNA sequences called introns (Fig 2-2). The initial RNA product of transcription from the DNA template has to be cleaved and the regions corresponding to the original exons reassembled to give the specific messenger RNA. Alternate splicing of the original RNA transcript is a mechanism by which cells can produce multiple products from a single gene. Alternate splicing relates to the process by which introns and exons are cleaved and separated during gene transcription. Different products can arise as a result of complete or incomplete inclusion or exclusion of specific exons and introns, resulting in novel codon reading frames. Tissue-specific alternate splicing explains the generation, from the same gene, of calcitonin in C cells of the thyroid and calcitonin-related gene product (CGRP) in nerve cells.

Regulatory sequences upstream from the coding region of the gene determine such factors as the cell specificity of expression of a gene and the rate at which the gene is transcribed within the cell.[9] Much of our understanding of the regulatory regions of the gene comes from "deletion experiments" in which segments of synthetically constructed genes are removed and the product expressed in an expression vector. Certain areas of the regulatory regions of the gene have been delineated to have universal sig-

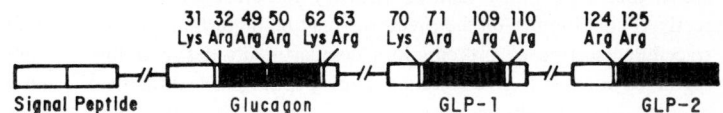

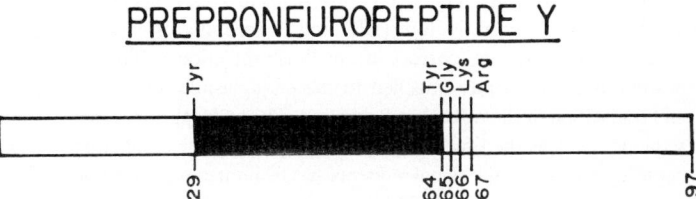

FIGURE 2–1. Schematic representation of preproglucagon and preproneuropeptide Y based on the cDNA structures. The signal sequence is denoted by cross-hatching at the amino-terminus, and potentially bioactive peptides generated by cleavage of the preprohormone are indicated by solid boxes. Potential cleavage sites marked by two basic amino acids in sequence are indicated. Glicentin and oxyntomodulin, which contain pancreatic glucagon with their sequence, are also shown.

nificance in terms of gene expression. One such sequence is the "TATA box," which can be found 25 to 30 nucleotides upstream from the site of initiation of transcription. The TATA box acts as a signal indicating the position downstream on the gene at which transcription should be initiated. Upstream from the TATA box is the tissue-specific enhancer, which is important for tissue-specific gene expression. Further upstream are regions of the gene that allow control of gene transcription in response to stimulation of the cell by external signals, such as steroids, peptide hormones, and neurotransmitters. While steroid hormones bind to intracellular receptors to form a complex that then interacts with these regulatory regions directly, peptide hormones and neurotransmitters need to first activate intracellular second message systems (see subsequent section).

In summary, a gene encoding a polypeptide hormone has two functionally distinct but interrelated units. The first is the transcriptional region, which is the segment of the gene that contains the sequence of the polypeptide hormone within its exons. The second functional unit, which lies upstream from the transcriptional region, contains the promoter or regulatory region that controls the site and rate at which messenger RNA is transcribed.

Synthesis of Gastrointestinal Peptides

Translation of the mRNA that is transcribed from a gene encoding a GI peptide (Fig 2-2) results in the synthesis of a large precursor

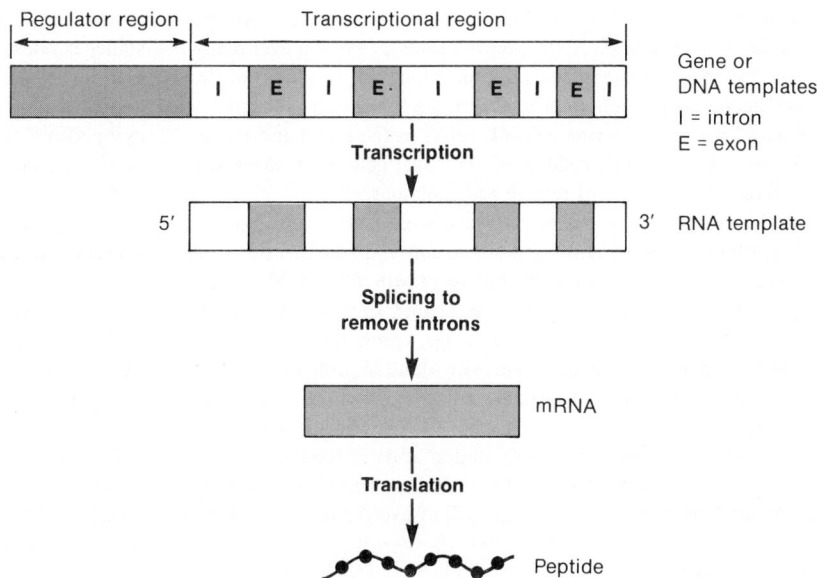

FIGURE 2–2. Schematic representation of the transcription and translation of a gene encoding a hypothetic gastrointestinal peptide.

molecule. There are multiple reasons for synthesizing large pre-cursor molecules rather than the primary hormonal product directly. The structure of the precursor may be important for intracellular sorting of proteins into compartments destined for regulated or constituitive secretion. Some peptides have difficulty crossing lipid membranes because they are not lipophilic; this property gives rise to a unique set of problems that must be overcome during transport of the peptide through the cell. Synthesis of secretory proteins[12] starts with the formation of a hydrophobic "leader" or "signal sequence." When the first few amino acid residues of the newly synthesized peptide chain appear from the ribosome, a signal recognition particle (SRP) attaches itself to this sequence and temporarily interrupts translation of the messenger RNA (mRNA). The SRP in turn binds to a docking protein on the endoplasmic reticulum (ER) and in so doing directs the nascent peptide to the correct intracellular membrane. The ribosome becomes firmly attached to the endoplasmic reticulum, and translation of the mRNA is reinitiated. The hydrophobic signal sequence crosses the lipid bilayer, dragging with it the elongating peptide chain. Once the signal sequence has facilitated translocation of the peptide across the lipid bilayer, it is clipped from the secretory peptide by enzymes on the inner surface of the endoplasmic reticulum. The newly formed peptide chain continues to traverse the membrane and, after synthesis is complete, becomes trapped within the lumen of the ER-Golgi apparatus.

Although most precursor molecules contain one copy of the peptide of interest, others contain multiple copies of the same molecule,[13] and some even encode for more than one peptide.[14,15] Precursor molecules usually undergo a wide variety of post-translational modifications during passage through the cell by the sequential action of a number of enzymes.[16] The molecule may be cleaved at specific sites, amino acid residues may be derived (e.g., sulfated or phosphorylated), cross-linking reactions may occur (e.g., development of disulfide bonds), and the peptide may undergo glycosylation.

Post-translational processing and modification of preprohor-mones offers another site at which hormone synthesis can be controlled and another means of generating different gene products, thereby leading to diversity of hormone expression. Different hormonal products of the same gene can be generated as a result of tissue-specific post-translational processing of the same precursor molecule. For example,[15] the preprohormone that will eventually give rise to pancreatic glucagon in the alpha cell (Fig 2-1) of the pancreatic islet is identical to that from which gut glucagon is derived within endocrine cells (L cells) in the ileum and colon. These two different products of the same gene have markedly different mechanisms of release and functions.

During passage of the newly synthesized peptide through the cell, folding and even subunit formation and dimerization can occur, as is the case with insulinlike growth factors. However, most GI peptides are single peptide chains, and when the signal peptide is removed by enzymatic cleavage, a prohormone is formed. The hormone proper is often buried within the prohormone (Fig 2-1), flanked by carboxyl-terminal and amino-terminal extensions, and is generated from the prohormone by a series of trypticlike cleavages. Frequently, two basic amino acids in sequence in the prohormone indicate the site of action of an endopeptidase (Fig 2-1 and Tables 2-1 and 2-2) that will cleave the precursor molecule.

An amino acid modification that is vital for biologic activity for many brain–gut peptides is amidation of the carboxyl-terminal amino acid residue.[17] The carboxyl-terminal flanking sequence in such a prohormone is joined to the hormone by a cleavage and amidation site.[17] This site typically consists of the carboxyl-terminal amino acid residue of the hormone to be, followed by a glycine residue and then two basic amino acids (Fig 2-1). During processing of this precursor molecule, a dibasic endopeptidase cleaves the molecule between the two basic amino acid residues, and a carboxypeptidase removes the remaining basic residue. At that stage, an amidating enzyme transforms the alpha amino group on the glycine residue into the amide group on the carboxyl-terminal amino acid residue of the hormone in question.

Tatemoto and Mutt[18] recently described a novel biochemical assay capable of identifying peptides that have an amidated carboxyl terminus. Because an amidated carboxyl terminus is a structural modification frequently found in brain–gut peptides that exhibit biologic activity, this technique has allowed the chemical identification of peptides that are most likely to have physiologic significance. This approach represents a reversal of the classical approach to peptide isolation, which required prior identification of a biologic action and then the laborious chemical purification of the peptide responsible.[3] To reflect their origins, peptides identified with this new assay were given chemical names[18] rather than the traditional names that described established biologic actions. Examples (Table 2-1) include "peptide with amino-terminal histidine and carboxyl-terminal isoleucine" (PHI) and "peptide with amino and carboxyl-terminal tyrosines" (PYY). The letters after the "P" for peptide are an international letter code (Table 2-2) for specific amino acids in the peptide chain (e.g., Y for tyrosine, H for histidine, and I for isoleucine).

Anatomy of the Gut–Endocrine System

Gastrointestinal peptides act in at least four distinct ways[16,19]— as endocrine, paracrine, neurocrine, and autocrine substances (Fig 2-3). An endocrine substance acts in the fashion of a classical hormone (i.e., a chemical substance released into the blood to be carried to a distant organ to exert its effects).[1] A paracrine substance is released locally to exert effects on cells in the immediate vicinity of the peptide's cell of origin.[19] A prototypic paracrine cell would be a subtype of the somatostatin cell, which has long, cytoplasmic processes that reach out from the base of the cell of origin to contact neighboring cells. A neurocrine substance is released from nerve endings and acts in the manner of a classical neurotransmitter or neuromodulator. Autocrine peptides are released by the same cell upon which they exert their biologic effects. For example, some small-cell carcinomas of the lung have been shown to synthesize and release gastrin-releasing polypeptide (GRP), which acts as an autocrine growth factor.[20] Paracrine, neurocrine, and autocrine mechanisms of action (Table 2-3) ensure that peptides are released in high concentrations locally without being diluted in a large intravascular space. This is efficient for conservation of peptide and is also a means by which very high concentrations of potent transmitter substances can be achieved locally without producing generalized systemic effects. There are many variations on these four standard themes. Thus, peptides

MECHANISMS OF ACTION OF GI PEPTIDES

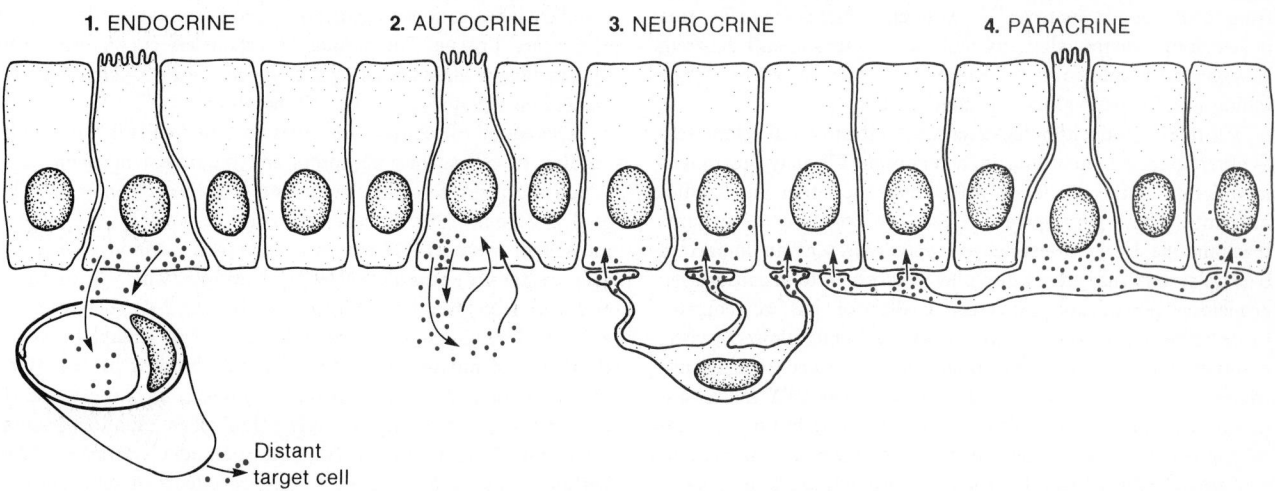

FIGURE 2–3. Modes of action of regulatory peptides illustrating endocrine, paracrine, neurocrine, and autocrine mechanisms.

released into the circulation as hormones can act as neuromodulators.[21] In turn, neuropeptides can be released from nerves directly into the bloodstream; this is the case with hypothalamic-releasing hormones, which are secreted into a local portal system to be carried to target cells in the anterior pituitary.[22]

Classical hormones, as opposed to paracrine substances, have distinct regional distributions within the gut. As a general rule, hormones that are released early in response to a meal are found high in the gastrointestinal tract. For example, gastrin, which is released rapidly after ingestion of a meal to stimulate acid secretion

while food is still in the stomach, is found in "G cells" in the gastric antrum and duodenum. The duodenum and upper jejunum are rich sources of many peptides, including secretin, cholecystokinin (CCK), and glucose-dependent insulinotropic peptide (GIP) all of which are released early after ingestion of a meal.[16] By contrast, although somatostatin is a hormone, it also acts as a neurotransmitter and as a paracrine substance; it is distributed in all regions of the gut and pancreas. This widespread distribution is more typical of paracrine substances. Insulin and glucagon are important regulators of glucose homeostasis and are found within

TABLE 2–3

Peptides Extracted From the Gastrointestinal Tract Together With Their Likely Role as Endocrine, Neurocrine, or Paracrine Substances

ENDOCRINE	NEUROCRINE	PARACRINE
Somatostatin†	Somatostatin†	Somatostatin†
Cholecystokinin (CCK)*†	Cholecystokinin (CCK)	Peptide YY†
Gastrin*		
Secretin*	Gastrin-releasing peptide (GRP)	
Insulin*	Opioids	
Glucagon*	Substance P	
Enteroglucagon	Vasoactive intestinal polypeptide	
Pancreatic polypeptide*	Neuropeptide Y (NPY)	
Neurotensin†	Neurotensin†	
Motilin*	Peptide HM (PHM and PHI)	
Glucose-dependent insulinotropic peptide (GIP)*	Pancreastatin	
	Galanin	
Peptide YY (PYY)	Motilin	
Urogastrone/epidermal growth factor	Peptide YY	

* Classical hormones with physiologic function.
† Some peptides may serve multiple functions.

the pancreatic islets. The release of these peptides is modulated by both circulating nutrients and gastrointestinal hormones released from the upper gut, such as GIP. Although pancreatic polypeptide is also found in the islets, its biologic function is still debated; however, a metabolic role for this peptide has been proposed (i.e., inhibition of hepatic glucose production).[21]

Peptides found within the distal small intestine and colon, such as enteroglucagon, neurotensin, and peptide YY, may function as modulators of the efficiency with which the upper gut handles nutrients. These peptides are released in response to nutrients reaching the lower intestine and may represent an important backup system that comes into play in response to malabsorption or maldigestion of food. The term "ileal brake" has been coined[23] to describe a constellation of events, including slowed gastric emptying and prolonged intestinal transit that occurs when nutrients bathe the ileal mucosa. Peptides such as PYY inhibit gut motility, enhancing the efficiency of nutrient digestion and absorption of digestive products by increasing nutrient–mucosa contact time.[24] Other peptides such as enteroglucagon may exert trophic effects on the small intestine,[16] which would serve to increase the absorptive surface of the small intestine in the face of malabsorption.

Although all neuropeptides do not have the same regional distribution, peptide-containing nerves do have distinct patterns of distribution and relationships with one another within the enteric nervous system.[25] It is likely that neuropeptides function as neuromodulators and neurotransmitters within the myenteric and submucous plexuses of the gut. Some peptides, such as substance P, may serve important functions in the transmission of the sensation of pain by sensory neurons. Although the enteric nervous system functions independently, it is greatly influenced by the autonomic nervous system. Parasympathetic preganglionic fibers enter the gut by way of the vagus and pelvic nerves, while sympathetic nerve fibers that innervate the gut arise within sympathetic ganglia. Many gut peptides have been colocalized with conventional neurotransmitters within nerves of the autonomic nervous system that innervate the gut. For example, neuropeptide Y (NPY) is colocalized with noradrenaline in a subpopulation of sympathetic nerve fibers that innervate the wall of blood vessels that supply the intestine. In contrast, other intrinsic gut nerves synthesize NPY apparently as a sole product.[21] It remains an interesting feature of the enteric nervous system that multiple peptides may be colocalized to the same nerve fiber.[25] There is evidence that different degrees of stimulation may preferentially release one or another neurotransmitter. Thus, electrical signals that vary in intensity or frequency may result in different patterns of release of neurotransmitters from nerve endings, resulting in quite different events being set into motion.[26]

Mechanisms of Release and Action of Gastrointestinal Peptides

Gastrointestinal peptides are stored in secretory granules within the cell and are extruded from their cell of origin by the process of exocytosis.[16] Exocytosis involves the fusion of the membrane lining the granule with the cell membrane and the release of the contents of the granule into the extracellular space. The peptide enters the intravascular space through fenestrations in the local capillaries. The peptide is carried in the circulation to the target organ and leaves the bloodstream by diffusion through similar capillary fenestrations to distribute itself in the extracellular space of the target tissue. The hormone exerts its effects on target cells by attaching to and interacting with specific, high-affinity receptors located on the surface of the cell membrane.

The action of peptide hormones on target cells is initiated by binding to cell-surface receptors and requires a mechanism by which the message can be transmitted to the cell interior. This goal is accomplished by the activation of a variety of second-messenger systems.[16] Some gastrointestinal hormones (e.g., the secretin family) stimulate adenylate cyclase, which leads to increased intracellular levels of cyclic AMP (Fig 2-4). The receptors are linked within the membrane[27] to the enzyme adenylate cyclase through a stimulatory guanine nucleotide–binding protein (Gs). Other receptors (e.g., neuropeptide Y) inhibit cAMP generations by interacting with adenylate cyclase through an inhibitory guanine nucleotide–binding protein (G_I). As such, levels of cyclic AMP within the cell represent the summated effects of multiple hormones acting on stimulatory and inhibitory receptors. Once activated, adenylate cyclase converts ATP to cyclic AMP, which, in turn, binds to the regulatory subunit of cyclic AMP–dependent protein kinase. When all four binding sites of the regulatory unit are occupied by cyclic AMP molecules, the catalytic subunit of the kinase is released in a bioactive form to phosphorylate target proteins that mediate a wide variety of biologic effects, including secretory events. Other hormone–receptor interactions activate changes in phospholipid metabolism within the cell membrane (Fig 2-5). Through another guanine nucleotide–binding (G) protein, hormones of this type[28] activate the membrane-bound enzyme phospholipase C, which converts phosphatidyl inositol bisphosphate to diacylglycerol and inositol trisphosphate (IP_3). Diacylglycerol activates protein kinase C, which phosphorylates specific protein substrates that then mediate the hormone's effects.[29] IP_3 releases ionized calcium from stores within the cell interior elevating the concentration of intracellular calcium, and this leads to the activation of calcium–calmodulin-dependent protein kinases.[29] The substrates for the phosphorylation reactions catalyzed by these two different kinases are diverse and include receptors, G proteins, cyclic AMP phosphodiesterases, phosphatases, ion channels, and so forth. The presence of multiple signal transduction mechanisms and diverse targets for phosphorylation allows for a complex interplay between second-messenger systems within the cell interior, leading to additive, potentiated, or inhibited responses.[30]

It is important to note that signals do not always have to be transmitted to the cell interior to alter cell function, particularly in the case of nerves.[31] Some receptors function as ion channels that open when agonists bind to them. Other receptors are linked directly to ion channels within the membrane by G proteins. The opening or closing of these channels alters the intracellular environment or the electrical potential of the cell membrane by modulating the passage across the cell membrane of ions such as calcium or potassium. Although most receptors remain on the surface of the cell after peptide agonists bind to them, some receptor–peptide complexes are internalized.[32] Although the exact purpose of receptor internalization is debated, it probably serves multiple functions, including the provision of a mechanism for degradation of the ligand and/or receptor. Internalization may also generate novel intracellular messengers that modulate cell

Cyclic AMP Pathway

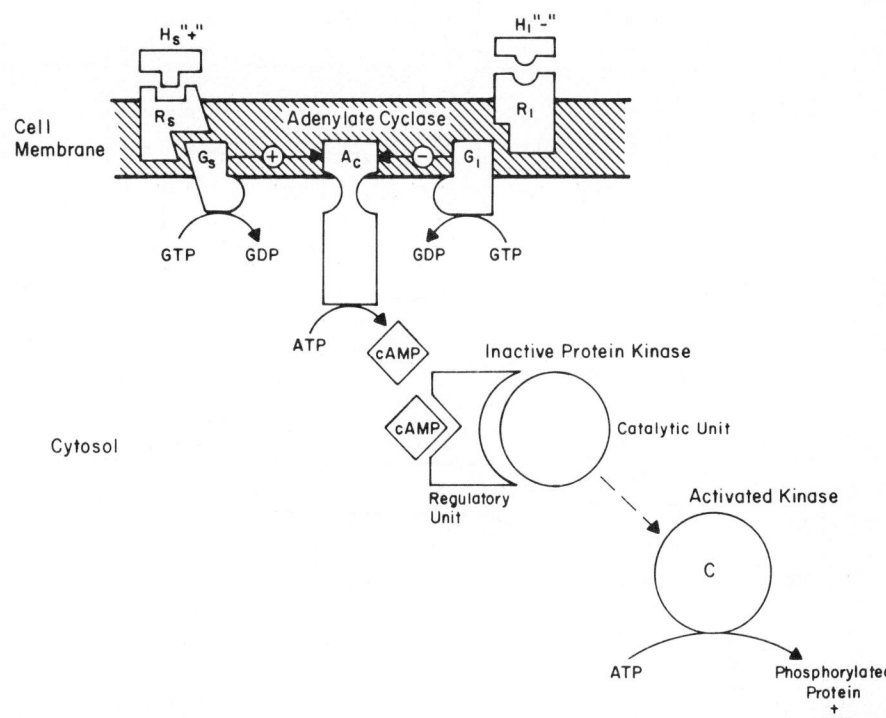

FIGURE 2-4. Intracellular second message systems: receptors mediating modulation of cyclic AMP levels.

functions. Examples of receptors that are internalized include those for insulin and epidermal growth factor (EGF). Both receptors exhibit tyrosine kinase activity, which is essential for receptor–ligand internalization and is a characteristic of many hormones that function as growth factors.[33]

Measurement of Gastrointestinal Peptides

As a result of the advances made in peptide chemistry,[5,6] brain–gut peptides became available in a highly purified state. This essential prerequisite permitted Yalow and Berson[34] to develop the concept of radioimmunoassay using insulin antibodies, radiolabeled insulin, and standard amounts of unlabeled insulin in a competitive binding assay. A standard curve could be generated by inhibiting the binding of radioactive insulin to the antiserum by the addition of increasing amounts of pure hormone. The addition of serum or a tissue extract that contained an unknown quantity of peptide also displaced the label from the antiserum. The amount of peptide in the unknown sample could be quantitated by comparing the resultant displacement of label with that caused by the addition of standard amounts of pure peptide. This new assay system proved capable of quantifying the minute amounts (10^{-12}M) of gastrointestinal peptides present in biologic fluids such as blood.

Although the theory of radioimmunoassay is easy to understand, its practice is made difficult by a number of potential pitfalls.[35] First, gastrointestinal hormones usually circulate in concentrations that are 1000-fold lower than those of conventional endocrine hormones such as insulin. Accordingly, antisera used to measure GI peptides must be of unusually high affinity. Second, gastrointestinal peptides are frequently unstable and subject to degradation by enzymes in tissues and in blood. Enzymatic degradation can be minimized by keeping blood at 4° C until it is centrifuged and the resultant plasma or serum stored at −70°C until assay. Alternatively, lyophilization of tissue extracts or serum may allow preservation of the peptides without the need for such stringent storage conditions. Other maneuvers that have proved helpful in decreasing degradation include the addition of protease inhibitors such as aprotinin. A third problem relates to specific and nonspecific interference in the assay due to inhibition of the binding of labeled peptide to antibody by substances other than the peptide being measured. Specific interference can occur when other peptides with a structural similarity to the hormone of interest interfere with accurate determination of the hormonal content of tissue and blood samples. As an example, the initial report of large amounts of gastrin in brain extracts was subsequently shown to reflect cross-reactivity of CCK in the gastrin radioimmunoassay.[36] Other nonspecific problems can arise when certain substances interfere with the separation of free label from that bound to the antibody. For example, the efficiency with which ion-exchange resins remove unbounded gastrin label is markedly inhibited by the use of the polyanion anticoagulant heparin.

Questions can arise as to how values obtained with a radioimmunoassay correlate with the biologic activity of a given peptide. For example, the measurement of a peptide with antisera generated against a region of the molecule that is not essential for biologic activity may not lead to information relevant to the physiologic function of the peptide as an endocrine hormone.[35] The significance

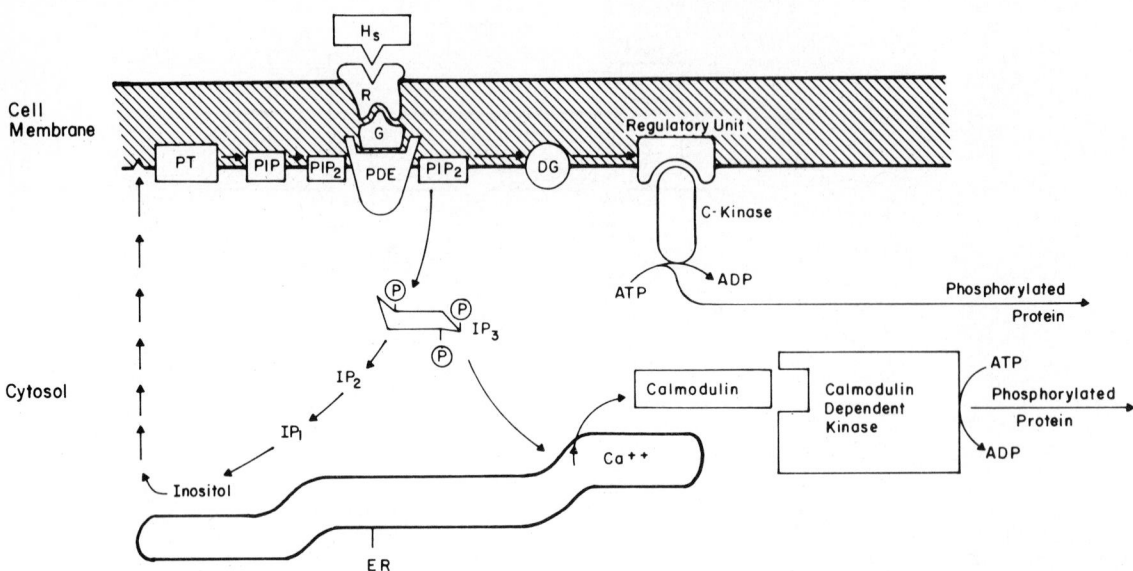

FIGURE 2–5. Intracellular second message systems: receptors mediating modulation of diacylglycerol (DG) and inositol trisphosphate (IP₃).

of this problem is well illustrated by cholecystokinin or gastrin, both of which require an intact carboxyl terminus for biologic activity. The carboxyl-terminal region of CCK is structurally similar to that of gastrin. Thus, cholecystokinin antisera directed against the carboxyl terminus may measure both CCK and gastrin.[36] Although amino-terminal cholecystokinin antisera do not cross-react with gastrin, they may measure biologically inactive amino-terminal fragments of CCK and, as such, will not accurately reflect biologic activity. This particular problem has been overcome by the use of a novel "in vitro" bioassay that makes use of the selective responsiveness of isolated pancreatic acini to CCK.[37] CCK is extracted and concentrated from plasma, then added to isolated acini to stimulate amylase release. The CCK content of the sample is determined by comparison of the amylase released by unknown samples with that obtained following addition of standard amounts of CCK. This assay system is both accurate and sensitive and gives a true measure of CCK bioactivity.

Irrespective of whether a bioassay or a radioimmunoassay is employed to quantitate levels of a gastrointestinal peptide, each system must be validated in terms of specificity, accuracy, and precision. Specificity can be evaluated by determining if structurally related and unrelated peptides will inhibit binding of labeled peptide to the antiserum. Accuracy is best quantitated by measuring recovery of known amounts of peptide added to a sample containing an unknown quantity of peptide. Precision is documented by demonstrated good agreement between multiple estimates of the sample in a single assay (intra-assay precision) or in multiple assays (inter-assay precision).

Methods have also been developed for tagging an antiserum raised against a particular GI peptide with a fluorescent label.[38] The tagged antiserum can then be used as a probe in immunohistochemical studies to localize and identify the cell of origin of that particular GI peptide (Fig 2-6). The application of this technique provided information to indicate that the same chemical messenger, or a close immunologic homologue, often could be found in both the brain and gastrointestinal tract. Thus, gut peptides have been identified in the intestine by use of antisera initially raised against a brain peptide, and neuropeptides have been identified by use of antisera raised against gut peptides (Table 2-3). The suffix "-like-immunoreactivity" was introduced to describe substances that were initially identified by use of immunochemical methods but whose structure had not been confirmed by chemical analysis (e.g., "gastrinlike immunoreactivity" in the brain). Peptides that were initially described in the gut by use of immunochemical means include somatostatin, substance P, neurotensin, enkephalin, and thyrotropin-releasing hormone (TRH).

GASTROINTESTINAL PEPTIDES

Many gastrointestinal peptides can be grouped as members of a family of structurally related peptides.[5,16,21] These families appear to have arisen by tandem gene duplication followed by a mutation of the progenitor gene, by alternative splicing of RNA, or by tissue-specific processing of a common preprohormone. The following discussion of the properties of individual peptides will begin with peptide families and then include peptides that are not, as of yet, identified as members of a distinct family.

The Gastrin–CCK Family

GASTRIN

Structure and Biosynthesis. Gastrin was the first gastrointestinal hormone to be isolated in sufficient purity and quantity to allow determination of its peptide sequence by classical

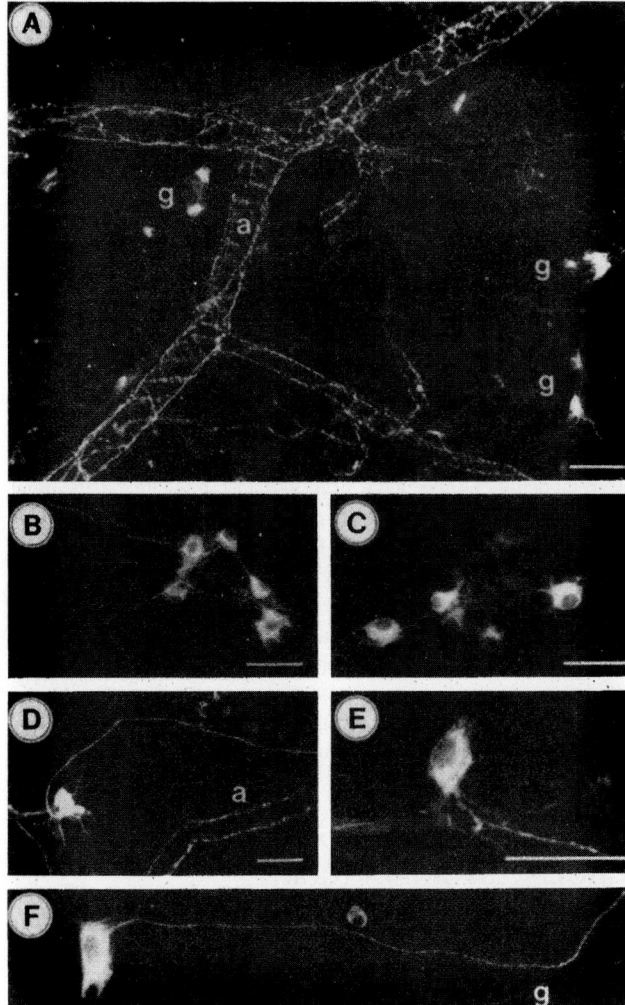

FIGURE 2-6. Nerve cell bodies with PP-like and NPY-like immunoreactivity in blood vessels and ganglia of submucous plexus of guinea pig ileum. **A,D,** NPY antiserum; **B,C,E,** antiavian PP; **F,** antirat PP. (Furness et al. Cell Tissue Res 1984;237:329.)

a minor form in the gastric antrum, it is the most abundant form in human duodenal mucosa.[16] A smaller biologically active carboxyl-terminal fragment, G_{14} or minigastrin, has also been identified in antral mucosa, gastrin-producing tumors, and plasma. The smallest biologically active fragment of gastrin to be identified in the antrum is the carboxyl-terminal hexapeptide (G_6). Larger forms of gastrin (component I and big big gastrin) have also been described. They may reflect intermediates generated during processing of the large precursor form. Biologically inactive amino-terminal fragments of gastrin[39] also have been identified, as have other apparently inactive forms generated by incomplete processing of the preprohormone. These include forms of G_{17} and G_{34} with a glycine extension at the carboxyl terminus.[40] Despite the discovery of a large number of molecular forms within tissues, G_{34} and G_{17} remain the predominant forms released into the circulation.[41]

As mentioned, structure–function studies have established that biologic activity resides within the carboxyl terminus.[16] Indeed, the carboxyl-terminal tetrapeptide amide of gastrin (G_4) mimics the full biologic activity of G_{17} and G_{34}, even though it is far less potent than the larger forms. Deamidation of the carboxyl-terminal phenylalanine residue results in substantial loss of biologic activity. Comparison of the biologic activity of different molecular forms of gastrin in vivo requires a consideration of both their intrinsic activity and the rate at which they are cleared from the circulation.[6] G_{17} and G_{14} have similar clearance rates and are approximately equipotent stimulants of acid secretion. In contrast, G_{34} has a disappearance half-life that is four to six times longer than that for G_{17}, which means that its apparent potency varies depending upon the method of administration of the peptide.[42] If the same molar doses of G_{34} and G_{17} are injected as bolus injections, G_{34} will appear more potent because it persists within the circulation about five times longer than G_{17}. However, when G_{17} and G_{34} are infused to achieve similar steady-state molar concentrations within the circulation, the two forms are equipotent.

Distribution, Release, and Metabolism. Gastrin has been localized to specific endocrine-type cells called G cells (Table 2-4) that lie midway between the neck and the base of the antral glands.[43] Lesser numbers of G cells occur in the small intestine, with the greatest concentration occurring in the duodenal mucosa. Although gastrin is not found in the adult pancreas, it can be found in the fetal pancreas where it has been proposed to play a role in islet cell growth.[44] Small quantities of true gastrin have also been found in the brain, particularly in the pituitary.[16]

The classical stimulant of gastrin release is an ingested meal,[16,46] and specific nutrients within the meal, such as amino acids, small peptides, and calcium ions, stimulate the release of gastrin by direct interaction with the G cell.[45] In contrast, other constituents of the meal, such as glucose and fat, do not stimulate gastrin release. When a large number of individual amino acids were tested,[46] the aromatic amino acids such as phenylalanine and tryptophan were found to be the most potent stimulants of gastrin release. Coffee is a potent stimulant of gastrin release, an effect that persists even after coffee is decaffeinated.[47] Although wine stimulates gastrin release, pure alcohol does not.[48] It is likely that small peptides and amino acids found within coffee and wine are the actual stimulants of gastrin release.

Some hormones and neurotransmitters, such as gastrin-releasing polypeptide (GRP), stimulate the release of gastrin,[16,49] while others, such as somatostatin, inhibit release.[50] GRP, which is the

chemical means.[6] Gastrin was also among the first gut peptides to have the structure of their genes determined.[10,11] The gene that encodes human gastrin was found to be about 4100 base pairs long, and the messenger RNA that is transcribed encodes a pre-prohormone of 101 amino acids. Preprogastrin consists of a "leader or signal" sequence of 21 amino acids, a 37-amino-acid intervening peptide, "big gastrin" (G_{34}), and a 6-amino-acid carboxyl-terminal extension. Big gastrin lies in position 59–92 within the preprohormone, and the carboxyl-terminal extension of 6 amino acids is joined to the carboxyl-terminal phenylalanine residue of G_{17} through three linking amino acid residues that form a prototypic cleavage and amidation sequence.[17] Sequential action of three enzymes results in an amidated phenylalanine residue at the carboxyl terminus, a structural modification that is essential for biologic activity.[6] Big gastrin contains within its carboxyl terminus (Table 2-1) the structure of little gastrin (G_{17}).

G_{17} (also called little gastrin or hexadecapeptide gastrin) is the most abundant form of gastrin in the human antrum. It is generated from the preprohormone within the G cell and is not "liberated" from G_{34} as a postsecretory event. Although G_{34} (big gastrin) is

TABLE 2–4
Gastrin Family—Cell of Origin and Likely Function

PEPTIDE	CELL OF ORIGIN	BIOLOGIC ACTION
Gastrin	"G" cell in antral and duodenal mucosa	1. Stimulates the stomach to secrete acid 2. Trophic to the gastric mucosa
Cholecystokinin	"I" or "CCK" cell in duodenal and jejunal mucosa	1. Stimulates secretion of pancreatic enzymes and contraction of the gallbladder 2. Trophic to the pancreas

mammalian equivalent of the amphibian peptide "bombesin," is the most potent stimulant of gastrin release identified in man.[49] GRP nerves may play a physiologic role in the release of gastrin and a pathophysiologic role in diseases such as G-cell hyperfunction.[51] Adrenergic mechanisms modulate gastrin release, although their role remains somewhat ill-defined.[16]

The role of the vagus and parasympathetic nervous system in gastrin release is complex. There appear to be tonic inhibitory fibers within the vagus, removal of which contributes to the hypergastrinemia seen after truncal vagotomy.[16] In keeping with this hypothesis, low doses of atropine enhance gastrin release in response to food.[52] Delineating the role of the vagus in gastrin release is made difficult because vagotomy also inhibits acid secretion,[53] which by itself has a major influence on gastrin release.[16] This relationship between acid secretion and gastrin release forms the basis for a negative feedback loop (i.e., gastrin stimulates acid secretion, which in turn inhibits gastrin release). Immediately after ingestion of a solid meal, free hydrogen ions within the stomach are buffered, removing a brake to gastrin release. When the buffering capacity of the food is overwhelmed or food leaves the stomach, the concentration of free hydrogen ions within the gastric lumen increases and gastrin release is inhibited. Somatostatin may act as a paracrine intermediary in this process by direct inhibition of G cells. Prolonged neutralization or inhibition of acid secretion in the stomach (as in atrophic gastritis) results in basal hypergastrinemia and a markedly enhanced gastrin response to food.[16]

The majority of gastrin released into the circulation after a meal is secreted by the gastric antrum as little gastrin.[41] As mentioned above, big gastrin forms a disproportionately large percentage of circulating gastrin relative to the amount released because of its slow rate of metabolism. After antrectomy, big gastrin is the predominant form released, an observation that is explained by the fact that it is the primary form in the residual duodenal mucosa.

The half-life of G_{17} in the circulation of man is approximately 7 minutes and that of G_{34} about 30 minutes.[54] G_{34} and G_{17} are fully metabolized in the circulation without interconversion. Although all vascular beds[55] play a role in the metabolism of gastrin, removing 20% to 25% of gastrin during one circulatory passage, the kidney may play a more important role in the metabolism of G_{34} as compared to G_{17}.[45] Two enzymes have been identified; one cleaves the amino terminus of hydrophobic residues,[56] while the other cleaves the carboxyl terminal dipeptide amide (asp-phe-

amide) from gastrin, thereby inactivating it.[57] Despite these observations, the role of these enzymes in gastrin metabolism remains to be delineated.

Biologic Actions. Gastrin exhibits a wide spectrum of biologic actions.[58] Although many of these effects are pharmacologic, gastrin is a potent physiologic stimulant of gastric acid secretion (Table 2-4).[58] Gastrin also exerts growth-promoting effects on the fundic mucosa, and the hypertrophic gastric folds that are seen in gastrinoma patients are a clinical reflection of this action.[59]

Gastrin interacts with other acid secretagogues (i.e., histamine and acetylcholine) such that removal of one of this trio makes the others less effective stimulants[60] of acid secretion (Fig 2-7). It has been proposed that the receptors for all three secretagogues or the second messengers interact with one another such that removal of one secretagogue decreases the response to the other secretagogues. Others have proposed histamine to be the final common pathway for acid secretion, a hypothesis that explains both the ability of H_2 blockers to inhibit all forms of stimulated acid secretion and their efficacy in the treatment of ulcers. This assumes that other secretagogues act upon a histaminocyte in the gastric mucosa stimulating release of histamine that then acts in a paracrine fashion. It may be that both systems (i.e., interacting receptors and second-message system versus a distinct histaminocyte) are operative. A recent model proposed by Soll and Berglindh[60] to explain these complex interactions is illustrated in Figure 2-7.

CHOLECYSTOKININ (CCK)

Structure and Biosynthesis. CCK was initially identified by its ability to stimulate contraction of the gallbladder.[3] The structure of CCK was found to be identical to that of pancreozymin, a peptide previously recognized for its ability to stimulate pancreatic enzyme secretion.[4] The carboxyl-terminal tetrapeptide amide sequence of CCK is essential for biologic activity and is identical in structure to the equivalent region of gastrin (Table 2-1). The presence of a sulfated tyrosine residue in the seventh position (counting unconventionally from the carboxyl terminus) largely determines the unique spectrum of biologic activity of cholecystokinin.[8]

The structure of the human gene for CCK has been delineated.[61] The cDNA is 345 base pairs long and encodes a preprohormone of 115 amino acids that contains a 20-amino-acid signal peptide, a 25-amino-acid linking region, a large form of CCK (CCK 58), and a 12-amino-acid carboxyl-terminal extension. As one might predict from the structure of the large precursor, multiple molecular forms have been identified. Although the initial form extracted from porcine intestine was 33 amino acids in length (CCK 33), the intestine also contains approximately equal amounts of a 39-amino-acid peptide (CCK 39). Smaller intermediate forms have been described, including CCK 25, CCK 22, CCK 18, CCK 8, CCK 7, and CCK 5.[16,62] In the dog, the predominant form of circulating CCK after duodenal perfusion of sodium oleate is reported to be CCK 58. In contrast, CCK 22 was found to be the predominant form in rats. In man, two forms predominate; one has elution characteristics similar to those of CCK 33, and the other appears to occupy an intermediate position between CCK

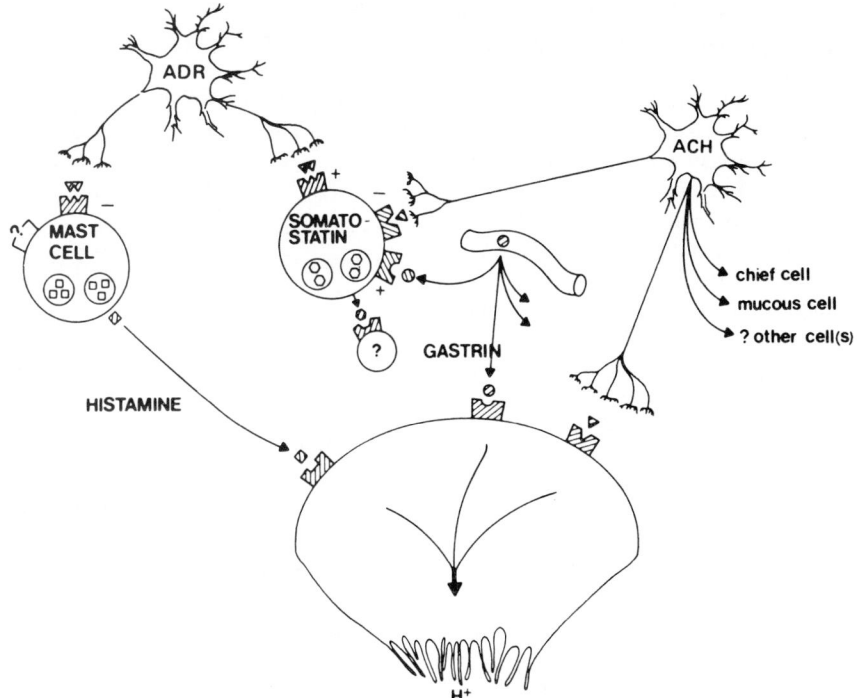

FIGURE 2–7. Model proposed by Soll and Berglindh for fundic mucosal regulatory pathways derived from studies with canine cells. Depicted is a model outlining a present view of the receptors and pathways regulating parietal cell function. Histamine, gastrin, and acetylcholine act in parallel on specific receptors on the parietal cell, while their actions are amplified by potentiating interactions. Gastrin, delivered by capillaries, also acts directly on receptors on the somatostatin cell to activate an inhibitory pathway. Gastrin receptors are probably also present on the stem cell and possibly on other cell types. Histamine is delivered from mast cells located in the lamina propria; canine fundic mast cells appear to have stimulatory adenosine and IgE receptors and inhibitory prostaglandin and B-adrenergic receptors. Other potentially important mast cell receptors remain to be established. Acetylcholine is delivered by postganglionic nerves to muscarinic receptors on the somatostatin cell that attenuate somatostatin release, and thus it dampens the pathway mediating somatostatin release. This "double negative" effect of acetylcholine at the somatostatin cell—inhibition of an inhibitor—serves to enhance the acid secretory response. Muscarinic receptors on other cell types may also modulate the acid secretory response, and many factors may influence acetylcholine delivery, but these elements remain to be elucidated. (Soll AH, Berglindh T. Physiology of the gastrointestinal tract. 1987:883.)

33 and CCK 8. CCK is synthesized and released from both nerve and endocrine cells and functions as both a classical neurotransmitter and a classical hormone.[36,62] In the brain, CCK 8 predominates, but larger forms have been identified.[36]

Distribution, Release, and Metabolism. CCK-containing cells (I cells) are most plentiful[43] in the mucosa of the human duodenum and upper jejunum; they are found in decreasing numbers as one progresses down the small intestine (Table 2-4). CCK-specific radioimmunoassays and an in vitro bioassay have demonstrated CCK release in response to ingestion of a mixed meal and have established that fat and protein are the most potent stimulants.[16,37] In man, amino acids are more potent stimulants than intact protein, with aromatic amino acids being the most potent.[16] In contrast, in rats, intact peptides and proteins are more potent stimulants than free amino acids.[37] As is the case with gastrin release, negative feedback loops control CCK release. A trypsin-sensitive protein (CCK-releasing peptide or CRP) secreted into the lumen of the duodenum interacts with the CCK cell to stimulate CCK release.[63] CCK, in turn, stimulates pancreatic enzyme secretion, and the trypsin released digests CRP, destroying its ability to stimulate the CCK cell. When trypsin is absent from the gut lumen (because of pancreatic destruction, diversion of pancreatic juice, or absorption of enzymes onto food particles), CRP escapes digestion and is able to stimulate the CCK cell to release more peptide. There is evidence that a second CCK-stimulating peptide may be synthesized by and released from the pancreas.[64] Neural reflexes do not seem to play a dominant role in CCK release.[16] Although vagotomy alters CCK release, this effect is probably secondary to the rapid gastric emptying that speeds the rate of delivery of nutrients to the duodenum and upper jejunum.

CCK is cleared rapidly from the circulation, and all capillary beds are presumed to play a role in its metabolism.[16] The relative importance of the liver in CCK metabolism varies depending upon the size of the molecular form under consideration.[65] Thus, the liver plays a disproportionately important role in the clearance of small forms of cholecystokinin, such as CCK 8 and CCK 4. Larger forms of cholecystokinin are not removed to any greater extent by the liver when compared with other vascular beds.

Biologic Actions. The major physiologic functions of CCK[16,62] are to stimulate the secretion of a pancreatic juice rich in pancreatic enzymes and to cause contraction of the gallbladder (Table 2-4). These dual effects result in the coordinated delivery of bile and pancreatic enzymes to the duodenum to optimize digestion of food. Several other effects[16] may be physiologic, including inhibition of gastric acid secretion (at least in some species), inhibition of gastric emptying, induction of satiety, and stimulation of growth of the exocrine pancreas (Table 2-5). However, as with most GI peptides, the spectrum of biologic actions is diverse, and the physiologic significance of many of the actions described in Table 2-5 remains unproved. CCK-containing neurons can be demonstrated in the myenteric plexus of Auerbach and the submucosal plexus of Meissner in the colon, a finding that supports a neuromodulator or neurotransmitter role.

The Secretin Family

SECRETIN

Structure and Biosynthesis. Secretin is a 27-amino-acid residue peptide (Table 2-1) that exhibits structural similarities to glucagon and enteroglucagon, vasoactive intestinal polypeptide and peptide HM (or PHI), growth hormone–releasing factor (GRF), and GIP.[16,66] Structure–function studies reveal that the whole molecule is required for full biologic activity.[5,16,66]

Distribution Release and Metabolism. Secretin is found in endocrine-type cells (S cells), which occur in greatest numbers in the duodenal mucosa (Table 2-6) and in decreasing numbers down the length of the jejunum.[43] The major stimulant of secretin release[67] is the entry of unbuffered hydrogen ions into the duodenum (Fig 2-8). Ingested nutrients are much less potent stimulants of secretin release, and their stimulating effects may well be related directly to their ability to stimulate acid secretion. However, oleate, bile salts, and alcohol have been noted to release secretin through mechanisms that are independent of their ability to stimulate acid. There is little or no evidence that secretin release is under the direct control of the autonomic nervous system.[16]

Secretin is cleared rapidly from the circulation and has a half-life of approximately 4 minutes in humans.[66] The kidney may have a disproportionately important role in the metabolism of secretin when compared with other gastrointestinal peptides; the liver, in contrast, appears to have little if any specific role in this process.

Physiologic Effects. The major physiologic action of secretin[66] is to stimulate the secretion of a bicarbonate-rich pancreatic juice, an action that is potentiated by CCK (Table 2-6). After ingestion of a meal, the entry of unbuffered hydrogen ions into the duodenum stimulates the release of secretin, which, in turn, stimulates the pancreas to secrete a high volume of bicarbonate-rich fluid. Pancreatic bicarbonate is secreted on a mole-for-mole basis relative to the amount of free hydrogen ions entering the intestine such that the acid entering the duodenum is accurately and rapidly neutralized. Secretin accounts for about 80% of the bicarbonate response of the pancreas to a meal,[68] and its release

TABLE 2–5
Some Biologic Effects of CCK

Gastrointestinal Secretion

Stimulates pancreatic enzyme secretion

Weak stimulation of pancreatic volume and bicarbonate (rat)

Weak stimulant of gastric acid secretion

Competitive antagonist of gastrin-stimulated acid (dogs, humans)

Stimulates hypertrophy and hyperplasia of pancreas

Increases intestinal lymph flow

Gastrointestinal Motility

Stimulates gallbladder contraction

Relaxes sphincter of Oddi

Decreases gastric emptying rate

Increases antral smooth muscle contraction

Possibly relaxes fundic smooth muscle in the gastric fundus

Decreases lower esophageal sphincter pressure

Possibly stimulates contraction of esophageal body

Increases small intestine motility and shortens transit time

Increases colonic motility

Hormone Release

Enhances insulin release

Increases pancreatic somatostatin output

Increases pancreatic polypeptide release

Increases GIP release

Releases calcitonin

Food Intake

Decreases when given centrally (cerebral ventricle)

(Modified from Walsh JH. Gastrointestinal hormones. In: Johnson, LR, ed. Physiology of the gastrointestinal tract. New York: Raven Press, 1989:183.)

ensures that the luminal environment of the small intestine is optimal for the action of pancreatic enzymes. Although secretin may play a role as an enterogastrone (i.e., as an inhibitor of gastric acid secretion and gastric motility) in some species,[69] it is unlikely to do so in man. Secretin, vasoactive intestinal polypeptide (VIP), and PHI (or peptide histidine methionine [PHM] in man) have all been shown to increase bicarbonate secretion from Brunner's glands in the duodenum.[70] Secretin and VIP are more potent in this regard than PHI or PHM. Other actions of secretin include stimulation of colonic mucus secretion, gastric pepsin secretion, inhibition of gastric secretion and motility, and inhibition of lower esophageal sphincter tone.[66] The physiologic significance of these actions is still debated.

GLUCOSE-DEPENDENT INSULINOTROPIC PEPTIDE (GIP)

Structure. GIP is a 42-amino-acid residue peptide (Table 2-1) that was first isolated as an apparent contaminant in natural preparations of cholecystokinin.[71] It exhibits marked homology with secretin, and, like secretin, the whole molecule is required

TABLE 2-6
Secretin Family—Cell of Origin and Likely Function

PEPTIDE	CELL OF ORIGIN	BIOLOGIC ACTION
Secretin	Endocrine cells (S) in duodenal and jejunal mucosa	Stimulates pancreatic secretion of fluid and bicarbonate
Vasactive intestinal polypeptide (VIP)	Nerve fibers throughout the GI tract	Controls blood flow Modulates function of GI sphincters Secretinlike action
Gastric inhibitory polypeptide (GIP)	Endocrine (K) cells in duodenal and jejunal mucosa	Stimulates secretion of insulin May inhibit secretion of acid
Glucagon	Alpha cells in the islet	Stimulates glycogenolysis, gluconeogenesis, and lipolysis
Enteroglucagon	"L" cells in ileal and colonic mucosa	Trophic effect on the small intestine

for full biologic potency. Multiple molecular forms exist, including a form larger than the 43-amino-acid peptide originally isolated.[72]

Distribution, Release, and Metabolism. GIP is localized (Table 2-6) to endocrine-type cells (K cells) in the villi and upper crypt region of the duodenal and jejunal mucosa.[43] This distribution contrasts with many other gut endocrine cells, which tend to be localized to the mid to lower regions of the gland or deep within the crypts.

Specific radioimmunoassays have been developed for GIP that exhibit little or no cross-reactivity with the other family members.[73] GIP is released in response to the ingestion of a meal, with all three major food groups (carbohydrates, fats, and protein) con-

tributing to this release.[72] However, glucose and the products of fat digestion are more potent stimulants of GIP release than free amino acids. Enzymatic digestion of complex nutrients is thus a prerequisite for stimulation of GIP release.[74] Beta-adrenergic agonists stimulate the release of GIP, while glucagon, insulin, somatostatin, and peptide YY all inhibit GIP release.[72]

As with other gastrointestinal peptides, GIP is cleared rapidly from the circulation, and almost all capillary beds are involved in metabolism. A specific role for the kidney has been suggested.

Biologic Actions. Although the peptide was initially identified based on its apparent ability to inhibit acid secretion,[71] the true physiologic function of GIP is to enhance insulin release[72,75] in response to carbohydrate meals (Table 2-6). Based on this finding, a name change was proposed[72] from "gastric inhibitory polypeptide" to "glucose-dependent insulinotropic polypeptide," retaining the initials "GIP." GIP appears to be responsible in large part for the potentiated insulin response that occurs when large amounts of glucose are ingested rather than infused intravenously. The body has developed several safeguards against the inappropriate stimulation of insulin release by GIP.[72,74,75] First, complex carbohydrates do not release GIP; GIP is released only when the ingested carbohydrate has been digested and is in a form that can be absorbed from the gut lumen.[74] Second, GIP will stimulate insulin release only if circulating glucose levels are elevated; it is incapable of stimulating insulin release when glucose levels are normal or low.[75]

VASOACTIVE INTESTINAL POLYPEPTIDE (VIP) AND PEPTIDE HISTIDINE METHIONINE (PHM)

Structure. In 1974, Said and Mutt identified a 28-amino-acid residue peptide based on its potent vasodilator properties.[76] They called the peptide vasoactive intestinal polypeptide (VIP) based on this property and the fact that it was first identified in the intestinal mucosa. When the gene was cloned,[14] VIP was found

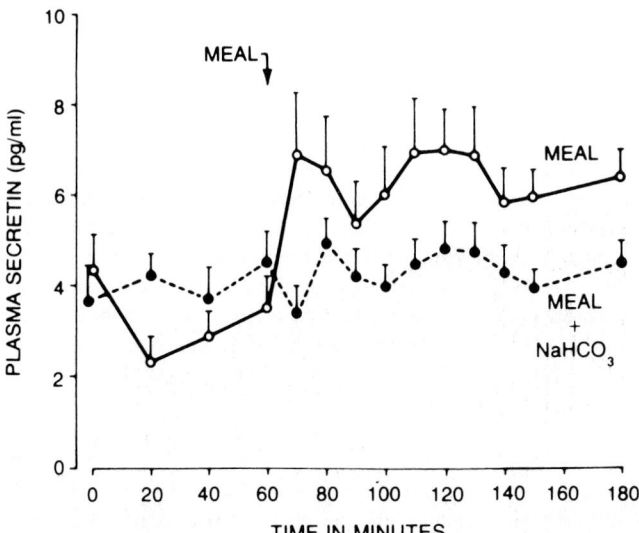

FIGURE 2-8. Comparison of the plasma secretin response to a test meal in normal human subjects when acid was allowed to enter the duodenum unbuffered and when *p*H was kept above 5.5 by intragastric infusion of bicarbonate.

to be contained within a large preprohormone that encoded a second structurally related peptide, peptide histidine isoleucine (PHI). In man (Table 2-1), this second peptide contains a methionine substitute for the isoleucine at the carboxyl-terminus (Figure 2-1) and is, as a result, called PHM. PHM and VIP share approximately 50% of their amino acid residues and may interact with the same receptor. This may explain their similar spectrum of biologic action. As with other members of the family, the whole VIP molecule is required for full potency.[77]

Distribution, Release, and Metabolism. It is apparent that VIP and PHI or PHM are not hormones but rather function as neuromodulators or neurotransmitters.[77,78] Although circulating VIP levels do not change with meals, pancreatic endocrine tumors (VIPomas) can synthesize and secrete large amounts of VIP into the circulation, resulting in profuse, often life-threatening watery diarrhea.[79]

VIP is cleared rapidly from the circulation and has a half-life in man of less than 1 minute.[77] This rapid clearance, which is typical of most neurotransmitters, probably serves as a protective mechanism ensuring that any VIP that escapes into the circulation as a result of overflow is rapidly removed.

Biologic Actions. VIP has a very wide spectrum of biologic actions.[77] As with most peptide neurotransmitters, trying to define how many of these actions are physiologic is extremely difficult. Currently, we do not have a delivery system that will accurately reproduce the concentrations of neurotransmitters seen at a synaptic junction. VIP does stimulate the secretion of a pancreatic juice rich in bicarbonate[77] and may be the neural equivalent of secretin (Table 2-6). VIP also acts through adenylate cyclase to increase cyclic AMP levels, thereby stimulating intestinal secretion; it remains to be determined if this is a physiologic function of VIP. VIP probably plays an inhibitory role in the control of intestinal motility through its ability to induce smooth muscle relaxation.[78] It may also play a role in relaxation of the lower esophageal sphincter and possibly the internal anal sphincter.[77,78] A role for VIP in the control of blood flow in multiple vascular beds (including the GI tract and brain) has been proposed based on its distribution and the fact that it is a potent vasodilator substance.[77,78] It also inhibits gastric acid and pepsin secretion and gastrin and somatostatin release.

GLUCAGON AND ENTEROGLUCAGON

Structure. Figure 2-1 shows the structure of human preproglucagon.[80] The signal sequence includes amino acids −20 to −1. Glicentin,[81] which is 69 amino acid residues in length, is the predominant form of gut glucagon produced by the enteroglucagon cell. It is composed of pancreatic glucagon with amino- and carboxyl-terminal extensions (Table 2-1). A second enteroglucagon, oxyntomodulin, has been identified and is 37 amino acid residues in length; it consists of pancreatic glucagon with a carboxyl extension of 8 amino acids. Tissue-specific processing of the precursor results in the production of pancreatic glucagon in the pancreas and glicentin and oxyntomodulin in the ileum and colon.[81] In the large precursor molecule, the carboxyl-terminal region beyond glicentin contains two glucagonlike peptides (GLP-1 and GLP-2).

Distribution, Release, and Metabolism. Pancreatic glucagon is a product of the alpha cell in the islet (Table 2-6), while glicentin and oxyntomodulin are products of L-type cells in the intestine. Enteroglucagon colocalizes with peptide YY in a subpopulation of L-type cells. In dogs, but not man, endocrine cells within the stomach produce true pancreatic glucagon.[43] Ingestion of a meal normally produces a small increase in enteroglucagon, a response that is markedly enhanced in patients with malabsorption.[16,82] Glucose stimulates enteroglucagon but inhibits pancreatic glucagon release, while intraluminal fat stimulates the release of both peptides.[82]

Biologic Actions. Although pancreatic and gut glucagon are members of the secretin family,[5,16] their spectrums of biologic action are relatively distinct (Table 2-6). Pancreatic glucagon is a metabolic hormone inducing glycogenolysis, lipolysis, gluconeogenesis, and ketogenesis.[16] Pancreatic glucagon also inhibits gut motility, intestinal absorption, gastrointestinal motility, pancreatic secretion, and lower esophageal sphincter tone.[16] Enteroglucagon likely functions as a trophic hormone stimulating growth of the small intestine.[82] In common with pancreatic glucagon, it inhibits gastric secretion and slows gastric emptying. The functions of the two glucagonlike peptides (GLP-1 and GLP-2) are unknown, but one may serve as an incretion enhancing insulin release.[83]

The Pancreatic Polypeptide Family

Structure and Biosynthesis. Pancreatic polypeptide (PP) is a 36-amino-acid residue peptide initially isolated as an apparent contaminant in chicken[84] and porcine[85] insulin preparations. Interaction between a polyproline helix and an alpha helix in the body of the molecule gives the peptide a distinctive globular shape.[86] Biologic activity of the molecule resides within the carboxyl-terminal hexapeptide, and an amidated carboxyl-terminal tyrosine residue is essential for biologic activity.[87]

The cDNA for human PP has been elucidated and found to contain four exons and three introns.[88] The gene encodes a preprohormone of 95 amino acid residues, within which the PP sequence is flanked at the amino terminus by a hydrophobic 29-amino-acid signal peptide and at the carboxyl terminus by a 27-amino-acid extension. These two extensions are joined to PP proper through classical tryptic cleavage sites (i.e., two basic amino acids in sequence). This basic structure is similar to that found in the NPY (Fig 2-1) and PYY precursors.[89,90] As with other GI peptides, PP occurs in multiple molecular forms.[91] This molecular heterogeneity largely reflects the synthesis and release of precursor molecules and their synthetic by-products.

Distribution, Release, and Metabolism. In man, PP cells are found on the periphery of the islets and in lesser numbers scattered throughout the acinar tissue of the exocrine pancreas.[43,91] PP cells have a unique distribution in the pancreas, being found within the pancreatic head and uncinate lobe. To some degree, the distribution of PP cells mirrors that of the pan-

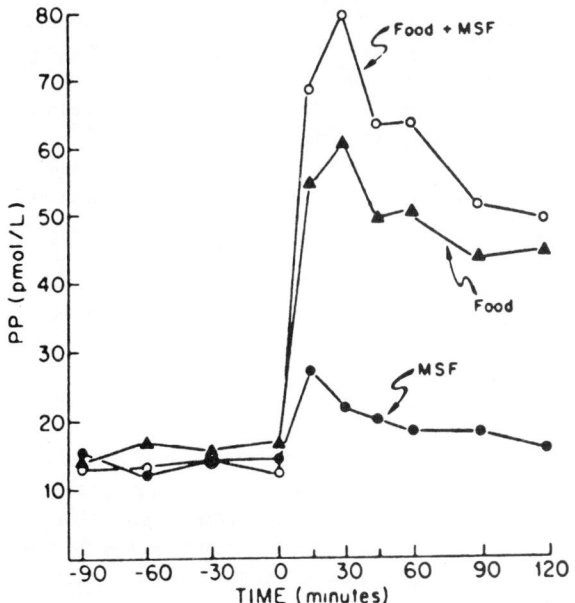

FIGURE 2–9. Comparison of the pancreatic polypeptide responses to modified sham feeding, intragastric instillation of homogenized food, and the combination of the two stimuli in normal subjects. (Taylor, et al. Gastroenterology 1978;75:432.)

creatic glucagon cells, which are found in highest concentrations in the body and tail of the pancreas.[43]

The PP response to a meal is readily measurable and is characteristically biphasic with an early peak followed by a prolonged plateau.[91] The first peak is largely neurally mediated and includes both cephalic–vagal and gastric phases (Fig 2-9). The cephalic-vagal phase is initiated by the sight, smell, and taste of food and is abolished by truncal vagotomy. The gastric phase is initiated by gastric distention and mediated through long vagovagal reflexes.[92] The prolonged plateau response represents a summated response to neural (predominately vagal–cholinergic) and hormonal stimulation modified by effects of circulating nutrients. Meals rich in protein or fat are the most potent stimulants of PP release; pancreaticobiliary secretions entering the duodenum may also contribute to PP release.[91]

In man, bovine PP has a metabolic half-life of about 7 minutes and is cleared from the circulation by all the body's vascular beds.[21,91] An important role for the kidneys in PP metabolism has been proposed based on the observation that patients with renal failure have elevated PP levels.[21,91]

Biologic Actions. Although many biologic actions of PP have been delineated, the exact physiologic role of the peptide is still debated (Table 2-7). PP is a potent inhibitor of pancreatic exocrine secretion, and infusion of exogenous PP to achieve blood levels similar to those seen after a meal inhibits pancreatic exocrine secretion, suggesting that this effect is physiologic.[93] PP may complete a series of negative feedback loops. First, PP is released by pancreaticobiliary secretions entering the duodenum and by CCK and then feeds back on the pancreas to inhibit pancreatic secretion.[91] Second, PP release is vagal–cholinergic-dependent, and PP may itself inhibit pancreatic exocrine secretion by inhibiting acetylcholine release from cholinergic nerve fibers.[94] A metabolic role for PP has also been proposed in that it inhibits hepatic glucose production.[95]

NEUROPEPTIDE Y

Structure and Biosynthesis. It has been deduced from the gene structure[89] that the preprohormone of human neuropeptide Y (NPY) is 97 amino acid residues in length and contains two tryptic cleavage sites (Fig 2-1). The action of proteolytic enzymes yields three peptides—a 28-amino-acid signal peptide, NPY proper, and a 30-amino carboxyl-terminal extension. The gene that encodes NPY has been localized to a chromosome (chromosome 7) separate from that which encodes PP (chromosome 17).

Distribution, Release, and Metabolism. NPY is the most abundant peptide isolated to date from the brain. The hypothalamic nuclei, which are particularly well innervated with NPY immunoreactive nerves, may serve as a site at which NPY regulates both sympathetic and parasympathetic activity.[96] There are at least two populations of NPY-immunoreactive nerves in the peripheral nervous system.[97] In one, NPY colocalizes with noradrenaline in sympathetic neurons that innervate blood vessels; in the other, NPY is found either as the only peptide or colocalized with other neuropeptides in the enteric nervous system. In addition to the gastrointestinal tract, a particularly rich innervation with NPY-immunoreactive nerves is seen in the heart, peripheral blood

TABLE 2–7
Pancreatic Polypeptide Family—Cell of Origin and Likely Function

PEPTIDE	DISTRIBUTION	BIOLOGIC ACTION
Pancreatic polypeptide	"PP" cells in pancreatic islet	Inhibits pancreatic secretion
		Decrease in hepatic glucose production
Neuropeptide Y	Nerve fibers in brain, spinal cord, enteric nervous systems	Vasoconstriction
		Stimulates food intake (central)
		Alters circadian rhythms (central)
Peptide YY	Endocrine (L) cells in ileocolonic mucosa	Inhibits pancreatic exocrine secretion
		Slows gastric emptying
		Inhibits intestinal transit

vessels, kidneys, spleen, eye, genital tract, biliary tree, respiratory tract, thyroid gland, and adrenal gland. NPY is released into the circulation during periods of extreme stress such as hypovolemic shock.

Biologic Actions. NPY produces a dose-dependent, slow, and sustained vasoconstriction (Table 2-7) in many peripheral arteries[98]; the magnitude of the response varies depending upon the vascular bed under investigation. Systemic administration of NPY induces a long-lasting increase in arterial blood pressure, secondary to sustained general vasoconstriction.[99] NPY is reported to be 24 times more potent than noradrenaline in reducing colonic blood flow and inhibiting colonic motility.[98] NPY also has numerous biologic effects[97] when injected centrally, including altered circadian rhythms, stimulation of food intake, induction of systemic hypotension, lowering of respiratory rate, decreased heart rate, and electroencephalogram synchronization.

PEPTIDE YY

Structure and Biosynthesis. Peptide YY was initially isolated from porcine duodenal mucosa[100] and given a chemical name based on the presence of a tyrosine residue at both the amino and carboxyl terminus (Y is the international sign for a tyrosine residue). The cDNA for rat PYY has been isolated[96] and shown to encode a preprohormone composed of a signal peptide, PYY itself, and a carboxyl-terminal extension.

Distribution, Release, and Metabolism. Although PYY was initially isolated from the duodenum, radioimmunoassay has demonstrated that PYY is present in highest concentration in the mucosa of the ileum and colon.[100] PYY cells are of two types; one is typically endocrine in nature, while the other has paracrine characteristics with basal cytoplasmic processes.[21,100] Although a paracrine role for PYY in the control of mucus secretion has been proposed,[100] it is also released into the circulation in response to a meal,[101] suggesting a true hormonal function. Fat and carbohydrates[21] are the most potent stimulants of peptide YY release. PYY has a short metabolic half-life similar to that of PP.[102]

Biologic Actions. PYY and NPY share many biologic actions. Thus, PYY and NPY are equipotent in terms of their vasoconstrictor effects[21,98,99] and probably act through a generic "NPY–PYY" receptor on smooth muscle cells. PYY is, like PP, a potent inhibitor of pancreatic secretion,[102] and it may be the "anti-CCK hormone" or "pancreatone" previously described in the ileocolonic mucosa (Table 2-7).

PYY exhibits characteristics typical of an enterogastrone[103] (i.e., a hormone released by fat to inhibit gastric acid secretion and slow gastric emptying). PYY inhibits cephalic-phase acid secretion over 90% while having little if any effect on the response to exogenous secretagogues, including bethanechol.[103] As such, PYY probably acts by inhibiting acetylcholine release from cholinergic nerve fibers (i.e., it may function as an endocrine neuromodulator).

It has also been suggested[21] that PYY mediates in part the "ileal brake" that comes into play when unabsorbed nutrients bathe the mucosa of the ileum and colon (Fig 2-10). The "ileal brake" describes a constellation of events[23] that serve to increase nutrient absorption by decreasing the rate of gastric emptying, hence slowing the delivery of nutrients to the already overburdened small intestine. PYY also slows intestinal transit, leading to increased efficiency of digestion and nutrient absorption by increasing nutrient–mucosal contact.

Opioid Peptides

Structure and Biosynthesis. In 1975,[104] two pentapeptides with opiate properties were isolated that differed from one another based on the presence of a methionine or leucine residue at the carboxyl-terminus (met-enkephalin and leu-enkephalin). There are now three known families of opioid peptides derived from three separate precursor molecules that are the products of three distinct genes.[105,106] The three opioid peptide precursors are proenkephalin A, proenkephalin B, and proopiomelanocortin.

Proopiomelanocortin, from which endorphin is generated, has 265 amino acids and a single met-enkephalin–related sequence within it. This large precursor molecule, which is largely restricted to the anterior pituitary, also contains the sequences for adrenocorticotropic hormone (ACTH) and melanocyte-stimulating hormone (MSH). Proenkephalin A is 263 amino acids long and contains four copies of met-enkephalin and one of leu-enkephalin, together with met-enkephalin Arg 6, Phe 7, and met-enkephalin

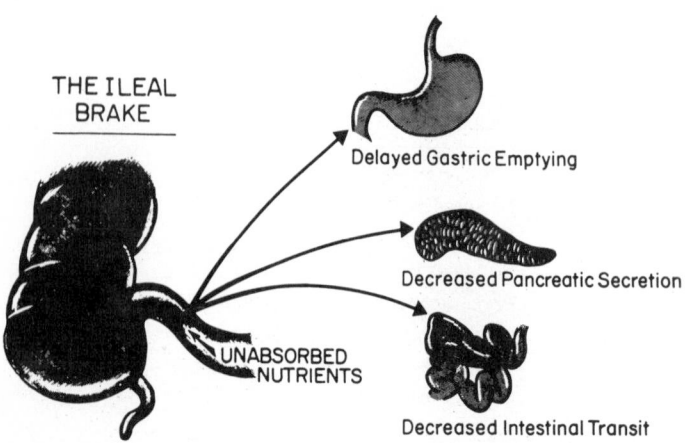

FIGURE 2–10. The "ileal brake" phenomenon describes the delayed gastric emptying and slowed intestinal transit that occur when unabsorbed nutrients bathe the ileal mucosa.

Arg 6, Gly 7, Leu 8. Each one of these opioid peptides is flanked within the precursor by two basic amino acids, which mark potential sites for trypticlike cleavage that liberates a wide variety of opioid peptides from this single precursor. It is apparent that tissue-specific processing of proenkephalin A results in the generation of specific opioidlike peptides in different tissues. In some tissues, products undergo amidation, yielding the opioid peptides amidorphin and metorphamide. Proenkephalin B has three copies of leu-enkephalin, each flanked within the precursor by pairs of basic amino acids. Again, tissue-specific processing of this precursor can yield a variety of opioid peptides, including dynorphin A and B or leu-enkephalin itself. Some of the family members that arise from these precursors are detected in highest concentrations outside the GI tract.[105,106] Thus, a general characteristic of the opioid precursor molecules is the presence within them of met- and/or leu-enkephalin sequences either as multiple copies or as a single copy. Although peptides with this sequence exhibit opioidlike activity, other products of these precursors also exhibit opioid agonist activity, even though they are structurally distinct from the enkephalins.

A wide variety of opioidlike peptides have been identified in the gastrointestinal tract, many of which are derived from the proenkephalin A gene.[107] Met-enkephalin and leu-enkephalin are abundant opioid peptides in the gut. In addition, octa and hepta forms of met-enkephalin have been identified in the gut by specific radioimmunoassay. Most of the enkephalinlike material in the gut is found in intrinsic nerves of the enteric nervous system. Although this material has been identified in both the myenteric and submucous plexuses, it is found in greatest concentration in the neurons of the myenteric plexus. The proenkephalin B–like peptide dynorphin is found in the gut and is released from the gut during peristalsis. However, dynorphin-containing neurons are less common than those containing the enkephalins. Although enkephalin-like peptides have been localized to endocrine-type cells, the data are less clear with respect to an endocrine origin for proenkephalin B–related peptides. Proopiomelanocortin-related peptides, including ACTH, alpha MSH, beta-lipotropin (beta LPH), and alpha- and beta-endorphins, have also been identified in the gut. Endorphinlike peptides have been colocalized with ACTH, alpha MSH, and corticotropin-releasing factor (CRF) within nerves in both myenteric and submucous plexuses.

Biologic Actions. In general, the opioid peptides act as neuromodulators (Table 2-8) inhibiting neuronal firing and decreasing the release of other neurotransmitters.[108] In myenteric neurons, opioid agonists hyperpolarize nerve cells by increasing K^+ conductance. Opioid peptides have been demonstrated to inhibit the release of acetylcholine, substance P, and noradrenaline. A variety of distinct opioid receptors have been identified in the myenteric plexus, including mu, delta, kappa, epsilon, and sigma receptors, stimulation of which gives rise to complex actions and interactions of endogenous opioids.[107,108] Although the net effect of opioid peptides on gut motility is to slow intestinal transit,[107] this event may be accompanied by either increased or decreased motility. The inhibition of transit is probably due to the interruption of the propulsive contractile activity in the intestine and/or an increase in tonic contraction, which increases the resistance to flow of chyme. The constipating effect of opioids is related to both decreased intestinal transit and increased fluid and electrolyte absorption.

An example of the complexity of responses to opioid agonists would be the differing effects opioids have on the lower esophageal

TABLE 2–8
Peptides That Do Not as Yet Belong to a Structurally Related Family—
Cell of Origin and Likely Function

PEPTIDE	CELL OF ORIGIN	BIOLOGIC ACTION
Somatostatin	Endocrine and paracrine cells (D) and nerves throughout the gut	Inhibits GI motility, inhibits exocrine and endocrine secretions
Motilin	Endocrine cells (M) in duodenal mucosa	Controls the interdigestive myoelectric complex
Neurotensin	endocrine (N) cells and nerves in ileum and colon	Inhibits gastric emptying
Substance P	Nerves in muscle coat of the gut	Stimulates the gut's smooth muscle
Gastrin-releasing peptide (GRP)	Nerves throughout the gut but particularly in the stomach	Stimulates release of gastrin
Urogastrone/epidermal growth factor	Endocrine cells in duodenal mucosa	Inhibits secretion of gastric acid
Opioids	Nerves throughout the gut	Inhibits GI motility and secretion
Pancreastatin	Nerves and endocrine cells of the gut	Inhibition of pancreatic and gastric secretion
Galanin	Enteric nerves	Inhibition of intestinal contraction

sphincter, depending on which types of opioid receptors are activated. Mu and kappa agonists relax the sphincter, while agonists that work through other receptors contract the lower esophageal sphincter. Like morphine, opioids are potent stimulants of sphincter of Oddi contraction; they also inhibit mucosal blood flow. Other studies suggest a role for opioid peptides in the regulation of insulin release and glucose homeostasis.[106] The effects of opioids on the release of other gastrointestinal peptides vary; they stimulate the release of some and inhibit others.[106]

Somatostatin

Structure and Biosynthesis. Somatostatin (SS) was initially isolated,[109] purified, and sequenced (Table 2-1) from half a million ovine hypothalami as a tetradecapeptide (SS-14; MW 1637). The isolation of SS-14 from the hypothalamus led to the generation of antibodies that were used to demonstrate somatostatinlike immunoreactivity in the GI tract.[110] The somatostatin that was initially isolated from the ovine and porcine hypothalamus was subsequently found to be identical to that isolated from the porcine intestine and pancreas. Larger forms of somatostatin, such as SS-28, have been identified in a variety of tissues.

The cDNA structure that encodes somatostatin has been determined[111] and found to encode a 116-amino-acid protein (MW 12,737) that contains SS-28 at its carboxyl-terminus. The same precursor molecule has been identified in both the brain and the gut. Pulse-chase experiments have confirmed that this is the precursor peptide from which the smaller biologically active somatostatin peptides are generated. The cDNAs for human and rat somatostatin show marked similarity[110,111] and encode preprohormones of identical size. Chromosomal mapping shows that the somatostatin gene resides on the long arm of chromosome 3.[112] Tetradecapeptide somatostatin (SS-14) lies within the carboxyl terminus of SS-28. SS-14 has a characteristic cyclic structure that is maintained by a disulfide bond within the body of the molecule. Amino acid residues 7 through 10, which lie between the two cysteine residues that form this bridge, are essential for biologic activity.[110]

Distribution. Somatostatin has been localized to nerves and two different non-neural cell types; one of these is endocrine in nature and the other possibly paracrine in that it exhibits long cytoplasmic extensions. The peptide is also widely distributed in the nerve cells in the brain and the enteric nervous system. Within the gut mucosa,[43] the somatostatin cell (D cell) can be either "open" and exposed to the luminal contents or "closed" with no luminal contact. D cells in the gastric antrum are of the open variety, while those in the fundus are closed. Somatostatin serves multiple functions, which are reflected in these different cell types; it is capable of acting as a neurotransmitter and neuromodulator, a true hormone, and a paracrine substance.[110,113] Within the intestine, 90% of the immunoreactivity is found in the mucosa (predominantly in endocrine and paracrine cells) and 10% in the muscle layers. Although SS-14 and SS-28 are both found in the intestinal mucosa, SS-14 is the predominant form in the fundus, antrum, pancreas, and the muscle layers of the intestine.

Somatostatin was initially held not to be a true hormone based on what we now know were difficulties in measuring somatostatin in serum and plasma due to enzymatic degradation of the labeled somatostatin.[110] However, subsequent studies involving extraction of the serum or the use of special assay conditions have shown that the ingestion of a meal does stimulate release of SS-14 and SS-28 into the circulation.[110,114] The gastrointestinal tract, which contains 70% of the body's somatostatin, is the main source of releasable peptide, with the stomach and duodenum being the main sites of release.[110] In dogs, fat and protein release somatostatin, while carbohydrates are much less potent. Nutrients may also modulate somatostatin release by stimulating acid release, which in turn releases somatostatin. Naloxone inhibits somatostatin release, suggesting involvement of endogenous opioids. Somatostatin release is stimulated by GRP and bombesin and may be suppressed by vagal–cholinergic inhibitory nerve fibers. However, much of the release data have been confounded by species differences,[110] differences in responses observed when agents are given "in vivo" or "in vitro,"[110,113] and differences dependent upon whether isolated glands or isolated cells are being studied.[113] Serotonin, epinephrine, cholecystokinin, and gastrin all stimulate somatostatin release from cultured cells.[113]

Somatostatin 14 is cleared rapidly from the circulation, with a half-life that ranges from ½ to 3 minutes.[110] The larger molecular form, SS-28, has a half-life that is about three to four times longer than that of SS-14. Somatostatin undergoes spontaneous degradation in serum, with 50% of the immunoreactivity in rat serum disappearing in about 15 minutes at 37°C. Within the circulation, it is probably cleared by endothelial peptidases in cell capillary beds of the body, although the exact enzymes involved have not been defined.[110]

Biologic Actions. Somatostatin has a wide spectrum of biologic activities in the gut, nearly all of which are inhibitory.[110] Somatostatin inhibits salivary, gastric, pancreatic, and biliary secretion and inhibits the release of a wide variety of gastrointestinal hormones, including gastrin, secretin, CCK, PP, GIP, motilin, insulin, and glucagon. Treatment of animals with somatostatin antisera results in enhanced postprandial release of gastrin, insulin, PP, parathyroid hormone, growth hormone, enteroglucagon, and calcitonin. Somatostatin inhibits smooth muscle contraction in the gut and gallbladder by inhibiting acetylcholine release from cholinergic fibers. In contrast, somatostatin may stimulate the early phase of gastric intestinal transit, inhibits intestinal secretion, and impairs absorption of a variety of nutrients. It also decreases splanchnic and portal blood flow. Important roles for somatostatin in feedback inhibition of acid secretion and in the local control of gastrin release (Fig 2-11) have been proposed.[115]

The recent development of a long-acting somatostatin analogue (SMS 201–995 or Sandostatin) represents the first effective use of a GI peptide as a therapeutic agent.[116] This analogue has 8 amino acid residues instead of 14, as in natural somatostatin. It is chemically modified to make it far more resistant to enzymatic degradation, thereby markedly prolonging its metabolic half-life in the body. Sandostatin has shown its efficacy in the treatment of gut endocrine tumors, markedly decreasing life-threatening diarrhea in the Verner–Morrison syndrome (VIPomas). This analogue also markedly reduces symptoms such as diarrhea and flushing in patients with metastatic carcinoid.

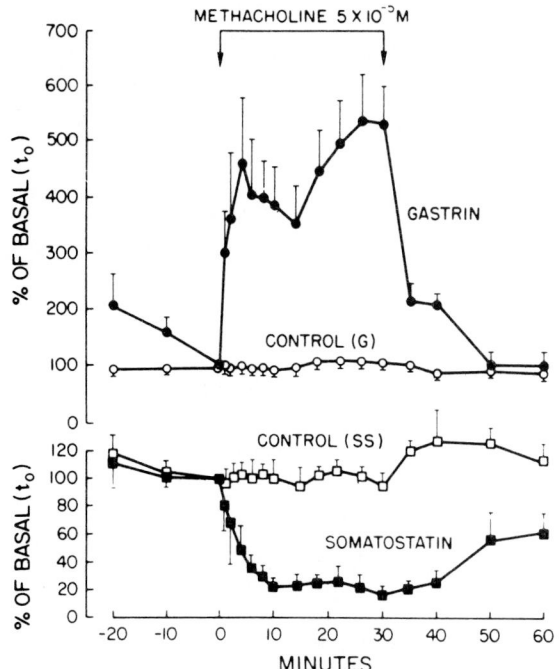

FIGURE 2–11. Reciprocal stimulation of gastrin release and inhibition of somatostatin release from the vascularly perfused stomach during methacholine infusion. (Saffour, et al. Am J Physiol 1980;238:495.)

Motilin

Structure. Motilin was initially isolated from extracts of porcine upper intestine based on its ability to stimulate gastric motor activity in antral and fundic pouches in dogs.[117] Although motilin was first identified as a 22-amino-acid peptide (Table 2-1) with a molecular weight of 2700, larger forms of motilin have been isolated.[118] In terms of structure–function relationships, the whole molecule appears necessary for biologic activity, because deletion of a single amino acid residue from either end of the molecule markedly reduces potency.[118]

Distribution, Release, and Metabolism. Motilin is present in highest concentrations in the mucosa of the duodenum and upper jejunum (Table 2-8) and is found in decreasing concentrations as one progresses down the small and large intestine.[43] Although motilin is normally seen within endocrine cells, a motilinlike peptide has also been identified in the brain, where it is present in highest concentrations in the pituitary and pineal glands.[118]

The pattern of release of motilin is somewhat atypical for most gastrointestinal hormones in that the peptide's release is inhibited in the dog after ingestion of a meal.[118–120] During the interdigestive period, motilin is released cyclically[118–120] in man and other species, with peptide concentrations peaking with phase III of the interdigestive myoelectric complex (IDMC) (Fig 2-12). Peak concentrations of motilin occur every 90 to 120 minutes when concentrations are two- to threefold higher than those observed during a nadir. Fluctuations in vagal tone may determine these rhythmic variations in motilin concentrations, given that vagal stimulation

causes release of motilin. Motilin release is also stimulated by pancreaticobiliary secretions entering the duodenum. In common with many other gastrointestinal peptides, motilin has a short half-life of about 5 minutes, and the kidneys may play an important role in its metabolism.[118]

Biologic Action. The fluctuations in motilin concentrations, which parallel the IDMC, suggests that the two may be causally related.[118–120] The IDMC, also known as the "house-keeper" potential, induces a wave of contractile activity that arises in a pacemaker high in the gastric fundus and "sweeps" down the intestine, clearing the lumen of undigested particulate matter.[118–120] The infusion of exogenous motilin induces premature phase 3 activity of the IDMC in the stomach and intestine, an effect that is blocked by the injection of atropine or antimotilin antisera.[120] In keeping with this last observation, infusion of motilin antiserum inhibits spontaneous IDMC activity. Erythromycin and its analogues[121] stimulate the IDMC by binding to the motilin receptor in the small intestine. Although infusion of large doses of motilin stimulates pancreatic exocrine secretion and smooth muscle contraction in the small intestine, gallbladder, sphincter of Oddi, and lower esophageal sphincter, these effects are probably pharmacologic.[118]

Substance P

Structure. Although substance P was initially described in the small intestine in 1931, its amino acid sequence was not determined until 1971.[122] Substance P is an undecapeptide, and the carboxyl-terminal tripeptide Gly-Leu-Met-NH_2 is common to a class of peptides referred to as tachykinins, which include the mollusk and amphibian peptides physalaemin, eledoisin, kassinin, and phyllomedusin.[123]

Distribution and Release. Substance P is widely distributed in the brain, spinal cord, and peripheral and enteric nervous systems.[123,124] Within the gastrointestinal tract, substance P concentrations are highest in the proximal small intestine and colon, where it can be colocalized with enkephalin in nerve fibers within the external muscle layer.[124] Rare endocrine cells have been described to contain substance P, and release of substance P has been described after a meal. Despite this observation, substance P is thought to function as a neurotransmitter rather than as a hormone.[123,125]

Biologic Actions. Substance P causes[123] contraction of gallbladder and intestinal smooth muscle and stimulates intestinal peristalsis (Table 2-8). It inhibits biliary secretion and intestinal absorption but stimulates basal pancreatic and intestinal exocrine secretion. Substance P also inhibits somatostatin release. It has direct effects on smooth muscle and indirect effects through stimulation of acetylcholine release.[123,125] Within the central nervous system (CNS), substance P functions as a neuromodulator controlling acetylcholine, dopamine, and serotonin release from nerves. In the peripheral and enteric nervous systems it is thought to play an important role in pain perception.[123,125]

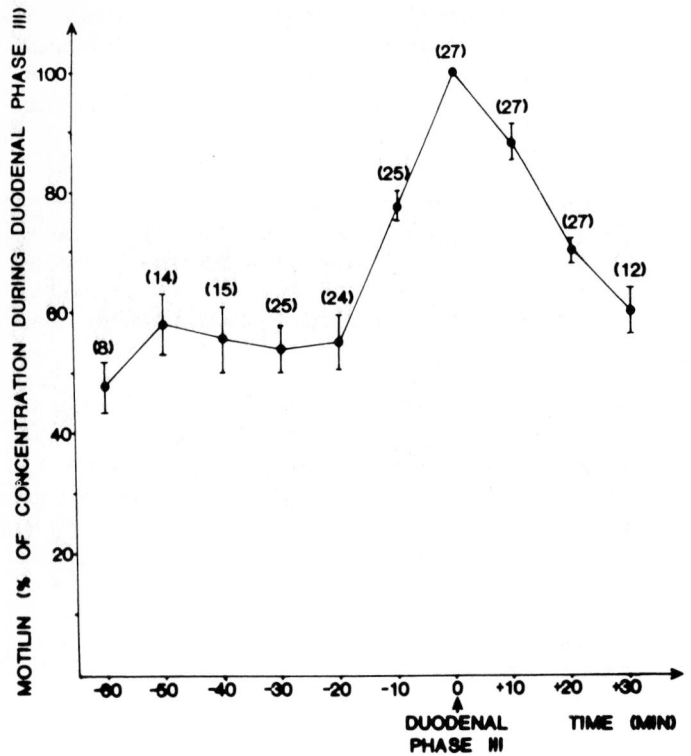

FIGURE 2–12. A peak in serum motilin concentrations occurs every 90–120 minutes and coincides with the onset of phase III of the interdigestive myoelectric complex. (Poitras, et al. Am J Physiol 1980;239:G215.)

Neurotensin

Structure. Neurotensin (NT) is a 13-amino-acid peptide (MW 1673) that was initially found as an apparent contaminant in substance P preparations.[126] It was identified based on its ability to produce vasodilation and hypotension. Smaller forms of NT have been identified in brain and gut extracts.[127] Biologic activity resides within the carboxyl terminus in that the NT 1–13 and 2–13 fragments exhibit equipotency, and an amino-terminal fragment (NT 1–9) exhibits less than 0.2% of the activity of the whole molecule.

Distribution, Release, and Metabolism. Neurotensin was initially isolated from the hypothalamus and subsequently localized to endocrine-type cells (N cells) in the ileal mucosa.[43] Eighty to ninety percent of NT in the body is found in the gut, predominantly in the distal jejunum and ileum.[127–129] Different amounts of peptide can be measured in tissues and in the circulation, depending upon whether amino-terminal– or carboxyl-terminal–specific neurotensin antisera are used in radioimmunoassays.[127–129] Neurotensin is released into the circulation in response to a meal, with fat being the most potent stimulant of release. Although jejunal and not ileal infusion of fat releases neurotensin by way of cholinergic-dependent mechanisms, ileal resection abolishes this response. Neural and hormonal signals from the upper gut are thought to be important factors stimulating release of neurotensin from cells within the ileal mucosa.[127–129]

The measured half-life of neurotensin varies depending upon whether amino- or carboxyl-terminal antisera are used to measure circulating levels.[127–129] When a carboxyl-terminal antiserum is used (which gives a truer measure of biologic activity), the half-life of neurotensin is about ½ minute. Half-lives are significantly longer when an amino-terminal antiserum is used, reflecting the slower clearance rates of amino-terminal fragments.

Biologic Actions. Neurotensin has many biologic actions (Table 2-8), including decreased tone in esophageal and intestinal sphincters, decreased intestinal peristalsis, inhibition of gastric acid secretion, delayed gastric emptying, decreased mucosal blood flow and intestinal secretion, and stimulation of pancreatic secretion.[127–129] Neurotensin induces contraction of the colon and defecation, a response that has been said to mimic the gastrocolic reflex. Although it relaxes the gallbladder in man, it causes transient contraction of the gallbladder in dogs. However, neurotensin is 50 times less potent than CCK in this regard. Neurotensin also stimulates the exocrine pancreas, potentiating secretory responses to secretin and CCK. Although a role for neurotensin as a physiologically important enterogastrone has been proposed, a definitive physiologic function for neurotensin is yet to be delineated.[128] Neurotensin release is markedly enhanced in patients with the dumping syndrome who exhibit rapid gastric emptying.

Gastrin-Releasing Peptide (GRP)

Structure and Biosynthesis. GRP is a heptacosapeptide (Table 2-1) that exhibits close structural homology to the amphibian peptide bombesin.[130] Indeed, GRP was first identified in man by the use of antisera directed against bombesin.[131] Two structurally related decapeptides have recently been isolated in the porcine intestine and spinal cord—neuromedin C and neuromedin B.[131]

Distribution and Release. GRP has been identified in the stomach, small intestine, and colon of most mammalian species.[132] Within these organs, GRP is largely restricted to nerves (Table 2-8), and the peptide does not appear to be released into the circulation. The peptide is widely distributed within nerves in the CNS and spinal cord.

Biologic Actions. GRP is a potent stimulant of the release of a large number of gastrointestinal peptides, including gastrin, PP, CCK, motilin, neurotensin, enteroglucagon, pancreatic glucagon, insulin, and somatostatin.[131] It is the most potent stimulant of gastrin release known in man. GRP also stimulates gastric acid secretion and pancreatic enzyme release and increases gut and gallbladder motility.[133] It is uncertain which of these effects are direct and which are mediated by other hormones released by GRP. Central and peripheral administration of GRP induces satiety.[134] In contrast to the satiety-inducing effects of CCK, GRP's effects are not dependent on the vagus. Central administration of GRP also inhibits acid secretion, induces hypoglycemia, and interferes with normal thermal regulation.[131-135] GRP, or a related peptide, is synthesized and released by small-cell carcinoma of the lung, where it functions as an autocrine growth factor.[136]

Epidermal Growth Factor (Urogastrone)

Structure. Urogastrone was initially identified in and isolated from urine based on its ability to inhibit acid secretion.[137] Epidermal growth factor (EGF) was isolated independently from the mouse salivary gland based on its ability to induce precocious eruption of teeth and early eyelid opening in newborn mice.[138] When the structure of urogastrone was determined, it was found to be similar to that of EGF.[139] Human urogastrone exists in two forms (alpha and beta) that differ by a single arginine substitution. Human beta urogastrone has 53 amino acid residues, as does mouse EGF; human EGF has 49. Human beta urogastrone and mouse EGF share 37 of their 53 amino acids and may be equivalent peptides.[140]

Distribution and Release. EGF and/or urogastrone can be localized immunochemically to the submandibular gland, thyroid, pancreas, duodenum, jejunum, and kidney.[140] Urogastronelike immunoreactivity has also been described in Brunner's glands, in serum, and in several body secretions, including urine, milk, and gastric and pancreatic juice. Serum levels of EGF are increased in pregnancy.[140]

Biologic Actions. EGF accelerates growth of a wide variety of normal tissues, including the liver and gut,[140] and it accelerates malignant growths, including some benign and malignant breast tumors. Receptors for EGF have been identified in the duodenum and jejunum, where they may mediate growth of the small intestine mucosa. Treatment of nutritionally deprived weaning rats with EGF induces growth of the GI tract and causes a significant increase in body weight. EGF also inhibits pentagastrin- and histamine-stimulated acid secretion.[141]

Pancreastatin

Structure. Pancreastatin was initially isolated as a 49-amino-acid residue peptide from porcine pancreatic extract with the use of Tatemoto and Mutt's novel assay.[142] Although the porcine form has a relatively unique primary structure, it nevertheless shares minor sequence homology with vasopressin (C-terminal Arg-Gly-NH$_2$) and gastrin (residues 34–38).[143] Bovine pancreastatin is 47 amino acids long with 74% sequence homology to the porcine form, while human pancreastatin contains 52 amino acid residues.[144,145] Pancreastatin is a product of a larger DNA message that encodes chromogranin A, a secretory protein present in many neuroendocrine cells.[144] Identical amino acid sequence homology exists between pancreastatin and the corresponding midportion of the chromogranin A peptide.

Distribution. Pancreastatin is distributed widely[145,146] throughout the central nervous system with high concentrations in the cortex, hypothalamus, hippocampus, and dorsal horn cells of the spinal cord. In addition, it has been localized to gonadotropic and thyrotropic cells of the anterior pituitary.[145] Pancreastatinlike immunoreactivity is described in adrenal medullary chromaffin cells (enterochromaffinlike cells in the medulla) and islet cells of the pancreas.[146,147] Not surprisingly, this distribution parallels that of chromogranin A, particularly in the nervous system and pancreas.

Actions. The name "pancreastatin" was derived from the ability of this peptide to inhibit glucose-stimulated insulin release in the perfused rat pancreas[148]; inhibition of second-phase insulin release was particularly marked. Although pancreastatin inhibits CCK-stimulated pancreatic exocrine secretion,[148,149] variable effects on amylase release have been reported. A carboxyl-terminal fragment (24–52) of human pancreastatin has been demonstrated to have biologic activity similar to that of the native peptide in terms of inhibition of CCK-stimulated pancreatic exocrine secretion and glucose-stimulated insulin secretion, indicating the importance of this part of the peptide for function.[149,150] Pancreastatin also inhibits histamine- and carbachol-stimulated acid secretion from isolated rabbit gastric glands[151] and canine parietal cells.[152]

Galanin

Structure. Galanin is a 29-amino-acid peptide initially isolated from the porcine intestine by use of the novel assay developed by Tatemoto and Mutt.[153] The name "galanin" is derived from the N- and C-terminal amino acid residues glycine and alanine. Unique in its full amino acid sequence, galanin does share some homology with other peptides; notably, its C-terminal tetrapeptide (-Tyr-Gly-Leu-Ala-NH$_2$) is similar to that of physalaemin (-Tyr-Gly-Leu-Met-NH$_2$) and substance P (-Phe-Gly-Leu-Met-NH$_2$).

Distribution. Galanin is widely distributed in nerves throughout the central and peripheral nervous systems. Galanin immunoreactivity has been reported in the brain[154] as well as in the nerves of the intestine[155] and pancreas.[156] In the enteric nervous system[157] of some mammals, galanin immunoreactivity is found in cell bodies of the myenteric ganglia. These cell bodies send processes to the circular muscle and submucous ganglia. Other nerve terminals supply submucosal vessels and mucosal cells.[157] Galanin colocalized with VIP and NPY in two distinct subpopulations of intrinsic enteric nerves.

Biologic Actions. In the gut, galanin stimulates contraction of intestinal smooth muscle directly.[153] It also inhibits stimulated acetylcholine release from the myenteric plexus in longitudinal muscle strips; it causes lower esophageal sphincter (LES) contraction and blocks sphincter relaxation.[158] Galanin inhibits bombesin-stimulated gastric acid output without affecting gastrin levels[159] and weakly inhibits stimulated amylase secretion from pancreatic acini.[160] Its other effects include stimulation of feeding,[156] inhibition of insulin and somatostatin secretion, and stimulation of secretion of glucagon.[161]

Miscellaneous Peptides

THYROTROPIN-RELEASING HORMONE (TRH)

Although TRH was initially isolated from the brain, TRH-like immunoreactivity has been identified in the gastrointestinal tract.[162] Exogenous TRH delays intestinal transit.

CALCITONIN GENE-RELATED PEPTIDE (CGRP)

CGRP has been localized to the enteric nervous system and may be found in endocrine cells.[163] Intravenous infusion of CGRP inhibits gastric acid secretion, an effect that is abolished by truncal vagotomy. CGRP stimulates the release of somatostatin, which may mediate the peptide's inhibitory effects on the stomach.

GUT HORMONES IN DISEASE

Despite the large number of GI peptides discovered to date, their primary interest to the clinician is their role in hormone-secreting tumor syndromes. Endocrine tumors of the gut are usually pancreatic in origin and give rise to a variety of clinical syndromes that are described in chapters 62 and 91. Although the role of gastrointestinal peptides in these syndromes is well defined, their role in other diseases is less clear. This is in part because control of gut function is characterized by redundancy; multiple gut hormones and neurotransmitters serve the same or similar functions. As such, loss of any single hormone may be difficult to detect, and its loss many have little clinical significance because three or four other peptides may serve a similar function. For this reason, investigation of the role of GI peptides in common diseases such as gallstones, motility disturbances, pancreatitis, and peptic ulcer disease remains in its infancy. However, peptide analogues are proving to be increasingly useful in the diagnosis and treatment of GI disease. An analogue of gastrin, pentagastrin, has become the agent of choice for gastric acid secretory tests, largely replacing histamine.[164] The synthetic octapeptide of CCK has proved to be a useful agent with which to stimulate contraction of the gallbladder in radiologic and ultrasound testing of gallbladder function. Secretin is a useful agent in pancreatic function tests and in provocative testing to diagnose gastrinoma.[164] Glucagon, because of its ability to relax smooth muscle, has found a widespread use in the endoscopy field to relax spastic regions of the colon, thereby allowing passage of the endoscope.[164] Relaxation of the duodenum with glucagon also aids cannulation of the pancreatic and bile duct during endoscopic retrograde cholangiopancreatography. Finally, the recent development of a potent somatostatin octreotide analogue has proved to be a milestone in gut endocrinology because it represents the first effective therapeutic agent derived from a natural gut peptide.[116] As mentioned earlier, this analogue markedly reduces symptoms in patients with metastatic carcinoids and can abolish the often incapacitating watery diarrhea seen in VIPoma patients.

The future of gastrointestinal endocrinology should bring a clearer understanding of the role of brain–gut peptides in the control of normal gut function and a delineation of their role in disease. The development of specific antagonists, such as those developed for CCK,[165] will prove to be a powerful tool to delineate physiologic function of individual peptides.

The reader is directed to Chapter 1, The Enteric Nervous System and its Extrinsic Connections; Chapter 3, The Brain–Gut Axis; Chapter 62, Zollinger–Ellison Syndrome; Chapter 91, Endocrine Neoplasms of the Pancreas.

REFERENCES

1. Bayliss WM, Starling EH. On the causation of the so called "peripheral reflex secretion of the pancreas." Proc R Soc Lond [Biol] 1902;69:352.
2. Edkins JS. On the chemical mechanisms of gastric secretion. Proc R Soc Lond [Biol] 1905;76:376.
3. Mutt V, Jorpes E. Hormonal polypeptides of the upper intestine. Biochem J 1971;125:57P.
4. Harper AA, Raper HS. Pancreozymin, a stimulant of the secretion of pancreatic enzymes in extracts of the small intestine. J Physiol 1943;102:115.
5. Mutt V. Hormonal peptides. In: Fidia Research Foundation Neuroscience Award Lectures, Vol 3. New York: Raven Press, 1989: 125.
6. Gregory RA, Tracy HJ. The constitution and properties of two gastrins extracted from hog antral mucosa. Gut 1964;5:103.
7. Mutt V, Jorpes J, Magnusson S. Structure of porcine secretin: The amino acid sequence. Eur J Biochem 1970;15:513.
8. Mutt V, Jorpes JE. Structure of porcine cholecystokinin—Pancreozymin. Eur J Biochem 1968;6:156.
9. Ellis J. Why is genetic engineering important and how has it come about. In: Murrell JC, Roberts LM, eds. Understanding genetic engineering. Chichester, England: Ellis Harwood, 1989:9.
10. Noyes B, Mearech M, Stein R, Agarwal K. Detection and partial sequence analysis of gastrin mRNA by using an oligodeoxynucleotide probe. Proc Natl Acad Sci USA 1979;76:1770.
11. Yoo O, Parel C, Agarwal K. Molecular cloning and nucleotide sequence of full-length cDNA coding for porcine gastrin. Proc Natl Acad Sci USA 1982;79:1049.
12. Weidmann M, Kurzchalia TV, Hartmann E, Rapoport TA. A signal sequence receptor in the endoplasmic reticulum. Nature 1987;328: 830.

13. Gubler U, Seeburg P, Hoffman BJ, Gage LP, Udenfriend S. Molecular cloning established pre-enkephalin as precursor of enkephalin containing peptides. Nature 1982;295:206.

14. Itoh N, Obata K-I, Yanaihara N, Okamoto H. Human pre-provasoactive intestinal polypeptide contains a novel PHI-27 like peptide, PHM-27. Nature 1983;304:547.

15. Tager HS, Steiner DF. Isolation of a glucagon containing peptide: Enteroglucagon primary structure of a possible fragment of proglucagon. Proc Natl Acad Sci USA 1973;70:2321.

16. Walsh JH. Gastrointestinal hormones. In: Johnson LR, ed. Physiology of the gastro-intestinal tract. New York: Raven Press, 1987:181.

17. Bradbury AF, Smyth DG. Enzyme-catalyzed peptide amidation. Eur J Biochem 1987;169:579.

18. Tatemoto K, Mutt V. Isolation of two novel candidate hormones using a chemical method for finding naturally occurring polypeptides. Nature 1980;285:417.

19. Feyrter F. Uber die These von den peripheren endokrinen (parakrinen). Drusen Acta Neurareg 1952;4:409.

20. Cuttilta F, Carney DN, Mulshine J, Moody TW, Fedorko J, Fischler A, Minna JD. Bombesin-like peptides can function as autocrine growth factors in human small cell–like CA. Nature 1985;316:823.

21. Taylor IL. The pancreatic polypeptide family: Pancreatic polypeptide, neuropeptide Y, and peptide YY. In: Makhlouf GM, ed. Handbook of physiology—The gastrointestinal system. II. Bethesda: American Physiology Society, 1989:476.

22. Lynch DR, Snyder S. Neuropeptides: Multiple molecular forms, metabolic pathways and receptors. Annu Rev Biochem 1986;55:773.

23. Read NW, McFarlane A, Kinsman RI, Bates TE, Blackhall NW, Farrar GBJ, Hall JC, Moss G, Morris AP, O'Neill B, Welch I, Lee Y, Bloom SR. Effect of infusion of nutrient solutions into the ileum and gastrointestinal transit and plasma levels of neurotensin and enteroglucagon. Gastroenterology 1983;86:274.

24. Pappas TN, Chang AM, Debas HT, Taylor IL. Peptide YY release by fatty acids is sufficient to inhibit gastric emptying in dogs. Gastroenterology 1986;91:1386.

25. Sundler F, Ekblad E, Hakanson R. Projections of enteric peptide-containing neurons in the fat. Arch Histol Cytol 1989;52(Suppl):181.

26. Pernaw J, Schwieler J, Kahan T, Kjemdahl P, Oberle J, Wallin BG, Lundberg JM. Influence of sympathetic discharge pattern on norepinephrine and neuropeptide Y release. Am J Physiol 1989;257:H866.

27. Neer EJ, Clopham DE. Roles of G protein subunits in transmembrane signalling. Nature 1988;333:129.

28. Berridge MS. Inositol trisphosphate and diacylglycerol: Two interesting second messengers. Annu Rev Biochem 1987;56:159.

29. Nishizuka Y. The molecular heterogeneity of protein kinase C and its implications for cellular regulations. Nature 1988;334:661.

30. Garner JD, Jensen RT. Cell membrane receptors for secretagogues on pancreatic acinar cells. In: Mutt V, ed. Advances in metabolic disorders, Vol II. New York: Academic Press, 1988:113.

31. Stevens CF. Channel families in the brain. Nature 1987;328:198.

32. Goldstein JL, Brown MS, Anderson RGW, Russell DW, Schneider WI. Receptor-mediated endocytosis: Concepts emerging from the LDL receptor system. Annu Rev Cell Biol 1985;1:1.

33. Sporn MB, Roberts AB. Peptide growth factors are growth multifunctional. Nature 1988;332:217.

34. Yalow RS, Berson SA. Immunoassay of endogenous plasma insulin in man. J Clin Invest 1960;39:1157.

35. Rehfeld JF. Radioimmunoassay problems for gut hormones in the eighties. In: Mutt V, ed. Advances in metabolic disorders, Vol II. New York: Academic Press, 1988:45.

36. Dockray G, Gregory R, Hutchison J. Isolation, structure, and biological activity of cholecystokinin octapeptides from sheep brain. Nature 1978;274:711.

37. Liddle R, Goldfine I, Williams J. Bioassay of plasma cholecystokinin in rats: Effects of food, trypsin inhibitor, and alcohol. Gastroenterology 1984;7:542.

38. Bishop AE, Bloom SR, Polak JM. Cytochemical techniques in work with gastrointestinal hormones. In: Mutt V, ed. Advances in metabolic disorders, Vol II. New York: Academic Press, 1988:11.

39. Dockray G, Walsh J. Amino terminal gastrin fragment in serum of Zollinger–Ellison syndrome patients. Gastroenterology 1975;68:222.

40. Sugano K, Aponte G, Yamada T. Identification and extended characterization of glycine-extended post-translational processing intermediates of progastrin in porcine stomach. J Biol Chem 1985;260:11724.

41. Dockray GJ, Taylor IL. Heptadecapeptide gastrin: Measurement in blood by specific radioimmunoassay. Gastroenterology 1977;71:971.

42. Walsh J, Isenberg J, Ansfield J, Maxwell V. Clearance and acid-stimulating action of human big and little gastrins in duodenal ulcer patients. J Clin Invest 1976;57:1125.

43. Solcia E, Capella C, Buffa R. Endocrine cells of the digestive system. In: Johnson LR, ed. Physiology of the gastrointestinal tract. New York: Raven Press, 1987:111.

44. Brand S, Anderson B, Rehfeld J. Complete tyrosine-O-sulphation of gastrin in neonatal pancreas. Nature 1984;309:456.

45. Dockray GJ, Gregory RA. Gastrin. In: Makhlouf GM, ed. Handbook of physiology and the gastrointestinal system. New York: Oxford University Press, American Physiology Society, 1989:311.

46. Taylor IL, Byrne N, Christie D, Ament M, Walsh JH. Effect of individual L-amino acids on gastric acid secretion and serum gastrin and pancreatic polypeptide release in humans. Gastroenterology 1982;83:273.

47. Feldman E, Isenberg J, Grossman M. Gastric acid and gastrin responses to decaffeinated coffee and a peptone meal. JAMA 1981;246:248.

48. Lenz HJ, Ferrari-Taylor J, Isenberg J. Wine and five percent ethanol are potent stimulants of gastric acid secretion in humans. Gastroenterology 1983;85:1082.

49. Walsh J, Maxwell V, Ferrari J, Varner A. Bombesin stimulates human gastric function by gastrin-dependent and independent mechanisms. Peptides 1981;2:193.

50. Creutzfeldt W, Arnold R. Somatostatin and the stomach. Exocrine and endocrine aspects. Metabolism 1978;27:1309.

51. Larson T, Sanchez J, Taylor IL. Bombesin induced tachyphylaxis markedly enhances gastrin release to a meal. Am J Physiol 1983;244:G652.

52. Feldman M, Richardson CT, Taylor I, Walsh JH. Effect of atropine on vagal release of gastrin and pancreatic polypeptide. J Clin Invest 1979;63:294.

53. Chan CB, Soll AH. Role of the cholinergic nervous system in acid secretion. Pharmacology 1988;37:17.

54. Walsh J, Debas H, Grossman M. Pure human big gastrin. Immunochemical properties, disappearance half time and acid-stimulating action in dogs. J Clin Invest 1984;54:477.

55. Strunz U, Walsh J, Grossman M. Removal of gastrin by various organs in dogs. Gastroenterology 1978;67:551.

56. Power DM, Bunnett N, Turner AJ, Dimaline R. Degradation of endogenous heptacapeptide gastrin by endopeptides 24:11 in the pig. Am J Physiol 1987;253:G33.

57. Walsh J, Laster L. Enzymatic deamidation of the C-terminal tetrapeptide amide of gastrin by mammalian tissues. Biochem Med 1973;8:432.

58. Gregory RA. Gastrin. In: Mutt V, ed. Advances in metabolic disorders, Vol II. New York: Academic Press, 1988:163.

59. Johnson LR. The trophic action of gastrointestinal hormones. Gastroenterology 1976;70:278.

60. Soll AH, Berglindh T. Physiology of isolated gastric glands and parietal cells: Receptors and effectors regulating function. In: Johnson LR, ed. Physiology of the gastrointestinal tract. New York: Raven Press, 1987:883.

61. Deschenes R, Lorenz L, Haun R, Roos B, Collier K, Dixon J. Cloning and sequence analysis of cDNA encoding rat prepro-cholecystokinin. Proc Natl Acad Sci USA 1984;81:726.

62. Mutt V. Cholecystokinin: Isolation structure and functions. In: Glass GBJ, ed. Gastrointestinal hormones. New York: Raven Press, 1980:169.

63. Lu L, Louie D, Owyang C. A cholecystokinin releasing peptide mediates feedback regulation of pancreatic secretin. Am J Physiol 1989;256:G430.

64. Iwai K, Fukuoka S, Fushiki T et al. Purification and sequencing of a trypsin-sensitive cholecystokinin-releasing peptide from rat pancreatic juice. Its homology with pancreatic secretory trypsin inhibitor. J Biol Chem 1987;262:8956.

65. Sakamoto T, Fujimura M, Newman J, Zhu X-G, Greiley G,

Thompson J. Comparison of hepatic elimination of different forms of cholecystokinin in dogs. J Clin Invest 1985;75:280.

66. Doyle HR, Lluis F, Rayford PL. Secretin. In: Thompson JC, ed. Gastrointestinal endocrinology. New York: McGraw-Hill, 1987:223.

67. Chey W, Lee Y, Hendricks J, Rhodes R, Tai H-H. Plasma secretin concentration in fasted and postprandial state in man. Am J Dig Dis 1978;28:981.

68. Chey WP, Kim MS, Lec KY, et al. Effect of rabbit anti-secretin serum on post-prandial secretion in dogs. Gastroenterology 1979;77:1268.

69. Chey W, Kim M, Lee K, Chang T. Secretin is an enterogastrone in the dog. Am J Physiol 1981;240:G239.

70. Isenberg J, Wallin B, Johansson C, Smedfors B, Mutt V, Tatemoto K, Emas S. Secretin, VIP, and PHI stimulate rat proximal duodenal surface epithelial bicarbonate secretion in vivo. Regul Pept 1984;8:315.

71. Jornvall H, Carlquist M, Kwank S, Otte SC, McIntosh CHS, Brown JC, Mutt V. Amino acid sequence and heterogeneity of gastric inhibitory polypeptide (GIP). FEBS Lett 1981;123:205.

72. Khalil T, Aluder G, Rayford PL. Gastric inhibitory polypeptide. In: Thompson JC, ed. Gastrointestinal endocrinology. New York: McGraw-Hill, 1987:248.

73. Kuzio M, Dryburgh J, Malloy K, Brown J. Radioimmunoassay for gastric inhibitory polypeptide. Gastroenterology 1974;66:357.

74. Rogers W, O'Dorisio T, Johnson S, Cataland S, Stradley R, Sherding R. Postprandial release of gastric inhibitory polypeptide and pancreatic polypeptide in dogs with pancreatic acinar atrophy. Correction of blunted GIP response by addition of pancreatic enzymes to a meal. Dig Dis Sci 1983;28:345.

75. Anderson D, Elahi D, Brown J, Tobin J, Andres R. Oral glucose augmentation of insulin secretion. Interactions of gastric inhibitory polypeptide with ambient glucose and insulin levels. J Clin Invest 1978;62:152.

76. Mutt V, Said SI. Structure of the porcine vasoactive intestinal octacosa peptide. Eur J Biochem 1974;42:581.

77. Said SI. Vasoactive intestinal peptide. In: Mutt V, ed. Advances in metabolic disorders, Vol II. New York: Academic Press, 1988:369.

78. Fahrenkrug J. Vasoactive intestinal peptide. In: Makhlouf GM, ed. Handbook of physiology: The gastrointestinal system. New York: Oxford University Press, American Physiology Society, 1989:611.

79. Bloom SR, Yiangou-Y, Polak JM. Vasoactive intestinal peptide secreting tumor. Pathophysiological and clinical correlations. Ann NY Acad Sci 1988;527:518.

80. Lund P, Goodman R, Dee P, Habener J. Pancreatic proglucagon cDNA contains two glucagon-related coding sequences arranged in tandem. Proc Natl Acad Sci USA 1982;79:343.

81. Conlon JM. Proglucagon-derived peptides: Nomenclature, biosynthetic relationships and physiological roles. Diabetologia 1988;31:563.

82. Buchan AMJ, Griffiths CJ, Morris JF, et al. Enteroglucagon cell hyperfunction in rat small intestine after gut resection. Gastroenterology 1985;88:8.

83. Fehmann HC, Goke B, Goke R, Traulman ME, Arnold B. Synergistic stimulatory effect of glucagon-like peptide-1 (7-36) amide and glucose-dependent insulin-releasing polypeptide on the endocrine rat pancreas. FEBS Lett 1989;252(1-2):109.

84. Kimmel J, Hayden LJ, Pollock HG. Isolation and characterization of a new pancreatic polypeptide hormone. J Biol Chem 1975;250:9369.

85. Chance RE, Moon NE, Johnson MG. Human pancreatic polypeptide (HPP) and bovine pancreatic polypeptide (BPP). In: Jaffee BM, Behman HR, eds. Methods of hormone radioimmunoassay. New York: Academic Press, 1979:657.

86. Blundell TL, Pitts JE, Tickle IJ, Wood SP, Wu CW. X-ray analysis (1.4 A resolution) of avian pancreatic polypeptide: Small globular protein hormone. Proc Natl Acad Sci USA 1981;78:4175.

87. Noelken ME, Chang PJ, Kimmel JR. Conformation and association of pancreatic polypeptide from three species. Biochemistry 1980;19:1838.

88. Leiter AB, Keutmann HT, Goodman RH. Structure of a precursor to human pancreatic polypeptide gene defines functional domains of the precursor. J Biol Chem 1985;260:13013.

89. Minth CD, Bloom SR, Polak JM, Dixon JE. Cloning, characterization,

and DNA sequence of a human cDNA encoding neuropeptide tyrosine. Proc Natl Acad Sci USA 1984;81:4577.

90. Leiter AB, Toder A, Wolfe HJ, Taylor IL, Cooperman S, Mandel G, Goodman RH. Peptide YY, structure of the precursor and expression in exocrine pancreas. J Biol Chem 1987;262:129.

91. Schwartz JW. Pancreatic polypeptide: A hormone under vagal control. Gastroenterology 85:1411-1425, 1983.

92. Taylor IL, Feldman M. Effect of cephalic-vagal stimulation on insulin, gastric inhibitory polypeptide, and pancreatic polypeptide release in humans. J Clin Endocrinol Metab 1982;55:1114.

93. Taylor IL, Solomon TE, Walsh HH, Grossman MI. Pancreatic polypeptide: Metabolism and effect on pancreatic secretion in dogs. Gastroenterology 1979;76:524.

94. Louie DS, Williams JA, Owyang C. Action of pancreatic polypeptide on rat pancreatic secretion: In vivo and in vitro. Am J Physiol 1985;249:G489.

95. Sun YS, Brunicardi FC, Druck P, Walfisch S, Berlin SA, Chance RE, Gingerich RL, Elahi D, Andersen DK. Reversal of abnormal glucose metabolism in chronic pancreatitis by administration of pancreatic polypeptide. Am J Surg 1986;151:130.

96. Allen JM, Bloom SR. Neuropeptide Y: A putative neurotransmitter. Neurochem Int 1986;8:1.

97. Lundberg JM, Terenius L, Hokfelt T, Goldstein M. High levels of neuropeptide Y in peripheral noradrenergic neurons in various mammals including man. Neurosci Lett 1983;42:167.

98. Hellstrom PM, Olerup O, Tatemoto K. Neuropeptide Y may mediate effects of sympathetic nerve stimulations on colonic motility and blood flow in the cat. Acta Physiol Scand 1985;124:613.

99. Dahlof C, Dahlof P, Lundberg JM. Neuropeptide Y (NPY): Enhancement of blood pressure increase upon alpha-adrenoceptor activation and direct pressor effects in pithed rats. Eur J Pharmacol 1985;109:289.

100. Tatemoto K. Isolation and characterization of peptide YY (PYY), a candidate gut hormone that inhibits pancreatic exocrine secretion. Proc Natl Acad Sci USA 1982;79:2514.

101. Taylor IL. Distribution and release of peptide YY in dog meal measured by specific radioimmunoassay. Gastroenterology 1985;88:731.

102. Pappas TN, Debas HT, Taylor IL. Peptide YY: Metabolism and effect on pancreatic secretion in dog. Gastroenterology 1985;89:1387.

103. Pappas TN, Debas HT, Taylor IL. The enterogastrone-like effect of peptide YY is vagally mediated in the dog. J Clin Invest 1986;77:49.

104. Hughes J, Smith TW, Kosterlitz HW, Fothergill LA, Morgan BA, Morris HR. Identification of two related pentapeptides from the brain with potent opiate agonist activity. Nature 1975;258:577.

105. Rossier J. Opioid peptides have found their roots. Nature 1982;298:221.

106. Terenius L, Hokfelt T. Opioid peptides in the gastrointestinal tract. In: Mutt V, ed. Advances in metabolic disorders, Vol II. New York: Academic Press, 1988:493.

107. Lord JAH, Waterfield AA, Hughes J, Kosterlitz HW. Endogenous opioid peptides: Multiple agonists and receptors. Nature 1977;267:495.

108. Smith AP, Lee NM. Pharmacology of dynorphin. Annu Rev Pharmacol Toxicol 1988;28:123.

109. Burgess R, Ling N, Butcher M, Guillemin R. Primary structure of somatostatin, a hypothalamic peptide that inhibits the secretion of pituitary growth hormone. Proc Natl Acad Sci USA 1973;70:684.

110. Lucey MR, Yamada T. Biochemistry and physiology of gastrointestinal somatostatin. Dig Dis Sci 1989;34:55.

111. Shen L-P, Rutter W. Sequence of the human somatostatin gene. Science 1984;224:168.

112. Naylor S, Sakaguchi A, Shen LP, Bell G, Rutter W, Shows T. Polymorphic human somatostatin gene is located on chromosome 3. Proc Natl Acad Sci USA 1983;80:2686.

113. Soll AH, Yamada T, Park J, Thomas LP. Somatostatin-like immunoreactivity from canine fundic mucosal cells in primary culture. Am J Physiol 1985;248:G184.

114. Chayvialle JA, Miyata M, Rayford PL, Thompson JC. Effects of intestinal, intragastric nutrients, and intraduodenal bile on plasma concentrates of immunoreactive somatostatin and vasoactive intestinal peptide in dogs. Gastroenterology 1980;79:844.

115. Saffouri B, Weir GC, Bitar KN, Makhlouf GM. Gastrin and so-

matostatin secretion by perfused rat stomach: Functional linkage of antral peptides. Am J Physiol 1980095.

116. O'Dorisio TM, Gaginella TS, Mekhjian HS, Rao B, O'Dorisio MS. Somatostatin and analogues in the treatment of vipoma. Ann NY Acad Sci USA 1988;527:528.

117. Brown J, Cook M, Dryburgh J. Motilin, a gastric motor activity stimulating polypeptide: The complete amino acid sequence. Can J Biochem 1973;51:533.

118. McIntosh CHS, Brown JC. Motilin. In: Mutt V, ed. Advances in metabolic disorders, Vol II. New York: Academic Press, 1988:439.

119. Itoh Z, Takeuchi S, Aizawa I, Mori K, Taminato T, Seino Y, Imura H, Yanaihara N. Changes in plasma motilin concentrations and gastrointestinal contractile activity in conscious dogs. Dig Dis 1978;23:929.

120. Itoh Z, Honda R, Hiwatashi K, Takeuchi S, Aizawa I, Takayananagi R, Couch E. Motilin-induced mechanical activity in the canine alimentary tract. Scand J Gastroenterol 1976;39(Suppl II):93.

121. Kondo Y, Torii K, Omura S, Itoh Z. Erythromycin and its derivatives with motilin-like biological activities inhibit the specific binding of motilin to duodenal muscle. Biochem Biophys Res Commun 1988;150:877.

122. Chang MM, Leeman SE, Niall HD. Amino-acid sequence of substance P. Nature 1971;232:86.

123. Walker JP, Thompson JC. Substance P. In: Thompson JC, ed. Gastrointestinal endocrinology. New York: McGraw-Hill, 1987:317.

124. Pearse AGE, Polak JM. Immunocytochemical localization of substance P in mammalian intestine. Histochemistry 1975;41:373.

125. Inverson LL. Substance P. Br Med Bull 1982;38:277.

126. Carraway R, Leeman SE. The isolation of a new hypotensive peptide, neurotensin, from bovine hypothalami. J Biol Chem 1973;248:6854.

127. Ferris CF. Neurotensin. In: Makhlouf GM, ed. Handbook of physiology-The gastrointestinal system. American Physiology Society 1989;559.

128. Thompson JC, Greeley GH Jr, Rayford TL, et al, eds. Neurotensin. In: Thompson JC, ed. Gastrointestinal endocrinology. New York: McGraw-Hill, 1987:300.

129. Olsen PS, Pedersen JH, Kirkegaard P, et al. Neurotensin inhibits meal-stimulated gastric acid secretion in man. Scand J Gastroenterol 1983;18:1073.

130. McDonald TJ, Jornvall H, Tatemoto K, et al. Identification and characterization of variant forms of the gastrin-releasing peptide (GRP). FEBS Lett 1983;156:349.

131. Greeley GH Jr, Newman J. Enteric bombesin-like peptides. In: Thompson JC, ed. Gastrointestinal endocrinology. New York: McGraw-Hill, 1987:322.

132. Walsh JH, Wong HC, Dockray GJ. Bombesin-like peptides in mammals. Fed Proc 1979;38:2315.

133. Miyata M, Rayford PL, Thompson JC. Hormonal and secretory effects of bombesin and duodenal acidification in dogs. Surgery 1981;87:209.

134. Stein LJ, Woods SC. Cholecystokinin and bombesin act independently to decrease food intake in the rat. Peptides 1981;1:431.

135. Tache Y, Marki W, Rivier J, et al. Central nervous system effect inhibition of gastrin secretion in the rat by gastrin-releasing peptide, a mammalian bombesin. Gastroenterology 1981;81:298.

136. Moody TW, Komn LY. The release of bombesin-like peptides from small cell lung cancer cells. Ann NY Acad Sci 1988;547:351.

137. Gregory RA. A new method for the preparation of urogastrone. J Physiol 1955;129:528.

138. Cohen S. Isolation of a mouse submaxillary gland protein growth accelerating incisor eruption and eyelid opening in the newborn animal. J Biol Chem 1962;237:1555.

139. Goodlad RA, Wright NA. Peptides and epithelial growth regulation. Experientia 1989;56(Suppl):180.

140. Walker JP, Townsend CM. Epidermal growth factor/urogastrone. In: Thompson JC, ed. Gastrointestinal endocrinology. New York: McGraw-Hill, 1981:337

141. Konturek SJ, Cieszkowski M, Joworek J, et al. Effects of epidermal growth factor on gastrointestinal secretions. Am J Physiol 1984;246:G580.

142. Tatemoto K, Enfedic S, Mutt V, Makk G, Feinster GJ, Barchas JD. Pancreastatin, a novel pancreatic peptide that inhibits insulin secretion. Nature 1986;324:476.

143. Nakano I, Funakoshi A, Miyasaka K, Ishida K, Makk G, Angwin P, Chang D, Tatemoto K. Isolation and characterization of bovine pancreastatin. Regul Pept 1989;25:207.

144. Konechi DS, Benedum UM, Gerdes HH, Huttner WB. The primary structure of human chromogranin A and pancreastatin. J Biol Chem 1987;262:17026.

145. Kar S, Bretherton-Watt D, Gibson SJ, Steel JH, Gentleman SM, Roberts GW, Valentino K, Tatemoto K, Ghatei MA, Bloom SR, Polak JM. Novel peptide pancreastatin: Its occurrence and codistribution with chromogranin A in the central nervous system of the pig. J Comp Neurol 1989;288:627.

146. Schmidt WE, Siegel EG, Lamberts R, Gallwitz B, Creutzfeldt W. Pancreastatin: Molecular and immunocytochemical characterization of a novel peptide in porcine and human tissues. Endocrinology 1988;123,1395.

147. Ishizuka J, Asada I, Poston GJ, Lluis F, Tatemoto K, Greeley GH, Thompson JC. Effect of pancreastatin on pancreatic endocrine and exocrine secretion. Pancreas 1989;4:277.

148. Funakoshi A, Miyasaka K, Nakamura R, Kitani K, Tatemoto K. Inhibitory effect of pancreastatin on pancreatic exocrine secretion in the conscious rat. Regul Pept 1989;25:157.

149. Funakoshi A, Miyasaka K, Nakamura R, Kitani K, Funakoshi S, Tamamura H, Fujii N, Yajima H. Bioactivity of synthetic human pancreastatin on exocrine pancreas. Biochem Biophys Res Commun 1988;156:1237.

150. Funakoshi A, Mimi A, Yasunami Y, Tateishi K, Funakoshi F, Tamamura H, Yajima H. Bioactivity of human pancreastatin and its localization in pancreas. Biochem Biophys Res Commun 1989;159:913.

151. Lewis JH, Zdon MJ, Adrian TE, Modlin IM. Pancreastatin: A novel peptide inhibitor of parietal cell secretion. Surgery 1988;104:1031.

152. DelValle J, Debas H, Tatemoto K, Yamada T. Pancreastatin directly inhibits gastric parietal cell activity. Gastroenterology 1987;92:1368.

153. Tatemoto K, Rokaeus A, Jornvall H, McDonald T, Mutt V. Galanin—A novel biologically active peptide from porcine intestine. FEBS Lett 1983;164:124.

154. Rokaeus A, Melander T, Hökfelt T, Lundberg JM, Tatemoto K, Carlquist M, Mutt V. A galanin-like peptide in the central nervous system and intestine of the rat. Neurosci Lett 1984;47:161.

155. Ekblad E, Rokaeus A, Hakanson R, Sundler F. Galanin nerve fibers in the rat gut: Distribution, origin and projections. Neuroscience 1985;16:355.

156. Dunning BE, Ahren B, Beith RC, Boettcher G, Sundler F, Taborsky GJ. Galanin: A novel pancreatic neuropeptide. Am J Physiol 1986;251:E127.

157. Furness JB, Costa M, Rokaeus A, McDonald TJ, Brooks B. Galanin—Immunoreactive neurons in the guinea-pig small intestine: Their projections and relationships to other enteric neurons. Cell Tissue Res 1987;250:607.

158. Rattan S, Goyal RK. Effect of galanin on the opossum lower esophageal sphincter. Life Sci 1987;41:2783.

159. Soldani G, Mengozzi G, Della Longa A, Intorre L, Martelli F, Brown DR. An analysis of the effects of galanin on gastric acid secretion and plasma levels of gastrin in the dog. Eur J Pharmacol 1988;154:313.

160. Ahren B, Andren-Sandberg A, Nilsson A. Galanin inhibits amylase secretion from isolated rat pancreatic acini. Pancreas 1988;3:559.

161. McDonald TJ, Dupre J, Tatemoto K, et al. Galanin inhibits insulin secretion and induces hyperglycemia in dogs. Diabetes 1985;34:192.

162. Leppaluoto J, Koivusala F, Kraama R. Thyrotropin-releasing factor: Distribution in neural and gastrointestinal tissues. Acta Physiol Scand 1978;104:175.

163. Fujimura M, Hancock MB, Cooper CW, et al. Immunocytochemical localization of calcitonin gene related peptide in pancreatic islet cells of the rat. Gastroenterology 1985;88:1390.

164. Walsh JH, Taylor IL. Pharmacology of gastrointestinal hormones. In: Bevan JA, Thomsen JH, eds. Essentials of pharmacology. Scranton: Rinehart, Harper and Row, 1983:530.

165. Liddle RA, Gertz BJ, Kanayama S, Beccaria L, Gettys TW, Taylor IL, Rushakoff RJ, Williams VC, Coker LD. Regulation of pancreatic endocrine functions by cholecystokinin. Studies with MK-239, a nonpeptide cholecystokinin receptor antagonist. J Clin Endocrinol Metab 1990;70:1312.

3

The Brain–Gut Axis

DAVID L. WINGATE
WENDY R. EWART

TWO NERVOUS SYSTEMS

The traditional concept of the neural control of the gut is similar to the concept of neural control of other body systems, which is that the property of control resides within the central nervous system (CNS) and is mediated through efferent nerves that connect the brain to the effector system. Within this framework, it has long been recognized that smooth muscle organs have a dual innervation, one being excitatory and the other inhibitory, and that this is necessary because smooth muscle exhibits spontaneous contractility that is tonic or phasic or both. For the digestive tract, it has been assumed that the parasympathetic (cholinergic) nerves are excitatory and the sympathetic (adrenergic) nerves are inhibitory; these two divisions were recognized many years ago by Langley[1] in his description of the autonomic nervous system (Fig 3-1A).

Langley, however, postulated a third division of the autonomic nervous system, the enteric division (Fig 3-1B). Although it seemed likely that the enteric division was responsible for the peristaltic reflex first described by Bayliss and Starling,[2] little attention was paid to the enteric nerves for many years, perhaps because there was a lack of experimental techniques that could be used to explore their function. Interest in the enteric nerves, comprising the intrinsic nerve plexuses of the gut wall, was awakened 3 decades later, in the 1960s, by the demonstration of enteric neural activity that was not blocked by either adrenergic or cholinergic antagonists—the nonadrenergic noncholinergic (NANC) nerves. This essentially negative description of enteric nerves did not survive for long, because the subsequent explosive growth of peptide chemistry and pharmacology, and of immunohistochemistry, has led to the positive identification of populations of enteric neurons characterized by different morphologies, different functions, and distinct neurochemistry.

We now recognize Langley's "enteric division" of the autonomic nervous system as the enteric nervous system (ENS).[3–5] It is a system of considerable complexity, composed of two principal layers that invest the entire digestive tube from esophagus to anus. The exact number of neurons in the human ENS is unknown, but estimates range from 10 million to 100 million; the ENS is said to have a neuronal population equivalent to that of the spinal cord. It was Langley who originally realized that the number of vagal efferent fibers (in humans, about 10,000) is very much less than the number of enteric neurons and that vagal commands must be mediated through enteric neurons; in other words, the autonomic nerves affect the gut by modulating the activity of the ENS rather than by direct innervation of gut effector systems.

It is now clear that the ENS differs from other divisions of the peripheral nervous system not only in its complexity but also in its autonomy. It responds to changes within the gut lumen by the initiation of coordinated programs of function that are appropriate to the altered conditions; of these programs the most prominent is the periodic activity of the gut, of which the motor component is the migrating motor complex (MMC).[6] Because of this autonomy, the ENS is considered to be the "gut brain"; the control that it exerts over the gut is analogous to the control that the CNS exerts over locomotor and behavioral activity.

The *brain–gut axis* refers to the functional connections between the CNS and ENS. This is not, as was once believed, merely the way in which the CNS controls an effector system; on the contrary, given the new perspectives on ENS function, the brain–gut axis has to be considered as the interaction between two autonomous control systems. At first sight, the gross morphologic disparities between the ENS and the CNS suggests that the notion that the two systems are in some way equivalent is mildly ludicrous. The control centers of the CNS are highly differentiated, with easily defined structural locations within a system that is anatomically condensed within a protected environment, and connected to effector systems through long and well-defined fiber tracts. In contrast, the ENS is diffuse with its neuronal elements in intimate relationship to the entire effector system; it appears to lack control centers for specific functions. If the CNS is like an egg in its shell, then the ENS resembles the filling in a sandwich; the former is a discrete structure, while the latter is no more than a layer. Yet appearances are deceptive, for there are important homologies between the two systems.

Structural Affinities Between the CNS and ENS

The ENS and the cerebral cortex share morphologic features that are not found in other parts of the nervous system. In both tissues, there is a reticular pattern of short fiber tracts between cell bodies. Glial cells are common to both; neurons and glial cells share a common embryonic origin that, in the case of the ENS, is the neural crest.[7] In both, neurons have short axons and dense synaptic

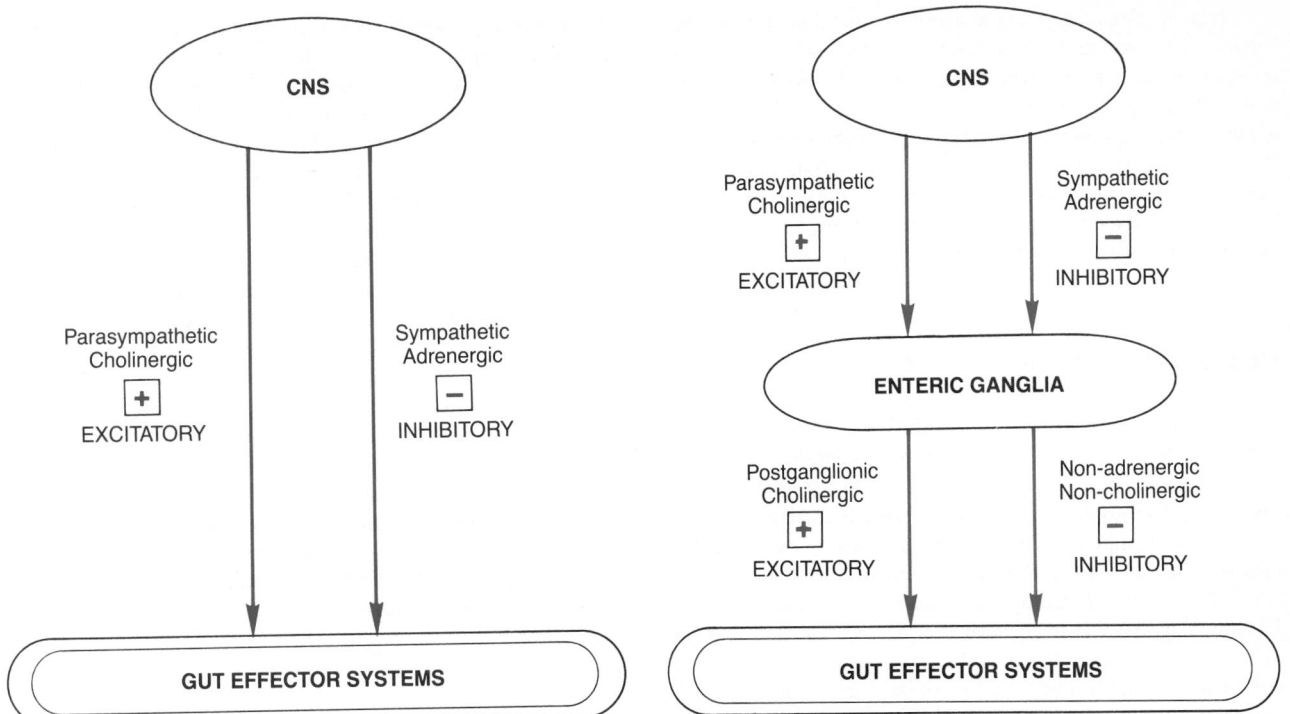

FIGURE 3–1. **A,** Classic concept of the efferent control of the gut by the central nervous system. According to this concept, gut effectors (e.g., smooth muscle, secretory cells) are directly innervated by the autonomic outflow from the CNS. **B,** With the discovery of the postganglionic nonadrenergic, noncholinergic (NANC) innervation of the gut, it was appreciated that it is the enteric ganglia, rather than the actual effector units, that are innervated by the autonomic outflow from the CNS.

neuropil, reflecting complex neuronal interactions. In both systems there appears to be a diffusion barrier between nerve tissue and blood; the blood–brain barrier of the CNS is paralleled by an apparent diffusion barrier in the structure of the enteric ganglia.

Chemical Affinities Between the CNS and ENS

The digestive tract is richer in neuropeptides, both in quantity and variety, than any other tissue outside the brain.[8] What is perhaps more remarkable is that the same species of neuropeptide seem to be shared between the CNS and ENS. Among the neuropeptides identified in both tissues are the opioids, somatostatin, cholecystokinin, and substance P. In addition, 5-hydroxytryptamine (5-HT) appears to act as a neurotransmitter in both the ENS[3] and the CNS. In the ENS, distinct populations of neurons have been identified by their neuropeptide content; specific combinations of neuropeptides appear to act as chemical codes.[8] The ENS, being essentially a monolayer, is more easily studied in this way; it is likely that CNS neurons will prove to possess similar attributes.

Functional Affinities Between the CNS and ENS

The functional similarities between the ENS and CNS are evident from both their integrated activity and their electrophysiology.

Neurons in both systems possess the property of altering their excitability with slow postsynaptic potentials that may be either excitatory with a lowered membrane potential or inhibitory with a raised membrane potential. This property confers considerable plasticity of function; the transmission of excitation through a neuronal network can thus be modulated by other neurons or by paracrine or even humoral chemical modulation.

At a higher level of integration, both systems are characterized by the phenomenon of periodicity in the absence of a sensory input; remarkably, in humans at least, these biorhythms have a similar periodicity of approximately 90 minutes. This is manifest in the gut as periodic motor and secretory activity[6] and in the CNS by the sleep cycle; in the former, maximal excitation is signaled by phase III of the MMC and in the latter by the phase of rapid eye movement (REM) sleep. There are differences as well as similarities that underline the absence of structural differentiation within the ENS. In the cerebral cortex, periodicity is synchronous in all areas, whereas within the ENS periodic cycle, different parts of the system will be in different phases of the cycle. Thus, all phases of periodic activity (phases I, II, and III) coexist within different regions of the small intestine at the same time.

At the level of integrated control, the role of the CNS in the regulation of locomotor activity and behavior is clearly established. It is not so well recognized that the ENS has similar functions in relation to the digestive tract, being responsible for the programmed activities seen in fasting and in response to food. The ENS also controls the motor response to noxious stimuli, in the form of adynamic ileus, and the gastrointestinal motor events that precede voiding either as vomiting or defecation.

Adynamic ileus highlights a significant functional difference between the two systems. Reference has already been made to the spontaneous activity of gastrointestinal smooth muscle, implying that control of gastrointestinal smooth muscle is inhibitory. Ileus is thus active inhibition and is in no way analogous to paresis of the locomotor system in the absence of CNS activity; the enteric equivalent of such paresis is excessive contractile activity, as may be demonstrated by the application of tetrodotoxin, a nerve poison, to isolated gut with intact intrinsic innervation.

Brain–Gut or Gut–Brain?

It is important to appreciate the revolution in our view of relationships between CNS and ENS. From being considered as merely part of the peripheral nervous system, increasing knowledge of the enteric nervous system has led to a steadily increasing appreciation of its complexity and autonomy. A few years ago, it was compared to "an intelligent terminal connected to a main-frame computer." Even this analogy may underestimate the role of the ENS; it is appropriate to consider it also as a brain, and thus the axis of communication between the two systems is at least bidirectional. Therefore, much of the afferent information passing from gut to brain appears to serve the purpose of keeping the CNS informed of events within the digestive system that have been initiated and controlled by the ENS. While the CNS may "command" a change of gut function in order to subserve the overall needs of the organism, the reverse is also true: the gut may "command" the CNS to modify the behavior of the organism in order to subserve the requirements of the digestive tract as in, for example, mechanisms of satiety. Because of the diverse functions controlled by the CNS, it is logical to consider it as the control center for all bodily functions; in relation to the ENS it is perhaps more appropriate to consider it as "primus inter pares" (first among equals).

ANATOMIC PATHWAYS

The Gut–Brain Axis: Afferent Pathways

The autonomic nerves provide the afferent trunks for signals from gut to brain; these comprise the parasympathetic vagus and pelvic nerves and sympathetic nerves that relay to the spinal cord through the prevertebral ganglia. That being said, there are important questions that remain to be answered. Among the possible anatomic routes for information transmission, which are physiologically—and pathophysiologically—important? Is sensory information from the gut preprocessed in the ENS before transmission to the CNS?

At present, only partial answers to these questions are possible. Of the possible pathways, only the vagal route is readily susceptible to study (Fig 3-2). The vagus appears to provide the main conduit of information from the foregut and midgut to the CNS, and this sensory traffic bypasses the ENS. Vagal neurons with sensory endings in the gut wall have their cell bodies in the nodose ganglion and make synaptic connections in the nucleus of the solitary tract (NTS) in the brain stem (Fig 3-3); this route, operated by single fibers without intermediate synapses is readily susceptible to both anatomic[9] and physiologic[10] study. In contrast, the route from the hindgut (colon) to the brain via the spinal cord is polysynaptic and not easily characterized but appears to be through the lumbar splanchnic and pelvic nerves via spinal afferents with cell bodies in the thoracolumbar and sacral dorsal root ganglia.

The sensory neurons that project directly to the brain stem or spinal cord are only part of the sensory innervation of the gut. The autonomy of the ENS with respect to the peristaltic reflex has always implied the existence of sensory neurons within the ENS; these have now been identified as belonging to the subgroup of AH Dogiel type II neurons within the myenteric plexus.[11]

Effectively, therefore, each of "the two brains" has an exclusive direct sensory input from the gut wall; both the CNS and the ENS are continuously and synchronously informed of events within the gut. Whether or not there are important afferent pathways from the ENS to the CNS remains to be determined, but the probability is that there are not.

Central Connections

As shown in Figure 3-2, the main relay station for the brain–gut axis is the dorsal vagal complex (DVC) within the brain stem; the main components of the DVC are NTS, where afferent vagal fibers arrive, and the dorsal motor nucleus of the vagus, which contains the cell bodies of vagal efferent neurons. The NTS also receives inputs from the facial and hypoglossal nerves.[12] In addition, the DVC contains interneurons that link the two nuclei and the cell bodies of neurons that project rostrally. The main rostral projections are to hypothalamus, via the parabrachial nucleus in the midbrain, and thence to the limbic system and cortex. Except for the cranial nuclei, all regions of the brain that receive inputs from the DVC also have efferent pathways to the DVC.

The Brain–Gut Axis: Efferent Pathways

The brain–gut efferent pathways that have been characterized are those that are routed through the DVC to vagal afferent fibers. The mapping of centers that appear to relay to the DVC has so far been accomplished by intracerebral microstimulation or microinjection. Studies with intracerebroventricular injection of different neuropeptides have shown activation or modulation of a variety of gastrointestinal secretory and motor functions,[13] but such experiments do not specify the loci affected by the stimulus. Anatomically focused studies have shown that three structures in the ventral forebrain—the paraventricular nucleus of the hypothalamus, the central nucleus of the amygdala, and the bed nucleus of the stria terminalis—appear to provide a continuous band of "prevagal neurons" with direct projections to the DVC[14]; these studies rely on foregut function as an index of activity, and there are no comparable studies relating to the midgut and hindgut.

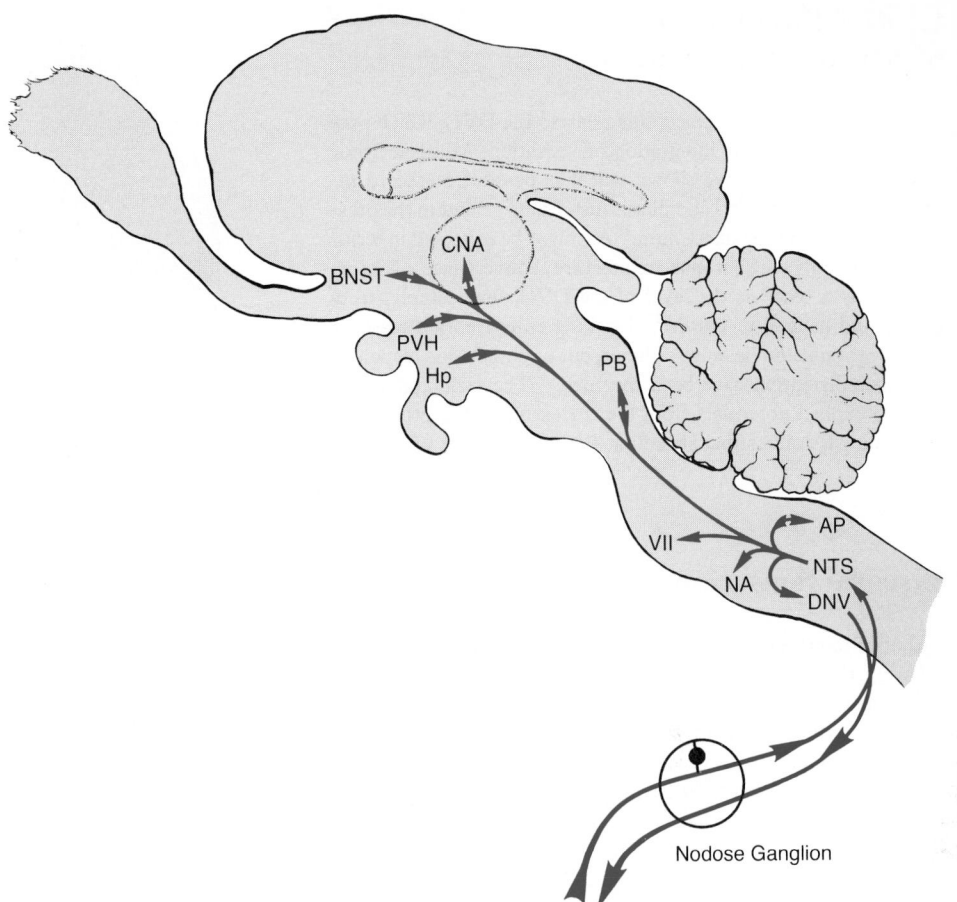

FIGURE 3–2. Schematic diagram of a sagittal section through the rat brain showing central connections of the vagal nerve in its function as part of the brain–gut axis. Sensory information from the gastrointestinal tract is passed centrally by the vagus nerve via the nodose ganglia (which contain the vagal afferent cell bodies) to the nucleus tractus solitarius (*NTS*). Information is disseminated from the NTS to various medullary nuclei, such as the area postrema (*AP*) and the dorsal nucleus of the vagus (*DNV*), which contains vagal motor neurons that supply the gastrointestinal tract, as do the nucleus ambiguus (*NA*) and the nucleus of the facial (*VII*) nerve. Sensory information is also passed from the NTS to higher centers, such as the parabrachial nucleus (*PB*), the hypothalamus (*Hp*), the paraventricular nucleus (*PVH*), the central nucleus of the amygdala (*CNA*), and the bed nucleus of the stria terminalis (*BNST*). Many of the nuclei that receive information from the dorsal vagal complex (*NTS* and *DNV*) also return efferent information to this complex. The direction of flow of information is indicated by arrows.

In the DVC, these prevagal neurons from higher centers join with interneurons from the afferent vagus in the NTS to synapse with the cell bodies of the efferent vagus. In this way the output from higher cerebral centers can influence the output of the vagovagal "reflex arc."

It is important to realize that the output of the efferent vagus nerve passes to the ENS, and not directly to effector units such as smooth muscle cells. With perhaps minor exceptions, the motor innervation of gastrointestinal smooth muscle is provided by the ENS. The efferent output from the CNS is therefore directed at modulation of ENS activity rather than at the activity of individual effector units.

SENSORY MECHANISMS

Modalities of Sensation: Enteroceptors

The precision with which conditions in the gut lumen and gut wall can be conveyed to the CNS and ENS is a function of the specificity of receptors for different types of stimuli.[15] Just as receptors for different modalities exist in the skin, there are sensory receptors responding to different stimuli within the digestive tract. These have been demonstrated for the most part by recording single-unit activity from primary vagal afferents and include mechanoreceptors, thermoreceptors, and chemoreceptors.[16–18] Such receptors signal conditions in the lumen adjacent to the mucosa but do not provide proprioceptive information on the state of the gut wall; this is provided by tension receptors within the muscle.[19,20] In this way, the CNS is continuously informed not only about conditions in the lumen but also about the motor response of the gut to them. Such mechanoreceptors have been shown, in acute studies in anesthetized animals, to modulate the output of the efferent vagus nerve via the afferent vagus nerve.[20,21] Furthermore, using an ingenious chronic nerve suture technique, it has been shown in conscious animals that vagal discharge varies with the intensity of gastric muscle contraction, so that the vagus nerve carries a representation of the different phases of fasting periodic activity.[22]

Mucosal receptors provide "preabsorptive" sensory information, but there is also evidence for vagal receptors in the liver that respond to changes in the blood and thus provide "postabsorptive" information.[23,24]

Central Integration of Sensory Information

Afferent fibers from enteroceptors relay to the DVC, which provides the first level of integration of sensation. Microelectrode studies in the DVC have shown that it is possible to record responses to gastric tonic[25] and phasic distention[26,32] and to the presence of glucose in the duodenum.[27] As might be expected in terms of the economy of neuronal architecture, convergence of information takes place at the level of the DVC, for example, from gastric and hepatic receptors.[28] Tracking enteroception rostrally from the brain stem is more difficult, but hypothalamic responses to gastric distention have been recorded.[29] The technique of recording evoked potentials from the cortex offers the promise of detecting gastrointestinal stimuli at the highest level of integration.[30,31]

Visceral Sensation

Although the responses that have been described are sensory and thus constitute "sensation" in neurophysiologic terms, this is not synonymous with cognition. It is clear that the CNS is continuously supplied with detailed information on the digestive tract—one study[25] showed that 50% of all units tested in the DVC responded to the stimulus of gastric distention—yet human experience informs us that little or, for most of the time, none of this information is projected into consciousness. Of the information provided by enteroceptors, probably only postprandial satiation is normally consciously perceived and then usually only as the cessation of the sensation of hunger. Even so, enteroception is not redundant; on the contrary, it is an essential requirement for the appropriate modulation of ENS activity by the CNS.

Cognitive visceral sensation, at least in humans, is virtually confined to the perception of discomfort and pain from the viscera and is discussed later in this chapter.

REGULATION OF MOTOR FUNCTION

Vagovagal Interaction

The vagovagal reflex arc represents the lowest level of gut–brain interaction (see Fig 3-3). Afferent signals arrive in the CNS at the level of the brain stem and provoke a discharge in the efferent vagus. It has already been pointed out that the afferent vagal neurons terminate in the NTS, which is adjacent to the motor nucleus of the vagus nerve (DMN) within the DVC. While there is evidence that a few vagal afferent fibers may terminate within the DMN, it is probable that, for the most part, this is a polysynaptic arc with one or more internuncial neurons between the NTS and the DMN and that this provides abundant opportunity for modulation from rostral control centers. Nonetheless, it is evident that the vagovagal route can, at the simplest level, operate as a reflex arc.

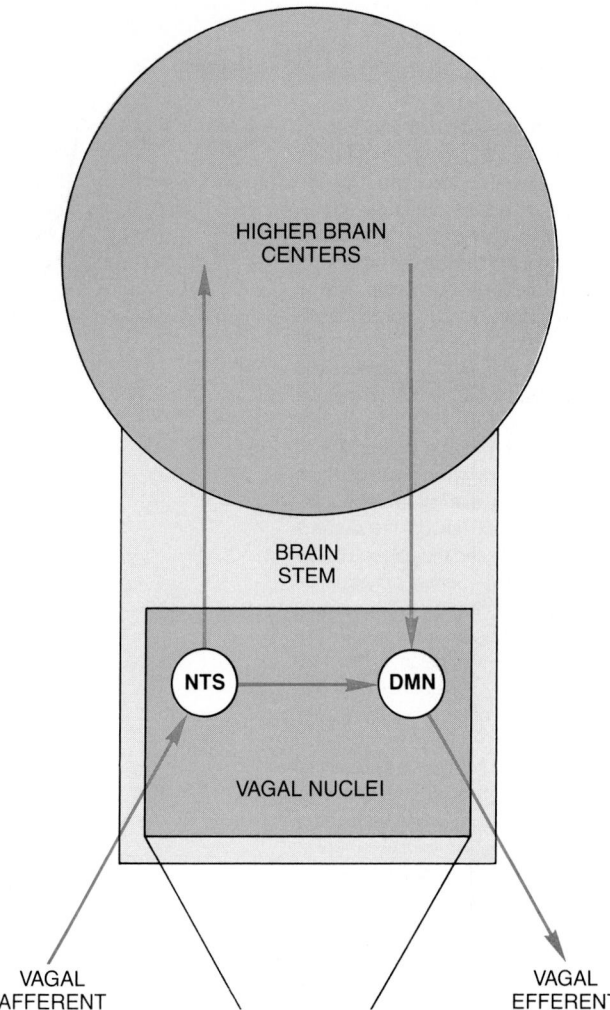

FIGURE 3–3. The brain stem is an important crossroads for information required in the control of gut function. Information from the gut is conveyed to the nucleus of the solitary tract (*NTS*). Connection by interneurons to the cell bodies of the dorsal motor nucleus (*DMN*) completes the vagovagal reflex pathway. However, the interposition of one or more interneurons between afferent and efferent vagal nuclei means that this is not a simple monosynaptic reflex; modulation of the traffic of information is possible at each synapse within the pathway. Information from the gut is transmitted onward toward higher centers through ascending tracts from the NTS (see Fig. 3-2); equally, descending commands modulate vagal outflow. Because of the tightly packed nuclei in the brain stem there is also intercommunication (not shown) between gut neurons, cardiovascular neurons, and neurons of some of the cranial nerves.

The motor response of the proximal digestive tract to food is programmed by the ENS but depends on the signal that food has been ingested. It has long been known, from clinical and experimental evidence, that the receptive relaxation of the gastric fundus to accommodate the bulk of a meal is vagally dependent and is abolished by vagotomy. It has recently been shown that neurons in the NTS respond to distention of the proximal stomach and that these responses are projected to the hypothalamus; moreover, these responses are abolished by vagotomy.[30] These data support the hypothesis that the loss of receptive relaxation of the proximal stomach following vagotomy is primarily a result of afferent denervation.

The importance of vagovagal innervation extends beyond the phenomenon of receptive relaxation. It has become clear that vagal afferents are the principal signaling system to the ENS, as well as to the CNS, of the arrival of nutrient in the gut; the initiation and maintenance of postprandial motor activity is dependent on the integrity of extrinsic vagovagal innervation. Hall and his coworkers[33] developed a technique for acute reversible vagal blockade in conscious dogs by cooling the vagus nerve; they have shown that in the postprandial state, acute vagal block causes the reversion of postprandial motility to the periodic activity normally seen only in fasting. Experiments with autotransplanted small intestine in dogs support these studies; in the transplants, which are extrinsically denervated, the normal motor postprandial response is greatly attenuated or absent.[34]

These data suggest that the sensory apparatus of the ENS, which provides the afferent limb of the peristaltic reflex, is not polymodal and does not have receptors that are chemosensitive. Vagovagal innervation provides a degree of sensory discrimination that is lacking within the ENS.

Central Regulation of Motor Function

Many experimental studies testify to the fact that it is possible to alter smooth muscle[14] or secretomotor[13] function in the gut by chemical or electrical stimulation of different areas of the brain. There have been numerous assertions that different areas of the brain are "involved in the control of the gut." Such studies do not clarify whether the putative control pathways operate under physiologic circumstances, and as evidence of the relative autonomy of the ENS accumulates, the probable physiologic significance of such mechanisms diminishes. There is evidence, which is considered in a later section, that higher control centers may be important in the mediation of gastrointestinal responses to stress.

One physiologic condition that must involve the CNS is the cephalic phase of digestion. However, it is possible that this is mediated at the level of the brain stem and does not require the intervention of higher centers within the CNS, since gustatory afferent fibers converge within the vagal territory of the DVC.[35,36] While there is undoubted convergence of gustatory afferents with vagal afferents at higher levels in the CNS,[37] there is no certainty that such pathways are involved in the normal control of gastrointestinal function; gustatory sensation is also important in the modification of behavior.

INTEGRATIVE PHYSIOLOGY OF BRAIN–GUT INTERACTION

Visceral Pain

As has already been remarked, visceral pain is the only common cognitive sensory modality within the abdominal viscera, the array of sensory modalities mediated by vagal receptors being unrepresented at the conscious level. It has long been believed, on the basis of experimental studies, that visceral pain arises from distention of the gut lumen.[38,39] Consciously perceived abdominal pain is not vagally transmitted, since subdiaphragmatic pain is abolished by injury to the cervical spinal cord. Visceral pain is mediated by visceral afferents traveling in the thoracolumbar splanchnic and pelvic nerves. The extrinsic visceral afferent nerve population is sparse,[40] and this is consistent with the poor somatotopic localization of distention pain.[41]

The mechanoreceptors of the abdominal viscera respond to distention but rarely produce the sensation of pain; thus it is important to distinguish between innocuous and noxious stimuli. It has been shown that distention of a segment of colon will reflexively induce relaxation of another segment of colon; the distention signal passes from the receptors in the affected segment to a prevertebral ganglion and thence back to the ENS in the responding segment.[42] One possible explanation of the difference between innocuous and painful stimuli is that the latter may be mediated by a subpopulation of mechanoreceptors that have a high threshold to distention and are not normally excited by physiologic changes in tension.[43] More intriguing is the possibility that the sensory threshold of the subpopulation of receptors that mediate pain is lowered by circumstances such as inflammation; many years ago, Wolf and Wolff[44] demonstrated that light and normally painless stimulation of the gastric mucosa became painful in the presence of mucosal inflammation. Such receptors have recently been characterized in the urinary bladder[45] but remain to be demonstrated within the gut.

No consideration of visceral pain can be complete without some mention of the pain perhaps mostly commonly encountered by gastroenterologists, which is due to the noxious effect of hydrochloric acid. Pain resulting from chemosensitivity has been studied very much less than the pain due to distention, owing to the difficulty of establishing reproducible human or animal test systems. Nevertheless, it has been shown that local injection of bradykinin will elicit pain[46] and that chemically induced pain is independent of motor events.[47]

Vomiting and Defecation

The expulsion of material from either end of the gastrointestinal tract requires close synchrony between somatic motor activity controlled by the CNS and enteric motor activity controlled by the ENS. The programs for such activity appear to be "hard wired"; they do not require training. On the contrary, training is required to prevent their uninhibited expression. No other physiologic events involve this type of synchrony between the two nervous systems. Few other physiologic events are as difficult to study; when spontaneous, their occurrence is unpredictable, and the considerable mechanical forces involved in the sequence of events often result in the stimulation of mechanical or electrical sensors.

VOMITING

Vomiting is a complex stereotypical motor event involving both the somatic and the visceral musculature.

The Vomiting Stimulus. The stimulus may be gastrointestinal (e.g., the ingestion of emetic substances, such as hypertonic saline) or central (motion sickness, psychogenic vomiting). Almost certainly gastrointestinal stimuli are conveyed to the CNS by vagal afferents, and all stimuli converge on the chemoreceptor trigger zone in the CNS.

The Visceral Response. Many years ago, Alvarez[48] noted that vomiting was accompanied by reverse peristalsis; more recently, such events have been characterized as "retrograde giant contractions" that have been shown to be an ENS motor program dependent on vagal efferent outflow.[49] Vomiting also appears to be accompanied by gastric motor dysrhythmias[50]; while the mechanism of this effect remains obscure, it is not due to a local noxious stimulus, since the arrhythmias can be produced by vection-induced motion sickness.

The Somatic Response. The act of retching involves coordination of the musculature of the abdominal wall, diaphragm, chest wall, and glottis, presumably temporally coordinated to coincide with the termination of reverse propulsion within the gut.

The Psychic Response. The psychic concomitants of nausea include the premonitory sensation of nausea, which may be prolonged or very brief, and the awareness of the somatic motor concomitants of retching. There is no evidence that the enteric component (retrograde propulsion) is represented by a conscious sensation, although it is possible that it underlies the sensation of nausea.

DEFECATION

Defecation is a similar stereotypical program, but considerably less is known about the nature of the CNS/ENS interaction; only the central psychic and peripheral motor events are clear, although it is known that the interaction is mediated through the spinal cord. Again, the program may be separated into discrete components.

The Colonic Stimulus. The presumed first event in defecation is filling of the rectum, for which the most effective stimulus seems to be the recent ingestion of a meal (the inappropriately termed *gastrocolic reflex*). The transit of feces requires propulsive motor activity, and there is evidence that this motor activity may often (but not invariably) include high-amplitude retrograde propagating contractions that occur rarely but probably accomplish the "mass movements" of the colon.

The Perineal Response. This involves both striated and smooth muscle. Rectal filling induces relaxation of the puborectalis sling and also evokes the rectoanal inhibitory reflex, which relaxes the internal anal sphincter. At this point, continence is maintained only by the contraction of the external anal sphincter.

The Psychic Response. The preceding events evoke the conscious desire to defecate ("call to stool"). In the untrained

(infants and the mentally subnormal), the somatic act of defecation automatically follows. In the trained individual, the urge may be resisted, and this will be followed shortly by reversion of perineal function to the continent mode, with the resumption of tonic contraction of the puborectalis and the internal sphincter after which the expulsion of stool is extremely difficult or impossible.

The Somatic Response. The act of voiding is a CNS program that involves raising intra-abdominal pressure by expiration against a closed glottis (Valsalva maneuver) and the automatic adoption of a squatting posture to decrease perineal and gluteal tone. It is not known to what extent contraction is an essential component of defecation, but to judge from the ease of defecation in colectomized patients with ileal pouches, the voiding force derives largely or entirely from the change in intra-abdominal pressure.

Satiety

The gastrointestinal function of digestion is preceded by the behavioral activity of ingestion. Ingestion is terminated by signals that arise during the ingestive/digestive process, and these signals constitute satiation and result in the cessation of ingestion. The question that arises is whether these signals originate in the gut and thus use the gut–brain axis.

The classic concept of ingestive behavior was that it was "under the control" of two hypothalamic centers with opposing functions, a lateral hypothalamic feeding center and a ventromedial satiety center; this idea of opposing influences was comparable to the view of gut function as being the result of opposing sympathetic and parasympathetic influences. The passage of time and the accumulation of discrepant data have shown this hypothesis to be relatively naive. It is obvious that ingestive behavior is dependent not only on the sensing of nutrient intake but also on the hedonistic effect of pleasant or unpleasant gustatory signals; it has been shown that gustatory signals converge with visceral vagal afferents at the level of the brain stem,[36] as well as at higher levels of the CNS.[35,37] The recognition that a number of gastrointestinal peptides are released into the plasma during ingestion raises the additional possibility that the gut–brain axis of satiety is not neural but humoral.

Three neuropeptides released on feeding have been implicated as potential satiety factors, but their actions on the CNS (which regulates ingestive behavior) do not appear to be humoral, but peripheral. These peptides are cholecystokinin (CCK), bombesin, and glucagon. In experimental animals, they do not cross the blood-brain barrier but will produce satiation when injected into the peritoneal cavity. The satiating effect of pancreatic glucagon is abolished by section of the hepatic vagus nerve.[51] Blunting the effect of CCK requires section of, at the least, the bilateral gastric branches of the vagus nerve.[52] Abolition of the effect of bombesin requires not only bilateral subdiaphragmatic vagal section but also ablation of much of the sympathetic supply to the gut.[53]

Taken together, all these data suggest that in experimental animals, the vagal link between gut and brain is an essential route for the transfer of satiety signals and that the vagal information is modulated at the receptor end by the local effect of neuropeptides. There are, however, problems with such a concept. The mode of interaction between peptides and the vagus nerve is not understood. More important, given the wide variation in humoral levels of peptide on the ingestion of food, it is not clear how the action of peptides in this way can mediate a quantitative effect such as satiety. It is possible to imagine that there is a relationship between the release of peptides and the volume of ingesta, but satiety is related to the caloric requirements of the animal and not merely to the volume.

Species differences pose problems in the investigation of behavior, and particularly so in the extrapolation of satiety research from laboratory animals to humans. The nutrient intake of humans is strongly conditioned by economic, cultural, and social determinants. Indeed, the prevalence of obesity in the relative prosperity of the developed world and of malnutrition and poverty elsewhere suggests that, in human society, satiety on the basis of gut–brain interaction is not the major determinant of caloric ingestion.

Sleep

It has already been pointed out that both the CNS and the ENS are dominated by biorhythms of similar periodicity, which are evident in the absence of sensory input. Possible interactions during sleep are therefore of particular interest since, under normal circumstances, both systems lack exogenous sensory stimuli during sleep. Sleep studies, however, require that the methods of monitoring do not interfere with normal sleep. CNS polysomnography allows normal sleep, but the same is less true of intubation of the upper gut with multilumen per oral perfused tubes.

The question of coincidence of the two biorhythms was raised by a study[54] that showed a possible interdependence between them; the authors suggested that it was thus likely that ENS periodic activity was governed centrally. The latter suggestion was reasonable at the time of the study, when there was little appreciation of the autonomy and complexity of ENS function; in fact, the data were equally consistent with the less plausible hypothesis that the REM–non-REM cycle was governed by the gut. Improved minimally invasive technology for the prolonged manometry of the gut has been developed, and with this a more recent study has shown that there appears to be no synchrony between CNS and ENS periodic activity; the CNS and the ENS appear to be governed by independent oscillators.[55] There is, moreover, a biorhythm of similar periodicity within the human rectum,[56] but not the human colon. The rectal motor complex (RMC) appears to be yet another independent oscillation, since it is not synchronized with the MMC.[57]

During sleep, motor activity in both the small bowel and the colon is diminished, and it increases on waking. In the colon, where there is no apparent periodicity of motor activity, the increased motor activity has no particular characteristic.[58,59] However, prolonged monitoring of gut motor activity in ambulatory subjects has shown a highly specific difference between waking and sleeping motor activity in the small bowel.[60] In the waking state, fasting motor activity is dominated by irregular contractions (phase II); quiescence (phase I) is of brief duration. During sleep,

however, phase II becomes greatly diminished or absent, so that the MMC cycle becomes virtually the alternation of phase I and phase III. This suggests that, in the waking state, CNS arousal activates irregular contractions. This is consistent with the hypothesis of vagal tone[61] during CNS arousal.

During sleep, periodicity in the ENS becomes dominant. If a meal is consumed late in the evening,[62] the normal postprandial response is abolished at the onset of sleep. The digestive process then appears to become periodic; while the expected postprandial activity is abolished, there is preservation of the prolonged phase II activity normally seen in the waking state. Digestion, transit, and perhaps gastric emptying are presumably all confined to phase II of the sleeping cycles, and the enhanced phase II persists through the night until digestion is completed. Thus it would appear that vagal efferent tone is required for the normal pattern of digestion; this is consistent with the effects of acute vagal blockade seen in dogs after feeding.[33]

Taken together, the available evidence suggests that sleep offers an opportunity to observe the function of the ENS when it is effectively uncoupled from the influence of the CNS. As will be seen, this may be important in determining the pathogenesis of enteric motor disorders.

Stress

If sleep represents the state in which the influence of the CNS on the gut is minimal, then stress is the opposite state, in which a perturbed CNS dominates gut function. The notion that stress alters gut function is not new, but systematic study of the phenomenon has been a relatively recent development. It has not proved easy to develop protocols for the controlled application of stressors in humans, or of reliable methods for measuring the effect of such stressors, not least because methods of measuring gut function are, of themselves, usually stressful.

There is, however, a considerable body of evidence on the mediation of stress in animals. Following Selye's original discovery, in 1938, that noxious stressors produce adrenal hypertrophy in rats, interest focused on the adenohypophysis, in the belief that the response was due to excess secretion of adrenocorticotropic hormone (ACTH). It was subsequently shown that the excess ACTH secretion was due to the release of corticotropin-releasing factor (CRF) from the hypothalamus. CRF was subsequently characterized as a 41-amino acid peptide and shown to regulate the physiologic release of ACTH.[63] In 1984, Tache and coworkers[64] showed that central administration of CRF altered gastric acid secretion in rats, and similar effects on motility were demonstrated by Bueno and Fioramonti in 1986.[65] The development of α-helical CRF, a specific antagonist of CRF, has allowed further refinement of the model. In 1987, Williams and associates[66] developed a sensitive method for the study of stress in rats using the technique of partial immobilization ("wrap restraint") to produce changes in gut transit, and these changes were blocked by pretreatment with α-helical CRF.

The question from the clinician that has to be answered is the extent to which the CRF axis mediates stress responses in the human gut; preliminary data on this topic are not supportive of a major role for CRF, since it has been shown that exogenous CRF administered to human volunteers in a dosage sufficient to evoke ACTH secretion does not affect gastric acid output.[67] However, it is important to note that exogenously administered CRF probably does not mimic the effect of central CRF. Perhaps more to the point, it remains to be determined whether the effects of centrally administered substances are mediated through the brain–gut axis or whether they are the effects of secondary changes in blood hormone levels. Within this context, the definition of periodic motor activity as an ENS-controlled program has been useful in the study of stress, since it offers a clear index of ENS function.

Studies on stressors in humans have used two principal modalities of experimental stressors, pain stress, which involves somatosensory pathways, and psychological stress, which uses the special senses. Usually pain is induced by the repeated immersion of one hand of the subject in ice water. Psychological stress usually takes the form of completing a task (e.g., calculation, verbal repetition, sorting) against a background of visual or auditory distraction. Both types of stressors can be shown to produce the expected somatic and subjective responses to stress.

As might be expected, such studies have been most profitable in those areas of the gut where the physiology is best understood. With the improved knowledge of the MMC, the small bowel provided a useful starting point, and a pilot study[68] in 1982 showed that mental stress appeared to inhibit periodic activity in some persons. An improved stressor protocol[69] showed that the effect could be reproducibly induced in all normal volunteers.

Gastric emptying has also been an obvious function for study. With one or two exceptions (such as mice exposed to loud music),[70] animal studies showed that stress delayed gastric emptying. This effect was confirmed in humans,[71] using a cold pain stressor. Investigation of the possible pathways responsible for this delay suggests the involvement of adrenergic and endogenous opioid[72] mechanisms; β-adrenoceptor mechanisms appear to mediate the delayed orocecal transit induced by the same stimulus.[73]

If it is postulated that brain–gut interaction is mediated through the neural networks of the ENS, it might be predicted that the effects of CNS perturbation will be slight or absent in regions of the gut where the intrinsic plexuses are relatively sparse. This is supported by two studies[74,75] that show that mental stressors that perturb intestinal function do not, apparently, affect the esophagus.

The one region of the gut where it is clear, from individual experience, that function is perturbed by stress is the colon, where altered defecation is the expected outcome. It has proved very difficult, to date, to add objective confirmation to this universal subjective perception. This is not due to lack of interest but to the difficulty of finding reproducible indices of human colonic function other than episodes of defecation; species variation in morphology and physiology render animal models of dubious value. Such studies as have been reported indicate discrepant results, showing either no effect of stress on colonic function[76,77] or stimulation by stress.[78,79] Useful progress in this field depends on the development of better methodology.

PATHOPHYSIOLOGY

From the preceding sections of this chapter, it is clear that the brain–gut axis is a topic that is attracting increased interest. Data are rapidly replacing speculation; an aspect of digestive physiology that was previously obscure is now being clarified. There can be little doubt that these new insights into physiology will extend to pathophysiology, and in particular to the syndromes that are currently categorized as "functional"; that is, conditions in which a disorder of function is apparent but the cause of the disorder remains obscure. It is not yet possible to define a systematic pathophysiology of the interaction between the CNS and the ENS but only to give some indication of where a little progress has been made and where more may be expected.

Postvagotomy Disorders

Dysfunction following truncal vagotomy has been attributed traditionally to disordered motor control of the stomach and pylorus by the vagus nerve. If our new perspective of the vagus as a nerve that is for the most part afferent is correct, then it would be expected that one consequence of vagotomy would be that the sensory stimulus in the gut of the arrival of food will not be conveyed to the ENS via the vagovagal link, producing an effect similar to that observed in dogs with acute vagal blockade.[33] This appears to be the case; one study in humans has shown attenuation of the upper gut response to food in vagotomized patients.[80]

Vagotomy is an interesting model for anatomic and functional disruption of the gut–brain axis; however, as the evidence that it is a procedure that leaves an unacceptable visceral sensitivity deficit increases, so does the clinical motivation for the procedure diminish with the development of effective alternative therapy for chronic ulcer disease.

Eating Disorders

The extent to which ordered eating depends on brain–gut interaction in humans remains to be clarified, and it is not yet clear whether malfunction of this interaction is part of the pathogenesis of morbid obesity or anorexia. Nevertheless, the therapeutic modality of attempting to modify eating behavior by producing spurious satiety signals has already been tried, using surgical procedures such as stapling or displacement of the lumen by a balloon. Perhaps the next step will be the use of medication to produce altered plasma levels of chemicals that signal satiety; CCK is a possible candidate.

Neuropathy

Clearly damage or dysfunction of one or other of the two nervous systems that are linked in the gut–brain axis may produce an altered interaction. Gastrointestinal dysfunction is well recognized in enteric neuropathies, which may be idiopathic, or a component of more generalized disorders such as diabetes mellitus and Chagas' disease. Dysfunction is equally recognized in CNS disorders such as Parkinson's disease and spinal injury. Systematic study of gut function in these conditions has, in general, not been carried out; possibly this will be stimulated with the growing realization that damage to one nervous system may alter the function of the other.

Irritable Bowel Syndrome

Because of the well-recognized relationship between stress and symptoms in the irritable bowel syndrome, this has been an obvious point of entry into the study of the pathophysiology of the brain-gut axis. Intermittent dysrhythmia of the small bowel provoked by mental stress[81] and by cholinergic stimulation[82] has been reported; it seems that such dysrhythmic episodes are confined to the waking state and thus are CNS dependent.[83] Colonic motor function may be similarly perturbed,[78,79] but the esophagus appears to be unaffected.[74,75] The difficulties of classifying irritable bowel syndrome, and of defining possible subgroups, need to be resolved to allow the study of homogeneous groups, but the possibilities for future study are evident, and it does seem clear that such functional disorders will assume growing importance as exemplars of this aspect of pathophysiology. Their importance as exemplars of disturbance of the brain-gut axis is underlined by the fact that they are the only group of disorders of gastrointestinal function that appear to be at least moderately susceptible to therapeutic modalities directed entirely at the CNS.[84]

The reader is directed to Chapter 1, The Enteric Nervous System and its Extrinsic Connections; Chapter 2, Gastrointestinal Hormones; Chapter 4, Smooth Muscle of the Gut; Chapter 7, Esophageal Motor Function; Chapter 8, The Physiology of Gastric Motility and Gastric Emptying; Chapter 9, Motility of the Small Intestine; Chapter 10, The Motor Function of the Colon; Chapter 11, Motility of the Biliary Tree; Chapter 27, Psychosocial Factors in the Care of Patients with Gastrointestinal Disease; Chapter 32, Approach to the Patient with Unexplained Weight Loss; Chapter 80, Irritable Bowel Syndrome; and the corresponding chapters in the Atlas.

REFERENCES

1. Langley JN. The autonomic nervous system, part I. Cambridge: W Heffer, 1921.
2. Bayliss WM, Starling EH. The movements of the small intestine. J Physiol (Lond) 1899;24:99.
3. Gershon M. The enteric nervous system. Ann Rev Neurosci 1981;4:227.
4. Wood JD. Physiology of the enteric nervous system. In: Johnson LR, ed. Physiology of the gastrointestinal tract. New York: Raven Press, 1981:1.
5. Furness JB, Costa M. The enteric nervous system. New York: Churchill Livingstone, 1987.
6. Wingate DL. Backwards and forwards with the migrating complex. Dig Dis Sci 1981;26:641.
7. Yntema CL, Hammond WS. The origin of enteric ganglia of trunk viscera from vagal neural crest in the chick embryo. J Comp Neurol 1954;101:515.
8. Costa M, Furness JB, Gibbins IL. Chemical coding of enteric neurones. In: Hokfelt T, Fuxe K, Pernow B, eds. Co-existence of neuronal messengers: a new principle in chemical transmission. Progr Brain Res 1986;68:217.
9. Kalia M, Sullivan JM. Brainstem projections of sensory and motor components of the vagus nerve. J Comp Neurol 1982;211:248.
10. Harding R, Leek BF. The locations and activities of medullary neurones associated with ruminant forestomach motility. J Physiol (Lond) 1971;219:587.
11. Hirst GDS, Holman ME, Spence I. Two types of neurones in the myenteric plexus of the guinea-pig duodenum. J Physiol (Lond) 1974;236:303.
12. Contreras RJ, Beckstead RM, Norgren R. Central projections of trigeminal, facial, glossopharyngeal, and the vagus nerves: an autoradiographic study in the rat. J Auton Nerv Sys 1982;6:303.
13. Tache Y. Peptidergic activation of brain-gut pathways. In: Goebell H, Singer MV, eds. Nerves and the gastrointestinal tract. Lancaster, England: MTP Press, 1989:315.
14. Hermann GE, Rogers RC. Extrinsic neural control of brainstem gastric vagovagal reflex circuits. In: Goebell H, Singer MV, eds. Nerves and the gastrointestinal tract. Lancaster, England: MTP Press, 1989:345.
15. Grundy D. Speculations on the structure/function relationship for vagal and splanchnic afferent endings supplying the gastrointestinal tract. J Auton Nerv Sys, 1988;22:175.
16. Clarke GD, Davison JS. Mucosal receptors in the gastric antrum and small intestine of the rat with afferent fibres in the cervical vagus. J Physiol (Lond) 1978;284:55.
17. Davison JS. Response of single vagal afferent fibres to mechanical and chemical stimulation of the gastric and duodenal mucosa in cats. Q J Exp Physiol 1972;57:405.
18. El-Ouazzani T. Thermoreceptors in the digestive tract and their role. J Auton Nerv Sys 1984;10:246.
19. Iggo A. Tension receptors in the stomach and urinary bladder. J Physiol (Lond) 1955;128:593.
20. Davison JS, Grundy D. Modulation of single vagal efferent fibre discharge by gastrointestinal afferents in the rat. J Physiol (Lond) 1978;284:69.
21. Grundy D, Salih AA, Scratcherd T. Modulation of vagal efferent fibre discharge by mechanoreceptors in the stomach, duodenum, and colon of the ferret. J Physiol (Lond) 1981;319:43.
22. Miolan P. Roman C. Discharge of efferent vagal fibres supplying gastric antrum: indirect study by nerve suture technique. Am J Physiol 1978;235:E366.
23. Adachi A. Thermosensitive and osmoreceptive afferent fibres in the hepatic branch of the vagus nerve. J Auton Nerv Sys 1984; 10:269.
24. Niijima A. The effect of D-glucose in the firing rate of glucose-sensitive vagal afferents in comparison with the effects of 2-deoxy-D-glucose. J Auton Nerv Sys, 1984, 10:255–260.
25. Ewart WR, Wingate DL. Cholecystokinin-octapeptide and the central representation of gastric mechanoreceptor activity in the rat. Am J Physiol 1983;244:G613.
26. Barber WD, Burks TR. Brain stem responses to phasic gastric distension. Am J Physiol 1983;245:G242.
27. Ewart WR, Wingate DL. The central representation of the arrival of glucose in the duodenum. Am J Physiol 1984;246:G750.
28. Appia F, Ewart WR, Pittam BS, Wingate DL. Convergence in the rat brainstem of sensory information from the abdominal viscera. Am J Physiol 1986;251:G169.
29. Jeanningros R. Modulation of lateral hypothalamic single unit activity by gastric and intestinal distension. J Auton Nerv Sys 1984;11:1.
30. Meunier P, Collet L, Duclaux R, Chery-Croze S. Cerebral evoked potentials after endo-rectal mechanical stimulation in humans. Dig Dis Sci 1987;32:921.
31. Frieling T, Enck P, Lubke JH, et al. Cerebral responses evoked by electrical stimulation of the rectosigmoid in normal subjects. Dig Dis Sci 1989;34:202.
32. Barber WD, Yuan CS, Burks TF. What does the proximal stomach tell the brain? In: Goebell H, Singer MV, eds. Nerves and the gastrointestinal tract. Lancaster, England: MTP Press, 1989:721.
33. Hall KE, El-Sharkawy TY, Diamant NE. Vagal control of canine postprandial upper gastrointestinal motility. Am J Physiol 1986;250:G501.
34. Sarr MG, Kelly KA. Myoelectric activity of the autotransplanted canine jejunoileum. Gastroenterology 1981;81:303.
35. Hamilton R, Norgren R. Central projection of gustatory nerves in the rat. J Comp Neurol 1984;222:560.
36. Hermann GE, Kohlerman NJ, Rogers RC. Hepatic-vagal and gustatory afferent interactions in the brainstem of the rat. J Auton Nerv Sys 1983;9:477.
37. Hermann GE, Rogers RC. Convergence of vagal and gustatory afferent input within the parabrachial nucleus of the rat. J Auton Nerv Sys 1985;13:1.
38. Bloomfield AL, Pollard WS. Experimental referred pain from the gastrointestinal tract: II. Stomach and duodenum. J Clin Invest 1931;13:353.

39. Bentley FH, Smithwick RG. Visceral pain produced by balloon distension of the jejunum. Lancet 1940;2:389.
40. Janig W, Morrison JFB. Functional properties of spinal visceral afferents supplying abdominal and pelvic organs with special emphasis on visceral nociception. In: Cervero F, Morrison JFB, eds. Visceral sensation. Prog Brain Res 1986;67:87.
41. Swarbrick ET, Hegarty JE, Bat L, et al. Site of pain from the irritable bowel. Lancet 1980;2:443.
42. Kreulen DL, Szurszewski JH. Reflex pathways in the abdominal prevertebral ganglia: evidence for a colo-colonic inhibitory reflex. J Physiol (Lond) 1979;295:21.
43. Blumberg H, Haupt P, Janig W, Kohler W. Encoding of visceral noxious stimuli in the discharge pattern of visceral afferent fibres from the colon. Pflugers Arch 1983;398:33.
44. Wolf S, Wolff HG. Pain arising from the stomach and mechanisms underlying gastric symptoms. Res Publ Assoc Nerv Ment Dis 1943;23:289.
45. Habler HJ, Janig W, Koltzenburg M. A novel type of unmyelinated chemosensitive response in the acutely-inflamed urinary bladder. Agents Actions 1988;25:219.
46. Guzman F, Braun C, Lim RKS. Visceral pain and pseudo-affective response to intraarterial injection of bradykinin and other algesic agents. Arch Int Pharmacodynam 1962;86:353.
47. Haupt P, Janig W, Kohler W. Response pattern of visceral afferent fibres supplying the colon upon chemical and mechanical stimuli. Pflugers Arch 1983;398:41.
48. Alvarez W. Reverse peristalsis in the bowel: a precursor of vomiting. JAMA 1925;95:1051.
49. Lang IM, Sarna SK, Condon RE. Gastrointestinal motor correlates of vomiting in the dog: quantification and characterisation as an independent phenomenon. Gastroenterology 1986;90:40.
50. Stern RM, Koch KL, Stewart WR, Lindblad IM. Spectral analysis of tachygastria recorded during motion sickness. Gastroenterology 197;92:92.
51. Geary N, Smith GP. Selective hepatic vagotomy blocks pancreatic glucagon's satiety effect. Physiol Behav 1983;31:391.
52. Smith GP, Jerome C, Cushin BJ, et al. Abdominal vagotomy blocks the satiety effect of cholecystokinin in the rat. Science 1981;213:1036.
53. Stuckey JA, Gibbs J, Smith GP. Neural disconnection of gut from brain blocks bombesin-induced satiety. Peptides 1985;6:1249.
54. Finch PM, Ingram DM, Henstridge JD, Catchpole BN. Relationship of fasting gastrointestinal motility to the sleep cycle. Gastroenterology 1982;63:605.
55. Kumar D, Idzikowski C, Soffer EE, et al. Do the brain and the gut sleep together? Gastroenterology 1988;94:A241.
56. Kumar D, Williams NS, Waldron D, Wingate DL: Prolonged manometric recording of anorectal motor activity in ambulant human subjects: evidence of periodic activity. Gut 1989;30:1009.
57. Kumar D, Thompson PD, Wingate DL: Absence of synchrony between the human small intestinal migrating motor complex (MMC) and rectal motor complex (RMC). Am J Physiol 1990;256:G171.
58. Narducci F, Bassoti G, Gasburri M, Morelli A. Twenty-four hour manometric recording of colonic motility in man. Gut 1987;28:17.
59. Soffer EE, Scalabrini P, Wingate DL: Prolonged ambulatory monitoring of human colonic motility. Am J Physiol 1989;255:G601.
60. Gill RC, Kellow JE, Wingate DL: The migrating motor complex (MMC) at home. Gastroenterology 1987;92:1405
61. Grundy D. Permissive regulations of gastrointestinal functions by the vagus nerve. In: Goebell H, Singer MV, eds. Nerves and the gastrointestinal tract. Lancaster, England: MTP Press, 1989:732.
62. Kumar D, Soffer EE, Wingate DL, et al. Modulation of the duration of human postprandial motor activity by sleep. Am J Physiol 1989;256:G851.
63. Rivier J, Rivier C, Vale W. Inhibition of adrenocorticotropic hormone secretion in the rat by immunoneutralisation of corticotropin-releasing factor. Science 1982;218:377.
64. Tache Y, Goto Y, Gunion M, et al. Inhibition of gastric acid secretion in rats and dogs by corticotropin-releasing factor. Gastroenterology 1984;86:281.
65. Bueno L, Fioramonti J. Effects of corticotropin-releasing factor, corticotropin, and cortisol on gastrointestinal motility in dogs. Peptides 1986;7:73.
66. Williams CL, Peterson JM, Villar RG, Burks TF. Corticotropin-releasing-factor directly mediates colonic responses to stress. Am J Physiol 1987;253:G562.
67. Beglinger C, Sieber C, Beltinger J, et al. Corticotropin-releasing hormone (CRH): lack of effect on gastric acid secretion in humans. In: Goebell H, Singer MV, eds. Nerves and the gastrointestinal tract. Lancaster, England: MTP Press, 1989:623.
68. McRae S, Younger K, Thompson DG, Wingate DL: Sustained mental stress alters human jejunal motor activity. Gut 1982;23:404.
69. Valori RM, Kumar D, Wingate DL: Effects of different types of stress and of "prokinetic" drugs on the control of the fasting motor complex in humans. Gastroenterology 1986;90:1890.
70. Bueno L, Gue M. Evidence for the involvement of corticotropin-releasing factor in the gastrointestinal disturbances induced by acoustic and cold stress in mice. Brain Res 1988;441:1.
71. Thompson DG, Richelson E, Malagelada J-R. Perturbation of gastric emptying and duodenal motility through the central nervous system. Gastroenterology 1982;83:1200.
72. Stanghellini V, Malagelada J-R, Zinsmeister AR, et al. Stress-induced gastroduodenal motor disturbances in man: possible humoral mechanisms. Gastroenterology 1983;85:83.
73. O'Brien JD, Thompson DG, Day SJ, et al. Perturbation of upper gastrointestinal transit and antroduodenal motility by experimentally-applied stress: the role of beta-adrenoceptor mediated pathways. Gut 1989;30:1530.
74. Soffer EE, Scalabrini P, Pope CE II, Wingate DL: Effect of stress on oesophageal motor function in normal subjects and in patients with the irritable bowel syndrome. Gut 1988 29:1591.
75. Ayres RCS, Robertson DAF, Naylor K, Smith CL. Stress and oesophageal motility in normal subjects and patients with irritable bowel syndrome. Gut 1989;30:1540.
76. Schang JC, Devroede G, Hebert M, et al. Effects of rest, stress, and food on myoelectrical spiking activity of left and sigmoid colon in humans. Dig Dis Sci 1988;33:614.
77. Frexinos J, Staumont G, Delvaux M, et al. Influence of cold water stress on colonic myoelectrical spiking activity in irritable bowel syndrome patients. In: Bueno L, Collins S, Junien J-L, eds. Stress and digestive motility. London: John Libby Eurotext, 1989:109.
78. Narducci F, Snape WJ, Battle WM, et al. Increased colonic motility during exposure to a stressful situation. Dig Dis Sci 1985;30:40.
79. Welgan P, Meshkinpout H, Beeler M. Effect of anger on colon motor and myoelectrical activity in irritable bowel syndrome. Gastroenterology 94;1988:1150.
80. Thompson DG, Ritchie HD, Wingate DL: Patterns of small intestinal motility in duodenal ulcer patients before and following vagotomy. Gut 1982;23:517.
81. Kumar D, Wingate DL: The irritable bowel syndrome: a paroxysmal motor disorder. Lancet 1985;2:973.
82. Kellow JE, Zinmeister AR, Phillips SF. Dysmotility of the small intestine in irritable bowel syndrome. Gut 1988;29:1236.
83. Kellow JE, Gill RC, Wingate DL: Prolonged ambulant recordings of small bowel motility demonstrate abnormalities in the irritable bowel syndrome. Gastroenterology 1990 (in press)
84. Creed F, Guthrie E. Psychological treatments of the irritable bowel syndrome: a review. Gut 1989;30:1601.

4

Smooth Muscle of the Gut

GABRIEL M. MAKHLOUF

The main function of smooth muscle of the gut is to mix and propel intraluminal contents to enable efficient digestion of food, progressive absorption of nutrients, and eventual evacuation of residues. This function is regulated by intrinsic electrical and mechanical properties of smooth muscle, such as the ability to maintain tone or undergo phasic contraction, and by alterations in these properties in response to hormonal and neural signals, particularly signals emanating from the enteric nervous system. A distinctive feature of physiologic regulation in the gut is that stimuli of hormonal release and neural activation arise within the lumen from the mechanical and chemical properties of food and digestive secretions.

STRUCTURE OF SMOOTH MUSCLE

Muscle Layers

Smooth muscle of the gut consists of a thin outer longitudinal layer and a thick, densely innervated circular layer; the layers derive their names from the orientation of the long axis of muscle cells in them. The layers are separated by laminar septa into bundles about 1 mm long, which probably act as contractile units. The muscle cells are embedded in a connective tissue matrix, a product of their synthetic and secretory activity consisting mainly of elastic and collagen fibrils. The layers include also glial cells, fibroblasts, and a distinctive population of fibroblastlike cells, the interstitial Cajal cells, described in a later section.

Muscle Cells: Membranes and Organelles

Single smooth muscle cells when fully relaxed are about 400 μm long and 5 μm wide. They are spindle-shaped and have a high surface area to volume ratio (1.5 $\mu m^2/\mu m^3$). Their plasma membranes consist of two specialized structures known as caveolae and dense bands.[1-3]

The *caveolae* are basket-shaped invaginations of the membrane, 70 nm wide and 120 nm deep, arranged in clusters (Fig 4-1). There are about 150,000 caveolae per cell, and they occupy about one third of the outer surface of the cell but constitute a much larger fraction of the surface of the plasma membrane. The bases of caveolae are surrounded by an abundant endoplasmic reticulum, the site of calcium storage and release in smooth muscle; the arrangement suggests that caveolae may be functional equivalents of transverse (T) tubules in striated muscle.

Clusters of caveolae are separated from each other by electron-dense structures, 1 to 2 μm long and 0.2 to 0.4 μm wide, called *dense bands* that occupy about one half of the surface of the cell (Figs 4-1 and 4-2). Dense bands are points of attachment of thin actin filaments; like dense bodies, their counterpart in the cytoplasm, they consist mainly of actinin, a protein that is a major component of the Z line in striated muscle. Intermediate 10-nm thick filaments, consisting mainly of desmin in visceral smooth muscle, link dense bands in the membrane to dense bodies in the cytoplasm and transmit force generated by the contractile apparatus within the cell to the entire surface of the cell (see Fig 4-2).[4] Some dense bands are juxtaposed to dense bands in adjacent cells; at these locations, called *intermediate junctions*, the intercellular space narrows to less than 30 nm and is filled with condensed extracellular matrix (see Fig 4-2). At other locations, dense bands in one cell are linked by collagen fibrils to dense bands in adjacent cells. Together, intermediate junctions and collagen fibrils anchor adjacent cells to each other, transmit force from one cell to the next, and couple the contractile apparatus of adjacent cells to the rest of the syncytium.

In some regions, patches of the plasma membrane of adjacent cells are closely apposed and the space between them is reduced to less than 3 nm; the space is bridged by intercellular channels that permit free movement of ions and small molecules. These patches, known as *gap junctions* or *nexuses*, are the most likely sites of electrical coupling between muscle cells.[1-3] Gap junctions also permit movement of intracellular regulatory molecules (e.g., cyclic AMP, inositol 1,4,5-trisphosphate [IP_3], Ca^{2+}), thus helping to propagate the signal from cell to cell. Gap junctions are abundant in circular muscle (about 250 per cell in guinea pig intestine) but appear to be rare or absent in longitudinal muscle and teniae coli.[1,2,5,6] It is not known why gap junctions are more abundant in circular muscle and whether this feature reflects other differences between circular and longitudinal muscle, such as differences in Ca^{2+} mobilization and signal transduction (see below). Despite their paucity in longitudinal muscle, electrical coupling between muscle cells in this layer appears to be well-maintained.

About 80% of the interior of the cell is occupied by dense bodies and contractile filaments; the remainder is occupied by various organelles, including nucleus, mitochondria, Golgi appa-

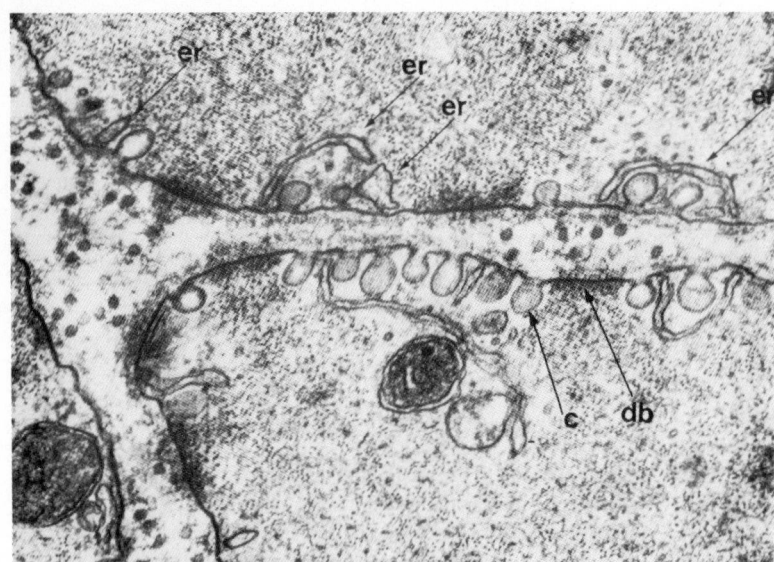

FIGURE 4–1. Surface organization of three adjacent muscle cells from circular muscle layer of guinea pig ileum. Clusters of basket-shaped caveolae, *c*, surrounded by endoplasmic reticulum, *er*, are separated from each other by dense bands, *db*; ×67,000. (From Gabella G. Structure of muscles and nerves in the gastrointestinal tract. In: Johnson LR, ed. Physiology of the gastrointestinal tract, ed 2. New York: Raven Press, 1987:335.)

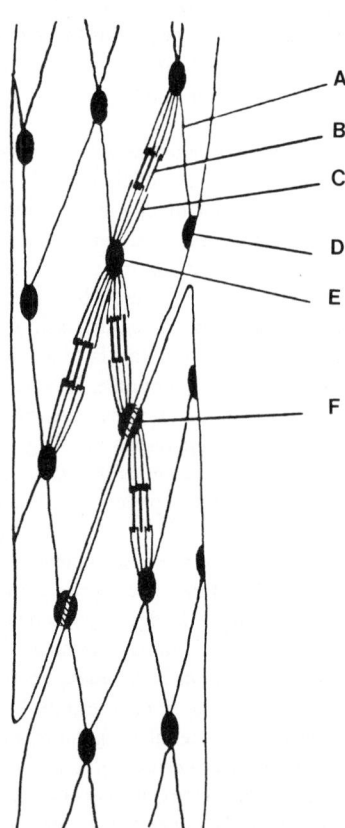

FIGURE 4–2. Organization of contractile and cytoskeletal apparatus in smooth muscle cells. Thin actin filaments, *c*, emerge from the poles of cytoplasmic dense bodies, *e*, and interdigitate with thick myosin filaments, *b*. Dense bodies, *d*, in the plasma membrane are connected to dense bodies, *e*, in the cytoplasm by intermediate filaments, *a*. When juxtaposed, dense bodies from adjacent cells can form close intermediate junctions, *f*. (Adapted from Murphy RA. Contraction of muscle cells. In: Berne RM, Levy MN, eds. Physiology ed 2. Washington, DC: CV Mosby, 1988:315.)

ratus, lysosomes, and rough and smooth endoplasmic reticulum. Mitochondria occupy 5% to 9% of cell volume and are found near the surface of the cell and at the poles of the nucleus. The *endoplasmic reticulum* occupies 2% of cell volume and is mostly located immediately beneath and parallel to the plasma membrane (see Fig 4-1). Evidence based on electron probe analysis of muscle cells[7] and on measurements of Ca^{2+} uptake and release in cells and microsomal fractions supports the notion that the endoplasmic reticulum is the site of Ca^{2+} storage and release.[8-10] However, there is also evidence that the endoplasmic reticulum consists of several functional compartments, only one of which is sensitive to IP_3, the membrane-derived messenger responsible for release of intracellular Ca^{2+}.[11] The mitochondria, considered a low-affinity, high-capacity store, can take up large amounts of Ca^{2+} but only after cell injury when cytosolic Ca^{2+} increases above maximal physiologic levels (> 1–5 μM).[12]

Contractile Apparatus: Thin and Thick Filaments

Three types of filaments can be distinguished in smooth muscle cells: thin actin filaments (5–7 nm), thick myosin filaments (15 nm), and intermediate desmin filaments (10 nm). Intermediate filaments link dense bodies in the cytoplasm to dense bands on the plasma membrane. Although the arrangement of thin, thick, and intermediate filaments and their attachment to cytoplasmic dense bodies lacks the order found in striated muscle, assemblies reminiscent of primitive sarcomeres can be distinguished (Figs 4-2 and 4-3).

Thin filaments consist of actin, a ubiquitous 42-kd globular protein (G-actin) that polymerizes to form two-stranded helical filaments (F-actin) of indeterminate length.[13] Inserted into the grooves of the actin helix is another protein, tropomyosin. Thin filaments have a distinct polarity; they appear to be inserted into

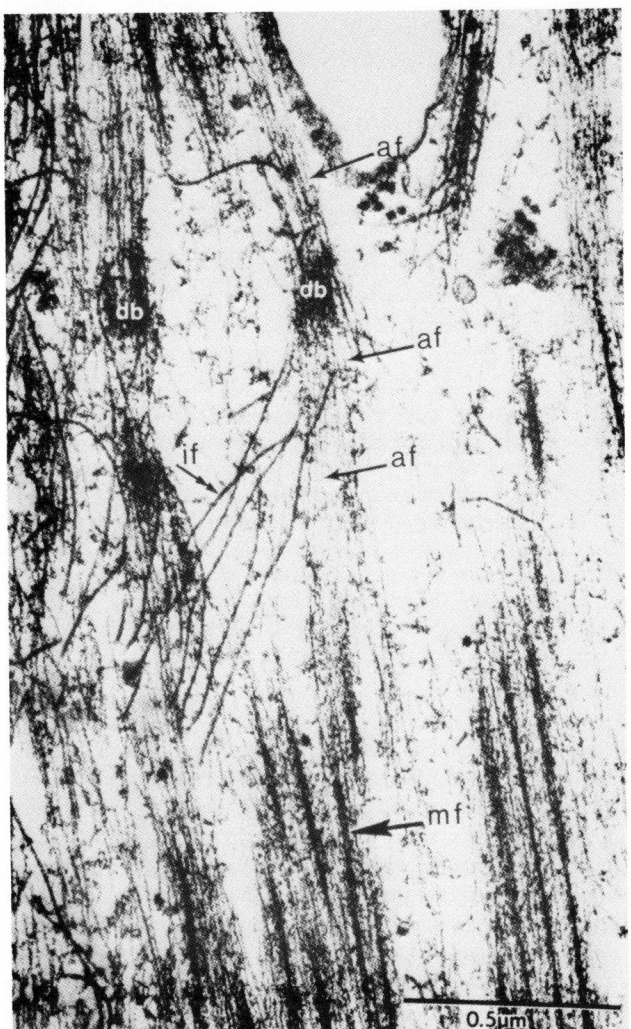

FIGURE 4–3. Organization of filaments in smooth muscle cells. Thin actin filaments, *af,* emerging from the poles of dense bodies, *db,* interdigitate with thick myosin filaments, *mf.* Intermediate filaments, *if,* associated with dense bodies are also shown. Section from a saponin-treated mesenteric vein by AV Somlyo. (From Hartshorne DJ. Biochemistry of the contractile process in smooth muscle. In Johnson LR, ed. Physiology of the gastrointestinal tract, ed 2. New York: Raven Press, 1987:423.)

or emerge from the poles of dense bodies and are arranged in bundles that run parallel to the long axis of the cells, their free ends surrounding and interdigitating with thick myosin filaments (see Figs 4-2 and 4-3).[1–3,14] The insertion of thin filaments in dense bodies is analogous to that found in Z disks of striated muscle cells; in effect, dense bodies may be viewed as dispersed fragments of Z discs held together and anchored to dense bands of the cell membrane by intermediate filaments.

Thick filaments are aggregates of myosin molecules, a complex 480-kd protein formed by the association of six different proteins.[13,15] These proteins are not covalently linked and can be dissociated from each other into a pair of *myosin heavy chains* and two pairs of *myosin light chains* (Fig 4-4). The heavy chains are coiled around each other to form a rigid insoluble α-helical core or tail. Each strand of the core terminates in a globular head

surrounded by two myosin light chains: a 20-kd regulatory chain and a 17-kd "essential" chain. Each globular head contains a binding site for actin and an *actin-activated Mg^{2+}*–adenosine triphosphatase (Mg^{2+}–ATPase). A hinge located at the junction of the globular head and core enables the head to rotate about the core. Another hinge in the core enables the globular heads to project laterally. The globular heads and the segments of the core between the two hinges are called *crossbridges* because they constitute a link or bridge between thick myosin and thin actin filaments.

The thick filaments are relatively few in number; three to five thick filaments are surrounded by and interdigitate with a much larger number of actin filaments. The ratio of thin to thick filaments is reflected in the relative content actin and myosin; visceral smooth muscle contains the same amount of actin as striated muscle (22–28 mg/g cell) but a lower amount of myosin (20 versus 62 mg/g cell).[13] Despite the low content of myosin, smooth muscle generates as much force as striated muscle (up to 6 kg/cm^2 of cross-sectional area).[4,16]

INTERACTION OF CONTRACTILE PROTEINS

The interaction of myosin and actin with hydrolysis of adenosine triphosphate (ATP) is the fundamental reaction whereby chemical energy is converted into mechanical energy in smooth muscle. The reaction generates force and induces shortening as a result of the sliding of overlapping, interdigitating thin and thick filaments.

Phosphorylation of Myosin Light Chain

An essential first step in smooth muscle contraction is phosphorylation of the 20-kd regulatory myosin light chain (MLC) by *myosin light chain kinase* (MLC kinase).[13,17–21] The steps leading to activation of this enzyme include the following: (1) increase in cytosolic free Ca^{2+} ($[Ca^{2+}]_i$), which occurs when the cell is stimulated; the increase results either from influx of Ca^{2+} into the cytosol by way of voltage-gated or ligand-gated Ca^{2+} channels or from release of Ca^{2+} into the cytosol from intracellular Ca^{2+} stores; (2) sequential binding of Ca^{2+} to the four binding sites on the regulatory protein, *calmodulin*; (3) the binding of Ca^{2+}-activated calmodulin to MLC kinase to form the active complex, Ca^{2+}–calmodulin–MLC kinase. Phosphorylation of the 20-kd MLC associated with the myosin head should be distinguished from phosphorylation of the myosin head itself (see below). Phosphorylation of MLC induces a conformational change in the myosin head that greatly enhances the ability of actin to activate myosin–Mg^{2+}–ATPase and bring about the hydrolysis of ATP bound to the myosin head.

Interaction of Myosin and Actin: The Crossbridge Cycle

The interaction of myosin and actin with hydrolysis of ATP occurs in a cycle the essential feature of which is a shift in the affinity

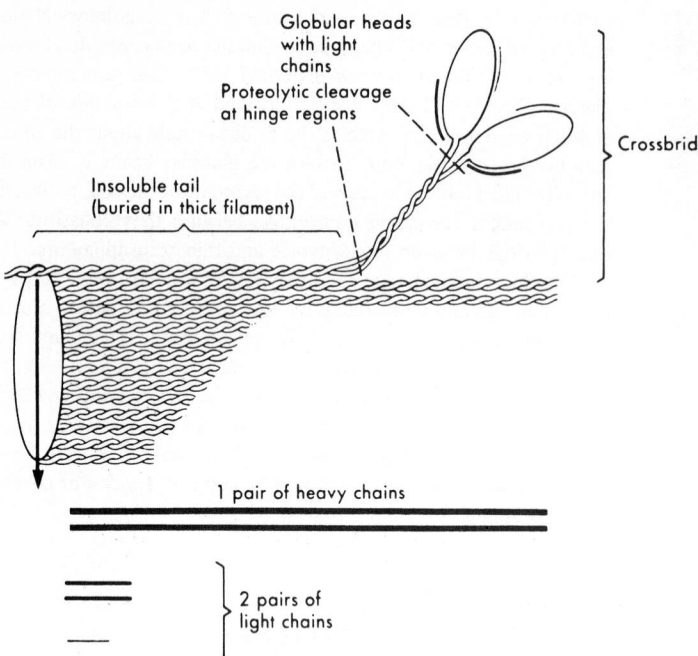

FIGURE 4–4. Component proteins of the myosin molecule. A crossbridge is shown projecting laterally from the main segment of the myosin core (tail). Each crossbridge consists of: (1) a pair of myosin heads each surrounded by a 17-kd and a 20-kd myosin light chain, and (2) a laterally projecting segment of the myosin core between the two hinge regions. The cores of many myosin molecules form thick filaments with several projecting crossbridges. (Adapted from Murphy RA. Contraction of muscle cells. In Berne RM, Levy MN, eds. Physiology, ed 2. Washington, DC: CV Mosby, 1988:315.)

of myosin for actin.[13] ATP, bound weakly to myosin, is hydrolyzed to adenosine diphosphate (ADP) and inorganic phosphate (P_i). The products of hydrolysis remain bound to the myosin head, and the energy released is stored in the myosin molecule, which, in this state, has a high affinity for actin. Upon release of ADP and P_i, ATP binds again to myosin, which reverts to a state of low affinity for actin.

Various models have been proposed to describe how the interaction between phosphorylated myosin heads and actin filaments could generate force, filament movement, and cell shortening.[13,22] According to the model illustrated in Figure 4-5, the myosin crossbridge (which includes the myosin head and associated MLCs together with a segment of the myosin core between the two hinges)

alternates between two conformations that have different affinities for actin. In one conformation, the myosin crossbridge is oriented such that its head makes a 90-degree angle with the actin filament; in this state, it has a low affinity for actin and is weakly bound to it. In the other conformation, the myosin crossbridge changes its orientation such that the head makes a 45-degree angle with the actin filament; in this state, it has a high affinity for actin and is tightly bound to it.

At the start of a cycle, the myosin crossbridge with ATP bound to the myosin head (myosin.ATP) is either detached or weakly bound to actin (Figs 4-5 and 4-6). Hydrolysis of ATP by myosin–Mg^{2+}–ATPase yields a myosin intermediate with the products of hydrolysis still bound to the myosin head (myosin.ADP.P_i). Release

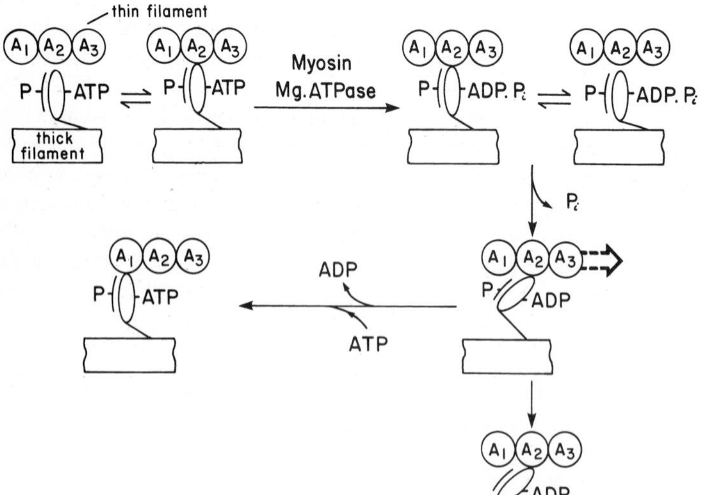

FIGURE 4–5. Interaction of myosin and actin filaments. At the start of the crossbridge cycle, the myosin head with ATP bound to it (myosin.ATP) is either detached or weakly attached to an actin molecule, A_2, in the thin filament. Hydrolysis of ATP by the myosin–Mg^{2+}–ATPase yields an intermediate with the products of hydrolysis still bound to it (myosin.ADP.P_i); the intermediate is either detached or weakly bound to the actin molecule. Release of P_i in the next step causes a transition from weak to strong binding of myosin and actin (actin.myosin.ADP) and a change from 90 degrees to 45 degrees in the angle of the myosin head. The strain imposed on the crossbridge by the change of angle is relieved when the actin molecule slides past the crossbridge. ADP is released slowly; the myosin head rebinds ATP (myosin.ATP) and reverts to a 90-degree angle facing the next actin molecule, A_1, for the start of another cycle. Dephosphorylation of the myosin light chain surrounding a bound myosin head yields a strongly attached, slowly cycling "latch" crossbridge. The interaction of only one myosin head in the crossbridge is illustrated. (Modified from Hartshorne DJ. Biochemistry of the contractile process in smooth muscle. In: Johnson LR, ed. Physiology of the gastrointestinal tract, ed 2. New York: Raven Press, 1987:423.)

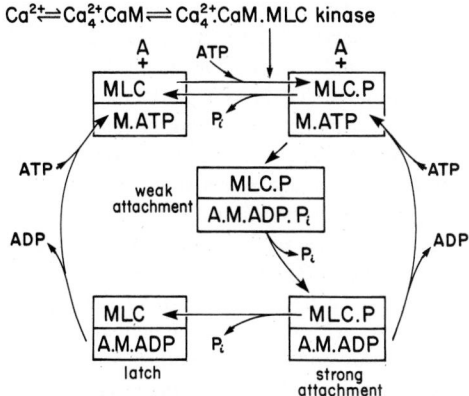

$Ca^{2+} \rightleftharpoons Ca_4^{2+}.CaM \rightleftharpoons Ca_4^{2+}.CaM.MLC \text{ kinase}$

FIGURE 4–6. Chemical reactions involved in contraction and relaxation. Phosphorylation of myosin light chain (MLC) by MLC kinase is a prerequisite for initiation of contraction in smooth muscle. MLC kinase is activated by a Ca^{++}–calmodulin complex. The sequence of attachment and detachment (cycling) of the crossbridges with hydrolysis of ATP bound to the myosin heads follows that illustrated in Figure 4–5. Relaxation occurs when cytosolic Ca^{++} decreases, causing a decrease in the activity of MLC kinase, dephosphorylation of MLC, and interruption of the crossbridge cycle. Dephosphorylation of MLC while the myosin head is still attached yields a "latch" crossbridge that detaches very slowly; the dephosphorylation of MLC is presumably mediated by an MLC phosphatase.

of P$_i$ from this intermediate is the force-generating step causing a transition from weak to strong binding of myosin and actin (actin.myosin.ADP) and a change from 90 degrees to 45 degrees in the angle of the myosin head. The change of angle imposes a strain on the crossbridge, which is relieved when the actin molecule slides past the crossbridge. In the next step, ADP is released from the myosin head. This step occurs slowly in smooth muscle and is rate-limiting with respect to the velocity of shortening. This means that, in smooth muscle, myosin remains bound to actin longer, generating more force with less consumption of energy than in striated muscle. Upon release of ADP, the myosin head is free to rebind ATP (myosin.ATP) and reverts to a 90-degree angle in which it is weakly bound to the next actin molecule for the start of another cycle.

The force generated by crossbridge cycling depends on the number of crossbridges acting in parallel. Because the crossbridges do not cycle in unison, the contraction induced by their concerted action is both slow and continuous. Force and shortening velocity depend on the stimulus in smooth muscle, which implies that, in smooth muscle, unlike striated muscle, both the number and cycling rate of activated crossbridges are regulated.

Crossbridge cycling ceases when the stimulus is withdrawn. Cytosolic Ca^{2+}, MLC kinase activity, and MLC phosphorylation revert to their resting levels and the dephosphorylated myosin crossbridges are arrested in a detached state characteristic of muscle relaxation.[16,23]

A different pattern of crossbridge cycling is observed during sustained (i.e., tonic) contraction of smooth muscle. Upon stimulation, there is initially a rapid increase in cytosolic Ca^{2+}, MLC kinase activity, MLC phosphorylation, and shortening velocity (reflecting crossbridge cycling rate); these events precede but are correlated with the increase in muscle tension.[16,19,23] Within seconds, despite continued stimulation, there is a rapid decrease in cytosolic Ca^{2+}, MLC phosphorylation, and shortening velocity to low suprabasal levels, while muscle contraction attains a peak and thereafter maintains a near steady state.

The state in which tension is maintained while Ca^{2+} levels, MLC phosphorylation, and shortening velocity are low has been called the *"latch"* state.[24] The state reflects a transition from a population of rapidly cycling crossbridges to a population of attached, noncycling or slowly cycling crossbridges. Force (sustained contraction) is maintained by "latch" bridges (i.e., crossbridges that become dephosphorylated while they are attached and, in this state, develop a slow detachment rate). This type of contraction is functionally useful in muscle that is required to maintain the dimensions of a hollow organ against imposed loads with minimal consumption of energy (less than 1% of the ATP consumption needed to sustain a comparable force in striated muscle).[16]

An alternative mechanism that does not depend on MLC phosphorylation or crossbridge cycling has been proposed to explain sustained tonic contraction. The mechanism is thought to depend on the binding of a segment (heavy meromyosin) of the myosin core to *caldesmon*, an elongated 150-kd protein associated with actin in the thin filament.[25,26] Caldesmon (molar ratio relative to actin 1:28) occupies the grooves between the actin double helix, its head piece located in register with tropomyosin. In vitro, its presence increases greatly the affinity of actin filaments for heavy meromyosin derived from smooth but not striated muscle. It is possible that the tight binding of the actin helix to the myosin core involves the phosphorylation of caldesmon by Ca^{2+}-dependent protein kinase C. This implies that sustained tonic contraction is mediated by a distinct Ca^{2+}-dependent mechanism involving the myosin core that is regulated differently from the Ca^{2+}-dependent cycle of contraction–relaxation controlled by myosin crossbridges.

Unlike tonic contraction, phasic contraction increases and decreases rapidly in phase with the influx and efflux of Ca^{2+}, driven by rhythmic changes in membrane potential and the opening and closing of voltage-gated ionic channels. A closer correlation is more likely to prevail during phasic activity between Ca^{2+} levels, MLC phosphorylation, crossbridge cycling rate, and contraction. Consequently, more energy is required to sustain phasic contraction; energy is saved, however, because phasic contractile activity is usually maintained in abeyance by a dominant inhibitory neural input (see below).

MOBILIZATION OF ACTIVATOR CALCIUM

Source of Activator Calcium

The concentration of Ca^{2+} in the cytosol is the essential determinant of smooth muscle activity. The cell mobilizes Ca^{2+} by various mechanisms to initiate, sustain, or terminate contraction. The mechanisms differ depending on the location of the muscle cell (e.g., in the circular or longitudinal muscle layer) and the type of stimulus (e.g., electrical or pharmacologic) resulting in Ca^{2+} mobilization. Differences in Ca^{2+} mobilization may reflect functional differences among types of smooth muscle that can sustain tonic, phasic, or both tonic and phasic contraction.

Two mechanisms have been identified that lead to an increase in cytosolic Ca^{2+} during contraction. In the first, interaction of a contractile agonist with a specific receptor on the plasma membrane generates a messenger that causes release of Ca^{2+} from intracellular stores. In the second, interaction of a contractile agonist with a specific receptor on the plasma membrane initiates the opening of agonist-gated or voltage-gated Ca^{2+} channels in the plasma membrane, directly, by way of release of second messengers or by causing depolarization of the plasma membrane. The first mechanism underlies tonic contraction and is demonstrable in muscle cells isolated from the circular muscle layer; the second underlies electrically driven phasic contraction and is demonstrable in muscle cells isolated from the longitudinal muscle layer. In the intact muscle syncytium, however, cells from both muscle layers can be electrically driven by rapid or slow depolarization of the plasma membrane (i.e., by slow waves and spike potentials) leading to opening of voltage-gated Ca^{2+} channels.

Outline of Transduction Pathway

The transduction of an external signal (neurotransmitter, hormone, autacoid, or drug) into an internal signal involves sequential activation of three membrane proteins: a receptor and a guanosine triphosphate (GTP)-binding protein (G protein) that couples the receptor to a specific effector enzyme; the latter acts on membrane-bound or cytoplasmic precursors to generate one or more regulatory signals (second messengers) (Fig 4-7).

Receptors consist of external, membrane-spanning and cytoplasmic domains with features that determine which specific ligand they bind (or agonist they recognize) and which G protein or membrane enzyme they activate.[27,28]

G proteins are a large family of closely related proteins that act as signal transducers.[29,30] Among these are G proteins that stimulate (G_s) or inhibit (G_i) adenylate cyclase activity and G proteins that stimulate (G_o or G_p) phospholipase C activity. G proteins are heterotrimeric with subunits designated α, β, and γ in order of decreasing mass. The α subunit (G_α), which serves to differentiate G proteins, contains a single, high-affinity binding site for GTP and possesses GTPase activity; the latter is crucial for terminating the action of G proteins. In the basal state, guanosine diphosphate (GDP) is tightly bound to the α subunit. The binding of a ligand to its receptor enables the ligand–receptor complex to interact with the G protein and stimulate the dissociation of GDP; this opens up a site that is rapidly filled with abundant cytoplasmic GTP. The binding of GTP to the ligand–receptor–G protein complex causes: (1) a decrease in the affinity of the ligand for the receptor and of the receptor for the G protein, thus freeing the receptor for a new cycle of ligand and G protein binding; and (2) a decrease in the affinity of the α subunit for the $\beta\gamma$ complex resulting in the dissociation of a mobile $G_\alpha.GTP$ complex, which activates the effector enzyme. The hydrolysis of GTP by the intrinsic GTPase activity of the $G_\alpha.GTP$ complex terminates the activity of the complex and enables the reassociation of the α, β, and γ subunits. The hydrolysis of GTP is slow, enabling prolonged activation of the effector enzyme. The various G proteins act as transducers that conduct and amplify the external signal and as adapters that allow the same receptor to be coupled to different effector enzymes.

The *effector enzyme* to which agonists capable of mobilizing intracellular Ca^{2+} in a variety of cells including muscle cells are coupled, is a specific *phospholipase C* that hydrolyzes *inositol phospholipids* located on the inner leaflet of the plasma membrane.[11,31-33] These phospholipids are products of sequential phos-

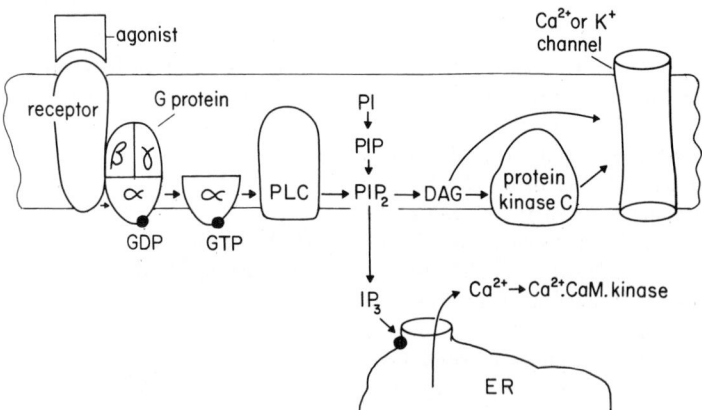

FIGURE 4–7. Signal transduction pathway for Ca^{++}-mobilizing agonists in smooth muscle cells. The sequence involves binding of an agonist to a specific receptor, activation of a transducing G-protein and binding of guanosine triphosphate (GTP) to its mobile α-subunit, activation of phospholipase C (PLC), and hydrolysis of membrane-bound inositol phospholipids. In circular muscle cells, the immediate substrate hydrolyzed by PLC is phosphatidylinositol 4,5-bisphosphate (PIP_2) yielding inosiol 1,4,5-trisphosphate (IP_3) and diacylglycerol (DAG) as second messengers. In longitudinal muscle cells, the main substrates hydrolyzed by PLC are phosphatidylinositol (PI) and phosphatidylinositol 4-monophosphate (PIP) yielding only diacylglycerol as second messenger. Diacylglycerol activates protein kinase C, translocating it from the cytosol to the plasma membrane. IP_3 diffuses through the cytosol to interact with an IP_3 receptor on the membrane of the endoplasmic reticulum causing release of Ca^{++} into the cytosol. Diacylglycerol either directly or by activation of protein kinase C regulates the activity of Ca^{++} and K^+ channels on the plasma membrane.

phorylation (i.e., addition of phosphate groups derived from ATP to positions 4 and 5 of the six-carbon ring of inositol) of *phosphatidylinositol* (PI) to *phosphatidylinositol monophosphate* (PIP) and *phosphatidylinositol 4,5-bisphosphate* (PIP$_2$). The latter is the immediate substrate (precursor) hydrolyzed by phospholipase C in most cells.

Second Messengers: IP$_3$ and Diacylglycerol

Hydrolysis of the inositol phospholipid, PIP$_2$, generates two messengers: (1) a water-soluble inositol phosphate, IP$_3$, which diffuses into the cytosol to interact with a specific receptor coupled to a Ca^{2+} channel located on a compartment of the endoplasmic reticulum, and (2) diacylglycerol (DAG), which activates the enzyme protein kinase C by increasing its affinity for Ca^{2+} and phospholipids and translocating it from the cytosol to the plasma membrane (see Fig 4-7).[31–35] IP$_3$ can be converted by sequential phosphorylation to IP$_4$, IP$_5$, or IP$_6$; these inositol phosphates, like IP$_3$, are eventually converted by sequential dephosphorylation to IP$_2$, IP$_1$, and inositol. DAG is hydrolyzed with release of arachidonic acid and monoacylglycerol; the metabolic products of the two messengers eventually merge to reconstitute PI.

One metabolic product of IP$_3$, *inositol 1,3,4,5-tetrakisphosphate* (IP$_4$), appears to be involved in regulating Ca^{2+} reuptake into the intracellular store.[11] Its action requires the simultaneous presence of IP$_3$. According to one hypothesis, IP$_4$ regulates reentry of Ca^{2+} from outside the cell into a compartment of the endoplasmic reticulum close to the plasma membrane, which, in turn, communicates with the IP$_3$-sensitive Ca^{2+}-depleted compartment (Fig 4-8).

The initial IP$_3$-induced release of Ca^{2+} is followed in many cell types by periodic release of smaller amounts of Ca^{2+} at intervals of 5 to 60 seconds.[11,36] It is not known whether the oscillations in cytosolic Ca^{2+} reflect oscillations in the level of IP$_3$. It is possible that initial release of Ca^{2+} by IP$_3$—a prerequisite for the subsequent oscillations of cytosolic Ca^{2+}—reflects Ca^{2+}-induced Ca^{2+} release from an IP$_3$-insensitive compartment. Like other second messengers (e.g., cyclic AMP), both IP$_3$ and Ca^{2+} can flow rapidly (about 10 μm/sec) through gap junctions to neighboring cells, propagating the intracellular signal and providing a means for sustained or oscillatory response of the tissue as a whole.

The *IP$_3$ receptor* on the endoplasmic reticulum has been characterized and found to be homologous to the "ryanodine" receptor, the Ca^{2+} channel of the sarcoplasmic reticulum in striated muscle.[37–39] The IP$_3$ receptor, like the "ryanodine" receptor, consists of four subunits surrounding a Ca^{2+} channel. Each subunit contains a large N-terminal domain on the cytoplasmic face of the endoplasmic reticulum, which probably includes the IP$_3$ binding site and the site for phosphorylation (inactivation of the channel) by cyclic AMP-dependent protein kinase (see Figs 4-7 and 4-8).

Identification of Steps in Signal Transduction

Several probes are useful in identifying specific steps in the signal transduction pathway. G proteins, including some coupled to phospholipase C, can be inactivated by exposure of cells to pertussis toxin, which induces nicotinamide adenine nucleotide (NAD)-dependent ADP-ribosylation of the α subunit. G proteins can be activated directly in intact muscle cells by NaF; G proteins can also be activated directly in permeabilized cells by nonhydrolyzable analogues of GTP, such as GTPγS; the effect of GTPγS is selectively blocked by GDPβS.[40] The cells are permeabilized by brief exposure to mild detergents to make the plasma membrane permeable to normally impermeant agents, and suspended in a

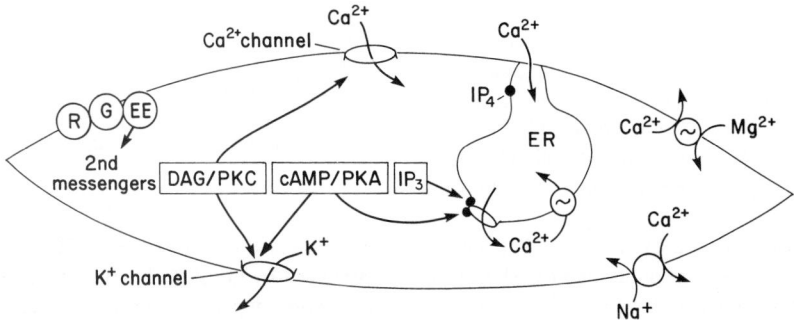

FIGURE 4-8. Messengers and ionic channels involved in the regulation of cytosolic Ca^{++}. Inositol 1,4,5-trisphosphate (IP$_3$) regulates Ca^{++} release from Ca^{++} stores (endoplasmic reticulum) in circular muscle cells. A Ca^{++}-ATPase pump and inositol 1,3,4,5-tetrakisphosphate (IP$_4$) are involved in Ca^{++} reuptake into the store. Diacylglycerol (DAG) either directly or by activation of protein kinase C (PKC) regulates the activity of Ca^{++} and K$^+$ channels, resulting in depolarization of the plasma membrane, opening of Ca^{++} channels, and Ca^{++} influx into the cytosol. Cyclic AMP-dependent protein kinase (kinase A) influences cytosolic Ca^{++} by (1) decreasing Ca^{++} release (by way of the IP$_3$ receptor/Ca^{++} channel) and increasing Ca^{++} uptake (by way of the endoplasmic Ca^{++} pump) in the endoplasmic reticulum, and (2) decreasing Ca^{++} influx by activating K$^+$ channels and hyperpolarizing the plasma membrane. A high affinity Ca^{++}-ATPase pump on the plasma membrane is chiefly responsible for dissipating Ca^{++} transients and maintaining resting Ca^{++} concentrations; a low affinity Ca^{++}/Na$^+$ exchanger on the plasma membrane comes into operation if Ca^{++} rises to supraphysiologic levels.

medium containing a cytosol-like concentration of Ca^{2+} (150 nM);[10,12] mildly permeabilized cells retain enough receptors to enable them to respond fully to appropriate agonists.[10,40] Exogenous IP_3 can gain access to the intracellular Ca^{2+} store in permeabilized cells, and its ability to interact with IP_3 receptors and induce Ca^{2+} release can be examined; the effect of IP_3 under these conditions is selectively blocked by heparin.[41]

Mobilization of Calcium in Cells of Circular Muscle Layer

The transduction pathway detailed above regulates a variety of processes in excitable and nonexcitable cells, including metabolism, secretion, cell proliferation, neural activity, and smooth muscle contraction. In the gut, the pathway is fully expressed in cells from the circular muscle layer of the stomach, intestine, gallbladder, and various sphincters including the lower esophageal sphincter, and appears to be particularly suited for the maintenance of tonic contraction. The various steps in this pathway have been examined in detail in dispersed muscle cells. Dispersion eliminates diffusion barriers and engenders a suspension of muscle cells devoid of neurons and other cell types; the cellular homogeneity of the suspension makes it possible to characterize receptors and intracellular messengers (cytosolic Ca^{2+}, products of inositol phospholipid metabolism, and cyclic nucleotides) in muscle cells and determine their coupling to mechanical response (contraction or relaxation).[9,10,42,43]

Exposure of cells derived from the circular muscle layer to a contractile agonist induces rapid contraction (shortening) accompanied by an increase in IP_3, cytosolic free Ca^{2+}, and net Ca^{2+} efflux.[9,10,43-45] The pattern of response consists of an initial peak of IP_3 and cytosolic Ca^{2+} (within 5 seconds) followed by a peak of Ca^{2+} efflux and contraction (within 15–30 seconds; Fig 4-9*A*). The peaks of IP_3, cytosolic Ca^{2+}, and contraction are followed by a lower sustained plateau, and the peak of Ca^{2+} efflux (reflecting extrusion of Ca^{2+} released from intracellular stores) is followed by slow reuptake of Ca^{2+} into the cell. The peak responses (IP_3, cytosolic Ca^{2+}, Ca^{2+} efflux, and contraction) are concentration-dependent and closely correlated with each other (see Fig 4-9*B*). Withdrawal of Ca^{2+} from the medium or addition of Ca^{2+} channel blockers has no effect on peak contraction, cytosolic Ca^{2+}, and Ca^{2+} efflux, but inhibits partly or completely these events during the plateau phase.

The pattern of response exhibited by muscle cells from the circular muscle layer implies that contractile agonists elicit contraction by way of G protein-coupled activation of a membrane-bound effector enzyme, phospholipase C, that hydrolyzes membrane-bound inositol phospholipids to generate a water-soluble second messenger, IP_3; the latter diffuses through the cytosol to interact with specific receptors on an IP_3-sensitive compartment of the endoplasmic reticulum to cause release of intracellular Ca^{2+}.

Studies using a variety of probes confirm the occurrence of this sequence. Sodium fluoride, which can directly activate G proteins in intact muscle cells, and $GTP\gamma S$, which can directly activate these proteins in permeabilized muscle cells, mimic closely the effects of receptor-linked agonists, causing contraction and an increase in cytosolic Ca^{2+} and IP_3 production.[45,46] In permeabilized

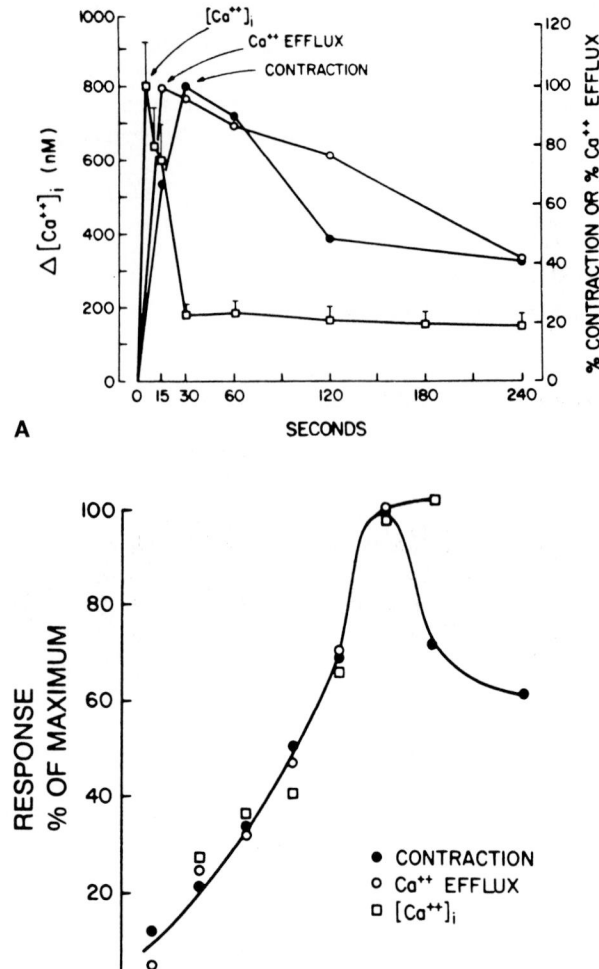

FIGURE 4–9. Time course, **A,** and stoichiometry, **B,** of contraction, increase in cytosolic Ca^{++} ($[Ca^{++}]_i$), and increase in net Ca^{++} efflux in smooth muscle cells isolated from guinea pig stomach in response to cholecystokinin-octapeptide (CCK-8). Similar results are obtained in muscle cells isolated from human stomach and intestine. (From Bitar KN, Bradford P, Putney JW Jr, Makhlouf GM. Cytosolic calcium during contraction of isolated mammalian gastric muscle cells. Science 1986;232:1143.)

muscle cells, the effects of $GTP\gamma S$, like those of agonists, are abolished by $GDP\beta S$. In these cells, exogenous IP_3 causes concentration-dependent contraction (EC_{50} 0.3 μM) and increase in cytosolic Ca^{2+}.[10,47] These responses to IP_3 and similar responses to $GTP\gamma S$ and receptor-linked agonists are inhibited by heparin, which is known to block IP_3-induced Ca^{2+} release.[41,46] In permeabilized muscle cells and in microsomal fractions containing endoplasmic reticulum derived from these cells, IP_3 but not other inositol phosphates, binds rapidly and saturably to specific IP_3 receptors; the binding of IP_3 is accompanied by release of Ca^{2+}.[47] Depletion of Ca^{2+} stores by repeated stimulation of permeabilized muscle cells suspended in Ca^{2+}-free medium with either IP_3 or a receptor-linked agonist abolishes the contractile response to both agents implying access to a common Ca^{2+} store.[9,10]

Mobilization of Calcium in Cells of Longitudinal Muscle Layer

Both the metabolism of inositol phospholipids and the source of Ca^{2+} responsible for contraction in cells isolated from the longitudinal muscle layer are markedly different. Exposure of these cells to a contractile agonist causes a concentration-dependent contraction and increase in cytosolic Ca^{2+} but not in net Ca^{2+} efflux.[44,47] Contraction and increase in cytosolic Ca^{2+} are abolished in Ca^{2+}-free medium or in the presence of Ca^{2+} channel blockers, implying that the source of Ca^{2+} responsible for contraction in these cells is extracellular. Sodium fluoride causes contraction in intact muscle cells, implying participation of a G protein in the pathway. In permeabilized muscle cells, however, receptor-linked agonists, GTPτS and IP_3 do not cause contraction or increase in cytosolic Ca^{2+}. Furthermore, in these cells and in microsomal fractions derived from them, there is little or no specific binding of IP_3.[47] Thus, although the cells can accumulate Ca^{2+} to the same extent as circular muscle cells, the stores do not contain receptors for and are not discharged by IP_3.

The pattern of inositol phospholipid metabolism suggests that IP_3 participates little or not at all in Ca^{2+} mobilization in longitudinal muscle cells. Despite equally high turnover of inositol phospholipids in both cell types,[45] the amount of IP_3 generated is minimal (3% of total inositol phosphates versus 50% in circular muscle cells), implying minimal hydrolyis of PIP_2. In contrast, inositol monophosphate (IP_1) and bisphosphate (IP_2) account for about 97% of total inositol phosphates, suggesting that in longitudinal muscle cells, PI and PIP are the major membrane phospholipids hydrolyzed by phospholipase C. Whether the effector enzyme or the G protein to which it is coupled is different in these cells is not known.

DAG is generated by hydrolysis of all membrane inositol phospholipids, whether the immediate substrate is PIP_2 (as in circular muscle cells), or PI and PIP (as in longitudinal muscle cells). Studies on isolated membrane patches suggest that DAG or DAG-activated protein kinase C may be responsible for Ca^{2+} influx into longitudinal muscle cells (see Figs 4-7 and 4-8). Mobilization of Ca^{2+} in longitudinal muscle cells could involve the following sequence. Interaction of a contractile agonist with a receptor coupled by way of a G protein to phospholipase C induces turnover of inositol phospholipids (mainly PI and PIP) and generation of DAG predominantly as second messenger; DAG activates protein kinase C, which, in turn, influences the activity of one or more ionic channels (see Figs 4-7 and 4-8). There is evidence that DAG can activate (open) voltage-gated Ca^{2+} channels and inactivate K^+ M-channels in smooth muscle cells.[48,49] Activation of Ca^{2+} channels carrying an inward current and inactivation of K^+ channels carrying an outward current depolarize the plasma membrane, causing further opening of voltage-gated Ca^{2+} channels and influx of Ca^{2+} into the cell.

Cytosolic Calcium Concentrations

Measurements of cytosolic Ca^{2+} using Ca^{2+}-sensitive fluorescent dyes were first made in muscle cells of the guinea pig and human stomach and subsequently confirmed in muscle cells of the longitudinal and circular muscle layers of the intestine in both species.[10,44] Resting (range 70 to 170 nM) and agonist-stimulated cytosolic Ca^{2+} concentrations were remarkably similar in cells isolated from the two muscle layers in both species. A two- to threefold increase in cytosolic Ca^{2+} (250–300 nM) induces half-maximal contraction and a four- to sixfold increase (800–1000 nM) induces maximal contraction in intact muscle cells. Exposure of permeabilized muscle cells to these concentrations of Ca^{2+} elicits similar degrees of contraction.

Periodic release of Ca^{2+} resulting in low-amplitude oscillations of cytosolic Ca^{2+} has been reported in vascular smooth muscle and may well occur in visceral smooth muscle.[50] According to one hypothesis, the oscillations are triggered by the initial Ca^{2+} transient independently of its source and reflect Ca^{2+}-induced Ca^{2+} release from IP_3-insensitive stores.[11] It is, therefore, likely that such oscillations will occur in both circular and longitudinal muscle cells.

Regulation of Cytosolic Calcium at Rest and During Relaxation

Smooth muscle cells, like other cells, possess efficient mechanisms to dispose of the Ca^{2+} transients that occur during contraction. In the resting state, the cells maintain low concentrations of Ca^{2+} in the cytosol despite large chemical (2 mM Ca^{2+} outside versus 100–200 nM Ca^{2+} inside the cell) and electrical (membrane potential -40 to -80 mV) gradients favoring the movement of Ca^{2+} into the cell. The gradient for Ca^{2+} is maintained because of low permeability of the plasma membrane to Ca^{2+} and the presence of efficient *Ca^{2+} extrusion* mechanisms in the plasma membrane and a *Ca^{2+} uptake* mechanism in the membrane of the endoplasmic reticulum, the site of Ca^{2+} storage in the cell.

The Ca^{2+} extrusion mechanisms in the plasma membrane[51] include: (1) a calmodulin-dependent *Ca^{2+}–Mg^{2+}–ATPase*, which acts as a high-affinity Ca^{2+} pump sustained by ATP hydrolysis; the pump responds to low concentrations of Ca^{2+} similar to those that occur during contraction (half-maximal velocity at 0.25 μM Ca^{2+}); and (2) a low-affinity, high-capacity *Na^+/Ca^{2+} exchanger* sustained by the Na^+ gradient across the plasma membrane; the exchanger responds to more drastic changes in cytosolic Ca^{2+} concentrations (half-maximal velocity at 1 to 5 μM Ca^{2+}; see Fig 4-8).

The Ca^{2+} uptake mechanism in the endoplasmic reticulum is also a high-affinity Ca^{2+}–ATPase pump, and it too participates in dissipating the Ca^{2+} transients occurring during contraction. Most of the Ca^{2+} required to replenish the endoplasmic Ca^{2+} store, however, enters the cell from the outside by way of voltage-gated Ca^{2+} channels that appear to have a privileged path to one compartment of the endoplasmic reticulum. Phosphorylation of the endoplasmic Ca^{2+} uptake pump by cyclic AMP-dependent protein kinase increases the activity of the pump and is partly responsible for the decrease in cytosolic Ca^{2+} induced by cyclic AMP-dependent relaxant agents (Fig 4-10).

Other mechanisms besides the Ca^{2+}-activated extrusion and uptake mechanisms participate in dissipating the Ca^{2+} transient and restoring the muscle cell to its resting, relaxed state. Where the Ca^{2+} transient is caused by influx of Ca^{2+} through voltage-

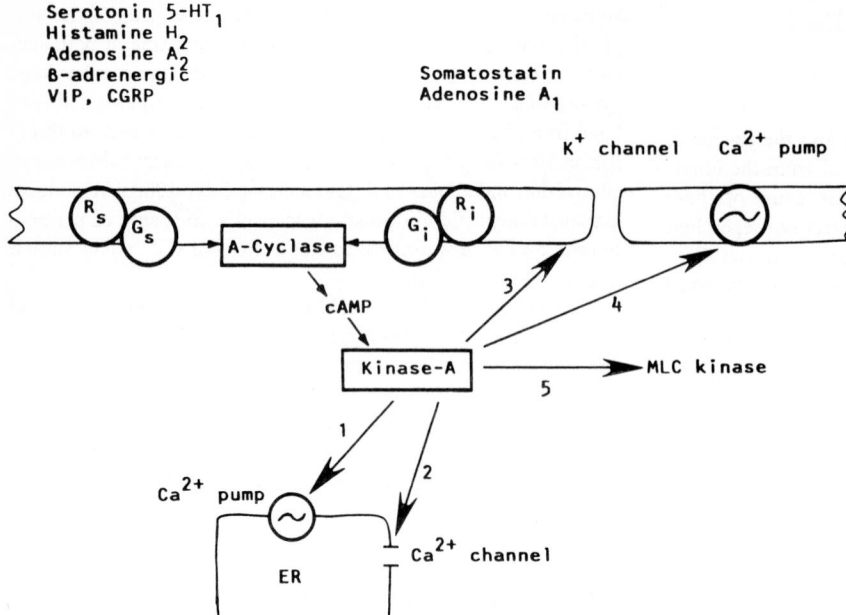

Serotonin 5-HT$_1$
Histamine H$_2$
Adenosine A$_2$
β-adrenergic
VIP, CGRP

Somatostatin
Adenosine A$_1$

K$^+$ channel   Ca^{2+} pump

FIGURE 4–10. Mechanisms of action of cyclic AMP-dependent protein kinase in causing smooth muscle relaxation. Stimulatory (R$_s$) and inhibitory (R$_i$) receptors coupled to stimulatory (G$_s$) or inhibitory (G$_i$) G-proteins determine the activity of membrane-bound adenylate cyclase and generation of cyclic AMP. Cyclic AMP-dependent protein kinase (kinase-A) can decrease the levels of cytosolic Ca^{++} by enhancing Ca^{++} uptake into the endoplasmic reticulum (*1*), inhibiting Ca^{++} release from the endoplasmic reticulum (*2*), opening Ca^{++}-activated K$^+$ channels, thus, hyperpoplarizing the plasma membrane and decreasing Ca^{++} influx into the cell (*3*), and possibly stimulating the activity of the Ca^{++}-ATPase pump on the plasma membrane (*4*). In addition, kinase-A by phosphorylating myosin light chain (MLC) kinase decreases its activity and, thus, lowers the sensitivity of contractile proteins to cytosolic Ca^{++}. The mechanisms of action of cyclic GMP-dependent protein kinase are probably similar.

gated Ca^{2+} channels after depolarization of the plasma membrane, repolarization (or hyperpolarization) of the membrane brought about by the opening of Ca^{2+}-activated K$^+$ channels interrupts further influx of Ca^{2+} into the cell. Some agents, in effect, induce relaxation by acting as agonists of various types of membrane K$^+$ channels (e.g., Ca^{2+}-activated or ATP-sensitive K$^+$ channels).[52–55]

Other agents such as the neuropeptide, vasoactive intestinal peptide (VIP), and β-adrenergic agonists cause relaxation by interacting with receptors coupled to adenylate cyclase[56,57] (see Figs 4-8 and 4-10). The resultant increase in cyclic AMP and *cyclic AMP-dependent protein kinase* activity leads to a decrease in cytosolic Ca^{2+} by: (1) inhibiting Ca^{2+} release from the endoplasmic reticulum and stimulating Ca^{2+} uptake by the endoplasmic Ca^{2+} pump;[58,59] and (2) stimulating the activity of membrane K$^+$ channels leading to hyperpolarization and interruption of further influx of Ca^{2+} into the cell (see Figs 4-8 and 4-10).[53,54] Thus, cyclic AMP-dependent mechanisms can reduce cytosolic Ca^{2+} whether the Ca^{2+} transient occurs as a result of release from intracellular stores or influx by way of voltage-gated Ca^{2+} channels. It is not certain whether the Ca^{2+} pump on the plasma membrane is also activated by cyclic AMP- or cyclic GMP-dependent protein kinase to aid in Ca^{2+} extrusion.[60]

In addition to influencing the level of cytosolic Ca^{2+}, cyclic AMP-dependent protein kinase can influence the action of Ca^{2+} by phosphorylating MLC kinase, thus decreasing its sensitivity to activation by the Ca^{2+}–calmodulin complex (see Fig 4-10).[61] Contraction induced in permeabilized muscle cells or muscle strips by changing the Ca^{2+} concentration in the medium is inhibited by addition of cyclic AMP or the regulatory component of cyclic AMP-dependent protein kinase, consistent with the existence of an additional mechanism involving the action rather than the mobilization of Ca^{2+}.[58,62]

ELECTRICAL PROPERTIES OF SMOOTH MUSCLE

Resting Membrane Potential

The resting membrane potential, defined as the steady-state potential at which the net flow of current (ions) across the plasma membrane is zero, varies from about −40 mV to −80 mV in muscle cells of the gut.[63,64] Graded differences in resting membrane potential exist between muscle cells in different regions (e.g., fundus, corpus, and antrum of the stomach) and between muscle cells located at different depths in the same region (e.g, cells near the myenteric border versus cells near the submucosal border of circular muscle in the antrum or colon).[64–67]

The membrane potential is largely determined by the activity of the Na$^+$-K$^+$ pump (Na$^+$-K$^+$-ATPase), which sets up diffusion gradients for K$^+$ (162 mM in versus 5 mM out) and Na$^+$ (136 mM out versus 14 mM in) across the membrane. The permeability of the membrane to K$^+$ is much greater than to Na$^+$, and the flow of K$^+$ ions down their electrochemical gradient creates a diffusion potential that is the major contributant to resting membrane potential. The flow occurs through passive K$^+$-selective channels that remain open at rest.[68]

In addition to setting up ionic gradients, the Na$^+$-K$^+$ pump is electrogenic, moving 3 Na$^+$ ions out of the cell for every 2 K$^+$ ions into the cell; the net outward flow of positive charge can contribute up to 30 mV to resting membrane potential. Variability in the direct contribution of this pump may account for regional differences in resting membrane potential. For example, the gradient in membrane potential between cells at the submucosal and myenteric borders of colonic circular muscle in the dog is abolished by the pump inhibitor, ouabain. A Cl⁻ pump, which maintains low Cl⁻ concentrations (55 mM) in the cell, can contribute up to 10 mV to resting membrane potential; its effect is partly offset by the tendency of Cl⁻ ions to diffuse out of the cell.

Gated Ion-Selective Channels

In addition to passive ion-selective channels, the plasma membrane contains ion-selective channels that can be regulated (i.e., gated) by membrane potential (voltage-gated) and by various humoral, hormonal, or neural agents (agonist- or ligand-gated). The channels are usually selective for one ion (e.g, K^+ or Ca^{2+}), although some allow the passage of more than one ion. The two main types of ion channel involved in the regulation of rhythmic activity of smooth muscle of the gut are highly selective for K^+ or Ca^{2+}. Pioneering studies on the properties of Ca^{2+} and K^+ channels were first done on muscle cells from amphibian stomach[69-71] and subsequently on muscle cells from various regions of the mammalian gut.[72-76]

Ion-selective channels exist in three main states: (1) a closed state, (2) an open activated state, which permits free diffusion of a specific ion, and (3) an open deactivated state, which does not permit free diffusion of the ion. The transition between the closed and open activated states is rapid; that between the open activated and deactivated states is slow.

The flow of ions in single channels can be measured in small patches of plasma membrane.[64,65,72,74] The patches can be electrically isolated by suction into the tip of a micropipette; there they form a tight seal, which makes it possible to record current flow in one or only a few channels in the patch. The patches can remain attached to the rest of the plasma membrane or become fully detached such that the inner (inside-out) or outer (outside-out) surface of the membrane faces the external medium. Each configuration has its advantages: inside-out patches are useful for examining the role of intracellular messengers; outside-in patches are useful for examining the influence of extracellular ions; and patches in the whole cell configuration are useful for examining the effect of ligands and second messengers. The use of patches has made it possible to characterize ion channels in terms of their ion selectivity, membrane density, activation and inactivation kinetics, voltage and ligand dependence, and dependence on changes in intracellular Ca^{2+}. The channels are electrically defined by their conductance (reciprocal of resistance) expressed in picosiemens (pS; i.e., by the amount of current flowing through the channel in response to an electrical gradient [current/voltage]).

Voltage-Gated Ca²⁺ Channels

Voltage-gated Ca^{2+} channels have been identified in muscle cells from the stomach and intestine of several mammals.[76-78] The channels carry the inward Ca^{2+} current responsible for the upstroke of the fast action potential. The channels are activated rapidly by depolarization of the plasma membrane to about −40 mV but are inactivated more slowly; inactivation occurs as a result of both

the entry of Ca^{2+} and membrane depolarization. The voltage range of activation (−40 to +10 mV) and inactivation (−60 to 0 mV) overlap, such that in the range of −40 to −50 mV some channels remain open and can carry a steady inward Ca^{2+} current.[77] The potential at which such a current might flow is close to resting membrane potential in some muscle cells and is usually attained during the plateau phase of a slow wave. Dihydropyridine Ca^{2+} channel agonists, such as BAY-k 8644, enhance the inward Ca^{2+} current by increasing the open-time probability of the channels, whereas dihydropyridine Ca^{2+} channel blockers, such as nifedipine, reduce the Ca^{2+} current by decreasing the number of active Ca^{2+} channels.[77,79] The channels are less sensitive to other types of Ca^{2+} channel blockers such as diltiazem and methoxyverapamil.

Voltage-Gated K⁺ Channels

Several types of K^+ channel have been identified in gastric and intestinal smooth muscle. The channels differ in their conductances, range of voltage activation, and Ca^{2+} sensitivity. The most widely distributed is a high conductance (100 pS in a physiologic K^+ gradient), Ca^{2+}-activated, voltage-sensitive K^+ channel.[73,75,78,80,81] Current through this channel flows outward and can be blocked by Ba^{2+} and tetraethylammonium (TEA). During resting conditions, when cytosolic Ca^{2+} concentrations are low (about 10^{-7} M), relatively few channels are open. Upon stimulation, the increase in cytosolic Ca^{2+} (by Ca^{2+} influx or Ca^{2+} release) induces a large negative shift in the range of voltage activation such that the channels become activated over a wide range of membrane potential negative and positive to 0 mV. A large number of channels are activated; these carry an outward current that drives membrane potential back toward the K^+ equilibrium potential (i.e., toward resting membrane potential). A stimulus that acts by inducing Ca^{2+} influx and membrane depolarization is, thus, terminated.

A second voltage-sensitive K^+ channel with lower conductance (50 pS) has also been identified.[74] The channel opens upon prolonged depolarization such as might occur during the plateau phase of slow waves or with ligand-induced depolarization.

A third K^+ channel has features similar to those found in K^+ channels of sympathetic neurons; these channels carry an outward current called the M-current.[53,82-84]

Nonselective Voltage-Gated Cationic Channels

High conductance channels (400–500 pS) with mixed selectivity for K^+ and Na^+ have also been identified. These channels carry an inward depolarizing current and are activated at membrane potentials negative to −70 mV. It is possible that current flowing through these channels is responsible for the depolarizing potential, known as "pacemaker potential" or "prepotential," that triggers slow waves in some regions of the gut.

Ligand-Gated Channels

Ligand-gated channels in smooth muscle cells have not been characterized to the same extent as voltage-gated channels. Ligands can activate channels directly or modulate the activity of voltage-gated channels either directly or by way of second messengers.

In smooth muscle undergoing tonic contraction or relaxation, contractile and relaxant agonists act mainly, if not exclusively, by way of second messengers (IP$_3$ or cyclic AMP) to induce release or sequestration of intracellular Ca^{2+}. In smooth muscle undergoing phasic contraction (i.e., contraction driven by rhythmic depolarization of the plasma membrane), the same agonists act to increase or decrease the influx of Ca^{2+} into the cell by way of ligand-gated and voltage-gated Ca^{2+} channels. In this type of muscle, muscarinic agonists depolarize the plasma membrane and cause an increase in inward Ca^{2+} current. In amphibian gastric muscle cells, the depolarization is accompanied by a decrease in membrane conductance that is consistent with suppression of an outward K$^+$ M-current.[83,84] In mammalian intestinal muscle cells, the depolarization is accompanied by an increase in membrane conductance, which appears to reflect increase in Ca^{2+} and other cationic inward current and suppression of an outward K$^+$ current carried by Ca^{2+}-activated K$^+$ channels.[85] There is evidence that the opening of Ca^{2+} channels and closure of K$^+$ channels are mediated by a second messenger, DAG, which activates protein kinase C (see Figs 4-7 and 4-8).[48,49] Conversely, β-adrenergic agonists and permeable analogues of cAMP inhibit phasic contraction by hyperpolarizing the plasma membrane and preventing further influx of Ca^{2+} into the cell.[53,59] The hyperpolarization reflects enhancement either of an M-current or of a current carried by Ca^{2+}-activated K$^+$ channels.

RHYTHMIC ELECTRICAL ACTIVITY OF SMOOTH MUSCLE

Relation of Ca^{2+} and K$^+$ Channels to Rhythmic Electrical Activity

Ca^{2+} channels and Ca^{2+}-activated K$^+$ channels constitute the electrical apparatus that sustains rhythmicity in smooth muscle. The Ca^{2+} sensitivity of K$^+$ channels links their activity to that of Ca^{2+} channels, creating the dynamic framework for rhythmic electrical activity. Activation of Ca^{2+} channels induces an inward flow of Ca^{2+} ions, which depolarizes the membrane and increases cytosolic Ca^{2+}. Depolarization and increase in cytosolic Ca^{2+} inactivate the Ca^{2+} channels and activate K$^+$ channels, inducing an outward flow of K$^+$ ions; suppression of the inward flow of Ca^{2+} ions and enhancement of the outward flow of K$^+$ ions restore resting membrane potential. Thus, cycles of membrane depolarization and repolarization can be engendered in all types of muscle, including isolated muscle cells. The cycles differ in speed, amplitude, and duration, depending on the relative proportions of Ca^{2+} and K$^+$ channels, modulation by neural and humoral agents, participation of other voltage-gated or ligand-gated channels, and coupling of muscle cells to each other and to pacemaker cells.

Fast Action (Spike) Potentials

In isolated muscle cells, only fast action potentials occur, either spontaneously or upon application of small depolarizing currents; slow waves are never seen.[64,69,74,77] Cell dispersion uncouples muscle cells from pacemaker regions responsible for slow wave activity and from other muscle cells in the syncytium, which normally acts as an electrical sink that tends to dissipate inward depolarizing currents. Accordingly, small inward currents can cause rapid and complete depolarization of isolated muscle cells, resulting in maximal activation of Ca^{2+} channels and rapid influx of Ca^{2+}. The depolarization and substantial increase in cytosolic Ca^{2+} inactivate the Ca^{2+} channels and induce massive activation of K$^+$ channels. The rapid depolarization and repolarization are characteristic of fast action potentials.

Fast action potentials (spike potentials) lasting 0.1 to 0.2 second can occur also in intact muscle.[64-67] The profile and mechanism underlying the occurrence of spike potentials are similar to that in isolated muscle cells. Spike potentials occur spontaneously in regions of the gut where resting membrane potential is either above (i.e., more positive than) a threshold of -30 mV or can be raised above that threshold by neural stimulation. In other regions, spike potentials occur only after the membrane has been depolarized by slow waves; fast oscillations superimposed on the plateau potential of these waves give way to spike potentials. Whether they occur spontaneously or are superimposed on slow waves, spike potentials are accompanied by muscle contraction. However, they are not essential for contraction, which can also be engendered by changes in the amplitude and duration of the plateau potential of slow waves.

Slow Waves: Profile

A typical slow wave consists of the following sequence: a rapid depolarization (upstroke), partial repolarization, a sustained plateau lasting several seconds, followed by complete repolarization to resting membrane potential (Fig 4-11).[65,67] In some regions, usually pacemaker regions, the upstroke is preceded by a slow, low-amplitude depolarization (prepotential or pacemaker potential), which may trigger the subsequent slow wave.

The amplitude, duration, and frequency of slow waves vary with the location of the muscle. Frequency decreases aborally in human and canine stomach (3–5 cycles/min in the corpus to 1.5 cycles/min in the antrum) and intestine (12 cycles/min in the duodenum, 7 cycles/min in the ileum, and 5–6 cycles/min in the proximal colon). The frequency gradient is continuous and intrinsic to each region; segments of intestine obtained sequentially along the main axis oscillate at progressively decreasing frequencies. In the canine stomach, the decreasing gradient in frequency is accompanied by an increasing gradient in resting membrane potential (from -51 mV in the corpus to -71 mV in the antrum) and in duration of plateau potential (from 5 seconds in the corpus to 20 seconds in the antrum). In addition, gradients in resting membrane potential and in the amplitude of plateau potential occur in the transverse direction (i.e., within the thickness of circular muscle).[66,86,87] The decrease in the amplitude of the plateau potential in the transverse direction reflects the decay of slow waves with

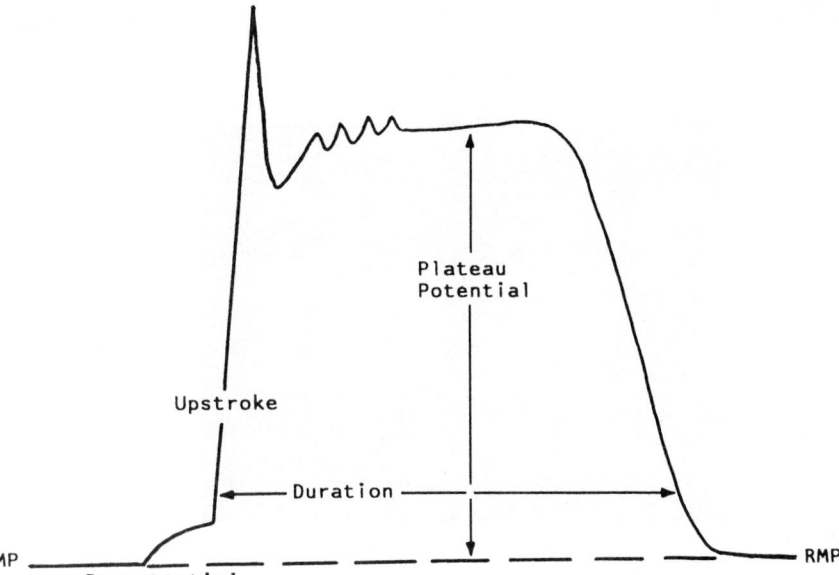

FIGURE 4–11. Profile of a typical slow wave. A slight depolarization (prepotential) of resting membrane potential (*RMP*) precedes and may trigger slow waves in some regions. A rapid upstroke is followed by partial repolarization, a plateau potential of variable duration on which may be superimposed small oscillations and/ or spike potentials, and complete repolarization.

increasing distance from the pacemaker regions at the borders of circular muscle.

Site of Origin of Slow Waves

Slow waves originate in pacemaker regions located at the myenteric and submucosal borders of circular muscle.[65–67,87,88] Where circular muscle is divided into bundles by septa, the pacemaker regions extend with the septa surrounding the muscle bundles. These regions contain a network of cells known as the *interstitial Cajal cells,* which may act as pacemakers capable of initiating rhythmic electrical activity.[89–91]

The interstitial Cajal cells are a distinctive population of fibroblastlike, stellate cells with large nuclei and an abundance of surface caveolae, mitochondria, and rough endoplasmic reticulum. The cells appear to make contact with muscle cells and nerve terminals. Single interstitial cells have been isolated from the submucosal border of circular muscle in the canine colon, and their electrophysiologic properties have been examined; the cells are spontaneously active, generate wavelike depolarizations analogous to slow waves in smooth muscle, and possess Ca^{2+} channels and Ca^{2+}-activated K^+ channels with properties similar to those found in muscle cells.[91] The abundance of mitochondria in these cells makes them susceptible to damage by dyes, such as methylene blue or rhodamine 123, that are preferentially taken up by mitochondria. Exposure of muscle tissue to these dyes disrupts and may even abolish slow waves.[92]

The activity of interstitial cells may not be uniform in all regions, as is evident from the decreasing frequency of slow waves aborally. In some regions (e.g., dog colon), slow waves initiated at the myenteric border differ in configuration and frequency from those initiated at the submucosal border.[87,88] In other regions, interstitial cells appear to be absent. Whether interstitial cells are essential for rhythmicity or whether rhythmic activity is an intrinsic property of muscle cells, which in some regions and species is driven or overridden by pacemaker cells, has not been settled.

The mechanism that triggers and, thus, sets the pace of slow waves is not known.

Propagation of Slow Waves

Slow waves originating in the myenteric and submucosal pacemaker regions propagate rapidly around circular muscle and throughout its thickness in both the transverse and long axis of the gut. Circumferential propagation is rapid and is facilitated by the peripheral networks of interstitial cells; propagation within the syncytium is facilitated by the abundance of gap junctions in circular muscle. Slow waves originating in the myenteric pacemaker region of circular muscle spread additionally to the longitudinal muscle.[87,93,94]

After they spread circumferentially, slow waves propagate in both oral and aboral directions as discrete rings of excitation capable of eliciting segmental contractions. Propagation in only one direction (i.e., oral or aboral) can occur provided: (1) the frequency gradient is steep and conduction velocity is fast enough to allow slow waves originating in a proximal segment to set the pace of slow waves in a more distal segment,[67] or (2) inhibitory neural input to one segment limits propagation to that segment.[95] Inhibitory neural input to muscle and pacemaker cells can hyperpolarize resting membrane potential and prevent the occurrence of a slow wave, or decrease plateau potential and prevent the development of a contraction. Inhibitory neural input appears to predominate normally, masking rhythmic electrical and contractile activity. This is most evident in the small intestine of the guinea pig where suppression of all neural input with tetrodotoxin or blockade of inhibitory neural input with the bee venom peptide, apamin, initiates slow waves with a mean frequency of 16 cycles/min.[96]

Ionic Basis of Slow Waves

The ionic mechanisms underlying slow wave activity are not well-understood and may differ from one region to another.[64–67] The

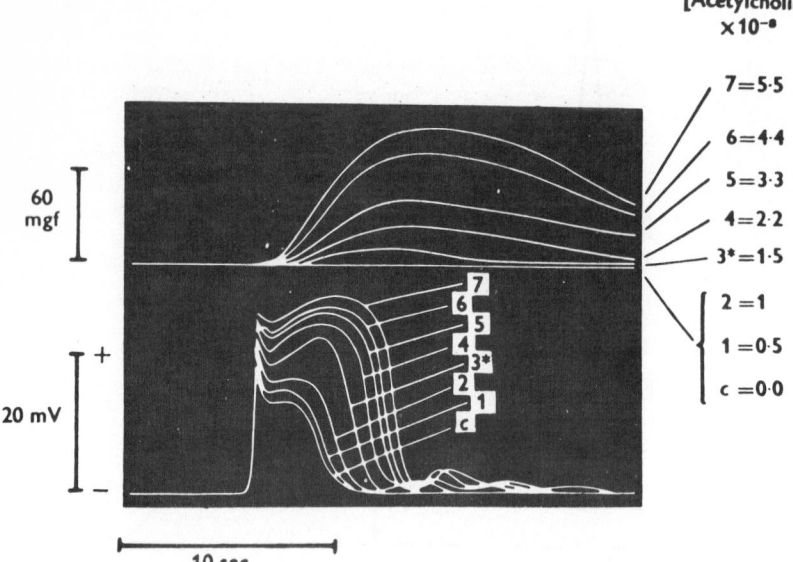

[Acetylcholine]
×10⁻⁸

7=5·5
6=4·4
5=3·3
4=2·2
3*=1·5
2=1
1=0·5
c=0·0

FIGURE 4–12. Relationship between amplitude and duration of plateau potential (*lower panel*) and corresponding contraction (*upper panel*) of longitudinal muscle of canine antrum in response to acetylcholine. (From Szurszewski JH. Mechanism of action of pentagastrin and acetylcholine on the longitudinal muscle of the canine antrum. J Physiol [Lond] 1975;252:335.)

rapid upstroke of the slow wave could reflect inward flow of current through channels of mixed cationic selectivity that are activated at high resting membrane potentials (-60 to -70 mV). Ca^{2+} currents appear to be involved also because the upstroke potential is reduced in the absence of Ca^{2+}. The plateau potential corresponds to the range at which Ca^{2+} channels are activated, and its amplitude reflects the combined activity of voltage-gated Ca^{2+} and K^+ channels. Ca^{2+}-activated K^+ channels appear to be the main type of K^+ channel involved in repolarization of the membrane.

Relation of Slow Waves to Phasic Contraction

The amplitude and duration of the plateau potential determine the magnitude of Ca^{2+} influx and can be modulated by stimulatory and inhibitory agents (Fig 4-12). Stimulatory agents (e.g., muscarinic agonists or cholecystokinin) increase the amplitude and duration of plateau potential, causing a concentration-dependent increase in cytosolic Ca^{2+} and contraction.[97,98,99,100] Spike potentials can be superimposed on plateau potentials, further augmenting cytosolic Ca^{2+} and contraction. In some regions (e.g., distal antrum and inner lamella of circular muscle in the small intestine), spike potentials appear to be necessary for contraction.[65,67,93,101]

Inhibitory agents decrease the amplitude and duration of plateau potential (or reduce the frequency of spike potentials) and prevent the development of contraction in association with a slow wave. Thus, neural input from the enteric nervous system can regulate electrical rhythmicity by influencing the generation, frequency, and propagation of slow waves, and contractile rhythmicity by modulating the amplitude and duration of plateau potential and the occurrence of spike potentials.

Regional Patterns of Slow Wave and Contractile Activity

The magnitude of resting membrane potential, the form, frequency and site of origin of slow waves, the occurrence and frequency of spike potentials, the extent of stimulatory or inhibitory neural input, and the mode of electromechanical coupling can be correlated with neuromuscular function of various regions in the gut. The results obtained in the dog, the most extensively studied species, parallel those obtained in humans.

STOMACH

The proximal-to-distal gradient in resting membrane potential of circular smooth muscle in the stomach has been noted above (Fig 4-13). Membrane potential in the orad segment or fundus is low (about -50 mV) and lies near or above the threshold for contraction.[65,102] Consequently, the segment is tonically contracted and is devoid of rhythmic electrical activity. However, slow waves can be generated in the fundus if resting membrane potential is rendered more negative by application of a hyperpolarizing current.[65] This implies that the ionic channels underlying electrical rhythmicity are present in smooth muscle of the fundus but have been inactivated by a low resting membrane potential. Conversely, the corpus, which is the site of spontaneous pacemaker activity in the stomach, can be rendered electrically quiescent by depolarization of its normally higher resting membrane potential.[99]

Small increases in stimulatory (depolarizing) or inhibitory (hyperpolarizing) neural input can tonically contract or relax the fundus, rendering this segment suitable for receiving (receptive relaxation) and discharging (tonic contraction) a meal into the corpus of the stomach.[102] The corpus can undergo both tonic and

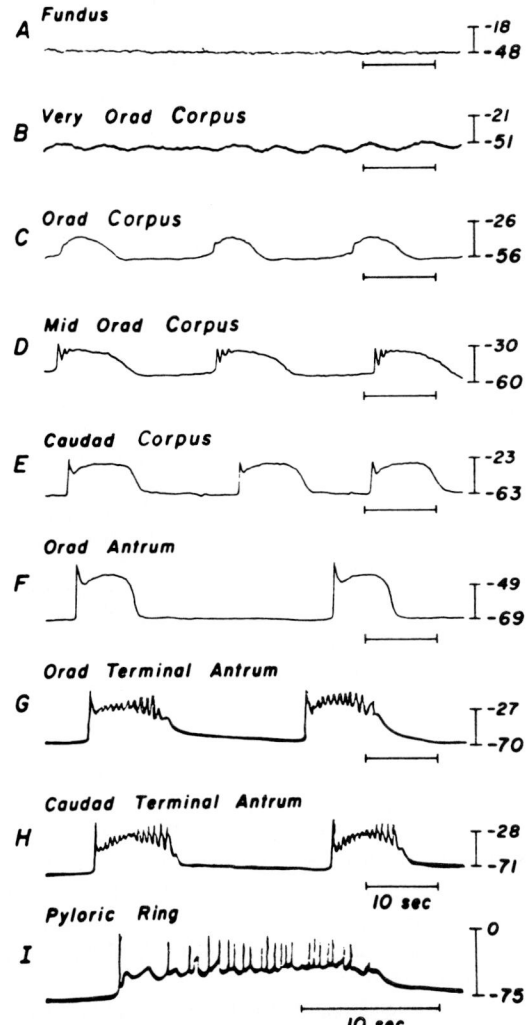

FIGURE 4–13. Gradient in resting membrane potential and profile of slow waves in various regions of canine stomach recorded with intracellular electrodes. From proximal to distal stomach, resting membrane potential is increasingly negative and slow wave duration is increasingly longer; the presence of potential oscillations and spike potentials is evident in the distal stomach and pylorus. (From Szurszewski JH. Electrical basis of gastrointestinal motility. In: Johnson LR, ed. Physiology of gastrointestinal tract, ed 2. New York: Raven Press, 1987:383.)

phasic contraction. Tonic contraction of the corpus, such as that induced by contractile agonists (e.g., acetylcholine), is mediated by release of intracellular Ca^{2+}; the decrease in resting membrane potential induced by these agonists is not sufficient to account for contraction (i.e., to open Ca^{2+} channels and induce Ca^{2+} influx; Fig 4-14).[99] Phasic contraction of the corpus, however, is determined by the amplitude and duration of plateau potential; here, small changes in amplitude and duration induced by contractile agonists result in substantial changes in the magnitude of phasic contraction.

Intrinsic pacemaker rhythm is highest in the orad corpus (5 cycles/min) and decreases progressively throughout the rest of the corpus, antrum, and pylorus. Slow waves originating in the

corpus propagate to and pace antral muscle. Slow waves originating in the distal antrum and pyloric sphincter have prolonged plateau potentials on which spike potentials are usually superimposed.

As a whole, the antrum has little tone and is best suited for propagation of slow waves and contractions originating in the corpus.[65,86,100,101] The electrical and mechanical properties of antral muscle vary with its depth. Close to the submucosal border, antral circular muscle undergoes both tonic and phasic contraction; at this location, phasic contraction induced by slow waves occurs at more negative membrane potentials.

Antral slow waves propagate aborally to the pyloric sphincter where they pace longitudinal muscle and the outer layer of circular muscle.[101] The slow waves decay before reaching muscle cells in the inner (i.e., submucosal) layer of circular muscle; muscle cells in this region are electrically quiescent and may be responsible for the intrinsic tone of the sphincter. Opening of the sphincter is probably mediated by an inhibitory (relaxant) neural reflex triggered by distention of the distal antrum; distention occurs when gastric contents are propelled aborally by phasic (peristaltic) contractions originating in the pacemaker region (i.e., corpus) of the stomach.

SMALL INTESTINE

In nearly all mammals, including humans, there is a decreasing gradient in slow wave frequency from duodenum to ileum. Despite earlier views, slow waves are now known to originate in a pacemaker region located at the myenteric border of circular muscle from where they propagate to the bulk of circular muscle and to longitudinal muscle.[93,94] Removal of a thin layer at the myenteric border of circular muscle abolishes slow waves in both longitudinal muscle and the bulk of circular muscle. Propagation around and in the long axis of the intestine occurs preferentially through circular muscle.

The configuration of slow waves in the small intestine is similar to that in the corpus of the stomach and consists of a rapid upstroke followed by a sustained plateau potential. The plateau potentials of slow waves recorded in the inner lamella, a thin layer of circular muscle located at the submucosal border, have spike potentials, whereas the plateau potentials of slow waves recorded in the thick outer lamella are devoid of spike potentials. Muscle cells in the inner lamella are smaller in size and have a lower mechanical threshold (−52 mV versus −42 mV). Phasic contraction in these cells occurs at a more negative plateau potential, and its magnitude is determined by the frequency of spike potentials, whereas the magnitude of phasic contraction in cells of the outer lamella is determined by changes in the amplitude of plateau potential. There is no evidence so far that slow waves recorded in the inner lamella originate from a separate pacemaker at the submucosal border (see section entitled "Colon").

Stimulatory and inhibitory neural input influences the amplitude of plateau potential and the frequency of spike potentials and, thus, determines the magnitude and occurrence of phasic contraction in the intestine. Nonetheless, a close scrutiny of the relation between plateau potential and circular muscle contraction shows that depolarization and the consequent influx of Ca^{2+} do

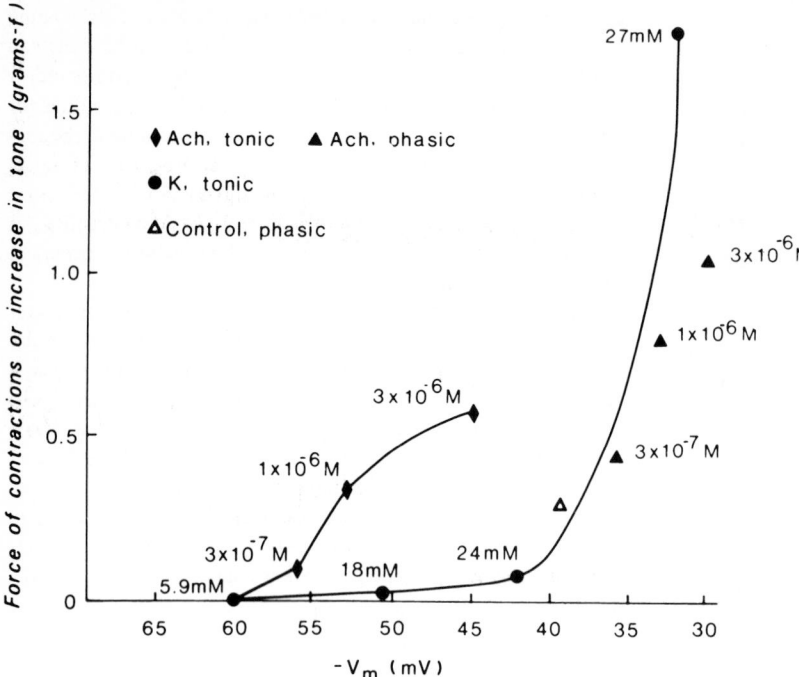

FIGURE 4-14. Comparative effects of acetylcholine and extracellular K^+ on membrane potential and contraction in circular muscle from the corpus of the canine stomach. Acetylcholine caused an increase in tonic contraction; the depolarization induced by acetylcholine does not exceed the threshold for opening of Ca^{++} channels, implying that the source of Ca^{++} for agonist-induced tonic contraction is intracellular. During slow wave activity, the magnitude of phasic contraction in response to acetylcholine correlates with the amplitude of plateau potential. Contraction induced by K^+ results from depolarization and influx of Ca^{++} and coincides with the pattern of phasic contraction induced by acetylcholine. (From Szurszewski JH. Electrical basis of gastrointestinal motility. In: Johnson LR, ed. Physiology of gastrointestinal tract, ed 2. New York: Raven Press, 1987:383.)

not fully account for contraction induced by contractile agonists, which, in addition, induce release of intracellular Ca^{2+}.[93]

COLON

Analysis of electrical activity in the colon and other regions has been greatly facilitated by the use of cross-sectional preparations that enable precise recording from muscle cells located at different depths.[66,87,88,95] From these records, it is clear that there is a decreasing gradient in resting membrane potential across circular muscle of the canine colon, from -80 mV in cells at the submucosal border to -45 mV in cells at the myenteric border (Fig 4-15). The gradient is abolished by ouabain and appears to reflect dif-

ferences in the contribution of an electrogenic Na^+–K^+–ATPase pump to resting membrane potential. Rhythmic electrical activity is mediated by two pacemaker regions, one located at the myenteric border, the other at the submucosal border and around septa surrounding bundles of circular muscle. Each pacemaker region generates slow waves with distinctive forms and frequencies that spread passively and summate in the bulk of circular muscle yielding waves of mixed form.[87,88]

Slow waves originating at the submucosal border and septa have a frequency of five to six cycles/min and a configuration similar to that found in the small intestine and corpus of the stomach; the waves consist of a rapid upstroke and a plateau potential of variable duration (3–15 seconds; see Fig 4-15).[87,103] The amplitude of the plateau potential decreases as the waves spread

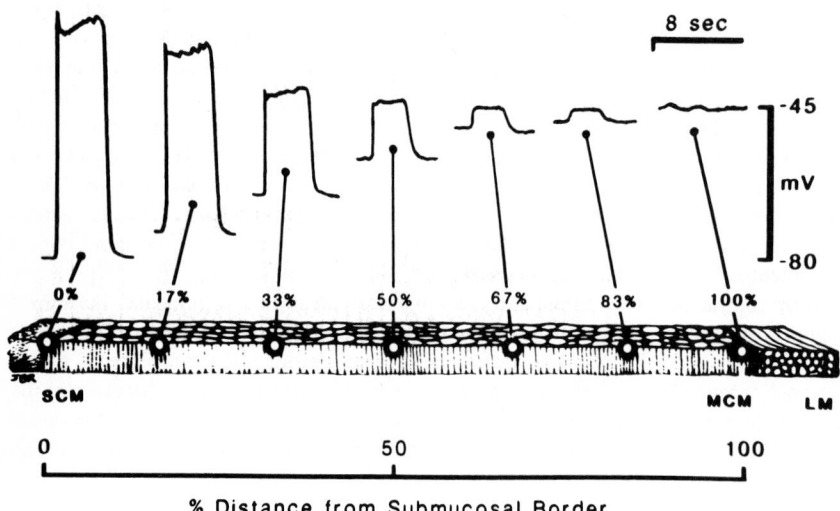

FIGURE 4-15. Records of slow waves obtained at various distances from the submucosal border of circular muscle in canine colon. Two gradients are evident: a decline in the amplitude of plateau potential from the submucosal (*SCM*) to myenteric (*MCM*) border is matched and offset by a decrease in resting membrane potential. The plateau potential during slow wave activity attains or exceeds threshold potential throughout the thickness of circular muscle. Slow waves with a different configuration originate at the myenteric border; as they propagate in circular muscle, they summate with slow waves originating at submucosal border. (From Smith TK, Reed BJ, Sanders KM. Origin and propagation of electrical slow waves in circular muscle of canine proximal colon. Am J Physiol 1987;252:C215.)

toward the myenteric border; the decrease in plateau potential is matched and offset by the decrease in resting membrane potential, such that the plateau potential is maintained at about −45 mV (i.e, close to the threshold for mechanical activity).

Slow waves originating at the myenteric border of circular muscle have a frequency of 17 cycles/min and a sinusoidal configuration (Fig 4-16).[66,87,88] The waves, called "myenteric potential oscillations," spread to and pace muscle cells in the longitudinal muscle layer. They also spread in circular muscle toward the submucosal border, their amplitude decreasing as a function of distance from the myenteric border (see Fig 4-16). The waves summate with waves originating at the submucosal border; the encounter boosts the plateau potential of waves that originate at the submucosal border and elicits contractions at the rate of six per minute. In longitudinal muscle, "myenteric potential oscillations" generate fast action potentials; the frequency of these fast transients and, thus, of longitudinal muscle contraction is regulated by neural input from the enteric nervous system. Fast action potentials are not generated in circular muscle and only rarely propagate from longitudinal to adjacent circular muscle cells.

Both stimulatory (cholinergic and noncholinergic) and inhibitory neural input is directed at both pacemaker regions where the density of innervation is highest.[95] It is probable that nerve fibers in both regions originate mainly in neurons of the myenteric plexus. Input from these neurons affects slow wave and phasic contractile activity in the same way it does in the small intestine.

Stimulus-Contraction Coupling in Syncytia: Tonic and Phasic Contraction

The signal transduction pathways described in isolated circular and longitudinal muscle cells regulate tonic contraction and relaxation of intact, syncytial muscle. Small depolarizations caused by hormonal or neural agonists are not sufficient to cause tonic contraction, except in some regions of the gut, such as the fundus of the stomach, where resting membrane potential is close to mechanical threshold (i.e., close to the membrane potential at which Ca^{2+} channels are presumed to open). In circular muscle of the intestine and corpus of the stomach, tonic contraction induced by agonists occurs at membrane potentials more negative than mechanical threshold, implying that the source of Ca^{2+} responsible for tonic contraction in these regions is intracellular (see Fig 4-14).[93,99] However, when either circular or longitudinal muscle is depolarized by a slow wave, relatively small changes in plateau potential imposed by the effect of an agonist are sufficient to induce Ca^{2+} influx and contraction. The contraction is phasic, coinciding with and determined by the amplitude of the plateau potential.

In some regions, spike potentials superimposed on plateau potentials produce the requisite depolarization for contraction. It is noteworthy that spike potentials are not seen in circular muscle of the colon,[87] small intestine (except for a thin inner lamella),[93] and corpus of the stomach.[99] In the proximal colon, slow waves

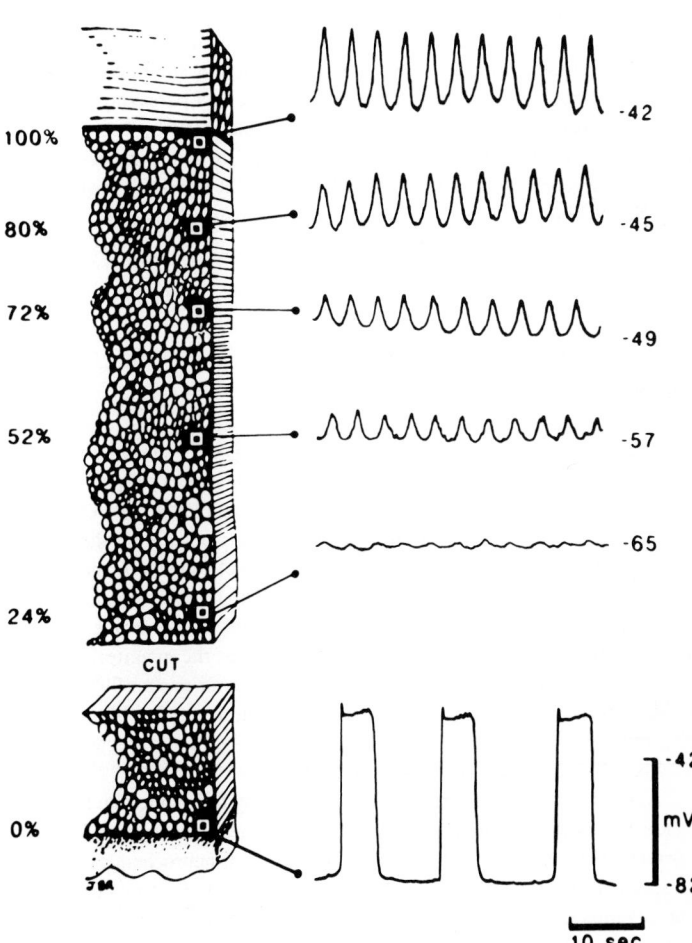

FIGURE 4–16. Records of slow waves obtained at various distances from the myenteric border of circular muscle in canine colon after removal of a thin strip of circular muscle from submucosal border. Configuration of slow waves originating in the pacemaker regions at the two borders are different. Slow waves originating at the myenteric border propagate through the thickness of circular muscle and to longitudinal muscle. (From Smith TK, Reed BJ, Sanders KM. Interaction of two electrical pacemakers in musculans of canine proximal colon. Am J Physiol 1987;252:C290.)

emanating from the pacemaker region at the myenteric border of circular muscle elicit spike potentials when they spread to the longitudinal muscle only. Spike generation appears to be more prevalent in longitudinal muscle and may be related to signal transduction pathways and channel characteristics in this muscle.

Relaxant hormonal or neural agonists act by way of cyclic AMP-dependent protein kinase to decrease cytosolic Ca^{2+}. They do so by enhancing sequestration of Ca^{2+} in intracellular stores,[58,59] a mechanism well-suited to relaxation of tonic contraction in circular muscle, or by reducing Ca^{2+} influx,[53,54] a mechanism well-suited to relaxation of phasic contraction in longitudinal and circular muscle (see Figs 4-8 and 4-10). The decrease in Ca^{2+} influx is a consequence of hyperpolarization of the plasma membrane resulting from activation of K^+ channels.

Hormonal and neural agonists can influence plateau potential and determine the occurrence of spike potentials by acting also on pacemaker cells. The cells are innervated by neurons of the myenteric plexus, and, like muscle cells, they possess voltage-gated Ca^{2+} channels and Ca^{2+}-activated K^+ channels and exhibit slow wave activity.[91]

NEURAL REGULATION OF SMOOTH MUSCLE

The intrinsic electrical and mechanical properties of smooth muscle are modulated by transmitters released from neurons of the myenteric plexus. These neurons constitute the final neural pathway regulating smooth muscle activity. Neurons of the submucosal plexus and extrinsic neurons of the sympathetic and parasympathetic systems influence smooth muscle mainly indirectly by acting on neurons of the myenteric plexus. Adrenergic neurons in pre- and paravertebral ganglia synapse with and inhibit the activity of cholinergic and noncholinergic neurons of the myenteric and submucosal plexus.

Topography of Neurons in the Myenteric Plexus

The neural organization of the myenteric plexus is well-conserved in mammals and has been extensively studied in guinea pig, rat, dog, and humans[104-106] (see ch 1). Neurons in this plexus project their fibers to other neurons in the plexus and to cells in the circular muscle layer; relatively few fibers project to cells in the longitudinal muscle layer. The fibers that make up the deep plexus close to the submucosal border of circular muscle are derived from neurons of the myenteric plexus. Excision of the myenteric plexus from segments of guinea pig intestine eliminates over 99% of the neurites in the underlying circular muscle layer, implying that muscle cells receive their innervation mainly—in some species exclusively—from the myenteric plexus.[107]

Advances in immunocytochemical and imaging techniques have made it possible to map the topography of these neurons and correlate their morphologic, electrophysiologic, and neurochemical properties, specifically their content of transmitters. Neurons of the myenteric plexus fall into two broad categories: those that contain *vasoactive intestinal peptide* (VIP) (40%–45%) and those

that contain *substance P* (SP) (40%–45%) with virtually no overlap between them.[106-108] VIP neurons contain a homologous peptide designated PHM in humans (peptide with N-terminal histidine and C-terminal methionine) and PHI in animals (peptide with N-terminal histidine and C-terminal isoleucine) derived from the same precursor, pre-pro-VIP. SP neurons contain a homologous peptide, substance K (SK), also known as neurokinin A (NKA), derived from the same precursor (β-pre-pro-tachykinin). Cholinergic neurons containing solely acetycholine are unlikely to constitute a distinct, large population, because VIP and SP neurons account for the great majority of neurons in the myenteric plexus. It is more likely that *acetylcholine* coexists with SP and SK in the same neurons.

The two main categories of neurons correspond to major roles for SP/SK/acetylcholine as excitatory transmitters and VIP/PHM or PHI as inhibitory (relaxant) transmitters. Subpopulations of neurons within these categories contain one or more of the following: *bombesin,* also known as gastrin-releasing peptide or GRP, *neuropeptide Y* (NPY), the opioid peptides, *dynorphin* and *[Met]enkephalin,* and *galanin.* A few neurons contain *gamma-aminobutyric acid (GABA),* serotonin, or *somatostatin.* Neurons that contain serotonin or somatostatin project their fibers exclusively within the myenteric plexus and can influence smooth muscle cells only indirectly by way of other neurons.

Transmitters present in the same or adjacent neurons may be released together or separately; the effect on a given target represents their combined influence, although in general the effect of one transmitter (e.g., VIP in VIP-containing neurons) is dominant. In addition, a variety of autacoids released from non-neural cells can influence muscle function. Among these are histamine, serotonin, eicosanoids (leukotrienes, prostaglandins, and thromboxanes), adenosine and adenosine 5'-triphosphate (ATP). There is no evidence that ATP is present in or released as a transmitter from neurons of the myenteric plexus; its presence in the interstitial fluid is more likely a product of metabolic activity of various cell types.[109]

Transmitters of the Myenteric Plexus: Pharmacologic Profile

Peptide and nonpeptide transmitters are released in passing from axonal varicosities in proximity of muscle cells. They diffuse across distances ranging from 20 to 100 nm to interact with receptors on muscle cells and adjacent nerve terminals. The presence of receptors on muscle cells and, therefore, the possibility of direct action can be determined in isolated muscle cells by measuring the binding of specific radioligands, the release of intracellular messengers (e.g., increase in cytosolic Ca^{2+}, IP_3, or cyclic nucleotides), or the mechanical response of the cell (i.e., contraction or relaxation).[9,43–45,56,110,111] The presence of receptors on neurons or their terminals and, therefore, the possibility of indirect, neurally mediated action of the transmitter on muscle cells require the use of innervated muscle strips; the neurally mediated component of mechanical response is identified by its sensitivity to blockade by neurotoxins.[110-112]

Transmitter substances can be classified pharmacologically in terms of their ability to : (1) cause direct contraction or relaxation of muscle cells, and (2) stimulate or inhibit the release of transmitters (i.e., acetylcholine, SP/SK, and VIP/PHI) in motor neurons (Fig 4-17). Thus, bombesin and CCK cause contraction in isolated muscle cells and innervated muscle strips; in the latter, they also elicit release of acetylcholine and SP.[113-116] Their effects in strips are partly neurally mediated and can be partly blocked by the axonal blocker, tetrodotoxin, or by a combination of muscarinic and tachykinin antagonists.

VIP and its homologues, PHI and PHM, cause relaxation of isolated muscle cells and of muscle strips.[56,117,118] GABA, acting by way of GABA-A receptors, causes relaxation in muscle strips but not isolated muscle cells. The relaxation in muscle strips is accompanied by release of VIP and can be blocked by VIP antagonists, and, therefore, can be attributed to GABA-induced release of VIP (see Fig 4-17).[119] Opioid peptides have an opposite effect: they cause a transient tonic contraction followed by phasic contractions in previously quiescent muscle strips. The transient tonic contraction is a direct effect of opioid peptides on muscle cells; this effect is demonstrable in isolated circular muscle cells.[120] The phasic contractions result from inhibition of background VIP release (i.e., opioid peptides suppress a dominant inhibitory [relaxant] neural influence mediated by VIP that normally masks phasic contractile activity).[118] In support of this notion, neutralization of background VIP with VIP antiserum or blockade of its effect with VIP antagonists induces phasic contractions in quiescent muscle strips. Addition of tetrodotoxin, which blocks stimulatory as well as inhibitory neural input, induces phasic contractions in various regions of the gut, implying that inhibitory neural input is normally dominant.

Galanin does not cause contraction or relaxation in isolated muscle cells by itself, but is capable of augmenting relaxation induced by VIP and β-adrenergic agonists.[121] Its potentiatory effect is accompanied by net efflux of K^+ from muscle cells and is suppressed by K^+ channel blockers. It is possible that release of galanin and VIP from the same or from separate neurons may be jointly responsible for "inhibitory junction potentials"; these rapid hyperpolarizations of resting membrane potential often accompany inhibitory neural input to muscle cells. Both VIP, acting by way of cAMP-dependent protein kinase, and galanin, acting by way

of opening of K^+ channels, can cause hyperpolarization and, thus, influence the generation, frequency, and plateau potential of slow waves and corresponding phasic contractions.

Transmitters of the Myenteric Plexus: Physiologic Profile

The pharmacologic profile of actions summarized above can serve as a framework for understanding the regulatory role of transmitters released from neurons of the myenteric plexus (see Fig 4-17). Excitatory motor neurons release one or both types of contractile transmitter: acetylcholine and the tachykinins, SP and SK.[122] Some transmitters (e.g., bombesin) stimulate, while others (e.g., NPY) inhibit release of acetylcholine and SP/SK from excitatory motor neurons. Inhibitory motor neurons release the relaxant transmitters, VIP with either PHI or PHM, depending on the species. Some transmitters (e.g., GABA) stimulate, while others (e.g., opioid peptides) inhibit the release of VIP from inhibitory motor neurons. Somatostatin acts indirectly on muscle cells, and its effect illustrates the interplay of various transmitters. Somatostatin inhibits the release of opioid peptides, which, in turn, inhibit the release of VIP. Thus, somatostatin eliminates the inhibitory restraint exerted by opioid neurons on VIP neurons, and its net effect is to enhance release of VIP (see section entitled "Physiologic Regulation of a Motor Function: The Peristaltic Reflex").

The following criteria must be fulfilled for a peptide present in neurons of the myenteric plexus to be identified as a transmitter:[111]

1. The presence of the peptide in nerve terminals close to the target cell should be demonstrable immunocytochemically; the target cell could be a muscle cell, an interstitial cell, or another neuron.
2. The peptide must be synthesized by myenteric neurons and released by physiologic stimuli (e.g., chemically or mechanically induced reflexes).

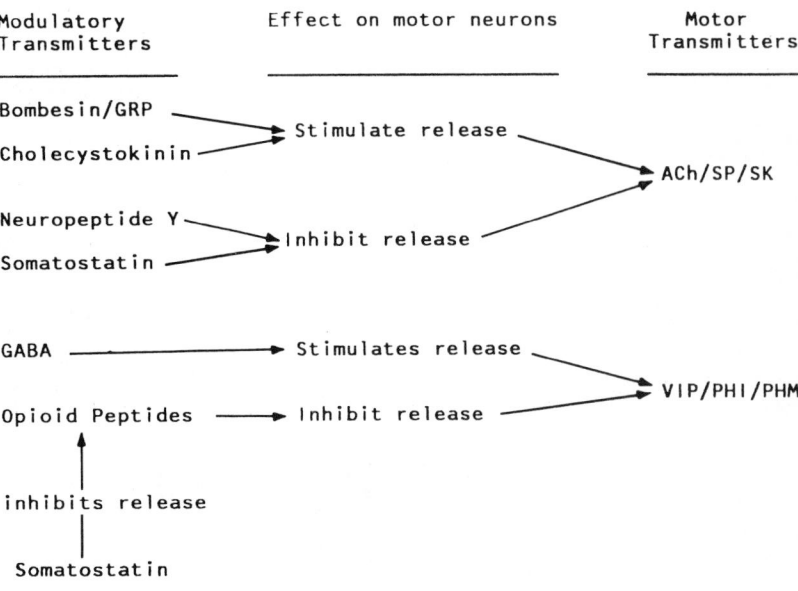

FIGURE 4-17. Effect of peptide and nonpeptide transmitters found in neurons of the myenteric plexus on release of transmitters from the two main populations of motor neurons: excitatory neurons containing acetylcholine (*ACh*), substance P (*SP*) and substance K (*SK*), and inhibitory (relaxant) neurons containing vasoactive intestinal peptide (*VIP*) with either peptide histidine isoleucine (*PHI*) in animals or peptide histidine methionine (*PHM*) in humans. Somatostatin inhibits release of opioid peptides, which, in turn, inhibit release of VIP/PHI/PHM; the net effect of somatostatin is increase in release of VIP/PHI/PHM (i.e., disinhibition or elimination of the inhibitory effect of opioid peptides).

3. Release of the peptide should be accompanied by an effect that can be mimicked by exogenous application of the peptide and that can be blocked by a specific antiserum or antagonist.
4. The effect and release of the peptide should be demonstrable in the context of a physiologic function, such as a peristaltic reflex.

These are minimal criteria, because often two or more peptides derived from the same or different precursors are colocalized and may be coreleased from the same neurons, producing pre- and postjunctional synergistic or inhibitory interactions that cannot be precisely mimicked by a single peptide. Nonetheless, the effects of the major transmitters in excitatory (acetylcholine, SP/SK) and inhibitory (VIP/PHI or PHM) motor neurons are dominant, while those of other colocalized peptide or nonpeptide transmitters are modulatory and generally subsidiary.

These criteria are fulfilled for two major peptide transmitters in motor neurons of the myenteric plexus, VIP/PHI, and SP/SK. The example of VIP is used here to demonstrate its role as relaxant motor transmitter.[111]

1. VIP and its homologues are unique among peptides of the myenteric plexus in their ability to cause relaxation in all regions of the gut, including the stomach, intestine, gallbladder, and sphincters.[56,117,118,123–126]
2. VIP is demonstrable immunocytochemically in neurons of the myenteric plexus, which innervate mainly circular muscle throughout the gut.
3. VIP is released in response to neural stimulation, and its release is accompanied by a proportional increase in relaxation.[117,118,123]
4. Neutralization of VIP with specific VIP antiserum or blockade of its effect with selective VIP antagonists inhibits neurally induced relaxation in all regions of the gut.[117,124–126]
5. Reflex activation of myenteric neurons by physiologic stimuli, such as stretch or distention, causes VIP release and

muscle relaxation; the latter is blocked by VIP antiserum and VIP antagonists.[127,128]

In considering the role of VIP, it should be noted that no other peptide or nonpeptide transmitter fulfills these criteria. For example, calcitonin gene-related peptide (CGRP) or neurotensin produces relaxation in some but not all regions of the gut. ATP has not been demonstrated histochemically in myenteric neurons, and there is no evidence that it is released as a transmitter from myenteric neurons. Furthermore, inactivation of ATP receptors with photoaffinity analogues of ATP or by desensitization does not affect neurally induced relaxation in most regions of the gut.[117]

Physiologic Regulation of a Motor Function: The Peristaltic Reflex

The role of motor neurons of the myenteric plexus in the regulation of a physiologic motor function is exemplified by the peristaltic reflex (Fig 4-18).[127,128] The reflex can be evoked by mucosal stroking (sensory receptors in mucosa) or by radial stretch (sensory receptors in circular muscle) and consists of two components: relaxation caudad and contraction orad to the site of the stimulus, referred to as descending relaxation and ascending contraction. A simple in vitro preparation consisting of a hollow or flat segment of intestine that can be stretched at the orad end to elicit only descending relaxation or at the caudad end to elicit only ascending contraction has made it possible to determine directly the type of transmitter released and its functional coupling to each component of the peristaltic reflex. Flat segments are particularly useful in examining the reflex in humans, which is identical in all respects to that in animals.[128] Thus, radial (i.e., circular muscle) stretch of the orad end of a segment causes descending relaxation accompanied by release of VIP; the relaxation can be blocked by VIP antiserum or VIP antagonists.[127,128] Caudad stretch, on the other

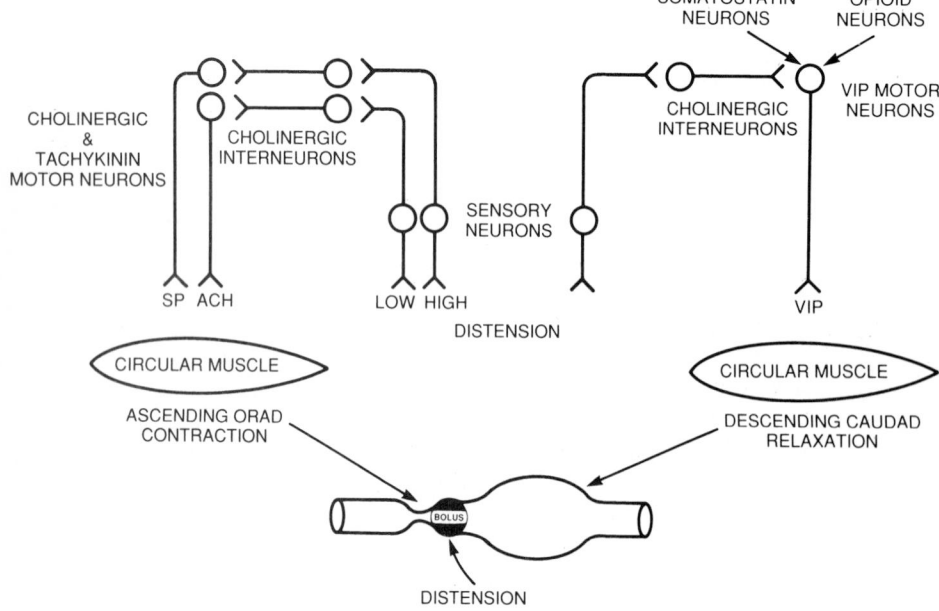

FIGURE 4–18. Regulation of peristaltic reflex by neurons of the myenteric plexus. The reflex has two components: ascending or orad contraction and descending or caudad relaxation. The stimulus (distention or mucosal stroking) is relayed by sensory neurons to cholinergic interneurons coupled to VIP neurons caudad and acetylcholine/tachykinin neurons orad. Although portrayed separately, acetylcholine and tachykinins (SP and SK) are probably present in the same neurons and released by different intensities of stimulation. Somatostatin and opioid neurons exert a modulatory influence on VIP neurons (see text for details). The pathways and transmitters mediating the reflex are identical in humans and animals.

hand, causes ascending contraction accompanied by release of acetylcholine, SP, and SK.[127-129] Contraction induced by low grades of stretch is preferentially inhibited by muscarinic antagonists; contraction induced by high grades of stretch is preferentially inhibited by tachykinin antagonists or antisera; a combination of muscarinic and tachykinin antagonists or antisera abolishes ascending contraction induced by all grades of stretch. Thus, transmitters present in the two major populations of motor neurons in the myenteric plexus regulate descending relaxation (VIP/PHI or PHM) and ascending contraction (acetylcholine and SP/SK).

Other neurons in the myenteric plexus participate in the peristaltic reflex by modulating the release of transmitters from motor neurons.[130] Opioid neurons exert a continuous restraint on VIP neurons. Consistent with this notion, naloxone enhances VIP release and descending relaxation. Release of opioid peptides decreases during descending relaxation, eliminating the restraint exerted by opioid neurons on VIP neurons. In contrast, release of somatostatin increases during descending relaxation, and this release is coupled to that of VIP, because neutralization of somatostatin with a specific somatostatin antiserum decreases both VIP release and descending relaxation. A neural circuit that describes the modulatory influence of opioid and somatostatin neurons on VIP motor neurons would operate as follows: a stimulus (e.g., stretch) relayed by myenteric sensory neurons activates somatostatin neurons, which, in turn, inhibit opioid neurons, eliminating their restraint on VIP neurons; elimination of the restraint exerted by opioid neurons enhances VIP release and descending relaxation. The circuit illustrates the notion of excitation by disinhibition (suppressing the influence of an inhibitor, in this instance, opioid peptides).

The two events that characterize the peristaltic reflex, descending relaxation and ascending contraction, underlie the opening and closing of various sphincters, including the lower esophageal, pyloric, choledochal ileocecal, and internal anal sphincters.[124-126] In these regions, also, there is strong evidence that VIP is the transmitter responsible for relaxation (i.e., opening of the sphincter). Acetylcholine and probably tachykinins participate in the closure of the sphincter.

HORMONAL REGULATION OF SMOOTH MUSCLE FUNCTION

Hormonal influences on smooth muscle activity are evident during and between meals. The example of *cholecystokinin* illustrates the interplay of hormonal and neural influences. Upon ingestion of a meal, cholecystokinin is released into the circulation from the upper small intestine, causing direct contraction of muscle cells in the gallbladder and neurally mediated relaxation of muscle cells in the sphincter of Oddi. Relaxation of the sphincter is accompanied by release of VIP and is blocked by VIP antiserum and VIP antagonists, implying that VIP is released by CCK from intramural neurons to cause relaxation.[126]

Motilin illustrates the participation of a hormone in the regulation of smooth muscle activity between meals. In humans and other mammals, cycles of electrical and contractile activity (described in greater detail in ch 8) recur at 1.5- to 2-hour intervals between meals. The cycles consist of four distinct phases, collectively known as the interdigestive myoelectric complex or migrating

motor complex; the cycles culminate in phase III, a 5- to 10-minute period of intense phasic contractile activity. Cycles typically begin in the stomach and migrate aborally throughout the small intestine; some cycles appear to begin in the small intestine. Motilin, a peptide released from enterochromaffin cells of the upper small intestine, appears to be responsible for initiating cycles that begin in the stomach. Peaks of motilin coincide with the onset of phase III in the stomach; neutralization of circulating motilin with motilin antiserum disrupts phase III activity, while infusion of motilin in concentrations that mimic circulating levels induces premature phase III activity.[131] Cycles that begin in the intestine are not controlled by motilin and may be regulated by input from intrinsic (myenteric) and extrinsic neurons. The neural and hormonal mechanisms that cause suppression of these cycles upon ingestion of a meal are not known.

HUMORAL REGULATION OF SMOOTH MUSCLE FUNCTION

In addition to neurotransmitters and circulating hormones, humoral agents produced by non-neural cells within the smooth muscle layer can influence smooth muscle activity. These include *histamine, serotonin, adenosine,* and various *eicosanoids* (prostaglandins, thromboxanes and leukotrienes). Receptors for most of these agents have been identified on smooth muscle cells of the gut.

Two types of receptors for serotonin, 5-HT$_2$ and 5-HT$_1$, coexist on smooth muscle cells of stomach and intestine; 5-HT$_2$ receptors mediate contraction by way of increase in cytosolic Ca^{2+}, and 5-HT$_1$ receptors mediate relaxation by way of increase in intracellular cAMP (see Fig 4-10).[132] The net effect of serotonin is contraction, reflecting the dominant influence of 5-HT$_2$ receptors. Similarly, two types of receptors for histamine, H$_1$ and H$_2$, coexist on smooth muscle cells of the stomach and intestine: H$_1$ receptors mediate contraction, and H$_2$ receptors mediate relaxation (see Fig 4-10).[133] The net effect of histamine is contraction, reflecting the dominant influence of H$_1$ receptors.

Two types of receptors for adenosine also coexist on smooth muscle cells of the intestine. Unlike receptors for histamine and serotonin, receptors for adenosine are coupled to a common pathway converging on adenylate cyclase: A$_2$ receptors mediate relaxation by way of increase in intracellular cAMP, and A$_1$ receptors block relaxation and the increase in cAMP (see Fig 4-10).[134] The net effect of adenosine is relaxation, reflecting the dominant influence of A$_2$ receptors (see Fig 4-10). Treatment of muscle cells with pertussis toxin (to inactivate the inhibitory G-protein, G$_i$) or with selective A$_1$ receptor antagonists eliminates the influence of A$_1$ receptors and enhances relaxation.

Finally, two types of receptors for peptido-leukotrienes have been identified in gastric muscle cells: a specific receptor for leukotriene C4 and a separate, common receptor for leukotrienes D4 and E4. All three leukotrienes cause contraction by way of increase in IP$_3$ and cytosolic Ca^{2+}.[135]

The influence of these agents, particularly histamine, serotonin, and eicosanoids, is likely to be most pronounced when smooth muscle is inflamed or hypersensitized by parasitic antigens.[136] The cells from which they are released lie in close proximity to muscle cells and to myenteric neurons and their terminals. Accordingly, the agents can act directly on muscle cells as well as indirectly by stimulating or inhibiting the release of neurotransmitters and, in this fashion, influence physiologic response.

The reader is directed to Chapter 1, The Enteric Nervous System and its Extrinsic Connections; Chapter 2, Gastrointestinal Hormones; Chapter 3, The Brain-Gut Axis; Chapter 7, Esophageal Motor Function; Chapter 8, The Physiology of Gastric Motility and Gastric Emptying; Chapter 9, Motility of the Small Intestine; Chapter 10, The Motor Function of the Colon; Chapter 11, Motility of the Biliary Tree; Chapter 54, Motility Disorders of the Esophagus; Chapter 60, Disorders of Gastric Emptying; Chapter 67, Dysmotility of the Small Intestine; Chapter 81, Motility Disorders of the Colon; Chapter 97, Postcholecystectomy Syndrome; and Chapter 128, Evaluation of Gastrointestinal Motility: Methodological Considerations.

REFERENCES

1. Gabella G. Structure of muscles and nerves in the gastrointestinal tract. In: Johnson LR, ed. Physiology of the gastrointestinal tract, ed 2. New York: Raven Press, 1987:335.
2. Gabella G. Structure of intestinal musculature. In: Wood JD, ed. Motility and circulation, vol II. Handbook of physiology, section 6: The gastrointestinal system. New York: American Physiological Society, Oxford University Press, 1989:103.
3. Gabella G. Quantitative morphological study of smooth muscle cells of the guinea-pig taenia coli. Cell Tissue Res 1976;170:161.
4. Murphy RA. Contraction of muscle cells. In: Berne RM, Levy MN, eds. Physiology, ed 2. Washington, DC: CV Mosby, 1988:315.
5. Frye GN, Devine CE, Burnstock G. Freeze-fracture studies of nexuses between smooth muscle cells. J Cell Biol 1977;72:26.
6. Gabella G, Blundell D. Gap junctions of the muscles of the small and large intestine. Cell Tissue Res 1981;219:469.
7. Somlyo AP, Somlyo AV, Shuman H. Electron probe analysis of vascular smooth muscle. J Cell Biol 1979;81:316.
8. Rayemakers L, Wuytack F, Batra S, Casteels R. A comparative study of the calcium accumulation by mitochondria and microsomes isolated from the smooth muscle of the guinea-pig taenia coli. Pflugers Arch 1977;368:217.
9. Bitar KN, Burgess GM, Putney JW Jr, Makhlouf GM. Source of activator calcium in isolated guinea pig and human gastric muscle cells. Am J Physiol 1986;250:G280.
10. Bitar KN, Bradford PJ, Putney JW Jr, Makhlouf GM. Stoichiometry of contraction and Ca^{2+} mobilization by inositol 1,4,5-trisphosphate in isolated gastric smooth muscle cells. J Biol Chem 1986;261:16591.
11. Berridge MJ, Irvine RF. Inositol phosphates and cell signalling. Nature 1989;341:197.
12. Burgess GM, McKinney JS, Fabiato A, Leslie BA, Putney JW Jr. Calcium pools in saponin-permeabilized guinea pig hepatocytes. J Biol Chem 1983;258:15336.
13. Hartshorne DJ. Biochemistry of the contractile process in smooth muscle. In: Johnson LR, ed. Physiology of the gastrointestinal tract, ed 2. New York: Raven Press, 1987:423.
14. Bond M, Somlyo AV. Dense bodies and actin polarity in vertebrate smooth muscle. J Cell Biol 1982;95:403.
15. Sobieszek A. Vertebrate smooth muscle myosin. Enzymatic and structural properties. In: Stephen NL, ed. The biochemistry of smooth muscle. Baltimore: University Park Press, 1977;413.
16. Murphy RA. Muscle cells of hollow organs. NIPS 1988;3:124.
17. Adelstein RS. Regulation of contractile proteins by phosphorylation. J Clin Invest 1983;72:1863.
18. Adelstein RS, Pato MD, Conti MA. The role of phosphorylation in regulating contractile proteins. Adv Cycl Nucl Res 1981;14:361.
19. Miller-Hance WC, Miller JR, Wells JN, Stull JT, Kamm KE. Biochemical events associated with activation of smooth muscle contraction. J Biol Chem 1988;263:13979.
20. Aksoy MO, Murphy RA, Kamm KE. Role of Ca^{2+} and myosin light chain phosphorylation in regulation of smooth muscle cells. Am J Physiol 1982;242:C109.
21. De Lanerolle P, Conti JR Jr, Tanenbaum M, Adelstein RS. Myosin phosphorylation, agonist concentration and contraction of tracheal smooth muscle. Nature 1982;298:871.
22. Eisenberg E, Hill TL. Muscle contraction and free energy transduction in biological systems. Science 1985;227:999.
23. Kamm KE, Stull JT. The function of myosin and myosin light chain kinase phosphorylation in smooth muscle. Annu Rev Pharmacol Toxicol 1985;25:593.
24. Dillon PF, Aksoy MO, Driska SP, Murphy RA. Myosin phosphorylation and cross-bridge cycle in arterial smooth muscle. Science 1981;221:495.
25. Marston SB. What is latch? New ideas about tonic contraction in smooth muscle. J Muscle Res Cell Motil 1989;10:97.
26. Kamm KE, Stull JT. Regulation of smooth muscle contractile elements by second messengers. Annu Rev Physiol 1989;51:299.
27. Lefkowitz RJ, Caron MG. Adrenergic receptors: Models for the study of receptors coupled to guanine nucleotide regulatory proteins. J Biol Chem 1988;263:4993.
28. Barnard EA. Separating receptor subtypes from their shadows. Nature 1988;335:381.
29. Casey PJ, Gilman AG. G protein involovement in receptor–effector coupling. J Biol Chem 1988;263:2577.
30. Gilman AG. G proteins: Transducers of receptor-generated signals. Ann Biochem 1987;56:615.
31. Berridge MJ, Irvine RF. Inositol trisphosphate, a novel second messenger in cellular signal transduction. Nature 1984;312:321.
32. Nishizuka Y. The role of protein kinase C in cell surface signal transduction and tumour promotion. Nature 1984;308:693.
33. Nishizuka Y. The molecular heterogeneity of protein kinase C and its implications for cellular regulation. Nature 1988;334:661.
34. Alkon DL, Rasmussen H. A spatial-temporal model of cell activation. Science 1988;239:998.
35. Rasmussen H, Takuwa Y, Park S. Protein kinase C in the regulation of smooth muscle contraction. FASEB J 1987;1:177.
36. Berridge MJ, Gallione A. Cytosolic calcium oscillators. FASEB J 1988;2:3074.
37. Gill DL. Receptor kinships revealed. Nature 1989;342:16.
38. Furuichi T, Yoshikawa S, Miyawaki A, Wada K, Maeda N, Mikoshiba K. Primary structure and function expression of the inositol 1,4,5-trisphosphate-binding protein P_{400}. Nature 1989;342:32.
39. Mignery GA, Sudhof TC, Takel K, De Camilli P. Putative receptor for inositol 1,4,5-triphosphate similar to ryanodine receptor. Nature 1989;342:192.
40. Kitazawa T, Kobayashi S, Horiuti K, Somlyo AV, Somlyo AP. Receptor-coupled permeabilized smooth muscle. Role of the phosphatidyl-inositol cascade, G-proteins and modulation of the contractile response to Ca^{2+}. J Biol Chem 1989;264:5339.
41. Kobayashi S, Somlyo AV, Somlyo AP. Heparin inhibits the inositol 1,4,5-trisphosphate-dependent but not the independent calcium release induced by guanine nucleotide in vascular smooth muscle. Biochem Biophys Res Comm 1988;153:625.
42. Bitar KN, Makhlouf GM. Receptors on smooth muscle cells: Characterization by contraction and specific antagonists. Am J Physiol 1982;242:G400.
43. Bitar KN, Bradford P, Putney JW Jr, Makhlouf GM. Cytosolic calcium during contraction of isolated mammalian gastric muscle cells. Science 1986;232:1143.
44. Grider JR, Makhlouf GM. Contraction mediated by Ca^{2+} release in circular and Ca^{2+} influx in longitudinal intestinal muscle cells. J Pharmacol Exp Ther 1988;244:432.
45. Murthy KS, Grider JR, Makhlouf GM. Different signal transduction in longitudinal and circular muscle cells: Specific generation of IP_3 in circular muscle. Gastroenterology 1989;96:356.
46. Murthy KS, Grider JR, Makhlouf GM. Distinct receptor-coupled G proteins mediate contraction in longitudinal and circular muscle cells of intestine. Gastroenterology 1990;98:377.
47. Murthy KS, Grider JR, Makhlouf GM. Contraction and calcium

release in circular muscle cells mediated by intracellular receptors for inositol 1,4,5-trisphosphate (IP$_3$). Gastroenterology 1989;96:356.

48. Clapp LH, Sims SM, Walsh VW Jr, Singer JJ. A diacylglycerol analogue suppresses both endogenous and isoproterenol-induced M-current in the same way as acetylcholine and substance P in isolated smooth muscle cells. J Gen Physiol 1988;92:51.

49. Vivaudou MB, Clapp LH, Walsh JV Jr, Singer JJ. Regulation of one type of Ca^{2+} current in smooth muscle cells by diacylglycerol and acetylcholine. FASEB J 1988;2:2497.

50. Weissberg PL, Little PJ, Bobik A. Spontaneous oscillations in cytoplasmic calcium concentration in vascular smooth muscle. Am J Physiol 1989;256:C951.

51. Carafoli E. Intracellular calcium homeostasis. Annu Rev Biochem 1987;56:395.

52. Castle NA, Haylett DG, Jenkinson DH. Toxins in the characterization of potassium channels. TINS 1989;12:59.

53. Sims SM, Singer JJ, Walsh JV Jr. Antagonistic adrenergic-muscarinic regulation of M current in smooth muscle cells. Science 1988;239:190.

54. Standen NB, Quayle JM, Davies NW, Brayden JE, Huang Y, Nelson MT. Hyperpolarizing vasodilators activate ATP-sensitive K$^+$ channels in arterial smooth muscle. Science 1989;245:177.

55. Kume H, Takai A, Tokuno H, Tomita T. Regulation of Ca^{2+}-activated K$^+$ channel activity in tracheal myocytes by phosphorylation. Nature 1989;341:152.

56. Bitar KN, Makhlouf GM. Relaxation of isolated gastric smooth muscle cells by vasoactive intestinal peptide. Science 1982;216:531.

57. Honeyman T, Merriam P, Fay FS. The effects of isoproterenol on adenosine cyclic 3':5'-monophosphate and contractility in isolated smooth muscle cells. Mol Pharmacol 1978;14:86.

58. Severi C, Grider JR, Makhlouf GM. Dual action of cyclic AMP-dependent relaxants: decrease in cytosolic Ca^{2+} and in Ca^{2+}-induced contraction. Gastroenterology 1987;92:1634.

59. Felbel J, Trockur B, Ecker T, Landgraf W, Hofmann F. Regulation of cytosolic calcium by cAMP and cGMP in freshly isolated smooth muscle cells from bovine trachea. J Biol Chem 1988;263:16764.

60. Rashatwar SS, Cornwell TL, Lincoln TM. Effects of 8-bromo-cGMP on Ca^{2+} levels in vascular smooth muscle cells: Possible regulation of Ca^{2+}-ATPase by cGMP-dependent protein kinase. Proc Natl Acad Sci USA 1987;84:5685.

61. De Lanerolle P, Nishikawa M, Yost DA, Adelstein RS. Increased phosphorylation of myosin light chain kinase after an increase in cyclic AMP in intact smooth muscle. Science 1984;223:1415.

62. Kerrick WGL, Hoar PE. Inhibition of smooth muscle tension by cyclic AMP-dependent protein kinase. Nature 1981;292:253.

63. Casteels R. Membrane potential in smooth muscle cells. In Bulbring E, Brading AF, Jones AW, Tomita T, eds. Smooth muscle: An assessment of current knowledge. Austin: University of Texas Press, 1981:105.

64. Sanders KM. Electrophysiology of dissociated gastrointestinal muscle cells. In: Wood JD, ed. Motility and circulation, vol I, Handbook of physiology, section 6: The gastrointestinal system. New York: American Physiological Society, Oxford University Press, 1989:163.

65. Szurszewski JH. Electrical basis of gastrointestinal motility. In: Johnson LR, ed. Physiology of gastrointestinal tract, ed 2. New York: Raven Press, 1987:383.

66. Sanders KM, Smith TK. Electrophysiology of colonic smooth muscle. In: Wood JD, ed. Motility and circulation, vol I, Handbook of physiology, section 6: The gastrointestinal system. New York: American Physiological Society, Oxford University Press, 1989:251.

67. Sanders KM, Publicover NG. Electrophysiology of gastric musculature. In: Wood J, ed. Motility and circulation, vol I, Handbook of physiology: The gastrointestinal system. New York: American Physiological Society, Oxford University Press, 1989:187.

68. Alberts B, Bray D, Lewis J, Raff M, Roberts K, Watson JD. Molecular biology of the cell. Garland Publishing, New York, 1983:291.

69. Walsh JV Jr, Singer JJ. Calcium action potentials in single freshly isolated smooth muscle cells. Am J Physiol 1980;239:C162.

70. Walsh JV Jr, Singer JJ. Voltage clamp of single freshly dissociated smooth muscle cells: Current–voltage relationships for three currents. Pflugers Arch 1981;390:207.

71. Singer JJ, Walsh JV Jr. Passive properties of the membrane of single freshly isolated smooth muscle cells. Am J Physiol 1980;239:153.

72. Benham CD, Bolton TB. Patch-clamp studies of slow potential-sensitive potassium channels in longitudinal smooth muscle cells of rabbit jejunum. J Physiol Lond 1983;340:469.

73. Benham CD, Bolton TB, Lang RJ, Takewaki T. Calcium-activated potassium channels in single smooth muscle cells of rabbit jejunum and guinea-pig mesenteric artery. J Physiol Lond 1986;371:45.

74. Bolton TB, Lang RJ, Takewaki T, Benham CD. Patch and whole-cell voltage clamp of single mammalian visceral and vascular smooth muscle cells. Experientia 1985;41:887.

75. Andreas C, Sanders KM. Ca^{2+}-activated K$^+$ channels of canine colonic myocytes. Am J Physiol 1989;257:C470.

76. Ganitkevich VY, Shuba MF, Smirnov SV. Potential-dependent calcium inward current in a single isolated smooth muscle cell of the guinea-pig taenia caeci. J Physiol Lond 1986;380:1.

77. Droogmans G, Callewaert G. Ca^{2+}-channel current and its modification by the dihydropyridine agonist BAY k8644 in isolated smooth muscle cells. Pflugers Arch 1986;406:259.

78. Mitra R, Morad M. Ca^{2+}- and Ca^{2+}-activated K$^+$ currents in mammalian gastric smooth muscle cells. Science 1985;229:269.

79. Bechem M, Hebisch S, Schramm M. Ca^{2+} agonists: New, sensitive probes for Ca^{2+} channels. TIPS 1988;9:257.

80. Singer JJ, Walsh JV Jr. Large conductance Ca^{2+} activated K$^+$ channels in smooth muscle cell membrane. Biophys J 1984;45:68.

81. Singer JJ, Walsh JV Jr. Characterization of calcium-activated potassium channels in single smooth muscle cells using the patch-clamp technique. Pflugers Arch 1987;408:98.

82. Brown DA, Adams PR. Muscarinic suppression of a novel voltage-sensitive K$^+$ current in a vertebrate neurone. Nature 1980;283:673.

83. Sims SM, Singer JJ, Walsh JV Jr. Cholinergic agonists suppress a potassium current in freshly dissociated smooth muscle cells of the toad. J Physiol (Lond) 1985;367:503.

84. Sims SM, Walsh JV Jr, Singer JJ. Substance P and acetylcholine both suppress the same K$^+$ current in dissociated smooth muscle cells. Am J Physiol 1986;251:C580.

85. Benham CD, Bolton TB, Lang RJ. Acetylcholine activates an inward current in single mammalian smooth muscle cell membranes. Nature 1985;316:345.

86. Bauer AJ, Sanders KM. Gradient in excitation–contraction coupling in canine gastric antral circular muscle. J Physiol (Lond) 1985;369:283.

87. Smith TK, Reed BJ, Sanders KM. Origin and propagation of electrical slow waves in circular muscle of canine proximal colon. Am J Physiol 1987;252:C215.

88. Sanders KM. Colonic electrical activity: Concerto for two pacemakers. NPS 1989;4:176.

89. Thuneberg L. Interstitial cells of Cajal. In: Wood JD, ed. Motility and circulation, vol I, Handbook of physiology, section 6: The gastrointestinal system. New York: American Physiological Society, Oxford University Press, 1989:349.

90. Kobayashi S, Furness JB, Smith TK, Pompolo S. Histological identification of the interstitial cells of Cajal in the guinea-pig small intestine. Arch Histol Cytol 1989;52:267.

91. Langton P, Ward SM, Carl A, Norell MA, Sanders KM. Spontaneous electrical activity of interstitial cells of Cajal isolated from canine proximal colon. Proc Natl Acad Sci USA 1989;86:7280.

92. Sanders KM, Burke EP, Stevens RJ. Effects of methylene blue on rhythmic activity and membrane potential in the canine proximal colon. Am J Physiol 1989;256:G779.

93. Hara Y, Kubota M, Szurszewski JH. Electrophysiology of the smooth muscle in the small intestine of some mammals. J Physiol (Lond) 1986;372:501.

94. Suzuki N, Prosser CL, Dahms V. Boundary cells between longitudinal and circular layers: Essential for electrical slow waves in cat intestine. Am J Physiol 1986;250:G287.

95. Smith TK, Reed BJ, Sanders KM. Electrical pacemakers of canine proximal colon are functionally innervated by inhibitory motor neurons. Am J Physiol 1989;256:C466.

96. Smith TK. Spontaneous junction potentials and slow waves in the circular muscle of isolated segments of guinea-pig ileum. J Auton Nerv Syst 1989;27:147.

97. El-Sharkawy TY, Morgan KG, Szurszewski JH. Intracellular activity of canine and human gastric smooth muscle. J Physiol (Lond) 1978;279:291.

98. Szurszewski JH. Mechanism of action of pentagastrin and acetyl-choline on the longitudinal muscle of the canine antrum. J Physiol (Lond) 1975;252:335.

99. Morgan KG, Szurszewski JH. Mechanisms of phasic and tonic actions of pentagastrin on canine gastric smooth muscle. J Physiol (Lond) 1980;301:229.

100. Morgan KG, Schmalz PF, Go VL, Szurszewski JH. Electrical and mechanical effects of molecular variants of CCK on antral smooth muscle. Am J Physiol 1978;235:E324.

101. Sanders KM, Vogalis F. Organization of electrical activity in the canine pyloric canal. J Physiol 1989;416:49.

102. Morgan KG, Muir TC, Szurszewski JH. The electrical basis for contraction and relaxation in canine fundal smooth muscle. J Physiol (Lond) 1981;311:475.

103. Smith TK, Reed BJ, Sanders KM. Interaction of two electrical pacemakers in muscularis of canine proximal colon. Am J Physiol 1987;252:C290.

104. Furness JB, Costa M. Identification of transmitters of functionally defined enteric neurons. In: Wood JD ed. Motility and circulation, vol I, Handbook of physiology, section 6: The gastrointestinal system, New York: American Physiological Society, Oxford University Press, 1989:387.

105. Costa M, Furness JB, Llewellyn-Smith IJ. Histochemistry of enteric nervous system. In: Johnson LR, ed. Physiology of the gastrointestinal tract, ed 2, New York: Raven Press, 1987:1.

106. Llewellyn IJ, Furness JB, Gibbins IL, Costa M. Quantitative ultra-structural analysis of enkephalin-, substance P-, and VIP-immuno-reactive nerve fibers in the circular muscle of the guinea pig small intestine. J Comp Neurol 1988;272:139.

107. Wilson AJ, Llewellyn-Smith IJ, Furness JB, Costa M. The source of the nerve fibres forming the deep muscular and circular muscle plexuses in the small intestine of the guinea-pig. Cell Tissue Res 1987;247:497.

108. Watchow DA, Furness JB, Costa M. Distribution and coexistence of peptides in nerve fibers of the external muscle of the human gastrointestinal tract. Gastroenterology 1988;95:32.

109. Furness JB, Costa M. Identification of gastrointestinal neurotrans-mitters. In: Bertaccini G, ed. Handbook of experimental pharmacology. Mediators and drugs in gastrointestinal motility. Berlin: Springer-Verlag, 1982;59:279.

110. Makhlouf GM, Grider JR. Receptors for gut peptides on smooth muscle cells of the gut. In: Makhlouf GM, ed. Neural and endocrine biology of the gut, vol 2, Handbook of physiology: The gastrointestinal system. New York: American Physiological Society, Oxford University Press, 1989:281.

111. Makhlouf GM, Grider JR, Schubert ML. Identification of physiological function of gut peptides. In: Makhlouf GM, ed. Neural and endocrine biology of the gut, vol 2, Handbook of physiology: The gastrointestinal system, New York: American Physiological Society, Oxford University Press, 1989:123.

112. Makhlouf GM. Enteric neuropeptides: Role in neuromuscular activity of the gut. Trends Pharmacol Sci 1985;6:214.

113. Micheletti R, Grider JR, Makhlouf GM. Identification of bombesin receptors on isolated muscle cells from human intestine. Regul Pept 1988;21:219.

114. Zetler G. Antagonism of the gut-contracting effects of bombesin and neurotensin by opioid peptides, morphine, atropine or tetrodotoxin. Pharmacology 1980;21:348.

115. Yau WM, Lingle PF, Youther ML. Interaction of enkephalin and caerulein on guinea pig small intestine. Eur J Pharmacol 1983;90:245.

116. Grider JR, Makhlouf GM. Regional and cellular heterogeneity of cholecystokinin receptors mediating muscle contraction in the gut. Gastroenterology 1987;92:175.

117. Grider JR, Cable MB, Said SI, Makhlouf GM. Vasoactive intestinal peptide: Relaxant neurotransmitter in tenia coli of the guinea pig. Gastroenterology 1985;89:36.

118. Grider JR, Makhlouf GM. Suppression of inhibitory neural input to colonic circular muscle by opioid peptides. J Pharmacol Exp Ther 1987;243:205.

119. Grider JR, Makhlouf GM. GABA neurons of the myenteric plexus facilitate the colonic peristaltic reflex: Receptor location and mode of action. Gastroenterology 1990;98:355.

120. Bitar KN, Makhlouf GM. Specific opiate receptors on isolated mammalian gastric smooth muscle cells. Nature 1982;297:72.

121. Grider JR, Makhlouf GM. The modulatory function of galanin: Potentiation of VIP-induced relaxation in isolated smooth muscle cells. Gastroenterology 1988;94:A157.

122. Souquet JC, Grider JR, Bitar KN, Makhlouf GM. Receptors for mammalian tachykinins on isolated intestinal smooth muscle cells. Am J Physiol 1985;249:G533.

123. Grider JR, Makhlouf GM. Prejunctional inhibition of vasoactive intestinal peptide release. Am J Physiol 1987;253:G7.

124. Biancani P, Walsh JH, Behar J. Vasoactive intestinal peptide. A neurotransmitter for lower esophageal sphincter relaxation. J Clin Invest 1984;73:936.

125. Biancani P, Walsh JH, Behar J. Vasoactive intestinal peptide: A neurotransmitter for relaxation of the rabbit internal anal sphincter. Gastroenterology 1985;89:867.

126. Wiley JW, O'Dorisio TM, Owyang C. Vasoactive intestinal peptide mediated CCK-induced relaxation of sphincter of Oddi. J Clin Invest 1988;81:1920.

127. Grider JR, Makhlouf GM. Colonic peristalic reflex: Identification of VIP as mediator of descending relaxation. Am J Physiol 1986;251: G40.

128. Grider JR. Identification of neurotransmitters regulating intestinal peristaltic reflex in humans. Gastroenterology 1989;97:1414.

129. Grider JR. Tachykinins as transmitters of ascending contractile component of the peristaltic reflex. Am J Physiol 1989;257:G709.

130. Grider JR, Makhlouf GM. VIP: Transmitter of inhibitory motor neurons of the gut. Ann NY Acad Sci 1988;527:369.

131. Hall KE, Greenber GR, El-Sharkawy TY, Diamant NE. Relationship between porcine motilin induced migrating motor complex-like activity, vagal integrity and endogenous motilin release in dogs. Gastroenterology 1984;87:76.

132. Kuemmerle JF, Martin DC, Murthy KS, Grider JR, Makhlouf GM. Serotonin (5-HT1) and (5-HT2) receptors co-exist and are coupled to different transduction pathways in intestinal muscle cells. Gastroenterology 1990;98:505.

133. Morini G, Impicciatore M, Grider JR, Makhlouf GM. Identification of distinct histamine H_1 and H_2 receptors on intestinal muscle cells by receptor protection with selective ligands. Gastroenterology 1989;96:A351.

134. McHenry L, Grider JR, Makhlouf GM. Coexistence of adenosine stimulatory (A_2) and inhibitory (A_1) receptors on intestinal muscle cells. Gastroenterology 1989;96:A334.

135. DeLegge MH, Murthy KS, Grider JR, Makhlouf GM. Identification of receptors and transduction pathways for peptidoleukotrienes (LTC4, LTD4 and LTE4) in isolated gastric muscle cells. Gastroenterology 1990;98:A344.

136. Vermillion DL, Ernst PB, Scicchitano R, Collins SM. Antigen-induced contraction of jejunal smooth muscle in the sensitized rat. Am J Physiol 1988;255:G701.

5

The Immune System

RICHARD P. MACDERMOTT
WILLIAM F. STENSON

INTRODUCTION

The mucosal immune system of the gastrointestinal tract represents one of the largest immunologic compartments in the body.[1] Host protection and defense is an essential function of the gastrointestinal tract immune system because of the continuous exposure of the intestine to a wide variety of bacterial, viral, and dietary antigens. Therefore, the mucosal immune system has developed a unique set of immunologic protective mechanisms and effector capabilities.[2] The gastrointestinal tract interfaces directly with the external environment (intestinal lumen). The mucosal immune system allows nutrients to cross this interface unimpeded and yet prevents entry of injurious agents.[1,3] Thus a critical function of the mucosal immune system is the ability to specifically recognize and neutralize infectious agents and injurious foreign antigens.[4,5] Discrimination between self and nonself is also vital, so that host tissues are not damaged during the expression of protective defense mechanisms. Advances in our understanding of immunologic and inflammatory processes in the intestine have provided new insights into the immunopathogenic mechanisms involved in autoimmune and chronic inflammatory gastrointestinal diseases.[6,7]

An effective immune response begins with the specific processing of antigens by macrophages, which endocytose large molecules and infectious organisms such as bacteria and viruses. The macrophages then break these molecules and organisms down so that appropriate size fragments can be generated for presentation to lymphocytes.[8] These processed antigenic fragments interact with major histocompatibility complex (MHC) class II determinants (glycoproteins that regulate immune cell interactions and are critical for cytotoxicity, antigen presentation, graft rejection, and lymphocyte differentiation) on the macrophage surface. The T cell receptor specifically recognizes Class II cell surface determinants in conjunction with antigen fragments on the macrophage. It is now clear that other cell types in addition to the macrophage have class II antigens on their surface and are capable of antigen presentation. The gastrointestinal tract in particular, has a number of different types of antigen-presenting cells, including epithelial cells and endothelial cells as well as dendritic cells (similar to Langerhans' cells found in the skin and lymphoid organs) and macrophages.

The presence of a variety of antigen-presenting cells further enhances the ability of the intestine to mount specific immune responses against the many different antigens to which it is exposed.[9,10] Specific antigen recognition is pivotal to the function of T cells, which both regulate immune responses through T helper cell function and serve as effector cells by carrying out T-cell-mediated cytotoxicity.

Cytokines produced by macrophages[11,12] and T cells induce B cells to produce antibodies that have specific antigen recognition capabilities. Antibodies have an antigen recognition site (combining site), which is composed of folded polypeptide chains that have defined areas in which the amino acid sequence varies greatly (variable regions) to provide antigen recognition specificity. Presentation of antigens to B cells initiates an orderly and precise genetic translocation by which genes that code for the variable regions are joined with genes that code for the constant regions of heavy and light chains of immunoglobulins. This results in the formation of a specific DNA, which produces a specific messenger RNA, which in turn allows a B cell to secrete an isotype and subclass defined antibody, specific for the initiating antigen. The normal gastrointestinal immune system has unique mechanisms that allow mucosal B cells to "switch" from predominantly IgM production to IgA production. Factors that promote the conversion from IgM production to IgA production are called *switch factors*.[13,14] A series of cell and cytokine-mediated regulatory events are involved in the production of IgA, which is the major mucosal protective immunoglobulin. Within the Peyer's patch, T-cell subsets produce specific B cell switch, differentiation and growth factors that regulate IgA production by B cells.[15]

T-cell recognition functions are controlled by the formation of a cell surface receptor with two polypeptide chains (α and β), which have variable regions. Sensitized T cells recognize specific antigens in conjunction with MHC class II molecules. Helper T lymphocytes are then stimulated by interleukin-1 release from antigen-activated macrophages.[12] Increased production of interleukin-2 by T cells further stimulates helper T cells to undergo cell cycle progression and clonal expansion.[16] Specific T cell help leads to enhanced production of immunoglobulins. Therefore, carefully regulated expansion by cytokines[17] of immunoglobulin-producing B cells in the mucosa occurs in response to specific infectious agents or stimulating antigens to provide a protective immune response.

GUT-ASSOCIATED LYMPHOID TISSUE AND HOMING OF LYMPHOBLASTS

An understanding of the gastrointestinal immune system requires appreciation of the unique structural and functional characteristics of the gut-associated lymphoid tissue (Fig 5-1). Gut-associated lymphoid tissue functions in the first line of defense against the large number of potentially injurious agents present within the gastrointestinal lumen. Follicle-associated epithelium contains microfold (M) cells, which are derived directly from undifferentiated immature epithelial stem cells in the crypts that surround Peyer's patches (see Fig 5-1). M cells cover the lymphoid follicles in the gastrointestinal tract and provide a site for the selective sampling of intraluminal antigens.[18] Clusters of M cells transport

microorganisms and large molecules into the underlying lymphoid tissues of Peyer's patches.[19]

Among the infectious agents known to undergo endocytosis and transport by M cells are reoviruses, cholera, and mycobacteria. Similarly, large molecules, including horseradish peroxidase, ferritin, and certain lectins are also absorbed by M cells. Among the characteristic morphologic features that differentiate M cells from absorptive epithelial cells is the presence of fewer, shorter, and wider microvilli.[20] Vesicles in the M cell cytoplasm transport antigens through the cell. The antigens then come into contact with lymphocytes and macrophages, which have migrated into an intercellular space or central hollow that indents into the M cell.[21] M cells themselves do not have class II antigens on their surface and they do not process or present antigens. The M cells thus primarily perform a transport function by moving selected antigens from the intestinal lumen so that subsequent macrophage processing and antigen presentation in the intestinal lymphoid follicles will initiate a specific mucosal immune response.

Activated lymphocytes from intestinal lymphoid follicles begin

Gut Associated Lymphoid Tissue

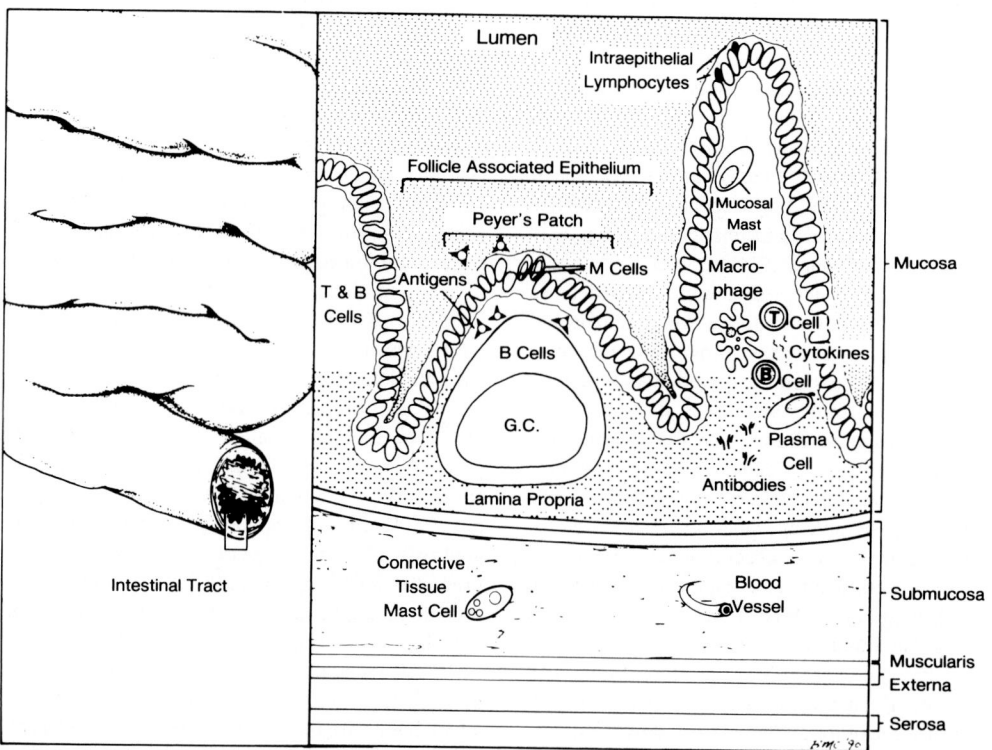

FIGURE 5–1. Gut Associated Lymphoid Tissue consists of the cells of the mucosal immune system located between the external environment (intestinal lumen) and the internal mileu of the host. Follicle-associated epithelial cells are located over Peyer's patch areas (animals) or lymphoid follicles (humans) in which immature germinal center cells, and B cells reside. Antigens from the intestinal lumen are transported through specialized epithelial cells called M cells. After being brought across the follicle-associated epithelium, the antigens come into contact with lymphocytes and macrophages. A subcompartment of T suppressor/cytotoxic lymphocytes called *intraepithelial lymphocytes* reside between absorptive epithelial cells. In animals, most intraepithelial lymphocytes bear the gamma/delta T cell receptor. Within the lamina propria, mature T cells, B cells, plasma cells and macrophages carry out cell-mediated immunologic processes including cytokine secretion, production of IgA, and phagocytosis. Two different types of mast cells (mucosal mast cells and connective tissue mast cells) are found in the mucosa and submucosa.

a "maturational journey" (Fig 5-2), whereby they leave the intestinal tract and migrate into afferent lymphatics that drain into mesenteric lymph nodes.[22,23] Lymphoctes then enter efferent lymphatics and pass through the thoracic duct into the peripheral blood (see Fig 5-2). During this process, the lymphocytes mature into T-cell and B-cell lymphoblasts. The B lymphocytes become surface IgA-bearing lymphoblasts after being promoted to switch their immunoglobulin isotype by regulatory ("switch") T cells within the Peyer's patch.[13,14,24] B lymphoblasts mature into IgA-secreting plasma cells after homing to mucosal sites. The homing of lymphoblasts results in mature B cells arriving at a variety of secretory sites[22,25] by interaction between specific "homing antigens"[26,27] on the surface of the lymphoblasts with "addressins,"[28] which are specific receptors on the surface of high endothelial venules (Fig 5-3). Thus, a selective recognition of lymphocyte-specific proteins by antigens on endothelial cells in specific organs regulates the distribution of lymphoid effector cells to the intestine and other mucosal secretory sites (see Fig 5-3).

Lymphoblasts recirculate or "home" to the sites of the original antigenic stimulation as well as to other mucosal secretory sites (Fig 5-4). In man, the cell interaction, adherence, and extravasation process is mediated by an 85 to 95 kD class of lymphocyte surface glycoproteins that define "homing receptors" for high endothelial venules and are present on normal human mucosal lamina propria lymphocyte populations.[26,27,29] IgA B cells preferentially migrate to mucosal secretory lymphoid sites, whereas T cells primarily home to peripheral lymph nodes. These differences in migration between B cells and T cells as well as differences in the migration of lymphoblasts based upon their tissue of origin are due to cell surface homing receptor interactions with high endothelial venules.[28]

Antigenic stimulation and chronic inflammation result in a rapid increase in the number of high endothelial venules (identified morphologically by their typical cuboid, plump appearance). Increase in the number of high endothelial venules is due to both enhanced differentiation as well as stimulation of proliferation.[26,27] Cytokines, including interleukin-1, interferon-γ, and tumor necrosis factor, increase lymphoblast adherence to endothelial cells, trigger the development of endothelial cell differentiation markers, and enhance the expression of endothelial adhesion molecules. Increased expression of adhesion molecules on endothelial cells allows an increase in the influx of antigen-specific, sensitized lymphocytes into areas of chronic inflammation or areas where cell-mediated host defense processes are needed. High endothelial venules increase in number in areas that are in close proximity to developing granulomas. The presence of high endothelial venules is thus closely associated with dense, lymphocytic infiltrates, particularly when the mononuclear cell-mediated processes are persistent. Although most studies to date have focused on the maturation and homing events related to lymphocytes,[26-29] it should be noted that the migration of granulocytes and macrophages is also regulated by interactions with similar endothelial cell adhesion molecules. Therefore, it is now clear that different cell surface receptors are involved in determining which lymphocytes become localized to both normal and inflamed intestine.

Following antigenic stimulation in the gastrointestinal tract, IgA lymphoblasts also circulate to a number of other mucosal secretory sites (see Fig 5-4) including breast, lung, and eye, where antigen-specific antibodies are secreted.[22,25] One piece of evidence supporting the importance of the common mucosal immune system is the finding that a breast-feeding mother can passively transfer secretory IgA in the breast milk to her nursing child. The breast

Maturational Journey

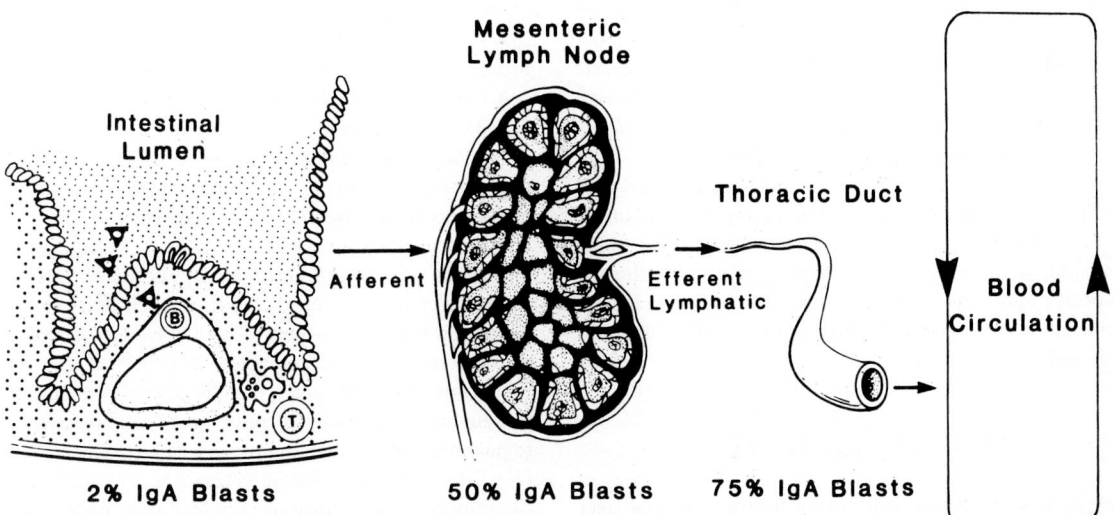

FIGURE 5-2. After sensitization to antigens transported across the epithelium through M cells from the intestinal lumen, immature B cells from lymphoid follicles (human) or Peyer's patches (animals) migrate from the intestine. During migration from the intestine through afferent lymphatics to the mesenteric lymph node, the percentage of lymphoblasts increases markedly. Lymphoblast maturation continues as the cells leave the mesenteric lymph nodes via the efferent lymphatics to enter the thoracic duct (IgA-bearing lymphoblasts increase from 2% to 50% to 75%). Lymphoblasts then circulate in the peripheral blood. The lymphoblasts also develop "homing" receptors that determine their selective recirculation back to secretory mucosal sites (See Figs. 5-3 and 5-4).

HOMING OF LYMPHOBLASTS

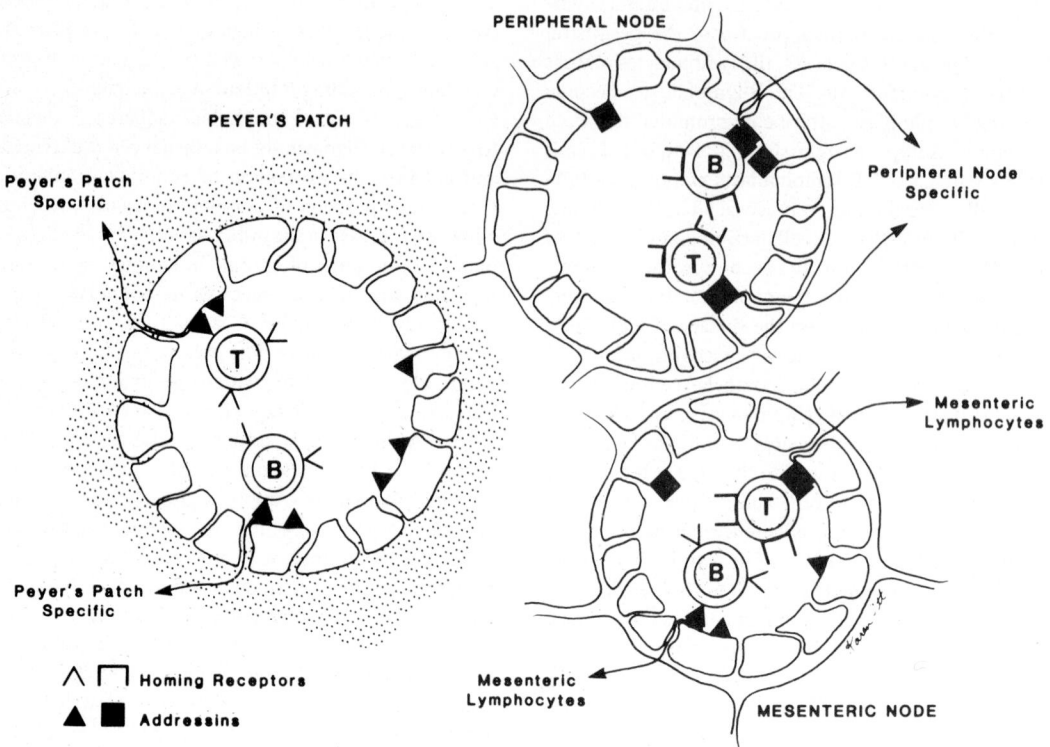

FIGURE 5–3. T cell lymphoblasts and B cell lymphoblasts develop specific "homing" receptors that allow their selective extravasation into secretory mucosal sites or peripheral lymph nodes. Lymphoblasts with homing receptors interact with the specific addressin molecules found on high endothelial ve-nules in Peyer's patch areas and then migrate into the surrounding mucosa as mucosal-specific lymphoblasts. In contrast, lymphoblasts with homing receptors specific for peripheral lymph node addressins migrate into peripheral lymph node tissue.

milk secretory IgA transferred to the infant has been shown to be specifically protective against bacteria or viruses found within the mother's gastrointestinal tract.[4] Homing of stimulated lymphoblasts to mucosal secretory sites thus allows the secretion into lung, breast, and eye fluids of protective antibodies directed against antigens within the gastrointestinal lumen. After lymphoblasts have "homed" to the gastrointestinal mucosa and have matured into effector cells, they provide protective immunity within the lamina propria. Thus, the intestinal immune system has distinct components that allow selective antigen sampling to occur with subsequent specific induction of immune responses that provide protection not only for the gastrointestinal tract but other mucosal surfaces as well.

IMMUNOGLOBULIN SECRETION

The major protective immune mechanism for the intestinal tract is the synthesis and secretion of dimeric IgA.[3,4,30,31] The intestine contains over 70% of the immunoglobulin-producing cells in the body.[1,32] Although IgG and IgM antibodies are also produced by lamina propria B cells within the normal intestine, the predominant antibody synthesized and secreted is IgA.[2–5] There are two IgA subclasses: IgA 1 and IgA 2 (Fig 5-5). In serum, less than 15%

of the IgA is IgA 2, whereas in external secretion up to 50% of IgA is IgA 2.[31,33] One possible explanation for the preferential production of IgA 2 in intestinal secretions is the observation that IgA 1 is easily cleaved by proteases produced by bacteria, whereas IgA 2 is more resistant to cleavage and thus may survive longer in the intestinal lumen.[34] Plasma cells produce IgA either in monomeric form or as a dimeric structure in which two IgA monomers are joined by a J (joining) chain. J chain is therefore also produced within the plasma cell.[32,33] J chain produces polymerization of both IgA and IgM. By subsequent interaction with secretory component on the epithelial cell basal surface, J chain participates in the transport of both polymeric IgA and IgM molecules across the intestinal epithelial cell.[32,35,36]

Secretory component is produced by epithelial cells and is present as a membrane receptor, which exhibits selective binding to polymeric immunoglobulins such as IgA, which contain J chain (Fig 5-6).[37–44] After initial interaction between polymeric IgA and the transmembrane form of secretory component (see Fig 5-6), the entire IgA-secretory component complex undergoes endocytosis into the basal side of the epithelial cell.[37–44] The polymeric IgA complexed with the membrane secretory component is then transported transcellularly (see Fig 5-6) in endoplasmic vesicles, which move to the apical surface of the epithelial cell where they fuse with the apical membrane and subsequently release the se-

Homing to Secretory Sites

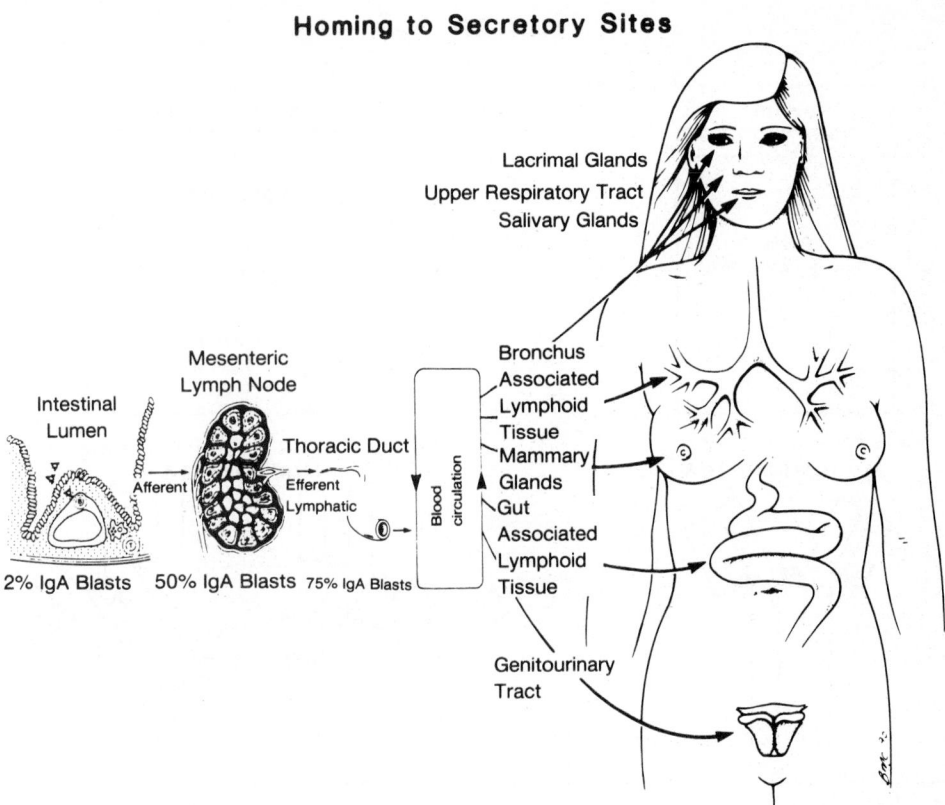

FIGURE 5–4. Homing to secretory sites is achieved by mature lymphoblasts after their maturational journey and the development of "homing" receptors. Antigen-specific IgA-secreting cells after antigenic stimulation in the intestine will "home" to lacrimal, upper respiratory, and salivary tissues in order to provide IgA-mediated, antigen-specific protection in the mouth and upper airway. Cells also home to the lung, where cells in the bronchus-associated lymphoid tissue carry out many of the same functional processes as gut-associated lymphoid tissue. Homing of IgA lymphoblasts to breast tissue allows antigen-specific IgA to be passively transferred to nursing infants. Homing of cells to the genitourinary tract helps provide IgA protective immunity for the kidneys, urinary tract, and female reproductive organs.

cretory component–IgA complex as an intact secretory IgA molecule into the intestinal lumen.[37-44]

Secretory component is synthesized in the rough endoplasmic reticulum of the epithelial cell (see Fig 5-6) and is then glycosylated in the Golgi complex.[40,41] Vesicles that contain secretory component then fuse with the basal membrane resulting in insertion of secretory component so that it can act as a receptor for J chain-containing polymeric IgA complexes.[42-44] Secretory component thus serves as a receptor for polymeric IgA, as well as an integral component of the transepithelial transport process of polymeric IgA, and also remains bound to polymeric IgA after its release into the external secretions.[37-44] Secretory component is also found by itself in mucosal secretions as a secreted glycoprotein not bound to polymeric immunoglobulins. Secretory component may serve to prevent proteolytic degradation of the secretory IgA molecule as well as to stabilize the structure of the polymeric IgA complex, thus providing an important protective function for secretory IgA, which is secreted into a hostile environment containing numerous proteolytic enzymes, bacteria, and other substances that could otherwise rapidly degrade it.[37-44]

In addition to being transported across epithelial cells into the intestinal lumen, IgA is also translocated across the hepatocyte or

bile duct epithelium (Fig 5-7) into the bile.[45,46] IgA in the bile is then carried into the duodenum. Important interspecies differences have been observed in that certain animals such as the rat and rabbit have IgA and secretory component as major components of their bile, whereas sheep, dogs, and man have much smaller amounts of IgA in their bile.[45,46] These differences in IgA translocation into bile appear to be related to the presence of secretory component on hepatocytes in rats and rabbits resulting in highly efficient movement of IgA into the bile, whereas secretory component is expressed only on biliary epithelium in man resulting in less efficient translocation of IgA.[45,46] The presence of secretory IgA in bile provides passive immunity and protection for both the biliary tract and the proximal parts of the small bowel.[45,46] A second implication of hepatobiliary secretion of IgA is that complexes of IgA and antigen can be transported into bile from the circulation. Hepatic removal of IgA-antigen complexes could provide a protective mechanism against absorbed substances including dietary antigens and bacterial products.

The major function of secretory IgA in host defense is protection against bacteria, viruses, and luminal antigens.[1,3,4,25] Secretory IgA prevents the adherence of bacteria to epithelial cells and thus prevents their effective colonization and multiplication.

Human IgA

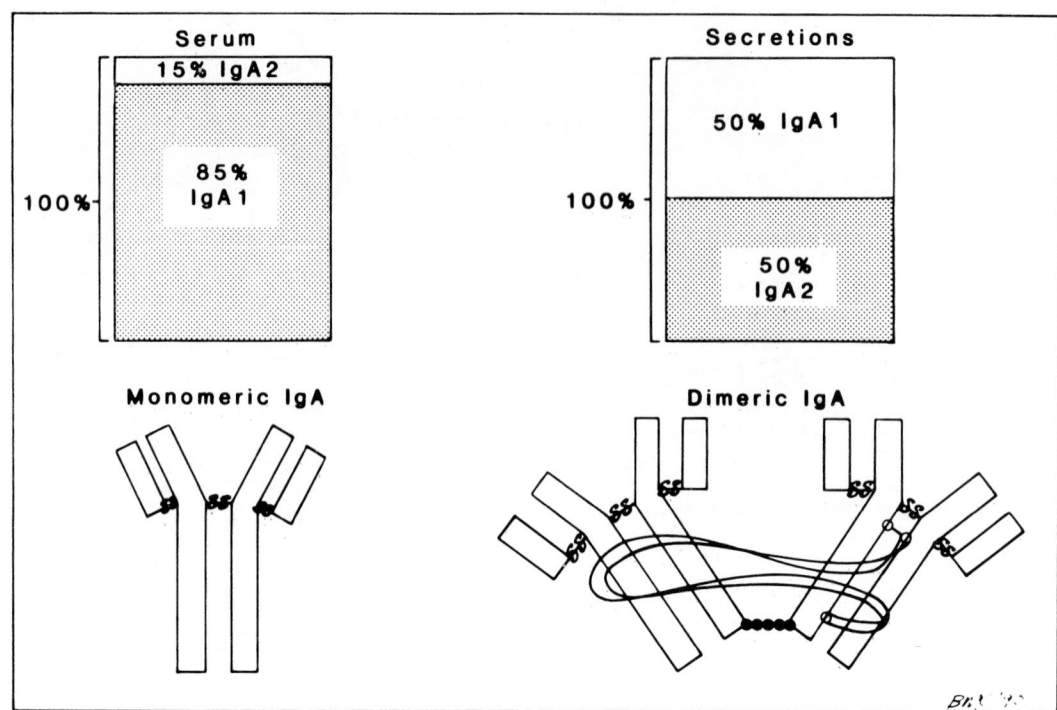

FIGURE 5–5. The IgA found in human serum is predominantly monomeric, whereas the IgA found in intestinal secretions is predominantly dimeric. Although 85% of the IgA in the serum is IgA subclass 1, only 50% of the IgA in external secretions is IgA subclass 1. Conversely, although only 15% of the IgA in the serum is IgA subclass 2, considerably more IgA subclass 2 (50%) is found in intestinal secretions.

In addition, secretory IgA neutralizes bacterial toxins and prevents their action on intestinal epithelial cells. The major antiviral properties of IgA are neutralization of viral activity and passive protective immunity. Secretory IgA also blocks the absorption of antigens from the gut and thus may be particularly important in disease states in which the mucosal barrier is broken. IgA does not activate complement and does not enhance cell-mediated opsonization or destruction of infectious organisms or antigens. This is in sharp contrast to other immunoglobulins such as IgG, which can also be secreted by B cells present in the intestine and which will initiate important complement-mediated and cell-mediated protective events within the intestine.

CELL-MEDIATED IMMUNITY IN MUCOSAL HOST DEFENSE

Although antibody secretion in general and IgA secretion in particular by B cells provide a protective mechanism of major importance for the intestine, a number of other cell types are also actively involved in effector capabilities, which play principal roles in host defense. Cell-mediated cytotoxicity is of particular importance in that there are intriguing differences in cytotoxic capabilities demonstrated by unique subcompartments of the intestinal immune system. Although it is well known that peripheral blood and splenic lymphocytes are excellent cytotoxic effector cells against cell line targets, intestinal lamina propria lymphocytes are very poor mediators of cell-mediated cytotoxicity in a variety of systems including spontaneous cell-mediated cytotoxicity, antibody-dependent cellular cytotoxicity, and cell-mediated lympholysis[47,48] However, small numbers of precursor natural killer, killer and cytotoxic T lymphocytes can be enriched from isolated lamina propria mononuclear cells.[49,50] Furthermore, lamina propria lymphocytes can be induced to mediate cell-mediated cytotoxicity by incubation with interleukin-2, interferon, lectins, and monoclonal antibodies directed against the T cell receptor.[49–53] Thus, there is in the intestine a set of lymphocytes that are cytotoxic effector precursor cells and can participate in host mucosal defense mechanisms when needed, without continuously causing damage to the surrounding tissue when not needed. Controlled activation of the intestinal immune system may be important in regulating cytotoxic effector cell function in the mucosa so that protection rather than destruction occurs. Thus, lymphocytes from a solid organ such as the intestine comprise a compartmentalized immune system that functionally differs from lymphocytes obtained from other sites such as the peripheral blood or the spleen.

Intraepithelial lymphocytes consist of a subcompartment of cells that are located between epithelial cells and are capable of mediating a number of different cellular cytotoxic functions.[54–57] Following the selective migration of this unique T-cell subset into areas between epithelial cells, most intraepithelial cells appear to subsequently reenter the lamina propria. Of particular interest is the observation in mice that intestinal intraepithelial lymphocytes

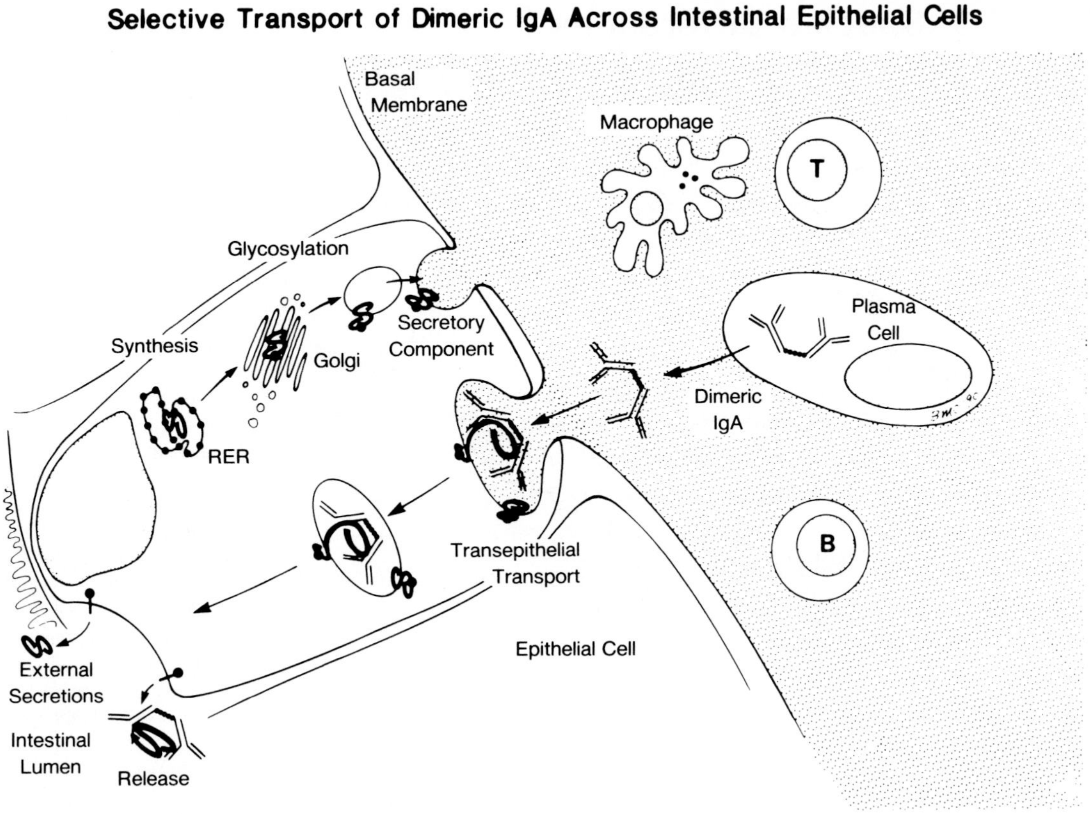

Selective Transport of Dimeric IgA Across Intestinal Epithelial Cells

FIGURE 5–6. Secretory component (also known as the polymeric immunoglobulin receptor) is synthesized in the rough endoplasmic reticulum, after which glycosylation occurs in the Golgi complex. Vesicles with secretory component then fuse with the basal membrane of the epithelial cell to form membrane-bound secretory component that functions as a receptor for the J chain-dimeric IgA complex. After synthesis and secretion of dimeric IgA in plasma cells, the two IgA monomers coupled by J chain interact with secretory component polymeric immunoglobulin receptor, on the basal membrane of the epithelial cell. The dimeric IgA secretory component complex is then transported through the epithelial cell cytoplasm in internalized endoplasmic vesicles. The endoplasmic vesicles then move to the apical membrane of the epithelial cell where fusion is followed by release of secretory IgA into the external secretions of the intestinal lumen.

include a distinct population of γ/δ-bearing T cells, which contain large amounts of proteases.[58,59] The fact that intestinal epithelia contain T γ/δ cells suggests specific homing of these cells to the epithelium and may indicate a specific role in regulatory, surveillance or protective functions by intraepithelial lymphocytes.[60] One of the ways in which intraepithelial lymphocytes may be involved in regulating immune responses is by the induction of MHC class II antigens on epithelial cells.[54] MHC class II antigens are present on normal human small intestinal epithelial cells but not normal human colonic epithelial cells.[61,62] In the presence of intestinal inflammation, increased amounts of interferon-γ are produced, and HLA class II expression is increased in both the small intestine as well as induced on colonic epithelial cells.[63–67] Enhanced HLA class II expression may then allow the increased presentation of antigens by epithelial cells.[9,10,68]

Although CD4 (helper) cells predominate in the lamina propria, CD8 (cytotoxic) cells represent 80% of the intraepithelial lymphocyte population.[54–56] Intraepithelial lymphocytes have been shown to release cytokines after immunologic stimulation or in response to parasitic infections.[56] Intraepithelial lymphocyte numbers are low in germ-free mice and increase with the development of normal bacterial flora. A marked increase in intraepi-

thelial lymphocytes occurs in parasitic infections.[56] Up to 60% of intraepithelial lymphocytes contain granules and are capable of mediating cytotoxicity in a number of different assays including antibody-dependent cellular cytotoxicity, spontaneous cell-mediated cytotoxicity, and T-cell-mediated cytotoxicity assays.[55,56] Thus, as a population, intraepithelial lymphocytes contain cells that have the ability to neutralize numerous infectious agents, including viruses as a first line host defense mechanism in the intestine.

Recent attention has focused on the cytokines (Fig 5-8) that regulate the cell-mediated immune system and are involved in the coordination and control of cell differentiation and proliferation of intestinal lymphocytes. Interleukin-1 is produced by macrophages in both the peripheral blood and the intestine and leads to the activation of T cells.[11,12] Production of interleukin-2 by T cells in turn stimulates both "helper" T cells and B cells to proliferate.[16,17] In the mouse, subpopulations of helper T cells have been identified, which differentially produce certain cytokines but not others. T_h1 cells but not T_h2 cells produce interleukin-2 and interferon-τ.[69] Both T_h1 and T_h2 cells produce interleukins-3 and granulocyte-macrophage colony stimulating factor.[69] T_h2 but not T_h1 cells produce interleukin-4 and interleukin-5.[69] It is therefore

Species Differences in
Hepatobiliary Transport of Dimeric IgA

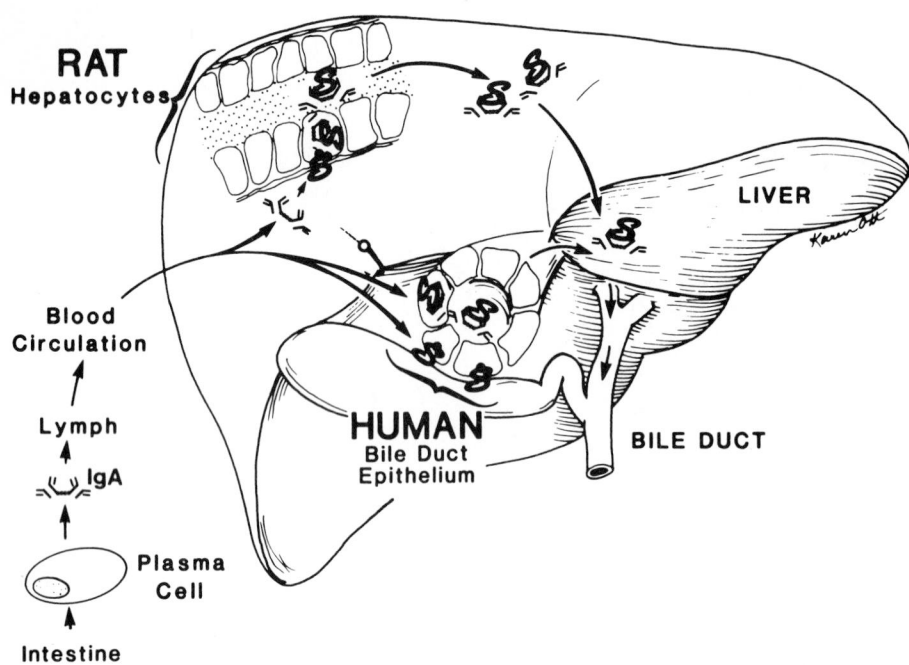

RAT
Hepatocytes

LIVER

Blood Circulation

Lymph

IgA

HUMAN
Bile Duct Epithelium

BILE DUCT

Plasma Cell

Intestine

FIGURE 5–7. IgA is translocated into bile where it can provide passive immunity and protection for both the biliary tract and proximal parts of the small bowel. There are species-dependent differences in the amount of IgA transported across the liver into the bile. In man, small amounts of IgA appear in the bile because only bile duct epithelial cells have secretory component present as a membrane receptor. Therefore, the total number of cells expressing secretory component in the human liver is small, and the amount of IgA present in human bile is low. In the rat, however, secretory component is synthesized by hepatocyes and is present on the hepatocyte membrane as a receptor. Consequently, large numbers of cells in the liver express secretory component leading to the highly efficient movement of dimeric IgA into the bile. In addition to dimeric IgA, complexes of antigen and IgA may also be transported into the bile from the circulation and may provide a mechanism for removal of absorbed bacterial products.

possible that unique subclasses of T cells may exert regulatory control in determining which cell-mediated functions are produced in the intestine.

Cytokines are involved in a series of stages of intestinal B cell development (Fig 5-8). Precursor intestinal B cells for IgA production are located in Peyer's patches.[70,71] "Switch" factors produced by T cells regulate the isotype switch from IgM to IgA expression.[13,14] "Switch" T cells, in conjunction with antigen presentation events within the Peyer's patch, promote this switch, resulting in "postswitched" B cells,[3,14] which can then be induced to terminally differentiate into IgA-secreting cells (Fig 5-8) by interleukin-4, interleukin-5, and interleukin-6.[15,72–77] T_h1 cells secrete cytokines, which in turn sustain their own growth. T_h1 cells are important in the early events of both T cell and B cell development through the production of interleukin-2 and interferon-γ.[69] T_h2 cells, on the other hand, utilize interleukin-4, to autoregulate proliferation and then produce a series of cytokines, including interleukin-4, interleukin-5, and interleukin-6, which markedly enhance immunoglobulin secretion.[72–77] Interleukin-4 and interleukin-5 induce resting B cells to become activated and also induce division and growth of activated B cells. Interleukin-6 is critical for the terminal differentiation of IgA plasma cells, resulting in the secretion of large amounts of IgA. The sequence of cytokine-mediated events that regulate B cell growth, differentiation, and development consists of a series of steps in which multiple cytokines work together (see Fig 5-8) to enhance the IgA immune response.[3,25,72–77] Cytokines are made by a number of different cell types including cells not classically part of the immune system. Furthermore, cytokines have major functional effects on a wide variety of immune and nonimmune cell types.

Another cell type that is important in host defense mechanisms

is the mast cell. Mast cells are found in all layers of the intestine and consist of two functionally and biochemically different cell types (see Fig 5-1) which vary in relative numbers depending upon location.[78] IgE receptor-bearing connective tissue mast cells participate in immediate type hypersensitivity reactions and contain large amounts of the proteoglycan heparin in their cytoplasmic granules.[79] Mucosal mast cells, on the other hand, contain an entirely different proteoglycan, chondroitin sulfate di-B, in their granules.[78,80] Another biochemical difference between connective tissue mast cells and mucosal mast cells is the type of proteases present in the two different subtypes of cells.[81] In some species, such as the rat, the presence of specific proteases distinguishes the two mast cell subtypes. Although mucosal mast cells do bear some IgE receptors, the number and density are much lower than what are present on connective tissue mast cells. A T-cell-derived cytokine, interleukin-3, supports the growth of bone marrow-derived mast cells, which are similar in characteristics to mucosal mast cells.[82] Interleukin-3, on the other hand, does not support the growth of connective tissue mast cells. Interestingly, disodium chromoglycate markedly inhibits mediator release by connective tissue mast cells but is ineffective against mucosal mast cells. Thus, within the human intestine there are two types of mast cells, both the extensively studied connective tissue mast cell and the more recently described mucosal mast cell. Depending upon the immunologic events or disease state, these different mast cell populations may perform specific regulatory and/or effector functions and thereby contribute significantly to host defense or inflammatory processes in the intestine.

Important interactions between nerves and mast cells occur in the gut, where they exist together in close proximity.[83] Extensive evidence has been provided, indicating that neuropeptides such

Regulation of IgA Synthesis and Secretion in the Intestine

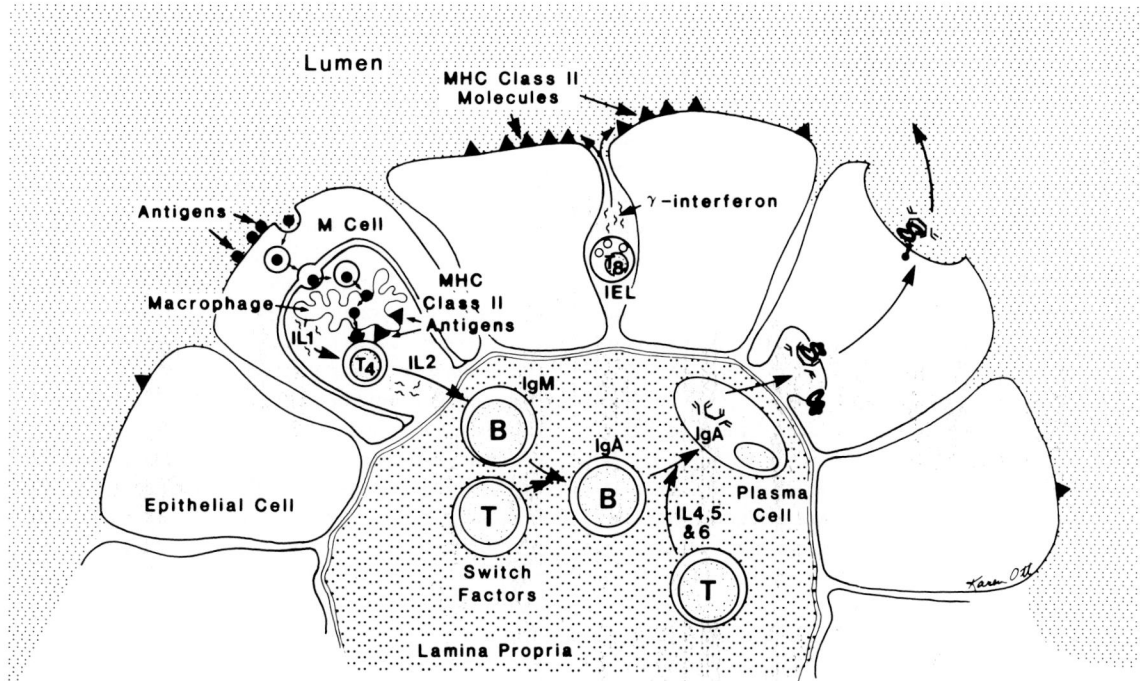

FIGURE 5–8. Antigens within the intestinal lumen are transported across specialized epithelial cells (M cells) into contact with underlying lymphoid cells. Antigen-induced activation of macrophages leads to secretion of interleukin-1 and activation helper T cells, wich secrete interleukin-2. Activation of intraepithelial lymphocytes and subsequent production of gamma interferon leads to enhanced production of MHC class II molecules by epitheilal cells. Increased numbers of MHC class II molecules on intestinal epithelial cells may lead to enhanced antigen presentation by intestinal epithelial cells with subsequent augmentation of antigen-specific IgA antibody production. The expansion of IgM-bearing B cells is regulated by switch factors that favor the development of IgA-bearing B cells. T cells secreting interleukin-4, interleukin-5, and interleukin-6 induce the differentiation and proliferation of B cells for subsequent maturation into plasma cells, which synthesize and secrete dimeric IgA with J chain. The dimeric IgA with J chain then interacts with secretory component receptor on the basal membrane of epithelial cells for subsequent secretion into the intestinal lumen.

as vasoactive intestinal peptide, substance P, and somatostatin can trigger histamine secretion by both connective tissue and mucosal mast cells.[83] However, in the rat, substance P induces histamine secretion by mucosal mast cells but not by connective tissue mast cells, indicating that important species differences may exist.

A central role of mast cells in host defense mechanisms is demonstrated by the immune response to parasitic infections. Mast cells mediate a wide variety of direct and indirect effects in the intestines of infected hosts.[78–83] Mast cell products are able to kill parasites directly, and perhaps more important, mediators produced by mast cells in response to parasitic infection increase vascular permeability and induce vasodilatation so that antibody- and complement-mediated host defense mechanisms take place more rapidly. Furthermore, some mediators released by mast cells are "chemo-attractants" and promote the recruitment, migration, and activation of a variety of different effector cell types, including lymphocytes, granulocytes, eosinophils, and macrophages, resulting in an increased cellular and humoral immune response mounted against parasitic organisms. Depletion of mast cells by steroids leads to a decreased immune response to intestinal parasites and increases the susceptibility to parasitic invasion of the host, thus demonstrating that mast cells play a pivotal role in intestinal host

defense. Mast cells also enhance complement and IgG receptor expression on eosinophils which potentiates antibody-dependent cytotoxic activity of eosinophils toward parasitic organisms such as *Schistosoma*.[84,85]

MECHANISMS OF INFLAMMATION IN THE GASTROINTESTINAL TRACT

Intestinal inflammation is an important component of host defense and is directed at eliminating potentially destructive bacteria, viruses, and other luminal agents. To date, there is no information suggesting that the regulation of inflammation in the gastrointestinal tract differs in any fashion from inflammatory mechanisms in other organ systems. Whereas normal inflammatory mechanisms in response to pathogens are essential for host survival, ongoing inflammation that is not adequately down-regulated can, over time, produce intestinal destruction.[6,7] Among the gastrointestinal diseases in which inflammation plays a significant role are reflux esophagitis, gastritis, pancreatitis, diverticulitis, sprue, Crohn's disease, ulcerative colitis, and a variety of infectious processes. During acute or chronic inflammatory processes, regeneration and healing mechanisms that serve to repair the damaged tissue are maximally augmented. As part of these reparative processes, the enhanced stimulation of collagen generation by chronic inflammation can lead to stricture formation[86] and intestinal obstruction.

The endoscopic picture of acute intestinal inflammation includes erythema and mucosal edema. This appearance is the same whether the initiating event is ischemia, radiation, a bacterial infection such as shigellosis, or inflammatory bowel disease. The similarity of the endoscopic and histologic appearances of these diseases of diverse etiology suggests that there is some final common pathway in the pathogenesis of intestinal inflammation. This final common pathway involves the activation of inflammatory cells, primarily neutrophils and macrophages, and the generation of soluble mediators of inflammation including prostaglandins, leukotrienes, platelet-activating factor, cytokines, histamine, and products of the complement cascade. Some of these mediators including histamine and prostaglandin E_2 are vasodilators and probably account for the hyperemia and erythema that are characteristic of intestinal inflammation. Other mediators including leukotriene B_4, platelet-activating factor, bradykinin, as well as prostaglandin E_2, enhance vascular permeability and account for the mucosal edema seen in acute inflammation.

Acute inflammatory events are marked by the influx of granulocytes into the intestine. Neutrophil influx is the major initial response to infectious organisms and other agents that cause cell injury.[87,88] In chronic inflammation, the cellular infiltrate contains a mixture of cells including granulocytes, lymphocytes, macrophages, eosinophils, and mast cells. These cells produce a number of inflammatory mediators that directly damage the surrounding tissue as well as cause further increases in inflammatory cell number by chemotaxis.[89-91] The infiltration of tissue with macrophages, granulocytes, and eosinophils is a nonspecific component of inflammation, and requires the presence of chemotactic mediators to promote the movement of inflammatory cells out of the blood stream and into the tissue.

Neutrophils are generally the first cell type with phagocytic capabilities to arrive at inflammatory sites.[92,93] There is a subsequent influx of monocytes that mature into macrophages.[94] Macrophages are involved in antigen processing and presentation events, destruction of offending agents, and resolution of the inflammatory process.[8,94] Although only small numbers of neutrophils are normally found within the intestinal tract, the circulating blood contains large numbers of neutrophils that can quickly adhere to endothelial cells and traverse blood vessels to arrive at mucosal sites.[92,93] It is likely that the initial attraction of granulocytes in increased numbers into the intestine is due to the release of chemotactic peptides produced by the activation of complement or the release of chemotactic mediators from macrophages.[95] The active recruitment of neutrophils and granulocytes results in increased inflammation within the tissue. This recruitment of acute inflammatory cells leads to the markedly increased production of mediators of inflammation. Indeed, certain inflammatory mediators, particularly prostaglandin E_2 and leukotriene B_4 have been shown to be elevated in intestinal inflammation by direct measurement in inflamed tissue and by rectal dialysis in vivo.[96-99] Large numbers of macrophages within the intestine may in turn lead to the increased production of cytokines such as interleukin-1 and tumor necrosis factor.[100]

Adhesion of granulocytes and monocytes to vascular endothelial surfaces is mediated by families of adhesion molecules including endothelial leukocyte adhesion molecule-1 (ELAM-1) and intracellular adhesion molecule-1 (ICAM-1).[101,102] The expression of these adhesive molecules by endothelial cells is enhanced by interleukin-1 and tumor necrosis factor. These adhesive proteins are augmented during inflammation and thus interaction of white cells with blood vessel walls is increased, allowing inflammatory cells to enter into the intestine in response to chemotactic agents from the gut lumen or mucosa. The insertion of pseudopods between endothelial cell junctions allows leukocytes to migrate into sites of both acute and chronic inflammation in response to a variety of chemotactic agents including bacterial products (FMLP),[103] components of the complement system $(C5_a)$,[104] and leukotriene B_4 (LTB_4).[95-97]

Chemotactic agents interact with receptors on leukocytes to cause activation and increased migration into the intestine. Neutrophils and macrophages within the mucosa are then able to protect against injurious agents such as bacteria. Neutrophils attach to bacteria (a process enhanced by coating of the bacteria with immunoglobulins and/or complement) and then phagocytose and kill the bacteria. Inflammatory cells also affect intestinal epithelium. The migration of granulocytes and macrophages between epithelial cells into the lumen causes breaks in the intercellular junctions and may participate in the production of altered intestinal permeability in inflammatory disorders of the intestine.[105,106]

Neutrophils, granulocytes, and eosinophils produce tissue damage not only by the release of proteases, but also by the release of large amounts of toxic oxygen metabolites.[91,107] The intestinal tract appears to have only small amounts of enzymes such as superoxide-dismutase and catalase, which provide protection against oxygen radical-induced damage.[108] Therefore, the enormous influx of phagocytic cells that produce large amounts of oxygen radicals may be particularly injurious to the intestinal tract. Nevertheless, the production of oxygen metabolites such as superoxide anion, hydroxyl radical, and hydrogen peroxide are critical components of the normal inflammatory response, because macrophages, granulocytes, and eosinophils utilize oxygen metabolites to kill bacteria.

After they have infiltrated the intestinal tract, neutrophils are end-stage resident cells and their death triggers reparative processes. Some neutrophils eventually migrate between epithelial cells and enter into the lumen of the intestine as part of an intestinal inflammatory reaction. This migration of neutrophils across the epithelium may indicate the presence of chemotactic peptides produced by bacteria within the intestinal lumen.[109] Macrophages are more likely to remain as constituent cells within the intestinal tract after the inflammatory process has resolved. Eosinophils are major producers of a number of granular enzymes and oxygen radicals and are particularly important in the immune response to parasitic infections. Indeed, eosinophils, in combination with IgE and mast cells, provide the major elements of natural host defense mechanisms against parasites.

AUTOIMMUNITY AND ORAL TOLERANCE

Central to our understanding of the processes that lead to the development of autoimmune diseases are the mechanisms that control the distinction of self from nonself. The central cell involved in antigen recognition and regulation of the immune response is the T cell. Considerable attention, therefore, has been given to understanding the role of T cells in autoimmune disease and, in particular, the ability to be tolerant to self-components through the elimination of self-reactive T cells. The ability to trigger immune responses directed against self-antigens is controlled by immune response genes, which determine class II antigen expression on cells of the immune system. Class II major histocompatibility complex molecules are centrally involved in the presentation of soluble antigens and therefore are essential in determining susceptibility to autoimmune disease. The antigens or infectious agents that lead to cross-reactivity provide the initiating factors that lead to development of self-reactive T cells. After an antigen-specific, self-reactive T cell receptor is formed, it in turn leads to the development of an immune response against itself.

Because the gastrointestinal tract must continuously mount immune responses against bacteria, viruses, and other antigens, molecular mimicry leading to activation of self-reactive T cells is a possible event in the development of autoimmune disease in genetically predisposed hosts. Furthermore, after the T cell has been activated, a variety of effector mechanisms can be brought into play. Cytokines not only can destroy host cells directly but they can also activate other cell types to mediate tissue damage. Furthermore, cytokines and interferon enhance class II antigen expression on cells such as epithelial cells, thus leading to further increased presentation of autoantigens or luminal antigens that could lead to molecular mimicry events. T-cell regulation of B cells through cytokines may lead to the generation of IgG autoantibodies, which, in turn, through activation of complement, may lead to the production of chemotactic factors and an increasing influx of a variety of cell types including macrophages, granulocytes, eosinophils, and others.

A great deal of information has also come from the treatment of autoimmune diseases in humans with cyclosporin A. Because cyclosporin A interferes with interleukin-2 synthesis and also blocks interleukin-2 receptor function, the effectiveness of cyclosporin A may primarily involve T-cell-mediated components of autoimmune disorders. The fact that cyclosporin A has been used with encouraging results in a number of different autoimmune disorders outside the gastrointestinal tract (uveitis, rheumatoid arthritis, and psoriasis) has provided further evidence for the importance of T cells in autoimmune disorders and has also led to its experimental use in certain gastrointestinal inflammatory disorders such as Crohn's disease.

Because the gastrointestinal tract contains a large number of antigens, including dietary proteins, which could lead to cross-reactivity and activation of self-reactive T cells, an important function of the gastrointestinal immune system is the generation of a state of tolerance to mucosal antigens. The gastrointestinal tract exhibits a fascinating example of a specific tolerance to orally ingested antigens, termed *oral tolerance*.[110] The administration of haptens orally can lead to hapten-specific unresponsiveness that results in the lack of both specific T-cell and B-cell responsiveness to those antigens. The ability of antigens in the gastrointestinal tract to induce a state of functional anergy is precise. The state of unresponsiveness or anergy holds only for the specific antigen that was presented orally to the gastrointestinal tract and is dependent upon the nature of the antigen. This allows the gastrointestinal tract to be exposed to and stimulated by diverse agents

and yet mount appropriate specific immune responses to defined infectious organisms, while rendering the host unresponsive to subsequent challenge by other antigens. It is not surprising that mechanisms to protect against the mounting of adverse immunologic reactions are present within the gastrointestinal tract. If this were not the case, numerous bacterial and viral antigens and food components could lead to frequent cross-reactive immunologic stimulatory events and result in intestinal autoimmune disorders. Likewise, many food substances might give rise to diverse and uncontrollable food-induced allergic reactions.

In experimental model systems, the induction of oral tolerance depends upon the type of antigen, the amount of antigen, the frequency of antigen sensitization, the type of animal being studied, and the particular immune response being evaluated.[110] The successful induction of oral tolerance may help prevent the initiation of autoimmune diseases. Interestingly, mice prone to the development of autoimmune disease exhibit defects in the induction of oral tolerance. There are, therefore, complex regulatory processes at work in the mucosal immune system which allow the development of a local protective mucosal immune response against pathogenic organisms, while at the same time preventing the development of adverse systemic autoimmune reactions to the same antigens.

An excellent example of a disease process that exhibits the adverse effects of altered immune function in the gastrointestinal system is gluten-sensitive enteropathy. In gluten-sensitive enteropathy the inflammatory infiltrate is primarily lymphocytic with B cells and IgA-containing plasma cells predominating in the lamina propria, combined with a particularly striking increase in the number of intraepithelial lymphocytes. Interestingly, increased numbers of intraepithelial lymphocytes appear within hours of gluten ingestion and thus represent an early event in the immunopathogenesis of gluten-sensitive enteropathy. Elevation in total serum IgA levels, circulating immune complexes, and an increased amount of autoantibodies, including antinuclear antibodies, antithyroid antibodies, and antiparietal cell antibodies in 20% to 30% of patients, has provided nonspecific evidence of possible ongoing autoimmune processes. Although IgA and IgG antigliadin antibodies have been noted in over 90% of gluten-sensitive enteropathy patients, the highest titers of the antibodies appear to be most strongly correlated with the extent and severity of intestinal damage and thus the levels may be secondary rather than primary in nature.[111,112]

Gluten-sensitive enteropathy is not a classic autoimmune disease, in that a dietary antigen found in cereal grains (gluten) causes the disease process, rather than a "self" antigen. The active component in gluten is gliadin, which is found in wheat, barley, rye, and oats. Thus, a well-defined foreign antigen, rather than resulting in tolerance, initiates ongoing host-destructive immune events that lead to villous flattening and hypertrophy of the intestinal crypts, associated with an intense inflammatory infiltrate.

Gluten-sensitive enteropathy occurs with increased frequency in first-degree relatives who have a 10% prevalence rate of latent, asymptomatic, biopsy-proven disease. Particular attention has focused on the strong association with certain histocompatibility antigens.[113-117] Seventy to 85 percent of patients with gluten-sensitive enteropathy bear HLA-B8[113] and HLA-DR3,[114,115] as opposed to 20% to 25% of the general population. An even stronger association has been shown with HLA-DQw2,[116] which occurs in over 90% of celiac sprue patients. It is possible that a specific gluten-sensitive enteropathy gene is in linkage disequilibrium with these markers and remains to be identified.[115-117] The strong association of gluten-sensitive enteropathy with defined histocompatibility antigens indicates that gluten-sensitive enteropathy is a human immunopathologic example of the genetic control of the immune response. The recently described ability of HLA class II antigens on intestinal epithelial cells to participate in antigen presentation raises the possibility that gliadin, in conjunction with defined epithelial cell surface histocompatibility antigens, may serve to initiate destructive recognition and cell-mediated effector mechanisms in gluten-sensitive enteropathy.[118] Thus, a genetically predetermined ability to present luminal antigens by epithelial cells may lead to a destructive immune response directed against the intestinal epithelium.

Nevertheless, the question still remains as to whether there are factors that initiate an immunologic cross-reactivity that allows gliadin to initiate pathogenic processes. One suggestion was that adenovirus 12 infection provides the initial sensitization process due to the homology of 8 of 12 amino acids residues, including an identical pentapeptide, between the adenovirus 12 Elb protein, and A-gliadin.[119] Adenovirus 12 is isolated from the human intestinal tract, and the Elb protein is expressed early in the infectious process providing the possibility that immunologic cross-reactivity could be initiated in hosts with a genetic predisposition.[119,120] However, the studies that to date have examined the potential role of adenovirus 12 sensitization and molecular mimicry in the induction of gluten-sensitive enteropathy are contradictory and this issue needs to be examined further.[121,122] Therefore, the question remains unresolved as to how patients with gluten-sensitive enteropathy initiate the immunologic recognition events that lead to their disease process. In this regard recent studies have focused on the intraepithelial lymphocyte.

Intraepithelial lymphocytes[54-56] are markedly increased in patients with gluten-sensitive enteropathy. Gluten challenge leads to a dose-dependent increase in intraepithelial lymphocytes in gluten-sensitive enteropathy patients. In recent studies, the percentage of intraepithelial lymphocytes expressing γ/δ T cell receptors was found to be disproportionately increased in untreated gluten-sensitive enteropathy, whereas disease specificity controls, including those with villous atrophy and tropical sprue, did not demonstrate this change.[123,124] Therefore, the increased numbers of a unique subclass of intraepithelial lymphocytes bearing a distinct form (γ/δ) of the T cell receptor[58-60] may provide important clues regarding the cell-mediated events that link a specific sensitizing antigen and cell surface HLA molecules on antigen-presenting epithelial cells. Gluten-sensitive enteropathy is an important human model of the genetic control of the immune response because the antigen (gliadin) is known, the target cell (intestinal epithelial cells) is known, and a unique subclass of T cells with marked cytotoxic potential (intraepithelial lymphocytes) is increased in the intestinal lesions.

ROLE OF MUCOSAL IMMUNE SYSTEM IN THE IMMUNE RESPONSE TO GASTROINTESTINAL VIRUSES

The development of a local antibody response to viruses in the gastrointestinal tract centers around secretory IgA. The most ef-

fective means of inducing a secretory IgA antibody response in the gastrointestinal tract is by exposure to either naturally occurring viruses or viral vaccines. A principal role of secretory IgA is to serve as a first line of defense against viral agents. In order to neutralize a virus in the gastrointestinal tract, antigen-specific secretory IgA molecules interfere with viral replication in the lumen, prevent mucosal penetration, and stop dissemination throughout the gastrointestinal epithelium. However, after viral infection becomes established, recovery is more complex and requires second-line defense mechanisms, including macrophages and IgG antibodies.

One of the clearest demonstrations of the importance of local immunization and the role of the secretory IgA system in protection against viral infections is provided by the study of poliovirus after immunization either parenterally with inactivated virus or orally with live attenuated virus.[125-127] Equivalent serum antibody responses are seen with the two routes of immunization. The initial antibody response is IgM, followed by IgG and finally by IgA. However, immunization by the oral route, but not by the parenteral route, produces significant levels of secretory IgA in gastrointestinal tract fluids.[125-127] The ability of the host to resist challenge with live virus correlates with secretory IgA levels in mucosal secretions. It is important to note that oral immunization produces significant titers of secretory IgA in both nasopharyngeal and gastrointestinal secretions. The development of significant titers of secretory IgA in nasopharyngeal secretions provides initial protection at the portal of entry and subsequent resistance to viral infection. This illustrates in a practical fashion the importance of the homing of cells stimulated by intestinal antigens to mucosal sites such as the nasopharynx. Therefore, the concept of a common mucosal immune system and diffuse production of antigen-specific antibodies at secretory mucosal surfaces in response to antigen in the gastrointestinal tract is elegantly demonstrated by the experiments with live attenuated polio vaccine.

Another aspect of mucosal immunology that is illustrated by immunization with poliovirus is that of increased stimulation of the immune system at the site of viral replication. When live attenuated poliovirus was instilled into the distal colons of patients with double-barreled colostomies and who thus had their colon separated physically from the remainder of the gastrointestinal tract, the highest titers of secretory IgA antibody were present in the immunized distal colon with lower titers of antibody in the rest of the gastrointestinal tract and no antibody in the nasopharynx.[125-127] Following tonsillectomy, antipolio antibodies in nasopharyngeal secretions diminish markedly. Therefore, regional lymphoid tissues play a major role in the amount of antibody produced, and the site of immunization determines the area in which the most marked immune response is seen.

Oral polio vaccination also illustrates the importance of a local secretory IgA immune response for the prevention of the carrier state. Parenteral vaccination with inactivated polio virus results in serum but not secretory antibodies. Although the parenterally immunized patient is adequately protected against the development of systemic infection, the live virulent polio virus can nevertheless persist in the intestinal tract and the patient can become a carrier of the virulent polio virus due to the absence of mucosally protective secretory IgA molecules.[125-127] In contrast, with oral vaccination using attenuated, avirulent polio virus, both serum and secretory antibodies are formed. The secretory IgA antibodies in the nasopharynx and intestinal tract, prevent the initial replication of the virulent polio virus and establish immunity by interfering with colonization. Thus with oral immunization, protective immunity prevents the patient from becoming a carrier for the virulent virus.[125-127]

Rotavirus infection demonstrates the importance of host factors in determining viral pathogenicity.[128,129] Both human and animal rotaviruses produce disease in children or young animals. Human rotaviruses produce diarrhea in infants primarily under 1 to 2 years of age and murine rotavirus produces disease in mice under 3 weeks of age. The reason for this age-related viral pathogenicity is that sufficient numbers of intestinal epithelial cells with specific binding sites for rotavirus must be available for the rotavirus to be able to replicate and cause clinical disease.[128,129] Because the number of specific binding sites on enterocytes declines significantly with increasing age, the replication of rotaviruses in the intestinal mucosa preferentially occurs in young children and young animals. After epithelial cells in the gastrointestinal tract become infected with rotavirus, the development of both specific antibodies and a specific cell-mediated immune response is necessary for effective elimination of the rotavirus-infected epithelial cells. The viral-specific antibody activity associated with destruction of virus-infected enterocytes is primarily IgG in nature. A single infection with rotavirus of a given strain produces protection against subsequent challenge with the same rotavirus strain. Locally produced IgG as well as IgA antibodies are involved in both clearance of the original virus and protection against subsequent viral challenges.

Reovirus infection has provided the opportunity to study in detail the mechanisms by which intestinal viruses enter the mucosa and spread to distant tissues.[130,131] Type I reovirus enters the host by way of a selective adherence to and penetration of membranous epithelial M (microfold) cells which are specialized epithelial cells that overlie Peyer's patches.[130] M cells transport a variety of antigens including viruses from the bowel lumen for subsequent processing and presentation by underlying macrophages and mononuclear cells.[18-21] Reovirus can then spread from Peyer's patches to the mesenteric lymph nodes and the spleen. M cells and Peyer's patches can therefore serve as a portal of entry for injurious viral pathogens including enteroviruses and reovirus.[130,131] Furthermore, bacteria such as salmonella have been found to be localized to Peyer's patches after presentation by way of the intestinal lumen. Thus viruses and also bacteria adhere to and are transported through the cytoplasm of M cells and endocytic vesicles to underlying Peyer's patches and may thus use normal cells of the immune system to gain access to and infect the host. The presence of an ongoing secretory IgA mucosal immune response can prevent adherence to and penetration of M cells by infectious agents. Vaccine strategies that interfere with the access of bacteria and viruses to M cells may be important in the future.

ROLE OF MUCOSAL IMMUNE SYSTEM IN THE IMMUNE RESPONSE TO GASTROINTESTINAL BACTERIAL PATHOGENS

Bacteria have several mechanisms by which they can circumvent and survive normal host defense mechanisms and carry out their pathogenic capabilities.[132] Adherence to the surface of intestinal epithelial cells determines the ability of bacteria to subsequently colonize and grow along the surface of the intestine and to then damage or destroy intestinal cells.[133] The ability of bacteria to penetrate and invade the mucosa as well as to release destructive cytotoxic molecules is particularly important for invasive organisms involved in colonic infectious processes.[133] On the other hand, bacteria in the small intestine commonly induce disease by the elaboration of enterotoxins that produce diarrhea without causing major destruction to the mucosa.

Although immunologic factors are critically important for normal host defense mechanisms against bacterial illnesses, a number of nonimmunologic defense mechanisms are present in the intestine and, if effective, either obviate the need for immunologic defense mechanisms or decrease the numbers of potentially pathogenic organisms to a small number so that immunologic defense mechanisms can lead to complete elimination of the potentially injurious bacteria. Acid in the stomach readily kills ingested organisms, and therefore achlorhydric patients are more prone to bacterial infections than patients with normal gastric acidity. Whereas many bacteria commonly survive in the stomach for longer periods of time, in achlorhydric patients mycobacteria are among the organisms most often associated with the loss of gastric acid. Similarly, other physiologic processes provide important host defense mechanisms. Normal gastrointestinal motility increases the movement of bacteria along the gastrointestinal tract. Thus, patients who have abnormal motility resulting in stasis, can develop small bowel bacterial overgrowth with resultant mucosal destruction. Mucus glycoproteins represent an important protective barrier by nonspecifically binding enterotoxins, by preventing interactions of infectious agents with enterocyte receptors, and by interfering with the attachment and proliferation of bacteria along the mucosal surface. Indeed the combination of gastric acidity, normal motility, and mucus production in large part accounts for the large numbers (up to 100 million) of potentially pathogenic bacteria required to successfully infect the normal volunteer subject by oral challenge.

Adherence to the epithelium provides bacteria with the ability to colonize and then multiply in the gastrointestinal tract.[133,134] Organisms adherent to epithelial cells directly damage underlying cells as well as decrease the effective surface area of the intestine. Invasive bacteria initially adhere to epithelial cells and then actively invade epithelial cells through a combination of endocytosis by the mast cell and penetration by the bacteria using flagellae, intracellular multiplication, toxin production, and lytic factors.[133,134] The production of toxins by bacteria leads to pathogenic effects through a variety of mechanisms, including massive activation of intestinal secretion, inhibition of protein synthesis by cytotoxic molecules and the induction of inflammation by chemotactic factors. Thus, the mucosal immune system must be able to protect against a number of different bacterial pathogenic mechanisms.

Secretory IgA antibodies inhibit the adherence of bacteria to epithelial cells, and thereby interfere with both colonization and multiplication.[133-136] Antibodies directed against adhesins present on pilli provide a mechanism to specifically protect against pathogenic organisms normally targeted to M cells and the follicle-associated epithelial tissue overlying Peyer's patches.[135,136] Because adhesins and attachment factors on isolated pilli are capable of inducing both primary and secondary immune responses, they are appropriate candidates for use as mucosal immunogens.

The immune response to invasive organisms is directed against bacterial cell wall lipopolysaccharides and plasmid-encoded polypeptides that function as virulence factors. Coating of invasive bacteria with antibodies directed against surface lipopolysaccharides enhances phagocytosis of the bacteria by granulocytes and macrophages, a major component of the cellular inflammatory response to these bacteria. Antibodies directed against virulence factors such as cytotoxins found within invasive organisms may interfere with mechanisms that would otherwise enhance the intracellular proliferation of invasive bacteria and also neutralize the toxic factors that they produce.

Bacteria that produce enterotoxins resulting in watery diarrhea are capable of activating a host-protective immune response directed against both the enterotoxins and the bacteria. Cholera vaccine induces secretory IgA antibodies that recognize the B subunit portion of cholera toxin as well as whole *Vibrios*.[137,138] The production of these antibodies provides evidence for a successful local mucosal immune response. Cholera toxin itself is an excellent mucosal immunogen and triggers both an intestinal secretory IgA response as well as a systemic IgG response.[137,138] Furthermore, cholera toxin is a very potent adjuvant for mucosal antigens and its combination with killed whole cell *Vibrios* results in long-term protective immunity in mucosally immunized vaccine recipients. Increased understanding of the normal mucosal immune response to bacteria as well as elucidation of mechanisms to induce protective immunity through the use of appropriately designed candidate vaccines is providing exciting advances in our ability to prevent infectious enteritis.

IMMUNE DEFICIENCY AND THE GASTROINTESTINAL TRACT

The role of the intact mucosal immune system is made particularly apparent by the study of immunodeficient patients, in whom the failure to produce an adequate immune response leads to a markedly increased susceptibility to infection.[139,140] Common variable immunodeficiency can result from defects that occur in any part of the B cell maturation pathway, as well as in regulatory cells involved in maintenance of a normal immune response. Patients may have macrophage antigen-processing defects, ineffective interactions between macrophages and T cells, decreased T cell help or cytokine deficiency, failure of the B cell to secrete antibody, immaturity of B cells, or failure of isotype switching as reasons for the development of common variable immunodeficiency.

Viral infections are not particularly increased in patients with decreased B cell activity.[139,140] Thus, an adequate cell-mediated immune system will protect against viral infections in a patient with decreased humoral immune responses. Pernicious anemia with achlorhydria is very common in immunoglobulin-deficient patients.[141,142] Colonization of the stomach with *Campylobacter pyloris* (Helicobacter) may cause pernicious anemia and achlorhydria in these patients. Nodular lymphoid hyperplasia with multiple small mucosal nodules containing lymphoid aggregates may occur in the stomach, rectum, or small intestine, or diffusely throughout the gastrointestinal tract in patients with immunodeficiency.[140,143] These nodules appear to be part of a compensatory, proliferative response by B cells to increase the number of plasma cells. The most common infection in common variable immunodeficiency is giardiasis, which often leads to chronic diarrhea and malabsorption due to invasion of the mucosa by the *Giardia* that directly damage

epithelial cells. Both gluten-sensitive enteropathy and inflammatory bowel disease can occur in patients with common variable immunodeficiency, thus demonstrating the importance of T cells and cell-mediated immune mechanisms in these disorders.

Selective IgA deficiency is the most common form of immunodeficiency and occurs in 1 to 2 of 1000 persons of European ancestry.[144,145] In IgA-deficient patients, there is an increased incidence of giardiasis, as well as gluten-sensitive enteropathy, inflammatory bowel disease, primary biliary cirrhosis, and other potentially autoimmune disorders.[144-148] Nevertheless, the mucosal immune system in general protects persons with IgA deficiency very well against the wide range of potential pathogens to which the intestine is exposed. The main reason for this is that IgM is substituted for IgA in the intestinal secretions of IgA-deficient patients.[149] IgM with J chain is efficiently transported across epithelial cells into the lumen, and specific IgM antibodies against different viral and bacterial pathogens have been documented in the saliva of persons who are IgA deficient. Thus, the mucosal immune system's protective mechanisms have sufficient backup systems so that the absence of only one line of defense does not significantly endanger the host.[150]

Acquired immunodeficiency syndrome (AIDS) patients develop infections due to a much wider array of agents. Infectious agents attack the gastrointestinal tract of a host who has impaired function of multiple arms of the immune system. In AIDS patients, *Candida albicans* can lead to esophagitis and dysphagia.[151] Protozoa such as *Cryptosporidium*[152,153] cause a severe chronic diarrheal illness associated with vomiting, malabsorption syndrome, and weight loss in AIDS patients. Parasites such as *Isospora belli*,[154] *Entamoeba histolytica*, and *Giardia* often present with diarrhea. *Mycobacterium avium intracellulare* causes systemic infection. Patients infected with this agent can present with severe ulceration of the stomach or involvement of the terminal ileum similar to that seen in Crohn's disease. Viral illnesses of the gastrointestinal tract are common in AIDS patients and include *Cytomegalovirus*, which can cause esophagitis, hepatitis, or a patchy diffuse ulceration similar to ulcerative colitis.[155,156] Herpes simplex virus can involve the esophagus, but more often involves the rectum with a severe proctitis. Herpes simplex may spread to the autonomic nerves and can lead to further symptoms outside the gastrointestinal tract. AIDS patients also develop bacterial infections including *Shigella*, *Salmonella*, and *Campylobacter*, all of which can lead to enteritis or colitis, and are particularly dangerous in the AIDS patient because of the possibility of systemic bacteremia.

CONCLUSION

Within the gastrointestinal tract, many different cell types contribute to the development of a successful mucosal immune response. M (microfold) cells within the follicle associated epithelium, overlie Peyer's patches and allow the attachment of specific viruses, bacteria, and antigens and their transport into contact with the underlying cells of the mucosal immune system. Immature cells within Peyer's patches (lymphoid follicles) are stimulated to recognize specific antigens, but rather than migrating directly to adjacent lamina propria, these cells migrate out of the gastrointestinal tract. Maturation and activation occur while the cells are traversing through the lymphatic system. After subsequent circulation of stimulated lymphoblasts in the peripheral blood, mature activated T cells and B cells "home" back to the intestine as specific effector cells.

The intraepithelial lymphocyte represents a unique subset of T cells that reside between intestinal epithelial cells and carry out specific cell-mediated cytotoxic effector functions. In addition to producing specific cytokines that regulate cell function, lamina propria and intraepithelial T cells also secrete nonspecific inflammatory mediators such as interferon-γ, which enhance antigen-presenting capabilities through the increased expression of class II MHC on epithelial cells and other cell types.

The intestine is fully capable of mounting an intense, protective inflammatory reaction in response to infectious agents or injurious substances. Antigen presentation by intestinal epithelial cells triggers the production of cytokines and subsequent inflammatory events. Antibodies leading to complement pathway activation, produce chemotactic factors and activate macrophages and granulocytes to produce inflammatory and cytotoxic molecules. Eosinophils and mast cells are important constituents in the intestine, particularly in the immune response to parasites. The final manifestations of intestinal inflammation are due in large part to the production of a wide variety of inflammatory mediators such as prostaglandins, leukotrienes, and platelet-activating factor.

The mucosal immune system must be able to separate self (autologous) components from foreign antigens. In the absence of appropriate self-recognition mechanisms, there may be formation of autoantibodies to intestinal components. Likewise, inappropriate T cell recognition of self components may lead to cell-mediated cytotoxic processes directed against specific intestinal target antigens. In order to prevent adverse immune reactions against dietary antigens or self components, oral tolerance is an important protective mechanism. The breakdown of tolerance after triggering by a viral or bacterial infection or other luminal antigens, may lead to autoimmune intestinal diseases. Specific antigen-recognition events in the intestine allow a protective immune response directed at eliminating potentially dangerous or noxious agents. Both nonimmune and immunologic mechanisms are involved in protecting against bacterial and viral infections of the intestine. Candidate oral vaccines must take into consideration the basic principles of the immune system's defense mechanisms. Immunodeficiency states demonstrate the importance of different arms of the mucosal immune system in the prevention of intestinal tract infections.

The reader is directed to Chapter 77, Inflammatory Bowel Disease; Chapter 103, Gastrointestinal Complications of the Acquired Immunodeficiency Syndrome; Chapter 107, Gastrointestinal Manifestations of Immunologic Disorders.

REFERENCES

1. Brandtzaeg P, Sollid L, Thrane P, et al. Lymphoepithelial interactions in the mucosal immune system. Gut 1988;29:1116.
2. Tomasi TB, Tan EM, Solomon A, et al. Characteristics of an immune system common to certain external secretions. J Exp Med 1965;121:101.
3. Mestecky J, McGhee JR. Immunoglobulin A (IgA): Molecular and cellular interactions involved in IgA biosynthesis and immune response. Adv Immunol 1987;40:153.
4. Hanson LA, Ahlstedt S, Anderson B, et al. The biologic properties of secretory IgA. J Reticuloendothel Soc 1980;28(suppl):1.
5. Underdown BJ, Schiff JM. Immunoglobulin A: Strategic defense initiative at the mucosal surface. Ann Rev Immunol 1986;4:389.
6. MacDermott RP, Stenson WF. Alterations of the immune system in ulcerative colitis and Crohn's disease. Adv Immunol 1988;42:285.
7. MacDermott RP, Stenson WF. The role of the immune system in inflammatory bowel disease. Immunol Allergy Clin North Am 1988;8:521.
8. Unanue ER, Allen PM. The basis for the immunoregulatory role of macrophages and other accessory cells. Science 1987;236:551.
9. Bland PW, Warren LG. Antigen presentation by epithelial cells of the rat small intestine. I. Kinetics, antigen specificity and blocking by antila antisera. Immunology 1986;58:1.
10. Bland PW, Warren LG. Antigen presentation by epithelial cells of the rat small intestine. II. Selective induction of suppressor T cells. Immunology 1986;58:9.
11. Dinarello CA, Mier JW. Lymphokines. N Engl J Med 1987;317:940.
12. Dinarello CA: Biology of interleukin-1. Fed Am Soc Exper Biol 1988;2:108.
13. Kawanishi H, Saltzman LE, Strober W. Mechanisms regulating IgA class-specific immunoglobulin production in murine gut-associated lymphoid tissues. I. T cells derived from Peyer's patches that switch IgM B cells to IgA B cells in vitro. J Exp Med 1983;157:433.
14. Kawanishi H, Saltzman L, Strober W. Mechanisms regulating IgA class-specific immunoglobulin production in murine gut-associated lymphoid tissues. II. Terminal differentiation of postswitch sIgA-bearing Peyer's Patch B cells. J Exp Med 1983;158:649.
15. Coffman RL, Shrader B, Carty J, et al. A mouse T cell product that preferentially enhances IgA production. I. Biologic characterization. J Immunol 1987;139:3685.
16. Smith KA. The interleukin 2 receptor. Adv Immunol 1988;42:165.
17. Miyajima A, et al. Coordinate regulation of immune and inflammatory responses by T cell-derived lymphokines. Fed Am Soc Exper Biol 1988;2:2462.
18. Owen RL, Jones AL. Epithelial cell specialization within human Peyer's patches: An ultrastructural study of intestinal lymphoid follicles. Gastroenterology 1974;66:189.
19. Wolf JL, Rubin DH, Finberg R, et al. Intestinal M cells: a pathway for entry of reovirus into the host. Science 1981;212:471.
20. Owen RL, Nemanic P. Antigen processing structures of the mammalian intestinal tract: An SEM study of lymphoepithelial organs. In: Becker RP, et al. Scanning electron microscopy, vol II. O'Hare, IL: Scanning Electron Microscopy, Inc, 1978:367–378.
21. Bockman DE, Cooper MD. Pinocytosis by epithelium associated with lymphoid follicles in the bursa of fabricius, appendix, and Peyer's patches. An electron microscopic study. Am J Anat 1973;136:455.
22. Bienenstock J, McDermott M, Befus D, et al. A common mucosal immunologic system involving the bronchus, breast and bowel. Adv Exp Med Biol 1978;107:53.
23. Dunkley ML, Husband AJ. Distribution and functional characteristics of antigen-specific helper T cells arising after Peyer's patch immunization. Immunology 1987;61:475.
24. Cebra JJ, Komisar JL, Schweitzer PA. C_H isotype "switching" during normal B-lymphocyte development. Ann Rev Immunol 1984;2:493.
25. Mestecky J. The common mucosal immune system and current strategies for induction of immune responses in external secretions. J Clin Immunol 1987;7:265.
26. Jalkanen S. Reichert RA, Gallatin WM, et al. Homing receptors and the control of lymphocyte migration. Immunol Rev 1986;91:39.
27. Jalkanen S. Streeter P, Lakey E, et al. Lymphocyte and endothelial cell recognition elements that control lymphocyte traffic to mucosa-associated lymphatic tissues. Monogr Allergy 1988;24:144.
28. Streeter PR, Berg EL, et al. A tissue-specific endothelial cell molecule involved in lymphocyte homing, Nature 1988;331:441.
29. Hamann A, Jablonski-Westrich D, Scholz KU, Duijvestijn A, Butcher EC, Thiele HG. Regulation of lymphocytes homing I. Alterations in homing receptor expression and organ-specific high endothelial venule binding of lymphocytes upon activation. J Immunol 1988;140:737:43.

30. Bull DM, Bienenstock J, Tomasi TB, Jr. Studies on human intestinal immunoglobulin A. Gastroenterology 1971;60:370.

31. Conley ME, Bartelt MS. *In vitro* regulation of IgA subclass synthesis. II. The source of IgA2 plasma cells. J Immunol 1984;133:2312.

32. Brandtzaeg P. Role of J chain and secretory component in receptor-mediated glandular and hepatic transport of immunoglobulins in man. Scand J Immunol 1985;22;111.

33. Conley ME, Delacroix DL. Intravascular and mucosal immunoglobulin A: Two separate but related systems of immune defense? Ann Intern Med 1987;106:892.

34. Gilbert JV, Plaut AG, Longmaid B. Inhibition of bacterial IgA proteases by human secretory IgA and serum. Ann NY Acad Sci 1983;409:625.

35. Brandtzaeg P, Prydz H. Direct evidence for an integrated function of J chain and secretory component in epithelial transport of immunoglobulins. Nature 1984;311:71.

36. Brandtzaeg P, Korsrud FR. Significance of different J chain profiles in human tissues: Generation of IgA and IgM with binding site for secretory component is related to the J chain expressing capacity of the total local immunocyte population, including IgG and IgD producing cells, and depends on the clinical state of the tissue. Clin Exp Immunol 1984;58:709

37. Mostov KE, Kraehenbuhl JP, Blobel G. Receptor-mediated transcellular transport of immunoglobulin: Synthesis of secretory component as multiple and larger transmembrane forms. Proc Natl Acad Sci USA 1 980;77:7257.

38. Mostov KE, Blobel G. A Transmembrane precursor of secretory component. The receptor for transcellular transport of polymeric immunoglobulins. J Biol Chem 1982;257:11816.

39. Mostov KE, Friedlander M, Blobel G. The receptor for transepithelial transport of IgA and IgM contains multiple immunoglobulin-like domains. Nature 1984;308:37.

40. Solari R, Kraehenbuhl JP. Biosynthesis of the IgA antibody receptor: A model for the transepithelial sorting of a membrane glycoprotein. Cell 1984;36:61.

41. Solari R, Kraehenbuhl JP. The biosynthesis of secretory component and its role in the transepithelial transport of IgA dimer. Immunol Today 1985;6:17.

42. Ahnen DJ, Brown WR, Kloppel TM. Secretory component: The polymeric immunoglobulin receptor. Gastroenterology 1985;89:667.

43. Mostov KE, Deitcher DL. Polymeric immunoglobulin receptor expressed in MDCK cells transcytoses IgA. Cell 1986;46:613.

44. Mostov KE, de Bruyn Kops A, Deitcher DL. Deletion of the cytoplasmic domain of the polymeric immunoglobulin receptor prevents basolateral localization and endocytosis. Cell 1986;47:359.

45. Delacroix DL, Hodgson HJF, McPherson A, et al. Selective transport of polymeric immunoglobulin A in bile. Quantitative relationships of monomeric and polymeric immunoglobulin A, immunoglobulin M and other proteins in serum, bile, and saliva. J Clin Invest 1982;70:230.

46. Delacroix DL, et al. The liver in the IgA secretory immune system. Dogs, but not rats and rabbits, are suitable models for human studies. Hepatology 1983;3(6):980.

47. MacDermott RP, Franklin GO, Jenkins KM, et al. Human intestinal mononuclear cells. I. Investigation of antibody-dependent, lectin-induced, and spontaneous cell-mediated cytotoxic capabilities. Gastroenterology 1980;78:47.

48. MacDermott RP, et al. Human intestinal mononuclear cells. II. Demonstration of a naturally occurring subclass of T cells which respond in the allogeneic mixed leukocyte reaction but do not effect cell-mediated lympholysis. Gastroenterology 1981;80:748.

49. MacDermott RP, et al. Deficient cell-mediated cytotoxicity and hyporesponsiveness to interferon and mitogenic lectin activation by inflammatory bowel disease peripheral blood and intestinal mononuclear cells. Gastroenterology 1986;90:6.

50. Targan S, et al. Isolation of spontaneous and interferon inducible natural killer like cells from human colonic mucosa: Lysis of lymphoid and autologous epithelial target cells. Clin Exp Immunol 1983;54:14.

51. Fiocchi C et al. Human intestinal mucosal mononuclear cells exhibit lymphokine-activated killer cell activity. Gastroenterology 1985;88:625.

52. Hogan PG, Hapel AJ, Doe WF. Lymphokine-activated and natural killer cell activity in human intestinal mucosa. J Immunol 1985;135:1731.

53. Shanahan R, Deem R, Nayersina R, et al. Human mucosal T-cell cytotoxicity. Gastroenterology 1988;94:960.

54. Cerf-Bensussan N, Quaroni A, Kurnick JT, Bhan AK. Intraepithelial lymphocytes modulate Ia expression by intestinal epithelial cells. J Immunol 1984;132:2244.

55. Cerf-Bensussan N, Guy-Grand D, Griscelli C. Intraepithelial lymphocytes of human gut: isolation, characterisation and study of natural killer activity. Gut 1985;26:81.

56. Ernst PB, Befus AD, Bienenstock J. Leukocytes in the intestinal epithelium: An unusual immunological compartment. Immunol Today 1985;6:50.

57. Cerf-Bensussan N, Jarry A, Brousse N, et al. A monoclonal antibody (HML-1) defining a novel membrane molecule present on human intestinal lymphocytes. Eur J Immunol 1987;17:1279.

58. Bonneville M, Janeway CA, Ito K, et al. Intestinal intraepithelial lymphocytes are a distinct set of gamma-delta T cells. Nature 1988;336:479.

59. Goodman T, Lefrancois L. Expression of the gamma-delta T-cell receptor on intestinal CD8+ intraepithelial lymphocytes. Nature 1988;333:855.

60. Janeway CA Jr, Jones B, Hayday A. Specificity and function of T cells bearing gamma-delta receptors. Immunol Today 1988;9:73.

61. Scott H, Brandtzaeg P, Solheim BG, et al. Relation between HLA-DR-like antigens and secretory component (SC) in jejunal epithelium of patients with coeliac disease or dermatitis herpetiformis. Clin Exp Immunol 1981;44:233.

62. Hirata I, Berrebi G, Austin LL, et al. Immunohistological characterization of intraepithelial and lamina propria lymphocytes in control ileum and colon and in inflammatory bowel disease. Dig Dis Sci 1986;31:593.

63. Selby WS, Janossy G, Mason DY, et al. Expression of HLA-DR antigens by colonic epithelium in inflammatory bowel disease. Clin Exp Immunol 1983;53:614.

64. McDonald GB, Jewell DP. Class II antigen (HLA-DR) expression by intestinal epithelial cells in inflammatory diseases of colon. J Clin Pathol 1987;40:312.

65. Scott H, Sollid LM, Fausa O, et al. Expression of MHC class II subregion products by jejunal epithelium in patients with coeliac disease. Scan J Immunol 1987;26:563.

66. Fais S, Pallone F, Squarcia O, et al. HLA-DR antigens on colonic epithelial cells in inflammatory bowel disease: I. Relation to the state of activation of lamina propria lymphocytes and to the epithelial expression of other surface markers. Clin Exp Immunol 1987;68:605.

67. Arnaud-Battandier F, Cerf-Bensussan N, Amsellem R, et al. Increased HLA-DR expression by enterocytes in children with celiac disease. Gastroenterology 1986;91:1206.

68. Mayer L, Shlien R. Evidence for function of Ia molecules on gut epithelial cells in man. J Exp Med 1987;166:1471.

69. Mosmann TR, Cherwinski H, Bond MW, et al. Two types of murine helper T cell clones. I. Definition according to profiles of lymphokine activities and secreted proteins. J Immunol 1986;136:2348.

70. Cebra JJ, Griffin PM, Lebman DA, et al. Perturbations in Peyer's patch B cell populations indicative of priming for a secretory IgA response. Adv Exp Med Biol 1988;216A:3.

71. Craig SW, Cebra JJ. Peyer's patches: An enriched source of precursors for IgA-producing immunocytes in the rabbit. J Exp Med 1971;134:188.

72. Bond MW, Shrader B, Mosmann TR, et al. A mouse T cell product that preferentially enhances IgA production. II. Physicochemical characterization. J Immunol 1987;139:3691.

73. Murray PD, McKenzie DT, Swain SL, et al. Interleukin-5 and interleukin-4 produced by Peyer's patch T cells selectively enhance immunoglobulin A expression. J Immunol 1987;139:2669.

74. Lebman DA, Griffin PM, Cebra JJ. Relationship between expression of IgA by Peyer's patch cells and functional IgA memory cells. J Exp Med 1987;166:1405.

75. Lebman DA, Coffman RL. The effects of IL-4 and IL-5 on the IgA response by murine Peyer's patch B cell subpopulations. J Immunol 1988;141:2050.

76. Harriman GR, Kunimoto DY, Elliott JF, et al. The role of IL-5 in IgA B cell differentiation. J Immunol 1988;140:3033.

77. Beagley KW, Eldridge JH, Kiyono H, et al. Recombinant murine IL-5 induces high rate IgA synthesis in cycling IgA-positive Peyer's patch B Cells. J Immunol 1988;141:2035.

78. Befus AD, Dyck N, Goodacre R, et al. Mast cell from the human intestinal lamina propria. Isolation, histochemical subtypes, and functional characterization. J Immunol 1987;138:2604.

79. Galli SJ, et al. Basophils and mast cells: Morphologic insights into their biology, secretory patterns, and function. Prog. Allergy 1981;34:1.

80. Ruoslahti E. Structure and biology of proteoglycans. Ann Rev Cell Biol 1988;4:229.

81. Irani AA, Schechter NM, Craig SS, et al. Two types of human mast cells that have distinct neutral protease compositions. Proc Natl Acad Sci USA 1986;83:4464.

82. Lee TD, Swieter M, Bienenstock J, et al. Heterogeneity in mast cell populations. Clin Immunol Rev 1985;4(2):143.

83. Bienenstock J, Denburg J, Scicchitano R, Stead R, Perdue M, Stanisz A. Role of neuropeptides, nerves and mast cells in intestinal immunity and physiology. Monogr Allergy 1988;24:134.

84. Gleich GJ, Adolphson CR. The eosinophilic leukocyte: Structure and function. Adv Immunol 1986;39:177.

85. Gleich GJ. Current understanding of eosinophil function. Hosp Pract 1988;23:137.

86. Graham MF, Diegelmann RF, et al. Collagen content and types in the intestinal strictures of Crohn's disease. Gastroenterology 1988;94:257.

87. Sandborg R, and Smolen J. Early biochemical events in leukocyte activation. Lab Invest 1988;59:300.

88. Schiffman E, et al. N-Formylmethionyl peptides as chemoattractants for leucocytes. Proc Natl Acad Sci USA 1975;72:1059.

89. Nathan CF. Secretory products of macrophages. J Clin Invest 1987;79:319.

90. Weissman G, et al. Release of inflammatory mediators from stimulated neutrophils. N Engl J Med 1980;303:27.

91. Fantone JC, Ward PA. Role of oxygen-derived free radicals and metabolites in leukocyte-dependent inflammatory reactions. Am J Pathol 1982;107:397.

92. Harlan JM. Leukocyte-endothelial interactions. Blood 1985;65:513.

93. Smith CW, et al. Recognition of an endothelial determinant for CD18-dependent human neutrophil adherence and transendothelial migration. J Clin Invest 1988;82:1746.

94. Johnston RB Jr. Monocytes and macrophages. N Engl J Med 1988;318:747.

95. Parker CW. Lipid mediators produced through the lipoxygenase pathway. Ann Rev Immunol 1987;5:65.

96. Sharon P, Stenson WF. Enhanced synthesis of leukotriene B4 by colonic mucosa in inflammatory bowel disease. Gastroenterology 1984;86:453.

97. Sharon P, Stenson WF. Metabolism of arachidonic acid in acetic acid colitis in rats. Similarity to human inflammatory bowel disease. Gastroenterology 1985;88:55.

98. Lauritsen K, Laursen LS, Bukhave K, Rask-Madsen J. Effects of topical 5-aminosalicylic acid and prednisolone on prostaglandin E2 and leukotriene B4 levels determined by equilibrium in vivo dialysis of rectum in relapsing ulcerative colitis. Gastroenterology 1988;91:837.

99. Lauritsen K, Laursen LS, Bukhave K, Rask-Madsen J. In vivo profiles of eicosanoids in ulcerative colitis, Crohn's colitis, and *Clostridium difficile* colitis. Gastroenterology 1988;95:11.

100. Le J, Vilcek J. Tumor necrosis factor and interleukin 1: Cytokines with multiple overlapping biological activities. Lab Invest 1987;56:234.

101. Bevilacqua MP, et al. Identification of an inducible endothelial-leukocyte adhesion molecule. ELAM-1. Proc Natl Acad Sci USA 1987;84:9238.

102. Dustin ML, Springer TA. Lymphocytes function-associated antigen-1 (LFA-1) interactions with intercelluar adhesion molecule-1 (ICAM-1) is one of at least 3 mechanisms for lymphocyte adhesion to cultured endothelial cells. J Cell Biol 1988;107:321.

103. Becker EL. The formylpeptide receptor of the neutrophil. A search and conserve operation. Am J Pathol 1987;129:16.

104. Muller-Eberhard HJ. Molecular organization and function of the complement system. Ann Rev Biochem 1988;57:321.

105. Nash S, Stafford J, Madara JL. Effects of polymorphonuclear leukocyte transmigration on the barrier function of cultured intestinal epithelial monolayers. J Clin Invest 1987;80:1104.

106. Madara JL, Stafford J. Interferon-Y directly affects barrier function of cultured intestinal epithelial monolayers. J Clin Invest 1988;83:724.

107. Babior BM. The respiratory burst of leukocytes. J Clin Invest 1984;73:599.

108. Grisham MB, MacDermott RP, Deitch EA. Antioxidant enzyme activities in the human colon. Gastroenterology 1989;96:A185.

109. Saverymuttu SH, Camilleri M, et al. Indium 111-granulocyte scanning in the assessment of disease extent and disease activity in inflammatory bowel disease. Gastroenterology 1986;90:1121.

110. Kagnoff MF. Oral tolerance. Monogr Allergy 1988;24:222.

111. Reunala T, et al. IgA anti-endomysial antibodies in dermatitis herpetiformis: Corrolation with jejunal morphology, gluten-free diet and anti-gliadin antibodies. Br J Dermatol 1987;117:185.

112. Levenson SD, et al. Specificity of antigliadin antibody in celiac Disease. Gastroenterology 1985;89:1.

113. Falchuck ZM, et al. Predominance of histocompatibility antigen HLA-B8 in patients with gluten-sensitive enteropathy. J Clin Invest 1972;51:1602.

114. Mearin ML, et al. HLA-DR phenotypes in Spanish coeliac children: Their contribution to the understanding of the genetics of the disease. Gut 1983;24:532.

115. Tolsi R, et al. Evidence that celiac disease is primarily associated with a DC locus allelic specificity. Clin Immunol Immunopathol 1983;28:395.

116. Corazza GR, et al. DR and non-DR Ia allotypes are associated with susceptibility to coeliac disease. Gut 1985;26:1210.

117. Alper CA, et al. Extended major histocompatibility complex haplotypes in patients with gluten-sensitive enteropathy. J Clin Invest 1987;79:251.

118. Kagnoff MF, et al. Celiac sprue: Corrolation with murine T-cell responses to wheat gliadin components. J Immunol 1982;129:2693.

119. Kagnoff MF, Raleigh K, Austin RK, et al. Possible role for a human adenovirus in the pathogenesis of celiac disease. J Exp Med 1984;160:1544.

120. Karagiannis JA, Priddle JD, Jewell DP. Cell-mediated immunity to a synthetic gliadin peptide resembling a sequence from adenovirus 12. Lancet 1987;1(8538):884.

121. Kagnoff MF, Paterson YJ, Kumar PJ, et al. Evidence for the role of a human intestinal adenovirus in the pathogenesis of coeliac disease. Gut 1987;28:995.

122. Howdle PD, et al. Lack of a serologic response to an E1B protein of adenovirus 12 in coeliac disease. Scand J Immunol 1989;24:282..

123. Brandtzaeg P, Bosnes B, Halstensen TS, et al. T lymphocytes in human gut epithelium preferentially express the alpha/beta antigen receptor and are often CD45/UCHL1-positive. Scand J Immunol 1989;30:123.

124. Spencer J, Isaacson PG, Diss TC, MacDonald TT. Expression of disulfide-linked and non-disulfide linked forms of the T cell receptor gamma/delta heterodimer in human intraepithelial lymphocytes. Eur J Immunol 1989;19:1335.

125. Ogra P, et al. Immunoglobulin response in serum and secretions after immunization with live and inactivated poliovaccine and natural infection. N Engl J Med 1968;279:893.

126. Ogra PL, Karzon DT. Poliovirus antibody response in serum and nasal secretions following intranasal inoculation with inactivated poliovaccine. J Immunol 1969;102:15.

127. Wolf JL, Cukor G, et al. Susceptibility of mice to rotavirus infection: Effects of age and administration of corticosteroids. Infect Immun 1981;33:565.

128. Ogra PL, Volovitz B, et al. Mucosal viral infections: Mechanisms of immunity and disease. Monogr Allergy 1988;24:266.

129. Greenberg HB, Offit PA, Shaw RD. Neutralization of rotaviruses in vitro and in vivo: Molecular determinants of protection and role in local immunity. In: Strober E, et al, ed. Mucosal Immunity and Infections at Mucosal Surfaces, New York: Oxford University Press, 1988:319.

130. Wolf JL, Kauffman S, et al. Determinants of reovirus interaction

with the intestinal M cells and absorptive cells of murine intestine. Gastroenterology 1983;85:291.

131. Wolf JL, Dambrauskas A, Sharpe H, et al. Adherence to and penetration of the intestinal epithelium by Reovirus type 1 in neonatal mice. Gastroenterology 1987;92:82.

132. Levine MM, Kaper JB, et al. New knowledge on pathogenesis of bacterial enteric infections as applied to vaccine development. Microbiol Rev 1983;47:510.

133. Boedeker E. Enterocyte adherence of *Escherichia coli*: Its relation to diarrheal disease (editorial). Gastroenterolgy 1982;83:489.

134. Boedeker E, Cheney C. Pili as adherence factors in *Escherichia coli* strain RDEC-1. In: Boedeker EC, ed. Attachment of Organisms to the Gut Mucosa, vol 1, Boca Raton, FL: CRC Press, 1984:101.

135. Cantey JR. Prevention of bacterial infections of mucosal surfaces by immune secretory IgA. Adv Exp Med Biol 1978;107:461.

136. McQueen C, Younushonis W, et al. Immune response to a live, model oral vaccine against enteropathogenic *E. coli: E coli* HB101 (strain M5) expressing the AF/R1 pilus. Gastroenterology 1986;90:1547.

137. Svennerholm AM, Sack A, et al. Intestinal antibody responses after immunisation with cholera B subunit. Lancet 1982;1:305.

138. Svennerholm AM, Jertborn M, et al. Mucosal antitoxic and antibacterial immunity after cholera disease and after immunization with a combined B subunit—whole cell vaccine. J Infect Dis 1984;149:884.

139. Brown WR, et al. Clinical, microbiological and immunological studies in patients with immunoglobulin deficiencies and gastrointestinal disorders. Gut 1972;13:441.

140. Ament ME, et al. Structure and function of the gastrointestinal tract in primary immunodeficiency syndromes. A study of 39 patients. Medicine 1973;52:227.

141. Twomey JJ, Jordan PH, Jarrold T, et al. The syndrome of immunoglobulin deficiency and pernicious anemia. A study of ten cases. Am J Med 1970;47:340.

142. Twomey JJ, Jordan PH, Laughter AH, et al. The gastric disorder in immunoglobulin-deficient patients. Ann Intern Med 1970;72:499.

143. Ranchod M, et al. Lymphoid hyperplasia of the gastrointestinal tract. A study of 26 cases and review of the literature. Am J Surg Pathol 1978;2:383.

144. Ammann AJ, Hong R. Selective Iga deficiency: Presentation of 30 cases and a review of the literature. Medicine 1971;60:223.

145. Burks AW Jr, Steel RW. Selective IgA deficiency. Ann Allergy 1986;57:3.

146. Crabbe PA, Heremans JF. Lack of gamma A-immunoglobulin in serum of patients with steatorrhea. Gut 1966;7:119.

147. Crabbe PA, Heremans JF. Selective IgA deficiency with steatorrhea. A new syndrome. Am J Med 1967;42:319.

148. Zinneman HH, Kaplan AP. The association of giardiasis with reduced intestinal secretory immolglobulin A. Dig Dis Sci 1975;125:207.

149. McClelland DBL, Shearman JC, Van Furth R. Synthesis of immunoglobulin and secretory component by gastrointestinal mucosa in patients with hypogammaglobulinaemia or IgA deficiency. Clin Exp Immunol 1979;25:103.

150. Plebani A, Mira E, Mevio E, et al. IgM and IgD concentrations in the serum and secretions of children with selective IgA deficiency. Clin Exp Immunol 1983;53:689.

151. Tavitian A, Raufman JP, Rosenthal LE. Oral candidiasis as a marker for esophageal candidiasis in the acquired immunodeficiency syndrome. Ann Intern Med 1986;104:54.

152. Pitlik S, Fainstein V, Garza D, et al. Human cryptosporidiosis: Spectrum of disease. Report of six cases and review of the literature. Arch Intern Med 1983;143:2269.

153. Wolfson JS, Richter JM, Waldron MA, et al. Cryptosporidiosis in immunocompetent patients. N Engl J Med 1985;312:1278.

154. DeHovitz JA, Pape JW, Boncy M, et al. Clinical manifestations and therapy of *Isospora belli* infection in patients with the acquired immunodeficiency syndrome. N Engl J Med 1986;315:87.

155. Freedman PG, Weiner BC, Balthazar EJ. Cytomegalovirus Esophagogastritis in a patient with acquired immunodeficiency syndrome. Am J Gastroenterol 1985;80:434.

156. Meiselman MS, Cello JP, Margaretten W. Cytomegalovirus colitis—report of the clinical, endoscopic and pathologic findings in two patients with the acquired immune deficiency syndrome. Gastroenterology 1985;88:171.

6

Epithelia: Biologic Principles of Organization

JAMES L. MADARA

All cavities within the alimentary tract, from the small ducts and acini of the pancreas to the gastric lumen, are lined by sheets of epithelial cells. Because these spaces link and, in fact, are contiguous with the external environment, it is obvious that one primary function of these epithelial linings is to act as a barrier. In this chapter, the generic structural organization of the gut wall and the biology of gut epithelial barriers are considered. Some areas relating to epithelial transport are briefly treated to emphasize interrelationships among epithelial transport, barrier function, and structure. Detailed reviews of active transport processes across specific epithelia are found in Chapters 12 through 16.

GENERIC ORGANIZATION OF THE GUT WALL

Figure 6-1 schematically depicts the architectural relationship of the epithelial barrier with other components of the gut wall. Although the diagram represents a cross section of the intestine, this general structural pattern is preserved throughout the esophagus, stomach, and appendix. These organs consist of four layers: the mucosa, the submucosa, the muscularis propria, and either a serosa or adventitia (see Fig 6-1). The mucosa consists of the surface epithelium, an underlying layer of loose connective tissue carrying nerves and vessels (lamina propria), and a thin layer of smooth muscle (muscularis mucosa). The mucosa also contains an array of lymphocytes, mast cells, macrophages, and, in disease states, polymorphonuclear leukocytes, all of which may be capable of modulating epithelial function. As detailed in subsequent chapters on the anatomy of individual organs (see ch 53, 59, 66, 76, and 93), organ-specific specializations in mucosal structure exist.

The mucosa is supported by an underlying layer of fibroconnective tissue aptly called the submucosa. The submucosa contains nerves, vessels, and lymphatics, which course to the mucosa. The submucosa, in turn, rests on the muscularis propria, which is composed of two, and sometimes three, layers and is also home to the myenteric plexus (see ch 1 for details of gut neurons). In most instances, organs are encased by a delicate layer of fibrofatty tissue, which supports a continuous layer of mesothelial cells (serosa). Where no serosa exists, such as in the esophagus, fibrofatty tissues of surrounding structures intimately interlace with the external portion of the muscularis propria. Such organs are said to have an adventitial, rather than a serosal, encasement.

In general, grasp biopsies retrieved endoscopically go no deeper than the muscularis mucosa, although thin wisps of submucosal tissues may occasionally be seen. Suction biopsies more consistently penetrate into the submucosa, although, here too, only the most superficial portion of the submucosa is obtained. Deeper portions of the wall appear in endoscopic samples by accident, such as in

an aggressive snare of a sessile mucosal lesion. Becoming familiar with both the general organizational pattern of gut and the interorgan variations that exist is of great benefit to physicians examining biopsies originating from the alimentary tract. For example, the extraordinarily thick muscularis mucosa underlying the lamina propria of the esophagus is not infrequently mistaken for the muscularis propria, leading to unwarranted concern of a biopsy-induced perforation.

CONSTRUCTING EPITHELIA: HOW ISOLATED CELLS BECOME INTEGRATED INTO SHEETS

To function properly as a barrier, single epithelial cells must assemble into a multicellular sheet (Fig 6-2). Here we consider the requirements for such higher organization: cytoskeletal stabilization of single cells, cell–cell adhesion, formation of cell–cell junctions, and the provision of a foundation by the basement membrane.

The Cytoskeleton: Stabilization of Cell Shape for Long-Term Cell–Cell Interactions

Interorgan differences in the structural stabilization of gut epithelial cells by the cytoskeleton largely represent variations on a single theme. Thus, we consider the cytoskeleton in the context of the villus absorptive cell of the small intestine, a cell type that has become an important model for studies of cytoskeletal structure and function in nonmuscle cells.

Of primary importance in stabilizing epithelial cell structure is provision of support for the apex of the cell that interfaces with the turbulent environment of the gut lumen (Fig 6-3). Most al-

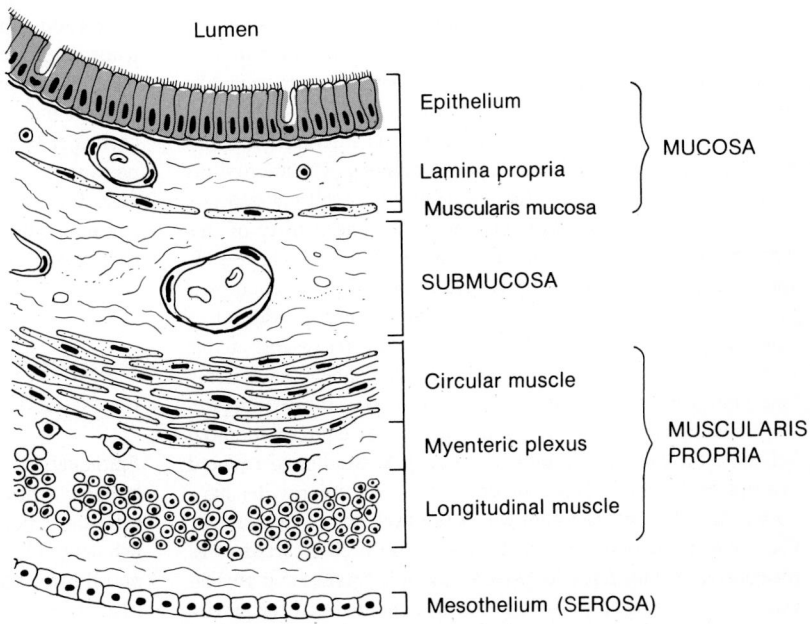

Lumen

Epithelium

Lamina propria

Muscularis mucosa

} MUCOSA

SUBMUCOSA

Circular muscle

Myenteric plexus

Longitudinal muscle

} MUSCULARIS PROPRIA

Mesothelium (SEROSA)

FIGURE 6–1. Generic organization of the gut wall.

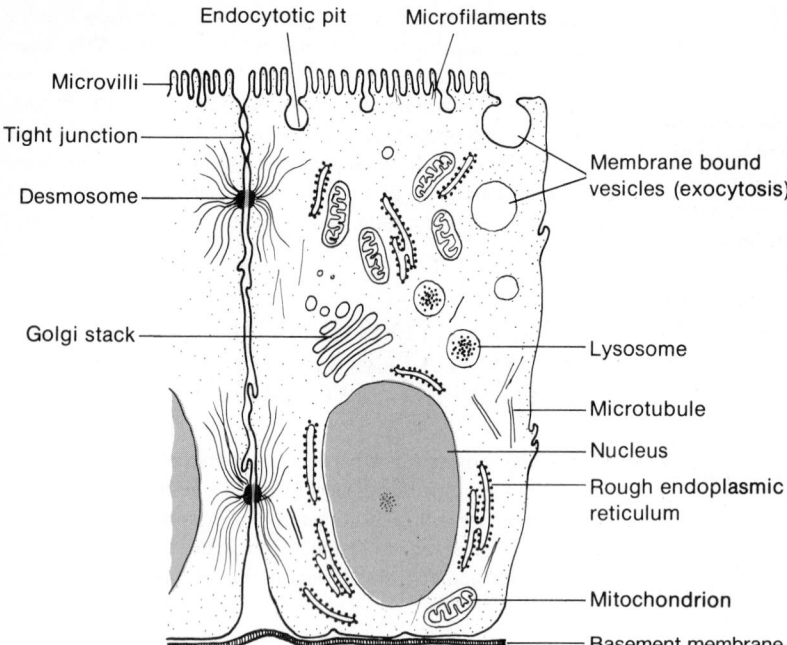

FIGURE 6–2. Generic organization of a gut epithelial cell.

imentary tract epithelia (esophageal squamous epithelia being the major exception) display microvillus projections on the apical surface. Microvilli may be short and less dense in cells undergoing substantial exocytosis of secretory vesicles (mucin-producing goblet and gastric foveolar cells) and in actively dividing cells, but microvilli are particularly well-formed in absorptive cells. A bundle of 20 to 30 microfilaments composed of F-actin resides in the core of such microvilli, and the bundle inserts into a dense cap of uncharacterized material at the extreme tip of microvilli.[1] Individual microfilaments are crosslinked to each other by fine filamentous structures (see Fig 6-3) consisting of filamin, a 68-kD actin-bundling protein, and villin, a 95-kd protein that can either bundle or sever F-actin microfilaments depending on intracellular Ca^{++} concentrations.[1] Additionally, the microfilament core is linked laterally to the plasma membrane of microvilli by a 110,000-dalton protein associated with a calcium-binding calmodulinlike protein. Because this protein possesses a myosin-like Mg^{++} ATPase activity (and is said to be a type 1 myosin), it is possible that force-transducing myosin–actin interactions could occur at this site and lead to microvillus swaying. The microvillus actin-bundle rootlets jut into the apical pole of the cell and associate with a terminal web of structural proteins. The density of this terminal web is most marked in cell types that do not have substantial exocytosis of secretory vesicles. Fine filaments, composed of classic or type II myosin, link adjacent rootlets. In addition, a heteromeric spectrinlike molecule (TW260/240) resides at this location and may be important in linking actin filaments and plasma membranes and in assisting in the stabilization of the cell surface. Columnar epithelial cells also generally display a circumferential belt of actin and myosin around their apex. Studies of isolated cell apices (termed brush borders, due to the microvilli) have shown that this belt can contract in the presence of micromolar Ca^{++} and millimolar ATP, and, thus, it has been referred to as the contractile ring. As is discussed below, it is possible that tension exerted by this ring on cell–cell contacts might modulate the barrier

function of epithelia. A thin F-actin cortex also wraps the basolateral pole of epithelial cells.

Cables composed of aggregates of 10-nm intermediate filaments course through the cells and function as support cables for structural buttressing.[2] Such tonofilament cables associate with plasma membranes at sites where specialized cell–cell junctions, termed desmosomes (see below and Figs 6-3 and 6-4), reside. From desmosomes, the cables loop through the terminal web and pass through the cytoplasm to associate with other desmosomes. These intermediate filaments are composed of keratin-type proteins.

The 25-nm-diameter microtubules, composed of tubulin, also course throughout the cell. Unlike tubulin, which is a highly conserved protein, various microtubule-associated proteins (MAPs) exist and differ between tissues. It is likely that tissue-specific microtubule functions are conferred by these MAPs. Experiments using agents that disrupt microtubule function have led to the conclusion that microtubules are not only important for structural support but are of major importance in directing vesicles to the correct sites within alimentary epithelial cells,[3] and, thus, are important in maintaining the biochemical asymmetry of the cell surface. For example, cultured intestinal epithelial cells direct the apical membrane protein aminopeptidase to the basolateral domain if microtubules are disrupted.

Adhesive Recognition of Neighboring Cells

Epithelial cells have at their disposal a diverse menu of mechanisms by which they can interact with their neighbors. Adhesive cell–cell interactions are the initial trigger allowing subsequent establishment of long-term cooperative interaction between cells. Uvomorulin, a protein present on the lateral surface of columnar epithelial cells, appears to be extremely crucial to initial cell–cell

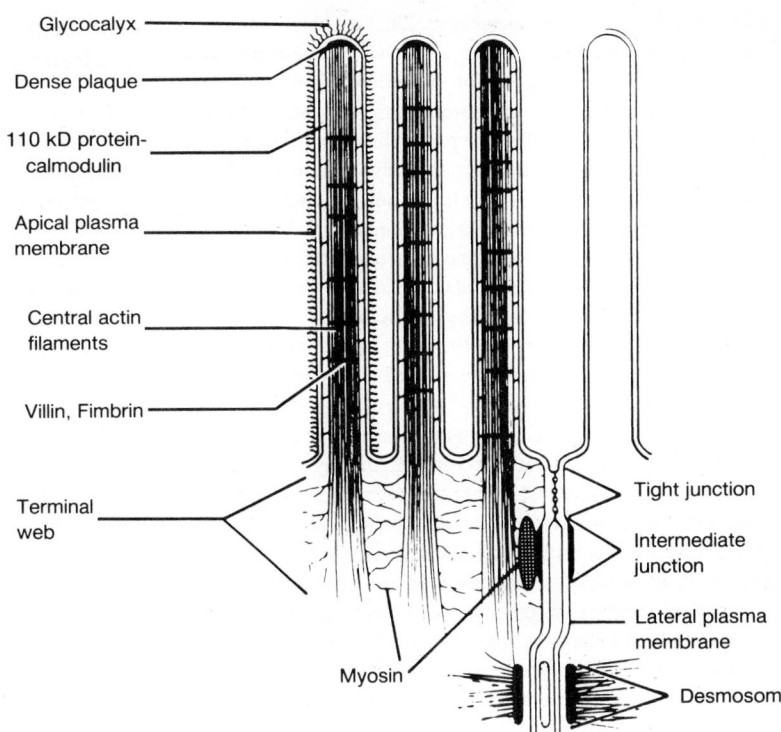

FIGURE 6–3. Organization of cytoskeleton in the apex of an absorptive cell.

recognition and adhesion.[4] Uvomorulin-based adhesion is homeotypic (i.e., based on uvomorulin–uvomorulin interactions) and is not represented by any particular morphologically defined junction. This adhesive protein belongs to a family of cell adhesion molecules (CAMs) and consists of a 120-kd glycoprotein that is both trypsin-sensitive and Ca^{++} dependent. Given the crucial role of this molecule in gut epithelial cell–cell adhesion, it would not be surprising if the dissolution of epithelial sheets into single epithelial cells, seen when extracellular Ca^{++} is depleted, is, in part, caused by interference with the uvomorulin–uvomorulin interactions between cells. For example, it has been shown, in cultured epithelia, that antibodies directed toward uvomorulin prevent both cell–cell adhesion and the development of junctional complexes (see below) between epithelial cells.[5]

Intercellular Junctions: Sealing the Paracellular Space and Stabilizing the Epithelial Monolayer

Aside from the squamous epithelium of the esophagus and perhaps a few enteroendocrine cells, alimentary epithelia have continuous circumferential intercellular tight junctions. These tight, or occluding, junctions are apically situated (see Fig 6-4). In thin sections viewed under the electron microscope, they appear as 100- to 300-nm-deep zones in which the plasma membranes from adjacent cells closely abut (Fig 6-5*A*). In fact, it appears that within this zone are a series of punctate fusions or "kisses" between these membranes. These fusion sites are transmitted in a linear anastomosing fashion around the apical pole of the cell and correspond to the netlike series of grooves or strands seen in replicated fracture faces of epithelial cells (see Fig 6-5*B*). Recognition of gasketlike

structural characteristics of the tight junction initially led to the concept that molecules could not leak between cells. In the 1970s, it became apparent that tight junctions were but relative barriers. The role of the tight junction in barrier function is discussed in more detail below (see section entitled "Epithelial Barriers"). At the cytoplasmic face at sites where tight junction kisses reside, lies a dense matrix, which, in part, likely consists of tight junction specific proteins such as the recently characterized proteins ZO-1 and cingulin.[6] ZO-1, the better characterized protein, is a peripheral membrane phosphoprotein with an apparent molecular size of 225 kd. It is unclear whether phosphorylation of this protein might lead to altered function of the tight junction, although differences in phosphorylation have been noted in cell lines that vary in junctional permeability. It is speculated that proteins such as ZO-1 may be involved in regulating tight junction permeability, perhaps by serving as a link between tight junction kiss sites and the cytoskeleton. Actin microfilaments appear to insert into the dense material adjacent to junctional kisses where ZO-1 is localized, providing the potential anatomic basis for direct cytoskeletal manipulation of the kiss sites.

Special note should be made of the peculiarities of the squamous epithelium of the esophagus. Unlike other alimentary epithelia, that lining the esophagus is multilayered ("stratified"). Current data suggest that most layers are relatively devoid of tight junctions and, where tight junctions do exist, they are discontinuous rather than circumferential. How does this epithelium barricade the paracellular space? It appears that these cells pack the paracellular space with secreted sheets of lipidlike material,[7] a unique strategy for barrier formation in the alimentary canal.

Directly below the tight junction lies a zone, termed the intermediate junction, in which the lateral membranes of adjacent cells parallel each other but do not touch. At this site, the previously mentioned perijunctional contractile ring of actomyosin resides and inserts into the plasma membrane. Directly below the intermediate junction lie desmosomes (see Fig 6-4). While several desmosomes belt the circumference of the cell at this site (referred to as the belt desmosome), desmosomes are also scattered over the basolateral surface of cells. The paracellular space is not obliterated at the site of desmosomes; rather, fine filaments (desmogliens) jut from the surface of each cell and overlap within the paracellular space. Extensions of these filaments jut from the cytoplasmic side of the membrane and associate with a dense disk of material (composed of desmoplakins) that is parallel to the membrane but removed from it by a distance of 8 to 10 nm. Intermediate filaments insert into this disk, further anchoring the cytoskeleton to the cell membrane as well as anchoring cells to neighboring cells.

Many epithelial cells, including gastric surface cells, pancreatic acinar cells, and undifferentiated crypt cells, display gap junctions[8] scattered on their basolateral membranes (see Fig 6-4). Gap junction-specific proteins have been isolated and characterized, and it appears there exists an organ-specific diversity in these proteins, which could allow for organ-specific regulation of these junctions. Gap junctions consist of aggregates of membrane particles, termed connexins, which behave as conduits to allow direct passage of ions and small molecules between the cytoplasm of adjacent cells. If a cell is "coupled" to its neighbor by way of gap junctions, one can inject a small hydrophilic fluorescent molecule in one cell and observe its passage into neighboring cells without entering the extracellular space. Gap junctions assist in coordination between cell within the epithelial sheet by allowing them to behave as syncytia with respect to transfer of small molecules.

Basement Membranes: The Foundation of Epithelia

All alimentary epithelia reside on a basement membrane of 20 to 40 nm in depth, which consists of a faintly fibrillar network and, in turn, rests on an underlying, complex extracellular matrix (see Fig 6-2). Although the basement membrane is only now being well-characterized in the alimentary tract,[9] it appears to be similar to basement membranes found elsewhere. Major elements of the basement membrane include: laminin, heparan sulfate proteoglycan, and type IV collagen,[10] however minor, but possibly important, constituents such as thrombospondin and entactin also exist. Laminin, a 850-kd glycoprotein, consists of an assembly of three chains: a straight A chain and two B chains, which helically wrap a portion of the A chain and flare off at an acute angle. This arrangement imparts a cross shape on rotary shadowed images of this molecule. Laminin exhibits specific binding sites for type IV collagen, heparan sulfate proteoglycan, cell surface laminin receptors, and entactin. In similar fashion, many matrix components display binding sites for several additional components,[11] adding to the complexity of interactions between the epithelial cell and its surrounding environment. The major proteoglycan of the basement membrane is heparan sulfate proteoglycan. Proteoglycans consist of long chains of glycosaminoglycans (such as heparan sulfate glycosaminoglycans) linked to a protein core. Hence, the structure of these massive molecules (molecular weight in excess of 10^6) is often likened to a test-tube brush: the bristles being the glycosaminoglycan extensions. Proteoglycans are likely act to or-

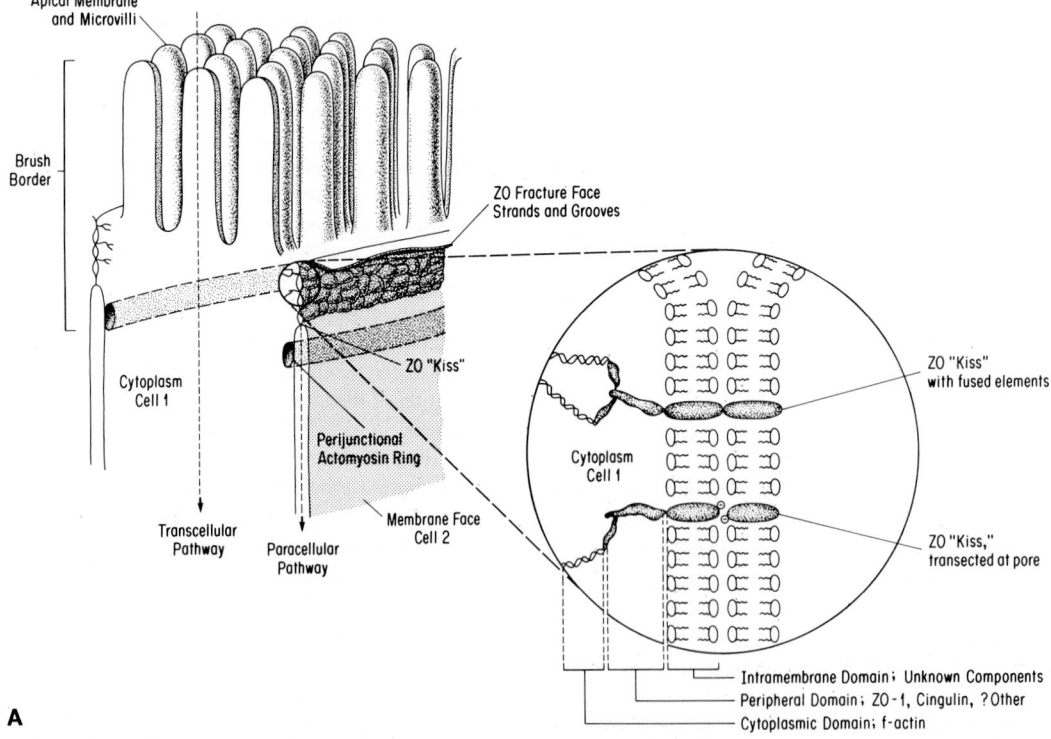

A

FIGURE 6–4. **A,** Schematic of the apical area of cell–cell contact: the junctional complex, which includes the important paracellular barrier, the tight junction or zonula occludentes. (From Madara JL. Loosening tight junctions: lessons from the intestine. J Clin Invest 83:1089, 1989).

(continued)

DESMOSOME

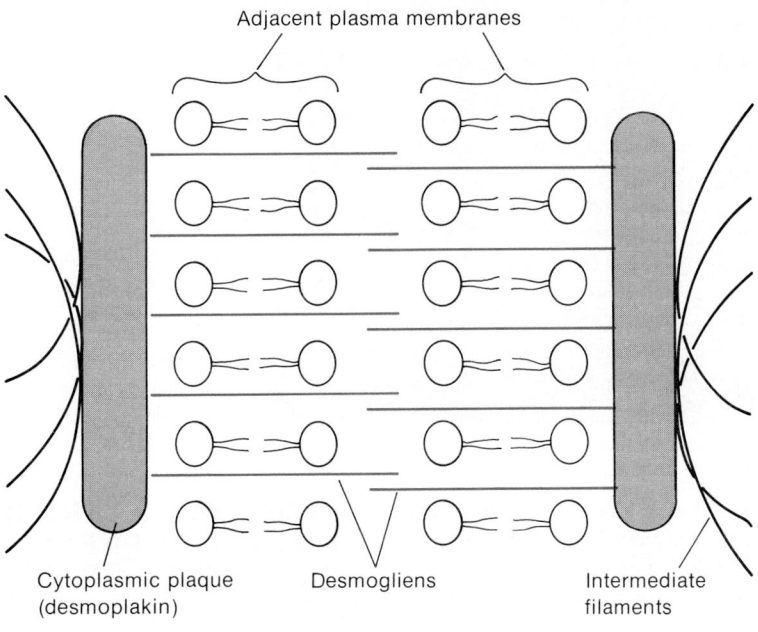

GAP JUNCTION

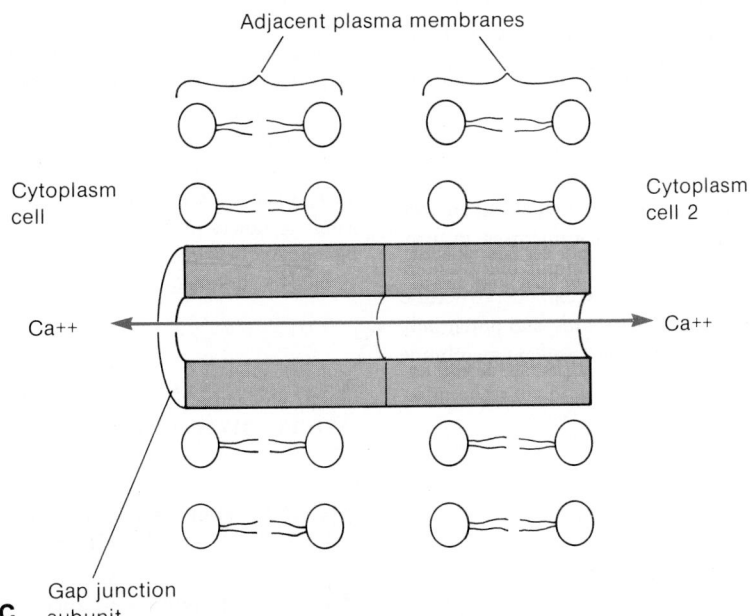

C

FIGURE 6–4. *(continued)* **B,** Schematic of desmosome; **C,** Schematic of gap junction.

ganize water within the basement membrane. That is, they not only serve to hydrate this environment due to their capacity to bind water, but they may be able to impart solute-sieving characteristics under conditions of bulk water flow. Type IV collagen originates as a triple-stranded helical molecule, which, unlike other collagens, does not have its propeptides sheared from it after deposition in the extracellular space. Partially as a result of this, collagen IV does not crosslink into dense fibrils, as many other collagen species do, but rather assumes a loose netlike structure by associating with other collagen IV molecules. This meshlike structure of collagen IV may well provide the basic structure to the basement membrane.

In addition to the specific components of the basement membrane mentioned above, other key elements are present in the remainder of the extracellular matrix. For example, the adhesive glycoprotein, fibronectin, not only exists in soluble plasma and cell-surface forms but also in a highly insoluble fibrillar form in the extracellular matrix. Fibronectin has binding sites for heparan, collagens, and epithelial cell surface receptors and serves as one link between the cell surface and the matrix underlying the basement membrane.

It is not clear if regional differences in basement membrane composition exist along the alimentary tract. Such issues are potentially of major importance because it has been shown repeatedly

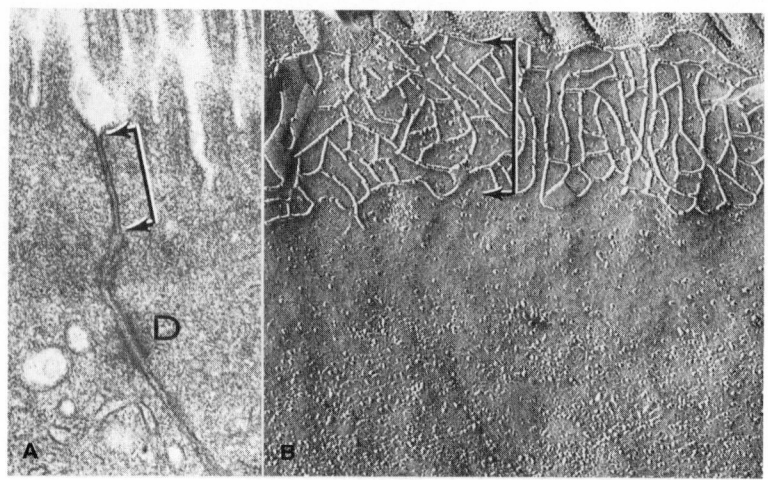

FIGURE 6–5. Thin section, **A,** and freeze fracture, **B,** electron microscopic appearance of the tight junction of an intestinal absorptive cell. In thin sections, the tight junction is a zone of close apposition between the lateral membranes of adjacent cells. By freeze fracture, strands—representing membrane-membrane "fusion" sites—are seen within the tight junction zone.

in several in vitro systems, as well as in a few in vivo ones, that basement membrane components can exert significant effects on epithelia including effects on proliferation, adhesion, migration, and differentiation[10] and perhaps even barrier function. For example, in stratified squamous epithelia, terminal differentiation of suprabasilar cells is actually triggered by the loss of contact with fibronectin that occurs as cells migrate up through the epithelium.[12] It is not yet clear which components of the alimentary epithelial basement membrane are contributed by epithelial cells and which are contributed by subepithelial cells such as fibroblasts. Many of the components of basement membranes have multiple binding sites.[13] For example, laminin can bind type IV collagen and heparan sulfate proteoglycan but also has a cell binding site. Basement membrane components bind to a family of epithelial cell surface molecules termed integrins, and it appears that integrins, in turn, can bind to cytoskeletal elements, such as F-actin, within the cell by way of linking proteins.[14] Through such associations, structural elements within the cell are able to connect with, and potentially be influenced by, events occurring within the basement membrane and even deeper in the extracellular matrix.

EPITHELIAL BARRIERS: HOW THE EPITHELIUM PREVENTS PERMEATION OF DIVERSE THREATS RANGING FROM H+ TO BACTERIA

This section addresses the question of how intraluminal threats are restricted to the lumen by the epithelial barrier (Fig 6-6). At various sites in the alimentary tract, threats such as H^+, chemotactic peptides, undigested potentially antigenic proteins, and bacteria reside. It is not surprising that the epithelial "barrier" consists of numerous components—some site-specific, some generalized. To discuss these barriers, we arbitrarily divide them into two major categories: those that are extrinsic to the epithelium (although in some instances produced by the epithelium) and those provided by the physical presence of the epithelium, which we arbitrarily categorize as intrinsic barriers.

Extrinsic Barriers: The Microenvironment Overlying Epithelia

MUCUS: BACTERIAL BARRIER, REDUCED SURFACE SHEAR

All alimentary epithelia are coated with a layer of mucus.

Most surfaces, including those of the stomach, the intestine, the biliary and pancreatic ducts, and the gallbladder, contain specialized cell types that synthesize, package, and release mucins. In the esophagus, however, mucins primarily are derived from small glands that lie under the epithelium and connect to the lumen by way of delicate ducts. Although the precise chemical nature of mucus varies throughout the alimentary tract, these various mucin molecules do, by definition, share common features.[15]

In one sense, mucus acts as a "barrier" simply by behaving as a viscous hydrated gel that undoubtedly attenuates shear forces that the epithelium would otherwise experience as particulates are driven down the alimentary tract by propulsive force. In addition, carbohydrate groups on mucin molecules have the potential for binding to bacterial surfaces and inhibiting direct epithelial-bac-

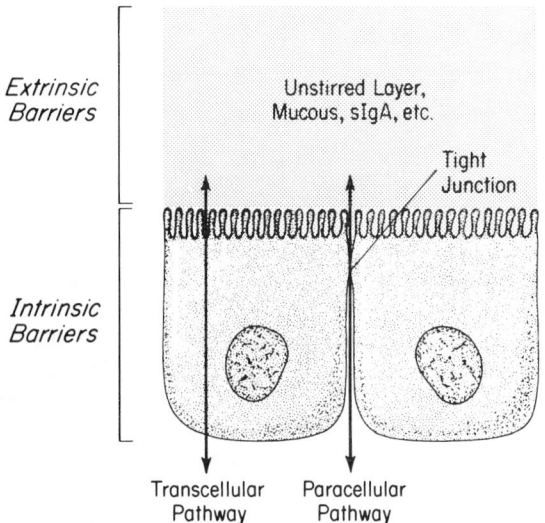

FIGURE 6–6. Schematic of gut epithelial barriers.

terial binding, which could lead to surface colonization.[15] In some instances, mucin carbohydrates specifically replicate epithelial carbohydrate binding sites to which bacteria can attach, presumably preventing colonization in a more specific fashion as well. Given their extensive glycosylation, mucins can crosslink several bacteria and also serve to aggregate bacteria. Such aggregation presumably aids in bacterial clearance by intestinal propulsive activity. The protective effects of mucin are further highlighted, in a teleologic fashion, by the fact that exposure of epithelial surfaces to threats such as bacterial toxins and noxious chemicals often results in a reflexive secretory release of mucins. Lastly, it has been noted that the diffusion coefficients of hydrophilic molecules are substantially lower in mucin than in free solution.[16] Some have suggested that such alterations would diminish contact between the epithelial surface and luminal threats such as hydrogen ions. However, given the depth of the mucin layer and the duration that luminal contents are in contact with the epithelium, small luminal molecules are likely to have sufficient time to equilibrate within the mucous gel.

UNSTIRRED LAYER: A "BARRIER" OF UNKNOWN PHYSIOLOGIC SIGNIFICANCE

Due to the propulsive movements of the alimentary tract, the lumen can be rather turbulent. There exists, however, a body of evidence suggesting that this turbulence or, more appropriately, this convective force does not extend to the epithelial surface.[17] The view is that the apical microenvironment of epithelial cells is still (i.e., unstirred), but, moving toward the lumen, one gradually achieves greater degrees of convection. Estimates of the depth of the unstirred layer range from 300 to 800 μm. One can imagine how important consideration of the unstirred layer is to investigators bent on achieving accurate kinetic data on epithelial transport systems; if surface convection is absent, one must depend on diffusive movement of molecules toward the epithelial surface. However, if uptake of the molecule by the epithelial transport system in question is more rapid than the diffusion to the epithelial surface, the concentration of the molecule at the epithelial surface would not be equivalent to the concentration of the molecule in the center of the lumen. Those interested in measuring the kinetics of uptake of various molecules by epithelial cells must confront this confounding issue of unstirred layers. Such considerations are particularly important when evaluating uptake of molecules such as lipids, which have permeability coefficients several orders of magnitude less in water than across lipid membranes (see the section entitled "Transcellular Pathway"). These considerations have led to what may be an erroneous conclusion that the unstirred layer plays a substantial role in physiologic barrier function. This remains to be shown. First, as with mucus, the exposure of luminal content to the epithelial surface is often long enough that substantial diffusive equilibration is likely to take place. Second, in absorptive epithelia, net inward water flow normally occurs after initiation of absorption, and this would establish inward convective movement at the epithelial surface. Lastly, recent physiologic measurements of unstirred layers suggest that they may be of much less significance in the unanesthetized state.[18] For example, it has been shown that, in the conscious rat, the unstirred layer of the small intestine is 100 μm or less, but this value dramatically increases with anesthesia alone or with anesthesia and laparotomy

to 200 μm and 600 μm, respectively.[18] While consideration of unstirred layers continues to be important to the investigator studying transport kinetics, it is less certain that the unstirred-layer phenomenon contributes substantially to epithelial barrier function.

SECRETORY IGA: A BARRIER TO ANTIGENS

In general, the epithelial surfaces in the alimentary tract are bathed by the immunoglobulin secretory IgA (see ch 5 for details). This molecule, by binding to luminal threats such as pathogenic bacteria or important antigens (e.g., cholera toxin), also acts as a "barrier." While of extreme importance in host defense, this is obviously a highly specific type of barrier that depends on antigenic sensitization. Secretory IgA binding to the surfaces of pathogens may not only impede pathogen–epithelial interactions over most of the epithelial surface but may actually enhance pathogen–epithelial interactions at selected sites such as at M-cells, a cell type responsible for the afferent limb of intestinal immunity (see ch 5).

SECRETED HCO₃⁻: A BUFFER BARRIER TO H⁺ IONS

Thus far, all of the "extrinsic barriers" discussed have their impact throughout the alimentary tract. However, other extrinsic barriers have regional distribution. A case in point is the net HCO_3^- secretion by epithelial surfaces that interface with acidic luminal compartments—the stomach and duodenum. Several microelectrode studies have shown that, while the pH of the gastric lumen may be 2 to 3, the pH at the surface of epithelial cells is at, or near, 7.[19] Initially, retarded diffusion of H⁺ on the basis of mucus and unstirred layers was thought to be the basis of this observation. However, as discussed above, such explanations were inadequate given the time over which diffusive equilibration of H⁺ within such "barriers" could occur. It has since been recognized that gastric surface foveolar cells (see ch 59) and duodenal villus absorptive cells (see ch 66) secrete HCO_3^- across the apical membrane and potentially assist in creating a microenvironment of neutral pH. This secretory process is an example of a highly specific and regionally localized extrinsic epithelial barrier.

HYDROPHOBIC LAYER: A PHYSICAL BARRIER TO IONS IN AQUEOUS SOLUTION

If one takes an epithelial surface such as that of the stomach or small intestine, blots off the surface with absorbent material, places a drop of water on the surface, and carefully measures the angle at which the drop of water intersects the surface, one can obtain a reasonable estimate of surface hydrophobicity.[20] This highly imaginative yet beautifully simple approach has been used by investigators to indicate that at least some alimentary epithelial surfaces are coated with a hydrophobic barrier extrinsic to the epithelial cells.[20] For example, a perfectly wetted surface would have a contact angle for water of 0 degrees, while an extremely nonwettable surface would have a contact angle of 108 degrees. Because the contact angle for aqueous solution on mammalian gastric mucosa is about 80 degrees, it has been concluded this is a very nonwettable, and thus hydrophobic, surface.[20] Questions remain, however, as to the extent to which such apparent barriers are induced by the method used to demonstrate them. Acceptance of this potentially important barrier and its distribution throughout the alimentary tract must await further development of the field.

Intrinsic Barriers: The Epithelium

One can gather from the discussion above that extrinsic barriers generally contribute in a relative, although in some instances regionally important, fashion to the overall barrier function of alimentary organs. As has been suspected since the last century when clear anatomic evidence of alimentary epithelial surfaces was described, it is the epithelial lining itself that principally allows for separation of luminal compounds from the subepithelial fluids. Classically, the barrier function of epithelia is discussed by considering the two pathways available to passive permeation: the *transcellular* pathway and the *paracellular* pathway (see Fig 6-6). Below, we follow this approach in discussion of passive transepithelial movement of hydrophilic solutes. However, the principles guiding movement of water and hydrophobic molecules across the epithelium are distinct from those governing movement of hydrophilic molecules. Hydrophobic compounds can cross epithelial cells directly by virtue of their solubility in the lipid bilayer of the plasma membrane. Physiologically, the most important transepithelial movement of hydrophobic compounds occurs during fat absorption (this process is discussed in ch 18). Water permeation is highly complex and is considered separately.

TRANSCELLULAR PATHWAY: A HIGHLY RESTRICTIVE PATHWAY FOR PASSIVE SOLUTE FLOW

To diffuse passively across a cell, an ion or other hydrophilic solute must interact with three barriers in series: the apical membrane, the cytosol, and the basolateral membrane (see Fig 6-6).

All epithelial cells are encased by a plasma membrane, which is the primary barrier isolating the cell interior from the environment. The general structural characteristics of the plasma membrane are shown in Figure 6-7. Like other biologic membranes, the plasma membrane consists of a lipid bilayer. Lipid bilayers severely restrict permeation of hydrophilic solutes and tend to preserve transmembrane gradients in ions. For example, the resistance to passive ion flow across model lipid bilayers ranges from 10^6 to 10^9 ohm-cm^2.[21] Similarly, as determined in osmotic experiments[22] using such model membranes, the reflection coefficients for NaCl, glucose, and sucrose approximate one. Reflection

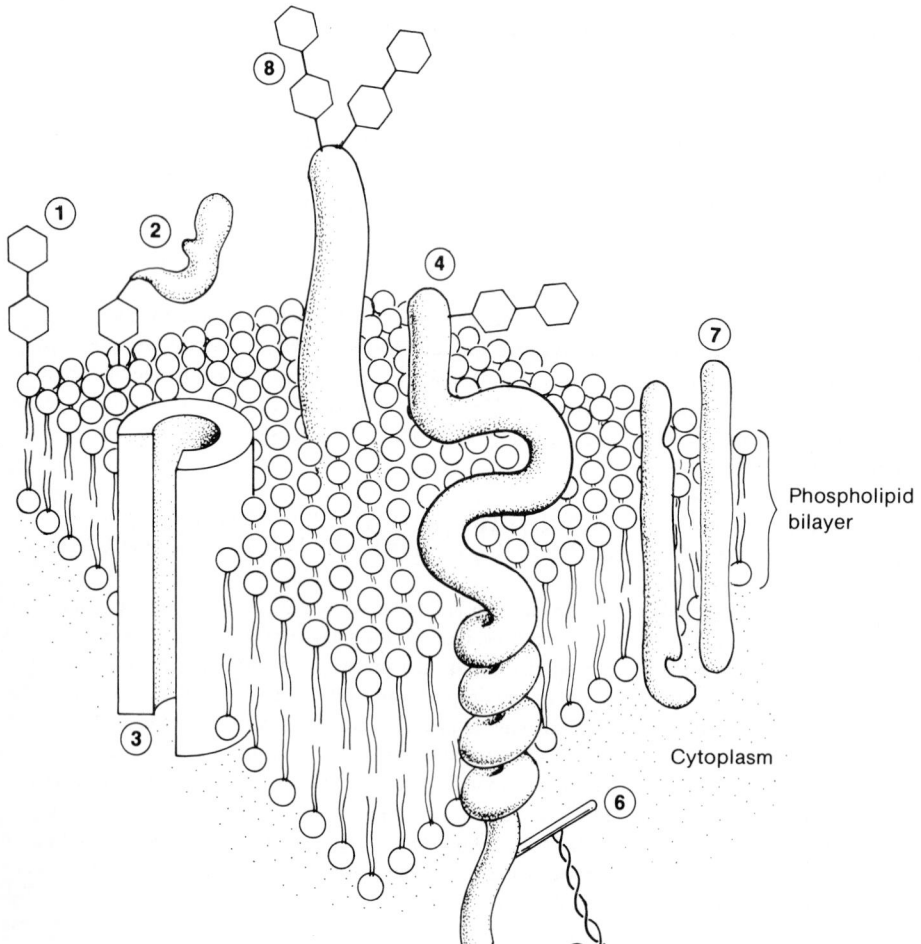

Phospholipid bilayer

Cytoplasm

FIGURE 6–7. Generic organization of the plasma membrane: (*1*) Glycolipid; (*2*) protein linked to phospholipid by way of oligosaccharide; (*3*) channel protein; (*4*) transmembrane protein with link to cytoskeleton (*5*), by way of a peripheral linking protein (*6*); (*7*) transport protein; (*8*) highly glycosylated protein.

coefficient refers to the ability of a barrier to prevent sieving, or "reflect," a molecule. A reflection coefficient of one means a barrier is totally impermeable to a molecule; an infinitely permeable barrier would have a reflection coefficient of zero. Biologic membranes (lipid bilayers plus integral membrane proteins) also have resistances that are very restrictive to passive ion flow, although less so than model lipid bilayers—in the range of 10^3 to 10^4 ohm-cm². Such resistance is very substantial when one considers that intact alimentary epithelia range in resistance from approximately 5×10^1 to 10^3 ohm-cm². This ability of a lipid membrane to retard passive flow of hydrophobic solutes is the basis of the ability of epithelial cells to maintain cytosolic ion concentrations far different from those in the interstitial space (e.g., Na^+ below 40 mM, K^+ above 100 mM, and Ca^+ in the nanomolar range). As indicated by the above data and as would seem ideal, the major component of ion movement across biologic membranes appears to be due to integral membrane proteins, presumably transporters and channels. In the absence of specific transport pathways, intact biologic membranes can be considered virtually impermeable to hydrophilic solutes .5 nm or greater in size. In contrast to hydrophilic solutes, hydrophobic molecules readily permeate the lipid bilayer. For example, saturated fatty acids are calculated to exhibit astounding permeability coefficients across jejunal epithelial cell microvillus membranes (10^6–10^7 cm/sec compared to 10^{-5}–10^{-6} cm/sec in aqueous solution).[23]

The building blocks of the membrane are highly hydrophobic molecules consisting of a hydrocarbon chain attached to a carboxyl group (fatty acid).[24] These carboxyl groups allow the fatty acid to form ester bonds with molecules, such as glycerol, which are endowed with hydroxyl groups. If all three hydroxyl groups of glycerol esterify with fatty acids, another hydrophobic molecule—triglyceride—results. However, if only two of the glycerol hydroxyl groups esterify with fatty acids (fatty acyl side chains) and the third is esterified to a hydrophilic compound such as phosphate, a hybrid molecule results that exhibits long hydrophobic side chains and a small hydrophilic "head" group (Fig 6-8). These amphipathic phospholipids, when in an aqueous environment, tend to self associate such that hydrophilic groups face water and hydrophobic groups face each other. This characteristic of amphipaths underlies the basic organization of biomembranes into lipid bilayers. Heterogeneity of phospholipids is accomplished by varying the length of acyl side chains, the degree of carbon–carbon bonding (single versus double) within these side chains, and the size of the "polar" head groups by addition of hydrophilic compounds such as choline, ethanolamine, and so forth. Along with the phospholipids, other amphipathic lipids, such as sphingomyelin, are present in the membrane as are sterols, such as cholesterol, and glycolipids. Differences in lipid composition between the external and internal half of the lipid bilayer exist, and this confers lipid asymmetry on the membrane.[11]

Intrinsic membrane proteins display hydrophobic domains at sites where they penetrate into the hydrophobic interior of the membrane (see Fig 6-7).[25] Less commonly, membrane proteins may anchor themselves to the membrane by attaching to a lipid moiety such as glycolipid (see Fig 6-7). Membrane proteins involved in translocation of ions or nutrients by channels or carrier mechanisms (chloride channel, sodium-glucose cotransporter) are thought to have large membrane-spanning segments perhaps arranged in helices that, based on alternating hydrophobic and hydrophilic sequences, have the potential to shuttle hydrophilic mol-

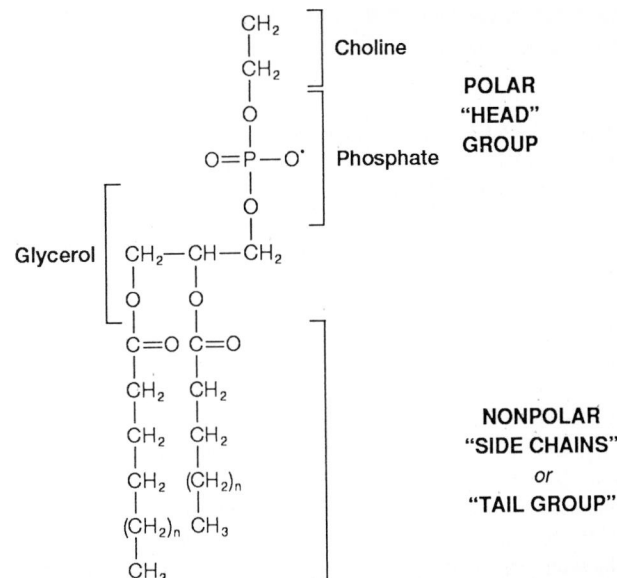

FIGURE 6–8. A glycerol molecule in which two hydroxyl groups esterify with fatty acids (hydrophobic portion) and the third esterifies with phosphate (giving a hydrophilic or polar "head"). Thermodynamically driven self-assembly of such amphipathic molecules into bilayer structures (Fig 6–7) confers stability to plasma membranes as barriers.

ecules across the membrane. One such protein is the product of the cystic fibrosis gene, which may represent either the Cl^- channel or, as is now thought, a regulatory element of the Cl^- channel. A model of the predicted protein product of this gene envisions 12 membrane-spanning helices clustered to form a transmembrane anion-selective channel with attached large polar cytoplasmic regulating regions.[26] Other integral membrane proteins that are predominately of importance in modifying the intraluminal environment (aminopeptidase, sucrase-isomaltose) often appear to be more superficially embedded in the membrane.[27] Because the mass of each individual protein is not uniformly distributed across the membrane, substantial asymmetry in protein composition also exists between the inner and outer leaflets of the membrane bilayer.[11]

The remaining barrier, other than the two plasma membranes, to restrict transcellular passive permeation is the cytosol. Because the cytosol has the characteristics of a hydrated gel, it is likely that the resistance afforded by this barrier is only marginally greater than that of free solution. For example, it is clear from single cell impalement studies that small injected tracers move freely about the cytosol but do not cross the plasma membrane. In contrast, application of even large tracers to the lumen of alimentary tract is followed by movement of tracer to the surface of the apical plasma membrane but generally not into the cytosol. One may conclude that plasma membranes are the key barriers that restrict the passive movement of hydrophilic solutes across cells. This is in keeping with the physical constraints to passive solute flow exhibited by model bilayers and biomembranes (outlined above).

In the 1960s, the observation that a variety of small hydrophilic solutes could passively leak across gut epithelia led to the conclusion that small transepithelial pores were scattered through this epithelium. However, it was wrongly assumed that molecules could not permeate across intercellular junctions (see section entitled "Paracellular Pathway"), and the language used to describe the location of these "pores" in the early literature incorrectly implies that the pores are transcellular.

PARACELLULAR PATHWAY: A MAJOR PATHWAY FOR PASSIVE SOLUTE PERMEATION

Although, as outlined above, plasma membranes tend toward high resistance, alimentary epithelia, with the exception of the esophagus, have either very low net resistance (50–100 ohm-cm^2) (i.e., they are leaky) or, at most, moderate levels of resistance (Table 6-1). It follows that the remaining pathway, the paracellular pathway, must largely be responsible for such leaks in these epithelia.

The paracellular pathway consists of the apical intercellular tight junction (see the section entitled "Intercellular Junctions") and the underlying paracellular space. When macromolecular tracers are applied to the alimentary tract lumen, they are restricted by the tight junction and do not enter the paracellular space. When the same tracers are applied from beneath the epithelium by vascular injection, they permeate throughout the paracellular space underlying the tight junction but, again, are restricted by the tight junction from crossing into the lumen.[6] Under most conditions, tight junctions are the rate-limiting barrier restricting passive movement of hydrophobic solutes through the paracellular space. When the subjunctional paracellular space is tightly collapsed, it may contribute to paracellular resistance in leaky epithelia such as the gallbladder and small intestine. In the baseline physiologic state, tight junctions may leak small quantities of molecules the size of mono- and disaccharides (fluxes on the order of 10^{-2} to 10^{-4} μM $\times$ cm^{-2} $\times$ hr^{-1}).[33] Such leakiness may be physiologically regulated and, under some conditions, greatly increased.

There may exist highly permeable foci within alimentary epithelia during health. For example, as dying adult cells slough from the surfaces of nonstratified alimentary epithelia, it is possible that barrier defects may exist, however transient. While, in aggregate, such sites would represent a minute fraction of the epithelial surface, it may be that these or similar low incidence defects could contribute substantially to the passive uptake of large solutes, which is known to occur in minute amounts.[34] A special case of

transepithelial transport of large solutes occurs in the region of Peyer's patches in the intestine. Here specialized epithelial cells, termed M cells, actively transport large, intact molecules from the lumen to underlying lymphoid cells. While such transfer is key to intestinal immunity (see ch 5), it is unlikely to represent more than a minute fraction of net transepithelial solute movement.

HOW DOES WATER FLOW ACROSS THE EPITHELIAL BARRIER?

Water movement across lipid membranes (i.e., transcellular water movement) is much less restricted than is that of hydrophilic solutes.[21] For example, the water diffusional permeability coefficient of model lipid bilayers is in the range of 2×10^{-5} to 2×10^{-2} cm/sec depending on the details of membrane composition.[22] It so happens this is the approximate range of water permeabilities in biologic membranes. Specific integral membrane proteins to handle water flow are not necessarily required to maintain transmembrane water movement. However, in some nonalimentary epithelia, such as urinary bladder, evidence for discrete, presumably proteinaceous, water channels does exist. Given this level of water permeability in the plasma membrane, it is not surprising that the cell interior is essentially isosmotic to the exterior.

How water permeates a biologic membrane is uncertain. However, given the equality of the diffusional and osmotic permeability coefficients for water moving across lipid bilayers,[22] it appears that water movement occurs as independent diffusional movement of individual molecules rather than as cooperative laminar flow. One picture that emerges from such studies and satisfies many of the observed features of water movement across membranes, is that water diffuses across the nonpolar portion of the outer membrane leaflet, dissolves in the central polar portion of the membrane in proportion to its molar fraction in the outer aqueous phase, and moves by diffusion across the inner leaflet (assuming an inwardly directed gradient favoring water movement).[22]

Because hydrophilic solutes the size of water can permeate tight junctions (see Paracellular Pathway above), it is also clear that water movement can occur across epithelia by the paracellular route. Although there is agreement that water crosses by both the transcellular and paracellular routes, the relative partitioning of water flow between these two pathways is controversial. One study that permits the quantification of the lower limit of paracellular water absorption during nutrient-driven absorption in rat small intestine provides evidence that approximately 50% of water absorption is likely to be paracellular in this physiologic state.[35] This figure was obtained by comparing clearance from the lumen of a paracellular marker by way of solvent drag with net volume flow or J_V. It can be concluded that even if the tight junction reflection coefficient for this paracellular marker were zero, approximately half (i.e., minimal estimate) of the J_V is paracellular. Data from other epithelia show that interepithelial differences in hydraulic conductivity, a measure of force-induced water flow, correlate reasonably well with paracellular resistance.[36] Similarly, correlations between hydraulic water permeability (determined at hydrostatic pressures that do not move water transcellularly: 24.4 cm H_2O) and transepithelial voltage gradients (an indirect measure of junctional permeability) correlate inversely and well over a wide variety of epithelia.[37] In aggregate, the above observations would argue that the paracellular pathway is a major route for

TABLE 6-1

Representative Examples of Transepithelial Electrical Resistance Along the Alimentary Tract of Mammals*

SITE	RESISTANCE (Ohm-cm^2)
Esophagus (rabbit)	1659[28]
Stomach (guinea pig)	99[29]
Small intestine	
Jejunum (rat)	65[30]
Ileum (rabbit)	100[31]
Colon (rabbit)	286[32]
Gallbladder (rabbit)	20[6a]

* *The figures noted are representative and vary somewhat from study to study and between species. They also do not correct for the amplification of surface area in various organs due to their complex surface geometry.*

water flow across epithelia when such flow is driven by hydrostatic or osmotic pressures. On the other hand, others have argued, based on clever experiments performed on amphibian gallbladder epithelium,[38] that the vast majority of water uptake across this epithelium is transcellular, not paracellular. In these studies, small changes in cell volume, in response to alteration of luminal fluid osmosity, were measured and used to calculate water permeability of the apical membrane. Reasoning that these measured permeabilities were so great (0.055 cm/sec) that paracellular water permeabilities would have to achieve almost impossible values to contribute substantially to transepithelial water movement, the authors concluded that water movement is largely transcellular. A potential flaw in these latter studies is that diffusional, not convectional, movement of water was measured (i.e., even though these values are occasionally referred to as "hydraulic conductivities," no units of force are expressed as would be required). This is a crucial issue because the diffusional water movement varies with the square of the pore radius (r^2) while convective (i.e., force-associated) water movement varies with the fourth power of the pore radius (r^4) as predicted by the Kedem-Katchalsky equation.[39] Although it is possible that paracellular pathways contribute little to diffusional water movement, paracellular pathways may be of greater importance in convective water flow. Moreover, convective water flow secondary to osmotic pressures generated by nutrient or ion transport or by countercurrent vascular flow in the lamina propria is likely to be the more physiologically significant type of transepithelial water movement in the alimentary tract. This very basic issue of the route of water flow across gut epithelia remains surprisingly open.

EPITHELIAL INJURY: HOW DOES THE EPITHELIAL BARRIER "BREAK"?

"Physiologic Injury": Diminished Cell Life Span Without Enhanced Epithelial Permeation

Epithelial injury is most readily apparent when gaps within the epithelium are present, such as in states of epithelial erosion or ulceration. However, the gut epithelia have such a remarkable ability to repair that premature death of individual epithelial cells due to "injury" does not necessarily result in breaks in epithelial continuity. Indeed, the life span of individual epithelial cells may be diminished by physiologic events, leading to the concept that epithelial "injury" spans a spectrum that extends into normal physiology.

Gut epithelial turnover occurs rapidly (on average, once a week) by a process of proliferation, migration, senescence, and sloughing. For example, gastric surface cells arise from the proliferative zone (gastric pit), migrate to the surface as they become differentiated foveolar cells, and ultimately slough into the lumen. By removing physiologic agents from the lumen, the half-life of epithelial cells can often be lengthened. For example, without exposure to products of the pancreatic and biliary secretion, intestinal absorptive cell life span is significantly prolonged. Similarly, the

half-life of individual molecules on the cell surface is modulated by the harshness of the physiologic environment. Sucrase-isomaltase on the absorptive cell brush border has a half-life of 6 hours in the presence of pancreatic proteases, but this is substantially prolonged in the absence of pancreatic secretion.[40] Such loss of cell surface proteins does not ultimately result in a protein-depleted cell surface because these lost or damaged components are constantly replaced by individual epithelial cells. Undoubtedly, lipids in the membrane are also turned over, but documentation of this is difficult given the proclivity of membrane lipids to exchange side chains under the influence of membrane phospholipases. Components of individual epithelial cells are turned over at rates that can be altered by normal physiologic events, and these events can also modulate the life span of the cell.

Another, more dramatic, type of physiologic epithelial "injury" has been described in the gut.[41] Due to physical trauma accompanying events such as gut motility, the usually highly restrictive apical plasma membrane of epithelial cells can transiently break down. In such instances, macromolecular tracers present in the lumen leak into and label the cytoplasm of these cells. These tracers do not appear to leak across the basolateral membrane, and there is no evidence to suggest such sites may be foci for transepithelial macromolecular leaks. Because these labeled cells subsequently remain in the epithelium and retain normal appearances for 48 hours, it appears such transient defects in apical membrane permeability are rapidly repaired. Experiments using cultured epithelial cells have similarly shown that, when scraped or trypsinized, plasma membranes can undergo a cycle of transient breakdown and rapid repair. Hence, transient plasma membrane breakdown and subsequent rapid repair might be considered a second variety of "physiologic injury."

Injury: Potential Mechanisms of Enhanced Permeation

As previously described, plasma membranes generally restrict passive flux of hydrophilic solutes unless specific uptake pathways are present. Furthermore, it is unlikely that the passive permeability of biomembranes to such solutes could be increased substantially for more than a transient period (seconds to minutes, such as occurs with rapid repair as described above) without resulting in cell death. This is because prolonged increases in plasma membrane permeation would likely lead to loss of intracellular regulatory elements, obliteration of the unique intracellular ionic environment, prolonged membrane depolarization, and influx of Ca^{++}, which, among other things, would activate cytoskeletal shearing proteins such as villin. It is only logical to suspect that disease states characterized by enhanced permeation of solutes, such as those in the size range of small peptides, are likely to have defects in paracellular permeability. Such enhanced paracellular permeability could result from either of two types of perturbations: (1) defective tight junction barrier function or (2) gross defects in the epithelium (erosions or ulcers) due to focal cell necrosis without concomitant epithelial resealing (i.e., a decrease in cell life span beyond that to which the epithelium can adapt by enhanced proliferation). That this second type of perturbation, which results in focal denudation of the epithelium would lead to increased epithelial permeation is intuitively obvious.

Injury in a Confluent Epithelium: Can Tight Junction Permeation Be Modulated?

It is clear that diseases exist in which the epithelium remains confluent but tight junction permeation to inert solutes, the size of disaccharides and larger, is enhanced. One example of such a disorder is celiac sprue.[42] Additionally, at least some of the protein-losing gastropathics may fall into this category as well, and it has recently been suggested that patients with Crohn's disease may exhibit a primary defect in tight junction permeability.[43] This provocative finding, which needs to be confirmed, stems from a study in which healthy relatives of a patient with Crohn's disease were found to have a defect in intestinal permeability to the inert tracer mannitol equal to that found in symptomatic patients.

It is unclear how tight junction permeability might be affected in such states. However, insights into the potential for alterations in tight junction barrier function come from recent evidence suggesting that this crucial barrier is physiologically regulated.[6,23,35] As outlined in detail in Chapter 14, active transepithelial transport of nutrients such as glucose occurs across villus absorptive cells. It appears that the presence of glucose within the lumen results in structural deformation of villus absorptive cell tight junctions and enhanced permeability of these junctions to molecules the size of amino acids and glucose (and perhaps substantially larger molecules). Precisely how glucose exposure leads to enhanced junctional permeability is unclear. The initial triggering event is activation of the Na^+-glucose cotransporter[43a] and that such activation may, in turn, induce enhanced cytoskeletal tension within the perijunctional ring of actin and myosin, which distorts the tight junction mechanically. As active transcellular absorption of Na^+ and water proceeds, a transepithelial osmotic gradient is thought to develop, which drives inward water movement across the tight junction. Because such altered tight junctions have abnormally low reflection coefficients for nutrient-sized molecules, substantial paracellular nutrient uptake by way of solvent drag may follow. If correct, this theory would explain why the intestine continues to absorb increasing amounts of nutrients from the lumen as luminal nutrient concentrations rise far above the concentration at which the Na^+-glucose cotransporter is saturated.[44] Most importantly, this phenomenon highlights not only how transcellular active transport events can be intertwined intimately with paracellular barrier function but also shows the plasticity that tight junction barrier function exhibits even in physiologic states. It is known that, in a variety of nonalimentary epithelia, classic intracellular mediators such as Ca^{++}, cAMP, and protein kinase C, as well as inflammatory mediators, can also affect tight junction structure or permeability.[33] Such modulation of tight junction permeability might underlie the abnormal epithelial permeability encountered in diseased, but still confluent, epithelia.

LOCAL CONSEQUENCES OF ENHANCED EPITHELIAL PERMEATION: MODULATION OF EPITHELIA BY SUBEPITHELIAL ELEMENTS

Gut epithelial function may be modulated by a host of local factors derived from nonepithelial sources. Specific examples of such in-fluences are provided in detail in chapters dealing with specific epithelia (chs 12–16). Here the point is made that such events may occur throughout the alimentary tract in the physiologic state and that subepithelial–epithelial interactions may be altered in states of enhanced epithelial permeation. Before dealing with the effects of enhanced permeation on these subepithelial–epithelial interactions, we describe examples of such interactions in health. Alimentary epithelia rest on a structurally complex lamina propria, which, as shown in Figure 6-9, contains many candidate elements that potentially could influence epithelial transport events or barrier function. Nerves, microvascular myofibroblasts, and a host of immune cells including mast cells, macrophages, and lymphocytes are within microns of epithelial cells. It is becoming increasingly clear that factors derived from such elements may profoundly affect epithelial function. These studies largely are performed by modulating one subepithelial component or by adding to an in vitro epithelial sheet one agent known to be produced by subepithelial components. While data derived from these studies provide a framework for our understanding of how subepithelial elements influence epithelia, it is likely the net effects of orchestrated subepithelial events on epithelial function will not be understood clearly for some time. Similarly, given the complex microenvironment of a gut epithelial cell, it is hard to know the precise range of concentrations of putative modulating factors the epithelial cell might encounter. Given that many such modulating factors are released in concentrated form close to epithelial cells (e.g., by exocytosis from nerve termini or from mast cells), it would not be surprising if epithelia detect concentrations of modulating elements far in excess of what would be predicted based on knowledge of average concentrations within the total extracellular water of the lamina propria. A few examples of such potential regulatory elements are discussed below.

Products of arachidonic acid metabolism, eicosanoids, are known to have profound effects on epithelia. For example, prostaglandin E_2 has effects ranging from promotion of healing of gastric epithelial injury[45] to eliciting electrogenic Cl^- secretion in the small and large intestine.[46] Although eicosanoids may have important effects on epithelia, they are chiefly produced by subepithelial cells.[47] Products of arachidonic acid metabolism generated by the lamina propria can be detected not only in health but may be markedly affected in disease. The stimuli to enhanced production may well be other mediators of inflammation that, in turn, could be elicited by enhanced epithelial permeability, which triggers a subepithelial immune response. For example, it appears that the subepithelial production of eicosanoids can be dramatically altered by inflammatory mediators such as bradykinin.[47]

Neurons of the enteric nervous system likewise produce a host of bioactive compounds, including peptides (vasoactive intestinal peptide [VIP], somatostatin, cholecystokinin [CCK], and so forth), catecholamines, and acetylcholine.[48] Moreover, termini from these nerves project to subepithelial positions often within 1 μm of epithelial cells. Compounds produced by neurons are known to influence epithelial functions ranging from acid secretion by gastric parietal cells to ion absorption by intestinal absorptive cells. Other examples of subepithelial influences on epithelial function include histamine, a product of mucosal mast cells, which produces a range of effects (e.g., induction of gastric acid secretion and intestinal Cl^- secretion) on alimentary epithelia. Mucosal mast cell activation in disease states subsequent to enhanced epithelial permeability must, therefore, be considered yet another important modulator of epithelial function that might arise locally.

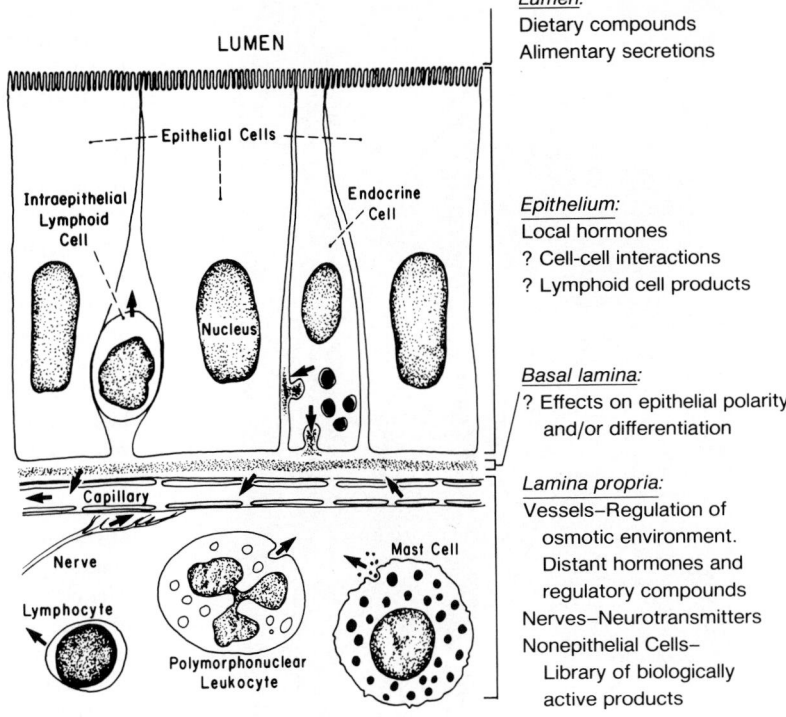

LUMEN

FIGURE 6-9. The gut epithelium is in close proximity to factors—vascular, neural, immune—that substantially influence epithelial function.

It is likely that enhanced epithelial permeation in disease states substantially modifies epithelial interactions with such subepithelial elements and, in doing so, further modifies epithelial function. Recruitment and activation of immune cells appear to follow enhanced permeation because chemoattractants (formylated peptides) and activators of immune cells (bacterially derived lipopolysaccharides, luminal antigens, and so forth) are present in the intestinal lumen. For example, in health, polymorphonuclear leukocytes (PMN) are rarely detected outside of vessels in the lamina propria. In contrast, in many forms of acute injury numerous PMN migrate into the epithelium, squeeze across intercellular tight junctions (Fig 6-10), and accumulate in gastric pits or intestinal crypts to form pit/crypt abscesses, a hallmark of active disease.[49] At least one class of compounds strongly chemotactic for PMN, N-formylated peptides-products of bacteria, undoubtedly is present normally in the lumen of the alimentary tract and probably is present in functionally significant concentrations in the colon. In fact, a degree of PMN transmigration may occur physiologically,[50] presumably driven by chemotactic luminal factors such as luminal N-formylated peptides. Not only might enhanced epithelial permeability, with subsequent leak of chemotactic compounds, promote intestinal inflammation, but the ensuing inflammatory process would lead to even greater epithelial permeability, perhaps even if individual epithelial cells were not destroyed. For example, data from a cultured model gut epithelium suggest that PMN transmigration across tight junctions can, by itself, result in enhanced tight junction permeation.[51]

HEALING OF EPITHELIAL WOUNDS: RESEALING BROKEN BARRIERS

When epithelial proliferation no longer keeps up with accelerated epithelial loss due to injury, a rent in the epithelial barrier ensues.

That is, erosions or even ulcers (underlying lamina propria and muscularis mucosa also destroyed) develop. To evaluate this situation in terms of the concepts outlined in this chapter, such an injury could be viewed as dramatic, focal expansion of the paracellular pathway associated with loss of the rate-limiting barrier to paracellular flow—the intercellular tight junction. Because the tight junction is the site at which the paracellular pathway normally reflects passive permeation to large hydrophilic solutes, it is obvious that in such states the barrier to even macromolecules is broken. The permeability coefficients within the wound to threatening lumen solutes such as macromolecules (including pancreatic proteases) and peptides (such as bacterially derived chemotactic N-formylated peptides) should largely be those exhibited by these molecules in free solution. The reflection coefficient at such sites can be assumed to be zero. In contrast, if a still confluent epithelium focally developed a disrupted tight junction in which the reflection coefficient to macromolecules also shifted to zero, the movement of luminal molecules inward would be slight in comparison with that observed in an open wound. In open epithelial wounds, the surface area exposed to unrestricted permeation—even if only 10 contiguous cell positions were lost—would be orders of magnitude greater than if two viable cells simply separated at the tight junction by a micron or so. Governed by Fick's first law of diffusional permeation, P_d directly relates to surface area, providing qualitative grounds for the intuitive realization that "small" breaks encompassing several cell widths expose subepithelial tissues to huge pulses over baseline of luminal solutes. As a result, transepithelial leaks of paracellular tracer molecules such as PEG-400 can increase by over 200% in patients with erosive intestinal disease,[43] even though the eroded surface may represent a minute percentage of the net intestinal surface area.

Once wounded, epithelia often respond by enhanced proliferation in an effort to replenish cells in the eroded area. An increased fraction of progenitor cells is stimulated to move through the S, G_2, and M phases of the cell cycle. However, because the

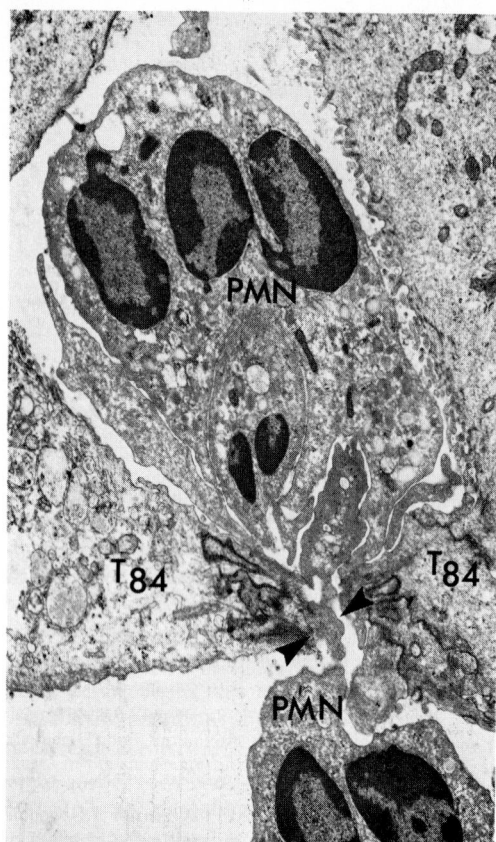

FIGURE 6-10. In an in vitro model of gut epithelial acute inflammation, neutrophils squeeze through an intercellular tight junction. This "impalement" leads to a transient increase in junctional permeability, a fall in transepithelial resistance. Mediators released from cells of the immune system or other subepithelial cells, such as fibroblasts, are also likely to influence epithelial transport and barrier functions, even in the absence of direct epithelial cell-immune cell contact, such as that seen here. (From Nash S, Stafford J, Madara JL. Effects of PMN transmigration on the barrier function of cultured intestinal epithelial monolayers. J Clin Invest 1987; 80:1104.

S phase of the cell cycle alone is 6 to 12 hours in length, the benefit of this proliferative response is not recognized for a period of hours. Although the stimuli for enhanced proliferation in gut epithelia are not precisely known, a variety of classic growth factors are likely involved. For example, it has been shown that epidermal growth factor (EGF) can stimulate DNA synthesis in the gastric mucosa of rodents.[52] Furthermore, when the major intraluminal source of EGF (salivary glands) is removed, healing of gastric and duodenal ulcerations is delayed and this delay can be reversed with the addition of either oral or parenteral EGF.[53] Other growth factors, such as transforming growth factor-alpha (TGFα) may also play a role in epithelial wound healing. In fact, recent evidence that shows that TGFα mRNA and TGFα/EGF receptor mRNA are expressed in gastric epithelial cells raises the interesting concept that epithelia might also produce their own growth factors in a regulated fashion.[54] Examples of epithelial growth responses to a variety of other growth factors abound[55] (growth hormone, thyroid hormones, CCK, gastrin, polyamines, and so forth). One is left with the conclusion that epithelial proliferation after wounding is influenced by a complex interactive set of growth promoting factors. Such factors could act directly (e.g., by binding surface re-

ceptors for growth factors) or indirectly (e.g., by modulating growth factor receptor expression or production of local growth factors).

As alluded to above, stimulated production of new epithelial cells requires, at the minimum, hours to increase the rate of epithelial cell renewal. In the short-term, reepithelialization of small wounds may also occur by the remarkable processes known as restitution.[56] Although the initial work in restitution was done in gastric epithelia,[56] it is clear that this process also occurs in the small and large intestine and the gallbladder and can be demonstrated in vivo as well as in vitro in a variety of species. The original observation was that, after rapid removal of the surface foveolar cells of the stomach by chemical means, epithelial barrier function, as assessed by resistance to passive ion flow, was reestablished in a time course too fast to be accounted for by enhanced cell division. Subsequently, it became apparent that gastric pit cells shouldering these surface wounds flattened and rapidly migrated to reseal the superficial defects. It is likely that this process of restitution is of utmost importance in daily resealing of subclinical epithelial injury as well as being important in disease states. This observation also partially explains why epithelial cells in states of acute injury often appear either cuboidal or flattened rather than columnar; restitution is attempting to keep pace with enhanced cell turnover. While the physiologic significance of restitution to epithelial resealing is well appreciated, the basic mechanistic principles underlying this response remain opaque. What signals the remaining viable epithelial cell that its neighbor is gone? How is this signal translated into a rapid, dynamic migratory response, which includes remolding of the cytoskeleton? When cells reapproximate, how do they reestablish surface polarity and normal phenotypes? What intracellular signals guide this repolarization? Answers to such questions will not only provide insights into restitution but also into the basic principles of how epithelial cells govern their form and movement.

How restituting cells or newly produced cells migrate over a denuded surface is also unclear. It is clear from experiments carried out in many other systems based on mammalian cells that directional migration, such as occurs in intestinal epithelial closure after wounding, generally requires extracellular signals. These experiments specifically suggest that extracellular matrix proteins are crucial in guiding cells during migration. For example, if cell binding sites for fibronectin are rendered inaccessible, epithelial migration after corneal injury is substantially impaired. Conversely, addition of fibronectin to the matrix enhances wound closure in this model.[57] Unfortunately, relatively little work is available in this area relating specifically to epithelial closure in the alimentary tract after wounding. Matrix components should also be crucial in organizing the subepithelial tissues in wounds that extend beyond the epithelium. Although beyond the scope of this chapter, organization of a provisional matrix for reepithelialization of a deep wound includes such key events as chemotaxis of fibroblasts by provisionally deposited collagen and fibronectin.[58]

Even nonmatrix elements in the lamina propria might influence epithelial resealing after injury. In a model of focal intestinal epithelial denudation, it has been shown that restitution is aided by myofibroblast-mediated contraction of the lamina propria.[59] This contractile event effectively diminishes the size of the defect to be reepithelialized.

During the early 1980s, a phenomenon termed "cytoprotection" was popularized.[60] Like restitution, the initial recognition of this phenomenon also occurred in gastric epithelia and subsequently it was also described throughout the intestine. The discovery was that exposure to low concentrations of compounds such as prostaglandins appeared to protect gastric epithelia from subsequent injury. Because the concentrations of prostaglandins used were too low to act by inhibiting gastric acid secretion, the term "cytoprotection" was created. This field received substantial study because it promised to unlock the secrets of how gut epithelial cells protect themselves from luminal threats such as H^+. However, cell injury in these early studies was largely judged by gross inspection of epithelial surfaces: without cytoprotection, hemorrhagic lesions were formed, but similar lesions did not occur in cytoprotected mucosae. Subsequent microscopic studies have revealed that surface epithelial cells were often equally injured in control and "cytoprotected" mucosae.[61] A major difference between control and cytoprotected groups appears to be vascular: "cytoprotection" prevented extravasation of red blood cells from subepithelial vessels. It is also clear that cytoprotection may reduce the depth of mucosal necrosis in some models, and this ultimately may have some clinical importance. Further studies of this phenomenon may also yield insights into the process of cell extravasation from mucosal vessels and perhaps the regulation of vascular flow in the mucosa. However, it is unclear that studies of cytoprotection will offer the substantial insights, once promised, into how epithelial cells regulate their intracellular environment.

SUMMARY

The gut epithelial barrier, which restricts passive permeation, is complex and dynamic. Maintenance of this barrier in health depends on the integrity of cellular plasma membranes and tight junctions as well as the elaboration of epithelial secretory products such as HCO_3^-. Focal denudation of this barrier results in permeation by a host of threatening luminal compounds including antigens, proteases, H^+, and factors chemotactic for inflammatory cells. By initiating inflammation and thus acting on subepithelial tissues, such factors can further influence epithelial transport and barrier function. Repair of epithelial injury is also complex, and both restitution and enhanced epithelial cell proliferation are likely to play major roles. Future studies need to be directed at examining the molecular mechanisms whereby such barriers are maintained and repaired.

The reader is directed to Chapter 12, Salivary Secretion; Chapter 13, Gastric Secretion; Chapter 14, Secretion and Absorption: Small Intestine and Colon; Chapter 15, Pancreatic Secretion; Chapter 16, Bile Secretion; Chapter 53, Esophagus: Anatomy and Structural Anomalies; Chapter 59, Stomach: Anatomy and Structural Anomalies; Chapter 66, Small Intestine: Anatomy and Structural Anomalies; Chapter 76, Colon: Anatomy and Structural Anomalies; and Chapter 93, Gallbladder and Biliary Tree: Anatomy and Structural Anomalies.

REFERENCES

1. Mooseker MS. Actin binding proteins of the brush border. Cell 1983;35:11.
2. Lazarides E. Intermediate filaments as mechanical integrators of cellular space. Nature (Lond) 1980;283:249.
3. Pavelka M, Ellinger A, Gangl A. Effect of colchicine on rat small intestinal absorptive cells. J Ultrastruct Mol Struct Res 1983;85:249.
4. Behrens J, Birchmier W, Goodman SG, Imhof BA. Dissociation of MDCK epithelial cells by monoclonal antibody anti-arc-1. J Cell Biol 1985;101:1307.
5. Imhof BA, Vollmers HP, Goodman SL, Birchmeier W, et al. Cell–cell interaction and polarity of epithelial cells: Specific perturbation using a monoclonal antibody. Cell 1983;35:667.
6. Madara J. Loosening tight junctions: Lessons from the intestine. J Clin Invest 1989;83:1089.
6a. Henin S, Cremasch T, Schettino G, et al. Electrical parameters in gallbladders of different species: their contribution to the origin of the transmural potential difference. J Membr Biol 1977;34:73.
7. Elias PM, Friend DS. The permeability barrier in mammalian epidermis. J Cell Biol 1975;65:180.
8. Bennett MVL, Goodenough DA. Gap junctions, electrotonic coupling and intercellular communication. Neurosci Res Program Bull 1978;16:383.
9. Wan Y, Wu T, Chang AE, Damjanov I. Monoclonal antibodies to laminin reveal the heterogeneity of basement membranes in the developing and adult mouse tissues. J Cell Biol 1984;98:971.
10. Ekblom P, Vestweber D, Kemler R. Cell matrix interactions and cell adhesion during development. Annu Rev Cell Biol 1986;2:27.
11. Rothman J, Lenard J. Membrane asymmetry. Science 1977;195:743.
12. Adams JC, Watt FM. Fibronectin inhibits the terminal differentiation of human keratinocytes. Nature 1989;340:307.
13. Roa CN, Margulies MK, Tralka TS, Terranova VP, Madri JA, Liotta, LA. Isolation of a subunit of luminin and its role in molecular structure and tumor cell attachment. J Biol Chem 1982;257:9840.
14. Burridge K, Fath K, Kelly T, Nickolls G, Turner C. Focal adhesions: Transmembrane junctions between the extracellular matrix and the cytoskeleton. Annu Rev Cell Biol 1988;4:487.
15. Neutra MR, Forstner JF. Gastrointestinal mucous: Synthesis, secretion and function. In: Johnson L, ed. Gastrointestinal physiology. New York:Raven Press, 1987:995.
16. Williams SE, Turnberg LA. Retardation of acid diffusion by pig gastric mucus: A potential role in mucosal protection. Gastroenterology 1980;79:299.
17. Westergaard H, Dietschy JM. Delineation of the dimensions and permeability characteristics of two major diffusion barriers to passive mucosal uptake in the rabbit intestine. J Clin Invest 1974;54:718.
18. Anderson BW, Levine AS, Levitt DG, Keupe M, Levitt M. Physiological measurement of luminal stirring in the perfused rat jejunum. Am J Physiol 1988;254:G843.
19. Flemstrom G, Kivilaakso E. Demonstration of a pH gradient at the luminal surface of rat duodenum in vivo and its dependence on mucosal alkaline secretion. Gastroenterology 1983;84:787.
20. Mills BA, Butler BD, Lichtenberger LM. Gastric mucosal barrier: Hydrophobic lining to the lumen of the stomach. Am J Physiol 1983;244:G561.
21. Finkelstein A, Cass A. Permeability and electrical properties of thin lipid membranes. J Gen Physiol 1968;52:145S.
22. Finkelstein A. The water and nonelectrolyte permeability of lipid bilayer membranes. J Gen Physiol 1976;68:127.
23. Madara JL, Pappenheimer JR. Structural basis for physiological regulation of paracellular pathways in intestinal epithelia. J Membr Biol 1987;100:149.
24. Thompson TE, Huang C. Dynamics of lipids in biomembranes. In: Andreoli TE, ed. Physiology of membrane disorders. New York: Plenum, 1978:27.
25. Lingappa VR. Intracellular traffic of newly synthesized proteins. J Clin Invest 1989;83:739.
26. Riordan JR, Rommens JM, Kerem B, et al. Identification of the cystic fibrosis gene: Cloning and characterization of complementary DNA. Science 1989;245:1066.
27. Brasitus TA, Schachter D, Mamouneas TG. Functional interactions of lipids and proteins in rat intestinal microvillus membranes. Biochemistry 1979;18:4136.
28. Orlando RC, Turjman NA, Tobey NA. Mucosal protection by sucralfate and its components in acid-exposed rabbit esophagus. Gastroenterology 1987;93:352.

29. Rutten MJ, Ito S. Morphology and electrophysiology of guinea pig gastric mucosal repair in vitro. Am J Physiol 1983;244:G171.
30. Okada YA, Irimajiri A, Inouye A. Electrical properties and active solute transport in rat small intestine II. Conductive properties of transepithelial routes. J Membr Biol 1977;31:221.
31. Frizzell RA, Schultz SG. Ionic conductances of extracellular shunt pathway in rabbit ileum. J Gen Physiol 1972;59:318.
32. Schultz SG, Frizzell RA, Nellans HN. Active sodium transport and the electrophysiology of rabbit colon. J Membr Biol 1977;33:351.
33. Madara JL. Tight junction dynamics: Is paracellular transport regulated? Cell 1988;53:497.
34. Walker WA. Intestinal transport of macromolecules. In: Johnson LR, ed. Physiology of the gastrointestinal tract. New York:Raven Press, 1981:1271.
35. Pappenheimer JR, Reiss KZ. Contribution of solvent drag through intercellular junctions to absorption of nutrients by the small intestine of the rat. J Membr Biol 1987;100:123.
36. Schultz SG. The role of paracellular pathways in isotonic fluid transport. Yale J Biol Med 1977;50:99.
37. Capuro C, Escobar E, Ibarra C, Porta M, Parishi M. Water permeability in different epithelial barriers. Biol Cell 1989;66:145.
38. Spring KR, Ericson A-C. Epithelial cell volume modulation and regulation. J Membr Biol 1982;69:167.
39. Kedem O, Katchalsky A. A physical interpretation of the permeability of biological coefficients of membrane permeability. J Gen Physiol 1961;45:143.
40. Alpers DH. The relation of size to the relative rates of degradation of intestinal brush border proteins. J Clin Invest 1972;51:2621.
41. McNeil PL, Ito S. Gastrointestinal cell plasma membrane wounding and healing in vivo. Gastroenterology 1989;96:1238.
42. Menzies IS, Lakar MF, Pounds R, et al. Abnormal intestinal permeability to sugars in villous atrophy. Lancet 1979;2:1107.
43. Hollander D, Vadhiem CM, Brettholtz E, Petersen GM, Delahunty TJ, Rotter JI. Increased intestinal permeability in patients with Crohn's disease and their relatives. Ann Intern Med 1986;105:883.
43a. Atisook K, Carlson G, Madara JL. Effects of phlorizin and sodium on glucose-elicited alterations of cell junctions in intestinal epithelia. Am J Physiol 1990;258:C77.
44. Holdsworth CD, Dawson AM. The absorption of monosaccharides in man. Clin Sci 1964;27:371.
45. Gilbert DA, Surawicz CM, Silverstein FE, et al. Prevention of acute aspirin-induced gastric mucosal injury by 15-R-15 methyl prostaglandin E$_2$. Gastroenterology 1984;86:339.
46. Kimberg DV, Field M, Johnson J, Henderson A, Gershon E. Stimulation of intestinal mucosal adenyl cyclase by cholera toxin and prostaglandins. J Clin Invest 1971;50:1218.
47. Lawson LD, Powell DW. Bradykinin-stimulated eicosanoid synthesis and secretion by rabbit ileal components. Am J Physiol 1987;252: G783.
48. Costa M, Furness JB, Llewellyn-Smith IJ. Histochemistry of the enteric nervous system. In: Johnson LR, ed. Physiology of the gastrointestinal tract, ed 2. New York:Raven Press, 1987:1.
49. Yardley JH. Pathology of idiopathic inflammatory bowel disease and relevance of specific cell findings: An overview. In: Recent developments in therapy of bowel disease. Myerhoff Center for Digestive Diseases at Johns Hopkins, Baltimore, 1986:3.
50. Trier H, Rytomaa T, Cederberg A, Kiviniemi K. Studies on the elimination of granulocytes in the intestinal tract of rat. Acta Pathol Microbiol Scand 1963;59:311.
51. Nash S, Stafford J, Madara JL. Effects of PMN transmigration on the barrier function of cultured intestinal epithelial monolayers. J Clin Invest 1987;80:1104.
52. Johnson LR, Guthrie PD. Stimulation of rat oxyntic gland mucosal growth by EGF. Am J Physiol 1980;238:645.
53. Konturek SJ, Dembinski A, Warzecha Z, Brzozowski T, Gregory H. Role of EGF in healing chronic gastroduodenal ulcers in rats. Gastroenterology 1988;94:1300.
54. Beauchamp RD, Barnard JA, McCutcheon CM, Cherner JA, Coffey RJ. Localization of TGF and its receptor in gastric mucosal cells. J Clin Invest 1989;84:1017.
55. Johnson LR. Regulation of gastrointestinal growth. In: Johnson LR, ed. Physiology of the gastrointestinal tract, ed 2. New York:Raven Press, 1987:301.
56. Svanes K, Ito S, Takeuchi K, Silen W. Restitution of the surface epithelium of the in vitro frog gastric mucosa after damage with hyperosmolar sodium chloride. Gastroenterology 1982;82:1409.
57. Colvin RB. Fibronectin in wound healing. In: Mosler DF, ed. Fibronectin. New York:Academic Press, 1987.
58. Alvarez OM. Pharmacological and environmental modulation of wound healing. In: Uitto J, Perejda AJ, eds. Connective tissue disease: Molecular pathology of the extracellular matrix. New York:Marcel Dekker, 1986:367.
59. Moore R, Carlson S, Madara JL. Villus contraction aids repair of intestinal epithelium after injury. Am J Physiol 1989;257:G274.
60. Silen W. What is cytoprotection of the gastric mucosa. Gastroenterology 1988;94:232.
61. Lacy ER, Ito S. Microscopic analysis of ethanol damage to rat gastric mucosa after treatment with a prostaglandin. Gastroenterology 1982;83:619.

B. MOTILITY

7

Esophageal Motor Function

PIERO BIANCANI
JOSE BEHAR

The esophagus is responsible for transporting food from the mouth to the stomach, preventing retrograde movement of esophageal or gastric contents, which may result in reflux of gastric secretions or regurgitation of food. It is a hollow tube closed at both ends by the upper esophageal sphincter (UES) and the lower esophageal sphincter (LES). Its lumen is lined with squamous mucosa, containing longitudinally oriented muscle fibers, and connected to the muscularis propria by a loose network of connective tissue fibers (submucosa). The muscularis propria consists of an inner circular muscle layer, with fibers oriented along the circumference of the tube, and an outer longitudinal layer, with fibers oriented along its axis. The pharynx and proximal esophagus contain striated muscle controlled entirely by the swallowing center, located in the brain stem, through the vagus nerves. The control mechanisms for the lower two thirds of the esophagus, which contain smooth muscle, are quite different from the striated portion. In the smooth muscle portion of the esophagus, peristalsis is controlled primarily by intrinsic neural networks located between the longitudinal and circular muscle layers (Auerbach's plexus) and in the submucosa (Meissner's plexus) and only modulated by central mechanisms in the swallowing center. However, myogenic factors may also play a role in peristalsis. Deglutition is the normal stimulus that initiates pharyngoesophageal motor activity and results in propulsion of the bolus from the pharynx to the stomach. Because of the high speed of contraction in the pharynx, deglutition has been studied by cinefluoroscopy, manometry, and combinations of both methods, whereas esophageal contractions, being slower, have been studied mainly by manometry alone.[1-3]

The major function of the esophagus is to serve as a conduit between the pharynx and the stomach. In humans and most mammals, the esophagus propels its contents in a caudad direction but only behaves as a passive conduit when orad transport occurs.[4,5] Esophageal function is complicated by the fact that the airways and digestive tract cross in the pharynx, and their respective contents must be kept separate. This requires precise control and coordination of swallowing and respiration, regulated by a rich innervation of pharyngeal muscles.[6,7]

Initiation of swallowing is voluntary, but continuation is reflexly mediated by sensory neurons with input to the swallowing center.

In preparation for swallowing, the bolus is gathered on the tongue and confined to the oral cavity by apposition of the soft palate to the posterior portion of the tongue. The voluntary portion of swallowing consists of closing the mouth and pressing the tip of the tongue against the palate while a progressive wave of contraction travels through the body of the tongue that squeezes the bolus toward the pharynx. Then follows a series of involuntary events consisting of transient suppression of respiration, during which the bolus slides to the base of the tongue and is pushed by the tongue toward the oropharynx, which is elevated and forced open. Posterior thrust of the tongue propels the bolus into the pharynx. The descending wave of pharyngeal peristalsis begins and continues through the open UES. A rapid series of events occur in the pharynx, namely, closure of the velopharyngeus to prevent reflux into the nose, closure of the larynx to prevent aspiration, pharyngeal peristalsis to clear the bolus out of the pharynx, and displacement of the larynx upward and forward to move out of the path of the bolus and to force open the cricopharyngeal region and the UES.[2]

Relaxation of the UES occurs immediately, almost simultaneously with the initiation of swallows, and has a very brief duration. The bolus is forcefully injected into the esophagus through the opened UES. A primary peristaltic wave is initiated in the pharynx and continues into the upper portion of the cervical esophagus. As the bolus enters into the body of the esophagus in upright subjects, it descends by gravity and is propelled by peristalsis. The relative contribution of gravity and peristalsis depends on bolus consistency. In the upright position, liquids travel faster by gravity than the peristaltic contraction that follows the swallow. In fact, liquids travel fast enough to impact on the closed LES. Once the peristaltic wave reaches the liquid bolus, the LES is opened and the bolus is pushed through the sphincter. Sometimes small amounts of fluid may remain in the distal esophagus behind the peristaltic wave. This may require a second contraction, unrelated to swallowing and originated by local esophageal distention (secondary peristalsis), to completely clear the esophagus. Solid boluses, on the other, hand are propelled by peristalsis even in the upright position, but their movement is helped by gravity. Progression of the bolus, however, does not outstrip peristalsis; the

---

119

bolus and the peristaltic wave move through the esophagus at the same speed. The bolus, propelled by the peristaltic contraction, forces the opening of the relaxed LES.

Since gastric contents are damaging to the esophageal squamous epithelium, esophageal function must be designed so that one-way flow of nutrients occurs, preventing reflux, except for occasional events such as vomiting or belching. The presence of tonic contraction in the UES and LES prevents or minimizes gastroesophageal reflux or esophagopharyngeal regurgitation. However, if gastroesophageal reflux occurs, the refluxed material is cleared by secondary peristalsis triggered by localized distention of the esophagus.

ANATOMY

Muscular Anatomy (Fig 7-1)

PHARYNX

The pharynx, connecting nose and mouth on the proximal end, to the esophagus and trachea on the distal end, is responsible for separating food and air as they go through this area. This requires fine motor control and is reflected by the complexity of this structure. The pharynx is a hollow cylinder, 12 to 14 cm long, extending from the base of the skull to the lower border of the cricoid cartilage and bordering posteriorly on the cervical spine. It consists of several distinct muscle groups and in its lower portion is supported anteriorly by several cartilages (arytenoid, cuneiform, corniculate, and cricoid). Traditionally, the pharynx has been divided into three segments:

1. The *nasopharynx* extends from the base of the skull, behind the soft palate, to the distal edge of the soft palate and is not part of the alimentary tract. Muscles located in the nasopharynx, however, contribute to elevating the soft palate and closing the nasopharyngeal passage during swallowing, thus preventing bolus entry into the nasal passage.
2. The *oropharynx* extends from the soft palate above to the base of the tongue and the level of the hyoid bone below and contains the upper border of the epiglottis, or the valleculae. In this area the respiratory and gastrointestinal tracts cross.
3. The *hypopharynx* extends from the valleculae at the base of the tongue to the lower border of the cricoid cartilage and contains the UES.

Muscle groups participating in deglutition are those of the soft palate, pharyngeal isthmus, tongue, hyoid bone, pharyngeal constrictors, and the muscles that elevate and displace the pharynx in a forward direction. They may be classified as *extrinsic* muscles, responsible for altering the shape of the pharynx and closing the airways, and *intrinsic* muscles, responsible for collapsing the lumen of the pharynx and propelling the bolus. The extrinsic muscles levator veli palatini, tensor veli palatini, palatoglossus, and others are located in the nasopharynx; together with the palatopharyngeus they raise and tense the soft palate and uvula and close the nasal

passage, preventing pressure generated in the mouth from being dissipated through the nose. When selective paralysis of these muscle occurs, as in poliomyelitis, the bolus is sometimes pushed into the nasopharynx.[8] The stylohyoid, styloglossus, palatopharyngeus, stylopharyngeus, digastric posterior, and other muscles located posteriorly cause elevation, while the geniohyoid, mylohyoid, digastric anterior, thyrohyoid, and other muscles located anteriorly cause forward displacement of the larynx and pharynx and contribute to opening the UES. Activation of these groups of muscles causes negative pressure to develop in the hypopharynx. The combination of the negative pressure in front of the bolus and positive pressure, caused by the tongue, palate, and proximal pharynx, in back of the bolus imparts to it a powerful forward movement,[3] resulting in high speed of injection of the bolus into the esophagus.[9] Based on evidence obtained from simultaneous pressure measurements and cinefluorography, it has been suggested that tongue driving pressure and the negative pressure generated in the pharyngoesophageal segment contribute significantly to the bolus driving force. When these components are absent or reduced in patients with tongue impairment or with laryngectomy, the transit of a food bolus is impaired.[3] When swallowing occurs, the thyroarytenoid, aryepiglottic, oblique arytenoid, and other muscles close the larynx, preventing food from entering the trachea.

The intrinsic muscles are the superior, middle, and inferior pharyngeal constrictors. These muscles overlap like tiles on a roof and insert into a collagenous sheet, the buccopharyngeal aponeurosis. In the upper pharynx this structure is attached to the prevertebral fascia by a median raphe, but distally the constrictors are vertically mobile in relation to the prevertebral fascia. This allows considerable axial movement during swallowing.[10] The inferior pharyngeal constrictor has two anatomic components: the thyropharyngeus, extending posteriorly from the thyroid cartilages and overlapping the middle constrictor, and the cricopharyngeus. The cricopharyngeus consists of a horizontal muscle loop surrounding the esophageal inlet and thus constituting part of the UES, and an oblique component on the posterior and proximal portion of the cricopharyngeus attaching to the median raphe. This arrangement creates a thin triangular area in the posterior aspect of the hypopharynx, which is called Killian's triangle. This area is structurally weak and likely to fail, producing outpouching of the mucosa through the muscular layer, called Zenker's diverticulum.[11] The term *cricopharyngeus muscle* commonly refers to the horizontal portion of the cricopharyngeus. The UES consists of the horizontal cricopharyngeus muscle and portions of the inferior constrictor. The sphincter is thus part of the pharynx. Some evidence suggests that muscles of the proximal esophagus do not contribute to UES function.[6,12]

UPPER ESOPHAGEAL SPHINCTER

The UES is functionally defined as a high-pressure zone, 2 to 4 cm wide, separating the pharynx from the body of the esophagus. There is some uncertainty about the muscles responsible for maintaining the high pressure, since the width of the horizontal cricopharyngeus accounts for only 1 to 1.5 cm of the UES. However, it appears that the UES high-pressure zone encompasses the cartilaginous hypopharynx, including the cricoid cartilage ante-

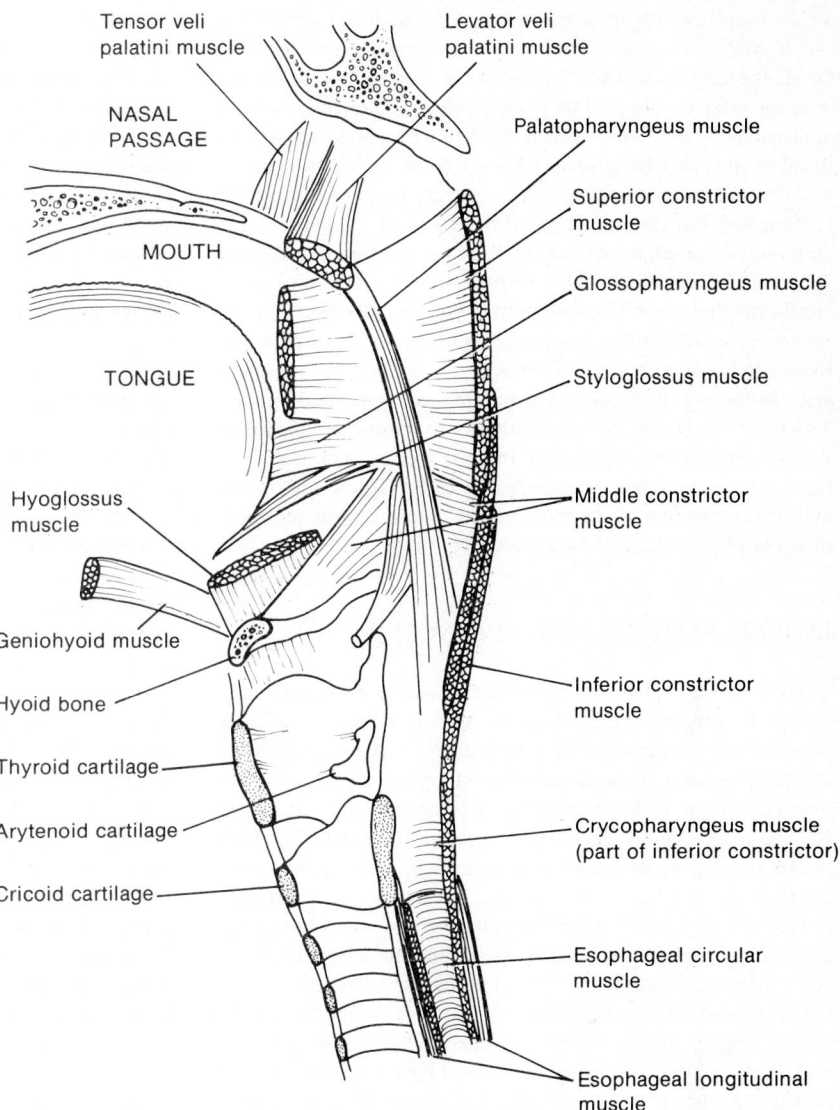

FIGURE 7–1. The pharynx comprises several distinct muscle groups, and in its lower portion it is supported anteriorly by several cartilages (arytenoid, cuneiform, corniculate and cricoid). Traditionally, the pharynx has been divided into three segments: (1) The nasopharynx, extending from the base of the skull, behind the soft palate, to the distal edge of the soft palate, is not part of the alimentary tract. Muscles located in the nasopharynx, such as the tensor veli palatini, levator veli palatini, and others, contribute to elevating the soft palate and closing the nasopharyngeal passage during swallowing, thus preventing bolus entry into the nasal passage. (2) The oropharynx extends from the soft palate above to the base of the tongue and the level of the hyoid bone below and contains the upper border of the epiglottis, or the valleculae. In this area the respiratory and gastrointestinal tracts cross. Muscles present in the orpharynx are responsible for bolus propulsion (middle constrictor and others) and for elevation (palatopharyngeus and others) and forward displacement (geniohyoid and others) of the pharynx. The hypopharynx extends from the valleculae at the base of the tongue to the lower border of the cricoid cartilage and contains the inferior constrictor muscle and the upper esophageal sphincter.

riorly and the cricopharyngeus and other components of the inferior pharyngeal constrictor. This conclusion is based on the following evidence: (1) The high-pressure zone extends from the laryngeal opening to the lower border of the cricoid cartilage, and thus the hypopharynx, including the oblique and horizontal fibers of the cricopharyngeus muscle, can account for the sphincter without including portions of the upper esophagus.[13] (2) In humans the area from the laryngeal opening (marked by the bottom of the air column on lateral radiographs of the pharynx) to the lower border of the cricoid cartilage is 3 to 3.5 cm, of which 0.5 to 1 cm is occupied by the arytenoid and interarytenoid muscles. The cricoid lamina extends an additional 2.5 cm distally, with the horizontal component of the cricopharyngeus overlapping the distal third of the cartilage. Thus, it appears that the hypopharynx together with the oblique and horizontal fibers of the cricopharyngeus muscle can account for the high-pressure zone present at the UES.[1,13–15] (3) Data obtained in experimental animals show good correlation between intraluminal pressure and electromyographic activity in the cricopharyngeus and inferior pharyngeal constrictor.[12]

ESOPHAGUS

The body of the esophagus is 18 to 25 cm in length, extending from the inferior border on the UES to the upper border of the LES. The length of the esophagus correlates with the subject's height and is generally longer in males than in females. It has a longitudinally oriented muscle layer in the muscularis mucosae and two muscle layers in the muscularis propria, the inner one oriented along the circumference (circular layer) and the outer one along the axis (longitudinal layer).

While the muscle in the muscularis mucosae is longitudinally oriented and smooth throughout the whole length of the esophagus, the muscularis propria is composed of striated muscle in the most proximal portion. Esophageal striated muscle has different histologic characteristics from other striated muscles. These differences include the type of motor innervation and end plates, the arrangement of the muscle fibers,[16–18] fiber diameter, and type of myosin adenosine triphosphatase.[19]

It is generally accepted that the junctional area between the striated and smooth muscle occurs in the middle third of the esophagus.[20] Data suggest that on the average the proximal 4.1 cm of the circular and the 5.1 cm of the longitudinal layers are entirely striated muscle. The point at which the circular layer is approximately half smooth and half striated muscle occurs 4.7 cm distal to the cricopharyngeus.[21] A 4- to 8-cm transition area (or middle third of the esophagus) has varying proportions of both striated and smooth muscle; the distal 10 to 14 cm consists exclusively of smooth muscle whose fibers are oriented in a circular or an elliptical direction.[22] This distribution is typical of the human esophagus, but there are considerable species differences in the relative proportions of striated and smooth muscle. A distribution similar to humans occurs in other primates, the cat, and the opossum. In the pig the esophagus is predominantly striated muscle, with a very short smooth muscle portion. In the dog and the sheep the esophagus is entirely striated. In some species, such as the rat, the striated muscle portion includes the LES.[23] Knowledge of the muscle composition of the esophagus is crucial for the interpretation of physiologic and pathophysiologic data.

LOWER ESOPHAGEAL SPHINCTER

There is some controversy about the existence of an anatomic sphincter distinct from the body of the esophagus. Human autopsies have shown an asymmetric thickened ringlike structure that angles obliquely upward from the lesser to the greater gastric curvature. The length of the thickened area along the lesser curvature is 2.3 cm, and it is 3.1 cm along the greater curvature. The LES proper is made up of complete muscle rings. Distally, however, the rings are split into two segments, one straddling the greater curvature and parallel to the sling fibers of the stomach and the other consisting of short "clasps" straddling the lesser curvature and connecting at an angle to the sling fibers.[24] The squamocolumnar junction is present within this structure. In similar studies on the esophagogastric junction of cats a clear correlation was found between the manometrically defined high-pressure zone and the thicker segment of circular muscle, with the squamocolumnar junction slightly distal to the high-pressure point.[25] The thickness of the circular muscle increases from the esophagus toward the LES, peaks at the in vivo high-pressure zone, and then decreases toward the stomach.

Electron microscopic studies reveal that the sarcolemma of the LES muscle has a greater number of evaginations than that of the esophageal muscle.[26,27] It is unclear, however, whether this morphologic feature has functional significance or whether it merely results from the tonically contracted state of the muscle. The LES muscle also contains more abundant mitochondria and a more developed endoplasmic reticulum than circular muscle from the esophageal body.[27]

Neural Anatomy

The esophagus has a rich network of intrinsic neurons in the submucosa (Meissner's plexus) and between the circular and longitudinal muscle layers (Auerbach's plexus). This network of enteric neurons is capable of producing secondary peristalsis in the smooth muscle portion even when the esophagus is separated from the central nervous system and isolated in an organ bath.[28] The enteric network receives instruction from, and sends signals to, the central nervous system via the vagi, adrenergic ganglia in the thoracic sympathetic chain, and the celiac ganglia.

The central regulation of the pharynx, esophagus, and LES arises from neurons located in the brain stem. The motor innervation includes somatic nerves supplying the striated muscle and autonomic nerves innervating the smooth muscle. The cell bodies of somatic motor nerves are located in the nucleus retrofacialis and the rostral portion of the nucleus ambiguus. Some of these nerves accompany the vagus, and others branch out into the pharyngeal nerve at the level of the nodose ganglion.[29-33] They end at the motor end plate of the striated muscle fibers. The transmitter released by these neurons is acetylcholine, acting through nicotinic cholinergic receptors in the end plate of the striated muscle fibers.[13] The somatic motor nerves supplying the pharyngeal muscles, including the UES, accompany the vagus nerve and branch out into the pharyngeal nerve at the level of the nodose ganglion. The majority of the nerves supplying esophageal striated muscle originate from the vagus nerve in the upper cervical region, but some are also found in the recurrent laryngeal nerve. These fibers are unmyelinated in their terminal portions.[17,34]

The autonomic parasympathetic preganglionic neurons innervating the smooth muscle of the esophagus and LES originate in the dorsal motor nucleus of the vagus nerve and in the nucleus ambiguus.[30,35,36] Their axons are carried in the vagus nerves, branch into the esophageal plexus, surrounding the body of the esophagus, and enter the esophagus at various levels. They travel within the esophageal body for some distance before synapsing on postganglionic neurons in the enteric esophageal plexuses.

The autonomic preganglionic sympathetic neurons originate in the intermediolateral columns of the spinal cord (segments T1–T10) and their preganglionic fibers enter the cervical, thoracic, and, possibly, celiac ganglia. Most preganglionic fibers pass through the greater splanchnic nerves and terminate in the celiac ganglia and then synapse with postganglionic neurons.[36,37] The majority of postganglionic axons originate in the celiac ganglia or reach the esophagus by way of perivascular fibers. Most postganglionic axons synapse in the myenteric or in the submucosal plexus, and very few innervate the smooth muscle directly.[13,37]

The intramural neurons are arranged in two networks, one between the circular and longitudinal muscle layers (Auerbach's or myenteric plexus) and the other between the circular layer and the submucosa (Meissner's or submucosal plexus). The myenteric plexus extends into the striated muscle of the esophagus,[17] and since muscle fibers in this portion of the esophagus receive direct motor input from extrinsic neurons, the function of the plexus is unclear. Perhaps the enteric neurons of this region may provide sensory output or may innervate esophageal glands.[13]

As in the rest of the gut, Auerbach's and Meissner's plexuses consist of a variety of interconnected neurons, capable of maintaining peristaltic function even in the absence of extrinsic input. At the turn of the century Bayliss and Starling[38-40] described descending relaxation in the intestine, which persisted when the intestine was extrinsically denervated by resecting vagal and mesenteric fibers. Langley and Magnus[41] reported that this reflex was maintained in vitro, in the absence of any extrinsic innervation. Based on this evidence the intrinsic neurons were believed to constitute a separate "enteric" division of the autonomic nervous system. Recently, it has become apparent that this enteric network is composed of a variety of neural cells containing numerous neuropeptides, which are also found in the brain. Peptides present in esophageal and LES neurons include vasoactive peptide (VIP),[42–46] neuropeptide Y, which is often present in neurons containing either VIP or catecholamines,[46,47] calcitonin gene-related peptide (CGRP),[48] substance P,[49,50] which is often present together with enkephalins,[51] and galanin.[52,53] This "brain–gut axis" is the equivalent of two computers connected by way of sympathetic and parasympathetic links but capable of processing signals independently of each other.

Sensory neurons from the entire esophagus run in the vagus nerve. In the lower esophagus they are also found in the splanchnic and thoracic sympathetic neurons. The cell bodies of the vagal fibers reside in the nodose ganglion, while those of the sympathetic fibers are found in the vertebral ganglia of the thoracolumbar region. CGRP has been found in esophageal sensory neurons, while other sensory neurons may contain acetylcholine or substance P.[48,50,54,55] Mechanoreceptors and thermoreceptors are present in the esophagus and LES.[13]

ESOPHAGEAL FUNCTIONS

Peristaltic (Propulsive) Function

OROPHARYNGEAL COMPONENTS (FIG 7-2)

Initiation of swallowing is voluntary, but continuation of swallowing is reflexly mediated by sensory neurons with input to the swallowing center located in the brain stem. In preparation for swallowing, a bolus of ingesta is first gathered on the tongue and confined to the oral cavity by apposition of the soft palate to the posterior portion of the tongue. With the mouth closed and the tip of the tongue pressed against the palate, a propulsive force travels through the body of the tongue and pushes the bolus toward the pharynx. This process is followed by transient suppression of respiration while the bolus slides on the base of the tongue and is pushed by the tongue toward the oropharynx, which is elevated and forced open by its anterior and posterior extrinsic muscles. Posterior thrust of the tongue propels the bolus into the pharynx with an action resembling a piston sliding into a cylinder. The descending wave of pharyngeal peristalsis begins and continues through the open UES. Within 1 to 2 seconds, the velopharyngeus closes to prevent reflux into the nose, the larynx closes to prevent aspiration, pharyngeal peristalsis clears the bolus out of the pharynx, and the larynx is displaced upward and forward to move it out of the path of the bolus and to force open the cricopharyngeal region and the UES.[6]

UPPER ESOPHAGEAL SPHINCTER (FIG 7-3)

The UES, or pharyngoesophageal (PE) segment, maintains closure of the proximal end of the esophagus and constitutes a further barrier to refluxed materials entering the pharynx. It also prevents air from entering into the esophagus, since intraesophageal pressure during inspiration is lower than pharyngeal pressure. In humans the UES exhibits an asymmetric pressure profile longitudinally[56,57] and radially.[12,58,59] There is a sharp increase in its upper part and

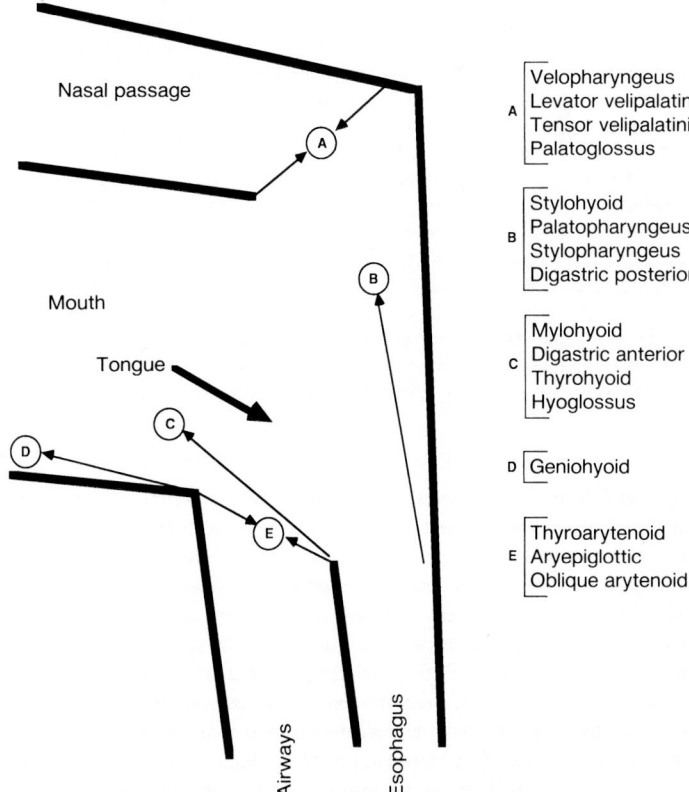

FIGURE 7–2. Muscle groups participating in deglutition may be classified as *extrinsic* muscles, responsible for altering the shape of the pharynx and closing the airways, and *intrinsic* muscles, responsible for collapsing the lumen of the pharynx and propelling the bolus. The extrinsic muscles levator veli palatini, tensor veli palatini, palatoglossus, and others are located in the nasopharynx; they raise and tense the soft palate and uvula and close the nasal passage, preventing pressure generated in the mouth from being dissipated through the nose. The stylohyoid, palatopharyngeus, stylopharyngeus, digastric posterior, and other muscles located posteriorly cause elevation, while the geniohyoid, mylohyoid, digastric anterior, thyrohyoid, and other muscles located anteriorly cause forward displacement of the larynx and pharynx and contribute to opening the upper esophageal sphincter. The thyroarytenoid, aryepiglottic, and oblique arytenoid muscles and others close the larynx, preventing food from entering the trachea. On swallowing, a rapid series of events occur in 1 to 2 seconds, namely closure of the velopharyngeus to prevent reflux into the nose, closure of the larynx to prevent aspiration, pharyngeal peristalsis to clear the bolus out of the pharynx, laryngeal upward and forward displacement to move the larynx out of the path of the bolus and to force open the cricopharyngeal region, and opening of the upper esophageal sphincter.[3,6,10,13]

Nasal passage

A — Velopharyngeus / Levator velipalatini / Tensor velipalatini / Palatoglossus

B — Stylohyoid / Palatopharyngeus / Stylopharyngeus / Digastric posterior

Mouth

Tongue

C — Mylohyoid / Digastric anterior / Thyrohyoid / Hyoglossus

D — Geniohyoid

E — Thyroarytenoid / Aryepiglottic / Oblique arytenoid

Airways

Esophagus

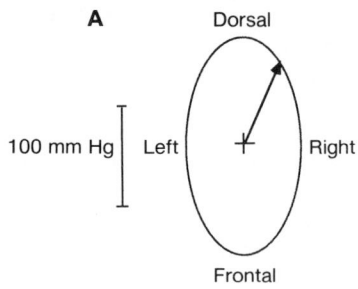

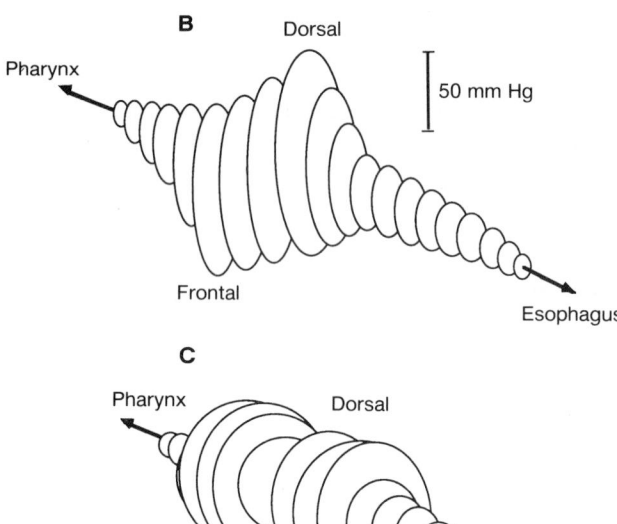

FIGURE 7–3. **A,** By using a multiple-pressure sensor oriented in different directions it is possible to measure pressure as a function of the radial orientation within the upper esophageal sphincter. In this sphincter pressure is highest in the frontal and dorsal direction and lowest in the lateral directions. **B,** As the probe is moved from the esophagus through the sphincter and into the pharynx a three-dimensional representation of the sphincter's pressure profile is obtained. In humans the upper esophageal sphincter exhibits an asymmetric pressure profile longitudinally and radially. The highest pressures occur in the anterior and posterior directions, the lowest occur laterally. Peak pressures occur at slightly different locations in the anterior and in the posterior direction. The highest peak in the frontal direction occurs orad to the highest peak in the dorsal direction. **C,** The asymmetry disappears in patients who have undergone laryngectomy, suggesting that it may be caused by squeezing of the esophagus against the laryngeal cartilages forming the anterior wall of the sphincter.[59]

a gradual decline in the lower part, and there is considerable radial asymmetry, with the highest pressures occurring in an anteroposterior direction and peak pressures occurring at slightly different locations in the anterior and in the posterior direction. In the anterior direction the peak pressure occurs 1 cm distal to the upper border of the high-pressure zone, while in the posterior direction it occurs 1 cm farther distally, that is, 2 cm distal to the upper border of the high-pressure zone.[59] The asymmetry disappears in patients who have undergone laryngectomy, suggesting that it may be caused by squeezing of the esophagus against the laryngeal cartilages forming the anterior wall of the sphincter.[59]

In normal subjects, different resting pressures have been recorded by different investigators[58–61] and by the same investigators using different techniques.[62] These resting pressures range between 40 and 100 mm Hg, with pressures in the lateral orientations being as low as 30% of the pressures in anterior or posterior orientations.

There has been controversy as to the exact anatomic components of the UES, and technical difficulties in obtaining accurate and reliable pressure measurements have contributed to this uncertainty. The sphincter relaxes rapidly and exhibits significant longitudinal excursions during swallowing, causing considerable confusion in the interpretation of pressure tracings obtained in awake subjects. In experimental animals, on the other hand, anesthesia affects the spike potentials associated with contraction of striated muscles. It is believed that the horizontal component of the cricopharyngeus participates in maintenance of the pressure barrier at the UES. This muscle, however, is approximately 1 cm wide, while the high-pressure zone spans 2 to 4 cm. Thus it is uncertain how pressure is generated in that portion of the high-pressure zone that extends beyond the limits of the cricopharyngeus.[12,13,59,63–67]

Elegant studies in the awake opossum[12] have shown that the cricopharyngeus and the inferior pharyngeal constrictor exhibit continuous electrical spike potentials, with firing frequency proportional to the resting tone present in the sphincter and relaxation occurring on abolition of the spike potential. The studies further noted that the abolition of spike potentials only reduced resting tone by half because some passive pressure was present as a result of the elasticity of the surrounding structures. Full relaxation occurred on contraction of the geniohyoid muscle, which caused forward displacement of the larynx and forced open the UES. There is no evidence to suggest that esophageal fibers distal to the cricopharyngeus are involved in maintenance of sphincter closure.

These findings have been confirmed in humans using a combination of videofluoroscopy and appropriate intraluminal manometry.[65] The high-pressure zone associated with the UES was found to span approximately 3 cm, but the width of the high-pressure zone with pressure greater than 25% of peak pressure averaged 1.6 cm, with its center located 1.1 cm distal to the vocal cords. On swallowing, the UES moved orad 2 to 3 cm, with extent of movement and opening size depending on the volume swallowed. Larger volumes are accommodated by greater axial excursions, wider opening, and prolonged opening interval. Peristaltic velocity in the pharynx, however, does not appear to be affected by bolus volume.

Deglutition evokes an almost immediate UES relaxation that briefly precedes pharyngeal contractions and within 2 seconds relaxes the LES. LES relaxation is observed as the peristaltic contraction appears within the mid-third of the esophagus.[68] The UES relaxes briefly (less than 1 second) and fully to pharyngeal or atmospheric pressures.

ESOPHAGEAL BODY (FIG 7-4)

Cinefluoroscopic studies of barium swallows have demonstrated that as an ingested bolus enters into the body of the esophagus it travels by gravity or peristaltic propulsion depending on its consistency. Liquids travel by gravity when a subject is in the upright position, faster than the peristaltic wave that follows. In fact, liquids

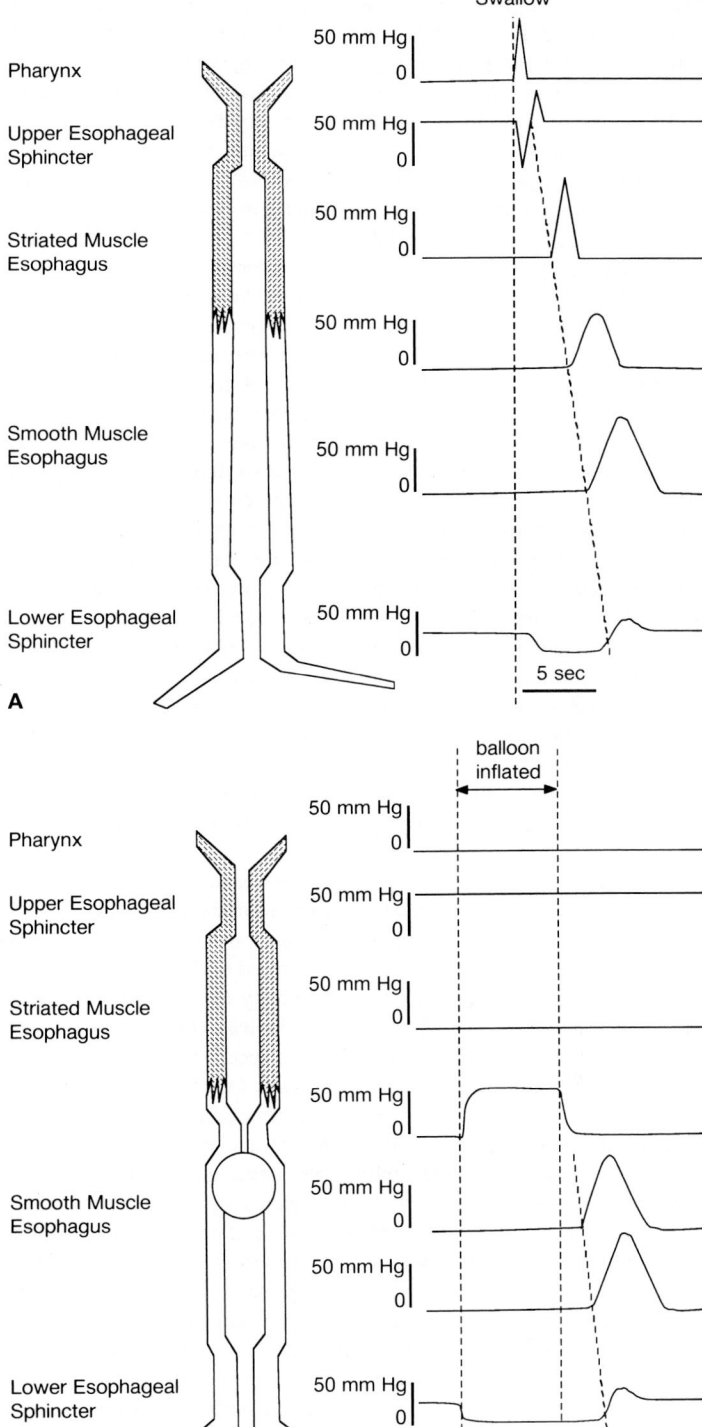

FIGURE 7–4. **A,** At rest the normal esophagus is quiescent without any spontaneous contractions while the sphincters are tonically contracted. Swallows trigger relaxation of the upper and lower esophageal sphincters and give rise to a peristaltic contraction. Each location along the esophageal axis contracts with latency that increases gradually from the upper esophagus to the lower esophageal sphincter. In the upper third of the esophagus contraction occurs within 1 to 2 seconds after swallowing; in the middle third, within 3 to 5 seconds; and in the lower third, between 5 and 8 seconds. The velocity of the peristaltic wave is slower in the striated muscle and faster in the smooth muscle segments of the esophagus. Contractions reach the smooth muscle segment within 2 seconds after the onset of the swallow, traveling at a speed of about 3 cm/sec; in the smooth muscle segment the velocity of propagation may be as fast as 5 cm/ sec. The contractions in the striated muscle segment are shorter (1–2 seconds), whereas in the smooth muscle segment they are of longer duration (4–7 seconds). Contractions in the distal one third of the esophagus are usually stronger (50 to 150 mm Hg) than those in the upper third (40 to 120 mm Hg), and both are stronger than those in the middle third (20 to 80 mm Hg), where they are relatively weak, probably occurring at the transition between the striated and smooth muscle esophagus. **B,** A similar sequence occurs in the smooth muscle esophagus during secondary peristalsis, which occurs when a bolus remains in the esophagus after ineffective primary peristalsis or when gastric contents reflux into the esophagus. Secondary peristalsis is believed to be caused by distention and can be demonstrated by inflating a balloon in the esophagus. On inflation, the esophagus contracts proximally to the balloon and relaxes distally, including the lower esophageal sphincter. This reflex was first discovered in the gut by Bayliss and Starling at the turn of the century. When the balloon is deflated peristalsis proceeds down the esophagus.

fall fast enough (within 2 seconds) to find the LES closed, causing distention of the distal esophagus and creating the radiologic appearance of the phrenic ampulla. Once the peristaltic contraction reaches the liquid bolus, it pushes the bolus through the relaxed LES. In a subject in the supine position the column of barium travels just ahead of the peristaltic wave. Small amounts of fluid may remain in the distal esophagus after the peristaltic wave.

Esophageal manometry shows that at rest the normal esophagus is quiescent without any spontaneous contractions, while the sphincters are tonically contracted. Resting pressure in the esophagus is therefore an approximate reflection of thoracic negative pleural pressures. These pressures vary, with the respiratory cycle becoming more negative during inspiration. Occasionally a 1- to 3-cm long high-pressure zone is present in mid-esophagus resulting from extrinsic compression by a vascular structure, possibly the aorta. Swallows trigger peristaltic contractions traveling along the entire length of the esophagus. Each location along the esophageal axis contracts with latency, which increases gradually from the upper esophagus to the LES. The latencies are site dependent and reproducible, constituting the esophageal gradient. In the upper third of the esophagus, contraction occurs within 1 to 2 seconds after swallowing; in the middle third, within 3 to 5 seconds; and in the lower third, between 5 and 8 seconds.

Complete propagation of the peristaltic contraction takes place after a swallow if a second swallow does not occur within at least 10 seconds after the first one. The complete peristaltic sequence is inhibited if a second swallow occurs within 8 seconds or less; a contraction may appear in the upper third of the esophagus (striated muscle) since it may occur before the second swallow is taken, but the peristaltic sequence is always inhibited in the lower two thirds of the esophagus.[69] After repeated swallows at short intervals, no contractions are observed in the entire esophagus until after the last swallow, which is followed by a high-amplitude contraction.[70] The inhibition of peristalsis by repeated swallows has been called "deglutitive inhibition." Deglutitive inhibition maintains the esophagus atonic during beer guzzling, which is performed by taking repeated swallows at very short intervals. The second swallow affects the motor response to the first; the first swallow, however, may also impair the response to the second if the two swallows are taken at short intervals.[71] Weak swallows may not evoke a full esophageal response; they may induce LES relaxation without esophageal contractions.[72] Occasionally, even in normal subjects, deglutition may evoke simultaneous contractions, occurring within a 5- to 10-cm segment.

The velocity of the peristaltic wave is slower in the striated muscle and faster in the smooth muscle segments of the esophagus. Contractions reach the smooth muscle segment within 2 seconds after the onset of the swallow, traveling at a speed of about 3 cm/sec. In the smooth muscle segment the velocity of propagation may be as fast as 5 cm/sec. Motility studies indicate that the size and viscosity of an ingested bolus affects the speed and force of the esophageal contractions. Increasing the size of the bolus slows its velocity and increases the force of the contractions Increased viscosity also increases the force of contraction and and decreases the speed of peristalsis.[73,74] Peristalsis is also affected by the temperature of the bolus, with warm boluses increasing its velocity and cold boluses reducing it.[75] Each contraction is preceded by a slight fall in pressure,[76] probably related to alterations in the respiratory pattern during swallowing. Then, pressures rise rapidly, usually peaking within 1 to 2 seconds from the onset of the contraction. Normal esophageal contractions have spikelike configurations, particularly in the striated muscle segment of the esophagus (upper third), but occasionally they may be biphasic in shape. The configuration of the pressure wave may vary depending whether the ingested bolus is liquid or solid, but it usually exhibits an initial hump or plateau before rising rapidly. The initial pressure change may simply reflect the pressure created in the esophagus by the presence of the bolus preceding the peristaltic wave. Motility studies with dry swallows reveal that the contractions in the striated muscle segment are shorter (1 to 2 seconds), whereas in the smooth muscle segment they are of longer (4 to 7 seconds) duration. Contractions in the distal one third of the esophagus are usually stronger (50 to 150 mm Hg) than those in the upper third (40 to 120 mm Hg), and both are stronger than those in the middle third

(20 to 80 mm Hg), where they are relatively weak, perhaps because of the transition between striated and smooth muscle esophagus. The force of the contractions can vary from segment to segment and even from swallow to swallow.[77]

LOWER ESOPHAGEAL SPHINCTER

At rest the LES is tonically contracted. The contraction is maintained by muscular mechanisms, even in the absence of neural input.[78,79] Passage of an ingested bolus is expedited by LES relaxation and by the force of peristaltic contractions. LES resistance to bolus transit is initially (within the first 2 seconds) caused by resting LES pressures. As the LES relaxes, it is passively forced open by the bolus, which has been propelled by the peristaltic wave. Although accurate measurements are difficult because of motion artifacts due to longitudinal esophageal movement during swallowing, it is estimated that the LES relaxes fully. LES relaxation occurs within 2 seconds of deglutition, at a time when the peristaltic wave appears in the mid-esophagus, that is, at the beginning of the smooth muscle segment. Within 1 second LES pressures fall to equal those of either the stomach or esophagus, depending on the location of the pressure sensor within the LES. Thus, when ingested boluses reach the LES, it is relaxed but closed. The bolus forces the LES open either with its own weight or with the aid of the peristaltic contraction. Deglutition induces an initial inhibition of the entire smooth muscle of the esophagus, and LES relaxation is part of this inhibitory response. After 5 to 7 seconds the LES recovers its initial pressure and then undergoes an aftercontraction. This contraction probably represents the end of the peristaltic pressure wave as it reaches the distal end of the esophagus. Circular muscle strips obtained from the LES exhibit relaxation only, whereas more proximal strips reveal relaxation followed by an aftercontraction, perhaps due to the presence of mixed LES and esophageal muscle fibers.[25]

Antireflux Function

In addition to propelling the bolus in a caudad direction, a second major function of the esophagus is to prevent or minimize retrograde movement of esophageal or gastric contents, which may result in reflux of gastric secretions or regurgitation of food. The esophagus accomplishes this function by creating an effective barrier consisting of a 3- to 5-cm long high-pressure zone at the LES that effectively separates the esophagus from the stomach. The junction is sealed by the LES circular muscle, which squeezes the mucosal folds together. The pressure in this segment ranges from 12 to 30 mm Hg above gastric pressures and exhibits radial and axial asymmetry, with highest pressures being present at the point of respiratory reversal,[80] where the esophagus crosses the diaphragm. This point separates the thoracic esophagus, where respiratory excursions decrease pressure with inspiration, from the abdominal esophagus, where pressures increase with inspiration, owing to compression of abdominal contents by the descending diaphragm.

Although LES pressures are affected by respiratory excursions, mid- or end-expiratory pressures are usually taken to be measures of LES strength. It is not well known whether the effectiveness of LES antireflux function depends on the amplitude of the pressures generated, on the length of the pressure barrier, or on combinations of these factors.[80-82] The accuracy of LES pressure measurement is also affected by changes in position, fasting, and time elapsed since the last meal. For instance, LES pressure transiently increases during phase III of the migrating myoelectric complex.[83] The composition of a meal may affect LES pressure. Fatty meals decrease LES pressure, whereas protein meals increase it.[84] The LES also has the ability to respond to increased intragastric pressure with a corresponding increase to prevent reflux. The ratio of LES to gastric pressure increases varies from 1.5 to 1.8, preventing the creation of a retrograde gastroesophageal pressure gradient. LES pressure increases occur almost simultaneously with increased gastric pressures and cholinergic fibers may participate in this arc reflex, since atropine blunts the LES response.

The LES is not an effective barrier at all times, even in healthy subjects. This is true particularly after meals[85] when reflux of gastric contents may occur as a result of a sudden, transient relaxation of the LES unrelated to swallowing. Once reflux takes place, the esophagus responds with a sweeping peristaltic contraction, which effectively clears the esophagus. The stimulus that triggers this "inappropriate" transient LES relaxation has not been defined, although several possibilities have been suggested. Transient LES relaxations occur more frequently during the postprandial state when the stomach accommodates the meal by a receptive relaxation of the fundus and the resultant distention relaxes the LES perhaps to facilitate belching. The "inappropriate" LES relaxation may therefore represent a silent belch.[86,87] These LES relaxations do not always occur after meals. For example, weak swallows can evoke LES relaxation without an esophageal response.[72] These observations in the human have also been demonstrated in the opossum, in which isolated and transient LES relaxations can be triggered by weak electrical stimuli to the vagus.[88]

Another mechanism by which the esophagus functions to prevent the injurious effect of reflux is by responding with segmental peristaltic contractions (secondary peristalsis) to clear the esophagus of any refluxed contents.[89,90] This response is similar to secondary peristalsis, which occurs as a result of distention by food, gas, and acid. It is not clear, however, if local esophageal distention is always necessary to trigger esophageal clearing in as much as acid by itself may evoke peristaltic contractions.[91] Once refluxed contents reach the upper esophagus, further retrograde movement is avoided by the high-pressure zone of the UES.[92] However, during deep sleep the UES pressure decreases, possibly resulting in reduced ability to prevent reflux at a time when the risk of reflux is higher.[93] The UES is capable of increasing its pressure in response to moderate esophageal distention with air,[94,95] but greater esophageal distention may result in sphincter relaxation in such a fashion as to mimic sphincter relaxation occurring with belching.[96]

CONTROL MECHANISMS

Pharynx

Mastication of food, mixing it with saliva and forming a bolus of a size and consistency appropriate for swallowing, occurs in the mouth under voluntary control. The presence of a bolus in the oropharynx activates a variety of receptors located at the base of the tongue, tonsils, soft palate, uvula, posterior pharyngeal wall, and larynx.[13,29,97] The afferents carrying the input to the swallowing center are believed to run in the maxillary branch of the trigeminal nerve, the glossopharyngeal nerve, and the superior laryngeal branch of the vagus nerve.[98,99] Continuation of deglutition in the pharynx and striated esophagus is under involuntary reflex control by motor nuclei in the "swallowing center." The swallowing center that controls the deglutition reflex is located in or near the nucleus solitarius in the brain stem. It is a functional center rather than a well-defined anatomic entity, since it is not identifiable by neuron type or exact location.[13,100,101] Afferent mucosal receptors, sensitive to pressure as well as taste, are present through the pharynx and larynx. They activate glossopharyngeal and vagal fibers to the swallowing center. Central recognition of the incoming sensory stimulus is believed to be accomplished by a pattern recognition system in the brain stem that identifies the stimulus as appropriate for swallowing and generates the required neuromuscular response.[101,102] The swallowing center then initiates a pattern of excitation and inhibition of medullary motor neurons, interacts with other brain stem centers, and coordinates cessation of breathing, initiation of swallowing, opening of the UES, and peristalsis in the striated portion of the esophagus.[29,103,104] Sensory loss in the oropharyngeal isthmus, pharynx, or larynx or local anesthesia is often associated with impairment of swallowing[105] or aspiration, suggesting that proper coordination of swallowing and respiration may depend in part on appropriate input from receptors located in the pharynx or larynx.[106] The sensory afferents are connected to motor nuclei in the brain stem by interneurons. Discrete motor input is distributed to all muscle groups in the pharynx, larynx, and soft palate, through motor fibers present in the glossopharyngeal and vagus nerves, except for the tensor veli palatini, which is innervated by the trigeminal nerve. The axons of the motor neurons to the pharyngeal muscles run through the vagi into the superior pharyngeal nerves, arising from the vagi at the level of the nodose ganglion. These form the pharyngeal plexus and control the pharyngeal muscles, including the cricopharyngeus and the upper portion of the esophagus.

Upper Esophageal Sphincter

Neural input to the UES is required for maintenance of high resting pressure and for precise coordination of relaxation with swallowing. In the opossum, sphincter tone is mediated through neural fibers present in the vagal trunks and originating in the nucleus ambiguus of the medulla.[107] Vagal transection abolishes activity in the cricopharyngeus and inferior pharyngeal constrictor muscles.[12] These muscles normally exhibit continuous spike activity, which is abolished by curare. Moreover, tone alters with changing firing frequency, indicating that motor neuron activity is responsible for maintenance of tonic muscle activity. Cessation of firing causes relaxation. Swallowing is further facilitated by forward displacement of the pharynx, which forces the sphincter to open.[12]

Resting tension in the UES is influenced by breathing as it increases during inspiration, when thoracic and esophageal resting pressures decrease.[93,108] Thus the change in pressure cannot be due to transmission of pressure from the body of the esophagus but probably results from reflex neural activity. In the opossum this increase is associated with increased spike activity in the cricopharyngeus and persists until stage III anesthesia, at which point activity of UES muscles is reduced or abolished.[12] The UES pressure is reduced during sleep[93] and increases in subjects under acute emotional stress.[109]

The effect of acid reflux or esophageal distention on the UES is controversial. Distention with small air-filled balloons[110] or injection of water or acid into the body of the esophagus causes an increase in UES pressure. The increase is greater when the bolus is closer to the UES and is greater for acid than for water or saline in normal persons.[111] In infants with gastroesophageal reflux the response to acid perfusion is not different from that of normal age-matched controls,[112] but in patients with esophagopharyngeal regurgitation[113] neither saline nor acid causes a significant increase in UES pressure. Increased UES pressure in response to acid perfusion or balloon distention of the proximal esophagus has been observed in the dog. In this species the response to acid increases with decreasing pH and with proximity of the distending balloon to the UES. The response to intraesophageal acid perfusion at all levels within the esophagus is abolished by bilateral blockade of the vagosympathetic trunks. The response to balloon distention of the distal esophagus is abolished, while response to distention of the proximal esophagus is only reduced.[95] These data suggest that the afferent pathways for the response to acid are found exclusively in the vagosympathetic trunks, presumably arising from branches of the recurrent laryngeal nerves. Responses induced by distention, at least in the proximal esophagus, may partly depend on another pathway.

Thus it is possible that reflux of small amounts of acid into the lower esophagus may not require contraction of the UES. More severe reflux, with acid into the upper esophagus, may elicit a protective contraction of the UES.[95]

Injection of air into the body of the esophagus, or distention by large balloons, however, relaxes the UES.[96] The relaxation facilitates expulsion of the air bolus by belching. The afferent mechanisms mediating discrimination between distention by fluid, causing contraction, or by air, causing relaxation, are unknown. It is possible that the spatial pattern and rapidity of esophageal distention may provide discrimination in the response to fluid or air.[65]

UES relaxation occurs during deglutition, belching, or vomiting. Relaxation during swallowing derives from two components: (1) inhibition of neural input arising from motor neurons in the brain stem, and resulting in cessation of spike activity in the muscles of the UES,[12,114,115] and (2) forceful opening of the UES resulting from elevation and forward displacement of the larynx by muscles of the oropharynx. (Stylohyoid, styloglossus, stylohyoid, palatopharyngeus, stylopharyngeus, digastric posterior, and other muscles located on the posterior aspect of the pharynx presumably contribute to elevation, while geniohyoid, myloyoid, digastric anterior, thyrohyoid, and other muscles located anteriorly contribute to forward displacement.) Inhibition of tonic muscle activity by itself is not sufficient to cause relaxation, and forceful opening of the sphincter is required to abolish resting pressure. Earlier investigators believed that resting UES pressure was entirely due to passive elasticity of the tissues constituting the sphincter.[63]

Pharyngeal peristalsis may force the bolus through the sphincter, even in the absence of forceful opening, while displacement of the larynx may force the UES open, even in the absence of cricopharyngeal inhibition. Nevertheless impairment of either relaxation or opening of the sphincter may affect smooth coordination of swallowing. Impairment of cricopharyngeal relaxation results in a prominent bar across the cricopharyngeal region (cricopharyngeal achalasia), while paralysis of the suprahyoid pharyngeal muscles may cause paralytic achalasia of the UES.[13]

Peristalsis in the Striated Muscle of the Esophagus (Fig 7-5)

Contraction of esophageal striated muscle is entirely dependent on neural input arising from neurons located in the nucleus ambiguus[30,35,116–118] and is centrally organized by sequential discharge of motor neurons controlling progressively distal segments in the body of the esophagus. Motor fibers course along the vagus, separating in the upper portion of the neck. These cholinergic fibers release acetylcholine and stimulate nicotinic cholinergic receptors located at the motor end plates of the striated muscle fibers. Bilateral vagotomy high in the neck, above the origin of the pharyngoesophageal fibers, completely abolishes peristalsis in this portion of the esophagus, while peristalsis in the smooth muscle portion can still be initiated by local distention.[13] Unilateral vagotomy, however has no effect. Furthermore, transection of the striated muscle segment does not affect the normal progression of the peristaltic contractions evoked by swallowing. Thus peristalsis in the striated muscle portion of the esophagus does not depend on the continuity of esophageal plexuses but is under central control.[119,120]

Other types of esophageal responses in the striated muscle portion also appear to be dependent on central control. This includes peristalsis in response to esophageal distention, that is, secondary peristalsis, the inhibition evoked by frequent swallows, and reverse peristalsis in ruminants.[121] Extrinsic denervation or bilateral cervical vagotomy eliminates the esophageal contractions evoked by esophageal distention in this segment. Furthermore, frequent swallows taken at very short intervals abolish the response of the striated muscle of the esophagus until the last swallow occurs.[70] Since the striated muscle is under direct central control, this swallow-induced inhibition probably originates in the swallowing center.

The strength of contraction in the striated muscle may be modulated by a variety of sensory inputs. These include bolus volume[73,122–125] and temperature.[75,126] An increase in volume augments the force and duration of the contractions while slowing the velocity of propagation. Warm boluses increase the force, whereas cold boluses decrease the force of the contractions. These effects may depend on afferent input to the central nervous system with subsequent modulation of vagal control of the striated esophageal fibers.[127]

Peristalsis in the Smooth Muscle of the Esophagus (see Fig 5)

Two hypotheses have been proposed to explain the control of peristalsis in the smooth muscle segment. In one it is proposed that peristalsis results from sequencing of motor neurons in the

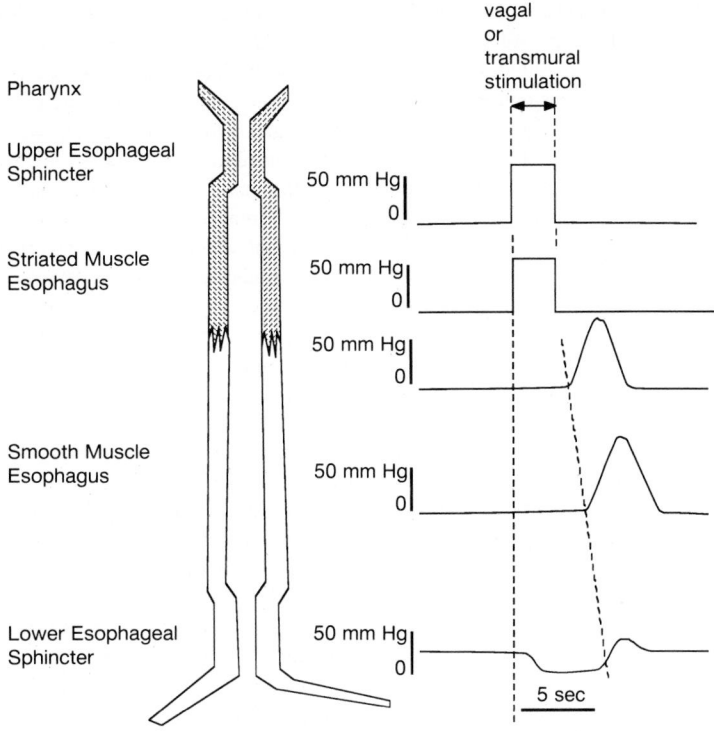

FIGURE 7–5. In the striated muscle portion of the esophagus, peristalsis is directly controlled by the central nervous system and sequencing of peristalsis occurs in the swallowing center. Motor neurons are activated sequentially—first those innervating the proximal striated esophagus, then those activating the more distal portion of the striated muscle. In the opossum, after division of the vagus at the cervical level, stimulation of the distal end, which activates simultaneously all vagal fibers, produces simultaneous contraction of the striated esophagus and relaxation of the lower esophageal sphincter. At the end of the stimulus peristalsis occurs in the smooth muscle esophagus. This suggests that whereas peristalsis in the striated esophagus is under central nervous system control, local mechanisms are responsible for peristalsis in the smooth muscle portion. However, even in the smooth muscle portion central input may regulate peristalsis. It has been shown that two types of vagal fibers may participate in smooth muscle peristalsis. Short latency fibers,[132] firing within 1 second of swallowing, coincide with the onset of inhibition in the esophagus and lower esophageal sphincter and may thus stimulate neurons that release inhibitory neurotransmitters; and long latency fibers discharging their impulses within 1 to 5 seconds, may coincide with the onset of contraction at various locations in the esophagus. These fibers may activate motor neurons to release excitatory neurotransmitters. It is possible that on swallowing the central nervous system mediates initial inhibition throughout the esophagus, via a nonsequential mechanism activating short latency fibers, resulting in hyperpolarization in the esophagus and relaxation in the lower esophageal sphincter. As hyperpolarization ends, sequential excitatory input through the long latency fibers causes sequential contraction and peristalsis in the smooth muscle esophagus.[138]

swallowing center that causes progressive stimulation of intramural cholinergic neurons.[128] This model, however, does not explain the occurrence of sequential peristaltic contractions on stimulation of the decentralized efferent vagus at the cervical level.[129] Furthermore, long latencies in response to field stimulation have been observed even in vitro, in muscle strips taken from the distal esophagus, while strips taken from the proximal esophagus exhibit shorter latencies.[130] The second hypothesis proposes that control of peristalsis may reside at least in part within peripheral mechanisms located in the intramural plexuses. This hypothesis is supported by the following findings:

1. Stimulation of decentralized vagal efferent nerves evokes peristalsis that is similar to the peristaltic wave produced by swallowing.[129,131]
2. Nerve conduction studies indicate that neural stimuli initiated by swallowing propagate with a speed of 5 to 6 m/sec and therefore reach the intramural neurons of the entire length of the esophagus at about the same time; yet the timing of the contractions reveals an aboral increment in latency with a peristaltic sequence.[132]
3. In vitro distal esophageal strips exhibit longer latencies than proximal strips.[130,133]
4. Esophageal transection at the level of the smooth muscle segment markedly affects the propagation of the peristaltic wave below the level of the transection, whereas transection of the striated esophagus does not affect the orderly transmission of peristalsis across the cut. This suggests that the integrity of the intramural mechanisms is essential for the normal progression of peristalsis in the smooth but not in the striated esophagus.[120]

Peripheral control is also illustrated by distention of the esophageal smooth muscle segment after extrinsic denervation.[28,134]

Peristalsis induced by balloon distention is always propagated in the caudad direction after extrinsic denervation with cervical vagotomy, and even in the isolated esophagus mounted in an organ bath. Esophageal peristalsis evoked by balloon distention is similar to that caused by swallowing, with a similar sequence of inhibition or hyperpolarization during distention followed by a latency period and contraction or depolarization after balloon deflation. Furthermore, repeated stimulation of the decentralized efferent vagal fibers at short intervals inhibits the esophageal responses, with contraction occurring only after the last stimulus.[135] This experimental model mimics deglutitive inhibition and suggests that the mechanism responsible resides in the intramural neurons.

Primary peristaltic waves in this segment are affected, however, by the presence of a bolus and by central mechanisms. The bolus modifies the speed, duration, and force of the contractions. Central mechanisms are also capable of modulating the occurrence and features of esophageal contractions, including the polarity of peristalsis, as occurs under some pathophysiologic conditions. Changing the parameters of vagal stimulation can drive the esophagus with peristaltic or antiperistaltic sequence with different speeds of propagation.[129]

The preganglionic fibers that mediate this control branch out from the thoracic vagus nerve, forming a plexus around the esophagus,[136] and then enter into the esophageal wall where they travel a few centimeters before synapsing with the myenteric neurons.[137] They arise from the dorsal motor nucleus and may synapse to the intramural neurons.[35,36] During swallowing, central regulation may be mediated by two types of vagal fibers: short latency fibers firing within 1 second may stimulate neurons that release inhibitory neurotransmitters, and long latency fibers discharging their impulses within 1 to 5 seconds, which may activate motor neurons to release excitatory neurotransmitters.[138,139] Central mechanisms also control the contractions of the longitudinal muscle layer. Swallowing induces peristaltic sequences with gradual activation from orad to caudad segments and a correspondent progressive increase in latencies.[140] Unlike the responses observed in the circular muscle layer,[129] stimulation of decentralized vagal efferent fibers causes simultaneous contractions in the longitudinal muscle layer. However, the functional role of this muscle layer on bolus transport has not been defined.

Esophageal peristalsis is characterized by a gradient with increasing latency of contractions along the length of the esophagus. Latency is the time interval between the swallow or electrical stimulus and the onset of contraction at a given site in the esophagus. In humans it is 2 seconds in the proximal smooth muscle esophagus and 5 to 7 seconds just above the LES. The nature of the latency gradient is controversial, but it can be changed by varying the parameters of vagal stimulation[129] or by pharmacologic manipulation of the esophageal contractions, suggesting that latency may result from the interaction between initial inhibition and subsequent excitation of esophageal smooth muscle. The muscarinic cholinergic antagonist atropine increases the latency, whereas the acetylcholinesterase inhibitor physostigmine decreases it.[139,141]

The data support the view that peristalsis is largely determined by neurally dependent esophageal gradients because the esophageal response to low-frequency electrical stimuli is sensitive to tetrodotoxin, an inhibitor of neurotransmission, and is aborally transmitted no matter where in the esophagus the stimulus is applied.[129] In contrast, the response to high-frequency stimuli that is tetro-

dotoxin resistant or myogenic tends to propagate in both directions from the stimulus site at a speed similar to that evoked by swallowing.[142] These findings suggest that myogenic propagation can occur but without strict polarity. The latencies are similar to neurally mediated peristalsis, suggesting that myogenic gradients may also contribute to peristalsis. Their contribution under physiologic conditions is unclear at this time.

Differences in resting membrane potential and potassium concentration along the esophagus may contribute to esophageal latency gradients. A gradual decrease in membrane potentials occurs along the esophagus, with muscle cells in the distal esophagus being less depolarized than those in the proximal esophagus.[143] Concurrently, a gradual decrease in potassium concentration is found between proximal and distal muscle cells and has been explained by increased permeability of the muscle to potassium.[144] The contribution of these myogenic properties to the progressive aboral change in latency has not been determined. Moreover, others have failed to confirm these observations and did not detect any membrane potential differences between proximal (8 cm above the LES) and distal (2 cm above the LES) smooth muscle esophagus.[133]

Preganglionic vagal fibers synapse with intramural excitatory neurons via activation of nicotinic receptors since the nicotinic ganglionic inhibitor hexamethonium blocks cervical vagal stimulation. The nature of the postganglionic intramural neurons varies with the animal species. It has been suggested that these neurons are exclusively inhibitory, using nonadrenergic noncholinergic transmitters. Stimulation of these neurons would result in an initial inhibition followed by a rebound contraction after cessation of the stimulus.[145] Studies in the opossum and cat, however, suggest that the inhibition occurring during the stimulus and the "off-contraction" occurring at the end of the stimulus are mediated by separate transmitters, if not by different neurons, although considerable species-related differences occur. The issue is complicated by experimental methodology since it is unclear how the esophageal response during various parameters of vagal and field stimulation mimics the response evoked by deglutition.

Swallowing causes a single contraction at each level of the esophagus following a given latency. Brief stimulations (1 second) of the efferent vagal fibers or of circular muscle strips also evoke a single contraction with a given latency.[146] On the other hand, the esophageal response induced by prolonged stimulation (5 to 20 seconds) is dissociated into an "on" contraction that occurs during the stimulus and an "off" contraction after the end of the stimulus. Since the act of swallowing is brief, it is conceivable that the "on" and "off" responses represent dissociations of one or more excitatory neurons during artificially prolonged stimulation. In addition, the "on" responses are not seen at lower stimulus frequencies, which are believed to elicit more representative physiologic events.[146] It is therefore unclear how the results of these experimental studies may relate to the esophageal response evoked by deglutition.

In the opossum, cholinergic and nonadrenergic noncholinergic excitatory neurons are responsible for the off-response; proximal segments are primarily controlled by cholinergic fibers and distal segments by noncholinergic motor neurons.[141] In the cat esophagus the off-response seems to be entirely under cholinergic control. The contractions induced by field stimulation in vitro[147,148] or by vagal stimulation[149] are blocked by atropine. Cholinergic fibers also contribute to the esophageal contractions of humans since atropine decreases the amplitude of pressure generated by swallowing.[150]

The hypothesis that esophageal smooth muscle response may result from two (or more) neurotransmitters is further supported by the finding that it is possible to dissociate esophageal inhibition and esophageal excitation by using selective antagonists. The initial inhibition is at least in part mediated by VIP-containing neurons that are present in the body of the esophagus.[151] Esophageal muscle strips tonically contracted with bethanechol relax during field stimulation; this neurally mediated (i.e., tetrodotoxin sensitive) relaxation is partially blocked by a selective VIP antiserum without affecting the force and duration of the off-contractions, which are blocked by atropine.[148]

Myogenic mechanisms responsible for esophageal smooth muscle contraction are different from those responsible for LES tone. Esophageal muscle is relaxed at rest and contracts in response to vagal or field stimulation with a brief and forceful contraction. This contraction is mediated almost exclusively by influx of extracellular calcium through voltage-dependent calcium channels, whereas the LES maintains spontaneous tone via calcium release from intracellular stores, probably through an inositol triphosphate-1,4,5-IP$_3$)–dependent mechanism.[152-154]

Lower Esophageal Sphincter

The LES exhibits spontaneous tone and myoelectrical activity that is characterized by continuous spike burst activity with or without short phasic contractions.[155,156] Spikes occur at a frequency of 15 to 40/min and may be associated with minicontractions, 5 to 15 mm Hg in amplitude. Partial relaxation of the LES is accompanied by complete cessation of electrical activity; therefore, there is substantial residual LES tension that is not accompanied by any detectable electrical activity. Phasic contractions and electrical spike activity become prominent after bethanechol or during phases II and III of the migrating myoelectrical complex. Feeding, barbiturates, and cholinergic antagonists abolish both electrical activity and associated contractions.

Basal LES pressures in vivo or basal circular muscle tension in vitro are maintained even in the absence of neural input.[78,157-159] Bilateral cervical vagotomy or denervation with the neural poison tetrodotoxin does not eliminate in vivo LES tension in most animal species, and in the opossum LES pressures do not change at all.[157] In vivo experiments, however, are usually performed in anesthetized animals. General anesthesia depresses LES pressure in the baboon,[160] suggesting that the neural input may be reduced or abolished in some of the in vivo experiments. Some evidence indicates the presence of a small neural contribution to the genesis or modulation of LES pressures in several animal species. Atropine reduces LES pressures in conscious humans[150,161] and dogs by 20% to 30%,[162] but similar doses of atropine do not affect LES pressures of conscious opossums and monkeys[150] or of anesthetized opossums and cats.[157-159] The precise nature of the contribution of the cholinergic input to LES pressure, however, is difficult to estimate because resting pressures may be modulated by excitatory and inhibitory influences. A decrease in tonic excitatory cholinergic input may enhance the tonic inhibitory effect. The dog LES appears to be the exception, with pressures being dependent on vagal tonic activity.[163,164] There also appears to be

a small adrenergic input to the genesis of LES pressure in the cat, where sympathetic nerves also mediate a reflex contraction.[158,159] The α-adrenergic blocker phentolamine decreases LES pressures by 25%, and a similar reduction is seen after administration of tetrodotoxin.[158,165] Since this neural poison blocks both excitatory and inhibitory innervation, the decrease in LES pressures suggests a true neural contribution to the genesis of LES tone. Furthermore, neural stimulation can evoke LES contraction in the opossum and cat. Electrical stimulation of the cervical afferent vagal fibers and of the splanchnic efferent nerves causes LES contraction during the period of stimulation. The LES responses to both types of stimulation are blocked by similar doses of phentolamine.[158,159,165,166] This reflex contraction could be the mechanism mediating the LES contraction in response to increases in abdominal pressures. Thus, some of the controversies surrounding the neural role in the genesis or modulation of LES pressures may be due to species differences.

The LES circular muscle is therefore the major determinant of LES tone, although the relative neurogenic contribution may vary with the animal species. Functionally this muscle is specialized with muscle strips from this region developing higher total and active forces than esophageal strips.[25,78,79] This distinctive contractility appears to be, at least in part, related to the ability of the LES muscle to handle calcium differently from esophageal circular muscle.[152,153,167] LES muscle maintains tension in a calcium-free environment for long periods of time even after esophageal strips are no longer capable of contraction in response to field stimulation or high concentrations of acetylcholine.[152,168] These findings suggest that the LES muscle can use calcium released from intracellular storage sites to maintain tonic contraction, and they are consistent with the histology and biochemistry of these muscles. The LES circular muscle has more abundant endoplasmic reticulum than the esophageal circular muscle.[27] Since the endoplasmic reticulum is believed to be the site of calcium stores, it is possible that the LES muscle may have larger calcium stores. There is substantial evidence that agonist-induced release of calcium from store sites is mediated by the second messenger 1,4,5-IP$_3$.[153] LES smooth muscle cells have greater concentrations of 1,4,5-IP$_3$ than esophageal smooth muscle cells.[154,168] It is thus possible that tonic contraction is maintained by greater 1,4,5-IP$_3$ turnover and steady calcium release from store sites. A higher 1,4,5-IP$_3$ concentration appears to be characteristic of other tonic muscles such as pyloric sphincter muscles. The LES contracts by aerobic mechanisms in vitro since gradual reduction of the oxygen concentration in the muscle bath causes a parallel decrease in muscle tension.[169] This is consistent with the more numerous mitochondria observed in this muscle.

Basal LES pressures are affected during fasting by the phase III of the migrating myoelectric complex (MMC), by certain esophageal contents, and by neurohormonal mechanisms activated during digestion. The phase III of the MMC begins in the LES, lasts for about 15 minutes, and is characterized mostly by an increase in short phasic contractions.[83] The control mechanisms have not been completely established, but they appear to be under vagal control and associated with a rise in circulating levels of the peptide motilin. The character of esophageal contents may also affect LES tone. In the anesthetized cat, distal esophageal acidification causes an increase in LES pressures.[170] The physiologic role of this response is unclear; it may be designed to tighten the sphincter to prevent further gastroesophageal reflux.

The inhibitory innervation that mediates LES relaxation on swallowing or as a result of gastroesophageal distention has been extensively studied.[166,171,172] LES relaxation induced by swallowing is mediated by the vagus nerve, which synapses with intramural inhibitory neurons. Electrical stimulation of decentralized efferent vagal fibers in vivo or field stimulation of LES muscle strips in vitro causes full relaxation with concomitant circular muscle hyperpolarization.[155,173] The vagus nerve uses acetylcholine as a ganglionic transmitter acting through both nicotinic and muscarinic receptors, since transmission is blocked by a combination of hexamethonium (nicotinic blocker) and atropine (muscarinic blocker). LES relaxation can be triggered by distention from both sides of the gastroesophageal junction. The relaxation evoked by esophageal distention is volume dependent since it disappears during inflation with small volumes but persists during inflation with large volumes.[174,175] The relaxation is unaffected by cervical vagotomy and is therefore mediated by intramural neurons. The intramural neurons of these reflexes use nonadrenergic noncholinergic inhibitory neurotransmitters because relaxation is not affected by adrenergic or cholinergic blockers. It is only antagonized by tetrodotoxin, which denervates smooth muscle without affecting its contractile function.[176] Evidence has been presented in support of VIP as one of the neurotransmitters of these neurons. The evidence almost fulfills the criteria required for VIP to be accepted as a neurotransmitter: namely, VIP-containing neurons have been demonstrated in the submucosal plexus by immunofluorescent methods[42–46]; VIP relaxes the LES in vivo and in vitro by direct muscle action since it is tetrodotoxin resistant[177–179]; electrical stimulation of in vitro LES muscle strips relax LES and release VIP in the muscle bath[179]; and specific VIP antiserum partially reduces the LES relaxation induced by VIP and evoked by vagal or field stimulation.[179,180] VIP, however, may not be the only neurotransmitter. There is some evidence that peptide histidine isoleucine (PHI) in the cat LES[181] and, to a lesser extent, CGRP in the opossum LES[182] may also participate as inhibitory neurotransmitters. Like VIP, PHI and CGRP relax the LES fully or in part by a direct action on the muscle.[181,182] PHI is of particular interest because it is derived from the same precursor as VIP and coexists with VIP in the same neurons.[183]

All of these peptides stimulate adenylate cyclase and increase the concentrations of cyclic adenosine monophosphate, which may be responsible for LES relaxation.[184–186] However, neurally mediated relaxation evoked by electrical stimulation of opossum LES strips appears to increase cyclic guanosine monophosphate formation,[187] suggesting that the neurotransmitter may be a still unknown peptide. More recently, it has been shown that VIP not only causes an increase in cyclic adenosine monophosphate concentrations in the cat LES but also reduces the levels of IP-3.[154] This cellular event may be responsible for LES relaxation since it would turn off calcium release from storage sites. High LES tension appears to be dependent on the gradual release of stored calcium that is elicited by IP-3.[153] It is unclear at this time how any of these biochemical changes are related to muscle relaxation induced by physiologic stimuli. Further studies are needed to define the neurotransmitter(s) and the intracellular pathways that mediate neurally evoked LES

The physiologic effects of gastrointestinal hormones or regulatory peptides on in vivo LES pressure have not been established. It has been difficult to demonstrate a role of any of the hormones studied during fasting or during meal digestion. This difficulty stems from the inability to release a given gastrointestinal hormone selectively and demonstrate a concomitant rise in LES pressures or to show increases in LES pressures during constant intravenous infusions of the hormone at levels similar to those observed circulating after a meal. However, the pharmacologic effects of these hormones and endogenous compounds are well established, including some of their mechanisms of action (Table 7-1). Gastrin causes LES contraction by direct muscle action since it is unaffected by tetrodotoxin.[188,189] Other hormones such as motilin, bombesin, pancreatic polypeptide, galanin, and substance P cause LES contraction when used in pharmacologic doses[190–196] In contrast, secretin, cholecystokinin, glucagon, gastric inhibitory peptide, VIP, PHI, CGRP, and neurotensin decrease in LES pressures, although significant species differences occur.[177,197–204] For instance, cholecystokinin causes LES relaxation in the human[197] and the cat[203] and LES contraction in the opossum.[204] It causes relaxation by stimulating the intramural noncholinergic nonadrenergic inhibitory neurons and causes contraction by direct muscle action.[203,204] Glucagon relaxes the human LES probably by direct action but contracts the cat LES by releasing catecholamines from the adrenal medulla.[177]

Some experiments however suggest a physiologic role for some hormones. Intravenous infusions of neurotensin in humans at or below the serum levels obtained postprandially cause a dose-de-

TABLE 7–1

Effects of Endogenous Compounds
on the Lower Esophageal Sphincter

COMPOUND	CONTRACTION	RELAXATION
Gastrin	+	
Cholecystokinin	+*	+†
Motilin	+	
Secretin		+
Glucagon	+†	+*
Vasoactive intestinal peptide		+
Peptide histidine isoleucine		+
Gastric inhibitory peptide		+
Pancreatic polypeptide	+	
Calcitonin–gene-related peptide		+
Somatostatin	–	–
Galanin	+	
Neurotensin		+
Substance P	+	
5-Hydroxytryptamine	+	
Acetylcholine	+ (m)	+ (n)
Phenylephrine	+ (alpha)	
Isoproterenol		+ (beta)
Dopamine		+*
Histamine	H1	H2
Prostaglandins		
E series		+
F series	+	

* *Opossum*
† *Cat*
m, Muscarinic; n, nicotinic

pendent decrease in pressures and may involve a cholinergic pathway.[205] Increases in the circulating levels of pancreatic polypeptide correlate with a rise in LES pressures after a protein meal and are abolished by duodenal exclusion to the meal.[194] Somatostatin has no effect on basal LES pressures but blocks the postprandial rise in LES pressures.[206] These observations suggest that meal-evoked rise in LES pressures is mediated by hormonal mechanisms since it is known that somatostatin inhibits hormonal release.[207,208] These findings support the belief that gastroduodenal hormones may play a physiologic role probably by regulating LES pressures during digestion of certain foodstuffs (fatty meals, chocolate, alcohol, and coffee) and during changes in gastroduodenal pH (acid or alkaline solutions) that may decrease or increase LES pressures in humans.[209,210]

The reader is directed to Chapter 1, The Enteric Nervous System and its Extrinsic Connections; Chapter 2, Gastrointestinal Hormones; Chapter 3, The Brain-Gut Axis; Chapter 4, Smooth Muscle of the Gut; Chapter 8, The Physiology of Gastric Motility and Gastric Emptying; Chapter 9, Motility of the Small Intestine; Chapter 10, The Motor Function of the Colon; Chapter 11, Motility of the Biliary Tree; Chapter 28, Approach to the Patient with Dysphagia; Chapter 29, Approach to the Patient with Chest Pain; Chapter 53, Esophagus: Anatomy and Structural Anomalies; Chapter 54, Motility Disorders of the Esophagus; and Chapter 55, Reflux Esophagitis.

REFERENCES

1. Cohen BR, Wolf BS. Cineradiographic and intraluminal pressure correlations in the pharynx and esophagus. In: Code CF, ed. Handbook of physiology, Alimentary canal, section 6, Motility, vol IV. Washington, DC: American Physiological Society, 1968;1841
2. Logemann JA. Swallowing physiology and pathophysiology. Otholaryngol Clin North Am 1988;21:613.
3. McConnel FMS. Analysis of pressure generation and bolus transit during pharyngeal swallowing. Laryngoscope 1988;98:71.
4. Lumsden K, Holden WS. The act of vomiting in man. Gut 1969;10:173.
5. Smith CC, Bizzee RK. Cineradiographic analysis of vomiting in the cat. Gastroenterology 1960;40:6544.
6. Atkinson M, Kramer P, Wyman SM, Ingelfinger FG. The dynamics of swallowing: I. Normal pharyngeal mechanisms. J Clin Invest 1957;36:581.
7. Ingelfinger FJ. Esophageal motility. Physiol Rev 1958;38:533.
8. Davenport HW. Physiology of the digestive tract. Chicago: Year Book Medical Publishers, 1977.
9. Mary DA, North PJ, Hunt JN. Scanning esophageal impedance probe for measurement of luminal cross section. Am J Physiol 1979;236:E545.
10. Palmer JB, Tanaka E, Siebens AA. Motions of the posterior pharyngeal wall in swallowing. Laryngoscope 1988;98:414.
11. Van Overbeck JJM. The hypopharyngeal diverticulum: endoscopic treatment and manometry. Amsterdam: Van Corcum Assen, 1976.
12. Asoh R, Goyal RK. Manometry and electromyography of the upper esophageal sphincter in the opossum. Gastroenterology 1978;74:514.
13. Goyal RK, Patterson WG. Esophageal motility. In: Woods JD, ed. Handbook of physiology–the gastrointestinal system II. Bethesda, MD: American Physiological Society, 1989:865.
14. Netter FH. Digestive tract. In: Oppenheimer E, ed., The Ciba collection of medical illustrations, vol 3. New York: Ciba Pharmaceutical Company, 1971.
15. Romanes GJ. Cunningham's textbook of anatomy. London: Oxford University Press, 1972.
16. Whitmore I. Oesophageal striated muscle arrangement and histochemical fibre types in guinea pig, marmoset macaque and man. J Anat 1982;134:685.
17. Whitmore I. The ultrastructural characteristics of oesophageal striated muscle in the guinea pig and marmoset. Cell Tissue Res 1983;234:365.
18. Whitmore I, Notman JA. A quantitative investigation into some ultrastructural characteristics of guinea oesophageal striated muscle. J Anat 1987;153:233.
19. Leese G, Hopwood D. Muscle fibretyping in the human pharyngeal constrictors and oesophagus: the effect of ageing. Acta Anat (Basel) 1986;127:77.
20. Arey LB, Tremaine MJ. The muscle content of the lower oesophagus of man. Anat Rec 1933;56:315.
21. Meyer GW, Austin RM, Brady CE, Castell DO. Muscle anatomy of the human esophagus. J Clin Gastroenterol 1986;8:131.
22. Lerche W. The esophagus and pharynx in action. Springfield, IL: Charles C Thomas, 1950.
23. Biancani P, Goyal RK, Phillips A, Spiro HM. Mechanics of sphincter action: studies on the lower esophageal sphincter. J Clin Invest 1973;52:2973.
24. Liebermann-Meffert D, Heberer M, Martinoli S, Allgoewer M. Are there muscular structures which may contribute to closure of the gastroesophageal junction? Scand J Gastroenterol 1981;suppl 67:123.
25. Biancani P, Zabinski M, Kerstein M, Behar J. Lower esophageal sphincter mechanics: anatomic and physiologic relationships of the esophagogastric junction of the cat. Gastroenterology 1982;82:468.
26. Seelig LL, Doody P, Brainard L, et al. Acetylcholinesterase and choline acetyltransferase staining of neurons in the opossum esophagus. Anat Rec 1984;209:125.
27. Christensen J, Roberts RL. Differences between esophageal body and lower esophageal sphincter in mitochondria of smooth muscle in opossum. Gastroenterology 1983;85:650.
28. Christensen J, Lund GF. Esophageal responses to distention and electrical stimulation. J Clin Invest 1969;48:408.
29. Doty RW. Neural organization of deglutition. In: Code CF, ed. Handbook of physiology, Alimentary canal, section 6, Motility, vol IV. Washington, DC: American Physiological Society, 1968:1861.
30. Fryscak T, Zenker W, Kantner D. Afferent and efferent innervation of the rat esophagus: a tracing study with horseradish peroxidase and nuclear yellow. Anat Embryol 1984;170:63.
31. Holstege G, Graveland G, Bijker-Biemond C, Schuddeboom I. Location of motoneurons innervating soft palate, pharynx, and upper esophagus: anatomical evidence for a possible swallowing center in the pontine reticular formation. Brain Behav Evol 1983;23:47.
32. Lawn AM. The localization in the nucleus ambiguus of the rabbit of the cells of origin of motor nerve fibers in the glossopharyngeal nerve and various branches of the vagus nerve by means of retrograde degeneration. J Comp Neurol 1966;127:293.
33. Sharoun SL, Barone FC, Wayner MJ, Jones SM. Vagal and gastric connection to the central nervous system determined by the transport of horseradish peroxidase. Brain Res Bull 1984;13:573.
34. Weisbrodt NW. Neuromuscular organization of esophageal and pharyngeal motility. Arch Intern Med 1976;136:524.
35. Barone FC, Lombardi DM, Ormsbee HS III. Effects of hindbrain stimulation on lower esophageal sphincter pressure in the cat. Am J Physiol 1984;247:G70.
36. Niel JP, Gonella J, Roman C. Localisation par la technique de marquage à la peroxydase des crops cellulaires des neurones ortho et parasympathiques innervant le sphincter oesophagien inférieur du chat. J Physiol Paris 1980;76:591.
37. Baumgarten MG, Lange W. Adrenergic innervation of the esophagus in the cat (Felis domestica) and rhesus monkey (Macacus rhesus). Z Fellorsch Mikrosk Anat 1969;95:529.
38. Bayliss WM, Starling EH. The movements and innervation of the small intestine. J Physiol (Lond) 1899;24:99.
39. Bayliss WM, Starling EH. The movements and innervation of the large intestine. J Physiol (Lond) 1900;26:107.
40. Bayliss WM, Starling EH. The movements and innervation of the small intestine. J Physiol (Lond) 1901;26:125.
41. Langley JN, Magnus R. Some observations on the movement of the

intestine before and after degenerative section of mesenteric nerves. J Physiol (Lond) 1904;33:34.

42. Alumets J, Schaffalitzky de Muckadell OB, Fahrenkrug J, et al. A rich VIP nerve supply is characteristic of sphincters. Nature 1979;280:155.

43. Aggestrup S, Uddman R, Sundler F, et al. Lack of vasoactive intestinal polypeptide nerves in esophageal achalasia. Gastroenterology 1983;84:924.

44. Berezin I, Allescher HD, Daniel EE. Ultrastructural localization of VIP-immunoreactivity in canine distal oesophagus. J Neurocytol 1987;16:749.

45. Christensen J, Rick GA, Soll DJ. Intramural nerves and interstitial cells revealed by the Champy-Maillet stain in the opossum esophagus. J Auto Nerv Syst 1987;19:137.

46. Wattchow DA, Furness JB, Costa M. Distribution and coexistence of peptides in nerve fibers of the external muscle of the human gastrointestinal tract. Gastroenterology 1988;95:32.

47. Wang YN, McDonald JK, Wyatt RJ. Immunocytochemical localization of neuropeptide Y–like immunoreactivity in adrenergic and non-adrenergic neurons of the rat gastrointestinal tract. Peptides 1987;8:145.

48. Rodrigo J, Polak JM, Fernandez L, et al. Calcitonin gene-related peptide immunoreactive and sensory motor nerves of the rat, cat, and monkey esophagus. Gastroenterology 1985;88:444.

49. Leander S, Brodin E, Hakanson R, et al. Neuronal substance P in the esophagus: distribution and effects on motor activity. Acta Physiol Scand 1982;115:427.

50. Christensen J, Williams TH, Jew J, O'Dorisio TM. Distribution of immunoreactive substance P in opossum esophagus. Dig Dis Sci 1989;34:513.

51. Wattchow DA, Furness JB, Costa M, et al. Distribution of neuropeptides in the human esophagus. Gastroenterology 1987;93:1363.

52. Melander T, Hokfelt T, Rokaeus A, et al. Distribution of galanin-like immunoreactivity in the gastrointestinal tract of several mammalian species. Cell Tissue Res 1985;239;253.

53. Sengupta A, Goyal RK. Localization of galanin immunoreactivity in the opossum esophagus. J Auton Nerv Syst 1988;22:49.

54. Green T, Dockray GJ. Calcitonin gene-related peptide and substance P in afferents to the upper gastrointestinal tract in the rat. Neurosci Lett 1987;76:151.

55. Sternini C, Reeve JR, Brecha N. Distribution and characterization of calcitonin gene-related peptide immunoreactivity in the digestive system of normal and capsaicin-treated rats. Gastroenterology 1987;3:852.

56. Sokol EM, Heitman P, Wolf BS, Cohen BR. Simultaneous cineradiographic and manometric study of the pharynx hypopharynx and cervical esophagus. Gastroenterology 1966;51:960.

57. Goyal RK, Sangree MH, Spiro HM. Pressure inversion point at the upper high pressure zone and its genesis. Gastroenterology 1970;59:754.

58. Winans CS. The pharyngoesophageal closure mechanism: a manometric study. Gastroenterology 1972;63:768.

59. Welch RW, Luckman K, Ricks PM, et al. Manometry of the normal upper esophageal sphincter and its alterations in laryngectomy. J Clin Invest 1979;63:1036.

60. Gerhardt D, Hewett J, Moeschberger M, et al. Human upper esophageal sphincter pressure profile. Am J Physiol 1980;239:G49.

61. Dodds WJ, Hogan WJ, Lyden SB, et al. Quantitation of pharyngeal motor function in normal human subjects. J Appl Physiol 1975;39:692.

62. Kahrilas PJ, Dent J, Dodds WJ, et al. A method for continuous monitoring of upper esophageal sphincter pressure. Dig Dis Sci 1987;32:121.

63. Doty RW, Bosma JF. An electromyographic analysis of reflex deglutition. J Neurophysiol 1956;19:44.

64. Isberg A, Nilsson ME, Schiratzki H. The upper esophageal sphincter during normal deglutition: a simultaneous cineradiographic and manometric investigation. Acta Radiol 1985;26:563.

65. Kahrilas PJ, Dodds WJ, Dent J, et al. Upper esophageal sphincter function during deglutition. Gastroenterology 1988;95:52.

66. Lund WS. A study of the cricopharyngeus sphincter in man and in the dog. Ann R Coll Surg Engl 1965;37:225.

67. Zaino C, Jacobsen HG, Lepow H, Osturk CH. The pharyngoesophageal sphincter. Springfield, IL: Charles C Thomas, 1970.

68. Code CF, Schlegel JF. Motor action of the esophagus and its sphincters. In: Code CF, ed. Handbook of physiology, Alimentary canal, section 6, Motility, vol IV. Washington, DC: American Physiological Society, 1968:1821.

69. Ask P, Tibbling L. Effect of time interval between swallows on esophageal peristalsis. Am J Physiol 1980;238:G485.

70. Meyer GW, Gerhardt DC, Castell DO. Human esophageal response to rapid swallowing: muscle refractory period or neural inhibition? Am J Physiol 1981;241:G129.

71. Vanek AW, Diamant NE. Responses of the human esophagus to paired swallows. Gastroenterology 1987;92:643.

72. Mittal RK, McCallum RW. Characteristics of transient lower esophageal sphincter relaxation in humans. Am J Physiol 1987;252:G636.

73. Dodds WJ, Hogan WJ, Reid DP, Stewart ET, Arndorfer RC. A comparison between primary esophageal peristalsis following wet and dry swallows. J Appl Physiol 1973;35:851.

74. Dooley CP, Schlossmacher B, Valenzuela JE. Effects of alterations in bolus viscosity on esophageal peristalsis in humans. Am J Physiol 1988;254:G8.

75. Winship DH, Viegas de Andrade SR, Zboralske FF. Influence of bolus temperature on human esophageal motor function. J Clin Invest 1970;49:243.

76. Vantrappen G, Hellemans J. Studies on the normal deglutition complex. Am J Dig Dis 1967;12:255.

77. Biancani P, Zabinski M, Behar J. Pressure, tension, and force of closure of the human lower esophageal sphincter and esophagus. J Clin Invest 1975;56:476.

78. Christensen J, Conklin JL, Freeman BW. Physiologic specialization at the esophagogastric junction in three species. Am J Physiol 1973;225:1265.

79. Christensen J, Freeman BQ, Miller JK. Some physiological characteristics of the esophagogastric junction in the opossum. Gastroenterology 1973;64:1119.

80. Welch RW, Gray JE. Influence of respiration on recordings of lower esophageal sphincter pressure in humans. Gastroenterology 1982;83:590.

81. Winans CS, Harris LD. Quantitation of lower esophageal sphincter competence. Gastroenterology 1967;52:773.

82. DeMeester TR, Lafontaine E, Joelsson BE, et al. Relationship of a hiatal hernia to the function of the body of the esophagus and the gastroesophageal junction. J Thorac Cardiovasc Surg 1981;82:547.

83. Dent J, Dodds WJ, Sekiguchi T, et al. Interdigestive phasic contractions of the human lower esophageal sphincter. Gastroenterology 1983;84:453.

84. Babka JC, Castell DO. On the genesis of heartburn: the effect of specific foods on the lower esophageal sphincter. Am J Dig Dis 1973;18:391.

85. Dent J, Dodds WJ, Friedman RH, et al. Mechanism of gastroesophageal reflux in recumbent asymptomatic human subjects. J Clin Invest 1980;65:256.

86. Creamer B. Oesophageal reflux. Lancet 1955;1:279.

87. McNally EF, Kelly JE, Ingelfinger FJ. Mechanism of belching: effects of gastric detension with air. Gastroenterology 1964;46:254.

88. Paterson WG, Rattan S, Goyal RK. Experimental induction of isolated lower esophageal sphincter relaxation in anesthetized opossums. J Clin Invest 1986;77:1187.

89. Fleshler B, Hendrix TR, Kramer P, Ingelfinger FJ. The characteristics and similarity of primary and secondary peristalsis in the esophagus. J Clin Invest 1959;38:110.

90. Helm JF, Dodds WJ, Riedel DR, et al. Determinants of esophageal acid clearance in normal subjects. Gastroenterology 1983;85:607.

91. Dodds WJ, Dent J, Hogan WJ, et al. Mechanisms of gastroesophageal reflux in patients with reflux esophagitis. N Engl J Med 1982;307:1547.

92. Kawasaki M, Ogura JH, Takenouchi S. Neurophysiologic observations of normal deglutition: I. Its relationship to the respiratory cycle: II. Its relationship to allied phenomena. Laryngoscope 1964;74:1747.

93. Kahrilas PJ, Dodds WJ, Dent J, et al. Effect of sleep, spontaneous

gastroesophageal reflux, and a meal on upper esophageal sphincter pressure in normal human volunteers. Gastroenterology 1987;92: 466.

94. Andreollo NA, Thompson DG, Kendall GP, Earlam RJ. Functional relationships between cricopharyngeal sphincter and oesophageal body in response to graded intraluminal distension. Gut 1988;29: 161.

95. Freiman JM, El-Sharkawy TY, Diamant NE. Effect of bilateral vagosympathetic nerve blockade on response of the dog upper esophageal sphincter (UES) to intraesophageal distention and acid. Gastroenterology 1981;81:78.

96. Kahrilas PJ, Dodds WJ, Dent J, et al. Upper esophageal sphincter function during belching. Gastroenterology 1988;91:133.

97. Shingai T, Shimada K. Reflex swallowing elicited by water and chemical substances applied in the oral cavity, pharynx, and larynx of the rabbit. Jpn J Physiol 1976;26:445.

98. Torvik A. Afferent connections to the sensory trigeminal nuclei, the nucleus of the solitaru tract and adjacent structures: an experimental study in the rat. J Comp Neurol 1956;106:51.

99. Bosma JF. Deglutition: pharyngeal stage. Physiol Rev 1957;37:275.

100. Donner MW, Bosma JF, Robertson DL. Anatomy and physiology of the pharynx. Gastrointest Radiol 1985;10:196.

101. Miller A. Deglutition. Physiol Rev 1982;62:129.

102. Larson C. Neurophysiology of speech and swallowing. In: Logeman J, ed. Relationship of speech and swallowing. New York: Thieme Statton, 1985.

103. Cherniack NS, Haxhiu MA, Mitra J, et al. Response of upper airway, intercostal and diaphragm muscle activity to stimulation of oesophageal afferents in dogs. J Physiol (Lond) 1984;349:15.

104. Jean A. Control of the central swallowing program by inputs from the peripheral receptors: a review. J Auton Nerv Syst 1984;10, 225.

105. Mathew OP, Abu-Osba YK, Thach BT. Genioglossus response to upper airway pressure changes: afferent pathways. J Appl Physiol 1982;52:445.

106. Sumi T. The activity of the brain stem respiratory neurons and spinal respiratory motor neurons during swallowing. J Neurophysiol 1963;26:466.

107. Yoshida Y, Miyazaki T, Hirano M, et al. Localization of efferent neurons innervating the pharyngeal constrictor muscles and the cervical esophagus muscle in the cat by means of the horseradish peroxidase method. Neurosci Lett 1981;22:91.

108. Scharoun SL, Barone FC, Wayner MJ, et al. Vagal and gastric connections to the central nervous system determined by the transport of horseradish peroxidase. Brain Res. Bull 1984;13:573.

109. Cook IJ, Dent J, Shannon S, Collins SM. Measurement of upper esophageal sphincter pressure: effect of acute emotional stress. Gastroenterology 1987;93:526.

110. Enzmann ER, Harell GS, Zboralske FF. Upper esophageal responses to intraluminal distension in man. Gastroenterology 1977;72:1292.

111. Gerhardt DC, Shuck TJ, Bordeaux RH, Winship DH. Human upper esophageal sphincter. Response to volume, osmotic, and acid stimuli. Gastroenterology 1978;75:268.

112. Sondheimer JM. Upper esophageal sphincter and pharyngoesophageal motor function in infants with and without gastroesophageal reflux. Gastroenterology 1983;85:301.

113. Gerhardt DC, Castell DO, Winship DH, Shuck TJ. Esophageal dysfunction in esophagopharyngeal regurgitation. Gastroenterology 1980;78:893.

114. Shipp T, Deatsch WW, Robertson K. Pharyngoesophageal muscle activity during swallowing in man. Laryngoscope 1970;80:1.

115. Van Overbeck JJM, Wit HP, Paping RHL, Segenhout HM. Simultaneous manometry and electromyography in the pharyngoesophageal segment. Laryngoscope 1985;95;582.

116. Andrew BL. The nervous control of the cervical esophagus in the rat during swallowing. J Physiol (Lond) 1956;134:729.

117. VanTrappen G, Hellemans J. Diseases of the esophagus. New York: Springer-Verlag, 1974.

118. Lawn AM. The localization, by means of electrical stimulation, of the origin and path in the medulla oblongata of the motor nerve fibers of the rabbit esophagus. J Physiol (Lond) 1964;174:232.

119. Roman C. Nervous control of peristalsis in the esophagus. J Physiol (Paris) 1966;58:79.

120. Janssens J, DeWever I, Vantrappen G, et al. Peristalsis in smooth muscle esophagus after transection and bolus deviation. Gastroenterology 1976;71:1004.

121. Stevens CE, Sellers AF. Rumination. In: Code CF, ed. Handbook of physiology, Alimentary canal, section 6, Bile, digestion, ruminal physiology, vol V. Washington, DC: American Physiological Society, 1968:2699.

122. Janssens JP, Valembois P, Hellemans J, et al. Studies on the necessity of a bolus for the progression of secondary peristalsis in the canine esophagus. Gastroenterology 1974;67:245.

123. Janssens J, Valembois P, Vantrappen G, et al. Is the primary peristaltic contraction of the canine esophagus bolus-dependent? Gastroenterology 1973;65:750.

124. Jordan PH, Longhi EH. Relationship between size of bolus and the act of swallowing on esophageal peristalsis in dogs. Proc Soc Exp Biol Med 1971;137:868.

125. Longhi EH, Jordan PH. Necessity of a bolus for propagation of primary peristalsis in the canine esophagus. Am J Physiol 1971;220: 609.

126. DeCarle DJ, Szabo AC, Christensen J. Temperature dependence of responses of esophageal smooth muscle to electrical field stimulation. Am J Physiol 1977;232:E432.

127. Roman C, Tieffenbach L. Activity of vagal efferent fibers innervating the baboon's esophagus. J Physiol (Paris) 1972;64:479.

128. Tieffenbach L, Roman C. The role of extrinsic vagal innervation in the motility of the smooth muscled portion of the esophagus: electromyographic study in the cat and baboon. J Physiol (Paris) 1972;64: 193.

129. Gidda JS, Cobb BW, Goyal RK. Modulation of esophageal peristalsis by vagal efferent stimulation in opossum. J Clin Invest 1981;68:1411.

130. Weisbrodt NW, Christensen J. Gradient of contractions in the opossum esophagus. Gastroenterology 1972;62:1159.

131. Rattan S, Gidda JS, Goyal RK. Membrane potential and mechanical responses of the opossum esophagus to vagal stimulation and swallowing. Gastroenterology 1983;85:922.

132. Gidda JS, Goyal RK. Swallow-evoked action potentials in vagal preganglionic efferents. J Neurophysiol 1984;52:1169.

133. Crist J, Suprenant A, Goyal RK. Intracellular studies of electrical membrane properties of esophageal circular smooth muscle in peristalsis. Gastroenterology 1987;92:987.

134. Diamant NE. Electrical activity of the cat smooth muscle esophagus: a study of hyperpolarizing responses. In: Daniel EE, ed. Proceedings of the Fourth International Symposium on Gastrointestinal Motility, Banff, Alberta, Canada. Vancouver: Mitchell, 1974:593.

135. Gidda JS, Goyal RK. Influence of successive vagal stimulation on contractions in esophageal smooth muscle of opossum. J Clin Invest 1983;71:1095.

136. Peden JK, Schneider MD, Bickel RD. Anatomic relations of the vagus nerves to the esophagus. Am J Surg 1950;80:32.

137. Kravitz JJ, Snape WJ, Cohen S. Effect of thoracic vagotomy and vagal stimulation on esophageal function. Am J Physiol 1978;234: E359.

138. Gidda JS. Control of esophageal peristalsis: viewpoints on digestive diseases. 1985;17:13.

139. Gidda JS, Buyniski JP. Swallow-evoked peristalsis in opossum esophagus: role of cholinergic mechanisms. Am J Physiol 1986;251: G779.

140. Sugarbaker DJ, Rattan S, Goyal RK. Swallowing induces sequential activation of esophageal longitudinal smooth muscle. Am J Physiol 1984;247:G515.

141. Crist J, Gidda JS, Goyal RK. Intramural mechanism of esophageal peristalsis: roles of cholinergic and non-cholinergic nerves. Proc Natl Acad Sci USA 1984;81:3595.

142. Sarna SK, Daniel EE, Waterfall WE. Myogenic and neural control systems for esophageal motility. Gastroenterology 1977;73:1345.

143. Decktor DL, Ryan JP. Transmembrane voltage of opossum esophageal smooth muscle and its response to electrical stimulation of intrinsic nerves. Gastroenterology 1982;82:301.

144. Schulze K, Conklin JL, Christensen J. A potassium gradient in smooth muscle segment of the opossum esophagus. Am J Physiol 1977;232: E270.

145. Christensen J. Motor functions of the pharynx and esophagus. In:

Johnson LR, ed. Physiology of the gastrointestinal tract, ed 2. New York: Raven Press, 1987:595.

146. Crist J, Gidda JS, Goyal RK. Characteristics of "on" and "off" contractions in esophageal circular muscle in vitro. Am J Physiol 1984;246:G137.

147. DeCarle DJ, Templeman DL, Christensen J. Responses of the circular layer of smooth muscle from the body to electrical field stimulation. In: Duthie HL, ed. Gastrointestinal motility in health and disease. Lancaster, England: MTP Press Ltd, 1978:513.

148. Behar J, Guenard V, Walsh JH, Biancani P. Vasoactive intestinal peptide and acetylcholine: Inhibitory and excitatory neurotransmitters in the cat esophagus. Am J Physiol 1989;257:G380.

149. Dodds WJ, Stef JJ, Stewart ET, et al. Responses of feline esophagus to cervical vagal stimulation. Am J Physiol 1978;235:E63.

150. Dodds WJ, Dent J, Hogan WJ, Arndorfer RC. Effect of atropine on esophageal motor function in humans. Am J Physiol 1981;240:G290.

151. Uddman R, Alumets J, Edvinsson L, et al. Peptidergic (VIP) innervation of the esophagus. Gastroenterology 1978;75:5.

152. Biancani P, Hillemeier C, Bitar KN, Makhlouf GM. Contraction mediated by Ca^{++} influx in the esophagus and by Ca^{++} release in the LES. Am J Physiol 1987;253:G760.

153. Hillemeier C, Bereiter D, Biancani P. Inositol triphosphate and phorbol 12-myristate 13-acetate-induced contraction in smooth muscle cells from esophagus, lower esophageal sphincter, and gastric fundus of cat. Gastroenterology 1987;92:1435.

154. Szewczak S, Behar J, Billett G, et al. VIP reduces resting phosphoinositide levels in the cat lower esophageal sphincter (LES). Gastroenterology 1989;96:A498.

155. Asoh R, Goyal RK. Electrical activity of the opossum lower esophageal sphincter in vivo: its role in the basal sphincter pressure. Gastroenterology 1978;74:835.

156. Holloway RH, Blank EL, Takahashi I, et al. Electrical control activity of the lower esophageal sphincter in unanesthetized opossums. Am J Physiol 1987;252:G511.

157. Goyal RK, Rattan S. Genesis of basal sphincter pressure: effect of tetrodotoxin on lower esophageal sphincter pressure in opossum in vivo. Gastroenterology 1976;71:62.

158. Behar J, Kerstein M, Biancani P. Neural control of the lower esophageal sphincter in the cat: studies on the excitatory pathways to the lower esophageal sphincter. Gastroenterology 1982;82:680.

159. Fournet J, Snape WJ, Cohen S. Sympathetic control of lower esophageal sphincter function in the cat: action of direct cervical and splanchnic nerve stimulation. J Clin Invest 1979;63:562.

160. Brown FC, Gideon RM, Voelker FA, Castell DO. Muscle function and structure of the esophagus of the baboon *(Papio anubis)*. Am J Vet Res 1978;39:1209.

161. Behar J, Kastendieck J. Studies on sphincter competence. Gastroenterology 1974;66:834.

162. Zwick R, Bowes KL, Daniel EE, Sarna SK. Mechanism of action of pentagastrin on the lower esophageal sphincter. J Clin Invest 1976;57:1644

163. Jennewein HM, Hummelt H, Meyer U, et al. The effect of vagotomy on the resting pressure and reactivity of the lower esophageal sphincter (LES) in man and dog. In: Vantrappen G, ed. Proceedings of the Fifth International Symposium on Gastrointestinal Motility. Herentals, Belgium: Typoff, 1976:186.

164. Price LM, El-Sharkawy TY, Mui HY, Diamant NE. Effect of bilateral cervical vagotomy on balloon-induced lower esophageal sphincter relaxation in the dog. Gastroenterology 1979;77:324.

165. DiMarino AJ, Cohen S. The adrenergic control of lower esophageal sphincter function: an experimental model of denervation supersensitivity. J Clin Invest 1973;52:2264.

166. Goyal RK, Rattan S. Nature of the vagal inhibitory innervation of the lower esophageal sphincter. J Clin Invest 1975;55:1119.

167. DeCarle DJ, Christensen J, Szabo AC, et al. Calcium dependence of neuromuscular events in esophageal smooth muscle of the opossum. Am J Physiol 1977;232:E547.

168. Biancani P, Billett G, Cooke P, et al. Experimental esophagitis affects inositol phosphates in the cat lower esophageal sphincter (LES). Gastroenterology 1989;96:A42.

169. Schulze-Delrieu K, Crane SA. Oxygen uptake and mechanical tension in esophageal smooth muscle from opossums and cats. Am J Physiol 1982;242:G258.

170. Reynolds JC, Ouyang A, Cohen S. A lower esophageal sphincter reflex involving substance P. Am J Physiol 1984;24646.

171. Christensen J. Motor functions of the pharynx and esophagus. In: Johnson LR, ed. Physiology of the gastrointestinal tract, ed 2. New York: Raven Press, 1987.

172. Goyal RK, Rattan S. Mechanism of the lower esophageal sphincter relaxation. Action of prostaglandin E$_1$ and theophylline. J Clin Invest 1973;55:337.

173. Zelcer E, Weisbrodt NW. Electrical and mechanical activity in the lower esophageal sphincter of the cat. Am J Physiol 1984;246:G243.

174. Paterson WG, Rattan S, Goyal RK. Lower esophageal sphincter responses to balloon inflation, deflation, and obstruction of the esophageal body. Gastroenterology 1986;90:1579.

175. Percy W, Schulze-Delrieu K, Shirazi S, VonDerau K. Spread of mechanical activity across the isolated gastroesophageal junction (JCT) of the opossum. Dig Dis Sci 1985;30:787.

176. Gershon MD. Effects of tetrodotoxin on innervated smooth muscle preparations. Br J Pharmacol Chemother 1967;29:259.

177. Behar J, Field S, Marin C. Effect of glucagon, secretin, and vasoactive intestinal polypeptide on the feline lower esophageal sphincter: mechanisms of action. Gastroenterology 1979;77:1001.

178. Rattan S, Said SI, Goyal RK. Effect of vasoactive intestinal polypeptide. Proc Soc Exp Biol Med 1977;155:40.

179. Biancani P, Walsh JH, Behar J. Vasoactive intestinal polypeptide: a neurotransmitter for lower esophageal sphincter relaxation. J Clin Invest 1984;73:963.

180. Goyal RK, Rattan S, Said SI. VIP as a possible neurotransmitter of non-cholinergic, non-adrenergic inhibitory neurons. Nature 1980;288:378.

181. Biancani P, Beinfeld, Hillemeier C, Behar J. Peptide histidine isoleucine: a second neurotransmitter for lower esophageal sphincter relaxation. Gastroenterology (In press).

182. Rattan S, Gonella P, Goyal RK. Inhibitory effect of calcitonin gene-related peptide and calcitonin on opossum esophageal smooth muscle. Gastroenterology 1988;94:284.

183. Lundberg JM, Fahrenkrug J, Larson O, Anggard A. Co-release of vasoactive intestinal polypeptide and peptide histidine isoleucine in relation to atropine-resistant vasodilation in cat submandibular salivary gland. Neurosci Lett 1984;52:37.

184. Magistretti PJ, Schorderet M. VIP and noradrenaline act synergistically to increase cyclic AMP in cerebral cortex. Nature 1984;308:280.

185. Borghi C, Nicosia S, Giachetti A, Said SI. Vasoactive intestinal polypeptide (VIP) stimulates adenylate cyclase in selected areas of rat brain. Life Sci 1979;24:65.

186. Kerwin RW, Pay S, Bhoola KD, Pycock CJ. Vasoactive intestinal polypeptide (VIP) sensitive adenylate cyclase in rat brain: regional distribution and localization on hypothalamic neurons. J Pharm Pharmacol 1980;32:561.

187. Torphy TJ, Fine CF, Burman M, et al. Lower esophageal sphincter relaxation is associated with increased cyclic nucleotide content. Am J Physiol 1986;251:G786.

188. Rattan S, Gidda JS, Goyal RK. Membrane potential and mechanical responses of the opossum esophagus to vagal stimulation and swallowing. Gastroenterology 1983;85:922.

189. Jensen DM, McCallum R, Walsh JH. Failure of atropine to inhibit gastrin-17 stimulation of the lower esophageal sphincter in man. Gastroenterology 1978;75:825.

190. Meissner AJ, Bowes KL, Zwick R, Daniel EE. Effect of motilin on the lower esophageal sphincter. Gut 1976;17:925.

191. Holloway RH, Blank E, Takahashi I, Dodds WJ, Layman RD. Motilin: a mechanism incorporating the opossum lower esophageal sphincter into the migrating motor complex. Gastroenterology 1985;89:507.

192. Mukhopadhyay AK, Kunnemann M. Mechanism of lower esophageal sphincter stimulation by bombesin in the opossum. Gastroenterology 1979;76:1409.

193. Corazziari E, Delle Fave G, Pozzessere C, et al. Effect of bombesin on lower esophageal sphincter in humans. Gastroenterology 1982;83:10-14.

194. Maher JW, Olinde AJ, McGuigan JE. Suppression of postprandial lower esophageal sphincter pressure and pancreatic polypeptide by duodenal exclusion. J Surg Res 1984;37:467.

195. Rattan S, Goyal RK. Effect of galanin on the opossum lower esophageal sphincter. Life Sci 1987;41:2783.

196. Mukhopadhyay AK. Effect of substance P on the lower esophageal sphincter of the opossum. Gastroenterology 1978;75:278.

197. Dodds WJ, Dent J, Hogan WJ, et al. Paradoxical lower esophageal sphincter contraction induced by cholecystokinin-octapeptide in patients with achalasia. Gastroenterology 1981;80:327.

198. Hogan WJ, Dodds WJ, Hoke SE, et al. Effect of glucagon on esophageal motor function. Gastroenterology 1975;69:160.

199. Sinar DR, O'Dorisio TM, Mazzaferri EL, et al. Effect of gastric inhibitory polypeptide on lower esophageal sphincter pressure in cats. Gastroenterology 1978;75:263.

200. Siegel SR, Brown FC, Castell DO, et al. Effects of vasoactive intestinal polypeptide (VIP) on lower esophageal sphincter in awake baboons: comparison with glucagon and secretin. Dig Dis Sci 1979;24:345.

201. Rosell S, Thor K, Rokaeus A, et al. Plasma concentration on neurotensin-like immunoreactivity (NTLI) and lower esophageal sphincter (LES) pressure in man following infusion of (Gln^4)-neurotensin. Acta Physiol Scand 1980;109:369.

202. Theodorsson-Norheim E, Thor K, Rosell S. Relation between lower esophageal sphincter (LES) pressure and the plasma concentration of neurotensin during intravenous infusion of neurotensin(1-13) and (Gln^4)-neurotensin(1-13) in man. Acta Physiol Scand (Suppl) 1983;515:29.

203. Behar J, Biancani P. Effect of cholecystokinin-octapeptide on lower esophageal sphincter. Gastroenterology 1977;73:57.

204. Dent J, Dodds WJ, Hogan WJ, et al. Effect of cholecystokinin-octapeptide on opossum lower esophageal sphincter. Am J Physiol 1980;239:G230.

205. Thor K, Rokaeus A. Studies on the mechanisms by which (Gln^4)-neurotensin reduces lower esophageal sphincter (LES) pressure in man. Acta Physiol Scand 1983;118:373.

206. Bybee DE, Brown FC, Georges LP, et al. Somatostatin effects on lower esophageal sphincter function. Am J Physiol 1979;237:E77.

207. Walsh JH. Gastrointestinal hormones. In: Johnson LR, ed. Physiology of the gastrointestinal tract, ed 2. New York: Raven Press, 1987:181.

208. Thor P, Krol R, Konturek SJ, et al. Effect of somatostatin on myoelectrical activity of small bowel. Am J Physiol 1978;235:E249.

209. Kaye MD. On the relationship between gastric pH and pressure in the normal human lower esophageal sphincter. Gut 1979;20:59.

210. Nebel OT, Castell DO. Kinetics of fat inhibition of the lower esophageal sphincter. J Appl Physiol 1973;35:6.

8

The Physiology of Gastric Motility and Gastric Emptying

JAMES H. MEYER

The stomach is a primary organ of digestion with many functions. In addition to its own secretion of intrinsic factor, acid, lipase, and proteases, its distention triggers reflexes that stimulate secretion of pancreatic enzymes and control intestinal motility. The stomach stores food not as a homogeneous mixture but in segregations that provide regions of varying pH and permit continuing digestion of starch by swallowed amylase near pH 7, while also initiating digestion of protein by pepsin at pHs below 5. It empties nutrients at tightly controlled rates that are slow enough to allow their efficient digestion and absorption from the small intestine and their frugal metabolic disposition after intestinal absorption. It fractures food into tiny particles, allowing them to pass on while retaining those which are larger and thus inherently less digestible. In view of these diverse and complex functions, it is little wonder that the stomach exhibits a vastly complex motility.

Scientists, driven by different clinical needs, are just beginning to grasp these complexities. There is an obvious need to understand symptomatic disorders of gastric motor function; but beyond this there are separate needs to know exactly how the stomach delivers drugs to drug-absorbing intestine or, so that better gastric operations can be devised, to know how the stomach contributes to digestion or ultimately controls rates of absorption and metabolism of nutrients. This review of gastric motor physiology is primarily intended as background for a clinical chapter on disorders of gastric emptying (ch 60) but will also deal with these other issues.

ANATOMY

The stomach is a J-shaped, almost conical bladder, with its apex terminating at the lower tip of the J in a 1-cm pyloric canal and its 8-cm base lying at the upper end of the J, under the diaphragm. The lesser curvature falls along the more medial, inner bend of the J, and the greater curvature falls along the lateral, outer aspect of the J curve. Its position is fixed by its attachments at its upper end to the esophagus (which is sheathed by the diaphragm) and at its lower end to the duodenum (which is anchored by ligaments and ducts). Between these two points of attachment, the stomach may dilate as it is filled with food so that the bottom of the J extends downward and the tip of the J becomes somewhat more U-shaped.

The walls of the stomach consist of smooth muscle fibers arrayed as an outer longitudinal layer, a median circular layer, and an inner oblique layer, but the circular layer predominates throughout. The oblique muscular layer is distinguishable only along the lesser curvature, near the cardia, and the longitudinal layer is prominent only along the greater and lesser curvatures of the distal two thirds of the stomach. The muscular walls are thicker in the distal portion of the stomach (the antrum and caudad corpus) than in the more proximal fundus and orad corpus.

At its distal apex, the stomach ends at the pyloric sphincter, a thickening of circular muscle layer 2 to 3 cm in length. The pylorus terminates in a septum of connective tissue that marks the gastroduodenal junction. Outer, longitudinal muscle fibers run from the antrum to this septum. Contractions of the circular muscle layers close the pyloric sphincter, while contractions of the longitudinal muscles open it. Closure of the pylorus is facilitated by a thick, redundant mucosa in the narrow pyloric canal.[1]

GASTRIC SMOOTH MUSCLE

Electromechanical Properties

The distal two thirds of the stomach (midcorpus to antrum) undergoes phasic contractions (i.e., vigorous contractions of high force over 10 seconds). These phasic contractions may be detected in a variety of ways. As they shorten circular muscle, they will deform strain gauges that have been surgically implanted along the serosal surface of stomachs in experimental animals. As they close the gastric walls, they can be discerned at fluoroscopy of contrast-filled stomachs, at gamma scintigraphy of nuclide-filled stomachs, or at real-time ultrasonography as rings of gastric narrowing. Similarly, the closure of gastric walls against intraluminal balloons, perfused, side-holed catheters, or intraluminal pressure transducers can be detected as localized increases in pressure. The proximal one third of the stomach (fundus and orad corpus) does not exhibit phasic contractions. Instead, it alters its tone (muscle fiber length) over many minutes or exhibits contractions of moderate force over 1 to 6 minutes. These slow contractions of medium amplitude cannot be discerned at fluoroscopy but have been detected by measuring changes in pressures within intraluminal balloons filled with constant volumes of air.[2] More recently, tone in the proximal stomach has been monitored in animals and human subjects[3] with an electronic barostat. This is an intraluminal balloon that is placed in the fundus; its volume is repeatedly and rapidly adjusted by sensitive electrical equipment to maintain a constant, low pressure against the walls of the fundus. The air volume needed to maintain this pressure is measured as an index of fundic volume (proportional to surrounding muscle length or tone).

Smooth muscle cells maintain negative transmembrane potentials with an electrogenic sodium pump. Fluctuations in this membrane potential, if large enough, alter calcium channels, creating

an inward flux of calcium. As calcium ions move inward into the cell, they trigger contraction of filaments of actomyosin. Gastric smooth muscle cells are interconnected by nexi or gap junctions (points of membrane fusions between cells), forming an electrical syncytium similar to that in the heart. Fluctuations in membrane potential at one point in the syncytium may then be conducted across membranes of adjacent cells in a wavelike pattern. If fluctuations of membrane potentials are large enough within this propagating wave, each cell will contract as the electrical wave crosses it, producing a similarly propagating wave of contractions.

Smooth muscle cells in various regions of the stomach have differing electrical behaviors (Fig 8-1) when examined as isolated cells in vitro.[4] These differences underlie regional differences in contractility. Muscle cells from the most proximal third of the stomach have smaller resting membrane potentials than cells from the more distal stomach, and the resting membrane potentials in

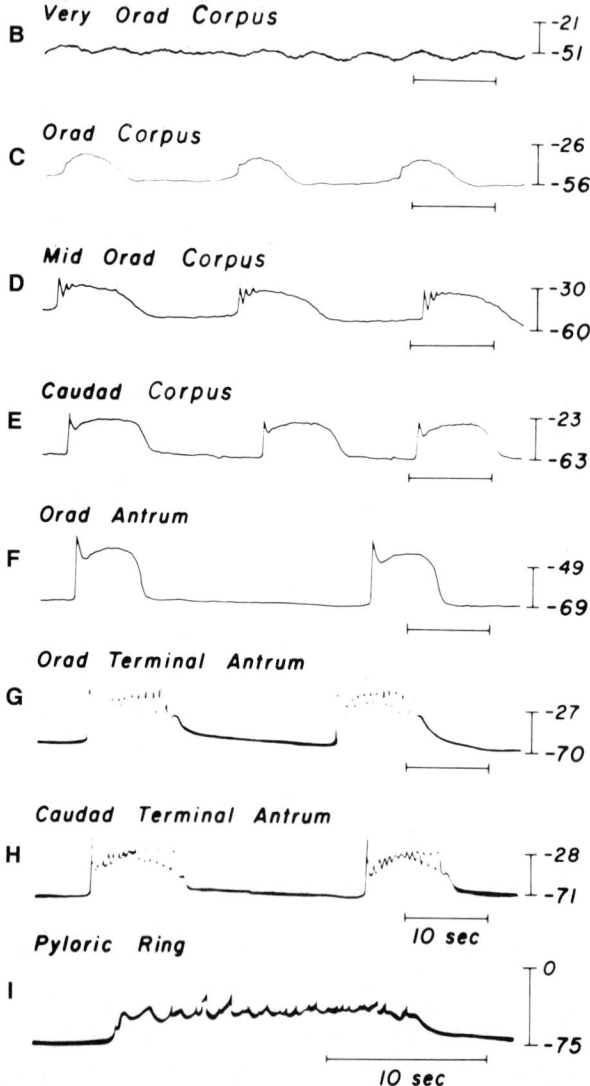

FIGURE 8–1. Intracellular resting membrane and spontaneous action or "plateau" potentials recorded in different regions of the canine stomach. (From Szurszewski JH. Electrical basis of gastrointestinal motility. In: Johnson LR, ed. Physiology of the gastrointestinal tract. New York: Raven Press, 1981:1435.)

the most proximal cells are stable and do not spontaneously fluctuate. Cells from the distal stomach have increasingly more negative resting membrane potentials as cells are examined from more and more distal sites. Moreover, the resting membrane potentials of these more distal cells are unstable, undergoing periodic, partial depolarizations. The magnitude of spontaneous voltage fluctuations becomes larger as cells which are more and more distal are examined. The frequencies of periodic fluctuations of membrane potential also vary among cells sampled from different regions of the distal two thirds of the stomach. The cycle frequency is highest in more proximal cells and lowest in more distal cells.

Fluctuations of membrane potential from the cells in the intact stomach with the highest periodicity are quickly conducted as a wave over neighboring, more distal cells with lower periodicities. Just as in the heart, gastric muscle cells with the highest frequency entrain and drive their slower neighbors. They are thus called the electrical pacesetter, and the waves of fluctuating electrical potentials that sweep out from them over their neighbors are called the pacesetter potential or the electrical control activity. The dominating cells with the highest frequency are found one third of the way down along the greater curvature of the stomach (Fig 8-2). If these cells are surgically removed, other cells with the next highest frequency become the pacesetter.[5] In humans, the pacesetter frequency is 3 cycles/min, but it is 5/min in dogs.

The pacesetter potential probably originates in cells between longitudinal and circular muscles, but its amplitude and conduction are reinforced and increased by circular muscle. Its conduction is seven times faster along the axis of circular muscle bundles than across the bundles.[6] The speed of conduction is doubled when

circular muscle is stretched in vitro by 25% to 50% of resting length, suggesting that the in vivo efficiency of conduction may increase as the stomach is distended with food. Because circumferential spread is considerably faster than downward spread, the wave of partial depolarization sweeps quickly around the stomach and then downward along the stomach as a ring that begins at midcorpus and sweeps over the antrum to the pylorus. Speed of conduction accelerates from 0.5 cm/sec to 4 cm/sec as the ringlike wave moves from midcorpus to antrum, and the magnitude of depolarization also changes from 0.5 mV to 2 mV as cells in the antrum are enveloped by the wave. The gastric pacesetter potential is seldom conducted across the pylorus into the duodenum because its propagation is quenched by the connective tissue septum between pylorus and duodenum.

If membrane potentials fluctuate enough, calcium channels are opened and the muscle cell contracts. A more sustained positive potential is associated with contraction, probably from a calcium current. These sustained, positive potentials with contractions are therefore variously called plateau potentials (because of their sustained duration), action potentials (because of their association with contractions), or electrical response activity (i.e., they represent a contractile response to the pacesetter or electrical control activity). The shape and duration of the plateau potential varies in different regions: it is steady and short (about 10 seconds) in muscle cells in the corpus but longer (20 seconds) and undulating in cells in the terminal antrum (Fig 8-1). Both the brief, regularly periodic pacesetter potentials and the more sustained, often undulating, less regular plateau potentials can be recorded by electrodes implanted into the serosal surface of the stomach in animals

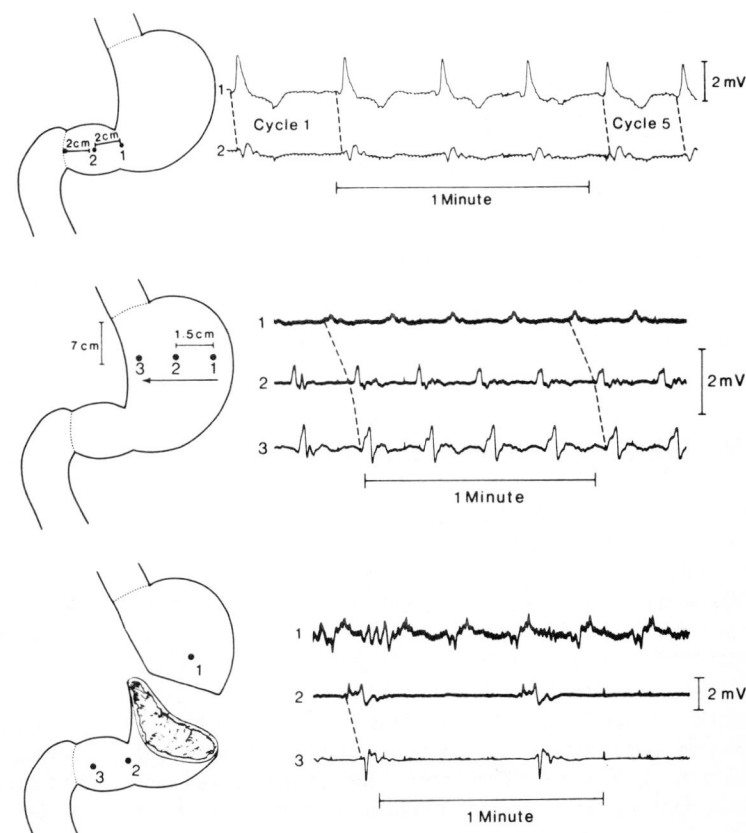

FIGURE 8-2. Pacesetter potentials measured during surgery on the human stomach. Top panel shows rapid progression of normal 3/min pacesetter potential along the terminal antrum. Middle panel illustrates normal, circumferential spread. In the bottom panel, transection of the stomach interrupted the dominance of the faster pacesetter from proximal stomach, so that a slower pacesetter at point #2 drives the antrum. (From Hinder RA, Kelly KA. Human gastric pacesetter potential. Site of origin, spread, and response to gastric transection and proximal gastric vagotomy. Am J Surg 1977;133:29.)

or by suction electrodes implanted endoscopically across the gastric mucosa into stomach muscle. In animals, the plateau or action potentials so recorded correspond temporally with recorded deformations of strain gauges also implanted on the serosal surface.[7]

As just indicated, the pacesetter potential will excite a contraction when the change in membrane voltage is great enough to open calcium channels. Because the pacesetter potential is larger in more distal cells of the antrum, contractions follow it more commonly here than more proximally, just as these isolated antral cells in vitro exhibit spontaneous contractions more commonly (Fig 8-1) than cells from the more proximal stomach. Similarly, the absence of pacesetter potentials in cells of the proximal third of the stomach accounts for the absence of phasic contractions there. Thus, regional contractility of the stomach is the direct outcome of cellular physiology of muscle in different regions. Even characteristics of the ringlike, peristaltic contractions that sweep the distal stomach are largely determined by the electrophysiologic properties of the muscle cells. Thus, the basic patterns of contractility are myogenic in origin.

How often a pacesetter potential will excite a contraction depends on the varying level of excitability of the muscle cell. Muscle cells may be made more or less likely to contract in response to a pacesetter potential by hormones that reach them from the general circulation and by neurotransmitters released at the locus of the muscle cell. Therefore, not every wave of pacesetter potentials results in contractions. For example, even though pacesetter waves continue to sweep the stomach, contractions of the antrum may be completely abolished when fat is in the small intestine; it is known that this inhibition is associated with the release of intestinal hormones into the bloodstream and with vagal inhibition (undoubtedly by neurotransmitters), which decrease the excitability of antral muscle cells. Conversely, antral contractility may be enhanced in response to vagovagal reflexes when the stomach is distended so that every pacesetter wave results in a wave of contractions that run along the entire stomach. Depending on local controls that modulate contractile responsiveness to the electrical pacesetter wave, contraction waves may begin in the midstomach and die out before sweeping the terminal antrum or, alternatively, involve only the terminal antrum. Despite the constant periodicity of pacesetter potentials (3/min in man), contractions may arise from 0 to a maximum of 3/min, depending on the modulation of muscular excitability by neurohormonal agents. Thus, *neurogenic* control may modify myogenic patterns.

Modulation by Regulatory Peptides

Many classic gastrointestinal (GI) hormones released from gastrointestinal mucosa into the bloodstream are now also known to be contained in and released from nerve endings near muscle cells. The actions of several of these regulatory peptides have been studied in vitro on isolated gastrointestinal smooth muscle cells.[8-13] To study stimulation of contractions (Table 8-1), the shortening of resting muscle cells can be measured when these agents are added singly, or in combination, to the cell bath at varying concentrations. Conversely, to study inhibition of contraction, agents can be added when suspended muscle cells are maximally shortened by octapeptide of cholecystokinin (CCK-8) already in the bath. This kind of in vitro testing is used to identify

TABLE 8-1

Efficacy of Mediators on Gastric Smooth Muscle Cells*

AGENT	EFFECTIVE CONCENTRATION (mol/liter)	INTERACTION
Contracting Agent		
Acetylecholine	10^{-12} to 10^{-7}	Atropine blocks
Gastrin-17	10^{-12} to 10^{-9}	
CCK-8	10^{-12} to 10^{-9}	Proglumide blocks
		Acetylcholine synergistic
Substance P	10^{-11} to 10^{-7}	Spantide blocks
Dynorphin	10^{-11} to 10^{-8}	
Met-enkephalin	10^{-10} to 10^{-8}	Naloxone blocks
Leu-enkephalin	10^{-8} to 10^{-6}	
Relaxing Agent		
VIP	10^{-10} to 10^{-7}	IBMX enhances
Secretin	10^{-9} to 10^{-6}	IBMX enhances
		Synergistic with VIP
Glucagon	Greater than secretin, weak compared with VIP	

* Most of these in vitro studies were performed with suspensions of antral muscle cells.

the presence of cell receptors and their sensitivity (affinity) to the agents and to study interactions between agonists. These studies indicate that at low physiologic concentrations, CCK and gastrin share the same receptor that stimulates contraction, acetylcholine stimulates contraction by way of a different receptor, and CCK and acetylcholine are synergistic. Vasoactive intestinal peptide (VIP), on the other hand, relaxes already contracted smooth muscle cells, an action shared at higher concentrations (lower receptor affinity) by its structural homologs, secretin and glucagon. There are also receptors to endorphins, enkephalins, and substance P, which are found at nerve endings and are probably neurotransmitters. How each agent alters the electromechanical properties of the cells is not well defined, but presumably the stimuli greatly heighten and the inhibitors reduce the spontaneous contractions of the cells.

Other scientists [4,14,15] have studied the action of hormones and neurotransmitters on electromechanical properties of muscle strips suspended in solutions in a way to allow measurement of both muscle tension and membrane potentials with cellular electrodes. Acetylcholine, gastrin, and cholecystokinin increase the duration and amplitude of the plateau potential while increasing simultaneously the duration and amplitude of contraction. Conversely, norepinephrine and neurotensin decrease the duration and amplitude of both the plateau potential and contraction. VIP antagonizes the effects of gastrin on amplitude and duration of plateau potentials and contractions. In addition, VIP inhibits spontaneous contractions or those stimulated by acetylcholine without altering membrane potential. These observations indicate that VIP has two separate modes of inhibition. Similarly, although both acetylcholine and gastrin augment duration and magnitude of plateau potentials and contractions, the fact that VIP reduces contractions to both agents while inhibiting the electrical response only to gastrin indicates that acetylcholine and gastrin stimulate contractions by different postreceptor pathways, a fact also implied by their synergism (potentiation).

NERVOUS CONTROL

Gastric Innervation

The stomach is innervated largely by way of the vagus nerves from which branches reach the stomach wall along the lesser curvature. Most vagal fibers are afferent nerves that originate in two kinds of gastric sensors. Stretch receptors, located in the gastric wall, increase their rate of discharge on passive distention of the stomach, but they may also fire during antral contractions that deform them. Free nerve endings in the mucosa are slowly adapting chemosensors. Long afferents run from the stomach to the brain stem. However, the persistence of some reflexes after vagal transection indicate that there also is an afferent nerve supply localized to the stomach. In addition to vagal afferent nerves,[16] there are mechanosensitive and chemosensitive afferent splanchnic nerves[17] along the gastrointestinal tract. Impulses from splanchnic afferents run along mesenteric nerves to prevertebral ganglia; eventually some of these impulses may reach the brain stem by way of the spinal cord.[18]

Vagal efferent nerves originate from cell bodies in the brain stem. These efferent nerves are of two types. When stimulated by interrupted current at low electrical frequencies, the low threshold fibers cause the stomach to increase its tone in the fundus, phasic contractions in the antrum, or resistance to flow in the pylorus (reduce pyloric diameter). In the antrum, this kind of excitation results in an increase in amplitude and duration of plateau potentials and a higher frequency of contractions after pacesetter potentials. These responses to low-frequency stimulation are blocked by atropine and by hexamethonium. Thus, they are excitatory fibers that are presumed to be parasympathetic, acetylcholinergic nerves acting primarily through intramural ganglia with which they synapse. A second group of efferent fibers is not stimulated at low frequency but responds to high-frequency current. These high-frequency fibers are inhibitory, relaxing fundic tone and decreasing antral contractions and pyloric resistance. Their inhibiting action is blocked neither by atropine nor by adrenergic blockers; hence they are termed noncholinergic, nonadrenergic nerves. They probably inhibit by releasing VIP near the gastric muscles. For example, when high-frequency stimulation of the peripheral cut ends of the vagus relaxes gastric muscle strips suspended in a tissue bath, VIP is simultaneously released into the bath,[19] and when the stomachs of anesthetized cats are made to relax by high-frequency stimulation, VIP is similarly released into gastric venous blood.[20]

The vagal branches also carry adrenergic, efferent nerves that originate in the thoracic spinal cord and commingle with vagal efferent fibers at the level of the esophageal plexus. Most efferent sympathetic supply enters the celiac ganglion and makes its way to the stomach along the celiac artery. Sympathetic efferents inhibit gastric contractions either by modulating activity in the myenteric plexus, where most fibers end, or through the release of norepinephrine along the muscles reached by some sympathetic fibers.

Like the rest of the gastrointestinal tract, the stomach has extensive submucosal and myenteric plexuses from which a great deal of programmed activity originates. Thus, many gastric reflexes remain after cutting vagal and/or splanchnic nerves (though some remaining are modified). Also, as in the rest of the gastrointestinal tract, intragastric nerves contain a variety of neurotransmitters such as VIP (most prominent), substance P, enkephalins, gastrin, and CCK.

Central Nervous Control

Although the vagal nerves originate in the brain stem in or near the nucleus ambiguous, it is quite clear that stimuli to other portions of the brain may influence gastric motility. The pathways are only partly known, but similar pathways may mediate abnormal responses in human neurologic and psychiatric disorders.

By rotating a drum around stationary subjects seated inside it, a form of motion sickness can be induced. The visual perception of the moving drum gives the subject an illusion of motion and in many individuals precipitates symptoms of motion sickness (sweating, nausea, salivation, dizziness, headache). When these subjects develop motion sickness, the pacesetter potentials in their stomachs are altered. During the motion sickness, pacesetters that fire more rapidly than 3/min arise in the more distal stomach where, because of their higher frequencies, they dominate, driving waves of pacesetter potentials in reverse toward the proximal stomach. There may be more than one such focus, so that the regular electrical pattern of the stomach is now chaotic. Consequently, contractile activity is frequently not peristaltic.[21] This disorganized pattern is analogous to fibrillation of the heart and is frequently called tachygastria. The response is an example of how stimuli to the visual cortex and higher brain centers somehow affect electrical stability of gastric muscle cell membranes.

Submersion of a hand in ice water or labyrinthine stimulation inhibits antral contractions after a solid meal in human volunteers,[22] and the labyrinthine stimulation slows gastric emptying of food. This response is associated with alterations in autonomic nervous controls (elevated pulse rate and blood pressure) and high levels of circulating norepinephrine and endorphins. Giving naloxone or beta adrenergic blockers prevents the change in antral motility. In dogs, acoustic stress alters contractile patterns of the fasting stomach but not the gut.[23] While heart rate and plasma cortisol levels are significantly elevated by the stress, the gastric response is blocked by bilateral truncal vagotomy. In rats, partial immersion into cold water stimulates gastric motility. High intracranial pressures also stimulate gastric motility.[24]

Some stresses induce the intracerebral release of corticotropin releasing factor (CRF), and others the release of thyrotropin releasing factor (TRF). Direct instillation of CRF or TRF into the cerebral ventricles or the nucleus ambiguous alters gastric motility, and these responses are blocked by truncal vagotomy.[25] On intracerebral injection in rats, some of these stress-induced responses are blocked by a specific CRF antagonist.[26] The many observations indicate a complex control of vagal nuclei by the cerebral cortex.

Gastrointestinal Reflexes

Several well-defined reflexes (Table 8-2) undoubtedly control gastric motility and gastric emptying in conscious man. However, it is probable that many other reflexes important to control of gastric emptying have, as yet, escaped definition.

Mechanical stimulation of the throat or distention of the esophagus in anesthetized animals relaxes the tone of the proximal stomach (i.e., pressure within inflated intragastric balloons drops). This response is abolished by vagal transection. It is thus a vagal reflex called receptive relaxation. It appears to be mediated by high-frequency, nonadrenergic, noncholinergic, VIP-releasing nerves.[27,28] The stomachs of normal, conscious, human volunteers relax when distended by instilled water; that is, intragastric pressures do not rise much until more than 500 ml are instilled.[29,30] By contrast, in human subjects who have undergone transection of the vagal trunks or of the vagal branches to the proximal stomach, intragastric pressures rise sharply after instillation of even 100-ml volumes. Thus, a gastric accommodation reflex to the proximal stomach is carried in the vagus nerves.

In anesthetized ferrets, distention of the proximal stomach, when transected from the antrum, excites antral peristalsis, increasing the percentage of pacesetter potentials that give rise to contractions.[31] This antral reflex is then abolished by vagally denervating the antrum. Similarly, in dogs and humans, truncal vagotomy diminishes antral peristalsis in response to gastric distention.[29,30,32] Such loss of antral contractility may underlie gastric stasis, which is seen in about 30% of patients who have had a truncal vagotomy (see ch 60).

Feedback inhibition of gastric emptying by nutrients in the small intestine is an important feature of normal alimentation (discussed more extensively later). It is not surprising, therefore, that several gastroenteric and enterogastric reflexes have been described that may provide some of this precise control. There are four enterogastric reflexes (Table 8-2): two to the fundus, two to the antrum. Distention of the duodenum (or colon), but not the proximal jejunum, reduces fundic tone[33,34] and antral peristalsis. This reflex to the fundus is abolished by vagal cooling (with cooling jackets placed around the vagal trunks under the skin in the neck) or by vagal transection.[34] Inhibition of antral peristalsis by duodenal distention is blunted by either vagotomy or splanchnicectomy and is completely abolished by both. Fat, acid, peptides, and tryptophan in the small intestinal lumen inhibit antral peristalsis. The degree of inhibition is reduced (but not abolished) by truncal vagotomy,[35] suggesting that this enterogastric reflex to the antrum is partially carried in the vagus nerves. Nutrients in the canine small intestine also relax the fundus, an effect abolished by vagal cooling or transection.[36]

Messages may also travel from stomach to small intestine. Distending the stomach with large volumes impedes the flow of liquids through the small intestine.[37] While this gastroenteric reflex is not affected by vagotomy, it is reduced by denervation of the small intestine.[38]

Enteropyloric reflexes have been proposed. The best documented of these is the increase of pyloric tone and isolated, phasic contractions of the pylorus in humans or dogs in response to instillation of acid into the duodenum.[39] Because atropine or hexamethonium block these responses in human subjects, but neither propranolol nor phentolamine do so, the effect of luminal acid is

TABLE 8–2
Pertinent Gastrointestinal Reflexes

NAME	STIMULUS	ACTION	PATHWAY	REFERENCE
Reflex relaxation	Stroking throat, distending esophagus	Relaxes gastric tone	Vagus NANC#	27, 28
Accommodation reflex	Distention of stomach	Relaxes gastric tone to maintain low pressures	Vagus NANC#	27, 28
Enterofundic reflex	Fat, protein in jejunum; sugar, protein in ileum	Relaxes fundic tone	Vagus	35
Enterofundic reflex	Duodeno-jejunal distention	Relaxes fundic tone	Vagus	34
Antral reflex	Distention of stomach	Stimulates antral peristalsis	Vagus	31
Enterogastric reflex	Nutrients or acid in contact with proximal gut mucosa*	Inhibits antral peristalsis	Vagus and splanchnics	32, 61
Enterogastric reflex	Duodeno-jejunal distention	Inhibits antral peristalsis	Vagus and splanchnics	33
Pyloric reflex	Acid and fat in contact with duodeno-jejunal mucosa*	Tonically narrows pylorus; increases frequency of pyloric phasic contractions	? Vagus	38, 40, 41
Gastroenteric reflex	Gastric distention, especially when food present in upper GI tract	Increases gut resistance to inflow	Mesenteric nerves	36, 37

* Action may also be mediated by GI hormones (see text). Most observations on pathways were deduced from nerve section or cooling; with the exception of receptive relaxation, accommodation, and antral reflexes, afferent and efferent limbs of reflex have not been established.
\# NANC = noncholinergic, nonadrenergic vagal efferent fibers.

undoubtedly mediated by cholinergic nerves. Fat in the proximal intestine also narrows the pylorus (increases tone) and induces isolated phasic contractions of the pylorus[40] by atropine-sensitive (neural) mechanisms.[41] Nevertheless, fat in the intestinal lumen is a potent releaser of both secretin and cholecystokinin, and both of these hormones stimulate pyloric contractions,[42] so the action of fat is ambiguous. Adding to this ambiguity is the suggestion that low concentrations of circulating CCK may contract the pylorus through atropine-sensitive (neural) mechanisms.[43]

HORMONAL CONTROL

The above difficulty in deciding whether fat stimulates pyloric contractions by way of nervous or hormonal pathways, or both, pertains to all regulation of gastric motility. Thus, there is a possible synergism or even a redundancy between neural and hormonal controls. Just as vagal, enterogastric reflexes may relax the fundus, so also do CCK, secretin, glucagon, and gastrointestinal insulin-releasing peptide (GIP) when injected intravenously.[44] As these hormones are released into the bloodstream by nutrients in the small intestine, it is likely that they act in concert with the vagal, enterogastric reflex to relax the fundus. Likewise, just as nutrients in the gut trigger an enterogastric reflex to the antrum to inhibit antral contractility, the nutrient-released hormones secretin, GIP, and glucagon also inhibit antral peristalsis. On the other hand, CCK is potently released by intestinal nutrients but excites antral contractility.

Most studies of hormonal control of gastric motility or gastric emptying have measured motility or gastric emptying of saline meals in conscious, fasting animals in response to an intravenous injection of a single hormone. By contrast, in the postprandial state, many hormones are released simultaneously when nervous mechanisms are also in play. It is therefore difficult to extrapolate from studies of individually infused hormones to estimate how hormones might control postprandial motility. However, specific receptor antagonists to CCK, such as proglumide or L364718, have now been given to fed animals or human subjects, and these agents appear to speed postcibal emptying of the stomach.[45–47] The results indicate a regulatory role of CCK in slowing gastric emptying, even in the presence of other circulating hormones and potently acting neural controls.

The majority of older studies on hormonal control employed unrealistically high doses of hormones, before reliable assays for circulating hormone and conceptual sophistication dictated more physiologic doses. Thus, their relevance to alimentary physiology is in question. Recently, however, two studies have employed tiny doses of secretin[48] or CCK[49] in human subjects, doses small enough to achieve the low concentrations of circulating hormone found postprandially. The low physiologic concentrations of each hormone inhibit gastric emptying. Both studies, therefore, support the idea that GI hormones normally contribute to the regulation of gastric emptying.

Because CCK stimulates peristaltic contractions of the antrum (Table 8-1), one would guess that CCK speeds rather than slows gastric emptying. But gastric emptying is controlled at multiple sites. CCK also relaxes the fundus and contracts the pylorus. Its

actions at these last two sites is what slows gastric emptying[50] despite increased antral contractility.

INTEGRATED RESPONSES

Terminal Antral Contractions

Contractions that reach the terminal antrum (i.e., its distal half) envelop the remaining antrum and pylorus in constant, stereotypical pattern as they sweep across it. The pylorus closes 2 to 3 seconds after the advancing contraction ring first reaches the antrum, an event that, in turn, occurs 2 to 3 seconds before the lumen of the terminal antrum is obliterated by its contraction. The constancy of this pattern has been established by cineradiography, real-time ultrasonography, and electrical monitoring with serosal strain gauges[51–53]; these methods have also established that the timing of pyloric closure relative to the advancing contraction wave does not vary despite wide variation in the types of meals, speeds of gastric emptying, and frequency or amplitude of antral contractions.[54]

Szurszewski[4] has suggested that the integration of terminal antral contraction with pyloric closure is myogenic. This invariable sequence can be explained by the nature of electromechanical coupling. There is a double peak in contractions as the pacesetter and later plateau potentials excite muscular contraction. In the more contractile or excitable muscle cells of the terminal antrum, an initial contraction of low and constant amplitude is triggered by the rapid change in membrane voltage at the front of the pacesetter potential (Fig 8-3). The plateau potential follows about 3 seconds after the initially rapid depolarization of the pacesetter; the strength and duration of the ensuing contraction vary with the magnitude and duration of this plateau potential (in turn controlled by several regulatory peptides). The small, constant amplitude of the initial contraction may not be detected readily by cineradiography or pressure transducers in the large antral lumen, but at the narrow pylorus, this small contraction is enough to close the pylorus in advance of the high-amplitude contraction wave.

Fluids are swept across the antrum and out the pylorus while the contraction wave descends onto the antrum, but flow ceases as the pylorus closes. In the final phase, the most distal antrum further narrows as the pylorus remains closed (Fig 8-3). During this final phase of antral contraction against a closed pylorus, the arrested fluid column in the lumen of the antrum is now forced backward (retropelled) as the terminal antral walls squeeze down to obliterate the lumen. In effect, this sequence of contraction provides a to-and-fro oscillation of gastric contents with each terminal antral contraction. As will be discussed, this pattern of movement may play a critical role in the ability of the stomach to empty solids.

The fact that the pylorus actually closes (i.e., entirely obliterates its lumen) is a conclusion from cineradiography or ultrasonography. Both methods trace the movement of luminal fluids. The arresting of forward motion has been taken as evidence of pyloric closure, an impression reinforced by the interruption of the radiopaque column of barium sulfate in the locus of the pylorus on

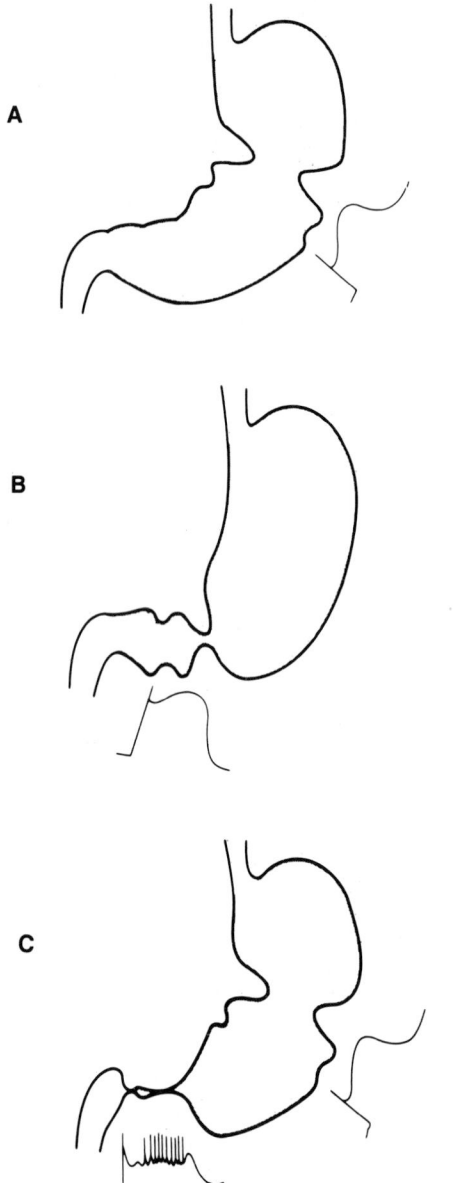

FIGURE 8–3. Schematic drawing of relation between action potentials and contractions. As depolarization sweeps over the distal stomach, there is some contraction at the initial depolarization, as well as a second, more vigorous contraction during the sustained, plateau or action potential. As the electrical events envelope the terminal antrum, the anatomically narrow pylorus clicks closed during the initial depolarization, just before the terminal antral lumen is obliterated by the deeper contractions during the later plateau potential. (From Szurszewski JH. Electrical basis of gastrointestinal motility. In: Johnson LR, ed. Physiology of the gastrointestinal tract. New York: Raven Press, 1981:1435.)

cineradiographs[50] and the apparent obliteration of the pyloric channel on ultrasonograms.[53,54] However, the anatomic resolution of either of these techniques is probably inadequate to say whether the pylorus was actually closed. The better spatial resolution of computed tomography has suggested that the (canine) pyloric canal narrows from 6.5 to about 2.5 mm but does not actually close.[55]

Ultrasonography has confirmed the intermittency of gastroduodenal fluid flows, especially frequent emptying of fluid for 2

to 3 seconds just in advance of the antral contraction wave. But gastric emptying of fluid is also often observed with this technique to start again as the pylorus opens well before the advance of the next wave into the antrum; similarly, episodes of duodenogastric reflux are observed without clear correspondence to duodenal or antral contractions near the pylorus.[56] The temporal patterns of flow indicate pressure transients generated by contractions in the more proximal stomach (or more distal duodenum in the case of reflux).

Gastroduodenal Coordination

Like the stomach, the duodenum has its own pacesetter potential that drives its contractions. The frequency of the duodenal pacesetter (11/min in humans, 18/min in dogs) is higher than the gastric pacesetter (3/min in man, 5/min in dogs). The two pacesetter potentials are insulated from each other by the fibrous portion of the pylorus. Nevertheless, there is some conduction of the gastric pacesetter across a few muscle fibers into the duodenum. In the dog, the duodenum contracts at variable rates but in modes of pacesetter frequency. The most prominent periodicity to duodenal contraction is 1 contraction/10.5 sec (or about once every third pacesetter). This frequency is close to the maximal antral frequency of 1 contraction/12 sec, so that a number of antral contractions over time will correspond to duodenal contractions. Nevertheless, the faster contracting duodenum also continues to contract between antral cycles. In fact, cineradiographic and ultrasonographic analyses suggest that duodenal contractions between antral cycles frequently obliterate the duodenal lumen, propelling contents in a stripping wave well beyond the pylorus and making room in the proximal duodenum again to receive gastric contents that will be expelled with the next antral wave.[46,57]

Similar to the small intestine as a whole, the duodenum exhibits a variety of contractions. Concentric contractions may obliterate the lumen but not propagate along the axis of the bowel, simply mixing intestinal contents at the fixed point of contraction; or contractions may obliterate the lumen and move down the bowel as a peristaltic ring (stripping wave), pushing chyme ahead of the wave. Nutrients in the intestinal lumen stimulate a predominance of nonpropagated, segmenting or mixing contractions, while intraluminal saline (gut distention) in the absence of nutrients promotes peristaltic activity. How far the contents of the proximal duodenum are swept into the distal duodenum or proximal jejunum to make room for fresh gastric contents depends on the proportion of peristaltic (versus segmenting) contractions in the duodenum between antral cycles. Thus, nutrients in the small intestine inhibit gastric emptying by directly altering gastric motility by way of neurohormonal arcs, but they may also slow gastric emptying by affecting gastroduodenal coordination, specifically, through the proportion of peristaltic waves.

Interdigestive and Fed Motilities

In fasting animals, the gastrointestinal tract undergoes cycles of contractions, with a cycle length of 90 to 120 minutes in man (Fig 8-4). Throughout most of this period, the gastrointestinal tract is relatively quiet. In the stomach, there are few contractions with

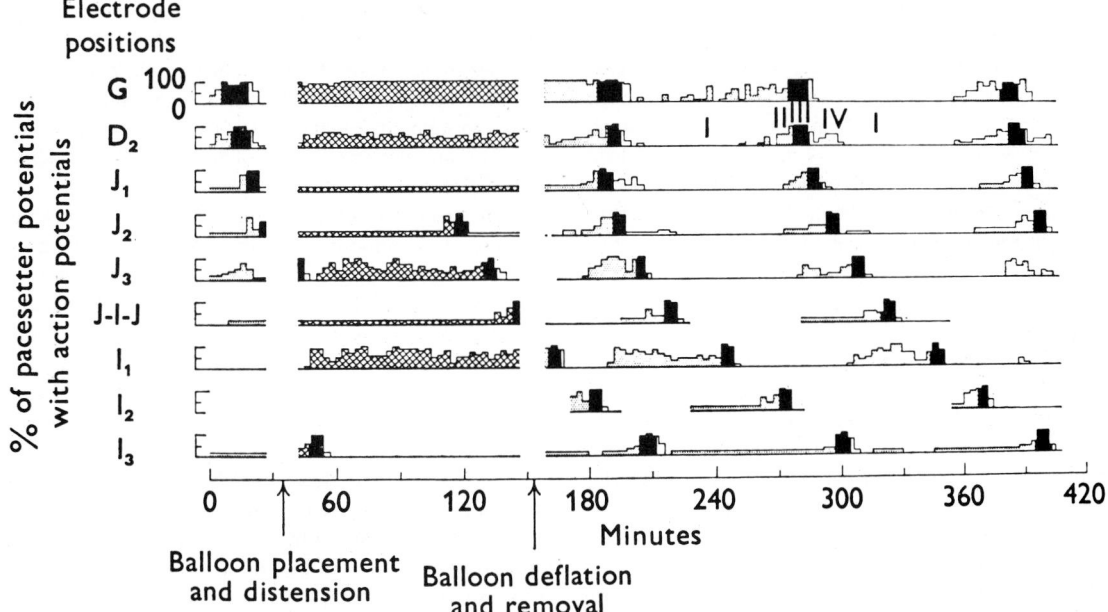

Electrode positions

Balloon placement and distension

Balloon deflation and removal

Minutes

FIGURE 8–4. Schematic representation of serosal electrical activity recorded by electrodes along the canine antrum (G), duodenum (D), jejunum (J), and ileum (I) during fasting and during balloon distension of the stomach. The right side of the figure (at 360 and at 420 minutes) illustrates typical cyclical activity during fasting. Note the long periods of quiescence of the antrum (phase I) between short bursts of intense activity (dark area, phase III), which propagate aborally into the small bowel. On the left of the figure, this cyclical, interdigestive or fasting activity is replaced by a "fed" pattern of continuous antral and small bowel contractions (cross-hatched areas) while the stomach is distended with an intragastric balloon. Earlier in this century, before the cyclical nature of the interdigestive motility was discovered in 1969, many scientists thought that bursts of antral contractility arising about every 2 hours were "hunger contractions." (From Code CF, Martlett JA. The interdigestive myoelectric complex of stomach and small bowel of dogs. J Physiol [London] 1975;246:289.)

each pacesetter wave, and even those contractions which are excited by pacesetter waves are weak and often die out before sweeping much of the stomach. This quiet phase is termed phase I of the interdigestive myoelectric cycle (IDMEC). In phase II, muscle contractions in the stomach begin to appear at an increasing frequency after each pacesetter, building to a crescendo of activity that is phase III. During phase III, which occurs every 90 to 120 minutes and lasts about 5 minutes, every pacesetter is followed by an especially forceful contraction that sweeps down the entire antrum, obliterating the antral lumen. Phase IV is a period of diminishing contractility between phase III and the next phase I. Each region of the gastrointestinal tract from the distal esophagus through the small intestine exhibits this temporal pattern of fasting motility, but the cycles are propagated in an aboral direction from esophagus to terminal ileum so that the crescendo of phase III activity sweeps sequentially from the stomach through the entire length of small intestine over a 90 to 120–minute interval of the cycle until the next cycle begins anew in the distal esophagus (Fig 8–4). The 5-minute bursts of crescendo, phase III activity that sweep along the gastrointestinal tract are commonly termed the migrating motor complex (MMC).

The control of the fasting cycles is complex. The hormone motilin seems to be an important stimulus of phase III. Thus, radioimmunoassays indicate that blood concentrations of motilin peak at the time the MMCs begin in the esophagus and stomach. If motilin secretion is suppressed or if motilin is removed by adsorbing it with antibodies, the intense, antral contractions that characterize phase III are replaced by intermittent, weaker contractions.[58,59] Because MMCs persist after vagal and splanchnic

nerve sectioning,[60] most authorities discount the role of nervous control in generating MMCs. But peaks in vagal efferent nerve traffic coincide temporally with the start of MMCs, and stressful stimuli may induce MMCs in the human duodenum.[61] Both observations suggest that nervous controls also participate in these cycles.

Carnivores and omnivores (dog, rat, man) develop a different motility pattern after eating and during fasting. The so-called fed pattern resembles the fasting phase II in that about half the pacesetter potentials are followed by submaximal contractions of antral muscles. Unlike the fasting or interdigestive motility, the fed pattern is not cyclical but is continuous as long as food remains in the stomach. Switching from fasting to a fed pattern (which does not happen in herbivores) is probably mediated, at least in part, by vagal nerves. Truncal vagotomy inhibits conversion of fasting to fed patterns in dogs and rats and shortens the time in which a fed pattern persists after a standard meal.[62,63] Similarly, acutely cooling the vagal trunks converts a typical fed pattern in dogs to one of cyclical bursts of activity with about the same periodicity as the fasting phase III (but without intermediary phases II and IV).[64]

The conversion of fasted to fed patterns in the stomach is a response to both gastric distention and the presence of nutrients within the gastrointestinal lumen. Nutrients work through their role in prolonging gastric distention and, as well, more directly stimulate a conversion to fed patterns. On reaching the small intestine, nutrients inhibit gastric emptying and thus can sustain gastric distention. Nutrient-free meals of saline only briefly remain in the stomach to distend it and only briefly evoke a fed pattern,[64] but equal volumes of milk produce a more sustained fed pattern because the nutrients in the milk inhibit gastric emptying to prolong gastric distention.[65] Because of its viscosity, polycarbophil (a synthetic polymer without nutrient value) is slowly emptied from the stomach yet sustains a fed pattern as long as it remains to distend the stomach.[66] On the other hand, only 17 ml of a medium-chain triglyceride evoke a prolonged fed pattern after instillation into the canine stomach.[67] Because this volume is too low by itself to stimulate a fed pattern, it is apparent that fat directly induces this pattern.

DeWever[67] fed dogs increasing volumes of the same dog food of modest fat content and noted a linear relation between the amount fed and the duration of the fed pattern, undoubtedly due to the duration over which food remained to distend the stomach. Extrapolating his data back to zero suggests that, in his dogs, more than a 100-ml volume of food would have been required to induce the conversion of a fasting to a fed pattern. In human subjects, the ingestion of as much as 200 ml of water does not disrupt the fasting motility pattern; indeed, it is unclear how large a volume is required in humans to disrupt fasting motility.[78]

As detailed below, the stomach in the fasting motility pattern empties liquids, drugs, or foreign bodies in a way much different from that of the stomach in a fed motility pattern.

Intestinal Feedback Inhibition

Gastric emptying of food is highly controlled by intestinal sensory mechanisms that respond to a variety of nutrients (Table 8-3). For the most part, these nutrients are products of digestion. Starch polymers inhibit gastric emptying in normal animals or human subjects about as much as isocaloric glucose,[68] and oligopeptides or proteins inhibit about as much as mixtures of their component amino acids,[69] probably because it is the end products of digestion (glucose or amino acids) that are actually detected by sensors along the bowel. In addition to nutrients, salts and other solutes that impart high osmolality to luminal contents inhibit gastric emptying. Acidity also inhibits emptying. Sensors to nutrients are

chemically specific. For example, tryptophan in the intestinal lumen strongly inhibits gastric emptying even at low concentrations that are much below body osmolality, whereas glycine inhibits gastric emptying effectively only at high luminal concentrations, much above body osmolality. In fact, glycine seems to be no more potent than solutions of electrolytes or mannitol at similarly high osmolality.

Until recently, most scientists believed that intestinal sensors were located primarily in the duodenum. It is becoming increasingly clear, however, that these sensors are arrayed over much of the small bowel. Thus, inhibition of gastric emptying is as great when glucose or sodium oleate is administered to the distal half of the canine intestine as when these inhibitors are confined to the proximal half of the bowel.[70,71] On the other hand, acid solutions inhibit canine gastric emptying when added to the proximal small bowel but do not do so when in the distal half of the intestine.[72]

Gastric emptying is controlled by feedback inhibition in a dose-related fashion. For example, in dogs or humans,[70,73] gastric emptying slows as the concentration of glucose in liquid meals is raised from 0.2 to 1.0 mol/L; but 1.0 mol/L is a maximally inhibiting dose, so that emptying is not further slowed as glucose concentrations in the meal are increased further. Within the dose range (0.2–1.0 mol/L), inhibition is such that the amount of glucose that enters the small intestine per minute is constant. For example, the volume of a meal of 0.25 mol/L glucose that empties over an hour is about four times the volume of a 1.0 mol/L glucose meal that empties in the same time interval. Similarly controlled is the gastric emptying of liquid meals that contain a range of concentrations of nutrients: as long as the caloric density (kJ/ml) is below a maximum of 4.2 kJ/ml, the stomach empties 4.2 kJ/min.[74]

Thus, over a considerable range, the load (amount/time) of nutrient is controlled independently from nutrient concentration. This control is accomplished by recruitment of sensors along the bowel (see Liquid Emptying, below). The control that limits the caloric entry of more complex meals is most likely the result of recruitment of a variety of sensors to the hydrolytic products of the individual dietary components (sugars, tryptophan, fatty acids).

Much evidence suggests that an array of sensors along the intestine controls gastric emptying by neural feedback. For example, we have already noted[36] that vagal blockade abolishes fundic relaxation in response to intestinal perfusion with sugars (see Gastrointestinal Reflexes). Similarly, the inhibition of antral contractions by fat in the intestinal lumen is much reduced, though not abolished, by truncal vagotomy.[32] On the other hand, many of these same nutrient inhibitors also release intestinal hormones. Thus, acids and fatty acids release secretin; fatty acids and amino acids (phenylalanine, tryptophan) release CCK; sugars and fatty acids release GIP and/or PYY; and so forth. All of these hormones can slow gastric emptying, so it is probable that control is achieved by some combination of neural and hormonal feedback. Because these hormones are released as nutrients contact hormonal cells along the intestinal mucosa, the level of hormone release achieved will depend on the length of mucosa contacted by the nutrient, that is, more and more hormonal response is recruited as more nutrients escape intestinal absorption to reach the more distal bowel.

The importance of this regulation of nutrient loads is readily illustrated by comparing alimentation in normal human subjects to that in patients who have had subtotal gastrectomies (with or without vagotomy) or patients who have had a truncal vagotomy

TABLE 8–3
Intestinal Inhibitors of Gastric Emptying

CLASS	SPECIFICITY
Acid	Titrateable (buffered) acid at pHs 1–5
	Enhanced pH effect below pH 2.5
Fat	Medium- and long-chain fatty acids; monolein also effective
Amino acids	Tryptophan highly potent in man & dog.
	Phenylalanine, histidine, cysteine in man; oligopeptides also effective
Sugars	Glucose effective, fructose less so, oligosaccharides also effective
Osmolytes	NaCl, KCl, mannitol, and so forth.
	Generally in proportion to concentration but much weaker than digestive products.
	Efficacy varies with different osmolytes.

with a pyloroplasty. By disrupting the normal muscular action of the pyloric sphincter and antrum and by interrupting vagal reflexes, these operations greatly diminish the ability of the stomach to regulate emptying of fluids. When normal subjects are given liquid meals of fat, protein, and sugar, gastric emptying is steady and so slow that all nutrients are just about completely digested and absorbed before reaching the midintestine.[75] Moreover, the rise in postcibal concentrations of plasma glucose is small, despite only a modest rise in plasma insulin. By contrast, the emptying of the same nutrient meals in patients who have had ulcer operations is initially precipitous. As a result, considerable amounts of fat and protein in the meal reach the distal ileum still undigested and unabsorbed.[76] Moreover, plasma glucose concentrations rise abruptly to abnormally high levels despite large increments in plasma insulin. Glucosuria and rebound hypoglycemia may follow.

CHARACTER OF GASTRIC EMPTYING DURING FASTING

Liquids

Schindlbeck[77] studied gastric emptying of endogenous secretions and found that emptying was greater in phase II–III than in phase I of the interdigestive myoelectric cycle (IDMEC). Oberle[78] characterized human gastric emptying of 50- or 200-ml drinks of water marked with the dye phenol red. Neither volume was large enough to convert the fasting motility pattern to a fed pattern. With drinks of either volume, the speed of gastric emptying varied (1) inversely with the interval between ingestion and the next MMC (phase III) and (2) directly with the motility of the antrum. Because the motility of the antrum is related to the temporal phases of the IDMEC, both correlations reflect the same relationship between time of ingestion in the IDMEC and the rate of emptying. Thus, the 50-ml drink emptied the fastest if ingested in late phase II or early phase III, less fast if ingested in early phase II, and least fast if ingested during phase I of the IDMEC. Similarly, the 200-ml drinks emptied faster if ingested during late phase II/early phase III than during early phase II. The 200-ml drinks emptied faster than the 50-ml drinks in each corresponding phase of the IDMEC.

The findings illustrate that fasting antral motility, especially MMCs (phase III), expels fluids from the stomach. Variations in fluid transit from the stomach with each phase of the IDMEC correspond to fasting transit in the small intestine, where MMCs clearly propel luminal contents.

Solids

Like liquids, solid beads or tablets are expelled with the powerful contractions of MMCs. In fact, plastic spheres of varying sizes and shapes from 1 to 7 mm empty more or less together during phase III of the IDMEC regardless of their size.[79–81] Based on these observations, many speculate that very large foreign bodies (like swallowed quarters or marbles) also empty from the fasting stomach with the powerful MMCs.

Obviously, the variable rates of gastric emptying of both liquids and solids with MMCs may affect the absorption profiles of orally ingested drugs. If drugs are ingested with small volumes of water during phase I, the time to peak blood levels will be longer than if they are ingested during later phase II/early phase III.

CHARACTER OF GASTRIC EMPTYING AFTER FEEDING

In man and other carnivores, the intermittent, fasting, interdigestive motility is replaced by a continuous fed pattern after a meal. In addition to this change of motor pattern, gastric emptying is also altered by eating.

Liquids

Unlike the situation under fasting conditions, where small volumes of water empty at rates that are sporadic and vary with the phase of the IDMEC, gastric emptying of larger liquid meals (300–800 ml) is a much more steady and reproducible process. Since the early observations of Hunt,[82] gastric emptying of liquids has been described most frequently as a simple exponential, that is, intragastric volume appears to decrease in a semilogarithmic fashion with time. Such a decay of gastric volume implies a "first-order kinetic," that is, milliliters emptied per minute is proportional to milliliters of meal volume ($-dv/dt=kv$, where v=intragastric meal volume, t=time, k=constant). The implication is that the speed of liquid emptying is determined by some volume-dependent variable, such as stretch of the gastric wall (to increase proximal muscular tone or reflexly trigger antral peristalsis) or the height of the liquid column in the stomach. In a truly first-order process (the most familiar example to many is radioactive decay of a radionuclide), the fraction of the original volume left at any given time after the meal is independent of the initial meal volume, or, in other words, fractional emptying is constant.

Only meals of water,[83] 0.15 mol/L NaCl,[84] or very dilute glucose[85] have met the criterion of constant fractional emptying. While meals of more concentrated glucose also empty in a curvilinear pattern, they do not meet this criterion. Thus, 300-ml meals of 11% glucose emptied at nearly the same rate of volume flow as 150-ml meals of 11% glucose[84] (i.e., fractional emptying was half that after the 150-ml meal). A major difference between water, saline, and very dilute glucose and concentrated glucose is that more concentrated nutrients inhibit gastric emptying by triggering feedback from intestinal sensors. With meals of more concentrated nutrients, there is a collision between the first-order driving forces in the stomach and inhibition from the intestine.

The curvilinear time-courses of gastric emptying of solutions of concentrated nutrients are probably the result of melding of two nearly linear phases of emptying: an initially rapid phase followed by a slow emptying phase. Thus, the rate of emptying of liquid nutrients is usually constant from 30 to 120 minutes after a meal but is almost always significantly slower than the emptying rate from 0 to 30 minutes.[86,87]

In man, the volume of glucose meals emptying from the stomach over 30 minutes decreases as the concentration of glucose in the meals increases.[73] However, most of the differences in speed of emptying of the meals of different concentrations of glucose arise in the first 5 minutes of the emptying time-course; after 5 minutes, the rates of emptying of meals of low or high concentrations are much the same. In other words, this regulation depends a great deal on the duration of the rapid emptying phase, and the latency from the start of emptying to the onset of the second, slow, constant phase depends on the concentration of the glucose.[87] These ideas about the relationships between the concentration of nutrient and the two phases of gastric emptying correspond quite well with many observations on the pattern of emptying of various liquid meals. Thus, at lower concentrations of glucose, the initially rapid emptying is more sustained and the overall time-course quite curvilinear, but at high-glucose concentrations, the initially rapid phase is very brief, almost indistinct, and the overall time-course is almost linear throughout.

A long length of small intestine (50% or more with glucose) participates in this dynamic feedback regulation (Fig 8-5).[70] Early after the meal, during the rapid emptying phase, the volume of glucose solution emptying into the bowel is large and therefore rapidly spreads along the intestine. Glucose is absorbed by active transport through saturable carriers. At saturation, absorption per centimeter of bowel is constant. How far glucose spreads down the gut with the initial surge of entering meal volume will thus depend on a balance between the rate of entry and the rate/cm of glucose absorption. The strength of intestinal inhibition depends on a summation of signals from glucose sensors along the bowel. This metering system for glucose along the bowel is the mechanism for greater feedback and earlier termination of the initially rapid emptying phase when the concentration of glucose is higher.

Indigestible Solids

In the 1970s, Kelly and co-workers studied canine gastric emptying of radiopacified 7-mm plastic spheres that served as facsimiles for food. At about the same time, others began to study gastric emptying of foods labeled with radionuclides. An early finding was that food is quickly fragmented and emptied as very small particles.[88] Because indigestible solids cannot undergo this fragmentation, interest in their emptying behavior waned. This subject, however, has been revisited in recent years by pharmaceutical scientists because of the increasing use of enterically coated medicines. Some of these medicines are simply enterically coated tablets of large size, while others are tiny beads (so-called multiparticulates). In gastroenterology, enteric-coated beads of pancreatin (Pancrease, Creon, and Cotazym-S) are examples of the latter. Clearly, it is important to know how characteristics such as size and density of these medicines affect their speed of delivery to the small intestine and hence their rate of absorption; or, in the case of enterically coated pancreatins, it is of interest to know whether these beads of enzymes actually are emptied along with food they are intended to digest. Unlike solid food, plastic spheres are not fragmented or partially digested in the stomach, so their emptying more narrowly reflects processes of gastric transit independent of digestion. Not surprisingly, therefore, observations from the recently intensified study of indigestible solids has shed considerable light on how food is emptied from the stomach.

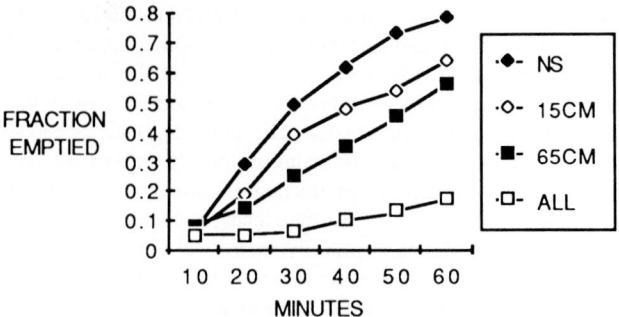

FIGURE 8–5. This figure depicts the fraction of 750 ml liquid meals that emptied from the canine stomach over 60 minutes. With meals of 0.15 mol/L of NaCl (NS) emptying was rapid, so that 80% emptied in 1 hour; but meals of 1.0 mol/L of glucose emptied slowly when the glucose (like the saline) had access to the whole small intestine (ALL). In other tests, the 1.0 mol/L glucose meals were diverted from the proximal small bowel at 15 (15 CM) or at 65 (65 CM) centimeters from the pylorus and replaced with saline. Confining the glucose to 15 or 65 cm of proximal small bowel abolished most of the inhibition from similar meals of glucose given access to the whole small intestine. The experiment indicates that the potent feedback inhibition from 1.0 mol/L glucose arises from the summation of signals from lengths of small bowel longer than 65 cm. (From Lin HC, Doty JE, Reedy TJ, Meyer JH. Inhibition of gastric emptying by sodium oleate depends on the length of gut exposed to the nutrient. Gastroenterology 1989;96:A304.)

The most remarkable of several of Kelly's findings[89] was that 7-mm spheres did not empty from the canine stomach in the presence of food, even while the food itself steadily emptied. Further investigation showed that the spheres were retained as long as the fed motility pattern persisted but that many spheres were subsequently emptied in boluses with the next few MMCs after the interdigestive pattern reappeared. On the other hand, Meyer[88] found that food emptied from the canine stomach predominantly as particles below 0.5 mm in diameter. Thus, the retention of 7-mm spheres but the passage of 0.5-mm particles of food indicated a selection by size. Unanswered were questions as to the cutoff size between 0.5 and 7 mm (i.e., objects below this size were emptied but above it were retained) and the similarity between the human and canine stomachs in these respects.

As shown by subsequent studies,[90,91] the food-filled canine stomach empties spheres 1 to 5 mm in diameter more and more slowly as diameter increases. All spheres 1 mm or less empty at about the same rate and more rapidly than radiolabeled food. Five-millimeter spheres hardly emptied at all while food was present. Thus, there is no discrete cutoff size; rather, the ease of emptying from the food-filled stomach is closely related to sphere diameter over a 1 to 5–mm range of diameters. Because the smallest spheres (especially those ≤1 mm) empty the fastest, it is unlikely that propulsion results directly from physical contact of the contracting walls of the stomach with the spheres (if that were the case, the larger spheres would be contacted by the closing antrum longer and more intensely, yet these emptied the least).

Further observations indicate that spheres more or less dense than 1 g/cm[3] empty more slowly than spheres of the same diameter with a density of 1 g/cm[3]. If the viscosity of gastric contents is raised by instilling a viscous polymer, even large, dense spheres are expelled rapidly.[91,92] Increased intragastric viscosity also changes the distribution of particles of expelled food so that large pieces are emptied.[91,93] The fact that sphere density and fluid viscosity affect how the spheres empty suggests very strongly that the spheres are carried out of the stomach by moving fluid in which they are suspended (discussed further in the last section of this chapter).

These fundamentals appear to apply to the human stomach, as well.

Enterically coated, large tablets (>10 mm) do not empty when food is present in the stomach, as evidenced by the fact that the rise in blood levels from ingested salicylate or erythromycin are greatly delayed when enterically coated tablets of these drugs are taken with food instead of under fasting conditions.[94] Radiolabeled spheres 1 mm in diameter empty faster than radiolabeled liver when the two are taken together, just as in dogs. Spheres 1.6 mm in size empty somewhat more slowly than liver, while 2.3- and 3.2-mm spheres empty much more slowly than liver, often after a prolonged period of no emptying.[95] Yet even larger objects (e.g., 2×6 mm pieces of tubing) are known to empty from the postcibal human stomach.[96] Just as in dogs, it seems as though there is no discrete cutoff by the human stomach but rather the ease of emptying varies with particle diameter. Particle density also seems to affect emptying from the human stomach. When taken together in the same meal, 1.6-mm spheres with a density of 2.0 g/cm^3 empty more slowly than spheres of the same size with a density of 1.0 g/cm^3.[95]

Digestible Solids

Digestible solids are reduced to small particles before they empty from the stomach. When radiolabeled chicken liver is ingested as 10-mm cubes along with steak by dogs with duodenal fistulas or intubated human subjects, the liver empties from the stomach as particles smaller than 1 mm.[88,97] In fact, in the dogs, the distribution of radiolabeled liver particles that empty is such that 95% of particles are smaller than 0.5 mm, and the distribution median is about .05 mm (50 μm) (Fig 8-6). If the canine pylorus and at least 3 cm of the distal antrum are resected (but not the pylorus alone or the antrum alone), the distribution of labeled food particles that empty from the stomach is converted to a bimodal one (Fig 8-6), with 70% of particles still in the normal mode but 30% of particles near the original size they were at ingestion.[88,98] Similarly, human patients with truncal vagotomy plus pyloroplasty empty radiolabeled liver particles in the normal size range (i.e., >90% were smaller than 1 mm), but patients with truncal vagotomy plus antrectomy empty about 30% of radiolabeled liver as particles > 1 mm.[97] Thus, the distal antrum and pylorus play an active role in the selective retention of meat particles larger than 1 mm.

Efficient digestion depends on the selective passage of very small food particles, because the large surface-to-mass of small particles facilitates enzymatic attack at the surfaces. The importance of this selective retention (or gastric sieving) for normal digestion has been illustrated by studies in dogs with fistulas at the midintestine.[99] Dogs were fed ^{14}C-labeled fat, either as a semiliquid fat in margarine or as a solid phase within the cells of chicken liver, and the percent of ^{14}C digested and absorbed by the midintestine was measured. In dogs with intact stomachs, virtually all liver particles reaching the midgut were smaller than 0.5 mm, and

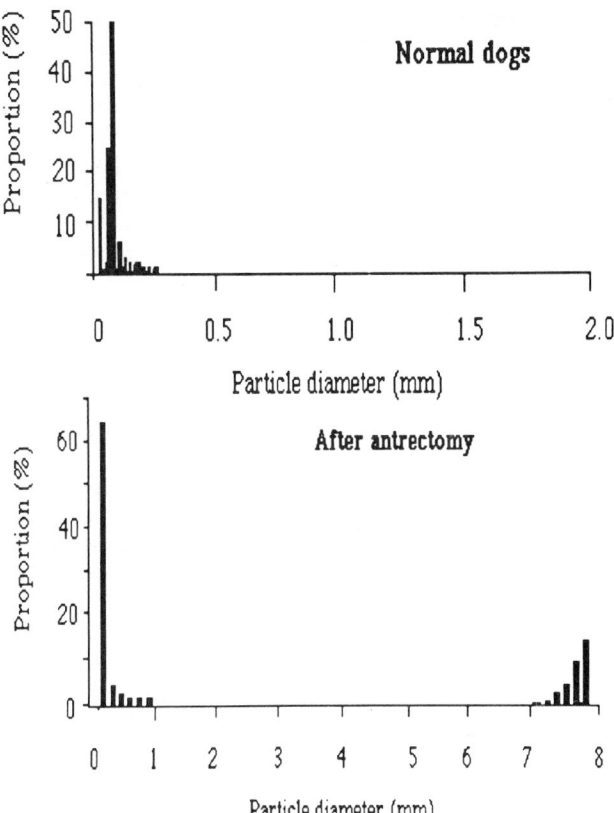

FIGURE 8–6. The size distributions of radiolabeled liver particles emptying from the normal canine stomach or the canine stomach after antrectomy. (From Meyer JH, Thomson JB, Cohen MB, Shadchehr A, Mandiolla S. Sieving of food by the canine stomach and sieving after gastric surgery. Gastroenterology 1979;76:804.)

these dogs absorbed 85% of the ^{14}C fat from the margarine and from the small liver particles. Dogs with truncal vagotomy plus antrectomy absorbed the liquid margarine normally, but they could digest and absorb only 43% of the fat from the liver. Only 15% of the fat was absorbed from liver particles larger than 0.5 mm, and nearly half the ingested liver reached the midintestine as particles larger than this size, observations that accounted for the poor overall absorption from the solid liver.

The time-course of gastric emptying of solid foods tends to be sigmoid in shape.[100–105] There is often an initial lag during which no solid food is emptied, followed by a prolonged linear phase, and finally, when the stomach is nearly empty, by a much slower phase. The predominately linear portion of the emptying curve suggests "zero order kinetics," that is, an emptying rate that is independent of meal volume (−dw/dt=k, where w=weight of solids in the stomach, t=time, and k= a constant).

An increasingly accepted idea is that the initial lag in the emptying of solid foods reflects the time required to reduce solid foods to particles ≤1 mm that are permitted to empty. Consistent with this idea are the observations in dogs or humans[88,104] that when chicken liver is fed as 0.25-mm particles labeled with one radionuclide and as 10-mm particles labeled with another nuclide in the same meal, the 0.25-mm particles empty promptly, without a lag and even a little more rapidly initially, while the 10-mm liver particles lag and then continue to empty somewhat more slowly than the 0.25-mm liver. In the dogs, both sizes of fed chicken liver empty from the stomach similarly distributed about a median particle diameter of .05 mm, so certainly the larger liver has to be more extensively reduced to this size than the smaller liver. Radiolabeled noodles[104] or radiolabeled cooked eggs[105] also empty faster than 10-mm ingested pieces of liver, and in vitro, both the noodles and the eggs are much more rapidly dispersed by peptic digestion than the liver. The difference between the emptying of the eggs and the liver is a longer lag for the liver, after which both foods empty at similar rates. Conversely, indigestible solids larger than 2 mm exhibit a very prolonged period of no emptying before they begin to slowly empty.[90,95] The differences between their emptying (i.e., long lag and slow emptying) and that of liver (shorter lags and faster, steady emptying phase) reflect how fragmentation and digestion of the meat to smaller particles shorten lag and speed emptying.

Solids empty from the stomach in a zero-order process, in contrast to first-order kinetics of liquid emptying. Determining kinetics with solid foods (in contrast to liquid meals of water or saline) is a difficult problem because it is hard to dissociate the propulsive forces of the stomach from the inhibitory effects of nutrients in the intestine in such studies with solids.[100] For example, if increasing the size of the meal actually increased gastric propulsion of food into the duodenum, the faster entry of nutrients into the intestine would trigger more feedback inhibition, and the real effect of meal volume on gastric motility would not be appreciated. To solve this problem, Moore[101] fed human subjects 20 g of radiolabeled liver with increasing amounts (25–875 g) of lettuce, a nearly zero-calorie bulking agent. He observed that the percent of liver emptied, or thus fractional emptying of the liver, over time is constant despite an 18-fold change of total meal weight, concluding that solid emptying is first-order, like liquid emptying. This conclusion, however, rests on the assumption that the radioliver and lettuce intermix completely, so that the emptying of the radiolabeled liver represents the emptying of the entire meal, an increasingly doubtful assumption (see Intragastric Distributions, below). Lin's approach to this problem[102] was to eliminate intestinal inhibition by diverting all chyme from duodenal fistulas in dogs. In his experiments, the fractional emptying of radiolabeled steak decreased, and grams per minute emptied remained constant, as the weight of ingested steak increased from 150 g to 600 g. By contrast, fractional emptying was constant (or thus, milliliters per minute emptied increased) as liquid meal volume was increased from 150 ml to 1200 ml in separate experiments in the same animals. This result indicates that solid emptying is fundamentally different (i.e., zero order) from first-order liquid emptying.

Inhibition of solid emptying by nutrients in the intestine is more potent in that solid emptying can be completely inhibited, whereas liquid emptying continues at a slow rate when the intestine is perfused with supramaximal doses of inhibitors. Various interpretations can be given to this set of observations. For example, liquids could be pulled by the force of gravity more readily, so that even with complete cessation of all gastric contractions, they would still trickle from the stomach, yet the slow outflow of liquid under these conditions is insufficient to carry particles of solids along. Alternatively, the motor activity that accomplishes the grinding of food to particles small enough to pass may be completely inhibited while some other muscular activity that propels material from the stomach continues even under complete intestinal inhibition of the former.

Dissociation Between Liquid and Solid Emptying

We have just discussed the evidence that indicates zero- versus first-order kinetics, respectively, for solids and liquids and the observations that solid emptying may be inhibited completely by nutrients while liquid emptying is not. Two other observations further support fundamental differences between liquid and solid emptying.

In either humans or dogs,[106,107] proximal gastric vagotomy accelerates the emptying of liquids (either saline or nutrients) but does not alter the gastric emptying of solids (7-mm spheres in dogs, radiolabeled liver in humans). On the other hand, truncal vagotomy (which denervates the antrum as well as the fundus) accelerates the emptying of liquids but may slow the emptying of solids in both species.[68,107–109]

Gue[110] has just reported that orally administered opioids have opposite effects on canine gastric emptying of water and radiolabeled liver. The kappa agonists, U-50488 and tifluadom, speed the gastric emptying of the liver while slowing emptying the water phase of the meal. How these agents produce this dissociation is unknown, but it is known that they stimulate both antral (Table 8-1) and pyloric contractions. Perhaps this latter action slows the flow of water while the former speeds the emptying of liver.

The fact that different processes govern liquid and solid transit is strongly indicated by all of these observations. Perhaps these fundamental differences account for the clinical observation that tests of gastric emptying of solids are more sensitive in detecting disease than those which measure emptying of liquids (see ch 60).

Fat

Like solids, fats constitute a phase separate from water, but unlike solids, fat is often fluid at body temperature, so that it can be fragmented into tiny spherules more easily. Yet these fat droplets may coalesce back into larger globules, a process that solid particles do not undergo. Fat is also considerably less dense (specific gravity about 0.92) than solid food (specific gravity about 1.2) or water (specific gravity = 1.0). This lower density allows fat to float as an unemulsified bulk phase upward, away from the antrum–pylorus. Even spherules of fat emulsified in the water phase will float slowly.

The emptying pattern of fat varies quite a bit, but on the average it empties at about the same rate as solid food, that is, considerably more slowly than the aqueous portion of the meal and after some lag. However, in individual tests, fat may empty more quickly or more slowly than the solid food phase, so it is likely that it empties independently from solid foods.[111,112] Despite a paucity of descriptive data on the emptying of fat, this is not a clinically irrelevant problem: How fat empties into the duodenum relative to aqueous or solid phases will in part determine how effectively orally administered pancreatin ameliorates steatorrhea in patients with pancreatic insufficiency.

The slower emptying of less dense fat (compared with water) is similar to the slower emptying of small plastic spheres of similarly low density,[90,92,95] so the idea that density determines how fat moves out of the stomach is most plausible. Slow emptying may reflect the floating of fat to the fundus,[111-114] where propulsive forces are less intense. In hydrodynamic theory (see below), fat droplets in an aqueous emulsion floating away from the central, fastest-moving portion of the water phase as it is ejected from the stomach could also explain the slower emptying of the fat relative to water. In contrast to the idea that the low density of fat determines its pattern of emptying, Cortot[115] observed that an indigestible and thus biologically inert fat (sucrose polyester) emptied from the human stomach almost as rapidly as water and much more rapidly than digestible triglyceride of the same low density. He suggested that the slower emptying of the triglyceride was due to its ability to inhibit specifically gastric emptying of fat by triggering inhibition from the intestine.

Intragastric Distribution

Postcibal gastric contents are not uniform. Even early in this century, Cannon[116] recognized at fluoroscopy that chunks of food resided in the proximal stomach early after eating, while the contents of the antrum were a gruel-like suspension of finer particles of food. Much more recently,[91] ratios of nuclide markers of fat and solid food deviated from unity in serial aspirates from the postcibal stomach, indicating a significant separation of phases throughout the period of emptying. With the early use of the gamma camera to study gastric emptying, scientists observed that foods were retained in the proximal stomach and that emptying of the proximal stomach paralleled emptying from the whole stomach, as antral activity stayed constant throughout most of the emptying period.[117]

Three very recent studies of the intragastric distribution of radiolabeled foods have suggested that distribution is dynamically controlled and that much of the initial lag phase of solid emptying results from the accumulation and retention of solid foods of intermediate particle sizes in the antrum.

Collins[118] examined the intragastric distribution over time of radioactivity when seated subjects were fed a hamburger meal that contained technetium-labeled liver. While there was considerable variation among the 13 subjects, the usual finding was that the technetium moved from proximal to distal stomach more rapidly than the technetium was emptied from the whole stomach, so that

radioactivity increased with time in the distal stomach (Fig 8-7). The lag phase, before technetium began to empty from the whole stomach, coincided with the buildup of antral radioactivity to a maximum, suggesting that passage from antrum to duodenum wa rate-limiting over more rapid passage from fundus to antrum.

Using similar techniques, Urbain[119] studied patterns of gastric distribution and emptying of technetium-labeled eggs, but in serial tests he varied the physical character of the labeled eggs so that in one test the eggs were fed as a water homogenate (liquid) and in the other tests, respectively, as 2.5-mm and 5.0-mm cu es (solid). Both liquid and solid eggs were initially retained in the fundus. However, the liquid eggs moved quickly from fundus to antrum, from which they were almost immediately passed into the duodenum, so that little radioactivity accumulated in the antrum. By contrast, the cubes of solid egg (the 2.5-mm and 5-mm cubes behaved similarly) were retained somewhat longer in the proximal stomach, and considerably more of their radioactivity (40% versus 16% with the liquid eggs) accumulated in the antrum, indicating that they were held up there longer than the liquid eggs. The lag in emptying from the total stomach was less with the liquid than the solid eggs.

Meyer[120] analyzed the intragastric distribution of simultaneously ingested 0.5–2.4-mm plastic spheres, labeled with indium, and of 10-mm cubes of technetium-liver. The plastic spheres passed more quickly from the proximal to the distal stomach than did the larger pieces of liver. Although both the liver and the smaller spheres emptied readily from the stomach, they usually emptied even more quickly from proximal to distal stomach, so that antral activity built up over time to 30% of total stomach counts. However, the 2.4-mm spheres hardly emptied at all from the whole stomach, yet they moved readily from proximal to distal stomach. As a result, antral activities of the 2.4-mm spheres accumulated to over 80% of total gastric activity.

The last two studies suggest that the proximal stomach selectively retains larger pieces of food (i.e., solid egg longer than liquid egg in Urbain's study and 10-mm liver longer than 0.5–2.5-mm spheres in Meyer's study), an idea consistent with Cannon's early fluoroscopic observations. All three studies suggest that the initial lag in emptying from the total stomach is the result of retention of particles of intermediate size in the antrum until they are reduced to particles ≤1 mm, which are then allowed to pass. Thus, liquid egg did not lag in emptying from the whole

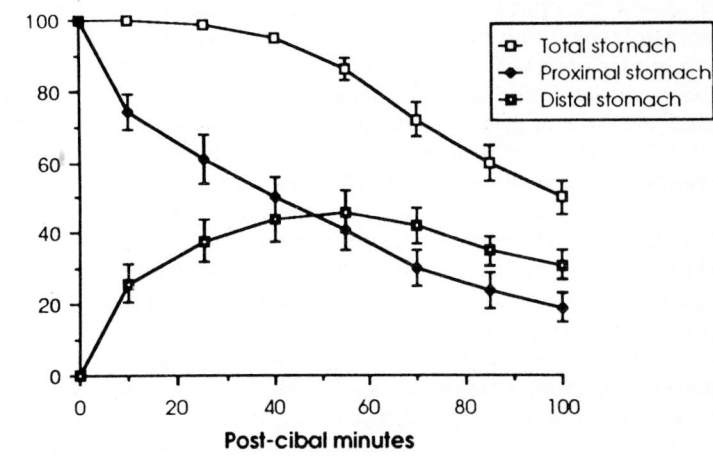

FIGURE 8–7. Distributions of radioactivity in human stomachs after a meal containing radiolabeled liver. During an initial 50 minute lag phase in which no liver emptied from the stomach, about half the ingested liver moved from proximal stomach to antrum, where radioactivity rose until the radioliver began to empty from the stomach. (From Collins PJ, Horowitz M, Chatterton BE. Proximal, distal and total stomach emptying of a digestible solid meal in normal subjects. Br J Radiol 1988;61:12.)

stomach and did not accumulate in the antrum in Urbain's study, while larger pieces of food lagged and were retained for a while in all three studies. In Meyer's study, the 2.5-mm spheres, which could not be further fragmented, hardly emptied (i.e., they lagged almost indefinitely) and therefore accumulated in much higher quantities in the antrum. Thus, the distal stomach is an even more selective sieve than the proximal stomach.

However, the ability of the proximal stomach to retain larger pieces of food selectively helps to explain the fact that the stomach can still sieve after distal gastric resection, that is, 70% of food particles enter the small intestine in the normal distribution of sizes (Fig 8-6). Probably as important is the potential for retention of parts of the meal in a chemical microclimate conducive to digestion. The pH high in the fundus is insulated by a floating layer of gastric and salivary mucus from lower pHs in the acid-secreting corpus.[121] Thus, the pH in balls of swallowed bread that are retained in the fundus remains near 7 so that there is extensive digestion of carbohydrate in the stomach by salivary amylase in this pH microclimate.[116] The floating of fat in the proximal stomach on top of a pH-insulating layer of gastric plus salivary mucus likewise may facilitate intragastric lipolysis[122] by pharyngeal and gastric lipases (gastric lipase is secreted from the proximal human stomach).

HOW DOES GASTRIC MOTILITY EMPTY THE STOMACH?

An unsolved problem in gastrointestinal motility is how to relate contractions to transit. While the problem is not unique to the stomach, this organ has idiosyncrasies that complicate the solution. Its conical shape frustrates intraluminal manometry because the walls of the more proximal stomach are increasingly away from the central axis where manometric probes are usually sited. Thus, more proximal manometric probes become less and less sensitive to phasic contractions.[123] This problem is worsened when gastric emptying is inhibited and the stomach is dilated from the presence of food in the intestine. Another problem is that the pyloric sphincter is so short that it is hard to site intraluminal probes within it to monitor its contractions, and the angulation of the pyloric tract further distorts manometric measurements.[124] This problem has been approached by short interspacing of multiple sensors or, more recently, by the use of a Dent manometric sleeve to straddle the pylorus.[39,40] Phasic contractions, which can be monitored conveniently by electrodes or pressure transducers, are only half the story; tonic shortening of luminal diameter may be a major driving force (i.e., in the fundus) or may contribute a major resistance to flow by narrowing the pyloric or duodenal canal. Tone is not easily measured and only recently has been examined by electronic barostat in the gastric fundus[3,36] or by videofluoroscopy to measure luminal diameter in the pylorus and duodenum.[125,126] The stomach is in series with the small intestine, which must receive gastric contents as they empty. The receptive capacity of the intestine depends not only on its tone and contractile patterns but also on its treatment of incoming fluids, electrolytes, and nutrients. Finally, gastric contents also move in response to gravitational forces, which are not easily measured. The fluid-filled stomach forms a J-shaped, vertical column that is supported by ligaments as much as by gastric muscle; the force of gravity in

such a column has not often been considered but is evidently important.

Gravity is a good illustration of how difficult it is to identify single forces that control gastric emptying while others operate simultaneously. The effect of gravity is normally so subtle that Thomas[127] completely dismissed it as a driving force of gastric emptying. Hunt[128] showed that human gastric emptying of liquid meals of glucose or acid was not different in the erect versus the supine or even the head-down position, but gastric emptying of saline was faster from the erect than from the supine position and slower from the head-down position. He concluded that gravity does operate but that intestinal feedback inhibition (to glucose or acid) normally slows emptying so much that even in the head-down position, where gravity impedes outflow, the stomach has the motor capacity to speed emptying to the slow rate permitted in the erect posture. However, when patients who have had a vagotomy plus pyloroplasty move from the supine to the erect posture, the change in speed of their gastric emptying of liquids is much greater than the changes Hunt observed in normal subjects,[68,129] because the operation interrupts both modulation by several neural reflexes and end organ response (the ability of the contracting pylorus to resist outflow). Evidently, gravitational flow of even nutrient-free saline is regulated to a large extent in normal subjects.

While it seems intuitively obvious that gastric transit must be controlled serially by the fundic tone, antral contractions, pyloric tone and contractions, and finally duodenal and intestinal reception, this idea has been difficult to establish. Part of the problem has been the redundancy of controlling mechanisms in the upper gastrointestinal tract, such that removing one portion of this serial chain of controls does not necessarily reveal the controlling capacity of the missing segment, as the other controlling regions take over the removed functions. The first hypothetical model of serial control was Kelly's two-component stomach. It is useful to review how this idea developed and why it is no longer adequate.

The Two-Component Stomach

Because peristaltic contractions of the antrum were easily recognizable at fluoroscopy or by balloon manometry, physiologists throughout most of this century focused on them as the major motive force in gastric emptying. This impression was deepened by work in animals with duodenal fistulas in which the emptying of gastric contents was observed to occur in spurts that coincided with antral contractions. Furthermore, Thomas[127] and others noted that nutrients in the intestine that inhibited gastric emptying also inhibited antral contractions. While pyloric reflexes were described as early as the 1930s, Crider[130] had shown that stenting the pylorus open did not alter the time-course of gastric emptying (a result more recently corroborated by Stemper[131]), and he considered therefore that gastric emptying was controlled entirely by antral contractility (in more modern times, this idea was reintroduced by Dooley[132]).

What most changed this line of thinking, which had dominated this century, was the development from the 1940s through the 1960s of a variety of operations on the human stomach for ulcers. These operations profoundly altered gastric emptying and provided the first clear model for a dissociation between liquid and solid emptying. Truncal vagotomy plus pyloroplasty reduced antral peristalsis and slowed gastric emptying of solids, but it sped the gastric emptying of liquids. Moreover, Staadas[29] showed that it altered gastric accommodation, raising intragastric pressure. Kelly, an abdominal surgeon at the Mayo Clinic, was working on electromechanical properties of the stomach and had already described the electrical quiescence of the fundus in contrast to the antrum, while Code, Dozois, Carlson, and others of his colleagues at the Mayo Clinic were working on the importance of terminal antral contractions on propulsion of spheres from the stomach. In this climate of evolving ideas, Kelly proposed that the fundus, by virtue of its tonic contractions, controlled intragastric pressures and thus the gastroduodenal pressure gradient that propelled fluids from the stomach, while the peristaltic contractions of the antrum controlled the gastric emptying of solids.[110]

At first, several different observations in dogs and human subjects supported this idea. Selective denervation of the proximal canine stomach (including the fundus) raised intragastric postcibal pressures and sped the emptying of saline but did not affect the emptying of spheres. Total gastric vagotomy also raised pressures and sped liquid emptying but slowed gastric emptying of spheres. Fundic resection raised gastric pressures and sped liquid emptying. Liquid nutrients could empty from the stomach during complete absence of antral contractions, implying that fundic tone drove the emptying (gravity was not considered).[133]

The explosive growth of studies on gastric emptying since the mid-1970s brought a variety of observations that indicate a greater complexity. The accelerating effects of total gastric or proximal gastric vagotomy on the emptying of liquids in humans are much greater when a pyloroplasty is added to the vagotomy.[134,135] This observation implies an additional regulating role of the pylorus. The ability of the pylorus to control flow was established by showing that flow through the pylorus at controlled transpyloric pressures is diminished in a dose-related fashion by fat or acid in the canine intestine and that this regulation is abolished by pyloroplasty.[37] Nutrient-responsive, postgastric resistances that could further modify fluid flows were also described.[37,136] The speeding of gastric emptying of fluids by truncal vagotomy plus pyloroplasty is much greater when human subjects are in the erect position as opposed to the supine position, [68,129] clearly a demonstration of the potent driving force of gravity. The proximal stomach is an important reservoir for solid foods, and it even has the ability to retain selectively larger pieces of food.[116–120] By contrast, fluids drop quickly in upright subjects from the proximal to the distal stomach, from which they are then expelled.[119] This, along with the preceding observation, indicates that the functions of the proximal and distal regions of the stomach cannot be relegated solely to the governance of liquid and solid emptying, respectively. Gastric fundoplication (an operation to treat gastroesophageal reflux, which functionally removes part of the fundus) speeds gastric emptying of both liquids and solids,[137] again implying that the fundus is a reservoir and propeller for both. While liquids may empty in the absence of antral contractions, under many circumstances their emptying can be correlated with antral contractions.[138–140] In experimental animals,[36] liquid emptying continues when the gastroduodenal pressure gradient is held by gastric and duodenal barostats to −2 cm of water (stomach lower), indicating that antral phasic contractions propel the fluid across the negative gradient. Furthermore, gastric emptying of liquids can be driven by electrically stimulated antral contractions.[140]

The importance of Kelly's two-component model is not much diminished by the fact that it is no longer adequate. It revolutionized thinking by introducing the idea that propulsion is a complex of both phasic and tonic contractions. It served as a focus for many subsequent investigations. Kelly's elucidation of the loss of fundic accommodation in the genesis of abnormally high gastric pressures and rapid liquid emptying, especially after proximal (but also after complete gastric) vagotomy, is unaltered by subsequent observation. Finally, his model forms the nucleus of an extended, multicomponent model that embraces many newer observations.

Multiple Components in Series

This model stresses the concerted action of the fundus, antrum, pylorus, and small intestine to propel chyme in a regulated fashion from the stomach. It is based not only on studies (already alluded to in the above) in animals of the regulatory capacities of each of these experimentally isolated segments, but also, and perhaps more important, on studies of normal gastric emptying that cross-correlate the spatial–temporal spread of phasic contractions, tone or diameter, and movement of chyme in all of these regions. Although difficult, this multivariate approach has been achieved by Ehrlein and co-workers[52,125,126,141] through concurrent videofluoroscopy, monitoring of phasic contractions by serosal strain gauges, inductographic recording of pyloric diameter, and the use of computers to integrate this variety of information.

Ehrlein has employed as controls viscous, but nutrient-free, liquid meals that contain hydroxyethylcellulose. Like 0.15 mol/L NaCl, these meals do not evoke much feedback regulation of the stomach, but unlike saline, they move slowly because of their viscosity, so that videofluroscopic recordings can be correlated during this form of slow motion with contractile and tonic events. He has compared the emptying of these control meals with emptying of meals of ethylcellulose to which he has added various nutrients to trigger feedback regulation.

All nutrient meals empty more slowly than the control, nutrient-free meal, but meals that contain oleic acid (fat) empty the slowest. Nutrient and non-nutrient meals are stored in the proximal stomach from which they are slowly pressed into the antrum. Antral diameter is smaller with the nutrient than with the non-nutrient meal, suggesting that nutrients are less vigorously pressed from the proximal stomach into the antrum. Antral motility is less pronounced after the nutrient meals than after the control meal. Pyloric diameter is smaller in the presence of nutrients, as is duodenal caliber. In the presence of nutrients, duodenal contractions are less vigorous, more segmenting, and less peristaltic than with control meals. These observations support the idea that all four regions work in concert to empty the stomach in a tightly controlled fashion.

Acceptance of this integrated, multicomponent model has been slow. For example, although it is certain that the pylorus can regulate gastric emptying,[37,142] many question its role in controlling gastric emptying under normal circumstances. Preventing pyloric closure by stenting or by pyloric myotomy alters little the overall speed of gastric emptying of liquid nutrients (although the initially rapid emptying phase is sped).[143] This lack of a major change after ablation of pyloric function is more a testimony of the ability of other controls to take over lost pyloric function than an irrefutable negation of the role of the pylorus, for if the stomach is also deprived of much of its reflex regulation by truncal vagotomy, then adding a pyloric myotomy to the vagotomy greatly speeds the emptying of liquids.[134,135,142,143] Similarly, the ability of the small intestine to resist gastric outflow has been demonstrated in a number of ways that isolate intestinal resistance from concurrent gastric and pyloric regulation[37,38,125,136,144]; intestinal control is difficult to demonstrate when all of these mechanisms operate together.[145]

Hydrodynamics: A Likely Link Between Solid and Liquid Emptying

Many people imagine that solids are propelled as the walls of a gastrointestinal organ squeeze down and close the lumen behind them, similar to the way the sigmoid colon expels feces. Such physical contact between the walls of the cavernous stomach and small pieces of food seems unlikely, even where the stomach narrows to small dimension in the terminal antrum, because pieces of food range from less than 20 mm when swallowed to .05 mm after trituration. The walls of the stomach do not have to make physical contact with food either to grind it or to expel it; they merely must move intragastric fluid in appropriate patterns to suspend and carry particles out of the stomach or even to break apart food particles. This idea that fluid movement is the mediator is called hydrodynamics.

One idea[146] is that fluid carries particles of suspended food or fat as it streams from the stomach, much in the way that a river carries suspended particles of sand. By this thesis, the sinking or floating of particles out of the fastest moving, central portion of the stream will slow their egress. High (or low) density and large diameter promote such sinking (or floating), so that only the smallest particles are propelled. High viscosity of gastric fluid retards sinking or floating and thus promotes emptying of larger particles.

In reality, however, fluid does not continuously stream from the stomach. We know from both ultrasonic and cineradiographic studies that forward fluid flow at the start of the terminal antral contraction (TAC) not only ceases with closure of the pylorus but also moves forcefully backward at the completion of the TAC. The second idea[147] is that the repeated pattern of TACs and the to-and-fro movement of gastric fluids associated with them are enough to grind food into small particles and to select only the smallest for expulsion.

Keller[147] speculated that under such to-and-fro movement of fluid in the terminal antrum, larger particles of food with higher inertia would be accelerated by forward flow much less than smaller particles of lower inertia. Significantly more small particles than larger particles would therefore be swept past the pylorus with each TAC, accounting for the selective gastric emptying of particles ≤1 mm. The larger particles that remain behind would be retropelled with fluid as the terminal antral lumen is obliterated at the end of the TAC. The sudden and forceful reversal of flow is associated with a fluid turbulence sufficient to break apart larger pieces of solid food and to emulsify fat, much in the same way that to-and-fro movement from a sonicator can break up and emulsify food or tissue. In this model, particles with higher diameter and density would have more inertia and therefore would be retained to be subsequently broken apart. Larger globules of low-density fat would float out of the terminal antrum, away from propulsive forces. By increasing the accelerating drag of forward-moving fluid, higher viscosity in gastric fluid would promote expulsion of larger particles.

Considerable credence to both hydrodynamic hypotheses is provided by recent studies of gastric emptying of indigestible solids. In these studies, spheres with larger diameters were retained longer, and spheres with low or high density emptied more slowly. Also, increasing the viscosity of gastric fluid promoted emptying of even large, dense spheres.[89-93] One might argue that spheres of large size were retained simply because their diameters approached or exceeded mean pyloric diameter. As the (canine) pylorus undergoes cycles of contraction, it narrows its luminal diameter from a maximum of 6.5 mm to a minimum of 2.5 mm.[55] These dimensions in and of themselves do not account for the observation that all spheres of 1 mm or less are emptied rapidly, while spheres from 1 mm to 5 mm are emptied more and more slowly as diameter increases. Even if pyloric diameter might account for such a selection by size, the effects of sphere density and fluid viscosity can be well explained only by some sort of hydrodynamic process.

Any hydrodynamic hypothesis must be able to account for dissociation of fluid from particle movements that are paradoxical. In Keller's inertial hypothesis, the rate of expulsion of solid particles is determined by the power of the TACs. Whatever their force and amplitude, TACs are limited to a maximum frequency (3/min in man, 5/min in dogs) and thus a maximum power. This limitation could well account for a zero-order kinetic or a fixed (maximal) rate of solid emptying. At low fluid volumes, fluids may also require TACs for emptying, but at progressively higher volumes, the tone (stretch) of the stomach (and/or the gravitational height of the fluid column) provides an increasing propulsive force that overrides the TACs, thus accounting for the first-order kinetic of fluid emptying. During maximal feedback inhibition of gastric emptying from nutrients in the intestine, antral peristalsis and thus TACs are abolished. Fluids continue to trickle from the stomach under the force of gravity and/or under the driving force of gastric tone. Velocity may be slowed enough under these circumstances to be inadequate to carry any but the very smallest particles of food. Furthermore, in the absence of the to-and-fro movement created by TACs, there may be too little fluid turbulence to break food apart. The same loss of power from TACs may characterize any pathologic condition in which the strength or frequency of TACs is much reduced (in diseases such as scleroderma, which reduces force and amplitude, or in gastric bradyrhythmias, which reduce frequency). After truncal vagotomy, increased gastric tone (from loss of relaxation and accommodation reflexes) may accelerate fluid emptying but, because of diminished force of TACs, slow solid emptying.

With its necessary dependence on the power of TACs, Keller's inertial, hydrodynamic model is more consistent with liquid–solid dissociations in health and disease and for that reason is more tenable than Amidon's model. Moreover, the ideas in the preceding paragraph are but an elaboration on Kelly's two-component model, which stressed the importance of TACs in the emptying of solids and the importance of (fundic) tone for the expulsion of liquids. With only the additional ideas that (1) under low intragastric volumes the TACs themselves also may propel liquids and (2) liquid outflow may be further modulated by pyloric and intestinal resistances, the multicomponent model is equally compatible with the Keller model. At the present time, the combination of the multicomponent and Keller models best accounts for all of the observations on gastric emptying and motility.

The reader is directed to Chapter 1, The Enteric Nervous System and its Extrinsic Connections; Chapter 2, Gastrointestinal Hormones; Chapter 3, The Brain-Gut Axis; Chapter 4, Smooth Muscle of the Gut; Chapter 7, Esophageal Motor Function; Chapter 9, Motility of the Small Intestine; Chapter 10, The Motor Function of the Colon; Chapter 11, Motility of the Biliary Tree; Chapter 59, Stomach: Anatomy and Structural Anomalies; Chapter 60, Disorders of Gastric Emptying; Chapter 64, Surgery for Peptic Ulcer Disease; Chapter 121, Gastrointestinal Radionuclide Imaging Procedures; and Chapter 128, Evaluation of Gastrointestinal Motility: Methodological Considerations.

REFERENCES

1. Schulze-Delrieu K, Wall JP. Determinants of flow across isolated gastroduodenal junctions of cats and rabbits. Am J Physiol 1983;245: G257.
2. Lind JF, Duthie HI, Schlegel JF, Code CF. Motility of the gastric fundus. Am J Physiol 1961;201:197.
3. Azpiroz F, Malagelada JR. Physiological variations in canine gastric tone measured by an electronic barostat. Am J Physiol 1985;248: G229.
4. Szurszewski JH. Electrical basis of gastrointestinal motility. In: Johnson LR, ed. Physiology of the gastrointestinal tract. New York: Raven Press, 1981:1435.
5. Hinder RA, Kelly KA. Human gastric pacesetter potential. Site of origin, spread, and response to gastric transection and proximal gastric vagotomy. Am J Surg 1977;133:29.
6. Publicover NG, Sanders KM. Myogenic regulation of propagation in gastric smooth muscle. Am J Physiol 1985;248:G512.
7. Valori RN, Collins SM, Daniel EE, et al. Comparison of methodologies of antroduodenal motor activities in the dog. Gastroenterology 1986;91:546.
8. Bitar KN, Jensen RT, Gardner JD, Makhlouf GM. Secretin, glucagon, and VIP receptors on smooth muscle cells. Physiological relevance. Gastroenterology 1982;82:1018.
9. Bitar KN, Makhlouf GM. Purinergic receptors on isolated smooth muscle cells: Potentiators of VIP relaxation. Gastroenterology 1982;82:1018.
10. Bitar KN, Makhlouf GM. Receptors on smooth muscle cells: Characterization by contraction and specific agonists. Am J Physiol 1982;242:G400.
11. Bitar KN, Makhlouf GM. Specific opiate receptors on isolated mammalian gastric smooth muscle cells. Nature 1982;297:72.
12. Bitar KN, Makhlouf GM. Relaxation of isolated smooth muscle cells by vasoactive intestinal peptide. Science 1982;216:531.
13. Louie D, Owyang C. Substance P receptors on isolated gastric smooth muscle cells. Dig Dis Sci 1984;29:49S.
14. Morgan KG, Schmalz PE, Szurszewski JH. The inhibitory effects of vasoactive intestinal peptide on the mechanical and electrical activity of the canine antral smooth muscle. J Physiol (Lond) 1978;282:437.
15. Morgan KG, Schmalz PF, Szurszewski JH. Electrical and mechanical effects of molecular variants of CCK on antral smooth muscle. Am J Physiol 1978;235:E324.
16. Mei N. Vagal glucoreceptors in the small intestine of the cat. J Physiol (Lond) 1978;282:485.
17. Perrin J, Crousilat J, Mei N. Assessment of true splanchnic glucoreceptors in the jejuno-ileum of the cat. Brain Res Bull 1981;7:625.
18. Jeanningros R, Mei N. Vagal and splanchnic effects at the level of the ventromedian nucleus of the hypothalamus (VMH) in the cat. Brain Res 1980;185:239.
19. Angel F, Schmalz PF, Morgan KG, Go VLW, Szurszewski JH. Innervation of the muscularis mucosa in the canine stomach and colon. Scand J Gastroenterol 1982;71(suppl):71.
20. Fahrenkrug J, Haglund U, Jodal M, Lundgren O, Olbe L, Schaffalitzky de Muckadell OB. Nervous release of vasoactive intestinal polypeptide in the gastrointestinal tract of cats: Possible physiological implications. J Physiol (Lond) 1978;284:291.
21. Stern RM, Kock KL, Stewart WR, Lindblad IM. Spectral analysis of tachygastria recorded during motion sickness. Gastroenterology 1987;92:92.
22. Stanghellini V, Malagelada J-R, Zinsmeister AR, et al. Effect of opiate and adrenergic blockers on the gut motor response to centrally acting stimuli. Gastroenterology 1984;87:1104.
23. Gue M, Fioramonti J, Frexinos J, et al. Influence of acoustic stress by noise on gastrointestinal motility in dogs. Dig Dis Sci 1987;32: 1411.
24. Livingston EH, Passaro EP, Garrick TR. Elevated intracranial pressure increases gastric contractility in the rat. Gastroenterology 1988;94:A255.
25. Garrick T, Buack S, Veiseh A, Tache Y. Thyrotropin-releasing factor (TRF) acts centrally to stimulate gastric contractility in rats. Life Sci 1987;40:648.
26. Tache Y, Kolve L, Stephans RL, Rivier J. Role of corticotropin-releasing factor (CRF) in postoperative surgery-induced inhibition of gastric emptying in the rat. Gastroenterology 1989;96:A499.
27. Jansson G. Extrinsic nervous control of gastric motility. An experimental study in the cat. Acta Physiol Scand 1969;326(suppl):1.
28. Martinson J, Muren A. Excitatory and inhibitory effects of vagus stimulation on gastric motility in the cat. Acta Physiol Scand 1963;57: 309.
29. Staadas J, Aune S. Intragastric pressure/volume relationship before and after vagotomy. Acta Chir Scand 1970;136:611.
30. Staadas JO. Intragastric pressure/volume relationship before and after proximal gastric vagotomy. Scand J Gastroenterol 1975;10: 129.
31. Andrews PLR, Grundy D, Scratcherd T. Reflex excitation of antral motility induced by gastric distension in the ferret. J Physiol (Lond) 1980;298:79.
32. Kelly KA, Code CF. Effect of transthoracic vagotomy on canine gastric electrical activity. Gastroenterology 1980;57:51.
33. Grundy D, Scratcherd T. A splancho-vagal component of the inhibition of gastric motility. In: Wienbeck M. Motility of the digestive tract. New York: Raven Press, 1982:39.
34. DePonti F, Azpiroz F, Malagelada JR. Reflex gastric relaxation in response to distension of the duodenum. Am J Physiol 1987;252: G595.
35. Schapiro H, Woodward ER. Pathway of the enterogastric reflex. Proc Soc Exp Biol Med 1959;101:407.
36. Azpiroz F, Malagelada J-R. Vagally mediated gastric relaxation induced by intestinal nutrients in the dog. Am J Physiol 1986;252: G727.
37. Miller J, Kauffman G, Elashoff J, Ohashi H, Carter D, Meyer JH. Search for resistances controlling gastric emptying of liquid meals. Am J Physiol 1981;241:G403.
38. Gregory RA. Some factors influencing the passage of fluid through intestinal loops in dogs. J Physiol (Lond) 1950;111:119.
39. Allescher H-D, Daniel EE, Dent J, Fox JET, Kostolanska F. Neural reflex of the canine pylorus to intraduodenal acid perfusion. Gastroenterology 1989;96:18.
40. Heddle R, Dent J, Read NW, et al. Antropyloroduodenal motor responses to intraduodenal lipid infusion in healthy volunteers. Am J Physiol 1988;254:G671.
41. Fraser R, Fone D, Horowitz M, et al. Pyloric motor response to intraduodenal lipid is sustained and atropine sensitive. Gastroenterology 1989;96:A157.
42. Fisher RS, Lipshutz W, Cohen S. The hormonal regulation of pyloric sphincter function. J Clin Invest 1973;52:1289.

43. Hasler W, Bowling B, Owyang C. Intaduodenal lipids induce pyloric contractions: Role of cholecystokinin and the cholinergic and opiate pathways. Gastroenterology 1989;96:A200.

44. Valenzuela JE. Effect of intestinal hormones and peptides on intragastric pressure in dogs. Gastroenterology 1976;71:766.

45. Shillabeer G, Davison JS. Proglumide, a cholecystokinin antagonist, increases gastric emptying in rats. Am J Physiol 1987;252:R353.

46. Decktor DL, Pendleton RG, Elnitsky AT, et al. Effect of metoclopramide, bethanechol and the cholecystokinin receptor antagonist, L-364718m on gastric emptying in the rat. Eur J Pharmacol 1988;147:313.

47. Fried M, Loechner C, Erlacher U, et al. Role of CCK in regulation of gastric emptying and pancreatic secretion in man. Gastroenterology 1989;96:A159.

48. Kleibeuker JH, Beekhuis H, Piers DA, et al. Retardation of gastric emptying of solid food by secretin. Gastroenterology 1988;94:122.

49. Liddle RA, Morita ET, Conrad CK, Williams JA. Regulation of gastric emptying in humans by cholecystokinin. J Clin Invest 1986;77:992.

50. Yamagishi T, Debas HT. Cholecystokinin inhibits gastric emptying by acting on both proximal stomach and pylorus. Am J Physiol 1978;234:E375.

51. Carlson HC, Code CF, Nelson RA. Motor action of the canine gastroduodenal junction: A cineradiographic, pressure, and electric study. Am J Dig Dis 1966;11:155.

52. Ehrlein HJ, Heisinger E. Computer analysis of mechanical activity of gastroduodenal junction in unanesthetized dogs. Q J Exp Physiol 1982;67:17.

53. King PM, Adam RD, Pryde A, McDicken WN, Heading RC. Relationships of human antroduodenal motility and transpyloric fluid movement: Non-invasive observations with real-time ultrasound. Gut 1984;25:1384.

54. King PM, Pryde A, Heading RC. Effect of alterations in test meal composition on episodic transpyloric fluid movement in humans. Dig Dis Sci 1988;33:1537.

55. Kumar D, Ritman EL, Malagelada J-R. Three dimensional imaging of the stomach: Role of pylorus in emptying of liquids. Am J Physiol 1987;253:G79.

56. King PM, Heading RC, Pryde A. Coordinated motor activity of the human gastroduodenal region. Dig Dis Sci 1985;30:219.

57. Friedman G, Wolf BS, Waye JD, Janowitz HD. Correlation of cineradiographic and intraluminal pressure changes in the human duodenum: An analysis of the functional significance of monophasic waves. Gastroenterology 1965;49:37.

58. Lee KY, Chang TM, Chey WY. Effect of rabbit antimotilin serum on myoelectric activity and plasma motilin concentrations in fasting dogs. Am J Physiol 1983;245:G547.

59. Poitras P, Steinbach JH, VanDeventer G, Code CF, Walsh JH. Motilin-independent ectopic fronts of the interdigestive myoelectric complex in dogs. Am J Physiol 1980;239:G215.

60. Saar MG, Spenser MP, Hakim NS, et al. Control of interdigestive patterns of the stomach and jejunum: Neural vs. hormonal. In: Singer MV, Goebell H. Nerves and the gastrointestinal tract. Lancaster, England: MTP Press Limited, 1989:399.

61. Stanghellini V, Malagelada J-R, Zinsmeister AR, et al. Stress-induced gastroduodenal motor disturbances in humans: Possible humoral mechanisms. Gastroenterology 1983;85:83.

62. Marik F, Code C. Control of the interdigestive myoelectric activity in dogs by the vagus nerves and pentagastrin. Gastroenterology 1975;69:387.

63. Wilen T, Gustavasson S, Jung B. Effects of a fatty meal on small bowel propulsion in intact and vagotomized rats. Eur Surg Res 1983;13:114.

64. Hall KE, El-Sharkay T, Diamant NE. Vagal control of postprandial upper gastrointestinal motility. Am J Physiol 1986;250:G501.

65. Code CF, Marlett JA. The interdigestive myoelectric complex of stomach and small bowel of dogs. J Physiol (Lond) 1975;246:289.

66. Russell J, Bass P. Canine gastric emptying of polycarbophil: An indigestible, particulate substance. Gastroenterology 1985;89:307.

67. DeWever I, Eeckhout C, Vantrappen G, Hellemans J. Disruptive effect of test meals on interdigestive motor complex in dogs. Am J Physiol 1985;235:E661.

68. Gulsrud PO, Taylor IL, Watts HD, Cohen MB, Meyer JH. How gastric emptying of carbohydrate affects glucose tolerance and symptoms after truncal vagotomy with pyloroplasty. Gastroenterology 1980;78:1463.

69. Stephens JR, Woolson RF, Cooke AR. Osmolyte and tryptophan receptors controlling gastric emptying in the dog. Am J Physiol 1976;231:848.

70. Lin HC, Doty JE, Reedy TJ, Meyer JH. Inhibition of gastric emptying by glucose depends on the length of the intestine exposed to the nutrient. Am J Physiol 1989;256:G404.

71. Lin HC, Doty JE, Reedy TJ, Meyer JH. Inhibition of gastric emptying by sodium oleate depends on the length of gut exposed to the nutrient. Gastroenterology 1989;96:A304.

72. Lin HC, Doty JE, Reedy TJ, Meyer JH. Inhibition of gastric emptying by acids depends on titratable acidity and the length of gut exposed to acid. Gastroenterology 1988;95:877.

73. Williams NS, Grossman MI, Meyer JH. Abnormalities of gastric emptying of liquids in duodenal ulcer disease. Dig Dis Sci 1986;31:943.

74. Hunt JN, Stubbs DF. The volume and energy content of meals as determinants of gastric emptying. J Physiol (Lond) 1975;215:209.

75. Borgstrom B, Dahlquist A, Lundh G, Sjovall J. Studies of intestinal digestion and absorption in the human. J Clin Invest 1957;36:1521.

76. Lundh G. Intestinal digestion and absorption after gastrectomy. Acta Chir Scand 1958;231(suppl):1.

77. Schindlbeck NE, Heinrich C, Muller-Lissner SA. Relation between fasting antroduodenal motility and transpyloric fluid movements. Am J Physiol 1989;257:G198.

78. Oberle RL, Chen TS, Lloyd C, Amidon GL, Barnett JL, Owyang C, Meyer J. The influence of the interdigestive migrating motor complex on gastric emptying of liquids. Gastroenterology 1988;94:A328.

79. Itoh T, Takeru H, Gardner CR, Caldwell L. Effect of particle size on gastric residence time of non-disintegrating solids in beagle dogs. J Pharm Pharmacol 1986;38:801.

80. Gruber P, Rubinstein A, Li VHK, et al. Gastric emptying of nondigestible solids in the fasted dog. J Pharm Sci 1987;76:117.

81. Meyer B, Beglinger C, Neumayer M, Stadler GA. Physical characteristics of indigestible solids affect emptying from the fasting stomach. Gut 1989;30:1526.

82. Hunt JN, Spurrell WR. The pattern of emptying of the human stomach. J Physiol (Lond) 1951;113:157.

83. Dubois A, Natelsonn B, Van Eerdewegh P, et al. Gastric emptying and secretion in the rhesus monkey. Am J Physiol 1977;232:E186.

84. McHugh PR, Moran TH. The accuracy of the regulation of caloric ingestion in the rhesus monkey. Am J Physiol 1978;235:R29.

85. Costill DL, Saltin B. Factors limiting gastric emptying during rest and exercise. J Appl Physiol 1979;236:254.

86. Hunt JN, Smith JL, Jiang CL. Effects of meal volume and energy density on the gastric emptying of carbohydrates. Gastroenterology 1985;89:1326.

87. Brener W, Hendrix TR, McHugh PR. Regulation of the gastric emptying of glucose. Gastroenterology 1983;85:76.

88. Meyer JH, Thomson JB, Cohen MB, Shadchehr A, Mandiolla S. Sieving of food by the canine stomach and sieving after gastric surgery. Gastroenterology 1979;76:804.

89. Hinder RA, Kelly KA. Canine gastric emptying of solids and liquids. Am J Physiol 1979;233:E335.

90. Meyer JH, Dressman J, Fink AS, Amidon G. Effect of size and density on gastric emptying of indigestible solids. Gastroenterology 1985;89:805.

91. Meyer JH, Gu YG, Dressman J, Amidon G. Effect of viscosity and flow rate on gastric emptying of solids. Am J Physiol 1986;250:G161.

92. Sirois PJ, Amidon GL, Meyer JH, Doty JE, Dressman JB. Size and density discrimination of nondigestible solids during gastric emptying in the canine. A hydrodynamic correlation. Am J Physiol 258:G65–G72.

93. Meyer JH, Doty JE. Multiple effects of guar on canine digestion and transit of solid foods. Am J Clin Nutr 1988;48:267.

94. Bogentoft C, Carlsson G, Ekenved G, Magnusson A. Influence of food on the absorption of acetylsalicylic acid from enteric-coated dosage forms. Eur J Clin Pharmacol 1978;14:351.

95. Meyer JH, Porter-Fink V, Elashoff J, Dressman J, Amidon GL. Human postcibal gastric emptying of 1–3 mm spheres. Gastroenterology 1988;94:1315.

96. Feldman M, Smith HJ, Simon TR. Gastric emptying of solid radioopaque markers: Studies in healthy subjects and diabetic patients. Gastroenterology 1984;87:895.

97. Mayer EA, Thomson JB, Jehn D, Reedy T, Elashoff J, Deveny C, Meyer JH. Gastric emptying of solid food and pancreatic and biliary secretions after solid meals in patients with nonresective ulcer surgery. Gastroenterology 1984;87:1264.

98. Hinder RA, San-Garde BA. Individual and combined roles of the pylorus and antrum in the canine gastric emptying of a liquid and a digestible solid. Gastroenterology 1983;84:281.

99. Doty JE, Meyer JH. Vagotomy and antrectomy impairs intracellular but not extracellular fat absorption in the dog. Gastroenterology 1988;94:50.

100. Moore JG, Christian PE, Brown JA, Brophy C, Datz F, Taylor A. Influence of meal weight and caloric content on gastric emptying of meals in man. Dig Dis Sci 1983;29:513.

101. Moore JG, Christian PE, Coleman RE. Gastric emptying of varying meal weight and composition in man: Evaluation by dual liquid- and solid-phase isotopic method. Dig Dis Sci 1981;26:16.

102. Lin HC, Kim BH, Doty JE, Meyer JH. Meal volume accelerated gastric emptying of liquids but not solids [Abstract]. Gastroenterology 1990;98:A371.

103. Collins PJ, Horowitz M, Cook DJ, Harding PE, Shearman DJC. Gastric emptying in normal subjects—A reproducible technique using a single scintillation camera and a computer system. Gut 1983;24:1117.

104. Weiner K, Graham LS, Reedy T, Elashoff J, Meyer JH. Simultaneous gastric emptying of two solid foods. Gastroenterology 1981;81:257.

105. Siegel JA, Urbain J-L, Adler LP, et al. Biphasic nature of gastric emptying. Gut 1988;29:85.

106. Lavigne ME, Wiley ZD, Martin P, Way LW, Sleisenger MH, MacGregor IL. Gastric, pancreatic, and biliary secretion, and the rate of gastric emptying after parietal cell vagotomy. Am J Surg 1979;138:644.

107. Wilbur BG, Kelly KA. Effect of proximal gastric, complete gastric, and truncal vagotomy on canine gastric electric activity, motility, and emptying. Ann Surg 1973;178:295.

108. MacGregor IL, Martin P, Meyer JH. Gastric emptying of solid food in normal man and after subtotal gastrectomy and truncal vagotomy with pyloroplasty. Gastroenterology 1977;72:206.

109. Kelly KA. Gastric emptying of liquids and solids: Roles of proximal and distal stomach. Am J Physiol 1980;239:G71.

110. Gue M, Fioramonti J, Honde C, et al. Opposite effects of kappa-opioid agonists on gastric emptying of liquids and solids in dogs. Gastroenterology 1988;95:927.

111. Meyer JH, Mayer EA, Jehn D, Gu YG, Fried M, Fink AS. Gastric processing and emptying of fat. Gastroenterology 1986;90:1176.

112. Jian R, Vigneron N, Najean Y, Bernier JJ. Gastric emptying and intragastric distribution of lipids in man. A new scintigraphic method of study. Dig Dis Sci 1982;27:705.

113. Chang CA, McKenna RD, Beck IT. Gastric emptying rate of water and fat phases of a mixed test meal. Gut 1968;9:420.

114. Roby DD, Brink KL, Place AR. Relative passage rates of lipid and aqueous digesta in penguin and petrel chicks: Formation of stomach oils. The Auk 1989;106:303.

115. Cortot A, Phillips SE, Malagelada JR. Parallel gastric emptying of nonhydrolyzable fat and water after a solid–liquid meal in humans. Gastroenterology 1982;82:877.

116. James AH. The nature of the gastric contents in man. In: The physiology of gastric digestion. London: Edward Arnold Publishers, 1957:1.

117. Barker MCJ, Cobden I, Axon ATR. Proximal stomach and antrum in stomach emptying. Gut 1979;20:309.

118. Collins PJ, Horowitz M, Chatterton BE. Proximal, distal and total stomach emptying of a digestible solid meal in normal subjects. Br J Radiol 1988;61:12.

119. Urbain J-L, Siegel JA, Charkes ND, et al. The two component stomach: Effects of meal particle size on fundal and antral emptying. Eur J Nucl Med 1989;15:254.

120. Meyer JH, Porter-Fink V, Graham LS, Dressman J, Amidon G. Proximal stomach also sieves. Gastroenterology 1988;94:A301.

121. Barlow AP, Hinder RA, DeMeester TR. Principles of 24-hour pH monitoring and its clinical application. Gastroenterology 1989;96:A27.

122. Place AR, Stoyan NC, Ricklefs R, Butler RG. The physiological basis and importance of stomach oil formation in Leach's Storm-Petrel. The Auk 1989;106:687.

123. You CH, Chey WY. Study of electromechanical activity of the stomach in humans and in dogs with particular attention to tachygastria. Gastroenterology 1984;86:1460.

124. Kaye MD, Mehta SJ, Showalter JP. Manometric studies of the human pylorus. Gastroenterology 1976;70:477.

125. Keinke O, Ehrlein HJ. Effect of oleic acid on canine gastroduodenal motility, pyloric diameter, and gastric emptying. Q J Exp Physiol 1983;68:675.

126. Keinke O, Schemann M, Ehrlein HJ. Mechanical factors regulating emptying of viscous nutrient meals. Q J Physiol 1984;69:781.

127. Thomas JE. Mechanics and regulation of gastric emptying. Physiol Rev 1957;37:453.

128. Hunt JN, Knox MT, Oginski A. The effect of gravity on gastric emptying with various test meals. J Physiol (Lond) 1965;154:270.

129. McKelvey STD. Gastric incontinence and postvagotomy diarrhea. Br J Surg 1970;57:741.

130. Crider JO, Thomas JE. A study of gastric emptying with the pylorus open. Am J Dig Dis 1937;4:295.

131. Stemper TJ, Cooke AR. Effect of a fixed pyloric opening on gastric emptying in the cat. Am J Physiol 1976;230:813.

132. Dooley CP, Reznick JB, Valenzuela JE. Variations in gastric and duodenal motility during gastric emptying of liquid meals in humans. Gastroenterology 1984;87:1114.

133. Rees WDW, Go VLW, Malagelada JR. Antroduodenal motor response to solid–liquid and homogenized meals. Gastroenterology 1979;76:1438.

134. Aeberhard P, Walther M. Results of a controlled randomized trial of proximal gastric vagotomy with and without pyloroplasty. Br J Surg 1978;65:634.

135. Clarke RJ, Alexander-Williams J. The effect of preserving antral innervation and of a pyloroplasty on gastric emptying after vagotomy in man. Gut 1973;14:300.

136. Williams NS, Miller J, Elashoff J, Meyer JH. Canine resistances to gastric emptying of liquids after ulcer surgery. Dig Dis Sci 1986;31:273.

137. Maddern GJ, Jamieson GG. Fundoplication enhances gastric emptying. Ann Surg 1985;201:296.

138. Stemper TJ, Cooke AR. Gastric emptying and relationship to antral contractile activity. Gastroenterology 1975;69:649.

139. Camilleri A, Malagelada J-R, Brown ML, et al. Relation between antral motility and gastric emptying of solids and liquids in humans. Am J Physiol 1985;249:G580.

140. Carr DH, Brooks FP. Vagally induced gastric antral contractions and gastric emptying of a liquid test meal. Q J Exp Physiol 1978;63:49.

141. Wulschke S, Ehrlein H-J, Tsiamitas C. The control mechanisms of gastric emptying are not overridden by motor stimulants. Am J Physiol 1986;251:G744.

142. Schulze-Delrieu K, Brown CK. Emptying of saline meals by the cat stomach as a function of pyloric resistance. Am J Physiol 1985;249:G725.

143. Hinder RA, Bremner CG. Relative role of pyloroplasty size, truncal vagotomy and milk meal volume in canine gastric emptying. Am J Dig Dis 1978;23:210.

144. Shirazi S, Schulze-Delrieu K, Brown CK. Duodenal resistance to the emptying of various solutions from the isolated cat stomach. J Lab Clin Med 1988;111:654.

145. Parr NJ, Baxter JN, Critchley M, Mackie CR. Small intestinal resistances and the gastroduodenal brake. Gut 1987;28:950.

146. Amidon GL. Fluid mechanics and intestinal transit [Letter]. Gastroenterology 1985;88:858.

147. Keller KH. Unpublished Presentation. Workshop on Gastric Emptying, Santa Monica, CA, February 1980.

9

Motility of the Small Intestine

WILLIAM L. HASLER

INTRODUCTION

The major function of the small intestine is to process and absorb nutrients so that they may be distributed to the rest of the body. The organized motor activity known to exist in the small intestine subserves this function by two basic contractile patterns, mixing and propulsion. These two patterns are seen after ingestion of a meal where chyme must be mixed with the bile and digestive enzymes to effect efficient digestion and propelled in a caudad direction to allow subsequent boluses from the stomach to be digested. Mixing and propulsion also occur under fasting conditions, which result in the cleansing of the small intestine of undigestible solids and sloughed enterocytes. Control of the motor activity of the small intestine involves multiple factors including extrinsic innervation of the bowel wall, innervation within the bowel wall itself, circulating hormones, and myogenic characteristics of intestinal smooth muscle. This chapter introduces the reader to the physiology of small intestinal motility. The first section discusses basic concepts of smooth muscle and neural anatomy and physiology that pertain specifically to motility of the small intestine. This is followed by a description of the known organized motor patterns responsible for mixing and propulsion of intestinal contents. Finally, the last section of this chapter discusses what is known about the ileocecal junction, a sphincteric region between the ileum and colon.

CHARACTERISTICS OF SMALL INTESTINAL SMOOTH MUSCLE

The small intestinal wall has two organized regions of muscle tissue, the muscularis externa and the muscularis mucosa. The muscularis externa consists of two layers oriented at 90-degree angles to each other, an outer longitudinal layer and an inner circular layer. The circular layer can be further subdivided into inner and outer layers. The muscularis externa is the major effector of contractile activity of the small intestine, and most of the discussion that follows concentrates on this region. The role of the muscularis mucosa is poorly understood and will not be discussed further.

Smooth muscle cells of the muscularis externa are spindle shaped with solitary nuclei. Their length is roughly 20 times greater than their width. In contrast to skeletal muscle, there are no obvious specialized regions for interaction with neural tissue. Intestinal smooth muscle cells are electrically active with a resting membrane potential of -40 to -80 mV, which is maintained by Na^+-K^+-ATPase activity.[1] Additionally, they exhibit spontaneous contractions, which can be activated by stretch.

Characteristics of the Intestinal Slow Wave

Alvarez and Mahoney were the first to characterize the rhythmic electrical activity of the small intestine.[2] Subsequent investigators have noted an ubiquitous oscillating fluctuation in membrane potential of 3 to 15 mV (referred to as the intestinal slow wave), which, in humans, cycles at a frequency of 11 to 12 per minute in the proximal small intestine (Fig 9-1). Extracellular electrodes have demonstrated the slow wave to be sinusoidal or to consist of a rapid biphasic deflection from the zero potential line. Intracellular electrodes have recorded the characteristic appearance of the intestinal slow wave as consisting of a rapid depolarization followed by a partial repolarization and a prolonged plateau phase of depolarization. The slow wave cycle terminates in a full repolarization to the resting membrane potential. Neural toxins, such as tetrodotoxin, do not abolish the intestinal slow wave, indicating its origin in smooth muscle or other non-neural tissue.

Slow waves determine both the frequency of intestinal contractions and their direction. However, for an intestinal contraction to occur, the membrane must reach a critical level of depolarization. Under quiescent conditions in vivo, the slow wave by itself does not often reach this level of depolarization, and no contractions occur, despite the presence of ongoing electrical slow wave activity. For most organized contractions to occur, the smooth muscle cell must be activated by neural or hormonal inputs, which evoke spike potentials that, in turn, induce membrane depolarization. Under some circumstances, spike potentials can be generated by intestinal smooth muscle even in the absence of neural input.[3] Electrical coupling between neighboring smooth muscle cells is close, thus, smooth muscle cells with the dominant pacemaker activity, usually with the highest slow wave frequency, entrain adjacent cells to the same frequency in a phenomenon termed *phase lock*. However, slow waves do not occur simultaneously at all locations. There is an orderly time lag in slow wave activity (phase lag) within a region of phase lock that determines the direction of propagation of the slow wave.[4] Under physiologic conditions, the phase lag occurs in a cephalad to caudad direction,

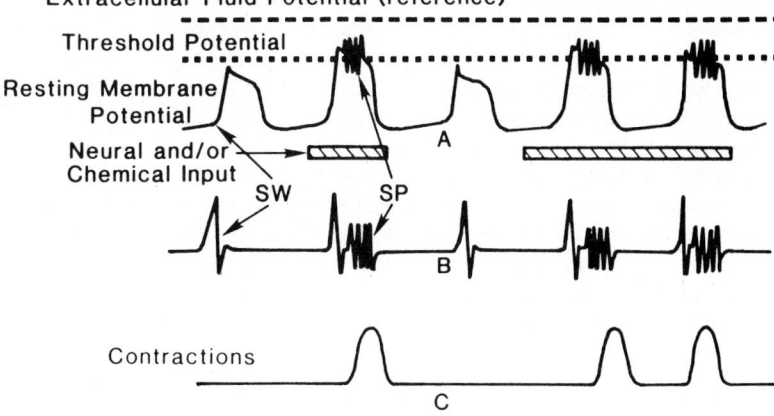

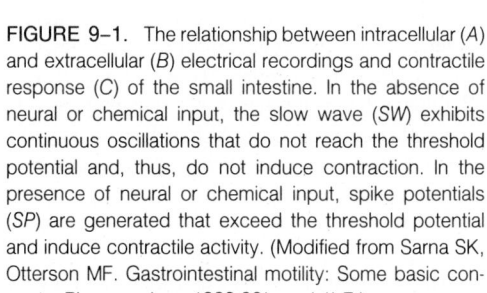

FIGURE 9–1. The relationship between intracellular (*A*) and extracellular (*B*) electrical recordings and contractile response (*C*) of the small intestine. In the absence of neural or chemical input, the slow wave (*SW*) exhibits continuous oscillations that do not reach the threshold potential and, thus, do not induce contraction. In the presence of neural or chemical input, spike potentials (*SP*) are generated that exceed the threshold potential and induce contractile activity. (Modified from Sarna SK, Otterson MF. Gastrointestinal motility: Some basic concepts. Pharmacology 1988;36(suppl 1):7.)

which ensures that contractile activity propagates aborally. In a normal person, the dominant pacemaker of the small intestine resides in the region from the pylorus to the ligament of Treitz.[5] The velocity of propagation of the slow wave is inversely related to the resistance of the smooth muscle tissue. The propagation velocity is much more rapid in the longitudinal axis (7–10 cm/s) than in the transverse axis (1 cm/s).[6]

Cellular Origins of the Intestinal Slow Wave

The origin of the small intestinal slow wave has been the subject of a great volume of investigation over the past 25 years, and a controversy has arisen as to which cell type initiates the rhythmic electrical activity. It was believed that the intestinal slow wave was generated in the longitudinal muscle layer and spread electrotonically to the circular layer. This was based on experiments on intestine from the cat and other species, which showed rhythmic depolarizations from isolated longitudinal muscle tissue but not circular tissue.[6–8] These observations were supported by in vitro experiments that demonstrated decreasing slow wave amplitude in the circular muscle layer with increasing distance from the junction of the longitudinal and circular layers.[9] However, these preparations have not always yielded consistent results. In some studies, only 20% of isolated preparations of longitudinal muscle generated slow waves.[10] Also, only certain regions of these preparations were capable of slow wave generation.[10,11] Finally, histologic examination of some of these preparations revealed the presence of fragments of myenteric plexus and circular smooth muscle, suggesting that the isolation procedure was incomplete.[12] Subsequent studies have indicated that maximal slow wave amplitude occurs either at the junction of the two muscle layers or in the outermost regions of the circular layer.[13] In recent studies, when more rigorous separation techniques were performed, no slow wave activity was detectable in longitudinal muscle while, in contrast, slow waves were consistently generated from the outermost cells of the circular layer.[14]

Cells known to reside at the junction of the two smooth muscle layers, the interstitial cells of Cajal, have been proposed as the initiators of the small intestinal slow wave. These cells are uninucleate with a thin surrounding cytoplasm, and they contain large quantities of mitochondria, indicating their high metabolic activity.[15] They also possess abundant caveoli on their surfaces, which are associated with prominent endoplasmic reticulum, inferring an active mechanism for membrane ion transport.[15] The interstitial cells of Cajal form close electrical contacts with smooth muscle cells from both muscle layers and are extensively innervated.[16,17] Special stains have demonstrated that these cells are distinct from neurons, glia, fibroblasts, and myocytes.[18] Evidence that the interstitial cells are the generators of the slow wave has been provided by a number of recent studies. In strips of smooth muscle from cat intestine, only those strips that contain interstitial cells generate rhythmic electrical activity.[19] Furthermore, intracellular recordings from interstitial cells of Cajal from canine colon reveal a cyclic electrical oscillation of 37 mV above a resting membrane potential of -70 mV occurring 4.6 times per minute.[20]

Effective propagation of the slow wave appears to require an intact muscularis externa. In cats, if a 1-mm-wide band of circular muscle is removed, the slow wave is propagated only 3 to 6 mm in a longitudinal direction.[21] When a band of longitudinal muscle greater than 5 mm is removed, slow wave propagation is abolished. Removal of smaller bands permits propagation albeit with reduced efficiency. Thus, for long distance slow wave propagation, both muscle layers are required.

Ionic Determinants of the Intestinal Slow Wave

The ion fluxes that define the small intestinal slow wave are complex and poorly understood. The intestinal slow wave is clearly an energy requiring process because metabolic inhibitors such as anoxia, cyanide, dinitrophenol, and pentachlorophenol can abolish rhythmic electric activity in intestinal muscle strips.[22,23] The requirement for an electrogenic sodium pump is suggested by the ability of ouabain to inhibit slow wave activity.[11,24,25] The intestinal slow wave also clearly depends on sodium flux as evidenced by studies showing abolition of the slow wave upon replacement of extracellular sodium with lithium, choline, sucrose, or Tris and enhanced slow wave amplitude upon intracellular iontophoresis of sodium.[24,25] Based on these results, Job theorized that influx of sodium occurs during depolarization while efflux of sodium, which depends on an electrogenic sodium pump, occurs during repolarization.[26] However, his experiments on whole muscle tissue showed that the potassium channel blocker tetraethylammonium chloride could slow the rates of depolarization and repolarization and suggested that potassium flux may play a role in slow wave electrogenesis. Job also noted calcium fluxes during the late repolarization phase of the slow wave cycle. Patch clamp studies of individual interstitial cells of Cajal demonstrated voltage-dependent inward and outward currents that could be elicited by depolarization.[27] The inward current resulted from the opening of membrane calcium channels, whereas a fraction of the outward current was due to calcium-activated potassium channels in the membrane. The specific role of each of these ionic currents in the genesis of the intestinal slow wave is not understood.

Electrical Coupling of Intestinal Smooth Muscle Cells

It is clear from the propagative characteristics of the intestinal slow wave that a high degree of electrical coupling exists between muscle cells in both muscle layers. In the circular muscle layer, discrete regions of cell contact are observed in which the outer leaflets of the cell membranes of adjacent muscle cells fuse to form a single leaflet. This structure, called the nexus, provides a pathway of low electrical resistance between cells.[28] Thus, in the circular layer, the nexus may represent the mechanism for phase lock of the slow wave. However, close electrical coupling is also seen in the longitudinal layer, but few or no nexus have been found in this layer. Thus, the structure responsible for electrical coupling in the longitudinal layer is unknown. In addition to electrical coupling within a muscle layer, there is also low-resistance coupling of the longitudinal to the circular layer. Microscopic studies of sections of small intestinal wall have revealed the presence of interconnecting bridges between the two layers.[29] It is likely that the interstitial cells of Cajal described above, with their extensive cellular contacts, may also provide a pathway for electrical conduction between the muscle layers.

Differences in the Slow Wave Between Proximal and Distal Small Intestine

Although phase lock between any two given intestinal muscle cells is generally very close, there tends to be some uncoupling of slow wave activity over the long distances encountered in the small intestine. This uncoupling, which is more pronounced in the distal intestine than in the duodenum, apparently results from the inability of cells in the distal intestine to be driven to the high slow wave frequencies of the proximal intestine. In experiments in which the intestine was cut into 1- to 2-cm lengths, each segment distal to the cut had a lower inherent slow wave frequency than the segment proximal to the cut.[30] In cats, the slow wave frequency decreases from 18 cycles per minute in the duodenum to 13 per minute in the ileum with a decrease in slow wave amplitude and an increase in variability of slow wave shape in the more distal intestine. In humans, the slow wave frequency decreases from 11 to 12 per minute in the duodenum to 7 to 8 per minute in the distal ileum.

In most species, the decrease in slow wave frequency from the duodenum to the ileum occurs in a stepwise rather than a continuous fashion. This results in areas of frequency plateau separated by regions of variable frequency (Fig 9-2). Frequency plateaus are more prominent in the proximal intestine. In the dog, there is a 60- to 70-cm plateau from the duodenum to the proximal jejunum, and, in the cat, there is a similar 30- to 50-cm plateau.[30] In contrast, in the distal ileum, frequency plateaus may be very short or even impossible to demonstrate. Although frequency plateaus have been demonstrated in many lower species, they have not been documented convincingly in humans.[31] The consequence of these plateaus is that, in the upper gut, there are long regions of slow wave coupling, which result in longer distances of propagation of individual contractions. In contrast, the uncoordinated slow waves of the distal ileum mandate contractions that propagate only very short distances (Fig 9-3).[32] By virtue of their uncoupling, the regions of variable frequency between frequency plateaus have been proposed as "mechanical stopcocks," which would act as brakes to long distance propulsion.[30] The motor correlate of these electrical observations is suggested by the data of Grivel and Ruckebusch who noted that one third of segmental contractions originating in the duodenum disappeared after travelling 60% of the length of dog intestine and 40% of the length of sheep intestine.[33]

In addition to the lower slow wave frequency in the distal intestine, there is also a decrease in slow wave velocity of propagation in distal compared to proximal intestine. In dogs and sheep, the slow wave velocity is 10 to 25 cm/min in the duodenum and 5 to 18 cm/min in the distal ileum.[34] This phenomenon, as well as the increase in slow wave uncoupling in the distal intestine, provides important physiologic advantages for efficient digestion. In the proximal intestine, it would be desirable to propel nutrients

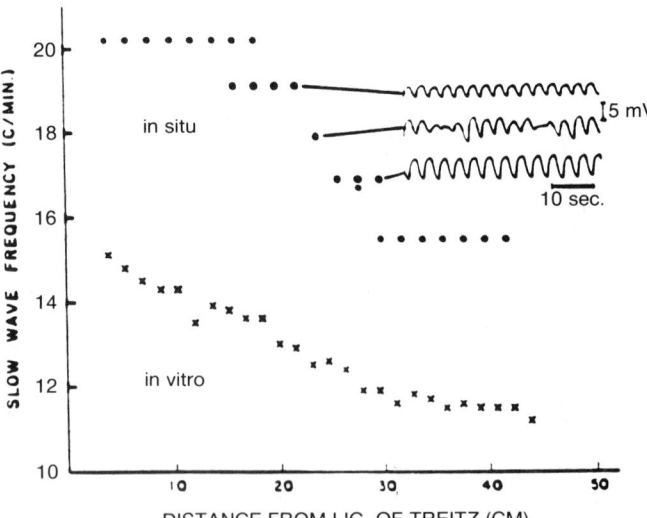

FIGURE 9–2. Recordings of slow-wave frequency from cat intestine in situ (●) or from short intestinal segments in vitro (×). The in situ recording illustrates the concept of frequency plateaus with abrupt decrements in slow-wave frequency aborally. Between the frequency plateaus are variable frequency regions where there is loss of phase lock of the slow wave. In vitro frequencies decrease in linear fashion without evidence of frequency plateaus. (Modified from Diamant NE, Bortoff A. Nature of the intestinal slow-wave frequency gradient. Am J Physiol 1969;216:301.)

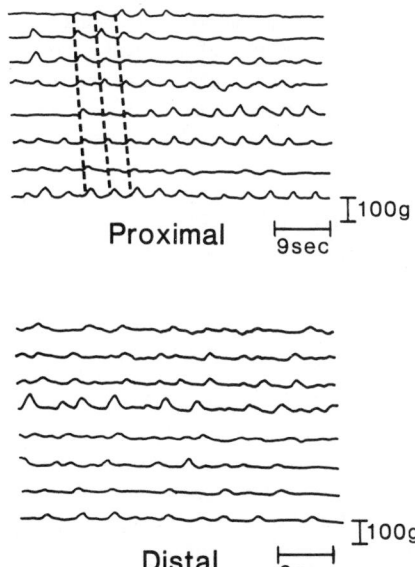

FIGURE 9–3. Postprandial spatial and temporal patterns of contraction in the proximal and distal small intestine. Contractions in the proximal intestine propagate over long distances due to extended regions of slow-wave phase lock; contractions in the distal intestine propagate only short distances due to uncoupling of slow-wave activity. (Modified from Sarna SK, Otterson MF. Small intestinal physiology and pathophysiology. Gastroenterol Clin North Am 1989;18:375.)

over a large surface area of mucosa for efficient digestion and absorption. In the distal intestine, it would be desirable for the propulsion to slow down to permit absorption of more slowly digested and absorbed substances such as fats, bile, and fat-soluble vitamins.

The structural basis for these decremental changes between the proximal and distal intestine is not known. There are no obvious quantitative or qualitative differences between nexus in the proximal and distal intestine.[35] However, it has been noted that the circular muscle cells are not as perpendicularly oriented to the longitudinal layer in the terminal ileum as are similar cells in the duodenum.[35] Also, mitochondria are less closely apposed to the cell membrane and the nucleus in circular smooth muscle cells of the ileum.[36] The functional effects of these anatomic differences are unknown.

Characteristics of Intestinal Spike Potential Activity

Whereas the slow wave controls the rate and direction of intestinal motor patterns, the presence of spike potentials or action potentials determines the presence and amplitude of individual phasic contractions. Excitatory agonists, such as acetylcholine, stimulate intestinal contractions by enhancing spike potential activity. Spike potentials are membrane depolarizations that, in contrast to the slow wave, are very short, usually only 10 to 100 milliseconds long with amplitudes of roughly 30 mV. Under most circumstances, they occur only during the plateau phase of depolarization, thus the frequency of intestinal phasic contractions is controlled by the

slow wave (see Fig 9-1). In contrast to the slow wave, spike potentials can occur in isolated sheets of both longitudinal and circular muscle and generally propagate only a very short distance, usually a few millimeters.[6] The ionic determinant of the spike potential appears to be membrane calcium flux because verapamil, removal of extracellular calcium, or replacement of calcium with other divalent ions such as manganese or cobalt abolishes spike potential activity.[25]

Contraction and Relaxation of Intestinal Smooth Muscle

Contractions in the small intestine are of two major types: phasic and tonic. In dogs and in humans, the vast majority of intestinal contractions are phasic and are controlled by spike potentials as described above. Tonic contractions lasting from 10 seconds to as long as 8 minutes are sometimes seen in the circular layer.[37,38] Tonic contractions are independent of slow wave activity, and, because they are mediated by agonist-induced release of intracellular calcium, removal of extracellular calcium or use of calcium channel blockers has no effect on them.

Relaxation of intestinal muscle may result from removal of a contractile stimulus or application of an active relaxant agent. In general, relaxant agonists are believed to act by way of cyclic AMP-dependent reduction in intracellular levels of calcium either by sequestration or reduction of membrane calcium flux.[39] The net effect of decreased intracellular calcium is decreased activation of the contractile apparatus.

Relative Roles of the Longitudinal and Circular Muscle Layers

The anatomically distinct physiologic functions of the longitudinal and circular muscle layers remain unclear. It is believed that the circular layer mediates both mixing and propulsion because occlusion of the lumen and displacement of gut contents require contraction of this layer. The most basic local contractile pattern of the small intestine is that of segmentation, which is predominantly a circular muscle phenomenon involving reciprocal inhibition and disinhibition of adjacent intestinal segments.[40] Although the longitudinal muscle probably does not have the same potent propulsive capabilities, contraction of this layer should theoretically shorten the gut and thereby facilitate longitudinal transit. Contraction of the longitudinal layer has also been proposed to increase luminal diameter, thereby facilitating the passage of a large bolus.[41] Macagno has postulated that intermittent contractions of the longitudinal layer are responsible for maximal exposure of the mucosa to the chyme.[42]

A major controversy has arisen as to whether contractions of the longitudinal layer occur simultaneously with or out of phase with those of the circular layer. A number of early investigators who performed direct observation of in vivo intestinal contractions believed that both muscle layers contracted simultaneously.[41,43,44] This was supported by the argument of Bortoff and Sachs that the electrotonic spread of electrical activity between the two layers mandates that both layers must depolarize at the same time.[9]

However, Trendelenburg noted a 90-degree phase lag between contractions of the circular and longitudinal layer in the guinea pig.[45] Other investigators demonstrated phase lags ranging from 90 to 270 degrees. In vivo experiments using serosal radiopaque markers showed that longitudinally oriented markers moved 164 degrees out of phase with transversely oriented markers.[46] Wood and Perkins theorized that these phenomena were a mechanical consequence of circular contraction causing a reciprocal passive, as opposed to active, relaxation of the longitudinal layer due to the noncompliance of the intestinal wall.[47] Thus, physical properties should prevent simultaneous activation of the two layers. Yokoyama and North, in studies of guinea pig ileum, noted independent contractions of the two layers at low intraluminal pressures and simultaneous contractions at higher intraluminal pressures.[48] Thus, the interrelation between the two layers remains unresolved.

INNERVATION OF SMALL INTESTINAL SMOOTH MUSCLE

The muscle layers of the small intestine are extensively innervated by extrinsic nerves relaying information to and from extraintestinal ganglia, the spinal cord, and the central nervous system and by intrinsic nerves within the intestinal wall itself. The major extrinsic supply to the small intestine is from the vagus and the splanchnic nerves. The major intrinsic innervation to the intestinal smooth muscle resides in the myenteric plexus at the junction of the longitudinal and circular layers and, to a lesser extent, in the submucous plexus along the luminal aspect of the circular layer. The number of intrinsic neurons in the gut greatly exceeds the number of fibers in the vagus or splanchnic nerves. In humans, it is believed that the enteric nervous system contains 10 to 100 million neurons compared to only 2000 efferent fibers in the vagus from the central

nervous system.[49] Investigators have concluded that the majority of reflex and control activities of the small intestine are directed by the intrinsic nerve plexus and that the extrinsic innervation serves only a modulatory function.

Extrinsic Innervation of the Small Intestine

The extrinsic innervation of the intestine can be divided conveniently into three categories: parasympathetic, sympathetic, and sensory. The majority of parasympathetic and sympathetic fibers terminate at the level of the myenteric plexus and form connections within the enteric ganglia, although some sympathetic axons are believed to terminate directly on sphincteric smooth muscle.

The vagus nerves contain four main groups of nerve fibers: preganglionic cholinergic nerves that supply excitatory neurons in the enteric plexus, preganglionic cholinergic nerves that supply inhibitory neurons in the myenteric plexus, sympathetic fibers from the cervical ganglia, and afferent fibers from the intestinal wall.[50] The efferent supply from parasympathetic cholinergic neurons acts principally on nicotinic receptors within the enteric ganglia (Fig 9-4).[51] Parasympathetic stimulation of the small intestine generally results in excitation. In dogs, vagal stimulation results in jejunal contraction by way of a cholinergic pathway.[52] The cell bodies of these efferent nerves reside predominantly in the dorsal motor nucleus of the vagus in the brain stem. Roughly 80% to 90% of the fibers in the vagus are afferent and synapse with neurons in the nodose ganglia.

The splanchnic nerves contain preganglionic and postganglionic sympathetic neurons as well as sensory fibers. The sympathetic innervation by the splanchnic nerves is different from the vagal parasympathetic innervation in that the neuronal cell bodies reside outside the gut wall in the prevertebral ganglia (celiac, and superior

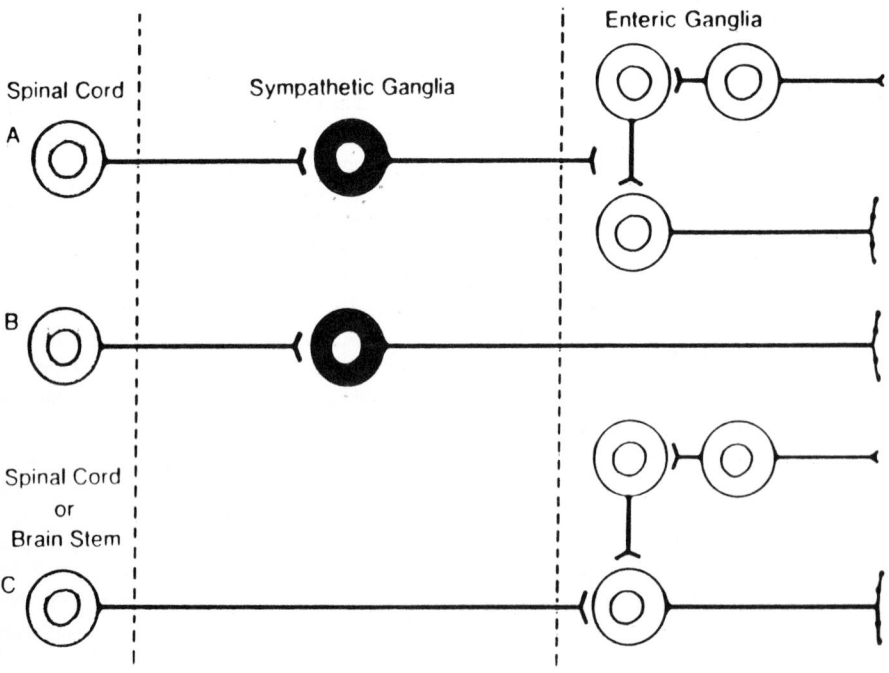

FIGURE 9–4. Representation of the relations of extrinsic sympathetic (*A,B*) and parasympathetic (*C*) innervation to the enteric nervous system. Most sympathetic innervation consists of preganglionic neurons, which synapse in the prevertebral ganglia, and postganglionic neurons, which project from the prevertebral ganglia to the enteric ganglia (*A*). Some sympathetic fibers project directly from the prevertebral ganglia to the smooth muscle in sphincteric regions (*B*). The parasympathetic fibers project directly from the spinal cord to the enteric ganglia (*C*). (Furness JB, Costa M. The enteric nervous system: An overview. In: Chey WY, ed. Functional disorders of the digestive tract. New York: Raven Press, 1983:47.)

and inferior mesenteric ganglia; see Fig 9-4). Preganglionic cholinergic neurons project from the spinal cord to the prevertebral ganglia where they synapse by way of nicotinic receptors. The postganglionic neurons, which are noradrenergic, project to the enteric ganglia by way of the splanchnic nerves. Noradrenergic innervation from the splanchnic nerves generally inhibits excitatory cholinergic transmission within the myenteric plexus.[53] The physiologic significance of these pathways is exemplified by the long inhibitory intestinal reflexes, which decrease motility by way of neural arcs involving the prevertebral ganglia.[54] Demonstration of the inhibitory effects of sympathetic innervation comes from in vivo studies showing that α_2-agonists, such as clonidine, delay intestinal transit and inhibit organized contractile patterns.[55] In addition to the classic neurotransmitters, both the vagus and splanchnic nerves contain numerous peptidergic fibers, such as somatostatin, substance P, cholecystokinin, neuropeptide Y, and the enkephalins.[56–60]

The small intestine is richly supplied with sensory fibers. Mechano-, chemo-, and thermoreceptors relay information by way of afferent fibers to the central nervous system. Sensory neurons of the small intestine have cell bodies within the myenteric and submucous plexus. The gut is also supplied by extrinsic sensory neurons with cell bodies within the dorsal root ganglia and sensory ganglia of the vagus.[61]

Intrinsic Innervation of the Small Intestine

The intrinsic nerves that control the motor activities of the small intestine reside predominantly in the myenteric plexus between the longitudinal and circular muscle layers. It is likely that the submucous plexus plays a smaller role. The density of neurons in the myenteric plexus is very high, ranging from 3,700 to 12,170 per square centimeter in the cat small intestine, or roughly that of the spinal cord.[62] The enteric nervous system has all the necessary elements for complete reflex activities, including sensory neurons, interneurons, and motor neurons and is thus capable of governing many of the physiologic motor patterns seen in the small intestine in the absence of extrinsic input. The structure of the enteric ganglia more closely resembles that of the central nervous system than of peripheral ganglia in that the only cell types present are neurons and glial cells. Blood vessels and connective tissue cells are absent, thus all nourishment for the neurons must come by way of diffusion through the interstitial fluid. Neurotransmitters released from axonal varicosities diffuse 20 to 100 nm to specific receptors on membranes of smooth muscle cells or other neurons.

The wiring of the enteric nervous system is complex and incompletely understood. In general, excitatory and inhibitory motor neurons project only 1 to 2 mm along the intestine with a few fibers running for 30 mm. Excitatory fibers in the longitudinal axis run in a cephalad direction, whereas inhibitory fibers project in a caudad direction. However, a number of the reflex responses of the intestine to local stimuli project to 100 cm or more, implying that an extensive array of interneuronal connections are involved in these responses.[63] Neurons in the myenteric plexus project most of their fibers to other myenteric neurons and to the circular muscle

layer, with a lesser number projecting to the submucous ganglia.[64] The longitudinal muscle layer is less well supplied with neurons and appears to receive fibers predominantly from excitatory motor neurons with little or no inhibitory input.[40] The circular muscle layer in humans has a thin dense plexus of nerve fibers at the junction of the outer and inner layers called the deep muscular plexus, which receives input from the myenteric plexus. The submucous ganglia are smaller than the myenteric ganglia and predominantly project to the intestinal mucosa. A few fibers project to the inner circular muscle layer or to the myenteric plexus.[65] Additional ganglia supply the muscularis mucosa and the blood vessels and extrinsic innervation of the intestine.

The excitatory neurons of the myenteric plexus are predominantly cholinergic, although many also appear to contain the tachykinins substance P and neurokinin A.[66] In rat intestinal longitudinal muscle strips, neural stimulation induces contraction that is incompletely blocked by the muscarinic antagonist atropine.[67] The atropine-resistant contraction has been demonstrated in many intestinal systems to be mediated by tachykinins. The inhibitory neurons predominantly contain vasoactive intestinal peptide (VIP). That VIP is the predominant relaxant substance in the enteric plexus is evidenced by the observations that VIP is released by neural stimuli and directly relaxes intestinal smooth muscle and that antagonists or antibodies to VIP prevent neurally mediated relaxation.[68–70] Additionally, a vast array of peptidergic neurons whose roles are very poorly understood has been demonstrated in the enteric ganglia.

The predominant neural influence on the small intestine under resting conditions is inhibitory. This was first demonstrated by Bayliss and Starling at the turn of the century when they noted that serosal application of a cocaine solution sufficient to induce local anesthesia induced a pattern of active, regular contractions.[41] In vitro studies of cat jejunum by Wood revealed that atropine, the local anesthetics procaine and xylocaine, and the neural toxin tetrodotoxin led to an increased percentage of slow waves accompanied by spiking activity.[3] It was concluded that phasic activity in the intestine is a myogenic phenomenon continuously inhibited by intrinsic neural pathways. Furthermore, these findings demonstrated that spike potentials of sufficient magnitude to induce contraction could be generated by intestinal smooth muscle alone.

LOCAL AND EXTENDED INTESTINAL REFLEXES

The most basic of the intestinal contractile patterns is that of segmentation. This pattern, which involves the alternate contraction and relaxation of adjacent segments of intestine, results in the mixing of intestinal contents but very little propagation. For effective mixing to occur, a contracting segment of intestine must be able to signal an adjacent segment to relax or vice versa. Segmentation is a local reflex that can be mediated solely by way of a neural pathway contained within the enteric nervous system. A number of more complex reflex activities of the small intestine are mediated by the enteric nervous system as well as the extrinsic nerves. These reflex activities allow the small intestine to respond to local stimuli from an adjacent segment of intestine or even a distant stimulus from another region of small intestine or another organ such as the stomach or colon.

Peristaltic Reflex

The phenomenon of peristalsis was first noted by gastrointestinal physiologists at the turn of the century. By fluoroscopic examination of cats fed a mixture of salmon and bismuth subnitrate, Cannon observed that the movement of the intestinal contents involved a combination of mixing nonpropulsive contractions, which divided the bolus, and aborally propulsive movements of peristalsis.[71] Mall first observed the peristaltic reflex, noting that when an object contacted the mucosa there was a constriction cephalad to the object associated with a simultaneous dilatation caudad to the object that together resulted in aboral propulsion.[71] Bayliss and Starling observed a strong tonic contraction cephalad to an intestinal luminal stimulus followed by numerous phasic contractions.[41] They noted that this reflex could be elicited by a broad range of stimuli including pinching the mucosa, application of hypertonic saline, and insertion of a solid bolus and that the reflex persisted in an externally denervated loop of intestine.

The peristaltic reflex consists of two phases, the contraction proximal to a luminal bolus known as the ascending contraction and the relaxation distal to the bolus known as the descending relaxation.[72] The peristaltic reflex requires sequentially timed motor activity of the circular and longitudinal layers, and this coordinated activity is controlled by intrinsic innervation. A neural model for the peristaltic reflex is the observation that stimulation of the myenteric plexus hyperpolarizes intestinal smooth muscle aborally and depolarizes the muscle orally.[73-75] The separate roles of the two muscle layers in the peristaltic reflex are not completely known. Wood noted that ascending contraction is associated with simultaneous contraction of the circular layer and relaxation of the longitudinal layer and that descending relaxation involves simultaneous contraction of the longitudinal layer and relaxation of the circular layer.[40] However, depending on the stimulus, the muscle layer responses may be more complex. In isolated guinea pig ileum distended to an intraluminal pressure of 0.5 to 1.5 cm H_2O, the only response is a change in longitudinal tension. At a pressure of 1.5 to 3.0 cm H_2O, the longitudinal tension increases further and is followed by an aborally propagating circular contraction.[76] Furthermore, the presence of an active descending relaxation phase has not been reproducibly demonstrated in whole animal preparations.[31]

To effect a peristaltic reflex, afferent sensory neurons must first be activated. Kosterlitz and Robinson have demonstrated that radial stretch of the intestinal wall is the most potent stimulus for induction of the reflex.[77] The primary location of the receptors that sense the radial stretch is believed to be in the mucosa because stripping the mucosa or applying topical anesthetics luminally abolishes the peristaltic reflex.[41] The presence of nonmucosal receptors has additionally been suggested by experiments in which chemical destruction of the mucosa by silver nitrate or tannic acid does not prevent the reflex.[78]

The mediators of the peristaltic reflex are the subjects of current investigation. The observation that the ascending contraction component of peristalsis can be blocked by atropine or the ganglionic blocker, hexamethonium, infers the involvement of both preganglionic and postganglionic cholinergic nerves in the pathway.[76] Tachykinin release may also be important for the ascending contraction.[79] Acetylcholine, substance P, and neurokinin A can all be released by radial stretch.[80,81] The final mediator of the descending relaxation is most likely VIP because VIP antisera and antagonists can block this response.[80] Other mediators that may modulate the peristaltic reflex include serotonin, which is released with luminal distention and lowers the threshold for the peristaltic reflex, and the opioid peptides, which inhibit VIP release.[82] The release of opioid peptides is inhibited during descending relaxation.[80]

Inhibitory Intestino-Intestinal Reflex

Extended reflex inhibition of small bowel motor activity was first described by Van Braam Houckgeest who observed that incision of the abdominal wall induced intestinal paralysis.[83] The intestino-intestinal reflex was subsequently characterized as a profound and extensive motor inhibition of up to several hundred centimeters of intestine usually induced by an abrupt stretching or dilation of a localized segment of intestinal wall.[84] In many lower species, the stimulus required is minimal, but, in dogs and humans, only the most vigorous distention elicits the reflex. In contrast to the peristaltic reflex, the receptor responsible for detecting the stimulus for the intestino-intestinal reflex does not reside in the mucosa because removal of the mucosa and submucosa does not abolish the reflex.[84] Instead, removal of the longitudinal muscle layer is necessary to prevent the reflex. In dogs, distention of an excluded but not extrinsically denervated intestinal segment to 50 mmHg abolishes spike activity in the excluded loop as well as in the intact but distant small intestine.[85] Sectioning of the splanchnic nerves prevents induction of the reflex. Other investigators have shown that an intact thoracolumbar spinal pathway is necessary for the reflex to occur because sectioning of the spinal cord below T7 abolishes it.[86] Accordingly, the inhibitory intestino-intestinal reflex depends on the extrinsic innervation of the small intestine. The clinical importance of the reflex is that, if there is distention due to a mechanical obstruction or other cause, the bowel responds with a decrease in motility and tone. Thus, the intestino-intestinal reflex may serve a protective function.

Extended Reflexes

While the peristaltic reflex provides an example of a local stimulus affecting local motor activity and the intestino-intestinal reflex provides an example of a local stimulus modifying local and distant motor activity, there are also a number of intestinal reflex responses in which only distant regions of the gut are affected. For example, motor activity of the small bowel may play a role in the regulation of gastric emptying. Duodenal distention results in reflex inhibition of gastric emptying by way of inhibition of gastric contractions (enterogastric reflexes) and stimulation of pyloric contractions (enteropyloric reflexes). These reflexes, which are independent of vagal activity, are discussed in greater detail in Chapter 8. Conversely, motility of the intestine may also be modified by stimuli from outside the small intestine. For example, ingestion of a meal results in an increase in myoelectric and motor activity in the distal ileum, a response known as the gastroileal reflex.[87-89] Also, an inhibitory colo-intestinal reflex has been described in which rectal distention retards small bowel transit and emptying of digesta into the cecum.[90] The mechanisms of these reflexes are incompletely studied.

An intriguing example of an extended intestinal reflex is the ileal brake mechanism. In normal volunteers, small bowel transit can be slowed by ileal perfusion of a lipid solution. Jejunal infusion of lipid does not have the same effect, verifying the specificity of the reflex.[91] This reflex is presumably a protective mechanism to prevent the distal intestine from being overwhelmed by a massive nutrient load. It can be prevented by infusion of the opioid antagonist, naloxone, suggesting that endogenous opioid peptides mediate the response.[92] The search for other hormonal mediators has centered on peptides known to be present in high concentration in the distal intestine such as peptide YY, neurotensin, and enteroglucagon.[91]

ORGANIZED MOTOR PATTERNS IN THE SMALL INTESTINE

Under physiologic conditions, the motility of the small intestine is characterized by organized motor patterns, which occur during the interdigestive period and after a meal. The interdigestive pattern known as the migrating motor (or myoelectric) complex (MMC) has been evaluated extensively over the past 25 years. Similarly, the fed pattern of intestinal motility seen after a meal has been the subject of numerous investigations. A number a specialized patterns have been described in the small intestine that occur infrequently during periods of health but are more common under pathologic conditions. These are discussed in a following section.

The Migrating Motor Complex in the Small Intestine

The existence of intermittent motor activity in the small intestine during fasting has been recognized for more than a century. Legros and Onimus in 1869 noted rhythmic activity in canine intestine.[93] A more complete description came in 1911 when Boldyreff observed 80-minute cycles of motor activity in the canine stomach and small intestine, which seemed to occur in relation to pancreatic and gastric secretion.[94] In 1969, Szurszewski noted a pattern of rhythmic myoelectric activity that propagated aborally during the interdigestive period.[95] Correlative motor phenomena during fasting were recorded by Carlson and coworkers and Code and Marlett. These phenomena came to be known as the interdigestive migrating motor (or myoelectric) complex (MMC).[96,97] In a number of mammalian species including humans, the MMC is a cyclic motor pattern that occurs during fasting and is abolished by ingestion of a meal, although in herbivorous ruminants and pigs disruption of the fasting pattern does not occur after a meal. Human MMCs occur every 84 to 112 minutes and consist of four separate phases (Fig 9-5).[98] Phase I is a period of motor quiescence, which lasts for 40% to 60% of the total cycle length. Phase II is a period of increasing but irregular contractions, which occupies 20% to 30% of the cycle. Phase II terminates in phase III, a 6- to 10-minute period of intense rhythmic contractions, which migrate aborally.[99] The maximal frequency of contractions during phase III is determined by the slow wave frequency of a segment of gut. Thus, the maximal contractile frequency is 3 cycles per minute in the stomach, 11 to 12 per minute in the duodenum, and 7 to 8 per minute in the ileum. The typical length of bowel in phase III is

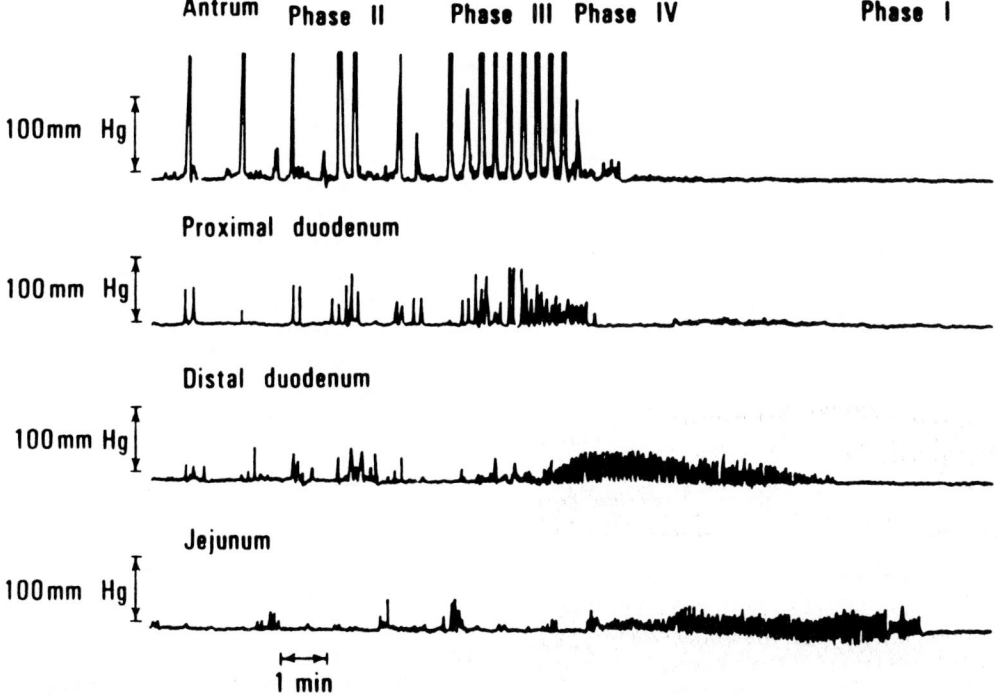

FIGURE 9–5. Manometric recording of the four phases of the human migrating motor complex (MMC) cycle from the stomach to the jejunum. (Rees WDW, Malagelada J-R, Miller LJ, Go VLW. Human interdigestive and postprandial gastrointestinal motor and gastrointestinal hormone patterns. Dig Dis Sci 1982;27:321.)

40 to 60 cm in the duodenum and decreases progressively to 5 to 10 cm in the ileum. The individual contractions of phase III propagate over longer distances than the contractions of phase II, suggesting that phase III is an intensely propulsive phase.[31] Phase IV, which lasts from 0% to 5% of the total cycle length, provides a transition phase from the intense motor activity of phase III to the quiescence of phase I. The transit time for an individual phase III complex approximates the cycle length of the MMC. As any given phase III is reaching the terminal ileum, a nascent phase III is developing in the proximal gut.

Although MMCs are nearly always present during the fasting period in healthy persons, there is extensive variation within a single cycle between the proximal and distal intestine as well as variability between cycles at different times of the day. In healthy volunteers, most phase III complexes originate in the gastroduodenal region, but up to one third may begin distal to the ligament of Treitz. Furthermore, of the complexes that begin in the proximal gut, only half propagate in a stable form beyond the midjejunum and only 10% reach the distal ileum.[100] Propagation velocity of phase III contractions decreases aborally from 4 to 6 cm/min in the duodenum to only 1 to 2 cm/min in the terminal ileum.[99] There is extensive diurnal variation in MMC cycling with complexes migrating two and a half times faster during the day but with higher contractile amplitudes during the night.[100,101]

The MMC of the upper gut is not an isolated phenomenon. There is associated contractile activity of the gallbladder and sphincter of Oddi, which cycles in phase with the intestinal complexes. Additionally, a number of secretory functions cycle in phase with the MMC. Gastric acid and pepsin secretions in the half hour before duodenal phase III are significantly greater than afterwards. Similarly, the release of bicarbonate, bile acids, bilirubin, and pancreatic enzymes such as amylase, lipase, and trypsin all increase in the 10 to 30 minutes before a duodenal phase III and

peak just before or during phase III activity (Fig 9-6).[102] The cycling responses are not affected by vagotomy. These observations suggest that the intestinal MMC is only a part of a larger cycling phenomenon involving all the visceral and solid organs in the upper abdomen.

The Fed Motor Pattern in the Small Intestine

In many species, including humans, ingestion of a meal results in the conversion of the normal fasting motor pattern to a characteristic fed pattern. In dogs, feeding induces predictable myoelectric and contractile changes, which peak within 10 to 20 minutes and persist for several hours depending on the characteristics of the meal.[103] Feeding interrupts the MMC simultaneously at all levels of the small intestine, suggesting the involvement of a neurohumoral mechanism rather than a local effect.[97] The myoelectric pattern seen after a meal consists of random bursts of spike potentials. The motor correlate is a series of ungrouped contractions of variable amplitude, which may be superimposed on small changes in tone (Fig 9-7).[104] In humans, these contractions consist of groups of one to three contractions separated by periods of motor quiescence lasting 5 to 40 seconds.[105] As in the fasting state, there is a decreasing gradient of contractile activity from the duodenum to the distal ileum, and the postprandial propagation velocity is greater in the proximal intestine.[103] The contractile pattern of the fed state serves both to mix and to propel intestinal contents after a meal. Dusdieker and Summers observed that 44% of individual contractions in the fed state do not propagate and that, of the contractions that do propagate, 90% propagate less than 30 cm and 66% less than 9 cm.[106] In humans, the fraction of individual contractions that are propagative in the fed state is intermediate between that seen in phase II and that of phase III in the interdigestive state.[31]

The duration of the fed motor pattern depends on both the caloric content and qualitative aspects of the meal ingested. In dogs, a mixed 450-kcal meal induces a fed pattern for more than 3 hours, and peanut oil, consisting mostly of 18-carbon-length triglycerides, induces the fed state for a much longer period than equicaloric amounts of sucrose or milk protein.[107] If calories in any form are increased, the duration of the fed pattern is correspondingly increased to 8 hours or more in the dog. In humans, the duration of the fed pattern is generally shorter, usually lasting no more than 4 hours. The threshold for induction of the fed state in humans is not known, but a meal of 345 to 395 kcal can disrupt MMC cycling for more than 90 minutes.[100]

The resumption of MMC cycling after completion of the postprandial period is a poorly understood phenomenon. Generally, the first MMC begins distal to the gastroduodenal region after completion of the fed state, implying that factors that initiate normal complexes during feeding are not yet operational and that factors that induce ectopic complexes resume the interdigestive pattern.[107,108] The mere presence of nutrients in the small intestine does not prevent resumption of MMC cycling. In dogs, continuous intraduodenal perfusion of a nutrient solution induces the fed motor pattern for only a finite time after which the fasting pattern returns.

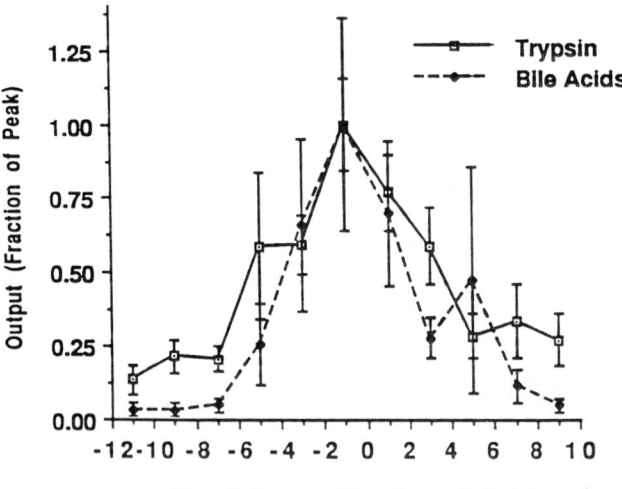

FIGURE 9–6. Relation of trypsin and bile acid output to the occurrence of phase III in the duodenum. Both trypsin and bile acid secretion peak 1 minute before the onset of duodenal phase III. (Modified from Keane FB, DiMagno EP, Dozois RR, Go VLW. Relationships among canine interdigestive exocrine pancreatic and biliary flow, duodenal motor activity, plasma pancreatic polypeptide, and motilin. Gastroenterology 1980;78: 310.)

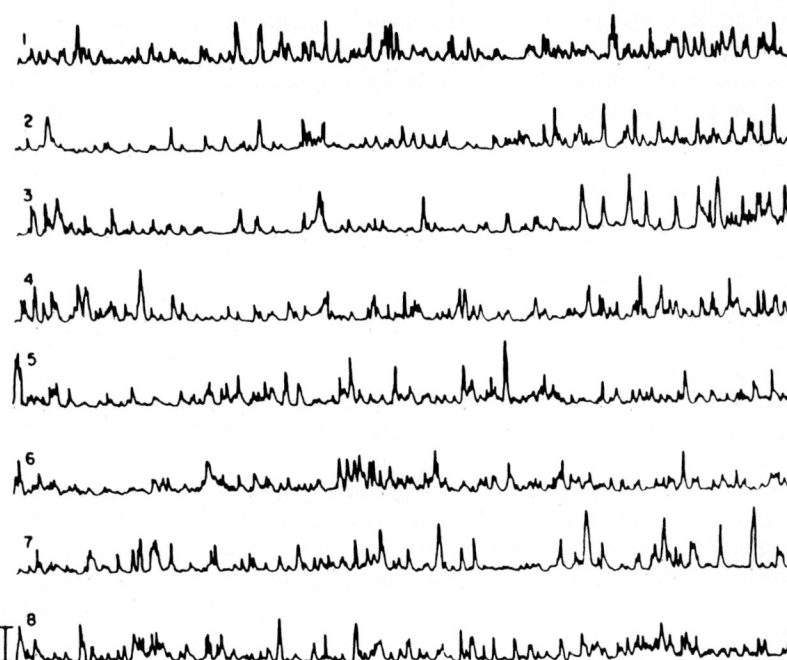

FIGURE 9–7. A typical fed motor pattern in the small intestine of a normal human volunteer. (Summers RW, Anuras S, Green J. Jejunal manometry patterns in health, partial intestinal obstruction, and pseudoobstruction. Gastroenterology 1983;85:1290.)

Transit of Small Intestinal Contents During the Fasted and Fed States

Transit of an intestinal bolus depends on both the pressure gradient generated by the intestinal smooth muscle and resistance to aboral propagation. Both the pressure gradient and resistance are determined by the caliber of the small intestinal lumen, the tone of the intestinal wall, and the presence and amplitude of intestinal phasic contractions. A number of techniques have been devised to measure small intestinal transit in humans, including migration of a radioactive technetium tracer or recovery of breath hydrogen or $^{14}CO_2$ after ingestion of unlabeled or ^{14}C-labeled lactulose. These techniques are comparable and reproducible for the most part, showing mean small intestinal transit times of 30 minutes to 3 hours in humans.[109,110] As expected from the manometric findings in both the fasted and fed states, transit in the upper small intestine tends to be more rapid than in the distal intestine. In rats, the transit time across the proximal half of the intestine is 30 minutes as compared to a total small intestinal time of 3 hours.[111] In contrast to the stomach where solids and liquids are handled quite differently, there is no difference in the small intestine. This was demonstrated by Malagelada in normal volunteers in which ^{131}I-fiber and ^{99m}Tc-DTPA-water were shown to be propelled through the small intestine at similar speeds.[112]

A number of investigators have attempted to correlate the known manometric findings of the MMC and the fed state with the more physiologically relevant movement of intestinal contents. Code and Schlegel combined cineradiographic techniques with simultaneous manometric pressure measurements to demonstrate that intestinal contents are effectively propelled ahead of the aborally propagating phase III.[113] They further noted that no radiopaque material remains after the phase III complex has passed. Thus, the MMC was termed the "intestinal housekeeper" because of its efficiency in cleaning the intestine. Additional radiographic

studies demonstrated that the transit of an inert opaque substance is four times as slow in phase I as in phase III and that 50% of the total flow occurs during phase III.[88] Bueno further observed that transit also occurs in phase II, with the most rapid propulsion during the transition from phase II to phase III.[34] The cineradiographic pattern of transit during phase III in humans is that of intermittent boluses of 4 to 5 cm in length separated by 1 to 2 cm intestinal contractions.[114] This pattern has also been shown in the rat. After a meal, the distribution of small bowel contents becomes more uniform. In dogs and humans, transit after a meal is more rapid than in the fasting state and shows some temporal and spatial fluctuations, although not as great as during the interdigestive period.[34,88] These findings from the study of intestinal transit and flow correlate well with manometric determinations of intestinal contractile activity.

Neural Regulation of the Fasting and Fed Small Intestinal Motor Patterns

The regulation of the fasting and fed motor patterns in the small intestine has been investigated intensively by gastrointestinal physiologists over the past 25 years. It has become apparent that the initiators of these organized complexes involve an intricate interaction of the extrinsic innervation of the intestine, the enteric nervous system, and humoral factors. Despite these studies, a clear definition of which factors are responsible for each pattern remains elusive.

NEURAL CONTROL OF THE MIGRATING MOTOR COMPLEX

The extrinsic innervation to the small intestine by way of the vagus and splanchnic nerves serves primarily to modulate rather than initiate migrating motor complex activity. Investigators have demonstrated that neither bilateral truncal vagotomy, removal of the superior and inferior mesenteric ganglia, total sympathectomy, nor complete extrinsic denervation of the small intestine prevent the cycling of the MMC.[115-119] However, in most instances of extrinsic denervation, there is alteration in the frequency or regularity of MMC cycling. After bilateral vagotomy, the frequency of MMC cycling is reduced in dogs.[115] Similarly, if the extrinsic nerves to the jejunum and ileum are severed, the frequency of MMC cycling decreases and the percentage of phase III complexes that propagate through to the terminal ileum is reduced.[120] This modulatory effect of the extrinsic nerve supply is illustrated by the clinical observation that the fraction of phase III complexes that propagate into the distal intestine in human patients with spinal cord transection above T3 is less than in control subjects.[121] The small intestine shows a lesser dependence on extrinsic innervation than the stomach and lower esophageal sphincter. Acute cooling of the vagus in dogs, a technique that effectively induces a reversible vagotomized state, eliminates phase III activity in the stomach and lower esophageal sphincter but has no effect on the small intestinal phase III activity.[122] The use of the vagal cooling technique has revealed that phase II and phase III in the small intestine are mediated by different neural pathways. In dogs, acute vagal cooling shortens or abolishes phase II activity without affecting phase III activity in the duodenum and jejunum but not the ileum.[123,124] These findings suggest a vagally mediated pathway for maintenance of phase II activity in the proximal small intestine and a vagally independent pathway for distal phase II activity and phase III activity.

The central nervous system can have profound effects on MMC cycling by way of the extrinsic innervation to the small intestine. Administration of an intense acoustic stress to normal volunteers abolishes jejunal MMC cycling for several hours.[125] Similarly, mental stress, such as participation in an active video arcade game or in an intense driving situation, can inhibit intestinal MMC cycling.[126] The ability of stress to disrupt MMC activity depends on the nature of the stressor and the time of day it is administered. For example, nocturnal stress induced by repetitively waking subjects from sleep does not modify MMC cycling despite the subjects' perception that the nocturnal stressor is considerably more obnoxious than the daytime stressors.[126] The mechanisms responsible for central nervous system modulation of MMC activity are unknown, however, a number of peptide mediators can modify MMC activity by way of central neural pathways. For example, intracerebroventricular administration of cholecystokinin decreases the frequency of MMC cycling, whereas intracerebroventricular somatostatin increases MMC frequency.[126]

The enteric nervous system coordinates the propagation of MMC cycling. Isolated denervated segments of small bowel exhibit spontaneous MMC activity that propagates aborally within the segment despite the absence of neural input from the extrinsic nerves or from the main segment of small intestine.[119] However, cycling in the excluded segment is out of phase with that of the main segment of small bowel, suggesting that continuity of the enteric nervous system is required for coordination of cycling from one region of intestine to the next. This is further exemplified by studies in which the small intestinal wall is transected into many segments and reanastomosed.[127] In these studies, MMC activity continues in each segment, however, each segment cycles independently from the others. If these animals are followed over

time, coordinated MMC cycling begins at 45 days and is complete within 100 days, suggesting that the enteric nervous system has the capability to regenerate connections that have been severed.[127] If, however, a segment of colonic wall is interposed between small intestinal segments, coordination does not resume even after 180 days, suggesting that enteric nerves show specificity for a given region of the gut.

The mechanisms involved in enteric nervous system control of MMC propagation have been studied by a number of investigators. In guinea pigs, longitudinal myomectomy with circumferential interruption of the myenteric plexus blocks propagation of 50% to 60% of phase III complexes.[128] If complete transection with reanastomosis is performed, only 20% of phase III complexes propagate across the transection. Most, but not all, of the intrinsic nerves regulating MMC propagation reside in the myenteric plexus. The deep muscular plexus and the submucous plexus appear to have some role in the maintenance of the MMC. Fox and Bass showed that serosal application of benzalkonium hydrochloride, which selectively destroys the myenteric ganglia, disrupts but does not abolish MMC cycling.[129]

Cholinergic as well as noncholinergic neural pathways are involved in maintenance of the intestinal MMC. In dogs, intravenous injections of the muscarinic antagonist, atropine; the ganglionic blocker, hexamethonium; or the neural toxin, tetrodotoxin, eliminate MMC activity.[130] If these compounds are administered by way of close intra-arterial injection, they prevent propagation of MMC activity distal to the site of injection.[131] These results suggest that both preganglionic and postganglionic cholinergic inputs are necessary for MMC propagation. Other mediators may play a role as well. Adrenoceptor antagonists disorganize but do not abolish MMC cycling. Immediately after transection and reanastomosis of the small intestine in guinea pigs, immunoreactivities for VIP, gastrin-releasing peptide, and somatostatin are markedly decreased distal to the anastomosis.[128] Recovery of MMC cycling after several weeks is associated with recovery of these immunoreactivities and evidence of nerve regrowth. This indirect evidence suggests the possibility that peptidergic nerves within the myenteric plexus contribute to the maintenance of coordinated MMC activity.

NEURAL CONTROL OF THE FED PATTERN

The extrinsic innervation of the small intestine plays a role in mediating, but is not required for the occurrence of, the fed motor pattern. Bilateral vagotomy, splanchnicectomy, mesenteric ganglionectomy, nor total extrinsic denervation prevent the induction of the fed motor pattern.[115,116] However, extrinsic denervation can modify the response to a meal. In dogs, bilateral vagotomy shortens the duration of the fed pattern, the regularity of interruption by meals of low caloric content, and the latency period from the time of ingestion to the onset of the fed pattern.[115,119,132] Furthermore, acute cooling of the vagus in dogs during the early postprandial period can convert the fed motor pattern to one containing intermittent phase III-like activity.[123,133] In the absence of continuity of the enteric nervous system, the extrinsic innervation alone is sufficient for the suppression of the fasting pattern in a distant region of intestine. If a nutrient solution is perfused into the lumen of an isolated loop of intestine that has not been extrinsically denervated, the fasting motor pattern can be disrupted in the unconnected main portion of the intestine.[134] Central nervous system modulation of the fed motor pattern is mediated through the extrinsic innervation to the gut. In dogs, the sight or smell of food can disrupt normal MMC cycling, suggesting a cephalic phase for induction of the fed motor pattern.[135] Intracerebroventricular injections of atropine and substance P decrease the duration of the fed state whereas intracerebroventricular injections of calcitonin, calcitonin gene-related peptide, neurotensin, neuropeptide Y, or enkephalin analogues actively induce intestinal phase III activity during the fed state.[136-140]

The enteric nervous system is also involved in the intestinal motor response to ingestion of a meal. Direct nutrient contact with the mucosa in one region of intestine induces a fed pattern in a distant region of intestine even after extrinsic denervation. However, Sarr and Kelly demonstrated that, when a dog with autotransplantation of the jejunoileum, which results in the transection of both extrinsic and intrinsic nerve supplies to the intestine, is fed proximal to the point of transection, there is no disruption of the normal MMC cycling distal to the transection.[119] Both extrinsic and intrinsic nerve supplies are required for a normal response to a meal, but either is capable of disrupting normal fasting motor activity. Atropine or hexamethonium abolishes motor activity in the fed state as well as during the MMC, underlining the importance of cholinergic innervation in this response.

Hormonal Regulation of the Fasting and Fed Intestinal Motor Patterns

A large number of peptide hormones and purported neurotransmitters can induce premature phase III activity in the small intestine when given exogenously. These include motilin, the motilin receptor agonist erythromycin, somatostatin, pancreatic polypeptide, morphine, substance P, metoclopramide, and histamine H_1-receptor agonists.[141-144] Some substances induce premature phase III cycling when given intraduodenally. In sheep, the serotonin receptor antagonist, methysergide, and also methylergonovine increase the frequency of phase III cycling, whereas cyproheptadine decreases the frequency of phase III occurrence, suggesting that serotonin receptors may be involved in the pacing of the MMC cycle.[145,146] However, for a peptide hormone or transmitter to satisfy the definition as a mediator or initiator of MMC activity, the phase III activity it generates should be physiologic in its location, duration, and propagation characteristics. Furthermore, any circulating peptide proposed as an initiator of phase III activity should cycle in phase with the endogenous MMC. Many of the compounds listed above do not satisfy these requirements. Mediators that best satisfy the requirements are discussed in following sections.

A number of compounds when given exogenously can inhibit fasting small intestinal motor activity and induce complexes that resemble the fed pattern. These include gastrin, cholecystokinin, insulin, glucagon, neurotensin, enkephalin analogues, and prostaglandin E_2.[115, 143,147-152] For any of these mediators to be considered as physiologic hormonal mediators of fed motor activity, they should inhibit MMC cycling, induce the fed pattern in the entire small intestine, be released during the fed period in a fashion that correlates with the duration of the fed state, and inhibit the cycling of purported humoral mediators of the MMC. To date, no peptide or transmitter has been discovered that satisfies all of these criteria. In dogs, cholecystokinin and gastrin inhibit MMC cycling but do not induce a motor pattern identical to the fed pattern nor do they prevent cycling of the peptide motilin, a purported mediator of MMC activity.[153,154] Although they are released postprandially, elevated levels of cholecystokinin and gastrin do not persist for the duration of the fed motor state. Certain nutrients, such as peanut oil, that induce a fed motor pattern do not induce release of peptides such as gastrin or insulin.[155] Conversely, certain nutrients, such as a low caloric glucose load, cause significant increases in circulating insulin but do not induce a fed pattern.[155] Peptides such as gastrin and cholecystokinin disrupt MMC cycling in the proximal intestine much more effectively than in the distal intestine, whereas a meal modifies the motor pattern throughout the entire intestine.[154] Similarly, the role of endogenous prostaglandins in the mediation of the fed state is unclear. Continuous indomethacin infusion induces a fed pattern in dogs, but infusion of prostaglandin E_2 also has significant disruptive effects on MMC cycling.[156] The effect of a meal on levels of the various prostaglandins in plasma and in the tissue is largely unknown. Neurotensin has been proposed as a mediator of the fed state and has been demonstrated to convert the fasting to the fed state along the entire small intestine of rats and humans.[151] Further investigation is required to determine if neurotensin is truly an important mediator of the fed state. No single peptide or transmitter candidate has yet been shown to be the primary mediator of the fed motor pattern. It is likely that a number of peptides act in concert with the enteric and extrinsic innervation of the gut to induce the fed state.

THE ROLE OF MOTILIN IN THE FASTING AND FED STATES IN THE SMALL INTESTINE

The peptide hormone, motilin, proposed by many investigators as the hormonal initiator of the MMC, comes closest to satisfying the requirements for such a mediator. Motilin is synthesized predominantly in the mucosa of the duodenum and proximal jejunum. Whether it is produced in enterochromaffin cells or in nonenterochromaffin endocrine cells is a matter of controversy.[157,158] Motilin has also been localized to the forebrain and cerebellum of the rat where it has been shown to release excitatory and inhibitory neurotransmitters.[159,160] Motilin immunoreactivity also has been detected in the vagus, however, its importance there is uncertain because vagotomy or vagal cooling do not modify plasma motilin levels.[161-163] Motilin is a 22-amino acid peptide that shows significant variation in sequence between species, suggesting possible differences in its physiologic role in different animals.

Motilin cycles in phase with endogenous MMC activity. In normal volunteers, endogenous phase III activity is immediately preceded by peak plasma motilin levels, which are at least 25 pM higher than the lowest levels seen in late phase I (Fig 9-8).[141,164] These findings have been confirmed by a number of investigators,[165-167] however, Sarna and coworkers have found that the peak in plasma motilin occurs after the initiation of duodenal phase III and believe that motilin peaking is caused by gastrointestinal contractile activity and not vice versa.[168] Nevertheless, motilin clearly cycles in phase with endogenous phase III activity.

Exogenous infusion of motilin induces physiologic MMC patterns. In normal volunteers, Vantrappen and coworkers reported that intravenous infusion of motilin to levels that mimicked peak levels seen during endogenous phase III activity induced premature

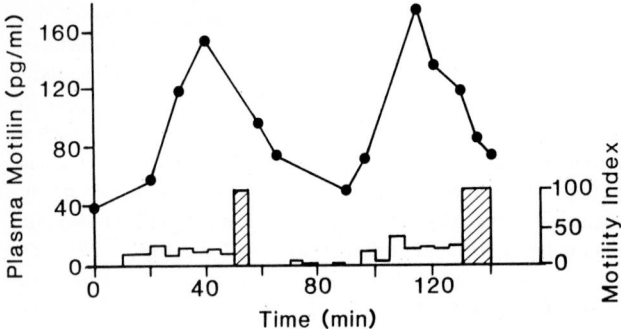

FIGURE 9-8. Relation of plasma motilin to intestinal phase II (*clear bars*) and phase III (*cross-hatched bars*) in a healthy volunteer. Plasma motilin rises throughout phase II to reach peak levels immediately before the onset of phase III. (You CH, Lee KY, Chey WY. Plasma motilin level and interdigestive motor complex in normal and abnormal states in man. In: Chey WY, ed. Functional disorders of the digestive tract. New York: Raven Press, 1983:213.)

phase III cycling in the stomach, which migrated aborally down the small intestine in 12 of 16 normal volunteers.[141] The phase III contractions were associated with increased intestinal transit, confirming their propulsive characteristics.[169] Itoh demonstrated that motilin-induced premature phase III activity was identical to endogenous phase III cycling in duration, amplitude, and migration velocity.[170] These observations were confirmed in a canine model by others.[166] In the dog, motilin-induced small intestinal phase III activity is not abolished by bilateral vagotomy but can be inhibited partially by atropine or hexamethonium and completely by the neural toxin, tetrodotoxin.[130,131] Motilin's actions in vivo are fully mediated by nerves by way of both cholinergic and noncholinergic pathways. It has been suggested that the noncholinergic component of the response to motilin is mediated by endogenous opioid peptides.[171] In vitro, motilin contracts smooth muscle strips from most mammalian species by stimulation of enteric nerves, although, in humans and rabbits, motilin may act directly on smooth muscle motilin receptors.[172]

The importance of motilin as the initiator of the MMC in the upper gut is suggested by experiments employing antisera to circulating motilin. Lee and coworkers reported that, in dogs, infusion of specific rabbit antisera to motilin in quantities sufficient to suppress circulating motilin levels to below those seen during endogenous phase I activity interrupts phase III cycling in the antrum, duodenum, and proximal jejunum with lesser effects on the ileum (Fig 9-9).[173] However, not all investigators have reproduced these findings. Borody and coworkers observed that motilin antiserum was capable only of inhibiting phase III activity induced by exogenous motilin but not endogenous phase III cycling.[174]

The role of motilin as the predominant initiator of MMC activity has been challenged by a number of physiologists who argue that not all spontaneous phase III activity is associated with increases in plasma motilin. However, most complexes that do not have associated rises in plasma motilin represent ectopic activity that begins distal to the antrum and duodenum.[175] Also, the distal jejunum and ileum are far less sensitive to the effects of motilin than the stomach and duodenum.[127,172] This is supported by motilin antisera infusion studies showing effective inhibition of MMC activity only at proximal sites.[173] Finally, in pigs, MMC cycling occurs at regular intervals associated with cyclic variations in plasma motilin, but neither intravenous motilin infusion nor motilin antisera modifies endogenous phase III activity.[176] These findings are most consistent with the conclusion that, in the pig, motilin is not important for MMC activity, but, in humans and dogs, motilin is a likely initiator of phase III activity in the stomach and proximal intestine. Propagation of proximal phase III complexes through the distal intestine or initiation of ectopic complexes in the distal intestine is mediated by pathways other than endogenous motilin release.

The endogenous stimuli that induce the cycling of motilin are poorly understood. The release of motilin is blocked by atropine or hexamethonium, suggesting regulation by a cholinergic pathway.[161] Stimulation of either the vagus or the nerve of Latarjet, which supplies the proximal gut, leads to an increase in plasma motilin in the portal and systemic circulation.[161,177] Motilin also is released by many stimuli that induce intestinal contractions.

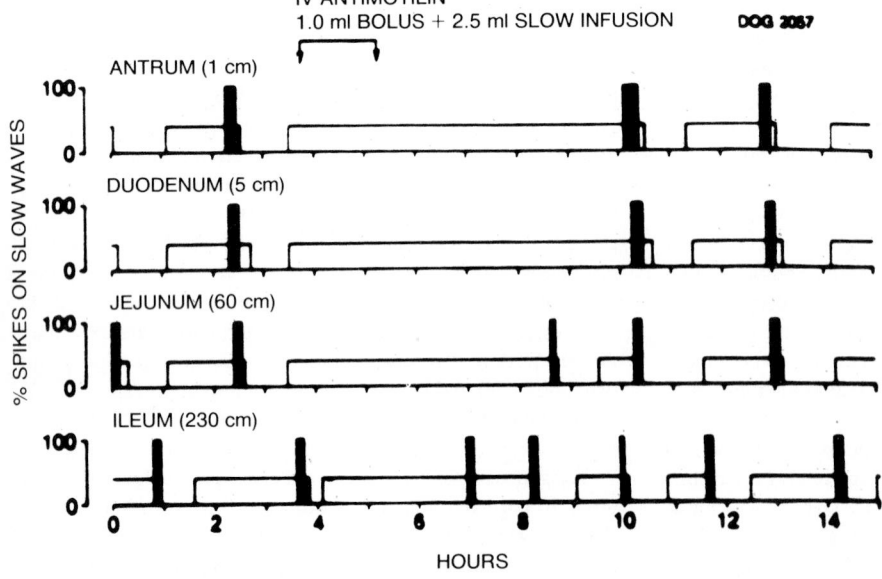

FIGURE 9-9. Effects of rabbit antimotilin serum on fasting motor activity in canine stomach and intestine. Antimotilin serum leads to prolonged disruption of phase III activity (*solid bars*) in the stomach and proximal intestine with only minimal effect on the ileum. (Lee KY, Chang T-M, Chey WY. Effect of rabbit antimotilin serum on myoelectric activity and plasma motilin concentration in fasting dog. Am J Physiol 1983;245:G547.)

These include cholinergic agonists such as urecholine and carbamylcholine. Similarly, morphine induces premature phase III activity followed by an increase in plasma motilin.[168] The investigation of physiologic stimuli that induce motilin release has often yielded inconsistent results. Motilin is released by duodenal alkalinization in dogs and duodenal acidification in humans.[166,178–180] Indeed, in healthy volunteers, intraduodenal perfusion of hydrochloric acid induces premature phase III activity.[181] Ingestion of a mixed meal suppresses plasma motilin, whereas ingestion of fat releases motilin.[153,179] In vitro and in vivo experiments have demonstrated release of motilin after exposure of duodenal mucosa to bile,[182] and diversion of bile from the intestine in the dog has been shown to delay spontaneous phase III activity. However, with bile discharge after a meal, motilin levels are suppressed.

Although motilin appears to be important in the initiation of intestinal fasting motor activity, it plays no significant role in the fed state. After ingestion of a meal, plasma levels of motilin fall to very low levels. If exogenous motilin is administered during the fed state, no phase III–like activity can be generated.[170] In the experiments of Lee and coworkers, the motility pattern seen after administration of motilin antisera resembled that seen during the fed state.[173] These results suggest that suppression of plasma motilin may be necessary for the fed state to occur.

THE ROLE OF SOMATOSTATIN AND PANCREATIC POLYPEPTIDE IN THE FASTING AND FED STATES IN THE SMALL INTESTINE

In addition to motilin, the only peptides known to cycle in phase with endogenous MMC activity are somatostatin and pancreatic polypeptide, both of which have been proposed as mediators of fasting motor activity.[102,183–185]

Somatostatin in the gastrointestinal tract is localized primarily to endocrine cells in the mucosa and to neurons in the enteric nervous system. Somatostatin exists in two molecular forms, of 14 and 28 amino acids, respectively. As stated above, some investigators have noted rises in plasma somatostatin levels in conjunction with duodenal phase III activity with the peaks occurring after peak plasma motilin levels. When given intravenously, somatostatin increases the frequency of intestinal phase III cycling to a maximum of one complex every 20 to 30 minutes (Fig 9-10).[183] This agrees with the clinical observation of accelerated MMC activity in patients with somatostatinomas who have been found to exhibit intestinal phase III cycling every 38 minutes.[186] However, these complexes are not physiologic in that they originate in the small intestine rather than in the lower esophageal sphincter or stomach. In fact, some studies have shown that spontaneous phase III activity as well as intravenous motilin-induced phase III cycling in the duodenum is inhibited by somatostatin.[174,187] Even as somatostatin accelerates MMC activity, it suppresses plasma motilin levels, verifying that motilin is not required for development of complexes in the more distal intestine.[168,174] Another important difference between somatostatin-induced and spontaneously occurring complexes is that the former consist only of alternating phase I and phase III activity and lack the long period of phase II activity seen with spontaneous patterns.[183] Whereas spontaneous and motilin-induced phase III activity results in acceleration of small intestinal transit, somatostatin infusion may delay transit as a result of its abilities to decrease the propagation velocity of intestinal contractions and to induce isolated or simultaneous contractions at multiple sites.[188] As with motilin, the proximal jejunum is more sensitive than the distal ileum to the effects of exogenous somatostatin.[189] These observations suggest that endogenous somatostatin is not the primary mediator of gastrointestinal MMC activity, although somatostatin-containing nerves within the enteric ganglia may function in the propagation of spontaneous phase III activity from the stomach into and down the small intestine.[183]

Somatostatin levels in the plasma rise significantly after a meal, especially one that is high in protein or fat.[190] In guinea pigs, increased intestinal intraluminal pressure is associated with release of somatostatin, suggesting that a bolus of chyme might have the same effect.[191] However, if somatostatin is infused during the fed state in low doses, there is a decrease in fed spike potential activity. At higher doses, some investigators have found that somatostatin inhibits the fed motor pattern and induces intermittent phase III activity similar to that seen after somatostatin infusion in the fasting

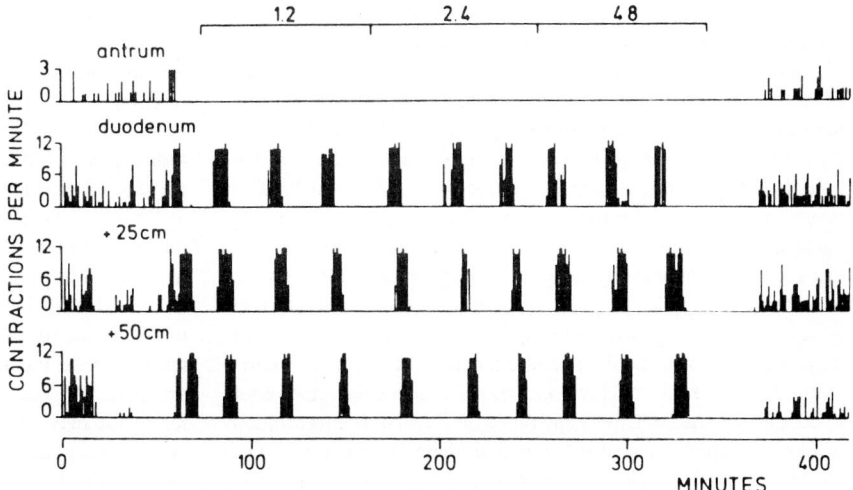

FIGURE 9–10. Effects of somatostatin infusion on fasting motor activity in human stomach and intestine. Somatostatin administration leads to suppression of gastric motor activity with development of alternating phase I and III activity in the small intestine with a period of 20 to 30 minutes. (Peeters TL, Janssens J, Vantrappen GR. Somatostatin and the interdigestive migrating motor complex in man. Regul Dept 1983;5: 209.)

state.[192] Although not all investigators have noted this phenomenon, somatostatin has been proposed as a possible contributor to the conversion of the fed pattern back to the MMC cycling seen during the interdigestive period.[174,187]

The circulating concentration of pancreatic polypeptide, a 36-amino acid peptide produced by the periduodenal pancreas, also fluctuates with intestinal MMC activity and peaks just before onset of phase III.[102] This peak in pancreatic polypeptide occurs earlier and decreases faster than the motilin peak.[102] After a meal, plasma pancreatic polypeptide increases fivefold.[193,194] The effects of exogenous pancreatic polypeptide on upper gut motility are not clear. Most investigators observe no effect on intestinal fasting motor activity when pancreatic polypeptide is infused to levels mimicking those seen in phase III.[193-195] At higher doses, which simulate those seen after a meal, exogenous pancreatic polypeptide can decrease[193] or inhibit[194,196] phase III cycling in the stomach and proximal intestine. One investigator has found an increase in spike potential activity similar to prolonged phase II cycling, which resembles but is not identical to the fed state.[193,194] This is associated with suppression of plasma motilin levels, suggesting that pancreatic polypeptide may act postprandially to regulate motilin levels in the plasma and thereby facilitate the initiation of the fed state.[194,196] Alternatively, pancreatic polypeptide may first inhibit upper gut phase III cycling and, thus, decrease release of motilin secondarily. The picture is clouded somewhat by studies showing that infusion of antisera to pancreatic polypeptide in the fed state has no effect on intestinal spike potential activity.[193]

THE ROLE OF OPIOID PEPTIDES IN THE FASTING AND FED STATES IN THE SMALL INTESTINE

Although they are not known to cycle in phase with MMC activity, the opioid peptides may play a pivotal role in the control of motor activity of the small intestine. Biosynthesis of enkephalins occurs in the myenteric plexus and α- and τ-endorphins have been identified in the small intestine as well.[197,198] Morphine is one of the substances known to induce premature phase III activity, although it acts only on the small intestine and not the stomach.[127,143,199] Morphine also stimulates phase III activity in the fed state.[199,200] Labyrinthine stimulation, which is known to induce phase III activity during the fed state, releases β-endorphin, suggesting a physiologic linkage between the two.[201,202] In contrast to the stimulatory effects of morphine, met-enkephalin can decrease spike potential amplitude in the fasting and fed states, suggesting that opioids with different receptor subtype specificities can have opposing effects.[143] One of the best known inhibitory effects of the opioids is the slowing of small intestinal transit,[203] most likely a result of an increased number of simultaneous, nonpropagating contractions.[40] The use of the opioid antagonist, naloxone, also has uncovered possible physiologic inhibitory and excitatory effects of endogenous opioids. In guinea pigs, intravenous administration of the opioid antagonist, naloxone, increases the frequency of peristaltic waves in the ileum and decreases the number of peristalsis-free intervals.[204] However, naloxone also delays the onset of duodenal phase III activity and raises the threshold concentration of motilin required to induce intestinal phase III cycling.[205] The above observations suggest that opioid peptides may be inter-

mediaries in the generation of intestinal phase III activity and may function in the recovery of phase III cycling after a meal.

THE ROLE OF MISCELLANEOUS MEDIATORS IN MOTOR ACTIVITY OF THE SMALL INTESTINE

There is a seemingly endless list of peptide and purported neurotransmitter mediators that have profound effects on small intestinal motility either in vivo or in vitro. A number of mediators, such as serotonin and cholecystokinin, have predominantly stimulatory effects,[34,206] while other mediators, such as secretin, GABA, and bombesin, have inhibitory effects.[206-208] Many compounds have both stimulatory and inhibitory effects depending on the experimental model employed, including gastrin, dopamine, peptide YY, bradykinin, and galanin.[209-215] The physiologic function of many of these mediators in the control of small intestinal motor activity has yet to be determined.

SPECIALIZED MOTOR PATTERNS IN THE SMALL INTESTINE

In addition to the fasting and fed motor patterns described above, there are a number of specialized motor patterns that are quite rare under normal physiologic circumstances but are more common in certain pathologic states. These contractile patterns involve disruption of the normal spike potential pattern or even disruption or abolition of intestinal slow wave activity and are, for the most part, intensely propulsive.

Giant Migrating Contractions

The presence of large individual contractile waves that propagate aborally down long segments of small intestine was noted by Bokai in experimental animals during hypoxia, anemia, gangrene, or immediately after death.[71] Similar activity was observed by Alvarez and Mahoney in the small intestine of animals after laparotomy in the absence of other intervention.[216] This activity was first termed *peristaltic rush* and has since been given many names, including prolonged propagated contractions, migrating action potential complexes, power contractions, and giant migrating contractions (GMC). In general, GMCs are two to three times greater in amplitude and four to five times longer in duration than individual phasic contractions in the intestine (Fig 9-11).[217] Each individual GMC may involve 20 to 30 cm of intestine and propagate at 1 cm/s.[218] GMCs generally begin in the mid-intestine or ileum during fasting and extend through to the ileocecal junction,[217,219] in contrast to phase III activity, which often does not propagate into the ileum. GMCs have been shown to be intensely propulsive of ileal contents and have been postulated as a physiologic mechanism to clean the ileum or to prevent colo-ileal reflux.[217,219] GMCs are quite rare, occurring at a frequency of only 0.03 times per hour, but they can be induced by noxious stimuli such as intravenous morphine, intragastric vinegar, ileal luminal perfusion of feces or short chain fatty acids, ionizing radiation, and infection

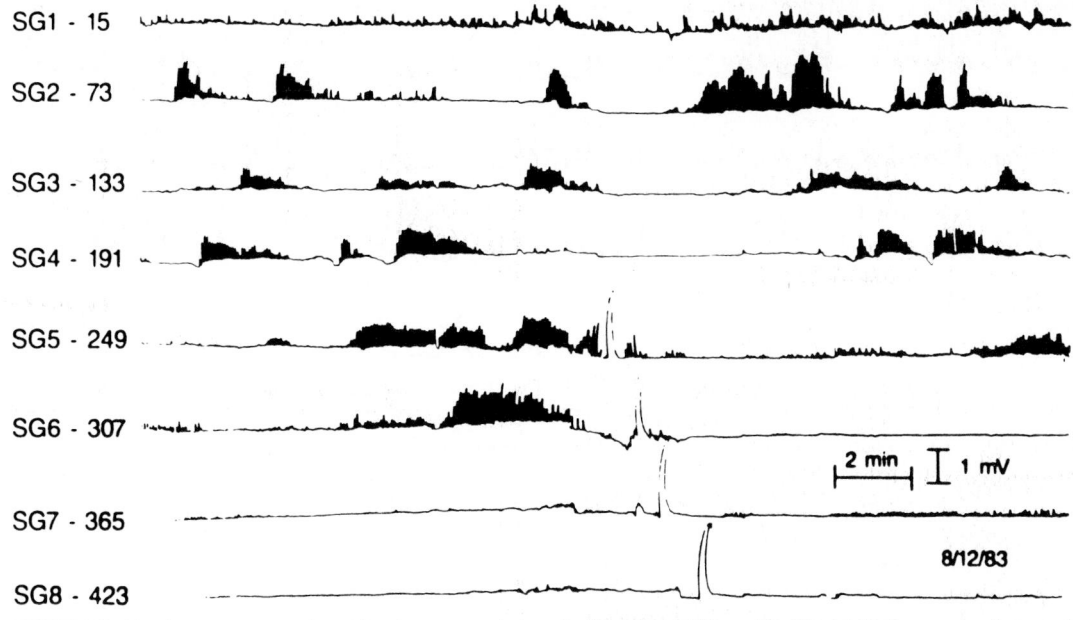

SG1 - 15

SG2 - 73

SG3 - 133

SG4 - 191

SG5 - 249

SG6 - 307

SG7 - 365

SG8 - 423

2 min   1 mV

8/12/83

FIGURE 9–11.   A spontaneous giant migrating contraction (GMC) originating in the middle of the canine small intestine. Recordings are from strain gauges from 15 to 423 cm distal to the pylorus. (Sarna SK. Giant migrating contractions and their myoelectric correlates in the small intestine. Am J Physiol 1987;253:G697.)

with *Vibrio cholerae, Clostridium perfringens, Clostridium difficile,* noninvasive *Escherichia coli, Shigella,* and *Trichinella spiralis.*[218,220] These observations suggest that GMCs are most commonly a response to pathologic conditions. The duration of a given GMC is generally longer than the duration of a single slow wave, suggesting a temporary dissociation from the normal slow wave regulation of phasic contractile activity.[217] In fact, myoelectric recordings reveal an intense burst of spike potential activity lasting 4 to 16 seconds, which obscures the slow wave.[218]

Other Aborally Migrating Specialized Contractile Patterns

In addition to the GMC, intense single contractile waves, which have been termed *individual migrating contractions,* may be seen during the fed period.[31] These complexes have amplitudes twice those of normal fed phasic contractions and have a duration of roughly two slow wave cycles. An extremely propagative pattern called the rapidly migrating contraction, which can migrate over a distance of 200 cm at a speed of greater than 30 cm/s also has been described.[221] In contrast to GMCs, these rapidly migrating contractions occur predominantly in the proximal small intestine and are associated with disruption or even abolition of the intestinal slow wave activity.[221] Sarna and Otterson have termed the disruption of slow wave activity *dysmyogenesia* and the absence of slow wave activity *amyogenesia.*

Intensely propagative contractions also occur in clusters. These have been termed *minute rhythm, migrating clustered contractions,* or *discrete clustered contractions (DCC).*[217,222] DCCs may occur in the fasted and fed states and consist of 3 to 10 contractions preceded and followed by 1 minute of motor quiescence. DCCs occur 5 to 10 times per hour and migrate at 5 to 10 cm/min.[219,222] They are effective at propulsion over distances of 2 to 40 cm and have been proposed along with GMCs as a physiologic mechanism to empty the terminal ileum.[217] DCCs also may be seen with increased frequency in irritable bowel syndrome or partial small bowel obstruction (Fig 9-12).[223]

Retrograde Peristaltic Contractions

The presence of orally migrating contractile patterns has been known for many decades. Alvarez observed retrograde propulsive activity in the intestine before vomiting.[224] Stewart observed, after the administration of emetic agents to cats, the occurrence of intense spike potential activity in the mid to distal small intestine, which migrates orally and reaches the duodenum immediately before the onset of vomiting.[225] Lang termed this phenomenon the *retrograde peristaltic contraction (RPC)* and noted an associated period of motor inhibition immediately before and after the RPC, which was followed by a series of phasic contractions and a subsequent motor inhibitory period (Fig 9-13).[226] The entire phenomenon could be abolished by prior vagotomy, but only the RPC itself could be prevented by atropine administration. In general, RPCs are associated with retching or vomiting but can occur in the absence of these somatomotor phenomena. Conversely, retching and vomiting can occur in the absence of RPC. It is likely the RPCs serve to empty the intestinal contents into the stomach so that they may be expelled during the act of vomiting. RPCs exhibit contractile amplitudes 1.3 to 1.8 times greater than normal phasic intestinal contractions and have durations two to four times longer. As with the aborally propagating, rapidly migrating contractions described above, RPCs migrate very rapidly, often up to 8 to 10 cm/s over distances in excess of 100 cm.[88] RPCs also are preceded by obliteration of intestinal slow wave activity before a burst of electrical activity, which migrates orally.[227]

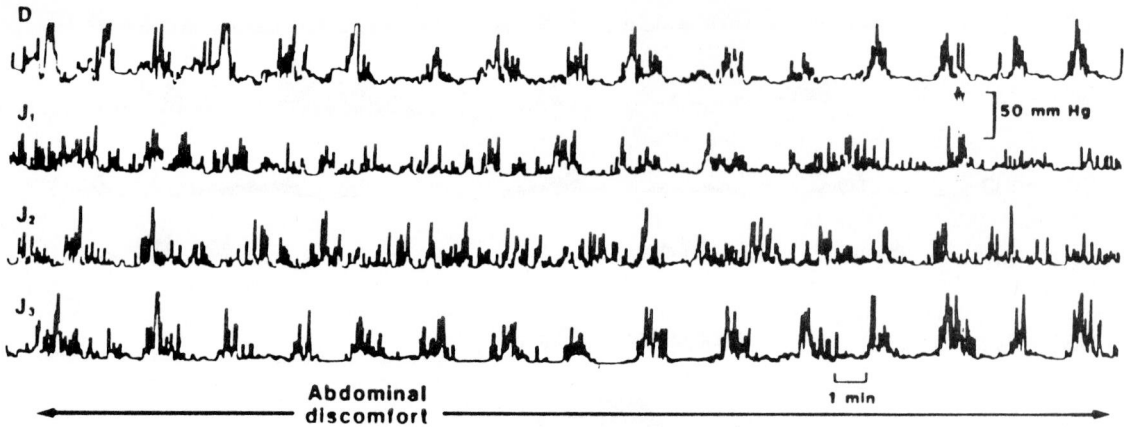

FIGURE 9–12. Discrete clustered contractions (DCC) occurring in the duodenum and jejunum of a human volunteer with a diagnosis of irritable bowel syndrome. In this instance, the DCCs were associated with the development of abdominal discomfort. (Kellow JE, Phillips SF. Altered small bowel motility in irritable bowel syndrome is correlated with symptoms. Gastroenterology 1987;92:1885.)

THE ILEOCECAL JUNCTION

At the terminus of the distal ileum is a structure known as the ileocecal junction (ICJ). This region of specialized smooth muscle and neural tissue has been postulated to control delivery of chyme from the terminal ileum into the cecum as well as to safeguard against reflux of fecal matter back into the ileum. The ICJ shares a number of properties with other sphincteric regions. Discrete thickening of the circular smooth muscle layer in the ICJ has been demonstrated in many species. The resting membrane potential of ICJ circular muscle is less negative (−43 mV) than that of the adjacent ileal circular smooth muscle (−62 mV).[228] Circular muscle

strips from the ICJ exhibit isometric tone that cannot be abolished by administration of neural toxins, indicating that increased tone is a myogenic property of ICJ.[229,230] The in vivo correlate is that, in many species, the ICJ represents a localized zone of high resting pressure. In the dog, manometric recordings show a resting pressure of 30 to 40 cm H_2O with phasic contractions that can exceed 100 cm H_2O.[231-233] This high-pressure zone spans a length of 2 cm in the dog, whereas the anatomic thickening of the smooth muscle layer only spans 0.5 cm, suggesting that the functional ICJ encompasses a greater expanse of distal small intestine than the anatomic one. In the human ICJ, Cohen and coworkers have described a 4-cm-long high-pressure zone with a magnitude of 20.3 mmHg.[234] Phasic contractions also have been noted in human ICJ. Intestinal slow wave activity migrates from the ileum into the ICJ in the cat and dog.[232,235] Similarly, in cats, spike potential activity migrates from the ileum across the ICJ into the colon. It is believed that the ICJ actively participates in over one half of the spontaneous migrating motor complexes in the dog,[232] although, in humans, the ICJ participates in very few MMC cycles.[236] High-amplitude, specialized, propulsive waves including the GMC and DCC activity pass from the ileum across the ICJ into the colon.[100,236] These are associated with bursts of spike potential activity in the ICJ smooth muscle.[100,236]

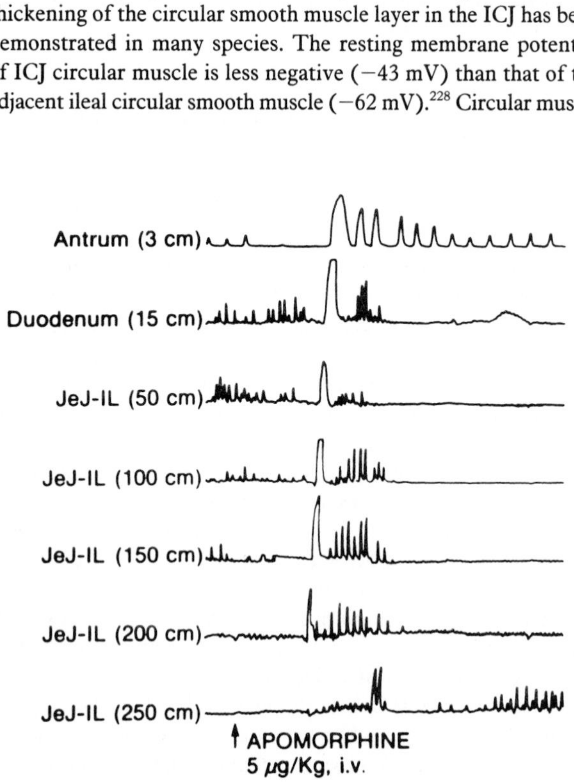

The ICJ is innervated intrinsically by the myenteric plexus and extrinsically by the vagus and superior and inferior mesenteric ganglia.[237,238] The extrinsic innervation is not responsible for resting tone in the ICJ because section of the vagus and splanchnic nerves has no effect.[238,239] Vagal innervation to the ICJ is associated with both stimulatory and inhibitory fibers because electrical stimulation can induce relaxation, contraction, or both.[240-242] Stimulation of the splanchnic nerves results in contraction of the ICJ, an effect that can be inhibited by α-adrenoceptor antagonists.[238-241,243] The intrinsic innervation of the ICJ is predominantly inhibitory. Electrical stimulation of isolated ICJ circular muscle strips induces relaxation.[229] Furthermore, use of the neural toxin, tetrodotoxin, increases the resting tension in the ICJ.[229] A structural correlate of these physiologic findings is that VIP-containing nerves are present in higher density in this region relative to the surrounding ileum.[244]

FIGURE 9–13. Induction of a retrograde peristaltic contraction in canine intestine by apomorphine. (Lang IM, Sarna SK, Condon RE. Gastrointestinal motor correlates of vomiting in the dog: Quantification and characterization as an independent phenomenon. Gastroenterology 1986;90:40.)

The physiologic role of the ICJ in the regulation of caudad and cephalad flow is incompletely understood. By radionuclide scanning, flow across the canine ICJ is maximal immediately before phase III activity during fasting.[245] In humans, relatively little flow can be correlated directly to different phases of the MMC.[236] In the fed state in dogs, flow across the ICJ peaks about 4 hours after a meal. It appears that motor activity of the ICJ increases after ingestion of a meal and, thus, participates in the gastroileal reflex.[232,246] The ability of the ICJ to act as a barrier has been shown by a number of investigators. Cannon noted significant resistance when attempting to reflux material from the colon cephalad into the ileum.[71] Studies in dog and human ICJ have demonstrated that colonic distention results in reflex contraction of the ICJ.[234,240,247,248] This response is not blocked by section of either vagal or pelvic nerves. In contrast, section of the splanchnic nerves blocks the reflex contraction, indicating the importance of the extrinsic sympathetic innervation in this reflex.[248] In addition to the smooth muscle and neural properties of the ICJ involved in this response, it is likely that the structure of the ICJ also plays an important role. The ICJ is maintained at a constant acute angulation at the point of insertion into the cecum by fibrous connections. If this fibrous tissue is severed such that this acute angulation is lost, the ICJ becomes incompetent to colonic distention and coloileal reflux results.[249] The role of the ICJ as a barrier to aboral flow from the intestine into the colon is far less clear. Early studies by Grutzner showed that the ICJ was incompetent to ileal flow of liquids.[71] Recent studies show reflex relaxation of the ICJ in response to distention of the terminal ileum in some studies and a reflex contraction in others.[240,247]

In humans and experimental animals, surgical excision of the ICJ results in increased bacterial counts in the ileum, suggesting that the ICJ serves as a barrier to coloileal reflux to maintain relative sterility in the ileum.[250] However, transit in the small intestine in vivo is minimally affected by excision of the ICJ, indicating that it is not a significant barrier to aboral flow.[251] However, if a long segment of small intestine is removed, excision of the ICJ results in marked acceleration of transit. Under conditions of high flow, the ICJ can serve as a barrier to aboral propagation.

A number of peptide mediators have been demonstrated to exert significant effects on the ICJ. Leucine enkephalin contracts the ICJ by way of direct actions on smooth muscle as well as by actions on intrinsic nerves in the ICJ.[252] Other opioid peptides contract the ICJ by way of direct myogenic actions as well as stimulation of intrinsic cholinergic nerves.[252] Substance P contracts the ICJ, whereas serotonin has a biphasic effect.[253,244] Neurotensin contracts cat ICJ by way of actions on adrenergic nerves.[255] Although these effects are potent, their physiologic significance is unknown.

The reader is directed to Chapter 1, The Enteric Nervous System and its Extrinsic Connections; Chapter 2, Gastrointestinal Hormones; Chapter 3, The Brain–Gut Axis; Chapter 4, Smooth Muscle of the Gut; Chapter 8, The Physiology of Gastric Motility and Gastric Emptying; Chapter 66, Small Intestine: Anatomy and Structural Anomalies; Chapter 67, Dysmotility of the Small Intestine; and Chapter 128, Evaluation of Gastrointestinal Motility: Methodological Considerations.

REFERENCES

1. Casteels R. Membrane potential in smooth muscle cells. In: Bulbring E, Brading AF, Jones AF, Tomita T, eds. Smooth muscle: An assessment of current knowledge. Austin: University of Texas Press, 1981:105.
2. Alvarez WC, Mahoney LJ. Action currents in stomach and intestine. Am J Physiol 1922;58:476.
3. Wood JD. Excitation of intestinal muscle by atropine, tetrodotoxin, and Xylocaine. Am J Physiol 1972;222:118.
4. Sarna SK. In vivo myoelectric activity: Methods, analysis and interpretation. In Wood JD, ed. Handbook of physiology, Section 6: The gastrointestinal system, Vol 1: Motility and circulation. Baltimore: American Physiological Society, Waverly Press, 1989:817.
5. Milton GW, Smith AWM. The pacemaking area of the duodenum. J Physiol 1956;132:100.
6. Daniel EE. The electrical activity of the alimentary tract. Am J Dig Dis 1968;13:297.
7. Connor JA, Kreulen D, Prosser CL, Weigel R. Interaction between longitudinal and circular muscle in intestine of cat. J Physiol 1977;273:665.
8. Kobayashi M, Nagai T, Prosser CL. Electrical interaction between muscle layers of cat intestine. Am J Physiol 1966;211:1281.
9. Bortoff A, Sachs F. Electrotonic spread of slow waves in circular muscle of small intestine. Am J Physiol 1970;218:576.
10. Connor J, Prosser CL, Weems WA. A study of pace-maker activity in intestinal smooth muscle. J Physiol 1974;240:671.
11. Kobayashi M, Prosser CL, Nagai T. Electrical properties of intestinal muscle as measured intracellularly and extracellularly. Am J Physiol 1967;213:275.
12. Bortoff A. Electrical transmission of slow waves from longitudinal to circular muscle. Am J Physiol 1965;209:1254.
13. Cheung DW, Daniel EE. Comparative study of the smooth muscle layers of the rabbit duodenum. J Physiol 1980;309:13.
14. Hara Y, Kubota M, Szurszewski JH. Electrophysiology of smooth muscle of the small intestine of some mammals. J Physiol 1986;372:501.
15. Thuneberg L. Interstitial cells of Cajal. In Wood JD, ed. Handbook of physiology, Section 6: The gastrointestinal system, Vol 1: Motility and circulation. Baltimore: American Physiological Society, Waverly Press, 1989:349.
16. Komuro T. Three-dimensional observation of the fibroblast-like cells associated with the rat myenteric plexus, with special reference to the interstitial cells of Cajal. Cell Tissue Res 1989;255:343.
17. Berezin I, Huizinga JD, Daniel EE. Interstitial cells of Cajal in the canine colon: A special communication network at the inner border of the circular muscle. J Comp Neurol 1988;273:42.
18. Prosser CL, Holzwarth MA, Barr L. Immunocytochemistry of the interstitial cells of Cajal in the rat intestine. J Auton Nerv Syst 1989;27:17.
19. Suzuki N, Ladd Prosser C, Dahms V. Boundary cells between longitudinal and circular layers: Essential for electrical slow waves in cat intestine. Am J Physiol 1986;250:G287.
20. Barajas-Lopez C, Berezin I, Daniel EE, Huizinga JD. Pacemaker activity recorded in interstitial cells of Cajal of the gastrointestinal tract. Am J Physiol 1989;257:C830.
21. Connor JA, Mangel AW, Nelson B. Propagation and entrainment of slow waves in cat small intestine. Am J Physiol 1979;237:C237.
22. Bortoff A. Slow potential variations of small intestine. Am J Physiol 1961;201:203.
23. Daniel EE, Honour AJ, Bogoch A. Electrical activity of the longitudinal muscle of dog small intestine studied in vivo using microelectrodes. Am J Physiol 1960;198:113.
24. Tamai T, Prosser CL. Differentiation of slow potentials and spikes in longitudinal muscle of cat intestine. Am J Physiol 1966;210:452.
25. Liu J, Prosser CL, Job DD. Ionic dependence of slow waves and spikes in intestinal muscle. Am J Physiol 1969;217:1542.
26. Job DD. Ionic basis of intestinal electrical activity. Am J Physiol 1969;217:1534.
27. Langton P, Ward SM, Carl A, Norell MA, Sanders KM. Spontaneous electrical activity of interstitial cells of Cajal isolated from canine proximal colon. Proc Natl Acad Sci 1989;86:7280.

28. Dewey MM, Barr L. Structure of vertebrate intestinal smooth muscle. In Code CF, ed. Handbook of physiology, Section 6, Alimentary canal, Vol 4, Motility. Baltimore: American Physiological Society, Waverly Press, 1968:1629.

29. Taylor AB, Kruelen D, Prosser CL. Electron microscopy of the connective tissues between longitudinal and circular muscle of the small intestine of cat. Am J Anat 1977;150:427.

30. Diamant NE, Bortoff A. Nature of the intestinal slow-wave frequency gradient. Am J Physiol 1969;216:301.

31. Sarna SK, Soergel KH, Harig JM et al. Spatial and temporal patterns of human jejunal contractions. Am J Physiol 1989;257:G423.

32. Sarna SK, Otterson MF. Small intestinal physiology and pathophysiology. Gastroenterol Clin North Am 1989;18:375.

33. Grivel M-L, Ruckebusch Y. The propagation of segmental contractions along the small intestine. J Physiol 1972;227:611.

34. Bueno L, Fioramonti J, Ruckebusch Y. Rate of flow of digesta and electrical activity of the small intestine in dogs and sheep. J Physiol 1975;249:69.

35. Daniel EE, Duchon G, Henderson RM. The ultrastructural basis for coordination of intestinal motility. Am J Dig Dis 1972;17:289.

36. Job DD, Griffing WJ, Rodda BE. A possible origin of intestinal gradients and their relation to motility. Am J Physiol 1974;226:1510.

37. Code CF, Rogers AG, Schlegel J, Hightower NC, Bargen JA. Motility patterns in the terminal ileum: Studies on two patients with ulcerative colitis and ileac stomas. Gastroenterology 1957;32:651.

38. Foulk WT, Code CF, Mrolock CG, Barzon JA. A study of the motility patterns and the basic rhythm in the duodenum and upper part of the jejunum of human beings. Gastroenterology 1954;26:601.

39. Severi C, Grider JR, Makhlouf GM. Dual action of cyclic AMP-dependent relaxants: Decrease in cytosolic Ca^{++} and in Ca^{++}-induced contraction. Gastroenterology 1987;92:1634.

40. Wood JD. Intrinsic neural control of intestinal motility. Annu Rev Physiol 1981;43:33.

41. Bayliss WM, Starling EH. The movements and innervation of the small intestine. J Physiol 1899;24:99.

42. Macagno E, Melville J, Christensen J. A model for longitudinal motility of the small intestine. Biorheology 1975;12:369.

43. Cannon WB. The mechanical factors of digestion. London: Arnold Press, 1911:135.

44. Bass P, Wiley JN. Electrical and extraluminal contractile-force activity of the duodenum of the dog. Am J Dig Dis 1965;10:183.

45. Trendelenburg P. Physiologische und pharmakologische Versuche uber die Dunndarmiperistaltik. Arch Exp Pathol Pharmakol 1917;81:55.

46. Tasaka K, Farrar JT. Mechanics of small intestinal muscle function in the dog. Am J Physiol 1969;217:1224.

47. Wood JD, Perkins WE. Mechanical interaction between longitudinal and circular axes of the small intestine. Am J Physiol 1970;218:762.

48. Yokoyama S, North RA. Electrical activity of longitudinal and circular muscle during peristalsis. Am J Physiol 1983;244:G83.

49. Furness JB, Costa M. Types of nerves in the enteric nervous system. Neuroscience 1980;5:1.

50. Bennett A, Stockley HL. The intrinsic innervation of the human alimentary tract and its relation to function. Gut 1975;16:443.

51. Furness JB, Costa M. The enteric nervous system: An overview. In Chey WY, ed. Functional disorders of the digestive tract. New York: Raven Press, 1983:47.

52. Martin JS, Innes DL, Tansy MF. A demonstration of vagal adrenergic vascular and motor influences in the small intestine of the dog. Surg Gynecol Obstet 1974;138:6.

53. Furness JB, Costa M. The adrenergic innervation of the gastrointestinal tract. Ergeb Physiol 1979;69:1.

54. Szurszewski JH, King BF. Physiology of prevertebral ganglia in mammals with special reference to inferior mesenteric ganglion. In Wood JD, ed. Handbook of physiology, Section 6: The gastrointestinal system, Vol 1: Motility and circulation. Baltimore: American Physiological Society, Waverly Press, 1989:519.

55. Ruwart MJ, Klepper MS, Rush BD. Clonidine delays small intestinal transit in the rat. J Pharmacol Exp Ther 1980;212:487.

56. Hokfelt T, Elfvin L-G, Elde R, Schultzberg M, Goldstein M, Luft R. Occurrence of somatostatin-like immunoreactivity in some peripheral noradrenergic neurons. Proc Natl Acad Sci 1977;74:3587.

57. Hokfelt T, Elfvin L-G, Schultzberg M, Goldstein M, Nilsson G. On the occurrence of substance P-containing fibers in sympathetic ganglia: Immunohistological evidence. Brain Res 1977;132:29.

58. Larsson L-I, Rehfeld J. Localization and molecular heterogeneity of cholecystokinin in the central and peripheral nervous system. Brain Res 1979;165:201.

59. Hokfelt T, Elfvin L-G, Schultzberg M. Immunohistochemical evidence of vasoactive intestinal polypeptide-containing neurons and nerve fibers in sympathetic ganglia. Neuroscience 1977;2:885.

60. Schultzberg M, Hokfelt T, Terenius L, et al. Enkephalin immunoreactive nerve fibers and cell bodies in sympathetic ganglia of the guinea-pig and rat. Neuroscience 1979;4:249.

61. Grundy D, Scratcherd T. Sensory afferents from the gastrointestinal tract. In Wood JD, ed. Handbook of physiology, Section 6: The gastrointestinal system, Vol 1: Motility and circulation. Baltimore: American Physiological Society, Waverly Press, 1989:593.

62. Leaming DB, Cauna N. A qualitative and quantitative study of the myenteric plexus of the small intestine of the cat. J Anat 1961;95:160.

63. Frantzides CT, Sarna SK, Matsumoto T, Lang IM, Condon RE. An intrinsic neural pathway for long intestino-intestinal inhibitory reflexes. Gastroenterology 1987;92:594.

64. Furness JB, Costa M. Identification of transmitters of functionally defined enteric neurons. In Wood JD, ed. Handbook of physiology, Section 6: The gastrointestinal system, Vol 1: Motility and circulation. Baltimore: American Physiological Society, Waverly Press, 1989:387.

65. Kirchgessner AL, Gershon MD. Projections of submucosal neurons to the myenteric plexus of the guinea pig intestine: In vitro tracing of microcircuits by retrograde and antegrade transport. J Comp Neurol 1988;277:487.

66. Llewellyn-Smith IJ, Furness JB, Gibbins IL, Costa M. Quantitative ultrastructural analysis of enkephalin-, substance P-, and VIP-immunoreactive nerve fibers in the circular muscle of the guinea pig small intestine. J Comp Neurol 1988;272:139.

67. Nowak TV, Harrington B. Evidence for diminished neuromuscular transmission in distal small intestine. J Pharmacol Exp Ther 1987;240:381.

68. Grider JR, Makhlouf GM. Prejunctional inhibition of vasoactive intestinal peptide release. Am J Physiol 1987;253:G7.

69. Biancani P, Walsh JH, Behar J. Vasoactive intestinal peptide. A neurotransmitter for lower esophageal sphincter relaxation. J Clin Invest 1984;73:963.

70. Wiley JW, O'Dorisio TM, Owyang C. Vasoactive intestinal peptide mediated CCK-induced relaxation of sphincter of Oddi. J Clin Invest 1988;81:1920.

71. Cannon WB. The movements of the intestines studied by means of the rontgen rays. Am J Physiol 1902;6:251.

72. Fiorenza V, Yee YS, Zfass AM. Small intestinal motility: Normal and abnormal function. Am J Gastroenterol 1987;82:1111.

73. Hirst GDS, Holman ME, McKirdy HC. Two descending nerve pathways activated by distension of guinea pig small intestine. J Physiol 1975;244:113.

74. Hirst GDS, McKirdy HC. A nervous mechanism for descending inhibition in guinea-pig small intestine. J Physiol 1974;238:129.

75. Yokoyama S, Ozaki T. Polarity of effects of stimulation of Auerbach's plexus on longitudinal muscle. Am J Physiol 1978;235:E345.

76. Kosterlitz HW, Robinson JA. Inhibition of the peristaltic reflex of the isolated guinea-pig ileum. J Physiol 1957;136:249.

77. Kosterlitz HW, Robinson JA. Reflex contractions of the longitudinal muscle coat of the isolated guinea-pig ileum. J Physiol 1959;146:369.

78. Ginzel KH. Investigations concerning the initiation of the peristaltic reflex in the guinea-pig ileum. J Physiol 1979;148:75P.

79. Costa M, Furness JB, Pullin CO, Bornstein J. Substance P enteric neurons mediate non-cholinergic transmission to the circular muscle of the guinea pig intestine. Naunyn Schmiedebergs Arch Pharmacol 1985;328:446.

80. Grider JR. Identification of neurotransmitters regulating intestinal peristaltic reflex in humans. Gastroenterology 1989;97:1414.

81. Grider JR. Tachykinins as transmitters of ascending contractile component of the peristaltic reflex. Am J Physiol 1989;257:G709.

82. Bulbring E, Crema A. The release of 5-hydroxytryptamine in relation to pressure exerted on the intestinal mucosa. J Physiol 1959;146:18.

83. Van Braam Houckgeest, JP. Untersuchungen uber Peristaltik des Magens und Darmkanals. Pflueger Arch Ges Physiol 6: 266, 1872.

84. Hukuhara TS, Nakayama S, Nanba R. Locality of receptors concerned with the intestino-intestinal extrinsic and intestinal muscular intrinsic reflexes. Jpn J Physiol 1960;10:414.

85. Da Cunha Melo J, Summers RW, Thompson HH, Wingate DL, Yanda R. Effects of intestinal secretagogues and distension on small bowel myoelectric activity in fasted and fed conscious dogs. J Physiol 1981;321:483.

86. Youmans WB. Innervation of the gastrointestinal tract. In Code CF, ed. Handbook of physiology, Section 6: Alimentary canal, Vol 4: Motility. Baltimore: American Physiological Society, Waverly Press, 1968:1655.

87. Douglas DM, Mann FC. The gastroileac reflex: Further experimental observations. Am J Dig Dis 1940;7:53.

88. Kerlin P, Zinsmeister A, Phillips S. Relationship of motility to flow of contents in the human small intestine. Gastroenterology 1982;82:701.

89. Kerlin P, Zinsmeister AR, Phillips SF. Motor responses to food of the ileum, proximal colon, and distal colon of healthy humans. Gastroenterology 1983;84:762.

90. Youle MS, Read NW. Effect of painless rectal distension on gastrointestinal transit of solid meal. Dig Dis Sci 1984;29:902.

91. Read NW, McFarlane A, Kinsman RI, et al. Effect of infusion of nutrient solutions into the ileum on gastrointestinal transit and plasma levels of neurotensin and enteroglucagon. Gastroenterology 1984;86:274.

92. Kinsman RI, Read NW. Effect of naloxone on feedback regulation of small bowel transit by fat. Gastroenterology 1984;87:335.

93. Legros C, Onimus E. Recherches experimentales sur les mouvements de l'intestin. J de l'Anat et Physiol 1869;6:37.

94. Boldyreff W. Einige neue Seiten der Tatigkeit des Pancreas. Ergeb Physiol 1911;11:121.

95. Szurszewski JH. A migrating electric complex of the canine small intestine. Am J Physiol 1969;217:1757.

96. Carlson GM, Bedi BS, Code CF. Mechanism of propagation of intestinal interdigestive myoelectric complex. Am J Physiol 1972;222:1027.

97. Code CF, Marlett JA. The interdigestive myoelectric complex of the stomach and small bowel of dogs. J Physiol 1975;246:289.

98. Rees WDW, Malagelada J-R, Miller LJ, Go VLW. Human interdigestive and postprandial gastrointestinal motor and gastrointestinal hormone patterns. Dig Dis Sci 1982;27:321.

99. Sarna SK. Cyclic motor activity: Migrating motor complex, 1985. Gastroenterology 1985;89:894.

100. Kellow JE, Borody TJ, Phillips SF, Tucker RL, Haddad AC. Human interdigestive motility: Variations in patterns from esophagus to colon. Gastroenterology 1986;91:386.

101. Kumar D, Wingate D, Ruckebusch Y. Circadian variation in the propagation velocity of the migrating motor complex. Gastroenterology 1986;91:926.

102. Keane FB, DiMagno EP, Dozois RR, Go VLW. Relationships among canine interdigestive exocrine pancreatic and biliary flow, duodenal motor activity, plasma pancreatic polypeptide, and motilin. Gastroenterology 1980;78:310.

103. McCoy EJ, Baker RD. Effect of feeding on electrical activity of dog's small intestine. Am J Physiol 1968;214:1291.

104. Reinke DA, Rosenbaum AH, Bennett DR. Patterns of dog gastrointestinal contractile activity monitored in vivo with extraluminal force transducers. Am J Dig Dis 1967;12:113.

105. Christensen J, Glover JR, Macagno EO, Singerman RB, Weisbrodt NW. Statistics of contractions at a point in the human duodenum. Am J Physiol 1971;221:1818.

106. Dusdieker NS, Summers RW. Patterns of smooth muscle contractions in the jejunum. Gastroenterology 1979;76:1126.

107. De Wever I, Eeckhout C, Vantrappen G, Hellemans J. Disruptive effect of test meals on interdigestive motor complex in dogs. Am J Physiol 1978;235:E661.

108. Bueno L, Rayner V, Ruckebusch Y. Initiation of the migrating myoelectric complex in dogs. J Physiol 1981;316:309.

109. Pressman JH, Hofmann AF, Witztum KF, et al. Limitations of indirect methods of estimating small bowel transit in man. Dig Dis Sci 1987;32:689.

110. Caride VJ, Prokop EK, Troncale FJ, Buddoura W, Winchenbach K, McCallum RW. Scintigraphic determination of small intestinal transit time: Comparison with the hydrogen breath technique. Gastroenterology 1984;86:714.

111. Lundqvist H, Jung B, Gustavsson S, Nilsson F, Lundqvist G. Analyses of small bowel propulsion, ileo-caecal passage and serum gastrin after truncal vagotomy. A methodological study in the rat with continuous intraduodenal infusion. Acta Chir Scand 1975;141:298.

112. Malagelada JR, Robertson JS, Brown ML, et al. Intestinal transit of solid and liquid components of a meal in health. Gastroenterology 1984;87:1255.

113. Code CF, Schlegel JF. The gastrointestinal housekeeper. In Daniel EE, ed. Gastrointestinal motility. Vancouver, BC: Mitchell Press, 1974:631.

114. Stevenson GW, Collins SM, Somers S. Radiological appearance of migrating motor complex of the small intestine. Gastrointest Radiol 1988;13:215.

115. Marik F, Code CF. Control of the interdigestive myoelectric activity in dogs by the vagus nerves and pentagastrin. Gastroenterology 1975;69:387.

116. Weisbrodt NW, Copeland EM, Moore EP, Kearley RW, Johnson LR. Effect of vagotomy on electrical activity of the small intestine of the dog. Am J Physiol 1975;228:650.

117. Marlett JA, Code CF. Effects of celiac and superior mesenteric ganglionectomy on interdigestive myoelectric complex in dogs. Am J Physiol 1979;237:E432.

118. Hashmonai M, Go VLW, Szurszewski JH. Effect of total sympathectomy and of decentralization on migrating complexes in dogs. Gastroenterology 1987;92:978.

119. Sarr MG, Kelly KA. Myoelectric activity of the autotransplanted canine jejunoileum. Gastroenterology 1981;81:303.

120. Heppell J, Kelly KA, Sarr MG. Neural control of canine small intestinal interdigestive myoelectric complexes. Am J Physiol 1983;244:G95.

121. Fealey RD, Szurszewski JH, Merritt JL, DiMagno EP. Effect of traumatic spinal cord transection on human upper gastrointestinal motility and gastric emptying. Gastroenterology 1984;87:69.

122. Diamant NE, Meri H, El-Sharkawy TY, Hall K. The vagus controls lower esophageal sphincter and gastric components of the migrating complex in the dog. Gastroenterology 1979;76:1122.

123. Chung SA, Diamant NE. Small intestinal motility in fasted and postprandial states: Effect of transient vagosympathetic blockade. Am J Physiol 1987;252:G301.

124. Hall KE, El-Sharkawy TY, Diamant NE. Vagal control of the migrating motor complex in the dog. Am J Physiol 1982;243:G276.

125. McRae S, Younger K, Thompson DG, Wingate DL. Sustained mental stress alters human jejunal motor activity. Gut 1982;23:404.

126. Valori RM, Kumar D, Wingate DL. Effects of different types of stress and of "prokinetic" drugs on the control of the fasting motor complex in humans. Gastroenterology 1986;90:1890.

127. Matsumoto T, Sarna SK, Condon RE, Cowles VE, Frantzides C. Differential sensitivities of morphine and motilin to initiate migrating motor complex in isolated intestinal segments. Regeneration of intrinsic nerves. Gastroenterology 1986;90:61.

128. Galligan JJ, Furness JB, Costa M. Migration of the myoelectric complex after interruption of the myenteric plexus: Intestinal transection and regeneration of enteric nerves in the guinea pig. Gastroenterology 1989;97:1135.

129. Fox DA, Bass P. Selective myenteric neuronal denervation of the rat jejunum. Differential control of the propagation of migrating myoelectric complex and basic electric rhythm. Gastroenterology 1984;87:572.

130. Ormsbee HS III, Telford GL, Mason GR. Required neural involvement in control of canine migrating motor complex. Am J Physiol 1979;237:E451.

131. Sarna S, Stoddard C, Belbeck L, McWade D. Intrinsic nervous control of migrating myoelectric complex. Am J Physiol 1981;241:G16.

132. Ruckebusch Y, Bueno L. Migrating myoelectrical complex of the small intestine. An intrinsic activity mediated by the vagus. Gastroenterology 1977;73:1309.

133. Hall KE, El-Sharkawy TY, Diamant NE. Vagal control of canine

postprandial upper gastrointestinal motility. Am J Physiol 1986;250:G501.

134. Schang JC, Angel F, Lambert A, Creener F, Aprahamian M, Grenier JF. Inhibition of canine duodenal interdigestive myoelectric complex by nutrient perfusion of jejunal and ileal Thiry-Vella loops. Gut 1981;22:738.

135. Steinbach JH, Code CF. Increase in the period of the interdigestive myoelectric complex with anticipation of feeding. In Christensen J, ed. Gastrointestinal motility. New York: Raven Press, 1980:247.

136. Fargeas MJ, Fioramonti J, Bueno L. Central muscarinic control of the pattern of small intestinal motility in rats. Life Sci 1987;40:1709.

137. Bueno L, Ferre JP, Fioramonti J, Honde C. Effects of intracerebroventricular administration of neurotensin, substance P and calcitonin on gastrointestinal motility in normal and vagotomized rats. Regul Pept 1983;6:197.

138. Fargeas MJ, Fioramonti J, Bueno L. Calcitonin gene-related peptide: Brain and spinal action on intestinal motility. Peptides 1985;6:1167.

139. Nitecki S, Szurszewski JH. The effect of central and peripheral administration of NPY on gastrointestinal myoelectrical activity in the dog. Gastroenterology 1988;94:A325.

140. Bueno L, Fioramonti J, Honde C, Fargeas MJ, Primi MP. Central and peripheral control of gastrointestinal and colonic motility by endogenous opiates in conscious dogs. Gastroenterology 1985;88:549.

141. Vantrappen G, Janssens J, Peeters TL, Bloom SR, Christofides ND, Hellemans J. Motilin and the interdigestive migrating motor complex in man. Dig Dis Sci 1979;24:497.

142. Itoh Z, Nakaya M, Suzuki T, Arai H, Wakabayashi K. Erythromycin mimics endogenous motilin in gastrointestinal contractile activity in the dog. Am J Physiol 1984;247:G688.

143. Konturek SJ, Thor P, Krol R, Dembinski A, Schally AV. Influence of methionine-enkephalin and morphine on myoelectric activity of small bowel. Am J Physiol 1980;238:G384.

144. Achem-Karem SR, Funakoshi A, Vinik AI, Owyang C. Dopaminergic regulation of the interdigestive migrating motor complex "independent" of motilin. Gastroenterology 1982;82:1005.

145. Ruckebusch Y, Bardon T. Involvement of serotonergic mechanisms in initiation of small intestine cyclic motor events. Dig Dis Sci 1984;29:520.

146. Ruckebusch Y. Enhancement of the cyclic motor activity of the ovine small intestine by lysergic acid derivatives. Mechanism and significance. Gastroenterology 1984;87:1049.

147. Weisbrodt NW, Copeland EM, Kearley RM, More EP, Johnson LR. Effect of pentagastrin on the electrical activity of the small intestine of the dog. Am J Physiol 1974;227:425.

148. Mukhopadhyay AK, Thor PJ, Copeland EM, Johnson LR, Weisbrodt NW. Effect of cholecystokinin on myoelectric activity of small bowel of the dog. Am J Physiol 1977;232:E44.

149. Bueno L, Ruckebusch M. Insulin and jejunal electrical activity in dogs and sheep. Am J Physiol 1976;230:1538.

150. Wingate DL, Pearce EA, Thomas PA, Boucher BJ. Glucagon stimulates intestinal myoelectric activity. Gastroenterology 1978;74:1152.

151. Al-Saffar A, Rosell S. Effects of neurotensin and neurotensin analogues on the migrating myoelectrical complexes in the small intestine of rats. Acta Physiol Scand 1981;112:203.

152. Konturek SH. Prostaglandins and gastrointestinal secretion and motility. Adv Exp Med Biol 1978;106:297.

153. Lee JY, Kim MS, Chey WY. Effects of a meal and gut hormones on plasma motilin and duodenal motility in dog. Am J Physiol 1980;238:G280.

154. Wingate DL, Pearce EA, Hutton M, Dand A, Thompson HH, Wunsch E. Quantitative comparison of the effects of cholecystokinin, secretin, and pentagastrin on gastrointestinal myoelectric activity in the conscious dog. Gut 1978;19:593.

155. Eeckhout C, De Wever I, Peeters T, Hellemans J, Vantrappen G. Role of gastrin and insulin in postprandial disruption of migrating complex in dogs. Am J Physiol 1978;235:E666.

156. Thor P, Konturek JW, Konturek SJ, Anderson JH. Role of prostaglandins in control of intestinal motility. Am J Physiol 1985;248:G353.

157. Heitz PU, Kasper M, Krey G, Polak JM, Pearse AGE. Immuno-

electron cytochemical localization of motilin in human duodenal enterochromaffin cells. Gastroenterology 1978;74:713.

158. Forssmann WG, Yanihara N, Helmstaedter V, Grube D. Differential demonstration of the motilin-cell and the enterochromaffin-cell. Scand J Gastroenterol 1976;11(Suppl 39):43.

159. Jacobowitz DM, O'Donohue TL, Chey WY, Chang TM. Mapping of motilin-immunoreactive neurons of the rat brain. Peptides 1981;2:479.

160. Nilaver G, Defendini R, Zimmerman EA, Beinfeld MC, O'Donohue TL. Motilin in the Purkinje cell of the cerebellum. Nature 1982;295:597.

161. Lee KY, Hyoung JP, Chang T-M, Chey WY. Cholinergic role on release and action of motilin. Peptides 1983;4:375.

162. Hall KE, Greenberg GR, El-Sharkawy TY, Diamant NE. Relationship between porcine motilin-induced migrating motor complex-like activity, vagal integrity, and endogenous motilin release in dogs. Gastroenterology 1984;87:76.

163. Lemoyne M, Wassef R, Tasse D, Trudel L, Poitras P. Motilin and the vagus in dogs. Can J Physiol Pharmacol 1984;62:1092.

164. You CH, Lee KY, Chey WY. Plasma motilin level and interdigestive motor complex in normal and abnormal states in man. In Chey WY, ed. Functional disorders of the digestive tract. New York: Raven Press, 1983:213.

165. Itoh Z, Takeuchi S, Aizawa I, et al. Changes in plasma motilin concentration and gastrointestinal contractile activity in conscious dogs. Am J Dig Dis 1978;23:929.

166. Lee KY, Chey WY, Tai HH, Yajima H. Radioimmunoassay of motilin: Validation of studies on the relationship between plasma motilin and interdigestive myoelectric activity of the duodenum of dog. Am J Dig Dis 1978;23:789.

167. Thomas PA, Kelly KA, Go VLW. Does motilin regulate interdigestive gastric motility? Dig Dis Sci 1972;24:577.

168. Sarna S, Chey WY, Condon RE, Dodds WJ, Myers T, Chang TM. Cause-and-effect relationship between motilin and migrating myoelectric complexes. Am J Physiol 1983;245:G277.

169. Ruppin H, Sturm G, Westhoff D, et al. Effect of 13-Nle-motilin on small intestinal transit time in healthy subjects. Scand J Gastroenterol 1976;11(Suppl 39):85.

170. Itoh Z, Honda R, Hiwatashi K, et al. Motilin-induced mechanical activity in the canine alimentary tract. Scand J Gastroenterol 1976;11(Suppl 39):93.

171. Fox JET. Motilin—An update. Life Sci 1989;35:695.

172. Strunz U, Domschke W, Mitznegg P, et al. Analysis of the motor effects of 13-norleucine motilin on the rabbit, guinea pig, rat, and human alimentary tract in vitro. Gastroenterology 1975;68:1485.

173. Lee KY, Chang T-M, Chey WY. Effect of rabbit antimotilin serum on myoelectric activity and plasma motilin concentration in fasting dog. Am J Physiol 1983;245:G547.

174. Borody TJ, Byrnes DJ, Titchen DA. Migrating myoelectric complexes and motilin in the dog. J Physiol 1981;320:62P.

175. Poitras P, Steinbach JH, VanDeventer G, Code CF, Walsh JH. Motilin-independent ectopic fronts of the interdigestive myoelectric complex in dogs. Am J Physiol 1980;239:G215.

176. Bueno L, Fioramonti J, Rayner V, Ruckebusch Y. Effects of motilin, somatostatin, and pancreatic polypeptide on the migrating myoelectric complex in pig and dog. Gastroenterology 1982;82:1395.

177. Lee KY, Chang TM, Chey WY. Effect of electrical stimulation of the vagus on plasma motilin concentration in the dog. Life Sci 1981;29:1093.

178. Dryburgh JR, Brown JC. Radioimmunoassay for motilin. Gastroenterology 1975;68:1169.

179. Mitznegg P, Bloom SR, Christofides N, et al. Release of motilin in man. Scand J Gastroenterol 1976;11(Suppl 39):53.

180. Mitznegg P, Bloom SR, Domschke W, Domschke S, Wunsch E, Demling L. Release of motilin after duodenal acidification. Lancet 1976;1:888.

181. Lewis TD, Collins SM, Fox JET, Daniel EE. Initiation of duodenal acid-induced motor complexes. Gastroenterology 1979;77:1217.

182. Domschke W, Lux G, Mitznegg P, Neeb S, Strowz U, Domschke S. Release of motilin in man by exogenous and endogenous bile. Gastroenterology 1979;76:1123.

183. Peeters TL, Janssens J, Vantrappen GR. Somatostatin and the in-

terdigestive migrating motor complex in man. Regul Pept 1983;5: 209.

184. Owyang C, Achem-Karem SR, Vinik AI. Pancreatic polypeptide and intestinal migrating motor complex in humans. Gastroenterology 1983;84:10.

185. Aizawa I, Itoh Z, Harris V, Unger RH. Plasma somatostatin-like immunoreactivity during the interdigestive period in the dog. J Clin Invest 1981;68:206.

186. Krejs GJ, Orci L, Conlon JM, et al. Somatostatinoma syndrome: Biochemical, morphologic, and clinical features. N Engl J Med 1979;301:285.

187. Ormsbee HS III, Koehler SL, Telford GL. Somatostatin inhibits motilin-induced interdigestive contractile activity in the dog. Am J Dig Dis 1978;23:781.

188. Johansson C, Efendic S, Wisen O, Uvnas-Wallensten S, Victor A, Weiner E. Effects of short-time somatostatin infusion on the gastric and intestinal propulsion in humans. Scand J Gastroenterol 1978;13: 481.

189. Hostein J, Janssens J, Vantrappen G, Peeters TL, Vanderweerd M, Leman G. Somatostatin induces ectopic activity fronts of the migrating motor complex via a local intestinal mechanism. Gastroenterology 1984;87:1004.

190. Krejs GJ. Physiological role of somatostatin in the digestive tract: Gastric acid secretion, intestinal absorption, and motility. Scand J Gastroenterol 1986;21(Suppl 119):47.

191. Donnerer J, Holzer P, Lembeck F. Release of dynorphin, somatostatin, and substance P from the vascularly perfused small intestine of the guinea-pig during peristalsis. Br J Pharmacol 1984;83:919.

192. Schippers E, Janssens J, Vantrappen G, Vanderweerd M, Peeters TL. Somatostatin induces ectopic activity fronts via a local intestinal mechanism during fed state or pentagastrin. Am J Physiol 1986;250: G149.

193. Thor PJ, Konturek JW, Konturek SJ. Pancreatic polypeptide and intestinal motility in dogs. Dig Dis Sci 1987;32:513.

194. Hall KE, Diamant NE, El-Sharkawy TY, Greenberg GR. Effect of pancreatic polypeptide on canine migrating motor complex and plasma motilin. Am J Physiol 1983;245:G178.

195. Janssens J, Hellemans J, Adrian TE, et al. Pancreatic polypeptide is not involved in the regulation of the migrating motor complex in man. Regul Pept 1982;3:41.

196. Janssens J, Vantrappen G, Peeters TL. The activity front of the migrating motor complex of the human stomach but not of the small intestine is motilin-dependent. Regul Pept 1983;6:363.

197. Schulz R, Wuster M, Simantov R, Snyder S, Herz A. Electrically stimulated release of opiate-like material from the myenteric plexus of the guinea pig ileum. Eur J Pharmacol 1977;41:347.

198. Davis TP, Culling AJ, Schoemaker H, Galligan JJ. Beta-endorphin and its metabolites stimulate motility of the dog small intestine. J Pharmacol Exp Ther 1983;227:499.

199. Telford GL, Hashmonai M, Moses AJ, Szurszewski JH. Morphine initiates migrating myoelectric complexes by acting on peripheral opioid receptors. Am J Physiol 1985;249:G557.

200. Sarna SK, Condon RE. Morphine-initiated migrating motor complexes in the fed state in the dog. Gastroenterology 1984;86:662.

201. Stanghellini V, Malagelada J-R, Zinsmeister AR, Go VLW, Kao PC. Stress-induced gastrointestinal motor disturbances in humans: Possible humoral mechanisms. Gastroenterology 1983;85:83.

202. Thompson DG, Richelson E, Malagelada J-R. Perturbation of gastric emptying and duodenal motility through the central nervous system. Gastroenterology 1982;83:1200.

203. Weisbrodt NW, Sussman SS, Stewart JJ, Burks TF. Effect of morphine sulfate on intestinal transit and myoelectric activity of the small intestine of the rat. J Pharmacol Exp Ther 1980;214:333.

204. Kromer W, Pretzlaff W. In vitro evidence for the participation of intestinal opioids in the control of peristalsis in the guinea pig small intestine. Naunyn Schmiedebergs Arch Pharmacol 1979;309:153.

205. Telford GL, Szurszewski JH. Blockade of migrating myoelectric complexes by naloxone. Gastroenterol Clin Biol 1983;7:717.

206. Gutierrez JG, Chey WY, Dinoso VP. Actions of cholecystokinin and secretin on the motor activity of the small intestine in man. Gastroenterology 1974;67:35.

207. Fargeas MJ, Fioramonti J, Bueno L. Central and peripheral action of GABAA and GABAB agonists on small intestine motility in rats. Eur J Pharmacol 1988;150:163.

208. Porreca F, Burks TF. Centrally administered bombesin affects gastric emptying and small and large bowel transit in the rat. Gastroenterology 1983;85:313.

209. Heilman RD, Lum BK. Studies on the intestinal relaxation produced by dopamine. J Pharmacol Exp Ther 1971;178:63.

210. Buell MG, Harding RK. Effects of peptide YY on intestinal blood flow distribution and motility in the dog. Regul Pept 1989;24:195.

211. Al-Saffar A, Hellstrom PM, Nylander G. Correlation between peptide YY-induced myoelectric activity and transit of small intestinal contents in rats. Scand J Gastroenterol 1985;20:577.

212. Belesin DB, Bogdanovic SB, Radmanovic BZ. The possible site of action of bradykinin on the peristaltic reflex of the isolated guinea pig ileum. Arch Int Pharmacodyn 1964;147:43.

213. Khairallah PA, Page IH. Effects of bradykinin and angiotensin on smooth muscle. Ann NY Acad Sci 1963;104:212.

214. Fox JE, McDonald TJ, Kostolanska F, Tatemoto K. Galanin: An inhibitory neural peptide of the canine small intestine. Life Sci 1986;39:103.

215. Fox JE, Brooks B, McDonald TJ, et al. Action of galanin fragments on rat, guinea-pig, and canine intestinal motility. Peptides 1988;9: 1183.

216. Alvarez WC, Mahoney LJ. Peristaltic rush in the rabbit. Am J Physiol 1924;69:211.

217. Kruis W, Azpiroz F, Phillips SF. Contractile patterns and transit of fluid in canine terminal ileum. Am J Physiol 1985;249:G264.

218. Sarna SK. Giant migrating contractions and their myoelectric correlates in the small intestine. Am J Physiol 1987;253:G697.

219. Quigley EMM, Phillips SF, Dent J. Distinctive patterns of interdigestive motility at the canine ileocolonic junction. Gastroenterology 1984;87:836.

220. Sarna SK, Otterson MF. Gastrointestinal motility: Some basic concepts. Pharmacology 1988;36(Suppl 1):7.

221. Sarna SK, Otterson MF. Small intestinal amyogenesia and dysmyogenesis induced by morphine and loperamide. Am J Physiol 1990;258: G282.

222. Summers RW, Anuras S, Green J. Jejunal manometry patterns in health, partial intestinal obstruction, and pseudoobstruction. Gastroenterology 1983;85:1290.

223. Kellow JE, Phillips SF. Altered small bowel motility in irritable bowel syndrome is correlated with symptoms. Gastroenterology 1987;92:1885.

224. Alvarez WC. Reverse peristalsis in the bowel, a precursor of vomiting. JAMA 1925;85:1051.

225. Stewart JJ, Burks TF, Weisbrodt NW. Intestinal myoelectric activity after activation of central emetic mechanism. Am J Physiol 1977;233: E131.

226. Lang IM, Sarna SK, Condon RE. Gastrointestinal motor correlates of vomiting in the dog: Quantification and characterization as an independent phenomenon. Gastroenterology 1986;90:40.

227. Lang IM, Marvig J, Sarna SK, Condon RE. Gastrointestinal myoelectric correlates of vomiting in the dog. Am J Physiol 1986;251: G830.

228. Kubota M. Electrical and mechanical properties and neuro-effector transmission in the smooth muscle layer of the guinea-pig ileocecal junction. Pflugers Arch 1982;394:355.

229. Conklin JL, Christensen J. Local specialization at the ileocecal junction of the cat and opossum. Am J Physiol 1975;228:1075.

230. Cardwell BA, Rubin MR, Snape WJ, Cohen S. Properties of the cat ileocecal sphincter muscle. Am J Physiol 1981;241:G222.

231. Kelley ML, Gordon EA, DeWeese JA. Pressure studies of the ileocolonic junctional zone of dogs. Am J Physiol 1965;209:333.

232. Quigley EMM, Phillips SF, Dent J, Taylor BM. Myoelectrical activity and intraluminal pressure of the canine ileocecal sphincter. Gastroenterology 1983;85:1054.

233. Quigley EM, Dent J, Phillips SF. Manometry of canine ileocolonic sphincter: Comparison of sleeve method to point sensors. Am J Physiol 1987;252:G585.

234. Cohen S, Harris LD, Levitan R. Manometric characteristics of the human ileocecal junctional zone. Gastroenterology 1968;54:72.

235. Ouyang A, Snape WJ, Cohen S. Myoelectric properties of the cat ileocecal sphincter. Am J Physiol 1981;240:G450.

236. Quigley EMM, Borody TJ, Phillips SF, Wienbeck M, Tucker RL, Haddad A. Motility of the terminal ileum and ileocecal sphincter in healthy humans. Gastroenterology 1984;87:857.

237. Hunter RH. The ganglionic tissue of the ileocecal junction. Ulster Med J 1936;5:54.

238. Elliot TR. On the innervation of the ileocolic sphincter. J Physiol 1904;31:157.

239. Rubin MR, Fournet J, Snape WJ, Cohen S. Adrenergic regulation of ileocecal sphincter function in the cat. Gastroenterology 1980;78:15.

240. Hinrichsen J, Ivy AC. Studies on the ileo-cecal sphincter of the dog. Am J Physiol 1931;96:494.

241. Jarrett RJ, Gazet JC. Studies in vivo of the ileo-caeco-colic sphincter in the cat and dog. Gut 1966;7:271.

242. Pahlin P-E, Kewenter J. The vagal control of the ileo-cecal sphincter in the cat. Acta Physiol Scand 1976;96:433.

243. Pahlin P-E, Kewenter J. Sympathetic nervous control of cat ileocecal sphincter. Am J Physiol 1976;231:296.

244. Ferri G-L, Adrian TE, Ghatei MA, et al. Tissue localization and relative distribution of regulatory peptides in separated layers from the human bowel. Gastroenterology 1983;84:777.

245. Spiller RC, Brown ML, Phillips SF, Azpiroz F. Scintigraphic measurements of canine ileocolonic transit: Direct and indirect effects of eating. Gastroenterology 1986;91:1213.

246. Kelley ML, DeWeese JA. Effects of eating and intraluminal filling on ileocolonic junctional zone pressures. Am J Physiol 1969;216:1491.

247. Kelley ML, Gordon EA, DeWeese JA. Pressure responses of canine ileocolonic junctional zone to intestinal distension. Am J Physiol 1966;211:614.

248. Pahlin P-E, Kewenter J. Reflexogenic contraction of the ileocecal sphincter in the cat following small or large intestine distention. Acta Physiol Scand 1975;95:126.

249. Kumar D, Phillips SF. The contribution of external ligamentous attachments to function of the ileocecal junction. Dis Colon Rectum 1987;30:410.

250. Richardson JD, Griffin WO. Ileocecal valve substitutes as bacteriologic barriers. Am J Surg 1972;123:149.

251. Singleton AO, Redmond DC, McMurray JE. Ileocecal resection and small bowel transit and absorption. Ann Surg 1964;159:690.

252. Bertiger G, Ouyang A, Reynolds JC, Cohen S. Evidence for a direct and indirect action of leucine enkephalin at the feline ileocecal sphincter. Life Sci 1988;42:1697.

253. Ouyang A, Vos P, Cohen S. Sites of action of mu-, kappa- and sigma-opiate receptor agonists at the feline ileocecal sphincter. Am J Physiol 1988;254:G224.

254. Rothstein RD, Johnson E, Ouyang A. Substance P: Mechanism of action and receptor distribution at the feline ileocecal sphincter region. Am J Physiol 1989;257:G447.

255. Rothstein RD, Ouyang A. Mechanism of action of neurotensin at the ileocecal sphincter region. Life Sci 1989;45:1475.

10

The Motor Function of the Colon

JAMES CHRISTENSEN

INTRODUCTION

The mammalian large intestine evolved to meet three major needs in animal physiology. The conservation of water, necessary for the adaptation to dry terrestrial environments, requires the existence of slow luminal flows and a permeable mucosa in the large intestine. The bacterial fermentation of dietary elements that are resistant to the digestive enzymes of the intestine, a means to increase nutritional efficiency in certain mammals, requires a colonic environment that fosters microbial growth and a mucosa that is permeable to the products of fermentation. The ability to control the delivery of the fecal mass, important to many mammals in defense against predation and in marking ranging territories, requires controlled timing of defecation. These needs may have diminished in humans, but the structures and processes that serve these needs survive.

All three requirements demand particular patterns of flow in the large intestine. Flow in the gastrointestinal tract results from the movements of its muscular walls. The patterns of wall movements (or contractions) vary among organs to provide the particular and different patterns of flow needed in each. Because flows and the wall movements differ among organs, the structures and the processes that accomplish these wall movements also differ.

There is no optimal animal model for the human large intestine. The organ varies enormously among species in its gross anatomy.[1] This tends to make tenuous the unqualified transposition of information obtained from the study of the bowel in an experimental animal to questions about the nature of bowel motility in humans. Still, all mammalian colons should be qualitatively alike. Species differences are likely to be differences of quantity or proportion.

The motor function of the large intestine has been examined quite extensively in the past few decades.[2-9] One can now discern systems and processes in which disturbances could account for the common and troublesome symptoms generally attributed to motor dysfunction of the bowel.

ANATOMY OF MOTOR STRUCTURES

Gross Anatomy

COMPONENT PARTS OF THE LARGE INTESTINE

The large intestine is often called by the name of one of its component parts, the colon. The large intestine is divided into five parts: the appendix, the cecum, the colon, the rectum, and the anal canal. These parts are anatomically and physiologically distinct. They should be kept in mind as separate structures.

The colon extends from the ileocolic junction to the rectosigmoid junction. It is divided into four regions: the ascending, transverse, descending, and sigmoid regions. Although the distinctions among these regions are somewhat arbitrary, this division is useful both physiologically and anatomically. The parts of the large intestine are partly delineated by points or loci. These points are the ileocolic junction, the hepatic flexure, the splenic flexure, and the rectosigmoid junction. All these parts and loci are shown in Figure 10-1.

DESCRIPTION OF THE COMPONENT PARTS OF THE LARGE INTESTINE

The cecum is a blind pouch beyond the ileocolic junction. The cecum and the appendix have a generous mesentery and are, therefore, quite mobile.

The ascending colon, extending from the ileocolic junction to the hepatic flexure, has no mesentery; the investing peritoneum holds it against the adjacent kidney and dorsal muscles. The transverse colon, extending from the hepatic flexure to the splenic flexure has a broad mesentery so that it generally loops below the interiliac line. The descending colon, extending from the splenic flexure to the upper aperture of the pelvis, lacks a mesentery so that the peritoneum holds it against the kidney and dorsal muscles. The sigmoid colon, extending from the pelvic aperture to the rectosigmoid junction, has a broad mesentery so that it often forms a loop that protrudes into the abdomen. The rectum extends from the rectosigmoid junction to the anal canal. About 6 to 8 cm above the anal canal, the peritoneum is reflected from the rectum to adjacent structures so that the distal rectum is extraperitoneal. The anal canal is surrounded by the striated musculature of the pelvic floor, including the external anal sphincter.

Structure of the Wall of the Large Intestine

The large intestinal wall, like the rest of the gut, has three major layers: the mucosa, the submucosa, and the muscularis propria. Each major layer has subdivisions.

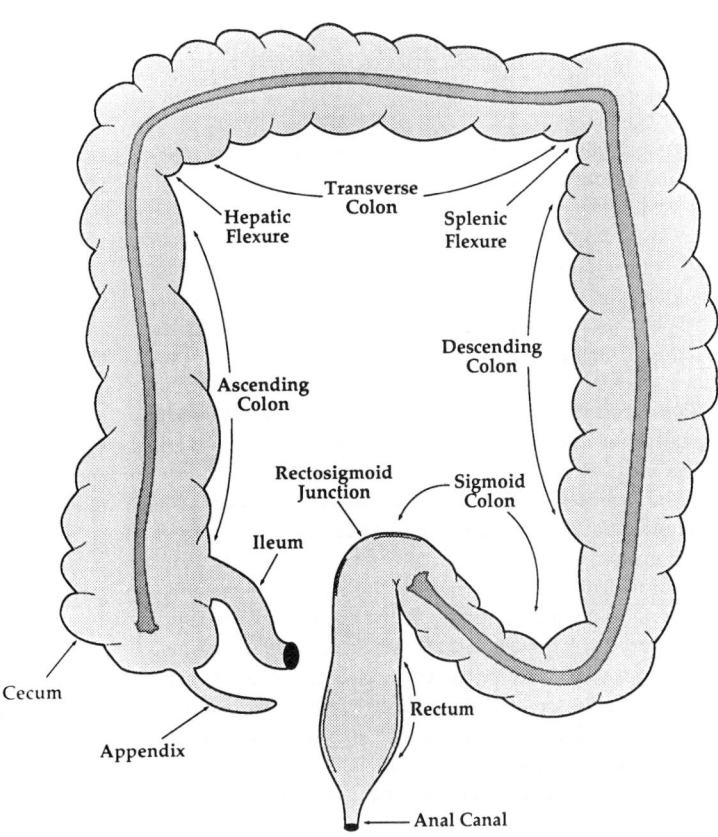

FIGURE 10–1. Gross anatomy of the large intestine.

The mucosa consists of the glandular epithelium, the lamina propria, and the muscularis mucosae. The epithelium, composed of absorptive cells and goblet cells with occasional enteroendocrine cells, is arranged with crypts, like those of the small intestine. It lies on the lamina propria, a loose stroma of connective tissue containing leukocytes and connective tissue cells. The muscularis mucosae is a thin sheet of smooth muscle in which the muscle fiber bundles extend in both the longitudinal and circumferential directions.

The submucosa constitutes about half the full wall thickness. It is a loose connective tissue stroma containing mainly connective tissue cells along with the ganglia of the submucous plexus of nerves.

The muscularis propria constitutes three layers. An inner thick muscle layer, with its fibers oriented circumferentially, and an outer thin muscle layer, with its fibers directed longitudinally, constitute most of the thickness of the muscularis. A very thin zone between them, the intermuscular zone, contains the ganglia of the myenteric plexus.

Innervation of the Large Intestine

The motility of the large intestine is controlled mainly by its nerves. The nerves constitute two general classes: those that lie wholly within the large intestine, the intrinsic nerves, and those that lie mainly outside it, the extrinsic nerves. These are a part of the enteric nervous system, the total nervous system of the gut. The enteric nervous system is a part of the autonomic nervous system. The enteric nerves supply the epithelium and the intramural vasculature of the large intestine, so they should not be considered to control only motor functions.

The intrinsic nerves of the large intestine lie mainly in two planes of the intestinal wall: the submucosa and the intermuscular space. The cell bodies (or perikarya) of the intrinsic nerves lie in these planes, from which nerve processes extend into the other layers of the intestinal wall.

In the submucosa, the perikarya lie in sparse, irregularly disposed clusters, the ganglia, which usually contain no more than about 10 perikarya. The perikarya make up about half the mass of a ganglion, the rest constituting the bodies of the glial cells, and a tangled net of glial processes and neuronal processes (axons and dendrites), the neuropil. The ganglia of the submucous plexus are joined together by bundles of nerve processes called the interganglionic fascicles or bundles. In the large intestinal submucous plexus, the ganglia lie in two layers, one close to the muscularis mucosae, called Meissner's plexus, and the other near the circular muscle layer, called Henle's or Schabadasch's plexus. These two layers are interconnected by interganglionic fascicles. The ganglia supply the mucosa as well as the circular muscle layer. The latter supply is provided through a dense mat of nerve cell processes that lies on the submucosal surface of the circular muscle layer. This mat of processes (or neurites) is associated with a dense mat of fibroblastlike cells, called interstitial cells. The network of neurites and interstitial cells is called the plexus submucosus extremus, and its position and density suggest that it controls the circular muscle layer on the face of which it lies.

Perikarya are also concentrated in ganglia in the intermuscular space to form the myenteric plexus. Here, the ganglia are much larger than they are in the submucosa, up to 100 nerve cells or more per ganglion. The ganglia are joined by thick interganglionic bundles, the ganglia and bundles forming the primary plexus of the myenteric plexus. The ganglia are regularly disposed so that they and the interganglionic fascicles form a fairly regular pattern. These interganglionic fascicles give smaller branches, bundles of neurites that ramify in the interstices of the primary plexus to form the secondary plexus. These, in turn, give still smaller branches of bundles of neurites to form a tertiary plexus that ramifies within the interstices of the secondary plexus. Branches extend from these plexus into the two main muscle coats on both sides of the intermuscular space.

Certain special cells, the interstitial cells, are associated intimately with the intrinsic nerves of the large intestine. They lie, in general, in a very close relationship to the axon terminals and the smooth muscle cells, but principally in two planes of the large intestinal wall. One plane is that of the plexus submucosus extremus, described above. The other plane is that of the myenteric plexus where they are associated with the tertiary plexus and, to some extent, with the branches that extend into the muscularis propria. These interstitial cells form cell-to-cell unions (gap junctions) with one another and with the muscle cells against which they lie, besides being in a very close relationship to terminal axons. These relationships suggest that they are involved in nerve-muscle communication. Evidence also suggests that they may be involved in the regulation of the rhythmicity of contraction of the muscular layers.

The extrinsic nerves to the large intestine represent the projection into the organ of axons from perikarya located outside the wall of the organ. These constitute two general classes, those arising from the brain and the caudal part of the spinal cord, the craniosacral nerves, and the thoracolumbar nerves, which supply the large intestine through the prevertebral ganglia (Fig 10-2).

The influence of the vagus extends to the level of the ascending colon. Most of the craniosacral innervation arises from the caudal part of the spinal cord, from levels S1 through S4. Processes from perikarya in the cord at this level form the pelvic and pudendal nerves. The pelvic nerves extend into the deep pelvis to form the pelvic plexus, which also receives nerves from the inferior mesenteric ganglion. This plexus sends branches, colonic nerves, to the rectosigmoid junction where they penetrate the longitudinal muscle layer to extend cephalad within the intermuscular plane over a long distance, and caudad to the level of the anal canal. These are the ascending colonic nerves or "shunt fascicles." Other perikarya in the sacral cord form the pudendal nerves, which supply somatic nerve fibers to the striated muscles of the pelvic floor and, probably, some autonomic nerve fibers to the distal large intestine.

The prevertebral ganglia receive preganglionic fibers from the central nervous system in the splanchnic nerves and supply postganglionic fibers to the gut by way of the paravascular mesenteric nerves. Those to the part of the organ supplied by the superior mesenteric ganglion follow the course of the corresponding artery, and those from the inferior mesenteric ganglion extend to the domain of that corresponding artery. The thoracolumbar supply to the part of the rectum beyond the distribution of the inferior mesenteric artery is not clear. It probably arises from the paravascular nerves.

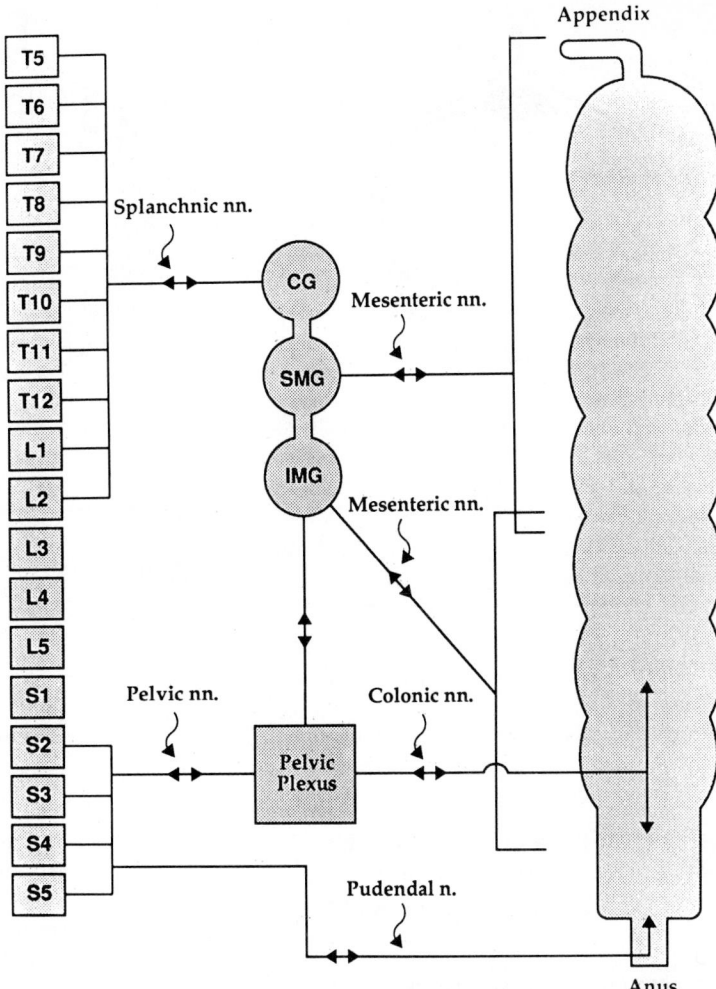

FIGURE 10–2. Extrinsic innervation of the large intestine. The blocks represent the levels of the spinal cord. *CG, SMG,* and *IMG* = the celiac, superior mesenteric and inferior mesenteric ganglia, respectively. *N* or *nn* = nerve or nerves.

Musculature Involved in Large Intestinal Motor Function

MUSCLES INTRINSIC TO THE WALL

The thin muscularis mucosae extends throughout the whole organ. Its location and the orientation of its muscle fibers suggest that it moves the mucosa about over the thick muscularis propria, a motion that would be allowed by the looseness of the submucosa.

The thickness of the circular layer of the muscularis propria is about the same throughout the large intestine except in the anal canal, where it broadens to form the internal anal sphincter. The orientation of its muscle fibers indicates that it is principally responsible for the lumen-occluding contractions that regulate the flow of the luminal contents.

The longitudinal layer of the muscularis propria is, throughout most of the large intestine, thickened to form three bundles, the teniae, with a very thin layer of such muscle between the teniae. At about the colorectal junction, the three teniae broaden and fuse so that the rectum is invested by a longitudinal muscle layer of uniform thickness (Fig 10-3). The teniae are equidistant from one another, one always lying along the line of the mesenteric insertion. Contraction of this layer must shorten the colon, but the process has had almost no description.

The teniae form longitudinal indentations or folds between which the walls of the organ bulge. In the circular muscle layer, thin rings of tonic contraction, spaced at irregular intervals of a few centimeters, indent the lumen to produce the external appearance of sacculation of the bulging intertenial walls (see Fig 10-3). These sacs are called haustra, and the indentations that define them are the haustral indentations or markings. They are vestigial at birth, becoming prominent later in infancy.[10]

MUSCLES EXTRINSIC TO THE WALLS

Muscles extrinsic to the large intestine are often ignored in the consideration of motility. Where a mesentery supports the organ, small bundles of smooth muscle occur at intervals to connect the organ to the posterior abdominal wall. The most prominent such bundle exists in the phrenicocolic ligament that holds the splenic flexure in position. Two other extrinsic muscles, the puborectalis and the anococcygeus, form loops about the cephalic and caudal parts of the rectum from the anterior and posterior pelvic walls. These extrinsic muscles presumably can alter the orientation of the large intestine within the abdomen.

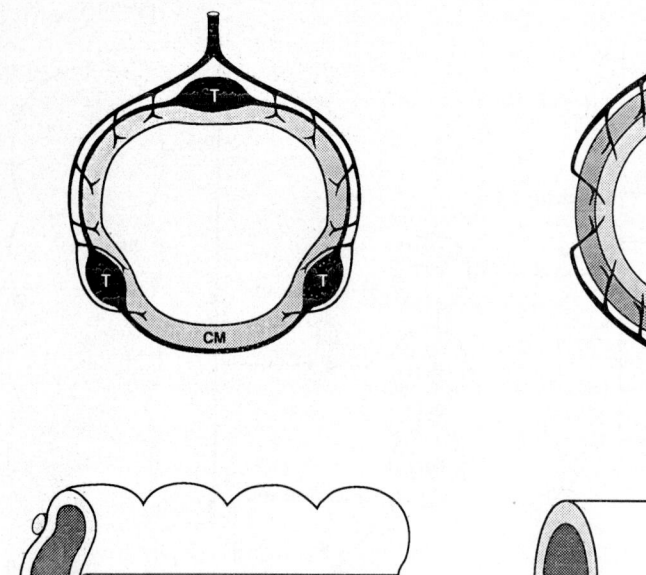

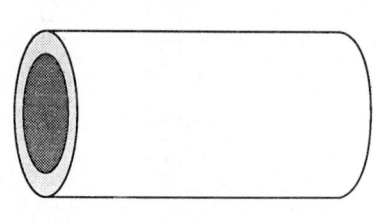

Taeniated Sacculated Part of the Large Intestine

Rectum

FIGURE 10–3. Diagram of the saccular part of the large intestine compared with the rectum. *T* = taenia. *LM* and *CM* = longitudinal and circular muscle layers, respectively. The cross-sectional diagrams show the distributions of arteries.

METHODS TO EXAMINE MOTOR FUNCTIONS IN THE LARGE INTESTINE

The observation of large intestinal motor function may involve the study of any of several processes. These include the flow of the luminal content, the motions of the circular muscle layer, the intraluminal pressure changes those motions cause, the behavior of pieces of muscle taken from the organ, and the electrical signals that accompany muscle contractions, both in the whole organ and in isolated strips of muscle.

Obviously, many different methods apply to the description of these interrelated functions. All methods have a use, but all have limitations in depicting the integrated process that the term "motility" designates. These methods include direct visual observation, radiographic observation, kymography, manometry, the direct recording of contractions in vivo and in vitro, and the recording of electrical events (electromyography) both in vivo and in vitro.

The direct visual observation of the large intestine exposed at operation suffers many limitations. The time of observation is restricted. The motions observed are probably affected profoundly by the drugs that must be used, by reflexes induced by the opening of the peritoneum and the handling of the viscera, and by the subnormal temperature. Little objectivity is possible in this obsolete approach.

Radiographic methods exclude such variables as drugs, reflexes, and body temperature. On the other hand, the low resolution of radiographic imaging allows the study only of the gross flow of the luminal content. The content observed is, to a variable degree, abnormal, being a radiopaque substance (in conventional radiography) or a radioactive isotope (in scintigraphy), in a solution or suspension that cannot always be assumed to behave like the usual luminal contents. Considerations of safety limit the time of observation in humans, and this may be important in the perception of the very slow processes. Objectivity and precise quantitation are hard to achieve. The most useful radiographic method has been the observation, by serial radiographs at intervals of hours to days, of the positions of tiny radiopaque plastic markers ingested along with food.

Kymography refers to the measurement of pressure and volume changes in balloons put into the large intestinal lumen. Contractions of the muscular wall presumably generate the pressure and volume changes recorded. Severe limitations have made this technique obsolete. A large balloon probably affects motility by exciting reflex responses. Its position cannot be firmly secured. It usually covers a segment of the organ several centimeters long so that spatial resolution is poor. Body motions that raise intraabdominal pressure can affect the volume and pressure in the balloon. The physical properties of the balloon, its elasticity or rigidity, affect the recorded functions. The use of small balloons circumvents some of these restrictions, but they may not fully sense contractions that fail to occlude the lumen, which are probably frequent in the colon.

Manometry, the recording of pressures from open-tip catheters (usually perfused very slowly with water), has found considerable application in the study of esophageal motility, but less in the study of the large intestine. The method lacks many of the restrictions of kymography. Its major limitation in the large intestine is the fact that an open tip detects the pressure in whatever sealed cavity it happens to lie. Thus, the spatial resolution is poor. It is the best method for the study of the behavior of the anal canal where the position of the open tip can be observed and controlled, and where the luminal occlusion produced by the anal sphincters is complete.

Miniature strain gauges, sewn to the wall of the gastrointestinal tract in animals, can detect contractions with high resolution and without most of the limitations described above. The technique, which has proved to be most useful in the small intestine, has had little application to the study of the behavior of the large intestine.

The recording of the activity of muscle strips taken from the gut, also much used to examine motility in the small intestine, has had much less use in the study of motor activity of the colon. The method cannot provide a picture of the action of the whole organ, but it can contribute to an understanding of how the colonic muscle is affected by the intrinsic nerves, by natural substances (like hormones and neurotransmitters), and by drugs.

Electromyography, the recording of the electrical signals that accompany contractions in muscle, fruitfully applied to examine motor functions of the stomach and small intestine, has been similarly instructive in the study of large intestinal motility. Its major limitation is that the signals recorded are not yet fully interpretable in terms of wall movements and intestinal flows. It has seen some application in humans, but technical problems have limited its usefulness in humans. It has proved more useful in animals, where one can record signals either from electrodes sewn to the whole organ or from excised muscle strips.

The preceding brief critique of methods might suggest that the limitations of the study techniques preclude any comprehensive understanding of how the large intestine operates. The methods, however, are complementary, and so they together provide a fairly clear global picture.

PATTERNS OF CONTRACTION AND FLOW IN THE LARGE INTESTINE

Overview of Large Intestinal Motor Function [11-23]

EXISTENCE OF DIFFERENT FUNCTIONAL UNITS

The large intestine, appearing anatomically to be a single organ, is functionally heterogeneous (i.e., its various parts exhibit quite different patterns of motor behavior). It is a series of functionally different units linked in series. No distinct operational margins separate these units.

Considering the whole of the large intestine, there are five functional units: the cecum, the right colon, the left colon, the rectum, and the anal canal.

The characteristic motor activity of the cecum does not much concern us because the human cecum is poorly developed. In many species (herbivores and omnivores that developed from herbivore ancestors), the cecum is very long, in some cases as long as all the rest of the large intestine (Fig 10-4). Obviously, such a long blind sac requires a controlled mechanism for its filling and emptying. Radiopaque markers have been seen to enter the cecum, pass toward its tip in an orderly fashion, reside there for a time, and then move out of the cecum, also in an orderly manner. This process, studied mostly in fowl, almost certainly involves a ring contraction of the circular muscle layer whose direction of movement is regulated.

The part of the large intestine strictly indicated by the term "colon" extends from the ileocecal junction to the rectosigmoid

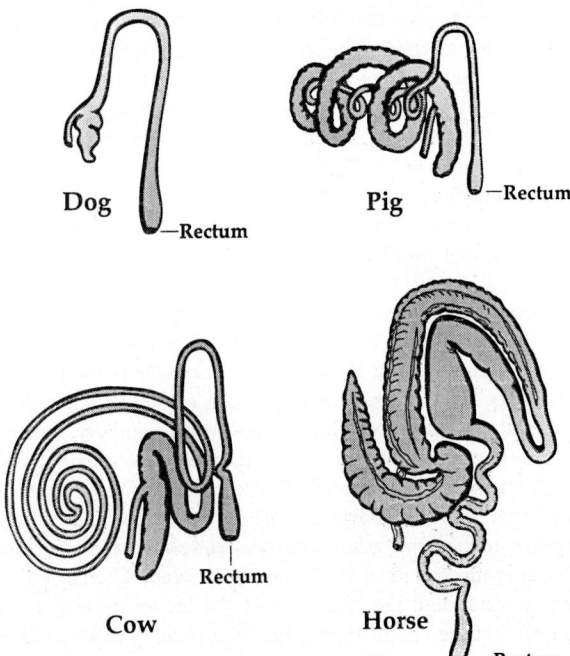

FIGURE 10–4. Large intestines of four common animals.

junction. Two functionally different units make up this anatomically homogeneous segment. The nature of peristalsis distinguishes them, as explained later.

The rectum differs from the colon mainly in the fact that its major form of contraction, lumen-occluding peristalsis, is infrequent, apparently being under the control of extrinsic nerves.

The anal canal differs from all other parts of the large intestine in that a strong tonic contraction, a contraction that occludes the lumen, is the dominant form of its motor activity.

FORMS OF CONTRACTIONS: PERISTALSIS AND TONIC CONTRACTIONS

The common term "peristalsis" is often applied imprecisely to all forms of gastrointestinal contractions. Contractions of the circular muscle, ring contractions, commonly occur as rhythmic events that move along the organ. In the more strict usage observed in this chapter, peristalsis refers to these events. Other ring contractions are not rhythmic but sustained and stationary. Such contractions are properly called tonic contractions. The longitudinal muscle layer also contracts. No adequate description of its pattern of contraction in the whole organ exists. Its contraction must produce sleeving of the organ, but this effect cannot yet be integrated into the overall picture of motor behavior.

Two Functional Units of the Colon

TWO PATTERNS OF RHYTHMIC PERISTALSIS

Observations of the colon exposed in animals at operation and radiographic studies long ago revealed gross patterns of flow and of rhythmic peristalsis that have since been confirmed and supported by other methods. The studies indicate that the colon constitutes two rather different functional segments. These are the proximal colon, from the ileocecal junction to about the hepatic flexure, and the distal colon, from about the hepatic flexure to the rectosigmoid junction.

In the proximal colon, the predominant pattern of contraction is rhythmic antiperistalsis (i.e., ring contractions of the circular muscle layer that move rhythmically from the neighborhood of the hepatic flexure toward the cecum). The contractions occur with a reasonably constant maximal frequency, 5 to 6 cycles per minute in most species, and with a rather constant velocity, 1 to 2 mm per second. Thus, the ring contractions lie several centimeters apart, following one another. Such activity is not stable. The contractions may occur intermittently or irregularly, but the fundamental period of 10 to 12 seconds, the stable velocity, and the antiperistaltic (or retrograde) direction seems to be present most of the time. The flows that are produced are accordingly retrograde, toward the cecum. Material entering the colon from the ileum is thus retained in the proximal colon. The closed ileocecal junction and the blind end of the cecum prevent their escape, so that the contractions exert a churning or mixing effect on the colonic contents. The contractions do not often appear to occlude the lumen fully, so they do not actually trap or confine the luminal content. Rather, the shallow contractions simply impart a retrograde vector at the surface of the fluid luminal mass. If such a pattern of motor activity were constant, the proximal colon would not readily empty. The fact that it does is explained by the observation that the antiperistaltic direction is not constant. It occasionally reverses, so that orthograde contractions, similar in frequency, velocity and depth, can empty the segment.

In the distal colon, the predominant pattern of contractions is rhythmic peristalsis, directed toward the anus. These rhythmic contractions resemble those of the proximal colon in maximal frequency, velocity, and magnitude or depth. They rarely move far, probably only a few centimeters, and they rarely occur at their maximal frequency. Like the rhythmic peristalsis of the proximal colon, that of the distal colon is not fully lumen-occluding. Rather, the ring contractions mainly indent or sweep the surface, imparting an orthograde vector to the fluid content, which is here rather more solid than it is in the proximal colon.

TONIC CONTRACTIONS IN THE COLON

Tonic contractions exist in the proximal and distal colon in the form of the narrow rings called the haustral markings. Once considered fixed structures, their origin as a tonic contraction of the circular muscle layer is evident from the fact that, in radiographs, they can be seen to disappear and reappear. Presumably, they serve to retard the axial flow of luminal contents that the rhythmic peristalsis induces. In their intermittent disappearance and reappearance, they may also forcibly knead the semisolid fecal mass and compress it. Kneading would be the only way to cause mixing of such a mass, and compression should help to expel water from it. Such effects are probably important in the extraction of water from the luminal contents.

The interaction of rhythmic peristalsis and the tonic contractions at the haustral markings can only be imagined. Radiographic observations suggest that the tonic contractions of the haustral markings overwhelmingly dominate. Rhythmic peristalsis is not usually evident with such methods. It seems likely that the study conditions greatly influence what is seen. Fasting (the usual condition for radiographic study), a foreign (and not necessarily inert) material in the colonic lumen, and a necessarily brief period of observation may all limit the ability to view the whole repertoire of motor functions.

The Rectum

Direct observations in animals long ago indicated that the rectum exhibits a pattern of motor behavior quite different from that of the colon. This idea finds support in later studies as well.

Rhythmic peristalsis seems to be absent from the rectum most of the time. Indeed, the lack of frequent movement is its prominent functional feature. A strong peristaltic contraction, moving slowly toward the anus, can be excited by electrical stimulation of the pelvic nerves in animals whose rectums are observed directly.

The human rectum in situ has received little study by methods that can be applied in the clinic. It contracts in defecation, as described later, and this is a peristaltic lumen-occluding contraction like that described with pelvic nerve stimulation in animals. At night, the rectum exhibits very prolonged and very powerful contractions at long intervals (D. Kumar, personal communication). It is not clear whether these are progressive in nature. They may be of the nature of tonic contractions, acting to prevent rectal filling in sleep. That idea remains conjectural.

The fixed folds of the rectum, the valves of Houston, are not contraction rings like the haustral markings of the colon, which they resemble superficially. The constancy of their presence and of their positions indicates this. Their histology further indicates that they are formed over bands of connective tissue, mainly at the level of the submucosa. Presumably, they serve to retard the flow of feces, but they are effaced by a solid fecal mass in defecation.

The Anal Canal[24–36]

A nearly constant ring contraction rather sharply defines the anal canal as distinct from the rectum. Complete luminal occlusion is achieved by contraction of the two sphincters that exist at this level (Fig 10-5). The internal anal sphincter, a thickening of the circular layer of smooth muscle that is continuous with that of the rectum, is tonically contracted most of the time except just before and during defecation. The loss of its tone at these times indicates that its operation is closely linked to motor events in the rectum and sigmoid colon. The external anal sphincter, a bundle of striated muscle just caudal to and outside the internal sphincter, exhibits a low level of tone most of the time. Its force of contraction can be raised voluntarily as the force of tone in the internal sphincter falls when defecation is imminent. This fact also indicates that its function is linked to that of the rectum and internal anal sphincter. The function of the anal sphincters is to prevent the escape of rectal contents except at convenient or desired times.

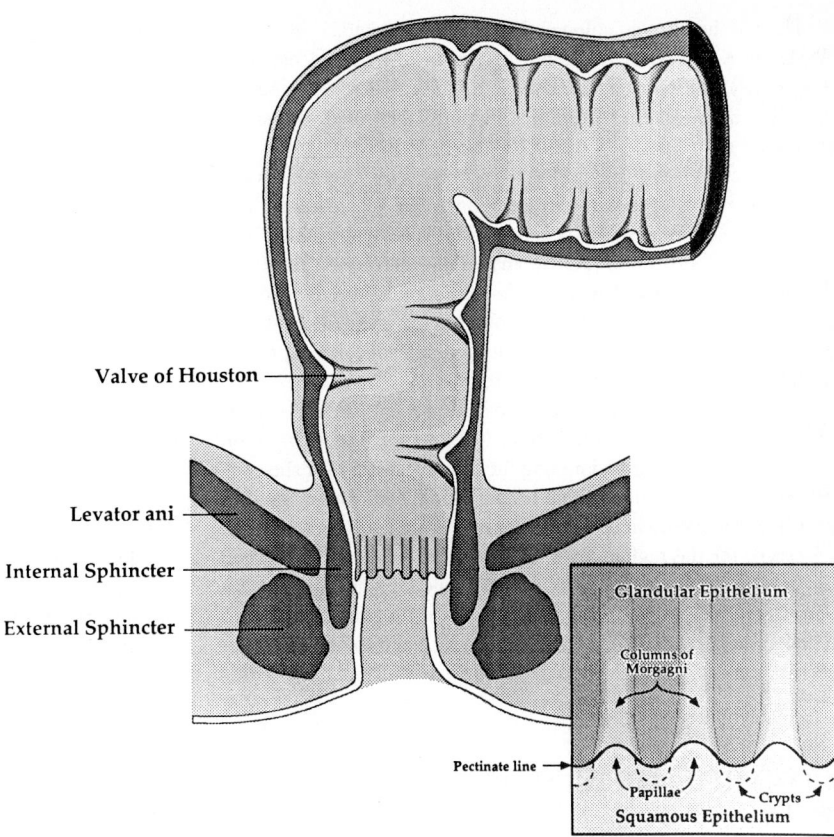

Valve of Houston

Levator ani

Internal Sphincter

External Sphincter

Glandular Epithelium

Columns of Morgagni

Pectinate line →

Papillae   Crypts

Squamous Epithelium

FIGURE 10–5. Anatomy of the rectum and anal canal.

FLOW OF THE LUMINAL CONTENTS IN THE LARGE INTESTINE

Most of the information given above about wall motions comes from studies in experimental animals observed under laboratory conditions. The behavior described must apply to humans, but it cannot be fully confirmed because of the limitations in methods that can be used in the clinic. Most human studies have involved the study of flow.

Flow, the function most readily examined in humans, reflects the patterns of wall motions. Many studies of flow, using radiopaque solutions and markers, have shown that flow patterns vary along the large intestine. They indicate that flow is overall very slow. The proximal colon retains material that enters from the ileum for many hours, where it is churned and mixed. A single meal arrives in the region after 4 to 6 hours, depending on the volume and composition of the meal. Radiopaque markers shaped differently for each meal and ingested with the three sequential meals of a single day, pool there and escape in random sequence, out of the order in which they were ingested. They may not escape completely for 72 hours or more, and while they are retained they drift in position, suggesting that the mixing that takes place is thorough. The retention and prolonged mixing take place in the whole ascending colon, more at the cecal end than at the caudal end. This reservoir function of the ascending colon is evident to the colonoscopist who commonly finds retained matter and fluid when the colonoscope tip rounds the hepatic flexure in an otherwise well-prepared large intestine.

Marker studies similarly show that the progress of the luminal content caudal to the hepatic flexure is different from that of the ascending colon. The fecal mass in this region has become more solid, the consequence of the extraction of water that has occurred during its prolonged residence in the ascending colon, and there appears to be relatively less mixing. The fecal mass moves very slowly in an orderly but intermittent pattern. The segmental contractions, the haustral indentations, form, disappear, and re-form at intervals of hours, at positions that are not at fixed points on the colonic wall. These segmental contractions can push the luminal content either cephalad or caudad.

A purely propulsive contraction, the mass movement, is an infrequently observed event that probably occurs only two or three times daily. It is a rather quick event in which, first, the stationary segmental indentations, the haustral markings, disappear abruptly. Immediately, a column of the fecal mass is moved caudad, after which the haustral markings reappear. The discrepancy between this pattern of flow and that which would be expected from the occurrence of rhythmic orthograde peristalsis in the left colon is not readily explained. Probably, rhythmic orthograde peristalsis is often present, but its contractions are too shallow and intermittent, and the fecal mass too solid, for the effect of the peristalsis to be expressed as a continuous flow. The mass movement, which seems to be the major means for the caudad translocation of the fecal mass, clearly depends on a mechanism different from that of rhythmic peristalsis. Such a flow would, however, be expected from the massive powerful peristaltic contraction that can be evoked experimentally in the distal colon in animals by pelvic nerve stimulation.

Flow in the sigmoid colon and rectum has received rather little attention. A reservoir function of the rectum is well-recognized. Apparently, the rectum fills slowly, because digital examination uncommonly reveals a rectum that is completely filled with stool. It may fill quite suddenly just before defecation. Clearly, the reservoir function is not confined to the rectum. The margin between the rectal reservoir and the descending colon is indistinct. The rectal reservoir can retain its contents for a very long time, as a consequence both of its inertia and of the barrier to emptying provided by the anal sphincter. The emptying of the reservoir, a process that seems to be, to some degree, independent of motor operations in more rostral parts of the large intestine, is the process of defecation, which is described later.

Thus, overall, the varied nature of the large intestine is evident from the observation of the flow of its contents. The right colon has largely a reservoir and mixing function, necessary for the concentration of the fecal mass that results from the massive extraction of water that occurs in that region. The rectum acts as a reservoir, necessary for the regulated expulsion of the fecal mass. Between the hepatic flexure and the rectosigmoid junction, the colonic walls very slowly propel the fecal mass, usually orthograde, and knead it to facilitate further the extraction of water and to deliver to the rectum a fecal mass of suitable and consistent plasticity.

CONTROL OF MOTOR FUNCTIONS

Virtually all that we know of the controls of contractions in the colon comes from studies in laboratory animals. Most experimental species have a large intestine with the structure typical of carnivores, one that lacks the teniae and haustra that characterize the colon in humans and other primates. Given the magnitude of the anatomic differences, it is possible that the controls are somewhat different, but the differences are probably quantitative rather than qualitative.

Rhythmic Peristalsis in the Large Intestine: The Basis of its Rhythmicity and Direction of Movement

SLOW WAVES: PACEMAKERS OF RHYTHMIC PERISTALSIS[37-53]

The motor behavior of gut muscle varies greatly from region to region. Spontaneous rhythmic contractions, usually considered to be the general behavior of all gastrointestinal muscle, in fact characterizes only certain regions: the gastric antrum, the small intestine, and parts of the large intestine. The esophagus, the gastric fundus, the rectum, and the sphincters of the gut exhibit other forms of motor behavior.

In those regions that exhibit rhythmic peristalsis, an electrical signal can be detected in the muscular wall that serves as a pacemaker for the contractions. The component parts of this electrical signal have received several names. The terms used here are those that have come to be most widely used to describe the phenomenon.

The signal differs in details among the organs that exhibit rhythmic peristalsis.

Electrodes applied to the circular muscle layer in vitro record signals, slow fluctuations in electrical potential. From a stable baseline, electrical potential recorded at a single point rises and falls rhythmically. A relatively rapid depolarization to a plateau potential is followed by a repolarization to the basal level. The whole event, lasting several seconds, recurs at a reasonably constant rate. This recurring event is called the electrical slow wave (Fig 10-6).

When the rhythmic contractions of the circular muscle layer of the colon are recorded along with the slow waves, the rhythmic contractions always occur simultaneously with slow waves. If the contraction is very strong, one or more very rapid electrical transients, spike depolarizations, occur on the plateau of the slow wave, but many contractions occur without the spike depolarizations. The burst of rapid electrical transients is called the spike burst.

The slow waves in the colon recur over and over, while the muscle responds to only a small proportion of them by exhibiting a contraction. From this, it is concluded that the slow wave is a pacemaker that runs continuously to restrict the occurrence of contractions to particular short intervals of time.

Records of slow waves from several electrodes spaced closely together along the colon show that slow waves do not occur simultaneously at the separate points. Rather, they occur sequentially at adjacent points, moving along the long axis of the colon (Fig 10-7). In moving, they have a vector. Because they also restrict the occurrence of a contraction to a particular interval in space, their vector imposes a direction on the contractions that they pace. Thus, the slow wave is a pacemaker that determines both the spatial and the temporal patterns of rhythmic contractions.

An analogy with the cardiac action potential is obvious. The difference is that, in the heart, every cardiac action potential produces a contraction. Only some do so in the colon, and it is usually a small proportion, although the slow waves run constantly.

The vector of the slow wave differs in the proximal colon and distal colon. In the right colon, from the ileocolic junction to about the hepatic flexure, slow waves are oriented such that the vector is toward the ileocolic junction most of the time. They occur at a frequency of five to six cycles per minute and move without break

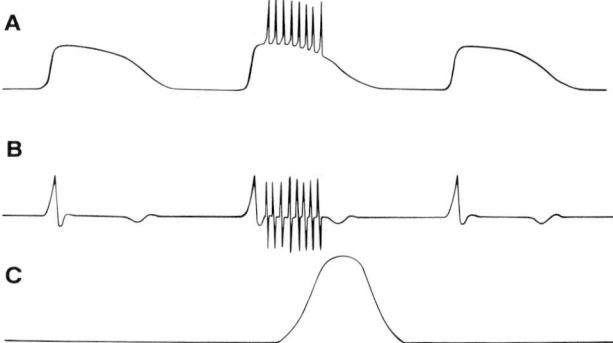

FIGURE 10–6. Diagram of three slow waves and a spike burst. **A** shows a record from an intracellular electrode. **B** shows the same record from an extracellular electrode. **C** shows the mechanical response of the muscle. The second slow wave carries a spike burst, which initiates a contraction.

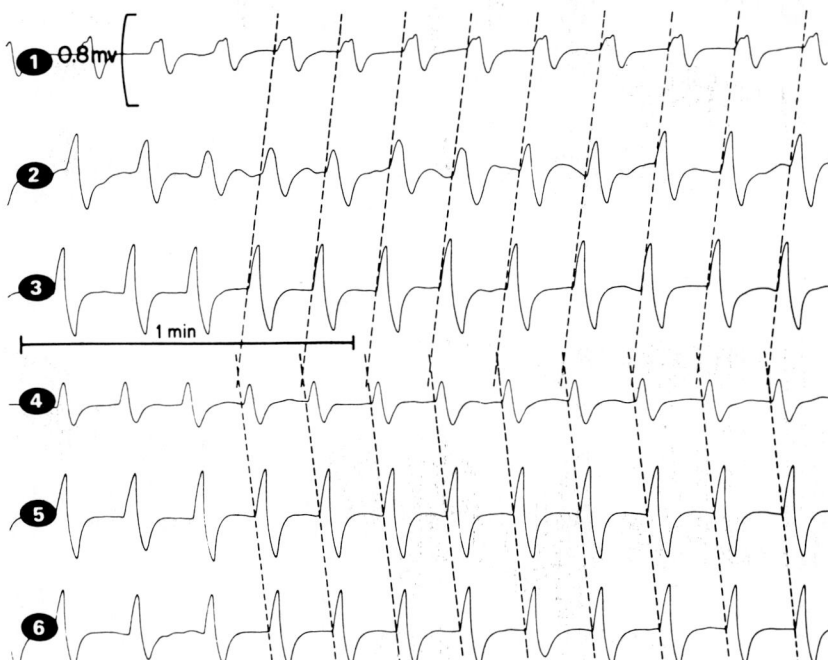

FIGURE 10–7. Slow waves recorded from the cat colon. Slow waves are recorded from six electrodes 1 cm apart in the ascending colon. *Dashed lines* show the temporal-spatial links of the slow waves. The signals arise from a pacemaker between electrodes 3 and 4. This record is devoid of spike bursts.

to the level of the ileocolic junction. This orientation of migration is not, however, constant. At intervals, slow waves reverse, to originate at the level of the ileocolic junction and sweep toward the hepatic flexure. It is as though the source point, away from which the slow waves spread, can move along the right colon, just as a wandering cardiac pacemaker can move. Thus, the slow wave mechanism explains the dominance of retrograde rhythmic peristalsis in the right colon and the retention of feces there. The capacity for reversal of polarity of slow waves also provides a means by which emptying of the region could take place.

In the left colon, the slow waves are oriented orthograde. Their frequency is about the same as in the right colon. Reversal of the vector seems to be rare. This vector is also consistent with the predominantly orthograde vector of rhythmic peristalsis in this region, and for the net orthograde flow.

ORIGIN OF SLOW WAVES AND SPIKE BURSTS[9,54]

The circular muscle layer of the colon was first thought to be the source of the slow waves, because slow waves were best recorded from electrodes applied to the submucosal surface of that layer or inserted into it. Hence, slow waves were once referred to as myogenic. It is now clear that they arise at the interface between the circular muscle layer and the submucosa. The plexus submucosus extremus, the plexus of neurites with abundant interstitial cells, lies on this surface. Evidence suggests that this plexus is actually involved in the generation and spread of the slow waves. The close linkages in this plexus between the neurites, the interstitial cells, and the superficial layer of circular muscle cells imply that the slow waves may arise in interactions of these three kinds of cells. The spread of slow waves through the muscle substance may take place in the gap junctions that join the muscle cells together.[55]

The spike burst, an infrequent event, is assumed to represent summed action potentials of the cells of the circular muscle layer as they contract. The fact that the muscle may contract without generating a spike burst is not surprising, because this is seen in the gastric antrum as well.

Nonrhythmic Peristalsis: Origin of the Mass Movement[56,57]

Mass movement seems to require a mechanism for nonrhythmic and highly intermittent peristalsis. A possible source for this has been revealed by colonic electromyography. Besides the slow waves and spike bursts, the colonic electromyogram exhibits another signal called the oscillation.[42] This signal is simultaneous with, but independent of, the slow waves. It is a high-frequency sinusoidal oscillation, much smaller in amplitude than the slow waves and of a much faster frequency, about 30 to 40 cycles per minute. It is intermittent, appearing in bursts, at its characteristic frequency, at intervals of minutes. These bursts move along the colon. They can move in both directions, but a caudad direction predominates. The oscillations carry spike bursts at times, each sinusoidal wave bearing a burst. The close spacing of the sinusoidal waves leads to spike bursts that are very prolonged, as long as the burst of oscillations, which may be 5 to 10 seconds or even more. When first observed,[42] this whole complex was called the migrating spike burst (Fig 10-8). Subsequently, it has received other names. A prolonged and powerful contraction accompanies these migrating spike bursts. The pattern of their occurrence suggests that these are the electrical expression of the intermittent nonrhythmic peristaltic contractions that accomplish mass movements. The oscillations arise at the outer face of the circular muscle layer, that which abuts the intermuscular space.

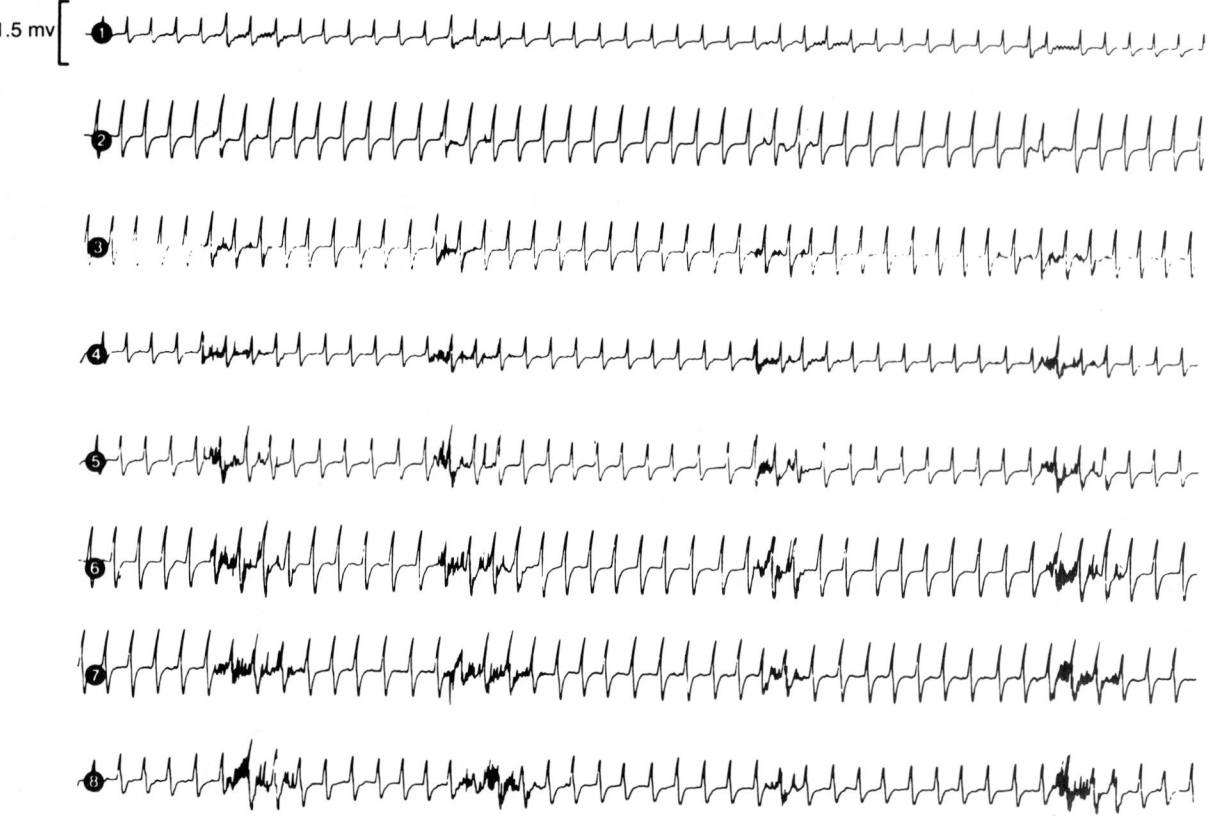

Proximal Colon–Normal

FIGURE 10–8. Colonic electromyogram containing a migrating spike burst. Slow waves are recorded from eight electrodes 2 cm apart from the cephalad half of the cat colon. Long bursts of rapid electrical transients recur at intervals of 1 to 1½ minutes, which progress distally. These are the migrating spike bursts.

Tone in Muscle Related to the Large Intestine

ORIGIN OF TONE IN SMOOTH MUSCLES OF THE LARGE INTESTINE

Tonic contraction in the large intestine characterizes the circular muscle layer at the haustral indentations and in the internal anal sphincter. The distinction between tonic and rhythmic smooth muscle in the gut is not absolute. Most smooth muscle exhibits some capacity for tonic contraction, and so the distinction is a matter of degree. But the distinction between tonic and rhythmic smooth muscle usually appears as though it were absolute, because smooth muscles exhibit either a high or a low capacity for tonic contraction. Those with a high capacity for tone correspondingly have a low capacity for rhythmic contraction. This implies that different mechanisms operate to generate the two kinds of contractions.

Tonic contraction must represent a maintained shortening of the muscle cells, because tone can be abolished by inhibitory drugs and by stimulation of inhibitory nerves. A maintained shortening of the contractile filament apparatus of the smooth muscle implies a concentration of calcium in the myoplasm that is maintained at a level sufficient to sustain the shortening. Evidence suggests that the internal calcium concentration in the internal anal sphincter is higher than that of rhythmic muscle of the large intestine, and similar observations have been made at the lower esophageal sphincter. This being the case, the question arises of the reason. Intracellular free calcium exists in a complex equilibrium with intracellular sites of calcium binding (mainly the smooth endoplasmic reticulum) and with the extracellular calcium, whose concentration is much greater. Thus, the myoplasmic concentration of free calcium could reflect several processes that affect this equilibrium, including the binding affinity at various intracellular storage sites and the fluxes of the ion across the cell membrane. These matters remain to be fully examined in tonic muscle of the large intestine.

The old teaching about the origin of tone in gut smooth muscle speculated that it occurs on the basis of a specialized innervation, either qualitative (a greater proportion of excitatory nerves) or quantitative (a denser total innervation). Neither postulate has found support in experimental evidence, although the morphology of the innervation of the internal anal sphincter remains to be adequately described.

ORIGIN OF TONE IN THE STRIATED MUSCLES THAT AFFECT LARGE INTESTINE FUNCTION

The actions of the external anal sphincter and the other striated muscles that make up the pelvic floor are related to bowel function only in defecation, but their normal operation is crucial to the process. The muscles resemble other somatic muscles in structure, although a thorough comparison remains to be made. They have a somatic innervation, like somatic muscle in general (i.e., the nerve cells that supply them lie in the anterior horns of the sacral cord). The cholinergic motor axons these cells provide traverse mainly the pudendal nerves. These axons terminate in motor end plates like those of all somatic muscle cells.

Tone in somatic muscle represents the constant excitation of the muscle by its somatic innervation (i.e., the source of tone is in the innervation rather than in the special properties of the striated muscle cells themselves).

The tone of the external anal sphincter has received the most study, but some degree of tone, probably less, characterizes the other striated muscles. This tone is not really constant, varying both spontaneously and in response to voluntary effort. It must be emphasized that this musculature, and its neural control, have received far less study than the analogous striated musculature at the other end of the gut, where striated muscles of the pharynx and neck also interface with gut smooth muscle. There may be some unique features of this pelvic floor musculature that remain to be found.

Autonomic Nerves: Their Regulation of Motor Function in the Large Intestine[58-70]

CLASSES OF THE NERVES: A GENERAL STATEMENT

Several different sets of terms find application to the description of the autonomic innervation of the gut. The adjectives *extrinsic* and *intrinsic* refer to the location of the nerve cell bodies, respectively outside and inside the large intestinal wall. The adjectives *thoracolumbar* and *craniosacral* refer to the levels at which tracts involving extrinsic nerves reach the central nervous system. Those tracts that connect to the cranial and sacral levels of the neuraxis are morphologically and functionally similar, hence the combined adjective. The same reasoning applies to those that join the spinal cord at thoracic and lumbar levels.

The adjectives *sympathetic* and *parasympathetic* are commonly used as synonyms for thoracolumbar and craniosacral, respectively. In the designation of functional types of motor fibers, adjectives describe the neurotransmitter released from the axon terminals. Thus, besides the familiar and specific terms, cholinergic and noradrenergic, there are newer specific terms, like dopaminergic and serotoninergic, and less specific terms, like peptidergic.

A major observation of the past 20 years is that the principal inhibitory innervation of gut smooth muscle is one whose transmitter is unknown.[40] Many candidate substances exist, but none has been established. The most prominent candidate neurotransmitters are some of the more than 20 biologically active peptides found in the gut wall, especially vasoactive intestinal polypeptide (VIP), and the purine nucleotides. Thus, terms like VIP-ergic and purinergic also appear. In fact, these important and cryptic inhibitory nerves may well include motor axons of several kinds, releasing several different candidate transmitter substances. The full identification of the transmitters of these inhibitory nerves constitutes a major contemporary challenge. Because no transmitter for these inhibitory nerves has yet been convincingly established, it seems best to use a noncommittal adjective to allude to them. They were called, when first discovered, the nonadrenergic noncholinergic inhibitory nerves, an awkward term that is most conveniently abbreviated to the NANC inhibitory nerves.

GENERAL NEURAL EFFECTS ON SMOOTH MUSCLE FUNCTION IN THE LARGE INTESTINE

Both the enhancement and the suppression of contractions can be effected in smooth muscle of the gut by the nerves that supply it. The effect is not one of the magnitude of contraction alone. In rhythmically active muscle, the effect may appear as well in the frequency of contractions or relaxations.

The effects are, in most cases, graded effects producing a range of responses from complete inhibition to maximal activity. In other cases, they are switch-effects, the response being all or none. This latter mode of operation characterizes the esophagus where nerves normally modulate a quite stereotyped, ungraded, and complex series of contractions and relaxations. An all-or-none effect seems, as well, to describe the similarly complex operations that take place in the most caudal parts of the large intestine and in the extraintestinal musculature in the process of defecation.

On the average, the nerves of the large intestine are inhibitory. The evidence for this broad statement is very simple. The toxin that makes the Pacific puffer fish poisonous is a neurotoxin, tetrodotoxin. This neurotoxin blocks the sodium channel that normally opens as the initial event in the neural action potential. Because the activation of smooth muscle does not require such a change in membrane permeability to sodium, the exposure of a smooth muscle preparation to tetrodotoxin selectively blocks neural effects. When tetrodotoxin is applied to muscle of the colon (of cat and other experimental animals), the colon is thrown into violent rhythmic contraction, approaching the maximum of which it is capable. This is the evidence that indicates that the effect of the nerves that supply the smooth muscle of the colon is, in the sum, tonic inhibition. This effect of tetrodotoxin on colonic muscle contrasts strikingly with its effect on muscle of other organs, where such excitation is not prominent.

If powerful sustained inhibition, exerted by the nerves, dominates the large intestinal smooth muscle for most of the time, contraction could come about either through disinhibition, the release of the tonic neurogenic inhibition, or by activation of excitatory nerves. Probably both mechanisms operate, but the consequence would be the same in both cases.

Intrinsic nerves can be selectively excited in vitro by the technique of electrical field stimulation of strips of the colon wall in vitro. The use of selective antagonists to the known neural transmitters in such studies can provide an indication of the kinds of nerves being stimulated. The limited studies of this sort that have been done in the large intestine indicate that the nerves capable of exciting the smooth muscle of the organ are largely cholinergic. Another kind of excitatory motor nerve was detected by this technique in human colonic tissue. It releases some transmitter that is not acetylcholine. All the inhibitory nerves revealed by this technique are NANC inhibitory nerves.

Adrenergic nerves are present in the colonic myenteric plexus where such fibers are conspicuous, but they are sparse in the muscle layers themselves. Norepinephrine inhibits the release of acetylcholine from this plexus. These two observations suggest that the function of the adrenergic innervation of the large intestine lies mostly in the regulation of the activity of the myenteric plexus.

Other kinds of nerves are present in the colon wall where they may serve sensory or internuncial functions. The evidence for the existence of such other classes of nerves constitutes morphologic or biochemical studies in which substances associated with nerves in general are sought in the colonic wall. These substances include VIP, gamma-aminobutyric acid (GABA), serotonin, somatostatin, Leu-enkephalin, and cholecystokinin.

NEURAL EFFECTS ON THE PATTERNS OF CONTRACTIONS IN RHYTHMIC MUSCLE OF THE LARGE INTESTINE

The patterns of origin and the spread of the electrical slow waves dictate the patterns of spread of the peristaltic contractions. These slow waves are not constant in respect to these patterns. Recent evidence indicates that the frequency of colonic slow waves is reduced by the stimulation of intrinsic nerves. This raises the possibility that the frequency and pattern of migration of peristaltic contractions may also be affected by intrinsic nerves.

NEURAL EFFECTS ON THE INTERNAL ANAL SPHINCTER

Tonic contraction of the internal anal sphincter is largely myogenic, as described above, representing a special property of the sphincteric muscle. The magnitude of the tonic contraction is graded. Enhancement of the force can be accomplished by excitatory cholinergic nerves, and a reduction by NANC nerves.

EXTRINSIC NERVES AND COLONIC MOTILITY

Electrical stimulation of the nerves that connect the large intestine to the central nervous system can be used to suggest the physiologic distribution of extrinsic nerves to the colon and the net effect of such nerves (which are always mixed in fiber content). The few such studies that have been done confirm conclusions about the distribution of extrinsic nerves made from anatomic studies, and about the effects of different classes of nerve fibers. Thus, lumbar sympathetic nerves go to all parts of the colon and exert both excitatory and inhibitory effects. The vagus is excitatory mainly to the right colon. The splanchnic nerves inhibit mainly the right colon. Excitatory and inhibitory effects result from electrical

stimulation of the hypothalamus and other parts of the brain known to contain nuclei related to the visceral autonomic innervation.

COLO-COLONIC REFLEXES

In the small intestine, a localized distention causes contraction above and relaxation below the level of distention. This peristaltic reflex makes use of intramural pathways in the myenteric plexus. Similar responses occur after localized stimulation in the colon, but they seem to be much more difficult to demonstrate, and they seem to differ among species. It seems likely that the reflex is not exactly like that in the small intestine. The reflex responses make use, in part, of the long tracts that exist in the shunt fascicles or ascending colonic nerves.

Hormonal Regulation of Large Intestinal Motor Function[71-73]

ENTERIC HORMONES

The enteric hormones, mostly polypeptides, are found in high concentration in the gut wall. They are potent in their actions on effector structures in the gut wall. These two facts suggest that they are synthesized, stored, and released locally to act either locally or after systemic circulation. Substances produced and acting locally are called paracrine agents, to distinguish them from substances that act only after systemic circulation, endocrine agents. There are many such substances, some excitatory and others inhibitory, and they affect the operation of the epithelium, intraneural nerves, blood vessels, and muscular tissues. Their actions may explain behavioral patterns of the gut, which do not find ready explanation in the known characteristics of the nerves or the effector tissues themselves.

In the large intestine, speculation on peptide function has been less rampant than elsewhere in the gut. Many enteric hormones are found in the large intestinal wall, and they exert powerful effects on the colonic muscle.

NONENTERIC HORMONES AND LARGE INTESTINAL MOTOR FUNCTION

Hormones that arise outside the gut itself might also affect large intestinal function. Cholecystokinin, a peptide released from the mucosa of the duodenum, is the principal systemic hormone thought to affect colonic motor function, mainly in respect to the excitation of the colonic muscle that follows eating.

Constipation is a well-known feature of pregnancy. The usual explanation for the constipation, a mechanical obstruction from the enlarged uterus, seems unlikely to be the whole reason, because constipation may occur early in pregnancy. Furthermore, the enlargement of the uterus occurs not so much in the pelvis, where the sacrum offers a rigid mass against which the soft rectum could be compressed, but more in the abdomen where the displacement of the soft anterior abdominal wall and other intraabdominal viscera should prevent passive occlusion of the colonic lumen. A better explanation could lie in the hormonal changes that occur in pregnancy. The pregnant state is associated with depressed smooth muscle function in other parts of the gut, and there is no reason to exclude the large intestinal muscle from such a depressant effect. A reduced closure force in the lower esophageal sphincter, delayed gastric emptying, and delayed emptying of the gallbladder all occur in pregnancy. The widespread changes could reflect a general effect of the gonadal hormones on the smooth muscle of the gut.

SOME INTEGRATED COLONIC FUNCTIONS

Defecation and Rectal Continence[36]

Defecation involves the coordinated operation of a variety of systems, some outside the large intestine. From this, it is clear that the central nervous system controls the process in part. The mechanism is largely known through observations in humans, rather than studies in animals, so the process can only be described in rather gross terms, not in details.

The rectum probably fills gradually. At some point, the sensation of the possibility for defecation arises from sensory receptors located in the wall of the large intestine. Mechanoreceptors, sensitive to distention and to motion, presumably are responsible. The location of these mechanoreceptors is not clear. The mucosa may contain such receptors as well as the deeper layers of the gut wall. Evidence of their presence has been demonstrated physiologically, but structural studies have failed to demonstrate a specific morphology. Their abundance or sensitivity is greater distally, at the lower end of the rectum, near the anal canal, than higher in the rectum.

Structures having the morphology of known cutaneous sensory receptors lie in the anal canal, in the part lined by squamous epithelium caudad to the pectinate line.[28,29] A very dense innervation lies here, with free nerve endings having the morphology of Golgi-Mazzoni, Krause's, Meissner's, Pacini's, and genital corpuscles. Such endings do not occur in the glandular mucosa above the pectinate line.

These anal canal receptors could be wholly responsible for the sensation of the readiness for defecation. When the rectum is filled, the anal canal is everted in the rostral direction. Receptors in the canal would thus be exposed to the pressure in the rectum and to the chemical constituents of its contents.

Relaxation, or loss of tone, of the internal anal sphincter results from rectal distention. This effect, clinically elicited as a test for the integrity of the innervation of the area, is mediated by NANC inhibitory nerves. The pathways for this reflex could be both central (involving extrinsic neural structures) and intrinsic to the gut wall. The response has a threshold and quickly reaches a maximum as the intensity of the stimulus is increased. Thus, it is more like a switch effect, an all-or-none response, than a graded response.

As the tone of the internal sphincter falls, the normal barrier to rectal evacuation disappears. A compensatory contraction in the striated muscle of the external anal sphincter can be induced to replace the barrier. This requires the activation of the somatic innervation that this muscle receives. Contraction of the external anal sphincter is a centrally mediated process and under voluntary control.

Contractions of the smooth muscle in the walls of the rectum and sigmoid colon follow the initiation of the defecatory reflex. These are involuntary contractions, mediated by the excitation of nerves. The powerful lumen-occluding contraction seems to resemble that which produces the mass movement that occurs in more rostral parts of the colon. It could have its origin in relation to the sinusoidal oscillations and spike bursts called the migrating spike burst described above, but this has not been demonstrated. This evacuating contraction seems not to develop immediately, only after the act of defecation has been initiated.

The act of defecation involves familiar voluntary maneuvers that include contraction of the abdominal wall muscles in straining against a closed glottis. The voluntary nature of such efforts, which depend on the perception of the need for defecation, indicate that the involved part of the central nervous system includes higher centers in the forebrain.

The urge to defecate can be resisted, and the action can be deferred. This involves mainly voluntary contraction of the external anal sphincter and other striated muscles of the pelvic floor, as well as conscious suppression of the urge to raise the intraabdominal pressure against a closed glottis. Such voluntary efforts constitute the mechanism of rectal continence.

Motor Response of the Large Intestine to Eating[72,74]

Motor activity in the large intestine increases for up to about an hour after eating. This effect, a matter of common experience that is supported by radiographic and manometric observations, is commonly called the gastrocolic reflex. This term is unfortunate, because it is inaccurate on three points. The stimulus does not arise from the stomach, the response is not confined to the colon, and its mechanism is not necessarily a neural reflex.

The source of the stimulus seems to be the small intestine, because exclusion of the esophagus and stomach from the food stream does not prevent the effect. The receptors initiating the response, whether chemoreceptors or mechanoreceptors, have not been localized more specifically.

The response is not confined to the colon, but concurrently affects the small intestine. The whole colon is involved in the response, that of the left colon somewhat exceeding that of the right.

The mechanism of the effect is obscure. If it is a neural reflex, the pathways do not require an intact vagus, an intact spinal cord, or intact splanchnic nerves. A better case can be made for the theory that the effect is hormonally mediated. The onset of the response is slow, and it exhibits an early peak and a later peak in magnitude. Current theories suggest cholecystokinin release as the mediator of the effect, and some have speculated about gastrin. Several other hormones, however, are released from the gut after eating, and these others seem to have been relatively left out of consideration. If the mechanism is hormonal, the hormone may act either on colonic muscle directly or on the nerves that supply the muscle. If the action of the hormone is on nerves, it could represent either the stimulation of excitatory nerves to the smooth muscle or the release of a tonic neurogenic inhibition.

Effects of the Emotions on Large Intestinal Motor Function

Anxiety is widely considered to affect the motor function of the large intestine. Furthermore, the anatomic and physiologic evidence that indicates that the forebrain is involved in defecation establishes a scientific substrate on which such a belief can be based. Direct experimental evidence for such an effect has been hard to obtain, however. Two problems restrict investigation of the question. First, anxiety and stress are difficult to define, to create, and to measure objectively. Second, the intact colon is not easily approached by motility-sensing methods that can be made objective and quantitative and that allow prolonged study. Hence, an effect of emotions on motor function in the large intestine remains to be fully demonstrated.

THERAPEUTIC AGENTS: THEIR EFFECTS ON COLONIC MOTOR FUNCTION

Autonomic Agonists and Antagonists[61,33,53,75]

Highly selective drugs that affect transmission at autonomic synapses find wide use in therapy. The α-adrenoceptor agonists used in vitro generally excite contractions in the circular muscle layer and inhibit them in the longitudinal layer. The β-adrenoceptor agonists and dopamine are inhibitory. The adrenoreceptor antagonists used in therapy in cardiovascular disease generally have no major effect on colonic motility.

Atropine and other antagonists of muscarinic cholinergic transmission inhibit contractions in the smooth muscle of the large intestine in vitro. In practice, they are often used in the attempt to treat symptoms presumed to represent abnormal colonic contractions. The objective evidence that they significantly depress colonic motility in reasonable therapeutic doses is not wholly convincing. The effect, if present at all, is rather small and transient, even in vitro.

Laxatives

Laxatives are among the most widely used drugs. Many are purely osmotic agents, increasing the bulk of the stool by increasing its water content. If such agents affect colonic motility, they do so only through the means by which the motility of the colon changes in response to an increased intraluminal volume. How motility changes with an increased load remains to be shown, and the mechanism of the effect remains unknown.

Other laxatives are considered to be "contact" or "irritant" agents, acting not through osmotic effects but through direct stimulation of contractions of the colonic neuromuscular system. "Natural" laxatives are among these, extracts of various plants (aloes, senna) that contain anthraquinones. The colonic bacteria degrade anthraquinones to produce a dark pigment that is taken up and retained by the mucosal macrophages to produce melanosis coli in long-term users of such agents. Furthermore, there is evidence that the prolonged abuse of such laxatives damages the cells of the colonic myenteric plexus, to produce the atonic colon of the "laxative colon." These observations indicate that some laxative components, perhaps the anthraquinones themselves, cross the colonic epithelium and affect the intramural nerves. It is unknown what kinds of nerves they affect, or how their function is altered.

Ricinoleic acid, 12-hydroxyoleic acid, is the laxative principal of castor oil. This substance has two actions that could explain its laxative effect. In very low concentrations in vitro, and in vivo, it interrupts the orderly spread of slow waves in the colon and disrupts the orderly progression of rhythmic peristalsis. It also stimulates the secretion of water by the colonic epithelium.

OPIATES[76]

The constipating effect of opiate drugs is familiar and commonly taken advantage of in therapy. Morphine excites contractions of colonic muscle in vitro. This excitation is due partly to the excitation of cholinergic motor nerves, partly to the suppression of NANC inhibitory nerves and partly to a direct excitation of the smooth muscle. Some of the excitatory effect probably also represents an action of morphine on control centers in the brain stem.

The reader is directed to Chapter 1, The Enteric Nervous System and its Extrinsic Connections; Chapter 2, Gastrointestinal Hormones; Chapter 3, The Brain–Gut Axis; Chapter 4, Smooth Muscle of the Gut; Chapter 25, Pharmacology of the Gastrointestinal Tract; Chapter 39, Approach to the Patient with Constipation; Chapter 76, Colon: Anatomy and Structural Anomalies; Chapter 80, Irritable Bowel Syndrome; Chapter 81, Motility Disorders of the Colon; and Chapter 85, Anorectal Diseases.

REFERENCES

1. Stevens CE. The Mammalian Digestive Tract. In: Comparative Physiology of the Vertebrate Digestive System. Cambridge: Cambridge University Press, 1988.
2. Bennett A. Symposium on colonic function. Pharmacology of colonic muscle. Gut 1975;16:307.
3. Christensen J. Motility of the colon. In: Johnson LR, ed. Physiology of the gastrointestinal tract. New York: Raven Press, 1981:445.
4. Christensen J. The colon. In: Christensen J, Wingate DL, eds. A guide to gastrointestinal motility. Bristol: Wright-PSG, 1983:198.
5. Christensen J. Motility of the colon. In: Johnson, LR, ed. Physiology of the gastrointestinal tract, ed 2. New York: Raven Press, 1987:665.
6. Connell AM. Motor action of the large bowel. In: Code CF, ed. Handbook of physiology, Section 6: Alimentary canal; Volume IV: Motility. Washington, DC: American Physiological Society, 1968: 2075.
7. Daniel EE. Symposium on colonic function. Electrophysiology of the colon. Gut 1975;16:298.
8. Garry RC. The movements of the large intestine. Physiol Rev 1934;14: 103.
9. Stach W. Der plexus entericus extremus des Dickdarmes und seine

Beziehungen zu den interstitiellen Zellen (Cajal). Z Mikrosk-Anat Forsch 1972;85:245.

10. Pace JL. The age of appearance of the haustra of the human colon. J Anat 1971;109:75.

11. Bayliss WM, Starling EH. The movements and the innervation of the large intestine. J Physiol (Lond) 1900;26:107.

12. Connell AM. The motility of the pelvic colon. II. Paradoxical motility in diarrhea and constipation. Gut 1962;3:342.

13. Connell AM, Lennard-Jones JE, Madanagopalan N. The distribution of faecal x-ray shadows in subjects without gastro-intestinal disease. Proc R Soc Med 1964;57:894.

14. Deller DJ, Wangel AG. Intestinal motility in man. I. A study combining the use of intraluminal pressure recording and cineradiography. Gastroenterology 1965;48:45.

15. Elliott TR, Barclay-Smith E. Antiperistalsis and other muscular activities of the colon. J Physiol (Lond) 1904;31:272.

16. Gramiak R, Ross P, Olmsted WW. Normal motor activity of the human colon: Combined radiotelemetric manometry and slow-frame cineroentgenography. Am J Roent Rad Ther Nucl Med 1971;113:301.

17. Hertz AF, Newton A. The normal movements of the colon in man. J Physiol (Lond) 1913;47:57.

18. Holdstock DJ, Misiewicz JJ, Smith T, Rowlands EN. Propulsion (mass movement) in the human colon and its relationship to meals and somatic activity. Gut 1970;11:91.

19. Holzknecht G. Die normale Peristaltik des Colon. Munch Med Wochenschr 1909;56:2401.

20. Kock NG, Hulten L, Leander L. A study of the motility in different parts of the human colon. Resting activity, response to feeding and to prostigmine. Scand J Gastroenterol 1968;3:163.

21. Misiewicz JJ, Connell AM, Pontes FA. Comparison of the effect of meals and prostigmine on the proximal and distal colon in patients with and without diarrhoea. Gut 1966;7:468.

22. Ritchie JA, Ardran GM, Truelove SC. Motor activity of the sigmoid colon of humans. A combined study by intraluminal pressure recording and cineradiography. Gastroenterology 1962;43:642.

23. Truelove SC. Movements of the large intestine. Physiol Res 1966;46:457.

24. Bouvier M, Gonella J. Nervous control of the internal anal sphincter of the cat. J Physiol (Lond) 1984;310:457.

25. Burleigh DE. Non-cholinergic non-adrenergic inhibitory neurons in human internal anal sphincter muscle. J Pharm Pharmacol 1983;35:258.

26. Costa M, Furness JB. The innervation of the internal anal sphincter of the guinea-pig. In: Daniel EE, ed. Proceedings of the Fourth International Symposium on Gastrointestinal Motility, Vancouver: Mitchell Press, 1974:681.

27. Denny-Brown D, Robertson EG. An investigation of the nervous control of defecation. Brain 1935;58:256.

28. Duthie HL, Bennett RC. The relation of sensation in the anal canal to the functional anal sphincter: A possible factor in anal continence. Gut 1963;4:179.

29. Duthie HL, Gairns FW. Sensory nerve-endings and sensation in the anal region of man. Br J Surg 1960;47:585.

30. Duthie HL, Watts JM. Contribution of the external anal sphincter to the pressure zone in the anal canal. Gut 1965;6:64.

31. Frenckner B, Euler C von. Influence of pudendal block on the function of the anal sphincters. Gut 1975;16:482.

32. Frenckner B, Ihre T. Influence of autonomic nerves on the internal anal sphincter in man. Gut 1976;17:306.

33. Friedmann CA. The action of nicotine and catecholamines on the human internal anal sphincter. Am J Dig Dis 1968;13:428.

34. Garrett JR, Howard ER, Jones W. The internal anal sphincter in the cat: A study of nervous mechanisms affecting tone and reflex activity. J Physiol (Lond) 1974;243:153.

35. Goligher JC, Hughes ESR. Sensibility of the rectum and colon: Its role in the mechanism of anal continence. Lancet 1951;1:543.

36. Phillips SF, Edwards DAW. Some aspects of anal continence and defaecation. Gut 1965;6:396.

37. Anuras S, Chien SM, Christensen J. Metabolic dependence of the electromyogram of the cat colon. Am J Physiol 1980;239(Gastrointest Liver Physiol):G173.

38. Anuras S, Christensen J. Effects of autonomic drugs on cat colonic muscle. Am J Physiol 1981;240:G361.

39. Caprilli R, Onori L. Origin, transmission and ionic dependence of colonic electrical slow waves. Scand J Gastroenterol 1972;7:65.

40. Christensen J. The controls of gastrointestinal movements: Some old and new views. N Engl J Med 1971;285:85.

41. Christensen J, Anuras S, Arthur C. Influence of intrinsic nerves on electromyogram of cat colon in vitro. Am J Physiol 1978;234:E641.

42. Christensen J, Anuras S, Hauser RL. Migrating spike burst and electrical slow waves in the cat colon: Effect of sectioning. Gastroenterology 1974;66:240.

43. Christensen J, Caprilli R, Lund GF. Electric slow waves in circular muscle of cat colon. Am J Physiol 1969;217:771.

44. Christensen J, Freeman BW. Circular muscle electromyogram in the cat colon: Local effect of sodium ricinoleate. Gastroenterology 1972;63:1011.

45. Christensen J, Hauser RL. Longitudinal axial coupling of slow waves in circular muscle of the cat colon. Am J Physiol 1971;221:1033.

46. Christensen J, Weisbrodt NW, Hauser RL. Electrical slow waves of the proximal colon of the cat in diarrhea. Gastroenterology 1972;62:1167.

47. Couturier D, Roze C, Couturier-Turpin MH, Debray C. Electromyography of the colon in situ: An experimental study in man and in the rabbit. Gastroenterology 1969;56:317.

48. Durdle NG, Kingma YJ, Bowes KL, Chambers MM. Origin of slow waves in the canine colon. Gastroenterology 1983;84:375.

49. El-Sharkawy TY. Electrical activity of the muscle layers of the canine colon. J Physiol (Lond) 1983;342:67.

50. Huizenga JD, Diamant NE, El-Sharkawy TY. Electrical basis of contractions in the muscle layers of the pig colon. Am J Physiol 1983;245:G482.

51. Huizenga JD, Stern H, Diamant NE, El-Sharkawy TY. The relationship between slow electrical oscillatory activity, spikes, and contractions in human colonic circular muscle. Gastroenterology 1984;86:1119.

52. Smith TK, Reed JB, Sanders KM. Interaction of two electrical pacemakers in muscularis of canine proximal colon. Am J Physiol 1987;252:C290.

53. Wienbeck M, Christensen J. Effects of some drugs on electrical activity of the isolated colon of the cat. Gastroenterology 1971;61:470.

54. Shearin NL, Bowes KL, Kingma YJ. In vitro electrical activity in canine colon. Gut 1978;20:780.

55. Gabella G, Blundell D. Gap junctions of the muscles of the small and large intestine. Cell Tissue Res 1981;219:469.

56. Ritchie JA. Movement of segmental constrictions in the human colon. Gut 1971;12:350.

57. Ritchie JA. Mass peristalsis in the human colon after contact with oxyphenisatin. Gut 1972;13:211.

58. Bianchi C, Beani L, Frigo GM, Crema A. Further evidence for the presence of non-adrenergic inhibitory structures in the guinea-pig colon. Eur J Pharmacol 1968;4:51.

59. Christensen J, Rick GA, Robison BA, Stiles MJ, Wix MA. Arrangement of the myenteric plexus throughout the gastrointestinal tract of the opossum. Gastroenterology 1983;85:890.

60. Christensen J, Stiles MJ, Rick GA, Sutherland J. Comparative anatomy of the myenteric plexus of the distal colon in eight mammals. Gastroenterology 1984;86:706.

61. Crema A, Del Tacca M, Frigo GM, Lecchini S. Presence of a non-adrenergic inhibitory system in the human colon. Gut 1968;9:633.

62. Fukai K, Fukuda H. The intramural pelvic nerves in the colon of dogs. J Physiol (Lond) 1984;354:89.

63. Furness JB. The presence of inhibitory nerves in the colon after sympathetic denervation. Eur J Pharmacol 1969;6:349.

64. Furness JB. An electrophysiological study of the innervation of the smooth muscle of the colon. J Physiol (Lond) 1969;205:549.

65. Gillespie JS. The electrical and mechanical responses of intestinal smooth muscle to stimulation of their extrinsic parasympathetic nerves. J Physiol (Lond) 1962;162:76.

66. Hulten L, Jodal M. Extrinsic nervous controls of colonic motility. Acta Physiol Scan (Suppl) 1969;335:21.

67. Jule Y. Nerve-mediated descending inhibition in the proximal colon of the rabbit. J Physiol (Lond) 1980;309:487.

68. Kuo DC, Hisamitsu T, De Groat WC. A sympathetic projection from

sacral paravertebral ganglion to the pelvic nerve and to postganglionic nerves on the surface of the urinary bladder and large intestine of the cat. J Comp Neurol 1984;226:76.

69. Rostad H. Colonic motility in the cat. II. Extrinsic nervous control. Acta Physiol Scand 1973;89:91.

70. Stach W. Uber die in der Dickdarmwand aszendierenden Nerven des Plexus pelvinus und die Grenze der vagalen und sakralparasympathetischen Innervation. Z Mikrosk-Anat Forsch 1971;84:65.

71. Bennett A, Misiewicz JJ, Waller SL. Analysis of the motor effects of gastrin and pentagastrin on the human alimentary tract in vitro. Gut 1967;8:470.

72. Connell AM, Logan CJH. The role of gastrin in gastroileocolic responses. Am J Dig Dis 1967;12:277.

73. Harvey RF, Read AE. Effect of cholecystokinin on colonic motility and symptoms in patients with the irritable-bowel syndrome. Lancet 1973;1:1.

74. Snape WJ Jr, Wright SH, Battle WM, Cohen S. The gastrocolic response: Evidence for a neural mechanism. Gastroenterology 1979;77: 1235.

75. Gagnon DJ, Devroede G, Belisle S. Excitatory effects of adrenaline upon isolated preparations of human colon. Gut 1972;13:654.

76. Sun EA, Snape WJ Jr, Cohen J, Renny A. The role of opiate receptors and cholinergic neurons in the gastrocolonic response. Gastroenterology 1982;82:689.

11

Motility of the Biliary Tree

JAMES P. RYAN

GALLBLADDER MOTILITY

Bile is a complex mixture of water and inorganic and organic solutes that is secreted continuously by the liver. During the interdigestive period, about one half of the hepatic bile is stored in the gallbladder, with the remaining flow delivered directly into the duodenum.[1] In addition to serving as a storage reservoir, it is now well recognized that the gallbladder undergoes cyclic periods of emptying and refilling during the interdigestive period. During the ingestion of a meal, the gallbladder undergoes a brief period of rapid emptying, followed by a more prolonged slower period of emptying. The purpose of this chapter is to review the changes in gallbladder and sphincter of Oddi motility necessary to promote the delivery of bile into the small intestine and to discuss the neural and hormonal factors believed to be involved in the control and regulation of biliary tract motility.

Interdigestive Period

"In the interdigestive period the resistance to bile flow through the sphincter of Oddi exceeds the pressure within the bile duct and, as a result, bile is diverted into the gallbladder. Because of the large absorptive capacity of the gallbladder, as well as the distensibility of the muscular sac, the intraluminal pressure remains low and only rarely are conditions suitable for the delivery of bile into the duodenum."[2] This quote from an earlier review on biliary tract motility reflected the popular belief that no significant motor activity occurs within the gastrointestinal tract during the interdigestive period. In more recent years, however, it has become evident that this assumption is not correct. Considerable data now exist to support the idea that during fasting the gastrointestinal tract exhibits a characteristic pattern of recurrent excitatory myoelectric activity that propagates distally from the esophagus to the terminal ileum and has been called the "migrating myoelectric complex" (MMC).[3-5] Associated with the increased myoelectric activity is an increased phasic contractile activity called the "migrating motor complex." It is believed that the function of this increased motor activity is to propel undigested residue from the proximal bowel to the terminal ileum, that is, that it serves a "housekeeping" function.[3]

In contrast to our knowledge of the motor activity of the stomach and small bowel during fasting, little is known concerning the motor activity of the gallbladder during the interdigestive period, particularly in humans. As noted, until recently it was generally believed that little or no gallbladder emptying occurred between meals. Any bile delivery into the duodenum during the interdigestive period was believed to be of hepatic origin.[6] However, recent work by Itoh and associates [7-11] and by other investigators[12-14] using animal models clearly indicates that the gallbladder evidences periods of increased rhythmic fluctuations in intraluminal pressure during the interdigestive period and that the pressure changes are associated with the intermittent delivery of bile into the duodenum.

In their initial study, Itoh and associates[7] simultaneously and continuously monitored the interdigestive contractile activity of the gallbladder, stomach, and proximal small bowel in conscious dogs by means of chronically implanted force transducers. A representative recording of the data they obtained is shown in Figure 11-1. They observed that the gallbladder regularly contracted in association with phase II of the MMC. Periodic gallbladder contractions also could be observed in the absence of any obvious increase in antral or duodenal motility. However, when all three contractile activities were present the rise in gallbladder pressure characteristically began within 1 to 2 minutes of the initiation of phase II contractile activity, reached a maximum within 5 minutes, and returned to basal levels prior to the cessation of motor activity in the antrum and duodenum. The magnitude of the gallbladder contraction during the interdigestive period did not differ significantly from that observed during the postprandial period.

These results demonstrate that the interdigestive period is characterized by periodic increases in the intraluminal pressure of the gallbladder. The authors assumed that the rise in pressure developed as a consequence of an increase in the contractile activity of the gallbladder. However, they could not rule out the possibility that periodic increases in sphincter of Oddi resistance contributed to the observed results. In an attempt to resolve this issue they measured the concentration of bilirubin and sodium in gallbladder bile during the interdigestive period and correlated the changes to the periodic contractile activity of the gallbladder.[8,9] Their findings are presented in Figure 11-2 and can be summarized as follows: (1) the bilirubin concentration increased during the interdigestive period, not in a linear fashion but in a series of stepped arcs; (2) the peak bilirubin concentration coincided with phase III of the antral and duodenal MMCs (shown by shaded line in Figure 11-2); (3) on termination of antral and duodenal motor activity bilirubin concentration first declined and then began to increase to

a higher concentration than in the previous cycle; and (4) gallbladder bile sodium concentrations decreased in parallel with bilirubin. Although the authors did not directly measure the bile input into the duodenum or gallbladder emptying, they concluded that their findings are best explained by assuming a cyclic pattern of gallbladder contraction and relaxation. They proposed that during relaxation there is a large inflow of hepatic bile into the gallbladder, with the result that there is a marked decrease in the concentration of sodium and bilirubin in the gallbladder bile.

Direct evidence that the rise in gallbladder pressure during the interdigestive period is associated with gallbladder contraction and the delivery of bile into the duodenum has been provided by Traynor and co-workers[14] and by Scott and colleagues.[13] Both groups reported a temporal relation between the transient elevation in gallbladder pressure that occurs during phase II of the MMC and the delivery of bile acids into the duodenum. Traynor and co-workers[14] used conscious dogs with chronic indwelling gallbladder and duodenal catheters to quantify gallbladder pressure and emptying and to relate these to the delivery of bile into the duodenum during the interdigestive period. They observed that during phase II of the MMC there was a transient increase in intragallbladder pressure that resulted in a 20% emptying of the gallbladder and the flow of bile into the duodenum. Scott and colleagues,[13] using a radiolabeled taurocholate infusion technique, were able to demonstrate that the bile acids delivered into the duodenum represented gallbladder and not hepatic bile. More recently, Takahashi and associates[15] have shown that gallbladder emptying in the opossum also evidences a cyclic pattern synchronous with phase II of the intestinal MMC.

It is now well documented that bile flow into the duodenum in humans also evidences a cyclic pattern during the interdigestive

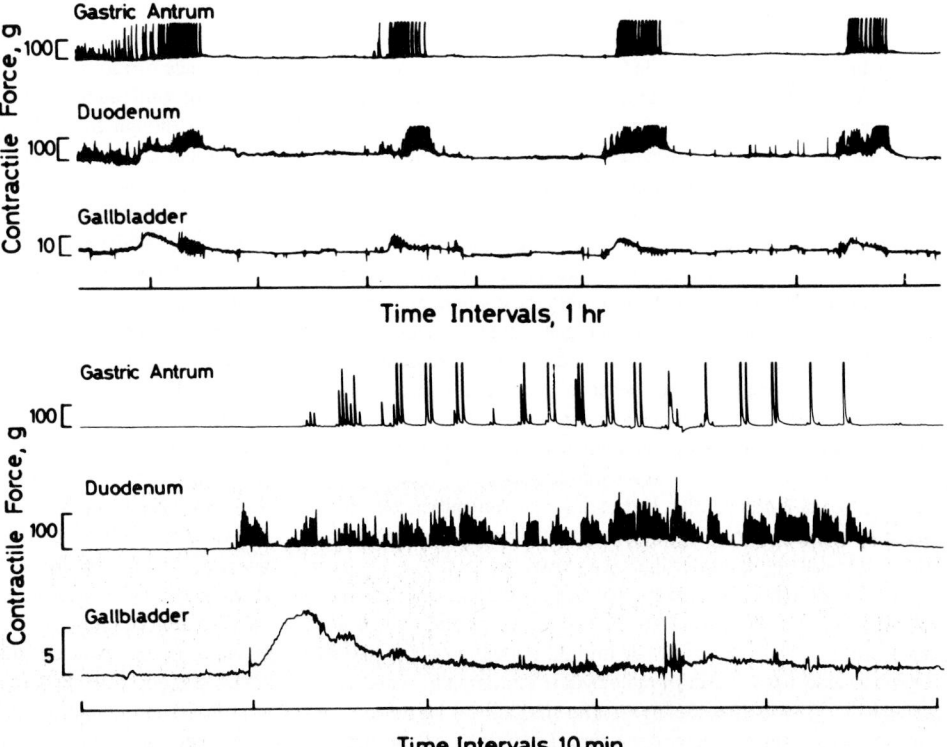

FIGURE 11–1. Interdigestive contractile pattern of the gastric antrum, duodenum, and gallbladder. Top figure represents data obtained over 8 hours; bottom figure shows data on an expanded time scale. Gallbladder contractions coincide with phase II of the MMC. (Itoh Z, Takahashi I. Periodic contractions of the canine gallbladder during the interdigestive state. Am J Physiol 1981;240:G183.)

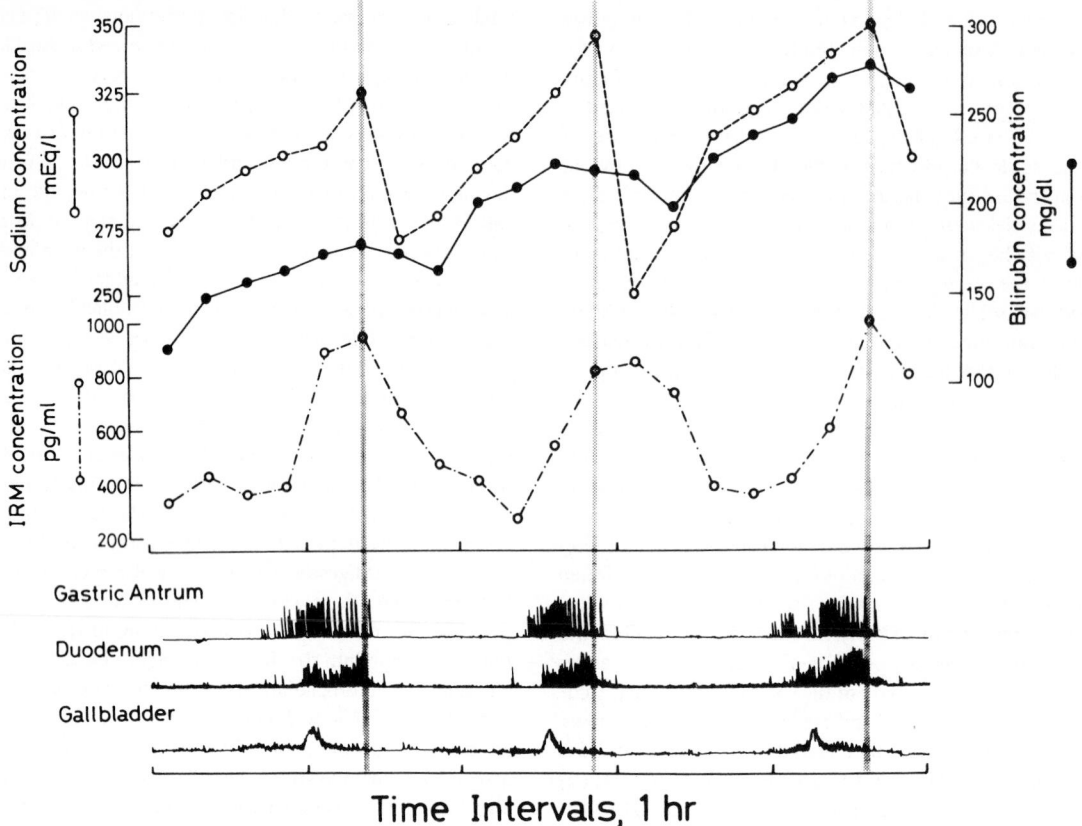

FIGURE 11–2. Interdigestive changes in gallbladder bilirubin and sodium concentration and their relation to the interdigestive contractile activity of the gastric antrum, duodenum, and gallbladder. *Shaded vertical line* indicates simultaneous occurrence of concentration and motor events. (Itoh Z, Takahashi I, Nakaya M, et al. Interdigestive gallbladder bile concentration in relation to periodic contraction of the gallbladder in the dog. Gastroenterology 1982;83:645.)

period.[6,16–19,19a] Although the initial studies established a close relationship between maximal bile flow into the duodenum and phase II of the intestinal MMC, the driving force was not believed to involve gallbladder contraction. Rather it was believed that the periodic choleresis represented either MMC-related increases in the hepatic secretion of bile or cyclic changes in the resistance to bile flow offered by the sphincter of Oddi. Support for this conclusion derived primarily from a study conducted by Peeters and co-workers.[6] These investigators examined the relationship between the MMC and bile acid output into the duodenum in normal subjects and in patients who had undergone cholecystectomy. They found that the pattern of bile flow did not vary significantly in the two groups, suggesting (at least to them) that contraction of the gallbladder is unlikely to be a major factor in the cyclic output of bile. Careful examination of their data, however, reveals that the amount of bile delivery to the duodenum was reduced significantly by cholecystectomy, suggesting that the gallbladder contributes at least in part to the periodic delivery of bile into the duodenum during the interdigestive period.

Although limited, recent studies support the concept that gallbladder contraction during the interdigestive period in humans contributes to the delivery of bile into the duodenum.[17,20–23] Svenberg and associates,[22] using a radionuclide scintigraphic technique, reported a 32% decrease in counts over the gallbladder during the interdigestive period, suggesting partial emptying of the organ.

The decrease in counts from the gallbladder was paralleled by the appearance of radioactivity in the duodenum, further suggesting a role for gallbladder emptying in the interdigestive period (Fig 11-3). Although Svenberg and associates provided evidence of gallbladder contraction during the interdigestive period, they did not examine the contractile pattern in relation to the intestinal MMC pattern. Studies by Kraglund and co-workers,[17] Toouli and associates,[23] Ovist and co-workers,[21] and Marzio and associates,[20] however, have clearly established that gallbladder emptying takes place during phase II of the intestinal MMC (Fig 11-4).

There appears to be little doubt that gallbladder emptying contributes to the intermittent flow of bile into the duodenum during the interdigestive period. What remains uncertain, however, are the factors responsible for the initiation of gallbladder emptying and the physiologic significance of periodic bile delivery into the small intestine. The gastrointestinal hormone motilin is considered by many investigators to play an important role in the initiation of gastric and intestinal MMC activity in several species, including humans.[7,24,25] The hormone evidences cyclic increases in circulating levels during the interdigestive period that parallel closely the development of phase III activity in the stomach and small bowel. In addition, the exogenous administration of motilin initiates the MMC pattern in all species examined to date.[22,26,27] The exogenous administration of motilin also has been reported to increase the phasic and tonic contractile activity of the gallbladder in a fashion

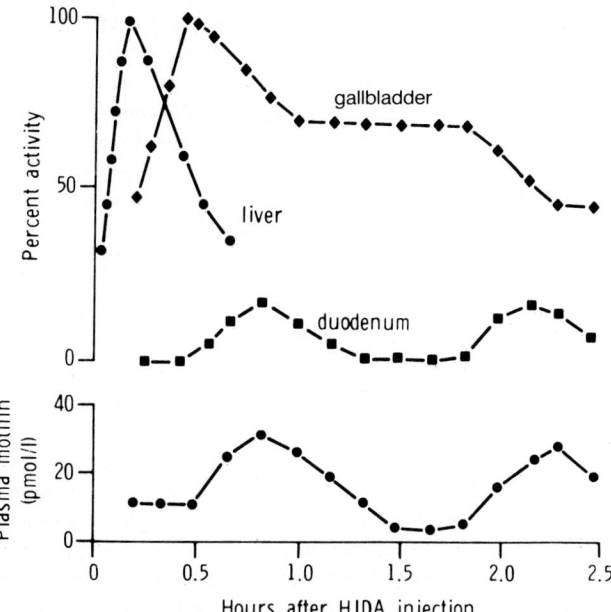

FIGURE 11–3. Time/activity curves over the liver, the gallbladder, and the duodenum after intravenous Tc-HIDA in a fasting human subject. Note increase in duodenal activity coincident with periodic partial "emptying" of the gallbladder. Note relation to changes in serum motilin levels. (Svenberg T, Christofides ND, Fitzpatrick ML, et al. Interdigestive biliary output in man: relationship to fluctuations in plasma motilin and effect of atropine. Gut 1982;23:1024.)

correlated with the appearance of phase III activity in the intestine, occurs after the period of increased gallbladder contractile activity (see Fig 11-3). This would suggest that factors other than motilin are involved in initiating the interdigestive contractile behavior of the gallbladder. However, one cannot rule out the possibility that the small rise in motilin levels observed before the onset of gallbladder emptying may in fact play a role in initiating the contraction. Indeed, Itoh and associates[7] have shown that exogenous motilin can produce gallbladder contraction at doses that have no effect on antral or duodenal motility. Clearly this is an issue that deserves further critical investigation.

The physiologic role of interdigestive gallbladder emptying remains unsettled. It has been proposed that it serves a "housekeeper function" and prevents the accumulation of microcrystals or debris in the concentrated bile during fasting.[12] The periodic mixing and emptying of bile may serve to prevent gallbladder stasis during fasting and thus decrease the likelihood of gallstone formation. Others have suggested that the periodic delivery of bile into the small intestine is necessary for the development of regularly occurring MMC cycles.[29,30] Further studies are necessary to test these hypotheses.

Finally, one topic that remains unsettled concerns the dynamics and factors responsible for filling of the gallbladder during the interdigestive period. Filling is generally believed to be a passive event that occurs as a consequence of the diversion of hepatic bile into a relaxed (low pressure) gallbladder.[2] The primary factor responsible for the diversion of bile is the resistance to bile flow offered at the sphincter of Oddi. Little is known about the dynamics of the filling process. While some investigators have suggested that the bile enters the gallbladder in a continuous uninterrupted manner,[31–33] others have reported that filling occurs in a stepwise fashion.[34] The significance of either type of filling pattern has not been determined. In addition the neurohumoral and/or physical properties of the gallbladder that contribute to the filling process remain unsettled. Davison and co-workers[35,36] have suggested that filling is augmented by activation of inhibitory neural inputs to the gallbladder. More recently, Cole and colleagues[37] have suggested that the mechanical properties of the gallbladder contribute to its ability to function as a storage organ. They demonstrated

similar to that seen during the interdigestive period.[7,12] These observations suggest that motilin may play an important physiologic role in the regulation of gallbladder contraction during the interdigestive period. Caution should be used, however, when making this assumption. Several exogenous substances in addition to motilin can induce MMC-like activity in the small intestine, but this does not mean that any of these substances play a significant physiologic role in the initiation of naturally occurring MMCs.[28] Also, in humans the peak rise in serum motilin levels, although well

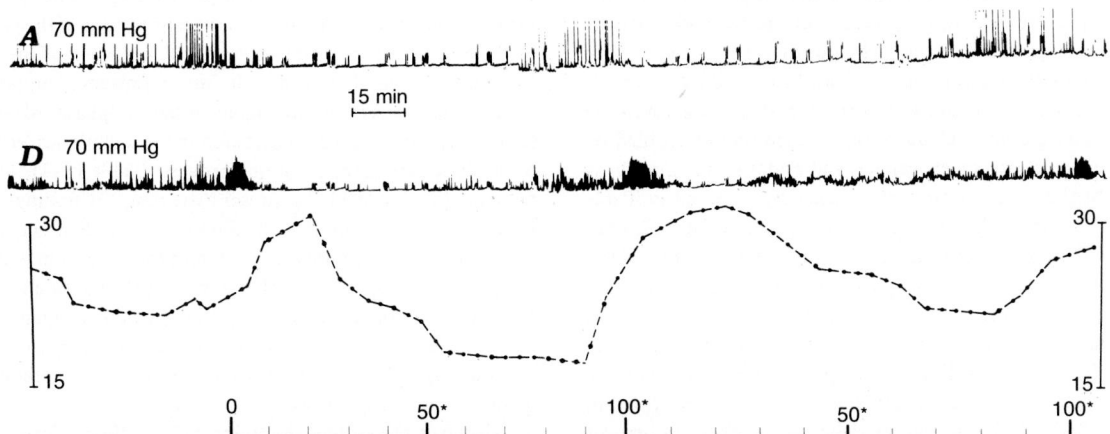

FIGURE 11–4. Intestinal manometry and gallbladder volume during two complete MMC cycles in a human subject. Gallbladder emptying occurs prior to phase III of the intestinal MMC. (*A* = antrum; *D* = proximal duodenum). (Marzio L, Nevi M, Capone F, et al. Gallbladder contraction and its relationship to the interdigestive duodenal motor activity in normal human subjects. Dig Dis Sci 1988;33:540.)

that the gallbladder adapts to distention by evidencing stress relaxation, an increase in compliance that permits further filling of the gallbladder with little additional change in pressure. It will be interesting to determine the biomechanical properties that contribute to the stress relaxation and to see how they may be altered with altered physiologic states.

Digestive Period

EVALUATION OF EMPTYING PATTERNS

An understanding of the factors that initiate and regulate gallbladder emptying during the digestive period depends in large part on the ability to accurately measure and quantify the emptying process. Until recently, the most frequently used technique involved opacification of the gallbladder with an oral cholecystographic agent and the monitoring of emptying with regularly spaced radiographs.[26,38–41] Estimates of gallbladder volume were obtained using planimetric measurements of the radiopaque areas. While this technique provided much useful data, the approach was limited because it provided only intermittent quantification of gallbladder "contraction," thus precluding any rigorous kinetic analysis of the emptying process. Another widely used approach involved marker infusion or aspiration systems that monitor the duodenal output of bile as an index of emptying.[42,43] Unfortunately, the method is not designed to measure events in the nonsteady state and cannot differentiate reliably between bile secreted from the liver and bile emptied from the gallbladder. Thus, until recently, the two most commonly used approaches provided the investigator with only an indirect measure of gallbladder emptying. Fortunately, in recent years, two noninvasive techniques, radionuclide cholescintigraphy and real-time ultrasonagraphy, have become available and have been used to provide continuous and quantitative information about the gallbladder emptying process in normal persons and in patients with a variety of pathophysiologic conditions.

Englert and Chiu[44] were among the first to appreciate that using a gamma-emitting, hepatocystic radionuclide in combination with continuous external recording by a scintillation counter could avoid many of the difficulties inherent in the methods used by previous investigators. With this technique they were able to define both the half-time of emptying ($t_{1/2}$) and the overall total percent of emptying. Since their initial report, several investigators have used cholescintigraphy to characterize the dynamics of gallbladder emptying in response to exogenous and endogenous stimuli. A summary of the results from these studies is presented in Table 11-1.[29,31,32,44–54] It can be seen that a wide variety of stimuli have been used. Differences in meal composition, volume, and caloric density, as well as differences in the doses of cholecystokinin (CCK) infused and the method of infusion (continuous vs. bolus) make it difficult to compare results. Nevertheless, a few generalities can be made. First, the gallbladder empties promptly in response to the ingestion of a meal or the infusion of CCK, generally within 2 minutes. Second, the decline in radioactivity over the area of interest decreases exponentially. This emptying pattern is consistent with observations made by other investigators using different techniques. Third, the percent emptied depends up the "physio-

logic" nature of the stimulus. Careful inspection of Table 11-1 reveals that stimuli that promote the continuous delivery of CCK into the peripheral circulation (constant infusion or feeding) actually result in a greater evacuation of the gallbladder (65%–85%) than does the bolus injection of CCK. It is clear that in the future, meal volume, composition, and caloric density will need to be standardized in order to compare data from different investigators. Also, the CCK hormone levels that result from such a meal will need to be determined. This latter information will permit the selection of a continuous infusion routine for CCK that most closely approximates the hormone levels after a meal. Only at this time will we be able to fully characterize the dynamics of gallbladder emptying under physiologic conditions.

Everson and associates[55] validated real-time ultrasonography as an alternative method for the noninvasive quantitation of gallbladder emptying in humans. With this technique, images of the greatest length, width, and anteroposterior dimension of the gallbladder are used to calculate volume at any given time prior to and after ingestion of a meal or administration of an exogenous cholecystokinetic agent (see reference 55 for specific details). The resultant data can be used to characterize the fasting volume (FV), residual volume (RV), percent emptied, and rate constant of emptying. A survey of the data obtained to date is presented in Table 11-2[17,47,55–69] and can be summarized as follows. First, the FV ranges from 10 to 50 mL, with the majority of investigators reporting fasting volumes of 20 to 30 mL. Second, changes in gallbladder volume can be detected almost immediately on stimulation. Third, gallbladder volume decreases exponentially. Fourth, both the ingestion of a meal and the continuous infusion of CCK produces an approximately 55% to 75% emptying of the gallbladder over a 30- to 45-minute period. The time to one-half of emptying ranges from 10 to 20 minutes.

The analysis of gallbladder emptying by real-time ultrasonography relies on the assumption that changes in calculated volume represent gallbladder contraction and emptying and do not represent changes in gallbladder geometry or movement of the organ. The validity of radionuclide scintigraphy relies on the correctness of the assumption that the decrease in the number of counts represents a decrease in volume. Clearly each technique relies heavily on assumptions that cannot be totally validated. A question arises therefore as to whether the different techniques provide different information with respect to the emptying pattern of the gallbladder or the kinetics of the emptying process. A review of the available literature reveals that each technique represents emptying as an exponential process, following an initial lag phase. More importantly, there is close agreement among the techniques with respect to the dynamics of the emptying process (Table 11-3). The values presented in Table 11-3 represent the range of findings reported in the literature. Note that the data on the percent emptying, the time to one half of emptying ($t_{1/2}$), and the time to maximal emptying (t_{100}) in response to either a meal or the continuous infusion of CCK are virtually identical regardless of the imaging technique. Thus, it seems that both real-time ultrasonography and radionuclide scintigraphy provide accurate, noninvasive methods for the quantification of gallbladder emptying.

Although the studies involving radionuclide scintigraphy and ultrasound provide useful information about the kinetics of the emptying pattern, they do not permit a characterization of the contractile activity of the gallbladder during the postprandial pe-

TABLE 11–1
Gallbladder Emptying Characteristics as Determined by Radionuclide Scintigraphy

STIMULUS	%E	T$_{1/2}$ (min)	T$_{100}$ (min)	REFERENCE
Fatty meal	64 ± 7		29.4 ± 2.5	45
CCK-8 (0.04 µg/kg bolus)	30 ± 10		20–30	46
Liquid meal	85 ± 3	10–15	60	46
CCK-8 (5 ng/kg/min)	80 ± 5	10–15	45–60	46
CCK (1.2 IDU/kg/hr)	82 ± 5	10.3 ± 0.7		46
Lundh meal		10.2 ± 1.5		47
CCK-8 (75 pM/kg/hr)		9 ± 1.4		47
CCK (0.02 IDU/kg/min)	85 ± 45	11 ± 1.0		48
Fatty meal	84 ± 3	18 ± 10	54 ± 13	44
CCK (11.7 IDU/kg/min)	78 ± 5	19 ± 11	46 ± 14	44
CCK (bolus)	32	60		44
CCK 8 (10 ng/kg/hr)	35 ± 11	15–20		32
20 (10 ng/kg/hr)	77 ± 5	15–20		32
40 (10 ng/kg/hr)	73 ± 7	15–20		32
CCK-8 (20 ng/kg bolus)	52 ± 10			32
Arachis oil	60–70	20 ± 3	40	49
CCK-8 (40 ng/kg bolus)	32 ± 14			50
CCK-8 (20 ng/kg bolus)	34 ± 24		10	51
CCK-8 (20 ng/kg bolus)	35 ± 17	10 ± 4		51a
CCK-8 (40 ng/kg bolus)	43 ± 26	11 ± 5		51a
CCK-8 (10 ng/kg bolus)	59 ± 4	11 ± 1		31
Liquid meal	78 ± 30	20	60	53
Solid meal	75 ± 68			53
Acetylcholine	39 ± 8	20	45	53
CCK-8 (5 ng/kg bolus)	82 ± 9.0	20	60	53
CCK (0.2 IDU/kg/min)	73 ± 2	11.3 ± 0.6		54
Meal	75	5.5 ± 0.7		29
	35	14 ± 1.0		29
Meal	76 ± 11	12–15	46 ± 9	
	83 ± 10	12–15	40 ± 10	

CCK, cholecystokinin; CCK-8, octapeptide of CCK.

riod. Data from nonhuman animal models obtained using strain gauges and pressure transducers, however, reveal a complex pattern of contractile activity.[12,14] For example, Traynor and associates[14] reported that the contractile activity of the canine gallbladder exhibits three distinct phases: phase I, an initial transient rise in pressure that returns to baseline; phase II, a prolonged period of tonic contraction; and phase III, a prolonged period of large amplitude phasic contractions (Fig 11-5). It has been suggested that the initial increase in tone and/or phasic activity promotes emptying, whereas the more dramatic increase in contractile activity during the latter stage of the postprandial period may serve to ensure the prompt delivery of recycled hepatic bile into the duodenum by restricting gallbladder filling.[29,30] While the validity of this hypothesis remains to be proven, it is clear that a complex relationship exists between gallbladder contraction and gallbladder emptying.

RESPONSE TO A MEAL: INTESTINAL PHASE

It has been known since the early years of this century that the presence of food in the small intestine promotes gallbladder emptying.[70–72] In 1928, Ivy and Oldberg[70] extracted from the upper small intestinal mucosa of the hog a substance that when injected intravenously into dogs caused contraction and evacuation of the gallbladder. They named the substance cholecystokinin ("that which excites or moves the gallbladder"). The experiments of Ivy and Oldberg, as well as the cross-circulation experiments of Houssay and Rubio,[73] firmly established the hormonal nature of the meal-induced stimulus. The subsequent isolation and purification of CCK was accomplished by Jorpes and Mutt[74–76] in the early 1960s. They identified the hormone as a linear polypeptide containing 33 amino acids (CCK-33). Since the initial isolation attempt it has become evident that CCK exists in several molecular

TABLE 11–2

Gallbladder Emptying Characteristics as Determined by Real-Time Ultrasonography

STIMULUS	FV (mL)	RV (mL)	%E	$T_{1/2}$ (min)	T_{100} (min)	REFERENCE
Liquid meal (35% fat)	16.7 ± 2.5	7.5 ± 1.9	55.5 ± 7.1		20–40	55
CCK (0.5 ng/kg/hr)	35–40	5	85	5	10	56
Liquid meal	11					57
Solid meal (25% fat)	26 ± 14		49 ± 26			17
Liquid meal (40% fat)	22	9	60		60	58
Mixed meal (40% fat)	23.7 ± 7.4					59
CCK-8 (0.02 ng/kg)			60.8 ± 15.8		37 ± 12	60
Mixed meal (high fat)			51.1 ± 15		45 ± 17	60
Mixed meal (low fat)			52.6 ± 13.8		34 ± 20	60
Mixed meal (no fat)			51.7 ± 22.0		35 ± 20	60
Lipomul	19.5 ± 2.3	5.6 ± 1.0	70 ± 5	10–20	30–40	61
Lundh meal	24.4 ± 2.1	9.6 ± 19	60	10–15		47
CCK-8 (75 pM/kg/hr)	28.2 ± 2.1	12.2 ± 1.6	58	10–15		47
Corn oil (male)	21.4 ± 3.2	5.8 ± 1.2	70 ± 7			62
Corn oil (female)	13.3 ± 2.1	48 ± 0.9	60 ± 6			62
CCK-8 (0.8 pM/kg/hr)	28.8 ± 2.4					63
(6.4 pM/kg/hr)	28.8 ± 2.4					63
						64
Mixed meal (40% fat)	17.2 ± 5.2	4.2 ± 1.8	74.1 ± 12.2			65
ID amino acid	18.5 ± 1.9	6.1 ± 1.2	68.1 ± 4.5			66
Corn oil			64		40	67
Lipomul (ID)	34.6 ± 6	11.5 ± 6	67	12	18	68
Lipomul (oral)	20.4 ± 2.2	7.5 ± 1.2	64	13	15	68
CCK-8 (0.5 ng/kg/hr)	23.0 ± 2.9	34 ± 0.5	85	6	10	69

FV, fasting volume; RV, residual volume; CCK, cholecystokinin; CCK-8, octapeptide of CCK.

forms. In addition to the CCK-33 molecule, a 39 amino acid polypeptide (CCK-39) and the carboxyl-terminal octapeptide (CCK-8; OP-CCK) fragment of the whole molecule also have been isolated and purified.[77,78] Initially it was proposed that CCK-8 is two to ten times more potent on a molar basis than CCK-33 in stimulating gallbladder contraction[79–87] and that it is the predominant molecular form of the hormone released into the circulation in response to a meal.[88–92] In recent years, however, several investigators have reported that the differences in biologic activity between CCK-8 and CCK-33 may be artifactual. Lamers and associates[85] were the first to report that CCK-8 and CCK-33 were equipotent in stimulating gallbladder contraction in vitro. Key to

their study was the addition of 1% albumin to all CCK-containing solutions to prevent adherence of the larger molecule to plastic or glass. In addition they reported that trypsinization of the CCK-33 molecule had no effect on either the biologic or immunologic activity of the molecule. They speculated that both CCK-8 and CCK-33 are important physiologic regulators of gallbladder motility. The studies of Solomon and associates[93] lend further support to the idea that the biologic activity of CCK-8 and CCK-33 are comparable. In an elaborate series of experiments involving both in vivo and in vitro experimental designs they were unable to demonstrate any significant difference in potency between CCK-8 and CCK-33. They proposed that the earlier finds of Hedner[84]

TABLE 11–3

Comparison of Gallbladder Emptying Characteristics as Determined by Real-Time Ultrasonography and Radionuclide Scintigraphy*

STIMULUS	ULTRASOUND			CHOLESCINTIGRAPHY		
	% Emptied	$T_{1/2}$ (min)	T_{100} (min)	% Emptied	$T_{1/2}$ (min)	T_{100} (min)
Test meal	50–70	10–20	40–60	60–80	10–20	30–60
CCK—continuous	60–85	10	40	75–85	10–20	40–60

* Represents range of values reported in the literature.

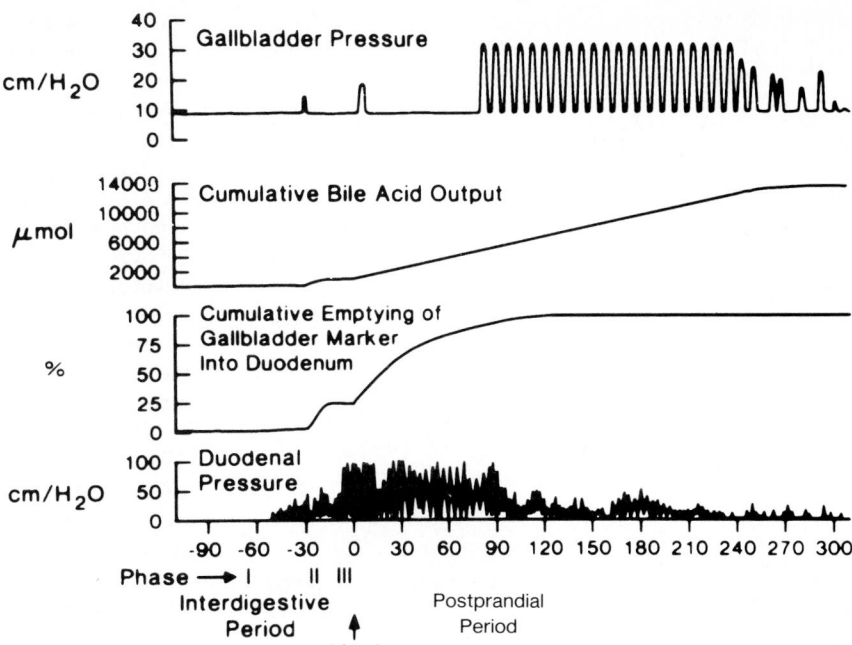

FIGURE 11-5. Schematic representation of the interdigestive (−90–0 min) and postprandial (0–300 min) gallbladder motility and emptying in the dog. (Traynor OJ, Dozois RR, DiMagno EP. Canine interdigestive and postprandial gallbladder motility and emptying. Am J Physiol 1984;246:G426.)

and others were artifactual due to the selective loss of CCK-33 from non-albumin-containing solutions. Such a loss would obscure the true potency of the larger molecular forms of CCK. Furthermore, they proposed that their data suggest an important role for CCK-33 in the physiologic regulation of gallbladder and pancreatic function.

As noted, several studies have suggested that CCK-8 is the major molecular form of the peptide in the circulation following a meal. In contrast, other investigators have reported that CCK-33 is the predominant circulating form of the molecule and have used this observation to support the hypothesis of Lamers and co-workers[85] and Solomon and associates[93] that CCK-33 contributes significantly to the physiologic regulation of gallbladder motility. Maton and his colleagues[94,95] demonstrated an equimolar elevation in the plasma concentrations of CCK-8 and CCK-33 after a fatty meal in humans. A similar observation was made by Chang and Chey.[96] Inoue and co-workers[97] found that pancreatic protein secretion in dogs in response to bombesin, a stimulant for CCK release, could be abolished by the prior administration of a CCK-33 specific antiserum. More recently, Sakamoto and associates[98] have reported that CCK-8 is partially inactivated by passage through the liver whereas the immunologic and biologic activity of CCK-33 remain unaffected. Furthermore, they reported that on a molar basis CCK-8 and CCK-33 were equipotent in affecting gallbladder contraction in vivo. Taken together the bioassay and radioimmunoassay data provide considerable support for the idea that CCK-33 is released in significant amounts in response to a meal and that the molecule has important biologic activities. In agreement with this idea is the recent report that CCK-8 and CCK-33 are virtually equipotent in their ability to bind to the CCK receptor on gallbladder smooth muscle.[99]

On a final note, there is a growing body of data obtained using molecular biology techniques that indicate that CCK is a heterogeneous molecule whose multiple molecular forms derive from a common precursor called preprocholecystokinin.[100] Indeed, re-

cent reports indicate that multiple molecular forms of the peptide can be identified in the intestinal mucosa and in the plasma of humans and that CCK-58 may be the most prevalent.[101] The physiologic implications of these findings are unknown and await further study. The full appreciation of the physiologic importance of the molecular variants awaits a more detailed understanding of the receptor activity of the molecules, as well as a clearer understanding of the release pattern of the variants and their biologic half-life.

Although it has long been proposed that gallbladder contraction in response to a meal in the small intestine is the result of fat-induced release of CCK, it has been only recently that this hypothesis has been tested directly and shown to be correct. In 1981, Wiener and associates[68] reported the development of a sensitive and specific radioimmunoassay for CCK and demonstrated a close correlation between the plasma levels of the hormone and the change in gallbladder volume that occurs in humans after either the oral or intraduodenal administration of a fatty meal (Fig 11-6). Regardless of the route of administration, the plasma levels of CCK increased significantly within 2 to 6 minutes and reached maximal levels within 16 minutes. The increase in CCK levels was followed closely by a significant decrease in gallbladder volume. Maximum gallbladder emptying occurred 2 minutes following the attainment of peak CCK levels. Because multiple physiologic mechanisms may be activated by the presence of fat in the stomach and small bowel it could be argued that the observed results represent two unrelated events and that fat-induced contraction is the result of other undefined mechanisms. Lilja and co-workers,[69] using the same radioimmunoassay system devised by Wiener and associates,[68] tested this possibility by correlating changes in plasma CCK concentrations to changes in gallbladder volume following the continuous infusion of CCK-33. They found the two events to be highly correlated. Gallbladder emptying was closely associated with increasing plasma CCK concentrations; sustained gallbladder contraction correlated with steady-state hormone lev-

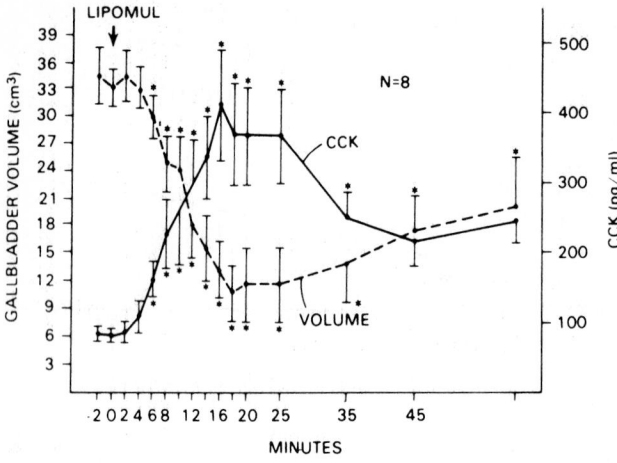

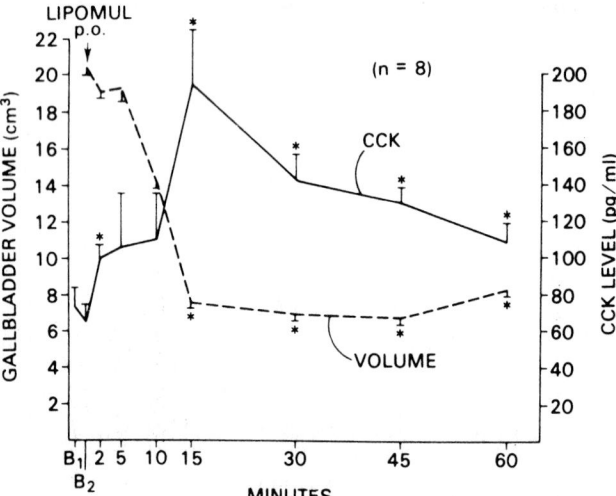

FIGURE 11–6. Changes in plasma CCK concentration and gallbladder volume in humans after intraduodenal (*top*) or intraduodenal (*bottom*) administration of a lipid meal. (Wiener I, Inoue K, Fagan CJ, et al. Release of CCK in man: correlation of blood levels with gallbladder contraction. Ann Surg 1981;194:321.)

els. Also, there was good correlation between decreasing CCK concentrations and gallbladder refilling. Since these early studies other investigators have shown that the endogenous release of CCK is associated with contraction and emptying of the gallbladder.[95,98,102–107] Finally, recent studies using the CCK-receptor antagonist loxiglumide indicate that CCK plays an important role not only in regulating meal-stimulated gallbladder contraction but also in determining the fasting volume of the gallbladder.[108–110] Thus, there is now good evidence to support the original hypothesis of Ivy and Oldberg that meal-induced gallbladder emptying occurs as the result of CCK-induced gallbladder contraction.

Although we have learned a great deal in recent years about the casual and temporal relationships between meal-induced increases in plasma CCK levels and gallbladder contraction, the site of action and the mechanism of action of the hormone has not been established. CCK stimulation of isolated muscle strips from guinea pigs and the rabbits is unaffected by adrenergic or cholinergic blockade or by tetrodotoxin.[2,87,111] These observations have

lead to the widely held belief that CCK acts directly at the level of the smooth muscle. However, there is now evidence from a number of species (including humans) to suggest that CCK may stimulate both the smooth muscle and postganglionic cholinergic neurons of the gallbladder.[11,112–114] In humans, for example, atropine has been reported to produce a rightward shift in the in vivo CCK–gallbladder contraction dose-response curve. While such a result may suggest that gallbladder contraction is mediated in part by CCK-induced acetylcholine release, one cannot rule out the possibility that atropine had an indirect effect by limiting the permissive effect of tonic cholinergic stimulation to the gallbladder or that atropine may have unmasked an inhibitory neural input to the gallbladder that antagonizes the excitatory actions of the hormone.

Also, little is known about the cellular mechanism of action of CCK on gallbladder smooth muscle. Studies performed in the mid 1970s suggested that CCK-induced gallbladder smooth muscle contraction was associated with changes in the intracellular concentrations of the cyclic nucleotides adenosine monophosphate (AMP) and guanosine monophosphate (GMP). Specifically, CCK was believed to alter calcium homeostasis within the cell via decreasing cyclic AMP levels and increasing cyclic GMP levels.[79,111,115,116] No additional studies are available to substantiate this hypothesis. In fact, a recent report indicates that CCK-stimulated gallbladder smooth muscle contraction is mediated via a calcium-phosphoinositide postreceptor coupling mechanism and that modulation of the cyclic AMP levels does not play a role.[117] Clearly, much work needs to be done before we can begin to identify the biochemical pathways activated in response to CCK stimulation.

Although the second messenger pathways involved in CCK-stimulated gallbladder contraction remain unsettled, there is clear evidence that both extracellular and intracellular stores of calcium are necessary for maximal force development.[117a,118] Ryan and associates[118,119] reported that CCK-induced contractions are reduced but not abolished by calcium channel blockers or by experimental protocols that depleted intracellular stores of calcium. Moreover, they have shown that CCK-mediated contractions are preceded by calcium-dependent increases in phosphorylation of the contractile protein myosin.[120] It is hoped that future investigators will expose the complexities of the CCK-receptor interaction that leads to the influx and mobilization of calcium.

In addition to CCK, other gastrointestinal peptides have been shown to affect the contractile behavior of the gallbladder. A summary of their effects is presented in Table 11-4.[6,10,11,76,86,87,121–165] With the exception of perhaps vasoactive intestinal peptide (VIP) and pancreatic polypeptide (PP), the physiologic importance of the peptides in gallbladder contraction remains unsettled.

Several investigators have reported that VIP is a potent inhibitor of basal and CCK-stimulated gallbladder contraction in vivo and in vitro.[87,158,159,161,162,166] Sundler and associates[114] reported the presence of VIP-containing nerve fibers in the smooth muscle layer of the feline and human gallbladder. This finding is significant since other investigators have postulated that VIP serves as a neurotransmitter and because of the recent report that vagal stimulation is associated with the appearance of VIP in the protal blood.[167,168] It may be that VIP acts locally to modulate the tone of the gallbladder and thus enhance filling during the interdigestive period. During the digestive period it may serve to modify the

TABLE 11–4
Summary of Excitatory and Inhibitory Stimuli to the Gallbladder

	REFERENCE
Excitatory	
Acetylcholine	87, 121–125
α-Adrenergic	6, 126, 127
Cholecystokinin	2
Gastrin	86, 87, 128–132
Histamine (H₁)	133–139
Motilin	10, 11, 140
Neurotensin	141
Prostaglandins	129, 142–145
Substance K	146
Substance P	147, 147a
Inhibitory	
Adenosine, ATP	148
β-Adrenergic	6, 126, 149–151
Histamine (H₂)	133–139
Pancreatic polypeptide	152–155
Secretin	156, 157
Vasoactive intestinal peptide	76, 123, 158–165

excitatory neurohumoral input to the gallbladder. These hypotheses remain to be tested.

Pancreatic polypeptide is a 36 amino acid peptide that is found in high concentrations in the pancreas.[155,169] Its release occurs following the delivery of fat into the duodenum and appears to involve both neural and hormonal factors. While considerable work still needs to be done, it appears as if PP may serve as an "anti-CCK" hormone and thus be involved in the negative feedback regulation of pancreatic and biliary tract function. It also has been proposed that the hormone may promote gallbladder filling. Lin and colleagues[170] were the first to report that in the dog PP has several effects that are directly opposite to those of CCK, including inhibition of pancreatic enzyme secretion, relaxation of the gallbladder, and contraction of the sphincter of Oddi. Similar findings have been reported for other species, including humans.[152,154] In each report the authors speculated that the hormone might play a physiologic role in the regulation of meal-stimulated pancreatic enzyme secretion and gallbladder emptying. The authors also suggested that the increased plasma levels of the hormone observed during the latter stages of digestion may promote postprandial filling of the gallbladder. A report by Conter and co-workers[153] supports this idea. Using the prairie dog as an animal model, they reported that the exogenous administration of PP significantly increased gallbladder filling following CCK-induced gallbladder contraction and that the enhanced filling was the result of a decreased intraluminal pressure. They proposed that gallbladder filling is not just a passive response to diminished CCK levels but also involves PP-mediated decreases in intraluminal pressure. These data strongly suggest that PP may be involved in the physiologic regulation of gallbladder emptying. It will be up to future investigators to test the validity of this assumption. Such information is necessary if we are to completely understand the complexity of the factors that affect both gallbladder contraction and relaxation. Moreover, in light of the recent observations that PP does not effect basal or CCK-stimulated gallbladder tension in vitro,[52,171] studies also should be aimed at determining the mechanism of action of the hormone.

In summary, the presence of food in the small intestine is associated with a prompt and significant emptying of the gallbladder. While there is little doubt as to the physiologic importance of CCK (and perhaps PP) in the regulation of this process, several questions remain unanswered. First, what other hormones or paracrine substances are physiologically important in the regulation of contraction and/or refilling? Second, is there a neural component to the intestinal phase of gallbladder contraction. Distention of the duodenum has been reported to promote gallbladder contraction, and this effect is reduced by vagotomy.[172,173] The decreased response after vagotomy could be caused by either impaired CCK release or interruption of an intestinal-biliary tract reflex.[174,175] Fried and associates[102] examined these alternatives by simultaneously measuring plasma CCK levels and gallbladder pressures in conscious dogs following the intraduodenal administration of a fatty meal before and after vagotomy. Truncal vagotomy significantly reduced the increase in gallbladder pressure but had no effect on the circulating levels of CCK. The authors suggested that the results could best be explained by assuming that vagotomy disrupts the integrity of a vagally mediated enterocholecystic reflex. The physiologic significance of an enterocholecystic reflex remains unknown. Whether it contributes significantly to the overall contractile activity of the gallbladder or whether the presence of an intact vagal input to the gallbladder modulates the response to CCK (or other hormones) stimulation remains an issue for further consideration. Finally, are there factors other than neural and hormonal inputs that might affect gallbladder emptying? This question is prompted by the recent observation that the presence of pancreatic enzymes and bile in the small intestine exerts a negative feedback effect on CCK release[175a,176–178] and that factors that lessen bile input into the small intestine enhance CCK release.[179,180] These results suggest that the extent of gallbladder contraction will be determined in part by the size of the bile salt pool delivered into the small intestine. It will be up to future investigators to determine whether conditions that interfere with the size and/or circulation of the bile acid pool are accompanied by alterations in the dynamics of the emptying process.

RESPONSE TO A MEAL: PREINTESTINAL STIMULI

It is generally proposed that the delivery of chyme into the small intestine serves as the stimulus for the initiation of gallbladder emptying. However, a careful review of literature indicates that the gallbladder begins to empty in advance of gastric emptying.[29,30,181–186] This would suggest the existence of "preduodenal" mechanisms that contribute to gallbladder contraction during the cephalic and/or gastric phases of digestion. Sham feeding has been reported to be associated with gallbladder emptying in both dog and humans.[184,185] Furthermore, this effect is eliminated by vagotomy or atropine, suggesting activation of excitatory cholinergic vagal fibers during the cephalic phase of digestion. Baxter and colleagues[30] examined the temporal and quantitative relationships between gastric and gallbladder emptying in normal patients and in patients with truncal vagotomy and pyloroplasty. They, too, observed that emptying of the gallbladder precedes gastric emptying and that the onset and extent of gallbladder emptying was significantly delayed in the vagotomized patients. This suggested to them the existence of a vagally mediated cephalic phase of contraction.

Although the available data strongly suggest that a cephalic phase of gallbladder contraction exists, one cannot rule out the possibility that stimuli from the gastric phase of digestion also influence gallbladder contraction. Indeed, distention of the antrum is known to evoke gallbladder contraction. While the results were initially attributed to the release of gastrin during the gastric phase of digestion,[63] Debas and Yamagashi[187] have provided strong evidence that antral distention-mediated contraction involves, at least in part, a neural reflex component. In a series of experiments in conscious dogs they examined the effect of graded antral distention with either an alkaline (pH 8.3) or acidic (pH 1.1) solution on gallbladder contraction. In both cases the extent of gallbladder contractions was directly related to the degree of antral distention. Because only distention with the alkaline solution was associated with an increase in serum gastrin levels the authors proposed the existence of a neurally mediated pylorocholecystic reflex. To test this hypothesis similar studies were performed in animals that had been atropinized and in animals that had undergone a truncal vagotomy. Each situation resulted in the complete elimination of antral-induced gallbladder contraction. The authors proposed that the results can be explained by postulating the existence of a cholinergic, vagovagal, pylorocholecystic reflex that contributes to gallbladder contraction during the gastric phase of digestion.

Neither the physiologic significance nor the exact contribution of cephalic and gastric influences to gallbladder emptying are known. Baxter and colleagues[30] have suggested that the delivery of gallbladder bile into the duodenum prior to the delivery of chyme may serve as an important physiologic mechanism for mobilizing the bile salt pool and returning some of the bile salts quickly into the enterohepatic circulation for continued secretion by the liver as needed. Others have suggested that activation of vagal cholinergic fibers is the primary factor responsible for the rapid component of gallbladder emptying.[185,188] In support of this latter idea are the numerous observations that vagotomy is associated with increased residual volumes and delayed and decreased emptying in response to the ingestion of a meal.

SPHINCTER OF ODDI MOTILITY

The sphincter of Oddi is a complex muscular structure that encircles the distal common bile duct and the ampulla of Vater. In humans, the major portion of the sphincter lies within the musculature of the duodenum and measures 4 to 6 cm in length. Once a point of considerable controversy, it is now well recognized that the sphincter of Oddi differs anatomically, embryologically, and functionally from the surrounding intestinal musculature.[2]

Numerous investigators have proposed that the sphincter remains closed between meals to ensure the delivery and storage of hepatic bile in the gallbladder and that following a meal the sphincter relaxes and allows gallbladder and hepatic bile to flow freely into the duodenum.[2,189] Under these circumstances the

sphincter is viewed as playing a passive role in the delivery of bile into the intestine. For the most part, the investigators used techniques that provided only an indirect measure of sphincter motility.[106,190–194] However, recent studies using techniques that directly evaluate sphincter of Oddi motility,[25,96,107,145,192,195–208] including electromyography, cineradiography, and endoscopic manometric techniques, indicate that the sphincter exhibits both tonic and phasic contractile activity and that it may play an active role in the dynamics of bile flow. The traditional view that the sphincter acts as a variable resistor to route hepatic bile into the duodenum or toward the gallbladder by alterations in sphincter tone must be coupled with the realization that the sphincter of Oddi also exhibits forceful spontaneous phasic contractions. Indeed, evidence is available that suggests that active peristaltic contractions within the sphincter may actually serve to promote bile delivery, that is, the sphincter may serve as a pump rather than as a resistor. For additional information on the sphincter of Oddi the reader is referred to review articles by Coelho and Moody,[209] Dodds and associates,[210] Sarles and colleagues,[189] and Steinberg.[211]

Interdigestive Period

In the interdigestive period, rhythmic fluctuations in duodenal bile acid delivery occur and are coordinated with the cyclic activity of the MMC in the duodenum. Evidence is available that suggests that the increased transsphincteric flow is due, at least in part, to active gallbladder contraction. Evidence also is available that supports the idea that alterations in the dynamics of sphincter of Oddi motility contribute quantitatively and qualitatively to the interdigestive flow pattern.[2] The increased transsphincteric flow may be achieved by either increasing or decreasing the peristaltic activity of the sphincter. The exact contribution of the sphincter appears to be species dependent.

The opossum has been used extensively to characterize the motor activity of the sphincter during the interdigestive period, after feeding, and in response to hormones.[19,205,207,212–221] Because the sphincter is mostly extraduodenal, it can be studied with minimal interference from the surrounding intestinal musculature. Using the opossum as an animal model, Toouli and co-workers[221] combined manometric, electromyographic, cineradiographic, and flow monitoring techniques simultaneously to characterize the pressure profile of the sphincter of Oddi in conscious animals and to relate the contractile activity to changes in common bile duct and sphincter of Oddi flow. They reported that the sphincter exhibited both a high pressure zone and rhythmic peristalitic contractions that originated in the proximal segment and migrated toward the duodenum. Electrical recordings from the sphincter showed that the contractions were preceded by slow waves with superimposed spike burst activity. Subsequent studies have shown these slow waves to be myogenic in origin and that the proximal to distal orientation of the contractile wave can best be explained by proposing a linear array of bidirectionally coupled relaxation oscillators, with the high-frequency pacemaker located in the most proximal segment of the sphincter.[19,216] During peristalsis, the sphincter contents were actively emptied into the duodenum while common bile duct filling was interrupted. On completion of the peristaltic wave, the common bile duct and the sphincter filled

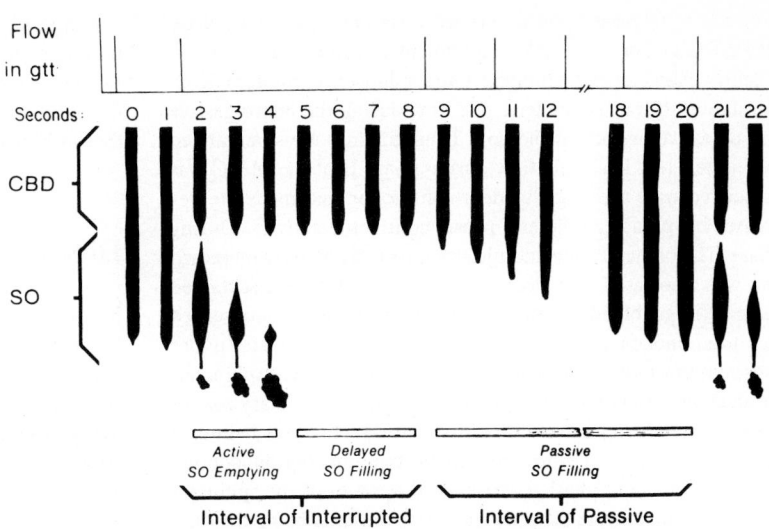

FIGURE 11–7. Diagrammatic representation of bile duct emptying. See text for details. (Toouli J, Dodds WJ, Honda R, et al. Motor function of the opossum sphincter of Oddi. J Clin Invest 1983;71:208.)

passively without any emptying of contrast material into the duodenum (Fig 11-7).

Toouli and associates[221] proposed that the sphincter acts as a peristaltic pump to promote bile flow into the duodenum. Consistent with this hypothesis is the observation that during the interdigestive period the sphincter exhibits cyclic changes in contractile frequency that are closely coupled to changes in bile flow rate.[222] Both the contractile activity and flow rate progress from a minimum during phase I of the interdigestive cycle to a maximum concurrent with phase III. Thus, it appears in the opossum that increased transsphincteric flow can be achieved by increasing the peristaltic contractile activity within the sphincter. This is consistent with the idea that the sphincter regulates flow by serving as a pump.

Rhythmic peristaltic contractions also have been recorded from the sphincter of Oddi in dogs and humans (see reference 223 for review table). In both species the sphincter is characterized by a baseline pressure above common bile duct pressure, on which phasic contractions are superimposed. Significant differences exist among laboratories with respect to the magnitude of the resting pressure and the amplitude of the phasic contractions (see reference 223 for summary table). It is now appreciated that the actual data recorded depends on the phase of the MMC cycle as well as on the characteristics of the manometric recording assembly.[210] There is good agreement, however, that the phasic contractions are peristaltic with the majority propagating toward the duodenum.[23,206,207,224] Figure 11-8 is an example of antegrade peristaltic contractions recorded from the sphincter of Oddi in humans.

As noted previously, bile delivery to the duodenum in dogs and humans during the interdigestive period also exhibits a cyclic pattern.[6,17,22,63,223] Unlike the opossum, peak bile flow occurs during phase II of the duodenal MMC cycle and is decreased in the

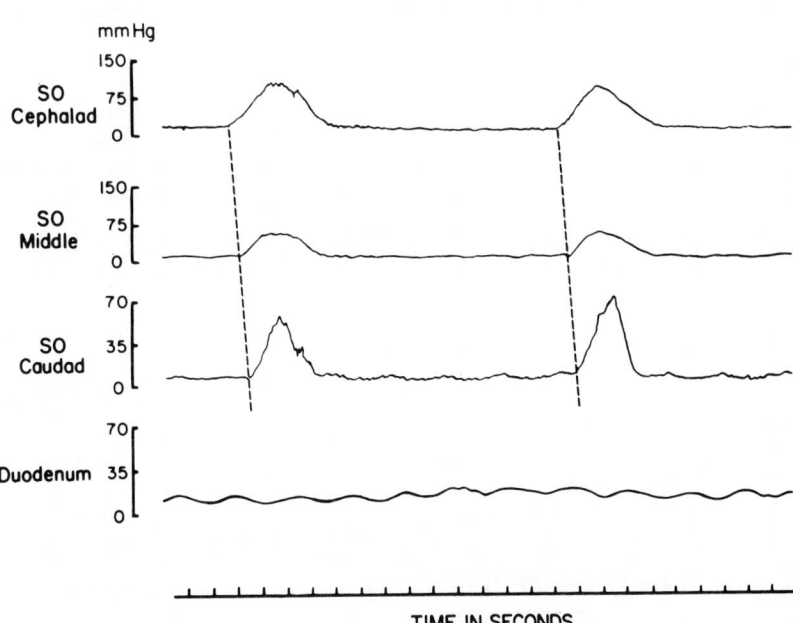

FIGURE 11–8. Manometric recording of phasic contractile activity within the sphincter of Oddi (*SO*) in humans. The contractions are antegrade in direction and occur independent of duodenal motor activity. *CBD,* common bile duct. (Toouli J, Hogan WJ, Geenen JE, et al. Action of cholecystokinin-octapeptide on sphincter of Oddi basal pressure and phasic wave activity in humans. Surgery 1982;92:497.)

presence of increased phasic activity within the sphincter (phase III). In an elaborate series of experiments, Scott and associates[185] recently characterized gallbladder and sphincter of Oddi motility in relation to transsphincteric bile flow during the interdigestive and digestive periods in the dog. Their findings are summarized in Figure 11-9. Peak bile flow during phase II of the MMC was associated with active gallbladder contraction and moderate decreases in sphincter tone and phasic contractile activity. During phase III, sphincter tone and phasic contractile activity increased and was associated with decreased bile flow, despite a sustained increase in gallbladder pressure. These researchers also observed that total duodenal bile acid delivery tended to be greater under those circumstances that eliminated the influence of the sphincter. From these observations they concluded that the primary role of the sphincter during the interdigestive period is to act as an output resistor that limits the flow of hepatic bile into the duodenum. Both the tonic and phasic contractile properties of the sphincter appear to contribute to the resistance, with the latter being critically important during phase III of the intestinal MMC. The authors could not rule out the possibility, however, that the delivery of bile into the duodenum across a sphincter that maintained a resting pressure higher than in the common bile duct (first half of MMC) might reflect a propulsive component to the phasic motor activity of the sphincter. While it is possible that the sphincter motor activity may serve two functions, they left little doubt that the primary function is to serve as a resistor to bile flow.

Relatively little is known about the motor dynamics of the sphincter of Oddi in humans as it relates to bile flow into the duodenum during the interdigestive period. It is known, however, that bile flow is cyclic and peaks during the latter part of phase II of the intestinal MMC and declines during phase III. Although the information is limited, there is evidence to suggest that the phasic contractile activity of the sphincter varies cyclically with the duodenal MMC. Torsoli and co-workers[127] have demonstrated that the frequency of contraction increases from a minimum of 2 per minute during phase I of the MMC cycle to 10 to 12 per minute coincident with phase III. It is tempting to speculate that the decreased transsphincteric flow during phase III of the MMC is a consequence of increased sphincter motor activity, suggesting that in humans the sphincter also serves the role of a resistor.

Digestive Period

Feeding is associated with the prompt and rapid delivery of bile into the duodenum. In addition to active gallbladder contraction, it is now appreciated that alterations in sphincter of Oddi tone and phasic contractile activity contribute to the postprandial delivery of bile.[210,211,225] The nature of the motility pattern depends on whether the primary role of the sphincter is to act as a pump or as a resistor. In the opossum, feeding is associated with an increase the phasic contractile activity of the sphincter,[215,226] and this is consistent with the hypothesis that the sphincter acts as a pump to promote the delivery of bile into the duodenum in this species.

In dogs and in humans the sphincter of Oddi is believed to regulate bile flow by acting as a variable resistor.[210,211,225] Thus it is not surprising that the response of the sphincter to feeding in these species is believed to involve a decrease in motor activity. Interestingly, few studies have directly examined this hypothesis. One such study by Scott and Diamant,[204] however, provides strong support for the idea of inhibition of sphincter motility during feeding (see Fig 11-9). In their study the sphincter evidenced an almost immediate decrease in tone and phasic contractile activity that lasted for only a brief period of time; this was followed by a slight increase in tone and the return of irregular phasic contractions. This pattern of activity was consistent with their finding that bile acid delivery into the duodenum was biphasic, with an immediate burst followed by a lower sustained rate of delivery.

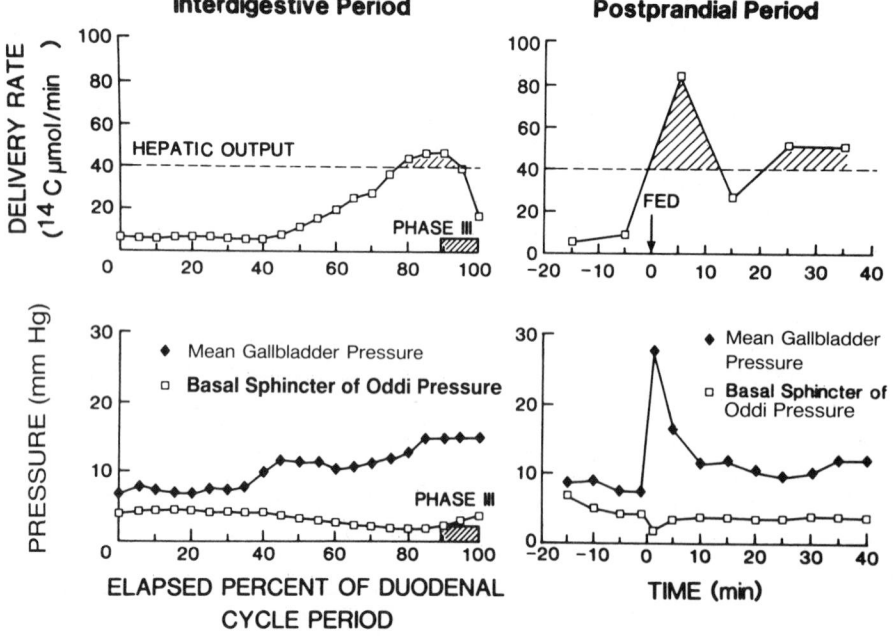

FIGURE 11-9. Summary of gallbladder and sphincter of Oddi (*SO*) pressures and bile delivery into the duodenum of dogs during the interdigestive and postprandial periods. (Scott RB, Diamant SC. Biliary motility associated with gallbladder storage and duodenal delivery of canine hepatic biliary output. Gastroenterology 1988;95:1069.)

They proposed that the degree of sphincter of Oddi relaxation (in combination with gallbladder contraction) regulates duodenal bile and delivery in the dog. Considering that the dynamics of bile flow in the dog closely resembles that of the human, it seems reasonable to suggest that the sphincter serves a similar role in humans.

HORMONAL CONTROL

As noted previously in this chapter, the hormone CCK plays an important physiologic role in the stimulation of bile delivery into the duodenum during the postprandial period. In addition to promoting gallbladder contraction, there is now considerable evidence that the hormone acts as the sphincter of Oddi.[210,211,225] Indeed, most of the insight into the behavior of the sphincter during feeding has been obtained from studies involving CCK rather than meal stimulation. Sandbloom and associates,[227] in 1939, were the first to demonstrate that the exogenous administration of CCK decreases the resistance to flow through the sphincteric region at the lower end of the common bile duct in dogs. Since that time numerous investigators have confirmed this observation in a number of animal species, including humans.[155,189,228]

In humans, as well as in cats and dogs, CCK decreases the resistance to bile outflow from the common bile duct into the duodenum by decreasing both the phasic and tonic contractile activity of the sphincter.[103,192,207,223,229,230] Behar and Biancani[80,231,232] have suggested that the inhibitory effect of CCK is the result of stimulation of nonadrenergic, noncholinergic inhibitory nerves that act on the sphincter muscle to produce a decrease in resistance and an increase in flow across the sphincter.

In contrast to the physiologic effect of CCK on the contractile activity of the sphincter of Oddi in cats, dogs, and humans and other primates, CCK increases the motility of the sphincter in rabbits, opossums, and prairie dogs.[203,212–214,217,233–235] In these animals CCK produces a dose-dependent increase in the frequency and force of the phasic contractions and augments bile flow into the duodenum. The increase in phasic contractions acts as a peristaltic pump that repeatedly clears the sphincter segment of bile, thus rendering it empty for filling from the common bile duct. The overall effect of an increase in phasic activity in these species is an accelerated rate of bile flow into the duodenum. The physiologic mechanisms responsible for the obvious species difference in the response of the sphincter of Oddi to CCK remain unsettled. As noted, Behar and Biancani[80,231,232] demonstrated that CCK decreases the resistance to flow across the feline sphincter of Oddi by stimulation of an inhibitory neural input to the muscle. They also demonstrated that CCK exerts a direct stimulatory effect on the sphincter muscle but that the inhibitory neural influences dominate under physiologic conditions. It has been proposed that in those species in which CCK exerts an inhibitory effect on sphincter activity the neurally mediated pathway is the predominant site of action of the hormone, whereas an excitatory response to CCK indicates a direct stimulation of the sphincteric smooth muscle.

As was the situation with the gallbladder, a variety of peptide hormones in addition to CCK have been reported to affect sphincter of Oddi motility. The physiologic significance of these observations, however, remain unsettled. Table 11-5 is a summary of the observations made to date.[2,131,189,195,209–211,214,222,234–243]

NEURAL CONTROL

Although myogenic mechanisms are believed to be primarily responsible for sphincter of Oddi tone and phasic contractile activity, there is increasing evidence that the contractile activity of the sphincter may be modulated by tonic excitatory and inhibitory neural inputs.[210,211,225] Potter and Mann[193,244] and Elman and McMaster[181] were among the first to demonstrate that the perception of food results in a decreased resistance to flow through the sphincter. Since then other investigators have demonstrated a cephalic phase to sphincter of Oddi relaxation, presumably mediated by the vagus nerve. Support for a role of the vagus nerve in modulating sphincter of Oddi tone comes from the observations that direct stimulation of efferent vagal fibers relaxes the sphincter of Oddi,[112] whereas vagotomy increases the resistance to flow through the sphincter.[186,237] These findings have led to the hypothesis that the vagus nerve exerts a predominantly tonic inhibitory input to the sphincter of Oddi.

Direct mechanical or electrical stimulation of the gallbladder also has been reported to initiate a reflex inhibition of the sphincter of Oddi that is independent of vagal pathways.[151,245,246] Other investigators have reported that vagotomy does not interfere with the cyclic nature of sphincter of Oddi activity in the fasting state.[247] These observations have led to the conclusion that extrinsic neural input via extramural autonomic ganglia, such as the celiac or superior mesenteric ganglia, also may be involved in the reflex regulation of sphincter of Oddi resistance.

It is now generally believed that the extrinsic neural inputs to the sphincter of Oddi mediate their actions via activation of intrinsic intramural neurons. Studies by Persson[21,248] and by Behar and Biancani[80,112,232,249–251] clearly demonstrate the existence of tonic excitatory and inhibitory intramural neural pathways. The makeup of the excitatory and inhibitory pathways is complex and appears to involve opiate containing neurons, serotonergic neurons, cholinergic excitatory neurons, and nonadrenergic, noncholinergic inhibitory neurons. Recent studies also suggest that the excitatory and inhibitory inputs may differ with the respect to the organization of their distribution. The excitatory cholinergic input is believed to be arranged in ascending pathways, whereas the inhibitory nerves

TABLE 11–5
Effect of Gastrointestinal Peptides on Sphincter of Oddi Motility

	REFERENCE
Excitatory	
Cholecystokinin	189, 209–211, 236
Secretin	195, 235, 237
Gastrin	131, 195, 214, 222, 234, 237, 238
Motilin	2, 189, 209–211, 239, 240
Inhibitory	
Cholecystokinin	2, 189, 209–211
Secretin	195, 236
Glucagon	195, 214, 222, 234
Peptide YY	241
Pancreatic polypeptide	242, 243

appear to descend in a proximal to distal orientation within the sphincter (Helm and colleagues, unpublished observation).

It is clear that the intramural neural input to the sphincter of Oddi is complex. At the present time the roles of the excitatory and inhibitory pathways remain unsettled. It has been suggested that the inhibitory neural input to the sphincter of Oddi serves to modify resting sphincter of Oddi tone and to mediate extrinsic neural and CCK-induced sphincter of Oddi relaxation during digestion. The role of the cholinergic excitatory input to the sphincter of Oddi remains even more speculative, but it may be involved in motilin-induced increases in sphincter motility during the interdigestive period and in determining the frequency and propagation characteristics of the phasic peristaltic contractions during the digestive period. Further studies are necessary if we are to fully understand the organization, operation, and function of the intramural neurons.

ABNORMALITIES OF BILIARY TRACT MOTILITY

Gallbladder

With the recent advent of noninvasive technologies for the determination of gallbladder emptying, it has become obvious that abnormal motility can be documented in a broad spectrum of patients. These include diabetics, patients who have undergone some forms of vagotomy, patients on total parenteral nutrition, patients with sprue, patients with hypercholesteremia, and pregnant women. Each of the above-mentioned conditions that leads to gallbladder stasis also results in an increased incidence of gallstone disease.

With the exception perhaps of pregnancy and hypercholesteremia, little is known about the underlying factors that contribute to the decreased motility of the gallbladder. Vagotomy and diabetes may alter emptying by disrupting the excitatory cholinergic innervation to the gallbladder.[30,53,174] Impaired postprandial emptying of the gallbladder in patients with sprue most likely reflects decreased CCK release from the atrophic intestinal mucosa.[49] The cause(s) of gallbladder enlargement and stasis in patients undergoing total parenteral nutrition remain a mystery but may be related to the unmasking of other factors that are associated with an increased risk of stasis such as ileal disease.[252]

In patients with cholesterol stones decreased gallbladder emptying may be due in part to alterations in the contractility of the gallbladder smooth muscle. Recent studies using ground squirrels and prairie dogs fed high-cholesterol diets clearly indicate that force development by the gallbladder decreases prior to stone formation and that the contractile response is decreased regardless of the agonist or its presumed mechanism of action.[253–256,256a,256b] Behar and associates[257] reported similar findings for gallbladder smooth muscle strips removed from humans. In their study, gallbladders exposed to bile with excess cholesterol contracted less forcefully than gallbladders removed from patients with black pigment stones. These findings are consistent with the general hypothesis that exposure of gallbladder smooth muscle to bile saturated with cholesterol alters the basic expression of the ex-

citation-contraction coupling process. The factors involved in the decreased contractility remain unresolved but may be related to changes in the isozyme pattern of the contractile protein actin[259] or to alterations in intracellular calcium storage or release.[257]

Pregnancy also is associated with a decrease in gallbladder emptying.[65,259] In contrast to patients with cholesterol gallstones, the decreased emptying that occurs during pregnancy appears not to reflect an overall decrease in smooth muscle contractility. Ryan[2,118] has reported that pregnancy decreases the in vitro contractile response of the guinea pig gallbladder to agonists that involve intracellular calcium in the excitation-contraction coupling process (CCK and acetylcholine) but has no effect on agonists that involve only extracellular calcium. The factors responsible for the decreased force development remain unsettled but may be related to the high circulating levels of progesterone.[65,252]

Sphincter of Oddi

As described in an earlier section of this chapter, the human sphincter of Oddi is characterized by a basal pressure that is generally 5 to 15 mm Hg above duodenal pressure and by phasic contractions that occur at a frequency of 4 to 5 per minute. With the advent of reliable manometric recording devices it has become obvious that populations of patients exist in whom sphincter motility is abnormal.[189,209–211] Generally, the motor abnormalities are broken down into four catagories: (1) increased basal pressure, (2) increased phasic contractile activity, (3) abnormal propagation of phasic contractions, and (4) paradoxic response to CCK. It has been proposed that each of these abnormal motility patterns may contribute to the biliary-type pain that is not infrequently experienced by patients who have no demonstrable mechanical cause for their discomfort.

The most common abnormality of sphincter dysfunction is increased basal pressure.[210] Increased tone can develop as a consequence of either anatomic (papillary stenosis) or functional (sphincter of Oddi dyskinesia) changes in sphincter performance. The distinction between the two entities is based on the fact that the increased basal pressure caused by stenosis does not decrease in response to smooth muscle relaxants such as amyl nitrate, CCK, or glucagon, whereas these agents significantly reduce the basal pressure in sphincter of Oddi dyskinesia. Increased sphincter tone may reduce bile flow by limiting passive bile flow across the sphincter.

Increased sphincter of Oddi phasic contractile activity, termed *tachyoddia*, has been reported to occur in 20% of patients suspected of having functional sphincter obstruction.[210,211] The phenomenon also occurs following the administration of morphine.[210] The increased contractile frequency is believed to reduce bile flow by causing a partial obstruction of the common bile duct.

In humans the majority of sphincter of Oddi phasic contractions propagate antegrade toward the duodenum.[207] The remainder of the contractions either occur simultaneously or propagate retrograde. There is some evidence from studies performed on the opossum that an increase in the retrograde activity of the phasic contractions decreases bile flow.[216] It has recently been reported that patients with retained common duct stones evidence increased retograde contractions and that this altered activity may favor common duct stasis and/or stone retention.[83] Two points should

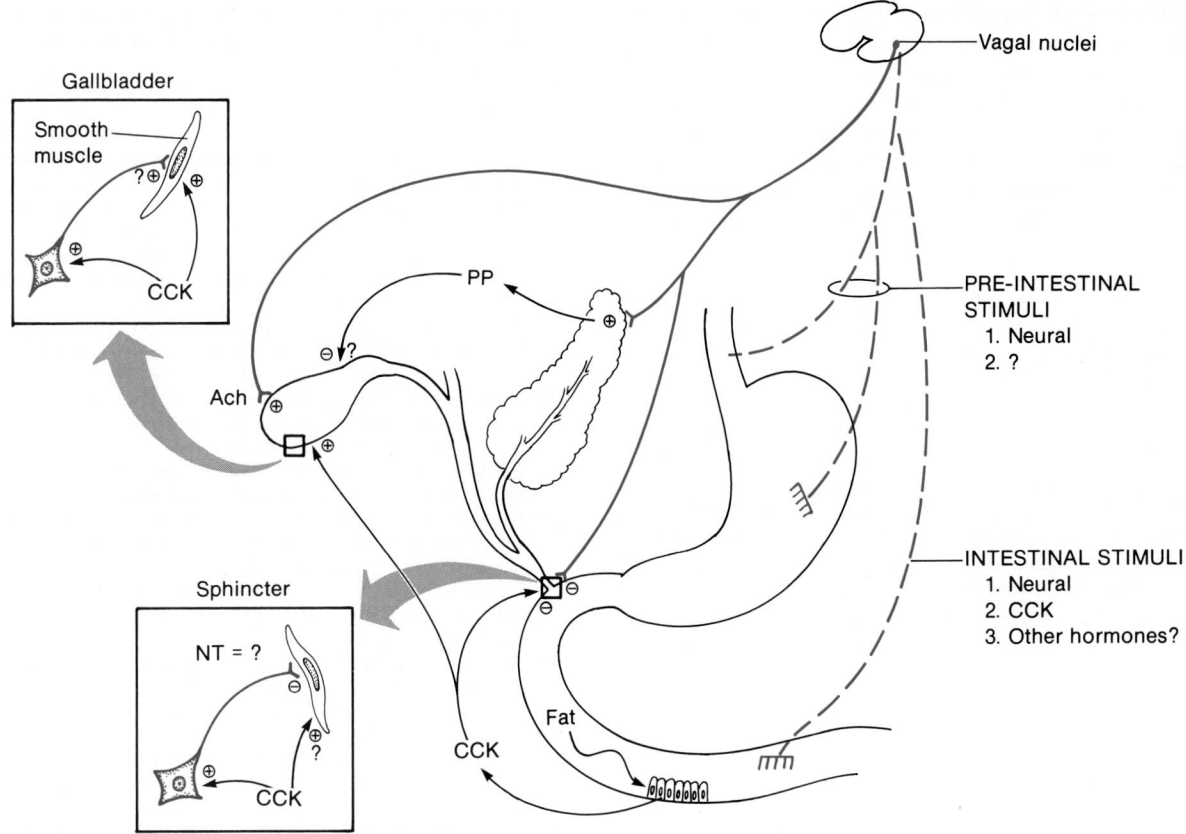

FIGURE 11-10. Schematic representation of the regulation of gallbladder emptying during the digestive periods. Acetylcholine and cholecystokinin cause gallbladder contraction and sphincter of Oddi relaxation. The inserts represent the proposed mechanism of action of acetylcholine and cholecystokinin at the gallbladder and the sphincter. Pancreatic polypeptide may be involved in the inhibitory feedback regulation of gallbladder contraction and sphincter of Oddi relaxation. The other factors responsible for the regulation of gallbladder emptying remain unknown.

be considered, however, when trying to define the role of retrograde contractions in affecting bile flow in humans. First, it remains to be determined whether the altered motility precedes stone formation or whether it is a result of the presence of stones in the lumen of the sphincter. Second, although decreased antegrade activity might limit flow during the interdigestive period in humans, flow during the digestive period may be less affected mainly because it occurs primarily between contractions.

In humans, the endogenous release or exogenous administration of CCK normally results in a decrease in the phasic and tonic contractile activity of the sphincter of Oddi. In some patients suspected of having obstructive sphincter of Oddi dysfunction, however, the exogenous administration of CCK elicits a paradoxic response—both the basal pressure and the contractile frequency increase, and the patient generally complains of upper abdominal pain.[230] It is presumed that a similar response occurs to the CCK released during the ingestion of a meal. The increased motor activity is believed to mimic sphincter obstruction, decrease bile flow, and lead to duct distention and pain. The paradoxic response to CCK may be related to alterations in the inhibitory innervation to the sphincter.[80] CCK is believed to relax the sphincter of Oddi by stimulation of nonadrenergic, noncholinergic inhibitory nerves whose actions tend to override any direct stimulatory effect of the peptide on the muscle. Any impairment of the inhibitory neuronal

input would unmask the excitatory effect of the hormone and lead to increased motor activity.

SUMMARY

Gallbladder emptying is an complex process involving gallbladder contraction and changes in the motor activity of the sphincter of Oddi. In those species in which the sphincter is believed to act as a pump, emptying is aided by an increase in the peristaltic contractile activity of the sphincter. In those species (including humans) in which the sphincter may serve as a variable resistor, decreases in sphincter tone and phasic contractile activity (sphincter relaxation) contribute to the flow of bile into the duodenum. There is little doubt that the regulation of gallbladder emptying during the interdigestive and digestive periods involves the interaction of neural, hormonal, and perhaps local factors. Unfortunately, very little is known about the different influences and how they interact to regulate gallbladder and sphincter of Oddi contraction and relaxation. While the role of CCK remains secure, there can be little doubt that other hormones must also be involved in the physiologic regulation of gallbladder emptying. It will be up to future investigators to combine the modern techniques available for monitoring gallbladder emptying with sensitive and specific radioimmunoassays for the different gastrointestinal hormones if we are to fully appreciate the hormonal regulation of biliary tract dynamics. More creative experimental designs also will be required if we are to define the role of the extrinsic and intrinsic nervous systems in regulating emptying. Figure 11-10 is a schematic representation of the factors believed to be involved in the control of gallbladder and sphincter of Oddi motility.

The reader is directed to Chapter 1, The Enteric Nervous System and its Extrinsic Connections; Chapter 2, Gastrointestinal Hormones; Chapter 3, The Brain–Gut Axis; Chapter 4, Smooth Muscle of the Gut; Chapter 7, Esophageal Motor Function; Chapter 8, The Physiology of Gastric Motility and Gastric Emptying; Chapter 9, Motility of the Small Intestine; Chapter 10, The Motor Function of the Colon; Chapter 93, Gallbladder and Biliary Tree: Anatomy and Structural Anomalies; Chapter 95, Diseases of the Biliary Tree; Chapter 113, Endoscopic Retrograde Cholangiopancreatography, Endoscopic Sphincterotomy and Stone Removal, Endoscopic Biliary and Pancreatic Drainage; and Chapter 128, Evaluation of Gastrointestinal Motility: Methodological Considerations.

REFERENCES

1. Lanzani A, Jazrawi RP, Northfield TC. Simultaneous quantitative measurements of absolute gallbladder storage and emptying during fasting and eating in humans. Gastroenterology 1987;92:852.
2. Ryan JP. Motility of the gallbladder and biliary tree. In: Johnson LR, ed. Physiology of the gastrointestinal tract. 2nd ed. New York: Raven Press, 1987.
3. Code CF, Schlegel JF. The gastrointestinal interdigestive housekeeper: motor correlates of the interdigestive myoelectric complex in the dog. In: Proceedings of the Fourth International Symposium on Gastrointestinal Motility. Banff, Alberta, Canada. Mitchell Press, Vancouver, 1974.
4. Code CF, Marlett JA. The interdigestive myoelectric complex of the stomach and small bowel of dogs. J Physiol Lond 1975;216:289.
5. Szurszewski JH. A migrating electric complex of the canine small intestine. Am J Physiol 1969;217:1757.
6. Peeters TL, Vantrappen G, Janssens J. Bile acid output and the interdigestive migrating complex in normals and in cholecystectomyzed patients. Gastroenterology 1980;79:678.
7. Itoh Z, Takahashi I. Periodic contractions of the canine gallbladder during the interdigestive state. Am J Physiol 1981;240:G183.
8. Itoh Z, Takahashi I, Nakaya M, et al. Interdigestive gallbladder bile concentration in relation to periodic contraction of gallbladder in the dog. Gastroenterology 1982;83:645.
9. Itoh Z, Takahaski I, Nakaya M, Suzuki T. Gallbladder bile concentration during the interdigestive state. Biomed Res 1983;4:269.
10. Suzuki T, Takahashi I, Itoh Z. Motilin and gallbladder: new dimensions in gastrointestinal physiology. Peptides 1981;2:229.
11. Takahashi I, Suzuki T, Aizawa I, Itoh Z. Comparison of gallbladder contractions induced by motilin and cholecystokinin in dogs. Gastroenterology 1982;82:419.
12. Matsumoto T, Sarna SK, Condon RE, et al. Canine gallbladder cyclic motor activity. Am J Physiol 1988;255:G409.
13. Scott RB, Eidt PB, Shaffer EA. Regulation of fasting canine duodenal bile acid delivery by sphincter of Oddi and gallbladder. Am J Physiol 1985;249:G622.
14. Traynor OJ, Dozois RR, DiMagno EP. Canine interdigestive and postprandial gallbladder motility and emptying. Am J Physiol 1984;246:G426.
15. Takahashi I, Kern MK, Dodds WJ, et al. Contraction pattern of opossum gallbladder during fasting and after feeding. Am J Physiol 1986;250:G227.
16. Hofmann AF. The enterohepatic circulation of bile acids in man. Clin Gastroenterol 1977;6:3.
17. Kraglund K, Hjermind J, Jensen FT, et al. Gallbladder emptying and gastrointestinal cyclic motor activity in humans. Scand J Gastroenterol 1984;19:990.
18. Small DM, Rapo S. The source of abnormal bile in patients with cholesterol gallstones. N Engl J Med 1970;283:53.
19. Shearin NL, Becker JM, Sharp SW. Analysis of intracellular slow waves recorded from opossum sphincter of Oddi. Gastroenterology 1984;86:1246A.
19a. Qvist N, Oster-Jorgensen E, Rasmussen L, et al. The relationship between gallbladder dynamics and the migrating motor complex in fasting healthy subjects. Scand J Gastroenterol 1988;23:562.
20. Marzio L, Neri M, Capone F, et al. Gallbladder contraction and its relationship to interdigestive duodenal motor activity in normal human subjects. Dig Dis Sci 1988;33:540.
21. Persson CGA. Excitatory effect of tetrodotoxin on an isolated smooth muscle organ. J Pharm Pharmacol 1971;23:986.
22. Svenberg T, Christofides ND, Fitzpatrick ML, et al. Interdigestive biliary output in man: relationship to fluctuations in plasma motilin and effect of atropine. Gut 1982;23:1024.
23. Toouli J, Bushell M, Stevenson G, et al. Gallbladder emptying in man related to fasting duodenal migrating motor contractions. Aust NZ J Surg 1986;56:147.
24. Lee KY, Chey WY, Tai HH. Radio-immunoassay of motilin: validation and studies on the relationship between plasma motilin and interdigestive myoelectric activity of duodenum of the dog. Am J Dig Dis 1978;23:789.
25. Beneventano TC, Rosen RG, Schein CJ. The physiological effect of acute vagal section on canine biliary dynamics. J Surg Res 1969;9:331.
26. Sturdivant RAL, Stern DH, Resin H, Isenberg JI. Effect of graded doses of octapeptide of cholecystokinin on gallbladder size in man. Gastroenterology 1973;64:452.
27. Takahashi I, Dodds WJ, Hogan WJ, et al. Effect of vagotomy on changes in gallbladder volume during fasting and after feeding on the conscious opossum. Gastroenterology 1984;186:1273A.
28. Sarna SK. Cyclic motor activity: migrating motor complex. Gastroenterology 1985;89:894.
29. Baxter JN, Grime JS, Critchley M, Shields R. Relationship between gastric emptying of solids and gallbladder emptying in normal subjects. Gut 1985;26:342.
30. Baxter JN, Grime JS, Critchley M, et al. Relationship between gastric emptying of a solid meal and emptying of the gallbladder before and after vagotomy. Gut 1987;28:855.
31. Kristnamurthy GT, Bobba VR, McConnell D, et al. Quantitative biliary dynamics: introduction of a new noninvasive scintigraphic technique. J Nucl Med 1983;24:217.
32. Sarva RP, Sheiner DP, VanThiel D, Yingvorapant N. Gallbladder function: method for measuring filling and emptying. J Nucl Med 1985;26:140.
33. Shaffer EA, McOrmand P, Duggan H. Quantitative cholescintigraphy: assessment of gallbladder filling and emptying and duodenogastric reflex. Gastroenterology 1980;79:899.
34. van der Linden W, Kempi V. Filling of the gallbladder as studied by computer-assisted Tc-99m HIDA scintigraphy. J Nucl Med 1984;25:292.
35. Davison JS, Al-Hassani M, Growe R, Burnstock G. The non-adrenergic, inhibitory innervation of the guinea pig gallbladder. Pflugers Arch 1978;377:43.
36. Davison JS, Al-Hassani M. The role of noncholinergic, nonadrenergic nerves in regulating the distensibility of the guinea pig gallbladder. In: Christensen J, ed. Gastrointestinal motility. New York: Raven Press, 1980.
37. Cole MJ, Shaffer EA, Scott RB. Gallbladder pressure, compliance, and hysteresis during cyclic volume change. Can J Physiol Pharmacol 1987;65:2124.
38. Boyden EA. Analysis of reaction of human gallbladder to food. Anat Rec 1928;40:147.

39. Edholm P. Gallbladder evacuation in the normal male induced by cholecystokinin. Acta Radiol 1960;53:257.

40. Herzog RJ, Nelson JA. The role of cholecystokinin in radiographic opacification of the gallbladder. Invest Radiol 1976;11:440.

41. Park CY, Pae YS, Hong SS. Radiologic studies on emptying of the human gallbladder. Am Surg 1970;96:869.

42. Brunner H, Northfield TC, Hoffman AF, et al. Gastric emptying and secretion of bile acids, cholesterol and pancreatic enzymes during digestion: duodenal perfusion studies in healthy subjects. Mayo Clin Proc 1974;49:851.

43. Levitt MO, Bond J. Use of constant perfusion techniques in the nonsteady state. Gastroenterology 1977;73:1450.

44. Englert E, Chiu VS. Quantitation analysis of human biliary evacuation with a radioisotopic technique. Gastroenterology 1966;50:506.

45. Bobba VR, Krishnamwurthy GT, Kingston E, et al. Gallbladder dynamics induced by a fatty meal in normal subjects and patients with gallstones. J Nucl Med 1984;25:21.

46. Fisher RS, Stelzer F, Rock E, Malmud LS. Abnormal gallbladder emptying in patients with gallstones. Dig Dis Sci 1982;27:1019.

47. Forgacs IC, Maisey MN, Murphy GM, Dowling RH. Influence of gallstones and ursodeoxycholic acid therapy on gallbladder emptying. Gastroenterology 1984;87:299.

48. Shaffer EA, Taylor PJ, Logan K, et al. The effect of progestin on gallbladder function in young women. Am J Obstet Gynecol 1984;148:504.

49. Maton PN, Selden AC, Fitzpatrick ML, Chadwick VS. Defective gallbladder emptying and cholecystokinin release in celiac disease. Gastroenterology 1985;88:391.

50. Krishnamurthy GT, Bobba VR, Kingston E. Radionuclide ejection fraction: a technique for quantitative analysis of motor function of the human gallbladder. Gastroenterology 1981;80:482.

51. Krishnamurthy GT, Bobba VR, Kingston E, Turner F. Measurement of gallbladder emptying sequentially using a single dose of ^{99m}Tc-labeled hepatobiliary agent. Gastroenterology 1982;83:773.

51a. Mackie CR, Baxter JN, Grime JS, et al. Gallbladder emptying in normal subjects: a data base for clinical cholescintigraphy. Gut 1987;28:137.

52. Lonovics J, Devitt P, Rayford PL, Thompson JC. Actions of VIP, somatostatin, and pancreatic polypeptide on gallbladder tension and CCK-stimulated gallbladder contraction in vitro. Surg Forum 1979;30:407.

53. Fisher RS, Rock E, Malmud LS. Cholinergic effects on gallbladder emptying in humans. Gastroenterology 1985;89:716.

54. Sylwestrowicz TA, Shaffer EA. Gallbladder function during gallstone dissolution. Gastroenterology 1988;95:740.

55. Everson GT, Braverman DZ, Johnson ML, Kern F Jr. A critical evaluation of real-time ultrasonography for the study of gallbladder volume and contraction. Gastroenterology 1980;79:40.

56. Lilja P, Fagan C, Wiener S, et al. Disappearance half-time of CCK-99% correlated with gallbladder volume in man. Gastroenterology 1981;80:1213A.

57. Campra JL, Caeiro T, Pitt HA. Dyskinesia and impaired gallbladder emptying in patients with Chagas' disease. Gastroenterology 1985;88:1653A.

58. Everson GT, Lawson MJ, McKinley C, et al. Gallbladder and small intestinal regulation of biliary lipid secretion during intraduodenal infusion of standard stimuli. J Clin Invest 1983;71:596.

59. Lawson M, Everson GT, Klingensmith W, Kern J Jr. Coordination of gastric and gallbladder emptying after ingestion of a regular meal. Gastroenterology 1983;85:866.

60. Worobetz LJ, Baker RJ, McCallum JA, et al. The effect of naloxone, morphine, and an enkephalin analogue on cholecystokinin octapeptide stimulated gallbladder emptying. Am J Gastroenterol 1982;77:509.

61. Mogadam M, Albarelli J, Ahmed SW, et al. Gallbladder dynamics in response to various meals: is dietary fat restriction necessary in the management of gallstones? Am J Gastroenterol 1984;79:745.

62. Thompson JC, Fried GM, Ogden WD, et al. Correlation between release of cholecystokinin and contraction of the gallbladder in patients with gallstones. Ann Surg 1982;195:670.

63. Gullo L, Bolondi L, Priori P, et al. Inhibitory effect of atropine on cholecystokinin-induced gallbladder contraction in man. Digestion 1984;29:209.

64. Ylostalo P, Kirkinen P, Heikkinen J, et al. Gallbladder volume and serum bile acids in cholestasis of pregnancy. Br J Obstet Gynecol 1982;89:59.

65. Everson GT, McKinley C, Lawson M, et al. Gallbladder function in the human female: effect of ovulatory cycle, pregnancy, and contraceptive steroids. Gastroenterology 1982;82:711.

66. Kern F Jr, Everson GT, DeMark B, et al. Biliary lipids, bile acids, and gallbladder function in human female: effects of pregnancy and the ovulatory cycle. J Clin Invest 1981;68:1229.

67. Hopman WPM, Jansen JBMJ, Rosenbusch G, Lamers CG. Effect of equimolar amounts of long-chain triglycerides and medium-chain triglycerides on plasma CCK and gallbladder contraction. Am J Clin Nutr 1984;39:356.

68. Wiener I, Inoue K, Fagan CJ, et al. Release of CCK in man: correlation of blood levels with gallbladder contraction. Ann Surg 1981;194:321.

69. Lilja P, Fagan CJ, Wiener I, et al. Infusion of pure CCK in humans: correlation between plasma concentration of CCK and gallbladder size. Gastroenterology 1982;83:256.

70. Isaza J, Jones DT, Dragstedt LR, Woodward ER. The effect of vagotomy on motor function of the gallbladder. Surgery 1971;70:616.

71. Ivy AC, Oldberg E. A hormone mechanism for gallbladder contraction and evacuation. Am J Physiol 1928;86:599.

72. Lin TM. Actions of gastrointestinal hormones and related peptides on motor function of the biliary tract. Gastroenterology 1975;69:1006.

73. Houssay BA, Rubio HH. La function de la vesicula biliar injertada y la hormona duodenocolecisto-quintica. Ren Soc Argent Biol 1932;8:369.

74. Jorpes JE. The isolation and chemistry of secretin and cholecystokinin. Gastroenterology 1968;55:157.

75. Jorpes JE, Mutt V. On the biological activity and amino acid composition of secretin. Acta Chem Scand 1961;15:1790.

76. Jorpes JE, Mutt V, Toczko K. Further purification of cholecystokinin and pancreozymin. Acta Chem Scand 1964;18:2408.

77. Kothary PC, Vinik AI, Owyjang C, Fiddian-Green RG. Immunochemical studies of molecular heterogeneity of cholecystokinin in duodenal perfusates and plasma in humans. J Biol Chem 1983;258:2856.

78. Rehfeld JF. Immunochemical studies on cholecystokinin: II. Distribution and molecular heterogeneity in the central nervous system and small intestine of hog and man. J Biol Chem 1978;253:4022.

79. Amer MS. Studies with cholecystokinin: II. Cholecystokinetic potency of porcine gastrins I and II and related peptides in three systems. Endocrinology 1969;84:1277.

80. Behar J, Biancani P. Effect of cholecystokinin and the octapeptide of cholecystokinin on feline sphincter of Oddi and gallbladder mechanisms of action. J Clin Invest 1980;66:1231.

81. Chowdhury JR, Berkowitz JM, Praissiman M, Fora JW. Interaction between octapetide-cholecystokinin, gastrin, and secretin on cat gallbladder in vitro. Am J Physiol 1975;229:1311.

82. Chowdhury JR, Berkowitz JM, Praissman M, Fora JW. Effect of sulfated and non-sulfated gastrin and octapeptide cholecystokinin on cat gallbladder in vitro. Experientia 1976;32:1173.

83. Davison JS, Najafi-Farashah A. Dibutryl cyclic GMP, a competitive inhibitor of cholecystokinin/pancreazymin and related peptides in the gallbladder and ileum. Can J Physiol Pharmacol 1981;59:1100.

84. Hedner P. Effect of the C-terminal octapeptide of cholecystokinin on guinea pig ileum and gallbladder in vitro. Acta Physiol Scand 1970;78:232.

85. Lamers CBHW, Poitras WP, Jansen JBMJ, Walsh JH. Relative potencies of cholecystokinin-33 and cholecystokinin-8 measured by radio-immunoassay and bioassay. Scand J Gastroenterol 1983;18(suppl 83):191.

86. Rubin B, Engel SL, Drungis AM, et al. Cholecystokinin-like activities in guinea pigs and in dogs of the C-terminal octapeptide of cholecystokinin. J Pharm Sci 1969;58:955.

87. Yau WM, Makhlouf GM, Edwards LE. Mode of action of cholecystokinin and related peptides on gallbladder muscle. Gastroenterology 1973;65:451.

88. Byrnes DJ, Henderson L, Borody T, Rehfeld JF. Radioimmunoassay of cholecystokinin in human plasma. Clin Chim Acta 1981;111:81.

89. Byrnes DJ, Borody T, Daskalopoulos G, et al. Cholecystokinin and

gallbladder contraction: effect of CCK infusion. Peptides 1981;2(suppl 2):259.

90. Calam J, Ellis A, Dockray GJ. Identification and measurement of molecular variants of cholecystokinin in duodenal mucosa and plasma: diminished concentrations in patients with celiac disease. J Clin Invest 1982;69:218.

91. Rehfeld JF, Holst JJ, Lindkaer Jenson S. The molecular notion of vascularly released cholecystokinin from the isolated prefused procine duodenum. Regul Pept 1982;3:15.

92. Walsh JH, Lamers CB, Valenzuala JE. Cholecystokinin-octapeptide-like immunoreactivity in human plasma. Gastroenterology 1982;82:438.

93. Solomon TE, Yamada T, Elashoff J, et al. Bioactivity of cholecystokinin analogues: CCK-8 is not more potent than CCK-33. Am J Physiol 1984;247:G105.

94. Maton PN, Selden AC, Chadwick VS. Large and small forms of cholecystokinin in human plasma: measurement using high pressure liquid chromatography and radioimmunoassay. Regul Pept 1982;4:251.

95. Maton PN, Selden AC, Fitzpatrick ML, Chadwick VS. Infusion of cholecystokinin octapeptide in man: relation between plasma cholecystokinin concentration and gallbladder emptying rate. Eur J Clin Invest 1984;14:37.

96. Chang TM, Chey WY. Radioimmunoassay of cholecystokinin. Dig Dis Sci 1983;28:456.

97. Inoue K, Baba N, Rayford PL. CCK antibody inhibits biologic actions of exogenous and endogenous CCK in dogs. Gastroenterology 1983;84:1194A.

98. Sakamoto T, Fujimura M, Newman J, et al. Comparison of hepatic elimination of different forms of cholecystokinin in dogs. J Clin Invest 1985;75:280.

99. Steigerwalt RW, Goldfine ID, Williams JA. Characterization of cholecystokinin receptors on bovine gallbladder membranes. Am J Physiol 1984;247:G709.

100. Eberlein GE, Eysslein VE, Hesse WH, et al. Detection of CCK-58 in human blood by inhibition of degradation. Am J Physiol 1987;253:G477.

101. Eysselein VE, Eberlein GE, Schaeffer M, et al. Characterization of the major molecular form of CCK in human intestine: CCK-58. Am J Physiol 1990;258:G253.

102. Fried GM, Odgen WD, Greeley G, Thompson JC. Correlation of release and actions of cholecystokinin in dogs before and after vagotomy. Surgery 1983;93:786.

103. Fried GM, Odgen WD, Sivierczek J, et al. Release of cholecystokinin in conscious dogs: correlation with simultaneous measurements of gallbladder pressure and pancreatic protein secretion. Gastroenterology 1983;85:1113.

104. Fried GM, Ogden WD, Fogan CJ, et al. Comparison of cholecystokinin release and gallbladder emptying in man and in women at estrogen and progesterone phases of the menstrual cycle. Surgery 1984;95:284.

105. Kerstens PJSM, Lamers CBHW, Jansen JBMJ, et al. Physiological plasma concentrations of cholecystokinin stimulate pancreatic enzyme secretion and gallbladder contraction in man. Life Sci 1985;36:565.

106. Spellman SJ, Shaffer EA, Rosenthal L. Gallbladder emptying in response to cholecystokinin. Gastroenterology 1979;77:115.

107. Thompson JC, Fried GM, Ogden WD, et al. Correlation between release of cholecystokinin and contraction of the gallbladder in patients with gallstones. Ann Surg 1982;195:670.

108. Malesci A, DeFazia C, Festorazzi S, et al. Effect of loxiglumide on gallbladder contractile response to cerulein and food. Gastroenterology 1990;98:1307.

109. Niederau C, Heindges T, Rovati L, Strohmeyer G. Effect of loxiglumide on gallbladder emptying in healthy volunteers. Gastroenterology 1989;97:1331.

110. Niederau C, Heindges T, Rovati L. Blockade of the CCK-receptor does not only abolish meal induced gallbladder emptying but increases fasting gallbladder volume in healthy humans. Gastroenterology 1989;96:365A.

111. Amer MS. Studies with cholecystokinin in vitro: III. Mechanism of the effect on the isolated rabbit gallbladder strip. J Pharmacol Exp Ther 1972;183:527.

112. Behar J, Biancani P. Effect of naloxone on the cat sphincter of Oddi: evidence for a physiological role of opiod peptides in the regulation of the sphincter of Oddi. In: Wienbeck M, ed. Motility of the digestive tract. New York: Raven Press, 1982.

113. Marzio L, DiGiammarco AM, Neri M, et al. Atropine antagonizes cholecystokinin and cerulein induced gallbladder evacuation in man: a real-time ultrasonographic study. Am J Gastroenterol 1985;80:1.

114. Sundler F, Alumets J, Hakanson R, et al. VIP innervation of the gallbladder. Gastroenterology 1977;72:1375.

115. Amer MS, Becvar WE. A sensitive in vitro method for the assay of cholecystokinin. J Endocrinol 1969;43:637.

116. Andersson KE, Andersson R, Hedner P. Cholecystokinetic effect and concentration of cyclic AMP in gallbladder muscle in vitro. Acta Physiol Scand 1972;85:511.

117. Takahashi S, Kurosawa S, Owyang C. Differential effects of carbachol and CCK on phosphoinositide turnover and adenylate cyclase system of the guinea pig gallbladder. Gastroenterology 1989;96:500A.

117a.Lee KY, Biancani P, Behar J. Calcium sources utilized by cholecystokinin and acetylcholine in the cat gallbladder smooth muscle. Am J Physiol 1989;256:G785.

118. Ryan JP. Calcium and gallbladder smooth muscle contraction in the guinea pig: effect of pregnancy. Gastroenterology 1985;89:1279.

119. Renzetti L, Wang MB, Ryan JP. Contribution of intracellular calcium to gallbladder smooth muscle contraction. Am J Physiol 1990;259:G1.

120. Dorst C, Wang MB, Ryan JP. Relationship between force, myosin phosphorylation, and crossbridge cycling rates in CCK and potassium stimulated gallbladder smooth muscle [Abstract]. Gastroenterology 1990;98:654.

121. Hedner P, Perrson H, Rossman G. Effect of cholecystokinin on small intestine. Acta Physiol Scand 1967;70:250.

122. Pallin B, Skoglund S. Neural and humoral control of gallbladder emptying mechanism in the cat. Acta Physiol Scand 1964;60:358.

123. Ryan J, Cohen S. Interaction of luminal volume and gastrointestinal hormone stimulation on gallbladder motor function. In: Vantrappen G, Agg H, eds. Fifth international symposium on gastrointestinal motility. Herentals, Belgium: Typoff Press, 1976.

124. Schoetz DJ Jr, Birkett DH, Williams LF. Gallbladder motor function in the intact primate: autonomic pharmacology. J Surg Res 1978;24:513.

125. Toouli J, Watts JM. In vitro motility studies on canine and human extrahepatic biliary tracts. Aust NZ J Surg 1971;40:380.

126. Persson CGA. Dual effects on the sphincter of Oddi and gallbladder induced by stimulation of the right splanchnic nerves. Acta Physiol Scand 1973;87:334.

127. Torsoli A, Corazziani E, Habib FI, et al. Frequencies and cyclical pattern of the human sphincter of Oddi phasic activity. Gut 1986;27:363.

128. Cameron AJ, Phillips SF, Summerskill WH. Effect of cholecystokinin, gastrin, secretin, and glucagon on human gallbladder in vitro. Proc Soc Exp Biol Med 1969;131:149.

129. Nakano M, McCloy RE, Gin AC, Nakano SK. Effect of protaglandins E_1, E_2, and F_{2a}, and pentagastrin on gallbladder pressure in dogs. Eur J Pharmacol 1975;30:107.

130. Praissman M, Fara JW, Berkowitz JN. Binding characteristics of the C-terminal octapeptide of cholecystokinin and gastrin to cat gallbladder tissue in vitro: comparison with isometric tension development. In: Bonfils S. Fromougeot P, Rosselin G, eds. Hormonal receptors in digestive tract physiology. New York: North Holland, 1977.

131. Toouli J, Watts JM. Actions of cholecystokinin-pancreozymin, secretin, and gastrin on extra-hepatic biliary tract motility in vitro. Ann Surg 1972;175:434.

132. Vagne M, Grossman MI. Cholecystokinetic potency of gastrointestinal hormones and related peptides. Am J Physiol 1968;215:881.

133. Gadacz TR. Effect of H_2 antagonists on gallbladder contraction. J Surg Res 1978;25:334.

134. Impiciatorre M. Occurrence of H_1 and H_2-histamine receptors in the guinea pig gallbladder in situ. Br J Pharmacol 1978;64:219.

135. LaMorte WW, Hingston SJ, Wise WE. pH-dependent activity of H_1 and H_2-histamine receptors in guinea pig gallbladder. J Pharmacol Exp Ther 1981;217:638.

136. Lennon F, Feeley TM, Clanachan AS, Scott GW. Effects of histamine

receptor stimulation on diseased gallbladder and cystic duct. Gastroenterology 1977;87:257.

137. Schoetz DJ Jr, Wise WE Jr, LaMorte WW, et al. Histamine receptors in primate gallbladder. Dig Dis Sci 1983;28:353.

138. Waldman DB, Zfas AM, Makhlouf GM. Stimulatory (H$_1$) and inhibitory (H$_2$) histamine receptors in gallbladder muscle. Gastroenterology 1977;22:932.

139. Wise WE Jr, LaMorte WW, Gaca JM, et al. Reciprocal H$_1$ and H$_2$-histamine receptors in guinea pig gallbladder. J Surg Res 1982;33:146.

140. Itoh Z. Effect of motilin on gastrointestinal motility. In: Bloom SR, Polak JM, eds. Gut hormones. Edinburgh: Churchill-Livingstone, 1981.

141. Sakamoto T, Mote L, Greeley GH Jr, et al. Effect of neurotensin on gallbladder contraction in dogs. Gastroenterology 1983;86:1229A.

142. Kotwall C, Lennon F, Clanachan AS, et al. Prostaglandins modulate human gallbladder motility. In: Ninth International Symposium on Gastrointestinal Motility. London: MTP Press, 1985.

143. Mroczka J, Baer HP, Scott GW. Effects of prostaglandins on isolated dog gallbladder and systic duct. In: Weinbick M, ed. Motility of the digestive tract. New York: Raven Press, 1982.

144. Nakata K, Osumi Y, Fujuwara M. Prostaglandins and the contractility of the guinea pig biliary system. Pharmacology 1981;22:24.

145. Thornell E, Svanik J, Wood JR. Effects of intraarterial PGE2 on gallbladder fluid transport, motility and hepatic bile flow in the cat. Scand J Gastroenterol 1981;16:1083.

146. Yau WM. Mode of stimulation of gallbladder contraction by substance K. Gastroenterology 1985;88:1637A.

147. Lonovics J, Varro V, Thompson JC. The effect of cholecystokinin and substance-P antagonists on cholecystokinin- and substance P–stimulated gallbladder contraction. Gastroenterology 1985;88:1637A.

147a. Mate L, Sakamoto T, Greeley GH Jr, Thompson JC. The effect of substance P on contractions of the gallbladder. Surg Gynecol Obstet 1986;163:163.

148. Naughton P, Baer HP, Clanachan AS, Scott GW. Adenosine and ATP effects on isolated guinea pig gallbladder. Pflugers Arch 1983;399:42.

149. Persson CGA. Adrenoreceptor functions in the cat choledochoduodenal junction in vitro. Br J Pharmacol 1971;42:447.

150. Persson CGA. Adrenergic, cholecystokinetic and morphine induced effects on extra-hepatic biliary motility. Acta Physiol Scand 1972;383(suppl):1.

151. Whitaker LR. The mechanism of the gallbladder. Am J Physiol 1926;178:411.

152. Adrian TE, Mitchenere P, Sagor GR, Bloom SR. Effect of pancreatic polypeptide on gallbladder pressure and hepatic bile secretion. Am J Physiol 1982;243:G204.

153. Conter RL, Roslyn JJ, DenBensten L, Taylor IL. Pancreatic polypeptide enhances post-contractile gallbladder filling in the prairie dog. Gastroenterology 1987;92:771.

154. Greenberg GR, McCloy RE, Chadwick VS, et al. Effect of bovine pancreatic polypeptide on basal pancreatic and biliary outputs in man. Dig Dis Sci 1979;24:11.

155. Lin TM, Chance RE. Spectrum of gastrointestinal actions of a new bovine pancreas polypeptide. Gastroenterology 1972;62:852A.

156. Ryan J, Cohen S. Interaction of gastrin I, secretin, and cholecystokinin on gallbladder smooth muscle. Am J Physiol 1976;230:553.

157. Ryan J, Cohen S. Pressure-volume response gastrointestinal hormones. Am J Physiol 1976;230:1461.

158. Jansson R, Steen G, Svanvik J. Effects of intravenous vasoactive intestinal peptide (VIP) on gallbladder function in the cat. Gastroenterology 1978;75:47.

159. Piper PJ, Said SI, Vane JR. Effects on smooth muscle preparations of unidentified vasoactive peptides from intestine and lung. Nature 1970;225:1144.

160. Ryan JP. Motility of the gallbladder and biliary tree. In: Johnson LR, ed. Physiology of the gastrointestinal tract. New York: Raven Press, 1981.

161. Ryan J, Cohen S. Effect of vasoactive intestinal peptide on basal and cholecystokinin induced gallbladder pressure. Gastroenterology 1977;73:870.

162. Ryan J, Ryave S. Effect of vasoactive intestinal polypeptide on gallbladder smooth muscle in vitro. Am J Physiol 1978;234:E44.

163. Said SI, Makhlouf GM. Vasoactive intestinal polypeptide: spectrum of biological actions. In: Chey WY, Brooks FP, eds. Endocrinology of the gut. Thorofare. NJ: CB Slack, 1974.

164. Said SI, Mutt V. Polypeptide with broad biological activity: isolation from small intestine. Science 1970;169:1217.

165. Said SI, Mutt V. Isolation from porcine intestinal wall of a vasoactive octacosa-peptide related to secretin and glucagon. Eur J Biochem 1973;28:199.

166. Jansson R. Effects of gastrointestinal hormones on concentrating function and motility in the gallbladder. Acta Physiol Scand 1979;456:1.

167. Bjorck S, Fahrenkrug J, Jivegard L, Svanvik J. Release of immunoreactive VIP from the gallbladder in response to vagal stimulation. Acta Physiol Scand 1986;128:639.

168. Schaffalitzky DM, Fahrenkrug J, Holst JJ. Release of vasoactive intestinal polypeptide by electrical stimulation of vagal nerves. Gastroenterology 1977;72:373.

169. Lonovics J, Devitt P, Watson LC, et al. Pancreatic polypeptide. Arch Surg 1981;116:1256.

170. Lin TM, Evans DC, Chance RE, Spray GF. Bovine pancreatic polypeptide: action on gastric and pancreatic secretion in dogs. Am J Physiol 1977;232:E311.

171. Pomeranz IS, Davison JS, Shaffer EA. In vitro effects of pancreatic polypeptide and motilin on contractility of human gallbladder. Dig Dis Sci 1983;28:539.

172. Amdrup BM, Griffith CA. The effect of vagotomy upon biliary function in dogs. J Surg Res 1970;10:209.

173. Fletcher DM, Clark CG. Changes in canine bile-flow and composition after vagotomy. Br J Surg 1969;56:103.

174. Debas HT, Konturek SJ, Grossman MD. Effect of extragastric and truncal vagotomy on pancreatic secretion in the dog. Am J Physiol 1975;228:1172.

175. Konturek SJ, Becker HD, Thompson JC. Effect of vagotomy on hormones stimulating pancreatic secretion. Arch Surg 1974;108:704.

175a. Gomez G, Lluis F, Guo YS, et al. Bile inhibits release of cholecystokinin and neurotension. Surgery 1986;100:363.

176. Gomez G, Upp JR, Lluis F, et al. Regulation of the release of cholecystokinin by bile salts in dogs and humans. Gastroenterology 1988;94:1036.

177. Green GM, Lyman RL. Feedback regulation of pancreatic enzyme secretion as a mechanism for trypsin-inhibitor-induced hypersecretion in rats. Proc Soc Exp Biol Med 1972;140:6.

178. Owyang C, Louie DS, Tatum D. Feedback regulation of pancreatic enzyme secretion: suppression of CCK release by trypsin. J Clin Invest 1986;77:2042.

179. Inoue K, Yazigi R, Watson LC, et al. Increased release of cholecystokinin after pancreatic duct ligation. Surgery 1982;91:467.

180. Weiner I, Walker JP, Greeley GJ Jr, et al. Increased release of cholecystokinin with intraduodenal fat after cholecystectomy in dogs. Surg Forum 1984;35:196.

181. Elman R, McMaster PD. The physiological variation in resistance to bile flow into the intestine. J Exp Med 1926;44:151.

182. Fisher RS, Rock E, Malmud LS. Gallbladder emptying in response to sham feeding in humans. Gastroenterology 1986;90:1854.

183. Fisher RS, Rock E, Malmud LS. Effect of meal composition on gallbladder and gastric emptying in man. Dig Dis Sci 1987;32:1337.

184. Puestow CB. The discharge of bile into the duodenum. Arch Surg 1931;23:1013.

185. Scott RB, Diamant SC. Biliary motility associated with gallbladder storage and duodenal delivery of canine hepatic biliary output. Gastroenterology 1988;95:1069.

186. Takahashi I, Dodds WJ, Hogan WJ, et al. Effect of vagotomy on biliary tract motor activity in the opossum. Dig Dis Sci 1988;33:481.

187. Debas HT, Yamagishi T. Evidence for a pyloro-cholecystic reflex for gallbladder contraction. Ann Surg 1979;190:170.

188. Yau WM, Youther ML. Modulation of gallbladder motility by intrinsic cholinergic neurons. Am J Physiol 1984;247:G662.

189. Sarles JC. Hormonal control of the sphincter of Oddi. Dig Dis Sci 1986;31:208.

190. Ashkin JR, Lyon DT, Shull SD, et al. Factors affecting delivery of bile into the duodenum in man. Gastroenterology 1978;74:560.

191. Daniels BT, McGlone FB, Job H, Sawyer RB. Changing concepts of common bile duct anatomy and physiology. JAMA 1961;178:394.

192. Ono K, Watanabe N, Suzuki K, et al. Bile flow mechanisms in man. Arch Surg 1968;96:869.

193. Potter MG. Observations of the gallbladder and bile during pregnancy at term. JAMA 1936;105:1070.

194. Wistown BW, Subramanian G, Van Hurtum RL, et al. An evaluation of ^{99m}TC-labeled hepatobiliary agents. J Nucl Med 1977;18:455.

195. Geenen JE, Hogan WJ, Dodds WJ, et al. Intraluminal pressure recording from the human sphincter of Oddi. Gastroenterology 1980;78:317.

196. Gerdes MM, Boydon EA. The rate of emptying of the human gallbladder in pregnancy. Surg Gynecol Obstet 1938;66:145.

197. Grossman MI. Gastrointestinal hormones: spectrum of actions and structure activity relations. In: Chey WY, Brooks FP, eds. Endocrinology of the gut. Thorofare, NJ: Charles B. Slack, 1975.

198. Ishioka T. Electromyographic study of the choledochoduodenal junction and duodenal wall muscle. Tohoku J Exp Med 1959;70:73.

199. Meshkinpour H, Mollot M, Eckerling GB, Bookman L. Bile duct dyskinesia: clinical and manometric study. Gastroenterology 1984;87:759.

200. Nebel OT. Manometric evaluation of the papilla of Vater. Gastrointest Endosc 1975;21:126.

201. Ono K. The discharge of bile into the duodenum and electrical activities of the muscle of Oddi and duodenum. Jpn J Smooth Muscle Res 1970;6:123.

202. Rosch W, Loch H, Demling L. Manometric studies during ERCP and endoscopic papillotomy. Endoscopy 1976;8:30.

203. Sarles JC, Midejean A, Devaux MA. Electromyography of the sphincter of Oddi. Am J Gastroenterol 1975;63:221.

204. Scott GW, Wlodizimierz JO. Resistance and sphincter-like properties of the cystic duct. Surg Gynecol Obstet 1979;149:177.

205. Takahashi I, Dodds WJ, Hogan WJ, Itoh Z. Effect of migrating myoelectric activity on the hepatic secretion of bile in the opossum. Gastroenterology 1984;86:1273A.

206. Tinker J, Cox AG. Gallbladder function after vagotomy. Br J Surg 1969;56:779.

207. Toouli J, Hogan WJ, Geenen JE, et al. Action of cholecystokinin-octapeptide on sphincter of Oddi basal pressure and phasic wave activity in humans. Surgery 1982;92:497.

208. Wyatt QP. The relationship of the sphincter of Oddi to the stomach, duodenum, and gallbladder. J Physiol 1967;193:225.

209. Coelho JCU, Moody GF. Certain aspects of normal and abnormal motility of the sphincter of Oddi. Dig Dis Sci 1987;32:86.

210. Dodds WJ, Hogan WJ, Geenen JE. Perspectives about function of the sphincter of Oddi. Viewpoints Dig Dis 1988;20:9.

211. Steinberg WM. Sphincter of Oddi dysfunction: a clinical controversy. Gastroenterology 1988;95:1409.

212. Becker JM, Moody FG. Effect of gastrointestinal hormones on the opossum biliary sphincter. Surg Forum 1978;24:400.

213. Becker JM, Moody FG. The dose/response effects of gastrointestinal hormones on the opossum biliary sphincter. Curr Surg 1980;65:60.

214. Becker JM, Moody FG, Zinsmeister AR. Effect of gastrointestinal hormones on the biliary sphincter of the opossum. Gastroenterology 1982;82:1300.

215. Coelho JCU, Gouma DJ, Moody FG, Schlegel JF. Effect of feeding on myoelectric activity of the sphincter of Oddi and the gastrointestinal tract in the opossum. Dig Dis Sci 1986;31:202.

216. Helm JE, Dodds WJ, Christensen J, Sarna S. Control mechanism of spontaneous in vitro contractions of the opossum sphincter of Oddi. Am J Physiol 1985;249:G572.

217. Honda R, Toouli J, Dodds WJ, et al. Relationship of sphincter of Oddi spike burst to gastrointestinal myoelectric activity in conscious opossums. J Clin Invest 1982;69:770.

218. Nakaya M, Kern MK, Dodds WJ, Hogan WJ. Evaluation of sphincter of Oddi basal pressure in awake opossums. Gastroenterology 1985;88:1515A.

219. Takahashi I, Honda R, Dodds WJ, et al. Effect of motilin on the opossum upper gastrointestinal tract and sphincter of Oddi. Am J Physiol 1983;245:G476.

220. Takahashi I, Dodds WJ, Itoh Z, et al. Influence of transsphincteric fluid flow in spike burst rate of the opossum sphincter of Oddi. Gastroenterology 1984;87:1292.

221. Toouli J, Dodds WJ, Honda R, et al. Motor function of the opossum sphincter of Oddi. J Clin Invest 1983;71:208.

222. Honda R, Toouli J, Dodds WJ, et al. Effect of enteric hormones on sphincter of Oddi and gastrointestinal myoelectric activity in fasted conscious opossums. Gastroenterology 1983;84:1.

223. Scott RB, Strasberg SM, El-Sharkway TY, Diamant NE. Fasting canine biliary secretion and the sphincter of Oddi. Gastroenterology 1984;87:793.

224. Carazziari E Torsoli A DeMasi E, et al. Frequency distribution of human sphincter of Oddi phasic activity. Gastroenterology 1984;86:1054A.

225. Takahashi I, Nakaya M, Suzuki T, Itoh Z. Postprandial changes in contractile activity and bile concentration in gallbladder of the dog. Am J Physiol 1982;243:G365.

226. Groh WJ, Takahashi I, Sarna S, et al. Computerized analysis of spike-burst activity of the upper gastrointestinal tract. Dig Dis Sci 1984;29:422.

227. Sandbloom P, Voegtlen WL, Ivy AC. The effect of CCK on the sphincter of Oddi. Am J Physiol 1935;93:175.

228. Cole WH. The development of cholecystography: the first fifty years. Am J Surg 1970;136:541.

229. Tanaka M, Ikeda S, Nakayama F. Change in bile duct pressure responses after cholecystectomy: loss of gallbladder as pressure reservoir. Gastroenterology 1984;87:1154.

230. Toouli J, Roberts-Thomson JC, Dent J, Lee J. Manometric disorders in patients with suspected sphincter of Oddi dysfunction. Gastroenterology 1985;8:1243.

231. Behar J, Biancani P. Role of cat sphincter of Oddi motor activity on transsphincteric flow. 1985. Gastroenterology 1985;88:1320A.

232. Behar J, Biancani P. Pharmacologic characterization of excitatory and inhibitory cholecystokinin receptors of the cat gallbladder and sphincter of Oddi. Gastroenterology 1987;92:764.

233. Pitt HA, Doty JE, DenBensten L, Kuchenbecker SL. Altered sphincter of Oddi phasic activity following truncal vagotomy. J Surg Res 1982;32:598.

234. Sarles JC, Bidart JM, Devaux MA, et al. Action of cholecystokinin and caerulin on the rabbit-sphincter of Oddi. Digestion 1976;14:415.

235. Sarles JC, Midejean A, Devaux MA. Electromyography of the sphincter of Oddi. Am J Gastroenterol 1975;63:221.

236. Lin TM, Spray GF. Effect of pentagastrin, cholecystokinin, caerulein and glucagon on the choledochal resistance and bile flow of dogs. Gastroenterology 1969;56:1178.

237. Nebel OT. Effect of enteric hormones on human sphincter of Oddi. Gastroenterology 1975;68:105A.

238. Raih TJ, Ashmore CS, Wilson FD, et al. Effect of enteric hormones on canine choledochal sphincter. Gastroenterology 1973;64:787A.

239. Behar J, Biancani P. Effects and mechanisms of action of motilin on the cat sphincter of Oddi. Gastroenterology 1988;95:1099.

240. Muller EL, Grace PA, Conter RL, et al. Influence of motilin and cholecystokinin on sphincter of Oddi and duodenal motility. Am J Physiol 1987;253:G679.

241. Grace PA, Muller EL, Conter RL, et al. Peptide YY inhibits sphincter of Oddi phasic wave activity in the prairie dog. Gastroenterology 1985;88:1356A.

242. Lin TM. Pancreatic polypeptide: Isolation, chemistry, and biological function. In: Glass GBJ, ed. Gastrointestinal hormones. New York: Raven Press, 1980.

243. Lin TM, Chance RE. Spectrum of action of bovine PP. In: Bloom SR, ed. Gut hormones. Edinburgh: Churchill Livingstone, 1978.

244. Potter JC, Mann FC. Pressure changes in the biliary tract. Am J Med Sci 1926;171:202.

245. Muller EL, Lewinski MA, Pitt HA. The cholecysto-sphincter of Oddi reflex. J Surg Res 1984;36:377.

246. Thune A, Thornell E, Svanvik J. Reflex regulation of flow resistance in the feline sphincter of Oddi by hydrostatic pressure in the biliary tract. Gastroenterology 1986;91:1364.

247. Suzuki T, Dodds WJ, Sarna SH, et al. Control mechanisms of sphincter of Oddi contraction rate in the opossum. Am J Physiol 1988;255:G619.

248. Persson CGA, Ekmon M. Effect of morphine, CCK, and sympathomimetics on the sphincter of Oddi and intramural pressure on the duodenum. Scand J Gastroenterol 1972;7:345.

249. Behar J, Biancani P. Neural control of the feline gallbladder. In: Christensen J, ed. Gastrointestinal motility. New York: Raven Press, 1981.

250. Behar J, Biancani P. Neural control of the sphincter of Oddi: a physiological role of 5 hydroxy-tryptamine in the regulation of basal sphincter of Oddi motor activity in the cat. J Clin Invest 1983;72: 551.

251. Behar J, Biancani P. Neural control of the sphincter of Oddi: physiologic role of enkephalins on the regulation of basal sphincter of Oddi motor activity in the cat. Gastroenterology 1984;86:134.

252. Roslyn JL, Pitt HA, Mann LL, et al. Gallbladder disease in patients on long-term parenteral nutrition. Gastroenterology 1983;84:148.

253. Doty JE, Pitt KA, Kuchenbecker SL, DenBensten L. Impaired gallbladder emptying before gallstone formation in the prairie dog. Gastroenterology 1983;85:168.

254. Fridhandler TM, Davison JS, Shaffer EA. Defective contractility in the ground squirrel and prairie dog during the early stages of cholesterol stone formation. Gastroenterology 1983;85:830.

255. Li YF, Weisbrodt NW, Moody FG, et al. Calcium induced contraction and contractile protein content of gallbladder smooth muscle after high cholesterol feeding of prairie dogs. Gastroenterology 1987;92:746.

256. Li YF, Moody FG, Weisbrodt NW, et al. Decrease of contractility of prairie dog muscle strips following cholesterol feeding. Surg Forum 1984;35:224.

256a. Meyer PD, DenBensten L, Gurll NJ. Effects of cholesterol gallstone induction on gallbladder function and bile salt pool size in the prairie dog model. Surgery 1978;83:559.

256b. Pitt HA, Doty JE, DenBensten L, Kuchenbecker SL. Stasis before gallstone formation: altered compliance or cystic duct resistance? Am J Surg 1982;143:144.

257. Behar J, Lee KY, Thompson WR, Biancani P Gallbladder contraction in patients with pigment and cholesterol stones. Gastroenterology 1989;97:1479.

258. Li YF, Weisbrodt NW, Moody FG. Actin and myosin isoforms in gallbladder smooth muscle following cholesterol feeding in prairie dogs. Gastroenterology 1989;96:300A.

259. Braverman DZ, Johnson ML, Kern F Jr. Effect of pregnancy and contraceptive steroids on gallbladder function. N Engl J Med 1980;302:362.

C. SECRETION AND ABSORPTION

12

Salivary Secretion

AARON LERNER
MARC A. ROSENTHAL
CHARLES LIEBOW
EMANUEL LEBENTHAL

The salivary glands represent a heterogenous group of exocrine glands that function in promoting the digestive process. These glands are very similar to the most studied of the exocrine glands, the pancreas, but although they receive a good deal of attention themselves, they have not been examined with the same intensity as the pancreas. One of the reasons why the pancreas has been so well studied, and why so many breakthrough concepts have evolved from our investigations of the pancreas, is the very homogeneity of this gland. The pancreas seems to have little anatomic heterogeneity in terms of function, biochemistry, and pathology and, excluding the nesting of islets of Langerhans, few regional differences. This homogeneity, along with the singular predominant function of protein secretion, has allowed macroscopic and biochemical generalizations about pancreatic function and the inferences made from these cells to generalizations about secretory and protein synthetic mechanisms in all cells.

The salivary glands do not possess this homogeneity, either within the same gland, within multiple glands from a single animal, or between species. This diversity of form and function has impeded progress in salivary gland studies but may provide a broader scope of responses against which to test hypotheses than is provided by the more stereotyped pancreas. In any event, this chapter will examine the salivary glands generally in comparison to the better characterized pancreas when this is possible. It will emphasize the role of salivary amylase and lingual lipase in digestion and pathophysiologic states.

The term "salivary glands" refers to a group of glands, including the parotid, submandibular, sublingual, and the "minor salivary" glands. The first three listed, the major glands, have a singular main duct each, whereas the minor glands have multiple openings.

ANATOMY

Comparison Among Glands

The major glands, the parotid, submandibular, and sublingual, are ducted glands, situated around the oral cavity. The parotid gland, the largest of the glands (about 25 g in man), lies between the mastoid process and the mandible lateral to the oropharynx. The parotid duct (Wharton's duct) opens from the cheek, opposite the second maxillary molar, after passing through the buccinator muscle. Passing through the body of the parotid gland itself are the facial nerve, the mandibular vein, and the carotid artery (from superficial to deep layers).

The submandibular gland, which, along with the parotid, accounts for almost 90% of the total production of saliva but is itself about half the size of the parotid, is in the submandibular fossa, nestled into a concavity in the lingual surface of the mandible near the second premolar and first molar. The gland extends from the mandible to the tongue, occupying the floor of the mouth. The posterior portion of the gland extends around the posterior border of the mylohyoid muscle. The submandibular duct (Stensen's duct) terminates through a small orifice on the caruncula sublingualis, a small papilla just lateral to the lingual frenum. Compared with the parotid, the duct orifice is quite small, consistent with the lighter, thinner nature of the duct. The duct extends posteriorly, arborizing from there, with branches extending all the way around the posterior border of the mylohyoid.

The sublingual gland is the smallest of the major glands (less than 4 g in man). It lies anterior to the submandibular gland, between the tongue (and genioglossus muscle) and the mandible and above the mylohyoid, with its anterior aspect bordering the anterior portion of the mandible. Unlike the parotid and the submandibular glands, the sublingual gland has no single convergent duct system. Instead, it has many (between 8 and 20) separate ducts opening independently either directly into the mouth or into the main submandibular duct. Those ducts opening directly into the mouth open on a crest of tissue, the plica sublingualis, which is lateral to the lingual frenula and contains the submandibular duct in its passage anterior to the sublingual glands. The smaller diameter and orifice of the submandibular and, especially, the sublingual glands, and the mixing of secretions of these two glands in the main submandibular duct, make study of the secretory process of these glands more difficult and interpretation and generalization of observations more ambiguous than for the pancreas or even the parotid. Although these difficulties have led to less frequent study of the submandibular and sublingual glands than of the pancreas and parotid, their varied functions may clarify many questions concerning the function of all exocrine glands.

The blood and nerve supplies of the various glands differ. The arterial supply of the parotid is from the external carotid artery, either directly or through short feeder vessels, and the venous drainage is into the external jugular, again either directly or through short tributaries. The arteries supplying the submandibular glands are branches of the facial and lingual arteries, with complementary veins following the arteries in a retrograde fashion. Similarly, the sublingual gland is supplied by vessels deriving from the sublingual and submental arteries. The sympathetic innervation of the parotid derives from the external carotid plexus. The sympathetic innervation of the submandibular and sublingual gland also derives from the external carotid plexus and from the facial artery plexus. The parasympathetic innervation of the parotid is from the glossopharyngeal and, possibly, the facial nerve through the otic ganglion and the auriculotemporal nerve. The submandibular and sublingual glands' parasympathetic innervation is from the facial nerve through the chorda tympani and submandibular ganglia to the secretomotor nerves. All glands share certain similarities in blood and nervous supply, but the submandibular and sublingual seem to share more.

Comparison with Pancreas and Other Exocrine Glands

DUCTS

The duct systems of the salivary glands offer some interesting comparisons, both among themselves and with the pancreas, in gross anatomy, microscopic morphology, and function. The parotid duct arborizes from a single collecting duct of significant diameter. This is similar to the pancreas, wherein one main duct (and possibly an accessory duct) conveys all the secretions directly into the digestive tract lumen. The pancreas is complicated by its coalescence with the bile duct, but prior to this union it carries a reasonably homogeneous fluid, as does the parotid duct. The submandibular duct is of much smaller diameter and is joined by many sublingual glands, producing a heterogeneous secretory

product. Those sublingual glands which do not coalesce with the submandibular duct open directly and individually into the oral cavity. The configuration of their ducts is comparable to that of the minor salivary glands, with multiple small-diameter short ducts.

The cells of all the ducts begin with intercalated ducts, composed of simple cuboidal epithelial cells that are less well differentiated than the other cells of the gland. They contain a few mitochondria, a few small secretory vesicles, and some organelles for protein synthesis. The cells are not packed with machinery for protein synthesis and storage, as are the acinar cells, though they seem to contain all the necessary equipment to carry on such activities at a limited rate. They also do not contain the specialized machinery for significant ion transport (e.g., abundant mitochondria, redundant folded plasma membranes, and excessive ATPase activity) that the striated ducts possess. Because of their undifferentiated appearance, their apparent high level of division, and their intermediate position between acini and more differentiated ducts, they have been postulated to fill the role of multipotentialed precursor cells for the acini and ducts. This role of progenitor cell has also led to the suggestion that they are the cells of origin in salivary carcinogenesis, just as the pancreatic duct and centroacinar cells are thought to be the cells that result in pancreatic cancer. Both hypotheses, that salivary intercalated ducts and the pancreatic ducts are the originating sites of human cancer, lack substantiating evidence.

The intercalated ducts contain a range of proteins, some common to the acini and others more unique to these cells. Amylase is contained in striated ducts in small quantities, along with ribonuclease and phosphatase. These same cells contain kallikrein, a serine protease involved in blood flow regulation. The striated ducts of the submandibular gland contain abundant supplies of epidermal growth factor and nerve growth factor. The parotid as well may contain a great deal of these peptides in some species. A number of other gastrointestinal regulatory peptides have been associated with salivary glands, including glucagon, insulin, somatostatin, gastrin, and vasoactive intestinal polypeptide (VIP).

ACINI

The glands vary in acinar staining properties and size of granules. The cells that stain pale blue with hematoxylin and eosin (i.e., basophilic) and have small granules generally produce thin, watery secretions and are called serous cells. Those which stain pink (i.e., eosinophilic) with large granules produce thick, viscous secretions containing high concentrations of glycoproteins and are called mucous cells. The parotid (and Ebner's) glands are composed almost entirely of serous cells (similar to the pancreas), the submandibular glands have much more serous than mucous cells, and the sublingual glands have the most mucous cells.

MYOEPITHELIUM

The myoepithelium represents an interesting anatomic and functional entity. It extends around acini in a fashion similar to the way in which a string bag surrounds potatoes, lying between the acinar cells and their basal lamina. These stellate cells, which constitute between 1% and 3% of the glandular volume, contain abundant thick and thin cytofilaments of myosin and actin that serve contractile functions with significant ATPase activity. They appear to function like muscles, providing for the coordinated and rapid expulsion of intraluminal saliva content, fulfilling the same role for saliva as the gallbladder serves for biliary secretion. These cells of epithelial, not muscle, origin are joined by gap junctions and desmosomes, providing electrical transmission between cells and coordinated contractile activity. The contraction of these cells can expel a transient stream of saliva at a considerable rate and provides the capability for rapid salivary response to insult.

DEVELOPMENT

The salivary glands derive from invaginations of the ectoderm. The ectodermal lining begins to thicken at certain places that then protrude into the mesodermal layer below. For each of the salivary glands, a cylindric cordlike projection initially develops and then begins to branch and bud. This branched, undifferentiated structure develops into the surrounding mesenchymal tissue. The structure next begins to separate and cavitate internally, forming a hollow duct. Lumen formation begins at the oral or surface point of initiation of growth and then proceeds quickly down into the duct and acini. Cells begin to differentiate after the lumen is formed. Central membranes are seen to thicken with the attachment of cytofilaments. Junctional complexes and desmosomes form, and these will provide the eventual tight junctions around the lumen. A terminal web of cytofilaments possessing myosin ATPase activity joins the junctional complexes. It is believed that these cytofilaments contract, pulling the unattached membranes apart and creating an opening bounded by the tight junctions. This opening begins to develop at the epithelial surface of the gland and tunnels its way down through the gland into the terminal buds. Cells of the salivary glands begin to differentiate as the salivary duct lumen develops.

It is tempting to hypothesize that duct formation stimulates cellular differentiation, but this has been shown not to be the case. Tissue culture of ductal anlagen continues to display cellular differentiation even in the absence of duct formation. It seems more reasonable to postulate that the first stage of cytodifferentiation is the formation of the cytoskeleton, desmosomes, and tight junctions. These structures lead to duct lumen formation, but the sequence of cytodifferentiation continues on from the formation of the terminal web. Once the cytofilaments establish cellular polarity, cellular differentiation progresses. The factors that determine why cells at the blind ends of the gland are differentiated into acinar cells, why those at the external end of the duct become duct cells, and why subacinar cells develop into myoepithelial cells are not known, but these factors seem partly dependent on hormones, mesenchymal interactions, and genetic programming. Mesenchymal elements contribute to cellular differentiation in the salivary glands, just as they contribute to the same process in the pancreas.

Comparison Between the Development of the Salivary Glands and That of the Pancreas

As the salivary gland grows and expands, the surrounding mesenchyme is forced outward, and this condensed mesenchyme forms the connective tissue capsule of the gland. Not all of the mesenchyme is forced out by the growing ectodermal gland cells, however, and the remaining cells form the connective tissue stroma of the gland and help direct its further differentiation. In the pancreas, it has been shown that all the different protein/peptide-secreting cells (i.e., exocrine cells, islet cells, duct cells) originate from one pluripotential stem cell of endodermal origin. The salivary glands appear to develop in the same manner, and this may explain how multiple products can be synthesized in the salivary gland and regulated independently. The development of cells of the salivary glands with exocrine and endocrine capability from the same anlagen cells, therefore, has precedence in the pancreas.

The development of the salivary glands and the pancreas is comparable despite the different germ layer of their origin. Their anatomy and general pattern of development are similar. Both grow from epithelial evaginations into the surrounding mesenchymal tissue. The mesenchymal tissue helps to direct their differentiation. One minor difference in their development is the method of duct lumen formation. As mentioned above, the salivary gland lumens develop by opening a space in the formed and arborized gland, while the pancreatic lumen forms continuously with the development of the gland.

The general similarities between the pancreas and salivary glands in structure, developmental pattern, and cytodifferentiation raise the possibility of similarities of genetic expression as well. However, although amylase is synthesized and secreted by both organs, in humans the pancreas and salivary glands utilize different amylase genes.

REGULATION

Neural

The salivary glands are controlled predominantly by the autonomic nervous system. Stimulation of the sympathetic or parasympathetic nerves to the salivary glands elicits salivary secretion. Sympathectomy results in virtually no major alteration of salivary gland function, whereas parasympathectomy leads to decreased secretion with glandular atrophy. This, along with the transient effect of sympathetic stimulation versus the prolonged effects with copious salivation produced by parasympathetic nerve stimulation, suggests that parasympathetic input is the main physiologic regulator of the salivary gland.

Salivary secretion is stimulated when neurohumoral agonists bind to acinar cell surface receptors and stimulate intracellular second messengers that activate the appropriate cellular mechanisms. Secretory receptors of the following variety have been identified: alpha-1, alpha-2, beta-1, and beta-2 adrenergic, muscarinic, dopaminergic, purine, vasoactive intestinal polypeptide, eledoisin, physalaemin, neurotensin, and substance P. These have been found in salivary glands of varying species, though all were not found within any one gland.

Catecholamines released by stimulation of the sympathetic nerves to the salivary glands and the circulating catecholamines are effective at the beta receptors and cause increased concentration of salivary potassium and bicarbonate, presumably through action on the ductal epithelium. Catecholamines also induce the secretion of saliva rich in amylase. One reason for the scantiness of the secretion induced by sympathetic stimulation in contrast to the copious volume elicited by parasympathetic agonists may be the vasoconstrictive action of catecholamines. Sympathetic activity by way of alpha receptors causes contraction of the acinar and ductal myoepithelial cells, leading to transient acceleration in the delivery rate of saliva to the oral cavity. The myoepithelial cell functions to prevent glandular distention that might occur as a result of increased intraluminal pressure during secretion.

The salivatory nuclei are excited by taste and tactile stimuli that depolarize the parasympathetic nerves and stimulate the salivary glands.[1] The neurotransmitters acetylcholine and vasoactive intestinal polypeptide are secreted from nerve terminals at the glandular epithelium. At rest, there is an impulse frequency from parasympathetic nerves of less than one per second. During feeding, the impulse rate increases to four to eight per second and can exceed eight per second in response to noxious stimuli. Maximal secretion from parasympathetic stimulation produces a volume five times greater than that produced by maximal sympathetic stimulation. The saliva elicited from parasympathetic activation is lower in concentrations of protein, potassium, and bicarbonate than that elicited by sympathetic nerve stimulation.

Hormonal

Along with neural regulation, hormonal control over salivary glands has also been observed. The hormones identified include estrogens, androgens, glucocorticoids, and peptide hormones.[2] By themselves, hormones cannot cause salivary secretion but are capable of modifying its constituents. The homeostatic proteases kallikrein, bradykinin, renin, tonin, aldosterone, and antidiuretic hormone have all been located in the granular ducts of the salivary glands.

A summary of the effects of hormone or hormonelike compounds on salivary content or secretion is as follows. Thyroxine has been shown to increase the sensitivity of salivary gland adrenergic beta receptors.[3] It has been noted that the salivary glands may be a target tissue for the androgen testosterone.[4] The peptides physalaemin and eledoisin stimulate secretion of salivary glands.[5] There are conflicting reports as to whether the gastrointestinal hormones secretin and cholecystokinin affect amylase secretion from the parotid.[5] Glucagon has been isolated from mouse and human submandibular glands, yet the role of salivary glucagon in glucose regulation has not been delineated. Renin[6] may mediate the secretory effect of alpha-adrenergic stimulation,[7] and through its release of angiotensin it may inhibit sodium transport by the secretory ducts.[8] This hormone has not been identified in human salivary gland tissue, however. Dilation of blood vessels in the submandibular gland after chorda tympani stimulation has been attributed indirectly to kallikrein, an enzyme hormone found in all three major human salivary glands whose secretion may be regulated by vasointestinal polypeptide (VIP).[9,10] Salivary kallikrein splits kininogen to form kinins, the most widely known being the vasodilator bradykinin. Kallikrein and renin secretion are induced mainly by alpha-adrenergic stimulation, while tonin secretion is elicited through beta-adrenergic activity. The function of these peptides is to control local blood flow and/or water and electrolyte transport.[11] Prostaglandin is postulated to control ductal electrolyte absorption.[4] Aldosterone is effective on salivary ductal epithelium and increases sodium absorption and potassium secretion. Antidiuretic hormone increases sodium absorption in ducts, thereby decreasing sodium concentration in saliva.[2]

Metabolism and Blood Flow

A maximally stimulated salivary gland in man can secrete its own weight in saliva every 10 minutes[1] at a rate of approximately one milliliter per minute per gram of gland. Secretory rates of this magnitude require a high blood flow to provide the nutrients, oxygen, electrolytes, and water necessary for salivation. This blood flow is almost 10-fold that supplied to an actively contracting skeletal muscle.

Vessels enter the hilus of the salivary glands, branch into the parenchyma, and form a separate capillary plexus around the acini and ducts, with the ductal capillary network more dense than that of the acini (Fig 12-1). The venous drainage courses with the arteries, exits the hilus, and empties into the external jugular vein. This vascular arrangement can be viewed as a portal network wherein the blood flows in a direction counter to that of salivary flow. The arterial blood supplies the ductal capillary network first, which then drains into the acinar plexus, forming a portal system. Such a model allows the ductal events to influence the acinar function.

Parasympathetic stimulation creates the demand for secretion, but the accepted mediators of vasodilatation are the noncholinergic neurotransmitters bradykinin and VIP. The list of potential contributors to vasodilatation may also be extended to include the accumulation of metabolites such as adenosine, lactic acid, and changes in osmolarity.[1]

The source of fluid for salivary secretion is provided by the circulation. Increased blood flow, arteriolar dilatation leading to increased capillary hydrostatic pressure, and perfused capillary density (capillary recruitment), which increases the surface area for fluid exchange, provide the enhanced capillary filtration rate necessary to meet the parasympathetic demand. In general, these cellular responses to neural stimulation and increase in glandular metabolism require increasing amounts of glucose and oxygen.

Message Transduction

Autonomic or circulating neurotransmitters elicit salivary secretion by one of two second messenger–mediated pathways that determine

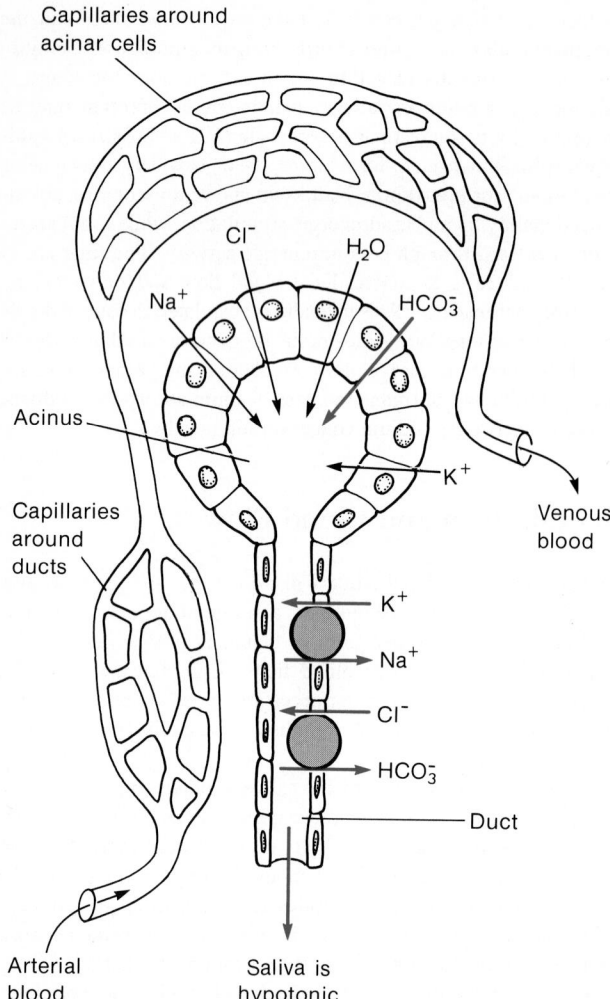

FIGURE 12–1. Schematic representation of salivary gland acinus, duct, and blood supply. The salivary gland blood supply flows countercurrent to the flow of saliva. The dense afferent capillary network absorbs ionic buildup in the interstitium by way of luminal reabsorption by the duct epithelium. These ions are transported to efferent capillaries surrounding the acinar cells and are transported or diffuse into the secretory cells. This arrangement helps maintain a hypotonic salivary secretion and a hypertonic primary fluid.

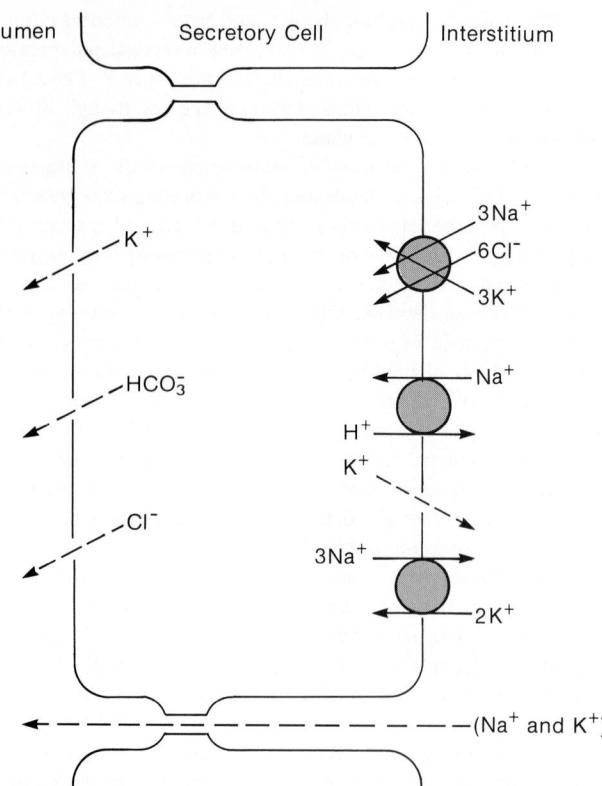

FIGURE 12–2. Diagram of a salivary gland acinar secretory cell and electrolyte transport. The darkened circle in the basolateral membrane is the Na^+/K^+ pump (sodium pump) that is ATPase driven and the driving force creating ion flow through the acinar cell. This pump removes three Na^+ ions from the cell while taking up two K^+ ions from the interstitium. The concentration gradients created by the sodium pump and the electrical potential difference across the membrane drive additional K^+ into the cytosol through an electroneutral symport in the basolateral membrane that has 1 Na^+/1 K^+/2 Cl^- stoichiometry. A basolateral Na^+/H^+ antiport balances the breakdown of carbonic acid. Downward sloping arrows depict ions moving down their concentration gradients. A flow of cations through a cation selective intercellular shunt pathway is driven by the electrically negative lumen. (Modified and redrawn from Johnson LR, ed. Physiology of the gastrointestinal tract, ed 2. New York: Raven Press, 1987:788.)

FLUID AND ELECTROLYTE SECRETION

Origin of Fluid

The acinar cells in the salivary glands secrete a primary fluid that is slightly hypertonic to plasma. It must be recognized that tonicity and ionic composition of the primary secretion vary between species and from salivary gland to salivary gland within a species. The individual glands are classified by the nature and content of the fluid secretion. The parotid and Ebner's glands secrete a thin, watery fluid, while the sublingual and submandibular gland secretion is more viscous because of a high mucinous content. The terms *serous*, *seromucous*, and *mucous* are used to describe the

the composition of secretion (stimulus-secretion coupling). The first pathway results in the production of cyclic AMP, and the other leads to an increase in cytosolic free calcium. A detailed description of these two separate signal transduction systems is provided elsewhere in this book (ch 15). The cyclic AMP–dependent pathway stimulates a primary salivary secretion rich in amylase (Fig 12-2). Stimulation of the salivary gland beta-adrenergic receptor activates the membrane-bound adenylate cyclase through a guanine nucleotide–binding protein. This enzyme catalyzes the conversion of ATP to cyclic AMP. As the intracellular concentration of cyclic AMP becomes elevated, a protein kinase is activated that phosphorylates proteins presumably secreted into the saliva. The other pathway, driven by the mobilization of intracellular calcium, produces a secretion of increased fluid volume.

amount of secretory proteins in the storage granules containing mucins.

The primary electrolytes are sodium, potassium, chloride, and bicarbonate. The concentrations of secreted solutes are regulated by the autonomic nervous system and the stimulus-secretion–coupled second messenger calcium. Secretion is dependent on the active transport of one or more of these solutes, with water following by osmosis.

The characteristics of the various membranes surrounding the cell determine the secretory mechanism of the salivary acinar cells (Fig 12-2). These components maintain cellular equilibrium in the following manner: the basolateral membrane contains a sodium pump, several carriers capable of exchanging ions, and one principal ion channel, the potassium channel. The carriers include an electroneutral sodium/potassium/chloride symport (cotransporter) and two electroneutral antiports, one involving sodium/hydrogen, the other chloride/bicarbonate. The apical membrane maintains a chloride-selective anion channel. The lateral intercellular spaces, constituting the largest area of plasma membrane, contain tight junctional complexes that are "leaky" but have a low permeability to anions.

Autonomic neurotransmitters cause an increase in cytosolic free calcium, leading to production of increased amounts of primary fluid. This occurs by stimulation of inwardly directed electroneutral sodium/potassium/chloride cotransport in a ratio of 1/1/2, respectively. Increased intracellular sodium stimulates the sodium pump, which results in the transfer of three sodium ions out of the cell in exchange for two potassium ions into the cytosol. Increased intracellular free calcium also increases membrane permeability by opening potassium channels, thus providing an exit for potassium to the interstitium. Chloride is maintained in the cytosol above electrochemical equilibrium by the symport mechanism and is expelled through anion-selective channels in the luminal membrane. The leakiness of the cation-selective tight junctions maintains the secreted anions in the lumen; the anions accumulate in sufficient concentration to attract cations into the lumen paracellularly. The pathway is completed by a sodium current that passes paracellularly through the tight junctions, from interstitium to the acinar lumen, with water following by osmosis (Fig 12-2).

A similar mechanism can be construed to explain the secretion of bicarbonate. The sodium/hydrogen antiport exchanges intracellular sodium for protons, resulting in the accumulation of bicarbonate in the cytosol. Whether by way of the luminal membrane anion (chloride) channel (which might be permeable to bicarbonate), a chloride/bicarbonate exchanger, or a sodium-dependent bicarbonate transporter, exit of bicarbonate would make secretion bicarbonate-rich instead of chloride-rich (Fig 12-2).[4]

Modification

As the primary secretion passes from the salivary gland to its destination in the oral cavity, it is modified by the ductal epithelium. The classical two-stage model presented by Thayson and colleagues in 1954[12] postulates that the secretory acinar epithelium produces, independent of secretory rate, a primary fluid that is slightly hypertonic. In the striated and excretory ducts, the fluid is altered by absorbing sodium and chloride while secreting po-

tassium and bicarbonate. Under cholinergic stimulation, water is relatively impermeable to the duct epithelium, and therefore the ducts do not absorb or add any volume to the saliva.

The absorptive ductal epithelial cell maintains an electrochemical gradient through luminal and basolateral membrane pumps, transporters, and ion channels (Fig 12-3). In the steady state, these cells maintain a duct lumen that is negatively charged with respect to the interstitium. Chloride is the only ion in electrochemical equilibrium, while the cell is actively absorbing sodium and secreting potassium and bicarbonate at rest. Luminal sodium conductance is controlled by a sodium-selective cation channel that maintains a steep sodium concentration gradient. Another mode by which sodium crosses the luminal membrane is through the electroneutral sodium/hydrogen antiport. The exchanged protons contribute to bicarbonate absorption, which stimulates

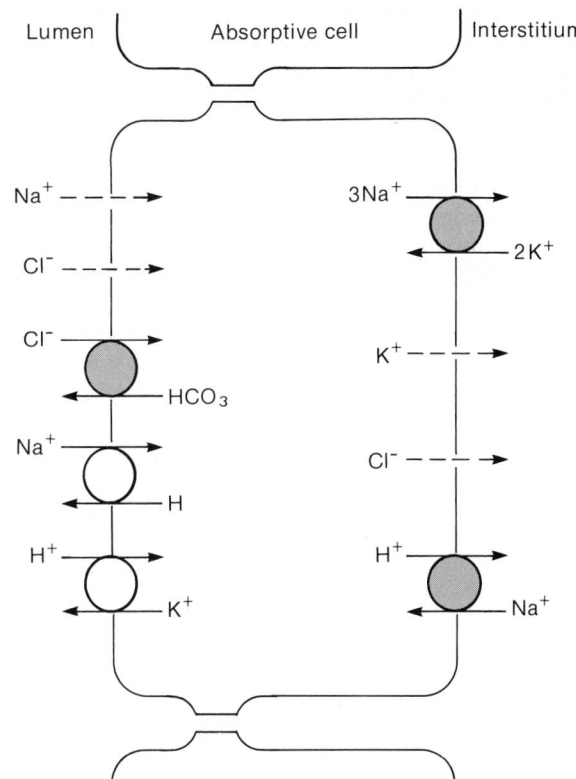

FIGURE 12–3. Model of a salivary gland absorptive duct epithelial cell and electrolyte transport. The basolateral Na^+/K^+ ATPase–driven pump (sodium pump) maintains low Na^+ and high K^+ intracellular concentrations. This creates a driving force for absorption. Cl^- enters the cell through a Cl^-/HCO_3^- antiport or a Cl^- channel. Na^+ is absorbed through a Na^+/H^+ antiport or a sodium channel. Cellular H^+ is replaced in exchange for K^+ through the luminal antiport. In addition, the secretory and absorptive activity of H^+ ions by the antiports is loosely coupled, providing pH control. Accumulated cystolic HCO_3^- enters the lumen in exchange for Cl^- by way of their respective antiports. Downward sloping arrows depict ions moving down their concentration gradients. The intercellular junctions are impermeable to ionic flow. Orchestration of these cellular components and the content of salivary secretion are dependent on the mix of sympathetic and parasympathetic regulation. (Modified and redrawn from Johnson LR, ed. Physiology of the gastrointestinal tract, ed 2. New York: Raven Press, 1987:803.)

the chloride/bicarbonate antiport to exchange bicarbonate for chloride. To maintain electroneutrality from the passive influx of sodium, a similar current of opposite charge is required. This anion flow is provided by a transcellular, anion-selective channel that allows entry of chloride ion. The chloride/bicarbonate antiport also provides entry of chloride in exchange for bicarbonate. A basolateral sodium pump exports three sodium ions to the interstitium while importing two potassium ions. This pump has been shown to operate at near maximum rates, and sodium entry through the luminal membrane is not a rate-limiting event in sodium transport.[4] The pump maintains low intracellular sodium and high potassium concentrations. A luminal potassium/hydrogen antiport provides the mechanism for the secretion of potassium. Bicarbonate is secreted in equimolar amounts but is absorbed as a consequence of the luminal sodium/hydrogen antiport. This makes net bicarbonate secretion less than that of potassium.

Transport of bicarbonate from the ducts is influenced by the body's acid/base status. Ductal secretion of potassium and bicarbonate is stimulated by metabolic alkalosis. In contrast, metabolic acidosis decreases potassium secretion, bicarbonate is retained, and sodium absorption is reduced.

The degree of hypotonicity of the saliva is inversely proportional to the rate of secretion when secretory rates are varied by cholinergic stimulation (Fig 12-4). That is, at low secretory rates, saliva has its lowest osmolality. The osmolality increases with increasing flow rate, approaching but never reaching the osmolarity of plasma. With the increasing secretory rate, the duct epithelium has less time to carry out ion exchange processes. The primary fluid, therefore, passes through less modified and is more similar to the primary secretion. At very low secretory rates in some glands, water can be absorbed from the duct through osmosis. This can cause an increase in osmolarity.

The secretory/absorptive patterns for the most common electrolytes are as follows: sodium and chloride concentrations both increase with increasing flow rates. When the secretory rate is low, sodium/chloride concentrations are low. As the secretory rate increases, their respective concentrations rise. Sodium approaches a peak concentration that is significantly less than its concentration in plasma. Chloride increases with increasing flow rates. Potassium remains constant over a wide range of flow rates, but it increases steeply at very low flow rates.

Bicarbonate concentrations vary in a more complex manner. At moderate to high secretory rates, bicarbonate concentrations are significantly higher in saliva than in the plasma as a result of bicarbonate secretion through the bicarbonate/chloride antiport. At low secretory rates, bicarbonate concentrations in secretion can actually fall below those of plasma. This is caused by the negative potential of the ductular lumen as compared with the interstitium. Although the bicarbonate concentration of saliva is below that of plasma, the electrochemical gradient still favors bicarbonate reabsorption. Thus, saliva at low flow rates is slightly acidic, whereas at maximal flow the fluid becomes more basic and approaches a pH of 8.

Duct Permeability

As the primary fluid moves down the duct system at low flow rates, it becomes more hypotonic, because the ducts remove more ions than they secrete. The movement of water is secondary to movement of the solutes. Under parasympathetic stimulation, ductal epithelium has relatively low water permeability. Therefore, even with an osmotic gradient that favors water flow out of the

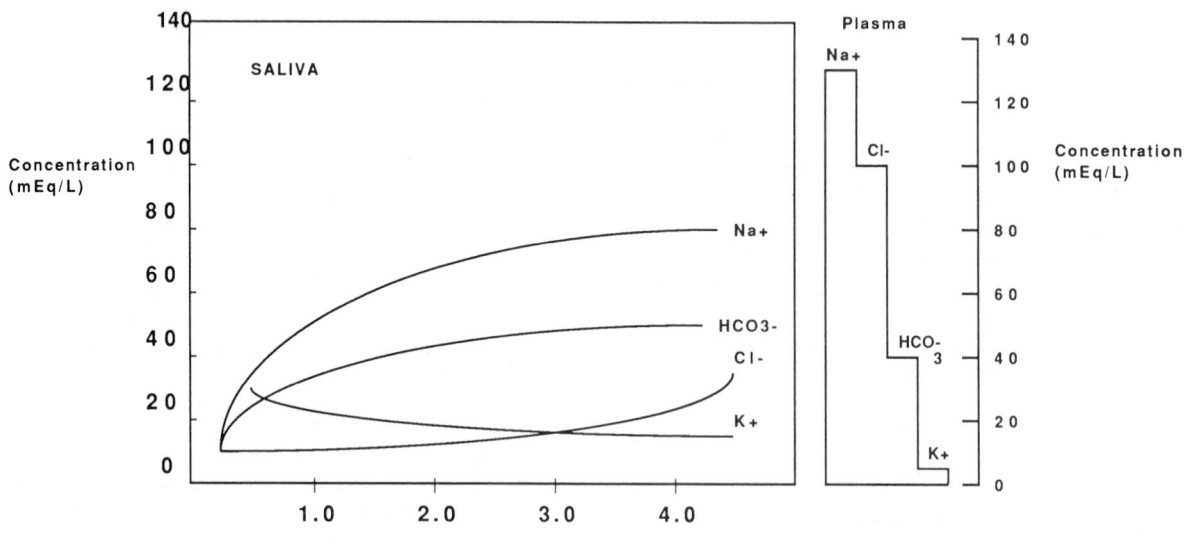

FIGURE 12–4. Average electrolyte concentrations of parotid saliva as a function of flow rate and compared with average plasma levels. At low flow rates, Na^+, Cl^-, and HCO_3^- levels are extremely hypotonic to plasma. At these flow rates, the K^+ concentration greatly exceeds its level in plasma or primary secretion. This is due to saliva spending a long time in the duct where Na^+–K^+ and Cl^-–HCO_3^- exchange can occur. As the salivary flow rate increases, the salivary content of sodium and chloride rises toward that of the primary secretion, potassium decreases toward levels in the primary secretion, and bicarbonate concentration stays above that of plasma. (Redrawn from Thaysen JH, Thorn NA, Schwartz IL, et al. Am J Physiol 1954;178:155.)

lumen, little water is reabsorbed because of this "impermeable" barrier.

Salivary duct electrolyte transport is under autonomic control.[13-15] The effect of simultaneous parasympathetic and sympathetic stimulation is greater than that of either system alone. The sodium/hydrogen antiport in the luminal membrane is thought to be the point of autonomic control. Both sympathetic and parasympathetic inputs stimulate the ductal epithelium to secrete potassium and bicarbonate to the same magnitude. The effect of parasympathetic stimulation is greater on the acinar cell; therefore, the potassium and bicarbonate concentrations after parasympathetic stimulation are lower in the final secretion. Sympathetic stimulation creates a primary secretion with proportionately more ductal ion exchange, yielding a final secretion richer in potassium and bicarbonate than that found under parasympathetic stimulation. Ducts also appear more permeable to water under sympathetic stimulation, allowing more water reabsorption and further concentration of saliva.

The luminal fluid, being hypotonic, creates a driving force that promotes water reabsorption. There is a small but finite water permeability across salivary gland ductal epithelium.[16,17] It has not been determined if this occurs through the tight junctions or the cell membrane.

Function and Diseases

Saliva performs many important functions in the oral cavity. It lubricates food and the oral and digestive tissues, maintaining mucous membrane integrity and aiding in soft-tissue repair. It maintains an ecologic balance by preventing bacterial aggregation. Salivary antibiotic activity causes lysis of oral bacteria and has antifungal and antiviral activity. Saliva also helps maintain a neutral to basic pH, which aids in maintaining dental integrity.[18]

DIGESTIVE ACTIVITY

The salivary digestive enzyme amylase (correlates to alpha-amylase in the pancreas) reduces starch by cleaving the internal alpha 1–4 linkages of the carbohydrate. Amylase is unable to hydrolyze the terminal alpha 1,4 linkages or alpha 1–6 linkages at branch points. This enzyme has activity in the pH range of 4 to 11, with an optimum level of 7. Amylase remains active in a bolus of food until the antrum of the stomach produces gastric acid to lower the pH below 4. The limited hydrolysis of starch by salivary amylase can reduce the average size of starch molecules greatly. This reduces food viscosity and promotes further digestion. Salivary amylase is discussed in detail in the second part of this chapter.

IMMUNOLOGIC ACTIVITY

Secretory IgA, synthesized in the plasma cells of the interstitium, passes through the duct epithelium and is secreted by binding to a secretory protein. IgA provides important local mucosal immunity from rhino and influenza viruses.[5]

XEROSTOMIA

Xerostomia is a symptom caused by lack of saliva in the oral cavity. Its most common cause is iatrogenic through the prescription of antidepressant, antihypertensive, and psychotropic drugs that inhibit salivary secretion. Other causes include any decreased peripheral stimulus of afferent input, disorders of saliva production, and restriction of salivary transport due to ductal stenosis with parenchymal destruction, as in sialadenitis. Finally, head and neck radiation therapy that encompasses any portion of the salivary glands will markedly reduce salivary production through irreversible acinar cell destruction.

Xerostomia has many negative effects on the gastrointestinal environment. There is a decrease in the pH of the oral cavity without salivary buffering. If teeth are present, this leads to an increased rate of dental caries. The lubrication, mastication, and digestion of food becomes difficult, and there can be altered taste sensation. This can lead to depression with poor nutrition and weight loss. An increase in opportunistic infection is also observed with xerostomia, the most common being candidiasis.

Salivary secretion has a dynamic composition, changing to varying demands. Salivary secretion adapts rapidly to foods of different composition. It can be extremely hypotonic to modify hypertonic foods, or it can be isotonic. It can be basic with a high buffering capacity to neutralize acids, or neutral in pH. Secretory rates can increase dramatically on demand, to the point that saliva can be injected into the oral cavity under significant pressure by the myoepithelium for protective lavage. Saliva can have a high or low content of digestive enzymes, depending on need. Its contribution to oral tissue integrity can also vary. Overall, it adapts rapidly as the front line of the digestive system.

PROTEIN AND MACROMOLECULAR SECRETION

A broad mix of proteins is secreted by the salivary glands, including amylase, mucins, lysozymes, proteases, lipases, immunoglobulins, and growth factors. The varied sites of synthesis and secretion of these products are summarized in Table 12-1, along with their known functions. Several factors have slowed the studies of salivary glands in comparison to those of the pancreas: there are multiple glands, and the function of one gland is not necessarily comparable to that of other glands; the glands secrete a wide variety of protein products, which, with the exception of amylase, are not as easily measured as pancreatic enzymes; there is significant regional heterogeneity for the site of protein secretion (i.e., whether acinar cells, duct cells, or a combination secrete the product), making it more difficult to generalize about secretion from salivary sources than about secretion from the pancreas; and the salivary glands are smaller than the pancreas with smaller ducts, making study of their formation more difficult. Although studies of salivary glands have often followed in the path of similar studies in the pancreas, the salivary glands offer some distinct advantages: duct cell activity can be examined more readily; secretion of products such as amylase by periacinar duct cells may serve as a marker for morphologic transition of a ductal cell to an acinar cell; salivary secretion is much more easily sampled than that of the pancreas; many blood-borne agents can be monitored in saliva (e.g., pharmacologic

TABLE 12–1
Salivary Proteins

PROTEIN	SOURCE	FUNCTION
Amylase	All glands, parotid	Starch digestion
Proline-rich proteins		Antibacterial, splits bacterial wall carbohydrates
Mucins	Submandibular	Lubricant
Lysozyme	Highest in parotid (up to 10% total protein). Also in submaxillary	Antimicrobial
Lipase	Ebner's glands	Long-chain triglyceride digestion
Peroxidase		
Kallikrein	Submandibular gland duct cells. Serum protein?	Bradykinin blood flow regulator. Protease?
Renin	Submandibular gland duct cells. Serum protein?	Blood flow regulator
Tonin	Submandibular gland duct cells. Serum protein?	Blood flow regulator
Blood group proteins	Submandibular and sublingual	?
Hormones		
EGF	Submandibular & parotid?	Stimulates growth of epithelium
NGF	Submandibular & parotid?	Stimulates development of neural tissue
Serum	Serum protein—antigenicly similar to blood proteins	?
Albumin		Antimicrobial, inhibits binding
Gamma globulin		

agents); and the production of growth factors by the submaxillary and other salivary glands can be studied directly. Much can be learned by studying the salivary glands, and their very heterogeneity may serve to increase our understanding of exocrine capabilities.

Secretion of protein products from the salivary glands seems to vary a great deal, with secretion coming from both acinar and duct cells into both saliva and blood, and with secretion deriving from typical zymogen granules (e.g., amylase, kallikrein, and tonin), from hypothesized microvesicles, or directly from the cytoplasm (e.g., growth factors). The source of some of these products, their handling, and the regulation of their individual secretion offer some fruitful models that could expand understanding of the mechanisms of exocrine secretion of proteins.

An example of the utility of studying salivary glands is provided by the data on secretion of kallikrein and tonin. These products are thought to be contained in the same granules, yet their secretion can be elicited by different secretagogues. Noradrenaline stimulates the release of only kallikrein, not tonin, while isoproterenol and theophylline stimulate release of both kallikrein and tonin. This seems to be analogous to the nonparallel secretion observed from pancreatic secretion in response to different secretagogues but seems to represent a more total separation of proteins than has been reported in the pancreas (i.e., no incremental secretion of one product during augmented secretion of another).

The partition of salivary products between duct lumen and blood can also serve as an excellent model for study of exocrine glands. Many pathways for movement of protein between acinar cell, duct cell, plasma, and duct lumen are possible, and evidence exists for almost all of them. The pathways include: (1) traditional release of protein from acinar cell into the lumen, where it stays until its passage into the mouth; (2) identical handling of protein, except that its source is duct or duct-transitional cells; (3) similar release into the lumen from acinar cells, but the passage of protein then, by specific or nonspecific means, across the duct into the extracellular and eventually into the vascular space; (4) same as (3), except that the original source is the duct cells; (5) direct basolateral release of proteins into the extracellular and vascular space, where the proteins stay; (6) basolateral release as in (5), with transport from serosa to duct lumen in an analogous manner but direction opposite to the transport discussed in (3); and (7) transport of proteins from nonsalivary sources into the duct through a process similar to that for basolaterally released salivary proteins discussed in (6). Secretion of various proteins is thought to occur primarily by one route or another. (For example, esteroproteases and growth factors are thought to be secreted mostly by duct cells in the mucosal direction with significant ductal reabsorption.) An extended discussion of the secretion of the two primary digestive enzymes secreted into the buccal cavity, salivary amylase and lingual lipase, follows. Some aspects of the secretion of these two enzymes have been the subject of recent reviews.[19,20]

Salivary Amylase

SYNTHESIS AND INTRACELLULAR LOCALIZATION

The salivary glands possess a subcellular structure similar to that of the exocrine pancreas. In the pancreas, the process of synthesis, packaging, storage, and secretion of the exocrine proteins takes 1 to 2 hours. A comparable chain of intracellular events in synthesis, processing, and secretion of the exportable acinar proteins occurs in the parotid.[21,22] The time course of the above intracellular steps, studied by pulse labeling with ^{3}H-leucine and monitored by radioautography, is as follows: the rough endoplasmic reticulum is labeled initially in 1 to 6 minutes, followed by the Golgi apparatus in 16 to 36 minutes, condensing vacuoles in 36 to 56 minutes, immature granules in 56 to 116 minutes, and mature storage granules in 116 to 356 minutes.[23] In comparison to the acinar pancreas, the intracellular processing rate of the secreted proteins is slower in the parotid with a more prolonged storage phase. The dynamic changes that the parotid acinar cell undergoes during the secretory cycle have been studied by Amsterdam and colleagues.[24,25] Secretion is paralleled by depletion of zymogen granules through fusion of the granule membrane with the acinar luminal membrane, followed by discharge of the contents. The whole process of secretion is completed within 2 hours. After secretion, the secretory granule membrane is resorbed into the cell. The formation of new granules involves synthesis of membrane protein de novo concomitantly with the synthesis of exportable proteins.

Recent studies have localized the amylase synthesis to the acinar cells of the human parotid. No salivary amylase mRNA has been found in ductal cells.[26,27] On the other hand, the salivary ductal system is capable of taking up salivary protein from the lumen.[28,29] Endocytosis of some secretory proteins, such as amylase or protein

B_1, from the saliva may be a significant function of these cells in physiologic or pathologic conditions.

STIMULUS-SECRETION COUPLING AND ITS REGULATION

More than 20 proteins have been identified in the rat parotid saliva,[30] including 4 isozymes of amylase, DNase, and RNase. The salivary glands also contain numerous physiologic active substances such as growth factors, vasoactive serine proteases, regulatory peptides, arylamidases, peroxidase, and kallikrein.[31] The same protein profile has been found in purified parotid secretory granule preparation.[32]

As noted above, the salivary glands are innervated by sympathetic and parasympathetic neurons, and stimulation of the former leads to a more concentrated volume of viscous secretion rich in exportable proteins, while a more diluted saliva is produced by stimulation of the latter.[33] As in other exocrine glands, stimulus-secretion coupling in the salivary glands involves a neurohumoral transmitter that specifically binds to corresponding cell-surface receptors. The agonist–receptor combination generates intracellular messenger pathways that result in protein or fluid secretion. The receptors are not equally and homogeneously distributed among the three salivary glands of the same species, and sometimes they are species-specific.[34] Table 12-2 summarizes the neuro-

TABLE 12–2
The Effect of Neurotransmitters on the Cellular Receptors of Rat Parotid Gland

	RECEPTOR	AGONIST	ANTAGONIST	NUMBER OF RECEPTORS/ CELL	RECEPTOR-STIMULATED CELLULAR EFFECT	REFERENCE
Beta	Adrenergic		[3]H] dihydroalprenolol	450 f mole/mg protein		35
Beta	Adrenergic	Pindolol	[125]I] iodohydroxybenzyl			36
Beta	Adrenergic	Isoprenaline			Amylase release	37
Beta$_1$	Adrenergic	Prenalterol		High number	Amylase release	38
Beta$_2$	Adrenergic	Terbutaline Salbutamol		Low number	Amylase release	38
Beta$_1$	Adrenergic		Metoprolol	Exist	Amylase release	39
Beta$_2$	Adrenergic		H35/25	Non/low no.		39
Alpha	Adrenergic		[3]H] dihydroergocryptine	15,000	K$^+$ release	40
Alpha	Adrenergic	Epinephrine	Phentolamine		Desensitization	41
Alpha$_1$	Adrenergic	Prazosin	[3]H] dihydro	7500	K$^+$ release	42
Alpha$_2$	Adrenergic	Prazosin	alpha-ergocryptine	7500	K$^+$ release	42
	Muscarinic		[3]H] quinuclidinyl benzilate	21,400	Protein and fluid release	43
	Muscarinic		[3]H] propylbenzylcholine mustard		Protein and fluid release	43
	Muscarinic	Methacholine Carbachol	[3]H] quinuclidinyl benzilate	23,000	K$^+$ release Ca influx	44 44
	Substance P	[125]I] Substance P		200	Amylase release	45
	Physalaemin	[125]I] Physalaemin		215	Amylase release	46
	Vasoactive intestinal peptide	[125]I] VIP		41,000	Amylase release	47

transmitter receptors and some of their characteristics. Recently it was shown that cyclic AMP and calcium are involved in protein secretions, and protein kinase C participates in salivary amylase secretions.[48-50] The intracellular pathways involved in salivary secretion have been described above.

AMYLASE GENETICS

In humans, amylase is produced mainly by the pancreas and the salivary glands. There are seven amylase genes;[51-55] two are pancreatic (AMY2A, AMY2B), three are salivary (AMY1A, AMY1B, AMY1C), and two are truncated pseudogenes (AMYP1, AMYP2). The AMY1 and AMY2 loci are closely linked and highly homologous. The nucleotide sequence homology in the coding region of salivary and pancreatic amylase cDNA is 98%, and the predicted sequences of 511 amino acids are 97% homologous.[56] The three salivary amylase genes do not differ within the 950 nucleotide regions that have been sequenced,[53] although there appear to be some electrophoretic dissimilarities of their products.[57] In spite of the close homology of the 5′ flanking region of the human amylase gene family, AMY1 and AMY2 genes are expressed with strict tissue specificity.[58] AMY1 is expressed only in the parotid, AMY2A only in the pancreas, and AMY2B mainly in the pancreas but also in the liver. Two endogenous genetic markers are present in the amylase gene family: one is a gamma-actin pseudogene situated in the 5′ regions of the five human amylase genes, and the second is a retroviral long terminal repeat (LTR) interrupting the actin sequences.[58,59] The presence of a poly A sequence at the 3′ terminus of the actin sequences associated with amylase genes indicates that the mechanism of insertion was by retroposition of an actin transcript. On the basis of the 89% sequence homology between the actin pseudogene and the functional gamma-actin gene, the time of origin of the pseudogenes has been estimated as approximately 23 million years ago.[58] Furthermore, because the actin sequences are inserted in the same position, upstream of exon A in all five amylase genes, it appears that the incorporation of actin preceded the separation of human salivary and pancreatic amylase genes. Additionally, the absence of the LTR sequence from only the AMY2B gene suggests that AMY2B separated from the other genes prior to insertion of the retroviral LTR.

BIOLOGIC AND BIOCHEMICAL DIFFERENCES BETWEEN SALIVARY AND PANCREATIC ISOAMYLASES

Salivary amylase differs from pancreatic amylase in several respects. The two proteins can be separated by ion-exchange chromatography, polyacrylamide gel electrophoresis, or isoelectric focusing.[60-62] Their molecular weights (55,000 for salivary and 62,000 for pancreatic amylase) as well as their amino acid compositions[63,64] are different. The isoenzymes of amylase can be further distinguished by their sensitivity to inhibitors. For example, an isolate from wheat inhibits 88% of salivary amylase but only 27% of the pancreatic isoenzyme.[65] The two amylases differ in their digestive capabilities: glucose is virtually absent from the digestion product of salivary isoamylase, whereas pancreatic isoamylase converts up to 30% of glycogen and starch to glucose. Finally, salivary isoamylase has a higher affinity for starch, while pancreatic amylase has a higher affinity for glycogen.[66]

PHYSIOLOGIC IMPORTANCE

During Development and Age Dependency. Pancreatic amylase is the key enzyme in carbohydrate digestion but is nearly absent in the first 4 to 6 months of life.[67] The alternate pathways for digestion are represented by the small bowel mucosal glucoamylase and by salivary and mammary amylases.[68] Salivary amylase is first detected at 20 weeks of gestation.[69] It is present in low quantities at birth and reaches one third of adult levels by 3 months of age.[70-72] Available data suggest that amylase activity increases with age in infancy.[73,74] During adulthood, a significant decrease of total protein may occur.[75] Although some have reported no significant difference in total protein between the young and old,[76] salivary amylase activity is decreased in the elderly in resting and stimulated parotid saliva.

Nutritional Aspects. The hydrolytic properties of the isoenzymes of human salivary amylase (1,4-glucan 4 glucanohydrolase EC 3.2.1.1) are important. When applied to glycogen and starch, the products are maltose, maltotriose, maltotetraose, pannose, and oligosaccharides of 5 to 10 glucose units. Maltotetraose and pannose are further digested to lower homologues. The percentage of conversion to these products is dependent on the substrate and is specific for each isoenzyme. Furthermore, contrary to pancreatic isoamylase, which has a higher affinity for glycogen, the salivary enzyme has increased affinity for starch.[66] These biochemical properties are biologically important, because salivary amylase plays a major part in carbohydrate digestion, especially early in life when the pancreatic amylase pathway is not functionally operative.[68] During nursing, the mammary amylase joins the salivary enzyme to function as a potential compensatory pathway for digestion of amylose, amylopectin, and glycogen.[77,78] Additionally, in congenital or acquired pancreatic insufficiency, the salivary mechanism of starch digestion may be the only one to operate physiologically. Infants in the first half year of life have physiologic pancreatic deficiency. Despite this, they tolerate starches and glucose polymers.[79,80] The ability to digest polymers of glucose represents a nutritional advantage, because glucose polymers with a high caloric density and low osmolarity are readily absorbed.[81] In the lumen of the midjejunum, distal ileum, and cecum, the isoamylases are of the pancreatic type.[82] By contrast, 15% of the total amylase in the duodenum is the salivary isoenzyme.[83] Fried and colleagues found that salivary amylase constituted 13.8 ± 3.9% of the total amylase output activity in the intestinal lumen, while 11% was generated in the intestine. Interestingly, 27% of the amylase was of the salivary type in achlorhydric subjects.[84] Below a gastric pH of 3.0, no activity of the salivary amylase type can be detected in the stomach.[74,84] Nutrients buffer the acid and protect the salivary enzyme from gastric inactivation.[74,85,86] Even in the young or premature infants, amylase activity can be demonstrated in the stomach and in the intestine after a meal when gastric pH is greater than 3.0.[74,80,87]

Salivary Amylase Body Compartmental Distribution. Human milk contains 1.2 to 1.5 g/dL of oligosaccharides ranging in length from penta to tetra-deca-saccharides.[88] To digest these carbohydrates as well as the carbohydrates in baby formula, infants need a mechanism of digestion other than by way of the pancreas, which is undeveloped at this age. Human milk amylase together with salivary amylase and mucosal glucoamylase provides this mechanism. Amylase is present in milk secreted by mothers of both preterm and term infants.[89,90] It has a pH optimum in the range of 4.5 to 7.5 but loses little activity at pH 3. It is resistant to the proteolytic action of pepsin,[77] and more than 95% of milk alpha amylase is of the salivary type rather than the pancreatic type.[91] Women with an inherited variant of salivary isoamylase express the same variant in their mother milk, supporting the hypothesis that the isoamylases of saliva and milk are products of the same gene. Furthermore, because salivary amylase has anti-infectious properties, human milk might inhibit the growth of certain microorganisms.[92]

Amniotic fluid contains amylase activity after the 14th week of gestation.[93] Both pancreatic and salivary isozymes are present thereafter. The amylase content is increased throughout gestation, with a rapid rise at 32 to 34 weeks, and the majority of this developmental increase appears to consist of the salivary amylase.[94] Amniotic amylase is produced by the fetus and not the mother.[60]

In normal persons, the serum amylase results from a mixture of pancreatic and salivary-type isoamylases, with the latter constituting 60% to 65% of the total amylase activity. In patients with chronic unexplained hyperamylasemia, the salivary-type amylase is the predominant serum isoamylase and results more often from metastatic tumors than from pancreatitis.[95,96] Isoamylase analysis provides information that might change the clinical diagnosis in 20% to 40% of hyperamylasemic patients.[97] Reference values for the salivary-type amylase serum level in different ages were reported by Skude.[98]

Salivary Amylase in Pathologic States. Following major maxillofacial surgery, a 10-fold increase of salivary serum amylase has been observed. This surge is transient and tends to disappear within 2 to 4 days. No change in serum pancreatic isoamylase is seen.[98]

Total serum amylase activity is within normal limits in the cystic fibrosis population, but there is an alteration in the isoamylase ratio such that pancreatic amylase is markedly decreased and the salivary counterpart is increased. This alteration is not detected in heterozygotes.[98] In babies with cystic fibrosis, the amylase activity in the duodenal aspirate increases dramatically after feeding.[99] This increase in duodenal amylase activity represents a mixture of salivary amylases from both the baby's saliva and the mother's milk.

Patients with chronic pancreatitis and chronic relapsing pancreatitis tend to have a moderately increased level of serum salivary amylase, whereas pancreatic carcinoma patients have a lower level compared to controls.[98] Sialolithiasis, salivary gland tumors, or aseptic inflammation of the salivary glands due to various drugs, may increase the activity of the salivary serum isoamylases.[98] Because iodine can be trapped and concentrated in salivary glands, therapeutic doses of iodine[131] can produce acute parotitis with enhanced amylase activity in the parotid saliva.[100]

Salivary-type isoamylase is produced by organs other than the salivary glands.[61] Thus, the increased serum salivary-type isoamylase seen in heroin addicts is thought to be derived in part from the lungs.[101] In addition, carcinoma of the lung has been associated with increased salivary-type amylase.[102,103]

Lingual Lipase

The human lipases represent an extensive family of enzymes responsible for lipid digestion and metabolism. The first site of lipid digestion occurs in the stomach, where lingual and gastric lipase join together and pretreat fat for final digestion by pancreatic lipase. A survey of the literature concerning the origin of preduodenal lipase activity in humans provides a confusing picture because of the variability of findings obtained by way of different types of studies.[104,105] Indeed, the very existence of lingual lipase has been questioned.[106]

LOCALIZATION

Roberts and colleagues[107] confirmed earlier studies[108,109] localizing lipase to lingual serous glands. Immunospecific staining was observed in all acinar cells of the rat serous von Ebner glands located beneath the circumvallate papilla of the tongue and in the demilunes of the lingual mucous glands. A comparable distribution was found in the human tongue.[108] The enzyme is localized in the apical zymogen granules of the acinar cells of the von Ebner glands.[107,110] It is important to note, however, that these studies are in discordance with another that found lipase activity to be missing from the human pharynx and the lingual area, including the circumvallate papillae.[106] Only rats and mice have a rich supply of lingual lipase, while in rabbits, guinea pigs, baboons, and humans, gastric lipase is the main lipase acting in the stomach. Aquatic mammals have equal lingual and gastric lipases.[111]

SECRETION

The lingual serous glands are similar to other exocrine glands in the subcellular localization of the enzymes to the zymogen of the acinar cells. However, despite a comparable mechanism of enzyme secretion, the potency of the different neurotransmitters is organ-specific. The regulation of lingual lipase secretion appears to be mediated principally by cholinergic pathways, in contrast to the beta-adrenergic stimulatory effect on amylase secretion from the parotid gland. However, in the rat,[110] lipase secretion is stimulated by isoprenaline, and bilateral resection of the glossopharyngeal nerves or bilateral sympathectomy leads to a 40% to 50% decrease in enzyme activity within a week.

Lingual lipase secretion can also be stimulated by the cholinergic agonist carbamylcholine chloride[112,113] and by cholecystokinin.[114] Beta-adrenergic agonists and the adenylate cyclase activator forskolin induce somewhat lower levels of secretion from lingual serous glands. The former effect appears to be mediated by beta 1-adrenoceptors.

GENETICS

The gene for rat lingual lipase has been cloned, and its structure has been predicted from the cDNA sequence.[115] It is a glycoprotein of approximately 52,000 kd. The mature enzyme consists of 377 amino acid residues and shares little homology with porcine pancreatic lipase. Some cloned human lipases have sequence homology with rat lingual lipase. Human lecithin–cholesterol acyltransferase is distinguished by a number of extended sequences of hydrophobic amino acids, one of which contains a hexapeptide identical with the interfacial binding segment of the active site of pancreatic lipase and is similar to the same site of lingual lipase.[116] A lipase gene from *Pseudomonas fragi* indicates some amino acid sequence homology around the reactive serine common to the lipases as mentioned above.[117] Finally, human gastric lipase was recently cloned and expressed in yeast.[118] This protein consists of a 379-amino-acid polypeptide with an unglycosylated molecular weight of 43,162. The N-terminal amino acid sequence of the human gastric lipase is homologous with the N-terminal sequence of rat lingual lipase, and the two enzymes have an overall amino acid sequence homology of 78%. Even greater homology may exist between human gastric and lingual lipase. The availability of yeast expressing human gastric lipase makes feasible the production of pharmaceutical quantities of this enzyme for use in human pancreatic insufficiency states.

BIOLOGIC ACTIVITY

Lingual lipase hydrolyzes long-chain triglycerides, which are the major components of dietary fat. The pH optimum of the purified rat enzyme is 4.0 and ranges from pH 2.0 to 8.0. In contrast to human pancreatic lipase, lingual lipase hydrolyzes triglycerides in emulsions and mixed micelles stabilized with both short-chain and long-chain lecithin and is inhibited only slightly by micellar concentrations of bile salts.[119] This suggests that lingual lipase biologic activity may extend from the site of secretion to the stomach and even into the upper small bowel. In contrast to pancreatic lipase, colipase has no effect on the interaction of lingual lipase with triglyceride.[120] Furthermore, lingual lipase preferentially attacks position 3 of the triglyceride, and medium-chain and polyunsaturated long-chain fatty acids are released in preference to saturated fatty acids.[121] The hydrolysis of triglycerides by lingual lipase is not affected by lecithin, as is the case for the pancreatic counterpart.[120] The resistance to acid and gastric enzymes makes lingual lipase an ideal candidate for fat digestion in the stomach.[122–125] In ruminants, 70% of dietary fat is absorbed in the absence of pancreatic lipase. By analogy, children with congenital or acquired absence of pancreatic lipase or severe pancreatic insufficiency might absorb 40% to 70% of ingested dietary fats.[126]

Mixed micelles of bile salts and phospholipids inhibit lipase—colipase-catalyzed hydrolysis of triacylglycerols. Free fatty acids can reverse this inhibition and reactivate lipase–colipase. The biologic relevance of these results is evident because the glyceride emulsion reaching the duodenum already contains free fatty acids as a result of the activity of lingual lipase in the stomach.[127] Recently, a membrane-disruptive effect of human milk capable of inactivating viral envelopes has been reported.[128] Antiviral activity in an infant's stomach may result from the activity of gastric and lingual lipases on milk triglycerides, causing the release of antiviral fatty acids.

DEVELOPMENTAL ASPECTS

The development of lingual lipase is the subject of a recent review by Hamosh.[129] Lingual lipase is present in the developing serous glands and is secreted to aid in fat digestion.[130] The importance of lingual lipase in neonatal gastric lipid digestion has been studied in rats.[131,132] Throughout the first 2 months of life, the total lipolytic activity in gastric mucosa was only 2% to 10% of that in lingual glands. During the suckling period, a close correlation between growth and lingual lipase activity has been demonstrated. Lipase hydrolyzes 50% to 60% of lipid in milk during the suckling period.

Furthermore, from the first day of life, the efficiency of dietary triglyceride hydrolysis is the same as later in life.

In humans, lingual lipase is detected before 26 weeks of gestation and has a high activity level at birth.[133,134] In preterm infants, lingual lipase may contribute significantly to fat digestion because duodenal lipolysis by pancreatic enzymes is poorly developed.[135] In adults, the main role of lingual lipase may be to act as an emulsifier by formation of more soluble lipids, thus providing a better substrate for pancreatic lipase. Because pancreatic function is decreased in the elderly,[136] this alternative mechanism for fat absorption may become more important.

PATHOBIOLOGIC IMPORTANCE OF LINGUAL LIPASE IN PANCREATIC INSUFFICIENCY

The contribution of nonpancreatic lipolytic activity to fat digestion becomes more significant under conditions of limited availability of pancreatic lipase. In cystic fibrosis, nonpancreatic lipase activity accounts for more than 90% of total lipolytic activity measured at the ligament of Treitz.[137] A comparable result has been obtained in patients with exocrine pancreatic insufficiency secondary to alcoholism.[138] The pH of the jejunum in patients with pancreatic insufficiency is lower than normal. This environment provides the prepancreatic lipases, which are acid-resistant, an optimal pH for lipid digestion.

> The reader is directed to Chapter 1, The Enteric Nervous System and its Extrinsic Connections; Chapter 2, Gastrointestinal Hormones; Chapter 13, Gastric Secretion; and Chapter 15, Pancreatic Secretion.

REFERENCES

1. Granger DN, Barrowman JA, Kvietys PR. Clinical gastrointestinal physiology. Eating, salivation, mastication, and deglutition. Philadelphia, WB Saunders, 1985:34.
2. Ten Cate AR. Oral histology development, structure and function, ed 3. New York: CV Mosby, 1989:312.
3. Nelson TE, Stouffer JE. Thyroxine modulation of epinephrine stimulated secretion of rat parotid alpha-amylase. Biochem Biophys Res Commun 1972;48:480.
4. Young JA, Cook DI, Van Lennep EW, et al. Secretion by the major salivary glands. In: Johnson LR, ed. Physiology of the gastrointestinal tract, ed 2. New York: Raven Press, 1987:773.
5. Seifert G, Miehlke A, Haubrich J, et al. Diseases of the salivary glands. New York: Thiem, 1986:27.
6. Bing J, Poulsen K. The renin system in mice. Acta Pathol Microbiol Scand 1971;79:134.
7. Michelakis AM, Menzie JW, Yoshida H. Sympathetic nervous system and renin release from submaxillary glands in vitro. Am J Physiol 1976;231:551.
8. Healy JF, Fraser PA, Young JA. Inhibition of sodium transport by angiotensin II in the main duct of the rabbit mandibular gland isolated and perfused in vitro: Pflugers Arch 1976;363:69.
9. Ellison SA. Proteins and glycoproteins of saliva. In: Coole CF, ed. Handbook of physiology, Sect 6, Vol 2. Alimentary Canal, Washington, DC: American Physiological Society, 1967:531.
10. Schachter M. Kinins—A group of active peptides. Annu Rev Pharmacol 1964;4:281.

11. Orstavik TB. The kallikrein-kinin system in exocrine organs. J Histochem Cytochem 1980;28:881.

12. Thayson JH, Thorn NA, Schwartz IL. Excretion of sodium, potassium, chloride and carbon dioxide in human parotid saliva. Am J Physiol 1954;178:155.

13. Young JA, von Lennep EW. The morphology of the salivary glands. New York: Academic Press, 1978.

14. Young JA, von Lennep EW. Transport in salivary and salt glands. Part I: Salivary glands. In: Giebisch G, ed. Membrane transport in biology, Vol 4B: Transport organs. Heidelberg: Springer-Verlag, 1979:563.

15. Cook DI, Young JA. Fluid and electrolyte secretion by salivary glands. In: Handbook of physiology, Sect 6: The gastrointestinal system. Bethesda, MD: American Physiological Society, 1989:1.

16. Schneyer LH. Sympathetic control of Na, K transport in perfused submaxillary main duct of rat. Am J Physiol 1976;230:341.

17. Schneyer LH. Parasympathetic control of Na, K transport in perfused submaxillary duct of the rat. Am J Physiol 1976;233:F22.

18. Mandel ID. The role of saliva in maintaining oral homeostasis. J Am Dent Assoc 1989;119:298.

19. Liebow C. Ontogeny of the oral cavity and its relationship to ontogeny of the gastrointestinal tract. In: Lebenthal E, ed. Human gastrointestinal development. New York: Raven Press, 1989:209.

20. Spearman TN, Butcher FR. Cellular regulation of amylase secretion by the parotid gland. In: Forte JG, ed. Handbook of physiology. The gastrointestinal system. Salivary, gastric, pancreatic and hepatobiliary secretion. Bethesda, MD: American Physiological Society, 1989:63.

21. Parks HF. Morphological study of the extrusion of secretory materials by the parotid glands of mouse and rat. J Ultrastruct Res 1962;6:449.

22. Bdolah A, Ben-Zvi R, Schramm M. The mechanism of enzyme secretion by the cell. II. Secretion of amylase and other proteins by slices of rat parotid gland. Arch Biochem Biophys 1964;104:58.

23. Castle JD, Jamieson JD, Palade GE. Radioautographic analysis of the secretory process in the parotid acinar cell of the rabbit. J Cell Biol 1972;53:290.

24. Amsterdam A, Ohad I, Schramm M. Dynamic changes in the ultrastructure of the acinar cell of the rat parotid gland during the secretory cycle. J Cell Biol 1969;41:753.

25. Amsterdam A, Schramm M, Ohad I, et al. Concomitant synthesis of membrane protein and exportable protein of the secretory granule in rat parotid gland. J Cell Biol 1971;50:187.

26. Morley DJ, Hodes JE, Calland J, et al. Immunohistochemical demonstration of ribonuclease and amylase in normal and neoplastic parotid glands. Hum Pathol 1983;14:969.

27. Morley DJ, Hodes ME. In situ localization of amylase mRNA and protein. An investigation of amylase gene activity in normal human parotid gland. J Histochem Cytochem 1987;35:9.

28. Hand AR, Coleman R, Mazariegas MR, et al. Endocytosis of proteins by salivary gland duct cells. J Dent Res 1987;66:412.

29. Lotti LV, Hand AR. Endocytosis of parotid salivary proteins by striated duct cells in streptozotocin-diabetic rats. Anat Rec 1988;221:802.

30. Robinovitch MR, Sreebny LM. Separation and identification of some of the protein components of rat parotid saliva. Arch Oral Biol 1969;14:935.

31. Garrett JR, Smith RE, Kidd A, et al. Kallikrein-like activity in salivary glands using a new tripeptide substrate, including preliminary secretory studies and observations on mast cells. Histochem J 1982;14:967.

32. Keller PJ, Robinovitch M, Ivenson J, et al. The protein composition of rat parotid saliva and secretory granules. Biochim Biophys Acta 1975;379:562.

33. Schneyer LH, Young JA, Schneyer CA. Salivary secretion of electrolytes. Physiol Rev 1972;52:720.

34. Gallacher DV. Are there purinergic receptors on parotid acinar cells? Nature 1982;296:83.

35. Au DK, Malbon CC, Butcher FR. Identification and characterization of beta adrenergic receptors in rat parotid membranes. Biochim Biophys Acta 1977;500:361.

36. Ludford JM, Talamo BR. Beta adrenergic and muscarinic receptors in developing rat parotid glands. Selective effect of neonatal sympathetic denervation. J Biol Chem 1980;255:4619.

37. Hata F, Ishida H, Kagawak, et al. Beta adrenoceptor alterations coupled with secretory response in rat parotid tissue. J Physiol (Lond) 1983;341:185.

38. Carlsoo B, Danielson A, Henriksson R, et al. Characterization of the rat parotid beta adrenoceptor. Br J Pharmacol 1981;72:271.

39. Fuller CM, Gallacher DV. Beta adrenergic receptor mechanisms in rat parotid glands: Activation by nerve stimulation and 3-isobutyl-1 methylxanthine. J Physiol (Lond) 1984;356:335.

40. Strittmatter WJ, Davis JN, Lefkowitz RJ. Alpha adrenergic receptors in rat parotid cells. I. Correlation of [^{3}H] dihydroergocryptine binding and catecholamine-stimulated potassium efflux. J Biol Chem 1977;252:5472.

41. Strittmatter WJ, Davis JN, Lefkowitz RJ. Alpha adrenergic receptors in rat parotid cells. II. Desensitization of receptor binding sites and potassium release. J Biol Chem 1977;252:5478.

42. Ito H, Hoopes MT, Baum BJ. K$^+$ release from rat parotid cells: An alpha$_1$ adrenergic mediated event. Biochem Pharmacol 1982;31:567.

43. Hootman SR, Picado-Leonard JM, Burnham DB. Muscarinic acetylcholine receptor structure in acinar cells of mammalian exocrine glands. J Biol Chem 1985;260:4186.

44. Putney JW Jr, Van De Wolle CM. The relationship between muscarinic receptor binding and ion movements in rat parotid cells. J Physiol (Lond) 1980;299:521.

45. Liang T, Cascieri MA. Specific binding of an immunoreactive and biologically active ^{125}I labeled n(1) acylated substance P derivative to parotid cells. Biochem Biophys Res Commun 1980;96:1793.

46. Putney JW Jr, Van De Walle CM, Wheeler CS. Binding of ^{125}I physalaemin to rat parotid acinar cells. J Physiol (Lond) 1980;301:205.

47. Inoue Y, Kaku K, Kaneko T, et al. Vasoactive intestinal peptide binding to specific receptors on rat parotid acinar cells induced amylase secretion accompanied by intracellular accumulation of cyclic adenosine 3′-5′ monophosphate. Endocrinology 1985;116:686.

48. Scott J, Baum BJ. Involvement of cyclic AMP and calcium in exocrine protein secretion induced by vasoactive intestinal polypeptide in rat parotid cells. Biochim Biophys Acta 1985;847:255.

49. Shimomura H, Terada A, Hashimoto Y, et al. The role of protein kinase C on amylase secretion from rat parotid gland. Biochem Biophys Res Commun 1988;150:1309.

50. McKinney JS, Rubin RP. Enhancement of cyclic AMP modulated salivary amylase secretion by protein kinase C activators. Biochem Pharmacol 1988;37:4433.

51. Nishide T, Nakamura Y, Emi M, et al. Primary structure of human salivary alpha-amylase gene. Gene 1986;41:299.

52. Horii A, Emi M, Tomita N, et al. Primary structure of human pancreatic alpha-amylase gene: Its comparison with human salivary alpha-amylase gene. Gene 1987;60:57.

53. Gumucio DL, Wiebauer K, Caldwell RM, et al. Concerted evolution of human amylase genes. Mol Cell Biol 1988;8:1197.

54. Handy DE, Larsen SH, Karn RC, et al. Identification of a human salivary amylase gene. Partial sequence of genomic DNA suggests a mode of regulation different from that of mouse, Amy 1. Mol Biol Med 1987;4:145.

55. Groot PC, Bleeker MJ, Pronk JC, et al. Human pancreatic amylase is encoded by two different genes. Nucleic Acids Res 1988;16:4724.

56. Nishide T, Emi M, Nakamura Y, et al. Corrected sequences of cDNAs for human salivary and pancreatic alpha amylases. Gene 1986;50:371.

57. Pronk JC, Frants RR, Jansen W, et al. Evidence of duplication of the human salivary amylase gene. Hum Genet 1982;60:32.

58. Samuelson LC, Wiebauer K, Gumucio DL, et al. Expression of the human amylase genes: Recent origin of a salivary amylase promoter from an active pseudogene. Nucleic Acids Res 1988;16:8261.

59. Emi M, Horii A, Tomita N, et al. Overlapping two genes in human DNA: A salivary amylase gene overlaps with a gamma-actin pseudogene that carries an integrated human endogenous retroviral DNA. Gene 1988;62:229.

60. Wolf RO, Taussig LM. Human amniotic fluid isoamylases: Functional development of fetal pancreas and salivary glands. Obstet Gynecol 1973;41:337.

61. Levitt MD, Ellis C, Engel RR. Isoelectric focusing studies of human serum and tissue isoamylases. J Lab Clin Med 1977;90:141.

62. Stephan J, Skrha J. Measurement of amylase isoenzymes in human sera and urine using a DEAE–cellulose mini-columnar method. Clin Chim Acta 1979;19:263.

63. Kam RC. The comparative biochemistry, physiology and genetics of animals' alpha-amylases. Adv Comp Physiol Biochim 1978;7:1.

64. Sky-Peck HH, Thuvasethakul P. Human pancreatic alpha-amylase. I. Purification and characterization. Am Clin Lab Sci 1977;7:298.

65. O'Donnell MD, Fitzgerald O, McGeeney KF. Differential serum amylase determination by use of inhibitor and design of a routine procedure. Clin Chem 1977;23:560.

66. Kaczmarek MJ, Rosenmund H. The action of human pancreatic and salivary isoamylases on starch and glycogen. Clin Chim Acta 1977;79:69.

67. Lebenthal E, Lee PC. Development of functional response in human exocrine pancreas. Pediatrics 1980;66:556.

68. Lebenthal E, Leung YK. Alternative pathways of digestion and absorption in the newborn. In: Lebenthal E, ed. Textbook of gastroenterology and nutrition in infancy, ed 2. New York: Raven Press, 1989:3.

69. Lebenthal E, Lee PC. Gastrointestinal physiologic considerations in the feeding of the developing infant. Ann Nestle spec edition—nutrition in early life. 1984:47.

70. Nicory C. Salivary secretion in infants. Biochem J 1922;16:387.

71. Lee PC, Nord KS, Lebenthal E. Digestibility of starches in infants. In: Lebenthal E, ed. Textbook of gastroenterology and nutrition in infancy, ed 1. New York: Raven Press, 1981:423.

72. Mobassaleh M, Montgomery RK, Biller JA, et al. Development of carbohydrate absorption in the fetus and neonate. Pediatrics 1985:75(Suppl):160.

73. Lourie RS. Rate of secretion of the parotid glands in normal children. Am J Dis Child 1943;65:455.

74. Hodge C, Lebenthal E, Lee PC, et al. Amylase in the saliva and in the gastric aspirates of premature infants: Its potential role in glucose polymer hydrolysis. Pediatr Res 1983;17:998.

75. Chauncey HH, Borkan GA, Wayler AH, et al. Parotid fluid composition in healthy aging males. In: Zelles T, ed. Saliva and salivation. Adv Physiol Sci New York: Pergamon Press, 1980;28:323.

76. Ben-Aryeh H, Shalev A, Szargel R, et al. The salivary flow rate and composition of whole and parotid resting and stimulated saliva in young and old healthy subjects. Biochem Med Metab Biol 1986;36:260.

77. Heitlinger LA, Lee PC, Dillon WP, et al. Mammary amylase: A possible alternate pathway of carbohydrate digestion in infancy. Pediatr Res 1983;17:15.

78. Lebenthal E. Role of salivary amylase in gastric and intestinal digestion of starch. Dig Dis Sci 1987;32:1155.

79. Lebenthal E, Lee PC, Heitlinger LA. Impact of the development of the gastrointestinal tract on infant feeding. J Pediatr 1983;102:1.

80. Murray RD, Kerzner B, Sloan HR, et al. Quantification of glucose polymer (GP) digestion by premature salivary amylase (SA). Pediatr Res 1985;19:228A.

81. Lebenthal E, Heitlinger LA, Lee PC, et al. Corn syrup sugars: In vitro and in vivo digestibility and clinical tolerance in infants with acute diarrhea. J Pediatr 1983;103:29.

82. Banks PA, Warshaw AL, Wolfe GZ, et al. Identification of amylase isoenzymes in intestinal contents. Dig Dis Sci 1984;29:297.

83. Skude G, Ihse I. Salivary amylase in duodenal aspirates. Scand J Gastroenterol 1976;11:17.

84. Fried M, Abramson S, Meyer JH. Passage of salivary amylase through the stomach in humans. Dig Dis Sci 1987;32:1097.

85. Malagelada JR, Longstrength GF, Summerskill HH, et al. Measurement of gastric functions during digestion of ordinary solid meals in man. Gastroenterology 1976;70:203.

86. Rosenblum JL, Irwin CL, Alpers DH. Human salivary amylase (SA) activity is protected at low pH by glucose polymers. Gastroenterology 1985;88:1559.

87. Heitlinger LA, Lee PC, Brooks SP, et al. Human amylases: Identification of pancreatic, salivary and mammary amylases in duodenal fluids. Gastroenterology 1982;82:1081.

88. Newburg DS, Daniel PF, O'Neill NE, et al. High performance liquid chromatography of neutral and acidic oligo-saccharides from human milk and colostrum. In: Hamosh M, Goldman AS, eds. Human lactation: Maternal–environmental factors. New York: Plenum Press, 1986:581.

89. Jones JB, Mehta NR, Hamosh M. Alpha amylase in preterm human milk. J Pediatr Gastroenterol Nutr 1982;1:43.

90. Hegardt P, Lindberg T, Borjesson J, et al. Amylase in human milk from mothers of preterm and term infants. J Pediatr Gastroenterol Nutr 1984;3:563.

91. Hamosh M. Enzymes in human milk: Their role in nutrient digestion, gastrointestinal function and nutrient delivery to the newborn infant. In: Lebenthal E, ed. Textbook of gastroenterology and nutrition in infancy, ed 2. New York: Raven Press, 1989:121.

92. Mellersh A, Clark A, Hofiz S. Inhibition of Neisseria gonorrhea A by normal human saliva. Br J Venereal Dis 1979;55:20.

93. Laxova R. Antenatal development of amylase in amniotic fluid. Prenat Diagn 1984;4:257.

94. Heitlinger LA. Intestinal and pancreatic enzymes in amniotic fluid and meconium: Content as an index of fetal maturity, well being, or disease. In: Lebenthal E, ed. Human gastrointestinal development. New York: Raven Press, 1989:521.

95. Levitt MD, Elis CJ, Meier PB. Extrapancreatic origin of chronic unexplained hyperamylasemia. N Engl J Med 1980;302:670.

96. Lehrner LM, Ward JC, Karn RC, et al. An evaluation of the usefulness of amylase isozyme differentiation in patients with hyperamylasemia. Am J Clin Pathol 1976;66:576.

97. Koehler DF, Eckfeldt JH, Levitt MD. Diagnostic value of routine isoamylase assay of hyperamylasemic serum. Gastroenterology 1982;82:887.

98. Skude G. On human amylase isoenzymes. Scand J Gastroenterol 1977(Suppl);12:1

99. Lindberg T, Skude G. Amylase in human milk. Pediatrics 1982;70:235.

100. Maier H, Bihl H. Effect of radioactive iodine therapy on parotid gland function. Acta Otolaryngol (Stockh) 1987;103:318.

101. Heffernon JJ, Smith WR, Berk JE, et al. Hyperamylasemia in heroin addicts: Characterization by isoamylase analysis. Am J Gastroenterol 1976;66:17.

102. Berk JE, Shimamura J, Fridhandler L. Tumor-associated hyperamylasemia. Am J Gastroenterol 1977;68:572.

103. Sudo K, Kanno T. Properties of the amylase produced in carcinoma of the lung. Clin Chim Acta 1976;73:1.

104. Salzman-Mann S, Hamosh M, Sivasubramanian KN, et al. Congenital esophageal atresia. Lipase activity is present in esophageal pouch and stomach. Dig Dis Sci 1982;27:124.

105. De Nigris SJ, Fink CS, Hamosh M, et al. Fat digestion: Species differences in the source of preduodenal lipolytic enzymes. Fed Proc 1985;44:811.

106. Moreau H, Laugier R, Gargouri Y, et al. Human preduodenal lipase is entirely of gastric fundic origin. Gastroenterology 1988;95:1221.

107. Roberts IM, Jaffe R. Lingual lipase: Immunocytochemical localization in the rat von Ebner gland. Gastroenterology 1986;90:1170.

108. Hamosh M, Burns WA. Lipolytic activity of human lingual glands (Ebner). Lab Invest 1977;37:603.

109. Hamosh M, Scow RO. Lingual lipase and its role in the digestion of dietary fat. J Clin Invest 1973;55:88.

110. Hamosh M. Rat lingual lipase: Factors affecting enzyme activity and secretion. Am J Physiol 1978;235:E416.

111. York CM, Yao J, Hamosh M, et al. Gastric lipase in the dog and seal: Implications for neonatal fat digestion. Fed Proc 1987;46:1084.

112. Field RB, Dromy R, Hand AR. Regulation of secretion of enzymes from von Ebner's gland of rat tongue. J Dent Res 1987;66:586.

113. Field RB, Hand AR. Secretion of lingual lipase and amylase from rat lingual serous glands. Am J Physiol 1987;253:G217.

114. Ruellan C, Moreau J, Bouisson M, et al. The Ebner glands: A pancreatic-like gland secreting an acid lipase. Secretory regulation in vitro. Int J Pancreatol 1988;3:293.

115. Docherty AJP, Bodmer MW, Angal S. Molecular cloning and nucleotide sequence of rat lingual lipase cDNA. Nucleic Acids Res 1985;13:1891.

116. McLean J, Fielding C, Drayna D, et al. Cloning and expression of

human lecithin–cholesterol acyltransferase cDNA. Proc Natl Acad Sci USA 1986;83:2335.

117. Kugimiya W, Otani Y, Hashimoto Y, et al. Molecular cloning and nucleotide sequence of the lipase gene from Pseudomonas fragi. Biochem Biophys Res Commun 1986;141:185.

118. Bodmer MW, Angal S, Yarranton GT, et al. Molecular cloning of a human gastric lipase and expression of the enzyme in yeast. Biochim Biophys Acta 1987;909:237.

119. Roberts IM, Montgomery RK, Carey MC. Rat lingual lipase: Partial purification, hydrolytic properties and comparison with pancreatic lipase. Am J Physiol 1984;247;G385.

120. Liao TH, Hamosh P, Hamosh M. Fat digestion by lingual lipase: Mechanism of lipolysis in the stomach and upper small intestine. Pediatr Res 1984;18:402.

121. Patton JS, Rigler MW, Liao TH, et al. Hydrolysis of triacylglycerol emulsions by lingual lipase—A microscopic study. Biochim Biophys Acta 1982;712:400.

122. Hamosh M. Lingual lipase. Gastroenterology 1986;90:1290.

123. Fink CS, Hamosh P, Hamosh M. Fat digestion in the stomach: Stability of lingual lipase in the gastric environment. Pediatr Res 1984;18;248.

124. Roberts IM, Hanel SI. Stability of lingual lipase in vivo: Studies of the iodinated enzyme in the rat stomach and duodenum. Biochim Biophys Acta 1988;960:107.

125. Roberts IM. Rat lingual lipase: Effect of proteases, bile, and pH on enzyme stability. Am J Physiol 1985;249:G496.

126. Hamosh M. A review. Fat digestion in the newborn: Role of lingual lipase and preduodenal digestion. Pediatr Res 1979;13:615.

127. Larsson A, Erlanson-Albertsson C. Effect of phosphatidylcholine and free fatty acids on the activity of pancreatic lipase–colipase. Biochim Biophys Acta 1986;876:543.

128. Isaacs CE, Thormar H, Pessolano T. Membrane-disruptive effect of human milk: Inactivation of enveloped viruses. J Infect Dis 1986;154:966.

129. Hamosh M, Hamosh P. Lingual and gastric lipases during development. In: Lebenthal E, ed. Human gastrointestinal development. New York: Raven Press, 1989:251.

130. Roberts IM, Nochomovitz LE, Jaffe R, et al. Immunocytochemical localization of lingual lipase in serous cells of the developing rat tongue. Lipids 1987;22:764.

131. Liao TH, Hamosh P, Hamosh M. Gastric lipolysis in the developing rat: Ontogeny of the lipases active in the stomach. Biochim Biophys Acta 1983;754:1.

132. Bitman J, Wood DL, Liao TH, et al. Gastric lipolysis of milk lipids in sucking rats. Biochim Biophys Acta 1985;834:58.

133. Hamosh M, Scanlon JW, Ganot D, et al. Fat digestion in the newborn: Characterization of lipase in gastric aspirates of premature and term newborns. J Clin Invest 1981;67:838.

134. Blackberg L, Hernell O, Fridrikzon B, et al. On the source of lipase activity in gastric contents. Acta Pediatr Scand 1977;66:473.

135. Smith LJ, Kaminsky S, D'Souza W. Neonatal fat digestion and lingual lipase. Acta Pediatr Scand 1986;75:913.

136. Langier R, Sarles H. The pancreas. Clin Gastroenterol 1985;14:749.

137. Abrams CK, Hamosh M, Hubbard VS, et al. Lingual lipase in cystic fibrosis. Quantitation of enzyme activity in the upper small intestine of patients with exocrine pancreatic insufficiency. J Clin Invest 1984;73:374.

138. Abrams CK, Hamosh M, Dutta SK, et al. Role of nonpancreatic lipolytic activity in exocrine pancreatic insufficiency. Gastroenterology 1987;92:125.

13

Gastric Secretion

DARYL F. DAUGHERTY
MICHAEL R. LUCEY
TADATAKA YAMADA

The stomach is a complex organ capable of secreting a great variety of products into the gastric lumen, vasculature, and interstitium. While hydrochloric acid is the paradigmatic gastric secretion, the stomach also secretes pepsinogen, mucus, bicarbonate, intrinsic factor, prostaglandins, regulatory peptides, and other chemical messengers. This chapter will discuss each of these, with particular emphasis on gastric acid secretion. We will attempt to integrate classical human and whole animal studies with more recent information gained at the cellular and molecular level and place this integrated model of acid secretion within the fabric of current clinical practice.

Although it may appear to be axiomatic that the stomach secretes hydrochloric acid, general acceptance of this fact came only quite recently after centuries of contention and controversy. Baron, in his review of this topic,[1] attributes to the seventeenth century Flemish physician Jean Baptiste van Helmont the first recognition that there was acid in gastric juice, which acted to cause digestion. He thought it was derived from the spleen. About the same time,

Sylvius, professor of medicine in Leyden, also proposed that gastric acid was a chemical digestive factor but thought it was secreted by the pancreas. Over the next period of more than a century there were numerous reports that acid was not present in gastric juices or, if acid was found, that it was a product of fermentation. Even the presence of secretions arising from the stomach was in doubt because many investigators asserted that gastric fluid was retained saliva. This issue was settled by William Beaumont, who demonstrated conclusively in 1825 and 1826 that Alexis St. Martin, a patient with a post-traumatic enterocutaneous fistula, secreted gastric juice that could dissolve food both inside and outside the stomach.[2] Beaumont sent bottles of this gastric juice to three chemists, all of whom showed it to be acidic. Baron gives credit to William Prout for the first qualitative and quantitative assessment of the composition of gastric juice in his paper of 1823 entitled "On the Nature of the Acid and Saline Matters Usually Existing in the Stomachs of Animals." Prout identified free hydrochloric acid in the gastric juice of rabbits, hares, horses, calves, dogs, and humans. In February 1824, two German workers, Tiedemann and Gmelin, unaware of Prout's work, reported to the French Academy their proof that gastric acid was hydrochloric acid. However, rival French workers reported that gastric acid was lactic acid, and this view held sway with many authorities throughout the nineteenth century, despite the work of Prout, Tiedemann, and Gmelin. Other workers who should be recognized are Schmidt, who, in a series of experiments in 1852, showed that HCl only was present in resting juice, and Dodds and Robertson, who, in 1930, demonstrated that the lactic acid in gastric juice was a product of fermentation.[3,4]

Study of the regulation of gastric acid secretion also has a long history. William Beaumont noted that "fear and anger suppressed secretion by the stomach."[2] Pavlov showed that sight and smell of food were powerful stimuli of gastric acid, and, introducing innervated and denervated gastric pouches, he established methods to study regulation of acid secretion that have prevailed for nearly a century.[5] In 1911, one of his colleagues, Bechterew, reported investigations into electrical stimulation of the frontal cortex as a stimulus of acid secretion, an effect inhibited by vagotomy.[6] In 1905, Edkins demonstrated that extracts of canine antral mucosa stimulated acid secretion when injected intravenously into dogs. This was due, he proposed, to the presence in the mucosa of a chemical stimulator of acid secretion, which he called gastrin.[7] Although similar observations were made by Lim in 1922,[8] studies of this mucosal factor were confounded by the presence of histamine, another powerful stimulus of acid secretion, in tissues under study.[9] Gastrin remained a hypothetical substance until 1964 and 1965, when Gregory and his colleagues, having purified it from hog antral mucosa, determined its structure and synthesized it in biologically active form.[10]

Inhibitory influences on acid secretion have been studied for many years also. Feng and colleagues in 1929 described a hormonally mediated inhibitor of acid secretion that was released when fat was placed in the duodenum. They called this putative hormone "enterogastrone."[11] Since then there have been many attempts to identify this agent, as we will discuss in a later section. While it is impossible in the space allotted here to highlight the discovery of each of the regulatory peptides implicated in acid secretion, special mention should be made of the isolation from ovine hypothalami of somatostatin, a powerful endocrine and exocrine inhibitor, by Brazeau in Guillemin's laboratory in 1973.[12]

Until the late 1970s, considerable controversy surrounded the relative roles of gastrin, acetylcholine, and histamine in mediating acid secretion. Some proposed that histamine was the final common pathway for acid stimulation. In a series of studies, Grossman and colleagues showed that these secretagogues potentiated the effects of each other (see below), and he proposed that there were individual receptors for these ligands on the parietal cell membrane.[13] Subsequently, Soll and colleagues confirmed this hypothesis by demonstrating receptor characteristics for gastrin, acetylcholine, and histamine on isolated canine parietal cells.[14,15] Recently, somatostatin receptors have also been identified on these cells.[16]

ANATOMY OF GASTRIC MUCOSA

A detailed understanding of gastric mucosal structure provides insight into the functional events occurring during gastric secretion. The epithelial lining of the stomach lumen consists of thick, vascular folds, or rugae, invaginated with microscopic gastric pits. Each pit opens into four to five gastric glands. The epithelial cells lining the gastric glands are highly specialized and quite different from the surface epithelial cells. Glands from the cardiac region of the stomach bridge the transition from esophageal squamous epithelium to gastric columnar epithelium. They contain mucous and endocrine cells and constitute less than 5% of the gastric gland area. The majority of gastric glands (75%) are from the oxyntic mucosa and are responsible for acid secretion (Fig 13-1). They include parietal, chief, mucous neck, endocrine, and enterochromaffin cells.[17] The pyloric glands cover the gastric antrum and pylorus and contain gastrin cells, mucous cells, and other endocrine cells. Each of these cell types has evolved into a highly specialized secretory cell that contributes to gastric secretion.

Cells

The parietal cell, or oxyntic cell, is the most distinctive cell of the gastric mucosa. It is generally found in the neck or isthmus of oxyntic glands bulging into the glandular lumen. The unstimulated parietal cell has prominent cytoplasmic tubulovesicles and an apical intracellular canaliculus lined with stubby microvilli. Upon stimulation, a dense meshwork of intracellular canaliculi rapidly forms while tubulovesicles disappear.[18,19] The canaliculi contain a large number of elongated microvilli formed by extensive microfilaments having a central cytoskeletal core of actin filaments stabilized by other proteins. It is across this apical canalicular surface that hydrochloric acid is secreted. Acid secretion is an active transport process and requires significant amounts of energy. In order to provide this energy, parietal cells have numerous mitochondria, which account for 30% to 40% of total cellular volume.[20] One prominent feature of parietal cells is their lack of the microvillous glycocalyx that is present on other cells in the gastric glands. Parietal cells are characterized by basolateral membrane folds that increase surface area for bicarbonate exchange. The functional importance of these features is discussed below.

Chief cells are pepsinogen-secreting exocrine cells found in the base or fundus of oxyntic glands. Zymogen granules containing proenzymes are located in the apical cytoplasm and release their

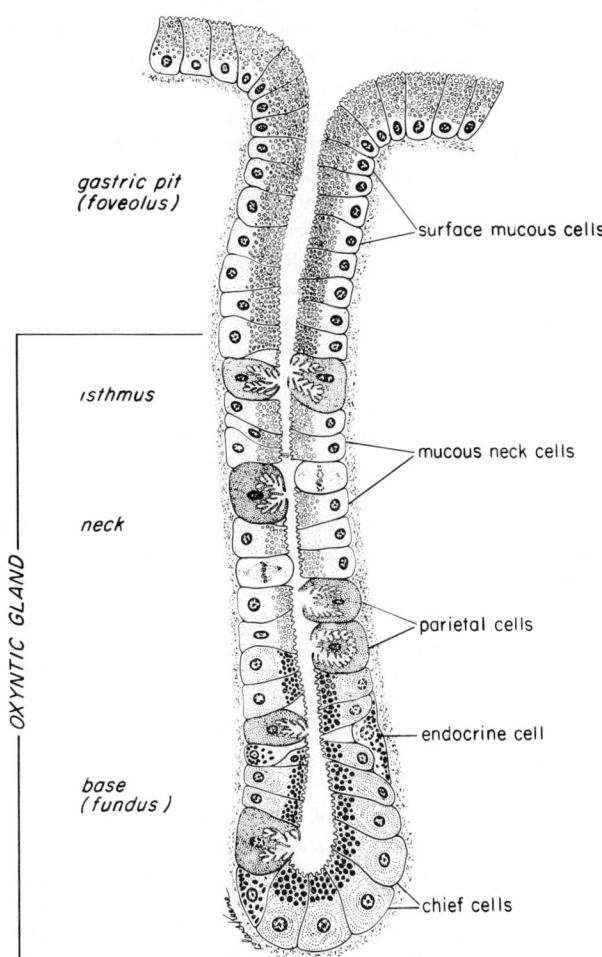

gastric pit
(foveolus)

surface mucous cells

OXYNTIC GLAND

isthmus

mucous neck cells

neck

parietal cells

endocrine cell

base
(fundus)

chief cells

FIGURE 13–1. Oxyntic gastric gland. (From Ito S. Functional gastric morphology. In: Johnson LR, ed. Physiology of the gastrointestinal tract. 2nd ed. New York: Raven Press, 1987:817.)

contents by exocytosis. The apical membrane has a few short microvilli covered by a thin coating of glycoprotein or glycocalyx. An abundant rough endoplasmic reticulum extends upward from the basal cytoplasm toward the apical granules. Functional characterization of chief cells has been aided in the recent past by the ability to obtain relatively pure populations of chief cells.

Mucous neck cells are located in the isthmus or neck region of oxyntic glands (Fig 13-1). A transition zone from mucous neck cells to surface mucous cells appears near the junction of gastric glands and gastric pits. The mucous neck cells are the stem cell precursors for all the gastric epithelial cells, including surface mucous, parietal, chief, and even endocrine cells.[21,22] Mucous neck cells differ in appearance from surface mucous cells. All mucous cells synthesize large amounts of mucin in prominent Golgi stacks, and these glycoproteins are transported by way of vesicles to large apical mucous granules. Mucous neck cells contain acidic glycoproteins (indicating sulfated forms), while surface mucous cells contain a neutral mucosubstance.[23,24] Mucous granules are larger and often paranuclear in mucous neck cells as compared with surface mucous cells. In addition, mucous neck cells have abundant ribosomes and moderate amounts of rough endoplasmic reticulum. Their function as both secretory cells and mucosal stem cells is

quite different from the presumed function of surface mucous cells in mucosal defense. Surface mucous cells line the gastric pits and cover all of the luminal surface of the stomach. They migrate up from the gastric pits and are continually replaced every 1 to 3 days.[25] They are thought to protect the stomach from injury by acid, pepsin, ingested materials, and pathogens by secreting mucus and bicarbonate to form a protective sheath. The apical portion of the surface mucous cell is packed with secretory granules. Short microvilli extend from the apical membrane and are covered by a glycocalyx. Secretion of granular mucus appears to occur by exocytosis, apical expulsion, and cell exfoliation.[26]

There are many different types of endocrine cells scattered throughout the gastric mucosa. The secretory products synthesized by these cells have important endocrine and paracrine effects on acid secretion. Immunohistochemical techniques have allowed for specific characterization of these cells based upon their secretory granule contents.[20,27] Gastric endocrine cells secrete gastrin, somatostatin, and enteroglucagon. Other morphologically distinct gastric endocrine cells may contain additional candidate hormones, but they await further characterization. Gastric endocrine cells can be classified as "open" cells, which have apical membranes in contact with the glandular lumen, or "closed" cells, which are located near the epithelial basement membrane and do not border on the lumen of the gland. The prototypical open endocrine cell is the gastrin (G) cell. The basilar portion of the cell is packed with secretory granules[28] from which gastrin is released by basilar exocytosis or emiocytosis,[29] consistent with the rapid postprandial appearance of the hormone in the bloodstream. The apical portion of the cell narrows until only a small microvillar border opens on the glandular lumen. The apical membrane may contain luminal receptors that can detect amino acids or their amine derivatives, which are thought to stimulate G cells during feeding.[30,31] The model of a closed gastric endocrine cell is the fundic somatostatin (D) cell. By immunohistochemical staining they can be seen to have long, slender processes that terminate on or near parietal and chief cells.[32] These processes presumably mediate the paracrine effect of somatostatin.

The primary cell containing mucosal histamine in the human and dog stomach is the mast cell.[33] Mast cells have been enriched from canine fundic mucosa and have been shown to contain characteristic dense granules that stain metachromatically.[34] Other species, including the rat, have histamine in endocrinelike cells that contain large granules and have the characteristic appearance of enterochromaffinlike cells.[35] The relative proportion of these two histamine cell types in man is not known. While in situ morphologic studies have not been definitive, it appears that these cells exist in the lamina propria in close proximity to the glandular cells.

Innervation

As is the case for the entire gastrointestinal tract, the stomach is innervated by both central and enteric nervous systems. This innervation mediates secretion and motor activity by way of efferent fibers and detects chemical or mechanical stimuli by way of afferent fibers. A full description of the enteric nervous system's structure and function is found in Chapter 1. Central efferents are carried by the parasympathetic vagal branches and the sympathetic greater splanchnic nerve.[36] Vagal preganglionic fibers arise from the dorsal motor nucleus of the brain stem and descend to the thorax, where they branch to form an esophageal plexus. These fibers merge into anterior and posterior vagal trunks just before they cross the diaphragmatic esophageal hiatus. The anterior trunk gives off a gastric branch that runs along the lesser curvature and supplies the anterior surface of the stomach down to the pylorus. Pyloric branches innervate the antrum, pylorus, and proximal duodenum. The posterior vagal trunk provides a similar gastric branch that supplies the posterior surface of the stomach. The preganglionic fibers synapse in intramural ganglionated plexuses. Postganglionic fibers may be final motor neurons or interneurons communicating with the enteric nervous system. Parasympathetic stimulation generally causes an increase in secretory and motor activity. Gastric sympathetic efferents emerge from spinal cord segments T5 through T9. These preganglionic fibers run along the greater splanchnic nerve and synapse in the celiac ganglion. Postganglionic axons extend to the stomach and enter it in association with blood vessels. These sympathetic fibers provide rich innervation to gastric blood vessels and the myenteric and submucous plexuses. In general, sympathetic stimulation causes a counterbalancing inhibition of gastric secretory and motor activity as well as constriction of blood vessels.

Afferent sensory neurons are exemplified by mucosal chemoreceptors and myenteric mechanoreceptors. These receptors communicate with both the central nervous system (CNS) and the enteric nervous system. Afferent nerve processes account for approximately 80% of vagal fibers and 20% of the greater splanchnic nerve's fibers.[37,38] The incoming information carried by these nerves is processed in central sensory nuclei and initiates neurally mediated gastric reflexes. Sensory neurons in enteric ganglia also initiate local reflexes such as gastric peristalsis. Cross talk between central and enteric fibers occurs continually in the enteric plexus as it modulates the effects of motor neurons.

Vasculature

Gastric mucosal blood flow maintains epithelial integrity and is an essential component of mucosal defense. The stomach receives its blood supply from the celiac axis by way of six major arteries. The right and left gastric arteries supply the lesser curvature and extend over the anterior and posterior surfaces of the stomach. In a similar fashion, the left and right gastroepiploic arteries supply the greater curvature. Short gastric arteries from the splenic artery perfuse the upper stomach, while the gastroduodenal artery serves the pyloroantral region. These arteries provide large arterioles that pierce the gastric muscle wall. The microvasculature of the stomach is illustrated in Figure 13-2. The entering arterioles provide smaller arterioles that extend to the submucosal plexus as well as to the muscle layers.[39] A capillary layer is present in the muscle and drains into the venous collecting system. The afferent arterioles supplying the submucosal plexus are innervated by sympathetic fibers coursing with the entering blood vessels. The submucosal arteriolar plexus does not communicate with the venous plexus directly but rather provides mucosal arterioles to the base of the gastric glands. The mucosal arterioles branch into capillaries that ascend perpendicularly between the glands to the epithelial surface. These ascending capillaries interconnect hori-

zontally so that they form a latticework around the gastric glands. Ascending capillaries receive bicarbonate secreted from the basolateral surface of stimulated parietal cells and carry it to the surface epithelium. This phenomenon has been termed the "alkaline tide." At the surface epithelium, the bicarbonate can assist in buffering any H^+ ion back-diffusion. At the mucosal surface, the fenestrated capillaries[40] empty into venules that drain into the submucosal venous plexus and efferent veins that follow the course of the primary arterial branches. This anatomic arrangement allows muscle layer blood flow to be in parallel with mucosal flow while submucosal flow is in series with the mucosa. Such a microvascular system would allow selective decreases in mucosal blood flow while muscular blood flow is maintained.

Mucosal blood flow has been shown to account for 70% to 80% of total gastric blood flow in both basal and stimulated states.[41,42] Previous studies using aminopyrine clearance techniques suggest that stimulation of acid secretion increases mucosal blood flow. However, interpretation of these results must be tempered by the knowledge that acid secretion affects aminopyrine clearance and may account for the apparent increase in mucosal blood flow.[43] Acid secretagogues appear to have no effect on mucosal blood flow with the use of recently developed indicator-dilution techniques. When gastric perfusion pressures are adequate, gastric acid secretion varies independently of blood flow.[44] These conclusions have challenged the long-held hypothesis[45] that secretagogue stimulation induces a parallel increase in acid secretion and mucosal blood flow.

The innervation of the gastric microvasculature reveals, in part, the mechanisms regulating mucosal blood flow. It appears that the submucosal arterioles are innervated by sympathetic nerve fibers.[46] When stimulated, these fibers constrict the arterioles and decrease mucosal blood flow temporarily.[47,48] After 3 to 4 minutes of prolonged sympathetic stimulation, flow increases.[49] This response has been described as "autoregulatory escape" from adrenergic vasoconstrictor influence.[50] Anatomic details[46] support these physiologic findings and suggest a regulatory function at the level of the submucosal arterioles.

REGULATION OF ACID SECRETION— IN VIVO STUDIES

The regulation of acid secretion can be subdivided into the supracellular influences that have been the focus of classical physiology since Beaumont and the cellular mechanisms that have been understood particularly in the last 10 years. This section will concentrate on supracellular influences and review in vivo studies of acid secretion.

Integrated Control Pathways

The integrated mechanisms that control acid secretion can be viewed as an arrangement of regulatory strata. These include neural control in two forms: long reflex or cephalovagal arcs and local intragastric reflex arcs. A second tier of control is exerted by humoral substances whether acting in an endocrine fashion such as gastrin or in a paracrine one such as histamine. Somatostatin may

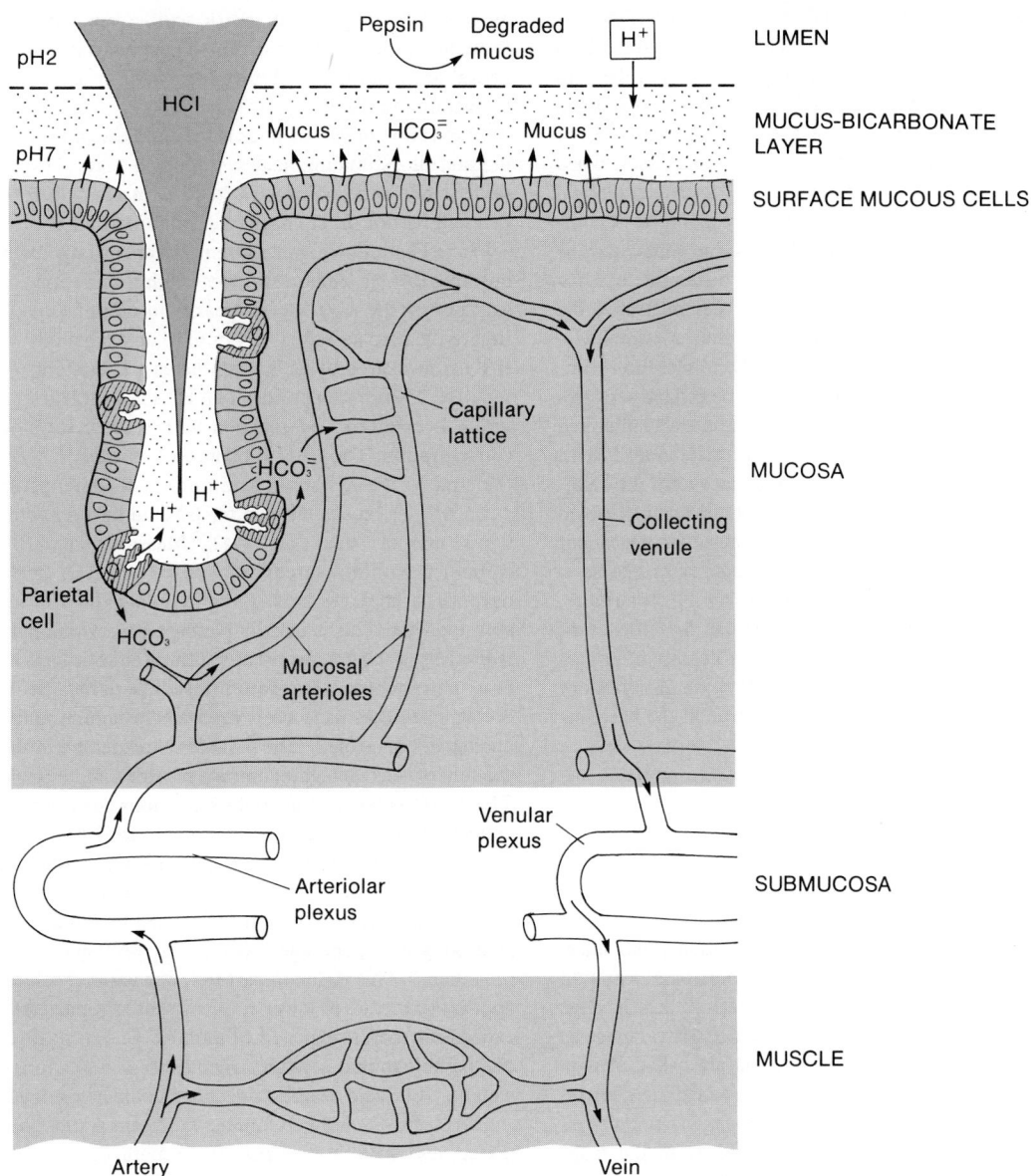

FIGURE 13–2. Gastric microvasculature. (Adapted from Guth PH, Leung FW. Physiology of the gastric circulation. In: Johnson LR, ed. Physiology of the gastrointestinal tract. 2nd ed. New York: Raven Press, 1987:1031; Koelz HR, Fimmel CJ, Garner A, et al. The stomach and duodenum. In Kern F, Blum AL, eds. The gastroenterology annual/3. New York: Elsevier, 1986:28.)

function as both an endocrine and a paracrine factor. The role of many such peptides remains uncertain. A further tier of regulation is the direct influence of chemical factors. This is typified by the action of amino acids and amines in stimulating gastrin release and by the effect of gastric acid in inhibiting gastrin release.

It will be apparent immediately that these strata are not distinct but closely intertwined—so intertwined that when discussing the phases of postprandial acid secretion, Grossman asserted that the individual contributions made by the various phases could not be distinguished.[51] Nevertheless, classical physiology has attempted to isolate and study various factors that influence acid secretion. From these studies it can be summarized that there are three prin-

cipal stimuli of acid secretion by the parietal cell, namely, histamine, acetylcholine, and gastrin. The principal inhibitory secretagogue appears to be somatostatin, although other chemical modulators, including peptides and prostaglandins, may also have a role.

When reviewing these in vivo studies, the following confounding facts should not be forgotten. (1) Acute responses should be distinguished from chronic adaptive changes. For example, the effect on gastrin and somatostatin cell number during acute achlorhydria differs from the changes seen in chronic achlorhydria.[52] By analogy, data in studies using vagotomy may signify the chronic adaptive response to achlorhydria rather than the effect of withdrawal of vagal innervation alone. (2) Acid secretagogues potentiate the response to one another. This central point, which is crucial to the understanding of studies of supracellular and cellular regulation, was first appreciated by Grossman. He defined a potentiated response as one in which the effect of two agents in combination is greater than the sum of their separate effects when administered alone. He demonstrated in dogs with Heidenhain pouches (see below) that the acid secretory response to a combination of Urecholine and gastrin and Urecholine and histamine greatly exceeded maximal response to gastrin, histamine, or Urecholine alone (Fig 13-3).[13] He subsequently demonstrated the corollary effect using antagonists of acid secretion. Metiamide, a histamine2 (H_2) receptor antagonist, inhibited acid secretion stimulated by histamine, pentagastrin, 2-deoxyglucose (which activates central vagal stimulation), and food. Atropine sulfate also inhibited the response to all of these stimulants except histamine.[53] With great perception, he deduced that there were receptors for histamine, gastrin, and acetylcholine on the parietal cell that interacted with one another. It is because of these interactions that one cannot predict the relative importance of each secretagogue on the basis of individual stimulation/inhibition studies in vivo. Furthermore, the phenomenon of potentiation is the basis for the efficacy of many of the acid-reducing therapies for peptic ulceration, in particular the use of H_2 antagonists. (3) Stimulatory and inhibitory influences are active simultaneously. This is true in the basal interprandial and the postprandial state.

Methods for Measurement of Acid Secretion

Animal studies in vivo have used dogs, rats, rabbits, and mice. There are great species differences, however, in both basal secretion and responsiveness to secretagogues.[54] Classical studies in dogs have used vascularly perfused isolated pouches of gastric mucosa. Fundic pouches with intact vagal innervation are called Pavlov pouches, and vagotomized fundic pouches are called Heidenhain pouches. It is assumed that secretion from a vagally innervated fundic pouch is an accurate index of secretion from the main stomach.[51] These gastric pouches have been used to define many

aspects of the regulation of gastric acid secretion, including cephalic influences, the role of gastrin, long cephalovagal and local reflex neural arcs, and the inhibitory feedback control of acid secretion by intraluminal acid.

Aspiration of gastric juice is the simplest and most widely used method of estimating acid secretion in man. To perform these tests, a fine-bore nasogastric tube is inserted into the most dependent part of the stomach under fluoroscopic control in a fasted subject. The following measurements are usually made: basal acid output (BAO), which estimates resting secretion, and maximal acid output (MAO) and/or peak acid output (PAO), which estimate the acid secretory response to an exogenous secretagogue. BAO is measured by aspirating the gastric contents for four consecutive 15-minute periods. The H^+ ion concentration of the aspirate is estimated by titration with a basic solution of known concentration. The BAO is expressed as mEq H^+ per hour and is the sum of the measured acid output in four unstimulated test periods. The expected range for BAO in healthy adult subjects is 0 to 11 mEq H^+/hour (Fig 13-4).[55] Measurement of BAO is usually combined with measurement of MAO or PAO. In this test, acid output is stimulated by a supraphysiologic dose of an exogenous secretagogue. This is usually pentagastrin, which may be administered by a subcutaneous or intramuscular injection (6 μg/kg) or by continuous intravenous infusion (6 μg/kg/hour). Other secretagogues that have been used are histamine and a histamine analogue—betazole.[17] The PAO is calculated by multiplying by 2 the sum of the two highest outputs recorded in the four test periods. The MAO is the sum acid output of four consecutive 15-minute collection periods. The expected range for PAO in healthy adult subjects is 10 to 63 mEq/hour (Fig 13-4).[55] MAO and PAO are a reflection of the total number of parietal cells, the so-called parietal cell mass,[56] which is influenced by gender, body weight, lean body mass, and age.[57] MAO and PAO are lower in women than men.[58] This is due in part to lower parietal cell mass but also appears to be due to lower sensitivity of that parietal cell mass to exogenous secretagogues.[58] Stimulated acid output in children is comparable to that in adults when expressed as a function of body weight,[59] but acid secretion declines in elderly subjects.[60]

BAO, MAO, and PAO under-represent actual basal and stimulated acid secretion because these methods do not account for acid lost through the pylorus, acid neutralization by gastric bi-

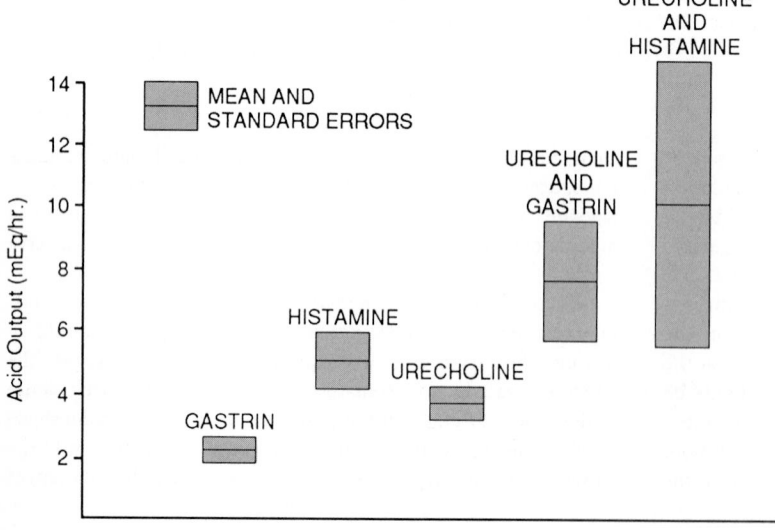

FIGURE 13–3. Maximal acid responses to gastrin extract, histamine, and Urecholine, alone and in combination in dogs with Heidenhain pouches. (From Gillespie IE, Grossman MI. Potentiation between Urecholine and gastrin extract and between Urecholine and histamine in the stimulations of Heidenhain pouches. Gut 1964;5:71.)

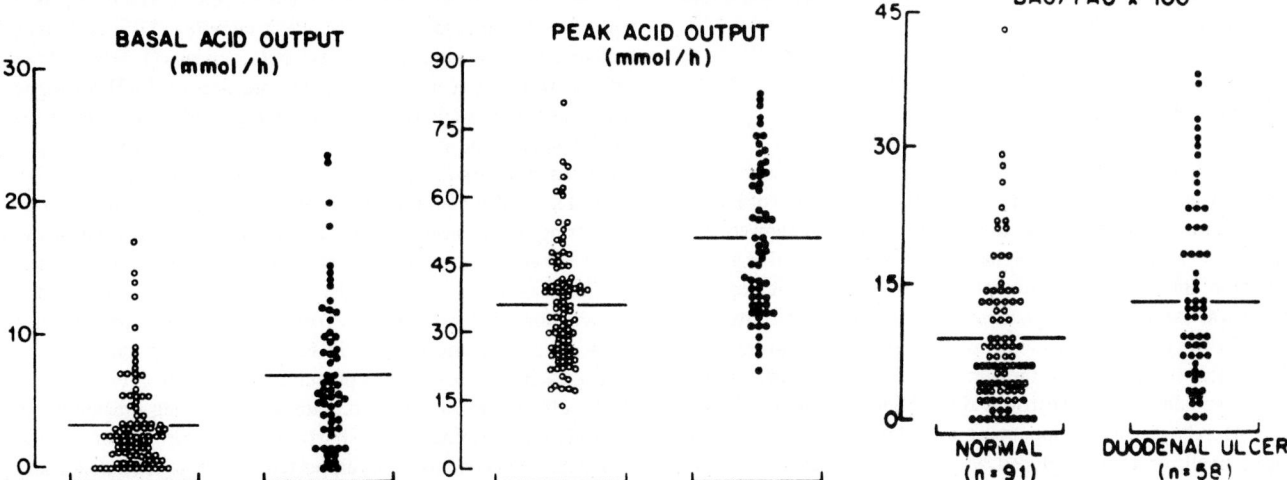

FIGURE 13–4. Basal acid output (*BAO*), peak acid output (*PAO*), and *BAO/PAO* ratio in 91 normal adult subjects (From Blair JA, Feldman M, Barnett C, Walsh JH, Richardson CT. Detailed comparison of basal and food-stimulated gastric acid secretion rates and serum gastrin concentrations in duodenal ulcer patients and normal subjects. J Clin Invest 1987;79: 582.)

carbonate and refluxed duodenal juice, and acid losses due to back-diffusion of H^+ through the gastric mucosa. Nonetheless, these measurements have proved useful in defining the pathophysiology of peptic ulcer disease[55] and have proved useful clinically in the diagnosis of Zollinger–Ellison syndrome.

Another method of estimating acid secretory ability was introduced by Fordtran and Walsh, using continuous in vivo intragastric titration.[61] By this means, the acid secretory response to the physiologic stimulation of ingested food is estimated. Continuous intragastric titration requires placement of a double-lumen tube into the most dependent part of the stomach, usually under fluoroscopic visualization. One lumen allows frequent sampling of small volumes (2–3 ml) of gastric contents. The pH of the sample is immediately measured and the gastric juice returned to the stomach. The port of the second tube is positioned 10 cm proximal to the sampling port and is used to infuse $NaHCO_3$. Throughout the study, gastric pH is maintained at an arbitrary value, usually 5.5, by infusion of $NaHCO_3$. A homogenized meal buffered to pH 5.5 is eaten. The amount of $NaHCO_3$ necessary to maintain the pH of the gastric juice at 5.5 is a measure of the postprandial acid secretory response. Because this is a cumbersome procedure, it has not gained widespread use outside specific research investigations. However, continuous intragastric titration has proved to be a useful method of measuring postprandial acid secretory responses.[62,63]

A different approach to studying continuous acid responses is to measure intragastric pH by use of an indwelling probe[64] or radiotelemetric capsule.[65] This does not estimate total H^+ concentration, because volume of gastric juice and buffering capacity are not accounted for. Further studies with these techniques will be required before their specific utility in man can be determined.

Basal or Interprandial Acid Secretion

Basal unstimulated acid secretion exhibits a circadian variation with greatest secretion at night and lowest in early morning.[66] This variation is not matched by changes in circulating serum gastrin

levels. It appears that vagal innervation is one of the principal regulatory factors controlling basal acid output. In man, vagotomy greatly reduces or abolishes interprandial acid secretion in patients with duodenal ulcer.[56,63,67] The caveats expressed above regarding the influence of potentiation, and chronic adaptive changes on studies of the effect of vagotomy on gastric endocrine and exocrine responses, are pertinent when interpreting these data, although vagotomy does not affect parietal cell number.[68] Thus, it is notable that twice-daily H_2 antagonist administration in duodenal ulcer patients reduces interprandial acid secretion, although it does not abolish it.[63] This suggests that H_2 receptor activation is also capable of influencing basal acid output. Because a dose–response study of the effect of H_2 antagonists on basal gastric acid secretion has not been performed, it is uncertain whether higher doses of H_2 antagonists would have a greater effect.[63] Nonetheless, it appears likely that basal interprandial acid secretion is due to a combination of cholinergic and histaminergic stimulation.

The cholinergic regulation of basal gastric acid secretion is complex. In dogs with gastric pouches, denervation of the antral pouch markedly reduces resting output of acid from both the main innervated stomach and the denervated fundic pouch but without changing plasma gastrin levels.[69] This suggests that there is a local interneuronal reflex arc innervated by the vagus and independent of plasma gastrin that carries acid-stimulatory signals from the antrum to the fundus. These data are mirrored in man, where the albeit small amount of basal acid secretion found in some vagotomized patients can be abolished by antrectomy plus vagotomy.[67]

Stimulated Acid Secretion

The physiologic stimulus for acid secretion is food. Traditionally, food-stimulated acid response has been described in three phases, namely, cephalic, gastric, and intestinal. These phases refer to site of origin of stimuli and do not imply mechanisms by which acid secretion is stimulated or inhibited. These phases occur concurrently and not consecutively. The acid secretory response at any instant represents the sum of all the stimulatory and inhibitory influences.

CEPHALIC PHASE

The recognition that the nervous system influences gastric acid secretion dates back to William Beaumont and the studies of Pavlov discussed in the historical section. In 1928, Farrell showed that the vagus was the sole gastrocephalic neural link involved in gastric secretion, and this observation still holds today.[70] The cephalic phase was estimated by Richardson and colleagues to contribute up to 50% of total postprandial acid.[71] These workers have studied the relative contribution of thought, sight, smell, and taste of food to the cephalic phase of gastric acid secretion in humans (Fig 13-5).[72] Merely discussing appetizing food for 30 minutes without sight, smell, or taste produced an average of 66% of the total cephalic response as estimated by the time-honored method of modified sham feeding. Serum gastrin levels were significantly increased also. Sight of food and smell of food alone, while still producing significant acid secretion and gastrin release, were considerably less potent stimuli than conversation. These data show by subtraction that taste is an important component of the cephalic phase also.

The mechanisms by which the senses stimulate acid secretion are less certain. As stated above, Bechterew induced acid secretion in dogs by electrically stimulating the frontal cortex. This effect was lost in vagotomized animals.[6] More recently, two forms of study have been used: electrical stimulation of various sites in the brain and injection of putative neuromodulatory substances into the brain. The putative ligands include (1) peptides, (2) classical neurotransmitters such as acetylcholine, GABA-ergic agonists, and catecholamines, and (3) prostaglandins. This subject has been reviewed by Tache.[73] A good example to consider is the tripeptide thyrotropin-releasing hormone (TRH). Stereotactic microinjection of TRH or a TRH analogue into specific sites of the medulla produced consistent stimulation of gastric acid secretion in rats.[74] Sensitive sites included the dorsal vagal complex (DVC), nucleus tractus solitarius (NTS), and dorsal motor nucleus (DMN). These effects were not seen following the injection of TRH analogue into other sites, such as the lateral, dorsal, and parvocellular reticular nuclei, the medial longitudinal fascicle, and the nucleus cuneatus, nor with injections of metabolites of TRH into sensitive sites. The DMN contains over 90% of the preganglionic neurons projecting to the stomach forming the descending branch of the vagus[75,76] and is intimately linked to a specific area overlying the NTS.[75] Vagotomy abolishes the acid secretory response to microinjection of TRH into the DVC.[74] Autoradiographic studies show a high concentration of TRH binding sites in the DVC.[77,78] Thus, Tache and co-workers postulate that release of endogenous TRH into the dorsal vagal complex activates long preganglionic neurons that terminate near short postganglionic neurons in the stomach. This conclusion is supported by previous studies using intracisternal or intracerebroventricular injections of TRH or TRH analogue, which showed that stimulation of acid secretion by these maneuvers depended on activation of parasympathetic outflow to the stomach and cholinergic pathways[79,80] and was independent of alterations in thyrotropin, gastrin, or catecholamine release.[79-81] Persuasive though these observations are, it is important to note that they have yet to be linked to any of the physiologic phenomena that we identify as the cephalic phase of gastric acid secretion. This should be said for all studies of intracerebral electrode stimulation or ligand injection.

There are many interrelated mechanisms by which cephalic-vagal input mediates the cephalic phase of stimulated acid secretion. Vagal innervation has a direct action on parietal cells. This was deduced from studies in dogs with antral and fundic gastric pouches. Denervation of the antral pouch reduced or abolished the serum gastrin response to sham feeding but did not abolish acid secretion by the vagally innervated fundic pouch.[69] Corroborative evidence for this mechanism is afforded by the demonstration of acetylcholine receptors on isolated canine parietal cells.

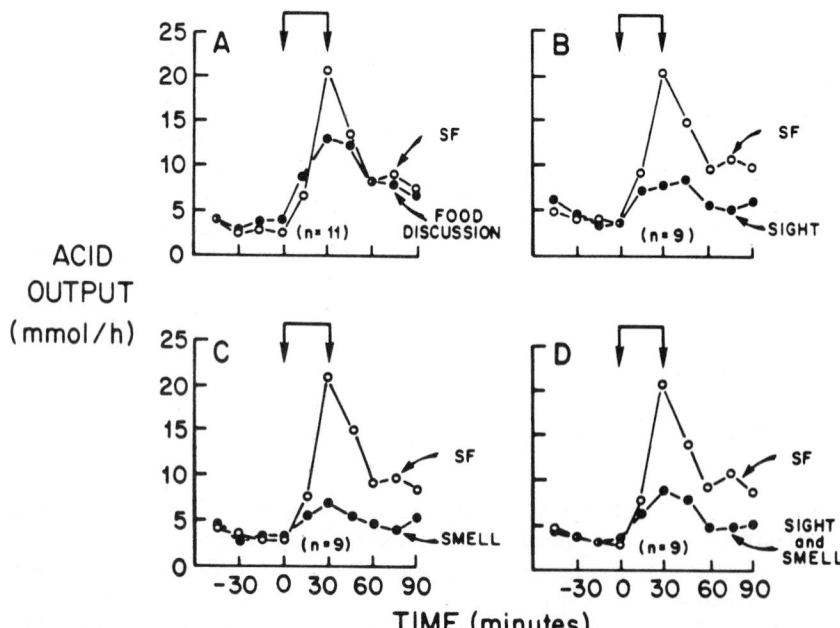

FIGURE 13–5. Mean gastric output in the same human subjects in response to sham feeding (SF), when compared with discussion of favorite foods (**A**), sight of appetizing food (**B**), smell of appetizing food (**C**), and a combination of sight and smell (**D**). (From Feldman M, Richardson CT. Role of thought, sight, smell, and taste of food in the cephalic phase of gastric acid secretion in humans. Gastroenterology 1986;90:428.)

A second pathway in the cephalic phase of gastric acid secretion is through release of circulating gastrin from the gastric antrum. The thought, sight, and smell of food and modified sham feeding increase serum gastrin levels.[72] Furthermore, isolated canine gastrin cells possess acetylcholine receptors. The plasma gastrin response to sham feeding in man is regulated by intragastric pH and is not observable when gastric pH is maintained at 2.5.[82] This effect is also atropine-sensitive. However, vagal control of postprandial gastrin release is complex. Low doses of atropine, a muscarinic antagonist, enhance rather than reduce the gastrin response to sham feeding[83,84] insulin-induced hypoglycemia,[85] or feeding.[86,87] Similarly, parietal cell vagotomy, while markedly reducing acid secretion, enhances gastrin release in response to sham feeding,[83,88] insulin-induced hypoglycemia,[89] or intragastric nutrient infusion. These effects are independent of changes in intragastric pH.[83,85] This suggests that the vagus carries cholinergic fibers that, in the absence of atropine, mediate either directly or indirectly an inhibitory control of gastrin release. Furthermore, studies in dogs with Heidenhain pouches and gastric fistulae demonstrate that truncal vagal denervation reduces gastrin release but elevates acid secretion by the pouch.[90] These data can be interpreted to suggest cholinergic release of a substance that can inhibit acid secretion independently of its effects on gastrin release. Although the nature of this substance has yet to be elucidated, somatostatin is one candidate.[87] However, Feldman and colleagues were unable to demonstrate a plasma somatostatin rise in human subjects during sham feeding[84]; thus, the role of somatostatin in regulating the cephalic–vagal control of gastric acid secretion, whether directly on the parietal cell or by inhibition of gastrin release, remains uncertain.

GASTRIC PHASE

When food enters the stomach, it initiates the gastric phase of acid secretion. This is usually divided into two components: a physical component due to distention of the stomach and a chemical component in which chemical effectors interact with gastric cells.

The acid secretory response to distention results from presumed stretch receptors in the gastric tissue. This response is the stereotypical long vasovagal reflex arc. Distention of the gastric fundus and corpus in man stimulates acid secretion. The effect is almost abolished by proximal gastric vagotomy and, at least in part, is independent of changes in serum gastrin levels.[91–93] Distention-induced acid secretion is a complex phenomenon in which antral and fundic responses can be viewed separately. Antral distention produces gastrin release in dogs[94] and man.[95] Debas called this the pyloro-oxyntic reflex. In dogs with antral and fundic pouches, this response was inhibited by antral acidification,[94] whereas in man, albeit with an intact stomach, it appeared to be independent of luminal pH.[95] In dogs, the pH sensitivity of the antral distention response required an intact cerebrovagal link to the antrum. In man, low-dose atropine, which inhibited the acid secretory response to antral distention, nonetheless enhanced the elevation of serum gastrin levels. This suggests that there is an atropine-sensitive inhibitory pathway restraining the gastrin response to antral distention. Fundic distention in dogs with vagally-innervated fundic pouches and vagally-innervated antral pouches produces gastrin release and acid secretion.[96] Both responses are lost when the antral pouch is maintained at pH 2.5. In contrast to the pyloro-oxyntic

reflex described above, this vasovagal reflex has been termed the oxyntopyloric reflex. There is a similar vagally-dependent acid stimulatory response to fundic distention in man.[91] However, it appears not to be mediated through elevated serum gastrin.

The roles of histamine and acetylcholine in mediating distention-induced acid secretion are unclear. As might be predicted from our knowledge of the potentiative interrelationship of the three principal secretagogues (gastrin, acetylcholine, and histamine [see above]), the acid response to gastric distention in man is abolished by vagotomy[97] or cimetidine.[98] However, this may indicate the facilitative effect of background secretion of these secretagogues only. Gastric release of either acetylcholine or histamine in response to distention has not been shown.

Food interacts with the gastric mucosa to cause acid secretion in a manner that is independent of stretch by the food bolus. There are at least four constituents of food that produce this stimulatory effect: peptic digests of proteins, ethanol, coffee, and calcium. Whole proteins are poor stimuli of gastric acid secretion, while peptic digests of the same proteins are effective.[99] The breakdown products of protein, amino acids, and amines produce acid secretion principally through the release of gastrin.[31,100,101] The aromatic amino acids phenylalanine and tryptophan are the most potent stimuli of gastric acid secretion and gastrin release in vivo.[102] Their amine derivatives may contribute significantly to this response.[31,100] Circulating gastrin is the principal mediator of postprandial gastric acid secretion. This has been demonstrated by studies in man in which the increment in plasma gastrin that occurred following an intragastric infusion of amino acids or ingestion of a protein-rich meal was reproduced with an intravenous infusion of gastrin, and a similar acid-secretory response to both endogenous and exogenous gastrin was observed.[62,101] Furthermore, these studies suggest that notwithstanding the cephalovagal component to gastrin release, it is the chemical response to protein breakdown products that is the principal stimulus for postprandial gastrin.[101]

While amines and amino acids can cause gastrin release by direct action on the G cell,[31,102] this phenomenon must be viewed within the larger orchestrated physiologic response to ingested nutrients. Nutrients stimulate the release of many peptides into circulation, including somatostatin, cholecystokinin (CCK), secretin, gastric inhibitory polypeptide (GIP), enteroglucagon, and peptide YY(PYY), which may influence acid secretion either directly or by affecting gastrin release. A summary of these actions is provided in Table 13-1. Based on studies in isolated rat stomachs, Makhlouf and co-workers have proposed that, within the gastric mucosa, gastrin release is controlled by a counterbalance of cholinergic and noncholinergic interneurons. In this model, cholinergic agonists stimulate gastrin indirectly by inhibiting somatostatin release and thus withdrawing the somatostatin-mediated restraint of gastrin release.[103] This pathway may also utilize a GABA-ergic interneuron.[104] In this model, noncholinergic stimulation activates gastrin release through neurocrine release of gastrin-releasing peptide (GRP). In support of this theory, Sugano and colleagues demonstrated a direct stimulatory response to both GRP and cholinergic agonists in isolated canine gastrin cells, implying the presence of receptors for each ligand on gastrin cells.[105]

Integrating this model with data derived from whole animal physiology has proved difficult. As described in the section on the cephalic phase of acid secretion, atropine enhances gastrin release in many circumstances, when, according to the in vitro model

TABLE 13–1
Peptides That Influence Gastric Acid Secretion

PEPTIDE	ACTION ON ACID SECRETION	TISSUE LOCALIZATION	ROUTE OF DELIVERY	SITE(S) OF ACTION	ACTIONS ON OTHER PEPTIDES	COMMENTS	REFERENCES
Definite							
Gastrin	Stimulatory	G cells—gastric antrum, duodenum	Endocrine	Direct on parietal cells, D cells	Stimulates SRIF release	Principal stimulatory hormone in postprandial acid response. Hypersecretion in Zollinger–Ellison syndrome	14, 62, 298
Somatostatin (SRIF)	Inhibitory	D cells—stomach, small bowel, pancreas, enteric neurons	Paracrine, probably endocrine, neurocrine, autocrine	Direct on parietal cells, G cells, D cells	Inhibits release of most gut peptides, including gastrin and insulin	Principal humoral restraint on gastric acid secretion both directly and through local inhibition of gastrin. Candidate-enterogastrone	12, 16, 133, 299
Gastrin-releasing peptide (bombesin)	Stimulatory	Gastric mucosal interneurons	Neurocrine	Direct action on G cells	Stimulates gastrin release and SRIF from isolated stomach	Unlikely to be a principal factor in postprandial gastrin release—may be significant interneuronal transmitter in cephalic phase	105, 174, 300
Probable							
Cholecystokinin (CCK)	Weak stimulant of basal secretion. Inhibitor of stimulated secretion	CCK cells in duodenum and jejunum	Uncertain ? endocrine	Direct action on parietal and D cells	Potent stimulus of SRIF release in vitro	No established physiologic role in gastric acid secretion. Candidate-enterogastrone	172, 300
Secretin	Uncertain. Inhibits acid secretion in some studies	In secretin(s) cells of small intestine, greatest abundance in duodenum	Uncertain ? endocrine	D cell. Secretin has no direct effects on parietal cells	Inhibits food-stimulated gastrin release. Causes paradoxical increase in serum gastrin in ZES. Stimulates SRIF release	No established physiologic role in gastric acid secretion. Candidate-enterogastrone	139, 140, 300, 301
Enteroglucagon (oxyntomodulin), glucagon, glicentin	Inhibitory	Stomach, small intestine, pancreas	Uncertain	D cell	Uncertain	Multiple products of glucagon gene can inhibit acid secretion in vitro. No established physiologic role. Candidate-enterogastrone	305–309

Agent	Effect on acid secretion	Source	Mode	Direct effect	Effect on gastrin release	Comments	References
Gastric inhibitory polypeptide (GIP)	Uncertain. Inhibits acid secretion in some studies	In K cells of small intestine, small quantities in gastric antrum	Uncertain ? endocrine	D cell: GIP has no direct effect on parietal or G cells	May inhibit gastrin release by stimulating SRIF release	Inhibits gastrin release by stimulating SRIF release. Candidate-enterogastrone. Physiologic role as glucose-dependent insulinotropic peptide	136, 302–304
Neurotensin	Inhibitory	N cell in ileal mucosa. Lesser amounts in proximal small bowel, stomach, colon. Neurotensin neurons in stomach	Presumed endocrine	Uncertain	Does not affect gastrin release	No established physiologic role in gastric acid secretion. Candidate-enterogastrone	133, 136, 300
Peptide YY (PYY)	Inhibitory	Endocrine cells of distal small intestine and colon	Presumed to be endocrine	Uncertain	Did not affect meal-stimulated gastrin in dogs	No established physiologic role in gastric acid secretion. Candidate-enterogastrone	137, 315, 316
Proposed							
Enterooxyntin	Stimulatory	Small intestinal mucosa	Endocrine	Uncertain	Uncertain	As yet poorly characterized entity	119–122
Enterogastrone	Inhibitory	Small intestine	Endocrine	Uncertain	Uncertain	Poorly characterized. Many candidates (see text)	
Gastrotropin (porcine ileal peptide)	Uncertain. Stimulatory in some studies	Nonendocrine cells of distal small bowel	Presumed by way of circulation	Uncertain. No direct effect on isolated canine parietal cells	Uncertain	No established physiologic role in gastric acid secretion. Candidate-enterooxyntin	119–122
Epidermal growth factor (EGF)	Inhibitory	Submandibular glands, Brunner's glands	Uncertain. May be luminal, endocrine, or paracrine	Presumed to be direct parietal	Did not affect insulin-stimulated gastrin release	No established physiologic role in gastric acid secretion. This applies also to other members of the EGF peptide family, such as TGF-α.	268, 317–319
Galanin	Inhibitory	Neurons	Neurocrine	Uncertain	Inhibits postprandial SRIF, neurotensin, and enteroglucagon but not gastrin	Physiologic significance unknown	321, 322
Calcitonin	Inhibitory	C cell of thyroid	Endocrine	Uncertain	Uncertain. Stimulates release of SRIF in some studies, not in others. No effect on postprandial serum gastrin	No established physiologic role in gastric acid secretion	310–312

(continued)

TABLE 13–1 (Continued)
Peptides That Influence Gastric Acid Secretion

PEPTIDE	ACTION ON ACID SECRETION	TISSUE LOCALIZATION	ROUTE OF DELIVERY	SITE(S) OF ACTION	ACTIONS ON OTHER PEPTIDES	COMMENTS	REFERENCES
Calcitonin gene-related peptides (CGRP) I and II	Inhibitory	Enteric neurons	Neurocrine	D-cell. CGRP has no direct effect on gastric parietal cells	Stimulates SRIF release in some studies. Did not affect meal-stimulated gastrin in dogs	No established physiologic role in gastric acid secretion; CGRP I and II have distinct effects in man	310, 311, 313, 314
Corticotropin-releasing factor (CRF)	Inhibitory	Neurons in gastrointestinal tract	Neurocrine	No direct effect on parietal cell	No effect on release of gastrin or SRIF	No established physiologic role in gastric acid secretion	320
Methionine–enkephalin (metenkephalin)	Stimulatory	Neuronal and endocrine cells throughout the gastrointestinal tract	Neurocrine	D-cells. ? direct effect on parietal cell	Does not stimulate gastrin release	No established physiologic role in gastric acid secretion	323, 324
Pancreastatin	Uncertain. Inhibits acid secretion in vitro	Gastric and duodenal mucosa	Uncertain ? endocrine ? paracrine	Uncertain ? direct on parietal cell	Inhibits SRIF release in some studies	Further studies necessary to determine if a physiologic role in gastric acid secretion exists	325, 326

described above, one would expect inhibition or no change. Furthermore, agents that block gastrin response to bombesin do not affect the gastrin response to food. Studies in man suggest also that β-adrenergic innervation may play a role in gastric acid secretion. Administration of terbutaline, a β₂ adrenoceptor agonist, enhances serum gastrin but inhibits acid secretion in response to intragastric infusion of a homogenized meal.[106] Thus, while it is likely that numerous neurohumoral mediators such as somatostatin, GRP, and cholinergic and adrenergic innervation are significant factors in postprandial gastrin release, we are not yet able to define their relative roles in the integrated physiology of gastrin release.

Studies in man have demonstrated either a modest acid stimulatory response[107,108] or no response[109] to direct intragastric infusions of pure alcohol. On the other hand, wine[107–109] and beer[107] are potent stimuli of acid secretion and serum gastrin. These effects are probably due to amines or amino acids in the beverage stimulating gastrin release and are not direct effects of the beverage's alcohol content.

Caffeine alone stimulates acid release in humans.[110] McArthur and colleagues showed that many household beverages were potent acid stimuli, including Tab, coffee, beer, and milk, each of which causes greater than 70% of pentagastrin-stimulated MAO.[111] Decaffeinated coffee was a potent stimulus also, showing that it is not only caffeine in coffee that is an acid stimulant. Unfortunately, these studies did not attempt to control for the cephalic phase of acid secretion, nor was gastrin measured. Consequently, one cannot draw conclusions as to the mechanisms that underlie these observations.

Oral ingestion of calcium carbonate stimulates gastrin release and acid secretion in humans.[112] This action is independent of acid-buffering capacity and is presumed to be an effect of dissociated calcium ions.

INTESTINAL PHASE

The entry of chyme into the small intestine initiates the intestinal phase of the acid secretory process. The primary stimulatory factors are distention[113,114] and proteins and their products of digestion.[113,114] Quantitating the significance of the intestinal phase to the stimulatory limb of acid secretion has proved controversial, perhaps because there are definite potentiation phenomena between the acid secretory response to intestinal nutrients and either gastrin or histamine.[115] Serum gastrin levels do not appear to mediate the intestinal phase of acid secretion in dogs[114] or man.[116] The acid stimulatory response to intestinal nutrients is preserved in vagotomized animals, indicating that, at least to some degree, circulating stimuli are involved.[117] This role may be filled in part by circulating amino acids, which have been shown to stimulate acid secretion without elevating serum gastrin.[118] In addition, there have been a number of attempts to isolate a distinct acid stimulatory peptide hormone—entero-oxyntin—from small bowel mucosa.[119,120] In one case (gastrotropin or porcine ileal peptide), this presumed moiety has been characterized[121] and cloned.[122] Unfortunately, this substance does not appear to be a true hormone because it lacks the signal peptide sequence characteristic of secreted peptide hormones, and, furthermore, the initially described stimulatory effect of this substance on acid secretion in vivo or in vitro could not be reproduced under more carefully controlled circumstances.[122]

Inhibition of Acid Secretion

CEPHALIC

One line of evidence that suggests that there may be cephalic inhibitory influence acting on gastric acid secretion comes from intracerebral microinjection studies. For example, inhibition of pentagastrin and meal-stimulated gastric acid secretion in the dog has been demonstrated by intracerebroventricular injection of calcitonin (CT), calcitonin gene-related peptide (CGRP), neurotensin (NT), β-endorphin, bombesin, and corticotropin-releasing factor (CRF).[123] There was no change in plasma gastrin, CT, CGRP, or CRF during these experiments. CGRP and bombesin, but not CT, NT, β-endorphin, or CRF, appeared to act independently of vagal integrity. Thus, it appears that vagal fibers carry inhibitory as well as stimulatory messages to the parietal cells. However, as with the cerebral microinjection studies in which gastric acid is stimulated, there are no data to indicate which, if any, of these observations are relevant to the cephalic phase of gastric acid secretion. In addition, the complex response of stimulated serum gastrin levels to low-dose atropine, described in detail in the section on cephalic stimulation of acid secretion, suggests that there are vagal inhibitory influences on gastrin release also.

GASTRIC

Just as vagal inhibitory fibers have been implicated in the cephalic acid secretory response, there appear to be vagally mediated inhibitory neural arcs involved in the acid secretory response to distention. Studies in dogs and man have led Debas and co-workers to conclude that antral distention, in addition to stimulating serum gastrin release, also results in release of an inhibitor of acid secretion.[94,124,125] Whether this effect is humoral or neurocrine is not clear, but it is dependent on an intact vagus.

Gastrin release in response to nutrients, sham feeding, and antral distention is inhibited by the presence of acid in the gastric antrum.[82,94,126] An intraluminal pH of 3 appears to be the threshold for initiating this response.[126] The mechanisms of this negative feedback loop are not certain but probably include release of somatostatin as a paracrine or endocrine inhibitor of gastrin.[127] There is evidence that gastric acid regulates both somatostatin release locally in the stomach in vitro[128] and postprandial circulating somatostatin in vivo.[129] An alternative mechanism for the inhibition of gastrin release at low intraluminal pH is that an acidic milieu causes amines to be protonated, and thus, as charged particles, they are not taken up by gastrin cells.[130] This cannot be the complete answer, however, because at pH 2.5, cephalovagal stimulation of gastrin is inhibited.[82] It is probable also that somatostatin acts directly upon the parietal cell to inhibit acid secretion[16] by way of either paracrine or endocrine pathways.[131]

INTESTINAL

As described in the historical review section, the observation that infusion of nutrients into the small intestine could inhibit acid secretion is an old one. Feng and colleagues proposed that fat infusion into the small bowel inhibited acid secretion by release from the small bowel mucosa of a circulating inhibitory hormone that they called enterogastrone.[11] There have been at least six candidate peptides for this role (somatostatin, neurotensin, GIP, PYY, secretin, and CCK) (see Table 13-1). It is probable that enterogastrone is not a single entity but a physiologic response to more than one circulating acid inhibitor. Somatostatin appears to be a major component of this response.[132] Seal and colleagues have shown that immunoneutralization of endogenous somatostatin by a specific monoclonal antibody abolishes the acid inhibitory response to intraduodenal fat infusion in rats.[133] In man, intraduodenal fat is a potent stimulus of somatostatin,[134] and postprandial somatostatin concentrations can inhibit acid secretion without affecting serum gastrin levels.[131] Each of the peptides listed as a potential enterogastrone has its proponents and its detractors. Thus, while immunoneutralization studies appear to implicate neurotensin as a distal small gut enterogastrone,[133] infusion of exogenous neurotensin required supraphysiologic doses to show an effect.[135] Similar arguments are made against GIP[136] and PYY.[137] Immunoneutralization experiments have suggested that GIP may be released by peptone and may thus act as a restraint on acid secretion in these circumstances.[138] Some authors have widened the definition of enterogastrone to include those hormones released by acidification of the duodenal bulb that inhibits acid secretion. Secretin is the obvious candidate for this function. Once again, the evidence to support such a function for endogenous secretin is in conflict.[139,140]

CELLULAR BASIS OF ACID SECRETION

Analysis of the regulatory effects of gastric secretagogues in vivo has provided important insight into the mechanisms of acid secretion in animals and man. Interactions between neurocrine, paracrine, and endocrine signals and their effects on the parietal cell ultimately must be studied in the intact organism. However, the complexity of the regulatory effects converging on the parietal cell makes integrated in vitro analysis a necessity. In vitro models of acid secretion have been developed and include gastric mucosa preparations, gastric glands, and isolated enriched parietal cells. Gastric endocrine cells affecting acid secretion have also been enriched and analyzed. These models have provided an understanding of the cellular events leading to acid secretion.

In Vitro Models

Isolated preparations of intact gastric mucosa allow study of secretory events while maintaining all of the mucosal cell types in their usual cellular environment. Cell polarity, tight junctions, gap junctions, desmosomes, and certain paracrine effects are maintained in such models. Physiologic neurocrine and endocrine effects are absent but can be mimicked by bathing one or both surfaces with the desired neurotransmitter or hormone. One such model, the isolated bullfrog mucosa, has been used to study histamine release and acid secretion.[141] Mucosal strips are bluntly dissected and mounted as a sheet between two sides of a leucite chamber. A flow-through system can be used to ensure rapid changes of the serosal solution.[142] Acid secretion into the mucosal solution is measured with a pH stat by maintaining the pH at 7.0 with isotonic 15 mM NaOH. Other types of mucosal studies use explants maintained in organ culture[143] or fragments of mucosa suspended in tissue culture solutions.[144] Studies using these types of models have been supplanted recently by gastric gland and isolated cell studies.

The initial steps in the preparation of glands[145] and cells[146] are similar. Gastric mucosa is bluntly dissected away from the submucosa, finely minced, then dispersed with pronase or crude collagenase. Viability of parietal cells obtained with this technique generally exceeds 95%, as judged by trypan blue exclusion.

Following digestion of gastric mucosa, glands can be separated from cells and debris by several sedimentation washes at unit gravity. The large size of the glands allows them to sediment rapidly, essentially free of nonglandular material. Separation of isolated cells can be achieved by velocity and density separation techniques. Counterflow elutriation is a velocity separation technique that separates cells predominantly on the basis of size.[146,147] Enriched fractions routinely contain 50% to 70% parietal cells that maintain both their viability and biologic activity. Antral G cells and fundic D cells have also been enriched by elutriation.[148] A second purification step using a density gradient can be added to enrich parietal or endocrine cells further.

Gastric secretion has been analyzed in different species with each of these models. Species variety may account for certain discrepant results occasionally observed with different models. Much of the analysis of cellular events controlling acid secretion has used canine gastric mucosal cells enriched by counterflow elutriation. The data obtained using canine cells can be correlated with the large body of data obtained with in vivo acid secretory studies in dogs. Moreover, canine parietal cells have several features in common with human parietal cells.

Indirect measures of parietal cell function have been developed to quantitate the biologic effect of various secretagogues and inhibitors. The development of these assays has made it possible to correlate binding of ligands with their functional effects. Oxygen consumption has been shown to correlate with HCl secretion in both in vivo[149] and ex vivo[150] studies. Oxygen consumption in isolated enriched parietal cells increases in response to gastrin, carbachol, and histamine, most likely reflecting the activity of the proton pump.[146] Glucose oxidation can also be used as a measure of parietal cell metabolic activity.[151] Morphologic transformation of parietal cells in response to secretagogues produces dramatic changes in cell appearance. Resting cells are filled with tubulovesicles, while stimulated cells rapidly develop a dense intracellular canalicular network communicating with the cell's apical surface. Nomarski optics can visualize this transformation in living cells, while fluorescent microscopy with acridine orange can show the accumulation of fluorescent dye in the newly generated acid spaces.[152] The accumulation of weak bases in membrane-bound acid spaces is the basis of the [14C] aminopyrine (AP) uptake assay.[15,153] Uncharged aminopyrine is lipid soluble and easily crosses cellular membranes. Upon entering an acidic compartment, aminopyrine is protonated and loses its lipid solubility. This sequestration of [14C] AP correlates with intracellular acid formation and is the most commonly used assay for parietal cell stimulation. Other methods involving measurement of the association of the proton pump with canalicular membranes are currently under study.

Receptors

Separation of gastric cells into highly enriched cell populations has made it possible to identify and characterize specific receptors on each cell type.[154] Purified cells maintain intact receptors through the separation procedure and bind radiolabeled ligands specifically. Binding of a ligand should correlate with a functional assay over the same dosage range to confirm that a specific cell type has biologically active receptors. An example of this would be the correlation of carbachol binding to parietal cells and the induction of aminopyrine uptake by carbachol. Once functional receptors have been demonstrated, they can be characterized in binding studies with available receptor agonists and antagonists. Further characterization of receptors has been achieved by solubilizing them from cell membranes and cross-linking them to specific radiolabeled ligands. The solubilized form of the receptor can be examined for size, subunit structure, or ligand-induced autophosphorylation. In addition, the receptors can be purified, their amino acid sequence analyzed, and their genes eventually cloned. This type of detailed structural analysis of gastric cell receptors is still in its infancy. As such structural data become available, they can be used to develop probes for functional studies investigating the intracellular mechanisms of ligand-receptor effects.

The question of whether acid secretagogues act directly or indirectly on parietal cells could be answered when isolated parietal cell preparations were developed. Initial studies showed that histamine, carbachol, and gastrin increased canine parietal cell oxygen uptake.[146,155] Later studies revealed that [14C] aminopyrine accumulation was also increased by each of these secretagogues.[14,15] In isolated rabbit gastric glands, somewhat different results were obtained in that AP accumulation could be demonstrated in response to histamine and carbachol but not to gastrin.[153] These differences may reflect species variability. For example, rabbits are known to feed continuously and, therefore, may not have developed the ability to marshall an acid secretory response to intermittent bolus feeding as mediated by gastrin. Alternatively, these differences may reflect differences in the methods of study. In recent experiments, DelValle and colleagues (personal communication) have demonstrated marked increases in intracellular Ca^{++} concentration upon administration of gastrin-17 in single isolated rabbit parietal cells, suggesting that gastrin receptors are, indeed, present on rabbit cells as well.

Isolated canine parietal cells have provided a useful in vitro model for studying the well-characterized in vivo acid secretagogue effect of histamine. In the parietal cell model, the biologic action of histamine is generally assayed in the presence of 0.1 mM isobutylmethylxanthine (IMX), a phosphodiesterase inhibitor. While IMX alone causes a small accumulation of aminopyrine, in combination with histamine a synergistic increase in AP uptake and cAMP generation is seen. Histamine responses are specifically blocked by metiamide or cimetidine, H_2 receptor antagonists. The dissociation constant (K_i) for cimetidine inhibition of histamine's AP effect is 1.0 mM.[15] Further studies of the parietal cell H_2 receptor have been complicated by rapid uptake and degradation of histamine.[156]

The presence of a specific muscarinic receptor on canine parietal cells is supported by specific blockade of carbachol's biologic effects with atropine. The dissociation constant for atropine inhibition of carbachol-induced AP uptake, 1.3 nM,[15] is consistent with dissociation constants observed with muscarinic receptors in other tissues. In addition to inducing oxygen uptake and aminopyrine accumulation in a dose-dependent manner, carbachol also produces a parallel increase in the turnover of membrane inositol phospholipids.[157] Pharmacologic studies indicate that the parietal cell muscarinic receptor may be of the M2 subtype[158] inasmuch as it has a very low affinity for the M1 receptor antagonist, pirenzepine, as compared with atropine. Rat parietal cells have also been shown to have M2 muscarinic receptors that stimulate AP uptake, increase inositol phospholipid turnover, and bind [N-methyl-3H] scopolamine.[159]

Gastrin receptors have been localized to isolated rat[160] and canine[14] parietal cells. Binding studies with purified parietal cells reveal specific binding that is rapid and saturable. Proglumide, a CCK/gastrin receptor blocker, inhibits both gastrin binding and stimulation of parietal cell function. Interestingly, CCK-8 is equipotent with G17 in displacing radioligand and in stimulating AP uptake.[14] This suggests that the parietal cell gastrin receptor binds and responds to either ligand in a similar fashion. The gastrin receptor has been characterized further by cross-linking studies in two species. In canine parietal cell membranes, cross-linking studies with ^{125}I-gastrin$_{2-17}$ revealed a single gastrin receptor with a molecular weight (MW) of 74,000.[161] Half-maximal inhibition of radiolabeled gastrin binding in these canine parietal cell preparations was 3×10^{-10}M, in agreement with the potency of gastrin in stimulating AP uptake.[14] Similar studies with detergent extracts of porcine gastric mucosal membranes using ^{125}I-[Nle^{15}] gastrin$_{2-17}$ as ligand resulted in the cross-linking of a binding protein of MW 78,000.[162] However, in contrast to the studies in canine parietal cells, 50% inhibition of binding required 2×10^{-6}M [Nle^{15}] gastrin$_{2-17}$. The apparent reduction in affinity may be an artifact of the extraction technique used. In both species, the receptor appears to be a single protein with no disulfide-linked subunits. These studies confirm the presence of a specific gastrin receptor on parietal cells. As described below, the gastrin receptor appears to be coupled to membrane inositol phospholipid turnover[157] and protein kinase C activation.[163]

The effects of somatostatin on isolated enriched canine parietal cells have recently been evaluated. Somatostatin dose-dependently inhibits histamine-induced AP uptake and cAMP production as well as pentagastrin-stimulated AP accumulation.[16] Somatostatin binding sites have been identified with the use of ^{125}I-[Leu^8-D-Trp^{22}-Tyr^{25}]somatostatin-28 as radioligand. Somatostatin-14 and -28 are equally potent at displacing bound ligand and at inhibiting AP accumulation. Scatchard analysis of the binding data revealed two binding sites with dissociation constants of 3.2×10^{-9} and 2.1×10^{-7} M, respectively. Crude membranes prepared from 95% to 100% pure parietal cells were incubated with ^{125}I-[Leu^8-D-Trp^{22}-Tyr^{25}]somatostatin-28 and cross-linked with disuccinimidyl suberate.[164] After solubilization, a single sharp band with no disulfide linkages was identified that corresponded to a membrane receptor of MW 99,000. These parietal cell somatostatin receptors could be activated by way of a direct paracrine effect mediated by long cytoplasmic processes extending from fundic mucosal D cells that appear to terminate on parietal cells.[32] Endocrine inhibition of acid secretion by postprandial serum somatostatin could also be mediated by way of these receptors.

The presence of other receptors on parietal cells has been suggested but awaits further confirmation. Prostaglandins E$_2$ (PGE$_2$) and I$_2$ inhibit histamine-stimulated AP accumulation and cAMP generation in enriched canine parietal cells.[165] These agents have no effect on aminopyrine uptake induced by gastrin, carbachol, or dibutyryl cAMP. Specific binding sites for PGE$_2$ have been demonstrated in porcine fundic mucosa[166,167] with subcellular membrane fractionation suggesting localization to the plasma membrane.[168] Prostaglandins have been shown to displace bound [³H]PGE$_2$ and inhibit histamine-stimulated AP uptake in isolated rabbit parietal cells.[169] Taken together, these findings strongly suggest the presence of prostaglandin receptors on parietal cells. The sympathetic arm of the autonomic nervous system might be expected to counterbalance the stimulatory effect of muscarinic receptors on acid secretion. While it is possible that β-adrenergic agonists may inhibit acid secretion by way of stimulation of somatostatin release[170] and inhibition of histamine release by fundic mucosal mast cells,[154,171] direct studies with parietal cells support the presence of stimulatory β-adrenergic receptors (Yokotani and colleagues, personal communication). The presence of parietal cell receptors for epidermal growth factor (EGF), secretin, glucagon, or opioid compounds has been suggested but requires further confirmation.

A schematic overview of the interactions of ligands and receptors involved in acid secretion is provided in Figure 13-6. The parietal cell has stimulatory receptors for gastrin, acetylcholine, and histamine. Several lines of evidence suggest that parietal cells in man may be exposed continuously to basal levels of acetylcholine and histamine. As noted above, gastrin can account for nearly all of the postprandial increase in gastric acid secretion.[62,101] The parietal cell also has inhibitory somatostatin receptors counteracting secretagogue effects. Vagal nerve fibers may enhance their acid stimulatory effect through stimulatory muscarinic receptors on G cells[105] and inhibitory muscarinic receptors on D cells.[170] Adrenergic fibers appear to stimulate D cell secretion and inhibit release by histamine-containing cells, thus counterbalancing vagal effects.[171] Gastrin and CCK stimulate both parietal cells and D cells.[172] GRP acts as a neurotransmitter that stimulates G cells,[173,174] while somatostatin may function as a paracrine G cell inhibitor.[175]

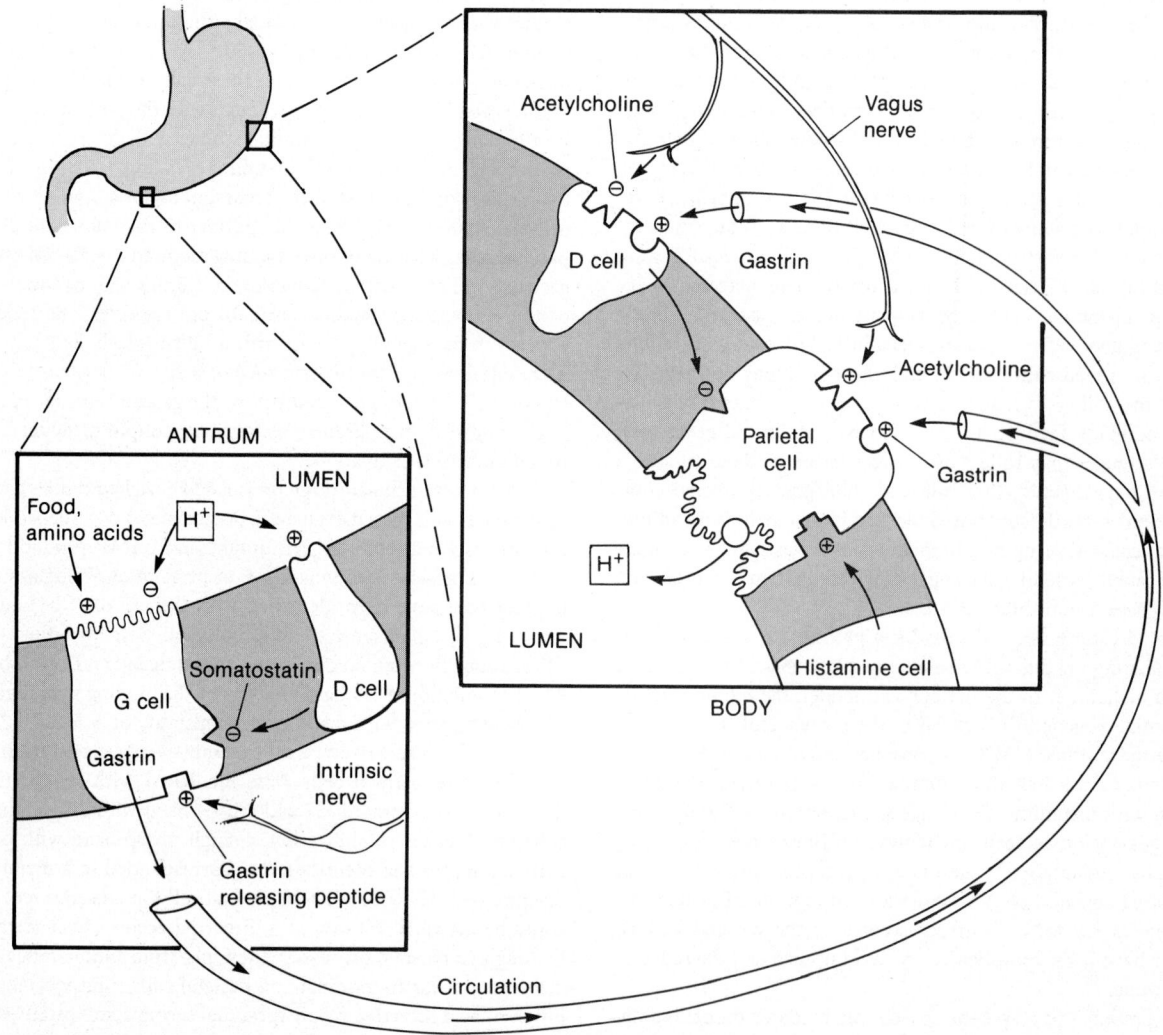

FIGURE 13–6. Regulation of gastric acid secretion. Major gastric mucosal ligand–receptor interactions regulating parietal cell HCl secretion are shown. *D cell,* somatostatin cell; *G cell,* gastrin cell. (Adapted from Feldman M. Acid and gastrin secretion in duodenal ulcer disease. The Regulatory Peptide Letter 1989;1:1.)

Further structural and functional analysis of each of these receptors will greatly enhance our understanding of gastric secretion.

Intracellular Signal Transduction

The interaction of acetylcholine, gastrin, or histamine with their respective parietal cell receptors induces a cascade of intracellular events culminating in acid secretion. The initial events involve changes in the concentration of intracellular second messengers, which subsequently result in the activation of protein kinases or increases in cytoplasmic Ca^{++} concentration ($[Ca^{++}]_i$). Two intracellular signal transduction pathways have been characterized in some detail and serve as generalized models for many cell types. Receptors linked to adenylate cyclase influence intracellular levels of cAMP. Such receptors are coupled to either inhibitory (G_i) or stimulatory (G_s) GTP binding proteins (Fig 13-7).[176,177] G_i attenuates adenylate cyclase activity, thereby decreasing cAMP levels. The ability of pertussis toxin to block selectively the actions of G_i has been used experimentally to dissect second messenger pathways. G_s, which increases adenylate cyclase activity and cAMP levels, can be stimulated selectively by cholera toxin. Increases in cytoplasmic cAMP levels result in activation of cAMP-dependent protein kinases and consequent phosphorylation of various intracellular proteins that, presumably, mediate the effects of the ligand–receptor interaction. A second major intracellular signal transduction cascade involves the turnover of membrane phospholipids, specifically the inositol phospholipids. Receptors are linked to this

pathway through a G protein that has yet to be characterized fully, and the initial events that are activated by occupancy of their receptor leads to phospholipase C–induced hydrolysis of phosphatidylinositol bisphosphate (PIP_2) to diacylglycerol (DAG) and inositol trisphosphate (IP_3).[178] IP_3 causes the release of Ca^{++} from intracellular stores, and DAG promotes the translocation of a Ca^{++}–phospholipid-dependent protein kinase (protein kinase C) from the cytoplasm to its active site on the cell membrane.[179,180] Increases in $[Ca^{++}]_i$ activate various calcium-dependent enzyme systems, such as the calmodulin kinases, and also promote the translocation and activation of protein kinase C.

Histamine's acid stimulatory action appears to be mediated by way of its ability to increase cAMP production in parietal cells.[181] This increase has been shown to parallel histamine's ability to stimulate aminopyrine uptake and oxygen consumption. Furthermore, histamine has been shown to increase cAMP-dependent protein kinase activity in enriched rabbit parietal cells.[182] The substrates for this enzyme activity have not been fully characterized, but they are thought to mediate the effects of histamine stimulation.[183] In contrast to histamine, neither carbachol nor gastrin has been reported to increase cAMP levels.[181]

The acid stimulatory actions of gastrin and carbachol appear to be mediated by Ca^{++}-dependent pathways. Gastrin and carbachol have been shown to have similar effects on membrane inositol phospholipid turnover in parietal cells. Both agents cause an apparent time-dependent decrease in phosphatidylinositol 4,5-bisphosphate (PIP_2) and an increase in the formation of IP_3.[157] These effects parallel increases in $[^{14}C]$ aminopyrine accumulation. The increase in IP_3 may mediate the mobilization of intracellular

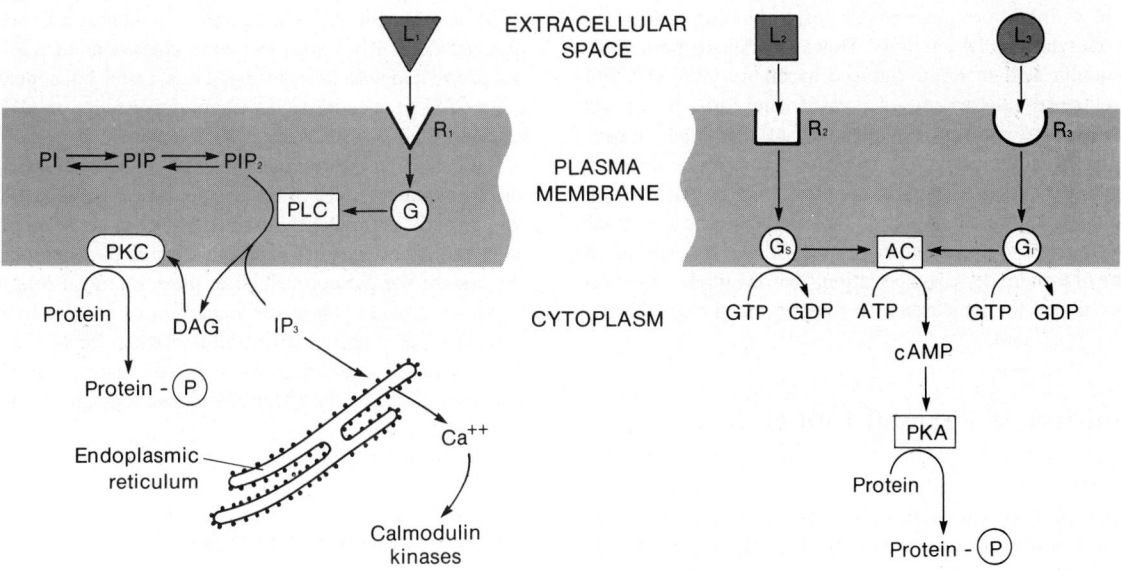

FIGURE 13–7. Signal transduction pathways in parietal cells. Ligands (*L*) interact with receptors (*R*) to initiate the target cell response. The left panel shows the membrane inositol phospholipid pathway activated by gastrin and acetylcholine (*L₁*). A guanine nucleotide binding protein (*G*) activates phospholipase C (*PLC*), which hydrolyzes phosphotidylinositol 4,5-bisphosphate (*PIP₂*) to diacylglycerol (*DAG*) and inositol 1,4,5-trisphosphate (*IP₃*). *DAG* activates protein kinase C (*PKC*), which phosphorylates (*P*) target proteins while IP₃ induces intracellular calcium mobili-

zation, which activates kinases as well. The right panel depicts the cAMP pathway used by histamine (*L₂*) and somatostatin (*L₃*) in parietal cells. The histamine receptor (*R₂*) acts through a stimulatory G protein (*Gs*), which activates adenylate cyclase (*AC*) and generates cAMP. Increased levels of cytoplasmic cAMP activate protein kinase A (*PKA*) and result in phosphorylation of parietal-cell effector proteins. The somatostatin receptor (*R₃*) activates an inhibitory G protein (*Gi*), which inhibits adenylate cyclase and decreases cAMP generation.

Ca^{++} observed in parietal cells stimulated with gastrin or carbachol. In the case of carbachol, increased $[Ca^{++}]_i$ may occur as a result of enhanced mobilization of Ca^{++} from intracellular stores or by way of influx of extracellular calcium across the cell membrane.[184-186] It is presumed that the elevated cytoplasmic Ca^{++} then activates several enzyme cascades, including the calmodulin kinase family and, in concert with diacylglycerol, the second product of PIP_2 breakdown, protein kinase C. Indeed, both gastrin and carbachol have been shown to increase membrane-associated protein kinase C activity.[163] The action of protein kinase C in parietal cells appears to be complex, however. Direct activation of protein kinase C with phorbol esters results in enhanced acid secretory activity, as quantified by uptake of aminopyrine. However, phorbol ester pretreatment may also decrease the stimulatory effects of subsequent treatment with carbachol and gastrin. This curious phenomenon appears to result from a protein kinase C–induced down-regulation of both cholinergic and gastrin receptors.[163] The mechanism for this effect has not been elucidated but may involve receptor phosphorylation.

The action of gastrin on parietal cells may not be accounted for solely by Ca^{++}-dependent mechanisms. In recent studies, Yokotani and colleagues[187] have demonstrated that gastrin may have a second inhibitory action on parietal cells mediated by way of G_i. Indeed, in the presence of pertussis toxin, gastrin's stimulatory action in parietal cells is greatly enhanced. Although gastrin has no inhibitory effect on basal cAMP accumulation in parietal cells, levels observed with forskolin stimulation are dose-dependently diminished by gastrin.

The mechanism by which somatostatin inhibits parietal cells has also been explored.[16] In the case of histamine-stimulated acid secretion, somatostatin appears to inhibit the generation of cAMP by way of an inhibitory guanine nucleotide–binding protein regulating adenylate cyclase activity. However, somatostatin is also able to inhibit acid secretion induced by dibutyryl cAMP. Furthermore, the stimulatory effects of gastrin and carbachol are also inhibited without altering the turnover of membrane inositol phospholipids or the activation of protein kinase C induced by these agents. Thus, somatostatin appears to act on parietal cells at a site distal to the activation of the intracellular signal transduction cascades. This action may be mediated by way of the induction of protein dephosphorylation,[188,189] the inhibition of cellular secretion,[190] or some other yet undetermined mechanism.

Regulation of Parietal Cell Genes

Stimulation of parietal cells induces several cellular events, including morphologic transformation, rapid changes in enzyme location and activity, and opening of ion channels. The resting parietal cell contains a collapsed canalicular system and cytoplasmic tubulovesicles containing the gastric proton pump H^+,K^+-ATPase. The stimulated cell rapidly develops a richly interdigitating intracellular canalicular system bulging with microvilli with concomitant loss of cytoplasmic tubulovesicles (Fig 13-8).[19,191] The microvilli have a central cytoskeletal core of actin filaments stabilized by other proteins.[192] These filaments appear to mediate the fusion of tubulovesicles with the canalicular system. This fusion translocates H^+,K^+-ATPase from vesicular membranes to the canalicular membrane,[193,194] where it actively pumps H^+ ions in

exchange for K^+. For each proton that is secreted, an intracellular OH^- ion is generated. This alkaline challenge is handled by carbonic anhydrase II (CAII)–mediated conversion of OH^- to HCO_3^-, which, in turn, is exchanged for Cl^- at the basolateral membrane (Fig 13-9). Obviously there are many proteins involved in generating and secreting gastric acid. Stimulation of parietal cells presumably involves not only activation of nascent proteins but also induction of the genes responsible for these effector molecules. The effect of acid secretagogues on the genes encoding these enzymes and structural proteins has recently been analyzed.

Induction of specific gene transcription has been studied in isolated canine parietal cells.[195] The cells were incubated in the presence of the three major secretagogues for varying lengths of time, and total cellular RNA was prepared for hybridization analysis. Significant increases in CAII RNA levels were induced with carbachol, gastrin, and histamine. Maximum stimulation was reached within 20 minutes for histamine and carbachol and within 60 minutes for gastrin. In order to determine whether the observed increases in mRNA levels were due to increased transcription or to decreased degradation, nuclear runoff experiments were performed and revealed increased transcription within 15 minutes for each agent. H^+,K^+-ATPase mRNA levels were also induced in the same fashion as CAII.[196] This coordinate induction of both enzymes could be blocked with competitive inhibitors of each secretagogue.

Because the role of CAII appears to be the catalysis of the reaction responsible for elimination of OH^- produced in the generation of H^+, increased transcription of CAII RNA in stimulated parietal cells could result as a secondary effect of the induction of H^+,K^+-ATPase. To explore this possibility, parietal cells were pretreated with omeprazole, an agent known to inactivate H^+,K^+-ATPase irreversibly.[197] Under these circumstances, carbachol still induced CAII RNA with the same kinetics as in cells that were not pretreated with omeprazole. Thus, carbachol appears to stimulate CAII gene expression without dependence on OH^- ion generation by H^+,K^+-ATPase.

Of particular interest in these gene expression experiments was the stimulatory effect of secretagogues on actin expression. Although actin is frequently used as a control housekeeper gene for such studies because its expression tends to remain constant, in the case of the parietal cell actin plays a crucial role in the acid secretory process. Thus, the induction of actin gene expression may serve as a particularly useful marker for acid secretion as opposed to H^+ generation. This type of analysis can elucidate at the molecular level the effect of acid secretagogues on parietal cell function.

Acid Secretory Process

The gastric epithelium secretes a fluid of nearly isotonic HCl by way of an active transport process. Acid is secreted at a pH of 0.8 while the parietal cell cytosolic pH is approximately 7.2. The parietal cell alone is responsible for this remarkable H^+ ion concentration gradient of 2.5 million–fold. Significant amounts of mitochondrial energy are required when the parietal cell is signaled to transform from a relatively quiet resting state to an actively secreting state. Dramatic changes in cellular membranes, cytoskeletal architecture, membrane ion conductances, and ATPase

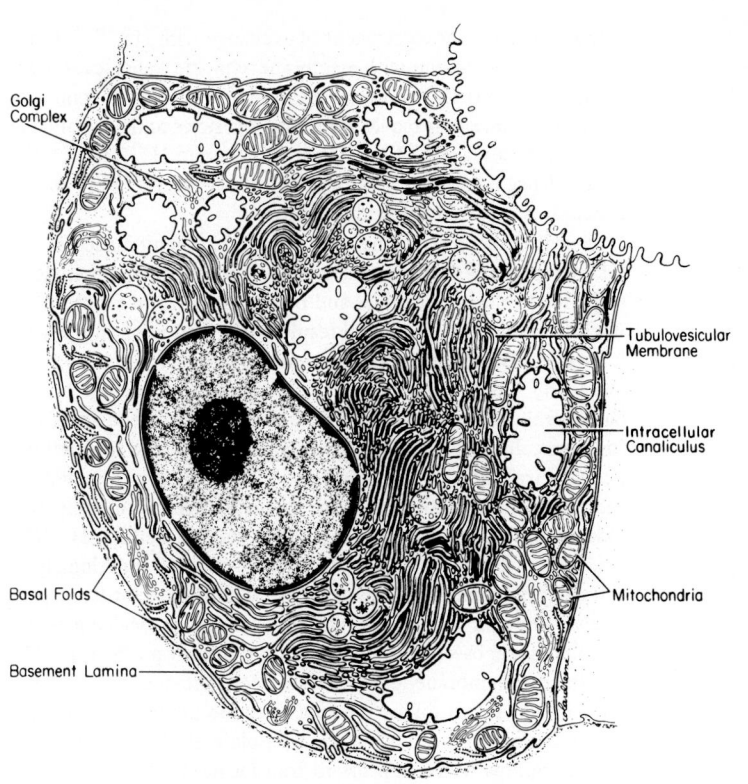

Golgi
Complex

Tubulovesicular
Membrane

Intracellular
Canaliculus

Mitochondria

Basal Folds

Basement Lamina

A PARIETAL CELL (Non-Secreting)

FIGURE 13–8. A, Resting nonsecretory parietal cell; **B,** Stimulated acid secretory parietal cell. See text for morphologic description of transition from the resting to the secretory state. (From Ito S. Functional gastric morphology. In: Johnson LR, ed. Physiology of the gastrointestinal tract. 2nd ed. New York: Raven Press, 1987:817.)

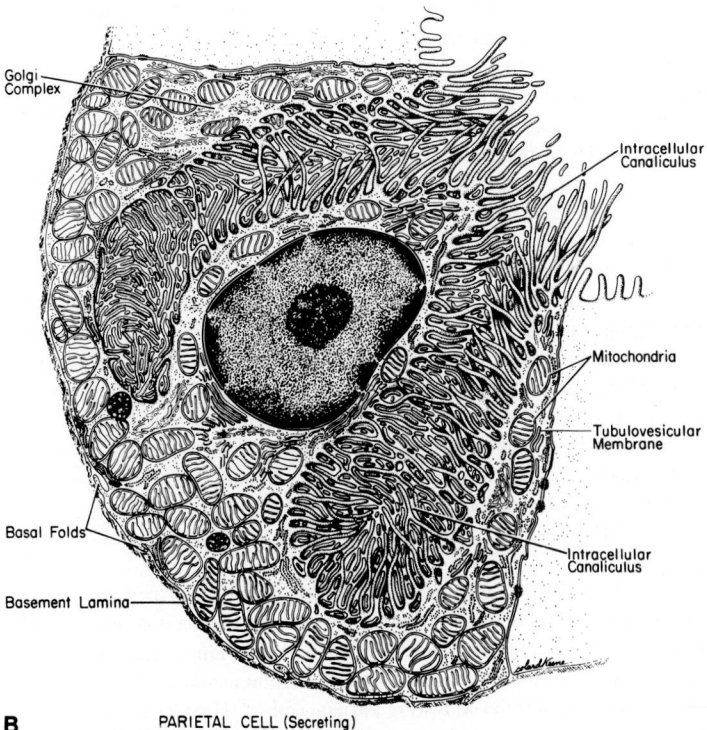

Golgi
Complex

Intracellular
Canaliculus

Mitochondria

Tubulovesicular
Membrane

Basal Folds

Intracellular
Canaliculus

Basement Lamina

B PARIETAL CELL (Secreting)

activities are only a portion of the events that accompany cell activation. Equally impressive is the compressed time frame over which these changes occur. These unique properties of the parietal cell provide a novel model for the study of active transport.

Stimulation of parietal cells induces formation of a dense apical meshwork of intracellular canaliculi packed with long microvilli.[198] The apical cell membrane surface area increases 5- to 10-fold after stimulation. This increases coincides with the disappearance

APICAL

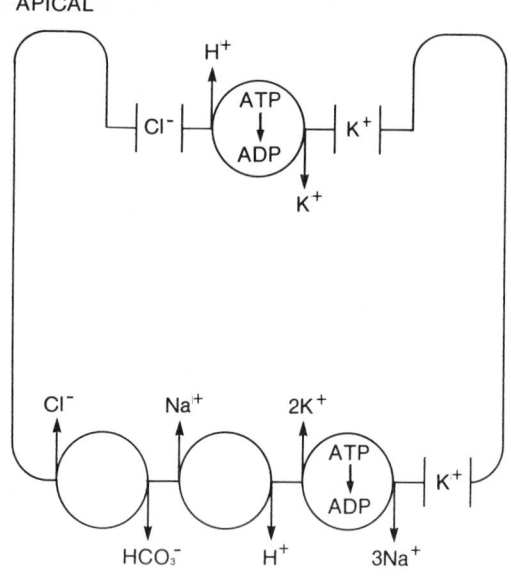

BASOLATERAL

FIGURE 13–9. Ion transport pathways in parietal cells. The apical membrane contains the H$^+$, K$^+$-ATPase pump as well as K$^+$ and Cl$^-$ conductances. The basolateral membrane also has a K$^+$ conductance as well as Cl$^-$/HCO$_3^-$ exchanges, Na$^+$/H$^+$ exchanges, and Na$^+$, K$^+$-ATPases to maintain cellular homeostasis during secretory and resting states.

of the majority of cytoplasmic tubulovesicles seen in the resting parietal cell. The mechanism of this increase in surface area appears to be fusion of tubulovesicles and apical membrane. Immunocytochemical studies with a monoclonal antibody to H$^+$,K$^+$-ATPase[193] demonstrate the translocation of the enzymes from tubulovesicles in the resting cell to the apical membranes in the stimulated cells, supporting the concept of secretagogue-induced membrane fusion and enzyme redistribution. The fusion of tubulovesicles with apical membrane is directed by cytoskeletal microfilaments composed of actin and other regulatory proteins. Membranes are recycled back to tubulovesicles as cells return to the resting state, and this process also appears to be mediated by actin-containing microfilaments.[192] These microfilaments anchor into apical membranes at regularly spaced intervals and are not seen in association with resting tubulovesicles. Cytochalasin, an agent that inhibits polymerization of actin, inhibits acid secretion.[199] Colchicine and vinblastine are also capable of inhibiting acid secretion.[200] These studies indicate the essential importance of actin-mediated H$^+$,K$^+$-ATPase translocation in the initiation of acid secretion.

Studies of H$^+$,K$^+$-ATPase activity have been performed on membrane vesicles obtained from both resting and stimulated parietal cells.[198] Vesicles from light microsomal membrane fractions, presumably containing the tubulovesicles, exhibit nearly all of the H$^+$,K$^+$-ATPase activity in resting parietal cells.[201] Heavier membrane vesicles associated with microfilaments contain the majority of H$^+$,K$^+$-ATPase activity in stimulated parietal cells. The membranes of these acid-secreting vesicles have a K$^+$-Cl$^-$ co-transport system that is lacking in membrane preparations from resting cells.[202] Other studies have confirmed that H$^+$,K$^+$-ATPase requires

extracellular K$^+$ for electroneutral exchange with H$^+$.[203,204] It appears that concomitant with membrane/enzyme translocation, associated K$^+$ and Cl$^-$ conductances are activated.[202] Opening of this conductance as it moves from tubulovesicles to the canalicular membrane allows H$^+$,K$^+$-ATPase to generate H$^+$. The K$^+$-Cl$^-$ conductance is intimately associated with H$^+$,K$^+$-ATPase and its function is required for acid secretion.

Several other ion channels are involved in maintenance of cellular homeostasis during acid secretion. A schematic representation of parietal cell conductances and pumps is shown in Figure 13-9. Each H$^+$ ion that is generated results in formation of an intracellular OH$^-$ ion which, in turn, reacts with CO$_2$ in a reaction catalyzed by CAII to form HCO$_3^-$. A mechanism located on the basolateral membrane permits the exchange of intracellular HCO$_3^-$ for extracellular Cl$^-$. This Cl$^-$ provides part of the intracellular pool for transport by the apical K$^+$-Cl$^-$ conductance system. A second mechanism located on the basolateral cell membrane provides for exchange of extracellular Na$^+$ for intracellular H$^+$. The Na$^+$/H$^+$ and Cl$^-$/HCO$_3^-$ exchanges are coupled functionally as cellular pH monitors handling excess acid or base loads, respectively. While physically separate, these exchange mechanisms act as a functional basolateral Na$^+$/Cl$^-$ co-transport mechanism. The basolateral membrane also has a K$^+$ conductance which allows intracellular K$^+$ to follow the concentration gradient. K$^+$ uptake by the parietal cell can occur via a basolateral Na$^+$/K$^+$-ATPase, or Na$^+$ pumps which appears to translocate 3 intracellular Na$^+$ for extracellular K$^+$. The net effect of these ion channels is to maintain cellular homeostasis in the face of HCl secretion. The osmotically active HCl generated in the canalicular lumen results in flow of H$_2$O across the cell. This flow leads to the formation of gastric fluid with acid secretion.

The gastric H$^+$,K$^+$-ATPase, or H$^+$ ion pump, has been studied in detail.[205] This membrane protein is a member of the ATPase family which includes Na$^+$/K$^+$- and Ca$^+$-ATPases. Structural homology between these family members suggests that they probably diverged from a common ancestor molecule.[206] The ATPases are proteins of approximately 1000 amino acids in length that are embedded in membranes such that there are 8 potential transmembrane domains. A long cytoplasmic portion of the molecule occurs in its midsection and contains the presumed ATP binding, phosphorylation, and energy transduction sites. It is presumed that the hydrophobic transmembrane domains of the molecule form the cation channel. The exact mechanism of action for this molecule is unknown, but it obviously requires sophisticated intramolecular communication. Presumed steps would include hydrolysis of ATP followed by phosphorylation of the enzyme. This would lead to conformational changes that open ion channels and allow energy transduction. If H$^+$ and K$^+$ ions are bound appropriately, they will be "pumped" across the transmembrane channel. The H$^+$,K$^+$-ATPase can be inactivated completely by omeprazole, a substituted benzimidazole. This compound will cyclize in the presence of acid and react with available sulfhydryl groups to form a covalent interaction that irreversibly inactivates the enzyme. The blockade of proton transport is virtually complete and has been used clinically as described in Chapter 61. Future advances should delineate the mechanism of action of H$^+$,K$^+$-ATPase and provide new approaches to the pharmacologic blockade of acid secretion.

OTHER GASTRIC SECRETORY PRODUCTS

Pepsinogen

Secretion of pepsinogen by the gastric mucosa occurs in response to food ingestion as described by Langley in 1886.[207] Pepsinogens are inactive proenzymes that are autocatalytically cleaved under acidic conditions to their active form, pepsin. The proenzyme is synthesized in exocrine chief cells found at the base of oxyntic glands as well as in mucous neck and mucous cells in cardiac, oxyntic, and pyloric glands.[208] Chief cells package pepsinogen in apical granules, where it is stored until the cells are stimulated. Stimulation of chief cells by various secretagogues induces exocytosis of granule contents into the glandular lumen. Concomitant stimulation of parietal cells provides the acidic luminal conditions needed for rapid production of pepsin, the major acid protease activity in the stomach. Pepsin is an aspartic protease that initiates protein digestion and is particularly active in proteolysis of collagen, a major protein component of meat. Peptides generated by the proteolytic activity of pepsin act as signals for secretion of digestive hormones such as gastrin and cholecystokinin. These peptide signals thus initiate the coordinated digestive response necessary for absorption of nutrients.

Pepsinogens have been electrophoretically separated into seven isozymogens.[209] Five fractions (1 to 5) that migrate toward the anode rapidly are immunologically similar and therefore have been named group I pepsinogens (PGI or PGA). Group II pepsinogens (fractions 6 and 7) migrate slightly slower in gels and are also antigenically similar (also called PGII or PGC). Both groups are active in acidic conditions (pH 2–3.5) and are inactivated at pH >5. Despite these similarities, there are many biochemical and immunochemical differences between PGI and PGII that are the subject of intense current investigation. The distribution of the two groups in gastrointestinal tissues also varies. While both groups are found in the gastric body, only group II pepsinogens are found in the gastric antrum, proximal duodenum, and Brunner's glands. The presence of different isozymogens could be due to multiple gene loci, multiple alleles at a single gene locus, alternate post-transcriptional processing of RNA, or post-translational modifications of primary gene products. Genetic analysis has revealed that the two groups have different gene loci. A human pepsinogen I gene has been isolated and sequenced,[210] and analysis of its chromosome 11 locus indicates the presence of multiple pepsinogen I genes.[211] This type of multigene protein polymorphism is quite rare and suggests that the pepsinogen gene complex is undergoing evolutionary gene duplication and selection. Other mechanisms of isozymogen diversity, such as post-translational modification, may also be active.

Stimulation of pepsinogen secretion has been analyzed in intact animals, gastric mucosal preparations, gastric glands, and isolated chief cells. Despite the use of different species in these models, certain generalizations about mechanisms of chief cell activation are supported by the data. Acetylcholine and its analogs appear to stimulate chief cells directly.[212] Studies with the muscarinic antagonists atropine and pirenzepine suggest that vagal stimulation of chief cells is mediated partially by way of M1 muscarinic re-ceptors.[213] Other neuronal mediators such as gastrin-releasing peptide (GRP) may also mediate vagal stimulation of pepsinogen secretion.[214] The adrenergic agonist isoproterenol has a stimulatory effect in vitro,[215] although the physiologic significance of this effect has not been demonstrated in intact animals. The ability of histamine to stimulate pepsinogen secretion remains controversial, and conflicting data preclude any definitive conclusion.[208] While gastrin stimulates chief cells only weakly, cholecystokinin (CCK-8) is a very potent stimulus of pepsinogen secretion in vitro.[216] The fact that peripherally administered CCK in vivo only weakly stimulates pepsinogen secretion may reflect CCK's function as a neurocrine, rather than endocrine, mediator of chief-cell stimulation. Alternatively, it may reflect the mixed effects of a direct stimulatory effect on chief cells and an indirect inhibitory effect such as might be mediated by CCK-induced somatostatin release. Secretin has been reported to stimulate pepsinogen secretion both in vivo[217] and in vitro.[218]

The intracellular signal transduction mechanisms activated by the various chief cell secretagogues have also been analyzed. Both isoproterenol and secretin appear to stimulate pepsinogen secretion by cAMP-mediated pathways.[208] Other secretagogues such as cholinergic agonists and CCK do not increase intracellular cAMP levels.[219] Current evidence is indirect but supports the presumption that these agents alter intracellular calcium.[218] If the second messenger pathways for these agents are analogous to those of other cellular models (e.g., parietal cells and pancreatic acini), they may involve membrane inositol phospholipid turnover with consequent increases in intracellular Ca^{++}. Hence, it appears that both cAMP- and Ca^{++}-mediated pathways are involved in pepsinogen secretion.

Pepsinogens are found not only in the gastric juice but also in serum,[220] urine, and seminal fluid.[221] Their physiologic role in nongastric fluids is currently unknown. Measurement of pepsinogens in these fluids is performed with specific radioimmunoassays.[220] Attempts to correlate serum pepsinogen groups with risk of peptic ulcer disease have proved to be of modest clinical value (see Chapter 61). Future advances in our understanding of pepsinogen physiology and pathophysiology may lend these measurements new clinical significance.

Mucus

Gastric epithelium is protected from acidic autodigestion in part by a mucous gel that covers the entire surface of the stomach. This gel acts as a barrier protecting the gastric mucosa from acid, pepsin, bile salts, alcohol, and other injurious agents. The barrier consists of an unstirred layer of mucus, bicarbonate, surface phospholipids, and water. A prominent pH gradient extending from the lumen (pH 2) to the epithelial cell surface (pH 7) is maintained by this gel.[222] Mucin, a high-molecular-weight glycoprotein, is secreted by surface mucous cells, mucous neck cells, and glandular mucous cells. Polymerization of mucin subunits by way of disulfide bonds is essential for the formation of the hydrated gel.[223] The precise structural organization and approximate molecular weight of mucin polymers are unknown. Two significantly different models of gastric mucin polymerization have been proposed and are described in other reviews.[224,225] The peptide backbone of mucin contains many serine, threonine, and proline residues (>40% mol), which serve as the amino acid anchors for the glycosyl residues that branch from the protein. Partial complementary DNA clones for mucin have been isolated recently,[226,227] and deduced peptide sequences confirm this amino acid preponderance. The mucin that is synthesized in the rough endoplasmic reticulum undergoes vesicular transport to the Golgi apparatus for glycosylation. The major portion of mucin is heavily glycosylated, while nonglycosylated or "naked" regions of the peptide are joined to other mucins by disulfide bridges. The initial peptide–carbohydrate linkage involves glycosidic bond formation between N-acetyl galactosamine and the hydroxyl groups of serine or threonine residues. This type of O-linked glycosylation involves addition of individual carbohydrate moieties (rather than transfer of preassembled oligosaccharides) to gradually lengthening chains.[228] Fucose, galactose, N-acetylglucosamine, and N-acetylgalactosamine make up over 95% of the sugar moieties in each chain.[229] Each mucin peptide contains up to several hundred linear or branched-chain oligosaccharides. This high carbohydrate content (>50% by weight) results in a highly viscoelastic substance that will expand when hydrated. These properties may be essential to the protective function that gastric mucus serves.

Intracellular transport of mucin proceeds through the cis-, medial-, and trans-Golgi cisternae before transfer to the apical mucous granule. Cytoplasmic transport vesicles presumably bud off Golgi membranes and transfer mucus molecules to their target organelles. Fusion of vesicle and granule membranes results in gradually enlarging mucus granules that ultimately pack the apical cytoplasm. Intact microtubules appear to be needed for transport of secretory granules from the Golgi apparatus to the cell surface. Basal secretion of mucus occurs continually throughout the life span of mucous cells.[230] In vitro pulse-labeling of human mucous granules reveals that intracellular transit and release occurs in 20 to 24 hours.[223] In contrast to basal secretion, stimulation of mucous cells results in fairly rapid fusion of granular and apical cell membranes or extrusion of mucous granule contents. In addition, fusion of subjacent mucous granules occurs to enhance the secretory response. This process is called compound exocytosis and results in a dramatically cavitated apical cell surface during stimulated secretion.

Study of the regulation of mucous cell secretion has been impeded by the inherent difficulties in quantitatively retrieving and measuring secreted mucus. Hydration of secreted mucus forms a viscous gel that adheres to mucosal cells. Attempts to quantify mucus secretion by morphologic methods,[231] release of radiolabeled glycoproteins,[232] and radioimmunoassay[233] have met with only limited success. Despite these limitations, several factors that affect mucin secretion have been identified and can be summarized. Cholinergic agonists stimulate secretion in at least a portion of gastric mucous cells, while adrenergic neurotransmitters do not appear to influence release of secretory granules. Gastrin and CCK may increase feline gastric luminal carbohydrate content, but the source of this presumed mucus secretion has not been determined.[234] Secretin has also been shown to increase carbohydrate content of secreted gastric mucus in man; however, the cellular origin of this effect also has not been established.[235] Prostaglandins E and F have been reported to stimulate release of soluble and insoluble mucin from gastric mucosa[236,237] with a resultant increase in mucous gel thickness. This increase may also be due to prostaglandin-induced bicarbonate secretion[238] creating an outward alkaline flow carrying previously secreted mucins from gastric

crypts and glands. After gastric mucosal injury has occurred, multiple inflammatory and immune cytokines may be present in the mucosa. It seems plausible that these factors might directly or indirectly stimulate mucous cell secretion as part of the reparative process.[223] Candidate secretagogues include leukotrienes, immune complexes, and mast cell histamine.

Mucous cells presumably have various receptors mediating stimulatory effects on their basolateral membrane. As of yet, however, no specific receptors have been demonstrated on these cells. The intracellular signals used by putative mucous cell receptors have been characterized only partially. Neither dibutyryl cyclic AMP nor phosphodiesterase inhibitors have been shown to stimulate release of mucin from intestinal mucous cells.[239] Conversely, a calcium ionophore has been shown to induce visible loss of mucus granules from guinea pig gastric mucosa and increase the thickness of the mucous gel.[240] Taken together, these results suggest that gastric mucous cells may be stimulated by secretagogues that use the calcium-mediated intracellular pathways. Much remains to be learned about the regulation of gastric mucous cell secretion in both the basal and stimulated states.

Bicarbonate

Gastric mucosal defense depends on a mucus–bicarbonate barrier coating the entire lumen of the stomach. This barrier exists as a gel containing a pH gradient that provides a neutral microenvironment at the epithelial surface. The gradient is generated by secretion of bicarbonate ions by gastric surface mucous cells. Uptake of bicarbonate at the basolateral membrane and secretion at the apical membrane are metabolically dependent processes.[241] Carbonic anhydrase, the enzyme responsible for HCO_3^- generation, has also been localized to the apical matrix and microvillar cores of surface epithelial cells.[242] Bicarbonate secretion appears to be mediated by a Cl^-/HCO_3^- exchange mechanism on the luminal surface of gastric epithelial cells.[243] In addition to active secretion, passive efflux of HCO_3^- presumably occurs by way of a paracellular route. Mucosal delivery of bicarbonate ions is enhanced by fenestrations of the capillaries supplying the epithelial cells.[40] The relative proportion of passive and active bicarbonate secretion in basal and stimulated states has been difficult to determine and depends on the type of model studied.

Several models have been used to measure gastric bicarbonate secretion. Mucosal membranes can be mounted in chambers and bathed with appropriate solutions.[244-246] Titration of luminal secretions is used to calculate HCO_3^- release. In vivo measurements have been performed in fundic and antral pouches and are described elsewhere.[247,248] Human gastric bicarbonate measurements have also been obtained with the use of two different approaches. The technique of Forssell and Olbe[249] involves rapid perfusion of the stomach (30 ml/min) with continuous measurement of pCO_2 and pH in the gastric aspirate. HCO_3^- and H^+ secretion can then be calculated by the Henderson–Hasselbach equation. This technique relies on the assumption that all luminal CO_2 results from neutralization of H^+ ions by HCO_3^-. Feldman has used a two-component model that calculates gastric bicarbonate secretion from measurements of gastric juice volume, H^+ concentration, and osmolality.[250] This model assumes a fixed relationship between the osmolality of plasma and gastric secretions such that a decrease in osmolality occurs only as a result of H^+/HCO_3^- neutralization. The latter method results in a higher calculation of gastric bicarbonate secretory rate (~ 2300 μEq/hr) than the former (~ 400 μEq/hr). Despite these quantitative differences, responses to various stimuli are qualitatively similar with both techniques.

Regulation of gastric bicarbonate secretion is an important component of gastric mucosal defense. Both sham feeding[251,252] and electrical stimulation of the vagus[253] induce gastric HCO_3^- secretion. This neural control mechanism is effectively blocked by atropine and benzilonium bromide. Intravenous infusion of cholinergic agents such as bethanechol also stimulates HCO_3^- and H^+ secretion.[250] The coordinate stimulation of acid and bicarbonate secretion by vagal transmitters is not reproduced by gastrin or histamine. Local regulation of bicarbonate secretion is initiated by the presence of luminal acid. Studies with both canine denervated pouches[254] and isolated frog mucosal strips[255] suggest that a humoral factor that stimulates bicarbonate secretion is released in response to luminal acid. Although exogenous prostaglandins have been shown to stimulate both gastric and duodenal HCO_3^- secretion, the physiologic role of endogenous prostaglandins in bicarbonate control is less clear.[241,256] Inhibition of gastric bicarbonate secretion has not been well characterized. In summary, the surface mucous cell appears to be stimulated to secrete HCO_3^- by vagal stimuli and luminal acid. Acid stimulation also results in delivery of bicarbonate from parietal cells to surface epithelium by ascending mucosal capillaries ("alkaline tide"). These regulatory controls ensure simultaneous secretion of gastric acid and bicarbonate.

Intrinsic Factor

Intrinsic factor (IF), a 45,000 MW glycoprotein present in gastric secretions, is essential for the absorption of cobalamin (Vitamin B_{12}) in the terminal ileum by receptor-mediated endocytosis. Its existence was first postulated by Castle in 1929.[257] In man, IF is synthesized and secreted by parietal cells.[258] Parietal cells are the source also in cats, rabbits, monkeys, guinea pigs, and oxen.[259] Intrinsic factor is a product of chief cells in rodents such as the rat and mouse, while its source in the pig is gastric mucous cells.[260,261] The structure of rat intrinsic factor, as deduced from a cDNA clone, indicates a primary amino acid sequence of 421 amino acids with a putative signal sequence of 22 amino acids.[261] The cobalamin-binding domain is thought to reside in the NH_2-terminal half of the protein.

IF is secreted in amounts far exceeding that which is necessary for cobalamin absorption.[262] Secretion of IF is stimulated by the same pharmacologic agents as acid secretion—pentagastrin, histamine, and cholinergic agonists,[263] yet this secretory response is not linked to acid secretion. For example, omeprazole does not alter basal or stimulated IF secretion in man,[264] nor does it alter absorption of labeled cobalamin.[265] The intracellular responses mediating IF secretion involve the cyclic AMP pathway when stimulated by histamine.[263] Whether pentagastrin and acetylcholine (which appear to act by way of Ca^{++}-phospholipid-dependent pathways when stimulating acid secretion) act in a similar fashion when stimulating IF secretion is unknown.

Inhibitory regulation of IF secretion is poorly understood. Somatostatin inhibits histamine- or pentagastrin-stimulated IF secretion in isolated guinea pig gastric glands.[266] Epidermal growth factor is reported to inhibit histamine-stimulated IF secretion in isolated rabbit gastric glands[267] and in man.[268] The physiologic significance of these observations is not known.

IF is resistant to digestion by gastric acid and proteolytic enzymes under normal circumstances. A rare kinship has been reported with cobalamin malabsorption due to an abnormal IF that was susceptible to acid and proteolysis.[269] There are rare cases also of absence of IF secretion in persons, usually children, with normal acid secretion.[270,271] Further discussion of the significance of IF in health and disease is presented in Chapter 20.

Prostaglandins

The role of prostaglandins in gastric acid secretion and mucosal defense has been an area of active research in the recent past. Prostaglandins are 20-carbon fatty acid derivatives that have diverse biologic activities and are produced in many different tissues. They are synthesized from arachidonic acid, a product of enzymatic cleavage of cell membrane phospholipids by phospholipases, particularly phospholipase A_2.[272] Cyclooxygenase rapidly metabolizes free arachidonic acid to cyclic endoperoxides, which are transformed to various prostaglandin subtypes by tissue-specific processing enzymes (Fig 13-10). Prostaglandins of the E type (PGE_2) and I type (PGI_2 or prostacyclin) are synthesized and secreted by the gastric mucosa of various species. The presence of these two predominant forms in homogenates of gastric mucosa has been confirmed by bioassay, radioimmunoassay, and gas chromatography–mass spectrometry. Biosynthetic studies using radiolabeled arachidonic acid has confirmed that gastric mucosa can synthesize both of these prostaglandins. The specific mucosal cell types synthesizing the various prostaglandins has not been identified for certain. While canine and rat parietal cell fractions appear to form several prostaglandin subtypes, other cells such as mucous and chief cells may synthesize prostaglandins as well.

Gastric prostaglandins are likely to have paracrine effects on other gastric mucosal cells. One example of this is direct inhibition of acid secretion by prostaglandins. Studies on canine parietal cells show that PGE_2 decreases [^{14}C] AP accumulation and cAMP production.[165] This effect appears to be mediated by way of prostaglandin receptors activating inhibitory guanine nucleotide-binding proteins.[273] Inhibition of parietal cells could be one effect of a prostaglandin-mediated negative feedback loop regulating gastric acid secretion. In addition to paracrine effects, prostaglandins may also function as luminal hormones. PGE_2 has been demonstrated in the gastric juice of several species, including human, cat, dog, and rat.[272] Secretion of PGE_2 into luminal fluid has been shown to be maximal during pentagastrin-stimulated acid secretion. The presence of prostaglandins in gastric juice and gastric mucosa might facilitate the diverse cytoprotective functions ascribed to these agents in addition to their antisecretory effects. These functions include stimulation of mucus and bicarbonate secretion, enhancement of mucosal blood flow, reduction in mucosal H^+ ion back-diffusion, and stimulation of mucosal cell turnover. Prostaglandins may thus function to mediate mucosal defense.

Conversely, prostaglandin deficiency may predispose to gastric mucosal injury. Cyclooxygenase inhibitors such as aspirin and nonsteroidal anti-inflammatory agents produce a spectrum of mucosal injuries in the stomach. Furthermore, immunization against prostaglandins has been shown to cause ulcers in rabbits.[274,275] Presumably, part of the etiology of these ulcerations is a decrease in prostaglandin-mediated mucosal defense. These observations

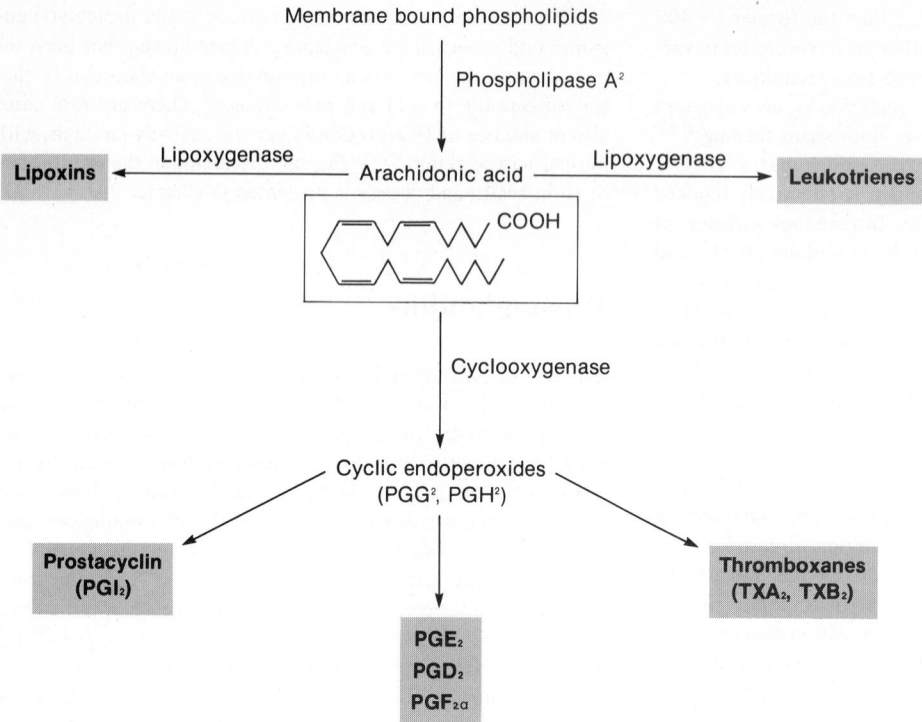

FIGURE 13–10. Pathways of arachidonic acid metabolism.

have served as the basis for the development of prostaglandins for use in treatment of acid/peptic diseases of the stomach, as reviewed in Chapter 61.

CLINICAL IMPLICATIONS OF GASTRIC SECRETION

As detailed above, gastric acid secretion is a well-studied process with a distinguished history involving many of the legendary names in gastrointestinal research, such as Beaumont, Pavlov, and Grossman. There are few bodily functions that have been examined so completely at both in vivo and in vitro levels. The importance of the stomach in processing food and initiating the digestive process is well established. Yet it must be remembered that humans without their stomachs can live normal lives when provided with Vitamin B_{12}. In this light, it is important to place the significance of gastric acid secretion in a clinical perspective.

Disorders Associated with Increased Acid Secretion

Chronic duodenal ulcer disease is the most common disorder associated with increased acid secretion. Feldman and his co-workers have demonstrated, in a large cohort of chronic duodenal ulcer patients, hypersecretion of acid, principally basal acid output.[55] This distinction between chronic duodenal ulcer patients and normal controls was confirmed[63] in 24-hour acid secretion by a combination of interprandial aspiration and postprandial in vivo titration. Basal interprandial acid secretion was higher in duodenal

ulcer patients than in normals, although the postprandial increase in H^+ secretion was of similar magnitude in both groups (Fig 13-11). Acid hypersecretion may thus be a factor in the etiology of chronic duodenal ulcers, because reducing daily acid secretion to normal levels is associated with ulcer healing.[63] This and the observation that duodenal ulcers are rare in achlorhydric subjects is the basis of the often repeated aphorism, "no acid, no ulcer." However, acid hypersecretion is obviously not the sole factor in the pathogenesis of chronic duodenal ulcers. Much attention has been directed toward the integrity of the mucosal barrier in these patients. At present, it is uncertain what role, if any, gastric mucus secretion, prostaglandin generation,[275] and bicarbonate secretion[276] play in the pathogenesis of peptic ulceration.

Zollinger–Ellison syndrome is a disorder in which there is autonomous hypersecretion of gastrin by an islet cell tumor usually situated in the pancreas. As a result, there is gross hypersecretion of acid in the basal state and a poor response to exogenous secretagogues. BAO is usually greater than 15 mmol/hr, and the ratio of BAO to MAO is usually greater than or equal to 0.6. These tests are useful in distinguishing hypergastrinemia due to Zollinger-Ellison syndrome from the more common situation in which serum gastrin levels are elevated as a consequence of achlorhydria.

Retained gastric antrum syndrome is a rare consequence of antrectomy and Billroth II gastrojejunostomy wherein the gastric secretions are directed away from a distal segment of unresected antrum. Because the antral segment is not in contact with the acidic gastric contents, the normal negative feedback loop in which gastrin release is inhibited at low intraluminal pH concentrations is not activated. This results in unrestrained secretion of gastrin and continuous stimulation of acid secretion. Some patients with retained antrum syndrome have recurrent peptic ulceration.

Antral G-cell hyperplasia is a rare disorder in which there is a moderate increase in basal serum gastrin levels but a markedly

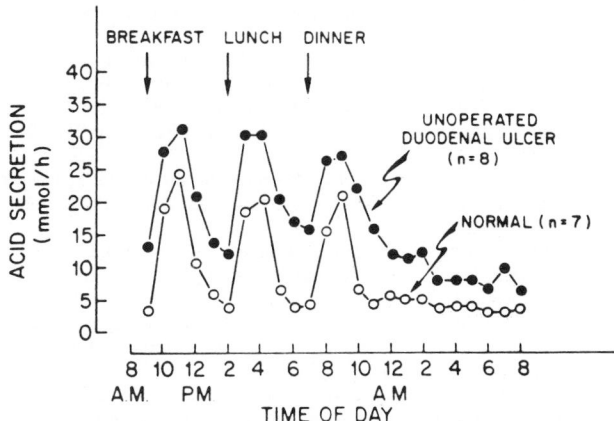

FIGURE 13–11. Mean hourly acid secretion during a 24-hour period in normal subjects and patients with unoperated duodenal ulcer. (From Feldman M, Richardson CT. Total 24-hour gastric acid secretion in patients with duodenal ulcer. Comparison with normal subjects and effects of cimetidine and parietal cell vagotomy. Gastroenterology 1986;90:540.)

excessive gastrin response to ingested food. This disorder is associated with acid hypersecretion and recurrent peptic ulceration.[277] This pattern must be distinguished from that which occurs in Zollinger–Ellison syndrome. Patients with antral G-cell hyperplasia do not have gastrin-secreting tumors. The pathogenetic mechanisms in antral G-cell hyperplasia are unclear and may include an increased density of G-cells and/or an increase in efficacy of the G-cell mass.[278]

Excess production of histamine is an unusual cause of gastric acid hypersecretion. It is found with systemic mastocytosis, foregut carcinoid tumors, and basophilic leukemia. Even rarer causes of significant hypersecretion are extensive resections of the small bowel and raised intracranial pressure.[279,280]

Disorders of Gastric Acid Hyposecretion

The most common hyposecretory disorder is chronic atrophic gastritis. This is accompanied by hypochlorhydria or achlorhydria. Because of the absence of gastric acid, the negative feedback control of gastrin release is interrupted, and these patients have elevated serum gastrin levels, frequently as high as 1000 pg/ml or more.[281] Therefore, such patients may be misdiagnosed, on the basis of hypergastrinemia, as having Zollinger–Ellison syndrome unless acid secretory studies are performed.

Chronic atrophic gastritis is often accompanied by an absence of intrinsic factor secretion. This leads to pernicious anemia, a disease characterized by failure of cobalamin absorption in the terminal ileum and megaloblastic anemia. These patients usually display circulating antibodies to intrinsic factor and parietal cells. Whether these antibodies have an etiopathogenetic role in inducing or maintaining intrinsic factor or acid hyposecretion is unknown, but some evidence suggests that they might.[282,283] There are rare cases, usually among children, of intrinsic factor hyposecretion in the presence of normal acid secretion.[270,271]

Reduced acid and pepsin secretion is often found in patients with gastric ulcers, gastric polyps, and gastric carcinoma. Hyposecretion of gastric acid is common following partial gastrectomy

or vagotomy procedures. A very rare cause of hypochlorhydria is the somatostatinoma syndrome (achlorhydria, diabetes mellitus, fat malabsorption, cholelithiasis), in which an endocrine tumor produces excessive amounts of somatostatin.[284]

Pharmacology of Acid Secretion

The advances in the pharmacology of suppression of acid secretion mirror the advances in physiologic understanding described in the foregoing sections. Pharmaceutical products that interact at almost all the stages of acid secretory regulation are available. Histamine type 2 receptor (H_2) antagonists are the prototypical acid secretory antagonists. These agents reduce but do not abolish stimulated acid secretion. Because of the influence of potentiation described in the foregoing sections, H_2 antagonists are able to reduce acid secretion in response to not only histamine but also pentagastrin and acetylcholine. They are very effective in promoting ulcer healing.

Selective muscarinic receptor antagonists (pirenzepine, telenzepine), the receptor responsible for mediating acetylcholine stimulus-secretion coupling in the parietal cell, are available. Like H_2 receptor antagonists, these agents are inhibitory across a spectrum of secretory stimuli, including pentagastrin, sham feeding, and insulin-induced hypoglycemia. They share similar acid secretory potency with H_2 antagonists and similar clinical efficacy in chronic duodenal ulcer disease also. Clinically useful selective antagonists of the gastrin receptor are not available at the present time.

Prostaglandins of the E and I series selectively inhibit histamine-stimulated parietal cell function in vitro. One mechanism for this effect of prostaglandin E analogues is their interaction with the pertussis toxin–sensitive, guanine nucleotide–binding regulatory protein of adenylate cyclase in the parietal cell basolateral membrane.[273] Prostaglandins of the E series are effective inhibitors of acid secretion in vivo also.[285] This action may also include a component due to prostaglandin-mediated release of somatostatin.[286] In addition, enprostil, a prostaglandin E agonist, inhibits serum gastrin levels.[285]

Direct interference with the parietal cell proton pump is possible with the use of substituted benzimidazoles (omeprazole), which inhibit acid secretion by blocking parietal cell H^+,K^+-ATPase.[287] These agents inhibit the acid secretory effects of all known stimuli.[287] They are the most powerful antisecretory agents available for use in man and are capable of producing an absolute achlorhydria.[288] When compared to cimetidine in patients with duodenal ulcers, they are more effective both in symptom relief and in producing ulcer healing.[289,290] Just as achlorhydria due to chronic atrophic gastritis–pernicious anemia causes a marked hypergastrinemia, so too omeprazole-induced achlorhydria is accompanied by sustained hypergastrinemia. The knowledge that gastrin is a growth-promoting hormone has raised concerns that long-term administration of omeprazole may promote gastric tumor formation, as is reported to occur in patients with pernicious anemia[291] or following gastric surgery for chronic duodenal ulcer.[292,293] Chronic administration of omeprazole in rats is reported to result in the development of gastric carcinoid tumors.[294] Whether chronic use of omeprazole and other H^+,K^+-ATPase inhibitors represents a clinically significant oncogenic risk has yet to be determined.

Somatostatin is a potent inhibitor of acid secretion and gastrin release. However, the naturally occurring 14-amino-acid peptide has a very short half-life in circulation and requires continuous intravenous infusion if it is to be clinically useful. Octreotide, a cyclic bridged octapeptide analogue of somatostatin, has a greatly extended half-life in the circulation and can be administered subcutaneously. It inhibits basal, meal-stimulated, and pentagastrin-stimulated acid secretion in man.[295,296] It has not been studied as a therapy for typical peptic ulcer disease, but its greatest value may be in the management of Zollinger–Ellison syndrome, because it inhibits gastrin release in addition to blocking acid secretion.[296,297]

The reader is directed to Chapter 1, The Enteric Nervous System and its Extrinsic Connections; Chapter 2, Gastrointestinal Hormones; Chapter 3, The Brain–Gut Axis; Chapter 6, Epithelia: Biologic Principles of Organization; Chapter 12, Salivary Secretion; Chapter 14, Secretion and Absorption: Small Intestine and Colon; Chapter 15, Pancreatic Secretion; Chapter 16, Bile Secretion; Chapter 59, Stomach: Anatomy and Structural Anomalies; Chapter 60, Disorders of Gastric Emptying; Chapter 61, Acid–Peptic Disorders; Chapter 62, Zollinger–Ellison Syndrome; Chapter 63, Tumors of the Stomach; Chapter 64, Surgery for Peptic Ulcer Disease; Chapter 65, Miscellaneous Diseases of the Stomach; and Chapter 129, Tests of Gastric and Exocrine Pancreatic Function and Absorption.

REFERENCES

1. Baron JH. The discovery of gastric acid. Gastroenterology 1979;78:1056.
2. Beaumont W. Experiments and observations on the gastric juice and the physiology of digestion. Plattsburgh. FP Allen, 1833. Reprinted in facsimile edition by The Classics of Medicine Library, 1980, Gryphon Editions, Birmingham, AL.
3. Dodds EC, Robertson JD. The origin and occurrence of lactic acid in human gastric contents with special reference to malignant and non-malignant conditions. Q J Med 1930;23:175.
4. Schmidt C. Die verdauungssafte und der stoffwechsel. Mitan U Leipz 1952:44.
5. Pavlov IP. The work of the digestive glands. Thompson WH (trans): London: Charles Griffen, 1902.
6. Bechterew W. Die functioneu der nervencentra. Drittes Heft: hemispharen des grosohirus. Jena: Gustav Fischer 1911. Quoted by Brooks FP. In: Code CF, ed. Central neural control of acid secretion. Handbook of physiology: Alimentary canal (Section 6, Vol II, Secretion). Washington, DC: American Physiological Society, 1967:805.
7. Edkins JS. On the chemical mechanism of gastric secretion. Proc R Soc Lond [Biol] 1905;756:376.
8. Lim RKS. The question of a gastric hormone. Q J Exp Physiol 1922;13:79.
9. Dale HH, Laidlaw PP. The physiological action of β-iminazolyl-ethylamine. J Physiol (Lond) 1910–1911;41:318.
10. Gregory RA. Isolation and chemistry of gastrin. In: Code CF, ed. Handbook of physiology: Alimentary canal. Washington, DC: American Physiological Society, 1967:827.
11. Feng T-P, Hou H-C, Lim RSK. On the mechanism of inhibition of gastric secretion by fat. Chin J Physiol 1929;3:371.
12. Lucey MR, Yamada T. Biochemistry and physiology of gastrointestinal somatostatin. Dig Dis Sci 1989;34(Suppl 1):5.
13. Gillespie IE, Grossman MI. Potentiation between urecholine and gastrin extract and between urecholine and histamine in the stimulations of Heidenhain pouches. Gut 1964;5:71.
14. Soll AH, Amirian DA, Thomas LP, Reedy TJ, Elashoff JD. Gastrin

15. Soll AH. Secretagogue stimulation of [^{14}C]aminopyrine accumulation by isolated canine parietal cells. Am J Physiol 1980;238:G366.
16. Park J, Chiba T, Yamada T. Mechanisms for direct inhibition of canine gastric parietal cells by somatostatin. J Biol Chem 1987;262:14190.
17. Feldman M. Gastric secretion in health and disease. In: Sleisenger MS, Fordtran JS, eds. Gastrointestinal disease, 4th ed. Philadelphia: WB Saunders, 1989:713.
18. Forte JG, Forte TM, Black JA, Okamoto C, Wolosin JM. Correlation of parietal cell structure and function. J Clin Gastroenterol 1983;5(Suppl 1):17.
19. Forte TM, Machen TE, Forte JG. Ultrastructural changes in oxyntic cells associated with secretory function: A membrane-recycling hypothesis. Gastroenterology 1977;73(4):941.
20. Ito S. Functional gastric morphology. In: Johnson LR, ed. Physiology of the gastrointestinal tract, 2nd ed. New York: Raven Press, 1987:817.
21. Matsuyama M, Suzuki H. Differentiation of immature mucous cells into parietal, argyrophil and chief cells in stomach grafts. Science 1970;169:385.
22. Lipkin M. Proliferation and differentiation of normal and diseased gastrointestinal cells. In: Johnson LR, ed. Physiology of the gastrointestinal tract, 2nd ed. New York: Raven Press, 1987:255.
23. Spicer SS, Katsuyama T, Sannes PL. Ultrastructural carbohydrate cytochemistry of gastric epithelium. Histochem J 1978;10:309.
24. Spicer SS, Sun DCH. Part II: The role of the mucous barrier in the defense of the stomach vs. peptic ulceration. Carbohydrate histochemistry of gastric epithelial secretions in dog. Ann NY Acad Sci 1967;140:762.
25. Stevens CE, Leblond CP. Renewal of the mucous cells in the gastric mucosa of the rat. Anat Rec 1953;115:231.
26. Zalewsky CA, Moody FG. Mechanisms of mucous release in exposed canine gastric mucosa. Gastroenterology 1979; 77:719.
27. Grube D, Forssmann WG. Morphology and function of the enteroendocrine cells. Horm Metab Res 1979;11:603.
28. Greider MH, Steinberg V, McGuigan JE. Electron microscopic identification of the gastrin cell of the human antral mucosa by means of immunocytochemistry. Gastroenterology 1972;63:572.
29. Orci L. Morphologic events underlying the secretion of peptide hormones. In: James VHT, ed. Endocrinology, Vol 2. Amsterdam: Excerpta Medica, 1977.
30. Lichtenberger LM, Delansorne R, Graziani LA. Importance of amino acid uptake and decarboxylation in gastrin release from isolated G cells. Nature 1982;295:698.
31. DelValle J, Yamada T. Amino acids and amines stimulate gastrin release from canine antral G-cells via different pathways. J Clin Invest 1990;85:139.
32. Larsson LI, Goltermann N, Demagistris L, Rehfeld JH, Schartz TW. Somatostatin cell processes as pathways for paracrine secretion. Science 1979;205:1393.
33. Soll A, Berglindh T. Physiology of isolated gastric glands and parietal cells: Receptors and effectors regulating function. In: Johnson LR, ed. Physiology of the gastrointestinal tract, 2nd ed. New York: Raven Press, 1987:883.
34. Soll AH, Lewin K, Beaven MA. Isolation of histamine-containing cells from canine fundic mucosa. Gastroenterology 1979;77:1283.
35. Soll AH, Lewin K, Beaven MA. Isolation of histamine-containing cells from rat gastric mucosa: Biochemical and morphologic differences from mast cells. Gastroenterology 1981;80:717.
36. Goyal RK, Crist JR. Neurology of the gut. In: Sleisenger MH, Fordtran JS, eds. Gastrointestinal disease, 4th ed. Philadelphia: WB Saunders, 1989:21.
37. Kuo DC, Krauthamer GM, Yamasaki DS. The organization of visceral sensory neurons in thoracic dorsal root ganglia (DRG) of the cat studied by horseradish peroxidase (HRP) reaction using the cryostat. Brain Res 1981;208:187.
38. Kuo DC, Yang CG, Yamasaki DS, Krauthamer GM. A wide field electron microscopic analysis of the fiber constituents of the major splanchnic nerve in cat. J Comp Neurol 1982;210:49.
39. Guth PH, Leung FW. Physiology of the gastric circulation. In:

Johnson LR, ed. Physiology of the gastrointestinal tract, 2nd ed. New York: Raven Press, 1987:1031.

40. Gannon B, Browning J, O'Brien P, Rogers P. Mucosal microvascular architecture of the fundus and body of human stomach. Gastroenterology 1984;86:866.

41. Cheung LY. Topical effects of 16,16 dimethyl prostaglandin E_2 on gastric blood flow in dogs. Am J Physiol 1980;238:G514.

42. Delaney JP, Grim E. Experimentally induced variations in canine gastric blood flow and its distribution. Am J Physiol 1965;208:353.

43. Holm L, Perry MA. Role of blood flow in gastric acid secretion. Am J Physiol 1988;254:G281.

44. Perry MA, Haedicke GH, Bulkley GB, Kvietys PR, Granger DN. Relationship between acid secretion and blood flow in the canine stomach: Role of oxygen consumption. Gastroenterology 1983;85:529.

45. Jacobson ED, Linford RH, Grossman MI. Gastric secretion in relation to mucosal blood flow studied by a clearance technique. J Clin Invest 1966;45:1.

46. Furness JB. The adrenergic innervation of the vessels supplying and draining the gastrointestinal tract. Z Zellforsch 1971;113:67.

47. Yano S, Fujiwara A, Ozaki Y, Harada M. Gastric blood flow responses to autonomic nerve stimulation and related pharmacological studies in rats. J Pharm Pharmacol 1983;35:641.

48. Reed JD, Sanders DJ, Thorpe V. The effect of splanchnic nerve stimulation on gastric acid secretion and mucosal blood flow in the anesthetized cat. J Physiol (Lond) 1971;214:1.

49. Jansson G, Kampp M, Lundgren O, Martinson J. Studies on the circulation of the stomach. Acta Physiol Scand 1966;68(Suppl 277):91.

50. Ross G. Escape of mesenteric vessels from adrenergic and nonadrenergic vasoconstriction. Am J Physiol 1971;221:1217.

51. Grossman MI. Neural and hormonal stimulation of gastric secretion of acid. In: Code CF, ed. Handbook of physiology: Alimentary canal. Washington, DC: American Physiological Society, 1967:837.

52. Koop H, Willemer S, Steinbech F, et al. Influence of chronic drug-induced achlorhydria by substituted benzimidazoles on the endocrine stomach in rats. Gastroenterology 1987;92:406.

53. Grossman MI, Konturek SJ. Inhibition of acid secretion in dog by metiamide—a histamine antagonist acting on H_2 receptors. Gastroenterology 1974;66:517.

54. Debas HT. Peripheral regulation of gastric acid secretion. In: Johnson LR, ed. Physiology of the gastrointestinal tract, 2nd ed. New York: Raven Press, 1987:931.

55. Blair JA, Feldman M, Barnett C, Walsh JH, Richardson CT. Detailed comparison of basal and food-stimulated gastric acid secretion rates and serum gastrin concentrations in duodenal ulcer patients and normal subjects. J Clin Invest 1987;79:582.

56. Card WI, Marks IN. The relationship between the acid output of the stomach following histamine stimulation and the parietal cell mass. Clin Sci 1960;19:147.

57. Baron JH. Lean body mass, gastric acid and peptic ulcer. Gut 1969;10:637.

58. Feldman M, Richardson CT, Walsh JH. Sex-related differences in gastrointestinal and parietal cell sensitivity to gastrin in healthy human beings. J Clin Invest 1983;71:751.

59. Christie DL, Ament ME. Gastric acid hypersecretion in children with duodenal ulcer. Gastroenterology 1976;71:242.

60. Venzant FR, Alvarez WC, Eusterman CB, Dunn HL, Berkson J. The normal range of gastric acidity from youth to old age. Arch Intern Med 1932;49:343.

61. Fordtran JS, Walsh JH. Gastric acid secretion rate and buffer content of the stomach after eating. Results in normal subjects and in patients with duodenal ulcer. J Clin Invest 1973;72:645.

62. Blair AJ III, Richardson CT, Walsh JH, Feldman M. Variable contribution of gastrin to gastric acid secretion after a meal in humans. Gastroenterology 1987;92:944.

63. Feldman M, Richardson CT. Total 24 hour gastric acid secretion in patients with duodenal ulcer. Comparison with normal subjects and effects of cimetidine and parietal cell vagotomy. Gastroenterology 1986;90:540.

64. Savarino V, Mela GS, Scalabrini P, et al. Twenty-four hour study of intragastric acidity in duodenal ulcer patients and normal subjects using continuous intraluminal pH-metry. Dig Dis Sci 1988;33:1077.

65. Colson RH, Walson BW, Fairclough PD, et al. An accurate, long term, pH-sensitive radiopill for ingestion and implantation. Biotelemetry Patient Monitoring 1981;8:213.

66. Moore JCT, Wolfe M. The relation of plasma gastrin to circadian rhythm of gastric acid secretion in man. Digestion 1973;9:97.

67. Gillespie IE, Clark DH, Kay AW, Tankel HI. Effect of antrectomy vagotomy with gastrojejunostomy and antrectomy with vagotomy on the spontaneous and maximal gastric acid output in man. Gastroenterology 1960;38:361.

68. Melrose AG, Russell RI, Dick A. Gastric mucosal structure and function after vagotomy. Gut 1964;5:546.

69. Tepperman BL, Walsh JH, Preshaw RM. Effect of antral denervation on gastrin release by sham feeding and insulin hypoglycaemia in dogs. Gastroenterology 1972;63:973.

70. Farrell JL. Contributions to the physiology of gastric secretion. The vagi as the sole efferent pathway of the cephalic phase of gastric secretion. Am J Physiol 1928;85:685.

71. Richardson CT, Walsh JH, Cooper KA, Feldman M, Fordtran JS. Studies of the role of cephalic-vagal stimulation in the acid secretory response to eating in normal human subjects. J Clin Invest 1977, 60:435.

72. Feldman M, Richardson CT. Role of thought, sight, smell and taste of food in the cephalic phase of gastric acid secretion in humans. Gastroenterology 1986;90:428.

73. Tache Y. Central nervous system regulation of gastric acid secretion. In: Johnson LR, ed. Physiology of the gastrointestinal tract, 2nd ed. New York: Raven Press 1987:911.

74. Stephans RL, Ishikawa T, Weiner H, Novin D, Tache Y. TRH analogue, RX77368, injected into dorsal vagal complex stimulates gastric secretion in rats. Am J Physiol 1988;254:G639.

75. Shapiro RE, Miselis RR. The central organization of the vagus nerve innervating the stomach of the rat. J Comp Neurol 1985;238:473.

76. Takayama K, Ishirawa N, Mura M. Sites of origin and termination of gastric vagus preganglionic neurons: An HRP study in the rat. J Auton Nerv Syst 1982;6:211.

77. Manaker S, Winokut A, Rostene WH, Rainbow TC. Autoradiographic localization of thyrotropin-releasing hormone receptors in the rat central nervous system. J Neurosci 1985;5:167.

78. Mantyl PW, Hunt SP. Thyrotropin-releasing hormone (TRH) receptors. Localization by light microscopic autoradiography in rat brain using $[^3H][3\text{-}ml\text{-}His^2]$ TRH as the radioligand. J Neurosci 1985;5:551.

79. Tache Y, Goto Y, Hamel D, Pekary A, Novin D. Mechanisms underlying intracisternal TRH-induced stimulation of gastric acid secretion in rats. Regul Pept 1985;13:21.

80. Tache Y, Lesiege D, Vale W, Collu R. Gastric hypersecretion by intracisternal TRH: Dissociation from hypophysiotropic activity and role of central catecholamine. Eur J Pharmacol 1985;107:149.

81. Tache Y, Vale W, Brown M. Thyrotropin-releasing hormone–CNS action to stimulate gastric acid secretion. Nature 1980;287:149.

82. Feldman M, Walsh JH. Acid inhibition of sham feeding–stimulated gastrin release and gastric acid secretion: Effect of atropine. Gastroenterology 1980;78:772.

83. Feldman M, Richardson CT, Taylor IL, Walsh JH. Effect of atropine on vagal release of gastrin and pancreatic polypeptide. J Clin Invest 1979;63:294.

84. Feldman M, Unger RH, Walsh JH. Effect of atropine on plasma gastrin and somatostatin concentrations during sham feeding in man. Regul Pept 1985;12:265.

85. Farooq O, Walsh JH. Atropine enhances serum gastrin responses to insulin in man. Gastroenterology 1975;68:662.

86. Walsh JH, Yalow RS, Berson SA. The effect of atropine on plasma gastrin in response to feeding. Gastroenterology 1971;60:16.

87. Lucey MR, Wass JAH, Fairclough PD, et al. Autonomic regulation of postprandial plasma somatostatin, gastrin and insulin. Gut 1985;26:683.

88. Feldman M, Dickerman RM, McClelland RN, Cooper KA, Walsh JH, Richardson CT. Effect of selective proximal vagotomy on food-stimulated gastric acid secretion and gastrin release in patients with duodenal ulcer. Gastroenterology 1979;76:926.

89. Stadil F, Rehfeld JF. Gastrin response to insulin after selective, highly selective and truncal vagotomy. Gastroenterology 1974;66:7.

90. Walsh JH, Csendes A, Grossman MI. Effect of truncal vagotomy on gastrin release and Heidenhain pouch acid secretion in response to feeding in dogs. Gastroenterology 1972;63:543.

91. Grotzinger U, Bergegardh S, Olbe L. Effect of atropine and proximal gastric vagotomy on the acid response to fundic distension in man. Gut 1977;18:303.

92. Strunz HT, Grossman MI. Effect of intragastric pressure on gastric emptying and secretion. Am J Physiol 1978;235:E552.

93. Soares EC, Zaterka S, Walsh JH. Acid secretion and serum gastrin at graded intragastric pressures in man. Gastroenterology 1977;72:676.

94. Debas HT, Konturek SJ, Walsh JH, Grossman MI. Proof of a pylorooxyntic reflex for stimulation of acid secretion in the dog. Gastroenterology 1974;66:526.

95. Schiller LR, Walsh JH, Feldman M. Distension-induced gastrin release and gastric acid secretion: Effects of luminal acidification and intravenous atropine. Gastroenterology 1980;78:912.

96. Debas HT, Walsh JH, Grossman MI. Evidence of oxyntopyloric reflex for release of antral gastrin. Gastroenterology 1975;68:691.

97. Cooke AR. Potentiation of acid output in man by a distension stimulus. Gastroenterology 1970;58:633.

98. Schoon IM, Olbe L. Inhibitory effect of cimetidine on gastric acid secretion vagally activated by physiological means in duodenal ulcer patients. Gut 1978;19:27.

99. Richardson CT, Walsh JH, Hicks MI, Fordtran JS. Studies on the mechanisms of food-stimulated gastric acid secretion in normal human subjects. J Clin Invest 1976;58:623.

100. Lichtenberger LM, Graziani LA, Dubinsky UP. Importance of dietary amines in meal-induced gastric release. Am J Physiol 1978;243:G341.

101. Feldman M, Walsh J, Wong HC, Richardson CT. Role of gastrin heptadecapeptide in the acid secretory response to amino acids in man. J Clin Invest 1977;61:308.

102. Taylor IL, Byrne WJ, Christie DL, Ament ME, Walsh JH. Effect of individual L-amino acids on gastric acid secretion and serum gastrin and pancreatic polypeptide release in humans. Gastroenterology 1982;83:273.

103. Schubert ML, Makhlouf GM. Regulation of gastrin and somatostatin secretion by intraneural neurones: Effect of nicotinic receptor stimulation with dimethyl-phenylpiperazinium. Gastroenterology 1982;83:626.

104. Harty RF, Franklin PA. Cholinergic mediation of gamma-aminobutyric acid-induced gastrin and somatostatin release from rat antrum. Gastroenterology 1986;91:1221.

105. Sugano K, Park J, Soll AH, Yamada T. Stimulation of gastrin release by bombesin and canine gastrin-releasing peptide. Studies with isolated canine G cells in primary culture. J Clin Invest 1987;79:935.

106. Thirlby RC, Richardson CT, Chew P, et al. Effect of terbutaline, a β2 adrenoceptor agonist, on gastric acid secretion and serum gastrin concentrations in humans. Gastroenterology 1988;95:913.

107. Singer MV, Lehman C, Eysselein VE, Calden H, Goebell H. Action of ethanol and some alcoholic beverages on gastric acid secretion and release of gastrin in humans. Gastroenterology 1987;93:1247.

108. Lenz HJ, Ferrari-Taylor J, Isenberg JI. Wine and five percent ethanol are potent stimulants of gastric acid secretion in humans. Gastroenterology 1983;85:1082.

109. Peterson WL, Barnett C, Walsh JH. Effect of intragastric infusion of ethanol and wine on serum gastrin concentration and gastric acid secretion. Gastroenterology 1986;91:1390.

110. Cano R, Isenberg JI, Grossman MI. Cimetidine inhibits caffeine-stimulated acid secretion in man. Gastroenterology 1976;78:1082.

111. McArthur K, Hogan D, Isenberg JI. Relative stimulatory effects of commonly ingested beverages on gastric acid secretion in humans. Gastroenterology 1982;83:199.

112. Levant JA, Walsh JH, Isenberg JI. Stimulation of gastric secretion and gastrin release by single oral doses of calcium carbonate in man. N Engl J Med 1973;289:555.

113. Konturek SJ, Radecki T, Kwiecien N. Stimuli for intestinal phase of acid secretion in dogs. Am J Physiol 1978;234:E64.

114. Kauffman GL Jr, Grossman MI. Serum gastrin during the intestinal phase of acid secretion in dogs. Gastroenterology 1979;77:26.

115. Debas HT, Slaft G, Grossman MI. Intestinal phase of gastric acid secretion: Augmentation of maximal response of Heidenhain pouch to gastrin and histamine. Gastroenterology 1975;68:691.

116. Isenberg JI, Ippoliti AF, Maxwell V. Perfusion of the proximal small intestine with peptone stimulates gastric acid secretion in man. Gastroenterology 1977;73:746.

117. Gregory RA, Ivy AC. The humoral stimulation of gastric secretion. Q J Exp Physiol 1941;31:111.

118. Isenberg JI, Maxwell V. Amino acids stimulate gastric acid secretion in man. N Engl J Med 1978;298:27.

119. Vagne M, Mutt V. Enterooxyntin: A stimulant of gastric acid secretion extracted from porcine intestine. Scand J Gastroenterol 1980;15:17.

120. Wider MD, Vinik AI, Heldsinger A. Isolation and partial characterization of an enterooxyntin from porcine ileum. Endocrinology 1984;115:1484.

121. Walz DA, Wider MD, Snow JW, Dass C, Desiderio DM. The complete amino acid sequence of porcine gastrotropin, an ileal protein which stimulates gastric acid and pepsinogen secretion. J Biol Chem 1988;263:14189.

122. Gantz I, Northwehr SR, Lucey MR, Sacchetini JE, DelValle J, Banaszak LJ, Gordon JT, Yamada T. Gastrotropin: Not an enterooxyntin but a member of a family of cytoplasmic hydrophobic ligand binding proteins. J Biol Chem 1989;264:20248.

123. Lenz HJ, Klapdor R, Hester SE, et al. Inhibition of gastric acid secretion by brain peptides in the dog. Role of the autonomic nervous system and gastrin. Gastroenterology 1986;91:905.

124. Soon-Shiong P, Debas HT. Pyloro-oxyntic neurohumoral inhibitory reflex of acid secretion. J Surg Res 1980;28:198.

125. Schoon IM, Bergegardh S, Grotzinger U, Olbe L. Evidence for defective inhibition of pentagastrin-stimulated gastric acid secretion by antral distension in the duodenal ulcer patient. Gastroenterology 1978;75:363.

126. Walsh JH, Richardson CT, Fordtran JS. pH dependence of acid secretion and gastrin release in normal and ulcer patients. J Clin Invest 1975;55:462.

127. Schubert ML, Edwards NF, Arimura A, Makhlouf GM. Paracrine regulation of gastric acid secretion by fundic somatostatin. Am J Physiol 1987;252:G485.

128. Schubert ML, Edwards NF, Makhlouf GM. Regulation of gastric somatostatin secretion in mouse by luminal acidity: A local feedback mechanism. Gastroenterology 1988;94:317.

129. Lucey MR, Wass JAH, Rees LH, Dawson AM, Fairclough PD. Relationship between gastric acid and elevated plasma somatostatin immunoreactivity after a mixed meal. Gastroenterology 1989;97:867.

130. Lichtenberger LM, Nelson AA, Graziani LA. Amine trapping: Physical explanation for the inhibitory effect of gastric acidity on postprandial release of gastrin. Gastroenterology 1986;90:1223.

131. Colturi TJ, Unger RH, Feldman M. Role of circulating somatostatin in regulation of gastric acid secretion, gastrin release and islet cell function. Studies in healthy subjects and duodenal ulcer patients. J Clin Invest 1984;74:417.

132. Lucey MR. Letter: Somatostatin as mediator of fat-induced inhibition of gastric functions. Gastroenterology 1988;95:1437.

133. Seal AM, Liu E, Buchan A, Brown J. Immunoneutralization of somatostatin and neurotensin. Effect on gastric acid secretion. Am J Physiol 1988;255:G40.

134. Lucey MR, Fairclough PD, Wass JAH, et al. Response of circulating somatostatin, insulin, gastrin, and GIP to intraduodenal infusion of nutrients in man. Clin Endocrinol 1984;21:209.

135. Mogard MH, Maxwell V, Sytnik B, Walsh JH. Regulation of gastric acid secretion by neurotensin in man. Evidence against a hormonal role. J Clin Invest 1987;80:1064.

136. Yamagishi T, Debas H. Gastric inhibitory polypeptide is not the primary mediator of the enterogastrone action of fat in the dog. Gastroenterology 1980;78:931.

137. Guo YS, Singh P, Gomez G, Greeley GH, Thompson JC. Effect of peptide YY on cephalic, gastric and intestinal phases of gastric acid secretion and a release of gastrointestinal hormones. Gastroenterology 1987;92:1202.

138. Wolfe M, Hocking M, Maico D, McGuigan J. Effects of antibodies

to gastric inhibitory peptide on gastric acid secretion and gastrin release in the dog. Gastroenterology 1983;84:941.

139. Kleibeuker J, Eysselein V, Maxwell V, Walsh JH. Role of endogenous secretin in acid-induced inhibition of human gastric function. J Clin Invest 1984;73:526.

140. You CH, Chey WY. Secretin is an enterogastrone in humans. Dig Dis Sci 1987;32:466.

141. Rangachari PK. Histamine release by gastric stimulants. Nature 1975;253:53.

142. Ekblad EBM, Licko V. Conservative and nonconservative inhibitors of gastric acid secretion. Am J Physiol 1987;253:G359.

143. Harty RF, Maico DG, McGuigan JE. Postreceptor inhibition of antral gastrin release by somatostatin. Gastroenterology 1985;88:675.

144. Wolfe MM, Short GM, McGuigan JE. β-adrenergic stimulation of gastrin release mediated by gastrin-releasing peptide in rat antral mucosa. Regul Pept 1987;17:133.

145. Berglindh T, Obrink KJ. A method for preparing isolated glands from the rabbit gastric mucosa. Acta Physiol Scand 1976;96:150.

146. Soll AH. The actions of secretagogues on oxygen uptake by isolated mammalian parietal cells. J Clin Invest 1978;61:370.

147. McEwen CR, Stallard RW, Juhos ET. Separation of biological particles by centrifugal elutriation. Anal Biochem 1968;23:369.

148. Yamada T. Isolation and primary culture of endocrine cells from canine gastric mucosa. In: Fleischer S, Fleischer B, eds. Methods in enzymology. 1990 (In press)

149. Moody FG. Oxygen consumption during thiocyanate inhibition of gastric acid secretion in dogs. Am J Physiol 1968;215:127.

150. Kowalewski K, Kolodej A. Relation between hydrogen ion secretion and oxygen consumption by ex vivo isolated canine stomach, perfused with homologous blood. Can J Physiol Pharmacol 1972;50:955.

151. Davidson WD, Klein KL, Kurokawa K, Soll AH. Instantaneous and continuous measurement of $^{14}CO_2$ by minute tissue specimens: An ionization chamber method. Metabolism 1981;30:596.

152. Berglindh T, DiBona DR, Ito S, Sachs G. Probes of parietal cell function. Am J Physiol 1980;238:G165.

153. Berglindh T, Helander HF, Obrink KJ. Effects of secretagogues on oxygen consumption, aminopyrine accumulation and morphology in isolated gastric glands. Acta Physiol Scand 1976;97:401.

154. Sanders MJ, Soll AH. Characterization of receptors regulating secretory function in the fundic mucosa. Annu Rev Physiol 1986;48:89.

155. Soll AH. The interaction of histamine with gastrin and carbamoylcholine on oxygen uptake by isolated mammalian parietal cells. J Clin Invest 1978;61:381.

156. Berglindh T. The mammalian gastric parietal cell in vitro. Annu Rev Physiol 1984;46:377.

157. Chiba T, Fisher SK, Junk P, Seguin EB, Agranoff BW, Yamada T. Carbamoylcholine and gastrin induce inositol lipid turnover in canine gastric parietal cells. Am J Physiol 1988;255:G99.

158. Rosenfeld GC. Pirenzepine (LS 519): A weak inhibitor of acid secretion by isolated rat parietal cells. Eur J Pharmacol 1983;86:99.

159. Pfeiffer A, Rochlitz H, Herz A, Paumgartner G. Stimulation of acid secretion and phosphoinositol production by rat parietal cell muscarinic M2 receptors. Am J Physiol 1988;254:G622.

160. Soumarmon A, Cheret AM, Lewin MJM. Localization of gastrin receptors in intact isolated and separated rat fundic cells. Gastroenterology 1977;73:900.

161. Matsumoto M, Park J, Yamada T. Gastrin receptor characterization: Affinity cross-linking of the gastrin receptor on canine gastric parietal cells. Am J Physiol 1987;252:G143.

162. Baldwin GS, Chandler R, Scanlon DB, Weinstock J. Identification of a gastrin binding protein in porcine gastric mucosal membranes by covalent cross-linking with iodinated $gastrin_{2,17}$. J Biol Chem 1986;261:12252.

163. Chiba T, Fisher SK, Agranoff BW, Yamada T. Autoregulation of protein kinase C activity in gastric parietal cells via down-regulation of muscarinic and gastrin receptors. Am J Physiol 1989;256:G356.

164. Park J, DelValle J, Yakabi K, Yamada T. Cross-linking of somatostatin receptors on canine gastric parietal cells (abstr). Biomed Res 1988;9(Suppl 1):93.

165. Soll AH. Specific inhibition by prostaglandins E_2 and I_2 of histamine-stimulated [^{14}C]aminopyrine accumulation and cyclic adenosine monophosphate generation by isolated canine parietal cells. J Clin Invest 1980;65:1222.

166. Tepperman B, Soper B. Prostaglandin E_2-binding sites and cAMP production in porcine fundic mucosa. Am J Physiol 1981;241:313.

167. Beinborn M, Netz S, Staar U, Sewing K-Fr. Enrichment and characterization of specific ^3H-PGE_2 binding sites in the porcine gastric mucosa. Eur J Pharmacol 1988;147:217.

168. Tepperman BL, Soper BD. Subcellular distribution of [^3H]-prostaglandin E_2 binding sites in porcine gastric mucosa. Prostaglandins 1983;25:425.

169. Seidler U, Beinborn M, Sewing K-F. Inhibition of acid formation in rabbit parietal cells by prostaglandins is mediated by the prostaglandin E_2 receptor. Gastroenterology 1989;96:314.

170. Yamada T, Soll AH, Park J, Elashoff J. Autonomic regulation of somatostatin release: Studies with primary cultures of canine fundic mucosal cells. Am J Physiol 1984;247:G567.

171. Soll AH, Toomey M. β-adrenergic and prostanoid inhibition of canine fundic mucosal mast cells. Am J Physiol 1989;256:G727.

172. Soll AH, Amirian DA, Park J, Elashoff JD, Yamada T. Cholecystokinin potently releases somatostatin from canine fundic mucosal cells in short-term culture. Am J Physiol 1985;248:G569.

173. Jain DK, Wolfe MM, McGuigan JE. Functional and anatomical relationships between antral gastrin cells and gastrin-releasing peptide neurons. Histochemistry 1985;82:463.

174. Schubert ML, Saffouri B, Walsh JH, Makhlouf GM. Inhibition of neurally-mediated gastrin secretion by bombesin anti-serum. Am J Physiol 1985;248:G456.

175. Yamada T. Local regulatory actions of gastrointestinal peptides. In: Johnson LR, ed. Physiology of the gastrointestinal tract, 2nd ed. New York: Raven Press, 1987:131.

176. Stryer L, Bourne HR. G proteins: A family of signal transducers. Annu Rev Cell Biol 1986;2:391.

177. Spiegel AM. G proteins in clinical medicine. Hosp Pract 1988;23:93.

178. Majerus PW, Connolly TM, Deckmyn H, Ross TS, Bross TE, Ishii H, Bansal VS, Wilson DB. The metabolism of phosphoinositide-derived messenger molecules. Science 1986;234:1519.

179. Berridge MJ, Irvine RF. Inositol trisphosphate, a novel second messenger in cellular signal transduction. Nature 1984;312:315.

180. Nishizuka Y. The molecular heterogeneity of protein kinase C and its implications for cellular regulation. Nature 1988;334:661.

181. Soll AH, Wollin A. Histamine and cyclic AMP in isolated canine parietal cells. Am J Physiol 1979;237(5):E444.

182. Chew CS. Parietal cell protein kinases. J Biol Chem 1985;260:7540.

183. Chew CS, Brown MR. Histamine increases phosphorylation of 27- and 40-kDa parietal cell proteins. Am J Physiol 1987;253:G823.

184. Negulescu PA, Machen TE. Release and reloading of intracellular Ca stores after cholinergic stimulation of the parietal cell. Am J Physiol 1988;254:C498.

185. Muallem S, Sachs G. Ca^{2+} metabolism during cholinergic stimulation of acid secretion. Am J Physiol 1985;248:G216.

186. DelValle J, Tsunoda Y, Williams JA, Yamada T. Regulation of $[Ca^{2+}]_i$ via secretagogue stimulation of isolated canine parietal cells (abstr). Gastroenterology 1989;95:A118.

187. Yokotani K, DelValle J, Park J, Yamada T. Dual stimulatory and inhibitory actions of gastrin in isolated canine gastric parietal cells (abstr). Gastroenterology 1989;96:A560.

188. Reyl FJ, Lewin MJM. Intracellular receptor for somatostatin in gastric mucosal cells: Decomposition and reconstitution of somatostatin-stimulated phosphoprotein phosphatases. Proc Natl Acad Sci USA 1982;79:978.

189. Hierowski MT, Liebow C, du Sapin K, Schally AV. Stimulation by somatostatin of dephosphorylation of membrane proteins in pancreatic cancer MIA PaCa-2 cell line. FEBS Lett 1985;179:252.

190. Green R, Shields D. Somatostatin discriminates between the intracellular pathways of secretory and membrane proteins. J Cell Biol 1984;99:97.

191. Ito S, Schofield GC. Studies on the depletion and accumulation of microvilli and changes in the tubulovesicular compartment of mouse parietal cells in relation to gastric acid secretion. J Cell Biol 1974;63:364.

192. Vial JD, Garrido J. Actin-like filaments and membrane rearrangement in oxyntic cells. Proc Natl Acad Sci USA 1976;73:4032.

193. Smolka A, Helander HF, Sachs G. Monoclonal antibodies against the gastric $(H^+ + K^+)$-ATPase. Am J Physiol 1984;245:G589.

194. Forte JG, Black JA, Forte TM, Machen TE, Wolosin JM. Ultrastructural changes related to functional activity in gastric oxyntic cells. Am J Physiol 1981;241:G349.

195. Campbell VW, DelValle J, Hawn M, Park J, Yamada T. Carbonic anhydrase II gene expression in isolated canine gastric parietal cells. Am J Physiol 1989;256:G631.

196. Campbell VW, Yamada T. Acid secretagogue-induced stimulation of gastric parietal cell gene expression. J Biol Chem 1989;264:11381.

197. Campbell VW, Yamada T. Regulation of H^+,K^+-ATPase Gene expression in canine gastric parietal cells by omeprazole. Gastroenterology 1988;94:A57.

198. Forte JG, Wolosin JM. HCl secretion by the gastric oxyntic cell. In: Johnson LR, ed. Physiology of the gastrointestinal tract, 2nd ed. New York: Raven Press, 1987:853.

199. Culp DJ, Forte JG. An enriched preparation of basolateral plasma membranes from gastric glandular cells. J Membr Biol 1981;59:135.

200. Kasbekar DK, Gordon GS. Effects of colchicine and vinblastine on in vitro gastric secretion. Am J Physiol 1979;236(5):E550.

201. Ganser AL, Forte JG. K^+-stimulated ATPase in purified microsome of bullfrog oxyntic cells. Biochim Biophys Acta 1973;307:169.

202. Wolosin JM, Forte JG. Stimulation of oxyntic cell triggers K^+ and Cl^- conductances in apical $(H^+ + K^+)$-ATPase membrane. Am J Physiol 1984;246:C537.

203. Sachs G, Chang HH, Rabon E, Schackmann R, Lewin M, Saccomani G. A non-electrogenic H^+ pump in plasma membranes of hog stomach. J Biol Chem 1976;251:7690.

204. Schackmann RA, Schwartz A, Saccomani G, Sachs G. Cation transport by gastric $H^+ + K^+$ ATPase. J Membr Biol 1977;32:361.

205. Sachs G. The gastric proton pump: The H^+, K^+-ATPase. In: Johnson LR, ed. Physiology of the gastrointestinal tract, 2nd ed. New York: Raven Press, 1987:865.

206. Shull GE, Lingrel JB. Molecular cloning of the rat stomach $(H^+ + K^+)$-ATPase. J Biol Chem 1986;261:16788.

207. Langley JN, Edkins JS. Pepsinogen and pepsin. J Physiol (Lond) 1886;7:371.

208. Hersey SJ. Pepsinogen secretion. In: Johnson LR, ed. Physiology of the gastrointestinal tract, 2nd ed. New York: Raven Press, 1987:947.

209. Samloff IM. Pepsinogens, pepsins, and pepsin inhibitors. Gastroenterology 1971;60:586.

210. Sogawa K, Fujii-Kuriyama Y, Mizukami Y, Ichihara Y, Takahashi K. Primary structure of human pepsinogen gene. J Biol Chem 1983;258:5306.

211. Taggart RT, Mohanda TK, Shows TB, Bell GI. Variable numbers of pepsinogen genes are located in the centromeric region of human chromosome 11 and determine the high-frequency electrophoretic polymorphism. Proc Natl Acad Sci USA 1985;82:6240.

212. Sanders MJ, Amirian DA, Ayalon A, Soll AH. Regulation of pepsinogen release from canine chief cells in primary monolayer culture. Am J Physiol 1983;245:G641.

213. Hirschowitz BI, Fong J, Molina E. Effects of pirenzepine and atropine on vagal and cholinergic gastric secretions and gastrin release and on heart rate in the dog. J Pharmacol Exp Ther 1983;225:263.

214. Skak-Nielsen T, Holst JJ, Nielsen OV. Role of gastrin-releasing peptide in the neural control of pepsinogen secretion from the pig stomach. Gastroenterology 1988;95:1216.

215. Koetz HR, Hersey SJ, Sachs G, Chew CS. Pepsinogen release from isolated gastric glands. Am J Physiol 1982;243:G218.

216. Kasbekar DK, Jensen RT, Gardner JD. Pepsinogen secretion from dispersed glands from rabbit stomach. Am J Physiol 1983;244:G392.

217. Berstad A, Petersen H. Dose-response relationship of the effect of secretin on acid and pepsin secretion in man. Scand J Gastroenterol 1970;5:647.

218. Raufman J-P, Kasbekar DK, Jensen RT, Gardner JD. Potentiation of pepsinogen secretion from dispersed glands from rat stomach. Am J Physiol 1983;245:G525.

219. Chew CS, Hersey SJ. Gastrin stimulation of isolated gastric glands. Am J Physiol 1982;242:G504.

220. Samloff IM, Liebman WM. Radioimmunoassay of group I pepsinogens in serum. Gastroenterology 1984;66:494.

221. Samloff IM, Liebman WM. Purification and immunochemical characterization of group II pepsinogens in human seminal fluid. Clin Exp Immunol 1972;11:405.

222. Allen A, Garner A. Mucus and bicarbonate secretion in the stomach and their possible role in mucosal protection. Gut 1980;21:249.

223. Neutra MR, Forstner JF. Gastrointestinal mucus: Synthesis, secretion, and function. In: Johnson LR, ed. Physiology of the gastrointestinal tract, 2nd ed. New York: Raven Press, 1987:975.

224. Carlstedt I, Sheehan JK. Macromolecular properties and polymeric structure of mucus glycoproteins. In: Mucus and mucosa (Ciba Found Symp 109). London: Pitman, 1984:157.

225. Allen A. Structure and function of gastrointestinal mucus. In: Johnson LR, ed. Physiology of the gastrointestinal tract. New York: Raven Press, 1981:617.

226. Gendler SJ, Buchell JM, Duhig T, Lamport D, White R, Parker M, Taylor-Papadimitriou J. Cloning of partial cDNA encoding differentiation and tumor-associated mucin glycoproteins expressed by human mammary epithelium. Proc Natl Acad Sci USA 1987;84:6060.

227. Gendler S, Taylor-Papadimitriou J, Duhig T, Rothbard J, Burchell J. A highly immunogenic region of a human polymorphic epithelial mucin expressed by carcinomas is made up of tandem repeats. J Biol Chem 1988;263:12820.

228. Schachter H. Glycoprotein biosynthesis. In: Horiwitz MI, Pigman W, eds. The glycoconjugate, Vol II. New York: Academic Press, 1978:87.

229. Fouad FM, Waldon-Edward D. Isolation and characterization of human and canine gastric mucosal glycoproteins and their degradation by proteases and acid hydrolases. Hoppe Seylers Z Physiol Chem 1980;361:703.

230. Neutra MR, Leblond CP. Radioautographic comparison of the uptake of galactose-H^3 and glucose-H^3 in the Golgi region of various cells secreting glycoproteins or mucopolysaccharides. J Cell Biol 1966;30:137.

231. Zalewsky CA, Moody FG, Allen M, Davis EK. Stimulation of canine gastric mucus secretion with intra-arterial acetylcholine chloride. Gastroenterology 1983;85:1067.

232. Neutra MR, Phillips TH, Phillips TE. Regulation of intestinal goblet cells in situ, in mucosal explants and in the isolated epithelium. In: Mucus and mucosa (Ciba Found Symp 109). London: Pitman, 1984:20.

233. Qureshi R, Forstner GC, Forstner JF. Radioimmunoassay of human intestinal goblet cell mucin. J Clin Invest 1979;64:1149.

234. Vagne M, Perret G. Regulation of gastric mucus secretion. Scand J Gastroenterol 1976;42:63.

235. Andre C, Lambert R, Descos F. Stimulation of gastric mucous secretions in man by secretin. Digestion 1972;7:284.

236. LaMont JT, Ventola AS, Maull EA, Szabo S. Cysteamine and prostaglandin $F_2\beta$ stimulate rat gastric mucin release. Gastroenterology 1983;84:306.

237. Seidler U, Knafla K, Rownatzki R, Sewing K-Fr. Effects of endogenous and exogenous prostaglandins on glycoprotein synthesis and secretion in isolated rabbit gastric mucosa. Gastroenterology 1988;95:945.

238. Kauffman G, Reeve JJ, Grossman MI. Gastric bicarbonate secretion: Effect of topical and intravenous 16,16-dimethyl-prostaglandin E2. Am J Physiol 1980;239:G44.

239. Roomi N, Laburthe J, Fleming N, Crother R, Forstner J. Cholera-induced mucin secretion from rat intestine: Lack of effect of cAMP, cycloheximide, VIP and colchicine. Am J Physiol 1984;247:G140.

240. Rutten MJ, Ito S. Ca^{2+}-ionophore stimulates mucus release from in vitro guinea pig gastric mucosa (abstr). Fed Proc 1985;44:618.

241. Flemstrom G. Gastric and duodenal mucosal bicarbonate secretion. In: Johnson LR, ed. Physiology of the gastrointestinal tract, 2nd ed. New York: Raven Press, 1987:1011.

242. Sugai N, Ito S. Carbonic anhydrase, ultrastructural localization in the mouse gastric mucosa and improvements in the technique. J Histochem Cytochem 1980;6:511.

243. Flemstrom G. Cl^- dependence of HCO_3^- transport in frog gastric mucosa. Ups J Med Sci 1980;85:303.

244. Mattsson H, Carlsson K, Carlsson E. Omeprazole is devoid of effect on alkaline secretion in isolated guinea pig antral mucosa. In: Allen A, Flemstrom G, Garner A, Silen W, Turnberg LA, eds. Mechanisms of mucosal protection in the upper gastrointestinal tract. New York: Raven Press, 1984:141.

245. Kuo YJ, Shanbour LL, Miller TA. Effects of 16,16-dimethyl prostaglandin E_2 on alkaline secretion in isolated canine gastric mucosa. Dig Dis Sci 1983;12:1121.

246. Machen TE, Silen W, Forte JG. Na^+ transport by mammalian stomach. Am J Physiol 1978;234:E228.

247. Grossman MI. The secretion of the pyloric glands of the dog. 21st Int Cong Physiol Sci 1959:226.

248. Kauffman GL, Reeve JJ, Grossman MI. Gastric bicarbonate secretion: Effect of topical and intravenous 16,16-dimethyl prostaglandin E_2. Am J Physiol 1980;239:G44.

249. Forssell H, Olbe L. Continuous computerized determination of gastric bicarbonate secretion in man. Scand J Gastroenterol 1985;20:767.

250. Feldman M. Gastric bicarbonate secretion in humans. J Clin Invest 1983;72:295.

251. Forssell H, Steinquist B, Olbe L. Vagal stimulation of human gastric bicarbonate secretion. Gastroenterology 1985;89:581.

252. Feldman M. Gastric H^+ and HCO_3^- in response to sham feeding in humans. Am J Physiol 1985;248:G188.

253. Nylander O, Fandriks L, Delbro D, Flemstrom G. Effects of vagal nerve stimulation of gastroduodenal HCO_3^- secretion in the cat in vivo. Acta Physiol Scand 1985;123:30A.

254. Konturek SJ, Bilski J, Tasler J, Laskiewicz J. Gastroduodenal alkaline response to acid and taurocholate in conscious dogs. Am J Physiol 1984;247:G149.

255. Heylings JR, Garner A, Flemstrom G. Regulation of gastroduodenal HCO_3^- transport by luminal acid in the frog in vitro. Am J Physiol 1984;246:G235.

256. Feldman M, Colturi TJ. Effect of indomethacin on gastric acid and bicarbonate secretion in humans. Gastroenterology 1984;87:1339.

257. Castle WB. Observations on the etiologic relationship of achylia gastrica to pernicious anemia. Am J Med Sci 1929;178:748.

258. Levine JS, Nakane PK, Allen RH. Immunocytochemical localization of human intrinsic factor: The non-stimulated stomach. Gastroenterology 1980;79:493.

259. Hoedemaeker PJ, Abels J, Wachters JJ, et al. Investigations about the site of production of Castle's gastric intrinsic factor. Lab Invest 1964;13:1394.

260. Hoedemaeker PJ, Abels J, Wachters JJ, et al. Further investigations about the site of production of Castle's gastric intrinsic factor. Lab Invest 1966;15:1163.

261. Dieckgraefe BK, Seetharam B, Banaszak L, Leykam JF, Alpers DH. Isolation and structural characterization of a cDNA clone encoding rat gastric intrinsic factor. Proc Natl Acad Sci USA 1988;85:46.

262. Jeffries GH, Sleisenger MH. The pharmacology of intrinsic factor secretion in man. Gastroenterology 1965;48:444.

263. Donaldson RM. Intrinsic factor and the transport of cobalamin. In: Johnson LR, ed. Physiology of the gastrointestinal tract, 2nd ed. New York: Raven Press 1987:959.

264. Kittang E, Aadland E, Schjowsby H. Effect of omeprazole on secretin of intrinsic factor, gastric acid and pepsin in man. Gut 1985;26:594.

265. Kittang E, Aadland E, Schjowsby H, Kohss K. The effect of omeprazole on gastric acidity and absorption of liver cobalamins. Scand J Gastroenterol 1987;22:156.

266. Oddsdottier M, Ballantyne GH, Adrien TE, Zdon MJ, Zucker KA, Modlin IM. Somatostatin inhibition of intrinsic factor secretion from isolated guinea pig glands. Scand J Gastroenterol 1987;22:233.

267. Rackoff PJ, Zdon MJ, Tyshkow M, Modlin IM. Epidermal growth factor (EGF) inhibits both intrinsic factor secretion and acid secretion in histamine-stimulated isolated gastric glands. Regul Pept 1988;21:279.

268. Elder JP, Ganguli PC, Gillespie IE, Gerring EL, Gregory H. Effect of urogastrone on gastric secretion and plasma gastrin levels in normal subjects. Gut 1975;16:887.

269. Yang T-M, Ducos R, Rosenberg AJ, et al. Cobalamin malabsorption in three siblings due to abnormal intrinsic factor that is markedly susceptible to acid and proteolysis. J Clin Invest 1985;76:2057.

270. Meeroff JC, Zagalsky D, Meeroff M. Intrinsic factor deficiency in adults with normal hydrochloric acid production. Gastroenterology 1981;80:575.

271. Carmel R. Gastric juice in congenital pernicious anaemia contains no immunoreactive intrinsic factor molecules: Study of three kindreds with variable ages at presentation, including a patient first diagnosed in adulthood. Am J Hum Genet 1983;35:67.

272. Whittle BJR, Vane JR. Prostanoids as regulators of gastrointestinal function. In: Johnson JR, ed. Physiology of the gastrointestinal tract, 2nd ed. New York: Raven Press, 1987:143.

273. Chen MCY, Amirian DA, Toomey M, Sanders MJ, Soll AH. Prostanoid inhibition of canine parietal cells: Mediation by the inhibitory guanosine triphosphate-binding protein of adenylate cyclase. Gastroenterology 1988;94:1121.

274. Olson GA, Leffler CW, Fletcher AM. Gastroduodenal ulceration in rabbits producing antibodies to prostaglandins. Prostaglandins 1985;29:475.

275. Redfern JS, Lee E, Feldman M. Effect of immunization with prostaglandin metabolites on gastrointestinal ulceration. Am J Physiol 1988;255:G723.

276. Feldman M, Barnett CC. Gastric bicarbonate secretion in patients with duodenal ulcer. Gastroenterology 1985;88:1205.

277. Glowniakl JV, Shapiro B, Vinik AI, Glaser B, Thompson NW, Cho KJ. Percutaneous transhepatic venous sampling of gastrin: Values in sporadic and familial islet-cell tumors and G-cell hyperfunction. N Engl J Med 1982;307:293.

278. Lewin KJ, Yang K, Ulich T, Elashoff JD, Walsh J. Primary gastrin cell hyperplasia: Report of five cases and review of the literature. Am J Surg Pathol 1984;8:821.

279. Mulvihill SJ, Pappas TN, Debas HT. Effect of increased intracranial pressure on gastric acid secretion. Am J Surg 1986;151:110.

280. Larson GM, Koch S, O'Dorisio TM, Osadchey B, McGraw P, Richardson JD. Gastric response to severe head injury. Am J Surg 1984;147:97.

281. McGuigan JE, Trudeau WI. Serum gastrin concentrations in pernicious anaemia. N Engl J Med 1970;282:358.

282. De Aizpurua JH, Ungar B, Tok B-H. Serum from patients with pernicious anaemia blocks gastrin stimulation of acid secretion by parietal cells. Clin Exp Immunol 1983;61:315.

283. Burman P, Mardh S, Norberg L, Karlsson FA. Parietal cell antibodies in pernicious anaemia inhibit H^+, K^+ adenosine triphosphatase, the proton pump of the stomach. Gastroenterology 1989;96:1434.

284. Krejs GJ, Orci L, Conlon JM, et al. Somatostatinoma syndrome. Biochemical, morphologic and clinical features. N Engl J Med 1979;301:285.

285. Mahachai V, Walker K, Sevelius H, Thompson ABR. Antisecretory and serum gastrin lowering effect of enprostil in patients with duodenal ulcer disease. Gastroenterology 1985;89:553.

286. Ligumsky M, Goto Y, Debas H, Yamada T. Prostaglandins mediate inhibition of gastric acid secretion by somatostatin in the rat. Science 1983;219:301.

287. Fellenius E, Berglindh T. Substituted benzimidazoles inhibit gastric acid secretion by blocking (H^+,K^+) ATPase. Nature 1981;290:159.

288. Sharma BK, Walt RP, Gomes M de FA, Wood EC, Logan LH. Optimal dose of oral omeprazole for maximal 24 hour decrease of intragastric acidity. Gut 1984;25:957.

289. Lauritsen K, Rune SJ, Bytzer P, et al. Effect of omeprazole and cimetidine on duodenal ulcer. A double blind comparative trial. N Engl J Med 1985;312:958.

290. Archambault AP, Pane P, Baily RJ, et al. Omeprazole (20 mg daily) versus cimetidine (1200 mg daily) in duodenal ulcer healing and pain. Gastroenterology 1988;94:1130.

291. Siurala M, Lehtola J, Ihamaki T. Atrophic gastritis and its sequelae. Scand J Gastroenterol 1974;9:441.

292. Lundegarde G, Adami HO, Helnich C, Zack M, Meirik O. Stomach cancer after partial gastrectomy for benign ulcer disease. N Engl J Med 1988;319:195.

293. Gaygill LPJ, Kirkham JS, Hill MJ, Northfield TC. Mortality from gastric cancer following gastric surgery for peptic ulcer. Lancet 1986;1:929.

294. Ekman L, Hansson E, Havu N, Carlson E, Lundberg C. Toxicological studies on omeprazole. Scand J Gastroenterol (Suppl)1985;108:53.

295. Whitehouse I, Beglinger C, Ruttiman G, Gyr K. Inhibition of pentagastrin-stimulated acid secretion after subcutaneous administration of a new somatostatin-analogue. Gut 1986;27:141.

296. Olsen JA, Loud FB, Christiansen J. Inhibition of meal stimulated gastric acid secretion by an octapeptide somatostatin analogue. SMS201-995. Gut 1987;28:464.

297. Kvols LK, Back M, Moertel CG, et al. Treatment of metastatic islet cell carcinoma with somatostatin analogue (SMS 201-995). Ann Intern Med 1987;107:162.

298. Walsh JH, Grossman MI. Gastrin. N Engl J Med 1975;292:1324.

299. Park J, Chiba T, Yokotani K, DelValle J, Yamada T. Somatostatin receptors on canine fundic D-cells. Evidence for autoregulation of gastric somatostatin. Am J Physiol 1989;257:G235.

300. Walsh JH. Gastrointestinal hormones. In: Johnson LR, ed. Physiology of the gastrointestinal tract, 2nd ed. New York: Raven Press, 1987: 181.

301. Wolfe MM, Reel GM, McGuigan JE. Inhibition of gastrin release by secretin is mediated by somatostatin in cultured rat antral mucosa. J Clin Invest 1983;72:1586.

302. Pederson RA, Brown JC. The inhibition of histamine, pentagastrin, and insulin stimulated gastric secretion by pure gastric inhibitory polypeptide. Gastroenterology 1972;62:393.

303. Wolfe MM, Reel GM. Inhibition of gastrin release by gastric inhibitory peptide is mediated by somatostatin. Am J Physiol 1986;250: G331.

304. Maxwell V, Shulhes A, Brown J, Solomon T, Walsh J. Effect of gastric inhibitory polypeptide on pentagastrin-stimulated acid secretion in man. Dig Dis Sci 1980;25:113.

305. Christiansen J, Holst J, Kalaja E. Inhibition of gastric acid secretion in man by exogenous and endogenous pancreatic glucagon. Gastroenterology 1976;70:688.

306. Peterson B, Christiansen J, Holst J. A glucose-dependent mechanism in jejunum inhibits gastric acid secretion: A response mediated through enteroglucagon? Scand J Gastroenterol 1985;20:193.

307. Dubrasquet M, Bataille D, Gesbach C. Oxyntomodulin (glucagon-37 or bioactive enteroglucagon): A potent inhibitor of pentagastrin-stimulated acid secretion in rats. Biosci Rep 1982;2:391.

308. Kirkegaard P, Moody A, Holst J, Loud F, Olsen F, Christiansen J. Glicentin inhibits gastric secretion in the rat. Nature 1982;297:156.

309. Jarrousse C, Audousset-Puech MP, Dubrasquet M, et al. Oxyntomodulin (glucagon-37) and its C-terminal octapeptide inhibit gastric acid secretion. FEBS Lett 1985;188:81.

310. Berlinger C, Born W, Tildebrand E, et al. Calcitonin gene-related peptides I and II and calcitonin: Distinct effects on gastric acid secretion in humans. Gastroenterology 1988;95:958.

311. Berlinger C, Koehler E, Born W, et al. Effect of calcitonin and calcitonin-gene-related peptide on pancreatic functions in man. Gut 1988;29:243.

312. Woloszcuk W, Reich-Hilscher B, Benke A, Dinstel K. Effect of infusion of salmon calcitonin on the secretion of somatostatin and gastrin in man. Horm Metab Res 1988;18:197.

313. Pappas J, Debas HT, Walsh JH, Rivier J, Tache Y. Calcitonin gene-related peptide-induced selective inhibition of gastric acid secretion in dogs. Am J Physiol 1986;250:G127.

314. Yamatani T, Kadowaki S, Chiba T, et al. Calcitonin gene-related peptide stimulates somatostatin release from isolated perfused rat stomach. Endocrinology 1986;118:2144.

315. Adrien TE, Savage AP, Sagor GR, et al. Effect of peptide YY on gastric pancreatic and biliary function in humans. Gastroenterology 1985;89:494.

316. Guo YS, Fujimura M, Lluis F, Tsong YI, Greeley GH, Thompson JC. Inhibitory action of peptide YY on gastric acid secretion. Am J Physiol 1987;252:G298.

317. Lewis JJ, Goldenring JR, Asher VA, Modlin IM. Effects of epidermal growth factor on signal transduction in rabbit parietal cells. Am J Physiol 1990;258:G476.

318. Hatt JF, Hanson PJ. Inhibition of gastric acid secretion by epidermal growth factor. Effects on cyclic AMP and on prostaglandin production in rat isolated parietal cells. Biochem J 1988;255:789.

319. Marti U, Burweu SH, Jones AL. Biological effects of epidermal growth factor, with emphasis on the gastrointestinal tract and liver: An update. Hepatology 1989;9:126.

320. Todisco A, Park J, Lezoche E, Debas H, Tache Y, Yamada T. Peripheral acid inhibitory action of corticotropin releasing factor: Mediation by nongastric means. Gastroenterology 1987;92:919.

321. Soldain G, Mengozii G, Della Louga A, Luttore L, Martelli F, Brown DR. An analysis of the effects of galanin on gastric acid secretion and plasma levels of gastrin in the dog. Eur J Pharmacol 1988;154: 313.

322. Bauer FE, Zintel Z, Kenney MJ, Calder D, Ghatei MA, Bloom SR. Inhibitory effect of galanin on postprandial gastrointestinal motility and gut hormone release in humans. Gastroenterology 1989;97:260.

323. Polak J, Bloom S, Sullivan SN. Enkephalin-like immunoreactivity in the human gastrointestinal tract. Lancet 1977;1:972.

324. Burks TF, Fox DA, Hirming LD, et al. Regulation of gastrointestinal function by multiple opioid receptors. Life Sci 1988;43:2177.

325. DelValle J, Fras AM, Tatemoto K, Yamada T. Characterization of pancreastatin-like immunoreactivity in porcine gastrointestinal tract. Gastroenterology 1988;94:A95.

326. Lewis JJ, Zdon MJ, Adrien TE, Modlin IM. Pancreastatin, a novel peptide inhibitor of parietal cell secretion. Surgery 1988;104:1031.

327. Koelz HR, Fimmel CJ, Garner A, Mendlein JD, Müller-Lissner SA. The stomach and duodenum. In: Kern F, Blum AL, eds. The gastroenterology annual/3. New York: Elsevier, 1986:28.

328. Feldman M. Acid and gastrin secretion in duodenal ulcer disease. Regul Pept Letter 1989;1:1.

14

Secretion and Absorption: Small Intestine and Colon

KIM E. BARRETT
KIERTISIN DHARMSATHAPHORN

The transport of water and electrolytes is a key function of the intestine and organs that drain into it, such as the liver and pancreas. This chapter focuses on water and electrolyte transport, and regulatory mechanisms of these processes, in the small intestine and colon.

The amount of water present in the intestine is of paramount importance for a variety of processes and accordingly is closely regulated. Digestion and absorption require water to maintain the fluidity of the luminal contents, to serve as a medium bringing digestive enzymes into contact with food particles, and to allow the diffusion of digested nutrients to the epithelial cells where absorption occurs. A large amount of water is secreted by various gastrointestinal organs to facilitate these processes. The daily fluid load varies according to the amount and type of meals taken but is usually about 9 liters, comprised of approximately 2000 ml of oral intake, 1500 ml of saliva, 2500 ml of gastric juice, 500 ml of bile, 1500 ml of pancreatic juice, and 1000 ml from the intestine itself. Most of the secreted fluid is absorbed downstream in association with nutrient absorption; water is also absorbed to follow active electrolyte absorption, the latter mechanism providing the "fine tuning" of the system. By the time a day's intestinal content reaches the colon, it is reduced to only 1500 to 2000 ml by these absorptive processes.[1] Most of this remaining fluid entering the colon is then absorbed, leaving only 100 ml or so to be excreted in the stool.[2] Thus, the intestine has a tremendous capacity for water absorption, although it should be mentioned that the capacity of the intestine to secrete water and electrolytes is at least as great as its capacity to absorb them. The fluid secreted under normal circumstances (1000 ml/day) can be augmented many times in the presence of toxins or endogenous secretagogues. The most dramatic example of this is in cholera, where secretion can amount to 10 to 20 liters of stool water a day.[3] Despite this vast reserve capacity, the intestine appears to have a relatively minor role in the normal physiologic regulation of water, electrolyte, and acid–base homeostasis. The importance of the intestine is more apparent in pathologic conditions that cause an alarming fluid and electrolyte loss. Anatomically, the marked ability of the intestine to secrete and absorb fluid and electrolytes probably results from the massive amplification of its surface area afforded by folds, villi, and microvilli (Fig 14-1).

Notwithstanding the large volumes involved in normal and even abnormal water transport by the intestine, water molecules are moved into and out of the lumen by passive processes. It is electrolytes that are transported by active processes, and therefore their movement plays a central role in the regulation of water absorption and secretion. The actively transported electrolytes cause water to move so that iso-osmolarity between the luminal and tissue compartments is maintained.

In other words, water transport is regulated indirectly by the regulation of electrolyte transport. Active electrolyte transport mechanisms usually drive the absorption (or secretion) of only one electrolyte across the epithelial cells. Each active transport mechanism is a transcellular process and is unidirectional; ions with the opposite charge and water follow the actively transported ion passively and paracellularly through the tight junction. For example, a common mechanism for water secretion in the intestine is in response to active chloride secretion by the crypt epithelial cells.

Electrolyte transport processes, both absorptive and secretory, are regulated by a variety of endogenous and exogenous factors. Endogenous regulatory factors are plentiful and include a broad variety of peptide hormones, neurotransmitters, and products of immunologic effector cells. Bacterial toxins are among the major exogenous factors affecting fluid and electrolyte secretion. Besides these endogenous and exogenous factors that directly affect the epithelial cell, food particles and nonabsorbable substances are also important. They contribute to the osmolarity of the luminal contents and thus affect passive water absorption or secretion by way of the tight junction. When these molecules remain in the intestinal lumen (e.g., lactose in lactase-deficient subjects), they decrease water absorption. The opposite is also true—when molecules are absorbed and leave the lumen, they increase water absorption.

Clinical applications of electrolyte transport physiology are mainly in the management of diarrhea. Knowledge regarding epithelial secretion may also be applicable to cystic fibrosis, a common

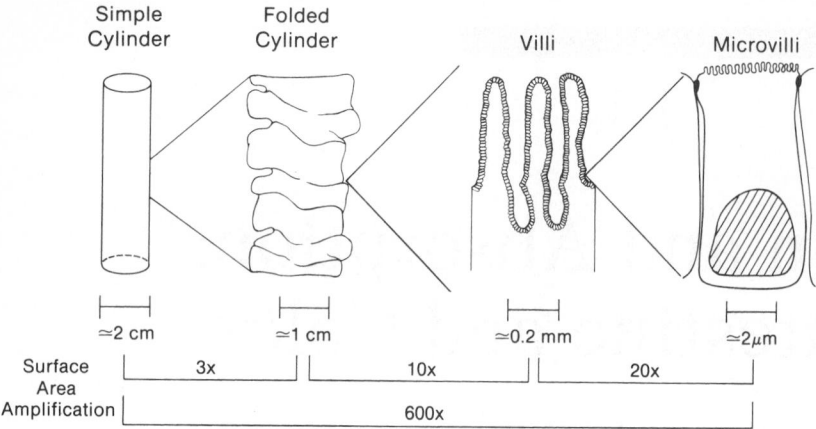

FIGURE 14–1. Amplification of the intestinal surface area by intestinal folds (plicae conniventes), villi, and microvilli. The numbers indicate the factor by which the surface area is amplified over a flat surface. Together, the folds, villi, and microvilli amplify the surface area by approximately 600-fold.

genetic disorder for which a Cl^- secretory defect has been implicated in the pathogenesis.

ANATOMIC CONSIDERATIONS

Epithelial Cells

The anatomy of the intestine provides insight into the complex functions of the epithelium and their regulation. Epithelial cells cover the surface of the gastrointestinal tract. Besides serving as a barrier between luminal and tissue compartments, these cells absorb nutrients, water, and electrolytes from the gut lumen; they also secrete water and electrolytes. The intestinal epithelium renews itself frequently, with the life span of differentiated epithelial cells in the intestine being only 4 to 7 days.[4,5] Analogous to stem cells of hematologic linages in the bone marrow, stem cells in the crypt region differentiate into a variety of cells with different functions, including absorptive cells, secretory cells, mucus-secreting cells (goblet cells), and possibly the endocrine cells that help to regulate the other epithelial cell types. Together, these cells form a continuous sheet of epithelium, under which, in the lamina propria and submucosa, are a number of other cell types, notably immunologic effector cells and nerve cells. The immune cells are quite active. They serve to continuously defend the epithelial barrier, a prominent portal of entry for a number of microorganisms and other antigenic substances. The immune cells may also coordinate defensive functions of the epithelium itself, by stimulation of mucus secretion by goblet cells and electrolyte secretion by crypt cells, for example. The unusually rich network of nerve cells forms the submucosal and myenteric plexuses. This neural network can coordinate the absorptive and secretory functions of epithelial cells in addition to controlling smooth muscle motility. The submucosal and myenteric plexuses function in a fashion that is largely independent of the central nervous system, although there is the potential for central feedback and/or control by way of the vagus nerve and sympathetic or parasympathetic ganglia. Epithelial function is also influenced by the local blood supply and vasculature.

In vivo, most intestinal transport phenomena involve both transcellular and paracellular processes. Therefore, the anatomic basis for transcellular and paracellular processes will be discussed briefly. Transcellular processes are active in nature and involve movement of nutrients or electrolytes across one membrane barrier, through the cell cytosol, and then across the opposite membrane. For nutrients, an absorptive process occurs, with uptake at the microvilli of the apical membrane and discharge on the basolateral, or bloodstream, side. Electrolytes, usually only one type per cell, are either absorbed or secreted, with net movement out of or into the lumen, respectively. The ability of specific epithelial cells to transport selectively and actively just one type of ionic species provides a simple controlling mechanism to drive vectorial transport of water. Once an electrically charged ion is transported across transcellularly, electrical neutrality is maintained by complementary paracellular transport of an oppositely charged ion, occurring by way of the intercellular tight junctions.

Each cell in the intestinal epithelium is linked to its neighbors, close to the apical surface, by structures known as tight junctions. These junctions link the cells together in much the same way as the plastic holder links the cans in a six-pack of beer. At the ultrastructural level, freeze-fracture techniques reveal that the tight junction is composed of a number of roughly parallel strands (Fig 14–2). The resistance of the epithelium to ion and water movement is dependent, among other things, on the number of these strands. In particularly permeable epithelia, the tight junction strand count is low, and the reverse is true for impermeable epithelia.[6–9] Water movement across the gastrointestinal epithelium occurs passively through the tight junction according to the osmotic gradient across the epithelium. Besides water, small molecules of molecular weight less than 300 and electrolytes that are not actively transported can also move through the tight junction. The plasma membrane of the epithelial cell, being a lipid bilayer, provides a barrier to the nonspecific movement of hydrophilic solutes (such as ions) unless specialized transport pathways are present. The tight junction, therefore, is the route for net movement of those substances which are not actively transported (such as water and charged ions that are counter to those being actively transported) to maintain the osmotic and electrical balance.[10–12] Thus, the gastrointestinal epithelium has the properties of a semipermeable membrane, with the tight junctions serving as selective pores. The restricted permeability of the tight junctions allows passive movement of water

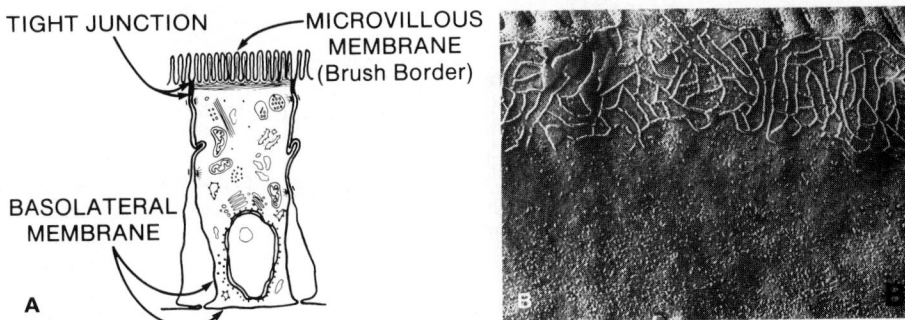

TIGHT JUNCTION — MICROVILLOUS MEMBRANE (Brush Border)

BASOLATERAL MEMBRANE

A

FIGURE 14–2. Tight junctions (occluding junctions). These structures seal the top of each epithelial cell to adjacent cells. **A,** The tight junction is localized to the apical pole of the cell and separates the apical (microvillous) membrane and basolateral membrane. **B,** Freeze fracture replicas of tight junctions on the lateral surface of a villous cell, demonstrating the network of tight junction strands. (Reprinted with permission from Madara J, Trier JR, Neutra MR. Structural changes in the plasma membrane accompanying differentiation of epithelial cells in human and monkey small intestine. Gastroenterology 1980;78:970. Copyright 1980 by The American Gastroenterological Association.)

and small molecules from one side of the epithelium to the other, according to the direction of the osmotic or chemical gradient.

In general, the permeability of tight junctions decreases distally through the intestine. The upper gut is therefore significantly more permeable than the colon to passive movement of fluids and electrolytes.[13,14] Variations of tight junction permeability also exist locally in the same segment of intestine, with the villous region being less permeable than the crypts. Indeed, it appears that most of the passive paracellular movement of water and electrolytes occurs in the crypt.[9] Recent studies have demonstrated that the cytoskeleton of the epithelial cells is somehow connected directly to the tight junction strands; furthermore, the number of strands increases with hypertonicity and is decreased by agents that disrupt the cytoskeleton.[15,16] It is likely, therefore, that tight junction permeability is not static, although the precise factors involved in its regulation are only beginning to be investigated.[17–21]

The intestine has a tremendous reserve capacity for both absorptive and secretory functions, having a surface area in man larger than a doubles tennis court (>200m²). The large surface area of the small intestine is achieved by intestinal folds, villi, and microvilli, as shown in Figure 14-1.[22–24] These structural features amplify the surface area tremendously. Because it does not have villi, the large intestine has a smaller amplification factor than the small intestine. In addition to the anatomic amplification of surface area, the motility of the intestine provides physiologic amplification. Contractions of the intestinal smooth muscle can increase or decrease the rate of flow of the luminal contents to ensure optimal contact time. Therefore, under normal circumstances, deficiency of mucosal absorptive function is rarely observed. On the other hand, the vast reserve capacity allows luminal toxins to cause excessive secretion readily. The absorptive and secretory functions of the intestine are unrelated and have different regulatory mechanisms. Therefore, the absorptive function may remain intact while the secretory function is excessively stimulated by toxins or other secretagogues. The belief that the crypt cells are responsible for secretion while the villous and surface cells are responsible for absorption provides a potential anatomic basis for these distinct functions.[25–29]

Regulatory Cells

Endocrine cells in the crypts, nerve cells in the submucosal and myenteric plexuses, the vagus nerve, and immune cells in the submucosa provide coordinated regulation of epithelial function. The absorptive and secretory functions of the epithelial cells are regulated by a large number of neurohumoral agents released from endocrine cells, nerve endings, and immune cells, as well as several classes of luminally active agents. Neurohumoral regulation can be of paracrine, neurocrine, endocrine, or immune nature, as illustrated in Figure 14-3. The endocrine cells located in the crypt region provide paracrine regulation of the local epithelium in addition to classical endocrine regulation of more distant cells.[30,31] The messengers (neurohumoral substances) contained in these cells are released in response to the luminal environment and relay a signal for coordinated reaction of both local and distant epithelial cells. Many of the messengers stimulate or inhibit electrolyte secretion, while others regulate electrolyte absorption. Neural elements provide neurocrine regulation.[32,33] As in the skin, nerve cells and nerve endings in the gut are in close proximity to the surface lining cells.[34,35] The neurones also innervate intestinal smooth muscle and may have an important role in coordinating epithelial transport with gut motility.[33,36,37] In addition, the central nervous system also plays a role in the regulation of fluid and electrolyte transport by way of the vagus nerve.[38,39] Besides paracrine and neurocrine regulation, endocrine regulation provides distant coordination between different portions of the gastrointestinal tract, or between the gut and other organs. This effect results from the release of peptides or neurotransmitters from endocrine cells and possibly nerve cells into the bloodstream. As stated above, constituents of the luminal content such as bile salts, fatty acids, and microbial toxins may also affect electrolyte transport function by direct actions on epithelial cells. With such a large number of potential regulatory mechanisms for ion transport, the precise physiologic contribution of each factor is difficult to determine and remains largely unclear.

Recently, the ability of cells of the immune system to control electrolyte transport has been investigated. The intestine is a par-

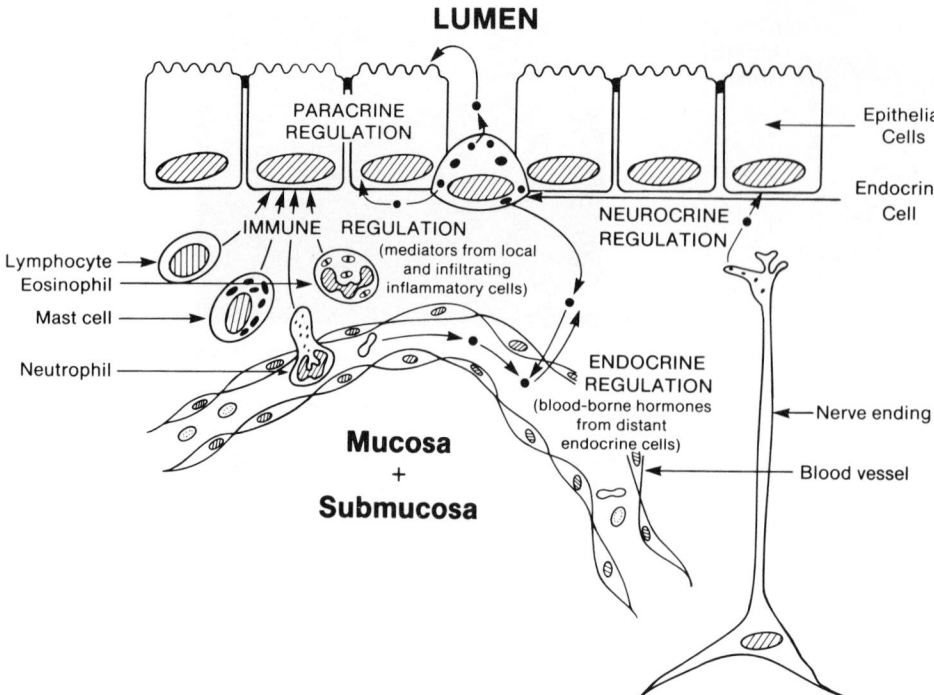

FIGURE 14–3. Neurohumoral and immune regulation of the intestinal epithelium. Endocrine cells in the crypt region release peptides or other substances across their basolateral membranes that regulate electrolyte-transporting cells nearby (paracrine regulation). These substances, or others from distant organs, can also enter the bloodstream to regulate distant parts of the epithelium (endocrine regulation). Nerve cells can release peptides or neurotransmitters from the nerve endings to regulate the epithelial cells or muscle cells (neurocrine regulation). Immunologic effector cells (mast cells, eosinophils, neutrophils, and lymphocytes) in the lamina propria can also be stimulated to release substances that regulate the epithelium (immune regulation).

ticularly rich repository of immunologic effector cells, consistent with its exposure to the external environment.[40,41] The immune system of the intestine, in common with other mucosal sites, has a number of specialized features. For example, IgA-bearing lymphocytes are prominent, and many plasma cells secrete this immunoglobulin. IgA is well suited to function in mucosal immunity in that it has modifications that permit it to be translocated across the epithelium and protect it from proteolytic cleavage in the gut lumen. Mast cells are also abundant in the lamina propria. These so-called mucosal mast cells have a striking morphologic, and possibly functional, association with gut neurons.[42] Neutrophils, eosinophils, and other inflammatory cells are also seen, although these cells may be more prominent in disease states. Although knowledge of how these diverse cell types can affect epithelial function is preliminary at present, findings in this area no doubt will have important implications for inflammatory bowel disease and other infectious or immune-related diseases of the gut. Modulation of such immune-mediated events may provide new therapeutic options. A variety of products released from mast cells, neutrophils, eosinophils, and lymphocytes have been shown to have effects on epithelial electrolyte secretion. Such actions may provide an underlying basis for diarrhea in immune-related diseases.

ELECTROLYTE TRANSPORT PATHWAYS

The preceding discussion has considered the significance of active and passive transport of ions and water across the epithelium as a whole. In this respect, passive transport of a substance occurs by way of the tight junctions (the paracellular route) and only in response to existing transepithelial electrochemical gradients. An active transport process in this setting would be one that requires energy and occurs in a transcellular fashion. We now turn to a discussion of these latter active processes in more detail. In fact, "active" transport of ions across the epithelium as a whole is actually made up of both active and passive processes at the membrane level.

In common with all cell types, the lipid environment of the plasma membrane interior of epithelial cells provides little solubility for charged species such as ions. This is a situation that is vital to life, because the regulation of cellular biochemistry is dependent on the tight control of intracellular ionic composition. Thus, ions are unable to passively diffuse through the lipid portion of the membrane into the cell interior. There are instead specialized proteins inserted into the membrane that can control ion movement in three main ways: active transport, secondary active transport, or passive transport. Again, it should be pointed out that while active transport at the transepithelial level must of necessity involve active transport at the transmembrane level, the former process will also involve secondary active and/or passive processes.

For ionic species, an important passive transmembrane transport process is through membrane pores, more commonly referred to as channels. These membrane-spanning proteins permit bidirectional flow of ions, with the direction of net movement dependent on the existing electrochemical gradient. Ion channels can be acutely regulated by cellular second messengers so that they are in an "open" configuration for a greater proportion of time, and they can display considerable selectivity for specific ions, probably through charged residues and because of steric considerations.

Active transport of ions implies movement against a concentration gradient. Clearly, such movement cannot occur by passive diffusion through membrane pores and therefore requires the input of cellular energy. The active transport pathway most frequently

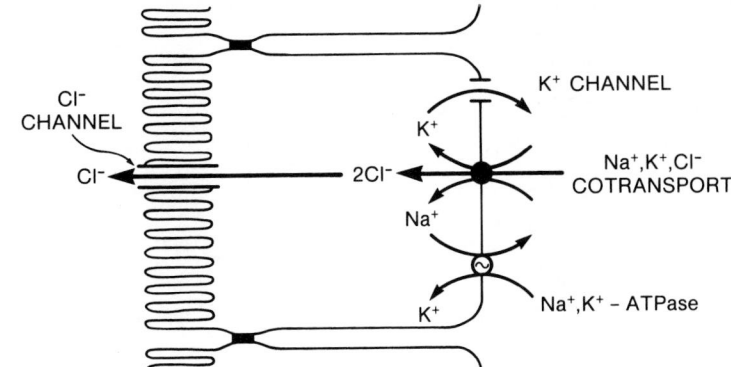

FIGURE 14–4. Chloride secretion. The Na^+,K^+,Cl^- cotransport on the basolateral membrane serves as the Cl^- uptake step with the Na^+,K^+-ATPase pump providing the driving force and recycling the Na^+. Excess K^+ is recycled by way of K^+ channels on the basolateral membrane, and chloride exits by way of a Cl^- channel on the apical membrane. Regulation of the Cl^- secretory process is at the level of the Cl^- channels and/or K^+ channels.

involved in epithelial ion transport is the Na^+,K^+-ATPase, which uses the energy from ATP hydrolysis to pump sodium ions out of the cell and potassium ions in. This pump is present in all cell membranes but, as will be discussed in more detail below, is expressed only on one side of polarized epithelia, permitting vectorial transport of solutes.

Finally, there is a type of transmembrane transport process that is passive in and of itself but operationally is a mix of active and passive processes. Such transport is referred to as secondary active transport because it takes advantage of the ionic gradients established by the active pumps to transport some ions, or other solutes, against a concentration gradient. This is achieved without the further input of metabolic energy because the transport of the energetically unfavored ion is linked to that of a species for which a large promoting concentration gradient exists. The proteins responsible for this linked transport are known as cotransporters and exchangers (or symports and antiports). An excellent example of a cotransport system is the Na^+-glucose cotransporter that is present in the apical membrane of small intestinal epithelial cells. This transporter moves glucose into the cell, against its concentration gradient, by taking advantage of the low intracellular sodium concentration established by the Na^+,K^+-ATPase. Thus, while the transport of the combination of sodium and glucose is itself passive, it relies secondarily on an active transport process.

At this point, some terms that will be used extensively should be defined. The term "transport mechanism" will be used in this chapter to refer to an active transport process that enables ions to move across the intestinal epithelium transcellularly. The term "transport pathway" refers to the specific membrane elements

that act as carriers, channels, or pumps in the cell membrane; "transport pathways" enable ions to move across the plasma membranes of an epithelial cell. Hence, "transport mechanisms" are comprised of a number of "transport pathways." In epithelial cells, each of these transport pathways is usually localized to only the apical or the basolateral membrane. This asymmetric sorting of the pathways provides for the vectorial nature of overall ion movement. It should be pointed out that similar electrolyte transport pathways and transport mechanisms may be shared by epithelial cells in many organs. This is particularly true for the gastrointestinal tract (including the stomach,[43] biliary tract,[44-46] and pancreas[47-49]), the kidney,[50] the respiratory tract,[51-55] the choroid plexus,[56-59] the sweat gland,[60-63] inner ear tissues,[64] and tissues of the eye.[65-67] Consequently, knowledge acquired from one cell system may be applicable to others.

In general, each active transport mechanism requires the participation of at least three transport pathways: an uptake step across one plasma membrane, an exit step across the other plasma membrane, and a pump that provides the energy. In the case in which the pump also serves as an uptake or exit step, only two transport pathways are required. The transport pathways constituting a number of intestinal transport mechanisms are shown in diagrammatic form in Figures 14-4 through 14-6. The various transport pathways present in a cell may also be called upon to maintain cellular volume and cytosolic water and ion concentrations.[68,69] One may consider an absorptive or secretory mechanism as a specialized function possessed by the epithelial cells. To exhibit a specialized transport mechanism, an epithelial cell must possess every electrolyte transport pathway required for the transport

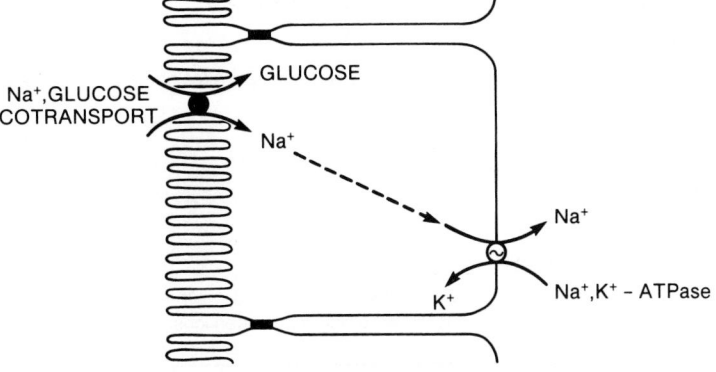

FIGURE 14–5. Na^+ and glucose absorption. A Na^+, glucose cotransport carrier on the apical membrane serves to bring glucose and Na^+ into the cell. Sodium is then pumped out by way of the Na^+,K^+-ATPase; glucose proceeds across the basolateral membrane by way of a specific facilitated transport carrier. Similar Na^+ cotransport mechanisms also exist for many amino acids, dipeptides, tripeptides, certain B vitamins, and bile salts.

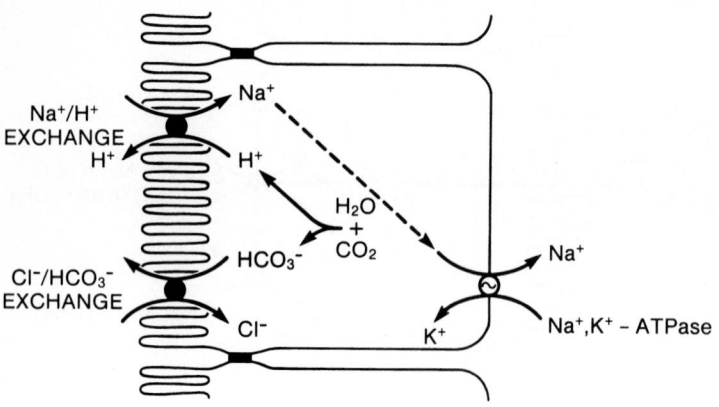

FIGURE 14–6. Electroneutral NaCl absorption. At the present, it is suggested that the electroneutral NaCl cotransport mechanism in the intestine results from a dual exchange system comprised of an Na^+/H^+ exchange and a Cl^-/HCO_3^- exchange working in concert. These exchange carriers serve to bring Na^+ and Cl^- across the apical membrane into the cell. Sodium is then pumped out by way of the Na^+,K^+-ATPase, with Cl^- following by way of an as-yet-unidentified Cl^- transport pathway.

process. Because most electrolyte transport pathways have been identified only recently, less is known about them than about the physiology of the overall transport mechanisms. At present, the participation of transport pathways in a large number of transport mechanisms is still being investigated. However, advances in experimental techniques, particularly the use of membrane vesicles, cultured cell lines, and patch clamp techniques, have allowed rapid progress in this area. An increasing number of pumps, carriers, and channels are being identified by these physiologic techniques.[70] Meanwhile, significant progress has also been made in the biochemical identification of the membrane proteins that serve as transport pathways.[71,72] Biochemical identification is important because it provides direct verification of the existence of a transport pathway, while verification by physiologic techniques is indirect. Furthermore, biochemical identification is a necessary step that paves the way for future studies of genetic regulation. The electrolyte transport pathways known to exist in gastrointestinal epithelia are summarized in Table 14-1, together with their possible participation in an absorptive or a secretory mechanism. Evidence that these transport pathways are regulated by peptides or neurotransmitters is accumulating rapidly and is providing important insight into the regulation of various transport mechanisms. Short-

TABLE 14–1
Electrolyte Transport Pathways, Their Participation in Transport Mechanisms, and Their Regulation

TRANSPORT PATHWAY	TRANSPORT MECHANISM IN WHICH THE PATHWAY PARTICIPATES	ENDOGENOUS REGULATION	REFERENCES
Transcellular Pathways			
Pumps			
Na^+, K^+-ATPase	All active transport mechanisms	Aldosterone or corticosteroid by affecting synthesis and insertion of the pump	76, 368
Ca^{++} and Mg^{++}-ATPases	Cellular handling of Ca^{++} and Mg^{++}	Unknown	73, 75
Carriers			
Na^+/H^+ exchange	Electroneutral NaCl absorption	Endogenous regulators that increase Ca^{++}-calmodulin	112, 369–375
Cl^-/HCO_3^- exchange	Electroneutral NaCl absorption and HCO_3^- secretion	Endogenous regulators that increase Ca^{++}-calmodulin	114, 115, 137
Na^+, K^+, Cl^- cotransport	Cl^- secretion	Unknown	108, 109, 376–378
Na^+, glucose cotransport	Glucose and Na^+ absorption	Unknown	91–97
Other Na^+ cotransports	Absorption of other nutrients	Unknown	102–107
Channels			
Na^+ channel	Electrogenic Na^+ absorption (colon only)	Aldosterone by increasing synthesis and insertion of the channel	119, 121, 379–383
Cl^- channel	Cl^- secretion	Endogenous regulators that increase cyclic AMP or cyclic GMP	384–388
K^+ channel	Cl^- secretion and possibly K^+ absorption and secretion	Endogenous regulators that increase cyclic AMP and cytosolic free Ca^{++}	134, 155, 389–393
Paracellular Pathways			
Tight junction	Allows oppositely charged ion and water to follow actively transported ions	Unknown, involves regulation of cytoskeleton	6, 17–21, 302–304

term regulation can be directed at pumps, carriers, or channels that participate in a given transport mechanism. In the longer term, cells can also adjust their transport capacity by increasing or decreasing the number of pumps, carriers, or channels, as well as receptors for the hormones that regulate those pathways, on the plasma membrane. Regulation of channels, because of the large capacity of these pathways as discussed below, is usually required for immediate or short-term adjustment. The discussion to follow will deal first with the properties of different types of transport pathways. Subsequently, this chapter will review how the arrangement of these transport pathways enables different portions of the gastrointestinal tract to carry out their specialized functions, and how such pathways are regulated.

Properties of Pumps, Carriers, and Channels

ATPase PUMPS

For active transport to occur, a pump is required to provide the necessary driving force for ion movement. In mammalian cells, ATPases appear to serve this energy-providing step. Among the ATPases, the Na^+,K^+-ATPase is the best understood, but other ATPases, such as the K^+,H^+-ATPase and Ca^{2+}- and Mg^{2+}-ATPase, have also been described.[73-76] In intestinal epithelial cells, the Na^+,K^+-ATPase pumps are localized basolaterally.[77,78] In the presence of Mg^{2+}, the Na^+,K^+-ATPase pump catalyzes outward movement of three Na^+ ions and inward movement of two K^+ ions at the expense of one ATP molecule per cycle.[76,79] Since more cation is pumped out than is replaced, a negative electrical potential is maintained intracellularly; the action of this ATPase pump also maintains a relatively low intracellular Na^+ concentration. Thus, the pump creates an electrochemical gradient favoring Na^+ influx by way of either Na^+ channels or the cotransport and exchange carriers for which Na^+ is required (Figs 14-4 through 14-6). The role of the Na^+,K^+-ATPase pump in active transport of nutrients and electrolytes has been well characterized. Most, if not all, active transport processes require the activity of this pump. This is supported by the fact that cardiac glycosides such as ouabain, which inactivate the pump, also inhibit every active transport mechanism currently known to exist in the intestine. Recently, two subunits of the Na^+,K^+-ATPase, alpha and beta, have been identified and biochemically characterized. Monoclonal antibodies have been developed against these subunits and may provide useful insight into their regulation, including that of synthesis of this important pump and its insertion into the basolateral membrane.[72,80-82]

Another ATPase pump that has received substantial attention is the K^+,H^+-ATPase pump.[74,83] It is present on the parietal cells of the gastric mucosa. Similar H^+-ATPase pumps have also been found in other acid-secreting epithelia and cellular organelles.[84-87] The pump has critical importance in H^+ secretory mechanisms in the stomach and kidney, but a role for it in the intestine has yet to be clarified. Other ATPases, including a number of Ca^{2+}- and Mg^{2+}-ATPases, are distributed on the membrane of cellular organelles as well as on the plasma membrane.[73,75] These ATPases are important in the regulation of cellular Ca^{2+} and Mg^{2+} distribution.

CARRIERS

A carrier is defined as either a cotransport carrier, also called a symport, or an exchange carrier, also called an antiport.[88,89] In the case of a cotransport carrier, the carrier protein binds to ions or other molecules on one side of the plasma membrane and shuttles them across to the other. In the case of an exchange carrier, an ion is transported in exchange for another ion (of the same electrical charge) on the opposite side of the plasma membrane. Even with a limited number of ATPase pumps, diversity of active transport mechanisms is possible because a large number of carriers serve to convert the energy provided by the pump into specialized functions. Because the carriers are integral parts of active transport mechanisms, they are called secondary active transport pathways. By themselves, these carriers are best described as facilitated transport pathways that allow certain ions to move across the plasma membrane faster than could be expected by simple diffusion along the existing electrochemical gradient. In sharp contrast with the pumps, which drive movement of a given ion across the plasma membrane in only one direction, the carriers are able to catalyze ion movement in both directions. The direction of movement depends on the existing electrochemical gradient. For a cotransport mechanism, the net chemical gradient is established by the concentrations of the molecules involved on each side of the membrane. For example, in the case of the Na^+-glucose cotransporter, the effective gradient can be calculated as the difference between the product of sodium and glucose concentrations on either side of the membrane. Therefore, by coupling the transport of the needed molecule, glucose, to that of Na^+, it is possible for the cell to move a desired molecule against its own chemical gradient and effectively use the energy provided by the Na^+,K^+-ATPase pump for this purpose. Accordingly, there are a large number of cotransport mechanisms that include Na^+, taking advantage of the favorable Na^+ gradient set up by the Na^+,K^+-ATPase pump.

The cotransport carriers or symports are major transport pathways for absorption of a wide variety of both nutrients and electrolytes by the intestine.[90] Of the nutrient-related carriers, the Na^+-glucose cotransport carrier has been studied most extensively (Fig 14-5).[91-98] In fact, the Na^+-glucose cotransport carrier is one of the few epithelial transport pathways that have been characterized biochemically.[99] The primary role of the Na^+-glucose cotransporter is nutrient absorption, but the process also brings in Na^+ and water and promotes positive electrolyte and water balance.[100,101] Besides glucose, many other food-derived products, including many amino acids, di- and tripeptides, vitamins, bile salts, and so forth, are taken up by cotransport mechanisms in association with Na^+.[93,102-107] Each mechanism involves a different and specific carrier protein. Intestinal cotransport carriers that deal only with electrolytes also exist.[108] Among these is the Na^+,K^+,Cl^- cotransport carrier, which participates in the Cl^- secretory mechanism (Fig 14-4).[109,110] Other cotransport pathways, such as a K^+,Cl^- cotransporter, have been postulated, but at the present time it is unclear what role they may play in the gut.[111]

The exchange carriers or antiports serve to carry a needed ion into the cell in exchange for a readily available intracellular ion. There are two major exchange carriers in the intestine, the Na^+/H^+ exchange[112,113] and Cl^-/HCO_3^- exchange pathways.[114,115] They are coupled in a so-called electroneutral NaCl absorptive process. The exchanges make good sense, because these pathways effectively exchange the waste product of respiration, CO_2 (which in the presence of carbonic anhydrase forms H^+ and HCO_3^-), for Na^+ and Cl^- (Fig 14-6). An exchange carrier that may be important for cellular Ca^{2+} homeostasis mediates Na^+/Ca^{2+} exchange.[116] This carrier moves Ca^{2+} out of the cells and keeps the intracellular Ca^{2+} concentration a few orders of magnitude lower than that usually found in the extracellular compartment.

CHANNELS

Ionic channels serve a similar but distinct function from that of carriers. While both systems are integral parts of transport mechanisms, the channel is a high flow system that is capable of moving a large number of ions rapidly. It also catalyzes the movement of only one kind of electrolyte.[117,118] When open, it allows large numbers of a selected ion to flow downstream according to the existing electrochemical gradient. The carrier system, on the other hand, moves smaller numbers of molecules, but it can do so against a chemical gradient as discussed above. One can compare a channel to a gate. Each channel on the plasma membrane, when open, allows 10^6 to 10^8 ions to move across per second. Because of its large capacity, the physicochemical characteristics of a channel approach those of a passive diffusion system that is not saturable. Also because of their capacity, ionic channels are probably the most important transport pathways for electrolytes. It is likely that the immediate actions of many peptides or neurotransmitters are the result of the opening or closing of ionic channels. Longer term regulation by neurohumoral agents can be achieved by altering the number of channels inserted in the membrane.[119-121] At the present time, the body of knowledge regarding ionic channels in the gastrointestinal tract is relatively small. However, the patch clamp technique, which is capable of detecting the opening and closing of single ion channels, is expected to expand information in this area rapidly. Specific ionic channels for Na^+, Cl^-, K^+, and Ca^{2+} have been described and will be reviewed briefly.

The existence of sodium channels has been known for some time. This has meant that these channels have been investigated more extensively than the others mentioned. There are at least two types of Na^+ channels, one of which functions in colonic and other epithelial Na^+ absorption, and another that serves as the acetylcholine receptor. The former Na^+ channel can be regulated by aldosterone and blocked by amiloride.[121,122] Many studies of this Na^+ channel prior to the availability of the patch clamp technique were indirect, using amiloride sensitivity as an indicator. The biochemistry of both types of Na^+ channel has recently been elucidated.[72,123-130] Indeed, for the acetylcholine receptor, the protein sequence, tertiary structure, and the regulatory structural gene have been identified.

Chloride channels have not yet been as well investigated. Their existence has been confirmed on the apical membrane of intestinal and other epithelial cells by the patch clamp technique. Patch clamp studies also suggest the presence of more than one type of Cl^- channel, one of which can be regulated by the cellular level of the nucleotide cyclic AMP.[131] The search for potent and specific blockers of Cl^- channels is currently in progress.[132,133] Once available, these Cl^- channel blockers may facilitate our understanding of electrolyte transport physiology. More important, they may have useful clinical applications, as discussed below.

Substantial evidence is available to confirm the existence of multiple K^+ channels in the gastrointestinal tract and their in-

volvement in the Cl^- secretory process (Fig 14-4).[134] K^+ channels are also likely to be involved in active K^+ absorption or secretion. At least two types of K^+ channels, one regulated by intracellular cAMP and another by Ca^{2+}-dependent effectors, are thought to be localized to the basolateral membrane of mucosal epithelial cells.[134] Their existence may soon be verified by patch clamp techniques, although technical difficulties with this approach exist because of their basolateral localization as opposed to the apical localization of chloride channels.

Lastly, the ability of Ca^{2+} channel blockers to inhibit certain secretory mechanisms in the intestine has provided suggestive evidence for the existence of Ca^{2+} channels in intestinal epithelia. Ca^{2+} transport in the intestine is relatively complex, and certain mechanisms attributed to Ca^{2+} channels may actually involve the Na^+/Ca^{2+} exchange carriers or a Ca^{2+}-ATPase. As is true for other ionic channels, definition of the precise role of Ca^{2+} channels in the intestine awaits further investigation with the patch clamp technique.

OTHER TRANSPORT PATHWAYS

Transport pathways for other ions, such as bicarbonate, sulfate, phosphate, organic ions, and divalent cations, are poorly defined, although on theoretical grounds they undoubtedly exist.[135-144] For bicarbonate, there may exist an HCO_3^- channel and an Na^+/HCO_3^- cotransport in addition to the Cl^-/HCO_3^- exchange carrier, and specific transport pathways for sulfate and phosphate have also been postulated. Discussion of these less well characterized pathways is, however, beyond the scope of this chapter.

ELECTROLYTE TRANSPORT MECHANISMS IN THE GASTROINTESTINAL TRACT

The preceding section dealt with the electrolyte transport pathways that serve as basic building blocks for electrolyte transport mechanisms. This section will discuss each major transport mechanism in the intestinal tract individually. Table 14-2 provides an overall view of electrolyte transport mechanisms in the small and large intestines. Transport functions exhibited by the intestinal tract are diverse. This diversity accommodates absorption of a broad range of nutrients and maintains proper amounts of fluid in the gut lumen. The small intestine is responsible for most of the absorption of nutrients and water. When needed, the intestine can absorb more water by delaying intestinal transit.

In contrast to the small intestine, the large intestine of man does not play a major role in absorbing nutrients but rather is important for the conservation of fluid and electrolytes. The colon actively absorbs most of the fluid and electrolytes presented to it.[145,146] Similar to the small intestine, the colon has a large secretory capacity that can be stimulated by luminal toxins or endogenous hormones. The colon can also absorb short-chain fatty acids that are produced by bacterial catabolism of unabsorbed carbohydrates. These nutrients may often account for up to 10% of the ingested calories.[147,148] Because the small and large intestines share a number of transport mechanisms, the discussion to follow is divided into secretory and absorptive mechanisms to minimize repetition.

TABLE 14–2
Electrolyte Transport Mechanisms and Their Distribution Along the Intestinal Tract

MAJOR TRANSPORT MECHANISMS	PATHOLOGIC CONDITION(S)*	DISEASES†
Small Intestine		
HCO_3^- secretion (mainly in proximal duodenum)	Decreased HCO_3^- secretion	Duodenal ulcer
Absorption of glucose and other nutrients in symport with Na^+	Decreased nutrient absorption	Osmotic diarrhea
Electroneutral NaCl absorption	Decreased NaCl absorption	Infectious diarrhea or other secretory diarrhea
Cl^- secretion	Excessive Cl^- secretion	Infectious diarrhea or other secretory diarrhea
Absorption of bile in symport with Na^+ (terminal ileum only)	Malabsorption of bile salts	Bile salt–induced diarrhea
Large Intestine		
Electrogenic Na^+ absorption	Decreased Na^+ absorption	Secretory diarrhea
Electroneutral NaCl absorption	Decreased NaCl absorption	Infectious diarrhea or other secretory diarrhea
Short-chain fatty acid absorption	Unknown	Unknown
Cl^- (and HCO_3^-) secretion	Excessive secretion	Infectious diarrhea or other secretory diarrhea

* *Pathologic conditions related to malfunction of the indicated transport mechanism, which may be either a decrease or increase in its activity.*
† *Diseases that may result from the pathologic condition noted.*

Secretory Mechanisms

Secretory mechanisms throughout the gastrointestinal tract center around the Cl^- ion. Hydrochloric acid is the major secretory product of the stomach. In other parts of the intestinal tract, the predominant ion secreted is either Cl^- or HCO_3^-.[135,145,149–151] Secretion of the latter ion may be related to and require the active secretion of Cl^-, as discussed below.[152–154]

INTESTINAL Cl^- SECRETION (ELECTROGENIC Cl^- SECRETION)

The components of the Cl^- secretory mechanism have been established reasonably well (Fig 14–4). The transcellular process is called electrogenic Cl^- secretion because the anion Cl^- is secreted by the intestinal epithelium without the active transport of an accompanying cation and without involving exchange with another anion. In the Cl^- secretory process, the cell takes up Cl^- from the bloodstream across the basolateral membrane by way of the Na^+,K^+,Cl^- cotransport pathway.[109,110] The Na^+,K^+-ATPase provides energy for this mechanism and recycles Na^+ while K^+ channels on the basolateral membrane allow for K^+ recycling.[110,155] Cl^- accumulates intracellularly above its electrochemical equilibrium. When Cl^- channels, which are normally closed, are opened, Cl^- can then exit across the apical membrane. In this secretory mechanism, the Cl^- ion is secreted actively and transcellularly, with Na^+, K^+, and water following passively by way of the tight junction. The sites of regulation by the intracellular messengers, cyclic AMP, cyclic GMP, and Ca^{2+}-dependent effectors, are at the Cl^- and/or K^+ channels.[110,155–157]

INTESTINAL HCO_3^- SECRETION

HCO_3^- is the predominant ion secreted by the biliary and pancreatic duct.[158–162] Recently, the importance of an HCO_3^- secretory mechanism in the proximal duodenum has been recognized. HCO_3^- secretion in these regions of the gut is important because of its possible role in mucosal defense against peptic ulcer formation (by way of H^+ ion neutralization).[163–167] Bicarbonate secretion is also important in other parts of the intestine.[149,168] The upper small intestine secretes more HCO_3^- than the lower portion. However, because of the acid load from the stomach, HCO_3^- is neutralized and free HCO_3^- content in the upper intestinal lumen is relatively low. Bicarbonate gradually becomes the predominant anion of the luminal content in the lower gut as a means to conserve Cl^- by way of the Cl^-/HCO_3^- exchange carrier.[152,153] At the present time, HCO_3^- secretory mechanisms have not been fully elucidated, and more than one mechanism may exist.[136] HCO_3^- secretion may occur by way of the Cl^-/HCO_3^- exchange carrier with the Cl^- secretory mechanism providing the intraluminal Cl^- for exchange.[154] Alternatively, HCO_3^- may be secreted across an apical membrane HCO_3^- channel, as postulated by some investigators. HCO_3^- could be either produced intracellularly by the action of carbonic anhydrase or possibly transported from the bloodstream by way of a carrier-mediated process. Other mechanisms for HCO_3^- secretion by the gastrointestinal epithelium that do not involve the Cl^-/HCO_3^- exchange pathway are likely, but they have yet to be explored in man.[136,138,169,170] As in the case of Cl^- secretion, HCO_3^- secretion also promotes increased secretion of cations and water by paracellular pathways.

Absorptive Mechanisms

Na^+ is the primary ion that drives water absorption in the intestine. In the small intestine, the cotransport of Na^+ with food-derived products and the electroneutral NaCl absorptive mechanism are jointly responsible for most, if not all, of the water and electrolyte absorption. The large intestine absorbs Na^+ avidly by way of both an Na^+ channel and an electroneutral NaCl absorptive mechanism in common with the small intestine.[171–179]

SODIUM-GLUCOSE COTRANSPORT AND SIMILAR SODIUM COTRANSPORT MECHANISMS IN THE SMALL INTESTINE

The absorption of nutrients, including carbohydrates, amino acids, dipeptides, tripeptides, fat, minerals, vitamins, and bile salts, is the key function of the small intestine. Many of these substances are absorbed by a cotransport pathway together with Na^+. Glucose is absorbed by way of an Na^+-glucose cotransport carrier on the apical membrane of the small intestinal epithelium (Fig 14-5).[91-93,97] Na^+ and glucose bind to the carrier, which then shuttles them from the outer surface of the apical membrane to the inner surface. Here, both transported species are released before the binding sites on the carrier return to the outer surface. Because transport carriers function in both directions, an appropriate electrochemical gradient must exist to provide a proper direction for the vectorial transport. The Na^+ gradient created by the Na^+,K^+-ATPase pump provides the needed energy for the absorptive direction. The glucose that accumulates in the cell then diffuses across the basolateral membrane by a facilitated transport pathway,[180] and the Na^+ is pumped out basolaterally by the Na^+, K^+-ATPase. The charge of the absorbed Na^+ promotes absorption of an anion by way of the paracellular pathway; Cl^- primarily serves this function. Water follows passively to keep the intercellular space iso-osmolar. The intestinal glucose transport mechanism therefore also drives water and electrolyte absorption.[101] The ability of this transport mechanism to promote positive electrolyte and water balance remains unaffected by most disease processes. This provides the basis for the clinical usage of glucose salt solution. The solution increases the activity of the transport mechanism, providing an approach to the management of diarrhea and dehydration by replacing electrolytes and water. Sucrose or starch (both of which yield glucose after digestion) can replace the glucose in the solution and provide similar results with the advantage of a lower initial osmotic load.[181]

Many other cotransport mechanisms for nutrients depend similarly on the Na^+ gradients across the apical membrane created by the Na^+,K^+-ATPase pump. Of the large numbers of these mechanisms that involve Na^+, most exist only in the small intestine. Cotransport of Na^+ and many amino acids, dipeptides, or tripeptides provides for the absorption of needed protein components.[102-107] Cotransport of Na^+ and certain B vitamins has been recognized.[106,182] Finally, ileal uptake of bile acids is also provided for by an Na^+ cotransport mechanism.[183]

ELECTRONEUTRAL Na^+ AND Cl^- ABSORPTION IN THE INTESTINE

An Na^+, Cl^- cotransport mechanism has been proposed to exist in the intestine because a significant portion of Na^+ absorption by this organ has been shown to require the presence of Cl^- and vice versa.[184-187] The mechanism is called electroneutral Na^+,Cl^- absorption to distinguish this mechanism from the electrogenic Na^+ absorptive mechanism discussed below. However, the interdependence of Na^+ and Cl^- transport has not been readily demonstrated in many studies of intestinal apical membrane vesicles, raising questions about the precise nature of this cotransport phenomenon.[188] The debate about the nature of this mechanism is likely to continue. In some instances, the so-called electroneutral

Na^+,Cl^- cotransport may be actually comprised of an Na^+/H^+ exchange working in concert with a Cl^-/HCO_3^- exchange mechanism.[112-115,137,189-191] This mechanism allows both Na^+ and Cl^- to enter the cell in exchange for H^+ and HCO_3^- (Fig 14-6). Protons and HCO_3^- are produced intracellularly by the action of carbonic anhydrase on CO_2. Sodium, which enters the cell, is pumped out by the Na^+,K^+-ATPase, with Cl^- following by way of another Cl^- transport pathway yet to be identified. Water then follows the absorbed ions by way of the tight junction. This Na^+,Cl^- cotransport mechanism appears to be widely distributed in the epithelium of the intestinal tract, including the small intestine, the proximal part of the large intestine, and the gallbladder. Interestingly, there is one report of congenital secretory diarrhea resulting from a defective jejunal Na^+/H^+ exchange pathway.[192]

ELECTROGENIC Na^+ ABSORPTION

Electrogenic Na^+ absorption is predominant in the colon.[179] The process is so named because absorption of the Na^+ ion, with a positive electrical charge, is unaccompanied by cation exchange or active anion cotransport. The Na^+ ion enters the cell by way of an Na^+ channel on the apical membrane. It is pumped out across the basolateral membrane by the Na^+,K^+-ATPase pump. Water and anion follow the absorbed Na^+ from the luminal side to the bloodstream side by way of paracellular routes.

Absorption and Secretion of Potassium, Calcium, and Other Ions

There are presumably specific transport mechanisms to handle other electrolytes, including potassium, calcium and other divalent cations, sulfate, phosphate, and organic anions.[135-144,193-199] In general, the body does not permit the absorption of important substances to occur in a totally passive fashion. Rather, mechanisms exist to regulate these processes and permit adaptation to changes in the environment. It is reasonable to assume that active transport processes exist for all of the important ions. Unfortunately, the transport mechanisms for many of these ions are poorly understood at the present time.

Only recently have active transport mechanisms for potassium in the intestine been recognized and investigated.[200-205] In the past, it was wrongly assumed that potassium simply leaked passively through the epithelial tight junction in response to existing gradients. Most investigators now believe that active transcellular mechanisms are the predominant means by which potassium is absorbed or secreted. Furthermore, active participation of the colonic mucosa in potassium homeostasis has also been emphasized.[202,205,206] However, the transport pathways involved in the potassium absorptive or secretory mechanisms have only been postulated.[205] For potassium absorption, it is possible that a K^+/H^+ exchange pathway serves to exchange intracellular H^+ for potassium. The accumulated potassium then might diffuse across the basolateral membrane by way of a potassium channel or other potassium carriers. For potassium secretion, either an increase in the Na^+,K^+-ATPase activity that pumps K^+ across the basolateral membrane into the cell or increased K^+ movement across the apical membrane may promote net movement of the ion into the lumen.

Luminal absorption of Ca^{2+} is regulated by Vitamin D and its metabolites, specifically 1,25 dihydroxy D_3.[195-197] Parathyroid hormone and calcitonin also influence Ca^{2+} transport.[198,199] Ca^{2+} in different intracellular pools serves different functions. Subcellular localization of calcium is conferred by association of the pools with different calcium-binding proteins, of which there are a number. Some of these calcium-binding proteins bind to newly absorbed Ca^{2+} and thus regulate Ca^{2+} absorption, while others bind free cytosolic Ca^{2+} and mediate cellular function.[207] Therefore, absorbed Ca^{2+} can be transported across the epithelial cell without affecting Ca^{2+}-mediated cellular events. It does not appear that Ca^{2+} absorbed from the lumen mixes with the pool that mediates epithelial cell functions. Consequently, the source of Ca^{2+} for Ca^{2+}-mediated cellular events is the bloodstream rather than the gut lumen. This Ca^{2+} must therefore enter the epithelial cells through the basolateral membrane. The transport processes involved at this site are thought to be an Na^+/Ca^{2+} exchange carrier,[116] a Ca^{2+}-ATPase,[73,75] or a Ca^{2+} channel.[208,209] In addition, a number of Ca^{2+}-ATPases may be very important in maintaining different intracellular compartments of Ca^{2+}.[73]

REGULATION OF ELECTROLYTE TRANSPORT

An understanding of the regulation of electrolyte transport mechanisms has the potential to be clinically useful. Therefore, a great deal of attention has been paid to the area of regulatory mechanisms. At the epithelial cell level, neurohumoral regulation has been widely investigated, and regulation by cells of the immune system has also been recognized recently. Our discussion will emphasize these aspects. Other factors that influence intestinal water and electrolyte transport are less well understood. They include regulation related to acid–base homeostasis, intestinal motility, intestinal permeability, oncotic pressure of the blood, arterial pressure, venous pressure, and luminal pressure. These factors will be discussed only briefly.

Neurohumoral Regulation of the Epithelial Cells

For the purpose of discussing peptide or neurotransmitter regulation, we can consider the intestine to be a self-modulated organ. The endocrine cells, nerve cells, and immune cells serve as sensors, while the regulatory peptides or neurotransmitters serve as messengers. Regulatory peptides or neurotransmitters are released in response to stimuli, and these substances serve to modulate and coordinate the functions of the intestine and other digestive organs.[210-214]

Significant advances have been made in recent years in our understanding of the mechanisms of action of the neurohumoral agents that regulate intestinal secretion or absorption. This is particularly true in the area of stimulus-secretion coupling. In the past, only cyclic AMP, cyclic GMP, and Ca^{2+} had been recognized as intracellular secondary messengers. Now, the roles of G-pro-

teins, calmodulin, products of phospholipid metabolism, products of arachidonic acid metabolism, and various protein kinases can be investigated directly. Preliminary evidence implies a role for all these cellular constituents in receptor-mediated events leading to electrolyte transport. These new developments allow a better and more complete understanding of the roles of secondary messengers in receptor-mediated regulation. The isolation of cellular organelles (e.g., endoplasmic reticulum, Golgi bodies, and so forth) has also facilitated our knowledge of the transport of ions and newly synthesized proteins such as channels, carriers, and pumps between different intracellular compartments. The combination of the increased understanding of these regulatory controls with the ongoing identification of basic transport pathways participating in a given transport mechanism should allow investigators to map the cellular regulatory events from the receptor to the final site of action (i.e., the transport pathway). Knowledge in this regard that has been obtained with, or can be directly applied to, intestinal cells is still quite limited, but as it is acquired it can be expected to have important clinical applications.

For practical purposes, receptor-mediated regulation of epithelial transport can be divided into three steps: (1) binding and activation of receptors by regulatory substances, (2) mobilization (synthesis, release, and so forth) of intracellular mediators (secondary messengers), and (3) activation and regulation of the cellular transport pathway.

RECEPTOR BINDING AND ACTIVATION BY REGULATORY SUBSTANCES

In most cases, endogenous regulatory peptides or neurotransmitters bind to and activate receptors on the basolateral membrane.[215] Bacterial toxins, in contrast, have their sites of action on the apical membrane.[157] The receptor recognizes the signal released by either sensor cells (endocrine cells, nerve cells, or immune cells) or microorganisms and initiates the biological event. A large number of regulatory peptides and neurotransmitters that modulate the transport function of epithelial cells have now been identified. The effects of these substances, together with the intracellular messenger(s) thought to be involved in their action, are summarized in Tables 14-3 and 14-4.[210-214] The precise physiologic role of each peptide or neurotransmitter cannot be clearly delineated at the present time. Some agents are active only at high doses in experimental models. Moreover, selective antagonists are available for only a few of the mediators listed.[216-224]

Activation of some receptor-mediated regulatory mechanisms has been applied clinically.[225] Drugs whose tertiary structures resemble peptides or neurotransmitters bind to their receptors and mimic their actions. Thus, opiates that have antisecretory properties, such as enkephalin derivatives, have been used in the treatment of diarrhea. Drugs displaying secretory properties have been employed in constipation. Some drugs were widely used before their mechanisms of action were well understood. A classic example is the use of synthetic opiates to treat diarrhea.

After binding to receptors, peptides and neurotransmitters mobilize a cascade of intracellular mediators, often referred to as secondary

TABLE 14–3
Intestinal Secretory Stimuli

SUBSTANCE	INTRACELLULAR MEDIATOR	REFERENCES
Endogenous Stimuli (Peptides, Neurotransmitters, and Products of Inflammation)		
Acetylcholine*	Ca^{++}-dependent effector	238, 261, 394–396
Histamine*	Ca^{++}-dependent effector	267, 268, 397–399
Serotonin	Ca^{++}-dependent effector	400–402
Substance P	Ca^{++}-dependent effector	403, 404
Neurotensin	Ca^{++}-dependent effector	403
Calcitonin	? Ca^{++}-dependent effector	198, 199, 404, 405
Cholecystokinin	? Ca^{++}-dependent effector	406–408
Prostaglandins*	Cyclic AMP	242, 409–412
Bradykinin†	Cyclic AMP	413, 414
Oxygen free radicals†	Cyclic AMP	281, 283
Platelet-activating factor†	Cyclic AMP	418
VIP*	Cyclic AMP	243, 244, 415–417
Secretin	Cyclic AMP	406, 408, 419
Glucagon	Cyclic AMP	408, 419–422
PHI	Cyclic AMP	423
Adenosine*	? Cyclic AMP	273, 424
Atrial natriuretic factor	Cyclic GMP	425
Gastrin	Unknown	408, 426
GIP	Unknown	408, 427
Vasopressin	Unknown	428
Motilin	Unknown	429
Bombesin	Unknown	405, 430
5-HPETE and 5-HETE	Unknown	266
Exogenous Stimuli (Microbial Enterotoxins and Luminally Active Agents)		
Bacterial Enterotoxins		
Vibrio cholerae	Cyclic AMP	242, 245, 431–436
Escherichia coli (heat-labile)	Cyclic AMP	435, 436
Salmonella	Cyclic AMP	437, 438
Campylobacter jejuni	Cyclic AMP	439–441
Escherichia coli (heat-stable)	Cyclic GMP	157, 247, 442, 443
Yersinia enterocolitica	Cyclic GMP	443, 444
Klebsiella pneumoniae	Cyclic GMP	443, 445
Clostridium difficile	Ca^{++}-dependent effector	446, 447
Other microbial enterotoxins	Unknown	448, 449
Bile Salts and Fatty Acids	Ca^{++}-dependent effector and ? cyclic AMP	337, 450–455
Pharmaceutical Agents		
Laxatives	Mostly unknown	

* The noted agents have been shown to regulate epithelial cells directly and, among endogenous secretory stimuli, may be of physiologic importance.
† Bradykinin, oxygen free radicals, and platelet-activating factor increase submucosal prostaglandin production, which may then cause an increase in epithelial cell cyclic AMP levels.

TABLE 14–4
Intestinal Absorptive Stimuli

SUBSTANCE*	REFERENCES
Endogenous Stimuli (Peptides and Neurotransmitters)†	
Alpha-adrenergic agonists	456–459
Dopamine	460, 461
Enkephalins and other opioids	321, 462–468
Somatostatin	469–472
Glucocorticoids	121, 368, 473–475
Angiotensin	476–478
Peptide YY and neuropeptide Y	479
Prolactin	480
Exogenous Stimuli (Luminally Active Agents)	
Nutrients	
(e.g., glucose, amino acids, dipeptides, tripeptides)	101–107
Pharmaceutical Agents	
Cyclo-oxygenase inhibitors (e.g., indomethacin, aspirin)	412, 481–486
Phenothiazines	248, 252, 253
Propranolol	457, 487, 488
Nicotinic acid and analogs	489
Chloroquine	490
Lithium	491, 492
Verapamil	493
Berberine	484, 495
Vinblastine	496
Colchicine	496

* *Intracellular mediators for the absorptive stimuli of the intestine are largely unknown, except for cyclo-oxygenase inhibitors, which inhibit prostaglandin synthesis. Other stimuli may affect the secretory mechanism anywhere in the cascade of regulation by cyclic nucleotides or calcium-dependent effectors.*

† *Except for alpha-adrenergic agonists, somatostatin, and glucocorticoids, which activate epithelial cells directly, the effects of the other named endogenous agents are most likely indirect by way of either local or central neural controls. Alpha-adrenergic agonists are probably of physiologic importance.*

messengers. The effects at the receptor level are often transduced by one of the guanine nucleotide-binding proteins known as G-proteins, which have been implicated in stimulus–response coupling in many cell types.[226] Some G-proteins may be directly linked to ionic channels,[227-230] but more commonly their role is to activate or inhibit synthesis of one or several secondary messengers.[226,231-236] Altered levels of these secondary messengers then regulate the various transport pathways to control absorptive or secretory processes in the intestinal epithelial cells. In contrast to the numerous receptor types, the number of intracellular mediators is relatively small. Many neurohumoral agents thus share similar amplifying events within the epithelial cell. A few major patterns of secondary messenger responses have been recognized in epithelia. They can be divided into two main groups, those mediated by cyclic nucleotides and those mediated by calcium-dependent effectors.[207,237-241]

For cyclic nucleotide-mediated mechanisms, cyclic AMP is more commonly called upon than cyclic GMP. Both, however, serve important roles in electrolyte transport. Increased cellular cyclic AMP or cyclic GMP stimulates Cl^- secretion by crypt cells and inhibits the neutral NaCl absorptive mechanism of surface or villous cells. The secretory response results directly from the action of the cyclic nucleotides in the secretory cells. The ability of cyclic nucleotides to directly inhibit NaCl absorption in absorptive cells is less clearly understood. Two important endogenous hormonal substances, prostaglandins and vasoactive intestinal polypeptide (VIP), have effects on the epithelium that are associated with activation of adenylate cyclase and an increase in cAMP production.[242-244] Exogenous substances may also act through this pathway. An example is cholera toxin, which causes ADP-ribosylation of the G_s protein (the regulatory subunit of the adenylate cyclase system).[245] ADP-ribosylation irreversibly sustains the G_s protein in an active form, leading to prolonged adenylate cyclase stimulation and elevated cellular cyclic AMP. A secretory response results. *Escherichia coli* heat-stable enterotoxin (ST_a), which increases guanylate cyclase activity and thus increases cellular cyclic GMP, also mediates a secretory response.[240,246,247] In this case, cyclic GMP rather than cyclic AMP stimulates chloride secretion and inhibits NaCl absorption.

Calcium-dependent effectors may activate a number of intracellular signaling mechanisms. Stimulation of the turnover of phospholipids such as phosphotidylinositol may generate the second messengers diacylglycerol and inositol trisphosphate.[248-251] The latter molecule can liberate calcium into the cytosol from intracellular stores, thereby activating calcium–calmodulin-dependent pathways, while calcium and diacylglycerol can act together to stimulate protein kinase C. The importance of the calcium–calmodulin complex in intestinal ion transport has been demonstrated by the observation that trifluoperazine and chlorpromazine, inactivators of the complex, have antidiarrheal properties.[252,253] In vitro studies have shown that calcium–calmodulin-dependent mechanisms can inhibit the activity of the apical Na^+/H^+ and Cl^-/HCO_3^- exchange carriers of surface and villous absorptive cells, resulting in an inhibition of NaCl absorption. Calcium mobilization can also be involved in the secretory responses of crypt cells, such as in the stimulation of chloride secretion by histamine and acetylcholine.

Besides the cyclic nucleotide and calcium-dependent effector mechanisms discussed above, the importance of arachidonic acid metabolites has recently been recognized. Arachidonic acid and products of its metabolism by way of the cyclo-oxygenase or lipoxygenase pathways (the latter normally considered a result of inflammation) may also be produced during phospholipid breakdown. Such mediators can affect electrolyte transport and should be considered secondary messengers. Finally, it is likely that most if not all of the secondary messengers described above mediate their action by activating a protein kinase or a phosphatase.[254-256] For example, cyclic AMP activates the cyclic AMP–dependent protein kinases,[257,258] cyclic GMP activates the cyclic GMP–dependent kinases, and diacylglycerol activates protein kinase C.[259] Because of the complexity of intestinal tissues, the roles of protein kinases and phosphatases remain to be investigated in isolated cell systems.

Pharmacologic interference with the cascade of secondary messengers has been applied successfully to treat secretory diarrhea. The use of trifluoperazine, a calmodulin inhibitor, is an example.[253] However, clinical application of knowledge in this area is still limited.

REGULATION OF CELLULAR TRANSPORT PATHWAYS

The final event regulated by receptor activation is at the transport pathway level, on either the basolateral or apical membrane. For short-term regulation, hormones and neurotransmitters can activate or inactivate an existing transport pathway by way of one of the secondary messengers. For example, cyclic AMP opens a cyclic AMP-dependent Cl^- channel on the apical membrane, causing Cl^- secretion.[110,258,260] Calcium-dependent effectors open a calcium-dependent K^+ channel on the basolateral membrane,[134,155,261] with the resulting K^+ exit creating a favorable electrical gradient for Cl^- secretion across the Cl^- channels on the apical membrane. Because opening of the apical Cl^- channels is the rate-limiting step, calcium-dependent mechanisms increasing intestinal Cl^- secretion are therefore synergistic with cyclic nucleotide–mediated mechanisms that open the Cl^- channels. Similar synergistic phenomena between cyclic nucleotide–mediated and calcium-mediated mechanisms have also been recognized in gastric acid secretion. Hence, short-term regulation of electrolyte transport resembles classical stimulus-secretion coupling, with activation of transport pathways being brought about by a cascade of secondary messengers. Electrolyte transport can also be regulated in the longer term. Some hormones, such as the steroids, can increase the number of pumps, carriers, or channels. For example, aldosterone increases Na^+ absorption in the colonic epithelium by increasing the number of Na^+ channels on the apical membrane and Na^+, K^+-ATPase pumps on the basolateral membrane.[121,122] Long-term regulation may also occur at the receptor level, with an increase or decrease in the number of receptors for a particular hormone leading to up- or down-regulation of the receptor-mediated event.

Only relatively recently have the transport pathways themselves been exploited as a site for therapeutic intervention. The effectiveness of omeprazole in inhibiting gastric acid secretion, by directly blocking H^+ secretion at the K^+, H^+-ATPase pump on the apical membrane, has stimulated interest in this area. In the intestine, blockage of the Cl^- exit pathway should inhibit intestinal secretion and diarrhea. Although drugs with this action are not currently available, successful development of potent and specific Cl^- channel blockers may provide a novel, targeted approach to the treatment of diarrhea in the future.[132,133]

Immune-Related Regulation of Epithelial Cells

The classical emphasis in the study of the regulation of intestinal electrolyte transport, as described above, has been to consider the effects of neurohumoral agents, such as peptides, neurotransmitters, and hormones. More recently, a number of investigators have begun to examine the participation of cells and cell products of the immune system in controlling the physiologic processes of the intestine, including electrolyte absorption and secretion. In particular, the ability of immunologic effector cells and their mediators to induce chloride secretion in several experimental models has been studied. In a number of intestinal diseases of presumed immunologic etiology, diarrhea is thought to result from the action of mediators released from inflammatory cell types. Such mediators may act directly at the epithelial level, or they may stimulate

production of secondary mediators (e.g., prostaglandins) from other mucosal cells, or they may promote intestinal secretion by interacting with the enteric nervous system. The complex pathways of interaction between inflammatory cells and intestinal physiology that are involved in immune-related electrolyte secretion are just beginning to be investigated.[41,262,263]

Several studies have defined a role for mast cell mediators in the promotion of chloride secretion. A number of substances released from activated mast cells can be shown to stimulate the epithelium and cause chloride secretion.[264–273] In the intact intestine of sensitized animals, a neuronal component of secretion can also be observed in antigen-stimulated tissues. Conversely, mast cell mediators may influence the in vitro intestinal secretion seen following electrical field stimulation.[274] This functional association between mast cells and nerves is mirrored by their morphologic association; mast cells and nerves can be shown by a variety of techniques to be in intimate contact in the intestinal mucosa, raising the potential for intercellular communication.[42,275]

Mast cell mediators that appear to affect electrolyte transport include histamine, adenosine, platelet activating factor, and eicosanoids such as leukotrienes, hydroxyeicosatetraenoic acids (HETEs), and prostaglandin D_2. Mast cells in the rat may also be a source of VIP, providing an example of a neurohumoral secretagogue that might be released in response to immunologic as well as physiologic stimulation.[276] Also in the rat, mast cell activation can induce epithelial sloughing at the villous tips, a process ascribed to the actions of a specific protease contained in the mast cell granules.[272] The selective loss of villous epithelium presumably would affect absorption but not secretion, changing the balance of electrolyte transport so that secretion predominates. The role of the mast cell in promoting diarrhea is further emphasized when we consider that diarrhea frequently accompanies systemic anaphylaxis.[277] Moreover, intestinal mast cell numbers, and evidence of mast cell activation, are increased in diseases where diarrhea is a feature, such as inflammatory bowel disease and parasitic infestation.[278]

Mast cells may also be important for their influence on other inflammatory cell types. Mast cells can synthesize a number of chemotactic factors that can stimulate the migration of neutrophils and eosinophils.[279] These cell types, too, can have effects on electrolyte transport. For example, neutrophils can stimulate chloride secretion, an effect that is possibly related to their ability to release reactive oxygen species such as hydrogen peroxide.[280,281] Migration of neutrophils across the epithelial barrier has been shown to lower its resistance temporarily.[282] Eosinophil products such as eosinophil peroxidase have been shown to have deleterious effects on the respiratory epithelium,[283] another secretory epithelium that shares a number of features with the intestinal epithelium. It is therefore likely that similar effects of eosinophil products will be observed in the gut, although this remains to be examined. To complete the circle, both neutrophils and eosinophils release substances that cause mast cell activation.[284] These histamine-releasing factors (so called because they are assayed by their ability to cause release of histamine, one mast cell product) have been identified as products of a number of different cell types in addition to neutrophils and eosinophils, such as lymphocytes, platelets, and monocytic cell lines. The existence of these factors may provide an amplification mechanism following mast cell mediator release. Overall, the multitude of potent mediators involved and the potential for extensive cellular interaction suggest that electrolyte secretion induced following immune system activation has the potential to be quite pronounced.

Other Factors that Influence Intestinal Water and Electrolyte Transport

There are a few other factors that may indirectly influence water and electrolyte transport by intestinal epithelial cells. Among these factors are acid-base homeostasis,[285-293] gastric and intestinal motility,[36,294-297] effects of flow rate and the unstirred water layer,[298-300] intestinal permeability,[301-304] oncotic pressure of the blood, arterial pressure, venous pressure, plasma volume and luminal pressure,[305-312] and the effects of physical and psychologic stress.[294,313,314] At our present level of knowledge, only intestinal motility appears to be an important factor clinically.[295-297] Retardation of the flow of intestinal contents achieved by the coordinated contraction of gastrointestinal smooth muscles may allow more contact time for absorption and decrease stool volume significantly.[295-297,315-319] The effectiveness of many antidiarrheal drugs, including synthetic opiates,[315,319-321] results mainly from their effect on gut motility. The effects of intestinal motility may additionally be integrated with neuronal, hormonal, or immunologic influences.[36,322]

Other factors listed above that influence electrolyte movement are not currently considered clinically important determinants of electrolyte transport in the intestine. This may simply reflect our lack of knowledge of the complex systems involved and their interrelationships. For example, intestinal permeability increases a great deal in diseases that cause mucosal injury, such as inflammatory bowel disease. Colonic permeability also increases when bile salts or fatty acids are present in the colon.[301] Theoretically, an increased intestinal permeability may allow the oncotic and hydrostatic pressures to have a more prominent effect on electrolyte secretion. Increased permeability may also allow a number of larger molecules, which normally are not absorbed, to diffuse across the intestinal mucosa more easily.

INTEGRATED ASPECTS OF FLUID AND ELECTROLYTE MOVEMENT IN VIVO

Up to this point, our discussion of intestinal electrolyte transport has been largely reductionist in nature. We have considered the various transport pathways that serve as the building blocks for intestinal transport mechanisms. Factors capable of influencing these mechanisms have also been covered, but essentially in isolation. The nature of the foregoing discussion largely reflects the current status of our knowledge regarding electrolyte transport. Most studies, of necessity, have focused on single aspects of electrolyte transport control and have tended to ignore other factors that may be operating in vivo. However, it is obvious that the net picture of electrolyte movement in vivo is the result of the influences of multiple controlling systems. The reasons for this complexity are not known, but the system has evolved presumably for

good reasons—perhaps to permit better "fine tuning" of electrolyte transport or to improve integration with other organ systems such as the cardiovascular and renal systems.

A survey of the literature reveals that few investigators in this modern era of molecular biology have been eager to tackle the complexities of electrolyte transport in vivo, especially in man, despite the fact that studies carried out in humans can presumably provide information that is directly applicable clinically. Our attempts here, therefore, to provide some insight into the integration of the control of fluid and of electrolyte movement must be preliminary and somewhat speculative in nature. However, it will be important in the future for investigators to continue to study such integration in both health and disease, because it is only by correctly identifying and quantitating the various factors that control the processes of electrolyte transport that we can begin to devise strategies to therapeutically alter such processes.

Integration of the influences controlling intestinal electrolyte transport can occur at three levels: at the cellular level, at the level of the epithelium as a whole, or when one considers the entire intestinal organ system. This concept of a three-level framework may aid discussion of electrolyte transport integration, and we will therefore consider each level in turn. At the cellular level, integration of responsiveness occurs because the epithelial cells have receptors for and are responsive to controlling agents that originate from the endocrine, neuronal, and immune elements of the intestine. The epithelial cells do not respond to these agents in isolation; rather, there is substantial interplay between mediators produced by the various controlling systems. For example, agents that can activate epithelial responses by mobilizing intracellular calcium (such as acetylcholine, a prototype neural stimulus) display marked synergism with those agents acting through cyclic nucleotides (such as prostaglandins, products of immunologic effector cells).[156,261] It appears likely that input to the epithelial cells from neurones provides a basal "tone" to the system. The cells are thus primed to respond more readily to increased levels of other hormonal or immunologic controlling substances. Evidence for the importance of this neurotransmitter-defined "tone" is provided by the observation that the secretory response of intestinal tissues to a wide variety of agents can be reduced markedly if the tissue is pretreated with blockers of neurotransmission, such as tetrodotoxin or atropine.[323-326] Thus, even for hormones and immune mediators that are known to have secretory effects directly at the epithelial level, the degree of neural input appears to be of paramount importance in setting the cellular sensitivity of the system.[32,327,328] Conversely, immunologic input may influence the ability of the epithelial cell to respond to neurotransmitters. The capacity of the intestinal epithelial cell to be placed in a state of readiness by the actions of one class of mediators, to then respond more markedly to another class, is analogous to the situation with gastric parietal cells that also respond synergistically to various combinations of stimuli.[329-331] At the intracellular level, the synergism observed when epithelial cells are presented with combinations of stimuli appears to relate to the different signal transduction mechanisms that are induced. Indeed, the need for integration between different controlling systems probably provides a rationale for the existence of the multiple intracellular mechanisms that promote electrolyte transport in epithelial cells.

One additional way in which electrolyte transport responses may be integrated at the cellular level relates to the actual distribution of the various transporter proteins that make up intestinal transport pathways. Essentially nothing is known of the factors that control localization of the different transporter proteins to specific areas of the intestine, although some recent studies have examined how the number of protein subunits constituting a transporter in a given epithelial cell can be up- or down-regulated to alter overall transport properties. A further degree of control can be obtained if the number of receptors for neurohumoral agents on the epithelial cells can be varied. In addition to the short-term synergistic interactions between different classes of mediators, some controlling agents may be able to alter chronically the responsiveness of epithelial cells to other substances. Hence, the control of epithelial cells is integrated both acutely and chronically, consistent with the requirement for the intestinal electrolyte transport system to respond to a variety of situations that may be either urgent (e.g., infection) or long term (e.g., dietary alterations) in nature.

At the epithelial level there appears to be coordination of the transcellular and paracellular responses of the epithelium.[302-304,332] For example, activation of Na^+-glucose cotransport in the intestine is apparently accompanied by a concomitant increase in tight junctional permeability, allowing an increase in the paracellular movement of ions and water. There is still a great deal to learn about the functioning of the tight junction, but one possible linkage for effects on paracellular and transcellular processes may lie at the level of intracellular messengers such as calcium. In other systems, calcium-related intracellular events appear to be associated with control of tight junctional events. Furthermore, the pathologic diarrhea that results when the intestine is exposed to elevated levels of bile salts (agents known to affect cellular calcium levels) is associated with both an increase in epithelial permeability and alterations in absorptive and secretory functions.

Epithelial function is also integrated in that the overall balance of electrolyte movement depends on the relative levels of absorption and secretion. Although absorptive and secretory processes are known to be localized to distinct cells, coordination between the functions of these cells is apparent (though not well understood). For example, agents that induce chloride secretion also inhibit neutral sodium and chloride absorption. In fact, this coordination is one of the factors that has made interpretation of electrolyte transport studies in intact tissue difficult. Although intestinal secretion was a topic of discussion in the 1930s, it was subsequently ignored by most investigators until the 1960s because, under normal circumstances, absorptive events predominate and totally obscure the secretory events.

It is important to keep in mind that the epithelium is not comprised solely of absorptive and secretory cell types. Under appropriate stimuli, as yet unknown, intestinal epithelial stem cells also differentiate into endocrine cells, goblet or mucous cells, M-cells, and Paneth cells.[23,24,211,333-335] Obviously, intraepithelial endocrine cells can communicate with the electrolyte-transporting cell types to provide paracrine regulation much as hormonal agents from more distant sites are involved. However, the potential communication between either absorptive or secretory cells and the other specialized epithelial cell types listed is only beginning to be investigated. The constant renewal of the intestinal lining suggests that the putative factors that influence the differentiation and growth of epithelial cell types should be extremely important in integrating the function of the epithelium as a whole.

At the organ level, our knowledge of the integration of electrolyte transport processes unfortunately becomes even more sparse. However, it is possible to envision readily how gut motility, blood flow, and distant endocrine glands might contribute to the overall process.[211-214,312,336] The local, sympathetic, and parasympathetic nervous systems are presumably also important, both because neurotransmitters can interact synergistically with other mediators at the cellular level and because the nervous system may be stimulated directly in response to a variety of situations in the intestine, leading to an effect on electrolyte transport as a secondary phenomenon. In this latter regard, the local network of neural elements in the gut (the submucosal and myenteric plexuses) appears to be of particular importance. Integration of the various systems at the organ level has been largely inferred from a variety of anecdotal clinical and experimental observations. For example, the electrolyte transport response in inflammatory and anaphylactic models can be substantially dependent on intact local neural function. This observation may be explained in part by the synergistic effects of neurotransmitters and other mediators, as discussed above. It may also result, however, from a possible role of the enteric nervous system as a central controlling element in the responsiveness to diverse substances. At least in animal models, the enteric nervous system appears to be capable of responding to inflammatory mediators such as platelet activating factor, histamine, kinins, and prostaglandins, because at least part of the secretory responses accompanying generation of these mediators by either allergic, inflammatory, or nociceptive stimuli is abolished by neural blockade.

Further evidence for integration between various intestinal systems and electrolyte transport is provided by the observation that, in many diarrheal states, particularly those induced by bacterial toxins or an excessive osmotic load, there is an increased rate of intestinal transit,[315,317,337] suggesting indirectly a close link, probably neurally mediated, between transport and motility functions. Contributions of gut motility are also recognized or implied in disease states such as dumping syndrome and diarrhea after vagotomy. Blood flow and related factors such as arterial, venous, and oncotic pressure and plasma volume presumably can also contribute to electrolyte transport control, although the mechanisms involved remain to be investigated. Rather more is known regarding how distant endocrine organs can affect electrolyte transport, because diarrhea is a well-recognized sequela of thyroid disease,[338] adrenal insufficiency, and endocrine tumors. Finally, the intestine may respond to overall acid–base status.[285-293,339] The influence of this last factor for the control of electrolyte transport is likely to be of minor significance, however, because the capacity of the intestine to correct acid–base imbalance in disease states is limited. Changes in electrolyte transport caused by alterations in acid–base imbalance are therefore thought to be secondary in nature rather than being primary compensatory homeostatic mechanisms.

In summary, it is clear that the overall status of fluid and electrolyte transport in the intestine is closely regulated at a variety of levels by a number of diverse, but integrated, influences. At present, our knowledge of the interplay between these controlling factors is largely theoretic, particularly at the organ level. One generalization that can be made (and one that is supported by some experimental evidence) is that the enteric nervous system appears to play a central role in coordinating the response of the intestine to diverse stimuli. The combination of reductionist studies with those carried out in intact tissues, and in vivo, should continue to yield further important information about the integration of the intestinal electrolyte transport system as a whole.

METHODS FOR THE STUDY OF INTESTINAL ELECTROLYTE TRANSPORT

No discussion of intestinal transport phenomena would be complete without a description of the experimental methods that have been employed to obtain the body of physiologic and pathophysiologic information detailed in this chapter. Many of these techniques have been mentioned above in passing; this section will seek to provide, in one place, a brief description of some of the many methods currently used by physiologists for the study of electrolyte transport both in vivo and in vitro.

In Vivo Techniques

In vivo perfusion techniques can be used to study water and electrolyte transport in healthy humans. The techniques are also widely used in whole animals. The two variants of this method are double-lumen perfusion and triple-lumen perfusion. Both techniques use nonabsorbable markers such as polyethylene glycol or polymeric dyes to calculate the amount of water absorbed or secreted between two points of an intestinal segment.[340,341] These in vivo perfusion techniques allow measurement of the rate of disappearance or appearance of a substance in the intestinal lumen. It is assumed that what disappears has been absorbed, and what appears has been secreted. In general, this assumption is valid, and the technique is quite useful for identification and study of absorptive or secretory phenomena. The techniques allow for the influence of most contributing factors, including gut motility and blood flow. Therefore, the results are representative of all factors involved. Perfusion studies have significant limitations when employed in the hope of elucidating the mechanisms involved in absorptive or secretory processes. Studies of these mechanisms can be better carried out with the in vitro techniques described below.

DOUBLE-LUMEN PERFUSION

A number of early studies of electrolyte transport used double-lumen perfusion. Using human volunteers, a double-lumen tube is inserted into the intestine by way of the mouth. The intestinal segment of interest may be occluded proximally by means of a balloon built into the tube (to prevent flow of intestinal contents into the test segment); in animal studies, the segment of intestine to be examined is usually isolated surgically. The infusate is instilled at the proximal port and the effusate is collected from the distal port. The use of nonabsorbable markers allows correction for incomplete collection of the effusate. The amount of water absorbed or secreted can be calculated from the relative concentrations of the nonabsorbable marker at the two ports. If water is absorbed, the concentration of the nonabsorbable marker in the effusate is increased compared with the infused concentration; if water is secreted, the marker is diluted. The amount of any electrolyte or other substance absorbed or secreted can also be calculated from the differences between the concentration entering the segment and the concentration collected distally once the amount of water absorption or secretion is known.

TRIPLE-LUMEN PERFUSION

Double-lumen perfusion is not ideal for human studies because the intestinal segment cannot be isolated surgically, and normal flow of intestinal contents from the upper tract may dilute the infusate. To compensate for this problem, a third lumen is introduced to sample the intestinal content after the infusate is mixed with the existing luminal contents (Fig 14-7).[340] This allows sampling of well-mixed contents between two points of an intestinal segment. Calculation of the amount of water and electrolyte absorbed between the two points follows the same principles used for the double-lumen perfusion technique.

In Vitro Techniques

In vitro techniques that use either isolated segments of the intestine, isolated enterocytes, or plasma membranes have been described. The relative advantages of each method arise mainly from their ability to exclude certain confounding factors. Isolated intestine stripped of the muscular layers excludes the effects of blood flow and motility. Isolated enterocytes exclude the influence of pre-existing peptides or neurotransmitters. Purified apical or basolateral membranes allow identification of transport pathways on either side of the plasma membrane. The disadvantages of each method are often the same as the advantages, resulting from the preparation's isolation from normal regulatory factors and the normal environment. The phenomena observed may therefore not be pertinent to whole organs.

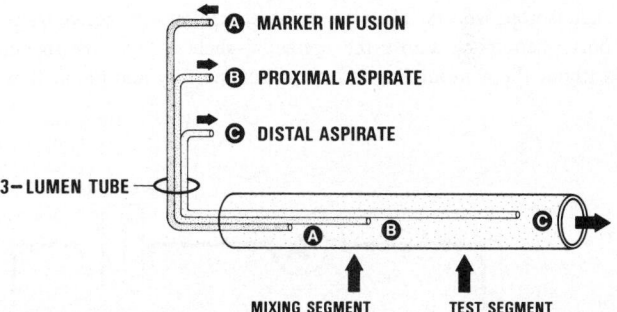

FIGURE 14–7. Triple-lumen perfusion. The technique is based on the same principles as double-lumen perfusion (see text) but allows correction for mixing of the infusate with normal intestinal contents. Rather than using the infusate as the starting point, the infusate (marker infusion) is allowed to mix with the intestinal contents in the mixing segment, between points A and B. At point B, the luminal contents are assayed, and the ionic compositions, and so forth, are taken as starting values (therefore corresponding to the infusion point in double-lumen perfusion). The test segment is therefore between points B and C. The amount of water or other substances absorbed from this segment can be calculated from the difference between B and C, using the proximal and distal aspirate samples. (Adapted from Moore EW. Gastroenterology—Liver disease teaching material. American Gastroenterology Association, Unit VII, Physiology of Intestinal Water and Electrolyte Absorption. Timonium, MD: Milner–Fenwick, Inc, 1976.)

EVERTED GUT SAC

This simple technique permits gross estimation of absorptive or secretory functions. A segment of the intestine is everted, tied at both ends, and suspended in the same solution that fills the sac.[342] The everted gut sac enlarges upon absorption and shrinks with secretion. The preparation retains most of the normal intestinal structure including local regulatory cells. With the exception of influences of blood flow and central nervous system (CNS) control, the phenomena observed should be pertinent to the whole intestine. One potential problem is that only those absorbed substances which are also able to penetrate the muscular layers and the serosa can be detected by this technique.

USSING CHAMBER

The Ussing chamber is designed to study active transport mechanisms. Transport processes occurring across the tight junctions, in a passive fashion, are not detected. In essence, the apparatus consists of two fluid-filled reservoirs separated by a piece of the isolated intestine or epithelium (Fig 14-8).[343,344] The mucosa or the luminal surface is bathed by the contents of one reservoir while the serosal or basolateral surface is bathed by the other. To eliminate any chemical gradient across the tissue, both surfaces are exposed to similar bathing solutions; to eliminate the electrical gradient, a voltage-clamp apparatus generates sufficient electrical current to constantly nullify the spontaneous electrical potential difference. The current required to achieve this state is called the short-circuit current and reflects the net amount of electrical charges carried by various transported ions. It can be used to monitor electrolyte transport activity once the ion transported is identified. By itself, the current does not identify the exact types of ion transported. Ion movement from one side of the intestine to the other can be identified directly and measured by the use of radioisotope tracers. The Ussing chamber allows the active transport phenomena across the epithelial sheet to be investigated without the confounding effects of gut motility and blood flow.

It is an excellent method to study a specific absorptive or secretory mechanism. The involvement of a given transport pathway (on the apical or basolateral membrane) in a transport mechanism can be inferred, provided that a specific inhibitor for the pathway exists. Similarly, the involvement of an intracellular mediator can be inferred if a specific inhibitor of that secondary messenger is available and found to inhibit the transport phenomenon. The Ussing chamber can also be modified so that stimulatory electrodes are included in the part of the chamber used to clamp the tissue. These electrodes can be used to activate nerves present in intact tissue preparations, enabling the investigation of neurocrine control of electrolyte transport.

MICROELECTRODES

Electrodes can be used to measure the concentrations of specific ions in the cell and the potential difference across the plasma membrane. The principle of the ion-selective electrode is similar to that of the pH electrode.[345–347] One can fill the tip of an electrode with an ion-selective substance, which only allows passage of a specific ion.[348] In the case of the pH electrode, only H^+ passes through the tip. Ion-selective substances for Na^+, K^+, Cl^-, and Ca^{2+} are available.[348,349] Because ions carry electrical charges, their movement results in an electrical current into the electrode. Because the amount of ion moving across the tip varies with its concentration gradient, comparison with known standards allows one to estimate the intracellular concentration of the ion of interest.

In addition to measurements of intracellular ionic concentrations, electrical potential difference across the plasma membrane (apical or basolateral) can be measured in single cells. This method allows estimation of the conductance across the membrane that may be attributed to an ionic channel or carrier. The advantage of the technique is that it allows studies to be carried out in single cells. This advantage is particularly important in the intestine, where different types of cells may exhibit different transport functions. The disadvantage is that the results are somewhat indirect. One must be cautious when interpreting results based on the elec-

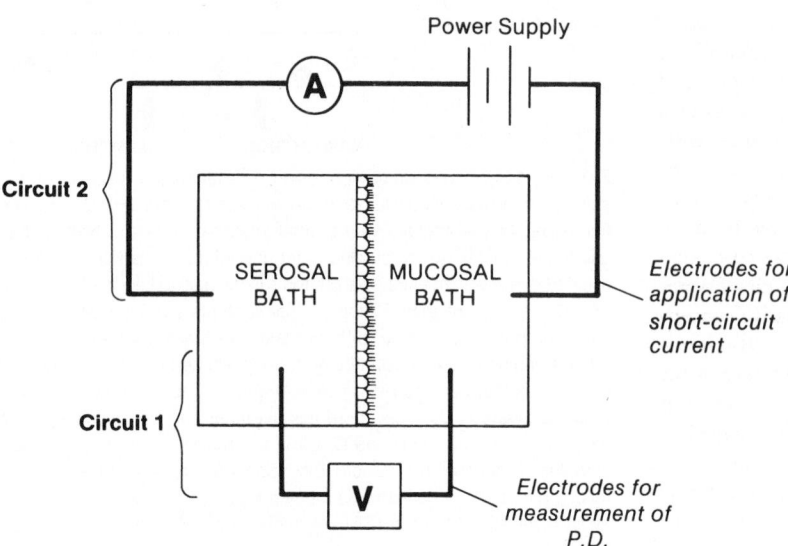

FIGURE 14–8. Ussing chamber. This device, shown here in diagrammatic form, can be used to quantitate active transport of ionic species. A piece of intestine or a sheet of epithelial cells is clamped between two baths containing a warmed, oxygenated, physiologic solution. Such tissues normally generate a small spontaneous potential difference (P.D.), apical side negative, reflective of ongoing electrolyte transport. This P.D. can be measured by the voltmeter, *V*, in circuit 1. During the experiment, the tissue is "short-circuited" by circuit 2, which applies an exactly sufficient amount of electrical current to nullify the spontaneous potential difference. Because there is no electrochemical gradient for paracellular, passive movement of ions between the baths under short-circuit conditions, the amount of current applied, measured at *A*, is wholly reflective of the net active transport of ions across the epithelium. In practice, circuits 1 and 2 are combined in a device known as a voltage clamp. Radioactive tracers can be placed in one bath and sampled from the opposite bath to determine the identity of the ion(s) being transported.

trical studies because many ions can exhibit the same electrical profile. Identification of the cell of interest in isolated intestine may also be problematic. Another method, electron probe microanalysis, also provides information about the intracellular content of ions, but the technique requires specialized equipment that is not readily available.[350]

PATCH CLAMP TECHNIQUES

The principle of the patch clamp technique is very similar to that of the ion-selective microelectrode. In this case, the tip of the electrode is sealed with a tiny patch of plasma membrane from the epithelial cell.[351] This tiny patch of plasma membrane, containing one or a few ionic channels of interest, acts like an ion-selective substance in an ion-selective microelectrode. When exposed to proper ion gradients, a small burst of electrical current can be detected if the ionic channel present in the patch opens. The study can be carried out with a cell-attached patch or an excised patch. Patch clamping is a direct method for verifying and studying ionic channels. It has therefore rapidly become an important and widely used technique.

RADIONUCLIDE UPTAKE AND EFFLUX STUDIES IN ISOLATED CELLS

Uptake of radionuclide into whole cells or efflux of radionuclide out of cells can be studied by use of isolated enterocytes. The techniques can verify whether a cotransport (symport) or ion exchange (antiport) mechanism is present. An ionic channel can also be detected readily. However, the method cannot differentiate a channel from a carrier directly. Activation or inhibition of these pathways by peptides or other compounds can also be tested.[109,134,260]

MEMBRANE VESICLES

The apical and basolateral membranes of intestinal epithelial cells can be isolated, separated, and purified on the basis of their different densities. The apical membrane is somewhat denser because it has an attached cytoskeleton. Enzyme markers, characteristic of each membrane, allow one to detect and estimate the extent of purification of the membrane preparations. The broken plasma membrane fragments, which contain the transport carriers, channels, or pumps, tend to seal as round vesicles. Radionuclide uptake and efflux studies can then be carried out with these vesicles in a manner similar to whole-cell studies.[88,352-354] The concentration of ions inside and outside the vesicle can be better controlled than in whole cells. Thus, shorter time courses can be studied more easily, and a better estimation of the stoichiometry of a given transport pathway can be obtained. Fluorescent dyes have also been widely applied for ion transport studies in membrane vesicles.[355] These dyes exhibit varying fluorescent characteristics depending on the concentration of the ion of interest, allowing ionic concentrations to be measured and monitored. Furthermore, membrane vesicles would be expected to be a better preparation for biochemical studies of transporter proteins.

CELL CULTURE

Cultured epithelial cells, especially continuous cell lines, exclude confounding factors introduced by the endocrine cells, nerve cells or nerve endings, and immune cells that are present in isolated tissue. A cultured line containing only one cell type serves as a better model for the study of transport mechanisms. Recently, a number of colonic cell lines have been successfully used to study Cl^- and mucus secretory mechanisms.[260,356-359] Many techniques mentioned above can be applied easily to cultured cells, including the Ussing chamber, radionuclide uptake and efflux, microelectrode, and patch clamp techniques. Cultured cells have the further advantages that mutants deficient or defective in specific transport pathways can be isolated and gene transfer techniques can be employed.[360] Application of all the mentioned techniques to cultured cells should provide results that are complementary to the studies of whole or isolated intestine. A combination of all the approaches described is likely to yield the most meaningful results.

IMPLICATION FOR DISEASE STATES

In clinical gastroenterology, knowledge obtained from the study of electrolyte transport physiology has been applied mainly to the management of hypersecretory states such as diarrhea.[361-363] Pharmacologic bypass of the secretory defect in cystic fibrosis is another current topic of investigation.[131,258,364]

Under normal circumstances, optimal contact time of the luminal contents with the epithelium ensures that absorptive processes predominate, based on both the reserve capacity of the absorptive surface and the ability of gastrointestinal motility functions to regulate the flow of the luminal contents. A deficiency of mucosal absorptive function is therefore rarely observed except in (1) patients with massive intestinal resection, (2) patients with diseases that form a submucosal barrier to the absorptive process, or (3) patients with diseases that destroy the absorptive cells. Some infectious or autoimmune processes affect villous cells more than crypt cells such that the balance between absorption and secretion is disturbed, resulting in diarrhea. The reserve capacity makes clinical deficiency of mucosal absorptive function uncommon, but it also allows luminal toxins to readily cause excessive secretion.

Diarrheas usually result from either retention of unabsorbed oral intake (osmotic diarrhea) or excessive secretion (secretory diarrhea). Fasting, or simple exclusion of the culprit unabsorbable substance, suffices to abolish osmotic diarrhea. Secretory diarrhea usually results from the actions of toxins produced by microorganisms, from unabsorbed bile salts or fatty acid in the colon, or from excessive release of endogenous regulatory substances. The pathologic processes usually mimic physiologic mechanisms. The primary action of both cholera toxin and the heat-stable toxin of *E. coli* is at the level of the epithelial cells, where the toxins stimulate Cl^- secretion and inhibit NaCl absorption by activating adenylate cyclase and guanylate cyclase, respectively. Some toxins, such as clostridium and shigella toxins, are cytotoxic to the epithelial cells or they may activate Ca^{2+}-dependent effector mechanisms. Bile salts and fatty acids activate Ca^{2+}-dependent effectors and they may also disrupt the epithelial barrier. Once these toxins, bile salts, or fatty acids reach the submucosa, they may have effects on both the immune system and the neural network. The resulting effects on intestinal secretion and gut motility may then lead to diarrhea. Endogenous sources of hormones may cause diarrhea when excessive amounts are released. Examples are endocrine tumors such as carcinoid tumors, medullary carcinoma of the thyroid, and VIPoma.

When discussing the treatment of secretory diarrhea, three basic approaches should be considered: (1) stimulation of the absorptive mechanism, which typically remains intact, and/or (2) inhibition of the excessive secretory function,[225,365] and (3) retardation of gastrointestinal transit. For the first approach, glucose–NaCl solutions have been successfully applied clinically to stimulate water absorption without affecting the secretory process. The latter two approaches may be applied by manipulating various receptor-mediated processes. Pharmacologic activation of receptors by drugs such as opiates, alpha$_2$-adrenergic agents, and somatostatin has been applied clinically and has proved effective in inhibiting secretion, stimulating absorption, and delaying gastrointestinal transit. Trifluoperazine is the only drug currently available for use that may interfere with a cellular secondary messenger pathway. In the future, new approaches aimed at the transporter proteins or receptors may become practical (e.g., direct inhibition of transport pathways such as the Cl$^-$ secretory pathway[132,133,366] or administration of synthetic receptors for toxins that can bind and inactivate the toxin).[367]

SUMMARY

This chapter has sought to describe how the transport of fluid and electrolytes is carried out in the small and large intestines. We have taken a reductionist approach, stressing how a limited number of transport systems are the building blocks for a variety of complex transport mechanisms. The transport systems may be common to a number of diverse epithelia and may also be present at various levels of the intestinal tract; it is their asymmetric assembly into the various transport mechanisms that defines the active transport processes that can be carried out by a given epithelial cell. We should also reiterate an important principle of intestinal electrolyte transport physiology—that water is not transported actively by the epithelium but rather follows passively to balance active ion movements. Hence, therapeutic strategies designed to regulate the transport of fluid into and out of the gut lumen must of necessity be directed at those factors which influence the transport of electrolytes. Such regulatory factors have been described in detail at both the extracellular (hormonal mediators, neurotransmitters, bacterial toxins) and intracellular (secondary messengers) level.

Finally, we have tried to integrate what is known of how the transport of electrolytes in the intestine works within the context of the organ as a whole. In particular, the interaction of transport physiology with neural activity and gut motility has been described. There is limited information available to date concerning the integration of electrolyte transport with other intestinal functions. It is to be expected that future studies of such integrated aspects of intestinal physiology will yield important data as to how the system operates in vivo and may also point the way to novel therapeutic strategies for diarrhea and other disorders of intestinal fluid balance.

The reader is directed to Chapter 6, Epithelia: Biologic Principles of Organization; Chapter 9, Motility of the Small Intestine; Chapter 10, The Motor Function of the Colon; Chapter 12, Salivary Secretion; Chapter 13, Gastric Secretion; Chapter 15, Pancreatic Secretion; Chapter 16, Bile Secretion; Chapter 17, Carbohydrate Assimilation; Chapter 18, Intestinal Lipid Absorption; Chapter 19, Protein Digestion and Assimilation; Chapter 20, Vitamins and Minerals; Chapter 37, Approach to the Patient with Ileus and Obstruction; and Chapter 38, Approach to the Patient with Diarrhea.

REFERENCES

1. Phillips SF, Giller J. The contribution of the colon to electrolyte and water conservation in man. J Lab Clin Med 1973;81:733.
2. Devroede GJ, Phillips SF. Conservation of sodium, chloride and water by the human colon. Gastroenterology 1969;56:421.
3. Phillips RA. Water and electrolyte losses in cholera. Fed Proc 1964;23:705.
4. Lipkin M, Sherlock P, Bell B. Cell renewal in stomach, ileum, colon and rectum. Gastroenterology 1963;45:721.
5. MacDonald WC, Trier JS, Everett NB. Cell proliferation and migration in the stomach, duodenum and rectum of man: Radioautographic studies. Gastroenterology 1964;46:405.
6. Gumbiner B. Structure, biochemistry, and assembly of epithelial tight junctions. Am J Physiol 1987;253:C749.
7. Claude P, Goodenough DA. Fracture faces of zonulae occludentes from "tight" and "leaky" epithelia. J Cell Biol 1973;58:390.
8. Madara JL, Dharmsathaphorn K. Occluding junction structure-function relationships in a cultured epithelial monolayer. J Cell Biol 1985;101:2124.
9. Marcial MA, Carlson SL, Madara JL. Partitioning of paracellular conductance along the ileal crypt-villus axis: A hypothesis based on structural analysis with detailed consideration of tight junction structure-function relationships. J Membr Biol 1984;80:59.
10. Farquhar MG, Palade GE. Junctional complexes in various epithelia. J Cell Biol 1963;17:375.
11. Fromter E, Diamond J. Route of passive ion permeation in epithelia. Nature 1972;235:9.
12. Schultz SG. The role of paracellular pathways in isotonic fluid transport. Yale J Biol Med 1977;50:99.
13. Davis GR, Santa Ana CA, Morawski SG, Fordtran JS. Permeability characteristics of human jejunum, ileum, proximal colon and distal colon: Results of potential difference measurements and unidirectional fluxes. Gastroenterology 1982;83:844.
14. Fordtran JS, Rector FC Jr, Ewton MF, Soter N, Kinney J. Permeability characteristics of the human small intestine. J Clin Invest 1965;44:1935.
15. Soybel DI, Ashley SW, DeSchryver-Kecskemeti K, Cheung LY. Effects of luminal hyperosmolality on cellular and paracellular ion transport pathways in Necturus antrum. Gastroenterology 1987;93:456.
16. Madara JL. Intestinal absorptive cell tight junctions are linked to cytoskeleton. Am J Physiol 1987;253:C171.
17. Bentzel CJ, Hainau B, Ho S, et al. Cytoplasmic regulation of tight junction permeability: Effect of plant cytokinins. Am J Physiol 1980;239:C75.
18. Mullin JM, O'Brien TG. Effects of tumor promoters on LLC-PK$_1$ renal epithelial tight junctions and transepithelial fluxes. Am J Physiol 1986;251:C597.
19. Palant CE, Duffey ME, Mookerjee BK, Ho S, Bentzel CJ. Ca^{2+} regulation of tight-junction permeability and structure in Necturus gallbladder. Am J Physiol 1983;245:C203.
20. Bakker R, Groot JA. cAMP-mediated effects of ouabain and theophylline on paracellular ion selectivity. Am J Physiol 1984;246:G213.

21. Burt JM. Block of intercellular communication: Interaction of intracellular H^+ and Ca^{2+}. Am J Physiol 1987;253:C607.

22. Moog F. The lining of the small intestine. Sci Am 1981;245:154.

23. Trier JS, Winter HS. Anatomy, embryology, and developmental abnormalities of the small intestine and colon. In: Sleisenger MH, Fordtran JS, eds. Gastrointestinal disease: Pathophysiology, diagnosis, management. 4th ed. Philadelphia: WB Saunders, 1989:991.

24. Trier JS, Madara JL. Functional morphology of the mucosa of the small intestine. In: Johnson LR, Christensen J, Jackson MJ, et al, eds. Physiology of the gastrointestinal tract. 2nd ed. New York: Raven Press, 1987:1209.

25. Donowitz M, Madara JL. Effect of extracellular calcium depletion on epithelial structure and function in rabbit ileum: A model for selective crypt or villus epithelial cell damage and suggestion of secretion by villus epithelial cells. Gastroenterology 1982;83:1231.

26. Hallback D-A, Jodal M, Sjoqvist A, Lundgren O. Evidence for cholera secretion emanating from the crypts: A study of villus tissue osmolarity and fluid and electrolyte transport in the small intestine of the cat. Gastroenterology 1982;83:1051.

27. MacLeod RJ, Hamilton JR. Absence of a cAMP-mediated antiabsorptive effect in an undifferentiated jejunal epithelium. Am J Physiol 1987;252:G776.

28. Roggin GM, Banwell JG, Yardley JH, Hendrix TR. Unimpaired response of rabbit jejunum to cholera toxin after selective damage to villus epithelium. Gastroenterology 1972;63:981.

29. Welsh MJ, Smith PL, Fromm M, Frizzell RA. Crypts are the site of intestinal fluid and electrolyte secretion. Science 1982;218:1219.

30. Polak JM, Buchan AMJ, Probert L, Tapia F, deMey J, Bloom SR. Regulatory peptides in endocrine cells and autonomic nerves: Electronimmunocytochemistry. In: Polak JM, Bloom SR, Wright NA, Daly MD, eds. Basic science in gastroenterology: Structure of the gut. Norwich: Page Bros, 1982:11.

31. Larsson LI, Goltermann N, De Magistris L, Rehfield JF, Schwartz TW. Somatostatin cell processes as pathways for paracrine secretion. Science 1980;205:1393.

32. Hubel KA. Intestinal nerves and ion transport: Stimuli, reflexes, and responses. Am J Physiol 1985;248:G261.

33. Wood JD. Enteric neurophysiology. Am J Physiol 1984;247:G585.

34. Bridges RJ, Rack M, Rummel W, Schreiner J. Mucosal plexus and electrolyte transport across the rat colonic mucosa. J Physiol 1986;376:531.

35. Andres H, Bock R, Bridges RJ, Rummel W, Schreiner J. Submucosal plexus and electrolyte transport across rat colonic mucosa. J Physiol 1985;364:301.

36. Greenwood B, Davison JS. The relationship between gastrointestinal motility and secretion. Am J Physiol 1987;252:G1.

37. Goyal RK, Crist JR. Neurology of the gut. In: Sleisenger MH, Fordtran JS, eds. Gastrointestinal disease: Pathophysiology, diagnosis, management. 4th ed. Philadelphia: WB Saunders, 1989:21.

38. Fogel R, Michelson G, Senler T, Marshall D, Brown T, Gaginella T. Central administration of benzodiazepines alters water absorption by the rat ileum in vivo. Gastroenterology 1987;93:330.

39. Fogel R, Kaplan RB, Arbit E. Central action of gamma-aminobutyric acid ligands to alter basal water and electrolyte absorption in the rat ileum. Gastroenterology 1985;88:523.

40. Heyworth MF, Jones AL, eds. Immunology of the gastrointestinal tract and liver. New York: Raven Press, 1988.

41. Elson CO, Kagnoff MF, Fiocchi C, Befus AD, Targan S. Intestinal immunity and inflammation: Recent progress. Gastroenterology 1986;91:746.

42. Stead RH, Tomioka M, Quinonez G, Simon GT, Felten SY, Bienenstock J. Intestinal mucosal mast cells in normal and nematode-infected rat intestine are in intimate contact with peptidergic nerves. Proc Natl Acad Sci USA 1987;84:2975.

43. Reenstra WW, Bettencourt JD, Forte JG. Mechanisms of active Cl^- secretion by frog gastric mucosa. Am J Physiol 1987;252:G543.

44. Rege RV, Moore EW. Evidence for H^+ secretion by the in vivo canine gallbladder. Gastroenterology 1987;92:281.

45. Poler SM, Reuss L. Protamine alters apical membrane K^+ and Cl^- permeability in gallbladder epithelium. Am J Physiol 1987;253:C662.

46. Scharschmidt BF, Van Dyke RW. Mechanisms of hepatic electrolyte transport. Gastroenterology 1983;85:1199.

47. O'Doherty J, Stark RJ. A transcellular route for Na-coupled Cl transport in secreting pancreatic acinar cells. Am J Physiol 1983;245:G499.

48. Petersen OH. Calcium-activated potassium channels and fluid secretion by exocrine glands. Am J Physiol 1986;251:G1.

49. Gasser KW, DiDomenico J, Hopfer U. Secretagogues activate chloride transport pathways in pancreatic zymogen granules. Am J Physiol 1988;254:G93.

50. Maxwell MH, Kleeman CR, Narins RG. Clinical disorders of fluid and electrolyte metabolism. 4th ed. New York: McGraw-Hill, 1988.

51. Smith PL, Welsh MJ, Stoff JS, Frizzell RA. Chloride secretion by canine tracheal epithelium: I. Role of intracellular cAMP levels. J Membr Biol 1982;70:217.

52. Goodman BE, Fleischer RS, Crandall ED. Evidence for active Na^+ transport by cultured monolayers of pulmonary alveolar epithelial cells. Am J Physiol 1983;245:C78.

53. Cullen JJ, Welsh MJ. Regulation of sodium absorption by canine tracheal epithelium. J Clin Invest 1987;79:73.

54. Welsh MJ, Smith PL, Frizzell RA. Chloride secretion by canine tracheal epithelium: II. The cellular electrical potential profile. J Membr Biol 1982;70:227.

55. Sano K, Voelker DR, Mason RJ. Effect of secretagogues on cytoplasmic free calcium in alveolar type II epithelial cells. Am J Physiol 1987;253:C679.

56. Saito Y, Wright EM. Bicarbonate transport across the frog choroid plexus and its control by cyclic nucleotides. J Physiol 1983;336:635.

57. Saito Y, Wright EM. Kinetics of the Na pump in the frog choroid plexus. J Physiol 1982;328:229.

58. Zeuthen T, Wright E. Epithelial potassium transport: Tracer and electrophysiological studies in choroid plexus. J Membr Biol 1981;60:105.

59. Wright EM. Active transport of anions across the choroid plexus. J Physiol 1974;240:535.

60. Bijman J, Quinton PM. Influence of calcium and cyclic nucleotides on beta-adrenergic sweat secretion in equine sweat glands. Am J Physiol 1984;247:C10

61. Sato K. Differing luminal potential difference of cystic fibrosis and control sweat secretory coils in vitro. Am J Physiol 1984;247:R646.

62. Quinton PM. Effects of some ion transport inhibitors on secretion and reabsorption in intact and perfused single human sweat glands. Pflugers Arch 1981;391:309.

63. Schulz IJ. Micropuncture studies in the sweat formation in cystic fibrosis patients. J Clin Invest 1969;48:1470.

64. Marcus DC, Marcus NY, Greger R. Sidedness of action of loop diuretic and ouabain on nonsensory cells of utricle: A micro-Ussing chamber for inner ear tissues. Hear Res 1987;30:55.

65. Reuss L, Reinach P, Weinman SA, Grady TP. Intracellular ion activities and Cl^- transport mechanisms in bullfrog corneal epithelium. Am J Physiol 1983;244:C336.

66. Hughes BA, Miller SS, Joseph DP, Edelman JL. cAMP stimulated the Na^+-K^+ pump in frog retinal pigment epithelium. Am J Physiol 1988;254:C84.

67. Candia OA, Grillone LR, Chu T-C. Forskolin effects on frog and rabbit corneal epithelium ion transport. Am J Physiol 1986;251:C448.

68. Eveloff JL, Warnock DG. Activation of ion transport systems during cell volume regulation. Am J Physiol 1987;252:F1.

69. Spring KR. Determinants of epithelial cell volume. Fed Proc 1985;44:2526.

70. Warnock DG, Greger R, Dunham PB, et al. Ion transport processes in apical membranes of epithelia. Fed Proc 1984;43:2473.

71. Chien S, Gargus JJ. Molecular biology in physiology. FASEB J 1987;1:97.

72. Wade JB, Lewis SA, eds. Current topics in membranes and transport. vol 20. Molecular approaches to epithelial transport. London: Academic Press, 1984.

73. Carafoli E, Zurini M. The Ca^{2+}-pumping ATPase of plasma membranes: Purification, reconstitution and properties. Biochim Biophys Acta 1982;683:279.

74. Forte JG, Machen TE, Obrink KJ. Mechanisms of gastric H^+ and Cl^- transport. Annu Rev Physiol 1980;42:111.

75. Haynes DH. Mechanism of Ca^{2+} transport by Ca^{2+}-Mg^{2+}-ATPase

pump: Analysis of major states and pathways. Am J Physiol 1983;244: G3.

76. Kaplan JH. Sodium ions and the sodium pump: Transport and enzymatic activity. Am J Physiol 1983;245:G327.

77. DiBona DR, Mills JW. Distribution of Na-pump sites in transporting epithelia. Fed Proc 1979;38:134.

78. Stirling CE. Radioautographic localization of sodium pump sites in rabbit intestine. J Cell Biol 1972;53:704.

79. Kirk KL, Halm DR, Dawson DC. Active sodium transport by turtle colon via an electrogenic Na-K exchange pump. Nature 1980;287: 237.

80. Schneider JW, Mercer RW, Caplan M, et al. Molecular cloning of rat brain Na,K-ATPase alpha-subunit cDNA. Proc Natl Acad Sci USA 1985;82:6357.

81. Pollack LR, Tate EH, Cook JS. Turnover and regulation of Na-K-ATPase in HeLa cells. Am J Physiol 1981;241:C173.

82. Schenk DB, Hubert JJ, Leffert HL. Use of a monoclonal antibody to quantify (Na+,K+)-ATPase activity and sites in normal and regenerating rat liver. J Biol Chem 1984;259:14941.

83. Wolosin JM. Ion transport studies with H+-K+-ATPase-rich vesicles: Implications for HCl secretion and parietal cell physiology. Am J Physiol 1985;248:G595.

84. Ives HE, Rector FC Jr. Proton transport and cell function. J Clin Invest 1984;73:285.

85. Gluck S. Al-Awqati Q. An electrogenic proton-translocating adenosine triphosphatase from bovine kidney medulla. J Clin Invest 1984;73:1704.

86. Brown D, Hirsch S, Gluck S. An H+-ATPase in opposite plasma membrane domains in kidney epithelial cell subpopulations. Nature 1988;331:622.

87. Zeidel ML, Silva P, Seifter JL. Intracellular pH regulation and proton transport by rabbit renal medullary collecting duct cells. Role of plasma membrane proton adenosine triphosphatase. J Clin Invest 1986;77:113.

88. Aronson PS. Identifying secondary active solute transport in epithelia. Am J Physiol 1981;240:F1.

89. Stein WD. Intrinsic, apparent, and effective affinities of co- and countertransport systems. Am J Physiol 1986;250:C523.

90. Freel RW, Goldner AM. Sodium-coupled nonelectrolyte transport across epithelia: Emerging concepts and directions. Am J Physiol 1981;241:G451.

91. Goldner AM, Schultz SG, Curran PF. Sodium and sugar fluxes across the mucosal border of rabbit ileum. J Gen Physiol 1969;53: 362.

92. Hopfer U, Nelson K, Perrotto J, Isselbacher KJ. Glucose transport in isolated brush border membrane from rat small intestine. J Biol Chem 1973;248:25.

93. Hopfer U. Membrane transport mechanisms for hexoses and amino acid. In: Johnson LE, Christensen J, Jackson MJ, et al, eds. Physiology of the gastrointestinal tract. 2nd ed. New York: Raven Press, 1987: 1499.

94. Baker RD. Intestinal sugar transport: Does the Na+ gradient provide all the energy. Am J Physiol 1986;250:G448.

95. Hudson RL, Schultz SG. Sodium-coupled sugar transport: Effects on intracellular sodium activities and sodium-pump activity. Science 1984;224:1237.

96. Karasov WH, Solberg DH, Diamond JM. What transport adaptations enable mammals to absorb sugars and amino acids faster than reptiles? Am J Physiol 1985;249:G271.

97. Murer H, Hopfer U. Demonstration of electrogenic Na+-dependent D-glucose transport in intestinal brush border membranes. Proc Natl Acad Sci USA 1974;71:484.

98. Karasov WH, Diamond JM. Adaptive regulation of sugar and amino acid transport by vertebrate intestine. Am J Physiol 1983;245:G443.

99. Hediger MA, Coady MJ, Ikeda TS, Wright EM. Expression cloning and cDNA sequencing of the Na+/glucose co-transporter. Nature 1987;330:379.

100. Fordtran JS, Ingelfinger FJ. Absorption of water, electrolytes, and sugars from the human gut. In: Code CF, ed. Handbook of physiology: Alimentary canal. Washington DC: American Physiological Society, 1968:1457.

101. Fordtran JS. Stimulation of active and passive sodium absorption by sugars in the human jejunum. J Clin Invest 1975;55:728.

102. Adibi SA, Morse EL, Masitamani SS, Amin PM. Evidence for two different modes of tripeptide disappearance in human intestine. J Clin Invest 1975;56:1355.

103. Adibi SA. Intestinal transport of dipeptides in man: Relative importance of hydrolysis and intact absorption. J Clin Invest 1971;50: 2266.

104. Alpers DH. Digestion and absorption of carbohydrates and protein. In: Johnson LR, Christensen J, Jackson MJ, et al, eds. Physiology of the gastrointestinal tract. 2nd ed. New York: Raven Press, 1987: 1469.

105. Curran PF, Schultz SG, Chez RA, Fuisz RE. Kinetic relations of the Na-amino acid interaction at the mucosal border of intestine. J Gen Physiol 1967;50:1261.

106. Rose RC. Intestinal absorption of water-soluble vitamins. In: Johnson LR, Christensen J, Jackson MJ, et al, eds. Physiology of the gastrointestinal tract. 2nd ed. New York: Raven Press, 1987:1581.

107. VanDyke RW. Mechanism of digestion and absorption of food. In: Sleisenger M, Fordtran JS, eds. Gastrointestinal disease: Pathophysiology, diagnosis, management. 4th ed. Philadelphia: WB Saunders, 1989:1062.

108. Lauf PK, McManus TJ, Hass M, et al. Physiology and biophysics of chloride and cation cotransport across cell membranes. Fed Proc 1987;46:2377.

109. Dharmsathaphorn K, Mandel KG, Masui H, McRoberts JA. Vasoactive intestinal polypeptide–induced chloride secretion by a colonic epithelial cell line: Direct participation of a basolaterally localized Na+,K+,Cl– cotransport system. J Clin Invest 1985;75:462.

110. Weymer A, Huott P, Liu W, McRoberts JA, Dharmsathaphorn K. Chloride secretory mechanisms induced by prostaglandin E1 in a colonic epithelial cell line. J Clin Invest 1985;76:1828.

111. Reuss L. Basolateral KCl co-transport in a NaCl-absorbing epithelium. Nature 1983;305:723.

112. Knickelbein R, Aronson PS, Atherton W, Dobbins JW. Sodium and chloride transport across rabbit ileal brush border: I. Evidence for Na-H exchange. Am J Physiol 1983;245:G504.

113. Murer H, Hopfer U, Kinne R. Sodium/proton antiport in brush-border-membrane vesicles isolated from rat small intestine. Biochem J 1976;154:597.

114. Liedtke CM, Hopfer U. Mechanism of Cl– translocation across intestinal brush border membrane: II. Demonstration of Cl–-OH– exchange and Cl– conductance. Am J Physiol 1982;242:G272.

115. Lowe AG, Lambert A. Chloride-bicarbonate exchange and related transport processes. Biochem Biophys Acta 1983;694:353.

116. Eisner DA, Lederer WJ. Na-Ca exchange: Stoichiometry and electrogenicity. Am J Physiol 1985;248:C189.

117. Stevens CF. Channel families in the brain. Nature 1987;328:198.

118. Stevens CF. Biophysical studies of ion channels. Science 1984;225: 1346.

119. Sariban-Sohraby S, Benos DJ. The amiloride-sensitive sodium channel. Am J Physiol 1986;250:C175.

120. Gunning R. Increased numbers of ion channels promoted by an intracellular second messenger. Science 1987;235:80.

121. Will PC, DeLisle RC, Cortright RN, Hopfer U. Introduction of amiloride-sensitive sodium transport in the rat colon by mineralocorticoids. Am J Physiol 1980;238:F261.

122. Will PC, Cortright RN, DeLisle RC, Douglas JG, Hopfer U. Regulation of amiloride-sensitive electrogenic sodium transport in the rat colon by steroid hormones. Am J Physiol 1985;248:G124.

123. Hartshorne RP, Catterall WA. The sodium channel from rat brain. J Biol Chem 1984;259:1667.

124. Kosower EM. A structural and dynamic molecular model for the sodium channel of Electrophorus electricus. FEBS Lett 1985;182: 234.

125. Kimmich GA, Randles J. An ATP- and Ca2+-regulated Na+ channel in isolated intestinal epithelial cells. Am J Physiol 1982;243:C116.

126. Palmer LG, Frindt G. Epithelial sodium channels: Characterization by using the patch-clamp technique. Fed Proc 1986;45:2708.

127. Grenningloh G, Rienitz A, Schmitt B, et al. The strychnine-binding

subunit of the glycine receptor shows homology with nicotinic acetylcholine receptors. Nature 1987;328:215.

128. Imoto K, Methfessel C, Sakmann B, et al. Location of a delta-subunit region determining ion transport through the acetylcholine receptor channel. Nature 1986;324:670.

129. Salkoff L, Butler A, Wei A, et al. Genomic organization and deduced amino acid sequence of a putative sodium channel gene in Drosophila. Science 1987;237:744.

130. Tamkun MM, Talvenheimo JA, Catterall WA. The sodium channel from rat brain: Reconstitution of neurotoxin-activated ion flux and scorpion toxin binding from purified components. J Biol Chem 1984;259:1676.

131. Frizzell RA, Rechkemmer G, Shoemaker RL. Altered regulation of airway epithelial cell chloride channels in cystic fibrosis. Science 1986;233:558.

132. Wangemann P, Wittner M, Di Stefano A, et al. Cl⁻-channel blockers in the thick ascending limb of the loop of Henle. Structure activity relationship. Pflugers Arch 1986;407(suppl 2):S128.

133. Montrose M, Randles J, Kimmich GA. SITS-sensitive Cl⁻ conductance pathway in chick intestinal cells. Am J Physiol 1987;253:C693.

134. McRoberts JA, Beuerlein G, Dharmsathaphorn K. Cyclic AMP and Ca²⁺-activated K⁺ transport in a human colonic epithelial cell line. J Biol Chem 1985;260:14163.

135. Flemstrom G, Garner G. Gastroduodenal HCO₃⁻ transport: Characteristics and proposed role in acidity regulation and mucosal protection. Am J Physiol 1982;242:G183.

136. Sullivan SK, Smith PL. Bicarbonate secretion by rabbit proximal colon. Am J Physiol 1986;251:G436.

137. Knickelbein R, Aronson PS, Schron CM, Seifter J, Dobbins JW. Sodium and chloride transport across rabbit ileal brush border: II. Evidence for Cl-HCO₃ exchange and mechanism of coupling. Am J Physiol 1985;249:G236.

138. Smith PL, Cascairo MA, Sullivan SK. Sodium dependence of luminal alkalinization by rabbit ileal mucosa. Am J Physiol 1985;249:G358.

139. Schron CM, Knickelbein RG, Aronson PS, Puca JD, Dobbins JW. pH gradient-stimulated sulfate transport by rabbit ileal brush-border membrane vesicles: Evidence for SO₄-OH exchange. Am J Physiol 1985;249:G607.

140. Schron CM, Knickelbein RG, Aronson PS, Dobbins JW. Evidence for carrier-mediated Cl-SO₄ exchange in rabbit ileal basolateral membrane vesicles. Am J Physiol 1987;253:G404.

141. Quamme GA. Phosphate transport in intestinal brush-border membrane vesicles: Effect of pH and dietary phosphate. Am J Physiol 1985;249:G168.

142. Karniski LP, Aronson PS. Formate: A critical intermediate for chloride transport in the proximal tubule. News in Physiological Sciences 1987;2:160.

143. Knickelbein RG, Aronson PS, Dobbins JW. Oxalate transport by anion exchange across rabbit ileal brush border. J Clin Invest 1986;77:170.

144. Kempson SA. Novel specific inhibitors of epithelial phosphate transport. News in Physiological Sciences 1988;3:154.

145. Sellin JH, De Soignie R. Ion transport in human colon in vitro. Gastroenterology 1987;93:441.

146. Hubel KA, Renquist K, Shirazi S. Ion transport in human cecum, transverse colon, and sigmoid colon in vitro: Baseline and response to electrical stimulation of intrinsic nerves. Gastroenterology 1987;92:501.

147. Bond JH, Currier BE, Buchwald H, Levitt MD. Colonic conservation of malabsorbed carbohydrate. Gastroenterology 1980;78:444.

148. Saunders DR, Wiggins HS. Conservation of mannitol, lactulose and raffinose by the human colon. Am J Physiol 1981;241:G397.

149. Dietz J, Field M. Ion transport in rabbit ileal mucosa: IV. Bicarbonate secretion. Am J Physiol 1973;225:858.

150. Davis GR, Santa Ana CA, Morawski S, Fordtran JS. Active chloride secretion in the normal human jejunum. J Clin Invest 1980;66:1326.

151. Sheerin HE, Field M. Ileal HCO₃ secretion: Relationship to Na and Cl transport and effect of theophylline. Am J Physiol 1975;228:1065.

152. Turnberg LA, Bieberdorf FA, Morawski SG, Fordtran JS. Interrelationships of chloride, bicarbonate, sodium and hydrogen transport in the human ileum. J Clin Invest 1970;49:557.

153. Davis GR, Morawski SG, Santa Ana CA, Fordtran JS. Evaluation of chloride/bicarbonate exchange in the human colon in vivo. J Clin Invest 1983;71:201.

154. Hubel KA. Bicarbonate secretion in rat ileum and its dependence on intraluminal chloride. Am J Physiol 1967;213:1409.

155. Mandel KG, McRoberts JA, Beuerlein G, Foster ES, Dharmsathaphorn K. Ba²⁺ inhibition of VIP- and A23187-stimulated Cl⁻ secretion by T₈₄ cell monolayers. Am J Physiol 1986;250:C486.

156. Cartwright CA, McRoberts JA, Mandel KG, Dharmsathaphorn K. Synergistic action of cyclic AMP and calcium mediated chloride secretion in a colonic epithelial cell line. J Clin Invest 1985;76:1837.

157. Huott PA, Liu W, McRoberts JA, Giannella RA, Dharmsathaphorn K. The mechanism of E. coli heat stable enterotoxin in a human colonic cell. J Clin Invest 1988;82:514.

158. Winterhager JM, Stewart CP, Heintze K, Petersen K-U. Electroneutral secretion of bicarbonate by guinea pig gallbladder epithelium. Am J Physiol 1986;250:C617.

159. Jones RS, Meyers WC. Regulation of hepatic biliary secretion. Annu Rev Physiol 1979;41:67.

160. Solomon TE. Control of exocrine pancreatic secretion. In: Johnson LR, Christensen J, Jackson MJ, et al, eds. Physiology of the gastrointestinal tract. 2nd ed. New York: Raven Press, 1987:1173.

161. Rose RC. Absorptive functions of the gallbladder. In: Johnson LR, Christensen J, Jackson MJ, et al, eds. Physiology of the gastrointestinal tract. 2nd ed. New York: Raven Press, 1987:1455.

162. Schultz I. Electrolyte and fluid secretion in the exocrine pancreas. In: Johnson LR, Christensen J, Jackson MJ, et al, eds. Physiology of the gastrointestinal tract. 2nd ed. New York: Raven Press, 1987:1147.

163. Quigley EMM, Turnberg LA. pH of the microclimate lining human gastric and duodenal mucosa in vivo. Studies in control subjects and in duodenal ulcer patients. Gastroenterology 1987;92:1876.

164. Flemstrom G. Gastric and duodenal mucosal bicarbonate secretion. In: Johnson LR, Christensen J, Jackson MJ, et al, eds. Physiology of the gastrointestinal tract. 2nd ed. New York: Raven Press, 1987:1011.

165. Flemstrom G, Garner A, Nylander O, Hurst BC, Heylings JR. Surface epithelial HCO₃⁻ transport by mammalian duodenum in vivo. Am J Physiol 1982;243:G348.

166. Flemstrom G, Jedstedt G, Nylander O. Beta-endorphin and enkephalins stimulate duodenal mucosal alkaline secretion in the rat in vivo. Gastroenterology 1986;90:368.

167. Rees WDW, Gibbons LC, Turnberg LA. Influence of opiates on alkali secretion by amphibian gastric and duodenal mucosa in vitro. Gastroenterology 1986;90:323.

168. Duffey ME. Intracellular pH and bicarbonate activities in rabbit colon. Am J Physiol 1984;246:C558.

169. Akiba T, Alpern RJ, Eveloff J, Calamina J, Warnock DG. Electrogenic sodium/bicarbonate cotransport in rabbit renal cortical basolateral membrane vesicles. J Clin Invest 1986;78:1472.

170. Soleimani M, Grassl SM, Aronson PS. Stoichiometry of Na⁺-HCO₃⁻ cotransport in basolateral membrane vesicles isolated from rabbit renal cortex. J Clin Invest 1987;79:1276.

171. Binder HJ. Absorption and secretion of water and electrolytes by small and large intestine. In: Sleisenger MH, Fordtran JS, eds. Gastrointestinal disease: Pathophysiology, diagnosis, management. 4th ed. Philadelphia: WB Saunders, 1989:1022.

172. Armstrong WM. Cellular mechanisms of ion transport in the small intestine. In: Johnson LR, Christensen J, Jackson MJ, et al, eds. Physiology of the gastrointestinal tract. 2nd ed. New York: Raven Press, 1987:1251.

173. Binder HJ, Sandle GI. Electrolyte absorption and secretion in the mammalian colon. In: Johnson LR, Christensen J, Jackson MJ, et al, eds. Physiology of the gastrointestinal tract. 2nd ed. New York: Raven Press, 1987:1389.

174. Binder HJ, ed. Mechanisms of intestinal secretion. New York: Alan R Liss, 1979.

175. Donowitz M, Welsh MS. Regulation of mammalian small intestinal electrolyte secretion. In: Johnson LR, Christensen J, Jackson MJ, et

al, eds. Physiology of the gastrointestinal tract. 2nd ed. New York: Raven Press, 1987:1351.

176. Robinson JWL, ed. Intestinal ion transport. Lancaster, U.K.: MTP Press, 1976.

177. Powell DW. Intestinal water and electrolyte transport. In: Johnson LR, Christensen J, Jackson MJ, et al, eds. Physiology of the gastrointestinal tract. 2nd ed. New York: Raven Press, 1987:1267.

178. Skadhage E, ed. Intestinal absorption and secretion. Lancaster, U.K.: MTP Press, 1984.

179. Grady GF, Duhamel RC, Moore EW. Active transport of sodium by human colon in vitro. Gastroenterology 1970;59:583.

180. Hopfer U, Sigrist-Nelson K, Ammann E, Murer H. Differences in neutral amino acid and glucose transport between brush border and basolateral plasma membrane of intestinal epithelial cells. J Cell Physiol 1976;89:805.

181. Mehta MN, Subramaniam S. Comparison of rice water, rice electrolyte solution, and glucose electrolyte solution in the management of infantile diarrhoea. Lancet 1986;1:843.

182. Alpers DH. Absorption of vitamins and divalent minerals. In: Sleisenger MH, Fordtran JS, eds. Gastrointestinal disease: Pathophysiology, diagnosis, management. 4th ed. Philadelphia: WB Saunders, 1989:1045.

183. Lucke H, Stange G, Kinne R, Murer H. Taurocholate-sodium cotransport by brush-border membrane vesicles isolated from rat ileum. Biochem J 1978;174:951.

184. Duffey ME, Turnheim K, Frizzell RA, Schultz SG. Intracellular chloride activities in rabbit gallbladder: Direct evidence for the role of the sodium-gradient in energizing "uphill" chloride transport. J Membr Biol 1978;42:229.

185. Frizzell RA, Dugas MC, Schultz SG. Sodium chloride transport by rabbit gallbladder: Direct evidence for a coupled NaCl influx process. J Gen Physiol 1975;65:769.

186. Frizzell RA, Field M, Schultz SG. Sodium-coupled chloride transport by epithelial tissues. Am J Physiol 1979;236:F1.

187. Nellans HN, Frizzell RA, Schultz SG. Coupled sodium-chloride influx across the brush border of rabbit ileum. Am J Physiol 1973;225:467.

188. Liedtke CM, Hopfer U. Mechanism of Cl^- translocation across small intestinal brush border membrane: II. Absence of Na^+-Cl^- cotransport. Am J Physiol 1982;242:G263.

189. Lubcke R, Haag K, Berger E, Knauf H, Gerok W. Ion transport in rat proximal colon in vivo. Am J Physiol 1986;251:G132.

190. Binder HJ, Foster ES, Budinger ME, Hayslett JP. Mechanism of electroneutral sodium chloride absorption in distal colon of the rat. Gastroenterology 1987;93:449.

191. Foster ES, Budinger ME, Hayslett JP, Binder HJ. Ion transport in proximal colon of the rat: Sodium depletion stimulates neutral sodium chloride absorption. J Clin Invest 1986;77:228.

192. Booth IW, Stange G, Murer H, Fenton TR, Milla PJ. Defective jejunal brush-border Na^+/H^+ exchange: A cause of congenital secretory diarrhea. Lancet 1985;1:1066.

193. Kikuchi K, Ghishan FK. Phosphate transport by basolateral plasma membranes of human small intestine. Gastroenterology 1987;93:106.

194. Mohrmann I, Mohrmann M, Biber J, Murer H. Sodium-dependent transport of P_i by an established intestinal epithelial cell line (CaCo-2). Am J Physiol 1986;250:G323.

195. Brautbar N, Levine BS, Walling MW, Coburn JW. Intestinal absorption of calcium: Role of dietary phosphate and vitamin D. Am J Physiol 1981;241:G49.

196. Favus MJ. Factors that influence absorption and secretion of calcium in the small intestine and colon. Am J Physiol 1985;248:G147.

197. Murer H, Hildmann B. Transcellular transport of calcium and inorganic phosphate in the small intestinal epithelium. Am J Physiol 1981;240:G409.

198. Gray TK, Bieberdorf FA, Fordtran JS. Thyrocalcitonin and the jejunal absorption of calcium, water and electrolytes in normal subjects. J Clin Invest 1973;52:3084.

199. Kisloff B, Moore EW. Effects of intravenous calcitonin on water, electrolyte, and calcium movement across in vitro rabbit jejunum and ileum. Gastroenterology 1977;72:462.

200. Smith PL, McCabe RD. Potassium secretion by rabbit descending colon: Effects of adrenergic stimuli. Am J Physiol 1986;250:G432.

201. Halm DR, Frizzell RA. Active K transport across rabbit distal colon: Relation to Na absorption and Cl secretion. Am J Physiol 1986;251:C252.

202. Hayslett JP, Binder HJ. Mechanism of potassium adaption. Am J Physiol 1982;243:F103.

203. Sullivan SK, Smith PL. Active potassium secretion by rabbit proximal colon. Am J Physiol 1986;250:G475.

204. Kliger AS, Binder HJ, Bastl C, Hayslett JP. Demonstration of active potassium transport in the mammalian colon. J Clin Invest 1981;67:1189.

205. Smith PL, McCabe RD. Mechanism and regulation of transcellular potassium transport by the colon. Am J Physiol 1984;247:G445.

206. Foster ES, Jones WJ, Hayslett JP, Binder HJ. Role of aldosterone and dietary potassium in potassium adaption in the distal colon of the rat. Gastroenterology 1985;88:41.

207. Donowitz M, Sharp GWG, eds. Mechanisms of intestinal electrolyte transport and regulation by calcium. New York: Alan R Liss, 1984.

208. Rink TJ. A real receptor-operated calcium channel. Nature 1988;334:649.

209. Tanabe T, Takeshima H, Mikami A, et al. Primary structure of the receptor for calcium channel blockers from skeletal muscle. Nature 1987;328:313.

210. Scott WN, Goodman DBP, eds. Hormonal regulation of epithelial transport of ions and water. Ann NY Acad Sci 1981;372:1.

211. Solcia E, Capella C, Buffa R, et al. Endocrine cells of the digestive system. In: Johnson LR, Christensen J, Jackson MJ, et al, eds. Physiology of the gastrointestinal tract. 2nd ed. New York: Raven Press, 1987:111.

212. Walsh JH. Gastrointestinal hormones and peptides. In: Johnson LR, Christensen J, Jackson MJ, et al, eds. Physiology of the gastrointestinal tract. 2nd ed. New York: Raven Press, 1987:181.

213. Walsh JH. Gastrointestinal peptide hormones. In: Sleisenger MH, Fordtran JS, eds. Gastrointestinal disease: Pathophysiology, diagnosis, management. 4th ed. Philadelphia: WB Saunders, 1989:78.

214. Laburthe M, Amiranoff B. Peptide receptors in the intestinal epithelium. In: Makhlouf GM, ed. Handbook of physiology: Neuroendocrinology of the gut. Bethesda, MD: American Physiological Society, 1989:215.

215. Dharmsathaphorn K, Harms V, Yamashiro DJ, Hughes RJ, Binder HJ, Wright E. Preferential binding of vasoactive intestinal polypeptide to basolateral membrane of rat and rabbit enterocytes. J Clin Invest 1983;71:27.

216. Pandol SJ, Dharmsathaphorn K, Schoeffield MS, Vale W, Rivier J. Vasoactive intestinal peptide receptor antagonist [4Cl-D-Phe^6, Leu^{17}]VIP. Am J Physiol 1986;250:G553.

217. Rosenblatt M. Peptide hormone antagonists that are effective in vivo. N Engl J Med 1986;315:1004.

218. Niederau C, Niederau M, Williams JA, Grendell JH. New proglumide-analogue CCK receptor antagonists: Very potent and selective for peripheral tissues. Am J Physiol 1986;251:G856.

219. Heinz-Erian P, Coy DH, Tamura M, Jones SW, Gardner JD, Jensen RT. [C-Phe^{12}]bombesin analogues: A new class of bombesin receptor antagonists. Am J Physiol 1987;252:G439.

220. Pan G-Z, Lu L, Qian J-M, Xue B-G. Bovine pancreatic polypeptide as an antagonist of muscarinic cholinergic receptors. Am J Physiol 1987;252:G384.

221. Gardner JD, Jensen RT. Cholecystokinin receptor antagonists. Am J Physiol 1984;246:G471.

222. Jensen RT, Murphy RB, Trampota M, et al. Proglumide analogues: Potent cholecystokinin receptor antagonists. Am J Physiol 1985;249:G214.

223. Dahl KD, Bicsak TA, Hsueh AJW. Naturally occurring antihormones: Secretion of FSH antagonists by women treated with a GnRH analog. Science 1988;239:72.

224. Holmdahl G, Hakanson R, Leander S, Rosell S, Folkers K, Sundler F. A substance P antagonist, [D-Pro^2, D-Trp^{7,9}]SP, inhibits inflammatory responses in the rabbit eye. Science 1981;214:1029.

225. Barrett KE, Dharmsathaphorn K. Pharmacological approaches to the therapy of diarrheal diseases. In: Field M, ed. Diarrheal diseases. New York: Elsevier Science Publishers, 1989 (in press)

226. Allende JE. GTP-mediated macromolecular interactions: The common features of different systems. FASEB J 1988;2:2356.

227. Nicoll RA. The coupling of neurotransmitter receptors to ion channels in the brain. Science 1988;241:545.

228. Sasaki K, Sato M. A single GTP-binding protein regulates K^+-channels coupled with dopamine, histamine and acetylcholine receptors. Nature 1987;325:259.

229. Andrade R, Malenka RC, Nicoll RA. A G protein couples serotonin and $GABA_B$ receptors to the same channels in hippocampus. Science 1986;234:1261.

230. Codina J, Yatani A, Grenet D, Brown AM, Birnbaumer L. The subunit of the GTP binding protein G_K opens atrial potassium channels. Science 1987;236:442.

231. Cockcroft S, Gomperts BD. Role of guanine nucleotide binding protein in the activation of polyphosphoinositide phosphodiesterase. Nature 1985;314:534.

232. Neer EJ, Clapham DE. Roles of G protein subunits in transmembrane signalling. Nature 1988;333:129.

233. Moss J. Signal transduction by receptor-responsive guanyl nucleotide-binding proteins: Modulation by bacterial toxin-catalyzed ADP-ribosylation. Clin Res 1987;35:451.

234. Gilman AG. Guanine nucleotide-binding regulatory proteins and dual control of adenylate cyclase. J Clin Invest 1984;73:1.

235. Fain JN, Wallace MA, Wojcikiewicz RJH. Evidence for involvement of guanine nucleotide-binding regulatory proteins in the activation of phospholipases by hormones. FASEB J 1988;2:2569.

236. Limbird LE. Receptors linked to inhibition of adenylate cyclase: Addition signaling mechanisms. FASEB J 1988;2:2686.

237. Donowitz M, Asarkof N. Calcium dependence of basal electrolyte transport in rabbit ileum. Am J Physiol 1982;243:G28.

238. Zimmerman TW, Dobbins JW, Binder HJ. Role of calcium in the regulation of colonic secretion in the rat. Am J Physiol 1983;244:G552.

239. Hubel KA, Callanan D. Effects of Ca^{2+} on ileal transport and electrically induced secretion. Am J Physiol 1980;239:G18.

240. Field M. Ion transport in rabbit ileal mucosa: II. Effects of cyclic $3',5'$-AMP. Am J Physiol 1971;221:992.

241. McCabe RD, Smith PL. Colonic potassium and chloride secretion: Role of cAMP and calcium. Am J Physiol 1985;248:G103.

242. Kimberg DV, Field M, Johnson J, Henderson A, Gershon E. Stimulation of intestinal mucosal adenyl cyclase by cholera enterotoxin and prostaglandins. J Clin Invest 1971;50:1218.

243. Schwartz CJ, Kimberg DV, Sheerin HE, Field M, Said SI. Vasoactive intestinal peptide stimulation of adenylate cyclase and active electrolyte secretion in intestinal mucosa. J Clin Invest 1974;54:536.

244. Waldman DB, Gardner JD, Zfass AM, Makhlouf GM. Effects of vasoactive intestinal peptide on rat colonic transport and adenylate cyclase activity. Gastroenterology 1977;73:518.

245. Gill DM. Mechanism of action of cholera toxin. Adv Cyclic Nucleotide Res 1977;8:85.

246. Brasitus TA, Field M, Kimberg DV. Intestinal mucosal cyclic GMP: Regulation and possible role in ion transport. Am J Physiol 1976;231:275.

247. Field M, Graf LH Jr, Laird WJ, Smith PL. Heat stable enterotoxin of *Escherichia coli*: In vitro effects of guanylate cyclase activity, cyclic GMP concentration, and ion transport in small intestine. Proc Natl Acad Sci USA 1978;75:2800.

248. Ilundain A, Naftalin RJ. Role of Ca^{2+}-dependent regulator protein in intestinal secretion. Nature 1979;279:446.

249. Nishizuka Y. Turnover of inositol phospholipids and signal transduction. Science 1984;225:1365.

250. Williamson JR, Cooper RH, Joseph SK, Thomas AP. Inositol trisphosphate and diacylglycerol as intracellular second messengers in liver. Am J Physiol 1985;248:C203.

251. Exton JH. Mechanisms of action of calcium-mobilizing agonists: Some variations on a young theme. FASEB J 1988;2:2670.

252. Rabbani GH, Greenough WB III, Holmgren J, Lonnroth I. Chlorpromazine reduces fluid-loss in cholera. Lancet 1979;1:410.

253. Smith PL, Field M. In vitro antisecretory effects of trifluoperazine and other neuroleptics in rabbit and human small intestine. Gastroenterology 1980;78:1545.

254. Hanks SK, Quinn AM, Hunter T. The protein kinase family: Conserved features and deduced phylogeny of the catalytic domains. Science 1988;241:42.

255. Shlatz LJ, Kimberg DV, Cattieu KA. Cyclic nucleotide-dependent phosphorylation of rat intestinal microvillus and basal lateral membrane proteins by an endogenous protein kinase. Gastroenterology 1978;75:838.

256. Shlatz LJ, Kimberg DV, Cattieu KA. Phosphorylation of specific rat intestinal microvillus and basal-lateral membrane proteins by cyclic nucleotides. Gastroenterology 1979;76:293.

257. Taylor SS, Bubis J, Toner-Webb J, et al. cAMP-dependent protein kinase: Prototype for a family of enzymes. FASEB J 1988;2:2677.

258. Schoumacher RA, Shoemaker RL, Halm DR, Tallant EA, Wallace RW, Frizzell RA. Phosphorylation fails to activate chloride channels from cystic fibrosis airway cells. Nature 1987;330:752.

259. Nishizuka Y. Studies and perspectives of protein kinase C. Science 1986;233:305.

260. Mandel KG, Dharmsathaphorn K, McRoberts JA. Characterization of a cyclic AMP-activated Cl^- transport pathway in the apical membrane of a human colonic epithelial cell line. J Biol Chem 1986;261:704.

261. Dharmsathaphorn K, Pandol S. Mechanism of chloride secretion induced by carbachol in a colonic epithelial cell line. J Clin Invest 1986;77:348.

262. Targan SR, Kagnoff MF, Brogan MD, Shanahan F. Immunologic mechanisms in intestinal diseases. Ann Intern Med 1987;106:853.

263. Miyajima A, Miyatake S, Schreurs J, et al. Coordinate regulation of immune and inflammatory responses by T cell–derived lymphokines. FASEB J 1988;2:2462.

264. Russell DA. Mast cells in the regulation of intestinal electrolyte transport. Am J Physiol 1986;251:G253.

265. Baird AW, Cuthbert AW, Pearce FL. Immediate hypersensitivity reactions in epithelia from rats infected with *Nippostrongylus brasiliensis*. Br J Pharmacol 1985;85:787.

266. Musch MW, Miller RJ, Field M, Siegel MI. Stimulation of colonic secretion by lipoxygenase metabolites of arachidonic acid. Science 1982;217:1255.

267. McCabe RD, Smith PL. Effects of histamine and histamine receptor antagonists on ion transport in rabbit descending colon. Am J Physiol 1984;247:G411.

268. Wasserman SI, Huott P, Barrett K, Beuerlein G, Kagnoff M, Dharmsathaphorn K. Immune-related intestinal Cl^- secretion: I. Effect of histamine on the T_{84} cell line. Am J Physiol 1988;254:C53.

269. Montzka DM, Smith PL, Fondacaro JD. Action of peptidoleukotrienes (PLTs) on electrolyte transport in rat small intestine. Gastroenterology 1987;92:1803.

270. Barrett KE. Immune-related intestinal secretion: Control of colonic chloride secretion by inflammatory mediators. In: MacDermott RP, ed. Inflammatory bowel disease: Current status and future approach. Amsterdam: Elsevier Science Publishers, 1988:377.

271. Perdue MH, Gall DG. Mucosal mast cells and the intestinal epithelium. In: Mestecky J, McGhee JR, Bienenstock J, Ogra PL, eds. Recent advances in mucosal immunology. New York: Plenum Publishing, 1987:645.

272. Perdue MH, Ramage JK, D'Inca R, et al. Mucosal changes during experimental inflammation in the rat. In: MacDermott RP, ed. Inflammatory bowel disease: Current status and future approach. Amsterdam: Elsevier Science Publishers, 1988:397.

273. Barrett KE, Cohn JA, Huott PA, Wasserman SI, Dharmsathaphorn K. Immune-related intestinal Cl^- secretion: II. Effect of adenosine on T_{84} cell line. Am J Physiol 1990;258:C902.

274. Wang YZ, Cooke HJ. Interaction of a mast cell inflammatory mediator with the enteric nervous system and the epithelium in guinea pig distal colon [Abstract]. Gastroenterology 1988;94:A487.

275. Bienenstock J, Tomioka M, Matsuda H, et al. The role of mast cells in inflammatory processes: Evidence for nerve/mast cell interactions. Int Arch Allergy Appl Immunol 1987;82:238.

276. Cutz E, Chan W, Track NS, Goth A, Said SI. Release of vasoactive intestinal polypeptide in mast cells by histamine liberators. Nature 1978;275:661.

277. Wasserman SI. Anaphylaxis. In: Middleton E, Reed CE, Ellis EF, eds. Allergy: Principles and practice. 2nd ed. St Louis: CV Mosby, 1983:689.

278. Barrett KE, Metcalfe DD. Mucosal mast cells and IgE. In: Heyworth MF, Jones AL, eds. Immunology of the gastrointestinal tract and liver. New York: Raven Press, 1988:65.

279. Metcalfe DD. Mast cell mediators with emphasis on intestinal mast cells. Ann Allergy 1984;53:563.

280. Bern MJ, Sturbaum CW, Karayalcin SS, et al. Immune system control of rat and rabbit colonic electrolyte transport. Role of prostaglandins and enteric nervous system. J Clin Invest 1989;83:1810.

281. Karayalcin SS, Sturbaum CW, Dixon MU, Powell DW. Hydrogen peroxide is the reactive oxygen species (ROS) which stimulates colonic electrolyte secretion. Gastroenterology 1988;94:A216.

282. Nash S, Stafford J, Madara JL. Effects of polymorphonuclear leukocyte transmigration on the barrier function of cultured intestinal epithelial monolayers. J Clin Invest 1987;80:1104.

283. Agosti JM, Ayars GH, Altman LC, Gleich GJ, Baker C, Loegering DA. Injurious effect of the eosinophil peroxidase-hydrogen peroxide-halide system on nasal epithelium. J Allergy Clin Immunol 1988;81:207.

284. Lichtenstein LM. Histamine-releasing factors and IgE heterogeneity. J Allergy Clin Immunol 1988;81:814.

285. Charney AN, Feldman GM. Systemic acid-base disorders and intestinal electrolyte transport. Am J Physiol 1984;247:G1.

286. Feldman GM, Charney AN. Effect of acute metabolic alkalosis and acidosis on intestinal electrolyte transport in vivo. Am J Physiol 1980;239:G427.

287. Feldman GM, Charney AN. Effect of acute respiratory alkalosis and acidosis on intestinal electrolyte transport in vivo. Am J Physiol 1982;242:G436.

288. Charney AN, Haskell LP. Relative effects of systemic pH, PCO_2, and HCO_3 concentration on colonic ion transport. Am J Physiol 1984;246:G159.

289. Kurtin P, Charney AN. Intestinal ion transport and intracellular pH during acute respiratory alkalosis and acidosis. Am J Physiol 1984;247:G24.

290. Wagner JD, Kurtin P, Charney AN. Effect of systemic acid-base disorders on colonic intracellular pH and ion transport. Am J Physiol 1985;249:G39.

291. Charney AN, Wagner JD, Birnbaum GJ, Johnstone JN. Functional role of carbonic anhydrase in intestinal electrolyte transport. Am J Physiol 1986;251:G682.

292. Kurtin P, Charney AN. Effect of arterial carbon dioxide tension on amiloride-sensitive sodium absorption in the colon. Am J Physiol 1984;247:G537.

293. Charney AN, Arnold M, Johnstone N. Acute respiratory alkalosis and acidosis and rabbit intestinal ion transport in vivo. Am J Physiol 1983;244:G145.

294. Cammack J, Read NW, Cann PA, Greenwood B, Holgate AM. Effect of prolonged exercise on the passage of a solid meal through the stomach and small intestine. Gut 1982;23:957.

295. Christensen J. Motility of the colon. In: Johnson LR, Christensen J, Jackson MJ, et al, eds. Physiology of the gastrointestinal tract. 2nd ed. New York: Raven Press, 1987:665.

296. Kerlin P, Zinsmeister A, Phillips S. Relationship of motility to flow of contents in the human small intestine. Gastroenterology 1982;82:701.

297. Weisbrodt NW. Motility of the small intestine. In: Johnson LR, Christensen J, Jackson MJ, et al, eds. Physiology of the gastrointestinal tract. 2nd ed. New York: Raven Press, 1987:631.

298. Levitt DG, Bond JH, Levitt MD. Use of a model of small bowel mucosa to predict passive absorption. Am J Physiol 1980;239:G23.

299. Harris MS, Dobbins JW, Binder HJ. Augmentation of neutral sodium chloride absorption by increased flow rate in rat ileum in vivo. J Clin Invest 1986;78:431.

300. Westergaard H, Holtermuller KH, Dietschy JM. Measurement of resistance of barriers to solute transport in vivo in rat jejunum. Am J Physiol 1986;250:G727.

301. Freel RW, Hatch M, Earnest DL, Goldner AM. Role of tight-junctional pathways in bile salt–induced increases in colonic permeability. Am J Physiol 1983;245:G816.

302. Pappenheimer JR, Reiss KZ. Contribution of solvent drag through intercellular junctions to absorption of nutrients by the small intestine of the rat. J Membr Biol 1987;100:123.

303. Pappenheimer JR. Physiological regulation of transepithelial imped-ance in the intestinal mucosa of rats and hamsters. J Membr Biol 1987;100:137.

304. Madara JL, Pappenheimer JR. Structural basis for physiological regulation of paracellular pathways in intestinal epithelia. J Membr Biol 1987;100:149.

305. Hakim AA, Papeleux CB, Lane JB, Lifson N, Yablonski ME. Mechanism of production of intestinal secretion by negative luminal pressure. Am J Physiol 1977;233:E416.

306. Norman DA, Atkins JM, Seelig LL Jr, Gomez-Sanchez C, Krejs GJ. Water and electrolyte movement and mucosal morphology in the jejunum of patients with portal hypertension. Gastroenterology 1980;79:707.

307. Humphreys MH, Earley LE. The mechanism of decreased intestinal sodium and water absorption after acute volume expansion in the rat. J Clin Invest 1971;50:2355.

308. Swabb EA, Hynes RA, Donowitz M. Elevated intraluminal pressure alters rabbit small intestinal transport in vivo. Am J Physiol 1982;242:G58.

309. Sjovall H, Butcher P, Martner J, Sellden H. Cardiac receptor modulation of blood flow and fluid transport in feline jejunum. Am J Physiol 1987;253:G116.

310. Swabb EA, Hynes RA, Decker RA, Tai Y-H, Donowitz M. Acute elevation of intraluminal hydrostatic pressure alters small intestinal but not rat colonic water transport and permeability. Gastroenterology 1979;76:1257.

311. Yablonski ME, Lifson N. Mechanism of production of intestinal secretion by elevated venous pressure. J Clin Invest 1976;57:904.

312. Granger DN. Intestinal microcirculation and transmucosal fluid transport. Am J Physiol 1981;240:G343.

313. Barclay GR, Turnberg LA. Effect of psychological stress on salt and water transport in the human jejunum. Gastroenterology 1987;93:91.

314. Barclay GR, Turnberg LA. Effect of cold-induced pain on salt and water transport in the human jejunum. Gastroenterology 1988;94:994.

315. Corbett CL, Thomas S, Read NW, Hobson N, Bergman I, Holdsworth CD. Electrochemical detector for breath hydrogen determination: Measurement of small bowel transit time in normal subjects and patients with the irritable bowel syndrome. Gut 1981;22:836.

316. Read NW, Cammack J, Edwards C, Holgate AM, Cann PA, Brown C. Is the transit time of a meal through the small intestine related to the rate at which it leaves the stomach? Gut 1982;23:824.

317. Read NW, Miles CA, Fisher D, et al. Transit of a meal through the stomach, small intestine, and colon in normal subjects and its role in the pathogenesis of diarrhea. Gastroenterology 1980;79:1276.

318. Meyer JH. Motility of the stomach and gastroduodenal junction. In: Johnson LR, Christensen J, Jackson MJ, et al, eds. Physiology of the gastrointestinal tract. 2nd ed. New York: Raven Press, 1987:613.

319. Schiller LR, Davis GR, Santa Ana CA, Morawski SG, Fordtran JS. Mechanism of the antidiarrheal action of codeine. Gastroenterology 1981;80:1275.

320. Bitar KN, Makhlouf GM. Selective presence of opiate receptors on intestinal circular muscle cells. Life Sci 1985;37:1545.

321. Dobbins J, Racusen L, Binder HJ. Effect of D-alanine methionine enkephalin amide on ion transport in rabbit ileum. J Clin Invest 1980;66:19.

322. Huizinga JD, Vermillion DL, Muller MJ, Collins SM. The effects of intestinal inflammation on smooth muscle function. In: MacDermott RP, ed. Inflammatory bowel disease: Current status and future approach. Amsterdam: Elsevier Science Publishers, 1988:403.

323. Eklund S, Brunsson I, Jodal M, Lundgren O. Changes in cyclic 3'5'-adenosine monophosphate tissue concentration and net fluid transport in the cat's small intestine elicited by cholera toxin, arachidonic acid, vasoactive intestinal polypeptide and 5- hydroxytryptamine. Acta Physiol Scand 1987;129:115.

324. Brunsson I, Sjoqvist A, Jodal M, Lundgren O. Mechanisms underlying the small intestinal fluid secretion caused by arachidonic acid, prostaglandin E_1 and prostaglandin E_2 in the rat in vivo. Acta Physiol Scand 1987;130:633.

325. Brunsson I, Sjoqvist A, Jodal M, Lundgren O. Mechanisms underlying the intestinal fluid secretion evoked by nociceptive serosal

stimulation of the rat. Naunyn Schmiedebergs Arch Pharmacol 1985;328:439.

326. Cooke HJ, Zafirova M, Carey HV, Walsh JH, Grider J. Vasoactive intestinal polypeptide actions on the guinea pig intestinal mucosa during neural stimulation. Gastroenterology 1987;92:361.

327. Nowak TV, Harrington B, Kalbfleisch JH, Amatruda JM. Evidence for abnormal cholinergic neuromuscular transmission in diabetic rat small intestine. Gastroenterology 1986;91:124.

328. Crampton JR, Gibbons LG, Rees WDW. Neural regulation of duodenal alkali secretion: Effects of electrical field stimulation. Am J Physiol 1988;254:G162.

329. Soll AH, Wollin A. Histamine and cyclic AMP in isolated canine parietal cells. Am J Physiol 1979;237:E444.

330. Soll AH, Berglindh T. Physiology of isolated gastric glands and parietal cells: Receptors and effectors regulating function. In: Johnson LR, Christensen J, Jackson MJ, et al, eds. Physiology of the gastrointestinal tract. 2nd ed. New York: Raven Press, 1987:883.

331. Soll AH, Walsh JH. Regulation of gastric acid secretion. Annu Rev Physiol 1979;41:35.

332. Powell DW. Barrier function of epithelia. Am J Physiol 1981;241:G275.

333. Smith AC, Podolsky DK. Biosynthesis and secretion of human colonic mucin glycoproteins. J Clin Invest 1987;80:300.

334. Specian RD, Neutra MR. Regulation of intestinal goblet cell secretion: I. Role of parasympathetic stimulation. Am J Physiol 1982;242:G370.

335. Neutra MR, O'Malley LJ, Specian RD. Regulation of intestinal goblet cell secretion: II. A survey of potential secretagogues. Am J Physiol 1982;242:G380.

336. Jodal M, Lundgren O. Countercurrent mechanisms in the mammalian gastrointestinal tract. Gastroenterology 1986;91:225.

337. Ladas S, Papanikos J, Arapakis G. Lactose malabsorption in Greek adults: Correlation of small bowel transit time with the severity of lactose intolerance. Gut 1982;23:968.

338. Culp KS, Piziak VK. Thyrotoxicosis presenting with secretory diarrhea. Ann Intern Med 1986;105:216.

339. Nellans HN, Frizzell RA, Schultz SG. Effect of acetazolamide on sodium and chloride transport by in vitro rabbit ileum. Am J Physiol 1975;228:1808.

340. Cooper H, Levitan R, Fordtran JS, Ingelfinger FJ. A method for studying absorption of water and solute from the human small intestine. Gastroenterology 1966;50:1.

341. Dupas J-L, Moreau M, Hofmann AF. Polymeric dyes: Useful non-absorbable reference markers for intestinal perfusion studies in animals. J Pharm Sci 1985;74:328.

342. Wilson TH, Wiseman G. The use of sacs of everted small intestine for the study of transference of substances from the mucosal to the serosal surface. J Physiol (Lond) 1954;123:116.

343. Ussing HH, Zerahan K. Active transport of sodium as the source of electric current in the short circuited frog skin. Acta Physiol Scand 1951;214:110.

344. Curran PF, Schultz SG. Transport across membranes: General principles. In: Code CF, ed. Handbook of physiology: Alimentary canal. Washington, DC: American Physiological Society, 1968:1217.

345. Fromter E. Viewing the kidney through microelectrodes. Am J Physiol 1984;247:F695.

346. Garcia-Diaz JF, Stump S, Armstrong W McD. Electronic device for microelectrode recordings in epithelial cells. Am J Physiol 1984;246:C339.

347. Gupta BL, Hall TA, Naftalin RJ. Microprobe measurement of Na, K and Cl concentration profiles in epithelial cells and intercellular spaces of rabbit ileum. Nature 1978;272:70.

348. Hixon DC. A guide to ion-selective electrodes. Nature 1988;335:279.

349. Chao AC, Armstrong W McD. Cl⁻-selective microelectrodes: Sensitivity to anionic Cl⁻ transport inhibitors. Am J Physiol 1987;253:C343.

350. Lechene C. Electron probe microanalysis of biological soft tissues: Principle and technique. Fed Proc 1980;39:2871.

351. Sakmann B, Neher E, eds. Single channel recording. New York: Plenum Press, 1983.

352. Gustin MC, Goodman DBP. Isolation of brush-border membrane from the rabbit descending colon epithelium. J Biol Chem 1981;256:10651.

353. Hopfer U. Isolated membrane vesicles as tools for analysis of epithelial transport. Am J Physiol 1977;233:E445.

354. Mircheff AK, van Os CH, Wright EM. Preparative scale isolation of basal-lateral plasma membranes from rat intestinal epithelial cells. Membr Biochem 1978;1:177.

355. Grover AK, Singh AP, Rangachari PK, Nicholls P. Ion movements in membrane vesicles: A new fluorescence method and application to smooth muscle. Am J Physiol 1985;248:C372.

356. Dharmsathaphorn K, Mandel KG, McRoberts JA, Tisdale LD, Masui H. A human colonic tumor cell line that maintains vectorial electrolyte transport. Am J Physiol 1984;246:G204.

357. Steele RE, Preston AS, Johnson JP, Handler JS. Porous-bottom dishes for culture of polarized cells. Am J Physiol 1986;251:C136.

358. Madara JL, Stafford J, Dharmsathaphorn K, Carlson S. Structural analysis of a human intestinal epithelial cell line. Gastroenterology 1987;92:1133.

359. Phillips TE, Huet C, Bilbo PR, Podolsky DK, Louvard D, Neutra MR. Human intestinal goblet cells in monolayer culture: Characterization of a mucus-secreting subclone derived from the HT 29 colon adenocarcinoma cell line. Gastroenterology 1988;94:1390.

360. Gargus JJ. Mutant isolation and gene transfer as tools in study of transport proteins. Am J Physiol 1987;252:C457.

361. Binder HJ. Net fluid and electrolyte secretion: The pathophysiological basis of diarrhea. Viewpoints Dig Dis 1980;12:2

362. Rosenthal LE, Pressman J, Dharmsathaphorn K. Development of new antidiarrheal medications. J Clin Gastroenterol 1983;5:131.

363. Fondacaro JD. Intestinal ion transport and diarrheal disease. Am J Physiol 1986;250:G1.

364. Berschneider HM, Knowles MR, Azizkhan RG, et al. Altered intestinal chloride transport in cystic fibrosis. FASEB J 1988;2:2625.

365. Fine KD, Krejs GJ, Fordtran JS. Diarrhea. In: Sleisenger MH, Fordtran JS, eds. Gastrointestinal disease: Pathophysiology, diagnosis, management. 4th ed. Philadelphia: WB Saunders, 1989:290.

366. Horvath PJ, Ferriola PC, Weiser MM, Duffey ME. Localization of chloride secretion in rabbit colon: Inhibition by anthracene-9-carboxylic acid. Am J Physiol 1986;250:G185.

367. Stoll BJ, Holmgren J, Bardhan PK, Huq I, Greenough WB III, Fredman P, Svennerholm L. Binding of intraluminal toxin in cholera: Trial of GM₁ ganglioside charcoal. Lancet 1980;2:888.

368. Field M. Corticosteroids, NaK-ATPase and intestinal water and electrolyte transport. Gastroenterology 1978;75:317.

369. Benos DJ. Amiloride: A molecular probe of sodium transport in tissues and cells. Am J Physiol 1982;242:C131.

370. Rocco VK, Cragoe EJ Jr, Warnock DG. N-ethoxycarbonyl-2-ethoxy-1,2-dihydroquinoline, amiloride analogues, and renal Na⁺/H⁺ antiporter. Am J Physiol 1987;252:F517.

371. Semrad CE, Chang EB. Calcium-mediated cyclic AMP inhibition of Na-H exchange in small intestine. Am J Physiol 1987;252:C315.

372. Sellin JH, De Soignie R. Ionic regulation of Na absorption in proximal colon: Cation inhibition of electroneutral Na absorption. Am J Physiol 1987;252:G100.

373. Binder HJ, Stange G, Murer H, Stieger B, Hauri H-P. Sodium-proton exchange in colon brush-border membranes. Am J Physiol 1986;251:G382.

374. Seifter JL, Aronson PS. Properties and physiologic roles of the plasma membrane sodium-hydrogen exchanger. J Clin Invest 1986;78:859.

375. Foster ES, Dudeja PK, Brasitus TA. Na⁺-H⁺ exchange in rat colonic brush-border membrane vesicles. Am J Physiol 1986;250:G781.

376. Hannafin J, Kinne-Saffran E, Friedman D, Kinne R. Presence of a sodium-potassium chloride cotransport system in the rectal gland of squalus acanthias. J Membr Biol 1983;75:73.

377. Musch MW, Orellana SA, Kimberg LS, et al. Na⁺-K⁺-Cl⁻ co-transport in the intestine of a marine teleost. Nature 1982;351:353.

378. O'Grady SM, Palfrey HC, Field M. Characteristics and functions of Na-K-Cl cotransport in epithelial tissues. Am J Physiol 1987;253:C177.

379. Noda M, Ikeda T, Suzuki H, et al. Expression of functional sodium channels from cloned cDNA. Nature 1986;322:826.

380. Li JH-Y, Cragoe EJ Jr, Lindemann B. Structure-activity relationships of amiloride analogs as blockers of epithelial Na channels: I. Pyrazine-ring modifications. J Membr Biol 1985;83:45.

381. Jorkasky D, Cox M, Feldman GM. Differential effects of corticosteroids on Na$^+$ transport in rat distal colon in vitro. Am J Physiol 1985;248:G424.

382. Will PC, Cortright RN, Groseclose RG, Hopfer U. Amiloride-sensitive salt and fluid absorption in small intestine of sodium-depleted rats. Am J Physiol 1985;248:G133.

383. Bastl CP, Binder HJ, Hayslett JP. Role of glucocorticoids and aldosterone in maintenance of colonic cation transport. Am J Physiol 1980;238:F181.

384. Peterson K-U, Reuss L. Cyclic AMP-induced chloride permeability in the apical membrane of Necturus gallbladder epithelium. J Gen Physiol 1983;81:705.

385. Welsh MJ. Anthracene-9-carboxylic acid inhibits an apical membrane chloride conductance in canine tracheal epithelium. J Membr Biol 1984;78:61.

386. Dubinsky WP, Monti LB. Solubilization and reconstitution of a chloride transporter from tracheal apical membrane. Am J Physiol 1986;251:C713.

387. Reinhardt R, Bridges RJ, Rummel W, Lindemann B. Properties of an anion-selective channel from rat colonic enterocyte plasma membranes reconstituted into planar phospholipid bilayers. J Membr Biol 1987;95:47.

388. Smith PL, Sullivan SK, McCabe RD. Concentration-dependent effects of disulfonic stilbenes on colonic chloride transport. Am J Physiol 1986;250:G44.

389. Latorre R, Miller C. Conduction and selectivity in potassium channels. J Membr Biol 1983;71:11.

390. Logothetis DE, Kurachi Y, Galper J, Neer EJ, Clapham DE. The subunits of GTP-binding proteins activate the muscarinic K$^+$ channel in heart. Nature 1987;325:321.

391. Schwarz TL, Tempel BL, Papazian DM, Jan YN, Jan LY. Multiple potassium-channel components are produced by alternative splicing at the Shaker locus in Drosophila. Nature 1988;331:137.

392. Papazian DM, Schwarz TL, Tempel BL, Jan YN, Jan LY. Cloning of genomic and complementary DNA from Shaker, a putative potassium channel gene from Drosophila. Science 1987;237:749.

393. Richards NW, Dawson DC. Single potassium channels blocked by lidocaine and quinidine in isolated turtle colon epithelial cells. Am J Physiol 1986;251:C85.

394. Isaacs PET, Corbett CL, Riley AK, Hawker PC, Turnberg LA. In vitro behavior of human intestinal mucosa: The influence of acetylcholine on ion transport. J Clin Invest 1976;58:535.

395. Tapper EJ, Powell DW, Morris SM. Cholinergic-adrenergic interaction of intestinal ion transport. Am J Physiol 1978;235:E402.

396. Zimmerman TW, Dobbins JW, Binder HJ. Mechanism of cholinergic regulation of electrolyte transport in rat colon in vitro. Am J Physiol 1982;242:G116.

397. Lee JS, Silverberg JW. Effect of histamine on intestinal fluid secretion in the dog. Am J Physiol 1976;231:793.

398. Fromm D, Halpern N. Effects of histamine receptor antagonists on ion transport by isolated ileum of the rabbit. Gastroenterology 1979;77:1034.

399. Linaker BD, McKay JS, Higgs NB, Turnberg LA. Mechanisms of histamine stimulated secretion in rabbit ileal mucosa. Gut 1981;22:964.

400. Beubler E, Bukhave K, Rask-Madsen J. Significance of calcium for the prostaglandin E$_2$-mediated secretory response to 5-hydroxytryptamine in the small intestine of the rat in vivo. Gastroenterology 1986;90:1972.

401. Zinner MJ, McFadden D, Sherlock D, Jaffe BM. Verapamil reversal of serotonin-induced jejunal secretion of water and electrolytes in awake dogs. Gastroenterology 1986;90:515.

402. Donowitz M, Charney AN, Heffernan JM. Effect of serotonin treatment on intestinal transport in the rabbit. Am J Physiol 1977;232:E85.

403. Kachur JF, Miller RJ, Field M, Rivier J. Neurohumoral control of ileal electrolyte transport: II. Neurotensin and substance P. J Pharmacol Exp Ther 1982;220:456.

404. Walling MV, Brasitus TA, Kimberg DV. Effects of calcitonin and substance P on the transport of Ca, Na and Cl across rat ileum in vitro. Gastroenterology 1977;73:89.

405. Barbezat GO, Reasbeck PG. Effects of bombesin, calcitonin, and enkephalin on canine jejunal water and electrolyte transport. Dig Dis Sci 1983;28:273.

406. Moritz M, Finkelstein G, Heshkinpour H, et al. Effect of secretin and cholecystokinin on the transport of electrolytes and water in human jejunum. Gastroenterology 1973;64:76.

407. Bussjaeger LJ, Johnson LR. Evidence for hormonal regulation of intestinal absorption by cholecystokinin. Am J Physiol 1973;224:1276.

408. Poitras P, Modigliani R, Bernier J-J. Effect of a combination of gastrin, secretin, cholecystokinin, glucagon, and gastric inhibitory polypeptide on jejunal absorption in man. Gut 1980;21:299.

409. Al-Awqati Q, Greenough WB III. Prostaglandins inhibit intestinal sodium transport. Nature 1972;238:26.

410. Bukhave K, Rask-Madsen J. Saturation kinetics applied to in vitro effects of low prostaglandins E$_2$ and F$_2$ concentrations on ion transport across human jejunal mucosa. Gastroenterology 1980;78:32.

411. Matuchansky C, Bernier JJ. Effect of prostaglandin E$_1$ on glucose, water and electrolyte absorption in the human jejunum. Gastroenterology 1973;64:1111.

412. Matuchansky C, Mary J-Y, Bernier J-J. Further studies on prostaglandin E$_1$-induced jejunal secretion of water and electrolytes in man, with special reference to the influence of ethacrynic acid, furosemide and aspirin. Gastroenterology 1976;71:274.

413. Lawson LD, Powell DW. Bradykinin-stimulated eicosanoid synthesis and secretion by rabbit ileal components. Am J Physiol 1987;252:G783.

414. Musch MW, Kachur JF, Miller RJ, Field M. Bradykinin-stimulated electrolyte secretion in rabbit and guinea pig intestine: Involvement of arachidonic acid metabolites. J Clin Invest 1983;71:1073.

415. Kane MG, O'Dorisio TM, Krejs GJ. Production of secretory diarrhea by intravenous infusion of vasoactive intestinal polypeptide. N Engl J Med 1983;309:1482.

416. Davis GR, Santa Ana CA, Morawski SG, Fordtran JS. Effect of vasoactive intestinal polypeptide on active and passive transport in the human jejunum. J Clin Invest 1981;67:1687.

417. Krejs GJ, Fordtran JS. Effect of VIP infusion on water and ion transport in the human jejunum. Gastroenterology 1980;78:722.

418. Hanglow AC, Bienenstock J, Dyck N, Perdue MH. Effects of platelet activating factor (PAF) on rat jejunal mucosa. Gastroenterology 1986;92:1424.

419. Hicks T, Turnberg LA. The effect of glucagon and secretin on salt and water transport in the human jejunum. Gut 1972;13:854.

420. Grander DN, Kvietys PR, Wilborn WH, Mortillaro NA, Taylor AE. Mechanism of glucagon-induced intestinal secretion. Am J Physiol 1980;239:G30.

421. Patel GK, Whalen GE, Soergel KH, Wu WC, Meade RC. Glucagon effects on the human small intestine. Dig Dis Sci 1979;24:501.

422. MacFerran SN, Mailman D. Effects of glucagon on canine intestinal sodium and water fluxes and regional blood flow. J Physiol 1977;266:1.

423. Anagnostides AA, Manolas K, Christofides ND, et al. Peptide histidine isoleucine (PHI): A secretagogue in porcine intestine. Dig Dis Sci 1983;28:893.

424. Dobbins JW, Laurenson JP, Forrest JN Jr. Adenosine and adenosine analogues stimulate adenosine cyclic 3',5'-monophosphate-dependent chloride secretion in the mammalian ileum. J Clin Invest 1984;74:929.

425. O'Grady SM, Field M, Nash NT, Rao MC. Atrial natriuretic factor inhibits Na-K-Cl cotransport in teleost intestine. Am J Physiol 1985;249:C531.

426. Bynum TE, Jacobson ED, Johnson LR. Gastrin inhibition of intestinal absorption in dogs. Gastroenterology 1971;61:858.

427. Helman CA, Barbezat GO. The effect of gastric inhibitory polypeptide on human jejunal water and electrolyte transport. Gastroenterology 1977;72:376.

428. Dennhardt R, Lingelbach B, Haberich FJ. Intestinal absorption under the influence of vasopressin: Studies in unanaesthetised rats. Gut 1979;20:107.

429. Kachel GW, Frase LL, Domschke W, Chey WY, Krejs GJ. Effect of 13-norleucin motilin on water and ion transport in the human jejunum. Gastroenterology 1984;87:550.

430. Kachur JF, Miller RJ, Field M, Rivier J. Neurohumoral control of

ileal electrolyte transport: I. Bombesin and related peptides. J Pharmacol Exp Ther 1982;220:449.

431. Al-Awqati Q, Cameron JL, Greenough WB III. Electrolyte transport in human ileum: Effect of purified cholera exotoxin. Am J Physiol 1973;224:818.

432. Banwell JG, Pierce NF, Mitra RC, et al. Intestinal fluid and electrolyte transport in human cholera. J Clin Invest 1970;49:183.

433. Field M, Fromm D, Al-Awqati Q, Greenough WB III. Effect of cholera enterotoxin on ion transport across isolated ileal mucosa. J Clin Invest 1972;51:796.

434. Powell DW, Binder HJ, Curran PF. Active electrolyte secretion stimulated by choleragen in rabbit ileum in vitro. Am J Physiol 1973;225:781.

435. Speelman P, Butler T, Kabir I, Ali A, Banwell J. Colonic dysfunction during cholera infection. Gastroenterology 1986;91:1164.

436. Hyun CS, Kimmich GA. Interaction of cholera toxin and *Escherichia coli* enterotoxin with isolated intestinal epithelial cells. Am J Physiol 1984;247:G623.

437. Peterson JW, Molina NC, Houston CW, Fader RC. Elevated cAMP in intestinal epithelial cells during experimental cholera and salmonellosis. Toxicon 1983;21:761.

438. Molina NC, Peterson JW. Cholera toxin-like toxin released by *Salmonella* species in the presence of mitomycin C. Infect Immun 1980;30:224.

439. Klipstein FA, Engert RF. Immunological relationship of the B subunits of *Campylobacter jejuni* and *Escherichia coli* heat-labile enterotoxins. Infect Immun 1985;48:629.

440. Ruiz-Palacios GM, Torres J, Torres NI, Escamilla E, Ruiz-Palacios BR, Tamayo J. Cholera-like enterotoxin produced by *Campylobacter jejuni:* Characterization and clinical significance. Lancet 1983;2:250.

441. Klipstein FA, Engert RF. Purification of *Campylobacter jejuni* enterotoxin. Lancet 1984;1:1123.

442. Guarino A, Cohen M, Thompson M, Dharmsathaphorn K, Giannella R. T$_{84}$ cell receptor binding and guanyl cyclase activation by *Escherichia coli* heat-stable toxin. Am J Physiol 1987;253:G775.

443. Rao MC, Orellana SA, Field M, Robertson DC, Giannella RA. Comparison of the biological actions of three purified heat-stable enterotoxins: Effects on ion transport and guanylate cyclase activity in rabbit ileum *in vitro.* Infect Immun 1981;33:167.

444. Rao MC, Guandalini S, Laird WJ, Field M. Effects of heat-stable enterotoxin of *Yersinia enterocolitica* on ion transport and cyclic guanosine 3'5' monophosphate metabolism in rabbit ileum. Infect Immun 1979;26:875

445. Klipstein FA, Engert RF, Houghten RA. Immunological properties of purified *Klebsiella pneumoniae* heat-stable enterotoxin. Infect Immun 1983;42:838.

446. Triadafilopoulos G, Pothoulakis C, O'Brien MJ, LaMont JT. Differential effects of *Clostridium difficile* toxins A and B on rabbit ileum. Gastroenterology 1987;93:273.

447. Hughes S, Warhurst G, Turnberg LA, Higgs NB, Giugliano LG, Drasar BS. *Clostridium difficile* toxin-induced intestinal secretion in rabbit ileum in vitro. Gut 1983;24:94.

448. Giannella RA, Gots RE, Charney AN, Greenough WB, Formal SB. Pathogenesis of salmonella-mediated intestinal fluid secretion. Gastroenterology 1975;69:1238.

449. Keusch GT, Grady GF, Mata LJ, McIver J. The pathogenesis of *Shigella* diarrhea: I. Enterotoxin production by *Shigella dysenteriae.* J Clin Invest 1972;51:1212.

450. Ammon HV, Phillips SF. Inhibition of ileal water absorption by intraluminal fatty acids: Influence of chain length, hydroxylation and conjugation of fatty acids. J Clin Invest 1974;53:205.

451. Binder HJ, Rawlins CL. The effect of conjugated dihydroxy bile salts on electrolyte transport in rat colon. J Clin Invest 1973;52:1460.

452. Bright-Asare P, Binder HJ. Stimulation of colonic secretion of water and electrolytes by hydroxy fatty acids. Gastroenterology 1973;64:81.

453. Mekhjian HS, Phillips SF, Hofmann AF. Colonic secretion of water and electrolytes induced by bile acids: Perfusion studies in man. J Clin Invest 1971;50:1569.

454. Schiller LR, Hogan RB, Morawski SG, et al. Studies of the prevalence and significance of radiolabeled bile acid malabsorption in a group of patients with idiopathic chronic diarrhea. Gastroenterology 1987;92:151.

455. Spiller RC, Brown ML, Phillips SF. Decreased fluid tolerance, accelerated transit, and abnormal motility of the human colon induced by oleic acid. Gastroenterology 1986;91:100.

456. Durbin T, Rosenthal L, McArthur K, Anderson D, Dharmsathaphorn K. Clonidine and lidamidine (WHR-1142) stimulate sodium and chloride absorption in the rabbit ileum. Gastroenterology 1982;82:1352.

457. Field M, McColl I. Ion transport in rabbit ileal mucosa: III. Effects of catecholamines. Am J Physiol 1973;225:852.

458. Hubel KA. Intestinal ion transport: Effect of norepinephrine, pilocarpine, and atropine. Am J Physiol 1976;231:252.

459. Laburthe M, Amiranoff B, Boissard C. Alpha-adrenergic inhibition of cyclic AMP accumulation in epithelial cells isolated from rat small intestine. Biochim Biophys Acta 1982;721:101.

460. Donowitz M, Cusolito S, Battisti L, Fogel R, Sharp GWG. Dopamine stimulation of active Na and Cl absorption in rabbit ileum. Interaction with alpha$_2$-adrenergic and specific dopamine receptors. J Clin Invest 1982;69:1008.

461. Donowitz M, Elta G, Battisti L, Fogel R, Label-Schwartz E. Effect of dopamine and bromocriptine on rat ileal and colonic transport: Stimulation of absorption and reversal of cholera toxin-induced secretion. Gastroenterology 1983;84:516.

462. Kachur JF, Miller RJ, Field M. Control of guinea pig intestinal electrolyte secretion by a delta-opiate receptor. Proc Natl Acad Sci USA 1980;77:2753.

463. McKay JS, Linaker BD, Turnberg LA. The influence of opiates on ion transport across rabbit ileal mucosa. Gastroenterology 1981;80:279.

464. Nishimura E, Buchan AMJ, McIntosh CHS. Autoradiographic localization of mu- and delta-type opioid receptors in the gastrointestinal tract of the rat and guinea pig. Gastroenterology 1986;91:1084.

465. Berschneider HM, Martens H, Powell DW. Effect of BW 942C, an enkephalinlike pentapeptide, on sodium and chloride transport in the rabbit ileum. Gastroenterology 1988;94:127.

466. Hautefeuille M, Brantl V, Dumontier A-M, Desjeux J-F. In vitro effects of beta-casomorphins on ion transport in rabbit ileum. Am J Physiol 1986;250:G92.

467. Stoll R, Ruppin H, Domschke W. Calmodulin-mediated effects of loperamide on chloride transport by brush border membrane vesicles from human ileum. Gastroenterology 1988;95:69.

468. Chang EB, Brown DR, Wang NS, Field M. Secretagogue-induced changes in membrane calcium permeability in chicken and chinchilla ileal mucosa: Selective inhibition by loperamide. J Clin Invest 1986;78:281.

469. Roberts WG, Fedorak RN, Chang EB. In vitro effects of the long-acting somatostatin analogue SMS 201-995 on electrolyte transport by the rabbit ileum. Gastroenterology 1988;94:1343.

470. Carter RF, Bitar KN, Zfass AM, Makhlouf GM. Inhibition of VIP-stimulated intestinal secretion and cyclic AMP production by somatostatin in the rat. Gastroenterology 1978;74:726.

471. Dharmsathaphorn K, Racusen L, Dobbins JW. Effect of somatostatin on ion transport in rat colon. J Clin Invest 1980;66:813.

472. Guandalini S, Kachur JF, Smith PL, Miller RJ, Field M. In vitro effects of somatostatin on ion transport in rabbit intestine. Am J Physiol 1980;238:G67.

473. Bastl CP, Barnett CA, Schmidt TJ, Litwack G. Glucocorticoid stimulation of sodium absorption in colon epithelia is mediated by corticosteroid IB receptor. J Biol Chem 1984;259:1186.

474. Levitan R, Ingelfinger FJ. Effect of d-aldosterone on salt and water absorption from the intact human colon. J Clin Invest 1965;44:801.

475. Bastl CP. Regulation of cation transport by low doses of glucocorticoids in in vivo adrenalectomized rat colon. J Clin Invest 1987;80:348.

476. Levens NR. Modulation of jejunal ion and water absorption by endogenous angiotensin after dehydration. Am J Physiol 1984;246:G700.

477. Levens NR, Peach MJ, Carey RM. Interactions between angiotensin peptides and the sympathetic nervous system mediating intestinal sodium and water absorption in the rat. J Clin Invest 1981;67:1197.

478. Levens NR, Peach MJ, Carey RM, Poat JA, Munday KA. Response of rat jejunum to angiotensin II: Role of norepinephrine and prostaglandins. Am J Physiol 1981;240:G17.

479. Friel DD, Miller RJ, Walker MW. Neuropeptide Y: A powerful modulator of epithelial ion transport. Br J Pharmacol 1986;88:425.

480. Mainoya JR. Effect of prolactin on fluid and NaCl absorption by the rat proximal and distal colon. Experientia 1979;35:1060.

481. Donowitz M, Wicks J, Sharp GWG. Drug therapy for diarrheal disease: A look ahead. Rev Infect Dis 1986;8(suppl 2):S188.

482. Smith PL, Blumberg JB, Stoff JS, Field M. Antisecretory effects of indomethacin on rabbit ileal mucosa in vitro. Gastroenterology 1981;80:356.

483. Powell DW, Tapper EJ, Morris SM. Aspirin-stimulated intestinal electrolyte transport in rabbit ileum in vitro. Gastroenterology 1979;76:1429.

484. Farris RK, Tapper EJ, Powell DW, Morris SM. Effect of aspirin on normal and cholera toxin–stimulated intestinal electrolyte transport. J Clin Invest 1976;57:916.

485. Ericsson CD, Evans DG, DuPont HL, Evans DJ Jr, Pickering LK. Bismuth subsalicylate inhibits activity of crude toxins of *Escherichia coli* and *Vibrio cholerae*. J Infect Dis 1977;136:693.

486. Campieri M, Lanfranchi GA, Bazzocchi G, et al. Treatment of ulcerative colitis with high-dose 5-aminosalicylic acid enemas. Lancet 1981;2:270.

487. Donowitz M, Charney AN, Hynes R. Propranolol prevention of cholera enterotoxin–induced intestinal secretion in the rat. Gastroenterology 1979;76:482.

488. Taub M, Bonorris G, Chung A, Coyne MJ, Schoenfield LJ. Effect of propranolol on bile acid– and cholera enterotoxin-stimulated cAMP and secretion in rabbit intestine. Gastroenterology 1977;72:101.

489. Turjman N, Gotterer GS, Hendrix TR. Prevention and reversal of cholera enterotoxin effects in rabbit jejunum by nicotinic acid. J Clin Invest 1978;61:1155.

490. Fogel R, Sharp GWG, Donowitz M. Chloroquine stimulates absorption and inhibits secretion of ileal water and electrolytes. Am J Physiol 1982;243:G117.

491. Feldman GM, Mann JJ, Charney AN. Effect of lithium ingestion on water and electrolyte transport in rat intestine. Gastroenterology 1981;81:892.

492. Pandol SJ, Korman LY, McCarthy DM, Gardner JD. Beneficial effect of oral lithium carbonate in the treatment of pancreatic cholera syndrome. N Engl J Med 1980;302:1403.

493. Donowitz M, Levin S, Powers G, Elta G, Cohen P, Cheng H. Ca²⁺ channel blockers stimulate ileal and colonic water absorption. Gastroenterology 1985;89:858.

494. Tai Y-H, Feser JF, Marnane WG, Desjeux J-F. Antisecretory effects of berberine in rat ileum. Am J Physiol 1981;241:G253.

495. Swabb EA, Tai Y-H, Jordan L. Reversal of cholera toxin-induced secretion in rat ileum by luminal berberine. Am J Physiol 1981;241:G248.

496. Notis WM, Orellana SA, Field M. Inhibition of intestinal secretion in rats by colchicine and vinblastine. Gastroenterology 1981;81:766.

15

Pancreatic Secretion

CHUNG OWYANG
JOHN WILLIAMS

INTRODUCTION

The pancreas is an organ with both exocrine and endocrine functions. The secretions of the exocrine pancreas, digestive enzymes and bicarbonate, affect the digestion and absorption of nutrients. The endocrine pancreas, on the other hand, releases hormones that regulate metabolism and the disposition of the breakdown products of food within the body. These combined exocrine and endocrine functions make the pancreas one of the most important and complex organs involved in the assimilation of food.

In the pancreas of humans and other mammals, the exocrine pancreas consists of clusters of acini that form lobules separated by loose connective tissue. Eighty percent or more of the pancreas consists of acini. Each individual acinus is a sphere composed of 20 to 50 pyramidal cells arranged with their broad bases around the circumference and their apices pointed toward a central lumen. Each acinus is drained by a ductule; the most proximal cells of the ductules extend into the lumen of the acinus and are called centroacinar cells. The ductules drain through a series of ducts with increasing caliber until the main ducts are reached.

Distributed within the pancreas are the islets of Langerhans, containing the cells of the endocrine pancreas. Morphologic studies have revealed both cell-to-cell contact between the exocrine and endocrine tissue and direct connections between the capillaries of the islets and the acini.[1,2,3] These morphologic arrangements may reflect a regulatory role for the islet hormones on the function of the exocrine pancreas and vice versa. Of the pancreatic hormones, glucagon[4,5] somatostatin,[6] and pancreatic polypeptide (PP)[7] have been shown to inhibit pancreatic exocrine secretion. Insulin, on the other hand, potentiates the stimulatory effect of cholecystokinin

(CCK) on pancreatic exocrine secretion.[8] In addition, exocrine pancreatic secretion can influence pancreatic hormone release.

FORMATION AND COMPOSITION OF PANCREATIC JUICE

The human pancreas secretes about 1 L of juice daily, consisting mostly of water, electrolytes, and digestive enzymes. The morphologic appearance of the different cells of the exocrine pancreas, as well as micropuncture studies, suggest that the acinar cells secrete digestive enzymes while the ductal cells are mainly responsible for electrolyte secretion that is rich in bicarbonate.[9] This thesis is further supported by experiments in which acinar or duct cells were selectively destroyed by administration of a toxin or a special diet to animals. Administration of alloxan, which destroys ductal but not acinar cells, results in diminished secretion of fluid and bicarbonate.[10] Ethionine administration, on the other hand, damages acinar cells with concomitant reduction in enzyme secretion, whereas secretion of fluid and electrolyte are relatively unaffected.[10]

Water and Electrolytes

Pancreatic electrolytes are secreted in a clear, alkaline fluid which is isosmotic with extracellular fluid. Current evidence suggests that water enters the juice passively along osmotic gradients established by active secretion of electrolytes or other solutes. The major cations in the pancreatic juice are Na^+ and K^+; both are secreted at concentrations similar to their plasma concentrations. The concentrations of both cations are constant and independent of secretory rates (Fig 15-1). The major anions in the pancreatic juice are HCO_3^- and Cl^-, the concentrations of which depend on

flow rates. As the flow rate increases, HCO_3^- concentration rises asymptotically, approaching a plateau value (150 mEq/L) at about 30% to 50% of the maximal secretory rate. The Cl^- concentration falls with increasing secretory rate reciprocally, so that the sum of the two anions remains constant and approximately equal to the sum of Na^+ and K^+ at all secretory rates. In humans and other animal species, the pancreatic juices also contain Ca^{+2} (1–2 mEq/L) and traces of Mg^{+2}, Zn^{+2}, HPO_4^{-2} and SO_4^{-2}.

Several theories have been postulated to explain the pattern of anion secretion in the pancreatic juice. The exchange diffusion hypothesis proposes that the principal anion secreted by the pancreas is HCO_3^- and, as the juice passes through the ductal system, HCO_3^- is exchanged for Cl^-. At low secretory rates, effective HCO_3Cl^- exchange can occur, producing a juice low in HCO_3^-; a high flow rate would not allow time for a large exchange of Cl^- for the secreted HCO_3^-. Another theory, the unicellular hypothesis, states that the juice extruded by the secreting cells contains both Cl^- and HCO_3^-, but the composition may vary according to the flow rates. A third proposal, the two component theory, hypothesizes that the juice collected may be a mixture of secretions from two cell types. One cell type (the centroacinar or ductular cell) secretes HCO_3^- and another (the acinar cell) secretes Cl^-. Each anion is secreted at different rates in response to secretagogues; when stimulated, the ductular cells add HCO_3^- to Cl^--rich juice from the acini.

Recent studies using micropuncture and microperfusion techniques provide information on the mechanism of ductal electrolyte secretion. In the cat pancreas, the concentration of Cl^- in the fluid obtained from interlobular ducts is 121 mM, similar to the Cl^- concentration in the extracellular fluid. After stimulation with secretin, the Cl^- concentration decreases to 46 mM in the main duct.[11] Split-drop microperfusion experiments[12] have demonstrated that the interlobular ducts are the major sites of secretin-stimulated fluid production, and the HCO_3^- in the pancreatic fluid is lost from the duct in exchange for Cl^-. Micropuncture studies in the rabbit pancreas indicate that, in the resting gland, the Cl^- concentration increases along the ductal tree to around 90 mM at the main duct, presumably reflecting HCO_3^-/Cl^- exchange in the small interlobular ducts. Stimulation with secretin reverses the gradient; Cl^- concentration decreases along the ductal tree with the largest fall in the small interlobular ducts.[13,14] Split-drop microperfusion experiments have shown that this results from the secretion of a HCO_3^--rich fluid by cells in the interlobular ducts, which are responsive to secretin stimulation. The interlobular ducts also contain a HCO_3^-/Cl^- antiport that is presumably saturated at high flow rates, allowing high HCO_3^- concentrations in the main pancreatic duct. Further evidence that HCO_3^- is secreted by the ductal cells comes from experiments using rats fed with a copper-deficient diet supplemented with D-penicillamine.[15] This diet destroys 98% of the acinar cells without effect on ductal cells. The pancreata from these animals do not respond to secretagogues of enzymes such as CCK. Secretin, however, significantly increases fluid and HCO_3^- secretion. In various animals and humans, HCO_3^- concentration in the pancreatic juice may be four times higher than that found in plasma fluid or extracellular fluids during active secretion. A potential difference across the pancreatic duct epithelium of several millivolts (lumen negative) suggests HCO_3^- is actively secreted.[16] However, recent studies suggest that secretion of HCO_3^- is not the primary chemical process. The main process is $Na^+:H^+$ exchange at the basal lateral membrane using the energy

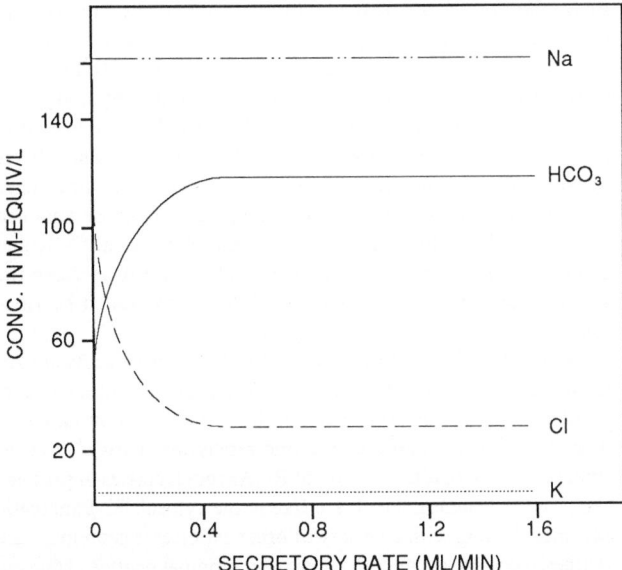

FIGURE 15-1. Relationship of secretory rate to electrolyte composition of pancreatic juice.

of the sodium gradient. Protons are delivered to the lumen by way of CO_2 diffusion across the ductal epithelium and subsequent hydration involving carbonic anhydrase.[17,18,19] The current view of the mechanisms involved in active electrolyte transport is depicted in Figure 15-2.

Enzymes

Depending on the species, the enzyme component of pancreatic juice is mixed in various proportions with the aqueous component. Human pancreatic juice contains protein at a concentration ranging from 0.7% to 10%. The majority of the proteins are enzymes and proenzymes; the remainder are plasma proteins, trypsin inhibitors, and mucoproteins. The four major enzyme groups are amylolytic, lipolytic, proteolytic, and nucleolytic (Table 15-1). The proteolytic enzymes, which include trypsinogen, chymotrypsinogen, procarboxypeptidase, and proaminopeptidase, account for the majority of enzymic proteins in the juice and are secreted as inactive proenzymes. After entering the intestinal lumen, trypsinogen is converted by enterokinase, an enzyme secreted by the duodenal mucosa, to the biologically active trypsin. Trypsin, in turn, autocatalytically activates trypsinogen and converts chymotrypsinogen and other proteolytic enzymes into their active forms.

Pancreatic juice also contains a low concentration of trypsin inhibitor, a polypeptide that, at pH of 3 to 7, combines with and inactivates trypsin in a 1:1 ratio. It also partially inhibits chymotrypsin. The presence of trypsin inhibitor in the pancreas is thought to protect the organ against autodigestion by small amounts active of trypsin within the pancreas. Because it is present in minute quantities in the juice, the proteolytic activity of fully activated juice in the intestinal lumen is not inhibited. In contrast to the proteolytic enzymes, amylase, lipase, and ribonuclease are

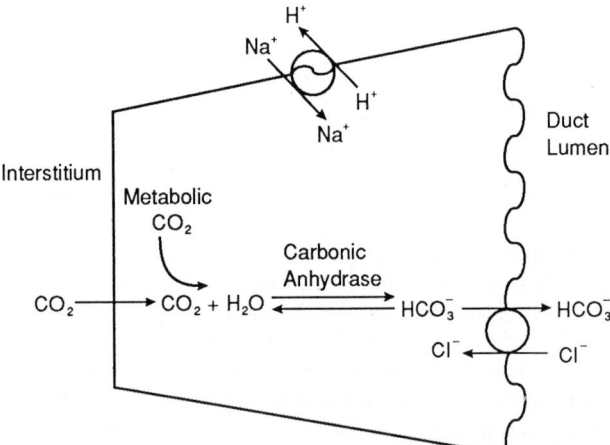

FIGURE 15-2. Intracellular mechanism responsible for pancreatic bicarbonate secretion. Bicarbonate in pancreatic juice is derived from CO_2 and H_2O supplied by diffusion from capillaries. Metabolic CO_2 contributes less than 5% of bicarbonate in juice. Under the influence of carbonic anhydrase, CO_2 reacts with H_2O intracellularly to form HCO_3^-, which is secreted into the juice. This process may be coupled with cellular uptake of Cl^-. H^+ resulting from production of HCO_3^- is transported out of the duct cell by a $Na^+:H^+$ exchange pump. This pump is indirectly coupled to the Na^+-K^+-ATPase found on the basolateral membrane of duct cell.

TABLE 15–1
Hydrolytic Enzymes Secreted by the Pancreas

Proteolytic Enzymes

Trypsinogen

Chymotrypsinogen

Proelastase

Procarboxypeptidase A

Procarboxypeptidase B

Amylolytic Enzyme

α-amylase

Lipolytic Enzymes

Lipase

Prophospholipase A_1, A_2

Nonspecific esterase

Nucleases

Deoxyribonuclease

Ribonuclease

---

secreted by the acinar cells in an active form. Pancreatic juice also contains a small-molecular-weight peptide called colipase (molecular weight 10,000), which is essential for optimal lipolysis.[20,21] It facilitates lipase action by binding with bile salt-lipid surfaces to increase the interaction of lipase with triglyceride.[22,23,24] In the presence of bile salts, colipase also lowers the optimum pH of lipase from 8.5 to 6.5, the normal pH in the proximal intestine.

Pancreatic enzymes are synthesized within acinar cells and packaged into zymogen granules.[25,26] The entire process from synthesis to the point at which enzymes are ready to be secreted into the lumen requires approximately 50 minutes. Total enzyme synthesis is estimated at 20 ng/g dry tissue/h, or, stated another way, 10 million enzyme molecules/acinar cell/min.[27] The controlling mechanism responsible for protein synthesis is largely unknown. Recent studies in rats demonstrate that CCK plays an important role in the regulation of gene expression of pancreatic enzymes.[28] Intraduodenal infusion of soybean trypsin inhibitor (SBTI) raises plasma CCK and also increases trypsinogen I and chymotrypsinogen β mRNA levels fivefold after 48 hours. In contrast, SBTI infusion has no effect on amylase mRNA levels. Similar effects on pancreatic enzyme mRNA levels are observed with intravenous infusion of CCK to plasma levels comparable to those obtained with SBTI. In addition to effects on gene regulation, CCK and other hormones exert posttranscriptional control to increase the synthesis of digestive enzymes as mRNA is translated by ribosomes.[29]

According to the classic model of Palade, amino acids are actively transported into the acinar cells and protein synthesis occurs in the ribosomes. The newly synthesized proteins eventually find their way to the rough endoplasmic reticulum (RER).[30] Recent studies indicate that translation of RNAs for all classes of proteins begins on polysomes, which are free in the cytosol.[31,32] Pancreatic enzymes,[33] along with a variety of other exportable proteins,[30] are synthesized proteins with an amino acid terminal peptide extension termed the *signal peptide*. This recognizes the endoplasmic membrane and allows for the attachment of the polysome to the membrane. Translation is temporarily halted when the signal peptide emerges from the ribosomal subunit and interacts with the signal recognition particle, which is associated with the large ribosomal subunit.[31] The protein–RNA complexes find their way to the endoplasmic reticulum membrane, where they interact with a membrane protein known as docking protein.[31] Interaction between the signal recognition particle and the docking protein permits the completion of translation, after which the ribosomal subunits, signal recognition particle, and RNA dissociate from the endoplasmic reticulum while the protein crosses the endoplasmic reticulum membrane into the cisternae. The need for the signal recognition particle–docking protein complex to form on the endoplasmic reticulum before translation of RNAs containing a signal peptide codon can be completed has important physiologic implications. This process ensures that potentially noxious proteins, such as proteinases, cannot access the cytosolic compartment. It also provides a mechanism for initial sorting of proteins not destined for export from those that must be processed by the endoplasmic reticulum-Golgi pathway and packaged for later secretion.[34] Inside the cisternae of endoplasmic reticulum, pancreatic secretory proteins undergo conformational changes, assuming tertiary and, in some cases, quaternary structure. These structural changes may account for the irreversible segregation of proteins within the RER. The transfer of pancreatic enzyme proteins from the endoplasmic reticulum to the Golgi complex occurs within 20 to 30 minutes of synthesis.[35] This is mediated by vesicles arising from pinched-off transitional elements of the RER, which act as transport containers for the secretory proteins.[35] Further modification and concentration in the Golgi complex occurs and may result, in part, from the interaction of the predominantly basic secretory proteins with polyanionic substances formed in the Golgi.[36] After their formation in the Golgi complex, secretory granules move to the apical portions of the acinar cell by a mechanism involving microtubules and remain there until an appropriate neurohormonal stimulus triggers exocytosis.

It is generally believed that pancreatic enzymes from a single cell are secreted in a fixed ratio, independent of the nature of the stimulus and of the rate of secretion, but determined at the time of synthesis. This phenomenon may be explained by the model proposed by Scheele and Palade,[37] which states that secretory proteins are mixed together in the zymogen granule and discharged in parallel. Under certain experimental conditions, however, there may be nonparallel secretion of pancreatic enzymes. In humans, increasing doses of CCK infusion results in pancreatic secretions characterized by greater response of lipase than chymotrypsin concentrations, both of which, in turn, are greater than amylase concentration.[38] Similar nonparallel secretion has been reported by Dagorn et al in rats[39] and humans.[40] Furthermore, intestinal perfusion with lysine in rabbits stimulates the preferential secretion of trypsinogen under some experimental conditions.[41] Injection of an extract of rat intestinal mucosa exposed to proteins or glucose causes selective pancreatic secretion of trypsin or amylase.[42] These observations suggest that the enzymic composition of the pancreatic juice may change in accordance with the composition of a meal. The mechanism(s) for the selective secretion of enzymes have not been defined. Chymodenin, a peptide extracted from porcine duodenal mucosa, is reported to stimulate specifically the pancreatic secretion of chymotrypsin in rabbits.[43] Nothing is known about factors that elicit the release of chymotrypsin, nor about the occasions when selective secretion of chymotrypsin occurs.

Nonparallel enzyme secretion also has been reported in isolated dispersed rat pancreatic acini.[44] CCK and carbachol induce a greater release of chymotrypsinogen than amylase or trypsinogen; secretion of all three enzymes is equally stimulated by secretin. Several possible explanations for nonparallel secretion have been proposed: (1) different rates of enzyme synthesis in response to different degrees of stimulation, (2) the existence of a soluble cytoplasmic pool of enzyme proteins that are in equilibrium with those contained in zymogen granules; and (3) differing enzymic content within populations of acinar cells. Recent morphologic studies show considerable differences in cell size in peninsular teleinsular acinar cells.[45] This, coupled with the observation that the enzyme content and the ratio of amylase to chymotrypsin varies widely among granules taken from the same animal,[46] supports the third hypothesis and suggests that nonparallel secretion is due to exocytosis from heterogeneous cells within the pancreas.[47]

Although much controversy exists regarding short-term deviations from parallel secretion, there is little doubt that long-term adaptation of enzymes to diet occurs in animals. Adaptation occurs in rats fed diets containing a preponderance of carbohydrate, protein, or fat as indicated by increased pancreatic content, mRNA, and rates of synthesis and secretion of the appropriate class of hydrolytic enzymes by the pancreas.[48] Moreover, the dietary effects are believed to be mediated by specific hormones. Insulin mediates the increased amylase synthesis while CCK released by protein increases the synthesis of proteases. Although such adaptive changes are unreported in humans, preferential secretion of lipase occurs in chronic renal failure associated with hypercholecystokinemia,[49] as consistent with the adaptive change found in animals receiving chronic administration of CCK.[50]

STIMULATION OF PANCREATIC SECRETION

Mediation of postprandial pancreatic secretion has been ascribed mainly to the hormones secretin and CCK and to vagovagal reflexes that activate cholinergic postganglionic neurons in the pancreas. Considerable knowledge has been gained about these classic regulatory mechanisms; however, the picture has become increasingly complicated by evidence suggesting that other regulatory peptide hormones and neurotransmitters are also involved.

Hormonal Mechanisms

SECRETIN

The intestinal hormone secretin is the most potent and efficacious stimulant of pancreatic fluid and bicarbonate secretion in humans and all other species tested. Duodenal pH is the major regulator of secretin release. The threshold value for secretin release and stimulation of pancreatic bicarbonate secretion is pH 4.5.[51,52] Below this pH, pancreatic bicarbonate output is related to the total amount of titratable acid presented to the duodenum. The increase in postprandial secretin levels in humans amounts to only a few picomolar[53,54] because of the buffering of an appreciable amount of acid produced in the stomach by food and the neutralization of the remaining acid entering the duodenum by pancreatico-biliary secretion. Thus, the pH of gastric chyme in the first portion of the duodenum is in the range of 4 to 5.0.[55] However, recent studies have demonstrated that dilute HCl infused into duodenum at a rate of 2 to 4 mmol/h can increase plasma secretin significantly in humans[53,56] and dogs.[57] In addition, H^+ bound to solid food particles may be a potent stimulus of pancreatic bicarbonate secretion.[58] The H^+ slowly diffusing from the particles stimulates pancreatic bicarbonate secretion by triggering H^+ receptors located in the more distal small intestine.

Nonacid factors may also play a role in the postprandial release of secretin. Among the major components of a mixed meal, fatty acids such as oleic acid and other digestive products of fat can increase plasma secretin levels[59] and pancreatic bicarbonate secretion.[60,61] Furthermore, bile in the upper small intestine can also stimulate the release of secretin.[62,63] However, the physiologic importance of these nonacid factors in the release of secretin is questionable, because postprandial plasma secretin does not increase in subjects who are either achlorhydric or in normal subjects in whom meal-induced acid secretion is neutralized with $NaHCO_3$.

Although the postprandial release of secretin into the circulation is rather small, the pancreas appears to be very sensitive to secretin. Secretin given in a dose range that mimics postprandial plasma secretin levels can stimulate pancreatic secretion of water and bicarbonate.[64,65] In addition, administration of secretin antiserum to conscious dogs greatly reduces the pancreatic bicarbonate response to a meal.[66] Thus, the small amount of secretin released postprandially appears sufficient to cause at least some of the bicarbonate secretory response. When secretin is given together with CCK[67] or with simultaneous vagal stimulation,[65,68,69] the full postprandial bicarbonate response is observed. This suggests that the synergistic effects of secretin with CCK or acetylcholine probably account for most of the postprandial bicarbonate secretion.

CHOLECYSTOKININ

CCK is the other gut hormone that plays an important role in pancreatic secretion. It is released by various hydrolytic products of digestion such as amino acids and fatty acids. In dogs, proteins do not stimulate pancreatic secretion,[70] whereas crude enzyme digests of protein that contain peptides and amino acids are effective stimulants of pancreatic enzyme secretion presumably by way of release of CCK.[71] Similarly, undigested fat is ineffective, but products of lipolysis such as fatty acids are the most potent stimulants of CCK release.[72]

Factors that influence CCK response to fatty acids include their chain length,[73,74] degree of saturation,[73] concentration, and total load.[74]

The mechanism by which nutrients stimulate the release of CCK is not clear, although it appears to be independent of cholinergic input. In species such as the rat where feedback inhibition of pancreatic enzyme secretion occurs,[75,76] CCK release may be controlled by the level of active intraluminal proteases.[77] Proteins, the major food stimulants of CCK secretion in the rat, may bind or inhibit intraluminal endopeptidases, which would otherwise inactivate the newly discovered "CCK-releasing peptide."[78]

Under fasting conditions, the plasma CCK levels are very low, averaging around 1 pM in humans.[79,80,81,82] After the ingestion of a protein- and fat-rich meal, the concentration increases to 6 to 8 pM within 10 to 30 minutes followed by a gradual decline to basal levels during the ensuing 3 hours.[81,82] It appears that several molecular forms of CCK are released into the circulation postprandially[83] including CCK33, CCK22, CCK12, and CCK8.[83] Their relative contribution to CCK activity of plasma in basal and stimulated states remains to be determined.

There appears to be little doubt that CCK plays an important role in the stimulation of pancreatic enzyme secretion during the postprandial state. Experiments have demonstrated that reproduction of meal-stimulated plasma CCK levels by exogenous infusion of CCK produces the same levels of pancreatic enzyme secretion as during postprandial state.[84] This indicates that endogenously released CCK is a major regulator of meal-induced pancreatic secretion. Further support for the physiologic role of CCK was obtained from in vivo studies investigating the effects of various CCK receptor antagonists. Administration of the potent CCK antagonists lorglumide or MK-329 produces a 50% to 60% inhibition of meal-stimulated pancreatic secretion in dogs.[85,86] Similar effects of these antagonists on meal-stimulated pancreatic secretion have been reported in humans.[87]

CCK can also stimulate fluid and bicarbonate secretion to some extent.[60,88] The effect on bicarbonate secretion is weak[89,90] but physiologically relevant because CCK potentiates the action of secretin on the pancreas. In contrast, in intact dogs[91,92] and humans,[67,84] CCK-stimulated pancreatic enzyme secretion is not potentiated by secretin.

OTHER HORMONES AND REGULATORY FACTORS

Many peptides and other factors have been shown to stimulate pancreatic enzyme secretion, but their physiologic role in the regulation of pancreatic secretion remains undetermined. These include gastrin, bombesin, and neurotensin.

In view of the structural similarity between CCK and gastrin, it is not surprising to find that gastrin, like CCK, also stimulates pancreatic enzyme secretion. In the dog, gastrin is about one third as effective as CCK on a molar basis in stimulating the pancreas to secrete enzyme.[41] Irrigation of a canine antral pouch with peptone and liver extracts at neutral pH stimulates pancreatic protein secretion, whereas irrigation with acidified solutions does not.[93,94] It is postulated that the stimulatory effects of the protein solution might be due to release of gastrin and that the inhibitory effects of acidification are due to suppression of gastrin release. This evidence, however, is indirect, and it is not known whether the postprandial increase in plasma gastrin is sufficient to produce significant stimulation of pancreatic secretion.

Bombesin (gastrin-releasing peptide in mammals), a polypeptide isolated from the skin of frogs and the human alimentary tract,[95,96] stimulates pancreatic secretions that contain small amounts of bicarbonate and high concentrations of enzymes in humans.[97] Bombesin can act directly on the pancreas because specific receptors have been identified on pancreatic acinar cells.[98] In addition, it has been suggested that bombesin exerts its stimulating effect on the exocrine pancreas indirectly by promoting the release of CCK from the small intestinal mucosa.[99] This is evidenced by the lack of stimulatory action of bombesin on pancreatic exocrine secretion after duodenectomy[100] and the release of CCK after intravenous infusion of bombesin.[101] Bombesin also has been reported to exert its effect by way of a cholinergic pathway in other systems.[102] However, recent in vivo studies in rats indicate that the action of bombesin in this species is probably direct because combined administration of atropine and proglumide did not affect pancreatic protein output stimulated by bombesin. The mechanism and physiologic role of bombesin in the stimulation of pancreatic enzyme secretion in humans are unknown.

Neurotensin, a hormone released by intestinal fatty acids,[103] has been shown to stimulate pancreatic secretion in dogs[103,104] and in humans.[105] This raises the interesting possibility that neurotensin may play a significant role in mediating pancreatic secretion stimulated by fat. However, exogenous infusion of neurotensin in doses that stimulate pancreatic secretion results in plasma levels much higher than those that occur after a normal meal.[103,105] In addition, neurotensin stimulates bicarbonate secretion but decreases enzyme secretion stimulated by secretin and cerulein (a CCK analogue) in humans.[105] These observations do not support neurotensin as a regulator of meal-stimulated pancreatic secretion.

Neural Mechanisms

PARASYMPATHETIC NERVOUS SYSTEM

The pancreas is innervated by parasympathetic and sympathetic nerve fibers. The parasympathetic fibers pass to the pancreas directly in the vagus nerves and indirectly through the celiac ganglion, splanchnic nerves, and, perhaps, through the intramural plexus of the duodenum.

The functional effect of vagal stimulation on the pancreas varies greatly with the species and with the experimental conditions.[106] In the dog and rabbit, vagal stimulation has little effect on secretory rate. It does produce an increase in the output of enzymes, but the increase is smaller in magnitude than with CCK stimulation. This response persists after the removal of the stomach and intestine, indicating a direct stimulatory effect on the pancreas. In the cat, stimulation of the vagus results in some increase in the rate of secretion not dependent on hormones. The secretion of enzymes is blocked by atropine, yet atropine has no effect on bicarbonate secretion. In the pig, vagal stimulation results in copious secretion of juice rich in enzymes and bicarbonate, even after the extirpation of the stomach and intestine.

In humans, the role of the vagi has not been clearly defined. Insulin-induced hypoglycemia, which is presumed to stimulate the vagus, augments secretin-stimulated pancreatic protein output.[107] Vagotomy reduces the bicarbonate-secretory response to exogenous hormones by about one quarter. Maximal enzyme secretion is not significantly affected, but the sensitivity of the pancreas to submaximal doses of CCK may be decreased.[108] Furthermore, vagotomy also reduces pancreatic enzyme responses to food[109] and to intestinal stimulants.[108] It seems that the cholinergic effects primarily modulate the actions of gut peptides on pancreatic secretion, but have no physiologically relevant effect on the release of CCK or secretin.[110,111]

In humans, volume receptors and osmoreceptors are known to be present in the duodenum. Stimulation of these receptors by distention or administration of a hyperosmolar solution elicits a pancreatic enzyme response mediated by way of cholinergic neurons.[112,113] In addition, increased firing rates in peripheral afferent vagal neurons and in central sites have been recorded after gastric distention[114] and intestinal perfusion with amino acids[115,116] and HCl.[117]

Recent studies indicate that intrapancreatic postganglionic cholinergic neurons regulate both enzyme and bicarbonate secretion. These neurons are activated by central input during the cephalic phase and by vagovagal reflexes initiated by gastric and intestinal phase stimulation. Acetylcholine released by the intrapancreatic neurons may act directly on acinar cells or potentiate the action of secretin on bicarbonate secretion from duct cells. The interaction between acetylcholine and CCK is additive. The enteropancreatic reflex is responsible for approximately 50% of postprandial enzyme secretion.[113]

SYMPATHETIC NERVOUS SYSTEM

Adrenergic innervation of the pancreas is mainly through the splanchnic nerves. In the pancreas, the majority of those fibers are distributed to the blood vessels and very few pass to the acini or ducts.[89] The splanchnic nerves are generally inhibitory for exocrine and endocrine pancreatic secretion because stimulation of the nerves usually decreases while splanchnicectomy increases the response to pancreatic stimulants.[89,118,119] The pancreatic inhibitory effect of splanchnic nerve stimulation appears to be synchronous with, and dependent on intense vasoconstriction caused by stimulation of α-adrenergic receptors on the blood vessels. In isolated guinea pig pancreatic acini, norepinephrine alone has no effect on the response to submaximal concentrations of CCK8.[120] On the other hand, epinephrine produces a modest stimulation of enzyme output in mouse[121] and rat[122] pancreas in vitro, and the stimulatory effect is inhibited by a β-receptor antagonists.[122] No clear pattern emerges from the large number of studies on regulation of exocrine pancreatic secretion by the sympathetic nervous system. It seems that the major role for adrenergic mechanism is in the inhibition of flow and bicarbonate secretion mediated at least in part by way of vasoconstriction.

PEPTIDERGIC NERVOUS SYSTEM

Recent immunocytochemical studies have revealed the presence of several peptides in nerve cell bodies or fibers in the pancreas. Among these, nerve fibers and cell bodies containing vasoactive intestinal polypeptide (VIP) are the most abundant.[123] The VIP fibers appear to surround the cell bodies of intrapancreatic ganglia and also innervate duct cells.[124]

In pigs, VIP is the neurotransmitter that mediates much of the bicarbonate secretory response to electrical stimulation of the vagus nerve.[125] Vagal stimulation after administration of atropine increases pancreatic venous outflow of VIP as well as pancreatic bicarbonate secretion, and these effects are blocked by somatostatin.[125] Furthermore, the time course of increased venous efflux of VIP and increased bicarbonate secretion after vagal stimulation are similar, and a specific VIP antiserum reduces the bicarbonate response to vagal stimulation.[124] The importance of intrapancreatic neuronal VIP as a regulator of pancreatic secretion may be species specific. VIP is only a weak partial agonist in humans.[126] In some species, VIP may also function to induce pancreatic vasodilation and increase blood flow in response to activation of the exocrine pancreas.[127]

Other peptidergic neurotransmitters that have been identified in the pancreas include the carboxyl terminal tetrapeptide of gastrin or CCK,[119,128] gastrin-releasing peptide,[129] substance P,[119,128] peptide histidine isoleucine (PHI),[130] neurotensin,[131] neuropeptide Y (NPY),[130,132] enkephalin,[119,128] and calcitonin gene-related peptide (CGRP).[90,133] Although some of these peptides (CCK/gastrin, substance P, gastrin-releasing peptide, PHI, neurotensin, CGRP) have been found to stimulate, and others (enkephalin, NPY) to inhibit exocrine pancreatic secretion in pharmacologic studies, the physiologic relevance of their effects on mediation of pancreatic secretion is unknown.

INTRACELLULAR CONTROL OF PANCREATIC SECRETION

Receptors

Most of the hormones and neurotransmitters discussed above as stimulating pancreatic secretion do so by directly regulating acinar and duct cells, but some may regulate indirectly by actions on nerves or blood vessels. It is important, therefore, to identify physiologic effects on isolated acinar and duct cells and localize high affinity receptors for each individual regulator to its target cell. Because of the great preponderance of acinar cells in the pancreas, a number of preparations of isolated acinar cells or pancreatic acini have been established. By using amylase secretion as a functional response, studies of agonists and antagonist action on secretion have indicated clearly the presence of specific receptors on acinar cells. These have been confirmed by binding studies with radiolabeled analogues and antagonists.[134,135] Moreover, in most cases, these receptors have been affinity labeled to establish their molecular size and, in some cases, solubilized with nondenaturing detergents and the protein molecules have been partially purified. Electron microscopic autoradiography has localized binding to the basolateral membrane domain, although bound ligand may be internalized subsequently by an energy-dependent process.[136] Through such studies, acinar cells of a variety of species, including humans, were shown to bear receptors for CCK, bombesin, acetylcholine, VIP, and secretin. Much less is known of duct cell receptors because of the relatively small number of these cells present in the pancreas and the difficulty in studying the physiologic function (i.e., ion transport) of isolated duct cells. Duct cells bear receptors for secretin and possibly VIP, CCK, and acetylcholine.

Receptors for pancreatic secretagogues are all believed to belong to the receptor family characterized structurally by seven hydrophobic transmembrane domains and functionally by their interaction with guanine nucleotide binding or G-proteins. This generalization is based on the fact that guanine nucleotides alter the binding properties of these pancreatic receptors and that the structures of other receptors known to interact with the same transmembrane signaling mechanisms as the pancreatic receptors are consistent with this model. The M3 subclass of muscarinic

receptor believed present in pancreas has been cloned from brain, and it is presumed that other receptors, such as those for CCK, secretin, and VIP, possess similar structure.

Structure-function studies with site-directed mutagenesis and chimeric receptors have established some general principles of function for this receptor family.[137] The transmembrane segments may form a pocket for the binding of small molecules such as acetylcholine while the extracellular amino terminal end and loops may also be important in the interaction with peptide molecules. The third cytoplasmic loop projecting between the fifth and sixth transmembrane domain is believed to interact with the appropriate G-protein while serine and threonine residues in the cytoplasmic carboxyl terminal tail may be involved with regulatory mechanisms such as desensitization and down-regulation by way of phosphorylation. The function of glycosylation on externally directed sites at the amino terminus is not yet well established, but these sites could play a role either in ligand binding or in intracellular processing of new receptors and insertion into the plasma membrane.

Transmembrane Signaling

While all membrane receptors are integral proteins spanning the lipid bilayer, the pancreatic secretagogue receptors convey information by interaction with G-protein. G-proteins are heterotrimeric proteins with unique α subunits and common $\beta\gamma$ subunits.[138,139] Acinar cells possess α_s and α_i subunits, which stimulate and inhibit adenylate cyclase, respectively. These subunits can be ADP-ribosylated by cholera toxin and pertussis toxin, which permanently activate or inhibit adenylate cyclase, respectively. In addition, acinar cells are believed to possess an analogous subunit, α_p, which activates phospholipase C.[140] A number of new α subunit isoforms are being discovered by molecular cloning techniques, and the full complement expressed in acinar and duct cells remains to be elucidated.

The α subunit possesses the guanine nucleotide binding site, which, in the resting state, is occupied by GDP. After the receptor binds its ligand, it interacts with the G-protein to catalyze the exchange of GTP for GDP. The GTP-α subunit dissociates from the $\beta\gamma$ complex and activates its effector (i.e., phospholipase C, adenylate cyclase). The system is amplified because the lifetime of the GTP-α complex is much longer than that of the hormone-receptor complex. Eventually, GTP is cleaved to GDP by an intrinsic GTPase activity, and the α subunit reassociates with $\beta\gamma$. It is because of this cycle that secretagogues activate GTPase activity in pancreatic membranes and that nonhydrolyzable analogues of GTP such as GTPγS activate adenylate cyclase or phospholipase C in pancreatic membranes or permeabilized acinar cells.[140,141]

The final component in transmembrane signaling is the membrane effector that generates the intracellular messenger. The two major effector enzymes in acinar cell membranes are the polyphosphoinositide specific phospholipase C, which cleaves phosphotidylinositol 4,5-bisphosphate producing 1,4,5-inositol trisphosphate (IP$_3$) and 1,2-diacylglycerol (DAG), and adenylate cyclase, which converts ATP to cyclic AMP (cAMP). These enzymes are presumed to be similar in structure and function to those expressed in a variety of cells. In the case of phospholipase C, multiple forms have recently been purified and cloned and

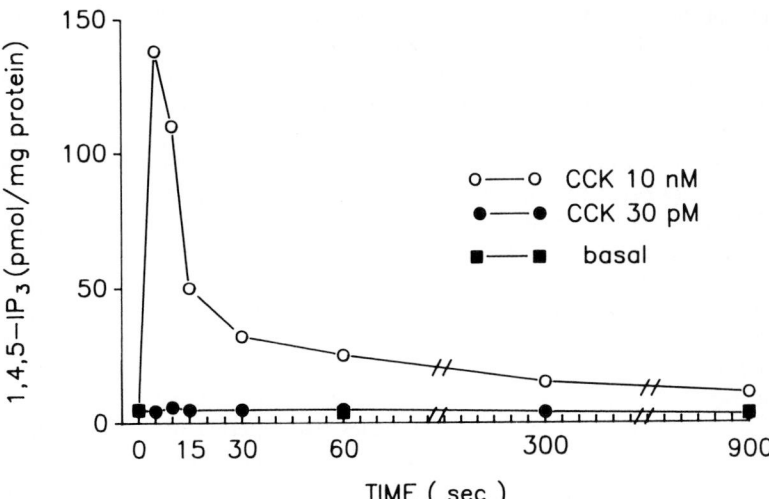

FIGURE 15–3. Time course of 1,4,5-IP$_3$ increase induced by CCK in rat pancreatic acini. (From Matozaki T, Williams JA. Multiple sources of 1,2-diacylglycerol in isolated rat pancreatic acini stimulated by cholecystokinin. J Biol Chem 1989;264:14729.)

shown to be expressed in a variety of tissues.[142] The importance of functional differences between the various molecular forms and whether they couple to the same or different G-proteins remains to be established. Adenylate cyclase has also been cloned, and its primary structure is consistent with its being an integral membrane protein with multiple membrane spanning domains, although the catalytic site is clearly intracellular.[143] Other membrane effectors in pancreas not yet well characterized may include phosphatidyl choline specific phospholipase C and D, phospholipase A$_2$, Na$^+$-H$^+$ ion exchanger, and various ion channels. However, these may be regulated by intracellular messengers rather than directly by G-proteins.

Intracellular Messengers

The major intracellular messengers involved in the regulation of pancreatic secretion are IP$_3$, Ca^{2+}, DAG, and cAMP.[135,144] The first three are predominant in the acinar cell and increase after the activation of phosphoinositide specific phospholipase C by CCK and acetylcholine while cAMP is the predominant messenger in duct cells and is activated by secretin.

Phosphotidylinositol (PI) and its polyphosphate derivatives phosphotidylinositol 4-phosphate (PIP) and phosphotidylinositol 4,5-bisphosphate (PIP$_2$) together form about 10% of membrane phospholipids. When acinar cells are stimulated with an analogue of acetylcholine, carbachol, or CCK, there is a rapid fall in prelabeled PIP$_2$ and PIP, an increase in DAG, and a delayed rise in phosphatidic acid.[145] This is interpreted as indicating the primary breakdown of phosphoinositides with production of diacylglycerol, which is subsequently converted to phosphatidic acid by DAG kinase. When the production of the water-soluble inositol phosphates is assessed after labeling with ^{3}H-inositol, IP$_3$, IP$_2$, IP, and I are all increased.[146,147] Because 1,4,5-IP$_3$ can only be produced by hydrolysis of PIP$_2$, this is presumed the primary event with further synthesis of PIP and PIP$_2$ from PI by the action of a PI kinase.

While production of IP$_3$ was initially measured by prelabeling with ^{3}H-inositol, it is now possible to measure the actual mass of cellular IP$_3$ by a competitive binding assay. Such measurements

show a rapid increase within 5 seconds in rat acini stimulated with CCK, carbachol, or bombesin (Fig 15-3). This 20- to 30-fold increase rapidly declines after 30 to 60 seconds to a smaller sustained plateau. Coincident with this rapid peak of IP$_3$ there is also a similar-sized, rapid increase in DAG (Fig 15-4) believed to arise simultaneously from the hydrolysis of PIP$_2$. In contrast to IP$_3$, however, DAG shows a larger secondary sustained increase. This latter increase may arise from the hydrolysis of PI or PC by distinct

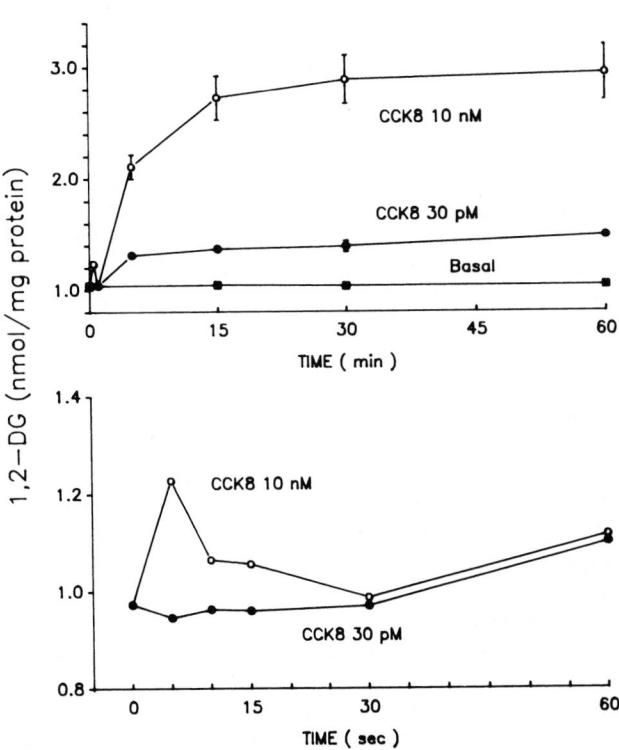

FIGURE 15–4. Time course of 1,2 diacylglycerol (DAG) increase induced by CCK in rat pancreatic acini. (From Matozaki T, Williams JA. Multiple sources of 1,2-diacylglycerol in isolated rat pancreatic acini stimulated by cholecystokinin. J Biol Chem 1989;264:14729.)

phospholipases.[148] Most importantly, it means that IP$_3$ and DAG can act as separate signals and are not necessarily in lockstep.

The IP$_3$ measured by the receptor binding is largely 1,4,5-IP$_3$ based on the characteristics of the binding protein. However, 1,4,5-IP$_3$ can also be phosphorylated further to produce 1,3,4,5-IP$_4$, which can be dephosphorylated to yield 1,3,4-IP$_3$. Whether a biologic role exists for these other inositol phosphates as well as the further degradation products (IP$_2$, IP$_1$) is not yet established.[149] In other cell types, IP$_4$ has been suggested to promote Ca^{2+} influx.

The established function of IP$_3$ is to bind to a receptor present on an intracellular Ca^{2+} store[150] and thereby release Ca^{2+} into the cytoplasm.[151] The morphologic identity of the Ca^{2+} sequestering organelle in pancreas is not yet clear. Earlier studies using oxalate to trap Ca^{2+} suggested rough ER was the major nonmitochondrial Ca^{2+}-sequestering organelle.[152] Recent studies have suggested that a more specialized organelle in pancreas called "calciosomes" might constitute the IP$_3$-sensitive Ca^{2+} store.[153] Microsomal vesicles prepared from acini have documented two different intracellular Ca^{2+} mobilization/storage mechanisms: one a Ca^{2+}-ATPase and the other a Ca^{2+}-H$^+$ exchanger coupled to a H$^+$ gradient established by an endosomal type H$^+$-ATPase.[152] These mechanisms coupled with another Ca^{2+}-ATPase present in the plasma membrane, which extrudes Ca^{2+} from the cell, are responsible for maintaining the intracellular Ca^{2+} concentration ([Ca^{2+}]$_i$) at about 100 nM.[154] IP$_3$, when injected into the cell or added to permeabilized acini or a microsomal vesicle fraction, can release some or all of the sequestered Ca^{2+}. There may also be communication between IP$_3$-sensitive and IP$_3$-insensitive Ca^{2+} stores. An IP$_3$ receptor of 260 kd has been isolated from brain and shows selectivity for 1,4,5-IP$_3$ as compared to other inositol phosphates. Although the presumption is that IP$_3$ activates a Ca^{2+} channel to release Ca^{2+}, it has been difficult to obtain direct evidence.

Much of the current knowledge regarding secretagogue-induced changes in acinar cell [Ca^{2+}]$_i$ has been obtained by using fluorescent Ca^{2+} probes such as quin 2 and fura-2.[155] These studies have been carried out initially on suspensions of cells or acini and on individual cells by microspectrofluorometry.[156,157,158] Such studies have shown that high concentrations of CCK, bombesin, and cholinergic analogues cause a rapid five- to tenfold increase of [Ca^{2+}]$_i$, which declines over a 2- to 5-minute period to a level slightly above basal (see Fig 15-4). This initial large increase is essentially independent of extracellular Ca^{2+}, while the small sustained plateau increase in [Ca^{2+}]$_i$ is absolutely dependent on extracellular Ca^{2+}. The initial increase shows a similar time course and dependence on secretagogue concentrations as does the rapid increase in IP$_3$ and is presumed to be dependent on IP$_3$ releasing intracellular Ca^{2+}. Much of this released Ca^{2+} is extruded from the cell as shown by earlier studies documenting an increased efflux of prelabeled ^{45}Ca^{2+} and a fall in total acinar Ca^{2+}.[154] All three of the major phospholipase C-activating secretagogues (CCK, acetylcholine, bombesin) access the same intracellular pool of Ca^{2+}, and, after maximal stimulation by one agonist, adding of another has no additional effect. Upon removal of the agonist, the IP$_3$-releasable intracellular pool refills over 2 to 10 minutes as Ca^{2+} is taken up from the medium and resequestered.[158]

The sustained increase in [Ca^{2+}]$_i$ and refilling of the intracellular Ca^{2+} pool both involve activation of a poorly understood Ca^{2+} entry mechanism.[159,160] Studies measuring ^{45}Ca^{2+} uptake and the influx of Mn^{2+}, which quenches intracellular fluorescence of fura-2, indicate that the phospholipase C-coupled secretagogues

increase Ca^{2+} influx two- to fourfold.[154] This influx mechanism is not voltage-dependent or sensitive to organic Ca^{2+} channel blockers such as D600 or nifedipine. It is blocked by La^{2+}, Ni^{2+}, Co^{2+} and is enhanced by alkaline and inhibited by acidic pH. Patch clamp studies have not yet defined a constituent channel. At this point, it is better defined as an entry mechanism. The mechanisms controlling Ca^{2+} influx are not yet defined but seem to be sensitive to the state of intracellular Ca^{2+} stores. The most direct evidence for this linkage comes from the finding in a number of cell types that the plant sesquiterpene, thapsigargin inhibits the microsomal Ca^{2+}-ATPase, releases intracellular Ca^{2+}, and activates the Ca^{2+} influx mechanism, bypassing the receptor and the generation of inositol phosphates.[161] That a sustained increase in [Ca^{2+}]$_i$ is important for sustained amylase release is demonstrated by the fact that La^{3+}, Ni^{2+}, and extracellular acidity all inhibit the sustained component of amylase release as does removal of Ca^{2+} from the medium.

Recording of [Ca^{2+}]$_i$ from individual cells of rat and mouse acini has revealed that low (physiologic) concentrations of CCK, ACh, and bombesin induce a different pattern of Ca^{2+} increase characterized by oscillations in [Ca^{2+}]$_i$.[162,163] After a lag of up to 1 or 2 minutes, [Ca^{2+}]$_i$ increases. Superimposed on any steady increase are phasic increases in Ca^{2+} of up to 100 to 250 nM in magnitude (Fig 15-5). These oscillations, which occur one to four times per minute in various studies, are relatively independent of extracellular Ca^{2+} and involve release and reuptake from the aforementioned intracellular Ca^{2+} stores. In the case of stimulation by CCK, oscillations occur over the physiologic 1- to 30-pM concentration range with a relatively constant frequency but an increasing amplitude with increasing CCK. [Ca^{2+}]$_i$ oscillations continue as long as the stimulus is present. The functional importance of [Ca^{2+}]$_i$ oscillations is not yet clear. Low agonist concentrations inducing Ca^{2+} oscillations also increase DAG and presumably activate protein kinase C.

Intracellular Messenger-Induced Secretion

The evidence to support the importance of Ca^{2+}, DAG, and cAMP as intracellular mediators regulating secretion was based on the ability of artificial changes in the level of each messenger to influence secretion.[144] In the case of Ca^{2+}, the discovery that certain antibiotics such as A23187 and ionomycin functioned as Ca^{2+} ionophores and could be used to increase Ca^{2+} influx and trigger secretion provided one of the cornerstones for the importance of [Ca^{2+}]$_i$ in this process. In the case of DAG, the discovery that certain phorbol esters could activate protein kinase C in a manner similar to DAG has led to extensive studies of the activation of this pathway.[164] Ca^{2+} ionophores and phorbol esters clearly stimulate acinar cell secretion, with their effects being additive or potentiative. There are species differences in the relative potency of these agents, but, in most cases, the combination of the two duplicates the effect of secretagogues such as CCK or carbachol.[165,166] In the case of cAMP, derivatives such as dibutyryl cAMP or 8Br-cAMP that are either lipophilic or phosphodiesterase-resistant have been used to activate the pathway normally initiated by secretin or VIP. In most species, cAMP derivatives alone have minimal effects on acinar cell secretion but potentiate the effects of agents working by way of Ca^{2+} and DAG.

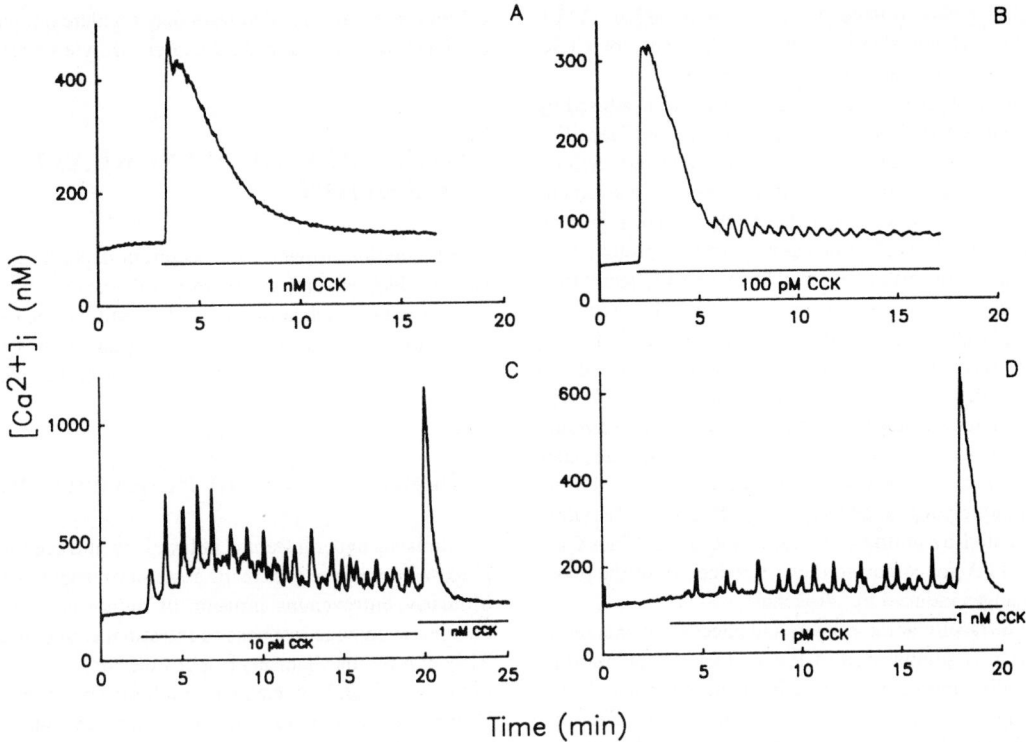

FIGURE 15–5. Increase in $[Ca^{2+}]_i$ in individual rat acinar cells in response to various concentrations of CCK (From Tsunoda Y, Stuenkel EL, Williams JA. Oscillatory mode of calcium signaling in rat pancreatic acinar cells. Am J Physiol 1990;258:C147.)

The quantitative importance of intracellular messengers is also shown by studies of permeabilized acini. When cells are suspended in an intracellularlike medium and permeabilized by electric shock, digitonin, or streptolysin, the addition of micromolar Ca^{2+} in the presence of Mg^{2+} and ATP can stimulate amylase release.[167,168,169] Activation of protein kinase C or addition of cAMP can further amplify Ca^{2+}-stimulated release.

Action of Intracellular Messengers

While the intracellular messengers active in pancreatic acinar cells have been identified and characterized, less is known about the mechanisms by which they act to induce granule exocytosis, fluid secretion, protein synthesis, and gene expression. Although other mechanisms may exist, all of the intracellular messengers activate protein kinases and phosphatases and thereby regulate the state of protein phosphorylation.[135] Furthermore, considerable data suggest that changes in the phosphorylation of regulatory proteins mediate the action of hormones and neurotransmitters in a variety of tissues.

Several Ca^{2+}-activated kinases and phosphatases have been identified in pancreatic acinar cells including Ca^{2+} calmodulin-activated type II[170] and III[171] kinases and myosin light chain kinase. The type III kinase is relatively specific for elongation factor 2, a 100-kd protein involved in ribosomal translation of mRNA. Upon phosphorylation of this factor, the efficiency of translation is greatly diminished. Myosin light chain kinase is relatively specific for myosin light chain, the phosphorylation of which is increased in acinar cells stimulated with CCK.[172] The type II kinase is a multifunctional kinase known to act on a number of proteins. It is a large multisubunit protein that undergoes autophosphorylation in a Ca^{2+}-dependent manner rendering the enzyme Ca^{2+} insensitive.[173] Thus, it can be viewed as a switch that might be activated by a large transient increase in $[Ca^{2+}]_i$. Protein kinase C (PKC), a Ca^{2+}/phospholipid/diacylglycerol-dependent protein kinase is known also to be present in acinar cells.[164,174] Recently, multiple isozymes of PKC have been identified,[175] although the functional significance of the isozymes is not yet clear. Acinar cells appear to express predominantly the type III or α form.[176] All forms of PKC require acidic phospholipids, diacylglycerol, and Ca^{2+} for activation. The Ca^{2+} dependence of these isozymes depends on both the lipid environment and substrate protein. Each molecule possesses a regulatory domain (which binds diacylglycerol or phorbol ester) and a catalytic domain. After treatment of acinar cells with active phorbol esters or, to a lesser extent, with CCK or carbachol, there is a translocation of PKC from cytoplasm to the membrane fraction,[177] and this translocation is taken to be a sign of "activation." Whether PKC is only active while membrane bound and, if so, which membranes are involved are not yet understood.

The known effects of cAMP are all mediated by cAMP-activated protein kinase. Binding of cAMP to a regulatory subunit results in dissociation and activation of a catalytic subunit. Isoforms of both regulatory and catalytic subunits exist. These have not been well characterized in pancreas, although the type II regulatory subunit, which is subject to autophosphorylation, is known to be present.[178] Activation of this kinase in situ can be estimated by homogenizing cells and measuring kinase activity without added cAMP and relating this to maximal activity with added cAMP. Such studies have shown that secretin and VIP, but not CCK, activate the kinase in guinea pig and rat pancreas.[179]

Substrate proteins, the phosphorylation of which is altered by secretagogues and intracellular messengers, have been identified by incubation of acini or lobules with ^{32}P to label intracellular ATP followed by separation of proteins by one- and two-dimensional electrophoresis. In rat and mouse acini, a major regulated particulate protein has been identified as ribosomal S6 protein.[180,181] The phosphorylation of this protein may be involved in facilitating protein synthesis and is enhanced by CCK, carbachol, secretin, and insulin. Its phosphorylation is regulated by a distinct S6 kinase, which, itself, is activated in part by second messenger-regulated kinases. Proteins that undergo phosphorylation in a similarly regulated fashion include elongation factor 2,[171] vitamin D-binding protein,[182] and myosin light chain.[172] Pancreatic secretagogues alter the phosphorylation of as many as ten other proteins.[166,183] Of the ten, some are uniquely regulated by $[Ca^{2+}]_i$, TPA, or cAMP, while others are regulated by multiple second messengers. When Ca^{2+} ionophore and TPA are combined they reproduce all of the phosphorylation changes induced by carbachol.

The role of intracellular messengers and effectors in pancreatic enzyme secretion is summarized in Figure 15-6. Stimulation of secretion normally involves synergetic interaction between intracellular messengers. In the case of acetylcholine and CCK, this includes interactions between Ca^{2+} and diacylglycerol-activated pathways. Agents such as VIP and secretin, which increase cAMP, add a further interaction at the postintracellular messenger level. Proteins localized on the granule and luminal plasma membrane as well as soluble and cytoskeletal proteins may be involved in exocytosis. In the case of pancreatic duct cells, the same intracellular messengers and kinases may regulate ion pumps, carriers, or channels involved in fluid and electrolyte secretion.

INHIBITION OF PANCREATIC SECRETION

The regulation of pancreatic secretion depends on a balance between inhibitory and stimulatory influences on the gland, which are exerted through hormones and the autonomic nervous system. While much has been written about pancreatic stimulation, less is known about the inhibitory influences on the pancreas.

Inhibitory Phase of Pancreatic Secretion

In humans, hyperglycemia induced by intravenous infusion of glucose inhibits the pancreatic secretory response to a test meal.[184] Similarly, intravenous infusion of amino acids inhibits human pancreatic enzyme response to intestinal amino acid perfusion.[185] Although the mechanisms responsible for these observations are unknown, secondary release of inhibitory hormones is postulated. Pancreatic glucagon exhibits characteristics consistent with such an inhibitory hormone. In most of the studies, glucagon inhibits pancreatic secretion stimulated by secretin and CCK, alone or in combination, or by ingestion of a test meal in dogs,[186-188] cats, rats,[189] and humans.[190] The inhibitory effect is characterized by reduction of volume of flow as well of bicarbonate and enzyme secretion. Pancreatic glucagon is secreted concomitantly with the hyperaminoacidemia observed after a high protein meal[191] or intestinally perfused amino acids.[189] This postprandial level of glucagon may be sufficient to inhibit secretin- or CCK-stimulated pancreatic secretion.[190] Another pancreatic hormone, somatostatin, may also play a role in the inhibition of pancreatic secretion. In humans, pharmacologic doses of somatostatin cause marked inhibition of CCK-stimulated pancreatic enzyme secretion and modest inhibition of secretin-stimulated bicarbonate secretion.[192] Studies in the perfused canine pancreas have demonstrated that somatostatin is released from the pancreas during perfusion with high concentrations of amino acids or glucose.[193] This peptide, in turn, may exert a paracrine inhibitory effect on the exocrine pancreas. Whatever the mechanism, the observations that hyperglycemia and hyperaminoacidemia induced by intravenous nutrient administration inhibit pancreatic secretion may provide a theoretical basis for "resting" the pancreas with hyperalimentation during severe acute pancreatitis.

Intrajejunal perfusion of hypertonic glucose (50%) produces dose-related inhibition of secretin-stimulated pancreatic fluid and bicarbonate secretion in humans.[194,195] Similar inhibition occurs with intraintestinal hypertonic (9%) sodium chloride infusion in dogs. The inhibitory effect of hypertonic glucose is reduced, but not abolished, by vagotomy. At least part of this inhibitory effect has been attributed to the release of enteric glucagon.[195] Infusion of oxyntomodulin (glucagon-37), a 37-amino acid, glucagon-containing peptide isolated from porcine lower intestine,[196] inhibits basal and cerulein-stimulated pancreatic secretion of bicarbonate and enzymes.[197] This intestinal glucagon is ten times more potent than pancreatic glucagon.

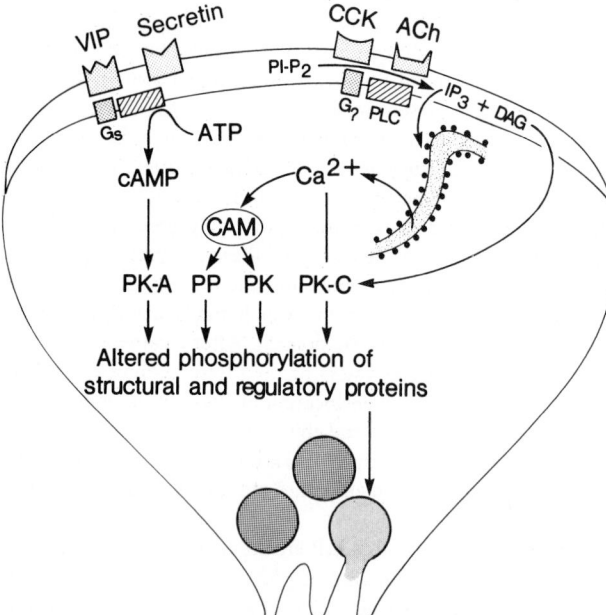

FIGURE 15–6. Schematic diagram of stimulus-secretion coupling of pancreatic acinar cell protein secretion. (From Williams JA, Burnham DB, Hootman SR. Cellular regulation of pancreatic secretion. In Forte J, ed. Handbook of physiology—The gastrointestinal system, III. Bethesda: American Physiological Society, 1989:419.)

Inhibitory control of pancreatic secretion by factors in the ileum and colon has been reported. Hage et al[198] demonstrated that infusions of oleic acid into the proximal colon of conscious dogs inhibits secretin-stimulated pancreatic secretion. Similar inhibitory effects have been observed in rats.[199,200] In the anesthetized cat, infusion of oleic acid or hypertonic glucose or saline into either the colon or terminal ileum inhibits secretin- or CCK-stimulated secretory volume, bicarbonate, and enzyme output from the pancreas.[201]

In humans, nutrients such as lipid in the colon inhibit CCK-stimulated pancreatic enzyme and bicarbonate output.[202] It is interesting to speculate that these late postprandial events may serve as physiologic signals to reduce exocrine pancreatic secretion after digestion and absorption of nutrients are completed. The inhibitory effect of nutrients in the distal gut on pancreatic secretion appears independent of the vagus and splanchnic nerves.[201] Cross circulation studies in the rat have shown a humoral factor mediates inhibition of pancreatic enzyme secretion induced by colonic perfusion of oleic acid. Harper used the term *pancreotone* to describe an inhibitory substance extracted from the colonic mucosa.[203] The function of pancreotone is abolished when the extract is preincubated with trypsin, demonstrating it is a peptide. PYY, a 36-amino acid peptide named for its amino and carboxyl terminal tyrosines, has been found to be present in abundance in the distal small intestine, colon, and rectum.[204-206] This peptide is released by fat and, to a lesser degree, protein in the distal gut or colon. Furthermore, the infusion of this peptide in dogs significantly inhibits basal and meal-stimulated pancreatic bicarbonate and enzyme secretion.[207] These observations support the hypothesis that PYY is at least a component of pancreotone.

Pancreatic polypeptide (PP), a peptide closely related to PYY, is another hormone that may play an important role in regulating pancreatic exocrine secretion. PP is localized in the islets of Langerhans and between the acinar cells of the exocrine pancreas.[208] Its only apparent physiologic actions are to inhibit pancreatic and biliary secretion. The secretion of PP is governed mainly by a cholinergic mechanism.[209] Postprandial release of PP is mediated by a long vagovagal reflex and short local cholinergic pathways.[209] Vagal cholinergic activity not only is the most powerful stimulant of PP release, it is also key to nearly all other stimulation of the PP cell.[209,210]

In both humans and dogs, infusion of physiologic concentrations of PP inhibits basal and stimulated pancreatic secretion.[7,211] In vivo, PP appears to act preferentially by inhibiting vagal stimulation,[212] while in vitro, PP inhibits pancreatic enzyme secretion by way of presynaptic modulation of acetylcholine release.[213] Because its secretion is under cholinergic control and it acts by interfering with cholinergic transmission, PP is an ideal candidate to modulate pancreatic secretion stimulated by the cholinergic enteropancreatic reflex. After ingestion of a meal, the enteropancreatic reflex is activated to stimulate pancreatic enzyme secretion and PP release. PP, in turn, inhibits cholinergic transmission and reduces pancreatic enzyme secretion. Thus, it is conceivable that PP may play an important role in the feedback regulation of pancreatic enzyme secretion activated by the enteropancreatic reflex.

In recent years, the list of peptides known to inhibit exocrine pancreatic secretion has expanded (Table 15-2). Little is known, however, about the mechanisms through which hormones or neurotransmitters inhibit pancreatic enzyme secretion. An important feature shared by these agents is the lack of direct inhibitory effect on pancreatic acinar cells. Many substances suppress pancreatic enzyme secretion in vivo but do not act directly on the acinar cell to suppress enzyme release. Based on recent in vitro studies, it appears that peptides such as PP,[213] somatostatin,[214] enkephalin,[215] and pancreastatin[216] inhibit pancreatic enzyme secretion by way of modulation of cholinergic transmission.

Feedback Regulation of Pancreatic Secretion

Much interest has been generated by a series of observations suggesting that the intraluminal action of pancreatic proteases plays an important role in regulating pancreatic enzyme secretion.[75,217,218,219] The underlying concept of feedback regulation of the pancreas is based primarily on studies in rats that show that diversion of pancreatic juice from the duodenum stimulates CCK release and thereby pancreatic enzyme secretion.[76] On the other hand, intraduodenal administration of trypsin or chymotrypsin inhibits the release of CCK and pancreatic enzymes.[76] This phenomenon is specific for activated proteases and is not observed with inactivated trypsin, amylase, lipase, or sodium bicarbonate. Subsequent studies demonstrated that intravenous infusion of proglumide or L364,718, a specific CCK receptor antagonist, abolishes the increase in pancreatic exocrine secretion evoked by

TABLE 15-2

Gastrointestinal Peptides That Inhibit Exocrine Pancreatic Secretion

PEPTIDE	MODE OF ACTION	MECHANISM
Glucagon	Endocrine/paracrine	Unknown
Somatostatin	Endocrine/paracrine	Unknown
Pancreatic polypeptide	Endocrine/paracrine	Inhibition of cholinergic transmission
Peptide YY	Endocrine/paracrine	Inhibition of cholinergic transmission
Neuropeptide Y	Neurocrine	Inhibition of cholinergic transmission
Enkephalin	Neurocrine	Inhibition of cholinergic transmission
Calcitonin gene-related peptide	Neurocrine	Unknown
Pancreastatin	Unknown	Inhibition of cholinergic transmission

diversion of bile-pancreatic juice.[76,220] These observations indicate that feedback inhibition of pancreatic secretion by trypsin is mediated by inhibition of CCK release or action.

The increased plasma CCK levels and pancreatic secretion after diversion of pancreatic juice appears to be mediated by a trypsin-sensitive substance secreted by the proximal small intestine that has been designated "CCK-releasing factor" (CCK-RF).[78] When trypsin is present, this peptide is cleaved and inactivated. This newly discovered CCK-RF may act as a mediator of pancreatic enzyme secretion in response to dietary protein intake in rats. Dietary protein in the intestine competes for the trypsin[77] that would otherwise inactivate CCK-RF. The resulting increase of CCK-RF in the intestinal lumen enhances CCK release and, thereby, stimulates pancreatic enzyme secretion. While this appears to be the principal mechanism regulating CCK release in rats, it is not known whether the same mechanism operates in other species.

In spite of several attempts to demonstrate a protease-sensitive feedback mechanism in humans, the issue has remained controversial until recently. Technical limitations in removing or blocking intraluminal protease activity have made studies in humans difficult. Using a different approach, it has been reported that intestinal administration of trypsin or chymotrypsin in humans suppresses CCK release and partially blocks the pancreatic response to intestinal administration of amino acids or oral ingestion of a test meal.[82,221] This supports the existence of feedback regulation of pancreatic enzyme secretion in humans.

Using an alternative approach, Dlugosz and colleagues,[222] and Hotz and colleagues[223] infused aprotinin, a trypsin inhibitor, intraduodenally and found no effect on basal pancreatic enzyme secretion. Similar findings were reported using the new trypsin inhibitor, FOY-305.[224] However, neither compound strongly inhibits human chymotrypsin. On the other hand, Liener and colleagues[225] demonstrated that Bowman-Birk SBTI, an inhibitor of chymotrypsin and elastase, markedly stimulates pancreatic enzyme secretion in humans. These observations suggest that not only trypsin, but also other proteases such as chymotrypsin and elastase should be removed to evoke pancreatic enzyme secretion in humans.

As noted above, postprandial pancreatic enzyme secretion is under both hormonal and neural control. Distention or administration of hyperosmolar solutions into the duodenum elicits pancreatic enzyme secretion without raising plasma CCK levels.[113] Furthermore, this stimulatory effect is inhibited by atropine, suggesting that it is cholinergically mediated. In contrast to amino acid-stimulated pancreatic enzyme secretion, pancreatic responses to stimulation by volume or osmolality in the duodenum are not suppressed by trypsin.[113] This indicates that feedback regulation of pancreatic secretion by trypsin is stimulus-specific and is mediated by inhibiting the release of CCK. The enteropancreatic reflex is unaffected by intraluminal proteases.

The existence of a feedback regulation of pancreatic enzyme secretion in humans may have important clinical implications. It is conceivable that in patients with chronic pancreatitis, decreased pancreatic enzyme secretion may result in elevated plasma CCK levels, reflecting a failure in the feedback modulation of CCK release. This, in turn, may cause hyperstimulation of the pancreas and produce pain. Thus, effective enzyme replacement therapy might reduce pancreatic stimulation, decrease intraductal pressure, and diminish pain. Indeed, large doses of pancreatic extract have been reported to reduce pain in some patients with chronic pancreatitis.[226,227] This exciting observation awaits more supporting data for confirmation.

PATTERNS OF SECRETION

Basal Secretion

Under basal conditions, pancreatic secretion occurs at very low rates, although a small amount of enzymes is always present in the pancreatic juice. Basal secretion of enzymes and bicarbonate is about 10% and 2% of maximal, respectively.[60] A pattern of cyclic change in basal pancreatic secretion has been demonstrated in dogs[228,229] and humans,[230,231] and this is characterized by brief increases in bicarbonate and enzyme secretion, which recur every 60 to 120 minutes during the interdigestive period. These bursts of pancreatic secretory activity are temporarily associated with periods of increased motor activity in the stomach and proximal intestine known as the interdigestive migrating motor complexes (IMMC).[228,229,230,231] Associated with bursts of pancreatic secretion are brief increases in gastric acid and biliary secretion.[230,231] In addition, plasma motilin and PP levels also fluctuate in phase with the IMMC.[231,232] The concentrations of pancreatic enzymes and bile acids during the transient surge of pancreatico-biliary secretion are similar to maximal postprandial outputs, although the concentrations diminish rapidly with the onset of type III duodenal motor activity.[231,232] It has been postulated that this cyclic secretion of pancreatic and biliary juice may be important in the digestion of residual food particles or cellular debris in the gastrointestinal tract during the interdigestive period.

The control of the cyclic patterns of pancreatic secretion is unclear. Bursts of increased acid secretion are unlikely to be the principal mediators for the cyclic changes in pancreatic secretion because removal of gastric acid by aspiration or through a fistula does not affect the pattern of interdigestive pancreatic secretion.[231,232,233] Recent studies have demonstrated that infusion of motilin prematurely initiates cyclic pancreatic secretion and shortens the periodicity between peaks.[234] Administration of motilin antiserum abolishes the cyclic pattern of pancreatic secretion.[235] In addition, cholinergic blockade with atropine also markedly decreases trypsin output and abolishes interdigestive motor activity. These observations suggest that both motilin and cholinergic pathways are important in the initiation of the cyclic pancreatic secretion that occurs during fasting.

Prandial and Postprandial Secretion

After ingestion of a meal, the exocrine pancreas is stimulated to secrete enzymes and bicarbonate. Total postprandial pancreatic output is approximately 60% to 70% of the output attained in response to maximal stimulation with intravenous infusion of CCK.[84] The stimulatory effect of a meal can be described by separating its components into cephalic, gastric, and intestinal phases (Table 15-3).

TABLE 15–3
Three Phases of Postprandial Pancreatic Secretion

PHASES	PERCENTAGE OF PANCREATIC RESPONSE (%)	STIMULANTS	MEDIATORS
Cephalic	25	Sight, smell, taste, eating	Vagal
Gastric	10	Distention	Vagal cholinergic
Intestinal	50–75	Amino acids	CCK, secretin
		Fatty acids	Enteropancreatic reflexes
		Ca^{++}, H^+	Other hormones (?)
		Distention	

CEPHALIC PHASE

In humans and experimental animals, pancreatic secretion rich in enzymes is stimulated by the sight, smell, and taste of appetizing food.[236,237] This cephalic effect in dogs amounts to 25% of the enzyme response to an ordinary meal.[238] In humans, the contribution of the cephalic phase to the postprandial pancreatic enzyme secretion appears to be larger and amounts to 50% of maximal responses induced by exogenous secretin and CCK.[239] The pancreatic response to sham feeding lasts only for the duration of feeding.[239]

The vagus appears to be important in the mediation of the cephalic phase because this phase can be completely abolished by vagotomy in rats.[240] It has also been shown that administration of an anticholinergic drug decreases[239] or abolishes[241] the pancreatic response to sham feeding in humans. The site of action of the efferent cholinergic fibers is probably directly on the pancreas, because vagal stimulation causes pancreatic secretion from the pancreas in dogs even when it is perfused extracorporeally[242] to eliminate any humoral effects of nerve stimulation. Sham feeding increases gastric acid secretion, but because pancreatic response to sham feeding occurs in patients who are achlorhydric,[237] it is unlikely that gastric acid secretion contributes significantly to the cephalic phase of pancreatic enzyme secretion.

GASTRIC PHASE

In dogs[243,244] and humans,[245] gastric distention increases the rate of pancreatic enzyme secretion. Gastric distention to a volume ranging from 250 to 400 ml with a balloon results in doubling of basal pancreatic protein output.[246] Although the actual contribution of the gastric phase to the total postprandial pancreatic secretion has not been determined in humans, the magnitude of the distention-induced pancreatic response in dogs is approximately 20% of the maximal CCK response over a range of distention from 300 to 1500 ml.[244] Both vagotomy and atropine reduce or abolish the pancreatic response to gastric distention,[245,246] suggesting that it is mainly mediated by vagal-cholinergic pathways. The mechanoreceptors appear to be located in the body of the stomach because distention of antral pouches does not stimulate pancreatic secretion whereas distention of the remaining stomach does.[246]

The presence of food in the stomach also releases antral hormones such as gastrin or gastric-releasing peptide, which can stimulate pancreatic secretion either directly or indirectly. However, this possibility is considered unlikely because a transplanted portion of pancreas does not respond to gastric distention in dogs.[246] Furthermore, distention of the intact stomach has only a slight effect on gastrin release in humans[247,248] and dogs.[249]

The stomach facilitates digestion by fractionating solid food into small particles and, further, by initiating digestion of dietary proteins and lipids by pepsin and gastric lipase, respectively.[250,251] In addition, gastric emptying is of obvious importance in determining the rate of delivery of acid and nutrients into the duodenum, thereby determining the pattern and magnitude of intestinal phase of pancreatic secretion. Accordingly, postprandial pancreatic enzyme secretion is frequently abnormal in patients after gastric surgery.[109,252]

INTESTINAL PHASE

The intestinal phase represents the most important phase of postprandial pancreatic secretion. In humans and animals, the delivery of food into the small intestine stimulates pancreatic enzyme secretion to about 70% of maximal.[109] The major hormonal mediators of the intestinal phase of pancreatic secretion are secretin and CCK. In addition, the intestinal mucosa also processes receptors for important vagal cholinergic reflexes that regulate both pancreatic bicarbonate and enzyme secretion.

The proximal intestine plays an important role in the stimulation of pancreatic bicarbonate secretion, primarily by the release of secretin. Although, duodenal pH is the major regulator for the release of secretin, nonacid factors such as fatty acids and bile may also participate. The physiology of secretin is discussed in a previous section.

Among the various hydrolytic products of digestion, amino acids and fatty acids are potent stimulants of enzyme secretion but have only a weak effect on water and bicarbonate secretion. Amino acid mixtures are more potent than fatty acids, and, of the amino acids, only phenylalanine, valine, and methionine stimulate enzyme secretion in humans,[253] whereas, in dogs, phenylalanine, leucine, and tryptophan as well as oligopeptides and casein are effective.[254] The pancreatic response to intestinal perfusion with amino acids above a concentration of 8 mM depends on the total load administered.[255] This dependence on load rather than concentration is due to exposure of longer segments of small intestine to amino acids at a concentration above a threshold value. In humans, the mechanisms responsible for pancreatic response to

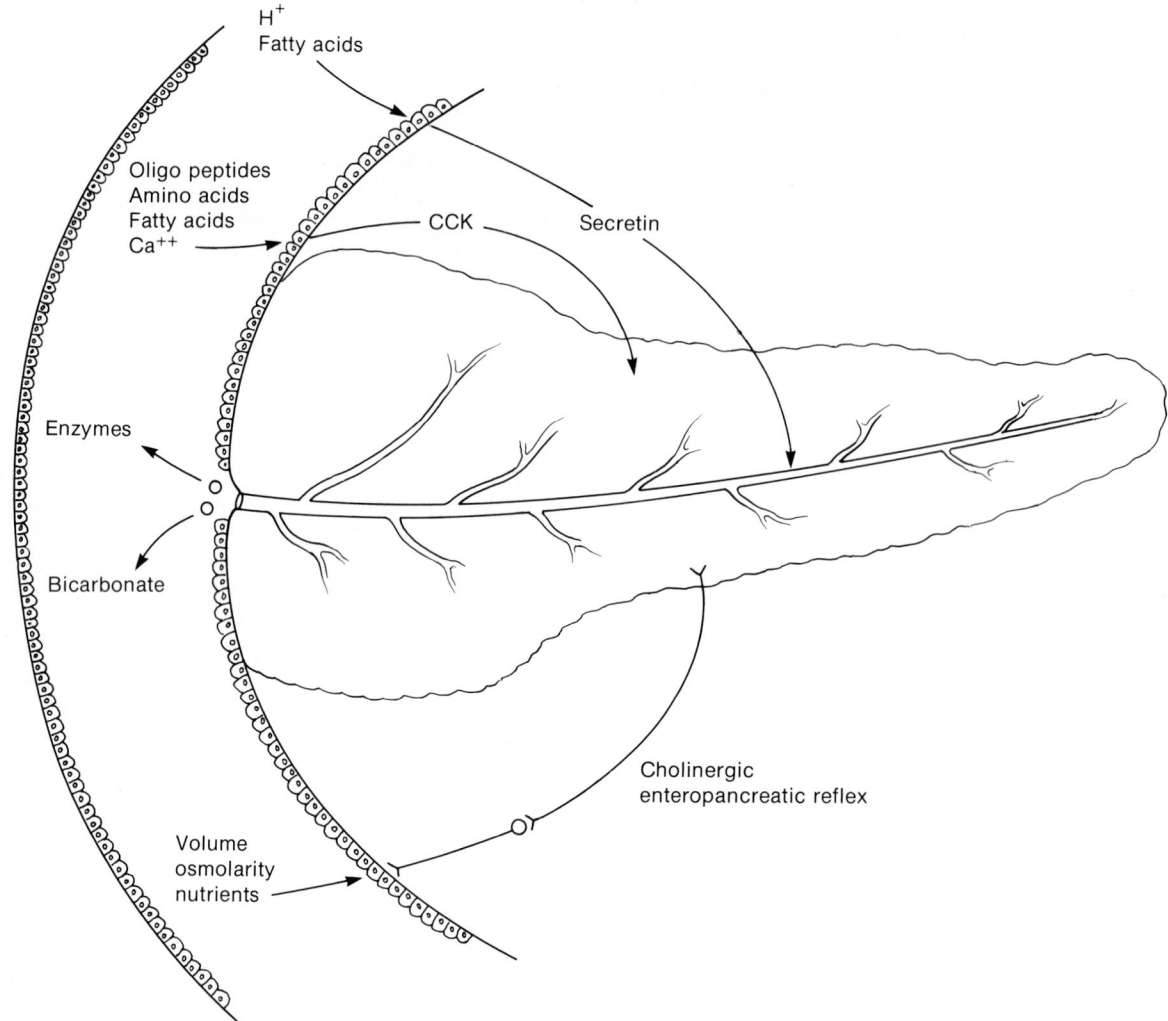

FIGURE 15–7. Intestinal phase of pancreatic enzyme secretion. Intestinal stimulants initiate enteropancreatic reflexes and release CCK, both of which act on pancreatic acinar cells to stimulate enzyme secretion. In addition, H⁺ and fatty acids release secretin, which stimulates bicarbonate secretion.

amino acids are confined to the duodenum and jejunum because no response is observed when amino acids were perfused into the ileum.[252]

Undigested fats are ineffective in stimulating pancreatic secretion, but fatty acids are potent pancreatic stimulants when present in micellar form.[61] Monoglycerides, the other product of lipolysis, also stimulate pancreatic secretion.[61,253] The chain length of fatty acids influences their potency in stimulating pancreatic secretion. In humans the order of potency is C18>C12>C8.[256] Other factors that influence pancreatic response to fatty acids include the degree of saturation,[257] the concentration and total load, and the concentration of bile salts relative to fatty acids.[256] In humans, intestinal perfusion of 10 mM monoolein produces a pancreatic enzyme output greater than that stimulated by intestinal amino acids and nearly equal to the maximal response to exogenous CCK.[258]

The release of CCK and the initiation of cholinergic enteropancreatic refluxes both appear to mediate the intestinal phase to pancreatic enzyme secretion. Plasma CCK levels increase after oral or intraduodenal administration of fat[79,80,81] and protein or amino acids.[81,82,259]

Administration of proglumide, a CCK receptor antagonist, partially inhibits pancreatic secretory responses to intestinally perfused amino acids and fat emulsions. Furthermore, increased firing rates in peripheral afferent neurons and in central sites have been recorded during intestinal perfusion with amino acids.[115,116,260] This finding, coupled with the observation that truncal vagotomy or administration of atropine markedly increases the latency of pancreatic secretory response to intestinal nutrients but not to CCK,[261,262] indicates participation of vagovagal cholinergic reflexes.

In contrast to amino acids and fatty acids, intestinal perfusion with isotonic glucose causes little or no pancreatic secretion in rats,[263] dogs,[254] or humans.[263] However, it is not known whether glucose potentiates other intestinal phase stimulants of pancreatic enzyme secretion such as by the release of insulin. Calcium, which is intimately involved in the action of CCK on pancreatic acinar cells, has a stimulatory action on the pancreas. In humans, intraduodenal perfusion of calcium solutions, in concentrations similar to those found in the duodenum after ingestion of a meal, stimulates pancreatic enzyme secretion and gallbladder contraction. Intraduodenal calcium concentration of 12 or 25 mmol induces pancreatic enzyme responses similar to the maximal enzyme output evoked by intravenous infusion of CCK.[266] Intestinal perfusion with $MgSO_4$,[265] $Mg Cl_2$[265] and $Zn SO_4$[266] also stimulates pancreatic enzyme secretion by mechanisms that are yet unknown.

The human duodenum contains receptors for volume and osmolality that mediate pancreatic enzyme secretion. Volume distention[113] or hyperosmolar solutions[113] in the duodenum elicit pancreatic enzyme secretion without raising plasma CCK levels. This enzyme secretion is inhibited by atropine, suggesting mediation by the cholinergic enteropancreatic reflex.[113] The volumes of saline required to induce pancreatic secretion are as low as 1 to 5 ml/min, in the range observed after meal ingestion in the duodenum postprandially. The degree of stimulation by volume- or osmoreceptor activation is 15% to 20% of the maximal enzyme response to CCK.[112] Factors involved in the mediation of the intestinal phase of pancreatic enzyme secretion are depicted in Figure 15-7.

The reader is directed to Chapter 1, The Enteric Nervous System and its Extrinsic Connections; Chapter 2, Gastrointestinal Hormones; Chapter 3, The Brain–Gut Axis; Chapter 6, Epithelia: Biologic Principles of Organization; Chapter 81, Motility Disorders of the Colon; Chapter 82, Diverticulitis; Chapter 83, Bacterial Infections of the Colon; Chapter 84, Malignant Tumors of the Colon; Chapter 85, Anorectal Diseases; Chapter 86, Miscellaneous Inflammatory and Structural Disorders of the Colon; Chapter 87, Pancreas: Anatomy and Structural Anomalies; Chapter 88, Acute Pancreatitis; Chapter 89, Chronic Pancreatitis; Chapter 90, Pancreatic Adenocarcinoma; Chapter 91, Endocrine Neoplasms of the Pancreas; Chapter 92, Congenital and Hereditary Disease of the Pancreas; Chapter 129, Tests of Gastric and Exocrine Pancreatic Function and Absorption.

REFERENCES

1. Ando S. A study of the vascular supply in the pancreas. Fukuoka Acta Med 1959;50:4247.
2. Henderson JR, Daniel PM. Portal circulation and their relation to counter current systems. Q J Exp Physiol 1978;63:355.
3. Fujita T, Watanabe Y. Effects of islet hormones upon the exocrine pancreas. In: Fujita T, ed. Gastro-entero-pancreatic endocrine system. A cell biological approach, Tokyo: Igaku Shoin, 1973:169.
4. Dyck WP, Texter EC, Lasater JM, et al. Influence of glucagon on pancreatic exocrine secretion in man. Gastroenterology 1970;58:532.
5. Fontana G, Costa PL, Tassari R, et al. Effect of glucagon on pure human exocrine pancreatic secretion. Am J Gastroenterol 1975;63:490.
6. Domschke S, Domschke W, Rosch W, et al. Inhibition of somatostatin of secretin-stimulated pancreatic secretion in man: A study with pure pancreatic juice. Scand J Gastroenterol 1977;12:59.
7. Greenberg GR, McCloy RF, Chadwick VS, et al. Effect of bovine pancreatic polypeptide on basal pancreatic and biliary outputs in man. Am J Dig Dis 1979;24:11.
8. Satio A, Williams J, Kanno T. Potentiation of cholecystokinin-induced exocrine secretion by both exogenous and endogenous insulin in isolated and perfused rat pancreata. J Clin Invest 1980;65;777.
9. Case RM. Pancreatic secretion: Cellular aspects. In: Duthe HL, Wormsley KG, eds. Scientific basis of gastroenterology, Edinburgh: Churchill Livingstone, 1979:163.
10. Grossman MI, Ivy AC. Effect of alloxan upon external secretion of the pancreas. Proc Soc Exp Biol Med 1946;63:62.
11. Lightwood R, Reber HA. Micropuncture study of pancreatic secretion in the cat. Gastroenterology 1977;72:61.
12. Mangoc JA, McSherry NR, Nausia-Arvanitakis S, et al. Transductal flexes of anions in the rat pancreas. Proc Soc Exp Biol Med 1974;146:321.
13. Reber H, Wolf CJ. Micropuncture study of pancreatic electrolyte secretion. Am J Physiol 1968;215:34.
14. Schulz I, Yamagata A, Weske M. Micropuncture studies on the pancreas of the rabbit. Pflugers Arch 1969;308:277.
15. Folsch UR, Creutzfeldt W. Pancreatic duct cells in rats: Secretory studies in response to secretin, cholecystokinin-pancreozymin and gastrin in vivo. Gastroenterology 1977;73:1053.
16. Case RM, Argent BE. Bicarbonate secretion by pancreatic duct cells: Mechanisms and control. In: Go VLW et al, eds. The exocrine pancreas, New York: Raven Press, 1986:213.
17. Swanson CH, Solomon AK. Micropuncture analysis of the cellular mechanisms of electrolyte secretion by the in vitro rabbit pancreas. J Gen Physiol 1975;65:22.
18. DePont JJHHM, Jansen JWCM, Kuijpers GAJ, et al. A model for pancreatic fluid secretion. In: Case RM et al, eds. Electrolyte and water transport across gastrointestinal epithelia. New York: Raven Press, 1982:11.
19. Scratcherd T, Hutson D, Case RM. Ionic transport mechanisms underlying fluid secretion by the pancreas. Philos Trans R Soc Lond 1981;296:167.
20. Borgstrom B, Erlanson-Albertsson C, Wieloch T. Pancreatic colipase: Chemistry and physiology. J Lipid Res 1973;20:805.
21. Erlanson C, Borgstrom B. Purification and further characterization of colipase from porcine pancreas. Biochim Biophys Acta 1972;217:400.
22. Borgstrom B, Erlanson C. Pancreatic lipase and colipase interactions and effects of bile salts and other detergents. Eur J Biochem 1973;37:60.
23. Borgstrom B, Donner J. Binding of bile salts to pancreatic colipase and lipase. J Lipid Res 1975;16:287.
24. Borgstrom B. On the interactions between pancreatic lipase and colipase and the substrate and the importance of bile salts. J Lipid Res 1975;16:411.
25. Palade GE. Intracellular aspects of the process of protein synthesis. Science 1975;189:347.
26. Gorelick FS, Jamieson JD. Structure-function relationship of the pancreas. In: Johnson LR, ed. Physiology of the gastrointestinal tract, ed 2. New York: Raven Press, 1987:1089.
27. Case RM. Pancreatic secretion: Cellular aspects. In: Duthie HL, Wormsley KG, eds. Scientific basis of gastroenterology. Edinburgh: Churchill Livingstone, 1979:163.
28. Rosewicz S, Lewis LD, Wang XY, Liddle RA, Logsdon CD. Pancreatic digestive enzyme gene expression: Effects of CCK and soybean trypsin inhibitor. Am J Physiol 1989;256:G733.
29. Steinhilber W, Poensgen J, Rausch U, Kern HF, Scheele GA. Translational control of anionic trypsinogen and amylase synthesis in rat pancreas in response to caerulein stimulation. Proc Natl Acad Sci USA 1988;85:6597.
30. Walter P, Gilmore K, Blobel G. Protein translocation across the endoplasmic reticulum. Cell 1984;38:5.
31. Meyer D, Krause E, Dobberstein B. Secretory protein translocation across membranes: The role of ducking protein. Nature 1982;297:647.
32. Gilmore R, Walter P, Blobel G. Protein translocation across the endoplasmic reticulum: Isolation and characterization of the SRP receptor. J Cell Biol 1982;95:470.
33. Schele G, Dobberstein B, Blobel G. Transfer of proteins across membranes: Biosynthesis in vitro of pretrypsinogen and trypsinogen by cell fractions of canine pancreas. Eur J Biochem 1978;82:593.
34. Caplan MJ, Rosenzweig SA, Jamieson JD. Processing and sorting of proteins synthesized in the endoplasmic reticulum. In: Andreoli TE et al, eds. Physiology of membrane disorders. New York: Plenum, 1986:273.
35. Jamieson JD, Palade GE. Intracellular transport of secretory proteins in the pancreatic exocrine cell. III. Dissociation of intracellular transport from proteins synthesis. J Cell Biol 1968;39:580.
36. Reggio HA, Palade GE. Sulfated compounds in the zymogen granules of the guinea pig pancreas. J Cell Biol 1978;77:288.
37. Scheele GA, Palade GE. Studies of the guinea pig pancreas. Parallel discharge of exocrine enzyme activities. J Biol Chem 1975;250:2660.

38. Sommer H, Schrezenmeir J, Kasper H. Output-dependent non-parallel enzyme secretion of the human pancreas. Hepatogastroenterology 1985;32:246.

39. Dagorn JC, Paradis D, Morriset J. Non-parallel response of amylase and chymotrypsinogen biosynthesis following pancreatic stimulation. Digestion 1977;15:110.

40. Dagorn JC, Sahel J, Sarles H. Non-parallel secretion of enzymes in human duodenal juice collected by endoscopic retrograde catheterization of the papilla. Gastroenterology 1977;73:42.

41. Wormsley KG. Pancreatic secretion: Physiological control. In: Duthie HL, Wormsley KG, eds. Scientific basis of gastroenterology, Edinburgh: Churchill Livingstone, 1979:199.

42. Felber JP, Dick J, de Kalbermattern N. Enteric control of the pancreas. In: Bloom SR, ed. Gut hormones, Edinburgh: Churchill Livingstone, 1978:310.

43. Adelson JW, Rothman SS. Chymodenin, a duodenal peptide: Specific stimulation of chymotrypsinogen secretion. Am J Physiol 1975;229:1680.

44. Majumdar AP, Dubick MA, Vesenka GD, et al. Non-parallel discharge of digestive enzymes from isolated pancreatic acini. Biochem Biophys Res Commun 1965;128:872.

45. Adelson JW, Miller PE. Heterogeneity of the exocrine pancreas. Am J Physiol 1989;256:G817.

46. Mroz EA, Lechene C. Pancreatic zymogen granules differ markedly in protein composition. Science 1986;232:871.

47. Adelson JW, Miller PE. Pancreatic secretion by non-parallel exocytosis: Potential resolution of a long controversy. Science 1985;24:993.

48. Wormsley KG, Goldberg DM. Progress report: The relationships of the pancreatic enzymes. Gut 1972;12:398.

49. Owyang C. Miller JL, DiMagno EP, et al. Gastrointestinal hormone profile in renal insufficiency. Mayo Clin Proc 1979;54:769.

50. Barrowman JA, Mayston PD. The trophic influence of cholecystokinin on the rat pancreas. J Physiol (Lond) 1974;238:73P.

51. Meyer JH, Way LW, Grossman MI. Pancreatic bicarbonate response to various acids in duodenum of the dog. Am J Physiol 1970;219:964.

52. Fahrenkrug J, Schaffalitzky de Muckadell OB, Rune SJ. pH threshold for release of secretin in normal subjects and in patients with duodenal ulcer and patients with chronic pancreatitis. Scand J Gastroenterol 1978;13:177.

53. Chey WY, Lee YH, Hendricks JG, et al. Plasma secretin concentrations in fasting and postprandial state in man. Dig Dis Sci 1978;23:981.

54. Schaffalitzky de Muckadell OB, Fahrenkrug J, Nielsen J, et al. Meal-stimulated secretin release in man: Effect of acid and bile. Scand J Gastroenterol 1981;16:981.

55. Rune SJ. pH in the human duodenum. Its physiological and pathophysiological significance. Digestion 1973;8:261.

56. Schaffalitzky de Muckadell OB, Fahrenkrug J. Secretion pattern of secretin in man: Regulation of gastric acid. Gut 1978;19:812.

57. Chang TM, Chey WY. Radioimmunoassay of cholecystokinin. Dig Dis Sci 1983;28:456.

58. Meyer JH, Fink AS. Pancreatic bicarbonate response to foodbound hydrogen ion along the gut. Gastroenterology 1984;87:587.

59. Watanabe S, Chey WY, Lee KY, Chang TM. Secretin is released by digestive products of fat in dogs. Gastroenterology 1986;90:1008.

60. Debas HT, Grossman MI. Pure cholecystokinin: Pancreatic protein and bicarbonate response. Digestion 1973;9:469.

61. Meyer JH, Jones RS. Canine pancreatic responses to intestinally perfused fat and products of digestion. Am J Physiol 1974;226:1178.

62. Lagerlof HO. Pancreatic secretion after introduction of bile salts into the duodenum. Acta Med Scand [Suppl] 1942;128:89.

63. Osnes M, Hanseen LE, Flaten O, et al. Exogenous pancreatic secretion and immunoreactive secretin release after intraduodenal instillation of bile in man. Gut 1978;19:180.

64. Schaffalitzky de Muckadell OB, Fahrenkrug J, Watt-Boolsen S, et al. Pancreatic response and plasma secretin concentration during infusion of low dose of secretin in man. Scand J Gastroenterol 1978;12:305.

65. You CH, Rominger J, Chey WY. Effects of atropine on the action and release of secretin in humans. Am J Physiol 1982;242:G608.

66. Chey WY, Kim MS, Lee KY, et al. Effect of rabbit antisecretin serum on postprandial pancreatic secretion in dog. Gastroenterology 1979;77:1268.

67. You CH, Rominger JM, Chey WY. Potentiation effect of cholecystokinin-octapeptide on pancreatic bicarbonate secretion stimulated by a physiological dose of secretin in humans. Gastroenterology 1963;85:40.

68. Brown JC, Harper AA, Scratcherd T. Potentiation of secretin stimulation of the pancreas. J Physiol (Lond) 1967;190:519.

69. Chey WY, Kim MS, Lee KY. Influence of the vagus nerve on release and action of secretin in dog. J Physiol (Lond) 1979;293:435.

70. Meyer JH, Kelly GA. Canine pancreatic responses to intestinally perfused proteins and protein digests. Am J Physiol 1976;231:682.

71. Wang CC, Grossman MI. Physiological determination of release of secretin and pancreozymin from intestine of dogs with transplanted pancreas. Am J Physiol 1951;164:527.

72. Meyer JH, Jones RS. Canine pancreatic responses to intestinally perfused fat and products of fat digestion. Am J Physiol 1974;226:1178.

73. Meyer JH. Release of secretin and cholecystokinin. In: Thompson JC, ed. Gastrointestinal hormones. Austin: University of Texas Press, 1974:475.

74. Malagelada JR, DiMagno EP, Summerskill WHJ, et al. Regulation of pancreatic and gallbladder functions of intraluminal fatty acids and bile acids in man. J Clin Invest 1976;58:493.

75. Green GM, Lyman RL. Feedback regulation of pancreatic enzyme secretion as a mechanism for trypsin inhibitor-induced hypersecretion in rats. Proc Soc Exp Biol Med 1972;140:6.

76. Louie DS, May D, Miller P, et al. Cholecystokinin mediates feedback regulation of pancreatic enzyme secretion in rats. Am J Physiol 1986;250:G252.

77. Liddle RA, Green GM, Conrad CK, et al. Proteins but not amino acids, carbohydrates or fats stimulate cholecystokinin secretion in the rat. Am J Physiol 1986;251:G243.

78. Lu L, Louie D, Owyang C. A cholecystokinin releasing peptide mediates feedback regulation of pancreatic secretion. Am J Physiol 1989;256:G430.

79. Byrnes DJ, Henderson L, Borody T, et al. Radioimmunoassay of cholecystokinin in human plasma. Clin Chim Acta 1981;111:81.

80. Jansen JBMJ, Lamers CBHW. Radioimmunoassay of cholecystokinin in human tissue and plasma. Clin Chim Acta 1983;131:305.

81. Liddle RA, Goldfine ID, Rosen MS, et al. Cholecystokinin bioactivity in human plasma. J Clin Invest 1985;75:1144.

82. Owyang C, Louie DS, Tatum D. Feedback regulation of pancreatic enzyme secretion in man: Suppression of cholecystokinin release by trypsin. J Clin Invest 1986;77:2042.

83. Cantor P, Rehfeld JF. The molecular nature of cholecystokinin in human plasma. Clin Chim Acta 1987;168:153.

84. Beglinger C, Fried M, Whitehouse I, et al. Pancreatic enzyme responses to a liquid meal and to hormonal stimulation. Correlation with plasma secretin and cholecystokinin levels. J Clin Invest 1985;75:1471.

85. Hosotani R, Chowdhury P, Rayford PL. L364,718, a new CCK antagonist inhibits postprandial pancreatic secretion and PP release in dogs. Dig Dis Sci 1989;34:462.

86. Konturek SJ, Tasler J, Cieszkowski M, et al. Effect of cholecystokinin receptor antagonist of pancreatic responses to exogenous gastrin and cholecystokinin and to meal stimuli. Gastroenterology 1988;94:1014.

87. Cantor P, Mortensen PE, Gjorup I, et al. Effect of the cholecystokinin receptor antagonist MK-329 on meal-stimulated pancreatic secretion in man. Digestion 1989;43:134.

88. Henriksen FW, Worning H. The interaction of secretin and pancreozymin on the exocrine pancreatic secretion in dogs. Acta Physiol Scand 1967;70:241.

89. Holst JJ. Neural regulation of pancreatic exocrine function. In: Go VLW et al, eds. The exocrine pancreas. New York: Raven Press, 1986:287.

90. Rosenfeld MG, Mermod J, Amara SG, et al. Production of a novel neuropeptide encoded by the calcitonin gene via tissue specific RNA processing. Nature 1983;304:129.

91. Beglinger C, Grossman MI, Solomon TE. Interaction between stimulants of exocrine pancreatic secretion in dogs. Am J Physiol 1984;246:G173.

92. Chey WY, Lee KY, Chang T, et al. Potentiating effect of secretin

on cholecystokinin-stimulated pancreatic secretion in dogs. Am J Physiol 1984;246:G248.

93. Preshaw RM, Cooke AR, Grossman MI. Stimulation of pancreation secretion by a humoral agent from the pyloric gland area of the stomach. Gastroenterology 1965;49:617.

94. Preshaw RM, Cooke AR, Grossman MI. Pancreatic secretion induced by stimulation of the pyloric gland area of the stomach. Science 1965;148:1347.

95. Erspamer V, Melchiorri P. Active polypeptides of the amphibian skin and their synthetic analogues. Pure Appl Chem 1973;35:463.

96. Polak JM, Hobbs S, Bloom SR, et al. Distribution of a bombesin like peptide in human gastrointestinal tract. Lancet 1976;1:1109.

97. Basso N, Gini S, Improta G, et al. External pancreatic secretion after bombesin infusion in man. Gut 1975;16:994.

98. Jensen RT, Moody T, Pert C, et al. Interaction of bombesin and litorin with specific membrane receptors on pancreatic acinar cells. Proc Natl Acad Sci USA 1978;75:6139.

99. Erspamer V, Improta G, Melchiorri P, et al. Evidence of cholecystokinin release by bombesin in the dog. Br J Pharmacol 1974;52:227.

100. Mennini C, Basso N, Minervini S, et al. Meccanismo di azione della bombesina sulla secrezione pancreatica: Perfusione di pancreas isolato di cane. Policlinico (Sez Chir) 1978;85:426.

101. Fender HR, Curtis PJ, Rayford PL, et al. Effect of bombesin on serum gastrin and cholecystokinin in dogs. Surg Forum 1976;37:4141.

102. Taylor IL, Walsh JH. Carter D, et al. Effects of atropine and bethanechol on bombesin stimulated release of pancreatic polypeptide and gastrin in dog. Gastroenterology 1979;77:714.

103. Konturek SJ, Jaworek J, Cieszkowski M, et al. Comparison of effects of neurotensin and fat on pancreatic stimulation in dogs. Am J Physiol 1983;244:G590.

104. Baca I, Feurle GE, Hass M, et al. Interaction of neurotensin, cholecystokinin and secretin in the stimulation of exocrine pancreas in the dog. Gastroenterology 1983;84:556.

105. Fletcher DR, Blackburn AM, Adrian TE, et al. Effect of neurotensin on pancreatic function in man. Life Sci 1981;29:2157.

106. Brooks FP. The neurohumoral control of pancreatic exocrine secretion. Am J Clin Nutr 1973;26:251.

107. Brooks FP, Manfredo M. The control of pancreatic secretion and its clinical significance. Am J Gastroenterol 1964;42:42.

108. Malagelada JR, Go VLW, Summerskill WMJ. Altered pancreatic and biliary function after vagotomy and pyloroplasty. Gastroenterology 1974;66:22.

109. MacGregor IL, Parent J, Meyer JH. Gastric emptying of liquid meals and pancreatic and biliary secretion after subtotal gastrectomy or truncal vagotomy and pyloroplasty in man. Gastroenterology 1977;72:195.

110. Chey WY, Kim MS, Lee KY. Influence of the vagus nerve on release and action of secretin in dog. J Physiol (Lond) 1979;293:435.

111. Fried GM, Ogden WD, Greeley G, et al. Correlation of release and actions of cholecystokinin in dogs before and after vagotomy. Surgery 1983;93:786.

112. Dooley CP, Valenzuela JE. Duodenal volume and osmoreceptors in the stimulation of human pancreatic secretion. Gastroenterology 1984;96:23.

113. Owyang C, May D, Louie DS. Trypsin suppression of pancreatic enzyme secretion. Gastroenterology 1986;91:637.

114. Andrews PLR, Grundy D, Scratcherd T. Vagal afferent discharge from mechanoreceptors in different regions of the ferret stomach. J Physiol (Lond) 1980;298:513

115. Jeanningros R. Vagal unitary responses to intestinal amino acid infusions in the anesthesized cat: A putative signal for protein induced satiety. Physiol Behav 1982;28:9.

116. Jeanningros R. Effect of intestinal amino acid infusions on hypothalamic single unit activity in the anesthetized cat. Brain Res Bull 1983;10:15.

117. Andrews CJH, Andrews WHH. Receptors activated by acid in the duodenal wall of rabbits. Q J Exp Physiol 1971;56:221.

118. Harper AA, Vass CCN. The control of the external secretion of the pancreas in cats. J Physiol (Lond) 1941;99:415.

119. Larsson L, Rehfield JF. Peptidergic and adrenergic innervation of pancreatic ganglia. Scand J Gastroenterol 1979;14:433.

120. Joehl RJ, Kelly GA, Nahrwold DL. Norepinephrine stimulates amylase release from pancreatic acini. J Surg Res 1983;34:543.

121. Kulka RG, Sternlight E. Enzyme secretion in mouse pancreas mediated by adenosine-3'-5'-cyclic phosphate and inhibited by adenosine-3''-phosphate. Proc Natl Acad Sci USA 1968;16:1123.

122. Pearson GT, Singh J, Petersen OH. Adrenergic nervous control of cAMP-mediated amylase secretion in the rat pancreas. Am J Physiol 1984;246:G563.

123. Larsson L, Fahrenkrug J, Holst JJ, et al. Innervation of the pancreas by vasoactive intestinal polypeptide (VIP) immunoreactive nerves. Life Sci 1978;22:773.

124. Holst JJ, Fahrenkrug J, Knuhtsen S, et al. Vasoactive intestinal polypeptide (VIP) in the pig pancreas: Role of VIPergic nerves in control of fluid and bicarbonate secretion. Regul Pept 1984;8:245.

125. Fahrenkrug J, Schaffalitzky de Muckadell OB, Holst JJ, et al. Vasoactive intestinal polypeptide in vagally mediated pancreatic secretion of fluid and HCO₃. Am J Physiol 1979;237:E535.

126. Domschke S, Domschke W, Rosch W, et al. Vasoactive intestinal peptide: A secretin-like partial agonist for pancreatic secretion in man. Gastroenterology 1977;73:478.

127. Inoue K, Kawano T, Shima K, et al. Effect of synthetic chicken vasoactive intestinal peptide on pancreatic blood flow and on exocrine and endocrine secretions of the pancreas in dogs. Dig Dis Sci 1983;28:724.

128. Larsson L. Innervation of the pancreas by substance P, enkephalin, vasoactive intestinal polypeptide and gastrin/CCK immunoreactive nerves. J Histochem Cytochem 1979;27:1283.

129. Moghimzadeh E, Ekman R, Hakanson R, et al. Neuronal gastrin-releasing peptide in the mammalian gut and pancreas. Neuroscience 1983;10:553.

130. Polak JM, Bloom SR. Regulatory peptides—the distribution of two newly discovered peptides: PHI and NPY. Peptides 1984;5(Suppl 1):79.

131. Feurle GE, Reinecke M. Neurotensin interacts with carbachol, secretin and caerulein in the stimulation of the exocrine pancreas of the rat in vitro. Regul Pept 1983;7:137.

132. Carlet F, Polak JM, Bloom SR, et al. Neuropeptide Y (NPY) localization in rat pancreas. J Pathol 1983;141:511.

133. Seifert H, Sawchenko P, Chesnut J, et al. Receptor for calcitonin gene-related peptide: Binding to exocrine pancreas mediates biological actions. Am J Physiol 1985;249:G147.

134. Gardner JD, Jensen RT. Secretagogue receptors on pancreatic acinar cells. In Johnson LR, ed. Physiology of the gastrointestinal tract, ed 2. New York: Raven Press, 1987:1109.

135. Williams JA, Burnham DB, Hootman SR. Cellular regulation of pancreatic secretion. In Forte j, ed. Handbook of physiology—The gastrointestinal system, III. Bethesda: American Physiological Society, 1989:419.

136. Williams JA, Bailey AC, Roach E. Temperature dependence of high affinity CCK receptors binding and internalization in rat pancreatic acini. Am J Physiol 1988;254:G513.

137. Kobilka BK, Kobilka TS, Daniel K, et al. Chimeric α_2, β_2-adrenergic receptors: Delineation of domains involved in effector coupling and ligand binding specificity. Science 1988;240:1310.

138. Gilman AG. G-proteins: Transducers of receptor-generated signals. Annu Rev Biochem 1987;56:617.

139. Neer EJ, Clapham DE. Roles of G-protein subunits in transmembrane signaling. Nature 1988;333:129.

140. Merritt JE, Taylor CW, Rubin RP, Putney JW Jr. Evidence suggesting that a novel guanine nucleotide regulatory protein couples receptors to phospholipase C in exocrine pancreas. Biochem J 1986;236:337.

141. Taylor CW, Merritt JE, Putney JW, et al. Effects of Ca²⁺ on phosphoinositide breakdown in exocrine pancrea. Biochem J 1986;238:765.

142. Rhee SG, Suh P-G, Rye S-H, et al. Studies of inositol phospholipid-specific phospholipase C. Science 1989;244:546.

143. Krupinski J, Coussen F, Bakalyar HA, et al. Adenylcyclase amino acid sequence possible channel-like or transporter-like structure. Science 1989;244:1558.

144. Hootman SR, Williams JA. Stimulus-secretion coupling in the pancreatic acinus. In: Johnson LR, ed. Physiology of the gastrointestinal tract, ed 2. New York: Raven Press, 1987:1129.

145. Orchard JL, Davis JS, Larson RE, et al. Effects of carbachol and pancreozymin (cholecyatokinin-octapeptide) on polyphosphoinositide metabolism in the rat pancreas *in vitro*. Biochem J 1984;217:281.

146. Trimble ER, Bruzzone R, Meehan CJ, Biden TJ. Rapid increases in inositol 1,4,5-trisphosphate, inositol 1,3,4,5-tetrakis phosphate and cytosolic free Ca^{2+} in agonist-stimulated pancreatic acini of the rat. Biochem J 1987;242:289.

147. Merritt JE, Taylor CW, Rubin RP, et al. Isomers of inositol triphosphate in exocrine pancreas. Biochem J 1986;238:825.

148. Matozaki T, Williams JA. Multiple sources of 1,2-diacylglycerol in isolated rat pancreatic acini stimulated by cholecystokinin. J Biol Chem 1989;264:14729.

149. Berridge MJ, Irvine RF. Inositol phosphates and cell signaling. Nature 1989;341:197.

150. Supattapone S, Worley PF, Baraban JM, et al. Solubilization, purification and characterization of an inositol trisphosphate receptor. J Biol Chem 1988;263:1530.

151. Streb H, Irvine RF, Berridge MJ, et al. Release of Ca^{2+} from a nonmitochondrial intracellular store in pancreatic acinar cells by inositol-1,4,5-trisphosphate. Nature 1983;306:67.

152. Schulz I, Thevenod F, Dehlinger-Kremer M. Modulation of intracellular free Ca^{2+} concentration by IP_3-sensitive and IP_3-insensitive nonmitochondrial Ca^{2+} pools. Cell Calcium 1989;10:325.

153. Volpe P, Krause KH, Hasimoto S, et al. "Calciosome," a cytoplasmic organelle: The inositol 1,4,5-trisphosphate-sensitive Ca^{2+} store of nonmuscle cells. Proc Natl Acad Sci USA 1988;85:1091.

154. Muallem S. Calcium transport pathways of pancreatic acinar cells. Annu Rev Physiol 1989;51:83.

155. Grynkiewicz G, Poenie G, Tsien RY. A new generation of Ca^{2+} indicators with greatly improved fluorescence properties. J Biol Chem 1985;260:3440.

156. Ochs DL, Korenbrot JT, Williams JA. Relation between free cytosolic calcium and amylase release by pancreatic acini. Am J Physiol 1985;249:G389.

157. Powers RE, Johnson PC, Houlihan MJ, et al. Intracellular Ca^{2+} levels and amylase secretion in Quin 2-loaded mouse pancreatic acini. Am J Physiol 1985;248:C535.

158. Stuenkel EL, Tsunoda Y, Williams JA. Secretagogue induced calcium mobilization in single pancreatic acinar cells. Biochem Biophys Res Commun 1989;158:863.

159. Muallem S, Pandol SJ, Beeker TG. Modulation of agonist activated calcium influx by extracellular pH in rat pancreatic acini. Am J Physiol 1989;257:G917.

160. Tsunoda Y, Stuenkel EL, Williams JA. Characterization of the sustained [Ca^{2+}] increase in stimulated pancreatic acinar cells and its relation to amylase secretion. Am J Physiol 1990;259:6792.

161. Putney JW, Takemura H, Hughes AR, et al. How do inositol phosphates regulate calcium signaling? FASEB J 1989;3:1899.

162. Yule DI, Gallacher DV. Oscillations of cytosolic calcium in single pancreatic acinar cells stimulated by acetylcholine. FEBS Lett 1988;239:358.

163. Tsunoda Y, Stuenkel EL, Williams JA. Oscillatory mode of calcium signaling in rat pancreatic acinar cells. Am J Physiol 1990;258:C147.

164. Nishizuka Y. The role of protein kinase C in cell surface signal transduction and tumor promotion. Nature 1984;308:693.

165. DePont JJHHM, Fleuren-Jakobs AMM. Synergistic effect of A23187 and phorbol ester on amylase secretion from rabbit pancreatic acini. FEBS Lett 1984;170:64.

166. Burnham DB, Munowitz P, Hootman SR, et al. Regulation of protein phosphorylation in pancreatic acini. Distince effects of Ca^{2+} ionophire A23187 and 12-O-tetradecanoyl-phorbol 13-acetate. Biochem J 1985;235:125.

167. Knight DE, Koh E. Ca^{2+} and cyclic nucleotide dependence of amylase release from isolated rate pancreatic acinar cells rendered permeable by intense electric fields. Cell Calcium 1984;5:401.

168. Kimura T, Imamura K, Eckhardt L, et al. Ca^{2+}-, phorbol ester-, and cAMP-stimulated enzyme secretion from permeabilized rat pancreatic acini. Am J Physiol 1986;250:G698.

169. Kitagawa M, Williams JA, De Lisle RC. Amylase release from streptolysin O permeabilized pancreatic acini. Am J Physiol 1990;259:G157.

170. Gorelick FS, Cohn JA, Freedmaqn SD, et al. Calmodulin-stimulated protein kinase activity from rat pancreas. J Cell Biol 1983;97:1294,

171. Nairn A, Bhagat B, Palfrey HC. Identification of calmodulin-dependent protein kinase III and its major M_r 100,000 substrate in mammalian tissues. Proc Natl Acad Sci USA 1985;82:7939.

172. Burnham DB, Soling H-D, Williams JA. Evaluation of myosin light chain phosphorylation in isolated pancreatic acini. Am J Physiol 1988;254:G130.

173. Miller SG, Kennedy MB. Regulation of brain type II Ca^{2+}/calmodulin-dependent protein kinase by autophosphorylation: A Ca^{2+}-triggered molecular switch. Cell 1986;44:861.

174. Noguchi M, Adachi H, Gardner JD, et al. Calcium-activated phospholipid-dependent protein kinase in pancreatic acinar cells. Am J Physiol 1985;248:G692.

175. Parker PJ, Kour G, Marais RM, et al. Protein kinase C—A family affair. Mol Cell Endocrinol 1989;65:1.

176. Wooten MW, Wrenn RW. Linoleic acid is a potent activator of protein kinase C type III-a isoform in pancreatic acinar cells; its role in amylase secretion. Life Sci 1988;153:67.

177. Machado-De Domenech E, Soling HD. Effects of stimulation of muscarinic and of b-catecholamine receptors on the intracellular distribution of protein kinase C in guinea pig exocrine glands. Biochem J 1987;242:749.

178. Mangeat PH, Chahinian H, Marchis-Mouren GJ. Characterization of the cyclic AMP-dependent protein kinase from rat pancreas, further purification of the catalytic subunit, substrate specificity, effect of the pancreatic heat stable inhibitor. Biochimie 1978;60:777.

179. Jensen RT, Gardner JD. Cyclic nucleotide dependent protein kinase activity in acinar cells from guinea pig pancreas. Gastroenterology 1978;75:806.

180. Jahn R, Soling HD. Phosphorylation of ribosomal protein S6 in response to secretagogues in the guinea pig exocrine pancreas, parotid and lacrimal gland. FEBS Lett 1983;153:71.

181. Freedman SD, Jamieson JD. Hormone-induced protein phosphorylation. I. Relationship between secretagogue action and endogenous protein phosphorylation in intact cells from exocrine pancreas and parotid. J Cell Biol 1982;95:903.

182. Wooten MW, Nel AE, Goldschmidt-Clermont PJ, Galbraith RM, Wrenn RW. Identification of the major endogenous substrate for the phospholipid/Ca^{2+}-dependent protein kinase in pancreatic acini as G_c (vitamin D-binding protein). FEBS Lett 1985;191:97

183. Burnham DB, Sung CK, Munowitz P, Williams JA. Regulation of protein phosphorylation in pancreatic acini by cyclic AMP-mediated secretagogues: Interaction with carbamylcholine. Biochem Biophys Acta 1988;969:33.

184. MacGregor IL, Daveney C, Way L, et al. The effects of acute hyperglycemia on meal stimulated gastric, biliary and pancreatic secretion serum gastrin. Gastroenterology 1976;70:197.

185. DiMagno EP, Go VLW, Summerskill WHJ. Intraluminal and postabsorptive effects of amino acids on pancreatic enzyme secretion. J Lab Clin Med 1973;83:241.

186. Dyck WP, Rudick J, Hoexter B, et al. Influence of glucagon on pancreatic exocrine secretion. Gastroenterology 1969;56:531.

187. Konturek SJ, Tasler V, Obtulowicz, W. Characteristics of inhibition of pancreatic secretion of glucagon. Digestion 1974;10:138.

188. Singer MV, Tiscornia OM, DeOliveiro JPM, et al. Effect of glucagon on canine exocrine pancreatic secretion stimulated by a test meal. Can J Physiol Pharmacol 1978;56:1.

189. Shaw HM, Heath TJ. The effect of glucagon on the formation of pancreatic juice and bile in the rat. Can J Physiol Pharmacol 1973;51:1.

190. Dyck WP, Texter EC, Lasater JM, et al. Influence of glucagon on pancreatic exocrine secretion in man. Gastroenterology 1970;58:532.

191. Müller WA, Faloona GR, Aquilar-Parada E, et al. Abnormal alpha-cell function in diabetes. N Engl J Med 1970;283:109.

192. Dollinger HC, Raptis S, Pfeiffer EF. Effects of somatostatin on exocrine and endocrine function stimulated by intestinal hormones in man. Horm Metab Res 1976;8:74.

193. Ipp E, Dobbs RE, Arimura A, et al. Release of immunoreactive somatostatin from the pancreas in response to glucose, amino acid, pancreozymin-cholestokinin, and tolbutamide. J Clin Invest 1977;60:760.

194. Harper AA. The control of pancreatic secretion. Gut 1972;13:308.
195. Dyck WP. Influence of intrajejunal glucose on pancreatic exocrine function in man. Gastroenterology 1971;60:864.
196. Bataille D, Coudray AM, Carlqvist M, et al. Isolation of glucagon-37 (bioactive enteroglucagon oxyntomodulin) from porcine jejuno-ileum. Isolation of the peptide. FEBS Letter 1982;146:73.
197. Biedzinski TM, Bataille D, Devaux MA, et al. The effect of oxyntomodulin (glucagon-37) and glucagon on exocrine pancreatic secretion in the conscious rat. Peptides 1987;8:967.
198. Hage G, Tiscornia O, Palasciano CT, et al. Inhibition of pancreatic exocrine secretion by intracolonic oleic acid infusion in the dog. Biomedicine 1974;21:263.
199. Laugier R, Sarles H. Action of oleic acid on the exocrine pancreatic secretion of the conscious rat: Evidence for an anticholecystokinin-pancreozymin factor. J Physiol 1977;271:81.
200. Demol P, Sarles H. Action of fatty acids on the exocrine pancreatic secretion of the conscious rats: Further evidence for a protein pancreatic inhibitory factor. J Physiol 1978;275:27.
201. Harrer AA, Hood AJC, Mushens J, et al. Inhibition of external pancreatic secretion by intracolonic and intraileal infusions in the cat. J Physiol 1979;292:445.
202. Owyang C, Green L, Rader DJ. Colonic phase of pancreatic and biliary secretion in man. Gastroenterology 1983;84:470.
203. Harper AA, Hood AJC, Mushens, et al. Pancreastone, an inhibitor of pancreatic secretion in extracts of ileal and colonic mucosa. J Physiol 1979;292:455.
204. El-Salhy MZ, Wilander E, Juntti-Berssren L, et al. The distribution and ontogeny of polypeptide YY (PYY)- and pancreatic polypeptide (PP)-immunoreactive cells in the gastrointestinal tract of rat. Histochemistry 1983;78:53.
205. Lundberg JM, Tatemotto K, Terenius LPM, et al. Localization of peptide YY (PYY) in gastrointestinal endocrine cells and effects on intestinal blood flow and motility. Proc Natl Acad Sci USA 1962;79:44.
206. Adrian TE, Ferri GL, Bacarese-Hamilton AJ, et al. Human distribution and release of PYY, a putative new gut hormone. Gastroenterology 1985;89:1070.
207. Pappas TN, Debas HT, Goto Y, et al. Peptide YY inhibits meal-stimulated pancreatic and gastric secretion. Am J Physiol 1985;248:G118.
208. Larsson LI, Sundler F, Hakanson R, Pancreatic polypeptide—A postulated new hormone: Identification of its cellular storage site by light and electron microscopic immunocytochemistry. Diabetologia 1986;12:211.
209. Schwartz TW. Pancreatic polypeptide: A hormone under vagal control. Gastroenterology 1983;85:1411.
210. Adrian TE, Bloom SR, Hermansen K, et al. Pancreatic polypeptide glucagon and insulin secretion from the isolated perfused canine pancreas. Diabetologia 1978;14:413.
211. Lin TM, Evans DC, Chance RE, et al. Bovine pancreatic peptide: Action on gastric and pancreatic secretion in dogs. Am J Physiol 1977;232:E311.
212. Putnam WS, Liddle RA, Williams JA. Inhibitory regulation of the rat exocrine pancreas by peptide YY and pancreatic polypeptide. Am J Physiol 1989;256:G698.
213. Jung G, Louie DS, Owyang C. Pancreatic polypeptide inhibits pancreatic enzyme secretion via a cholinergic pathway. Am J Physiol 1987;253:G706.
214. Wiley J, Owyang C. Somatostatin inhibits cyclic AMP mediated cholinergic transmission in the myenteric plexus. Am J Physiol 1987;253:G607.
215. Louie DS, Chen HT, Owyang C. Inhibition of exocrine pancreatic secretion by opiates is mediated by suppression of cholinergic transmission: Characterization of receptor subtypes. J Pharmacol Exp Ther 1988;246:132.
216. Herzig KH, Tatemoto K, Owyang C. Pancreastatin inhibits pancreatic enzyme secretion by pre-synaptic modulation of acetylcholine release. Gastroenterology 1988;94:A184.
217. Booth AN, Robbins DJ, Ribelin WE, et al. Effect of raw soybean meal and amino acids on pancreatic hypertrophy in rats. Proc Soc Exp Biol Med 1960;104:681.
218. Lyman RL. The effect of raw soybean meal and trypsin inhibitor diets on the intestinal and pancreatic nitrogen in the rat. J Nutr 1957;62:285.
219. Lyman RL, Lepkovsky S. The effect of raw soybean meal and trypsin inhibitor diets on pancreatic enzyme secretion in the rat. J Nutr 1957;62:265.
220. Louie DS, Liang JP, Owyang C. Characterization of a new CCK antagonist, L364,718: In vitro and in vivo studies. Am J Physiol 1988;255:G261.
221. Slaff J, Jacobson D, Tillman CR, et al. Protease-specific suppression of pancreatic exocrine secretion. Gastroenterology 1984;87:44.
222. Dlugosz J, Folsch UR, Creutzffeldt W. Inhibition of intraduodenal trypsin does not stimulate exocrine pancreatic secretion in man. Digestion 1983;26:197.
223. Hotz J, Ho SB, Go VLW, et al. Short term inhibition of duodenal tryptic activity does not affect human pancreatic, biliary, or gastric function. J Lab Clin Med 1983;101:488.
224. Adler G. Mullenhoff A, Bozkurt T, et al. Effect of a proteinase inhibitor (FOY-305) on pancreatic secretion and plasma CCK in human. Digestion 1986;35:3.
225. Liener IE, Goodale RL, Deshmukh A, et al. Effect of a trypsin inhibitor from soybeans (Bowman-Birk) on the secretory activity of the human pancreas. Gastroenterology 1988;94:419.
226. Isaksson G. Ihse IH. Pain reduction by an oral pancreatic enzyme preparation in chronic pancreatitis. Dig Dis Sci 1983;28:97.
227. Slaff JI, Wolfe MM, Toskes PP. Elevated fasting cholecystokinin level in pancreatic exocrine impairment: Evidence to support feedback regulation. J Lab Clin Med 1985;105:282.
228. DiMagno EP, Hendricks JC, Go VLW, et al. Relationships among canine fasting pancreatic dust pressure and duodenal phase III motor activity—Boldyreff revisited. Dig Dis Sci 1979;24:689.
229. Hoh Z, Takahashi I, Nakaya M, et al. Variation in canine exocrine pancreatic secretory activity during the interdigestive state. Am J Physiol 1981;241:G98.
230. Vantrappen GR, Peeters TL, Janssens J. The secretory component of the interdigestive migrating motor complex in man. Scand J Gastroenterol 1979;14:663.
231. Owyang C, Achem-Karam SR, Vinik AI. Pancreatic polypeptide and intestinal migrating motor complex in humans. Effect of pancreaticobiliary secretion. Gastroenterology 1983;84:10.
232. Keane FB, DiMagno EP, Dozois RR, et al. Relationship among canine interdigestive exocrine pancreatic and biliary flow, duodenal motor activity, plasma pancreatic polypeptide and motilin. Gastroenterology 1980;78:10.
233. Chen MH, Gaffee SN, Magee DF, et al. Cyclic changes of plasma pancreatic polypeptide and pancreatic secretion in fasting dogs. J Physiol (Lond) 1983;341:453.
234. Magee DF, Naruse S. The role of motilin in periodic interdigestive pancreatic secretion in dogs. J Physiol (Lond) 1984;355:441.
235. Lee KY, Shiratori K, Chen YF, et al. Role of motilin on the mechanism of interdigestive pancreatic secretion in dog. Dig Dis Sci 1985;30:980.
236. Sarles H, Dani R, Prezelin G, et al. Cephalic phase of pancreatic secretion in man. Gut 1968;9:214.
237. Novis BM, Bank S, Marks IN. The cephalic phase of pancreatic secretion in man. Scand J Gastroenterol 1971;6:417.
238. Solomon T, Grossman MI. Vagal control of pancreatic exocrine secretion. In: Brooks FP, Evers PW, eds. Nerves and the gut. Thorofare, New Jersey: Charles B. Slack, 1976.
239. Defillipi C, Solomon TE, Valenzuela JE. Pancreatic secretory response to sham feeding in humans. Digestion 1982;23:217.
240. Alphin RS, Lin TM. Effect of feeding and sham feeding on pancreatic secretion of the rat. Am J Physiol 1959;197:260.
241. Anagostideo A, Chadwick, Selden VS, et al. Sham feeding and pancreatic secretion. Evidence for direct vagal stimulation of output. Gastroenterology 1984;87:109.
242. Bergman RN, Miller RE. Direct enhancement of insulin secretion by vagal stimulation of the isolated pancreas. Am J Physiol 1973;225:481.
243. Blair EL, Brown JC, Harper AA, et al. A gastric phase of pancreatic sercretion. J Physiol (Lond) 1966;184:812.
244. Vagne M, Grossman MI. Gastric and pancreatic secretion in response to gastric distension in dogs. Gastroenterology 1969;57:300.

245. White TT, McAlexander RA, Magee DF. The effect of gastric distension on duodenal aspirates in man. Gastroenterology 1963;44:48.

246. White TT, Lundh G, Magee DF. Evidence for the existence of a gastropancreatic reflex. Am J Physiol 1960;198:725.

247. Soares EC, Zaterka S, Walsh J. Acid secretion and serum gastrin at graded intragastric pressures in man. Gastroenterology 1977;72:676.

248. Schiller LR, Walsh JH, Feldman M. Distension induced gastrin release. Effects of luminal acidification and intravenous atropine. Gastroenterology 1980;78:912.

249. Strunz UT, Grossman, MI. Effect of graded increases in intragastric pressure on gastrin release and acid secretion in intact dogs. Gastroenterology 1977;72:1137.

250. Freeman HJ, Kim YS. Digestion and absorption of protein. Annu Rev Med 1978;29:99.

251. Hamosh M, Klaeveman HL, Wolf RO, et al. Pharyngeal lipase and digestion of dietary triglyceride in man. J Clin Invest 1975;55:908.

252. DiMagno EP, Go VLW, Summerskill WHJ. Intraluminal and postabsorptive effects of amino acids on pancreatic enzyme secretion. J Lab Clin Med 1973;82:241.

253. Go VLW, Hofmann AF, Summerskill WHJ. Pancreozymin bioassay in man based on pancreatic enzyme secretion: Potency of specific amino acids and other digestive products. J Clin Invest 1970;45: 1158.

254. Wang CC, Grossman MI. Physiological determination of the release of secretin and pancreozymin from intestine of dogs with transplanted pancreas. Am J Physiol 1951;164:527.

255. Meyer JH, Kelly GA, Spingola LJ, et al. Canine gut receptors mediating pancreatic responses to luminal L-amino acids. Am J Physiol 1976;231:669.

256. Malagelada JR, DiMagno EP, Summerskill WHJ, et al. Regulation

257. of pancreatic and gallbladder functions by intraluminal fatty acids and bile acids in man. J Clin Invest 1976;58:493.

257. Meyer JH. Release of secretin and cholecystokinin. In: Thompson JC, ed. Gastrointestinal hormones. Austin: University of Texas Press, 1975:475.

258. Malagelada JR, Go VLW, DiMagno EP, et al. Interactions between luminal bile acids and digestive products on pacreatic and gallbladder function. J Clin Invest 1973;52:2160.

259. Izzo RS, Brugge WR, Praissman M. Immunoreactive cholecystokinin in human and rat plasma: Correlation of pancreatic secretion in response to CCK. Regul Pept 1984;9:21.

260. Sharma KN, Nasset ES. Electrical activity in mesenteric nerves after perfusion of gut lumen. Am J Physiol 1962;202:725.

261. Singer MV, Solomon TE, Wood J, et al. Latency of pancreatic enzyme response to intraduodenal stimulants. Am J Physiol 1980;238:G23.

262. Mayer EA, Thompson JB, Jehn D, et al. Gastric emptying and sieving of solid food and pancreatic and biliary secretion after solid meals in patients with truncal vagotomy and antrectomy. Gastroenterology 1982;83:184.

263. Demol P, Sarles H. Action of fatty acids on the exocrine pancreatic secretion of the conscious rat: Further evidence for a protein pacreatic inhibitory factor. J Physiol (Lond) 1978;275:27.

264. Holtermuller KH, Malagelada JR, McCall JT, et al. Pancreatic, gallbladder and gastric responses to intraduodenal calcium perfusion in man. Gastroenterology 1976;70:693.

265. Malagelada JR, Holtermuller KH, McCall JT, et al. Pancreatic, gallbladder and intestinal responses to intraluminal magnesium salts in man. Am J Dig Dis 1978;23:481.

266. Inoue K, Fried GM, Wiena I, et al. Effect of divalent cations on gastrointestinal hormone release and exocrine pancreatic secretion in dogs. Am J Physiol 1985;248:G28.

16

Bile Secretion

RICHARD H. MOSELEY

The biliary tract and its contents represent the interface between the disciplines of hepatology and gastroenterology. Bile formation is essential for normal intestinal lipid digestion and absorption, the excretion of lipid-soluble xenobiotics and endogenous toxins, and cholesterol homeostasis, the latter as a result of both bile acid synthesis from cholesterol and biliary cholesterol excretion. Bile may also serve an important immunologic role in the intestine by transporting immunoglobulin A (IgA). Therefore, a discussion of bile formation is not to be considered incongruous with the focus of this text and, instead, may serve to illustrate the somewhat artificial divisions between the two disciplines. Hepatocytes, like other secretory epithelial cells, are polarized cells with functional and structural differences between their basolateral (sinusoidal) and apical (canalicular) surface domains. However, in contrast to current understanding of the mechanisms governing secretion and absorption in the stomach and the intestinal tract, as discussed in the previous chapters, our understanding of the cellular mechanisms behind water and solute transport in the liver was, until recently, relatively limited. This was, in large part, the result of the inability of traditional techniques used to study transport phenomena to define events occurring at the level of the canaliculus. With the advent of techniques to selectively isolate canalicular and sinusoidal plasma membrane vesicles[1-3] and the development of short-term cultured isolated hepatocyte couplets,[4,5] considerable progress has been made in defining these mechanisms. A complete understanding of bile secretion that rivals, for example, the state of knowledge concerning gastric acid secretion has still not been achieved. Yet, in this chapter, the diverse pieces of information that collectively define what is known about this critical hepatobiliary function are provided.

BILE COMPOSITION

Bile is a complex fluid, isosmotic with plasma, composed primarily of water, inorganic electrolytes, and organic solutes, such as bile acids, phospholipids, cholesterol, and the bile pigments (Table 16-1). The relative proportions of the major organic solutes of bile are illustrated in Figure 16-1. The volume of bile excreted after cholecystectomy has been estimated to be between 500 and 600 ml/day.[6]

Bile acids (or bile salts) are the major organic solutes in bile. Bile acids present in bile are derived from two sources: (1) primary bile acids (cholic and chenodeoxycholic acid in humans) are syn-

thesized from cholesterol in the liver; and (2) secondary bile acids (deoxycholic, lithocholic, and ursodeoxycholic acid in humans) are produced from primary bile acids by intestinal bacteria (Fig 16-2). Bile acids consist of two components that determine their physiologic and physicochemical properties: (1) a steroid (cyclopentenophenanthrene) nucleus with its hydroxyl substituents; and (2) an aliphatic side chain. All of the major mammalian primary bile acids contain a 3- and a 7-hydroxyl substituent, which greatly increase water solubility, or hydrophilicity.[7] The terminal carboxylic acid group of the side chain is modified after the synthesis of the primary bile acids, and during the hepatic phase of the enterohepatic cycling of the secondary bile acids, by enzymatic conjugation, by way of a bile acid-coenzyme A intermediate, to glycine or taurine. Conjugation with taurine is the preferred pathway, and intracellular taurine depletion, resulting from decreased endogenous synthesis, poor dietary intake, or decreased hepatic uptake by way of a Na^+-dependent carrier,[8] may alter the proportions of bile acid conjugates in bile and affect bile flow. Conjugation also enhances the hydrophilicity of bile acids (taurine > glycine) as well as the acidic strength of the side chain (lowered pKa), both features decreasing their ability to traverse cell membranes by passive diffusion in their transit down the biliary tract and small intestine.[7] Furthermore, glycine and taurine conjugates of bile acids demonstrate selective resistance to hydrolysis by pancreatic enzymes during small intestinal transit.[9] The net effect of conjugation to glycine or taurine is to permit bile acids to accumulate at an intraluminal concentration in the small intestine high enough to facilitate fat digestion and absorption.

Sulfation and glucuronidation of bile acids are minor metabolic pathways except in cholestatic disorders where urinary elimination of bile acids predominates.[10,11] An exception to this rule is the sulfation of lithocholate, the secondary bile acid formed from bacterial modification of chenodeoxycholate in the intestine.

The presence of hydrophilic (the hydroxyl substituents and the amide linkage on the aliphatic side chain) and lipid-soluble or hydrophobic (the steroid nucleus) regions allows conjugated bile salts to act as amphiphilic molecules that form micelles (or polymolecular aggregates) above a critical micellar concentration.[12] Bile salt micelles can, in turn, solubilize other biologically important amphiphilic solutes, such as cholesterol and phospholipids, to form mixed micelles. This detergentlike property of bile acids is important in stabilizing the physical state of bile and in promoting fat digestion and absorption.[12]

Bile acid synthesis from cholesterol is an example of a negative feedback system, although the nature of the regulation at a molecular and biochemical level is not well understood. Microsomal 7-hydroxylation of cholesterol is thought to be the rate-limiting enzymatic step in bile acid synthesis.[13] Gallstone dissolution therapy with chenodeoxycholate suppresses bile acid synthesis and, therefore, increases plasma cholesterol levels.[14] In contrast, ursodeoxycholate (UDCA) does not suppress bile acid synthesis, and plasma cholesterol levels are unchanged with chronic therapy with this bile acid.[14]

As shown in Table 16-1, the predominant biliary cation is sodium and the concentrations of inorganic electrolytes in bile are similar to plasma concentrations. The inorganic electrolytes are largely responsible for the osmotic activity of bile because the osmotic activity of most of the organic solutes, such as bile acids, is lost by aggregation into mixed micelles.[15]

TABLE 16-1
Composition of Hepatic Bile

COMPONENT	CONCENTRATION (mmol)
Electrolytes	
Na^+	141–165
K^+	2.7–6.7
Cl^-	77–117
HCO_3^-	12–55
Ca^{2+}	2.5–6.4
Mg^{2+}	1.5–3.0
Organic Anions	
Bile acids	3–45
Bilirubin	1–2
Lipids	
Lecithin	140–810 (mg/dl)
Cholesterol	97–320 (mg/dl)
Proteins	2–20 (mg/ml)
Peptides and Amino Acids	
Glutathione	3–5
Glutamate	0.8–2.5
Aspartate	0.4–1.1
Glycine	0.6–2.6

(Data from Boyer JL. Mechanisms of bile secretion and hepatic transport. In: Andreoli TE, Hoffman JF, Fanestil DD, Schultz SG, eds. Physiology of membrane disorders, ed 2. New York: Plenum, 1986:609; obtained from measurements of human, rat, and rabbit bile.)

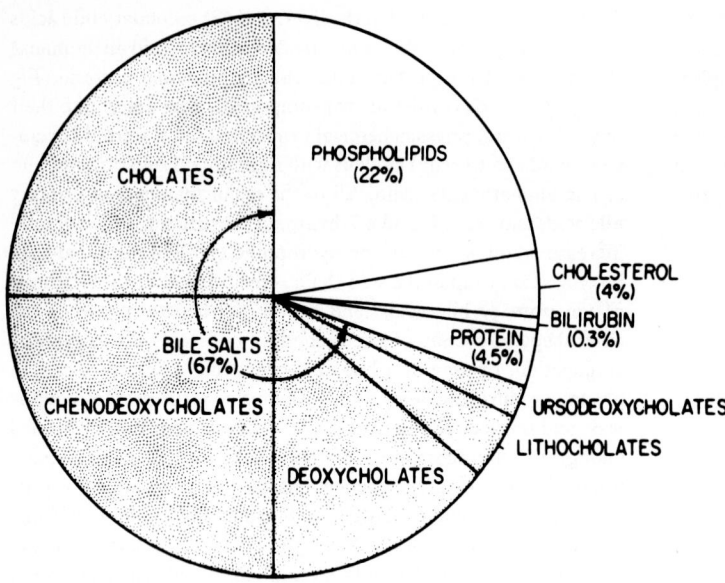

FIGURE 16–1. Typical solute composition (weight percentage) of hepatic and gallbladder bile in healthy humans. (From Carey MC, Cahalane MJ. Enterohepatic circulation. In: Arias IM, Jakoby WB, Popper H, Schachter D, Shafritz DA, eds. The liver: biology and pathobiology, ed 2. New York: Raven Press, 1988:574.)

MORPHOLOGIC CONSIDERATIONS

Critical to an understanding of bile secretion is a familiarity with the anatomy and ultrastructure of the bile secretory apparatus. As illustrated in Figure 16-3, neighboring hepatocytes, typically arranged in single-cell-thick plates, are joined by junctional complexes that serve to demarcate the canalicular space, approximately 1 μm in diameter, from the basolateral, or sinusoidal, domain. Adjacent plates of hepatocytes are separated by the hepatic sinusoids, lined by sinusoidal endothelial cells with several characteristic ultrastructural features.[16] Slender processes extending from the cell body contain pores (fenestrae), arranged in so-called sieve plates, which allow direct contact between plasma and the sinusoidal membrane of the hepatocyte. Thus, unlike other endothelia, sinusoidal endothelial cells lack an underlying basal lamina. This feature is thought to facilitate the transfer of protein-bound solutes from the sinusoid to the space of Disse and, subsequently, to the hepatocyte as well as the excretion of, for example, lipoproteins from the hepatocyte to the sinusoid.

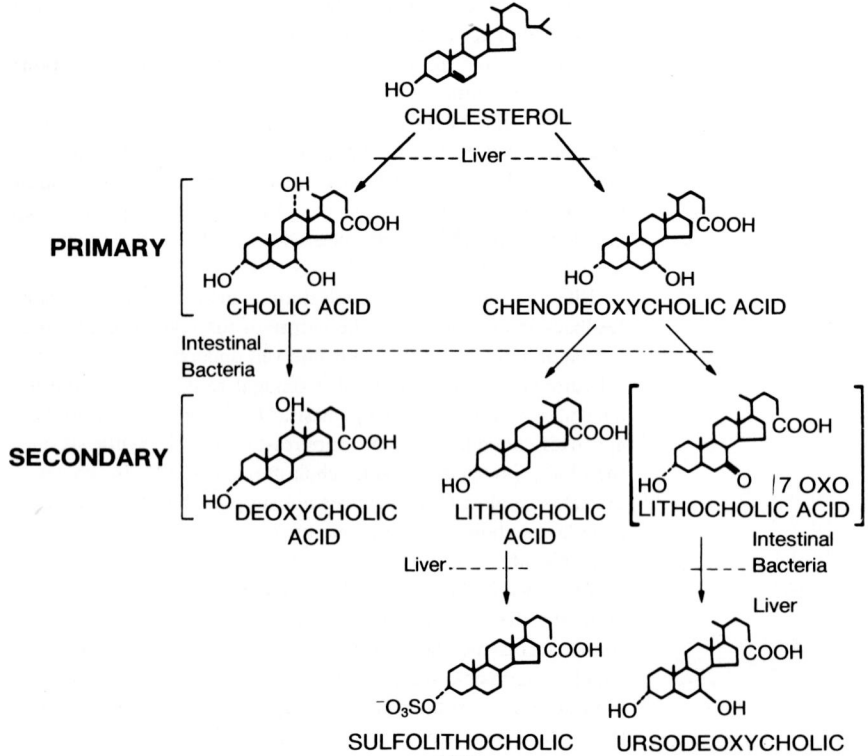

FIGURE 16–2. Major primary and secondary bile acids with sites of synthesis and metabolism. (From Carey MC, Cahalane MJ. Enterohepatic circulation. In: Arias IM, Jakoby WB, Popper H, Schachter D, Shafritz DA, eds. The liver: biology and pathobiology, ed 2. New York: Raven Press, 1988:576.)

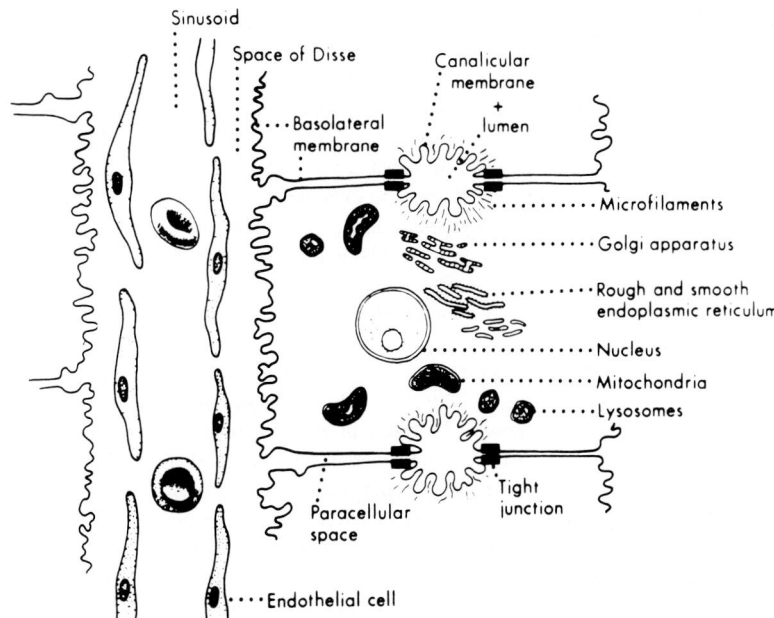

FIGURE 16–3. Structural features of the bile secretory apparatus. (From Schwartz CC. Hepatic metabolism. In: Kelley WN, ed. Textbook of internal medicine. Philadelphia: JB Lippincott, 1989:472.)

As discussed above, differences in the structure and function of the sinusoidal and canalicular membrane define the hepatocyte as a polarized cell. The canalicular membrane is notable for a high sialic acid content and a higher cholesterol:phospholipid and a lower phospholipid:sphingomyelin molar ratio than the sinusoidal domain.[1] As a result of these differences in lipid composition, the canalicular domain has significantly less membrane lipid fluidity than the sinusoidal domain.[17] This lipid composition also confers on the canalicular membrane a relative resistance to the detergent actions of bile acids. Morphologically similar to other transporting epithelia, the surface area of the sinusoidal and canalicular membranes is increased by microvilli. However, the ratio between the surface area of microvilli to effaced canalicular membrane is less than one tenth that observed in the enterocyte brush border.[18] Major alterations in canalicular microvilli occur with intra- and extrahepatic forms of cholestasis, including reduction in the number of microvilli and the development of giant microvilli secondary to edema and bleb formation that occlude the canalicular lumina to varying degrees.[19]

Functionally, the sinusoidal membrane is primarily involved in the bidirectional exchange of solutes, containing uptake mechanisms for amino acids, glucose, and organic anions, such as bile acids, fatty acids, and bilirubin, receptor-mediated endocytotic processes, Na^+,K^+-ATPase and glucagon-stimulatable adenylate cyclase activity, and export processes for albumin, lipoproteins, and clotting factors.[20] In contrast, the predominant function at the canalicular membrane surface is bile secretion, although limited reabsorptive capacity has been demonstrated recently.[21,22] Certain membrane enzymes are selectively localized to the canalicular domain, including alkaline phosphatase, leucine aminopeptidase, and γ-glutamyl transpeptidase.[20]

From adjacent canaliculi, bile enters small terminal bile ductules, the canals of Hering, consisting of fusiform cells in close association with neighboring hepatocytes. These short channels, in turn, traverse the limiting plate to form, successively, larger ductules and intralobular bile ducts, composed of cuboidal epi-

thelial cells. Interlobular bile ducts, ranging in size from 30 to 40 μm, convey bile eventually to the extrahepatic bile duct, the gallbladder (if present), and the duodenum.[18] Intralobular bile ducts are supplied by a peribiliary plexus, derived from the hepatic artery, which subsequently enters the sinusoids by way of portal vein branches.[23,24] This peribiliary plexus may provide a pathway not only for solutes to be extracted from bile and recirculate to hepatocytes but also for solutes, such as ceruloplasmin,[25] to be taken up by bile duct epithelial cells and directly secreted into bile without undergoing hepatocytic processing.

The junctional complexes that join adjacent hepatocytes consist of several discrete structures. The function of the tight junctions (zonulae occludens) as a blood–bile barrier is presented later in this chapter (see section entitled Paracellular Pathway). Generally located distal to the tight junction is the nexus or gap junction. One of the proposed functions for gap junctions is mediation of intercellular communication under physiologic conditions. Gap junctional communication may be regulated by several cytoplasmic factors, including intracellular pH, calcium, and calmodulin.[26] Biochemical studies have shown that isolated rat liver gap junctions contain a major 27-kd nonglycosylated protein that may function as the cell–cell channel.[27,28] Spot and belt desmosomes, involved in cell-to-cell adhesion, are also found in the junctional complex. These structures may serve a bridging function, maintaining contact between hepatocytes during pathologic situations that interfere with the function of gap junctions.[29]

Actin-containing microfilaments are numerous in the pericanalicular cytoplasm where they insert into the canalicular microvilli as well as into the junctional complex to form a pericanalicular web.[30] Several points of evidence support a role of these cytoskeletal elements in bile formation. Coordinated and periodic contractions of canaliculi, responsive to intracellular Ca^{++} and taurocholate, have been observed in isolated hepatocytes.[31–33] Inhibitors of calmodulin, such as trifluoperazine, and cytochalasin B and phalloidin, inhibitors of actin microfilaments, decrease contractile activity.[32–34] These latter two agents decrease bile flow in experimental animals,[35,36] cytochalasin exhibiting an immediate effect and phalloidin exerting a delayed effect that parallels an increase in the thickness of the pericanalicular microfilament network.[37] Phalloidin-induced alterations in microfilament function also increase junctional complex permeability.[38] The 17α-alkyated anabolic steroid, norethandrolone, associated with drug-induced cholestasis in humans,[39] induces changes in experimental animals similar to those observed with cytochalasin B,[40] and increases in number and density of hepatocyte microfilaments have been observed in human cholestasis.[41] Thus, microfilaments may play a role in overall bile formation, and dysfunction of these cytoskeletal elements may lead to cholestasis.

A variety of vesicular transport processes in cells are dependent on the integrity of microtubules. The role of these noncontractile cytoskeletal elements, composed of tubulin, in bile formation has been less well studied, in part because they are less abundant than microfilaments. Vesicular transport is an energy-dependent process mediated, in part, by the microtubule-associated ATPase, kinesin,[42] present in abundance in hepatocytes. Microtubule inhibitors, such as colchicine and vinblastine, have been shown to inhibit bile acid-induced choleresis without affecting basal bile flow.[37] Biliary lipid and IgA secretion also appear to be affected by microtubule dysfunction.[43,44] It should be recognized, however, that several of these agents, including cytochalasin B, colchicine, and phalloidin, have effects on the plasma membrane as well, and the relevance of these various experimental findings to bile formation and cholestasis in humans remains to be established.

The Golgi complex is also preferentially located at the canalicular pole of the hepatocyte. As discussed below, several points of evidence support a role for intact Golgi function in intracellular processes involved in bile secretion. In addition, bile acids have been shown to interact with another intracellular organelle, the smooth endoplasmic reticulum. Monohydroxylated bile acids, such as lithocholate and its conjugates, appear to increase cytosolic calcium concentrations by stimulating the release of calcium from intracellular stores in the smooth endoplasmic reticulum.[45–47] Permeabilization of this intracellular compartment may play a role in the inhibition of bile secretion seen with these hepatotoxic bile acids.

PHYSIOLOGIC CONSIDERATIONS

Early work in hepatobiliary physiology established the sensitivity of bile flow to metabolic inhibitors and temperature changes and the significantly higher bile secretory pressure compared with sinusoidal perfusion pressure.[48] Thus, in contrast to the passive, hydrostatic forces governing glomerular filtration by the kidney, bile formation by hepatocytes is considered to be an osmotic process involving the active secretion of inorganic and organic solutes into the canalicular lumen, followed by passive water movement. In this important respect, hepatic bile secretion can be characterized by the same processes found in more conventional secretory epithelia.

Canalicular bile formation is classically measured using metabolically inert solutes, such as erythritol and mannitol, which are assumed to enter bile passively only at the level of the canaliculus and not undergo modification by biliary ductular cells. Using these markers, canalicular bile formation has been traditionally divided

into two components (Fig 16-4): (1) bile acid–dependent bile flow (BADBF), defined as the slope of the line relating canalicular bile flow to bile salt excretion; and (2) bile acid–independent bile flow (BAIBF), attributed to the active secretion of inorganic electrolytes and other solutes and defined as the extrapolated *y*-intercept of this line. Experimental evidence suggests that in some, if not all, species the relationship between bile flow and bile salt output is curvilinear and cannot be represented by the single regression line illustrated in Figure 16-4.[49] Whether BAIBF is only overestimated or cannot be experimentally measured at all remains to be established. Although these two components are discussed separately in the following sections, BAIBF and BADBF should be viewed as interrelated rather than independent components of bile flow.

Bile Acid–Dependent Bile Formation

There are two hypotheses to explain the apparent linear relation between bile acid secretion rates and bile flow. Because bile acids are in a micellar form in bile, bile acids or, more accurately, their accompanying counterions, may provide an osmotic driving force for water and electrolyte movement.[50] In support of this hypothesis is the observation that bile acids that either do not form micelles or have a high critical micellar concentration have a greater choleretic action than physiologic bile acids[51] and the finding that other osmotically active organic anions in bile have a choleretic effect proportional to the osmotic load.[52] However, the osmotic activity of a bile acid does not always correlate with its choleretic properties. Another way in which bile acids may affect bile flow is by alterations in the transport of other solutes into bile. In support of this mechanism are observations that UDCA produces a hypercholeresis associated with a marked increase in biliary bicarbonate secretion[53] and that dehydrocholate can induce a choleresis before its appearance in bile.[54]

Bile acids have also been shown to influence the biliary secretion of other organic anions, such as bilirubin.[55] This effect was previously thought to be the result of sequestration of the organic anion into mixed micelles formed by bile acids, creating a "micellar sink" that would reduce the effective concentration of organic

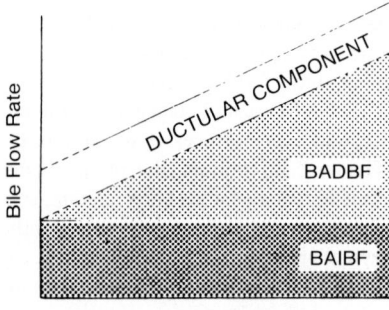

FIGURE 16–4. Schematic representation of the components of bile flow. *BADBF*, bile acid–dependent bile flow; *BAIBF*, bile acid–independent bile flow. (From Moseley RH. Mechanisms of bile formation in cholestasis: Clinical significance of recent experimental work. Am J Gastrol 1986;81: 731. Copyright by American College of Gastroenterology.)

anions in canalicular bile as well as decrease their reabsorption and, thereby, enhance their net excretion.[56] However, more recent data suggest that bile acids may interact, in some manner, with the canalicular transport processes for these organic anions.[57]

SINUSOIDAL BILE ACID TRANSPORT

It has been well established that sinusoidal uptake of conjugated bile acids, such as taurocholate, is primarily mediated by a secondary active transport process driven by the inwardly directed Na^+ gradient maintained by Na^+,K^+-ATPase activity (see Frimmer and Ziegler[58] for review). Determinants for the efficient Na^+-dependent cotransport of bile acids at the sinusoidal surface include position and number of hydroxyl groups on the steroid moiety as well as length and charge of the side chain.[59-61] Whereas albumin enhances hepatic bile acid uptake,[62,63] the exact mechanism for this "albumin effect" remains undefined, although a conformational change in albumin due to interaction with the hepatocyte membrane[64] appears to be more likely than a specific membrane albumin receptor.[64,65] The sinusoidal bile acid carrier exhibits a broad substrate specificity that includes electroneutral steroids (such as ouabain and progesterone), cyclic oligopeptides (such as phalloidin, somatostatin analogues, and cyclosporine) and a wide variety of xenobiotics.[58] Hepatic uptake of amatoxins, the toxic bicyclic octapeptides of toadstools of the genus *Amanita,* the cause of most accidental mushroom poisonings, is also mediated by the sinusoidal bile acid carrier.[66] The uptake of unconjugated bile acids appears to be mediated by a Na^+-independent process involving nonionic diffusion,[61] although a hydroxyl/bile acid exchange has been proposed as a mechanism for the Na^+-independent uptake of cholate.[67]

Several studies have been performed to identify the sinusoidal bile salt transport system using photoaffinity labeling techniques, and at least two polypeptides with apparent molecular weights of 54,000 and 48,000 may be involved in bile salt uptake.[68-70] Recent evidence suggests that the 54-kd protein may mediate Na^+-independent bile acid transport,[71] whereas the 48-kd protein is the Na^+-dependent bile acid symport.[72]

Serum bile acids are frequently elevated in patients with cirrhosis. Whether this is the result of hemodynamic alterations and the reduced liver cell mass observed in cirrhosis (the "intact cell hypothesis"[73]) or dysfunction at the level of the individual hepatocyte (the "sick cell hypothesis"[74]) has been examined in an experimental model of cirrhosis. Bile acid uptake was, in fact, decreased,[75] although this was most likely the result of impaired Na^+,K^+-ATPase activity, the driving force for bile acid uptake, rather than an abnormality of the sinusoidal bile acid transport protein.[76]

INTRACELLULAR EVENTS

The mechanism for intracellular transport of bile acids from sinusoidal to canalicular poles of hepatocytes is not well understood. Intracellular binding of bile acids has been proposed as both a mechanism for hepatic transport and a protective mechanism against potential toxic effects of free bile acids. Two unrelated families of cytosolic proteins with high affinity for bile acids have been identified, characterized, and purified, namely ligandins (45-

to 50-kd dimers)[77] and Y' proteins (33- to 36-kd monomers).[78,79] Ligandins are glutathione S-transferases that bind bile acids and bilirubin at a nonsubstrate, high affinity site.[80] Recently, Y' bile acid binders have been shown to possess 3α-hydroxysteroid dehydrogenase activity.[81] Because the enzyme can bind bile acids at the active site without biotransformation, the enzyme may serve a dual role: reduction of 3-oxo-bile acids and cytosolic bile acid binding under normal redox conditions.[81]

On the basis of morphometric studies of endoplasmic reticulum, Golgi apparatus, and the pericanalicular cytoplasm after bile acid–induced choleresis, a vectorial vesicular transport of bile acids across the hepatocyte has been proposed.[82,83] Additional support for this view is derived from autoradiographic and immunoperoxidase studies that demonstrate a preferential localization of bile acids[84] and bile acid analogues[85,86] in Golgi and smooth endoplasmic reticulum. High affinity binding sites for taurocholate have been identified in Golgi,[87] and taurocholate transport by Golgi vesicles has been demonstrated to have characteristics, such as Na^+-independence, that distinguish it from bile acid uptake at the sinusoidal membrane.[88] Recently, intracellular cotransport of taurocholate and bilirubin glucuronides from the endoplasmic reticulum to the canalicular membrane by way of a microtubule-dependent process was demonstrated.[89] Despite all these observations, morphologic evidence of exocytosis of bile acid–loaded vesicles at the canalicular membrane has not, to date, been reported. Nevertheless, the kinetics of biliary secretion of taurocholate[90] are more consistent with vesicular transport than a process that depends on random diffusion through the hepatocyte cytosol.

CANALICULAR BILE ACID TRANSPORT

Canalicular excretion represents the rate-limiting step in hepatic transport of bile acids.[91] The maximum secretory rate of bile acids, however, does not conform to the classic definition of a transport maximum (T_m), because experimental administration of bile acids above this maximum results in decreased bile acid secretion.[92] This characteristic of bile acid transport is referred to as the secretory rate maximum (SR_m).[92] The cause for this decline is unclear, although depletion of canalicular membrane phospholipid and a resulting increase in the cholesterol:phospholipid ratio, a critical determinant of membrane lipid fluidity, may be involved.[93]

Studies with isolated canalicular membrane vesicles have demonstrated that the excretion of taurocholate is mediated by a saturable transport process driven, in part, by the physiologic intracellular negative membrane potential.[94,95] This canalicular bile acid transport system preferentially transports trihydroxylated and conjugated dihydroxylated bile acids, but not oxo bile acids.[96] Because conjugation confers a higher negative charge, this preference for conjugated species favors the electrogenic driving forces and is consistent with the observation that negatively charged bile acids are more efficiently secreted by the intact liver than uncharged or positively charged bile acid derivatives.[59] In addition, the canalicular bile acid transport system may also share substrate specificity with other amphipathic solutes, such as sulfobromophthalein (BSP),[96] although the hepatic secretory mechanism for bile acids is distinct from that for other organic anions.[97] Further studies, using a photoreactive taurocholate analogue, indicate that canalicular bile salt excretion is mediated by a 100-kd glycoprotein,[98,99] with a thiol group present at or near the active site.[100] Preliminary

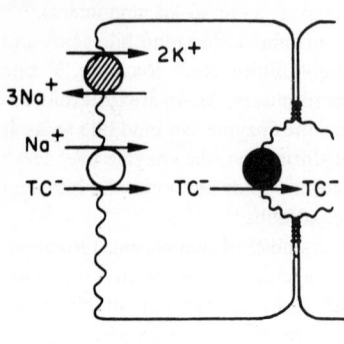

NORMAL LIVER   OBSTRUCTIVE CHOLESTASIS

FIGURE 16–5. Schematic representation of the effect of extrahepatic obstruction on hepatocyte bile acid transport processes. For discussion, see text. *TC⁻*, taurocholate. (From Fricker G, Landmann L, Meier PJ. Extrahepatic obstructive cholestasis reverses the bile salt secretory polarity of rat hepatocytes. J Clin Invest 1989;84:876, by copyright permission of the American Society for Clinical Investigation.)

findings suggest that this canalicular-specific protein is ontogenically regulated, perhaps accounting for the decreased rates of bile flow and bile salt secretion observed during the neonatal period.[101]

Thus, canalicular secretion of anionic bile acids may be primarily mediated by passive facilitated diffusion down an energetically favorable electrochemical gradient. However, alternative mechanisms may exist for carrier-mediated secretion at the canalicular membrane. Using an animal model with an autosomal recessive defect in the hepatic transport of bilirubin, separate transport systems for the biliary secretion of sulfated and unsulfated bile acids have been recently identified.[102] In addition, reversal of this polarity for bile salt secretion may also occur, as has been recently demonstrated in an experimental model of extrahepatic cholestasis.[103] In this study, redistribution of functionally active canalicular bile salt transport protein to the sinusoidal membrane surface was observed after bile duct ligation.[103] As illustrated in Figure 16-5, bile acid efflux mediated by the membrane potential-sensitive canalicular bile salt transport protein located on the sinusoidal membrane might prevent hepatocytes in cholestatic disorders from accumulating toxic concentrations of bile

acids. Delayed reestablishment of normal bile secretory polarity could well provide an explanation for the high levels of serum bile acids temporarily observed even after relief of extrahepatic biliary obstruction.[104]

ONTOGENY OF BILE ACID TRANSPORT

Immaturity of hepatic excretory function exists during infancy and may account, in part, for the increased susceptibility to total parenteral nutrition (TPN)-induced and sepsis-associated cholestatic liver disease.[105,106] A deficient number or slower translocation rate of the specific carrier that mediates sinusoidal Na^+-bile acid cotransport during postnatal development limits bile acid uptake.[107,108] The ability of hepatocytes to take up and conjugate bile acids parallels a rapid increase in cytosolic bile acid binding proteins.[109] Preliminary studies suggest that canalicular transport of bile acids is, also, not fully developed at birth.[110]

Bile Acid–Independent Bile Formation

ELECTROLYTE TRANSPORT

In contrast to information regarding BADBF, there is less known concerning the hepatocellular mechanisms underlying BAIBF. Inhibition of Na^+,K^+-ATPase activity does not appear to have a significant effect on BAIBF[111,112] and indirect evidence points to a primary role for bicarbonate transport.[111–113] In other epithelia, such as the pancreas, bicarbonate transport has been attributed to $Na^+:H^+$ exchange (or antiport) activity.[114] After the identification and characterization of sinusoidal $Na^+:H^+$ exchange[115,116] and canalicular $Cl^-:HCO_3^-$ exchange,[117] a model has been proposed (Fig 16-6) in which these two transport processes are functionally coupled, by way of cytosolic carbonic anhydrase, to generate net biliary bicarbonate secretion.[118,119] Support for this model has come primarily from studies examining the effects of certain cholestatic and choleretic agents on membrane transport. Thus, ethinyl estradiol, which causes a diminution in BAIBF,[120] has also been

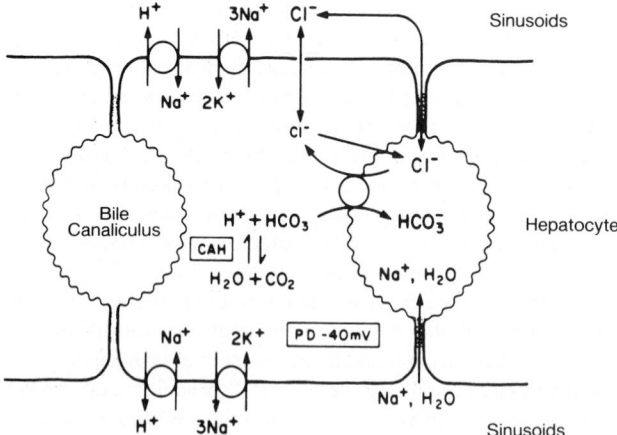

FIGURE 16–6. Model of bile acid–independent bile formation. For discussion of the model, see text. *PD* = potential difference with respect to the extracellular space; *CAH*, cytosolic carbonic anhydrase. (From Moseley RH, Meier PJ, Aronson PS, Boyer JL. Na-H exchange in rat liver basolateral but not canalicular plasma membrane vesicles. Am J Physiol 1986;250: G35.)

shown to inhibit Na^+:H^+ exchange activity,[121] whereas UDCA, which results in a bicarbonate-rich choleresis,[53,122] stimulates Na^+:H^+ exchange activity.[123] In addition, inhibitors of Na^+:H^+ exchange activity, such as amiloride, and acetazolamide, an inhibitor of carbonic anhydrase, produce a concentration-dependent inhibition of UDCA-stimulated bile flow and biliary bicarbonate output.[124-126]

However, inorganic electrolytes may not provide a sufficient driving force for BAIBF, because their biliary secretion depends primarily on passive diffusion and solvent drag.[127] This has led to the alternative suggestion that organic anions, at present unidentified, may provide a major driving force for canalicular BAIBF.[127,128] The tripeptide, glutathione (γ-L-glutamyl-L-cysteinylglycine; GSH) may fulfill this role. GSH is present in bile in high concentrations (see Table 16-1), and, as a result of intrabiliary catabolism of GSH by γ-glutamyl transpeptidase located on the luminal membranes of bile ductule cells as well as the bile canalicular membrane,[129] the concentration of this solute in the canalicular lumen may be substantially higher than that measured in excreted bile.[130] At concentrations that exceed free (nonmicelle associated) bile acids and bile pigments, GSH may generate a potent osmotic driving force for canalicular bile formation. Because biliary secretion of GSH is a carrier-mediated process,[131] the requirement that the solute providing the driving force for BAIBF not be governed by passive diffusion or solvent drag is met. Additional indirect evidence supports a role for GSH in BAIBF, including the strong correlation of GSH excretion with drug-induced changes in BAIBF[132] and with ontogenic changes in bile formation.[133] Recent studies suggest, however, that in addition to GSH, other unidentified solutes may also contribute to BAIBF.[134]

CHOLEHEPATIC SHUNT PATHWAY

The mechanism by which UDCA produces a hypercholeresis is of importance in that similar mechanisms may govern basal bile formation or bile formation in response to physiologic bile acids. Alternative models have been proposed to explain the bicarbonate-rich hypercholeresis observed with UDCA. Unconjugated bile acids secreted into canalicular bile may be protonated by a hydrogen ion generated by carbonic anhydrase activity in biliary ductular cells.[135] Passive absorption of the bile acid by the choleangiocyte into the periductular capillary plexus results in presentation of the bile acid at the sinusoidal membrane for another intrahepatic cycle. The primary difference between this cholehepatic shunt pathway and stimulation of bile formation at the level of the hepatocyte is in the origin of biliary bicarbonate. In the former, biliary bicarbonate arises from carbonic anhydrase activity present in biliary ductular cells, whereas in the latter, the source of biliary bicarbonate is the hepatocyte. Observations consistent with this hypothesis include the finding that inhibition of the UDCA-stimulated increase in bile flow and biliary HCO_3^- secretion is associated with a decrease in the percentage of unconjugated UDCA in bile, replaced by UDCA glucuronides.[136] Furthermore, recent studies using isolated hepatocyte couplets failed to demonstrate a hypercholeresis with UDCA when compared with taurocholate, suggesting that the effect of UDCA involves processes more distal to the hepatocyte secretory unit, such as the bile ductules or ducts.[137]

Paracellular Pathway

Tight junctions (zonulae occludens) serve as a barrier to unrestricted movement of solutes from the space of Disse to the canalicular lumen. With freeze-fracture electron microscopy, the tight junction appears as a set of continuous, anastomosing intramembrane strands or fibrils in the outwardly facing cytoplasmic leaflet[138] (Fig 16-7). The number of freeze-fracture strands lying in parallel at the zonula occludens (ZO) correlate with the transepithelial electrical resistance.[139] Compared with other epithelia, hepatic tight junctions are composed of an intermediate number of strands,[140] although the number of strands may be highly variable within the same hepatocyte tight junction.[141] This barrier for entry into bile appears to possess a net negative charge, because the paracellular movement of negatively charged solutes from blood to bile is impaired.[142] In contrast, greater than 90% of the sodium present in bile may result from flux across this selective permeability barrier.[127] Whether negatively charged species, such as conjugated bile acids, secreted across the canalicular membrane are retained in the canalicular lumen by this property remains a matter of speculation. However, support for this hypothesis comes from a study demonstrating regurgitation of negatively charged solutes from bile into blood across this barrier in an experimental model of cholestasis.[143]

Evidence that the paracellular pathway is important in normal bile formation largely rests with studies that demonstrate alterations in tight junction permeability in experimental models of in-

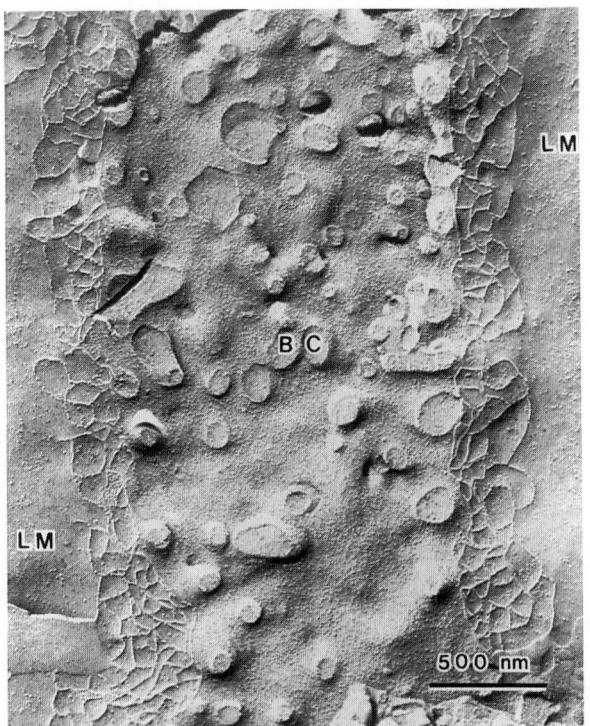

FIGURE 16-7. Freeze-fracture replica of the tight junction of the hepatocyte. Magnification × 23,325. *BC*, bile canaliculus; *TJ*, tight junction; *LM*, lateral cell membrane. (From Boyer JL. Tight junctions in normal and cholestatic liver: does the paracellular pathway have functional significance. Hepatology 1983;3:615.)

trahepatic cholestasis. Examples include cholestasis produced by hypocalcemic perfusions,[144] and by the administration of ethinyl estradiol,[145] bile acids,[146] and microfilament toxins.[36] Physiologic regulation of tight junction permeability by hormones that act by way of alterations in membrane phosphoinositides and intracellular calcium has been recently demonstrated, although these permeability changes most likely play only a minor role in overall bile formation in the normal animal.[147]

Extrahepatic cholestasis may also alter tight junction permeability. The morphologic features of tight junctions observed in patients with extrahepatic bile duct obstruction closely resemble those seen after bile duct ligation in experimental animals,[148,149] where functional disruption of the permeability barrier, reflected by the penetration of large proteins, such as horseradish peroxidase, into bile, has been demonstrated.[150] Of note, a 220-kd protein, called ZO-1, associated with the cytoplasmic surface of the tight junction has been identified in hepatocytes and other epithelia.[151] Although the function of ZO-1 in the tight junction remains unknown, a role in the assembly or organization of the zonula occludens is suggested by studies demonstrating that bile duct ligation results in alterations in the immunostaining pattern of ZO-1 at the tight junction.[152] Given the seemingly ubiquitous nature of this structural component of the tight junction, cholestatic liver injury may also be the reflection of similar changes in tight junction permeability in biliary epithelial cells, although, to date, this issue has not been explored.

Bilirubin Transport

The steps involved in the transhepatocytic movement of bilirubin, another major organic solute in bile, are discussed in detail in Chapter 41. It is important to recognize, however, that hyperbilirubinemia, although frequently encountered in cholestasis, can result from a selective defect in the hepatic handling of bilirubin.

Biliary Excretion of Drugs

Bile secretion provides an excretory pathway for organic lipophilic drugs, because these solutes are poorly filtered at the glomerulus

and minimally secreted by the renal tubule.[153] Furthermore, many of these lipid-soluble agents first undergo biotransformation to more water-soluble solutes by the hepatic mixed function oxidase system.[153] A specific example of a biliary excretory mechanism for drugs that has received considerable attention is the multidrug transport protein known as P-glycoprotein or P170, a 170-kd protein encoded by the MDR1 gene.[154] Originally described in tumor-derived tissue culture systems resistant to cytotoxic hydrophobic agents, such as vinblastine, vincristine, and daunomycin, this ATP-dependent drug efflux system has been localized to the canalicular membrane and the apical surface of biliary epithelial cells lining small biliary ductules.[155] This selective localization suggests that this membrane transport protein may serve as a pathway for the detoxification of physiologic metabolites and chemotherapeutic agents. Preliminary studies demonstrate that this canalicular membrane protein preferentially transports weakly charged 400- to 900-d amphipaths, but does not mediate bile acid efflux into the canalicular lumen.[156] In addition, bile duct ligation results in loss of the protein from the canalicular membrane, possibly rendering hepatocytes more susceptible to cell injury and death.[156]

Biliary Lipid Secretion

The major functions of bile acids within the biliary tract are to promote endogenous lipid secretion and to stabilize the physicochemical state of bile.[12] Biliary output of nonesterified cholesterol and phosphatidylcholine (lecithin), the two major lipids in bile, has been shown to be curvilinearly related to bile acid output.[157] As illustrated in Figure 16-8, lecithin secretion exceeds cholesterol secretion. The fatty acid composition of biliary lecithin (predominantly palmitoyl-linoleyl and -oleyl lecithins) distinguishes it from other cellular sources of lecithin.[158] Lecithin is minimally soluble in aqueous solutions, and cholesterol is essentially insoluble. It was classically held that biliary cholesterol solubility was maintained by association with bile salt–lecithin mixed micelles. However, at low bile salt secretion rates, such as during fasting, the concentration of cholesterol in bile approaches maximum metastable cholesterol solubility, and studies suggest that cholesterol is transported, instead, as a nonmicelle (phospholipid) vesicle.[159] It has been suggested that these phospholipid vesicles are the pri-

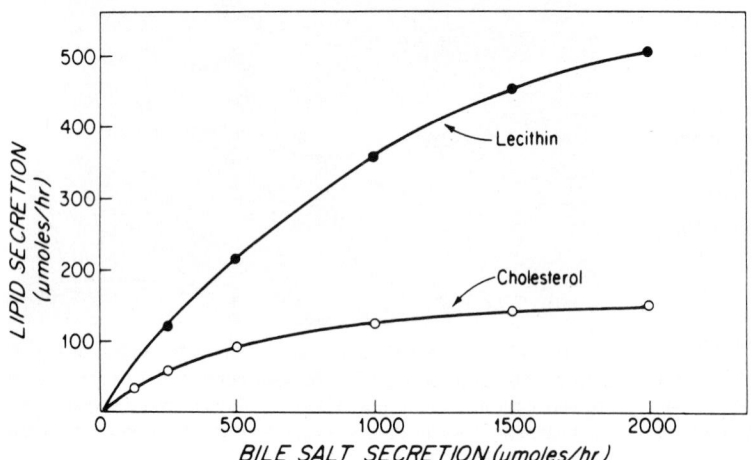

FIGURE 16–8. Influence of bile salt excretion rates on lecithin and cholesterol secretion rates. (From Carey MC, Cahalane MJ. Enterohepatic circulation. In: Arias IM, Jakoby WB, Popper H, Schachter D, Shafritz DA, eds. The liver: biology and pathobiology, ed 2. New York: Raven Press, 1988:599.)

mary form of canalicular cholesterol secretion.[159,160] The mechanism(s) of biliary lipid secretion and the coupling to bile acid excretion remain largely speculative, although recent evidence demonstrating a dependence on microtubule integrity is consistent with a intracellular vesicular pathway for micelle-forming bile salts and associated phospholipid and cholesterol.[161]

Although the mechanisms are poorly understood, the initiating event in the pathogenesis of cholesterol cholelithiasis may involve disruption of the coupling of biliary cholesterol excretion to simultaneous secretion of phospholipid and bile acids. Only 20% of biliary cholesterol in humans appears to be newly synthesized, suggesting that cholesterol excretion into bile is largely independent of cholesterol synthesis.[162] However, in obesity, increased biliary secretion is linked to increased whole body cholesterol synthesis, although it is unclear whether the liver or some extrahepatic site is the origin of the additional newly synthesized cholesterol or, if it is an extrahepatic source, how such cholesterol is ultimately secreted into bile.[163] Recent evidence suggests that the activity of acyl coenzyme A: cholesterol acyltransferase (ACAT), which catalyzes the esterification of cholesterol, may regulate biliary cholesterol secretion by controlling the availability of "metabolically active" free (nonesterified) cholesterol for transport into bile.[163,164] Age has been positively correlated with cholesterol secretion rate and negatively correlated with bile acid synthesis, perhaps offering an explanation for age as a risk factor for cholesterol gallstone formation.[165] Although the mechanism is equally unclear, increased biliary lipid secretion has been demonstrated in patients with celiac sprue.[166] Conversely, decreased biliary secretion of cholesterol, phospholipids, and bile acids occurs in advanced alcoholic cirrhosis and chronic cholestatic syndromes, such as primary biliary cirrhosis.[167,168] Because of a disproportionate decrease in biliary cholesterol secretion in alcoholic cirrhosis, bile is relatively unsaturated with cholesterol[169] and the incidence of cholesterol gallstones, in contrast to pigment gallstones, is low.[170] On the other hand, cholesterol gallstones occur frequently in chronic cholestatic disorders.[170]

Biliary Protein Secretion

In humans, biliary protein concentrations of between 0.02 and 5.3 g liter^{-1} have been reported in hepatic bile, and up to 5.5 g liter^{-1} in gallbladder bile, thus accounting for less than 5% of total biliary solids.[171] Plasma proteins, primarily albumin; hepatocellular enzymes, derived from the outer leaflet of the canalicular membrane and lysosomes; and several proteins peculiar to bile have been identified in bile. In contrast to biliary lipid secretion, the rate of bile acid excretion has no effect on net biliary protein secretion. Simple diffusion by way of the paracellular pathway may account for the presence in bile of certain proteins, such as carcinoembryonic antigen and α_1-acid glycoprotein.[172,173] Alternative mechanisms involving fluid phase and receptor-mediated endocytosis are responsible for transhepatocytic movement of proteins into bile either directly (e.g., polymeric IgA[174]), or indirectly, after interaction with the Golgi complex or its associated system of lysosomes and smooth endoplasmic reticulum (e.g., apolipoproteins[175]). A transepithelial route across bile duct epithelium for ceruloplasmin has been suggested and may account for the transfer of proteins previously thought to reach bile by way of the paracellular route.[25] Furthermore, biliary secretion of IgA in humans may be mediated by biliary ductular cells rather than hepatocytes.[176]

The functional significance of biliary proteins remains largely a matter for speculation. High biliary concentrations of secretory IgA specifically support an immunologic role for this protein. The osmotic activity of biliary proteins has been proposed as a driving force for BAIBF,[177] and a role for biliary proteins in the pathogenesis of cholelithiasis merits serious consideration. Defects in the exocytotic discharge of lysosomal enzymes and contents into bile may be involved, in some manner, in the pathogenesis of hepatic overload states, such as hemochromatosis and Wilson's disease. Apolipoproteins present in bile may play a specific role in biliary lipid secretion.[175]

Acinar Heterogeneity

Up to this point, this discussion has largely ignored the acinar concept of hepatic structure and function as proposed by Rappaport,[178] in which the metabolic and transport processes of a given hepatocyte are determined by the location of the hepatocyte within the hepatic acinus, arbitrarily divided into three zones (Fig 16-9). Zone 1 hepatocytes are located around the terminal portal venule and are exposed to the highest solute concentrations; zone 2 hepatocytes occupy a region intermediate to that of zones 1 and 3; and zone 3 hepatocytes surround the terminal hepatic venule. According to the acinar model, bile flows from pericentral cells toward the interlobular portal tracts. Morphologic and physiologic studies indicate functional differences between acinar zones in the contribution to bile flow. Bile canalicular diameter is smaller in pericentral than in periportal cells and preferentially increases during bile acid-induced choleresis.[179] The Golgi complex and associated cytosol comprise approximately 5% of periportal he-

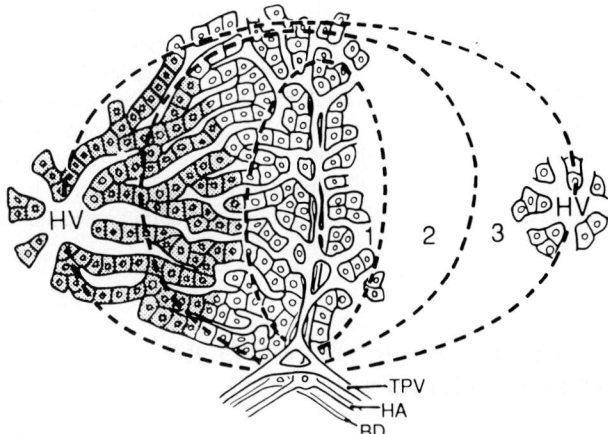

FIGURE 16-9. The hepatic acinus. The acinar axis is formed by the terminal branch of the portal vein (*TPV*), hepatic artery (*HA*), and bile ductule (*BD*). Blood enters the sinusoids in zone 1 and flows sequentially through zone 2 and zone 3, where it exits the acinus by way of the terminal branch of the hepatic vein (*HV*). (From Traber PG, Chianale J, Gumucio JJ. Physiologic significance and regulation of hepatocellular heterogeneity. Gastroenterology 1988;95:1131.)

patocytes but only 2% of pericentral hepatocytes.[82] A decreasing periportal to pericentral concentration gradient for bile acid uptake has been established within the hepatic acinus suggesting that, under physiologic conditions, zone 1 hepatocytes are primarily involved in bile salt transport.[180,181] However, zone 3 hepatocytes are also capable of transporting bile acids.[181] Therefore, during periods of increased bile acid load, distal hepatocytes may be progressively recruited for bile acid transport. Biliary excretion of bile acids may, on the other hand, be delayed in zone 3 hepatocytes.[181,182] Whether this difference results from the heterogeneous distribution of intracellular processes for bile acid transport, such as the presence of greater amounts of cytosolic bile acid-binding proteins in pericentral cells,[183] or heterogeneous transport rates at the canalicular membrane remains to be determined. The effects of selective damage of the periportal or pericentral cells by allyl alcohol or bromobenzene, respectively, suggest that pericentral hepatocytes contribute primarily to BAIBF.[184] However, more direct methods are required to validate the hypothesis that there are zonal differences in the contribution of hepatocytes to the bile salt-dependent and -independent fractions of bile secretion.

Ductular Events

The presence of secretory activity in biliary epithelial cells has been established by a number of studies: (1) water and electrolyte secretion has been demonstrated in isolated extrahepatic bile ducts both in situ[185] and in vitro;[186] (2) choleresis induced by secretin[187] and other hormones,[188] and, possibly, by neurogenic stimuli[189] appears to be at the level of the biliary ductules or ducts; and (3) induction of bile ductular cell hyperplasia by chronic biliary obstruction results in a profound increase in basal bile flow and responsiveness to secretin choleresis.[190] A clinical correlation of the secretory activity of the biliary epithelia can be found in the increased response to secretin and increased bile flow observed in patients with chronic liver diseases associated with ductular proliferation.[191] Similarly, choleresis has been reported in patients with congenital dilatation of the intrahepatic biliary tree.[192] Vasoactive intestinal peptide (VIP) has recently been shown to produce a bicarbonate-rich choleresis at the ductular level.[193] Conversely, somatostatin, by way of inhibition of choleretic hormone release,[194] inhibits bile flow either by enhancing ductular reabsorption or by inhibiting ductular secretion of a bicarbonate-rich electrolyte fraction of bile.[195] Alternatively, somatostatin may have an effect on canalicular bile flow and bile acid output independent of ductular effects.[196]

GALLBLADDER STRUCTURE AND FUNCTION

The physiologic functions of the gallbladder include: (1) concentration and storage of bile during interdigestive periods; (2) evacuation by smooth muscle contraction in response to cholecystokinin (CCK); (3) moderation of hydrostatic pressure within the biliary tract; (4) bile acidification; and (5) absorption of organic components of bile.[197]

Although not essential for bile secretion, the gallbladder serves to concentrate bile up to tenfold. This concentrative process is largely the result of electroneutral sodium-coupled chloride transport and passive water movement.[197] The exact mechanism remains controversial, with experimental evidence supporting either coupled NaCl entry[198,199] or a $Na^+:H^+$ and $Cl^-:HCO_3^-$ exchange operating in parallel.[200,201] An alternative model has also been proposed in which short-chain fatty acids, particularly butyrate, can substitute to varying degrees for HCO_3^- in a double-exchange system.[202] The result of this concentrative process is the formation of gallbladder bile, isotonic to plasma and composed of higher concentrations of sodium, bile salts, potassium, and calcium and lower concentrations of chloride and bicarbonate than hepatic bile.[203]

Net fluid and electrolyte absorption by the gallbladder appears to be under hormonal regulation. Vasoactive intestinal polypeptide (VIP), present in neurons innervating gallbladder mucosa,[204] and serotonin inhibit net fluid and electrolyte movement, reversing absorption to secretion.[205,206] In contrast, α-adrenergic ganglionic blockage of neuronal release of VIP increases the rate of net water absorption.[207]

Transport processes for certain amino acids and sugars are present, as well, in gallbladder mucosa.[208] In contrast, despite the considerable concentration gradient for bile salts and bile pigments, the absorption of highly ionized organic solutes such as taurocholate, sulfobromophthalein (BSP), and iodipamide, is minimal.[209] In acute cholecystitis, increased permeability to water and to highly ionized solutes has been demonstrated, and enhanced absorption of iodipamide may account for the nonvisualization of the gallbladder that occurs in this setting.[210] Accelerated absorption of bile salts resulting from bacterial deconjugation or gallbladder mucosal injury may be a factor in gallstone formation.[197] Conversely, absorption of cholesterol by the gallbladder, by preventing supersaturation and precipitation, may protect against gallstone formation.[211]

Mucus is released by exocytosis of secretory granules in the apical portion of gallbladder epithelial cells.[212] Gallbladder mucin synthesis and release are markedly accelerated in animal models of cholesterol cholelithiasis before crystal and stone formation.[213,214] Formation of an insoluble mucin–bilirubin complex may provide a nidus for cholesterol monohydrate nucleation.[215]

ENTEROHEPATIC CIRCULATION

It is best to consider bile acid secretion as a cyclic flow of molecules anatomically limited to the hepatocyte, biliary tree, small intestine, enterocyte, and portal blood, known as the enterohepatic circulation (Fig 16-10). Intestinal conservation of bile acids is approximately 90% efficient, reflecting the additive effects of both passive and active reabsorptive processes. Although other endogenous and exogenous substances undergo enterohepatic cycling, such as the bacterial reduction products of bilirubin, vitamin D_2, vitamin B_{12}, antibiotics (e.g., ampicillin), and other drugs (e.g., warfarin), the enterohepatic circulation of bile acids assumes primary physiologic importance.[12] The bile acid pool cycles 5 to 15 times daily through this pathway.[216]

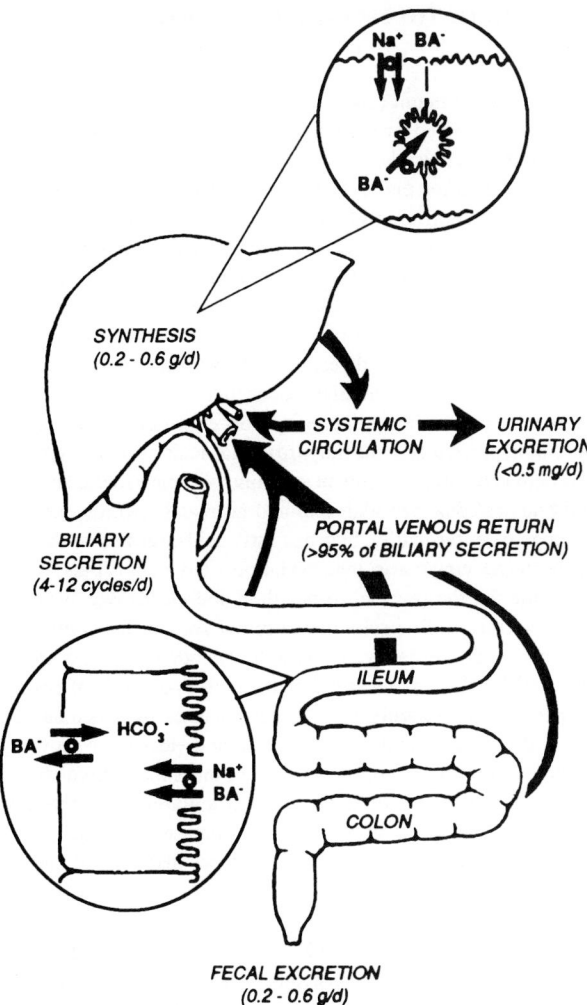

FIGURE 16–10. Enterohepatic circulation of bile salts showing typical kinetic values for healthy humans.

Intraluminal Events

A full discussion of the role of bile acids in fat digestion and absorption can be found in other chapters. It is worthwhile merely to reiterate that the function of bile acids in the small intestine is directly related to their amphipathic structure and their tendency to form mixed micelles with cholesterol and lecithin. Although bile acid micelles solubilize lipolytic products in their lipophilic interior, by a process termed micellar solubilization, and promote lipase activity, bile salts are not essential for normal triglyceride digestion and absorption.[217] In contrast, bile acid deficiency severely impairs the absorption of cholesterol and the fat-soluble vitamins.[217]

Bile acids in the intestinal lumen may fulfill other physiologic and pathophysiologic roles. Bile acids may complex Fe^{2+} in the duodenum and, by inhibiting precipitation, enhance intestinal absorption. Reflux of duodenal bile into the stomach occurs continuously even in the presence of a competent pyloric sphincter resulting in a concentration of bile acids on the order of 0.05 to

0.17 mM.[12] After pyloroplasty, bile salt concentrations may be great enough to solubilize mucosal cell membrane lipids to form mixed micelles and compromise normal gastric mucosal barriers.[12]

Intestinal Transport

Passive absorption occurs throughout the small intestine and is dependent on intestinal pH and bile acid structure. The most hydrophobic bile acids (glycine-conjugated dihydroxy bile acids) are passively absorbed in the more acidic environment of the duodenum, where the fraction present in protonated form is greatest.[7] Bile acids are transported across the ileal brush border membrane by a Na^+-dependent secondary active transport process (i.e., the accumulation of bile acid within the enterocyte against its electrochemical gradient is driven by the inwardly directed Na^+ gradient maintained by a basolateral Na^+,K^+-ATPase).[218] Photoaffinity labeling studies of bile salt-binding proteins in the small intestinal brush border membrane suggest that the transport system for bile salts in small intestine is different from that in liver.[219] Active transport favors trihydroxy (cholic acid) over dihydroxy (chenodeoxycholic acid) bile acids, and conjugated over unconjugated species.[216] As in the liver, this transport process is not fully operative at birth,[220] and the inability to conserve bile salts may contribute to the diminished bile salt pool size and "physiologic steatorrhea" of the immediate postnatal period.[221] Postnatal development may be dependent, in part, on increasing plasma levels of endogenous corticosteroids.[222,223]

At the basolateral membrane of the ileum, bile acid leaves the enterocyte by a Na^+-independent anion exchange process,[224] which may involve 54-kd and 59-kd proteins.[225] Absorption of bile acids occurs solely into portal blood resulting in a concentration on the order of 0.01 to 0.02 mM. The concentration of chenodeoxycholate in portal vein blood is greater than that of cholate, owing to the more rapid absorption and the more efficient conservation of chenodeoxycholate.[226] Bile acids in portal blood are predominantly bound, by way of hydrophobic interactions, to albumin, although a small fraction are bound to lipoproteins, particularly high-density lipoproteins.[227] Uptake by the liver, completing the enterohepatic cycle, is typically expressed as fractional extraction (FE) or "first pass" extraction, equivalent to the percentage of bile acids removed during a single passage through the hepatic acinus. The FE is related to bile acid structure and albumin binding, and, in general, is greatest for the hydrophilic bile acids and least for the lipophilic, protein-bound bile acids.[13] Thus, the FE is about 80% to 90% for conjugated cholate, 70% to 80% for conjugated chenodeoxycholate, 70% for unconjugated cholate, 60% for unconjugated chenodeoxycholate, and 50% for unconjugated UDCA.[216]

The small fraction of bile acids that escape active or passive absorption in the small intestine undergo bacterial modification in the colon by way of: (1) deconjugation; (2) dehydrogenation of a hydroxyl group, typically the 7-hydroxyl group, to form an oxo bile acid; (3) 7-dehydroxylation; and (4) epimerization of a hydroxyl group. Secondary bile acids so formed are also reabsorbed to varying degrees, depending on their physicochemical properties, their interaction with luminal constituents, and the permeability characteristics of the colon. Lithocholate and deoxycholate, formed from the 7-dehydroxylation of chenodeoxycholate and cholate, respectively, are the major fecal bile acids in humans. Approximately one third of the deoxycholate formed in the colon is absorbed. The colonic absorption of lithocholate is, however, less efficient. Once absorbed, deoxycholic and ursodeoxycholic acid are conjugated in the liver with glycine or taurine; lithocholate, in addition, undergoes sulfation.[228] This is most likely a protective mechanism from lithocholate hepatotoxicity because the sulfates of lithocholate do not undergo intestinal absorption and further enterohepatic cycling.[229] The administration of chenodeoxycholate to animal species without the capacity for lithocholate sulfation during drug trials of this agent resulted in the accumulation of lithocholic acid in the enterohepatic circulation and subsequent cirrhosis.[230] The enterohepatic circulation of deoxycholate may be important in cholesterol cholelithiasis, because there is an inverse relationship between the concentration of deoxycholate in bile and the degree of cholesterol saturation.[231] Secondary bile acids formed from bacterial dehydrogenation and epimerization undergo hepatic biotransformation so that the major bile acids in human bile are the glycine and taurine conjugates of the two primary bile acids, cholic and chenodeoxycholic acid, and their three secondary bile acid derivatives, deoxycholic, lithocholic, and ursodeoxycholic acid, and the sulfated glycine and taurine conjugates of lithocholate.

CLINICAL CORRELATES

Cholestasis

A detailed discussion of cholestasis, best defined as bile secretory failure, is beyond the scope of this chapter, and the interested reader is referred to several recent reviews of the subject.[232–234] In brief, cholestasis can be further categorized as either a functional defect in bile formation at the level of the hepatocyte (intrahepatic cholestasis) or an obstruction to bile flow within the biliary tract (extrahepatic cholestasis). Frequent causes of extrahepatic cholestasis include choledocholithiasis, pancreatic and periampullary carcinoma, biliary strictures, and pancreatitis. Based on what is known about normal bile formation, several mechanisms can be identified that may play a role in the pathogenesis of intrahepatic cholestasis, including alterations in sinusoidal membrane function and composition, alterations in cytoskeletal organization and function, alterations in tight junction permeability, and impairment of canalicular membrane structure and function. No single mechanism can explain the development of cholestasis in all clinical settings, and multiple mechanisms may be involved in any given disorder. Regardless of the mechanism of cholestasis, the net effect is retention of solutes, including bile acids, bilirubin, and cholesterol, which are preferentially excreted into bile under normal conditions. The decreased biliary excretion of bile acids into the small intestine reduces the concentration of bile acids to levels below those required for normal fat digestion and absorption, and steatorrhea and deficiencies in the fat-soluble vitamins may result. Jaundice results from the retention of bilirubin. Defective cholesterol excretion, in turn, leads to the formation of xanthelasma, xanthomas, and alterations in the erythrocyte membrane leading to target and spur cell formation. Sulfation and glucuronidation of bile acids, particularly chenodeoxycholyl conjugates,[235] increases in cholestasis, and the renal route of elimination becomes predominant.[10,11]

Defects in Intestinal Transport

Diseases of the ileum (e.g., Crohn's disease, ileal resection or bypass) characterized by defective absorption of bile salts may give rise to either a cholerrheic enteropathy or a steatogenic enteropathy. The critical factor that determines which of these two conditions predominates appears to be the length of the distal ileal segment affected by disease or resection.[12] In disorders involving greater than 100 cm of ileum, as measured from the ileocecal valve, hepatic synthesis of new bile salts cannot compete with intestinal loss to maintain a critical concentration of bile salts in the proximal small intestine for normal fat digestion and absorption, and steatorrhea with or without fatty acid diarrhea occurs. In disorders with lesser degrees of involvement, increased concentrations of bile salts in the colon, particularly the dihydroxy bile acids chenodeoxycholate and deoxycholate,[236] result in net fluid and electrolyte secretion, and bile acid diarrhea with minimal fat malabsorption occurs. In steatogenic enteropathy, hydroxy fatty acids, formed in the colon by bacterial enzymatic hydroxylation of dietary lipids, are responsible for the reversal of net fluid and electrolyte absorption to net secretion. Bile salts play a minor role in this condition, if any, because free deoxycholate and chenodeoxycholate are precipitated by the low fecal pH that exists as a result of bacterial fermentation and alkali loss.[237] The mechanism by which bile acids and hydroxy fatty acids alter net fluid and electrolyte movement in the colon remains controversial, but most likely involves both increased mucosal permeability and stimulation of active anion secretion.[238] The response to bile salt sequestrants, such as cholestyramine, helps to differentiate these two disorders of intestinal bile salt malabsorption.[239]

Additional consequences of the steatorrhea caused by severe bile acid malabsorption include (1) increased colonic absorption of dietary oxalate with subsequent hyperoxaluria and oxalate nephrolithiasis;[240] and (2) cholesterol cholelithiasis.[241]

Idiopathic bile acid catharsis has been defined as a chronic diarrheal illness characterized by: (1) bile acid malabsorption; (2) lack of association with other forms of ileal dysfunction; and (3) response to cholestyramine.[242,243] Histologic studies demonstrating subtotal villous atrophy with crypt hyperplasia in the ileum are consistent with the hypothesis that a relative lack of ileal bile acid transport proteins is responsible for the bile acid malabsorption observed in this disorder.[244] Immunologic abnormalities may also occur, including the presence of serum autoantibodies, circulating immune complexes, and hypocomplementemia.[244] The diagnosis is established by the response to cholestyramine and the recently described [75]SeHCAT (23-selena-25-homocholyltaurine) test, in which abdominal γ-counting is performed after the oral administration of this radioactive taurocholate analogue.[245] Retention of less than 34% of the administered dose after 3 days had a 94% sensitivity and 100% specificity in the detection of bile acid loss.[245] Measurements of bile acid absorption, such as the [75]SeHCAT test, may become standard tests in the diagnostic evaluation of patients with nonfatty, watery diarrhea of unknown origin.

Congenital defects in intestinal bile acid transport have been documented.[246] Ultrastructural examination of the ileal mucosa in affected individuals presenting with congenital diarrhea, steatorrhea, and growth failure revealed no significant abnormality.[246] In addition, transient bile acid malabsorption has been reported to occur in children with infectious gastroenteritis.[247]

Defects in Biotransformation

Disorders associated with acidic duodenal pH, such as Zollinger-Ellison syndrome[248] or exocrine pancreatic insufficiency,[249] result in greater passive absorption of bile acids, particularly glycine conjugates, or their intraluminal precipitation as bile acid crystals. This leads to decreases in the concentration of intraluminal bile acids available for fat digestion, contributing, in part, to the steatorrhea seen with these disorders. Rarely, bile acid enteroliths may form as a result of intraluminal precipitation. In small bowel bacterial overgrowth, bile acids undergo bacterial deconjugation and dehydroxylation to form unconjugated deoxycholate and lithocholate, which are absorbed passively by nonionic diffusion. Intraluminal bile salt concentration is again compromised by this "short circuiting" of the enterohepatic circulation, and steatorrhea may supervene. Clinically, moderate elevations in serum levels of unconjugated bile acids may be detected in small bowel bacterial overgrowth.[250] Abnormalities in the cholyl-^{14}C-glycine breath test, in which glycine released by bacterial deconjugation is absorbed and measured as [14]CO_2 in expired air, can also be observed[251] but are difficult to differentiate from disorders of bile acid absorption.

Exocrine pancreatic insufficiency may interfere with normal enterohepatic cycling of bile acids by additional mechanisms. In patients with alcoholic pancreatitis[252] and cystic fibrosis,[253] increased fecal bile acid excretion, reversed by oral pancreatic enzyme administration, appears to be the result of a combination of effects, including bile salt binding to maldigested protein, carbohydrate, fibers, and other food residues.[254]

Defects in Enterohepatic Circulation Dynamics

The enterohepatic circulation should be conceptually regarded as the result of coordinated actions of mechanical pumps, the gallbladder and the small intestine; chemical pumps, the transport systems of the hepatocyte and the enterocyte; and valves, the sphincter of Oddi and the ileocecal valve.[12] Thus, the dynamics of the enterohepatic circulation are influenced by alterations in either the gallbladder or the small intestine. Rapid intestinal transit results in increased cycling frequency and delayed intestinal transit decreases cycling frequency.[255] Celiac sprue alters the dynamics of the enterohepatic circulation by way of a neuroendocrine mechanism. Reductions in CCK release from intestinal mucosa and impaired gallbladder emptying, reversed by a gluten-free diet, have been observed,[256,257] leading to infrequent cycling of the bile acid pool and stagnation of bile within the biliary tree.[258] An example of an extreme neurohumoral imbalance affecting the enterohepatic circulation is the syndrome associated with somatostatinomas. Elevated plasma immunoreactive somatostatin levels lead to inhibition of CCK-induced gallbladder contraction and bile stasis, accounting for the clinical manifestations of cholesterol gallstones and steatorrhea.[259]

Despite removal of a major storage pool of bile acids, cholecystectomy has little effect on the enterohepatic circulation. Increased dehydroxylation of cholic to deoxycholic acid with a normal or expanded deoxycholic acid pool has been described, consistent with increased exposure of the bile acid pool to colonic bacterial modifications.[260] However, bile acid malabsorption and increased fecal loss do not appear to result from this apparent augmented passage of bile acids into the colon, and bile acids are not thought to be a causative factor in postcholecystectomy diarrhea.[261]

Defects in Synthesis

Continuous bile acid synthesis from cholesterol is required to maintain the bile acid pool in the enterohepatic circulation. The maximal rate of synthesis is on the order of 4 to 6 g/day.[262] The importance of bile acid synthesis in health is evident if one considers the effects of a cessation in synthesis. Fecal loss would not be repleted, cholesterol would not be excreted, BADBF would stop, and fat-soluble substances would not be absorbed.[13]

Patients with cirrhosis have a diminished total bile salt pool, primarily reflecting a reduction in cholate pool size by way of a selective defect in microsomal 12α-hydroxylation of cholate precursors.[263,264] Impaired conversion of cholate to deoxycholate leading to a reduction in deoxycholate pool size[265] and increased synthesis of sulfated primary bile acids[235] have also been reported in cirrhotic patients.

Cerebrotendinous xanthomatosis (CTX) is a rare inherited defect in bile acid synthesis characterized by progressive neurologic disturbances, premature atherosclerosis, cataracts, and tendinous xanthomas.[266] Low plasma cholesterol but elevated plasma cholestanol levels are the result of mitochondrial 26-hydroxylase deficiency, an enzyme involved in cholesterol side-chain oxidation.[267] Bile acid synthesis is decreased in this disorder, preferentially affecting chenodeoxycholate levels. Loss of bile acid feedback inhibition of cholesterol synthesis leads to the formation of cholestanol, which accumulates in myelin. Hydroxylation of cholesterol to form bile alcohols, which are conjugated to glucuronides and excreted in bile and urine, accounts for the low cholesterol levels.[268] Treatment with chenodeoxycholate suppresses the biochemical abnormalities and may improve neurologic symptoms.[266]

Zellweger syndrome is a rare and fatal autosomal recessive disorder associated with multiple craniofacial dystoses, central nervous system abnormalities, generalized hypotonia, hepatomegaly, and renal cysts.[269] The absence of peroxisomes, single membrane-limited cytoplasmic organelles, in the liver and kidney is responsible for defective β-oxidation of long-chain fatty acids and bile acids;[270] prenatal diagnosis is possible.[271]

Serum Bile Acids

Serum bile acid levels are a direct reflection of the enterohepatic circulation, because they are determined not only by hepatic uptake but also by intestinal absorption. During fasting, the major portion of the bile acid pool is stored in the gallbladder, although delivery into the duodenum and intestinal reabsorption continue. After meal-induced gallbladder contraction, delivery of bile acids into the small intestine is dramatically increased. Thus, the early phase of the normal postprandial elevation in serum bile acid levels consists primarily of the most lipophilic bile acids (glycine conjugates of chenodeoxycholic and deoxycholic acid), reflecting passive absorption in the proximal small intestine.[13] The abnormal elevation in unconjugated bile acid levels occurring in small bowel bacterial overgrowth as a result of enhanced passive absorption was discussed previously. Active absorption in the distal ileum accounts for the 2-hour postprandial peak, consisting predominantly of conjugates of cholic acid.[13] As a consequence, in ileal disorders associated with defects in transport (see above), postprandial elevation of cholyl conjugates is blunted.[216] Spill-over of bile acids into the systemic circulation is determined by the fractional extraction of the individual bile acids, as discussed above. Hepatic uptake mechanisms normally operate far below saturation, and serum bile acid levels are, therefore, largely independent of load.[216] In patients with liver disease, defects in the hepatic phase of the enterohepatic circulation may result from reduced hepatic extraction, portosystemic shunting, or a combination of these two mechanisms.[216] Reduced hepatic extraction, in turn, may reflect both decreased fractional extraction from portal blood and decreased systemic clearance. A potential contributory factor in the reduction of hepatic uptake of bile acids in chronic liver disease may be loss of the fenestrations in the sinusoidal endothelium[272] or basal lamina formation,[273] restricting the transfer of albumin-bound bile acids from the sinusoid to the space of Disse. The use of serum bile acid determinations in the assessment of patients with suspected liver disease is discussed in Chapter 42.

The reader is directed to Chapter 6, Epithelia: Biologic Principles of Organization; Chapter 11, Motility of the Biliary Tree; Chapter 18, Intestinal Lipid Absorption; and Chapter 41, Approach to the Patient with Jaundice.

REFERENCES

1. Meier PJ, Sztul ES, Reuben A, et al. Structural and functional polarity of canalicular and basolateral plasma membrane vesicles isolated in high yield from rat liver. J Cell Biol 1984;98:991.
2. Inoue M, Kinne R, Tran T, et al. Rat liver canalicular membrane vesicles: isolation and topological characterization. J Biol Chem 1983;258:5183.
3. Blitzer BL, Donovan CB. A new method for the rapid isolation of basolateral plasma membrane vesicles from rat liver: characterization, validation and bile acid transport studies. J Biol Chem 1984;259:9295.
4. Graf J, Gautam A, Boyer JL. Isolated rat hepatocyte couplets: a primary secretory unit for electrophysiologic studies of bile secretory function. Proc Natl Acad Sci USA 1984;81:6516.
5. Gautam A, Ng OC, Boyer JL. Isolated rat hepatocyte couplets in short-term culture: structural characteristics and plasma membrane reorganization. Hepatology 1987;7:216.
6. Boyer JL, Bloomer JR. Canalicular bile secretion in man: studies utilizing the biliary clearance of ^{14}C-mannitol. J Clin Invest 1974;54:773.
7. Hofmann AF. Chemistry and enterohepatic circulation of bile acids. Hepatology 1984;4:4S.
8. Bucuvalas JC, Goodrich AL, Suchy FJ. Hepatic taurine transport: a Na^+-dependent carrier on the basolateral plasma membrane. Am J Physiol 1987;253:G351.
9. Huijghebaert SM, Hofmann AF. Pancreatic carboxypeptidase hydrolysis of bile acid–amino acid conjugates: selective resistance of glycine and taurine amidates. Gastroenterology 1986;90:306.
10. Stiehl A. Bile salt sulphates in cholestasis. Eur J Clin Invest 1974;4:59.
11. Back P, Spaczynski K, Gerok W. Bile acid glucuronides in urine. Hoppe-Seyler's Z Physiol Chem 1974;335:749.
12. Carey MC, Cahalane MJ. Enterohepatic circulation. In: Arias IM, Jakoby WB, Popper H, Schachter D, Shafritz DA, eds. The liver: biology and pathobiology, ed 2. New York: Raven Press, 1988:573.
13. Hofmann AF. Bile acids. In: Arias IM, Jakoby WB, Popper H, Schachter D, Shafritz DA, eds. The liver: biology and pathobiology, ed 2. New York: Raven Press, 1988:553.
14. Fromm H. Gallstone dissolution therapy: current status and future prospects. Gastroenterology 1986;91:1560.
15. Wheeler HO, Ramos OL. Determinants of the flow and composition of bile in the unanesthetized dog during constant infusion of sodium taurocholate. J Clin Invest 1960;39:161.
16. Knook DL, Wisse E, eds. Sinusoidal liver cells. Amsterdam: Elsevier/North Holland, 1982.
17. Schachter D. Fluidity and function of hepatocyte plasma membranes. Hepatology 1984;4:140.
18. Jones AL, Schmucker DL, Renston RH, et al. The architecture of bile secretion: a morphological perspective of physiology. Dig Dis Sci 1980;25:609.
19. Philips MJ, Poucell S, Patterson J, Valencia P. The liver: an atlas and text of ultrastructural pathology. New York: Raven Press, 1987:101.
20. Meier PJ. Transport polarity of hepatocytes. Sem Liver Dis 1988;8:293.
21. Ballatori N, Moseley RH, Boyer JL. Sodium gradient dependent L-glutamate is localized to the canalicular domain of liver plasma membranes: studies in rat liver sinusoidal and canalicular membrane vesicles. J Biol Chem 1986;261;6216.
22. Moseley RH, Ballatori N, Murphy SM. Na^+-glycine cotransport in canalicular liver plasma membrane vesicles. Am J Physiol 1988;255:G253.
23. Burkel WE. The fine structure of the terminal branches of the hepatic arterial system of the rat. Anat Rec 1970;167:329.
24. Rappaport AM. The microcirculatory hepatic unit. Microvascular Res 1973;6:212.
25. Kressner MS, Stockert RJ, Morell AG, et al. Origins of biliary copper. Hepatology 1984;4:867.
26. Spray DC, Bennett MVL. Physiology and pharmacology of gap junctions. Annu Rev Physiol 1985;47:281.
27. Hertzberg EL. Antibody probes in the study of gap junctional communication. Annu Rev Physiol 1985;47:305.
28. Zimmer DB, Green CR, Evans WH, et al. Topological analysis of the major protein in isolated intact rat liver gap junctions and gap junction-derived single membrane structures. J Biol Chem 1987;262:7751.
29. Saez JC, Bennett VL, Spray DC. Carbon tetrachloride at hepatotoxic levels blocks reversibly gap junctions between rat hepatocytes. Science Wash DC 1987;236:967.
30. Oda M, Price VM, Fisher MM, et al. Ultrastructure of bile canaliculi, with special reference to the surface coat and the pericanalicular web. Lab Invest 1974;31:314.
31. Philips MJ, Oshio C, Miyairi M, et al. A study of bile canalicular contractions in isolated hepatocytes. Hepatology 1982;2:763.
32. Watanabe S, Philips MJ. Ca^{2+} causes active contraction of bile canaliculi: direct evidence from microinjection studies. Proc Natl Acad Sci USA 1984;81:6164.
33. Miyairi M, Oshio C, Watanabe S, et al. Taurocholate accelerates bile canalicular contractions in isolated rat hepatocytes. Gastroenterology 1984;87:788.
34. Watanabe S, Miyairi M, Oshio C, et al. Phalloidin alters bile canalicular contractility in primary monolayer cultures of rat liver. Gastroenterology 1983;85:245.
35. Philips MJ, Oda M, Mak E, et al. Microfilament dysfunction as a possible cause of intrahepatic cholestasis. Gastroenterology 1975;69:48.
36. Dubin M, Maurice M, Feldmann G, et al. Phalloidin-induced cholestasis in the rat: relation to changes in microfilaments. Gastroenterology 1978;75:450.
37. Dubin M, Maurice M, Feldmann G, et al. Influence of colchicine and phalloidin on bile secretion and hepatic ultrastructure in the

rat: possible interaction between microtubules and microfilaments. Gastroenterology 1980;79:646.

38. Elias E, Hruban Z, Wade JB, et al. Phalloidin-induced cholestasis: a microfilament-mediated change in junctional complex permeability. Proc Natl Acad Sci USA 1980;77:2229.

39. Ishak KG, Zimmerman HJ. Hepatotoxic effects of the anabolic/androgenic steroids. Semin Liver Dis 1987;7:230.

40. Philips MJ, Oda M, Funatsu K. Evidence for microfilament involvement in norethandrolone-induced intrahepatic cholestasis. Am J Pathol 1978;93:729.

41. Adler M, Chung KW, Schaffner F. Pericanalicular hepatocytic and bile ductular microfilaments in cholestasis in man. Am J Pathol 1980;98:603.

42. Vale RD, Reese TS, Sheetz MP. Identification of a novel force-generating protein, kinesin, involved in microtubule-based motility. Cell 1985;42:39.

43. Gregory DH, Vlahcevic ZR, Prugh MF, et al. Mechanisms of secretion of biliary lipids: role of a microtubular system in hepatocellular transport of lipids in the rat. Gastroenterology 1978;74:93.

44. Goldman IS, Jones AL, Hradek GT, et al. Hepatocyte handling of immunoglobulin A in the rat: the role of microtubules. Gastroenterology 1983;85:130.

45. Combettes L, Dumont M, Berthon B, et al. Release of calcium from the endoplasmic reticulum by bile acids in rat liver cells. J Biol Chem 1988;263:2299.

46. Combettes L, Berthon B, Doucet E, et al. Characteristics of bile acid-mediated Ca^{2+} release from permeabilized liver cells and liver microsomes. J Biol Chem 1989;264:157.

47. Anwer MS, Engelking LR, Nolan K, et al. Hepatotoxic bile acids increase cytosolic Ca^{++} activity of isolated rat hepatocytes. Hepatology 1988;8:887.

48. Brauer RW, Leong GF, Holloway RJ. Mechanics of bile secretion: effect of perfusion pressure and temperature on bile flow and bile secretion pressure. Am J Physiol 1954;177:103.

49. Balabaud C, Kron KA, Gumucio JJ. The assessment of the bile salt-nondependent fraction of canalicular bile water in the rat. J Lab Clin Med 1977;89:393.

50. Sperber I. Secretion of organic anions in the formation of urine and bile. Pharmacol Rev 1959;11:109.

51. O'Maille ERL, Kozmary SV, Hofmann AF, et al. Differing effects of norcholate and cholate on bile flow and biliary lipid secretion in the rat. Am J Physiol 1984;246:G67.

52. Erlinger S. Physiology of bile secretion and enterohepatic circulation. In: Johnson LR, ed. Physiology of the gastrointestinal tract. New York: Raven Press, 1987:1557.

53. Dumont M, Erlinger S, Uchman S. Hypercholeresis induced by ursodeoxycholic acid and 7-ketolithocholic acid in the rat: possible role of bicarbonate transport. Gastroenterology 1980;79:82.

54. Soloway RD, Hofmann AF, Thomas PJ, et al. Triketocholanoic (dehydrocholic) acid: hepatic metabolism and effect on bile flow and biliary lipid secretion in man. J Clin Invest 1973;52:715.

55. Goresky CA, Haddad HH, Kluger WS, et al. The enhancement of maximal bilirubin excretion with taurocholate-induced increments in bile flow. Can J Physiol Pharmacol 1974;52:389.

56. Scharschmidt BF, Schmid R. The micellar sink: a quantitative assessment of the association of organic anions with mixed micelles and other macromolecular aggregates in rat bile. J Clin Invest 1978;62:1122.

57. Binet S, Delage Y, Erlinger S. Influence of taurocholate, taurochenodeoxycholate, and taurodehydrocholate on sulfobromophthalein transport into bile. Am J Physiol 1979;236:E10.

58. Frimmer M, Ziegler K. The transport of bile acids in liver cells. Biochim Biophys Acta 1988;947:75.

59. Anwer MS, O'Maille ERL, Hofmann AF, et al. Influence of side-chain charge on hepatic transport of bile acids and bile acid analogues. Am J Physiol 1985;249:G479.

60. Bellentani S, Hardison WGM, Marchegiano P, et al. Bile acid inhibition of taurocholate uptake by rat hepatocytes: role of OH groups. Am J Physiol 1987;252:G339.

61. Van Dyke RW, Stephens JE, Scharschmidt BF. Bile acid transport in cultured rat hepatocytes. Am J Physiol 1982;243:G484.

62. Forker EL, Luxon BA. Albumin helps mediate the removal of taurocholate by rat liver. J Clin Invest 1981;67:1517.

63. Blitzer BL, Lyons L. Enhancement of Na^{+}-dependent bile acid uptake by albumin: direct demonstration in rat basolateral liver plasma membrane vesicles. Am J Physiol 1985;249:G34.

64. Horie T, Mizuma T, Kasai S, et al. Conformational change in plasma albumin due to interaction with isolated rat hepatocyte. Am J Physiol 1988;254:G465.

65. Stremmel W, Potter BJ, Berk PD. Studies of albumin binding to rat liver plasma membranes: implications for the albumin receptor hypothesis. Biochim Biophys Acta 1983;756:20.

66. Kroncke KD, Fricker G, Meier PJ, et al. α-Amanitin uptake into hepatocytes: identification of hepatic membrane transport systems used by amatoxins. J Biol Chem 1986;261:12562.

67. Blitzer BL, Terzakis C, Scott KA. Hydroxyl/bile acid exchange: a new mechanism for the uphill transport of cholate by basolateral liver plasma membrane vesicles. J Biol Chem 1986;261:12042.

68. von Dippe P, Drain P, Levy D. Synthesis and transport characteristics of photoaffinity probes for the hepatocyte bile acid transport system. J Biol Chem 1983;258:8890.

69. Wieland T, Nassal M, Kramer W, et al. Identity of hepatic membrane transport systems for bile salts, phalloidin and antamanide by photoaffinity labeling. Proc Natl Acad Sci USA 1984;81:5232.

70. Kramer W, Bickel U, Buscher HP, et al. Bile-salt binding polypeptides in plasma membranes of hepatocytes revealed by photoaffinity labeling. Eur J Biochem 1982;129:13.

71. Fricker G, Hugentobler G, Meier PJ, et al. Identification of a single sinusoidal bile salt uptake system in skate liver. Am J Physiol 1987;253:G816.

72. Ananthanarayanan M, von Dippe P, Levy D. Identification of the hepatocyte Na^{+}-dependent bile acid transport protein using monoclonal antibodies. J Biol Chem 1988;263:8338.

73. Wood AJJ, Villeneuve JP, Branch RA, et al. Intact hepatocyte theory of impaired drug metabolism in experimental cirrhosis in the rat. Gastroenterology 1979;76:1358.

74. Villeneuve JP, Wood AJJ, Shand DG, et al. Impaired drug metabolism in experimental cirrhosis in the rat. Biochem Pharmacol 1978;27:2577.

75. Reichen J, Hoilien C, Le M, et al. Decreased uptake of taurocholate and ouabain by hepatocytes isolated from cirrhotic rat liver. Hepatology 1987;7:67.

76. Krahenbuhl S, Meier-Abt PJ, Reichen J. Taurocholate transport by liver plasma membrane vesicles is not altered in cirrhotic rats. J Hepatology 1989;9:1.

77. Kaplowitz N. Physiological significance of glutathione S-transferases. Am J Physiol 1980;239:G439.

78. Sugiyama Y, Yamada T, Kaplowitz N. Newly identified bile acid binders in rat liver cytosol: purification and comparison with glutathione S-transferases. J Biol Chem 1983;258:3602.

79. Stolz A, Sugiyama Y, Kuhlenkamp J, et al. Identification and purification of a 36-kDa bile acid binder in human hepatic cytosol. FEBS Lett 1984;177:31.

80. Sugiyama Y, Stolz A, Sugimoto M, et al. Evidence for a common affinity binding site on glutathione S-transferase B for lithocholic acid and bilirubin. J Lipid Res 1984;25:1177.

81. Stolz A, Takikawa H, Sugiyama Y, et al. 3α-hydroxysteroid dehydrogenase activity of the Y' bile acid binders in rat liver cytosol: identification, kinetics, and physiologic significance. J Clin Invest 1987;79:427.

82. Jones AL, Schmucker DL, Mooney JS, et al. A quantitative analysis of hepatic ultrastructure in rats during enhanced bile acid secretion. Anat Rec 1978;192:277.

83. Jones AL, Schmucker DL. Mooney JS, et al. Alterations in hepatic pericanalicular cytoplasm during enhanced bile secretory activity. Lab Invest 1979;40:512.

84. Lamri Y, Roda A, Dumont M, et al. Immunoperoxidase localization of bile salts in rat liver cells: evidence for a role of the Golgi apparatus in bile salt transport. J Clin Invest 1988;82:1173.

85. Suchy FJ, Balistreri WF, Hung J, et al. Intracellular bile acid transport in rat liver as visualized by electron microscope autoradiography using a bile acid analogue. Am J Physiol 1983;245:G681.

86. Goldsmith MA, Huling S, Jones AL. Hepatic handling of bile salts and protein during intrahepatic cholestasis. Gastroenterology 1983;84:978.

87. Simon FA, Fleischer B, Fleischer S. Subcellular distribution of bile

acids, bile salts, and taurocholate binding sites in rat liver. Biochemistry 1984;23:6459.

88. Simon FA, Fleischer B, Fleischer S. Two distinct mechanisms for taurocholate uptake in subcellular fractions from rat liver. J Biol Chem 1984;259:10814.

89. Crawford JM, Gollan JL. Hepatocyte cotransport of taurocholate and bilirubin glucuronides: role of microtubules. Am J Physiol 1988;255:G121.

90. Hacki W, Paumgartner G. Determination of the biliary dead space using ^{14}C-taurocholate as a marker. Experientia 1973;29:1091.

91. Reichen J, Paumgartner G. Uptake of bile acids by perfused rat liver. Am J Physiol 1976;231:734.

92. Hardison WGM, Hatoff DE, Miyai K, et al. Nature of bile acid maximum secretory rate in the rat. Am J Physiol 1981;24:G337.

93. Yousef IM, Barnwell S, Gratton F, et al. Liver cell membrane solubilization may control maximum secretory rate of cholic acid in the rat. Am J Physiol 1987;252:G84.

94. Inoue M, Kinne R, Tran T, et al. Taurocholate transport by rat liver canalicular membrane vesicles: evidence for the presence of an Na$^+$-independent transport system. J Clin Invest 1984;73:659.

95. Meier PJ, Meier-Abt AS, Barrett C, et al. Mechanisms of taurocholate transport in canalicular and basolateral rat liver plasma membrane vesicles: evidence for an electrogenic canalicular organic anion carrier. J Biol Chem 1984;259:10614.

96. Meier PJ, Meier-Abt AS, Boyer JL. Properties of the canalicular bile acid transport system in rat liver. Biochem J 1987;242:465.

97. Alpert S, Mosher M, Shanske A, et al. Multiplicity of hepatic excretory mechanisms for organic anions. J Gen Physiol 1969;53:238.

98. Ruetz S, Fricker G, Hugentobler G, et al. Isolation and characterization of the putative canalicular bile salt transport system of rat liver. J Biol Chem 1987;262:11324.

99. Ruetz S, Hugentobler G, Meier PJ. Functional reconstitution of the canalicular bile salt transport system of rat liver. Proc Natl Acad Sci USA 1988;85:6147.

100. Griffiths JC, Sies H, Meier PJ, et al. Inhibition of taurocholate efflux from rat hepatic canalicular membrane vesicles by glutathione disulfide. FEBS Lett 1987;213:34.

101. Novak DA, Suchy FJ. Postnatal expression of the canalicular bile acid transport system in rat liver (Abstract). Hepatology 1987;7:1037.

102. Kuipers F, Enserink M, Havinga R, et al. Separate transport systems for biliary secretion of sulfated and unsulfated bile acids in the rat. J Clin Invest 1988;81:1593.

103. Fricker G, Landmann L, Meier PJ. Extrahepatic obstructive cholestasis reverses the bile salt secretory polarity of rat hepatocytes. J Clin Invest 1989;84:876.

104. Accatino L, Conteras A, Fernandez S, et al. The effect of complete biliary obstruction on bile flow and bile acid excretion: postcholestatic choleresis in the rat. J Lab Clin Med 1979;93:706.

105. Whitington PF. Cholestasis associated with total parenteral nutrition in infants. Hepatology 1985;5:693.

106. Rooney JC, Hill DJ, Danks DM. Jaundice associated with bacterial infection in the newborn. Am J Dis Child 1971;122:39.

107. Suchy FJ, Courchene SM, Blitzer BL. Taurocholate transport by basolateral plasma membrane vesicles isolated from developing rat liver. Am J Physiol 1985;248:G648.

108. Suchy FJ, Bucuvalas JC, Goodrich AL, et al. Taurocholate transport and Na$^+$-K$^+$-ATPase activity in fetal and neonatal rat liver plasma membrane vesicles. Am J Physiol 1986;251:G665.

109. Stolz A, Sugiyama Y, Kuhlenkamp J, et al. Cytosolic bile acid binding protein in rat liver: radioimmunoassay, molecular forms, developmental characteristics and organ distribution. Hepatology 1986;6:433.

110. Sippel CJ, Ananthanarayanan M, Suchy FJ. Ontogenic expression of the canalicular bile acid transport system (Abstract). Hepatology 1989;10:620.

111. van Dyke RW, Stephens JE, Scharschmidt BF. Effects of ion substitution on bile acid-dependent and independent bile formation by rat liver. J Clin Invest 1982;70:505.

112. Anwer MS, Hegner D. Role of inorganic electrolytes in bile acid independent canalicular bile formation. Am J Physiol 1983;244:G116.

113. Hardison WGM, Wood CA. Importance of bicarbonate in bile salt independent fraction of bile flow. Am J Physiol 1978;235:E158.

114. Schulz I. Bicarbonate transport in the exocrine pancreas. Ann NY Acad Sci 1980;341:191.

115. Arias IM, Forgac M. The sinusoidal domain of the plasma membrane of rat hepatocytes contains an amiloride-sensitive Na$^+$/H$^+$ antiport. J Biol Chem 1984;259:5406.

116. Moseley RH, Meier PJ, Aronson PS, et al. Na–H exchange in rat liver basolateral but not canalicular plasma membrane vesicles. Am J Physiol 1986;250:G35.

117. Meier PJ, Knickelbein R, Moseley RH, et al. Evidence for carrier-mediated chloride:bicarbonate exchange in canalicular rat liver plasma membrane vesicles. J Clin Invest 1985;75:1526.

118. Scharschmidt BF, van Dyke RW. Mechanisms of hepatic electrolyte secretion. Gastroenterology 1983;85:1199.

119. Moseley RH, Boyer JL. Mechanisms of electrolyte transport in the liver and their functional significance. Semin Liver Dis 1985;5:122.

120. Gumucio JJ, Valdivieso V. Studies on the mechanisms of ethinyl estradiol impairment of bile flow and bile salt excretion in the rat. Gastroenterology 1971;61:339.

121. Arias IM, Adachi Y, Tran T. Ethinyl estradiol cholestasis: a disease of the sinusoidal domain of hepatocyte plasma membrane (Abstract). Hepatology 1983;3:872.

122. Kitani K, Kanai S. Effect of ursodeoxycholate on the bile flow in the rat. Life Sci 1982;31:1973.

123. Moseley RH, Ballatori N, Smith DJ, et al. Ursodeoxycholate stimulates Na$^+$:H$^+$ exchange in rat liver basolateral plasma membrane vesicles. J Clin Invest 1987;80:684.

124. Lake JR, van Dyke RW, Scharschmidt BF. Effects of Na$^+$ replacement and amiloride on ursodeoxycholic acid-stimulated choleresis and biliary bicarbonate secretion. Am J Physiol 1987;252:G163.

125. Renner EL, Lake JR, Cragoe EJ, et al. Ursodeoxycholic acid choleresis: relationship to biliary HCO$_3^-$ and effects of Na$^+$-H$^+$ exchange inhibitors. Am J Physiol 1988;254:G232.

126. Garcia-Marin JJ, Dumont M, Corbic M, et al. Effect of acid–base balance and acetazolamide on ursodeoxycholate-induced biliary bicarbonate secretion. Am J Physiol 1985;248:G20.

127. Graf J. Canalicular bile salt-independent bile formation: concepts and clues from electrolyte transport in rat liver. Am J Physiol 1983;244:G233.

128. Klos C, Paumgartner G, Reichen J. Cation–anion gap and choleretic properties of rat bile. Am J Physiol 1979;236:E434.

129. Ballatori N, Jacob R, Boyer JL. Intrabiliary glutathione hydrolysis: a source of glutamate in bile. J Biol Chem 1986;261:7860.

130. Ballatori N, Truong AT, Ma AK, et al. Determinants of glutathione efflux and biliary GSH/GSSG ratio in perfused rat liver. Am J Physiol 1989;256:G482.

131. Inoue M, Kinne R, Tran T, et al. The mechanism of biliary secretion of reduced glutathione: analysis of transport process in isolated rat-liver canalicular membrane vesicles. Eur J Biochem 1983;134:467.

132. Ballatori N, Clarkson TW. Biliary transport of glutathione and methylmercury. Am J Physiol 1983;244:G435.

133. Ballatori N, Clarkson TW. Developmental changes in the biliary excretion of methylmercury and glutathione. Science 1982;216:61.

134. Ballatori N, Truong AT. Relation between biliary glutathione excretion and bile acid-independent bile flow. Am J Physiol 1989;256:G22.

135. Yoon YB, Hagey LR, Hofmann AF, et al. Effect of side-chain shortening on the physiologic properties of bile acids: hepatic transport and effect on biliary secretion of 23-nor-ursodeoxycholate in rodents. Gastroenterology 1986;90:837.

136. Lake JR, Renner EL, Scharschmidt BF, et al. Inhibition of Na$^+$/H$^+$ exchange in the rat is associated with decreased ursodeoxycholate hypercholeresis, decreased secretion of unconjugated ursodeoxycholate, and increased ursodeoxycholate glucuronidation. Gastroenterology 1988;95:454.

137. Gautam A, Ng OC, Strazzabosco M, et al. Quantitative assessment of canalicular bile formation in isolated hepatocyte couplets using microscopic optical planimetry. J Clin Invest 1989;83:565.

138. Gumbiner B. Structure, biochemistry, and assembly of epithelial tight junctions. Am J Physiol 1987;253:C749.

139. Claude P, Goodenough DA. Fracture faces of zonulae occludentes from "tight" and "leaky" epithelia. J Cell Biol 1973;58:390.

140. Friend DS, Gilula NB. Variations in tight and gap junctions in mammalian tissues. J Cell Biol 1972;53:758.

141. LaGarde S, Elias E, Wade JB, et al. Structural heterogeneity of hepatocyte "tight" junctions—a quantitative analysis. Hepatology 1981;1:193.
142. Bradley SE, Herz R. Permselectivity of biliary canalicular membrane in rats: clearance probe analysis. Am J Physiol 1978;235:E570.
143. Cotting J, Zysset T, Reichen J. Biliary obstruction dissipates bioelectric sinusoidal–canalicular barrier without altering taurocholate uptake. Am J Physiol 1989;256:G312.
144. Reichen J, Berr F, Le M, et al. Characterization of calcium deprivation-induced cholestasis in the perfused rat liver. Am J Physiol 1985;249:G48.
145. Forker EL. The effect of estrogen on bile formation in the rat. J Clin Invest 1969;48:654.
146. Reichen J, Le M. Taurocholate, but not taurodehydrocholate, increases biliary permeability to sucrose. Am J Physiol 1983;245:G651.
147. Lowe PJ, Miyai K, Steinbach JH, et al. Hormonal regulation of hepatocyte tight junctional permeability. Am J Physiol 1988;255:G454.
148. Robenek H, Herwig J, Themann H. The morphologic characteristics of intercellular junctions between normal human liver cells and cells from patients with extrahepatic cholestasis. Am J Pathol 1980;100:93.
149. Easter DW, Wade JB, Boyer JL. Structural integrity of hepatocyte tight junctions. J Cell Biol 1983;96:745.
150. Metz J, Aoki A, Merio M, et al. Morphologic alterations and functional changes of interhepatocellular junctions induced by bile duct ligation. Cell Tissue Res 1977;182:229.
151. Stevenson BR, Siliciano JD, Mooseker MS, et al. Identification of ZO-1: a high molecular weight polypeptide associated with the tight junction (zonula occludens) in a variety of epithelia. J Cell Biol 1986;103:755.
152. Anderson JM, Glade JL, Stevenson BR, et al. Hepatic immunohistochemical localization of the tight junction protein ZO-1 in rat models of cholestasis. Am J Pathol 1989;134:1055.
153. Levine WG. Biliary excretion of drugs and other xenobiotics. Prog Drug Res 1981;25:362.
154. Gottesman MM, Pastan I. The multidrug transporter, a double edged sword. J Biol Chem 1988;263:12163.
155. Thiebaut F, Tsuruo T, Hamada H, et al. Cellular localization of the multidrug-resistance gene product P-glycoprotein in normal human tissues. Proc Natl Acad Sci USA 1987;84:7735.
156. Kamimoto K, Gatmaitan Z, Arias IM. The function of Gp170, the multi drug resistance gene product, in bile canaliculi (Abstract). Hepatology 1988;8:1277.
157. Wagner CI, Trotman BW, Soloway RD. Kinetic analysis of biliary lipid excretion in man and dog. J Clin Invest 1976;57:473.
158. Balint JA, Kyriakides EC, Spitzer HL, et al. Lecithin fatty acid composition in bile and plasma of man, dogs, rats, and oxen. J Lipid Res 1965;6:96.
159. Pattinson BR, Chapman BA. Distribution of biliary cholesterol between mixed micelles and nonmicelles in relation to fasting and feeding in humans. Gastroenterology 1986;91:697.
160. Somjen GJ, Gilat T. Changing concepts of cholesterol solubility in bile. Gastroenterology 1986;91:772.
161. Crawford JM, Berken CA, Gollan JL. Role of the hepatocyte microtubular system in the excretion of bile salts and biliary lipid: implications for intracellular vesicular transport. J Lipid Res 1988;29:144.
162. Schwartz CC, Berman M, Vlahcevic ZL, et al. Multicompartmental analysis of cholesterol metabolism in man: characterization of the hepatic bile acid and biliary cholesterol precursor sites. J Clin Invest 1978;61:408.
163. Turley SD, Dietschy JM. The metabolism and excretion of cholesterol by the liver. In: Arias IM, Jakoby WB, Popper H, Schachter D, Shafritz DA, eds. The liver: biology and pathobiology, ed 2. New York: Raven Press, 1988:617.
164. Stone BG, Erickson SK, Craig WY, et al. Regulation of rat biliary cholesterol secretion by agents that alter intrahepatic cholesterol metabolism: evidence for a distinct biliary precursor pool. J Clin Invest 1985;76:1773.
165. Einarsson K, Nilsell K, Leijd B, et al. Influence of age on secretion of cholesterol and synthesis of bile acids by the liver. N Engl J Med 1985;313:277.
166. Vuoristo M, Miettinen TA. Increased biliary lipid secretion in celiac disease. Gastroenterology 1985;88:134.
167. von Bergman K, Mok HYI, Hardison WGM, et al. Cholesterol and bile acid metabolism in moderately advanced stable cirrhosis of the liver. Gastroenterology 1979;77:1183.
168. Kesaniemi YA, Salaspuro MP, Vuorsito M, et al. Biliary lipid secretion in chronic cholestatic liver disease. Gut 1982;23:931.
169. Angelin B, Einarsson K, Ewerth S, et al. Biliary lipid composition in patients with portal cirrhosis of the liver. Scand J Gastroenterol 1980;15:849.
170. Bouchier IAD. Post-mortem study of the frequency of gallstones in patients with portal cirrhosis of the liver. Gut 1969;10:705.
171. Reuben A. Biliary proteins. Hepatology 1984;4:46S.
172. Thomas P, Zamcheck N. Role of the liver in clearance and excretion of circulating carcinoembryonic antigen (CEA). Dig Dis Sci 1983;28:216.
173. Thomas P, Toth CA, Zamcheck N. The mechanism of biliary excretion of α_1-acid glycoprotein in the rat: evidence for a molecular weight-dependent, nonreceptor-mediated pathway. Hepatology 1982;2:800.
174. LaRusso NF. Proteins in bile: how they get there and what they do. Am J Physiol 1984;247:G199.
175. Sewell RB, Mao SJT, Kawamoto T, et al. Apolipoproteins of high, low, and very low density lipoproteins in human bile. J Lipid Res 1983;24:391.
176. Nagura H, Smith PD, Nakane PK, et al. IgA in human bile and liver. J Immunol 1981;126:587.
177. Kakis G, Yousef IM. Protein composition of rat bile. Can J Biochem 1978;56:287.
178. Rappaport AM. The structural and functional unit in the human liver (liver acinus). Anat Rec 1958;130:673.
179. Layden TJ, Boyer JL. Influence of bile acids on bile canalicular morphology and the lobular gradient in canalicular size. Lab Invest 1978;39:110.
180. Jones AL, Hradek GT, Renston RH, et al. Autoradiographic evidence for hepatic lobular concentration gradient of bile acid derivative. Am J Physiol 1980;238:G233.
181. Groothuis GMM, Hardonk MJ, Keulemans KPT, et al. Autoradiographic and kinetic demonstration of acinar heterogeneity of taurocholate transport. Am J Physiol 1982;243:G455.
182. Baumgartner U, Miyai K, Hardison WGM. Greater taurodeoxycholate biotransformation during backward perfusion of rat liver. Am J Physiol 1986;251:G431.
183. Redick JA, Jakoby WB, Baron J. Immunohistochemical localization of glutathione S-transferases in livers of untreated rats. J Biol Chem 1982;257:15200.
184. Gumucio JJ, Balabaud C, Miller DL, et al. Bile secretion and liver cell heterogeneity in the rat. J Lab Clin Med 1978;91:350.
185. Strasberg SM, Petrunka CN, Ilson RG. The contribution of the extrahepatic bile ducts to bile formation. Can J Physiol Pharmacol 1976;54:757.
186. Chenderovitch J. Secretory function of the rabbit common bile duct. Am J Physiol 1972;223:695.
187. Wheeler HO, Mancusi-Ungaro PL. Role of bile ducts during secretin choleresis in dogs. Am J Physiol 1966;210:1153.
188. Nahrwold DL, Shariatzedeh AN. Role of the common bile duct in formation of bile and in gastrin-induced choleresis. Surgery 1971;70:147.
189. Kaminsky DL, Dorighi J, Jellinek M. Effect of electrical vagal stimulation on canine hepatic blood flow. Am J Physiol 1974;227:487.
190. Alpini G, Lenzi R, Sarkozi L, et al. Biliary physiology in rats with bile ductular cell hyperplasia: evidence for a secretory function of proliferated bile ductules. J Clin Invest 1988;81:569.
191. Lenthall J, Reynolds TB, Donovan AJ. Excessive output of bile in chronic hepatic disease. Surg Gynecol Obstet 1970;130:243.
192. Turnberg LA, Jones EA, Sherlock S. Biliary secretion in a patient with cystic duct dilatation of the intrahepatic biliary tree. Gastroenterology 1968;54:1155.
193. Nyberg B, Einarsson K, Sonnenfeld T. Evidence that vasoactive intestinal peptide induces ductular secretion of bile in humans. Gastroenterology 1989;96:920.
194. Lewis MH, Baker AL, Ipp E, et al. Effect of somatostatin on de-

terminants of bile flow in unanesthetized dogs. Ann Surg 1982;195: 97.

195. Rene E, Danzinger RG, Hofmann AF, et al. Pharmacologic effect of somatostatin on bile formation in the dog: enhanced ductular reabsorption as the major mechanism of anticholeresis. Gastroenterology 1983;84:120.

196. Magnusson I, Einarsson K, Angelin B, et al. Effects of somatostatin on hepatic bile formation. Gastroenterology 1989;96:206.

197. Rose RC. Absorptive functions of the gallbladder. In: Johnson LR, ed. Physiology of the gastrointestinal tract, ed 2. New York: Raven Press, 1987;1455.

198. Ericson A-C, Spring KR. Coupled NaCl entry into *Necturus* gallbladder epithelial cells. Am J Physiol 1982;243:C140.

199. Larson M, Spring KR. Bumetanide inhibition of NaCl transport by *Necturus* gallbladder. J Membr Biol 1983;74:123.

200. Reuss L, Costantin JL. Cl$^-$/HCO$_3$ exchange at the apical membrane of *Necturus* gallbladder. J Gen Physiol 1984;83:801.

201. Weinman SA, Reuss L. Na$^+$–H$^+$ exchange and Na$^+$ entry across the apical membrane of *Necturus* gallbladder. J Gen Physiol 1984;83: 57.

202. Petersen K-U, Wood JR, Schulze G, et al. Stimulation of gallbladder fluid and electrolyte absorption by butyrate. J Membr Biol 1981;62: 183.

203. Dietschy JM. Water and solute movement across the wall of the everted rabbit gallbladder. Gastroenterology 1964;47:395.

204. Sundler F, Alumets J, Hakanson R, et al. VIP innervation of the gallbladder. Gastroenterology 1977;72:1375.

205. Jansson R, Steen G, Svanvik J. Effects of intravenous vasoactive intestinal peptide (VIP) on gallbladder function in the cat. Gastroenterology 1978;75:47.

206. Donowitz M, Tai Y-H, Asarkof N. Effect of serotonin on active electrolyte transport in rabbit ileum, gallbladder, and colon. Am J Physiol 1980;239:G463.

207. Bjorck S, Jansson R, Svanvik J. Adrenergic influence on concentrating function in the feline gallbladder. Gut 1982;23:1019.

208. Mirkovitch V, Sepulveda F, Menge H, et al. Active amino-acid and sugar uptake by gall bladder epithelium in dog, guinea-pig and man. Pflugers Arch 1975;355:319.

209. Ostrow JD. Absorption by the gallbladder of bile salts, sulfobromophthalein, and iodipamide. J Lab Clin Med 1969;74:482.

210. Ostrow JD. Absorption of organic compounds by the injured gallbladder. J Lab Clin Med 1971;78:255.

211. Neiderhiser D, Harmon C, Roth H. Absorption of cholesterol by the gallbladder. J Lipid Res 1976;17:117.

212. Wahlin T, Bloom GD, Carlsoo B. Histochemical observations with the light and the electron microscope on the mucosubstances of the normal mouse gallbladder epithelial cells. Histochemistry 1974;42: 119.

213. Lee SP, LaMont JT, Carey MC. The role of gallbladder mucus hypersecretion in the evolution of cholesterol gallstones: studies in the prairie dog. J Clin Invest 1981;67:1712.

214. Lee SP. Hypersecretion of mucus glycoprotein by the gallbladder epithelium in experimental cholelithiasis. J Pathol 1981;134:199.

215. Smith BF, LaMont JT. Bovine gallbladder mucin binds bilirubin in vitro. Gastroenterology 1983;85:707.

216. Paumgartner G. Serum bile acids: physiological determinants and results in liver disease. J Hepatology 1986;2:291.

217. Porter HP, Saunders DR, Tytgat G, et al. Fat absorption in bile fistula man. Gastroenterology 1971;60:1008.

218. Wilson FA. Intestinal transport of bile acids. Am J Physiol 1981;241: G83.

219. Kramer W, Burckhardt G, Wilson FA, et al. Bile salt-binding polypeptides in brush-border membrane vesicles from rat small intestine revealed by photoaffinity labeling. J Biol Chem 1983;258:3623.

220. de Belle RC, Vaupshas V, Vitullo BB, et al. Intestinal absorption of bile salts; immature development in the neonate. J Pediatr 1979;94: 472.

221. Watkins JB, Szczepanik P, Gould JB, et al. Bile salt metabolism in the human premature infant. Gastroenterology 1975;69:706.

222. Little JM, Lester R. Ontogenesis of intestinal bile salt absorption in the neonatal rat. Am J Physiol 1980;239:G319.

223. Barnard JA, Ghishan FK. Methylprednisolone accelerates the ontogeny of sodium–taurocholate cotransport in rat ileal brush border membranes. J Lab Clin Med 1986;108:549.

224. Weinberg SL, Burckhardt G, Wilson FA. Taurocholate transport by rat intestinal basolateral membrane vesicles: evidence for the presence of an anion exchange transport system. J Clin Invest 1986;78:44.

225. Lin MC, Weinberg SL, Kramer W, et al. Identification and comparison of bile acid-binding polypeptides in ileal basolateral membrane. J Membrane Biol 1988;106:1.

226. Ahlberg J, Angelin B, Bjorkhem I, et al. Individual bile acids in portal venous and systemic blood serum of fasting man. Gastroenterology 1977;73:1377.

227. Kramer W, Buscher H-P, Gerok W, et al. Bile salt binding to serum components: taurocholate incorporation into high-density lipoproteins revealed by photoaffinity labeling. Eur J Biochem 1979;102:1.

228. Cowen AE, Korman MG, Hofmann AF, et al. Metabolism of lithocholate in healthy man. I. Biotransformation and biliary excretion of intravenously administered lithocholate, lithocholylglycine, and their sulfates. Gastroenterology 1975;69:59.

229. Cowen AE, Korman MG, Hofmann AF, et al. Metabolism of lithocholate in healthy man. II. Enterohepatic circulation. Gastroenterology 1975;69:67.

230. Schwenk M, Hofmann AF, Carlson GL, et al. Bile acid conjugation in the chimpanzee: effective sulfation of lithocholic acid. Arch Toxicol 1978;40:109.

231. Hofmann AF, Lachin JM. Biliary bile acid composition and cholesterol saturation. Gastroenterology 1983;84:1075.

232. Reichen J, Simon FR. Cholestasis. In: Arias IM, Jakoby WB, Popper H, Schachter D, Shafritz DA, eds. The liver: biology and pathobiology, ed 2. New York: Raven Press, 1988:1105.

233. Duffy MC, Boyer JL. Pathophysiology of intrahepatic cholestasis and biliary obstruction. In: Ostrow JD, ed. Bilirubin, bile pigments and jaundice. New York: Marcel Dekker, 1986:333

234. Philips MJ, Poucell S, Oda M. Biology of disease: mechanisms of cholestasis. Lab Invest 1986;54:593.

235. Stiehl A, Ast E, Czygan P, et al. Pool size, synthesis, and turnover of sulfated and nonsulfated cholic acid and chenodeoxycholic acid in patients with cirrhosis of the liver. Gastroenterology 1978;74:572.

236. Chadwick VS, Gaginella TS, Carlson GL, et al. Effect of molecular structure on bile acid-induced alterations in absorptive function, permeability, and morphology in the perfused rabbit colon. J Lab Clin Med 1979;94:661.

237. McJunkin B, Fromm H, Sarva RP. Factors in the mechanism of diarrhea in bile acid malabsorption: fecal pH—a key determinant. Gastroenterology 1981;80:1454.

238. Binder HJ, Sandle GI. Electrolyte absorption and secretion in the mammalian colon. In: Johnson LR, ed. Physiology of the gastrointestinal tract, ed 2. New York: Raven Press, 1987:1389.

239. Hofmann AF, Poley JR. Cholestyramine treatment of diarrhea associated with ileal resection: factors influencing response. N Engl J Med 1969;281:397.

240. Dowling RH, Rose GA, Sutor DJ. Hyperoxaluria and renal calculi in ileal disease. Lancet 1971;1:1103.

241. Heaton KW, Read AE. Gallstones in patients with disorders of the terminal ileum and disturbed bile salt metabolism. Br Med J 1969;3: 494.

242. Thaysen EH, Pedersen L. Idiopathic bile acid catharsis. Gut 1976;17: 965.

243. Thaysen EH. Idiopathic bile acid diarrhea reconsidered. Scand J Gastroenterol 1985;20:452.

244. Popovic OS, Kostic KM, Milovic VB, et al. Primary bile acid malabsorption: histologic and immunologic study in three patients. Gastroenterology 1987;92:1851.

245. Sciarretta G, Vicini G, Fagioli G, et al. Use of 23-selena-25-homocholyltaurine to detect bile acid malabsorption in patients with ileal dysfunction or diarrhea. Gastroenterology 1986;91:1.

246. Heubi JE, Balistreri WF, Fondacaro JD, et al. Primary bile acid malabsorption: defective in vitro ileal active bile acid transport. Gastroenterology 1982;83:804.

247. Jonas A, Arigad S, Diver-Haber A, et al. Disturbed fat absorption following infectious gastroenteritis in children. J Pediatr 1979;95: 366.

248. Go VLW, Poley JR, Hofmann AF, et al. The disturbances of fat digestion induced by acid jejunal pH due to gastric hypersecretion in man. Gastroenterology 1970;58:638.

249. Regan PT, Malagelada J-R, DiMagno EP, et al. Reduced intraluminal bile acid concentrations and fat maldigestion in pancreatic insufficiency: correction by treatment. Gastroenterology 1979;77:285.

250. Setchell KDR, Harrison DL, Gilbert JM, et al. Serum unconjugated bile acids: qualitative and quantitative profiles in ileal resection and bacterial overgrowth. Clin Chim Acta 1985;152:297.

251. Thaysen EH. Diagnostic value of the ^{14}C-choylglycine breath test. Clin Gastroenterol 1977;6:227.

252. Dutta SK, Anand K, Gadacz TR. Bile salt malabsorption in pancreatic insufficiency secondary to alcoholic pancreatitis. Gastroenterology 1986;91:1243.

253. Watkins JG, Tereyak AM, Szcepanik P, et al. Bile salt kinetics in cystic fibrosis: influence of pancreatic enzyme replacement. Gastroenterology 1977;73:1023.

254. Birkner HJ, Kern F. In vitro adsorption of bile salts to food residues, salicylazosulphapyridine and hemicellulose. Gastroenterology 1974;67:237.

255. Hardison WGM, Tomaszewski N, Grundy SM. Effect of acute alterations in small bowel transit time upon the biliary excretion rate of bile acids. Gastroenterology 1979;76:568.

256. Calam J, Ellis A, Dockray G. Identification and measurement of molecular variants of cholecystokinin in duodenal mucosa and plasma: diminished concentrations in patients with celiac disease. J Clin Invest 1982;69:218.

257. Maton PN, Selden AC, Fitzpatrick ML, et al. Defective gallbladder emptying and cholecystokinin release in celiac disease: reversal by gluten-free diet. Gastroenterology 1985;88:391.

258. Low-Beer TS, Heaton KW, Pomare EN, et al. The effect of coeliac disease upon bile salts. Gut 1973;14:204.

259. Krejs GJ, Orci L, Conlon JM, et al. Somatostatinoma syndrome: biochemical, morphologic and clinical features. N Engl J Med 1979;301:285.

260. Almond HR, Vlahcevic ZR, Bell PCC, et al. Bile acid pools, kinetics and biliary lipid composition before and after cholecystectomy. N Engl J Med 1973;289:1213.

261. Fromm H, Tunuguntla AK, Malavolti M, et al. Absence of significant role of bile acids in diarrhea of a heterogeneous group of postcholecystectomy patients. Dig Dis Sci 1987;32:33.

262. Dowling RH, Mack E, Small DM. Effects of controlled interruption of the enterohepatic circulation of bile salts by biliary diversion and by ileal resection on bile salt secretion, synthesis, and pool size in the rhesus monkey. J Clin Invest 1970;49:232.

263. Vlahcevic ZR, Buhac I, Farrar JT, et al. Bile acid metabolism in patients with cirrhosis. I. Kinetic aspects of cholic acid metabolism. Gastroenterology 1971;60:491.

264. Patterson TE, Vlahcevic ZR, Schwartz CC, et al. Bile acid metabolism in cirrhosis. VI. Sites of blockage in the bile acid pathways to primary bile acids. Gastroenterology 1980;79:620.

265. Knodell RG, Kinsey MD, Boedeker EC, et al. Deoxycholate metabolism in alcoholic cirrhosis. Gastroenterology 1976;71:196.

266. Berginer VM, Salen G, Shefer S. Long-term treatment of cerebrotendinous xanthomatosis with chenodeoxycholic acid. N Engl J Med 1984;311:1649.

267. Oftebro H, Bjorkhem I, Stormer FC, et al. Cerebrotendinous xanthomatosis: defective liver mitochondrial hydroxylation of chenodeoxycholic acid precursors. J Lipid Res 1981;22:632.

268. Hosita T, Yasuhara M, Une M, et al. Occurrence of bile alcohol glucuronides in bile of a patient with cerebrotendinous xanthomatosis. J Lipid Res 1980;21:1015.

269. Bowen P, Lee CSN, Zellweger H, et al. A familial syndrome of multiple congenital defects. Bull Johns Hopkins Hosp 1964;114:402.

270. Goldfischer S, Moore CL, Johnson AB, et al. Peroxisomal and mitochondrial defects in the cerebro-hepato-renal syndrome. Science 1973;182:62.

271. Moser AE, Singh I, Brown FR, et al. The cerebrohepatorenal (Zellweger) syndrome: increased levels and impaired degradation of very-long-chain fatty acids and their use in prenatal diagnosis. N Engl J Med 1984;310:1141.

272. Horn T, Christoffersen P, Henriksen JH. Alcoholic liver injury: defenestration in noncirrhotic livers—a scanning electron microscopic study. Hepatology 1987;7:77.

273. Orrego H, Medline A, Blendis LM, et al. Collagenization of the Disse space in alcoholic liver disease. Gut 1979;20:673.

D. NUTRITION

17

Carbohydrate Assimilation

WARD A. OLSEN
MARK L. LLOYD

Within the past few years the techniques of modern cell and molecular biology have been applied to study the mechanisms responsible for intestinal carbohydrate digestion and absorption. As a consequence of these studies, our knowledge of these processes has grown substantially in a very short time. In this chapter carbohydrate assimilation is reviewed and recent advances are highlighted. The carbohydrates in the human diet, the mechanisms of their digestion and absorption, and the enzyme and transport proteins responsible for these processes are discussed. Finally some well-characterized examples of alterations in carbohydrate digestion and absorption are presented.

DIETARY CARBOHYDRATE

Carbohydrate is the major source of calories in the human diet, accounting for some 1700 kcal/d. Total carbohydrate intake is similar in different populations, although there are regional differences in the type of carbohydrate ingested, especially in the proportions of starch and sucrose. More starch is consumed in underdeveloped countries than in developed countries where sucrose replaces a considerable portion of starch calories.[1] Lactose is the third major source of dietary carbohydrate, with age-related as well as geographic differences in intake.

Starch is the form in which carbohydrate is stored in plants, with cereal grains and roots serving as the usual dietary source. It is stored within the cell walls of plants as a mixture of two very large polymers of glucose—amylose and amylopectin in roughly a 1:3 ratio. Table 17-1 is a list of some common sources of starch. The molecular size of amylose ranges between 100 and 1000 kd, and the structure consists of straight chains of glucose molecules joined in α-1,4 linkages; that is, the first carbon of one glucose is joined to the fourth carbon of the next glucose. Amylopectin is the larger (100-fold on the average) and more complex molecule (Fig 17-1). It consists of chains of α-1,4-linked glucoses that branch at approximately every 25 glucose residues. The branching chains are attached by α-1,6 linkages, as shown in the figure. Glycogen is the equivalent of amylose in animals, but it is not an important substrate for intraluminal digestion because the polymer has largely been converted to glucose before ingestion. A variety of starch hydrolysates containing oligosaccharides of varying lengths are produced and used in enteral diet formulations and as sweeteners in processed foods.

Sucrose, ordinary table sugar, is a disaccharide consisting of glucose joined to fructose in an α-1,2 linkage. Sucrose is largely purified from sugar cane and the sugar beet and consumed in varying amounts as a sweetening agent. Lactose, a disaccharide with galactose joined to glucose in β-1,4 linkage, is the sugar of milk and provides an important source of calories for the suckling animal and for many humans beyond the age of infancy. Lactose is present in ice creams and many milk-derived foods such as cheese. It is also frequently added to processed foods.

A variety of carbohydrate polymers, usually structural components of plants, contain bonds that cannot be hydrolyzed by pancreatic or intestinal carbohydrases and consequently cannot be absorbed. They can, however, be hydrolyzed to varying extent by enzymes of colonic bacteria as discussed in Chapter 72. These together with related noncarbohydrate polymers (principally lignin) constitute "dietary fiber." In industrialized societies, dietary fiber is largely removed in the processing of food, whereas in underdeveloped societies substantial amounts of dietary fiber may be consumed. Fiber may have a variety of physiologic effects, some of which may be beneficial. Foods containing higher amounts of dietary fiber are increasingly popular in Western countries for a variety of reasons, which range from management of constipation to prevention of cancer. The relationship of dietary fiber to human disease is an area that requires further study. Table 17-2 is a summary of the major constituents of dietary fiber and the degree to which they can be metabolized by colonic bacteria.

Several smaller carbohydrates (oligosaccharides) are indigestible also. Some like stachyose and raffinose are present in common foods such as beans and other legumes. Because they are readily metabolized by colonic bacteria they may cause increased flatus and loose stools. Other oligosaccharides such as lactulose and lactitol are used therapeutically as treatment for hepatic encephalopathy and constipation.

Cereal Products

Prepared breakfast foods

Grits

Rice

Breads

Bread

Crackers

Pasta

Tortillas

Pancakes

Waffles

Starchy Vegetables

Corn

Potatoes

Peas

Navy beans

Lentils

INTRALUMINAL DIGESTION OF STARCH

Since the small intestine is not capable of transporting carbohydrates more complex than monosaccharides, dietary disaccharides and polysaccharides must be cleaved to monomeric form. While oligosaccharides and disaccharides are directly hydrolyzed by membrane-bound enzymes of the enterocyte, starch is first digested by secreted amylase to products more appropriate for brush-border enzymes.

Synthesis and Secretion of Amylase

Proteins with α-amylase activity are secreted by both salivary gland and pancreatic tissue. The amylases from the two organs differ somewhat in molecular size (54.5 kd for human pancreatic enzyme and 56 kd for human salivary enzyme)[2] but are closely related. Both appear to be synthesized with cleavable signal sequences, and the two proteins are 94% homologous when the structures predicted by nucleotide sequencing of cDNAs are compared.[3] Although salivary amylase is probably not important in starch digestion in health, it has been suggested that it may be important in patients with pancreatic insufficiency and possibly also during the first year of life when secretion of pancreatic amylase may be limited.[4] Although free salivary amylase is inactivated by the acid pH of the stomach, the presence of starch substrate and hydrolytic products seems to protect the active site of the enzyme until the safety of the more neutral pH of the intestine is reached.[5] Amylase synthesis and secretion are under control by complex neural and hormonal mechanisms that are regulated by food ingestion (see chs 12 and 15).

Starch Hydrolysis

Pancreatic and salivary amylases are potent endoglucosidases and readily attack the internal α-1,4 bonds of both amylose and amylopectin, but the α-1,6 bonds of amylopectin are resistant. The external α-1,4 bonds and those that are adjacent to the α-1,6 bonds are also resistant. Thus, as shown in Figure 17-1, amylose can be cleaved to generate the disaccharide maltose and the trisaccharide maltotriose. Little glucose is generated, however, because of the resistance of the external bonds. Amylopectin is cleaved to maltose and maltotriose but also to a group of branching oligosaccharides of varying size (averaging between 5 and 10 glucose residues) called the α-limit dextrins. Although it has been suggested that pancreatic amylase adsorbed to the intestinal surface is important in starch hydrolysis,[6] it is clear that the concentration of the enzyme

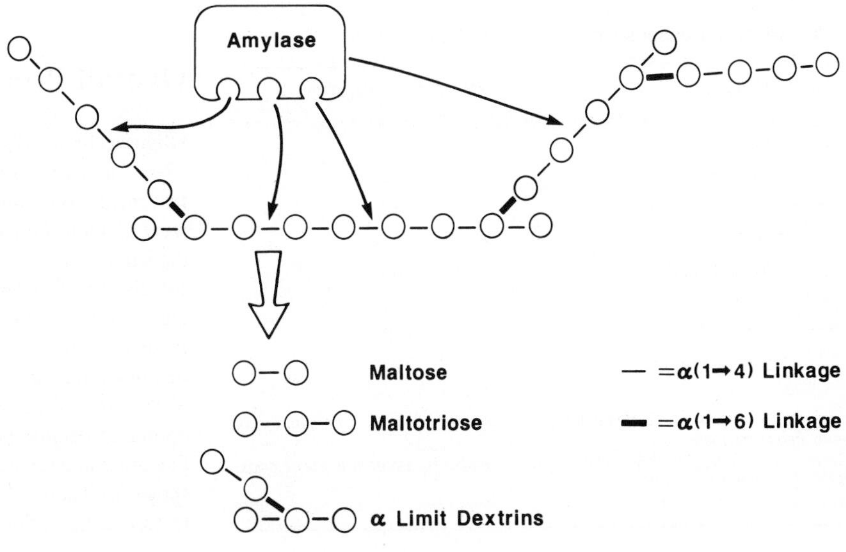

FIGURE 17–1. Amylopectin digestion. The arrows indicate bonds susceptible to cleavage by salivary and pancreatic amylase.

TABLE 17–2
Dietary Fiber

FIBER	STRUCTURE	COLONIC METABOLISM
Cellulose	Glucose polymer (β-1,4 linked)	Moderate
Hemicelluloses	β-1,4-linked sugars (mannose, galactose especially)	Moderate
Lignins	Aromatic polymers (not carbohydrate)	None
Pectins	Galacturonic acid polymers	Extensive
Gums/mucilages	Complex polysaccharides containing galactose, mannose, glucuronic acid, and other sugars	Extensive

in luminal fluid is more than sufficient to hydrolyze dietary starch in humans.[7,8] Intubation studies in volunteers given a test meal containing soluble starch suggest rapid hydrolysis with much of the process complete in the proximal intestine.[7,8] Surprisingly, however, the starch in ordinary meals may be digested much more slowly with great differences from food to food. When different foods, each containing similar amounts of carbohydrate, are fed, the blood glucose response varies widely, as indicated in Table 17-3, presumably because of differences in the rates of starch hydrolysis. Indeed, measurements of breath hydrogen excretion and ileal contents after test meals confirm differences in assimilation of starch from different sources and suggest that 2% to 20% of dietary starch is malabsorbed in healthy persons.[9,10] The reasons for the varying bioavailability of dietary starch are incompletely understood.[11] Clearly processing and preparation of food is important as removal of plant cell wall (fiber), processing to smaller particles, and boiling (by breaking plant cell walls) all increase the availability of starch.[11] In addition, the protein content of food may affect the availability of its starch. Amylase inhibitors in plants have been identified, and these substances may conceivably limit hydrolysis of starch from certain foods.[11,12] The protein fraction of certain grains (gluten) also seems to inhibit absorption of the carbohydrate of bread[9] for reasons that are not yet clear.

TABLE 17–3
Blood Glucose Response to 50 Grams of Carbohydrate

FOOD	GLYCEMIC INDEX*
Glucose	100
Cornflakes	80
Instant potatoes	80
Rice	72
White bread	69
Corn	59
Oatmeal	49
Kidney beans	29

* *Glycemic index is area under the 2-hour glucose curve as a percentage of response to glucose.*
Data from Jenkins DJA, Wolwer TMS, Taylor RH, Barber H. Glycemic index of foods. Am J Clin Nutr 1981;34:362.

BRUSH-BORDER DIGESTION

Subsequent digestion of the hydrolytic products of starch (maltose, maltotriose, and α-limit dextrins) as well as sucrose and lactose occurs on the brush-border membrane of the mature enterocyte. This membrane is a highly specialized organelle with the appropriate hydrolytic enzymes in proximity to transport mechanisms for the monosaccharide products of hydrolysis. This proximity may help to ensure maximal rates of absorption of released monosaccharides.[13] The brush-border hydrolases are large, heavily glycosylated proteins with 30% to 40% of the mass of the human proteins accounted for by carbohydrate chains.[14] The biologic role of the carbohydrate chains remains uncertain. As shown in Figure 17-2, the hydrolases are anchored to the lipid core of the brush-border membrane, usually via a sequence of hydrophobic amino acids embedded in the membrane. This anchor segment appears to cross the membrane only once and is the only intracellular portion of the peptide. The segment is connected via a 2.5- to 5-nm stalk to globular domains containing the active sites.[15] The globular domains have been visualized by electron microscopy and resemble pairs of lollipops or dumbbells stuck onto the membrane surface.[16,17] These and other studies suggest that brush-border hydrolases are generally organized in the brush-border membrane in homodimeric form, that is, they exist in pairs, each attached to the membrane, as illustrated in Figure 17-2.

Overall Process

Oligosaccharide digestion is summarized in Tables 17-4 through 17-6. These processes occur relatively rapidly, and studies in which test meals containing soluble starch, sucrose, maltose, or lactose were given to human volunteers indicate that most carbohydrate digestion and absorption has occurred before the meal has reached the distal half of small intestine.[7,18] Table 17-6 shows the specific enzymatic activities of the major carbohydrases in homogenates from proximal human intestinal biopsy specimens.[19] The table demonstrates that lactase activity is considerably lower than that of the other disaccharidases even in a population in which developmental decline in lactase is uncommon. Most adult humans, like other mammals, have substantially lower levels of lactase than shown in Table 17-6, and hydrolysis is the rate-limiting step in lactose assimilation.[20] It is interesting that glucose, the major

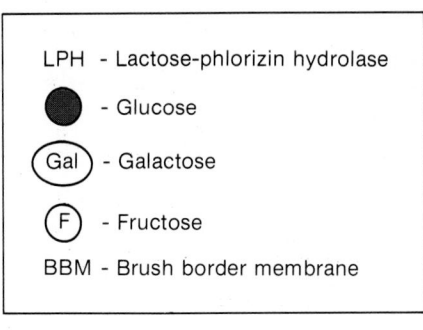

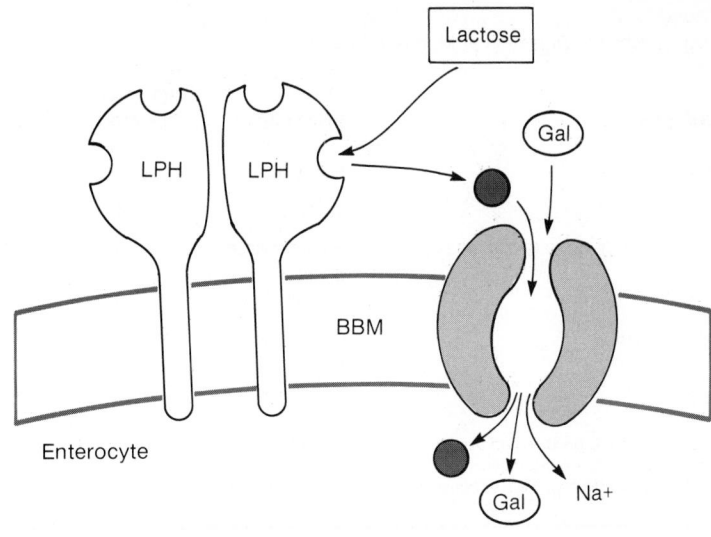

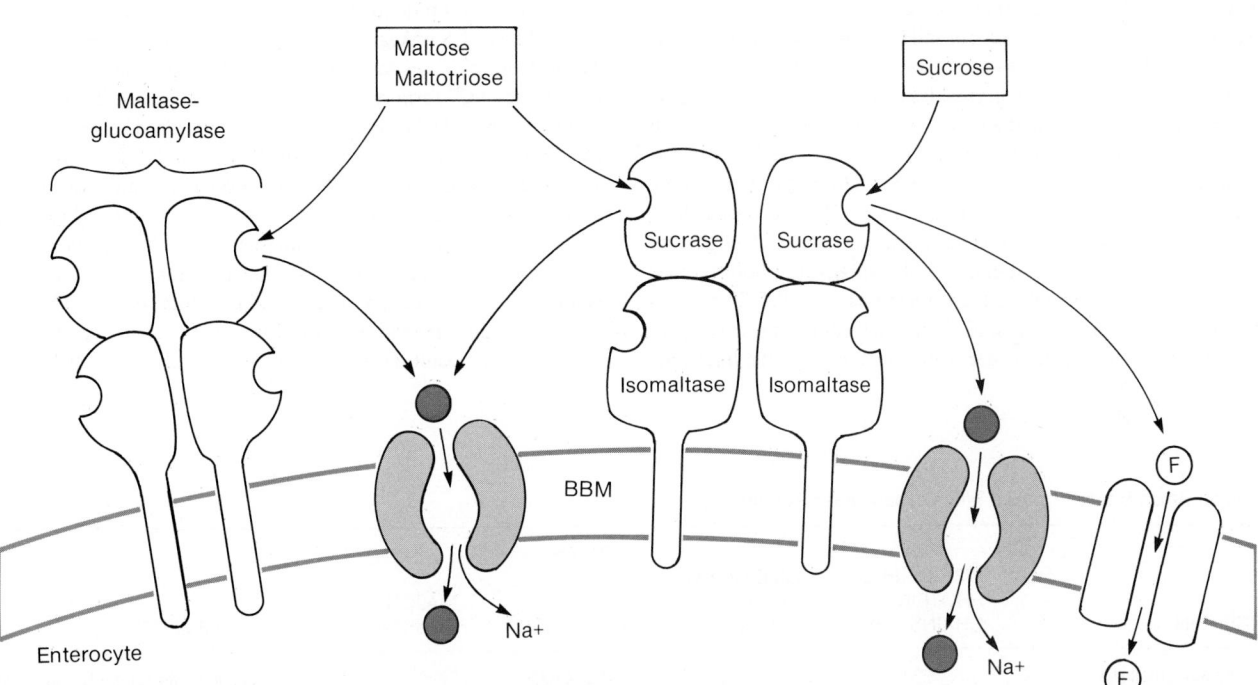

FIGURE 17–2. Brush-border carbohydrases. The upper panel illustrates the hydrolysis of lactase by lactase-phlorizin hydrolase and the uptake of the monosaccharide products by the sodium/glucose co-transporter. The lower panel illustrates the hydrolysis of maltose and maltotriose by one of the two similar active sites of maltase-glucoamylase and sucrose by the sucrase site of sucrase-isomaltase. Monosaccharide product transport is via the co-transporter and the fructose transporter.

product of oligosaccharide hydrolysis, inhibits lactose hydrolysis (end-product inhibition).[21] Thus, lactose malabsorption from slow hydrolysis is very common. Sucrose, on the other hand, is hydrolyzed faster than absorption of its monosaccharide products, especially fructose, can occur, and monosaccharide absorption occurs as rapidly from sucrose as from an equivalent glucose/fructose mixture.[22] Thus, product absorption, not hydrolysis, is the rate-limiting step in sucrose assimilation and monosaccharides, particularly fructose, accumulate within the intestinal lumen in segmental perfusion studies with sucrose in human volunteers.[22] Hydrolysis of glucose oligosaccharides also occurs more rapidly than product absorption,[20] and glucose can be readily found within the intestinal lumen after a starch meal,[7,23] an observation that cannot be accounted for by the action of amylase on starch.

TABLE 17–4

Oligosaccharide Digestion at Mucosal Surface

SUBSTRATE	ENZYMES	BONDS CLEAVED*	K_m (mM)	PRODUCTS
Sucrose	Sucrase	Glcα1-2Fru	20	Glucose, fructose
Lactose	Lactase	Galβ1-4Glc	18	Glucose, galactose
Linear α-1,4 glucose oligomers (G$_{2-9}$)†	Glucoamylase Sucrase Isomaltase	Glcα1-4Glc	1–4	Glucose
α-Limit dextrins	Glucoamylase Sucrase	Glcα1-4Glc	1–4	Glucose, oligosaccharide with terminal α1,6-linked glucose
	Isomaltase	Glcα1-6Glc	5–11	Glucose, maltotriose

* Glycosidic linkage indicated using the following convention: Glc = glucose, Fru = fructose, Gal = galactose; numbers indicate carbon atoms involved in the bond, and α or β indicate the configuration.
† (G$_{2-9}$) indicates oligomers of between 2 and 9 glucose residues.

As indicated in Table 17-4, lactose and sucrose are cleaved by single enzymes—lactase and the sucrase subunit of sucrase-isomaltase. The hydrolytic products are the glucose and galactose moieties of lactose and the glucose and fructose moieties of sucrose. Hydrolysis of the products of amylase digestion of starch can be catalyzed by the several α-glycosidases of the brush border: glucoamylase, isomaltase, and sucrase; and the contribution of each enzyme is not yet completely clear. The process begins with the sequential cleavage of α-1,4 linked glucoses from the nonreducing end of the dextrins, as shown in Figure 17-3. Glucoamylase, which has maximal activity for oligomers containing between 5–9 glucose residues,[24] may play a predominate role initially, but both sucrase and isomaltase will catalyze these reactions as well.[25] The α-1,4 glucose oligomers in processed foods or formulas are also good substrates for the brush-border α-glucosidases, but the high-mo-

lecular-weight polymers of starch are not. A glucosidase that hydrolyzes α-limit dextrins has been purified from pig intestine[26,27] and named α-limit dextrinase, but it may very well be glucoamylase.[28] The α-1,6 linkages of α-limit dextrins resist cleavage until the adjacent glucoses in 1,4 linkages at the nonreducing end have been removed,[25] forming the tetrasaccharide shown in Figure 17-3. The α-1,6–linked residue must then be removed before digestion can continue. Isomaltase will hydrolyze α-1,6 bonds as well as α-1,4 bonds and appears crucial in digestion of the tetrasaccharide,[25] although glucoamylase does possess at least some ability to cleave α-1,6 bonds.[24,29] It should be pointed out that although isomaltase will hydrolyze isomaltose in a test tube and thus acquired its name, isomaltose is not encountered in the intestinal lumen. The maltotriose product is readily cleaved by either sucrase or glucoamylase, and the resultant maltose can be hydrolyzed by any one of

TABLE 17–5

Human Brush-Border Proteins With Carbohydrase Activity

PROTEIN	SIZE OF PRO-PROTEIN CHAINS (kd)	SIZE OF BB PROTEIN CHAINS (kd)	SITE OF PRO-PROTEIN CLEAVAGE	MAJOR SUBSTRATES	COMMENTS
Sucrase-isomaltase	231		Extracellular		Active site on each chain; size estimates from reference 72; size estimates vary between laboratories
Sucrase		145		Sucrose	
Isomaltase		151		α-Limit dextrins	
Lactase-phlorizin hydrolase	215	160	Intracellular		Single chain contains both sites (reference 45)
Lactase				Lactose	
Phlorizin hydrolase				Glycosylceramides	
Glucoamylase	335	335	None	α-1,4-Linked glucose oligomers	Single chain contains two sites with similar specificities; pro-protein cleaved in some species
Trehalase		75 (in rabbit)	Undetermined	Trehalose	Studies done with rabbit not human protein

TABLE 17–6
Carbohydrase Activity in Human Intestinal Biopsy Specimens

ENZYME	SPECIFIC ACTIVITY (units/g protein)	
	Mean	Standard Error of Mean
Sucrase	49	3.5
Isomaltase	64	4.4
Total maltase	179	11.0
Lactase	29	2

One unit of enzymatic activity hydrolyzes 1 μmol of substrate per minute under standard assay conditions. Lactase activity in these subjects was higher than in many other adult populations: the population studied was Danish, and none of the subjects had the relatively low lactase levels found in most adult humans and other mammals.
Data from Asp N-G, Gudmand-Hoyer E, Andersen B, et al. Distribution of disaccharidases, alkaline phosphatase, and some intracellular enzymes along the human small intestine. Scand J Gastroenterol 1975;10:745.

the α-glucosidases, especially sucrase and glucoamylase.[24,25] The maltotriose and maltose derived from initial starch digestion by amylase are handled in a similar way.

Brush-Border Carbohydrases

Sucrase-isomaltase is, by far, the best studied disaccharidase. The protein and its mRNA are present throughout the small intestine, although in reduced amounts in the distal ileum and not at all in colon or stomach.[30] Studies suggest that the sucrase-isomaltase gene is closely related to the gene coding for a lysosomal α-glucosidase, which shares considerable homology with sucrase-isomaltase.[31,32] Surprisingly, the lysosomal glucosidase has been demonstrated in enterocyte brush border by immunocytochemistry,[33] but a physiologic role in carbohydrate assimilation seems doubtful. Sucrase-isomaltase consists of two peptide chains, one of which contains the sucrase catalytic site, the other the isomaltase site. Sucrase will not only hydrolyze sucrose but also sequentially cleave glucoses from the nonreducing end of glucose oligosaccharides linked by α-1,4 bonds, including maltose, maltotriose, and α-limit dextrins.[25] Sucrase does not cleave the α-1,6 bonds of isomaltose, however. Although isomaltase shares much of the substrate specificity of sucrase, including the ability to cleave maltose and maltotriose and to remove glucoses from the nonreducing ends of α-limit dextrins, it will not cleave sucrose. It is essential, however, in the cleavage of the α-1,6 bond. From studies with sucrase-isomaltase and its separated sucrase and isomaltase components, Gray and colleagues have concluded that sucrase and isomaltase have differing specificities for α-limit dextrins of varying size and that both enzymes participate in complementary fashion in the hydrolysis of α-limit dextrins.[25]

In addition to substrate specificity, the enzymes share a number of other characteristics suggesting that they are closely related. These characteristics include sodium activation of both enzymes[34] and considerable overlap in inhibitor specificities.[35] The enzymatic mechanisms for both are also similar. Concomitant with hydrolysis of disaccharide, both generate small amounts of oligosaccharides (transglycosylation), which are ultimately cleaved.[36] Kinetic analyses of both enzymes have demonstrated a ping-pong bi-bi (two

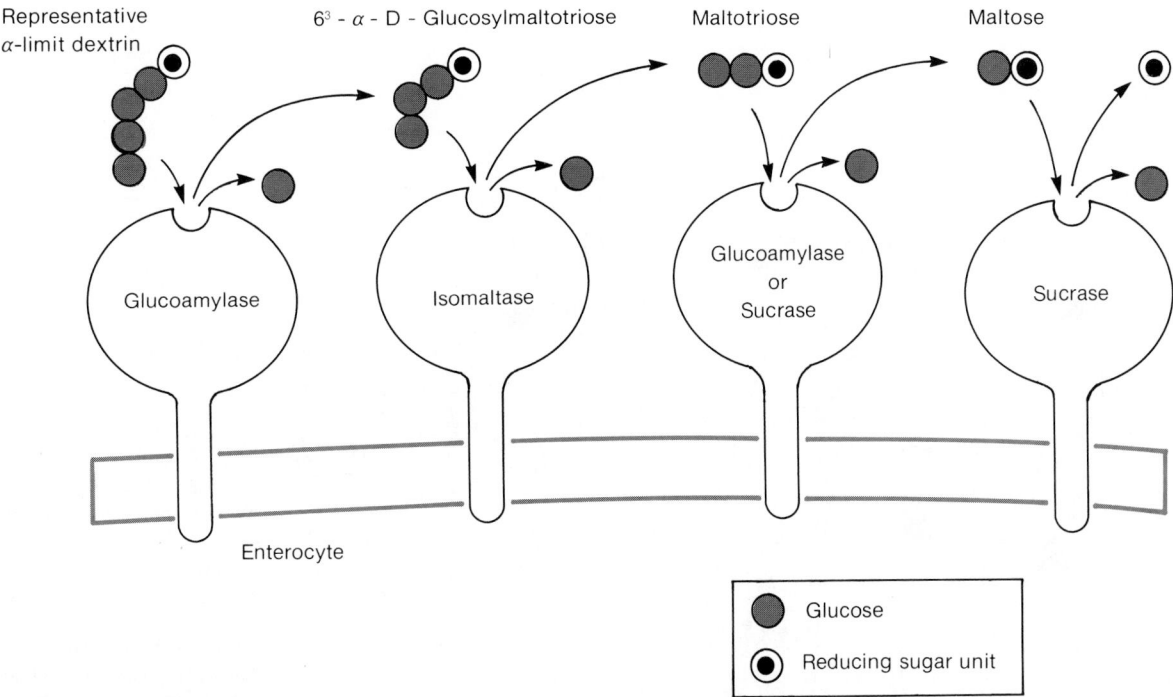

FIGURE 17–3. Brush-border hydrolysis of α-limit dextrins. Terminal glucoses are cleaved sequentially from the nonreducing ends by several enzymes with α-glucosidase activity, especially glucoamylase, to form the inter mediate product, 6³-α-D-glucosylmaltotriose. This tetrasaccharide contains an α-1,6 linkage that must be hydrolyzed by the isomaltase subunit of sucrase-isomaltase before further digestion can proceed.

substrates, two products with only one substrate bound to the catalytic site at one time) for transglucosidation and ordered uni-bi (one substrate, two products) for hydrolysis only.[35] Cleavage of the glycosidic bond occurs between carbon 1 of the glucosyl moiety and the glycosidic oxygen,[36] and aspartic acid groups within both active sites appear to be important in catalysis.[37,38] Cogoli and Semenza have proposed that the mechanism of both enzymes involves binding of the glycosyl moiety and protonation of the glycosidic oxygen followed by schism of the glycosidic bond with formation of an oxocarbonium ion in the glucosyl moiety temporarily stabilized by a carboxylate group in the active site of the enzyme.[39] The recent sequencing of sucrase-isomaltase precursor cDNA has revealed a high degree of amino acid homology between the sucrase and isomaltase domains[40] that supports the evolutionary hypothesis proposed by these investigators.[41] Semenza suggested that the sucrase-isomaltase gene arose from an ancestral gene coding for a single peptide chain capable of hydrolyzing both maltose and isomaltose. This gene was partially duplicated, resulting in a gene coding for a long peptide with two identical active sites. Subsequent point mutations or deletions changed one active site to a sucrase. Interestingly, the sea lion has a double isomaltase that cleaves maltose and isomaltose but not sucrose.[42]

Human intestine contains three β-galactosidases: a lysosomal enzyme with an pH optimum of 4.5, a cytosolic enzyme that hydrolyzes synthetic β-galactosides, but not lactose, perhaps derived from a lactase precursor (see section on biosynthesis of lactase-phlorizin hydrolase), and an enzyme with a pH optimum of 6.0 that is five times as active against lactose as against cellobiose or synthetic substrates.[43,44] The latter enzyme is the brush-border lactase responsible for dietary lactose digestion. Curiously, the protein responsible for lactase activity contains an independent site that hydrolyzes phlorizin to phloretin and glucose, and the protein is commonly called lactase-phlorizin hydrolase. Recently it has been established that both catalytic sites are carried on the same polypeptide chain[45] (see section on the biosynthesis of lactase-phlorizin hydrolase). Although the physiologic substrates of phlorizin hydrolase are unknown, they may be the glucosylceramides and lactosylceramides present in fat globules of milk.[33] The post-weaning decline in lactase activity is discussed later in this chapter.

Glucoamylase is an exoglucanase that cleaves α-glucoside bonds at the nonreducing end of glucose oligomers.[29] Sucrose is not hydrolyzed, suggesting that a reducing end is important, but maltose is hydrolyzed. The human enzyme prefers linear α-1,4 glucose oligomers with between 5 and 9 residues (K_m of 1.0–1.5 mM) and will hydrolyze α-1,6 bonds, although more slowly.[24]

Trehalase is a curious brush-border enzyme in that its only known substrate, trehalose, is an unusual dietary constituent. Trehalose consists of two glucose moieties joined by glycosidic linkage at the two anomeric carbons and is found in yeast, young mushrooms, and insects. Surprisingly, substantial amounts of the enzyme are present in the intestine.

Synthesis and Processing of Brush-Border Hydrolases: General Concepts

The brush-border hydrolases are synthesized on polysomes bound to the cytoplasmic surface of endoplasmic reticulum and like other membrane proteins must be transported to their final destination. Their journey is accompanied by a variety of events, some of which are illustrated by Figure 17-4. These events are often studied in biosynthetic experiments using techniques illustrated in Figures 17-5 and 17-6. In these experiments, enterocytes are briefly ex-

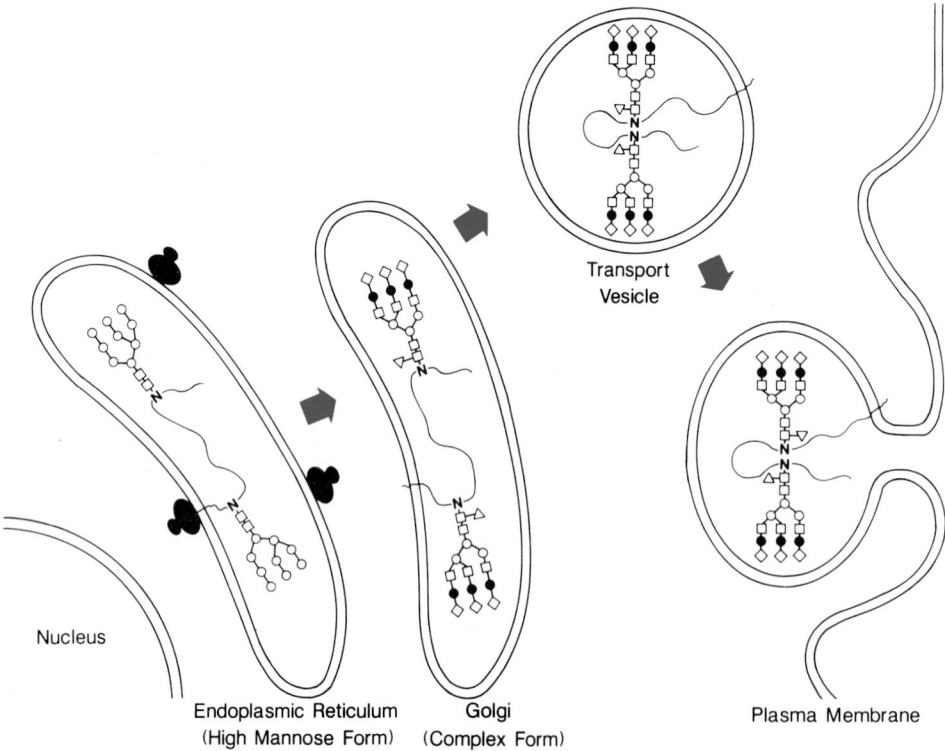

FIGURE 17–4. Asparagine-linked glycosylation of membrane proteins. N = nitrogen of asparagine; □ = N-acetylglucosamine; ○ = mannose; ● = galactose; ◇ = sialic acid; △ = fucose. This scheme is simplified in that it omits three glucose residues that are present on the carbohydrate chain at initial transfer to the peptide but rapidly removed. This figure is adapted from concepts reviewed in reference 46.

Transport Vesicle

Nucleus

Endoplasmic Reticulum (High Mannose Form)

Golgi (Complex Form)

Plasma Membrane

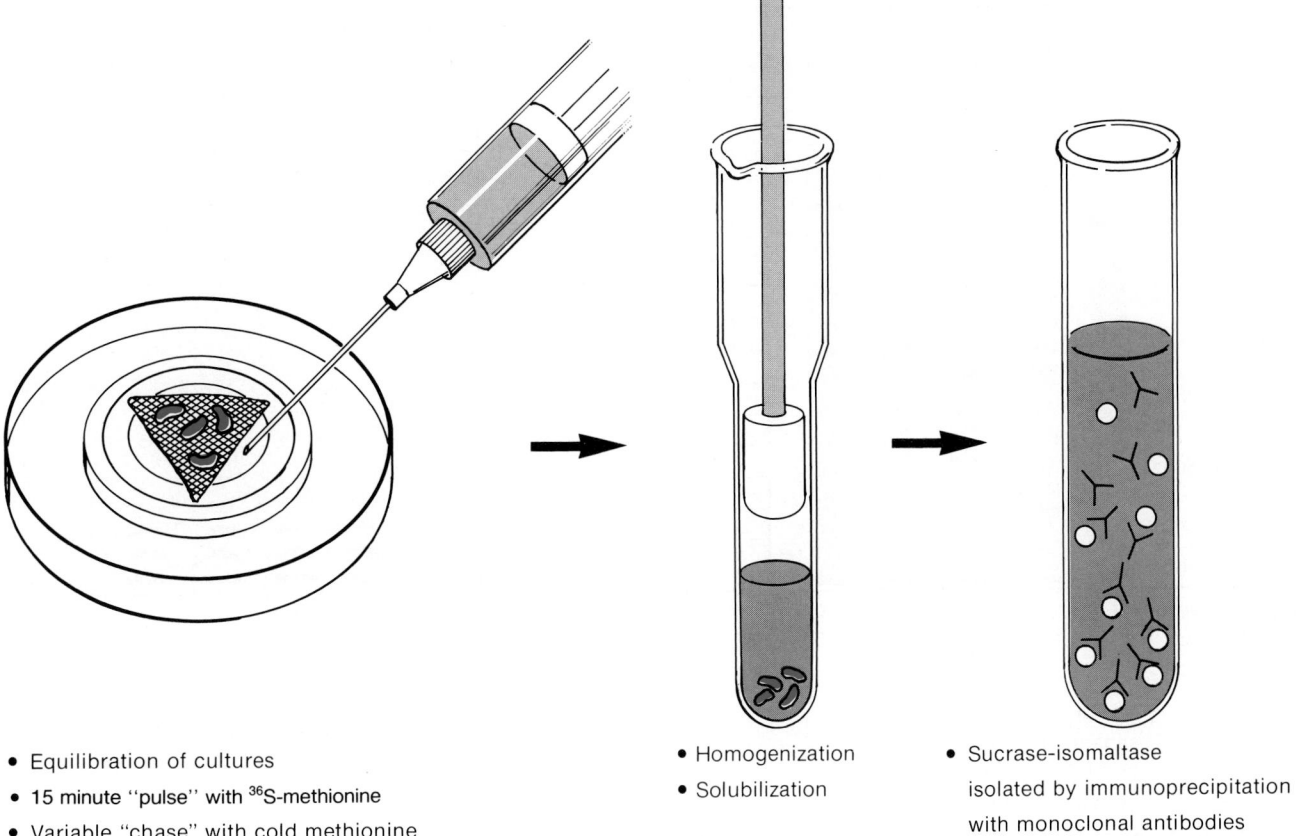

- Equilibration of cultures
- 15 minute "pulse" with ^{36}S-methionine
- Variable "chase" with cold methionine

- Homogenization
- Solubilization

- Sucrase-isomaltase
  isolated by immunoprecipitation
  with monoclonal antibodies

FIGURE 17–5. Study of the biosynthesis of brush-border hydrolases in organ-cultured small intestine. Sucrase-isomaltase is illustrated as a typical brush-border carbohydrase.

posed to radioactive amino acid, usually ^{35}S-methionine, to label newly synthesized proteins ("pulse"). The radioactive amino acid is removed and replaced with nonradioactive amino acid ("chase") so that proteins synthesized at a single point in time can be identified. Either polyclonal or monoclonal antibodies can be used to isolate proteins by immunoprecipitation or immunoadsorption, and changes in the molecular size of the peptide can be determined by sodium dodecyl sulfate-polyacrylamide gel electrophoresis (SDS-PAGE). Since SDS imparts a similar charge to peptide chains, migration in the gel is a function of molecular size alone. The radioactive peptide can be readily detected by exposing the gels to x-ray film (autoradiography or fluorography).

During translation the peptide chain is translocated across the membrane of the endoplasmic reticulum and into the endoplasmic reticulum lumen but remains attached to the membrane, in general by a short hydrophobic anchor segment that is embedded in the bilayer. The association with membrane persists through the functional life of the protein. Very early in its life the nascent peptide undergoes initial N-linked glycosylation within the lumen of the endoplasmic reticulum, probably as translation and translocation are proceeding. A good review of N-linked glycosylation has been published[46] and should be consulted for a detailed description of these events. Oligosaccharide structures rich in mannose are transferred en bloc from a lipid-linked precursor to asparagines of the polypeptide with the formation of an N-glycosidic linkage between N-acetylglucosamine of the oligosaccharide and the amide

nitrogen of asparagine. Not all asparagines are involved, however. They must occur in the sequence Asn-X-Ser or Asn-X-Thr where X represents almost any amino acid, but even when the correct sequences are present glycosylation may not occur. Since initial glycosylation probably occurs co-translationally, it should not be surprising that the earliest detectable precursors of brush-border proteins are already glycosylated. The early carbohydrate chains are rich in mannose, and the structure of the "high mannose" glycoproteins is shown in Figure 17-4. These "high mannose" chains can be readily removed experimentally with a specific glycosidase, endo-β-N-acetyl-glucosaminidase(endo H for short). Endo H has proven very useful in research because it can be used to determine whether or not a glycoprotein contains unprocessed "high mannose" chains.

The newly synthesized membrane-bound protein then moves to and through the Golgi apparatus where further modifications may occur. Transport is believed to occur in vesicles that pinch off from one membrane and fuse with the next. As the proteins traverse the Golgi stack, the N-linked carbohydrate chains are modified by enzymes located in different compartments. Mannose residues are partially removed and different monosaccharides added in sequence: N-acetylglucosamine, fucose, and finally galactose. Although sialic acid is a terminal sugar of the carbohydrate chains of many glycoproteins and may be present in brush-border proteins of suckling animals,[47] it is much less abundant in purified carbohydrases isolated from older animals.[14] The Golgi apparatus

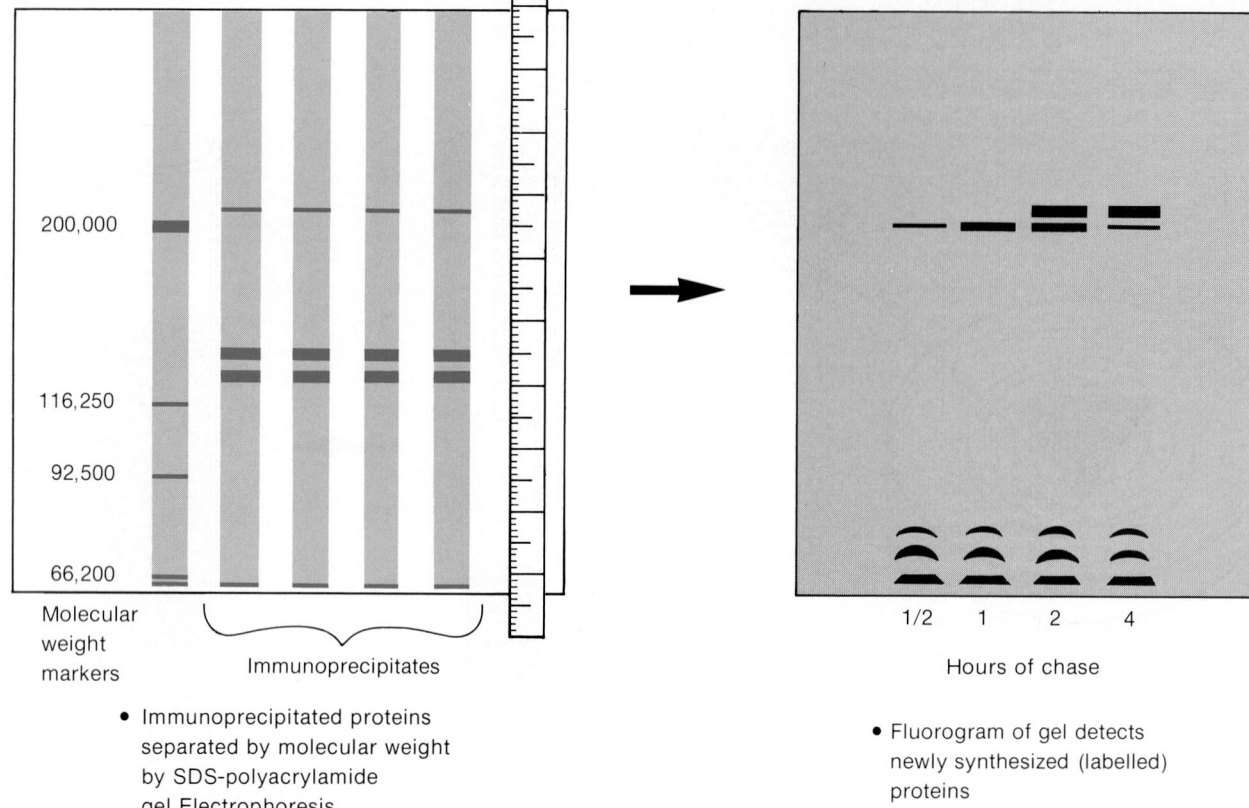

Molecular
weight
markers

Immunoprecipitates

Hours of chase

- Immunoprecipitated proteins
  separated by molecular weight
  by SDS-polyacrylamide
  gel Electrophoresis

- Fluorogram of gel detects
  newly synthesized (labelled)
  proteins

FIGURE 17–6. Study of biosynthesis of sucrase-isomaltase: separation by molecular size and detection of radioactive forms. The fluorogram demonstrates the conversion of "high mannose" sucrase-isomaltase to the complex glycosylated form. Note that no proteolytic cleavage to brush-border form occurs in organ culture because pancreatic proteases are absent. Nonradioactive sucrase and isomaltase can be seen with protein staining in the left panel.

appears to be also the site of another type of glycosylation, O-linked glycosylation, in which N-acetylgalactosamine is attached to serine or threonine residues via an O-glycosidic linkage to the hydroxyl groups of serine or threonine. Subsequent chain enlargement follows by a sequence of glycosyl transfer reactions. Most brush-border hydrolases including human sucrase-isomaltase and glucoamylase appear to have O-linked as well as N-linked chains,[14,48] although pig glucoamylase is a possible exception.[49] Much less is known about the structure of the O-linked chains. Differences in processing of carbohydrate chains may well account for some of the species-dependent and developmentally dependent differences in molecular size of individual hydrolases. For example, brush-border hydrolases are smaller in the human fetus than in the adult and correspond in size to those expressed in Caco-2 cells, a cell line derived from a human colon cancer.[50] The carbohydrate chains are apparently not involved in the targeting of the hydrolases for the brush-border membrane, but they may provide conformational stability since alterations produced with tunicamycin and castanospermine that inhibit N-linked glycosylation and initial trimming of N-linked chains, respectively, lead to rapid degradation of newly synthesized hydrolases.[49,51]

Further processing of the glycoprotein may include proteolytic cleavage of peptide chains either within the cell or after incorporation into the brush-border membrane. Immune electron microscopic studies of intracellular localization of a brush-border carbohydrase have demonstrated reaction product in the major

biosynthetic sites: endoplasmic reticulum, Golgi apparatus, subapical vesicles presumably headed for the brush border, and finally the brush border. The precise mechanism and route of transport of newly synthesized hydrolases are still somewhat controversial. Some investigators have identified soluble early-labeling forms and have suggested that they might be precursors,[52] but it may be that they represent fragments dislodged from membranes during tissue preparation. Others have postulated that brush-border hydrolases interact first with basolateral membrane and then reach the brush-border membrane. These suggestions were based on cell fractionation experiments that suggested apparent flow of labeled peptide from the Golgi complex to the basolateral membrane and then to the brush-border membrane.[53–55] Immune electron microscopic studies of the localization of sucrase-isomaltase do not support this concept, however,[56] and suggest that brush-border hydrolases move instead directly from Golgi apparatus to their destination. The findings in the cell fractionation experiments may reflect the known difficulties in isolation of highly purified intracellular membrane fractions. Thus, contamination of the basolateral membrane fractions with Golgi and transport vesicle membranes containing newly synthesized hydrolases might explain the experimental results. Further studies of the route taken by these hydrolases need to be done before firm conclusions can be drawn.

Electron microscopic studies have also identified a brush-border hydrolase within lysosomal structures,[56,57] a finding that suggests the possibility that some newly synthesized hydrolases are shunted directly to lysosomes without ever reaching the brush border. Indeed, there is recent direct experimental support for this suggestion.[58] It may be that this apparent shunt constitutes a post-translational regulator mechanism.[59] Travel of brush-border hydrolases to their destination occurs at different rates with a more leisurely pace for the carbohydrases than the peptidases. The extra time required for carbohydrase movement is involved in getting from endoplasmic reticulum to Golgi apparatus.[60] Figure 17-7 illustrates the different times required for sucrase-isomaltase and aminooligopeptidase to move to the brush-border membrane in human intestine.

The stalk segment of brush-border hydrolases is susceptible to cleavage by intraluminal proteases, and the rapid turnover of these proteins appears to be the consequence of cleavage by pancreatic proteases. Using a double isotope method for studying protein turnover in vivo, Alpers studied brush-border proteins separated according to molecular size and showed that the large-molecular-weight proteins (including the hydrolases) turned over more rapidly than low-molecular-weight proteins.[61] He and his colleagues subsequently showed that in the absence of pancreatic secretion, the large proteins turn over as slowly as the smaller ones,[62,63] presumably since they are no longer clipped off the membrane. Thus in contrast to the fate of many proteins that are degraded within the cell of origin, the brush-border membrane hydrolases appear to be first removed from the cell and then degraded within the intestinal lumen.

Biosynthesis of Sucrase-Isomaltase

Figure 17-8 is a summary of the major steps in the processing of this protein. Sucrase-isomaltase has been studied intensively over the past few years using the techniques of modern cellular and molecular biology. Although the brush-border form of the protein comprises two peptide chains, it has been known for some time that it is synthesized as a single-chain precursor that contains both active sites.[54,64] Cleavage is not required for enzyme activity, and both enzymatic sites are fully active in the precursor molecule. The structure of the precursor protein (pro-sucrase-isomaltase) has been primarily studied in the rabbit. Although only portions of the peptide chain have been directly sequenced, the complete amino acid structure has been determined indirectly by sequencing the complementary DNA (cDNA) synthesized from sucrase-isomaltase mRNA.[40] Pro-sucrase-isomaltase appears to consist of 1827 amino acids with a very short hydrophilic segment at the N-terminus, probably the intracellular domain, followed by a hydrophobic segment of 20 amino acids that is believed to serve as the membrane-anchoring segment, crossing the membrane once. A segment rich in serine and threonine (therefore possibly carrying O-linked carbohydrate chains) follows, probably representing the stalk. The stalk is followed by the catalytic domains for isomaltase and for sucrase. These catalytic domains have considerable amino acid homology, which is interpreted as evidence of partial gene duplication in the phylogenetic development of the protein. Nineteen Asn-X-Ser/Thr sequences, potential N-glycosylation sites, were identified, 12 of which were located in the sucrase domain. Recently a cDNA encoding much of the N-terminus of human sucrase-isomaltase has been isolated[65] and shown to have considerable homology with the rabbit cDNA. This probe was used to assign the human gene to chromosome 3, probably on the long arm. Cell-free translation of mRNA encoding rabbit[66] and rat[67] sucrase-isomaltase has also been performed to study the earliest biosynthetic events. The rabbit peptide is synthesized as a 200-kd peptide in the absence of membranes and as a 220-kd high-mannose glycoprotein sequestered within vesicles when translation was performed in the presence of microsomal vesicles.[66] No evidence of a cleavable signal peptide has been found so that presumably the hydrophobic anchor itself is the signal sequence involved in initiating translocation across the membrane.

FIGURE 17–7. Asynchronous arrival of digestive hydrolases at the brush-border membrane. Fluorograms of radiolabeled sucrase-isomaltase (*SI*) and aminooligopeptidase (*AOP*) from pulse chase experiments with human intestine are shown. Panel A demonstrates detection of an immature (high mannose) SI with a molecular size of 204,000 daltons (204 kd) in intracellular membranes within 30 minutes of chase. At 90 minutes, there has not yet been conversion to the more complex glycosylated form (228,000 daltons) (228 kd) nor transfer to the brush-border membrane. Panel B demonstrates detection of an immature AOP at 30 minutes, complex glycosylated AOP at 60 minutes, and transfer to the brush-border membrane by 90 minutes. (Burke T, Lloyd M, Lorenzsonn V, Olsen W. Synthesis and intracellular processing of aminooligopeptidase by human intestine. Gastroenterology 1988;94: 1426.)

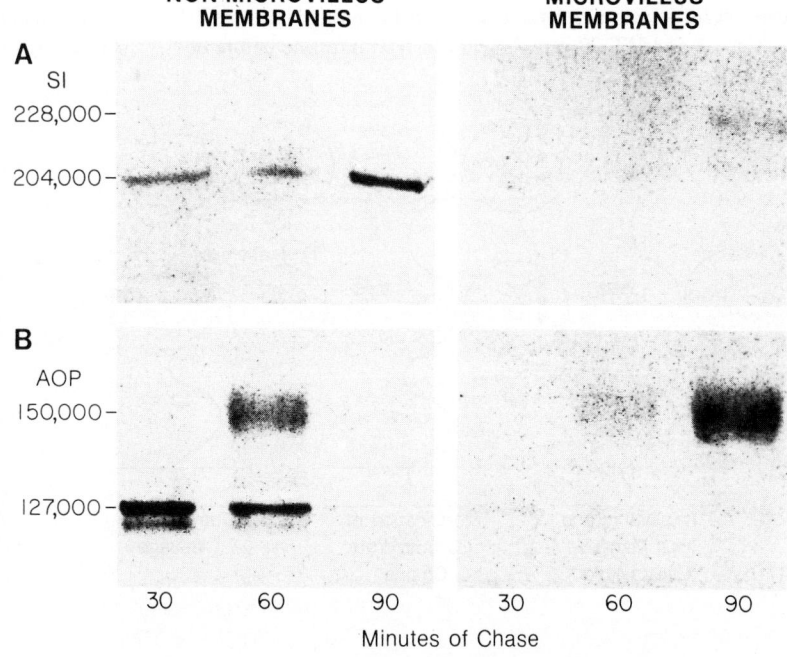

NON-MICROVILLUS MEMBRANES / MICROVILLUS MEMBRANES

A
SI
228,000–
204,000–

B
AOP
150,000–
127,000–

30   60   90   30   60   90

Minutes of Chase

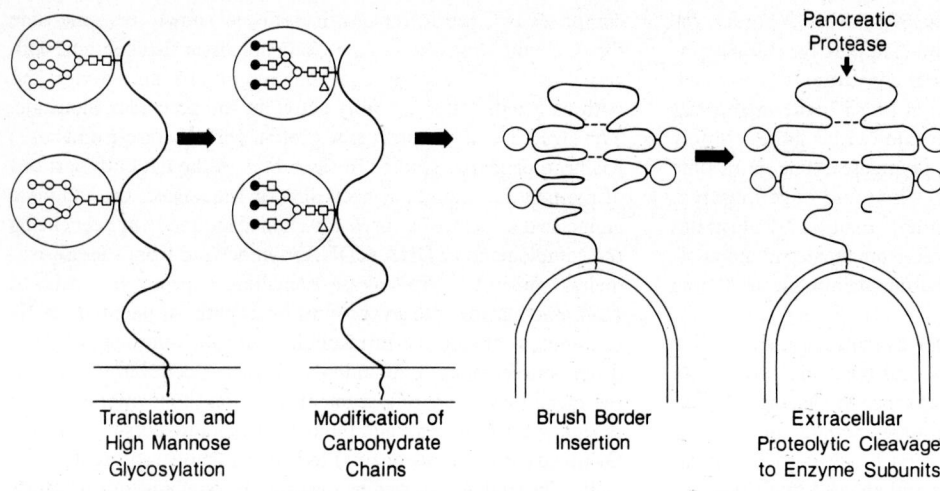

FIGURE 17-8. Intracellular processing of sucrase-isomaltase. Dotted lines indicate noncovalent bonds. Other symbols are the same as for Figure 17-4.

Translation and High Mannose Glycosylation — Modification of Carbohydrate Chains — Brush Border Insertion — Extracellular Proteolytic Cleavage to Enzyme Subunits

The synthesis and processing of the protein have been extensively studied in a variety of systems, including organ-cultured intestine from pig[68–70,51] and human,[71,72] human colon cancer cells HT-29 and Caco-2,[73,50] and in whole animals.[54,64,74] The results of these kinds of experiments have been remarkably similar. Pro-sucrase-isomaltase is first identifiable as a high-mannose endo H–sensitive glycoprotein 205 to 240 kd in molecular size, depending on the species. In organ-cultured human intestine the 205-kd high-mannose protein can be recognized within a few minutes of labeling with conversion within 3 hours to a 225-kd form that contains highly processed, endo H–resistant carbohydrate chains.[71] The high-mannose precursor, at least in the pig, is not fully enzymatically active,[75] but the mature form has full sucrase and isomaltase activity.[76–78] The mature precursor is then transferred to and incorporated into the brush-border membrane, where it is rapidly cleaved by pancreatic proteases to the two subunit chains of sucrase and isomaltase.[54,64] The importance of the pancreas in this cleavage has been very clearly established since only the pro-protein is synthesized in the absence of pancreatic secretions. This has been shown by studies with ligation of the pancreatic duct,[76] with heterotopic intestinal transplantation,[77] in organ-cultured intestine,[71,79] in Caco-2 and HT-29 cells,[50,73] and in fetal intestine before de-

velopment of pancreatic proteases.[78] Although trypsin appears to be responsible for cleavage of the human protein,[72] the responsible protease in rat is not clear, with evidence that either elastase[54] or trypsin[72] is primarily involved. It may be that cleavage of the protein should be regarded as the first step in its degradation rather than a part of its biosynthetic processing. Despite proteolytic cleavage, the two subunit chains of sucrase and isomaltase remain firmly attached to each other because of noncovalent forces, probably hydrophobic and/or electrostatic,[15] and attached to the membrane via the hydrophobic anchor of the isomaltase subunit.[80]

Biosynthesis of Lactase-Phlorizin Hydrolase

Figure 17-9 summarizes the major steps in the processing of this protein. Full-length cDNAs coding for rabbit and for human lactase-phlorizin hydrolase have been cloned and isolated[45] and the human gene has been localized to chromosome 2.[81] Nucleic acid sequencing to deduce the primary structure of the protein provided

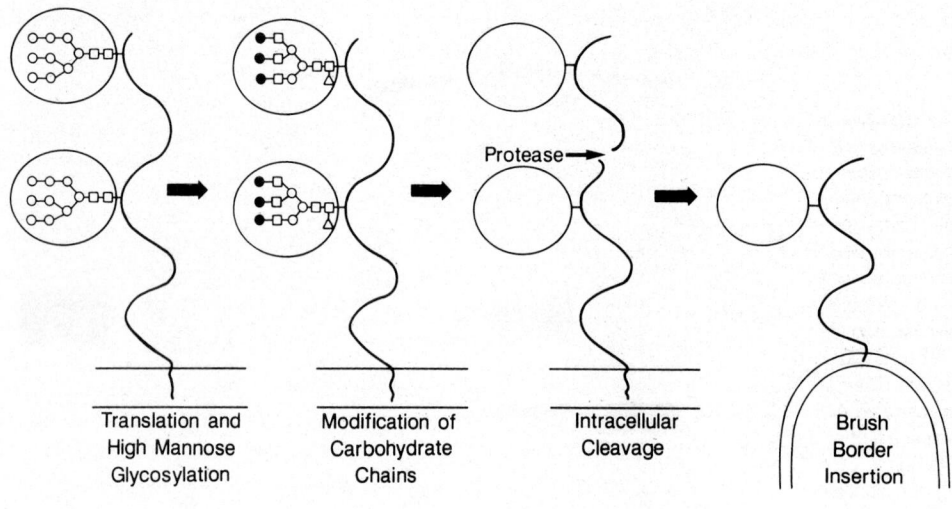

FIGURE 17-9. Intracellular processing of lactase-phlorizin hydrolase. Symbols are the same as for Figure 17-4.

Translation and High Mannose Glycosylation — Modification of Carbohydrate Chains — Intracellular Cleavage — Brush Border Insertion

a large amount of new information about its biosynthesis.[45] The protein is remarkably different from pro-sucrase-isomaltase, although the size (1927 amino acids) and number of potential N-linked glycosylation sites are similar. The primary peptide product begins with a 19 amino acid sequence at the N-terminus with the characteristics of a cleavable signal peptide so that it is presumably removed shortly after transport into the endoplasmic reticulum, leaving pro-lactase-phlorizin hydrolase associated with the membrane. (Thus the original peptide is called a "pre-pro-protein".) The signal peptide is followed by a large (847 amino acids) sequence that must also be removed during processing since sequences of the mature peptide are not found within this segment but only in the stretch of 1060 amino acids that follows it. So unlike sucrase-isomaltase where the two chains remain together even after cleavage, prolactase appears to lose a very large segment in the process. Also unlike mature sucrase-isomaltase where the active sites lie in separate chains, lactase-phlorizin hydrolase contains both active sites (i.e., lactase and phlorizin hydrolase) within the single peptide chain remaining. Finally the mature peptide contains a hydrophobic sequence of sufficient length to span the membrane in helical form so that it is almost certainly the anchoring sequence; but unlike the hydrophobic segment in sucrase-isomaltase, it is present near the carboxy terminus. Thus lactase-phlorizin hydrolase and sucrase-isomaltase appear to be attached to the brush-border membrane from opposite ends.

These findings correlate well with observations from biosynthetic experiments using pulse/chase techniques in Caco-2 cells[50] and in organ-cultured human,[82] suckling rat,[83] and pig[84] intestine. These studies demonstrated synthesis of a high-mannose high-molecular-weight precursor that undergoes further processing of carbohydrate chains and then cleavage to the size found in the brush-border membrane. Since the cleavage to brush-border size occurred in the absence of pancreatic enzymes, one can conclude that pancreatic proteases are not involved in the process. Because a signal peptide would probably have been cleaved before lactase could be identified, it is reasonable to believe that the initial high-molecular-weight precursor in biosynthetic experiments corresponds to the pro-protein deduced from the cDNA sequence. Presumably cleavage to mature peptide corresponds to the postulated removal of the "pro" segment. Unlike brush-border sucrase-isomaltase, mature lactase-phlorizin hydrolase appears as a single band on SDS-PAGE under reducing conditions so that its chains are of one size. Until the cDNA sequencing work it was thought possible that there were two separate chains that happened to be of identical size. Naim and colleagues have reported that in organ-cultured human intestine a 215-kd high-mannose protein can be detected within minutes of exposure to labeled methionine with conversion to the mature size (160 kd) within several hours.[82] Although the mature protein contained highly processed endo H–resistant carbohydrate chains, no complex-glycosylated precursor protein was identified in those experiments, although the studies in the pig suggest that cleavage takes place after complex glycosylation of the precursor has occurred.[84] Studies in human explants have shown that cleavage occurs intracellularly,[82] but in rat it may occur at the brush border. Büller and colleagues have reported studies where appearance of the labeled protein was followed in endoplasmic reticulum–Golgi and microvillus membrane fractions.[83] Their studies suggest that cleavage in the rat occurs in the microvillus membrane in a two-step process possibly catalyzed by an integral endopeptidase.[85]

Biosynthesis of Glucoamylase

Glucoamylase possesses two distinguishable active sites with similar substrate specificities, suggesting the possibility of duplication of an ancestral maltase gene, and, like sucrase-isomaltase, appears to be anchored to the brush-border membrane via a hydrophobic domain near the N-terminus.[17] Unlike sucrase-isomaltase, however, there appear to be major species-related differences in the protein. Although the brush-border protein in pig and rat consists of different-sized subunits, the human brush-border form is a single, very large peptide (355 kd by SDS-PAGE under reducing conditions),[50] much larger than either of the two subunits reported in other animals, suggesting that the human peptide is not split. This suggestion was confirmed in extensive biosynthetic studies reported by Naim and colleagues.[86] These investigators also found a large-sized (335 kd by SDS-PAGE) glucoamylase in human brush-border membrane and compared it with the size of the peptide synthesized by explants. Newly synthesized glucoamylase was first detected as a high-mannose 285-kd polypeptide that was subsequently converted to an endo H–resistant 335-kd form. Thus human glucoamylase does not undergo proteolytic cleavage in its processing. In contrast to other brush-border hydrolases, Naim and associates suggest that the human protein is not organized in dimeric form. The situation is different in the pig where the brush-border membrane contains 135- and 125-kd subunits of glucoamylase in addition to a considerable amount of a 245-kd molecule.[29] Biosynthetic studies in vitro indicated that it is the 245-kd peptide that is synthesized by pig intestine,[79] which is then presumably converted to subunit form by pancreatic proteases after insertion into the brush-border membrane. Thus in the pig glucoamylase is processed much like sucrase-isomaltase (although the cleavage must occur more slowly since considerable pro-glucoamylase is found in the brush border). Possibly differences in the extent of glycosylation[86] account for the differences in susceptibility to proteolytic cleavage between the human and pig proteins. Finally, the rat protein may differ entirely. Cell-free translation experiments suggest that the primary translational product in the rat is surprisingly small (145 kd), prompting the authors to suggest that the two mature subunits in the brush border arise from only minor proteolytic modifications of the precursor.[67]

Biosynthesis of Trehalase

Little is known about the synthesis and processing of trehalase. The protein has been purified from the intestine of several species including rabbit where its subunit molecular weight by SDS-PAGE is 75 kd.[87] Unlike the other brush-border carbohydrases, trehalase resists removal from the membrane by the protease papain and must be solubilized by detergent,[88] suggesting it might interact with the membrane in a different way. Recently it was reported to be solubilized by a phosphatidylinositol-specific phospholipase C, suggesting that it is bound to the membrane through phosphatidylinositol.[89]

TABLE 17–7
Monosaccharide Transport Mechanisms

MECHANISM	LOCATION	SIZE OF TRANSPORTER (kd)	Na$^+$ COUPLING
Diffusion	BBM	—	No
	BLM	—	No
Sodium/glucose co-transporter	BBM	73	Yes
Basolateral glucose transporter	BLM	?57	No
Fructose transporter	BBM	Undetermined	No

BBM, brush-border membrane; BLM, Basolateral membrane.

MONOSACCHARIDE TRANSPORT

Although there have been exciting advances over the past 25 years in our understanding of the mechanism by which glucose and galactose are actively transported across the small intestinal epithelium, it is important to recognize that nonsaturable transport also occurs, probably in large part by simple diffusion driven by concentration gradients. This component may contribute significantly to overall absorption in view of the relatively high concentrations of monosaccharide within the intestinal lumen after carbohydrate meals.[23] The nonsaturable component of carbohydrate transport can be demonstrated in studies using both highly purified brush-border vesicles as well as intact mucosa, thus demonstrating that it does not solely represent paracellular movement. The bulk of absorbed hexose is transported intact into the portal vein, indicating that it is not metabolized within the enterocyte.[90] Intestinal monosaccharide transport is summarized in Table 17-7.

The Sodium/Glucose Co-Transporter and Active Hexose Transport

Progress in understanding of membrane transport mechanisms at the molecular level has been slow until recently since the function of transporters removed from membrane for purification and study is difficult to assay. It has been known for some time that the enterocyte accumulates glucose and galactose despite unfavorable concentration gradients because of the presence of a sodium/glucose co-transporter located in the brush-border membrane, as shown in cartoon form in Figure 17-10. Some of the characteristics of the co-transporter are listed in Table 17-8. The concept that active hexose transport is driven by a sodium gradient was originally formulated by Crane based on studies of the effects of sodium ion on sugar uptake by intact tissue[91,92] and extended by the work of Schultz and Zalusky, who examined the effects of hexose on sodium transport and movement of electrical charges beginning in the early 1960s.[93] The evidence to support the concept is far too extensive to review here, and the interested reader is urged to consult several recent reviews.[94–96] A particularly elegant confirmation of the Crane hypothesis was the observation by Hopfer and colleagues that isolated brush-border membrane vesicles retained the glucose transporter and that creation of a sodium gradient across the membrane greatly stimulated glucose entry.[97] Subsequently it was recognized that in the presence of sodium a membrane potential as well as a sodium gradient could energize glucose transport (i.e., electrogenic co-transport).[98] Thus the downhill electrochemical sodium gradient is believed to drive the movement of glucose (and a positive charge) across the brush-border membrane. Hydrolysis of adenosine triphosphatase (ATP) by the sodium-potassium ATPase of the basolateral membrane is responsible for the maintenance of a low intracellular sodium concentration and the electrically negative cytoplasm, thus ultimately providing the energy for glucose transport. Although originally the transporter was viewed as a mobile carrier, it may possibly function as a gated pore with translocation the result of a confirmational change of the transporter.[99] As shown in Table 17-9, the

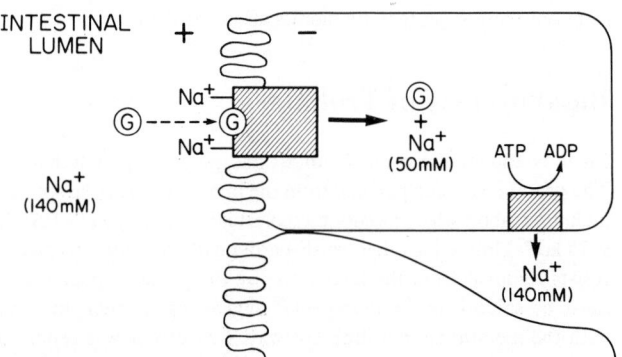

FIGURE 17–10. Mechanism of uphill transport of glucose and galactose. Sodium/glucose co-transporter is shown in the brush-border membrane with sites for Na$^+$ and hexose. Sodium-potassium ATPase, the Na$^+$ pump, is shown in the basolateral membrane, energized by ATP hydrolysis. The stoichiometry of Na$^+$:glucose co-transport is controversial.

TABLE 17–8
Some Functional Characteristics of the Intestinal
Sodium/Glucose Transporter

Saturable: K$_m$ for D-glucose of 2–3 mM in rabbit brush-border membrane vesicles[99]

Stereospecific: affinity for D-glucose but not L-glucose

Specificity for sodium ion

Inhibition by phlorizin

TABLE 17–9
Specificity of Sodium/Glucose Co-Transporter

INHIBITOR	UPTAKE (%)
None	100
D-Glucose	11
α-Methyl-D-glucopyranoside	22
D-Galactose	31
3-0-Methylglucoside	71
D-Mannose	94
L-Glucose	96

The effects of different monosaccharides on uptake of α-methyl-D-glucopyranoside by brush-border membrane vesicles are given as a percentage of uptake with no inhibitor.
Data adapted from Ikeda TS, Hwang E-S, Coady MJ, et al. Characterization of a Na⁺/glucose co-transporter cloned from rabbit small intestine. J Membrane Biol 1989;110:87.

transporter has affinity for a number of sugars besides glucose. The table shows the effects of a variety of monosaccharides on the uptake of a glucose derivative transported by the sodium/glucose transporter. Monosaccharides that inhibit uptake interact with the transporter. Thus galactose is also believed transported by this mechanism, but mannose and L-glucose are not. The effect of fructose is not shown, but fructose does not interact with the transporter either.

The transporter has been purified as a 75-kd polypeptide and functionally reconstituted into phosphatidyl choline:cholesterol liposomes where it demonstrated sodium-dependent, phlorizin-inhibitable glucose transport.[100] Also recently, a nearly full-length cDNA for the rabbit co-transporter has been cloned and sequenced[101] and the cloned mRNA expressed as functional transporter in *Xenopus* oocytes[102] and COS-7 cells.[103] The cDNA codes for a 662 amino acid peptide (predicted size of 73 kd) with no recognized homologies to sodium-independent glucose transporters.[104–106] Unlike the brush-border hydrolases, only two potential N-linked glycosylation sites were identified, although transporter function in transfected COS-7 cells was markedly reduced with tunicamycin, an inhibitor of N-linked glycosylation, suggesting that the limited glycosylation, nonetheless, may be important to the protein.[103] The polypeptide is believed to span the membrane 11 times based on hydrophobic analysis and contains two highly charged hydrophilic segments perhaps important in glucose binding. The predicted size of the peptide is in agreement with the previous identification of a 75-kd peptide as the transporter by fluorescein isothiocyanate labeling.[107,108] Recent radiation inactivation studies suggest that the transporter is organized in the brush-border membrane as a homotetramer with four independent, identical subunits each containing a site for sodium and a site for glucose.[109] The gene for the human transporter has been assigned to chromosome 22.[110]

The Basolateral Glucose Transporter

Glucose and galactose exit the enterocyte via a transporter on the basolateral plasma membrane into the lamina propria from which they are taken up by the capillary network of the villus. The existence of this transporter has been demonstrated best in studies of monosaccharide movement across purified basolateral membrane.[111,112] Stereospecific and saturable hexose uptake has been demonstrated in this fashion. The observation that this uptake is not affected by sodium gradients implies that it is a facilitated transport system much like that of red blood cells. The transporter has an affinity for galactose as well as glucose,[112] suggesting that it is also responsible for galactose exit from the cell. Recent studies have identified a protein similar to a glucose transporter in liver membrane that may turn out to be the basolateral transporter. Thorens and colleagues showed that a cDNA probe encoding the liver glucose transporter hybridized with an intestinal mRNA and that an antibody to the liver protein recognized a 61-kd protein in a membrane fraction from intestine.[106] The protein deduced from the cDNA structure contains 522 amino acids with a calculated mass of 57 kd. Only one potential site for N-linked glycosylation was identified, and hydropathy plots disclosed 12 hydrophobic segments that presumably cross the membrane.

Fructose Absorption

Fructose is transported across the brush-border membrane by another transporter not coupled to sodium. Early studies suggested that fructose absorption is not sodium dependent,[113] although absorption rates were found to exceed those of diffusion of comparably sized monosaccharides.[114] Studies of portal vein blood after fructose instillation into human jejunum suggest that the unexpectedly high absorption cannot be attributed to metabolic conversion to glucose or lactate.[114] Clear evidence of a distinct fructose transport system was found by Sigrist-Nelson and Hopfer, who demonstrated saturable but not sodium-dependent uptake into brush-border membrane vesicles.[115] Uptake of fructose was slower than glucose, but faster than L-glucose or mannitol and could not be shown to be affected by other potential substrates, including phlorizin, an inhibitor of the sodium/glucose co-transporter. Thus fructose is transported across the brush-border membrane by facilitated diffusion. Whether a fructose transporter also exists on the basolateral membrane is unknown.

REGULATION OF BRUSH-BORDER CARBOHYDRASES AND TRANSPORTERS

An enormous literature exists, largely descriptive, that deals with physiologic or pathologic changes in the levels of intestinal carbohydrase or monosaccharide transport function. Considerable work is required before a coherent concept of the regulation of these functions can be realized. Rather than present an exhaustive review of the literature, we have chosen to focus on a few well-characterized topics relative to regulation of the assimilation of carbohydrates.

Developmental Changes

Although amylase secretion is low under the age of 1,[116] it apparently increases with starch ingestion[117] so that starch intolerance is rarely a problem in infancy.[118] In humans, the brush-border carbohydrases develop during fetal life and are present at high levels at birth.[119] The mechanism of regulation of sucrase-isomaltase during development of the human embryo has been studied using a rabbit cDNA probe that recognizes the human mRNA.[120] A close correlation between enzymatic activity and sucrase-isomaltase mRNA was found, suggesting that developmental control of expression of the gene in humans is pretranslational. In other species such as rabbit and rat although lactase levels are high at birth, levels of other hydrolases remain low until weaning when they increase dramatically. Changes in mRNA levels appear to account also for the post-weaning increase in sucrase-isomaltase, at least in the rabbit.[121] The major developmental change in intestinal carbohydrases is, of course, the changes that occur in lactase and phlorizin-hydrolase levels. A post-weaning decline in lactase activity occurs in essentially all mammals. The changes have been most thoroughly studied in the rat where lactase appears late in gestation and reaches a peak at 2 to 3 days after birth. Levels remain high until weaning begins (about 14 days after birth) and fall to adult levels (approximately 10% of adult levels) by 21 days of age.[122] In humans, lactase activity increases during gestation, reaching a maximum at birth,[119] and, in most populations declines during infancy, with lactose malabsorption present in a majority by the age of 5. In some groups the disappearance of lactase does not occur until the teen years. Developmental decline of lactase is not simply an adaptation to a missing substrate since the enzyme declines even when weaning is prevented.[123] Luminal factors seem to be of some importance however, since the decline is considerably postponed in intestinal isografts implanted under the skin.[124] Although developmental changes in disaccharidases are influenced by hormones, especially corticosterone and thyroxine, the hormonal effects appear to be permissive rather than primary.[125] On the basis of studies in rats, three hypotheses have been proposed to account for developmental decreases in lactase. Tsuboi and colleagues suggest that the increase in enterocyte migration rate (and consequent decrease in life span) which occurs at weaning accounts for the fall in lactase activity—i.e., less time for lactase to accumulate in the brush-border membrane.[126] Jonas and co-workers, on the other hand suggest a more specific change as they found that weaning resulted in less incorporation of labeled amino acid into brush-border lactase relative to other brush-border proteins suggesting a decrease in the rate of synthesis of the protein.[127] Recently a poor correlation between lactase specific activity and mRNA levels has been demonstrated in pigs, rats, rabbits, and humans, suggesting that the presumed decline in lactase synthesis may be a change at the translational or post-translational level.[128,129] A post-translational alteration is supported by another study that suggests that pro-lactase may not be efficiently cleaved to the brush-border form in adult rats.[130] Perhaps both changes in cell migration and a specific biosynthetic alteration account for the fall in enzyme levels. Clearly more research will be required to understand fully developmental regulation of lactase. Whatever the mechanism, developmental decline in lactase occurs in most humans, resulting in lactose intolerance. A percentage of persons in all racial groups retain lactase throughout life, and in some groups a majority of persons retain lactase as discussed in Chapter 72. It has been suggested that low prevalence of lactose malabsorption among certain human groups arose because of selective nutritional pressures over a long period that gave an advantage to adult lactose absorbers.[131]

Dietary Regulation

It is not surprising that the small intestine is very responsive to changes in food consumption, and alterations in carbohydrase and transport function occur with both qualitative and quantitative changes in the diet. Changes in the time of meals synchronize diurnal changes in brush-border function.[132-136] In rats, at least, levels of disaccharidases and transport function increase prior to feeding, persist during the feeding period, and fall thereafter. The circadian rhythm in intestinal sucrase activity has been studied using an antibody recognizing sucrase-isomaltase and shown to reflect differences in the amount of enzyme protein.[137] Although these studies that used labeled precursor incorporation techniques suggested that the rate of synthesis of sucrase-isomaltase remained constant, there were dramatic changes in the degradation of the protein with very rapid degradation occurring after feeding (half-life as short as 2.5 hours) but essentially no degradation in the hours before feeding. Presumably these changes are mediated by changes in the secretion of pancreatic proteases that appear to be responsible for the surface removal of the carbohydrases as discussed earlier.

The intestinal mucosa is particularly vulnerable to starvation, with experimental animals losing 50% of mucosal protein in 6 days of starvation.[138] The decrease in protein reflects both a decrease in the numbers of enterocytes and a decrease in the protein content of each enterocyte. Since starvation (as well as other dietary manipulations) affects the mass of total proteins in the mucosa, it is important to measure changes in a particular function in relation to the whole gut rather than just to total protein of sampled tissue. Starvation results in loss of several brush-border carbohydrases,[139] although lactase seems curiously resistant.[140] Studies in vivo suggest that semistarvation results in large reductions in the V_{max} for glucose and galactose largely because of the reduced numbers of enterocytes but also because of a decrease in the apparent affinity of the transporter for its substrates.[141]

The presence or absence of carbohydrate in the diet is known to affect the brush-border carbohydrases. The enzymatic activity of sucrase falls with carbohydrate restriction[142-145] and increases with sucrose feeding.[142,143] Although most studies have been conducted in rats, it is clear that sucrose restriction and refeeding has similar effects in humans.[144] The regulation of carbohydrases does not appear to be substrate specific. Thus low- and high-starch diets affect levels of sucrase, maltase, and lactase,[146,147] and sucrose or lactose refeeding after carbohydrate restriction stimulates both sucrase and lactase activities.[148] These dietary manipulations not only change the enzymatic activity of the brush-border hydrolases but also alter the rate of disaccharide hydrolysis in vivo.[149] Increases in dietary carbohydrate, however, do not increase brush-border peptidase activity[150,151] and may actually lower it. The presence or absence of carbohydrate in the diet appears to also increase or decrease monosaccharide transport,[149,152] suggesting some coordination of carbohydrase and transporter regulation. There have been surprisingly few studies of the mechanism by which carbohydrate substrate regulates carbohydrase and transporter levels. Regulation largely involves changes in the mass of enzyme protein and not in catalytic efficiency[146,153,154] and occurs through changes in rates of carbohydrate synthesis, as shown by isotope incorporation studies.[146,153,155] Understanding of the mechanisms that regulate intestinal carbohydrases should increase rapidly when the tools of molecular genetics are applied to this area.

Pathologic Regulation

Because there are multiple steps in the synthesis and intracellular processing of brush-border membrane proteins, it would not be surprising if defects in any one of several steps were to lead to deficiency of a functional protein. As discussed in Chapter 72, clinical examples of such defects are being discovered. It also seems evident that extensive small intestinal disease of any sort might affect the function of the brush-border membrane. These disorders are also discussed in Chapter 72. A few conditions appear to increase, not decrease, brush-border function and have consequently been studied extensively. One example is diabetes mellitus, which increases the activity of brush-border carbohydrases as well as other hydrolases.[156] Although largely studied in experimental animals, carbohydrase levels are believed to be increased in the human disease as well.[157] Sucrase-isomaltase has been the only hydrolase studied at the protein level, and its increase in the diabetic brush-border membrane appears to be the result of both a decrease in degradation of the protein[158] and a stimulation of synthesis.[159] Intraluminal factors do not account entirely for the effect since diabetes enhances intestinal carbohydrase activity even in segments excluded from luminal continuity.[160] Membrane transport systems are also altered in experimental diabetes with increased active transport of glucose and galactose as well as amino acids.[161,162] Kinetic studies of the monosaccharide effects have shown increases in V_{max} of transport, suggesting the presence of more transporters in diabetes,[162] observations consistent with recent studies of phlorizin binding to assay the transporters.[163] Localization of the alteration to the brush-border membrane was firmly established by Hopfer, who found enhanced glucose transport in brush-border membrane vesicles from diabetic rats.[164]

Alcoholic pancreatic insufficiency in humans[165] and spontaneous pancreatic insufficiency in mice[63] and dogs[166] are associated with elevated carbohydrase levels. These observations may result because of the importance of pancreatic proteases in the physiologic removal of carbohydrases from the brush border,[63] with diminished removal in pancreatic disease allowing their accumulation in the membrane.

Increases in intraluminal proteases may have the opposite effect of decreasing intestinal carbohydrase activity. Low disaccharidase levels have been recognized in intestinal bacterial overgrowth in humans[167,168] and also in experimental animals.[169,170] Increased carbohydrase degradation by bacterial proteases appears to be the mechanism for these observations,[169–171] although the possibility that bacterial overgrowth also inhibits synthesis of the proteins has yet to be examined.

The possible therapeutic inhibition of carbohydrate assimilation has been studied as a means to treat diabetes and obesity. An inhibitor of pancreatic amylase isolated from kidney beans[12] was marketed as a "starch blocker" with some success in the early 1980s. Although the commercially available product was ineffective in inhibiting starch digestion in humans,[172,173] it is possible that higher doses might be able to inhibit starch hydrolysis in vivo.[174] In other studies several potent α-glycosidase inhibitors have been isolated from microorganisms and have been shown to be effective in decreasing carbohydrate absorption in humans.[175,176] Significant inhibition of carbohydrate absorption by any of these agents would, in all likelihood, lead to symptoms of carbohydrate malabsorption. Thus, further studies are required before any of these approaches result in a safe and clinically useful means of decreasing the absorption of carbohydrate calories.

The reader is directed to Chapter 6, Epithelia: Biologic Principles of Organization; Chapter 12, Salivary Secretion; Chapter 15, Pancreatic Secretion; Chapter 18, Intestinal Lipid Absorption; Chapter 19, Protein Digestion and Assimilation; Chapter 20, Vitamins and Minerals; Chapter 21, General Nutritional Principles; Chapter 48, Approach to the Patient Requiring Nutritional Supplementation; and Chapter 72, Specific Mucosal Protein Deficiency States.

REFERENCES

1. MacDonald I. Carbohydrates. In: Shils ME, Young UR, eds. Modern nutrition in health and disease. 7th ed. Philadelphia: Lea & Febiger, 1988:38.
2. Stiefel DJ, Keller PJ. Preparation and some properties of human pancreatic amylase including a comparison with human parotid amylase. Biochim Biophys Acta 1973;302:345.
3. Nakamura Y, Ogawa M, Nishide T, et al. Sequences of cDNAs for human salivary and pancreatic α-amylases. Gene 1984;28:263.
4. Hodge C, Lebenthal E, Lee PC, Topper W. Amylase in the saliva and in the gastric aspirates of premature infants: its potential role in glucose polymer hydrolysis. Pediatr Res 1983;17:998.
5. Rosenblum JL, Irwin CL, Alpers DH. Starch and glucose oligosaccharides protect salivary-type amylase activity at acid pH. Am J Physiol 1988;254:G775.
6. Ugolev AM. Influence of the surface of the small intestine on enzymatic hydrolysis of starch by enzymes. Nature 1960;188:588.
7. Dahlqvist A, Borgstrom B. Digestion and absorption of disaccharides in man. Biochem J 1961;81:411.
8. Fogel MR, Gray GM. Starch hydrolysis in man: an intraluminal process not requiring membrane digestion. J Appl Physiol 1973;35:263.
9. Anderson IH, Levine AS, Levitt MD. Incomplete absorption of the carbohydrate in all-purpose wheat flour. N Engl J Med 1981;304:891.
10. Stephen AM, Haddad AC, Phillips SF. Passage of carbohydrate into the colon: direct measurements in humans. Gastroenterology 1983;85:589.
11. Snow P, O'Dea K. Factors affecting the rate of hydrolysis of starch in food. Am J Clin Nutr 1981;34:2721.
12. Marshall JJ, Lauda CM. Purification and properties of phaseolamin, an inhibitor of alpha-amylase, from the kidney been *Phaseolus vulgaris*. J Biol Chem 1975;250:8030.
13. Malath P, Ramaswamy K, Caspary WF, Crane RK. Studies in the transport of glucose from disaccharides by hamster small intestine in vitro: I. Evidence for a disaccharidase-related transport system. Biochim Biophys Acta 1973;307:613.
14. Kelly JJ, Alpers DH. Blood group antigenicity of purified human intestinal disaccharidases. J Biol Chem 1975;248:8216.
15. Semenza G. Anchoring and biosynthesis of stalked brush-border membrane proteins: glycosidases and peptidases of enterocytes and renal tubuli. Ann Rev Cell Biol 1986;2:255.
16. Cowell GM, Tranum-Jensen J. Sjostrom H, Noren O. Topology and quaternary structure of pro-sucrase/isomaltase and final-form sucrase/isomaltase. Biochem J 1986;237:455.
17. Norén O, Sjoström H, Cowell GM, et al. Pig intestinal microvillar maltase-glucoamylase: structure and membrane insertion. J Biol Chem 1986;261:12306.
18. Gray GM, Ingelfinger FJ. Intestinal absorption of sucrose in man: the site of hydrolysis and absorption. J Clin Invest 1965;44:390.
19. Asp N-G, Gudmand-Hoyer E, Andersen B, et al. Distribution of disaccharidases, alkaline phosphatase, and some intracellular enzymes

along the human small intestine. Scand J Gastroenterol 1975;10: 745.

20. Gray GM, Santiago NA. Disaccharide absorption in normal and diseased human intestine. Gastroenterology 1966;51:489.

21. Alpers DH, Cote MN. Inhibition of lactose hydrolysis by dietary sugars. Am J Physiol 1971;221:865.

22. Gray GM, Ingelfinger FJ. Intestinal absorption of sucrose in man: interrelation of hydrolysis and monosaccharide product absorption. J Clin Invest 1966;45:388.

23. Olsen WA, Ingelfinger FJ. The role of sodium in intestinal glucose absorption in man. J Clin Invest 1968;47:1133.

24. Kelly JJ, Alpers DH. Properties of human intestinal glucoamylase. Biochim Biophys Acta 1973;315:113.

25. Gray GM, Lally BC, Conklin KA. Action of intestinal sucrase-isomaltase and its free monomers on an α-limit dextrin. J Biol Chem 1979;254:6038.

26. Taravel, FR, Datema R, Woloszczuk W, et al. Purification and characterization of a pig intestinal α-limit dextrinase. Eur J Biochem 1983;130:147.

27. Rodriguez IR, Taravel FR, Whelan WJ. Characterization and function of pig intestinal sucrase-isomaltase and its separate subunits. Eur J Biochem 1984;143:575.

28. Dahlqvist A, Semenza G. Disaccharidases of small-intestinal mucosa. J Pediatr Gastroenterol Nutr 1985;4:857.

29. Sorensen SH, Norén O, Sjöström H, et al. Amphiphilic pig intestinal microvillus maltase/glucoamylase: structure and specificity. Eur J Biochem 1982;126:559.

30. Leeper LL, Henning SJ. Development and tissue distribution of sucrase-isomaltase mRNA in rats. Am J Physiol 1990;258:652.

31. Freund J-N, Heilig R, Lehner N, Raul F. The gene for intestinal sucrase-isomaltase as member of a gene family. Cell Mol Biol 1989;35:313.

32. Hoefsloot LH, Hoogeveen-Westerveld M, Kroos MA, et al. Primary structure and processing of lysosomal α-glucosidase: homology with the intestinal sucrase-isomaltase complex. EMBO J 1988;6:1697.

33. Leese HJ, Semenza G. On the identity between the small intestine enzymes phlorizin hydrolase and glycosylceramidase. J Biol Chem 1973;248:8170.

34. Auricchio S, Semenza G, Rubino A. Multiplicity of human intestinal disaccharidases: II. Characterization of the individual maltases. Biochim Biophys Acta 1965;96:498.

35. Semenza G, Von Balthazar A-K. Steady-state kinetics of rabbit-intestinal sucrase: kinetic mechanism, Na$^+$ activation, inhibition by *tris* (hydroxymethyl) aminomethane at the glucose subsite. Eur J Biochem 1974;41:149.

36. Zagalak B, Curtius H. The mechanism of the human intestinal sucrase action. Biochem Biophys Res Commun 1975;62:503.

37. Quaroni A, Semenza G. Partial amino acid sequences around the essential carboxylate in the active sites of the intestinal sucrase-isomaltase complex. J Biol Chem 1976;251:3250.

38. Quaroni A, Gershon E, Semenza. Affinity labeling of the active sites in the sucrase-isomaltase complex from small intestine. J Biol Chem 1974;249:6424.

39. Cogoli A, Semenza G. A probable oxocarbonium ion in the reaction mechanism of small intestinal sucrase and isomaltase. J Biol Chem 1975;250:7802.

40. Hunziker W, Spiess M, Semenza G, et al. The sucrase-isomaltase complex: primary structure, membrane-orientation, and evolution of a stalked, intrinsic brush-border protein. Cell 1986;46:227.

41. Semenza G. The sucrase-isomaltase complex, a large dimeric amphipathic protein from the small intestinal brush-border membrane: emerging structure-function relationships. In: Ahlberg P, Sundelof L-O, eds. Structure and Dynamics of Chemistry. Stockholm: Almquist Wikesell Intl, 1978.

42. Wacker H, Aggeler R, Kretchmer N, et al. A two-active site one-polypeptide enzyme: the isomaltase from sea lion small intestinal brush-border membrane: the possible phylogenetic relationship with sucrase-isomaltase. J Biol Chem 1984;259:4878.

43. Asp NG, Berg NO, Dahlqvist A, et al. The activity of three different small intestinal β-galactosidases in adults with and without lactase deficiency. Scand J Gastroenterol 1971;6:755.

44. Gray GM, Santiago NA. Intestinal β-galactosidases: I. Separation and characterization of three enzymes in normal human intestine. J Clin Invest 1969;48:716.

45. Mantei N, VJilla M, Enzler T. Complete primary structure of human and rabbit lactase-phlorizin hydrolase: implications for biosynthesis, membrane anchoring and evolution of the enzyme. EMBO J 1988;7: 2705.

46. Kornfeld R, Kornfeld S. Assembly of asparagine-linked oligosaccharides. Ann Rev Biochem 1985;54:631.

47. Kraml J, Kolinska J, Kadlecova L, et al. Analytical isoelectric focusing of rat intestinal brush-border enzymes: postnatal changes and effect of neuraminidase in vitro. FEBS Lett 1983;151:193.

48. Herscovics A, Quaronia A, Bugge B, et al. Partial characterization of the carbohydrate units of intestinal sucrase-isomaltase. Biochem J 1981;197:511.

49. Danielsen EM, Cowell GM. Biosynthesis of intestinal microvillar proteins: processing of N-linked carbohydrate is not required for surface expression. Biochem J 1986;240:777.

50. Hauri H-P, Sterchi EE, Bienz D, et al. Expression and intracellular transport of microvillus membrane hydrolases in human intestinal epithelial cells. J Cell Biol 1985;101:838.

51. Danielsen EM, Cowell GM. Biosynthesis of intestinal microvillar proteins: further characterization of the intracellular processing and transport. FEBS Lett 1984;166:28.

52. Cezard JP, Conklin KA, Das BC, Gray GM. Incomplete intracellular forms of intestinal surface membrane sucrase-isomaltase. J Biol Chem 1979;254:8969.

53. Quaroni A, Kirsch K, Weiser MM. Synthesis of membrane glycoproteins in rat small-intestinal villus cells: effect of colchicine on the redistribution of L (1,5,6-^{3}H) fucose-labelled membrane glycoproteins among Golgi, lateral basal and microvillus membranes. Biochem J 1979;182:203.

54. Hauri H-P, Quaronia A, Isselbacher KJ. Biogenesis of intestinal plasma membrane: post-translational route and cleavage of sucrase-isomaltase. Proc Natl Acad Sci USA 1979;76:5183.

55. Hauri H-P. Biosynthesis and transport of plasma membrane glycoprotein in the rat intestinal epithelial cell. CIBA Symp 1983;95: 13225.

56. Lorenzsonn V, Korsmo H, Olsen WA. Localization of sucrase-isomaltase in the rat enterocyte. Gastroenterology 1987;92:98.

57. Hauri H-P, Roth J, Sterchi EE, et al. Transport to cell surface of epithelial sucrase-isomaltase is blocked in a patient with congenital sucrase-isomaltase deficiency. Proc Natl Acad Sci USA 1985;82: 4423.

58. Matter K, Hauri H-P. Transport of intestinal brush-border enzymes to lysosomes by a direct intracellular pathway. J Cell Biol 1988;107: 566a.

59. Fransen JA, Ginsel LA, Hauri H-P, et al. Immunoelectron microscopical localization of a microvillus membrane disaccharidase in the human small-intestinal epithelium with monoclonal antibodies. Eur J Cell Biol 1985;38:6.

60. Danielsen E, Cowell G. The intracellular transport of aminopeptidase N and sucrase-isomaltase occurs at different rates pre-Golgi but at the same rate post-Golgi. FEBS Lett 1985;190:69.

61. Alpers DH. The relation of size to the relative rates of degradation of intestinal brush-border proteins. J Clin Invest 1972;51:2621.

62. Alpers DH, Tedesco FJ. The possible role of pancreatic proteases in the turnover of intestinal brush-border proteins. Biochim Biophys Acta 1975;401:28.

63. Kwong WKL, Seetharam B, Alpers DH. Effect of exocrine pancreatic insufficiency on small intestine in mouse. Gastroenterology 1978;74: 1277.

64. Hauri HP, Quaroni A, Isselbacher KJ. Monoclonal antibodies to sucrase-isomaltase: probes for the study of postnatal development and biogenesis of the intestinal microvillus membrane. Proc Natl Acad Sci USA 1980;77:6629.

65. Green F, Edwards Y, Hauri H-P, et al. Isolation of a cDNA probe for a human jejunal brush-border hydrolase, sucrase-isomaltase, and assignment of the gene locus to chromosome 3. Gene 1987;57:101.

66. Ghersa P, Huber P, Semenza G, et al. Cell-free synthesis, membrane integration, and glycosylation of pro-sucrase-isomaltase. J Biol Chem 1986;261:7969.

67. Alpers DH, Helms D, Seetharam S, et al. In vitro translation of

intestinal sucrase-isomaltase and glucoamylase. Biochem Biophys Res Commun 1986;134:37.

68. Danielsen EM, Skovbjerg H, Norén O, Sjöström H. Biosynthesis of intestinal microvillar proteins; nature of precursor forms of microvillar enzymes from Ca⁺⁺-precipitated enterocyte membranes. FEBS Lett 1981;132:197.

69. Danielsen EM. Biosynthesis of intestinal microvillar proteins: pulse-chase labelling studies on aminopeptidase N and sucrase-isomaltase. Biochem J 1982;204:639.

70. Danielsen EM, Cowell GM, Poulsen SS. Biosynthesis of intestinal microvillar proteins: role of the Golgi complex and microtubules. Biochem J 1983;216:37.

71. Lloyd ML, Olsen WA. A study of the molecular pathology of sucrase-isomaltase deficiency: a defect in the intracellular processing of the enzyme. N Engl J Med 1987:316, 438.

72. Naim HY, Sterchi EE, Lentze MJ. Biosynthesis of the human sucrase-isomaltase complex: differential O-glycosylation of the sucrase subunit correlates with its position within the enzyme complex. J Biol Chem 1988;263:7242.

73. Trugnan G, Rousset M, Chantret I. The post-translational processing of sucrase-isomaltase in HT-29 cells in a function of their state of enterocytic differentiation. J Cell Biol 1987;104:1199.

74. Grand RJ, Montgomery RK, Perez A. Synthesis and intracellular processing of sucrase-isomaltase in rat jejunum. Gastroenterology 1985;88:531.

75. Sjöström H, Norén O, Danielsen EM. Enzymatic activity of "high mannose" glycosylated forms of intestinal microvillar hydrolases. J Pediatr Gastroenterol Nutr 1985;4:980.

76. Sjöström H, Norén O, Christiansen L, et al. A fully active, two-active site, single-chain sucrase-isomaltase from pig small intestine. J Biol Chem 1980;255:11332.

77. Montgomery RK, Sybicki MA, Forcier AG, et al. Rat intestinal microvillus membrane sucrase-isomaltase is a single high molecular weight protein and fully-active enzyme in the absence of luminal factors. Biochim Biophys Acta 1981;661:346.

78. Skovbjerg H. High molecular weight pro-sucrase-isomaltase in human fetal intestine. Pediatr Res 1982;16:948.

79. Danielsen, EM, Sjöström H, Norén O, et al. Biosynthesis of intestinal microvillar proteins: characterization of intestinal explants in organ culture and evidence for the existence of pro-forms of the microvillar enzymes. Biochem J 1982;202:647.

80. Brunner J, Hauser H, Braun H, et al. The mode of association of the enzyme complex sucrase-isomaltase with the intestinal brush-border membrane. J Biol Chem 1979;254:1821.

81. Kruse TA, Bolund LH, Grzeschik K-H, et al. The human lactase-phlorizin hydrolase gene is located on chromosome 2. FEBS Lett 1988;240:123.

82. Naim HY, Sterchi, EE, Lentze MJ. Biosynthesis and maturation of lactase-phlorizin hydrolase in the human small intestinal epithelial cells. Biochem J 1987;241:427.

83. Büller HA, Montgomery RK, Sasak WV, et al. Biosynthesis, glycosylation, and intracellular transport of intestinal lactase-phlorizin hydrolase in rat. J Biol Chem 1987;262:17206.

84. Danielsen EM, Skovbjerg H, Norén O, Sjöström H. Biosynthesis of intestinal microvillar proteins: intracellular processing of lactase-phlorizin hydrolase. Biochem Biophys Res Commun 1984;122:82.

85. Ahnen DJ, Singleton JR, Hoops TC, Kloppel TM. Post-translational processing of secretory component in the rat jejunum by a brush-border metalloprotease. J Clin Invest 1986;77:1841.

86. Naim HY, Sterchi EE, Lentze MJ. Structure, biosynthesis, and glycosylation of human small intestinal maltase-glucoamylase. J Biol Chem 1988;263:19709.

87. Yokota K, Nishi Y, Takesue Y. Purification and characterization of amphiphilic trehalase from rabbit small intestine. Biochim Biophys Acta 1986;881:405.

88. Sasajima K, Kawachi T, Shigeaki S, Sugimura T. Purification and properties of α,α-trehalase from the mucosa of rat small intestine. Biochim Biophys Acta 1975;403:139.

89. Takesue Y, Yokota K, Nishi Y, et al. Solubilization of trehalase from rabbit renal and intestinal brush-border membranes by a phosphatidylinositol-specific phospholipase C. FEBS Lett 1986;201:5.

90. Rich-Denson C, Kimura RE. Evidence in vivo that most of the intraluminally absorbed glucose is absorbed intact into the portal vein and not metabolized to lactate. Biochem J 1988;254:931.

91. Crane RK, Miller D, Bihler I. The restrictions on possible mechanisms of intestinal active transport of sugars. In: Kleinzeller A, Kotyk A, eds. Membrane transport and metabolism. London: Academic Press, 1961:439.

92. Crane RK. Hypothesis for mechanism of intestinal active transport of sugars. Fed Proc 1962;21:891.

93. Schultz SG, Zalusky R. Ion transport in isolated rabbit ileum: II. The interaction between active sodium and active sugar transport. J Gen Physiol 1964;47:1043.

94. Hopfer U. Membrane transport mechanisms for hexoses and amino acids in the small intestine. In: Johnson LR, ed. Physiology of the gastrointestinal tract. 2nd ed. New York: Raven Press, 1987:1499.

95. Semenza G, Kessler M, Hosang M, et al. Biochemistry of the Na⁺, D-glucose transporter of the small intestinal brush-border membrane: state of the art in 1984. Biochim Biophys Acta 1984;779:343.

96. Freel RW, Goldner AM. Sodium-coupled nonelectrolyte transport across epithelia: emerging concepts and directions. Am J Physiol 1981;241:G451.

97. Hopfer U, Nelson K, Perrotto J, Isselbacher KJ. Glucose transport in isolated brush-border membrane from rat small intestine. J Biol Chem 1973;248:25.

98. Murer H, Hopfer U. Demonstration of electrogenic Na⁺-dependent D-glucose transport in intestinal brush-border membranes. Proc Natl Acad Sci USA 1974;71:484.

99. Hopfer U, Groseclose R. The mechanism of Na⁺-dependent D-glucose transport. J Biol Chem 1980;255:4453.

100. Peerce BE, Clarke RD. Isolation and reconstitution of the intestinal Na⁺/glucose co-transporter. J Biol Chem 1990;265:1731.

101. Hediger MA, Coady MJ, Ikeda TS, Wright EM. Expression, cloning and cDNA sequencing of the Na⁺/glucose co-transporter. Nature 1987;330:379.

102. Ikeda TS, Hwang E-S, Coady MJ, et al. Characterization of a Na⁺/glucose co-transporter cloned from rabbit small intestine. J Membrane Biol 1989;110:87.

103. Birnir B, Lee HS, Hediger MA, Wright EM. Expression and characterization of the intestinal Na⁺/glucose co-transporter in COS-7 cells. Biochim Biophys Acta 1990;1048:100.

104. Mueckler M, Caruso C, Baldwin SA, et al. Sequence and structure of a human glucose transporter. Science 1985;229:941.

105. Birnbaum MJ, Haspel HC, Rosen OM. Cloning and characterization of a cDNA encoding the rat brain glucose-transporter protein. Proc Natl Acad Sci USA 1986;83:5784.

106. Thorens B, Sarkar HK, Kaback HR, Lodish HF. Cloning and functional expression in bacteria of a novel glucose transporter present in liver, intestine, kidney, and β-pancreatic islet cells. Cell 1988;55:281.

107. Peerce BE, Wright EM. Conformational changes in the intestinal brush-border sodium-glucose co-transporter labeled with fluorescein isothiocyanate. Proc Natl Acad Sci USA 1984;81:2223.

108. Peerce BE, Wright EM. Sodium-induced conformational changes in the glucose transporter of intestinal brush borders. J Biol Chem 1984;259:14105.

109. Stevens BR, Fernandez A, Hirayama B, et al. Intestinal brush-border membrane Na⁺/glucose co-transporter functions in situ as a homo-tetramer. Proc Natl Acad Sci USA 1990;87:1456.

110. Hediger MA, Budarf ML, Emanuel BS, et al. Assignment of the human intestinal Na⁺/glucose co-transporter gene (SGLT1) to the q11.2 → qter region of chromosome 22. Genetics 1989;4:297.

111. Murer H, Hopfer U, Kinne-Saffran E, Kinne R. Glucose transport in isolated brush-border and lateral-basal plasma-membrane vesicles from intestinal epithelial cells. Biochim Biophys Acta 1974;345:170.

112. Wright EM, Van Os CH, Mircheff AK. Sugar uptake by intestinal basolateral membrane vesicles. Biochim Biophys Acta 1980;597:112.

113. Guy MJ, Deren JJ. Selective permeability of the small intestine for fructose. Am J Physiol 1971;221:1051.

114. Holdsworth CD, Dawson AM. Absorption of fructose in man. Proc Soc Exp Biol Med 1965;118:142.

115. Sigrist-Nelson K, Hopfer U. A distinct D-fructose transport system in isolated brush-border membrane. Biochim Biophys Acta 1974;367:247.

116. Klumpp TG, Neale AV. The gastric and duodenal contents of normal infants and children. Am J Dis Child 1930;40:1215.

117. Zoppi G, Andreotti G, Pajno-Ferrara F, et al. Exocrine pancreas function in premature and full-term neonates. Pediatr Res 1972;6:880.

118. Grand RJ, Watkins JB, Torti FM. Development of the human gastrointestinal tract: a review. Gastroenterology 1976;70:790.

119. Auricchia S, Rubino A, Murset G. Intestinal glycosidase activities in the human embryo, fetus, and newborn. Pediatrics 1965;35:944.

120. Sebastio G, Hunziker W, O'Neill B, et al. The biosynthesis of intestinal sucrase-isomaltase in human embryo is most likely controlled at the level of transcription. Biochem Biophys Res Commun 1987;149:830.

121. Sebastio G, Hunziker W, Ballabio A, et al. On the primary site of control in the spontaneous development of small-intestinal sucrase-isomaltase after birth. FEBS Lett 1986;208:460.

122. Doell RG, Kretchmer N. Studies of small intestine during development: I. Distribution and activity of β-galactosidase. Biochim Biophys Acta 1962;62:353.

123. Henning SJ. Postnatal development: coordination of feeding, digestion and metabolism. Am J Physiol 1981;241:G199.

124. Yeh K-Y, Holt PR. Ontogenic timing mechanism initiates the expression of rat intestinal sucrase activity. Gastroenterology 1986;90:520.

125. Montgomery RK, Sybicki MA, Grand RJ. Autonomous biochemical and morphological differentiation in fetal rat intestine transplanted at 17 and 20 days of gestation. Dev Biol 1981;87:76.

126. Tsuboi KK, Kwong LK, Neu J, Sunshine P. A proposed mechanism of normal intestinal lactase decline in the postweaned mammal. Biochem Biophys Res Commun 1981;101:645.

127. Jonas MM, Montgomery RK, Grand RJ. Intestinal lactase synthesis during postnatal development in the rat. Pediatr Res 1985;19:956.

128. Freund J-N, Duluc I, Raul F. Discrepancy between the intestinal lactase enzymatic activity and mRNA accumulation in sucklings and adults: effect of starvation and thyroxine treatment. FEBS Lett 1989;248:39.

129. Sebastio G, Villa M, Sartorio R, et al. Control of lactase in human adult-type hypolactasia and in weaning rabbits and rats. Am J Hum Genet 1989;45:489.

130. Nsi-Emvo E, Launay J-F, Raul F. Is adult-type hypolactasia in the intestine of mammals related to changes in the intracellular processing of lactase? Cell Molec Biol 1987;33:335.

131. Simoons FJ. The geographic hypothesis and lactose malabsorption: a weighing of the evidence. Dig Dis 1978;23:963.

132. Saito M. Daily rhythmic changes in brush-border enzymes of the small intestine and kidney in the rat. Biochim Biophys Acta 1972;286:212.

133. Saito M, Murakami E, Suda M. Circadian rhythms in disaccharidases of rat small intestine and its relation to food intake. Biochim Biophys Acta 1976;421:177.

134. Nishida T, Saito M, Suda M. Parallel between circadian rhythms of intestinal disaccharidases and food intake of rats under constant lighting conditions. Gastroenterology 1978;74:224.

135. Stevenson NR, Ferrigni F, Panicky K, et al. Effect of changes in feeding schedule on the diurnal rhythms and daily activity levels of intestinal brush border enzymes and transport systems. Biochim Biophys Acta 1975;406:131.

136. Stevenson NR, Fierstein JS. Circadian rhythms of intestinal sucrase and glucose transport: cued by time of feeding. Am J Physiol 1976;230:731.

137. Kaufman MA, Korsmo HA, Olsen WA. Circadian rhythm of intestinal sucrase activity in rats: mechanism of enzyme change. J Clin Invest 1980;65:1174.

138. Steiner M, Bourges HR, Freedman LS, Gray SJ. Effect of starvation on the tissue composition of the small intestine in the rat. Am J Physiol 1968;215:75.

139. McNeill LK, Hamilton JR. The effect of fasting on disaccharidase activity in the rat small intestine. Pediatrics 1971;47:65.

140. Yamada K, Goda T, Bustamante S, Koldovsky O. Different effect of starvation on activity of sucrase and lactase in rat jejunoileum. Am J Physiol 1983;244:G449.

141. Debnam ES, Levin RJ. Effects of fasting and semistarvation on the kinetics of active and passive sugar absorption across the small intestine in vivo. J Physiol 1975;252:681.

142. Blair DGR, Yakimets W, Tuba J. Rat intestinal sucrase: II. The effects of rat age and sex and of diet on sucrase activity. Can J Biochem 1963;41:917.

143. Deren JJ, Broitman A, Zamcheck N. Effect of diet upon intestinal disaccharidases and disaccharide absorption. J Clin Invest 1967;46:186.

144. Rosenweig NS, Herman RH. Control of jejunal sucrase and maltase activity by dietary sucrose or fructose in man: a model for the study of enzyme regulation in man. J Clin Invest 1968;47:2253.

145. Rosenweig NS, Herman RH. Time response of jejunal sucrase and maltase activity to a high sucrose diet in normal man. Gastroenterology 1969;56:500.

146. Tsuboi KK, Kwong Yamada K, et al. Nature of elevated rat intestinal carbohydrase activities after high-carbohydrate feeding. Am J Physiol 1985;249:G510.

147. Goda T, Yamada K, Bustamante S, Koldovsky O. Dietary-induced rapid decrease of microvillar carbohydrase activity in rat jejunoileum. Am J Physiol 1983;245:G418.

148. Goda T, Bustamante S, Koldovsky O. Dietary regulation of intestinal lactase and sucrase in adult rats: quantitative comparison of effect on lactose and sucrose. J Pediatr Gastroenterol Nutr 1985;4:998.

149. Leichter J, Goda T, Bhandari SD, et al. Relation between dietary-induced increase of intestinal lactase activity and lactose digestion and absorption in adult rats. Am J Physiol 1984;247:G729.

150. McCarthy DM, Nicholoson JA, Kim YS. Intestinal enzyme adaptation to normal diets of different composition. Am J Physiol 1980;239:G445.

151. Raul F, Simon PM, Kedinger M, et al. Effect of sucrose refeeding on disaccharidase and aminopeptidase activities of intestinal villus and crypt cells in adult rats. Biochim Biophys Acta 1980;630:1.

152. Karasov WH, Pond RS, Solberg DH, Diamond JM. Regulation of proline and glucose transport in mouse intestine by dietary substrate levels. Proc Natl Acad Sci USA 1983;80:7674.

153. Cezard JP, Broyart JP, Cuisinier-Gleizes P, Mathieu H. Sucrase-isomaltase regulation by dietary sucrose in the rat. Gastroenterology 1983;84:18.

154. Goda T, Bustamante S, Thornburg W, Koldovsky O. Dietary-induced increase in lactase activity and in immunoreactive lactase in adult rat jejunum. Biochem J 1984;221:261.

155. Riby JE, Kretchmer N. Effect of dietary sucrose on synthesis and degradation of intestinal sucrase. Am J Physiol 1984;246:G757.

156. Olsen WA, Rogers L. Jejunal sucrase activity in diabetic rats. J Lab Clin Med 1971;77:838.

157. Tandon RK, Sriuastava LM, Pandey SC. Increased disaccharidase activity in human diabetics. Am J Clin Nutr 1975;28:621.

158. Olsen WA, Korsmo H. The intestinal brush-border membrane in diabetes: studies of sucrase-isomaltase metabolism in rats with streptozotocin diabetes. J Clin Invest 1977;60:181.

159. Olsen WA, Perchellet E, Malinowski RL. Intestinal mucosa in diabetes: synthesis of total proteins and sucrase-isomaltase. Am J Physiol 1986;250:G788.

160. Olsen WA, Korsmo H. Enhancement of intestinal sucrase activity in experimental diabetes: the role of intraluminal factors. J Lab Clin Med 1975;85:832.

161. Crane RK. An effect of alloxan-diabetes on the active transport of sugars by rat small intestine, in vitro. Biochim Biophys Res Commun 1961;4:436.

162. Olsen WA, Rosenberg IH. Intestinal transport of sugars and amino acids in diabetic rats. J Clin Invest 1970;49:96.

163. Fedorak RN, Gershon MD, Field M. Induction of intestinal glucose carriers in streptozocin-treated chronically diabetic rats. Gastroenterology 1989;96:37.

164. Hopfer U. Diabetes mellitus: changes in the transport properties of isolated intestinal microvillus membranes. Proc Natl Acad Sci USA 1975;72:2027.

165. Arvanitakis C, Olsen WA. Intestinal mucosal disaccharidases in chronic pancreatitis. Am J Dig Dis 1974;19:417.

166. Batt RM, Bush BM, Peter TJ. Biochemical changes in the jejunal mucosa of dogs with naturally occurring pancreatic insufficiency. Gut 1979;20:709.

167. Coello-Ramirez P, Lifschitz F. Enteric microflora and carbohydrate intolerance in infants with diarrhea. Pediatrics 1972;49:233.

168. Giannella R, Rout W, Toskes P. Jejunal brush-border injury and impaired sugar and amino acid uptake in the blind loop syndrome. Gastroenterology 1974;67:965.

169. Jonas A, Flanagan D, Forstner G. Pathogenesis of mucosal injury in the blind loop syndrome: brush-border enzyme activity and glycoprotein degradation. J Clin Invest 1977;60:1321.

170. Jonas A, Krishnan C, Forstner G. Pathogenesis of mucosal injury in the blind loop syndrome: release of disaccharidases from brush-border membranes by extracts of bacteria obtained from intestinal blind loops in rats. Gastroenterology 1978;75:791.

171. Riepe SP, Goldstein J, Alpers DH. Effect of secreted *Bacteroides* proteases on human intestinal brush-border hydrolases. J Clin Invest 1980;66:314.

172. Bo-Linn GW, SantaAnna CA, Morawski SG, Fordtran JS. Starch blockers—their effect on calorie absorption from a high starch meal. N Engl J Med 1982;307:1413.

173. Carlson GL, Li BUK, Bass P, Olsen WA. A bean alpha-amylase inhibitor formulation (starch blocker) is ineffective in man. Science 1983;219:393.

174. Layer P, Carlson GL, DiMagno EP. Partially purified white bean amylase inhibitor reduces starch digestion in vitro and inactivates intraduodenal amylase in humans. Gastroenterology 1985;88:1895.

175. Jenkins DJA, Taylor RH, Goff DU, et al. Scope and specificity of acarbose in slowing carbohydrate absorption in man. Diabetes 1981;30:951.

176. Taylor RH, Barker H, Bowey EA, Canfield JE. Regulation of the absorption of dietary carbohydrate in man by two new glycosidase inhibitors. Gut 1986;27:1471.

18

Intestinal Lipid Absorption

NICHOLAS O. DAVIDSON
ARTHUR M. MAGUN

Dietary lipid represents a major caloric source in most Western cultures. In addition to the 120 to 150 g of lipid consumed each day, the small intestine must process 40 to 50 g of biliary lipid together with small amounts contributed by sloughed mucosal cells and bacteria. Over the past decade, tremendous advances have been made in understanding how this process is coordinated with such efficiency. In addition, widespread attention given the "diet–heart" question has renewed investigation into the role of the small intestine as an active participant in systemic lipoprotein metabolism. This review will provide a current account of the integrated processing of lipid by the small intestine, starting with the sequential *intraluminal events*, which encompass emulsification, lipolysis, and micellar uptake. Attention will then be focused on *intracellular events* within the small intestinal enterocyte, which result in vectorial delivery of lipid for reassembly. Finally, the process of *intestinal lipoprotein assembly and secretion* will be reviewed in order to provide an integrated picture of intestinal lipid processing prior to its secretion into the aqueous milieu of the lymph and plasma compartments.

INTESTINAL LIPID BALANCE

The major form of dietary lipid consumed each day is long-chain ($>C_{14}$) triglyceride together with smaller amounts (up to 10 g/d)

of phospholipid (lecithin). The predominant sources of intraluminal lecithin arise from biliary secretion (10–20 g/d) and membrane phospholipid from desquamated intestinal cells. Additionally, most Americans consume 200 to 500 mg of cholesterol daily, which, in conjunction with large fluxes of biliary cholesterol (1–2 g/d), constitutes a major source of the body's daily metabolic requirements for this sterol. Additionally, various plant sterols (principally β-sitosterol) and shellfish sterols may be substantial dietary components. Other complex lipids such as waxes, lipovitamins (A, D, E, K), hydrophobic xenobiotics (including potentially toxic insecticides and preservatives), and lipid-soluble by-products of commercial food processing are also ingested each day. Absorption of these various intestinal lipids is highly distinctive both in terms of overall efficiency (>95% coefficient of absorption for triglyceride and <5% for β-sitosterol) and the underlying physiologic parameters regulating uptake, intracellular processing, and secretion.

INTRALUMINAL LIPID DIGESTION

Intestinal lipid digestion is a complex, multistep process dependent, first, on effective dispersion of fat into a stable form with a large surface area (emulsification). Second, several lipolytic enzymes become sequentially adsorbed to this emulsion and, under appropriate conditions, mediate digestion of the long-chain triglyceride, phospholipid, and sterol ester bonds (lipolysis). Lipolysis additionally involves important phase transitions, the controlled, sequential evolution of which is integral to the successful completion of both digestion and solubilization of lipid. These lipolytic products subsequently undergo incorporation into aggregated mixtures of bile salts and biliary lecithin for delivery to the microvillus membrane of the villus cell (micellar uptake). Micellar uptake therefore requires that the aqueous milieu of the small bowel lumen be traversed, and consideration will be given below to the physical and apparent barriers limiting this process.

Intragastric Events

Topographically, lipid digestion begins in the stomach with initiation of emulsification. The interaction of triglyceride droplets with dietary and other intraluminal sources of lecithin is a key step in providing stability to the crude lipid emulsion resulting from the shearing action of gastric peristalsis. Proteolytic fragments resulting from peptic digestion additionally stabilize the emulsion. The properties of such emulsions have been characterized both in vivo[1] and in vitro using both phase equilibria and ^{13}C magnetic resonance spectroscopy.[2] Studies of the initial properties of a model emulsion consisting of triglyceride, phospholipid, cholesterol, and water predict a surface layer of lecithin containing approximately 3% triglyceride by weight together with small amounts of cholesterol.[2] The bulk of the triglyceride is sequestered within the core of this emulsion and exists as a homogeneous oil phase. An important consideration is that in this conformation, important quantities of surface triglyceride would be accessible to lipase digestion. Additionally, the rapid exchange that occurs between core and surface triglyceride continuously allows new substrate to be exposed to lipase, facilitating the efficient initiation of lipid digestion.

Intragastric lipolysis is of substantial quantitative importance in both humans and experimental animals. Intragastric lipase activity has been demonstrated (in gastric contents) from premature neonates as early as 26 weeks' gestation[3] and in adults (from mucosal biopsy) up to 80 years of age, although enzyme activity decreases in subjects older than 60 years.[4] Estimates based on studies in ruminants and extrapolated to recent data in human subjects where total recoverable gastric lipase activity has been quantitated[4-6] suggest that normal intragastric lipolysis may account for 20% to 30% of total intraluminal lipid digestion. As will be discussed below, in situations in which a relative or absolute decrease in pancreatic lipase secretion is encountered, this proportion may rise to over 90%. Earlier evidence suggested that possibly two separate lipases were detectable in human gastric contents, namely, lingual lipase[7] and a gastric lipase principally of fundic origin.[4,6] In the rat, lingual lipase is secreted from acinar cells of serous von Ebner glands lying beneath the circumvallate papillae[7] and has been identified by immunohistochemical staining within demilune cells of the lingual mucous glands.[7] Lingual lipase has been characterized extensively in mice, rats, and various ruminants[8] and appears to be the major, if not sole, source of preduodenal lipase in these species. Definitive proof of its importance in human gastric lipolysis, however, has yet to be demonstrated. Of interest in this regard is the recent finding that lipase

activity in tissue supernatants from numerous regions of the tongue (including von Ebner glands), pharynx, and upper gastrointestinal tract from two human organ donors demonstrated activity almost exclusively in the gastric fundus, with less than 0.015% of total gastric lipase activity attributable to a lingual source.[4] Thus, numerous earlier reports characterizing the functional properties of the "lipase" found in human gastric contents[3,9-11] must be viewed with caution in regard to the precise tissue origin of the enzyme. Species considerations may be of some relevance in analyzing the results of these previous studies.[8,12] Evidence indicates ~78% homology between the deduced amino acid sequence of rat lingual lipase (RLL)[13] and human gastric lipase (HGL) based on their recently cloned cDNAs.[14] Specifically, both cDNAs predict peptides of 377 (RLL) and 379 (HGL) amino acids with a deduced M_r of 42564 and 43162, respectively, for the unglycosylated translation products.[13,14] Both HGL and RLL are extensively (15%-20%) glycosylated, and neither bears homology to porcine pancreatic lipase except for a hydrophobic hexapeptide sequence: Ile—Gly—His—Ser—Leu—Gly; this sequence is found in both RLL and HGL as Val—Gly—His—Ser—Gln—Gly and is speculated to be involved in attachment of lipase to its substrate at an interface.[13] It is speculated therefore that the RLL gene is expressed exclusively in rat (but not human) von Ebner glands while a closely analogous, and perhaps evolutionarily related, gene is expressed in human (but not rat) gastric fundic cells.

Intragastric lipolysis differs in several important respects from small intestinal lipolysis. Based on assay of human gastric contents[3,15] and biopsy of gastric fundic cells,[4,6] preduodenal lipase activity displays a broad pH range with an optimum of ~4 to 5.5 and preferential activity against the Sn-3 position long-chain fatty acid ester bond of triglyceride. Since there is product inhibition of lipolytic activity, the major gastric lipolytic products are diglyceride and fatty acid. Activity of the purified enzyme in vitro is inhibited in the presence of bile salts,[15] and a similar effect could be demonstrated following addition of bile salts to human gastric aspirates,[3] particularly in concentrations above 5 mM. This suggests that intragastric lipolysis is sensitive to interfacial denaturation, although it bears emphasis that at bile salt concentrations typically encountered in neonates, that is, ~1 to 2.0 mM, a situation in which intragastric lipolysis may assume particular significance, little inhibitory effect on lipolysis would be predicted.[3] In addition to its low pH optimum and inactivation by bile salts, preduodenal lipase is resistant to pepsin and requires no cofactors.[16] By contrast, at neutral to alkaline pH and in the presence of bile salts, preduodenal lipase is rapidly and extensively degraded by pancreatic proteases,[17] making it unlikely that it would function effectively in the upper small intestine under normal circumstances.

Intragastric lipolysis, then, encompasses a process by which crude dietary lipid undergoes emulsification and initiation of lipolysis. As alluded to above, this contribution to lipid digestion may assume particular importance in neonates where a developmental deficiency in pancreatic lipase secretion is compensated for by preduodenal lipase secretion that results in intragastric lipolysis of 60% to 70% dietary triglyceride.[18] These findings are consistent with the maintenance of approximately 50% triglyceride absorption in children with congenital absence of pancreatic lipase.[19,20] Additionally, patients with cystic fibrosis and exocrine pancreatic insufficiency typically exhibit quite variable degrees of steatorrhea.[21] Measurement of preduodenal lipase activity in five such patients suggested that this source accounted for more than

90% of the total lipase activity measurable at the ligament of Treitz.[21] A notable contributor to the apparent preservation of preduodenal lipase activity in these subjects was the low postprandial intraluminal pH of ~4.0 to 5.0, presumably reflecting decreased bicarbonate secretion, which would permit continued lipolysis by gastric (but not pancreatic) lipase.[21]

At a pH of 5.0 to 6.0, essentially all the liberated fatty acid will remain protonated and, together with diglyceride, become dissolved in the oil phase of the triglyceride emulsion. This emulsion, containing partially digested triglyceride and its lipolytic products, then enters the small intestine where the bulk of intraluminal fat digestion will take place.

Small Intestinal Events

Several key events related to the physicochemical environment of the upper small intestine act in concert to augment the rate and extent of luminal lipolysis. First, at duodenal pH (6.0–7.5), the fatty acids released by intragastric lipolysis lose their protons and become ionized, migrating to the surface of the emulsion, where, as charged particles, they assist in emulsification and, equally importantly, help anchor colipase to the triglyceride emulsion.[2] As will be reviewed below, this is an essential step in initiating pancreatic lipase digestion. Second, following a variety of hormonal stimuli, gallbladder contraction occurs, resulting in the entrance of bile into the duodenum. The combination of alkaline pH, adequate Ca^{++}, bile salts, and lecithin in the presence of lipolytic enzymes initiates a dynamic and dramatic cascade of events.

Lipolytic enzymes (Table 18-1)[19–46] encounter the triglyceride emulsion resulting from gastric processing of ingested fats, and in the presence of appropriate cofactors, ionic conditions and pH, they produce a vigorous acceleration of intraluminal lipolysis. Pancreatic lipase-colipase is secreted from acini in an equimolar stoichiometry. Effective activation of pancreatic lipase requires several interdependent steps. First, following clearing of the lipid emulsion from adsorbed protein by bile salts the colipase-lipase enzyme complex becomes attached to the triglyceride emulsion through colipase physically anchoring lipase in an appropriate configuration to expose its active site. This anchoring is achieved by colipase binding both directly to the triglyceride emulsion and also indirectly through micelle formation with bile salts, which then bind to the emulsion surface. These interactions are augmented by the presence of ionized fatty acid.[25–29] Pancreatic lipase activity in vitro is inhibited by bile salts and phospholipid. Bile salt inhibition can be viewed as occurring by the same mechanism as described previously by which bile salts generally desorb surface protein (including lipase) from the lipid emulsion. This inhibitory process is specifically reversed by colipase.

Colipase-dependent anchoring of lipase to the lipid emulsion is further enhanced by phospholipase A_2 digestion of the phospholipid on the surface of the lipid emulsion, thus allowing exposure of the triglyceride core to the colipase-lipase complex. Phospholipase A_2 digestion requires bile salts and Ca^{++} for activation, and this may further assist colipase-lipase–mediated triglyceride lipolysis by providing a mechanism for removal of the lipolytic products. As previously described, dietary and biliary phospholipid play an important role in stabilizing the crude triglyceride emulsion. The major intraluminal phospholipid is phosphatidylcholine (lecithin), which is unabsorbable intact and requires hydrolysis by phospholipase A_2, yielding a mole of fatty acid and a mole of lysolecithin per mole of substrate. Lysolecithin has a high aqueous solubility and undergoes rapid diffusion and uptake while the newly generated long-chain fatty acid will undergo micellar solubilization and participate in lipolytic product phase formation.

Sterol and lipovitamin esters are largely sequestered within the oily core of the triglyceride emulsion and undergo hydrolysis of their fatty acid ester bond through the actions of cholesterol esterase.[34,35] Bile salts are an obligatory component of this reaction, serving both as an essential enzyme cofactor and as a vehicle for effective solubilization of the extremely hydrophobic sterol and lipovitamin alcohols.

The dynamic aspects of intraluminal fat digestion have been elucidated recently in a series of elegant in vitro and in vivo studies. With the use of mixtures of triglyceride, pancreatic lipase, colipase, and bile salts in a buffered solution at duodenal pH (~6.5), researchers have demonstrated the existence of at least two sequential product phases of triglyceride lipolysis as visualized by light microscopy.[47] The initial products were contained within a lamellar liquid crystalline phase composed of a shell of birefringent calcium soaps (Ca^{++}:fatty acid, 1:2) encapsulating an oily core of unhydrolyzed triglyceride. When a similar analysis conducted at pH 5.0 was used, no visible product phases were visible,[1] suggesting that at intragastric pH the resultant minimal ionization of the liberated fatty acids becomes limiting in calcium-soap formation. Formation of this calcium-soap phase can be preserved in vitro by performing incubations in the absence of bile salts,[1] suggesting that this may be a transient, intermediate phase of intraluminal lipolysis. In the presence of bile salts, a second phase is formed, the composition of which varies continuously as a function of the molar ratio of lipolytic products to bile salts. This phase continuum is referred to as the viscous isotropic phase and is composed largely of monoglyceride and protonated fatty acid in a 1:1 molar ratio.[47] Attempts at obtaining finer resolution of this process have met with mixed success. Transmission electron microscopy has been used to study micelle formation and structure,[48] but these studies suffer from the disadvantages of fixation artifacts and the inability to halt lipolysis completely. More recently this process has been visualized successfully in vivo by means of freeze-fracture using a jet of liquid propane to fix tissue and intraluminal contents instantaneously.[49] The results of representative in vitro and in vivo studies are illustrated below. The initial products of lipolysis, visible 5 minutes after lipase addition in vitro, appear as spherical vesicles of 11- to 30-nm diameter (Fig 18-1). As lipolysis proceeds to completion, lamellar products accumulate at the surface of unhydrolyzed triglyceride emulsions. In the presence of physiologic, micellar concentrations of bile salts, multilamellar product phases and lamellar product vesicles could also be detected in vitro, with product vesicles averaging 50 to 250 nM in diameter. A similar situation was encountered in vivo, wherein, following intraluminal lipid instillation, rough multilamellar product appears initially (Fig 18-2) giving way to an abundance of product vesicles as bile salts enter the intestinal lumen and result in micellar solubilization of lipolytic products for delivery to the microvillus membrane. The layered, multilamellar phase in both in vitro and in vivo systems is proposed as corresponding to the viscous isotropic phase previously described at the light microscope level.[47] It is proposed that as lipolysis proceeds in the upper small intestine, the lipolytic

TABLE 18–1
Small Intestinal Lipolysis: Lipases Present in Humans

ENZYME	TISSUE ORIGIN	STRUCTURAL FEATURES	FUNCTIONAL CHARACTERISTICS	IMPORTANCE
Pancreatic lipase	Pancreatic acini	1.4 Kb mRNA encodes a preenzyme of 465 AA, secreted as mature peptide of 449 AA (M_r = 49,558).[22,23] It is evolutionarily linked to hepatic lipase but divergent from lipoprotein lipase.[24]	In absence of colipase, pH is optimum at 8.0 to 9.0 and activity is inhibited by bile salts >5–10 mM.[25,26] In presence of colipase pH is optimum at 6.0 to 6.5. It is irreversibly denatured at pH <4.0. Activity is increased 40% to 50% by colipase and directed principally against Sn-1,3 positions of triglyceride. There is little activity against sterol esters, phospholipid, or monoglyceride. 1 mol triglyceride is lipolyzed to produce 1 mol β-(Sn-2) monoglyceride, 2 mol fatty acids.[25,26]	Major lipolytic enzyme of humans. Isolated congenital lipase deficiency reportedly[19,20] results in 50% triglyceride malabsorption (gastric lipase may compensate).[21] In health, secreted in approximately 1000-fold molar excess, providing huge functional reservoir of activity.
Pancreatic colipase	Pancreatic acini	336 base pair open reading frame encoding 112 AA procolipase. Removal of —NH_2 terminal pentapeptide following signal peptide cleavage converts procolipase into its active form (M_r-10,111). It is unclear whether this is mediated by thrombin or tryptic cleavage or another protease with specificity for Arg—Gly.[27,28]	Bile salts clear triglyceride emulsion from adsorbed protein/peptic fragments and form micellar aggregates with colipase that assist in directly anchoring coenzyme to the emulsion.[29] Ionized fatty acids further assist in anchoring colipase to triglyceride. Lipase then binds to colipase in a configuration that exposes its active site and allows lipolysis to proceed.	Specific, although not obligate, cofactor for pancreatic lipase action. Isolated colipase deficiency is reported, resulting in approximately 50% triglyceride malabsorption.[30]
Pancreatic phospholipase A_2	Pancreatic acini	Synthesized as a pre-propeptide and secreted as propeptide, requiring tryptic cleavage of —NH_2 terminal 7AA. Mature peptide is 124 AA,[22] M_r ~13,640	Absolute requirement for Ca^{++}. It hydrolyzes phospholipids at the Sn-2 position,[31] producing lysophospholipid and fatty acid.	Removal of phospholipid envelope from triglyceride emulsion enhances lipase-colipase action.
Pancreatic cholesterolesterase	Pancreatic acini	May be similar/identical to human breast milk lipase. It is secreted as an inactive monomer, requiring trihydroxy bile salts for polymerization to a tetramer of M_r ~400,000.[32]	Absolute requirement for bile salts. Broad substrate affinity includes triglyceride, sterol, and vitamin esters.[33–35] It is immunologically detected within human enterocytes,[36] where it is speculated to catalyze the reverse reaction (i.e., acylation of cholesterol, ?-retinol). Its importance in overall scheme of human triglyceride digestion is unclear.	Sterol and lipovitamin absorption. It is unclear whether it exerts a regulatory role.[37–39] No congenital deficiency states have been reported.
Human breast milk lipase	Lactating mammary gland	Identical N terminal sequence to pancreatic cholesterol esterase. Predicted nonglycosylated M_r of 65,000 to 75,000,[40] with glycosylated M_r ~100,000.[41] It is definitively demonstrated to be synthesized in mammary gland.[42]	Neutral-alkaline pH optimum; stable at acid pH; absolute requirement for bile salts.[43] Activity is against triglyceride, cholesteryl, and retinyl ester. It catalyzes retinol acylation ? within enterocyte.[44]	Detectable at 26 weeks' gestation. It is an important contributor to lipolysis in neonate.[45,46] It may be important in vitamin A metabolism.

products (monoglyceride and fatty acid) initially accumulate to form rough, multilamellar phases (viscous isotropic phase). The density and size of these phases will vary as a result of divalent cation and bile salt concentration. In the presence of bile salts above critical micellar concentration, lipolytic products will be partitioned into mixed micelles whose size will reflect the proportions of bile salt to lipolytic product. This process is represented schematically in Figure 18-3. The concordance of the results of in vitro analyses with in vivo experiments indicates the likelihood that this phase transition complex occurs physiologically in humans.

Knowledge of the physical behavior of lipid complexes in mixtures of known composition make it likely that the dynamic aspects of human intestinal lipolysis will soon be accessible to direct study.

Micellar Uptake and Delivery of Lipolytic Products to the Brush Border

The presence of adequate luminal concentrations of conjugated bile salts is an important factor governing the effective solubili-

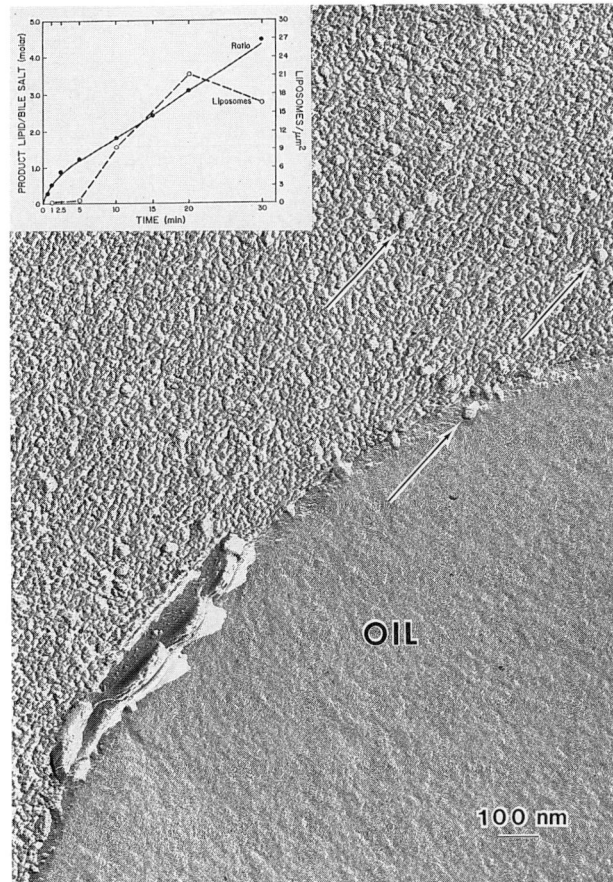

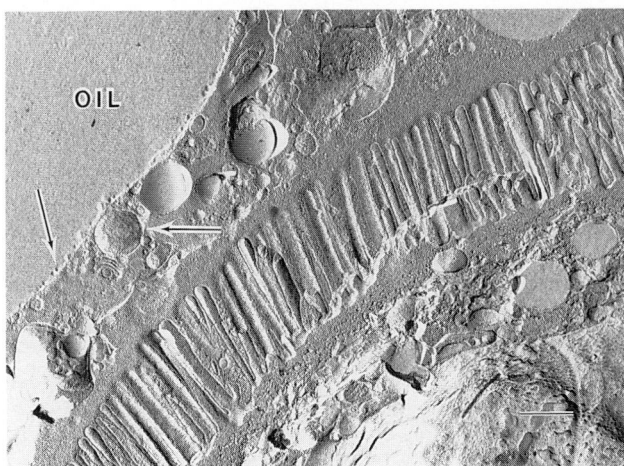

FIGURE 18–2. Morphology of intestinal lipid digestion in vivo. In the view shown, lamellar product vesicles (*arrows*) are seen adjacent to a large triglyceride droplet (*oil*). The product phases are demonstrated to be in close proximity to the enterocyte brush border. (The bar equals 500 nM.) (From Rigler M, Honkanen RE, Patton JS. Visualization by freeze fracture, in vitro and in vivo, of the products of fat digestion. J Lipid Res 1986;27:836.)

FIGURE 18–1. Ultrastructural (freeze fracture) morphology of early in vitro lipolytic products. A triglyceride emulsion (oil) was incubated in the presence of purified pancreatic lipase, colipase, and micellar concentrations (4 mM) of bile salts. The arrows show production of product lamellae and liposomes 10 minutes after lipase addition. The insert shows the rate of vesicle (liposome) production at the indicated ratios of lipolytic product to bile salts over 30 minutes. (From Rigler M, Honkanen RE, Patton JS. Visualization by freeze fracture, in vitro and in vivo, of the products of fat digestion. J Lipid Res 1986;27:836.)

zation of lipolytic products. The important functional characteristic of bile salts in this regard is their tendency to undergo spontaneous aggregation into negatively charged particles called micelles. The concentration at which this occurs is a distinctive property of each species of bile salt and is referred to as the critical micellar concentration. Lipolytic products and phospholipid (biliary lecithin) become incorporated into these aggregates, producing mixed micelles. The more hydrophobic products of lipolysis partition preferentially into the core of these micelles and traverse the aqueous medium of the intestinal lumen by virtue of micellar solubilization. Examples of lipids that are critically dependent on this mechanism include cholesterol, fat-soluble vitamins, and plant sterols.[50] In the absence of bile salts at effective micellar concentrations—either as a result of low intraluminal concentrations (e.g., from biliary obstruction) or because of bacterial deconjugation (e.g., bacterial overgrowth) or abnormal small intestinal acidity (e.g., acid hypersecretory states)—absorption of these hydrophobic compounds is reduced virtually to zero. By contrast, absorption of fatty acids and monoglycerides is facilitated by but not exclu-

sively dependent on micellar solubilization. The major practical evidence for this is the observation that triglyceride malabsorption is relatively mild (<30%) in patients with total biliary obstruction[51] in whom lipolysis would be expected to proceed normally but micellarization of lipolytic products would be absent. The explanation for this observation resides in the phase equilibria produced following triglyceride digestion, in which, in the absence of bile salts, fatty acids and monoglycerides exist as a lamellar, viscous isotropic phase from which presumably monomeric fatty acid can be delivered to the brush-border membrane for uptake.

The importance of effective solubilization of lipolytic products within the bulk luminal contents is one component of the process by which diffusional barrier resistance to mucosal uptake may be overcome. In regard to lipid absorption, diffusion of hydrophobic molecules through this aqueous medium and presentation in sufficient concentrations at the brush-border membrane is a major rate-limiting process. Several hypotheses have been proposed to describe the functional and physical properties of this intestinal diffusional barrier. As a result of the mechanical configuration of the small intestine, its luminal contents are inconsistently mixed and propulsion is regionally variable. These observations have given rise to a number of proposals to explain the behavior of solutes within the bulk phase of luminal contents. One explanation, the unstirred layer hypothesis, predicts that contents in the center of the lumen will be ideally mixed while contents at the outermost region of the loop (i.e., closest to the brush-border membrane) will be functionally "unstirred." Several attempts have been made at indirect quantification of this unstirred layer,[52,53] and the implicit assumption is that differences in absorption may be produced by changes in the physical (or functional) dimensions of this barrier. Quantitation of this unstirred layer, which is physically composed of a dense mucous layer overlying the brush-border glycocalyx[54] has produced figures for the rat in the range of 100 to 1100 μM,[55] depending on the length of intestine used, the flow rate of perfusate, and the effective rate of luminal stirring.[52] By contrast, the laminar

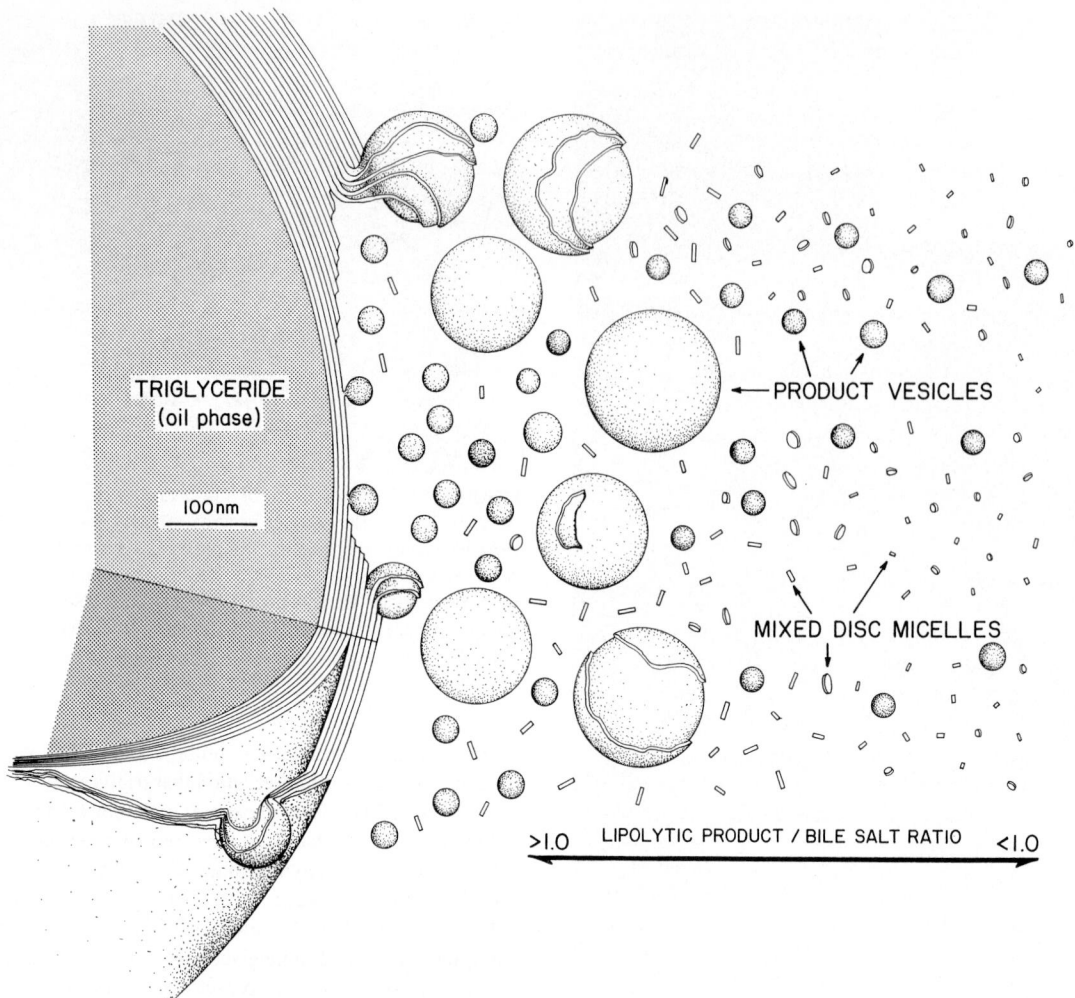

FIGURE 18–3. Accumulation of lipolytic (LP) product lamellae and their subsequent dispersion into vesicles. The figure illustrates schematically the formation of product vesicles whose density and size varies as a function of the LP/bile salt ratio. At high LP/bile salt ratios, large LPs are obtained while discoidal structures of high flotation density are obtained at higher bile salt/LP ratios. (From Rigler M, Honkanen RE, Patton JS. Visualization by freeze fracture, in vitro and in vivo, of the products of fat digestion. J Lipid Res 1986;27:836.)

flow model[53] predicts that solutes would be mixed by a physical process dependent on their relative position with respect to an ideal central axis of vectorial flow. The essential difference resides in the assumption that the laminar flow model has fixed physical dimensions derived from direct determination of solute movement relative to fluid movement in both longitudinal and horizontal axes and, additionally, determination of epithelial versus luminal resistance to solute movement. However, most determinations of unstirred layer thickness are produced by calculations that allow it to vary so as to fit the observed differences in net absorption. Recent studies[53] have provided considerable support for the laminar flow hypothesis by demonstrating that absorption of a variety of probes was independent of luminal volume, the assumption being that it is unlikely that the unstirred layer would systematically alter to the exact dimensions necessary in each setting. These results obtained in perfused jejunal loops will need direct confirmation in the unmanipulated gut but, nevertheless, provide a useful

framework for establishing the basis for luminal resistance to solute movement.

A recent observation provides insight into another mechanism for assimilation of fats that supersedes either of the above hypotheses.[56,57] Workers have demonstrated that intestinal brush-border membranes contain a heparin-like binding site that mediates specific, saturable, and heparin-displaceable binding of pure pancreatic cholesterol esterase (100-kDa peptide) and pancreatic lipase but not amylase or ribonuclease. The implications of this novel finding are that the immobilization of lipolytic enzymes at the brush-border membrane would obviate the necessity to invoke elaborate mechanisms for lipolytic products to traverse the aqueous diffusion barrier. These workers postulate that in situ lipolysis of cholesteryl ester or triglyceride would release fatty acids, mono-glyceride, and free cholesterol in direct proximity to the brush-border membrane where they would undergo rapid uptake.

Other factors that may be important considerations in regulating luminal lipid delivery for uptake are the pH of luminal bulk contents and the possible existence of an acid microclimate at the brush-border surface.[58] Abnormally acidic conditions within the bulk luminal contents will impair micelle formation (since the pKa of bile salts will be exceeded) and result in protonation of liberated fatty acids. Additionally, at pH values more acidic than 4.0, pancreatic lipase is irreversibly denatured. The combination of these factors will prevent normal lipid digestion and absorption to varying degrees. The importance of a local acid microclimate at the brush-border membrane was investigated with respect to the uptake of fatty acid from nonmicellar solutions.[59] These studies demonstrated no significant difference in monomer concentration, solubility, or mucosal uptake of oleic acid at pH 5.5 or 6.5, suggesting that the physiologic impact of a local acid microclimate on the behavior of fatty acids (and particularly with respect to their degree of protonation/ionization which is highly pH dependent) is probably negligible.[59]

Lipolysis and Uptake of Medium-Chain Triglyceride

A triglyceride with fatty acyl groups of 6 to 12 carbon chain lengths is referred to as medium-chain triglyceride. Its luminal and intracellular metabolism differs in several respects from that of long-chain triglyceride. First, medium-chain triglyceride forms more expanded surface films as emulsions than does long-chain triglyceride,[2] thus facilitating intragastric lipolysis. Second, as a result of their intrinsically higher aqueous solubility, medium-chain fatty acids released by both intragastric and small intestinal lipolysis are effectively absorbed by both gastric and small intestinal epithelium and undergo rapid transepithelial delivery. Third, medium-chain fatty acids do not become activated to their CoA-derivative[60] for reassembly into complex lipid (see below for comparison with long-chain fatty acids) but rather undergo direct secretion into the portal vein, where they become bound to albumin for transport to the liver.[61] Last, although intrinsically more susceptible to lipase digestion than long-chain triglyceride, it is speculated that a proportion of medium-chain triglyceride may be absorbed directly, without prior lipolysis. Direct proof of this in humans is lacking, however.

Bile Salt Absorption

It is axiomatic that intestinal lipid absorption does not involve pinocytotic uptake of intact micelles. However, the factors involved in regulating bile salt absorption and the mechanisms by which intraluminal bile salt concentrations are preserved in health have received relatively little attention. Details of the physical structure alterations that accompany micellar lipid delivery to the brush-border membrane are beginning to be explored.

As currently viewed, micellar lipid delivery involves the disgorgement of micellar contents at the brush-border membrane for uptake. Conjugated bile salts, as monomers, are passively absorbed throughout the upper small intestine and, owing to the efficient processes of hepatic uptake following portal vein delivery and reexcretion into bile, become rapidly available again to participate

in micellar lipid solubilization. In addition to passive uptake through the small intestine, an active Na^+-coupled uptake process is present in the mature ileum, which retrieves greater than 95% intraluminal bile salts. The carrier for this process has not been identified in human ileum but may be analogous to a 48- to 49-kDa peptide identified in rat hepatic sinusoidal membranes[62] that may be developmentally regulated.[63]

Colonic Events

Unabsorbed long-chain fatty acids that enter the colon are not absorbable by this organ and undergo a series of bacterial modifications (principally hydroxylation). In health, no undigested triglyceride is found in the stool and the "normal" fecal fat estimate of ~approximately 7 g/d reflects the cumulative total excretion of saponification products (i.e., fatty acids) that arise principally from membrane phospholipid and bacteria. It is likely, therefore, that estimates of normal triglyceride fractional absorption (>95%) may underestimate the astonishing efficiency of this process. Short-chain fatty acids, by contrast, are the principal aqueous solute in colonic contents, with a total concentration of 100 to 240 mM,[64] over 90% of which is accounted for by acetic, propionic, and n-butyric acids. Short-chain fatty acids arise from bacterial fermentation of unabsorbed carbohydrate and may be an important energy source for colonocytes in health and disease.[65] In addition, human fecal matter contains approximately 500 mg bile salts and a smaller quantity, 200 to 500 mg, of cholesterol and its bacterial degradation products cholestanol and cholestanone.[63] Bile salts are principally deconjugated and dehydroxylated in the colon, and, in health, a balance is maintained between these daily fecal losses and de novo bile salt synthesis by the liver.[65]

Brush-Border Membrane Events

The mechanism of long-chain fatty acid uptake across the intestinal microvillus membrane is incompletely understood. Although it is likely that a favorable concentration gradient exists for passive diffusion of these lipophiles, other evidence suggests the presence of a specific carrier. Studies using purified rat jejunal microvillus membranes have identified an affinity-purified ligand specific for long-chain fatty acid.[66] This ligand, referred to as the microvillus membrane fatty acid–binding protein (MVM-FABP), appears to be a homogeneous peptide M_r of 40,000 that co-elutes exclusively with long-chain fatty acid following molecular exclusion chromatography; by contrast, incubation with either phospholipid or cholesteryl ester failed to produce a co-elution pattern. Antisera raised against the MVM-FABP peptide demonstrated immunolocalization of reaction products in apical portions of jejunal villi and partially suppressed uptake of fatty acid in vitro by isolated microvillus membrane preparations. These data, together with kinetic evidence suggesting that long-chain fatty acid uptake is saturable, heat sensitive, trypsin inactivated, and competitive, indicate that a specific carrier is involved. Other work[67] has indicated antigenic homology of the jejunal MVM-FABP to a 40-kDa peptide isolated from rat liver plasma membranes (LPM-FABP). Further work[68] indicates that a 40-kDa peptide expressing shared antigenic epitopes with the MVM-FABP is found in cardiac myocytes and adipocytes, and these researchers speculate that facilitated uptake of fatty acids in these tissues is mediated by a similar or identical membrane protein. Taken together, it is likely that this 40-kDa peptide represents a gene or gene family widely expressed in the membranes of tissues transporting long-chain fatty acids. Furthermore, this gene is likely to be part of a highly conserved family since a similar-sized peptide with fatty acid affinity has been identified in the membranes of bacteria and yeast.[69] Although no specific membrane carrier has been identified for monoglyceride or cholesterol, recent work has raised the interesting possibility that the MVM-FABP may be involved in mediating uptake of these lipids.[70] The evidence for this is based on both substrate competition and MVM-FABP antibody inhibition of lipid uptake in vitro. Clearly, this important area needs additional investigation. In particular, it will be important to determine whether adaptive regulation occurs for these membrane-bound transporters, as has been demonstrated for other nutrient transport systems.[71]

INTRACELLULAR EVENTS IN LIPID REASSEMBLY

Intracellular Transport of Long-Chain Fatty Acids

Following brush-border membrane uptake, long-chain fatty acids and monoglyceride must be translocated across the aqueous cytosolic compartments of the enterocyte and delivered to the smooth endoplasmic reticulum for incorporation into complex lipid. This process of directed intracellular trafficking is believed to be facilitated by fatty acid–binding proteins (FABPs). Intestinal mucosa was first demonstrated to have cytosolic fatty acid–binding activity in studies performed over 15 years ago.[72] Since then, much has been learned about the biology of long-chain FABPs.

Mammalian enterocytes express genes for two cytosolic FABPs, referred to as intestinal or I-FABP and liver or L-FABP.[73] The titles refer to the organ from which each gene product was initially isolated. These FABP genes are part of a immediate gene family that includes at least one other member, namely, a myocardial FABP or H-FABP.[74,75] Collectively, the cytosolic FABPs are members of a larger, supergene family that includes several vitamin A–binding proteins in addition to other proteins whose function is as yet unknown.

The principal FABPs in small intestinal mucosa are I-FABP and L-FABP. The mRNAs encoding these proteins are highly abundant, accounting for 2% to 3% of total intestinal translation products and representing 1% to 2% of soluble cytosolic protein mass.[76–79] L-FABP and I-FABP structures were initially deduced from the nucleotide sequence of their cloned complementary DNAs.[80,81] L-FABP mRNA encodes a 127 residue peptide of M_r 14273 while I-FABP mRNA encodes a slightly larger peptide of 132 residues and M_r 15124,[71] with over 80% nucleotide and amino acid homology between rat and human genes.[73,82] The gene for L-FABP is located on human chromosome 2, while the I-FABP gene is located on human chromosome 4.[82] Analysis of the primary translation products[80,81] in addition to peptide sequencing of the

—NH_2 terminus of L-FABP[83] reveal acetylated methionine residues in both I-FABP and L-FABP. In addition, co-translational cleavage experiments using pancreatic microsomes failed to produce the cleavage/translocation characteristic of peptides synthesized with a signal sequence that are destined to enter the secretory apparatus of the cell. The general conclusion of these experiments, therefore, is that both of these cytosolic FABPs are synthesized as obligate intracellular peptides and not destined for export.

Tissue distribution of these two cytosolic FABPs differs, with I-FABP mRNA essentially confined to the small intestinal enterocyte. Normalizing transcript abundance to that in small intestine (100%), less than 8% of the small intestinal signal was present in colon, while stomach and liver demonstrated 2% to 4% of the intestinal signal.[84] By contrast, L-FABP was expressed in the liver to 50% to 70% of the level found in the small intestine. L-FABP mRNA was found additionally in stomach and colon, both tissues expressing 2% to 6% of the level of mRNA found in small intestine.[84] Regulation of the biosynthesis of these two FABPs has been studied using a variety of techniques. Earlier studies demonstrated that the cytosolic concentration of immunoassayable "fatty acid–binding protein" was increased in a gradient from villus to crypt and proximal to distal small intestine.[76] Since the antibody used to assay this intestinal immunoreactive FABP cross-reacted with hepatic cytosolic FABP, the findings of these earlier studies suggest that intestinally located L-FABP (rather than I-FABP) may be subject to regulation by the availability of luminal substrate.[76] More recently the developmental expression of these two cytosolic FABPs has been examined in the rat and a striking pattern of tissue-specific regulation demonstrated.[84] There was a coordinated increase in mRNA abundance for both L-FABP and I-FABP in intestinal mucosa following birth, with detectable levels at day 19 of gestation. Peak levels of mRNA abundance were observed in adult small intestine. With the use of complementary approaches of cDNA hybridization and classic protein turnover kinetics, it has been established that L-FABP mRNA abundance and translatable activity is higher in the jejunum of female as compared with male rats.[78,79] However, the turnover of newly synthesized L-FABP in female rats was also faster than in males, producing no net effect on steady-state cytosolic L-FABP concentrations. By contrast there was no effect of gender on either the cytosolic concentration or translatable activity of I-FABP. Clofibrate, a hypolipidemic agent with a variety of effects on hepatic fatty acid metabolism, produced a twofold elevation of intestinal L-FABP mRNA and protein concentration but no effect on I-FABP. Thus a consensus of data supports the hypothesis that these two cytosolic FABPs are independently regulated and probably play distinct roles in intracellular fatty acid metabolism. More recently, both L-FABP and I-FABP have been expressed in *Escherichia coli* and their structure and ligand-binding affinities directly determined.[85–87] L-FABP has a binding capacity of 2 mol fatty acid per mole of protein while I-FABP binds in a 1:1 stoichiometry. Further studies demonstrated that L-FABP exhibits higher affinity for polyunsaturated fatty acids than saturated species while I-FABP exhibited broadly similar affinity for saturated and polyunsaturated fatty acids. These data support the general concept that intracellular FABPs within the enterocyte may serve to target substrate fatty acid to selective compartments for incorporation into triglyceride, phospholipid, or cholesteryl or retinyl esters. Fatty acids entering the enterocyte from the basolateral membrane (plasma derived) are believed to be metabolically distinct from fatty acids absorbed across the brush border.[88] The precise role of L-FABP and I-FABP in maintaining such ordered polarity in fatty acid use remains to be elucidated. It has recently been speculated that the differences in ligand-binding stoichiometry, underlying mechanisms of conformational interaction, and pH sensitivity may be correlated with their distinctive physiologic role in enterocyte fatty acid trafficking.[87]

Intracellular Transport of Sterols

Intestinal absorption and metabolic processing of dietary and biliary sterols—principally cholesterol—is a major component of the body's homeostatic control mechanisms for regulating sterol uptake. In addition, the intestine is the portal of entry of the fat-soluble vitamins (A, D, E, and K) and elaborate conservation mechanisms have evolved to ensure constant availability of these essential nutrients, particularly vitamin A.

These hydrophobic molecules are currently postulated to traverse the lipid bilayer of the brush border by passive diffusion. From the perspective of regulating intracellular cholesterol traffic, the enterocyte receives the bulk of its daily flux of cholesterol from luminal sources (dietary and biliary) but is also capable of de novo cholesterol synthesis from 2 carbon units. In addition, the intestinal cell expresses low-density lipoprotein (LDL) receptors on its basolateral membrane,[89] thus facilitating endocytotic uptake of circulating plasma LDL. The interactions of these various sources of intestinal cholesterol will be considered in more detail below. Cholesterol that partitions into the lipid bilayer of brush border is present in at least two metabolically distinct forms.[90] There is a small, readily mobilized pool and a separate less readily accessible pool, in proportions of approximately 1:3. Cholesterol delivery to a variety of intracellular locations is facilitated by means of its 1:1 stoichiometric association with a specific carrier protein[91] referred to as sterol carrier protein-2 (SCP_2). In earlier publications this protein was referred to as the nonspecific lipid transfer protein, but at least partial immunologic identity between the two peptides has been confirmed[92] and their amino acid sequence is closely homologous, although not identical.[93] Details of the association kinetics between different membrane-bound pools of free cholesterol and SCP_2, however, are currently unknown. SCP_2 has been purified to homogeneity from bovine and rat liver, appearing as a monomeric peptide of M_r 13,500.[94] Several lines of evidence indicate it is distinct from a peptide earlier referred to as "sterol carrier protein."[95] Antisera raised to this protein have been used to detect immunologically cross-reactive material in a variety of intracellular organelles from both villus and crypt cells.[96] The majority of intestinal SCP_2 mass appeared in mitochondria with only small amounts detected in brush-border membranes. Other studies have demonstrated that exogenously added SCP_2 enhanced cholesterol esterification in vitro using isolated intestinal microsomes,[97] suggesting that intestinal SCP_2 may serve an analogous role to that postulated in both the liver[95] and adrenal[98] where alterations in steroidogenesis and cholesterol use have been shown to be critically dependent on SCP_2 availability. In addition, SCP_2 is involved in the facilitated conversion of several microsome-located precursors to their eventual end product, cholesterol.[94] Thus SCP_2 is intimately involved with both cholesterol synthesis and its ultimate metabolic targeting either to membrane cholesterol or for esterification. Currently, little is known about the regulation of SCP_2 gene expression, although recent work in cultured rat adrenocortical cells[98] suggests that its synthesis may be translationally regulated by changes in steroidogenesis induced by adrenocorticotropic hormone (ACTH) or dibutyryl cyclic adenosine monophosphate (AMP).

Intracellular Transport and Metabolism of Vitamin A

All mammals require vitamin A for effective cell growth and differentiation. Two major sources of this nutrient are available: carotenoids, principally β-carotene from plants, and retinyl esters derived from animal tissues. Carotenoids must be converted, following uptake into the enterocyte, into retinol, a two-step procedure involving cleavage by 15,15′dioxygenase to yield two molecules of retinaldehyde, which is subsequently reduced to retinol.[99] Dietary retinyl esters must first undergo hydrolysis to retinol prior to absorption and, although clear details are lacking, the evidence suggests that both β-carotene and retinol are absorbed into the enterocyte by passive diffusion.

The intestine synthesizes specific binding protein(s), which provide a mechanism by which cellular vitamin A is stored and delivered for esterification prior to secretion in the form of retinyl ester. There are at least six cellular vitamin A–binding proteins, including cellular retinol-binding protein (CRBP), cellular retinol-binding protein II (CRBP II), cellular retinaldehyde-binding protein (CRABP), cellular retinaldehyde-binding protein II (CRABP II), cellular retinal-binding protein (CRALBP), and the interstitial retinol-binding protein (IRBP). The latter two vitamin A–binding proteins are located exclusively in the eye, and all members of this family are distinct from the serum retinol-binding protein RBP.[100] Together these proteins form part of a supergene family with at least eleven known members, including I-FABP, L-FABP, H-FABP, adipocyte 422 protein, and myelin P_2 protein. The two principal intracellular vitamin A–binding proteins of relevance to the intestine are cellular retinol-binding protein (CRBP) and cellular retinol-binding protein II (CRBP II). These two peptides exhibit extensive amino acid and nucleotide homology, and both genes are located on human chromosome 3.[101] The tissue distribution of the two mRNAs, however, is distinct, with CRBP II gene expression virtually confined to the enterocyte,[102] while CRBP is widely distributed among vitamin A–responsive cells and CRBP immunoreactivity in the gut is confined to submucosal and lamina propria staining.[103] CRBP II is abundantly expressed, representing approximately 1% soluble protein in rat jejunum and 0.4% soluble protein in human proximal small bowel.[104] The highest levels were detected in villi of the proximal small bowel, illustrating a striking gradient both vertically (villus to crypt) and horizontally (jejunum to ileum). Studies further suggest that CRBP II undergoes developmental regulation with peak mRNA abundance just prior to birth, at 21 days of gestation in the rat.[102] This finding would be compatible with cellular retinol flux undergoing changes temporally related to morphologic differentiation of the villus-crypt axis. It is clear from recent studies in which the retinoic acid receptor gene has been cloned and sequenced[105] that this new member of the steroid/thyroid hormone receptor gene family may function as a vertebrate morphogen. Further studies directed at elucidating the structure of its intestinal homolog may well provide important insights into the factors controlling cellular maturation and differentiation.

Retinol is secreted by the enterocyte in the form of retinyl ester, predominantly in the hydrophobic core of triglyceride-rich lipoproteins. The mechanism by which intestinal retinol undergoes esterification has been the subject of considerable debate. Potential mechanisms include the reversible action of pancreatic cholesterol esterase, microsomal conversion employing acyl CoA cholesterol acyl transferase (ACAT), or acyl CoA retinol acyl transferase (ARAT).[106] The latter two enzymes have been favored because of the observed fatty acid specificity of the esterification reaction as evidenced by gas liquid chromatographic analysis of both human and rat lymph retinyl esters.[99] Recent studies[107,108] have indicated that when retinol is presented as a complex with CRBP II, microsomes are able to use endogenous acyl donors and synthesize retinyl esters with strikingly similar fatty acid composition to that described for rat lymph. Moreover, retinol–CRBP II complexes were unavailable for acyl-CoA directed esterification, while retinol complexed to albumin was effectively esterified in an acyl-CoA–driven reaction. The rates of retinyl ester production by rat intestinal microsomes using this (acyl CoA–independent) novel mechanism were calculated to be over 1 μmol/d, which is more than sufficient to meet physiologic requirements. Taken together, these observations suggest that a potentially major function of CRBP II may be to direct intestinal retinol to an appropriate milieu for esterification.[107,108] Specifically, this would involve retinol being targeted to a non acyl-CoA–driven reesterification process, thus permitting distinct metabolic compartmentalization. Although this remains to be shown directly, presumably this mechanism would avoid competition between retinol and other intracellular lipid components (e.g., cholesterol) for acyl-CoA donors.

Intestinal Cholesterol Metabolism

From the perspective of the body's economy of cholesterol, intestinal cholesterol absorption and processing assume a major role since dietary and biliary sources together provide between 1 and 2 g cholesterol that enters the intestinal lumen each day. Biliary cholesterol is essentially all free sterol, while 10% to 20% of dietary cholesterol is present as cholesteryl ester that must undergo hydrolysis prior to absorption. Cholesterol is absorbed by passive diffusion, its delivery to the brush-border lipid bilayer being facilitated by micellar diffusion.

Free cholesterol in the intestinal brush-border membrane exists in both a slowly exchangeable and a rapidly exchangeable form.[90] Treatment of membrane vesicles with papain or sodium deoxycholate failed to release substantial quantities of the residual (slowly exchangeable) cholesterol, indicating that the slowly miscible membrane cholesterol pool is not sequestered within the glycocalyx or nonspecifically trapped within vesicles of limited pore size. The conclusion from this work is that membrane cholesterol may be associated with some protein component capable of mediating specific interactions with sterol acceptors, such as SCP$_2$. From the brush border, cholesterol is transported, presumably by SCP$_2$ and potentially other acceptor proteins (but not L-FABP or I-FABP, which have no sterol-binding affinity[95]), to the smooth endoplasmic reticulum for reesterification. Although

small amounts (up to 25%) of cholesterol may be secreted from the enterocyte and transported in mesenteric lymph as free cholesterol, the overwhelming bulk of intracellular cholesterol that is destined for export undergoes reesterification. There has been considerable debate over the years as to the principal enzyme responsible for physiologic regulation of intestinal cholesterol esterification. The two candidate enzymes are pancreatic cholesterol esterase and acyl-CoA:cholesterol acyltransferase (ACAT). In favor of the former is the demonstration by immunohistochemical staining that a reactive product is detectable within villus enterocytes using antisera raised against pancreatic cholesterol esterase.[109] More recently[36] this finding has been extended to an immunoelectronmicroscopic demonstration that pancreatic cholesterol esterase (or an immunoreactive fragment) is located within endocytotic vesicles in the human small intestine. Furthermore, in vitro evidence suggests that this enzyme that mediates cholesteryl ester hydrolysis within the lumen of the gut demonstrates a reversal of this activity at a pH of 5.0 to 6.0.[37] It is postulated that the multimeric form of luminal pancreatic cholesterol esterase ($M_r \sim 400,000$) becomes internalized by the enterocyte where it facilitates cholesterol esterification.[109] Convincing studies have been presented showing that pancreatic duct diversion, which removes all luminal sources of cholesterol esterase, effectively reduces both absorbed cholesteryl ester mass and the properties of free to esterified cholesterol transported in mesenteric lymph.[38] This maneuver additionally depletes immunohistochemically detectable enzyme from within rat enterocytes.[109] Other studies, by contrast, have demonstrated that intestinal ACAT activity can account for all the esterified cholesterol transported by human and rat mesenteric lymph.[110] Moreover, a consensus of both in vivo and in vitro studies supports a role for ACAT based on (1) its intracellular location and presence in high concentrations in jejunal villus cells; (2) the presence of both a horizontal (jejunal > ileal) and vertical (villus > crypt) gradient of enzyme activity; and (3) the consistent increase of intestinal ACAT activity following dietary cholesterol augmentation.[111] Recent attempts to resolve the question of which enzyme is functionally responsible for intestinal cholesterol esterification have used the experimental ACAT inhibitor 58-035 in an attempt to suppress the intracellular activity of one or other (but not both) potential mediators of cholesterol esterification.[38,39] The data were insufficiently conclusive to resolve the issue one way or another, suggesting that the enterocyte may employ more than one metabolic route for cholesterol esterification. Possibly differences in the mode of cholesterol delivery to different intracellular pools may define in part which esterification mechanism is used.

The enterocyte receives the bulk of its cholesterol from luminal sources. However, the cell expresses specific LDL receptors and is also capable of internalizing LDL by non-receptor-mediated pathways in proportions of approximately 3:2.[112] Thus circulating plasma LDL may provide cholesterol for intestinal metabolism. Studies in the rat estimate that approximately 10% of the total LDL removed each day by receptor-dependent pathways was accounted for by the small bowel.[112] A further source of cholesterol is from de novo synthesis, and in this respect the enterocyte is second only to the liver on a per organ basis as a synthetic source of cholesterol. A series of elegant experiments conducted over the past few years has elucidated much important information concerning the physiologic relationships between the various sources of intestinal cholesterol and the metabolic fate of each. Based on a consensus of such studies, the following general comments can be made. First, the small intestine is a major synthetic source of cholesterol with estimates of approximately 25% of the total daily synthesis accounted for by this organ in the rat,[113] and in animals such as the guinea pig and hamster (whose cholesterol metabolism more closely resembles that of the human) values may be substantially higher.[114] Opinion varies as to the location and cell type most actively involved in cholesterol synthesis. Most of the disagreement is likely due to methodologic variation, but studies using ^3H_2O as the preferred substrate to measure sterol synthesis[115] or immunocytochemical localization of 3-hydroxy-3-methylglutaryl coenzyme A reductase (HMG CoA reductase), the rate-limiting enzyme of cholesterol biosynthesis,[116] are in general agreement that the ileum is more active than the duodenum and that cells of the lower and middle thirds of the villus are more active than cells at the villus tip. Second, cholesterol biosynthesis is inducible in the small bowel by removing or interfering with luminal cholesterol uptake (either by drug therapy such as cholestyramine or by bile elimination that removes luminal cholesterol and bile salts). Both of these general maneuvers result in a compensatory increase of intestinal cholesterol synthesis.[114] By contrast, intestinal cholesterol synthesis is unaltered or incompletely suppressed in the rat by dietary cholesterol augmentation.[117] This apparent paradox is resolved by the observation that the balance of intracellular cholesterol is maintained in this setting by the up-regulation of ACAT and increased secretion of cholesteryl ester.[114] There appear to be species considerations of relevance to the question of whether intestinal cholesterol biosynthesis may be directly regulated by dietary cholesterol. Studies in canine intestine suggest the presence of sensitive feedback inhibition,[118] while studies in humans have demonstrated no effect of dietary cholesterol augmentation on intestinal cholesterol synthesis.[119] Third, the integrated relationship between these parameters is unresolved since studies have shown that neither intestinal cholesterol synthesis rates nor intracellular ACAT activity is related to the rate at which the enterocyte internalized plasma LDL,[114,117] while other studies have suggested that circulating plasma lipoprotein cholesterol may directly affect intestinal HMG CoA reductase and ACAT specific activity.[120] Studies in hypercholesterolemic human subjects suggest that jejunal HMG CoA reductase activity is lower in these subjects than in controls and is lowered further by lovastatin therapy.[121]

Taken together, the available evidence suggests that there exist several discrete metabolic compartments for intestinal cholesterol. Absorbed (luminal) cholesterol appears to regulate ACAT activity, and it is speculated that this may be the preferred substrate. Newly synthesized cholesterol clearly plays an important part in delivering cholesterol for cell membrane biosynthesis but is not clearly related to the dietary-related export demands of the enterocyte. Whether de novo synthesized cellular cholesterol is targeted for esterification by a particular enzyme is unknown at present. Finally, the factors that regulate LDL internalization and the role that this source plays in the traffic of intracellular cholesterol are currently unresolved and together form a focus of active investigation.

Studies in humans have suggested that dietary cholesterol may be a major factor in conferring increased risk of atherosclerosis in Western society. Although clear evidence concerning physiologic regulation is lacking, studies have suggested that humans absorb about 50% of their dietary cholesterol and that (medications such as cholestyramine aside[122]) this rate is unrelated to hyperlipidemic phenotype[122] or circulating LDL cholesterol levels.[123]

Studies have suggested that cholesterol absorption in certain subjects may be related to the phenotype for apolipoprotein E (apo E),[124] a finding of some interest since apo E is synthesized predominantly by the liver and in several extrahepatic tissues but notably not by the small intestine.

In addition to cholesterol, humans consume plant sterols (phytosterols) and shellfish sterols that are related to cholesterol but contain minor structural modifications. β-sitosterol, for example, which is the major phytosterol consumed by humans, differs by a single ethyl substitution at C24. The biologic importance of these sterols has been recognized recently, principally as a result of the observation that they are variably absorbed by normal human subjects.[125] Furthermore, their abnormal absorption in subjects with phytosterolemia may provide a clue to how the normal intestine discriminates between cholesterol and other sterol molecules that closely resemble it. A systematic study of the abnormal absorption of such sterols in a subject with sitosterolemia[126] revealed a generalized abnormality in the ability of the gut to discriminate between these related phytosterols and shellfish sterols. Other studies suggest that β-sitosterol is an ineffective substrate for intestinal ACAT.[127] The accumulation of intracellular free phytosterols would therefore provide one mechanism that would limit absorption of these compounds under normal circumstances. Other recent studies show that plant sterols may displace cholesterol from micelles competitively, thus reducing intestinal uptake.[128,129]

Intestinal Triglyceride Synthesis and Metabolism

Triglyceride is the most abundant lipid processed by the intestine and is almost quantitatively absorbed by the enterocyte following intraluminal lipolysis. Approximately 75% of absorbed luminal fatty acids are resynthesized into triglyceride and secreted by the enterocyte as lipoprotein.[130,131] The remaining 25% serve as a substrate for phospholipid and other intracellular lipid resynthesis events or undergo transport to the liver bound to albumin via the portal vein.[61,132,133] The intestine also synthesizes and secretes triglyceride during fasting, with estimates of 10% to 40% of circulating plasma triglyceride being derived from the intestine following an overnight fast.[134]

There are two major synthetic pathways for triglyceride synthesis in the enterocyte, as illustrated in Figure 18-4. The glycerol-3-phosphate pathway is the major synthetic route during periods of limited availability of luminal monoglyceride and fatty acid.[134,135] α-Glycerophosphate CoA acyltransferase, which catalyzes triglyceride synthesis via the glycerol-3-phosphate pathway, is predominantly associated with rough rather than smooth endoplasmic reticulum.[136] The substrates for triglyceride synthesis via this pathway, glycerol-3-phosphate and lysolecithin, are derived from glucose metabolism (dihydroxy-acetone phosphate) and bile, respectively.[134,137] The importance of biliary phospholipid as a substrate for triglyceride synthesis is highlighted by the fact that 75% of the fatty acids in infused lecithin are incorporated into secreted triglyceride during fasting.[138]

When triglyceride is ingested and luminal 2-monoglyceride and free fatty acids are present in abundance, the glycerol-3-phosphate pathway is inhibited and the monoacylglycerol pathway becomes the predominant route of triglyceride synthesis.[130,139] The mech-

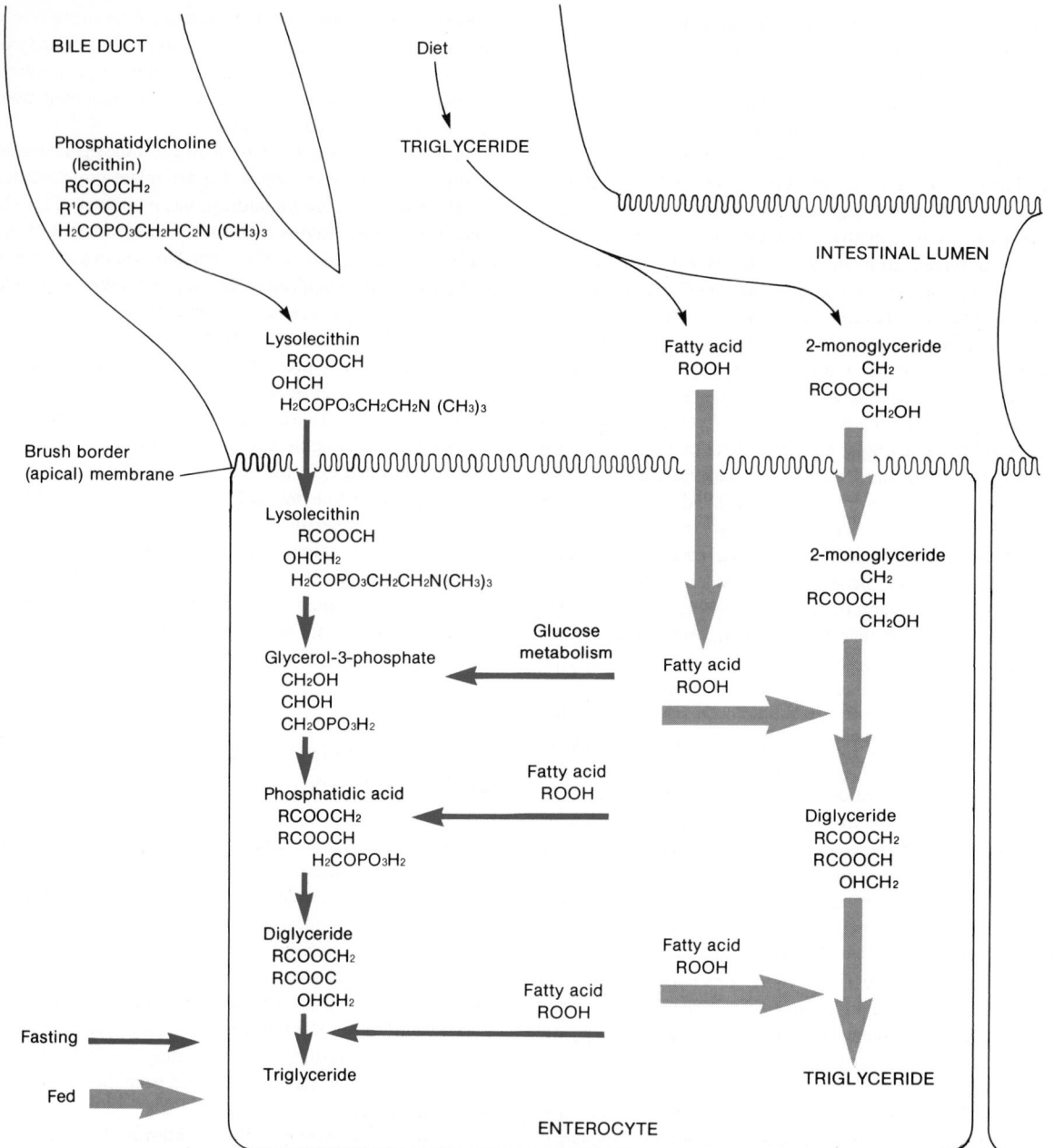

FIGURE 18–4. Intestinal triglyceride biosynthesis. Triglyceride is synthesized within enterocytes via two major pathways. During fasting, triglyceride is synthesized via the glycerol-3-phosphate pathway from the products of glucose metabolism and hydrolyzed lysolecithin (*blue arrows*). In the fed state, triglyceride is synthesized from absorbed 2-monoglyceride and fatty acids (*red arrows*).

anism for this inhibition is not known. The intracellular location of the enzymes catalyzing triglyceride synthesis in the monoacylglycerol pathway are located in the smooth endoplasmic reticulum, in contrast to the location of the enzymes of the glycerol-3-phosphate pathway. These enzymes are collectively referred to as triglyceride synthetase, and they include acyl CoA-synthetase and monoglyceride and diglyceride acyltransferase.[140] Although the liver also contains monoacylglycerol acyl transferase, the intestinal form of the enzyme appears to be distinct based on substrate specificity, thermolability, and susceptibility to various detergents.[141] The intestinal enzyme is stereospecific in that almost 90% of 2-monoacylglycerol is converted into sn 1,2-diacylglyc-

erol.[142] The diglyceride formed from 2-monoacylglycerol appears to be in a separate intracellular pool from diglyceride synthesized via the glycerol-3-phosphate pathway, as based on in vitro incubation studies.[133,143]

Intestinal Phospholipid Synthesis and Metabolism

Phospholipids, particularly phosphatidylcholine (lecithin), are essential components of cell membranes. Lecithin is also a key component of lipoproteins, providing a surface coat for the inner core of triglyceride and cholesteryl ester. There are two major synthetic pathways for phospholipid in the enterocyte (Fig 18-5): (1) the phosphatidic acid–phosphorylcholine pathway[144-146] and (2) reacylation of absorbed lysolecithin.[138,144] A third pathway found in the liver in which phosphatidylethanolamine is methylated is not an important intestinal phospholipid synthetic pathway.[147]

The substrates for lecithin synthesis via the phosphatidic acid pathway are glycerol-3-phosphate derived from glucose metabolism and lysolecithin hydrolysis and CDP-choline derived from biliary and dietary choline.[138,145,148] Lecithin synthesis via the reacylation pathway involves the enzyme lysophosphatidylcholine acyl transferase, which transfers a fatty acid back onto lysolecithin to form lecithin.[137] The highest specific activity of the enzyme is in the villous tips of the proximal intestine.[149] Choline phosphotransferase, the enzyme catalyzing the transfer of choline onto diglyceride in the phosphatidic acid pathway, has a specific activity less than that of lysophosphatidylcholine acyl transferase in the tips of the villi but equal to it in the crypts.[149]

It is unclear as to which pathway is quantitatively more important for intestinal phospholipid synthesis. Lysophosphatidylcholine acyl transferase is more responsive to lipid feeding than choline phosphotransferase,[150] suggesting that the lysolecithin reacylation pathway may be more important postprandially. During periods of fasting and low levels of luminal lecithin, the phosphatidic acid–phosphorylcholine pathway is the main synthetic route.[138,148] Postprandially, with higher levels of both biliary and dietary lysolecithin available, there is increased synthesis of lecithin via the reacylation pathway (see Fig 18-5). During very high rates of experimental lecithin infusion into the lumen of the rat intestine, lymphatic chylomicron-phospholipid was exclusively derived from the infused lecithin via the reacylation pathway.[148] It is likely, however, that this experimental model is not physiologic and that during postprandial periods, the intraluminal concentration of lecithin is such that both pathways are operative.[148]

INTESTINAL LIPOPROTEIN ASSEMBLY AND SECRETION

Enterocyte Morphology and Lipoprotein Assembly Overview

The morphology of the intracellular events occurring during lipid absorption has been well studied in both human and rat intestine (Fig 18-6).[151-153] Serial electron micrographic studies reveal that 5 to 10 minutes following lipid instillation into the intestinal lumen, large droplets of lipid form near the microvillus membrane. These lipid droplets are resynthesized triglyceride in and adjacent to the smooth endoplasmic reticulum. During lipid absorption, rough endoplasmic reticulum membranes decrease in both size and number while smooth endoplasmic reticulum increases, suggesting the active involvement of smooth endoplasmic reticulum in the process of lipid absorption.[151] The enzymes involved in triglyceride and phospholipid synthesis are located in the smooth and rough endoplasmic reticulum.[149] It is possible that there are two pools of intracellular triglyceride, one destined for chylomicron secretion

derived from the 2-monoglyceride pathway and the other derived from the phosphatidic acid pathway, which may not be destined for chylomicron secretion.[133] The exact intracellular location and relative size of these pools of triglyceride is unclear (Fig 18-7).

Apolipoprotein synthesis occurs in the rough endoplasmic reticulum.[154] Apolipoproteins are believed to be transferred from the rough endoplasmic reticulum onto newly synthesized lipid, as evidenced by the decrease in apo B immunostaining in the rough endoplasmic reticulum together with a corresponding increase in apo B immunostaining in the smooth endoplasmic reticulum following lipid feeding.[154] The distribution of apolipoproteins within the enterocyte is such that, during fasting, about 90% of apolipoprotein is not bound to lipoprotein, but remains associated with the endoplasmic reticulum.[155] Lipid feeding mobilizes 5% to 10% of this apolipoprotein from the non-lipoprotein-bound pool onto newly assembled lipoproteins.[155,156] The mechanism by which apolipoproteins associate with lipids to form nascent intracellular lipoproteins is not known. Other studies have suggested that microtubules may be involved in intracellular lipid transport, although precise details are somewhat unclear.[157]

The Golgi apparatus membranes, which are generally located close to the nucleus of the cell, become filled with lipid droplets corresponding in size to chylomicrons and very low density lipoprotein (VLDL)–like particles following lipid feeding (see Figs 18-6 and 18-7). In the liver, lipid and apolipoproteins are added to nascent lipoproteins in Golgi organelles, and it is likely that similar remodeling occurs in the intestinal enterocyte.[158] Golgi organelles are believed to be precursors to secretory vesicles, which are larger vesicles filled with lipid droplets of varying size representing nascent forms of intracellular lipoproteins prior to secretion.[152] These secretory vesicles fuse with the basolateral membranes and release nascent lipoproteins into the extracellular space and mesenteric lymph.[152,153] The rate-limiting step during chylomicron formation and secretion appears to be the rate at which luminal triglyceride is absorbed and not the rate of apolipoprotein synthesis.[155,159] There does not appear to be a difference in secretion rates of apolipoprotein in proximal as compared with distal small intestine in rats,[159] although distal intestine has been shown to transport lipid more slowly than proximal intestine.[159] In humans, following lipid infusion directly into the jejunum and ileum, no morphologic differences in the enterocytes of the jejunum as compared with ileum are seen, suggesting that fat absorption and lipid secretion in the proximal and distal bowel is similar.[160]

Regulation of Intestinal Apolipoprotein Gene Expression

Apolipoproteins are the protein components of lipoproteins, the vehicles by which water-insoluble lipid is transported through the aqueous medium of plasma. Plasma lipoproteins exist in several distinct subclasses and are conventionally separated and identified by virtue of their distinctive physical and functional characteristics. A brief overview of human plasma lipoprotein classification is presented in Table 18-2.

There are at least six apolipoprotein genes whose presence in the small intestine has been demonstrated either by immunologic detection of the final gene product and/or by cDNA hybridization to an appropriate-sized transcript (Table 18-3). Of these apolip-

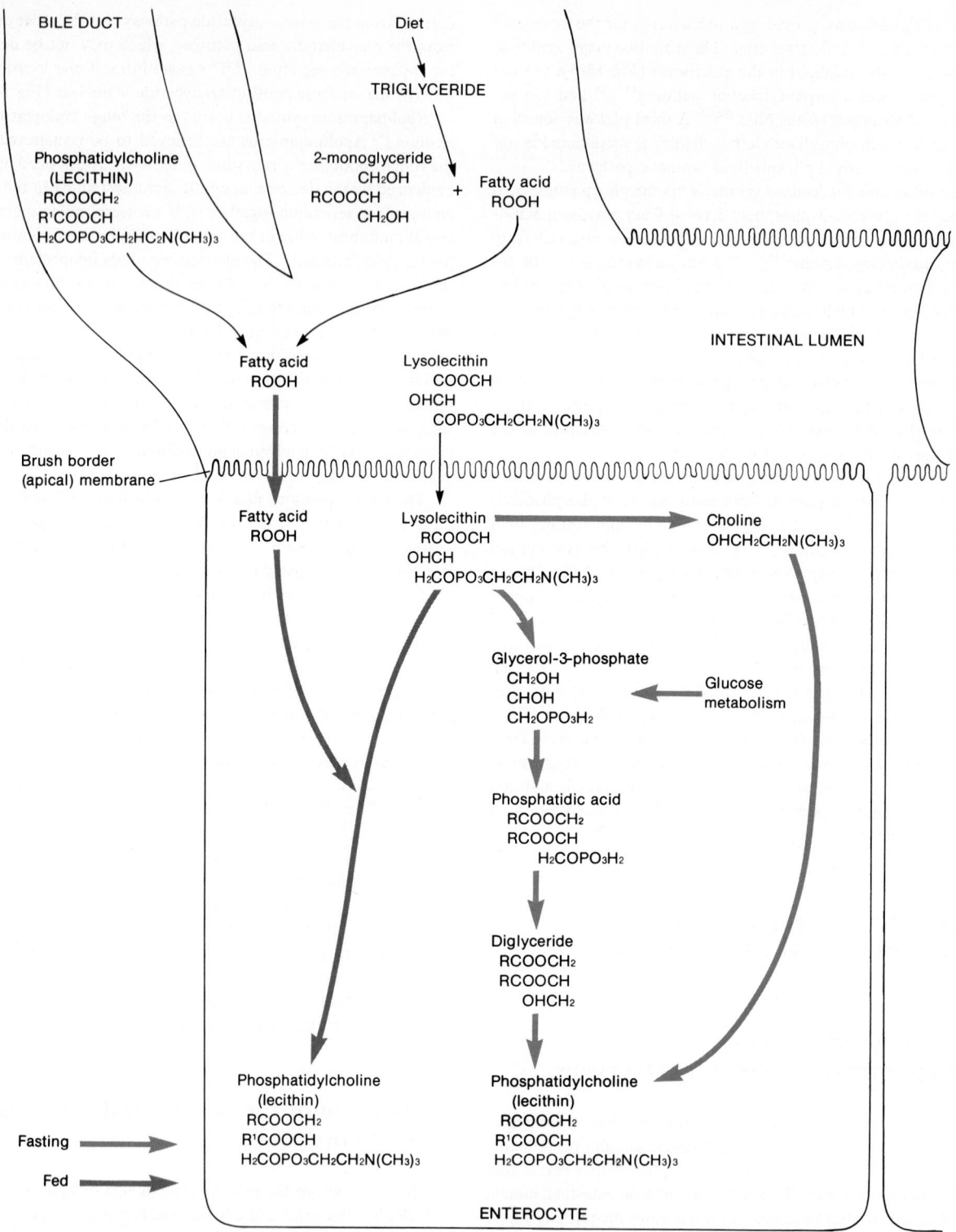

BILE DUCT

Diet

TRIGLYCERIDE

Phosphatidylcholine
(LECITHIN)
RCOOCH$_2$
R^{1}COOCH
H$_2$COPO$_3$CH$_2$HC$_2$N(CH$_3$)$_3$

2-monoglyceride
CH$_2$OH
RCOOCH   +   Fatty acid
CH$_2$OH   ROOH

INTESTINAL LUMEN

Fatty acid
ROOH

Lysolecithin
COOCH
OHCH
COPO$_3$CH$_2$CH$_2$N(CH$_3$)$_3$

Brush border
(apical) membrane

Fatty acid
ROOH

Lysolecithin
RCOOCH
OHCH
H$_2$COPO$_3$CH$_2$CH$_2$N(CH$_3$)$_3$

Choline
OHCH$_2$CH$_2$N(CH$_3$)$_3$

Glycerol-3-phosphate
CH$_2$OH
CHOH
CH$_2$OPO$_3$H$_2$

Glucose
metabolism

Phosphatidic acid
RCOOCH$_2$
RCOOCH
H$_2$COPO$_3$H$_2$

Diglyceride
RCOOCH$_2$
RCOOCH
OHCH$_2$

Phosphatidylcholine
(lecithin)
RCOOCH$_2$
R^{1}COOCH
H$_2$COPO$_3$CH$_2$CH$_2$N(CH$_3$)$_3$

Phosphatidylcholine
(lecithin)
RCOOCH$_2$
R^{1}COOCH
H$_2$COPO$_3$CH$_2$CH$_2$N(CH$_3$)$_3$

Fasting

Fed

ENTEROCYTE

FIGURE 18–5. Intestinal phospholipid biosynthesis. Phospholipid is synthesized within the enterocyte via two pathways. During fasting, biliary lecithin and the products of glucose metabolism serve as substrates in the glycerol-3-phosphate pathway (*blue arrows*). Addition of biliary-derived choline to diglyceride results in the formation of phosphatidylcholine (lecithin). In the fed state, lecithin is synthesized from the reacylation of absorbed lysolecithin (*red arrows*) and by ongoing synthesis via the glycerol-3-phosphate pathway.

oprotein genes, there are three expressed at high levels of abundance (apo A-I, apo A-IV, and apo B) that will be discussed in particular detail. Excellent reviews of the molecular genetics of apolipoproteins[161–163] and structure-function/evolutionary aspects of apolipoprotein genes[164] have been published recently, and these topics will not be discussed extensively here. Apolipoprotein gene structure in mammals shows a high degree of conservation, with four of the six genes expressed in human small intestine showing

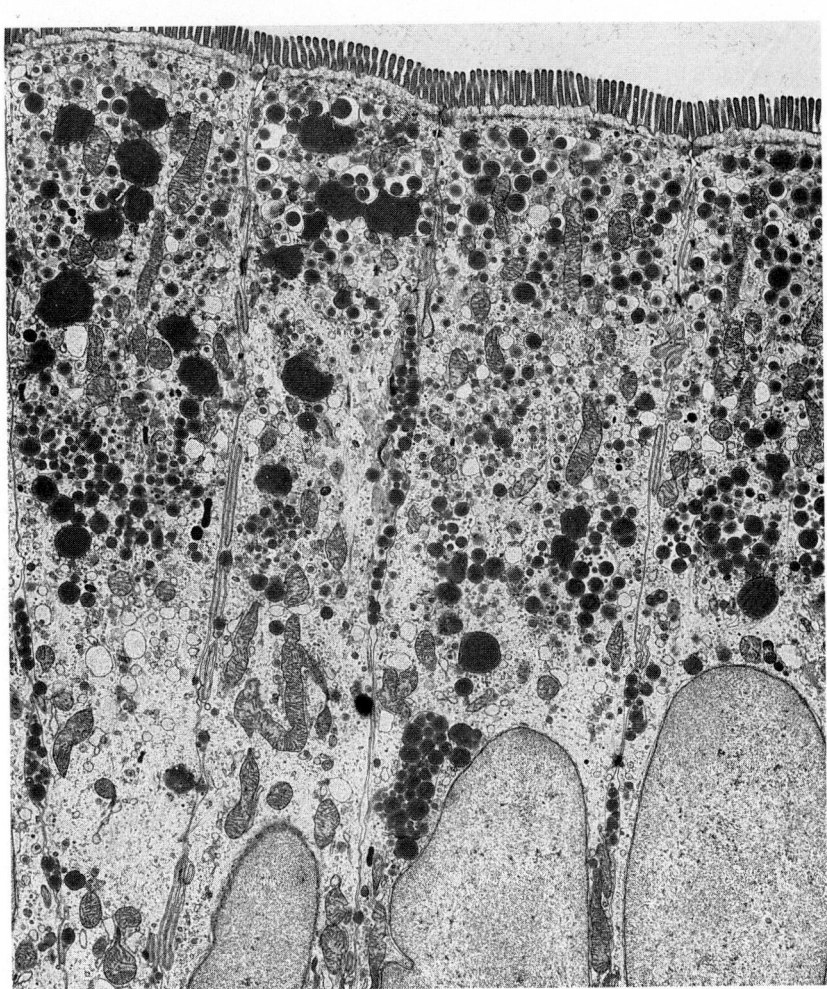

FIGURE 18–6. Intestinal absorptive cells following lipid feeding. This electron micrograph, taken 2 hours following lipid feeding, shows the apical cytoplasm to be engorged with osmiophilic droplets bounded by smooth endoplasmic reticulum. Golgi zones and intercellular spaces contain chylomicron-sized particles (×8000). (From Sabesin SM, Frase S. Electron microscopic studies of the assembly, intracellular transport, and secretion of chylomicrons by rat intestine. J Lipid Res 1977;18:496.)

distinct similarities (structure of the apo B gene and predicted structure of the apo D gene are quite different). The major apolipoproteins demonstrate such structural conservation that they are predicted to have arisen from a common ancestral gene.[165] The basic organization is a four-exon, three-intron gene structure, the exception being apo A-IV, which lacks an intron in the 5′ noncoding region of the corresponding mRNA.[166] The observed structural similarity in the genes reflects structural conservation noted in the gene products where multiple repeats of 22 amino acids confer a marked α-helical amphipathic secondary structure that contributes to their essential function as lipid-binding proteins.[167,168] An additional feature is that, similar to most proteins destined for export, all the intestinal apolipoproteins are synthesized with signal peptides,[165] which are cotranslationally cleaved, while the stable post-translational forms of both apo A-I and apo A-II mRNA contain an additional prosegment that undergoes extracellular cleavage.[169,170]

Apo A-I is an abundant intestinal mRNA coding for approximately 1% to 2% of newly synthesized protein in the rat.[169] In humans, apo A-I is the major protein component of high-density lipoprotein (HDL) and is the principal cofactor for the enzyme lecithin-cholesterol acyl transferase (LCAT), which is responsible for plasma cholesterol esterification.[171,172] A number of studies suggest that the intestine synthesizes approximately half of the body's daily input of this apolipoprotein.[173] Recent attention given

the importance of HDL as a "protective factor" against atherosclerosis and, in particular, recent evidence demonstrating that ambient serum levels of apo A-I may be an even more potent predictive factor[174] have focused attention on factors that influence the biosynthesis of apo A-I. Studies in the rat suggest that apo A-I is synthesized throughout the small intestine, with highest levels noted in the proximal jejunum with a gradient reaching a nadir in the terminal ileum.[175] Further studies in the rat demonstrated that intestinal apo A-I synthesis and mRNA content are unaltered following either acute triglyceride feeding or sustained exposure (3 to 6 weeks) to diets containing widely discrepant quantities, 0% to 30% by weight, triglyceride.[176] Additionally, there are no effects on intestinal apo A-I synthesis of diets composed of butter fat or corn oil and no effect of dietary cholesterol augmentation suggesting that, at least in this species, intestinal apo A-I gene expression appears to be largely constitutive with respect to alterations in dietary lipid flux. Apo A-I synthesis demonstrates regional sensitivity to the removal of biliary lipid components with no effect noted in the jejunum but marked suppression in the ileum.[175] The molecular basis and physiologic consequences of this regional heterogeneity are unknown. Intestinal apo A-I gene expression undergoes marked induction developmentally with an increase in mRNA abundance occurring at birth, presumably with the onset of suckling,[177] while subsequent levels of mRNA appear to remain relatively constant until adulthood. Researchers have demonstrated

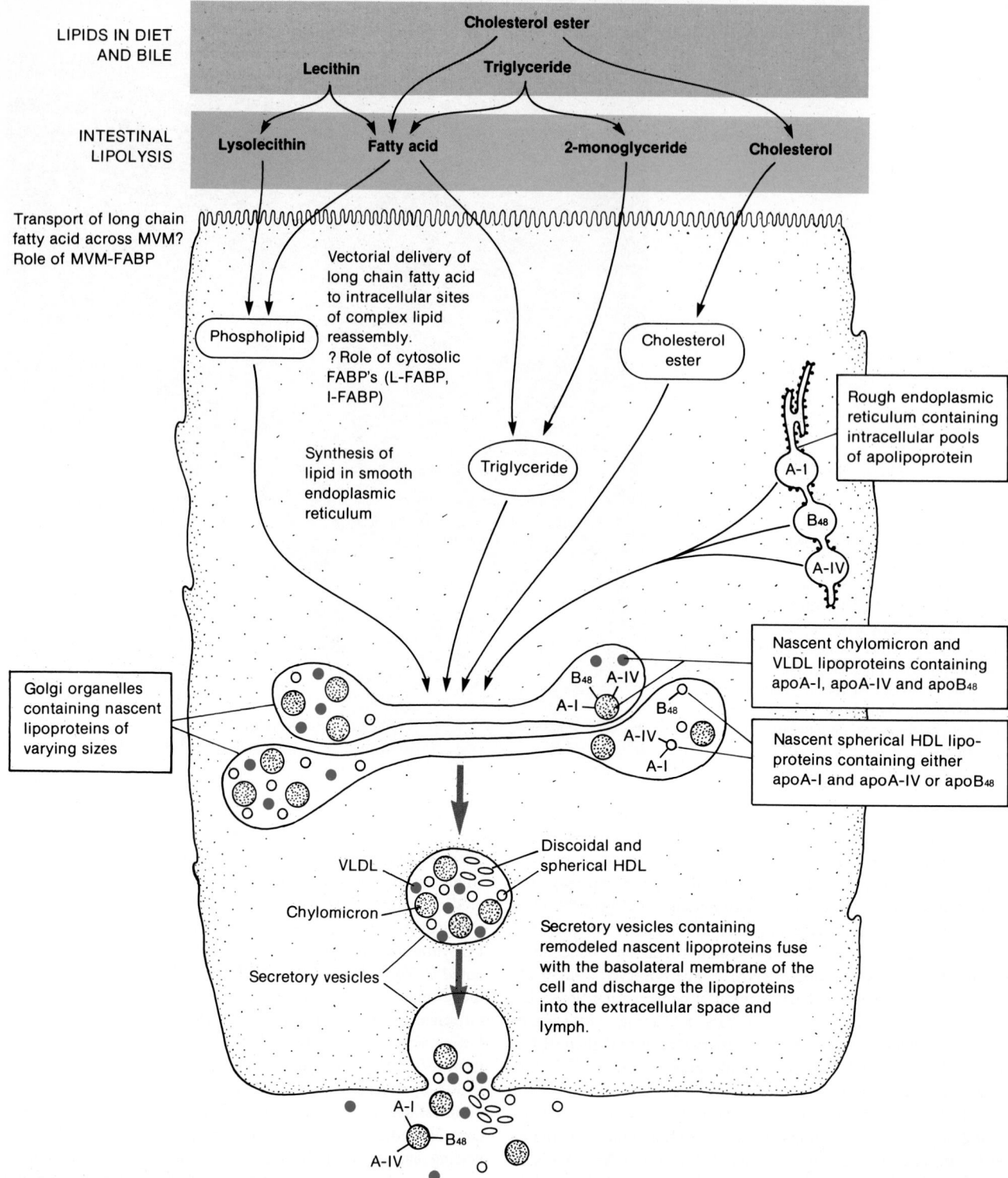

FIGURE 18–7. Intracellular pathways of intestinal lipoprotein assembly. Luminal lipids are absorbed across the microvillus membrane and transported to the smooth endoplasmic reticulum, where they serve as substrates for the synthesis of triglyceride, lecithin, and cholesterol ester—the lipids of nascent lipoproteins. Apolipoproteins from the rough endoplasmic reticulum are mobilized during lipoprotein formation onto lipid to form nascent lipoproteins in Golgi organelles. Lipoproteins are remodeled in the Golgi secretory vesicles. The secretory vesicles fuse with the basolateral membrane of the enterocyte and release the content nascent lipoproteins into the lymph.

TABLE 18–2
Human Plasma Lipoprotein Subclasses

SUBCLASS	SIZE	TISSUE ORIGIN	LIPID COMPOSITION	PROTEIN COMPOSITION	METABOLISM
Chylomicrons	>100 nM	Intestine	Triglyceride with smaller amounts of free cholesterol, cholesteryl ester, and phospholipid	Apo A-I, A-II, A-IV, B_{48}; acquire apo E and C apoproteins following secretion into lymph	Major vehicle for transport of dietary triglyceride and fat-soluble vitamins. Converted to chylomicron remnant following lipolysis of core triglyceride by lipoprotein lipase, for which apo CII is an obligate cofactor. Liberated surface protein components arising as a result of lipolytic shrinkage (apo A-I, A-II, A-IV) fuse with phospholipid, forming high-density lipoproteins (HDL).
Chylomicron remnants	≈100 nM	See above	Triglyceride; relatively enriched in free cholesterol and cholesteryl ester compared with chylomicrons	Apo E, B_{48}	Largely cleared by liver but uptake demonstrated to a smaller extent in a number of peripheral tissues, including bone marrow. Role of a distinct receptor is possible, but this requires confirmation.
Very low density lipoproteins (VLDL)	30–90 nM	Liver	Triglyceride with smaller amounts of free cholesterol, cholesteryl ester, and phospholipid	Apo B_{100}, E, Cs	Major vehicle for transport of endogenous triglyceride. They are converted to VLDL remnants and intermediate density lipoproteins (IDL) by lipolytic actions of lipoprotein and hepatic lipase. Some VLDL remnants are cleared by liver, but most are converted to IDL in circulation. Surface protein components are liberated as a result of lipolytic shrinkage and contribute to plasma HDL pool.
Intermediate density lipoproteins	30–60 nM	See above	Triglyceride/cholesteryl ester with smaller amounts of free cholesterol and phospholipid	Apo B_{100}, E	Small amounts are taken up by LDL receptor (apo B, E receptor). Most are converted to LDL via continued intravascular lipolysis of core triglyceride.
Low density lipoproteins (LDL)	≈20 nM	See above	Cholesteryl ester with smaller amounts of triglyceride, free cholesterol, phospholipid	Apo B_{100}	Major transporter of plasma cholesterol. They are taken up by LDL (apo B, E) receptor, which is expressed on all cells.
High-density lipoproteins	8–12 nM	Intestine Liver Plasma compartment	Phospholipid with smaller amounts of free cholesterol and cholesteryl ester and minor amounts of triglyceride	Apo A-I, A-II, A-IV, E	Synthesized directly by intestine and liver. They arise also as a result of intravascular catabolism of chylomicrons and VLDL. They participate in a variety of lipid exchange reactions and are probably involved in cholesterol mobilization from cells (so-called reverse cholesterol transport). Details of their catabolic fate, however, are unclear. No consensus on whether an HDL receptor exists.

that intestinal apo A-I gene expression may be sensitive to alterations in thyroid hormone status, with such changes being mediated at a translational or post-translational level.[178]

Apo A-IV is another abundant intestinal mRNA species, coding for up to 3% of newly synthesized protein.[179,180] Its distribution in plasma differs from apo A-I and indeed all the other members of this gene family in that it circulates largely unbound to lipoproteins, although approximately 25% of the plasma apo A-IV in

TABLE 18–3
Human Intestinal Apolipoproteins*

APOLIPO-PROTEIN	CHROMOSOMAL LOCALIZATION	MATURE PEPTIDE LENGTH (AA)†	LIPOPROTEIN DISTRIBUTION	FUNCTION	MAJOR SITE(S) OF EXPRESSION
A-I	11	243	CM, HDL	Cofactor for lecithin cholesterol acyltransferase (LCAT)	Intestine, liver
A-IV	11	377	CM, HDL, d > 1.21	Unknown, possible cofactor for LCAT	Intestine (liver)
B	2	B_{100} 4536	VLDL, LDL	Prerequisite for normal cellular triglyceride secretion. Apo B_{100} mediates LDL-receptor binding.	Liver§
		B_{48} 2152	CM, VLDL		Intestine§
C-II	19	79	CM, VLDL, HDL	Cofactor for lipoprotein lipase (LPL)	Liver, intestine
C-III	11	79	CM, VLDL, HDL	Unknown role in hepatic CM and VLDL remnant uptake	Liver, intestine
D	3	169	HDL	Complex formation involving plasma cholesteryl ester exchange and LCAT action	Adrenal, kidney (intestine)

* *Abbreviations used: CM, chylomicrons; VLDL, very low density lipoprotein; HDL, high-density lipoprotein; d > 1.21, lipoprotein free fraction; LDL, lipoprotein lipase; LCAT, lecithin cholesterol acyl transferase.*

† *All the apolipoproteins are synthesized with signal peptides ranging in length from 18 to 27 amino acids. Additionally the stable intracellular post-translational products of both apo A-I and apo A-II mRNA are preproteins with a 6 (apo A-I) or 5 (apo A-II) amino acid pro-piece that undergoes extracellular cleavage.*

§ *Apo B_{100} mRNA is present in both human intestine and liver. The mRNA undergoes a tissue-specific modification producing an in-frame stop codon in the intestinal but not hepatic transcript, resulting in translation of a truncated species (apo B_{48}), which is colinear with the —NH_2 terminus of apo B_{100}.[192,193]*

Apo A-II and C-I may be minor intestinal apolipoproteins; there is conflicting evidence for their presence in adult human intestine (see references 164, 181–187).

humans is associated with HDL.[181] Its regulation within enterocytes is also distinct from apo A-I in that it is responsive to changes in cellular triglyceride flux.[175,179] Synthesis rates and mRNA abundance of both jejunal and ileal apo A-IV have been found to double within 4 to 6 hours of a fat bolus,[179] although under both fasting and postprandial conditions the proximal-distal gradient of both synthesis rates and mRNA abundance are maintained. Further studies demonstrated striking developmental induction of intestinal apo A-IV mRNA abundance with a greater than 20-fold increase occurring at birth, followed by a gradual decline over the ensuing 14 days.[177] The intestine is the major synthetic and secretory source of apo A-IV, and although no specific function has yet been attributed to this protein, studies suggest that it may act as a potential cofactor for LCAT, but not as effectively as apo A-I.[182]

Apo C-III is a minor intestinal apolipoprotein whose mRNA codes for less than 0.5% total protein synthesis.[183] Its gene is localized on chromosome 11 between and in a reverse orientation to the apo A-I and apo A-IV genes.[184] Apo C-III probably functions in regulating the hepatic uptake of remnant lipoprotein particles, although precise details are not completely understood. Studies have demonstrated that, like apo A-IV, apo C-III is regulated following increases in intestinal triglyceride flux with accumulation of both mRNA and its translational product.[183,184]

Apo A-II,[185] apo C-I, and apo C-II[186,187] are minor intestinal apolipoproteins whose regulation has not been studied extensively. Apo D mRNA codes for a protein whose function is as yet incompletely understood but that is found in human plasma in association with HDL. This mRNA has been demonstrated in human intestine.[188] No information is available concerning its regulation.

Apo B is synthesized in mammalian enterocytes and hepatocytes as an obligate component of triglyceride-rich lipoproteins (chylomicrons and VLDL). Based on a centile score in human plasma, two major molecular forms of apo B are found, respectively apo B_{100} M_r ~512 kd and apo B_{48} (unglycosylated) ~M_r ~241 kd.[189] The structural properties of the apo B gene are distinct from the other apolipoproteins in that, first, it is larger (43 kb) and second, of its 29 exons, exon 26 is the longest mammalian coding sequence yet identified (7572 bases).[190,191] Another unusual feature makes the biology of apo B of particular interest. As currently viewed, apo B is the product of a single gene that in humans is transcribed into a message encoding apo B_{100} in the liver and apo B_{48} in the intestine.[192] The mechanism by which a single gene gives rise to two separate products has recently been elucidated.[193] The primary apo B_{100} transcript undergoes a co- or post-transcriptional modification producing conversion of a single nucleotide from a C in apo B_{100} mRNA to a U in apo B_{48} mRNA.[193] This change modifies codon 2153 in the human apo B_{100} cDNA sequence from CAA, which codes for glutamine, to TAA, which specifies a stop.[193] Remarkably, the stop codon is not present in the genome, indicating that this conversion involves alteration of an mRNA—a phenomenon without precedent in eukaryotes. Studies suggest that this mechanism may be under hormonal regulation, since the rat liver, which synthesizes both forms of apo B, can be shown to synthesize virtually only apo B_{48} following administration of tiiodothyronine.[194] Studies have further demonstrated that the mechanism for this switch involves a modification of apo B_{100} mRNA analogous to that described previously in the intestine. It is currently unresolved as to whether there is complete organ-specific partitioning of this gene-processing phenomenon in adult tissues. Studies have shown that fetal human intestine synthesizes both apo B_{100} and apo B_{48}, with a developmentally regulated switch occurring late in gestation.[195]

Despite its evident requirement in the assembly and secretion of triglyceride-rich lipoproteins, studies have shown that intestinal apo B synthesis is not regulated in response to dietary triglyceride augmentation.[196] Researchers, however, have demonstrated that intestinal apo B gene expression may be regulated by various components of bile.[197] Specifically, studies have shown that intestinal apo B synthesis is decreased in the rat following removal of biliary lipid and reexpressed following introduction of various components such as fatty acids and bile salts. The postulated mechanism appears to be provision of substrate (fatty acid) for microsomal triglyceride assembly that presumably reaches a threshold level at which intestinal apo B synthesis is reexpressed. Augmentation of triglyceride flux above this putative threshold produces no further change in apo B synthesis. Apo B gene expression also undergoes developmental regulation with a pattern in the rat distinct from either apo A-I or apo A-IV.[198] Following an increase at birth, there is a decline until day 8 when a second increase occurs, followed by a second decline to a nadir at 24 to 35 days of age. Following this second decline, there is an increase to adult levels. The mechanism(s) underlying these changes is unknown.

The major evidence that apo B is essential to the process of triglyceride-rich lipoprotein secretion has emanated from studies in humans afflicted with syndromes of defective chylomicron assembly and secretion in which there is abnormal apo B gene expression (see Table 18-3). The prototype of such syndromes is abetalipoproteinemia, an autosomal recessive condition characterized by mild fat malabsorption and several systemic abnormalities, including ataxia, acanthocytosis, and retinitis pigmentosa.[199] Parents of such subjects are obligate heterozygotes but manifest normal levels of plasma apo B and no evidence of fat malabsorption. Studies on the intestine of two homozygous subjects with abetalipoproteinemia revealed an absence of immunoreactive apo B,[200] a finding in contrast to the recent report of quantitatively normal amounts of immunoreactive apo B_{48} (and apo B_{100}) epitopes in another patient with this disorder.[201] The heterogeneity of abetalipoproteinemia is further exemplified by the apparent divergence of reports of both absent[202] and normal[203] apo B_{48} synthesis by intestinal explant cultures. Studies in the liver of two subjects with abetalipoproteinemia revealed the presence of *increased* amounts of apo B mRNA and detectable apo B_{100} mass.[204] Although it has not been excluded that there may be a post-translational abnormality producing a defective apo B_{100} protein, convincing studies have been presented based on restriction fragment length polymorphism, to suggest that abetalipoproteinemia may involve a genetic defect distinct from the apo B gene.[205] Studies have also been presented to suggest that the molecular basis for abetalipoproteinemia is distinct from a genetically distinct entity referred to as hypobetalipoproteinemia.[206] The distinguishing features in hypobetalipoproteinemia include autosomal codominant inheritance and the presence of low plasma apo B levels in obligate heterozygotes. Studies have shown a sevenfold *decrease* in hepatic apo B_{100} mRNA levels (compared with a sixfold increase in abetalipoproteinemia) and reduced amounts of intracellular apo B_{100} mass.[206] The conclusion from these studies is that hypobetalipoproteinemia may represent a translational abnormality with either an unstable or an abnormal mRNA.

A number of other syndromes have been described of hypocholesterolemia, varying degrees of fat malabsorption, and inability to assembly/secrete triglyceride-rich lipoproteins from enterocytes and/or hepatocytes.[207-211] These are summarized in Table 18-4[199-211] and collectively form the basis for investigating the molecular details of apo B assembly, processing, and its requisite involvement in chylomicron secretion.

Characterization of Intracellular Intestinal Lipoproteins

Lipoproteins are multimolecular aggregates of lipid and protein whose configuration allows the transport of intensely hydrophobic lipid through the aqueous milieu of both cellular cytosol and plasma compartments. The apolar lipid core of the particle contains triglyceride and cholesterol ester, and the surface coat is composed of cholesterol, lecithin, and apolipoproteins. The intestine has been shown to assemble and secrete chylomicrons, VLDL, and HDL and perhaps LDL (see Fig 18-7).

Chylomicrons (80–500 nm) are assembled during periods of lipid absorption and can be visualized easily on electron micrographs taken during lipid absorption. Chylomicrons have been isolated from within intestinal Golgi organelles. Intracellular chylomicrons are composed of 13% to 25% protein and 75% to 85% lipid,[155,176,212] two thirds of which is triglyceride. In contrast, extracellular chylomicron composition (lymph and plasma) is greater than 95% lipid, 90% of which is triglyceride.[213,214] The major apolipoproteins on the surface of intracellular chylomicrons are apo B_{48}, apo A-I, and apo A-IV. These proteins are synthesized within the enterocyte.

VLDL-sized particles (25–80 nm) are assembled in the enterocyte during fasting and lipid feeding. Approximately 15% of intracellular VLDL is apolipoprotein, and these proteins are apo B_{48}, apo A-I, and apo A-IV. As with chylomicrons, the lipid moiety of VLDL is largely triglyceride and phospholipid.[212] The compositional resemblance of chylomicrons and VLDL to each other suggests that these particles represent a size continuum of the same type of lipoprotein whose volume varies relative to the availability of intracellular triglyceride.[215] Evidence has been presented to support the hypothesis of separate pathways for chylomicron and VLDL assembly, based on the demonstration of chylomicrons and VLDL in different Golgi organelles,[216] together with other studies showing selective inhibition of chylomicron secretion despite persistent VLDL secretion.[217]

LDL particles have been isolated from within enterocytes and partially characterized.[155] The particles contain newly synthesized apo A-IV and apo B and trace amounts of apo A-I. The lipid composition is 40% phospholipid and 31% triglyceride. In rats administered galactosamine, which profoundly reduces hepatic synthesis of lipoproteins, there appear to be intestinally derived LDL particles in mesenteric lymph.[218]

HDL particles, although too small to be seen in electron micrographs of unfractionated enterocytes, have been isolated and characterized from within Golgi vesicles of rat enterocytes.[219] Intracellular HDL particles have been visualized as spherical 6- to 13-nm sized particles. Compositional analysis has revealed two distinct populations, one containing both apo A-I and A-IV, the other containing apo B_{48} as the surface apolipoprotein. The par-

TABLE 18-4
Syndromes of Defective Chylomicron and VLDL Secretion

SYNDROME	AUTOSOMAL INHERITANCE	PLASMA			FAT MALABSORPTION	GUT APO B	LIVER APO B	COMMENTS
		Apo B	Cholesterol	Triglyceride				
Abetalipoproteinemia	Recessive					Molecular basis unknown. Divergent reports of apo B_{48} synthesis reported as normal or absent.[202,203] Apo B protein reported as either normal[201,204] or undetectable.[200] Fat-filled enterocytes.	mRNA sixfold increased—detectable apo B_{100} protein.[204]	Acanthocytosis. Neurologic sequelae from vitamin E deficiency. Retinitis pigmentosa.[199]
Homozygotes		0/very low	Low	Low	+			
Heterozygotes		N/increased	Normal	Normal	−			
Hypobetalipoproteinemia	Codominant					Unknown apo B status. Fat-filled enterocytes.	mRNA sevenfold decreased. Apo B_{100} protein reduced but detectable.[206]	Distinction from ABL based on parenteral phenotype. Clinically milder than ABL, with later onset.[206]
Homozygotes		0/very low	Low	Low	+			
Heterozygotes		Low	Low	Low	−			
Normotriglyceridemic abetalipoproteinemia	Unknown	>90% reduction; only apo B_{48} detectable	Low	Normal	± (10 g/d on "normal" US diet)	Presumed normal. No fat-filled enterocytes.[207]	Presumed defective apo B_{100} synthesis and/or secretion.[207]	Ataxic. 1% acanthocytosis. No retinitis pigmentosa. Plasma triglyceride increases tenfold after meal.[207]
Apo B_{100} deficiency	Recessive	>90% reduction; only apo B_{48} detectable	Low	Low	+	Unknown. Fat-filled enterocytes.[208]	Presumed defective apo B_{100} synthesis and/or secretion.[208]	Acanthocytosis. Neurologic sequelae. No retinitis pigmentosa.[208]
Anderson's disease	Recessive	Reduced to 50% normal	Low	Low	+	Increased apo B protein, probably apo B_{48}. Fat-filled enterocytes.[209]	Unknown	No neurologic sequelae. No acanthocytosis. No retinitis pigmentosa.[209]
Chylomicron retention disease	Recessive	Reduced to 80% normal	Reduced to 40% normal	Normal	+	Increased apo B protein, probably apo B_{48}. Fat-filled enterocytes.[210,211]	Macroglobular steatosis. Unknown apo B status.[210,211]	Neurologic findings present. No retinitis pigmentosa. 5% acanthocytosis in one of eight cases. Disease may be identical to Anderson's disease.[210,211]

ticles are composed of 70% protein and 30% lipid, half of which is phospholipid. Whether the HDL particles that contain apo B_{48} are metabolic precursors to chylomicrons is not known, and the fate of these apo B_{48} containing HDL is under investigation. Mesenteric lymph contains a population of discoidal and spherical HDL particles, which have both been shown to be secreted from the intestine.[220,221] Discoidal particles make up about 50% of fasting lymph HDL; these particles are apo A-I and phospholipid-enriched relative to plasma HDL. Apo A-I on these HDL particles is metabolically derived by de novo intestinal synthesis. Metabolic labeling experiments provide good evidence that discoidal HDL particles are synthesized within rat enterocytes and do not simply reflect lipolytic products of triglyceride-rich lipoproteins or ultracentrifugation artifacts.[221] Spherical lymph HDL particles are also relatively protein and phospholipid enriched compared with plasma HDL particles and contain core cholesterol ester suggestive of an intestinal source (i.e., ACAT derived) rather than a plasma (i.e., LCAT derived) source, as evidenced by the high saturated to unsaturated fatty acid ester ratio.[221] These spherical particles resemble intracellular HDL particles. Further evidence that newly synthesized HDL particles are secreted by the intestine comes from examination of the specific activity of lipoprotein phospholipid following administration of choline-labeled bile lecithin.[222] The phospholipid of lymph HDL has a lower specific activity than VLDL phospholipid, consistent with HDL particles being derived from a distinct synthetic pathway from VLDL particles.[222]

Mesenteric Lymph Lipoproteins

Studies in the rat have characterized the principal species of intracellular apolipoproteins. Following secretion into the lymph compartment, several alterations occur in their composition, largely as a result of passive exchange of surface protein components with lipoproteins in lymph.[213] It is likely, although currently unproven, that a similar situation pertains in humans. Rat mesenteric lymph chylomicrons and human chyluric chylomicrons have been found to demonstrate a striking degree of homology in their apolipoprotein composition.[213] Thus, in addition to apo B_{48}, apo A-IV, and A-I, both human and rat lymph-derived chylomicrons contain substantial quantities of albumin, apo E, and apo C. In addition, human chyluric and pig intestinal lymph[223] chylomicrons contain a peptide of a size compatible with apo B_{100},[224] suggesting either that apo B_{100} transfers onto lymph chylomicrons or, more likely, that hepatic VLDL (containing apo B_{100}), which is secreted into the cisterna chyli, contaminate the chylomicron fraction.

The presence of discoidal HDL in mesenteric lymph and in perfusates from rat liver, but not in plasma, suggests that this form of lipoprotein is secreted directly into lymph. It is postulated that discoidal HDL becomes rapidly converted to a spherical morphology following the action of lecithin cholesterol acyltransferase (LCAT), which converts free cholesterol to cholesteryl ester and thus enriches the core of these particles with hydrophobic lipid.[221] During fasting, 75% to 85% of lymph apo A-I is in the HDL fraction.[156,225,226] Essentially all apo B in fasting lymph is in the chylomicron-VLDL fraction.[156] During lipid feeding, 25% to 50%

of apo A-I and 67% to 100% of apo B in lymph is in chylomicrons and VLDL.[156,227]

Effects of Lipid on Intestinal Lipoprotein Assembly and Secretion

EFFECT OF TRIGLYCERIDE ON APOLIPOPROTEIN SYNTHESIS AND SECRETION

There is no experimental consensus regarding the possible regulatory effect of triglyceride feeding on human intestinal apolipoprotein synthesis. The most current studies suggest that only apo A-IV synthesis, but not apo A-I or apo B_{48} synthesis, is increased by *acute* triglyceride feeding.[175,179,196,228] *Chronic* triglyceride feeding has also been shown not to increase synthesis of apo A-I or apo B_{48}.[176] Older studies using immunofluorescence or immunoperoxidase staining of apo A-I,[225] apo A-IV, or apo B[229,230] have shown an increase in intracellular apolipoprotein content in response to triglyceride feeding, which can be interpreted as being consistent with increased synthesis. It may be the case, however, that alterations in intracellular location of apolipoproteins, as occurs during lipid absorption, may account for differences in staining characteristics. To place these qualitative findings in perspective, reports of enterocyte apolipoprotein content after lipid absorption have shown increased, decreased, or unchanged apo A-I and apo B content.[175,229,231,232] Taken together, available evidence suggests that only apo A-IV gene expression is responsive to alterations in mucosal triglyceride flux.

Secretion of apolipoproteins A-I, A-IV, and B into the lymph, as distinct from intracellular content or synthesis, increases during lipid feeding.[225,227–234] During lipid absorption, however, lymph flow rates and transfer of proteins from plasma to lymph increases,[226,227,233,235] making conclusions about enterocyte synthesis, based on lymph apolipoprotein measurements, difficult to interpret. Different approaches to examine the effect of lipid on intestinal apolipoprotein secretion have been attempted. In patients with chyluria, in which intestinal lymph is directly secreted into urine, there is an increase of apo A-I and apo A-IV following lipid feeding.[223,236] Examination of human thoracic lymph after lipid feeding has shown an increase in secretion of pro-apo A-I.[237] However, when plasma apolipoprotein levels are experimentally reduced in rats treated with ethinyl estradiol only apo A-IV increases in lymph during triglyceride absorption,[238] suggesting that the observed postprandial increases in apo A-I and apo B_{48} may be due to plasma filtration. Thus, the issue of increased intestinal secretion versus plasma filtration of apo B_{48} and apo A-I is still unsettled.

The results of recent studies may provide a unifying hypothesis to account for the apparently conflicting observations of increased lymph apolipoprotein secretion without accompanying changes in intestinal apolipoprotein synthesis rates following a fatty meal.[155] These studies demonstrate a large intracellular pool of apo A-I and apo B that is principally microsomal and not associated with lipoprotein. Following a fatty meal, a significant shift occurs, increasing by twofold to threefold the lipoprotein-associated fractions of both apolipoproteins, which are then destined for export, while producing minimal changes (<10%) in the total intracellular pool size of apolipoproteins.[155]

EFFECT OF TRIGLYCERIDE ON LIPOPROTEIN COMPOSITION

The fatty acid composition of chylomicron triglyceride mirrors the composition of luminal triglyceride in the intestinal lumen.[214,239,240] The size of secreted chylomicrons is affected by both the quantity and type of lipid being absorbed. The more triglyceride that is absorbed, the larger the chylomicrons.[240] The composition of the triglyceride forming the newly synthesized chylomicron also affects the size of chylomicrons. In general, chylomicrons increase in size as the lipids in the chylomicron become less saturated.[240] When saturated fats, such as palmitate, are fed, smaller chylomicrons are secreted into lymph than when unsaturated fatty acids are fed,[215] although a more recent study has not been able to corroborate the effect of palmitate on chylomicron size.[227] The presence of unsaturated fatty acids also affects the composition of chylomicrons in that there is less apo B_{48} on chylomicrons containing unsaturated triglyceride.[227] Interestingly, during active lipid absorption, uptake of free fatty acids from plasma into the enterocyte and incorporation of these fatty acids into newly synthesized triglyceride is increased.[88]

Triglyceride feeding affects not only the triglyceride component of lipoproteins but also the phospholipids. The fatty acid composition of lymph lipoprotein phospholipids at least partially reflects the fatty acids present in the intestinal lumen. This observation is consistent with the concept that phospholipids are in part derived from luminal triglyceride during triglyceride feeding.[222] Phospholipids are also synthesized de novo during triglyceride feeding,[222,241] suggesting that both reacylation of absorbed lysolecithin and the phosphatidic acid–CDP-choline pathways contribute to lipoprotein phospholipid. Triglyceride feeding also increases the phospholipid in lymph HDL.[222]

EFFECT OF BILE DIVERSION AND FASTING

Reduced intestinal lipid flux has been produced experimentally using a combination of bile diversion combined with fasting. The lack of biliary lipid, bile salts, and exogenous luminal lipid reduces triglyceride output in lymph by 85% and results in almost total disappearance of VLDL from Golgi organelles.[226] Apo A-I synthesis in jejunal enterocytes following bile diversion is similar to that observed in fasted animals, although ileal enterocytes exhibit lower rates of synthesis.[175] Reinfusion of bile salts alone fails to prevent the decrease in ileal apo A-I synthesis. By contrast, apo B_{48} synthesis is dramatically suppressed in both jejunal and ileal enterocytes following bile diversion and reexpressed in jejunal but not ileal enterocytes following intraluminal administration of sodium taurocholate.[196] Further studies demonstrated that the bile salt–dependent reexpression of apo B biosynthesis in rat enterocytes could be reproduced by infusion of lysolecithin or fatty acid alone and that this regulation is at a translational or post-translational level since total apo B mRNA abundance is unaltered.[197] Studies examining intestinal microsomal triglyceride concentration

indicated a relationship between reexpression of jejunal apo B biosynthesis and microsomal triglyceride content, suggesting that a threshold level of triglyceride may be required for the stable elaboration of intestinal apo B_{48}.[197] Consistent with the dramatically reduced secretion of triglyceride following bile diversion, intestinal synthesis of apo A-IV is also reduced (Nicholas O. Davidson, unpublished observation). The phospholipid composition of lymph HDL during bile diversion is similar to that of non–bile-diverted controls, suggesting that intestinal HDL phospholipid is not derived from exogenous sources.[222]

In the absence of dietary fat, the intestine contributes 11% to 40% of the total plasma triglyceride,[215,242–244] 10% to 15% of apo B, 50% of plasma apo A-I, and close to 100% of apo A-IV.[173,245] Under fasting conditions intracellular apolipoprotein and VLDL particles can be localized to enterocytes and newly synthesized apolipoprotein can be isolated from enterocytes and lymph.[154,176,246,247,250] Intestinal VLDL and HDL are also found in lymph during fasting, the lipid presumably arising from bile and sloughed, digested enterocytes.

EFFECT OF PHOSPHOLIPID

Absorbed phospholipid comes from the bile (10–20 g/d) and from exogenous dietary phospholipid (5–10 g/d). In addition to absorbed phospholipid, endogenous sources of lipoprotein phospholipid include de novo synthesized lecithin and the preformed intracellular pool of phospholipids. Lecithin is the predominant phospholipid in lipoproteins.

Lecithin infusion results in intracellular synthesis of both triglyceride and lecithin and incorporation of these lipids into secreted lipoproteins. Infusion of lecithin alone (without triglyceride) leads to newly synthesized triglyceride and consequent VLDL secretion.[222,251] Most of the infused phospholipid is reassembled into triglyceride via the intracellular hydrolysis of lysolecithin to glycerol-3-phosphate and subsequent reassembly to triglyceride via the phosphatidic acid pathway, as shown in Figure 18-6.[137,252] Infusion of triglyceride along with phospholipid similarly leads to newly synthesized chylomicron triglyceride, which is in part derived from the infused lecithin. Approximately 75% of the fatty acids in infused lecithin is found in lymph triglyceride.[251] Addition of lecithin during high rates of triglyceride infusion increases lymph triglyceride secretion, suggesting that adequate amounts of phospholipid need to be available to serve as the surface coat for newly synthesized triglyceride to be secreted as a chylomicron.[253] On the other hand, if biliary lecithin is eliminated during high-dose triglyceride infusion, the effect on lipoprotein phospholipid is variable. Some researchers have found a decrease,[253–255] while others report no change.[222] At normal rates of triglyceride infusion, there is no decrease in lymph phospholipid secretion following bile diversion.[222,253] Interestingly, infusion of lecithin decreases cholesterol secretion.[255]

In fasting animals, the phospholipid compositions of VLDL and HDL in lymph are similar and resemble the phospholipids contained in bile.[222] Elimination of bile (which contains 16:0 fatty acids) significantly decreases the 16:0 species from lymph lipoproteins in fasted animals.[222] In triglyceride-fed animals, the phospholipid compositions of both VLDL and HDL mirror the fatty acids in the infused triglyceride.[222] Bile diversion does not significantly affect the composition of lipoprotein phospholipid in fed animals.

EFFECT OF CHOLESTEROL FEEDING

Only a small percentage of cholesterol recovered in lymph is of exogenous origin.[239] In general, the consequence of increased dietary cholesterol is increased cholesterol content in all lymph lipoproteins. In monkeys, during the experimental infusion of diets with a high cholesterol content, there is an increase in thoracic duct total lymph cholesterol mass.[256] Amounts of both free and esterified cholesterol increase, although there is preferential esterification of the absorbed (luminal) cholesterol in the lymph chylomicron and VLDL fractions, which leads to a greater proportional rise in esterified cholesterol relative to free cholesterol in the lymph.[257] In rats chronically fed diets containing high levels of cholesterol, mesenteric lymph cholesterol redistributes to an intermediate-density lipoprotein fraction (1.006–1.030 g/mL), in which there appears a particle that is triglyceride and cholesteryl ester enriched, with apo A-I and apo B as the major apolipoproteins.[258] Alterations in the composition of ingested triglyceride may affect cholesterol absorption in the rat. Animals fed large concentrations of unsaturated fatty acids demonstrate increased cholesterol absorption, the apparent excess being recovered in the lymph VLDL fraction.[187] These results, however, have not been substantiated in a recent series of controlled studies in human subjects.[122]

Metabolic Fate of Intestinal Lipoproteins

The small intestine synthesizes and secretes a variety of lipoprotein particles, principally triglyceride-rich lipoproteins-chylomicrons and VLDL, and HDL (see also Table 18-2). The metabolic fate of each is distinct and has been the focus of considerable investigation. Chylomicrons enter the lymphatic circulation through fenestrations in the capillary endothelium and immediately undergo a series of modifications to their surface protein composition. Nascent intracellular intestinal chylomicrons contain principally (pro) apo A-I, apo A-IV, and apo B_{48} as surface protein components. On entering the lymph compartment, apo E, apo C-II, and apo C-III transfer from the surface of (filtered) plasma HDL by passive exchange, a process during which chylomicron apo A-I, apo A-IV, and phospholipid is transferred into HDL.[259] Apo A-IV is transferred largely (50%–75%) into the lipoprotein-free fraction of lymph and plasma[234] where it displays fractional turnover kinetics distinct from HDL-associated apo A-IV.[260] As previously described, apo A-I is synthesized and secreted in the form of a stable propeptide containing a 6 amino acid prosegment.[169] This prosegment, terminating with paired glutamine rather than paired basic residues,[169] is cleaved extracellularly in both lymph and plasma compartments by a metal-dependent protease.[261] The biologic importance of this conversion process is unclear since both pro apo A-I and the mature apo A-I peptide associate, with similar

affinity, with an identical spectrum of lipoproteins in vitro.[261] There is evidence to suggest that the proteolytic conversion of pro apo A-I to apo A-I may be defective in Tangier disease,[262] although the balance of evidence points to other defects in the Tangier apo A-I gene.[263] The metabolic fate of chylomicron surface apolipoproteins A-I and A-IV appears to be distinctive. These apolipoproteins are speculated to contribute substantially to the circulating pool of HDL apolipoprotein. In view of the importance of HDL as an epidemiologic marker of coronary artery disease susceptibility,[174] increased understanding of the physiologic parameters governing chylomicron surface catabolism will be of clinical importance. Once the surface exchange reactions have been completed (note that apo B_{48} does not participate in these reactions and therefore can be used as a marker of an intestinally derived lipoprotein) chylomicrons are transported to the capillary beds of peripheral tissues where the core triglyceride undergoes hydrolysis mediated by lipoprotein lipase.[264] Apo C-II is a critical cofactor in activating lipoprotein lipase and its deficiency is associated with severe hypertriglyceridemia and chylomicron accumulation.[265] Apo C-II is synthesized in both liver and intestine in human subjects and circulates predominantly with triglyceride-rich lipoproteins.[266] Following catabolism of the core triglyceride, the resulting chylomicron particle undergoes substantial modification, resulting in loss of most of the surface apolipoproteins, with the notable exception of apo E and apo B_{48}. This particle is referred to as a chylomicron remnant and is transported to a number of sites, including the liver where it is postulated to bind to a putative receptor. The available evidence suggests that apo E may be the cognate ligand.[267] This receptor displays characteristics distinct from the LDL (apo B, E) receptor.[267] Furthermore, metabolic studies in subjects with homozygous familial hypercholesterolemia, and an appropriate animal model in which there is also virtually complete deficiency of LDL receptors, demonstrate normal chylomicron uptake, further supporting the hypothesis that at least two populations of lipoprotein receptors recognize apo E-containing particles.[268,269] Recent studies have identified several apo E-binding peptides in canine liver membranes, and immunologic screening has revealed the presence of several peptides in the range of 56 to 59 kDa.[270] Further analysis has revealed that the 56-kDa peptides are the α- and β-subunits of a mitochondrial F_1-adenosine 5′ triphosphatase while the identity of the 59-kDa peptide is unknown.[270] Other, very recent, work has identified a cell surface receptor that displays resemblance to both the LDL (apo B, apo E) receptor and epidermal growth factor precursor.[271] This peptide, which may be the apo E receptor, has an estimated molecular mass of 503 kDa and is translated from a 15-kb transcript.[270] Interestingly, the tissue distribution of this transcript (liver > brain > lung > intestine) suggests that this receptor—if indeed it functions as a chylomicron remnant receptor—may play a more widespread role in tissue cholesterol delivery than previously supposed. Hepatic uptake of triglyceride-rich lipoprotein remnant particles is also modulated by the presence of C apolipoproteins on the lipoprotein surface. Substantial inhibition of remnant uptake occurs with particles containing apo C-II, particularly isoform 2.[272] This finding, based on in vitro studies in the perfused rat liver, has been extended to a recent study of chylomicron catabolism in subjects with apo C-III–A-I deficiency, in whom chylomicron catabolism was unusually rapid.[273]

The regulation of plasma HDL metabolism is distinct from chylomicron and LDL metabolism and, as yet, no conclusive evidence has been presented to support the existence of an HDL receptor. Plasma HDL arises as a result of direct secretion from both the liver[274] and the intestine[219] as well as its generation from the catabolism of triglyceride-rich lipoproteins.[259]

The reader is directed to Chapter 6, Epithelia: Biologic Principles of Organization; Chapter 12, Salivary Secretion; Chapter 13, Gastric Secretion; Chapter 14, Secretion and Absorption: Small Intestine and Colon; Chapter 15, Pancreatic Secretion; Chapter 16, Bile Secretion; Chapter 17, Carbohydrate Assimilation; Chapter 19, Protein Digestion and Assimilation; Chapter 20, Vitamins and Minerals; Chapter 21, General Nutritional Principles; and Chapter 48, Approach to the Patient Requiring Nutritional Supplementation.

REFERENCES

1. Patton JS, Vetter RD, Hamosh M, et al. The light microscopy of triglyceride digestion. Food Microstructure 1985;4:29.
2. Carey MC, Small DM, Bliss CM. Lipid digestion and absorption. Ann Rev Physiol 1983;45:651.
3. Hamosh M, Scanlon JW, Ganot D, et al. Fat digestion in the newborn: characterization of lipase in gastric aspirates of premature and term infants. J Clin Invest 1981;67:838.
4. Moreau H, Laugier R, Gargouri Y, et al. Human preduodenal lipase is entirely of gastric fundic origin. Gastroenterology 1988;95:1221.
5. Gooden JM, Lascelles AK. Relative importance of pancreatic lipase and pregastric esterase in lipid absorption in calves 1–2 weeks of age. Aust J Biol Sci 1973;26:625.
6. Abrams CK, Hamosh M, Lee TC, et al. Gastric lipase: localization in the human stomach. Gastroenterology 1988;95:1460.
7. Roberts IM, Jaffe R. Lingual lipase: immunocytochemical localization in the rat von Ebner gland. Gastroenterology 1986;90:1170.
8. DeNigris SJ, Hamosh M, Kasbekar DK, et al. Lingual and gastric lipases: species differences in the origin of prepancreatic digestive lipases and in the localization of gastric lipase. Biochim Biophys Acta 1988;959:38.
9. Hamosh M, Scow RO. Lingual lipase and its role in the digestion of dietary fat. J Clin Invest 1973;55:88.
10. Hamosh M, Klaeveman HL, Wolf RO, et al. Pharyngeal lipase and digestion of dietary triglyceride in man. J Clin Invest 1975;55:908.
11. Hamosh M. A review: fat digestion in the newborn: role of lingual lipase and preduodenal digestion. Pediatr Res 1979;13:615.
12. Hamosh M. Lingual lipase [Editorial]. Gastroenterology 1986;90:1290.
13. Docherty AJP, Bodmer MW, Angal S, et al. Molecular cloning and nucleotide sequence of rat lingual lipase cDNA. Nucl Acids Res 1985;13:1891.
14. Bodmer MW, Angal S, Yarranton GT, et al. Molecular cloning of a human gastric lipase and expression of the enzyme in yeast. Biochim Biophys Acta 1987;909:237.
15. Gargouri Y, Pieroni G, Riviere C, et al. Kinetic assay of human gastric lipase on short- and long-chain triacylglycerol emulsions. Gastroenterology 1986;91:919.
16. Bernback S, Hernell O, Blackberg L. Bovine pregastric lipase: a model for the human enzyme with respect to properties relevant to its site of action. Biochim Biophys Acta 1987;922:206.
17. Roberts IM, Hanel SI. Stability of lingual lipase in vivo: studies of the iodinated enzyme in the rat stomach and duodenum. Biochim Biophys Acta 1988;960:107.
18. Smith LJ, Kamisky S, D'Souza SW. Neonatal fat digestion and lingual lipase. Acta Paediatr Scand 1986;175:313.
19. Sheldon W. Congenital pancreatic lipase deficiency. Arch Dis Child 1964;39:268.
20. Muller DPR, McCollum JPK, Trompeter RS, et al. Studies on the mechanism of fat absorption in congenital isolated lipase deficiency. Gut 1975;16:838.
21. Abrams CK, Hamosh M, Hubbard VS, et al. Lingual lipase in cystic fibrosis: quantitation of enzyme activity in the upper small intestine of patients with exocrine pancreatic insufficiency. J Clin Invest 1984;73:374.
22. Kerfelec B, LaForge KB, Puigserver A, et al. Primary structures of canine pancreatic lipase and phospholipase A_2 messenger RNAs. Pancreas 1986;1:430.
23. Lowe ME, Rosenblum JL, Strauss AW. Cloning and characterization of human pancreatic lipase cDNA. J Biol Chem 1989;264:20042.
24. Datta S, Luo CC, Li WH, et al. Human hepatic lipase: cloned cDNA sequence, restriction fragment length polymorphisms, chromosomal localization and evolutionary relationships with lipoprotein lipase and pancreatic lipase. J Biol Chem 1988;263:1107.
25. Borgstrom B. The importance of phospholipids, pancreatic phospholipase A2 and fatty acid for the digestion of dietary fat. Gastroenterology 1980;78:954.
26. Blackberg L, Hernell O, Olivecrona T. Hydrolysis of human milk fat globules by pancreatic lipase: role of colipase, phospholipase A_2 and bile salts. J Clin Invest 1981;67:1748.
27. Borgstrom B, Erlanson-Albertsson C, Wielock T. Pancreatic colipase: chemistry and physiology. J Lipid Res 1979;20:805.
28. Lowe ME, Rosenblum JL, McEwan P, et al. Cloning and characterization of the human colipase cDNA. Biochemistry 1990;29:823.
29. Donner J, Spink JH, Borgstrom B, et al. Interactions between pancreatic lipase, colipase and taurodeoxycholate in the absence of triglyceride substrate. Biochemistry 1976;19:5413.
30. Hildebrand H, Borgstrom B, Bekassy A, et al. Isolated colipase deficiency in two brothers. Gut 1982;23:243.
31. Dijkska BW, Drenth J, Kalk KH. Active site and catalytic mechanism of phospholipase A2. Nature 1981;289:604.
32. Hyun J, Treadwell DC, Vahouny GV. Pancreatic juice cholesterol esterase: studies on molecular weight and bile salt induced polymerization. Arch Biochem Biophys 1972;152:233.
33. Lombardo D, Guy O, Figarella L. Purification and characterization of a carboxyl ester hydrolase from human pancreatic juice. Biochim Biophys Acta 1978;527:142.
34. Lombardo D, Fauvel J, Guy O. Studies on the substrate specificity of a carboxyl ester hydrolase from human pancreatic juice: I. Action on carboxyl esters, glycerides and phospholipids. Biochim Biophys Acta 1980;611:136.
35. Lombardo D, Guy O. Studies on the substrate specificity of a carboxyl ester hydrolase from human pancreatic juice: II. Action on cholesterol esters and lipid-soluble vitamin esters. Biochim Biophys Acta 1980;611:147.
36. Lechene de la Porte P, Abouakil N, LaFont H, et al. Subcellular localization of cholesterol ester hydrolase in the human intestine. Biochim Biophys Acta 1987;920:237.
37. Gallo LL, Bennett-Clark S, Myers S, et al. Cholesterol absorption in rat intestine: role of cholesterol esterase and acyl coenzyme A: cholesterol acyltransferase. J Lipid Res 1984;25:604.
38. Bennett-Clark S, Tercyak AM. Reduced cholesterol transmucosal transport in rats with inhibited mucosal acyl CoA:cholesterol acyltransferase and normal pancreatic function. J Lipid Res 1984;25:148.
39. Gallo LL, Wadsworth JA, Vahouny GV. Normal cholesterol absorption in rats deficient in intestinal acyl coenzyme A:cholesterol acyltransferase activity. J Lipid Res 1987;28:381.
40. Abouakil N, Rogalska E, Bonicel J, et al. Purification of pancreatic carboxylic-ester hydrolase by immunoaffinity and its application to the human bile salt–stimulated lipase. Biochim Biophys Acta 1988;961:299.
41. Wang CS. Human milk bile salt–activated lipase: further characterization and kinetic studies. J Biol Chem 1981;256:10918.
42. Blackberg L, Angquist KA, Hernell O. Bile salt–stimulated lipase in human milk: evidence for its synthesis in the lactating mammary gland. FEBS Lett 1987;217:37.
43. Freed LM, York CM, Hamosh P, et al. Bile salt–stimulated lipase of human milk: characteristics of the enzyme in the milk of mothers of premature and full-term infants. J Pediatr Gastroenterol Nutr 1987;6:598.

44. O'Connor CJ, Yaghi B. A rapid and sensitive separation of retinol and retinyl palmitate using a small, disposable bonded-phase column: kinetic applications. J Lipid Res 1988;29:1693.

45. Blackberg L, Lombardo D, Hernell O, et al. Bile salt–stimulated lipase in human milk and carboxyl ester hydrolase in pancreatic juice. FEBS Lett 1981;136:284.

46. Hernell O, Blackberg L. Digestion of human milk lipids: physiologic significance of sn-2 monoacylglycerol hydrolysis by bile salt–stimulated lipase. Pediatr Res 1982;16:882.

47. Patton JS, Carey MC. Watching fat digestion: the formation of visible product phases by pancreatic lipase is described. Science 1979;204:145.

48. Takahasui Y, Mizunuma T. Cytochemistry of fat absorption. Int Rev Cytol 1984;89:115.

49. Rigler MW, Honkanen RE, Patton JS. Visualization by freeze fracture, in vitro and in vivo, of the products of fat digestion. J Lipid Res 1986;27:836.

50. Thompson ABR, Dietschy JM. Intestinal lipid absorption: major extracellular and intracellular events. In: Johnson LR, ed. Physiology of the gastrointestinal tract. New York: Raven Press, 1981:1147.

51. Porter HP, Saunders DR, Tytgat G, et al. Fat absorption in bile fistula man: a morphological and biochemical study. Gastroenterology 1971;60:1008.

52. Westergaard H, Holtermuller KH, Dietschy JM. Measurement of resistance of barriers to solute transport in vivo in rat jejunum. Am J Physiol 1986;250:G727.

53. Levitt MD, Kneip JM, Levitt DG. Use of laminar flow and unstirred layer models to predict intestinal absorption in the rat. J Clin Invest 1988;81:1365.

54. Smithson KW, Millar DB, Jacobs LR, et al. Intestinal diffusion barrier: unstirred water layer or membrane surface mucous coat? Science 1981;214:1241.

55. Levitt MD, Fetzer CA, Kneip JM, et al. Quantitative assessment of luminal stirring in the perfused small intestine of the rat. Am J Physiol 1987;252:G325.

56. Bosner MS, Gulick T, Riley DJS, et al. Receptor-like function of heparin in the binding and uptake of neutral lipids. Proc Natl Acad Sci USA 1988;85:7438.

57. Bosner MS, Gulick T, Riley DJS, et al. Heparin-modulated binding of pancreatic lipase and uptake of hydrolyzed triglycerides in the intestine. J Biol Chem 1989;264:2021.

58. Lucas ML. Determination of acid surface pH in vivo in rat proximal jejunum. Gut 1983;24:734.

59. Chijiiwa K, Linsheer WG. Mechanism of pH effect on oleic acid and cholesterol absorption in the rat. Am J Physiol 1987;252:9506.

60. Brindley DN, Hubscher G. The effect of chain length on the activation and subsequent incorporation of fatty acid into glyceride by the small intestinal mucosa. Biochim Biophys Acta 1966;125:92.

61. McDonald GB, Weidman M. Partitioning of polar fatty acids into lymph and portal vein after intestinal absorption in the rat. Q J Exp Physiol 1987;72:153.

62. Ananthanarayanan M, Von Dippe P, Levy D. Identification of the hepatocyte Na$^+$-dependent bile acid transport protein using monoclonal antibodies. J Biol Chem 1988;263:8338.

63. Suchy FJ, Ananthanarayanan M, Bucuvalas JC, et al. An antibody to a developmentally regulated 48-kDA liver plasma membrane protein inhibits taurocholate uptake by isolated rat hepatocytes. Gastroenterology 1988;94:A596.

64. Harig JM, Soergel KH, Komorowski RA, et al. Treatment of diversion colitis with short-chain fatty acid irrigation. N Engl J Med 1989;320:23.

65. Davidson NO, Samuel P, Lieberman S, et al. Measurement of bile acid production in hyperlipidemic man: does phenotype or methodology make the difference? J Lipid Res 1981;22:620.

66. Stremmel W, Lotz G, Strohmeyer G, et al. Identification, isolation and partial characterization of a fatty acid-binding protein from rat jejunal microvillous membranes. J Clin Invest 1985;75:1068.

67. Stremmel W, Strohmeyer G, Borchard F, et al. Isolation and partial characterization of a fatty acid-binding protein in rat liver plasma membranes. Proc Natl Acad Sci USA 1985;82:4.

68. Sorrentino D, Stump D, Potter BJ, et al. Oleate uptake by cardiac myocytes is carrier mediated and involves a 40-Kd plasma membrane fatty acid–binding protein similar to that in liver, adipose tissue and gut. J Clin Invest 1988;82:928.

69. Berk PD, Potter BJ, Stremmel W. Role of plasma membrane ligand-binding protein in the hepatocellular uptake of albumin-bound organic anions. Hepatology 1987;7:165.

70. Stremmel W. Uptake of fatty acids by jejunal mucosal cells is mediated by a fatty acid–binding membrane protein. J Clin Invest 1988;82:2001.

71. Diamond JM, Karasov WH. Adaptive regulation of intestinal nutrient transporters. Proc Natl Acad Sci USA 1987;84:2442.

72. Ockner RK, Manning JA, Poppenhausen RB, et al. A binding protein for fatty acids in cytosol of intestinal mucosa, liver, myocardium and other tissues. Science 1972;177:56.

73. Gordon JI, Lowe JB. Analyzing the structures, functions and evolution of two abundant gastrointestinal fatty acid–binding proteins with recombinant DNA and computational techniques. Chem Phys Lipids 1985;38:137.

74. Heuckeroth RO, Birkenmeier EH, Levin MS, et al. Analysis of the tissue-specific expression, developmental regulation, and linkage relationships of a rodent gene encoding heart fatty acid–binding protein. J Biol Chem 1987;262:9709.

75. Bass NM, Manning JA. Tissue expression of three structurally different fatty acid–binding proteins from rat heart muscle, liver and intestine. Biochem Biophys Res Commun 1986;137:929.

76. Ockner RK, Manning JA. Fatty acid–binding protein in small intestine: identification, isolation, and evidence for its role in cellular fatty acid transport. J Clin Invest 1974;54:326.

77. Ockner RK, Manning JA. Fatty acid–binding protein: isolation from rat liver, characterization, and immunochemical quantification. J Biol Chem 1982;257:7872.

78. Bass NM, Manning JA, Ockner RK, et al. Regulation of the biosynthesis of two distinct fatty acid–binding proteins in rat liver and intestine: influence of sex difference and of clofibrate. J Biol Chem 1985;260:1432.

79. Bass NM, Manning JA, Ockner RK. Turnover and short-term regulation of fatty acid–binding protein in liver. J Biol Chem 1985;260:9603.

80. Gordon JI, Alpers DH, Ockner RK, et al. The nucleotide sequence of rat liver fatty acid–binding protein mRNA. J Biol Chem 1983;258:3356.

81. Alpers DH, Strauss AW, Ockner RK, et al. Cloning of a cDNA encoding rat intestinal fatty acid–binding protein. Proc Natl Acad Sci USA 1984;81:313.

82. Sweetser DA, Birkenmeier EH, Klisak IJ, et al. The human and rodent intestinal fatty acid–binding protein genes: a comparative analysis of their structure, expression and linkage relationships. J Biol Chem 1987;262:16060.

83. Takahashi K, Odani S, Ono T. Isolation and characterization of the three fractions (DE-I, DE-II and DE-III) of rat liver Z-protein and the complete primary structure of DE-II. Eur J Biochem 1983;136:589.

84. Gordon JI, Elshourbagy N, Lowe JB, et al. Tissue specific expression and developmental regulation of two genes coding for rat fatty acid–binding proteins. J Biol Chem 1985;260:1995.

85. Lowe JB, Sacchettini JC, Laposata M, et al. Expression of rat intestinal fatty acid–binding protein in *Escherichia coli*: Purification and comparison of ligand binding characteristics with that of *Escherichia coli*-derived rat liver fatty acid–binding protein. J Biol Chem 1987;262:5931.

86. Sacchettini JC, Gordon JI, Banaszak LJ. The structure of crystalline *Escherichia coli*-derived rat intestinal fatty acid–binding protein at 2.5: a resolution. J Biol Chem 1988;263:5815.

87. Cistola DP, Sacchettini JC, Banaszak LJ, et al. Fatty acid interactions with rat intestinal and liver fatty acid–binding proteins expressed in *Escherichia coli*: a comparative ^{13}C NMR study. J Biol Chem 1989;264:2700.

88. Gangl A, Ockner RK. Intestinal metabolism of plasma free fatty acids: intracellular compartmentation and mechanisms of control. J Clin Invest 1975;55:803.

89. Pittman RC, Attie AD, Carew TE, et al. Tissue sites of catabolism of rat and human low density lipoproteins in rats. Biochim Biophys Acta 1982;710:7.

90. Bloj B, Zilversmit DB. Heterogeneity of rabbit intestine brush-border plasma membrane cholesterol. J Biol Chem 1982;257:7608.

91. Chanderbhan R, Noland BJ, Scallen TJ, et al. Sterol carrier protein$_2$: delivery of cholesterol from adrenal lipid droplets to mitochondria for pregnenolone synthesis. J Biol Chem 1982;257:8928.

92. Teerlink T, Poorthuis BJHM, Van Der Krift TP, et al. Measurement of phosphatidylcholine transfer protein in rat liver and hepatomas by radioimmunoassay. Biochim Biophys Acta 1981;665:74.

93. Pastuszyn A, Noland BJ, Bazan JF, et al. Primary sequence and structural analysis of sterol carrier protein-2 from rat liver: homology with immunoglobulins. J Biol Chem 1987;262:13219.

94. Noland BJ, Arebalo RE, Hansbury E, et al. Purification and properties of sterol carrier protein$_2$. J Biol Chem 1980;255:4282.

95. Scallen TJ, Noland BJ, Gavey KL, et al. Sterol carrier protein-2 and fatty acid–binding protein: separate and distinct physiological functions. J Biol Chem 1985;1985:4733.

96. Kharroubi A, Wadsworth JA, Chanderbhan R, et al. Sterol carrier protein$_2$–like activity in rat intestine. J Lipid Res 1988;29:287.

97. Gallo LL, Myers S, Vahouny GV. Rat intestinal acyl coenzyme A: cholesterol acyl transferase properties and localization. Proc Soc Exp Biol Med 1984;177:188.

98. Trzeciak WH, Simpson ER, Scallen TJ, et al. Studies on the synthesis of sterol carrier protein-2 in rat adrenocortical cells in monolayer culture. J Biol Chem 1987;262:3713.

99. Goodman DS, Blaner WS. Biosynthesis, absorption and hepatic metabolism of retinol. In: The retinoids, vol 2. New York: Academic Press, 1984:1.

100. Chytil F, Ong DE. Intracellular vitamin A–binding proteins. Ann Rev Nutr 1987;7:321.

101. Demmer LA, Birkenmeier EH, Sweetser DA, et al. The cellular retinol-binding protein II gene: sequence analysis of the rat gene, chromosomal localization in mice and humans, and documentation of its close linkage to the cellular retinol-binding protein gene. J Biol Chem 1987;262:2458.

102. Li E, Demmer LA, Sweetser DA, et al. Rat cellular retinol-binding protein: II. Use of a cloned cDNA to define its primary structure, tissue-specific expression, and developmental regulation. Proc Natl Acad Sci USA 1986;83:5779.

103. Crow JA, Ong DE. Cell-specific immunohistochemical localization of a cellular retinol-binding protein (type two) in the small intestine of rat. Proc Natl Acad Sci USA 1985;82:4707.

104. Ong DE, Page DL. Cellular retinol-binding protein (type two) is abundant in human small intestine. J Lipid Res 1987;28:739.

105. Giguere V, Ong ES, Segui P, et al. Identification of a receptor for the morphogen retinoic acid. Nature 1987;330:624.

106. Helgerud P, Petersen LB, Norum KR. Retinol esterification by microsomes from the mucosa of human small intestine: evidence for acyl-coenzyme A retinol acyltransferase activity. J Clin Invest 1983;71:747.

107. Ong DE, Kakkad B, MacDonald PN. Acyl-CoA–independent esterification of retinol bound to cellular retinol-binding protein (type II) by microsomes from rat small intestine. J Biol Chem 1987;262:2729.

108. MacDonald PN, Ong DE. Evidence for a lecithin–retinol acyltransferase activity in the rat small intestine. J Biol Chem 1988;263:12478.

109. Gallo LL, Chiang Y, Vahouny GV, et al. Localization and origin of rat intestinal cholesterol esterase determined by immunocytochemistry. J Lipid Res 1980;21:537.

110. Clark SB. Mucosal coenzyme A–dependent cholesterol esterification after intestinal perfusion of lipids in rats. J Biol Chem 1979;254:1534.

111. Suckling KE, Stange EF. Role of acyl-CoA:cholesterol acyltransferase in cellular cholesterol metabolism. J Lipid Res 1985;26:647.

112. Spady DK, Turley SD, Dietschy JM. Receptor-independent low-density lipoprotein transport in the rat in vivo: quantitation, characterization, and metabolic consequences. J Clin Invest 1985;76:1113.

113. Turley SD, Andersen JM, Dietschy JM. Rates of sterol synthesis and uptake in the major organs of the rat in vivo. J Lipid Res 1981;22:551.

114. Stange EF, Suckling KE, Dietschy JM. Synthesis and coenzyme A-dependent esterification of cholesterol in rat intestinal epithelium. J Biol Chem 1983;258:12868.

115. Dietschy JM, Spady DK. Measurement of rates of cholesterol synthesis using tritiated water. J Lipid Res 1984;25:1469.

116. Li AC, Tanaka RD, Callaway K, et al. Localization of 3-hydroxy-3-methylglutaryl CoA reductase and 3-hydroxy-3-methylglutaryl CoA synthase in the rat liver and intestine is affected by cholestyramine and mevinolin. J Lipid Res 1988;29:781.

117. Stange EF, Dietschy JM. Cholesterol synthesis and low-density lipoprotein uptake are regulated independently in rat small intestinal epithelium. Proc Natl Acad Sci USA 1983;80:5739.

118. Gebhard RL, Prigge WF. In vivo regulation of canine intestinal 3-hydroxy-3-methylglutaryl coenzyme A reductase by cholesterol, lipoprotein and fatty acids. J Lipid Res 1981;22:1111.

119. Betteridge DJ, Krone W, Middleton C, et al. Regulation of sterol synthesis in human intestinal mucosa. Eur J Clin Invest 1980;10:227.

120. Purdy BH, Field FJ. Regulation of acylcoenzyme A cholesterol acyltransferase and 3-hydroxy-3-methylglutaryl coenzyme A reductase activity by lipoproteins in the intestine of parabiont rats. J Clin Invest 1984;74:351.

121. Freeman ML, Prigge WF, Hunninghake DB, et al. Intestinal HMG-CoA reductase activity is low in hypercholesterolemic patients and is further decreased with lovastatin therapy. J Lipid Res 1988;29:839.

122. McNamara DJ, Davidson NO, Samuel P, et al. Cholesterol absorption in man: effect of administration of clofibrate and/or cholestyramine. J Lipid Res 1980;21:1058.

123. McNamara DJ, Kolb R, Parker TS, et al. Heterogeneity of cholesterol homeostasis in man: response to changes in dietary fat quality and cholesterol quantity. J Clin Invest 1987;79:1729.

124. Kesaniemi YA, Ehnholm C, Miettinen TA. Intestinal cholesterol absorption efficiency in man is related to apoprotein E phenotype. J Clin Invest 1987;80:578.

125. Connor WE, Lin DS. Absorption and transport of shellfish sterols in human subjects. Gastroenterology 1981;81:276.

126. Gregg RE, Connor WE, Lin DS, et al. Abnormal metabolism of shellfish sterols in a patient with sitosterolemia and xanthomatosis. J Clin Invest 1986;77:1864.

127. Field FJ, Mathur SN. β-sitosterol: esterification by intestinal acylcoenzyme A:cholesterol acyltransferase (ACAT) and its effect on cholesterol esterification. J Lipid Res 1983;24:409.

128. Ikeda I, Tanaka K, Sugano M, et al. Inhibition of cholesterol absorption in rats by plant sterols. J Lipid Res 1988;29:1573.

129. Ikeda I, Tanaka K, Sugano M, et al. Discrimination between cholesterol and sitosterol for absorption in rats. J Lipid Res 1988;29:1583.

130. Kayden H, Senior JR, Mattson F. The monoglyceride pathway of fat absorption in man. J Clin Invest 1967;11:1695.

131. Mattson FH, Volpenhein RA. The digestion and absorption of triglycerides. J Biol Chem 1964;239:2772.

132. Brown JL, Johnston JM. The utilization of I- and 2-monoglycerides for intestinal triglyceride biosynthesis. Biochim Biophys Acta 1964;84:448.

133. Mansbach CB II, Parthasarathy S. A re-examination of the fate of glyceride-glycerol in neutral lipid absorption and transport. J Lipid Res 1982;23:1009.

134. Popper DA, Shiau YF, Reed M. Role of small intestine in pathogenesis of hyperlipidemia in diabetic rats. Am J Physiol 1985;249:G161.

135. Kennedy E. Biosynthesis of complex lipids. Fed Proc 1961;20:934.

136. Higgins JA, Barnett RJ. Fine structural localization of acyltransferases. J Cell Biol 1971;50:102.

137. Parthasarathy S, Papasani SV, Ganguly J. The mechanism of intestinal absorption of phosphatidylcholine in rats. Biochem J 1974;140:503.

138. Scow R, Stein Y, Stein O. Incorporation of dietary lecithin and lysolecithin into lymph chylomicrons in the rat. J Biol Chem 1967;242:4919.

139. Polheim D, David JSK, Schultz FM, et al. Regulation of triglyceride biosynthesis in adipose and intestinal tissue. J Lipid Res 1973;14:415.

140. Rao A, Johnston JM. Purification and properties of triglyceride synthetase from the intestinal mucosa. Biochim Biophys Acta 1966;125: 465.

141. Coleman R, Haynes E. Monoacylglycerol acyltransferase. J Biol Chem 1986;261:224.

142. Coleman RA, Walsh JP, Millington DS, et al. Stereospecificity of monoacylglycerol acyltransferase activity from rat intestine and suckling rat liver. J Lipid Res 1986;27:158.

143. Johnston JM, Rao GA, Lowe PA. The separation of the x-alpha glycerophosphate and monoglyceride pathways in the intestinal biosynthesis of triglycerides. Biochim Biophys Acta 1967;137:578.

144. Nilsson A. Intestinal absorption of lecithin and lysolecithin by lymph fistula rats. Biochim Biophys Acta 1967;137:578.

145. Noma A. Studies on the phospholipid metabolism of the intestinal mucosa during fat absorption. J Biochem 1964;56:522.

146. Coleman R, Bell RM. Evidence that biosynthesis of phosphatidylethanolamine, phosphatidylcholine and triacylglycerol occurs on the cytoplasmic side of microsomal vesicles. J Cell Biol 1978;76:245.

147. Vance JE, Vance DE. The role of phosphatidylcholine biosynthesis in the secretion of lipoproteins from hepatocytes. Can J Biochem Cell Biol 1985;63:870.

148. Mansbach C II. The origin of chylomicron phosphatidylcholine in the rat. J Clin Invest 1977;60:411.

149. Mansbach C II. Complex lipid synthesis in hamster intestine. Biochim Biophys Acta 1973;296:386.

150. Mansbach C II. Effect of fat feeding on complex lipid synthesis in hamster intestine. Gastroenterology 1975;68:708.

151. Cardell RR Jr, Badenhausen S, Porter K. Intestinal triglyceride absorption in the rat. J Cell Biol 1967;34:123.

152. Tytgat GN, Rubin CE, Saunders DR. Synthesis and transport of lipoprotein particles by intestinal absorptive cells in man. J Clin Invest 1971;50:2065.

153. Sabesin SM, Frase S. Electron microscopic studies of the assembly, intracellular transport, and secretion of chylomicrons by rat intestine. J Lipid Res 1977;18:496.

154. Christensen NJ, Rubin CE, Cheung MC, et al. Ultrastructural immunolocalization of apolipoprotein B within human jejunal absorptive cells. J Lipid Res 1983;24:1229.

155. Magun AM, Mish B, Glickman RM. Intracellular apoA-I and apoB distribution in rat intestine is altered by lipid feeding. J Lipid Res 1988;29:1107.

156. Alpers DH, Lock DR, Lancaster N, et al. Distribution of apolipoproteins A-I and B among intestinal lipoproteins. J Lipid Res 1985;26:1.

157. Reaven EP, Reaven GM. Distribution and content of microtubules in relation to the transport of lipid. J Cell Biol 1977;75:559.

158. Higgins JA, Fieldsend JK. Phosphatidylcholine synthesis for incorporation into membranes or for secretion as plasma lipoproteins by Golgi membranes of rat liver. J Lipid Res 1987;28:268.

159. Wu AL, Bennett Clark S, Holt PR. Transmucosal triglyceride transport rates in proximal and distal rat intestine in vivo. J Lipid Res 1975;20:494.

160. Surawicz CM, Levine DS, Saunders DR, et al. Comparison of human jejunal and ileal fat absorption by electron microscopy. Gastroenterology 1988;94:1376.

161. Breslow JL. Human apolipoprotein molecular biology and genetic variation. Ann Rev Biochem 1985;54:699.

162. Hegele RA, Breslow JL. Apolipoprotein genetic variation in the assessment of atherosclerosis susceptibility. Genet Epid 1987;4:163.

163. Humphries SE. DNA polymorphisms of the apolipoprotein genes: their use in the investigation of the genetic component of hyperlipidaemia and atherosclerosis. Atherosclerosis 1988;72:89.

164. Li W-H, Tanimura M, Luo C-C, et al. The apolipoprotein multigene family: biosynthesis, structure, structure-function relationships, and evolution. J Lipid Res 1988;29:245.

165. Luo C-C, Li W-H, Moore MN, et al. Structure and evolution of the apolipoprotein multigene family. J Mol Biol 1986;187:325.

166. Boguski MS, Birkenmeier EH, Elshourbagy NA, et al. Evolution of the apolipoproteins: structure of the rat apo A-IV gene and its relationship to the human genes for apo A-I, C-III and E. J Biol Chem 1986;261:6398.

167. Boguski MS, Elshourbagy N, Taylor JM, et al. Rat apolipoprotein

168. Boguski MS, Elshourbagy N, Taylor JM, et al. Comparative analysis of repeated sequences in rat apolipoproteins A-I, A-IV, and E. Proc Natl Acad Sci USA 1985;82:992.

169. Gordon JI, Smith DP, Andy DH, et al. The primary translation product of rat intestinal apolipoprotein A-I mRNA is an unusual preproprotein. J Biol Chem 1982;257;971.

170. Gordon JI, Budelier KA, Sims E, et al. Biosynthesis of human preproapolipoprotein A-II. J Biol Chem 1983;258:14054.

171. Glomset JA. The plasma lecithin cholesterol acyltransferase reaction. J Lipid Res 1968;9:155.

172. Fielding CJ, Shore VG, Fielding PE. A protein cofactor of lecithin, cholesterol acyltransferase. Biochem Biophys Res Commun 1972;46: 1493.

173. Wu A-L, Windmueller HG. Relative contributions by liver and intestine to individual plasma apolipoproteins in the rat. J Biol Chem 1979;254:7316.

174. Maciejko JJ, Holmes DR, Kottke BA, et al. Apolipoprotein A-I as a marker of angiographically assessed coronary artery disease. N Engl J Med 1983;309:385.

175. Davidson NO, Glickman RM. Apolipoprotein A-I synthesis in rat small intestine: regulation by dietary triglyceride and biliary lipid. J Lipid Res 1985;26:368.

176. Davidson NO, Magun AM, Brasitus TA, et al. Intestinal apolipoprotein A-I and B-48 metabolism: effects of sustained alterations in dietary triglyceride and mucosal cholesterol flux. J Lipid Res 1987;28: 388.

177. Elshourbagy NA, Boguski MS, Liao WSL, et al. Expression of rat apolipoprotein A-IV and A-I genes: mRNA induction during development and in response to glucocorticoids and insulin. Proc Natl Acad Sci USA 1985;82:8242.

178. Davidson NO, Carlos RC, Drewek MJ, et al. Apolipoprotein gene expression in the rat is regulated in a tissue-specific manner by thyroid hormone. J Lipid Res 1988;29:1511.

179. Apfelbaum TF, Davidson NO, Glickman RM. Apolipoprotein A-IV synthesis in rat intestine: regulation by dietary triglyceride. Am J Physiol 1987;252:G662.

180. Gordon JI, Bisgaier CL, Sims HF, et al. Biosynthesis of human preapolipoprotein A-IV. J Biol Chem 1984;259:468.

181. Lefevre M, Roheim PS. Metabolism of apolipoprotein A-IV. J Lipid Res 1984;25:1003.

182. Steinmetz A, Utermann G. Activation of lecithin:cholesterol acyltransferase by human apolipoprotein A-IV. J Biol Chem 1985;260: 2258.

183. Blaufuss MC, Gordon JI, Schonfeld G, et al. Biosynthesis of apolipoprotein C-III in rat liver and small intestinal mucosa. J Biol Chem 1984;259:2452.

184. Haddad IA, Ordovas JM, Fitzpatrick T, et al. Linkage, evolution and expression of the rat apolipoprotein A-I, C-III, and A-IV genes. J Biol Chem 1986;261:13268.

185. Gordon JI, Budelier KA, Sims HF, et al. Biosynthesis of human preproapolipoprotein A-II. J Biol Chem 1983;258:14054.

186. Lenich C, Brecher P, Makrides S, et al. Apolipoprotein gene expression in the rabbit: abundance, size, and distribution of apolipoprotein mRNA species in different tissues. J Lipid Res 1988;29:755.

187. Schonfeld G, Grimme N, Alpers D. Detection of apolipoprotein C in human and rat enterocytes. J Cell Biol 1980;86:562.

188. Drayna D, Fielding C, McLean J, et al. Cloning and expression of human apolipoprotein D cDNA. J Biol Chem 1986;261:16535.

189. Kane JP, Hardman DA, Paulus HE. Heterogeneity of apolipoprotein B: isolation of a new species from human chylomicrons. Proc Natl Acad Sci USA 1980;77:2465.

190. Blackhart BD, Ludwig EM, Peirotti VR, et al. Structure of the human apolipoprotein B gene. J Biol Chem 1986;261:15364.

191. Knott TJ, Pease RJ, Powell LM, et al. Complete protein sequence and identification of structural domains of human apolipoprotein B. Nature 1986;323:734.

192. Cladaras C, Hadzopoulou-Cladaras M, Nolte RT, et al. The complete sequence and structural analysis of human apolipoprotein B-100:

A-IV contains 13 tandem repetitions of a 22-amino acid segment with amphipathic helical potential. Proc Natl Acad Sci USA 1984;81: 5021.

relationship between apo B-100 and apo B-48 forms. EMBO J 1986;5: 3495.

193. Powell LM, Wallis SC, Pease RJ, et al. A novel form of tissue-specific RNA processing produces apolipoprotein B-48 in intestine. Cell 1987;50:831.

194. Davidson NO, Powell LM, Wallis SC, et al. Thyroid hormone modulates the introduction of a stop codon in rat liver apolipoprotein B messenger RNA. J Biol Chem 1988;263:13482.

195. Glickman RM, Rogers M, Glickman J. Apolipoprotein B synthesis by human liver and intestine in vitro. Proc Natl Acad Sci USA 1986;83:5296.

196. Davidson NO, Kollmer ME, Glickman RM. Apolipoprotein B synthesis in rat small intestine: regulation by dietary triglyceride and biliary lipid. J Lipid Res 1986;27:30.

197. Davidson NO, Drewek MJ, Gordon JI, et al. Rat intestinal apolipoprotein B gene expression: evidence for integrated regulation by bile salt, fatty acid and phospholipid flux. J Clin Invest 1988;82:300.

198. Demmer LA, Levin MS, Elovson J, et al. Tissue-specific expression and developmental regulation of the rat apolipoprotein B gene. Proc Natl Acad Sci USA 1986;83:8102.

199. Gotto AM, Levy RI, John K, et al. On the protein defect in abetalipoproteinemia. N Engl J Med 1971;284:813.

200. Glickman RM, Green PHR, Lees RS, et al. Immunofluorescence studies of apolipoprotein B in intestinal mucosa: absence in abetalipoproteinemia. Gastroenterology 1979;76:288.

201. Dullaart RPF, Speelberg B, Schuurman H-J, et al. Epitopes of apolipoprotein B-100 and B-48 in both liver and intestine: expression and evidence for local synthesis in recessive abetalipoproteinemia. J Clin Invest 1986;78:1397.

202. Levy E, Marcel YL, Mine RW, et al. Absence of intestinal synthesis of apolipoprotein B-48 in two cases of abetalipoproteinemia. Gastroenterology 1987;93:1119.

203. Bouma ME, Beucler I, Pessah M, et al. Description of two different patients with abetalipoproteinemia: synthesis of a normal-sized apolipoprotein B-48 in intestinal organ culture. J Lipid Res 1990;31:1.

204. Lackner KJ, Monge JC, Gregg RE, et al. Analysis of the apolipoprotein B gene and messenger ribonucleic acid in abetalipoproteinemia. J Clin Invest 1986;78:1707.

205. Talmud PH, Lloyd JK, Muller DP, et al. Genetic evidence from two families that the apolipoprotein B gene is not involved in abetalipoproteinemia. J Clin Invest 1988;82:1803.

206. Ross RS, Gregg RE, Law SW, et al. Homozygous hypobetalipoproteinemia: a disease distinct from abetalipoproteinemia at the molecular level. J Clin Invest 1988;81:590.

207. Malloy MJ, Kane JP, Hardman DA, et al. Normotriglyceridemic abetalipoproteinemia. J Clin Invest 1981;67:1441.

208. Herbert PN, Hyams JS, Bernier DN, et al. Apolipoprotein B-100 deficiency. Intestinal steatosis despite apolipoprotein B-48 synthesis. J Clin Invest 1985;76:403.

209. Bouma M-E, Beucler I, Aggerbeck L-P, et al. Hypobetalipoproteinemia with accumulation of an apoprotein B-like protein in intestinal cells. J Clin Invest 1986;78:398.

210. Levy E, Marcel Y, Deckelbaum RJ, et al. Intestinal apo B synthesis, lipids, and lipoproteins in chylomicron retention disease. J Lipid Res 1987;28:1263.

211. Roy CC, Levy E, Green PHR, et al. Malabsorption, hypocholesterolemia, and fat-filled enterocytes with increased intestinal apoprotein B: chylomicron retention disease. Gastroenterology 1987;92:390.

212. Swift LL, Soule PD, Gray ME, et al. Intestinal lipoprotein synthesis: comparison of nascent Golgi lipoproteins from chow-fed and hypercholesterolemic rats. J Lipid Res 1984;25:1.

213. Green PHR, Glickman RM. Intestinal lipoprotein metabolism. J Lipid Res 1981;22:1153.

214. Zilversmit DB. The composition and structure of lymph chylomicrons in dog, rat, and man. J Clin Invest 1969;48:2079.

215. Ockner RH, Hughes FB, Isselbacher KJ. Very low density lipoproteins in intestinal lymph: origin, composition, and role in lipid transport in the fasting state. J Clin Invest 1969;48:2079.

216. Mahley RW, Bennett BD, Morre J, et al. Lipoproteins associated with the Golgi apparatus isolated from epithelial cells of rat small intestine. Lab Invest 1971;25:435.

217. Tso P, Drake DS, Black DD, et al. Evidence for separate pathways of chylomicron and very-low density lipoprotein assembly and transport by rat small intestine. Am J Physiol 1984;247:G599.

218. Black DD, Tso P, Weidman S, et al. Intestinal lipoproteins in the rat with D-(+)-galactosamine hepatitis. J Lipid Res 1983;24:977.

219. Magun AM, Brasitus TA, Glickman RM. Isolation of high density lipoproteins from rat intestinal epithelial cells. J Clin Invest 1985;75:209.

220. Green PHR, Tall AR, Glickman RM. Rat intestine secretes discoid high density lipoprotein. J Clin Invest 1978;61:528.

221. Forester GP, Tall AR, Bisgaier CL, et al. Rat intestine secretes spherical high density lipoproteins. J Biol Chem 1983;258:5938.

222. Patton GM, Bennett Clark S, Fasulo JM, et al. Utilization of individual lecithins in intestinal lipoprotein formation in the rat. J Clin Invest 1984;73:231.

223. Black DD, Davidson NO. Intestinal apolipoprotein synthesis and secretion in the suckling pig. J Lipid Res 1989;30:207.

224. Green PHR, Glickman RM, Saudek CD, et al. Human intestinal lipoproteins. J Clin Invest 1979;64:233.

225. Glickman RM, Green PHR. The intestine as a source of apolipoprotein A1. Proc Natl Acad Sci USA 1977;74:2569.

226. Bearnot HR, Glickman RM, Weinberg L, et al. Effect of biliary diversion on rat mesenteric lymph apolipoprotein A-I and high density lipoprotein. J Clin Invest 1982;69:210.

227. Renner F, Samuelson A, Rogers M, et al. Effect of saturated and unsaturated lipid on the composition of mesenteric triglyceride-rich lipoproteins in the rat. J Lipid Res 1986;27:72.

228. Gordon JI, Smith DP, Alpers DH, et al. Cloning of complementary deoxyribonucleic acid encoding a portion of rat intestinal preapolipoprotein AIV ribonucleic acid. Biochemistry 1982;21:5424.

229. Schonfeld G, Bell E, Alpers DH. Intestinal apoproteins during fat absorption. J Clin Invest 1978;61:1539.

230. Green PHR, Lefkowitch JH, Glickman RM, et al. Apolipoprotein localization and quantitation in the human intestine. Gastroenterology 1982;83:1223.

231. Alpers DH, Lancaster N, Schonfeld G. The effects of fat feeding on apolipoprotein AI secretion from rat small intestinal epithelium. Metabolism 1982;31:784.

232. Rachmilewitz D, Albers JJ, Saunders DR. Apoprotein B in fasting and postprandial human jejunal mucosa. J Clin Invest 1976;57:530.

233. Imaizumi K, Havel RJ, Fainaru N, et al. Origin and transport of the A-I and arginine-rich apolipoproteins in mesenteric lymph of rats. J Lipid Res 1978;19:1038.

234. Bisgaier CL, Sachdev OP, Megna L, et al. Distribution of apolipoprotein A-IV in human plasma. J Lipid Res 1985;26:11.

235. Wollin A, Jacques LB. Plasma protein escape from the intestinal circulation to the lymphatics during fat absorption. Proc Soc Exp Med Bio 1972;142:1114.

236. Green PHR, Glickman RM, Riley JW, et al. Human apolipoprotein A-IV. J Clin Invest 1980;65:911.

237. Ghiselli G, Schaefer EJ, Light JA, et al. Apolipoprotein A-I isoforms in human lymph: effect of fat absorption. J Lipid Res 1983;24:731.

238. Krause BR, Sloop CH, Castle CK, et al. Mesenteric lymph apolipoproteins in control and ethinyl estradiol-treated rats: a model for studying apolipoproteins of intestinal origin. J Lipid Res 1981;22:610.

239. Whyte M, Goodman DS, Karmen A. Fatty acid esterification and chylomicron formation during fat absorption in rat: III. Positional relations in triglycerides and lecithin. J Lipid Res 1965;6:233.

240. Feldman EB, Russell BS, Chen R, et al. Dietary saturated fatty acid content affects lymph lipoproteins: studies in the rat. J Lipid Res 1983;24:967.

241. Arvidson GAE, Nilsson A. Formation of lymph chylomicron phosphatidylcholines in the rat during the absorption of safflower oil or triolein. Lipids 1972;7:344.

242. Risser TR, Reaven GM, Reaven EP. Intestinal contribution to secretion of very low density lipoproteins into plasma. Am J Physiol 1978;234:E277.

243. Holt PR, Dominguez AA. Triton-induced hyperlipidemia: a model for studies of intestinal lipoprotein production. Am J Physiol 1980;238:G453.

244. Cenedella RJ, Crouthamel WG, Mengoli HF, et al. Intestinal versus hepatic contribution to circulating triglyceride levels. Lipids 1974;9:35.

245. Windmueller HG, Wu AL. Biosynthesis of plasma apolipoproteins

by rat small intestine without dietary or biliary fat. J Biol Chem 1981;256:3012.

246. Glickman RM, Kilgore A, Khorana J. Chylomicron apoprotein localization within rat intestinal epithelium: studies of normal and impaired lipid absorption. J Lipid Res 1978;19:260.

247. Glickman RM, Khorana J, Kilgore A. Localization of apolipoprotein B in intestinal epithelial cells. Science 1976;193:1254.

248. Mak KM, Trier JS. Lipoprotein particles in the jejunal mucosa of postnatal developing rats. Anat Rec 1979;194:491.

249. Jones AL, Ockner RK. An electron microscopic study of endogenous very low density lipoprotein production in the intestine of rat and man. J Lipid Res 1971;12:580.

250. Berendsen P. Sites of lipoprotein production in the small intestine of the unsuckled and suckled newborn rat. Anat Rec 1979;195:15.

251. Beil U, Grundy SM. Studies of plasma lipoproteins during absorption of exogenous lecithin in man. J Lipid Res 1980;21:525.

252. Breckenridge WC, Yeung SKF, Kuksis A. Biosynthesis of triacylglycerols by rat intestinal mucosa in vivo. Can J Biochem 1976;54:145.

253. Tso P, Balint JA, Simmonds WJ. Role of biliary lecithin in lymphatic transport of fat. Gastroenterology 1977;73:1362.

254. O'Doherty PJA, Kakis G, Kuksis A. Role of luminal lecithin in intestinal fat absorption. Lipids 1973;8:249.

255. Bennett Clark S. Chylomicron composition during duodenal triglyceride and lecithin infusion. Am J Physiol 1978;235:E183.

256. Klein RL, Rudel LL. Cholesterol absorption and transport in thoracic duct lymph lipoproteins of nonhuman primates: effect of dietary cholesterol level. J Lipid Res 1983;24:343.

257. Klein RL, Rudel LL. Effect of dietary cholesterol level on the composition of thoracic duct lymph lipoproteins isolated from nonhuman primates. J Lipid Res 1983;24:357.

258. Riley JW, Glickman RM, Green PHR, et al. The effect of chronic cholesterol feeding on intestinal lipoproteins in the rat. J Lipid Res 1980;21:942.

259. Tall AR, Green PHR, Glickman RM, et al. Metabolic fate of chylomicron phospholipids and apoproteins in the rat. J Clin Invest 1979;64:977.

260. Ghiselli G, Krishnan S, Beigel Y, et al. Plasma metabolism of apolipoprotein A-IV in humans. J Lipid Res 1986;27:813.

261. Edelstein C, Gordon JI, Toscas K, et al. In vitro conversion of proapoprotein A-I to apoprotein A-I. Partial characterization of an extracellular enzyme activity. J Biol Chem 1983;258:11430.

262. Gordon JI, Sims HF, Lentz SR, et al. Proteolytic processing of human preproapolipoprotein A-I. J Biol Chem 1983;258:4037.

263. Breslow JL. Human apolipoprotein molecular biology and genetic variation. Ann Rev Biochem 1985;54:699.

264. Eckel RH. Lipoprotein lipase: a multifunctional enzyme relevant to common metabolic diseases. N Engl J Med 1989;320:1060.

265. Breckenridge WC, Little JA, Steiner G, et al. Hypertriglyceridemia associated with deficiency of apolipoprotein C-II. N Engl J Med 1978;298:1265.

266. Myklebost O, Williamson B, Markham AF, et al. The isolation and characterization of cDNA clones for human apolipoprotein CII. J Biol Chem 1984;259:4401.

267. Hui DY, Brecht WJ, Hall EA, et al. Isolation and characterization of the apolipoprotein E receptor from canine and human liver. J Biol Chem 1986;261:4256.

268. Kita T, Goldstein JL, Brown MS, et al. Hepatic uptake of chylomicron remnants in WHHL rabbits: a mechanism genetically distinct from the low density lipoprotein receptor. Proc Natl Acad Sci USA 1982;79:3623.

269. Scott J. Unravelling atherosclerosis. Nature 1989;338:118.

270. Mahley RW, Hui DY, Innerarity TL, et al. Chylomicron remnant metabolism: role of hepatic lipoprotein receptors in mediating uptake. Arteriosclerosis 1989;9(suppl I):1-14.

271. Herz J, Hamann U, Rogne S, et al. Surface location and high affinity for calcium of a 500-kd liver membrane protein closely related to the LDL-receptor suggest a physiological role as lipoprotein receptor. EMBO J 1988;7:4119.

272. Quarfordt SH, Michalopoulos G, Schirmer B. The effect of human C apolipoproteins on the in vitro hepatic metabolism of triglyceride emulsions in the rat. J Biol Chem 1982;257:14642.

273. Ginsberg HN, Le N-A, Goldberg IJ, et al. Apolipoprotein B metabolism in subjects with deficiency of apolipoproteins CIII and AI. J Clin Invest 1986;78:1287.

274. Hamilton RL, Williams MC, Fielding C, et al. Discoidal bilayer structure of nascent high density lipoproteins from perfused rat liver. J Clin Invest 1976;58:667.

19

Protein Digestion and Assimilation

DENNIS J. AHNEN

Protein digestion in the intestine occurs by a highly efficient and coordinated series of hydrolytic steps. Both dietary proteins and proteins secreted into the intestine are cleaved initially to oligopeptides and small numbers of free amino acids by proteases secreted by the stomach and pancreas. A series of membrane-bound oligopeptidases located on the intestinal brush border then cleave the oligopeptides further to amino acids and di- and tripeptides, which are absorbed into the enterocyte by specific transport systems of the brush border. Another family of peptidases located in the cytosol of the enterocytes cleaves the absorbed di- and tripeptides to free amino acids. Within the enterocyte, amino acids are available for protein synthesis by the cell, but the majority diffuse into the lamina propria and are cleared predominantly by the portal circulation. The overall scheme of protein digestion is illustrated in Figures 19-1 and 19-2.

Digestion and assimilation of proteins differ from the intestinal handling of lipids and carbohydrates in two major ways. Unlike fats, dietary proteins and their hydrolytic products are largely hydrophilic and do not require bile acid micelles for solubilization. In addition, as a result of the enormous structural diversity of amino acids, and thus proteins, larger families of hydrolases and transport systems are necessary for efficient assimilation of proteins than are required for fats or carbohydrates.

DIETARY PROTEINS

Dietary Intake and Requirements

The average American diet contains 70 to 100 g of protein per day, well in excess of the recommended daily allowance (RDA, 0.8 g/kg/d). The RDA for protein is above the minimal requirements for maintenance of positive nitrogen balance in healthy individuals (around 0.4 g/kg/d).[1,2] Dietary protein assimilation is the only source of the nine essential amino acids that are required

for protein synthesis but cannot be synthesized in human tissues[2] (Fig 19-3). Adequate intake of nonprotein calories (84–105 kilojoules per gram dietary protein) is also required to prevent amino acid utilization for energy and allow normal protein synthesis.

Digestibility of protein is affected by the type of protein and its state of processing prior to ingestion. In general, plant proteins are less digestible than animal proteins.[3] High proline content in proteins such as gluten or casein reduces their digestibility. Cooking food generally denatures proteins and makes them more digestible; however, heat can also cause the formation of covalent bonds within or between some proteins and reduce their digestibility.[4]

In addition to dietary protein, significant amounts of endogenous proteins are presented to the intestine for digestion and absorption. Twenty to thirty grams of protein flow into the intestinal lumen each day by way of salivary gland, gastric, biliary, pancreatic, and intestinal secretions.[5] Desquamation of enterocytes adds about another 30 g of protein per day to the intestinal lumen.[6]

Protein Structure

The multiplicity of systems for hydrolysis and transport of proteins is due to the large diversity of protein structure. Proteins are composed of 21 common amino acids (Fig 19-3). Amino acids are linked to form polypeptides and proteins by peptide bonds

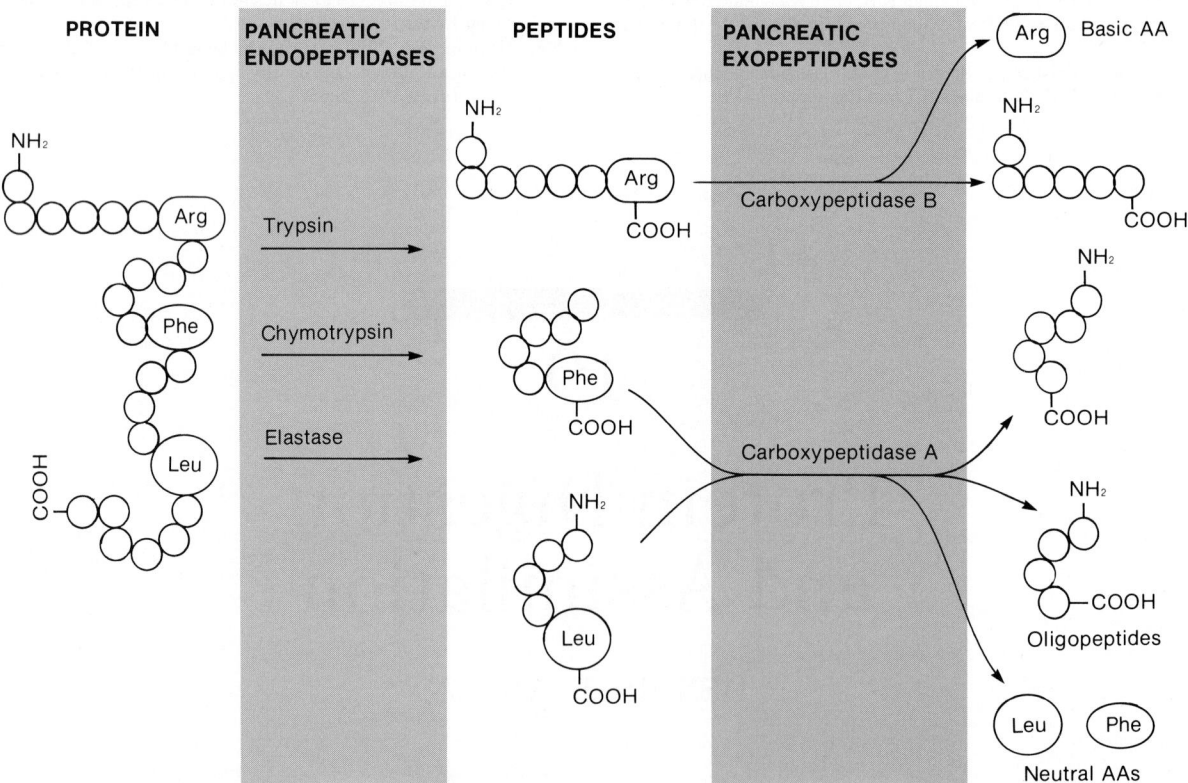

FIGURE 19–1. Intraluminal digestion of proteins by pancreatic proteases. Pancreatic endopeptidases (trypsin, chymotrypsin, elastase) cleave internal peptide bonds of proteins. Each of the endopeptidases has a different substrate specificity (see text for details). The peptide products of endopeptidase digestion are then acted upon by the pancreatic ectopeptidases (carboxypeptidases A and B). The carboxypeptidases cleave the carboxyterminal amino acid from the peptides. The products of pancreatic proteolysis are about 30% neutral and basic amino acids and 70% oligopeptides.

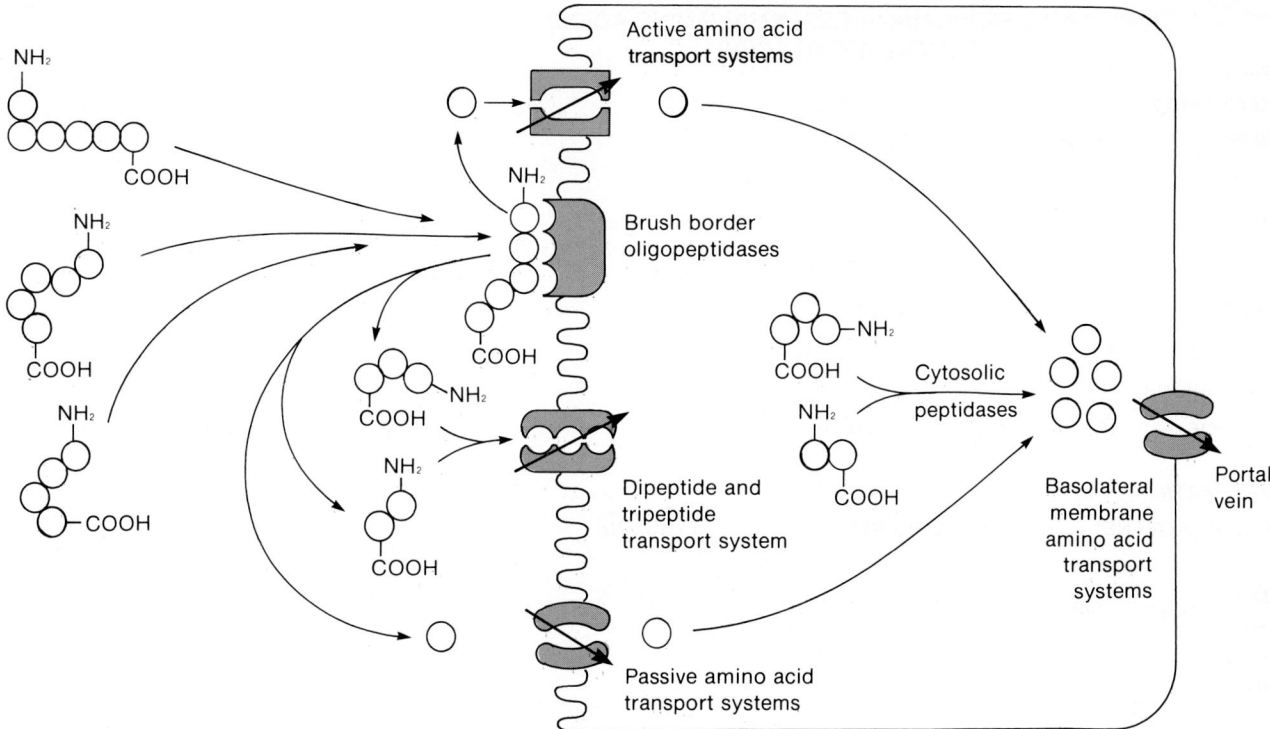

FIGURE 19–2. Hydrolysis of oligopeptides and absorption of amino acids and di- and tripeptides by the enterocyte. The oligopeptides produced by pancreatic proteolysis of proteins are further hydrolyzed by a family of brush border oligopeptidases to free amino acids, dipeptides, and tripeptides. Amino acids are absorbed across the microvillar membrane by both Na^+-dependent active (*upward arrow*) transport systems and passive (*downward arrow*) transport systems (facilitated and simple diffusion). Dipeptides and tripeptides are absorbed by at least one separate active transport system. Absorbed dipeptides and tripeptides are hydrolyzed to amino acids by a family of cytosolic peptidases. Amino acids exit the enterocyte across the basolateral membrane largely by passive transport systems.

that couple the alpha-carboxyl group of one amino acid residue to the alpha-amino group of another residue. The great diversity of protein structure and function is largely derived from the variability in the amino acid side chains (see Fig 19-3). With two exceptions, all of the common amino acids are primary alpha amino acids, which means that the carboxyl and amino groups are attached to the same carbon atom. The imino acids proline and hydroxyproline contain an imino nitrogen rather than a primary amino group; thus, they are handled differently from the other amino acids (see below). The 21 common amino acids can be divided into three groups on the basis of their charge (neutral, basic, and acidic; Fig 19-3). Certain amino acids play specific roles in protein structure. N-linked carbohydrates are added to only asparagine residues, O-linked carbohydrates are added to either serine or threonine; proline is frequently found at sites of a major turn in the protein orientation; and series of hydrophobic (aromatic and long-chain aliphatic) amino acids are found in the membrane-spanning domain of transmembrane proteins.

The enormous variety of possible amino acid combinations (400 possible dipeptides, 8000 tripeptides, 160,000 tetrapeptides, and so forth) is responsible for the functional and antigenic heterogeneity of proteins. Multiple types of hydrolytic enzymes with varied substrate specificity are necessary for the complete and efficient digestion of the entire array of proteins and peptides. Similarly, multiple transport systems for amino acids and small peptides are necessary for efficient absorption of the range of amino acids and small peptide products of protein hydrolysis.

PROTEIN DIGESTION

Protein digestion occurs through a series of coordinated hydrolytic steps. Initial hydrolysis of proteins occurs in the intestinal lumen and is mediated by a family of soluble proteases and peptidases. The final hydrolysis of oligopeptides is mediated by integral membrane hydrolases located in the enterocyte microvillar membrane.

Intraluminal Proteolysis

Intraluminal proteolysis of dietary proteins is initiated in the stomach by the action of pepsins and is completed in the small intestine by the action of pancreatic proteases. In the stomach, emulsification and acid denaturation release dietary protein in forms that are more susceptible to proteases. Gastric proteolysis is mediated by a family of acid proteases (the pepsins).[7-9] The two major pepsins (pepsins I and II) are synthesized, stored, and secreted by chief cells as inactive precursors (pepsinogen I and II). Pepsinogen secretion is closely related to acid secretion and is increased by gastrin, histamine, and vagal stimulation. At acidic pH, the pepsinogens are converted to pepsins by autocatalytic cleavage of an oligopeptide from the N-terminal end of the precursor. The cleavage results in a decrease in the isoelectric point of the molecules from 3.7 to 1 and a marked increase in their enzymatic activity.

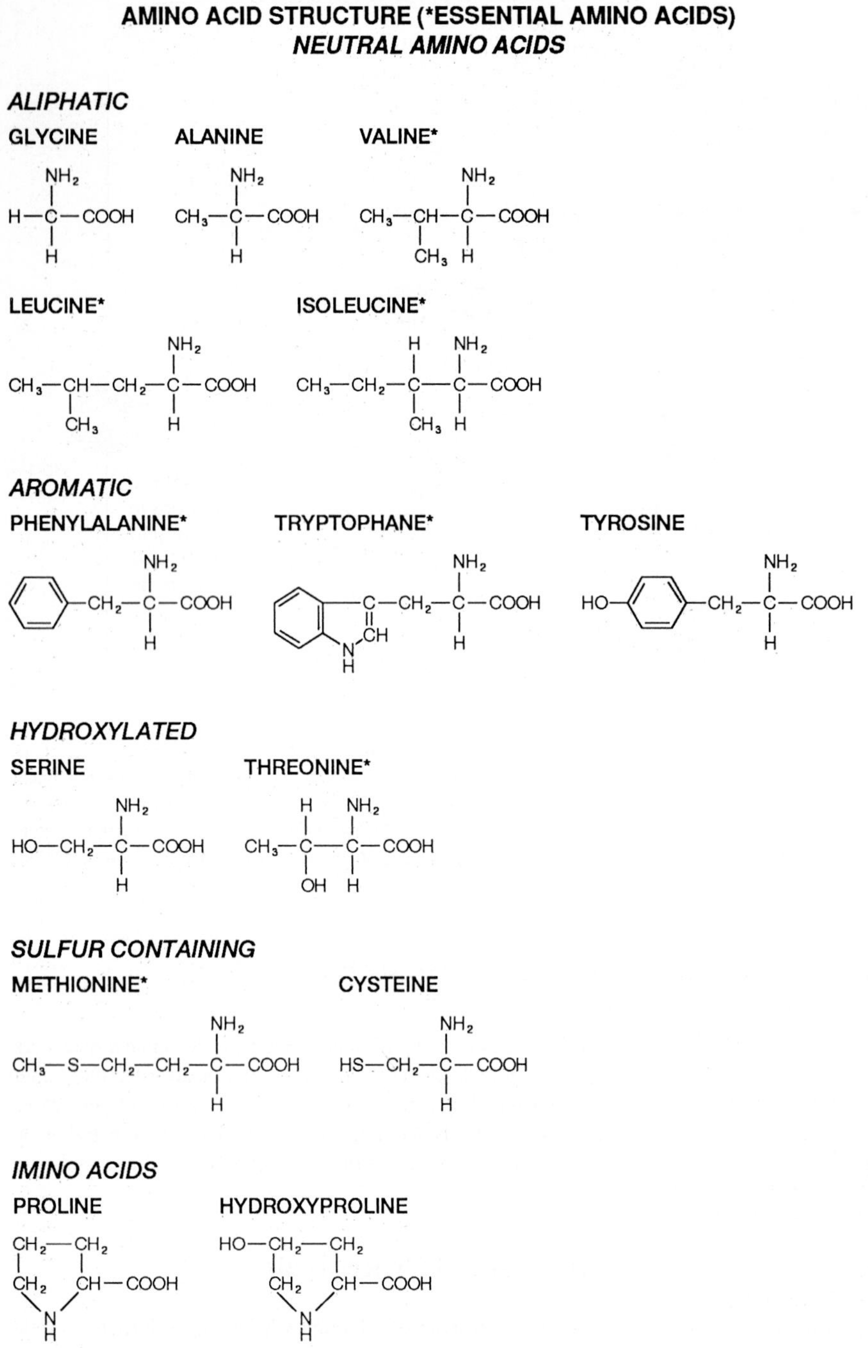

AMINO ACID STRUCTURE (*ESSENTIAL AMINO ACIDS)
NEUTRAL AMINO ACIDS

ALIPHATIC

GLYCINE ALANINE VALINE*

LEUCINE* ISOLEUCINE*

AROMATIC

PHENYLALANINE* TRYPTOPHANE* TYROSINE

HYDROXYLATED

SERINE THREONINE*

SULFUR CONTAINING

METHIONINE* CYSTEINE

IMINO ACIDS

PROLINE HYDROXYPROLINE

FIGURE 19–3. The variability in primary structure of the 21 common amino acids is responsible for the great diversity of protein structure and function. The eight essential amino acids are indicated by the asterisk. The amino acids can be divided on the basis of charge into neutral, basic, and acidic groups. The neutral amino acids are subdivided into aliphatic, aromatic, hydroxylated, sulfur-containing, and imino groups. Two molecules of the sulfur-containing amino acid cysteine can combine by disulfide bonds to form cystine (cysteine and cystine are counted as a single amino acid).

(continued)

The substrate specificity of pepsins I and II is similar and broad. It includes most neutral amino acids, but the highest activity occurs at peptide bonds involving aromatic or large aliphatic amino acids. The hydrophobic nature of these amino acids is thought to be the common feature responsible for the specificity of the pepsins.

Gastric proteolysis is dependent on acid secretion and is proportional to residence time in the stomach because the pepsins are maximally active at pH 1–3 and rapidly inactivated at pH above 4.5. Thus, proteolysis by these enzymes generally ceases when food enters the neutral pH melieu of the duodenum. Overall, gastric proteolysis results in release of only a small proportion (10%–15%) of ingested amino acids and is not essential for protein digestion. Individuals with achlorhydria or total gastrectomy usually have normal protein digestion and absorption; apparently the proteolytic mechanisms available in the intestine can compensate for the lack of pepsin activity. The major products of gastric proteolysis are large, nonabsorbable peptides that are further hydrolyzed by pancreatic proteases in the proximal small bowel.

HYDROLYSIS BY PANCREATIC PROTEASES

The bulk of intraluminal proteolysis in the gut is mediated by pancreatic proteases acting by way of a highly ordered series of

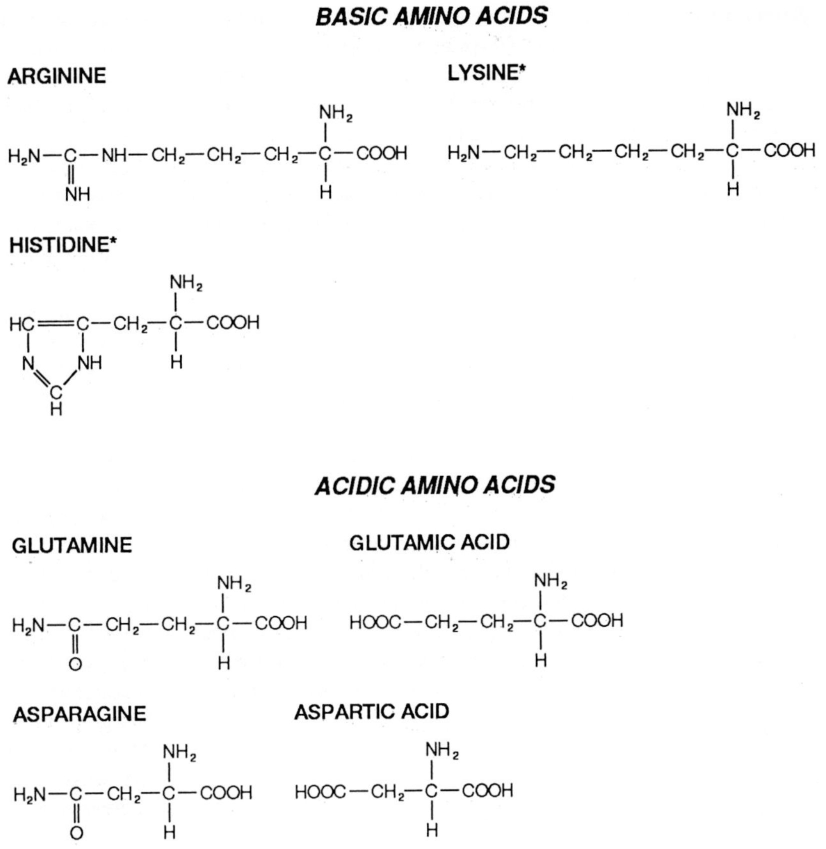

BASIC AMINO ACIDS

ARGININE

$H_2N-C-NH-CH_2-CH_2-CH_2-\overset{\overset{\displaystyle NH_2}{|}}{\underset{\underset{\displaystyle H}{|}}{C}}-COOH$

$\underset{\displaystyle NH}{\|}$

LYSINE*

$H_2N-CH_2-CH_2-CH_2-CH_2-\overset{\overset{\displaystyle NH_2}{|}}{\underset{\underset{\displaystyle H}{|}}{C}}-COOH$

HISTIDINE*

$HC=C-CH_2-\overset{\overset{\displaystyle NH_2}{|}}{\underset{\underset{\displaystyle H}{|}}{C}}-COOH$

ACIDIC AMINO ACIDS

GLUTAMINE

$H_2N-\underset{\underset{\displaystyle O}{\|}}{C}-CH_2-CH_2-\overset{\overset{\displaystyle NH_2}{|}}{\underset{\underset{\displaystyle H}{|}}{C}}-COOH$

GLUTAMIC ACID

$HOOC-CH_2-CH_2-\overset{\overset{\displaystyle NH_2}{|}}{\underset{\underset{\displaystyle H}{|}}{C}}-COOH$

ASPARAGINE

$H_2N-\underset{\underset{\displaystyle O}{\|}}{C}-CH_2-\overset{\overset{\displaystyle NH_2}{|}}{\underset{\underset{\displaystyle H}{|}}{C}}-COOH$

ASPARTIC ACID

$HOOC-CH_2-\overset{\overset{\displaystyle NH_2}{|}}{\underset{\underset{\displaystyle H}{|}}{C}}-COOH$

FIGURE 19–3. *(Continued)*

events. The pancreas secretes three endopeptidases (trypsin, chymotrypsin, and elastase) that are capable of cleaving internal peptide bonds and two carboxypeptidases (carboxypeptidase A and B) that cleave the carboxy-terminal amino acid of peptides.[1,10,11]

Structural and sequence analyses have demonstrated that the pancreatic endopeptidases are related. They are all neutral proteases that are inactivated at acid *p*H and they all have a reactive serine residue that forms part of the active site of the enzyme. The pancreatic carboxypeptidases (A and B) are also structurally related; they are both zinc-dependent metalloproteases.

All of the pancreatic proteases are synthesized, stored in zymogen granules, and secreted as inactive precursors.[11] Pancreatic protease secretion is increased by both endocrine (cholecystokinin [CCK], secretin, gastrin) and neural (acetylcholine, vasoactive intestinal polypeptide [VIP]) stimulation.[12] Studies in isolated acinar cells have identified a variety of other pancreatic exocrine secretagogues (bombesin, substance P, calcitonin gene-related peptide [CGRP]).[13,14] All of the stimuli of pancreatic exocrine secretion appear to act through specific acinar cell surface receptors and mediate pancreatic enzyme secretion through activation of one of two cellular pathways. The actions of acetylcholine, CCK, bombesin, and substance P are mediated by Ca^{++}-dependent intracellular signal transduction mechanisms, while VIP and CGRP effects are mediated by increased cellular cyclic AMP.[14]

Upon secretion into the small bowel, the pancreatic proenzymes are themselves activated by a series of proteolytic events depicted in Figure 19-4. Within the intestinal lumen, trypsinogen is activated by way of the proteolytic cleavage of a hexapeptide from its amino terminus. Proteolytic activation of trypsinogen is mediated by en-

teropeptidase, an integral endopeptidase of enterocyte microvillar membrane. Trypsin is then capable of cleaving additional molecules of trypsinogen to trypsin, as well as the other inactive enzymes (chymotrypsinogen, proelastase, and procarboxypeptidases A and B) to their active counterparts (chymotrypsin, elastase, and carboxypeptidases A and B).

The five pancreatic proteases have a complementary array of substrate specificities and act in a coordinated manner to hydrolyze

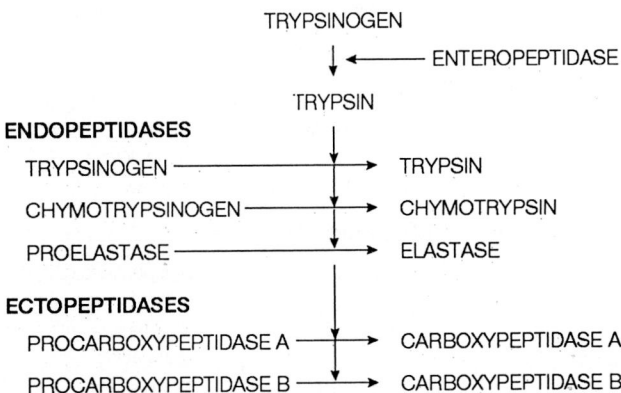

FIGURE 19–4. Intraluminal activation of pancreatic proteases. Upon secretion into the intestinal lumen, trypsinogen is activated to trypsin by proteolytic cleavage by enteropeptidase. Trypsin then cleaves and activates additional molecules of trypsinogen and the proenzymes of the other endo- and ectopeptidases to active proteases.

dietary proteins efficiently.[10] Initially, the proteins are cleaved by the pancreatic endopeptidases (trypsin, chymotrypsin, elastase), each of which has a different substrate specificity. The resultant peptides are the preferred substrates for the pancreatic carboxypeptidases (see Fig 19-1). For example, trypsin preferentially cleaves internal peptide bonds adjacent to basic amino acids (arginine, lysine), resulting in small peptides with basic amino acids at their carboxyl-terminus. These peptides are the preferred substrate for carboxypeptidase B, which cleaves the carboxyl-terminal basic amino acid from the peptide. In an analogous manner, chymotrypsin preferentially cleaves internal peptide bonds adjacent to neutral aromatic amino acids (phenylalanine, tryptophane, tyrosine), and elastase cleaves internal peptide bonds adjacent to aliphatic neutral amino acids (glycine, leucine, and so forth), producing peptides with neutral amino acids at their carboxy-terminus. These peptides in turn are the preferred substrates for carboxypeptidase A, which cleaves the neutral carboxyl-terminal amino acid from them.

Intraluminal hydrolysis results in the conversion of dietary protein to oligopeptides (60%–70% of total amino nitrogen) and free neutral and basic amino acids (30% of total amino nitrogen). The free amino acids can be absorbed efficiently without further modification. The oligopeptides are suitable substrates for hydrolysis by the membrane-bound oligopeptidases of the enterocyte brush border.

BRUSH BORDER HYDROLYSIS OF OLIGOPEPTIDES

The oligopeptide products of intraluminal proteolysis are further hydrolyzed by a family of oligopeptidases that are integral membrane proteins of the enterocyte brush border (see Fig 19-2). The brush border hydrolases include endopeptidases that cleave internal bonds and ectopeptidases that cleave amino acids or dipeptides from the ends of oligopeptides (see Table 19-1). The brush border hydrolases that have been described thus far share many features.[15–22] They are synthesized by enterocytes as large integral membrane glycoproteins (molecular weight range 90–300 kd) with short anchoring segments. They are synthesized and core-glycosylated in the rough endoplasmic reticulum. The carbohydrate side chains are modified in both the endoplasmic reticulum and the Golgi apparatus. The glycoproteins are subsequently transported to the brush border where they accumulate. Synthesis of the brush border peptidases is regulated during differentiation. The enzymes are not present in the crypt, initial synthesis is normally detected at the crypt–villus junction, and the enzyme content in the brush border increases as the cells migrate up the villus. In rats, a high-protein diet increases brush border peptidase activity (substrate stimulation),[23] and certain amino acids can inhibit aminopeptidase activity (product inhibition).[24]

Enteropeptidase was the initial brush border endopeptidase identified.[15,16] It cleaves trypsinogen to trypsin and initiates the sequence of pancreatic protease activation described above (see Fig 19-4). Recently, a family of brush border neutral endopeptidases[21,25,26] that are capable of hydrolyzing protein substrates has been identified (Table 19-1). Endopeptidase 24.11 is the best characterized of the neutral endopeptidases. It preferentially cleaves peptide bonds adjacent to internal hydrophobic amino acids. At least two other neutral endopeptidases have been identified in the brush border.[25] The endogenous substrates for the neutral endopeptidases in the intestine are not known; hence, their relative importance from a nutritional standpoint is unclear. They may become critically important in states of exocrine pancreatic insufficiency.

At least six different ectopeptidases with a broad range of substrate specificities are present in the enterocyte brush border (Table 1). Two aminopeptidases (aminopeptidase N and aminopeptidase A) cleave the N-terminal amino acids from oligopeptides (C²–

TABLE 19-1
Brush Border Peptidases

ENZYMES	ENDOGENOUS SUBSTRATE(S)	PRODUCTS
Endopeptidases		
Enteropeptidase	Trypsinogen	Trypsin
Endopeptidase 24.11	Unknown—cleaves at internal hydrophobic amino acids	Peptides
Neutral endopeptidases	Unknown	Peptides
Ectopeptidases		
Aminopeptidase N	Oligopeptides (C2–C6) with neutral N-terminal amino acids	Neutral amino acids, dipeptides, tripeptides
Aminopeptidase A	Oligopeptides (C2–C6) with acidic N-terminal amino acids	Acidic amino acids, dipeptides, tripeptides
Dipeptidyl peptidase IV	Oligopeptides containing pentultimate PRO, ALA at N-terminus	Dipeptides
Folate conjugase	Polyglutamated folates	Pteroylglutamic acid
Gly-Leu peptidase	Dipeptides	Amino acids
Asp-Lys peptidase	Dipeptides	Amino acids

C[6]) having neutral and acidic N-terminal amino acids, respectively.[27-33] Dipeptidyl aminopeptidase IV cleaves a dipeptide from the amino terminus of peptides containing a proline or alanine in the penultimate position.[34-36] This enzyme is likely to play an important role in digestion of proline-containing peptides, because these peptides are not readily cleaved by pancreatic or the other brush border hydrolases. Folate conjugase cleaves all but the final glutamyl residue from the polyglutamyl forms of folic acid.[37] Two dipeptidases (Gly-Leu peptidase and zinc-stable Asp-Lys peptidase) cleave dipeptides containing neutral and charged N-terminal amino acids, respectively.[38] The action of the brush border hydrolases is illustrated in Figure 19-2.

ABSORPTION OF DI- AND TRIPEPTIDES AND AMINO ACIDS

The final products of brush border hydrolysis are free amino acids and di- and tripeptides that are absorbed by way of a family of transport systems of the enterocyte brush border.

Peptide Absorption

Significant di- and tripeptide absorption occurs across the microvillar membrane.[39-41] The most convincing evidence for dipeptide transport comes from studies in patients with inherited defects in amino acid transport systems.[42] Patients with Hartnup disease (defect in neutral amino acid transport) and cysteinuria (defect in basic amino acid transport) do not become amino acid-deficient and can absorb the affected amino acids efficiently when they are delivered in the form of dipeptides.[42,43] Dipeptides containing proline and glycine are more resistant to hydrolysis by the brush border dipeptidase and appear to be absorbed preferentially as dipeptides.[44] The nutritional importance of the dipeptide transport system is suggested by intestinal perfusion studies demonstrating that many amino acids are absorbed faster as dipeptides than as free amino acids. However, the relative physiologic importance of free amino acid versus di- and tripeptide transport in vivo is not yet known.[41,45,46]

The total number of microvillar membrane peptide transporters has not yet been determined. At least one active peptide transport system that is distinct from the amino acid transporters described below has been identified.[47] Recent evidence suggests that in contrast to active amino acid transport, peptide transport is not directly Na$^+$-coupled but may be linked to proton (H$^+$) transport.[48] Energy for this peptide transport system could be derived from the inward proton gradient generated by the Na$^+$–H$^+$ exchanger in the brush border. In this model, the observed Na$^+$ requirement for peptide transport would be explained by the Na$^+$ dependence of the Na$^+$–H$^+$ exchanger.

Within the enterocyte, the bulk of absorbed di- and tripeptides are hydrolyzed to free amino acids by a family of cytosolic peptidases that are capable of hydrolyzing a broad range of di- and tripeptides.[39,49,50] Three of the cytosolic peptidases (one tripeptidase and two dipeptidases) have been characterized partially (see Table 19-2). Amino tripeptidase cleaves the N-terminal amino acid from tripeptides, resulting in free amino acid and dipeptide

TABLE 19-2
Cytosolic Peptidases in the Enterocyte

ENZYMES	ENDOGENOUS SUBSTRATES	PRODUCTS
Amino tripeptidase	Tripeptides	Dipeptides, amino acids
Amino dipeptidase	Dipeptides	Amino acids
Prodipeptidase	Dipeptides containing proline	Amino acids

products.[51] Dipeptides are hydrolyzed by at least two enzymes; amino dipeptidase has a broad specificity for dipeptides,[52] and prodipeptidase (prolidase) plays a special role because it is one of the few peptidases that cleave peptide bonds involving imino acids (proline, hydroxyproline).[53]

Some dipeptides escape intracellular hydrolysis and are transported across the basolateral membrane intact. The overall nutritional importance of intact peptide absorption is not clear. In the rat, the magnitude of intact peptide transport into the portal circulation varies with the type of protein absorbed and ranges from 0% to 30% of absorbed luminal nitrogen.[54] Intact absorption of small amounts of larger peptides and proteins (albumin, intrinsic factor, IgG) is not nutritionally significant but may be very important immunologically in both the production of an immune response as well as the tolerance to dietary antigens (see ch 5).

Amino Acid Absorption

Amino acids are transported across the small intestinal epithelium in two stages: predominantly active uptake across the microvillar membrane and predominantly passive release into the interstitium across the basolateral membrane.

Amino Acid Uptake Across the Microvillar Membrane

Transport of amino acids across the microvillar membrane is mediated by a family of transporters with overlapping specificity[55] (see Table 19-3). The generally accepted convention for naming amino acid transport systems uses letters that indicate the specificity of the transporter. Uppercase letters are used for Na$^+$-dependent transporters and lowercase letters are used for Na$^+$-independent systems. The bulk of nutrient amino acids are transported across the microvillar membrane by at least five Na$^+$-dependent secondary active transport systems. For each of the Na$^+$-dependent transport systems, Na$^+$ uptake is coupled to the uptake of a group of amino acids—three for subsets of neutral amino acids, one for acidic amino acids, and one for basic amino acids. Na$^+$-independent facilitated diffusion transport systems for amino acids that are analogous to those present in nonepithelial cells are also present in the microvillar membrane of the enterocyte.

The three Na$^+$-dependent active transport systems for subsets of neutral amino acids are specifically adapted for absorption of

TABLE 19–3
Amino Acid Transport Systems of the Enterocyte Brush Border

TRANSPORT SYSTEM	AMINO ACID SPECIFICITY	TYPE OF TRANSPORT
NBB (neutral brush border)	Neutral amino acids	Na-dependent active
PHE (phenylalanine)	Hydrophobic amino acids (phenylalanine, methionine)	Na-dependent active
IMINO	Proline, hydroxyproline	Na-dependent, active
X_{GA}^- (glutamate, aspartate)	Acidic amino acids	Active, Na cotransport, K countertransport
Y^+ (lysine)	Basic amino acids	Na-dependent, active
y^+ (lysine)	Basic amino acids	Facilitated diffusion
L (leucine)	Neutral amino acids	Facilitated diffusion
Diffusion	All amino acids	Passive diffusion

luminal amino acids.[56] The neutral brush border (NBB) transporter has broad specificity for most neutral amino acids and is quantitatively the most important of the Na^+-dependent transporters. This transporter has been shown to be responsible for up to 70% of the total transport of some neutral amino acids. The phenylalanine (PHE) carrier preferentially transports phenylalanine and methionine, and the IMINO carrier exclusively transports imino acids such as proline and hydroxyproline. These systems are present on polar cells with brush borders (enterocytes, renal tubular cells). The transport maximum for uptake of these amino acids is 5 to 10 mmolar, so they are efficient only when luminal concentrations of amino acids are relatively high. During fasting, other amino acid transporters become more important. The energy for these Na^+-dependent transport systems is derived from the action of Na^+,K^+-ATPase at the basolateral membrane, which maintains the low intracellular Na^+ concentration and electronegativity of the enterocyte interior. This allows Na^+ to be transported down an electrochemical gradient from the intestinal lumen to the cell interior. The general scheme of Na^+-dependent secondary active amino acid transport is depicted in Figure 19-5.

Acidic amino acids (glutamic acid, aspartic acid) are transported by a system ($X^-_{G,A}$) that appears to be more complex than that of neutral amino acids.[57,58] In addition to the cotransport of Na^+ and acidic amino acids, this system mediates the countertransport of K^+ or H^+.

Basic amino acids and cysteine appear to be handled by at least two separate brush border carriers.[59,60] Both an Na^+-dependent secondary active transport system (Y^+) and an Na^+-independent facilitated diffusion transport system (y^+) have been identified in the rat small intestine.

Na^+-independent facilitated diffusion of neutral amino acids is mediated by a transport system (L for leucine; the uppercase abbreviation is an exception to the standard convention) that is found in all animal cells.[56] Finally, all amino acids can be absorbed by passive diffusion.

It is clear that there are several different systems for transport of neutral amino acids, and the interactions between the systems are not completely understood. For the neutral amino acid alanine, the NBB transport is quantitatively the most important, accounting for about 70% of total transport; the L system handles about 20%, and 10% is absorbed by simple diffusion.

AMINO ACID UPTAKE ACROSS THE BASOLATERAL MEMBRANE

During feeding, the amino acid requirements of the cell can be met easily by the luminal absorption of amino acids and dipeptides described above. During fasting, however, it is likely that amino acid uptake across the basolateral membrane from the circulation becomes more important.

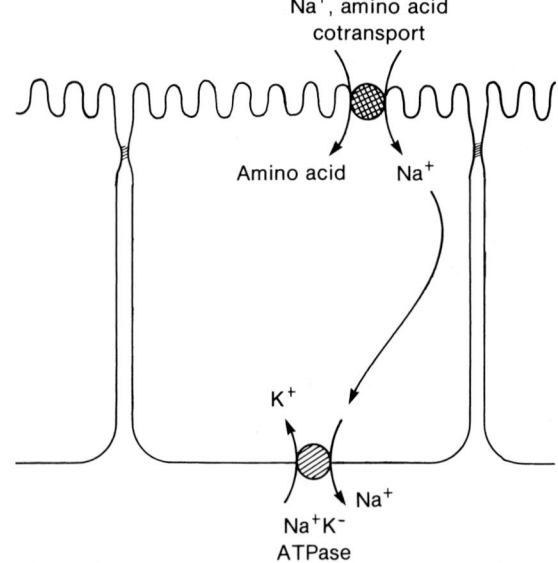

FIGURE 19–5. Na^+-dependent active transport of amino acids across the enterocyte brush border. Na^+-amino acid cotransport is mediated by a family of carriers in the enterocyte microvillar membrane. The energy for transport is derived from Na^+, K^+ ATPase-mediated Na^+, K^+ countertransport at the basolateral membrane of the cell, which generates a downhill electrochemical Na^+ gradient across the microvillar membrane. Na^+ transport down its electrochemical gradient is coupled to amino acid transport into the enterocyte. The activity of the NBB, PHE, IMINO, and Y^+ transport systems of the microvillar membrane is consistent with this model. The $X^-_{G,A}$ (glutamate, aspartate) transport system and the peptide transport system appear to be more complex (see text for details).

The enterocyte basolateral membrane contains amino acid transporters analogous to the classical types found in other cell types (Table 19-4) and distinct from the specialized transporters (NBB, IMINO, PHE) of the microvillar membrane. Two Na$^+$-dependent active transporters for neutral amino acids, the A (alanine) and the ASC (alanine, serine, cysteine) pathways, have been found in enterocyte basolateral membranes.[56,61] Uptake by these systems has been detected at low substrate concentrations such as during fasting.

INTRACELLULAR METABOLISM OF AMINO ACIDS

Although the large majority of absorbed dietary amino acids are released unaltered into the portal circulation, the enterocyte is dependent on the intracellular amino acid pool for protein synthesis and at times for an energy source.

Glutamine and glutamic acid appear to be handled by the enterocyte in a manner different from that of other amino acids. They are the only amino acids that are taken up consistently from the circulation by the small intestinal mucosa.[62–64] While other amino acids retained by the enterocyte are used primarily for protein synthesis, glutamine and glutamic acid are metabolized substantially and used as a major energy source. Deamidization of glutamine by enterocytes is also a significant source of ammonia that is released into both the circulation and the intestinal lumen to be taken up and utilized by other tissues.[65] The mechanism for the preferential uptake of glutamine is not yet defined, but it is likely that active transport occurs at the basolateral as well as the apical membrane of the enterocyte.

Amino Acid Exit Across the Basolateral Membrane

During feeding, the intracellular amino acid concentration is high, and transport out of the cell occurs primarily by simple or facilitated diffusion down the amino acid gradient across the basolateral membrane (see Table 19-4). Na$^+$-independent facilitated diffusion is mediated by the L system, which has a broad specificity for neutral amino acids.[56,61] As described above, this transport system is also present on the brush border and accounts for a small fraction of amino acid uptake at that site. In contrast, the L system is a major exit pathway from the enterocyte, accounting for about half of the transport alanine out of the cell. All amino acids can exit the cell by simple diffusion, and this pathway accounts for the other half of alanine transport out of the cell.

CLINICAL IMPLICATIONS OF PROTEIN DIGESTION AND ABSORPTION

Efficiency of Protein Assimilation

Despite the multiplicity of steps necessary for protein digestion and absorption and the great diversity of amino acid structure, overall protein assimilation is very efficient. This is due to the broad array of potent hydrolases and high-capacity transport systems with their overlapping and coordinated specificities that are described above. Over 95% of the total luminal protein (70–100 g of dietary intake, 20–30 g of endogenous secretions, 20–30 g from desquamated cells) is absorbed by the small intestine.[66] More than half of normal protein digestion and absorption occurs in the duodenum and jejunum; the remainder occurs in the ileum.[67] In contrast to the disaccharidases, the brush border peptidases continue to be expressed in as high or higher concentrations in the ileum as in the duodenum and jejunum.[68] Only about 1 to 3 g of protein enter the colon; more of the protein in stool (5–9 gm) is from bacteria than from dietary sources.

In general, the proteins in the diet and those from endogenous secretions are hydrolyzed in the same manner. There are, however, some endogenous proteins that are notably resistant to intestinal hydrolysis and depend on this resistance for their function. Cobalamin absorption is dependent on the hydrolytic resistance of intrinsic factor.[69] The polymeric immunoglobulin receptor mediates the transcellular transport of polymeric IgA and IgM into intestinal secretions.[70] The ectoplasmic domain of the receptor (secretory component) is secreted in complex with the immunoglobulin and increases the resistance of IgA to proteolysis by pancreatic enzymes.[70]

There are also specific functions for digestive proteases other than dietary protein hydrolysis. Pancreatic proteases are necessary for cleavage of R proteins bound to cobalamin so that intrinsic factor can bind to the vitamin and subsequently mediate its ab-

TABLE 19–4
Amino Acid Transport Systems of the Enterocyte Basolateral Membrane

TRANSPORT SYSTEM	AMINO ACID SPECIFICITY	TYPE OF TRANSPORT	ROLE
A (alanine)	Short-chain neutral amino acids	Na-dependent, active	Uptake pathway
ASC (Ala, Ser, Cys)	3- and 4-carbon neutral amino acids	Na-dependent, active	Uptake pathway
L (leucine)	Neutral amino acids cysteine, glutamine	Facilitated diffusion	Exit pathway
Diffusion	All amino acids	Passive diffusion	Exit pathway

sorption.[68] Pancreatic proteases play a role in both the post-translational processing and degradation of brush border constituents, such as by cleaving the single-chain precursor of sucrase- α-dextrinase into its two subunits after insertion into the microvillar membrane and by removing and inactivating sucrase- α-dextrinase and other disaccharidases from the brush border.[71] The increased quantity of brush border sucrase and maltase activity in pancreatic insufficiency probably results from decreased degradation of these enzymes. Pancreatic proteases may also function in the pathogenesis of some enteroviral infections. Attachment of rotaviruses to the enterocyte appears to require proteolytic cleavage of constituents of the outer capsule of the virus.[72]

Clinical Syndromes of Impaired Protein Assimilation

Both inherited and acquired defects of steps in each of the stages of protein digestion and absorption have been identified.

HEREDITARY DEFECTS

Many specific inherited defects in protein assimilation undoubtedly have gone undetected because of the redundancy of the mechanisms for digestion and absorption of these nutrients. Defects at critical steps in the process can, however, result in major nutritional consequences.[73]

Inherited defects in portal and lymphatic flow (hepatic vein stenosis, intestinal lymphangiectasia, hereditary lymphedema) can result in intestinal protein loss that overwhelms the normal small bowel capacity for digestion and absorption, thus producing the syndrome of protein-losing enteropathy.

Cystic fibrosis is the most common genetic disorder of the pancreas (1 per 2000 births) and is the leading cause of malabsorption in children. It is inherited as an autosomal recessive trait and results in abnormally viscous pancreatic secretions, ductal obstruction, and subsequent destruction of ducts and acinar cells. About 90% of patients with cystic fibrosis have exocrine pancreatic insufficiency.

Specific deficiencies of the key enzymes responsible for intraluminal activation of pancreatic proteases (enteropeptidase and trypsinogen) result in neonatal malabsorption and failure to thrive. If recognized, these deficiencies respond well to pancreatic enzyme therapy.

Several specific defects in the amino acid transporters are known. *Hartnup syndrome* is a rare (1/100,000 live births) autosomal recessive defect in neutral amino acid transport across the microvillar membranes of the enterocyte and renal tubular cell. The transport defect causes aminoaciduria, but the intestinal defect is usually compensated for by the other neutral amino acid and dipeptide transporters. When dietary protein intake is low, however, a pellegralike state due to deficiency of tryptophane and its end product nicotinamide may result.

Cystinuria is an autosomal recessive defect in the transport of cystine and basic amino acids in the intestine and renal tubule. The intestinal transport defect is compensated for by the other transporters, and the only clinical manifestation is cystine crystal formation and nephrolithiasis.

Iminoglycinuria is an autosomal recessive defect in transport of glycine and imino acids (proline, hydroxyproline). The defect is usually fully compensated for by other transport systems in the intestine; thus, it rarely causes symptoms.

In contrast to the other amino acid transport defects that affect brush border uptake, *lysinuric protein intolerance* is characterized by a defect in the exit of basic amino acids across the basolateral membrane of enterocytes and renal tubular cells. During fasting, this defect is not compensated for by other transporters; thus, patients with this disorder present with failure to thrive, nausea, vomiting, diarrhea, and growth retardation in infancy at the time of initiation of cows' milk.

Deficiency of the cytosolic peptidase prodipeptidase (prolidase) results in impaired hydrolysis of di- and tripeptides containing proline. The resultant proline deficiency causes abnormal collagen metabolism.

ACQUIRED DEFECTS

The clinical features and specific diseases causing malabsorption are discussed in detail in Chapters 71–75. As with the hereditary defects, acquired disorders occur at each stage of protein assimilation.

Delivery of excessive protein to the gut that may occur in hypertrophic gastropathy or other protein-losing enteropathies can overwhelm the capacity of the normal intestine for protein assimilation.

Exocrine pancreatic insufficiency is by far the most common cause of defective intraluminal proteolysis. Chronic pancreatitis and malignancy are the most common causes of exocrine pancreatic insufficiency. Defects in gastric proteolysis occur (achlorhydria, gastric resection), but they are usually compensated for by pancreatic proteolysis and do not cause protein malabsorption.

Acquired defects in brush border hydrolysis of oligopeptides and the transport of amino acids and di- and tripeptides are usually the result of diffuse injury to the enterocyte with villous atrophy. The spectrum of disorders producing partial and total villous atrophy is presented in Chapter 71.

> The reader is directed to Chapter 14, Secretion and Absorption: Small Intestine and Colon; Chapter 21, General Nutritional Principles; Chapter 47, Approach to Gastrointestinal Problems Associated with Common Clinical Conditions; Chapter 71, Celiac Disease; and Chapter 72, Specific Mucosal Protein Deficiency States.

REFERENCES

1. Silk DBA, Grimble GK, Rees RG. Protein digestion and amino acid and peptide absorption. Proc Nutr Soc 1985;44:63.
2. Adibi SA, Gray SJ. Intestinal absorption of essential amino acids in man. Gastroenterology 1967;52:837.
3. Fleming C. Parenteral and enteral nutrition. In: Kelley WN, ed. Textbook of internal medicine. Philadelphia: JB Lippincott, 1988: 722.
4. Alpers DH. Digestion and absorption of carbohydrates and proteins. In: Johnson LR, ed. Physiology of the gastrointestinal tract, ed 2. New York: Raven Press, 1987:1469.

5. Freeman HJ, Sleisenger MH, Kim YS. Human protein digestion and absorption: Normal mechanisms and protein-energy malnutrition. Clin Gastroenterol 1983;12:357.

6. Gardner MG. L-amino acid and peptide absorption from partial digests of proteins in isolated rat small intestine. J Physiol 1978;284:83.

7. Whitecross DP, Armstrong C, Clark AD, Piper DW. The pepsinogens of human gastric mucosa. Gut 1973;14:850.

8. Foltmann B. Gastric proteinases—Structure, function, evolution and mechanism of action. In: Campbell PN, Marshal RD, eds. Essays in biochemistry. New York: Academic Press, 1981:52.

9. Samloff IM. Pepsins, peptic activity, and peptic inhibitors. J Clin Gastroenterol 1981;3:91.

10. Rinderknecht H. Pancreatic secretory enzymes. In: Go VLW, Brooks FP, DiMagno EP, Gardner JD, Lebenthal E, Scheele GA, eds. The exocrine pancreas: Biology, pathobiology, and diseases. New York: Raven Press, 1986:163.

11. Rinderknecht H. Activation of pancreatic zymogens. Dig Dis Sci 1986;31:314.

12. Solomon TE. Control of exocrine pancreatic secretion. In: Johnson LR, ed. Physiology of the gastrointestinal tract, ed 2. New York: Raven Press, 1987:1173.

13. Gardner JD, Jensen RT. Secretogogue receptors on pancreatic acinar cells. In: Johnson LR, ed. Physiology of the gastrointestinal tract, ed 2. New York: Raven Press, 1987:1109.

14. Hootman SR, Williams JA. Stimulus-secretion coupling in the pancreatic acinus. In: Johnson LR, ed. Physiology of the gastrointestinal tract, ed 2. New York: Raven Press, 1987:1129.

15. Hermon-Taylor J, Perrin J, Grant DAW, et al. Immunofluorescent localisation of enterokinase in human small intestine. Gut 1987;18:259.

16. Grant DAW, Hermon-Taylor J. The purification of human enterokinase by affinity chromatography and immunoadsorption. Biochem J 1976;155:243.

17. Kenny AJ, Maroux S. Topology of microvillar membrane hydrolases of kidney and intestine. Physiol Rev 1982;62:91.

18. Danielsen M, Cowell GM, Noren O, Sjostrom H. Biosynthesis of microvillar proteins. Biochem J 1984;221:1.

19. Hauri H-P, Sterchi EE, Bienz D, et al. Expression and intracellular transport of microvillus membrane hydrolases in human intestinal epithelial cells. J Cell Biol 1985;101:838.

20. Ahnen DJ, Mircheff AK, Santiago NA, Yoshioka C, Gray GM. Intestinal surface amino-oligopeptidase. Distinct molecular forms during assembly in intracellular membranes in vivo. J Biol Chem 1983;258:5940.

21. Kenny AJ, Fulcher IS. Microvillar endopeptidase, an enzyme with special topological features and a wide distribution (Ciba Foundation Symposium 95). In: Brush border membranes. London: Pitman Books, 1983:12.

22. Danielsen EM, Cowell GML. Biosynthesis of intestinal microvillar proteins. Eur J Biochem 1985;152:493.

23. Nordstrom C. Release of enteropeptidase and other brush border enzymes from the small intestine wall in the rat. Biochim Biophys Acta 1972;289:376.

24. Cheeseman CL, Smyth DH. Interaction of amino acids, peptides, and peptidases in the small intestine. Proc R Soc Lond Biol 1975;190:149.

25. Guan D, Yoshioka M, Erickson RH, Heizer W, Kim YS. Protein digestion in human and rat small intestine: Role of new neutral endopeptidases. Am J Physiol 1988;255:G212.

26. Song IS, Yoshioka M, Erickson RH, et al. Identification and characterization of brush-border membrane-bound neutral metalloendopeptidases from rat small intestine. Gastroenterology 1986;91:1234.

27. Ferraci H, Maroux S. Rabbit intestinal aminopeptidase N. Purification and molecular properties. Biochim Biophys Acta 1980;599:448.

28. Tobey N, Heizer W, Yeh R, Huang TI, Hoffner C. Human intestinal brush border peptidases. Gastroenterology 1985;88:913.

29. Kim YS, Brophy EJ, Nicholson JA. Rat intestinal brush border membrane peptidases. J Biol Chem 1976;251:3206.

30. Gray GM, Santiago NA. Intestinal surface amino-oligopeptidases. I. Isolation of two weight isomers and their subunits from rat brush border. J Biol Chem 1977;252:4922.

31. Kania RK, Santiago NA, Gray GM. Intestinal surface amino-oligopeptidases. II. Substrate kinetics and topography of the active site. J Biol Chem 1977;252:4929.

32. Bella AM Jr, Erickson RH, Kim YS. Rat intestinal brush border membrane dipeptidyl-aminopeptidase. IV. Kinetic properties and substrate specificities of the purified enzyme. Arch Biochem Biophys 1982;218:156.

33. Kim YS, Brophy SJ. Rat intestinal brush border membrane peptidases. I. Solubilization, purification, and physicochemical properties of two different forms of the enzyme. J Biol Chem 1976;251:3199.

34. Erickson RH, Bella AM Jr, Brophy EJ, et al. Purification and molecular characterization of rat intestinal brush border membrane dipeptidyl aminopeptidase IV. Biochem Biophys Acta 1983;756:258.

35. Auricchio S, Greco L, de Vizia B, Buonocore V. Dipeptidylaminopeptidase and carboxypeptidase activities of the brush border of rabbit small intestine. Gastroenterology 1978;75:1073.

36. Kenny AJ, Booth AC, George SG, et al. Dipeptidyl peptidase IV, a kidney brush border serine peptidase. Biochem J 1976;157:169.

37. Reisenauer AM, Krumdieck CL, Halsted CH. Folate conjugase: Two separate activities in human intestine. Science 1977;198:196.

38. Tobey N, Heizer W, Yeh R, et al. Human intestinal brush border peptidases. Gastroenterology 1985;88:913.

39. Adibi SA, Kim YS. Peptide absorption and hydrolysis. In: Johnson LR, ed. Physiology of the gastrointestinal tract. New York: Raven Press, 1981:1073.

40. Silk DBA. Peptide transport. Clin Sci 1981;60:607.

41. Matthews DM. Intestinal absorption of peptides. Physiol Rev 1975;55:537.

42. Wellner D, Meister A. A survey of inborn errors of amino acid metabolism and transport in man. Annu Rev Biochem 1980;50:911.

43. Asatoor AM, Cheng B, Edwards KDG, Lant AF, et al. Intestinal absorption of two dipeptides in Hartnup disease. Gut 1970;11:380.

44. Rajendran VM, Ansari SA, Harig JA, et al. Transport of glycyl-L-proline by human intestinal brush border membrane vesicles. Gastroenterology 1985;89:1298.

45. Silk DBA, Hegarty JE, Fairclough PD, Clark ML. Characterization and nutritional significance of peptide transport in man. Ann Nutr Metab 1982;26:337.

46. Rosen-Levin EM, Smithson KW, Gray GM. Complementary role of surface hydrolysis and intact transport in the intestinal assimilation of di- and tripeptides. Biochim Biophys Acta 1980;629:126.

47. Matthews DM, Gundy RW, Taylor E, Burston D. Influx of two dipeptides glycylsarcosine and L-glutamyl-L-glutamic acid into hamster jejunum in vitro. Clin Sci Mol Med 1979;56:15.

48. Ganapathy V, Leibach FH. Is intestinal peptide transport energized by a proton gradient? Am J Physiol 1985;249:G153.

49. Kim YS, Kim YW, Sleisenger MH. Studies on the properties of peptide hydrolases in the brush-border and soluble fractions of small intestinal mucosa of rat and man. Biochim Biophys Acta 1974;370:283.

50. Heizer WD, Kerley RL, Isselbacher KJ. Intestinal peptide hydrolases: Differences between brush border and cytoplasmic enzymes. Biochim Biophys Acta 1972;264:450.

51. Doumeng G, Maroux S. Amino tripeptidase, a cytosol enzyme from rabbit intestinal mucosa. Biochem J 1979;177:801.

52. Noren O, Sjostrom H, Josephsson L. Studies on soluble dipeptidase from pig intestinal mucosa. I. Purification and specificity. Biochim Biophys Acta 1973;327:446.

53. Sjostrom H, Noren O. Structural properties of pig intestinal proline dipeptidase. Biochim Biophys Acta 1974;351:177.

54. Gardner MG. Absorption of intact peptides—Studies on transport of protein digests and dipeptides across rat small intestine in vitro. Q J Exp Physiol 1982;67:629.

55. Hopfer U. Membrane transport mechanisms for hexoses and amino acids in the small intestine. In: Johnson LR, ed. Physiology of the gastrointestinal tract, ed 2. New York: Raven Press, 1987:1499.

56. Stevens BR, Kaunitz JD, Wright EM. Intestinal transport of amino acid and sugars: Advances using membrane vesicles. Annu Rev Physiol 1984;46:417.

57. Berteloot A. Characteristics of glutamic acid transport by rabbit

intestinal brush border membrane vesicles. Effects of Na^+, K^+, and H^+-gradients. Biochim Biophys Acta 1984;775:129.

58. Corcelli A, Storelli C. The role of potassium and chloride ions on the Na^+/acidic amino acid co-transport system in rat intestinal brush border membrane vesicles. Biochim Biophys Acta 1983;732:24.

59. Cassano G, Leszcynska B, Murer H. Transport of L-lysine by rat intestinal brush border membrane vesicles. Pflugers Arch 1983;397:114.

60. Wolfram S, Giering H, Scharrer E. Na^+-gradient dependence of basic amino acid transport into rat intestinal brush border membrane vesicles. Comp Biochem Physiol [A]1984;78A:475.

61. Hopfer U, Sigrist-Nelson K, Ammann E, Murer H. Differences in neutral amino acid and glucose transport between brush border and basolateral plasma membrane of intestinal epithelial cells. J Cell Physiol 1976;89:805.

62. Windmueller HG, Spaeth AE. Identification of ketone bodies and glutamine as the major respiratory fuels in vivo for post absorptive rat small intestine. J Biol Chem 1978;253:69.

63. Windmueller HG, Spaeth AE. Respiratory fuels and nitrogen metabolism in vivo in small intestine of fed rats. J Biol Chem 1980;255:107.

64. Bradford NM, McGivan JD. The transport of alanine and glutamine into isolated rat intestinal epithelial cells. Biochim Biophys Acta 1982;689:55.

65. Weber FL, Veach GL. The importance of small intestine in gut

ammonium production in the fasting dog. Gastroenterology 1979;77:235.

66. Allison JB, Bird JWC. Elimination of nitrogen from the body. In: Munro HN, Allison JB, eds. Mammalian protein metabolism. New York: Academic Press, 1964:483.

67. Chung YC, Kim YS, Shadchehr A, et al. Protein digestion and absorption in human small intestine. Gastroenterology 1979;76:1415.

68. Triadou N, Bataille J, Schmitz J. Longitudinal study of the human intestinal brush border membrane proteins. Gastroenterology 1983;85:1326.

69. Seetharam B, Alpers DH. Cellular uptake of cobalamin. Nutr Rev 1985;43:97.

70. Ahnen DJ, Brown WR, Kloppel TM. Secretory component: The polymeric immunoglobulin receptor. What's in it for the hepatologist and gastroenterologist. Gastroenterology 1985;89:667.

71. Alpers DH, Tedesco FJ. The possible role of pancreatic proteases in the turnover of intestinal brush border proteins. Biochim Biophys Acta 1975;401:28.

72. Rodger SM, Schnagl R, Holmes IH. Further biochemical characterization including the detection of surface glycoproteins of human, calf, and simian rotaviruses. J Gen Virol 1977;35:403.

73. Randolph LM, Rotter JI. Hereditary disorders of the gut and liver. In: Kelley WN, ed. Textbook of internal medicine. Philadelphia: JB Lippincott, 1988:630.

20

Vitamins and Minerals

CHARLES M. SCHRON

The intraluminal events and cellular mechanisms required for the intestinal absorption of minerals and vitamins are the primary focus of this chapter. Important clinical consequences (e.g., anemia, bone disease) often result from the malabsorption of certain minerals (e.g., iron, calcium) and vitamins (e.g., folate, cobalamin). In view of the physiologic importance of these minerals and vitamins, special attention will be given to their absorption. With the exception of pernicious anemia or specific drug effects, mineral or vitamin malabsorption does not usually occur as an isolated abnormality. Instead, mineral or vitamin malabsorption often accompanies disease processes that affect specific portions of the small intestine. Therefore, whenever possible the site of absorption along the length of intestine will be emphasized to assist the clinician in understanding the pathophysiology of commonly encountered disease processes.

ABSORPTION OF WATER-SOLUBLE VITAMINS

Folic Acid (Pteroylglutamic Acid, PteGlu)

SOURCES

For adults, a folate intake of 3 μg/kg/d (or 200 μg/d), which is largely obtained from the consumption of vegetables and fruits, is sufficient to avoid the consequences of folate deficiency.[1] The folates normally present in the diet are mostly (75%) polyglutamates, that is, pteroylpolyglutamate or $PteGlu_n$.[2] In vivo perfusion studies suggest that the absorption of PteGlu$_n$ is comparable to that of monoglutamate folate, that is, PteGlu.[3] However, when different food sources are compared, the bioavailability of folate varies widely,[4] suggesting that other factors influence absorption. For example, a folate-binding protein endogenous to human or cow's milk apparently increases the bioavailability of milk folate by retarding the rate of absorption, thus avoiding high blood levels that would otherwise enhance renal excretion.[5,6]

INTESTINAL ABSORPTION (FIG 20-1)

Hydrolysis of Polyglutamate Folates. Although dietary folates are largely PteGlu$_n$, only PteGlu appears in the portal blood following a meal.[7] The accumulation of PteGlu$_n$ deconjugation products in the intestinal lumen suggests hydrolysis of PteGlu$_n$ to PteGlu prior to intestinal absorption.[8] In humans, the enzyme that catalyzes this reaction, pteroylpolyglutamate hydrolase (or folate conjugase), is an integral membrane protein[9] present on jejunal, but not ileal, brush borders.[10] This enzyme, which is maximally active at pH 5.5, is a zinc-activated exopeptidase that cleaves successive glutamate residues from the carboxy terminus of PteGlu$_n$, yielding PteGlu.[9] A comparison of the maximal velocities (V_{max}) for hydrolysis of PteGlu$_n$ and transport of PteGlu (V_{max} = 320 and 1.4 pmol per milligram of protein per minute, respectively) suggests that transport is the rate-limiting step for absorption.[11]

Intestinal Absorption of Folic Acid. The monoglutamyl form of dietary folate is absorbed in the jejunum by a saturable (i.e., carrier-mediated) process that is maximal at a luminal pH between 5.5 and 6.0.[12] When the luminal pH exceeds 6.5, concentrative folate uptake is not observed.[12] Recordings of the pH at the luminal surface documented a brush-border acid microclimate (luminal pH 5.8) in proximal jejunum.[13] Since this pH is significantly below the pH of the enterocyte interior (pH 6.8),[14] an outwardly directed OH$^-$ gradient (or inwardly directed H$^+$ gradient) is present under physiologic conditions.

Studies in rabbit jejunal brush-border membrane vesicles demonstrated that an outwardly directed OH$^-$ gradient (pH$_{inside}$ 7.7, pH$_{outside}$ 5.5) markedly stimulates PteGlu uptake compared with uptake in the absence of a pH gradient (pH$_{inside}$ 5.5, pH$_{outside}$ 5.5) and that this gradient is required for the transient accumulation of PteGlu at concentrations greater than at equilibrium ("uphill" transport).[15] Under these pH conditions, PteGlu is predominantly in the anionic form and uptake is saturable. In contrast, PteGlu uptake by ileal brush-border membrane vesicles is similar in the presence or absence of a pH gradient. These data, which were confirmed in human intestinal brush-border membrane vesicles,[16] are consistent with the primacy of the jejunum in folate absorption and provide evidence for carrier-mediated PteGlu:OH$^-$ exchange (or phenomenologically indistinguishable H$^+$:PteGlu co-transport).[15] The same carrier also transports reduced and methylated forms of PteGlu.[17,18] Since an inwardly directed Na$^+$ gradient does not stimulate PteGlu uptake by jejunal brush-border membrane vesicles,[15] the Na$^+$ dependence of PteGlu transport observed by some investigators[19] may be secondary to dual exchange, that is, the parallel operation of brush-border Na$^+$:H$^+$ and PteGlu:OH$^-$ exchangers.

Intracellular Processing, Transport Across Basolateral Membrane, and Delivery to Peripheral Tissues. At low, but not high, luminal PteGlu concentrations, most of the absorbed PteGlu is reduced and methylated to 5-methyltetrahydrofolate.[20] A carrier on the basolateral membrane transports 5-methyltetrahydrofolate and PteGlu to the serosal surface,[21] where the vitamin enters the portal circulation. Between 60% and 70% of serum folate is bound to either low-affinity, high-capacity (albumin) or high-affinity, low-capacity binding proteins.[22]

The reduced and methylated folates are largely (80%) taken up by peripheral tissues.[23] In contrast, PteGlu is preferentially bound by a high-affinity folic acid–binding protein[24] for delivery to the liver.[25] PteGlu is reduced and methylated in the liver and distributed to peripheral tissues by secretion into bile and reabsorption by the intestine (i.e., folate enterohepatic cycle) (Fig 20-2).[23] Folate stores from senescent erythrocytes are also returned to the liver for redistribution to peripheral tissues via the enterohepatic cycle. This "salvage pathway" is capable of meeting 10% to 20% of the minimal folate requirements during periods of folate deprivation.[23]

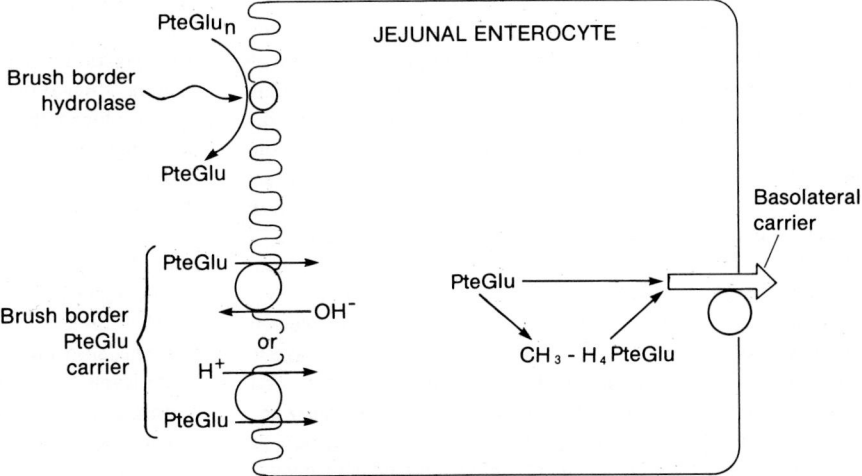

FIGURE 20–1. Digestion and absorption of dietary folate by the jejunal enterocyte. Dietary folate (pteroylpolyglutamate or PteGlu$_n$) is hydrolyzed to the monoglutamate form (PteGlu) by a brush-border hydrolase and absorbed by carrier-mediated PteGlu:OH$^-$ exchange or H$^+$: PteGlu cotransport. At physiologic concentrations, most of the absorbed PteGlu is reduced and methylated to 5-methyltetrahydrofolate (CH$_3$–H$_4$PteGlu). Transport of PteGlu and CH$_3$–H$_4$PteGlu across the basolateral membrane is also carrier mediated. See text for details.

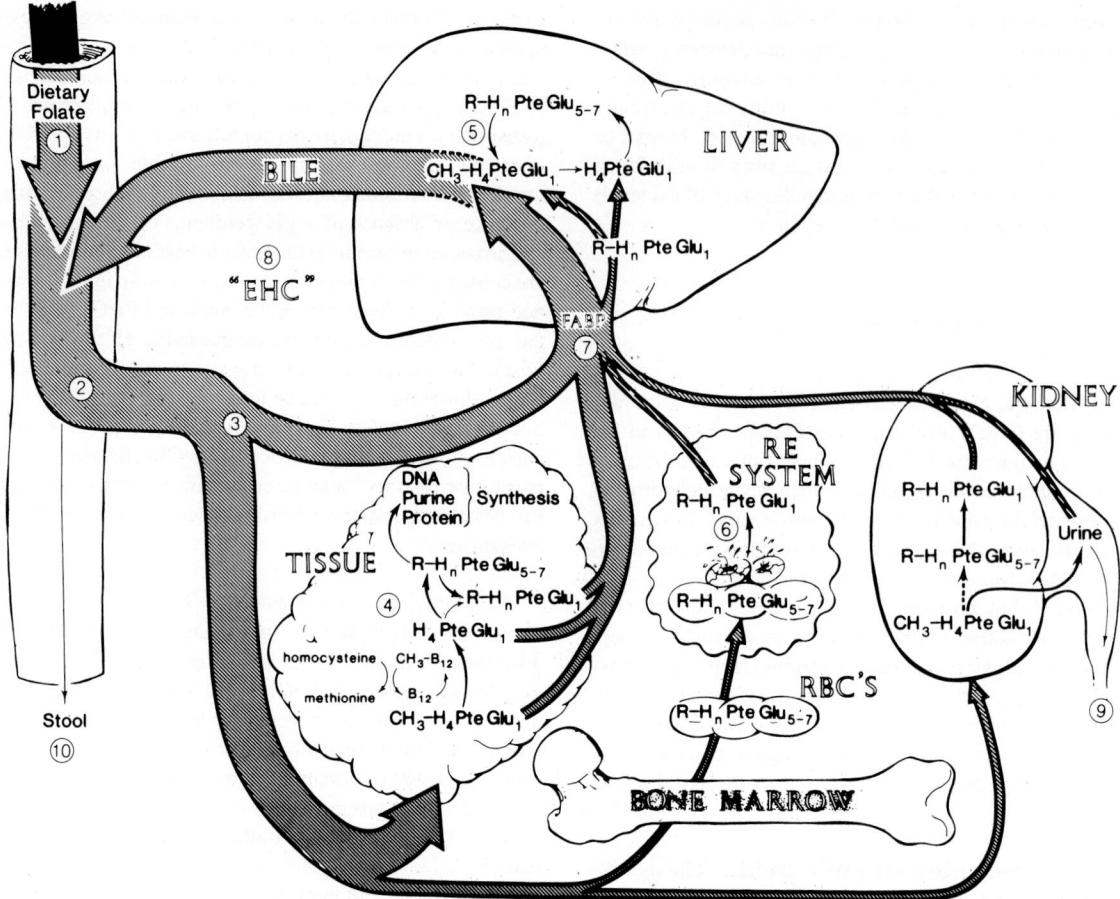

FIGURE 20–2. Enterohepatic circulation of folate. Dietary folate (step 1) is taken up by the jejunal enterocyte (step 2) and delivered into the portal circulation (step 3). Reduced and methylated folates ($CH_3H_4PteGlu$) are delivered to peripheral tissues for intracellular demethylation and conversion to polyglutamates (step 4). Polyglutamates are important for cellular retention of folates (storage function) and compared with monoglutamates are more effective cofactors for folate-dependent enzymes (biochemical function). Hepatic monoglutamates are derived from two sources: (1) hydro-lysis of polyglutamates within the liver (step 5) and (2) reticuloendothelial hydrolysis of polyglutamates from senescent red blood cells (step 6) with return to the liver of monoglutamates bound to plasma folic acid binding protein (abbreviated FABP; step 7). Secretion into bile of $CH_3H_4PteGlu$ permits redistribution of folate to peripheral tissues (i.e., enterohepatic cycle, step 8). (From Steinberg SE. Mechanisms of folate homeostasis. Am J Physiol 1984;246: G319.)

DISORDERS OF FOLATE HOMEOSTASIS

A number of drugs, such as amethopterin (methotrexate), pyrimethamine (antimalarial), trimethoprim (antibiotic), and triamterine (K^+-sparing diuretic), interfere with folate use by inhibiting dihydrofolate reductase, the intracellular enzyme that reduces dihydrofolate to biologically active tetrahydrofolate.[26] In addition, these drugs[27–29] compete with PteGlu for transport by the jejunal brush-border folate carrier. Other drugs also compete with dietary folate for the specialized processes required for the absorption of this vitamin. For example, sulfasalazine (Azulfidine) lowers serum folate levels by competitively inhibiting brush-border pteroyl-polyglutamate hydrolase[30,31] and PteGlu transport.[32] In women taking oral contraceptives, the malabsorption of PteGlu$_n$ suggests inhibition of pteroylpolyglutamate hydrolase.[33] However, oral contraceptives rarely result in folate deficiency, presumably because of normal PteGlu absorption.[33] Similarly, absorption of PteGlu$_n$, but not PteGlu, is impaired in human zinc deficiency.[34]

Certain anticonvulsants, such as phenytoin (Dilantin), primi-done, and carbamazepine, lower serum folate levels (30% to 90% of patients) and on rare occasions (<1%) are associated with megaloblastic anemia.[35] Phenytoin has been reported to inhibit PteGlu$_n$ deconjugation,[36] but this has not been confirmed by other investigators.[37] Regardless of possible effects on deconjugation, phenytoin inhibits the absorption of PteGlu,[38] the end product of deconjugation. Since phenytoin is a relatively strong base, a phenytoin-induced alkalinization of the luminal fluid might reduce the transmembrane pH gradient that is the driving force for brush-border PteGlu:OH$^-$ exchange (or H$^+$:PteGlu cotransport). Similarly, diseases that secondarily alkalinize the brush-border acid microclimate are associated with impaired folate absorption, such as celiac disease[39] and atrophic gastritis.[40] In atrophic gastritis, folate malabsorption is not of sufficient magnitude to lower serum folate levels.[40] In contrast, the reduced bicarbonate output that characterizes pancreatic insufficiency acidifies luminal contents and enhances folate absorption.[41]

Since the proximal small intestine is the site where pteroyl-polyglutamate hydrolase and the brush-border PteGlu carrier are localized, diseases affecting this portion of small intestine are commonly associated with folate deficiency. For example, the diffuse mucosal injury of celiac disease markedly depresses pteroyl-polyglutamate hydrolase activity[42] and impairs folate absorption. On the other hand, conditions that require jejunal resection rarely lead to folate deficiency, perhaps secondary to compensatory changes in the remnant ileum ("intestinal adaptation"). In rats, ileal adaptation includes expression of the jejunal brush-border folate carrier.[43]

Folate deficiency is common in malnourished alcoholics. While direct effects of luminal alcohol on the acid microclimate or membrane structure can impair folate absorption, the adequacy of nutrient intake immediately prior to admission correlates better with tests of intestinal PteGlu absorption.[44] After normalization of PteGlu absorption on a hospital diet, the reinstitution of alcohol did not affect PteGlu absorption in 5 of 7 patients tested,[44] suggesting that in most patients alcohol alone is not sufficient to cause folate malabsorption.

Cobalamin (Vitamin B$_{12}$)[45,46]

NOMENCLATURE AND STRUCTURE

The cobalamin molecule consists of a cobalt atom in the center of a planar corrin ring with a dimethyl benzimidazole and ribose phosphate below the ring (Co-α group) and a variable ligand above the ring (Co-β group). The first cobalamin to be purified was cyanocobalamin, which was named vitamin B$_{12}$. In mammalian tissues, the predominant cobalamin species are hydroxycobalamin, methylcobalamin, and adenosylcobalamin.[47] Therefore, the preferred terminology for this vitamin is the generic term *cobalamin.*

DIETARY SOURCES

Bacteria and protozoa, but not mammalian tissues, synthesize cobalamin and a variety of inactive cobalamin analogues. Although microorganisms are the ultimate source of cobalamins, human dietary cobalamin requirements are met almost exclusively by the consumption of animal products, namely meat and eggs. Daily intake of 0.5 to 1.0 μg of cobalamin per day is sufficient to avoid the consequences of cobalamin deficiency.[48] Since cobalamin stores approximate 2 to 3 mg, vegetarians require years before body stores are depleted and manifestations of cobalamin deficiency develop.

COBALAMIN ABSORPTION (FIG 20-3)

Gastric Phase. The absorption of cobalamin begins in the stomach where acid, and perhaps pepsin, liberates dietary methylcobalamin and adenosylcobalamin from ingested food sources.[49] The parietal cells of the stomach are also required for the synthesis and secretion of intrinsic factor, a cobalamin-binding protein. However, in the acidic environment of the stomach, cobalamin preferentially binds to endogenous R proteins of salivary origin.[50,51] The R proteins are a family of antigenically related glycoproteins that are present in a variety of body fluids. Unlike intrinsic factor, the R proteins have high affinity for biologically active and *inactive* cobalamin analogues.

The quantity of intrinsic factor secreted into the gastric lumen greatly exceeds that required for the subsequent absorption of dietary cobalamin.[52] Intrinsic factor secretion is under the same hormonal control mechanisms that regulate acid secretion. Cyclic adenosine monophosphate agonists that stimulate acid secretion (e.g., histamine) also stimulate intrinsic factor secretion.[45] Conversely, the H$_2$ receptor antagonist cimetidine inhibits intrinsic factor secretion.[53] Although dog pancreas synthesizes and secretes intrinsic factor,[54] the relevance of these findings to humans has not been determined.

Proximal Small Intestinal Phase. In the duodenum and jejunum, the salivary R proteins are partially degraded by pancreatic proteases and the bound cobalamin is released as free cobalamin into the lumen.[50,51] Under the pH conditions that prevail in the small intestine, intrinsic factor has high affinity for biologically active cobalamin.[55,56] In contrast, cobalamin analogues of bacterial origin that have even minor changes in the corrin ring or Co-α ligand do not bind to intrinsic factor. Since binding to intrinsic factor is a required step prior to ileal absorption, absorption of biologically inactive and potentially harmful cobalamin analogues is largely avoided.[55] With the binding of cobalamin, intrinsic factor undergoes a conformational change[57] that renders the protein resistant to proteolysis.[58]

Ileal Phase. High-affinity receptors for the intrinsic factor–cobalamin complex[56] are located in pits between adjacent brush-border microvilli of ileal enterocytes.[59] The limited capacity of the gut to absorb cobalamin (only 1 to 2 μg of a given dose) is a direct consequence of the relative paucity of these receptors (approximately 300 per enterocyte[60]). In humans, these receptors are present along the entire length of ileum,[61] which comprises the distal half of the small intestine.

The binding of the intrinsic factor–cobalamin complex to the ileal receptor does not require the cobalamin moiety.[56] These data, and studies with antibodies that block either binding of cobalamin to intrinsic factor or binding of the complex to the ileal receptor,[62] suggest that intrinsic factor has functionally separate binding domains for cobalamin and the ileal receptor. The cloning of the rat gene encoding gastric intrinsic factor[63] will enable the structure-function studies necessary to confirm this model.

Attachment of the macromolecular complex to the ileal receptor proceeds by a rapid, temperature-insensitive mechanism that requires divalent cations (Ca^{2+}, Mg^{2+}) but not metabolic energy.[64,65] Since the receptor does not bind free cobalamin or R protein–bound cobalamin, binding is highly specific.[56,65] Internalization of the entire complex has been suggested[66] but not confirmed morphologically.[67] After a delay that lasts for hours, newly absorbed cobalamin appears in the portal circulation bound to another cobalamin–binding protein, transcobalamin II.[68] Transcobalamin II delivers cobalamin to body tissues for cellular uptake by receptor-mediated endocytosis.[69]

In the plasma, excess cobalamin and inactive cobalamin analogues are bound by the plasma R protein transcobalamin III for hepatic uptake and secretion into bile.[70] The hepatic secretion of cobalamin approximates 4 μg/d[71] and provides an effective mechanism for disposing of inactive cobalamin analogues. Thus, as

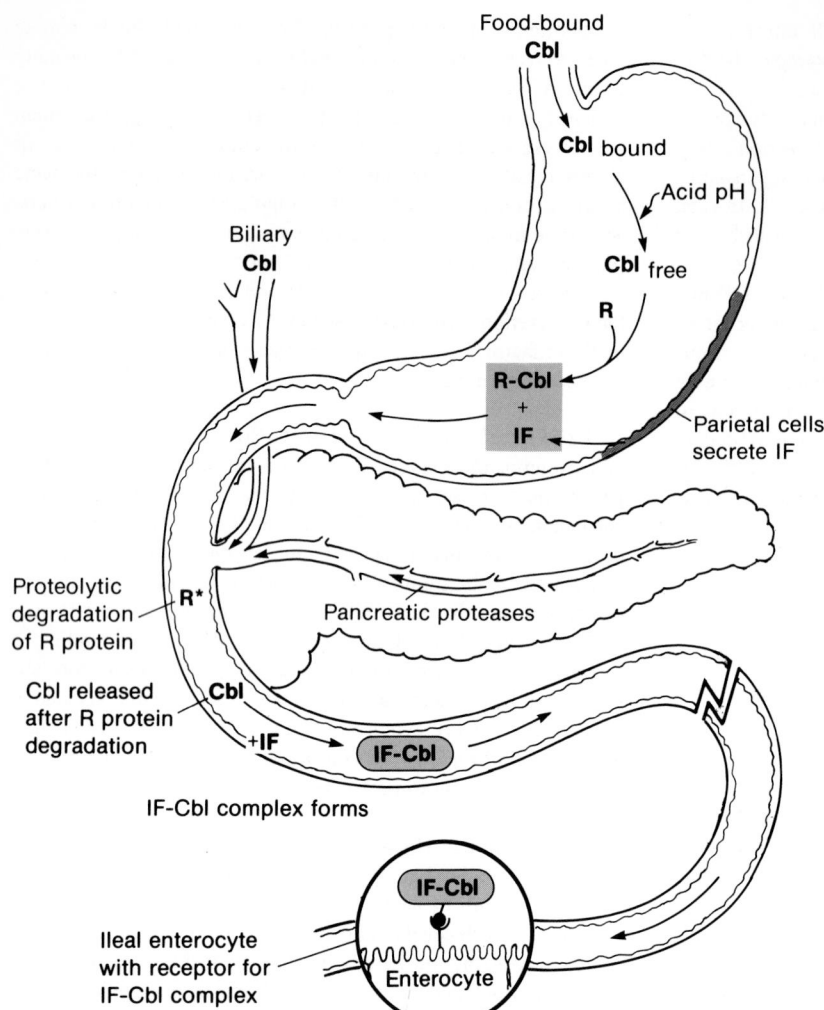

FIGURE 20–3. Sequential steps in the absorption of cobalamin. See text for details.

with folate, enterohepatic cycling plays an important role in cobalamin homeostasis.

TESTS OF COBALAMIN LEVELS AND ABSORPTION

In the late 1970s, the radioassays that were available for measuring serum cobalamin sometimes gave spuriously normal results, even in patients with untreated pernicious anemia. While the currently available test kits have eliminated this problem, other conditions can still affect the serum cobalamin level.[72,73] For example, in folate deficiency, serum cobalamin levels are moderately depressed but quickly return to values that reflect the true cobalamin status of the patient after folate supplementation.[74] Whether the administration of folate supplements to cobalamin-deficient patients can similarly raise cobalamin levels, thereby obscuring the correct diagnosis, has not been evaluated. However, it is known that folate supplements can mask the hematologic changes typically observed in cobalamin deficiency.[75,76] Although serum cobalamin levels normally decline in the geriatric population, serum cobalamin values usually remain within the normal range. As a consequence, a borderline low serum cobalamin value should not be attributed to

a patient's advanced age without further investigation. This is particularly important since a low serum cobalamin value can precede the onset of anemia and macrocytosis[77] and is sometimes the only laboratory abnormality in patients with neuropsychiatric sequelae of cobalamin deficiency.[78]

The most widely used test of cobalamin absorption is the Schilling test. In stage I of the Schilling test, the patient ingests radiolabeled crystalline cobalamin. Two hours later, a 1000-μg flushing dose of unlabeled cobalamin is administered parenterally, displacing the previously absorbed, radiolabeled cobalamin from tissue stores and plasma into urine. The results of a 24-hour urine collection are then expressed as a percentage of the dose ingested (usually 10%–20%). If absorption of cobalamin is abnormal, the test is repeated with intrinsic factor (stage II Schilling test). If the test result is still abnormal, the stage II Schilling test may be repeated after a trial of antibiotics to treat possible bacterial overgrowth. An inadequate urine collection (14% of patients), or the presence of renal disease, invalidates the urinary measurement as a method of assessing the adequacy of intestinal cobalamin absorption.

Since cobalamin is required for the enzymatic conversion of methylmalonic acid to succinic acid, urinary methylmalonic acid levels are elevated in patients with cobalamin deficiency. Initial reports indicate that measurement of urinary methylmalonic acid levels by gas chromatography-mass spectrometry is highly sensitive and specific for cobalamin deficiency.[79,80] Further clinical trials are in progress.

DISORDERS OF COBALAMIN ABSORPTION

The differential diagnosis of cobalamin malabsorption (Table 20-1) requires an appreciation for the many organ systems, and multiple steps, involved in cobalamin absorption. The different patterns of test results (serum cobalamin, Schilling test) associated with these diverse disorders are summarized in Table 20-2.

Gastric. In the complete absence of intrinsic factor secretion, as in pernicious anemia or following total gastrectomy, dietary and biliary cobalamin ($\approx$1 and 4 μg/d, respectively) are malabsorbed, hastening the onset of vitamin deficiency. Unlike vegetarians, these patients typically manifest the clinical signs of deficiency within 3 to 6 years.[45] In such patients, tests of cobalamin absorption are corrected by simultaneous administration of intrinsic factor (i.e., normal stage II Schilling test).

Pernicious anemia typically affects elderly (>60 years old) whites of European descent, but it is not restricted to this racial

TABLE 20–1
Differential Diagnosis of Cobalamin Malabsorption

I. Disorders of Gastric Phase
  A. Absence of biologically active intrinsic factor
    1. Pernicious anemia (adult or juvenile form)
    2. Total gastrectomy
    3. Secretion of abnormal intrinsic factor
      a. Fails to bind to ileal receptor
      b. Susceptible to proteolytic degradation
    4. Congenital absence of intrinsic factor
  B. Inadequate release of food-bound cobalamin
    1. Surgical operations reducing gastric acid
    2. Atrophic gastritis
    3. H_2 blockers
II. Disorders of Proximal Small Intestinal Phase
  A. Impaired proteolytic degradation of R proteins
    1. Pancreatic exocrine insufficiency
    2. Zollinger-Ellison syndrome
  B. Competition for uptake of luminal cobalamin
    1. Stasis with bacterial overgrowth
    2. Fish tapeworm *Diphyllobothrium latum*
III. Disorders of Ileal Phase
  A. Diminished or absent ileal receptors
    1. Surgical resection or bypass
    2. Abnormal mucosa
      a. Crohn's disease
      b. tropical sprue
      c. celiac sprue
      d. severe cobalamin deficiency
      e. HIV infection
  B. Abnormal translocation of cobalamin across ileal enterocyte
    1. Inherited defect in transileal transport (Immerslund-Gräsbeck syndrome)
    2. Drugs (*p*-aminosalicylic acid, biguanides)
    3. Transcobalamin II deficiency, congenitally absent or defective

Modified with permission from Kapadia CR, Donaldson RM Jr. Disorders of cobalamin (vitamin B$_{12}$) absorption and transport. Ann Rev Med 1985; 36:93.

group.[81] The disease is characterized by atrophy of the oxyntic mucosa, achlorhydria, and absence of intrinsic factor secretion. Serum antibodies[62] directed against intrinsic factor are common ($\approx$70%) and include (1) an IgG antibody that prevents binding of cobalamin ("blocking" or "type I") and (2) an IgG, or less commonly IgM, antibody that interferes with binding of the intrinsic factor–cobalamin complex to the ileal receptor ("binding" or "type II"). These antibodies are relatively specific for pernicious anemia.[45] If sufficient quantities of these antibodies are present in the intestinal lumen, cobalamin absorption tests do not normalize even with exogenous intrinsic factor.[82] Rarely, intrinsic factor may be functionally absent, owing to the secretion of an abnormal molecule that either fails to bind to the ileal receptor or is highly susceptible to degradation by acid-pepsin.[83]

Patients with atrophic gastritis, or those who have undergone acid-reducing operations for peptic ulcer disease, may present with low serum cobalamin levels but normal tests for absorption of crystalline cobalamin (i.e., a normal stage I Schilling test).[84,85] The likely mechanism for cobalamin deficiency in such patients is impaired release of food-bound cobalamin secondary to diminished acid-pepsin secretion. Similarly, 11 of 12 patients receiving H_2 blockers[86] had diminished absorption of food-bound cobalamin.[87] Malabsorption of food cobalamin can even occur when gastric function is apparently normal.[88]

Proximal Small Intestine. Proteolytic degradation of R proteins is required to release cobalamin into the lumen for binding to intrinsic factor.[50,51] In pancreatic insufficiency, diminished secretion of proteolytic enzymes impairs R protein degradation.[51] As a consequence, the Schilling test, which is performed in the fasting state, is abnormal in 50% of patients with pancreatic insufficiency.[89] However, food is a stimulus for pancreatic secretion, even in patients with pancreatic insufficiency. If radiolabeled crystalline cobalamin is administered with a meal, a test condition that more closely approximates absorption of dietary cobalamin, cobalamin absorption is often normal.[90] Thus, patients with pancreatic insufficiency rarely develop cobalamin deficiency despite abnormal Schilling tests. Impaired R protein degradation is also the likely mechanism for cobalamin malabsorption in patients with the Zollinger-Ellison syndrome. In this syndrome, gastric acid hypersecretion lowers intraduodenal pH, inactivating pancreatic proteolytic enzymes. With correction of intraduodenal acidification, cobalamin absorption returns to normal.[91]

Certain bacterial species, such as *Escherichia coli* and *Bacteroides fragilis*, and the fish tapeworm *Diphyllobothrium latum*, take up cobalamin even when the vitamin is bound to intrinsic factor.[92] Intestinal conditions that predispose to stasis (e.g., jejunal diverticula, strictures, or scleroderma) are associated with bacterial overgrowth. When cobalamin deficiency complicates these conditions, test results of cobalamin absorption return to normal levels following antibiotic therapy.

Ileal. Since the capacity of the intestine to absorb cobalamin is limited, and directly related to the number of ileal receptors, ileal disease and/or surgical resection is commonly associated with cobalamin malabsorption. In patients with clinically quiescent Crohn's disease, a history of an ileal resection exceeding 50 cm is invariably associated with an abnormal Schilling test.[93] Similarly, malabsorption of cobalamin occurs in 60% of patients with tropical sprue, a condition that commonly involves the ileum.[45] Although

TABLE 20–2
Patterns of Test Results in Disorders of Cobalamin Absorption

SERUM COBALAMIN	SCHILLING TEST Stage I	SCHILLING TEST Stage II	MECHANISM	DIFFERENTIAL DIAGNOSIS
Low	Abnormal	Normal	Decreased intrinsic factor secretion	Pernicious anemia
				Total gastrectomy
				Congenital absence of intrinsic factor
			Abnormal intrinsic factor	Decreased ileal binding
				Susceptible to proteolysis
Low	Normal		Inadequate intake	Vegetarian diet
			Impaired release of food-bound cobalamin	Atrophic gastritis
				Acid-reducing operations
				H_2 blockers
				Normal gastric function
Normal (rarely low)	Abnormal	Abnormal	Impaired R protein degradation	Pancreatic insufficiency
				Zollinger–Ellison syndrome
Low	Abnormal	Abnormal	Decreased ileal receptors	Ileal disease or resection
			Antibody to intrinsic factor secreted into lumen	Pernicious anemia
			Reversible ileal abnormality secondary to cobalamin deficiency	Pernicious anemia (25% of untreated patients)
			Competition for cobalamin uptake	Bacterial overgrowth

celiac sprue is usually limited to the proximal small intestine, severe cases involve the ileum and are associated with cobalamin malabsorption.[45] Infection with the human immunodeficiency virus (HIV) is associated with low serum cobalamin levels in 15% of patients with AIDS and 7% of those merely infected with the virus.[93a] In these patients, the Schilling test is invariably abnormal, despite the coadministration of intrinsic factor and pancreatic enzymes.[93a] These results suggest an ileal defect in the absorption of cobalamin, the likely cause of which is an HIV-associated enteropathy.

The small intestinal mucosa is an actively proliferating epithelium. Since cell replication requires cobalamin, severe vitamin deficiency often results in a reversible abnormality of the ileal mucosa that secondarily impairs cobalamin absorption.[94] In untreated pernicious anemia, 25% of patients will have an abnormal Schilling test that fails to correct with intrinsic factor.[73] After cobalamin treatment, the ileal abnormality resolves and cobalamin absorption normalizes with intrinsic factor (i.e., normal stage II Schilling test).[94]

OTHER WATER-SOLUBLE VITAMINS

The translocation of other water-soluble vitamins across the apical membrane of the enterocyte involves separate Na^+-dependent (ascorbic acid, biotin, riboflavin, pantothenic acid) and Na^+-independent (thiamine, dehydroascorbic acid) carrier-mediated mechanisms. Niacin and the B_6 vitamins (pyridoxine, pyridoxal, pyridoxamine) are absorbed by passive diffusion. The essential features that characterize the absorption of these vitamins are summarized in Table 20-3[95–106] and Figure 20-4. The clinical syndromes classically associated with deficiencies of ascorbic acid, niacin, and thiamine are scurvy, pellagra, and beriberi, respectively. Deficiencies of biotin, riboflavin, and the B_6 vitamins give rise to a variety of dermatologic (dermatitis, stomatitis, glossitis) and neurologic manifestations.

ABSORPTION OF FAT-SOLUBLE VITAMINS

The absorption of fat-soluble vitamins requires micellar solubilization by bile salt micelles. Diseases that reduce the surface area available for intestinal absorption, or lower intraluminal bile salt concentrations thus impairing micellar solubilization, are often associated with malabsorption of fat-soluble vitamins. The inclusion within the bile salt micelle of products of fat digestion, that is, monoglycerides and fatty acids ("swelling amphiphiles"), permits greater solubilization of nonpolar lipids (fat-soluble vitamins).[107] However, this is not an absolute requirement for the absorption of fat-soluble vitamins. Thus, pancreatic insufficiency is not as commonly associated with clinically significant malabsorption of fat-soluble vitamins as are other causes of steatorrhea.

Vitamin D[108,109]

SOURCES AND INTESTINAL ABSORPTION

In the skin, previtamin D_3 is formed from the precursor molecule 7-dehydrocholesterol by a reaction that requires ultraviolet light.

TABLE 20–3
Intestinal Transport of Water-Soluble Vitamins

WATER-SOLUBLE VITAMIN	DIETARY FORM	SITE OF METABOLISM (IF ANY)	ABSORBED MOIETY	MECHANISM OF BRUSH-BORDER TRANSPORT	SODIUM-DEPENDENT	REFERENCES
Vitamin C	Ascorbic acid	—	Same	Carrier	Yes	95, 96, 97
	Dehydroascorbic acid	—	Same	Carrier	No	98
Biotin	Biotin	—	Same	Carrier	Yes	99, 100
Vitamin B_2 (riboflavin)	Flavin mononucleotide (FMN)	Brush border	Riboflavin	Carrier	Yes	96
Pantothenic acid	Coenzyme A	Lumen	Pantothenic acid	Carrier	Yes	101
Thiamine	Thiamine	—	Same	Carrier	No	102
Niacin	Nicotinamide adenine dinucleotide (NAD)	Brush border	Nicotinamide	Passive	—	103, 104
Vitamin B_6	Pyridoxamine-5-phosphate (PMP)	Lumen	Pyridoxamine	Passive	—	105, 106
	Pyridoxal-5-phosphate (PLP)	Lumen	Pyridoxal	Passive	—	105, 106
	Pyridoxine	—	Same	Passive	—	105, 106

After a thermal rearrangement that converts previtamin D_3 to vitamin D_3, vitamin D_3 binds to a vitamin D–binding protein for transport in the circulation. The amount of endogenous vitamin D_3 synthesis is directly proportional to sunlight exposure, which varies among persons and is seasonal. Although endogenous synthesis of vitamin D_3 is usually sufficient to meet minimum daily requirements, the diet provides additional sources of vitamin D, primarily from fortified milk and bread. Vitamin D, like other lipid-soluble compounds, requires bile acid micelles for intraluminal solubilization and absorption by the enterocyte. Newly absorbed vitamin D is incorporated into chylomicrons for delivery into the circulation (via the lymphatics) and uptake by the liver. A significant enterohepatic circulation for the vitamin has been suggested but was recently refuted.[110]

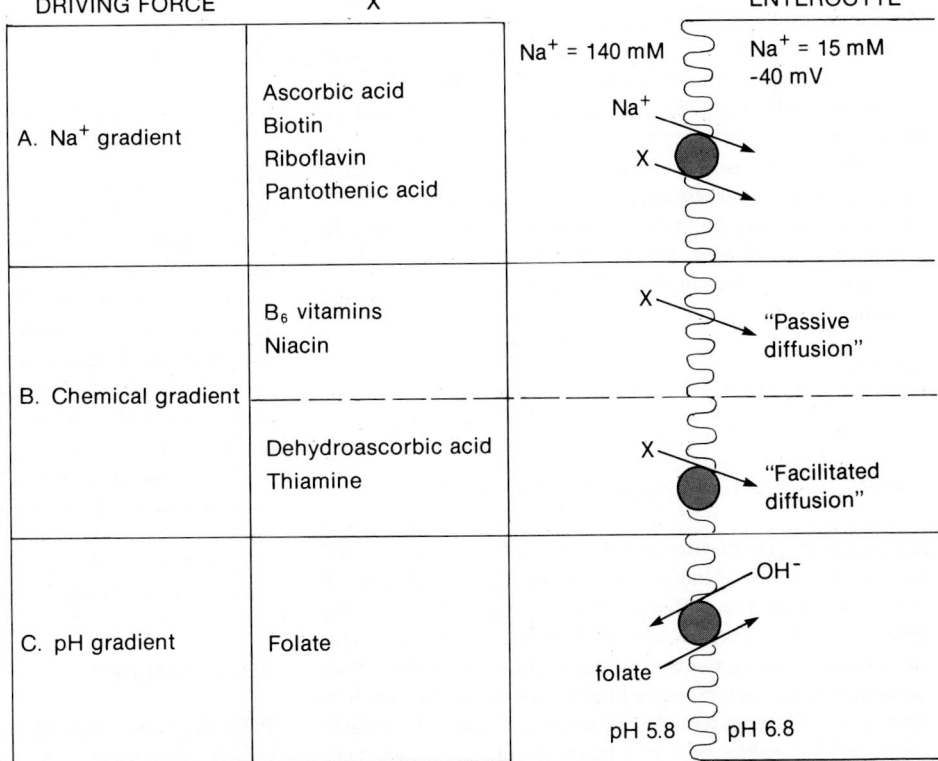

FIGURE 20–4. Driving forces for the absorption of water-soluble vitamins across the brush-border membrane. **A,** Na^+ gradient. A favorable electrochemical gradient for Na^+ is the driving force for Na^+-dependent transport of ascorbic acid, biotin, riboflavin, and pantothenic acid by separate brush-border carriers. **B,** Chemical gradient. A concentration gradient (lumen > intracellular) drives passive (B_6 vitamins, niacin) or facilitated (thiamine, dehydroascorbic acid) diffusion of many water-soluble vitamins. **C,** pH gradient. An electrochemical gradient across the brush-border membrane favors outwardly directed OH^- movement (or inwardly directed H^+ movement). A carrier on the brush border couples OH^- (or H^+) flux to monoglutamate folate (PteGlu) transport by PteGlu:OH^- exchange (or H^+:PteGlu cotransport).

METABOLISM

In the liver, vitamin D_3 is 25-hydroxylated to biologically inactive $25(OH)D_3$, the predominant circulating form of vitamin D. The kidney is the principal site where $25(OH)D_3$ is either 1-hydroxylated to the active steroid hormone, $1,25(OH)_2D_3$, or 24-hydroxylated to $24,25(OH)_2D_3$. The vitamin D status of a person determines whether the synthesis of $1,25(OH)_2D_3$ or $24,25(OH)_2D_3$ prevails. This step in the metabolism of vitamin D is closely regulated by circulating levels of $1,25(OH)_2D_3$ and parathyroid hormone that inhibit or stimulate synthesis of $1,25(OH)_2D_3$, respectively. In all target tissues including the intestine, the physiologic effects of $1,25(OH)_2D_3$ are mediated by binding to a high-affinity, low-abundance intracellular receptor. The hormone-receptor complex localizes to the nucleus, interacts with chromatin, and stimulates transcription of specific genes. The intestinal effects of $1,25(OH)_2D_3$ relate primarily to Ca^{2+} absorption. The enzymes required for the catabolism of $1,25(OH)_2D_3$ are present both in the target organ (intestine) and in the organ where the hormone is synthesized (kidney).

DISORDERS OF VITAMIN D HOMEOSTASIS[111,112]

Vitamin D deficiency impairs mineralization of newly formed bone, resulting in osteomalacia (adults) or rickets (children). Since osteomalacia further predisposes patients with osteoporosis to pathologic fractures, this condition warrants diagnosis and treatment. An abnormally low $25(OH)D_3$ level, together with biochemical or histologic evidence of vitamin D deficiency, is an indication for treatment with physiologic doses of vitamin D. Biochemical evidence for vitamin D deficiency would include a 24-hour urinary Ca^{2+} of <100 mg/day ($\downarrow$ intestinal absorption), a high parathyroid hormone level, or elevated alkaline phosphatase or urinary hydroxyproline levels ($\uparrow$ bone resorption). During vitamin D treatment, urinary and serum Ca^{2+} should be followed closely to avoid potentially serious complications of vitamin D therapy (hypercalcemia, hypercalciuria $\rightarrow$ nephrolithiasis). Age-associated osteoporosis that is not complicated by osteomalacia and postmenopausal osteoporosis do not benefit from vitamin D treatment. Prolonged (>2 years) treatment with high doses of the cholesterol-lowering agent cholestyramine can also induce osteomalacia secondary to vitamin D malabsorption.[113]

Vitamin K[114]

SOURCES AND INTESTINAL ABSORPTION

The total body pool of vitamin K is remarkably small (50 to 100 μg). Rapid turnover of this pool necessitates the daily absorption of 1 μg/kg to maintain adequate levels. Like vitamin D, daily requirements for vitamin K are met from endogenous and exogenous sources, that is, synthesis of menaquinones by colonic flora (vitamin K_2) and dietary intake of phylloquinones (vitamin K_1), respectively. The important dietary sources of vitamin K_1 include green leafy vegetables and, to a lesser extent, meats and dairy products. The small intestine normally absorbs 30% to 70% of the 300 to 500 μg of vitamin K_1 ingested daily, a quantity sufficient to meet minimum daily requirements. Nevertheless, approximately half of hepatic vitamin K stores are menaquinones of bacterial origin. Since healthy subjects on vitamin K-deficient diets do not develop deficiency unless bowel-sterilizing antibiotics are administered concurrently,[115] bacterial menaquinones are not only biologically available but, under certain circumstances, are also physiologically important.

METABOLISM

After intestinal absorption, vitamin K is taken up largely by the liver and accumulated in the microsomal fraction. In the liver, vitamin K is a required cofactor for the enzymatic γ-carboxylation of glutamic acid residues on vitamin K-dependent coagulation proenzymes (Factors II, VII, IX, and X) and other proteins involved in coagulation and fibrinolysis (proteins C, S, M, and Z).

DISORDERS OF VITAMIN K HOMEOSTASIS

A prolongation of the prothrombin time, which is correctible with vitamin K, is the chief clinical manifestation of vitamin K deficiency. Since critically ill patients are often anorectic and being treated with broad-spectrum antibiotics, such patients are particularly susceptible to developing clinically significant vitamin K deficiency.[116] More sensitive tests of vitamin K nutriture, such as measurement of abnormal prothrombin levels, detect subclinical vitamin K deficiency in approximately 30% and 60% of patients with inflammatory bowel disease[117] and primary biliary cirrhosis,[118] respectively.

Vitamin A[119]

SOURCES AND INTESTINAL ABSORPTION

The term *retinoid* refers to naturally occurring compounds having vitamin A activity (retinol, retinoic acid) and active or inactive synthetic analogues. Dietary sources of vitamin A include plant carotenoid pigments, e.g. β-carotene, and retinyl esters from animal tissues. Dietary retinyl esters are hydrolyzed to retinol by pancreatic and intestinal brush-border esterases prior to uptake from the gut lumen. Retinol is also obtained from the vitamin precursor, β-carotene, following transport of β-carotene across the apical membrane of the enterocyte and intracellular processing, which includes enzymatic cleavage to two molecules of retinaldehyde and reduction to retinol. The absorbed retinol binds to retinol-binding protein type II (CRBP II), which is uniquely localized to the villus absorptive cell.[120] Re-esterification to retinyl esters, incorporation into chylomicrons, and delivery into the lymphatics completes the intestinal absorption of the vitamin.

METABOLISM

Following hepatic uptake from chylomicron remnants, long-chain retinyl esters are stored in hepatocytes and hepatic fat storage cells (Ito cells). Hepatic delivery of vitamin A to target tissues is highly regulated, requiring hydrolysis to retinol and binding to retinol-binding protein, a plasma transport protein synthesized in the liver. Glomerular filtration and renal catabolism of retinol-binding protein is reduced by formation of a complex with another circulating protein, transthyretin (or "prealbumin"). Cell-surface receptors for retinol-binding protein apparently mediate the uptake of retinol by target tissues.

In contrast, retinoic acid, the other naturally occurring compound with vitamin A activity, is transported in the circulation bound to albumin. Body stores of retinoic acid are negligible compared with retinol.

DISORDERS OF VITAMIN A HOMEOSTASIS

Although retinoids are important in cell differentiation and proliferation, the clinical effects of vitamin A deficiency relate primarily to the role of retinol as a precursor of the visual pigment rhodopsin. Clinical findings, termed *xerophthalmia*, range from night blindness to corneal ulceration and irreversible blindness. Vitamin A deficiency is particularly common in impoverished sections of the world. In Southeast Asia alone, 500,000 new cases of xerophthalmia occur each year, with half progressing to blindness. Less commonly, a hypervitaminosis state can occur secondary to self-medication or overuse of prescription supplements. The syndrome is characterized by signs and symptoms of increased intracranial pressure (headache, nausea, and vomiting), mucocutaneous lesions, and skeletal pain.[121] Rarely, hepatic injury with portal hypertension can supervene. Synthetic retinoids are currently being used in the treatment of a variety of dermatologic conditions, such as 13-*cis*-retinoic acid (Accutane) for severe cystic acne.

Vitamin E[122,123]

SOURCES AND INTESTINAL ABSORPTION

Vitamin E (α-tocopherol) is widely distributed in grains, vegetables, and meats. The luminal phase of absorption requires intraluminal bile salts for micellar solubilization[124] and pancreatic esterases to hydrolyze vitamin E esters.[125] Vitamin E is then absorbed across the brush-border membrane of the enterocyte by passive diffusion.[126] Like other fat-soluble vitamins, vitamin E is packaged into chylomicrons and delivered into the mesenteric lymphatics.

METABOLISM

Vitamin E is stored primarily in the liver and adipose tissue. After hepatic uptake, the vitamin is returned to the circulation bound to lipoproteins (VLDL, HDL, and in the fasting state, LDL). Therefore, serum vitamin E levels vary in parallel with serum lipid levels and, to correct for hyperlipidemia, are expressed as the ratio of vitamin E to total lipid. Vitamin E probably functions as an antioxidant, protecting membrane lipids from free radical damage, particularly in neural and muscle tissues.

DISORDERS OF VITAMIN E HOMEOSTASIS

In children with chronic cholestasis, vitamin E deficiency is common (50%–75%) and associated with retinopathy and a progressive neurologic disorder (cerebellar ataxia, loss of deep tendon reflexes, and diminished vibratory and position sense). Vitamin E deficiency, along with similar neurologic findings, is often found in untreated patients with abetalipoproteinemia, which is an inborn error of metabolism characterized by absence of abetalipoprotein B, inability to secrete chylomicrons, and steatorrhea.

As with the other fat-soluble vitamins, malabsorption of vitamin E in adults occurs when fat absorption is adversely affected by diminished absorptive surface area (Crohn's disease, short bowel syndrome, radiation enteritis) or impaired micellar solubilization secondary to decreased bile salt concentration (ileal disease, intrahepatic or extrahepatic obstruction). Malabsorption must be present for years to deplete body stores and develop the full-blown neurologic abnormalities that characterize childhood cholestasis.[123] Nevertheless, in primary biliary cirrhosis, biochemical evidence of vitamin E deficiency is not uncommon ($\approx$13% incidence), even in patients with early asymptomatic disease.[127] The possibility that vitamin E deficiency contributes to the neurologic dysfunction sometimes seen in this disorder constitutes a rationale for vitamin E supplementation.[122] If vitamin K deficiency is also present, this should be corrected first since vitamin E may displace vitamin K from bile salt micelles, thus worsening the vitamin K deficiency and the associated coagulopathy.

ABSORPTION OF MINERALS

Iron

SOURCES

Dietary iron consists of heme and nonheme iron. Regardless of the iron status of the person, heme iron from hemoglobin or myoglobin is more efficiently absorbed than nonheme iron.[128] In iron deficiency, 35% of heme iron but only 20% of nonheme iron is absorbed. Comparable figures in the iron-replete subject are 15% and 2% for the absorption of heme and nonheme iron, respectively. Analysis of the iron content of a variety of meats and seafoods suggests that 30% to 60% is heme iron. In contrast, vegetables, grains, and fruits contain only nonheme iron, largely in the form of ferric salts. Overall, the quantity of nonheme iron in the diet exceeds that of heme iron.[128] In the adult male, iron losses in desquamated epithelium (skin, villus enterocytes) and intestinal secretions approximate 1 mg/d.[129] With menstrual bleeding and pregnancy, women have additional losses of 3 to 60 mg/month and 500 mg during pregnancy. Intestinal absorption of dietary iron is highly regulated to compensate for these losses and maintain iron balance.

INTESTINAL ABSORPTION

Luminal Factors. The physicochemical form of nonheme iron depends on intraluminal dietary constituents and has a major influence on intestinal absorption.[129] Ferric iron (Fe^{3+}) salts are relatively insoluble when the luminal pH exceeds pH 3.0. Hence, absorption of Fe^{3+} requires the formation of soluble complexes within the acidic environment of the stomach. In contrast, ferrous iron (Fe^{2+}) remains soluble even at pH 8.0. Various low molecular weight substances (sugars, amino acids, citrate, ascorbate) chelate intraluminal iron, enhancing solubility and promoting absorption. Other agents (carbonates, oxalates, phosphates, vegetable phytates, tannates) form insoluble complexes with iron and inhibit absorption. Bile contains ascorbic acid, which maintains the more soluble Fe^{2+} in the reduced state, and other substances that chelate luminal iron, thus enhancing absorption. These luminal factors do not influence absorption of heme iron, which enters the enterocyte as the intact metalloporphyrin.

Intestinal Factors. Iron is absorbed predominantly in the duodenum and jejunum, where absorption increases in response to iron deficiency.[130] Iron absorption occurs in two stages: (1) two thirds of the iron is absorbed over 30 to 60 minutes (rapid phase) and (2) the remainder is absorbed over 12 to 24 hours (slow phase). According to one hypothesis, the first step in absorption involves binding of intraluminal iron to high-affinity sites on the brush-border membrane.[131] At least in iron deficiency, the translocation of iron across the brush border is carrier mediated.[131] An alternative hypothesis involves secretion of the iron-binding protein transferrin and endocytic uptake of the iron-transferrin complex by the enterocyte. Since both mechanisms may be operative, these hypotheses are not mutually exclusive. However, the absence of transferrin receptors on duodenal microvilli argues against receptor-mediated endocytic uptake of iron-transferrin complexes. The intracellular processing of newly absorbed iron for delivery to the circulation is highly regulated. Involvement of one or more iron-binding proteins is likely, but the identity of the putative protein(s) has not been established. Competition for binding to this protein(s) may explain inhibition of iron uptake by other trace metals (cadmium, lead, cobalt, manganese). Conversely, in iron deficiency, enhanced iron absorption is accompanied by enhanced absorption of these trace metals. More recently, a central role for macrophages within the lamina propria and iron-secreting goblet cells has been postulated.[132]

Regulation. Within cells, iron is stored primarily as ferritin, a hollow spherical protein housing up to 4500 iron atoms. Although serum ferritin is an indicator of body iron stores, this acute phase reactant is also elevated in a variety of inflammatory conditions. In the circulation, iron binds to transferrin, a plasma protein, for delivery to hepatocyte storage sites and the erythroid marrow. Although iron absorption is closely regulated by rates of erythropoiesis and tissue iron stores, absorption does not always correlate with transferrin saturation, hemoglobin concentration, serum iron, or transferrin levels. Thus, the precise factors that regulate intestinal iron absorption are unknown.[129,133]

DISORDERS OF IRON HOMEOSTASIS[129,134]

Deficiency. Iron deficiency develops in three sequential stages: (1) depletion of storage iron (↓ serum ferritin); (2) decrease in circulating iron (↓ serum iron, ↑ iron-binding capacity, ↓ transferrin saturation); and (3) tissue effects, primarily impaired he-

matopoiesis (hypochromic, microcytic anemia). Effects on other iron-containing compounds, such as muscle myoglobin and mitochondrial cytochromes (adenosine triphosphate [ATP] production), may explain those clinical cases where the sensation of weakness is disproportionate to the degree of anemia. Iron deficiency also impairs synthesis of biogenic amines and alters immune responses. However, the clinical correlates of these effects are difficult to assess. In children who are iron deficient, diminished disaccharidase activity, and resulting lactose malabsorption, is correctible with iron repletion.

Causes of iron deficiency include bleeding (menstrual, gastrointestinal), urinary losses secondary to intravascular hemolysis, pregnancy, inadequate intake (vegetable diet deficient in heme iron), and intestinal malabsorption. Gastrointestinal causes of decreased iron absorption include diseases affecting (celiac disease, Crohn's disease, Whipple's disease) or bypassing (partial gastrectomy with Billroth II anastomosis) the proximal small intestine. Decreased acid production (H_2 blockers, achlorhydria, surgery for peptic ulcer disease) impairs absorption of nonheme ferric iron.

Overload. Excessive gastrointestinal absorption is the primary abnormality in the autosomal recessive, HLA-related disorder idiopathic hemochromatosis. With ineffective erythropoiesis (e.g., homozygous thalassemia or sideroblastic anemia), intestinal iron absorption is enhanced and commonly results in parenchymal iron overload.[133]

Calcium

SOURCES[136]

Dietary intake of Ca^{2+} approximates 500 to 1000 mg/d and is derived largely ($\approx$75%) from milk and related dairy products. Dietary Ca^{2+} from other animal products is protein bound and must be released from these protein complexes prior to intestinal absorption. Vegetables and grains are relatively poor dietary sources of Ca^{2+}, because organic anions (phytate, oxalate, alginate, uronate) endogenous to plants form insoluble complexes with Ca^{2+}, reducing bioavailability. Indeed, a high-fiber diet may impair the absorption of Ca^{2+} from other dietary sources. Since obligatory endogenous losses in stool and urine approximate 250 mg/d, approximately 30% of the dietary load must be absorbed to maintain positive Ca^{2+} balance.

INTESTINAL ABSORPTION[135,137]

Luminal Factors. Calcium salts are ionized at the acidic pH that normally prevails in the stomach. In the ionized form, Ca^{2+} is readily available for intestinal absorption. Many different Ca^{2+} salts (e.g., lactate, chloride, gluconate, carbonate, and sulfate) are used as dietary supplements, and all have equal bioavailability in normal subjects.[138] However, patients with achlorhydria have decreased acid output, which might impair Ca^{2+} absorption. In addition, the most widely used Ca^{2+} supplement, Ca^{2+} carbonate, is also an antacid. As a consequence, Ca^{2+} carbonate is poorly

TABLE 20–4
Luminal Factors Affecting Intestinal Ca^{2+} Absorption

DECREASED ABSORPTION	NO EFFECT	INCREASED ABSORPTION
Plant components	Phosphate	Medium-chain triglycerides
Cellulose	Pectin	Lactose
Uronic acid	Ascorbic acid	Amino acids
Alginate	Citric acid	Lysine
Phytate (organic phosphate)	High-protein diet	Arginine
Oxalate		Tryptophan
Long-chain fatty acids (formation of insoluble soaps)		Drugs
Alcohol		Penicillin
Drugs		Chloramphenicol
Glucocorticoids		Neomycin
Anticonvulsants (phenytoin)		
Tetracycline		
Antacids		

Data from Birge SJ, Avioli LV. Pathophysiology of calcium absorptive disorders. In: Andreoli TE, Hoffman JF, Fanestil DD, Schultz SG, eds. Clinical disorders of membrane transport processes. 2nd ed. New York: Plenum Publishing Co, 1987; and Allen LH. Calcium bioavailability and absorption: a review. Am J Clin Nutr 1982;35:783.

absorbed by fasting patients with achlorhydria.[139] Since impaired acid production is common in elderly patients, Ca^{2+} preparations that maintain gastric acidity (e.g., Ca^{2+} citrate) may be better absorbed in this patient population. Other luminal factors influencing intestinal Ca^{2+} absorption are listed in Table 20-4.

Intestinal Factors. While the duodenum manifests the greatest Ca^{2+} flux per unit length, all small intestinal segments absorb Ca^{2+}.[140] When adjusted for transit time and the relative lengths of different segments, both the jejunum and ileum contribute substantially to overall Ca^{++} absorption.[135] At least in rats, Ca^{2+} absorptive mechanisms are also present in cecum and colon.[141]

The transcellular transport of Ca^{2+} from lumen to serosa involves three separate steps (Fig 20-5). First, Ca^{2+} movement across the brush-border membrane of the enterocyte proceeds down a favorable electrochemical gradient by a carrier-mediated process (i.e., facilitated diffusion). Second, Ca^{2+} is shuttled through the cell cytosol to the basolateral membrane in a sequestered state that protects the cell from the potential toxicity of high Ca^{2+} concentrations. Third, Ca^{2+} is extruded from the cell across the basolateral membrane against an unfavorable electrochemical gradient by the Ca^{2+}-ATPase pump. The relative contribution, and even the existence, of basolateral Na^+/Ca^{2+} exchange is controversial.[142] At high luminal Ca^{2+} concentrations (above 5–10 mM), the lumen to serosa flux of Ca^{2+} is not saturable, suggesting diffusion.

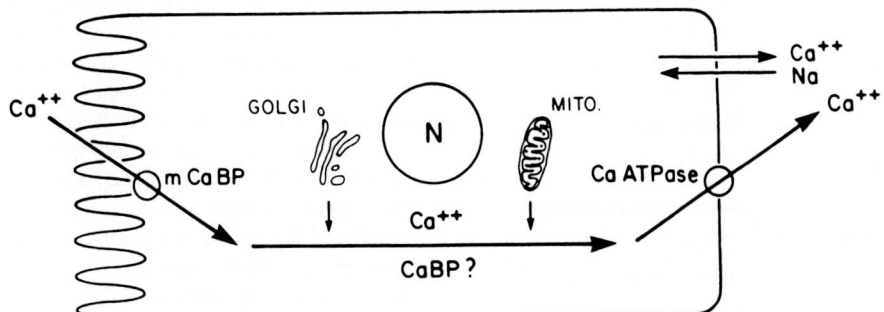

FIGURE 20–5. Transcellular transport of calcium involves three steps. First, facilitated diffusion (i.e., carrier mediated) across the brush border membrane down a favorable electrochemical gradient (*downwardly directed arrow*). Second, shuttling of Ca^{++} through the cytosol, perhaps bound to calbindin D, a vitamin D–dependent protein, or another calcium-binding protein (CaBP). Third, uphill transport across the basolateral membrane against a steep electrochemical gradient (*upwardly directed arrow*) by the Ca^{++}-ATPase pump. Basolateral Na^+/Ca^{++} exchange is depicted, but its role is controversial. (From Birge SJ, Avioli LV. Pathophysiology of calcium absorptive disorders. In: Andreoli TE, Hoffman JF, Fanestil DD, Schultz SG, eds. Clinical disorders of membrane transport processes. 2nd ed. New York: Plenum Publishing, 1987.)

Hormonal Regulation. Intestinal Ca^{2+} absorption is closely regulated by the biologically active metabolite of vitamin D, $1,25(OH)_2D_3$. $1,25(OH)_2D_3$ stimulates each step in the transcellular absorption of Ca^{2+}. First, $1,25(OH)_2D_3$ enhances the facilitated diffusion of Ca^{2+} ($K_m = 1.5$ mM) across the brush-border membrane,[143] perhaps by altering membrane lipid composition and fluidity.[144] These brush-border effects of $1,25(OH)_2D_3$ are not contingent on de novo protein synthesis.[143] Second, $1,25(OH)_2D_3$ induces synthesis of a high-affinity, intracellular Ca^{2+} binding protein, calbindin D, that is postulated to function in the cytosolic transfer of Ca^{2+} from the apical to the basolateral pole of the enterocyte.[145] A shuttle-like function for calbindin D is supported by the strong correlation between calbindin D concentration and Ca^{2+} transport[146] and the effects of calbindin D on Ca^{2+} diffusion in vitro.[147] Third, $1,25(OH)_2D_3$ stimulates ATP-dependent Ca^{2+} transport across the basolateral membrane,[148] either by enhancing Ca^{2+}–ATPase pump activity directly or by raising calbindin D levels, which secondarily stimulates the Ca^{2+} pump.[149]

DISORDERS OF CALCIUM ABSORPTION[135] (TABLE 20-5)

Increased Absorption. Pregnancy[150] and lactation are physiologic states associated with enhanced Ca^{2+} absorption. In some patients with sarcoidosis, intestinal absorption of Ca^{2+} is increased secondary to elevated levels of $1,25(OH)_2D_3$.[151] Whether the hypercalcemia that complicates other granulomatous diseases (e.g., coccidioidomycosis, histoplasmosis, berylliosis, and tuberculosis) is causally related to elevated $1,25(OH)_2D_3$ levels is not known. Patients with recurrent renal calculi often have idiopathic hypercalciuria on the basis of either "absorptive" (increased intestinal absorption secondary to inappropriately high $1,25(OH)_2D_3$ levels[152]) or "resorptive" (decreased renal reabsorption) defects. In patients with "resorptive" defects, increased renal Ca^{2+} losses leads to the sequential development of secondary hyperparathyroidism, enhanced production of $1,25(OH)_2D_3$, and stimulation of intestinal absorption of Ca^{2+}.

Increased intestinal Ca^{2+} absorption can occur without apparent changes in vitamin D metabolism. For example, despite reduced levels of $1,25(OH)_2D_3$, Ca^{2+} absorption is increased in diabetes mellitus.[135,153] Somewhat more complex, and controversial, is the mechanism of increased intestinal Ca^{2+} absorption in severe phosphate depletion. Hypophosphatemia increases synthesis of $1,25(OH)_2D_3$. However, in an animal model, vitamin D deficiency does not prevent the stimulatory effects of phosphate depletion on intestinal Ca^{2+} absorption, suggesting a vitamin D–independent mechanism.

Enhanced intestinal Ca^{2+} absorption can also be drug induced. In the past, the milk-alkali syndrome was a frequent cause of hypercalcemia and chronic renal failure secondary to aggressive treatment of peptic ulcer disease with milk and antacids. Increased intestinal Ca^{2+} absorption was a direct consequence of the increased dietary load imposed by excessive milk intake. In vitamin D intoxication,[154] intestinal Ca^{2+} absorption is enhanced even though renal conversion of $25(OH)D_3$ to $1,25(OH)_2D_3$ is suppressed by hypercalcemia. Presumably, an interaction of pharmacologic levels of $25(OH)D_3$ with the intestinal $1,25(OH)_2D_3$ receptor increases Ca^{2+} absorption. The modest stimulatory effect of pharmacologic doses of estrogens on intestinal Ca^{2+} absorption is mediated by reduced bone resorption and secondary hyperparathyroidism.[155]

Decreased Absorption. In elderly subjects, intestinal Ca^{2+} absorption is normally decreased as a consequence of diminished production of $1,25(OH)_2D_3$ and, possibly, an impaired intestinal response to vitamin D.[156] In this situation, Ca^{2+} supplementation is recommended to maintain a daily intake of 1500 mg and retard the resulting age-related loss of cortical bone.[111] Osteomalacia, secondary to Ca^{2+} malabsorption, is common when diseases diffusely involve the small bowel, reducing the surface area available for Ca^{2+} absorption (e.g., Crohn's disease, tropical sprue, and celiac disease).[157] In ileal disease, interruption of the bile salt enterohepatic circulation reduces the bile salt pool size, impairing micellar solubilization. As a consequence, Ca^{2+} absorption is further reduced by intraluminal binding of dietary Ca^{2+} to unabsorbed fatty acids and malabsorption of fat-soluble vitamin D. Similarly, in chronic cholestasis, impaired micellar solubilization leads to decreased intestinal Ca^{2+} absorption and osteomalacia. Osteomalacia is also a frequent (25%) late complication of surgery for peptic ulcer disease, particularly after subtotal gastrectomy and gastrojejunostomy.[157] Postulated mechanisms include reduced intake and/or malabsorption of vitamin D and Ca^{2+}.[158]

Intestinal Ca^{2+} absorption can be affected by nonintestinal diseases, drugs, and nutritional factors. In hypoparathyroidism, the reduction in parathyroid hormone decreases renal conversion of $25(OH)D_3$ to $1,25(OH)_2D_3$, resulting in diminished intestinal Ca^{2+}

TABLE 20–5
Conditions Associated With Altered Intestinal Ca^{2+} Absorption

INCREASED ABSORPTION	DECREASED ABSORPTION
Physiologic States	**Physiologic States**
Pregnancy	Aging
Lactation	
	Intestinal Diseases
Disease States	Reduced surface area
Increased $1,25(OH)_2D_3$ Levels	Crohn's disease
Granulomatous diseases	Celiac
Sarcoid	Tropical sprue
Coccidioidomycosis	Short bowel syndrome
Histoplasmosis	Impaired micellar solubilization
Berylliosis	Chronic cholestasis
Tuberculosis	Ileal disease
Idiopathic hypercalciuria	Gastric surgery
Hyperparathyroidism	
	Nonintestinal Diseases
Normal $1,25(OH)_2D_3$ Levels	Hypoparathyroidism
Diabetes mellitus	Hyperthyroidism
	Chronic renal failure
Drug or Nutritional	Renal tubular acidosis
	Nephrotic syndrome
Hypophosphatemia	
Milk-alkali syndrome	**Drug or Nutritional**
Vitamin D intoxication	Chlorothiazide diuretics
Estrogens	Magnesium deficiency

absorption. Similarly, in hyperthyroidism, increased bone resorption raises serum Ca^{2+} levels[159] and suppresses parathyroid hormone secretion.[159,160] As a result, serum levels of $1,25(OH)_2D_3$ are reduced[160] and Ca^{2+} absorption diminished in hyperthyroidism. Absorption of Ca^{2+} is also decreased in chronic renal failure by mechanism(s) that are not fully understood. Vitamin D–resistant Ca^{2+} malabsorption has been described in patients with the classic type of renal tubular acidosis and the nephrotic syndrome.[135] In renal tubular acidosis, alkali treatment corrects the absorptive defect, suggesting an inhibitory effect of systemic acidosis on Ca^{2+} absorption.

Drug-induced malabsorption of Ca^{2+} occurs with anticonvulsants (particularly phenytoin), glucocorticoids, and chlorothiazide diuretics. Phenytoin and glucocorticoids probably inhibit intestinal Ca^{2+} absorption directly and are listed among the luminal factors affecting Ca^{2+} absorption (see Table 20-4). The primary effect of chlorothiazide diuretics is stimulation of Ca^{2+} reabsorption in the distal nephron, which suppresses parathyroid hormone secretion and reduces renal production of $1,25(OH)_2D_3$. Nutritional deficiencies of vitamin D or minerals (iron or magnesium) also impair intestinal Ca^{2+} absorption. The mechanism by which magnesium deficiency gives rise to impaired Ca^{2+} absorption is discussed below.

Magnesium

SOURCES

Magnesium is widely available in cereals, vegetables, and meats.[162] Since Mg^{2+} is a component of chlorophyll, green vegetables are a particularly rich source. The intake of Mg^{2+} varies widely, but averages 200 to 300 mg/d. Although this is below the recommended dietary allowance of 300 to 400 mg/d, the latter recommendations are based on balance studies using older, less reliable analytical methods.[161] Gastric, biliary, and pancreatic secretions are additional sources of luminal Mg^{2+}. Normally, all of the endogenously secreted Mg^{2+} but only 20% to 70% of the dietary Mg^{2+} is absorbed.[162]

ABSORPTION

In normal adults, Mg^{2+} is absorbed throughout the small intestine by a mechanism that is saturable at low luminal concentrations (Mg^{2+} $K_m \approx 5.0$ mM).[163,164] This mechanism is functionally absent in children with primary hypomagnesemia, a rare genetic disorder characterized by defective intestinal Mg^{2+} transport.[164] At high luminal Mg^{2+} concentrations, Mg^{2+} is absorbed by passive diffusion.[164] Unabsorbed fatty acids inhibit Mg^{2+} absorption by formation of insoluble complexes.

REGULATION

In the serum, Mg^{2+} is 30% protein bound, with the rest being freely ionized. The ionized fraction is filtered by the glomerulus and largely reabsorbed in the thick ascending limb of the loop of Henle. Renal tubular reabsorption is directly proportional to dietary intake and constitutes an important mechanism for maintaining Mg^{2+} homeostasis.[161]

DEFICIENCY

Diagnosis. Certain conditions, such as K^+ depletion or starvation, deplete tissue Mg^{2+} levels without affecting serum concentrations. Hence, many investigators concluded that the serum Mg^{2+} concentration does not accurately predict the adequacy of Mg^{2+} stores.[162] However, in human and animal models of experimental Mg^{2+} deficiency, the serum Mg^{2+} level is a reliable indicator of tissue levels.[161] The hallmarks of experimental Mg^{2+} deficiency are hypomagnesemia, hypokalemia, and hypocalcemia. In early Mg^{2+} deficiency, hypocalcemia is related to inhibition of exchange between bone Ca^{2+} and serum Mg^{2+}. As the Mg^{2+} deficiency progresses, secretion of parathyroid hormone is impaired, decreasing renal production of $1,25(OH)_2D_3$ and as a consequence, intestinal absorption of Ca^{2+}. Ca^{2+} and vitamin D supplementation do not correct the resulting hypocalcemia.

Etiology. Gastrointestinal disorders that reduce the absorptive surface area of the small intestine or cause malabsorption of fatty acids (forms insoluble complexes) are commonly associated with Mg^{2+} deficiency and include Crohn's disease, celiac disease, tropical sprue, and intestinal resection. Inadequate intake (alcoholism, protein–calorie malnutrition), endocrine disorders (hyperaldosteronism, hyperthyroidism), and renal causes must also be considered in the differential diagnosis.[161]

Zinc

SOURCES

The average diet provides 10 to 15 mg/d of zinc, which is just sufficient to meet the recommended dietary allowance. Seafood and meat products are the most important dietary sources of zinc. The bioavailability of zinc from vegetable sources is reduced by plant phytates and perhaps, fiber. As with Ca^{2+}, the consumption of foods rich in phytates (beans, corn) inhibits zinc absorption from other sources.[166]

ABSORPTION

Luminal Factors. Interestingly, the binding of zinc within the intestinal lumen can either facilitate (EDTA, certain amino acids) or retard (phytate) the absorption of zinc.[165] The ability of selective amino acids (i.e., lysine, cysteine, and glycine) to chelate and promote the absorption of luminal zinc is a possible explanation for the stimulatory effect of high-protein diets on intestinal zinc absorption. Similarly, the greater bioavailability of zinc from human milk as compared with cow's milk may relate to differences in zinc-binding proteins (lactoferrin in human milk, casein in cow's milk) or the digestibility of constituent proteins.[165] When the ratio of iron to zinc exceeds 1:1, nonheme iron inhibits absorption of inorganic (sulfate salt), but not dietary (seafood) zinc.[167] This observation may be important with respect to multivitamin formulations having mineral supplements.

Intestinal Factors. Although zinc is absorbed throughout the small intestine, rates of absorption are greater in jejunum, compared with ileum or duodenum.[168] Transport across the apical membrane of the enterocyte is carrier—mediated (K_m = 0.38 mM[169]) and responsive to bodily needs for zinc. In zinc deficiency, the maximal velocity of the carrier increases twofold.[169] Within the enterocyte, zinc binds to an inducible protein, metallothionein, the levels of which are proportional to dietary zinc and copper intake. The transfer of mucosal zinc across the basolateral membrane is carrier—mediated[170] and *inversely* proportional to intracellular metallothionein levels. Therefore, induction of metallothionein by dietary copper may explain inhibition of zinc absorption and vice versa.

REGULATION

In the plasma, 80% of zinc is loosely bound to albumin and available for transfer to peripheral tissues.[165] The remainder of plasma zinc is tightly bound to α_2-macroglobulin. Under conditions of dietary zinc excess, the major route of zinc excretion is the small intestine.[171]

DEFICIENCY

Since the plasma zinc level does not accurately reflect total-body zinc stores, the diagnosis of zinc deficiency is difficult.[172] Physiologically, zinc is an important cofactor for over 100 intracellular metalloenzymes. Hence, the clinical manifestations of zinc deficiency are protean, ranging from growth retardation, hypogonadism, impaired taste acuity, alopecia, and bullous pustular dermatitis to immunologic defects and neuropsychiatric manifestations.[173] Nutritional deficiency, alcoholism (inadequate intake, hyperzincuria), small intestinal diseases (reduced absorptive surface area, e.g., Crohn's disease), chronic renal failure, and acrodermatitis enteropathica, an inherited disorder of zinc absorption, are among the diverse clinical situations associated with zinc deficiency.[173]

Other Minerals

Like other minerals, copper absorption is enhanced (amino acids, citrate, phosphate, gluconate) or retarded (ascorbate, phytate, fiber, bile) by luminal formation of soluble or insoluble complexes, respectively.[165] The mutual antagonism that was mentioned previously between the absorption of zinc and copper is one of the many interactions in the absorption of trace metals.[174]

In recent years, nutritional importance has been attached to certain ultratrace elements, such as chromium, molybdenum, and selenium.[175] For other ultratrace elements (e.g., arsenic, nickel, and silicon), nutritional significance is implied from animal studies.[175]

LOCALIZATION OF MINERAL AND VITAMIN ABSORPTION TO SPECIFIC REGIONS OF SMALL INTESTINE (FIG 20-6)

With the exception of cobalamin, the proximal small intestine is more important than the ileum in the absorption of water-soluble vitamins. Indeed, the jejunum is the exclusive site for carrier-mediated folate absorption. The absorption of calcium, zinc, and iron also occurs preferentially, but not exclusively, in the proximal small intestine. Similarly, absorption of fat-soluble vitamins takes place largely in the proximal small intestine. In contrast, the stomach and ileum are of paramount importance in the absorption of cobalamin. In mineral and vitamin homeostasis, the only function of the colon is to provide an additional source of vitamin K (bacterial phylloquinones). Therefore, at least with respect to the absorption of minerals and vitamins, the statement made by Spiro[176] over a decade ago is still essentially correct: "The small intestine, after all, provides the main reason for the existence of the gut; all the rest is prologue or epilogue, for man can live without his stomach or his esophagus, and may thrive without his colon, but

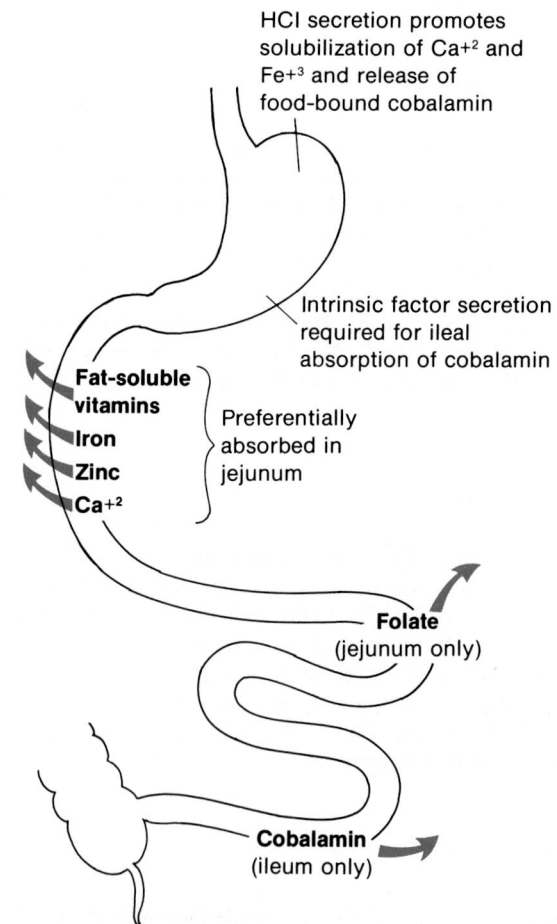

FIGURE 20–6. The localization of vitamin and mineral absorption to specific regions of the small intestine.

hidden in the darkest interior lie the two mysteries of liver and small intestine without which life is not possible."

The reader is directed to Chapter 14, Secretion and Absorption: Small Intestine and Colon; Chapter 17, Carbohydrate Assimilation; Chapter 18, Intestinal Lipid Absorption; Chapter 19, Protein Digestion and Assimilation; Chapter 20, Vitamins and Minerals; Chapter 21, General Nutritional Principles; and Chapter 47, Approach to Gastrointestinal Problems Associated with Common Clinical Conditions.

REFERENCES

1. Herbert V. Recommended dietary intakes (RDI) of folate in humans. Am J Clin Nutr 1987;45:661.
2. Butterworth CE Jr, Santini R Jr, Frommeyer WB Jr. The pteroylglutamate components of American diets as determined by chromatographic fractionation. J Clin Invest 1963;42:1929.
3. Halsted CH. The intestinal absorption of folates. Am J Clin Nutr 1979;32:846.
4. Tamura T, Stokstad ELR. The availability of food folate in man. Br J Haematol 1973;25:513.
5. Tani M, Fushiki T, Iwai K. Influence of folate-binding protein from bovine milk on the absorption of folate in gastrointestinal tract of rat. Biochim Biophys Acta 1983;757:274.
6. Tani M, Iwai K. Some nutritional effects of folate-binding protein in bovine milk on the bioavailability of folate to rats. J Nutr 1984;114:778.
7. Baugh CM, Krumdieck CL, Baker HJ, Butterworth CE Jr. Studies on the absorption and metabolism of folic acid: I. Folate absorption in the dog after exposure of isolated segments to synthetic pteroylpolyglutamates of various chain lengths. J Clin Invest 1971;50:2009.
8. Halsted CH, Baugh CM, Butterworth CE Jr. Jejunal perfusion of simple and conjugated folates in man. Gastroenterology 1975;68:261.
9. Chandler CJ, Wang TT, Halsted CH. Pteroylpolyglutamate hydrolase from human jejunal brush borders: purification and characterization. J Biol Chem 1986;261:928.
10. Chandler CJ, Harrison D, Buffington CAT, Halsted CH. Functional specificity of jejunal brush-border folate hydrolase. Gastroenterology 1989;96:A81.
11. Reisenauer AM. Folate transport by pig intestinal brush-border vesicles. In: Cooper BA, Whitehead VM, eds. Pteridines and folic acid derivatives. New York: de Gruyter, 1986:551.
12. Strum WB. Enzymatic reduction and methylation of folate following pH-dependent, carrier-mediated transport in rat jejunum. Biochim Biophys Acta 1979;554:249.
13. Lucas ML, Blair JA. The magnitude and distribution of the acid microclimate in proximal jejunum and its relation to luminal acidification. Proc R Soc Lond [A] 1978;200:27.
14. Kurtin P, Charney AN. Intestinal ion transport and intracellular pH during acute respiratory alkalosis and acidosis. Am J Physiol 1984;247:G24.
15. Schron CM, Washington C Jr, Blitzer BL. The transmembrane pH gradient drives uphill folate transport in rabbit jejunum: direct evidence for folate:OH⁻ exchange in brush-border membrane vesicles. J Clin Invest 1985;76:2030.
16. Said HM, Ghishan FK, Redha R. Folate transport by human intestinal brush-border membrane vesicles. Am J Physiol 1987;252:G229.
17. Selhub J, Powell GM, Rosenberg IH. Intestinal transport of 5-methyltetrahydrofolate. Am J Physiol 1984;246:G515.
18. Schron CM, Washington C Jr, Blitzer BL. Anion specificity of the jejunal folate carrier: effects of reduced folate analogues on folate uptake and efflux. J Membr Biol 1988;102:175.
19. Eilam Y, Ariel M, Jablonska M, Grossowicz N. On the mechanism of folate transport in isolated intestinal epithelial cells. Am J Physiol 1981;240:G170.
20. Olinger EJ, Bertino JR, Binder HJ. Intestinal folate absorption: II. Conversion and retention of pteroylmonoglutamate by jejunum. J Clin Invest 1973;52:2138.
21. Said HM, Redha R. A carrier-mediated transport for folate in basolateral membrane vesicles of rat small intestine. Biochem J 1987;247:141.
22. Wagner C. Folate-binding proteins. Nutr Rev 1985;43:293.
23. Steinberg SE. Mechanisms of folate homeostasis. Am J Physiol 1984;246:G319.
24. Kamen BA, Caston JD. Purification of folate binding factor in normal umbilical cord serum. Proc Natl Acad Sci USA 1975;72:4261.
25. Fernandes-Costa F, Metz J. Role of serum folate binders in the delivery of folate to tissues and to the fetus. Br J Haematol 1979;41:335.
26. Lambie DG, Johnson RH. Drugs and folate metabolism. Drugs 1985;30:145.
27. Selhub J, Rosenberg IH. Folate transport in isolated brush-border membrane vesicles from rat intestine. J Biol Chem 1981;256:4489.
28. Zimmerman J, Selhub J, Rosenberg IH. Competitive inhibition of folate absorption by dihydrofolate reductase inhibitors, trimethoprim and pyrimethamine. Am J Clin Nutr 1987;46:518.
29. Zimmerman J, Selhub J, Rosenberg IH. Competitive inhibition of folic acid absorption in rat jejunum by triamterene. J Lab Clin Med 1986;108:272.
30. Halsted CH, Gandhi G, Tamura T. Sulfasalazine inhibits the absorption of folates in ulcerative colitis. N Engl J Med 1981;305:1513.
31. Reisenauer AM, Halsted CH. Human jejunal brush-border folate conjugase: characteristics and inhibition by salicylazosulfapyridine. Biochim Biophys Acta 1981;659:62.
32. Zimmerman J, Selhub J, Rosenberg IH. Drug-folate interactions in intestinal folate absorption: comparison of sulfasalazine, phenytoin, and salicylates. Gastroenterology 1985;88:1643.
33. Necheles TF, Snyder LM. Malabsorption of folate polyglutamates associated with oral contraceptive therapy. N Engl J Med 1970;282:858.
34. Tamura T, Shane B, Baer MT, et al. Absorption of mono- and polyglutamyl folates in zinc-depleted man. Am J Clin Nutr 1978;31:1984.
35. Rivey MP, Schottelius DD, Berg MJ. Phenytoin-folic acid: a review. Drug Intell Clin Pharm 1984;18:292.
36. Rosenberg IH, Streiff RR, Godwin HA, Castle WB. Impairment of intestinal deconjugation of dietary folate. Lancet 1968;2:530.
37. Bernstein LH, Gutstein S, Weiner S, Efron G. The absorption and malabsorption of folic acid and its polyglutamates. Am J Med 1970;48:570.
38. Gerson CD, Hepner GW, Brown N, et al. Inhibition by diphenylhydantoin of folic acid absorption in man. Gastroenterology 1972;63:246.
39. Kitis G, Lucas ML, Bishop H, et al. Altered jejunal surface pH in coeliac disease: its effect on propranolol and folic acid absorption. Clin Sci 1982;63:373.
40. Russell RM, Krasinski SD, Samloff IM, et al. Folic acid malabsorption in atrophic gastritis: possible compensation by bacterial folate synthesis. Gastroenterology 1986;91:1476.
41. Russell RM, Dhar GJ, Dutta SK, Rosenberg IH. Influence of intraluminal pH on folate absorption: studies in control subjects and in patients with pancreatic insufficiency. J Lab Clin Med 1979;93:428.
42. Halsted CH, Beer WH, Chandler CJ, et al. Clinical studies of intestinal folate conjugases. J Lab Clin Med 1986;107:228.
43. Said HM, Redha R, Tipton W, Nylander W. Folate transport in ileal brush-border membrane vesicles following extensive resection of proximal and middle small intestine in the rat. Am J Clin Nutr 1988;47:75.
44. Halsted CH, Robles EA, Mezey E. Decreased jejunal uptake of la-

beled folic acid (^{3}H-PGA) in alcoholic patients: roles of alcohol and nutrition. N Engl J Med 1971;285:701.

45. Kapadia CR, Donaldson RM Jr. Disorders of cobalamin (vitamin B$_{12}$) absorption and transport. Ann Rev Med 1985;36:93.

46. Donaldson RM Jr. Intrinsic factor and the transport of cobalamin. In: Johnson LR, ed. Physiology of the gastrointestinal tract. 2nd ed. New York: Raven Press, 1987:959.

47. Linnell JC. The fate of cobalamin in vivo. In: Babior BM, ed. Cobalamin: biochemistry and pathophysiology. New York: John Wiley & Sons, 1975:287.

48. Baker SJ, Mathan VI. Evidence regarding the minimal daily requirement of dietary vitamin B$_{12}$. Am J Clin Nutr 1981;34:2423.

49. Cooper BA, Castle WB. Sequential mechanisms in the enhanced absorption of vitamin B$_{12}$ by intrinsic factor in the rat. J Clin Invest 1960;39:199.

50. Allen RH, Seetharam B, Podell ER, Alpers DH. Effect of proteolytic enzymes on the binding of cobalamin to R protein and intrinsic factor: in vitro evidence that a failure to partially degrade R protein is responsible for cobalamin malabsorption in pancreatic insufficiency. J Clin Invest 1978;61:47.

51. Marcoullis G, Parmentier Y, Nicolas JP, et al. Cobalamin malabsorption due to non-degradation of R proteins in the human intestine: inhibited cobalamin absorption in exocrine pancreatic insufficiency. J Clin Invest 1980;66:430.

52. Jeffries GH, Sleisenger MH. The pharmacology of intrinsic factor secretion in man. Gastroenterology 1965;48:444.

53. Binder HJ, Donaldson RM Jr. Effect of cimetidine on intrinsic factor and pepsin secretion in man. Gastroenterology 1978;74:371.

54. Batt RM, Horadagoda NU, McLean L, et al. Identification and characterization of a pancreatic intrinsic factor in the dog. Am J Physiol 1989;256:G517.

55. Kolhouse JF, Allen RH. Absorption, plasma transport, and cellular retention of cobalamin analogues in the rabbit. J Clin Invest 1977;60:1381.

56. Mathan VI, Babior BM, Donaldson RM Jr. Kinetics of the attachment of intrinsic factor-bound cobamides to ileal receptors. J Clin Invest 1974;54:598.

57. Gräsbeck R. Intrinsic factor and the transcobalamins with reflections on the general function and evolution of soluble transport proteins. Scand J Clin Lab Invest [Suppl] 1967;95:7.

58. Abels J, Schilling RF. Protection of intrinsic factor by vitamin B$_{12}$. J Lab Clin Med 1964;64:375.

59. Levine JS, Allen RH, Alpers DH, Seetharam B. Immunocytochemical localization of the intrinsic factor–cobalamin receptor in dog ileum: distribution of the intracellular receptor during cell maturation. J Cell Biol 1984;98:1111.

60. Donaldson RM Jr, Small DM, Robins S, Mathan VI. Receptors for vitamin B$_{12}$ related to ileal surface area and absorptive capacity. Biochim Biophys Acta 1973;311:477.

61. Hagedorn CH, Alpers DH. Distribution of intrinsic factor–vitamin B$_{12}$ receptors in human intestine. Gastroenterology 1977;73:1019.

62. Schade SG, Abels J, Schilling RF. Studies on antibody to intrinsic factor. J Clin Invest 1976;46:615.

63. Dieckgraefe BK, Seetharam B, Banaszak L, et al. Isolation and structural characterization of a cDNA clone encoding rat gastric intrinsic factor. Proc Natl Acad Sci USA 1988;85:46.

64. MacKenzie IL, Donaldson RM Jr. Effect of divalent cations and pH on intrinsic factor–mediated attachment of vitamin B$_{12}$ to intestinal microvillous membranes. J Clin Invest 1972;51:2465.

65. Donaldson RM Jr, MacKenzie IL, Trier JS. Intrinsic factor–mediated attachment of vitamin B$_{12}$ to brush borders and microvillous membranes of hamster intestine. J Clin Invest 1967;46:1215.

66. Kapadia CR, Serfilippi D, Voloshin K, Donaldson RM Jr. Intrinsic factor–mediated absorption of cobalamin by guinea pig ileal cells. J Clin Invest 1983;71:440.

67. Levine JS, Nakane PK, Allen RH. Immunocytochemical localization of intrinsic factor–cobalamin bound to the guinea pig ileum in vivo. Gastroenterology 1982;82:284.

68. Chanarin I, Muir M, Hughes A, Hoffbrand AV. Evidence for intestinal origin of transcobalamin II during vitamin B$_{12}$ absorption. Br Med J 1978;1:1453.

69. Sennett C, Rosenberg LE, Mellman IS. Transmembrane transport of cobalamin in prokaryotic and eukaryotic cells. Annu Rev Biochem 1981;50:1053.

70. Burger RL, Schneider RJ, Mehlman CS, Allen RH. Human plasma R-type vitamin B$_{12}$–binding proteins: II. The role of transcobalamin I, transcobalamin III, and the normal granulocyte vitamin B$_{12}$–binding protein in the plasma transport of vitamin B$_{12}$. J Biol Chem 1975;250:7707.

71. Green R, Jacobsen DW, Van Tonder SV, et al. Enterohepatic circulation of cobalamin in the nonhuman primate. Gastroenterology 1981;81:773.

72. Fairbanks VF, Elveback LR. Tests for pernicious anemia: serum vitamin B$_{12}$ assay. Mayo Clin Proc 1983;58:135.

73. Fairbanks VF, Wahner HW, Phyliky RL. Tests for pernicious anemia: the "Schilling test." Mayo Clin Proc 1983;58:541.

74. Sheppard K, Ryrie D. Changes in serum levels of cobalamin and cobalamin analogues in folate deficiency. Scand J Haematol 1980;25:401.

75. Conley CL, Krevans JR. Development of neurologic manifestations of pernicious anemia during multivitamin therapy. N Engl J Med 1951;245:529.

76. Vilter CF, Vilter RW, Spies TD. The treatment of pernicious anemia and related anemias with synthetic folic acid: I. Observations on the maintenance of a normal hematologic status and on the occurrence of combined system disease at the end of one year. J Lab Clin Med 1947;32:262-73.

77. Carmel R. Pernicious anemia: the expected findings of very low serum cobalamin levels, anemia, and macrocytosis are often lacking. Arch Intern Med 1988;148:1712.

78. Lindenbaum J, Healton EB, Savage DG, et al. Neuropsychiatric disorders caused by cobalamin deficiency in the absence of anemia or macrocytosis. N Engl J Med 1988;318:1720.

79. Matchar DB, Feussner JR, Millington DS, et al. Isotope-dilution assay for urinary methylmalonic acid in the diagnosis of vitamin B$_{12}$ deficiency. Ann Intern Med 1987;106:707.

80. Norman EJ, Martelo OJ, Denton MD. Cobalamin (vitamin B$_{12}$) deficiency detection by urinary methylmalonic acid quantitation. Blood 1982;59:1128.

81. Carmel R, Johnson CS. Racial patterns in pernicious anemia. N Engl J Med 1978;298:647.

82. Schade SG, Feick P, Muckerheide M, Schilling RF. Occurrence in gastric juice of antibody to a complex of intrinsic factor and vitamin B$_{12}$. N Engl J Med 1966;275:528.

83. Cooper BA, Rosenblatt DS. Inherited defects of vitamin B$_{12}$ metabolism. Ann Rev Nutr 1987;7:291.

84. King CE, Leibach J, Toskes PP. Clinically significant vitamin B$_{12}$ deficiency secondary to malabsorption of protein-bound vitamin B$_{12}$. Dig Dis Sci 1979;24:397.

85. Dawson DW, Sawers AH, Sharma RK. Malabsorption of protein bound vitamin B$_{12}$. Br Med J 1984;288:675.

86. Steinberg WM, King CE, Toskes PP. Malabsorption of protein-bound cobalamin but not unbound cobalamin during cimetidine administration. Dig Dis Sci 1980;25:188.

87. Aymard JP, Aymard B, Netter P, et al. Haematological adverse effects of histamine H$_2$-receptor antagonists. Med Toxicol 1988;3:430.

88. Carmel R, Sinow RM, Siegel ME, Samloff M. Food cobalamin malabsorption occurs frequently in patients with unexplained low serum cobalamin levels. Arch Intern Med 1988;148:1715.

89. Toskes PP, Hansell J, Cerda J, Deren JJ. Vitamin B$_{12}$ malabsorption in chronic pancreatic insufficiency: studies suggesting the presence of a pancreatic "intrinsic factor." N Engl J Med 1971;284:627.

90. Henderson JT, Warwick RRG, Simpson JD, Shearman DJC. Does malabsorption of vitamin B$_{12}$ occur in chronic pancreatitis? Lancet 1972;2:241.

91. Shimoda SS, Saunders DR, Rubin CE. The Zollinger-Ellison syndrome with steatorrhea: II. The mechanisms of fat and vitamin B$_{12}$ malabsorption. Gastroenterology 1968;55:705.

92. Schjönsby H. The mechanism of vitamin B$_{12}$ malabsorption in blind-loop syndrome. Scand J Gastroent 1973;8:97.

93. Lenz K. The effect of the site of lesion and extent of resection on duodenal bile acid concentration and vitamin B$_{12}$ absorption in Crohn's disease. Scand J Gastroenterol 1975;10:241.

93a. Harriman GR, Smith PD, Horne MK, et al. Vitamin B$_{12}$ malabsorption in patients with acquired immunodeficiency syndrome. Arch Int Med 1989;149:2039.

94. Carmel R, Herbert V. Correctable intestinal defect of vitamin B_{12} absorption in pernicious anemia. Ann Intern Med 1967;67:1201.

95. Levine M. New concepts in the biology and biochemistry of ascorbic acid. N Engl J Med 1986;314:892.

96. Rose RC. Transport of ascorbic acid and other water-soluble vitamins. Biochim Biophys Acta 1988;947:335.

97. Rose RC. Intestinal absorption of water-soluble vitamins. In: Johnson LR, ed. Physiology of the gastrointestinal tract. 2nd ed. New York: Raven Press, 1987:1581.

98. Bianchi J, Wilson FA, Rose RC. Dehydroascorbic acid and ascorbic acid transport systems in the guinea pig ileum. Am J Physiol 1986;250: G461.

99. Said HM, Redha R, Nylander W. A carrier-mediated, Na^+ gradient-dependent transport for biotin in human intestinal brush-border membrane vesicles. Am J Physiol 1987;253:G631.

100. Sweetman L, Nyhan WL. Inheritable biotin-treatable disorders and associated phenomena. Ann Rev Nutr 1986;6:317.

101. Fenstermacher DK, Rose RC. Absorption of pantothenic acid in rat and chick intestine. Am J Physiol 1986;250:G155.

102. Casirola D, Ferrari G, Gastaldi G, et al. Transport of thiamine by brush-border membrane vesicles from rat small intestine. J Physiol 1988;398:329.

103. Henderson LM. Niacin. Ann Rev Nutr 1983;3:289.

104. Baum CL, Selhub J, Rosenberg IH. The hydrolysis of nicotinamide adenine dinucleotide by brush-border membranes of rat intestine. Biochem J 1982;204:203.

105. Ink SL, Henderson LM. Vitamin B_6 metabolism. Ann Rev Nutr 1984;4:455.

106. Merrill AH Jr, Henderson JM. Diseases associated with defects in vitamin B_6 metabolism or utilization. Ann Rev Nutr 1987;7:137.

107. Shiau Y-F. Lipid digestion and absorption. In: Johnson LR, ed. Physiology of the gastrointestinal tract. 2nd ed. New York: Raven Press, 1987:1527.

108. Audran M. The physiology and pathophysiology of vitamin D. Mayo Clin Proc 1985;60:851.

109. Henry HL, Norman AW. Vitamin D: metabolism and biological actions. Ann Rev Nutr 1984;4:493.

110. Clements MR, Chalmers TM, Fraser DR. Enterohepatic circulation of vitamin D: a reappraisal of the hypothesis. Lancet 1984;1:1376.

111. Sewell KL. Modern therapeutic approaches to osteoporosis. Rheum Dis Clin North Am 1989;15:583.

112. Alden JC. Osteoporosis—a review. Clin Ther 1989;11:3.

113. Knodel LC, Talbert RL. Adverse effects of hypolipidaemic drugs. Med Toxicol 1987;2:10.

114. Olson RE. The function and metabolism of vitamin K. Ann Rev Nutr 1984;4:281.

115. Frick PG, Riedler G, Brögli H. Dose response and minimal daily requirement for vitamin K in man. J Appl Physiol 1967;23:387.

116. Alperin JB. Coagulopathy caused by vitamin K deficiency in critically ill, hospitalized patients. JAMA 1987;258:1916.

117. Krasinski SD, Russell RM, Furie BC, et al. The prevalence of vitamin K deficiency in chronic gastrointestinal disorders. Am J Clin Nutr 1985;41:639.

118. Kaplan MM, Elta GH, Furie B, et al. Fat-soluble vitamin nutriture in primary biliary cirrhosis. Gastroenterology 1988;95:787.

119. Goodman DS. Vitamin A and retinoids in health and disease. N Engl J Med 1984;310:1023.

120. Crow JA, Ong DE. Cell-specific immunohistochemical localization of a cellular retinol-binding protein (type two) in the small intestine of rat. Proc Natl Acad Sci USA 1985;82:4707.

121. Russell RM, Boyer JL, Bagheri SA, Hruban Z. Hepatic injury from chronic hypervitaminosis A resulting in portal hypertension and ascites. N Engl J Med 1974;291:435.

122. Sokol RJ. The coming of age of vitamin E. Hepatology 1989;9:649.

123. Sokol RJ. Vitamin E deficiency and neurologic disease. Ann Rev Nutr 1988;8:351.

124. Gallo-Torres HE. Obligatory role of bile for the intestinal absorption of vitamin E. Lipids 1969;5:379.

125. Muller DPR, Manning JA, Mathias PM, Harries JT. Studies on the intestinal hydrolysis of tocopheryl esters. Int J Vitam Nutr Res 1976;46:207.

126. Hollander D, Rim E, Muralidhara KS. Mechanism and site of small intestinal absorption of α-tocopherol in the rat. Gastroenterology 1975;68:1492.

127. Muñoz SJ, Heubi JE, Balistreri WF, Maddrey WC. Vitamin E deficiency in primary biliary cirrhosis: gastrointestinal malabsorption, frequency and relationship to other lipid-soluble vitamins. Hepatology 1989;9:525.

128. Monsen ER, Hallberg L, Layrisse M, et al. Estimation of available dietary iron. Am J Clin Nutr 1978;31:134.

129. Conrad ME. Iron absorption. In: Johnson LR, ed. Physiology of the gastrointestinal tract. 2nd ed. New York: Raven Press, 1987:1437.

130. Muir A, Hopfer U. Regional specificity of iron uptake by small intestinal brush-border membranes from normal and iron-deficient mice. Am J Physiol 1985;248:G376.

131. Muir WA, Hopfer U, King M. Iron transport across brush-border membranes from normal and iron-deficient mouse upper small intestine. J Biol Chem 1984;259:4896.

132. Refsum SB, Schreiner BBI. Regulation of iron balance by absorption and excretion: a critical review and a new hypothesis. Scand J Gastroenterol 1984;19:867.

133. Finch CA, Huebers H. Perspectives in iron metabolism. N Engl J Med 1982;306:1520.

134. Dallman PR. Biochemical basis for the manifestations of iron deficiency. Ann Rev Nutr 1986;6:13.

135. Birge SJ, Avioli LV. Pathophysiology of calcium absorptive disorders. In: Andreoli TE, Hoffman JF, Fanestil DD, Schultz SG, eds. Clinical disorders of membrane transport processes. 2nd ed. New York: Plenum Publishing Company, 1987:121.

136. Allen LH. Calcium bioavailability and absorption: a review. Am J Clin Nutr 1982;35:783.

137. Wasserman RH, Fullmer CS. On the molecular mechanism of intestinal calcium transport. In: Dintzis FR, Laszlo JA, eds. Mineral absorption in the monogastric GI tract. New York: Plenum Press, 1989:45. (Advances in experimental medicine and biology; vol 249.)

138. Patton MB, Sutton TS. The utilization of calcium from lactate, gluconate, sulfate and carbonate salts by young college women. J Nutr 1952;48:443.

139. Recker RR. Calcium absorption and achlorhydria. N Engl J Med 1985;313:70.

140. Birge SJ, Peck WA, Berman M, Whedon GD. Study of calcium absorption in man: a kinetic analysis and physiologic model. J Clin Invest 1969;48:1705.

141. Favus MJ, Kathpalia SC, Coe FL, Mond AE. Effects of diet calcium and 1,25-dihydroxyvitamin D_3 on colon calcium active transport. Am J Physiol 1980;238:G75.

142. Nellans HN. Intestinal sodium-dependent calcium transport: role for Na:Ca exchange? In: Donowitz M, Sharp GW, eds. Mechanisms of intestinal electrolyte transport and regulation by calcium. New York: Liss, 1984:209.

143. Rasmussen H, Fontaine O, Max EE, Goodman DBP. The effect of 1-hydroxyvitamin D_3 administration on calcium transport in chick intestine brush-border membrane vesicles. J Biol Chem 1979;254:2993.

144. Brasitus TA, Dudeja PK, Eby B, Lau K. Correction by 1-25-dihydroxycholecalciferol of the abnormal fluidity and lipid composition of enterocyte brush-border membranes in vitamin D–deprived rats. J Biol Chem 1986;261:16404.

145. Kretsinger RH, Mann JE, Simmonds JG. Model of the facilitated diffusion of calcium by the intestinal calcium binding proteins. In: Norman AW, Schaefer K, Herrath DV, Grigoleit HG, eds. Vitamin D: chemical, biochemical, and clinical endocrinology of calcium metabolism. Berlin: de Gruyter, 1982:233.

146. Bronner F, Pansu D, Stein W. An analysis of intestinal calcium transport across the rat intestine. Am J Physiol 1986;250:G561.

147. Feher JJ. Facilitated calcium diffusion by intestinal calcium-binding protein. Am J Physiol 1983;244:C303.

148. Ghijsen WEJM, Van Os CH. 1α,25-dihydroxyvitamin D-3 regulates ATP-dependent calcium transport in basolateral plasma membranes of rat enterocytes. Biochim Biophys Acta 1982;689:170.

149. Walters JRF. Calbindin-D$_{9k}$ stimulates the calcium pump in rat enterocyte basolateral membranes. Am J Physiol 1989;256:G124.

150. Heaney RP, Skillman TG. Calcium metabolism in normal human pregnancy. J Clin Endocr 1971;33:661.

151. Bell NH, Stern PH, Pantzer E, et al. Evidence that increased circulating 1α,25-dihydroxyvitamin D is the probable cause for abnormal calcium metabolism in sarcoidosis. J Clin Invest 1979;64:218.

152. Kaplan RA, Haussler MR, Deftos LJ, et al. The role of 1α,25-dihydroxyvitamin D in the mediation of intestinal hyperabsorption of calcium in primary hyperparathyroidism and absorptive hypercalciuria. J Clin Invest 1977;50:756.

153. Frazer TE, White NH, Hough S, et al. Alterations in circulating vitamin D metabolites in the young insulin-dependent diabetic. J Clin Endocrinol Metab 1981;53:1154.

154. Paterson CR. Vitamin-D poisoning: survey of causes in 21 patients with hypercalcaemia. Lancet 1980;1:1164.

155. Gallagher JC, Riggs BL, DeLuca HF. Effect of estrogen on calcium absorption and serum vitamin D metabolites in postmenopausal osteoporosis. J Clin Endocrin Metab 1980;51:1359.

156. Gallagher JC, Riggs BL, Eisman J, et al. Intestinal calcium absorption and serum vitamin D metabolites in normal subjects and osteoporotic patients. J Clin Invest 1979;64:729.

157. Sitrin M, Meredith S, Rosenberg IH. Vitamin D deficiency and bone disease in gastrointestinal disorders. Arch Intern Med 1978;138:886.

158. Imawari M, Kozawa K, Akanuma Y, et al. Serum 25-hydroxyvitamin D and vitamin D-binding protein levels and mineral metabolism after partial and total gastrectomy. Gastroenterology 1980;79:255.

159. Burman KD, Monchik JM, Earll JM, Wartofsky L. Ionized and total serum calcium and parathyroid hormone in hyperthyroidism. Ann Intern Med 1976;84:668.

160. Bouillon R, Muls E, De Moore P. Influence of thyroid function on the serum concentration of 1,25-dihydroxyvitamin D$_3$. J Clin Endocrinol Metab 1980;51:793.

161. Shils ME. Magnesium in health and disease. Ann Rev Nutr 1988;8:429.

162. Wester PO. Magnesium. Am J Clin Nutr 1987;45:1305.

163. Brannan PG, Vergne-Marini P, Pak CYC, et al. Magnesium absorption in the human small intestine: results in normal subjects, patients with chronic renal disease, and patients with absorptive hypercalciuria. J Clin Invest 1976;57:1412.

164. Milla PJ, Aggett PJ, Wolff OH, Harries JT. Studies in primary hypomagnesaemia: evidence for defective carrier-mediated small intestinal transport of magnesium. Gut 1979;20:1028.

165. Cousins RJ. Absorption, transport, and hepatic metabolism of copper and zinc: special reference to metallothionein and ceruloplasmin. Physiol Rev 1985;65:238.

166. Solomons NW, Jacob RA, Pineda O, Viteri F. Studies on the bioavailability of zinc in man: II. Absorption of zinc from organic and inorganic sources. J Lab Clin Med 1979;94:335.

167. Solomons NW, Jacob RA. Studies on the bioavailability of zinc in humans: effects of heme and nonheme iron on the absorption of zinc. Am J Clin Nutr 1981;34:475.

168. Lee HH, Prasad AS, Brewer GJ, Owyang C. Zinc absorption in human small intestine. Am J Physiol 1989;256:G87.

169. Menard MP, Cousins RJ. Zinc transport by brush-border membrane vesicles from rat intestine. J Nutr 1983;223:1434.

170. Oestreicher P, Cousins RJ. Zinc uptake by basolateral membrane vesicles from rat small intestine. J Nutr 1989;119:639.

171. Wastney ME, Aamodt RL, Rumble WF, Henkin RI. Kinetic analysis of zinc metabolism and its regulation in normal humans. Am J Physiol 1986;251:R398.

172. Solomons NW. On the assessment of zinc and copper nutriture in man. Am J Clin Nutr 1979;32:856.

173. Prasad AS. Clinical manifestations of zinc deficiency. Ann Rev Nutr 1985;5:341.

174. Mills CF. Dietary interactions involving the trace elements. Ann Rev Nutr 1985;5:173.

175. Nielsen FH. Ultratrace elements in nutrition. Ann Rev Nutr 1984;4:21.

176. Spiro H. Visceral viewpoints: the rough and the smooth—some reflections on diet therapy. N Engl J Med 1975;293:83.

21

General Nutritional Principles

FREDERICK H. OPPER
WILLIAM D. HEIZER

Human nutrition is the study of food and drink requirements for maintenance, growth, activity, healing, reproduction, and lactation.[1] This discipline, now essential to the care of patients, cannot be understood apart from metabolism. Metabolism is the sum of a highly integrated network of chemical reactions enabling cells to synthesize macromolecules from small molecules (anabolism) and to extract energy, reducing power, and new substrate by converting large molecules into smaller ones (catabolism).[2]

Evidence that dietary factors are implicated in the prevention and modification of many diseases, including coronary artery disease and malignancies, has heightened public awareness of nutrition.[3] Nutrition information of varied quality is disseminated in newsletters, magazines, and other media, but the "medical establishment" is occasionally criticized for perceived ignorance or indifference about nutritional matters. We now have unprecedented ability to support ill patients nutritionally by enteral and parenteral routes in both hospital and outpatient settings. The significant impact on medical care of knowledge in nutrition mandates that all physicians rendering patient care master a core of nutritional principles as surely as they master anatomy and physiology.

CONTROL OF APPETITE

The drive to eat is basic, primitive, and essential to survival. It is difficult to separate the physiology of human eating behavior from the nonphysiologic factors influencing food intake, and no unifying theory of appetite regulation has achieved general acceptance.[4] Hunger is defined as a desire or need for food.[1] Appetite may be defined as a sensation that makes one want to eat a particular food, and palatability as the quality of a food that evokes appetite.[5] Satiety is a sensation intermediate between the relief of hunger and the discomfort that ultimately limits overeating.[6]

Human body mass is controlled by the balance of energy intake and output. Appetite regulation is the key factor in energy intake. Several models exist for the control systems that regulate energy balance in humans, and two merit brief mention. The *set point* concept is based on accepted models for the control of vital body processes, such as temperature and osmolarity. It assumes the presence of an energy sensor that operates in a feedback manner to adjust energy intake and expenditure to maintain a predetermined, fixed body mass.[7-9] Although humans tend to change their metabolic rates to oppose departure from an established normally maintained weight, the observation that both men and experimental animals can be made obese by voluntary ingestion of a high-fat, palatable diet argues against the set point hypothesis.[10] Furthermore, the proposed sensor has not been identified. The *buffer theory* postulates a mechanism similar to physiologic acid–base buffering. This is a system that works to minimize rapid changes in the steady state; thus, it is a coarser control mechanism than the set point. Because it postulates no sensor or feedback loop, such a system can only minimize the magnitude of an imbalance between nutrient ingestion and need; it cannot correct the imbalance completely.[11]

The control of eating is complex and multifactorial. There are peripheral satiety signals, including taste and smell as well as mechanical and neurohumoral responses arising in the gastrointestinal tract. Although peripheral signals ultimately relay information to the brain, there also appears to be a central satiety system acting directly at the brain.

Central Nervous System Factors in Eating Control

HYPOTHALAMUS

The hypothalamus is largely responsible for integrating impulses involved in appetite regulation. Early work focused on the ventromedial hypothalamus (VMH) as a satiety center and the lateral hypothalamus (LH) as a feeding center.[12,13] Further research has shown that these areas are more complex than initially appreciated.

The VMH is associated with a serotonergic (raphe nuclei) tract and a ventral adrenergic bundle, while the LH, aside from receiving projections of the ventral adrenergic bundle, is associated with the dopaminergic nigrostriatal tract. These tracts appear to influence related areas of the brain, such as those involved in pleasure or reward, and the results of lesioning may be partly related to interference with these pathways.[14,15] Because VMH lesions result in hyperinsulinemia and increased vagal tone, autonomic imbalance has also been proposed to explain the hyperphagia and weight gain following VMH destruction.[16] Lesions of the LH may produce their aphagic effect by lowering the body weight set point.[17]

APPESTATS

Various factors have been proposed as determinants of appetite control. These appestats have included glucose, amino acids, adipose stores, and heat. Although each of these putative appestats has some experimental support, none has been able to withstand close scrutiny or become widely accepted.[14,15]

NEUROTRANSMITTERS AND NEUROPEPTIDES

Even oversimplified models of neurotransmitter involvement in central nervous system (CNS) appetite regulation are complex.[18] Dopaminergic tracts supplying the lateral hypothalamic feeding area appear to be vital in initiating feeding, probably through interactions with endogenous opioid peptides.[14] Norepinephrine systems are involved in both promoting feeding behavior[14,19] and, by way of serotonin interactions, inducing satiety.[15] An increase in brain serotonin levels following carbohydrate ingestion is a proposed mechanism by which the macronutrient content of the meal is sensed by the brain.[20] According to this proposal, insulin secretion provoked by a carbohydrate-containing meal decreases the plasma concentration of large neutral amino acids (leucine, valine, isoleucine) that normally compete with tryptophan for active transport across the blood–brain barrier. The increased tryptophan results in increased serotonin production.

The octapeptide of cholecystokinin (CCK-8) is the major form of this peptide in the brain of most species.[21] The hormone appears to be synthesized in both the CNS and peripheral tissue, and both may play a role in the control of eating. Evidence for a central satiety effect comes from lateral ventricular infusion of antibody to CCK, which produces increased feeding in sheep.[21,22] The effects of peripheral cholecystokinin on feeding behavior are considered later.

Insulin's role in appetite control is unclear. Insulin receptors are present in the brain, and the hormone is normally present in the cerebral spinal fluid, although the concentration changes far more slowly than in the plasma.[23] Insulin decreases feeding when administered into the central nervous system or peripherally under conditions that prevent hypoglycemia.[23] Although hypoglycemia stimulates feeding, chronically elevated CNS insulin levels suppress feeding. This observation suggests that insulin may function to provide the brain with information regarding the size of body adipose tissue stores.[23]

Peripheral Factors in Eating Control

From the lips to the colon, the digestive tract functions as a large neurosensory organ to interact with ingested food. Pregastric stimuli (mouth and throat) and hedonic qualities of food (taste, smell, and appearance) contribute to feeding and satiety, but they are not the only important peripheral factors. For example, rats with fistulae preventing ingested food from entering the stomach will eat almost continuously.[15] Gastric distention is an important satiety signal, but the mechanism is controversial. Vagal afferent receptors in the gastric wall as well as humoral mechanisms may be involved.[24] Bombesin is a likely humoral candidate.[24] Studies involving infusion of food into the small intestine of sham-fed animals indicate that there are satiety mechanisms arising distal to the stomach.[24]

The postprandial rise in cholecystokinin may be a satiety signal to the CNS because peripherally administered CCK has a dose-related inhibitory effect on feeding in several species, including humans, both lean and obese. However, convincing evidence for a similar effect of endogenously released CCK has not yet appeared.[25,26] Vagotomy appears to abolish the satiety-inducing effect of exogenously administered CCK in both rats and humans.[25] In one study, patients with bulimia had decreased postprandial plasma cholecystokinin levels as well as subjectively decreased postprandial satiety. Tricyclic antidepressants, which are used to treat bulimia, increase postprandial cholecystokinin levels and subjective satiety.[27] CCK has not been proved in humans to either produce weight loss or inhibit the ingestion of highly palatable foods.[25] Furthermore, no orally active form of the hormone is available.

Psychosocial Factors in Eating Control

Numerous psychosocial factors affect eating, including stress, social influence, palatability, and cognitive calculations. These factors may be of paramount importance because there are observed human feeding behaviors that cannot be explained with the current knowledge regarding physiologic mechanisms of appetite regulation. Stress, for example, is most often considered to be an appetite suppressant. Yet stress often increases food intake in the dieting and nondieting obese individual.[28] Palatability is influenced by both culture and biology and is a powerful factor in feeding behavior. Both variety and palatability of food influence the amount eaten. Thus, the palatability of food influences the experience of hunger, and a highly preferred food can rekindle the desire to eat, even in the period of postprandial satiety.[29] Social factors powerfully influence eating behavior. Thus, individuals often yield to the pressures of an insistent host or ingrained admonitions not to "waste" food and eat despite having no sensation of hunger. Conversely, eating is routinely avoided or delayed despite hunger in situations where it is not socially acceptable to eat. Finally, cognitive considerations combine to make dieters eat virtually independently of hunger and satiety signals. At least for short periods of time, they can override biologic cues to follow prescribed dietary rules designed to alter body weight.

Perhaps Garrow aptly expressed the difficulty of understanding human eating behavior when he wrote, "Even if we knew exactly the neurophysiology of the hypothalamus, and the neural and endocrine signals which it receives, there is little reason to suppose that the effect of these signals would be seen in eating behavior in man after the monstrous bureaucracy of his intellect has scrambled the message."[6]

ENERGY REQUIREMENTS

The study of the interconversion of energy and work is "thermodynamics," from the Greek words for "movement of heat." The first law of thermodynamics establishes that energy can be converted from one form to another but never created or destroyed. The second law codifies the observation that energy always flows from a high potential level to a lower potential level. An extension of the second law is that entropy, a tendency toward disorder and randomness, is always increasing.[30] This randomness to which all spontaneous reactions lead underlies the necessity for living things to burn fuels continuously to preserve order.

We ingest chemical energy in the form of carbohydrates, fats, and proteins and oxidize these compounds primarily to carbon dioxide and water, liberating heat, the most disordered form of energy. Fortunately, a good portion of the chemical energy released from food is temporarily trapped by the body in other forms of chemical energy, largely as high-energy phosphate bonds of adenosine triphosphate (ATP) and other substances. In this easily accessible form, the energy is used to power chemical reactions necessary for life, including everything from the muscular movements of breathing and walking to the transmission of electrical impulses required for thought. In these reactions, the chemical energy of the phosphate bond is also converted to heat.

Measurement of Energy Expenditure

Energy (heat) is measured in kilocalories (kcal) or kilojoules (kJ), the international unit. One kilocalorie is the amount of heat required to raise the temperature of one kilogram of water by one degree centigrade. A kilocalorie is 4.183 kilojoules.

Because energy cannot be created or destroyed, all heat produced by the body is either stored in the body or released. Humans in a steady state maintain a stable mean body temperature within narrow limits; therefore, heat production equals heat loss.[31] Heat production can be measured directly or indirectly. For direct calorimetry, a subject is sealed in an insulated room, and water circulated through pipes in the walls picks up heat produced by the subject. Heat production is calculated from the temperature change and volume of the water.

Indirect calorimetry makes use of the fact that the amount of heat produced when food is oxidized by the body, or burned in a calorimeter, is proportional to the amount of CO_2 produced and O_2 consumed. Therefore, by accurately measuring the volume of O_2 ($\dot{V}O_2$) used and CO_2 ($\dot{V}CO_2$) produced, energy expenditure (EE) can be calculated by use of the modified Weir formula, as follows:

$$EE \text{ (kcals/day)} = [3.9 \, (\dot{V}O_2 \, \text{l/min})$$

$$+ 1.1 \, (\dot{V}CO_2 \, \text{l/min})] \times 1440 \, \text{min/day}^{[32]}$$

If 24-hour urinary nitrogen (UN) is measured, the complete Weir formula can be used to adjust for the fact that humans do not oxidize proteins completely to nitrogen oxides:

EE (kcals/day) = [3.941 ($\dot{V}O_2$ l/min) + 1.106 ($\dot{V}CO_2$ l/min)]

$$\times \; 1440 \; min/day - 2.17 \; UN \; g/day \; ^{33}$$

However, this adjustment seldom changes the calculated energy expenditure by more than 2%.[32,33]

Reliable measurement of energy expenditure by indirect calorimetry requires accurate equipment, an experienced operator, and meticulous attention to detail. Results generally correlate well with direct calorimetry as long as the subject is in steady state.[33-35]

Indirect calorimetry can also be used to estimate the amount of carbohydrate, fat, and protein the body is oxidizing at the time of the measurement. On oxidation, the three substrates yield different ratios of $\dot{V}CO_2$ produced per $\dot{V}O_2$ consumed. This ratio, the respiratory quotient (RQ), is 0.7 for fat and 1.0 for carbohydrate. The RQ for protein can vary from less than 0.75 to more than 0.95, depending on the relative amount of the nitrogen oxidized to creatinine, urea, or ammonia.[36,37] A healthy, nonfasted subject on a typical diet will have an RQ of 0.8 to 0.85.[31] During prolonged fasting, when the fuel being used is predominantly stored fat, the RQ will approach 0.7, and it will reach 1.0 when a healthy subject is given enough carbohydrate to supply total energy needs. When an even larger amount of carbohydrate is given, some is converted to fat. Because this conversion has an RQ of infinity, the combination of carbohydrate oxidation and lipid synthesis at high carbohydrate loads produces an RQ greater than 1.[38,39] If urinary nitrogen is measured and the patient is in steady state, indirect calorimetry permits calculation of the percentage of energy expenditure arising from oxidation of each of the three fuels—carbohydrate, fat, and protein. These calculations are particularly sensitive to errors in measurement of gas volumes as well as other errors.[36,37,39]

In clinical practice, gas exchange for indirect calorimetry is usually measured for a brief period, 5 to 15 minutes, while the patient is resting. Daily energy expenditure is extrapolated from this "snapshot." Although this extrapolation introduces potential error, the resting energy expenditure (REE) thus measured in a resting patient in steady state with regard to substrate oxidation and clinical status is generally considered reliable.[35-37,39] In some research settings, energy expenditure has been measured continuously for hours to days with use of a canopy over the patient's head and continual monitoring of gas exchange.

Doubly labeled water has recently been introduced as a way to measure energy expenditure in free-living subjects over a period of days. The technique is based on the observation that oxygen and hydrogen undergo differential elimination from the body water.[40] When water is labeled with ^2H and ^{18}O, the ^{18}O is eliminated in both carbon dioxide and water, whereas the ^2H is eliminated only in water. The difference between the two elimination rates is proportional to carbon dioxide production. If the RQ is known, based on the composition of ingested food, then $\dot{V}O_2$ can be calculated and energy expenditure can be determined by the Weir formula.[41-44] Improvements in mass spectrometry have made the technique feasible for clinical practice. Despite sources of possible error, including variations in RQ and changes in body water pool size, results appear to be comparable in terms of precision and accuracy to other methods of measuring energy expenditure in healthy subjects as well as in hospitalized patients receiving total parenteral nutrition (TPN).[41-48]

Components of Energy Expenditure

The total energy requirement in humans is the sum of basal energy expenditure (BEE); energy expenditure of activity (EEA); diet-induced thermogenesis (DIT), which was formerly called specific dynamic action of food; and cold-induced thermogenesis (CIT), also known as nonshivering thermogenesis.

BASAL ENERGY EXPENDITURE (BEE) AND RESTING ENERGY EXPENDITURE (REE)

Basal energy expenditure (BEE) is the energy expenditure of an individual who is healthy, at rest mentally and physically 12 to 18 hours after a meal, and in a neutral thermal environment.[6] Conditions for BEE are difficult to meet, and, by definition, they are not possible for sick persons. Resting energy expenditure (REE) is similar to BEE except that measurements are taken 2 to 4 hours after a light meal as opposed to fasting.[6] The term is applied to measurements of energy expenditure in resting patients. In nutrition support literature, the terms *basal energy expenditure (BEE)*, *basal metabolic rate (BMR)*, *basal energy requirement (BER)*, and *resting energy expenditure (REE)* are often used interchangeably. REE accounts for approximately 65% to 70% of daily energy expenditure for most healthy adults.[49] Energy expenditure falls below BEE during sleep and hypotension.

Compared with the euthyroid state, the REE is increased in hyperthyroidism and decreased in hypothyroid states.[36] Other hormones can also increase metabolic rate, including growth hormone, male sex hormones, epinephrine, and norepinephrine.[50] Hypothermia reduces metabolic rate, a fact that is used to advantage during cardiopulmonary bypass. Conversely, the rate increases approximately 12% for each degree centigrade increase in core body temperature. Prolonged fasting or decreased food intake significantly reduces REE out of proportion to the loss of lean body mass. This response has survival advantages when food supplies are limited or sporadic, but it also diminishes the rate at which obese individuals lose weight by fasting or dieting.

Resting energy expenditure decreases slightly with age. The lower fat-free mass as well as the higher incidence of brain dysfunction (the CNS consumes 20% of REE) in the elderly probably account for the decline in REE. In healthy adults with normal physical and mental functioning, age has only minimal if any influence on REE.[11,49] On a weight basis, children have higher metabolic rates because of the energy cost of growth. Higher REEs for men compared with women having similar body weights appear to reflect more lean body weight per kilogram in men, because the influence of sex is negligible if fat-free mass is used to estimate REE.[11,49]

Body surface area, as proposed by Rubner in 1883, does not appear to be the determining factor in resting metabolism. Rather, most authors agree that active body mass approximated by fat-free mass or lean body mass is the proper reference for energy expenditure.[6,11,51,52] Fat-free mass refers to the total mass of the body minus the total mass of fat. Lean body mass is nearly synonymous and refers to the total mass of the body minus the adipose tissue, which is comprised mostly of fat with about 15% water and 2% protein.[11,49] The methods for measuring body composition as well as their advantages and disadvantages are shown in Table

TABLE 21–1
Techniques to Determine Body Composition

	ADVANTAGES	DISADVANTAGES
Density	Apparatus inexpensive	Subject cooperation necessary for underwater weighing technique
	Estimates LBM and fat simultaneously	
	Nonhazardous	Unsuitable for young children, elderly
	Can be repeated frequently	Error from intestinal gas
^{40}K counting	No hazard	Instrument expensive
	Minimal subject cooperation	Proper calibration necessary
	Can be repeated frequently	Problem in interpretation in subjects with K deficiency
Metabolic balance	No hazard	Measures only change in body composition
	Suitable for many elements	Meticulous subject cooperation
	Can detect small changes in body content (<1%)	Metabolic ward expensive
		Error from unmeasured skin losses
		Many laboratory analyses needed
Neutron activation	Minimal subject cooperation	Apparatus very expensive
	Body content Ca, P, N, Na, Cl	Calibration very difficult
		Radiation exposure
Creatinine excretion	No hazard	Meticulous subject cooperation
	Estimate of muscle mass	Influenced by diet, collection time critical
		Day-to-day variation (c.v. 5–10%)
Fat-soluble gases	Direct estimate of body fat	Cyclopropane, xenon, ^{85}Kr
		Apparatus expensive
		Long equilibration time
Dilution methods	Estimate body fluid volumes	Radiation exposure (some materials)
	Inexpensive	Blood samples needed (some materials) (some require several samples)
	Great variety: Na, K, Cl(Br), H$_2$O	
		Incomplete equilibration Na, K; overestimation by D$_2$O, THO; value for ECF depends on method used; 18O assay requires elaborate equipment
Anthropometry	Cheap	Poor precision in obese subjects and in those with firm s.c. tissue
	Direct estimate of body fat, muscle mass	
		Regional variation in subcutaneous fat layer; uncertainty ratio s.c. fat/total fat*
Radiography, photon densitometry	Bone density, volume, muscle widths	Limited regions
		Radiation exposure
CT scan	Organ size, configuration; s.c. fat; intraperitoneal, pericardial fat, bone	Instrument expensive
		Radiation exposure
Ultrasound	Organ size	Poor definition subcutaneous fat layer
	No hazard	
Electrical conductivity (TOBEC)	No hazard	Expensive
Bioelectrical impedance	No hazard	Electrode placement critical
	Inexpensive	

* *This ratio varies from 0.04 to 0.43 among various mammals. There are only two reports for humans: in one newborn infant the ratio was 0.42, and in one adult it was 0.32. Recent observations by CT scan suggest that the ratio of intra-abdominal fat to subcutaneous fat varies considerably in adults.*
(From Forbes GB. Body composition: Influence of nutrition, disease, growth, and aging. In: Shils ME, Young VR, eds. Modern nutrition in health and disease, ed 7. Philadelphia: Lea and Febiger, 1988:533.)

21-1. Even lean body mass is quite heterogeneous in its metabolic requirements. Brain and liver together constitute only 4% to 5% of total body weight yet account for about 40% of REE. Muscle, which usually constitutes 35% to 40% of body weight, is responsible for only 20% of REE.[49]

Because of the importance of REE, numerous methods have been proposed for estimating REE when direct or indirect calorimetry is not practical. A persuasive argument can be made for estimating REE based on total body weight alone. However, large amounts of adipose tissue, because of its small contribution to metabolism on a per unit weight basis, can make estimates based on weight inaccurate. Nevertheless, weight is easily and accurately measured, and the sizes of most body compositional variables (lean body mass, fat-free mass, body surface area, weight) are highly interrelated.[49,53] Furthermore, when combinations of variables are used to estimate REE, they give results comparable to weight alone. Kleiber's law,[54] a popular method for estimating REE based on weight, states that the mean metabolic rate of mammals is 70 times the three-quarter power of body weight:

$$MR = 70 \times weight^{0.75}$$

where MR = metabolic rate in kcal/day.

In clinical practice, REE is most often estimated by the Harris–Benedict equations, which are based on weight, height, age, and sex. These formulas were derived in the early 1900s from indirect calorimetry data on healthy subjects.[55]

$$BEE \ (men) = 66 + (13.7 \times W) + (5 \times H) - (6.8A)$$

$$BEE \ (women) = 655 + (9.5 \times W) + (1.8 \times H) - (4.7A)$$

W = actual or usual weight in kilograms
H = height in centimeters
A = age

ENERGY EXPENDITURE OF ACTIVITY (EEA)

This component of the energy requirement equation varies with body weight and with the duration and intensity of activity. Intense activity can raise energy expenditure to more than 15-fold above resting levels. Activity usually constitutes 25% to 30% of total daily energy expenditure. The net metabolic cost of exercise is the gross cost minus the cost of whatever else the individual would have been doing if not exercising.[6] For example, if a 200-pound man runs 5.5 miles in 1 hour, he has expended 850 calories. Sitting or standing, he still would have used about 120 calories over that time period. Hence, the true net energy expenditure from the exercise was about 730 calories. For hospitalized patients, it is common practice to add 20% of BEE for EEA for bed-bound patients and 30% for ambulatory patients.[56]

DIET-INDUCED THERMOGENESIS

Diet-induced thermogenesis (DIT), also called specific dynamic action (SDA) and thermic effect of food (TEF), describes the heat generated after eating in excess of basal metabolism. The effect is also observed after intravenous administration of nutrients and reflects the combined energy cost of transport, metabolism, and storage as well as digestion and absorption of nutrients. The absolute magnitude of DIT increases as meal size (kcals) increases. The magnitude of DIT as a percentage of ingested calories varies with the nutrient ingested and the state of the subject. Normally, DIT consumes 12% to 20% of the energy in ingested protein, 6% to 12% of carbohydrate energy, 2% to 3% of fat energy, and about 6% to 10% of the total energy in a typical American diet. The percentage is less in individuals who are hypermetabolic, fasting, or obese. The contribution of DIT can safely be ignored in most hospitalized patients.[32,57] The lower energy cost of assimilating

fat versus carbohydrate and protein gives rise to the concept that a fat calorie is more fattening than a carbohydrate or protein calorie.

The concept of diet-induced thermogenesis bears on body weight regulation in yet another way. It is useful to consider that DIT consists of an obligatory component, described above, and an adaptive component. The adaptive component, which is more theoretic and controversial, is a proposed mechanism by which mammals can "waste" excess energy in order to maintain a constant body weight despite fluctuating amounts of energy intake,[58] a concept initially called "luxus consumption." Why should such a "wasteful" system as adaptive DIT evolve? Rothwell and Stock propose that adaptive DIT allows an animal to consume large quantities of poor-quality foods, for example foods low in protein, and dispose of excess energy while obtaining sufficient protein or other essential nutrients.[59] It has been proposed that heat production for both adaptive DIT and cold-induced thermogenesis involves brown adipose tissue and skeletal muscle.[60]

COLD-INDUCED THERMOGENESIS (CIT)

Mammals exposed to cold increase their heat production by increasing muscle activity (shivering thermogenesis) and by a non-shivering thermogenic mechanism (CIT) that eventually obviates the need for shivering.[36] Possibly, CIT and adaptive DIT depend on the unique properties of brown fat, which is anatomically discrete and readily identified in some mammals. In humans, brown fat is dispersed, and the amount is uncertain but probably significant. The mitochondria of brown fat possess the unique potential for uncoupling ATP synthesis from respiration. Proposed mechanisms for this involve increased proton conductance of the inner mitochondrial membrane.[61] Because the formation of ATP is uncoupled, the rate at which substrates can be oxidized is not dependent on the availability of ADP precursor. Hence, the reaction can continue at high rates, generating large amounts of heat.[61] Other tissues, especially skeletal muscle, may also play a role in CIT and adaptive DIT.

Energy Sources

Energy balance studies show that normal humans can extract 9 kcal of energy per gram of dietary fat, 4 kcal/g of fiber-free dietary carbohydrates, and 4 kcal/g of dietary protein. Bomb calorimetry of the same nutrients gives somewhat greater values, especially for proteins. This is because humans do not absorb and retain 100% of ingested nutrients and cannot oxidize the nitrogen in protein completely. The amount of energy supplied by a specific pure fat, carbohydrate, or protein may differ substantially from the averages above. Thus, pure glucose yields 3.7 kcal/g, while the dextrose used clinically, which is hydrated glucose, yields 3.4 kcal/g. Because dietary fiber is by definition not digestible, it is considered to provide no calories. This concept must be modified based on new evidence that short-chain fatty acids produced from dietary fiber by the activity of colonic bacteria are absorbed and used for energy.[62] Normally, humans derive energy principally from carbohydrates and fats.

Glucose has been the obvious choice for an intravenous calorie source because of its well-understood metabolism[63] and early studies demonstrating a protein-sparing effect.[64] The introduction of safe intravenous fat emulsions, now available in 10% and 20% concentrations, has permitted administration of a more balanced intravenous calorie supply as well as prevention of essential fatty acid deficiency. Other lipids are being investigated for intravenous use, including medium-chain triglycerides (MCT), mixtures of MCT and long-chain lipids, and structured lipids in which each triglyceride molecule contains fatty acids of two or three different chain lengths. These products may prevent some of the potentially harmful effects of current lipid emulsion, such as immune suppression and reticuloendothelial system blockade (see section on Lipids in Nutritional Support). Other intravenous energy sources have been tried and rejected, including fructose and the alcohols: ethanol, sorbitol, and xylitol.[63]

Estimation of Energy Requirements

When an individual's caloric intake maintains a steady weight, he or she is said to be in energy balance. A calorie excess is reflected in weight gain, primarily as adipose tissue (approximately 1 pound per 3500 excess kilocalories), and caloric insufficiency is manifested as weight loss.

To estimate total daily energy requirements of healthy individuals, the previously described formula can be employed (energy expenditure = REE + EEA + DIT + CIT). The REE (resting energy expenditure) and EEA (energy expenditure of activity) can be estimated as described previously on the basis of published tables.[57] DIT (diet-induced thermogenesis) can be estimated at 10% of REE CIT (cold-induced thermogenesis) will be negligible for healthy individuals in temperate environments.

For patients, an additional factor, the energy expenditure of stress, may have to be added to the right side of the energy equation above. Stresses such as bone fractures, fever, and inflammation increase heat production. This may be partially offset by decreased activity (EEA) and food intake (DIT).[57] Many guidelines for estimating energy requirements of patients have been published, but the results do not correlate well with actual measurements of energy expenditure.[65–67] The specifics of changes in metabolism and energy requirements with stress will be discussed later in this chapter. The practical aspects of determining energy goals for patients are discussed in Chapter 48.

PROTEIN REQUIREMENTS

Proteins constitute nearly 16% of human body weight, and nitrogen makes up 2.6% of body weight.[64] Proteins are functionally diverse, serving as enzymes, carriers, receptors, and hormones, as well as serving important roles in immunity, blood coagulation, and structure. Body proteins have widely different half-lives and fractional turnover rates. This great diversity is determined by the sequence of up to 22 amino acids joined by peptide bonds in the protein polymer. The sequence determines the location of sites for covalent attachment of carbohydrate and ultimately the protein's three-dimensional configuration and specific function.

Amino acids are present in the body as components of proteins and in free amino acid pools. The free amino acids are in a dynamic state with those becoming incorporated into tissue proteins, undergoing catabolic reactions, and being used for the synthesis of other nitrogen-containing compounds such as purine bases.[68] When tissue protein undergoes breakdown, the amino acid may be returned to the free pool (Fig 21-1).[8]

Protein Quality

Among the great variety of dietary proteins, some support homeostasis and growth better than others. These differences in protein "quality" derive from several characteristics, most importantly the amino acid content. Nonessential amino acids are those whose corresponding keto acids can be synthesized by the body, which then converts them to the amino acid, usually during the course of carbohydrate metabolism. Hence, it is not essential that these amino acids be consumed in the diet. Essential amino acids must be consumed in the diet because the keto acids from which they are made cannot be synthesized by the body. The eight amino acids essential for healthy adult humans are phenylalanine, tryptophan, leucine, isoleucine, lysine, threonine, valine, and methionine.[64,69] The nutritional quality of a protein is dependent on its content of essential amino acids.

Many in vitro and in vivo indices have been designed to describe the quality of a protein. The "chemical score" or "amino acid score" is based on comparing the protein in question to an "ideal" protein whose amino acid composition provides all essential amino acids in optimal concentrations. The essential amino acid concentrations in one gram of any given protein source can be compared to the ideal protein and expressed as percentages. The "limiting amino acid," that essential amino acid present in the lowest percentage compared to the "ideal protein," determines the protein's "chemical score."[68]

All protein sources are not equally well absorbed. True digestibility, equivalent to absorption, is the percent of ingested protein nitrogen absorbed after subtracting from fecal nitrogen the amount excreted on a protein-free diet. True digestibility ranges from 97% to 99% for the protein in meat, milk, and eggs to 75% for the protein in potatoes and navy beans.[70,71]

The biologic value of a protein is the percent of absorbed nitrogen that is retained for growth and maintenance. The range is broad (e.g., 94% for egg protein and 42% for wheat gluten).[65,70,71] The bioavailability of a protein can be affected by the usual method of preparation. For example, some lysine is lost by heating in the presence of reducing sugars, and oxidation of a protein with sulfur dioxide can cause loss of methionine. Lysine and cysteine residues may react when exposed to alkali treatment, forming lysinoalanine, which is toxic.[68] Food preparation can also enhance bioavailability, as exemplified by the inactivation by heating of trypsin inhibitor, naturally present in soybeans.[72] The proteins of egg, milk, fish, red meat, and poultry are high in biologic value.

Because mammals have no capability of storing amino acids for later use, it is necessary to ingest all of the amino acids required for protein synthesis nearly simultaneously, but not necessarily at the same meal. In this regard, it is noteworthy that combinations of foods have developed that commonly combine either low- and high-quality proteins (e.g., cereal and milk) or two "incomplete" protein sources that then supply all the amino acids necessary for protein synthesis (e.g., rice and beans or rice and fish).

MAMMALIAN PROTEIN METABOLISM

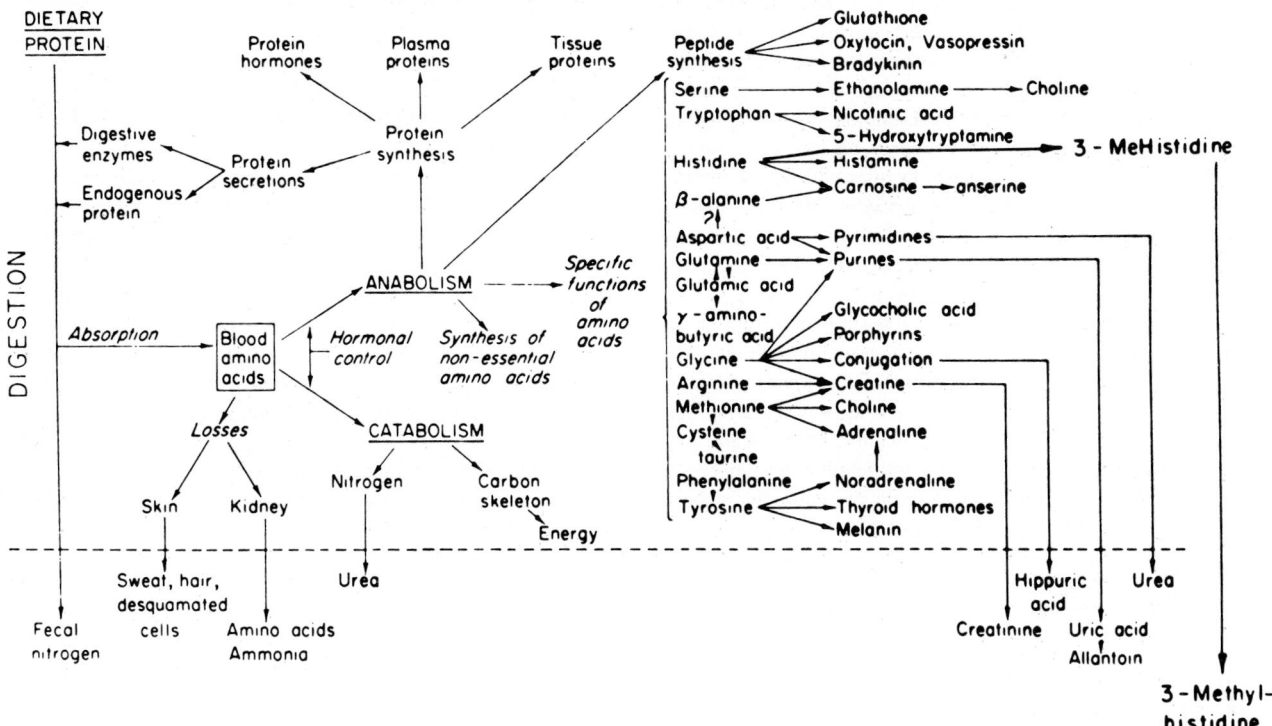

FIGURE 21–1. General features of mammalian protein metabolism. (Munro HN. An introduction to biochemical aspects of protein metabolism. In: Munro HN, Allison JB, eds. Mammalian Protein Metabolism. New York: Academic Press, 1964:32.)

Nitrogen Losses

Each type of body protein is in a state of constant flux, some molecules being degraded while new ones are forming. Normal daily protein turnover is 1% to 2% of total body protein and results largely from the degradation of muscle protein. Most of the amino acids released are reused for synthesis of new proteins, while most of the remaining amino acids are transaminated and the resulting carbon skeletons oxidized as a calorie source. The nitrogen is excreted as nitrogenous wastes primarily in the urine in the form of urea, creatinine, porphyrins, ammonia, and uric acid. The relative proportions of these compounds vary with protein and calorie intake, but normally urea accounts for approximately 80% of urinary nitrogen. For a healthy person with no nitrogen intake, urinary nitrogen will reach a low level of approximately 2 mg per kcal of BEE or about 37 mg/kg body weight.

Fecal nitrogen losses result from unabsorbed dietary protein as well as the proteins that are not reabsorbed from intestinal secretions and shedding. The amount of endogenous protein that normally enters the intestinal lumen is approximately 50 g/day, but estimates vary from 25 to 200 g/day. Mucosal shedding accounts for most of this, followed in decreasing order by pancreatic juice, gastric juice, saliva, and bile. Absorption of both exogenous and endogenous protein is so efficient that fecal nitrogen is only 1 to 2 g/day in the absence of decreased absorption or abnormal secretion by the intestine. Other sources of nitrogen loss include intact skin, 0.3 g/day, and minor losses from nasal secretions, semen, menstrual fluid, and hair cuttings. Therefore, in addition to urinary losses, a total of 1 to 3 g/day of nitrogen is lost from

fecal and other sources.[57] Several factors may increase nitrogen losses, including strenuous physical activity, cold exposure, protein-losing diseases of the kidney and intestinal tract, and the elevated metabolic rate associated with disease processes.[31]

Nitrogen Balance

Nitrogen balance is the difference between intake and output. It is a useful measurement, although it gives no indications of the rates of synthesis or degradation of body proteins. If nitrogen balance is positive, then retention exceeds loss, and this implies new growth or replacement of wasted body protein. One gram of nitrogen is the equivalent of approximately 30 grams of hydrated lean body mass. Unlike fat and carbohydrate, amino acids consumed in excess are not stored. Instead, the carbon skeletons are burned as fuel and the amino groups excreted as nitrogenous waste. Negative nitrogen balance is an indication that protein catabolism exceeds anabolism. It may occur when poor-quality protein is ingested for a long period of time, when calorie or protein intake is substantially below normal, and when stress hypercatabolism is severe. Most healthy adults are in nitrogen equilibrium in which absorbed nitrogen equals excreted nitrogen. Slight positive nitrogen balance occurs with weight gain (e.g., after an illness or with cessation of dieting). As a general rule, well-nourished adults do not attain a positive nitrogen balance without an increase in adipose tissue,[68] but successful body builders are undoubtedly exceptions to this rule. Any weight loss that is not entirely attributable to fluid loss is accompanied by negative nitrogen balance.

Nitrogen balance is very dependent on energy intake as well as protein intake,[68] partly reflecting the fact that formation of a peptide bond requires hydrolysis of three high-energy phosphate bonds.[57] The relationships between nitrogen balance and the intake of energy and protein are influenced by several factors, including the subject's age, health, and nutritional state and the calorie source. It has been stated that a positive energy balance (i.e., subject getting more calories than he or she is burning) of about 2 calories per kilogram per day is required for a positive nitrogen balance. However, it has been shown that when adequate amino acids are infused, hospitalized patients can achieve positive nitrogen balance while they remain in negative energy balance.[73]

Most normal adults can maintain nitrogen equilibrium by ingesting 0.5 g/kg body weight/day of high-quality protein. The range of recommended intake for adults is 0.5 g/kg/day (WHO/FAO/UNU Committee, 1985)[68,74] to 0.8 g/kg/day (National Research Council RDA, 1989).[75,76] The recommended amounts include a margin of safety that is estimated to allow for a decrease in efficiency of nitrogen utilization from egg protein at levels above

3 g of nitrogen per day and for the fact that average dietary protein has only 75% of the biologic value of egg protein.[68,77]

Conditions Requiring Increased Protein

Infancy is a time of intense growth, and, accordingly, protein requirements per unit body weight are increased compared with the adult. The normal infant also requires a higher proportion of essential to nonessential amino acids.[78] The growth spurt of adolescence, the only extrauterine time that growth velocity increases, occurs between ages 10 and 13 for American females and ages 12 and 15 for American males and contributes about 15% of final adult height and 50% of adult weight.[79] Guidelines for protein and calorie needs in infancy, childhood, and adolescence are summarized in Table 21-2.

The nutritional demands of a normal pregnancy average 80,000 kilocalories (300 kcal/day) and 950 g of protein (3.5 g/day).[80]

TABLE 21–2
Recommended Allowances of Reference Protein and U.S. Dietary Protein

CATEGORY	AGE (YEARS) OR CONDITION	WEIGHT (KG)	DERIVED ALLOWANCE OF REFERENCE PROTEIN* (g/kg)	(g/day)	RECOMMENDED DIETARY ALLOWANCE (g/kg)†	(g/day)	AVERAGE ENERGY ALLOWANCE (KCAL)§ Multiples of REE	Per kg	Per Day‖
Both sexes	0–0.5	6	2.20‡		2.2	13		108	650
	0.5–1	9	1.56		1.6	14		98	850
	1–3	13	1.14		1.2	16		102	1300
	4–6	20	1.03		1.1	24		90	1800
	7–10	28	1.00		1.0	28		70	2000
Males	11–14	45	0.98		1.0	45	1.70	55	2500
	15–18	66	0.86		0.9	59	1.67	45	3000
	19–24	72	0.75		0.8	58	1.67	40	2900
	25–50	79	0.75		0.8	63	1.60	37	2900
	51+	77	0.75		0.8	63	1.50	30	2300
Females	11–14	46	0.94		1.0	46	1.67	47	2200
	15–18	55	0.81		0.8	44	1.60	40	2200
	19–24	58	0.75		0.8	46	1.60	38	2200
	25–50	63	0.75		0.8	50	1.55	36	2200
	51+	65	0.75		0.8	50	1.50	30	1900
Pregnancy	1st trimester			+1.3		+10			+0
	2nd trimester			+6.1		+10			+300
	3rd trimester			+10.7		+10			+300
Lactation	1st 6 months			+14.7		+15			+500
	2nd 6 months			+11.8		+12			+500

* *Data from WHO (1985).*
† *Amino acid score of typical U.S. diet is 100 for all age groups, except young infants. Digestibility is equal to reference proteins. Values have been rounded upward to 0.1 g/kg.*
‡ *For infants 0 to 3 months of age, breastfeeding that meets energy needs also meets protein needs. Formula substitutes should have the same amount and amino acid composition as human milk, corrected for digestibility if appropriate.*
§ *In the range of light to moderate activity, the coefficient of variation is ±20%.*
‖ *Figure is rounded.*
(Adapted from Recommended dietary allowances, ed 10. Washington, DC: National Academy Press, 1989.)

The U.S. National Research Council's Recommended Dietary Allowances (RDA) for protein during pregnancy are 60 g/day, representing a 10 g/day increase over the RDA for nonpregnant women ages 25 and above.[75]

For lactating women over age 25 averaging 850 ml of milk output daily, a protein intake of 65 g/day in the first 6 months and 62 g/day in the second 6 months are recommended by the National Research Council.[75] Slightly lower values are recommended for younger women.[75] The increased protein requirements with stress are discussed later in this chapter, and practical aspects of determining protein goals for patients are discussed in Chapter 48.

VITAMIN AND MINERAL REQUIREMENTS

Vitamins

Vitamins, organic compounds required for normal metabolism, cannot be synthesized by the body in quantities required for growth and maintenance and must be obtained in the diet or by specific supplementation. They are required in only microgram or milligram quantities, which is consistent with their general role as catalysts.

Vitamins are conveniently divided into water-soluble and fat-soluble groups. In contrast to fat-soluble vitamins (A,D,E, and K), the water-soluble vitamins are not associated with dietary lipids, and most are not stored in the body in large quantities. This predisposes humans to earlier development of deficiency states of the water-soluble vitamins. The water-soluble vitamins generally contain nitrogen and are components of coenzymes.[64] They encompass Vitamin C and the B-complex group. The B-complex group can be classified into three subgroups: (1) energy-releasing (thiamine, niacin, riboflavin, pantothenic acid, biotin), (2) hematopoietic (folate and Vitamin B_{12}), and (3) other (pyridoxine).

Minerals

Essential mineral elements can be defined as inorganic nutrients that have demonstrable functions in living organisms. To be classified as essential, a mineral should meet several criteria: (1) it is present in the healthy tissues of different living things at comparable concentrations, (2) withdrawal of the element leads to reproducible abnormalities of physiology and/or structure, (3) the abnormalities are associated with a specific biochemical change that is prevented and/or cured by providing the nutrient.[81,82] High toxicity does not preclude essentiality but may delay recognition of an element's essential nature, as in the case of fluoride and selenium.[82] As knowledge of physiology and nutrition expands along with increases in sensitivity and accuracy of analytic methods, the list of essential elements should continue to grow and possibly encompass some elements currently regarded as "contaminants."

Essential macrominerals, required in quantities of >100 mg per day, include sodium, potassium, chloride, calcium, phosphorus, magnesium, and sulfur. The essential microminerals needed in quantities much smaller than 100 mg per day include iron, copper, fluoride, iodine, cobalt, zinc, manganese, molybdenum, and chromium. Possible essential microminerals include tin, nickel, silicon, selenium, and vanadium. Listed as trace contaminants, but not excluded as essential, are lead, cadmium, mercury, arsenic, strontium, boron, aluminum, and lithium.

The essential microminerals serve as required cofactors for vital metalloenzymes. They are present at tissue concentrations as low as 10^{-9} M, yet they are required for life. The relative abundance of elements in living organisms tends to reflect the relative amounts of the elements in the oceans more closely than those in the earth's crust, an observation with possible evolutionary implications.[82]

The absorption and metabolism of vitamins and minerals is further discussed in Chapter 20. Management of deficiencies is discussed in Chapter 48.

The Recommended Dietary Allowances (RDA)

The Recommended Dietary Allowances (RDA) are recommendations that have been published by the Food and Nutrition Board since 1941. They are defined as "the levels of intake of essential nutrients that on the basis of scientific knowledge are judged by the Food and Nutrition Board to be adequate to meet the known nutritional needs of practically all healthy persons."[75] These recommendations are followed in setting policy for a wide range of programs, including school lunches, clinical dietetics, menu planning and food procurements, food programs, food labeling, and food and nutrition information and education. The last published recommendations are from 1989.[75]

The RDAs, which are intended for healthy populations, are higher than required for the average healthy individual in order to provide a margin of safety for population variability, but they may be lower than required for patients who are sick or depleted. The recommendations provide amounts to ensure against clinical deficiency. They do not state an ideal or optimum level of intake, although future recommendations may do so.

The RDAs (Recommended Dietary Allowances) are distinct from the U.S. RDAs (Recommended Daily Allowances), which are formulated by the U.S. Food and Drug Administration and are based on the highest amount of each nutrient recommended by the 1968 RDA from the Food and Nutrition Board.[57] The U.S. RDA is defined for people over age 4 who are not pregnant or lactating and is used for food labels.

ENERGY METABOLISM—PATHWAYS AND REGULATION

Living organisms require a continuous supply of energy from their environment to power reactions necessary for maintenance, movement, and growth. The reactions by which the chemical energy in fat, carbohydrate, and protein is liberated by oxidation and captured constitute many of the pathways of intermediary metabolism.

Part of the energy released by the oxidation of foodstuffs is trapped by linking these reactions to the formation of high-energy phosphate bonds, primarily ATP, the principal energy currency of biologic systems. ATP turns over rapidly because it is continuously formed and immediately used to power in vivo energy-requiring (endergonic) reactions. It is not used as a depot for energy storage; in fact, it would take over 600 kg of ATP to store the energy equivalent to 1 kg of fat.[49]

Carbohydrates and fats are the major substrates for energy production, with proteins making a small contribution. Following hydrolysis of carbohydrates to simple sugars, fats to fatty acids and glycerol, and proteins to amino acids, most of these small molecules are converted to the acetyl unit of acetyl CoA, generating a small amount of ATP in the process. Thus, acetyl CoA is a common breakdown product of the three macronutrients. Acetyl CoA, carrying most of the chemical energy of the original macronutrients, enters the citric acid cycle and oxidative phosphorylation, which are the final common pathways in the oxidation of food molecules (Fig 21-2).[2] Many amino acids enter the citric acid cycle as alpha-ketoglutarate or oxaloacetate rather than as acetyl CoA.

Carbohydrate Metabolism

Carbohydrates, which constitute most of earth's organic matter, are important sources of metabolic fuel. In the U.S., carbohydrates normally account for about 50% of ingested calories. Approximately 60% of this is complex carbohydrate, primarily starch, and most of the rest is sucrose and lactose.[49] They all undergo hydrolysis to yield glucose and other simple sugars. Most cells can metabolize

glucose irreversibly to carbon dioxide and water with the release of energy. Erythrocytes are a major exception because they do not possess the mitochondria necessary to proceed beyond the anaerobic catabolism of glucose. Nevertheless, glucose is essential for erythrocytes. These cells and the brain normally use about 40 and 140 g of glucose per day, respectively.[83]

Humans store carbohydrate in the form of glycogen, a branching, long-chain polymer of glucose molecules with water and electrolytes between the chains. It is found in most tissues but stored to a significant degree only in the liver and skeletal muscle. Because of its water content, glycogen is an inefficient and quantitatively insignificant form of energy storage, yielding about 1 kcal per gram. Rather, the primary function of glycogen in the liver, about 150 g in a normal adult, is to serve as a ready source of glucose for maintaining blood glucose levels. This is essential to the health of glucose-dependent tissues between meals and during exercise. The glycogen in skeletal muscle cells serves as a glucose supply for the muscle cell's own energy needs and not for maintenance of blood glucose levels. The "altruistic" export of glucose from the liver's glycogen supply is dependent on the enzyme glucose-6-phosphatase, not present in muscle or brain, which cleaves phosphorus from the phosphorylated glucose molecule, enabling glucose to leave the cell.[2] The muscle can indirectly contribute to blood glucose by release of lactate, pyruvate, and glucogenic amino acids, which can be converted to glucose in the liver and kidney by the process of gluconeogenesis.

GLYCOLYSIS

Glycolysis is a nearly universal pathway by which glucose is converted to pyruvate with concomitant production of ATP. This vital sequence of reactions takes place in the cytosol and does not require oxygen. The process grosses four ATPs and nets two ATPs per molecule of glucose. The pyruvate generated is a major metabolic junction (Fig 21-3). Under anaerobic conditions, pyruvate can be reduced to lactate with concomitant oxidation of NADH to NAD^+. It can also be transaminated to form the amino acid alanine. Because this reaction is reversible, it serves as a route by which amino acids can enter other pathways. Pyruvate can enter the mitochondria and undergo carboxylation to oxaloacetate, one of the intermediates in the Krebs cycle. Finally, pyruvate can undergo oxidative decarboxylation to acetyl CoA, which has several possible fates as well (Fig 21-3).[2] Thiamine is a necessary coenzyme in this reaction that is catalyzed by the pyruvate dehydrogenase complex. Also, the vitamin pantothenic acid is a component of the acyl carrier protein CoA.

Hormones interact to regulate the glycolytic pathway as well as the other components of carbohydrate metabolism. Glucagon has an inhibitory effect on glycolysis by decreasing the concentration of fructose-2,6,-bisphosphate.[84,85] Insulin accelerates glycolysis in the liver, thereby increasing acetyl CoA, a precursor for fatty acid synthesis. Insulin's main hepatic action opposes the hyperglycemic effect of glucagon on the liver.[85,86]

THE CITRIC ACID CYCLE

The citric acid cycle (tricarboxylic acid cycle, Krebs cycle), a series of reactions in the mitochondria, is the final common pathway

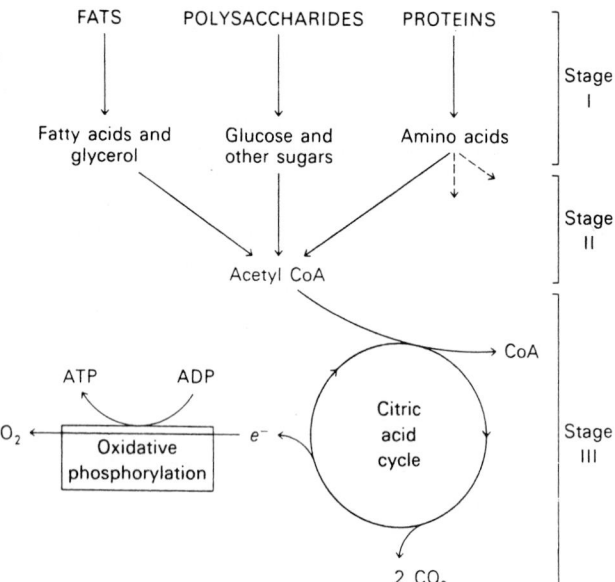

FIGURE 21–2. Stages in the extraction of energy from foodstuffs. (Stryer L. Biochemistry, ed 3, p 325. New York: WH Freeman, 1988. Reprinted with permission.)

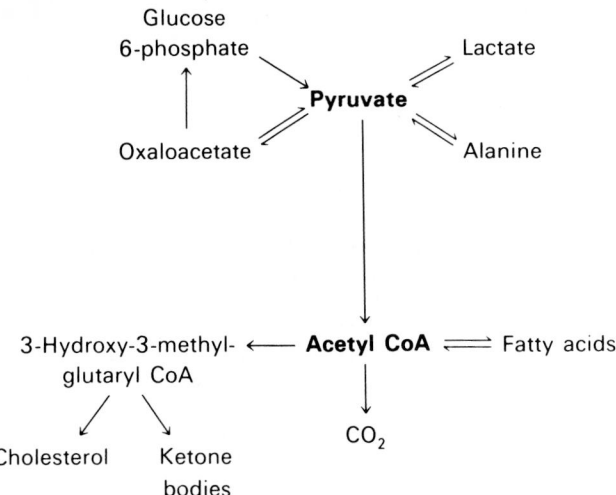

FIGURE 21-3. Major metabolic fates of pyruvate and acetyl CoA in mammals. (Stryer L. Biochemistry, ed 3, p 633. New York: WH Freeman, 1988. Reprinted with permission.)

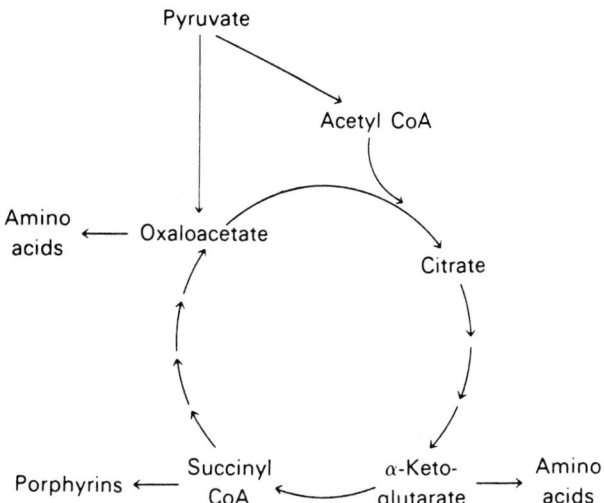

FIGURE 21-4. Biosynthetic roles of the citric acid cycle. Intermediates drawn off for biosyntheses (shown by dashed arrows) are replenished by the formation of oxaloacetate from pyruvate. (Stryer L. Biochemistry, ed 3, p 387. New York: WH Freeman, 1988. Reprinted with permission.)

for the oxidation of fuel molecules. Carbohydrates, lipids, and some amino acids enter the cycle after being metabolized to acetyl CoA, which is then completely oxidized to carbon dioxide. Vital biosynthetic intermediates are produced by the cycle, and it plays a major role in gluconeogenesis, lipogenesis, and amino acid transamination and deamination. The cycle runs only under aerobic conditions. As acetyl CoA is oxidized, electrons are transferred to form NADH and $FADH_2$, which in turn transfer the electrons to the respiratory chain in the inner mitochondrial membrane, generating ATP in the process. The vitamins riboflavin and niacin are important components of $FADH_2$ and NADH, respectively. Thiamine is required for alpha-ketoglutarate dehydrogenase function.

While glycolysis (anaerobic respiration) yields a net of only two ATPs per molecule of glucose, aerobic metabolism (citric acid cycle and oxidative phosphorylation) yields 36 ATPs for each molecule of glucose oxidized. Because the main function of the citric acid cycle is energy production, it is not surprising that the cycle rate is dependent on the cell's requirement for ATP. Key enzymes, including citrate synthase, isocitrate dehydrogenase, and alpha-ketoglutarate dehydrogenase, are activated by substances that signify a low energy state, such as adenosine diphosphate (ADP), NAD^+, and FAD.

The citric acid cycle also provides valuable intermediates for the biosynthesis of amino acids and porphyrins (Fig 21-4). Under conditions of oxaloacetic acid use for amino acid biosynthesis, the pyruvate carboxylase reaction that generates oxaloacetic acid from pyruvate replenishes oxaloacetic acid for continued cycle operation.[2]

OXIDATIVE PHOSPHORYLATION

Mitochondria perform the vital function of coupling transfers of high-energy electrons to the generation of ATP from ADP and inorganic phosphate, a process known as oxidative phosphorylation. The process is carried out by respiratory assemblies located in the inner mitochondrial membrane. Briefly stated, electrons from

NADH or $FADH_2$ flow through the chain in stepwise manner from relatively electronegative components to oxygen, which serves as the final electron receptor. Electron carriers contained in the assemblies include the cytochromes, a class of iron-containing hemoproteins (Fig 21-5). As electrons are transferred down the chain, protons are pumped out of the mitochondria, generating a transmembrane electric potential. It is the return flow of protons into the mitochondrial matrix that allows for the synthesis of ATP by the phosphorylation of ADP.[2] The most important determinant of the rate of oxidative phosphorylation is the level of ADP. Higher levels signify low energy levels and the need for ATP synthesis.[2]

GLUCONEOGENESIS

Gluconeogenesis is the synthesis of glucose from noncarbohydrate precursors. It occurs primarily in the liver, but the kidneys can produce glucose at about 10% of the hepatic rate. Precursors for gluconeogenesis are lactate from anaerobically contracting muscles and from erythrocytes, glycerol from adipose tissue, and some amino acids derived from dietary protein or lean body mass catabolism. The reactions of gluconeogenesis take place partly in the mitochondria and partly in the cytosol and use six high-energy phosphate bonds to synthesize one glucose molecule from two molecules of pyruvate.

The mitochondrial enzyme pyruvate carboxylase, which forms oxaloacetate from pyruvate, is a key control point in that it is activated by acetyl CoA, another product of pyruvate metabolism (see Fig 21-3). Therefore, when there is sufficient acetyl CoA for energy production by way of the citric acid cycle and oxidative phosphorylation, pyruvate may be converted to oxaloacetic acid for gluconeogenesis. Oxaloacetate that is synthesized in the mitochondria cannot traverse the mitochondrial membrane. However, in the presence of sufficient ATP it is converted to malate, which is transported to the cytosol, reconverted to oxaloacetate, and used for gluconeogenesis. Pyruvate carboxylase is bound to biotin, a B

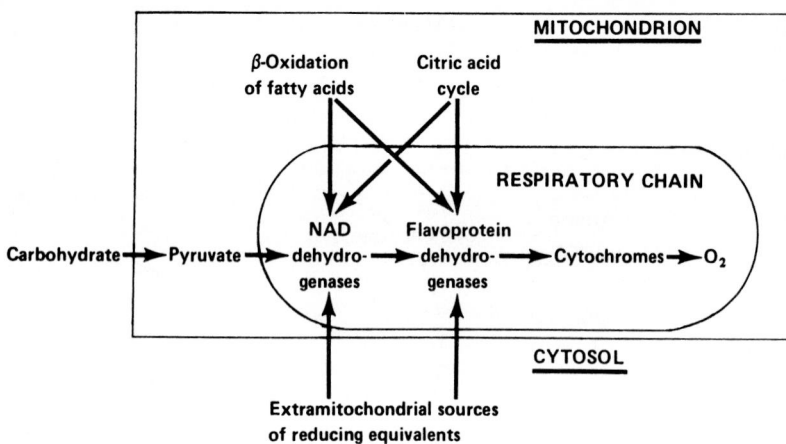

FIGURE 21–5. The major sources of reducing equivalents and their relationship to the mitochondrial respiratory chain. The main extramitochondrial source is NADH formed in glycolysis. (Mayes PA. Oxidative phosphorylation and mitochondrial transport systems. In: Murray RK, Granner DK, Mayes PA, Rodwell VW, eds. Harper's biochemistry, ed 21. Norwalk, CT: Appleton & Lange, 1988:108.)

vitamin that is essential for transferring carbon dioxide (from bicarbonate) to pyruvate. Thus, gluconeogenesis from lactate requires niacin and biotin, whereas gluconeogenesis from amino acids requires niacin and Vitamin B_6.

The enzymes of the gluconeogenesis pathway are regulated in a reciprocal fashion to the enzymes of the glycolytic pathway. In general, the enzymes for gluconeogenesis are active when cellular energy is high and ATP is abundant, while glycolytic enzymes are active when glucose is abundant.[85,86] Gluconeogenesis is stimulated directly or indirectly by glucagon, glucocorticoids, catecholamines, decreased insulin levels, and increases in precursors, such as lactate, amino acids, and glycerol.

CORI CYCLE

The Cori cycle is a mechanism by which part of the burden for supplying energy to vigorously exercising muscle is shifted to the liver (Fig 21–6). Skeletal muscle contracting under anaerobic conditions develops an excess of NADH because of the lack of oxygen, which serves as the ultimate acceptor of high-energy electrons. In order for glycolysis to continue, an alternative to oxidative phosphorylation is required to regenerate NAD^+ from NADH. This is accomplished by the action of lactate dehydrogenase, which catalyzes the reduction of pyruvate to lactate and the concomitant oxidation of NADH to NAD^+. Lactic acid, which is a metabolic dead end and must be oxidized back to pyruvate in order to be metabolized further, diffuses into the blood and is oxidized primarily in the liver to pyruvate. In the liver, pyruvate is reconverted

to glucose by the energy-requiring gluconeogenic pathway, and the glucose may be exported for use again by skeletal muscle. The operation of this cycle in cancerous tissue is wasteful of energy, and it is referred to as a futile cycle.

PROTEIN METABOLISM

Intracellular Proteolysis

The hydrolysis of intracellular proteins is a complex, highly regulated process that is not well understood. Intracellular proteases play an essential role in normal protein catabolism and in the accelerated proteolysis that occurs during infection, trauma, and other stress. They also function to degrade foreign protein ingested by the cell, abnormal protein made in the cell, and enzymes.[87–89] Although lysosomal proteases (cathepsins) are the most thoroughly characterized, significant proteolysis occurs in many cellular compartments, including plasma membranes, mitochondria, and the cytosol.[88,90] ATP-dependent protease systems have been identified and may be important for hydrolysis of muscle protein.[91] In one, ATP is required to conjugate ubiquitin to specific proteins, and only ubiquitin-conjugated substrates are degraded by the system.[90,91] Other proteases require ATP as an allosteric activator.[90] Amino acids released by intracellular proteolysis may be reused for protein synthesis or further metabolized.

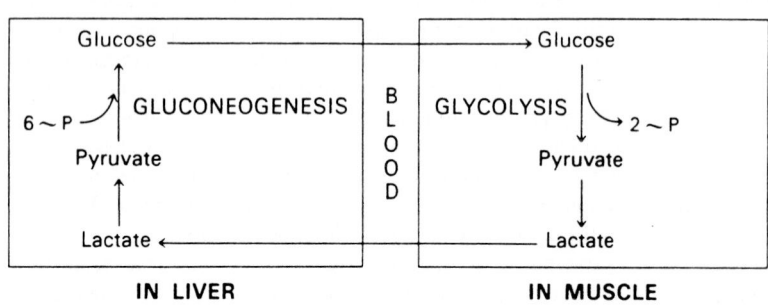

FIGURE 21–6. The Cori cycle. Lactate formed by active muscle is converted into glucose by the liver. This cycle shifts part of the metabolic burden of active muscle to the liver. (Stryer L. Biochemistry, ed 3, p 445. New York: WH Freeman, 1988. Reprinted with permission.)

Amino Acid Degradation

Amino acids that are not used for protein synthesis are deaminated. Their carbon skeletons are transformed into citric acid cycle intermediates and oxidized for energy or used for synthesis of glucose, ketone bodies, or fatty acids.[2] Amino acids can be categorized according to the fates of their carbon skeletons after deamination. Glucogenic amino acids are degraded to products that may be used for glucose synthesis. The ketogenic amino acids are degraded to acetyl CoA or acetoacetyl CoA, which give rise to ketone bodies. Glucoketogenic amino acids can follow either pathway.[2]

The nitrogen of degraded amino acids is converted to urea by way of a series of steps, including transamination, oxidative deamination, and the urea cycle. Aminotransferases (transaminases) catalyze the transfer of an amino group from an amino acid to a ketoacid to form a different ketoacid and amino acid. The prosthetic group pyridoxal phosphate derived from pyridoxine (Vitamin B_6) is vital to the function of all aminotransferases.[2] Glutamate transferases transfer the nitrogen of amino acids to alpha-ketoglutarate to form glutamate, which is then oxidatively deaminated by glutamate dehydrogenase. Glutamate is the only amino acid in human tissue that undergoes oxidative deamination at an appreciable rate, so it acts as a funnel for the nitrogen from amino acids.[92] In the liver, this enzyme is allosterically activated by adenosine diphosphate (ADP) and guanosine diphosphate (GDP) and inhibited by adenosine triphosphate (ATP) and guanosine triphosphate (GTP), a mechanism that accelerates oxidation of amino acids when cellular energy is low.[2] The glutamate dehydrogenase reaction is reversible, yielding ammonia and alpha-ketoglutarate from glutamate. Ammonia, a toxic compound, is converted to urea by enzymes constituting the urea cycle. The urea cycle reactions up to and including the formation of citrulline occur in the mitochondria, while the final three reactions resulting in the formation of urea take place in the cytosol. Carbamoyl-phosphate synthase catalyzes the most important step in the entry of the ammonium ion into the urea cycle. This reaction requires two molecules of ATP, rendering it virtually irreversible.[2] The enzyme is activated by N-acetylglutamate, which is present in increased levels after amino acid or protein feeding.[64]

Role of Specific Organs

In the metabolism of amino acids there are important interactions between organs, especially liver, skeletal muscle, kidney, brain, and intestine (Fig 21-7).

LIVER

The liver is the site of synthesis for urea and plasma proteins. It is the main site of catabolism for the essential amino acids, with the exception of the branched-chain amino acids (leucine, isoleu-

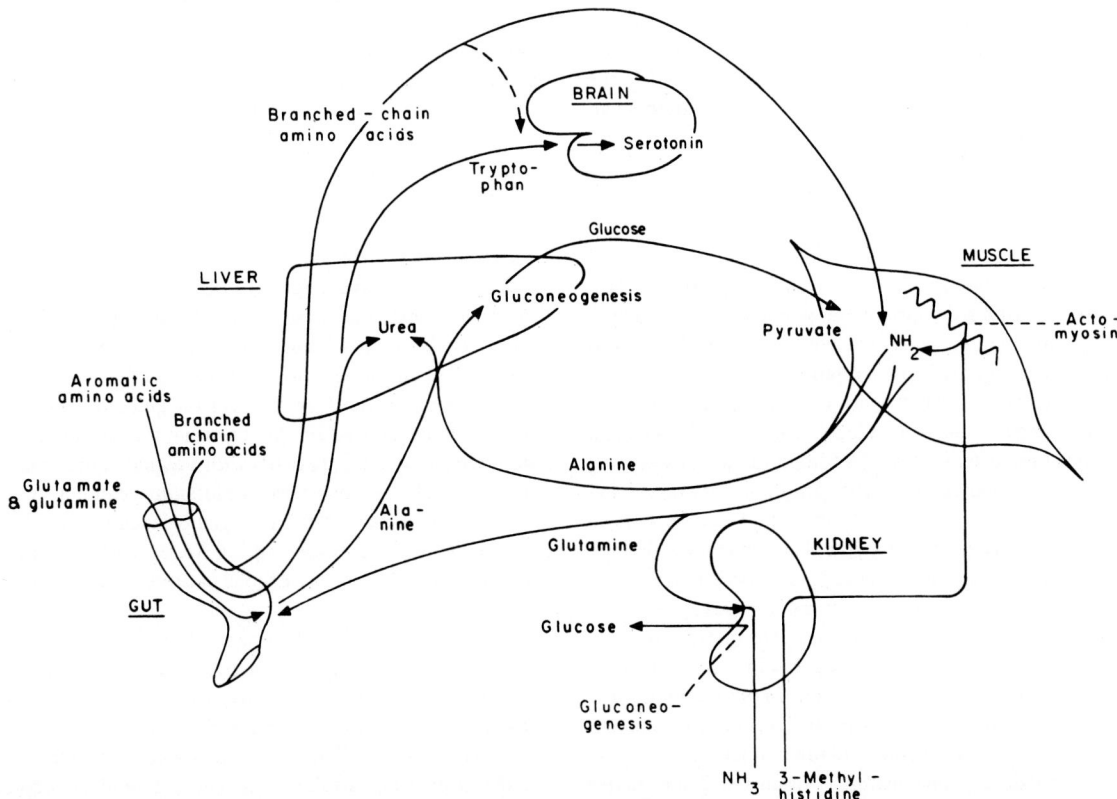

FIGURE 21–7. Interactions of organs in the metabolism of some major amino acids. (Munro HN. Interactions of the liver and muscle in the regulation of metabolism in response to nutritional and other factors. In: Arias IM, Popper H, Schachter D, et al, eds. The liver: Biology and pathobiology, p 677. New York: Raven Press, 1982.)

cine, and valine), which are degraded in muscle and kidney. The liver adjusts the rate of metabolism of the amino acids it receives by way of the portal vein to meet the needs of the organism.[93] Dogs fed large amounts of meat rapidly degrade over half of the incoming amino nitrogen to urea.[93] When intake of an essential amino acid exceeds requirements, specific degradative enzymes are induced, probably triggered by elevated peripheral blood levels of the amino acid.[68] The preferred fuel for the liver is keto acids derived from amino acid degradation.[2]

SKELETAL MUSCLE

Skeletal muscle, which constitutes approximately 45% of adult body weight,[68] preferentially takes up the branched-chain amino acids (isoleucine, leucine, and valine) after each meal and is the primary site of metabolism for these amino acids. Although these three constitute only 8% of dietary amino acids, they make up 60% of the amino acids in the systemic circulation.[64,93] When muscle proteins are catabolized, the branched-chain amino acids undergo transamination, yielding alanine, glutamine, and branched-chain keto acids. The keto acids are used by the muscle as fuel, while alanine and glutamine are exported and taken up predominantly by the liver and intestine, respectively.[64] These two amino acids account for more than 50% of the total amino acid nitrogen released from muscle.[92–94] Hence, alanine, and glutamine that is converted to alanine in the intestinal mucosa, serves to transport nitrogen from the periphery to the liver for urea formation while also furnishing carbon skeletons in the form of pyruvate for gluconeogenesis. Some of the glutamine leaving the muscle is taken up by the kidney and deaminated to yield ammonia and glutamate. Histidine is methylated to 3-methylhistidine after incorporation into muscle protein. Because 3-methylhistidine is excreted in the urine without being reused for synthesis, it has been used as an index of muscle protein catabolism.[68]

BRAIN

The brain uses the carbon skeletons derived from glucose metabolism and the nitrogen from circulating ammonium ions to synthesize nonessential amino acids. The concentration of free nonessential amino acids in the brain is relatively stable and does not change rapidly with changes in plasma amino acid concentrations. Nevertheless, changes in the plasma level of amino acids can affect brain function. Amino acids may affect brain function by serving as neurotransmitters and precursors of neurotransmitters. For example, serotonin, which is derived from tryptophan, appears to be a mood elevator. The precursor tryptophan competes with other large neutral amino acids (phenylalanine, tyrosine, valine, isoleucine, and leucine) for entry into the central nervous system. Because the activity of tryptophan hydroxylase, the rate-limiting enzyme in serotonin synthesis, is limited by the availability of tryptophan, it can be concluded that changes in plasma amino acid concentrations can result in changes in the level of serotonin and other neurotransmitters in the brain and brain function.[20,95] A possible role in hepatic encephalopathy is discussed below under branched-chain amino acids. Gamma-aminobutyric acid (GABA), the decarboxylation product of glutamate, is an inhibitory neu-

rotransmitter in the central nervous system. Glycine and glutamine may also be neurotransmitters or neurotransmitter precursors.[2,96,97]

Ammonia produced in the brain by deamination of amino acids is detoxified by glial cells, which use it to produce glutamine from glutamate by way of the enzyme glutamine synthetase.[98,99]

INTESTINE

The intestinal mucosa plays an important role in interorgan nitrogen exchange and fuel metabolism in both normal and catabolic states. Glutamine is vital to this role. This nonessential glucogenic amino acid is the most abundant amino acid in whole blood as well as in the skeletal muscle pool, making up about half of the whole body pool of free amino acids.[99] It is the preferred energy source of small intestinal mucosa,[100,101] which uses glutamine from both luminal and arterial sources. The presence of glutamine or glutamate in the lumen decreases the concurrent use from the blood.[101]

In the postabsorptive state, the gut uses glutamine for fuel and releases ammonia, alanine, and citrulline into the portal circulation. The ammonia is used for ureagenesis or glutamine synthesis by the liver, and a portion of the citrulline is metabolized to arginine in the kidneys.[99,100] The kidneys also take up glutamine, the major substrate for renal ammoniagenesis, and release alanine, which can be metabolized by the liver to glucose.[99] Ammonia released by the intestine into the portal blood as a result of glutamine metabolism may play a role in hepatic encephalopathy.[99–101]

The intestinal mucosa also appears to serve as a barrier to entry into the bloodstream of dietary glutamate that is neurotoxic. Failure of this function in the face of very large glutamate loads has been implicated in the upper torso and facial burning and pressure sensation known as the Chinese restaurant syndrome.[102,103]

Branched-Chain Amino Acids

The branched-chain amino acids (BCAAs) leucine, isoleucine, and valine may have a special role in metabolism during hypercatabolic stress and hepatic encephalopathy. In hypercatabolic states, skeletal muscle protein is rapidly hydrolyzed to yield branched-chain amino acids, which are used by the muscle as fuel; alanine, which is used by the liver for gluconeogenesis; and glutamine, which is used by the intestinal mucosa for fuel. By providing hypercatabolic patients with adequate quantities of BCAA along with glucose and perhaps glutamine, catabolism of skeletal muscle may be slowed and nitrogen balance improved. The ultimate benefit of administering BCAA-enriched enteral and parenteral products to hypercatabolic patients remains unsettled.[104–108]

Hepatic encephalopathy is associated with an abnormal amino acid profile in the peripheral blood. Concentrations of methionine and aromatic amino acids (phenylalanine, tyrosine, and tryptophan) are greater than normal, while the concentrations of BCAA are less than normal. This pattern is probably initiated by a decrease in the circulating insulin level, which stimulates catabolism of skeletal muscle protein. The BCAAs released from muscle protein are oxidized by muscle cells for fuel, while the methionine and aromatic amino acids accumulate because they are not metabolized by the diseased liver. The pattern of decreased BCAA concentration and increased aromatic amino acid concentration favors entry of aromatic amino acids into the brain, leading to the accumulation of false neurotransmitters, octopamine and phenylethanolamine.[109] If this hypothesis is correct, then nutritional products deficient in methionine and aromatic amino acids and enriched with BCAA should enable patients with hepatic encephalopathy to tolerate increased amounts of protein while improving or at least not adversely affecting the patient's neurologic status.[110] Trials of such products intravenously and orally in hepatic encephalopathy have yielded conflicting results.[111-115] Some investigators have found improvements in encephalopathy, although not necessarily correlated with improved amino acid ratios in the serum. Others have documented normalization or improvements in plasma amino acid ratios without improvement in encephalopathy.[111-115]

LIPID AND FATTY ACID METABOLISM

The lipids are a heterogeneous group of compounds with the common property of being soluble in organic solvents. Important functions of lipids include compact storage and transport of metabolic energy, maintenance of cell membrane structural integrity, and provision of thermal insulation in the subcutaneous tissue and electrical insulation in neural tissue. Vitamins A, D, E, and K are lipids. Although lipids include fats, waxes, phospholipids, glucolipids, and numerous other compounds, the primary lipids involved in energy metabolism are triacylglycerols (triglycerides, neutral fats). Adipose tissue, which consists of approximately 80% triglyceride, is distributed subcutaneously over the entire body. There are also large depots in the pericardial, perirenal, and mesenteric areas. Adipose tissue serves as a cushion for body organs as well as a storehouse for long-chain fatty acids.

Fat is transported to adipose tissue in the form of triglyceride-rich chylomicrons and very-low-density lipoproteins (VLDL) made in the intestinal mucosal cells and hepatocytes, respectively. In adipose tissue, the chylomicrons and VLDL particles adhere to the capillary walls long enough for a portion of their triglyceride to be hydrolyzed to free fatty acids and glycerol by lipoprotein lipase (LPL). This enzyme is attached to the luminal surface of the capillary endothelium. Most of the free fatty acids released are vectored into the adipocytes, where they are re-esterified to triglycerides for storage. Insulin facilitates lipid storage by inducing LPL and by increasing glucose entry into adipocytes, where it is converted to the glycerol-3-phosphate that serves as a substrate for triglyceride synthesis.[116-118] Lipoprotein lipase activity is present in the capillaries of all tissues that store or use fatty acids. The enzyme appears to respond differently to various stimuli depending on the tissue in which it is located.[118] This difference may help direct fat storage during pregnancy to the hips and thighs for use later to support lactation.

Fat is removed from adipocytes when triglyceride is hydrolyzed to glycerol and free fatty acids by an intracellular, hormone-sensitive lipase. This lipase is activated by glucagon and catecholamines by way of cyclic AMP–dependent mechanisms. Its activity is also increased by growth hormone, glucocorticoids, and thyroid hormone and is decreased by insulin.[116-118] The long-chain fatty acids released from adipose tissue enter the circulation where they bind to albumin and are taken up primarily by the liver.

Fatty Acid Metabolism (Beta Oxidation)

Long-chain fatty acids are activated to fatty acid acyl CoA by way of the enzyme acyl CoA synthetase on the outer mitochondrial membrane. The long-chain acyl CoA is transferred to a carrier molecule, carnitine. The resulting acyl carnitine traverses the inner mitochondrial membrane by the activity of a translocase. Once in the mitochondrial matrix, carnitine is removed and the long-chain acyl CoA is reformed. In the mitochondria, the enzyme complex known as "fatty acid oxidase" catalyzes the sequential removal of two carbon fragments from the carboxyl end of the long-chain acyl CoA molecule. Each cycle of this beta oxidation reaction yields acetyl CoA, NADH, and $FADH_2$. Each acetyl CoA molecule yields 12 ATPs when oxidized by way of the citric acid cycle and oxidative phosphorylation. The $FADH_2$ and NADH molecules yield two and three ATPs, respectively, by oxidative phosphorylation. If it is not oxidized, the acetyl CoA generated by beta oxidation can combine with two other molecules of acetyl CoA to form the cholesterol and ketone body precursor 3-hydroxy-3-methylglutaryl CoA, or it can be transported to the cytosol for fatty acid synthesis (see Fig 21-3).[2]

Regulation of Fatty Acid Oxidation

The oxidation of fatty acids is regulated by substrate availability, which in turn is related to the energy needs of the organism. During starvation, lipid-mobilizing hormones, including epinephrine, norepinephrine, glucagon, and adrenal steroids, stimulate the release of fatty acid and glycerol from adipose tissue. Insulin antagonizes the effects of these hormones with a potent antilipolytic action.[119] Beta oxidation is inhibited by a high energy charge.[2,119] For example, the enzyme carnitine acyl transferase I, which catalyzes the transfer of carnitine to fatty acid acyl CoA and thereby controls the entry of fatty acid into the mitochondrial matrix, is inhibited by malonyl CoA, a molecule whose presence signifies abundant fuel supplies.

Ketone Bodies

Ketone bodies are an important fuel source in certain metabolic states associated with a high rate of fatty acid oxidation, such as starvation or uncontrolled diabetes mellitus. They are synthesized from acetyl CoA predominantly in the mitochondria of the liver, released into the blood, and taken up by extrahepatic tissues. Some tissues, especially renal cortex and cardiac muscle, employ ketone bodies as a preferred fuel. Ketone bodies are a water-soluble transport form of acetyl units, which the body uses for energy production when there is a deficiency of available carbohydrate.[2]

Fatty Acid Synthesis

The biosynthesis of fatty acids is a stepwise process occurring in the cytosol and mediated by fatty acid synthase, a multienzyme complex embodied in a single polypeptide chain. It elongates the molecule by sequential additions of two carbon units and stops with the formation of palmitic acid, a 16-carbon fatty acid.[2] The formation of malonyl CoA from acetyl CoA is the committed step in fatty acid biosynthesis and the most important site of regulation.[2] The enzyme that catalyzes this step, acetyl CoA carboxylase, is stimulated by citrate. Citrate is abundant when there is an abundance of ATP and acetyl CoA, conditions appropriate for fat synthesis. Palmitoyl CoA, the end product of fatty acid synthesis, antagonizes the activation of acetyl CoA carboxylase by citrate.[2]

Essential Fatty Acids

Essential fatty acids cannot be synthesized by the body, and therefore they must be provided in the diet to prevent a deficiency state. They are important constituents of cell membranes[120] and precursors of the eicosanoids. They are also involved in the transport and oxidation of cholesterol. Linoleic acid is the principal essential fatty acid in humans. Its chemical structure is C_{18}:2n-6, signifying that it is 18 carbons in length and has two double bonds, the first of which is between the sixth and seventh carbons from the methyl end. The most important fatty acids in nature are cis-isomers, meaning the two hydrogens at the double bond are on the same side of the chain. Vegetable oils (corn, soybean, sunflower, peanut, cottonseed) are rich sources of linoleic acid.[120,121] Arachidonic acid (C_{20}:4n-6) is a precursor of eicosanoids, prostaglandins, leukotrienes, prostacyclins, and thromboxanes, but it is not considered essential because humans can synthesize it from linoleic acid.[120,121]

Alpha linolenic acid (C_{18}:3n-3) has many metabolic properties similar to those of linoleic acid. Despite arguments to the contrary, the essentiality of the n-3 (omega-3) family is now widely accepted, and deficiency states have been described.[122–126] The omega-3 fatty acids are present in high concentrations in cell membranes of the retina, cerebral cortex, and spermatozoa.[124]

Linoleic acid deficiency induces an elevated triene/tetraene ratio, a characteristic plasma lipid pattern that is a sensitive test for essential fatty acid deficiency.[127] This occurs because eicosatrienoic acid, a fatty acid containing three double bonds (a "triene"), is formed when oleic acid (C_{18}:1) substitutes as substrate for the enzyme system that normally elongates linoleic acid. Concomitantly, formation of arachidonic acid (a tetraene), which is the usual product of linoleic acid elongation, is reduced.

Despite the usual presence of large amounts of essential fatty acids in adult adipose tissue, individuals on fat-free parenteral nutrition may develop plasma lipid changes of essential fatty acid deficiency in less than 10 days of continuous feeding.[128] The continuously elevated insulin levels during TPN apparently inhibit lipolysis in patients who are not hypercatabolic, preventing the release of essential fatty acids stored in adipose tissue.

Human diets that provide at least 1% to 2% of total calories as essential fatty acids appear to be adequate, although estimates of infant requirements vary from 0.55% to 6% of calories.[120,121,129] The optimal level of consumption of essential fatty acids and

other unsaturated fats is not yet determined. The American Heart Association has recommended for adults that dietary fat contribute no more than 30% of total calories and that about two thirds of that should be unsaturated, but no more than 10% polyunsaturated.[130–132]

Fish (Marine) Oil

Epidemiologic studies have indicated a possible healthful effect of omega-3 polyunsaturated fatty acids found in marine animals.[133,134] In one study, an average daily intake of only 30 g of fish appeared to provide a protective effect against coronary heart disease independent of known risk factors.[134] Substantial amounts of omega-3 fatty acids are found in commonly eaten fish such as herring, salmon, bluefish, and tuna.[124]

In sufficient doses, fish oil will prolong bleeding time and decrease the production of the proaggregating substance thromboxane A_2.[135,136] The significant hypotriglyceridemic effects of fish oils have been confirmed repeatedly in healthy subjects as well as in various hyperlipidemic states,[135–139] but the long-term effects may be less striking.[140] Effects on serum cholesterol and LDL levels have been variable.[124,141] Animal models suggest that fish oils have an inhibitory effect on coronary arthrosclerosis and intimal hyperplasia.[124] Omega-3 fatty acids generally suppress cellular inflammatory responses by changing the end products of leukotriene synthesis.[124,140,142,143] Dietary supplementation with fish oil has been shown to suppress the production by monocytes of the polypeptide cytokines interleukin-1 and tumor necrosis factor, suggesting an additional mechanism whereby fish oils may exert an anti-inflammatory effect.[144] Controlled clinical studies suggest possible beneficial effects of fish oil in rheumatoid arthritis, psoriasis, atopic dermatitis,[142,145–147] essential hypertension,[124,142,148] and in the prevention of postcoronary angioplasty restenosis in men.[149] At the 5- to 10-g per day doses used in many clinical studies, fish oils should be considered pharmacologic agents. Side effects include bloating, weight gain from the additional fat calories, Vitamin E deficiency, superficial hematomas, diarrhea, and worsening of glucose control in diabetics.[121,140,148,150]

Lipids in Nutritional Support

LIPIDS AND INFECTION

Lipids are not merely sources of nonglucose calories, because they have important modulatory effects on the immune system. Animal and human studies describe deleterious immunologic effects of the currently used intravenous fat emulsions that contain vegetable oil, possibly as a result of the high concentration of linoleic acid. Lipid-related dysfunctions that have been documented include reduced antibody production, inhibition of neutrophil chemotaxis, impaired phagocytosis, and depressed reticuloendothelial system function resulting in decreased bacterial clearance and enhanced bacterial virulence.[151]

Fat influences immune responsiveness in two ways—structural changes and chemical or functional alterations.[152,153] Incorporation of omega-6 polyunsaturated fatty acids, such as linoleic, increases cell membrane fluidity, which may affect cytoskeletal organization, distribution, and movement of cell-surface proteins and cellular transport of nutrients and hormones.[151-154] These changes may influence many functions, including cellular protein synthesis, antigen capping, and the rate of cell division.[151,152] Excessive lipid loads may decrease reticuloendothelial system (RES) clearance capacity, perhaps secondary to the uptake and accumulation of "oil droplets" by the RES.[151]

Intravenous and dietary products rich in linoleic acid may also affect immune responses by influencing the type and quantity of eicosanoid metabolites. Thus, an increase in linoleic acid leads to an increase in its metabolite arachidonic acid in membranes and results in increased prostaglandin and leukotriene production.[151,153] How increased eicosanoid production may account for immune dysfunction is not clear, but several mechanisms have been proposed. One postulate is that administration of linoleic acid favors prostaglandin E_2 production, which decreases immune function by several mechanisms, including inhibition of lymphocyte proliferation and lymphokine secretion, inhibition of natural killer cell activity, and suppression of interleukin-1 production.[151,155] The use of the omega-3 marine oils has a theoretic advantage over conventional lipid sources because they favor prostaglandin E_3 production, which has less immunosuppressive potency than prostaglandin E_2. Furthermore, the omega-3 fatty acids and their metabolites have inhibitory effects on linoleic acid metabolism, including the conversion of arachidonic acid to prostaglandin.[155] Studies of burned guinea pigs fed enterally with omega-3 fatty acids support the hypothesis that the omega-3 series does not produce the adverse immune effects seen with linoleic acid administration.[155]

STRUCTURED LIPIDS

The currently employed intravenous lipid emulsions contain vegetable oils, predominantly soybean and safflower. These are long-chain triglycerides (LCTs), because their fatty acid components are 16 or 18 carbons in length. Medium-chain triglycerides (MCTs) are composed mostly of fatty acids, with 8 or 10 carbons found in coconut and palm kernel oil.[156]

MCTs have important enteral uses because they are more efficiently absorbed than LCTs when bile salt concentration, small bowel surface area, or pancreatic lipase activity is limiting. In addition, the fatty acids released from MCTs are absorbed by way of the portal system rather than by way of the lymphatics, making MCT useful in diseases that obstruct intestinal lymphatics.

MCTs are also being investigated for intravenous use because they have several advantages over LCTs as a nonglucose energy source. While LCTs are slowly cleared from the blood and tend to deposit as fat, MCTs are rapidly cleared because of their smaller size and greater solubility. Also, medium-chain fatty acids do not require carnitine for transport into the mitochondria. Beta oxidation of medium-chain fatty acids is very rapid and in catabolic states may be able to supply enough ketone bodies for muscle fuel to reduce muscle protein catabolism.[156-159] Furthermore, MCTs do not seem to impair reticuloendothelial system function.[157,160] However, MCTs do not provide essential fatty acids, and their oxidation may be too rapid. For example, administration of 100%

MCT parenterally to animals has resulted in narcosis and coma as well as essential fatty acid deficiency.[151,156-158]

Two methods for combining the beneficial properties of MCTs and LCTs in one product are being investigated. The simplest method consists of emulsions of various proportions of MCT and LCT (physical mixtures). The other method involves structured lipids (structured triglycerides), products in which individual triglyceride molecules may have fatty acids of two or three different chain lengths esterified to the three glycerol carbons. To make structured lipids, mixtures of MCTs and LCTs are hydrolyzed and re-esterified to produce randomly mixed triglycerides. Further variation is possible by including several types of LCTs in the original mixture, for example fish oil (omega-3) as well as vegetable oil (omega-6).[160]

BODY COMPOSITION AND ENERGY STORES

Body Composition

The major body components are lean tissue and fat. Lean tissue, the most metabolically active component, is defined in any of several ways that yield somewhat different results. Lean body mass (LBM) is the sum of all the body's tissues minus the adipose tissue, while fat-free mass (FFM) is the sum of all the body's tissues minus the total body fat. The difference between the two lies in the fact that fat and adipose tissue are not synonymous. Fat is triglyceride, while adipose tissue is about 80% fat, 2% protein, and 18% water. This distinction becomes important in the obese patient in whom the loss of large amounts of adipose tissue is not the equivalent of losing pure fat.[6] Another conceptually related term is body cell mass (BCM), defined as "the homogeneous energy-exchanging, work-performing moiety of body tissue measurable by the total exchangeable potassium."[161] It includes all the cellular components of the muscle, viscera, and nerves and makes up 35% to 45% of the body weight in normal males and 30% to 40% in females.[161] Extracellular mass (ECM) is defined as a heterogeneous group of tissues and fluids supporting the BCM.[161] Thus, the lean body mass (LBM) is composed of the BCM and the ECM. In starvation states, extracellular mass is proportionally increased and body cell mass is decreased.

Energy Stores

Adipose cells store fat in the form of triglycerides, a very efficient means of energy storage. Not only do triglycerides yield about 9 kcal per gram when oxidized, but also their main advantage is that they represent a relatively anhydrous energy store.[162] In contrast, body glycogen is a quantitatively insignificant energy store because it is a gel with 2 to 4 g of water per gram of glycogen.[162] The total energy stored in the form of blood glucose, liver glycogen (about 100 g), and muscle glycogen (about 200–500 g) in a normal 75-kg man is 1200 to 2400 kcal, barely a single day's energy supply.[162,163] The adipose tissue in that same individual would supply 2 months of basal energy needs.[162]

RESPONSE TO STARVATION

A normal resting person requires about 1400 to 1800 kcal per day or about 1 kcal per minute.[162,164] Approximately 20% of resting energy use is consumed by the brain, which requires an uninterrupted energy supply because it is unable to store energy substrates. Under normal conditions the brain's principal fuel is glucose, and in the resting state it consumes two thirds of the circulating glucose supply and about 45% of the oxygen.[165] Acute interruption of the brain's glucose or oxygen results in rapid mental status alteration, followed in a few minutes by neuronal death. The liver and viscera use about 30% of basal caloric requirements, the kidneys 10%, and the heart 5%.[162]

The human body is remarkably adapted for surviving long periods without food. Healthy, resting individuals of normal weight receiving no calories or protein can survive for 60 to 70 days, while a heavily muscled, obese person may survive as long as 12 months under the same conditions.[162,163,165] At the time of death from starvation, total body protein has usually declined about 30% and energy stores have declined much more. If the rates of nitrogen loss and energy consumption occurring during the first few days of fasting continued unabated, these body composition changes and death would occur much sooner than actually happens. Prolonged survival is dependent on adaptive changes that occur during starvation.

In 1912, Francis Benedict performed a now classic study of a healthy 40-year-old man who fasted for 31 days and lived about half that time in a calorimeter.[166] He noted a marked shift after a few days of fasting to the use of fat for calories and also noted a progressive decrease in urinary nitrogen excretion, representing the body's metabolic shift to conserve protein.[166] For a more extensive review of human starvation studies, as well as a detailed account of the effects of 168 days of "semistarvation" on healthy volunteers, the reader is referred to the work of Ancel Keys and colleagues.[167]

Early Starvation (1–7 Days)

In the response to starvation, progressive shifts occur over time in the type and amounts of fuel used. Changes begin in the postabsorptive period (e.g., after an overnight fast), at which point hepatic glycogen is decreasing and gluconeogenesis is increasing. Unlike glycogen in the liver, glycogen contained in skeletal muscle is unavailable to support blood glucose levels because muscle lacks the enzyme glucose-6-phosphatase. After 15 to 24 hours of fasting, blood glucose levels may fall slightly because of continued glucose use by peripheral organs.[168] This causes diminished insulin secretion and increased glucagon and growth hormone levels. Such altered hormonal ratios influence hepatic enzyme systems to inhibit glycolysis and oxidation of three carbon intermediates in the Krebs cycle while activating gluconeogenic pathways and mobilizing free fatty acids from adipose tissues.[163] Because insulin is an inhibitor of muscle breakdown, decreased insulin levels remove a barrier to proteolysis.[168] After 24 hours of fasting, gluconeogenesis will have supplanted hepatic glycogenolysis as the principal means of hepatic glucose production.

After 48 to 72 hours of starvation, the brain and erythrocytes become reliant upon gluconeogenesis. A fraction of the glucose is synthesized from non-nitrogenous substrates, namely, 18 to 20 g of glycerol released daily from the mobilization of 180 to 200 g of triglyceride, as well as lactate and pyruvate from the metabolism of muscle glycogen.[162] However, amino acids from the breakdown of muscle protein provide most of the gluconeogenic substrate. At this stage of starvation, approximately 75 g per day of muscle protein is catabolized to make glucose.[162] Because muscle is about 20% protein, this 75 g represents a loss of about two thirds of a pound of muscle tissue daily. If protein loss continued at this rate, it would require only about 2 weeks for a normal-weight adult to use up 30% of his or her skeletal muscle and die.

The production of glucose at the expense of muscle protein provides a radically altered fuel supply to the starved body. A large quantity of alanine is formed in the muscle by transamination between pyruvate derived from glucose and the amino groups of branched-chain amino acids (Fig 21-8).[160] The alanine is transported to the liver, where its carbon skeleton is reconverted to glucose. This glucose–alanine cycle does not provide for the net formation of new glucose molecules. However, it is postulated that some of the pyruvate in muscle is formed from amino acids rather than glucose.[168] In either case, the glucose–alanine cycle functions to transport nitrogen groups from the periphery to the liver for urea formation and excretion.[169] Glutamine is also released in large quantities by the skeletal muscle. It serves as fuel for the intestine, and it is the key nitrogen transporter and gluconeogenic substrate for the kidneys. Not only are the branched-chain amino acids extensively catabolized in muscle cells, but their levels are increased in the circulation. They are believed to be inhibitors of proteolysis.[168]

During the first week of starvation, the metabolic rate falls by as much as 10% to 15%.[166] This steadily decreasing rate is the result of both altered metabolism and decreased body mass. Changes in thyroid hormone activity may play a role, because

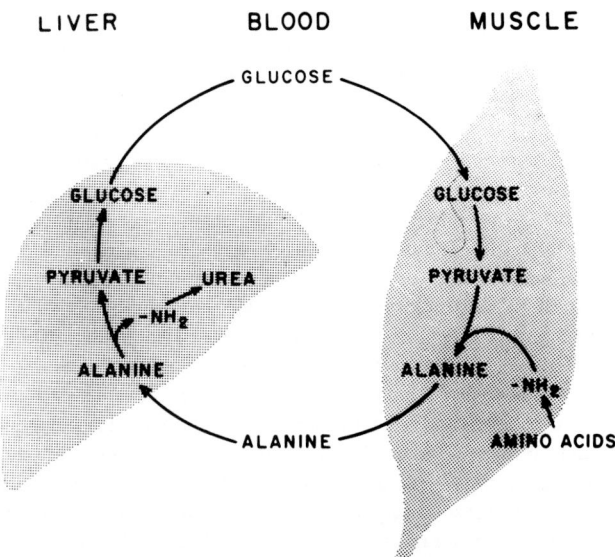

FIGURE 21–8. The glucose–alanine cycle. Glucose released by the liver is taken up by muscle, where it is converted to pyruvate and transaminated to form alanine. The alanine thus synthesized is released by muscle and taken up by the liver, where its carbon skeleton is reconverted to glucose, thus completing the cycle. (Felig P. The glucose–alanine cycle. Metabolism 1973;22:179.)

serum T3 declines rapidly as a result of conversion to metabolically inactive reverse T3 in peripheral tissue.[170,171] Furthermore, starvation may decrease tissue sensitivity to T3.[171] The physical torpor that accompanies starvation also reduces energy expenditure.[162,167]

Perhaps the most significant metabolic substrate alteration in early starvation is the development of mild ketoacidosis. The liver begins production of ketone bodies as it shifts to gluconeogenesis and to dehydrogenation of long-chain fatty acids as a source of energy, under the influence of low insulin levels and permissive levels of glucagon, thyroid hormone, and glucocorticoids.[162] The blood levels of acetoacetate and beta-hydroxybutyrate gradually increase during the first week of starvation and persist until fat supplies become depleted. The ketone-oxidizing enzymes in the brain are already active after an overnight fast,[163] and by 7 days ketone bodies make up 65% to 75% of the brain's fuel. Ketones provide 30% to 40% of total caloric requirements after a few days of starvation.[172]

Late Starvation (1–4 Weeks)

As starvation continues and ketones supply more of the brain's fuel, there is less reliance on hepatic gluconeogenesis and therefore less proteolysis. After 2 weeks of starvation, muscle proteolysis is decreased from 75 g per day to 20 to 30 g per day and urinary nitrogen excretion drops to 3 to 5 g per day.[162] Beta-hydroxybutyrate is an important signal to reduce muscle proteolysis.[162,172] In long-term starvation, protein synthetic capability is limited because of a decreased amino acid pool. Therefore, the starving organism cannot respond well to rapid changes in environmental stimuli.

The blood glucose concentration in starvation stabilizes at mildly depressed values and remains at that level until death.[162] Renal gluconeogenesis, primarily using glutamine as a substrate, plays a substantial role in supporting blood glucose late in starvation. Early in starvation, glucose production by gluconeogenesis is approximately 90% hepatic and 10% renal, while in late starvation renal gluconeogenesis accounts for about 45% of the total. A small amount of glucose, about 10 to 15 g per day, can also be produced from acetoacetate derived from fatty acids.[173-175]

Some investigators conclude that the renal handling of glutamine also contributes to acid–base balance (Fig 21-9). In the fed state, nitrogenous waste is disposed of primarily as urea. During prolonged starvation, large amounts of base are needed to neutralize approximately 100 mEq per day of keto acids. Glutamine arriving in the kidney from muscle is hydrolyzed by glutaminase, yielding ammonia (NH_3) and glutamate. The glutamate is deaminated by glutamate dehydrogenase, yielding a second NH_3 molecule and a keto acid that is used for renal gluconeogenesis. The NH_3 molecules are protonated and leave the body as NH_4+. Other glucogenic amino acids can be used by the kidney in similar fashion.[168] Others question whether the protonation of NH_3 can significantly contribute to acid–base balance.[176]

The metabolic changes in skeletal muscles, including proteolysis, are vital to survival in starvation. Muscle is normally fueled by glucose and fatty acids. In starvation, the decreased insulin levels and increased growth hormone levels inhibit the uptake of glucose from blood, and fatty acids become the principal fuel source.

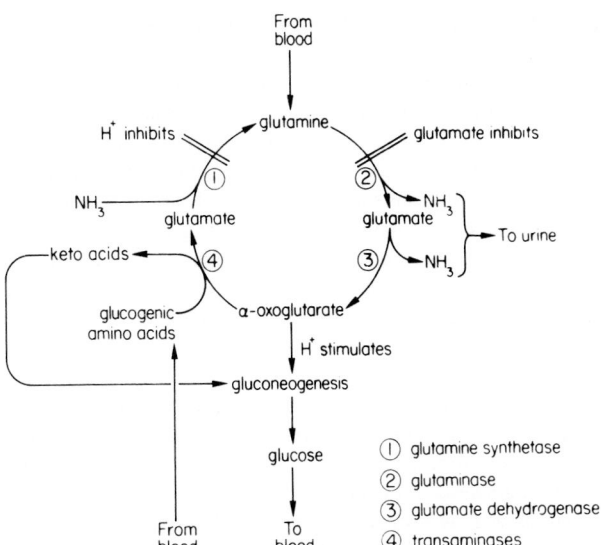

FIGURE 21–9. Relationship between gluconeogenesis and ammonia production in the kidney. (Banks P, Bartley W, Birt LM. *The biochemistry of the tissues,* ed 2. London: John Wiley & Sons, 1976. Reprinted with permission.)

Many hormones help orchestrate the adaptations occurring during starvation. The lowered insulin level that persists throughout starvation inhibits amino acid uptake by muscles and glucose uptake by muscles and adipose tissue and stimulates gluconeogenesis, lipolysis, and proteolysis. Glucagon levels rise early in starvation but return to prefasting levels after 3 to 4 weeks of starvation.[168] Glucagon facilitates amino acid release from muscle and uptake by the liver. It inhibits glycolysis, activates gluconeogenesis, and stimulates fatty acid oxidation and ketone body synthesis.[172,177] Growth hormone, which is elevated in adults and children with prolonged protein–calorie malnutrition, enhances lipolysis and protein synthesis.[168] Cortisol levels also increase with protein depletion. This hormone promotes gluconeogenesis by decreasing protein synthesis and augmenting hepatic uptake and utilization of amino acids.[168] The increased conversion of active T3 to inactive reverse T3 during starvation lowers the resting metabolic rate and promotes a reducing environment that inhibits the formation of phosphoenolpyruvate and may be a mechanism for decreasing proteolysis.[168,170,171]

The hallmark of starvation is progressive weight loss. The rate of weight loss is greatest early in starvation because the early weight loss is a mixture of glycogen (1 kcal/g), lean tissue (1 kcal/g), and adipose tissue (9 kcal/g), with a caloric equivalent of only about 2000 kcal per kilogram. Once the adaptive mechanisms come into play, fat becomes the major fuel source, and the weight lost has a caloric equivalent of approximately 8000 kcal per kilogram.[167,168] Normal human beings generally do not survive weight losses much greater than about 40%.[168]

Protein–Energy Malnutrition

Protein–energy malnutrition (PEM) results when needs for protein, energy sources, or both are not satisfied by the diet.[178,179]

Within the spectrum of PEM, three clinical types of severe malnutrition are classically distinguished: kwashiorkor, marasmus, and marasmic kwashiorkor.[179] These states are distinguished largely on subjective clinical grounds, although various classifications have been proposed based on the presence of edema and weight for age.[178] Kwashiorkor, named by the Ga tribe of Ghana to denote the disease the older child acquires after the birth of the next baby, is predominantly a protein deficiency out of proportion to energy intake, which is low. Edema is always present and is usually accompanied by hypoalbuminemia and loss of lean body mass and often hepatomegaly, dyspigmentation of the hair and skin, and psychologic changes.[178] Marasmus is primarily an energy deficiency. The striking features are marked deficits in weight and, to a lesser extent, height.[178] The typical infant is emaciated with a large-appearing head, staring eyes, and shrunken trunk, limbs, and buttocks. Marasmic kwashiorkor has clinical features of marasmus and kwashiorkor. Edema and lean body mass atrophy are present as well as stunted growth and other features of the two conditions, such as skin and hair changes, psychologic changes, and fatty liver.

In all forms of PEM, one of the most prominent features is weakness, decreased physical strength and endurance far exceeding the degree of weight loss. The weakness is an important factor in the development of pneumonia, which is frequently the terminal event in PEM.

Effect of Malnutrition on the Gastrointestinal Tract

The organs of the digestive system are very active metabolically; hence, it is not surprising that structural and functional features are substantially altered by protein–energy malnutrition. Effects on the stomach include gastric mucosal atrophy and hypochlorhydria.[180] As a result, the antimicrobial gastric acid barrier is probably impaired, as evidenced by increased bacterial and yeast counts in duodenal aspirates.[180]

In chronic severe PEM, the exocrine pancreas undergoes marked morphologic and structural changes. Acinar cell atrophy, marked diminution in zymogen granules, and cystic dilatations of the pancreatic ducts have been shown in humans with severe PEM.[181] Although bicarbonate production and the volume of secretions are not altered, enzyme output is severely decreased in PEM, even after stimulation by secretin and pancreozymin.[180,181] This exocrine impairment appears to be largely reversible with nutritional repletion.[182] An interesting form of chronic calcific pancreatitis, possibly caused by childhood malnutrition occurring years earlier, affects young people in developing countries.[181] The pathogenesis may involve blockage of pancreatic ducts by inspissated mucus or laminated secretions that subsequently calcify. The etiology is unclear; however, speculation has centered on childhood PEM with additional interfering factors such as trace element deficiency or cyanogenic glycoside consumption in cassava.[183,184]

Excess fat in the liver is a frequent feature of kwashiorkor, but the cause is uncertain.[185–187] There is also a decreased production of conjugated bile acids.[180]

During PEM, both adults and children manifest structural and functional disturbances of the small intestine, including a substantial decrease in mass. The intestinal wall becomes thin, and there is mucosal atrophy with flat spruelike villi, usually most dramatic in kwashiorkor.[188] In addition to decreased brush border height, there is a decrease in the rates of cell proliferation in the crypts and migration along the crypt–villus axis.[189] Intestinal motility is reduced, and a prolonged transit time can be demonstrated even in the presence of diarrhea.[180] A striking feature is an overgrowth of facultative and anaerobic bacteria and yeast,[180,188] which may secondarily worsen intestinal function. There are marked decreases in absorption of glucose and D-xylose in protein deficiency.[171,179,180] Lactose and other disaccharide intolerances often contribute to the diarrhea.[180,190,191] Fat malabsorption may result from bile salt deficiency, lipase deficiency, and impaired enterocyte function.[180] Protein absorption appears to be better preserved but also may be abnormal.[180] As a result of poor sanitation, pathologic bacteria and parasites frequently contribute to the diarrhea seen in malnourished individuals. Intestinal mucosal function is diminished by deficiencies of specific nutrients, including B_{12}, folate, niacin, and zinc.

Discussion of the immunologic effects of malnutrition is beyond the scope of this section. How much of the well-established association between famine and pestilence is due to poor sanitation and how much is the result of weakness, immunologic deficiency, or other effects of malnutrition is unclear.

METABOLIC RESPONSE TO SEPSIS

General Response to Infection

The invasion of the body by microorganisms leads to a highly predictable, stereotyped series of metabolic, biochemical, and hormonal responses. The magnitude of these responses depends on patient variables, including age, function of vital organs, nutritional status, immunologic memory, associated disease processes, and extent, duration, and nature of infection.[192] Although the infected patient is often anorectic and not eating, the response to infection supersedes the normal energy- and protein-sparing response to starvation.

The acute phase of infection, characterized by fever, hypermetabolism, leukocytosis, activation of various immunologic reactions, and secretion of hormones and endogenous mediators, is initiated by substances released from macrophages.[193] The hypermetabolism consists of an increase in anabolism and an even greater increase in catabolism. It has been aptly termed "septic autocannibalism."[194] Catabolism provides energy and substrate molecules for the synthesis of specialized proteins and cells needed for the host defensive system. The infected patient enters a state of negative nitrogen balance, weight loss, loss of intracellular constituents, and unalterable lipolysis. In starvation, proteolysis is curtailed by the hepatic synthesis of ketone bodies for use as an energy source, but this adaptation does not occur in generalized infection.[192,193]

Protein and Amino Acid Metabolism in Infection

In systemic infections there is rapid mobilization of amino acids contained in functional proteins, especially of skeletal muscle but also of all other organs, including heart, gut, and liver.[193] An increased catabolism of extracellular proteins, including acute-phase reactants, coagulation system proteins, and complement system proteins, also occurs.[193,195–197]

The endogenous peptide mediator interleukin-1 (IL-1) activates skeletal muscle proteases and also increases hepatocyte uptake of amino acids.[193,198–203] The branched-chain amino acids of skeletal muscle are metabolized within the muscle cell for energy while transamination generates glutamine and alanine. As a result, plasma alanine and glutamine content is increased while the branched-chain amino acid concentration is decreased.[193] Glutamine is taken up and metabolized by the kidney at an accelerated rate, providing additional ammonium ion for excretion to help maintain acid–base balance in the face of the acidosis that frequently accompanies sepsis.[192] Alanine is captured by the liver for gluconeogenesis, and its nitrogen contributes to the increased ureagenesis of sepsis.[204] Plasma concentrations of phenylalanine, tryptophan, and proline are also often increased in sepsis.[205,206] Much of the increased tryptophan is rapidly shunted into degradative pathways, and the metabolic products are excreted in the urine.[205] Elevated proline levels in patients with surgical sepsis correlated positively with lactate levels and inversely with total peripheral resistance and oxygen consumption, and plasma proline concentration has been proposed as a prognostic indicator.[206]

Anabolic activity is also increased in sepsis, although it is overshadowed by catabolism and the resultant negative nitrogen balance. The anabolism builds the arsenals of body defenses, including phagocytes, peptide hormones, and other mediators (interleukins, monokines, lymphokines), intracellular proteins (metallothionein, ferritin, hemosiderin), immunoglobulins, complement and coagulation system proteins, and acute-phase reactant glycoproteins (haptoglobin, ceruloplasmin, fibrinogen, C-reactive protein).[193]

Fat and Carbohydrate Metabolism in Infection

Fat is a major fuel source in infected patients, even when exogenous carbohydrates are administered. However, plasma lipid concentrations are very variable.[207] There is increased production of fatty acids and triglycerides by the liver. Despite hepatic uptake of free fatty acids, ketosis in the absence of exogenous carbohydrate is diminished, in contrast to the accelerated ketogenesis of fasting.[208] Hyperinsulinemia is the most likely explanation for this hypoketonemic state.[208]

Sepsis is generally marked by hyperglycemia secondary to both a relative insulin resistance and gluconeogenesis, primarily in the liver. Gluconeogenesis is favored by the hormonal milieu (elevated glucagon, catecholamines, glucocorticoids, and growth hormone) combined with ready availability of the necessary substrates, including lactate, alanine and other glucogenic amino acids, pyruvate, and glycerol.[204,205] These conditions induce gluconeogenesis, as well as enhanced glycolysis, despite hyperinsulinemia.[204] Infusion studies of normal volunteers using cortisol, glucagon, and epinephrine demonstrated additive and synergistic interactions that simulated many of the metabolic responses observed in sepsis and trauma.[209] Total synthesis of glucose by the liver may approach or exceed 500 g per day. Unlike starvation, hepatic glucose production in sepsis is not completely suppressed by exogenous glucose.[210]

Substrate cycling involves simultaneous activity of opposing, nonequilibrium reactions ultimately requiring expenditure of ATP and resulting in heat production without changing the concentration of substrate or product.[211] There is evidence for increased substrate cycling in glycolytic–gluconeogenic and triglyceride–fatty acid pathways during highly catabolic states such as trauma, sepsis, and burns.[212,213] It seems unlikely that this represents "futile" cycling, which is wasteful of precious energy stores. It is more likely that these are useful adaptive responses, but the benefits remain to be documented.[212]

Hormone and Hormonelike Mediators

Other hormones and hormonelike substances are important in the nutritional aspect of sepsis. In contrast to cortisol, which rises rapidly with the onset of fever and drops abruptly when the fever abates, aldosterone rises and falls more gradually. The retention of excess water in sepsis is partly due to aldosterone secretion, not infrequently accompanied by inappropriate antidiuretic hormone (ADH) secretion.[193,205]

In addition to its role in protein metabolism, IL-1 also affects the concentrations of plasma divalent cations during infection. IL-1 stimulates the liver to synthesize metallothioneins, which are cysteine-rich proteins with a high affinity for heavy metals. The increased intracellular metallothioneins allow hepatocytes to sequester zinc, depriving invading organisms of this trace element, which is essential for rapid microbial metabolism. IL-1 similarly mediates the sequestration of iron in tissue stores of hemosiderin and ferritin, making it unavailable for use by infecting microorganisms.[193,198,201,214–217] Copper seems to be important in proper immune system function, and IL-1 increases hepatic secretion of the copper-containing protein ceruloplasmin.[198,201] IL-1 stimulates other portions of the acute-phase response, such as fibrinogen and C-reactive protein production by hepatocytes and the release of lactoferrin by neutrophils.[193,198,201] IL-1 enhances immunoglobulin production by B lymphocytes and stimulates IL-2 production by T lymphocytes.[193,201] IL-2 also enhances immune function.[193,218]

Cachectin, or tumor necrosis factor (TNF), is a peptide produced by endotoxin-activated macrophages. It has been proposed as the primary cytokine mediating many of the responses to gram-negative sepsis, including hypotension, metabolic acidosis, hypoglycemia, fever, and hyperkalemia.[219–221] Studies of protein metabolism in febrile states suggest that TNF may be the principal catabolic monokine.[199] Furthermore, TNF decreases synthesis of anabolic enzymes in adipose tissue and, like IL-1, stimulates acute-phase protein expression.[199,221,222]

Vitamin Alterations in Infection

There is increased use of some vitamins during generalized infection. In patients with baseline poor nutritional status, an acute infection can occasionally unmask classic vitamin deficiency states, including beriberi, pellagra, and scurvy.[193] The adrenal cortex and neutrophils are normally rich in Vitamin C, but the accelerated steroidogenesis and phagocytosis associated with infection can deplete them.[193]

Antimicrobials used to treat infection may have unfavorable effects on vitamin metabolism. Isoniazid treatment for tuberculosis can result in pyridoxine deficiency as a result of inhibition of pyridoxine-dependent enzyme reactions and as a result of loss of isoniazid pyridoxal hydrazone complex in the urine.[223–225] Isoniazid can also cause niacin deficiency, possibly secondary to its effects on pyridoxine. Broad-spectrum antibiotics can decrease synthesis of Vitamin K by altering colonic microflora.[224] Trimethoprim can cause folate deficiency,[193] and tetracycline has been reported to reduce the concentration of Vitamin C in leukocytes.[225] Neomycin can cause a reversible B_{12} malabsorption as well as decreased serum Vitamin A concentration.[225] Many other antibiotic–vitamin interactions are described in the literature.[223–225]

Immune cell function is influenced by vitamins, including effects of Vitamin C, folate, and B vitamins on phagocytic cells and Vitamins A, D, and E and several B vitamins on macrophages and lymphocytes.[193] These, among others, are reasons to be certain that patients with infection are not vitamin-deficient. However, the efficacy, if any, of vitamin supplementation in excess of the U.S. RDA for patients with infection and other catabolic conditions remains unsettled. A randomized, controlled study strongly supported the use of Vitamin A supplements in children with severe measles.[225a] Data, mostly derived from studies of traumatized animals, suggest that higher doses of Vitamins A and C and some B vitamins may be beneficial. There is evidence that thiamine deficiency occurs frequently in intensive care unit patients and correlates with the likelihood of a fatal outcome.[226] On the other hand, vitamin supplementation during acute illness may not be without risk. For example, 1,25,dihydroxyvitamin D inhibits proliferation of T lymphocytes, possibly due, in part, to down-regulation of IL-1 production by monocytes.[227]

Minerals and Trace Elements

During systemic infections, intracellular elements, including potassium, phosphorus, magnesium, sulfur, and zinc, are lost in the urine in proportion to the loss of nitrogen.[193] If diarrhea occurs, losses of potassium, magnesium, and zinc are increased disproportionately.[193] Serum electrolytes may also reflect the results of increased ADH or aldosterone. The effects of IL-1 in decreasing zinc and iron availability while increasing copper levels have been discussed. Theoretically, administration of exogenous iron or zinc may thwart the antimicrobial effect of reduced serum iron and zinc.[214–217]

METABOLIC RESPONSE TO TRAUMA

The metabolic response to injury shares many features with the body's response to infection. Both conditions are characterized by hypermetabolism, negative nitrogen balance, hyperglycemia, and reliance upon fat as the major energy source.

Cuthbertson divided the metabolic response to long-bone fractures into two phases, ebb and flow.[228] Moore has since divided the flow phase into catabolic and anabolic phases.[229] The ebb phase occurs immediately after the trauma and is usually short-lived (12–24 hours). It is characterized by hyperglycemia, elevated lactic acid, and reduced blood pressure, oxygen consumption, and body temperature. The restoration of tissue perfusion marks the beginning of the catabolic phase. This lasts from days to weeks, depending on variables such as severity of injury, medical intervention, and premorbid health of the patient. This phase is characterized by catabolism, heat production, negative nitrogen balance, and hyperglycemia.[228,229] It ends after volume deficits are corrected, infection is controlled, pain is eliminated, and oxygenation is restored. At this point, net anabolism may occur, resulting in slow reaccumulation of protein followed by the reaccumulation of body fat.

Energy Metabolism in Trauma

The degree of elevation of metabolic rate in the catabolic portion of the flow phase is usually related to the severity of injury and the person's size.[192] There appears to be an intrinsic upper limit to metabolic rate because it rarely exceeds twice the normal basal rate regardless of the extent of injury.[31] During the period of hypermetabolism, a temporary resetting of the hypothalamic thermoregulatory set point is generally responsible for a 1° to 2°C elevation of body temperature known as the "post-traumatic fever."[230] Because the central temperature set point is higher, the comfort temperature for an injured patient is elevated, and elevating the ambient temperature will decrease the energy requirement.[31]

Glucose Metabolism in Trauma

The altered carbohydrate metabolism in trauma is similar to that in infection.[231] Hyperglycemia may occur in the ebb phase and persist despite normal or elevated plasma insulin concentrations throughout the flow phase.[192] The elevated concentrations of glucose and other solutes contribute to an increased plasma osmolality, which may play a role in restoring postinjury blood volume.[231]

Studies of burned or wounded tissues show exuberant uptake of glucose with up to 80% converted to lactate.[232] The accelerated glucose uptake correlates with the degree of inflammatory cellular infiltrate present.[231–233] Traditionally attributed to anaerobic glycolysis resulting from poor local tissue perfusion, the increased glucose consumption and lactate production by injured tissue has been shown to occur even in the presence of adequate oxygen (aerobic glycolysis), but the mechanism is unknown.[231,234]

Protein Metabolism in Trauma

Many of the changes of protein metabolism in the injured patient are similar to the changes in sepsis. Despite the reliance upon fat as the major energy source, a net catabolism of 300 to 500 g per day of lean body cell mass serves to provide amino acids. Approximately 80% of these amino acids are used for gluconeogenesis, and about 20% are used directly for energy.[235] The increased gluconeogenesis from amino acids results in accelerated ureagenesis and urinary nitrogen excretion. The source of most of the catabolized protein is skeletal muscle. The gluconeogenesis in trauma, as in sepsis, does not cease with the infusion of carbohydrates, as it would in simple starvation.[236] Nevertheless, postinjury nutrient deprivation contributes to the negative nitrogen balance, and it can be markedly reduced or eliminated by appropriate energy and protein intake.[231,237]

There is controversy regarding the effects of trauma on the metabolism of specific amino acids, especially the branched-chain amino acids. Alanine and glutamine constitute only 12% of muscle protein, but they make up 50% to 60% of amino acids released into the plasma by muscle. Conversely, branched-chain amino acids make up 15% of muscle protein but only 6% of the amino acids released. The most likely explanation is that within muscle tissue, branched-chain amino acids donate amino groups to alpha-ketoglutarate, yielding glutamate that is released from the muscle and branched-chain keto acids that are metabolized in the muscle for fuel.[192] In addition to carrying amino groups from the periphery to the liver and kidney, glutamine serves as a major energy source for the lymphocytes and fibroblasts constituting the cellular infiltrate at the site of injury.[231]

Despite the fact that a postinjury patient is in a state of negative nitrogen and energy balance with reduced plasma concentrations of important minerals and vitamins, most wounds proceed to heal, a phenomenon termed "biological priority of wound healing."[229,230]

Multisystem Organ Failure (MOF)

Major advances in both initial resuscitation and intensive care treatment have increased patient survival after catastrophic illness. This has led to the evolution of a high-morbidity process known as multisystem organ failure (MOF). MOF is often characterized by the sequential failure of anatomically and physiologically distinct organs, likened to a biologic domino effect.[238,239] Although systemic infection can initiate MOF, the lack of positive blood cultures in up to 50% of patients with this hyperdynamic, hypermetabolic syndrome has led in the past to its being named "nonbacteremic clinical sepsis."[240] MOF appears to be the clinical manifestation of the ultimate inflammatory response that results from the cascade of events activated by invading microorganisms and tissue injury or necrosis.[241,242] These events may be mediated by way of the integration of classic neuroendocrine factors with other soluble protein and lipid mediators.[240,243] Several proposed mediators include interleukin-1, prostacyclin, thromboxane, opioids, tumor necrosis factor, and complement proteins.[243] Despite increased knowledge of the role of humoral mediators in producing the altered metabolism associated with MOF, the observed defect in oxygen use, so fundamental to visceral organ failure, remains undefined.[238,239]

The lung is usually the first organ to fail in MOF, followed often by the liver and kidneys.[240] Pre-existing disease such as cirrhosis or renal insufficiency adversely affects the reserve capacity of the organ and can influence the order of organ failure.[238] Failure of two organ systems plus the kidneys is nearly always fatal.[238]

The average hospital cost for a patient with MOF exceeds $100,000.[240] Avoiding shock states prior to organ failure through aggressive fluid resuscitation, as well as monitoring hemodynamics and oxygen delivery, may prevent MOF.[239] A major factor in the pathogenesis of MOF is the inability of the failing gastrointestinal tract to exclude systemic access to virulent intestinal microflora.[243] An attempt to maintain mucosal integrity with enteral nutrition does not appear to influence the incidence of postseptic MOF or mortality,[244] but further studies to examine the effect of preserving mucosal integrity are under way.

INTESTINAL ADAPTATION

After small-bowel resection, adaptive changes occur that affect all layers of the remaining small intestine and colon. The dominant change is mucosal hyperplasia without hypertrophy. Villous height and crypt depth are increased. There are increased numbers of epithelial cells per unit length of villus and crypt, and the intestinal remnant lengthens and dilates.[245,246] These changes are more pronounced after resection of jejunum than ileum and are most marked just distal to the anastomosis.[245]

The small intestinal mucosa is normally in dynamic equilibrium between cell production at the base of the crypt and cell extrusion at the tip of the villus.[247] The rapidly dividing, immature cells in the crypt lose the ability to divide as they migrate onto the villus, where they differentiate into mature columnar cells.[245] Mechanisms regulating cell renewal are unclear, but cell division in the crypts may be controlled in feedback fashion by the number of cells on the villus. In addition to intrinsic regulation of intestinal epithelial renewal, a number of extrinsic factors influence intestinal adaptation, as shown in Figure 21-10.[247]

Intraluminal Factors

Adaptation is enhanced by substances in the lumen, including endogenous secretions and exogenous nutrients. Both gastric and duodenal juices have been shown to stimulate ileal hyperplasia in rats.[248] Pancreaticobiliary secretions have a more marked trophic effect on distal small bowel than bile alone.[247,249,250]

The presence of food in the lumen, even if not absorbed sufficiently to contribute to overall nutrition, is important in intestinal adaptation.[239] Thus, hyperphagia and the resulting increased chyme in the gut are associated with intestinal hyperplasia,[246] while diminished luminal nutrients (due to surgical exclusion of a bowel segment, starvation, or use of TPN) result in structural and functional atrophy.[246,247] Glucose or amino acids perfused through isolated bowel loops prevent hypoplasia in some species. Animal

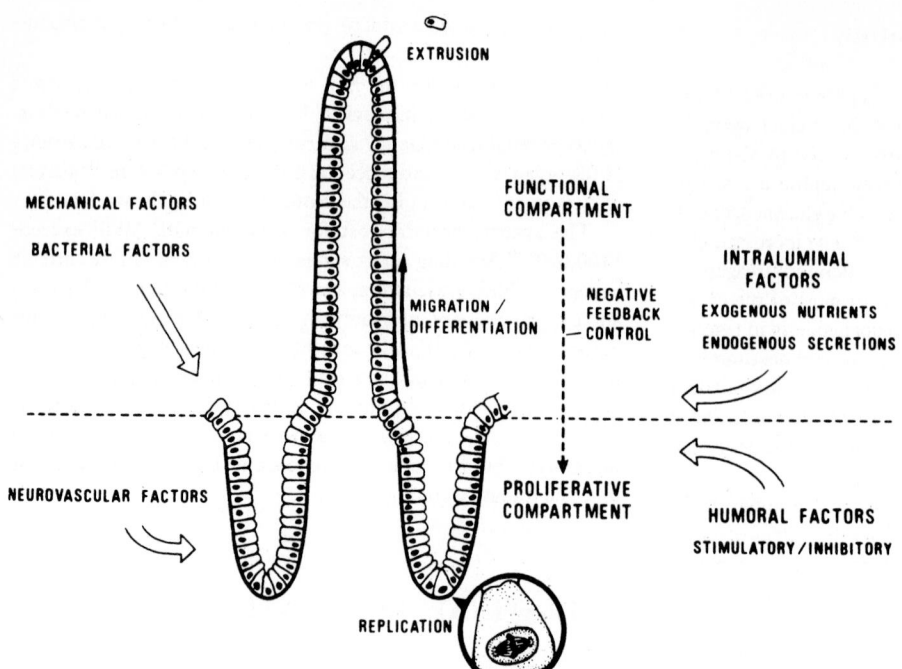

FIGURE 21–10. Schematic representation of the intrinsic and extrinsic mechanisms regulating cell proliferation in the enteric epithelium. (Williamson RC, Chir M. Intestinal adaptation. II. N Engl J Med 1978;298:1444. Reprinted with permission.)

studies suggest that long-chain triglycerides given intragastrically promote small-bowel adaptation after resection.[245] However, perfusion with non-nutritive substances can also stimulate cell proliferation in isolated bowel, indicating a role for mechanical stimulation.[247] In general, the more complex the nutrient substrate, the greater the stimulus. The special role of glutamine as a fuel for enterocytes was reviewed earlier. Dietary fiber stimulates intestinal adaptation, possibly as a result of its fermentation to short-chain fatty acids, which are important fuel sources, especially for colonic cells.[251,252]

Hormonal Factors

Many hormones appear to have trophic effects on intestinal epithelium. Intraluminal factors alone can't account for the jejunal hyperplasia seen after distal enterectomy or for the ileal hyperplasia seen after surgical diversion of gastroduodenal and pancreaticobiliary contents to the cecum.[247] Evidence to support a role for humoral factors in intestinal adaptation is presented in vascular parabiosis experiments in which intestinal resection in one animal results in intestinal adaptive changes in the nonresected partner.[246] Enteroglucagon, which is present in endocrine cells in the distal small intestine and to a lesser degree in the colon, is regarded as the leading candidate for the "growth hormone to the small intestine."[253] Its release is stimulated by intraluminal carbohydrate and long-chain triglycerides.[253] Any type of intestinal "shortening" would enhance the delivery of these nutrients to the distal intestine, with the resultant release of enteroglucagon and subsequent enhancement of mucosal growth.[246] Enteroglucagon levels are elevated both basally and postprandially in patients with small-bowel resections.[246,253] A direct relationship has been demonstrated between enteroglucagon plasma levels and cellular proliferation in diverse experimental models, including small-bowel bypass, partial

enterectomy, pancreaticobiliary diversion, and cold-induced hyperphagia.[246]

Gastrin has been suggested as a trophic stimulant for the entire digestive tract, excluding only the esophagus and gastric antrum, but the preponderance of data indicate that it is not trophic to the jejunoileum.[246,247,254] Cholecystokinin (CCK), which is structurally related to gastrin, has a trophic effect on the jejunoileum in animals, but secretin may be a necessary cofactor for this effect.[246] Epidermal growth factor (EGF) has a trophic action on duodenal and small-bowel mucosa and the gastric oxyntic gland mucosa in adult rats when given enterally.[246,255] Future investigation may reveal a role in intestinal adaptation for other peptides, including neurotensin, bombesin, pancreatic polypeptide (PP), gastric inhibitory polypeptide (GIP), vasoactive intestinal polypeptides (VIP), and motilin.[246]

Mechanical and Neurovascular Factors

Mechanical stimulation from dilation, pressure, or local motility disturbances may play a minor role in intestinal adaptation. This is supported by reports of local mucosal hypertrophy on either side of intestinal anastomoses.[247]

Proliferative rates of crypt cells are influenced by neural stimulation. Alpha-adrenergic stimulation increases intestinal epithelial cell mitotic activity and migration rate.[256] All forms of sympathectomy (chemical, surgical, and immunologic) as well as beta-adrenergic stimuli inhibit cellular proliferation.[256] Electrical stimulation of mesenteric nerves or use of cholinergic drugs increases the mitotic rate in intestinal crypts, whereas total abdominal vagotomy reduces cell proliferation.[247,256] The intimate relationship between blood vessels and autonomic innervation obscures the precise role of each in these phenomena.

DIETARY FIBER

Hugh Trowell, working in East Africa, related the bulky stools of Africans to their dietary fiber intake and proposed that dietary factors contributed to chronic diseases.[257] Later, Denis Burkitt lent supportive data as well as credence to the fiber hypothesis.[257] This hypothesis proposes that consumption of a diet high in fiber and unrefined carbohydrate is protective against many Western diseases, including colon cancer, appendicitis, diverticulosis, constipation, varicose veins, and obesity.[258]

Definition of Fiber

Dietary fiber is an umbrella term encompassing a heterogeneous group of substances that generally includes plant polysaccharides and lignin that are resistant to hydrolysis by the digestive enzymes of man.[259] It consists of the structural and matrix components of plant cell walls, primarily cellulose, hemicellulose pectins, and lignin. Cellulose is a polymer of glucose beta 1–4 and the main structural component of plant cell walls. Hemicellulose consists of branched polymers of pentose and hexose sugars. Lignin is a noncarbohydrate cell wall material that is highly resistant to degradation. Other noncellulose polysaccharides include pectins, which are complex mixtures of colloidal polysaccharides, and several polysaccharides not associated with the cell wall, including mucilages and gums. The heterogeneity of dietary fiber has inspired numerous classification schemes, including ones based on source, chemistry, and structure, water solubility, detergent solubility, physiochemical properties, and physiologic actions. Some fiber undergoes digestion by colonic bacteria; therefore, dietary fiber is not limited to substances that are recoverable in the feces. The term "crude fiber" was commonly used until the early 1970s. It refers to the residue of plant material that remains when food is extracted by dilute acids and alkalies. Although crude fiber is the measurement still referred to in most food tables, it is of little use in human nutrition studies because it underestimates by 80% to 90% the amount of material in foods that is undigestible by human digestive enzymes.[260]

Physical Properties

The physical properties of dietary fiber that play a significant role in determining its physiologic effects can be grouped into several broad categories, namely, hydratability (water-holding capacity), viscosity, ion exchange properties, and adsorptive capacity. Hydratability relates to a fiber's ability to form viscous gels. It is a function of the physical and chemical composition of the fiber, including particle size and the age of the plant, and the chemical properties of the surrounding solvent.[261,262] The water-holding capacity of a particular fiber may be important in reducing colonic transit time.[259] The various dietary fibers, especially lignins and pectins, have significant capacity to bind and exchange ions, particularly calcium, iron, magnesium, zinc, and phosphorus. The magnitude and significance of these effects vary with the species studied, types and amounts of fiber used, and duration of the studies.[261] Dietary fiber can adsorb materials such as bile salts, proteins, and bacterial cells.[261] Lignin, a common component of foods and grains, has the greatest bile salt binding potential.

Digestibility by Colonic Bacteria

Pectins and other noncellulosic polysaccharides are degraded by colonic bacteria, yielding volatile fatty acids such as acetic, propionic, and butyric, which are used as the preferred energy substrate of colonocytes. The absorption of these substances can constitute a significant percentage of daily energy intake in individuals consuming high-fiber diets.[62,259] In general, the water-insoluble fibers such as wheat bran and bagasse are less subject to fermentation in the colon than are the water-soluble fibers such as vegetable fiber, pectins, and gums.

Actions of Fiber in the Gastrointestinal Tract

The physiologic effects of dietary fiber on gastrointestinal function are dependent on their physicochemical properties (Table 21-3). The effects of the dietary fibers are complex because of their heterogeneity and the changes in luminal environment along the gastrointestinal tract. Furthermore, combinations of fibers may have effects that differ from individual purified preparations, and the same purified fiber can have different effects depending on how finely or coarsely it is ground.

Dietary fiber affects most segments of the gastrointestinal tract. Fiber increases chewing time, and this results in increased salivary and gastric juice flow, which in turn decreases dental plaque as well as appetite and caloric intake.[261] The rate of gastric emptying, and therefore the rate of digestion and absorption, is influenced by fiber components. Guar gum and pectins increase the viscosity of the chyme and slow gastric emptying, while particulate fibers such as wheat bran appear to promote more rapid gastric emptying.[260]

Intestinal transit time and stool bulk are inversely related. Dietary fiber usually reduces mouth-to-anus transit time but can actually increase it depending on the fiber source and other factors.[263,264] Particle size is important because coarse wheat bran produces a greater increase in stool bulk and greater decrease in transit time than finely ground bran.[260] The mechanism by which fiber decreases colonic transit time is not known, but possibilities include a primary action on colonic motor activity and an increase in colonic peristalsis secondary to increased fecal bulk.[263,264] A relatively nondegradable fiber such as bran increases stool bulk largely through its water-holding capacity. Fermentable fibers such as pectin and guar gum do not make as great a direct contribution to stool bulk and are recovered in stool in small amounts relative to nondegraded fibers. However, because the degradable fiber encourages proliferation of colonic bacteria, a larger portion of the fecal mass will be composed of bacteria.[261] Although the total number of bacteria can be affected by diet, there is no convincing evidence that dietary changes produce major changes in the composition of colonic microflora.[265,266]

TABLE 21-3
Physicochemical, Physiologic and Clinical Aspects of Fiber

PHYSICOCHEMICAL PROPERTY	TYPE OF FIBER	PHYSIOLOGIC EFFECT	CLINICAL IMPLICATION
Viscosity	Gums, mucilages, pectins	↓ Gastric emptying, ↑ mouth to cecum transit, ↓ rate of small intestinal absorption (e.g., of glucose, bile acids)	Dumping syndrome Diabetes Hypercholesterolemia
Particle formation and water-holding capacity	e.g., Wheat bran, pentosan content, polysaccharide–lignin mixtures	↑ Gastric emptying, ↓ mouth to cecum transit, ↓ total GI transit time, ↓ Colonic intraluminal pressure, ↑ fecal bulk	Peptic ulcer Constipation Diverticular disease Dilute potential carcinogens
Adsorption and nonspecific effects	Lignin, pectin mixed fibers	↑ Fecal steroids output ↑ fecal fat and N losses (small)	Hypercholesterolemia Cholelithiasis
Cation exchange	Acidic polysaccharides (e.g., pectins)	↑ Small intestinal losses of minerals (±), trace elements (±), heavy metals	Negative mineral balance, probably compensated for by colonic salvage, antitoxic effect
Antioxidant	Lignin (reducing phenolic groups)	↓ Free radicals in digestive tract	Anticarcinogenesis?
Degradability (colonic bacteria)	Polysaccharides (free of lignin)	↑ Gas and SCFAs production, ↓ cecal pH	Flatus, energy production

(SCFA = short-chain fatty acids)
(Modified from Eastwood MA, Strasberg SM. Am J Clin Nutr 32;364–367, 1979. Copyright Am J Clin Nutr American Society for Clinical Nutrition and Kay RM, Strasberg SM. Clin Invest Med 1:9–24, 1978. As appears in Jenkins DJ. Dietary fiber in Shils ME, Young VR (eds). Modern nutrition in health and disease, ed 7. Philadelphia: Lea and Febiger, 1988:52.)

Preventive and Therapeutic Roles

Available data support the contention that some amount of fiber is essential for normal intestinal function. However, the hypothesis that adequate dietary fiber intake is necessary to prevent a variety of Western ailments has not been proved.

Epidemiologic studies suggesting a correlation between low-fiber diets and increased rates of colonic cancer are confounded by other nutritional factors.[262,267–270] Some of the mechanisms by which dietary fiber is postulated to prevent colon carcinoma include: decrease in colonic transit time, which decreases the time that colonic mucosa is exposed to carcinogens, adsorption of carcinogenic sterols or other carcinogens by fiber, dilution of potential carcinogens by increasing stool volume, and alteration of the relative number of anaerobic and aerobic bacteria in the colon.

Colonic diverticulosis has been attributed to low dietary fiber consumption. Black Africans are reported to have a much lower prevalence of diverticulosis (20 cases per 12,000 subjects) than blacks in other countries.[261] The prevailing hypothesis is that diverticula are the result of high, localized, intraluminal pressures and that increased luminal bulk decreases intraluminal pressures by maintaining a larger diameter lumen and eliminating closed segments during contractions. Although treatment of patients who have recurrent diverticulitis or painful diverticulosis with increased fiber intake appears to relieve symptoms,[270–273] the ability of high fiber intake to prevent diverticular formation is unproved.

The epidemiologic evidence to support a role for dietary fiber in preventing cholelithiasis is difficult to analyze because the known risk factors for cholelithiasis, such as obesity and hyperglycemia, are more prevalent in Western populations where a low-fiber diet is consumed. Several studies have suggested that wheat bran promotes the formation of a less lithogenic bile by expanding the pool of bile salts, increasing the amount of chenodeoxycholic acid in the bile salt pool, and decreasing the levels of deoxycholic acid in the pool.[259,261] Other studies suggest that only specific dietary fibers (e.g., pectins, but not lignins or oat bran) are capable of lowering the lithogenic index in normal subjects.[261]

Twenty-five percent of the American population 20 years of age or older have serum cholesterol levels at or above 6.21 mmol/L and are at high risk for developing coronary heart disease.[274] Anderson and colleagues demonstrated a 19% drop in total cholesterol when 100 g of oat bran or 100 g of dried beans were added daily to the typical Western diet of 20 hypercholesterolemic patients.[275] Water-soluble fibers appear to have a much greater lipid-lowering effect than water-insoluble fibers.[276,277] Psyllium, a water-soluble, gel-forming fiber, lowers serum cholesterol when added to a typical 40%-fat Western diet[274,277] and has an additive cholesterol lowering effect when used as an adjunct to the American Heart Association's Step I diet (30% of total calories from fat, 300 mg cholesterol).[274] The mechanisms for these effects are not known; however, available evidence suggests that soluble fibers increase fecal excretion of bile acids, decrease intestinal absorption of fatty acids and cholesterol by interfering with micelle formation, and decrease hepatic cholesterol synthesis as a secondary effect of their short-chain fatty acid fermentation products. Recent work comparing the effects of oat bran versus a low-fiber wheat supplement on serum cholesterol suggests that the hypolipidemic effects may be due primarily to a displacement of fats from the diet rather than to direct effects of the oat bran.[278,279]

High-fiber diets improve diabetic control even when they contain up to 20% more carbohydrate than control diets.[280,281] The use of fiber-containing carbohydrates is now advocated by major diabetes associations. Fiber plays a role in determining a food's glycemic index, which is a numerical indication of the food's effect on blood glucose levels. As shown below, the glycemic index is calculated by expressing the blood glucose response area resulting from eating a food as a percentage of the blood glucose response area given by a reference food, either glucose or bread, containing the same amount of carbohydrate.

Glycemic Index

$$= \frac{\text{Blood glucose response area for test food}}{\text{Blood glucose response area for reference food}} \times 100$$

Many foods high in soluble fiber have low glycemic indices. The flatter blood glucose curves resulting from high-fiber foods imply that they represent a slower release form of carbohydrate. The viscous fibers such as pectins, guar, tragacanth, and leguminous seeds (beans) appear to be the most effective in stabilizing blood glucose, possibly by delaying gastric emptying and slowing absorption in the small intestine.[259,281]

Treatment of irritable bowel syndrome with a high-fiber diet has produced conflicting results.[261] Because there are groups of patients who clearly seem to benefit symptomatically from increased dietary fiber, most gastroenterologists agree that a trial is warranted. It has been suggested that those patients whose major symptom is constipation will be the ones most likely to benefit from increased fiber intake.[261]

Several studies have shown that bran supplements are effective in preventing constipation in the elderly.[282,283] Hull and colleagues reported that the use of high fiber in a geriatric population nearly eliminated the use of laxatives, at a savings of $44,000 in one year.[283] The "bulk" of available data strongly favor the use of fiber, especially the insoluble ones, in the prophylaxis and treatment of constipation.

Hemorrhoids are common in Western countries but are extremely rare in rural areas of developing countries.[284] It is postulated that straining at stool causes engorgement of the vascular cushion lining the distal rectum and anal canal, making them more vulnerable to shearing stress. The passage of hard fecal masses through the anal canal exacerbates these shearing forces and displaces the vascular cushion caudally, where it may be trapped temporarily by contraction of the anal sphincter.[284] As in the case of diverticular disease, most gastroenterologists favor a trial of fiber for hemorrhoids.

Adverse Effects of Fiber Consumption

The consumption of a high-fiber diet is generally safe and well tolerated. The possible adverse effects of excess fiber ingestion follow logically from the preceding discussions. Bloating and flatulence are perhaps the most common and annoying side effects. There have been reports of obstruction of the esophagus and small intestine, an event more likely to occur when the extensively hydratable pectins, gums, and hydrophilic colloids are ingested with insufficient liquid.[261] Both small-bowel and sigmoid volvuli have been reported in conjunction with high fiber intake, although very rarely.[261]

Despite some initial and continuing concern, increasing dietary fiber intake does not seem to result in long-term mineral and trace element depletion in populations eating adequate diets.[258,260] Although fibers will bind minerals, including calcium, magnesium, and zinc, in vitro, the intraluminal environment modifies this interaction, enhancing binding in some cases and inhibiting it in others.[285] The effects of fiber on minerals and trace elements are of greatest concern in populations whose diets may be unbalanced in the relative proportion of fiber and micronutrients. Subjects at greatest risk include children, the elderly, and populations of less developed countries.[261] Zinc deficiency seen in Iran, where a dietary staple is an unleavened bread high in fiber and phytate, is one such adverse interaction.[259,261]

Silica, which is associated with cereal fibers, especially millet, may play a role in the etiology of esophageal cancer. High intake of fiber-associated silica has been found in Northern China, South Africa, and Iran, all areas of high incidence for esophageal cancer.[259]

Optimal Daily Intake of Fiber

The optimal daily intake of fiber is controversial. One panel of experts concluded that a healthy adult should ingest about 25 to 35 g per day or 10 to 13 g per 1000 kcal. The panel held that the fiber should be derived from a well-chosen diet rather than fiber supplements and would ideally provide a 3:1 insoluble-to-soluble fiber ratio.[261]

OBESITY

Obesity, long a national obsession for cosmetic reasons, is now established as a cause of excess morbidity and mortality.[286] Americans annually spend more than 30 billion dollars on drugs, foods (including soft drinks), and literature related to losing weight.

Obesity is defined as excess body fat. There is a strong, although by no means perfect, correlation between body fat and body weight in adults.[287] The most frequently used method for expressing weight independent of stature is weight/height^2, which is termed Quetelet's index or body mass index (BMI).[288,289] Desirable weight is that associated with the lowest mortality rate. The average weight of Americans is about 10% above the desirable level.[290]

Risks of Obesity

Although the harmful effects appear to vary in a continuous manner with the degree of obesity, some find it helpful to categorize obese individuals as overweight, obese, or morbidly obese (Table 21-4). Based on 1976–1980 National Health and Nutrition Examination Surveys (NHANES), it is estimated that about 26% of U.S. adults, or 34 million people, are overweight and 12.4 million are severely overweight.[291]

The relationship between weight and mortality from all causes is illustrated in Figure 21-11. Increased mortality rates observed

TABLE 21–4

Criteria for Classification as Overweight, Obese, and Morbidly Obese

	% ABOVE DESIRABLE WEIGHT	BODY MASS INDEX
Overweight	>10	>25 kg/m²
Obesity	>20	>35 kg/m²
Morbid obesity	>100 or >100 pounds above desirable weight	

in the lowest weight groups in such studies are partially, if not totally, accounted for by individuals with undetected disease on entry into the study and smokers who tend to be thinner and have higher mortality rates.[290,292] The data suggest that being overweight is more risky for men than for women (Fig 21–11). Increased mortality in obesity is largely mediated by an increase in obesity-induced risk factors for cardiovascular disease, namely, hypertension, hypercholesterolemia, and diabetes.[293–296] However, studies of large numbers of individuals followed for up to 26 years reveal that obesity is associated with excess cardiovascular disease and mortality even in the absence of these three risk factors.[296–299]

Fat around the waist (android pattern, male pattern, upper body obesity, apple shape) is a greater health risk than the same amount of fat on the hips and thighs (gynecoid pattern, female pattern, lower body obesity, pear shape). It appears that the increased risk is associated with both intra-abdominal fat and subcutaneous fat around the waist. A waist-to-hip circumference ratio provides a simple method for quantitating fat distribution, and several methods for making the measurements have been published. An acceptable technique is to measure waist circumference at the umbilicus and hip circumference where it is greatest. The risks of hypertension, hypercholesterolemia, diabetes, cardiovascular disease, stroke, and premature mortality increase significantly as the waist/hip ratio approaches and exceeds 1.0 for men and 0.8 for women.[299–303]

Obesity is also associated with increased risks of stroke, gallstones, gout, osteoarthritis, pulmonary dysfunction, and certain cancers, including breast, uterus, ovary, and colon.[304]

Because some people smoke cigarettes as a method of controlling weight, the relative risk of smoking and obesity is important. Within every weight group, the overall mortality rate of smokers is approximately twice that of nonsmokers. Nonsmokers who are about 40% above average weight have mortality rates comparable to average-weight smokers.[305]

Is obesity a cause of disease and early mortality, or is there merely an association? Although there is still much to be learned, there is now sufficient evidence, particularly from studies of the Framingham population, that obesity is one of the causes of diabetes and cardiovascular disease and that weight reduction reduces an individual's risk of acquiring these diseases.[286,306,307] Thus, the 1988 U.S. Surgeon General's Report on Nutrition and Health concluded that a reduction in the average weight of the general population would improve the nation's health![286]

Causes of Obesity

On a thermodynamic level, the cause of all obesity is unequivocal: more food energy is ingested and absorbed than is oxidized and dissipated as heat. The excess energy is stored as fat. Obesity is not caused by a difference in absorption. On the same diet, obese and nonobese individuals absorb the same percentage of ingested energy.[308] As a group, the nonobese may eat a diet higher in fiber, and because much of the energy in dietary fiber cannot be assimilated by humans, in this sense the nonobese may absorb a lower percentage of ingested energy. However, it should be noted that dietary fiber is not counted in the caloric value of foods.

On a less basic level, virtually nothing is known with certainty about the cause of obesity. The confusing and conflicting results of studies investigating the etiology of obesity may indicate that there are many types of obesity with different etiologies. Poor study designs and inadequate numbers of patients have also played a role in the confusion. There is substantial evidence that inheritance and physiologic mechanisms are at least partly responsible for obesity, and this should caution against simplistic assumptions about why obese patients are overweight and why their attempts to lose weight frequently fail.[309–311]

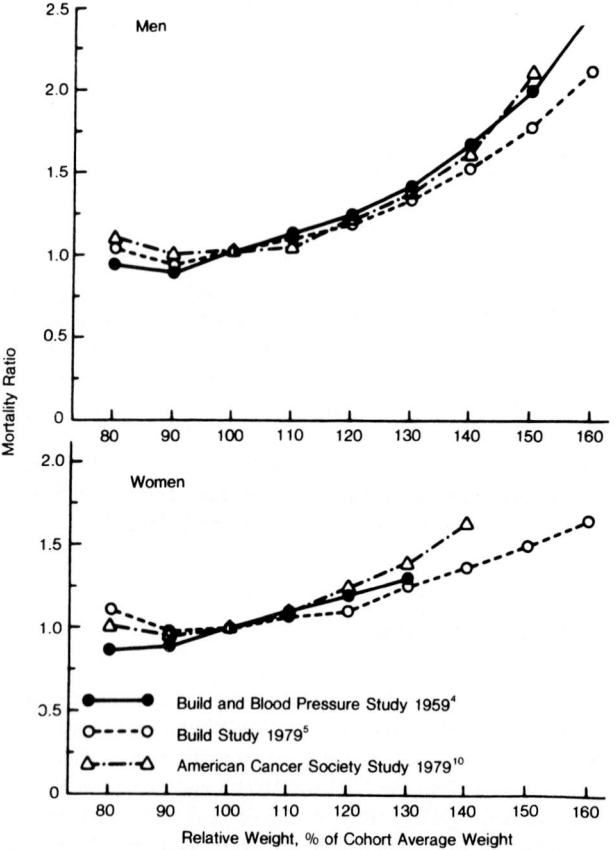

FIGURE 21–11. Mortality ratios for all ages combined, by relative weight. Results from three largest studies that provided relative weights are presented in relation to death rate of those of average weight within each cohort. (Manson JE, Stampfer MJ, Henekens CH, Willett WC. Body weight and longevity. JAMA 1987;257:357.)

Treatment of Obesity—Theoretic Considerations

Weight can be lost only by creating a negative energy balance—more calories out than in. Unless the laws of thermodynamics are proved incorrect, this fact will never change, no matter how many billions of dollars are spent on fad diets and diet books. The weight that is lost should have the same composition as the excess weight that is stored, about 25% lean and 75% fat tissue.[312] Tissue of this composition has approximately 7000 kcal/kg. Any weight loss in excess of 1 kg per 7000 kcal of energy deficit can be accomplished only by losing tissue that is more than 25% lean, which is not good, or by losing water, which is not helpful. A brief period, 2 to 3 days, of rapid weight loss will occur with any diet that decreases the amount of carbohydrate intake. This is due to utilization of stored glycogen, which is approximately 75% water.

Of all of the ways in which a negative energy balance can be achieved, the only practical methods are a decrease in energy intake and/or an increase in thermogenesis by physical activity and by diet-induced thermogenesis. The other methods bear brief mention.

ENERGY ABSORPTION

Efforts to decrease absorption have included jejunoileal bypass, which has been totally abandoned as too risky, and "starch blockers," orally ingested inhibitors of pancreatic amylase, which are ineffective. A nonabsorbable fat, Olestra, is currently being reviewed by the Food and Drug Administration (1989). Assuming it is eventually marketed, it remains to be seen whether obese people will use it in place of ordinary fat and whether they will lose weight. Another "fat substitute," Simplesse, is not in the same class because it is a modified protein and is absorbed. However, it is said to taste and feel like fat but yields only 4 kcal/g instead of 9 kcal/g. Because dietary fiber is by definition nonabsorbable material in the diet, a high-fiber diet is currently the most effective way to decrease absorption of ingested food.

Efforts to increase resting energy expenditure (REE), if successful, would pay off handsomely, because REE makes up 70% to 75% of total daily energy expenditure. Suggestions that REE is increased for many hours following active exercise have been refuted.[313] Because lean tissue is the most metabolically active body component, exercise that increases muscle mass will increase REE. However, in practice, it has been difficult to prove that obese individuals can significantly increase their REE by this method.[314] A number of drugs that can increase energy expenditure have been investigated. Dinitrophenol, which uncouples oxidative phosphorylation, was abandoned because of toxicity. Triiodothyronine (T_3) was unacceptable because it induced marked loss of lean body mass. Sympathomimetic drugs are being tested. Caffeine

and nicotine appear to increase REE by a small percentage. To be useful, a thermogenic drug must be not only effective but also safe for indefinite use if the weight loss is to be maintained. There are no likely candidates at this time.

SURGERY

Adipose tissue can be removed by excision and liposuction. These are painful, expensive, and potentially dangerous methods, and they are not permanent because new fat cells can be recruited from the remaining subcutaneous stromal tissue.

Treatment of Obesity—Practical Considerations

Weight loss that is not permanent, at least lasting for several years, seems of little practical benefit. The few long-term follow-up studies published, primarily involving participants in university and other expensive weight loss programs, are very discouraging.[315,316] However, the percentage of people in the general population who try to lose weight and succeed in permanently doing so is not known and may be substantial. Therefore, health care providers should not be discouraged from counseling patients about proper weight management. In doing so, it should be recognized that of all possible approaches to losing weight, only three are practical: (1) reduction of energy intake with an emphasis on lowering fat and increasing fiber in the diet, (2) increasing energy expenditure by physical activity, and (3) increasing diet-induced thermogenesis by ingesting a larger percentage of energy as carbohydrate. All appropriate weight reduction plans emphasize permanent changes in both eating and exercise habits, not dieting and exercising for temporary weight loss. It is important to help the overweight individual understand that once thinner, the body will *always* require fewer calories than those currently ingested. The eventual weight is entirely determined by the individual's permanent eating and activity, not by temporary losses achieved by dieting. For this reason, it is most practical and sensible for overweight individuals to achieve a new weight equilibrium as dictated by the change in eating habits they feel they can live with comfortably.

The fact that a physician would encourage dietary and activity changes may be enough to motivate some people with mild to moderate obesity to modify their habits and lose weight. When there is motivation to lose weight, factual information, especially about ways to reduce dietary fat while eating a well-balanced diet, may be all some individuals need. Others will benefit from joining more formal programs. Characteristics of a desirable weight loss program are outlined in Table 21-5.

THE IMPORTANCE OF DECREASING DIETARY FAT

Several lines of evidence support the contention that eating less fat is the single most effective strategy for reducing weight. Most obvious is the fact that fat provides more calories per gram than any other nutrient. In addition, fat produces less diet-induced thermogenesis and less adaptive thermogenesis than carbohydrate

TABLE 21-5
Characteristics of a Desirable Weight Loss Program

Nutrition instruction
Behavior modification
Calorie intake not below 1000 kcal/day for women and 1200 kcal/day for men
Acceptable foods
Weight loss not exceeding 1 kg/week
Diet that is sufficient in all nutrients except energy
Exercise at least 3 days/week for 20–30 minutes
Habits encouraged and continued for life

and protein. Excess carbohydrate intake stimulates thermogenesis, while excess fat ingestion does not. On ingestion of pure fat, carbohydrate, and protein, 3%, 10% to 25%, and 25% of the ingested calories are burned as diet-induced thermogenesis, respectively. Therefore, fat calories eaten in excess of energy needs are more likely to be deposited as fat than are excess carbohydrate or protein calories, which are more likely to be oxidized and dissipated as heat.[317-320]

Clinical studies indicate that these concepts have practical application. In a crossover study, women who were eating to satiety lost weight when the "hidden" fat content of the food served was reduced.[321] The case for decreasing fat ingestion for weight control has been summarized and popularized, if somewhat overstated, in the popular book, *The T-Factor Diet.*[322]

In practice, obese patients must be cautioned that as far as weight is concerned, one fat or oil is as bad as another. Eating food fried in vegetable oil instead of lard will help lower cholesterol but not weight. The patient must learn to recognize, buy, cook, eat, and enjoy foods with less fat. In choosing between foods, the patient should read labels and choose those foods with the least content of fat per serving and not be as concerned about the calories per serving or percentage of calories supplied by fat. How successful an individual obese person will be in decreasing fat ingestion may depend on the intensity of his or her inherited or acquired taste preference for fat.

BEHAVIOR MODIFICATION

Introduction of behavior modification methods into weight loss programs has been associated with a decreased attrition rate, decreased negative emotional responses to treatment, increased cost-effectiveness, and somewhat improved long-term maintenance of weight loss. The traditional psychologic approach to obesity was to investigate the tensions, hostility, insecurity, or other emotional difficulties that might be expressed as overeating. The behavior therapy approach is based on the assumption that eating behavior is acquired and maintained by environmental events and can be changed by appropriate manipulation of the environment. Thus, obese people seem to eat in response to many inappropriate cues, such as television, cooking, anxiety, or boredom. If eating can be limited to specified times and a particular place, then the obese person may regain control of his or her eating. The emphasis in behavior therapy is on learning more about circumstances in which a person eats particular foods and how those circumstances can be changed.[323]

VERY LOW CALORIE DIETS

Fasting is the quickest way to lose weight, averaging .54 kg/day, but causes disproportionate loss of lean tissue. Attempts to preserve the rapid weight loss while avoiding the excess loss of lean body mass have resulted in a number of very low calorie diet (VLCD) plans, sometimes designated protein-sparing modified fast (PSMF). These diets provide 300 to 800 kcal/day. The earliest commercial version of these diets, which was deficient in several essential amino acids and not routinely supplemented with vitamins and minerals, was associated with more than 50 deaths. More recently marketed products are rich in high-quality proteins, are variable in carbohydrate content, and contain recommended daily amounts of vitamins and minerals. They are marketed under various names, including the Cambridge diet and Optifast. They do not appear to be associated with major complications when used under adequate supervision. How well these diets prevent excess wasting of lean body mass is controversial. In the hope of enhancing long-term success, the products are used in conjunction with behavior modification principles and a gradual return to ordinary food. Some programs return participants to the low calorie liquid diet when weight begins to increase. Weight loss on VLCD averages about 20 kg in 12 weeks.[324,325] These weight loss programs are very expensive, there is a high dropout rate, and recent studies reveal that 30 to 60 months after completing these programs, most people who lost weight have regained most of it.[326-329] The most appropriate use of these diets is for those few patients in whom very rapid weight loss is indicated for medical reasons.

SURGERY

A number of mechanical methods have been used for restricting food intake in the obese. The most widely used is surgery to create a small gastric pouch (10–15 ml), usually accomplished by a vertical banded gastroplasty or by gastric stapling and a gastrojejunal bypass. Dramatic weight loss with reversal of diabetes and other obesity-associated conditions can be achieved, but the risks are significant and the results are not necessarily permanent. Jaw wiring can be done with less immediate risk, but it is not a long-term option and is virtually never used in the U.S. Use of gastric balloons (artificial bezoars) received a brief flurry of enthusiasm but was abandoned when randomized, controlled clinical trials indicated no benefit of this expensive and temporary method.

DRUG THERAPY

Anorectic drugs include those with stimulant properties, such as amphetamines and phentermine, which act on adrenergic receptors in the brain to decrease hunger, and those without stimulant properties, such as fenfluramine, which promote the release of serotonin and enhance satiety. Randomized, controlled trials have yielded conflicting results, but a substantial proportion of them have demonstrated significantly greater weight loss in participants on anorectic drugs versus those on placebo. However, the only long-term follow-up study showed that those who took the drug regained significantly more weight when it was discontinued than did the control group. As a result, their final weight after 1 year was greater than that of the control group.[330]

Few physicians would be able to evaluate the teaching materials, cookbooks, and popular books that deal with weight loss. Help is available in the form of a recent publication in which qualified nutritionists have rated many such publications.[331]

The reader is directed to Chapter 17, Carbohydrate Assimilation; Chapter 18, Intestinal Lipid Absorption; Chapter 19, Protein Digestion and Assimilation; Chapter 20, Vitamins and Minerals; and Chapter 48, Approach to the Patient Requiring Nutritional Supplementation.

REFERENCES

1. Stedman's medical dictionary, ed 23. Baltimore: Williams & Wilkins, 1976.
2. Stryer L. Biochemistry, ed 3. New York: WH Freeman, 1988.
3. The Surgeon General's Report on Nutrition and Health. Washington, DC: US Department of Health and Human Services (Public Health Service), Publication No. 88-50210, 1988:275.
4. Campbell RG, Hashim SA, Van Itallie TB. Studies of food-intake regulation in man. N Engl J Med 1971;285:1402.
5. Yudkin J. Nutrition and palatability with special reference to obesity, myocardial infarction, and other diseases of civilisation. Lancet 1963;7295.
6. Garrow JS. Energy balance and obesity in man, ed 2. Amsterdam: Elsevier, North Holland Biomedical Press, 1978.
7. Mrosovsky N, Powley TL. Set points for body weight and fat. Behav Biol 1977;20:205.
8. Keesey RE. Physiological regulation of body weight and the issue of obesity. Med Clin North Am 1989;73:15.
9. Keesey RE. The body weight set-point. What can you tell your patients? Postgrad Med 1988;83:114.
10. Wirtshufler D, Davis JD. Set points, settling points, and the control of body weight. Physiol Behav 1977;19:75.
11. Garrow JS. Energy balance and obesity in man. Amsterdam: North Holland Publishing Co, 1974.
12. Anand BK, Brobeck JR. Hypothalamic control of food intake in rats and cats. Yale J Biol Med 1951;24:123.
13. Powley TL, Laughton W. Neural pathways involved in the hypothalamic integration of anatomic responses. Diabetologia 1981;20:378.
14. Morley JE, Levine AS. The central control of appetite. Lancet 1983;i:398.
15. Levin BE. Neurological regulation of body weight. CRC Crit Rev Clin Neurobiol 1987;2:1.
16. Grossman SP. Contemporary problems concerning our understanding of brain mechanisms that regulate food intake and body weight. In: Stunkard AJ, Stellar E, eds. Eating and its disorders. New York: Raven Press, 1984:5.
17. Keesey RE, Corbett SW. Metabolic defense of the body weight set-point. In: Stunkard AJ, Stellar E, eds. Eating and its disorders. New York: Raven Press, 1984:87.
18. Morley JE, Levine AS, Gosnell BA, Billington CJ. Neuropeptides and appetite: Contribution of neuropharmacological modeling. Fed Proc 1984;43:2903.
19. Marino LA, DeBellis MD, Leibowitz SF. Alpha-2 adrenergic receptors in the paraventricular nucleus mediate feeding induced by norepinephrine and clonidine. Abstracts of the Society for Neurosciences 1983;9:467.
20. Wurtman RJ. Neurotransmitters, control of appetite and obesity. In: Winick M, ed. Control of appetite. New York: John Wiley & Sons, 1988:27.
21. Yalow RS, Eng J, Strauss E. The role of CCK-like peptides in appetite regulation. In: Levine R, Luft R, eds. Advances in metabolic disorders. San Diego, CA: Academic Press, Inc, 1983;10:435.
22. Baile CA, McLaughlin CL, Della-Fera MA. Role of cholecystokinin and opioid peptides in control of food intake. Physiol Rev 1986;66:172.
23. Woods SC, Porte D. The role of insulin as a satiety factor in the central nervous system. In: Levine R, Luft R, eds. Advances in metabolic disorders. San Diego, CA: 1983;10:457.
24. Smith GP. The peripheral control of appetite. Lancet 1983;2:88.
25. Smith GP, Gibbs J. The satiating effect of cholecystokinin. In: Winick M, ed. Control of appetite. New York: John Wiley & Sons, 1988:27.
26. Kissileff HR, Pi-Sunyer FX, Thornton J, Smith GP. C-terminal octapeptide of cholecystokinin decreases food intake in man. Am J Clin Nutr 1981;34:154.
27. Geracioti TD, Liddle RA. Impaired cholecystokinin secretion in bulimia nervosa. N Engl J Med 1988;319:683.
28. Herman CP, Polivy J. Psychological factors in the control of appetite. In: Winick M, ed. Control of appetite. New York: John Wiley & Sons, 1988:41.
29. Blundell JE, Hill AJ. Analysis of hunger: Inter-relationships with palatability, nutrient content and eating. In: Hirsch J, Van Itallie TB, eds. Recent advances in obesity research: IV. London: John Libbey and Co, 1985:118.
30. Asimov I. Order! Order! In: Asimov on physics. Garden City, NY: Doubleday & Co, 1976:128.
31. Wilmore DW. The metabolic management of the critically ill. New York: Plenum Medical Book Co, 1977.
32. Weir JB. New methods for calculating metabolic rate with special reference to protein metabolism. J Physiol 1949;109:1.
33. Head CA, McManus CB, Seitz S, Grossman GD, Staton GW, Heymsfield SB. Simple and accurate indirect calorimetry system for assessment of resting energy expenditure. J Parenter Enteral Nutr 1984;8:45.
34. Feurer I, Mullen JL. Bedside measurement of resting energy expenditure and respiratory quotient via indirect calorimetry. Nutr Clin Pract 1986;1:43.
35. Dietrich KA, Romero MD, Conrad SA. The technique of measuring energy expenditure at the bedside. J Crit Ill 1989;14:65.
36. Kinney JM. Energy metabolism: Heat, fuel and life. In: Kinney JM, Jeejeebhoy KN, Hill GL, Owen OE, eds. Nutrition and metabolism in patient care. Philadelphia: WB Saunders, 1988:3.
37. Livesey G, Elia M. Estimation of energy expenditure, net carbohydrate utilization, and net fat oxidation and synthesis by indirect calorimetry: Evaluation of errors with special reference to the detailed composition of fuels. Am J Clin Nutr 1988;47:608.
38. Elia M, Livesey G. Theory and validity of indirect calorimetry during net lipid synthesis. Am J Clin Nutr 1988;47:591.
39. Feurer ID, Mullen JL. Measurement of energy expenditure. In: Rombeau JL, Caldwell MD, eds. Parenteral nutrition, Vol 2. Clinical nutrition. Philadelphia: WB Saunders, 1986:224.
40. Lifson N, McClintock R. Theory of use of turnover rates of body water for measuring energy and material balance. J Theor Biol 1966;12:46.
41. Schoeller DA. Measurement of energy expenditure in free-living humans by using doubly labeled water. J Nutr 1988;118:1278.
42. Schoeller DA. Energy expenditure from doubly labeled water: Some fundamental considerations in humans. Am J Clin Nutr 1983;38:999.
43. Schoeller DA, Van Santen E. Measurement of energy expenditure in humans by doubly labeled water method. J Appl Physiol 1982;53:955.
44. Schoeller DA, Webb P. Five-day comparison of the doubly labeled water method with respiratory gas exchange. Am J Clin Nutr 1984;40:153.
45. Coward WA, Prentice AM. Letter: Isotope method for the measurement of carbon dioxide production rate in man. Am J Clin Nutr 1985;41:659.
46. Schoeller DA. Letter: Reply to letter from Coward and Prentice. Am J Clin Nutr 1985;41:659.
47. Schoeller DA, Ravussin E, Schutz Y, Acheson KJ, Baertschi P, Jequier E. Energy expenditure by doubly labeled water: Validation in humans and proposed calculation. Am J Physiol 1986;250:R823.
48. Schoeller DA, Kushner RF, Jones PJ. Validation of doubly labeled water for measuring energy expenditure during parenteral nutrition. Am J Clin Nutr 1986;44:291.
49. Owen OE. Regulation of energy and metabolism. In: Kinney JM, Jeejeebhoy KN, Hill GL, Owen OE, eds. Nutrition and metabolism in patient care. Philadelphia: WB Saunders, 1988:35.
50. Guyton AC. Textbook of medical physiology. Philadelphia: WB Saunders, 1986:846.
51. Kinney JM. Food as fuel: The development of concepts. In: Shils ME, Young VR, eds. Modern nutrition in health and disease, ed 7. Philadelphia: Lea & Febiger, 1988:516.
52. Cunningham JJ. A reanalysis of the factors influencing basal metabolic rate in normal adults. Am J Clin Nutr 1980;33:2372.
53. Owen OE, Holup JL, D'Alessio DA, et al. A reappraisal of the caloric requirement of men. Am J Clin Nutr 1987;46:875.
54. Kleiber M. The fire of life: An introduction to animal energetics. New York: John Wiley & Sons, 1961.
55. Michel L, Serrano A, Malt RA. Nutritional support of hospitalized patients. N Engl J Med 1981;304:1147.

56. Kinney J, Long CL. Tissue composition of weight loss in surgical patients. Ann Surg 1969;168:459.

57. Alpers DH, Clouse RE, Stenson WF. Manual of nutritional therapeutics. Boston: Little, Brown, 1983.

58. Rothwell NJ, Stock MJ. Diet-induced thermogenesis. In: Girardier L, Stock MJ, eds. Mammalian thermogenesis. New York: Chapman and Hail, 1983:208.

59. Rothwell NJ, Stock MJ. Thermogenesis: Comparative and evolutionary considerations. In: Cioff LA, ed. The body weight regulatory system: Normal and disturbed mechanisms. New York: Raven Press, 1981.

60. Dulloo AG, Miller DS. Obesity: A disorder of the sympathetic nervous system. World Rev Nutr Diet 1987;50:1.

61. Nicholls DG, Locke RM. Thermogenic mechanisms in brown fat. Physiol Rev 1984;64:1.

62. Ruppin H, Bar-Meir S, Soergel KH, Wood CM, Schmitt MG. Absorption of short-chain fatty acids by the colon. Gastroenterology 1980;78:1500.

63. Woolfson AM. Energy and nitrogen requirements. In: Woolfson AM, ed. Biochemistry of hospital nutrition. Edinburgh: Churchill Livingstone, 1986:140.

64. Jeejeebhoy KN. Nutrient metabolism. In: Kinney JM, Jeejeebhoy KN, Hill GL, Owen OE, eds. Nutrition and metabolism in patient care. Philadelphia: WB Saunders, 1988:60.

65. Foster GD, Know LS, Dempsey DT, Mullen JL. Caloric requirements in total parenteral nutrition. J Am Coll Nutr 1987;6:231.

66. Roza AM, Shizgal HM. The Harris-Benedict equation reevaluated: Resting energy requirements and the body cell mass. Am J Clin Nutr 1984;40:168.

67. Daly JM, Heymsfield SB, Head CA, et al. Human energy requirements: Overestimation by widely used prediction equation. Am J Clin Nutr 1985;42:1170.

68. Munro HN, Crim MC. The proteins and amino acids. In: Shils ME, Young VR, eds. Modern nutrition in health and disease, ed 7. Philadelphia: Lea & Febiger, 1988:1.

69. Laidlaw SA, Kopple JD. Newer concepts for the indispensable amino acids. Am J Clin Nutr 1987;46:593.

70. Allison JB. Biological evaluation of proteins. Physiol Rev 1955;35:664.

71. Bressani R. Human assays and applications. In: Bodwell CE, ed. Evaluation of proteins for humans. Westport, CT: AVI Publishing Co, 1977:81.

72. KaKade ML, Hoffa DE, Liener IE. Contribution of trypsin inhibitors to the deleterious effects of unheated soybeans fed to rats. J Nutr 1973;103:1772.

73. Shaw SN, Elwyn DH, Askanazi J, et al. Effects of increasing nitrogen intake on nitrogen balance and energy expenditure in nutritionally depleted adults receiving parenteral nutrition. Am J Clin Nutr 1983;37:930.

74. WHO/FAO/UNU Report: Energy and protein requirements. WHO Technical Report Series, No. 724, 1985.

75. Recommended dietary allowances, ed 10. Washington, DC: National Academy Press, 1989.

76. Monsen ER. The 10th edition of the recommended dietary allowances: What's new in the 1989 RDAs? J Am Diet Assoc 1989;89:1748.

77. Callaway DH, Margen H. Variation in endogenous nitrogen excretion and dietary nitrogen utilization as determinants of human protein requirement. J Nutr 1971;101:204.

78. Heird WC, Cooper A. Nutrition in infants and children. In: Shils ME, Young VR, eds. Modern nutrition in health and disease, ed 7. Philadelphia: Lea & Febiger, 1988:944.

79. Gong EJ, Heald FP. Diet, nutrition and adolescence. In: Shils ME, Young VR, eds. Modern nutrition in health and disease, ed 7. Philadelphia: Lea & Febiger, 1988:969.

80. Whitehead RG. Pregnancy and lactation. In: Shils ME, Young VR. Modern nutrition in health and disease, ed 7. Philadelphia: Lea & Febiger, 1988:931.

81. Cotzias GC. Role and importance of trace substances in environmental health. In: Hemphill DD, ed. Proceedings of the First Annual Conference on Trace Substances in Environmental Health. Columbia, MO: University of Missouri, 1967:5.

82. Frieden E. A survey of the essential biochemical elements. In: Frieden E, ed. Biochemistry of the essential trace elements. New York: Plenum Press, 1984:1.

83. McDonald I. Carbohydrates. In: Shils ME, Young VR, eds. Modern nutrition in health and disease, ed 7. Philadelphia: Lea & Febiger, 1988:38.

84. Hers HG, Van Schuftingen E. Fructose 2,6-bisphosphate 2 years after its discovery. Biochem J 1982;206:1.

85. Mayes PA. Regulation of carbohydrate metabolism. In: Murray RK, Granner DK, Mayes PA, Rodwell VW, eds. Harper's biochemistry. Norwalk, CT: Appleton and Lange, 1988:186.

86. Devlin JT, Horton ES. Hormone and nutrient interaction. Philadelphia: Lea & Febiger, 1988:570.

87. Mortimer GE. Intracellular protein catabolism and its control during nutrient deprivation and supply. Annu Rev Nutr 1987;7:539.

88. Bond JS, Butler PE. Intracellular proteases. Annu Rev Biochem 1987;56:333.

89. Horl WH, Wanner C, Schollmeyer P. Proteinases in catabolism and malnutrition. J Parenter Enteral Nutr 1987;11:98s.

90. Beynon RJ, Bond JS. Catabolism of intracellular protein: Molecular aspects. Am J Physiol 1986;20:C141.

91. Fagan JM, Waxman L, Goldberg AL. Skeletal muscle and liver contain a soluble ATP+ ubiquitin-dependent proteolytic system. Biochem J 1987;243:335.

92. Rodwell VW. Catabolism of amino acid nitrogen. In: Murray RK, Granner DK, Mayes PA, Rodwell VW, eds. Harper's biochemistry. Norwalk, CT: Appleton and Lange, 1988:271.

93. Elwyn DH, Parikh HC, Shoemaker WC. Amino acid movements between gut, liver, and periphery in unanesthetized dogs. Am J Physiol 1968;215:1260.

94. Wharen J, Felig P, Hagenfeldt TL. Effect of protein ingestion on splanchnic and leg metabolism in normal man and in patients with diabetes mellitus. J Clin Invest 1976;57:987.

95. Fernstrum JD, Wurtman RJ. Brain serotonin content: Physiological regulation by plasma neutral amino acids. Science 1972;178:419.

96. Zapsalis C, Beck RA. Food chemistry and nutritional biochemistry. New York: John Wiley & Sons, 1985:935.

97. Wills ED. Biochemical basis of medicine. Bristol:John Wright and Sons, 1985:412.

98. Lowenstein JM. Ammonia production in muscle and other tissues: The purine nucleotide cycle. Physiol Rev 1972;52:382.

99. Souba WW. Interorgan ammonia metabolism in health and disease: A surgeon's view. J Parenter Enteral Nutr 1987;11:569.

100. Souba WW, Smith RJ, Wilmore DW. Glutamine metabolism by the intestinal tract. J Parenter Enteral Nutr 1985;9:608.

101. Windmueller HG. Glutamine utilization by the small intestine. Adv Enzymol Relat Areas Molec Biol 1982;53:202.

102. Olney JW. Excitotoxic amino acids: Research applications and safety implications. In: Filer LJ, Garattini S, Kare MR, Reynolds WA, Wurtman RJ, eds. Glutamic acid: Advances in biochemistry and physiology. New York: Raven Press, 1979:287.

103. Schaumberg HH, Byck R, Gerstl R, Mashman JH. Monosodium glutamate: Its pharmacology and role in the Chinese restaurant syndrome. Science 1969;163:82c.

104. Bower RH, Muggia-Sullam M, Vallgren S, et al. Branched chain amino acid–enriched solutions in the septic patient. Ann Surg 1986;203:13.

105. Sax HC, Talamini MA, Fischer JE. Clinical use of branched chain amino acids in liver disease, sepsis, trauma, and burns. Arch Surg 1986;121:358.

106. Desai SP, Bistrian BR, Palombo JD, Moldawer LL, Blackburn GL. Branched chain amino acid administration in surgical patients. Arch Surg 1987;122:760.

107. Lundholm K, Bennegard K, Wickstrom I, Lindmark L. Is it possible to evaluate the efficacy of amino acid solutions after major surgical procedures or accidental injuries? Evaluation in a randomized and prospective study. J Parenter Enteral Nutr 1986;10:29.

108. Brennan MF, Cerra F, Daly JM, et al. Report of a research workshop: Branched chain amino acids in stress and injury. J Parenter Enteral Nutr 1986;10:446.

109. Fisher JE, Baldessarini RJ. False neurotransmitters and hepatic failure. Lancet 1971;2:75.

110. Cerra FB, McMillen M, Angelico R, et al. Cirrhosis, encephalopathy and improved results with metabolic support. Surgery 1983;94:612.

111. Eriksson LS, Conn HO. Branched chain amino acids in the management of hepatic encephalopathy: An analysis of variants. Hepatology 1989;10:228.

112. Naylor CD, O'Rourke K, Detsky AS, Baker JP. Parenteral nutrition with branched chain amino acids in hepatic encephalopathy. Gastroenterology 1989;97:1033.

113. Berlin JA, Chalmers TC. Meta-analysis of branched chain amino acids in hepatic encephalopathy. Gastroenterology 1989;97:1043.

114. Alexander WF, Spindel E, Harty RF, Cerda JJ. The usefulness of branched chain amino acids in patients with acute or chronic encephalopathy. Am J Gastroenterol 1989;84:91.

115. Blackburn GL, O'Keefe SJ. Nutrition in liver failure. Gastroenterology 1989;97:1049.

116. Shafrir JE, Bergman M, Felig P. The endocrine pancreas: Diabetes mellitus. In: Felig P, Baxter JD, Broadus AE, Frohman LA, eds. Endocrinology and metabolism, ed 2. New York: McGraw-Hill, 1987: 1043.

117. Ganong WF. Review of medical physiology, ed 13. Norwalk, CT: Appleton and Lange, 1987:253.

118. Rebuffe-Scrive M, Enk L, Crona N, et al. Fat cell metabolism in different regions in women. J Clin Invest 1985;75:1973.

119. Third JL, Bremner WF. Lipid and lipoprotein metabolism. In: Fischer JE, ed. Surgical nutrition. Boston: Little, Brown, 1983:213.

120. Hariharan K. Essential fatty acids. Indian Pediatr 1988;25:67.

121. Friedman Z. Essential fatty acids revisited. Am J Dis Child 1980;134: 406.

122. Spielmann D, Bracco U, Traitler H, et al. Alternative lipids in usual w6 PUFAS: Gamma-linolenic acid, alpha linolenic acid, stearidonic acid, EPA, etc. J Parenter Enteral Nutr 1988;12:111s.

123. Anderson GJ, Connor WE. On the demonstration of omega-3 essential-fatty-acid deficiency in humans. Am J Clin Nutr 1989;49: 585.

124. Gorlin R. The biological actions and potential clinical significance of dietary omega-3 fatty acid. Arch Intern Med 1988;148:2043.

125. Holman RT, Johnson SB, Hutch TT. A case of human linolenic acid deficiency involving neurological abnormalities. Am J Clin Nutr 1982;35:617.

126. Holman RT, Johnson SB, Hatch TF. Human linolenic acid deficiency (reply to letter). Am J Clin Nutr 1982;36:1254.

127. Holman RT. Essential fatty acid deficiency. In: Holman RT, ed. Progress in the chemistry of fats and other lipids. Oxford: Pergamon Press, 1968:275.

128. Wene JD, Connor WE, DenBesten L. The development of essential fatty acid deficiency in healthy men fed fat-free diets intravenously and orally. J Clin Invest 1975;56:127.

129. Carroll KK. Essential fatty acids: What level in the diet is most desirable? Adv Exp Med Biol 1977;83:535.

130. Grundy SM, Bilheimer D, Blackburn H. Rationale of the diet-heart statement of the American Heart Association. Report of Nutrition Committee. Circulation 1982;65:839A.

131. Report of the National Cholesterol Education Program Expert Panel on detection, evaluation, and treatment of high blood cholesterol in adults. Arch Intern Med 1988;148:36.

132. Gwynne JT, Lawrence MK. Current concepts in the evaluation and treatment of hypercholesterolemia. Mod Med 1989;57:126.

133. Bang HO, Dyerberg J, Nielsen AB. Plasma lipid and lipoprotein pattern in Greenlandic West-Coast Eskimos. Lancet 1971;ii:1153.

134. Kromhaut D, Bosschieter EB, de Lezenne Coulander C. The inverse relation between fish consumption and 20-year mortality from coronary heart disease. N Engl J Med 1985;312:1205.

135. Dyerberg J, Bang HO, Stofferson E, Moncada S, Vane JR. Eicosapentanoic acid and prevention of thrombosis and atherosclerosis? Lancet 1978;ii:11.

136. Dyerberg J, Bang HO. Hemostatic function and platelet polyunsaturated fatty acids in Eskimos. Lancet 1979;ii:433.

137. Fehily AM, Burr ML, Phillips KM, Deadman NM. The effect of fatty fish on plasma lipid and lipoprotein concentrations. Am J Clin Nutr 1983;38:349.

138. Bronsgeest-Schoute HC, Van Gent CM, Luten JB, Ruiter A. The effect of various intakes of W3 fatty acids on the blood lipid composition in healthy human subjects. Am J Clin Nutr 1981;34:1752.

139. Phillipson BE, Rothrock DW, Connor WE, Harris WS, Illingworth DR. Reduction of plasma lipids, lipoproteins, and apoproteins by dietary fish oils in patients with hypertriglyceridemia. N Engl J Med 1985;312:1210.

140. Schectman G, Kaul S, Cherayil GD, Lee M, Kissebah A. Can the hypotriglyceridemic effect of fish oil concentrate be sustained? Ann Intern Med 1989;110:346.

141. Harris WS, Dujovne CA, Zucker M, Johnson B. Effects of a low saturated fat, low cholesterol fish oil supplement in hypertriglyceridemic patients. Ann Intern Med 1988;109:465.

142. Yetiv JZ. Clinical applications of fish oil. JAMA 1988;260:665.

143. Lee TH, Hoover RL, Williams JD, et al. Effect of dietary enrichment with eicosapentaenoic and docosahexanoic acids on *in vitro* neutrophil and monocyte leukotriene generation and neutrophil function. N Engl J Med 1985;312:1219.

144. Endres S, Ghorbani R, Kelley VE, et al. The effect of dietary supplementation with n-3 polyunsaturated fatty acids on the synthesis of interleukin-1 and tumor necrosis factor by mononuclear cells. N Engl J Med 1989;320:265.

145. Kremer JM, Jubiz W, Michalek A, et al. Fish-oil fatty acid supplementation in active rheumatoid arthritis. Ann Intern Med 1987;106: 497.

146. Bittiner SB, Tucker WF, Cartwright I, Bleher SS. A double blind, randomized, placebo-controlled trial of fish oil in psoriasis. Lancet 1988;ii:378.

147. Bjorneboe A, Soyland E, Bjoraebo GE, et al. Effect of dietary supplementation with eicosapentanoic acid in the treatment of atopic dermatitis. Br J Dermatol 1987;117:463.

148. Knapp HR, Fitzgerald GA. The antihypertensive effects of fish oil. N Engl J Med 1989;320:1037.

149. Dehmer GJ, Popma JJ, Van Den Berg EK, et al. Reduction in the rate of early restenosis after coronary angioplasty by a diet supplemented with n-3 fatty acids. N Engl J Med 1988;319:733.

150. Glauber H, Wallace P, Griver K, Brechtel G. Adverse effect of omega-3 fatty acids in non–insulin-dependent diabetes mellitus. Ann Intern Med 1988;108:663.

151. Wan JM, Teo TC, Babayan VK, Blackburn GL. Invited comment: Lipids and the development of immune dysfunction and infection. J Parenter Enteral Nutr 1988;12:43s.

152. Erickson KL. Dietary fat modulation of immune response. Int J Immunopharmacol 1986;8:529.

153. Hwang D. Essential fatty acids and immune response. FASEB J 1989;3:2052.

154. Palmblad J, Gyllenhammar H. Effect of dietary lipids on immunity and inflammation. APMIS 1988;96:571.

155. Trocki O, Heyd TJ, Waymack JP, Alexander JW. Effects of fish oil on postburn metabolism and immunity. J Parenter Enteral Nutr 1987;11:521.

156. Babayan VK. Medium chain triglycerides and structured lipids. Lipids 1987;22:417.

157. Mascioli EA, Bistrian BR, Babayan VK, Blackburn GL. Medium chain triglycerides and structured lipids as unique non-glucose energy sources in hyperalimentation. Lipids 1987;22:421.

158. Heird WC, Grundy SM, Hubbard VS. Structured lipids and their use in clinical nutrition. Am J Clin Nutr 1986;43:320.

159. Birkhahn RH. Invited comment: The role of synthetic compounds in clinical nutrition. J Parenter Enteral Nutr 1988;12:89s.

160. Mascioli EA, Babayan VK, Bistrian BR, Blackburn GL. Novel triglycerides for special medical purposes. J Parenter Enteral Nutr 1988;12:127s.

161. Moore FD, Olesen KH, McMurrey JD, Parker VH, Ball MR, Boyden CM. The body cell mass and its supporting environment. Philadelphia: WB Saunders, 1963.

162. Cahill GF. Starvation: Some biological aspects. In: Kinney JM, Jeejeebhoy KN, Hill GL, Owen OE, eds. Nutrition and metabolism in patient care. Philadelphia: WB Saunders, 1988:193.

163. Hoffer LJ. Starvation. In: Shils ME, Young VR, eds. Modern nutrition in health and disease. Philadelphia: Lea & Febiger, 1988:774.

164. Cahill GF. Starvation in man. N Engl J Med 1970;282:668.

165. Young VR, Scrimshaw NS. The physiology of starvation. Sci Am 1971;225:14.

166. Benedict FG. A study of prolonged fasting. Washington, DC: Carnegie Institute of Washington, No. 203, 1915.

167. Keys A, Brozek J, Henschell A, Mickelsen O, Taylor HL. The biology

of human starvation. Minneapolis: The University of Minnesota Press, 1950.

168. Levenson SM, Seifter E. Starvation: Metabolic and physiologic responses. In: Fischer JE, ed. Surgical nutrition. Boston: Little, Brown, 1983.

169. Felig P. The glucose-alanine cycle. Metabolism 1973;22:179.

170. Vagenakis A, Burger A, Portnay GI, et al. Diversion of peripheral thyroxine metabolism from activating to inactivating pathways during complete fasting. J Clin Endocrinol Metab 1975;41:191.

171. Wimpfheimer C, Saville E, Voirol MJ, Danforth E, Burger AG. Starvation-induced decreased sensitivity of resting metabolic rate to triiodothyronine. Science 1979;205:1272.

172. Owen E. Starvation. In: Degrout LJ, Besser GM, Cahill GF, et al, eds. Endocrinology. Philadelphia: WB Saunders, 1989:2282.

173. Owen OE, Trapp VE, Skutches CL, et al. Acetone metabolism during diabetic ketoacidosis. Diabetes 1982;31:242.

174. Reichard GA, Haff AC, Skutches CL, Paul P, Holroyde CP, Owen OE. Plasma acetone metabolism in the fasting human. J Clin Invest 1979;63:619.

175. Reichard GA, Skutches CL, Hoeldtke RD, Owen OE. Acetone metabolism in humans during diabetic ketoacidosis. Diabetes 1986;35:668.

176. Atkinson DE, Camien MN. The role of urea synthesis in the removal of metabolic bicarbonate and the regulation of blood pH. Curr Top Cell Regul 1982;21:261.

177. Marliss EB, Aski TT, Unger RH, Soeldner JS, Cahill GF. Glucagon levels and metabolic effects in fasting man. J Clin Invest 1970;49:2256.

178. Torun B, Viteri FE. Protein-energy malnutrition. In: Shils ME, Young VR, eds. Modern nutrition in health and disease, ed 7. Philadelphia: Lea & Febiger, 1988:746.

179. Alleyn GA, Hay RW, Picou DI, Stanfield JP, Whitehead RG. Protein-energy malnutrition. London: Edward Arnold Ltd, 1977.

180. Viteri FE, Schneider RE. Gastrointestinal alterations in protein-calorie malnutrition. Med Clin North Am 1974;58:1467.

181. Dune PR, Moore DJ, Forstner GG. The role of the pancreas: Malnutrition and the exocrine pancreas. In: Walker-Smith JA, McNeish AS, eds. Diarrhoea and malnutrition in childhood. London: Butterworths, 1980.

182. Tondon BN, Banks PA, George PK. Recovery of exocrine pancreatic function in adult protein-calorie malnutrition. Gastroenterology 1970;58:358.

183. Pitchumoni CL. Special problems of tropical pancreatitis. Clin Gastroenterol 1984;13:941.

184. Nwokolo C, Oli J. Pathogenesis of juvenile tropical pancreatitis syndrome. Lancet 1980;i:456.

185. Tai da Rocha-Afodu J. The liver in kwashiorkor. Scand J Gastroenterol 1986(Suppl);124:9.

186. Schaffner F, Thaler H. Nonalcoholic fatty liver disease. Prog Liver Dis 1986;8:283.

187. Achord JL. Nutrition, alcohol, and the liver. Am J Gastroenterol 1988;83:244.

188. Lifshitz F, Teichberg S, Wapnir RA. Malnutrition and the intestine. In: Tsang RC, Nichols BL, eds. Nutrition and child health: Prospectives for the 1980's. New York: Alan R Liss, 1981:1.

189. Hamilton JR. The effect of malnutrition on gut structure, function, and healing after injury. In: Walker-Smith JA, McNeish AS, eds. Diarrhoea and malnutrition in childhood. London: Butterworths, 1980:23.

190. Tandon BN, Magotra ML, Saraya AK, Ramalingaswami V. Small intestine in protein malnutrition. Am J Clin Nutr 1968;21:813.

191. Herskovic T. Protein malnutrition and the small intestine. Am J Clin Nutr 1969;22:300.

192. Souba WW, Wilmore DW. Diet and nutrition in the care of the patient with surgery, trauma, and sepsis. In: Shils ME, Young VR, eds. Modern nutrition in health and disease, ed 7. Philadelphia: Lea & Febiger, 1988:1306.

193. Beisel WR. Metabolic response to infection. In: Kinney JM, Jeejeebhoy KN, Hill GL, Owen OE. Nutrition and metabolism in patient care. Philadelphia: WB Saunders, 1988:605.

194. Cerra FB, Siegel JH, Coleman B, Border JR, McNamy R. Septic autocannibalism. A failure of exogenous nutritional support. Ann Surg 1980;192:570.

195. Douglas RG, Shaw JH. Metabolic response to sepsis and trauma. Br J Surg 1989;76:115.

196. Goldstein SA, Elwyn DH. The effects of injury and sepsis on fuel utilization. Annu Rev Nutr 1989;9:445.

197. Shaw JH, Wolfe RR. Energy and protein metabolism in sepsis and trauma. Aust N Z J Surg 1978;57:41.

198. Dinarello CA. Biology of interleukin-1. FASEB J 1988;2:108.

199. Pomposelli JJ, Flores BS, Bistrian BR. Role of biochemical mediators in clinical nutrition and surgical metabolism. J Parenter Enteral Nutr 1988;12:212.

200. Dinarello CA, Mier JW. Lymphokines. N Engl J Med 1987;317:940.

201. Dinarello CA. Interleukin-1. Rev Infect Dis 1984;6:51.

202. Clowes GH, George BC, Villee CA, Saravis CA. Muscle proteolysis induced by a circulatory peptide in patients with sepsis or trauma. N Engl J Med 1983;308:545.

203. Beisel WR. Mediators of fever and muscle proteolysis. N Engl J Med 1983;308:586.

204. Beisel WR, Wannemacher RW. Gluconeogenesis, ureagenesis, and ketogenesis during sepsis. J Parenter Enteral Nutr 1980;4:277.

205. Beisel WR. Magnitude of the host nutritional responses to infection. Am J Clin Nutr 1977;30:1236.

206. Cerra FB, Caprioli J, Sigel JH, McMenamy RR, Border JR. Proline metabolism in sepsis, cirrhosis, and general surgery. Ann Surg 1979;190:577.

207. Beisel WR, Fiser TH. Lipid metabolism during infectious illness. Am J Clin Nutr 1970;23:1069.

208. Watters JM, Wilmore DW. Role of catabolic hormones in the hypoketonaemia of injury. Br J Surg 1986;73:108.

209. Bessey PQ, Watters JM, Aoki TT, Wilmore DW. Combined hormonal infusion simulates the metabolic response to injury. Ann Surg 1984;200:264.

210. Long C, Kinney JM, Geiger JW. Nonsuppressibility of gluconeogenesis by glucose in septic patients. Metabolism 1976;25:193.

211. Wolfe RR, Herndon DN, Jahoor F, Miyoshi H, Wolfe M. Effect of severe burn injury on substrate cycling by glucose and fatty acids. N Engl J Med 1987;317:403.

212. Katz J, Rognstad R. Futile cycles in the metabolism of glucose. Curr Top Cell Regul 1976;10:237.

213. Hue L. The role of futile cycles in the regulation of carbohydrate metabolism in the liver. Adv Enzym Relat Areas Molec Biol 1981;52:247.

214. Beisel WR. Iron nutrition: Immunity and infection. Resident and Staff Physician 1981;May:37.

215. Beisel WR. Trace elements in infectious processes. Med Clin North Am 1976;60:831.

216. Letendre ED, Holbein BE. Ceruloplasmin and regulation of transferrin iron during Neisseria meningitidis infection in mice. Infect Immun 1984;45:133.

217. Ampel NM, Van DB, Aguirre MA, Willis DG, Popp RA. Resistance to infection in murine beta-thalassemia. Infect Immun 1989;57:1011.

218. Michie HR, Eberlein TJ, Spriggs DR, Manogue KR, Cerami A, Wilmore DW. Interleukin-2 initiates metabolic responses associated with critical illness in humans. Ann Surg 1988;208:493.

219. Tracey KJ, Beuthea B, Lowry SF, et al. Shock and tissue injury induced by recombinant human cachectin. Science 1986;234:470.

220. Michie HR, Manogue KR, Spriggs DR. Detection of circulating tumor necrosis factor after endotoxin administration. N Engl J Med 1988;318:1481.

221. Beutler B. The presence of cachectin/tumor necrosis factor in human disease states. Am J Med 1988;85:287.

222. Perlmutter DH, Dinarello CA, Punsal PI, Colten HR. Cachectin/tumor necrosis factor regulates hepatic acute-phase gene expression. J Clin Invest 1986;78:1351.

223. Yosselson S. Drugs and nutrition. Drug Intell Clin Pharm 1976;10:8.

224. Roe DA. Drug induced nutritional deficiencies, ed 2. Westport, CT: AVI Publishing Co, 1985.

225. Ovesen L. Drugs and vitamin deficiency. Drugs 1974;18:278.

225a. Hussey GD, Klein M. A randomized controlled trial of Vitamin A in children with severe measles. N Engl J Med 1990;323:160.

226. Cruickshank AM, Telfer AB, Shenkin A. Thiamine deficiency in the critically ill. Intensive Care Med 1988;14:384.

227. Tsoukas CD, Watry D, Escoban S, et al. Inhibition of interleukin-1 production by 1,25 dihydroxyvitamin D3. J Clin Endocrinol Metab 1989;69:127.

228. Cuthbertson DP. Observations on the disturbance of metabolism produced by injury to the limbs. Q J Med 1932;1:233.

229. Moore FD. Bodily changes during surgical convalescence. Ann Surg 1953;137:289.

230. Wilmore DW, Orcutt TW, Mason AD, Pruitt BA. Alterations in hypothalamic function following thermal injury. J Trauma 1975;15:697.

231. Gann DS, Amaral JF, Caldwell MD. Metabolic response to injury, stress and starvation. In: Davis JH, Drucker WR, Foster RS, Ganelli RL, Gana DJ, Pruitt BA, Sheldon GF, eds. Clinical surgery. St. Louis: CV Mosby, 1987:337

232. Wilmore DW, Aulick LH, Mason AD, Pruitt BA. Influence of the burn wound on local and systemic responses to injury. Ann Surg 1977;186:444.

233. Turinsky J. Glucose metabolism in the region recovering from burn injury. Endocrinology 1983;113:1370.

234. Caldwell MD, Shearer J, Morris A, Mastrofrancisco B, Henry W, Albina JE. Evidence for aerobic glycolysis in lambda-carageenan wounded skeletal muscle. J Surg Res 1984;37:63.

235. Duke JH, Jorgensen SB, Broell JR, Long CL, Kinney JM. Contribution of protein to caloric expenditure following injury. Surgery 1970;68:168.

236. Kinney JM. Energy requirements in injury and sepsis. Acta Anaesthesiol Scand 1974(Suppl);55:15.

237. Cuthbertson DP. The metabolic response to injury and its nutritional implications: Retrospect and prospect. J Parenter Enteral Nutr 1979;3:108.

238. Fry DE. Multiple system organ failure. Surg Clin North Am 1988;68:107.

239. Scholten DJ. Multiple organ failure syndrome. Presented at The A.S.P.E.N. Thirteenth Clinical Congress, February 1989.

240. DeCamp MM, Demling RH. Posttraumatic multisystem organ failure. JAMA 1988;260:530.

241. Cerra FD. Hypermetabolism, organ failure, and metabolic support. Surgery 1987;101:1.

242. Goris RJ, Te Boekhorst TP, Nuytinck JK, Gimbrere JS. Multiple-organ failure. Arch Surg 1985;120:1109.

243. Carrico CJ, Meakins JL, Marshall JC, Fry D, Maier RV. Multiple-organ-failure syndrome. Arch Surg 1986;121:196.

244. Cerra FB, McPherson JP, Konstantinides NN, Teasely KM. Enteral nutrition does not prevent multiple organ failure syndrome after sepsis. Surgery 1988;104:727.

245. Williamson RC, Chir M. Intestinal adaptation (first of two parts). N Engl J Med 1978;298:1393.

246. Bristol JB, Williamson RC. Nutrition, operations and intestinal adaptation. J Parenter Enteral Nutr 1988;12:299.

247. Williamson RC, Chir M. Intestinal adaptation (second of two parts). N Engl J Med 1978;298:1444.

248. Altmann GG, Leblond CP. Factors influencing villus size in the small intestine of adult cats as revealed by transposition of intestinal segments. Am J Anat 1970;127:15.

249. Altmann GG. Influences of bile and pancreatic secretions on the size of intestinal villi in the rat. Am J Anat 1971;132:167.

250. Dowling RH, Gleeson MG. Cell turnover following small bowel resection and by-pass. Digestion 1973;8:176.

251. Koruda MJ, Rolandelli RH, Settle RG, Saul SH, Rombeau JL. The effect of pectin-supplemented elemental diet on bowel resection. J Parenter Enteral Nutr 1986;10:343.

252. Koruda MJ, Rolandelli RH, Settle RG, Zimmaro DM, Rombeau JL. Effect of parenteral nutrition supplemented with short-chain fatty acids on adaptation to massive small bowel resection. Gastroenterology 1988;95:715.

253. Bloom SR, Polak JM. Enteroglucagon and the gut hormone profile of intestinal adaptation. In: Robinson JW, Dowling RH, Riecken EO, eds. Mechanisms of intestinal adaptation. Lancaster:MTP Press, 1982:189.

254. Johnson LR. Role of gastrointestinal peptides in intestinal adaptation. In: Robinson JW, Dowling RH, Riecken EO, eds. Mechanisms of intestinal adaptation. Lancaster: MTP Press, 1982:201.

255. Dembinski A, Gregory H, Korturek SJ, Polanski M. Trophic action of epidermal growth factor on the pancreas and gastroduodenal mucosa in rats. In: Robinson JW, Dowling RH, Riecken EO, eds. Mechanisms of intestinal adaptation. Lancaster: MTP Press, 1982:281.

256. Levine GM, Kotler DP, Yezdimir EA. Luminal nutrition obviates sympathectomy-induced intestinal atrophy. In: Robinson JW, Dowling RH, Riecken EO, eds. Mechanisms of intestinal adaptation. Lancaster: MTP Press, 1982:311.

257. Burkitt D. Foreword. In: Valhouny GV, Kritchevsky D, eds. Dietary fiber. New York: Plenum Press, 1986:IX.

258. Trowell H. Dietary fibre: A paradigm. In: Trowell H, Burkitt D, Heaton K, eds. Dietary fibre, fibre-depleted foods and disease. London: Academic Press, 1985:1.

259. Trowell H, Southgate DA, Wolever TM, Leeds RA, Gassul MA, Jenkins DJ. Dietary fibre redefined. Lancet 1976;i:1967.

260. Jenkins DJ. Carbohydrates. In: Shils ME, Young VR, eds. Modern nutrition in health and disease, ed 7. Philadelphia: Lea & Febiger, 1988:52.

261. Kritchevsky D. Dietary fiber. Annu Rev Nutr 1988;8:301.

262. Dietary fiber and health—A report by The Council on Scientific Affairs, American Medical Association. JAMA 1989;262:542.

263. Eastwood M. Dietary fiber. In: Olson RE, Broquist HP, Crichester CO, Darby WJ, Kolbye AC, Stalvey RM, eds. Present knowledge in nutrition, ed 5. Washington, DC: The Nutrition Foundation, Inc, 1984:156.

264. Read NW. Dietary fiber and bowel transit. In: Valhouny GV, Kritchevsky D, eds. Dietary fiber. New York: Plenum Press, 1986:81.

265. Salyers AA. Diet and the colonic environment: Measuring the response of human colonic bacteria to changes in the host's diet. In: Valhouny GV, Kritchevsky D, eds. Dietary fiber. New York: Plenum Press, 1986:119.

266. Eastwood M, Brydon WG. Physiological effects of dietary fibre on the alimentary tract. In: Trowell H, Burkitt D, Heaton K, eds. Dietary fibre, fibre-depleted foods and disease. London: Academic Press, 1985:105.

267. Willett WC, MacMahon B. Diet and cancer—An overview. N Engl J Med 1984;310:697.

268. Cranston D, McWhinnie D, Collin J. Dietary fiber and gastrointestinal disease. Br J Surg 1988;75:508.

269. Jacobs LR. Fiber and colon cancer. Gastroenterol Clin North Am 1988;17:747.

270. Kritchevsky D. Diet, nutrition and cancer. Cancer 1986;58:1830.

271. Brodribb AJ. Treatment of symptomatic diverticular disease with a high fibre diet. Lancet 1977.664.

272. Painter NS, Almeida AZ, Colebourne KW. Unprocessed bran in treatment of diverticular disease of the colon. Br Med J 1972;2:127.

273. Painter NS. Diverticular disease of the colon. S Afr Med J 1982;61:1016.

274. Bell LP, Hectorne K, Reynolds H, Balm TK, Hunninghake DB. Cholesterol-lowering effects of psyllium hydrophilic mucilloid. JAMA 1989;262:3419.

275. Anderson JW, Story L, Sieling B, Chen WJ, Pero MS, Story J. Hypocholesterolemic effects of oat-bran or bean intake for hypercholesterolemic men. Am J Clin Nutr 1984;40:1146.

276. Ullrich IM. Evaluation of a high fiber diet in hyperlipidemia: A review. J Am Coll Nutr 1987;6:19.

277. Anderson JW, Zettwoch N, Feldman T, Tietyen-Clark J, Oeltgen P, Bishop CW. Cholesterol lowering effects of psyllium hydrophilic mucilloid for hypercholesterolemic men. Arch Intern Med 1988;148:292.

278. Swain JF, Rouse IL, Curley CB, Sacks FM. Comparison of the effects of oat bran and low-fiber wheat on serum lipoprotein levels and blood pressure. N Engl J Med 1990;322:147.

279. Connor WE. Dietary fiber—Nostrum or critical nutrient. N Engl J Med 1990;322:193.

280. Jenkins DJ, Wolever TM, Jenkins AL, Thompson LU, Rao AV, Francis T. The glycemic index: Blood glucose response to foods. In: Valhouny GV, Kritchevsky D, eds. Dietary fiber. New York: Plenum Press, 1986:167.

281. Simpson HC, Simpson RW, Lousley S, Carter RD, Greekie M, Hockaday TM, Man JI. A high carbohydrate leguminous fibre diet improves all aspects of diabetic control. Lancet 1981;i:1.

282. Stephen A. Constipation. In: Trowell H, Burkitt D, Heaton K, eds. Dietary fibre, fibre-depleted foods and disease. London: Academic Press, 1985:133.

283. Hull C, Greco RS, Brookside DL. Alleviation of constipation in the elderly by dietary fiber supplementation. J Am Geriatr Soc 1980;28: 410.

284. Burkitt D. Varicose veins, haemorrhoids, deep-vein thrombosis and pelvic phleboliths. In: Trowell H, Burkitt D, Heaton K, eds. Dietary fibre, fibre-depleted foods and disease. London: Academic Press, 1985:317.

285. Kelsay JL. Update on fiber and mineral availability. In: Valhouny GO, Kritchevsky D, eds. Dietary fiber. New York: Plenum Press, 1986:361.

286. The Surgeon General's Report on Nutrition and Health. Summary and recommendations. Washington, DC: U.S. Department of Health and Human Services. DHHS Publication No. 88-50211, 1988.

287. Webster JD, Hesp R, Garrow JS. The composition of excess weight in obese women estimated by body density, total body water, and total body potassium. Hum Nutr Clin Nutr 1984;38C:299.

288. Garrow JS, Webster J. Quetelet's Index (W/H$_2$) as a measure of fatness. Int J Obes 1985;9:147.

289. Keys A, Fidanza F, Karvonen MJ, Kimura N, Taylor HL. Indices of relative weight and obesity. J Chronic Dis 1972;25:329.

290. Manson JE, Stampfer MJ, Henekens CH, Willett WC. Body weight and longevity. JAMA 1987;257:353.

291. Kral JG, Heymsfield S. Morbid obesity definitions, epidemiology, and methodological problems. Gastroenterol Clin North Am 1987;16: 197.

292. Lew EA, Garfinkel L. Variations in mortality by weight among 750,000 men and women. J Chronic Dis 1979;32:563.

293. Gordon T, Kannel WB. Obesity and cardiovascular disease: The Framingham study. J Chronic Dis 1974;27:103.

294. Haines AP, Imeson JD, Meade TW. Skinfold thickness and cardiovascular risk factors. Am J Epidemiol 1987;126:86.

295. Smoak CG, Burke JL, Webber LS, Harsha DW, Srinivasan SR, Berenson GS. Relation of obesity to clustering of cardiovascular disease risk factors in children and young adults. The Bogalusa Heart Study. Am J Epidemiol 1987;125:364.

296. Peiris AN, Sothmann MS, Hoffman RG, et al. Adiposity, fat distribution, and cardiovascular risk. Ann Intern Med 1989;110:867.

297. Hubert HB, Feinleib M, McNamara PM, Castelli WP. Obesity as an independent risk factor for cardiovascular disease: A 26-year follow-up of participants in the Framingham Heart Study. Obes Cardiovasc Dis 1983;67:968.

298. Hubert HB. The nature of the relationship between obesity and cardiovascular disease. Int J Cardiol 1984;6:268.

299. Larsson B. Obesity and prospective risks for associated diseases. In: Vague J, Vague PH, Ebling FJ, et al, eds. Metabolic complications of human obesities. New York: Elsevier Science Publishers, 1985.

300. Kissebah AH, Vydelingum N, Murray R, Evans DJ, Hartz AJ, Kalkhoff RK, Adams PW. Relation of body fat distribution to metabolic complications of obesity. J Clin Endocrinol Metab 1982;54:254;

301. Lapidus L, Bengtsson C, Larsson B, Pennert K, Rybo E, Sjostrom L. Distribution of adipose tissue and risk of cardiovascular disease and death: A 12-year follow-up of participants in the population study of women in Gothenburg, Sweden. Br Med J 1984;289:1257.

302. Bjorntorp P. Obesity and the risk of cardiovascular disease. Ann Clin Res 1985;17:3.

303. Raison J, Buy-grand B. Body fat distribution in obese hypertensives. In: Vague J, Vague PH, Ebling FJ, et al, eds. Metabolic complications of human obesities. New York: Elsevier Science Publishers, 1985: 67.

304. Mann GV. The influence of obesity on health. N Engl J Med 1974;29: 178.

305. Garrison RJ, Feinleib M, Castelli WP, McNamara PM. Cigarette smoking as a confounder of the relationship between relative weight and long-term mortality. JAMA 1979;249:2199.

306. MacMahon SW, Wilcken DEL, MacDonald GJ. The effect of weight reduction on left ventricular mass. A randomized control trial in young, overweight, hypertensive patients. N Engl J Med 1986;314: 334.

307. Hubert HB, Eaker ED, Garrison RJ, Castelli WP. Life-style correlates of risk factor change in young adults: An 8-year study of coronary heart disease risk factors in the Framingham offspring. Am J Epidemiol 1987;125:812.

308. Boer JOD, Van Es AJH, Van Raaij JMA, Hautvast JGAJ. Energy requirements and energy expenditure of lean and overweight women, measured by indirect calorimetry. Am J Clin Nutr 1987;46:13.

309. Stunkard AJ, Sorensen TIA, Hanis C, Teasdale TW, Chakraborty R, Schull WJ, Schulsinger F. An adoption study of human obesity. N Engl J Med 1986;314:193.

310. Bogardus C, Lillioga S, Ravussin E, Abbott W, Zawadzki JK, Young A, Knowler WC, Jacobowitz R, Moll PP. Familial dependence of the resting metabolic rate. N Engl J Med 1986;215:96.

311. Roberts SB, Savage J, Coward WA, Chew B, Lucas A. Energy expenditure and intake in infants born to lean and overweight mothers. N Engl J Med 1988;318:461.

312. Garrow JS. Measurement of energy stores. Obesity and related diseases. New York: Churchill-Livingstone, 1988:25.

313. Freedman-Akabas S, Colt E, Kissileff HR, Pi-Sunyer FX. Lack of sustained increase in VO$_2$ following exercise in fit and unfit subjects. Am J Clin Nutr 1985;41:545.

314. Hill JO, Schlundt DG, Sbrocco T, Sharp T, Pope-Cordle J, Stetson B, Kaler M, Heim C. Evaluation of an alternating-calorie diet with and without exercise in the treatment of obesity. Am J Clin Nutr 1989;50:248.

315. Wing RR, Jeffery RW. Outpatient treatments of obesity: A comparison of methodology and clinical results. Int J Obes 1979;3:261.

316. Stunkard AJ. Conservative treatments of obesity. Am J Clin Nutr 1987;456:1142.

317. Acheson KJ, Schultz Y, Bessard T, Anantharaman K, Flatt JP, Jequier E. Glycogen storage capacity and de novo lipogenesis during massive carbohydrate overfeeding in man. Am J Clin Nutr 1988;48:240.

318. Flatt JP. Dietary fat, carbohydrate balance, and weight maintenance: Effects of exercise. Am J Clin Nutr 1987;45:296.

319. Schultz Y, Flatt JP, Jequier E. Failure of dietary fat intake to promote fat oxidation: A factor favoring the development of obesity. Am J Clin Nutr 1989;50:307.

320. Danforth E. Diet and obesity. Am J Clin Nutr 1985;41:1132.

321. Lissner L, Levitsky DA, Strupp BJ, Kalwarf HJ, Roe DA. Dietary fat intake and the regulation of energy intake in human subjects. Am J Clin Nutr 1987;46:886.

322. Katahn M. The T-Factor Diet. New York: WW Norton and Co, 1989.

323. Stunkard AJ. Behavioral management of obesity. Med J Aust 1985;142:S13.

324. Smuller JW, Wadden TA, Brownell KD. Popular and very low-calorie diets in the treatment of obesity. In: Frankle RT, Yang MU, eds. Obesity and weight control. Rockville, MD: Aspen Publishers, 1988:133.

325. Owen OE. Obesity. In: Kinney JM, Jeejeebhoy KN, Hill G, Owen OE, eds. Nutrition and metabolism in patient care. Philadelphia: WB Saunders, 1988:167.

326. Andersen T, Stockholm K, Backer O, Quaade F. Long-term (5-year) results after either horizontal gastroplasty or very-low-calorie diet for morbid obesity. Int J Obes 1988;12:277.

327. Hovell M, Koch A, Hofstetter R, Sipan C, Vaucher P, Dellinger A, Borok G, Forsythe A, Felitti V. Long-term weight loss maintenance: Assessment of a behavioral and supplemented fasting regimen. Am J Public Health 1988;78:663.

328. Wadden T, Stunkard A, Liebschutz J. Three-year follow-up of the treatment of obesity by very low calorie diet, behavior therapy, and their combination. J Consult Clin Psychol 1988;56:925.

329. Wadden TA, Van Itallie TB, Blackburn GL. Responsible and irresponsible use of very-low-calorie diets in the treatment of obesity. JAMA 1990;263:83.

330. Craighead LW, Stunkard AJ, O'Brien RM. Behavior therapy and pharmacotherapy for obesity. Arch Gen Psychiatry 1981;38:763.

331. Berkowitz SA, ed. National weight control resource directory. Oakland, CA: Society for Nutrition Education and the American Dietetic Association, 1988.

E. MISCELLANEOUS

22

Gastrointestinal Blood Flow

KAREN D. CRISSINGER
D. NEIL GRANGER

The ultimate function of the gastrointestinal tract is to assimilate nutrients and water from the external environment and make them available for cells throughout the body. While the mucosal epithelium is largely responsible for extracting nutrients from the external environment, the blood and lymph circulations provide the conduit for transfer of absorbed nutrients and water to the entire body. The vascular supply to the gastrointestinal mucosa is particularly well suited for the absorptive and secretory functions of this tissue in that it allows for a high rate of blood flow, has a large exchange surface area, and exhibits characteristics that allow for easy permeation of nutrients and water, while largely retaining proteins within the plasma compartment. This chapter summarizes current concepts regarding circulatory control and function in the gastrointestinal tract during normal physiologic conditions and reviews current knowledge about pathophysiologic mechanisms of intestinal injury resulting from periods of inadequate perfusion (i.e., ischemia).

ANATOMY OF THE GASTROINTESTINAL CIRCULATION

Extramural Vessels

In humans, the major arteries supplying the stomach and intestines are the celiac, the superior mesenteric, and the inferior mesenteric arteries. The celiac artery supplies the stomach, the first portion of the duodenum, a portion of the pancreas, and the liver. The superior mesenteric artery (SMA) supplies the remainder of the pancreas and duodenum, and the jejunum, ileum, and colon through two thirds of the transverse segment.

The inferior mesenteric artery supplies the remainder of the colon and rectum, except the distal rectum, which is supplied by way of rectal arteries arising from the internal iliac arteries. Along the mesenteric border of the intestine, arterial and venous branches form multiple arcades, anastomose with one another, and provide

a pathway for collateral blood flow. The arcades give rise to vasa recta, which branch to encircle the intestine and ultimately pierce the circular muscle.[1-3]

Venous drainage from the stomach, pancreas, and intestines is into the portal vein, except for the distal rectum, which drains into the internal iliac veins. The vessels that drain the intestines course within the mesentery, except those vessels supplying retroperitoneal portions.[1-3]

Lymph vessels are closely associated with the arteries supplying the stomach and intestines, ultimately draining into the intestinal lymph trunk to the cisterna chyli, and then into the systemic circulation by way of the thoracic duct to the left subclavian vein.

In humans, the lymphatic drainage of the distal portion of the intestines is by way of the left lumbar lymph trunk, which empties into the cysterna chyli separate from the drainage of the proximal gut.[1-3]

Intramural Vessels/Microcirculation

STOMACH

In the human stomach, submucosal arterioles break up into capillaries at the base of the gastric glands, pass perpendicularly through the mucosa, form a luminal capillary network, and drain into mucosal venules at, and only at, the most luminal level of the lamina propria (Fig 22-1). These venular branches converge on infrequent mucosal collecting venules, which pass directly to the submucous venous plexus, without receiving any direct capillary tributaries within the mucosa.[4]

SMALL INTESTINE

The major intramural arterial vessels are located in the deep submucosal plexus. Both arteries and veins in the deep submucosal plexus undergo extensive self-anastomosis. The capillaries of the

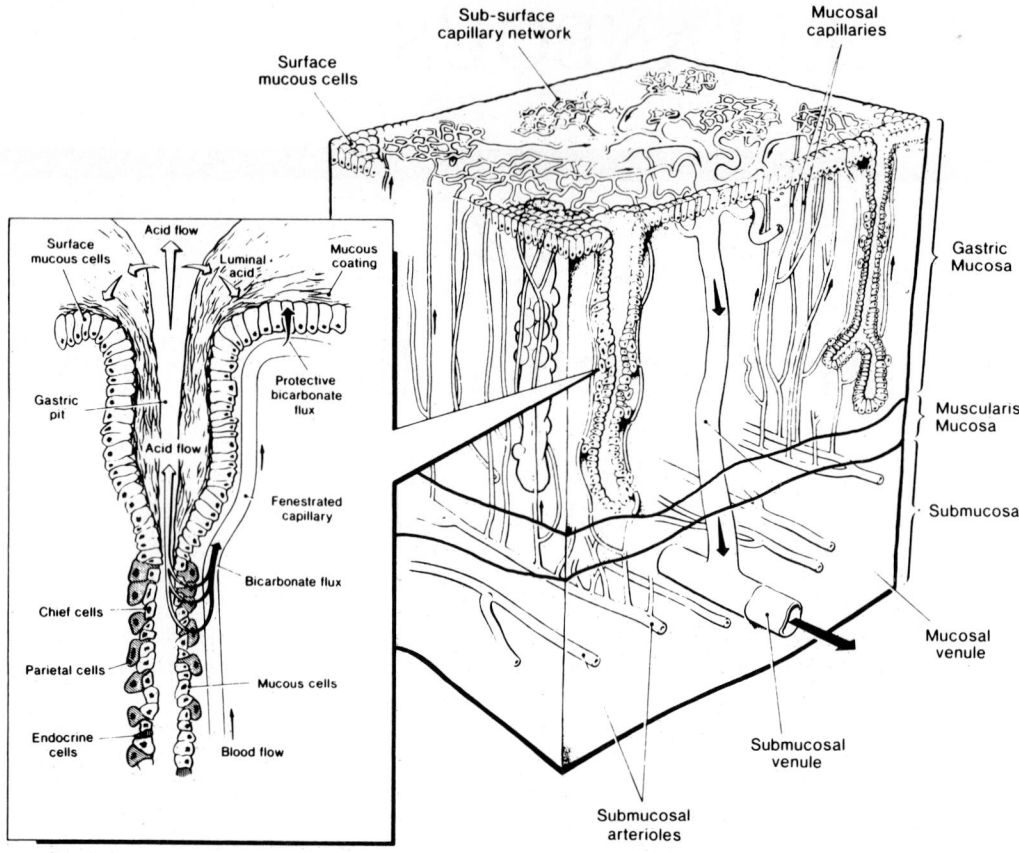

FIGURE 22–1. Schematic diagram of the vascular organization in gastric mucosa (*right*) and the proposed mechanism for vascular transport of HCO_3^-, toward the surface mucous cells, from deeper within the mucosa (*inset left*). (From Gannon B, Browning J, O'Brien P, Rogers P. Mucosal microvascular architecture of the fundus and body of human stomach. Gastroenterology 1984;86:866.)

muscular, submucosal, and mucosal layers are supplied by branches from the submucosal vascular network.[1,2]

Villous microvascular architecture varies considerably among species (Fig 22-2).[5] Human villi contain single, eccentrically located arterioles, which pass to the villus tip, break up in a fountainlike pattern, and anastomose with eccentrically located venules that start about 15% of villus height below the tip. A tuft pattern of blood supply, derived from the tubular capillary plexus surrounding the epithelium of the crypts, supplies the basal 70% to 80% of the villus and also drains into the venule high in the villus (Fig 22-3).[2,6]

Anatomic requirements for countercurrent exchange include the presence of countercurrent flow of blood and a short arteriole-to-capillary distance. Although the existence of countercurrent exchange within the villi has been proposed,[7] controversy remains about whether these requirements are met in human villi.[5]

COLON

The colonic mucosa is devoid of villi, and the arterioles and their capillary branches pass to the epithelial surface between the crypts to form a network of capillary plexus around the crypts. The colonic capillaries are much closer to the epithelial cells than are the villus capillaries in the small intestine.[8]

Intramural Lymphatic Circulation

The gastric lymphatics normally begin as a plexus of vessels immediately superficial to, within, and below the muscularis mucosae. The upper two thirds of the gastric lamina propria is normally devoid of lymphatics.[9]

Small intestinal lymphatic vessels begin as centrally located, blind-ended vessels (lacteals) in villi and are emptied when smooth muscle in the core of the villus contracts. These initial lacteals, which are similar in size to venous capillaries but with open endothelial intercellular junctions, few pericytes, and tenuous basement membranes, drain into a submucosal plexus connected with the collecting lymphatics.

The lymphatics leave the intestine at the mesenteric border and pass through the mesentery in association with blood vessels.[2,10]

Colonic lymphatics begin at the level of the muscularis mucosae, are smaller and more sparsely distributed than those in the small intestine, and do not penetrate higher than the bases of the crypts in humans.[11]

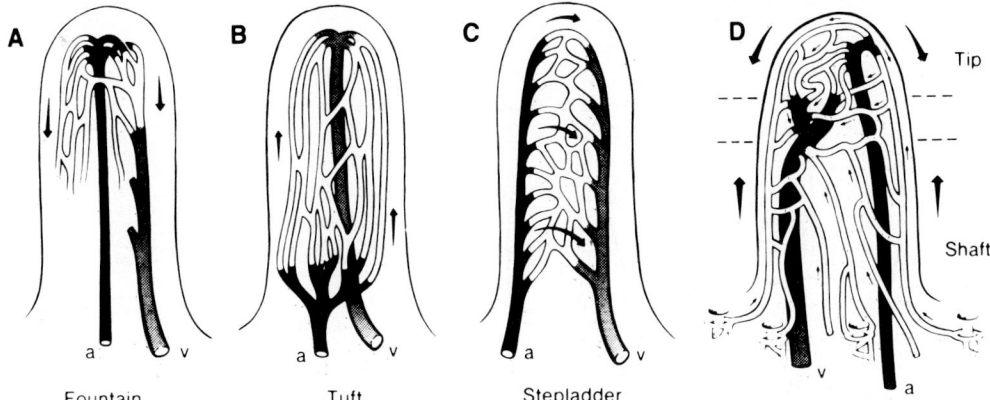

FIGURE 22–2. Models of mucosal microcirculation of the intestine. **A, B, C,** "Fountain," "tuft," and "stepladder" patterns of villus blood supply. **D,** Dual pattern comprising both "fountain" and "tuft" components. *a* = arteriole, *v* = venule, *large arrows* = principal direction(s) of capillary blood flow in each pattern. (**A** through **D** from Gannon BJ. The co-existence of fountain and tuft patterns of blood supply in individual intestinal villi of rabbit and man: resolution of an old controversy. Bibl Anat 1981;20:130.)

TECHNIQUES FOR MEASUREMENT OF BLOOD FLOW

There are at least 30 techniques available for measurement of gastrointestinal perfusion. Although none fulfills the criteria outlined by Jacobson[12] for the ideal method (i.e., safe, noninvasive, continuous, quantitative, accurate, reproducible, measures intramural distribution, and does not alter blood flow), all of these methods do appear to provide a useful measure of tissue perfusion in the splanchnic circulation.

Techniques Measuring Total Organ Blood Flow

The *venous outflow technique* directly measures blood flow by way of timed collections of venous blood. It is the gold standard of blood flow measurement against which other techniques are validated. It is easy, accurate, and allows repeated (or continuous with a drop counter) measurement of blood flow. The major disadvantage is that this technique cannot be used in the clinical setting or in chronic animal studies. It also measures only total flow, giving no information on flow distribution to different layers or regions in an organ. Furthermore, the organ or segment under study must be drained by a single vein.[13]

Blood flow measurement using *electromagnetic flow probes* is based on the principle of electromagnetic induction by flowing blood. It requires cannulation of a vessel or placement of a perivascular sensor to measure volume flow or flow velocity. This technique allows continuous, instantaneous, and quantitative measurement of flow. The perivascular sensors leave the vessel intact, don't interfere with flow, permit flow measurement in situ, and can be used in acute or chronic animal studies. The major disadvantages of this technique are its invasiveness and the need to occlude the vessel to obtain zero flow calibration. Finally, flow must be temporarily interrupted to insert a cannulating flow probe;

or the perivascular cuff may disturb the nervous supply surrounding the vessel during its placement.[14]

The *pulsed Doppler technique* for measuring blood flow involves placement of a single piezoelectric crystal that emits a 20-mHz ultrasonic signal. The same crystal receives the reflected signal from passing blood cells in the interval between ultrasonic pulses. The major advantages include continuous measurements, chronic implantation of multiple flow probes in small animals, minimal interference of vessels during placement of the crystals, and the capability of determining zero flow electronically. The disadvantages of this technique are the necessity for surgical implantation and the inability to measure volume flow quantitatively (although percentage change in flow can be calculated accurately).[15,16]

Techniques Measuring Fractionated Blood Flow

Measurement of blood flow with *radioactive microspheres* is based on the assumption that the number of microspheres trapped in an organ is proportional to blood flow. In the intestinal circulation, the microsphere technique has long been used to measure intramural distribution of blood flow. Although this method has no clinical applicability, it has been widely used in animals to study blood flow to organs without manipulation of the vessels supplying those organs. Disadvantages of the technique, however, are that only single measurements of flow in time can be made, flow may be underestimated due to arteriovenous shunting of spheres or movement of spheres after injection due to vasodilation, and microspheres may be impeded from reaching some tissues in series-coupled vascular beds if the size of the spheres exceeds 12 μm.[17–20]

The *aminopyrine clearance method* capitalizes on the fact that aminopyrine is a weak base, which is freely permeable in tissues at pH 7 and above. At a pH less than 3, however, it dissociates and is no longer permeable. In the stomach, it is cleared from gastric mucosal blood, diffuses into the gastric lumen, and becomes

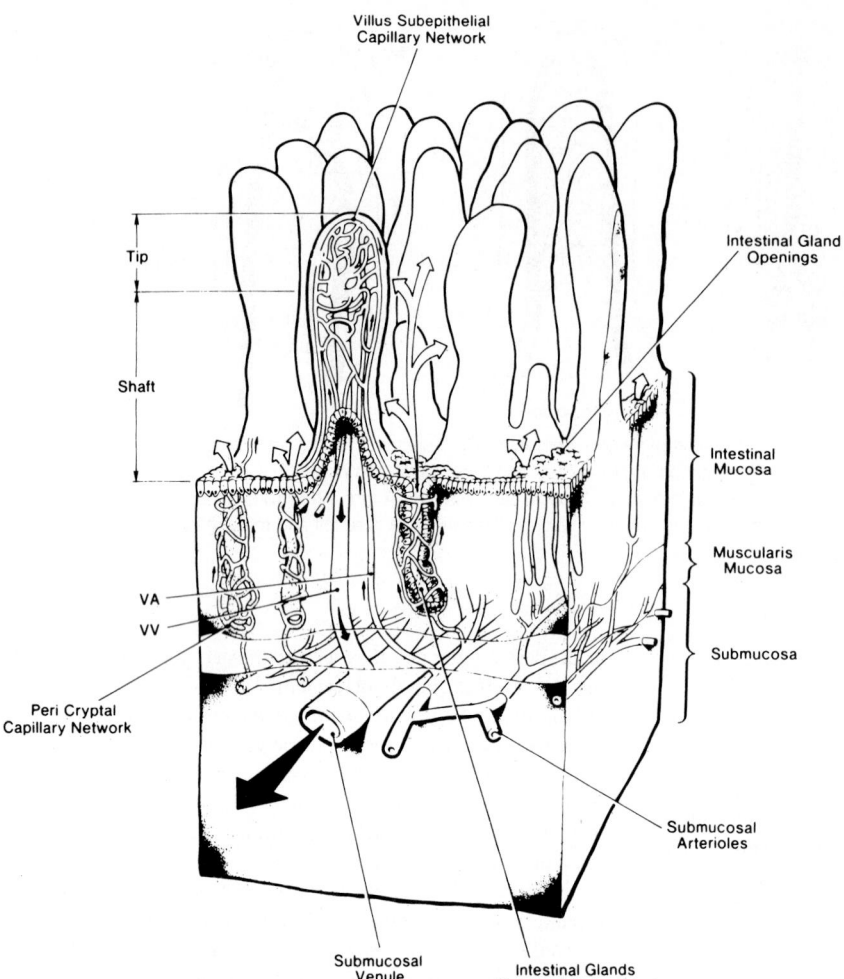

Villus Subepithelial
Capillary Network

Tip

Shaft

VA
VV

Peri Cryptal
Capillary Network

Intestinal Gland
Openings

Intestinal
Mucosa

Muscularis
Mucosa

Submucosa

Submucosal
Arterioles

Submucosal
Venule

Intestinal Glands
(Crypts of Lieberkuhn)

FIGURE 22–3. Model of mucosal microcirculatory patterns typical of human and rabbit small intestine. (Modified from Frasher WG Jr, Wayland H. Repeating modular organization of the microcirculation of cat mesentery. Microvasc Res 1972;4:62.)

"trapped" by way of dissociation at a pH of 3 in the gastric lumen. Gastric mucosal clearance of aminopyrine should provide an accurate estimate of gastric mucosal blood flow if: (1) aminopyrine is completely cleared by the gastric mucosa from the circulation in a single passage, (2) aminopyrine is not actively transported into the gastric lumen, and (3) clearance of aminopyrine is blood flow limited. The major advantages of this technique are that it measures gastric mucosal (rather than total) blood flow, it provides a continuous measurement of blood flow, it can be used in unanesthetized animals and humans, and it provides simultaneous acid secretory data. It has been used extensively for studying the relationship of mucosal blood flow to gastric acid secretion during the administration of various agents. Major disadvantages of this technique include significant metabolism of ^{14}C-aminopyrine within the body, dependence of the clearance calculation on the volume of acid secretion, and significant overestimation of blood flow at high rates of blood flow, suggesting that aminopyrine clearance measures a combination of blood flow and parietal cell activity.[21-23]

Inert gases rapidly diffuse into tissues due to their high lipid solubility. The rate of elimination of an inert gas from a tissue is flow-limited, and, therefore, flow rates in whole organs or parts of organs can be estimated from the rate of washout of radioactive isotopes of inert gases ([133]xenon and [85]krypton). An inert gas may be introduced into a tissue by way of the intravascular route or by injecting it directly into the tissue. In the intestine, the gas may be placed into the intestinal lumen or into the peritoneal space. The major advantages of this technique are that no sampling of blood or tissue is necessary and clinical applications are possible. Disadvantages include the fact that it is a discontinuous measurement of blood flow, flow must be constant during the entire measurement period (15 minutes), trauma to the microvasculature may occur from injection into the tissue, and countercurrent exchange may significantly affect mucosal blood flow estimates in the small intestine.[24,25]

The *technique of iodoantipyrine clearance* is based on the assumption that this highly diffusible tracer distributes in tissue as a function of the rate of blood flow to the tissue. The major advantages of this method are that the spatial resolution is so well defined that blood flow can be measured even in single villi, it is minimally affected by the countercurrent exchange mechanism, regional flow and microscopic anatomy can be closely correlated, and there is no need for anesthesia or surgery before measuring blood flow. Major disadvantages include the need for biopsy specimens, blood flow measurement is discontinuous, fluid in the lumen leads to underestimation of blood flow due to diffusion of iodoantipyrine into this compartment, and radioactive material must be used.[26-28]

The *hydrogen gas clearance technique* is based on the principle that the disappearance of hydrogen, a highly diffusible, biologically inert gas, from a perfused tissue is determined by the rate of venous outflow from that tissue. A 3% hydrogen–20% oxygen mixture is inhaled, and a platinum electrode (which can be affixed to an endoscope) that is in contact with the tissue surface generates a current proportional to the hydrogen concentration in the tissue. The advantages of this technique are its clinical applicability to the stomach and colon without the need for anesthesia or laparotomy and the capability of using a nontoxic, nonradioactive marker. Also, no tissue destruction or vessel cannulation is required. The disadvantages are that it provides discontinuous measurement of flow, and blood flow must be constant during the 15- to 30-minute measurement period. The platinum electrode may alter blood flow due to tissue compression or mechanical stimulation. Countercurrent exchange limits its application in the small intestine of some species. Finally, the spatial (depth) resolution of the technique remains uncertain.[27,29–33]

Laser Doppler velocimetry works on the principle that light scattered by moving red cells undergoes a shift in frequency such that the mean Doppler frequency provides an estimate of blood flow. Fiber optic guides, which conduct laser light to the tissue and return scattered light back to a photodetector, are placed directly on the tissue of interest. The advantages of the technique are that it provides a continuous measurement and it is unaffected by countercurrent exchange in the small intestine. It also can be used clinically by way of endoscopy without the need for anesthesia or surgery. There are, however, major difficulties associated with this method. The depth resolution has not been clarified, with some investigators finding a resolution of 0.5 to 1.0 mm, while others give a value greater than 3 mm, which roughly corresponds to total intestinal thickness. Another problem with this method is that it does not provide a measure of blood flow in absolute units. There is also difficulty in maintaining constant optic coupling between the probe and tissue due to peristalsis. Finally, blood flow may be altered due to tissue compression or mechanical stimulation by the flow probe.[27,30,34–38]

In vivo microscopy allows direct visualization of microvessels and photometric measurement of red blood cell velocity. Blood flow is calculated from measurements of vessel cross-sectional area and red blood cell velocity. The upper limit of vessel diameter for accurate measurement of velocities is about 70 μm. Advantages of the technique are (1) the capability of correlating intestinal vascular responses to specific types, sizes, and tissue locations of microvessels and (2) the capability of determining flow to discrete layers or regions in an organ. Disadvantages of the technique include the need for anesthesia, the necessity of surgical manipulation and exteriorization of the tissue, and optical resolution, which can limit the accurate determination of vessel diameter and red cell velocity.[39,40]

BASAL HEMODYNAMICS AND OXYGENATION

Blood Flow

Recently hydrogen gas clearance has become available as a noninvasive means to measure gastric and colonic blood flow endo-scopically in humans. Laser Doppler flowmetry is also amenable to measurement of changes in gastric and colonic blood flow, although absolute units and spatial resolution remain to be clarified. Experimental animals are used extensively to study gastrointestinal blood flow, with possible applications to human disease states. Table 22-1 summarizes basal values of total and fractionated blood flow obtained in several commonly used experimental animals. One must be cognizant that widely variable values have been obtained within a given experimental preparation or model.

Oxygenation

In recent years, measurements of indices of oxygenation have become commonplace in studies relating blood flow to gastrointestinal function and pathology. The most frequently monitored parameter is tissue oxygen uptake, which can be estimated from the product of blood flow and arteriovenous oxygen difference. In addition, a limited number of studies have used measurements of tissue oxygen tension as an index of tissue oxygenation. Table 22-2 lists representative values for resting arteriovenous oxygen difference, oxygen uptake, and tissue pO_2 (where available).

BLOOD FLOW REGULATION

Intrinsic Control

Blood flow in the gastrointestinal tract is normally maintained within narrow limits and changes in response to various functional stimuli. This ability to modulate blood perfusion in accordance with the moment-to-moment demands of the tissue has been attributed to intrinsic vasoregulatory systems. Several regulatory mechanisms have been proposed to explain vascular phenomena such as pressure–flow autoregulation and functional hyperemia in the gastrointestinal tract. However, of these, metabolic, myogenic, and hormonal mechanisms are considered to be of greatest physiologic significance. The following section summarizes the available data that implicate intrinsic factors in the regulation of gastrointestinal blood flow and the specific mechanisms that have been invoked to explain these vascular phenomena.

Pressure–flow autoregulation has been demonstrated in the stomach,[75,76] small intestine,[59,77–85] and colon.[44,45,86–88] Autoregulation of blood flow in the gastrointestinal tract during fasting is not the intense phenomenon observed in kidney and brain; however, the results of several studies indicate that the intensity of autoregulation increases during periods of enhanced functional activity (Fig 22-4).[46] Furthermore, it appears that the autoregulatory ability of the more metabolically active mucosal region of the intestines exceeds that of the whole organ.[89] The correlation between metabolic rate and autoregulatory ability does not appear to apply to the neonate because autoregulation of blood flow is less intense (or absent) in the more metabolically active neonatal intestine than adult intestine.[67,90] Recent work suggests that autoregulation in the intestine is an endothelium-dependent phenomenon.[91]

Although blood flow is not perfectly regulated over an arterial pressure of 100 mmHg to 50 mmHg, oxygen uptake remains within

TABLE 22–1
Resting Blood Flow Values and Transmural Distribution (ml $\times$ min^{-1} $\times$ 100 g^{-1})

SPECIES	AREA MEASURED	STOMACH	SMALL INTESTINE	LARGE INTESTINE	REFERENCES
Human	Total wall		8–77	8–44	41–43
	Mucosa-submucosa*†	38–77	7–103	9–55	32, 41–43
	Muscle-serosa†		5–38	10–34	43, 44
Dog	Total wall	20–45	30–80	30–74	44–53
	Mucosa-submucosa*‡	23–110	58–87	91–112	29, 30, 33, 53
	Muscle-serosa	13–24	27–49	12–48	44, 53
Cat	Total wall	26–32	20–78	11–39	38, 42, 43, 54–57
	Mucosa-submucosa‡	35–42	42–119	13–58	42, 43, 56, 58
	Muscle-serosa		7.5–18	1.1–17	42, 43, 56
Rat	Total wall	32–118	68–346	29–87	59–63
	Mucosa-submucosa*‡§	23–136	75–140	30–41	28, 31, 32, 63
	Muscle-serosa	2	2.5–7.5	1–5	63
Piglet					
1 day	Total wall		40–128	22–53	64–66
	Mucosa-submucosa‡		50–78		66
	Muscle-serosa		20–38		66
3 day	Total wall	75–140	55–188	33–118	64, 65, 67–69‖
	Mucosa-submucosa‡		95–237		68, 69‖
	Muscle-serosa		15–95		68, 69‖
2 week	Total wall		49–96	35–52	70, 71‖
	Mucosa-submucosa‡		57–102		‖
	Muscle-serosa		43–49		‖
1 mo	Total wall		27–57	19–49	64, 66, 67‖
	Mucosa-submucosa‡		30–60		66
	Muscle-serosa		10–20		66

* *H$_2$ gas clearance.*
† *Inert gas washout.*
‡ *Radioactive microspheres.*
§ *Iodo$^{(14)}$ Cantipyrine.*
‖ *Data also from Crissinger KD, Granger DN. Unpublished data from experiments in Crissinger and Granger.[66]*

normal limits over the same range of pressures.[45,46] This "autoregulation" of gastrointestinal oxygen uptake is often cited as evidence that tissue oxygenation is the controlled variable rather than blood flow. As arterial pressure is reduced, vascular resistance falls while perfused capillary density rises. These changes enhance both the convective and diffusive exchange of oxygen during the reduced pressure state. As a result, tissue oxygen tension tends to remain above the level at which oxygen availabilty limits mitochondrial oxygen consumption. Mathematical models of intestinal oxygen exchange predict that the contribution of capillary recruitment exceeds that of vasodilation in maintaining normal tissue oxygenation during acute hypotension.[92]

Reactive hyperemia is a term used to describe the overshoot in blood flow that occurs after release of arterial occlusion. All regions of the gastrointestinal tract exhibit a reactive hyperemia after brief (less than 5 minutes) periods of arterial occlusion.[93] The magnitude and duration of the hyperemic response are related to the extent and duration of the arterial occlusion, suggesting that the vascular response is caused by metabolite accumulation and oxygen deficiency. The ability of the intestine to repay the oxygen debt in-

curred during vascular occlusions is largely determined by which vessel is occluded (i.e., artery or vein). With arterial occlusion, there is inadequate repayment of the oxygen debt, and the magnitude of the deficit is proportional to the duration of arterial occlusion.[94] Venous occlusions are associated with an overpayment of oxygen in the postocclusion period, the magnitude of which is related to the duration of occlusion. It is suggested that arterial occlusions depress, while venous occlusions enhance, intestinal oxygen utilization. Increasing basal intestinal oxygen consumption by intraenteric placement of nutrients prolongs the reactive hyperemic response and increases the oxygen payback-to-debt ratio.[95] Laser Doppler studies indicate that mucosal and total blood flow consistently show reactive hyperemia in response to a 60-second occlusion, but the muscularis externa does not.

Alterations in arterial blood gases and hematocrit also affect gastrointestinal blood flow. Arterial hypoxemia increases blood flow and elicits capillary recruitment in denervated intestinal preparations.[96,97] The vasodilation and increased perfused capillary density tend to minimize the reduction in oxygen uptake induced by the limited oxygen delivery. When blood flow is held constant,

TABLE 22–2
Resting Values for Arteriovenous Oxygen Content Difference (ml O_2/100 ml),
Oxygen Uptake (ml $\times$ min^{-1} $\times$ 100 g^{-1}), and Tissue pO_2 (mmHg)

SPECIES	PARAMETER	STOMACH	SMALL INTESTINE	LARGE INTESTINE	REFERENCES
Dog	A–V O_2 difference	3.0–3.7	3.5–4.5	3.0–4.4	37, 46, 47, 50–52
	Oxygen uptake	1.0–1.5	1.5–2.2	1.56–1.68	37, 45–47, 49–52, 73
Cat	A–V O_2 difference		4.6		55
	Oxygen uptake		1.4		55
Rat	A–V O_2 difference		4.5		59
	Oxygen uptake		4.8		59
	Villous pO_2		14–17		40, 74
	Muscle pO_2		21–26		40, 74
Piglet					
1 day	A–V O_2 difference		3.4–3.8		64, 65
	Oxygen uptake		2.9–4.3		64, 65
3 day	A–V O_2 difference		3.1–4.2		64, 65, 67, 69
	Oxygen uptake		2.0–2.9		64, 65, 67–69
2 week	A–V O_2 difference		3.3–4.8		64, 65
	Oxygen uptake		2.4–3.0		64, 65
1 mo	A–V O_2 difference		4.3–4.5		64, 67, 72
	Oxygen uptake		1.8–2.4		64, 67, 72

the intestine maintains oxygen consumption within 48% of control during arterial hypoxemia. However, when both blood flow and capillary density are free to increase, oxygen uptake remains within 26% of control despite the hypoxia. As with hypoxia, there is marked relaxation of resistance vessels during hypercapnia.[97] Unlike hypoxia, the precapillary sphincters constrict and capillary density decreases with hypercapnia. Alterations in arterial hematocrit also influence gastrointestinal blood flow and oxygenation.[47–49] There is an inverse linear correlation between intestinal blood flow and hematocrit, and a direct linear correlation between the arteriovenous oxygen difference and hematocrit in both in-

testine and stomach. The relationship between intestinal oxygen uptake and hematocrit is parabolic (Fig 22-5),[47] showing a maximal uptake at a hematocrit of 48.7% (optimal hematocrit). Intraenteric placement of nutrients increases the optimal hematocrit to 57.1%. In stomach, the optimal hematocrit is 38.2% under resting conditions, and it increases to 45.7% during pentagastrin stimulation. In the neonate, intestinal blood flow and oxygen uptake are unaltered by alterations in hematocrit over a range between 10% and 54%, indicating that increases in oxygen extraction play a major role in maintaining a normal rate of oxygen utilization when intestinal oxygen delivery is reduced by lowering the hematocrit.[98]

Venous pressure elevation has proved to be a useful perturbation for determining whether metabolic or myogenic mechanisms are involved in local vasoregulation. The metabolic hypothesis predicts that acute venous hypertension should cause vasodilation and an increased capillary density as a result of reduced blood flow and vasodilator accumulation. According to the myogenic hypothesis,

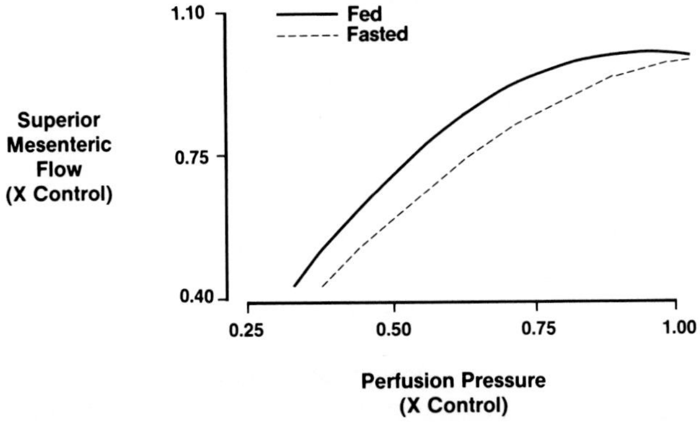

FIGURE 22–4. Responses of intestinal blood flow to step reductions in perfusion pressure in fed (*solid line*) versus fasted (*dashed line*) dogs, demonstrating an increased intensity of autoregulation during enhanced functional activity. (From Granger HJ, Norris CP. Intrinsic regulation of intestinal oxygenation in the anesthetized dog. Am J Physiol 1980;238: H836.)

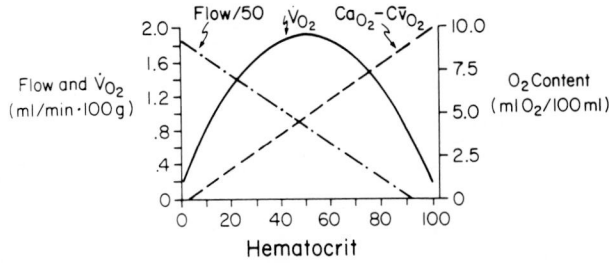

FIGURE 22–5. Effect of hematocrit on canine intestinal blood flow, oxygen consumption ($\dot{V}_{O_2}$), arterial O_2 content, and arteriovenous O_2 difference ($Ca_{O_2} - C\bar{v}_{O_2}$). (From Shepherd AP, Riedel GL. Optimal hematocrit for oxygenation of canine intestine. Circ Res 1982;51:233.)

vascular resistance increases and capillary density decreases during venous pressure elevation due to a rise in intravascular (intramural) pressure at the arteriolar and precapillary sphincter levels (Fig 22-6).[93] Studies of the stomach, small intestine, and colon in adult animals indicate that vascular resistance rises in response to venous pressure elevation,[44,45,54,70,86-88,98-104] findings that are consistent with a myogenic mechanism. In newborns, the intestinal vasculature dilates, rather than constricts, in response to venous hypertension, suggesting that metabolic factors are dominant in the hypermetabolic neonatal intestine.[64] The vasoconstriction elicited by acute venous hypertension in adult intestine results from a rise in precapillary (arteriolar) resistance while postcapillary resistance falls.[105] Capillary exchange capacity increases in the stomach and the colon but decreases in the small intestine, during venous hypertension.[93] These observations are consistent with the view that metabolic factors exert a greater influence on precapillary sphincters in the stomach and colon while myogenic factors dominate in the small intestine. In spite of the intense capillary derecruitment initiated by venous hypertension in the small intestine, oxygen extraction rises disproportionately to the fall in blood flow, and, consequently, oxygen consumption rises.[94] The elevated intestinal oxygen utilization during venous hypertension has been attributed to increased villous motility.[106] There are conflicting reports regarding the influence of enhanced oxidative metabolism on the vascular responses to venous pressure elevation. Some investigators have observed that an increased oxygen demand significantly reduces or abolishes the rise in vascular resistance,[46,88] while others note an exaggerated resistance response to venous pressure elevation.[107] However, there is uniform agreement that acute venous hypertension alters the distribution of blood flow within the bowel wall.[54,108]

As venous pressure is elevated, the percentage of total blood flow directed to the mucosa-submucosa is reduced, while the muscularis receives a larger fraction. These observations indicate that the constriction of arteriolar and precapillary sphincter smooth muscles elicited by venous hypertension takes place in the mucosa-submucosa layers and that the vasculature of the muscularis dilates in response to venous hypertension.

In contrast to the increased vascular resistance and reduced blood flow produced by acute venous pressure elevation, chronic portal hypertension is associated with intense vasodilation in the entire gastrointestinal tract.[109] Elevated circulating levels of glucagon and bile acids contribute significantly to the hyperdynamic circulation of chronic portal hypertension. A reduced sensitivity of the intestinal vasculature to norepinephrine and vasopressin also appears to play a role in mediating the hyperemia. Chronic portal hypertension does not alter intestinal oxygen consumption or intramural blood flow distribution.

Postprandial hyperemia is a term used to describe the increase in blood flow that occurs in response to a meal. The anticipatory/ingestion phase of digestion is characterized by transient increases in heart rate, cardiac output, and aortic pressure, while gastrointestinal blood flow is either unchanged or slightly increased.[110-114] These transient hemodynamic responses appear to be mediated by activation of the sympathetic nervous system because they can be attenuated by adrenergic blocking agents.[112] In conscious animals, blood flow to the stomach and proximal bowel increases 30 to 90 minutes after ingestion of a meal.[110-117] Blood flow to the ileum increases 45 to 120 minutes postprandially, while colonic blood flow generally does not increase.[115,117] Transient decreases in distal colon blood flow have been observed 30 minutes after a meal, and the response was attributed to tonic contractions pro-

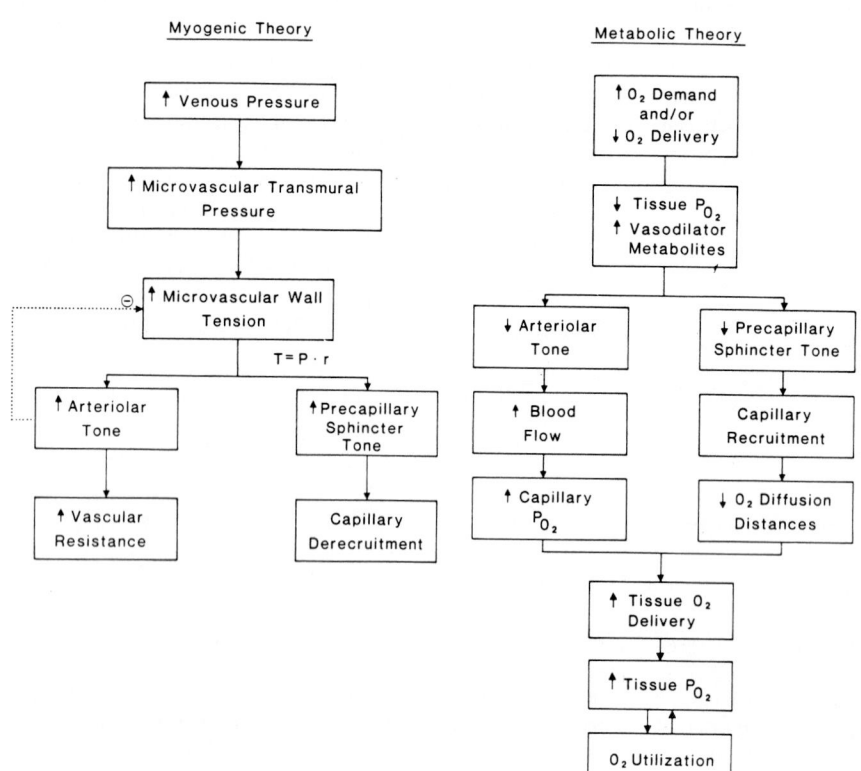

FIGURE 22-6. Metabolic and myogenic theories of intestinal blood flow regulation. (From Granger DN, Perry MA, Kvietys PR, et al. Metabolic, myogenic and hormonal factors in local regulation of alimentary tract blood flow. In: Koo A, Lam SK, Smaje LH, eds. Microcirculation of the alimentary tract. Singapore: World Scientific, 1983:131.)

duced by the gastrocolic reflex.[117] Blood flow in the SMA of conscious animals typically increases by 25% to 130% after ingestion of a meal.[110-112,118] The splanchnic vasodilation may last for 4 to 7 hours, depending on the nature and quantity of the meal.[119,120] A smaller increase (10%–60%) in blood flow is observed in isolated bowel segments after intraluminal placement of digested food or nutrient solutions.

It remains unclear whether the postprandial hyperemia is confined only to those bowel segments that are exposed to chyme. In general, placement of nutrient solutions into one of two isolated segments in anesthetized animals increases blood flow to the segment containing the nutrient, while not affecting blood flow to the adjacent segment.[121-124] However, in conscious animals, ingestion of a meal produces a hyperemia in distal bowel segments that are not yet exposed to chyme, suggesting that the hyperemia is a diffuse phenomenon.[60] The intramural responses to nutrient absorption are generally confined to the mucosal layer.[117,124-126] In some instances, blood flow to the external muscle layer falls after intraluminal placement of nutrients.[127] Studies in the rat small intestine suggest that the postprandial hyperemia occurs uniformly in all layers of the bowel wall.[128]

Considerable effort has been devoted to defining the luminal stimuli responsible for the postprandial hyperemia. Although mechanical stimulation of the mucosa elicits a hyperemia, chyme per se does not appear to produce the degree of mechanical stimulation necessary to increase intestinal blood flow. Similarly, luminal placement of undigested food does not elicit a hyperemia, while digested food significantly increases blood flow.[122] The latter observation indicates that hydrolytic products of food digestion initiate the hyperemia. The rise in luminal osmolality that often accompanies a meal has received some attention, particularly in view of the fact that the intestinal vasculature dilates significantly in response to an increase in plasma osmolality.[129]

Normally, the osmolality of intestinal chyme varies between 220 and 320 mOsm/kg, yet lumen osmolalities in excess of 1500 mOsm/kg are needed to increase gut blood flow.[121,130] A similar argument has been advanced to negate a role for pH changes in the postprandial hyperemia in jejunum and ileum (i.e., gut blood flow increases only when luminal pH falls below 2.5).[131]

Bile appears to play an important role in postprandial intestinal hyperemia. Ten percent gallbladder bile (the steady-state concentration in proximal bowel in the early postprandial period) does not increase jejunal blood flow, yet it appears to render glucose and long chain fatty acids vasoactive.[132] Thirty-three percent gallbladder bile renders both short chain fatty acids (caproic acid) and amino acids vasoactive, while further enhancing glucose-induced hyperemia. Although intraluminal placement of endogenous or synthetic bile lacks a direct vasoactive effect in the jejunum, bile more than doubles blood flow in the ileum.[122,133] Bile acids are largely responsible for the bile-induced hyperemia. This assertion is supported by the observation that cholestyramine abolishes the vasodilatory effects of endogenous bile on ileal blood flow.[133]

Ingestion of protein-rich meals in humans or gastric placement of protein in conscious rats produces marked increases in splanchnic blood flow. In isolated loops of proximal small bowel, a protein-rich diet (64%) increases blood flow by the same extent as a carbohydrate-rich diet (68%).[134] Although hydrolyzed proteins are well known to induce a postprandial hyperemia, the specific hydrolytic products of protein digestion that mediate the response remain unknown. When postprandial concentrations of 16 different amino acids and 3 peptides are placed in the bowel lumen, blood flow fails to increase.[122] It has been suggested that fragments cleaved off protein molecules during hydrolysis may possess amino acid sequences similar to those found in vasoactive regulatory peptides normally produced in the intestinal mucosa.[135]

After a meal, the luminal concentration of glucose fluctuates between 28 and 222 mmol. At these concentrations, glucose usually produces only a slight hyperemia (5%–10%) in dog and cat small intestine.[121,122,136,137] An 18% to 21% increase in blood flow is produced by glucose in rat small bowel.[138] Glucose analogues have been used to define the contribution of absorptive and oxidative processes in the carbohydrate-induced hyperemia.[139] Analogues of glucose that are neither transported nor metabolized (e.g., 2-deoxyglucose) do not increase blood flow, but 3-O methylglucose, which is transported but not metabolized, produces a hyperemia that is about one third that produced by glucose.

Solubilized long chain fatty acids appear to be the most potent luminal stimulus of the postprandial intestinal hyperemia. Oleic acid (10–20 mmol) solubilized in 10% gallbladder bile produces a 20% to 60% increase in intestinal blood flow.[121,132,140]

Relatively little is known about the vascular response of the gut to luminal placement or ingestion of other dietary lipids. Short chain fatty acids (e.g., caproic acid) do not alter blood flow even in the presence of 10% gallbladder bile. Although lipids produce the greatest intestinal hyperemia, the vascular responses elicited by protein and carbohydrate are not insignificant in that the three major dietary components of food (fats, proteins, and carbohydrates) appear to act synergistically on blood flow when placed in the bowel lumen (Fig 22-7).[141]

MODULATORS OF INTRINSIC VASOREGULATION

A number of chemical and physical factors have been proposed to explain intrinsic vasoregulatory phenomena in the gastrointestinal tract. These factors generally fall into one of three major categories: (1) myogenic factors, (2) chemicals directly linked to oxidative metabolism, and (3) vasoactive peptides, hormones, and autacoids. The myogenic theory has been invoked to explain both pressure–flow autoregulation and the responses to venous pressure elevation in the intestine and stomach. The myogenic theory is based on the assumption that vascular wall tension is a controlled variable. According to this concept, arteriolar tension receptors modulate vascular smooth muscle tone in response to changes in microvascular transmural pressure. In accordance with the Laplace relationship, resistance vessels should dilate when vascular transmural pressure is decreased and should constrict when it is increased. The myogenic theory predicts that vascular resistance should fall when arterial pressure is reduced. Similarly, this mechanism predicts the rise in intestinal vascular resistance that occurs during acute venous pressure elevation (Fig 22-8).[54]

Because the intensity of all intrinsic vasoregulatory phenomena described in the gastrointestinal tract are significantly influenced by the oxidative requirements of the tissue, metabolic factors have received much attention. According to the metabolic theory of blood flow regulation, vascular resistance and precapillary sphincter tone are linked to the metabolic status of the tissue. Any condition that reduces oxygen delivery, increases oxygen demand, or

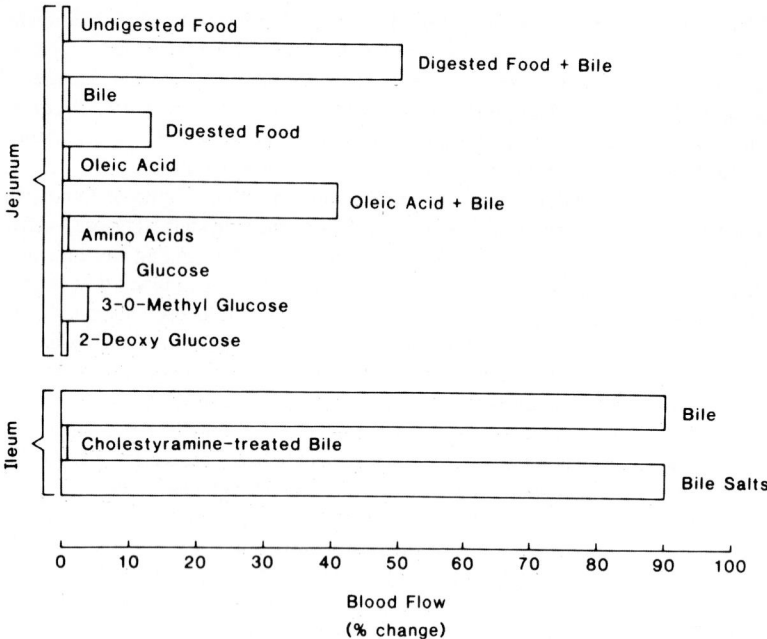

FIGURE 22-7. Effects of intraluminal placement of various constituents of chyme on intestinal blood flow. (From Granger DN, Kvietys PR, Parks DA, Benoit JN. Intestinal blood flow: relations to function. Surv Dig Dis 1983;1:217.)

both leads to a reduction in tissue oxygen tension and an accumulation of vasodilator metabolites in the immediate perivascular space. These changes cause relaxation of arteriolar and precapillary sphincter smooth muscle. The resulting increases in blood flow and capillary recruitment serve to stabilize capillary pO_2, increase the surface area for O_2 exchange, and decrease the capillary-to-cell diffusion distance. The ultimate effect of these changes is to maintain cell pO_2 above the critical level at which O_2 availability limits energy metabolism. The metabolic theory has been invoked to explain the vascular responses during pressure–flow autoregulation, reactive hyperemia, arterial hypoxemia, postprandial hyperemia, and venous pressure elevation.

Both adenosine and tissue oxygen tension have been proposed as mediators of metabolic vasoregulatory responses in the gastrointestinal tract. Adenosine is a powerful vasodilator when infused into the splanchnic circulation. Adenosine accumulation in venous blood has been demonstrated during reactive and postprandial hyperemias in the small bowel. The role of adenosine in local vasoregulation has been assessed using substances such as theophylline (competitive antagonist), the enzyme adenosine deaminase (converts adenosine to inosine), and dipyridamole (an inhibitor of adenosine reuptake). These agents attenuate or completely abolish the vasodilation associated with reductions in arterial pressure, release of an arterial occlusion, and absorption of nutrients.[142,143] For example, adenosine deaminase completely prevents the absorptive hyperemia induced by glucose-oleic acid test meal in the rat small intestine.[142] Similarly, 8-phenyltheophylline abolishes pressure–flow autoregulation and reduces the reactive hyperemic response by 50% in the SMA of anesthetized cats.[144] There is considerably less information regarding the role of tissue oxygen tension in intrinsic vasoregulation. Mucosal pO_2 falls by about 50% during the absorption of glucose in the proximal small bowel, and the hyperemic response is quantitatively and temporally related to the fall in mucosal pO_2.[128] Taurocholic acid produces a similar fall (58%) in mucosal pO_2 and 65% increase in blood flow in the ileum. Cholic acid does not affect either mucosal pO_2 or blood flow when placed in the ileal lumen. There is also a large body of indirect evidence that the degree of tissue oxygenation influences intestinal vasoregulation. For example, at any given oxygen uptake, the magnitude of the postprandial hyperemia is larger if the resting oxygen extraction (arteriovenous oxygen difference) is high, which indicates that the vascular response is influenced by the prevailing tissue oxygen tension.[82]

Most of the hormones and peptides produced in the gastroin-

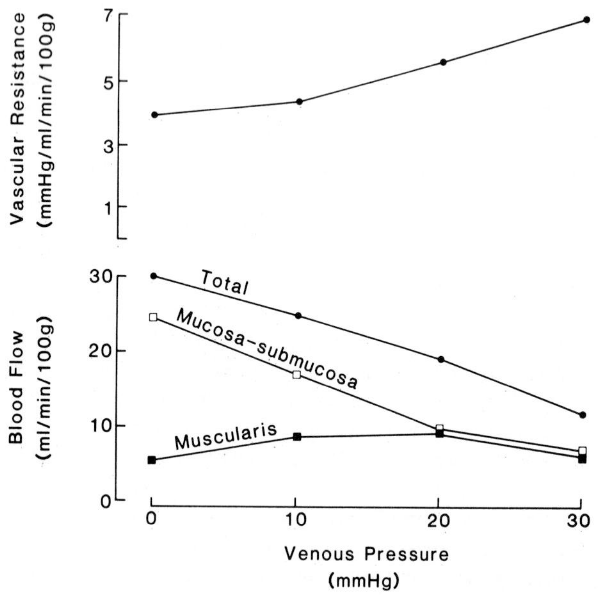

FIGURE 22-8. Intestinal vascular responses to acute venous hypertension in cats. The increase in vascular resistance and decrease in blood flow during acute venous pressure elevation is consistent with the myogenic theory of intrinsic vasoregulation. (Data from Granger DN, Richardson PDI, Taylor AE. Volumetric assessment of the capillary filtration coefficient in the cat small intestine. Pflugers Arch 1979;381:25.)

testinal mucosa are vasodilators when infused into the splanchnic circulation. Because many of these substances are also released into the mucosal interstitium in response to a meal, it has been proposed that peptides and hormones mediate postprandial hyperemia. This hypothesis has received less attention in recent years because of studies that demonstrate that gastrointestinal peptides and hormones are not vasoactive when infused into arterial blood at concentrations that are measured postprandially. Cholecystokinin, secretin, gastrin, and neurotensin do not produce vasodilation when infused, either alone or in combination, into the arterial supply of the proximal bowel to achieve postprandial levels.[145] However, in the distal ileum, neurotensin significantly increases blood flow at postprandial concentrations.[146] Although vascular infusion studies tend to argue against a role for gastrointestinal hormones and peptides in postprandial hyperemia, these experiments do not exclude the possibility that these peptides vasodilate by a paracrine or neurocrine action (see ch 2). This concept has been addressed using immunoneutralization.[147] Intravenous administration of antiserum directed against vasoactive intestinal peptide (VIP) produces a dose-related suppression of the absorptive hyperemia induced by luminal placement of bile-oleic acid. Antisera against cholecystokinin or substance P have no effect on absorptive hyperemia. These results indicate that VIP, which is released from mucosal neurons, mediates at least a fraction of postprandial hyperemia by acting as a paracrine agent.

A variety of endogenous autacoids also have been implicated as local paracrine mediators in the regulation of intestinal blood flow. These substances are diversified in regard to structure and overall biologic activity, but they appear to have at least one property in common (i.e., vasodilation of the gastrointestinal vasculature). Three members of this diversified group have been studied relative to mediation of the postprandial hyperemia (i.e., serotonin, histamine, and prostaglandins). Feeding or acid perfusion of the duodenum produces an elevation in portal blood levels of serotonin.[148] However, a serotonin antagonist, methysergide, does not reduce the magnitude of postprandial hyperemia. Intrajejunal placement of a mixed meal increases blood flow by 30%, a response that is attenuated by pretreatment with an H_1-receptor antagonist, tripelennamine, but not with metiamide, an H_2-receptor antagonist.[149] Because tripelennamine also blocks the food-induced increase in oxygen uptake, it remains unclear whether histamine directly dilates the vasculature during postprandial hyperemia or whether the blunted response to H_1-receptor blockade reflects a reduction in oxidative metabolism. Studies in rat and dog jejunum suggest that endogenous prostaglandins may also play a role in postprandial hyperemia. The cyclooxygenase inhibitors, indomethacin and mefenamic acid, greatly enhance food-mediated increases in blood flow and oxygen uptake, while arachidonic acid attenuates these responses.[150-152] Thus, the available data suggest that prostaglandins are produced during the postprandial state and these cyclooxygenase products tend to limit the increase in blood flow, either by inhibiting oxidative metabolism or by a direct vasoconstrictor action.

Extrinsic Control

Blood flow within the gastrointestinal tract is also influenced by extrinsic neurohumoral factors. Because the splanchnic organs receive approximately 25% of the cardiac output and contain approximately 25% of the total blood volume at rest, neurohumoral control of the splanchnic vascular bed can be an important component in the overall reflex control of the circulation, especially during periods of stress, such as exercise and shock.[153]

Neural control of intestinal blood flow is predominantly by way of sympathetic noradrenergic nerves.[154] Extrinsic cholinergic nerves from the vagus do not supply the intestinal vasculature,[155,156] but the myriad, extravascular actions of parasympathetic stimulation in the gastrointestinal tract may indirectly affect blood flow. A local, intramural, vasodilatory nervous pathway also appears to exist within the intestine, which causes an increase in intestinal blood flow after local electrical stimulation or mechanical stimulation of the mucosa.[157,158] This response is blocked by tetrodotoxin or lidocaine, but not by autonomic denervation.

Autoregulatory escape (Fig 22-9)[72] is a phenomenon in which stimulation of sympathetic nerves or intraarterial infusion of norepinephrine produces an initial intense vasoconstriction and fall in blood flow, followed by a return ("escape") of blood flow toward baseline levels, despite continued nerve stimulation or norepi-

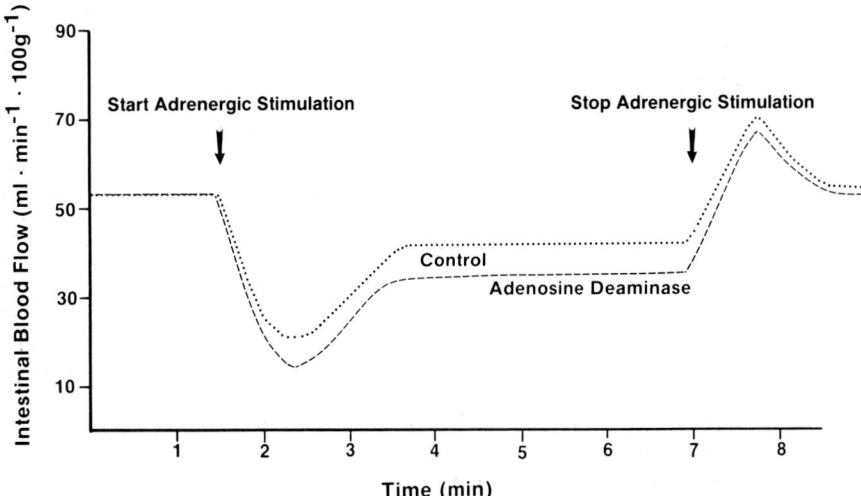

FIGURE 22-9. Autoregulatory escape from adrenergic stimulation in autoperfused piglet small intestine. Adenosine deaminase (degrades adenosine) pretreatment reduced the steady-state escape response to norepinephrine infusion, while pretreatment with chlorpheniramine (an H_1 blocker) had no effect. (Data from Crisinger KD, Kvietys PR, Granger DN. Autoregulatory escape from norepinephrine infusion: Roles of adenosine and histamine. Am J Physiol 1988;245:G560.)

nephrine infusion. Discontinuation of stimulation/infusion results in a poststimulatory hyperemia. Autoregulatory escape was first described in the intestine by Folkow and coworkers in 1964,[159] but the mechanism of the escape phenomenon is not completely understood. It occurs only in arteriolar smooth muscle and not in venous smooth muscle.[159] It is unaltered by β-receptor blockade[160] and administration of atropine.[161] In developing animals, there appears to be an age-related maturation in the ability of the intestine to escape from nerve stimulation or norepinephrine infusion, because the intestine of swine less than 2 weeks of age does not undergo autoregulatory escape from these stimuli.[162]

Three mechanisms commonly invoked to explain autoregulatory escape include: (1) redistribution of blood flow from the mucosa to the submucosa, (2) adaptation of adrenergic receptors to continued nerve stimulation, and (3) accumulation of vasodilator metabolites. The first possibility of redistribution of blood flow has not been substantiated, as demonstrated by in vivo microscopic studies in which the vessels that initially constrict subsequently relax during the steady-state escape phase.[163]

Adaptation of adrenergic receptors is also unlikely, because infusion of norepinephrine during the steady-state escape phase of sympathetic nerve stimulation leads to a further vasoconstriction and a second escape.[160]

The most popular theory used to explain autoregulatory escape is that vasodilator metabolites accumulate during the initial vasoconstrictor phase, leading to arteriolar dilation and a consequent restoration of blood flow toward normal.[160,164-166] The metabolic theory of intestinal vasoregulation states that tissue metabolism and arteriolar smooth muscle constitute a local control system that provides the necessary coupling between blood flow and tissue nutritional requirements. Any condition causing an imbalance between oxygen supply and demand produces an outpouring of metabolites into the interstitial fluid. The metabolites diffuse to the arterioles and precapillary sphincters to cause vasodilation and capillary recruitment.

The increased blood flow and/or oxygen extraction restore oxygen supply to a level compatible with tissue oxygen demand.[167] Consistent with this theory is experimental evidence that the propensity for blood flow to escape from sympathetic vasoconstriction is significantly greater in the metabolically active mucosa than in the muscularis.[168]

Adenosine appears to play at least a partial role in autoregulatory escape (see Fig 22-9),[72] while a role for histamine[72,161] and prostaglandins[161] has not been substantiated. Recent evidence also implicates a possible role for vasodilatory peptidergic neurons in effecting autoregulatory escape after sympathetic nerve stimulation but not during infusion of norepinephrine.[169] One neurotransmitter substance produced by these fibers is vasoactive intestinal polypeptide.[147]

Circulating vasoactive substances that affect gastrointestinal blood flow include adrenergic agents, vasopressin, and angiotensin. Norepinephrine, a predominantly α-adrenergic receptor stimulant causes intestinal vasoconstriction, a decrease in capillary density, and a reduction in oxygen uptake.[166,170,171] With continuous intraarterial infusion, the intense initial vasoconstriction is followed by return of blood flow toward control levels despite continued norepinephrine infusion (see discussion of autoregulatory escape above). Epinephrine can cause either α-receptor-mediated vasoconstriction (high doses) or β-receptor-mediated vasodilation (low doses), as well as a variable response in oxygen uptake.[166,172,173]

Both vasopressin and angiotensin II are potent physiologic vasoconstrictors that reduce blood flow and increase vascular resistance in all gastrointestinal organs. They cause generalized vasoconstriction, with disproportionate (selective) reduction in mesenteric blood flow at doses that have been measured in pathophysiologic states of hypotension.[174] Vasopressin causes a decrease in capillary density and a reduction in intestinal oxygen uptake, while angiotensin II reduces or does not affect[175] splanchnic oxygen uptake. The renin–angiotensin and vasopressin systems appear to have overlapping mechanisms to maintain resting intestinal vascular tone, because blockade of both systems is necessary to alter this tone.[176,177] Both pressor systems are also involved in the intestinal vasoconstrictor response to hemorrhage and hypovolemia, and significant attenuation of this increase in vascular resistance occurs only when both systems are blocked simultaneously,[178,179] even in the presence of an intact sympathetic system. Furthermore, angiotensin does not affect the mesenteric circulation indirectly through activation of the sympathetic nervous system or by promoting vasopressin release, but rather plays a physiologically important direct role in the control of mesenteric blood flow after volume depletion.[180] (A complete review and discussion of the effects of vasoactive agents, including physiologic and pharmacologic vasoconstrictors and vasodilators, on splanchnic oxygen uptake can be found in Kvietys and Granger.[175])

Oxygen Uptake–Blood Flow Relationship: Functional Implications

Considerable attention has been devoted to the interaction between gastrointestinal blood flow and oxygen uptake, and the relevance of this interaction to mucosal function and integrity. Figure 22-10 depicts the relationship observed between intestinal blood flow and oxygen uptake when blood flow is altered with a pump or by way of graded reductions in perfusion pressure.[55] Oxygen uptake remains virtually constant over a wide range of blood flows (blood flow independent), and it is compromised only when blood flow reaches a critically low level. Below this critical blood flow, oxygen uptake is blood flow dependent. Resting blood flow in the small intestine, stomach, and colon is usually greater than the critical blood flow at which oxygen uptake is blood flow dependent.[45,50,175,181]

The reduction in oxygen uptake that occurs when blood flow falls below a critical level can be explained in terms of the normal relationship between mitochondrial oxygen consumption and cell pO_2. This relationship predicts that oxygen uptake remains constant over a wide range of cell pO_2 and it is reduced only when cell pO_2 falls to a critically low level (the critical pO_2). The resting cell pO_2 is normally well above the critical pO_2. There is evidence indicating that graded reductions in blood flow produce concomitant reductions in cell pO_2 without altering oxygen uptake in the stomach.[175] However, at very low blood flows, the rate of oxygen diffusion to the cells is so low that the intracellular pO_2 falls below the critical level required to maintain normal oxidative metabolism. Thus, the reduction in oxygen uptake observed at low blood flows may simply reflect a depression in oxidative metabolism due to a limited availability of oxygen.

A number of conditions alter the relationship between oxygen uptake and blood flow such that oxygen uptake is dependent on

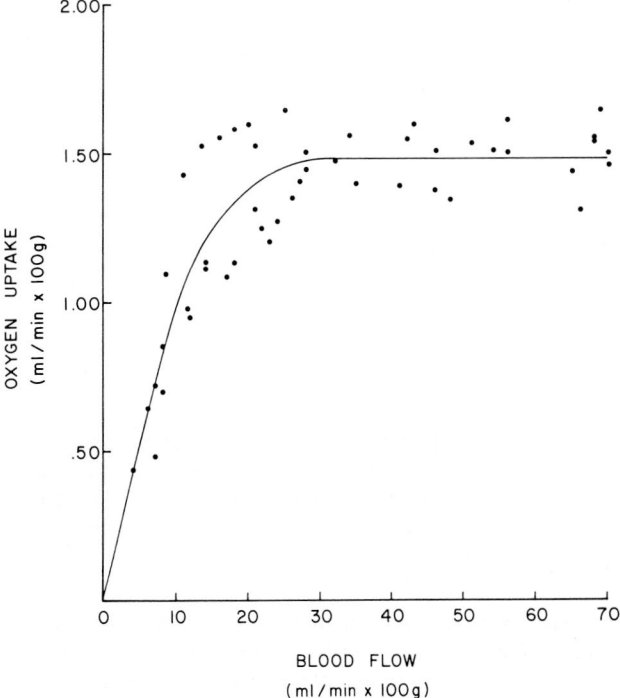

FIGURE 22–10. Relationship between intestinal blood flow and oxygen uptake in feline jejuno-ileum when blood flow is altered with a pump or by way of graded reductions in perfusion pressure. (From Granger DN, Kvietys PR, Perry MA. Role of exchange vessels in the regulation of intestinal oxygenation. Am J Physiol 1982;242:G570.)

blood flow even when it is increased above normal. These include luminal distention,[182] alterations in hematocrit,[183] and devascularization.[86] All of these conditions presumably result in a severe reduction in tissue oxygenation (cell pO_2 falls below the critical pO_2) in discrete or generalized regions of the stomach or gut. Luminal distention and devascularization reduce tissue oxygenation by compromising blood flow, while low hematocrits limit oxygen delivery even at high blood flows. Normal physiologic conditions can also influence the relationship between oxygen uptake and blood flow. Stimulation or inhibition of oxidative me-

tabolism shifts the plateau of the blood flow–oxygen uptake curve upward and downward, respectively (Fig 22-11).[175] It has been shown that stimulation of intestinal motility or enhancement of active transport raises the plateau of the blood flow–oxygen uptake curve.[184] Conversely, decreasing the temperature of isolated bowel segments lowers the plateau. Another important aspect of the blood flow–oxygen uptake relationship in the small bowel is that it predicts the influence of blood flow reductions on oxygen-requiring processes such as absorption and secretion. For example, it has been shown that the reductions in glucose absorption produced by graded decrements in blood flow parallel the decline in oxygen uptake,[185] suggesting that oxygen availability limits solute transport when cell pO_2 falls below the critical level.

Many vasodilators tend to increase intestinal oxygen uptake irrespective of their effects on oxidative metabolism. These observations have been attributed to the use of preparations in which oxygen uptake depends on blood flow. If vasodilators are infused into these preparations, the increase in oxygen uptake would be expected to parallel the increase in blood flow. Vasodilators do not alter oxygen uptake in preparations in which oxygen uptake is independent of blood flow unless an effect is exerted on oxidative metabolism. In general, vasoconstrictors decrease oxygen uptake in preparations exhibiting either a normal or abnormal relationship between blood flow and oxygen uptake, unless the agent enhances oxidative metabolism. Vasoconstrictors that do not affect oxidative metabolism would be expected to decrease oxygen uptake by simply moving down the normal blood flow–oxygen uptake curve.

Another important determinant of the rate of oxygen exchange across capillaries is the effective capillary density. The number of capillaries perfused at any given time determines the flux of oxygen out of the capillary and into the tissue through an effect on diffusion parameters (i.e., surface area available for exchange and capillary-to-cell diffusion distances). Thus, one would expect that alterations in capillary density may affect oxygen uptake. The expected influence of capillary density on the relationship between blood flow and oxygen uptake is shown in Figure 22-12. If capillary density within an organ is increased, the minimum blood flow required to attain the plateau of the blood flow–oxygen uptake curve would be lower (i.e., the curve would be shifted to the left) due to an increased capillary surface area and a reduced capillary-to-cell diffusion distance.[175]

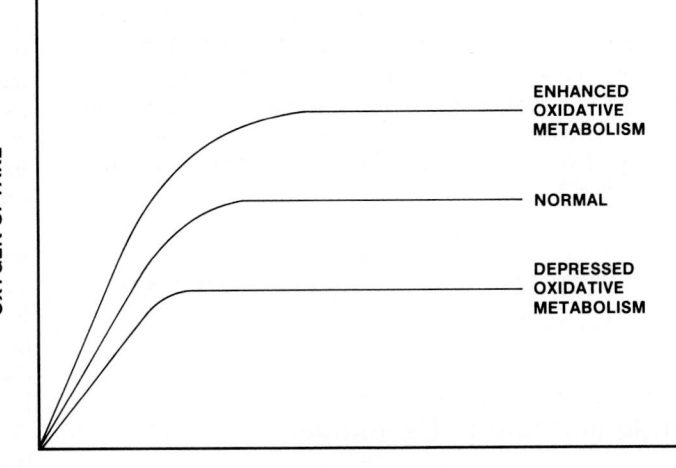

FIGURE 22–11. Relationship between blood flow and oxygen uptake during stimulation or inhibition of oxidative metabolism. (From Kvietys PR, Granger DN. Vasoactive agents and splanchnic oxygen uptake. Am J Physiol 1982;243:G1.)

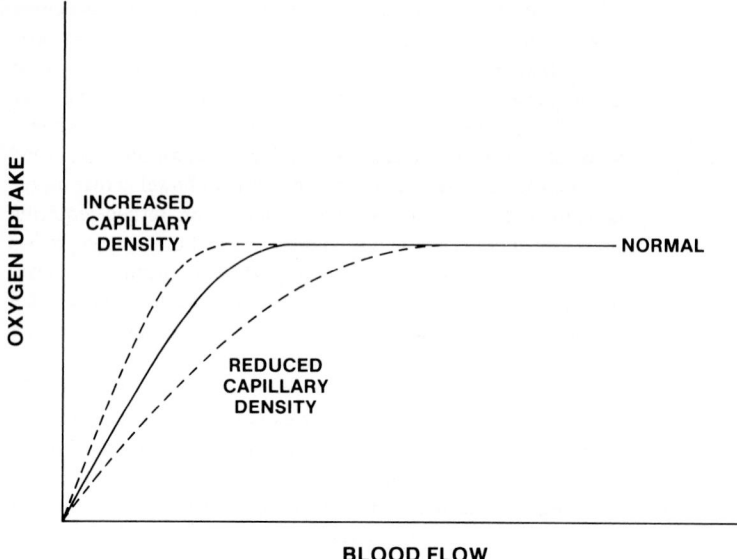

FIGURE 22–12. Relationship between oxygen uptake and blood flow under conditions of increased or reduced perfused capillary density. (From Kvietys PR, Granger DN. Vasoactive agents and splanchnic oxygen uptake. Am J Physiol 1982;243:G1.)

The relationship between blood flow and oxygen uptake has also been useful in explaining some of the reported observations regarding the influence of blood flow on gastric acid secretion.[186] The production of gastric acid is an energy-consuming process that results in an increase in gastric oxygen uptake. The consistent finding that acid secretion and oxygen consumption are highly correlated raises the question of whether acid secretion in the stomach depends on blood flow. The answer to this question largely depends on the surgical preparation employed. In some preparations, a number of vessels supplying the stomach are occluded, and the end result is flow-dependency of oxygen uptake. In this situation, an increase or decrease in blood flow is associated with a corresponding change in acid secretion. However, in normally perfused preparations, acid secretion and blood flow exhibit a relationship similar to that observed between oxygen consumption and blood flow. That is, acid secretion depends on blood flow at low blood flows and it is independent of blood flow at higher flow rates. This explains why vasoconstrictors generally tend to reduce gastric acid output and why some vasodilators (acid secretagogues) increase acid output while others (nonsecretagogues) do not. The controversy regarding the relationship between gastric acid output and blood flow cannot be entirely resolved on the basis of tissue oxygenation. Most of the reports that demonstrate a relationship between blood flow and acid secretion have relied on the aminopyrine clearance technique for measurement of blood flow. However, it is well recognized that aminopyrine clearance more accurately reflects acid output by the stomach rather than blood flow to it (see section entitled "Techniques for Measurement of Blood Flow").

PHYSIOLOGY OF MICROVASCULAR EXCHANGE

Principles of Transcapillary Fluid and Solute Exchange

It can be estimated that approximately 1.5 L of fluid and 45 g of protein are filtered across microvessels in the gastrointestinal tract each day. Several characteristic features of the gastrointestinal microcirculation account for its ability to exchange such large amounts of fluid and protein.[187] In comparison to other tissues (e.g., skeletal muscle), the gastrointestinal tract has a high capillary density and, consequently, a large surface area for exchange. The capillaries found in the mucosa are generally of the fenestrated type. These fenestrations greatly enhance the hydraulic conductivity of the capillaries and provide an enormous pore area for exchange. Gastrointestinal capillaries are highly permeable to small solutes, yet they are relatively impermeable to macromolecules. This allows for the maintenance of a constant interstitial volume by restricting colloids to the intravascular compartment, yet facilitates the transport of absorbed solutes (e.g., glucose) and water between the intravascular and extravascular spaces. The objective of this section is to describe the factors that determine the rate and direction of fluid and protein movement across gastrointestinal capillaries and to discuss how these factors interact during periods of excess fluid filtration and during net mucosal fluid absorption or secretion. The basic concepts regarding capillary fluid filtration are discussed in terms of the Starling hypothesis (i.e.,

$$Jv = Kfc \, [\, (\, Pc - Pt \,) - \sigma(\, \pi p - \pi t \,) \,]$$

where Jv is the rate of net transcapillary fluid movement [when Jv is positive the capillaries are filtering, and when Jv is negative the capillaries are absorbing fluid], Kfc is the capillary filtration coefficient, Pc is the capillary hydrostatic pressure, Pt is the interstitial fluid pressure, σ is the capillary osmotic reflection coefficient, πp is the plasma oncotic pressure, and πt is the tissue oncotic pressure).

Net capillary fluid filtration rate (Jv) is generally assumed to equal the rate of lymph flow when the tissue is in an isovolumetric state (i.e., interstitial volume is neither increasing nor decreasing). In the absence of active transport across the mucosa, lymph flow in the stomach and intestine ranges between 0.03 and 0.10 ml·min^{-1}·100 g tissue^{-1}.[188] A number of conditions are known to modify lymph flow in the gastrointestinal tract. Conditions that increase Pc or decrease either σ or πp generally result in an increase in lymph flow (Jv). Lymph flow increases by as much as 30 times control after acute portal hypertension or acute hypoproteinemia.[70,189–191] Histamine,[95] bradykinin,[192,193] glucagon,[194] cholecystokinin,[195,196] secretin,[195,197] and prostaglandin E₁[198] have been shown to increase intestinal lymph flow. Vasoconstrictors generally tend to reduce lymph flow, presumably by decreasing Pc and Kfc. Mucosal fluid absorption in the intestine increases lymph flow, while acid secretion in the stomach decreases lymph flow. As in other tissues, the interstitial-to-lymphatic hydrostatic pressure gradient appears to be the primary determinant of gastrointestinal lymph flow.[199] This view is supported by the observation that intestinal lymph flow is highly correlated to steady-state interstitial fluid pressure.[70]

Capillary filtration coefficient (Kfc) measurements provide a direct estimate of the transcapillary hydraulic conductance. Kfc is influenced by both the size and number of pores in each capillary as well as by the number of perfused capillaries. Kfc relates net fluid filtration (or absorption) rate to the pressure gradient across the microvascular barrier. Values ranging between 0.05 and 0.15 ml·min⁻¹·mmHg⁻¹·100 g tissue⁻¹ have been reported for the stomach and small bowel.[188] In general, vasodilators increase, while vasoconstrictors decrease, Kfc. These responses are usually interpreted to indicate that vascular elements controlling perfused capillary density (precapillary sphincters) relax or constrict in response to the vasoactive agents. Although most of the responses produced by vasoactive drugs can be attributed to increased microvascular surface area, some agents and conditions appear to increase Kfc by increasing capillary permeability. These include hemorrhagic shock,[200] histamine,[95] bradykinin,[193] glucagon,[194] and arterial hypoxemia.[201] Intestinal Kfc decreases, while gastric Kfc increases, when portal pressure is acutely elevated. The different responses to portal hypertension have been explained by dominance of myogenic control mechanisms in the intestine and metabolic control mechanisms in the stomach. In the intestine, the greatest reduction in Kfc occurs between portal pressures of 0 and 15 mmHg.[188] The myogenic reduction in filtering surface area serves to protect the intestine against edema formation after sudden elevations in venous pressure by attenuating the increase in capillary filtration rate.

Capillary pressure (Pc) is the major force favoring fluid filtration across gastrointestinal capillaries. The resting value of Pc in intestine ranges between 15.5 and 17.0 mmHg at normal portal pressures.[59,81,202] When arterial pressure is increased, only 5% to 10% of the pressure increment is transmitted to the capillaries. Venous pressure elevation has a more profound effect, with 70% of the pressure increment transmitted to the capillaries.[70,81] The different responses to arterial and venous pressure elevation reflect the high pre-to-postcapillary resistance ratio in normal intestine. In general, vasodilators increase Pc while vasoconstrictors decrease Pc due to changes in precapillary resistance.[188]

Interstitial fluid pressure (Pt) has been estimated using indirect approaches in both stomach and small intestine. At portal pressures between 0 and 5 mmHg, Pt ranges between −3.0 and 0 mmHg in the small intestine.[188] When portal pressure exceeds 5.0 mmHg, Pt is consistently positive. A resting value of 0.5 mmHg has been reported for the stomach. Studies in a variety of organs indicate that the value of Pt is determined by the interstitial volume. The relationship between interstitial volume and pressure indicates that, at normal tissue hydration, small changes in interstitial volume result in large changes in interstitial pressure. When the tissue becomes edematous, a considerable volume of fluid can accumulate in the interstitial spaces without altering Pt.[70] Thus, there are two distinct regions to the interstitial compliance curve (Fig 22-13),[187] (i.e., a low compliance region at Pt between −3 and 3 mmHg [portal pressure less than 15 mmHg] and a high compliance region at Pt greater than 3 mmHg [portal pressure greater than 15 mmHg]). The transition from low to high compliance is associated with a corresponding increase in interstitial hydraulic conductivity (Lp) as illustrated in Figure 22-13.[187] Pt increases in the intestine during intraarterial infusion of glucagon[194] or bradykinin,[192] and during mucosal fluid absorption.[203] Cholera toxin–induced fluid secretion,[204] arterial hypotension,[205] and sympathetic stimulation[206] are associated with a reduction of Pt in the small intestine.

Osmotic reflection coefficient (σ) of gastrointestinal capillaries to plasma proteins has been estimated using lymphatic protein flux data. Because fenestrated capillaries are permeable to plasma proteins, only part of the oncotic pressure generated by proteins is actually exerted across the capillary membrane. The osmotic reflection coefficient describes the fraction of the total oncotic pressure generated across the capillary membrane. Impermeant proteins generate 100% of their maximum oncotic pressure and σ = 1. Experimentally derived values of σ for total plasma proteins indicate that 78%, 92%, and 85% of the total oncotic pressure is

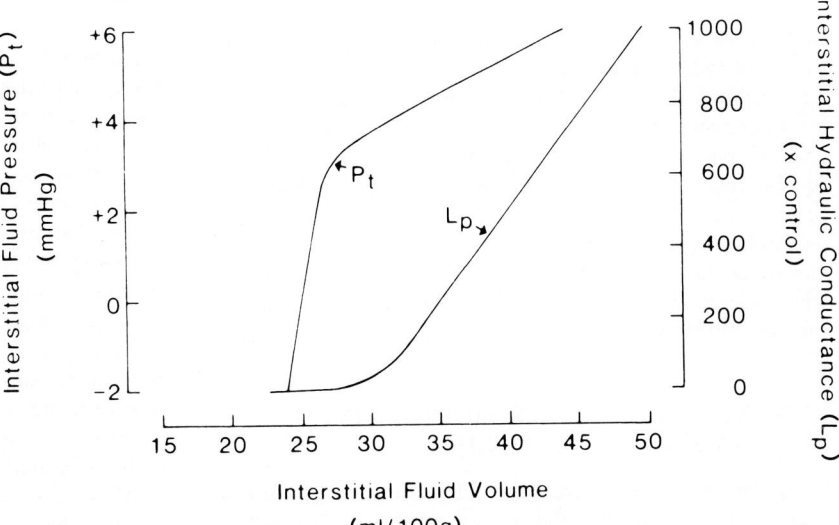

FIGURE 22–13. Steady-state relationship between intestinal interstitial fluid volume, interstitial fluid pressure, and interstitial hydraulic conductance. (From Granger DN, Kvietys PR, Perry MA, Barrowman JA. The microcirculation and intestinal transport. In: Johnson LR, ed. Physiology of the gastrointestinal tract, ed 2. New York: Raven Press, 1987:1671.)

transmitted across the capillary wall in stomach, small intestine, and colon, respectively.[188] Osmotic reflection coefficients for endogenous macromolecules of varying sizes (37–120 A) have been determined in stomach, small intestine, and colon.[207] Estimates of pore sizes and distributions have been derived from the σ data for different sized solutes. A small population of pores ranging between 46 and 53 A radius and large pores ranging between 180 and 250 A radius have been predicted for capillaries in the stomach, small intestine, and colon. A variety of agents and conditions have been shown to reduce σ and consequently increase microvascular permeability. These include histamine, bradykinin, *Escherichia coli* endotoxin, glucagon, hypertonic glucose, ischemia–reperfusion, Goldblatt hypertension, and lipid absorption.[207] Most conditions that increase microvascular permeability to plasma proteins do so by increasing the dimensions of the large pores. It is of particular interest that a normal physiologic event such as lipid absorption is associated with increased vascular permeability.[195] The mechanism underlying the lipid-induced increase in permeability remains undefined; however, neurotensin is a viable candidate because this peptide increases intestinal vascular permeability when infused into the arterial supply to achieve postprandial concentrations.[208]

Transcapillary oncotic pressure gradient ($\Delta\pi$) in stomach, small intestine, and colon normally ranges between 11 and 13 mmHg.[188] To obtain these estimates, it is assumed that lymph provides a valid reflection of interstitial fluid, and, therefore, lymph oncotic pressure is used to estimate interstitial oncotic pressure. Because the reflection coefficient is greater than zero in gastrointestinal capillaries, a change in capillary filtration rate should alter $\Delta\pi$, the magnitude of the change depending on capillary surface area, the reflection coefficient, lymph flow, and interstitial compliance. The transcapillary oncotic pressure gradient increases if Pc is increased and $\Delta\pi$ decreases if microvascular permeability is increased. Net fluid absorption is generally associated with an increase in $\Delta\pi$ because protein free fluid enters the mucosal interstitium.[209] Likewise, active (e.g., cholera toxin–induced) secretion is associated with a reduction in $\Delta\pi$ because protein-free fluid is moved from the interstitium to the bowel lumen.[210]

Interaction of Capillary and Interstitial Forces

In the nonabsorbing small intestine or nonsecreting stomach, the balance of hydrostatic and oncotic forces governing transcapillary fluid exchange favors net filtration of fluid from vascular to extravascular compartments. To maintain a constant interstitial volume, the rate of transcapillary fluid filtration is balanced by an equal outflow of fluid by the lymphatics. However, when fluid accumulates in the interstitium by way of the blood or lumen, the interstitial forces readjust in an effort to minimize the increase in interstitial volume. The following section describes how the interstitial forces and lymph flow interact during periods of enhanced capillary filtration, net fluid absorption, and net fluid secretion.

ENHANCED CAPILLARY FILTRATION AND EDEMA SAFETY FACTORS

If capillary pressure is increased or plasma oncotic pressure is reduced, the rate of capillary fluid filtration increases. The resulting fluid accumulation within the mucosal interstitium causes interstitial fluid pressure and lymph flow to increase and interstitial oncotic pressure to fall. These changes oppose further filtration of fluid out of the capillaries, and, eventually, a new steady state is achieved with a more hydrated interstitium. For small imbalances in intravascular forces, extravascular forces are able to limit edema formation. The resistance to edema formation resulting from readjustment of interstitial forces and lymph flow has been referred to as the "edema safety factor." In the small intestine, the total safety factor against edema ranges between 12 and 15 mmHg.[70] Increments in capillary pressure or reductions in plasma oncotic pressure below 15 mmHg can be opposed by the safety factors. It has been estimated that increases in lymph flow and interstitial fluid pressure and the reduction in interstitial oncotic pressure contribute equally to the total edema safety factor in the small intestine.[70]

If capillary pressure is increased or plasma oncotic pressure is reduced by more than 15 mmHg, there is unrestrained fluid accumulation in the intestinal mucosa, and, ultimately, interstitial fluid enters the bowel lumen.[70,211] The terms "filtration secretion" and "secretory filtration" have been used to describe this process. Filtration secretion can be induced by acute portal hypertension, increased intraenteric pressure, plasma dilution, lymphatic obstruction, and conditions or agents that increase capillary permeability or pressure or both. Filtration secretion does not occur with imbalances in capillary forces less than 15 mmHg (threshold value) for two reasons: a low mucosal hydraulic conductance and a low mucosal interstitial fluid pressure.[211] When net capillary filtration pressure, [(Pc − Pt) − σ(πp − πt)], exceeds the threshold value, sustained net capillary filtration occurs. The increased capillary filtration causes mucosal interstitial fluid pressure to increase. When Pt increases by more than 5 mmHg, large channels are opened in the mucosal membrane at the villous tips.[212] The width of the intercellular channels between mucosal epithelium, which is 8 to 10 A under normal conditions, increases to an extent sufficient to allow molecules greater than 37 A radius (albumin) to enter the lumen and the hydraulic conductance of the mucosal membrane increases. Ultrastructurally, the changes in the mucosal membrane vary from widening of the mucosal intercellular space during plasma volume expansion to villous tip erosion. The increased mucosal hydraulic conductance allows for filtration secretion to proceed at rates exceeding $1.0\ ml \cdot min^{-1} \cdot 100$ g tissue^{-1} at a portal pressure of 30 mmHg. If the mucosal fluid pressure remains at 5 mmHg, the mucosal hydraulic conductance would be ~$0.20\ ml \cdot min^{-1} \cdot mmHg^{-1} \cdot 100\ g^{-1}$, a value that is 2000 times greater than that reported for normal mucosa.[213] With filtration secretion, the composition of the secreted fluid closely resembles that of lymph, suggesting that the process represents an exudation of interstitial fluid into the bowel lumen.

Active, solute-coupled fluid secretion is characterized by an intact mucosal barrier with either chloride or NaCl secretion providing the driving force for interstitium-to-lumen fluid movement. Unlike filtration secretion, the active secretions are devoid of plasma proteins, supporting the contention that the mucosal membrane is intact. As the protein-free fluid is secreted into the lumen, the mucosal interstitium becomes dehydrated, causing tissue oncotic pressure to increase and interstitial fluid pressure to fall. Assuming a normal (low) interstitial compliance, a 5% reduction in interstitial volume due to active secretion should produce a greater than 2.0 mmHg reduction in Pt and a greater than 0.5 mmHg increase in πt. The reduction in Pt leads to a concomitant reduction in lymph flow.[204,210,214] The changes in interstitial forces tend to enhance capillary filtration, which, in turn, serves to provide the fluid necessary for the active pump. This view of the changes associated with active secretion is supported by observations that lacteal pressure[204] and total lymph flow[210,215] decrease or fall to zero during intestinal secretion induced by cholera toxin, vasoactive intestinal polypeptide, or theophylline. Most secretagogues are vasodilators in the splanchnic circulation; thus, their secretions are generally associated with increases in Pc (1–2 mmHg) and Kfc (25%–50%).[216] The enhanced net filtration pressure, coupled to the elevated Kfc, should further increase capillary filtration rate. Therefore, the fluid requirements of the active secretory process are met by alterations in capillary and interstitial forces and increased capillary exchange capacity.

Active, solute-coupled fluid absorption initiates a series of physical changes in the mucosal interstitium, which, ultimately, facilitates the removal of absorbed fluid by way of blood and lymph capillaries. Fluid absorption in the small intestine is associated with an increase in mucosal interstitial volume.[187,215,217] There is a positive linear correlation between interstitial volume and net fluid absorption rate such that a doubling of interstitial volume is predicted at absorption rates greater than 1.8 ml·min^{-1}·100 g^{-1}. Several physiologic consequences of the interstitial volume expansion occur during net fluid absorption. These include an increased hydraulic conductance of the interstitial matrix, increased interstitial fluid pressure, and reduction in interstitial oncotic pressure.[187,188] Because mucopolysaccharides tend to immobilize interstitial fluid, the hydraulic conductance of the interstitium is quite low. However, interstitial hydraulic conductivity increases to approximately 100 times the nonabsorptive value at an absorption rate of 1.0 ml·min^{-1}·100 g^{-1}, and it increases 1000 fold at a rate of 2.0 ml·min^{-1}·100 g^{-1}. Such profound changes in interstitial conductivity should allow small hydrostatic pressure gradients within the mucosal interstitium to move large amounts of fluid between epithelia and microvessels (blood and lymph).

The most important physiologic consequences of the interstitial volume expansion associated with fluid absorption are increased interstitial fluid pressure and decreased interstitial oncotic pressure. These changes enhance the removal of absorbed fluid from the lamina propria by (1) opposing further capillary filtration and converting filtering capillaries to absorbing capillaries, and (2) providing an increased hydrostatic pressure gradient for lymphatic filling. Interstitial hydrostatic pressure increases by as much as 5 mmHg at high absorption rates, while interstitial oncotic pressure is reduced by 2 to 7 mmHg.[218] The magnitude of the changes in Pt and πt depends on net fluid absorption rate (Fig 22-14).[219] At absorption rates less than 0.30 ml·min^{-1}·100 g^{-1}, interstitial oncotic pressure is minimally reduced, while Pt increases significantly. However, at higher absorption rates πt decreases by as much as 6 to 7 mmHg.

The rise in interstitial fluid pressure produced by net fluid absorption should lead to an increased rate of intestinal lymph formation. During absorption, lymph flow can increase by as much as 20 times control.[209,220] The magnitude of the rise in lymph flow appears to be influenced by the rate of fluid absorption. The dependence of lymph flow on absorption rate presumably results from the fact that interstitial volume and, consequently, interstitial fluid pressure are directly related to absorption rate. The relative fraction of absorbed fluid that is removed from the mucosal interstitium by the lymphatics and capillaries is also influenced by net fluid absorption rate. Only at low absorption rates does the

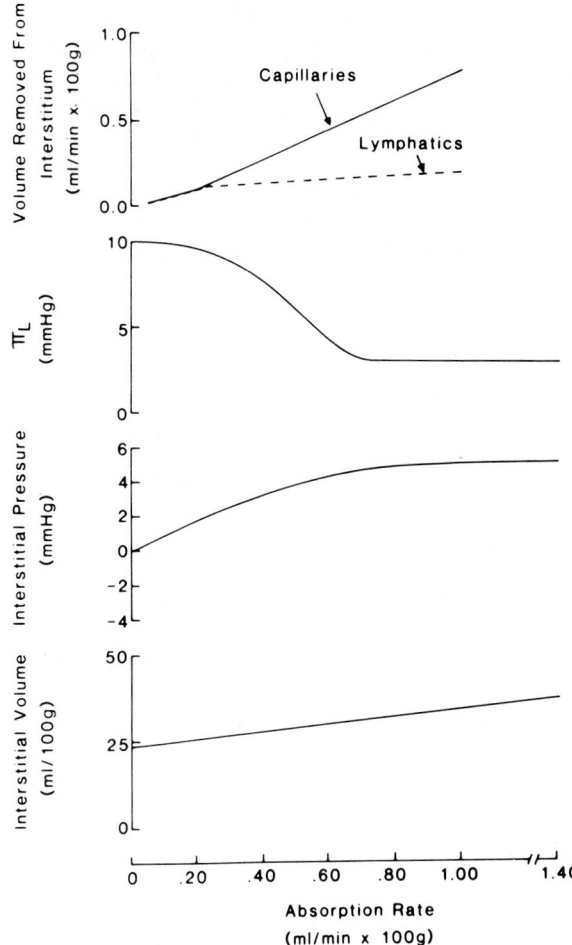

FIGURE 22–14. Steady-state relationships between intestinal fluid absorption rate, interstitial volume, interstitial fluid pressure, lymph oncotic pressure, and the rate of removal of absorbed fluid by intestinal capillaries and lymphatics. (From Kvietys PR, Granger DN. Role of microcirculation in intestinal transmucosal fluid transport. In: Koo A, Lam SK, Smaje LH, eds. Microcirculation of the alimentary tract. Singapore: World Scientific, 1983:247.)

lymphatic contribution exceed 50%. At absorption rates greater than 0.20 ml·min^{-1}·100 g^{-1}, the capillaries are the major route for removal of absorbed fluid from the interstitium, accounting for up to 85% of the total volume removed.[209]

Although the changes in interstitial forces induced by interstitial volume expansion is the primary event leading to vascular removal of absorbed fluid, alterations in capillary pressure, surface area, and permeability appear to modify this response. Capillary pressure generally increases during net fluid absorption because of the well-documented intestinal hyperemia elicited by food ingestion or placement of nutrients into the bowel lumen. Glucose absorption, which elicits a relatively small hyperemia (10%–15%), is associated with a ~1.0-mmHg increase in Pc, while lipid absorption doubles blood flow and produces a 2.5-mmHg increase in Pc. The larger increment in Pc produced by micellar lipid may account for the diminished fluid absorptive capacity during lipid absorption.[203]

Several studies demonstrate an effect of nutrient absorption on intestinal capillary filtration coefficient.[184,203,221] Kfc increases by 100% during glucose absorption, an effect that has been attributed to capillary recruitment. However, lipid absorption produces a significantly greater rise in Kfc (200%), which is caused by both an increase in microvascular permeability and capillary recruitment.[222] The fact that hydraulic conductance increases during absorption is of physiologic importance because Kfc determines the imbalance in transcapillary forces required to move a given volume of absorbed fluid from interstitium to blood.

Although intestinal vascular permeability is not altered during absorption of glucose or electrolytes, fat absorption is associated with a pronounced reduction in the osmotic reflection coefficient (0.92–0.70).[195] The reduction in the reflection coefficient significantly lowers the effective absorptive force generated by the transcapillary oncotic pressure gradient during fat absorption. The reduction in net capillary absorptive force is partially compensated by the large increase in Kfc.[222]

In the nonabsorptive state, there is a small (0.30 mmHg) imbalance of forces across the capillary wall that favors net fluid filtration into the interstitium (Fig 22-15).[203] To maintain normal interstitial volume, the rate of capillary filtration is balanced by an equal outflow of fluid by way of the lymphatics. Perfusion of the intestinal lumen with a glucose–electrolyte solution leads to net transmucosal fluid absorption and a rise in interstitial volume (Fig 22-16).[203] Interstitial volume expansion produces an increase in interstitial hydrostatic pressure (2.0 mmHg) and a reduction in interstitial oncotic pressure (1.8 mmHg). Associated with the changes in interstitial forces are an increase in capillary pressure (1.1 mmHg) and a doubling of capillary hydraulic conductance. Because vascular permeability is not altered by glucose absorption, the capillary reflection coefficient remains the same. The absorption-induced changes in capillary and interstitial forces modify the balance of pressures across intestinal capillaries to produce a net absorptive force of 2.3 mmHg. This force, coupled to the elevated capillary hydraulic conductance, drives 82% of the ab-

sorbed fluid into the capillaries. Intestinal lymph flow also increases during glucose absorption because of increased lymphatic filling caused by the rise in interstitial hydrostatic pressure. The enhanced lymph flow removes the remaining 18% of absorbed fluid from the mucosal interstitium.

Lipid absorption, compared with glucose absorption, is associated with greater increments in lymph flow, capillary filtration coefficient, capillary pressure, and interstitial fluid pressure, yet a smaller reduction in the transcapillary oncotic pressure gradient,[203,222] even though the rate of fluid entry into the mucosal interstitium (net fluid absorption rate) is comparable for the two nutrients. The different responses of capillary and interstitial forces to glucose and lipid absorption may be explained by the fact that lipid absorption produces a greater hyperemic response and is associated with an increase in microvascular permeability. A major consequence of the response to lipid absorption is that a significantly greater portion of the absorbed fluid leaves the mucosal interstitium by way of the lymphatics. Enhanced formation of lymph during lipid absorption is physiologically advantageous because it allows for greater convective transport of chylomicrons from the mucosal interstitium to the systemic circulation.[223]

PHYSIOLOGY AND BIOCHEMISTRY OF ISCHEMIA

General Considerations

Ischemic damage to the intestine occurs when splanchnic blood flow falls to a level at which delivery of oxygen and other nutrients

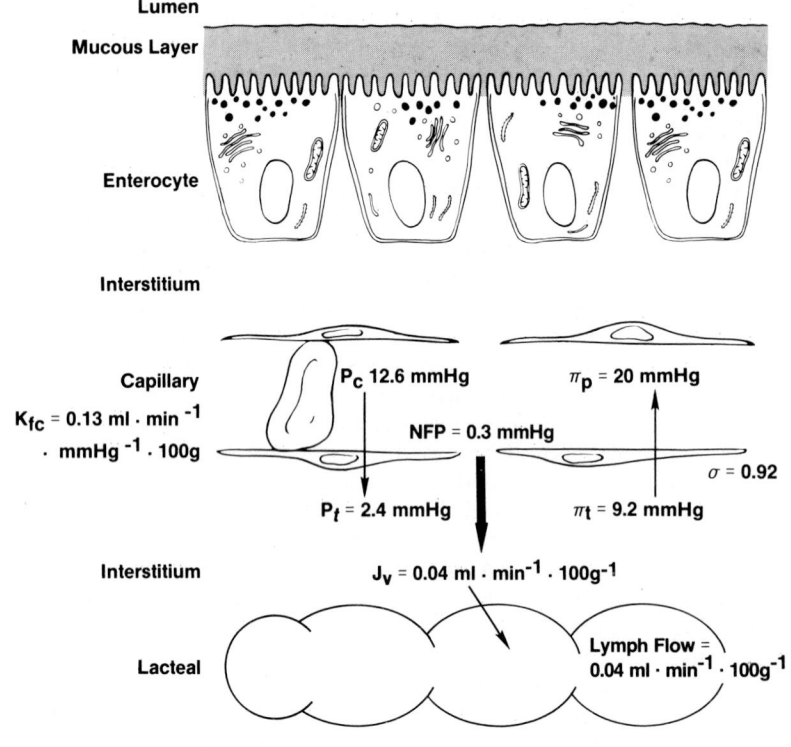

FIGURE 22–15. Starling forces and capillary membrane parameters in the small intestine under control (nontransporting) conditions. J_v, net capillary filtration rate; K_{fc}, capillary filtration coefficient; P_c, capillary pressure, P_t, interstitial fluid pressure; σ, capillary reflection coefficient; π_p, plasma oncotic pressure, π_t, interstitial oncotic pressure. (Adapted from Granger DN, Perry MA, Kvietys PR, Taylor AE. Capillary and interstitial forces during fluid absorption in the cat small intestine. Gastroenterology 1984;86:262.)

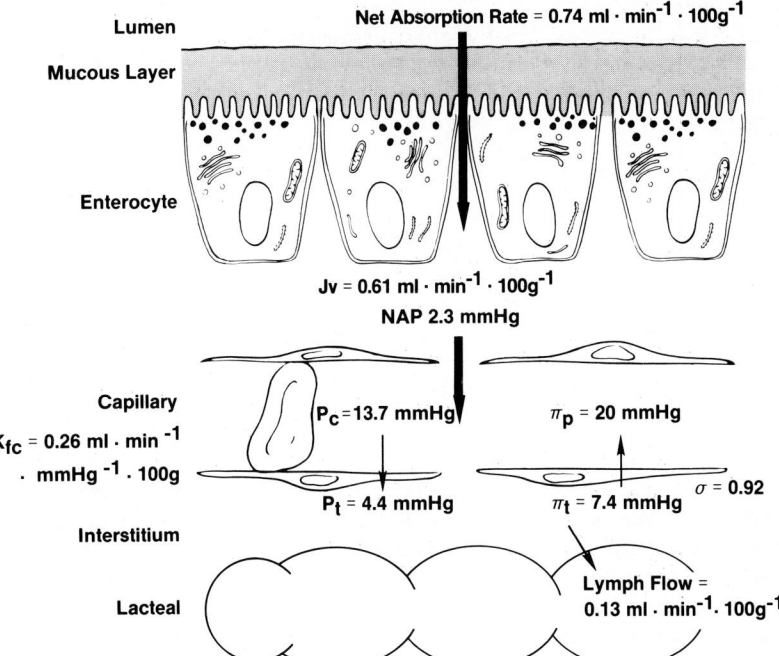

FIGURE 22–16. Effects of net fluid absorption on Starling forces and capillary membrane parameters in the small intestine. NAP, net capillary absorptive pressure; J_v, net capillary filtration rate; K_{fc}, capillary filtration coefficient; P_c, capillary pressure, P_t, interstitial fluid pressure; σ, capillary reflection coefficient; π_p, plasma oncotic pressure, π_t, interstitial oncotic pressure. (Adapted from Granger DN, Perry MA, Kvietys PR, Taylor AE. Capillary and interstitial forces during fluid absorption in the cat small intestine. Gastroenterology 1984;86:262.)

is insufficient to maintain oxidative metabolism and, hence, cell integrity. Reduced blood flow to the gastrointestinal tract may occur during generalized "nonocclusive" ischemia (circulatory shock, congestive heart failure [especially those treated with cardiac glycosides]), and in occlusive disorders (emboli, atherosclerosis, thrombosis) that primarily involve the mesenteric circulation. The mortality of acute mesenteric ischemia in adults has been reported at 70% to 90%,[224] due primarily to the difficulty in early diagnosis before bowel infarction occurs. Surgical intervention (embolectomy, intestinal resection)[225] and local intraarterial infusion of vasodilators (e.g., papaverine)[226] are used to treat acute mesenteric ischemia, but the mortality of this disease continues to be significant. Experimental nonocclusive mesenteric ischemia in dogs has been treated successfully with intravenously administered selective mesenteric vasodilators (urotensin I, sauvagine, and corticotropin-releasing factor),[227] thus potentially obviating the risk of an indwelling angiographic catheter, but the use of these drugs in humans remains to be investigated.

Mesenteric ischemia also appears to play a role in necrotizing enterocolitis (NEC), a disease that predominately affects the ileum and colon of premature infants, averages 40% mortality, and can result in short bowel syndrome and intestinal strictures. The pathogenesis of NEC is unknown, but enteral alimentation, infectious agents/immune factors, and mesenteric ischemia/tissue hypoxia have been invoked frequently as primary initiators of the disease.[228,229]

Alterations of Intestinal Morphology With Ischemia

The response of the intestine to decreased blood flow can range from no damage to transmural necrosis,[230] and a gradient of sen-

sitivity to ischemic injury has been demonstrated from the villus tips to the muscularis.[230–232] Mesenteric ischemia is associated with characteristic mucosal lesions, which progress from subepithelial edema within 30 minutes after total vascular occlusion, to loss of epithelial cells along the villus after 1 hour of total occlusion, to total loss of villi after 2 hours of occlusion.[230,231] Within 30 to 60 minutes of total mesenteric artery occlusion, changes indicative of cellular failure appear (mitochondrial vacuolization and decreased oxygen uptake, loss of ATP, and release of lysosomal enzymes).[231]

Changes in Vascular and Mucosal Permeability With Ischemia

Increases in the capillary filtration coefficient and microvascular permeability in the small intestine have been observed after ischemia.[205] The osmotic reflection coefficient of ileal capillaries to plasma proteins decreases after 1 hour of ischemia and reperfusion, indicative of increased vascular permeability. Furthermore, the increase in permeability is derived from an increased size of large (200 Å) pores, while the small pore (50 Å) population is unaffected. Thus, in the intestine, the increase in capillary filtration coefficient observed after ischemia and reperfusion is not solely a result of increased capillary surface area.

Increases in mucosal permeability induced by ischemia and reperfusion have been estimated based on the clearance of solutes ranging from 700 to 70,000 Daltons.[71,233] The ischemia–reperfusion-induced increases in mucosal permeability depend on both the duration and severity of the ischemic insult (Fig 22-17).[234] Mucosal permeability increases significantly after 1 to 2 hours of mesenteric artery occlusion in adult animals. In developing intestine, there is a similar correlation between the duration of isch-

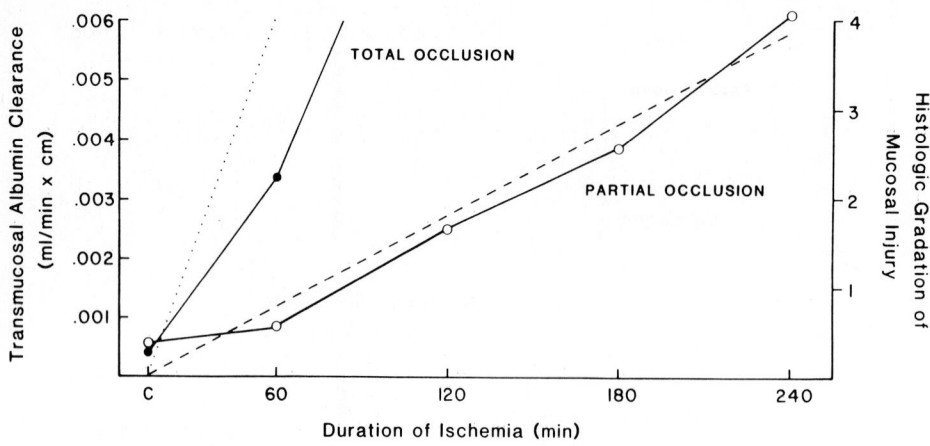

FIGURE 22–17. Comparison of quantitative morphologic data (*dotted* and *broken lines*) of Chiu and coworkers[230] and mucosal albumin clearance results (*solid lines*) from Parks and coworkers.[234] (From Parks DA, Grogaard B, Granger DN. Comparison of partial and complete arterial occlusion models for studying intestinal ischemia. Surgery 1982;92:896.)

emia and the magnitude of the increase in clearance of [51]chromium EDTA (358 Daltons) during reperfusion.[235] The extent of reperfusion-induced injury in the absence of luminal nutrients is similar among age groups of young swine (from 1 day to 1 month old), but perfusion of the ileal lumen with cow milk-based formula causes a significantly larger increase in reperfusion-induced injury in 1 day olds compared to all older age groups (Fig 22-18).[235]

Blood Flow, Oxygenation, and Ischemic Injury

Ischemic injury to the intestine occurs when blood flow is reduced to a level at which delivery of oxygen and other nutrients to the tissue is compromised. Although the correlation of tissue pO₂, mucosal blood flow, and mucosal injury has not been investigated, reduction of blood flow to levels that do not affect oxygen uptake is not associated with any evidence of mucosal damage in adult

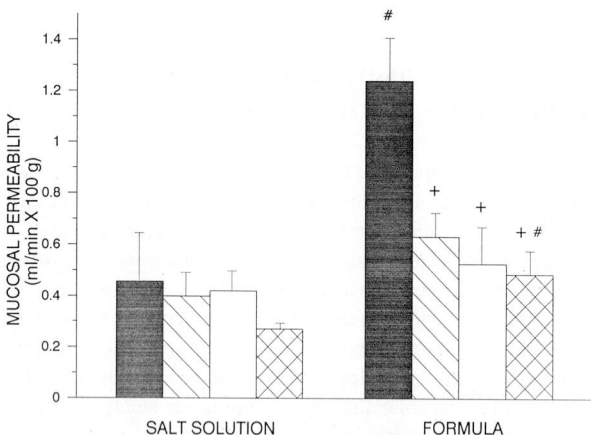

FIGURE 22–18. Comparison of ^{51}Cr-labeled EDTA clearance among age groups of developing piglets during reperfusion after 60 minutes of total intestinal ischemia in ileal loops perfused with a balanced salt solution versus predigested cow milk–based formula. (1 day old = *solid*, 3 day old = *hatched*, 2 wk old = *empty*, and 1 mo old = *cross-hatched bars*). + indicates *p* < 0.05 versus 1-day-old values and # shows *p* < 0.05 versus salt solution within an age group. (From Crissinger KD, Granger DN. Mucosal injury induced by ischemia and reperfusion in the piglet intestine: Influences of age and feeding. Gastroenterology 1989;97:920.)

animals.[73] Furthermore, substantial increases in mucosal albumin clearance are not seen until the blood flow falls to levels where oxygen consumption is reduced by approximately 50% (Fig 22-19).[73] In the neonatal intestine, which has a limited capacity to maintain oxygen uptake during reductions in perfusion pressure,[67] arterial hypoxia,[236] hemorrhage,[65] and the combined stresses of hypoxemia and feeding,[68] one might predict that the neonatal intestine may be more vulnerable to mucosal injury induced by ischemic cardiovascular stress than is the intestine of older animals.

The importance of collateral blood flow in prevention of intestinal ischemia is well recognized in humans,[237–239] and adult animals.[56,240,241] Intestinal collateral blood flow may occur by way of anastomotic connections at several levels of vessel branching, including the main arterial trunks (celiac, superior, and inferior mesenteric arteries),[56,237] extramural vessels (arterial arcades, marginal arteries),[241,242] and intramural vascular plexus located within the intestinal wall itself.[237,242] Quantitative studies in adult animals have demonstrated that collateral channels among the major arterial trunks and between adjacent bowel segments both play a role in prevention of intestinal ischemia. In the adult cat, perfusion through collateral vessels after occlusion of the SMA maintains flow to the small intestine and proximal colon to within 30% to 65% of preocclusion flow.[56] However, the efficiency of collateral perfusion by way of the celiac and inferior mesenteric arteries is substantially lower in dogs after SMA occlusion.[240] In adjacent segments of canine small bowel, collateral vessels maintain blood flow in one segment at approximately 55% of its control level when the artery to that segment is totally occluded. The percentage of collateral flow attributed to extramural vessels is 67%; that attributed to intramural vessels is 33%.[241] In developing piglet intestine, after occlusion of a distal branch of the SMA, total wall and mucosal/submucosal blood flow falls by 70% in 1-day-old animals, compared with a 25% fall in 1 month olds.[66] This finding suggests that newborn intestine may be at greater risk from ischemic injury than adult intestine due to poorly developed and inefficient collateral blood vessels.

Possible Mechanisms of Injury/Villous Necrosis

Ischemic injury in the intestine appears to be either primarily or secondarily related to the effects of tissue hypoxia. In some species,

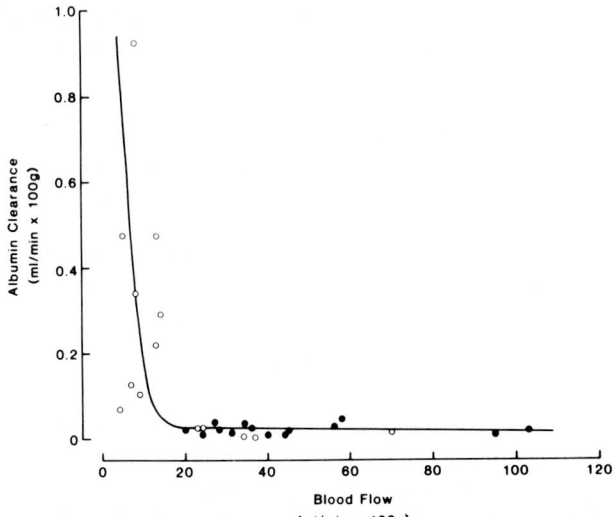

FIGURE 22-19. Relationship between blood flow (control period = *closed circles*; ischemic period = *open circles*) and mucosal albumin clearance during reperfusion of canine jejunum (*left panel*). The *right panel* shows the relationship between intestinal oxygen consumption during control (*single closed circle with error bar*) and ischemia and mucosal albumin clearance during reperfusion of canine jejunum. Substantial increases in albumin clearance were not seen unless blood flow was reduced below 20 ml·min^{-1}·100 g^{-1} or oxygen consumption was reduced to approximately half the control values. (From Bulkley GB, Kvietys PR, Parks DA, et al. Relationship of blood flow and oxygen consumption to ischemic injury in the canine small intestine. Gastroenterology 1985;89:852.)

the hypoxic stress induced by ischemia is exacerbated by the presence of a countercurrent exchange mechanism.[7] A role for hypoxia is supported by the observation that mucosal injury is markedly attenuated by intraluminal perfusion with oxygenated saline during ischemia induced by hypotension,[243] while perfusion with nitrogenated saline does not attenuate injury. Possible mechanisms of mucosal injury induced by tissue hypoxia include (1) depletion of high-energy phosphates necessary to produce protective substances, such as mucus, leading to increased susceptibility to the action of intraluminal proteases;[244] (2) accumulation of histamine, leading to increased microvascular permeability;[245] (3) production of metabolic acidosis, leading to release of lysosomal enzymes and cellular digestion;[246] (4) conversion of xanthine dehydrogenase to xanthine oxidase, an enzyme that can produce cytotoxic oxygen-derived free radicals during reoxygenation;[247] and (5) attraction of circulating granulocytes into the mucosa or activation of resident leukocytes within the mucosa with release of neutrophilic proteases and oxidants to initiate or propagate mucosal injury.[248]

It has been demonstrated that changes in the intestinal mucosa induced by circulatory shock lead to an increased vulnerability to the digestive action of trypsin and chymotrypsin. Inhibition of pancreatic proteases by aprotinin[249] or previous ligation of the pancreatic ducts[250] significantly attenuates ischemic mucosal injury. In addition, an intraluminal injection of trypsin exacerbates mucosal injury.[249] The digestive action is caused by enzymes already present along the intestinal wall before shock, because removal of the pancreas has no effect if the animal is subjected to shock immediately after pancreatectomy.[251] Inhibition of pancreatic elastase and bile salts, both of which contribute to the loss of protective brush border glycoproteins,[252,253] decreases mucosal injury. It has been proposed that if impairment of mesenteric blood flow prevents the steady regeneration of these brush border glycoproteins, the mucosa becomes accessible to the digestive action of the pancreatic endopeptidases present along the intestinal wall and lumen.[244] It

is generally believed, however, that pancreatic proteases are not the primary mediators of ischemic injury in the small bowel.

A possible role for histamine in the pathogenesis of mucosal injury during intestinal ischemia arises from its known capability to increase microvascular permeability to macromolecules[245,254] and the finding that the concentration of histamine in plasma is elevated after reperfusion of ischemic intestine.[255] Furthermore, inhibition of diamine oxidase, a histamine-catabolizing enzyme present in large quantities in the superficial epithelial cells of the intestinal mucosa, reduces survival in dogs[256] and rabbits[257] subjected to intestinal ischemia. It appears unlikely, however, that histamine is a mediator of ischemic injury to the small intestine, based on the failure of H$_1$- and H$_2$-receptor antagonists to attenuate the increased vascular permeability resulting from ischemia and reperfusion of the intestine.[200] Histamine is also a potent vasodilator, and this effect should decrease, rather than increase, mucosal injury resulting from mesenteric ischemia.[172]

Because most lysosomal enzymes have an acid pH optimum, it has been postulated that ischemia-induced metabolic acidosis may stimulate the release of hydrolytic enzymes from lysosomes. Elevated plasma levels of lysosomal enzymes have been reported in association with acute mesenteric ischemia.[246] Although it has also been postulated that massive doses of corticosteroids in shock attenuates the hypoxia-induced lability of lysosomal membranes,[246] there are no well-controlled studies demonstrating a beneficial effect of corticosteroid treatment in shock. The reperfusion-induced increase in microvascular permeability after mesenteric ischemia is also not attenuated by pretreatment with methylprednisolone.[200]

A role for reactive oxygen metabolites in the pathogenesis of injury associated with reperfusion of the ischemic bowel has received considerable attention during the last 10 years. Reactive oxygen metabolites play an important role in normal cellular metabolism, most notably as intermediates in mitochondrial and microsomal electron-transport systems.[258] Greater than 90% of the molecular oxygen consumed by most cells is reduced by the mitochondrial electron transport chain to form water, with the remaining oxygen metabolized to reactive oxygen species. Under normal conditions, tissues are protected from these oxygen-derived free radicals by the action of certain antioxidant enzymes and scavengers.

In adult animals, the digestive system is particularly well-endowed with the enzymatic machinery capable of generating significant quantities of reactive oxygen metabolites. For example, the intestine and liver are the richest sources of xanthine oxidase,[259] an enzyme that catalyzes the production of both superoxide and hydrogen peroxide. Xanthine oxidase activity in the small intestine is primarily located within the mucosa, with a gradient of activity from villous tip to base.[260] In addition, the intestine contains a large resident population of phagocytic cells (neutrophils, eosinophils, macrophages), which, when activated, produce considerable quantities of superoxide, hydrogen peroxide, and hypochlorous acid.[261] Oxidants generated by either xanthine oxidase or activated phagocytes can injure cells by a variety of mechanisms. These include lipid peroxidation, degradation of the extracellular matrix, protein and carbohydrate decomposition, and DNA strand breakage.[258] Cellular enzymatic defense mechanisms against these oxidants include superoxide dismutase, which dismutates the superoxide anion to hydrogen peroxide and oxygen; and catalase and glutathione peroxidase, which detoxify hydrogen peroxide.[262] Another important oxidant defense is reduced glutathione, which serves both as a cosubstrate for the glutathione peroxidase–catalyzed decomposition of hydrogen peroxide and as a free radical scavenger.[258]

A large amount of experimental data support the hypothesis that reactive oxygen metabolites mediate the microvascular and mucosal permeability changes after reperfusion of the ischemic intestine and stomach in adult animals.[248,263–267] Increased intestinal vascular permeability produced by ischemia–reperfusion injury is not attenuated by antihistamines, indomethacin, or methylprednisolone, arguing against a role for histamine, prostaglandins, and lysosomal enzymes in this injury.[200] On the other hand, superoxide dismutase (scavenges superoxide anions), catalase (detoxifies hydrogen peroxide), and dimethylsulfoxide (scavenges hydroxyl radicals and decomposes hypochlorous acid) attenuate the vascular permeability changes observed after reperfusion of the ischemic intestine.[263]

A role for xanthine oxidase in the increased vascular permeability and morphologic changes induced by reperfusion has been proposed based on the following observations: (1) attenuation of injury by pretreatment with allopurinol or pterin aldehyde, inhibitors of xanthine oxidase;[264,268,269] (2) increased vascular and mucosal permeability during intraarterial infusion of hypoxanthine/xanthine oxidase, a superoxide anion generating system;[270] (3) attenuation of injury by soybean trypsin inhibitor, a substance that prevents the conversion of xanthine dehydrogenase to xanthine oxidase;[265] and (4) attenuation of reperfusion injury by administration of a tungsten-supplemented, molybdenum-deficient diet, which inactivates xanthine oxidase.[271] In the intestine of developing piglets, however, the total absence of xanthine dehydrogenase/oxidase precludes its role in intestinal ischemia–reperfusion injury.[272]

Evidence to support a role for granulocyte-mediated injury after ischemia and reperfusion is also accumulating. Ischemia may lead to neutrophil activation, release/production of neutrophilic oxidants (superoxide, hydrogen peroxide, hypochlorous acid, N-chloramines) and proteases, and subsequent tissue injury[261,273–275](Fig 22-20). A 5- to 7-fold increase in myeloperoxidase activity (an index of granulocyte number) occurs during ischemia, while reperfusion induces an 18-fold increase in myeloperoxidase activity in feline intestine.[266] Both neutrophil depletion and prevention of neutrophil adherence significantly attenuate the increased intestinal microvascular permeability induced by ischemia and reperfusion in cat intestine,[248] suggesting that neutrophils,

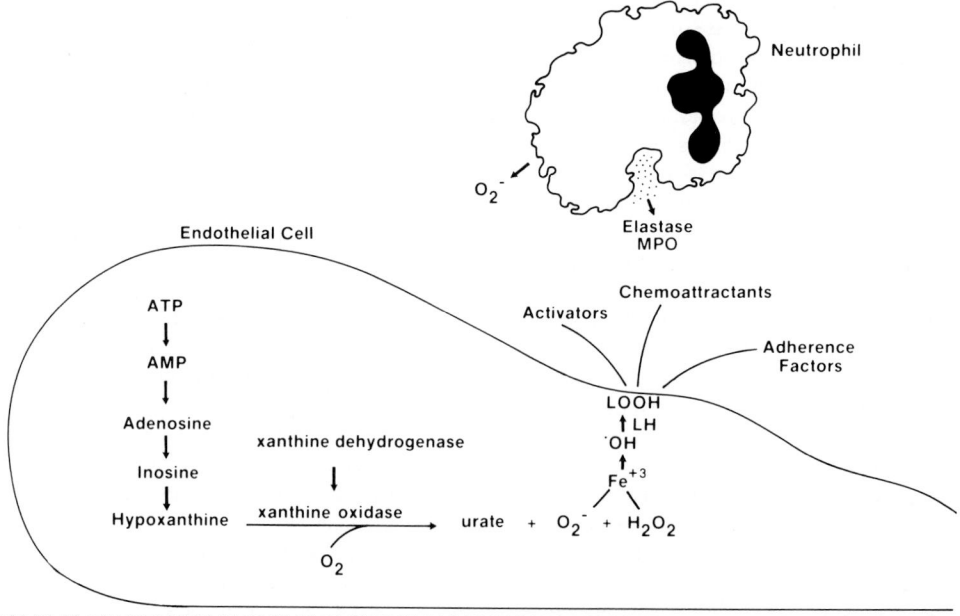

FIGURE 22-20. Proposed interaction between xanthine oxidase–derived oxidants, neutrophil infiltration, and microvascular injury following reperfusion of the ishemic intestine. (From Zimmerman BJ, Grisham MB, Granger DN. Mechanisms of oxidant-mediated microvascular injury following reperfusion of the ischemic intestine. In: Simic MG, Taylor KA, Ward JF, Von Sonntag C, ed. Oxygen radicals in biology and medicine.

which migrate into the mucosa, mediate the injury produced by reperfusion of the ischemic bowel.

It has also been proposed that xanthine oxidase-derived oxidants may serve as chemoattractants for granulocytes in postischemic adult intestine. Allopurinol (an inhibitor of xanthine oxidase),[261] superoxide dismutase (a superoxide scavenger and inhibitor of neutrophil adherence),[261] catalase (a scavenger of hydrogen peroxide),[276] deferoxamine (an iron-chelator),[276] dimethylthiourea (a hydroxyl-radical scavenger),[276] and MoAb IB$_4$ (a monoclonal antibody inhibitor of neutrophil adherence)(unpublished observations) all inhibit reperfusion-induced granulocyte accumulation into the small intestine.

Newborn swine intestine contains significantly fewer resident granulocytes than that of older animals, a fact that does not support the postulation that newborn piglet intestine is more vulnerable to oxidant-induced injury.[272] This lower number of resident granulocytes in the mucosa does not, however, preclude the possibility of a role for injury induced by resident granulocytes and those recruited into the tissue during ischemic or other stresses.

Finally, platelet activating factor (PAF) has recently received considerable attention as a possible mediator of injury induced by ischemia and reperfusion as well as in inflammatory lesions of the bowel.[277,278] PAF is an ether phospholipid that can be synthesized upon immunologic or nonimmunologic stimulations in a variety of cell types, such as basophils, neutrophils, eosinophils, macrophages, monocytes, platelets, and vascular endothelial cells.[279-282] Its multiple effects may contribute to mucosal injury during ischemia. It is a potent activator of vascular smooth muscle cells,[283] endothelial cells,[284-286] and inflammatory cells[287] in vitro. Neutrophils exposed to PAF develop chemotaxis, generate superoxide radicals, increase their turnover of arachidonic acid, and undergo aggregation and degranulation.[288-290] In vivo, PAF induces localized accumulation of leukocytes.[291] PAF also dramatically increases vascular permeability and causes extravasation of plasma into the tissue.[292-294] However, because of these multiple effects it is very difficult to determine PAF's actual mechanism of action in producing mucosal injury after ischemia.

PAF has been postulated to play a role in experimental ischemic enterocolitis,[277] but because it induces significant hypotension in all species in which it has been tested, the effect of PAF in some studies may be simply related to this hypotension-induced mesenteric ischemia. However, PAF levels do increase severalfold in dog small intestine during ischemia and reperfusion.[295] PAF antagonists protect the small intestine against ischemia–reperfusion injury,[296] and they have recently been shown to attenuate adherence of leukocytes to mesenteric venular endothelium induced by ischemia and reperfusion in the intestine.[297]

The reader is directed to Chapter 1, The Enteric Nervous System and its Extrinsic Connections; Chapter 2, Gastrointestinal Hormones; Chapter 3, The Brain-Gut Axis; Chapter 4, Smooth Muscle of the Gut; Chapter 7, Esophageal Motor Function; Chapter 8, The Physiology of Gastric Motility and Gastric Emptying; Chapter 9, Motility of the Small Intestine; Chapter 10, The Motor Function of the Colon; Chapter 11, Motility of the Biliary Tree; Chapter 12, Salivary Secretion; Chapter 13, Gastric Secretion; Chapter 14, Secretion and Absorption: Small Intestine and Colon; Chapter 15, Pancreatic Secretion; Chapter 16, Bile Secretion; Chapter 108, Vascular Ectasias, Tumors, and Malformations; Chapter 109, Vascular Insufficiency; and Chapter 122, Angiography.

REFERENCES

1. Warwick R, Williams PL, eds. Gray's anatomy, ed 36. Philadelphia: WB Saunders, 1980:1338.
2. Casley-Smith JR, Gannon BJ. Intestinal microcirculation: Spatial organization and fine structure. In: Shepherd AP, Granger DN, eds. Physiology of the intestinal circulation. New York: Raven Press, 1984:9.
3. Wheaton LG, Sarr MG, Schlossberg L, Bulkley GB. Gross anatomy of the splanchnic vasculature. In: Granger DN, Bulkley GB, eds. Measurement of blood flow: Applications to the splanchnic circulation. Baltimore: Williams & Wilkins, 1981:9.
4. Gannon B, Browning J, O'Brien P, Rogers P. Mucosal microvascular architecture of the fundus and body of human stomach. Gastroenterology 1984;86:866.
5. Gannon BJ. The co-existence of fountain and tuft patterns of blood supply in individual intestinal villi of rabbit and man: Resolution of an old controversy, Bibl Anat 1981;20:130.
6. Frasher WG Jr, Wayland H. Repeating modular organization of the microcirculation of cat mesentery. Microvasc Res 1972;4:62.
7. Jodal M, Lundgren O. Countercurrent mechanisms in the mammalian gastrointestinal tract. Gastroenterology 1986;91:225.
8. Kvietys PR, Wilborn WH, Granger DN. Effects of net transmucosal volume flux on lymph flow in the canine colon. Structural–functional relationship, Gastroenterology 1981;81:1080.
9. Listrom MB, Fenoglio-Preiser CM. Lymphatic distribution of the stomach in normal, inflammatory, hyperplastic, and neoplastic tissue. Gastroenterology 1987;93:506.
10. Granger DN, Kvietys PR, Perry MA, Barrowman JA. The microcirculation and intestinal transport. In: Johnson LR, ed. Physiology of the gastrointestinal tract, ed 2. New York: Raven Press, 1987: 1671.
11. Fenoglio CM, Kaye GI, Lane N. Distribution of human colonic lymphatics in normal, hyperplastic, and adenomatous tissue. Gastroenterology 1973;64:51.
12. Jacobson ED. Criteria for an ideal method of measuring blood flow to a splanchnic organ. In: Granger DN, Bulkley GB, eds. Measurement of blood flow: Applications to the splanchnic circulation. Baltimore: Williams & Wilkins, 1981:5.
13. Larsen KR, Moody FG. Selection of appropriate methodology for the measurement of blood flow in the gut. In: Granger DN, Bulkley GB, eds. Measurement of blood flow: Applications to the splanchnic circulation. Baltimore: Williams & Wilkins, 1981:514.
14. Charbon GA, Van Der Mark F. Use of electromagnetic flowmeters for the study of splanchnic blood flow. In: Granger DN, Bulkley GB, eds. Measurement of blood flow: Applications to the splanchnic circulation. Baltimore: Williams & Wilkins, 1981:125.
15. Haywood JR, Shaffer RA, Fastenow C, et al. Regional blood flow measurement with pulsed Doppler flowmeter in conscious rat. Am J Physiol 1981;241:H273.
16. Van Orden DE, Farley DB, Fastenow C, Brody MJ. A technique for monitoring blood flow changes with miniaturized Doppler flow probes. Am J Physiol 1984;247:H1005.
17. Dregelid E, Haukaas S, Amundsen S, et al. Microsphere method in measurement of blood flow to wall layers of small intestine. Am J Physiol 1986;250:G670.
18. Maxwell LC, Shepherd AP, McMahan CA. Microsphere passage through intestinal circulation: Via shunts or capillaries? Am J Physiol 1985;248:H217.
19. Maxwell LC, Shepherd AP, Riedel GL. Vasodilation or altered perfusion pressure moves 15-μm spheres trapped in the gut wall. Am J Physiol 1982;243:H123.
20. Maxwell LC, Shepherd AP, Riedel GL, Morris MD. Effect of microsphere size on apparent intramural distribution of intestinal blood flow. Am J Physiol 1981;241:H408.
21. Kauffman GL, Grossman MI. Use of aminopyrine clearance as a measure of gastric mucosal blood flow. In: Granger DN, Bulkley GB, eds. Measurement of blood flow: Applications to the splanchnic circulation. Baltimore: Williams & Wilkins, 1981:203.
22. Holm-Rutili L, Berglindh T. Pentagastrin and gastric mucosal blood flow. Am J Physiol 1986;250:G575.
23. Sack J, Spenney JG. Aminopyrine accumulation by mammalian gastric glands: An analysis of the technique. Am J Physiol 1982;243: G313.
24. Lundgren O. Use of inert gas washout for studying blood flow and

flow distribution in the intestine. In: Granger DN, Bulkley GB, eds. Measurement of blood flow: Applications to the splanchnic circulation. Baltimore: Williams & Wilkins, 1981:227.

25. Gharagozloo F, Bulkley GB, Zuidema GD, et al. The use of intraperitoneal xenon for early diagnosis of acute mesenteric ischemia. Surgery 1984;95:404.

26. Dugas MC, Wechsler RL. Validity of iodoantipyrine clearance for measuring gastrointestinal tissue blood flow. Am J Physiol 1982;243: G155.

27. Granger DN, Kvietys PR. Recent advances in measurement of gastrointestinal blood flow. Gastroenterology 1985;88:1073.

28. Hudson D, Scremin OU, Guth PH. Measurement of regional gastroduodenal blood flow with iodo(^{14}C)antipyrine autoradiography. Am J Physiol 1985;248:G539.

29. Ashley SW, Cheung LY. Measurements of gastric mucosal blood flow by hydrogen gas clearance. Am J Physiol 1984;247:G339.

30. Gana TJ, Huhlewych R, Koo J. Focal gastric mucosal blood flow by laser-Doppler and hydrogen gas clearance: A comparative study. J Surg Res 1987;43:337.

31. Leung FW, Guth PH, Scremin OU, et al. Regional gastric mucosal blood flow measurements by hydrogen gas clearance in the anesthetized rat and rabbit. Gastroenterology 1984;87:28.

32. Murakami M, Moriga M, Miyake T, Uchino H. Contact electrode method in hydrogen gas clearance technique: A new method for determination of regional gastric mucosal blood flow in animals and humans. Gastroenterology 1982;82:457.

33. Soybel DI, Wan YL, Ashley SW, et al. Endoscopic measurements of canine colonic mucosal blood flow using hydrogen gas clearance. Gastroenterology 1987;92:1045.

34. Ahn H, Lindhagen J, Nilsson GE, et al. Assessment of blood flow in the small intestine with laser Doppler flowmetry. Scand J Gastroenterology 1986;21:863.

35. Ahn H, Lindhagen J, Lundgren O. Measurement of colonic blood flow with laser Doppler flowmetry. Scand J Gastroenterol 1986;21: 871.

36. DiResta GR, Kiel JW, Riedel GL, et al. Hybrid blood flow probe for simultaneous H_2 clearance and laser-Doppler velocimetry. Am J Physiol 1987;253:G573.

37. Kiel JW, Riedel GL, Shepherd AP. Local control of canine gastric mucosal blood flow. Gastroenterology 1987;93:1041.

38. Kvietys PR, Shepherd AP, Granger DN. Laser-Doppler, H_2 clearance, and microsphere estimates of mucosal blood flow. Am J Physiol 1985;249:G221.

39. Bohlen HG. In vivo microscopy of the intestinal microcirculation. In: Granger DN, Bulkley GB, eds. Measurement of blood flow: Applications to the splanchnic circulation. Baltimore: Williams & Wilkins, 1981:89.

40. Bohlen HG. Intestinal tissue pO$_2$ and microvascular responses during glucose exposure. Am J Physiol 1980;238:H164.

41. Forrester DW, Spence VS, Walker WF. The measurement of colonic mucosal-submucosal blood flow in man. J Physiol (Lond) 1980; 299:1.

42. Hulten L, Jodal M, Lindhagen J, Lundgren O. Colonic blood flow in the cat and man as analyzed by an inert gas washout technique. Gastroenterology 1976;70:36.

43. Hulten L, Lindhagen J, Lundgren O. Sympathetic nervous control of intramural blood flow in the feline and human intestines. Gastroenterology 1977;72:41.

44. Kvietys PR, Granger DN. Regulation of colonic blood flow. Fed Proc 1982;41:2106.

45. Kvietys PR, Miller T, Granger DN. Intrinsic control of colonic blood flow and oxygenation. Am J Physiol 1980;128:G478.

46. Granger HJ, Norris CP. Intrinsic regulation of intestinal oxygenation in the anesthetized dog. Am J Physiol 1980;238:H836.

47. Shepherd AP, Riedel GL. Optimal hematoctrit for oxygenation of canine intestine. Circ Res 1982;51:233.

48. Kiel JW, Shepherd AP. Optimal hematocrit for canine gastric oxygenation. Am J Physiol 1985;256:H472.

49. Kiel JW, Riedel GL, Shepherd AP. Effects of hemodilution on gastric and intestinal oxygenation. Am J Physiol 1989;256:H171.

50. Bulkley GB, Kvietys PR, Perry MA, Granger DN. Effects of cardiac tamponade on colonic blood flow and oxygenation. Am J Physiol 1983;244:G604.

51. Kvietys PR, Granger DN. Relation between intestinal blood flow and oxygen uptake. Am J Physiol 1982;242:G202.

52. Perry MA, Bulkley GB, Kvietys PR, Granger DN. Regulation of oxygen uptake in resting and pentagastrin-stimulated canine stomach. Am J Physiol 1982;242:G565.

53. Chou CC, Grassmick B. Motility and blood flow distribution within the wall of the gastrointestinal tract. Am J Physiol 1978;235:H34.

54. Granger DN, Richardson PDI, Taylor AE. Volumetric assessment of the capillary filtration coefficient in the cat small intestine. Pflugers Arch 1979;381:25.

55. Granger DN, Kvietys PR, Perry MA. Role of exchange vessels in the regulation of intestinal oxygenation. Am J Physiol 1982;242: G570.

56. Premen AJ, Banchs V, Womack WA, et al. Importance of collateral circulation in the vascularly occluded feline intestine. Gastroenterology 1987;92:1215.

57. Kvietys PR, Smith MS, Grisham MB, Manci EA. 5-Aminosalicylic acid protects against ischemia/reperfusion-induced gastric bleeding in the rat. Gastroenterology 1988;94:733.

58. Groenbech JE, Matre K, Stangeland L, Svanes K, Varhaug JE. Gastric mucosal repair in the cat: Role of the hyperemic response to mucosal damage. Gastroenterology 1988;95:311.

59. Anzueto L, Benoit JN, Granger DN. A rat model for studying the intestinal circulation. Am J Physiol 1984;246:G56.

60. Hernandez LA, Kvietys PR, Granger DN. Postprandial hemodynamics in the conscious rat. Am J Physiol 1986;251:G117.

61. Ulrich-Baker MG, Hollwarth ME, Kvietys PR, Granger DN. Blood flow responses to small bowel resection. Am J Physiol 1986;251: G815.

62. Tuma RF, Vasthare US, Irion GL, Wiedeman MP. Considerations in use of microspheres for flow measurements in anesthetized rat. Am J Physiol 1986;250:H137.

63. Benoit JN, Womack WA, Korthuis RJ, Wilborn WH, Granger DN. Chronic portal hypertension: Effects on gastrointestinal blood flow distribution. Am J Physiol 1986;250:G535.

64. Crissinger KD, Kvietys PR, Granger DN. Developmental intestinal vascular responses to venous pressure elevation. Am J Physiol 1988;254:G658.

65. Crissinger KD, Granger DN. Intestinal blood flow and oxygen consumption: Responses to hemorrhage in the developing piglet. Pediatr Res 1989;26:102.

66. Crissinger KD, Granger DN. Characterization of intestinal collateral blood flow in the developing piglet. Pediatr Res 1988;24:473.

67. Nowicki PT, Miller CE. Autoregulation in the developing postnatal intestinal circulation. Am J Physiol 1988;254:G189.

68. Szabo JS, Mayfield SR, Oh W, Stonestreet BS. Postprandial gastrointestinal blood flow and oxygen consumption: Effects of hypoxemia in neonatal piglets. Pediatr Res 1987;21:93.

69. Nowicki PT, Stonestreet BS, Hansen NB, Yao AC, Oh W. Gastrointestinal blood flow and oxygen consumption in awake newborn piglets: Effect of feeding. Am J Physiol 1983;245:G697.

70. Mortillaro NA, Taylor AE. Interaction of capillary and tissue forces in the cat small intestine. Circ Res 1976;39:348.

71. Grogaard B, Parks DA, Granger DN, et al. Effects of ischemia and superoxide radicals on mucosal albumin clearance in the dog intestine. Am J Physiol 1982;242:G448.

72. Crissinger KD, Kvietys PR, Granger DN. Autoregulatory escape from norepinephrine infusion: Roles of adenosine and histamine. Am J Physiol 1988;254:G560.

73. Bulkley GB, Kvietys PR, Parks DA, et al. Relationship of blood flow and oxygen consumption to ischemic injury in the canine small intestine. Gastroenterology 1985;89:852.

74. Bohlen HG. Intestinal mucosal oxygenation influences absorptive hyperemia. Am J Physiol 1980;239:H489.

75. Lutz J, Beister J. The reactions of gastric vascular bed to venous and arterial pressure elevation. Pflugers Arch 1971;330:230.

76. Holm-Rutili L, Perry M, Granger DN. Autoregulation of gastric blood flow and oxygen uptake. Am J Physiol 1981;241:G143.

77. Hanson KM. Hemodynamic effects of distension of the dog small intestine. Am J Physiol 1973;225:456.

78. Hanson KM, Johnson PC. Evidence for local arterio-venous reflex in intestine. J Appl Physiol 1962;17:509.

79. Hinshaw LB. Arterial and venous pressure–resistance relationships in perfused leg and intestine. Am J Physiol 1962;203:271.

80. Johnson PC. Autoregulation of intestinal blood flow. Am J Physiol 1960;199:311.

81. Johnson PC, Hanson KM. Effect of arterial pressure on arterial and venous resistance of intestine. J Appl Physiol 1962;17:503.

82. Norris CP, Barnes GE, Smith EE, Granger HJ. Autoregulation of superior mesenteric flow in fasted and fed dogs. Am J Physiol 1979;237:H174.

83. Scott JB, Dabney JM. Relation of gut motility to blood flow in the ileum of the dog. Circ Res 1964;14:234.

84. Texter EC, Schwartz MS, Vanderstrappen M, Haddy FJ. Relationship of blood flow to pressure in the intestinal vascular bed. Am J Physiol 1962;202:253.

85. Granger DN, Mortillaro NA, Perry MA, Kvietys PR. Autoregulation of intestinal capillary filtration rate. Am J Physiol 1982;243:G475.

86. Granger DN, Kvietys PR, Mailman D, Richardson PDI. Intrinsic regulation of functional blood flow and water absorption in canine colon. J Physiol 1980;239:G516.

87. Hanson KM, Johnson PC. Pressure–flow relationships in isolated dog colon. Am J Physiol 1967;212:574.

88. Kvietys PR, Granger DN. Effects of solute-coupled fluid absorption on blood flow and oxygen uptake in dog colon. Gastroenterology 1981;81:450.

89. Lundgren O, Svanvik J. Mucosal hemodynamics in the small intestine of the cat during reduced perfusion pressure. Acta Physiol Scand 1973;88:551.

90. Buckley NM, Brazeau P, Frasier ID. Intestinal and femoral blood flow autoregulation in developing swine. Biol Neonate 1986;49:229.

91. Randall MD, Hiley CR. Detergent and methylene blue affect endothelium-dependent vasorelaxation and pressure–flow relations in rat blood perfused mesenteric arterial bed. Br J Pharmacol 1988;95:1081.

92. Granger DN, Granger HJ. Systems analysis of intestinal hemodynamics and oxygenation. Am J Physiol 1983;245:G786.

93. Granger DN, Perry MA, Kvietys PR, et al. Metabolic, myogenic and hormonal factors in local regulation of alimentary tract blood flow. In: Koo A, Lam SK, Smaje LH, eds. Microcirculation of the alimentary tract. Singapore: World Scientific, 1983:131.

94. Mortillaro NA, Granger HJ. Reactive hyperemia and oxygen extraction in the feline small intestine. Circ Res 1977;41:859.

95. Mortillaro NA, Granger DN, Kvietys PR, et al. Effects of histamine and histamine antagonists on intestinal capillary permeability. Am J Physiol 1981;240:G381.

96. Shepherd AP. Intestinal oxygen consumption and 86Rb extraction during arterial hypoxia. Am J Physiol 1978;234:248.

97. Svanvik J, Tyllstrom J, Wallentin J. The effects of hypercapnia and hypoxia on the distribution of capillary blood flow in the denervated intestinal vascular bed. Acta Physiol Scand 1968;74:543.

98. Holzman IR, Tabata B, Edelstone DI. Effects of varying hematocrit on intestinal oxygen uptake in neonatal lambs. Am J Physiol 1985;248:G432.

99. Johnson PC. Myogenic nature of increase in intestinal vascular resistance with venous pressure elevation. Circ Res 1959;6:992.

100. Johnson PC. Myogenic and venous-arteriolar responses in intestinal circulation. In: Shepherd AP, Granger DN, eds. Physiology of the intestinal circulation. New York: Raven Press, 1984:49.

101. Johnson PC, Hanson KM. Capillary filtration in the small intestine of the dog. Circ Res 1966;19:766.

102. Shepherd AP. Myogenic responses of intestinal resistance and exchange vessels. Am J Physiol 1977;233:H547.

103. Shepherd AP, Riedel GL. Effects of pulsatile pressure and metabolic rate on intestinal autoregulation. Am J Physiol 1982;242:H769.

104. Hanson KM, Moore FT. Effects of intraluminal pressure in the colon on its vascular pressure–flow relationships. Proc Soc Exp Biol Med 1969;131:373.

105. Johnson PC. The myogenic response. In: Bohr DF, Somlyo AT, Sparks HV, eds. Handbook of physiology; Section II, Cardiovascular system; Vol II, Vascular smooth muscle. Bethesda: American Physiological Society, 1980:409.

106. Womack WA, Tygart PK, Mailman D, et al. Villous motility: Relationship to lymph flow and blood flow in jejunum. Gastroenterology 1988;94:977.

107. Shepherd AP. Intestinal blood flow autoregulation during foodstuff absorption. Am J Physiol 1980;239:H156.

108. Davis MJ, Gore RW. Capillary pressures in rat intestinal muscle and mucosal villi during venous pressure elevation. Am J Physiol 1985;249:H174.

109. Benoit JN, Granger DN. Chronic portal hypertension and splanchnic circulation. Semin Liver Dis 1986;6:287.

110. Fronek K, Fronek A. Combined effect of exercise and digestion on hemodynamics in conscious dogs. Am J Physiol 1970;218:555.

111. Fronek K, Stahlgren LH. Systemic and regional hemodynamic changes during food intake and digestion in non-anesthetized dogs. Circ Res 1968;23:687.

112. Vatner SF, Franklin D, Van Citters RL. Mesenteric vasoactivity associated with eating and digestion in the conscious dog. Am J Physiol 1970;219:170.

113. Vatner SF, Franklin D, Van Citters RL. Coronary and visceral vasoactivity associated with eating and digestion in conscious dogs. Am J Physiol 1970;219:1380.

114. Vatner SF, Patrick TA, Higgins CB, Franklin D. Regional circulatory adjustments to eating and digestion in conscious unrestrained primates. J Appl Physiol 1974;36:524.

115. Bond JH, Prentiss RA, Levitt MD. The effects of feeding on blood flow to the stomach, small bowel, and colon of the conscious dog. J Lab Clin Med 1979;93:594.

116. Burns GP, Schenk WG. Effect of digestion and exercise on intestinal blood flow and cardiac output. Arch Surg 1969;98:790.

117. Gallavan RH, Chou CC, Kvietys PR, Sit SP. Regional blood flow during digestion in the conscious dog. Am J Physiol 1980;238:H220.

118. Snape WJ, Jr, Wright SH, Battle WM, Cohen S. The gastrocolic response: Evidence for a neural mechanism. Gastroenterology 1979;77:1235.

119. Chou CC. Splanchnic and overall cardiovascular hemodynamics during eating and digestion. Fed Proc 1983;42:1658.

120. Fara JW. Postprandial mesenteric hyperemia. In: Shepherd AP, Granger DN, eds. Physiology of the intestinal circulation. New York: Raven Press, 1984:99.

121. Chou CC, Burns TD, Hsieh CP, Dabney JM. Mechanism of local vasodilation with hypertonic glucose in the jejunum. Surgery 1972;71:380.

122. Chou CC, Kvietys P, Post J, Sit SP. Constituents of chyme responsible for postprandial intestinal hyperemia. Am J Physiol 1978;235:H677.

123. Van Heerden PO, Wagner HM, Jr, Kaihora S. Intestinal blood flow during perfusion of the jejunum with hypertonic glucose in dogs. Am J Physiol 1968;215:30.

124. Yu YM, Yu LC, Chou CC. Distribution of blood flow in the intestine with hypertonic glucose in the lumen. Surgery 1975;78:520.

125. Chou CC, Hsieh CP, Yu YM, et al. Localization of mesenteric hyperemia during digestion in dogs. Am J Physiol 1976;230:583.

126. Pawlik W, Fondacaro JD, Jacobson ED. Metabolic hyperemia in the canine gut. Am J Physiol 1980;239:G12.

127. Shepherd AP, Riedel GL. Laser-Doppler blood flowmetry of intestinal mucosa hyperemia induced by glucose and bile. Am J Physiol 1985;248:G393.

128. Chen HI, Yeh FC, Ho W. Direct effects of nitroglycerin on the resistance, exchange and capacitance functions of canine intestinal vasculature. J Pharmacol Exp 1981;218:497.

129. Levine SE, Granger DN, Brace RA, Taylor AE. Effect of hyperosmolality on vascular resistance and lymph flow in the cat ileum. Am J Physiol 1978;234:H14.

130. Kvietys P, Pittman R, Chou CC. Contribution of luminal concentration of nutrients and osmolality to postprandial hyperemia in dogs. Proc Soc Exp Biol Med 1976;152:659.

131. Chou CC, Hsieh CP, Burns TD, Dabney JM. Effects of lumen pH and osmolarity on duodenal blood flow and motility. Gastroenterology 1971;60:648.

132. Kvietys PR, Gallavan RH, Chou CC. Contribution of bile to postprandial intestinal hyperemia. Am J Physiol 1980;238:G284.

133. Kvietys PR, McLendon JM, Granger DN. Postprandial intestinal hyperemia: Role of bile salts in the ileum. Am J Physiol 1981;241:G469.

134. Siregar H, Chou CC. Relative contribution of fat, protein, carbo-

hydrate, and ethanol to intestinal hyperemia. Am J Physiol 1982;242:G27.

135. Gallavan RH, Jr, Chou CC. Possible mechanisms for the initiation and maintenance of postprandial intestinal hyperemia. Am J Physiol 1985;249:G301.

136. Valleau JD, Granger DN, Taylor AE. Effect of solute-coupled volume absorption on oxygen consumption in the cat ileum. Am J Physiol 1979;236:E198.

137. Varro V, Csernay L, Szarvas F, Blaho G. Effect of glucose and glycine solution on the circulation of the isolated jejunal loop in the dog. Am J Dig Dis 1967;12:60.

138. Proctor KG. Contribution of hyperosmolality to glucose-induced intestinal hyperemia. Am J Physiol 1985;248:G521.

139. Sit SP, Nyhof P, Gallavan R, Jr, Chou CC. Mechanisms of glucose-induced hyperemia in the jejunum. Proc Soc Exp Biol Med 1980;163:273.

140. Kvietys PR, Wilborn WH, Granger DN. Effect of atropine on bile-oleic acid-induced alterations in dog jejunal hemodynamics, oxygenation, and net transmucosal water movement. Gastroenterology 1981;80:31.

141. Granger DN, Kvietys PR, Parks DA, Benoit JN. Intestinal blood flow: Relations to function. Surv Dig Dis 1983;1:217.

142. Proctor KG. Possible role for adenosine on local regulation of absorptive hyperemia in rat intestine. Circ Res 1986;59:474.

143. Granger HJ, Norris CP. Role of adenosine in local control of intestinal circulation in the dog. Circ Res 1980;46:764.

144. Lautt WW. Autoregulation of superior mesenteric artery is blocked by adenosine antagonism. Can J Physiol Pharmacol 1986;64:1291.

145. Premen AM, Kvietys PR, Granger DN. Postprandial regulation of intestinal blood flow: Role of gastrointestinal hormones. Am J Physiol 1985;249:G250.

146. Harper SL, Barrowman JA, Kvietys PR, Granger DN. Effect of neurotensin on capillary permeability and blood flow. Am J Physiol 1984;247:G161.

147. Rozsa Z, Jacobson ED. Capsaicin-sensitive nerves are involved in bile-oleate induced intestinal hyperemia. Am J Physiol 1989;256:G476.

148. Black JW, Fisher EW, Smith AN. The effects of precursors of 5-hydroxytryptamine on gastric secretion in anesthetized dogs. J Physiol (Lond) 1959;146:10.

149. Chou CC, Siregar H. Role of histamine H_1- and H_2-receptors in postprandial intestinal hyperemia. Am J Physiol 1982;243:G248.

150. Gallavan RH, Jr, Chou CC. Prostaglandin synthesis inhibition and postprandial intestinal hyperemia. Am J Physiol 1982;242:G140.

151. Mangino MJ, Chou CC. Arachidonic acid and postprandial intestinal hyperemia. Am J Physiol 1984;246:G521.

152. Proctor KG. Differential effect of cyclooxygenase inhibitors on absorptive hyperemia. Am J Physiol 1985;249:H755.

153. Rowell LB, Johnson JM. Role of the splanchnic circulation in reflex control of the cardiovascular system. In: Shepherd AP, Granger DN, eds. Physiology of the intestinal circulation. New York: Raven Press, 1984:153.

154. Furness JB, Costa M. Types of nerves in the enteric nervous system. Neuroscience 1980;5:1.

155. Kewenter J. The vagal control of the jejunal and ileal motility and blood flow. Acta Physiol Scand (Suppl 65) 1965;251:1.

156. Tibblin S, Burns GP, Hahnloser PB, Schenk WG. The influence of vagotomy on superior mesenteric artery blood flow. Surg Gynecol Obstet 1969;129:1231.

157. Biber B, Fara J, Lundgren O. Intestinal vasodilatation in response to transmural electrical field stimulation. Acta Physiol Scand 1973;87:277.

158. Biber B, Lundgren O, Svanvik J. Studies on the intesinal vasodilatation observed after mechanical stimulation of the mucosa of the gut. Acta Physiol Scand 1971;82:177.

159. Folkow B, Lewis DH, Lundgren O, et al. The effect of graded vasoconstrictor fibre stimulation on the intestinal resistance and capacitance vessels. Acta Physiol Scand 1964;61:445.

160. Ross G. Escape of mesenteric vessels from adrenergic and non-adrenergic vasoconstriction. Am J Physiol 1971;221:1217.

161. Greenway CV, Scott GD, Zink J. Sites of autoregulatory escape of blood flow in the mesenteric vascular bed. J Physiol (Lond) 1976;259:1.

162. Buckley NM, Jarenwattananon M, Gootman PM, Frasier ID. Autoregulatory escape from vasoconstriction of intestinal circulation in developing swine. Am J Physiol 1987;252:H118.

163. Guth PH, Ross G, Smith E. Changes in intestinal vascular diameter during norepinephrine vasoconstrictor escape. Am J Physiol 1976;230:1466.

164. Fasth S, Hulten L, Nordgren S. Adjustments of hepatic and small intestine blood flow on selective vasoconstrictor fibre stimulation. Acta Physiol Scand 1980;110:343.

165. Shepherd AP, Granger HJ. Autoregulatory escape in the gut: A systems analysis. Gastroenterology 1973;65:77.

166. Shepherd AP, Pawlik W, Mailman D, et al. Effects of vasoconstrictors on intestinal vascular resistance and oxygen extraction. Am J Physiol 1976;230:298.

167. Granger DN, Richardson PDI, Kvietys PR, Mortillaro NA. Intestinal blood flow. Gastroenterology 1980;78:837.

168. Shepherd AP, Riedel GL. Intramural distribution of intestinal blood flow during sympathetic stimulation. Am J Physiol 1988;255:H1091.

169. Remak G, Hottenstein OD, Jacobson ED. Peptidergic nerves are involved in norepinephrine-induced vasoconstriction, but not in escape from norepinephrine. Gastroenterology 1989;96:A412.

170. Richardson PDI, Granger DN, Kvietys PR. Effects of norepinephrine, vasopressin, isoproterenol, and histamine on blood flow, oxygen uptake, and capillary filtration coefficient in the colon of the anesthetized dog. Gastroenterology 1980;78:1537.

171. Shepherd AP, Mailman D, Burks TF, Granger HJ. Effects of norepinephrine and sympathetic stimulation on extraction of oxygen and ^{86}Rb in perfused canine small bowel. Circ Res 1973;33:166.

172. Pawlik W, Shepherd AP, Jacobson ED. Effects of vasoactive agents on intestinal oxygen consumption and blood flow in dogs. J Clin Invest 1975;56:484.

173. Pawlik WW, Shepherd AP, Mailman D, et al. Effects of dopamine and epinephrine on intestinal blood flow and oxygen uptake. Adv Exp Med Biol 1976;75:511.

174. Rocha E, Silva M, Rosenberg M. The release of vasopressin in response to haemorrhage and its role in the mechanism of blood pressure regulation. J Physiol (Lond) 1969;202:535.

175. Kvietys PR, Granger DN. Vasoactive agents and splanchnic oxygen uptake. Am J Physiol 1982;243:G1.

176. McNeill JR, Wilcox WC, Pang CCY. Vasopressin and angiotensin: Reciprocal mechanisms controlling mesenteric conductance. Am J Physiol 1977;232:H260.

177. McNeill JR. Redundant nature of the vasopressin and renin–angiotensin systems in the control of mesenteric resistance vessels of the conscious fasted cat. Can J Physiol Pharmacol 1983;61:770.

178. Pang CCY. Effect of vasopressin antagonist and saralasin on regional blood flow following hemorrhage. Am J Physiol 1983;245:H749.

179. McNeill JR. Intestinal vasoconstriction following diuretic-induced volume depletion: Role of angiotensin and vasopressin. Can J Physiol Pharmacol 1974;52:829.

180. Suvannapura A, Levens NR. Local control of mesenteric blood flow by the renin–angiotensin system. Am J Physiol 1988;255:G267.

181. Kvietys PR, Navia CA, Premen AJ, Granger DN. Quantitative assessment of the two-component model of intestinal circulation. Am J Physiol 1986;251:G446.

182. Ohman U. Blood flow and oxygen consumption in the feline small intestine: Responses to artificial distention and intestinal obstruction. Acta Chir Scand 1976;142:329.

183. Shepherd AP, Riedel GL. Intestinal oxygen uptake versus blood flow relationship and optimal hematocrit for O_2 transport. Fed Proc 1981;40:491.

184. Kvietys PR, Perry MA, Granger DN. Intestinal capillary exchange capacity and oxygen delivery-to-demand ratio. Am J Physiol 1983;245:G635.

185. Varro V, Blaho G, Cserney L, et al. Effect of decreased local circulation on the absorptive capacity of the small intestine in the dog. Am J Dig Dis 1965;10:170.

186. Holm L, Perry MA. Role of blood flow in gastric secretion. Am J Physiol 1988;254:G281.

187. Granger DN, Kvietys PR, Perry MA, Barrowman JA. The microcirculation and intestinal transport. In: Johnson LR, ed. Physiology of the gastrointestinal tract, ed 2. New York: Raven Press, 1987:1671.

188. Granger DN, Barrowman JA. Microcirculation of the alimentary tract. I. Physiology of transcapillary fluid and solute exchange. Gastroenterology 1983;84:846.

189. Richardson PDI, Granger DN, Mailman D, Kvietys PR. Permeability characteristics of colonic capillaries. Am J Physiol 1980;239:G300.

190. Kvietys PR. Microcirculation of the large intestine. In: Mortillaro NA, ed. Physiology and pharmacology of the microcirculation. Orlando: Academic Press, 1984:77.

191. Granger DN, Parker RE, Quillen EW, et al. Lymph flow transients. In: Malek P, Bartos V, Weissleder H, Witte M, eds. Lymphology. Stuttgart: G. Thieme, 1979:61.

192. Barrowman JA, Perry MA, Kvietys PR, et al. Effects of bradykinin on intestinal transcapillary fluid exchange. Can J Physiol Pharmacol 1981;59:786.

193. Granger DN, Richardson PDI, Taylor AE. The effects of isoprenaline and bradykinin on capillary filtration in the cat small intestine. Br J Pharmacol 1979;67:361.

194. Granger DN, Kvietys PR, Wilborn WH, et al. Mechanism of glucagon-induced intestinal secretion. Am J Physiol 1980;239:G30.

195. Granger DN, Perry MA, Kvietys PR, Taylor AE. Permeability of intestinal capillaries: effects of fat absorption and gastrointestinal hormones. Am J Physiol 1982;242:G194.

196. Turner SG, Barrowman JA. Intestinal lymph flow and lymphatic transport of protein during fat absorption. Q J Exp Physiol 1977;62:175.

197. Lawrence JA, Bryan D, Roberts KB, Barrowman JA. Effect of secretin on intestinal lymph flow and composition in rat. Q J Exp Physiol 1981;66:297.

198. Granger DN, Shackleford JS, Taylor AE. Prostaglandin E₁ induced filtration secretion in the feline ileum. Am J Physiol 1979;236:E788.

199. Nicoll PA, Taylor AE. Lymph formation and flow. Annu Rev Physiol 1977;39:73.

200. Granger DN, Rutili G, McCord JM. Superoxide radicals in feline intestinal ischemia. Gastroenterology 1981;81:22.

201. Perry MA, Shepherd AP, Kvietys PR, Granger DN. Effects of hypoxia on feline intestinal capillary permeability. Am J Physiol 1985;248:G272.

202. Granger DN, Perry MA, Kvietys PR, Taylor AE. A new method for estimating intestinal capillary pressure. Am J Physiol 1983;244:G341.

203. Granger DN, Perry MA, Kvietys PR, Taylor AE. Capillary and interstitial forces during lipid absorption in the cat small intestine. Gastroenterology 1984;86:262.

204. Lee JS. Lymph pressure in intestinal villi and lymph flow during fluid secretion. In: Hargens AR, ed. Tissue fluid pressure and composition. Baltimore: Williams & Wilkins, 1981:165.

205. Granger DN, Sennett M, McElearney P, Taylor AE. Effect of local arterial hypotension on cat intestinal capillary permeability. Gastroenterology 1980;79:474.

206. Granger DN, Barrowman JA, Harper SL, et al. Sympathetic stimulation and intestinal capillary fluid exchange. Am J Physiol 1984;247:G279.

207. Taylor AE, Granger DN. Exchange of macromolecules across the circulation. In: Renkin EM, Michel CC, eds. Handbook of physiology, microcirculation. Washington, DC: American Physiological Society, 1984:467.

208. Harper SL, Barrowman JA, Kvietys PR, Granger DN. Effect of neurotensin on capillary permeability and blood flow. Am J Physiol 1984;247:G161.

209. Granger DN, Taylor AE. Effects of solute-coupled transport on lymph flow and oncotic pressures in cat ileum. Am J Physiol 1978;235:E429.

210. Granger DN, Mortillaro NA, Taylor AE. Interactions of intestinal lymph flow and secretion. Am J Physiol 1978;232:E13.

211. Yablonski ME, Lifson N. Mechanism of production of intestinal secretion by elevated venous pressure. J Clin Invest 1976;57:904.

212. Granger DN, Cook BH, Taylor AE. Structural locus of transmucosal albumin efflux in canine ileum: A fluorescence study. Gastroenterology 1976;71:1023.

213. Fordtran JS, Rector FC, Ewton MF, et al. Permeability characteristics of the human small intestine. J Clin Invest 1965;44:1935.

214. Granger DN, Cross R, Barrowman JA. Effects of various secreta- gogues and human carcinoid serum on lymph flow in the cat ileum. Gastroenterology 1982;83:896.

215. Granger DN, Mortillaro NA, Kvietys PR, et al. Role of the interstitial matrix during intestinal volume absorption. Am J Physiol 1980;238:G183.

216. Cedgard S, Hallback DA, Jodal M, et al. The effects of cholera toxin on intramural blood flow distribution and capillary hydraulic conductivity in the cat small intestine. Acta Physiol Scand 1978;102:148.

217. Katz JA, Sellers L, Banoris G, Golden S. Studies on the extravascular albumin of rats. In: Rothschild M, Waldmonn P, eds. Plasma protein metabolism. New York: Academic Press, 1970:129.

218. Granger DN. Intestinal microcirculation and transmucosal fluid transport. Am J Physiol 1981;240:G343.

219. Kvietys PR, Granger DN. Role of microcirculation in intestinal transmucosal fluid transport. In: Koo A, Lam SK, Smaje LH, eds. Microcirculation of the alimentary tract. Singapore: World Scientific, 1983:247.

220. Barrowman JA. Physiology of the gastrointestinal lymphatic system. Cambridge: Cambridge University Press, 1978:126.

221. Shepherd AP. Intestinal capillary blood flow during metabolic hyperemia. Am J Physiol 1979;237:E548.

222. Granger DN, Korthuis RJ, Kvietys PR, Tso P. Intestinal microvascular exchange during lipid absorption. Am J Physiol 1988;255:G690.

223. Tso P, Pitts V, Granger DN. Role of lymph flow in intestinal chylomicron transport. Am J Physiol 1985;249:G21.

224. Boley SJ, Brandt LJ. Selective mesenteric vasodilators: A future role in acute mesenteric ischemia? Gastroenterology 1986;91:247.

225. McCready RA, Hollier LH, Pairolero PC. Superior mesenteric artery embolus. South Med J 1984;77:789.

226. Boley SJ, Feinstein FR, Sammartano R, et al. New concepts in the management of emboli of the superior mesenteric artery. Surg Gynecol Obstet 1981;153:561.

227. MacCannell KL, Newton CA, Lederis K, et al. Use of selective mesenteric vasodilator peptides in experimental nonocclusive mesenteric ischemia in the dog. Gastroenterology 1986;90:669.

228. Kliegman RM, Fanaroff AA. Necrotizing enterocolitis. N Engl J Med 1984;310:1093.

229. Holzman IR, Brown DR. Necrotizing enterocolitis: A complication of prematurity. Semin Perinatol 1986;10:208.

230. Chiu CJ, McArdle AH, Brown R, et al. Intestinal mucosal lesions in low-flow states. I. A morphological, hemodynamic and metabolic reappraisal. Arch Surg 1970;101:478.

231. Haglund U, Lundgren O. Reactions within consecutive vascular sections of the small intestine of the cat during prolonged hypotension. Acta Physiol Scand 1972;84:151.

232. Robinson JWL, Mirkovitch V. The roles of intraluminal oxygen and glucose in the protection of the rat intestinal mucosa from the effects of ischemia. Biomed 1977;27:60.

233. Kingham JGC, Whorwell PJ, Loehry CA. Small intestinal permeability: Effects of ischaemia and exposure to acetyl salicylate. Gut 1976;17:354.

234. Parks DA, Grogaard B, Granger DN. Comparison of partial and complete arterial occlusion models for studying intestinal ischemia. Surgery 1982;92:896.

235. Crissinger KD, Granger DN. Mucosal injury induced by ischemia and reperfusion in the piglet intestine: Influences of age and feeding. Gastroenterology 1989;97:920.

236. Nowicki PT, Miller CE, Haun S. Effects of arterial hypoxia and isoproterenol on in vitro postnatal intestinal circulation. Am J Physiol 1988;255:H1133.

237. Michels NA, Siddharth P, Kornblith PL, Parke WW. Routes of collateral circulation of the gastrointestinal tract as ascertained in a dissection of 500 bodies. Int Surg 1968;49:8.

238. Meyers MA. Griffiths' point: Critical anastomosis at the splenic flexure. Am J Roentgenol 1976;126:77.

239. Saegesser F, Loosli H, Robinson JWL, Roenspies U. Ischemic diseases of the large intestine. Int Surg 1981;66:103.

240. Molstad C, Granger HJ. Collateral circulation in the splanchnic vasculature. Fed Proc 1981;40:491.

241. Bulkley GB, Womack WA, Downey JM, et al. Characterization of

segmental collateral blood flow in the small intestine. Am J Physiol 1985;249:G228.

242. Cho KJ, Schmidt RW, Lenz J. Effects of experimental embolization of superior mesenteric artery branch on the intestine. Invest Radiol 1979;14:207.

243. Ahren C, Haglund U. Mucosal lesions in the small intestine of the cat during low flow. Acta Physiol Scand 1973;88:541.

244. Bounous G. Acute necrosis of the intestinal mucosa. Gastroenterology 1982;82:1457.

245. Guth PH, Hirabayashi K. The effect of histamine on microvascular permeability in the muscularis externa of rat small intestine. Microvasc Res 1983;25:322.

246. Haglund UK, Lundholm O, Lundgren O, Schersten O. Intestinal lysosomal enzyme activity in regional simulated shock: Influence of methylprednisolone and albumin. Circ Shock 1977;4:27.

247. Parks DA, Granger DN. Xanthine oxidase: Biochemistry, distribution, and physiology. Acta Physiol Scand (Suppl) 1986;548:87.

248. Hernandez LA, Grisham MB, Twohig B, et al. Role of neutrophils in ischemia-reperfusion-induced microvascular injury. Am J Physiol 1987;253:H699.

249. Bounous G, Hampson LG, Gurd FN. Cellular nucleotides in hemorrhagic shock. Relationship of intestinal metabolic changes to hemorrhagic enteritis and the barrier function of intestinal mucosa. Ann Surg 1964;160:650.

250. Bounous G, Brown RA, Mulder DS, et al. Abolition of "tryptic enteritis" in the shocked dog. Arch Surg 1965;91:372.

251. Crowell JW. Oxygen transport in the hypotensive state. Fed Proc 1970;29:1848.

252. Bounous G, Menard D, De Medicis E. Role of pancreatic proteases in the pathogenesis of ischemic enteropathy. Gastroenterology 1977;73:102.

253. Bounous G, Proulx J, Konok G, et al. The role of bile and pancreatic proteases in the pathogenesis of ischemic enteropathy. Int J Clin Pharmacol Biopharm 1979;17:317.

254. Fox J, Galey F, Wayland H. Action of histamine on the mesenteric microvasculature. Microvasc Res 1980;19:108.

255. Kobold EE, Thal AP. Quantitation and identification of vasoactive substances liberated during various types of experimental and clinical intestinal ischemia. Surg Gynecol Obstet 1963;117:315.

256. Kusche J, Stahlknecht CD, Richter H, et al. Diamine oxidase activity and histamine release in dogs following acute mesenteric artery occlusion. Agents Actions 1977;7:81.

257. Kusche J, Lorenz W, Stahlknecht C, et al. Intestinal diamine oxidase and histamine release in rabbit mesenteric ischemia. Gastroenterology 1980;80:980.

258. Freeman BA, Crapo JD. Free radical and tissue injury. Lab Invest 1982;47:412.

259. Batelli MG, Della Corte E, Stirpe F. Xanthine oxidase type d (dehydrogenase) in the intestine and other organs of the rat. Biochem J 1972;126:747.

260. Pickett JP, Pendergrass RE, Bradford WD, Elchlepp JG. Localization of xanthine oxidase in rat duodenum: Fixation of sections instead of blocks. Stain Tech 1970;45:35.

261. Granger DN, Hernandez LA, Grisham MB. Reactive oxygen metabolites: Mediators of cell injury in the digestive system. Viewpoints Dig Dis 1986;18:13.

262. Marklund SL, Westman NG, Lundgren E, Roos G. Copper- and zinc-containing superoxide dismutase, manganese-containing superoxide dismutase, catalase, and glutathione peroxidase in normal and neoplastic human cell lines and normal human tissues. Can Res 1982;42:1955.

263. Granger DN, Hoellwarth ME, Parks DA. Ischemia-reperfusion injury: Role of oxygen-derived free radicals. Acta Physiol Scand (Suppl) 1986;548:47.

264. Granger DN, McCord JM, Parks DA, Hoellwarth MA. Xanthine oxidase inhibitors attenuate ischemia-induced vascular permeability changes in the cat intestine. Gastroenterology 1986;90:80.

265. Parks DA, Granger DN, Bulkley GB, Shah AK. Soybean trypsin inhibitor attenuates ischemic injury to the feline small intestine. Gastroenterology 1985;89:6.

266. Grisham MB, Hernandez LA, Granger DN. Xanthine oxidase and neutrophil infiltration in intestinal ischemia. Am J Physiol 1986;251:G567.

267. Smith SM, Grisham MB, Manci EA, et al. Gastric mucosal injury in the rat. Role of iron and xanthine oxidase. Gastroenterology 1987;92:950.

268. Parks DA, Bulkley GB, Granger DN, et al. Ischemic injury in the cat small intestine: Role of superoxide radicals. Gastroenterology 1982;82:9.

269. Parks DA, Granger DN. Ischemia-induced vascular changes: Role of xanthine oxidase and hydroxyl radicals. Am J Physiol 1986;250:G749.

270. Parks DA, Shah AK, Granger DN. Oxygen radicals: Effects of intestinal vascular permeability. Am J Physiol 1984;247:G167.

271. Parks DA, Granger DN. Role of oxygen radicals in gastrointestinal ischemia. In: Rotilio G, ed. Superoxide and superoxide dismutase in chemistry, biology, and medicine. Amsterdam: Elsevier, 1986: 614.

272. Crissinger KD, Grisham MB, Granger DN. Developmental biology of oxidant-producing enzymes and antioxidants in the piglet intestine. Pediatr Res 1989;25:612.

273. Weiss SJ. Tissue destruction by neutrophils. N Engl J Med 1988;320: 365.

274. Henson PM, Johnston RB. Tissue injury in inflammation. Oxidants, proteinases, and cationic proteins. J Clin Invest 1987;79:669.

275. Zimmerman BJ, Grisham MB, Granger DN. Mechanisms of oxidant-mediated microvascular injury following reperfusion of the ischemic intestine. In: Simic MG, Taylor KA, Ward JF, Von Sonntag C, eds. Oxygen radicals in biology and medicine. New York: Plenum, 1988;881.

276. Zimmerman BJ, Granger DN. Role of hydrogen peroxide, iron, and hydroxyl radicals in ischemia/reperfusion-induced neutrophil infiltration. Physiologist 1988;31:A229.

277. Sun X, Hsueh W. Bowel necrosis. An investigation of secondary mediators in its pathogenesis. Am J Pathol 1986;122:231.

278. Eliakim R, Karmeli F, Razin E, Rachmilewitz D. Role of platelet-activating factor in ulcerative colitis. Enhanced production during active disease and inhibition by sulfasalazine and prednisolone. Gastroenterology 1988;95:1167.

279. Chignard M, LeCouedic JP, Tence M, et al. The role of platelet-activating factor from human monocyte. Int Arch Allergy Appl Immunol 1979;70:245.

280. Arnoux B, Duval D, Benveniste J. Release of platelet-activating factor (PAF-acether) from alveolar macrophages by the calcium ionophore A23187 and phagocytosis. Eur J Clin Invest 1980;10:437.

281. Camussi G, Aglietta M, Coda R, Bussolino F. Release of platelet-activating factor and histamine. II. The cellular origin of human PAF: Monocytes, polymorphonuclear neutrophils and basophils. Immunology 1981;42:191.

282. Camussi G, Aglietta M, Malavasi F, et al. The release of platelet-activating factor from human endothelial cells in culture. J Immunol 1983;131:2397.

283. Doyle VM, Creba JA, Ruegg UT. Platelet-activating factor mobilises intracellular calcium in vascular smooth muscle cells. FEBS Lett 1986;197:13.

284. Bussolino F, Aglietta M, Sanavio F, et al. Alkyl-ether phosphoglycerides influence calcium fluxes into human endothelial cells. J Immunol 1985;135:2748.

285. Brock TA, Gimbrone MA. Platelet activating factor alters calcium homeostasis in cultured vascular endothelial cells. Am J Physiol 1986;250:H1086.

286. D'Humieres S, Russo-Marie F, Vargaftig BB. PAF-acether-induced synthesis of prostacylin by human endothelial cells. Eur J Pharmacol 1986;131:13.

287. Benveniste J, Henson PM, Cochrane CG. Leukocyte-dependent histamine release from rabbit platelets. The role of IgE, basophils and a platelet-activating factor. J Exp Med 1972;136:1356.

288. O'Flaherty JT, Wykle RL, Miller CH, et al. 1-O-alkyl-sn-glyceryl-3-phosphorylcholines. A novel class of neutrophil stimulants. Am J Pathol 1981;103:70.

289. Shaw JO, Pinckard RN, Ferrignini KS, et al. Activation of human neutrophils with 1-O-hexadecyl octadecyl-2-acetyl-sn-glyceryl-3 phosphorylcholine (platelet activating factor). J Immunol 1981;127: 1250.

290. Ingraham L, Coates T, Allen J, et al. Metabolic, membrane, and

functional responses of human polymorphonuclear leukocytes to platelet-activating factor. Blood 1982;59:1259.

291. Dillon PK, Fitzpatrick MF, Ritter AB, Duran WN. Effect of platelet-activating factor on leukocyte adhesion to microvascular endothelium. Time course and dose–response relationships. Inflammation 1988;12:563.

292. Wedmore CV, Williams RJ. Platelet-activating factor (PAF), a secretory product of polymorphonuclear leukocytes, increases vascular permeability in rabbit skin. Br J Pharmacol 1981;74:916P.

293. Humphrey DM, McManus LM, Hanahan DJ, Pinckard RN. Morphological basis of increased vascular permeability induced by acetyl glyceryl ether phosphorylcholine. Lab Invest 1984;50:16.

294. Handley DA, Arbeeny CM, Lee ML, et al. Effect of platelet-activating factor on endothelial permeability to plasma macromolecules. Immunopharmacology 1984;8:137.

295. Filep J, Herman F, Braquet P, Mozes T. Increased levels of platelet activating factor in blood following intestinal ischemia in the dog. Biochem Biophys Res Commun 1989;158:353.

296. Tagesson C, Lindahl M, Otamiri T. BN 52021 ameliorates mucosal damage associated with small intestinal ischaemia in rats. In: Braquet P, ed. Ginkgolides: Chemistry, biology, pharmacology and clinical perspectives. Barcelona: JR Prous Science, 1988:553.

297. Kubes P, Granger DN. Neutrophil adherence during ischemia and reperfusion: Role of platelet activating factor. Am J Physiol 1990;259:G300.

23

Growth and Development in the Gastrointestinal Tract

MARK W. BABYATSKY
DANIEL K. PODOLSKY

The structural and functional integrity of the mature gastrointestinal tract is the product of a complex developmental program of intricate mechanisms for the constant self-renewal of the mucosal surface, which continues throughout life. During embryonic and fetal life, the gastrointestinal tract and its accessory organs develop from a single nondescript tubular structure to the specialized constituent organs, which exhibit their unique structural, cellular, and functional specificities by the time of parturition. While important characteristics in architectural organization are similar along the length of the gastrointestinal tract, regional specialization is inherent to this development. The gastrointestinal tract remains highly dynamic throughout a person's lifetime with a continuing, if regionally variable, cycle of cellular proliferation, differentiation, and senescence. Disruption of the normal sequence of developmental evolution in utero leads to a wide spectrum of anatomic disorders usually manifest during infancy. An appreciation of the mechanisms of ongoing self-renewal and maturation and their regulation is integral to an understanding of the pathogenesis of a number of disorders including both neoplastic and non-neoplastic diseases. This chapter first considers the macroscopic and microscopic maturation of the gastrointestinal tract. This is followed by discussion of functional maturation and its regulation and finally a summary of the processes controlling homeostasis of the epithelium in the adult.

EMBRYOLOGY AND HISTOGENESIS

The human gastrointestinal tract can first be distinguished in the 4th week of gestation when infolding creates an endoderm-lined tubular structure extending from esophagus to cloaca. The nascent gastrointestinal tract is joined in its ventral region to the yolk stalk and allantois, which remain outside of the embryo. During development, the gastrointestinal tract can be divided into foregut, midgut, and hindgut reflecting roughly those structures supplied by celiac, superior mesenteric, and inferior mesenteric arteries, respectively.[1] The foregut includes the esophagus, stomach, duodenum (to the level of the ampulla of Vater), liver, pancreas, and biliary tract. The midgut extends from the mid-second portion of the duodenum to the proximal transverse colon. The hindgut includes the distal transverse colon as well as the remaining large intestine to the proximal anal canal.

Esophagus

The foregut and the respiratory tracts are initially a single tube at the cephalad end of the primordial gastrointestinal tract. However, subsequent development includes longitudinal division of this structure leading to separation of respiratory and foregut structures, with the esophagus occupying a dorsal position by the 2nd month of gestation. The intimate relationship between the developing esophagus and tracheobronchial structures contributes to the potential for developmental anomalies involving connections between the esophagus and trachea.

The esophagus is distinguishable from the stomach as early as the 4th week of gestation.[2] Rapid cephalad extension of the esophageal anlage leads to an elongated structure, which achieves its mature length relative to other structures by the 7th week of gestation. At the same time, rapid proliferation of the endodermal lining leads to near or actual occlusion of the lumen. Recanalization occurs through vacuolization of the endodermal cells, which reestablishes the lumen by the 8th week of gestation. A similar sequence of mucosal proliferation, luminal obliteration, and subsequent reestablishment of the lumen through vacuolization is found throughout the gastrointestinal tract (see below). Failure of recanalization may be a factor in the development of esophageal stenosis or atresia, which can be seen in association with tracheoesophageal fistulas.

The esophagus is initially covered with a simple, cuboidal epithelium. In the 5th week of gestation, two layers of these cuboidal cells, as well as occasional neuroblasts dispersed in a developing layer of circular smooth muscle, are present.[3] The external longitudinal layer of muscle develops in a process discrete from the inner layer of circular muscle and is first appreciated during the 8th week. As noted above, the epithelium becomes vacuolated in the 7th week of gestation, leading to the formation of a longitudinal channel, which forms the lumen when the vacuolization process is complete in the 8th week. In the 10th week of gestation, the esophageal epithelium is ciliated, but subsequent proliferation and maturation lead to a stratified squamous epithelium typical of the adult esophagus by the 22nd week of gestation.[4] Superficial glands may be found as early as the 18th week of gestation, but the deep mucosal glands characteristically found in the mature esophagus are rare before birth and appear to develop during postnatal life. Myenteric plexus can be demonstrated by the 10th week with mature ganglion cells found by the 13th week of gestation.[3]

The mature esophagus is a muscular organ throughout its length. Striated muscle present in the upper esophagus is derived from the caudal branchial arches and is innervated through branches of the vagi. The smooth muscle present in the distal two thirds of the esophagus derives its innervation from the splanchnic plexus.

Stomach and Duodenum

The stomach forms as a fusiform dilatation of the foregut in the neck of the 4-week-old embryo (Fig 23-1A).[5] As it grows, the stomach descends into the abdomen by the 7th week of gestation. The gastric walls grow at disparate rates, creating the characteristic asymmetric shape as the dorsal border (which becomes the greater curvature) grows more rapidly than the ventral border (see Fig 23-1B). During the 6th week, the stomach undergoes a 90-degree clockwise rotation along its longitudinal axis so that the dorsal border lies to the left and the ventral border or lesser curvature lies on the right (see Fig 23-1C). As a result of this rotation, the left and right vagi largely supply the anterior and posterior areas

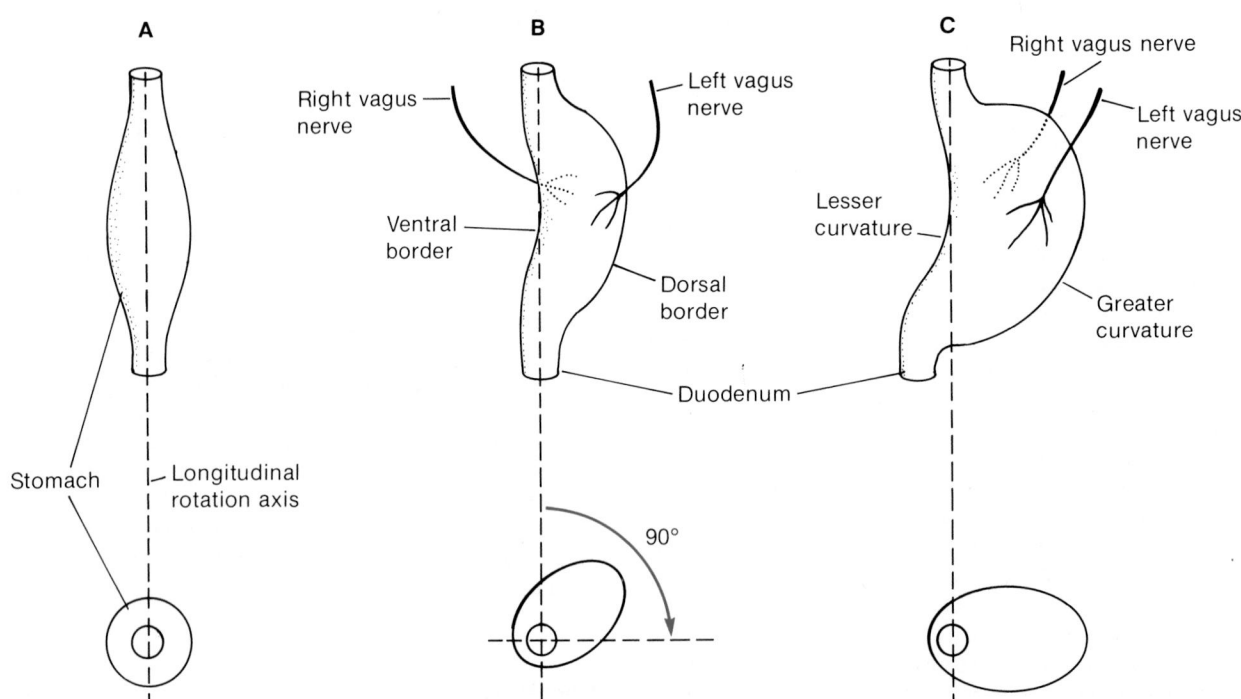

FIGURE 23–1. Schematic representation of the positional changes of the stomach. **A,** The stomach at four weeks. **B,** Rapid growth of the dorsal border resulting in asymmetry. **C,** Following a 90-degree clockwise rotation along the longitudinal axis, the left and right vagus nerves supply the anterior and posterior stomach, respectively. (Adapted from Sadler TW, ed. Langman's medical embryology. Baltimore: Williams & Wilkins, 1985.)

of the stomach, respectively. The pyloric region of the stomach can be identified by the 3rd month of gestation.[6]

The duodenum forms from the caudal foregut and cephalad midgut, which meet and fuse just distal to the area that becomes the ampulla of Vater. The duodenum grows rapidly, rotating to the right at the time of gastric rotation, thus creating a "C" loop in its retroperitoneal position by the 6th week of gestation. During this period of rapid growth, the duodenal lumen is also temporarily obliterated by proliferation of the epithelium but is reestablished through the process of vacuolization by the 8th week. Failure of this recanalization results in duodenal stenosis or atresia.

The dorsal mesentery initially extends from the distal esophagus to the cloaca, but the ventral mesentery is found only from distal esophagus to the end of the foregut region of the duodenum. After gastric rotation, the ventral mesentery extends from the lesser curvature to the liver and includes the falciform ligament, which attaches to the anterior abdominal wall. The dorsal mesentery, in contrast, extends to the left as the omental bursa, which envelops the spleen and covers the pancreas.

In gastric histogenesis, the stomach is initially lined by a stratified columnar epithelium comprised of two to three cell layers in the 7th week of gestation.[7] Gastric pits are rare at this time but thereafter increase in number, initially in the region of the lesser curvature, followed by the greater curvature in the 8th week and finally in the antral and cardiac regions by the 10th to 11th weeks. The glands first develop mucous neck cells followed by parietal and chief cells.[8] Enteroendocrine cells can be detected by the 8th week of gestation, and the fully differentiated spectrum of endocrine cell types can be detected by the 10th week.[9] The deeper pyloric glands form between the 11th and 13th weeks. Circular smooth muscle appears in the 8th and 9th weeks of development.

Pancreas

The liver, biliary tract, and pancreas share closely connected origins in outpouchings or buds from the foregut. The pancreas emerges in the 4-week-old embryo as ventral and dorsal buds from the proximal duodenum (Fig 23-2*A* and *B*). The ventral pancreatic bud is a component of the hepatic diverticulum, which appears between the 3rd and 4th weeks of gestation and encompasses the primordia of the liver and bile ducts as well as the ventral pancreas. As the duodenum grows and rotates, the ventral bud migrates around the duodenum to join the dorsal bud, contributing to the formation of the uncinate process and inferior region of the pancreatic head (see Fig 23-2*C*). Tissue arising from the dorsal bud forms the remainder of the gland. The duct of Wirsung, primarily derived from the dorsal bud, is fused with the ducts of the ventral pancreas and serves as the dominant pancreatic duct emptying at the ampulla of Vater (see Fig 23-2*D*). The accessory duct of Santorini may also persist. Incomplete fusion of the two ductal systems results in pancreas divisum, which may contribute to development of recurrent pancreatitis in later life.

On a histologic level, the pancreas first emerges at the end of the 8th week of gestation as a collection of primitive epithelial tubules. These structures become branched, and their ends become surrounded by "cell buds" from which mature pancreatic acini develop. Endocrine cells are apparent in developing islets during the 10th week. During the 4th month of gestation, a lobular ar-

rangement of the pancreas can first be recognized, leading to the compact structure of the mature pancreas.[10]

Small Intestine and Colon

During the 5th week of gestation, the tubular midgut portion of the intestinal tract, which is joined to the yolk sac by the vitelline duct, elongates rapidly, extending into the body stalk in the ventral dimension. The vitelline duct, which normally becomes obliterated before birth, occasionally persists as a Meckel's diverticulum. The area cephalad to the duct constitutes the small intestine from the junction of foregut and midgut in the duodenum to the proximal ileum. The segment distal to the duct forms the remaining components of the midgut to midtransverse colon. Between the 5th and 10th weeks, the small intestine extends through the umbilicus, as the result of further elongation. During this period of rapid elongation, the midgut rotates 90 degrees around the superior mesenteric artery present in the dorsal mesentery. This rotation brings the proximal midgut to the right and the distal midgut to the left (Fig 23-3*A*). Subsequently, the midgut reenters the abdominal cavity in the 10th week of gestation. During the process in which the midgut reenters the abdomen, it undergoes a further 180-degree rotation (for a total rotation of 270 degrees; see Fig 23-3*B*). The proximal jejunum enters first and occupies the left side of the abdomen, and the ileum settles into the right side.

When the midgut reenters the abdominal cavity, the cecal swelling enters last, locating temporarily in the right upper quadrant just caudal to the right lobe of the liver (see Fig 23-3*C*). Between the 3rd and 5th months of gestation, the cecum descends into the right iliac fossa and becomes fixed to the posterior wall of the abdomen (see Fig 23-3*D*). As the liver increases in size, the ascending colon and hepatic flexure become distinct from the transverse colon. The descending colon loses its mesentery and becomes anchored to the abdominal wall, leaving the sigmoid in its more caudal position on a mesentery.

The rectum arises independently from the remaining large intestine as a subdivision of the cloaca, which is separated from the urogenital sinus by the urorectal septum. The urorectal septum reaches the cloacal membrane during the 7th week of gestation, forming the perineum (Fig 23-4). During the 8th week, the rectum fuses with the colon, and the cloacal membrane forms the anal membrane, which is lost during the 9th week to establish communication with the amniotic space.

Both the small and large intestine are initially lined by a simple cuboidal epithelium. In a process analogous to that found in more proximal regions of the gastrointestinal tract, epithelial proliferation during the 6th and 7th weeks may lead to actual occlusion of the lumen, especially in proximal areas. The lumen is reestablished in the 9th and 10th week, and a simple columnar epithelium is again found by the 12th week of gestation.

Villi form first in the proximal intestine during the 9th week, and villi emerge in successively more distal regions over the ensuing days. Villus formation appears to be complete by the end of the 3rd month of gestation. The mechanism of villus formation in humans is unclear, but in the stratified epithelium of the near-term fetal rat small intestine and colon, secondary lumina are identified, which are thought to play a crucial role in the formation of the villi.[11] These lumina are found surrounding the main lumen and are joined by continuous tight junctions. The secondary lumina

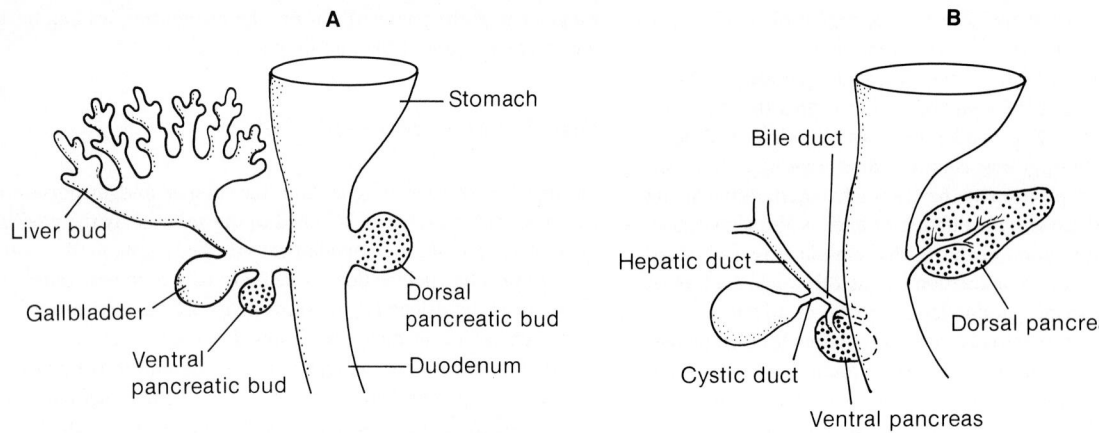

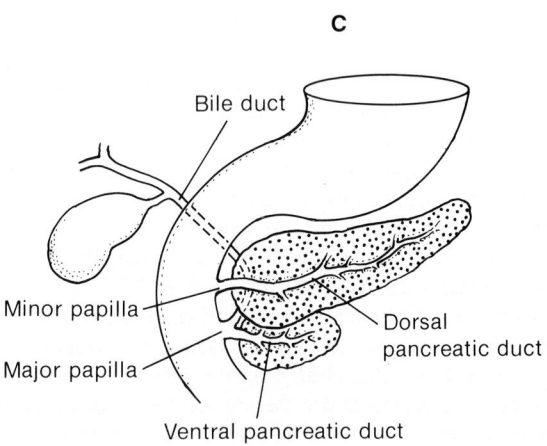

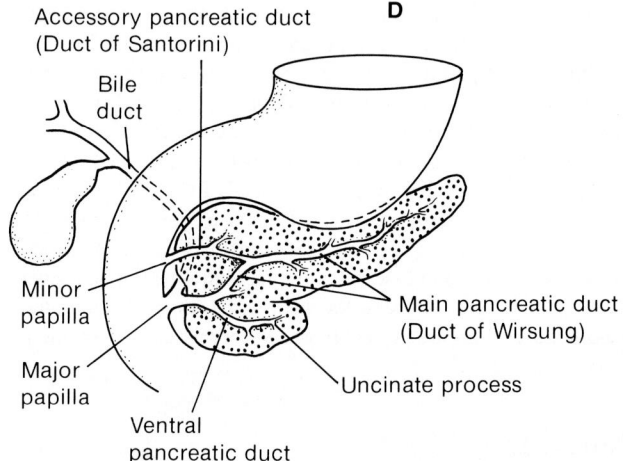

FIGURE 23–2. Successive stages in the maturation of the pancreas. **A,** The pancreas at 4 weeks. Note the location of the ventral bud arising form the primitive hepatobiliary system (hepatic diverticulum). **B,** The pancreas at 5 weeks. Note the rapid growth and elongation of the dorsal bud. **C,** The pancreas at 6 weeks. Note the migration of the ventral pancreatic bud to join the inferior portion of the dorsal bud. **D,** The pancreatic ductal system at 6 weeks. The main pancreatic duct joins the bile duct to enter the duodenum at the major papilla. The accessory pancreatic duct enters the duodenum at the minor papilla. (Adapted from Sadler TW, ed. Langman's medical embryology. Baltimore: Williams & Wilkins, 1985.)

enlarge and eventually fuse with the main lumen, leaving a villus outpouching. Crypt formation begins in the 10th to 12th weeks of gestation and also appear in a proximal to distal temporal sequence. Brunner's glands appear later in the 13th and 14th weeks.

The four cell types found within the intestinal epithelium (absorptive columnar, goblet, enteroendocrine, and Paneth's cells) appear to arise from a common progenitor cell present in the mid to high crypt (see below). Recent studies using both chimeric and transgenic mice and a number of cellular markers have demonstrated that the crypts in mature animals are clonal products of single progenitor cells (i.e., all cells in a single crypt appear to arise from a single stem cell).[12] However, related observations suggest that during initial development crypts are, in fact, polyclonal and that entrenchment of a single stem cell must be established during development through competitive mechanisms, which are as yet unknown.

The intestinal tube is initially surrounded by a layer of mesoderm that ultimately forms connective tissue, muscle, and serosa.

As in gastric mucosa, enteroendocrine cells can be detected by the 8th week of gestation, with early differentiation of the various cell types. The circular muscle layer can be discerned by the 8th week, followed closely by the emergence of the longitudinal muscle layer. The muscularis mucosa develops later but is present throughout the bowel by the 20th week of gestation. Auerbach's plexus can be found by the 9th week, and Meissner's plexus can be found by the 13th week. Peyer's patches emerge later, at approximately the 20th week.[13]

The histogenesis of the colon is similar to that of the small intestine. Interestingly, colonic villi, not found in the term infant, appear during embryonic life (10 to 12 weeks) but subsequently disappear during the second trimester.

The molecular mechanisms controlling formation of the different organs of the gastrointestinal tract are not understood. Recent observations suggest that mammalian homologues of the homeobox gene family initially recognized to control body segmentation in *Drosophila melanogaster* may be important in this

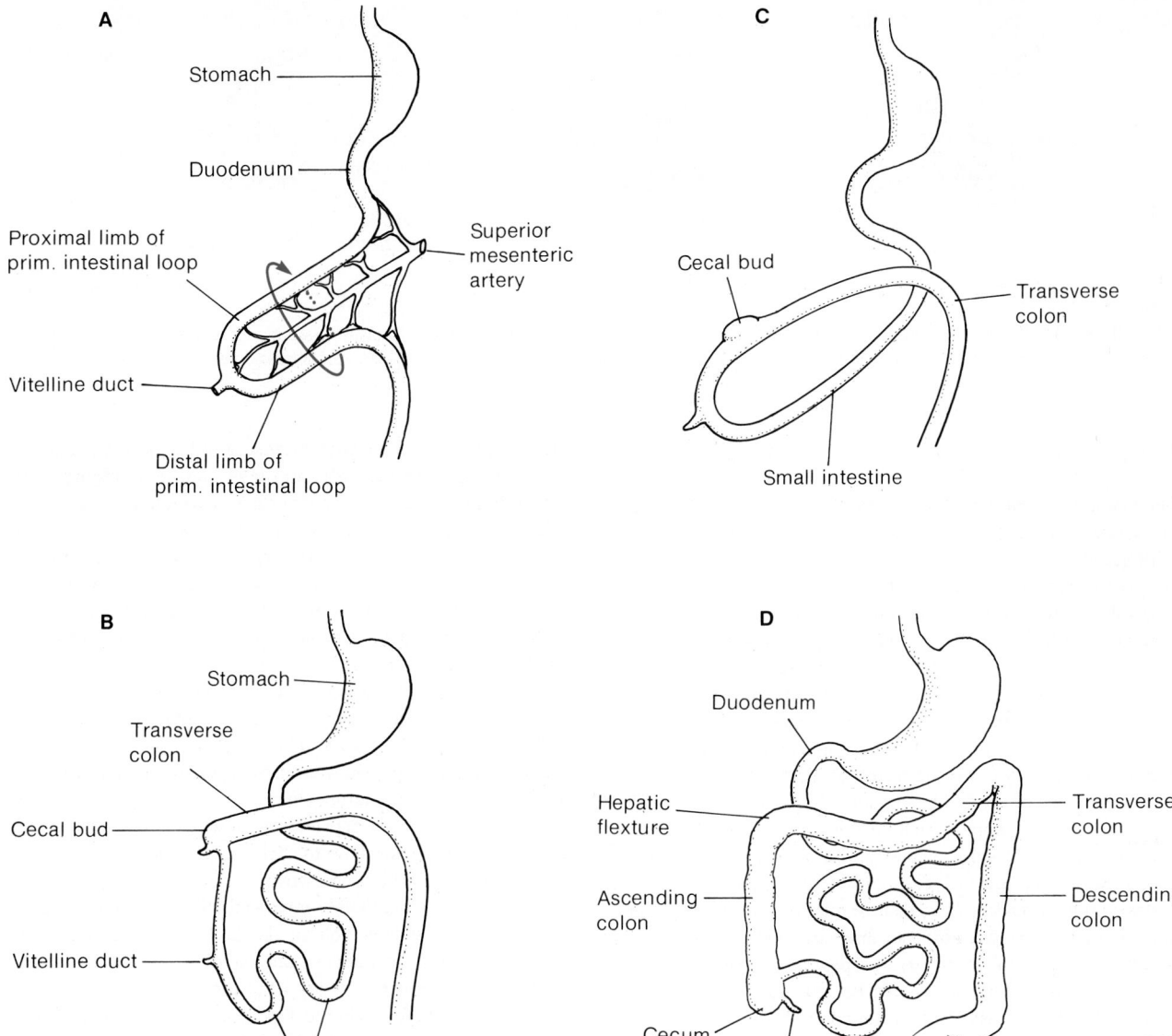

FIGURE 23–3. Migration of the intestinal loops. **A,** The intestine after a 90-degree rotation around the axis of the superior mesenteric artery, the proximal loop on the right and the distal loop on the left. **B,** The intestinal loop after a further 180-degree rotation. Note that the transverse colon passes in front of the duodenum. **C,** Position of the intestinal loops after reentry into the abdominal cavity. Note the elongation of the small intestine with formation of the small intestine loops. **D,** Final position of the intestines following descent of the cecum into the right iliac fossa. (Adapted from Sadler TW, ed. Langman's medical embryology. Baltimore: Williams & Wilkins, 1985.)

process.[14] Homeobox-family genes have also been characterized recently in mouse[15] and human[16] models. Transgenic mice created using Hox-l.4, a mouse homeoboxlike gene, are expressed at elevated levels in embryonic gut and are associated with alterations in the development of the mouse colon, which lead to the appearance of megacolon.[17]

FUNCTIONAL MATURATION

While the structural features of the gastrointestinal tract are well developed by the end of the second trimester, functional maturation continues throughout fetal gestation and into postnatal life. In general, human gastrointestinal functional development is precocious, with appearance of a wide spectrum of capabilities well in advance of the time that they are needed. In contrast, many functional activities of other animal species occur only when dictated by the stimulus of weaning (altricial development).[18] Development of many absorptive and enzymatic activities in rodents coincide with weaning—a process that begins in the 3rd week of life. However, much of our knowledge of gastrointestinal tract functional development has been gained through study of rodent and other animal models, and, therefore, these are also considered in the discussion below.

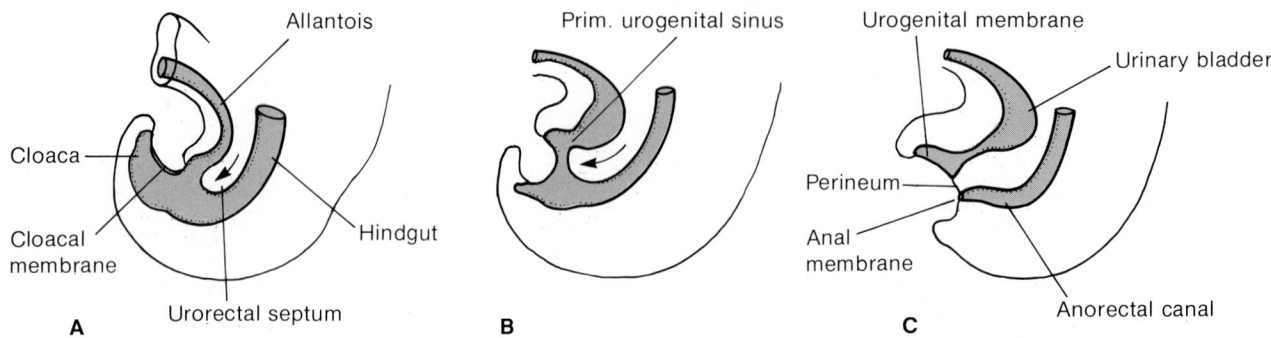

FIGURE 23–4. Successive stages of development of the cloacal region. The urorectal septum grows toward the cloacal membrane to form the perineum by 8 weeks' gestation. (Adapted from Sadler TW, ed. Langman's medical embryology. Baltimore: Williams & Wilkins, 1985.)

Esophagus

Fetal swallowing has been noted as early as the 16th to 17th weeks of gestation in humans.[19] The rate of fetal swallowing increases with gestational age, reaching 450 ml of amniotic fluid daily in the presence of a mean amniotic fluid volume of 850 ml at term.[19] The role of swallowing in the control of amniotic fluid volume remains unclear.[20] For the first 12 hours after birth, swallowing is poorly coordinated, with both a high peristaltic rate and frequent, nonperistaltic, simultaneous contractions throughout the length of the esophagus.[21] Postprandial reflux and regurgitation are common in the human neonate.[22] Lower esophageal sphincter (LES) pressure is only 2.5 mmHg at birth but increases to adult levels by 3 to 6 weeks of age.[23] This functional immaturity in the LES mechanism at birth appears to be shared by other animal species. The opossum esophagus demonstrates an age-dependent rise in LES pressure and increasing responsiveness of LES pressure to gastrin.[24] It has been suggested that the relatively low LES pressure in the newborn may result from an absence of mature or functional receptors for gastrin, insofar as this peptide appears to play an important role in maintenance of LES tone and adequate circulating and tissue levels have been found in the newborn.

Stomach

Gastric secretory function is not fully developed at birth in either humans or rats. The gastric mucosa of most animals, including humans, is capable of secreting some acid before birth.[25] In the rat, differentiation of gastric epithelial cells, including the appearance of parietal cells containing microvilli, is found in the final days of gestation. However, basal acid secretion is minimal until the neonatal rat begins to ingest solid food. By day 40 of life, basal acid secretion matches the adult level in the rat.[26] In humans, production rates for acid are less than 50% of adult values during the first 3 months of life and reach mature levels only after the age of 2 years.[27]

By the end of gestation, the rat appears to be capable of some response to all of the usual stimulants of gastric acid secretion, including gastrin, histamine, and an acetylcholine analogue (carbomylcholine).[28] However, this responsiveness is limited, and the animal appears to be relatively insensitive to gastrin before weaning.[28] Humans exhibit a similar relative insensitivity to gastrin in the neonatal period. Gastrin insensitivity has been attributed to both fewer gastrin receptors and lower intrinsic activity of the receptors present in the neonate than those found in the mature infant and adult.[29] Nearly normal gastric acid response to cholinergic stimulation has been demonstrated at birth,[30] while the gastric secretory response to histamine[31] is less than that observed in later life in a manner similar to that observed for gastrin.

Secretion of pepsinogen and peptic activity can be detected in parallel with acid secretion in the near-term rat stomach. In humans, pepsinogen secretion has been found to be less than 50% of adult levels during the first 3 months of life but slowly rises to full activity by age 2 years. The mucous neck cell may be the primary source of pepsinogen in the neonate, in contrast to the older infant in whom mature chief cells, which appear after birth, are the major source of pepsinogen. Gastric pepsinogen secretion also appears to be responsive to cholinergic stimulation at an earlier age than that observed for gastrin or histamine stimulation in a manner similar to that found for parietal cell acid secretory activity. Intrinsic factor is detectable in the gastric mucosa by the 14th week of gestation in humans and rapidly increases after birth, achieving mature levels by day 10 of life.[27]

Gastrin can be found in the duodenal mucosa by the 11th week of gestation and has been localized to antral cells by the 19th to 20th weeks of gestation in humans.[32] In the rat, tissue levels rise slowly in the postnatal period until weaning, when antral gastrin levels rise dramatically.[33] However, neonatal hypergastrinemia has been found in humans,[34] dogs,[35] and rats[36] soon after birth. The presence of hypergastrinemia in association with the apparent limited functional response to gastrin has led to the concept that the neonatal mucosa may lack adequate numbers of gastrin receptors or, alternatively, that receptors remain "immature." However, neonatal hypergastrinemia itself may simply result from secretion of insufficient acid to inhibit gastrin release. Hypergastrinemia could also reflect insensitivity to somatostatin, which serves to modulate gastrin inhibition in the mature individual. Although administration of somatostatin does not inhibit gastrin release on day 10 or day 15 in the rat, it does lower gastrin levels by day 18, suggesting that the antral mucosa is capable of response to somatostatin before the time of weaning.[36]

Many of the maturational changes observed in the stomach of laboratory animal species occur at the time of weaning.[37] However, some of these associations may be coincidental, and it appears that many ontogenetic functional changes can occur in the absence of weaning. Although the rate of increase and the maximum tissue levels are somewhat lower in the unweaned animal, temporally antral gastrin levels rise at the same age in weaned and unweaned rats.[33] Subsequently, serum gastrin levels also fall at the same age in weaned and unweaned rats.[29] (The effects of diet on functional maturation are discussed in more detail in the section entitled "The Small Intestine.")

In the rat, concentrations of free cortisone rise immediately before the onset of the weaning and reach a peak during the weaning process.[38] In the rat neonate, injection of ACTH or glucocorticoids causes a precocious rise in gastric pepsinogen levels,[39] premature appearance of gastrin receptors,[40] an earlier rise in antral gastrin levels, and an earlier induction of acid secretion responsive to histamine, carbachol, and pentagastrin (Fig 23-5).[38] Conversely, adrenalectomy delays the rise in antral gastrin levels and the development of gastrin receptors by almost a week, although delayed development does occur despite adrenalectomy, and eventually achieves normal levels. These maturational delays can be prevented by administration of corticosterone. Sensitivity to the effect of glucocorticoids appears to be present for a limited time interval. No effects of corticosteroid on subsequent gastric functional maturation are observed in the rat when administered after the 3rd week of life. Thyroxine also causes a precocious rise in pepsinogen activity,[41] an effect that is additive to that of glucocorticoid. Estrogens reduce food intake, acid secretion, serum gastrin levels, and the number of gastrin receptors in the female or castrated male rat. However, the functional significance of this in humans is unknown.[42]

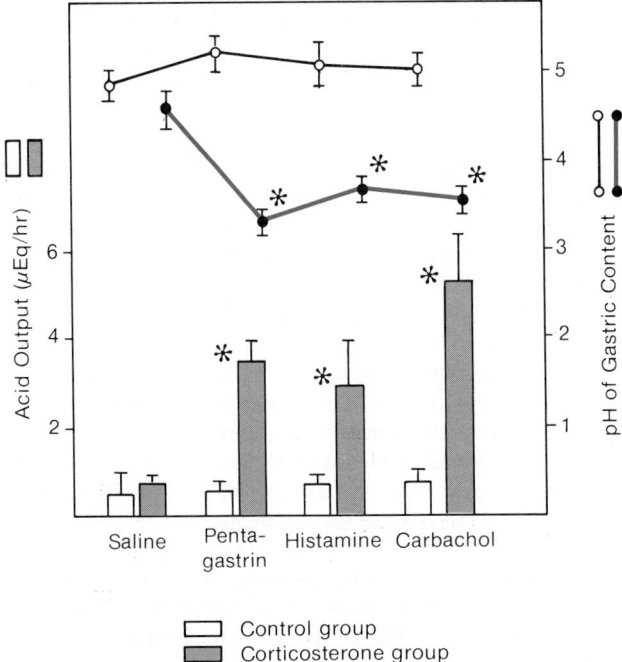

FIGURE 23–5. Gastric acid secretion in rats: effect of corticosterone on the response to pentagastrin (250 mg/kg), histamine (10 mg/kg), or carbachol (40 mg/kg). Rats were injected with 200 mg/kg corticosterone acetate on day 8, and secretory testing was done on day 12. Each point or bar represents mean (±) SE of means of six observations. *$P < 0.05$ compared with controls injected with 1% methylcellulose on day 8 instead of corticosterone. (From Ikezaki M, Johnson LR. Development of sensitivity to different secretagogues in the rat stomach. Am J Physiol 1983;244: G165.)

The Small Intestine

The ontogeny of small intestinal function has received more attention than that of any other part of the gastrointestinal tract. Study of this topic can be divided into (1) the development of digestive function, including hydrolysis and absorption of various nutrients and (2) effects of diet, hormones, peptide growth factors, and bacterial colonization on these processes.

CARBOHYDRATE DIGESTION AND ABSORPTION

Lactase activity may be detected early in fetal life, with measurable, if low, levels present before the 12th week of gestation in humans (Table 23-1).[43] Significant increase in this activity occurs after the 24th week, and a late gestational surge is observed throughout the entire third trimester. In rodents, this burst of activity is observed only at the end of the third trimester. After birth, the rat, as well as a number of other mammals, has high lactase levels, which fall at the time of weaning in association with a change from a diet rich in maternal milk lactose to a laboratory diet rich in sucrose and starch as primary carbohydrate source.

Humans also demonstrate high lactase activity at birth, but the decrease in activity does not correlate well temporally with weaning, and humans are the only known species in which lactase activity does not uniformly fall in the postweaning period. Paradoxically, disaccharidase activities, such as sucrase, maltase, isomaltase, and trehalase, which should be physiologically unnecessary before weaning, are already present by the 10th week of gestation at 60% to 70% of human adult levels (see Table 23-1). Glucoamylase, a microvillus enzyme, has been detected as early as the 10th week of gestation in a manner similar to that found with the disaccharidase activities. Seventy percent of adult levels are achieved by the 26th to 34th weeks of gestation.[44] Salivary amylase can be detected in the 20th week of gestation and increases with fetal age.[45] Proximal to distal gradients for lactase and the other glucosidase activities can be demonstrated in the 17th week of gestation with maximal activities in the proximal jejunum and progressively less of these enzymatic activities along the more distal portions of the small intestine.[46,47]

In contrast to humans, induction of adult levels of these disaccharidase activities is only observed during postnatal weaning in rodents. In the rat, maltase activity is low in the first 2 postnatal weeks but increases 5- to 10-fold in the 2 weeks after weaning.[48] Sucrase, isomaltase, and trehalase are undetectable before weaning but rise to adult levels by the 4th week of life. This pattern differs, as noted above, from the precocious pattern of human development in which activity of the α-glucosidases rises during fetal life and reaches adult levels by term.[49]

Pancreatic amylase activity has been demonstrated in the human fetus as early as the 22nd week of gestation but reaches only 10% of adult levels by term.[50] Although the secretory apparatus for pancreatic amylase appears to be mature by the time of parturition, only small amounts of pancreatic amylase are detectable in the small intestinal lumen of the rat during the first 2 postnatal weeks. In the human newborn, pancreatic amylase remains low for 4 to 6 months after birth; adult levels are achieved by 2 years of age.[50] Other sources of amylase may play important functional roles during the human neonatal period. These include intestinal glu-

TABLE 23-1
Specific Activities of Disaccharidases in the Mid-jejunum of Developing Human Fetuses

GESTATIONAL AGE (wk)	LACTASE (μm/g/min)	SUCRASE (μm/g/min)	MALTASE (μm/g/min)	ISOMALTASE (μm/g/min)
10–14	6.1 ± 2.2	52.1 ± 15.1	129.2 ± 37.6	10.1 ± 2.9
14–16	7.2 ± 3.7	62.1 ± 35.0	138.7 ± 57.3	10.3 ± 5.5
16–24	7.6 ± 2.5	80.7 ± 28.0	172.1 ± 62.3	13.5 ± 4.4

Adapted from Antonowicz I, Chang SK, Grand RJ. Development and distribution of lysosomal enzymes and disaccharidases in human fetal intestine. Gastroenterology 1974;67:51 © by Williams & Wilkins, 1974.

coamylase activity, which is present at 50% to 100% of adult levels at birth.[51] Salivary amylase has been detected in gastric aspirates of premature infants[52,53] and may play a role in polysaccharide digestion in early life. In addition, maternal mammary amylase is present in milk and probably aids in the breakdown of starch in the neonate.[54]

Uptake of glucose against a concentration gradient is demonstrable in both jejunum and ileum at the 11th to 19th weeks of gestation in the human.[55] Active sodium-dependent transport can be demonstrated by the 19th day of gestation in fetal rat ileum.[56] The longitudinal gradient in the level of glucose transport, well-documented in the mature intestine, is present early in development. Higher levels are present in the jejunum than in the ileum by the 11th to 19th week in the human fetus.[57,58]

Hexose transport increases in the first few days after birth in both experimental animal and humans. While a peak in transport activity is observed on the 10th day in the rat,[59] the maximal capacity for glucose absorption continues to increase in humans. However, the rate of glucose absorption in infants is comparable to that observed in adults at low glucose loads. The increase in absorptive capacity may reflect either an increase in the number of transporters or an increased efficiency of the transporters present.[60] Development of galactose transport parallels that of glucose and uses the same sodium-dependent carrier. However, galactose uptake is competitively inhibited by glucose uptake.[57]

PROTEIN DIGESTION AND ABSORPTION

The pancreas secretes inactive forms of proteolytic enzymes that are activated after cleavage of trypsinogen to trypsin by enterocyte-derived enterokinase. Subsequently, trypsin acts on the other precursor pancreatic proteolytic enzymes to facilitate their activation. The pancreas appears to be functionally immature in its capacity for protease synthesis and secretion during the early neonatal period in a manner similar to that observed for amylase. It is unclear whether synthesis or secretion of proenzymes is rate limiting in the neonatal pancreas. Trypsin activity is occasionally demonstrable in the 16-week-old fetus.[61] Morphologically, mature zymogen granules can be demonstrated as early as the 20th week of gestation in the human fetus. When enterokinase is added to the pancreatic extracts, maximal tryptic activity can be shown at approximately the 24th week of gestation.[62] Trypsin and chymotrypsin activities depend on activation of enterokinase, and its activity is only 6% of adult levels in the 26th to 30th week of

gestation and remains at 20% of adult levels even at the time of parturition.[48,63]

Microvillar dipeptidase enzymes, which complete peptide digestion, are detected throughout the length of the small intestine in the 11-week-old fetus.[64] Adult levels of dipeptidase activity have been demonstrated in the 14- to 16-week-old fetus.[65] As noted for other microvillar hydrolases, concentrations of dipeptidases are generally found on a longitudinal gradient with highest levels in the proximal intestine. Leucine aminopeptidase is an exception to this general organization and is found in an opposite differential distribution with distal activity twice that of proximal activity in the 16th week of gestation.[66]

In the rat, very small amounts of trypsin and chymotrypsin, as well as lipase and amylase (see below), are found in the small bowel lumen during the first 2 postnatal weeks but increase dramatically with weaning during the 3rd postnatal week.[67] However, chymotrypsin, carboxypeptidase, and enterokinase activities are much lower than those found in the adult.[48] At 1 month of age, no stimulation of trypsin and minimal stimulation of chymotrypsin can be shown in response to CCK or secretin administration,[48,68] suggesting that regulatory controls remain incompletely developed, even when the pancreas has acquired the capacity for nearly mature levels of protease production. Brush border and cytosolic peptidases are present at adult levels in the neonate and aid in proteolysis in neonatal life.[69]

Active amino acid transport has been demonstrated in fetal tissue. Uptake of L-alanine against a concentration gradient has been demonstrated in everted gut sacs from 11- to 19-week-old fetuses.[70] Indeed, at the time of birth, levels appear to be essentially equivalent to the adult. However, detailed information on the uptake of amino acids across the spectrum of amino acid transporters is limited, and it is possible that differential patterns of expression occur.[71]

In the fetus and neonate, macromolecular transport plays an important role in the digestion of both proteins and lipids. At least in experimental animals, the small intestinal epithelium appears to be more permeable to amino acids and peptides in the immediate postnatal period than in the mature intestine. Macromolecular tracers infused into amniotic fluid or the intestinal lumen late in gestation are absorbed into enterocytes of humans, monkeys, guinea pigs, and rats. This process does not take place by a paracellular pathway but, instead, reflects a high rate of pinocytosis.[72] The rat small intestine is capable of pinocytosis by the 19th or 20th day of gestation.[73] This process is extremely active in the first 2 postnatal weeks and decreases dramatically with weaning.[74] Sites of absorption of different proteins vary in the rat. Intact immunoglobulins are transported in the jejunum but not the ileum by way of IgG-receptor complexes on the jejunal enterocytes.[75] Nutritional proteins undergo pinocytosis in the ileum in a nonspecific manner.[76] Pinocytosis of both nutritional proteins and immunoglobulins decreases at weaning, although the adult rat can still absorb small amounts of intact protein.[77] In parallel with the extensive use of pinocytosis, enterocytes exhibit high levels of lysosomal proteases, such as cathepsins and other peptidases, during the first 2 postnatal weeks, but these levels fall thereafter. These intracellular enzymes provide a mechanism for protein digestion before the maturation of the mechanisms necessary for production and secretion of pancreatic proteolytic enzymes.[78]

Differences in the microvillar membrane surface have been demonstrated between neonate and adult animals. The neonatal microvillar membrane is more fluid than the adult membrane, perhaps accounting for increased penetration of antigens and organisms through the newborn GI surface.[79] Surface glycoconjugates, which may be involved in the attachment of certain bacteria and antigens, are also different in newborn and adult animals. Thus, *N*-acetylglucosamine, which is a site for *Shigella* toxin binding, appears in higher concentration in newborns, while *N*-acetylgalactosamine, which contributes to binding of *Vibrio cholerae*, is not detectable in the newborn microvillus membranes.[80] Two common food antigens, β-lactoglobulin and bovine serum albumin, bind more avidly to newborn membranes, perhaps contributing to the increased antigen uptake found in the newborn period. Cortisone or thyroxine injections have been shown to modulate both membrane fluidity and glycoconjugate composition.[81]

Intact proteins are also absorbed in premature and term human infants during the first few months of life.[82] Macromolecules may continue to cross the healthy adult small intestine, but the amounts are extremely low compared to those observed in the newborn. Imperfect barrier function during the first months of life may play an important role in conferring either tolerance or sensitivity to a number of dietary proteins.

LIPID DIGESTION AND ABSORPTION

Lipase has been detected in pancreatic extracts of human fetuses in the 16th week of gestation.[83] While levels rise significantly during the third trimester, in the 32nd week of gestation lipase activity remains only 50% of term levels, which are themselves only 10% of the levels found in adults.[48] The human neonate also has lingual lipase activity, which rises to adult levels by 2 years of age.[68] The relatively low levels of lipase may contribute to the presence of unhydrolyzed triglycerides in the feces of neonates. In the human, as in the rat, lingual lipase and maternal milk lipase both aid in neonatal fat digestion.[84] A lipase of gastric origin has been recognized in infants with esophageal atresia. However, the precise role of this activity in digestion is unknown.[85]

Lingual lipase is produced in the serous glands of the tongue and appears to aid in the digestion of milk triglycerides in neonatal rats, mainly through hydrolysis in the stomach.[84,86] In the rat, lingual lipase is present in very small amounts at birth and increases markedly at weaning.[85] Maternal milk lipase also plays a role in fat digestion. The relative importance of these lipases in the economy of dietary lipid remains controversial.

TABLE 23–2

Relationship Between Pancreatic Lipase Activity and Fat Intake in Newborn and Adult Rats

AGE	PANCREATIC LIPASE (μ/g)	FAT INTAKE (kJ/100 g wt/24 hr)
Suckling, 10 days old	200	25.536
Adult	1700	10.584

From Hamosh M. A review. Fat digestion in the newborn: Role of lingual lipase and preduodenal digestion. Pediatr Res 1979;13:615.

Synthesis of bile acids from cholesterol and conjugation with taurine and glycine can be demonstrated in human liver organ culture in vitro obtained from fetuses in the 15th week of gestation.[87] Biliary secretion can be demonstrated as early as the 22nd week of gestation.[88] Bile acid reabsorption also occurs but does not appear to reflect the presence of the specific active transport present in adult ileum and may instead result from nonspecific processes including pinocytosis and increased intestinal permeability.

Both secretion and reabsorption of bile acids are lower in suckling rats than in adults. Most importantly, bile acid concentrations are initially too low to facilitate the formation of micelles.[84] In the neonatal period, before the maturation of bile acid secretion and reabsorption, as well as the mature production of pancreatic lipase, the suckling rats' small intestine has increased permeability to lipid, which may be absorbed intact as triglyceride.[89]

The lipoproteins required for chylomicron production are abundant in the small intestine of the suckling rat, and chylomicrons can be formed and presumably transported into lymphatic channels.[90]

After weaning, the dietary content of fat decreases, pancreatic lipase activity matures (Table 23-2), and fewer large lipid particles are seen in the enterocyte. Ileal bile acid absorption also begins at this time, reaching adult capacity after 1 month in the rat.[91] In human neonates, bile acid synthesis is present at relatively high levels (Table 23-3). However, ileal resorptive mechanisms are not yet mature, and a reduction in the actual bile acid pool results.[92] In premature infants, this reduction is even more severe (see Table 23-3) so that 10% to 20% of fat intake in formula-fed premature infants may not be absorbed.[93] During the first 4 to 6 weeks of human life, intraluminal bile acid levels increase as absorptive mechanisms mature, leading to improved lipid absorption.

TABLE 23–3

Bile Salt Synthesis in Premature and Newborn Infants

AGE	CHOLIC ACID POOL (mg/m²)	CHOLIC ACID SYNTHESIS (mg/m²/day)
Premature	85 ± 20	34 ± 6
Full-term	290 ± 36	110 ± 20
Adult	600 ± 20	190 ± 25

From Hamosh M. A review. Fat digestion in the newborn: Role of lingual lipase and preduodenal digestion. Pediatr Res 1979;13:615.

VITAMINS AND MINERALS

Copper, iron, magnesium, and zinc are all absorbed by the suckling rat small intestine in increased amounts, but rates of absorption decline to normal during the weaning period.[94,95] Lead, cadmium, radium, plutonium, barium, and other toxic heavy metals are also absorbed more easily in the suckling than adult rat. Active transport of calcium occurs throughout the rat small intestine and colon before weaning but appears to depend on mechanisms distinct from those in the mature mucosa. This absorption is uniform throughout the intestine and does not require vitamin D, in contrast to the vitamin D-dependent uptake mechanisms concentrated in the duodenum that appear in the 4th postnatal week.[94,96]

Human neonates absorb iron, copper, calcium and zinc well.[97,98] They also absorb lead more efficiently than adults.[99] Although the mechanisms remain uncertain, these processes clearly can facilitate lead intoxication. Inadequate bone mineralization is a common problem in premature human infants. This is not thought to result from a lack of absorptive capacity but an insufficient supply of calcium in maternal or formula milk, insofar as simple calcium supplementation corrects the calcium imbalance.[18]

Vitamin absorption in the newborn has not been extensively studied. Impaired absorption of fat-soluble vitamins is present in neonates and likely reflects the same pattern of impaired absorption of all lipids. Vitamin B_{12} absorption has been demonstrated in the rat neonate.[100] Folate absorption is impaired in the human neonate and infant compared to the adult.[101] Recently, biotin transport was found to be higher in the ileum than in the jejunum of suckling rats, equal in both parts of the small intestine in weanlings, and higher in the jejunum than the ileum of adult rats.[102]

MODULATION OF INTESTINAL MATURATION

Role of Diet. During weaning, a process that is temporally determined in most species but widely variable in humans, the infant GI tract is exposed to a dramatic change in dietary composition. Maternal milk is high in fat and low in carbohydrate, while a "conventional" diet generally includes relatively high amounts of carbohydrate and low fat content. Furthermore, the dominant carbohydrate source changes from lactose to a more varied mixture, usually dominated by sucrose and starch. As discussed earlier, many of the maturational changes of the small intestine occur at the same time as weaning, leading to the supposition that dietary composition is an important factor contributing to these ontogenic changes. While this relationship may be important in the rodent, in humans it appears that dietary factors are not essential to the expression of many functional activities that emerge before the weaning process. Interestingly, lactase exhibits an accelerated surge before parturition, which suggests that the birth process (and possibly hormonal factors related to it) rather than dietary challenge regulate expression of this activity.

Even in rodents, the importance of dietary components in triggering changes in various activities during weaning may be limited, and it has been found that similar changes occur at almost the same time in rats prevented from weaning.[103] Early weaning has been associated with precocious maturation, but premature weaning also elevates glucocorticoid levels, and these too can result in precocious digestive tract maturation (see below).[54] Other observations that suggest that dietary factors do not play a major role in small intestinal development have been obtained through studies using intestinal explants. Despite subsequent implantation into the kidney,[104] subcutaneous space,[105] or culture in vitro,[106] the normal pattern of functional maturation has been observed. Further, rat ileum that is bypassed by surgical implantation at 12 to 14 days of age has been found to express sucrase and maltase activity in the normal temporal framework.[107] It should also be noted that intestinal explants from 6-day-old rats cultured in the absence of hormones cannot be induced to precocious expression of sucrase or maltase.[107] Finally, as noted, human ontogeny is poorly coordinated with weaning, removing diet as a primary candidate for human ontogenetic control.

While dietary factors may not fundamentally regulate the temporal sequence of gastrointestinal development, they may be able to modulate the process. Thus, humans or rats fed a diet high in maltose or sucrose exhibit increased maltase or sucrase activity, but not lactase activity.[108] Similarly, feeding lactose appears to increase the level of brush border membrane lactase in rats.[109] In the rabbit, increased oral nutrition results in precocious maturation of the small intestine, as evidenced by lower lactase and higher sucrase activity in the brush border membrane, which is associated with accelerated weight gain. However, the contribution of glucocorticoid or other factors has not been excluded.[110] Malnourished suckling rats display delayed patterns of mucosal enzyme development, which can be reversed by refeeding.[111] Interestingly, in experimental studies, bypassed segments maintain high levels of lactase activity while decreased lactase activity is found in segments of the intestine left in continuity.[107] Clinically, a high-protein diet has been reported to stimulate greater pancreatic secretion of trypsin and lipase in premature infants.[112]

Although nutrients in the diet appear to have a limited impact on intestinal maturation, other substances present in food, especially maternal milk, may have an effect on these processes. Pig,[113] rabbit,[114] and dog[115] neonates in their first 24 hours postpartum experience greater increases in small intestine weight, size, and DNA or protein content when fed colostrum than when fed an artificial diet. In the rat, neonates fed colostrum were also found to have increased small intestinal DNA content and synthesis, although intestinal weight was not significantly different from that of neonatal rats fed mature milk.[116] In guinea pigs, no differences between natural and artificial feeding were found in full-term neonates. However, a trophic effect of colostrum was found in this species in the premature animal.[116] Thus, the time frame in which factors in colostrum or breast milk exert an effect on gastrointestinal tract development may vary among different animal species.[117]

These observations suggest that constituents present in the diet other than conventional nutrients may play a role in modulating functional maturation. What are the potential growth factors contained in breast milk? Epidermal growth factor (EGF) has been demonstrated in high concentrations in human, mouse, and rat milk.[118–121] The concentration of EGF is greater in colostrum than in mature milk.[122] Interestingly, the near-term infant and rat neonate have been reported to have high concentrations of EGF receptors throughout the enterocyte population. However, the number of EGF receptor appears to decline markedly after birth. Recently, it has been shown that EGF is present throughout the lumen of the GI tract of the rat and is present at higher levels in the intestinal lumen of suckling than of adult rats. These levels directly correlate with the milk intake, implicating milk as an important source of EGF in the suckling period.[123]

In addition to EGF, human milk also contains a mitogenic compound that resembles nerve growth factor, although its role in digestive development remains unclear.[124] Somatomedin-C, a peptide with insulinlike activity also known as insulinlike growth factor type II (IGF-II), is found in human milk and colostrum. The peptide is protein-bound but released after treatment with acid.[125] Insulin, too, is found in both colostrum and milk, and, if administered to a neonate mouse, premature development of sucrase activity has been observed.[126] Furthermore, glucocorticoids and thyroxine, which may play important roles in gastrointestinal maturation (see below), are present in human milk, although not in physiologically significant quantities.[127] Formula containing varying amounts of corticosterone has been shown to result in intestinal expression of sucrase and maltase activity in adrenalectomized rats only when the formula contains a concentration of corticosterone considerably higher than that found in maternal milk.[128] This concentration produces a serum level similar to that of 18- to 20-day-old control rats, when sucrase and maltase activities are normally expressed.

Hormones and Peptide Growth Factors. Although nutrients in the diet may modify some ontogenic changes of the gastrointestinal tract, hormones and peptide growth factors may play a more direct role. Among these factors, glucocorticoids have the most well-documented impact on intestinal development. Tissue concentrations of free corticosterone rise 48 hours before the appearance of the enzymatic changes associated with weaning (Fig 23-6).[38] This observation suggests that weaning may promote development indirectly through induction of changes in corticosteroid concentration. In addition, administration of glucocorticoids to

rats or mice during the suckling period results in premature decreases in pinocytosis, lactase levels, and lysosomal hydrolases, as well as premature increases in sucrase, maltase, trehalase, peptidase, pancreatic and salivary amylase, pepsinogen, and gastrin receptor levels.[18] The spectrum of effects suggests that glucocorticoid modifies functional development throughout the gastrointestinal tract. The effect of glucocorticoids can also be found when intestinal mucosal explants are exposed in vitro in the absence of other confounding factors.

Age appears to be an important determinant of the response to glucocorticoids.[129] Glucocorticoids have been found to accelerate the rate of cellular proliferation of the suckling, but not the adult rat.[130] The concentration of glucocorticoid receptors in the intestinal mucosa peaks at the time of weaning in the rat,[131] and hypophysectomy is associated with decreased intestinal sucrase activity in suckling rats, which can be normalized by administration of cortisone. Glucocorticoid levels rise at 12 to 14 days of age in the rat, but intestinal enzyme levels do not respond to glucocorticoid administration after 16 to 17 days. Similarly, enzyme levels are not stimulated by glucocorticoids in rats adrenalectomized after 17 to 18 days of age.[132] Thus, there appears to be a "window" period when glucocorticoids can influence small intestinal maturation. Although adrenalectomy slows the rate of enzymatic changes at weaning in the rat, the changes begin at approximately the same time and eventually reach the same levels as those of sham-operated controls.[133] These studies suggest that these changes may be genetically programmed and glucocorticoids are not essential. Genetic programming would explain the preservation of the normal temporal development of sucrase, lactase, maltase, and β-galactosidase activity in fetal rat or mouse intestine when transplanted into an adult.

In humans, prenatal administration of glucocorticoids decreases the incidence of necrotizing enterocolitis in the neonate, a disease

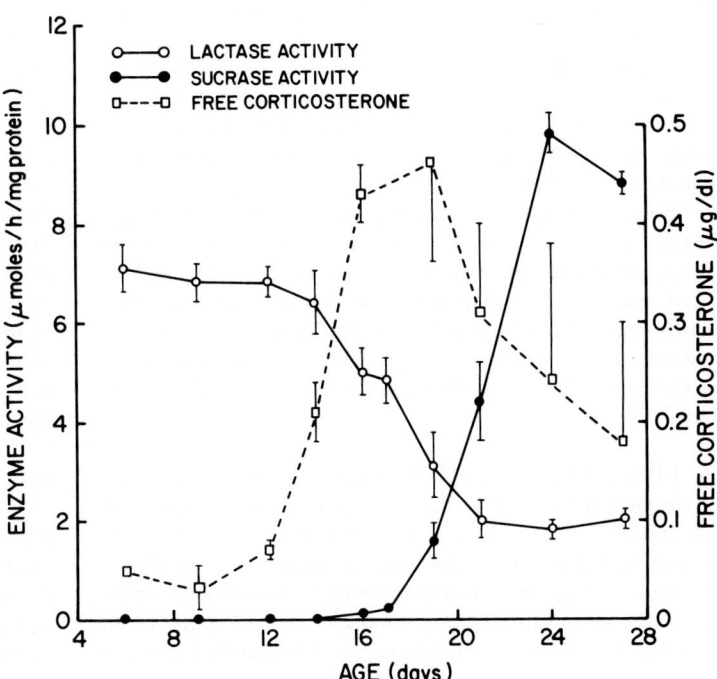

FIGURE 23–6. Development of activity of lactase and sucrase in jejunal mucosa as compared with free corticosterone in plasma. Values are given as means (±) SE for five rats. Absence of error bars indicates SE was smaller than symbol. (From: Henning SJ. Plasma concentrations of total and free corticosterone during development in the rat. Am J Physiol 1978;235:E451.)

associated with intestinal immaturity.[134] Glucocorticoids also influence the differentiation of human fetal intestine in organ culture.[135] Mothers who receive glucocorticoids in late pregnancy have been found to deliver neonates with higher bile salt pool size than neonates of the same age born to mothers who were not treated.[136]

Thyroxine has also been found to affect intestinal maturation, but interpretation of the mechanism is difficult because thyroxine leads to increased glucocorticoid levels.[137,138] Although hypothyroidism prevents or delays intestinal maturation, it also abolishes the developmental rise of corticosterone.[139] Further, the maturational delay in the expected rise in sucrase and related activity in hypothyroid fetuses can be reversed by administration of glucocorticoids without the addition of thyroxine.[131] However, thyroxine may still be important in certain aspects of gastrointestinal maturation. Administration of cortisone results in only partial restoration of reduced jejunal lactase activity after hypophysectomy; thyroxine fully restores this decline in the absence of any effect on corticosterone levels.[140]

As noted above, EGF is present in colostrum and maternal milk in many animal species, including humans. At weaning, the concentration of EGF in mouse maternal milk decreases[141] and endogenous sources of EGF increase markedly.[142] Although a number of workers have suggested that EGF may have important trophic effects throughout the gastrointestinal tract, the imprecise temporal relationship of declining maternal milk EGF concentrations to the augmented production from endogenous sources indicates that EGF is unlikely to play an essential role in the regulation of developmental changes. While EGF has been found to result in premature appearance of intestinal sucrase activity, alkaline phosphatase, and trehalase activities when administered before weaning, the effect is much smaller than that observed when glucocorticoids are given.[143] In addition, EGF administered orally has been shown to increase cell growth in the intestine and pancreas of neonatal rats,[144] although much of the administered (and endogenous) growth factor was undoubtedly degraded by proteolytic enzymes.

Bombesin, also known as gastrin-releasing peptide, stimulates gastric, colonic, and pancreatic cell growth in suckling rats.[145,146] A bombesinlike compound has been found in the breast milk of some mammals.[147] However, a physiologic role for bombesin in intestinal maturation has not been proven.

Exogenous insulin administered to suckling mice causes premature maturation of the small intestine.[148] Endogenous insulin levels rise during the weaning period in the rat,[149] although no clear role has been established for insulin in the maturation of the gastrointestinal tract. Prostacyclin (PGI_2) prematurely increases sucrase and maltase activity in suckling rats, and these effects occur even in the absence of glucocorticoids in adrenalectomized rats.[150,151]

Effect of Bacterial Colonization. Colonization of the gastrointestinal tract of human neonates occurs within a few days of delivery.[152] Therefore, gut bacteria have no role in fetal development but may play a role in postnatal development. Disaccharidase activity of germ-free rats is higher than that of control rats after weaning. In addition, introducing cecal contents of control rats into the small intestine causes disaccharidase levels to decrease to normal levels.[153] The intestinal wall of the germ-free rat is also considerably thinner with shallower crypts and a smaller mucosal surface area than control rats.[154] The importance of the response of the intestinal tract to the appearance of gut flora in its development remains unclear.

The Colon

Functional maturation of the colon has not been studied extensively. The fetal rat colon is capable of actively transporting glucose and alanine.[155] Administration of glucocorticoids to the fetal rat colon enhances sodium absorption, an effect not seen in the rat small intestine.[156] Calcium, strontium, and magnesium are also absorbed in the colon at much higher rates in suckling than in adult rats.[157,158]

GROWTH AND DIFFERENTIATION IN THE MATURE GI TRACT

Cellular Components

Undifferentiated stem cells are present throughout the gastrointestinal tract. In the small intestine, there is emerging appreciation of two classes of stem cells. By the 2nd postnatal week in rats, each crypt appears to be a monoclonal population derived from a single stem cell anchored approximately five cell positions from the base of the crypt.[12] This gives rise, directly or indirectly, to the four cell lineages present, the Paneth's cell (which migrates downward), the goblet, the enteroendocrine, and the most abundant columnar absorptive cell.[159] The latter three cell lines, which migrate up the villus, are thought to be the direct product of committed stem cells that derive from the anchored stem cell. The committed stem cells retain proliferative activity and reside in the middle zone of the crypt.[12]

An analogous organization may be present at other sites along the length of the gastrointestinal tract. In the stomach, neck cells located in the middle third of the gastric glands serve as stem cells for the mucus-secreting cells. They probably also differentiate into the specialized gastric, parietal, chief, G, and zymogen cells. In the esophageal mucosa, where the epithelium is squamous and stratified, proliferative stem cells are present in the basal layer and produce the squamous, nonproliferating cells that migrate to the luminal surface.[160]

The adult villus columnar cell in the small intestine undergoes significantly greater differentiation than its fetal counterpart. In early fetal life, columnar cells contain short microvilli and large glycogen deposits.[11] During later fetal life, the organelles of the columnar cells differentiate with the appearance and subsequent disappearance of the meconium corpuscle system and the apical tubular system. Columnar cells exhibit still further morphologic evolution during continued gestation, including a reduction in glycogen content, appearance of smooth endoplasmic reticulum, and the development of tall, uniform microvilli.[161] The mature villus cell is a highly polarized cell with a well-organized complex of endosomal compartments and markedly different apical and basolateral surface membranes. Furthermore, a gradient of functional differentiation is present in enterocytes along the vertical axis of the villus.

In the adult gastrointestinal tract, more than 10 distinct enteroendocrine cell types have been identified by their secretory products. In the stomach, the mucous neck cell is thought to be the stem cell for the enteroendocrine cell. The primary enteroendocrine cells in the gastric antrum are the G cell, which secretes gastrin, and the D cell, which secretes somatostatin. The gastric fundus also contains the A cell, which secretes enteroglucagon, and the argentaffin cell, which secretes serotonin and histamine. The small intestine contains enteroendocrine cells that migrate toward the villus tip, differentiating during this migration, as evidenced by an increase in the number of cytoplasmic granules and a progressive loss of the ability to divide.[162] Innovative studies using transgenic mice that express intestinal specific transgene products due to the presence of villus specific intestinal fatty acid binding protein promoters have demonstrated fundamental heterogeneity of enteroendocrine cell populations.[12,163,164] Differential expression of different products was seen among enteroendocrine cells in a single villus. Colonic enteroendocrine cells originate in the crypt base and demonstrate slow renewal, at least in rectal mucosa.[165]

As noted, Paneth cells appear to derive from stem cells in the middle zone of the crypt. The products of these cells are not completely known but include lysozyme, and it is likely that the Paneth cells contribute to the host mucosal defense system.[166] Paneth cells do not divide,[167] but migrate to the base of the crypt where they degenerate and are phagocytosed.

Tuft (caveolated) cells, first described in mouse gastric mucosa in 1955,[168] are widely distributed in the gastrointestinal tract.[169] Recognized by distinctive caveolae invaginating the apical surface between individual long microvilli, they appear to be highly differentiated cells that, in the small intestine, arise from stem cells in the lower parts of the crypts and migrate to be extruded in the villus. In mouse colon, tuft cells have an estimated turnover time of 8.2 days.[170] Although their function is unclear, tuft cells contain an extensive vesicular network consistent with a role in absorption. Recent recognition of these cells in two human colon carcinoma cell lines should enable further investigation of their function and structure.[171]

In addition to the cell types noted above, the intestinal mucosa contains the intestinal distinctive M cell, which is restricted to the dome epithelium overlying the lymphoid follicles of Peyer's patches in the ileum.[172] These cells appear to be important in sampling the antigenic milieu in the lumen. Ironically, they also appear to be the avenue of infection for a number of viral agents that can breach the mucosal barrier (e.g., reoviruses). Cells resembling adult M cells are first identified overlying lymphocyte aggregates in the distal small intestine in the 17th week of gestation, and their appearance is temporally related to the appearance of these lymphoid aggregates.[173] The M cell contains surface membranes with microfolds instead of microvilli and abundant vesicles, which may play a role in the transport of luminal antigens, mi-

croorganisms, and other macromolecules to the underlying lymphoid tissue.[174,175]

Cell Kinetics

The epithelium of the gastrointestinal tract undergoes rapid turnover in which cell production in zones of proliferation is usually balanced by cell extrusion, creating a steady state under normal conditions.[176] True growth occurs when the rate of cell proliferation is greater than the rate of cell loss. Only a selective population of cells in the gastrointestinal tract retain proliferative capability. The compartmentalization of proliferating populations and the zonal concentration of the nonproliferating cells committed to terminal differentiation are features shared by all regions of the luminal gastrointestinal tract. The kinetics of cell proliferation have been largely defined through analysis of labeled mitotic frequencies after administration of ^{3}H-thymidine to identify the fractional mitotic index. This analysis allows determination of the lengths of the constituent component phases of the cell cycle (S phase or DNA synthesis, G_1, a premitotic latent period, M mitosis, and G_2 a pre-DNA synthesis latent period; Table 23-4). Pulse labeling mucosal explants further permits estimation of mucosal turnover rates as cohorts of labeled cells complete mitosis and emerge from the zone of proliferation to traverse the vertical distance to surface mucosa before subsequent loss.

ESOPHAGUS

As a stratified squamous epithelium, the esophageal mucosa differs from that of the rest of the intestinal tract. However, as in other parts of the gastrointestinal tract, proliferation in the esophagus occurs in the basal layer. Turnover of the esophageal squamous epithelium takes 4 to 5 days in rats and mice, longer in humans.[179] After cell division, one daughter cell may remain in the basal layer, one may migrate toward the esophageal lumen, or both may migrate. The life span of the basal cell in the esophagus is 80 hours in rats and mice and approaches 8 days in humans.[180] The rate of cellular proliferation in the esophagus is approximately one third that of the jejunum.[177] This squamous epithelium is penetrated at irregular intervals by papillae of the lamina propria.

Mucous glands similar to those found in the cardia of the stomach are found at the level of the cricoid cartilage beneath the epithelium. Having no secretory or absorptive functions, the esophageal mucosa serves mainly in a protective capacity and, thus, has no specialized cells.

STOMACH

The stomach serves mostly as a secretory organ and contains many more specialized cell types than the esophagus. The body and fundus are lined by mucus-secreting cells extending into gastric pits with long glands extending deep into the gastric mucosa. These glands are lined by parietal cells, which secrete acid and intrinsic factor, and chief cells, which secrete pepsinogen. The mucous

TABLE 23-4
Summary of Kinetic Parameters in Human Gastrointestinal Mucosa*

	LABELING INDEX (%)†	MITOTIC INDEX (%)‡	T_{G_2} (hr)	T_S (hr)	T_{G_1} (hr)	T_M (hr)	T_C (hr)§	T MIGRATION (hr)
Esophagus				10–20		0.79–1.57		102–202
Stomach								
Cardia	13.1	1.3						
Fundus	4.2–14	0.8–1.0	2–4	7.1–10	62		48–72	
Antrum	12.8–15.2	1.4						
Small Intestine								
Duodenum		2.36				1.1	48–54	120–144
Jejunum				1.5		1.1	42–48	
Ileum								72
Colon	12–18		1–6	11–20	14	1	40	72–92
Rectum	18–25		2	9–14			24–48	

* *Data adapted from References 162, 177, 178.*
† *Percentage of total cell population labeled with tritiated thymidine.*
‡ *Percentage of mitotic figures in total cell population measured.*
§ *Cell cycle duration.*

neck cells lie in the middle third of the gastric glands.[181] The gastric antrum contains deeper gastric pits than the rest of the stomach and contains cells that secrete an alkaline mucus. Enteroendocrine cells are predominantly found in the middle portion of the gastric glands among the mucous-secreting cells in the antrum, body, and fundus.

The mucous neck cells, the principal proliferating cells of the stomach, migrate to the luminal surface where most differentiate into mucus-secreting cells. The cell population above the zone of proliferation for the gastric mucous-epithelial cell is replaced every 2 to 3 days in humans.[178] Migration rates from the proliferative zone in the glandular neck to the surface are comparable to those in small and large bowel.[182] During development in the first 4 postpartum weeks, rates of DNA synthesis are markedly higher, but fractional cell loss is lower, leading to significant mucosal growth.

Parietal cells are incapable of dividing and are replaced by migrating cells that differentiate.[183] They appear to have long life spans (e.g., 90 days in the mouse).[184] Most G (gastrin) cells located in the antrum are derived from mitosis of other G cells, although some may arise from differentiation of other gastric cells.[185] G-cell turnover has been found to vary widely between animal species. In the mouse, cell turnover of G cells is 2 to 4 months; in the hamster, G cells, which arise mostly from mucous neck cells and migrate into the lower glands, turn over every 10 to 15 days.[186]

SMALL INTESTINE

The small intestinal mucosa is comprised of villi, which project into the lumen, and the surrounding crypts of Lieberkühn, which project away from the luminal surface. The crypts and villi are lined by a single layer of columnar cells.[187] As they migrate, the columnar cells differentiate into the other small intestinal cell types. Enteroendocrine cells also migrate toward the villus tip. Mature goblet cells are located in the upper crypts and villi, while immature oligomucous cells are limited to the crypts. Paneth cells are located at the base of the crypts.[188] Transitional cells (i.e., cells with features common to columnar and goblet cells) are also found in the crypts.[162] At birth, crypts are populated by the progeny of several uncommitted stem cells. However, by the end of 2nd postnatal week, a selection process of unknown mechanism, which has been termed "purification," occurs so that a single stem cell dominates and subsequently the cell population in a single crypt are clonal in origin.[189] Progeny from that crypt migrate up adjacent villi (Fig 23-7).[12,189] Insofar as most villi are surrounded by 4 to 10 crypts, villi are comprised of linear stripes of cells of different "parentage" (see Fig 23-7). The latter may be literally true in the context of X-linked genes in females, which undergo random X-activation creating mosaicism for those gene products.

As noted above, in the organization of the intestinal crypt, true stem cells are present at a fixed position in the mid to lower crypt cell, and a zone of actively proliferating progeny are clustered just above in the midzone of the crypt. Columnar cells migrate from the crypt base to the villus tip in 5 to 6 days in the proximal human small intestine[187] and 3 days in the human ileum. On mean, these cells migrate one to two cell positions per hour.[190] However, a few scattered cells may remain for weeks after pulse-labeling with ^{3}H-thymidine. The shorter time for migration in the distal than proximal small intestine may be secondary to the proximal to distal villus height–crypt depth gradient (i.e., the progressive decline in crypt depth and villus size through the length of the small intestine).[191] The cell cycle of the human small intestine basal crypt cell takes about 10 hours. However, great variability exists; those cells that survive for weeks remain in a prolonged G_2 or G_0 (resting) phase. Paneth and neuroendocrine cells have cell cycles that last for several days.[162]

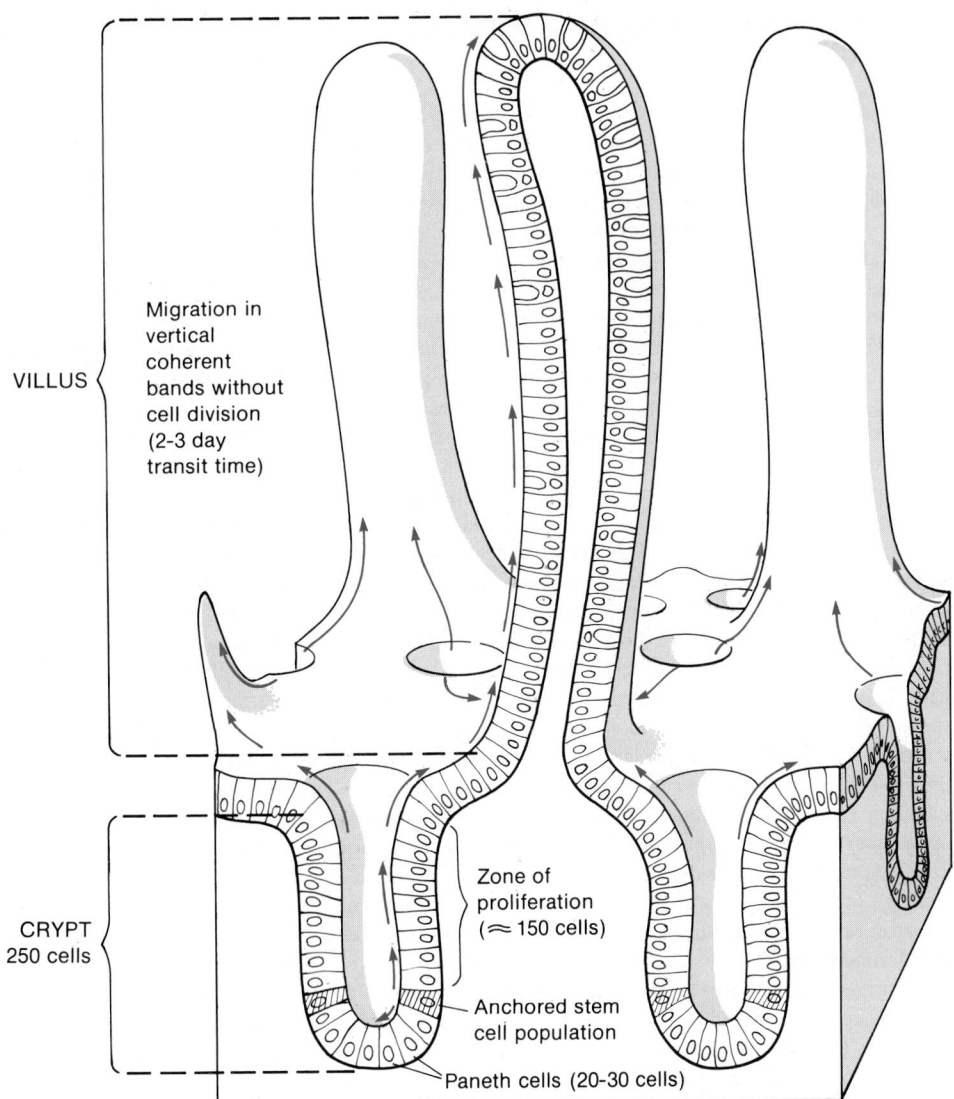

FIGURE 23–7. Schematic representation of the crypt–villus relationship in the adult mouse small intestine. Six to fourteen crypts surround each villus base, less proximally, more distally in the ileum (horizontal gradient). The lower five cell positions contain a total of 40 to 50 cells with an average cycle time of 26 hours and containing 20 to 30 nonproliferative Paneth cells. Anchored stem cells exist at the fifth position with maximal rates of proliferation. Cells migrate from this position toward both the villus tip and the crypt base (the Paneth cells). The upper portion of the crypt contains proliferating cells that undergo upward migration; 275 cells are delivered to the villus base from each crypt. This migration occurs in strict vertical coherent bands toward the villus tip, where the cells are extruded.

VILLUS

Migration in vertical coherent bands without cell division (2-3 day transit time)

Zone of proliferation (≈ 150 cells)

Anchored stem cell population

CRYPT 250 cells

Paneth cells (20-30 cells)

COLON

The colon has a flat surface without villi, and cells appear to be extruded directly from the flat surface into the bowel lumen. The proliferative zone is found in the basal half of the colonic crypts. Less is known directly about the organization of stem cells and the zones of proliferation and differentiation in the colon than the small intestine. However, observations made in mice and colon tumors support a similar arrangement for colon and small intestine (i.e., an anchored stem cell that gives rise to clonal populations of cells in a single crypt and the presence of a larger number of committed but proliferatively competent cells in the mid-portion of the crypt). The latter are presumed to give rise to the several cell types found in the normal colonic epithelium, most notably columnar absorptive cells and goblet cells. This suggestion is supported by the demonstration of clonality in colonic crypts and colonic tumors using techniques to identify mosaicism of expression of X-linked markers in females[192] and more recently RFLP analysis.[193] The validity of the analogy is also supported circum-

stantially by the apparent close ontogenetic similarity between colonic and intestinal epithelia with the identification of several colon cancer derived cell lines (e.g., CaCo₂, HT-29) that recapitulate the entire spectrum of small intestinal epithelial cellular constituents when their growth conditions are properly manipulated.

The proliferative zone lies in the bottom of the colonic crypt, with migration to the luminal surface taking 3 to 8 days in humans[194] and 2 to 3 days in rodents.[195] Much variability exists in the size and shape of the colon crypts along the length of the colon, as well as in the duration of the cell cycles of the proliferating crypt cell.[196] Approximately 15% to 20% of cells in the crypt appear to be involved in DNA synthesis at any one time. In humans, the cell cycle duration varies from 58 hours in the descending colon to 25 hours in the cecum. This is due to variability in the G_1 phase of the cell cycle.[197] Cells migrate at somewhat less than one cell position per hour. Enteroendocrine cells undergo cell renewal more slowly, and populations appear to turn over in 35- to 100-day intervals.[198]

CELL KINETICS IN GASTROINTESTINAL DISORDERS

A brief consideration of alterations of cell kinetics in a selected spectrum of gastrointestinal disorders is informative. In inflammatory or destructive lesions of the intestinal tract, the mucosa responds by either proliferation or atrophy. In the esophagus, injury due to reflux esophagitis leads to increased tritiated thymidine incorporation in the proliferative basal layer and results in a thickened basal layer in the involved portion of the esophagus.[199] In the stomach, stress-induced gastric erosions are associated with a decrease in gastric epithelial mitosis and thymidine labeling,[200] while pernicious anemia is linked with an increase in thymidine labeling, migration, and proliferation of gastric epithelial cells.[180] Ethanol also decreases the depth of gastric pits within 4 hours in dog stomach, but mitotic activity increases at 20 to 24 hours with a prompt renewal of normal gastric mucosa. In the small intestine, ethanol decreases crypt and villus cell number and is associated with shorter villi in the jejunum. In contrast, ileal crypts reveal increased mitotic and thymidine kinase activity and increased cell number as a response to injury induced by alcohol.[201] In the mucosa of patients with duodenal ulcer disease, a fall in thymidine incorporation and mitosis occurs, and this decrease in proliferation has been implicated in the pathogenesis of peptic ulcerations.[202] In the colon, repeated radiation injury leads to cell death. In mice with surviving cells, formation of larger crypts with higher labeling indices than those found in control mice have been noted.[203] Irradiation also results in altered epithelial cell morphology with appearance of cuboidal epithelial cells and a decreased mitotic rate in humans.[204] Bypassing the colon experimentally leads to a decrease in proliferation with fewer cells per crypt, although the life span of the crypt epithelial cell is the same in both bypassed and normal colon.[205]

Disorders of the gastrointestinal tract that are precursors to malignancy are associated with varying degrees of altered cell proliferation. In Barrett's epithelium, for example, intestinal metaplasia is found, and an increase in tritiated thymidine incorporation occurs at the base of the villuslike columnar epithelium.[206] A similar pattern is observed in atrophic gastric mucosa, with a selective increase in mitotic activity found in those glands demonstrating intestinal metaplasia.[207] In colonic adenomas, progressive expansion of the proliferative zone to the luminal surface has been demonstrated. In addition, abnormal retrograde migration from the mucosal surface occurs, a pattern that becomes more accentuated in colonic carcinoma. In the mucosa of patients with Gardner's syndrome or familial polyposis, progressive expansion of the proliferative compartment occurs to the extent that mitosis may be seen anywhere in the mucosa.[208] Expansion of the proliferation zone compartment toward the lumen has also been noted in ulcerative colitis.[209] Higher rates of proliferation appear to persist during remission in the colonic mucosa of patients with ulcerative colitis.

In colon carcinomas of the rat, proliferation is no longer confined to discrete zones, and cells proliferate in nearly all portions of the carcinomas.[210] The neoplastic cells demonstrate a longer proliferative cell cycle due to an increase in duration of the G_1 phase, as well as more variability in duration of the S and G_2 phases. Reduced epithelial cell loss and longer life cycles of the neoplastic cells lead to a change in the steady state and growth of the tumor.

Regulation of Proliferation and Differentiation

The functional importance of the constant cycle of proliferation, differentiation, and senescence in the gastrointestinal tract is not entirely clear but may reflect a necessary means of protection from the constant exposure of mucosal cells to potentially injurious factors present in the lumen. Rapid replacement of the mucosal cells could be especially important in the colon where the luminal contents have been demonstrated to include potent mutagens and carcinogenic substances. The high rate of cell turnover requires an exquisite regulatory mechanism to maintain mucosal homeostasis. Cell loss, cell proliferation, and cellular commitment to differentiation must be balanced precisely. Undoubtedly, a large series of factors modulate this balance including nutrients and other factors present in the lumen as well as proteins and hormones produced within the mucosa and more distant sites.

In contrast to other tissues in the body, the nutritional requirements of the gastrointestinal tract mucosa itself may potentially be obtained directly from dietary components in the lumen. Luminal substances include both direct nutrients and other factors that could regulate growth and differentiation by direct effects on the absorptive cells before systemic circulation or by stimulation of systemic factors, (e.g., trophic hormones), as well as through modulation of motor activity. It has been suggested that the gradient in villus height and crypt depth that is present in the small intestine reflects the important contribution of luminal nutrient concentration on mucosal growth. The greater villus height and crypt depth found in the proximal small intestine could result, in part, from the exposure to higher concentrations of nutrients, local growth factors, and pancreaticobiliary secretory products than those present in the more distal intestine. Indeed, when ileal and jejunal loops are transposed, the gradient can be reversed and the transposed ileal segment is found to exhibit increased villus size while the distally placed jejunal segment contains smaller villi.[211,212]

The role of luminal factors in maintenance of mucosal growth has been examined through the use of Thiry-Vella loops in which intestinal segments with their neurovascular connections remaining intact are removed from continuity with the remainder of the bowel and the two ends brought to the abdominal wall.[213,214] These loops may be used to study local effects of a variety of factors and more particularly to assay directly the importance of luminal substances on mucosal growth and proliferation. After formation of Thiry-Vella loops from either jejunal or ileal segments, hypoplasia of the intestinal mucosa is observed.[215] Further, when liquid elemental diets have been administered into the bypassed segments in the dog,[216] mucosal hyperplasia has been observed. However, it should be noted that comparable nutrient effects were not observed in similar studies performed in rabbits.[217]

Small intestinal resection leads to hypertrophy and dilatation in the remaining small bowel, with epithelial cell hyperplasia, villus growth, increased cell migration rates, and increased absorptive capacity.[218–221] Local nutrition may be important in the development of postresection hyperplasia; dogs fed intravenously after jejunal resection do not show the same adaptive proliferative response observed in dogs fed orally.[222] Intravenous feeding was also associated with decreased pancreatic secretion[223] and reduced levels of several gastrointestinal hormones.[224] The latter observations suggest that luminal nutrients may exert their trophic actions directly or indirectly through stimulation of hormones and other peptides as well as neural mediators, which modulate mucosal growth (neurocrine regulation). This concept is supported by the observation of gastric hypersecretion after small intestinal resection in the dog,[225] rat,[226] and human,[227] indicating that trophic factors such as gastrin could play a role in the adaptive response to small intestine resection by way of local (paracrine regulation) or systemic (hormonal regulation) action.

Other observations suggest that the importance of luminal nutrients and other luminal factors may be limited. Hyperplasia has been observed in ileal mucosa after resection of the colon.[228] Similarly, distal small bowel resection has been associated with hyperplasia of the more proximal small bowel,[229] and resection of distal or proximal small bowel can result in hyperplasia of the gastric mucosa.[230] Indeed, the mucosal hypoplasia observed in Thiry-Vella loops may be reversed by partial resection of any of the small intestine remaining in continuity.[215] Additional evidence supporting the concept that systemic factors may be more important than the direct effect of the luminal contents is derived from the study of paired rats in which cutaneous or vascular connections have been established. In these studies, mucosal hyperplasia has been observed in the small bowel of unoperated rats when connected to rats undergoing small bowel resection.[231]

Glucose stimulates cell production and mucosal hyperplasia of the proximal small intestine when infused into surgically prepared sacs.[232] However, in the same system, galactose, methyl-glucoside, and sodium chloride, which are actively transported but not metabolized by the small bowel mucosa, have the same trophic effect as glucose. Mannose, which is not actively transported or metabolized by the small intestine, does not increase cell production or cause mucosal hyperplasia. These studies have led to the notion that the active transport workload itself may be the stimulus for growth in response to some luminal factors—the "functional workload" hypothesis.[232] Support for this hypothesis has been obtained from experiments in which the effects of carbohydrate infusions into intact small intestine were examined. Direct infusions of disaccharides and, to a much smaller extent, monosaccharides increased mucosal mass in rat small intestine, but this trophic response did not occur if the "functional workload" was eliminated by prior substrate hydrolysis.

The importance of local nutrition in the regulation of intestinal growth is further discounted by the results of a series of experiments in which amino acid incorporation was studied.[233] Orally administered labeled amino acids were found to be incorporated into the nonproliferating surface villus absorptive cells of the small bowel mucosa. However, little incorporation of amino acids was observed in the proliferative zone of the crypt unless amino acids were provided by an intravenous route. These observations demonstrate a differential economy between the functionally active but mitotically inert differentiated villus cells and the actively proliferating crypt compartment. These results are consistent with the observation that luminal nutrients can lead to villus hypertrophy but not true mucosal hyperplasia.

It has been suggested that fiber within the diet has an important effect on mucosal proliferation. When cellulose is added to a low-fiber synthetic diet, an increase in DNA synthesis and content in gastric and colonic mucosa ensues, regardless of the protein or carbohydrate content of the diet.[234] Guar and pectin, two fibers that are poor bulking agents, are stimulants of growth in the colon, indicating that the effect of fiber on growth is not simply through bulk.[235] Kaolin, an excellent bulking agent, does not appear to have any effect on mucosal growth.[236] Fibers that cause fermentation appear to stimulate colonic mucosal growth more than those that are inert, possibly mediating their effect through a decrease in luminal pH in the colon.[237] The proliferative effect of refeeding fermentable dietary fiber to starved rats is not seen in germ-free rats, indicating that the products of intestinal fermentation, and not fiber itself, stimulate intestinal growth.[238]

The polyamines spermidine, spermine and their precursor, putrescine, are present in the diet and synthesized in the gut lumen. After ligation of the small intestine in the rat, the concentrations of luminal polyamines increase markedly in the proximal bowel where a large increase in mucosal growth is also observed.[239] Thus, polyamines may contribute to the longitudinal gradient of growth noted in the small intestine.[240] Moreover, infusion of dietary polyamines prevents the decrease in gastric and small intestinal weight, DNA, RNA, and protein content normally observed after antrectomy.[241] The trophic effect of polyamines on the gastric mucosa is independent of their ability to stimulate gastrin release insofar as comparable trophic effects are found after antrectomy.[242]

Ornithine decarboxylase is the enzyme controlling the rate-limiting step in the formation of the polyamines spermine and spermidine. The activity of this enzyme is increased by many gastrointestinal proteins, by food,[243] after partial resection,[244] and during lactation.[245] Difluoromethylornithine (DFMO), an inhibitor of ornithine decarboxylase activity, decreases the proliferative response to lactation,[245] intestinal obstruction,[246] and feeding.[247] In response to feeding or refeeding, an increase in ornithine decarboxylase predominantly in nondividing villus cells near the luminal surface has been noted.[248] In contrast, EGF leads to increased ornithine decarboxylase activity throughout the entire length of the crypt-villus unit.[249] Therefore, certain growth factors may increase ornithine decarboxylase activity in stem cells and influence intestinal growth through this mechanism. Polyamine synthesis and subsequent cellular proliferation after refeeding of cultured gastrointestinal crypt cells appears to be regulated by a calcium-activated, calmodulin-dependent process vital for proliferation of crypt cells in culture.[250] In addition to nutrients, a number of gastrointestinal proteins with potential growth-modulating properties are present in the intestinal lumen and might exert some or most of any growth regulation effects through interaction with the luminal mucosal surface. The protein, EGF, has been suggested to interact with the intestinal luminal surface. EGF is synthesized in the salivary glands and Brunner's glands of the duodenum, a distribution consistent with the notion that this protein could contribute to the proximal to distal horizontal gradient of villus-height crypt depth found in the small intestine.[251] Further, EGF is not present in serum in physiologically important amounts.

Gastrin has also been demonstrated in the intestinal lumen in large amounts.[252] Gastrin, too, is synthesized in the proximal gastrointestinal tract, with highest production in the gastric antrum and smaller quantities in the duodenum and pancreas. When gastrin is infused into the ileum through a catheter, mucosal hyperplasia has been observed downstream from the catheter in the absence of demonstrable elevation of serum gastrin levels. However, when the same amount of gastrin was infused into the stomach, the peptide was degraded and no trophic effect was observed in either the gastric or small intestinal mucosa.[253] These studies suggest that gastrin may not be present in sufficient quantities in the lumen under physiologic conditions to play an important role in regulating mucosal growth and proliferation.

Prostaglandins appear to promote small intestinal and gastric proliferation and growth, but some studies indicate that they may actually have an inhibitory effect on growth in the colon.[254,255] Nonetheless, rats treated for 48 hours with 16,16-dimethylprostaglandin E_2 exhibit an increase in gastric and small intestinal weight, as well as an increase in ^{3}H-thymidine incorporation into the mucosa of the duodenum and colon.[255,256] Prostaglandin delivered by a gastric feeding tube produces an increase in antral weight and in small intestine weight and length.[257] A similar study shows increased mucosal thickness throughout the digestive tract, but most marked in the antrum, after administration of exogenous prostaglandins.[258] Prostaglandins are thought to prevent gastric injuries caused by alcohol, acid, hypertonic saline, and alkali at doses below those required to inhibit acid secretion, a concept termed "cytoprotection."[259] Prostaglandin E also prevents ethanol-induced decreases in gastric mucosal DNA, RNA, and protein content.[260]

PANCREATIC AND BILIARY SECRETIONS

A number of proteins with potential or actual trophic action on the intestinal mucosa synthesized by the endocrine pancreas are also found in exocrine pancreatic secretions. These include gastrin, insulin, and glucagon. The concentration of these proteins present in pancreatic secretions decreases along the length of the small intestine in parallel with the proximal to distal gradient of growth in the small intestine. Diversion of pancreatic and biliary secretions into the ileum causes ileal mucosal hyperplasia in the rat.[261,262] However, displacement of these secretions into the distal ileum does not result in hypoplasia or decreased growth of crypts or villi in those areas of the proximal intestine removed from exposure to the pancreatic and biliary secretions.[263]

SYSTEMIC FACTORS

A number of nongastrointestinal hormones are thought to play a role in maintenance of intestinal growth. Hypophysectomy results in a decrease in weight, mitotic activity, villus height, and diameter of the small intestine in experimental animals.[264] Hypophysectomy also decreases the incorporation of thymidine and orotic acid into DNA and RNA in the intestinal mucosa and leads to reduced rates of protein synthesis.[265] Hypophysectomy results in atrophy of both parietal and chief cells in the gastric mucosa.[266] However, it should be noted that hypophysectomy also markedly decreases appetite and food intake and may exert some of its effects through its impact on some of the luminal factors discussed above. Moreover, the various pituitary hormones removed by hypophysectomy may affect intestinal growth indirectly by other, as yet unknown, influences on various gastrointestinal proteins. It has been demonstrated that serum gastrin levels decrease by 60%,[267] in parallel with antral gastrin content. which also is decreased by 80% after hypophysectomy. Small intestinal secretin content is also diminished in this setting.[268]

Adrenalectomy results in gastric and intestinal atrophy, but to a less marked degree than hypophysectomy.[269] ACTH and glucocorticoids inhibit cell proliferation in the stomach and, to a lesser extent, in the duodenum.[270] In other regions of the small intestine, glucocorticoids increase digestive and absorptive functions but decrease cell proliferation.[271] Of note, glucocorticoids increase antral gastrin levels in the rat and prevent the decrease in antral gastrin content that occurs in hypophysectomized rats.[272] It appears that corticosteroids promote the manifestations of functional differentiation while inhibiting proliferative activity.

Growth hormone stimulates growth of most tissues during development. Growth hormone does stimulate mitosis in the duodenal crypts of hypophysectomized or thyroidectomized rats[273] and leads to increased pancreatic DNA, and RNA content and weight in hypophysectomized rats.[274] However, growth hormone also leads to increased food intake, small intestinal secretin content,[268] and serum and antral gastrin levels[267] in hypophysectomized rats. Antral G-cell proliferation and an increase in antral gastrin content has been noted in patients with acromegaly.[275] Thus, the effects of growth hormone on gastrointestinal growth may be effected through intermediate modulation of a number of other growth factors.

Thyroxine causes an increase in pancreatic weight and RNA content, but not DNA content.[276] However, thyroxine does not increase the mitotic activity of duodenal crypts in hypophysectomized rats unless growth hormone is also administered.[276]

GI PEPTIDES

Gastrin, the most potent stimulant of gastric acid secretion is thought to have important trophic effects on the gastrointestinal tract. Exogenous gastrin stimulates the growth of mucosa throughout the entire gastrointestinal tract except for the esophagus and, possibly, the gastric antrum, where most of the peptide is produced. Gastrin has no trophic effects outside of the intestinal tract, and, within the intestinal tract, its effects appear to be limited to the mucosa.[277] In the stomach, gastrin increases the parietal cell population due to a shortening of the time of differentiation of fundic stem cells into parietal cells.[278] Pentagastrin also increases thymidine kinase activity in the rat gastric mucosa.[279] The number of neuroendocrine cells but not chief cells is increased by gastrin in the stomach.[280] Administration of a pentagastrin leads to increased RNA, DNA, or protein content in the pancreas of both normal[281,282] or hypophysectomized[283] rats.

Gastrin stimulates the production of its own receptors as evidenced by a direct correlation between serum gastrin levels and gastrin binding capacity.[284] Proglumide, a competitive inhibitor of gastrin binding to its receptor which is derived from glutaramic acid, inhibits the trophic actions of gastrin on the stomach, duodenum, and colon.[285] Cholecystokinin (CCK) also competes for binding to the gastric receptor,[286] and secretin blocks the gastrin receptor in a noncompetitive manner.[284]

A number of observations suggest that, at physiologic concentrations, systemic gastrin does exert trophic effects on gastrointestinal mucosa. Intravenous infusions of gastrin, which maintain serum gastrin concentrations similar to those expected after a meat meal lead to increased DNA synthesis.[287] Gastrin-17 and gastrin-34, the two most abundant forms of endogenous gastrin, are equal to pentagastrin in effecting increased DNA synthesis and content in duodenal and gastric mucosa.[288] Serum gastrin levels also parallel gastrointestinal growth responses after antrectomy or dietary manipulations.[233] Studies with omeprazole, a H^+-K^+-ATPase inhibitor, indicate that marked increases in serum and antral gastrin levels caused by this blocker are associated with increased parietal, chief, and mucous cell number by 25% to 30%, and a fivefold increase in gastric neuroendocrine cell number and thymidine incorporation.[289] High doses of omeprazole have been noted to induce gastric endocrine cell carcinoids in rats, which may reflect the effect of growth stimulation due to persistently elevated gastrin concentrations.[290]

Recent studies show that trophic responses in the gastrointestinal tract are muted when ornithine decarboxylase activity is inhibited by DFMO.[291] This observation is consistent with the concept that polyamine synthesis is necessary for cellular response to gastrin and other peptide mediators. Pentagastrin does not induce ornithine decarboxylase activity, but it does appear to induce spermine/spermidine N-acetyltransferase and thus polyamine interconversion and might regulate the rate of putrescine production in this way.[292]

CCK is structurally and functionally related to gastrin, differing only in the location and sulfation of its tyrosine residue.[293] CCK and its family of related peptides have low affinity for receptors controlling gastric acid secretion and high affinity for receptors regulating gallbladder contraction and pancreatic enzyme secretion. CCK may also possess trophic effects on the pancreas leading to increased pancreatic size and weight,[294] and its DNA content.[295] Cerulein, a CCK analogue isolated from the skin of amphibians, increases pancreatic somatostatin content and release while having no effect on insulin or glucagon content or secretion.[296]

Physiologically, infusion of amino acids and hydrochloric acid into the rat duodenum, which elevate CCK and secretin levels, increases pancreatic weight, DNA, RNA, and protein content.[297] This provides indirect evidence that endogenous forms of these two peptides are responsible for the trophic effects on the pancreas. Soybean trypsin inhibitor has been used to study the effects on endogenous CCK that result from its ability to prevent feedback inhibition of CCK release. Although interpretations of the effects of soybean trypsin inhibitor are complicated by its ability to alter other factors that may potentiate the effects of CCK on pancreatic growth, administration of soybean trypsin inhibitor does result in pancreatic growth.[298] A recent study indicates that the mechanism of CCK's trophic action on the pancreas may involve induction of ornithine decarboxylase gene expression.[299] Thus, polyamine synthesis may provide a common pathway for the expression of at least some of the gastrointestinal peptides. At low doses, CCK octapeptide has no effect on the growth of gastric or duodenal mucosa. Paradoxically, CCK inhibits the trophic effects of gastrin on these tissues at higher doses.[300] CCK, itself, may have a direct trophic effect on murine gallbladder epithelia.[301]

Secretin also stimulates pancreatic growth, although to a lesser extent than CCK.[302] When secretin is administered in combination with CCK, pancreatic growth response is greater than that observed with either individual peptide, indicating the possible existence of synergistic action.[303] Secretin inhibits the secretory and trophic effects of gastrin in a manner similar to CCK.[304] Secretin inhibits gastrin's stimulation of DNA synthesis and content in gastric, duodenal, and colonic mucosa.[305,306]

Vasoactive intestinal peptide (VIP) is structurally related to secretin. VIP similarly inhibits the effect of pentagastrin on markers of gastric and colonic mucosal proliferation but does not appear to have any significant intrinsic trophic effects. VIP also has no effect on growth of pancreatic acinar cells in vitro.[307]

Gastrin-releasing peptide (GRP), which is homologous to the amphibian peptide, bombesin, can stimulate clonal growth of cultured small cell lung cancer cells[308] and has been shown to be produced by a human small cell lung cancer line.[309] In the gastrointestinal tract, GRP stimulates antral gastrin cell (G-cell) proliferation[310] and increases gastric and colonic mucosal DNA content,[311] as well as pancreatic growth.[312] Its effects may be partly or completely mediated through stimulation of gastrin release from the G-cell.[313]

Neurotensin, a tridecapeptide widely distributed throughout the gastrointestinal tract and also known as neuropeptide Y, is a member of the pancreatic polypeptide family secreted by the N-cell. The N-cell is found in all parts of the small intestine and colon but has its highest density in the ileum.[314] Neurotensin has been shown to stimulate pancreatic growth and to increase small intestinal mucosal weight, DNA, and protein content in the rat. However, neurotensin did not appear to have any effect on mucosal growth in the colon.[315] Neurotensin appeared to stimulate mucosal growth throughout the small intestine, and the magnitude of the trophic effect was much greater than that of gastrin. In this same study, neurotensin was noted to increase sucrase, maltase, and alkaline phosphatase content of the small intestine. The latter effect was more pronounced in mucosa from the proximal intestine than the distal small bowel.[315] Neurotensin also stimulates thyroxine release in rats[316] and insulin and glucagon release in dogs.[317] However, none of these hormones demonstrates a trophic effect on gastrointestinal growth of the magnitude observed after administration of neurotensin. Neurotensin has been found to bind the same receptor site as peptide-YY (see below) in small intestinal epithelial cells. However, these receptors have a greater affinity for peptide-YY than neurotensin. Neurotensin (and peptide-YY) have been shown to decrease VIP or prostaglandin-stimulated cAMP levels in rat jejunal epithelial cells.[318]

Peptide YY, a 36-amino acid polypeptide originally found in high concentrations in enteroendocrine cells of the small intestine and colon,[319] is predominantly synthesized in the pancreas.[320] Serum levels correlate with enterocyte proliferation, and, when the effect of EGF on plasma levels of gastrin, enteroglucagon, and peptide YY were correlated with gut proliferation, only peptide YY levels were significantly elevated by EGF, indicating a possible role for peptide YY in the modulation of gastrointestinal proliferation.[321]

As noted above, concentrations of EGF in serum are very low. Nevertheless, intravenous EGF does stimulate epithelial cell proliferation in humans, chickens, and mice.[322] Exogenous EGF stimulates DNA, RNA, and protein content of the gastric mucosa but does not stimulate growth of duodenal or colonic mucosa.[323] EGF is synthesized in both salivary and Brunner's glands. Within 1 week after surgical excision of submandibular glands, rats demonstrate lower jejunal and ileal but not colonic RNA and DNA content than sham-operated controls.[324] A number of investigations have suggested the presence of specific receptors for EGF in intestinal epithelial cells including both microvillar and basolateral surfaces. The presence of receptors in microvillus membrane preparations detected through binding of the labeled ligand has lent support to the notion that luminal EGF may regulate intestinal epithelial growth. However, more recent studies using immuno-histochemistry have localized the receptors to the basolateral surface.[325] It is possible that EGF present in the lumen may interact with these basolateral receptors after initial uptake from the lumen. In addition, EGF stimulates gastrin promoter activity[326] and may exert some of its trophic effects by stimulation of gastrin.

Over the past several years, two additional classes of peptides, initially identified through their ability to stimulate or augment anchorage independent growth of nontransformed fibroblasts and designated transforming growth factors α and β (TGFα and TGFβ) have been recognized to have potent effects on proliferation of many epithelial cell types. TGFα, structurally homologous to EGF, has been found to stimulate thymidine incorporation in many cell types.[327] Recent studies have demonstrated production of TGFα by intestinal epithelial cells in the rat.[328] TGFα has also been found in gastric and colonic mucosa. TGFα appears to be mediated through the same receptor that binds EGF.[329] It is possible that the physiologically relevant ligand of the receptor previously thought to specify EGF is, in fact, TGFα. In contrast, TGFβ, a peptide structurally unrelated to either EGF or TGFα, has been found to inhibit proliferative activity of many cell types including intestinal crypt cells.[330] TGFβ is also produced by intestinal epithelial cells.[328]

The presence of both TGFα and TGFβ and their receptors in crypt and villus cell populations suggest that the mechanisms of self-regulation (autocrine control) and local cellular regulation (or paracrine control) may be important in controlling mucosal proliferation and differentiation. Paracrine communication in which cells secrete peptide factors that are recognized by nearby cells may be an especially important mechanism for coordinating proliferation with cell loss. Autocrine control in which the cell secretes a factor recognized by receptors on its own surface may provide an important mechanism for self-correction through down-regulation of surface receptors.

Somatostatin is located throughout the intestinal tract and pancreas and inhibits the release of many gastrointestinal peptides, including gastrin.[331] It also inhibits the action of gastrin and other gut peptides at their target cell. Therefore, in addition to inhibition of gastrin release, somatostatin inhibits stimulation of gastric mucosal growth by both endogenous[332] and exogenous[333] gastrin. It also inhibits pancreatic secretion[334] and gastric acid secretion.[335] Pancreatic DNA, protein, and enzyme content are decreased after administration of somatostatin.[336] Further, somatostatin reduces the trophic effect of cerulein on the pancreas.[337] It is still unclear whether somatostatin exerts its inhibitory effects on gastrointestinal growth solely through its inhibition of gastrointestinal peptides or if it has direct effects on mucosal growth of its own.

High serum enteroglucagon levels have been found in a number of conditions associated with growth of the small bowel: adaptation after intestinal resection,[338] celiac sprue,[339] and tropical sprue.[340] Serum enteroglucagon levels correlate with the rate of crypt cell production in the distal small bowel, but not the colon.[341] Despite correlations of enteroglucagon levels and mucosal growth, no evidence exists that enteroglucagon directly stimulates growth. Pancreatic glucagon's effects on gastrointestinal growth are not well understood. While glucagon has been shown to increase DNA synthesis and content in gastric and colonic mucosa,[342] another

study shows that exogenous glucagon decreases villus height along the rat small intestine.[343]

Molecular cloning of glucagon and proglucagon has led to a better understanding of the molecular relationships between glucagon, enteroglucagon, and a number of related products of the proglucagon gene.[344] Enteroglucagon, also known as gut glucagonlike immunoreactivity (GLI), consists of a family of peptides that bind to antibodies against the central portion of the glucagon molecule. Oxyntomodulin, containing 37 amino acids, and glicentin, containing 69 amino acids, share the same c-terminus and are thought to be the main gastrointestinal GLIs in the rat and human.[345] These various peptides result from differential splicing during transcription of the glucagon gene, which also produces a number of additional products including glucagonlike peptide I (GLP-I), glucagonlike peptide II (GLP-II) and intervening peptides IP-I and IP-II. While GLP-I appears to have an important role in regulation of insulin in the pancreas where GLP-I is selectively produced, it is possible that GLP-II has a significant effect on intestinal mucosal proliferation where it is selectively produced. The biologic activities of IPI and IPII are unknown. With the recognition of these selected gene products, the effects of glucagon on gastrointestinal mucosal growth must be reassessed.

The gastrointestinal tract represents a dynamic model for the study of cell and tissue development, growth, and differentiation. Although recent insights into newly described growth factors and mechanisms of cell-to-cell communications and interactions have allowed much greater understanding of the regulation of intestinal growth and development, the precise signals controlling these processes, as well as the specific pathways of events such as cell migration, adhesion, renewal, extrusion, and transformation, await further definition.

The reader is directed to Chapter 2, Gastrointestinal Hormones; Chapter 6, Epithelia: Biologic Principles of Organization; Chapter 24, Neoplasia of the Gastrointestinal Tract; and Chapter 74, Short Bowel Syndrome.

REFERENCES

1. Moore KL. The developing human: Clinically oriented embryology, ed 3. Philadelphia: WB Saunders, 1982;197.
2. Grand RJ, Watkins JB, Torti FM. Development of the human gastrointestinal tract: A review. Gastroenterology 1976;50:790.
3. Smith RB, Taylor IM. Observations of the intrinsic innervation of the human foetal oesophagus between the 10mm and 140mm crown-rump length stages. Acta Anat 1972;81:127.
4. Johns BAE. Developmental changes in the oesophageal epithelium in man. J Anat 1952;86:431.
5. Sadler TW. Digestive System. In: Sadler TW, ed. Langman's medical embryology. Baltimore: Williams & Wilkins, 1985:224.
6. Bremner CG. Studies on the pyloric muscle. I. The embryology of the pyloric muscle. S Afr J Surg 1968;6:79.
7. Nishimura H, ed. Atlas of human prenatal histology. Tokyo: Igaku-Shoin, 1983.
8. Salenius P. On the ontogenesis of the human gastric epithelial cells. Acta Anat 1962;50(Suppl 46):1.

9. Facer P, Bishop AE, Cole GA, et al. Developmental profile of chromogranin, hormonal peptides, and 5-hydroxytryptamine in gastrointestinal endocrine cells. Gastroenterology 1989;97:48.

10. Lui HM, Potter EL. Development of the human pancreas. Arch Pathol 1962;74:439.

11. Colony PC. Successive phases of human fetal intestinal development. In: Kretchmer N, Minkowki A, eds. Nutritional adaptation of the gastrointestinal tract of the newborn, New York: Vevey/Raven Press, 1983:3.

12. Gordon JI. Intestinal epithelial differentiation: New insights from chimeric and transgenic mice. J Cell Biol 1989;108:1187.

13. Cornes JS. Number, sign and distribution of Peyer's patches in the human small intestine. Gut 1965;6:225.

14. Gehring WJ. Homeoboxes in the study of development. Science 1987;236:1245.

15. Wolgemuth DJ, Viviano CM, Gizang-Ginsberg E, et al. Differential expression of the mouse homeobox-containing gene Hox-1.4 during male germ cell differentiation and embryonic development. Proc Natl Acad Sci USA 1987;84:5813.

16. Simeoni A, Mavilio F, Acampora D. Two human homeobox genes c1 and c8: Structure analysis and expression in embryonic development. Proc Natl Acad Sci USA 1987;84:4914.

17. Wolgemuth DJ, Behringer RR, Mostoller MP, Brinster RL, Palmiter RD. Transgenic mice over-expressing the mouse homeobox-containing gene Hox 1.4 exhibit abnormal gut development. Nature 1989;337:464.

18. Henning SJ. Functional development of the gastrointestinal tract. In: Johnson LR, ed. Physiology of the gastrointestinal tract, ed 2. New York: Raven Press, 1987:285.

19. Pritchard JA. Fetal swallowing and amniotic fluid volume. Obstet Gynecol 1966;28:606.

20. Abramovich DR. The volume of amniotic fluid and factors affecting or regulating this. In: Fairweather DVI, Eskes TKAB, eds. Amniotic fluid. Amsterdam: Excerpta Medica, 1973:29.

21. Gryboski JD. The swallowing mechanism of the neonate. I. Esophageal and gastric motility. Pediatrics 1965;35:445.

22. Ketel HG, Ziegra SR. Regurgitation in the full-term infant: A controlled clinical study. Am J Dis Child 1961;103:749.

23. Gryboski JD, Thayer WR Jr, Spiro HM. Esophageal motility in infants and children. Pediatrics 1963;31:382.

24. Cohen S. Developmental characteristics of lower esophageal sphincter function: A possible mechanism for infantile chalasia. Gastroenterology 1974;67:252.

25. Deren JS. Development of structure and function in the fetal and newborn stomach. Am J Clin Nutr 1971;24:144.

26. Christie DL. Development of gastric function during the first month of life. In: Lebenthal E, ed. Textbook of gastroenterology and nutrition in infancy. New York: Raven Press, 1981:109.

27. Agunod M, Yamaguchi N, Lopez R, et al. Correlative study of hydrochloric acid, pepsin, and intrinsic factor secretion in newborns and infants. Am J Dig Dis 1969;14:400.

28. Ikezaki M, Johnson LR. Development of sensitivity to different secretagogues in the rat stomach. Am J Physiol 1983;244:G165.

29. Takeuchi K, Okabe S, Johnson LR. Mucosal gastrin receptor V. Development in newborn rats. Am J Physiol 1981;240:G163.

30. Seidel ER, Johnson LR. Ontogeny of the gastric mucosal muscarinic receptor and sensitivity to carbachol. Am J Physiol 1984;246:G550.

31. Ackerman SH. Ontogeny of gastric acid secretion in the rat: Evidence for multiple response systems. Science 1982;217:75.

32. Larsson LI, Hakanson R, SjÜberg NO, et al. Fluorescence histochemistry of the gastrin cell in fetal and adult man. Gastroenterology 1975;68:1152.

33. Lichtenberger L, Johnson LR. Gastrin in the ontogenetic development of the small intestine. Am J Physiol 1974;227:390.

34. Rogers IM, Davidson DC, Lawrence J, Ardill J, Buchanan KD. Neonatal secretion of gastrin and glucagon. Arch Dis Child 1974;49:1974.

35. Mallow MH, Morriss FH, Denson SE, et al. Neonatal gastric motility in dogs: Maturation and response to pentagastrin. Am J Physiol 1979;236:E562.

36. Johnson LR. Effects of somatostatin and acid on inhibition of gastrin release in newborn rats. Endocrinology 1984;114:743.

37. Johnson LR. Functional development of the stomach. Annu Rev Physiol 1985;47:199.

38. Henning SJ. Plasma concentrations of total and free corticosterone during development in the rat. Am J Physiol 1978;235:E451.

39. Ikezaki M, Johnson LR. Development of sensitivity to different secretagogues in the rat stomach. Am J Physiol 1983;244:G165.

40. Peitsch W, Takeuchi K, Johnson LR. Mucosal gastrin receptor VI. Induction by corticosterone in newborn rats. Am J Physiol 1981;240:G442.

41. Kumegawa M, Takuma T, Hosoda S, Kunii S, Kauda Y. Precocious induction of pepsinogen in the stomach of suckling mice by hormones. Biochem Biophys Acta 1978;543:243.

42. Johnson LR, Peitsch W, Takeuchi K. Mucosal gastrin receptor VIII. Sex-related differences in binding. Am J Physiol 1982;243:G469.

43. Antonowicz I, Chang SK, Grand R. Development and distribution of lysosomal enzymes and disaccharidases in human fetal intestine. Gastroenterology 1974;67:51.

44. Antonowicz I, Lebenthal E. Developmental pattern of small intestinal enterokinase and disaccharidase activities in the human fetus. Gastroenterology 1977;72:1299.

45. Lebenthal E, Lee PC. Alternative pathways of digestion and absorption in early infancy. J Pediatr Gastroenterol Nutr 1984;3:1.

46. Newcomer AD, McGill DB. Distribution of disaccharidase activity in the small bowel of normal and lactose-deficient subjects. Gastroenterology 1966;51:481.

47. James PS, Smith MW, Tivey DR. Single-villus analysis of disaccharidase expression by different regions of the mouse intestine. J Physiol 1988;401:533.

48. Rubino A, Zimbalatti F, Auricchio S. Intestinal disaccharidase activities in adult and suckling rats. Biochem Biophys Acta 1964;92:305.

49. Mobassaleh M, Montgomery RK, Biller JA, Grand RJ. Development of carbohydrate absorption in the fetus and neonate. Pediatrics 1985;75(Suppl):160.

50. Zoppi G, Andreotti G, Pajno-Ferrara F, et al. Exocrine pancreas function in premature and full term neonates. Pediatr Res 1972;6:880.

51. Lebenthal E, Lee PC. Glucoamylase and disaccharidase activities in normal subjects and in patients with mucosal injury of the small intestine. J Pediatr 1980;97:389.

52. Murray R, Kerzner B, Sloan H, et al. Quantification of glucose polymer digestion by premature salivary amylase (Abstract). Pediatr Res 1985;19:228A.

53. Hodge C, Lee PC, Topper W, et al. Digestion of corn syrup sugars in neonates: Importance of salivary amylase and gastric hydrolysis. Pediatr Res 1983;17:998.

54. Lebenthal E, Lee PC. Review article. Interactions of determinants in the ontogeny of the gastrointestinal tract: A unified concept. Pediatr Res 1983;17:19.

55. Koldovsky O, Heringova A, Jirsova V, et al. Transport of glucose against a concentration gradient in everted sacs of jejunum and ileum of human fetuses. Gastroenterology 1965;48:185.

56. Thomson ABR, Keelan M. The development of the small intestine. Can J Physiol Pharmacol 1986;64:13.

57. Lebenthal E, Tucker NT. Carbohydrate digestion: Development in early infancy. Clin Perinatology 1986;13:37.

58. Gall DG, Perdue M, Chung M. Postnatal development of glucose transport in the proximal small intestine of the rabbit. J Pediatr Gastroenterol Nutr 1983;2:127.

59. Younoszai MK, Lynch A. In vivo D-glucose absorption in the developing rat small intestine. Pediatr Res 1975;90:130.

60. Younoszai MK. Jejunal absorption of hexose in infants and children. J Pediatr 1974;85:446.

61. Keene MFL, Hewer EE. Digestive enzymes of the human fetus. Lancet 1929;1:767.

62. Lieberman J. Proteolytic enzyme activity in fetal pancreas and meconium. Gastroenterology 1966;50:183.

63. Ibrahim J. Trypsinogen und enterokinase beim menschlichen neugerborenen und embryo. Biochem Zeitschr 1909;23:24.

64. Lindberg T. Intestinal dipeptidases: Characterization, development, and distribution of intestinal dipeptidases of the human foetus. Clin Sci 1966;30:505.

65. Rubino A, Perno M, La Torretta G, et al. Studies on intestinal hydrolysis of peptides. II. Dipeptidase activity toward L-glutaminyl-L-proline and glycyl-L-proline in the small intestine of the human fetus. Pediatr Res 1969;3:313.

66. Jirosva V, Koldovsky O, Heringova A, et al. The development of the functions of the small intestine of the human fetus. Biol Neonate 1965;9:44.

67. Robberecht P, Deschodt-Lanckman M, Camus J. Rat pancreatic hydrolysis from birth to weaning and dietary adaptation after weaning. Am J Physiol 1971;221:376.

68. Lebenthal E, Lee PC. Development of functional response in human exocrine pancreas. Pediatrics 1980;66:556.

69. Auricchio S, Stellato A, De Vizia B. Development of brush border peptidases in human rat small intestine during fetal and neonatal life. Pediatr Res 1981;15:991.

70. Levin RJ, Koldovsky O, Hoskova J, et al. Electrical activity across human foetal small intestine associated with absorption processes. Gut 1968;9:206.

71. Rubino A. Absorption of amino acids and peptides during development. Mod Probl Paediatr 1975;15:201.

72. Colony PC, Neutra MR. Macromolecular transport in the fetal rat intestine. Gastroenterology 1985;89:294.

73. Williams RM, Beck F. A histochemical study of gut maturation. J Anat 1969;105:487.

74. Clark SL. The ingestion of proteins and colloidal materials by columnar absorptive cells of the small intestine in suckling rats and mice. J Biophys Biochem Cytol 1959;4:41.

75. Walker WA, Isselbacher KJ. Uptake and transport of macro-molecules by the intestine. Possible role in clinical disorders. Gastroenterology 1974;67:531.

76. Gonnella PA, Neutra MR. Membrane-bound and fluid-phase macromolecules enter separate paralysosomal compartments in absorptive cells of suckling rat ileum. J Cell Biol 1984;99:909.

77. Walker WA, Cornell R, Davenport LM, Isselbacher KJ. Macromolecular absorption. Mechanism of horseradish peroxidase uptake and transport in adult and neonatal rat intestine. J Cell Biol 1972;54:195.

78. Dickson JJ, Messer M. Intestinal neuraminidase activity of suckling rats and other mammals: Relationship to the sialic acid content of milk. Biochem J 1978;170:407.

79. Pang KY, Bresson JL, Walker WA. Development of gastrointestinal surface VIII. Lectin identification of carbohydrate differences. Am J Physiol 1987;252:G685.

80. Israel EJ, Walker WA. Development of intestinal mucosal barrier function to antigens and bacterial toxins. Adv Exp Med Biol 1987;216A:673.

81. Baumann H, Chu FF. Altered composition of membrane glycoconjugates in rat hepatoma tissue culture cells after desamethasone treatment or in vivo growth. Cancer Res 1979;39:3540.

82. Eastham EJ, Lichauco T, Grady MI, Walker WA. Antigenicity of infant formulas: Role of immature intestine on protein permeability. J Pediatr (St Louis) 1978;93:561.

83. Tachibana T. Phsyiological investigation of the fetus. 4. Lipase in pancreas. Jap J Obstet Gynecol 1928;11:92.

84. Hamosh M. Oral lipases and lipid digestion during the neonatal period. In: Lebenthal E, ed. Textbook of gastroenterology and nutrition in infancy. New York: Raven Press, 1981:445.

85. Sauraux B, Girard-Globa A. Development of pancreatic enzymes in fetal and suckling rats with emphasis on lipase and colipase. J Dev Physiol 1982;4:121.

86. Hamosh M. A review. Fat digestion in the newborn: Role of lingual lipase and preduodenal digestion. Pediatr Res 1979;13:615.

87. De Bell ER, Brown A, Blacklow NR, et al. Organ culture of fetal liver—a new model system. Pediatr Res (Abstract) 1973;7:292.

88. Bongiovanni AM. Bile acid content of gallbladder of infants, children, and adults. J Clin Endocrinol 1965;25:678.

89. Berendson PB, Blanchette-Mackie EJ. Milk lipid absorption and chylomicron production in the suckling rat. Anat Rec 1979;195:397.

90. Mak KM, Trier JS. Lipoprotein particles in the jejunal mucosa of postnatal developing rats. Anat Rec 1979;194:491.

91. Little JM, Lister R. Ontogenesis of intestinal bile salt absorption in the neonatal rat. Am J Physiol 1980;239:G319.

92. Watkins JB. Lipid digestion and absorption. Pediatrics 1985;75(Suppl):151.

93. Watkins JB. Role of bile acids in the development of the enterohepatic circulation. In: Lebenthal E, ed. Textbook of gastroenterology and nutrition in infancy. New York: Raven Press 1981:167.

94. Gallagher ND, Mason R, Foley KE. Mechanisms of iron absorption and transport in neonatal rat intestine. Gastroenterology 1973;64:438.

95. Mills CF, Davies NT. Perinatal changes in the absorption of trace elements. In: Development of mammalian absorptive processes. Ciba Found Symp, New York: Excerpta Medica 1961;70:247.

96. Batt ER, Schachter D. Developmental pattern of some intestinal transport mechanisms in newborn rats and mice. Am J Physiol 1969;216:1064.

97. Dostal LA, Toverud SV. Effect of vitamin B_3 on duodenal calcium absorption in vivo during early development. Am J Physiol 1984;246:G528.

98. Oettinger L Jr, Mills WB, Hahn PF. Iron absorption in premature and full term infants. J Pediatr 1954;45:320.

99. Ziegler EE, Edwards BB, Jensen RL, et al. Absorption and retention of lead by infants. Pediatr Res 1978;12:29.

100. Boass A, Wilson TH. Development of mechanisms for intestinal absorption of vitamin B_{12} in growing rats. Am J Physiol 1963;204:101.

101. Shojania AM, Hornady G. Folate metabolism in newborn and during early infancy I. Absorption of pteroylglutamic (folic) acid in newborns. Pediatr Res 1970;4:412.

102. Said HM, Redah R. Ontogenesis of the intestinal transport of biotin in the rat. Gastroenterology 1988;94:68.

103. Henning SJ. Postnatal development. Coordination of feeding, digestion, and metabolism. Am J Physiol 1981;241:G199.

104. Kendall K, Jumawan J, Koldovsky O. Development of jejunoileal differences of lactase, sucrase, and beta-galactosidase in isografts of fetal rat intestine. Biol Neonate 1979;36:204.

105. Leapman SB, Deutsch AA, Grand RJ, Folkman J. Transplantation of fetal intestine: Survival and function in a subcutaneous location in adult animals. Ann Surg 1974;179:109.

106. De Ritis G, Falchuk FM, Trier JS. Differentiation and maturation of cultured fetal rat jejunum. Dev Biol 1975;45:304.

107. Tsuboi KK, Kwong LK, Ford WDA, Colby T, Sunshine P. Delayed ontogenic development in the bypassed ileum of the infant rat. Gastroenterology 1981;80:1550.

108. Raul F, Kedinger M, Simon PM, et al. Comparative in vivo and in vitro effect of mono- and di-saccharides on intestinal brush border enzyme activities in suckling rats. Biol Neonate 1981;39:200.

109. Lebenthal E, Sunshine P, Kretchmer N. Effect of prolonged nursing on the activity of intestinal lactase in rats. Gastroenterology 1973;64:1136.

110. Gall DG, Chung M. Effect of body weight on postnatal development of the proximal small intestine of the rabbit. Biol Neonate 1982;42:159.

111. Hamilton JR, Guiraldes E, Rossi M. Impact of malnutrition on the developing gut: Studies in suckling rats. J Pediatr Gastroenterol Nutr 1983;2(Suppl I):S151.

112. Lebenthal E, Choi TS, Lee PC. The development of pancreatic function in premature infants after milk based and soy based formulas. Pediatr Res 1981;15:1240.

113. Stoddart RW, Widdowson EM. Changes in the organs of pigs in response to feeding for the first 24 h after birth. III. Fluorescence histochemistry of the carbohydrates of the intestine. Biol Neonate 1976;28:272.

114. Hall RA, Widdowson EM. Response of the organs of rabbits to feeding during the first days after birth. Biol Neonate 1979;35:131.

115. Heird WC, Schwarz SM, Hansen IH. Colostrum-induced enteric mucosal growth in beagle puppies. Pediatr Res 1984;18:512.

116. Berseth CL, Lichtenberger LM, Morriss FH Jr. Comparison of the gastrointestinal growth-promoting effects of rat colostrum and mature milk in newborn rats in vivo. Am J Clin Nutr 1983;37:52.

117. Walker WA, Sheard NF. The role of breast milk in the development of the gastrointestinal tract. Nutr Rev 1988;46:1.

118. Klagsbrun M. Human milk stimulates DNA synthesis and cellular

proliferation in cultured fibroblasts. Proc Natl Acad Sci USA 1978;75:5057.

119. Shing YW, Klagsbrun M. Human and bovine milk contain different sets of growth factors. Endocrinology 1984;115:273.

120. Grueters A, Alm J, Laksmaman J, Fisher DA. Epidermal growth factor in mouse milk during early lactation: Lack of dependency on submandibular glands. Pediatr Res 1985;19:853.

121. Thornburg W, Matrisian L, Magun B, Koldovsky O. Gastrointestinal absorption of epidermal growth factor in suckling rat. Am J Physiol 1984;246:G80.

122. Read LC, Upton FM, Francis GL, et al. Changes in the growth-promoting activity of human milk during lactation. Pediatr Res 1984;18:133.

123. Schanders RP, Grimes J, Davis D, Rao RK, Koldovsky O. EGF content in the gastrointestinal tract of rats: Effect of age and fasting on feeding. Am J Physiol 1989;256:G856.

124. Levi-Montalcini R, Booker B. Excessive growth of the sympathetic ganglia evoked by a protein isolated from mouse salivary glands. Proc Natl Acad Sci USA 1960;46:373.

125. Baxter RC, Zaltsman Z, Turtle JR. Immunoreactive somatomedin-C/insulin-like growth factor I and its binding protein in human milk. J Clin Endocrinol Metab 1984;58:955.

126. Menard D, Malo C, Calvert R. Insulin accelerates the development of intestinal brush border hydrolytic activities of suckling mice. Dev Biol 1981;85:150.

127. Koldovsky O, Thornburg W. Review: Hormones in milk. J Pediatr Gastroenterol Nutr 1987;6:172.

128. Yeh K-Y, Yeh M, Holt PR. Induction of intestinal differentiation by systemic and not by luminal corticosterone in adrenalectomized rat pups. Endocrinology 1989;124:1898.

129. Yeh K-Y, Moog F. Hormonal influences on the growth and enzymic differentiation of the small intestine of the hypophysectomized rat. Growth 1978;42:495.

130. Herbst JJ, Sunshine P. Postnatal development of the small intestine of the rat. Pediatr Res 1969;3:27.

131. Henning SJ, Ballard PL, Kretchmer N. A study of the cytoplasmic receptors for glucocorticoid in intestine of pre- and post-weanling rats. J Biol Chem 1975;250:2073.

132. Henning SJ, Leeper LL. Coordinate loss of glucocorticoid responsiveness by intestinal enzymes during postnatal development. Am J Physiol 1982;242:G89.

133. Martin GR, Henning SJ. Enzymic development of the small intestine: Are glucocorticoids necessary? Am J Physiol 1984;246:G695.

134. Bauer CR, Morrison JC, Poole WB, et al. A decreased incidence of necrotizing enterocolitis after prenatal glucocorticoid therapy. Pediatrics 1984;73:682.

135. Menard D, Arsenault P. Influence of hydrocortisone on the development of human fetal small intestine in organ culture. J Steroid Biochem 1984;20:1429.

136. Watkins JB. Role of bile acids in the development of the enterohepatic circulation. In: Lebenthal E, ed. Gastroenterology and nutrition in infancy. New York: Raven Press, 1981:167.

137. Malinowskz KW, Chan WS, Nathanielskz PW, Hardy RN. Plasma adrenocorticosteroid changes during thyroxine-induced accelerated maturation of the neonatal rat intestine. Experientia 1974;30:61.

138. D'Agostino JB, Henning SJ. Role of thryoxine in coordinated control of corticosterone and CBG in postnatal development. Am J Physiol 1982;242:E33.

139. Yeh K-Y, Moog F. Influence of the thyroid and adrenal glands on the growth of the intestine of the suckling rat and on the development of intestinal alkaline phosphatase and disaccharidase activities. J Exp Zool 1977;200:337.

140. Yeh K-Y, Moog F. Intestinal lactase activity in the suckling rat: Influence of hypophysectomy and thyroidectomy. Science 1974;182:77.

141. Beardmore JM, Richards RC. Concentrations of epidermal growth factor in mouse milk throughout lactation. J Endocrinol 1983;96:287.

142. Byyny RL, Orth DN, Cohen S. Radioimmunoassay of epidermal growth factor. Endocrinology 1972;90:1261.

143. Calvert R, Beaulieu JF, Menard D. Epidermal growth factor accel-erates the maturation of fetal mouse intestinal mucosa in utero. Experientia 1982;38:1096.

144. Puccio F, Lehy T. Oral administration of epidermal growth factor in suckling rats stimulates cell DNA synthesis in fundic and antral gastric mucosae as well as in intestinal mucosa and pancreas. Regul Pept 1988;20:53.

145. Lehy T, Puccio F, Chariot J, Labeille D. Stimulating effect of bomesin on the growth of gastrointestinal tract and pancreas in suckling rats. Gastroenterology 1986;90:1942.

146. Puccio F, Lehy T. Bombesin ingestion stimulates epithelial digestive cell proliferation in suckling rats. Am J Physiol 1984;256:G328.

147. Jahnke GD, Lazarus LH. A bombesin immunoreactive peptide in milk. Proc Natl Acad Sci USA 1984;81:578.

148. Menard D, Malo C, Calvert R. Insulin accelerates the development of intestinal brush border hydrolytic activities of suckling mice. Dev Biol 1981;85:150.

149. Blazqies E, Montoya E, Quijada CL. Relationship between insulin concentrations in plasma and pancreas of foetal and weanling rats. J Endocrinol 1970;48:553.

150. Neu J, Hoffman RG, Crim WN. Prostaglandin-mediated effects on growth and markers of biochemical development in the rat. Pediatr Res 1983;17:537.

151. Neu J, Crim WN, Hodge NC. Prostaglandins stimulate disaccharidase activity in adrenalectomized suckling rats. Pediatr Res 1985;19:228A.

152. Simon GL, Gorbach SL. Intestinal flora in health and disease. Gastroenterology 1984;86:174.

153. Reddy BS, Wostmann BS. Intestinal disaccharidase activities in the growing germ-free and conventional rats. Arch Biochem Biophys 1966;113:609.

154. Gordon HA, Bruchorer-Kardoss E. Effect of normal microbial flora on intestinal surface area. Am J Physiol 1961;201:175.

155. Potter GD, Schmidt KL, Lester R. Glucose absorption by in vitro perfused colon of the fetal rat. Am J Physiol 1983;245:G424.

156. Meneely R, Ghishan FK. Intestinal maturation in the rat: The effect of glucocorticoids on sodium, potassium, water and glucose absorption. Pediatr Res 1982;16:775.

157. Meneely R, Leeper L, Ghishan FK. Intestinal maturation: In vivo megnesium transport. Pediatr Res 1982;16:295.

158. Batt ER, Schachter D. Developmental pattern of some intestinal transport mechanisms in newborn rats and mice. Am J Physiol 1969;216:1064.

159. Cheung H, Leblond CF. Origin, differentiation, and renewal of the four main epithelial cell types in the mouse small intestine. V. Unitarian theory of the origin of the four epithelial cell types. Am J Anat 1974;141:537.

160. Cameron IL, Gosslee DG, Pilgrim C. The spatial distribution of dividing and DNA-synthesizing cells in the mouse epithelium. J Cell Comp Physiol 1965;66:431.

161. Moxey PC, Trier JS. Development of villous absorptive cells in the human fetal small intestine: A morphologic and morphometric study. Anat Rec 1979;195:463.

162. Lipkin M. Proliferation and differentiation of normal and diseased gastrointestinal cells. In: Johnson LR, ed. Physiology of the gastrointestinal tract, ed 2. New York: Raven Press, 1987:255.

163. Sweetser DA, Hauft SM, Hoppe PC, Birkenmeier EH, Gordon JI. Transgenic mice containing intestinal fatty acid-binding protein-human growth hormone fusion genes exhibit correct regional and cell-specific expression of the reporter gene in their small intestine. Proc Natl Acad Sci USA 1988;85:9611.

164. Sweetser DA, Birkenmeier EH, Hoppe PC, McKeel DW, Gordon JI. Mechanisms underlying generation of gradients in gene expression within the intestine: An analysis using transgenic mice containing fatty acid binding protein-human growth hormone fusion genes. Genes Dev 1988;2:1318.

165. Peschner EE, Lipkin M. An autoradiographic study of the renewal of argentaffin cells in human rectal mucosa. Exp Cell Res 1966;43:661.

166. Trier JS, Lorennzsonn V, Groehler K. Pattern of secretion of Paneth cells of the small intestine of mice. Gastroenterology 1967;53:240.

167. Deschner EE. Observations on the Paneth cell in human ileum. Exp Cell Res 1967;47:624.

168. Jarvi OH, Keyrilainer O. On the cellular structures of the epithelial

invasions in the glandular stomach of mice caused by intramural application of 20-methylcholanthrene. Acta Pathol Microbiol Scand 1955;111(Suppl):72.

169. Isomaki AM. A new cell type (tuft cell) in the gastrointestinal mucosa of the rat. Acta Pathol Microbiol Scand 1973;240(Suppl):1973A.

170. Tsubouchi S, Leblond CP. Migration and turnover of enteroendocrine and caveolated cells in the epithelium of the descending colon, as shown by radioautography after continuous infusion of 3H-thymidine into mice. Am J Anat 1979;156:431.

171. Barkla DH, Whitehead RH, Foster H, Tutton PJM. Tuft (caveolated) cells in two human colon carcinoma cell lines. Am J Pathol 1988;132:521.

172. Owen RL, Jones AL. Epithelial cells specialization within human Peyer's patches: An ultrastructural study. Gastroenterology 1977;72:440.

173. Moxey PC, Trier JS. Specialized cell types in the human fetal small intestine. Anat Rec 1978;191:269.

174. von Rosen L, Podjaski B, Bettmann I, Otto H. Observations on the ultrastructure and function of the so-called 'microfold' or 'membranous' cells by means of peroxidase as a tracer. An experimental study with special attention to the physiological parameters of resorption. Virchows Arch (Pathol Anat) 1981;390:289.

175. Wolf JL, Rubin DH, Finberg R, et al. Intestinal M cells: A pathway for entry of retrovirus into the host. Science 1981;212:471.

176. Creamer B, Shorter RG, Banforth J. The turnover and shedding of epithelial cells. I. The turnover in the gastrointestinal tract. Gut 1961;2:110.

177. Bell B, Almy TP, Lipkin M. Cell proliferation kinetics in the gastrointestinal tract of man. III. Cell renewal in the esophagus, stomach, and jejunum of a patient with treated pernicious anemia. J Natl Cancer Inst 1967;38:615.

178. Lipkin M, Sherlock B, Bell B. Cell proliferation kinetics in the gastrointestinal tract of man. II. Cell renewal in stomach, ileum, colon and rectum. Gastroenterology 1963;45:721.

179. Marques-Pereira JP, Leblond CP. Mitosis and differentiation in the stratified squamous epithelium of the rat esophagus. Am J Anat 1965;117:73.

180. Lipkin M. Growth and development of gastrointestinal cells. Annu Rev Physiol 1985;47:175.

181. Messier R. Radioautographic evidence for the renewal of the mucous cells in the gastric mucosa of the rat. Anat Rec 1960;136:242.

182. McDonald C, Trier JS, Everett B. Cell proliferation and migration in the stomach, duodenum, and rectum of man. Gastroenterology 1964;46:405.

183. Willems G, Galand P, Vansteenkiste Y. Cell population kinetics of zymogen and parietal cells in the stomachs of mice. Z Zellforsch Mikrosk Anat 1972;134:505.

184. Ragins H, Wincze F, Liu SM. The origin of gastric parietal cells in the mouse. Anat Rec 1968;162:99.

185. Lehy T, Willems G. Population kinetics of antral gastrin cells in the mouse. Gastroenterology 1976;71:614.

186. Fugimoto S, Kawai K, Hattori T, Fujita S. Tritiated thymidine autoradiographic study on origin and renewal of gastrin cells in pyloric area of hamsters (Abstract). Gastroenterology 1979;76:1136.

187. Hermos JA, Mathan M, Trier JS. DNA synthesis and proliferation by villous epithelial cells in fetal rats. J Cell Biol 1971;50:255.

188. Cheng H, Merzel J, Leblond CP. Renewal of Paneth cells in the small intestine of the mouse. Am J Anat 1969;126:507.

189. Wilson TJG, Ponder BAJ, Wright NA. Use of a mouse chimeric model to study cell migration patterns in the small intestinal epithelium. Cell Tissue Kinet 1985;18:333.

190. Shorter RG, Moertel CG, Titus JL, Reitemeier RJ. Cell kinetics in the jejunum and rectum of man. Am J Dig Dis 1964;9:760.

191. Altmann GG, Leblond CP. Factors influencing villous size in the small intestine of adult rats as revealed by transportation of intestinal segments. Am J Anat 1976;127:15.

192. Griffiths DFR, Davies SJ, Williams D, Williams GT, Williams ED. Demonstration of somatic mutation and colonic crypt clonality by X-linked enzyme histochemistry. Nature 1988;333:461.

193. Fearon ER, Hamilton SR, Vogelstein B. Clonal analysis of human colorectal tumors. Science 1987;238:193.

194. Lipkin M, Bell B, Sherlock P. Cell proliferation kinetics in the gas-

trointestinal tract of man. I. Cell renewal in colon and rectum. J Clin Invest 1963;42:767.

195. Messier B, Leblond CP. Cell proliferation and migration as revealed by radioautography after injection of thymidine-111[3] into rats and mice. Am J Anat 1960;106:247.

196. Sunter JP, Watson AJ, Wright NA, Appleton DR. Cell proliferation at different sites along the length of the rat colon. Virchows Arch (Cell Pathol) 1979;32:75.

197. Messier B. Renewal of the colonic epithelium of the rat. Am J Dig Dis 1960;5:833.

198. Deschner EE, Lipkin M. An autoradiographic study of the renewal of argentaffin cells in human rectal mucosa. Exp Cell Res 1966;43:661.

199. Ismael-Beigi F, Pope CE II. Distribution of histologic changes of reflux. Gastroenterology 1974;66:1109.

200. Kim Y, Kerr RJ, Lipkin M. Cell proliferation during the development of stress erosions in mouse stomach. Nature 1967;215:1180.

201. Baraona E, Pirsla RC, Lieber CS. Small intestinal damage and changes in cell population produced by ethanol ingestion in the rat. Gastroenterology 1974;66:226.

202. Zagorulko MP, Puzyrev AA. On proliferation of the epithelium of the duodenal mucosa in ulcerative disease. Arkh Patol 1974;36:31.

203. Hamilton E. Cell proliferation and ageing in mouse colon. I. Repopulation after repeated x-ray injury in young and old mice. Cell Tissue Kinet 1978;11:423.

204. Gelfand MD, Tepper M, Katz LA, et al. Acute irradiation proctitis in man. Development of eosinophilia in crypt abscesses. Gastroenterology 1968;54:401.

205. Rijke RPC, Gait R, Langendoen NJ. Epithelial cell kinetics in the descending colon of the rat. II. The effect of experimental bypass. Virchows Arch (Cell Pathol) 1979;31:23.

206. Herbst JJ, Berenson MM, Weser WC, et al. Cell proliferation in Barrett's esophageal epithelium. Clin Res 1976;24:168A.

207. Liavag I. Mitotic activity of the gastric mucosa. Acta Pathol Microbiol Scand 1968;72:43.

208. Lightdale C, Lipkin M, Deschner E. In vivo measurements in familial polyposis: Kinetics and location of proliferating cells in colonic adenomas. Cancer Res 1982;42:4280.

209. Bleiberg H, Mainguet P, Galand P, et al. Cell renewal in the human rectum. In vitro autoradiographic study on active ulcerative colitis. Gastroenterology 1970;58:85.

210. Makela P, Nossal G. Autoradiographic studies on the immune response. II. DNA synthesis among single antibody-producing cells. J Exp Med 1962;115:231.

211. Altmann GV, Leblond CP. Factors influencing villous size in the small intestine of adult rats as revealed by transposition of intestinal segments. Am J Anat 1970;127:15.

212. Gronqvist B, Engstrom B, Grimelius L. Morphological studies of the rat small intestine after jejunoileal transposition. Acta Chir Scand 1971;141:208.

213. Vella L. Neues verfahren zur gewinnung reinen darmsaftres und festsellung seiner physiologischen eigenschaften. Moleschotts Uptersuchungen zur Naturlehre 1882;13:40. Cited in: Markowitz J, Archibald J, Downie HG, eds. Experimental surgery. Baltimore: Williams & Wilkins, 1964:143.

214. Stringel G, Uauy R. A model to study the direct effect of diet on early intestinal growth and maturation using Thiry-Vella loops. J Pediatr Surg 1988;23:80.

215. Hanson WR, Rijke RPC, Plaisier HM, et al. The effect of intestinal resection on Thiry-Vella fistulae of jejunal and ileal origin in the rat: Evidence for a systemic control mechanism of cell renewal. Cell Tissue Kinet 1975;8:135.

216. Jacobs LR, Taylor BR, Dowling RH. Effect of luminal nutrition on the intestinal adaptation following Thiry-Vella bypass in the dog (Abstract) Clin Sci Mol Med 1975;49:26.

217. Keren DF, Elliot HL, Brown GD, Yardley JH. Atrophy of villi with hypertrophy and hyperplasia of Paneth cells in isolated (Thiry-Vella) ileal loops in rabbits. Gastroenterology 1970;58:208.

218. Booth CC, Evans KI, Meuzies T, Street DF. Intestinal hypertrophy following partial resection of the small bowel of the rat. Br J Surg 1959;46:403.

219. Nygaard K. Resection of the small intestine in rats. III. Morphological changes in the intestinal tract. Acta Chir Scand 1967;13:233.

220. Bury KD. Carbohydrate digestion and absorption after massive resection of the small intestine. Surg Gynecol Obstet 1972;135:177.

221. Weser E, Hernandez MH. Small bowel adaptation after intestinal resection in the rat. Gastroenterology 1971;60:69.

222. Feldman EJ, Dowling RH, McNaughton J, Peters TJ. Effects of oral versus intravenous nutrition on intestinal adaptation after small bowel resection in the dog. Gastroenterology 1976;70:712.

223. Johnson LR, Schanbacker LM, Dudrick SJ, Copeland EM. Effect of long-term parenteral feeding on pancreatic secretion and serum secretin. Am J Physiol 1977;233:E524.

224. Johnson LR, Copeland EM, Dudrick SJ, Lichtenberger LM, Castro GA. Structural and hormonal alterations in the gastrointestinal tract of parenterally fed rats. Gastroenterology 1975;68:1177.

225. Wickbom G, Lander JH, Bushkin FL, McGuigan JE. Changes in canine gastric acid output and serum gastrin levels following small intestinal resection. Gastroenterology 1975;69:448.

226. Cardis DT, Roberts M, Smith G. The effect of small bowel resection on gastric acid secretion in the rat. Surgery 1969;65:292.

227. Frederick PL, Sizyer JS, Osborne MP. Relation of the massive bowel resection to gastrin secretion. N Engl J Med 1965;272:509.

228. Wright HK, Poskitt T, Cleveland JC. The effect of total colectomy on morphology and absorptive capacity of the ileum in the rat. J Surg Res 1969;9:301.

229. Nygaard K. Small bowel resection and by-pass. In: Dowling RH, Rieckin EO, eds. Intestinal adaptation. Stuttgart: FK Schattaeuer, Verlag, 1974:47.

230. Winborn WB, Seeling LL Jr, Nakayama H, Weser E. Hyperplasia of gastric glands after small bowel resection in the rat. Gastroenterology 1982;66:384.

231. Loran MR, Carbone JV. The humoral effect of intestinal resection on cellular proliferation and maturation in parabiotic rats. In: Sullivan MF, ed. Gastrointestinal radiation injury. Amsterdam: Excerpta Medica, 1968:127.

232. Clarke RM. "Luminal nutrition" versus "functional work-load" as controllers of mucosal morphology and epithelial replacement in the rat small intestine. Digestion 1977;15:411.

233. Johnson LR. Regulation of gastrointestinal mucosal growth. Physiol Rev 1988;68:456.

234. Sircar B, Johnson LR, Lichtenberger LM. Effect of synthetic diets on gastrointestinal mucosal DNA synthesis in rats. Am J Physiol 1983;244:G327.

235. Jacobs LR, Lupton JR. Effect of dietary fibers on rat large bowel mucosal growth and cell proliferation. Am J Physiol 1984;246:G378.

236. Dowling RH, Riecken EO, Lows JW, Booth CC. The intestinal response to high bulk feeding in the rat. Clin Sci 1967;32:1.

237. Jacobs LR, Lupton JR. Dietary wheat bran lowers colonic pH in rats. J Nutr 1982;112:592.

238. Goodlad KA, Ratcliffe B, Fordham JP, Wright NA. Does dietary fiber stimulate intestinal epithelial cell proliferation in germ free rats? Gut 1989;30:820.

239. Seidel ER, Haddox MK, Johnson LR. Polyamines in the response to intestinal obstruction. Am J Physiol 1984;246:G649.

240. Dembinski AB, Yamaguchi T, Johnson LR. Stimulation of mucosal growth by a dietary amine. Am J Physiol 1984;247:G352.

241. Seidel ER, Haddox MK, Johnson LR. Ileal mucosal growth during intraluminal infusion of ethylamine or putrescine. Am J Physiol 1985;249:G434.

242. Lichtenberger LM, Graziani LA, Dubinsky WP. Importance of dietary amines in meal-induced gastrin release. Am J Physiol 1982;243:G341.

243. Russell DH, Durie BGM. Ornithine decarboxylase—a key enzyme in growth. Prog Cancer Res Ther 1978;8:43.

244. Luk GP, Baylin SB. Polyamines and intestinal growth—increased polyamine biosynthesis after jejunectomy. Am J Physiology 1983;245:G656.

245. Yang P, Balin SB, Luk GD. Polyamines and intestinal growth: Absolute requirement for ODC activity in adaptation and lactation. Am J Physiol 1984;247:G553.

246. Seidel ER, Maddox MK, Johnson LR. Polyamines in the response to intestinal obstruction. Am J Physiol 1984;245:G649.

247. Seidel ER. Hormonal regulation of postprandial ornithine decarboxylase activity. Am J Physiol 1986;251:G460.

248. Fitzpatrick LR, Wang P, Johnson LR. Effect of refeeding on poly-

amine biosynthesis in isolated enterocytes. Am J Physiol 1986;250:G709.

249. Fitzpatrick LR, Wang P, Johnson LR. Effect of epidermal growth factor on polyamine synthesizing enzymes in rat enterocytes. Am J Physiol 1987;252:G209.

250. Gintz DD, Seidel ER. Polyamine-dependent growth and calmodulin-regulated induction of ornithine decarboxylase. Am J Physiol 1989;256:G342.

251. Vishen MH, Lyn-Cook LE, Raasch RH. Effects of intraluminal epidermal growth factor on mucosal proliferation in the small intestine of adult rats. Gastroenterology 1986;91:1134.

252. Uvnas-Wallenstein K. Occurrence of gastrin in gastric juice, in antral secretion and in perfusate of cats. Gastroenterology 1977;73:487.

253. Johnson LR, Guthrie PD, Dudrick SJ. Effects of luminal gastrin on the growth of rat intestinal mucosa. Gastroenterology 1981;81:71.

254. Alpers DH, Philpott GW. Control of DNA synthesis in normal rabbit colonic mucosa. Gastroenterology 1975;G19:951.

255. Derubertis FR, Craven PA. Early alterations in rat colonic mucosal cyclic nucleotide metabolism and protein kinase activity induced by 1,5 methylhydrazine. Cancer Res 1980;40:45.

256. Gilbertson TJ, Ruwait MJ, Stryd RP, et al. Partial characterization of the gastrointestinal weight changes produced in the fetal rat by 16,16-dimethylprostaglandin E_2. Prostaglandins 1983;26:745.

257. Johansson C, Alg A, Kollberg B, et al. Trophic actions of oral E_2 prostaglandins on the rat gastrointestinal mucosa. In: Samuelsson B, Paoletti R, Ramwell P, eds. Advances in prostaglandin, thromboxane, and leukotriene research, Vol 12. New York: Raven Press, 1983:403.

258. Reinhart WH, Muller O, Holter F. Influence of long-term 16,16-dimethyl prostaglandin E_2 treatment on the rat gastrointestinal mucosa. Gastroenterology 1983;85:1003.

259. Robert A, Nezamis JE, Lancaster C, Hanchar AJ. Cytoprotection of prostaglandins in rats: Prevention of gastric necrosis produced by alcohol, HCl, NaOH, hypertonic NaCl, and thermal injury. Gastroenterology 1979;77:433.

260. Miller TA, Gum ET, Guinn EJ, Henagan JM. Prostaglandin prevents alterations in DNA, RNA, and protein in damaged gastric mucosa. Dig Dis Sci 1982;27:776.

261. Weser E, Drummond A, Tawil T. Effects of octapeptide cholecystokinin, secretin, and glucagon on intestinal mucosal growth in parenterally nourished rats. Dig Dis Sci 1981;26:406.

262. Miazza BM, Levan H, Vaja S, Dowling RH. Effect of pancreaticobiliary diversion on jejunal and ileal structure and function in the rat. In: Robinson JWL, Dowling RH, Riecken EO, eds. Mechanisms of intestinal adaptation. Lancaster, United Kingdom: MTP, 1982:467.

263. Altmann GG. Influence of bile and pancreatic secretions on the size of intestinal villi in rats. Am J Anat 1971;133:391.

264. Jacobson ED, Magnani TJ. Some effects of hypophysectomy on gastrointestinal function and structure. Gut 1964;5:1964.

265. Leviton R, Havivi E. Effect of hypophysectomy on amino acid, thymidine, and orotic acid incorporation into the mucosa of the small bowel. Can J Biochem 1970;48:828.

266. Baker BL, Abrams GD. Effect of hypophysectomy on the cytology of the fundic glands of the stomach and on the secretion of pepsin. Am J Physiol 1954;177:409.

267. Enochs MR, Johnson LR. Effect of hypophysectomy and growth hormone on serum and antral gastrin levels in the rat. Gastroenterology 1976;70:727.

268. Dorchester JEC, Haist RE. The secretin content of the intestine in normal and hypophysectomized rats. J Physiol (Lond) 1952;N8:188.

269. Crean GP. The endocrine system and the stomach. Vitam Horm 1963;21:215.

270. Rasanen T. Fluctuations in the mitotic frequency of the glandular stomach and intestine of the rat under the influence of ACTH, glucocorticoids, stress and heparin. Acta Physiol Scand 1963;58:211.

271. Scott JR, Batt M, Maddison YE, Peters TJ. Differential effect of glucocorticoids on structure and function of adult rat jejunum. Am J Physiol 1981;241:G306.

272. Sander LD, Enochs MR, Johnson LR. Effects of ACTH and the

adrenals on serum and antral gastrin levels in the rat. Proc Soc Exp Biol Med 1978;158:609.

273. Leblond CP, Carriere RM. The effect of growth hormone and thyroxine on the mitotic rate of the intestinal mucosa of the rat. Endocrinology 1955;56:261.

274. Sesso A, Valeri V. Nucleic acid patterns in the pancreas of hypophysectomized rats after administration of growth hormone and of thyroxine. Exp Cell Res 1958;14:201.

275. Pearse AGC, Bussolati G. Immunofluorescence studies of the distribution of gastrin cells in different clinical states. Gut 1970;11:646.

276. Eartly H, Leblond CP. Identification of the effects of thyroxine mediated by the hypophysis. Endocrinology 1954;54:249.

277. Johnson LR, Aures D, Hakanson R. Effect of gastrin on the in vivo incorporation of ^{14}C-leucine into protein of the digestive tract. Proc Soc Exp Biol Med 1969;132:996.

278. Willems G, Lehy T. Radioautographic and quantitative studies on parietal and peptic cell kinetics in the mouse. Gastroenterology 1975;69:416.

279. Majumdar APN. Effect of pentagastrin on DNA synthesis and thymidine kinase activity in gastric mucosa of rats. Horm Res 1983;15:37.

280. Hakanson R, Ekelund M, Sundler F. Activation and proliferation of gastric endocrine cells. In: Falkner S, Hakanson R, Sundler F, eds. Evolution and tumor pathology of the neuroendocrine system. New York:Elsevier, 1984:371.

281. Mayston PD, Barrowman JA. The influence of chronic administration of pentagastrin on the rat pancreas. Q J Exp Physiol 1971;56:113.

282. Solomon TE, Morriset J, Wood JG, Bussjaeger LJ. Additive interaction of pentagastrin and secretion on pancreatic growth in rats. Gastroenterology 1987;92:429.

283. Mayston PD, Barrowman JA. The influence of chronic administration of pentagastrin on the pancreas in hypophysectomized rats. Gastroenterology 1973;64:391.

284. Takeuchi K, Speir GR, Johnson LR. Mucosal gastrin receptor binding specificity. Am J Physiol 1980;239:G395.

285. Johnson LR, Guthrie PD. Proglumide inhibition of trophic action of pentagastrin. Am J Physiol 1984;246:G62.

286. Johnson LR, Grossman MI. Analysis of inhibition of acid secretion by cholecystokinin in dogs. Am J Physiol 1970;218:550.

287. Ryan GP, Copeland EM, Johnson LR. Effects of gastrin on vagal denervation on DNA synthesis in canine fundic mucosa. Am J Physiol 1978;235:E32.

288. Johnson LR, Guthrie PD. Stimulation of DNA synthesis by big and little gastrin (G-34 and G-17). Gastroenterology 1976;71:599.

289. Hakanson RH, Blom E, Carlsson H, et al. Hypergastrinemia produces trophic effects in stomach but not in pancreas and intestines. Regul Pept 1986;13:225.

290. Larssen H, Carlsson E, Mattson H, et al. Plasma gastrin and gastrin enterochromaffin-like cell activation and proliferation. Gastroenterology 1986;90:391.

291. Seidel ER, Tabata K, Dembinski AB, Johnson LR. Attenuation of the trophic response to gastrin after inhibition of ornithine decarboxylase. Am J Physiol 1985;249:G16.

292. Seidel ER, Snyder RG. Pentagastrin induction of spermine/spermidine N^1-acetyltransferase and mucosal polyamines. Am J Physiol 1989;256:G16.

293. Johnson LR, Stening GF, Grossiman MI. The effect of sulfation on the gastrointestinal action of caerulein. Gastroenterology 1970;58:208.

294. Rothman SS, Wells H. Enhancement of pancreatic enzyme synthesis by pancreozymin. Am J Physiol 1967;213:215.

295. Mainz DL, Black O, Webster PD. Hormonal control of pancreatic growth. J Clin Invest 1973;52:2300.

296. Yamada T, Brunstedt J, Solomon T. Chronic effects of caerulein and secretin on the endocrine pancreas of the rat. Am J Physiol 1983;244:G541.

297. Temler RS, Dormand CA, Simone E, Morel B. The effect of feeding soybean trypsin inhibitor and repeated injections of cholecystokinin on rat pancreas. J Nutr 1984;114:1083.

298. Johnson LR, Dudrick SJ, Guthrie PD. Stimulation of pancreatic growth by intraduodenal amino acids and HCl. Am J Physiol 1980;239:G400.

299. Rosewicz S, Lewis LD, Liddle RA, Logsdon CD. Effects of cholecystokinin on pancreatic ornithine decarboxylase gene expression. Am J Physiol 1988;255:G818.

300. Johnson LR, Guthrie PD. Effect of cholecystokinin and 16,16-dimethyl prostaglandin E_2 on RNA and DNA of gastric and duodenal mucosa. Gastroenterology 1976;70:59.

301. Lamote J, Putz P, Willems G. Effect of cholecystokinin-octapeptide, caerulein, and pentagastrin on epithelial cell proliferation in the murine gallbladder. Gastroenterology 1982;83:371.

302. Dembinski AB, Johnson LR. Stimulation of pancreatic growth by secretin, caerulein, and pentagastrin. Endocrinology 1980;106:323.

303. Solomon TE, Peterson H, Elaskoff J, Grossman MI. Interactin of caerulein and secretin on pancreatic size and composition in the rat. Am J Physiol 1978;235:E714.

304. Stanley MD, Coalson RE, Grossman MI, Johnson LR. Influence of secretin and pentagastrin on acid secretion and parietal cell numbers in rats. Gastroenterology 1972;63:264.

305. Johnson LR, Guthrie PD. Secretin inhibition of gastrin-stimulated deoxyribonucleic acid synthesis. Gastroenterology 1974;67:601.

306. Johnson LR, Guth PD. Effect of secretin on colonic DNA synthesis. Proc Soc Exp Biol Med 1978;158:521.

307. Logsdon CD. Stimulation of pancreatic acinar cell growth by CCK, epidermal growth factor, and insulin in vitro. Am J Physiol 1986;251:G487.

308. Sporn MB, Roberts AB. Autocrine growth factors and cancer. Nature 1985;313:745.

309. Reeve JR Jr, Cuttitta F, Vigna SR, et al. Multiple gastrin-releasing peptide gene-associated peptides are produced by a human small cell lung cancer line. J Biol Chem 1988;263:1928.

310. Lehy T, Accary JP, Labeille D, Dulrasquet M. Chronic administration of bombesin stimulates antral gastrin cell proliferation in the rat. Gastroenterology 1983;84:914.

311. Johnson LR, Guthrie PD. Regulation of antral gastrin content. Am J Physiol 1983;245:G725.

312. Dange C. Hajri A, Lhoste E. Aprahamian M. Comparative effect of chronic bombesin, gastrin-releasing peptide and caerulein on the rat pancreas. Regul Pept 1988;20:141.

313. Saffouri B, DuVal JW, Makhlouf GM. Stimulation of gastrin secretion in vitro by intraluminal chemical: Regulation by intramural cholinergic and noncholinergic neurons. Gastroenterology 1984;87:557.

314. Helmstaedter V, Taugner CH, Feurle GE, Forssmann WG. Localization of neurotensin-immunoreactive cells in the small intestine of man and various mammals. Histochemistry 1977;53:35.

315. Wood JG, Hoang HD, Bussjaeger LJ, Solomon TE. Neurotensin stimulates growth of small intestine in rats. Am J Physiol 1988;255:G813.

316. Folkers K, Chang D, Humphries J, et al. Synthesis and activities of neurotensin and its acid and amide analogs. Possible natural occurrence of Gln4-neurotensin. Proc Nat Acad Sci USA 1976;73:3833.

317. Ukai M, Inoue I, Hatsu T. Effect of somatostatin on neurotensin-induced glucagon release and hyperglycemia. Endocrinology 1977;100:1284.

318. Servin AL, Youyer-Fessard C, Balasubramaniam A, Pierre SS, Laburthe M. Peptide-YY and neuropeptide-Y inhibit vasoactive intestinal peptide-stimulated adenosine 3′,5′-monophosphate production in rat small intestine: Structural requirements of peptides for interacting with peptide-YY-preferring receptors. Endocrinology 1989;124:692.

319. El-Salhy M, Wilander E, Juntti-Berggrenl, Grimelius L. The distribution and ontogeny of polypeptide YY and pancreatic polypeptide-immunoreactive cells in the gastrointestinal tract of rats. Histochemistry 1983;78:53.

320. Leiter AB, Toder A, Taylor IL, et al. Identification of the pancreas as the major site of peptide YY mRNA synthesis using a cloned cDNA probe. (Abstract) Gastroenterology 1987;92:1499.

321. Goodlad RA, Ghatei MA, Domin J, Bloom SR, Gregory H, Wright NA. Plasma enteroglucagon, peptide YY and gastrin in rats deprived of luminal nutrition and after urogastroine-EGF administration. A proliferative rate for PYY in the intestinal epithelium. Experientia 1989;45:168.

322. Cohen S, Taylor JM. Epidermal growth factor: Chemical and biological characterization. Recent Prog Horm Res 1974;30:533.

323. Johnson LR, Guthrie PD. Stimulation of rat oxyntic gland mucosal growth by epidermal growth factor. Am J Physiol 1980;238:G45.

324. Li AKC, Schattenkerk ME, Huffman RG, Ross JS, Malt RA. Hypersecretion of submandibular saliva in male mice: Trophic response in small intestine. Gastroenterology 1983;84:949.

325. Scheving LA, Shiurba RA, Nguyen TD, Gray GM. Epidermal growth factor receptor of the intestinal enterocyte. Localization to laterobasal but not brush border membrane. J Biol Chem 1989;264:1735.

326. Godley JM, Brand SJ. Regulation of the gastrin promoter by epidermal growth factor and neuropeptides. Proc Natl Acad Sci USA 1989;86:3036.

327. Coffey RJ, Derynck R, Wilcox JN, Bringman TS, Goustin AS, Moses HL, Pittelkow MR. Production and auto-induction of transforming growth factor a in human keratinocytes. Nature 1987;328:817.

328. Koyama S, Podolsky DK. Differential expression of transforming growth factors α and β in rat intestinal epithelial cells: Mirror-image gradients from crypt to villus. J Clin Immunol 1989;83:1768.

329. Derynck R. Transforming growth factor α. Cell 1988;54:1988.

330. Kurokowa M, Lynch K, Podolsky D. Effects of growth factors on an intestinal epithelial cell line: Transforming growth factor β inhibits and stimulates differentiation. Biochem Biophys Res Commun 1987;142:775.

331. Saffouri B, Weir G, Bitar K, Makhlouf GM. Gastrin and somatostatin secretion by perfused rat stomach: Functional linkage of antral peptide. Am J Physiol 1980;238:G495.

332. Lehy T, Accary JP, Labeille D, Dubrasquet M. Chronic administration of bombesin stimulates antral gastrin cell proliferation in the rat. Gastroenterology 1983;84:914.

333. Lehy T, Dubrasquet M, Brazeau P, Bonfils S. Inhibitory effect of prolonged administration of long-acting somatostatin on gastrin-stimulated fundic epithelial cell growth in the rat. Digestion 1982;24:246.

334. Boden G, Switz MC, Owen OT, Ersa-Koumar N, Landor JH. Somatostatin suppresses secretin and pancreatic exocrine secretion. Science 1975;190:163.

335. Konturek SJ, Tasler J, Ciezkowski M, Coy DN, Schally AV. Effect of growth hormone release inhibiting hormone on gastric secretion, mucosal blood flow, and serum gastrin. Gastroenterology 1976;70:737.

336. Morisset J, Genik P, Solomon TE. Effects of chronic administration of somatostatin on rat exocrine pancreas. Regul Pept 1982;4:49.

337. Morriset J. Somatostatin: A potential antigrowth factor for the exocrine pancreas. Regul Pept 1984;10:11.

338. Bloom SR, Polak JM. The hormonal pattern of intestinal adaptation. A major role for enteroglucagon. Scand J Gastroenterol 1982;17(Suppl 74):93.

339. Besterman HS, Bloom SR, Sarson DL, et al. Gut hormone profile in coeliac disease. Lancet 1978;1:785.

340. Besterman HS, Cook GC, Sarson DL, et al. Gut hormones in tropical malabsorption. Br Med J 1979;2:1252.

341. Goodlad RA, Al-Mukhtar MYT, Ahatei MA, Bloom SR, Wright NA. Cell proliferation, plasma enteroglucagon and plasma gastrin levels in starved and refed rats. Virchows Arch (Cell Pathol) 1983;43:55.

342. Johnson LR. New aspects of the trophic action of gastrointestinal hormones. Gastroenterology 1977;72:788.

343. Lorenz-Meyer H, Menge H, Riecken EO. Functional and morphological studies on intestinal mucosa of the rate under chronic glucagon application. Res Exp Med 1977;170:181.

344. Blache P, Kervran A, Martinez J, Bataille D. Development of an Oxyntomodulin/Glicentin c-terminal radioimmunoassay using a "thiol-maleoyl" coupling method for preparing the immunogen. Anal Biochem 1988;173:151.

345. Blache P, Kervran A, Batille D. Oxynto-modulin and glicentin: Brain-gut peptides in the rat. Endocrinology 1988;123:2782.

24

Neoplasia of the Gastrointestinal Tract

C. RICHARD BOLAND
ANDREW P. FEINBERG

THE CELLULAR BIOLOGY OF TUMOR DEVELOPMENT CARCINOGENESIS: AN INTRODUCTION

The gastrointestinal tract, including the hollow organs of the gut, pancreas, liver, and biliary tree, is the site of more cancers and cancer mortality than any other organ system in the body. However, there is no simple explanation to unify the etiology of all gut tumors. One of the most notable features of international cancer epidemiology is the wide variability of tumor incidence by organ site. For example, an esophageal cancer belt extends from Northeast China, through Soviet Central Asia, and into Northern Iran.[1] In portions of these regions, the incidence of squamous cell carcinoma of the esophagus is over 100 times higher than in adjacent low-incidence regions. In the United States, threefold to fourfold differences in incidence of esophageal cancer may be found simply based on sex and race.[2] In Japan, the incidence of gastric carcinoma is approximately 10 times higher than it is in the United States. Conversely, colorectal cancer occurs less commonly in Japan but is the most frequently occurring gastrointestinal malignancy in North America and in Western Europe. These marked differences in cancer risk do not seem to be based entirely on racial or genetic factors. When persons migrate from a high-incidence region to a low-incidence region, the organ-specific rates of some cancers change to match that of the new region, usually within two generations. Collectively, the epidemiologic observations strongly suggest the importance of environmental factors in gastrointestinal carcinogenesis.

Laboratory models using chemical carcinogens have been developed for the esophagus, stomach, pancreas, and large intestine and have provided substantial insight into the mechanisms by which dietary factors can produce cancer. The focus in this chapter is on the cellular and molecular mechanisms responsible for the generation of solid tumors in the gut. Additional details on specific factors influencing carcinogenesis will also be found in the chapters addressing cancer in individual organs of the gut. Carcinogenesis in the liver and biliary tree may be mediated by different mechanisms from those operative in the lumenal gut and will not be addressed here.

The Cell Cycle

In order to appreciate carcinogenesis in the gastrointestinal tract, one must first understand how proliferation and differentiation are regulated in the epithelial unit.[3] Because it is lined with squamous epithelium, the esophagus is somewhat different from the remainder of the gut (with the exception of the anus). The proliferative region in esophageal mucosa is in the basal layer, and daughter cells migrate to the surface where they differentiate, flatten, and form a tight barrier impermeable to lumenal contents. Absorption does not occur in the esophagus. The squamous epithelium of the esophagus replicates very slowly, with a replacement rate of approximately 7 days in mice and somewhat slower than this in humans. Most esophageal cancers are squamous cell carcinomas derived from the basal layers; adenocarcinomas arise from foci of epithelial metaplasia.

Gastric epithelium is more complex, having a number of specialized elements, including mucous cells, parietal cells, chief cells, endocrine cells, and Paneth cells. It is not clear whether there is more than one variety of stem cell in the stomach; however, a single proliferating pool of undifferentiated cells can be found in the mid and lower portions of the gastric gland. Cell turnover varies widely depending on the region of the stomach, the cell type, and the species. Specialized cells, such as parietal cells and chief cells, do not appear to proliferate rapidly. It is not clear which cell pool is responsible for adenocarcinomas of the stomach.

The epithelium of the small intestine is also complex and includes a variety of absorptive, secretory, and endocrine cells. The proliferative zone is confined to the small intestinal crypt region, while the villus is composed exclusively of mature cells. Although it is difficult to determine the turnover time in the stomach and small intestine, it appears to take 48 to 72 hours for a cell containing newly synthesized DNA to become fully mature and to be extruded into the lumenal stream. For a variety of reasons, adenocarcinoma of the small intestine is rare.

The large intestine is the most extensively studied epithelium in the gastrointestinal tract and consists of a simple crypt unit made up primarily of absorptive cells and mucin-secreting goblet cells. The proliferative region is confined to the lower two thirds of the crypt, and the daughter cells differentiate and migrate toward the lumenal surface. The turnover time for colonic epithelium in humans is somewhat longer than it is in the proximal gastrointestinal tract, requiring 3 to 4 days in the colon and 4 to 8 days in the rectum.

The cell replication cycle consists of five phases.[4] Resting cells not involved in active replication may be in either G_0 or G_1. G_1 represents the postmitotic period prior to the initiation of new DNA synthesis as the cell prepares to divide. The cell may spend a variable period of time in G_1. Cells not involved in replication may be referred to arbitrarily as resting in the G_0 phase. After receiving the signal to divide, cells enter a phase of active DNA synthesis, the S phase. Following the duplication of the entire genome, the cell is tetraploid and is briefly in the G_2 phase prior to entering mitosis (M phase). After cell division, the cell reenters the G_1 phase. As the genome becomes more complex with tumor progression, the S phase and M phases may be prolonged, altering the apparent fraction of cells involved in replication. This complicates a direct comparison of the proliferative activity of tumors with that of normal tissue.

Cellular proliferation is central to neoplasia but is frequently misunderstood. An apparent paradox is that the rate of proliferation is generally equal to or greater in the stem cell pool of normal epithelium than in solid tumors derived from the same tissue. Some of the confusion derives from the different means of measuring proliferation. Two commonly used measures are the mitotic index and the labeling index. The mitotic index (MI) is a measure of the number of mitoses observed in a population of cells. Although this would seem to be a reasonable measure of proliferative activity, the number of mitoses seen in a histologic section is a function of a product of the number of cells in the proliferative pool and the duration of mitosis. Thus, when mitosis is prolonged, as it often is in cancer, there may be an increase in the MI without a true increase in proliferative rate. The labeling index (LI) is determined by the number of cells that incorporate ^{3}H-thymidine into DNA. This estimates the number of cells actively involved in DNA synthesis, or in the S phase of the cell cycle. The LI is a more accurate measure of proliferative activity than the MI. Of interest, many, and perhaps most, cells in a solid tumor are not actively involved in proliferation and will not grow if one attempts to grow them in culture.

Regulation of Proliferation

Classically, cancer is recognized as a disease of unregulated growth, but it is important to recall that tumor cells do not necessarily proliferate more rapidly than their nonneoplastic counterparts. Neoplastic stem cells give rise to cells that fail to differentiate properly, and a larger proportion of their progeny are capable of additional proliferation. Thus, cancer is a problem associated with failure of differentiation and accumulation of excessive numbers of stem cells. However, an enhanced rate of cell turnover is characteristic of premalignant or high-risk tissues, and considerable attention has been focused on this process.[3-5] Furthermore, cell proliferation may play a role in the stepwise expression of the malignant phenotype by the clonal expansion of selected cells.

The signal that triggers cellular proliferation of the gut is not known. Furthermore, the regulation of DNA replication and cell division is undoubtedly complex. However, several factors have been identified that accompany the process of proliferation and provide some insight into its regulation. First, the polyamines spermidine and spermine are present in all mammalian cells, enter into noncovalent interactions with nucleic acids and other molecules, and are required for cell proliferation.[5] Polyamines are derived from the conversion of arginine and methionine to ornithine, and the subsequent generation of the immediate polyamine precursor putrescine requires the activity of ornithine decarboxylase (ODC). This is of particular importance because compounds that inhibit the activity of ODC can be used to inhibit the expansion of a proliferating pool of cells. ODC inhibitors have been shown to inhibit the appearance and growth of tumors in experimental animals.

Cell proliferation in the colon is mediated in part by eicosanoids. Inhibition of prostaglandin synthesis increases cell proliferation in the rat colon, and administration of prostaglandin E_2 or its intracellular messenger, cyclic adenosine monophosphate (AMP), suppresses proliferative activity.[6] The tumor-promoting phorbol ester 12-O-tetradecanoyl phorbol-13-acetate (TPA) stimulates proliferative activity in colonic mucosa, presumably by activating protein kinase C. The bile salt deoxycholate (DOC) may stimulate colonic epithelial proliferation through the same mechanism, by increasing membrane inositol phospholipid turnover and release of diacylglycerol from the cell membranes.[7] The stimulation of colonic epithelial cell proliferation by bile salts (see ch 84) also involves the generation of superoxide radicals at the epithelial surface, since antioxidants and free radical scavengers can abolish bile acid–mediated proliferation.[8] Polyunsaturated fatty acids can also induce ODC activity and deoxyribonucleic acid (DNA) synthesis in the colon, much in the manner of bile salts. When fatty acids are oxidized, the primary products are significantly more active in stimulating mucosal proliferation, which suggests a collaborative mechanism involving bile salts and fatty acids.[9]

Manipulation of the extracellular calcium concentration can play a role in colonic epithelial proliferation. The addition of supplemental dietary calcium produces a contraction of the proliferative pool in the colons of patients at risk for familial colonic cancer,[10] and the growth of explanted colonic tissues can be inhibited by increasing the calcium concentration within a physiologic range.[11] The implications of this for colon cancer are discussed in more detail in Chapter 84.

Peptide growth factors also participate in the regulation of gastrointestinal epithelial growth. Receptors for gastrin have been found on the surface of normal and malignant gastric epithelial cells, and gastrin stimulates proliferation in both tissues.[12] Gastric achlorhydria brings about a change in the flora and chemical environment of the gastric lumen that facilitates the production of carcinogens. By stimulating proliferation, the hypergastrinemia that accompanies achlorhydria cooperates with the carcinogenic milieu and makes acid-reducing maneuvers (atrophic gastritis, vagotomy with antrectomy, and possibly the long-term suppression of acid secretion) high-risk settings for the development of gastric cancer (see ch 63).

In like manner, receptors for epidermal growth factor (EGF) are present on colonic epithelial cells, and EGF stimulates their proliferation.[13] Although it is not known if there are disease states associated with elevated levels of EGF, it has been shown that the *erb* B oncogene encodes for a protein homologous to the EGF receptor, and this gene is amplified in certain gastrointestinal cancers. This is discussed in more detail later in the chapter.

As previously mentioned, malignant transformation is not a simple matter of increased cellular proliferation, but an increase in proliferative activity is often seen in epithelium at high risk to develop cancer. For example, abnormal patterns of cell replication have been demonstrated throughout normal-appearing colonic crypts among persons with colorectal neoplasms or at very high risk for developing them.[14] Similarly, inflammatory bowel disease, in which there is an enhanced rate of cell turnover, is associated with an increased risk of dysplasia and carcinoma. In the same vein, chronic atrophic gastritis and epithelial metaplasia in the esophagus (Barrett's esophagus) all demonstrate elevated labeling indices and proliferative activity, and these tissues are at heightened risk for cancer. It is not clear why most hyperproliferative states in the gastrointestinal tract are associated with increased rates of cancer, whereas psoriasis, which is arguably the most hyperproliferative disease state in humans, is not associated with an increased risk of skin cancer. Thus it would appear that synergistic factors are required in the setting of enhanced cellular proliferation to produce neoplastic transformation.

Chemical Carcinogenesis

Carcinogenesis classically begins with damage to DNA; however, epigenetic mechanisms may be critical starting points in some forms of cancer. There are three primary mechanisms for damaging DNA: radiation (including ultraviolet radiation, ionizing electromagnetic radiation such as x-rays and gamma rays, and particle radiation, such as electrons, alpha particles, heavy ions, etc.), viral oncogenesis, and chemical carcinogenesis (Table 24-1). As an internal organ, the gastrointestinal tract tends not to be exposed to sufficient radiation to make it a major factor in gastrointestinal carcinogenesis. However, very high doses of x-rays administered under unusual circumstances have been implicated in some instances of intestinal carcinogenesis. Viral oncogenesis has been well documented in a number of nonhuman tumor models but has not been proven in the genesis of any human gastrointestinal tumors. Chemical carcinogenesis is believed to be the most important mechanism involved in initiating neoplasia in the gastrointestinal tract because of its access by ingestion to the gut mucosa.

Chemical carcinogens are rarely present in our diet in their active forms. Typically, "proximate carcinogens" are highly reactive, short-lived chemical compounds that bind nucleic acids, proteins, and other macromolecules near the site of their generation. Chemical carcinogens usually have a narrow range of host and tissue specificity. The microbial flora of the gastrointestinal tract and mucosal enzymes are important factors in the activation (and inactivation) of many carcinogens. For example, an extract made from cycad nuts, cycasin, produces intestinal tumors when administered to most rodents.[15] This compound is a glycoside that must be hydrolyzed by intestinal bacteria to produce methylazoxymethanol (MAM), which is unstable and spontaneously de-

TABLE 24–1
Carcinogenic Agents

Radiation Injury

Ultraviolet radiation

   Especially important for skin

   Most important wavelengths 290–320 nm

Ionizing radiation

   Electromagnetic radiation: x-rays, gamma rays

Particulate radiation

   Electrons, protons, neutrons, alpha particles, heavy ions

Viral Oncogenesis

Proven in numerous animal systems

Implicated in some human tumors

   Papillomavirus—genital cancer

   Epstein-Barr virus—Burkitt's lymphoma, nasopharyngeal carcinoma

   Hepatitis B virus—hepatoma

   Human T cell leukemia viruses

Chemical Carcinogens

Implicated role in a wide spectrum of cancers, including digestive, oral, pulmonary, urinary, cutaneous, and hematologic malignancies

Complex relationships between host and environment involved

Numerous defensive or protective mechanisms at work

---

duce colon cancer after parenteral injection. A more stable compound, dimethylhydrazine (DMH), has been synthesized to study colon carcinogenesis in the laboratory. After absorption in the gut, this procarcinogen undergoes oxidation and hydroxylation in the liver, giving rise to the less stable MAM. Thus, the activities of cycasin and DMH both require specific activation by the intestinal flora or host tissue. It is not surprising, therefore, to learn that certain rodent species do not develop intestinal tumors in response to DMH; in fact, one species resistant to intestinal cancers regularly develops leukemia in response to this compound.[16]

Nitrosamines are believed to be important in carcinogenesis of the esophagus and stomach. Methylbenzylnitrosamine (MBN) is a potent carcinogen that requires microsomal cytochrome P450 activation to be mutagenic (i.e., to damage DNA). During oxidation to benzaldehyde, a reactive methylator is generated that can form O^6-methylguanine adducts in target tissues. These adducts have been shown to induce DNA mutations that lead to cancer. Strain-dependent organ specificity is noted with this carcinogen; MBN produces esophageal tumors in the rat, lung cancers in the mouse, and buccal cheek pouch tumors in the hamster. The mechanism for organ specificity may be demonstrated by measurement of the conversion of MBN to the proximate carcinogen benzaldehyde by mucosal enzyme preparations. Rat esophageal microsomes readily convert MBN to benzaldehyde, whereas gastric microsomal preparations cannot. Rats develop esophageal, but not gastric, tumors.

By manipulating the diet, one can increase or decrease the numbers of esophageal tumors produced in rats with this carcinogen[17] (Table 24-2). For example, rats rendered zinc deficient by a number of different dietary manipulations show a significant increase in carcinogen-induced esophageal cancers. The ability to metabolize MBN to benzaldehyde is increased twofold in the esophageal microsomes from zinc-deficient rats as compared

composes, giving rise to a reactive carbonium ion capable of methylating nucleic acids (Fig 24-1). Cycasin does not give rise to tumors in germ-free rodents, since they lack the necessary glycosidases produced by the intestinal flora. For the same reason, cycasin is only active when administered orally, and does not pro-

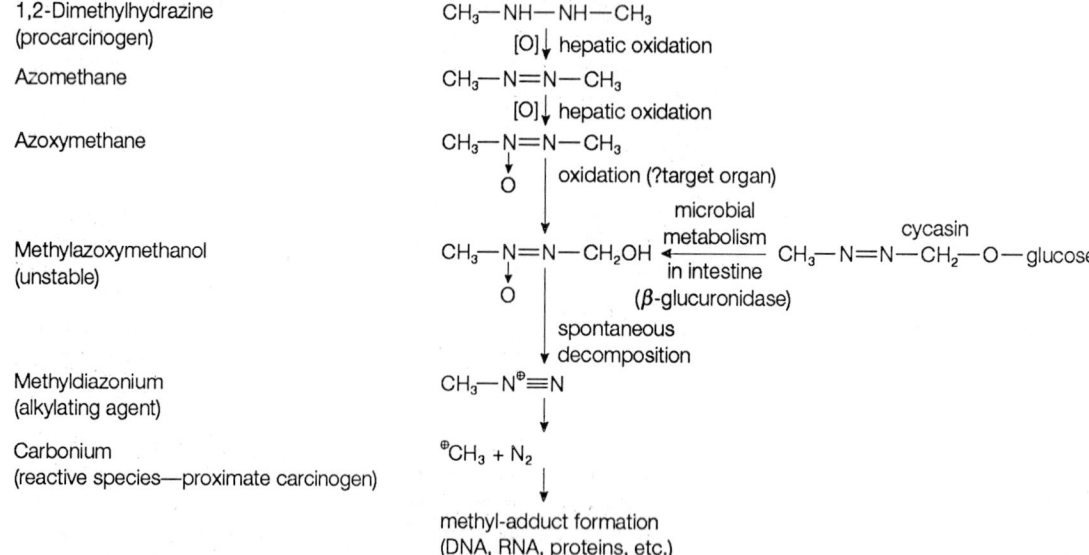

FIGURE 24–1. Metabolic activation of the carcinogen dimethylhydrazine (DMH). This metabolic scheme demonstrates the activation of the procarcinogen DMH through a series of oxidations, some of which occur in the liver and some of which occur at the target organ. An unstable compound is generated that gives rise to a carbonium ion that is the reactive species. DMH is an effective colonic carcinogen whether administered orally (and absorbed from the gut) or given parenterally (and taken up by the liver directly). Cycasin is a carcinogen only if administered orally, assuming the presence of intestinal β-glucuronidase of bacterial origin. The removal of glucose from cycasin gives rise to the unstable compound methylazoxymethanol. (Modified from Lamont JT, O'Gorman TA. Experimental colon cancer. Gastroenterology 1978;75:1157.)

TABLE 24–2
Environmental Modification of Chemical Carcinogenesis:
Methylbenzylnitrosamine-Induced Rat Esophageal Cancer

DIETARY MODIFICATION	APPARENT MECHANISM	MODIFICATION IN CARCINOGENESIS
Zinc deficiency	Increased activation of proximate carcinogen by cytochrome P450 in esophageal microsomes	Increase in tumor production
Disulfiram, saffroles	Diminished metabolism of proximate carcinogen in the esophagus; twofold to fivefold increase in carcinogen activation by hepatic microsomes	Twofold to fivefold increase in tumor production
Ellagic acid	Unchanged activation of carcinogen in esophagus; reduction of O^6-methylguanine formation (cancer-producing mutation), but no change in 7-methylguanine adduct formation (not carcinogenic); selective protection of DNA	Reduction in tumor production

with those from controls. The rate of O^6-methylguanine adduct formation is similarly increased in the zinc-deficient animals.[18] To highlight the specificity of this complex process, zinc deficiency actually reduces tumor formation by other chemical carcinogens (e.g., 3-methylcholanthrene and others). Dietary zinc deficiency and environmental exposure to nitrosamines have been implicated in the very high incidence of esophageal cancer in China. The rodent model provides a possible mechanism by which a dietary factor may accelerate the activation of a procarcinogen. It is important to note that two factors are required to promote carcinogenesis in this setting: (1) exposure to a critical concentration of procarcinogen and (2) a critical degree of nutrient deficiency.

The MBN-induced model of esophageal carcinoma in the rodent has yielded additional insights into possible dietary manipulation of cancer risk. A naturally occurring plant phenol, ellagic acid, when added to the diet of zinc-replete MBN-treated rats reduces the incidence of carcinogen-induced tumors by 30% to 50%. Of particular interest is that ellagic acid does not alter the ability of esophageal microsomes to activate MBN but selectively blocks the ability of the activated or "proximate" carcinogen to form the O^6-methylguanine DNA adducts critical for carcinogenesis.[19,20]

Certain other compounds such as disulfiram and saffroles increase the production of esophageal tumors twofold to fivefold in the MBN model. Pretreatment of the animals with these drugs to increase tumor production actually diminishes the metabolism of the carcinogen by esophageal microsomes but increases carcinogen activation by hepatic microsomes. Thus carcinogens activated in the liver may enter the circulation and produce cancer at a distant site.[21] However, the complexities of carcinogen metabolism (i.e., differential induction of activating and inactivating enzymes in different tissue) leave other possible explanations for the interpretation of these findings.

Some potential carcinogens may be inactivated by microsomal drug-metabolizing enzymes, and it has been suggested that the high activity of mixed function oxidases in the small intestinal mucosa provides protection against carcinogens produced in the digestion of food. The substrates presented to the mucosa represent ingested materials that not only have been subjected to intralumenal digestion but also have been modified further by bacterial enzymes elaborated by the resident flora in the intestine. The microbial environment differs among species and individuals and varies in a predictable way throughout the gastrointestinal tract. As a result, bacterial β-glucuronidases can release carcinogenic aglycones from stable water-soluble glycosides in the intestine, and in the distal intestine nitroreductase can produce other mutagenic products from the fecal contents. The generation of these toxic materials is balanced by inactivating enzymes produced in the mucosa. Furthermore, many of the mucosal enzymes are inducible in the presence of the appropriate substrates. Therefore, as indicated above, the mechanism responsible for modifying susceptibility to carcinogenesis is complex and may involve activation of procarcinogens, inactivation of proximate carcinogens, protection of DNA from adduct formation, or other mechanisms such as those involved in DNA repair.

Tumor Progression

In the case of the gastrointestinal tract, it is generally assumed that chemical mechanisms initiate the process of carcinogenesis. Since the carcinogens are delivered by the lumenal contents of the gut, the entire mucosal surface is exposed and DNA adduct formation occurs in a very large number of cells. However, this exposure results in no immediate phenotypic changes in the epithelium. Indeed, gastrointestinal tract cancer is typically a disease of later adult life despite the continuous exposure of the gut to carcinogens almost from birth. In laboratory animal models of cancer where the administration of carcinogen is precisely determined, there is a long delay between the administration of carcinogen and the appearance of tumors. Thus, the evolution and progression of a tumor appears to involve multiple steps.

Studies performed several decades ago by applying coal tar to mouse skin gave rise to the traditional concepts of initiation and promotion in carcinogenesis.[22] The repeated application of the carcinogen coal tar produced papillomas on the mouse skin. This property made coal tar a "complete carcinogen." However, a single application of coal tar was insufficient to produce tumors. If a single dose of coal tar was applied as an "initiating agent" and was followed by the repeated application of a nonmutagenic "tumor promoter" (croton oil), skin tumors were produced. Repeated application of tumor promoter alone did not produce tumors, and if the sequence were reversed and tumor promoter were applied before the initiating agent, no tumors were produced. Furthermore, it was found that the actions of the initiating agent were permanent. Even if a long period of time were permitted to elapse between the application of the initiator and the promoter, tumors could be produced. Therefore, two properties were attributed to coal tar. The first of these, initiation, was the result of a permanent mutagenic injury to the stem cells of the epidermis. However, this was not sufficient, in and of itself, to produce papillomas. A second property was present in coal tar and croton oil that was epigenetic and did not require mutagenicity. This property has been called "tumor promotion" since it facilitates the expression of the neoplastic phenotype in appropriately initiated cells. At the time these experiments were conducted, it was not possible to identify initiated cells by any morphologic abnormality, but these cells could be induced to neoplastic transformation by the application of agents that were not themselves complete carcinogens.

The traditional concept of initiation and promotion appears to be inadequate to explain the complexities of carcinogenesis that have become apparent with the advancement of molecular biologic techniques. A variety of oncogene mutations, genetic deletions, and chromosomal rearrangements have been found in a large percentage of gastrointestinal cancers; however, none of these abnormalities appears in the earliest stages of neoplasia, such as in very small adenomas of the colon. This raises the possibility that some epigenetic mechanisms may occur early in the natural history of neoplasia and that mutations may accrue sequentially during tumor progression. Therefore, during instances in which the precise application of the mutagenetic carcinogen is identified (as in the case of experimental models), one can discuss carcinogenesis in terms of the traditional periods of "initiation" and "promotion" (or "postinitiation"). The human gastrointestinal tract is exposed to carcinogens beginning in infancy. The entire mucosal "field" is therefore subject to chemical mutation as a function of procarcinogen content of the diet, deactivation of these by host and microbial mechanisms in the intestine, and factors that protect and repair DNA.

Additional factors that increase the likelihood of tumor development are present in the gut lumen. Cellular proliferation may be an essential part of neoplastic progression because it permits the clonal expansion of a critically mutated cell. Proliferation in normal tissue is linked to a process of cellular differentiation in which one of the progeny of a stem cell retains its ability to proliferate and the other either terminally differentiates or undergoes a limited number of additional divisions. Under normal circumstances, the generation of new cells is perfectly balanced with the loss of senescent cells, so that the total cell number remains constant. Enhanced proliferation occurs in response to cell injury and increased cell loss. Proliferation slows during periods of reduced cell loss. However, the equation is skewed in neoplasia. Mutations induced by chemical carcinogens may give rise to changes in cell behavior. The loss of a critical protein required for cell survival might be a lethal mutation. In other instances, a mutation may have no impact on the ability of the cell to survive. In exceptional circumstances, a chance mutation might actually increase the ability of the cell to undergo additional proliferation. The emergence of an "immortalized" clone of cells (an in vitro concept that has yet to be tested directly in humans) represents the beginning of neo-

plastic transformation. The initiation-promotion model is an attempt to conceptualize data obtained in the study of carcinogenesis in skin. Although gastrointestinal carcinogens in experimental models appears to fit this theoretical model, it is not clear how applicable the cutaneous model is in other organ systems.

Neoplastic transformation is not strictly a problem of increased proliferative rate; it is a failure of a population of cells to restrain its proliferation. The stem cell pool in normal epithelium has a proliferative rate that is greater than that observed in most solid neoplasms, but the resulting normal daughter cells do not increase the pool of proliferating cells. However, transformed cells give rise to an ever-increasing pool of cells capable of proliferating, and these cells continue to divide even after they have moved out of the normal proliferative zone.

Most tumors are monoclonal, that is, they have derived from the clonal expansion of a single transformed cell.[23] The clonal expansion of a single transformed cell gives rise to a benign neoplasm (Fig 24-2, steps 1–2). Malignant conversion represents the acquisition of additional cell behavior that underlies the "adenoma to carcinoma" sequence (step 3). Tumor progression involves genomic instability of a neoplasm, resulting in tumor cell heterogeneity and ultimately giving rise to malignant invasion and metastasis. The mechanisms that underlie each of these steps have not yet been elucidated.

After neoplastic transformation, a clone of cells that has acquired the ability to undergo indefinite proliferative expansion is produced. This may be mediated by the activation of genes that are required for normal cell growth. Oncogene activation may be seen in benign neoplasms and has been demonstrated best by discrete point mutations in the *ras* gene.[13] Three separate single nucleotide base mutations in the *ras* gene produced by chemical carcinogens may be sufficient to explain its transforming activity.[22] The mutated *ras* gene product is a signal-transduction protein that retains its guanosine triphosphatase activity and substrate specificity but appears to have undergone a critical change in its regulatory domain so that it is not properly inhibited by normal feedback mechanisms.

During normal cell renewal, one cell retains the ability to proliferate and stays in the stem cell zone, while the other migrates away and undergoes differentiation. By contrast, the progeny of a transformed cell may all retain the ability to divide. Accordingly, cells will accumulate to the degree that the rate of new cell production exceeds the rate of extrusion. Since neoplastic cells do not differentiate normally, they do not become senescent and detach from the basement membrane. Thus, clonal expansion may be associated with accumulation of cells in a tumor even in the absence of an increase in the absolute rate of proliferation.

Importantly, although cells in a benign neoplasm may undergo a subtle change in morphology (such as in benign tubular adenomas or dysplasias), they are incapable of penetrating the basement membrane in order to invade or metastasize. However, the expanding pool of cells develop "genomic instability" by which nuclear changes (either mutations, chromosomal rearrangements, or other modifications of the genome) occur in the daughter cells. This process is usually slow, and for unknown reasons, some dysplastic or adenomatous lesions may remain small and benign for an indefinite period, whereas other lesions undergo "malignant conversion" (step 3 in the scheme of Fig 24-2). Malignant conversion can be acquired through a number of different mechanisms,

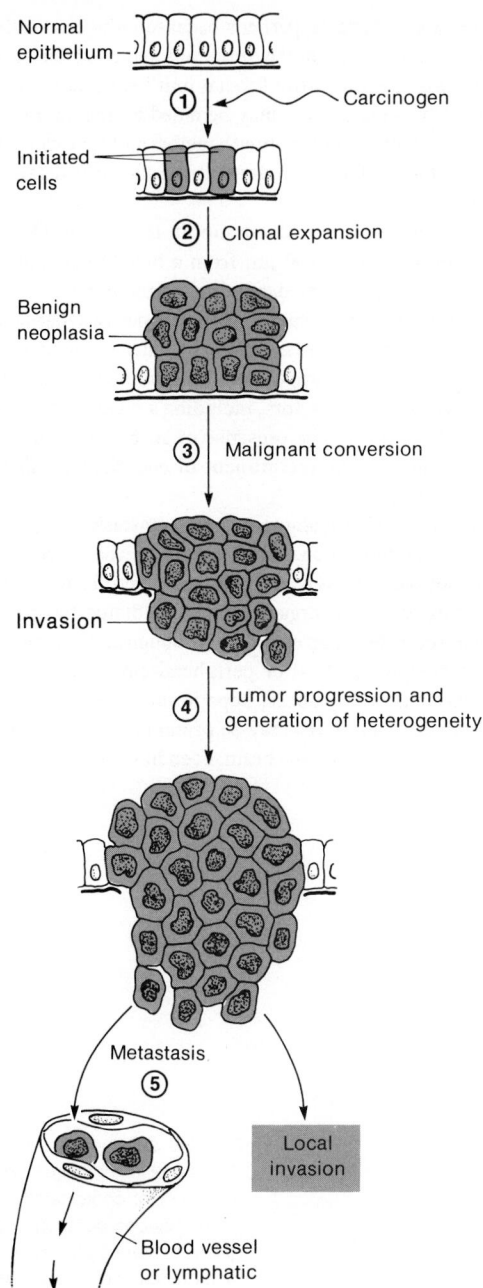

Normal epithelium

① Carcinogen

Initiated cells

② Clonal expansion

Benign neoplasia

③ Malignant conversion

Invasion

④ Tumor progression and generation of heterogeneity

Metastasis ⑤

Local invasion

Blood vessel or lymphatic

FIGURE 24–2. Tumor progression. This scheme illustrates the natural history of carcinogenesis. The first step represents a genotoxic event caused by a carcinogen. When a critical number of genes is mutated (the specific site and number remain speculative) a cell becomes neoplastic (step 1). Clonal expansion gives rise to a benign neoplasm (step 2). Unless additional events occur, a benign neoplasm may grow indefinitely without becoming malignant. However, if additional events occur, cells appear within a benign neoplasm that are capable of malignant behavior, such as invasion and metastasis. It is not clear whether malignant conversion (step 3) involves exclusively genetic or epigenetic steps, or a combination of these. A malignant neoplasm may invade locally and damage the host and surrounding organs. However, the genome of the malignant neoplasm is intrinsically unstable, and, in spite of its monoclonal origin, the cancer becomes more heterogeneous with time (steps 4 and 5). Clinically, the generation of tumor cell heterogeneity increases the likelihood of metastasis to one or more distant sites.

but the process requires cells to secrete proteases that digest type IV collagen in the basement membrane.[24,25] This permits the expanding cell pool to invade the underlying connective tissue. The size of the tumor that accumulates on the lumenal surface is related to ongoing proliferative rate and rate of cell loss. The sheer size of the tumor is less important than the invasive activity that occurs at the basement membrane. This principle has directed the pathologists' attention to the relationship between neoplastic cells and the basement membrane in an adenomatous polyp in making the distinction between carcinoma in situ and invasive cancer. In addition to the secretion of type IV collagenase, malignant cells become mobile and are able to migrate through the underlying muscle, fat, and serosa. In fact, many of the characteristics of malignant cells are similar to those seen in fetal cells, such as the ability to move through tissue planes and migrate to distant sites. In the case of malignant cells, however, there do not appear to be specific targets sites to which the cells may "home" and differentiate.

After malignant conversion, specific tumors may assume uncharacteristic behavior patterns. For example, a basal cell carcinoma of the skin has intrinsically different behavior than a cutaneous malignant melanoma, even taking into account the differences in the tumor size. Similarly, a small cancer of the pancreas has a different natural history than a similar-sized lesion in the colon and is far more likely to have metastasized by the time it has reached 2 to 3 cm in diameter than tumors found elsewhere in the gut. These differences in tumor behavior are explained by different rates and directions of "tumor progression."

The acquisition of specific malignant characteristics results from tumor cell heterogeneity (step 4 in Fig 24-2). The mechanism that permits tumor cell heterogeneity is unknown but may involve the loss of nuclear regulatory elements that normally inhibit the expression of specific genes or are involved in the repair of genomic mutations. Although tumors are characteristically monoclonal in origin, the processes of malignant conversion and tumor progression eventually result in the generation of enormous chromosomal and phenotypic diversity within a tumor.[26] For example, in an adenocarcinoma, many of the individual cells are either slow growing or in a terminal state. The rest of the cells may have different proliferative rates and different degrees of intrinsic "malignancy." Those cells with greater proliferative capacity or special survival characteristics will overgrow the slower growing pool of cells. Thus, cells from different sites in a single tumor may have entirely different biologic characteristics. Furthermore, cells from a single tumor examined at different points in time will demonstrate increasing proliferative rates and invasive capabilities as more aggressive groups of cells selectively expand their numbers. For these reasons, tumor progression usually emerges slowly with the gradual selection of more aggressive cells within a tumor mass.

The Biology of Tumor Metastasis

The metastasis of tumor cells is not a random or accidental process. For a tumor to metastasize, it must degrade the basement membrane and associated matrix components, migrate through the subtending connective tissue, enter into a lymphatic or blood vessel, migrate away from the parent tumor, avoid a gauntlet of naturally occurring defensive mechanisms, lodge at a distant site, emigrate from the vessel, and effectively colonize elsewhere (Fig 24-3).[27,28] Metastasis generally occurs as a late event in the natural history of a tumor, because time is required for the gradual evolution of clonal cells with all of the above properties.

The characteristics required for metastasis are quite specific. A malignant neoplasm, for example, may acquire the ability to digest the basement membrane and slowly expand into the submucosa, making it, by definition, malignant, but it may not acquire other properties required for entry into the circulation or survival in a distant organ. Such a tumor is pathologically malignant and may become a bulky mass, but there may be a relatively long period of time during which it can be detected and successfully removed. Alternatively, a highly metastatic clone of cells emerging from a malignant tumor may give rise rapidly to a large number of metastatic units, and the host may suffer a brisk and relentless downhill clinical course.

As mentioned above, tumor biologists do not have sufficient insight into this process to predict the clinical source by studying tumor cells in vitro. Tumor cells are frequently present in the portal and peripheral circulation at the time of colectomy for a colon cancer.[29,30] Yet, the presence of cytologically identifiable tumor cells in the circulation has no prognostic significance because most of these cells are incapable of growing at a distant site and are susceptible to cytolysis by natural killer lymphocytes and other immunologic mechanisms. Clumps of cells appear to be more likely to survive as a metastasis, perhaps because individual cells in the clump have only some of the functions required for successful metastasis whereas the entire "social unit" is capable of growing independently. This process may be aided by the ability of some tumor cells to secrete tumor growth factors and/or express growth factor receptors.[31] This is discussed in additional detail later in the chapter.

Tumor cells require a blood supply to survive. Oxygen can normally diffuse 100 to 200 μm from a blood vessel, or roughly only 4 to 10 cell diameters, depending on the tumor. Tumors can stimulate the growth of capillaries (i.e., neovascularization) to facilitate their growth at either primary or metastatic sites. Tumor-associated angiogenesis appears to be mediated by a variety of different tumor growth factors, including a recently characterized "angiogenesis factor." The presence of such growth factors may be demonstrated by the recruitment of endothelial cells to form capillaries in vitro.

The sites to which malignant cells metastasize may appear to be a random phenomenon, based purely on the blood supply of an organ, but the process is actually more complicated, and tumor cell targeting to distant organs may be mediated by specific cell membrane receptors. For example, although tumor cells may be present in the portal blood or peripheral circulation at the time of removal of a colon cancer, hepatic metastases occur only in some instances. Metastases may be present in the lung, bone, and other distant sites such as the brain, even in the absence of hepatic

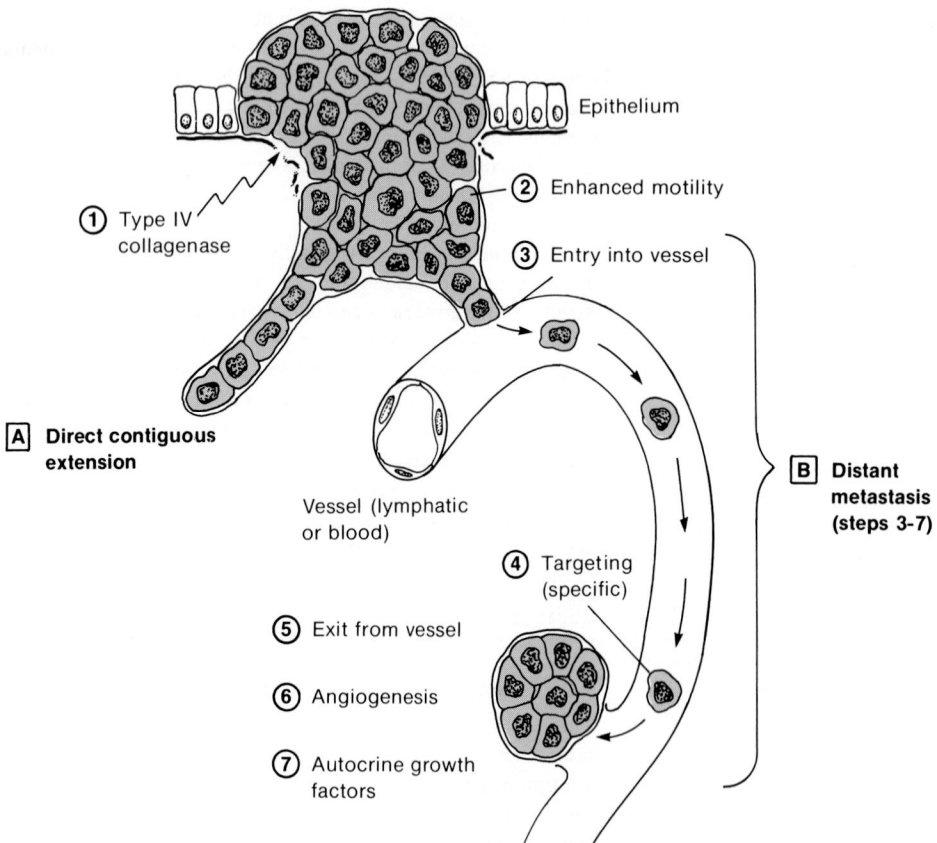

FIGURE 24–3. Tumor metastasis. Successful tumor metastasis requires a number of coordinated events to occur. Specific collagenases are required to transgress the basement membrane (step 1). The tumor may grow by direct contiguous extension into surrounding organs (A). Alternatively, tumor cells may enter a vascular structure for distant metastasis to occur (B). The spread of malignant cells is enhanced by the development of cellular motility (step 2). Access to a vascular structure is permitted by the expansion of the growing tumor, the motile cells, and the in-growth of blood vessels, which is stimulated by angiogenesis factors (steps 3 and 6). Entry into the circulation is not sufficient to ensure distant metastasis. Specific targeting mechanisms and adaptations that would enhance survival at a distant site are required for distant metastatic spread (see text).

metastases. In these instances, it would appear that the tumor cells migrated through the hepatic sinusoids without establishing a malignant deposit in the liver.

On the basis of studies in a murine melanoma model, it appears that not all cells in a primary tumor have identical metastatic potential.[32] From a primary tumor it is possible to clone cells that have enhanced capacity for metastasis and propensity to metastasize to specific organs. For example, certain of the cloned cells form lung metastases, whereas others do not. When the metastatic colonies are removed from the lungs, their numbers expanded in culture and reinjected by tail vein, with each successive cycle, a larger number of pulmonary metastases is produced.

The propensity of the highly metastatic cell line to grow in the lung appears to result from a specific interaction between the injected cells and the pulmonary capillary bed. Thus, lung lesions are seen even after left ventricular injection of the cells (in which the lung is not the first capillary bed) or after transplantation of lung tissue to a subcutaneous location. Using the same technique, other cell lines can be developed with an enhanced propensity to metastasize to the liver or specific sites within the brain.[32]

Site-specific metastasis appears to be mediated by cell surface membrane glycoproteins. Removal of the glycoproteins from the above-mentioned tumor cells interferes with the specificity of metastasis. Furthermore, by fusing membrane vesicles from metastatic to nonmetastatic cells, it is possible to confer homing specificity to the recipient cells.

The behavior of metastatic colon cancer has been pursued more recently using both syngeneic[33] and athymic[34] mouse models. By injecting cells of modest metastatic potential into the wall of the colon, occasional hepatic metastases may be produced. However, when the metastatic tumor cells from the liver are grown in culture and reinjected into colonic tissue, enhanced ability to metastasize to the liver may be detected. If the hepatic metastases are recovered, expanded in culture, and reinjected into colonic tissues, progressively more metastatic cell lines are selected. Attempts are being made to identify the factors that mediate enhanced metastatic ability and site-specific metastasis in colorectal cancer.

Role of Diet in Gastrointestinal Carcinogenesis

As discussed in the previous sections, carcinogenesis and tumor progression may be considered as a series of steps. Certain of these steps may be viewed as the effects of exogenous factors applied to the epithelial cell, whereas others are more closely related to host cell characteristics and their responses to external agents. In the case of the gastrointestinal tract, diet appears to be the most important, albeit not the only, exogenous factor. The environment experienced by epithelial cells is modified by secretions into the gastrointestinal tract, and, very importantly, the microbial flora. These factors may even be interrelated, as the resident flora is in part dependent on host secretions, which may themselves be modified by dietary factors (Fig 24-4).

Although the steps involved in carcinogenesis and tumor progression may be interrelated, each of them has distinct areas of regulation that may be influenced by dietary factors. The lumenal contents undergo major modifications as they progress through the gastrointestinal tract. Therefore, each portion of the gut must be considered in the context of its own unique environment. For example, the esophagus is exposed to dietary contents that have undergone a minimum of digestive modification. Thus, it is more susceptible to the effects of highly reactive dietary constituents that require minimal activation. The flora of the esophageal lumen is primarily a reflection of that which contaminates food. The

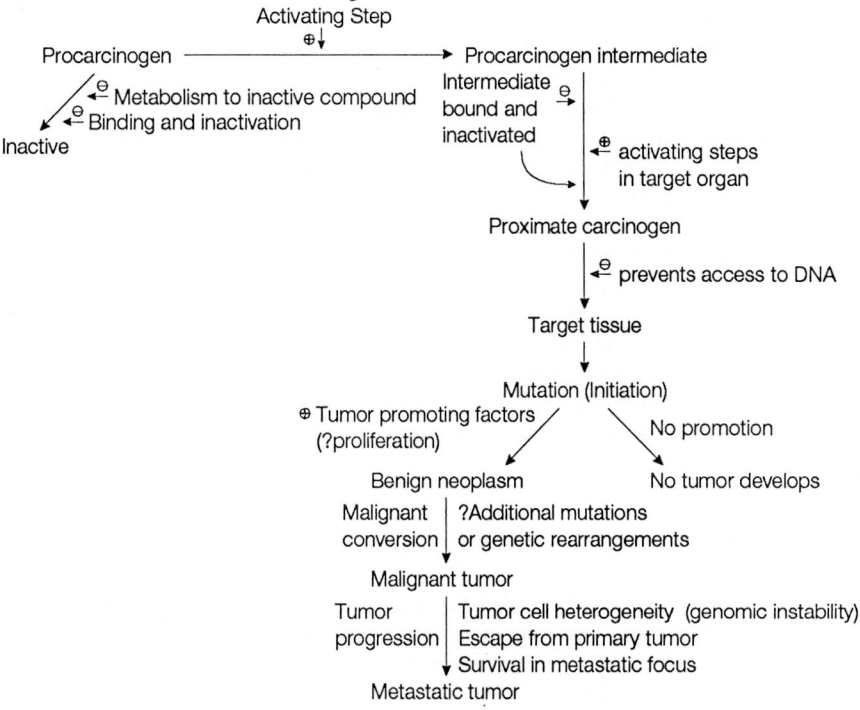

FIGURE 24-4. Potential sites for the modification of carcinogenesis. Procarcinogens may undergo metabolic activation or inactivation by the contents of the gut lumen or by the mucosa; mucosal metabolizing capacity may be modified by dietary factors as described in the text. This process may be complicated, since procarcinogens may be activated in one organ and have its target at a distant site. As discussed in the text, some agents may prevent access of the proximate carcinogen to DNA or may modify repair mechanisms. Moreover, carcinogenesis may be inhibited after the establishment of mutated cells, and it may be possible to modify tumor progression once these processes are better understood.

interaction between food and the esophagus is very brief; therefore, it is not surprising that disease states associated with increased risk for esophageal neoplasia include those that involve stasis (achalasia) or gastroesophageal reflux (e.g., Barrett's esophagus).

The secretion of hydrochloric acid in the gastric lumen eliminates a large proportion of the bacterial flora contaminating food. The low pH restricts the variety of chemical reactions that may occur in the stomach; however, it favors the generation of certain nitrosamines in the presence of nitrites and complex amines. The development of achlorhydria dramatically alters the lumenal environment of the stomach and increases the likelihood of carcinogenesis. The gastric flora changes, with a marked increase in gram-negative rods and anaerobic bacteria. The presence of nitrate reductase of microbial origin favors the conversion of dietary nitrates to nitrites, which are then available for the generation of carcinogenic nitrosamines.[35] Also, certain substances, including nitrates, are absorbed from the stomach, enter into the circulation, and are resecreted by the salivary glands. This "enterosalivary" circulation increases the exposure of the mouth, esophagus, and stomach to those substances.

After acidification, the bacterial content of the chyme drops, and with the addition of bicarbonate by the small intestinal, biliary, and pancreatic secretions, the small intestine is exposed to an entirely different milieu. In addition, the small intestinal mucosa is endowed with enzymes that inactivate highly reactive molecular species. These two factors are believed to be important in the low incidence of cancer seen in the small intestine.

The colon, like the stomach, is exposed to intestinal contents for longer periods of time. The bacterial concentration rises from approximately 10^3 organisms/mL in the stomach to more than 10^{12} organisms/mL in the colon. A variety of bacterial enzymes is present in fecal material that may activate procarcinogens. Furthermore, as fluid and electrolytes are removed from stool, the residual contents are concentrated and prolonged contact between the lumenal contents and the epithelium and stool occurs.

Aside from their direct actions as tumor-initiating agents, dietary constituents may have indirect effects on tumor promotion and tumor progression. For example, dietary fiber inhibits tumor production in experimental animals. The addition of fiber to the diet reduces fecal pH, and this may inhibit the generation of carcinogens as well as the formation or bioavailability of compounds that participate in tumor promotion or progression. Butyric acid, a short-chain fatty acid produced on fermentation of nonabsorbed carbohydrate in the feces, is a "differentiating agent" in vitro that has been hypothesized to interfere with tumor development, perhaps by inhibiting tumor promotion.[36] The supplementation of the diet with nondigestible fiber enhances the production of this and other volatile fatty acids in the stool. This area is in need of additional exploration, but it highlights the fact that carcinogenesis is a sequential process that potentially may be interrupted at several key points, once the mechanism of each step is understood better.

The Role of Genetics in Carcinogenesis

Host susceptibility, presumably mediated by genes, plays a role in carcinogenesis. Genetic susceptibility to cancer appears to be inherited by mechanisms that produce discrete, organ-specific risk. For example, xeroderma pigmentosum is a hereditary deficiency of any one of several enzymes in the skin involved in repairing ultraviolet light–induced damage to DNA. Thus, ordinary exposure to light results in an extraordinary number of mutations and a very high rate of skin cancer in patients with this disease. There are very few examples of genetic diseases predisposing to cancer for which the enzymatic defect has been worked out so carefully. Familial adenomatous polyposis is an inherited disorder in which the gastrointestinal tract develops countless benign neoplasms early in life, some of which will undergo malignant conversion. Although the gene responsible for this disorder has been located on the long arm of chromosome 5, the gene product and the mechanism resulting in the development of adenomatous polyposis is unknown. Elucidation of this process will shed insight into mechanisms of neoplasia because it appears to mediate an early event in neoplastic transformation. The lesion in polyposis is probably limited to an initiating event, and malignant conversion may be no different than that occurring sporadically. This is contrasted to the cancer family syndromes of Lynch (Lynch syndrome I and II).[37] Persons with this genetic syndrome do not develop polyposis, but virtually every gene carrier develops cancer. In this disease, the critical lesion may be in accelerated tumor promotion or very rapid malignant conversion of initiated tissues. By examining the stages of carcinogenesis outlined in Figure 24-2, one may imagine that genetic lesions may occur at any step that would result in an increased risk of cancer. In the future, gastrointestinal carcinogenesis may be traced to a series of abnormal enzyme activities such as seen in the example of skin cancer, or perhaps defective structural genes, yet to be described.

Drug Resistance in Gastrointestinal Neoplasia

In spite of intensive efforts by numerous investigators, gastrointestinal cancer remains highly resistant to systemic chemotherapy. There are numerous mechanisms that underlie this vexing clinical problem. To begin with, the proliferative rate of gastrointestinal cancers is not predictably greater than it is for stem cells of normal tissues. As a result, chemotherapeutic approaches using antimetabolites will not selectively kill gastrointestinal tumor cells. Thus, effective levels of drugs used for treatment of gastrointestinal malignancies produce unacceptable systemic toxicity.

Cells in many tissues throughout the body contain a surface membrane glycoprotein, termed *P-glycoprotein*, which is responsible for elimination of toxic compounds. P-glycoprotein, normally expressed in gastrointestinal tissues, may be amplified in certain tumor cells, rendering them resistant to multiple chemotherapeutic agents.[38] Such cells have a growth advantage over other neoplastic or even normal cells when reexposed to chemotherapeutic agents. This is one reason why an apparent initial response to a chemotherapeutic agent may not confer prolonged survival.

Oncodevelopmental Tumor Markers

There has been a long and persistent search for cellular markers that are specific for neoplastic transformation. Neoplasia is characterized by a long latent period during progression from the earliest events to the emergence of a clinically recognizable cancer. The immortalized characteristic of neoplastic tissues, the limited differentiation, and the ability to invade basement membranes and migrate to distant sites are shared by cancer cells and fetal tissues. Thus, it is not surprising that most tumor markers are also expressed in embryonic tissues. No markers are expressed in tumors from all organs, and organ-specific markers are rarely found in all tumors from a given organ, or even uniformly expressed throughout a single tumor. Thus, no protein has been identified whose expression is either a necessary or sufficient component of the malignant phenotype.

Nonetheless, a variety of markers that shed light on tumor cell biology have been described. For example, carcinoembryonic antigen (CEA) is a glycoprotein normally expressed on the microvillar membranes of the epithelium in the stomach and intestine. Because of the strict vectorial expression of this glycoprotein toward the gastrointestinal lumen by differentiated cells, only a tiny amount of CEA is shed into the blood during the turnover of senescent cells. However, because tumor cells may lose their polarity, CEA gains access to the circulation as it is shed from the tumor cell membranes.[39] Thus, a normally expressed glycoprotein may be used as a tumor marker, but since the aberrant location of CEA expression does not occur until after malignant conversion, plasma CEA levels are not an effective marker of early neoplastic disease.

A number of blood group antigens are expressed on gastrointestinal epithelial cells, including the ABO and Lewis antigens. In the distal colon, blood group antigens are expressed during early, but not late, fetal life. These blood group activities are reexpressed in neoplastic tissue.[40] This phenomenon has been reported in gastric, breast, pancreatic, and urinary tract tumors and many other malignancies. The reappearance in neoplastic tissue of antigenic structures normally expressed in the fetus suggests a functional role for these carbohydrate antigens in oncofetal cellular behavior. Glycosylation is essential for normal function of the fibroblast growth factor receptor, and the EGF receptor expressed by certain tumor cell lines appears to carry an unexpectedly large proportion of tumor-associated carbohydrate antigens.[41] It is possible that the expression of these carbohydrate antigens on the growth factor receptors mediates neoplastic behavior.

Mucins are the principal glycoproteins secreted by gastrointestinal epithelium. They are highly glycosylated and have been found to comprise several tumor-associated antigens linked to gastrointestinal epithelium.[42] Tumor-associated mucin antigens have been found in premalignant tissues, including adenomatous polyps of the colon[43] and dysplasia in the setting of ulcerative colitis.[44] The oncodevelopmental form of mucin also appears in histologically normal colonic epithelium after the administration of carcinogens to rodents. Mucin-type carbohydrate structures expressed in upper gastrointestinal tract epithelium also appear to correlate with metaplastic and neoplastic changes in Barrett's esophagus.[45] Mucins do not readily enter the blood, and as such, are not serologic markers of neoplasia. However, modifications in mucin synthesis accompany the earliest stages of gastrointestinal tract neoplasia, and thus these glycoproteins may serve as useful tools in mapping the behavior of dedifferentiating epithelia.

THE MOLECULAR GENETICS OF TUMOR DEVELOPMENT

Cancer is a disease of somatic genes. While this may seem obvious to the contemporary scientist, it is worth reviewing the rationale

for this statement, since it has not always been widely accepted. First and foremost, cancer cells beget cancer cells, generally irreversibly. Second, as Ames and co-workers showed in bacteria, most mutagens are carcinogens and most carcinogens are mutagens.[46] The lack of complete correlation, however, considerably frustrates regulatory agencies and reveals that cancer is not simply a disease of mutation. Third, cancer-prone strains of animals develop malignancy at high frequency, presumably because of a genetic predisposition. Similarly, many hereditary syndromes in humans predispose to cancer. Fourth, both DNA and RNA viruses cause tumors in animals. Finally, tumors possess chromosomal alterations. Boveri first noticed mitotic abnormalities in tumor cells and proposed in 1914 that cancer is a genetic disease.[47] By modern standards, Boveri's conclusion is unsurprising, but his ideas were dismissed in his own day. Thus, one should not forget that ideas out of the mainstream of research in our own time may nevertheless be correct.

While the genetic nature of cancer is well established, it has been possible only in the past decade to begin to determine the molecular alterations in DNA. The purpose of this section is to review the contribution of each type of molecular alteration to cancer of the gastrointestinal tract. Of the following types of molecular alteration, the emphasis will be on those malignancies about which we know the most: (1) point mutation, or a change in a single nucleotide; (2) DNA rearrangement, the molecular equivalent of a specific chromosomal translocation; (3) DNA amplification, the reduplication of a gene or cluster of genes; (4) DNA deletion, or the loss of a specific gene; and (5) alterations in DNA methylation. The gastrointestinal tumors about which we know the most at the molecular level are colorectal cancer and stomach cancer, because they are common in the regions from which the studies emerge—colorectal cancer in the United States and Europe and gastric cancer in Japan. Pancreatic cancer has only recently been studied in a systematic way, and extremely little is known about the molecular genetics of esophageal and small bowel cancer.

Mutation

While the existence of animal tumor viruses has been known for decades, a surprising observation by Stehelin and colleagues[48] 15 years ago provided insight into the genesis of human malignancy. They had been studying Rous sarcoma virus (RSV), an RNA virus that replicates itself from RNA to DNA with reverse transcriptase and then incorporates the proviral DNA into the DNA of the host genome. These investigators found that the transforming gene of RSV has a homologue in normal cells.[48] Thus, RSV must have been created by a nontransforming retrovirus that transduced, or picked up during the proviral stage, a normal host sequence, which then became a transforming gene (oncogene) in the retrovirus. Shih and associates,[49] on learning of this experiment, reasoned that humans could develop cancer without the participation of an exogenous retrovirus if they simply mutated the normal cellular homologue of an oncogene. In order to confirm this hypothesis, they transferred, by a process termed *transfection*, DNA from tumors into normal recipient cells and showed that the transfected DNA transformed a particular murine cell line termed *NIH 3T3*. Transformation means that the cells are no longer contact inhibited; rather, they pile up, assume a malignant-looking morphology, and form tumors when injected into nude mice. Thus, transformation is the in vitro correlate of malignancy, but it is not identical to malignancy, which is generally far more complex. Later, several laboratories identified a transforming oncogene, using this technique, in a human bladder carcinoma cell line alternately termed *EJ* or *T24*. The transforming oncogene in EJ/T24 is the cellular homologue of the Harvey murine sarcoma virus, v-Ha-*ras*. The cellular oncogene in EJ/T24, called c-Ha-*ras*, resulted from a single point mutation in the coding region of an otherwise harmless endogenous gene.[50-52]

When the c-Ha-*ras* mutation in EJ/T24 was discovered, there was an intense effort by many laboratories to identify similar mutations in primary human tumors. This search could be conducted without cloning the gene from each tumor, because of a fortuitous molecular structure, in which a specific Msp I restriction endonuclease site is changed whenever the EJ/T24 mutation occurs. By examining a large number of human tumors including colorectal cancers for this Msp I site, the c-Ha-*ras* mutation was shown to occur infrequently, in 5% or fewer gastrointestinal tumors.[53] However, additional members of the *ras* gene family were discovered through transfection experiments, and mutations on these proved to be more prevalent. In particular, c-Ki-*ras*, homologous to the Kirsten murine sarcoma virus, is mutated in many solid tumors.[54]

A recent technologic development called the polymerase chain reaction (PCR), permits in vitro amplification of a target DNA sequence to allow DNA analysis on small amounts of material. This has led to several comprehensive surveys for *ras* and other oncogene mutations in gastrointestinal tumors. As many as 40% of colorectal cancers,[55,56] and more than 80% of pancreatic cancers, when examined by PCR, show a mutation in c-Ki-*ras*.[57] The normal and abnormal functions of *ras* genes still are understood only partly. Normal *ras* genes are involved in signal transduction at the cell membrane, and the *ras* protein interacts with a second protein called guanosine triphosphatase activating protein.[58] Despite the relatively high frequency of c-Ki-*ras* mutation in colorectal and pancreatic carcinoma, it is not 100% as it is in experimental carcinogen–induced animal tumors.[59] Thus, these cancers in humans cannot be due entirely to the mutation of cellular oncogenes.

A peculiar transforming gene has been found by transfecting stomach carcinoma DNA into fibroblasts. DNA from 2 of 37 tumor samples transformed NIH 3T3 cells,[60] and the gene responsible, termed *hst* for human stomach, encoded basic fibroblast growth factor.[61] Oddly, some examples of normal stomach[60] and leukocyte[62] DNA also transform recipient cells by an activated *hst* gene. It is still not clear whether the *hst* mutation plays a role in gastrointestinal carcinoma, whether normal cells can contain the mutation without becoming transformed, or whether in vitro transformation with this oncogene is at least in part an artifact of transfection.

DNA Rearrangement

A quantum jump in basic understanding of mitotic abnormalities in cancer was made by Nowell and Hungerford,[63] who observed an abnormal chromosome in chronic myelogenous leukemia (CML). This abnormality was later found to represent a reciprocal translocation between chromosomes 9 and 22 that is virtually pathognomonic of CML.[64] We now know that this translocation causes the juxtaposition of a gene on chromosome 22, with c-*abl*,

a cellular oncogene on chromosome 9 homologous to the Abelson murine leukemia virus. The translocation creates a chimeric RNA message, leading to an abnormally large *abl* protein.[65] A similar discovery was made regarding Burkitt's lymphoma, which is characterized by a reciprocal translocation between chromosomes 8 and 14 that juxtaposes the immunoglobulin heavy-chain gene constant region and c-*myc*, the cellular homologue of the avian leukosis virus oncogene.[66] This DNA rearrangement may cause deregulated expression of c-*myc*.

Despite the comparatively great understanding of the molecular nature of DNA rearrangements in leukemia and lymphoma, very little is known about the role of DNA rearrangement in solid tumors. Part of the reason for this ignorance is that, while leukemias and lymphomas characteristically show specific translocations that virtually define the subtype of disease, solid tumors show more generalized and nonspecific chromosomal translocations. With a few exceptions such as in Ewing's sarcoma, most solid tumors are not characterized by a specific chromosomal rearrangement.[67] Nevertheless, an interesting translocation in a colorectal cancer has been found in the course of DNA transfection studies. One cancer in more than 50 studied showed a specific translocation involving fusion of a tyrosine kinase gene and a gene for tropomyosin.[68] Presumably, the rearrangement enhances or alters the tyrosine kinase activity, a known pathway for cellular transformation. Also, rearrangements of a histocompatibility gene were recently reported in two of 12 colon tumors,[69] but this observation has not yet been confirmed by other laboratories.

DNA Amplification

DNA amplification has attracted considerable experimental interest as a factor in carcinogenesis for two reasons. First, it is a known mechanism of drug resistance. For example, resistance to methotrexate can be caused by amplification of the gene for dihydrofolate reductase.[70] Second, gene amplification appears to play an important role in the progression of some solid tumors. For example, a homologue of c-*myc* termed N-*myc* is amplified in most advanced neuroblastomas and is even predictive of disease progression.[71]

Many tumor cell lines show either extra minichromosomes, called double minutes (DMs), or long homogeneously staining insertions in chromosomes called homogeneously staining regions (HSRs). Both DMs and HSRs are caused by gene amplification. Thus, tumor cell lines have been surveyed by many laboratories for amplified cellular oncogenes. Colon carcinoma cell lines with oncogene amplification include SW480, with an amplified and mutated c-Ki-*ras*,[72] COLO201 and COLO205 with amplified c-*myb*,[73] and COLO320, a neuroendocrine colon tumor line with amplified c-*myc*.[74] However, oncogene amplification appears much more commonly in cultured cells than in primary tumors. Only 2 of 31 colorectal cancers examined systematically showed oncogene amplification, and both of these involved c-*myc*.[75] One stomach cancer showed amplification of *hst*,[76] and several showed amplification of genes for other growth factors or their receptors.[77-79]

An interesting technique allows discovery of amplified genes in a given DNA sample, without prior knowledge of the gene being assayed. DNA from the tissue is denatured into single strands in vitro and then reannealed. Only DNA present in relatively high copy number (such as amplified sequences) will reanneal efficiently. The DNA is then treated with an enzyme that removes all but the reannealed double-stranded DNA.[80] Using this technique, the multiple drug resistance (MDR) gene was recently identified.[81] While the technique has been applied to the study of gastrointestinal tumors without success, recent improvements in the method will permit detection of as few as seven copies of a gene,[82] and thus it may soon become possible to learn of amplified genes that were previously unrecognized.

DNA Deletion

Through a combination of astute clinical observation and careful epidemiologic study, Knudson proposed that some human cancers arise by a recessive mechanism, in which inactivation of both alleles of a gene causes cancer. Loss of the first allele could occur as a dominantly inherited trait, transmitted vertically in the germ line. It would then require an inactivating mutation or deletion of the second allele to eliminate expression of the gene product. Individuals with an inherited "first hit" would be at risk of multiple tumors occurring at an early age, while persons with sporadically occurring tumors would generally acquire only a single malignancy at a later age, since they would need to develop two mutations in a given somatic cell lineage to develop cancer.[83] Thus, a recessive tumor gene could be manifest in two ways. It would be present as a dominant trait in some families, and it could be deleted in both familial and sporadically occurring tumors.

A paradigm for Knudson's hypothesis is Wilms' tumor, for which some children with aniridia (absent iris) and other malformations are predisposed. Such children usually have a visible cytogenetic deletion involving chromosomal band 11p13, representing loss of the first Wilms' tumor allele in the germ line.[84] An indirect way to detect deletion of a recessive tumor gene is through the use of restriction fragment length polymorphisms (RFLPs). These are functionally insignificant variations in DNA sequence present in the general population but that happen to alter specific restriction endonuclease sites in the genome. Thus, the two alleles of a given locus will be cleaved into fragments of distinguishably different size. Using RFLPs, one can determine whether one of the alleles at a specific locus has been deleted in a tumor. In the case of Wilms' tumor, polymorphic markers on the short arm of chromosome 11 reveal that sporadically occurring tumors have lost a portion of chromosome 11.[85] Using RFLPs, many laboratories have now shown loss of specific chromosomal regions in a variety of sporadically occurring malignancies, including bladder,[86] lung,[87] renal,[88] breast,[89] and endocrine tumors.[90,91]

An important clue for gastrointestinal tumors was provided by a patient with familial adenomatous polyposis (FAP) and multiple congenital anomalies who had an interstitial deletion on the long arm of chromosome 5.[92] Presumably, the patient had lost several genes on chromosome 5, including the FAP gene. Based on that report, the FAP gene was later mapped in families to chromosome 5.[93,94] Also, RFLP analysis showed loss on chromosome 5 in sporadically occurring colorectal cancers.[95] Thus, the FAP gene could be a common recessive tumor gene in colorectal cancer. A systematic study of allelic loss in colorectal cancer revealed, however, that chromosome 5 is deleted comparatively infrequently when compared with other chromosomal regions in only about one third

of tumors.[96] By comparison, losses on chromosomes 17 and 18 both occur in at least two thirds of these tumors.[96] *p53*, a known tumor suppressor gene on chromosome 17 was mutated in two colorectal carcinomas, suggesting that it represents the critical gene lost on chromosome 17.[97] Recently, a gene on chromosome 18 termed DCC (deleted in colorectal carcinoma) was cloned and found to be mutated or lost in tumors with chromosome 18 loss. Interestingly, this gene is homologous to N-CAM, a cellular adhesion molecule, suggesting a role in tumor metastasis.[98]

Perhaps even more important than the frequency of allelic losses is the fact that all three of the above genetic deletions, on chromosomes 5, 17, and 18, occur relatively late in carcinogenesis. They are not present in smaller adenomas, which may lead to adenocarcinoma, but are only seen in relatively large adenomas or carcinomas.[96,99] However, by the Knudson model, there should not be any progression toward malignancy until both alleles of the candidate gene are lost. Even patients with familial colorectal cancer do not show early loss of alleles. For example, two colorectal cancers from a patient with FAP showed allelic loss on chromosome 18: one of the cancers showed allelic loss on chromosome 17, but neither showed loss on chromosome 5.[96] This patient would thus fit a model in which FAP was transmitted as a dominant mutation and did not function as a recessive tumor gene, while allelic losses on chromosomes 17 and 18 were involved in tumor progression rather than its initiation. Of course, RFLPs may be too insensitive a measure of loss of the FPC gene.

Recently, allelic losses were seen in 41% of gastric cancers on chromosome 13,[100] which harbors the retinoblastoma gene. Whether gastric cancer involves the retinoblastoma gene or another recessive gene on chromosome 13 has yet to be determined. The subcellular localization of oncogenes implicated in gastrointestinal neoplasia is shown in Figure 24-5.

Alterations in DNA Methylation

Laennec, an early 19th century pathologist, first noted that cancer cells show properties normally expressed by cells of other tissues or at other stages of development.[101] In contemporary parlance, cancer involves the abnormal expression of normal cellular genes. Direct measures suggest that expression of several percent of the genome is altered in malignancy.[102,103] One way in which gene expression is normally controlled is through alterations in DNA methylation, a covalent modification of the base cytosine. Expressed genes generally are hypomethylated at specific cytosine residues within or surrounding the gene, and those sites are methylated in nonexpressing tissues. The pattern of DNA methylation is heritably preserved during cell division within a given tissue.[104] Many laboratories have examined DNA methylation in cancer, with varying results. Increases, decreases, and no change in DNA methylation have all been reported.[105] This variation is due in part to the lack of comparison in many studies of primary tumors to adjacent normal material of the same histologic type, since DNA methylation varies in a tissue-specific manner. In a direct comparison of primary colorectal cancers to adjacent normal mucosa, a wide variety of genes showed substantial hypomethylation.[106] These include the gamma-globin gene,[107] normally hypomethylated only in blood precursor cells, and the gamma-crystallin gene,[107] normally hypomethylated only in embryonic lens. It appears that

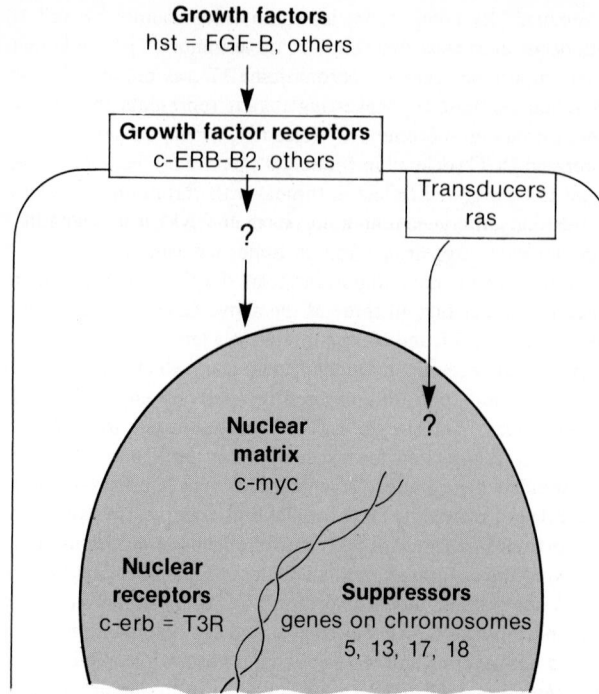

FIGURE 24–5. A proposed scheme for the actions of some oncogenes. Oncogenes are modified cellular genes that participate in the production of the malignant phenotype. Introduction of any of these genes into the unstable but nontransformed rat fibroblast cell line NIH 3T3 is sufficient to produce the malignant phenotype. Of note, oncogenes may encode for secreted growth factors, membrane-associated receptors, or nuclear proteins, and many have tyrosine kinase activity.

approximately one third of single copy genes are hypomethylated in colorectal cancer.[107]

What distinguishes hypomethylation from the other types of DNA alteration is its ubiquity (in that all colorectal cancers appear hypomethylated) and its early onset. Indeed, the smallest adenomas are equally hypomethylated as the most advanced carcinomas.[108] The methylation changes involve cellular oncogenes,[109] and thus it is possible that one mechanism by which cellular oncogenes may be activated in cancer is by hypomethylation and abnormal expression. However, the hypomethylated genes in tumors are not necessarily expressed, and there are other ways by which methylation might be playing a role in carcinogenesis. For example, when cells are treated with a drug that causes hypomethylation in vitro, they show decondensation of centromeric heterochromatin and chromosomal rearrangements.[110] Thus, methylation changes might cause genetic instability, leading to other genetic alterations in cancer. Interestingly, patients with Lynch syndrome (non–polyposis familial colorectal cancer) appear to show an altered level of DNA methylation in their normal colonic mucosa, although only a very small number of patients have been studied to date.[108]

Gastric and esophageal cancers are also hypomethylated, as are all other human tumors that have been systematically examined.[111] Thus, DNA methylation appears to be a general property of human malignancy. Proving a direct role for DNA methylation in carcinogenesis will be quite difficult, however, since the changes are so widespread in the genome and they occur so early.

A novel model system[112] for early transformation may allow identification of the hypomethylated genes expressed prior to transformation. Cells are treated with a drug that causes hypomethylation in vitro and then isolated prior to transformation. Pretransformed cells committed to transformation but still phenotypically normal are isolated, and the genes that are activated in these cells can then be identified.[112]

Molecular Markers

The knowledge that cellular oncogenes play an important role in carcinogenesis has tempted many investigators to directly measure oncogene expression in a variety of tumors. The assumption underlying these studies is that abnormal oncogene expression per se is responsible for carcinogenesis or, at the very least, might serve as an important molecular marker of disease. However, the significance of such comparisons is unclear for two reasons. First, cellular oncogenes are important in normal cellular function, and since biochemical, morphologic, and kinetic properties of the cancer cell differ from normal, oncogene expression might also change, as a consequence rather than as a cause of malignancy. Second, change in expression alone of a gene is weak evidence for a pathogenetic role, in the absence of a defined molecular alteration in the gene.

Studies of *ras* oncogene expression in gastrointestinal cancer appear contradictory.[113,114] Attempts to correlate oncogene expression with disease progression have also been disappointing. For example, c-*myc* expression is elevated in some colorectal tumor cell lines,[115,116] but expression is unrelated to the clinical stage or grade of disease.[117] When several oncogenes were examined systematically in colorectal cancer, no correlation between expression and in vitro properties were seen for c-Ha-*ras*, c-Ki-*ras*, N-*ras*, c-*myb*, c-*fos*, and *p53*.[118] One study showed a relationship between oncogene expression and certain morphologic characteristics but also showed a lack of correlation with clinical stage or histologic grade.[119] Expression of c-Ha-*ras* may give the same information as measurement of mucin production (a putative marker of differentiation) but does not seem to be related to tumorigenicity or aggressiveness of the tumor.[120] Thus, while oncogenes play an important role in gastrointestinal neoplasia, measurement of expression is probably no more useful than biochemical markers, whose use is also quite limited at present.

Multistep Transformation

How can the many types of DNA alteration observed in human gastrointestinal tumors be reconciled and a causal role be ascribed to any one of them? The answer to this question is partly epidemiologic. Causality is generally defined by the following three criteria: (1) the putative cause must occur with high frequency in association with the disease; (2) the cause must precede the disease; and finally, (3) the mechanism must be sufficiently understood to rule out alternative explanations for the association. If each type of DNA alteration in colorectal cancer for which the data are most complete is reviewed, then a molecular model of carcinogenesis can be constructed. Point mutation of c-Ki-*ras* occurs frequently and appears mechanistically relevant, but the mutations do not appear to be present in small adenomas (an early stage of neo-

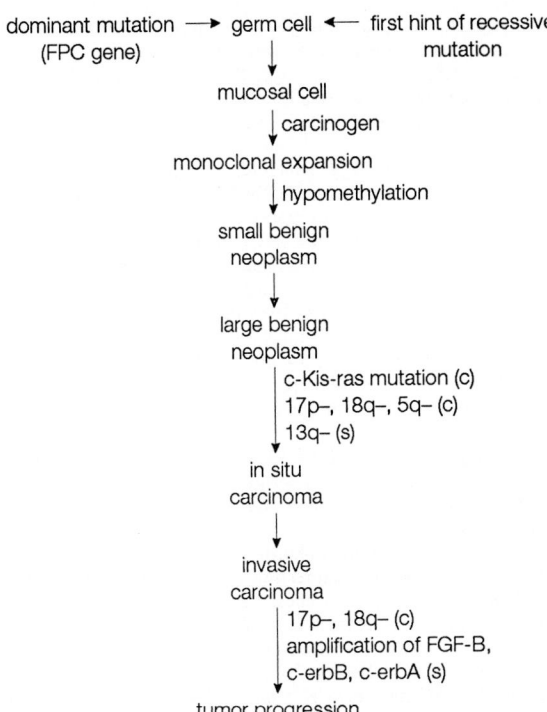

dominant mutation ⟶ germ cell ⟵ first hint of recessive
(FPC gene) mutation

mucosal cell
↓ carcinogen
monoclonal expansion
↓ hypomethylation
small benign
neoplasm
↓
large benign
neoplasm
↓ c-Kis-ras mutation (c)
17p–, 18q–, 5q– (c)
13q– (s)
in situ
carcinoma
↓
invasive
carcinoma
↓ 17p–, 18q– (c)
amplification of FGF-B,
c-erbB, c-erbA (s)
tumor progression

FIGURE 24–6. Relationship between oncogenes and normal cellular genes. Protooncogenes, the normal cellular homologs of animal tumor viruses, subserve normal cellular functions. Alterations in a protooncogene could lead to neoplastic growth by increasing the production of growth factors, altering the growth factor receptor to enhance its response to ligand binding, modifying the signal transduction apparatus, or altering nuclear gene regulation. Tumor suppressor genes are those whose loss promotes transformation and may normally inhibit cell growth. *c,* colorectal; *s,* stomach.

plasia). Gene deletions, as detected by allelic loss using RFLPs, occur much more frequently than point mutation. Many chromosomes show allelic losses, but they, too, appear relatively late in tumorigenesis, after adenomas have already developed. For example, in one colon cancer, allelic loss on chromosome 17 was complete, while in the same tumor, only half the cells had lost alleles on chromosome 18.[96] Thus, loss of a gene on chromosome 18 can occur even after a carcinoma has developed. In the tumor described, a gene on chromosome 18 must have been lost in a single original cell within a tumor already manifesting chromosome 17 loss, but clonal overgrowth of that cell's descendants was only half complete. Therefore, the gene on chromosome 18 did not actually cause the colorectal cancer. There are similar examples in which chromosome 17 appears to be involved after the development of the cancer.[96] The high frequency of allelic loss on chromosomes 17 and 18 in colorectal cancer supports a causal role for recessive tumor genes on those chromosomes, but there may be other explanations. Perhaps there is a gene on chromosome 17 or 18 whose loss or inactivation in one copy promotes neoplastic progression. This would represent neither a traditional dominant or recessive alteration.

Hypomethylation fulfills the first two epidemiologic criteria for causality. It occurs earliest and apparently in all cases. However, the mechanism by which hypomethylation might play a role in carcinogenesis has not yet been established.

The multiple genetic alterations in colorectal carcinogenesis are not as confusing as they might appear, however (Fig 24-6). Twenty years ago, Doll proposed that there are four to five sequential events in the complete development of a colorectal cancer, based on life table analysis.[121] Thus, the earliest change may be a change in DNA methylation. This could confer clonal expression of a cell and permit adenomatous growth. Roughly coincident with malignant conversion, a mutation in c-Ki-*ras* or a loss of a gene on chromosomes 5, 17, or 18 may take place. With tumor progression, the cancer invades and eventually metastasizes; the other genetic alterations that have not yet taken place (e.g., c-Ki-*ras* mutation and deletions on chromosomes 5, 17, and 18) may also occur, conferring on the cells an even greater ability to survive and expand in the normal host environment. Colorectal cancers, like most solid tumors, are hyperdiploid and aneuploid, and thus altered dosage of a large number of genes may play a cumulative role in neoplastic progression.

Another, perhaps more intriguing, explanation of multiple genetic changes is the possibility that chromosomal instability may underlie tumor progression. It has recently been found that losses of chromosomes 5, 17, and 18, as well as hyperploidy (an increase in chromosome number), are nonrandomly associated in colorectal cancer. Thus, for example, tumors that lose chromosome 17 are also more likely to lose chromosomes 5 and 18, as well. In addition, this apparent chromosomal instability is much more frequent in distal colorectal cancers than in proximal tumors, perhaps explaining differences in the biologic behavior of these tumors.[122]

From a public health standpoint, eventual understanding of the earliest events in neoplasia, and, in particular, whether they might promote chromosomal instability and tumor progression, may provide the greatest opportunity for innovations in prevention and treatment of neoplasia.

The reader is directed to Chapter 2, Gastrointestinal Hormones; Chapter 6, Epithelia: Biologic Principles of Organization; Chapter 23, Growth and Development in the Gastrointestinal Tract; Chapter 49, Genetic Counseling for Gastrointestinal Patients; Chapter 57, Esophageal Tumors; Chapter 63, Tumors of the Stomach; Chapter 70, Tumors and Other Neoplastic Diseases of the Small Intestine; Chapter 84, Malignant Tumors of the Colon; Chapter 90, Pancreatic Adenocarcinoma; and Chapter 91, Endocrine Neoplasms of the Pancreas.

REFERENCES

1. Schottenfield D. Epidemiology of cancer of the esophagus. Semin Oncol 1984;11:92.
2. Ziegler RG, Morris LE, Blot WJ, et al. Esophageal cancer among black men in Washington, D.C.: II. Role of nutrition. JNCI 1981;67:1199.
3. Lipkin M. Proliferation and differentiation of normal and diseased gastrointestinal cells. In: Johnson LR, ed. Physiology of the gastrointestinal tract. 2nd ed. New York: Raven Press, 1987:225.
4. Pardee AB. Principles of cancer biology: biochemistry and cell biology. In: De Vita VT Jr, Hellman S, Rosenberg SA, eds. Cancer: principles and practice of oncology. 2nd ed. Philadelphia: JB Lippincott, 1985:3.

5. Pegg AE. Polyamine metabolism and its importance in neoplastic growth and as a target for chemotherapy. Cancer Res 1988;48:759.
6. Craven PA, Saito R, DeRubertis FR. Role of local prostaglandin synthesis in the modulation of proliferative activity of rat colonic epithelium. J Clin Invest 1983;72:1365.
7. Craven PA, Pfanstiel J, DeRubertis FR. Role of activation of protein kinase C in the stimulation of colonic epithelial proliferation and reactive oxygen formation by bile acids. J Clin Invest 1987;79:532.
8. Craven PA, Pfanstiel J, DeRubertis FR. Role of reactive oxygen in bile salt stimulation of colonic epithelial proliferation. J Clin Invest 1986;77:850.
9. Bull AW, Nigro ND, Marnett LJ. Structural requirements for stimulation of colonic cell proliferation by oxidized fatty acids. Cancer Res 1988;48:1771.
10. Lipkin M, Newmark H. Effect of added dietary calcium on colonic epithelial cell-proliferation in subjects at high risk for familial colonic cancer. N Engl J Med 1985;313:1381.
11. Lipkin M, Friedman E, Winawer SJ, et al. Colonic epithelial cell proliferation in responders and nonresponders to supplemental dietary calcium. Cancer Res 1989;49:248.
12. Johnson LR. Regulation of gastrointestinal mucosal growth. Physiol Rev 1988;68:456.
13. Buckley I. Oncogenes and the nature of malignancy. Adv Cancer Res 1988;50:71.
14. Lipkin M. Phase 1 and phase 2 proliferative lesions of colonic epithelial cells in diseases leading to colonic cancer. Cancer 1974;34:878.
15. LaMont JT, O'Gorman TA. Experimental colon cancer. Gastroenterology 1978;75:1157.
16. Diwan BA, Meier H, Blackman KE. Genetic differences in the induction of colorectal cancer by 1,2-dimethylhydrazine in inbred mice. JNCI 1977;59:455.
17. Barch DH, Kuemmerle SC, Hollenberg PF, et al. Esophageal microsomal metabolism of N-nitrosomethylbenzylamine in the zinc-deficient rat. Cancer Res 1984;44:5629.
18. Barch DH, Fox CC. Dietary zinc deficiency increases the methylbenzylnitrosamine-induced formation of O^6-methylguanine in the esophageal DNA of the rat. Carcinogenesis 1987;8:1461.
19. Mandal S, Shivapurkas N, Superczynski M, et al. Inhibition of methylbenzylnitrosamine-induced esophageal tumors in rats by ellagic acid [Abstract]. Proc Am Assoc Cancer Res 1986;27:4.
20. Barch DH, Fox CC. Selective inhibition of methylbenzylnitrosamine-induced formation of esophageal O^6-methylguanine by dietary ellagic acid in rats. Cancer Res 1988;48:7088.
21. Mehta R, Labuc GE, Archer MC. Induction and suppression of N-nitrosomethylbenzylamine activation by microsomes from rat liver and esophagus. JNCI 1984;72:1443.
22. Yuspa SH, Poirier MC. Chemical carcinogenesis: from animal models to molecular models in one decade. Adv Cancer Res 1988;50:25.
23. Woodruff MFA. Tumor clonality and its biological significance. Adv Cancer Res 1988;50:197.
24. Mullins DE, Rohrlich ST. The role of proteinases in cellular invasiveness. Biochim Biophys Acta 1983;695:117.
25. Friedman EA, Buset M, Winawer SJ. Tumor promoter–enhanced destruction of noninvasive human benign colon tumor cells by co-cultivated carcinoma cells. Digestion 1988;40:197.
26. Nicholson GL. Tumor cell instability, diversification, and progression to the metastatic phenotype: from oncogene to oncofetal expression. Cancer Res 1987;47:1473.
27. Schirrmacher V. Cancer metastases: experimental approaches, theoretical concepts, and impacts for treatment strategies. Adv Cancer Res 1985;43:1.
28. Weiss L. Random and nonrandom processes in metastasis and metastatic inefficiency. Invasion Metas 1983;3:193.
29. Griffiths JD, McKinna JA, Rowbotham HD, et al. Carcinoma of the colon and rectum: circulating malignant cells and five-year survival. Cancer 1973;31:226.
30. Salsbury AJ. The significance of the circulating cancer cell. Cancer Treat Rev 1975;2:55.
31. Heldin CH, Belsholtz C, Claesson-Welch L, et al. Subversion of growth regulatory pathways in malignant transformation. Biochim Biophys Acta 1987;907:219.
32. Liotta LA. Mechanisms of cancer invasion and metastasis. In: DeVita

VT Jr, Hellman S, Rosenberg SA, eds. Important Advances in Oncology 1985. Philadelphia: JB Lippincott, 1985:28.
33. Bresalier RS, Hujanen ES, Raper SE, et al. An animal model for colon cancer metastasis: establishment and characterization of murine cell lines with enhanced liver metastasizing ability. Cancer Res 1987;47:1398.
34. Bresalier RS, Raper SE, Hujanen ES, et al. A new animal model for human colon cancer metastasis. Int J Cancer 1987;39:625.
35. Mirvish SS. The etiology of gastric cancer: Intragastrin nitrosamide formation and other theories. JNCI 1983;71:629.
36. Augeron C, Laboisse CL. Emergence of permanently differentiated cell clones in a human colonic cancer cell line after treatment with sodium butyrate. Cancer Res 1984;44:3961.
37. Boland CR, Troncale FJ. Familial colonic cancer without antecedent polyposis. Ann Intern Med 1984;100:700.
38. Mukhopadhyay T, Batsakis JG, Kuo MT. Expression of the *mdr* (P-glycoprotein) gene in chinese hamster digestive tracts. JNCI 1988;80:269.
39. Ahnen DJ, Nakane PK, Brown WR. Ultrastructural localization of carcinoembryonic antigen in normal intestine and colon cancer: abnormal distribution of CEA on the surfaces of colon cancer cells. Cancer 1982;49:2073.
40. Itzkowitz SH, Yuan M, Fukushi Y, et al. Lewis^x- and sialylated Lewis^x-related antigen expression in human malignant and non-malignant colonic tissue. Cancer Res 1986;46:2627.
41. Basu A, Murthy U, Rodeck U, et al. Presence of tumor-associated antigens in epidermal growth factor receptors from different human carcinomas. Cancer Res 1987;47:2531.
42. Boland CR, Montgomery CK, Kim YS. Alterations in human colonic mucin occurring with cellular differentiation and malignant transformation. Proc Natl Acad Sci USA 1982;79:2051.
43. Boland CR, Montgomery CK, Kim YS. Cancer associated mucin alterations in benign colonic polyps. Gastroenterology 1982;82:664.
44. Boland CR, Lance P, Levin B, et al. Abnormal goblet cell glyco-conjugates in rectal biopsies associated with an increased risk of neoplasia in patients with ulcerative colitis: early results of a prospective study. Gut 1984;25:1364.
45. Shimamoto C, Weinstein WM, Boland CR. Glycoconjugate expression during upper gastrointestinal metaplasia and neoplasia: the relationship between normal and metaplastic columnar epithelium in the esophagus. J Clin Invest 1987;80:1690.
46. Ames BN, Durston WE, Yamasaki E, Lee FD. Carcinogens are mutagens: a simple test system combining liver homogenates for activation and bacteria for detection. Proc Natl Acad Sci USA 1973;70:2281.
47. Boveri T. Zur Frage der Maligner Tumoren. Jena, Germany: Fisher, 1914.
48. Stehelin D, Varmus HE, Bishop JM, Vogt PK. DNA related to the transforming gene(s) of avian sarcoma virus is present in normal avian DNA. Nature 1976;260:170.
49. Shih C, Shilo BZ, Goldfarb MP, et al. Passage of phenotypes of chemically transformed cells via transfection of DNA and chromatin. Proc Natl Acad Sci USA 1979;76:5714.
50. Parada LF, Tabin CJ, Shih C, Weinberg RA. Human EJ bladder carcinoma oncogene is homologue of Harvey sarcoma virus *ras* gene. Nature 1982;297:474.
51. Santos E, Tronick SR, Aaronson SA, et al. T24 human bladder carcinoma oncogene is an activated form of the normal human homologue of BALB- and Harvey-MSV transforming genes. Nature 1982;298:343.
52. Goldfarb M, Shimizu K, Perucho M, Wigler M. Isolation and preliminary characterization of a human transforming gene from T24 bladder carcinoma cells. Nature 1982;296:404.
53. Feinberg AP, Vogelstein B, Droller MJ, et al. Mutation affecting the 12th amino acid of the c-Ha-*ras* oncogene product occurs infrequently in human cancer. Science 1983;220:1175.
54. Pulciani S, Santos E, Lauver AV, et al. Oncogenes in solid human tumors. Nature 1982;300:539.
55. Forrester K, Almoguera C, Han K, et al. Detection of high incidence of K-*ras* oncogenes during human colon tumorigenesis. Nature 1987;327:298.
56. Bos JL, Fearon ER, Hamilton SR, et al. Prevalence of *ras* gene mutations in human colorectal cancers. Nature 1987;327:293.

57. Almoguera C, Shibata D, Forrester K, et al. Most human carcinomas of the exocrine pancreas contain mutant c-K-*ras* genes. Cell 1988;53: 549.

58. Adari H, Lowy DR, Willumsen BM, et al. Guanosine triphosphatase activating protein (GAP) interacts with the p21 *ras* effector binding domain. Science 1988;240:518.

59. Zarbl H, Sukumar S, Arthur AV, et al. Direct mutagenesis of Ha-*ras*-1 oncogenes by N-nitroso-N-methylurea during initiation of mammary carcinogenesis in rats. Nature 1985;315:382.

60. Sakamoto H, Mori M, Taira M, et al. Transforming gene from human stomach cancers and a noncancerous portion of stomach mucosa. Proc Natl Acad Sci USA 1986;83:3997.

61. Yoshida T, Miyagawa K, Odagiri H, et al. Genomic sequence of *hst*, a transforming gene encoding a protein homologue to fibroblast growth factors and the int-2-encoded protein. Proc Natl Acad Sci USA 1987;84:7305.

62. Sakamoto H, Yoshida T, Nakakuki M, et al. Cloned *hst* gene from normal human leukocyte DNA transforms NIH3T3 cells. Biochem Biophys Res Commun 1988;151:965.

63. Nowell PC, Hungerford DA. A minute chromosome in human granulocytic leukemia. Science 1960;132:1197.

64. Rowley JD. A new consistent chromosomal abnormality in chronic myelogenous leukemia identified by quinacrine fluorescence and Giemsa staining. Nature 1973;243:290.

65. Heisterkamp N, Stam K, Groffen J, et al. Structural organization of the *bcr* gene and its role in the Ph' translocation. Nature 1985;315:758.

66. Taub R, Kirsch I, Morton C, et al. Translocation of the c-*myc* gene into the immunoglobulin heavy chain locus in human Burkitt lymphoma and murine plasmacytoma cells. Proc Natl Acad Sci USA 1982;79:7837.

67. Mitelman F. Catalog of chromosome aberrations in cancer. New York: Alan R. Liss, 1988.

68. Martin-Zanca D, Hughes SH, Barbacid M. A human oncogene formed by the fusion of truncated tropomyosin and protein tyrosine kinase sequences. Nature 1986;319:743.

69. Bar-Eli M, Battifora H, Cline MJ. Alterations of class I HLA genes in human colon cancers. Hum Genet 1988;78:86.

70. Schimke RT, Alt FW, Kellems RE, et al. Amplification of dihydrofolate reductase genes in methotrexate-resistant cultured human mouse cells. Cold Spring Harbor Symp Quant Biol 1978;42:649.

71. Seeger RC, Brodeur GM, Sather H, et al. Association of multiple copies of the N-*myc* oncogene with rapid progression of neuroblastomas. N Engl J Med 1985;313:1111.

72. McCoy MS, Toole JJ, Cunningham JM, et al. Characterization of a human colon/lung carcinoma oncogene. Nature 1983;302:79.

73. Alitalo K, Winqvist R, Lin CC, et al. Aberrant expression of an amplified c-*myb* oncogene in two cell lines from a colon carcinoma. Proc Natl Acad Sci USA 1984;31:4534.

74. Alitalo K, Schwab M, Lin CC, et al. Homogeneously staining chromosomal regions contain amplified copies of an abundantly expressed cellular oncogene (c-*myc*) in malignant neuroendocrine cells from a human colon carcinoma. Proc Natl Acad Sci USA 1983;80:1707.

75. Yokota J, Yamamoto T, Toyoshima K, et al. Amplification of c-*erb* B-2 oncogene in human adenocarcinomas in vivo. Lancet 1986;1: 765.

76. Yoshida MC, Wada M, Satoh H, et al. Human HST1 (HSTF1) gene maps to chromosome band 11q13 and coamplifies with the INT2 gene in human cancer. Proc Natl Acad Sci USA 1988;35: 4861.

77. Yokota J, Yamamoto T, Toyoshima K, et al. Amplification of c-*erb* B-2 oncogene in human adenocarcinomas in vivo. Lancet 1986;1: 765.

78. Fukushige S, Matsubara K, Yoshida M, et al. Localization of a novel v-*erb* B-related gene, c-*erb* B-2, on human chromosome 17 and its amplification in a gastric cancer cell line. Mol Cell Biol 1986;6:955.

79. Yokota J, Yamamoto T, Miyajima N, et al. Genetic alterations of the c-*erb* B-2 oncogene occur frequently in tubular adenocarcinoma of the stomach and are often accompanied by amplification of the v-*erb* A homologue. Oncogene 1988;2:283.

80. Roninson IB. Detection and mapping of homologous, repeated and amplified DNA sequences by DNA renaturation in agarose gels. Nucleic Acids Res 1983;11:5413.

81. Roninson IB, Chin JE, Choi KG, et al. Isolation of human *mdr* DNA sequences amplified in multidrug-resistant KB carcinoma cells. Proc Natl Acad Sci USA 1986;83:4538.

82. Fukumoto M, Shevrin DH, Roninson IB. Analysis of gene amplification in human tumor cell lines. Proc Natl Acad Sci USA 1988;85: 6846.

83. Knudson AG. Genetics of human cancer. Ann Rev Genet 1986;20: 231.

84. Francke U, Holmes LB, Atkins L, Riccardi VM. Aniridia-Wilms' tumor association: evidence for specific deletion of 11p13. Cytogenet Cell Genet 1979;24:185.

85. Fearon ER, Vogelstein B, Feinberg AP. Somatic deletion and duplication of genes on chromosome 11 in Wilms' tumors. Nature 1984;309:176.

86. Fearon ER, Feinberg AP, Hamilton SH, Vogelstein B. Loss of genes on the short arm of chromosome 11 in bladder cancer. Nature 1985;318:377.

87. Yokota J, Wada M, Shimosato Y, et al. Loss of heterozygosity on chromosomes 3, 13, and 17 in small-cell carcinoma and on chromosome 3 in adenocarcinoma of the lung. Proc Natl Acad Sci USA 1987;84:9252.

88. Zbar B, Brauch H, Talmadge C, Linehan M. Loss of alleles of loci on the short arm of chromosome 3 in renal cell carcinoma. Nature 1987;327:721.

89. Ali IU, Lidereau R, Theillet C, Callahan R. Reduction to homozygosity of genes on chromosome 11 in human breast neoplasia. Science 1987;238:185.

90. Mathew CGP, Smith BA, Thorpe K, et al. Deletion of genes on chromosome 1 in endocrine neoplasia. Nature 1987;328:524.

91. Larsson C, Skogseid B, Oberg K, et al. Multiple endocrine neoplasia type 1 gene maps to chromosome 11 and is lost in insulinoma. Nature 1988;332:85.

92. Herrera L, Kakati S, Gibas L, et al. Brief clinical report: Gardner syndrome in a man with an interstitial deletion of 5q. Am J Med Genet 1986;25:473.

93. Bodmer WF, Bailey CJ, Bodmer J, et al. Localization of the gene for familial adenomatous polyposis on chromosome 5. Nature 1987;328:614.

94. Leppert M, Dobbs M, Scambler P, et al. The gene for familial polyposis coli maps to the long arm of chromosome 5. Science 1987;238:1411.

95. Solomon E, Voss R, Hall V, et al. Chromosome 5 allele loss in human colorectal carcinomas. Nature 1987;328:616.

96. Law DJ, Olschwang S, Monpezat J-P, et al. Concerted nonsyntenic allelic loss in human colorectal carcinoma. Science 1988;241:961.

97. Baker SJ, Fearon ER, Nigro JM, et al. Chromosome 17 deletions and p53 gene mutations in colorectal carcinomas. Science 1989;244: 217.

98. Fearon ER, Cho DR, Nigro JM, et al. Identification of a chromosome 18q gene that is altered in colorectal cancers. Science 1990;247:49.

99. Vogelstein B, Fearon ER, Hamilton SR, et al. Genetic alterations during colorectal tumor development. N Engl J Med 1988;319:525.

100. Motomura K, Nishisho I, Takai S, et al. Loss of alleles at loci on chromosome 13 in human primary gastric cancer. Genomics 1988;2: 180.

101. Pitot HC. Fundamentals of oncology. New York: Marcel Dekker, 1981.

102. Grady LJ, Campbell WP. Non-repetitive DNA transcription in mouse cells grown in tissue culture. Nature 1973;243:195.

103. Scott MRD, Westphal KH, Rigby PWJ. Activation of mouse genes in transformed cells. Cell 1983;34:557.

104. Razin A, Rigg AD. DNA methylation and gene function. Science 1980;210:604.

105. Hoffman RM. Altered methionine metabolism, DNA methylation and oncogene expression in carcinogenesis. Biochim Biophys Acta 1984;738:49.

106. Feinberg AP, Vogelstein B. Hypomethylation distinguishes genes of some human cancer from their normal counterparts. Nature 1983;301:89.

107. Goelz SE, Vogelstein B, Hamilton SR, Feinberg AP. Hypomethylation of DNA from benign and malignant human colon neoplasms. Science 1985;228:187.

108. Feinberg AP, Gehrke CW, Kuo KC, Ehrlich M. Reduced genomic

5-methylcytosine content in human colonic neoplasia. Cancer Res 1988;48:1159.

109. Feinberg AP, Vogelstein B. Hypomethylation of *ras* oncogenes in primary human cancers. Biochem Biophys Res Commun 1983;111:47.

110. Schmid M, Grunert D, Haff T, Engel W. 5-Azacytidine-induced undercondensations in human chromosomes. Cytogenet Cell Genet 1983;36:554.

111. Feinberg AP. The molecular genetics of DNA methylation in colorectal cancer. In: Augenlicht L, ed. Cell and molecular biology of human colon cancer. Boca Raton, FL: CRC Press, 1989, pp. 187–198.

112. Rainier S, Feinberg AP. Capture and characterization of 5-aza-2'-deoxycytidine-treated C3H 10T½ cells prior to transformation. Proc Natl Acad Sci USA 1988;85:6384.

113. Hand PH, Thor A, Wunderlich D, et al. Monoclonal antibodies of predefined specificity detect activated *ras* gene expression in human mammary and colon carcinomas. Proc Natl Acad Sci USA 1984;81:5227.

114. Tanaka T, Slamon DJ, Battifora H, Cline MJ. Expresion of p21 *ras* oncoproteins in human cancers. Cancer Res 1986;46:1465.

115. Erisman MD, Scott JK, Watt RA, Astrin SM. The c-*myc* protein is constitutively expressed at elevated levels in colorectal carcinoma cell lines. Oncogene 1988;2:367.

116. Untawale S, Blick M. Oncogene expression in adenocarcinomas of the colon and in colon tumor–derived cell lines. Anticancer Res 1988;8:1.

117. Erisman MD, Litwin S, Keidan RD, et al. Noncorrelation of the expression of the c-*myc* oncogene in colorectal carcinoma with recurrence of disease or patient survival. Cancer Res 1988;38:1350.

118. Trainer DL, Kline T, McCabe FL, et al. Biological characterization and oncogene expression in human colorectal carcinoma cell lines. Int J Cancer 1988;41:287.

119. Monnat M, Tardy S, Saraga P, et al. Prognostic implications of expression of the cellular gene *myc*, *fos*, Ha-*ras* and Ki-*ras* in colon carcinoma. Int J Cancer 1987;40:293.

120. Augenlicht LH, Augeron C, Yander G, Laboisse C. Overexpression of *ras* in mucous-secreting human colon carcinoma cells of low tumorigenicity. Cancer Res 1987;47: 3763.

121. Doll R. The age distribution of cancer: implications for models of carcinogenesis. J R Statist Soc Series A 1971;134:133.

122. Delattre P, Olschwang S, Law DJ, et al. Multiple genetic alterations distinguish distal from proximal colorectal cancer. Lancet 1989;2: 353.

25

Pharmacology of the Gastrointestinal Tract

PAUL B. WATKINS

The ability of the gastrointestinal tract to absorb nutrients efficiently from our diet is obviously essential for life. An often overlooked function of the gastrointestinal (GI) tract is to provide an impermeable barrier to the many other substances that may be harmful to us. In fact, the GI tract is the major barrier between us and our environment. It has been estimated that the surface area of the digestive tract in contact with lumenal contents is about 200 m²,[1] or approximately the size of a doubles tennis court. By comparison, the surface area of the aerated portions of the lung has been approximated to be 70 m², and the surface area of our skin has been approximated to be 2 m².

Our food commonly contains natural toxins, such as those produced by some plants to render them inedible to insects. Many synthetic toxins are also present, either as intentional additives, such as dyes and preservatives, or as contaminants, such as insecticides and chemical waste. Airborne particulate matter, including products of internal combustion, is also swallowed frequently after it is trapped in our nasal sinuses or bronchial tree.

Finally, many of the most potentially injurious compounds that may be present in the GI tract do not pass through the esophagus. Bile can contain toxins, mutagens, and carcinogens not ingested but produced by the liver from less reactive compounds. Potentially harmful substances can also be generated in the gut lumen by enteric flora or by the epithelial cells lining the digestive tract.

The vast majority of medications used in clinical medicine are administered orally. With few exceptions, their usefulness depends on their ability to traverse the barrier of the GI tract. Thus, defeating the barrier function of the gut is a major challenge for the pharmaceutical industry. This chapter provides a broad overview of the current understanding of how the gut interacts with drugs; more complete reviews of this topic are available elsewhere.[2,3] Although this discussion focuses entirely on drugs, the concepts involved apply to all molecules that may appear in the gut. The majority of medications in use today are, in fact, derivatives of naturally occurring substances that may be normally present in our diet in small quantities.

FUNCTIONAL ANATOMY OF THE GASTROINTESTINAL BARRIER

In many ways, absorption along the GI tract appears to behave as if the digestive tract were a tube made of lipid. According to this model, substances must be nonpolar and soluble in lipid to traverse the wall of the gut. On the other hand, efficient absorption can occur only if the substance is delivered to the gut wall in a dispersed, diffusible form. This generally means that the substance must be water-soluble because water makes up the vast majority of the lumenal contents of the gut. These opposing properties of being both lipid- and water-soluble are possessed by weak acids and weak bases.[4] At any given moment, a proportion of the weak acid or base in solution is ionized and, therefore, polar and dissolvable in the aqueous phase; the remainder is nonionized and is, therefore, more lipid-soluble. The ratio of nonionized to ionized species at equilibrium is a function of the dissociation constant of the acid or base (K_a or K_b). Even if only a small fraction of the acid or base is in the lipid-soluble (nonionized) form, efficient absorption into the body can occur because, as the nonionized species diffuses from the gut lumen (and is removed from the serosal surface by blood flow), it is replaced by freshly associated acid or base in proportion to the dissociation constant. This is schematically shown in Figure 25-1 for the hypothetical electrolyte XY.

Many oral medications are weak acids or weak bases. In most circumstances, an acid becomes ionized by losing a hydrogen ion, whereas a base becomes ionized by gaining a hydrogen ion. In biologic systems, a base or an acid can be considered to be weak if its degree of dissociation varies with the changes in pH normally encountered in the digestive tract.[4] The degree of association or dissociation of these compounds is directly related to the pH of the medium as predicted by the Henderson-Hasselbalch equation. This equation is usually written as Equation I below but can also be written as Equation II.

$$pH = pKa + \log \frac{[X]}{[XH]} \qquad (I)$$

$$\frac{[X]}{[XH]} = 10^{(pH-pKa)} \qquad (II)$$

Gut Wall

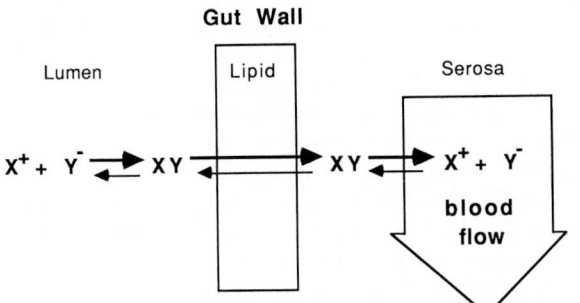

FIGURE 25–1. Absorption of a hypothetical electrolyte (*XY*). The electrolyte (*XY*) is dissolvable in the aqueous phase of the gut lumen in its dissociated, ionized form (*X*$^+$, *Y*$^-$). These ions are in equilibrium with the associated, nonionized form (*XY*), which is lipid-soluble and can traverse the lipid membranes of the gut wall. After entering the serosa, the electrolyte is again in equilibrium with its dissociated ions, which are continually removed in the portal blood. This results in continued absorption of the electrolyte without obtaining equilibrium across the gut wall.

Equation II tells us that the degree of ionization of a weak base or weak acid (X) is related to the logarithms of both the dissociation constant of the compound (pKa) and the hydrogen ion concentration in the solution (pH). At neutral pH (7.0), the Henderson-Hasselbalch equation predicts that a weak acid with pKa of 5 or a weak base with pKa of 9 will have the associated, lipid-soluble species present in a ratio of 1:100 with the ionized water-soluble species at neutral pH as shown below.

Weak acid:

$$\frac{[X^-]}{[XH]} = 10^{(7-5)} = 10^2$$

Weak base:

$$\frac{[X]}{[XH^+]} = 10^{7-9} = 10^{-2}$$

The pH of the GI tract varies along its length, and, therefore, the concentration of the nonionized (absorbable) species varies as a function of location.[5] Osterhout[6] is generally credited with developing the "pH partition hypothesis," which predicts that the rate of absorption of weak acids and bases will vary at different locations within the GI tract. In the acidic environment of the stomach, weak bases are largely in their ionized state and, therefore, not readily absorbed. Weak acids, however, are primarily associated and more readily absorbed. Aspirin is a weak acid having significant absorption in the stomach. After absorption through the hypothetical lipid layer of the gut wall, aspirin enters the neutral pH of the body fluids and is reionized. Because the reionized aspirin is not diffusible through the lipid membrane, appreciable back diffusion of aspirin into the gut lumen should not occur. Aspirin absorption from the gut lumen, therefore, continues without attaining equilibrium of exchange across the hypothetical lipid wall.

The pH of lumenal contents rises after they have traversed the pyloris but does not attain neutrality. The pH of proximal jejunum appears to range from 4.5 to 6.0, and the lumenal contents gradually become more alkaline toward the terminal ileum (pH 7.0).[5] According to the pH partition hypothesis, weak acids should be better absorbed in the proximal small intestine than in the distal small intestine, and weak bases should be more efficiently absorbed in the ileum than the proximal intestine. In general, this appears to be the case. However, due to the enormous surface area of the small bowel, significant absorption can occur even if a seemingly trivial fraction of a compound is in the associated, lipid-soluble state. Furthermore, partitioning of a drug between aqueous and lipid phases is never absolute, and small proportions of polar drugs dissolve in lipids.

The longitudinal pH gradient in the GI tract has important implications in the design of pharmaceuticals. For example, because aspirin-induced gastric injury appears to result, at least in part, from absorption of the drug into the gastric mucosal cells, some newer nonsteroidal antiinflammatory agents have been designed as weak bases. This results in decreased absorption in the stomach. On the other hand, it may be desirable to design some drugs as weak acids to enhance their absorption in the stomach. This approach may be useful in the future design of drugs that inhibit gastric acid production or that enhance cytoprotection. Finally, pharmaceutical companies have taken advantage of the gut's longitudinal pH gradient to "target" some drugs to the distal small bowel and colon. For example, the presumed active moiety of Azulfidine (sulfasalazine) in the treatment of ulcerative colitis is 5-ASA (see the section entitled "Role of Enteric Flora in Gut Metabolism"). A form of 5-ASA that is undergoing clinical trials has a coating that should dissolve only at the alkaline pH of the distal small bowel.

If the gut behaved as a lipid tube and the pH partition hypothesis were correct, the pKa alone should predict the relative absorption of any weak acid or base in a given portion of the GI tract. The actual absorption of many drugs, however, deviates considerably from these predicted values. In general, weak acids seem to be more efficiently absorbed and weak bases less efficiently absorbed than predicted.[4] It is clear that the lipid tube model is not sufficient to explain many aspects of drug absorption. Other features of the gut must be considered.

Aqueous Phase

The lumenal content of the GI tract is mostly water and, therefore, represents an "aqueous phase." Optimal absorption of a compound requires more than just its dispersion in the lumenal contents, as might occur with mixing. The drug must actually be dissolved in the aqueous phase. This is because the rate of flow of lumenal contents falls as a drug approaches the mucosal surface, forming a stationary aqueous layer adjacent to the microvillous border of the enterocytes, termed the "unstirred water layer." Fish swimming in a rapidly flowing river directly experience this concept. The velocity of the water current decreases as the fish swim down toward the river bottom and approaches zero as the fish reach the river bed. Adjacent to the river bed, the water is stationary, and molecules move in the water by brownian motion only. This concept of the unstirred water layer also applies in the GI tract, although with far more complexity. The GI tract undergoes peristalsis, which results in mixing of the lumenal contents and tends to disrupt the unstirred water layer. On the other hand, the GI tract contains a mucous layer that logically impedes mixing and promotes maintenance of the unstirred water layer. The situation is further complicated by the fact that the mucosal surface of the GI tract is not flat, but contains folds, villi, and microvilli. For all of these reasons, the thickness of the unstirred water layer in the GI tract (estimated to be 100–300 μm[7]) appears to vary depending on location and depending on the physiologic state of the gut. Drugs must be dissolved in the aqueous phase to diffuse passively through the unstirred layer.

The potential importance of the unstirred water layer is illustrated by the normal absorption of lipids. The primary function of the micelles formed by the bile acids is as water-soluble carriers for lipids otherwise incapable of traversing the unstirred layer. Absorption of fat-soluble vitamins largely depends on lumenal bile acids, presumably for this reason. It is likely that diffusion through the unstirred layer also limits the rate of absorption of many lipophilic drugs.

The effect of the unstirred water layer does not alone explain the relatively enhanced absorption of weak acids compared to that of weak bases previously mentioned. To account for these observations, Hogben et al[8] postulated that there exists a region adjacent to the microvillous border that has a pH significantly lower than the main bulk of the lumenal contents. A region of acidic pH

directly adjacent to the mucosal surface has been measured directly using micro pH probes[4,9] and the existence of this "acid microclimate"[8] is generally (but not universally) accepted. Although its precise dimensions are unknown, the acid microclimate appears to make up only a small portion of the thickness of the unstirred layer. A sodium/hydrogen ATPase capable of generating the acid microclimate has been identified in enterocyte apical membranes, and recent evidence suggests that a Na^+,K^+–ATPase may also be involved.[10] It is assumed that the glycocalix of the microvilli and mucus somehow maintain the acid microclimate by preventing the otherwise rapid diffusion of hydrogen ions into the intestinal lumen.

The clinical significance of the acid microclimate remains unclear. It has been claimed that the ability to maintain the acid microclimate is significantly diminished in celiac sprue and Crohn's disease, and this loss of acidity has been invoked as an explanation for the poor absorption of folate (a weak acid) sometimes seen in these conditions.[11] The oral absorption of some weak bases, such as trimethoprim, propranolol, and quinidine, is increased in some malabsorption syndromes, and this may also reflect loss of the acid microclimate.[9] It has also been postulated that the acid microclimate facilitates the breakdown of micelles after they have traversed the unstirred layer.[12] If this is true, alterations in the acid microclimate associated with GI disease may contribute to steatorrhea.

Paracellular Route

Some clinically useful drugs remain ionized at the full range of pH encountered along the GI tract (i.e., they are strong electrolytes). The lipid tube hypothesis is not satisfactory in explaining absorption of these compounds. For these ions to be absorbed, they must traverse the enterocyte monolayer either through the cell membranes or through spaces in the intercellular junctions. The enterocytes lining the GI tract are attached near the apical surfaces by tight junctions, which are contiguous around the entire apical circumference of the enterocyte. This structure has been compared to a six-pack of beer or soda, where the cans represent enterocytes and the plastic attaching rings are the tight junctions.[13] The arrangement is characteristic of most polarized epithelia in the body, including renal tubular epithelia. Tight junctions[14] are not perfect seals but have varying degrees of permeability to ions depending on the location of the epithelium. The intercellular junctions in the small bowel are quite ion-permeable compared to those present in the colon, gallbladder, and other tissues. Studies of tight junctions have suggested that ions pass through channels or gates. In some cases, cations appear to traverse the junctions more readily than identically sized anions, suggesting that the area surrounding the tight junctions possesses a negative charge.

It remains unclear as to what extent most drugs are absorbed through the paracellular pathway (pathway A in Fig 25-2). Although many drugs have diameters less than the estimated dimensions of the tight junction channels present in the small bowel, most ionized drugs are hydrated with water, greatly increasing their effective size and limiting their access to the paracellular route. Therefore, many and perhaps most ionized molecules are absorbed into the body by traversing the apical membrane of the enterocyte and not by the paracellular pathway.

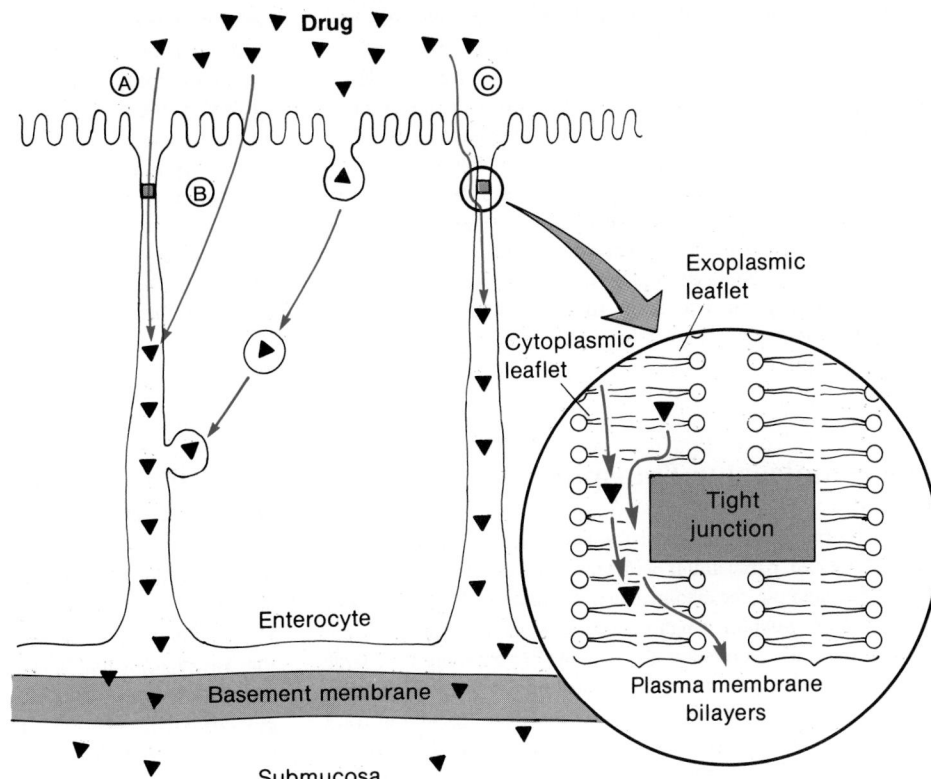

FIGURE 25–2. Schematic representation of the transepithelial movement of drugs. Drugs that encounter the apical surface of the gut epithelia can enter the body by several routes: (**A**) the paracellular route, which involves traversing the tight junctions; (**B**) transcytosolic migration, which involves movement of the drug from the apical to the basolateral membrane by diffusion or by cytosolic carrier proteins; (**C**) lateral diffusion within the cytoplasmic leaflet of the plasma membrane bilayer; and (**D**) transcytosis. Route 3 is possible because, although the tight junction prevents a lateral diffusion of drugs from apical to basolateral membrane in the exoplasmic leaflet, this diffusion is not inhibited by the tight junction if drugs enter the cytoplasmic leaflet of the bilayer. The relationship of the tight junctions to the exoplasmic and cytoplasmic leaflets is schematically shown in the magnified insert.

Transcellular Route

There are large differences between the composition of the apical and basolateral membranes of enterocytes.[15] The unique composition of the apical membrane probably confers properties that improve its integrity as a barrier. For example, the apical membrane is known to be significantly less fluid than the basolateral membrane.[15]

The mechanisms involved in the transcellular migration of drugs during absorption are not well known. Uptake from the lumen may involve simple dissolution of lipid-soluble drugs into the apical membrane. Alternatively, pores may exist in the apical membrane that allow passage of small molecules into the enterocyte. In addition, many selective transport mechanisms exist in the apical membrane that may be used by drugs. For example, peptides appear to be removed actively from the gut lumen by transport proteins present in the apical membrane. Recent experiments indicate that captopril, an angiotensin-converting enzyme inhibitor, is actively transported out of the gut lumen and that this absorption is inhibited in the presence of peptides.[16] These observations suggest that the absorption of captopril may be mediated by one or more peptide transporters present in the apical membrane. Fatty acid uptake from the GI lumen appears to involve a transport protein present in the apical membrane[17] that may also transport some drugs. Finally, the apical membrane has been shown to contain transport systems that apparently function to pump into the gut lumen substances present in the enterocyte (see the section entitled "Secretion of Drugs by the Gut"). It may be possible for these transport mechanisms to work "in reverse" when the lumenal concentration of a transported substance is very high,

as would occur after an oral dose of a drug. For example, quaternary ammonium compounds are actively secreted across the gut epithelium into the lumen by a carrier-mediated active transport process present in enterocytes[18]; however, absorption of these ions can occur, apparently, by the same transport mechanism if the lumenal concentration is sufficiently high.[18]

Once they traverse into the apical membrane, most drugs appear to reach the basolateral surface of the enterocyte by way of the cytosol (pathway B in Fig 25-2). Weak acids dissociate after traversing the apical membrane as the result of the neutral pH of the cytosol, and the resulting ions may be sufficiently water-soluble to diffuse to the basolateral membrane. However, lipid-soluble drugs traverse the enterocyte, presumably by binding soluble cytosolic proteins. This may be the mechanism by which some fluorescent lipid probes are able to equilibrate rapidly throughout all the internal membranes of polarized epithelial cells after they are introduced into the apical membrane. The fatty acid binding protein is an example of an abundant cytosolic protein that is probably involved in the binding and intracellular transport of fatty acids and may also function in the transport of some drugs.[19]

It is theoretically possible for a drug to diffuse from the apical membrane of the enterocyte to the basolateral membrane without entering the cytosol. The current understanding of polarized epithelia is that domain-specific proteins and lipids are present only in the outer lipid layer (the "exoplasmic leaflet") of the plasma membrane bilayer.[14,20] The inner lipid layer (the "cytoplasmic leaflet") of the bilayer is believed to have an identical composition in basolateral and apical membranes. Lateral diffusion and mixing of apical and basolateral constituents of the exoplasmic leaflet appear to be prevented by the tight junctions (schematically shown in Fig 25-2). However, the tight junction does not appear to be a barrier to diffusion within the cytoplasmic leaflet. For example, certain fluorescent lipids diffuse rapidly from the apical to basolateral domains only if they are introduced into the cytoplasmic leaflet.[20] Hence, a lipid-soluble drug that enters the apical membrane from the gut lumen need only be segregated to the cytoplasmic leaflet of the bilayer (by passive diffusion or by way of transport proteins) to diffuse laterally to the basolateral membrane. There is no direct evidence that this pathway (shown as C in Fig 25-2) is important in the absorption of drugs. Nonetheless, its recent discovery should prompt a reexamination of drugs whose absorption is presumed to occur through paracellular channels simply because they have not been detected within enterocytes during absorption.

Macromolecular Transport

Many observations of intestinal absorption are not adequately explained by the paracellular and transcellular routes explained above. For example, the mammalian neonate is capable of absorbing intact immunoglobulins (high-molecular-weight proteins) present in maternal milk. Adults are also capable of absorbing very large molecules. A dramatic example is botulinum toxin, which has a molecular weight of 900,000 and is lethal when ingested in trace amounts. Particulate matter, such as starch granules and asbestos fibers, can also be absorbed into the body through the GI tract. In part, such absorption of large molecules and particles is likely to be due to transcytosis. This process results from the pinching off of the apical membrane around a particle, forming a cytoplasmic vesicle. The intracellular vesicle can migrate, presumably by an active process, to the basolateral membrane where exocytosis of the enclosed particle or macromolecule can occur. Transcytosis (depicted as pathway D in Fig 25-2) has been invoked to explain the carrier-mediated absorption of vitamin B_{12} in the terminal ileum, but the extent to which this occurs in the remainder of the GI tract is unclear.

An alternate hypothesis to explain absorption of macromolecules has been termed "persorption."[21] The enterocyte population is in a constant state of flux such that enterocytes move from the crypt up the villus, ultimately to be sloughed from the villus tip. It is speculated that, as enterocytes detach from the villus tip, there is transient direct contact between portions of the basement membrane and the lumenal contents, providing an avenue for relatively nonspecific absorption of even large molecules and particles. Persorption has never been demonstrated in vivo, thus it is unclear at present whether it is a significant route of absorption.

The Immune System

The immune system may function to limit absorption of potentially harmful compounds. In laboratory animals, absorption of the carcinogens 7,12-dimethylbenzanthracene (DMBA)[22] and 2-acetylaminofluorene (AAF)[23] was significantly reduced after animals were immunized actively or passively to these agents. This appears to result from secretion of xenobiotic-specific IgA into the gut lumen, with the subsequent formation of IgA-xenobiotic complexes that are poorly absorbed.[23] Although most potentially harmful substances are not immunogenic by themselves, covalent binding to proteins present in the gut lumen, as may result from the action of enteric flora,[24] could produce immunologically active moieties. However, there is no evidence that antibodies are normally produced to xenobiotics present in the diet. Nonetheless, an exciting possibility is the development of oral vaccines that would limit absorption of selected xenobiotics. For example, immunization might reduce the health threat of some insecticides commonly present in our food. Although it is possible that the immune system plays a significant role in limiting absorption of certain xenobiotics present in low concentrations in our diet, it seems unlikely that absorption of most drugs is significantly influenced by immunologic responses.

The Effect of Gastrointestinal Physiology on Drug Absorption

The absorption of a drug can be influenced dramatically by lumenal and physiologic factors not appreciated by discussion of anatomic factors alone. First, the GI tract is a dynamic organ with motility that varies according to time of the day and in response to certain drugs, diseases, or the consumption of food. These alterations in gut physiology can have profound effects on the absorption of drugs. For example, the rate at which a drug is passed from the stomach into the duodenum may vary greatly depending on the motility status of the gut at the time the drug is ingested. If a drug is taken in the fasting state just before a migrating motor complex, it is conceivable that an intact tablet could be carried to a distal location in the small bowel; the same pill taken moments later could remain in the stomach for a prolonged period (see ch 8).

Concomitant administration of drugs with food can alter dramatically their rate of absorption for a number of reasons.[25,26] For example, splanchnic blood flow increases by up to 50% during feeding. This should result in more rapid removal of drug from the basolateral surface of the enterocyte and accelerated absorption of drugs that diffuse readily through the unstirred water layer and the enterocytes. Ingestion of fats with drugs can also influence their absorption because fat delays gastric emptying. Furthermore, because fat may float in the aqueous phase of the stomach and, therefore, empty from the stomach last, lipid-soluble drugs may partition into the lipid phase and be delayed further in leaving the stomach. Alternatively, fat may improve the absorption of some drugs by stimulating gallbladder contraction, thereby providing bile acid micelles to transport lipid-soluble drugs through the unstirred layer. Cyclosporine A is administered in an olive oil solution, presumably for this reason. Drugs that rely on nutrient transport systems for uptake may also have decreased absorption when taken with a meal. For example, captopril uptake may rely on a peptide transporter; lumenal peptides may compete for binding and uptake of this drug. This may explain partly why absorption of captopril has been reported to decrease by up to 30% when taken with meals.[16] Finally, many drugs can bind substances found in the diet, hindering their absorption.[26,27]

Gastric acid, digestive enzymes, and bile can alter dramatically the bioavailability of drugs. Erythromycin, for example, is inactivated by gastric acid and, therefore, must be administered in an enteric-coated form to retard its dissolution in the stomach. Peptide drugs, such as insulin, are readily digested and cannot be administered orally. Some investigators have attempted to administer peptide hormones orally by enclosing them in small membrane vesicles (liposomes), which may sequester the drug partially from digestive enzymes.[5] Bile may be crucial to the absorption of some lipophilic drugs. As discussed above, the absorption of the immunosuppressive agent cyclosporin A is significantly enhanced by the presence of bile in the GI lumen.[28]

Summary

The GI tract is a highly sophisticated and successful barrier between us and our environment. For most drugs, this barrier appears to consist of gut lumenal factors and the properties of the single layer of epithelial cells that line the GI tract. Absorption of individual drugs can be influenced dramatically by the unstirred water layer and acid microclimate that exist on the lumenal surface of the gut. Absorption is not limited to drugs with lipid solubility; efficient absorption of permanently ionized drugs also occurs. Such absorption may involve the paracellular route or may occur through transcellular routes dependent on apical membrane transporters or pores. Transcytosis and persorption may account for the absorption of larger molecules and particles into the GI tract. The effects of diet, GI physiology, and splanchnic blood flow are complex. It is often difficult to predict for a given drug whether administration with meals will enhance or decrease its absorption.

THE METABOLIC BARRIER OF THE GI TRACT

The majority of drugs, once absorbed from the GI tract, enter the portal venous system and pass through the liver before they enter the systemic circulation. It is widely assumed that the drug-metabolizing capability of the liver evolved, at least in part, as a mechanism to protect the body from potentially harmful substances that overcome the barrier of the gut. In most instances, the metabolites generated from drugs by the liver are less biologically active and more readily excreted from the body than the parent drugs. However, some drugs and other apparently innocuous compounds may be converted through liver metabolism into toxins, mutagens, and carcinogens. These metabolites may be excreted into bile and are, therefore, reintroduced into the GI tract. Alternatively, metabolites may appear in hepatic venous blood for subsequent metabolism or elimination by the kidney, lung, liver, or gut. In either case, metabolism by the liver often results in a significant drop in the systemic availability of the parent drug, an effect referred to as "first pass elimination." Some drugs have little if any first pass elimination, and the parent compound leaves the liver unchanged.

The enterocyte, in addition to providing a sophisticated anatomic barrier, is also capable of metabolizing drugs. It is likely that the contribution of intestinal metabolism to the overall metabolism and first pass elimination of drugs has been underestimated in the past. Many of the drug-metabolizing enzymes present in intestinal mucosa are identical or closely related to those that have been characterized in the liver. To understand intestinal drug metabolism, it is necessary to review briefly drug-metabolizing systems that have been well characterized in the liver.

Hepatic Drug Metabolism

The liver is capable of performing a wide variety of enzymatic modifications of drugs. These reactions have traditionally been divided into two groups: phase 1 reactions, which result in a direct modification of the primary structure of the drug, and phase 2 reactions, which involve covalent binding (conjugation) to polar ligands such as glucuronic acid, sulfate, glutathione, or amino acids. The conjugation of a drug greatly enhances its water solubility, allowing it to be excreted in the urine and, when excreted into the bile, preventing its reabsorption from the gut. The terms phase 1 and phase 2 refer to the fact that often, but not always, drugs must first be subjected to phase 1 metabolism before they can be conjugated. Phase 1 and phase 2 enzymes of various types are present in the cytosol of the hepatocyte, but most identified forms are embedded in or attached to the endoplasmic reticulum. Knowledge of the membrane-bound drug-metabolizing enzymes is extensive, in part because techniques are available that allow rapid isolation of the internal membrane or "microsomal" fraction from whole liver. It has been possible, therefore, to study metabolism of any drug by simply adding it to a test tube containing liver microsomes. Such studies have revealed that microsomes are capable of performing phase 1 and phase 2 reactions on a vast array of structurally diverse drugs, largely mirroring drug metabolism occurring in the liver in vivo.

Reactions catalyzed by microsomal phase 1 enzymes are predominantly oxidations involving insertion of molecular oxygen, usually in the form of a hydroxyl group. The majority of these reactions depend on a large multigene family of enzymes called the "cytochromes P-450." This rather cumbersome term derives from the biochemical similarity between the enzymes and the mitochondrial cytochromes and from the fact that, under certain experimental conditions, these enzymes maximally absorb light of approximately 450 nm wavelength. The "P" is believed to have stood for "pigment," referring to the fact that these enzymes contain heme and are, therefore, red in color. Like hemoglobin, another heme-containing protein, cytochromes P-450 bind molecular oxygen, which is the source of the oxygen atom required for hydroxylation.

There has been a dramatic increase in knowledge of the cytochromes P-450 over the last decade.[29] Several factors have contributed to the intense interest in these enzymes. First, the cytochromes P-450 catalyze the metabolism of many endogenous compounds, such as steroid hormones, in addition to drugs. Furthermore, the reactions they catalyze are often rate-limiting in the inactivation and elimination of drugs. Second, they are the liver enzymes most responsible for generating toxic, mutagenic, and carcinogenic metabolites from more harmless compounds. Third, these enzymes appear to be both inducible and inhibitable, providing a model for the study of gene regulation. Finally, purification of the cytochromes P-450 has, in general, been easier than that of the other drug-metabolizing enzymes. This is because the cytochromes P-450 are abundant, representing up to 25% of the total protein present in liver microsomes prepared from animals that have been pretreated with certain inducers. Moreover, these enzymes generally retain their catalytic properties (and their red color) as they are purified.

Over 15 individual cytochromes P-450 have been purified from rat liver microsomes, and over 12 cytochromes P-450 have been purified from human liver microsomes. Many of the genes coding for these enzymes have been cloned and sequenced, and the data obtained indicate that many of the hepatic cytochromes P-450 are highly conserved in mammalian species. On the basis of the amino acid sequences derived from the corresponding cDNAs, the liver cytochromes P-450 can be divided into gene families.[30] This enzyme family appears to have diverged from a single precursor enzyme roughly 1.5 billion years ago.

The liver's ability to metabolize a vast array of structurally diverse drugs results in large part from several properties of the cytochromes P-450. First, the multiple forms of cytochrome P-450 present in the liver can differ dramatically from each other in structure and ability to metabolize individual drugs. Second, mammalian liver often contains subfamilies of these enzymes whose members are highly homologous to each other in terms of amino acids sequence but differ subtly in their abilities to bind and metabolize drugs. Third, a single cytochrome P-450 appears to be able to bind and metabolize multiple drugs with structural similarities. Finally, in some cases, the liver has the ability to make more ("induce") rapidly just the right cytochrome P-450 necessary to metabolize a drug presented to it. Table 25-1 lists some human liver cytochromes P-450 that have been partially characterized regarding substrate specificity and regulation.

There are marked differences among patients in their ability to perform phase 1 liver metabolism of some drugs; this may reflect corresponding differences in the liver content and the catalytic activity of specific forms of cytochrome P-450. For example, the ability to hydroxylate the antihypertensive medicine, debrisoquine (formerly used widely in Europe), is deficient in approximately 10% of the population, and this has been shown to result from genetic defects in a single form of cytochrome P-450 (P-450IID; see Table 25-1).[31] This selective defect does not affect other phase 1 or phase 2 enzymes, thus most other medications are metabolized normally. Inherited defects in other forms of cytochrome P-450 also appear to be common in patients, and these individual defects may help to determine the variable therapeutic responses to many medications.[32]

In general, phase 2 enzymes have not been as well characterized as have the cytochromes P-450. The best studied phase 2 enzymes are the uridine 5'-diphosphate (UDP)-glucuronyl transferases and the glutathione S-transferases, which catalyze conjugation to glucuronic acid and glutathione, respectively. Conjugation to glucuronic acid always results in greatly enhanced water solubility; for this reason, glucuronide conjugates are usually readily excreted into urine. Glucuronide conjugates are also often excreted into the bile and, because they are usually poorly absorbed in the gut, appear in the stool. Endogenous substances, such as bilirubin, undergo conjugation to glucuronic acid as an important part of normal physiology. Conjugation may not detoxify some substances completely. The partially metabolized drugs may still remain capable of covalent binding to hepatic proteins and thereby induce damage to the liver. As with the cytochromes P-450, the UDP-glucuronyl transferases appear to be a multigene family of microsomal enzymes, some of which are inducible.[33] In some cases, their regulation appears to be linked with that of the cytochromes P-450. For example, when animals are treated with phenobarbital,

TABLE 25-1

Characteristics of Some Human Liver P-450s

P-450	DRUG	PROBABLE INDUCERS
IA2	Phenacetin[71-73]	Cigarette smoke[74]
	Caffeine[72,75,76]	Charcoal broiled foods[77]
	Theophylline[72,76]	
IIC*	Mephenytoin[78]	None identified
	Hexobarbital[79,80]	
	Diazepam[81]	
	Tolbutamide[79]	
	Sulfinpyrazone[82]	
	Phenylbutazone[83]	
IID*	Debrisoquine[78]	None identified
	Dextromethorphan[84]	
	Metoprolol[85]	
	Other β blockers[32]	
	Perhexiline[86]	
	Amitriptyline[87]	
	Other neuroleptics[32]	
	Encainide[88]	
	Codeine[89]	
IIE1	Acetaminophen[90]	Ethanol[91]
	Ethanol[92]	Isoniazid[93]
IIIA*	Erythromycin[94,95]	Glucocorticoids[94,95]
	Nifedipine[96,97]	Rifampicin[94,98]
	Cyclosporine[98-100]	
	Steroids[97,101]	
	Midazolam/triazolam[102]	
	Lidocaine[103]	

* *Multiple subfamily members exist, which may have differing catalytic properties.*

3-methylcholanthrene, or glucocorticoids, induction of the characteristic cytochromes P-450 is associated with induction of specific glucuronyl S-transferases. This coordinated response usually results in the increased capacity of the liver to detoxify and eliminate the inducer. Human liver UDP-glucuronyl transferases appear to be similar to those described in animals, although little work has been done at the molecular level. Genetic defects in human bilirubin UDP-glucuronyl transferase have been recognized, and it is likely that polymorphisms in these enzymes also exist.

The glutathione S-transferases are multiple enzymes present in both the cytosol and endoplasmic reticulum of the hepatocyte.[34] Because conjugation to glutathione occurs through its nucleophilic thiol group, it conjugates only to molecules possessing an electrophilic center. Electrophiles are, in general, dangerous to the cells because they are capable of indiscriminate binding to cellular components. Conjugation to glutathione, therefore, almost always results in detoxification. Most electrophiles metabolized by the glutathione S-transferases are generated from less harmful substances by the liver, often as a result of reactions catalyzed by the cytochromes P-450. It appears that some of the glutathione S-transferases may be inducible in animals by many of the medications that induce the cytochromes P-450 and the UDP-glucuronyl transferases. Glutathione S-transferases have two subunits, each reflecting expression of multiple distinct genes. In human liver, three distinct families of glutathione S-transferases have been identified, and it appears that there are allelic variations in the population.[34] The activities of these enzymes are, therefore, likely to vary among individuals, and this may have important clinical implications for cancer risk and aging.

In summary, it is clear that the liver has developed a highly effective system of enzymes to detoxify and facilitate the elimination of the vast array of structurally diverse compounds that may threaten the body. This is accomplished in large part by the phase 1 and phase 2 enzymes, which derive from complex multigene families. In some instances, the liver responds to a drug or other substance by increasing its ability to detoxify and eliminate it; this appears to involve coordinate and selective induction of phase 1 and phase 2 enzymes. In patients, genetic factors play an important role in determining the liver's ability to metabolize a drug, and inherited defects in the structure or regulation of individual enzymes appear to be common.

Intestinal Drug Metabolism

Enterocytes contain both phase 1 and phase 2 drug-metabolizing enzymes. Detoxification at the level of the intestine is probably necessary, in part, because potentially harmful ingested substances (especially highly lipophilic substances) may enter the systemic circulation through lymphatic drainage and, therefore, may not traverse the portal vein to the liver. However, the contribution of the intestine to "first pass" metabolism of drugs is believed to be small for several reasons. First, most drugs detected in mesenteric lymph during absorption also enter the systemic circulation through the portal vein and liver. The proportion of the drug that bypasses the liver is generally very small because lymph flow is far slower than that of the portal blood. Thus, metabolism in the enterocyte does not seem necessary. Second, the systemic availability of most drugs appears to be explained adequately by liver first pass metabolism combined with variable absorption from the GI tract. Finally, the ability of enterocytes (or of various subcellular fractions prepared from enterocytes) to metabolize drugs usually appears to be small compared to the liver.

In spite of these considerations, it is likely that metabolism of drugs at the level of the intestine is more significant than has been appreciated previously. First, the concentration of a drug in the enterocyte after absorption from the gut lumen may exceed greatly that subsequently present in the hepatocyte. High capacity enzymes could, therefore, metabolize a large amount of drug even at the low enzyme concentrations thought to be present in the enterocyte. Furthermore, once a drug gains access to the enterocyte, it may not be transported passively into the body because the surface area of the basolateral membrane is considerably less than that of the apical membrane (due to the latter's microvilli). This might result in back diffusion of the parent compound into the intestinal lumen, where uptake may occur again, resulting in repeated exposure of parent drug to intestinal enzymes. Finally, metabolites of drugs generated within the enterocyte can be secreted back into the gut lumen in nonabsorbable form. This would provide a useful

mechanism for handling conjugated metabolites that remain reactive and have a potential for toxicity inside the body. For example, when naphthol and benzene are placed into loops of rat intestine in vitro, conjugated naphthol and phase 1 and phase 2 metabolites of benzene appear in the gut lumen.[35,36] Similar experiments have shown that the antidiarrhea drug loperamide is N-demethylated by intestinal phase 1 enzymes, and the metabolites appear to be secreted into the gut lumen.[37] Because these polar metabolites largely appear in the stool, the intestinal metabolism of these compounds is unappreciated if only portal and systemic blood measurements are obtained. It is difficult to design studies to assess the contribution of intestinal metabolism to the in vivo disposition of drugs, because metabolites present in the gut lumen or stool may be generated in other organs and excreted into the gut through biliary or nonbiliary pathways (see the section entitled "Secretion of Drugs by the Gut"). Nonetheless, it is likely that metabolism at the level of the intestine contributes significantly to the bioavailability of many drugs.

Molecular characterization of the drug-metabolizing enzymes present in intestine has lagged behind that of the enzymes present in the liver. However, many, but not all, of the genes coding for enzymes involved in hepatic drug metabolism are also expressed in the intestine. As in the liver, most investigation in the intestine has centered on cytochromes P-450, UDP-glucuronyl transferases, and glutathione S-transferases.

The original belief that the enterocyte contained only cytochromes P-450 identical or similar to those inducible by 3-methylcholanthrene in the liver (also termed "P-448") is incorrect. Rat small bowel also contains cytochromes that are inducible by 3-methylcholanthrene, phenobarbital, and glucocorticoids, and these enzymes are indistinguishable from some of their liver counterparts.[38–40] However, in rat liver, multiple closely related cytochromes P-450 are induced by 3-methylcholanthrene or phenobarbital, whereas only one enzyme in each of the respective gene families has been identified in rat enterocytes.[38,39] Multiple glucocorticoid-inducible cytochromes P-450 are present in rat enterocytes, and these are major phase 1 enzymes present in untreated animals.[40] Human jejunal mucosa has been shown to contain a cytochrome P-450 that is indistinguishable from a major P-450IIIA enzyme present in human liver.[40] This enzyme appears to be the major cytochrome P-450 present in human jejunum; however, the corresponding hepatic form accounts for less than 25% of the total cytochrome P-450 present in liver.[40] It is likely that identical or similar genes coding for cytochromes P-450 are expressed in intestine and liver, but there are clearly organ-specific differences in the expression of some of these enzymes.

The vertical distribution of the P-450IIIA enzyme along the villus in human small bowel is shown in Figure 25-3. This enzyme is undetectable in villus crypt cells. The enterocyte concentration of P-450IIIA appears to increase as enterocytes migrate up the villus to the tip. The location of cytochrome P-450 is appropriate for metabolism of drugs present in the gut because absorption is believed to occur almost exclusively in the upper part of the villus. There are several mechanisms whereby drug metabolites may appear in the gut lumen after they are generated in enterocytes. First, immunohistochemistry suggests that the highest concentration of cytochrome P-450 is in the apical half of the enterocyte (see Fig 25-3). This location, combined with the large surface area of the apical microvilli, would favor passive diffusion of metabolites into the gut lumen rather than toward the serosa. Second,

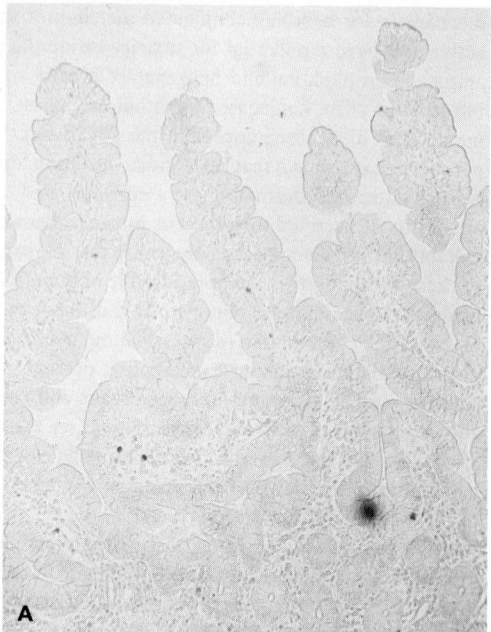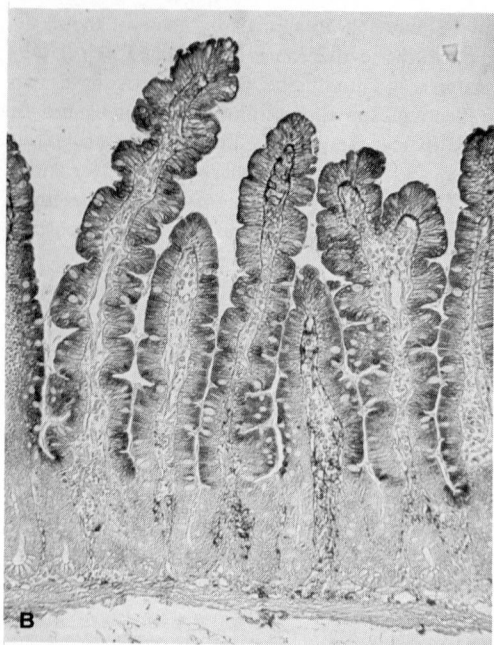

FIGURE 25–3. Distribution of cytochrome P-450IIIA. Formaline-fixed human small bowel mucosa was subjected to immunoperoxidase staining after preincubation with preimmune rabbit serum, **A,** and serum obtained from the rabbit after immunization with purified cytochrome P-450IIIA, **B.** No staining is evident in the intestinal crypts (*c*) and the most intense staining is evident near the tips of the villi. Within each enterocyte, immunoreactive protein appears to be most abundant in the apical one-third of the cytosol. (From Kolars J, Austin L, Dobbins WO, Wrighton SA, Watkins PB. Heterogeneity of cytochrome P-450 III expression in glucocorticoid inducible rat gut epithelia. Gastroenterology, 1989;96(5)A 264.)

the apical membrane is known to contain transporters capable of actively pumping compounds from the inside of the enterocyte into the gut lumen (see the section entitled "Secretion of Drugs by the Gut"). Third, metabolites may be carried into the lumen within the enterocytes as they are sloughed from the tip of the villus. Finally, it is possible that the enterocytes may remain metabolically active after sloughing from the villus tip[41] and continue to metabolize drugs while mixing with lumenal contents. This event has been discounted largely because, in the process of leaving the basement membrane of the villus, enterocytes appear to be dying on the basis of histologic characteristics. There is, however, no obvious reason why these enterocytes should die immediately because villus tip cells appear to obtain most of their nutrients from the gut lumen and not from the systemic circulation. Recently, investigators have reported the purification of viable gut epithelial cells from normal human stool specimens,[42] suggesting that at least some exfoliated enterocytes may not be dead and may be capable of continuing drug metabolism in the gut lumen. This would provide the theoretical advantage of placing the enterocyte outside the unstirred water layer and in more direct contact with the lipophilic compounds most likely to be substrates for the cytochrome P-450 enzyme system. In addition, cell death or malignant transformation due to formation of reactive metabolites in exfoliated cells would not threaten the health of the body. However, at present, the existence of such wandering metabolic "factories" in the intestinal lumen remains hypothetical.

The catalytic activity of intestinal cytochromes P-450 appears to be influenced by normal dietary constituents. For example, removal of iron or selenium from the diet for even a few hours

appears to result in a dramatic drop in the catalytic activity of intestinal cytochromes P-450 in rats.[43,44] Furthermore, when healthy volunteers are maintained on a semisynthetic diet, there is a significant fall in the catalytic activity of some cytochromes P-450 assayed in intestinal mucosal biopsies.[45] In rats, certain vegetable matter and polycyclic hydrocarbons that result from charcoal broiling can induce intestinal activities of cytochromes P-450 that have been associated with activation of procarcinogens,[46,47] raising concern that charcoal broiled foods may predispose humans to cancer as well.

In rats some of the cytochromes P-450 present in the colon are similar to those present in the small bowel and liver.[48] However, the regulation of individual cytochromes P-450 may not be identical in the colon and the small bowel. For example, rat colonic mucosa contains a cytochrome P-450 that is indistinguishable from a glucocorticoid-inducible enzyme present in rat intestine and liver, but the colonic enzyme does not appear to be inducible by systemically administered glucocorticoids.[49]

The existence of phase 2 reactions in intestinal mucosa was established over three decades ago. Gut mucosa or subcellular preparations of enterocytes have been demonstrated to conjugate model drugs with glucuronic acid, sulfate, glutathione, and amino acids, essentially encompassing the range of such reactions known to occur in the liver.[50] However, to date, there has been little work attempting to characterize intestinal phase 2 enzymes on a molecular basis. Indirect evidence suggests that the UDP-glucuronyl tranferases and glutathione S-tranferases present in intestine are identical or similar to some of those present in the liver. For example, rats that have a genetic defect in liver bilirubin UDP-glucuronyl transferase (Gunn rats) are also deficient in the ability to conjugate bilirubin in the intestinal mucosa. Induction characteristics of the intestinal and liver UDP-glucuronyl transferases also appear to be similar in the rat.[51] In humans, immunochemical analysis of liver and enterocyte microsomes has suggested that some, but not all, of the UDP-glucuronyl transferases are present in both organs.[52] These observations suggest that, as with phase 1 enzymes, organ-specific differences exist in the expression of the phase 2 enzymes.

Glutathione S-transferases are abundant in epithelial cells lining the small bowel but are present in low concentrations in the stomach and colon of rats.[53] This may explain, in part, the relatively low incidence of spontaneous malignancy in the small bowel compared to stomach and colon. Little work has been done to characterize glutathione S-transferases present in the human gut.

In summary, the intestine appears to have many, but not all, of the phase 1 and phase 2 enzymes that are present in the liver. It is likely that many drugs are metabolized by these enzymes after absorption, and that the metabolites generated either enter the body or are secreted back into the gut lumen. P-450IIIA enzymes appear to be the major phase 1 enzymes present in intestine, and this may account, in part, for the poor oral bioavailability characteristic of drugs metabolized by these enzymes, such as erythromycin and cyclosporine A (see Table 25-1). The small bowel's well-known resistance to spontaneous malignancy may be due, at least in part, to its efficient detoxification machinery. It is likely that polymorphisms in catalytic activity of intestinal drug-metabolizing enzymes similar to those described in human liver will be found in the future. Many nongenetic factors including normal dietary constituents also influence the activity of intestinal drug-metabolizing enzymes.

Role of Enteric Flora in Gut Metabolism

The GI tract is inhabited by a diverse array of bacteria capable of metabolizing many of the drugs used in clinical medicine.[54–56] While the acid environment of the stomach and the peristalsis in the small bowel largely restrict bacteria to the colon, organisms are present in jejunum with increasing concentrations through the ileum. It has often been difficult to determine the contribution made by gut flora to metabolism of drugs because elimination of the gut flora results in confounding variables. For example, animals raised from birth in germ-free environments have significant reductions in portal blood flow and alterations in intestinal morphology. Alternatively, the use of broad-spectrum antibiotics to reduce acutely the numbers of bacteria present in the gut may influence absorption and metabolic capabilities due to the chemical properties of the antibiotics themselves.

Drug metabolism by enteric flora can have several consequences. Enteric flora may metabolize drugs to inactive metabolites. Digitalis, for example, can be metabolized by intestinal flora to nonabsorbable and less bioactive metabolites.[57] This may be the reason why patients who have been placed on broad-spectrum antibiotics can have significant elevations in their serum digitalis levels.[57]

Reactions catalyzed by enteric flora may also produce compounds that are more bioactive than the parent compounds. This fact is used in normal physiology. For example, dietary quinones

are converted to vitamin K by bacteria normally present in the colon. Deficiency of this fat-soluble vitamin has been observed in patients treated with prolonged courses of broad-spectrum antibiotics, presumably on the basis of reduced bacterial quinone conversion. In some cases, the effectiveness of a drug appears to be critically dependent on its metabolism by enteric flora. The antiplatelet effect of sulfinpyrazone, for example, is apparently due exclusively to a sulfide metabolite produced by colonic flora.[58] The existence of enteric flora is also used in the targeted delivery of drugs. An example of this is Azulfidine (sulfasalazine) (Fig 25-4), a medication used commonly in the treatment of ulcerative colitis. This compound contains sulfa and salicylate moieties covalently linked by a diazo bond. Azulfidine itself appears to have no antiinflammatory activity and is poorly absorbed from the small bowel. However, the diazo bond is cleaved by enteric flora present in the colon, releasing the active salicylate.[59] The flora necessary for activation of Azulfidine are probably also present in low concentrations in the distal ileum, but the relatively rapid transit of lumenal contents through this region of the gut may prevent a significant therapeutic effect in ileal Crohn's disease. Sulfasalazine has a variety of common side effects, which has limited the usefulness of this agent in some patients. Because it appears that most side effects result from the sulfa moiety, various attempts are

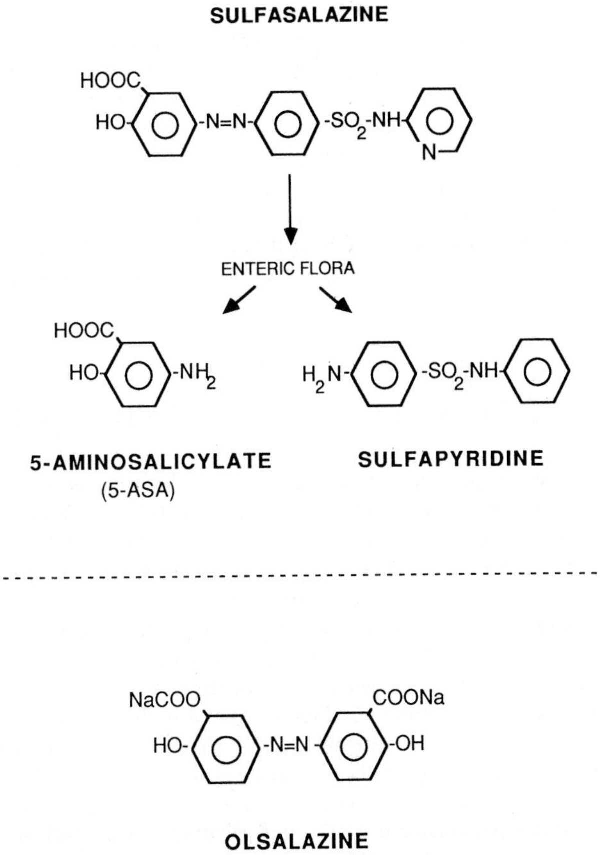

FIGURE 25–4. The fate of orally ingested sulfasalazine. Bacteria present predominantly in the colon catalyze reduction of the diazo bond, resulting in the pharmacologically active moiety 5-ASA and sulfapyridine. Also shown is the chemical formula for an experimental drug, olsalazine, which is designed to undergo similar metabolism by colonic flora, liberating two active salicylate moieties.

being made to develop alternate preparations that target delivery of salicylate to the colon. One such compound is olsalazine, which is two salicylate moieties linked with a diazo bond (see Fig 25-4).

Gut flora may produce toxic metabolites from drugs, resulting in adverse drug reactions. A slow release formulation of L-dopa was found to cause toxicity in some patients with Parkinson's disease. This appears to have been the result of toxic metabolites of L-dopa formed by colonic bacteria.[60]

Many of the bacteria present in the distal small bowel and colon are capable of deconjugating the products of phase 2 metabolism. Deconjugation routinely occurs in the colon, which is impermeable to many of the liberated drugs. However, deconjugation by enteric flora may result in significant enterohepatic cycling of some drugs.[61] Finally, there are considerable differences among people in the types of bacteria inhabiting the gut. These differences, which appear to reflect both genetic and nongenetic factors such as age and diet,[54] may account, in part, for interpatient differences in the response to some medications.

Summary

The GI tract has a large variety of metabolic capabilities that only partially resemble those present in the liver. Because the metabolites generated may not enter the body, the significance of drug metabolism by the enterocyte and enteric flora is likely to be far greater than is appreciated. This "preabsorptive metabolism"[62] undoubtedly represents an important component of the digestive tract's function as the major barrier between humans and the environment. These metabolic capabilities presumably evolved to handle the small quantities of potential toxins likely to be encountered in the diet. In light of these observations, the success of oral drug therapy may depend on overwhelming natural host defenses.

SECRETION OF DRUGS BY THE GUT

Compounds present in sinusoidal blood can be extracted by hepatocytes and excreted in bile either unchanged or as metabolites. If a compound undergoes conjugation and is excreted in bile, it is usually not readily absorbed in the gut and, therefore, is eliminated in stool. Nonbiliary pathways provide for the excretion of drugs into the lumen of the GI tract. As discussed previously, the intestine is capable of both phase 1 and phase 2 metabolism, and the resulting metabolites can be excreted directly into the lumen. Furthermore, because there appears to be little resistance to diffusion of substances from the enterocyte into mucosal blood, it would be logical to assume that drugs or their metabolites could diffuse passively from the subepithelial blood vessels into the enterocytes for subsequent elimination into the GI tract. However, passive diffusion of a drug from mucosal blood into the gut lumen is less likely to occur than diffusion in the opposite direction,[63,64] partially because medications present in systemic blood are generally in lower concentrations than those attained in the lumen of the gut after oral administration. Diffusion from mucosal blood vessels is further hindered by the frequent binding of drugs to plasma proteins. In

the liver, large pores (fenestrations) are present in the sinusoidal endothelium, which allow plasma proteins to leave the blood space (sinusoid) and make direct contact with the hepatocyte. Fenestrations are also present in the endothelia of intestinal capillaries, but these contain a membrane or diaphragm that is likely to hinder the diffusion of protein-bound drug. Even if the identical concentration of diffusible (free) drug were present in both the lumen and the submucosa of the gut, diffusion into the enterocyte occurs more rapidly through the apical membrane because the surface area of its microvilli greatly exceeds that of the basolateral membrane. Furthermore, some drugs appear to move into the enterocyte from the lumen by active transport mechanisms that favor transport in one direction.

In spite of these considerations, some drugs appear to be significantly eliminated from the body by secretion across the enterocyte into the gut lumen. For example, quaternary amines and nonionized amines are actively pumped across the mucosal epithelium into the intestinal lumen.[18,65] In some cases, drugs excreted into the gut may be reabsorbed almost completely. Oral administration of nonabsorbable binding resins, including polysulfated sucrose or cholestyramine, can accelerate greatly the removal of such drugs and other compounds from the body by preventing their reabsorption.[65]

A recent major breakthrough in understanding the excretory functions of the gut is the discovery that the multidrug resistance (MDR) gene is normally expressed in the enterocytes of intestinal. mucosa. The MDR gene[66–68] was discovered as a result of cancer research. Some cancers initially responsive to chemotherapeutic agents become resistant to the effects of these drugs after repeated therapeutic courses. Cancer cells that become resistant to chemotherapy with a single drug, often become resistant to many other chemotherapeutic agents as well, including some to which they may not have been exposed. Development of this resistant phenotype is closely associated with enhanced expression of the MDR gene. This gene codes for a 170-kd protein, termed P-170 or P-glycoprotein. P-170 is present in the plasma membranes of resistant cancer cells and has structural homology to other proteins known to act as membrane transporters. It appears that P-170 confers resistance to multiple chemotherapeutic agents by acting as a versatile pump, removing these drugs from the interior of the cell. It was initially hoped that only cancer cells expressed the MDR gene, so that antibodies to P-170 could be used to target cytotoxic agents selectively to malignant tissue. However, when antibodies to this protein were used in immunohistochemical analyses of various human tissues, it was discovered that this gene is also normally expressed in biliary canaliculi, small intestine, and colon, as well as in pancreas, placenta, renal tubules, adrenals, and in the blood–brain barrier.[69] The multidrug resistance gene product, P-170, is expressed in human enterocytes exclusively in the brush border membranes and is not detected on the basolateral surface (Fig 25-5). It is logical to assume that this protein normally functions as a pump to prevent absorption of many potentially injurious compounds that may appear in our diet.

The presence of P-170 in the apical domains of biliary epithelia may confer protection to the biliary tree from the reactive molecules excreted by, and often produced by, the liver. It also seems highly likely that P-170 functions to excrete potential toxins, including phase 1 and phase 2 metabolites, that either are generated in the enterocyte or diffuse into the enterocyte from the systemic circulation. It may be that the active excretion by the gut of qua-

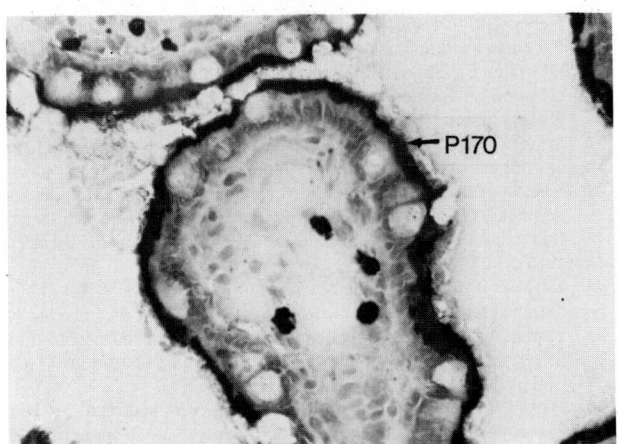

FIGURE 25–5. Immunohistochemical localization of P-170 in human duodenal mucosa. Formaline-fixed duodenal mucosa was subjected to immunoperoxidase staining after reaction with a monoclonal antibody that selectively recognizes the product of the multidrug resistance gene (P-170). Shown is the tip of a single villus. P-170 is exclusively located on the apical membrane of the enterocytes and appears as the dark band outlining the villus. (From Thiebaut F, Tsuruo T, Hamada H, Gottesman MM, Pastan I, Willingham MC. Cellular localization of the multidrug-resistance gene product P-glycoprotein in normal human tissues. Proc Natl Acad Sci 1987;84:7735.)

ternary ammonium compounds and noncharged amines[18] reflects the activity of P-170. The MDR gene appears to be part of a family of genes, and it is possible that other related transport proteins may be present in the GI tract. P-170 may be inducible in the biliary canaliculi by some of the compounds known to induce phase 1 and phase 2 enzymes,[70] suggesting that it may also be part of a coordinated response to large loads of potentially harmful substances encountered in the diet.

There are many potentially important clinical implications of MDR gene expression in the gut, but research is just beginning in this area. For example, the normal expression of the MDR gene in gut epithelia may explain the well-known resistance of GI adenocarcinomas to chemotherapy.[69] Verapamil tightly binds P-170, and it is likely that many other drugs are capable of transport by this system. If so, important drug interactions may result from competition for P-170 transport into, or out of, the body.

ALTERNATE ROUTES FOR DRUG ADMINISTRATION

Many potentially useful drugs cannot be administered orally because they cannot permeate the gut barrier. Rectal, nasal, or sublingual administrations provide alternate routes to the body for some drugs. The direct application of the drug to the mucosa circumvents gastric acid, digestive enzymes, and the unstirred water layer. In addition, the metabolic capability of the mucosa in these regions of the gut appears to be lower than in the small bowel. It is difficult, however, to obtain sustained release of medication through the nasal sinuses or sublingual mucosa. Many drugs are also not effectively administered through rectal mucosa; in humans, much of the venous drainage of the rectum enters the portal vein and is subject to "first pass" liver metabolism. For these reasons, relatively few drugs are used commonly in clinical medicine that are not given orally.

SUMMARY

The clinical efficacy of drugs generally relies on their ability to gain access to the body after oral administration. This means that they must defeat complex anatomic and metabolic systems that have evolved in the gut to protect against potentially harmful substances present in the environment. Many potentially useful medications never reach the pharmacist's shelf because of poor or erratic absorption from the gut. These drugs may be either degraded by stomach acid or cleaved into inactive components by digestive enzymes. Those that survive the hostile environment of the bulk phase of the gut must cross the unstirred water layer. This means that successful drugs must be either water-soluble or capable of interacting with soluble elements present in the gut lumen, such as bile acid micelles. The acid microclimate adjacent to the apical membrane of the enterocyte appears to provide an additional barrier to the absorption of weak bases.

Upon presentation to the apical membrane of the enterocyte, drugs must gain access to the body by either paracellular migration through the tight junctions or by transcellular routes. The latter may involve incorporation into the apical membrane by random dissolution in the lipid bilayer, binding to membrane-bound transport proteins, or passing through membrane pores. Subsequent translocation from the apical to basolateral membranes may involve migration through the enterocyte cytosol by active or passive forces, or possibly translocation within the cytoplasmic (inner) leaflet of the plasma membrane. Drugs that enter the enterocyte may be metabolized by a complex system of phase 1 and phase 2 enzymes, which appear to be similar to some of the corresponding enzymes in the liver. In at least some cases, drugs or their metabolites present in the enterocyte can be excreted back into the gut lumen, perhaps as a result of the action of apical transport proteins, such as the multidrug resistance gene product P-170. The enteric flora are also capable of metabolizing some drugs or their metabolites. Such metabolism may liberate conjugated drugs for reabsorption or may result in metabolites that are more inert or more biologically active than the parent drug.

The components of this sophisticated barrier are not static but may change in a given individual. The unstirred water layer and acid microclimate appear to be altered by physiologic perturbations of the gut and by certain diseases. The metabolic capabilities of the mucosa and enteric flora appear to be sensitive to changes in diet and are also likely to have genetic determinants. The nature of the gut barrier can vary considerably among individuals and, over time, in a single individual. The rational design of safe and effective oral medications will only be possible after complete characterization of the basic components of the gut barrier. This should remain an active area of investigation for the future.

The reader is directed to Chapter 6, Epithelia: Biologic Principles of Organization; and Chapter 50, Approach to the Patient with Drug or Alcohol Dependency.

REFERENCES

1. Wilson ITH. Intestinal absorption. Philadelphia: WB Saunders, 1962: 67.
2. Rozman K, Hanninen O, eds. Gastrointestinal toxicology. New York: Elsevier, 1986.
3. Csaky TZ, ed. Pharmacology of intestinal permeation, vols I and II. New York:Springer-Verlag, 1984.
4. Jackson MJ. Drug transport across gastrointestinal epithelia. In: Johnson LR, ed. Physiology of the gastrointestinal tract, vol 2. New York: Raven Press, 1987:1597.
5. Wilson ITH. Intestinal absorption. Philadelphia: WB Saunders, 1962: 130.
6. Osterhout WJV. Is living protoplasm permeable to ions? J Gen Physiol 1925;8:131.
7. Westergaard H, Dietschy JM. Delineation of the dimensions and permeability characteristics of the two major diffusion barriers to passive mucosal uptake in the rabbit intestine. J Clin Invest 1974;54:718.
8. Hogben CAM, Tocco D, Brodie BB, Schauker LS. On the mechanism of intestinal absorption of drugs. J Pharmacol Exp Ther 1959;125: 275.
9. Lucas M. The surface pH of the intestinal mucosa and its significance in the permeability of anions. In: Csaky TZ, ed. Pharmacology of intestinal permeation, vol II. New York: Springer-Verlag, 1984:121.
10. Iwatsubo T, Sugiyama Y, Miyamoto Y, et al. Effects of phenothiazine derivatives on the microclimate-pH in the rat jejunum. J Pharm Sci 1988;77:586.
11. Lucas ML, Cooper BT, Lei FH, et al. Acid microclimate in coeliac and Crohn's disease: A model for folate malabsorption. Gut 1978;19: 735.
12. Shian YF, Levine GM. pH dependence of micellar diffusion and dissociation. Am J Physiol 1982;239:G177.
13. Diamond JM. Channels in epithelial cell membranes and junctions. Fed Proc 1978;37:2639.
14. Gumbiner B. Structure, biochemistry, and assembly of epithelial tight junctions. Am J Physiol 1987;253:C749.
15. Csaky TZ, ed. Pharmacology of intestinal permeation, vol I. New York: Springer-Verlag, 1984:289.
16. Hu M, Amidon GL. Passive and carrier-mediated intestinal absorption components of captopril. J Pharm Sci 1988;77:1007.
17. Stremmel W. Uptake of fatty acids by jejunal mucosal cells is mediated by a fatty acid binding membrane protein. J Clin Invest 1988;82: 2001.
18. Lauterbach F. Intestinal permeation of organic bases and quaternary ammonium compounds. In: Csaky TZ, ed. Pharmacology of intestinal permeation, vol II. New York: Springer-Verlag, 1984:271.
19. Sweetser DA, Heuckeroth R, Gordon JI. The metabolic significance of mammalian fatty acid binding proteins: Abundant proteins in search of a function. Annu Rev Nutr 1987;7:337.
20. van Meer G, Simons K. Lipid polarity and sorting in epithelial cells. J Cell Biochem 1988;36:51.
21. Volkheimer G. Persorption of particles, physiology and pharmacology. Adv Pharmacol Chemother 1977;14:163.
22. Moolton FL, Capparell NJ, Boger E, Mahathalang P. Induction of antibodies against carcinogenic polycyclic aromatic hydrocarbons. Nature 1978;272:614.
23. Silbart LK, Keren DF. Reduction of intestinal carcinogen absorption by carcinogenic-specific secretory immunity. Science 1989;243:1462.
24. Larsen GL, Bakke JE. Enterohepatic circulation in formation of propachlor (2-chloro-N-isopropylacetanilide) metabolites in the rat. Xenobiotica 1981;11:473.
25. Melander A, Lalka D, McLean A. Influence of food on the presystemic metabolism of drugs. Pharmacol Ther 1988;38:253.
26. Welling PG. Interactions affecting drug absorption. Clin Pharmacokinet 1984;9:404.
27. D'Arcy PF, McElnay JC. Drug interactions in the gut involving metal ions. Rev Drug Metab Drug Interact 1985;5:83.
28. Tredger JM, Naoumov NV, Steward CM, et al. Influence of biliary T tube clamping on cyclosporine pharmacokinetics in liver transplant recipients. Transplant Proc 1988;20(2):512.
29. Guengerich FP. Characterization of human microsomal cytochrome P-450 enzymes. Annu Rev Pharmacol Toxicol 1989;29:241.
30. Nebert DW, Adesnik M, Coon MJ, et al. The P450 gene superfamily: Recommended nomenclature. DNA 1987;6(1):1.
31. Gonzalez FJ, Shoda RC, Kimura S, et al. Characterization of the common genetic defect in humans deficient in debrisoquine metabolism. Nature 1988;331:442.
32. Jacqz E, Hall SD, Branch RA. Genetically determined polymorphisms in drug oxidation. Hepatology 1986;6(5):1020.
33. Siest G, Antoine B, Fournel S, Magdalou J, Thomassin J. The glucuronosyltransferases: What progress can pharmacologists expect from molecular biology and cellular enzymology? Biochem Pharmacol 1987;36(7):983.
34. Ketterer B. Detoxification reactions of glutathione and glutathione S-transferases. Xenobiotica 1986;16:957.
35. Koster A, Noordhoek J. Glucuronidation in isolated perfused rat intestinal segments after mucosal and serosal administration of 1-naphthol. J Pharmacol Exp Ther 1983;266:533.
36. Hietanen E. Oxidation and subsequent glucuronidation of 3,4-benzopyrene in everted intestinal sacs in control and 3-methylcholanthrene-pretreated rats. Pharmacology 1980;21:233.
37. Miyazaki H, Nambu K, Hashimoto M. Loperamide in rat intestines: A unique disposition. Life Sci 1982;30:2203.
38. Goldstein JA, Linko P. Differential induction of two 2,3,7,8-tetrachlorodibenzo-p-dioxin-inducible forms of cytochrome P-450 in extrahepatic versus hepatic tissues. Mol Pharmacol 1984;25:185.
39. Traber PG, Chianale J, Florence R, Kim K, Wojcik E, Gumucio JJ. Expression of cytochrome P450b and P450e genes in small intestinal mucosa of rats following treatment with phenobarbital, polyhalogenated biphenyls, and organochlorine pesticides. J Biol Chem 1988; 263(19):9449.
40. Watkins PB, Wrighton SA, Schuetz EG, Molowa DT, Guzelian PS. Identification of glucocorticoid-inducible cytochromes P-450 in the intestinal mucosa of rats and man. J Clin Invest 1987;80:1029.
41. Nienstedt W, Harri M-P, Hartiala K. Intestinal absorption and metabolism of androstenedione in the dog. Steroids Lipids Res 1972;3: 193.
42. Albaugh GP, Iyeugar V, Lohani A, Schatzkin A, Nair PP. Recovery and isolation of exfoliated intestinal tract cells from fresh human stools by counterflow elutriation. J Cell Biol 1988;107(6):575a.
43. Hoensch H, Woo CH, Raffin SB, Schmid R. Oxidative metabolism of foreign compounds in rat small intestine: Cellular localization and dependence of dietary iron. Gastroenterology 1976;70:1063.
44. Pascoe GA, Sakai-Wong J, Soliven E, Correia MA. Regulation of intestinal cytochrome P-450 and heme by dietary nutrients. Biochem Pharmacol 1983;32(20):3027.
45. Hoensch HP, Steinhardt HJ, Weiss G, Haug D, Maier A, Malchow H. Effects of semisynthetic diets on xenobiotic metabolizing enzyme activity and morphology of small intestinal mucosa in humans. Gastroenterology 1984;86:1519.
46. Pantuck EJ, Hsiao K-C, Loub WD, Wattenberg LW, Kuntzman R, Conney AH. Stimulatory effect of vegetables on intestinal drug metabolism in the rat. JPET 1976;128:278.
47. Pantuck EJ, Hsiao K-C, Kuntzman R, Conney AH. Intestinal metabolism of phenacetin in the rat: Effect of charcoal-broiled beef and rat chow. Science 1975;187:744.
48. Oshinsky RJ, Strobel HW. Drug metabolism in rat colon: Resolution of enzymatic constituents and characterization of activity. Mol Cell Biochem 1987;75:51.
49. Kolars J, Austin L, Dobbins WO, Wrighton SA, Watkins PB. Heterogeneity of cytochrome P-450 III expression in glucocorticoid inducible rat gut epithelia. Gastroenterology 1989;96(5):A264.
50. Laitinen M, Watkins JB. Mucosal biotransformations. In: Rozman K, Hanninen O, eds. Gastrointestinal toxicology. New York: Elsevier, 1986:169.
51. Koster AS, Schirmer G, Bock KW. Immunochemical and functional characterization of UDP-glucuronosyltransferases from rat liver, intestine and kidney. Biochem Pharmacol 1986;35:3971.
52. Peters WHM, Jansen PLM. Immunocharacterization of UDP-glucuronyltransferase isoenzymes in human liver, intestine, and kidney. Biochem Pharmacol 1988;37:564.
53. Siegers C-P, Riemann D, Thies E, Younes M. Glutathione and GSH-dependent enzymes in the gastrointestinal mucosa of the rat. Cancer Lett 1988;40:71.

54. Rowland IR. Reduction by the gut microflora of animals and man. Biochem Pharmacol 1986;35:27.

55. Smith RV. Metabolism of drugs and other foreign compounds of intestinal microorganisms. World Rev Nutr Diet 1978;29:60.

56. Remmel RP, Goldman P. Xenobiotics, the intestinal flora, and carcinogenesis. In: Rydstrom J, Montelius J, Bengtsson M, eds. Extrahepatic drug metabolism and chemical carcinogenesis. New York: Elsevier, 1983:283.

57. Lindenbaum J, Rund DG, Butler VP, Tse-Eng D, Sha JR. Inactivation of digoxin by the gut flora: Reversal by antibiotic therapy. N Engl J Med 1981;305:789.

58. Strong JA, Oates J, Sembi J, Renwick AG, George CF. Role of the gut flora in the reduction of sulfinpyrazone in humans. J Pharmacol Exp Ther 1984;230:726.

59. Peppercon MA, Goldman P. The role of intestinal bacteria in the metabolism of salicylazosulfapyridine. J Pharmacol Exp Ther 1972;181:555.

60. Sandler M, Karoum F, Ruthven CRJ, Calne DB. M-hydroxyl phenylacetic acid formation for L-dopa in man: Suppression by neomycin. Science 1969;166:1417.

61. Walsh CT, Feierabend JF, Levine RR. The effect of lincomycin on the excretion of diethylstilbestrol and its ureterotrophic effects in rats. Life Sciences 1975;16(11):1683.

62. Routledge PA, Shand DG. Presystemic drug elimination. Annu Rev Pharmacol Toxicol 1979;19:447.

63. Gwilt PR, Comer S, Chaturvedi PR, Waters DH. The influence of diffusional barriers of presystemic gut elimination. Drug Metab Dispos 1988;16:521.

64. Minchin RF, Ilett KF. Presystemic elimination of drugs: Theoretical considerations for quantifying the relative contribution of gut and liver. J Pharm Sci 1982;71:458.

65. Israili ZH, Dayton PG. Enhancement of xenobiotic elimination: Role of intestinal excretion. Drug Metab Rev 1984;15:1123.

66. Moscow JA, Cowan KH. Multidrug resistance. J Natl Cancer Inst 1988;80:14.

67. Croop JM, Gros P, Housman DE. Genetics of multidrug resistance. J Clin Invest 1988;81:1303.

68. Gottesman MM, Pastan I. The multidrug transporter, a double-edged sword. J Biol Chem 1988;263:12163.

69. Thiebaut F, Tsuruo T, Hamada H, Gottesman MM, Pastan I, Willingham MC. Cellular localization of the multidrug-resistance gene product P-glycoprotein in normal human tissues. Proc Natl Acad Sci USA 1987;84:7735.

70. Burt RK, Thorgeirsson SS. Coinduction of MDR-1 multidrug-resistance and cytochrome P-450 genes in rat liver by xenobiotics. J Natl Cancer Inst 1988;80:1383.

71. Sesardic D, Boobis AR, Edwards RJ, Davies DS. A form of cytochrome P450 in man, orthologous to form d in the rat, catalyses the O-deethylation of phenacetin and is inducible by cigarette smoking. Br J Clin Pharmacol. 1988;26:363.

72. Butler MA, Iwasaki M, Guengerich FG, Kadlubar FF. Human cytochrome P-450PA (P-450IA2), the phenacetin O-deethylase, is primarily responsible for the hepatic 3-demethylation of caffeine and N-oxidation of carcinogenic arylamines. Proc Natl Acad Sci USA 1989;86:7696.

73. Distlerath LM, Reilly PE, Martin MV, Davis GG, Wilkinson GR, Guengerich FP. Purification and characterization of the human liver cytochromes P-450 involved in debrisoquine 4-hydroxylation and phenacetin O-deethylation, two prototypes for genetic polymorphism in oxidative drug metabolism. J Biol Chem 1985;260:9057.

74. Pantuck EJ, Hsiao K-C, Maggio A, Nakamura K, Kuntzman R, Conney AH. Effect of cigarette smoking on phenacetin metabolism. Clin Pharmacol Ther 1974;15:9.

75. Ratanasavanh D, Berthou F, Dreano Y, Mondine P, Guillouzo A, Riche C. Methylcholanthrene but not phenobarbital enhances caffeine and theophylline metabolism in cultured adult human hepatocytes. Biochem Pharmacol 1990;39:85.

76. Campbell ME, Grant DM, Inaba T, Kalow W. Biotransformation of caffeine, paraxanthine, theophylline, and theobromine by polycyclic aromatic hydrocarbon-inducible cytochrome(s) P-450 in human liver microsomes. Drug Metabolism and Disposition 1987;15:237.

77. Conney AH, Pantuck EJ, Hsiao K-C, Garland WA, Anderson KE, et al. Enhanced phenacetin metabolism in human subjects fed charcoal-broiled beef. Clin Pharmacol Ther 1976;20:633.

78. Gut J, Meier UT, Catin T, Meyer UA. Mephenytoin-type polymorphism of drug oxidation: Purification and characterization of a human liver cytochrome P-450 isozyme catalyzing microsomal mephenytoin hydroxylation. Biochim Biophys Acta 1986;884:435.

79. Brian WR, Srivastava PK, Umbenhauer DR, Lloyd RS, Guengerich FP. Expression of a human liver cytochrome P-450 protein with tolbutamide hydroxylase activity in Saccharomyces cerevisiae. Biochemistry 1989;28:4993.

80. Knodell RG, Dubey RK, Wilkinson GR, Guengerich FP. Oxidative metabolism of hexobarbital in human liver: Relationship to polymorphic S-mephenytoin 4-hydroxylation. J Pharmacol Exp Ther 1988;245:845.

81. Bertilsson L, Henthorn TK, Sanz E, Tybring G, Sawe J, Villen T. Importance of genetic factors in the regulation of diazepam metabolism: Relationship to S-mephenytoin, but not debrisoquin, hydroxylation phenotype. Clin Pharmacol Ther 1989;45:348.

82. Miners JO, Foenander T, Wanwimolruk S, Gallus AS, Birkett DJ. The effect of sulphinpyrazone on oxidative drug metabolism in man: Inhibition of tolbutamide elimination. Eur J Clin Pharmacol 1982;22:321.

83. Pond SM, Birkett DJ, Wade DN. Mechanisms of inhibition of tolbutamide metabolism: Phenylbutaxone, oxyphenbutazone, sulfaphenazole. Clin Pharmacol Ther 1977;22:573.

84. Dayer P, Leeman T, Striberni R. Dextromethorphan O-demethylation in liver microsomes as a prototype reaction to monitor cytochrome P-450 dbl activity. Clin Pharmacol Ther 1989;45:34.

85. Lennard MS, Silas JH, Freestone S, Trevethick J. Defective metabolism of metoprolol in poor hydroxylators of debrisoquine. Br J Clin Pharmacol 1982;14:301.

86. Morgan MY, Reshef R, Shah RR, Oates NS, Smith RL, Sherlock S. Impaired oxidation of debrisoquine in patients with perhexiline liver injury. Gut 1984;25:1057.

87. Mellstrom B, Sawe J, Bertilsson L, Sjoqvist F. Amitriptyline metabolism: Association with debrisoquin hydroxylation in nonsmokers. Clin Pharmacol Ther 1986;39:369.

88. Woosley RL, Roden DM, Dai GH, Wang T, Altenbern D, Oates J, Wilkinson GR. Coinheritance of the polymorphic metabolism of encainide and debrisoquin. Clin Pharmacol Ther 1986;39:282.

89. Yue QY, Svensson J-O, Alm C, Sjoqvist F, Sawe J. Codeine O-demethylation cosegregates with polymorphic debrisoquine hydroxylation. Br J Clin Pharmacol 1989;28:639.

90. Raucy JL, Lasker JM, Lieber CS, Black M. Acetaminophen activation by human liver cytochromes P450IIE1 and P450IA2. Arch Biochem Biophys 1989;271:270.

91. Tsutsumi M, Lasker JM, Shimizu M, Rosman AS, Lieber CS. The intralobular distribution of ethanol-inducible P450IIE1 in rat and human liver. Hepatology 1989;10:437.

92. Lasker JM, Raucy J, Kubota S, Bloswick BP, Black M, Lieber CS. Purification and characterization of human liver cytochrome P-450-ACL. Biochem Biophys Res Commun 1987;148:232.

93. Wrighton SA, Thomas PE, Molowa DT, Haniu M, Shively JE, Maines SL, Watkins PB, Parker G, Mendez-Picon G, Levin W, et al. Characterization of ethanol-inducible human liver N-nitrosodimethylamine demethylase. Biochemistry 1986;25:6731.

94. Watkins PB, Murray SA, Winkelman LG, Heuman DM, Wrighton SA, Guzelian PS. The erythromycin breath test as an assay of glucocorticoid-inducible liver cytochromes P-450. J Clin Invest 1989;83:688.

95. Watkins PB, Wrighton SA, Maurel P, Schuetz EG, Mendez-Picon G, Parker GA, Guzelian PS. Identification of an inducible form of cytochrome P-450 in human liver. Proc Natl Acad Sci USA 1985;82:6310.

96. Gonzalez FJ, Schmid BJ, Umeno M, McBride OW, Hardwick JP, Meyer UA, Gelboin HV, Idle JR. Human P450PCN1: Sequence, chromosome localization, and evidence through cDNA expression that P450PCN1 is nifedipine oxidase. DNA 1988;7:79.

97. Guengerich FP, Martin MV, Beaune PH, Kremers P, Wolff T, Waxman DJ. Characterization of rat and human liver microsomal cytochrome P-450 forms involved in nifedipine oxidation, a prototype for genetic polymorphism in oxidative drug metabolism. J Biol Chem 1986;261:5051.

98. Combalbert J, Fabre I, Fabre G, Dalet I, Derancourt J, Cano JP, Maurel P. Metabolism of cyclosporin A: IV. Purification and identification of the Rifampicin-inducible human liver cytochrome P-450 (Cyclosporin A Oxidase) as a Product of P450IIIA Gene subfamily. Drug Metabolism and Disposition 1989;17:197.

99. Aoyama T, Yamano S, Waxman DJ, Lapenson DP, Meyer UA, Fischer V, Tyndale R, Inaba T, Kalow W, Gelboin HV, et al. Cytochrome P-450 hPCN3, a novel cytochrome P-450 IIIA gene product that is differentially expressed in adult human liver. cDNA and deduced amino acid sequence and distinct specificities of cDNA-expressed hPCN1 and hPCN3 for the metabolism of steroid hormones and cyclosporine. J Biol Chem 1989;264:10388.

100. Kronbach T, Fischer V, Meyer UA. Cyclosporine metabolism in human liver: Identification of a cytochrome P-450III gene family as the major cyclosporine-metabolizing enzyme explains interactions of cyclosporine with other drugs. Clin Pharmacol Ther 1988;43:630.

101. Waxman DJ, Attisano C, Guengerich FP, Lapenson DP. Human liver microsomal steroid metabolism: Identification of the major microsomal steroid hormone 6 beta-hydroxylase cytochrome P-450 enzyme. Arch Biochem Biophys 1988;263:424.

102. Kronbach T, Mathys D, Umeno M, Gonzalez FJ, Meyer UA. Oxidation of midazolam and triazolam by human liver cytochrome P450IIIA4. Mol Pharm 1989;36:89.

103. Bargetzi MJ, Aoyama T, Gonzalez FJ, Meyer UA. Lidocaine metabolism in human liver microsomes by cytochrome P450IIIA4. Clin Pharmacol Ther 1989;46:521.

26

The Gastrointestinal Microflora

KENNETH H. WILSON

The human gastrointestinal microflora consists of around 10^{14} (one hundred trillion) bacterial cells representing some 30 genera and 500 species. Our flora is thought to be unique to humans. There is very little overlap between the species found in the human alimentary tract and those found in the gut of an unrelated animal such as the mouse or pig.[1-3] It seems intuitively obvious that the presence of an extremely complex ecosystem specially adapted to live within the human host must have a significant impact on our health, and there is ample evidence supporting this view. However, we have little ability to manipulate the flora for the benefit of the host. The technology to work with most of these organisms has been evolving for only about 30 years, and only a relatively small group of workers has been conducting research in this area. Furthermore, the recent advances in biotechnology have not yet had a major impact on this field of research, where the possible applications seem astounding. It is probably fair to say that our understanding of the intestinal flora is in its infancy. We will review in this chapter what is known of the makeup of this microflora and its interactions, both favorable and unfavorable, with the host. Because the bacteria found in the colon outnumber the rest of the intestinal flora by at least 100,000 to 1, and there are almost 100 times as many species found in the colon as elsewhere in the gut, we will focus largely on the colonic flora. This chapter will cover the makeup of the flora and its metabolic activities. Because the flora's most important function is probably to protect the host from pathogens, we will cover bacterial interactions at length. Until recently, our knowledge of these interactions consisted of a morass of disjointed experimental observations. However, it has proved possible to make physical and corresponding mathematical models of the colonic ecosystem. These models have allowed us to begin to understand the processes involved.

COMPOSITION OF THE FLORA

The organisms found in the gastrointestinal (GI) tract can be divided into two groups: (1) organisms that are ingested and simply pass through the GI tract and (2) organisms that maintain a stable population without being ingested.[4] Although the former group includes some significant pathogens, it is not the subject of this discussion. The latter organisms are the true colonizers of the gut and are responsible for the failure of most transient organisms to colonize. The colonizers have been variously called the "normal" flora, the indigenous flora, and the autochthonous flora.[5] The term "normal" implies that we know what is normal and what is not; because this is not the case, most serious investigators avoid the term.

Methodologic Considerations

Bacteriology is sometimes thought of as a discipline that was mastered in the last century and is now simple and routine. This is not the case. Unless one pays close attention to the methods used to study the gut flora, the literature is an obscure morass of contradictory observations. Most of the bacteria in the GI tract are found in the colon. If one performs a microscopic count of the organisms found in a fecal specimen or in colonic contents, one will almost invariably find around 10^{11} organisms per milliliter, or five to ten times this amount (up to 10^{12}) per gram of dry weight. The redox potential of colonic contents is around -250 mV; the environment is highly anaerobic. Therefore, the vast majority of these organisms are fastidious anaerobes and will not grow unless cultured on specialized media under strictly anaerobic conditions. By using careful methodology, one can show that nearly all of the organisms counted through the microscope are in fact viable.[5-7] Identification of most isolates from the colonic flora requires around 100 analytical observations,[8] and only a handful of laboratories in the world are able to do this accurately. Many studies reporting the composition of the colonic flora under various conditions describe a recovery of 10^9 to 10^{10} viable cells per milliliter. Recovery rates in this range usually reflect culture conditions that select against the 90% to 99% of organisms that are fastidious anaerobes. The composition of the remaining 1% to 10% of organisms, selected solely on the basis of their ability to grow under harsh conditions, is of dubious significance. Much of the work on the colonic flora is therefore potentially misleading. An attempt has been made to base this chapter only on work done using valid methods.

Another problem encountered in dealing with the gut flora has to do with the sheer number of organisms present. When nonselective isolation techniques are used, an organism present at a population size of 10^7 (ten million) per milliliter, and thus representing only 0.01% of the flora, would not be detected by randomly picking colonies. For that reason, efforts have been made to culture the flora on selective media. Although there can be no assurance that a selective medium for streptococci, for example, actually recovers streptococci with anything approaching 100% efficiency, this type of approach has given an indication of the kinds of organisms found in relatively small numbers in the GI tract. One slight disadvantage to the use of selective media is that these media have been devised mostly for use in an anaerobic chamber, an environment that is less anaerobic than a roll tube, so viable counts are slightly lower.

The stomach and small bowel are more sparsely populated than the colon, and the bacteria found in these locations are less fastidious than the colonic flora. The ecosystem is also much less complex at these sites, and for these reasons bacteriologic methods are less of a concern.

The statistical analysis of data presents yet another methodologic problem. The difference between the gastric flora and the colonic flora is obvious and does not require statistical analysis. However, the comparison of colonic microfloras from two individuals or from two sites in the colon is usually exceedingly difficult and subtle. I.J. Good has developed a powerful approach known as "lambda analysis"[6] to compare the overall similarity of two floras. The method is an application of Monte Carlo analysis, and because of its complexity, it requires a computer.* Despite its usefulness, lambda analysis can miss significant differences among the less numerous members of the flora. These differences may be tested by other more routine methods such as the Student's *t*-test. However, the test must be applied over and over because

there are so many genera and species to compare. It is difficult to see the meaning of "$P<.001$" when 100 comparisons have been made in the same paper. Furthermore, given the extreme variability of the flora, any statistical test may lack the power to find important differences. Many of these issues have not yet been addressed adequately.

Another difficulty with statistical analysis of population sizes of bacteria in the gut is that they are not distributed normally, while most statistical tests assume that data are normally distributed. One way to deal successfully with this problem is to convert data to $\log_{10}$ form, a procedure that normalizes the distribution.[9]

The Oral Flora

Only in recent years have we begun to realize the complexity of the oral flora. The composition of the flora varies from place to place in the mouth. Thus, tooth surfaces, the buccal mucosa, the surface of the tongue, and the pharynx all have a different and characteristic flora that is composed of organisms that adhere most efficiently to these surfaces.[10] Most of the genera of bacteria found in the more distal GI tract can also be found in the mouth, but the species tend to be quite different. This was first known for the streptococci, where there is practically no overlap between the species found in the mouth and those found in the colon.[11] The largest numbers of bacteria and the most complex flora are to be found in the gingival crevices, where conditions are anaerobic and rapid dilution by saliva is less of a factor. Here, bacteria grow as densely as in the colon. It is difficult to say what is a "natural" flora for the gingival crevice, because toothbrushing is an artifact of our culture. If one stops brushing his teeth, the subgingival flora gradually becomes more and more complex, and eventually gingivitis ensues.[12] The microflora to be found here consists of hundreds of species and subspecies of mostly anaerobic bacteria, largely of the same genera as those found in the colon (see below), but again most isolates can be differentiated clearly from colonic bacteria, as seen in Table 26-1. Because most bacteria are killed as they pass through the stomach and never appear in the colonic flora, it must be concluded that the oral flora is important locally in the mouth but has little significance for the rest of the GI tract.

The Gastric Flora

Unless *Helicobacter pylori* is present, the microflora of the stomach is generally sparse. Only relatively acid-resistant organisms survive for any length of time, so bacterial counts are usually low, in the range of 0 to 100 colony-forming units (CFU) per milliliter. *Lactobacillus*, *Candida*, *Streptococcus viridans*, *Neisseria*, *Staphylococcus* (coagulase-negative), and *Peptostreptococcus* are the genera best represented. Bacteriologic counts are significantly higher in the achlorhydric stomach. Snepar and colleagues have shown that treatment with antacids or cimetidine also raises bacterial counts 10- to 100-fold.[13] Most of the organisms found in the stomach very likely represent the most acid-resistant components of the oral flora and do not actually colonize the stomach.

H. pylori on the other hand, is a true gastric colonizer. It is not certain whether *H. pylori* should be considered part of the indigenous flora or a pathogen. The fact that it is nearly always associated with histologic gastritis has suggested to some that it is a

---

* Space does not permit a full description of this method, but a computer program written in Fortran is available from W.E.C. Moore at Virginia Polytechnic Institute.

TABLE 26–1

Comparison of Bacteroides Found in the Gingival Crevice
With Those Found in Feces

ORAL BACTEROIDES	FECAL BACTEROIDES
B. intermedius (homology group 8944)	B. vulgatus
B. oralis	B. uniformis
B. pneumosintes	B. thetaiotaomicron
B. denticola	B. distasonis
B. gingivalis	B. fragilis
B. M1	B. ovatus
B. oris	B. hypermegas
B. intermedius (homology group 4197)	B. capillosus
	B. furcosus
B. gracilis	B. eggerthii
	Unnamed—15 types

Data from Holdeman LV, Cato EP, Moore WEC. Human fecal flora: Variation in bacterial composition within individuals and a possible effect of emotional stress. Appl. Environ Microbiol 1976;32:359; Moore WEC, Holdeman LV. Human fecal flora: The normal flora of 21 Japanese–Hawaiians. Appl Microbiol 1974;27:961.

TABLE 26–2

Composition of the Fecal Flora* Organisms Found
to Make up 1% or More of the Flora

GENUS	PERCENTAGE OF FLORA	
	Holdeman and Moore	Finegold et al
Bacteroides	30	56
Eubacterium	26	14
Bifidobacterium	11	4
Peptostreptococcus	9	4
Fusobacterium	8	0.1
Ruminococcus	4	9
Clostridium	2	2
Lactobacillus	2	1
Unclassifiable	2	—
Streptococcus	2	6
Facultative gram-negatives	0.5	0.1
Propionibacterium and Actinomyces	0.3	0.6
Staphylococcus	0.1	0.01
Coprococcus	0.1	0.1
Acidaminococcus	—	0.2

* *Organisms found to make up 0.1% or more of the flora.*
Moore WEC, Holdeman LV. Human fecal flora: The normal flora of 21 Japanese–Hawaiians. Appl Microbiol 1974;27:961; Finegold SM, Sutter VL, Mathisen GE. Normal indigenous intestinal flora. In: Human intestinal microflora in health and disease. New York: Academic Press, 1983:3.

pathogen. There is no doubt that it actually causes the gastritis (see ch 61). However, the indigenous flora is known to cause infiltration of the lamina propria with inflammatory cells at other levels of the gastrointestinal tract.[2] Lack of these inflammatory cells is one of the peculiarities of the germfree state. It is therefore not safe to assume that the presence of inflammatory cells indicates a pathologic response. Furthermore, most patients with histologic gastritis are asymptomatic. The presence of *H. pylori* is also associated with peptic ulcer disease, an unquestionably pathologic state. Whether or not it causes duodenal ulcers remains to be determined.

Flora in the Small Intestine

The numbers and types of bacteria found in the small intestine depend, in part, on the flow rate of intestinal contents. When stasis occurs, the small intestine may contain an extensive, complex flora. (This abnormal state of small bowel overgrowth will be discussed in a later chapter.) Normally, flow is brisk enough to wash bacteria through to the distal ileum and colon before the bacteria multiply. Although the numbers of bacteria found in the upper small bowel vary over a wide range from person to person, the density of bacteria is always a minuscule fraction of what is found in the colon. The duodenum and jejunum are often sterile but contain on the average 10^2 (range, $0–10^4$) organisms per milliliter.[14–17] Anaerobes only slightly outnumber facultative organisms; streptococci, lactobacilli, yeasts, and staphylococci are found. The proximal ileum may also be sterile, but on the average, 10^3 (range, $0–10^5$) organisms of the same types found in the jejunum are present. In the proximal small bowel, clostridia, bacteroides and coliforms are normally either absent or present in exceedingly small numbers. In the distal ileum, these organisms are among the

predominant types, and the bacterial count averages around 10^5 to 10^6 (range, $10^3–10^9$) per milliliter.

Colonic Flora

Prior to the Apollo lunar landing, there was a great deal of concern that astronauts could bring novel microbes back from the moon. In order to detect these alien organisms, it was considered necessary to know the human flora in detail. For this reason, exhaustive studies were done, largely by Moore, Holdeman, and colleagues at Virginia Polytechnic Institute (VPI), to describe the human colonic microflora. Many of the species of anaerobes found in the human colon were first described by these investigators. Their work could be described as a "gold standard" with which other studies of the predominant colonic flora can be compared.[6,7,18] Recovering an average of 94% of the microscopic count, they identified 1147 fecal isolates from 20 Japanese–Hawaiians. Ninety-five percent of viable bacteria belonged to 15 genera, as shown in Table 26–2. A subsequent study revealed that the flora of astronauts was not significantly different from that of Japanese–Hawaiians and that by statistical inference 400 to 500 species of bacteria were present.

Finegold, Sutter, and others at the Wadsworth Veterans Administration Medical Center studied the fecal flora in an effort to determine whether the composition of the flora correlated with risk of colon carcinoma. Their methods differed from those of the group at VPI in that they used an anaerobic chamber rather than roll tubes, and they used selective as well as nonselective media. They studied 141 individuals from a variety of cultural groups consuming a variety of diets.[14,19,20] The results of these studies have been reviewed in detail.[14] About 35% of cells counted microscopically were recovered and identified. Despite the differences in techniques and the potential bias of the Wadsworth data against extremely oxygen-sensitive organisms, their results (Table 26-2) were very similar to those of the group at VPI. The most noticeable difference is in the relatively large proportion of the flora identified as bacteroides by the Wadsworth group. Their use of selective media allowed them to detect organisms present in small numbers, for example *Butyrivibrio, Megasphaera, Sarcina, Veillonella, Staphylococcus,* and *Bacillus* species as well as yeasts. There was again a large variation in the composition of the flora between individuals; the investigators did not specifically look at the stability of an individual's flora. The flora of patients with colon cancer was not impressively different from the flora of controls. With the exception of *Escherichia coli,* no gram-negative facultative organism was found in the majority of subjects. *Candida albicans* and staphylococci were also detected in a minority.

Overall, well-done studies of the human colonic flora agree with one another and show that 98% or more of the organisms present in the colon are strict anaerobes, and that nearly the entire colonic flora consists of organisms with very little invasive potential under normal circumstances. Most ubiquitous high-grade pathogens, such as *Clostridium tetani, C. botulinum,* meningococcus, *Cryptococcus,* pneumococcus, and so forth, never appear in the tabulation of indigenous human flora. The potential pathogens that do appear, for instance *Staphylococcus aureus* and *Clostridium difficile,* are present in very low numbers as long as the microflora is not disturbed by antibiotics. While there is great variation among people in the composition of their colonic flora, the flora of a given individual remains quite stable over time.[6,21] Indeed, workers at VPI were often able to recognize a fecal donor by a bacteriologic examination of his specimen. There is little change in the makeup of the flora as one proceeds from cecum to rectum.[18] Comparisons of the composition of the flora adherent to the colonic wall with that of the flora in the lumen have so far not shown any significant differences.[22–24] Despite the variability of the flora from individual to individual, there has been no convincing demonstration that most of the major components of the flora vary significantly among human populations.

Factors That Alter the Composition of the Flora

Although the intestinal microflora forms a stable ecosystem, it is possible to alter this system. Probably the most effective way known to do this is to administer antibiotics. The effects depend on the antibiotics used and the schedule of dosing[25] and range from little change to nearly total annihilation of the entire flora. Because antibiotics can affect more than the composition of the flora, this subject will be discussed later in the chapter after the functioning of the flora has been presented.

At the most proximal end of the alimentary tract, the oropharynx tends to become colonized with gram-negative bacteria in ill patients. The likelihood of colonization increases with the severity of illness so that a person admitted to an intensive care unit usually is colonized.[26] In these patients, adhesion to epithelial cells appears to be a mechanism by which the gram-negatives colonize.[27] The mechanisms for this phenomenon may involve other less studied factors (e.g., decreased dependence on adhesion of the entire mouth ecosystem because of stasis [decreased salivary flow]). Gram-negatives also colonize the oropharynx of alcoholics. Colonization by *C. albicans* from the mouth to the distal esophagus increases dramatically with impaired cell-mediated immunity. The frequent presence of plaques of the organism on the mucosal surfaces strongly suggests that *C. albicans* maintains a population in this high-flow area by adhering to epithelial cells. The effect of cell-mediated immunity on adhesion to the mucosal surfaces is not well understood.

The major factor that can change the composition of gastric flora is decreased acidity. This subject was discussed above. Increased colonization of the hypochlorhydric stomach can lead to reflux of bacteria into the oropharynx.[28] The effects of stasis on the flora of the small bowel will be discussed in a later chapter.

The colonic flora has been studied under many conditions, and while it has been possible to show the effects of various manipulations on various species as a whole, only antibiotic treatment has been shown to cause wholesale shifts in the major populations.

The idea that host immunity could play a role in determining the composition of the flora has great intuitive appeal. There is no basis either in common sense or in experimental work to suggest that serum antibodies have any effect on populations within the intestinal lumen. Intraluminal or "coproantibodies," however, are a different matter. Clearly, IgA antibody can decrease the population size of *Vibrio cholerae* in the mouse cecum.[29] The major antibody class within the cecum is secretory IgA (see ch 5). These antibodies are not complement-fixing and therefore are not cidal; they probably have their effect by decreasing adhesion. As shown below, bacterial species within the colon are probably often in a delicate balance, and it seems likely that altered adhesion could alter this balance. However, there is little experimental work to substantiate a major role of immunoglobulins in determining the composition of the flora. Studies of human flora in immunoglobulin-deficient patients[30,31] have not settled the question. Interestingly, the effects of the flora on the immune system have been much easier to demonstrate. One remarkable defect of the germfree state is the nearly complete absence of any kind of antibodies.[32] It has been easy to demonstrate that humans as well as animals develop antibodies directed at components of the intestinal flora.[33–36] In some cases, these antibodies cross-react with antigens of pathogens.[37,38] Thus, our flora appears to be responsible for "natural antibodies."

Many studies have been done to determine the effects of diet on the composition of the colonic flora.[39] While it has been easy to show a major effect on rodent flora,[40] results have not been so striking with human flora. Most studies have concentrated on the effects of varying the amounts of meat and fiber in the diet. Taken as a whole, the results indicate that a few bacterial species may be sensitive to diet, but the bulk of the predominant flora is made up of bacteria that are not affected. For example, Moore and colleagues[41] looked at extreme changes in diet with subjects eating four diets, including a normal western diet and a diet of unpolished boiled rice, salt, unsweetened tea, and vitamins. They found that of 20 species in the predominant flora, only three varied with diet. Holdeman and colleagues showed that people in anger/stress situations develop unusually high populations of *Bacteroides uniformis*.[6] In these people, *B. uniformis* may make up as much as 30% of the colonic flora. It has been suggested that the rise in this population may be due to increased bile flow.

METABOLISM

Because of the sparseness of the flora in the proximal GI tract, its metabolic activities are quantitatively insignificant compared with those of the colonic flora. A compendium of the metabolic reactions that the colonic flora can perform is beyond the scope of this chapter. Each of the hundreds of species present has a characteristic set of metabolic capabilities; these capabilities allow the bacteria to be classified and identified. The subject is probably more complicated than metabolism in all the rest of the human body combined. Not only can bacteria be found that are able to carry out almost any reaction that occurs in a mammalian cell, but these organisms can also carry out more exotic metabolic processes, such as production of short-chain fatty acids, hydrogen gas, and ammonia; reduction of sulfate to sulfide; reduction of nitrate to nitrite; and hydrolysis of cellulose. Some individuals are even colonized with organisms that derive their energy from reducing CO_2 to methane gas.[42,43] In this section we will cover broadly the important metabolic functions of the flora.

Carbohydrate Metabolism

Most of the members of the colonic flora are capable of fermenting carbohydrates,[8] and as mentioned above, competition for carbon sources appears to be a major mechanism controlling the composition of the flora. Large amounts of carbohydrate enter the cecum from the ileum. These consist largely of the oligosaccharide moieties of gastrointestinal mucin, chondroitin sulfate and hyaluronic acid from desquamated colonic epithelial cells, and plant polysaccharides such as cellulose, hemicellulose, pectins, and sugars that are not degraded by digestive enzymes or absorbed.[44] The colonic flora utilizes most of the carbohydrate that enters the colon,[45,46] while protein and amino acids are broken down much less extensively. The breakdown of complex carbohydrates and the details of competitive interactions promise to be very complicated. Bacteria in general are not able to transport oligosaccharides to an intracellular location, so carbohydrates must be broken down into mono- or disaccharides before entry into the cell. It is known that many members of the predominant flora make enzymes capable of hydrolyzing the specific glycosidic linkages found in the carbohydrates involved.[44,47-52] Bacteria seem to adapt one of two strategies: they either (1) produce extracellular enzyme or (2) utilize cell-associated enzymes in the periplasmic space.[44,47,53,54] In the case of cellulose degraders, the organisms attach to cellulose particles and secrete cellulase into pockets created between the organism and the particle.[55] Many of the predominant bacteroides are able to break down a variety of plant carbohydrates, a factor that may help to explain the stability of the flora in the face of a varying diet.[44] Another factor contributing to this stability may be the relatively large amount of mucin present in the ecosystem. Being of host origin, this substance does not vary as much as

dietary carbohydrate. Studies so far have found relatively few species involved in this process, and all are present in small numbers.[56,57] The reported finding that 1% of the flora is capable of utilizing mucin seems at odds with the large amount of mucin present. The organisms identified as being able to degrade mucin so far have been unable to utilize other carbon sources. Some organisms, for instance *C. difficile*, require a carbohydrate but do not produce hydrolases[46]; perhaps this lack explains the ecologic disadvantage of *C. difficile*. The gut flora metabolizes monosaccharides by a variety of pathways, giving volatile fatty acids (VFAs), CO_2, and H_2 as end products.[43,58-60] The VFAs appear to be important for the host. In other monogastric animals, up to a third of the energy requirement of the host is met by absorbing VFAs from the colon.[61] The human colon absorbs both protonated and ionic VFAs.[62,63] Colonic epithelial cells are able to utilize VFAs as a carbon source, and up to 75% of these cells' energy consumption can be attributed to their use of n-butyrate.[64] After a diverting colostomy, the segment with no fecal flow is subject to develop a colitis that is responsive to infusions of VFAs.[65] Some bacteria are able to utilize VFAs,[66] and this may be yet another factor accounting for the stability of the flora, because VFA concentrations vary over a narrow range in the colon.[67] In individuals colonized with *Methanobrevibacter smithii*, methane is also produced, although this organism does not metabolize carbohydrate.[42,43]

Nitrogen Metabolism

While the colonic flora depletes 90% or more of the available carbohydrates, the concentration of proteins in the colon is little different from the concentration in the distal ileum.[45,46] This fact indicates that amino acids are not used as extensively as sugars for energy metabolism, although it does not necessarily indicate that proteins are not extensively broken down. It may be that proteins are broken down to produce new extracellular enzymes. Some bacterial species are highly proteolytic, and the flora as a whole does produce its own proteolytic activity.[68,69] Furthermore, the presence of branched-chain VFAs in colonic contents probably indicates that branched-chain amino acids are broken down by the gut bacteria. It is believed that a better studied similar ecosystem, the rumen, may give some clues about the nature of nitrogen metabolism in the colon. Most ruminal bacteria do not require amino acids for growth but do require ammonia.[70] When amino acids are used for growth, they are generally deaminated first, and the ammonia is used to synthesize amino acids. It has also been shown that some colonic anaerobes also preferentially utilize ammonia even when amino acids or proteins are made available.[71] Many isolates from human colon (*e.g.*, *Peptostreptococcus productus* and *Clostridium beijerinckii*) are capable of generating ammonia from urea.[72,73] Indeed, about 25% of urea in humans appears to be broken down in the gut to form 3 to 4 g of ammonia per day, and the ammonia concentration in the colon is more than adequate to support the nitrogen requirement of bacteria.

Steroid Metabolism

The human host synthesizes and secretes four bile acids—taurocholate, taurochenodeoxycholate, glycocholate, and glycochenodeoxycholate. These acids are secreted in bile and are involved in absorption of fats. Most are reabsorbed in the terminal ileum and recirculated to the liver, but about 130 to 650 mg per day escape to the colon, where the flora metabolizes them extensively. The deconjugation of bile acids (removal of taurine and glycine groups) goes essentially to completion. The flora is then able to generate at least 15 to 20 different secondary bile acids from cholate and chenodeoxycholate. These secondary bile acids are to some extent reabsorbed to enter the enterohepatic circulation. The advantage of this arrangement to the host is not known, nor is it obvious that the ability to transform bile acids is to the advantage of most of the bacteria involved. However, secondary bile acids inhibit many bacteria (a fact that can sometimes be used to quickly differentiate oral flora from colonic flora). Colonic bacteria may benefit ecologically from their bile acid conversions. Bile acid metabolism has already been covered in detail in Chapter 16.

In the past decade it has become apparent that the colonic flora metabolizes a wide range of steroid substrates. (For an excellent review of this topic, the reader is referred to Bokkenheuser and Winter.[74]) Steroid hormones also undergo enterohepatic circulation. While bile acids are conjugated to taurine and choline, other steroids are conjugated to glucuronide and sulfate. The gut flora is able to deconjugate these steroids[75] and to transform them in a variety of reactions. *Eubacterium lentum* is particularly active at steroid metabolism. It is capable of 21-dehydroxylation,[76] 16α-dehydroxylation,[77] and 3α-hydroxyl epimerization.[76] This organism is also capable of the reductive degradation of digoxin.[78] *Bacteroides fragilis* and *Bifidobacterium adolescentis* are capable of C-20 reduction,[79] a reaction that prevents 21-dehydroxylation. A variety of gram-positive anaerobes have been shown to reduce the keto group at the 3 position of ring A in 3-ketosteroids.[80] *B. fragilis* has been shown to reduce the 17-keto group of estrone to make estradiol,[81] a reversible reaction. Some strains of clostridia have been found to reduce the 17-keto groups of progestins.[82] Finally, side-chain cleavage of 17-hydroxysteroids has been shown to occur. In one example of this conversion, a clostridium was shown to convert cortisol to the androgen androstene.[83] It has been suggested that alterations in steroid metabolism by the colonic flora may explain pregnancies in women treated with antibiotics while taking the birth control pill.[84] Except for the metabolism of digoxin, however, the importance of these reactions to the host remains unknown.

Metabolic Disease of the Host

The colonic flora may actually cause metabolic disease in the host. D-lactic acidosis is an example of this situation.[85–87] A prerequisite for this disorder appears to be a shortened small bowel, leading to entry into the colon of nutrients that are normally not present. In response to the presence in the colon of carbohydrates normally absorbed by the small bowel, non–spore-forming gram-positive organisms overgrow and generate large amounts of D-lactic acid that are absorbed systemically. The resulting acidosis usually presents as mental status alteration. A second metabolic disease in which the colonic flora appears to be involved is methylmalonic aciduria,[88] an inherited disorder of propionyl coenzyme A. The metabolic defect responds to antibiotic treatment, probably because the major source of propionic acid in humans is the gut flora.

Metabolism of Drugs

Drugs are also metabolized by the gut flora. In the case of Vitamin K, the pharmacologic agent is synthesized. Most species of the genus *Bacteroides* are able to do this as well as many eubacteria and *Enterobacteriaceae*.[89] At least in the rat, significant amounts of Vitamin K are absorbed through the colonic mucosa.[90] The role of bacterial Vitamin K in human metabolism is not certain, but given the association of Vitamin K deficiency with antibiotic therapy, it is possible that Vitamin K synthesized in the gut may be used in malnourished hospitalized patients.

Other agents are broken down in the gut. Some anaerobes, particularly of the genus *Bacteroides*, synthesize beta-lactamases, and these enzymes can be measured in colonic contents during therapy with antibiotics.[91] The beta-lactamase can then decrease activity of penicillins in the colonic lumen. Metronidazole and other nitroimidazoles, on the other hand, possess no antimicrobial properties until activated by anaerobes.[92] Sulfasalazine, used in the treatment of ulcerative colitis, is also inactive until the colonic flora cleaves a nitro bond yielding sulfapyridine and the active moiety, 5-aminosalicylate.[93] As mentioned above, digoxin is reduced in some subjects by the colonic flora, and this reaction may consume almost half of the dose administered. Numerous other reactions have been described for food additives.[94] For instance, the toxicity of Laetrile is due to the release of cyanide by the colonic flora.

SUPPRESSION OF PATHOGENS

As noted above, none of the organisms making up the predominant anaerobic flora is a particularly efficient pathogen. Probably the most important function of the colonic microflora is to suppress populations of other bacteria that are more pathogenic. Not only are the potential pathogens within the flora (*e.g.*, Enterobacteriaceae, *Streptococcus faecalis*) kept to low numbers, but other organisms (*e.g.*, *C. difficile* and *Pseudomonas aeruginosa*) ingested even in large numbers are totally unable to establish any population. This suppression is possible because the interactions of bacteria in the colon are fundamentally competitive, and our flora has evolved over the millennia to include the best competitors. The indigenous flora's efficiency at suppression is illustrated by the fact that every enteric pathogen studied to date has the ability either to adhere to small bowel mucosa or to penetrate gut epithelial cells (see chs 68, 69, 83). None has succeeded in competing directly with the gut flora to establish a population within the lumen. Because of the availability of a proven continuous-flow culture model of mouse flora and the great usefulness of germfree animals, most of what we know about bacterial interactions in the gut has been learned from studying mice. Although the relevance of our knowledge of mouse flora has been debated, it is likely that the principles involved in bacterial competition within the mouse gut hold for interactions in the human gut as well.

In the mid 1950s, Bohnhoff and colleagues[95] and Freter[96] independently described the findings that *Vibrio cholerae* (not normally pathogenic for mice) and *Salmonella typhimurium* colonized experimental animals more efficiently than usual after the animals had been treated with antibiotics. In both instances, the investigators correctly concluded that antibiotics were acting on the colonic flora, which normally suppressed these pathogens. Suppression of bacteria by the indigenous flora has been termed "bacterial antagonism," "bacterial interference," and "colonization resistance" by various investigators and has been rediscovered several times.[97,98]

Initial attempts to investigate this phenomenon further focused on the role of *E. coli*, an indigenous organism that suppresses many different pathogens in the digestive tract. However, the work of Dubos,[1] Bryant,[99] and others made it clear that *E. coli* was normally only a very minor part of the colonic flora and that the bulk of the biomass within the colon was made up of fastidiously anaerobic organisms. The detailed bacteriologic work of Syed and colleagues[100] and Freter and Abrams[2] indicated that mouse flora was extremely complex and that most of the suppressive effect of the colonic flora could be attributed to the anaerobes. The work of van der Waaij,[98] Berg,[101] and Ducluzeau and colleagues[102] lent further credence to this concept. The study of Freter and Abrams also suggested that the cecal flora of mice did not function normally without a full complement of species; nearly 100 distinguishable cecal isolates administered to germfree mice only partially normalized the animals. While most suppression is exerted by the predominant anaerobic flora, it also appears that similar organisms compete. Thus, Freter and Abrams found that for suppressing *Shigella flexneri*, 100 anaerobes alone are less efficient than 100 anaerobes plus *E. coli*. By the same token, a nontoxigenic strain of *C. difficile*, if administered first, is able to suppress a toxigenic strain and prevent colitis,[103] and two strains of *E. coli* compete against one another in the digestive tract.[104,105] As with *C. difficile*, the strain of *E. coli* administered first (the resident) has an advantage over the invader. Other examples of bacterial interactions may seem more idiosyncratic. For instance, Ducluzeau and colleagues showed that a collection of three clostridia is able to suppress *S. flexneri*.[106] *Escherichia coli* is able to suppress *C. difficile* by about a log in the gnotobiotic mouse.[107] Except for the study by Freter and Abrams, which dealt with a complex flora, most of this work must be interpreted cautiously. Nearly any organism inoculated into the germfree mouse will attain a population of around 10^9 per milliliter. Just because organism *x* at this population density can suppress another does not mean that it could still do so after the entire flora had suppressed organism *x*.

The control mechanisms by which organisms are suppressed are difficult to study in the intact animal. The best documented in vitro model is that of Freter and colleagues.[108] The system has been under development since 1962, when Hentges and Freter compared the ability of various strains of bacteria to antagonize *S. flexneri* in the gut of the gnotobiotic mouse with their ability to antagonize it in various in vitro systems. In vitro suppression was comparable to in vivo suppression only when organisms were grown in continuous-flow (CF) culture[109] and not, for instance, in static broth cultures. Later work showed that if mouse flora was inoculated into a CF culture within an anaerobic chamber, the culture maintained the entire ecosystem in equilibrium for months.[108] The model was continuously colonized with anaerobic species in about the same proportions as the conventional mouse; showed colonization resistance; suppressed resident *E. coli* strains; and, when administered to germfree mice, the CF culture contents

conventionalized them in every respect. The CF culture model has also been useful for investigating the mechanisms of interaction between *C. difficile* and the colonic flora.[46] Similar models have been used to study human flora,[110,111] but no model for human flora has yet been documented as carefully as Freter's. Because of the simultaneous development of a highly detailed understanding of bacterial competition in chemostats (a type of CF culture), it has been possible to develop a theoretic basis for understanding bacterial competition as it occurs in the colon.[112] It presently seems reasonable to look at the colonic flora as a complex group of organisms that compete for nutrients, most often for carbohydrates. Bacterial strains maintain colonization at the expense of other strains by (1) their high affinity[113] for the growth-limiting substrates (in other words, they deplete the substrates so that other organisms cannot grow fast enough to keep from being washed out) and (2) their ability to adhere to the gut wall. The predominant flora further improves its competitive edge by elaborating metabolic by-products that interfere with their competitors. These by-products include volatile fatty acids,[114,115] H_2S,[113] and possibly secondary bile acids.[116]

There is little evidence to support two popular concepts about the interactions of bacteria in the gut. The first is the idea of the "ecologic niche." As noted before, there is no good evidence that the human flora varies from one site to another in the colon. Admittedly, this may be because we do not have the tools yet to look at microenvironments, but unless one is talking about adhesion, the concept is presently too vague to be of much use. The second concept is that bacteriocins play a significant role in an organism's fitness in the gut. Bacteriocins are antibioticlike substances produced by one strain that are active against other strains of bacteria. Currently, evidence suggests that bacteriocins are not important in determining the outcome of bacterial competition in the gut. Although there may be a tendency for colicin-producing strains of *E. coli* to persist in the human GI tract,[117] in controlled studies of gnotobiotic animals colonized with a bacteriocin producer and a bacteriocin-sensitive strain, the producer has no noticeable advantage.[118,119]

How much of the discussion above directly applies to the human flora? Presently we know little more about the ability of human flora to suppress pathogens than we knew about the ability of mouse flora in 1956. Humans challenged with large oral inocula of *Candida albicans*[120] or *Pseudomonas aeruginosa*[121] show colonization resistance. However, *P. aeruginosa* can colonize people given antibiotics. Treatment with antibiotics also facilitates colonization by *C. difficile*[122] and *E. coli*.[4] Treatment with cefoxitin leads to increases in the populations of facultative organisms such as enterococcus and *E.coli* that one would expect to be suppressed normally by the predominant flora.[123] The cefoxitin study was intended to show an effect of antibiotics on colonization resistance but failed to do so, possibly because of poor timing of the challenge inoculum, which consisted of a poorly colonizing strain of *E. coli*. Cefoxitin also facilitates colonization by antibiotic-resistant organisms not normally found in the human flora. These findings are a strong indication that control mechanisms are at work in the human flora. The fact that the control mechanisms are similar to those for mouse flora is suggested by the finding that *E. coli* is probably suppressed by lack of a carbon source in human flora as well.[124] Human flora appears to remain stable when introduced into CF culture,[110,111] but the data supporting a CF culture model are much less complete than those supporting the use of mouse flora in CF culture.

EFFECTS OF ANTIBIOTICS ON THE FLORA

The literature on the effects of antibiotics on the composition of the colonic flora is often difficult to interpret. Most studies either do not document efficiency of culture methods at all or report the effect of antibiotics on the 1% to 10% of the flora that is relatively easy to grow. Many studies classify organisms only to the genus level or identify them simply as anaerobes or gram-negative facultative bacteria. This approach may be very misleading. Because the organisms present in small numbers are known to be suppressed by the more numerous bacteria, elimination of the species accounting for 90% of the anaerobic biomass would be followed by an increase of the remaining species to take their place. Therefore, most studies concluding that an antibiotic does not have a significant effect on the flora should be viewed with skepticism. Despite these methodologic problems, the effects of antibiotics are often very clear cut.

Work in mice preceded studies of human flora, and in some cases information on animals still exceeds our knowledge of the effects of antibiotics on the human flora. Administration of antibiotics rapidly alters the composition of mouse flora and induces changes similar to the germfree state.[25] Thus, treatment of animals with many types of antibiotics makes them susceptible to colonization with organisms that are not normally found in the intestinal tract. The ceca of antibiotic-treated animals rapidly dilates, and the increase in size is due to a rise in water content. Ceca in antibiotic-treated rodents may reach a remarkable size (15% or more of body weight); there is no similar change in humans. Related to this change, mice given some antibiotics develop loose stools just as humans do. A possible explanation for the diarrhea is that gastrointestinal mucin, which is normally hydrolyzed by the flora, accumulates in the lumen.[125] Mucin molecules carry large numbers of negative charges. As a result, cations associated with mucin are not absorbed normally and create an osmotic load. Feeding germfree animals a chloride exchange resin partially corrects this defect.[126] A similar approach to antibiotic-associated diarrhea in humans has not yet been tried. A final effect of antibiotics on animals is the appearance of antibiotic-resistant strains in the intestinal flora.[127] All of these effects vary with the type and dose of antibiotic given.

The literature on the effects of antibiotics on the composition of human flora is voluminous. Table 26-3 summarizes some of these effects; for an extensive review see the work by Finegold and colleagues.[125] Antibiotics known to be highly active against individual components of the flora (*e.g.,* penicillin) sometimes have little effect on the composition of the flora. At first this may seem surprising, but there are likely explanations for this observation. One cause of this discrepancy is that antibiotics reach the lumen of the colon in varying amounts, but this fact does not

TABLE 26–3
Effect of Antibiotics on Components of the Colonic Flora

ANTIBIOTIC*	EFFECTS ON FLORA†						
	Anaerobes				Facultatives		
	GNR‡	GPC	GPR	CLOS	GNB	STR	YST
Penicillin[135]	0	0	0	0			
Ampicillin[136]	− − −	− − −	− − −	− − −	− −	− −	
Piperacillin§[137]	Anaerobes as a whole¶		−		−	0	++
Cefoxitin[137]	Anaerobes as a whole¶		0		++	++	+
Cefoperazone‖[137§,138]	− − −	− − −	− − −	− − −	− − −	− −	+++
Imipenem[139§-141]	0	0	0	0	0	+	+
Aztreonam[137]	Anaerobes as a whole¶		0		− −	+	0
Clindamycin[135,142]	− − −		−		0	0	
Ciprofloxacin[143]	0		0		− − −	−	
Polymyxin B[136]	Anaerobes as a whole¶		0		− − −	0	
Neomycin[136]	Anaerobes as a whole¶		0		0		−

* References from which data are taken.
† + = 2 log increase; − = 2 log decrease; 0 = little or no effect.
‡ GNR = gram-negative rods (fusobacteria, bacteroides); GPC = gram-positive rods (peptostreptococci); GPR = gram-positive non–spore-forming rods (eubacteria, bifidobacteria, and lactobacilli); CLOS = clostridia; GNB = Enterobacteriaceae; STR = Streptococcus fecalis; YST = yeast.
§ Study with recovery of 10^{11} or more organisms per milliliter.
‖ Cefoperazone is secreted in bile and reaches extremely high concentrations in intestinal contents.
¶ Anaerobes not classified.

totally explain the paradox. Perhaps just as important, efforts to correlate antibiotic effects on the flora with in vitro sensitivity data have not taken into account the method of testing sensitivity. The standard method of performing these tests is to induce organisms to multiply at their maximal growth rate and to expose them to various antibiotics looking for complete inhibition of growth. This approach is not totally relevant to the colonic flora in two regards. First, it is known that antibiotics having a major inhibitory effect on rapidly growing bacteria may have a minimal effect on slowly growing organisms[128]; the organisms in the colon are thought to grow slowly. Second, even a slight slowing of the growth rate would be expected to have a major effect on the population size of an organism colonizing the gut. More work needs to be done to clarify the roles of all these variables.

Because antibiotics can grossly alter the composition of the flora, these drugs can probably affect all the functions of the flora and bring about a condition analogous to the germfree state. Increases in water content and in osmotic pressure have been observed in the intestinal lumen[125] By suppressing organisms that degrade digoxin, antibiotic administration may lead to digoxin toxicity. Neomycin, a drug used for treating hepatic encephalopathy, has been shown to decrease the production of ammonia by the colonic flora[129] An examination of Table 26-3 will show that some antibiotics, for instance cefoxitin, may lead to an increase in certain bacterial populations. This is undoubtedly because organisms such as yeasts, the enterococcus, and enteric gram-negatives are normally suppressed by other more numerous populations that are eliminated by the antibiotics. It also becomes possible for new strains of bacteria to implant in the GI tract once the controlling flora has been removed. The most obvious example, oral thrush, can be seen with the naked eye. It is now clear that *C. difficile* is often not an endogenous infection but that spores from the environment are ingested and may implant in the intestinal tract of the antibiotic-treated patient[130,131] *Clostridium botulinum* may colonize not only infants who do not have a complete flora but also the adult patient who receives antibiotics[132] *P. aeruginosa*, not normally a member of the microflora, may colonize people who have been receiving antibiotics[121] It is very likely that the intestinal tract of antibiotic-treated patients is the major reservoir of the antibiotic-resistant gram-negative hospital flora, because most normal subjects do not harbor large numbers of antibiotic-resistant organisms.

a necessary energy source for the colonic mucosal cells. The breakdown of the complex carbohydrates allows cations associated with these large molecules to be absorbed, a process that leads to more efficient absorption of water. The flora also not only generates urea but breaks it down to form ammonia, a process that may have pathologic consequences in patients with hepatic failure. The bacteria in the gut metabolize both bile acids and steroid hormones in complex ways, although the full significance of these reactions has thus far eluded us. Vitamin K is produced and may be absorbed in large enough quantities to sustain the host during the fasting state. Drugs are metabolized, thus altering the pharmacodynamics. Food additives are metabolized. Mutagenic compounds are synthesized by the flora and are associated with a risk of colonic cancer[133] In the face of altered physiology, bacterial activities can become very detrimental to the host. For instance, after small bowel bypass surgery, the normal metabolic patterns can change so that large enough amounts of D-lactate can be produced to make the host severely acidotic. In small bowel stasis there is overgrowth of anaerobes normally found only in the colon, with resultant diarrhea.

One must wonder whether overall our flora helps or hinders us. The germfree animal grows larger and lives longer than its conventional counterpart[134] The logical conclusion is that the microflora competes with the host and we would be better off germfree. But this conclusion would be warranted only in a germfree world. A germfree animal's chance encounter with *C. difficile* or *C. botulinum* is likely to be a lethal event, while neither organism can colonize the conventional animal. The germfree animal also does not have naturally protective antibodies and does not respond normally to new antigens. The advantage of having a microflora is that it prepares us to face a world of hostile microbes.

The reader is directed to Chapter 5, The Immune System; Chapter 16, Bile Secretion; Chapter 56, Esophageal Infections; Chapter 61, Acid-Peptic Disorders; Chapter 68, Small Intestine: Infections with Common Bacterial and Viral Pathogens; Chapter 69, Chronic Infections of the Small Intestine; Chapter 71, Celiac Disease; Chapter 73, Bacterial Overgrowth; Chapter 74, Short Bowel Syndrome; Chapter 83, Bacterial Infections of the Colon; Chapter 99, Intraabdominal Abscesses and Fistulas; and Chapter 127, Microbiologic Studies.

OVERALL INTERACTION OF THE MICROFLORA WITH THE HOST

The size and complexity of the ecosystem within dictates a complicated interaction with the host. Thus, the flora is constantly crossing the mucosal barrier and translocating to regional lymph nodes where it interacts with the immune system to stimulate antibody production as well as cell-mediated immunity. It has been suggested that this process is also responsible for some inflammatory diseases such as arthritides. The flora forms an impenetrable network that prevents potentially pathogenic bacteria from colonizing the intestinal tract. The metabolic interactions with the host are extensive. Breakdown of carbohydrates leads to production of short-chain fatty acids that are to some extent absorbed as an energy source for the host. These fatty acids are also

REFERENCES

1. Dubos R, Schaedler RW, Costello R, Hoet P. Indigenous, normal and autochthonous flora of the gastrointestinal tract. J Exp Med 1965; 122:67.
2. Freter R, Abrams GD. Function of various intestinal bacteria in converting germfree mice to the normal state. Infect Immun 1972; 6:119.
3. Moore WEC, Moore LVH, Cato EP, Wilkins TD, Kornegay ET. Effect of high-fiber and high-oil diets on the fecal flora of swine. Appl Environ Microbiol 1987;53(7):1638.
4. Cohen IR, Norins LC. Natural human antibodies to gram-negative bacteria: Immunoglobulins G, A, and M. Science 1966;152:1257.
5. Aranki A, Syed SA, Kenny EB, Freter R. Isolation of anaerobic bacteria from human gingiva and mouse cecum by means of a simplified glove box procedure. Appl Microbiol 1969;17:568.

6. Holdeman LV, Cato EP, Moore WEC. Human fecal flora: Variation in bacterial composition within individuals and a possible effect of emotional stress. Appl Environ Microbiol 1976;32:359.

7. Moore WEC, Holdeman LV. Human fecal flora: The normal flora of 21 Japanese–Hawaiians. Appl Microbiol 1974;27:961.

8. Holdeman LV, Cato EP, Moore WEC. Anaerobic laboratory manual. Blacksburg, VA: Virginia Polytechnic Institute and State University, 1977.

9. Best WR. On the logarithmic transformation of intestinal bacterial counts. Am J Clin Nutr 1970;23:1608.

10. Gibbons RJ, van Houte J. Bacterial adherence in oral microbial ecology. Annu Rev Microbiol 1975;29:19.

11. Skinner FA. Quesnel LB. Streptococci. New York: Academic Press, 1978.

12. Moore LVH, Moore WEC, Cato EP, Smibert RM, Burmeister JA, Best AM, Ranney R. Bacteriology of human gingivitis. J Dent Res 1987;66(5):989.

13. Snepar R, Poporad GA, Romano JM, Kobasa WD, Kaye D. Effect of cimetidine and antacid on gastric microbial flora. Infect Immun 1982;36(2):518.

14. Finegold SM, Sutter VL, Mathisen GE. Normal indigenous intestinal flora. In: Hentges DJ, ed. Human intestinal microflora in health and disease. New York: Academic Press, 1983:3.

15. Justesen T, Nielsen OH, Jacobsen IE, Lave J, Rasmussen SN. The normal cultivable microflora in upper jejunal fluid in healthy adults. Scand J Gastroenterol 1984;19:279.

16. Plaut AG, Gorbach SL, Nahas L, Weinstein L, Spanknebel G, Levitan R. Studies of intestinal microflora. III. The microbial flora of human small intestinal mucosa and fluids. Gastroenterology 1967;53(6):868.

17. Gorbach SL, Plaut AG, Nahas L, Weinstein L, Spanknebel G, Levitan R. Studies of intestinal microflora. II. Microorganisms of the small intestine and their relations to oral and fecal flora. Gastroenterology 1967;53(6):856.

18. Moore WEC. Anaerobes as normal flora: Gastrointestinal tract. In: Finegold SM, McFadzean JA, Roe FJC, eds. Metronidazole: Proceedings of the International Conference. Princeton, NJ: Exerpta Medica, 1977:222.

19. Finegold SM, Sutter VL, Sugihara PT, Elder HA, Lehmann SM, Phillips RL. Fecal microbial flora in Seventh Day Adventist populations and control subjects. Am J Clin Nutr 1977;30:1781.

20. Finegold SM, Attebery HR, Sutter VL. Effect of diet on human fecal flora: Comparison of Japanese and American diets. Am J Clin Nutr 1974;27:1456.

21. Zubrzycki L, Spaulding EH. Studies on the stability of the normal human fecal flora. J Bacteriol 1962;83:968.

22. Edmiston CE Jr, Avant GR, Wilson FA. Anaerobic bacterial populations on normal and diseased human biopsy tissue obtained at colonoscopy. Appl Environ Microbiol 1982;43(5):1173.

23. Croucher SC, Houston AP, Bayliss CE, Turner RJ. Bacterial populations associated with different regions of the human colon wall. Appl Environ Microbiol 1983;45(3):1025.

24. Nelson DP, Mata LJ. Bacterial flora associated with the human gastrointestinal mucosa. Gastroenterology 1970;58(1):56.

25. Savage DC, Dubos R. Alterations in the mouse cecum and its flora produced by antibacterial drugs. J Exp Med 1968;128:97.

26. Johanson WG, Pierce AK, Sanford JP. Changing pharyngeal bacterial flora of hospitalized patients: Emergence of gram-negative bacilli. N Engl J Med 1969;281:1137.

27. Johanson WG Jr, Woods DE, Chaudhun T. Association of respiratory tract colonization with adherence of gram-negative bacilli to epithelial cells. J Infect Dis 1979;139:667.

28. Atherton ST, White DJ. Stomach as source of bacteria colonising respiratory tract during artificial ventilation. Lancet 1978;2:968.

29. Freter R. Coproantibody and bacterial antagonism as protective factors in experimental enteric cholera. J Exp Med 1956;104:419.

30. Brown WR, Savage DC, Dubois RS, Alp MH, Mallory A, Kern F Jr. Intestinal microflora of immunoglobulin-deficient and normal human subjects. Gastroenterology 1972;62:1143.

31. Parkin DM, McClelland BL, O'Moore RR, Percy-Robb IW, Grant IWB, Shearman DJC. Intestinal bacterial flora and bile salt studies in hypogammaglobulinemia. Gut 1972;13:182.

32. Hashimoto K, Handa H, Umehara K, Sasaki S. Germfree mice reared on an "antigenfree" diet. Lab Anim Sci 1978;28:38.

33. Brown WR, Lee EM. Radioimmunologic measurements of naturally occurring bacterial antibodies. I. Human serum antibodies reactive with *Escherichia coli* in gastrointestinal and immunologic disorders. J Lab Clin Med 1973;82:125.

34. Brown WR, Lee E. Radioimmunological measurements of bacterial antibodies. II. Human serum antibodies reactive with *Bacteroides fragilis* and *Enterococcus* in gastrointestinal and immunological disorders. Gastroenterology 1974;66:1145.

35. Foo MC, Lee A. Immunological response of mice to members of the autochthonous intestinal microflora. Infect Immun 1972;6:525.

36. Carter PB, Plllard M. Host responses to "normal" microbial flora in germfree mice. J Reticuloendothel Soc 1971;9:580.

37. Foo MC, Lee A, Cooper GN. Natural antibodies and the intestinal flora of rodents. Aust J Exp Biol Med 1974;52:321.

38. Robbins JB, Myerwotz RL, Whisnant JK, Argaman M, Schneerson R, Handzel ZT, Gotschlich EC. Enteric bacteria cross-reactive with *Neisseria meningitidis* groups A and C and *Diplococcus pneumoniae* types I and II. Infect Immun 1972;6:651.

39. Hentges DJ. Does diet influence human fecal microflora composition? Nutr Rev 1980;38(10):329.

40. Wilkins TD. Microbiological considerations in interpretation of data obtained with experimental animals. In: Bruce WR, ed. Banbury report 7: Gastrointestinal cancer: Endogenous factors. Cold Spring Harbor Press, Cold Spring Harbor, NY, 1981:3.

41. Moore WE, Cato EP, Good IJ, Holdeman LV. The effect of diet on the human fecal flora. In: Bruce WR, ed. Banbury report 7: Gastrointestinal cancer: Endogenous factors. Cold Spring Harbor Press, Cold Spring Harbor, NY, 1981:11.

42. Miller TL, Wolin MJ. Stability of *Methanobrevibacter smithii* populations in the microbial flora excreted from the human large bowel. Appl Environ Microbiol 1983;45(1):317.

43. Wolin MJ, Miller TL. Carbohydrate fermentation. In: Hentges DJ, ed. Human intestinal microflora in health and disease. New York: Academic Press, 1983:147.

44. Salyers AA, Leedle JA. Carbohydrate metabolism in the human colon. In: Hentges DJ, ed. Human intestinal microflora in health and disease. New York: Academic Press, 1983:129.

45. Vercellotti JR, Salyers AA, Bullard WS, Wilkins TD. Breakdown of mucin and plant polysaccharides in the human colon. Can J Biochem 1977;55:1190.

46. Wilson KH, Perini F. Role of competition for nutrients in suppression of *Clostridium difficile* by the colonic microflora. Infect Immun 1988;56:2610.

47. Salyers AA, O'Brien M. Cellular location of enzymes involved in chondroitin sulfate breakdown by *Bacteroides thetaiotaomicron*. J Bacteriol 1980;143:772.

48. Salyers AA, Vercellotti JR, West SEH, Wilkins TD. Fermentation of mucins and plant polysaccharides by *Bacteroides* from the human colon. Appl Environ Microbiol 1977;33:319.

49. Salyers AA, West SEH, Vercellotti JR, Wilkins TD. Fermentation of mucins and plant polysaccharides by anaerobic bacteria from the human colon. Appl Environ Microbiol 1977;34:529.

50. Salyers AA, Gherardini F, O'Brien M. Utilization of xylan by two species of human colonic *Bacteroides*. Appl Environ Microbiol 1981b;41:1065.

51. Wedekind KJ, Mansfield HR, Montgomery L. Enumeration and isolation of cellulolytic and hemicellulolytic bacteria from human feces. Appl Environ Microbiol 1988;54:1530.

52. Dekker J, Palmer JK. Enzymatic degradation of the plant cell wall by a *Bacteroides* of human fecal origin. J Agric Food Chem 1981;29:480.

53. Berg JO. Cellular localization of glycoside hydrolases in *Bacteroides fragilis*. Curr Microbiol 1981;5:13.

54. Salyers AA. *Bacteroides* of the human lower intestinal tract. Annu Rev Microbiol 1984;38:293.

55. Kauri T, Kushner DJ. Role of contact in bacterial degradation of cellulose. Fed Euro Microbiol Soc Microbiol Eco 1985;31:301.

56. Miller RS, Hoskins LC. Mucin degradation in human colon ecosystems. Fecal population densities of mucin-degrading bacteria estimated by a "most probable number" method. Gastroenterology 1981;81(4):759.

57. Bayliss CE, Houston AP. Characterization of plant polysaccharide- and mucin-fermenting anaerobic bacteria from human feces. Appl Environ Microbiol 1984;48(3):626.

58. Wolin MJ. Fermentation in the rumen and human large intestine. Science 1981;213:1463.

59. Allison MJ. Production of branched-chain volatile fatty acids by certain anaerobic bacteria. Appl Environ Microbiol 1978;35:872.

60. Bryant MP. Nutritional features and ecology of predominant anaerobic bacteria of the gastrointestinal tract. Am J Clin Nutr 1974;27:1313.

61. Wrong OM, Edmonds CJ, Chadwick VS. Short-chain organic acids. In: Wrong OM, Edmonds CJ, Chadwick VS, eds. The large intestine: Its role in mammalian nutrition and homeostasis. New York: John Wiley & Sons, 1981:113.

62. Ruppin H, Bar-Meir S, Soergel KH, Wood CM, Schmitt MG Jr. Absorption of short chain fatty acids in the colon. Gastroenterology 1980;78:1500.

63. McNeil NI, Cummings JH, James WPT. Short chain fatty acid absorption by the human large intestine. Gut 1978;19:819.

64. Roediger WEW. Role of anaerobic bacteria in the metabolic welfare of the colonic mucosa in man. Gut 1980;21:793.

65. Harig JM, Soergel KH, Komorowski RA, Wood CM. Treatment of diversion colitis with short-chain fatty acid irrigation. N Engl J Med 1989;320:23.

66. Allison MJ, Bryant MP, Doetsch RN. A volatile fatty acid growth requirement for cellulolytic cocci of the bovine rumen. Science 1958;128:474.

67. Cummings JH. Short chain fatty acids in the human colon. Gut 1981;22(9):763.

68. Macfarlane GT, Cummings JH, Allison C. Protein degradation by human intestinal bacteria. J Gen Microbiol 1986;132:1647.

69. Macfarlane GT, Allison C, Gibson SAW, Cummings JH. Contribution of the microflora to proteolysis in the human large intestine. J Appl Bacteriol 1988;64:37.

70. Hespell RB, Smith CJ. Utilization of nitrogen sources by gastrointestinal tract bacteria. In: Hentges DJ, ed. Human intestinal microflora in health and disease. New York: Academic Press, 1983:167.

71. Takahashi M, Benno Y, Mitsuoka T. Utilization of ammonia nitrogen by intestinal bacteria from pigs. Appl Environ Microbiol 1980;39:30.

72. Suzuki K, Benno Y, Mitsuoka T, Takebe S, Kobashi K, Hase J. Urease-producing species of intestinal anaerobes and their activities. Appl Environ Microbiol 1979;37(3):379.

73. Wozny MA, Bryant MP, Holdeman LV, Moore WEC. Urease assay and urease-producing species of anaerobes in the bovine rumen and human feces. Appl Environ Microbiol 1977;33:1097.

74. Bokkenheuser VD, Winter J. Biotransformation of steroids. In: Hentges DJ, ed. Human intestinal microflora in health and disease. New York: Academic Press, 1983:215.

75. Van Eldere J, Robben J, DePauw G, Merckx R, Eyssen H. Isolation and identification of intestinal steroid-desulfating bacteria from rats and humans. Appl Environ Microbiol 1988;54(8):2112.

76. Bokkenheuser VD, Winter J, Dehazya P, Kelly WG. Isolation and characterization of human fecal bacteria capable of 21-dehydroxylating corticoids. Appl Environ Microbiol 1977;34:571.

77. Calvin HI, Lieberman S. Studies on the metabolism of 16α-hydroxyprogesterone in humans. Conversion to urinary 17-isopregnanolone. Biochemistry 1962;1:639.

78. Lindenbaum J, Rund DG, Butler VP Jr, Tse-Eng D, Saha JR. Inactivation of digoxin by the gut flora: Reversal by antibiotic therapy. N Engl J Med 1981;305:789.

79. Winter J, Cerone-McLernon AM, O'Rourke S, Bokkenheuser VD, Ponticorvo L. Formation of 20-dihydrosteroids by anaerobic bacteria. J Steroid Biochem 1982;17:661.

80. Bokkenheuser VD, Winter J, Dehazya P, De Leon O, Kelly WG. Formation and metabolism of tetrahydrodeoxycorticosterone by human fecal flora. J Steroid Biochem 1976;7:837.

81. Jarvenpaa P, Kosunen T, Fotsis T, Adlercreutz H. In vitro metabolism of estrogens by isolated intestinal microorganisms and by human faecal microflora. J Steroid Biochem 1980;13:345.

82. Bokkenheuser VD, Winter J, Mosenthal AC, Mosbach EH, McSherry CK, Ayengar NKN, Andrews AW, Lebherz WB III, Pienta RJ, Wallenstein S. Fecal steroid 21-dehydroxylase, a potential marker for colorectal cancer. Am J Gastroenterol 1983;78:469.

83. Bokkenheuser VD, Morris GN, Ritchie AE, Holdeman LV, Winter J. Biosynthesis of androgen from cortisol by a species of *Clostridium* recovered from human fecal flora. J Infect Dis 1984;149(4):489.

84. Bokkenheuser VD, Winter J, Cohen BI, O'Rourke S, Mosbach EH. Inactivation of contraceptive steroid hormones by human intestinal clostridia. J Clin Microbiol 1983;18:500.

85. Oh MS, Phelps KR, Traube M, Barbosa-Saldivar JL, Boxhill C, Carroll HJ. D-lactic acidosis in a man with the short-bowel syndrome. N Engl J Med 1979;301(5):249.

86. Stolberg L, Rolfe R, Gitlin N, Merritt J, Mann L Jr, Linder J, Finegold S. D-lactic acidosis due to abnormal gut flora. Diagnosis and treatment of two cases. N Engl J Med 1982;306(22):1344.

87. Halverson J, Gale A, Lazarus C, Avioli LV. D-lactic acidosis and other complications of intestinal bypass surgery. Arch Intern Med 1984;144:357.

88. Bain MD, Borriello SP, Tracey BM, Jones M, Reed PJ, Clamers RA, Stacey TE. Contribution of gut bacterial metabolism to human metabolic disease. Lancet 1988;140:1078.

89. Ramotar K, Conly JM, Chubb H, Louie TJ. Production of menaquinones by intestinal anaerobes. J Infect Dis 1984;150(2):213.

90. Hollander D, Muralidhara KS, Rim E. Colonic absorption of bacterially synthesized vitamin K_2 in the rat. Am J Physiol 1976;230:251.

91. Rolfe RD, Finegold SM. Intestinal β-lactamase activity in ampicillin-induced, *Clostridium difficile*-associated ileocecitis. J Infect Dis 1983;147(2):227.

92. Goldman P. Drug therapy: Metronidazole. N Engl J Med 1980;303:1212.

93. Peppercorn MA, Goldman P. The role of intestinal bacteria in the metabolism of salicylazosulfapyridine. J Pharmacol Exp Ther 1972;181:555.

94. Goldman P. Biochemical pharmacology and toxicology involving the intestinal flora. In: Hentges DJ, ed. Human intestinal microflora in health and disease. New York: Academic Press, 1983:241.

95. Bohnhoff M, Drake BL, Miller CP. Effect of streptomycin on susceptibility of the intestinal tract to experimental *Salmonella* infection. Proc Soc Exp Biol Med 1954;86:132.

96. Freter R. Fatal enteric cholera infection in the guinea pig achieved by inhibition of normal enteric flora. J Infect Dis 1955;97:57.

97. Shinefield HR, Ribble JC, Boris M, et al. Bacterial interference: Its effect on nursery-acquired infection with *Staphylococcus aureus*. I. Preliminary observations on artificial colonization of newborns. Am J Dis Child 1963;105:146.

98. van der Waaij D, Berghuis-de Vries JM, Lekkerkerk-van der Wees JEC. Colonization of the digestive tract in conventional and antibiotic-treated mice. J Hygiene 1971;69:405.

99. Bryant MP, Robinson IM. An improved nonselective culture medium for ruminal bacteria and its use in determining diurnal variation in numbers of bacteria in the rumen. J Dairy Sci 1961;44:1446.

100. Syed SA, Abrams GD, Freter R. Efficiency of various intestinal bacteria in assuming normal functions of enteric flora after association with germfree mice. Infect Immun 1970;2:376.

101. Berg RD. Antagonism among the normal anaerobic bacteria of the mouse gastrointestinal tract determined by immunofluorescence. Appl Environ Microbiol 1978;35:1066.

102. Ducluzeau R, Dubos F, Hudault S, Nicolas JL, Dabard J, Raibaud P. Microbial barriers against enteropathogenic strains in the digestive tract of gnotoxenic animals. Application to treatment of *Clostridium difficile* diarrhea in the young hare. Recent Advances in Germfree Research. Proceedings of the VII international symposium on gnotobiology. Tokai U Press 1981;135.

103. Wilson KH, Sheagren JN. Antagonism of toxigenic *Clostridium difficile* by nontoxigenic *C. difficile*. J Infect Dis 1983;147:733.

104. Ozawa A, Freter R. Ecologic mechanism controlling growth of *Escherichia coli* in continuous-flow cultures and in the mouse intestine. J Infect Dis 1964;114:235.

105. Duval-Iflah Y, Raibaud P, Rousseau M. Antagonisms among isogenic strains of *Escherichia coli* in the digestive tracts of gnotobiotic mice. Infect Immun 1981;34:957.

106. Ducluzeau R, Ladire M, Callue D, Raibaud P, Abrams GD. Antagonistic effect of extremely oxygen-sensitive clostridia from the mi-

croflora of conventional mice and of *Escherichia coli* against *Shigella flexneri* in the digestive tract of gnotobiotic mice. Infect Immun 1977;17:415.

107. Wilson KH, Freter R. Interactions of *Clostridium difficile* and *E. coli* with microfloras in continuous-flow cultures and gnotobiotic mice. Infect Immun 1986;54:354.

108. Freter R, Stauffer E, Cleven D, Holdeman LV, Moore WEC. Continuous-flow cultures as in vitro models of the ecology of large intestinal flora. Infect Immun 1983;39:666.

109. Hentges DJ, Freter R. In vivo and in vitro antagonism of intestinal bacteria against *Shigella flexneri*. J Infect Dis 1962;110:30.

110. Zubrzycki L, Spaulding EH. Application of the continuous flow culture method to studies on the normal human fecal flora. Bacteriol Proc 1957;57:101.

111. Miller TL, Wolin MJ. Fermentation by the human large intestine microbial community in an *in vitro* semicontinuous culture system. Appl Environ Microbiol 1981;42:400.

112. Freter R, Brickner H, Fekete J, Vickerman MM, Carey KE. Survival and implantation of *Escherichia coli* in the intestinal tract. Infect Immun 1983;39:686.

113. Freter R, Brickner H, Botney M, Cleven D, Aranki A. Mechanisms that control bacterial populations in continuous-flow culture models of mouse large intestinal flora. Infect Immun 1983;39:676.

114. Bohnhoff M, Miller CP, Martin WR. Resistance of the mouse's intestinal tract to experimental *Salmonella* infection. J Exp Biol Med 1964;120:805.

115. Hentges DJ, Maier BR. Inhibition of *Shigella flexneri* by the normal intestinal flora. III. Interactions with *Bacteroides fragilis* in vitro. Infect Immun 1972;6:168.

116. Floch MH, Binder JJ, Filburn B, Gershengoren W. The effect of bile acids on intestinal microflora. Am J Clin Nutr 1972;25:1418.

117. Branche WC Jr, Young VM, Robinet HG, Massey ED. Effect of colicin production on *Escherichia coli* in the normal human intestine. Proc Soc Exp Biol Med 1963;114:198.

118. Ikari NS, Kenton DM, Young VM. Interaction in the germfree mouse intestine of colicinogenic and colicin-sensitive microorganisms. Proc Soc Exp Biol Med 1969;130:1280.

119. Craven JA, Miniats OP, Barnum DA. Role of colicins in antagonism between strains of *Escherichia coli* in dual-infected gnotobiotic pigs. Am J Vet Res 1971;32:1775.

120. Krause W, Matheis H, Wulf K. Fungaemia and funguria after oral administration of *Candida albicans*. Lancet 1969;1:598.

121. Wilson KH, Sheagren JN, Freter R. Population dynamics of ingested *Clostridium difficile* in the gastrointestinal tract of the Syrian hamster. J Infect Dis 1985;151:355.

122. Buck AC, Cooke M. The fate of ingested *Pseudomonas aeruginosa* in normal persons. J Med Microbiol 1969;2:521.

123. Barza M, Giuliano M, Jacobus V, et al. Effect of broad-spectrum parenteral antibiotics on "colonization resistance" of intestinal microflora of humans. Antimicrob Agents Chemother 1987;31:723.

124. Guiot HF. Role of competition of substrate in bacterial antagonism in the gut. Infect Immun 1982;38:887.

125. Finegold SM, Sutter VL, Mathisen GE. Normal indigenous intestinal flora. In: Hentges DJ, ed. Human intestinal microflora in health and disease. New York: Academic Press, 1983:3.

126. Asano T. Modification of cecal size in germfree rats by long-term feeding of anion exchange resin. Am J Physiol 1969;(4):911.

127. Spika JS, Waterman SH, Soo Hoo GW, St. Louis ME, Pacer RE, James SM, Bisset ML, Mayer LW, Chiu JY, Hall B, Greene K, Potter ME, Cohen ML, Blake PA. Chloramphenicol-resistant *Salmonella newport* traced through hamburger to dairy farms. N Engl J Med 1987;316:565.

128. Cozens RM, Tuomanen E, Tosch W, Zak O, Suter J, Tomasz A. Evaluation of the bactericidal activity of B-lactam antibiotics on slowing growing bacteria cultured in the chemostat. Antimicrob Agents Chemother 1986;29:797.

129. Weber FL Jr, Fresard KM, Lally BR. Effects of lactulose and neomycin on urea metabolism in cirrhotic subjects. Gastroenterology 1982;82:213.

130. Heard SR, O'Farrell S, Holland D, Crook S, Barnett J, Tabaqchali S. The epidemiology of *Clostridium difficile* with use of a typing scheme: Nosocomial acquisition and cross-infection among immunocompromised patients. J Infect Dis 1986;153:159.

131. Wust J, Sullivan NM, Hardegger U, Wilkins TD. Investigation of an outbreak of antibiotic-associated colitis by various typing methods. J Clin Microbiol 1982;16:1096.

132. Sonnabend WF, Sonnabend OA, Grundler P, Ketz E. Intestinal toxicoinfection by *Clostridium botulinum* type F in an adult. Lancet 1987;1:357.

133. Wilkins TD, van Tassel RL. Production of intestinal mutagens. In: Hentges DJ, ed. Human intestinal microflora in health and disease. New York: Academic Press, 1983:265.

134. Luckey TD. Germfree life. New York: Academic Press, 1963.

135. Heimdahl A, Lindqvist L, Nord CE. Effects of phenoxymethylpenicillin, clindamycin, and tinidazole on the anaerobic oral, throat and colon flora in man. Scand J Infect Dis 1980;24:204.

136. Hazenberg MP, van de Boom M, Bakker M. Binding to faeces and influence on human anaerobes of antimicrobial agents used for selective decontamination. Antonie van Leeuwenhoek 1983;49:111.

137. Barza M, Giuliano M, Jacobus V, et al. Effect of broad-spectrum parenteral antibiotics on "colonization resistance" of intestinal microflora of humans. Antimicrob Agents Chemother 1987;31:723.

138. Mulligan ME, Citron DM, McNamara BT, et al. Impact of cefoperazone therapy on fecal flora. Antimicrob Agents Chemother 1982;22:226.

139. Wexler HM, Finegold SM. Impact of imipenem/cilastatin therapy on normal fecal flora. Am J Med 1985;78:41.

140. Nord CE, Kager L, Philipson A. Impact of imipenem/cilistatin therapy on fecal flora. Eur J Clin Microbiol 1984;3:475.

141. Welkon CJ, Long SS, Gilligan W. Effect of imipenem-cilastatin therapy on fecal flora. Antimicrob Agents Chemother 1986;29:741.

142. Kager L, Liljeqvist L, Malmborg AS, et al. Effects of ampicillin plus sulbactam on bowel flora in patients undergoing colorectal surgery. Antimicrob Agents Chemother 1982;22:208.

143. Enzensberger R, Shah PM, Knothe H. Impact of oral ciprofloxacin on the fecal flora of healthy volunteers. Infection 1985;13:273.

II

Approaches to Common Gastrointestinal Problems

27

Psychosocial Factors in the Care of Patients with Gastrointestinal Disease

DOUGLAS A. DROSSMAN

If the only tool you have is a hammer, you tend to treat everything as if it were a nail.[1]
A. Maslow

Physicians recognize that the medical model (i.e., focusing on the organic origins of illness) is not sufficient to understand many clinical occurrences or to make meaningful diagnoses or treatment plans. Medical *illness* (the experience of ill health or bodily dysfunction) and its clinical consequences are not fully explained by known *disease* (abnormalities in structure and function of organs and tissues).[2] It is best understood in terms of a multifactorial model of causation that assumes a complex interplay of biologic, psychologic, and sociologic variables (Fig 27-1). The Biopsychosocial Model,[3-5] derived from general systems theory,[6] specifies that an individual consists of and participates in multiple interrelated systems extending from the molecule to the organ, the person, the two-person system, the family, and the society within which he or she lives. Therefore, illness and disease are framed within and related to a more comprehensive system. For example, the physician, by giving steroids for control of inflammatory bowel disease, elicits a change at the patient's cellular level, such as impaired leukocyte function, which has the potential to affect the organ (abscess formation), the individual (sepsis/shock), the family (threatened loss of the "breadwinner"), or the community (major health care costs through an extended hospitalization).[7]

Consider the following actual cases:

1. Two patients have peptic ulcer disease.
   A. Mr. H. repeatedly visits his physician for epigastric pain that limits his ability to work. Endoscopies either are normal or show superficial erosions.
   B. Mr. L. is hospitalized for the second time with massive gastrointestinal bleeding secondary to an ulcer. He reports no pain.
2. Ms. A., disabled with a 20-year history of chronic abdominal pain, received a celiac plexus nerve block and for the first time became pain-free. On her first return to the clinic, while still without pain, she entered the room slowly, being assisted by her husband. When asked why this was neces-

sary, they looked at each other and she said, "We just don't want to take chances." Two weeks later she began seeing a neurologist for unexplained episodes of recurrent syncope.
3. Ms. S. visits the emergency room with symptoms of severe abdominal pain. Her medical record indicates a history of other somatic complaints leading to extensive evaluations at major medical centers. She now demands relief and challenges her physicians to make a diagnosis. The x-ray and blood studies are negative. A nondiagnostic emergency laparotomy is performed.
4. Mr. and Mrs. F. have their 16-year-old daughter hospitalized for anorexia nervosa. The staff note that while professing their commitment to help, the parents are reluctant to become involved in family work and resist efforts directed toward their daughter's health. Further evaluation indicates considerable intrafamily conflict, which is ameliorated when attention is diverted to the daughter's illness. Three months after discharge the patient is rehospitalized.
5. Ms. J., a young black woman from a rural community, gets into an altercation with another woman, who is acknowledged in the community to have special powers ("root worker"). An incantation is made by the other woman, who states that Ms. J. will die. Three days later, the patient begins to laugh at a joke and has a cardiac arrest. The autopsy is nondiagnostic, and it is presumed she died from an arrhythmia.
6. Mr. D. is diagnosed to have Stage III gastric carcinoma and is given a 6 to 12–month prognosis. He refuses chemotherapy and joins a group that "cures" cancer through meditation and imagery techniques. His family and physicians acknowledge that he is "denying" the illness. He survives two and one half years.

In example #1, a nociceptive experience like peptic ulcer is evaluated and modified by prior experience and psychosocial fac-

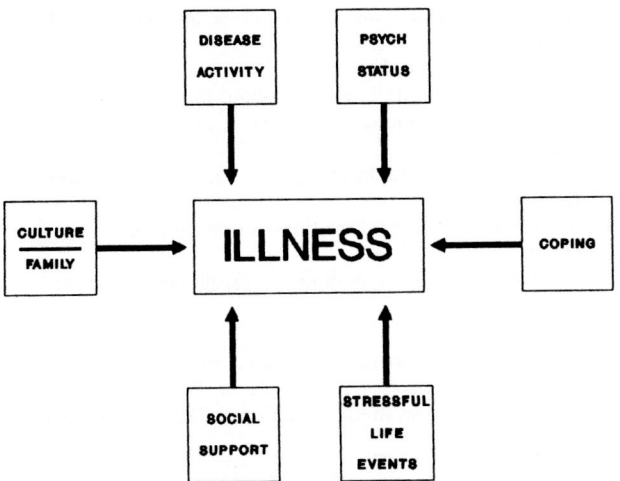

FIGURE 27–1. The multidetermined nature of human illness.

tors leading to variation among individuals in the perception and reporting of pain.[8] If one explores these factors, one may determine why Mr. L. reports no pain while Mr. H., with less evidence of disease, has chronic severe pain. With case #2, the psychosocial "benefits" of the sick role may be greater than what is obtained from relief of symptoms.[9] With case #3, a patient's demands for diagnosis and relief of pain affects the physician's judgment.[10] With case #4, psychologic stability in a malfunctioning family system (enmeshing) may occur by diverting attention to the child's illness.[11] With case #5, culturally determined personal belief systems can affect the degree of autonomic arousal, thereby producing a psychophysiologic response including cardiac arrest.[12] Finally, as in case #6, psychologic or environmental events may alter immune-mediated host response to disease.[13]

Understanding the biopsychosocial relationships in disease and illness, as shown here, optimizes diagnosis and patient care by integrating the data into a more understandable form. In contrast, a disease-centered model of illness may place "blinders" on the physician so that psychosocial data either are not recognized or are perceived as irrelevant.

RELATIONSHIP OF BIOLOGICAL AND PSYCHOSOCIAL FACTORS IN GASTROINTESTINAL ILLNESS

While it is recognized that psychosocial factors affect gastrointestinal (GI) illness, until recently scientific support has lagged behind this clinical awareness.[14] This has been in part because: (1) physicians have been trained in a medical model that has ignored the psychosocial aspects of illness, (2) research in human behavior and its physiologic relationships requires multidisciplinary methodology, and (3) the data are more difficult to measure and interpret.[15] The scientific evidence supporting the association between psychosocial variables and gastrointestinal illness is briefly discussed; a more comprehensive review is found elsewhere.[5]

Healthy subjects frequently report abdominal discomfort or bowel dysfunction when they are upset or distressed,[16] and psychophysiologic studies confirm these observations. It is well established in animals and man that stressful stimuli can produce

disturbances in intestinal vascularity, secretion, motility, and pain perception. It is also possible that physiologic disturbances in bowel function may affect central nervous system (CNS) function. This may be indicated by interactions between the CNS and the enteric nervous system or its neuroendocrine associations. Peptides such as vasoactive intestinal polypeptide (VIP), substance P, cholecystokinin, and the enkephalins, to name a few, are found in bowel and brain and appear to have integrated activities on intestinal function and behavior. For example, exogenous administration of cholecystokinin inhibits feeding activity and elicits postprandial satiety in several animals.[17] A recent study found that bulimic patients fail to have the normal postprandial rise in serum cholecystokinin,[18] suggesting that the regulation of cholecystokinin may play a role in the expression of a behavioral disorder. Similarly, the opiate peptides, which modulate pain perception, also have a pronounced effect on intestinal motility. Full understanding of the complexity of these associations is yet to be delineated.

Recent data also indicate that stress and other psychosocial factors affect how physiologic disturbances are perceived and acted upon. In a study of patients with gastroesophageal reflux disease, acute psychologic stress produced reports of greater reflux pain and greater autonomic arousal and anxiety. However, there was no change in the degree of acid reflux (*p*H probe), indicating that the greater pain reporting was due to a stress-induced alteration in the perception of the symptoms.[19]

The decision to seek health care also appears to be affected by psychosocial factors. The degree of psychosocial disturbance in irritable bowel syndrome (IBS) has been shown to affect health care utilization.[20,21] Furthermore, the patient's perception of ill health with inflammatory bowel disease may be at least as important as disease activity in determining physician visits and hospitalizations.[22] These and other data[5] provide evidence that biologic and psychosocial processes interact to create the illness experience and its clinical outcomes.

Another intriguing relationship involves the effect of psychosocial factors on disease activation. Epidemiologic studies in humans have supported the influence of disordered social structures, pressured life-styles, and stressful life events on the onset of many diseases.[5] The traditional model for stress research involves the induction of acute gastric erosions in rats and chronic gastrointestinal lesions in monkeys in response to restraint and conditioned anxiety. While studies have not completely explained the biologic mechanisms underlying these relationships, there is evidence that psychosocial factors may alter physiologic, endocrine, and immune function, thereby making the organism more or less susceptible to disease.[23]

Like many other physiologic systems, the immune system is sensitive to environmental influences by way of the CNS. The capacity of rats to cope with their environment can influence tumor growth and mortality or their susceptibility to infections. Using a Pavlovian conditioning model for altering immune function, Ader and Cohen have been able to delay the development of murine lupus erythematosus in NZB-NZW hybrid mice.[24] Recently, MacQueen and colleagues used a similar model to condition rat mucosal mast cells to secrete more protease II when rats were given an audiovisual cue linked to the injection of egg albumin than when these stimuli were given noncontingently.[25] Human studies support a relationship between stressful life events and in vitro alterations in immune function. In one prospective study,[26] 15 men whose wives had advanced breast cancer showed a poorer blastogenic response to mitogens after their wives' deaths than before bereavement. In a study of psychiatric inpatients, distressed (as measured by a depression scale) patients had significantly poorer DNA repair of their irradiated leukocytes than their non-distressed patient counterparts.[27] The authors proposed that altered psychosocial states may effect carcinogenesis through alterations in DNA repair, in addition to having indirect effects on immune surveillance of mutant cells. These studies indicate a relationship between transient altered psychosocial states and in vitro modification of immune response through behavioral conditioning. While further work is needed to determine the clinical relevance of these findings, they provide the groundwork to explain how psychosocial factors may affect health.

Once disease is established, sociocultural norms (explanatory models)[28] and family beliefs, as well as personality, environmental stress, and an individual's previous experiences, affect how the patient will react to illness. These reactions and possibly the activity of the disease may be modified or "buffered" by the development of particular coping strategies, by social support, and by the physician–patient interaction. Therefore, it behooves clinicians to assess psychosocial factors that may contribute to any illness experience and to use this information in order to improve clinical outcome. This chapter will now focus on how clinicians can take into account psychosocial factors in medical practice. I will describe how psychosocial data can be obtained, organized, and prioritized and used in treatment.

OBTAINING PSYCHOSOCIAL DATA: THE INTERVIEW

The medical interview is the *process* of obtaining data to diagnose, treat, and determine prognosis. It is a natural form of inquiry, though all too often the physician's style can interfere with the accurate collection of data. Observe the following hypothetical example:*

Interview #1

Patient is seated looking down and with shoulders slumped as the physician enters the room and sits down.

1. DOCTOR: Mr. . . .uh. . .(*looks at chart*). . .Jones? How can I help you?
PATIENT: (*Speaking slowly, looking down*) Well, it's this aching. . .right here. . .(*points to upper abdomen*). . .and diarrhea. . . .I've had it for weeks and. . .(*briefly looks up at doctor*)
2. DOCTOR: (*Writing in chart*). . .Epigastric pain and diarrhea. . .any other symptoms?
PATIENT: Well, this achi. . .this "pain" makes me not want to eat. . .and I'm sick to my stomach and tired. . . .I live alone now, and. . .

---

* Excerpted from Drossman DA: "Maximizing the Interview," a videotape produced by Medical Sciences Teaching Laboratory, University of North Carolina, Chapel Hill, NC, 1988.

3. DOCTOR: Hmmm. . .does eating cause the pain *and* give you diarrhea?
PATIENT: Uh, maybe, I guess.
4. DOCTOR: Can you tell me more about the diarrhea?
PATIENT: Well, it's loose. . .(*pause*). . .uh. . .what do you want to know?
5. DOCTOR: How often do you go?. . .and is there any blood in the stool?
PATIENT: About two or three times a day. No, I don't see any blood.
6. DOCTOR: Any other symptoms. . .fever, weight loss, or vomiting?
PATIENT: . . .Yes. . .
7. DOCTOR: (*More hurried*) Well, fever, weight loss, or what?
PATIENT: Don't think I've had any fever. I've lost about 10 pounds, and I'm so tired. . .don't feel like doing anything.

Later, in the interview:
8. DOCTOR: Well, it seems like you've had these symptoms for a while. What I'd like to do now is examine you and then order some tests. . .to make sure there's nothing serious. . .but from what you've said, I don't think that'll be the case. Uh. . .is there anything you know that could be causing this?. . .Are you under any stress?
PATIENT: Well, I'm having a lot of pressure at work. . .
9. DOCTOR: (*Smiles, closes chart*) I can understand that.

Later, the physician obtained blood and stool samples, ordered a small-bowel series, and performed a small-bowel biopsy and flexible sigmoidoscopy. The results were negative and the doctor reassured the patient and gave him a diagnosis of irritable bowel syndrome.

This physician believed he obtained enough data to make a medical diagnosis. But the questioning style raises some doubt as to the accuracy and completeness of the medical and psychosocial data. Table 27-1 describes several interviewer behaviors that can influence the quality of the data. Several items relating to this physician's style are to be noted.

1. He does not know the patient's name when he greets him (1).
2. Writing in the chart interferes with attention to the patient (2).
3. He interrupts (2–4,7).
4. He restates the patient's "aching" as "pain" (2).
5. He asks vague (4) and multiple closed-ended questions (3,5,6,7) that seem to confuse the patient. In general, closed-ended questions are less efficient than a combination of open and closed questions in obtaining medical information.[29]
6. He does not attend to or acknowledge the patient's nonverbal communication (poor eye contact, slumped posture) (1).
7. He does not respond to the patient's verbal cues relating to psychosocial issues (2,7).
8. He maintains control of the interview, focusing on disease-related questions, without eliciting the patient's agenda (2–7).
9. He gives a mixed message about the etiology of the illness (i.e., he plans to order tests, though prematurely reassures the patient) (8).
10. He "probes" for psychosocial factors only after the medical data are obtained, implying that the problem is psychologic (8).

TABLE 27–1
Physician Behaviors Influencing Accurate Data Collection

BEHAVIOR	FACILITATES	INHIBITS
Nonverbal		
Clinical environment	Private, comfortable	Noisy, physical barriers
Eye contact	Frequent	Infrequent or constant
Body posture	Direct, open, relaxed	Body turned, arms folded
Head nodding	Helpful if well timed	Infrequent, excessive
Body proximity	Close enough to touch	Too close or too distant
Facial expression	Interest, empathy, understanding	Preoccupation, boredom, disapproval
Touching	Helpful when used to communicate empathy	Insincere if not appropriate or properly timed
Verbal		
Question forms	Open-ended to generate hypotheses	Rigid or stereotyped style
	Closed-ended to test hypotheses	Multiple choice or leading questions ("You didn't . . . ?")
	Use of patient's words	Use of unfamiliar words
	Fewer questions and interruptions	More questions and interruptions
Question style	Nonjudgmental	Judgmental
	Follows lead of patient's earlier responses	Follows preset agenda or style
	Uses a narrative thread	HPI → PMH → ROS → Psych
	Appropriate silence	Frequent interruptions
	Appropriate reassurance	Premature or unwarranted reassurance
	Elicits psychosocial data in a sensitive and skillful manner	Ignores psychosocial data or uses "probes"

11. He communicates a lack of interest in exploring psychosocial issues (9).

Consider the differences with a different style of interview:

Interview #2

1. DOCTOR: Hello, Mr. Jones (*handshake*). I'm Dr. Smith. How can I help you?
2. PATIENT: (*Speaking slowly*) Well, it's this aching. . .right here. . .(*points to upper abdomen*). . .and diarrhea. . . .I've had it for weeks and (*briefly looks up at doctor who is attentive*). . .I just feel bad.
DOCTOR: So, you have aching and diarrhea. . .anything else?
3. PATIENT: Well, I don't feel like eating. . .and I'm sick to my stomach and tired.
DOCTOR: (*After brief pause*) Yes. . .
4. PATIENT: (*Continues*). . .I've lost 10 pounds since this began. . .(*pause*). . .and it keeps me from working.
DOCTOR: (*Speaking more slowly*) So this is affecting your work. . .
5. PATIENT: Yes. . .(*briefly looks up as if to say something and then quickly down*). . .I worry if it's something serious.
DOCTOR: (*Nods, maintains silence*)
6. PATIENT: (*Continuing*) I live alone now. . .(*long silence, nervously looks up and then down*)
DOCTOR: (*Leans forward slightly, looking concerned; speaks slowly and deliberately*) Mr. Jones, you seem a bit tense now. Is there anything else you'd like to tell me?
7. PATIENT: (*Looking down*) Well, (*pause*) I had a roommate who had similar symptoms. . .(*pause*)
DOCTOR: (*Speaking more softly*) So you thought you may have caught something? (*Patient nervously looks up and then down*). . .(*pause*). . .Why do you think that?
8. PATIENT: Well, he was a very close friend. . .(*long silence, begins to wipe eye and then continues*). . .first they didn't know what was wrong. . .then they found he had AIDS (*starts to sob*).
DOCTOR: (*Physician moves closer; then a long period of silence*) I can understand how difficult this has been for you. You've lost someone very close to you and are also concerned about your own health, and it's all affecting your ability to work. . .(*pause*). . .I'd now like to ask you a few more questions about your illness and then I'll examine you. Whatever we find, we'll need to talk more about what can be done to help you. Is there anything else you'd like to tell me?
9. PATIENT: (*Looks up*) No. . .(*brief smile*). . .thank you, Doctor.

In this interview, the physician obtained additional data that expand the differential diagnosis: the patient may have been exposed to AIDS, and depression, relating to fears of acquiring the disease and/or the loss of his close friend, may also be contributing to the illness. All these possibilities will need to be addressed.

As noted in Table 27-1, several facilitative behaviors used by this physician are worthy of comment.[30]

1. He readjusts the tempo of his questioning to match that of the patient (4,6,7).
2. He uses silence and brief facilitating statements to encourage the patient to elaborate (3,5).
3. He uses nonverbal behaviors to communicate interest and support (1,6).
4. He encourages the patient to elaborate without introducing bias by restating his earlier responses (2,4,7).

5. He elicits psychosocial data by facilitation rather than direct inquiry (e.g., probing). This is accomplished nonverbally (e.g., silence, attentiveness) (5) and by a more open-ended interview style that encourages the patient to elaborate on previous cues (4,7).

6. He acknowledges (and validates) the patient's mood disturbance (6).

7. He obtains simultaneously both psychosocial and medical data. This is done through more open-ended inquiries that explore the symptoms and their psychosocial context.

8. He ends by summarizing the patient's concerns and commits himself to help regardless of cause (8). This facilitates the development of a therapeutic relationship.

Guidelines for Interview Technique

These vignettes illustrate several important guidelines derived from research and clinical observation about the medical interview.

1. The physician strives to understand the illness from the patient's perspective and then uses medical knowledge to reorient the data into disease-related and behavioral categories.[31]

2. The physician needs to use a flexible technique. For example, more open-ended questions are used, as in this case, for patients with unexplained or chronic symptoms, but more directed questions may be needed in an emergency situation. Also, as in this example, the physician may need to slow his pace to permit the more passive or inhibited patient to elaborate. However, the physician must take a more directive role for the garrulous or controlling patient so as not to lose sight of the goal of obtaining the needed information for diagnosis and treatment.

3. The psychosocial and biomedical data are obtained more efficiently when elicited concurrently rather than sequentially.[30,32] Aside from saving time, this approach yields quality information, because the patient doesn't need to shift back and forth between two dimensions that are actually experienced in an integrated fashion. Furthermore, the patient learns to accept the legitimacy of this association and of the physician's interest in hearing about it. It is a frequent error of students and physicians who exhibit poor interview technique to avoid discussion of psychosocial issues by overcontrolling the questions.[32,33]

4. Addressing the patient's thoughts, concerns, and emotional state facilitates the development of a therapeutic relationship. In one study, the physician's openness to communication and caring behavior were shown to be major factors in the patient's compliance, satisfaction, and decision to continue the therapeutic relationship.[34]

UNDERSTANDING THE DATA

Once the medical and psychosocial data are obtained, their relative contributions to the current illness must be determined. The physician should address several questions (Table 27-2) in order to

TABLE 27-2
Questions to Consider When Obtaining and Using Psychosocial Data

1. Does the patient have acute or chronic illness?
2. What is the patient's life history of illness?
3. Why is the patient coming now?
4. What are the patient's perceptions and expectations?
5. Does the patient exhibit abnormal illness behavior?
6. What is the impact of the illness?
7. Is there a psychiatric diagnosis?
   a. Depression
   b. Anxiety disorder
   c. Somatization—somatoform disorder
   d. Factitious disorder
8. Are there cultural or ethnic influences?
9. How does the family interact around the illness?
10. What are the patient's other psychosocial resources?
11. How far do you go in the workup?
12. When do you call the psychiatric consultant?

prioritize the psychosocial data. Their importance will vary among patients and with the same patient over time.

Does the Patient Have Acute or Chronic Illness?

Regardless of etiology, the longer illness is present, the more likely psychosocial processes contribute to the patient's behavior, and these processes must be considered in treatment and prognosis. For example, medical patients with long-standing *unexplained* pain symptoms are unlikely to have a specific medical disease diagnosed, and psychologic assessment usually identifies contributing psychosocial factors.[35] Also, patients with chronic gastrointestinal disease may develop a variety of psychosocial responses (e.g., depression, interference with activities, increased illness behaviors, increased social support, financial compensation, and decreased home and work responsibilities) that may exacerbate their illness and interfere with their motivation to develop healthier behaviors.

What Is the Patient's Life History of Illness?

The *frequency* of other physical complaints, present and past, and the frequency of health care visits for these complaints are important diagnostic and prognostic indicators. Patients with life histories of illnesses and physician visits are more likely to have stresses, personality factors, and social circumstances that will require behavioral interventions for improvement.

Why Is the Patient Coming Now?

When the clinical presentation is not a medical emergency, it is important to determine what other factors influenced the patient's decision to seek medical care. These factors are not always volunteered and often must be elicited in a skillful and sensitive manner. For example, asking, "Why did you come now?" may be interpreted as more rejecting than "Was there anything else that led you to see me?" Table 27-3[36] lists reasons why patients may seek medical care and offers suggestions for treatment.

What Are the Patient's Perceptions and Expectations?

CASE EXAMPLE[7]

A 27-year-old homemaker has had chronic, moderately active ulcerative colitis for 13 years. Colonoscopy on two recent occasions showed high-grade epithelial dysplasia; she refused colectomy. After several unsuccessful attempts to "educate" her as to the reasons for the procedure, the physician asked what she believed would happen if she underwent surgical treatment. For the first time she expressed the fear that she would be unable to have children; she and her husband were childless. When these unrealistic fears were addressed, she consented.

This vignette illustrates the importance of identifying patient misperceptions or unrealistic expectations that may interfere with treatment. As another example, many patients with chronic illness

TABLE 27-3
Why Is the Patient Coming to the Doctor?

REASON	PHYSICIAN'S APPROACH
Recent symptom exacerbation	Identify exacerbating factors (e.g., by way of a patient diary).
	Encourage patient to modify them.
Fear of serious disease	Determine underlying concerns (e.g., recent family death or GI illness, prodding by spouse, media exposure of illness).
	Offer reassurance.
	Avoid premature or false reassurance ("There's nothing wrong . . . it's nerves").
Environmental stressor(s)	Identify stressor(s).
	Determine patient's insight and ability to work toward changing stressor(s).
	Determine best treatment approach:
	Wait expectantly for resolution,
	Counsel patient,
	Suggest stress-reduction techniques (exercise, relaxation training, hypnosis),
	Refer for psychologic counseling.
Psychologic distress	Is there a psychiatric diagnosis?
	Anxiety
	Depression
	Somatization
	Consider pharmacologic intervention:
	Antidepressant
	Antianxiety agent
	Psychiatric consultation as needed.
Functional impairment	Determine change in functional status.
	Set treatment goal to be improved function, not relief of symptoms.
"Hidden agenda"	Determine the hidden agenda:
	Narcotics
	Laxative abuse
	Disability
	Keep sick role privileges (work/home)
	Clarify your role and the limits of your treatment.
Social/cultural factors	Determine if:
	Physician visits for social support
	There are cultural effects (e.g., "roots," folk remedies)
	There is a need to legitimize to family/friends
	Adapt treatment to be consistent with patient beliefs or expectations:
	Set up brief, regular appointments.
	Permit "folk" remedies if not harmful.

Modified from Drossman DA. Treatment of the patient with irritable bowel syndrome. In: Bayless T, ed. Current therapy in gastroenterology and liver disease. Toronto: BC Decker, 1989; 166–170.

harbor unrealistic expectations for cure, even though the symptoms have been present for years. The physician must encourage patients to state their expectations in order to work toward realistic treatment goals.

Important questions to ask include: "What do you think is causing this problem?" "What are your concerns or fears about this illness?" "What kind of treatments do you think you should receive?" and "What do you hope I will be able to do for you?"[37] The patient who bypasses these questions by saying, "That's why I came to you" or "You're the doctor" is not taking the proper degree of responsibility for his/her health care and will need to be re-educated (see below).

Does the Patient Exhibit Abnormal Illness Behavior?

The varying patterns of how symptoms are perceived, evaluated, and acted upon are designated as illness behaviors.[38-40] This is determined by current and prior experiences with illness and its benefits; the attitudes and behaviors of family, friends, culture, and society; and the patient's personality, current psychologic state, and coping style. As with the case of Ms. A, when the patient's behavior is perceived by the physician to be inconsistent with clinical expectations, *abnormal* illness behavior[41,42] should be considered. Blackwell[43] lists several diagnostic features: (1) disability disproportionate to detectable disease, (2) a relentless search for validation of disease, (3) placement of control and responsibility for health care with the physician, (4) a sense of entitlement to be cared for by others, (5) a tendency to avoid health-promoting roles, (6) adoption of and (7) display of behaviors oriented toward sustaining the "sick role"[9] (e.g., exemption from work or family obligations, avoidance of stressful situations, gratification of needs through a dependent relationship with a physician). Regardless of disease etiology, successful treatment of abnormal illness behaviors will require behavioral interventions by the physician or other health care professionals.

What Is the Impact of the Illness?

For any illness, the physician must decide whether, when, and to what degree medical or behavioral intervention is necessary. Particularly for chronic illness, this decision is best made when the illness is understood in the context of its effects on the patient's daily life. For example, the patient with chronic pain who begins to decrease activity (e.g., no longer able to work) will require more intervention than the patient with pain who can maintain daily activities. The impact of the illness is evaluated by its effects on physical (ambulation, body care), psychologic (cognitive, affective, sexual), and social (e.g., vocational management, recreation) functioning.

Is There a Psychiatric Diagnosis?

Psychologic illnesses, such as depression and anxiety, are the most common diagnoses seen in primary care medical practice.[44,45] These disorders, as either the cause or result of chronic illness, will modify the patient's experience of medical disease. In either situation, their recognition is essential for proper treatment, which may also include psychopharmacologic agents such as antidepressant or antianxiety agents or behavioral forms of treatment.

DEPRESSION

Depression, or affective disorder, can be an ambiguous term and is best understood as existing on a clinical continuum: from a normal emotional response, to real or threatened loss (the "blues"), to a more intense expression of a mood (depressive symptoms), to a collection of signs and symptoms (syndrome of depression), to a more severe state associated with neurochemical and pathophysiologic disturbance (disease). Similarly, the diagnostic categories and the type of therapeutic interventions for depression (e.g., "tincture of time," counseling, pharmacotherapy) are determined by the degree and persistence of the disorders on this continuum.

There is a close relationship between depression and gastrointestinal complaints.[46] First, the intestinal tract responds physiologically to alterations in mood[5] (e.g., it is common for patients with depression to report constipation). Second, patients with chronic gastrointestinal diseases have a high prevalence (>30%) of depression, possibly for several reasons: loss of autonomy, loss of bodily or daily function, fear or embarrassment, possible separation from friends, family and work, and fear of possible death. Finally, depression is a common underlying determinant of functional gastrointestinal symptoms. In fact, symptoms such as anorexia, weight loss, abdominal pain, and constipation are used as diagnostic criteria for depression in standardized self-report depression inventories and standardized interviews.

With regard to identifying primary depression, the Diagnostic and Statistical Manual of Mental Disorders—Revised (DSM-III-R)[47] lists diagnostic criteria. The medical physician should first consider *Major Depression, Single (296.2x) or Recurrent (296.3x)*. Major depression is characterized by at least 2 weeks of one or more episodes of depressed mood or diminished interest or pleasure in activities and associated symptoms that include change in weight, sleep disturbance, psychomotor retardation, loss of energy, feelings of worthlessness or inappropriate guilt, decreased concentration, and recurrent thoughts of death. A more chronic (>2 years) disturbance of depressed mood with these same associated symptoms is called *Dysthymia (300.40)*. Finally, *Depressive Disorder Not Otherwise Specified (300.40)* includes patients with depressive features that do not meet more specific criteria for a mood disorder.

In establishing any of these diagnoses, it is important to exclude other conditions that can present with the same clinical features. These include other medical or psychiatric (e.g., dementia) disorders, uncomplicated bereavement, and drugs that may mimic or exacerbate an affective disorder. In medical practice, these would include corticosteroids, cimetidine, alcohol, benzodiazepines, and a variety of antihypertensive agents (alpha methyldopa, propranolol, reserpine, clonidine).

Particularly for medical patients, primary depression may be manifested atypically[48] (e.g., "masked" depression), with the patient focusing more on somatic complaints such as chronic pain[49,50] than on mood disturbance. Therefore, the physician who considers only somatic etiologies would overlook a prevalent and possibly treatable psychiatric disorder,[44,48] particularly if associated symptoms of sadness, sleep disturbance, and anhedonia are assumed to be secondary to some yet-to-be-determined physical disease.

CASE EXAMPLE: DEPRESSION PRESENTING AS CHRONIC PAIN

Ms. L., a 54-year-old retired civil service worker, has a long-standing history of pelvic and abdominal pain, nausea, lack of energy, and sleep disturbance. She reports crying spells, feelings of worthlessness, and a sense that life is not worth living, all of which she relates to her pain. Medical evaluations and surgeries have consistently been nondiagnostic. She has a history of frequent emergency room visits for pain medication and is on disability.

Using the previously described interview style, the physician determined that the patient had a traumatic childhood history. She lost her father at age 10 and then experienced sexual abuse from her alcoholic stepfather. (Upon discussing these events, the patient clutched her abdomen and reported pain). Dysmenorrhea began at the time of menarche, and over the next 20 years pain episodes eventuated in appendectomy, hysterectomy, and cholecystectomy. She vehemently denied a role for these previous experiences in her current illness and urgently requested further diagnostic evaluation and medication for control of the pain.

A previous history of loss[51,52] and physical/sexual abuse[53,54] is common among patients presenting to referral centers for chronic pain syndromes. Psychologic assessments of these patients reveal a high prevalence of depression.[49,50] Depending on the severity of the depression, treatment may include psychologic therapy by the medical physician, psychiatrist, or other health care professional, antidepressants, or electroconvulsive therapy (ECT).

Ms. L. was informed that her long-standing history of pain and the negative studies to date preclude further extensive diagnostic evaluation; the focus should now be on treatment and adaptation to her chronic disorder. She was offered psychologic counseling to help her cope with the condition and refused. Ms. L. was also told that whatever the etiology of her pain, antidepressant medication provides a means of achieving pain control as well as relief of associated depressive symptoms such as fatigue and poor sleep.

She was started on 50 mg of doxepin, which was increased to 150 mg over 3 weeks. Monthly follow-up visits oriented toward improvement in function were scheduled. The sleep disturbance, fatigue, and sense of hopelessness improved, though she continued to report pain.

In this case, the patient had clinical evidence for *Dysthymic Disorder (300.40)* and benefited from antidepressants.[55] However, the long-standing history of pain and chronic illness precluded complete pain relief. Treatment was directed toward improved function and adaptation to the chronic illness.

ANXIETY DISORDER

CASE EXAMPLE

Ms. J., a 25-year-old secretary, has a 7-year history of irritable bowel syndrome characterized by abdominal cramps and diarrhea. She reports an increase in the frequency and severity of these symptoms over the previous 2 years, which has caused her to quit work and to severely restrict social activities and travel outside of the home. She feared that during an attack she would not be able to get to the bathroom in time. Upon further questioning, she reported that her IBS attacks have also been associated with feelings of panic: impending doom, palpitations, dizziness, "suffocation," and feeling out of control.

Like depression, anxiety denotes a broad spectrum of phenomena ranging from normal emotions to psychiatric syndromes. In either form, it is an unpleasant emotion accompanied by a sense of impending threat or danger from an unknown or irrational source. (When the source is known and realistic, the experience is called "fear.") It can be associated with a specific stimulus (e.g., phobia) or not (e.g., "free-floating" anxiety). When the anxiety becomes intense, frequent, and pervasive, or begins to disrupt mental and physical function, it requires clinical intervention.

Anxiety is associated with autonomic activation ("flight-fight" response), and symptoms of breathlessness, palpitations, chest or abdominal discomfort, diaphoresis, and diarrhea are common. Given these symptoms, it is the medical physician's role to consider the possibility of an anxiety episode in the differential diagnosis. If present, the physician should then determine if the episode is appropriate for the circumstances or represents a more disruptive and pervasive disorder requiring treatment.

The anxiety disorders can be diagnosed using DSM-III-R criteria.[56] *Panic Disorder (300.01)* is probably the most common anxiety disorder leading to medical visits, although it may be given other diagnoses (e.g., hyperventilation syndrome, functional hypoglycemia). It is characterized by recurrent unexpected episodes of panic associated with at least four of the following symptoms: shortness of breath, dizziness, palpitations, trembling, sweating, choking, nausea, depersonalization, paresthesias, flushes or chills, chest pain, fear of dying, and feeling out of control. When these episodes are associated with an avoidance of places or situations, the diagnosis is *Panic Disorder with Agoraphobia (300.21)*. Other medical conditions (e.g., hyperthyroidism, true hypoglycemia, partial complex seizures, cardiac disease with arrhythmias, pulmonary embolism) and, importantly, drug usage or withdrawal (e.g., amphetamines, caffeine, cocaine, marijuana, over-the-counter appetite suppressants, allergy medicines, and bronchodilators) must be excluded before a diagnosis of *Panic Disorder* can be made.

The high family prevalence and recent evidence for possible abnormalities in CNS function by way of noradrenergic, GABA, or benzodiazepine receptors[57] suggest a strong biologic contribution to anxiety disorder and its pathophysiology and treatment. Recently, benzodiazepines have been shown effective in short-term treatment,[58] but there is risk of withdrawal rebound. The tricyclic antidepressants are also effective[59] and are favored for long-term use. Behavioral treatments, such as relaxation response exercises with respiratory control and cognitive maneuvers designed to improve the patient's sense of control, also can help reduce the frequency and severity of panic attacks.[60]

Ms. J. was diagnosed as having *Panic Disorder with Agoraphobia* concurrent with irritable bowel. Panic disorder may be a specifically treatable subset of patients with irritable bowel.[61]

She was placed on alprazolam with prompt resolution of her panic episodes. After several weeks, she was switched to imipramine and began a 5-week course of relaxation training and cognitive-behavioral therapy to increase her sense of control during the episodes. After 6 months the antidepressants were stopped and she has continued to do well.

Several other anxiety disorders should be considered in medical patients.

Generalized Anxiety Disorder (300.02) is diagnosed when patients have chronic unrealistic or excessive anxiety about life circumstances (such as finances or health) usually associated with increased motor tension, autonomic hyperactivity, and increased vigilance. *Simple (300.29) or Social (300.23) Phobias* are characterized by persistent fear of an object or one or more situations. *Post-traumatic Stress Disorder (309.89)* is diagnosed when the patient has persistence or re-experiencing of a traumatic event outside the range of usual experience. Finally, *Obsessive Compulsive Disorder (300.30)* is diagnosed when the patient has either recurrent or persistent disease (obsessions) or repetitive behaviors in response to the obsession (compulsion). Treatment should be initiated when the disorder becomes pervasive or when there is impairment of social or occupational function.

SOMATIZATION—SOMATOFORM DISORDER

Somatization is the tendency to experience and communicate psychologic distress as somatic symptoms that the patient misinterprets as signifying serious physical illness.[62] Somatization can be situation-specific (e.g., "medical student syndrome"), present itself during times of anxiety, and can be influenced by cultural factors. For example, "imagined pain" in response to an anxiety-provoking situation is more likely to be reported by Western subjects than by Chinese or Scandinavians,[63] and Jews and Italians in Western society are more likely to report pain than Anglo-Americans and Irish.[64]

When somatization is associated with frequent health care visits and an unwillingness to be reassured in the presence of nondiagnostic evaluations, and psychologic determinants are presumed to contribute, a *Somatoform Disorder*[65] should be considered. These patients are at high risk for unneeded and possibly harmful diagnostic and therapeutic interventions.

CASE EXAMPLE

Ms. R. is a 46-year-old woman referred for evaluation of nausea, vomiting, abdominal bloating, and inability to tolerate most foods. She presents with a large packet of medical records and x-rays. She also sees a neurologist for unexplained syncope and an internist for a collagen disease that is difficult to diagnose. There is a past history of laminectomy for back pain, hysterectomy for chronic pelvic pain, and dilatations by a urologist for "urethral syndrome." Current medications include propranolol for "click-murmur" syndrome, alprazolam for "nerves," aspirin with codeine for migraine headaches, hydrochlorothiazide for "body swelling," a nonsteroidal anti-inflammatory agent for joint pain, and estrogen replacement.

Ms. R. has *Somatization Disorder (300.81)* characterized by a history of numerous physical complaints beginning early in life. Diagnosis is based on identifying at least 13 items from a large list of gastrointestinal, musculoskeletal, cardiopulmonary, pseudoneurologic, sexual, and female reproductive symptoms. Other somatoform disorders to consider among medical patients with negative medical evaluations include:

1. *Conversion Disorder (300.11):* Loss of physical functioning.
2. *Hypochondriasis (300.70):* Characterized by a history of at least 6 months' preoccupation with the fear of having a seri-

ous disease. It is based on an overinterpretation of physical signs or sensations as evidence for physical illness.
3. *Somatoform Pain Disorder (307.80):* At least a 6-month preoccupation with an unexplained pain.
4. *Undifferentiated Somatoform Disorder (300.70):* At least a 6-month history of one or more physical complaints (e.g., fatigue, loss of appetite, GI complaints) that do not fit with other *Somatoform* diagnoses.

With all categories, patients having medical or psychiatric (e.g., *Panic Disorder*) diagnoses (or who take drugs; see *Panic Disorder*) that explain these symptom items are excluded.

Treatment usually involves behavioral interventions that attempt to minimize the patient's tendency to communicate by way of bodily complaints[66] (see below).

FACTITIOUS DISORDER

Patients with factitious disorders simulate illness (e.g., ingest anticoagulants or blood, produce false elevation of temperature) in a manner not likely to be discovered.[67] Unlike malingering, where patients consciously feign illness for obvious gain (e.g., to obtain drugs, exemption from work, disability), the motives in these patients are more enigmatic: usually to assume or maintain the sick role.

CASE EXAMPLE

Ms. P., a 43-year-old nurses' aide, was hospitalized for evaluation of unexplained diarrhea, nausea, and vomiting. She is obese and also has difficult-to-treat type II diabetes mellitus. She requires hospitalization several times a year for dehydration and poor metabolic control.

On this hospitalization she was found to have a hypokalemic hypochloremic metabolic alkalosis, mild dehydration, and mild hyperglycemia. Stool volume was 800 ml/day and after fasting was still increased at 550 ml/day. A solid-phase gastric emptying study was abnormally delayed. Computerized tomography (CT) scan, upper endoscopy, and colonoscopy were negative. She received intravenous rehydration and was discharged on insulin, metoclopramide, and clonidine in an attempt to control her vomiting and diarrhea. On follow-up clinic visit 2 weeks later, her stool sample tested positive for phenolphthalein. She denied use of laxatives.

This patient, having *Factitious Disorder with Physical Symptoms (301.51)*, represents an important subgroup of gastroenterology patients: those with laxative-induced factitious diarrhea.[68,69] Generally, these patients are women who often work in health-related fields. A large proportion are younger women with eating disorders who take laxatives and/or diuretics to "control" body size. Another group, usually older women, take laxatives for less clear reasons, although in some manner they derive benefits from being ill.

Their surreptitious behavior often gets them extensively evaluated before the diagnosis is suspected. They are often referred to medical centers. In one series, 9 of 27 patients referred for evaluation of unexplained diarrhea were found to be surreptitious laxative users.[70]

Because all patients initially deny use of laxatives, diagnosis usually is based on detecting the offending substance by stool examination. Phenolphthalein-containing laxatives (e.g., Ex-Lax,

Correctol) turn pink with alkalinization of the stool or urine. The anthraquinones (e.g., senna, cascara) cause melanosis coli, which can be detected at sigmoidoscopy, and the osmotic laxatives (e.g., sodium phosphate) may be detected by stool analysis. Finally, if the patient is endangering her life, a room search may be ethically justified.

Disclosure of the findings must be done in a nonpunitive manner and only when the diagnosis is fully assured. It is best to identify the problem as a difficult-to-control compulsive disorder that requires treatment rather than to confront the patient for having unacceptable behavior. If, as is often the case, the patient refuses psychiatric help, the medical physician can continue to monitor the medical status. Patients who exhibit depressive features may benefit from antidepressant medication.

Are There Cultural or Ethnic Influences?

Explanatory models of illness are a useful framework to identify the meaning that a particular illness experience holds for an individual. As with Ms. J., explanatory models based on cultural or ethnic beliefs may modify clinical illness or even patient interactions with traditional health care systems. This information may not be volunteered to traditional health care professionals, although it may exist in many ethnic populations, including blacks, Hispanics, native Americans, and Gypsies.[71]

CASE EXAMPLE

Ms. Y., a 65-year-old woman admitted for prolonged fever and weight loss, was eventually found to have ulcerative colitis and chronic myelocytic leukemia. Diagnostic evaluation was complicated by the patient's repeated requests to have all diagnostic procedures discussed between the chief of each consultation service and her family (consisting of 20 to 30 members).

This patient's behavior was understood in the context of her being a Gypsy, a member of a cohesive cultural group possessing medical sophistication and a strong directive to negotiate only with the "big" doctor (baro). The problem was resolved by having the ward attending physician, the person acknowledged with the most authority, arrange for daily conferences with the family at the end of each day.

The physician must maintain a high index of suspicion for cultural effects and inquire about the patient's beliefs of the onset, pathophysiology, expected course, and desired or expected treatment.[28] Furthermore, to limit the meaning of illness and its treatments to biomedical processes excludes the possibility of simple and effective interventions. On one occasion, the author was able to eliminate a patient's chronic abdominal pain believed to be due to "roots" (voodoo) by engaging the activities of a root worker.

How Does the Family Interact Around the Illness?

The family provides the structure within which we learn about and interact around illness. For the most part, early experiences with illness are associated with appropriate family responses (to provide some attention and support with an orientation toward recovery and health), which carry through to adult life. However, undue focus on illness during childhood may affect later illness behaviors and the capacity for a healthy life-style. For example, patients with irritable bowel during childhood recalled having more school absences and physician visits and receiving more toys and other "rewards" when ill than persons without illness, other medical patients, or persons with IBS who did not see physicians.[72,73]

The previous case report of Mr. and Mrs. F. and their 16-year-old child describes a "psychosomatic family" in which the participants are closely attached to the illness as a means of maintaining family harmony. Minuchin[11] believes this occurs in emotionally linked ("enmeshed") families that do not effectively manage intrafamilial stresses. Instead, when family tensions arise, the afflicted child (having a disease such as diabetes, asthma, inflammatory bowel disease, or anorexia nervosa) becomes conditioned to divert attention from family distress by focusing on the activated illness. These children may have difficulty achieving autonomy and separating psychologically from the family environment, and these behaviors may be carried out into the adult family. Therefore, it is important to understand how the patient interacts with the family around the illness and vice versa. If the patient is married, the husband and wife should at some time be seen together, and inquiry should be made about how the spouse perceives and responds to the patient's illness. If healthy family behaviors are seen, then the family members can be recruited into helping the patient toward recovery.

What Are the Patient's Other Psychosocial Resources?

Psychosocial factors that promote health also need to be identified. For example, availability of social support such as church, recreational clubs, and community organizations directly affects a patient's perception of coping and plays a role in "buffering" the adverse effects of stress on physical and mental illness. Patients with good social support experience a better sense of control over their illness and report lower stress levels than occur in the absence of social support.[74] Coping, defined as "efforts, both action-oriented and intrapsychic, to manage (i.e., master, tolerate, minimize) environmental and internal demands and conflicts, which tax or exceed a person's resources,"[75] is another mediating psychosocial factor that helps to promote health. The perception of available social support and good coping strategies is of prognostic benefit.

How Far Do You Go in the Workup?

The decision to do additional diagnostic studies is based on the biologic and psychosocial data obtained from the initial evaluation. Abnormal findings (e.g., blood in stool, fever, abnormal liver chemistries, abdominal mass) ultimately determine whether further tests are needed. It is also important to consider tests with regard to their safety, their cost-effectiveness, whether the results will affect treatment, and, ultimately, the benefit to the patient. A common pitfall is to overdo diagnostic studies when the diagnosis is uncertain, particularly if the patient is insistent for the doctor to "do something." As a general rule, if the initial evaluation is negative, a patient with chronic unexplained symptoms ("functional disorder") is unlikely to have a new diagnosis made over several years of follow-up study.[76] However, it is also important to remain vigilant to new findings that will require further assessment.

When Do You Call the Psychiatric Consultant?

When psychologic factors are considered to strongly contribute to the illness (regardless of the medical diagnosis), a psychiatric consultation should be considered. Examples include (1) when a psychiatric diagnosis that would benefit from specific treatment is suspected, (2) situations in which the patient's level of psychosocial functioning is seriously impaired in the absence of a reasonable medical explanation, and (3) when invasive diagnostic or therapeutic strategies are being considered based on patient symptom reports and without substantial support from the medical data.

PSYCHOSOCIAL TREATMENT

Setting Up a Therapeutic Physician–Patient Relationship

In recent decades, the physician–patient relationship has begun to change from one in which the physician always assumes a dominant role to a more flexible arrangement, depending on the clinical context.[77] While the physician must take charge of medical emergencies, with chronic disease or illnesses in which psychosocial difficulties are predominant, the physician needs to encourage a relationship based on shared responsibility. This approach offsets the tendency for patients to assume more passive and dependent roles that impair psychologic growth, and it ameliorates the tendency for the physician to assume too much responsibility for patients' health care. A therapeutic physician–patient relationship is accomplished when the physician (1) elicits and validates the patient's beliefs, concerns, and expectations, (2) offers empathy when needed, (3) clarifies patient misunderstandings, (4) provides education, and, finally, (5) negotiates with the patient the plan of treatment.[30]

Modify Abnormal Illness Behaviors

Patients will vary in the degree to which abnormal illness behaviors affect the illness. The greater their influence, the more likely the patient will not respond to reassurance and traditional biomedical-oriented interventions. Several strategies to modify abnormal illness behaviors can be incorporated into the treatment plan.[5,43,78,79]

ACCEPT THE PATIENT'S DEFINITION OF THE ILLNESS WITHOUT CHALLENGING ITS REALITY

Because abnormal illness behaviors relate to the disparity between the patient's suffering and the degree of detectable pathology, the patient may perceive the absence of a biomedical etiology as an implication that the illness is imagined. This may lead the patient to request further diagnostic evaluation that is not indicated. It takes skill to address this issue in a manner that is consistent with the physician's assessment yet doesn't challenge the patient's reality. For example, consider the patient who urgently requests that an unneeded CT scan be done to rule out cancer. Rather than trying to "convince" the patient that "nothing is wrong" (by pathologic standards), the physician should acknowledge the patient's (and physician's) concern that cancer not be overlooked. Then, the physician should firmly state that, based on the clinical data, this test is not indicated but would be done if. . .(e.g., certain laboratory tests become abnormal, and so forth). It is also important to avoid ambiguous behaviors that feed into patient doubts or fears (e.g., to order studies "just to be sure"). This approach should be supported by continuing to show interest and being available through routine follow-up appointments.

LIMIT DISCUSSION OF PSYCHOLOGIC ISSUES TO WHAT THE PATIENT IS ABLE OR WILLING TO ACCEPT

Patients with abnormal illness behavior are unable or unwilling to report feeling states or acknowledge a relationship between psychologic stresses and their symptoms.[80,81] Therefore, offering "insight" about the possible role of psychologic factors in the illness is usually rejected by the patient. It is best to reframe the discussion to be consistent with the patient's frame of reference. For example, if a behavioral intervention or use of a psychoactive drug is indicated, the rationale can be explained as a means of helping the patient cope with the psychologic distress or dysfunction encumbered by the illness.

INCREASE PATIENT CONTROL OVER THE SYMPTOMS

Patients with chronic, unexplained, or psychosocially determined illness often give up the responsibility for their health care (e.g., by decreasing physical activity and relying upon prescription medication for relief of symptoms). Patients should be encouraged to develop self-initiated treatments such as progressive physical exercise and relaxation techniques and to distract themselves from focusing on illness by developing hobbies or returning to work.

I often find it helpful to have the patient keep a diary that identifies the intensity and quality of the symptoms and the environmental factors (e.g., diet, stress, activity, and so forth) that cause symptom flare-ups.[82] This approach encourages the patient to take control by finding the triggers of symptom onset and by determining possible strategies that will ameliorate future occurrences. The physician becomes more of an advisor and facilitator.

USE ATTENTION TO REINFORCE HEALTHY BEHAVIORS

The patient with abnormal illness behavior receives certain needs (e.g., attention, privileges) by focusing on symptoms and communicating suffering. These maladaptive behaviors are reinforced in the medical setting, where health care professionals are trained to respond supportively to illness-contingent behaviors. The physician must modify these responses by refocusing attention toward healthier behaviors. Generally, this involves minimizing diagnosis and symptomatic treatment and rewarding the patient's ability to adapt to and function in the presence of the illness. Some examples follow:

1. Do not ask how the patient feels; ask what the patient has accomplished (despite the symptoms). This reinforces the patient's need to increase activity and divert attention from the illness.
2. When the patient reports information relating to the illness or suffering, maintain a neutral manner and do not ask the patient to elaborate. If the information suggests a need for further medical evaluation, act accordingly. Most often, this is not the case, so when the patient finishes, redirect the inquiry toward management: "I see, and have you still been able continue your household activities?"
3. Use nonverbal reinforcement when the patient reports healthy behaviors. For example, if the patient shifts the discussion to mention how he/she has taken on new activities, encourage the patient to elaborate by leaning forward, nodding, and smiling.
4. Do not set the patient up to fail. If the patient proposes the idea of beginning an exercise program or taking on a new hobby, do not say, "That's a great idea, I'm sure you can do it." If the task is not done, the patient may perceive himself to be a failure. You might instead say, "Given your pain, it will be a difficult task, but well worth the effort. I'm pleased to hear that you're thinking of ways to get yourself better."

This same approach can be used in therapy involving the family, where relatives are taught to selectively encourage the patient's efforts to cope with the symptoms while ignoring relapses of illness reporting.

TIME MANAGEMENT

At the end of a visit, it is not unusual for a patient to occasionally bring up new symptoms. The physician may feel a bit resentful of staying late but usually accedes in order to permit the patient the opportunity to air his/her concerns. However, if this pattern occurs repeatedly, the physician should consider whether the behavior reflects certain psychosocial issues (e.g., concerns about loss or rejection, need to be in control, somatization). If so, this pattern can be corrected by setting up a "contract" for regular visits (e.g., 20 minutes every 4 weeks) in which the patient is requested to bring up the most important concerns first. When the appointment is about to end, the patient should be reminded that there are about 5 minutes left, and he/she should summarize. If time runs out and the patient continues to talk, the physician can indicate nonverbally that the visit has ended (e.g., close up the chart, shift to get up) and mention that what isn't finished can be brought up the next time. If the patient still continues to speak, the physician can quietly state that the visit has ended and begin to stand up. If the physician is consistent in this approach, the patient will accept the time-structured visit, provided the physician maintains a commitment to continuing care.

Pharmacotherapy

Psychopharmacologic agents may be indicated for treatment of a primary psychiatric disorder or as an adjunct to medical treatment in patients with gastrointestinal complaints.

ANTIDEPRESSANTS

The tricyclic antidepressants (TCA) and the monamine oxidase inhibitors (MAOI) are the principal agents used for treatment of major depressive disorder but are also indicated for patients with chronic pain (by way of excitation of corticofugal pain inhibitory pathways),[55,83] panic attacks,[59] or eating disorders,[84] or for depressive symptoms associated with medical illness. Regardless of disease etiology, their use should also be considered for patients who exhibit "vegetative" signs of depression: poor appetite and weight loss, sleep disturbance, decreased energy and libido (activities subserved by central brain monoamine function), or deterioration in functional status (e.g., inability to work or maintain usual social or home management activities).

The choice of an antidepressant will often depend on its known side effects. The tertiary amine class of TCA drugs (e.g., amitriptyline, doxepin) has theoretic benefit in providing pain control (by way of facilitation of endogenous serotonin release). They also help promote sleep and can be given as a single nighttime dose. Desipramine and nortriptyline have less anticholinergic and sedative effects. A new agent, fluoxetine, appears to have fewer side effects in general and may not cause weight gain or fluid retention. The MAOIs (e.g., tranylcypromine, phenelzine) are second-line agents that are generally safe but require the patient to restrict certain drugs (e.g., decongestants) and tyramine-containing foods (e.g., fermented cheeses, wine, beer, processed meats). Patients can be worked up to full therapeutic levels over 2 to 3 weeks and maintained for 3 to 6 months. A poor clinical response often relates to the tendency for physicians to use relatively low dosages or not to initiate appropriate dosage increases.[85]

ANXIOLYTICS

The most frequently used agents for treatment of anxiety are the benzodiazepines (e.g., diazepam, lorazepam, alprazolam). Their amelioration of the behavioral consequences of fear and anxiety make them effective for short-term treatment of acute anxiety, and they may be prescribed as an adjunct for patients with stress-induced flare-ups of bowel disturbance. The benefit of benzodiazepines for patients with chronic anxiety disorders must be balanced with the long-term risks: sedation, drug interactions, habituation, and symptom rebound upon withdrawal. Overall, their benefit in treating patients with chronic gastrointestinal disturbances remains to be proved. Furthermore, they may be contraindicated for patients with chronic pain and depression. They have the potential to decrease serotonin levels and lower pain thresholds and, by stimulation of gamma-aminobutyric acid (GABA) receptors, may actually contribute to depression.[86] Newer antianxiety agents such as buspirone, which do not act on the benzodiazepine receptor, may have fewer short- and long-term side effects.[87]

ANTIPSYCHOTIC DRUGS

Also called major tranquilizers or neuroleptics, the phenothiazines (e.g., chlorpromazine) and butyrophenones (e.g., haloperidol) produce improvement in disordered thought, perception, and behavior in psychotic patients. They have limited value in treating medical patients, although they have been used for nighttime sedation and to treat acute episodes of agitation or the effects of alcohol withdrawal.

OPIATES

These agents have little or no role in treating patients with chronic pain or psychosocial disorders because of their potential for abuse and dependency.

Behavioral Treatments

Behavioral treatments generally are safe, noninvasive, and cost-effective methods that can be performed by psychologists, behaviorally trained social workers, nurses, and physicians. Efficacy data from controlled clinical trials relating to patients with gastrointestinal disorders are limited. However, studies involving patients with chronic pain suggest that these techniques may help to: (1) reduce anxiety levels, (2) teach patients how to engage in health-promoting behaviors, (3) give the patient greater responsibility ("ownership") and control in the treatment, and (4) improve pain control.

GENERALIZED TREATMENTS

Generalized behavioral treatments include stress management and methods of relaxation to elicit a state of passive relaxation. The *relaxation response* is associated with reduced sympathetic nervous system activity and muscle relaxation. It can be facilitated through a variety of ancillary techniques, including *biofeedback, meditation,* and *autogenic training*. The process is relatively simple and generally requires: (1) a quiet and comfortable environment and (2) the ability of the person to focus on an image, word, or phrase, thereby removing distractions. A modification of the relaxation response is *systematic desensitization*, a method of "defusing" phobic responses. The patient exposes him/herself to a series of increasingly fearful situations until the dysfunctional response is ameliorated. This technique has been successfully used in a patient with protracted vomiting.[88] Cognitive–behavioral therapy is effective for patients with bulimia[89] and other compulsive disorders. It involves: (1) identifying stressors, (2) recognizing thoughts

that increase distress, and (3) learning new ways of coping with the stress by restructuring the thoughts.

SPECIFIC BEHAVIORAL TREATMENTS

Biofeedback is a technique in which physiologic activity is monitored and unconscious physiologic information is provided by audio or visual instruments so that the patient can gain control over these functions. The technique is effective for fecal incontinence.[90,91] *Transcutaneous nerve stimulation (TENS Unit), physical exercise,* and *acupuncture* are methods often used for control of chronic pain. Their effects may be due to stimulation of inhibitory pain pathways or release of endogenous opioids.

BEHAVIORAL MODIFICATION

Withdrawal From Narcotics
Narcotic abuse is a common problem for patients with chronic pain and other functional disorders. Efforts to gradually reduce narcotic medication on an outpatient basis or to maintain the patient on a fixed dose of medication are usually unsuccessful. My approach, as modified from Fordyce,[79] involves gradual reduction of medication that is given on a noncontingent basis in the inpatient setting. The patient must understand and agree to all aspects of the following protocol, except for the percentage and timing of the dose reduction:

1. The patient's medication requirement (given orally) and the dosage interval are observed over a 48 to 72–hour period.
2. Upon beginning withdrawal, the patient's required daily dose is converted to methadone or another long-acting narcotic to avoid the "soar–crash" effect on blood levels of shorter acting narcotics.
3. The drug is administered in a fixed volume, color, and taste-masked vehicle (e.g., total volume of 10 ml in cherry-flavored syrup base) to minimize visual or taste cues of dosage reduction.
4. A short dose frequency is used to sustain blood levels (q.6h. is sufficient for methadone), and the medication is given on a noncontingent (i.e., fixed frequency) basis.
5. A tricyclic antidepressant is begun for pain control.
6. The active drug dose is gradually reduced by 10% every 1 to 3 days while maintaining the same volume.
7. Clonidine 0.1 mg twice daily is given to minimize physiologic withdrawal effects.
8. Recreational activity including daily physical exercise is continued throughout the hospitalization.

Bowel Retraining
Bowel retraining can be recommended for patients with habit constipation due to poor bowel training or laxative abuse. The technique assumes that the patient has lost the normal physiologic response to the "call to stool" and there is no underlying organic disturbance in bowel function:

1. All stimulant laxatives are discontinued.
2. The patient is prescribed daily a high-fiber diet or fiber supplement and an osmotic cathartic (e.g., milk of magnesia or lactulose).

3. The patient establishes a 15- to 20-minute distraction-free period (usually in the morning) to sit on the commode.
4. Prior to this time, the patient eats breakfast and drinks coffee or tea to stimulate the bowels.
5. While on the commode, the patient should read for relaxation and, if a smoker, may have a cigarette. There should be no obligation to "perform"; the effort is to identify a time at which bowel function can naturally resume.
6. If the patient does not have a bowel movement in 72 hours, an enema is taken.

Psychotherapy

Referral for psychotherapy should be made when: (1) the patient is diagnosed as having a treatable psychiatric disorder (e.g., major depression, panic disorder, psychosis), (2) the illness has impaired the patient's psychologic or social functioning, or (3) the patient is motivated to improve his/her psychologic condition and to find ways to achieve stress reduction or improve coping strategies. Psychologic treatment must be seen by the patient as relevant to personal needs and as part of an overall treatment plan. The patient who is referred after a negative medical evaluation or who goes to "prove I'm not crazy" is not likely to be helped.

The form of psychotherapy chosen can be individualized. For the psychologically minded patient, insight-oriented therapy may be considered. The patient with limited finances who is able to share personal thoughts with others may benefit from group therapy. Crisis intervention (three to five sessions designed to get the patient over a particularly difficult period) can help the patient who experiences identifiable causes for recent exacerbation. Family or marital counseling is indicated when difficulties in the family interaction contribute to the illness state or to the patient's maladaptive behavior.

Physician Considerations

Patients who have unexplained complaints or underlying psychosocial disturbances can be taxing to physicians, particularly when they don't "fit" a medical diagnosis and do not respond to traditional treatment. Their potential effects upon physician judgment and behavior can be understood in terms of the generic issues that they raise:

DIAGNOSTIC UNCERTAINTY

Physicians are uncomfortable with diagnostic uncertainty[92] and strive to make a pathologic diagnosis, expecting that such knowledge will make the patient's illness understandable and easily treatable. However, the largest proportion of patients seen by gastroenterologists have symptoms with "no known structural or metabolic causes"[93] (i.e., functional disorders), and follow-up studies for several years are equally unrevealing.[76] Lack of diagnostic certainty after an adequate evaluation should alert the physician to consider other (particularly psychosocial) determinants of the illness. Assuming the patient is at no immediate risk, it is

wiser to accept a diagnosis of "functional" disorder and refocus efforts from diagnosis to identifying and modifying the factors that exacerbate the illness.

WITH NO DISEASE, IS THE ILLNESS REAL?

It has been said, "To have pain is to have certainty; to hear about pain is to have doubt."[94] Patients can surmise when the physician does not believe that their complaints are legitimate. The absence of a pathologic diagnosis does not preclude the degree of discomfort and suffering that these patients experience; it merely requires the physician to focus on symptoms management and adaptation.

DON'T REACT

Some patients develop controlling or overdependent relationships, demand counterproductive services from physicians (e.g., for unneeded narcotics, disability), or become adversarial when physicians too quickly expect them to become symptom-free. It is important to understand these behaviors as part of the patient's illness. Physicians can use their inner thoughts and feelings (e.g., "What is it about this patient's behavior that makes me angry?") as barometers and reduce the tendency to overreact (e.g., to blame or stigmatize patients as "crocks," "turkeys," or "gomers"). "Furor medicus" describes the response of physicians to demanding patients (like Ms. S.) who may heighten physician feelings of uncertainty, ineffectiveness, or failure. In one study,[10] emergency room patients having multiple previous operations and demanding behaviors when compared to patients with acute emergencies were overmedicated and received more unneeded and potentially harmful procedures. The physicians in the study acknowledged suspending their usual clinical judgment to respond to the patients' insistent behavior. While it is important to remain vigilant to new diagnostic and therapeutic possibilities, the decision to undertake them should be based on objective assessment of the data rather than patient demands. When in doubt, "Don't just do something, stand there!"[78]

RESET TREATMENT GOALS

Despite some patients' expressed intent to be well, adaptations develop that, at least in the beginning, interfere with clinical improvement, and some patients never get better. The physician must reset treatment goals from cure to coping with chronic illness. The patient can be informed that it is unrealistic to expect rapid and complete relief when the condition has existed for so long, but it is reasonable to work toward improvement in sleep or functional status *despite* the symptoms.

SET PERSONAL LIMITS

Each physician must determine the commitment to make for patients who may be demanding of time and energy. The frequency and length of office visits should be established and adhered to. Some patients take a dependent, regressed role in the physician-patient relationship and place responsibility for treatment with the physician. Here, the physician must encourage the patient to take an active role in the health care (e.g., to make choices in the treatment). Not only will the patient develop a more mature health-oriented behavior, but the burden of responsibility is lifted from the physician. Finally, some physicians feel unable or unwilling to work on improving the psychosocial aspects of the illness.[95] When indicated, appropriate referral is recommended.

The reader is directed to Chapter 29, Approach to the Patient with Chest Pain; Chapter 32, Approach to the Patient with Unexplained Weight Loss; Chapter 33, Approach to the Patient with Nausea and Vomiting; Chapter 34, Approach to the Patient with Abdominal Pain; Chapter 38, Approach to the Patient with Diarrhea; Chapter 80, Irritable Bowel Syndrome; Chapter 130, Psychiatric Evaluation and Management in Gastrointestinal Illness; and the corresponding chapters in the Atlas.

REFERENCES

1. Brody H, Sobel DS. A systems view of health and disease. In: Lee PR, Estes CL, Ramsay NB, eds. The nation's health. San Francisco: Boyd & Fraser Publishing, 1984:73.
2. Reading A. Illness and disease. Med Clin North Am 1977;61:703.
3. Engel GL. The need for a new medical model: A challenge for biomedicine. Science 1977;196:129.
4. Engel GL. The clinical application of the biopsychosocial model. Am J Psychiatry 1980;137:535.
5. Drossman DA. The physician and the patient: Review of the psychosocial gastrointestinal literature with an integrated approach to the patient. In: Sleisenger MH, Fordtran JS, eds. Gastrointestinal disease: Pathophysiology, diagnosis, management. Philadelphia: WB Saunders, 1989:3.
6. Von Bertalanffy L. General system theory. New York: Braziller, 1968.
7. Drossman DA. Psychosocial aspects of ulcerative colitis and Crohn's disease. In: Kirsner JB, ed. Inflammatory bowel disease. Philadelphia: Lea & Febiger, 1988:209.
8. Loeser JD. Perspectives on pain. In: Proceedings of the First World Conference on Clinical Pharmacology and Therapeutics. London: MacMillan, 1980:313.
9. Parsons T. The social system. New York: Free Press of Glencoe, 1951.
10. Devaul RA, Faillace LA. Persistent pain and illness insistence—A medical profile of proneness to surgery. Am J Surg 1978;135:828.
11. Minuchin S. Psychosomatic families: Anorexia nervosa in context. Cambridge: Harvard University Press, 1978.
12. Engel GL. Psychologic stress, vasodepressor (vasovagal) syncope, and sudden death. Ann Intern Med 1978;89:403.
13. Ader R. Psychoneuroimmunology. New York; Academic Press, 1981; 1–661.
14. Mitchell CM, Drossman DA. Letter: Survey of the AGA membership relating to patients with functional gastrointestinal disorders. Gastroenterology 1987;92:1282.
15. Drossman DA. Clinical research in the functional digestive disorders. Gastroenterology 1987;92:1267.
16. Drossman DA, Sandler RS, McKee DC, Lovitz AJ. Bowel patterns among subjects not seeking health care. Use of a questionnaire to identify a population with bowel dysfunction. Gastroenterology 1982;83:529.
17. Smith GP. Satiety effect of gastrointestinal hormones. In: Beers RF Jr, Bassett EG, eds. Polypeptide hormones. New York: Raven Press, 1980:413.
18. Geracioti TD Jr, Liddle RA. Impaired cholecystokinin secretion in bulimia nervosa. N Engl J Med 1988;319:683.
19. Pulliam TJ, Bradley LA, Dalton CB, Salley AN, Richter JE. Role of psychological stress in gastroesophageal reflux disease (GERD). Gastroenterology 1989;96:A401.
20. Drossman DA, McKee DC, Sandler RS, et al. Psychosocial factors in the irritable bowel syndrome. A multivariate study of patients and nonpatients with irritable bowel syndrome. Gastroenterology 1988;95:701.
21. Whitehead WE, Bosmajian L, Zonderman AB, Costa PT Jr, Schuster MM. Symptoms of psychologic distress associated with irritable bowel syndrome. Comparison of community and medical clinic samples. Gastroenterology 1988;95:709.
22. Drossman DA, Patrick DL, Mitchell CM, Zagami EW, Appelbaum MI. Health related quality of life in inflammatory bowel disease: Functional status and patient worries and concerns. Dig Dis Sci 1989; 34:1379.
23. Dorian B, Garfinkel PE. Stress, immunity and illness—A review. Psychol Med 1987;17:393.
24. Ader R, Cohen N. Behaviorally conditioned immunosuppression and murine systemic lupus erythematosus. Science 1982;215:1534.
25. MacQueen G, Marshall J, Perdue M, Siegel S, Bienenstock J. Pavlovian conditioning of rat mucosal mast cells to secrete rat mast cell protease II. Science 1989;243:83.
26. Schleifer SJ, Keller SE, Camerino M, Thornton JC, Stein M. Suppression of lymphocyte stimulation following bereavement. JAMA 1984;250:374.
27. Kiecolt-Glaser JK, Stephens RE, Lipetz PD, Speicher CE, Glaser R. Distress and DNA repair in human lymphocytes. J Behav Med 1985;8:311.
28. Rosen G, Kleinman A. Social science in the clinic: Applied contributions from anthropology to medical teaching and patient care. In: Carr JE, Dengerink HA, eds. Behavioral science in the practice of medicine. New York: Elsevier, 1983:85.
29. Roter DL, Hall JA. Physicians' interviewing styles and medical information obtained from patients. J Gen Intern Med 1989;2:325.
30. Lipkin M. The medical interview and related skills. In: Branch WT, ed. Office practice of medicine. Philadelphia: WB Saunders, 1987.
31. Morgan WL Jr, Engel GL. The approach to the medical interview. In: Morgan WL Jr, Engel GL, eds. The clinical approach to the patient. Philadelphia: WB Saunders, 1969:26.
32. Platt FW, McMath JC. Clinical hypocompetence: The interview. Ann Intern Med 1979;91:898.
33. Smith RC. Teaching interviewing skills to medical students: The issue of "countertransference". J Med Educ 1988;59:582.
34. Dimatteo MR, Prince LM, Taranta A. Patients' perceptions of physicians behavior: Determinants of patient commitment to the therapeutic relationship. J Community Health 1979;4:280.
35. Buccini R, Drossman DA. Chronic idiopathic abdominal pain. Curr Concepts Gastroenterol 1988;12:3.
36. Drossman DA. Treatment of the patient with irritable bowel syndrome. In: Bayless T, ed. Current therapy in gastroenterology and liver disease. Toronto: BC Decker, 1989; 166–170.
37. Barsky AJ. Hidden reasons some patients visit doctors. Ann Intern Med 1981;94:492.
38. Mechanic D. The concept of illness behavior: Culture, situation and personal predisposition. Psychol Med 1986;16:1.
39. Mechanic D. The concept of illness behavior. J Chron Dis 1962;15: 189.
40. McHugh S, Vallis TM. Illness behavior: A multidisciplinary model. New York: Plenum Press, 1986:1.
41. Pilowsky I. A general classification of abnormal illness behaviors. Br J Med Psychol 1978;51:131.
42. Pilowsky I. Abnormal illness behavior. Br J Med Psychol 1969;42: 347.
43. Blackwell B, Gutmann M. The management of chronic illness behaviour. In: McHugh S, Vallis TM, eds. Illness behavior: A multidisciplinary model. New York: Plenum Press, 1986:401.
44. Katon W. Depression: Relationship to somatization and chronic medical illness. J Clin Psychiatry 1984;45:4.
45. Marshland DW, Wood M, Mayo F. Content of family practice: II. Diagnosis by disease category and age/sex distribution. J Fam Pract 1976;3:37.

46. Drossman DA. Depression and the gastrointestinal disorders. Clinical Advances in the Treatment of Depression 1987;1:8.

47. American Psychiatric Association. Mood disorders. In: Diagnostic and statistical manual of mental disorders—revised. Washington, DC: American Psychiatric Association, 1987:213.

48. Davis TC, Nathan RG, Cash MN. Diagnosing depression in primary care: A practical, interdisciplinary review and a call for change. South Med J 1986;79:1273.

49. Hendler N. Depression caused by chronic pain. J Clin Psychiatry 1984;45:30.

50. Kramlinger KG, Swanson DW, Maruta T. Are patients with chronic pain depressed? Am J Psychiatry 1983;140:747.

51. Hill OW, Blendis L. Physical and psychological evaluation of 'non-organic' abdominal pain. Gut 1967;8:221.

52. Drossman DA. Patients with psychogenic abdominal pain: Six years' observation in the medical setting. Am J Psychiatry 1982;139:1549.

53. Walker E, Katon W, Harrop-Griffiths J, Holm L, Russo J, Hickok LR. Relationship of chronic pelvic pain to psychiatric diagnoses and childhood sexual abuse. Am J Psychiatry 1988;145:75.

54. Drossman DA, Leserman J, Nachman G, et al. Sexual and physical abuse among women with functional and organic gastrointestinal disorders. Ann Int Med, in press.

55. Hameroff SR, Weiss JL, Lerman JC, et al. Doxepin's effects on chronic pain and depression: A controlled study. J Clin Psychiatry 1984;45:47.

56. American Psychiatric Association. Anxiety disorders. In: Diagnostic and statistical manual of mental disorders—revised. Washington, DC: American Psychiatric Association, 1987:235.

57. Anixter WL. Panic disorder and agoraphobia: An update for primary care physicians. N C Med J 1988;49:507.

58. Ballenger JC, Burrows GD, DuPont RL. Alprazolam in panic disorder and agoraphobia: Results from a multicenter trial. I. Efficacy in short-term treatment. Arch Gen Psychiatry 1988;45:413.

59. Liebowitz MR. Imipramine in the treatment of pain disorders and its complications. Psychiatr Clin North Am 1985;8:37.

60. Tyrer P. Treating panic. Psychological treatments are preferable to drug treatments. Br Med J 1989;298:201.

61. Lydiard RB, Laraia MT, Howell EF, Ballenger JC. Can panic disorder present as irritable bowel syndrome? J Clin Psychiatry 1986;47:470.

62. Lipowski ZJ. Somatization: The concept and its clinical application. Am J Psychiatry 1988;145:1358.

63. Moore R, Miller ML, Weinstein P, Dworkin SF, Liou HH. Cultural perceptions of pain and pain coping among patients and dentists. Community Dent Oral Epidemiol 1986;14:327.

64. Zborowski M. Cultural response to pain. J Soc Issues 1952;8:16.

65. American Psychiatric Association. Somatoform disorders. In: Diagnostic and statistical manual of mental disorders—revised. Washington, DC: American Psychiatric Association, 1987:255.

66. Ford CV. The somatizing disorders. Psychosomatics 1986;27:327.

67. American Psychiatric Association. Factitious disorder. In: Diagnostic and statistical manual of mental disorders—revised. Washington, DC: American Psychiatric Association, 1987:315.

68. Cummings JH, Sladen GE, James OFW, Sarner M, Misiewics JJ. Laxative-induced diarrhoea: A continuing clinical problem. Br Med J 1974;537.

69. Ewe K, Kerbach U. Factitious diarrhea. Clin Gastroenterol 1986;15:723.

70. Read NW, Krejs GJ, Read MG, Santa Ana CA, Morawski SG, Fordtran JS. Chronic diarrhea of unknown origin. Gastroenterology 1980;78:264.

71. Thomas JD. Gypsies and American medical care. Ann Intern Med 1985;102:842.

72. Lowman BC, Drossman DA, Cramer EM, McKee DC. Recollection of childhood events in adults with irritable bowel syndrome. J Clin Gastroenterol 1987;9:324.

73. Whitehead WE, Winget C, Fedoravicius AS, Wooley S, Blackwell B. Learned illness behavior in patients with irritable bowel syndrome and peptic ulcer. Dig Dis Sci 1982;27(3):202.

74. Cohen S, Syme SL. Issues in the study and application of social support. In: Cohen S, Syme SL, eds. Social support and health. New York: Academic Press, 1985.

75. Lazarus RS, Folkman S. Stress, appraisal and coping. New York: Springer Publishing Co, 1984:1.

76. Svendsen JH, Munck LK, Andersen JR. Irritable bowel syndrome: Prognosis and diagnostic safety. A 5-year follow up study. Scand J Gastroenterol 1985;20:415.

77. Szasz TS, Hollender MH. The basic models of the doctor-patient relationship. Arch Intern Med 1956;97:585.

78. Drossman DA. The problem patient: Evaluation and care of medical patients with psychosocial disturbances. Ann Intern Med 1978;88:366.

79. Fordyce WE. Behavioral methods in medical practice. In: Karasu TB, Steinmuller RI, eds. Psychotherapeutics in medicine. New York: Grune & Stratton, 1978:83.

80. Keltikangas-Jarvinen L. Concept of alexithymia: I. The prevalence of alexithymia in psychosomatic patients. Psychother Psychosom 1985;44:132.

81. Papciak AS, Feuerstein M, Belar CD, Pistone L. Alexithymia and pain in an outpatient behavioral medicine clinic. Int J Psychiatry Med 1986;16:347.

82. Shimberg EF. Relief from IBS. New York: M. Evans and Co, 1988:1.

83. Ward NG, Bloom VL, Friedel RO. The effectiveness of tricyclic antidepressants in the treatment of coexisting pain and depression. Pain 1979;7:331.

84. Herzog DB, Brotman AW, Bradburn IS. Treating eating disorders with antidepressants. Aust Paediatr J 1988;24:169.

85. Cakkues AL, Popkin MK. Antidepressant treatment of medical-surgical inpatients by nonpsychiatric physicians. Arch Gen Psychiatry 1987;44:157.

86. Hendler N. The anatomy and psychopharmacology of chronic pain. J Clin Psychiatry 1982;43:15.

87. Rakel R. Assessing the efficacy of antianxiety agents. Am J Med 1987;82(suppl 5A):1.

88. Latimer PR, Malmud LS, Fisher RS. Gastric stasis and vomiting: Behavioral treatment. Gastroenterology 1982;83:684.

89. Leitenberg H, Rosen JC. Cognitive-behavioral treatment of bulimia nervosa. Prog Behav Modif 1988;23:11.

90. Latimer PR. Biofeedback and behavioral approaches to disorders of the gastrointestinal tract. Psychother Psychosom 1981;36:200.

91. Whitehead WE, Schuster MM. Behavioral approaches to the treatment of gastrointestinal motility disorders. Med Clin North Am 1981;65:1397.

92. Fox RC. Training for uncertainty. In: Merton R, Reader D, Kendall T, eds. The student physician. Cambridge: Harvard University Press, 1957:207.

93. Mitchell CM, Drossman DA. Survey of the AGA membership relating to patients with functional gastrointestinal disorders. Gastroenterology 1987;92:1282.

94. Scarry E. The body in pain: The making and unmaking of the world. New York: Oxford University Press, 1985.

95. Strain JJ, Hamerman D. Ombudsmen (medical-psychiatric) rounds. An approach to meeting patient-staff needs. Ann Intern Med 1978;88:550.

28

Approach to the Patient with Dysphagia

DONALD O. CASTELL

INTRODUCTION

The word "dysphagia" is derived from the Greek *phagia* (to eat) and *dys* (with difficulty). It specifically refers to the sensation of food being hindered in its normal passage from the mouth to the stomach. Patients with dysphagia most frequently complain that food "sticks," "hangs-up," "gets caught," or "just won't go down right." They may occasionally complain of some associated pain, but the symptom of dysphagia should not be used interchangeably with odynophagia, or pain on swallowing. The importance of the clinical history in suggesting the etiology of esophageal causes of dysphagia cannot be overstated. When Schatzki first described the lower esophageal ring that bears his name, he asserted that a careful history should give the physician a strong suspicion of the right diagnosis in 80% to 85% of patients with dysphagia. Although Schatzki was referring to what we now classify as esophageal dysphagia, that statement helps to emphasize the critical importance of the medical history in clarifying the cause of this symptom.[1]

GLOBUS

A generally accepted clinical "truth" is that dysphagia almost always indicates the presence of an organic dysfunction. It is important, therefore, not to confuse dysphagia with "globus hystericus," the sensation of a lump, fullness, or "tickle" in the throat. Globus is usually a more constant symptom that typically does not interfere with swallowing and, in fact, may be relieved during deglutition. As the name implies, globus hystericus has long been considered a symptom occurring in patients having hysterical personality traits. This is probably not an appropriate indictment since psychologic evaluations have revealed an increase in depression[2] and obsessive-compulsive tendencies[3] in patients with globus, but little evidence of hysterical traits. Thus, the term *globus* or globus sensation is preferable.

It is also important to recognize that symptoms consistent with the diagnosis of globus might also occur in patients with organic esophageal disease. The diagnosis of globus should never be made without a thorough investigation for a lesion in the pharynx, larynx, or neck. A hypertensive upper esophageal sphincter (UES) has

been described in association with the globus sensation in some patients.[4] The true importance of this observation, however, is not clear at present because older manometric techniques, as used in a study of only nine patients, record UES pressure values of questionable accuracy. It has also been suggested that increases in UES pressure might occur in some globus patients secondary to reflux of gastric acid into the upper esophagus. Some patients with gastroesophageal reflux present with a variety of complaints, including chronic cough, hoarseness, and globus sensation.[5] Laryngeal abnormalities typically found with reflux, such as inflammation of the vocal cords, may also be associated. Specific testing for reflux with intraesophageal pH monitoring may confirm this diagnosis and the symptoms may resolve with appropriate antireflux therapy. These observations support the conclusion that a diagnosis of globus is appropriate only after organic esophageal pathology has been excluded, particularly gastroesophageal reflux.

CLASSIFICATION

Dysphagia is usually readily divided into two distinct syndromes, that produced by abnormalities affecting the finely tuned neuromuscular mechanism of the striated muscle of the mouth, pharynx, and upper esophageal sphincter (oropharyngeal dysphagia), and that due to any one of the variety of disorders affecting the smooth muscle esophagus (esophageal dysphagia).

Oropharyngeal dysphagia is usually described as an inability to initiate the act of swallowing. It is a *transfer* problem, due to impaired ability to transfer food from mouth to upper esophagus or due to an impaired oral preparatory phase. Affected patients present with a variety of complaints including food sticking in the throat, difficulty initiating a swallow, nasal regurgitation, and coughing during swallowing. They may also complain of dysarthria or may display nasal speech because of associated muscle weaknesses. A wide variety of local, neurologic, and muscular diseases can produce oropharyngeal dysphagia (Table 28-1). Usually, the dysphagia is only one of the manifestations of a relatively obvious disease process and does not pose a diagnostic problem.[6]

A variety of neuromuscular (motility) defects or mechanical obstructing lesions can cause esophageal dysphagia (Table 28-2), producing difficulty with the *transport* of ingested material down

TABLE 28-1
Abnormalities Causing Oropharyngeal Dysphagia

A. Neuromuscular diseases
  Central nervous system (CNS)
    Cerebral vascular accident (brain stem or pseudobulbar palsy)
    Parkinson's disease
    Wilson's disease
    Multiple sclerosis
    Amyotrophic lateral sclerosis
    Brain stem tumors
    Tabes dorsalis
    Miscellaneous congenital and degenerative disorders of CNS
  Peripheral nervous system
    Bulbar poliomyelitis
    Peripheral neuropathies (diphtheria, botulism, rabies, diabetes mellitus)
  Motor end plate
    Myasthenia gravis
  Muscle
    Muscular dystrophies
    Primary myositis
    Metabolic myopathy (thyrotoxicosis, myxedema, steroid myopathy)
    Amyloidosis
    Systemic lupus erythematosus
B. Local structural lesions
  Inflammatory (pharyngitis, abscess, tuberculosis, syphilis)
  Neoplastic
  Congenital webs
  Plummer-Vinson syndrome
  Extrinsic compression (thyromegaly, cervical spine hyperostosis, lymphadenopathy)
  Surgical resection of the oropharynx
C. Motility disorders of the upper esophageal sphincter (UES)
  Hypertensive UES ("globus," "spasm")
  Hypotensive UES (esophagopharyngeal regurgitation)
  Abnormal UES relaxation
    Incomplete relaxation (Cricopharyngeal achalasia; CNS lymphoma; Cricopharyngeal bar)
    Premature closure (Zenker's diverticulum?)
    Delayed relaxation (familial dysautonomia)

the esophagus. Careful analysis of the history usually allows the physician to categorize patients into one of these two main groups.

PATHOPHYSIOLOGIC CONSIDERATIONS

Normal swallowing involves both voluntary and involuntary skeletal muscle activity. In the *oral phase*, solid food is first prepared by the muscles of the jaw, face, and tongue into a bolus of suitable size and consistency. With the initiation of swallowing the lips are closed, the front of the oral cavity is sealed by the tip of the tongue, the mandible is fixed, and the hyoid bone is elevated. The bolus is contained within a trough created by the muscles of the tongue. The reflex (involuntary) actions of swallowing then take over and continue until the bolus has been transferred to the upper esophagus, less than 1 second later.[7-11] This is the *pharyngeal phase* of swallowing. The swallowing center in the medulla can be activated by either the cerebral cortex (voluntary swallowing) or by afferent impulses from the mouth and oropharynx (reflex swallowing). After the swallowing center is activated, the entire

sequence of the involuntary swallowing mechanism is played out to produce the transfer of the bolus from the oropharynx to the esophagus.

The swallowing reflex involves sensory input to the medullary swallowing center by way of the V, X, and XI cranial nerves and motor activity transmitted through the V, VII, IX, X, and XII cranial nerves. Respiration is inhibited centrally and the airway is closed by a series of muscular actions that produce elevation of the larynx under the base of the tongue, approximation of the true and false vocal cords, infolding of the aryepiglottic folds and the epiglottis in concert with further elevation and anterior displacement of the larynx.[12] These actions have recently been shown to result in orad movement of the UES during swallowing.[13]

Disorders of the Pharyngeal/UES Pressure Dynamics

Swallowing difficulties are not uncommon and represent a major cause of disability in patients with neurologic and neuromuscular disorders and in the elderly.[14] Pharyngeal dysphagia is a nonspecific symptom that may result from dysfunction in the complex mechanism of contraction and relaxation of the pharynx and UES. Abnormal function of the UES has been described in a variety of conditions,[15-17] but case reports have been few in number and all too often the manometric data upon which the definition of abnormality has been based were derived by methods now considered to be obsolete and invalid.

Pharyngeal dysphagia may occur in a variety of neurologic abnormalities, including acute stroke, amyotrophic lateral sclerosis,

TABLE 28-2
Etiology of Esophageal Dysphagia

A. Neuromuscular (motility) disorders
  Most common
    Achalasia
    Scleroderma
    Diffuse esophageal spasm
  Other associated motility abnormalities
    Nutcracker esophagus
    Hypertensive lower esophageal sphincter
    Vigorous achalasia
    Nonspecific esophageal motility disorders
  Other secondary motility disorders
    Other collagen disorders
    Chagas' disease
B. Mechanical lesions—intrinsic
  Most common
    Peptic stricture
    Lower esophageal (Schatzki's) ring
    Carcinoma
  Other
    Esophageal webs
    Esophageal diverticula
    Benign tumors
    Foreign bodies
C. Mechanical lesions—extrinsic
  Vascular compression
  Mediastinal abnormalities
  Cervical osteoarthritis

Huntington's disease, Parkinson's disease, myasthenia gravis, and muscular disorders such as polymyositis and myotonic dystrophy.[18-20] In these patients, swallowing disorders may contribute to life-threatening aspiration. Objective studies of the swallowing mechanism in these patients suffer from the lack of adequate technology for pharyngeal and UES manometry and from insufficient information on normal physiologic parameters, particularly for patients in the age groups afflicted by many of these neurologic and neuromuscular disorders.

An assortment of other possible abnormalities of pharyngeal/UES function are described in the medical literature. Increased resting UES pressure has been described in "spasm" of the cricopharyngeus, associated with a "hypopharyngeal bar" seen radiographically, in patients with globus sensation and in patients with hiatal hernia and reflux.[15,21,22] Lower UES pressures have been reported in patients with esophagopharyngeal reflux, many of whom had chronic heartburn.[23,24] Three types of abnormality in UES relaxation may occur: incomplete relaxation, delayed relaxation, and premature closure.[25,26] The term *cricopharyngeal achalasia* has been used to refer to all these abnormalities but is perhaps better reserved specifically for the disorder of incomplete relaxation.

Cricopharyngeal achalasia has been described as an isolated phenomenon in children[27,28] and in adults secondary to cerebrovascular accident affecting the brain stem, bulbar poliomyelitis, stiff-man syndrome, thyrotoxic myopathy, oculopharyngeal muscular dystrophy, and sometimes partial or total laryngectomy.[15,29] A review of adult patients with cricopharyngeal achalasia reveals that it is primarily a problem of the elderly.[28] Patients with familial dysautonomia (Riley-Day syndrome) may have a number of disturbances related to autonomic function, including sucking and swallowing difficulty, which is usually present from birth.[30] Radiologic studies have shown delayed opening of the cricopharyngeus with normal pharyngeal motor activity.[31] No manometric evidence for incoordination of this type has been reported.

Zenker's diverticulum is an outpouching of one or more layers of the esophageal wall located immediately above the upper esophageal sphincter. The earliest symptoms may be transient preesophageal dysphagia. When the pharyngeal sac becomes large enough to retain food, patients develop the more classic symptoms of persistent cough, fullness in the neck, gurgling in the throat, postprandial regurgitation, and aspiration. Some diverticula become so large that patients must perform various maneuvers such as applying pressure on the neck and repeatedly coughing to empty them. These sacs can become large enough to produce a visible mass in the neck or to obstruct the esophagus by compression.

The pathogenesis of these diverticula is controversial. Both radiographic and manometric studies of patients with Zenker's diverticula have suggested that premature closure of the cricopharyngeus plays a role. Careful manometric studies have not so far resolved this issue, since groups of patients have been reported in which all,[32] some,[33] or none,[34] showed premature UES closure. There has been general agreement that UES resting pressure is, if anything, lower than normal. A recent manometric study using more refined techniques has failed to show any discoordination between pharyngeal contraction and UES relaxation.[34] In addition, there has never been a report of a patient with premature closure of the UES without an associated diverticulum who subsequently developed one.

Disorders of Esophageal Smooth Muscle

Esophageal dysphagia can result from a variety of structural or neuromuscular defects in the smooth muscle portion of the esophagus and the lower esophageal sphincter. Conceptually, dysphagia is likely with either of two generic mechanisms. The first is that which is due to any condition producing obstruction to luminal flow, including rings, strictures, carcinoma, extrinsic masses, and muscular contractions in the esophageal body (diffuse spasm) or LES (achalasia). The second mechanism for esophageal dysphagia is failure of peristalsis (achalasia; scleroderma) or disruption of the normal peristaltic progression (diffuse spasm). Further details of pathophysiology will be discussed with specific conditions.

HISTORY AND PHYSICAL EXAMINATION

As noted, the patient with oropharyngeal dysphagia usually describes trouble initiating a swallow; he or she has difficulty in the transfer of food from the mouth or pharynx back into the esophagus. Associated phenomena include nasal regurgitation, coughing during swallowing, dysarthria, and nasal speech due to palate weakness. Other features that may be present and that should be important diagnostic clues are the presence of a speech disorder or any evidence of cranial nerve deficits, limb weakness, and changes in sleep pattern, including sleep apnea or recent onset of snoring. Dysphagia is usually only part of the symptom complex in patients with oropharyngeal dysphagia, and the primary diagnosis is usually apparent. Other symptoms may include the recent onset of a stroke or the development of weakness due to some kind of muscular disease. This is in contrast to esophageal dysphagia in which dysphagia is usually the prominent manifestation.

Motility defects of the hypopharynx are usually mild or moderate and are due to progressive weakness of the functions of the mouth and pharynx combined with atrophy of the musculature. The patient can usually compensate for these abnormalities, except in sleep, when labial spill of saliva occurs. When the patient is questioned, fatigue may be an important symptom noted. Gradually progressive pharyngeal dysphagia resulting from progressive muscular impairment may lead to changes in dietary preferences or prolonging of meals. Obviously, any patient presenting with oropharyngeal dysphagia deserves a careful neurologic examination and evaluation of the pharynx and larynx, including direct laryngoscopy.

When approaching the patient with apparent esophageal dysphagia, a careful evaluation of the history is equally important. Three important questions are particularly crucial: (1) What kind of food (liquid or solid) produces the symptom? (2) Is the dysphagia intermittent or progressive? (3) Is there associated heartburn? On the basis of these symptoms, it is often possible not only to identify the etiology as either a mechanical or neuromuscular defect but also to postulate which of the three major causes in each of these two subdivisions is the more likely diagnosis. An algorithm for the historical aspects of the common causes of esophageal dysphagia is shown in Figure 28-1. The additional associated symptoms of chest pain and nocturnal coughing can be valuable additions to this diagnostic approach.[35]

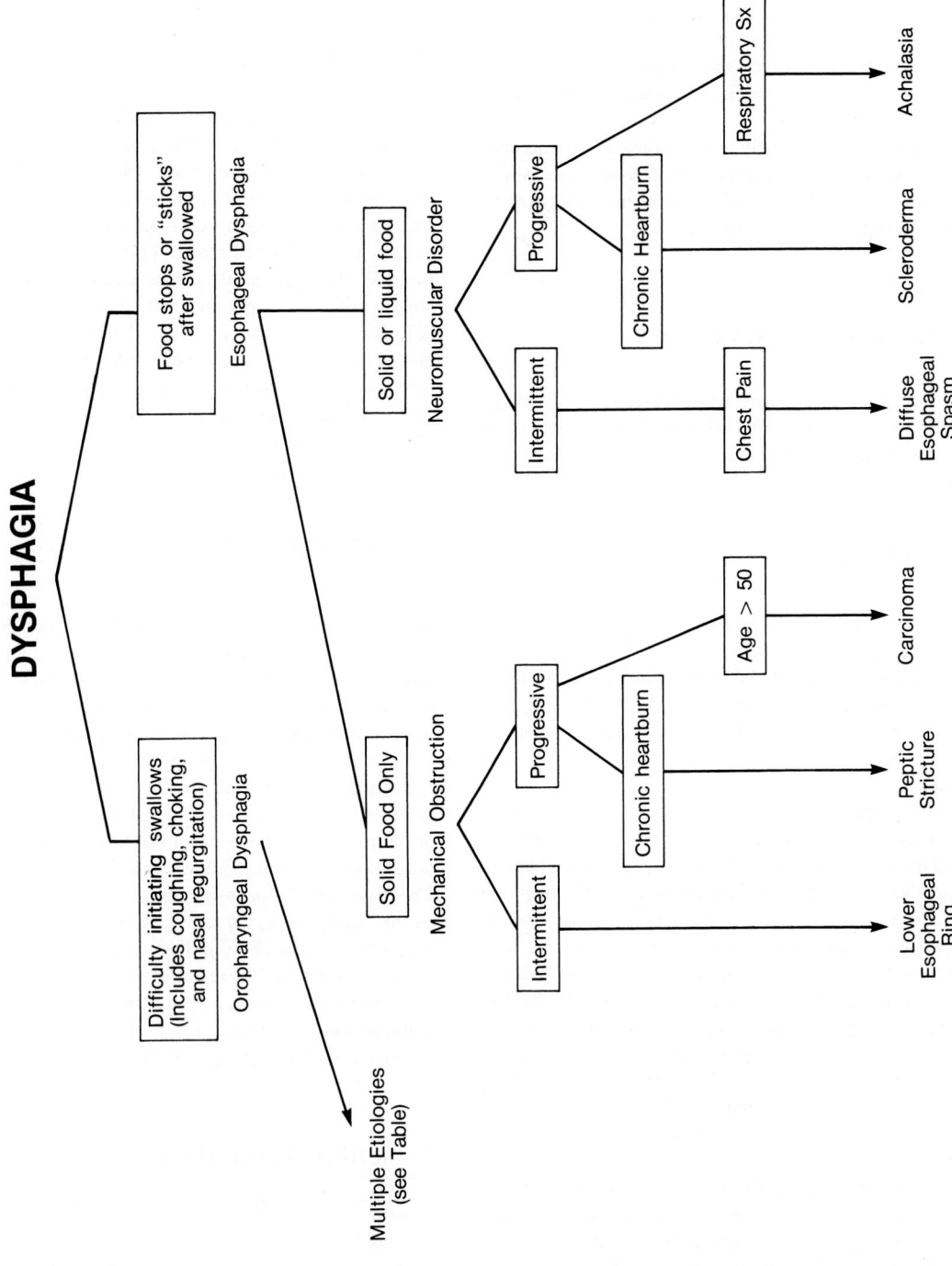

FIGURE 28–1. Diagnostic algorithm indicating the important aspects of the patient's history, distinguishing important subdivisions and specific etiologic possibilities in patients presenting with dysphagia.

Patients with motility disorders usually complain of slowly progressive dysphagia for both liquids and solids from the onset. Conversely, patients with mechanical obstruction usually have dysphagia initially for solids only and more progressive symptoms, although the onset is occasionally sudden. The exception is the lower esophageal ring, in which the dysphagia is not usually progressive.

The site at which the patient localizes his or her symptoms is of limited value. Whereas symptoms in the epigastric or retrosternal areas frequently correspond to the site of obstruction, dysphagia localized by the patient to the neck is frequently referred from below.[36]

Physical examination is usually not revealing in patients with esophageal dysphagia, with the exception of scleroderma, in which other manifestations of CREST syndrome (calcinosis, Raynaud's, sclerodactyly, telangiectasia) may be present.

CLINICAL PRESENTATION

The clinical presentation of patients with oropharyngeal dysphagia is discussed in the previous section. Details of clinical aspects of conditions causing esophageal dysphagia are discussed below.

Rings and Webs

Patients who have only *intermittent dysphagia for solids* most frequently are noted to have either rings or webs. A mucosal ring at the junction of the esophageal and gastric mucosa is commonly referred to as a Schatzki's ring or B ring. Microscopically, the mucosa of the upper surface of the ring is stratified squamous epithelium (esophageal) with columnar epithelium (gastric) on its underside.

Although the incidence of B rings is reported to be up to 14%, most are asymptomatic. Symptoms generally occur only when the intraluminal diameter is less than 13 mm.[37] Symptomatic patients have a distinctive clinical history. Characteristically, the dysphagia is episodic and not progressive. The first episode usually occurs while the person is eating a hurried meal and notes that a bolus of food has stuck in the lower esophagus. This is frequently a piece of steak, and is called *steakhouse syndrome*. Bread is another food that frequently precipitates symptoms. The patient can occasionally force the bolus through by drinking liquids, but frequently must regurgitate to relieve the obstruction. After doing so, he or she is usually able to continue the meal without difficulty. Dysphagia that occurs every day is not likely to be caused by a lower esophageal ring.

The diagnosis can essentially be made by this history, although barium studies are needed to confirm this impression. The radiographic study usually shows the typical thin, symmetric invagination in the distal 3 to 5 cm of the esophagus (Fig 28-2A). It is crucial to recognize the importance of distending the barium-filled distal esophagus by having the patient perform a Valsalva maneuver and possibly including a solid bolus during the examination to clearly identify the lesion. Further endoscopic identification may be desired.

The other ring of the lower esophagus is called a muscular, contractile, or A ring. These occur less frequently than B rings and are rarely symptomatic. When present, symptoms are identical with those of B rings. In contrast to mucosal rings, muscular rings appear on barium esophagrams as broad constrictions a few centimeters above the squamocolumnar junction.

Peptic Stricture

If the solid food dysphagia is clearly progressive, then the major differential diagnosis is between peptic esophageal stricture and carcinoma. Patients with peptic stricture usually have a long antecedent history of heartburn and chronic antacid use combined with intermittent dysphagia, although some patients have dysphagia as their presenting complaint. This solid food dysphagia is progressive. Radiographically, these strictures are smooth, vary in length, and usually present in the lower third of the esophagus (Fig 28-2B). Evaluation should always include endoscopy with biopsy and cytology to exclude carcinoma. A peptic stricture located more proximally in the esophagus strongly suggests a diagnosis of Barrett's esophagus, metaplastic changes (columnar epithelium) in the mucosa secondary to chronic reflux esophagitis.

Esophageal Carcinoma

Patients with squamous carcinoma of the esophagus differ from those with peptic stricture in several ways. As a group, the cancer patients are older and have a history of rapidly progressive dysphagia. They frequently do not have the long history of heartburn, but the chance association of reflux may occur. The exception to this rule is the patient with Barrett's esophagus secondary to chronic reflux disease who develops an adenocarcinoma in the metaplastic epithelium. Patients with esophageal cancer frequently have anorexia and have a more significant weight loss than the severity or duration of their dysphagia would support. Heavy alcohol and tobacco use are associated with esophageal squamous carcinoma. The diagnosis of esophageal carcinoma can be strongly suggested by the history alone, but radiography is the main method of initial diagnosis (see Fig 28-2C). The tumors may be infiltrative, polypoid, or ulcerative. These patients should all undergo endoscopy with biopsy and cytology to confirm the diagnosis. Recently, CT scanning has been shown to be useful to identify the extent of the lesion around the esophagus and to evaluate potential resectibility.

Vascular Anomalies

Several vascular anomalies produce dysphagia by compression of the esophagus. The most common complete vascular rings reported to cause dysphagia are, in order of frequency, (1) double aortic arch, (2) right aortic arch with retroesophageal left subclavian artery and left ligamentum arteriosum, and (3) right aortic arch with mirror-image branching and left ligamentum arteriosum. The most common incomplete rings are (1) retroesophageal right aberrant subclavian artery (arteria lusoria) and (2) anomalous left

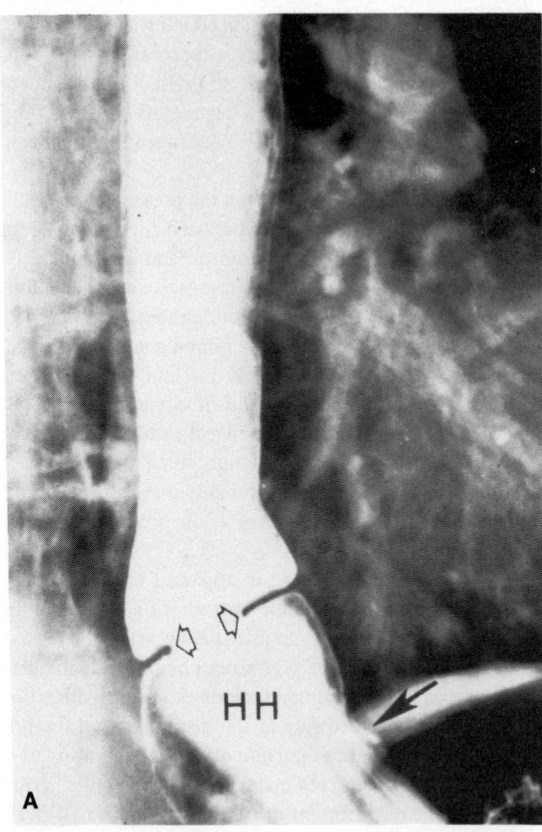

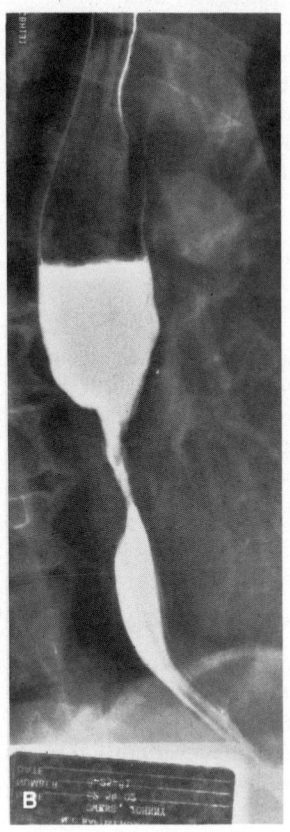

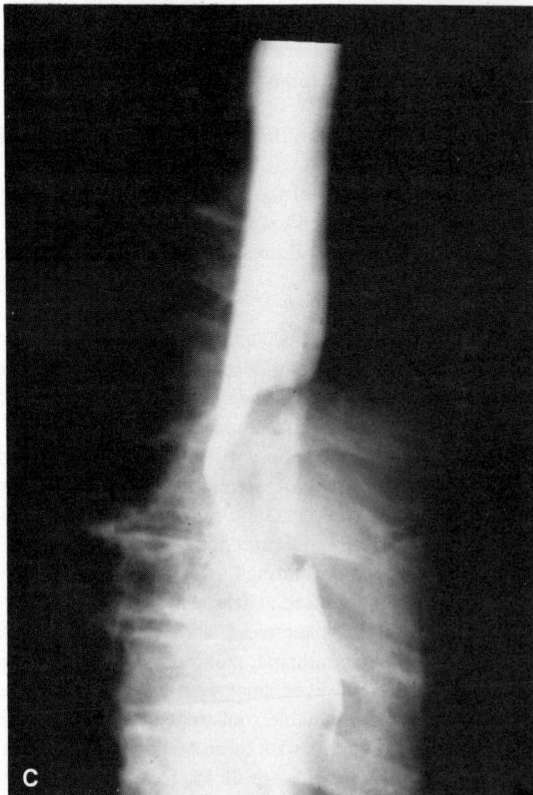

FIGURE 28–2. **A,** Barium swallow in a patient with a typical lower esophageal B ring (Schatzki's ring). Arrow indicates level of the diaphragm, and identifies the hiatal hernia (*HH*). **B,** Typical barium swallow appearance in a patient with peptic stricture of a distal esophagus. **C,** Barium swallow from a patient with esophageal squamous carcinoma.

pulmonary artery. The dysphagia associated with these lesions (so-called *dysphagia lusoria*) usually presents early in childhood, although occasionally symptoms may present in the adult.

The incidence of arteria lusoria is about 0.75%, but clinically important obstructive manifestations are unusual. When present, the dysphagia is usually a constant, daily problem, described as a temporary arrest of a solid bolus beneath the manubrium.

Dysphagia Aortica

Dysphagia aortica includes impingement upon the thoracic esophagus by a massive thoracic aortic aneurysm or compression of the anatomically restricted distal esophagus between a rigid atherosclerotic aorta posteriorly and the heart or the ventral margin of the esophageal hiatus anteriorly. As expected, this is a disorder of the elderly with the average age at diagnosis in the 70s.

Cervical Hypertrophic Osteoarthropathy

Dysphagia secondary to compression of the esophagus by hypertrophic spurs of the anterior portion of cervical vertebrae is unusual, considering the frequency of cervical osteoarthritis. The most common complaint is difficulty swallowing solid foods, but patients also complain of odynophagia, a foreign-body sensation, cough, hoarseness, or an urge to clear the throat. Diagnosis can be made by barium esophagram (lateral view), although careful endoscopy should be performed to exclude intraluminal pathology.

Mediastinal Abnormalities

Dysphagia may occur owing to a variety of pathologic processes resulting in mediastinal adenopathy, including bronchial carcinoma and sarcoidosis.

Achalasia

If the patient has dysphagia for liquids as well as solids, a motility disorder is the most likely cause.[38] More specific details on esophageal motility disorders are provided in Chapter 54. Idiopathic achalasia is an esophageal motility disorder characterized clinically by slowly progressive dysphagia and regurgitation of ingested foods. There are two major defects in achalasia: (1) obstruction of the esophagogastric junction and (2) abnormal esophageal peristalsis. Based on early radiographic studies, the obstruction was initially felt to be due to spasm of the cardia or lower esophageal sphincter (LES); hence the term *cardiospasm*. Later, manometric studies showing absence of relaxation of the LES with swallowing resulted in the term *achalasia*. Currently available manometric techniques have shown that the LES abnormality is indeed dual.

Motility studies often demonstrate increased resting LES pressures that display incomplete relaxation, producing a considerable functional obstruction. In addition, there is aperistalsis of the esophageal body. The pathophysiology involves a defect in the innervation of the esophagus and LES due to degeneration of ganglion cells in Auerbach's plexus. A specific etiologic agent has not been demonstrated.

There are significant variations in the presentation of achalasia. The majority of patients present between the age of 20 and 40, although the disease occurs in children and in the elderly. The most common initial complaint is progressive dysphagia for either liquids or solids. Regurgitation of undigested food that had been eaten many hours previously is a common complaint, particularly at night when it may result in aspiration and nocturnal coughing. Patients may occasionally complain of odynophagia early in the course of the disease. Gastroesophageal reflux is rare because of the "superprotective" LES, although some patients describe a symptom similar to heartburn, probably due to the marked dilatation and stasis in the esophagus or acidic products from bacterial fermentation of retained food.[39]

Diagnosis of achalasia is often apparent on routine chest radiograph; likely findings include absence of a gastric air bubble, mediastinal widening with a double shadow created by the dilated esophagus, and evidence of aspiration pneumonia. Characteristic features on barium esophagram include esophageal dilatation with a smoothly tapered narrowing at the distal end and the presence of a fluid level in the upper portion due to the retention of esophageal secretions and ingested material. The "beaklike" symmetric narrowing of the distal end of the esophagus helps to differentiate achalasia from the more ragged appearance of carcinoma in the distal end of this organ.

Manometry is the preferred method to make the diagnosis of achalasia and reveals the following:

1. Absence of peristalsis in the body of the esophagus ("aperistalsis")
2. Incomplete relaxation of the LES
3. Hypertensive LES (> 45 mm Hg) ("cardiospasm")
4. Elevated intraesophageal pressure (greater than intragastric pressure)

The diagnosis of idiopathic achalasia should not be considered conclusive until a thorough endoscopic evaluation of the esophagogastric junction has been made, including a retroflexed view from within the stomach to rule out infiltrating carcinoma of the cardia. The ability of the endoscope to easily "pop through" the tight LES and the absence of nodularity or mucosal defects are important findings to help exclude cancer in this area mimicking achalasia. Unfortunately, the presence of the characteristic x-ray, motility, and endoscopic findings of achalasia may occasionally be seen in carcinoma-induced achalasia syndromes that have been associated with gastric, pancreatic, and oat cell (bronchogenic) carcinoma as well as lymphoma, making the need for endoscopy even more crucial.[40] However, since even biopsies can be negative, the history may be a valuable tool to separate this entity from primary achalasia. Patients with these "secondary achalasia" syndromes are usually over the age of 55, have a short duration of dysphagia (< 1 year), and present with significant weight loss (greater than 15 pounds).

Progressive Systemic Sclerosis (PSS)

The other major motility disorder that presents with slowly progressive dysphagia for liquids and solids is that seen with PSS or scleroderma. Esophageal involvement occurs in more than 80% of patients with PSS and correlates best with the presence of Raynaud's phenomenon.[41,42] A similar association of Raynaud's and esophageal dysfunction is seen in mixed connective tissue disease (MCTD).

The motility defects are marked diminution of peristalsis in the lower two thirds (smooth muscle) of the esophagus and hypotension of the LES, but with normal contraction pressures in the upper one third (striated muscle) and a normal UES. Dysphagia may be a major complaint, but heartburn is usually a more prevalent symptom, separating these patients from those with achalasia. Severe reflux results in stricture in up to 40% of these patients.[43]

Chagas' Disease

South American trypanosomiasis, or Chagas' disease, caused by infestation with *Trypanosoma cruzi* represents an infectious process in which the chronic esophageal form presents symptoms and laboratory findings indistinguishable from achalasia. This disease, which occurs in Central and South America, may be associated with megacolon, megaduodenum, or megaureter.

Diffuse Esophageal Spasm (DES) and Related Syndromes

Symptomatic diffuse esophageal spasm is a disorder of esophageal motility associated clinically with dysphagia or chest pain. It is important to stress that this diagnosis should not be made without clinical symptoms because the radiographic, and even some of the motility, findings can be seen in asymptomatic persons. The cause of the disorder is unknown, although the functional abnormalities of the esophagus suggest both muscular and neural defects.

A number of observations suggest that DES and achalasia are related: (1) a positive methacholine (Mecholyl) test may occur in both conditions; (2) manometric transformation from DES to achalasia has been documented; and (3) many patients have manometric components of both diseases, most typical in those patients with a diagnosis of "vigorous achalasia."

The dysphagia of DES usually occurs with liquids or solid food, and is variable. It is usually intermittent and nonprogressive, and occasionally associated with pain—features separating it from the other motility disorders. Patients may report that a variety of factors may precipitate dysphagia or chest pain, including ingesting hot or cold foods or carbonated beverages, or being exposed to stress.

The barium esophagram reveals simultaneous, nonperistaltic contractions with resultant segmentation of the barium column. This has led to a variety of descriptive terms that attempt to depict the spectrum of findings from mild serration of the margin of the esophagus ("tertiary contractions") to frank subdivision of the esophageal outline ("rosary bead esophagus") to marked tortuosity of the esophagus ("corkscrew esophagus"). No distal beaking or dilatation is noted.

The manometric findings are shown below:

A. Major findings
1. Increased simultaneous (nonperistaltic) contractions (> 10% of wet swallows)
2. Intermittent normal peristalsis
B. Associated abnormalities
1. Repetitive wave peaks (> 2 peaks/wave)
2. Increased duration of contractions (> 6 sec)
3. Spontaneous contractions
4. High amplitude (> 180 mm Hg) contractions
5. Lower esophageal sphincter defects
   a. Increased resting pressure
   b. Incomplete relaxation

A number of other abnormalities of esophageal motility are frequently identified in patients presenting with dysphagia or chest pain that cannot be easily categorized into the more traditional diagnoses discussed above. The symptom patterns in these patients—intermittent dysphagia and chest pain or both—are similar to those in patients with DES. Some of these entities are described here.

NUTCRACKER ESOPHAGUS

Brand and colleagues first reported the finding of manometric patterns characterized by high amplitude peristaltic contractions in patients with noncardiac chest pain.[44] Benjamin and coworkers confirmed these observations and coined the term "nutcracker esophagus" for these strong peristaltic contractions in patients with dysphagia or chest pain or both.[45] Subsequently, this manometric diagnosis has been identified in large numbers of similar patients with reports from many areas of the United States.[46–49]

The nutcracker esophagus represents the prototype of newer esophageal motility abnormalities now recognized as a result of improved technology and better understanding of the range of normal esophageal pressures. By definition, the nutcracker esophagus is a descriptive term for the manometric finding in a patient with chest pain or dysphagia of distal esophageal peristaltic pressures greater than the upper limit of normal, best defined as average pressures greater than 180 mm Hg with durations frequently greater than 6.0 seconds.

HYPERTENSIVE LOWER ESOPHAGEAL SPHINCTER

Code and colleagues first described the manometric finding of hypertensive lower esophageal sphincter in patients with chest pain or dysphagia or both.[50] It is characterized by resting lower esophageal sphincter pressure exceeding the upper limit of normal (usually > 45 mm Hg) associated with normal sphincter relaxation and with normal peristalsis in the body of the esophagus. The majority of these patients also demonstrate the high amplitude peristaltic contractions seen in the nutcracker esophagus. Radiographic and scintigraphic studies usually have found normal esophageal function without bolus retardation at the level of the lower esophageal sphincter. Manometric studies using a more quantitative assessment of sphincter relaxation have revealed some degree of abnormality of relaxation of the lower esophageal sphincter in these patients.[51]

VIGOROUS ACHALASIA

In patients with vigorous achalasia, the manometric features show a combination of those expected for both diffuse esophageal spasm and achalasia. The features of achalasia that may be found include an increased resting LES pressure or incomplete relaxation, whereas the features of DES are simultaneous, repetitive contractions in the body of the esophagus. This combination differs from DES with LES abnormality in that patients with DES intermittently have normal peristaltic waves. In patients with vigorous achalasia, peristalsis is absent and only nonpropagated (simultaneous) waves are found.

NONSPECIFIC ESOPHAGEAL MOTILITY DISORDERS

A variety of other abnormalities may be found during esophageal motility testing in patients with dysphagia or chest pain. Also, these patients have no evidence of other systemic disease to explain the motility abnormalities. The manometric tracings in these patients show a variety of nonspecific findings that do not occur during wet swallows in normal subjects. These may include increased percentage of nontransmitted contractions (> 20%), prolonged duration of contractions (longer than 6 seconds), triple-peaked contractions, retrograde contractions, average distal esophageal contraction amplitudes less than 30 mm Hg, or the combination of absent distal peristalsis with normal LES function. The term *nonspecific esophageal motility disorder* (NEMD) is often used to categorize these manometric findings.

ASSESSMENT

Traditionally the preferred diagnostic test in patients with oropharyngeal dysphagia is a barium swallow. Because of the rapid sequence of pressure changes and movement of anatomic structures in this region, special techniques must be employed for adequate study. Videotaping of a series of swallows with radiographic projections in the anteroposterior and lateral directions provide imaging information that can be replayed at slower speed for careful diagnostic assessment. The videotaped sequences at 30 frames per second can be assessed separately to identify abnormalities of movement of the various anatomic structures and muscle activities in the mouth, pharynx, and UES. A "modified" barium swallow is performed with the addition of thick barium and a solid bolus, usually a small marshmallow. These techniques improve the overall assessment of the ability of the patient to normally transfer food from mouth to esophagus.

Older manometric technologies are grossly inadequate for proper study of pressure events in this area. This has led to the general consensus that pharyngeal/UES manometry is of little or no value in the study of the normal process of swallowing or in patients with swallowing disorders. The technologic limitations of catheters used in the past have included the measurement of pressure limited by either infused systems that would underestimate pharyngeal contractions and might provide pressure distortion in studying sitting patients or recording orifices directed in one orientation that could not properly measure asymmetric UES contraction. In addition, the rapid sequence of changes in pressures occurring during the act of swallowing have made the manual analysis of the timing of these pressure events difficult. Because of these technical deficiencies, it has been the consensus of investigators in this field that radiographic studies are the preferred, if not the only, effective technique for studying pharyngeal/UES interrelationships during swallowing.

The development of improved techniques for measuring pharyngeal and UES pressures and pressure dynamics during swallowing has now allowed more quantitative assessment of these functions in health and disease. By the use of entire solid state transducer systems or the combination of solid state pharyngeal transducers and sleeve recording sensors spanning the UES, more accurate pressures and coordination sequences during swallowing are obtainable. With the development of on-line computer analysis of the rapid pressure changes occurring in this area with swallowing, the technology has advanced to a stage at which subtle changes in pressure dynamics can be identified and categorized.

Evaluation of the patient with esophageal dysphagia should begin with a barium swallow as the initial screening test. It is particularly important to ask the radiologist to give a solid bolus (usually a marshmallow) to assess the ability of the patient to swallow solids. If the initial barium swallow suggests an obstructing lesion in the esophagus, endoscopy and possibly biopsy should follow. If, on the other hand, the radiograph is negative or otherwise suggests a motility disorder, an esophageal motility study should be performed. A more detailed discussion on esophageal manometrics studies is presented in Chapter 128. A radionuclide esophageal emptying study of a solid meal can be helpful to provide quantitation of transit function throughout the esophagus (Fig 28-3).

THERAPEUTIC CONSIDERATIONS

Pharyngeal Dysphagia

Therapeutic manipulations in patients with impaired swallowing due to pharyngeal dysphagia include altering the patient's head position and body position and altering the food consistency and bolus size. Based on the observations made during the modified barium swallow these positional and mechanical modifications are individualized to help overcome the patient's swallowing deficit. Through consultation with a speech pathologist a rehabilitation program can be developed. Additional techniques such as thermal stimulation for assisting these patients are being developed. Thermal stimulation uses the principle that lowering the temperature of the pharyngeal mucosa enhances the sensory aspects of the pharyngeal reflex during swallowing. This is accomplished by

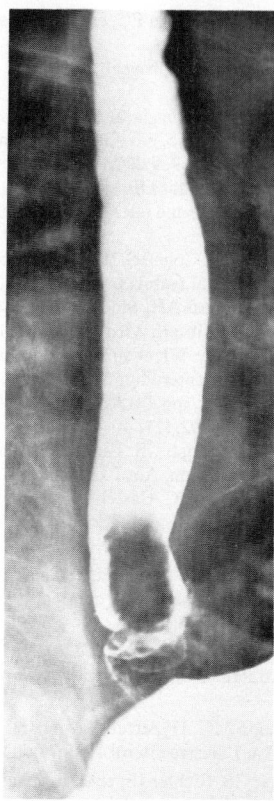

FIGURE 28–3. Barium swallow showing temporary delay in the passage of a solid bolus (marshmallow) in a patient with an obscure lower esophageal ring.

gentle application of cold to the anterior faucial arch by way of a small iced mirror as usually employed for indirect laryngoscopy.

The role of cricopharyngeal myotomy in the treatment of patients with pharyngeal dysphagia is controversial. Over the years, it has been used primarily in patients with pharyngoesophageal (Zenker's) diverticula. Myotomy has been advocated on the basis of manometric studies, suggesting that premature closure of the UES is an important factor in the pathogenesis of Zenker's diverticulum.[50] The universal acceptance of cricopharyngeal myotomy in the management of this condition has little justification based upon the manometric data available today.

Myotomy is believed by many clinicians to benefit patients with disorders included under the term *cricopharyngeal achalasia.* The mechanism of pharyngeal/UES dysfunction in many of these cases may actually be due to inadequate pharyngeal contraction or discoordination of the pharynx and UES that have not been detected because of inadequate manometric techniques. Although "hypertonicity" of the UES has been suggested, this finding has rarely been confirmed. Patients with a variety of neurologic disorders, including stroke and degenerative conditions, present with pharyngeal dysphagia. Studies in small groups of patients have revealed good to excellent results of cricopharyngeal myotomy in the majority of these patients with the following conditions: stroke, motor neuron disease, head trauma, polio, and neoplastic or post-surgical nerve injury.[32,52,53]

Recent cineradiographic studies have revealed that myotomy produces considerable change in the motor function of the pharyngoesophageal segment, not restricted to the UES alone.[54] One study using preoperative manometry in a group of only 18 patients with pharyngeal dysphagia has resulted in the suggestion that manometry is the preferred method to evaluate pharyngeal dysphagia and that myotomy should be considered for patients with a motility disorder of the pharyngeal phase of swallowing characterized by any of the following: (1) inadequate pharyngeal contraction pressures, (2) pharyngeal/UES incoordination, or (3) incomplete UES relaxation.[52]

Esophageal Dysphagia

Specific details of the treatment of patients with esophageal motility disorders are presented in Chapter 54.

The reader is directed to Chapter 7, Esophageal Motor Function; Chapter 29, Approach to the Patient with Chest Pain; Chapter 53, Esophagus: Anatomy and Structural Anomalies; Chapter 54, Motility Disorders of the Esophagus; Chapter 55, Reflux Esophagitis; Chapter 56, Esophageal Infections; Chapter 57, Esophageal Tumors; Chapter 58, Miscellaneous Diseases of the Esophagus; Chapter 128, Evaluation of Gastrointestinal Motility: Methodological Considerations.

REFERENCES

1. Schatzki R. Panel discussion on diseases of the esophagus. Am J Gastroenterol 1959;31:117.
2. Pratt LW, Tobin WH, Gallagher R. Globus hystericus—office evaluation by psychological testing with the MMPI. Laryngoscope 1976;86:1540.
3. Puhakka H, Lehtenen V, Aalto T. Globus hystericus—a psychosomatic disease? J Laryngol Otol 1976;90:1021.
4. Watson WC, Sullivan SN. Hypertonicity of the cricopharyngeal sphincter: A cause of globus sensation. Lancet 1974;2:1417.
5. Ossakow SJ, Elta G, Colturi T. Esophageal reflux and dysmotility as the basis for persistent cervical symptoms. Ann Otol Rhinol Laryngol 1987;96:387.
6. Hurwitz AL. Oropharyngeal dysphagia. Am J Dig Dis 1975;20:313.
7. Bosma JF, Donner MW, Tanaka E, Robertson D. Anatomy of the pharynx pertinent to swallowing. Dysphagia 1986;1:23.
8. Bosma JF. Deglutition; pharyngeal stage. Physiol Rev 1967;37:275.
9. Doty RW, Bosma JF. An electromyographic analysis of reflex deglutition. J Neurophysiol 1956;19:44.
10. Doty RW. Neural organisation of deglution. In: Code CF, ed. Handbook of physiology. Section 6. Alimentary canal, vol IV. Washington DC: American Physiological Society 1968:1861.
11. Miller AJ. Neurophysiological basis of swallowing. Dysphagia 1986;1:91.
12. Shiff T, Deatsch WW, Robertson K. Pharyngoesophageal muscle activity during swallowing in man. Laryngoscope 1970;80:1.
13. Isberg A, Nilsson ME, Schiratzki H. Movement of the upper esophageal sphincter and a manometric device during deglutition. Acta Radial Diag 1985;86:381.
14. Siebens H, Trupe E, Siebens A, et al. Correlates and consequences of eating dependency in institutionalized elderly. J Am Geriatr Soc 1986;34:192.
15. Vantrappen G, Hellmans J. Diseases of the esophagus. New York: Springer-Verlag, 1974:399.

16. Palmer ED. Disorders of the cricopharyngeus muscle; a review. Gastroenterology 1976;71:510.
17. Gerhardt DC, Winship DH. Cricopharyngeal disorders. In: Cohen S, Soloway RD, eds. Diseases of the esophagus. New York: Churchill Livingstone, 1982:121.
18. Gordon C, Hewer RL, Wade DT. Dysphagia in acute stroke. Br Med J 1987;295:411.
19. Mayberry JF, Atkinson M. Swallowing problems in patients with motor neuron disease. J Clin Gastroenterol 1986;8:233.
20. Schultz AR, Niemtzow P, Jacobs SR, Naso F. Dysphagia associated with cricopharyngeal dysfunction. Arch Phys Med Rehabil 1979;60:381.
21. Watson WC, Sullivan SN. Hypertonicity of the cricopharyngeal sphincter; a cause of globus sensation. Lancet 1974;2:1417.
22. Hunt PS, Connell AM, Smiley TB. The cricopharyngeal sphincter in gastric reflux. Gut 1970;11:303.
23. Stanciu C, Bennett JR. Upper esophageal yield pressures in normal subjects and patients with gastroesophageal reflux. Thorax 1974;29:459.
24. Gerhardt DC, Castell DO, Winship DH, Schuck TJ. Esophageal dysfunction in esophagopharyngeal regurgitation. Gastroenterology 1980;78:893.
25. Kilman WJ, Goyal RK. Disorders of pharyngeal and upper esophageal sphincter motor function. Arch Intern Med 1976;136:592.
26. Hurwitz AL, Nelson JA, Haddad JK. Oropharyngeal dysphagia. Manometric and cineradiographic esophagraphic findings. Am J Dig Dis 1975;20:313.
27. Reichert TJ, Bluestone CD, Stool SE, et al. Congenital cricopharyngeal achalasia. Ann Otol 1977;86:603.
28. Roed-Peterson K. The pharyngoesophageal sphincter. Dan Med Bull 1979;26:275.
29. Hellmans J, Agg HO, Pelemans W, VanTrappen G. Pharyngoesophageal swallowing disorders and the pharyngoesophageal sphincter. Med Clin North Am 1981;65:1149.
30. Riley CM. Familial dysautonomia. Adv Pediatr 1957;5:157.
31. Marguilies SI, Bruut PW, Donner MW, Silbiger ML. Familial dysautonomia, a cineradiographic study of the swallowing mechanism. Radiology 1968;90:107.
32. Ellis FH, Corzier RE. Cervical esophageal dysphagia. Ann Surg 1981;194:279.
33. Logemann JA. Criteria for studies of treatment for oral-pharyngeal dysphagia. Dysphagia 1987;1:193.
34. Knuff TE, Benjamin SB, Castell DO. Pharyngoesophageal (Zenker's) diverticulum: A reappraisal. Gastroenterology 1982;82:734.
35. Cattau EL, Castell DO. Symptoms of esophageal dysfunction. In: Stollerman GH, ed. Advances in Internal Medicine, vol 27. Chicago: Year Book Medical Publishers, 1982:147.
36. Castell DO, Knuff TE, Brown FC, et al. Dysphagia. Gastroenterology 1979;76:1015.
37. Schatzki R. The lower esophageal ring. Am J Roentgenol 1963;90:805.
38. Pope CE. Heartburn, dysphagia, and other esophageal symptoms. In: Sleisenger MH, Fordtran JS, eds. Gastrointestinal disease, ed 4. Philadelphia: WB Saunders, 1989:200.
39. Smart HL, Foster PN, Evans DF, et al. Twenty-four hour oesophageal acidity in achalasia before and after pneumatic dilatation. Gut 1987;28:883.
40. Tucker HJ, Snape WJ, Cohen S. Achalasia secondary to carcinoma: Manometric and clinical features. Ann Intern Med 1978;89:315.
41. Treacy WL, Baggenstoss AH, Slocumb CH, Code CF. Scleroderma of the esophagus. Ann Intern Med 1963;59:351.
42. Cohen S, Laufer I, Snape WJ, et al. The gastrointestinal manifestations of scleroderma. Gastroenterology 1980;79:155.
43. Zamost BJ, Hirschberg J, Ippoliti AF, et al. Esophagitis in scleroderma. Gastroenterology 1987;92:421.
44. Brand DL, Martin D, Pope CE. Esophageal manometrics in patients with angina-like chest pain. Am J Dig Dis 1977;22:300.
45. Benjamin SB, Gerhardt DC, Castell DO. High amplitude, peristaltic esophageal contractions associated with chest pain and/or dysphagia. Gastroenterology 1979;77:478.
46. Herrington JP, Burns TW, Balart LA. Chest pain and dysphagia in patients with prolonged peristaltic contractile duration of the esophagus. Dig Dis Sci 1984;29:134.
47. Traube M, Abibi R, McCallum RW. High amplitude peristaltic esophageal contractions associated with chest pain. JAMA 1983;250:2655.
48. Orr WC, Robinson MG. Hypertensive peristalsis in the pathogenesis of chest pain. Am J Gastroenterol 1982;77:604.
49. Katz PO, Dalton CB, Richter JE, et al. Esophageal testing in patients with non-cardiac chest pain and/or dysphagia. Ann Intern Med 1987;106:593.
50. Code CF, Schlegel JF, Kelley ML, et al. Hypertensive gastroesophageal sphincter. Mayo Clin Proc 1986;35:391.
51. Waterman DC, Dalton CB, Ott D, et al. The hypertensive lower esophageal sphincter: What does it mean? Clin Res 1988;36:14A.
52. Bonavina L, Khan NA, DeMeester TR. Pharyngoesophageal dysfunctions. Arch Surg 1985;120:541.
53. David VC. Relief of dysphagia in motor neuron disease with cricopharyngeal myotomy. Ann Roy Coll Surg Engl 1985;67:229.
54. Ekberg O, Lindgren S. Effect of cricopharyngeal myotomy on pharyngoesophageal function: Pre- and postoperative cineradiographic findings. Gastrointest Radiol 1987;12:1.

29

Approach to the Patient with Chest Pain

TIMOTHY T. NOSTRANT

INTRODUCTION

Recurring chest pain is a common problem for the internist. It ranks only behind abdominal pain as the most frequent reason for urgent office evaluation.[1] Chest pain ranks fourth behind upper respiratory tract infection, family illnesses, and abdominal pain as a cause for missed work.[2] Chest pain requiring emergency evaluation is presumed to be cardiac in origin because of the life-threatening nature of myocardial ischemia and the belief that other forms of chest pain are rare or unimportant. Cardiac catheterization has clearly shown that coronary artery disease with myocardial ischemia is not the only cause of typical or atypical angina pectoris. Of the 500,000 patients undergoing coronary angiography for presumed cardiac pain yearly, 30% will have normal epicardial coronary arteries.[3-5] Coronary artery vasospasm or small vessel disease will be found and presumed as the cause for chest pain in only a small proportion of those patients with normal epicardial vessels.[6,7] Antianginal medications are continued despite normal coronary arteries, and no further evaluation is done.[5] Long-term follow-up of patients with normal coronary arteries and chest pain reveals both good and bad news. In one study of 821 patients, morbidity and mortality were very low (0.2% and 0.3%, respectively).[4] Nevertheless, these patients underwent drastic life-style changes that included decreasing or eliminating work and requiring repeat coronary care unit admissions. Fifty percent of patients were either partially or totally disabled, and most of them still considered the heart as their pain source.[3-5] Fifty percent of these patients were continued to be placed on antianginal programs despite the absence of cardiac disease.[3-7] Most of these medications had significant cardiovascular, genitourinary, and gastrointestinal side effects. Thus an aggressive approach to determine the specific source for chest pain would seem warranted.[8,9]

The esophagus is presumed to be the major cause of noncardiac chest pain. Ward and colleagues reported a follow-up study of patients with noncardiac chest pain after esophageal testing.[10] They divided the patients into three groups. The first group had negative esophageal testing. The second and third groups both had an esophageal pain source, but only the third group was informed of the results. Observation of these patients revealed that more than 90% continued with chest pain. Both the first and second groups continued to believe the heart was the source for their chest pain (45%), and each required frequent office visits and admissions (60%). The third group thought the esophagus was the source for pain (45%) and rarely the heart (4%). These patients required fewer visits and admissions (30%), and they believed esophageal evaluation was important. Mortality was low and equal among the groups in this short-term study. Thus both disability and resource use may be decreased by an aggressive evaluation of patients with noncardiac chest pain.

CAUSES OF CHEST PAIN

The major causes for chest pain are listed in Table 29-1. Pleuropulmonary disease will not be addressed since chronic chest pain is rarely seen with these conditions.

Cardiac Pain

Myocardial ischemia is the cause of chest pain in most patients with cardiac angina. Chest pain occurs when oxygen supply cannot meet demand. Since the heart maximally extracts oxygen at rest, increased coronary blood flow must supply increased oxygen demands. Minor changes in coronary artery radius will markedly alter oxygen supply since coronary blood flow is inversely related to the fourth power of the vessel's radius.[11,12] When intraluminal diameters are reduced by 70%, myocardial vessels are dilated to the maximum and increased blood flow cannot occur. When blood flow cannot meet oxygen demand, chest pain occurs secondary to accumulation of toxic metabolites and is transmitted predominantly through the dorsal spinal roots T_1–T_5.[12-14]

There are multiple causes for increased myocardial oxygen consumption that include blood flow and extravascular factors. Working on an inclined surface, using the arms rather than the legs, and rapidly moving to maximal exercise all increase oxygen demands.[15-17] Emotional distress, cold weather, food ingestion, and pulmonary infection are additional contributing factors. Severe valvular heart disease, hypertension, or dilated cardiomyopathies may decrease coronary blood flow in the presence of normal coronary arteries.[13-17]

TABLE 29–1
Causes of Chest Pain

Cardiac Pain

Coronary artery disease

Pericardial pain

Valvular heart disease

Dissecting aortic aneurysm

Esophageal Chest Pain

Symptomatic gastroesophageal reflux without esophagitis

Reflux esophagitis

Acid-induced esophageal dysmotility

Esophageal dysmotility

Nonesophageal Gastrointestinal Sources

Acid peptic disease

Biliary colic and biliary dyskinesia

Chest Wall Pain

Ribs and their articulations

    Tietze's syndrome and costochondritis

    Precardial catch, slipping rib, and rib tip syndromes

Myofascial disorders

    Pectoralis major muscle

    Pectoralis minor muscle

    Sternalis muscle

Psychosomatic Illnesses

Hyperventilation

Aerophagia

Panic attack

All heart pain cannot be explained by factors that are associated with increased oxygen demands, decreased coronary blood flow, or decreased oxygen delivery. Classic examples of these are pericardial pain, pain from dissecting aneurysm, and pain from mitral valve prolapse. Mechanical rubbing of the pericardial surfaces and distention of the aortic wall are the presumed causes of chest pain in pericarditis and dissecting aortic aneurysm, respectively.[12–14] No specific mechanism has been proven as the cause for chest pain in mitral valve prolapse, although altered pain perception is considered to be a major contributor.[18]

Esophageal Chest Pain

The role of the esophagus in producing chest pain is becoming increasingly appreciated. The disorders associated with esophageal chest pain have been more clearly defined with the advent of sophisticated esophageal function testing, including 24-hour pH and pressure monitoring. What has been elusive is the mechanism(s) by which these disorders produce chest pain. The potential mechanisms of esophageal chest pain are listed in Table 29-2.

SYMPTOMATIC GASTROESOPHAGEAL REFLUX AND GASTROESOPHAGEAL REFLUX DISEASE

The mechanisms producing chest pain during esophageal acid exposure still remain controversial. Acid-induced dysmotility was initially believed to be the major cause of esophageal pain. Siegel and Hendrix demonstrated increased esophageal amplitude and duration of contraction with acid exposure.[19] Simultaneous and spontaneous contractions were seen in most patients during acid infusion. Other investigators have not been able to reproduce this.[20,21] Although diffuse esophageal spasm has been reported during spontaneous acid reflux in some patients, most studies show that simultaneous or multipeaked waves are very infrequent during acid infusion.[22–24] In addition, changes in amplitude and duration of esophageal contraction have been identical in both normal subjects and reflux patients during acid infusion.[22] These changes in manometric parameters were also poorly correlated with chest pain. Recently, 24-hour simultaneous ambulatory esophageal pH and motility monitoring has shown that spontaneous acid-induced chest pain is infrequently associated with esophageal dysmotility ($< 10\%$).[25]

Other mechanisms by which acid can induce chest pain include acid-induced esophageal inflammation, acid stimulation of che-

TABLE 29–2
Mechanisms of Esophageal Chest Pain

Symptomatic Gastroesophageal Reflux and Gastroesophageal Reflux Disease

Acid-induced dysmotility

Chemoreceptor stimulation by acid

Acid-induced esophageal inflammation

Acid distention of the esophagus

Coronary ischemia

Esophageal ischemia

Alkaline reflux

Osmoreceptor stimulation (food induced)

Unrelated to Gastroesophageal Reflux Esophageal Inflammation

Esophageal infection

Pill-induced esophagitis

Neoplasm-Induced Chest Pain

Inflammatory pain

Nerve and bone involvement

Esophageal Dysmotility

Achalasia

Diffuse esophageal spasm

Nutcracker esophagus

Hypertensive lower esophageal sphincter

Secondary

Psychosomaticism and esophageal pain

moreceptors, acid distention of the esophagus, coronary ischemia, and potentially esophageal ischemia. The occurrence of esophagitis appears to correlate best with the positional type of acid reflux and the length of acid exposure time. Physiologic reflux occurs predominantly after meals and is quickly eliminated by peristalsis and neutralized by saliva. Reflux in the supine position is rare and short-lived in normal subjects.[26,27] Patients with pathologic reflux have three patterns of abnormal reflux. The first pattern is an exaggeration of the postprandial pattern seen in normal subjects. Esophagitis is rare (< 10%), and heartburn is less pronounced.[26,27] The two other positional patterns of reflux are supine reflux and reflux in both the upright and supine positions (i.e., combined reflux). Duration of acid exposure is much greater, and this is the major feature separating this group from the group with reflux in the upright position. Esophagitis occurs in 50% of patients with supine or combined reflux. Symptoms are more common and severe in these two groups. Orlando and co-workers have shown that continued exposure to acid at low pH produces esophageal squamous layer damage and loss of the normal impermeability to hydrogen ions and other molecules.[28] Passage of hydrogen ions to potential acid-sensitive chemoreceptors is facilitated by esophagitis and may be an explanation for the increased incidence of chest pain in patients with esophagitis.[28,29] Lacey and colleagues found that all 25 symptomatic chest pain patients had pain reproduction during infusion of solutions with pH 1.0 but only 50% had pain with solutions of pH greater than 2.5.[30] Although acid-induced pain secondary to chemoreceptor stimulation is presumed to be the cause of pain in patients with acid reflux, direct proof for acid passage through the squamous layer without visible damage is still needed since 30% to 60% of patients will have a normal esophagus by endoscopy.[31,32] Other factors that may influence duration of acid exposure and subsequent back-diffusion of acid are acid clearance mechanisms, salivary neutralization of acid, and the interaction of acid, pepsin, and other barrier breakers.

Reflux-induced esophageal distention may be another mechanism producing chest pain. Distention of the esophagus has been documented after acid exposure.[33] Balloon distention of the esophagus can produce chest pain in both patients with chest pain and normal subjects.[34,35] Incapacitating pain can be seen in those patients who undergo esophageal cooling or have impairment of belching; both of which are associated with esophageal distention at the time of pain.[33,36] The role of esophageal distention secondary to acid reflux in causing chest pain requires further investigation.

The importance of coexistent coronary artery disease in patients with acid-induced pain should not be overlooked. Intraesophageal acid infusion can produce ST-T wave changes consistent with myocardial ischemia.[37] However, direct proof that these ST-T wave changes are secondary to coronary ischemia and that coronary artery disease is more common in those with acid-induced ST-T wave changes is still wanting. Small vessel or microvessel cardiac angina has been hypothesized as a cause for acid-induced pain based on pacing studies showing decreased vasodilator reserve in patients with chest pain. Studies by Yakshe and associates have shown decreased coronary blood flow and increased coronary sinus resistance in 50% of patients with a presumed esophageal source for chest pain.[38] The provocative agents used to induce chest pain included acid infusion and all standard provocative agents. Studies to elucidate the mechanisms of esophageal chest pain are needed to answer the question of whether esophageal chest pain is coming from the esophagus or is simply cardiac pain from small vessel disease.

Esophageal wall ischemia is the most recent addition to a long list of possible mechanisms for noncardiac chest pain. Overall, esophageal blood flow is increased with esophagitis, although selective blood flow reduction to the mucosa/submucosa cannot be excluded.[39] A selective decrease in mucosal blood flow could hamper effective hydrogen ion buffering. Blood flow measurements during acid infusion in the intact esophagus have not been done. MacKenzie and co-workers studied the rate of esophageal rewarming after cold water challenge in nine patients with diffuse esophageal spasm and nutcracker esophagus and compared the results with those found in 21 normal subjects.[40] The distal esophagus was perfused with water at 7°C for 30 seconds at a rate of 2 mL/s. The temperature of the cooled esophageal wall was measured continuously with a thermocouple during and after this cold water challenge. The time to rewarm the esophageal wall was significantly longer in patients than in normal subjects (90 vs. 44 seconds), and in only one patient was the result within the range of time in normal subjects. Age or sex had no effect on the rewarming rates. Since studies of rewarming rates in patients with Raynaud's phenomenon directly correlated with blood flow,[41] esophageal ischemia was presumed to be the cause of the prolonged rewarming rates seen in patients with dysmotility. Whether ischemia is important in acid-induced chest pain requires further investigation. Selective measurements of mucosal and submucosal blood flow during acid infusion or provoked dysmotility will help to resolve this controversy.

Acid alone is not the only culprit in postprandial esophageal chest pain. Barrier breakers such as bile salts and pancreatic enzymes increase esophageal acid penetration.[42,43] Simultaneous reflux of acid and duodenal juice has been documented in patients with acid reflux. Patients with combined acid and alkaline reflux are more symptomatic, and combined reflux may partially account for treatment failure in some patients with reflux esophagitis.[42,44]

NON-ACID-INDUCED ESOPHAGEAL INFLAMMATION

Esophageal infection and pill-induced esophageal inflammation may cause noncardiac chest pain. Esophageal infection is most frequently seen in the context of immunosuppression either related to the primary disease or to medication (corticosteroids, antineoplastic medications). Pain is acute in onset, constant, and poorly relieved by standard anti-acid treatment. *Candida* species, herpes simplex, and cytomegalovirus are the most common organisms found. A high index of suspicion for infection should be maintained and esophageal biopsy and cytology performed in all immunocompromised patients with nonresponsive chest pain.

Pills and capsules are common causes of esophagitis. Antibiotics (tetracycline, doxycycline), anti-inflammatory medications, potassium supplements, and ferrous sulfate are the usual offenders.[45-47] Highly caustic coatings, direct medication injury, and poor esophageal clearance of pills can lead to acute inflammation.[45-49] Taking medications at bedtime or without fluids is a common preceding event. Capsules and pills are usually cleared slowly in the mid and distal esophagus.[48,49] These areas correspond to areas of diminished peristalsis by both esophageal radiography and manometrics and are frequently the site of inflammation observed in pill-induced esophagitis. Pain is immediate, intense, and incapacitating. History and gastrointestinal endoscopy will confirm the diagnosis. Treatment is supportive, although acid reduction is used frequently as an adjunct. Ulcer healing and symptoms are more closely correlated in patients with pill-induced esophagitis than in patients with acid reflux–induced ulceration and symptoms.[45-49]

Osmolarity and direct esophageal irritation may be responsible for food-induced chest pain.[50,51] High osmolar liquids are more likely to produce heartburn than isotonic solutions, even if hydrogen content is equal. Dilution decreases the frequency of symptoms. Neither osmolality nor pH could account for symptoms with some liquids such as tomato juice or highly spiced solutions. Direct stimulation of chemoreceptors or direct esophageal irritation may be responsible for production of pain.

NEOPLASM-INDUCED CHEST PAIN

Neoplastic involvement of the esophagus can lead to esophageal ulceration, producing pain by mechanisms similar to acid reflux. Pain is more localized and can radiate to the back or spine in a position directly behind the anterior chest pain. Malignant involvement of the trachea and thoracic spine can produce pain by direct nerve and bone involvement.

ESOPHAGEAL MOTILITY DISORDERS

Abnormalities of esophageal motility were first reported as a cause for anginal chest pain in the 1930s. Diffuse esophageal spasm is the label given to the frequent simultaneous contractions and multipeaked waves commonly seen in this patient group.[52] With the widespread use and refinement of esophageal manometric systems, simultaneous, nonperistaltic contractions (tertiary contractions) are found to occur not infrequently in the distal two thirds of the esophagus in all normal subjects.[53,54] The occurrence of simultaneous contractions at night, during stressful situations, and with increasing age in asymptomatic normal subjects raises doubts about the pathophysiologic significance of these manometric findings. Despite this, diffuse esophageal spasm is still the most common diagnosis given to patients with anginal chest pain after the physician has ruled out the heart as a source of pain.[52]

The development of reliable motility recording instruments ushers in a new era of esophageal testing. Low-compliance tubing with precision low-friction pumping systems allows measurement of pressure almost equal to direct strain gauge recorders.[53,54] Normal values for amplitude of contraction vary from 30 to 180 mm, with higher values seen in the elderly.[52-54] Duration of contraction is less affected by age and averages less than 5 seconds in most patients. Values greater than 7 seconds are considered abnormal. Contraction waves are usually single, but double-peaked waves are seen in normal subjects.[53,54] Using these manometric criteria, investigators have found several groups of esophageal motility disorders to be associated with noncardiac chest pain. These include achalasia, diffuse esophageal spasm, high-amplitude peristalsis (nutcracker esophagus), and the hypertensive lower esophageal sphincter. In addition, about 40% of patients with chest pain and esophageal dysmotility cannot be classified into the four major

groups and are given the diagnosis of nonspecific esophageal dysmotility.[52-54] However, it is not known if nonspecific esophageal dysmotility is responsible for the chest pain reported by these patients.

Primary Esophageal Motor Disorders. These entities and their specific manometric requirements are discussed fully in Chapter 54. Only their mechanism of chest pain production is discussed here.

Achalasia. Despite the fact that dysphagia is the predominant symptom, chest pain is present in over 50% of patients with achalasia.[55,56] It is both an early and a late phenomenon. Early in the course of disease, high-amplitude simultaneous contractions and absence of contractions after swallowing are both common and correlate with chest pain. Pain late in the course of achalasia should alert the physician to the occurrence of complications such as stasis ulceration and cancer.

Diffuse Esophageal Spasm. Simultaneous contractions in the smooth muscle portion of the esophagus are the sine qua non of this diagnosis. Amplitude and duration of contraction can be normal or high.[52] With modern manometric techniques, this diagnosis is becoming increasingly uncommon (< 10%) as a cause for esophageal chest pain.[52,57]

The Nutcracker Esophagus. Brand was the first to describe the entity of peristaltic contractions of high amplitude in patients with chest pain.[34,58] Forty-one percent of patients in this initial study had peristaltic waves with a mean amplitude of contraction greater than the mean plus 2 SD of the control population.[59] Benjamin was the first to coin the term *nutcracker esophagus*. Studies from multiple centers have confirmed the high incidence of this finding in patients with noncardiac chest pain.[54,59-61] The cause of chest pain is unknown, although increased wall tension and excessive reactivity to pain have been proposed as mechanisms.[59-62] The high incidence of nutcracker esophagus in psychiatric populations raises the specter of psychosomaticism as a factor causing chest pain.[63,64] Since most patients are asymptomatic when their motility disorder is identified, this manometric abnormality may only serve as a marker for patients who have noncardiac chest pain caused by other mechanisms such as intermittent high-pressure waves, marked increased duration of contractions, or complete loss of contraction (nonresponse). These motility abnormalities may only be seen during chest pain and be produced by unknown stimuli. These comments also pertain to patients with diffuse esophageal spasm and hypertensive lower esophageal sphincter.

Hypertensive Lower Esophageal Sphincter. Hypertensive lower esophageal sphincter is defined by sphincter pressures exceeding the mean plus 2 SD of the normal population.[57,65,66] A lower esophageal sphincter pressure greater than 45 mm Hg is usually required for the diagnosis.[57,65,66] Hypertensive lower esophageal sphincter is rarely a pure entity, and increased lower esophageal sphincter pressures are found in 30% of patients with nutcracker esophagus.[57] Patients with chest pain rarely have only hypertensive lower esophageal sphincter (4%), and dysphagia is the most common symptom in this group.

Psychosomaticism and Chest Pain. The role of the psyche in the production of chest pain is a frequently accepted but unproven cause for chest pain. Emotional stress was recognized as an important cause of chest pain in the late 19th century. Both Clouse and colleagues[63] and Richter and associates[64] have shown a high incidence of psychiatric illnesses in patients with high amplitudes of contraction and nutcracker esophagus, respectively. Both of these results were based on structured psychiatric interviews. Unfortunately the psychological inventory does not take into account the effects of long-term chest pain and its associated disability on the scales for depression, anxiety, and pain perception. Evaluation of patients with motility disorders before the onset of pain and at variable intervals during the disease will allow more accurate determination of cause or effect of chest pain.

More direct proof for the role of altered pain perception in patients with chest pain comes with a recent study of esophageal balloon distention.[8,9] Richter and associates found that 60% of patients with chest pain had reproduction of their pain with graded balloon distention of the mid esophagus.[8,9,64] These patients also had their chest pain at lower balloon volumes ($\leq$ 9 mL in 83%) than the control subject who had chest discomfort (10 mL). These authors proposed increased pain perception as the basis for pain. Clouse and colleagues have extended this theory to a controlled trial of medications that can decrease pain perception (antidepressants).[67] Increased response rates to antidepressants in patients with chest pain when compared with placebo and the absence of manometric changes with successful treatment indicated a potential psychological cause for pain. Preliminary studies using measurable means to increase psychic stress (discordant sounds, difficult intellectual tasks) also gives credence to the role of psychic stress in producing chest discomfort.[8,9,68] Follow-up studies are eagerly awaited.

Nonesophageal Gastrointestinal Causes for Chest Pain

PEPTIC ULCER DISEASE

Peptic ulcer disease can present as subxyphoid and anterior chest pain. Based on the high incidence of positive Bernstein examinations in patients with peptic ulcer disease, reflux of acid is the presumed cause. A 2.5-fold increase over normal subjects in the incidence of reflux changes in distal esophageal biopsy specimens is also seen in ulcer patients.[69] Other mechanisms such as abnormal esophageal motility, gastric dysmotility, and changes in pain perception with illness have not been fully studied.

BILIARY COLIC AND BILIARY DYSKINESIA

The pain of cystic or common bile duct obstruction is quite characteristic. It usually begins as midepigastric pain that can have substernal components owing to T3 to T6 spinal innervation. The pain is intermittent and occurs predominantly after meals. Nocturnal onset of pain is not uncommon. The pain builds to its maximum in less than 30 minutes and can last for 15 minutes to 6 hours without discernable complications. The pain usually begins and ends rapidly. Pain is due to common bile or cystic duct distention and has been reproduced by balloon distention of these structures.[70] Coronary blood flow and blood pressure can be decreased and heart rate increased after experimental distention of the biliary duct.[71] Therefore, critical coronary artery disease should

always be kept in mind as a coexistent problem in patients with bile duct disease who present with central chest pain. All forms of intermittent chest pain require exclusion of gallstones as a pain source. Mere presence of gallstones does not indicate that biliary colic is a source for chest pain. Biliary scintiscanning during pain will usually provide evidence of duct obstruction or poor gallbladder emptying as a mechanism for pain.

Biliary dyskinesia refers to a syndrome of biliary colic without gallstones or other hepatobiliary cause for pain. Abnormal bile duct motility and/or increased sphincter of Oddi pressures producing functional bile duct obstruction have been implicated as the cause for pain. Biliary dyskinesia and biliary colic secondary to stones produce similar types of pain and functional obstruction with distention of the common bile duct as the proposed mechanism.[72,73] An increased incidence of coronary artery spasm and esophageal dysmotilty has been observed in this group of patients.[74] Whether biliary dyskinesia is a true entity is still controversial and should be considered in the differential diagnosis of chest pain only as a remote possibility. Proof for its role in human chest pain will most likely come from treatments aimed at directly reducing sphincter of Oddi pressures and eliminating biliary dysmotility. Preliminary studies with endoscopic sphincterotomy have shown significant short- and long-term success in decreasing symptoms in patients with increased sphincter of Oddi pressures and recurrent biliary colic.[72,73]

Chest Wall Syndromes

The causes of musculoskeletal chest pain are listed in Table 29-1. Although the exact prevalence of chest wall pain as a source for chest pain is unknown, a rate of 10% has been reported.[75] Subdivision of chest wall pain into articulation and myofascial disorders allows better appreciation of the mechanisms causing chest pain.

RIBS AND THEIR ARTICULATIONS

Tietze Syndrome and Costochondritis. Tietze syndrome is a benign condition characterized by painful, nonsuppurative swelling of anterior chest wall cartilage.[76] This syndrome usually occurs in the second to fourth decade and has an equal sex distribution. As many as 10% of patients evaluated for chest pain have been diagnosed with this condition.[75] A single tender and painful swelling of any of the left costal cartilages (T2 especially) is most commonly described. Inflammation of the cartilage is rarely found even on biopsy, despite the common assumption that swelling is secondary to inflammation with edema. Upper respiratory tract infection preceding pain is common, and trauma secondary to prolonged coughing is a proposed mechanism. Conventional radiographs are usually not helpful, although computed tomography has shown bulbous enlargement and ventral angulation of the costochondral junctions.[77,78] The diagnosis is made clinically, and the frequency of Tietze syndrome is declining with the increasing recognition of noninflammatory causes of chest wall pain.[77,78]

Costochondritis is similar to Tietze syndrome, although it more commonly affects multiple junctions with frequent symmetry. Involvement of the lower rib junctions is more common than in Tietze's syndrome. Inflammation is not seen here. Cervical strain with "fibrositis" is the most common quoted reason for pain.[79] Sternal infection should be a major differential diagnosis.

Precordial Catch, Slipping Rib, and Rib Tip Syndromes.   These three entities represent the least common causes of rib articulation chest wall pain.[79-81] All of these syndromes can be produced by trigger points in the pectoralis major muscle, and trigger points should be carefully excluded by physical examination. Precordial catch or "Texidor's twinge" is a sudden stabbing or needle-like inframammary pain that occurs in young, healthy patients.[80] Patients seek relief with breath holding or shallow breathing. Pain is transient and does not radiate. Bird reported that the pain lasted less than 1 minute in 80% of patients.[82] Pain is most commonly a single event or occurs in well-spaced episodes, although a small percentage can have frequent attacks. The cause of the pain is unknown, but the brief duration, association with inspiration, and consistent left-sided location makes pinching or tethering of pleuropericardial structures the most likely cause.

Slipping rib and rib tip syndrome most commonly affect middle-aged persons.[80] The male-to-female ratio of the incidence of these disorders is equal. Overriding of ribs with associated tenderness is found in one half of reported cases. Pain is reproduced by palpation at one or more points along the rib costal margin, which separates it from other noninflammatory muscle pains. Movement is a common precipitant for pain. Lying or turning over in bed, prolonged sitting, stretching or reaching, bending forward, or coughing are the most common aggravating factors in order of frequency. Assurance is the best treatment, but injection therapy may also be helpful.

MYOFASCIAL DISORDERS

Any of the chest wall muscles can produce pain with the major focus of pain remote from the origin of pain. The muscle tissues are subject to continuous wear and tear to a greater extent than bones, joints, or nerves, but these other tissues have received much more attention from physicians.

To understand muscular pain, it is important to define certain terms. The first is *active myofascial trigger point*. This refers to a pattern of pain at rest or during motion that is specific to that muscle. Active trigger points are always tender and produce active restriction of motion. In addition to motion restriction, active trigger points produce muscular weakness and referred pain on compression. Autonomic dysfunction such as decreased sweating and excess pilomotor activity is common in the zone of referred pain.[83] In association with active trigger points, *associated myofascial trigger points* can develop secondary to compensatory overload. The associated trigger points are specific to each active trigger point. *Latent myofascial trigger points* refer to points that are tender but are not associated with spontaneous pain. These latent trigger points possess all of the other characteristics of active trigger points. Latent trigger points can become active through trauma or even by association with other active trigger points. This composite of latent trigger points becoming active, producing referred pain secondary to activation of associated trigger points and pain referral to distant points specific for each muscle, is the basis of long-term muscular pain.[84-86]

The prevalence of active and latent trigger points is unknown. Sola and co-workers found latent trigger points in the shoulder girdle of 54% of female and 45% of male subjects.[87] Referred pain was seen in 5%. The subjects in this study were asymptomatic young adults. The incidence is assumed to increase with age, although this still lacks proof.

The cost of unrecognized myofascial pain makes it one of the major causes of workers' compensation and industrial work losses.[88] Chronic use of analgesics as well as medications for presumed but unproven visceral sources is costly and associated with a considerable incidence of nephropathy.[89,90]

The mechanisms responsible for trigger points are still debated.[90-92] The major reason for lack of physician acceptance is the lack of correlation of symptoms with actual muscle pathology.[93-98] It has been hypothesized that trigger points began as areas of nerve hyperirritability that progressed to a histologically demonstrable dystrophy.[91-102] High levels of tissue neurotransmitters, high tissue metabolic demands, and poor tissue circulation have been shown in trigger point areas.[103-105] Muscular spasm as a cause for trigger points is untenable since it is frequently absent in the affected areas.[105,106] Contractures of muscle fibers could occur if muscle fibers were disrupted in such a way that their sarcoplasmic reticulum released its calcium permanently.[105,106] Progressive muscle damage would occur to continued metabolic demands but impeded circulation secondary to persistent muscle contraction. The chronic stress of sustained contracture could increase strain to complementary muscle groups, repeating the vicious cycle. This permanent histologic change could explain the relative failure of treatment in long-standing myofascial pain. In addition, the response to stretching can be explained by its effect of breaking the cycle of sustained contraction in areas not yet permanently damaged.[104,105]

Pectoralis Major Muscle.   This is the muscle group prescribed in 1936 by Edeiken and Wolerth as the cause for persistent chest pain after myocardial infarction.[91,107,108] Five trigger point areas with specific pain patterns have been described.[109] A clavicular trigger point can produce pain over the anterior deltoid muscle but usually does not go into the anterior chest. Active trigger points in the intermediate sternal area most commonly produce left precordial pain and pain down the inner aspect of the left arm. The medial sternal attachment of the pectoralis major muscle can refer pain to the sternum without crossing the midline. Costal and abdominal insertions of the pectoralis muscle can cause breast tenderness with nipple sensitivity and intolerance to clothing in this area. All of these symptoms are more common in women than men. Variability from hour to hour and day to day is common with pectoralis major pain, which usually differentiates it from the more consistent limitation imposed by cardiac angina. Disruption of sleep is common.[110,111] Entrapment of chest wall lymphatics can lead to breast engorgement and tenderness. Relief with local treatment confirms the diagnosis.

Pectoralis Minor Muscle.   It is difficult to differentiate pectoralis minor muscle pain from pain induced by the pectoralis major muscle.[109] Involvement of this muscle more closely mimics myocardial ischemia than involvement of the pectoralis major muscle. Inspiration may increase the pain if the upper chest musculature is used. The patient may note pain with forward and upward movement of the arm or reaching backward with the arm at shoulder levels. Because involvement of this muscle may cause entrapment of the neurovascular apparatus of the upper extremity, paresthesias, radial pulse loss, muscular weakness, and differential temperature changes can occur.[109]

Sternalis Muscle. The referred pain from sternalis muscle involvement closely mimics myocardial ischemia. It is present in the midline with little radiation laterally. It is severe and often frightening. It is usually unaffected by movement, and this feature makes its appreciation difficult. Pain usually stops at the elbow if pain radiation to the arm occurs. This is different than pectoralis major pain, which frequently goes to the hand. Trigger points can be anywhere from the manubrium to the xiphoid process but are more common in the upper two thirds of the sternum. Pain can be on either side of the sternum or in the midline. Entrapments have not been attributed to this muscle.[109,110]

Hyperventilation/Aerophagia/ Panic Disorders

Recurrent hyperventilation is a common stress-related condition of modern society.[112] The myriad of symptoms of hyperventilation range from annoying dizziness to the frightening sensations of palpitations and chest pressure. Patients most commonly present with a combination of light-headedness, dizziness, dyspnea, and chest pain. Fatigue is also common, and phobias are frequent. The classic symptoms of perioral and peripheral paresthesias, muscle cramping, and anxiety are less common and directly relate to the severity of the acid–base disturbance.[112,113] Difficulty in recognizing this constellation of symptoms and signs stems from the fact that the full-blown complex is not always present and isolated symptoms can be produced by coronary artery disease, esophageal dysfunction, and skeletal muscle spasm. Organic disease itself can precipitate hyperventilation that only produces an exaggeration of the disease symptoms. An example of this is chest pressure in a patient with known coronary artery stenosis.

Chest pain secondary to hyperventilation mimics angina pectoris. It can be associated with ectopic arrhythmias that can occur at rest. Many investigators have shown a significant incidence of hyperventilation in patients being evaluated for chest pain. Wheatley found hyperventilation as the cause for chest pain in 27 of 95 patients sent for evaluation of chronic chest discomfort. Fifteen of these 27 patients had clear-cut angina pectoris as their primary complaint but had no demonstrable coronary artery disease.[114]

There are at least four mechanisms producing chest pain in hyperventilation.[112,113] The first is clearly musculoskeletal, producing a continuous dull aching that can last for days. This pain is believed to be due to increased intercostal tone produced by chronic hypocapnia secondary to exaggerated respiratory activity.[112,113] A second factor is sympathetic hyperactivity, which has also been demonstrated in hyperventilation. Common manifestations of this include heightened peripheral vasoconstriction (cold, clammy palms) and increased myocardial contractility (sensation of thumping). The third factor in hyperventilation is a true respiratory alkalosis.[112,113] Increased arterial pH is associated with a shift in the oxygen dissociation curve to the left and decreasing serum phosphate levels. Decreased oxygen and tissue energy stores

in conjunction with heightened demands from increased sympathetic activity can produce tissue hypoxia. Dizziness, paresthesias, decreased attention span, and disorientation are directly correlated with increased arterial pH and may be manifestations of tissue hypoxemia. The last mechanism of chest pain in hyperventilation involves the effects on the cardiovascular system from chronic overbreathing. Ischemic electrocardiographic findings are common with hyperventilation and exercise.[115,116] Since fixed coronary artery disease is not found in most patients with angina and hyperventilation, these changes were considered falsely positive for coronary ischemia. Recent studies have documented an impaired myocardial oxygen supply and coronary vasospasm in patients with chronic hyperventilation.[117,118] This could produce true myocardial ischemia with normal coronary arteries. Documented ischemic changes with coronary vasospasm have been reported in chronic hyperventilation.[115,116,118] This form of vasospasm has a slow onset, occurring only after 3 to 8 minutes of hyperventilation.[118] The mechanism for this delay is not known, but a minimum respiratory alkalosis of 7.54 is required.[118]

Aerophagia often accompanies hyperventilation. Esophageal and gastric distention can produce left anterior chest pain that radiates to the neck and left shoulder. Known as the Magenblase syndrome, this distention can produce chest pain that is aggravated by maneuvers that increase diaphragmatic and abdominal pressure such as bending, twisting, lying down, or deep breathing.[112,113,119] Pain produced in this manner can start a vicious cycle of hyperventilation, increased abdominal pressure, and increased chest pain. Belching and flatus commonly relieve these symptoms.

In addition to gastric distention, colonic distention can also produce chest pain. Air entrapment most commonly occurs in the splenic or hepatic flexures.[119,120] The location of gas accumulation in these flexures is related to their posterior location and their relative fixed position. Left precordial pain occurs, but left upper abdominal pain is more common with splenic flexure gas accumulation.[120] Exercise is not a usual provocative maneuver, and pain can occur at any time. Anxiety, dyspnea, and increased emotional lability are common accompaniments. Pain can improve with passage of flatus, and eating may decrease the pain if it stimulates defecation. Associated symptoms of both the Magenblase syndrome and the splenic flexure syndrome are diffuse abdominal distention, belching, associated flatus, and vague dyspepsia. Radiographic demonstration of gaseous distention and pain reproduction following palpation of the area of trapped gas supports the diagnosis.

It is important to remember that inflammatory diseases of the upper gastrointestinal tract can produce the syndromes outlined above. Reflux esophagitis can produce aerophagia since swallowing air to push acid back into the stomach is a frequent, learned behavior in patients with acid reflux.[27] Slow intestinal transit with bacterial overgrowth and the increasing number of gastrointestinal dysmotility syndromes can also produce excessive intestinal gas and distention. As diagnostic sophistication increases, organic dysfunction of the gastrointestinal tract is likely to displace the exaggerated response to stress as a more common cause for these painful syndromes.

The last form of psychologically induced chest pain is the panic disorder. Recent studies have suggested that at least one third of patients with chest pain and normal coronary arteries have panic disorder.[121-123] Many patients with panic disorder are labeled as "cardiac neurotics" and are given little help to treat their illness.

Panic disorder is characterized by frequent periods of intense fear or discomfort (at least three attacks in 3 weeks). These periods of panic are accompanied by at least four of the following: shortness of breath, smothering, choking, palpitations, tachycardia, chest pain or discomfort, sweating, faintness, dizziness, unsteadiness, feelings of depersonalization, paresthesias, flushes or chills, and fear of dying, going crazy, or losing control. None of these symptoms can be sustained by any organic disease or stimulant. Beitman and associates found by questionnaire that 59% of 74 patients with atypical or nonanginal chest pain and no coronary artery disease had panic disorder.[121] More remarkably, more than 50% of patients with atypical or nonanginal chest pain and coronary artery disease had panic disorder. This study raises two intriguing questions. The first is: Can panic disorder cause chest pain? The second question is: Does angiographic coronary artery disease denote the cause for the chest pain if panic disorder is present? Answers to these questions will come from studies of patients with panic disorder for cardiovascular and esophageal dysfunction and also by examining the incidence of panic disorder in patients with true angina and coronary artery disease. In anticipation of future studies, clinicians should consider panic disorder in patients with atypical or nonanginal chest pain that cannot be explained by organic causes since this diagnosis implies that treatment with antidepressants may have a higher likelihood of success than treatment with antianginal medications.[122,123]

HISTORY

Interviewing the patient with chest pain will define the cause of chest pain in over 90% of patients.[124] The first priority in history taking is to differentiate anginal from nonanginal chest pain. Even when physicians diagnose typical angina, close questioning will reveal many nonanginal components to the pain. The high incidence of normal coronary arteries (up to 30%) in patients diagnosed as having typical angina underscores the need for better interviewing skills.[120] It should not be surprising that the percentage of normal coronary arteries climbs to 80% in patients with atypical anginal symptoms. It is of upmost importance to ask first about nonanginal pain before going on to ask questions detailing true angina.[124]

The first question to ask is is this chest pain one or more different chest discomforts? This is crucial since questions and answers should be directed to each type of chest pain separately. The following points summarize the questions asked to define nonanginal chest pain.

Criteria for Diagnosis

DURATION OF PAIN

Most physicians agree that a recurrent chest pain that lasts for hours or days is not chronic cardiac angina. It is important to differentiate if the time period of chest pain described is truly continuous or punctuated by multiple episodes of short duration pains that come together. Typical angina secondary to coronary artery disease or coronary vasospasm rarely lasts longer than 30 minutes or shorter than 1 to 2 minutes.[124] If pain lasts more than 30 minutes, it is essential to ask whether the pain is accompanied by palpitations. True angina can be prolonged by tachycardia. The supine position can exaggerate the duration of chest pain because of increased myocardial oxygen demands secondary to increased venous return.[124] Patients with true angina rarely lie down since this position increases pain.[124] Both musculoskeletal pain and pain secondary to gastric distention will also be increased with the supine position but frequently last longer than 30 minutes. Chest pains that last only a few seconds (< 5) should be considered nonanginal unless the patient has learned to rest immediately with the onset of pain. Furthermore, pain duration per pain episode is crucial. Pain that lasts for a few minutes but is made up of repeated episodes of pain each lasting less than 5 seconds is nonanginal in origin.

RESPIRATORY MOVEMENT CRITERIA

Pain with breathing is considered nonanginal chest pain. However, hyperventilation can produce chest pain that is long lasting.[112,113] The key question for chest pain and breathing is not whether the pain increases with breathing but whether one deep breath will bring on or worsen the pain.[14,125]

ARM AND TRUNK MOVEMENT CRITERIA

Single arm or trunk movements will not bring on true angina. This provocative maneuver is rarely volunteered by the patient and must be asked for by the physician. Repeated arm movements may precipitate true angina by increasing myocardial oxygen demands.[17] It is important, therefore, to examine the effects of single and repeated arm movements in eliciting chest pain. Movements associated with increased chest wall tension such as isometrics will also increase nonanginal chest pain but do not precipitate true angina.[112,113,124–127]

CHEST TENDERNESS CRITERIA

Angina should not be reproduced or worsened by local pressure, that is, chest tenderness should not be present at the site of chest pain. The sole exception to this is referral of angina pain to areas of previous trauma. The mechanism for this has been attributed to facilitation of pain impulses at the thoracic spinal cord.[14] Under these circumstances, angina has been reported to occur at the top or side of the head.[112,113,124,128]

BODY POSITION CRITERIA

If the patient reports that lying down relieves the pain within less than 5 seconds, the pain is not anginal and most likely represents chest wall pain. Pain, however, will be relieved with continued rest no matter what the position. The key question is how long it takes for relief in the supine position.

FACTORS THAT INDUCE AND RELIEVE PAIN

If the pain is brought on immediately with stooping or bending, it is rarely cardiac angina. Esophageal pain secondary to reflux or pain with gas entrapment can be brought on by stooping, bending, or any movement that increases intra-abdominal pressure such as abdominal compression or tight clothes. A sensation of abdominal fullness is common, and passage of gas either by mouth or rectum will relieve the pain. Pain with acid reflux is relieved with sitting or assuming the upright position. Relief, however, is delayed and closely correlates with acid clearance. Acid reflux–induced pain will stimulate an increase in the rate of swallowing, presumably in an effort to neutralize the acid. Pain relieved immediately or brought on immediately with position change is most commonly musculoskeletal in origin. However, pain related to body position should be classified as nonanginal only if it is brought on by positional change without concomitant exercise.

Pain that is relieved with swallowing one or two times is nonanginal. Precipitation by cold water and relief with warm liquids also mean that the pain is noncardiac in origin. Pain precipitated by cold weather can be true angina, particularly if coupled with exercise. Predictable precipitation with exercise is almost always true angina. The patient who relates that he can bring on his pain reproducibly by working with his hands over his head or walking to the mailbox is suffering from coronary pain. Pain that is prevented with a slow warm-up period followed by exercise is also true angina.

Use of antacids with relief is also considered a sign of acid reflux–induced pain. Unfortunately 5% of patients with true angina may also get relief with antacids.[128] Whether this is angina precipitated by acid is not yet established. Relief is not immediate in true angina and usually takes 3 to 4 minutes. Immediate relief with swallowing antacids or water should suggest an esophageal source.

MISCELLANEOUS POINTS

In addition to the clinical features listed above, there are other signs that are also helpful. Pain that is sharply localized so that the patient points to it with one finger is not related to ischemic pain. Patients with true angina will rarely use one finger to locate pain if asked where the pain is but may use one finger if asked to "point to the pain."

Since it is assumed that cardiac pain is mediated by chemical mediators, the onset of pain to the maximum point should be gradual. Pain that is at its maximum from its outset is safely considered nonanginal.

The presence of left inframammary pain is presumptive evidence of nonanginal pain. It is commonly associated with other nonanginal features such as local tenderness, muscle spasm, and onset with sudden muscle movement or hyperventilation.[129]

Another feature in nonanginal pain is posterior neck radiation of pain.[128] Radiation of pain to the anterior neck is frequently seen in patients with cardiac pain, while posterior cervical radiation is more common in patients with normal coronary arteries.[117,118] Pain that begins in the low anterior or posterior chest and radiates to the posterior neck should first be considered esophageal. Pain that goes to the occiput is rarely anginal unless there has been previous head trauma to this area. A follow-up session after the patient has had time to assess duration of pain and the effects of local pressure, respiration, and arm movements on the pain will be very useful. A summary of clinical features differentiating noncardiac from cardiac chest pain is presented in Table 29-3.

PHYSICAL EXAMINATION

Physical examination is important primarily in the evaluation of cardiac and musculoskeletal sources for chest pain. Esophageal or other gastrointestinal disorders rarely produce any significant findings except for midepigastric tenderness with peptic ulcer disease and possibly an inspiratory halt with palpation of the right upper quadrant secondary to acute cholecystitis. Nonspecific

TABLE 29–3
Clinical Features Differentiating Noncardiac
From Cardiac Chest Pain

Myocardial Pain

Chest pressure lasting less than 30 minutes

Pain continuous and not intermittent stabs

Pain provoked by exercise and relieved with warm-up

Pain is mid upper sternal in location (not left inframammary)

Radiation to front of neck/jaw

Gradual onset and offset (>30 seconds)

Not reproduced with chest pressure

Esophageal Pain

More common postprandially and in supine position (relieved with upright position)

Relieved with antacids (<30 seconds) and can last more than 30 minutes

Low substernal location with movement upward (signified by hand moving upward)

Radiation to back and posterior neck

Associated with regurgitation (not universal)

Bending and stooping can bring on pain (almost instantly)

Musculoskeletal Pain

Brought on with arm movement (one)

Point tenderness with trigger points

Well-localized pain

Radicular components

Inspiration can bring on pain (single)

History of trauma or overuse

Hyperventilation/Aerophagia/Panic Disorder

Anxiety with feeling of loss of control

Fear feelings precede chest discomfort

Perioral and peripheral paresthesias

Abdominal gas with distention common

Increased diaphragm and abdominal pressure increase pain

Relieved with belching

findings of autonomic hyperactivity (sweating, peripheral vaso-constriction) and agitation are common to all causes of chest pain and reflect primarily the intensity and duration of pain.

Acute Severe Pain

The severity of pain will usually dictate the order of the physical examination. Intense substernal pain mandates a rapid cardiovascular evaluation. Physical examination during acute myocardial infarction reveals a patient in significant distress. The skin is cool, and the patient may have diaphoresis. Blood pressure and pulse are usually elevated secondary to increased sympathetic tone. Decreased blood pressure or pulse usually indicates a complication of myocardial infarction such as a extensive myocardial necrosis with cardiac failure or significant bundle branch block. Inferior wall damage can produce hypotension and bradycardia due to stimulation of diaphragmatic vagal efferents. Asymmetry of the arterial pulses and a new aortic insufficiency murmur may indicate aortic dissection in a middle-aged man suffering from hypertension. Palpation may reveal a third or fourth heart sound consistent with decreased ventricular compliance and increased left atrial pressures. Signs of congestive heart failure such as pulmonary congestion or a third heart sound are usually indicative of transmural infarction. Mitral murmurs can indicate papillary dysfunction.

Subacute Chest Pain

Less intense pain or pain present after a cardiovascular source has been excluded can be evaluated in a more leisurely manner but with the same thoroughness. Most of the physical examination is directed at the musculoskeletal system. Four maneuvers appear to be the most useful in detecting acute chest wall pain. The first is a firm palpation of the sternum, left and right parasternal junctions, the intercostal spaces, the ribs, and the inframammary area. A complete examination of the pectoralis major, including its attachments, is crucial. This should include palpation and firm pressure on the humeral, clavicular, and lower costal attachments of this muscle. Abducting the arm will allow muscle stretch and better muscle definition. Muscle twitching with pressure and relief of pain and twitching with continued increased pressure are consistent with muscular contraction as the source of pain. The next technique to examine the pectoralis muscle group is horizontal flexion of the arm. With this maneuver, the arm is flexed across the anterior chest and steady, prolonged traction is applied horizontally. During this traction, the head is rotated to the ipsilateral shoulder as far as possible. Both arms are examined in this way. The third test position is called the "crowing rooster." The patient extends the neck while the physician standing behind the patient exerts traction on the upper arms by pulling them backward and slightly superiorly. This maneuver will usually bring out pain secondary to sternalis and pectoralis muscle involvement. The last maneuver is application of pressure to the top of the head. This increases tension in all intercostal and rib musculature and may reproduce the patient's spontaneous pain. The goal of palpation and of all of these maneuvers is to elicit the patient's own pain. It has been shown that atypical chest wall pain can be reproduced in over 90% of patients by using these techniques.[79,126,129]

In addition to proving that pain is coming from a musculoskeletal source, muscular entrapment of nerves, vessels, and lymphatics must be excluded. Common nerve entrapments are produced by cervical osteoarthritis and the thoracic outlet syndrome. Horizontal flexion of the arm and pressure to the top of the head may induce increased pain radiating to the arm, decreased arm muscle strength, and decreased mobility if nerve entrapment is present. Assuming the military position (shoulders back, chest out) may also induce these changes. Sympathetic nerve entrapment could produce Raynaud's phenomenon.[126,129] Arterial pulses should be examined to exclude subclavian artery involvement, producing decreased arterial pulses. Worsening pain and color changes with exercise can also be seen. Edema or dilated veins may also be present if venous compression occurs. Adson's maneuver may be required to bring out vascular involvement. Chin elevation and rotation of the head to the involved side with adduction of the arm will elicit evidence of nerve or vessel involvement.

Cervical osteoarthritis may induce signs and symptoms similar to thoracic outlet syndrome. Involvement of the posterior and anterior cervical muscles is more common, and posterior head involvement is almost universal. Head compression is the most useful test to produce this pain.

Physical examination in patients with hyperventilation/aerophagia is usually nonspecific. Excessive belching and abdominal distention with anxiety is almost always present. Perioral and peripheral paresthesias are common clues. Since all of these signs can be nonspecific, exclusion of acute angina pectoris or myocardial infarction is mandatory.

DIAGNOSTIC STRATEGIES

Evaluation of Anginal Chest Pain

MYOCARDIAL ISCHEMIA

The first strategy in differential diagnosis is to define anginal versus nonanginal chest pain. The incidence of abnormal coronary arteries or coronary vasospasm in patients with true angina is approximately 90%, while the incidence in patients with atypical chest pain is only 15%.[130] It is rare for any disease other than true myocardial ischemia to present as true angina with no atypical features. Although true angina has been reported with both esophageal and musculoskeletal diseases, coexistent coronary artery disease can be seen in up to 50% of patients in age groups in which esophageal and musculoskeletal causes for chest pain are common.[131,132] This underlies the importance of a complete cardiovascular evaluation in patients with both true angina and atypical anginal syndromes.

The questions are not should coronary artery disease be excluded but how far should one go to do so and also if coronary artery disease is found, is it the cause of the chest pain? Exercise stress testing is commonly used to exclude coronary artery disease but carries a sensitivity of only 64% and a specificity of 89%.[130,133]

In a young population, the incidence of false negativity can be as high as 40%.[130,133] Stress testing does exclude multivessel disease to a reasonable degree (85%) but cannot be used to exclude single-vessel disease (44% sensitivity).[130,133] Exercise stress testing cannot be used to exclude coronary artery disease in patients with true angina or in any high-risk patient with atypical anginal pain.

Radionuclide testing offers both anatomic and functional cardiac evaluation. Assessment of myocardial perfusion during exercise with thallium-201 is the most sensitive and specific of the radionuclide studies. An overall sensitivity of 80% and a specificity of 90% with a positive predictive value of 85% are the usual quoted figures.[130,134] This sensitivity and specificity can be increased if adequate cardiac stress (> 250 pressure-rate product) can be achieved. Radionuclide ventriculography offers functional evaluation of the heart. Regional dyskinesia or a 10% drop in global ejection fraction is seen in patients with myocardial ischemia.[130,134] Unfortunately the sensitivity and specificity of ventriculography is less than stress thallium-201 examination.[128,130,134] Newer radionuclide approaches and positron emission tomographic scanning may offer greater sensitivity but are still experimental.[130] The best current approach to rule out a coronary source in patients with atypical chest pain is thallium-201 testing. If the result of this examination is negative, coronary artery disease can be safely excluded (< 5% false negatives) if adequate cardiac stress (> 250 pressure-rate product) is achieved.

Coronary artery catheterization should only be used in patients with atypical chest pain if thallium-201 testing with adequate cardiac stress is positive or in patients who cannot achieve adequate cardiac stress. A frequently used substitute is thallium scanning after administration of dipyridamole. Dipyridamole is a coronary vasodilator that enhances blood flow differences during thallium scanning. Its sensitivity and specificity approach that of thallium scanning with adequate stress.[130] Cardiac catheterization should be performed in patients with typical angina even if thallium-201 testing is negative. If significant coronary artery obstruction is found (> 75% narrowing), angina is generally considered to be due to coronary artery disease. A positive thallium-201 scan in this situation offers confirmation of decreased perfusion with myocardium at risk. A negative coronary arteriography does not exclude cardiac angina unless ergonovine testing is performed to exclude coronary vasospasm. Reproduction of the patient's chest pain with ergonovine without demonstrable coronary vasospasm is highly predictive of esophageal dysmotility.[58,135]

Evaluation of Noncardiac Chest Pain

ESOPHAGEAL CHEST PAIN

The major goal of esophageal function testing is to correlate esophageal dysmotility or acid reflux with chest pain. Unfortunately, esophageal sources for chest pain frequently produce sporadic pain that is rarely present at the time of baseline manometric or pH testing. The gold standard to prove that the esophagus is the pain source is the presence of acid or esophageal dysmotility at the time of chest pain. For these reasons, esophageal provocation as a form of "stress testing" has evolved as a functional test of

the esophagus. The ideal esophageal provocation test should have a high positive predictive value and should be safe and easy to administer. Multiple provocative tests have been developed, including food and ice water swallows,[136-138] intraesophageal acid infusion,[139,140] and systemic injections of bethanechol,[141-143] edrophonium,[144,145] ergonovine,[146-148] and pentagastrin.[149,150] A review of these tests will allow the most logical approach to esophageal function testing.

Standard Provocative Tests

Food and Temperature Provocation. Many patients note that certain foods or cold liquids bring on their chest pain. Mellow showed that food ingestion could produce esophageal dysmotility that was not evident in baseline examinations.[151] This dysmotility was enhanced if bethanechol was administered concurrently (55 μg/kg). The rate of positive examinations in patients with food-induced symptoms was 100% while standard esophageal manometry was negative in all of these patients. Esophageal manometry in normal subjects did not differ before or after food or bethanechol administration. Low-temperature liquids can also incite chest pain.[136,138] Unlike food ingestion, which enhances nonperistaltic contractions and incomplete sphincter relaxation, ice water most commonly produces chest pain and a complete absence of motor activity in affected persons.[138] Modeling the provocative test around the situations that induce spontaneous pain requires serious future study.

Systemic Provocative Agents. Systemic administration of provocative agents is the current standard method for inducing pain in patients with chronic chest pain and presumed esophageal dysmotility. Pentagastrin was used because of its ability to induce repetitive contractions and high-amplitude waves in patients with achalasia and diffuse esophageal spasm.[149,150] The use of this agent in unselected patients with presumed esophageal pain is low (< 10%).[150] This may be due to the low incidence of achalasia and diffuse esophageal spasm in patients with chest pain (12%).[57,150] Ergonovine, the standard agent for provoking coronary vasospasm, has also been used in patients with esophageal dysfunction.[135,148] Coronary arteriography and vasospasm testing before ergonovine is used is considered necessary because of reported myocardial infarction following use of this agent.[135]

Bethanechol also induces motor abnormalities in patients with documented primary esophageal motility disorders such as achalasia and diffuse esophageal spasm.[51,139] Subcutaneous injection of bethanechol at doses of 40 to 50 μg/kg has induced chest pain in 12% to 33%.[142,143] Nostrant and co-workers[141] reported that bethanechol given as a bolus of 50 μg/kg and then repeated 15 minutes later increased the diagnostic yield to 77%. Patients were chosen by having true angina and normal coronary angiograms/stress radionuclide studies prior to entering the study. All parameters of esophageal motility (amplitude of contraction, duration of contraction or abnormal contractions) had a positive predictive value for chest pain. This means that patients with abnormally increased parameters (> mean + 2 SD) had chest pain (90%). However, only duration of contraction had a high negative predictive value (100%), implying no chest pain in patients with a normal duration of contraction. Bethanechol produced pain at the injection site in all patients but had no serious side effects. Fifteen of 154 patients were given atropine for relief of postinjection symptoms. Cardiac monitoring is required for all patients with known cardiac disease, but the test can safely be done to evaluate esophageal dysfunction even in patients with known coronary artery disease if coronary artery disease is not critical or considered the source for chest pain.[141]

The most common provocative agent used in esophageal function testing today is edrophonium hydrochloride.[57,144,145] Edrophonium is a cholinesterase inhibitor used in the diagnosis of myasthenia gravis. At a dose of 80 μg/kg it produces an increase in all esophageal parameters in normal and patient populations.[152] Benjamin and colleagues,[152] in their pioneering work, compared acid infusion, edrophonium (80 μg/kg), bethanechol (40 μg/kg SC), and pentagastrin (6 μg/kg SC) as provocative agents for esophageal chest pain.[152] All patients had chest pain that was believed not to be cardiac in origin. Separation into true angina and nonanginal chest pain was not done. None of the provocative agents induced chest pain frequently. Edrophonium induced chest pain in the highest percentage of patients (18%). The authors concluded that edrophonium was the test of choice based on the higher yield of positive examinations and a lower incidence of side effects. The rate of significant side effects in patients given edrophonium in this study was 38% and similar to the previously reported bethanechol study.[57,152] Currently the choice of provocative agent still remains unsettled and future studies defining and comparing patients based on pretest likelihood of esophageal disease are needed.

Acid Perfusion. Since its introduction in 1958 by Bernstein and Baker, acid infusion has been used to detect patients with presumed gastroesophageal reflux and acid-induced chest pain.[139,140] If heartburn is the endpoint, the sensitivity and specificity of this test approaches 80%.[140] Anginal chest pain may also be induced by acid.[139,140] The use of intraesophageal acid infusion in this situation is variable (7%–64%).[139,153,154] A false-positive rate of 10% was seen in normal controls and patients with peptic ulcer disease.[69] The test is long for both patient and physician if performed in the original way, and it loses only a small amount of specificity if modified to a single acid infusion. This simplification greatly reduces the duration of testing and may increase its widespread use in patients with chest pain.[153]

Usefulness of Standard Provocative Agents. Katz and associates' report of their experience with 910 patients with noncardiac pain is representative of most clinical investigators in this field.[57] Baseline esophageal motility was abnormal in 28%. Twenty-seven percent of the total patient group had their chest pain reproduced with provocation, defining the esophagus as the source of pain. Reproduction of chest pain was similar in the groups with and without baseline motility abnormalities. Only a small percentage had acid-induced pain (7%), while most had pain after edrophonium administration. The limitations of standard testing are based on a lack of a "gold standard" for esophageal pain. All of the current provocative agents can stimulate gastric, intestinal, colonic, and biliary motility, thus putting into question the source of pain. Acid infusion can also potentially induce myocardial ischemia.[37,38] The last major question is whether induced pain is the same as spontaneous pain. Final decisions on esophageal pain await further investigations into the pathophysiology of chest pain and further studies in patients with chest pain using prolonged monitoring techniques.

New Provocative Test

Esophageal Balloon Distention. Recent studies on esophageal balloon distention as a provocative test have led to renewed interest in this old standby for esophageal function testing.[8,9,155] Barish and co-workers[155] demonstrated abnormal sensory perception in patients with chest pain consistent with a psychological causation for chest pain. In addition, they found a high incidence of irritable bowel complaints in patients with chest pain induced by balloon dilatation. The addition of esophageal balloon distention to acid infusion and provocative esophageal stimulation increased the proportion of patients with induced chest pain from 24% to 48%.[155] Other investigators have not documented the usefulness of balloon distention.[156]

Ambulatory 24-Hour pH and Pressure Monitoring. Both of these techniques are still in their infancy, although 24-hour pH monitoring is gaining rapid acceptance as the standard test for acid reflux–induced chest pain. Two large studies of ambulatory pH and pressure monitoring have shown a greater incidence of acid-induced chest pain than previously reported.[25,154] Twenty-two of 92 chest pain episodes (24%) were associated with intraesophageal pH of less than 4.0, while only 5 episodes (7%) were associated with abnormal motility. A total of 36% of the painful events could be explained by abnormal motility or acid reflux. The cause of pain in the other 64% of chest pain events remains elusive.

Radionuclide Esophageal Emptying. The role of radionuclide scanning to measure esophageal emptying is well established for gastric emptying disorders, but its role in esophageal emptying has only recently been studied.[157-159] The attraction of this test lies in the speed of its performance, the quantifiable results, and its noninvasive nature. Several studies using the technique of scanning esophageal areas of interest have shown abnormalities in movement where conventional radiology and manometry were normal.[158] Decaestecker and colleagues,[158] in a review of 150 patients, found that radionuclide esophageal transit offered little more than standard manometry in achalasia.[159] However, both manometry and radionuclide scanning found a significant number of abnormalities not detected by the other test. Concordance of the two tests was 71%, while discordance was 29%. The major positive advantage of manometry was in patients with nutcracker esophagus and hypertensive lower esophageal sphincter. Overall sensitivity in detecting esophageal dysmotility was 73% for radionuclide esophageal transit, 83% for esophageal manometry, and 30% for barium studies.[158] The major future use of this technique will be in assessing treatment response in a noninvasive manner and offering a true first "esophageal function test."[157,159]

Diagnostic Strategy for Esophageal Chest Pain. After myocardial ischemia is excluded either clinically or by cardiac evaluation, esophageal function testing should be performed to decrease long-term disability and decrease medical resource overuse. If the patient presents with classic pyrosis and has no risk factors for cancer (advanced age, heavy alcohol/smoking, gastrointestinal bleeding, or dysphagia), a treatment trial is most appropriate. Patients with risk factors would require endoscopic evaluation. If the patient does not respond to mechanical antireflux measures and H₂ receptor antagonists, further evaluation is required. Standard esophageal manometrics with provocative testing with both acid infusion and a systemic provocative agent for dysmotility is the next step. Acid infusion should be continued for a minimum of 30 minutes before calling the test negative. Saline perfusion before or after acid infusion increases specificity but is not required. Chest pain and not heartburn should be the diagnostic end point. The choice of systemic provocative agent is still moot, with both bethanechol (50 μg/kg $\times$ 2) and edrophonium (80 μg/kg) having almost equal diagnostic efficacy and similar rates of side effects. Edrophonium might be the first choice in patients with known but clinically insignificant coronary artery disease because of the concern over paradoxic vasoconstriction with bethanechol in atherosclerotic coronary arteries.[8,9] It also offers a quicker examination. Bethanechol would be most useful in the patient with normal coronary arteries because of its increased sensitivity. Ergonovine for esophageal dysmotility would also be appropriate in those patients with chest pain reproduced by ergonovine during cardiac catheterization if coronary vasospasm is not seen. Esophageal dysmotility is found in most of these patients (80%) and has been documented in our laboratory with simultaneous esophageal manometrics and cardiac catheterization in patients with ergonovine-induced chest pain. Twenty percent of patients had simultaneous coronary spasm and esophageal dysmotility during testing, underlining the need for cardiac catheterization before or at the time of esophageal testing if ergonovine is used.

MUSCULOSKELETAL CHEST PAIN

History and physical examination is the standard diagnostic strategy for chest wall pain. Electromyography, nerve conduction velocity, and Doppler flow studies are used to exclude significant muscle, nerve, or vascular entrapment. Relief of pain with involved muscle stretching and vasocoolant spraying confirms the diagnosis.

HYPERVENTILATION/AEROPHAGIA/PANIC DISORDER

History and physical examination will point to the diagnosis. Exclusion of cardiac disease is foremost since many of the symptoms of hyperventilation can be reproduced by myocardial ischemia. A controlled hyperventilation trial will establish the diagnosis and allow the patient to recognize the association of symptoms with excessive breathing.[113,114] Known cardiovascular or cerebrovascular disease, as well as sickle cell anemia or baseline hypoxemia, are relative contraindications to hyperventilation testing.

THERAPEUTIC CONSIDERATIONS

Ischemic Heart Disease

Primary prevention and reduction in risk for myocardial infarction should be the goals of treatment.[130,134] Nitroglycerin, in its many forms, is still the mainstay of treatment for acute cardiac angina. Prophylactic use is most beneficial since it allows an increase in physical activity. Tolerance is common and can be diminished by intermittent use.[130,134,160] Since myocardial ischemia can be silent and occurs in the early morning, continuous treatment with a long-acting nitroglycerin preparation should be seriously considered even during pain-free intervals.[160]

Calcium-blocking agents are increasing in popularity as primary treatment for angina pectoris.[130,161] This group of medications increases blood flow to the entire myocardium through relaxation of arterioles and large vessels.[134] Nifedipine produces significant tachycardia, hypotension, and pedal edema. Verapamil and diltiazem decrease heart rate and can exacerbate conduction defects and bradyarrythmias. All of these agents can increase congestive heart failure.

β-Adrenergic blockers are also effective antianginal medications.[130,134] They are particularly useful in exercise-induced chest pain in patients without congestive heart failure. Their primary use is as adjuncts to nitroglycerin and nifedipine to control heart rate.

The choice of surgery or angioplasty is individual but should be a serious consideration in patients who do not respond to medical treatment or who are at high risk for extensive myocardial damage (i.e., triple-vessel disease, proximal left anterior descending artery stenosis).[162-168]

Esophageal Chest Pain

TREATMENT OPTIONS

Therapeutic options in patients with documented esophageal pain are much less clear than those with myocardial ischemia.[8,9] Much of the problem stems from prior trials of treatment in patients with the umbrella diagnosis of "diffuse esophageal spasm." Newer subgroups of motility disorders, such as nutcracker esophagus and hypertensive lower esophageal sphincter, will need to be studied separately to design effective treatment. In addition to these problems, exclusion of gastroesophageal acid reflux is mandatory since treatment with nitroglycerin, β-blockade, and, particularly, calcium-blocking agents, can increase gastroesophageal reflux and decrease acid clearance, potentially leading to worsening pain.[8,9,169]

Nitrates. The effectiveness of nitroglycerin in esophageal dysmotility relates to relaxation of smooth muscle. Although response can be dramatic in individual patients, overall effectiveness in this patient population has yet to be proven. Chest pain after eating may be alleviated with preprandial administration of nitroglycerin.[170,171]

Anticholinergics. Like nitrates, anticholinergics may have significant individual effectiveness but are not useful in the vast majority of patients.[8,9] A short-term trial is appropriate (1 to 2 weeks) but should not be continued unless objective response is documented. Patient diaries before and after treatment are extremely useful.

Anxiolytics/Antidepressants/Behavioral Modification. The high incidence of psychiatric disorders or abnormal psychological profiles in patients with esophageal dysmotility has prompted evaluation of these medications for esophageal pain. Clouse and associates,[67] in a controlled trial, have shown decreased symptom scores in patients treated with antidepressants. No effect on esophageal pressure or duration of contraction was seen in patients successfully treated with antidepressants. Biofeedback may hold some promise for stress-induced symptoms, but controlled studies with defined forms of esophageal dysmotility are needed.

Calcium-Blocking Agents. The use of calcium-blocking agents is based on smooth muscle relaxation. Amplitude of contraction is decreased with nifedipine but requires a dose (30 mg) that produces significant side effects.[169] Controlled trials with nifedipine have been disappointing.[171–173] Controlled and uncontrolled studies with diltiazem have shown both no effect and dramatic response.[174] To date, all studies are quite preliminary and like the medications noted previously, a therapeutic trial is reasonable but should be stopped if no response is seen.

Esophageal Bougienage, Pneumatic Dilatation, and Esophageal Myotomy. All of these measures are considered a last resort. Bougienage and pneumatic dilatation may be effective on an individual basis but should be reserved to those patients with dysphagia as their primary or predominant symptom.[175,176] Patients with dysphagia and hypertensive lower esophageal sphincter with documented food delay at the gastroesophageal junction on scintigraphy may well be suited to this treatment. Treatment of chest pain alone with any of these modalities is limited. Esophagomyotomy should be reserved for the rare patient whose life style is severely compromised and who has failed other treatments, including bougienage and pneumatic dilatation.[177]

APPROACH TO TREATMENT OF ESOPHAGEAL DYSMOTILITY

Documentation is crucial here. Intermittent symptoms can best be controlled with reassurance and short-acting agents such as nitroglycerin or sublingual calcium-blocking agents. Tranquilizers are a useful adjunct only in patients with clear-cut stress-induced symptoms. Use of long-term medical treatment should be reserved for those patients with distressing continuous symptoms. It is important to tell the patient that medical treatment can be effective in controlling symptoms but is unlikely to be curative.

APPROACH TO TREATMENT OF GASTROESOPHAGEAL REFLUX

The treatment of symptomatic gastroesophageal reflux and reflux-induced esophagitis is covered in chapter 55. H$_2$ receptor antagonists are the mainstay of treatment and have been clearly shown to be effective treatment for both acid-induced symptoms and acid-induced inflammation when compared with placebo. Symptoms respond better to treatment than does inflammation. H$_2$ receptor antagonists will be effective in relieving symptoms in over 80% of patients if treatment is continued for 12 weeks. Erosions and ulcerations are more difficult to heal, with response rates of 50% with large ulcers.[178] Treatment may need to be more prolonged

or continuous. Relapse of symptoms is rapid after discontinuing medication, with 75% relapsing in the first 6 months.[178] Reintroduction of treatment the second time is usually as effective as the first. Nocturnal dosing is usually inadequate, and more frequent dosing (two or four times a day) with stronger agents (ranitidine, 150 or 300 mg) or famotidine (20 or 40 mg) may be necessary to control symptoms and/or inflammation. The use of sucralfate is primarily as an adjunct in patients with documented inflammation[179,180]; its use for reflux symptoms without inflammation needs documentation. Metoclopramide and bethanechol, both alone and in combination with H$_2$ receptor antagonists, are effective for symptoms and/or inflammation.[179,181] These prokinetic agents alone are equally effective as H$_2$ receptor antagonists in patients with esophagitis.[181] Side effects from these medications usually limit their role. Newer prokinetic agents (domperidone, cisapride) do increase esophageal and gastric emptying in higher doses (20–30 mg), but documentation of their use in acid-reflux treatment is still preliminary. Omeprazole, a substituted benzimidazole, has been approved for use in refractory esophagitis and severe esophagitis at initial presentation.[182,183] Omeprazole covalently binds to hydrogen-potassium adenosine triphosphatase selectively in the parietal cell and essentially eliminates acid secretion by that cell for prolonged periods.[184] Higher and more rapid rates of esophageal healing compared with standard doses of H$_2$ receptor antagonists have been shown. Long-term safety has not been documented, and maintenance therapy with this medication is not recommended at this time.

Surgery is usually reserved for patients who experience treatment failure. Recalcitrant esophagitis is the usual reason for surgical correction. It is important to remember that continuous reflux symptoms without esophagitis can be as incapacitating as esophageal inflammation and may require antireflux surgery. A common example of this is the heavy laborer with severe symptoms when lifting but no inflammation on endoscopy. Esophageal surgery in experienced hands carries a low morbidity and mortality. Ten-year breakdown rates are acceptable, and recurrent symptoms/inflammation are low.[185] Fundoplication has the best response rate, while posterior gastropexy (Hill procedure) has the least.[185] The key to any successful antireflux procedure is the choice of the surgeon who performs it.

Musculoskeletal Chest Pain

The treatment of acute muscular pain and chronic musculoskeletal pain is markedly different. Although warmth and analgesia (particularly nonsteroidal anti-inflammatory medications) are useful for acute muscular pain, they are rarely helpful in the long-term management of chronic pain and many analgesics have significant gastrointestinal toxicity. Stretch and vasocoolant spray are the basis of treatment in all patients with chronic musculoskeletal pain. Stretch is the essential component but is not easily accomplished unless spraying precedes the stretching. Each of the major muscle groups (pectoralis major, pectoralis minor, and sternalis) should be examined and trigger points located. Active or latent trigger points may decrease movement, and vasocoolant spraying may allow a full range of motion. Multiple treatment sessions may be required. Both before and after a treatment session, moist warm packs should be applied to the involved muscles to decrease muscle tension and post-treatment muscle soreness. Moist heat is preferable to dry heat to allow full skin stretching with exercise. Moist heating pads may be all that is required when previously active trigger points become active again. Heat treatment applied over 2 to 3 days may replace stretch and spray techniques. The basis of all of these techniques involves spinal inhibition by skin afferents and direct effects on trigger points.[91]

Reasons for failure are many but most commonly involve inadequate stretching technique, noncorrection of spinal or posture perpetuating factors, or inadequate post-treatment maintenance. The efforts of both a dedicated physiatrist and physical therapist are invaluable.

As pain subsides, restriction of motion secondary to active muscular contraction may prevent further treatment and diminish response. Reactivation of trigger points is more common here. In addition, stretching of certain muscles, such as the sternalis muscle, is limited or impossible. Injection techniques in addition to stretch and spray methods may be necessary for many chronic chest pain syndromes. Injection with procaine 0.5% diluted from 2% with isotonic saline is most commonly used because of its efficacy, its low systemic side effects, its low cost, and its reasonable duration of action. Epinephrine should be avoided since it can increase pain from active trigger points. Dry needling without injection may also be effective in some cases. After injection is completed, stretch and spray should always be done for maximum effect.[91]

In addition to the standard stretching, vasocoolant spraying, and injection techniques, alternative treatments may afford increased success. These include ischemic compression, massage, and ultrasound. Ischemic compression applies force in a sustained fashion to inactivate trigger points. This is especially useful in muscles that are relatively thin and overlie the bone, such as the sternalis. Acupuncture may work in this fashion as well. Massage and ultrasound produce their benefit by heating muscles and improving stretch.

Corrective actions in posture are extremely helpful for chest wall pain. A slouched posture with the head and shoulders projected forward puts the pectoralis major muscle at strain. Standing straight expands the anterior chest and improves muscle stretch. A similar condition is produced by sitting in reclining chairs. A lumbar support will produce the same effect as standing straight.

A coordinated approach involving the internist, physiatrist, and pain specialist will give the best overall results in patients with chest wall pain.

Hyperventilation/Aerophagia/ Panic Disorder

The major diagnostic and therapeutic maneuver in patients with hyperventilation is to provoke the patient's symptoms with the hyperventilation trial. This allows symptom correlation with excessive breathing. Breathing awareness, relaxation techniques, and altered breathing patterns will be useful for this group of patients. Lum has shown that conversion from thoracic to abdominal breathing will allow the respiratory center to adjust to higher levels of $PaCO_2$.[186] β-blockers have been used to decrease sympathetic tone.[186] Palpitations but not fatigue might be helped by this treatment.

Reassurance is the best method to alleviate symptoms. Lum reported that 70% of 640 patients treated by the above techniques were completely asymptomatic and 20% to 25% of the remainder improved.[187] Approximately one third required more than one to two revisits. Only 10% of patients experienced recurrences over the next 6 to 24 months, and these were controllable by rebreathing techniques. Since hyperventilation can be a chronic recurring problem, strong physician support at least initially is recommended.

The patient with aerophagia offers similar but frequently more difficult treatment problems. Postprandial symptoms can usually be managed with small frequent meals, preferably avoiding caffeine and other stimulants. Since symptoms are decreased in the standing position and exercise after meals improves gastric emptying, this should be encouraged. Partial relief with simethicone-containing antacids is a temporary solution. Recognition of the role of air swallowing and exclusion of gastrointestinal motility disorders should be the goal of both patient and physician. Recognizing the coexistence of hyperventilation with aerophagia will help the patient connect excessive breathing with air swallowing. A logical and compassionate approach will frequently be rewarded with success.

> The reader is directed to Chapter 54, Motility Disorders of the Esophagus; and Chapter 55, Reflux Esophagitis.

REFERENCES

1. Katon W, Vitalliano DD, Russo J, et al. Panic disorder: epidemiology in primary care. J Fam Pract 1986;23:233.
2. Mayou R. The patient with angina: symptoms and disability. Postgrad Med J 1973;49:250.
3. Kemp HG, Vokonas PS, Cohn PF, et al. The anginal syndrome associated with normal coronary arteriograms: report of a six year experience. Am J Med 1973;54:735.
4. Wielgosz AT, Fletcher RH, McCants CB, et al. Unimproved chest pain in patients with minimal or no coronary disease: a behavioral phenomenon. Am Heart J 1984;108:67.
5. Ockene IS, Shay MJ, Alpert JS, et al. Unexplained chest pain in patients with normal coronary arteriograms: a follow-up of functional status. N Engl J Med 1980;303:1249.
6. Cannon RO, Leon MB, Watson R, et al. Chest pain and "normal" coronary arteries—role of small coronary arteries. Am J Cardiol 1985;55:50B.
7. Cannon RO, Bonow RO, Bacharach SL, et al. Left ventricular dysfunction in patients with angina pectoris, normal epicardial coronary arteries and abnormal vasodilator reserve. Circulation 1985;71:218.
8. Richter JE, Castell DO. Esophageal disease as a cause of noncardiac chest pain. Adv Intern Med 1988;33:311.
9. Richter JE, Bradley LA, Castell DO. Esophageal chest pain: current controversies in pathogenesis, diagnosis and therapy. Ann Intern Med 1989;110:66.
10. Ward BW, Wu WC, Richter JE, et al. Long-term follow-up of symptomatic status of patients with noncardiac chest pain: is diagnosis of esophageal etiology useful? Am J Gastroenterol 1987;82:215.
11. Aohel FL, Nordstrom LA, Nelson RR, et al. The rate pressure product as an index of myocardial oxygen consumption in patients with angina pectoris. Circulation 1978;57:549.
12. Donat WE. Chest pain: cardiac and noncardiac causes. Clin Chest Med 1987;8:241.

13. Christie LA, Conti CR. Systematic approach to the evaluation of angina-like chest pain. Am Heart J 1981;102:897.

14. Sampson JJ, Cheitew M. Pathophysiology and differential diagnosis of cardiac pain. Prog Cardiovasc Dis 1971;13:507.

15. Schneider RR, Seckler SG. Evaluation of acute chest pain. Med Clin North Am 1981;65:53.

16. Astrand PO. Quantification of exercise capability. Prog Cardiovasc Dis 1976;19:51.

17. Henry JA, Montuschi E. Cardiac pain referred to site of previously experienced somatic pain. Br Med J 1978;2:1605.

18. Joyner CR, Cornman CR. The mitral value prolapse syndrome: clinical features and management. In: Frankl WS, Brest AW, eds. Valvular heart disease: comprehensive evaluation and management. Philadelphia: FA Davis, 1986:233.

19. Siegel CI, Hendrix TR. Esophageal motor abnormalities induced by acid perfusion in patients with heartburn. J Clin Invest 1963;42:686.

20. Atikinson M, Bennett JR. Relationship between motor changes and pain during esophageal acid perfusion. Am J Dig Dis 1968;13:346.

21. Tuttle SG, Rufin F, Bettarello A. The physiology of heartburn. Ann Intern Med 1961;55:292.

22. Richter JE, Johns DN, Wu WC, et al. Are esophageal motility abnormalities produced during the intraesophageal acid perfusion test? JAMA 1985;253:1914.

23. Swamy N. Esophageal spasm: clinical and manometric response to nitroglycerin and long-acting nitrates. Gastroenterology 1977;72:23.

24. Kjellen A, Tibbling L. Oesophageal motility during acid-provoked heartburn and chest pain. Scand J Gastroenterol 1985;20:937.

25. Peters LJ, Maas L, Petty D, et al. Spontaneous noncardiac chest pain: evaluation by 24-hour ambulatory esophageal motility and pH monitoring. Gastroenterology 1988;94:878.

26. Johnston LF, DeMeester TR. Twenty-four hour pH monitoring of the distal esophagus: a quantitative measure of gastroesophageal reflux. Am J Gastroenterol 1974;62:325.

27. DeMeester TR, Wang CI, Wernly JA, et al. Technique, indications and clinical use of 24-hour esophageal pH monitoring. J Thoracic Cardiovascular Surg 1980;79:656.

28. Orlando RC, Powell DW, Carney CN. Pathophysiology of acute acid injury in rabbit esophageal epithelium. J Clin Invest 1981;68:286.

29. Carney CN, Orlando RC, Powell DW, et al. Morphologic alterations in early acid-induced epithelial injury of the rabbit esophagus. Lab Invest 1981;45:198.

30. Lacey SJ, Operkun AR, Larkai E, et al. Sensitivity of the esophageal mucosa to pH in gastroesophageal reflux disease. Gastroenterology 1989;96:683.

31. Richter JE, Castell DO. Gastroesophageal reflux: pathogenesis, diagnosis and therapy. Ann Intern Med 1982;97:93.

32. Robinson MG, Orr WC, McCallum R, et al. Do endoscopic findings influence response to H$_2$ antagonist therapy for gastroesophageal reflux disease. Am J Gastroenterol 1987;82:519.

33. Kahrilas PJ, Dodds WJ, Hogan WJ. Dysfunction of the belch reflex. Gastroenterology 1987;93:818.

34. Richter JE, Barish CF, Castell DO. Abnormal sensory perception in patients with esophageal chest pain. Gastroenterology 1986;91:845.

35. Barish CF, Castell DO, Richter JE. Graded esophageal balloon distention: a new provocative test for noncardiac chest pain. Dig Dis Sci 1986;31:1292.

36. Kaye MD, Kilby AE, Harper PC. Changes in distal esophageal function in response to cooling. Dig Dis Sci 1987;32:22.

37. Mellow MH, Simpson AG, Watt L, et al. Esophageal acid perfusion in coronary artery disease: induction of myocardial ischemia. Gastroenterology 1983;83:306B.

38. Yakshe PN, Cattau EL, Cannon RO, et al. Role of provocative testing in differentiating esophageal and cardiac pain in patients with microvascular angina and esophageal motility disorders. Gastroenterology 1989;96:975.

39. Bass BL, Schweitzer EJ, Harmon JW, et al. H$^+$ back diffusion interferes with intrinsic reactive regulation of esophageal mucosal blood flow. Surgery 1984;96:404.

40. Mackenzie J, Land D, Belch J. Esophageal ischemia in motility disorders associated with chest pain. Lancet 1988;2:592.

41. Tindell H, Tooke JE, Menys VC, et al. Effect of dazoxiben, a thromboxane synthetase inhibitor on skin blood flow following cold challenge in patients with Raynaud's phenomena. Eur J Clin Invest 1985;15:20.

42. Pellegrini CA, Demelstier TR, Wernly JA, et al. Alkaline gastroesophageal reflux. Am J Surg 1978;125:177.

43. Lillemore KD, Johnson JF, Harmon JW. Alkaline esophagitis: a comparison of the ability of components of gastroesophageal contents to injure the rabbit esophagus. Gastroenterology 1983;85:621.

44. Matikainen M, Laatikainen T, Kalima T, et al. Bile acid composition and esophagitis after total gastrectomy. Am J Surg 1982;143:196.

45. Kikendall JW, Friedman AC, Oyewole AM, et al. Pill-induced esophageal injury: case reports and review of the medical literature. Dig Dis Sci 1983;28:174.

46. Agha FP, Wilson JAP, Nostrant TT. Medication-induced esophagitis. Gastrointestinal Radiol 1986;11:7.

47. Coates A, Nostrant T, Wilson JAP, et al. Nonsteroidal anti-inflammatory medication–induced esophagitis: case reports and review of the literature. S Med J 1986;9:1094.

48. Bailey RT, Bonavina L, McChesney L, et al. Factors influencing the transit of gelatin capsules in the esophagus. Drug Intell Clin Pharm 1987;21:282.

49. Russel LD, Hill LD, Holmes ER, et al. Radionuclide transit: a sensitive screening test for esophageal dysfunction. Gastroenterology 1981;8:887.

50. Lloyd DA, Borda IT. Food-induced heartburn: effect of osmolality. Gastroenterology 1981;80:741.

51. Price SF, Smithsau KW, Castell DO. Food sensitivity in reflux esophagitis. Gastroenterology 1978;75:240.

52. Richter JE, Castell DO. Diffuse esophageal spasm: a reappraisal. Ann Intern Med 1984;100:242.

53. Clouse RF, Staiano A. Contraction abnormalities of the esophageal body in patients referred for manometry: a new approach to manometric classification. Dig Dis Sci 1983;28:784.

54. Richter JE, Wu WC, Johns DN, et al. Esophageal manometry in 95 healthy adult volunteers: variability of pressures with age and frequency of abnormal contractions. Dig Dis Sci 1987;32:583.

55. Vantrappen G, Janssen J, Hellemans SJ, et al. Achalasia, esophageal spasm and related motility disorders. Gastroenterology 1979;76:450.

56. Clouse RA. Motor disorders of the esophagus. In: Sleisenger MH, Fordtran JS, eds. Gastrointestinal disease, pathophysiology, diagnosis and treatment. Philadelphia: WB Saunders, 1989:567.

57. Katz PO, Dalton CB, Richter JE, et al. Esophageal testing of patients with noncardiac chest pain and/or dysphagia. Ann Intern Med 1987;106:513.

58. Brand DL, Martin D, Pope CE. Esophageal manometrics in patients with angina-like chest pain. Am J Dig Dis 1977;22:300.

59. Benjamin SB, Gerhardt DC, Castell DO. High-amplitude, peristaltic esophageal contractions associated with chest pain and/or dysphagia. Gastroenterology 1979;77:478.

60. Traube M, Abibi R, McCallum RW. High-amplitude peristaltic esophageal contractions associated with chest pain. JAMA 1983;250:2655.

61. Herrington JP, Burns TW, Balart LA. Chest pain and dysphagia in patients with prolonged peristaltic contractile duration of the esophagus. Dig Dis Sci 1984;29:134.

62. Orr WC, Robinson MG. Hypertensive peristalsis in the pathogenesis of chest pain. Am J Gastroenterol 1982;77:604.

63. Clouse RE, Lustman PJ. Psychiatric illnesses and contraction abnormalities of the esophagus. N Engl J Med 1982;309:1337.

64. Richter JE, Obrecht WF, Bradley LA, et al. Psychological similarities between patients with nutcracker esophagus and irritable bowel syndrome. Dig Dis Sci 1986;31:131.

65. Code CF, Schlegel SF, Kelley ML, et al. Hypertensive gastroesophageal sphincter. Mayo Clin Proc 1960;35:391.

66. Garrett JM, Godwin DH. Gastroesophageal hypercontracting sphincter. JAMA 1969;108:993.

67. Clouse RE, Lustman PJ, Eckert TC, et al. Low-dose trazodone for symptomatic patients with esophageal contraction abnormalities—a double-blind placebo-controlled trial. Gastroenterology 1987;92:1027.

68. Young LD, Richter JE, Anderson KO, et al. The effects of psychological and environmental stressors on peristaltic esophageal contraction in healthy volunteers. Psychophysiology 1987;24:132.

69. Behar J, Biancani P, Sheahan DG. Evaluation of esophageal tests in the diagnosis of reflux esophagitis. Gastroenterology 1967;71:9.

70. Doran F. Sites of pain referred from the common bile duct. Br J Surg 1967;54:599.

71. Cullen M, Reese H. Myocardial circulatory changes measured by clearance of ^{24}Na; effect of common bile duct distension on myocardial circulation. J Appl Physiol 1953;5:28.

72. Geenan JE, Hogan WS, Dodds WJ, et al. The efficacy of endoscopic sphincterotomy after cholecystectomy in patients with sphincter of Oddi dysfunction. N Engl J Med 1989;320:82.

73. Steinberg WM. Sphincter of Oddi dysfunction: a clinical controversy. Gastroenterology 1988;95:1409.

74. Ravdin IS. Reflexes originating in the common duct giving rise to pain simulating angina pectoris. Ann Surg 1942;115:1055.

75. Wolfe E, Stern S. Costosternal syndrome: its frequency and importance in differential diagnosis of coronary heart disease. Arch Intern Med 1976;136:189.

76. Tietze A. Veber eine eigenartige hallfung von fallen mit dystrophie der rippen knorpel. Berl Klin Wochenschr 1921;58:829.

77. Edelstein G, Levitt RG, Slaker DP, et al. Computed tomography of Tietze syndrome. J Comput Assist Tomogr 1984;8:20.

78. Sain AK. Bone scan in Tietze's syndrome. Clin Nucl Med 1978;3:470.

79. Fam AG, Symthe HA. Musculoskeletal chest wall pain. J Can Med Assoc 1985;133:379.

80. Wright JT. Slipping rib syndrome. Lancet 1980;2:632.

81. Miller AJ, Texidor TA. "Precordial catch" neglected syndrome of precordial pain. JAMA 1955;159:1364.

82. Sparrow MJ, Bird EL. "Precordial catch": a benign syndrome of chest pain in young persons. N Z Med J 1978;88:325.

83. Travell J, Berry C, Bigelow NH. Effects of referred somatic pain on structures in the reference zone. Fed Proc 1944;3:49.

84. Mense S, Schmidt RF. Muscle pain: which receptors are responsible for the transmission of noxious stimuli. In: Rose FC, ed. Physiological aspects of clinical neurology. Oxford, 1977:345.

85. Melzack R, Wall PD. Pain mechanisms: a new theory. Science 1965;150:971.

86. Procacci P, Zoppi M. Pathophysiology and clinical aspects of visceral and referred pain. Pain [Suppl] 1981;1:6.

87. Sola AE, Rodenberger ML, Geity BB. Incidence of hypersensitive areas in posterior shoulder muscles. Am J Phys Med 1955;34:585.

88. Bonica JJ. Neurophysiologic and pathologic aspects of acute and chronic pain. Arch Surg 1977;112:750.

89. Goldberg M, Murray TG. Analgesic associated nephropathy. N Engl J Med 1978;299:716.

90. Reynolds MD. Myofascial trigger point syndromes in the practice of rheumatology. Arch Phys Med Rehabil 1981;62:111.

91. Travell JG, Simons DG. Background and principles. In: Travell JG, Simons DG, eds. Myofascial pain and dysfunction—a trigger point manual. Baltimore: Williams & Wilkins, 1983:12.

92. Melzack R, Stillwell DM, Fox EJ. Trigger points and acupuncture points for pain: correlations and implications. Pain 1977;3:3.

93. Kendall HO, Kendall FP, Wadsworth GE. Muscle testing and function. Baltimore: Williams & Wilkins, 1971.

94. Inman VT, Saunders JB. Referred pain from skeletal structures. J Nerv Ment Dis 1944;99:660.

95. MacDonald AJR. Abnormally tender muscle regions and associated painful movements. Pain 1980;8:197.

96. Simons DG. Muscle pain syndromes: I and II. Am J Phys Med 1975;54:289 and 55:15.

97. Bennett RM. Fibrositis: does it exist and can it be treated? J Musculoskel Med 1984;1:57.

98. Symthe HA. "Fibrositis" as a disorder of pain modulation. Clin Rheum Dis 1979;5:823.

99. Awald EA. Interstitial myofibrositis: hypothesis of the mechanism. Arch Phys Med 1973;54:440.

100. Travell J. Introductory comments. In: Rajan C, ed. Connective Tissues Transactions of the 5th Conference. New York: Josiah-Macy Jr Foundation, 1954:12.

101. Fassbender HG. Pathology of rheumatic diseases. New York: Springer Verlag, 1975:303.

102. Popelianskii IU, Zaslauskii ES, Vesolusrii VP. Medicosocial significance, etiology, pathogenesis and diagnosis of nonarticular disease of soft tissue of the limb and back. Vopr Rheum 1976;3:38.

103. Marbach JJ. Arthritis of the temporomandibular joint. Am Fam Physician 1979;19:131.

104. Kraft GH, Johnson EW, Laban MM. The fibrositis syndrome. Arch Phys Med 1968;49:155.

105. Simons DG, Travell JG. Myofascial trigger points: a possible explanation. Pain 1981;10:106.

106. Stenger RJ, Spiro D, Scully RE, et al. Ultrastructural and physiological alterations in ischemic skeletal muscle. Am J Pathol 1962;40:1.

107. Edeiken J, Wolferth CC. Persistent pain in the shoulder region following myocardial infarction. Am J Med Sci 1936;191:201.

108. DeMaria AN, Lee G, Amsterdam G, et al. The anginal syndrome with normal coronary arteries. JAMA 1980;244:826.

109. Travell JJ, Simons DG. The pectoralis major muscle. In: Travell JJ, Simons DG, eds. Myofascial pain and dysfunction—a trigger point manual. Baltimore: Williams & Wilkins, 1986:576.

110. Moldofsky H, Scarisbrick P. Induction of neurasthenic musculoskeletal pain syndrome by selective sleep deprivation. Psychosom Med 1976;38:35.

111. Moldofsky H, Scarisbrick P, England R, et al. Musculoskeletal symptoms and non REM sleep disturbance in patients with "fibrositis syndrome" and healthy subjects. Psychosom Med 1975;37:341.

112. Magarian GJ. Hyperventilation syndromes: infrequently recognized common expressions of anxiety and stress. Medicine 1982;61:219.

113. Magarian CJ. Noncardiac causes of angina-like chest pain. Prog Cardiovasc Dis 1986;29:65.

114. Wheatley CE, Hyperventilation syndrome: a frequent cause of chest pain. Chest 1975;68:195.

115. Lary D, Goldschlager N. Electrocardiographic changes during hyperventilation resembling myocardial ischemia in patients with normal coronary arteriograms. Am Heart J 1974;87:383.

116. Jacobs WF, Battle WE, Ronen JA. False-positive ST-T wave changes secondary to hyperventilation and exercise: cine angiographic correlation. Ann Intern Med 1974;81:479.

117. Neill WA, Hattenhauer M. Impairment of myocardial oxygen supply due to hyperventilation. Circulation 1975;52:854.

118. Rasmussen K, Bagger JP, Bottzauw B, et al. Prevalence of vasospastic ischemia induced by the cold pressor test or hyperventilation in patients with severe angina. Eur Heart J 1984;5:354.

119. Roth JLA. The symptom patterns of gaseousness. Ann NY Acad Sci 1968;150:109.

120. Freeman LJ, Nixon PEG. Chest pain and the hyperventilation syndrome—some aetiological considerations. Postgrad Med 1985;61:957.

121. Beitman BD, Basha I, Flaker G, et al. Angina or nonanginal chest pain: Panic disorder or coronary artery disease. Arch Intern Med 1987;147:1548.

122. Bass C, Wade C. Chest pain with normal coronary arteries: a comparative study of psychiatric and social morbidity. Psychol Med 1984;14:51.

123. Mukerji V, Beitman BD, Alpert MA, et al. Panic attack in chest pain patients with angiographically normal coronary arteries. J Anxiety Disord 1987;1:41.

124. Constant J. The clinical diagnosis of nonanginal chest pain: the differentiation of angina from nonanginal chest pain by history. Clin Cardiol 1983;6:11.

125. Buda A, Levene DL. The influence of inspiration on angina pectoris: a clue to right coronary artery disease. Am Heart J 1976;92:537.

126. Kremer RM, Ahlquist RE. Thoracic outlet syndrome. Am J Surg 1975;130:612.

127. Levene DL. Some helpful hints. In: Levene DL, ed. Chest pain: an integrated diagnostic approach. Philadelphia: Lea & Febiger, 1977:183.

128. McElroy JB. Angina pectoris with coexisting skeletal pain. Am Heart J 1973;66:196.

129. Epstein SE, Gerber LH, Borer JS. Chest wall syndrome: a common cause of unexplained cardiac pain. JAMA 1979;241:2793.

130. Roberts R. Ischemic heart disease. In: Kelley WN, ed. Textbook of internal medicine. Philadelphia: JB Lippincott, 1989:144.

131. Svensson O, Stenport G, Tibbling L, et al. Oesophageal function and coronary angiograms in patients with disabling chest pain. Acta Med Scand 1978;204:173.

132. Alban-Davies H, Jones DB, Rhodes J, et al. Angina-like esophageal

pain: differentiation from cardiac pain by history. J Clin Gastroenterol 1985;7:477.

133. Beller GA, Gibson RS. Sensitivity specificity and prognositc significance of noninvasive testing for occult or known coronary disease. Prog Cardiovasc Dis 1987;29:241.

134. Williams ES, Willerson JT. Approach to the patient with chest pain. In: Kelley WN, ed. Textbook of internal medicine. Philadelphia: JB Lippincott, 1989:374.

135. Eastwood GL, Weyner BH, Dickerson J, et al. Use of ergonovine to identify esophageal spasm in patients with chest pain. Ann Intern Med 1981;94:768.

136. Respass JC, Ingelfinger FJ, Kramer P, et al. Effect of cold on esophageal motor function. Am J Med 1952;20:955.

137. Catalano CJ, Bozymski EM, Orlando RC. Temperature dependent symptoms in a patient with esophageal motor disease. Gastroenterology 1983;85:1407.

138. Meyer GW, Castell DO. Human esophageal response during chest pain induced by swallowing cold liquids. JAMA 1981;246:2057.

139. Hewson EG, Sinclair JW, Dalton CB, et al. Acid perfusion test: does it have a role in the assessment of noncardiac chest pain. Gut 1989;30:305.

140. Richter JE, Castell DO. Gastroesophageal reflux: pathogenesis, diagnosis and therapy. Ann Intern Med 1982;97:93.

141. Nostrant TT, Sams J, Huber T. Bethanechol increases the diagnostic yield in patients with esophageal chest pain. Gastroenterology 1986;91:1131.

142. Cole MJ, Paterson WG, Beck IT, et al. The effect of acid and bethanechol stimulation in patients with symptomatic hypertensive peristaltic (nutcracker) esophagus. J Clin Gastroenterol 1986;8:223.

143. Mellow M. Symptomatic diffuse esophageal spasm: manometric follow-up and response to cholinergic stimulation and cholinesterase inhibition. Gastroenterology 1977;73:237.

144. Richter JE, Hackshaw BT, Wu WC, et al. Edrophonium: a useful provocative test for esophageal chest pain. Ann Intern Med 1985;103:14.

145. London RC, Ouyang A, Snape WJ, et al. Provocation of esophageal pain by ergonovine or edrophonium. Gastroenterology 1981;81:10.

146. Koch KL, Curry C, Feldman RL. Ergonovine-induced esophageal spasm in patients with chest pain resembling angina pectoris. Dig Dis Sci 1982;27:1073.

147. Dalab JJ, Dast AM, Alban-Davies H, et al. Coronary and peripheral artery responses to ergometrine in patients susceptible to coronary and esophageal spasm. Br Heart J 1981;45:181.

148. Alban-Davies H, Kaye MD, Rhodes J, et al. Diagnosis of esophageal spasm by ergometrine provocation. Gut 1982;23:89.

149. Eckardt VF, Kruger J, Holtermuller KH, et al. Alteration of esophageal peristalsis by pentagastrin in patients with diffuse esophageal spasm. Scand J Gastroenterol 1975;10:475.

150. Orlando RC, Bozymski EM. The effects of pentagastrin in achalasia and diffuse esophageal spasm. Gastroenterology 1979;77:472.

151. Mellow MH. Esophageal motility during food ingestion: a physiologic test of esophageal motor function. Gastroenterology 1983;85:570.

152. Benjamin SB, Richter JE, Cordova CC, et al. Prospective manometric evaluation with pharmacologic provocation of patients with suspected esophageal motility dysfunction. Gastroenterology 1983;84:893.

153. Wranne D, Areskog M, Tibbling L. The acid perfusion test as differential diagnostic aid in patients with chest pain. Acta Med Scand 1981;209(suppl):59.

154. Janssens J, Vantrappen G, Ghillebert G. Twenty-four hour recording of esophageal pressure and pH in patients with noncardiac chest pain. Gastroenterology 1986;90:1978.

155. Barish CF, Castell DO, Richter JE. Graded esophageal balloon distention: a new provocative test for noncardiac chest pain. Dig Dis Sci 1986;31:1292.

156. Baylis JH, Kountz R, Trounce JR. Observations on distention of the lower end of the esophagus. Q J Med 1955;94:143.

157. Blackwell JN, Hannan WJ, Adam RD, et al. Radionuclide transit studies in the detection of oesophageal dysmotility. Gut 1983;24:421.

158. Decaestecker JS, Blackwell JN, Adam RD. Clinical value of radionuclide esophageal transit measurement. Gut 1986;27:659.

159. Benjamin SB, O'Donnell JK, Hancock J, et al. Prolonged radionuclide transit in "nutcracker esophagus." Dig Dis Sci 1983;28:775.

160. Silverman KJ, Grossman W. Angina pectoris: Natural history and strategies for evaluation and management. N Engl J Med 1984;310:1712.

161. Feldman RL. A review of medical therapy for coronary artery spasm. Circulation 1987;75(suppl V):V-96.

162. Luchi RJ, Scott SM, Deupree RH, et al. Comparison of medical and surgical treatment for unstable angina pectoris. N Engl J Med 1987;316:977.

163. Roberts KB, Califf RM, Harrell JR, et al. The prognosis for patients with new onset angina who have undergone cardiac catheterization. Circulation 1983;68:970.

164. Coronary artery surgery study (CASS). A randomized study of coronary artery bypass surgery: survival data. Circulation 1983;68:639.

165. Bolli R. Bypass surgery in patients with coronary artery surgery: indications based on the multicenter randomized trials. Chest 1987;91:760.

166. Hurst JW. Percutaneous transluminal coronary angioplasty: a word of caution. Circulation 1987;75:902.

167. Smith B, Kennedy JW. Thrombolysis in the treatment of acute transmural myocardial infarction. Ann Intern Med 1987;106:414.

168. Roberts R. Acute myocardial infaction. In: Kelley WN, ed. Textbook of internal medicine. Philadelphia: JB Lippincott, 1989:152.

169. Traube M, McCallum RW. Calcium channel blockers and the gastrointestinal tract. Am J Gastroenterol 1984;79:892.

170. Kikendall JW, Mellow MH. Effect of sublingual nitroglycerin and long-acting nitrate preparations on esophageal motility. Gastroenterology 1980;79:703.

171. Bortolotti M, Labo G. Clinical and manometric effects of nifedipine in patients with esophageal achalasia. Gastroenterology 1981;80:39.

172. Richter JE, Dalton CB, Buice RG, et al. Nifedipine: a potent inhibitor of contractions in the body of the human esophagus: studies in healthy volunteers and patients with the nutcracker esophagus. Gastroenterology 1985;89:549.

173. Davies HA, Lewis MJ, Rhodes J, et al. Trial of nifedipine for prevention of oesophageal spasm. Digestion 1987;36:81.

174. Spurling TJ, Cattau EL, Hirszel R. A double-blind crossover study of the efficacy of diltiazem on patients with esophageal motility dysfunction. Gastroenterology 1985;88:1596.

175. Winters C, Artnak EJ, Benjamin SB, et al. Esophageal bougienage in symptomatic patients with the nutcracker esophagus. JAMA 1984;252:363.

176. Ebert EC, Ouyang A, Wright SH, et al. Pneumatic dilation in patients with symptomatic diffuse esophageal spasm and lower esophageal dysfunction. Dig Dis Sci 1983;28:481.

177. Horton ML, Goff JS. Surgical treatment of nutcracker esophagus. Dig Dis Sci 1986;31:878.

178. Koeltz NR, Birchler R, Bretholz A, et al. Healing and relapse of reflux esophagitis during treatment with ranitidine. Gastroenterology 1986;91:1198.

179. Castell DO. Medical therapy for reflux esophagitis: 1986 and beyond. Ann Intern Med 1986;104:112.

180. Elsburg L, Beck B, Stubgaard M. Effect of sucralfate on gastroesophageal reflux in esophagitis. Hepatogastroenterology 1985;32:181.

181. Lieberman DA, Keefe EB. Treatment of severe reflux esophagitis with cimetidine and metoclopramide. Ann Intern Med 1984;104:21.

182. Hetzel DJ, Dent J, Reed WD, et al. Healing and relapse of severe peptic esophagitis after treatment with omeprazole. Gastroenterology 1988;95:903.

183. Vantrappen G, Rutgeerts MD, Schurmans P, et al. Omeprazole is superior to ranitidine in short-term treatment of ulcerative reflux esophagitis. Dig Dis Sci 1988;33:523.

184. Naesdal J, Bodemar G, Walan A. Effect of omeprazole, a substituted benzimidazole, on 24-hour intragastric acidity in patients with peptic ulcer disease. Scand J Gastroenterol 1984;19:916.

185. Brand DL, Eastwood IR, Martin D, et al. Esophageal symptoms, manometry, and histology before and after antireflux surgery. Gastroenterology 1979;76:1393.

186. Lum LC. Hyperventillation: the tip of the iceberg. J Psychosom Res 1975;19:375.

187. Lum LC. The syndrome of chronic habitual hyperventilation. In: Hill OW, ed. Modern trends in psychosomatic medicine. London: Buttersworth, 1976:196.

30

Approach to the Patient with Gross Gastrointestinal Bleeding

GRACE H. ELTA

INTRODUCTION

Gastrointestinal (GI) bleeding is a common clinical problem requiring more than 300,000 hospitalizations annually in the United States. The rate of hospitalization for upper GI bleeding has been estimated at 150 patients per 100,000 population per year.[1] Lower GI bleeding is much less common, although incidence figures are not available. Mortality rates from upper GI hemorrhage have been stable at 8% to 10% over the last 40 years. In view of our aging population and the higher mortality of bleeding in the elderly, this may represent a slight improvement in mortality.[2-4] The mortality from lower gastrointestinal (LGI) bleeding appears to have significantly improved, and this has been attributed to superior diagnostic techniques.[5] In contrast, the improved accuracy in diagnosis afforded by the widespread use of upper endoscopy has not been shown to alter the outcome from UGI bleeding.[6-8] The majority of bleeding episodes from both UGI and LGI sources resolve spontaneously. However, among patients with persistent or recurrent bleeding, mortality is high, and they may require invasive interventional techniques. Hopefully, early and accurate diagnosis in the patients with severe bleeding will facilitate therapeutic maneuvers leading to lower mortality. Despite the increasing armamentarium of the therapeutic endoscopist and angiographer, it is important to remember that the cornerstone of management for GI hemorrhage remains rapid assessment of the patient with appropriate resuscitation. The patient must be hemodynamically stabilized before diagnosis, therapy, and prevention of rebleeding can begin.

CLINICAL PRESENTATION

The presentation of gastrointestinal bleeding depends on its acuity and the location of its source. Chronic GI blood loss may present with unsuspected iron deficiency anemia or occult blood in stools found on routine screening examinations. Patients with more severe chronic or unrecognized GI bleeding may present with symptoms of anemia, such as pallor, dizziness, angina, or dyspnea. Acute GI bleeding usually has a much more obvious presentation. Bleeding from the upper GI tract often presents with hematemesis or bloody vomitus. This may be recent bleeding causing bright red vomitus or previous bleeding resulting in a coffee-ground appearance. Melena consists of black, tarry, loose, or sticky malodorous stool due to degraded blood in the intestine and generally indicates an upper GI source, although it may originate in the right colon. Other causes of black stool, such as iron or bismuth ingestion, should be ruled out. Hematochezia is bright red blood from the rectum. It may be mixed with stool and generally indicates a lower gastrointestinal lesion. When hematochezia is due to an upper GI source, it indicates that there is massive hemorrhage.

PATIENT ASSESSMENT

The first step in assessment of the bleeding patient is to determine the urgency of the situation. Agitation, pallor, hypotension, and tachycardia may indicate shock requiring immediate volume replacement. Patients with severe blood loss may actually have bradycardia rather than tachycardia due to vagal slowing of the heart.[9] Shock occurs when blood loss approaches 40% of blood volume. If there is no evidence for hypotension, then orthostatic vital signs will help diagnose lesser degrees of intravascular volume depletion. Postural hypotension of 10 mm Hg or greater usually indicates at least a 20% reduction in blood volume. In the acutely bleeding patient, intravenous access should be established. If the patient has signs of shock or continued bleeding, a large-bore central intravenous line is useful. Blood samples for assessment of hematocrit, platelets, coagulation factors, and blood typing and crossmatching should be taken immediately.

The initial hematocrit obtained in a patient with acute bleeding poorly reflects the degree of blood loss. Because the hematocrit is expressed in terms of red blood cell volume as a percent of total blood volume, it will not drop until blood volume has been restored. This repletion of blood volume from extravascular fluid begins immediately but takes 24 to 48 hours to equilibrate completely. Therefore, in the acutely bleeding patient, close attention to blood pressure, pulse, and gross evidence of ongoing bleeding is better in evaluating blood loss than are laboratory tests. In contrast, the hematocrit accurately reflects the degree of anemia in patients with chronic blood loss, although the severity of iron deficiency, reflected by microcytic indices and low serum iron, is a better indicator of the chronicity of bleeding.

RESUSCITATION

Patients with severe acute GI bleeding require admission to an intensive care unit. Fragile patients with a history of cardiopulmonary disease may require measurement of capillary wedge pressure. Intravascular volume should be repleted with normal saline to prevent the consequences of shock while blood is being crossmatched for transfusion. This allows adequate circulation of the remaining red blood cells. The oxygen-carrying capacity of blood can be maximized by administration of supplemental oxygen. In rapidly bleeding patients, oxygen availability is markedly decreased during early hemorrhage, reflecting primarily a decreased cardiac output. The decreased oxygen-carrying capacity of the blood due to a decrease in hemoglobin is less important. A metabolic acidosis has been measured in patients with acute hemorrhage, reflecting poor tissue perfusion.[10] Close attention to vital signs, urine output, and central vascular pressure is mandatory.

The specific criteria that define when a patient requires transfusion vary with the age of the patient, the presence of concomitant cardiopulmonary disease, and the presence of continued bleeding. In general, the hematocrit should be maintained above 30% in elderly patients and above 20% in young, healthy patients. With continued evidence of bleeding, the decision to transfuse cannot be based on hematocrit alone. Unstable vital signs and gross evidence of active bleeding (i.e., hematemesis, bright red blood per nasogastric aspirate, or hematochezia) are better requisites for transfusion. The hematocrit is a poor index for following the patient's need for additional transfusions. The plasma volume after acute GI bleeding is often overexpanded by intravenous fluids; thus, the immediate post-transfusion hematocrit may underestimate the final value. The overuse of transfusions is probably more common than underuse, significantly increasing the likelihood of transmitting infection.

In general, packed red blood cells are the preferred form of blood transfusion. Whole-blood transfusions should be reserved for the unusual circumstances of massive blood loss and rapid high-volume replacement, which increase the need for coagulation factor replacement. Preferably, blood volume has already been replenished with saline by the time banked blood is available. The use of packed cells also spares components for the blood bank. If coagulation tests are abnormal, as is the case in many patients with cirrhosis, fresh frozen plasma and platelets may also have to be administered. Even patients with initially normal coagulation factors and platelet count eventually need plasma and platelet transfusions when they are transfused repeatedly. Patients who require massive transfusions (>3000 ml) should receive warmed blood to prevent decreases in body temperature.[11] Rarely in massively transfused patients, calcium supplementation may be necessary to counter the effects of calcium-binding agents in banked blood.

LOCATION OF BLEEDING

In obvious upper GI bleeding that presents with hematemesis, a nasogastric tube should be placed to further assess the rate of ongoing blood loss. When upper GI bleeding is only suspected, as in the patient with melena or with a history of previous epigastric

symptoms or disease, a nasogastric tube aspirate demonstrating blood confirms the upper tract as the source. Not infrequently, however, there may be a negative nasogastric aspirate in duodenal bleeding presenting with melena due to a competent pylorus that prevents duodenogastric reflux.[12] Therefore, a negative nasogastric aspirate does not preclude the upper gut as the bleeding source. Melena usually indicates an upper GI source (above the ligament of Treitz), although bleeding may be from the small bowel or proximal colon. Melena occurs when hemoglobin is converted to hematin or other hemochromes by bacterial degradation. This can be produced experimentally by ingestion of as little as 100 to 200 ml of blood.[13] If the volume of a lower GI hemorrhage is too small to cause hematochezia yet large enough to supply enough hemoglobin for degradation, and if colonic motility is sufficiently slow, bleeding from either small bowel or proximal colon may cause melena. This is an uncommon occurrence, because small bowel bleeding is rare and colonic sources either bleed slowly, causing hemoccult positive stools, or bleed rapidly enough to cause hematochezia. Another indication of an upper GI source of bleeding is a mildly elevated blood urea nitrogen (BUN) level. Some of this azotemia is caused by absorption of blood, but the experimental ingestion of blood results in lower elevations in BUN of shorter duration, suggesting that part of the azotemia is secondary to hypovolemia.[14] Testing for occult blood in nasogastric aspirates is rarely necessary because the blood is often obvious. The one occasion in which occult blood testing is helpful is when a coffee-ground aspirate appearance may be produced by some foods. In addition, a simple positive test for occult blood may merely indicate nasogastric tube trauma. When occult testing of gastric aspirates is utilized, it is important not to rely on standard stool kits that may be falsely negative in acidic solutions.[15]

Hematochezia usually indicates a lower GI source. However, 11% of patients with rapid bleeding from an upper source pass bright red blood per rectum because of rapid gastrointestinal transit.[16] Therefore, placement of a nasogastric tube and even performance of an endoscopic examination should be considered if there is any clinical question of bleeding location in a patient with hematochezia.

ACUTE UPPER GASTROINTESTINAL BLEEDING

Upper GI bleeding is a common clinical problem, causing 10,000 to 20,000 deaths per year in the United States. The stability of the mortality rate over several decades has been interpreted as an improvement in mortality because our population is aging.[17] Thirty percent of hospital discharges for UGI bleeding occur in patients over 65 years.[1] Approximately 80% of upper GI bleeding episodes are self-limited and require only supportive therapy.[18] Mortality in patients with continued or recurrent bleeding is 30% to 40%.[18,19]

Prognostic Indicators of Outcome of UGI Bleeding

Several factors that are predictive of a poor prognosis in UGI bleeding have been identified. The most important of the prognostic indicators is the cause of bleeding. Variceal hemorrhages have much higher rebleeding and mortality rates than other diagnoses. Mortality from variceal hemorrhage during the initial hospitalization is at least 30%, with rebleeding rates of 50% to 70%.[20] Improvement in mortality rates from variceal bleeding would lower the overall mortality of UGI bleeding because varices account for approximately 10% of all bleeding episodes.[21]

Stigmata of recent bleeding, such as active arterial spurting, oozing of blood, visible vessel, or fresh or old blood clot, observed during endoscopy, are important predictors of outcome in peptic ulcer bleeding (Fig 30-1*A–C*; Color Fig 1). Visible vessels are described endoscopically as an elevated dark red, blue, or grey mound that protrudes from the ulcer crater and is resistant to washing. The endoscopic diagnosis of a visible vessel has been validated by pathologic correlation in a group of gastric ulcer patients who required surgical resection.[22] The predictive value of all bleeding stigmata, including visible vessels, remains controversial.[23] Most believe that the presence of a visible vessel in an ulcer crater at endoscopy predicts an increased risk for requiring surgical intervention and increased mortality.[24] Ulcers with visible vessels have up to a 50% incidence of rebleeding compared with no observed rebleeding in patients with no stigmata of recent bleeding.[25] When endoscopy is performed within 6 to 24 hours of admission, visible vessels are found in 20% to 50% of bleeding

ulcers. Other stigmata of bleeding, such as clot, black eschar, or oozing, appear to be less common (18%–20%) and are associated with a lower incidence (6%–8%) of rebleeding.[22,25] It has been suggested that bleeding stigmata have greater significance with gastric than with duodenal ulcers.[26] The identification of predictors of recurrent hemorrhage would seem to be important in directing the need for supportive measures, such as intensive care unit observation, therapeutic endoscopic techniques, and early surgical intervention. Endoscopic coagulation techniques have been reported to lower mortality in patients with ulcers that have stigmata of recent bleeding.[27]

Other important prognostic indicators include:

1. The severity of the initial bleed as assessed by transfusion requirement, bright red blood in the nasogastric aspirate, or presence of hypotension (Table 30-1).[28]
2. The age of the patient: elderly patients (>60 years) have been shown to have higher mortality than their younger counterparts,[12] although this indicator may not be independent from concomitant disease.
3. The presence of concomitant disease (e.g., chronic renal failure).
4. Onset of bleeding during hospitalization has a mortality of

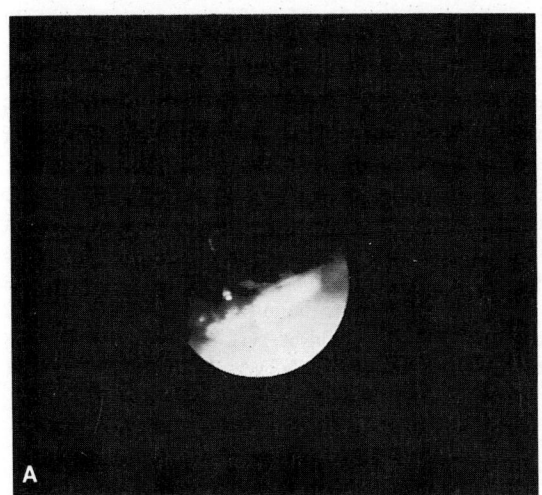

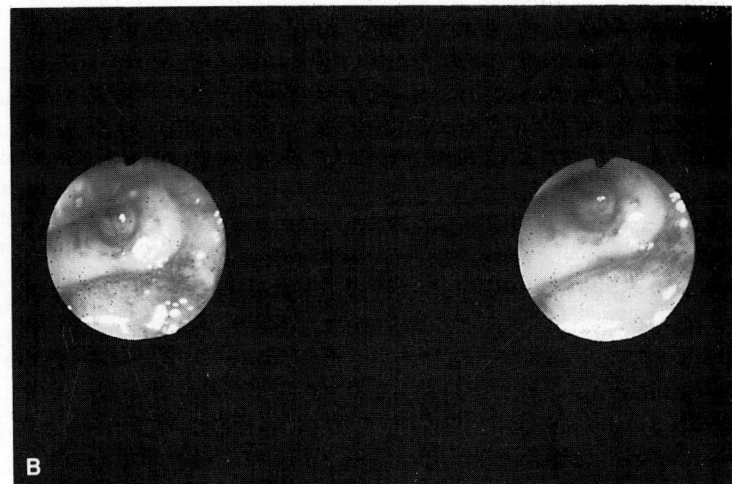

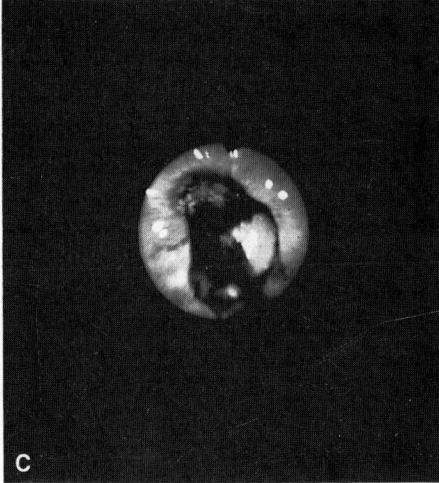

FIGURE 30–1. (See Color Fig 1) Three endoscopic pictures of stigmata of hemorrhage. **A,** Arterial spurting from a gastric ulcer crater. **B,** Visible vessel in a duodenal alcer that is not actively bleeding. **C,** Adherent blood clot obscuring most of this duodenal ulcer base.

TABLE 30–1
Prognostic Value of the Severity of UGI Bleeding

NG ASPIRATE	STOOL COLOR	MORTALITY (%)
Clear	Red, brown, black	10
Coffee grounds	Brown or black	10
	Red	20
Red blood	Black	10
	Brown	20
	Red	30

33% to 44% compared with only 7% to 12% in patients who start to bleed prior to admission.[29]

5. Patients with giant ulcers (diameter > 2.0 cm) have reported mortality rates as high as 40%.[30]

6. Patients requiring emergency surgery have a surgical mortality as high as 30% compared with 10% for those undergoing elective surgery.

ETIOLOGIES OF UGI BLEEDING

The three major causes of upper GI bleeding are peptic ulcer disease, gastritis (or gastric erosions), and varices (Table 30–2). The distribution of etiologies varies depending on the patient population studied. For example, large urban centers or Veterans Administration Hospitals may have more variceal hemorrhages because of the increased number of patients with cirrhosis. In all endoscopic series, no diagnosis is made in 10% to 15% of patients, and as many as 20% to 30% have more than one diagnosis.[31] The patients with no endoscopic diagnosis have an excellent prognosis.

Peptic Ulcer Bleeding

Duodenal, gastric, and stomal ulcers account for about 50% of UGI bleeding episodes (see ch 61 and ch 62). Although several effective therapies have been developed for peptic ulcer disease over the past 15 years, this has had little if any impact on hospitalization rates for bleeding ulcers.[32] Perhaps the reason for this is that ulcers not infrequently bleed without prior history of peptic symptoms.[33] Also, there may actually be an increase in UGI bleeding in the elderly, caused by the widespread use of nonsteroidal anti-inflammatory drugs (NSAIDs) and aspirin.[34] Anatomically, ulcers that are located high on the lesser curve of the stomach or on the posteroinferior wall of the duodenal bulb are more likely to rebleed.[35] Bleeding tends to occur when an ulcer erodes into the lateral wall of a vessel. The vessel often loops up to the floor of the crater and commonly protrudes with an aneurysmal dilatation. An eccentric breach in a vessel is more likely to be associated with continued or recurrent bleeding than is a transected vessel because retraction contraction of a severed vessel is an important mechanism of hemostasis.[22] It is the patients with continued or recurrent ulcer bleeding that have increased mortality. Therapy

is therefore directed at both cessation of bleeding and prevention of recurrent bleeding.

CESSATION OF BLEEDING: NONENDOSCOPIC METHODS

Multiple trials using various pharmacologic agents have failed to demonstrate any improvement in survival in UGI bleeding. There have been over 25 randomized controlled studies using histamine H2 antagonists in the management of UGI hemorrhage.[36–41] An analysis of pooled results in over 2500 patients suggests that treatment may reduce rates of surgery and death by 20% and 30%, respectively, although these reductions were only marginally significant.[42] Practically, because even a moderate reduction in mortality is still desirable and because H2 blockers are without significant toxicity, these agents are commonly administered to patients with ulcer bleeding despite the lack of proven efficacy. Other drugs, such as somatostatin,[43] prostaglandins,[44] tranexamic acid (an antifibrinolytic agent),[45,46] and intravenous vasopressin,[47] have also not proved to alter the course in bleeding ulcer patients.

Because of the failure of medical therapy, the emphasis in treating persistent ulcer hemorrhage is on endoscopic therapy or surgical intervention. Emergency surgery has an increased mortality, so endoscopic methods are usually attempted prior to surgery. If hemorrhage is not stopped or if it recurs, surgery should be considered early, because mortality increases as the patient becomes more unstable. Peptic ulcer bleeding is effectively treated with surgery, and this is safer than other therapeutic alternatives such as angiography. Intra-arterial vasopressin is not effective in bleeding from ulcers in contrast to bleeding from gastritis, presumably because of the large size of the bleeding vessel in peptic ulcer disease.[48] Embolization via an angiographic catheter with Gelfoam or coils can be successful but requires significant expertise and has considerable complications.[49] Therefore, this should be reserved for the patient who is too unstable to undergo surgery. The type of surgery that should be performed for the bleeding patient remains controversial. Simple oversewing can be performed

TABLE 30–2
Final Diagnoses of Cause of Upper GI Bleeding in 2225 Patients

DIAGNOSES	% OF TOTAL DIAGNOSES
Duodenal ulcer	24.3
Gastric erosions	23.4
Gastric ulcer	21.3
Varices	10.3
Mallory-Weiss tear	7.2
Esophagitis	6.3
Erosive duodenitis	5.8
Neoplasm	2.9
Stomal ulcer	1.8
Esophageal ulcer	1.7
Miscellaneous	6.8

Modified from Silverstein FE, Gilbert DA, Tedesco FJ. The national ASGE survey on upper gastrointestinal bleeding. Gastrointest Endosc 1981;27:73.

quickly, and it effectively stops bleeding. However, many surgeons choose to perform an acid-reducing procedure at the same time to prevent further ulcers. This decision must be individualized, depending on the underlying condition of the patient and the history of the peptic disease.

CESSATION OF BLEEDING: ENDOSCOPIC METHODS

Endoscopic control of bleeding should be tried on patients with continued or recurrent hemorrhage from peptic ulcer disease. Endoscopic methods can be divided into two types: thermal and nonthermal. They are described in detail in Chapter 134. Nonthermal methods are less well studied and remain experimental at this time. They include injection of sclerosing agents, as in sclerotherapy for varices, or injection of vasoconstrictors such as epinephrine.[50] A controlled study of epinephrine injection has shown an improvement in initial hemostasis, transfusion requirement, and the need for emergency surgery.[51] Other nonthermal methods that have been tried without significant success are sprays of clotting factors, tissue glues, and crystalline collagen.[52-54]

Thermal methods are better studied and are more widely used. These include the neodymium-yttrium aluminum garnet (Nd-YAG) laser, the heater probe, and electrocoagulation. The multipolar electrocoagulation probe (Bicap) has replaced monopolar electrocoagulation because of its reduced depth of tissue injury.[55] It is a small mobile unit that can be used in the intensive care or emergency unit setting. This technique uses direct probe pressure to tamponade the bleeding vessel, and then the tissue temperature is raised to coagulate and seal the vessel. Results of controlled trials are somewhat contradictory but, in general, show at least temporary cessation of bleeding.[56] A similar technique that uses pure thermal energy is the heater probe. It appears to be similar in efficacy to the Bicap device.[57] It is likely that these two relatively simple techniques will gain wider usage. The Nd-YAG laser is as effective as the heater probe and Bicap; numerous trials have shown probable success for the Nd-YAG laser in stopping active hemorrhage.[58,59] However, its immobility, requirement for trained support personnel, and the marked equipment expense reduce its attractiveness.

PREVENTION OF RECURRENT HEMORRHAGE

Acid-reducing pharmacologic therapy remains of uncertain benefit in preventing ulcer rebleeding.[42] The rationale is to prevent clot dissolution and allow healing of the underlying lesion. In vitro data show that coagulation and platelet function are better at neutral pH.[60] Although clot is not dissolved by acid, it is dissolved by gastric juice, suggesting that pepsin degradation may be important.[61] Because the activity of pepsin is pH dependent, it is reasonable to assume that clot will not dissolve if gastric juice pH is high.[62] The clinical importance of this in vitro data is unclear; there appears to be only slight, if any, reduction in rebleeding rates from gastric and duodenal ulcers with acid-reducing therapy.[42] Either clot dissolution is not important in rebleeding or insufficient acid reduction is achieved with standard therapy.[63] The potent hydrogen–potassium ATPase inhibitor omeprazole, which is ca-

pable of raising gastric pH to near-neutral levels, has not been studied for prevention of rebleeding. Despite the lack of firm proof of efficacy, H2 blockers and antacids are commonly used in this setting because of their potential to help and their lack of toxicity.

The prevention of rebleeding by therapeutic endoscopic methods in high-risk ulcers with stigmata of bleeding remains controversial.[64] First, there is the problem of identifying which stigmata signify high risk.[25] The literature available to date suggests that only visible vessels are of sufficient risk of rebleeding to be treated prophylactically and other stigmata are not.[24] Second, therapeutic endoscopy adds to both the risk of the endoscopic procedure and its cost. Further trials in ulcer patients with bleeding stigmata are needed to examine the effect of prophylactic therapeutic endoscopy on survival, transfusion requirement, and hospital costs.

UGI Hemorrhage from Gastritis or Gastric Erosions

Gastritis is often defined differently by the endoscopist than by the pathologist (see ch 61). Histologically, gastritis is defined by epithelial distortion and inflammatory cell infiltrate, which may be chronic (predominantly plasma cells) or acute (polymorphonuclear cells). There may be biopsy evidence of severe histologic gastritis with normal endoscopic appearances.[65] Clearly, this type of gastritis is not associated with UGI hemorrhage. Endoscopically, gastritis is defined by the gross appearance of mucosal hemorrhages, erythema, and erosions. An erosion is technically a break in the mucosa that does not cross muscularis mucosae. Practically, most endoscopists define an erosion as either an area of adherent hemorrhage or a defect in the mucosa with a necrotic base that is less than 3 to 5 mm and is without significant depth. This type of erosive gastritis may be the cause of UGI bleeding and has several different causes.[66]

GASTRITIS DUE TO DRUGS

Drug-induced gastritis due to aspirin or other nonsteroidal anti-inflammatory drugs (NSAIDs) is very common. Almost all normal volunteers challenged with aspirin develop mild hemorrhagic gastritis involving the proximal or entire stomach within 24 hours.[67] The bleeding associated with this acute damage is minimal and only rarely clinically apparent. If the aspirin is continued, adaptation and healing occur. A smaller percentage of individuals chronically exposed to NSAIDs will go on to develop either chronic erosive gastritis, predominantly involving the antrum, or frank ulcer disease.[68] This common type of erosive gastritis is usually a self-limited disease that heals rapidly after removal of the offending agent. Interventional treatments such as therapeutic endoscopy or surgery are very rarely required. Bleeding from NSAIDs usually resolves spontaneously, although H2 blockers, antacids, or sucralfate are commonly administered. The marginal efficacy of these drug therapies in the treatment of bleeding from erosive gastritis and from ulcer disease is presumably the same.

A more important issue in the management of NSAID-gastropathy is prophylaxis. Prostaglandins, which have recently become available in the United States, have been shown effective in prevention of acute gastritis due to NSAIDs.[69] It is less clear whether they are also effective in preventing the chronic damage or hemorrhage that is clinically more important. Prophylactic treatment with H2 blockers appears effective in duodenal disease but not in the stomach.[70] Sucralfate has not been well studied for this indication, although it is reportedly effective.[71] The efficacy of antacid prophylaxis is unknown. It remains unclear who should receive prophylaxis, because most patients on NSAIDs do not develop significant UGI bleeding, and routine prophylaxis with prostaglandins would be extremely expensive and has some side effects. It seems reasonable to recommend co-treatment with prostaglandins or other agents in the patient who has already demonstrated significant UGI bleeding and yet requires continued NSAID intake. Another alternative is to change the NSAID to a less damaging agent such as enteric-coated aspirin. This has been shown to cause fewer ulcers and less gastritis in both normal volunteers and patients with chronic rheumatic diseases.[72] Although less well studied to date, it has been suggested that the nonacetylated salicylates may also be gastric-sparing.[73]

An uncommon cause of drug-induced erosive gastritis is that associated with hepatic artery pump chemotherapy. This may cause hemorrhagic gastritis, duodenitis, and frank ulcer disease.[74] The pathogenesis is presumably due to direct tissue injury from the chemotherapeutic agents or from ischemia due to catheter placement. Little is known about management of this entity.

GASTRITIS RELATED TO ALCOHOL INTAKE

It is generally thought that alcohol ingestion can cause hemorrhagic gastritis. In animal models, absolute alcohol causes severe hemorrhagic gastritis, although lower doses of intragastric alcohol can actually produce adaptive cytoprotection.[75] These lower doses are closer to those obtained in human alcohol use. Furthermore, a history of alcohol intake in the previous 72 hours was not more common in patients presenting with UGI hemorrhage than in controls in one study.[76] Perhaps some of the alcohol-induced gastritis observed clinically is actually due to portal hypertension in patients with alcoholic liver disease. Portal hypertension has been shown to predispose to alcohol induction of gastritis in laboratory animals.[77] The histologic picture of alcoholic hemorrhagic gastritis is one of a predominance of subepithelial hemorrhages and edema with little evidence of inflammatory infiltrate.[78] At least one fourth of the patients in this study also had portal hypertension, again clouding the issue of how much damage is due to direct alcohol injury versus the effect of portal hypertension. The bleeding from alcoholic gastritis is similar to that seen in drug-induced gastritis, because it is usually self-limited and rarely requires invasive intervention.

Portal hypertension is also associated with "gastritis" or portal gastropathy. This has been described as a diffuse erythematous reticular pattern of gastric mucosa.[79] Presumably, a more severe variant of portal gastropathy is the vascular ectasias that may be present throughout the stomach or have an antral predilection.[80] Clinically, the second most common cause of UGI bleeding in patients with chronic liver disease is erosive gastritis.[81] It is not uncommon for the endoscopist to see chronic hemorrhagic mucosa in patients with portal hypertension who are undergoing frequent sclerotherapy sessions. Bleeding is usually not a management problem in these patients. This type of "gastritis" responds poorly to treatment with H2 blockers and sucralfate,[82] although portal systemic shunting in the unusual patient who has continued significant blood loss is reported to be effective.[83] Propranolol has been used effectively to decrease rebleeding in portal gastropathy and has decreased endoscopic evidence of gastritis in a controlled study.[84]

STRESS GASTRITIS

An important type of gastritis that causes major hemorrhages is that associated with stress. It occurs in intensive care unit patients with respiratory failure, hypotension, sepsis, renal failure, thermal burns, peritonitis, jaundice, and neurologic trauma.[85] The risk of bleeding in an individual patient varies with the number of such conditions.[86] Endoscopic evidence of gastritis is found in almost all intensive care unit patients, although only 2% to 10% of these patients have significant bleeding.[87] All treatment modalities for significant bleeding from stress gastritis are associated with high failure rates and significant morbidity. Endoscopic therapy is usually the first and safest choice in treatment, although it has not been specifically studied in gastritis bleeding. The presence of multiple bleeding sites will preclude its use in some patients. In contrast to bleeding ulcers, angiographic control of gastric mucosal bleeding reportedly has a good success rate, perhaps because of the small vessel size in these superficial lesions. Intra-arterial vasopressin controls hemorrhage in 80% to 90% of the successfully catheterized gastritis patients. Unfortunately, even skilled angiographers can only catheterize 75% of patients.[88] Intravenous infusion of vasopressin has not been as well studied but is also reported to be effective.[89] Operative mortality is extremely high for patients bleeding from stress gastritis, and rebleeding after surgery is common; thus, surgery is reserved as a last alternative.[90,91]

Currently, the major emphasis in the management of stress gastritis is prophylaxis. All patients ill enough to be in an intensive care unit should receive prophylaxis. Routine use of high-dose antacids,[92] H2 blockers,[93] or sucralfate[94] in patients at risk has been shown to decrease the bleeding incidence. Some authors have shown lesser degrees of bleeding with antacids than with intravenous H2 blockers. This suggests that the time below a pH of 4 may be crucial, because antacids are dosed in a titratable manner according to the gastric aspirate pH.[95] This raises the possibility of using continuous infusion H2 blocker to maintain a high gastric pH, although this has not been studied in a controlled fashion.[96] Many studies have used heme-positive gastric aspirates as evidence for gastric bleeding rather than overt bleeding. Clearly, it is only overt bleeding that is important clinically. A review of multiple studies using overt blood loss as an endpoint found intravenous cimetidine equally as effective as antacid titration.[97] Because high-dose antacids cause considerable side effects and nursing inconvenience, intravenous H2 blockers and sucralfate are more popular. Sucralfate per nasogastric tube appears as effective as high-dose antacids.[98] Recent data suggest that agents that improve mucosal defense without altering intragastric pH, such as sucralfate, may result in lower rates of nosocomial pneumonia in patients on respirators.[99] It is hypothesized that gastric bacterial overgrowth occurs with acid-reducing therapy and that endotracheal intubation allows a pathway for colonization of the respiratory tract.

Esophageal Varices

The first episode of UGI hemorrhage from esophageal varices has a mortality of 30% to 50%, and two thirds of these patients die within a year.[20] These bleak mortality figures may have improved slightly in recent studies,[100] although a variable delay in trial entry makes comparison of mortality rates between studies difficult.[101] This high mortality attests to the difficulty in both the management of acute variceal bleeding and the prevention of further bleeding. It also may explain why so many therapeutic alternatives have been proposed. The majority of patients with varices have underlying cirrhosis; this contributes to the high mortality, because ~40% die from associated medical problems. It has been estimated that one fourth to one third of patients with cirrhosis will hemorrhage at least once from varices.[102] Despite the increasing array of therapeutic options for treatment of variceal hemorrhage, there has been little if any change in long-term survival.[103]

DETERMINANTS OF VARICEAL RUPTURE

Portal hypertension must be present with pressures of 12 mm Hg or greater in order for varices to develop. However, the level of pressure elevation does not correlate with the risk of rupture.[104] Indeed, portal pressures may be similar in patients with no evidence of varices and in those with large varices. It appears that once a threshold portal pressure that permits varices is present, other factors control their formation and their risk for rupture. It has been suggested that direct measurement of intravariceal pressure may correlate better with risk of hemorrhage.[105]

Esophagitis has not been shown to predispose to variceal bleeding, even though intuitively it seems reasonable that erosions on top of esophageal varices may erode a vessel. This remains somewhat controversial at present.[106] It is important to note that gastroesophageal reflux as measured by pH probe is not more common in patients with a history of variceal bleeding than in controls.[107]

The best predictor of variceal hemorrhage is the size of the varices. Several studies have shown that large varices are more likely to bleed than small ones.[108] Wall tension is a factor of diameter and wall thickness, so that it is not surprising that larger varices are more likely to rupture. There are several ways to grade variceal size. Some endoscopists use a 1 to 4 scale, depending on the degree of protrusion in the esophageal lumen. Others prefer an estimated measurement of variceal height by comparing them to an open forceps width.[109] Another endoscopic finding of value in predicting variceal bleeding is the appearance of the vessel wall. The color of varices is thought to be predictive of impending hemorrhage. The red color sign is due to microtelangiectasia of the varix. Variants of this sign are red wale marks that look like whip marks; cherry red spots, 2 mm in diameter; hemocystic spots, which are round, crimson projections greater than 4 mm that look like blood blisters; and diffuse redness. (2) The "fundamental" color of the varices is also of predictive value.[106] All of the red color signs and a blue color to one varix are thought to be risk factors for bleeding. The presence of cutaneous vascular spiders also correlates with the risk of hemorrhage from esophageal varices.[110] A prognostic index for variceal hemorrhage using three variables (i.e., variceal size, red wale marks, and a modified Child's

classification of the underlying liver disease) was able to identify subsets of patients with one-year incidences of bleeding ranging from 6% to 76%.[108] The value of these predictors for variceal rupture depends on the usefulness of prophylactic therapy for variceal bleeding.

MANAGEMENT OF ACUTE VARICEAL HEMORRHAGE

Variceal bleeding is often the most rapid type of UGI hemorrhage. Therefore, the emphasis in acute management is on resuscitation. Over 90% of variceal bleeding episodes cause a drop in the hematocrit below 30% and require transfusions. However, as is the case with other etiologies of UGI hemorrhage, 70% to 80% resolve without specific intervention. Urgent endoscopy is indicated in patients with a suspected variceal source, because both the treatment of the acute bleeding episode and the prevention of recurrent bleeding are different from those in patients with bleeding from other UGI causes. One half to two thirds of patients with cirrhosis who present with bleeding will have a nonvariceal source, and many of these patients have more than one lesion.[111] This makes early endoscopy mandatory to determine the site and cause of bleeding.

In the acutely bleeding patient, intravenous vasopressin is often begun as soon as the diagnosis is clear. Early controlled studies using intra-arterial or intravenous bolus vasopressin appeared to show efficacy,[112,113] although lower transfusion requirements and decreased mortality were not demonstrated. Subsequently, several studies showed that peripheral intravenous vasopressin was as effective as intra-arterial vasopressin.[114] A more recent study comparing intravenous vasopressin with placebo was not able to show any therapeutic benefit with this therapy, raising the question of whether any mode of delivery is effective.[115] A compilation of multiple studies using vasopressin showed that hemorrhage was stopped in 54% of 185 episodes of bleeding, yet only 53% of the 170 patients who received vasopressin survived.[116] Despite this lack of proven efficacy, vasopressin is commonly used. The usual dose is 0.2 to 0.4 U/min, although high-dose therapy (1.0–5 U/min) has been advocated.[117] Complications from vasopressin are primarily cardiovascular and increase with higher doses. Sublingual or intravenous nitroglycerin administered concomitantly with vasopressin significantly decreases the complication rate of vasopressin.[118,119] Surprisingly, the control of bleeding with this combination therapy is superior to that achieved with vasopressin alone. Perhaps this added benefit comes from reducing portal venous resistance and portal venous pressure. Medical alternatives to vasopressin for control of variceal hemorrhage include somatostatin and a synthetic analog of vasopressin, terlipressin.[120,121] Although somatostatin has been shown to decrease variceal pressure,[122] it has not proved successful in clinical trials of variceal bleeding.[123] Recently, it has been suggested that pharmacologic constriction of the lower esophageal sphincter with metoclopramide may arrest variceal hemorrhage from the distal 2 cm of esophagus.[124,125]

When supportive medical therapy and vasopressin/nitroglycerin infusion fail to stop variceal bleeding, the next step in management is urgent sclerotherapy: the endoscopic injection of a sclerosing agent into or next to the bleeding varix. If a skilled endoscopist is not available or, rarely, if the bleeding is too rapid to permit endoscopy, balloon tamponade is indicated. In uncontrolled trials, emergent sclerotherapy has a reported success rate for control of bleeding of 85% to 90%,[126] and similar efficacy has been shown in a controlled trial.[127] However, when examined as a spin-off question in the Copenhagen study, urgent sclerotherapy was not more effective than medical therapy for the cessation of bleeding.[128] When compared with balloon tamponade, sclerotherapy is more effective and may even improve survival.[129] Complications from both therapies were comparable in this study, although sclerotherapy is generally considered safer.

Balloon tamponade with the Sengstaken–Blakemore (SB) tube or the Linton–Nachlas (LN) balloon is effective in achieving hemostasis in 70% to 90% of cases.[130–132] Unfortunately, hemostasis is often temporary, with rebleeding occurring in 30% to 50% of patients when the balloon(s) is deflated. The LN tube is a single balloon device that fits in the gastric fundus, while the SB tube has both a gastric and esophageal balloon. Comparison of these two tubes suggests that the SB tube may be more effective in obtaining permanent hemostasis of esophageal varices, while the LN tube is more effective in gastric varices.[133] An adapted SB tube with an esophageal aspiration port or the Minnesota tube with a built-in esophageal port is probably the most popular device (Fig 30-2).[134] Balloon tamponade has a 10% to 30% complication rate, including esophageal perforation, aspiration pneumonia, malfunction requiring replacement, chest pain, gastric erosion, and agitation.[135] Endotracheal intubation prior to balloon insertion has been recommended to decrease complications.[136]

Percutaneous transhepatic obliteration of varices via angiographic catheterization of the portal vein and embolization using Gelfoam and thrombin has an 80% to 90% success rate for cessation of bleeding.[137,138] For several reasons this technique has not become popular. First, there is a 20% complication rate. Second, it requires the presence of a skilled invasive angiographer. Third, there is a high incidence of rebleeding (65% at 5 months), suggesting that this technique may be considered only for acute management of variceal hemorrhage.[139] Lastly, more readily available, safer, and at least equally effective modalities are current options.

Surgical shunting of portal blood to the systemic circulation for control of ongoing hemorrhage from varices is usually reserved for patients resistant to other therapies. Mortality from these emergency shunts is as high as 50% to 80%. This has dampened enthusiasm for this procedure.[140] This is in contrast to the use of surgery for the prevention of recurrent variceal bleeding. Although a better survival rate for emergency shunting has been reported,[141] this study may include patients that would be controlled with other simpler techniques at other centers. Staplegun transection of the esophagus has been advocated as the simplest type of emergency surgery for active variceal bleeding.[142] In contrast to surgical shunts, this does not complicate any further consideration of liver transplantation.

PREVENTION OF RECURRENT VARICEAL HEMORRHAGE

One third of patients surviving a variceal hemorrhage will rebleed within 6 weeks.[20] Death due to bleeding occurs in 40% to 60% of these patients. Therefore, prevention of recurrent hemorrhage is an important part of therapy. Therapies for prophylaxis include sclerotherapy, surgical shunts, and possibly propranolol, although there is some question of proven efficacy with each of these.[143] An improvement in mortality is particularly difficult to demonstrate, although a compilation of seven randomized trials suggests efficacy for sclerotherapy.[100] The difficulty in improving survival despite decreased rebleeding rates suggests that the risk of dying is better correlated to the severity of the underlying liver disease than to rebleeding.

Sclerotherapy has been shown to be superior to medical management for the prevention of rebleeding.[144] The risk of rebleeding is greatest in the first few weeks after initiation of a sclerotherapy regimen prior to obliteration of the varices.[145] When compared with surgical shunts, sclerotherapy is as effective in the long-term prevention of rebleeding, although early rebleeding, prior to obliteration, is higher with sclerotherapy.[146] There is no agreement on the best method of variceal injection, intravariceal versus paravariceal, with or without the benefit of an oversleeve, amount or type of sclerosant used at each session, and so on (see ch 133). It is also unclear what is the best timing schedule for sclerotherapy. In general, the more aggressive the sclerotherapy regimen in terms of timing and sclerosant, the faster obliteration is achieved with lower rebleeding rates.[147] However, these aggressive regimens also have higher complication rates. Since new varices may form, these patients will require follow-up endoscopy with sclerotherapy performed as necessary on monthly to yearly intervals for the rest of their lives. Despite the success of sclerotherapy in the prevention of rebleeding, long-term morbidity and mortality are improved only slightly if at all.[148–150] This appears to be a recurrent theme in the management of variceal hemorrhage. Even when bleeding

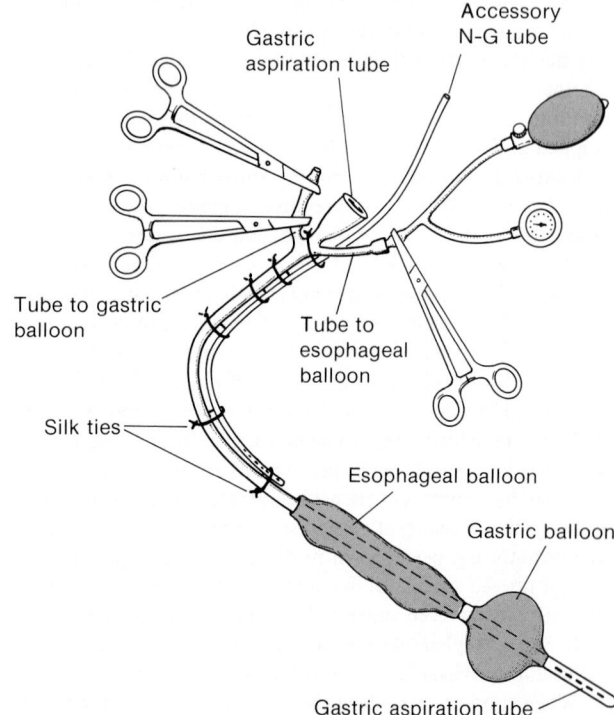

FIGURE 30–2. Modified Sengstaken-Blakemore tube. There also is the Minnesota tube which has a built-in esophageal port. (Redrawn from Jensen DM, Machicado GA. Diagnosis and treatment of severe hematochezia. The role of urgent colonoscopy after purge. Gastroenterology 1988;95:1569.)

is controlled, the patient goes on to die of other complications of his liver disease.

Propranolol has been proposed for the prevention of rebleeding in patients who have already presented with variceal hemorrhage.[151] Propranolol decreases portal pressures in both laboratory animals and humans,[152] although the response is not uniform.[153] Despite an early favorable report on the efficacy of β_1-blockade in prevention of rebleeding in patients,[151] subsequent studies did not confirm this therapeutic benefit.[154,155] A controlled trial of β_1-blockade versus sclerotherapy showed higher rebleeding rates in the patients on metoprolol.[156] Selective β_1 and β_2 agents are as effective as propranolol in decreasing portal pressures.[157,158] The use of selective β_2-blockade may prevent the impairment in cardiac compensatory mechanisms, thereby making these agents more desirable.[159] However, unless further studies show therapeutic efficacy for β_1-blockade in general, it is unlikely that there will be enthusiasm for this type of preventive treatment.

Surgical shunts decompress the portal system by diverting blood into the systemic circulation. Several types of shunts have been used, including the end-to-side portacaval, side-to-side portacaval, mesocaval, and splenorenal (Figs 30-3 and 30-4). Multiple studies have confirmed their efficacy in preventing rebleeding.[160] Unfortunately, 10% to 40% of patients suffer encephalopathy postoperatively. This led to the development of the distal splenorenal, or Warren, shunt, which spares portal blood flow to the liver. The proponents of this shunt report lower rates (4%–15%) of encephalopathy.[161] This has been confirmed in some controlled trials,[162,163] although other studies of nonselective versus distal splenorenal shunts have shown similar rates of operative mortality, late mortality, incidence of encephalopathy, and shunt occlusion.[164–166] It appears that the incidence of encephalopathy is related more to the severity of underlying liver disease than to the type of surgery performed. Some surgeons reserve the selective shunt for patients with preserved hepatopedal (intestine-to-liver) blood flow, although this may be unnecessary. The side-to-side portacaval shunt is usually recommended for patients with intractable ascites because of the increased morbidity and mortality associated with the distal splenorenal shunt in this group of patients.[167] Despite the efficacy of all shunts in preventing rebleeding, controlled trials have not shown improved mortality.[168–170] A randomized comparison of surgical shunt versus sclerotherapy showed similar survival and efficacy for the prevention of variceal rebleeding, with sclerotherapy having lower costs.[146] Therefore, most physicians currently favor sclerotherapy as the initial therapy, with surgery reserved for the patients who fail an adequate attempt at variceal obliteration.

Two other surgical methods of portal decompression have been used. The Sugiura procedure involves esophageal transection with paraesophagogastric devascularization.[171] Many modifications of this esophageal transection and devascularization procedure exist. Sugiura's results in nonalcoholic liver disease have been excellent, but other surgeons have experienced high rebleeding rates.[172] A newer procedure that has not been extensively studied is splenopneumonopexy.[173,174] This can be performed in patients with diffuse splanchnic venous thrombosis when other alternative shunts are not technically possible. It involves resection of part of the left diaphragm with apposition of the abraded surfaces of the spleen and left lung to allow decompressive collaterals to form.

Hepatic transplantation is the accepted treatment for otherwise healthy patients with end-stage liver disease. When these patients present with bleeding varices, management of the bleeding should avoid abdominal operations that make transplantation more difficult.

PROPHYLACTIC TREATMENT TO PREVENT VARICEAL HEMORRHAGE

Because 30% of cirrhotics will experience variceal hemorrhage, and the mortality of even one episode is very high, prevention is important. Prophylactic portal caval shunts have been shown to prevent bleeding successfully but do not improve survival.[175,176] The benefit of not bleeding may be offset by the operative morbidity and mortality, and this surgical treatment has completely fallen out of favor. Less invasive methods of prophylactic therapy include sclerotherapy and propranolol. It was hoped that identification of a high-risk group of cirrhotics for variceal bleeding, those with large varices with red color signs, would select a subset of patients who would benefit from preventive sclerotherapy. Unfortunately, this does not appear to be the case. Despite initial promising results with prophylactic sclerotherapy,[177] subsequent studies have not confirmed its efficacy.[178,179] Propranolol is the least invasive therapy of the prophylactic alternatives and therefore the most attractive. Again, results of controlled trials have been controversial.[103] The three studies that report a beneficial effect are certainly promising.[180–182] Whether this relatively complication-free treatment will be truly beneficial in the long run remains to be proved.

Gastric Varices

Gastric varices usually accompany esophageal varices, although they may occur alone.[183] They are located in the gastric fundus and are best appreciated endoscopically on a retroflexed view. They are a much less common cause of variceal hemorrhage than esophageal varices but are important to recognize as the source of bleeding because their management is different. When gastric varices are prominent and associated with minimal to absent esophageal varices, one must consider splenic vein thrombosis as the etiology of the increased venous pressures. Angiography may verify this diagnosis. These patients are best treated with simple splenectomy, which adequately decompresses their varices. Such patients have an excellent prognosis because of the lack of underlying liver disease.[184,185] Splenic vein thrombosis may occur as a complication of pancreatitis due to contiguous inflammation from the body and tail of the pancreas.[186]

More commonly, bleeding gastric varices are associated with large esophageal varices and are due to underlying liver disease. The acute management of bleeding gastric varices is similar to esophageal varices except that sclerotherapy has been poorly studied. Although success has been reported in a small number of patients,[187] it has been suggested that sclerotherapy has a higher complication rate in gastric mucosa, raising the question of whether it should be used at all.[188,189] Other alternatives for acute management include balloon tamponade, decompressive surgery, or β-blockade.

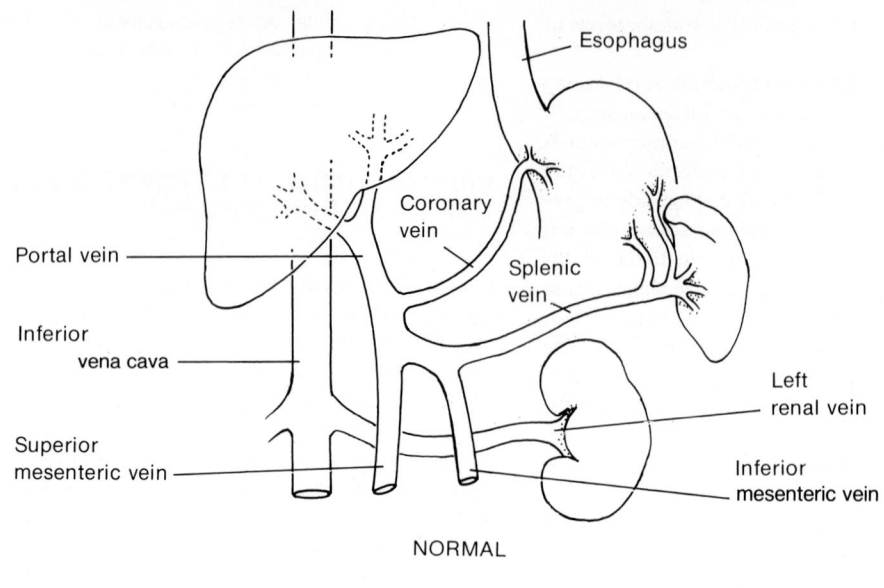

NORMAL

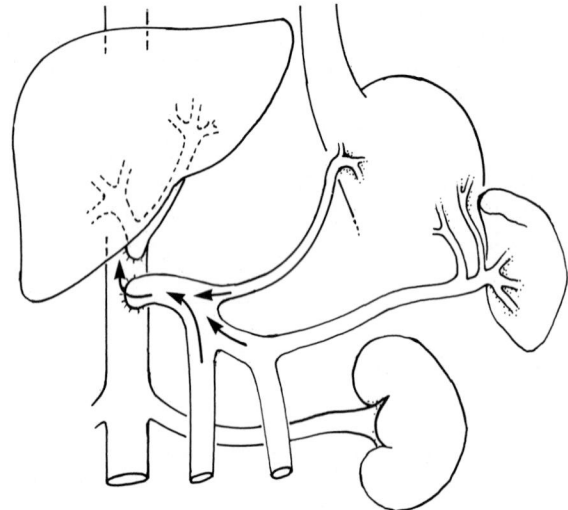

END-TO-SIDE PORTACAVAL SHUNT

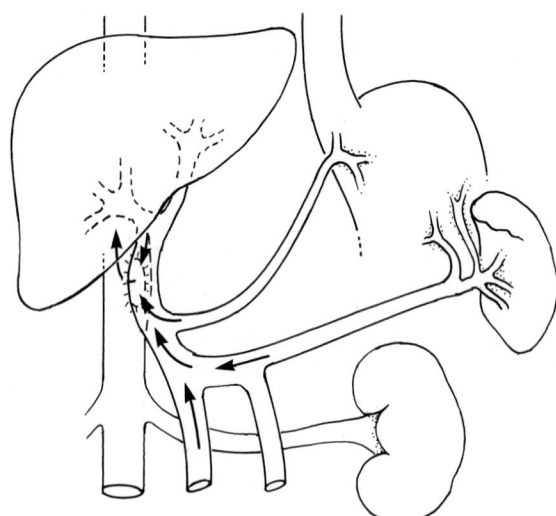

SIDE-TO-SIDE PORTACAVAL SHUNT

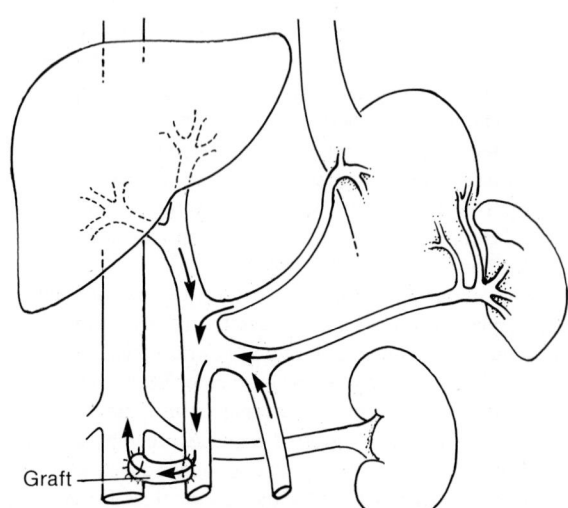

SIDE-TO-SIDE MESOCAVAL SHUNT

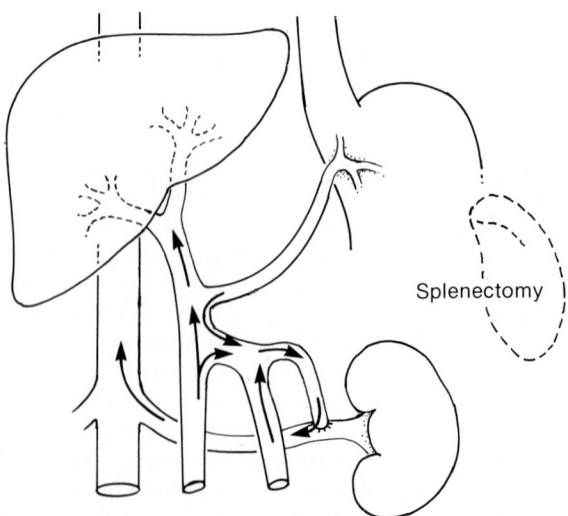

END-TO-SIDE SPLENORENAL SHUNT

FIGURE 30–3. Diagramatic illustration of the end-to-side portacaval, side-to-side portacaval, mesocaval, and proximal splenorenal shunts.

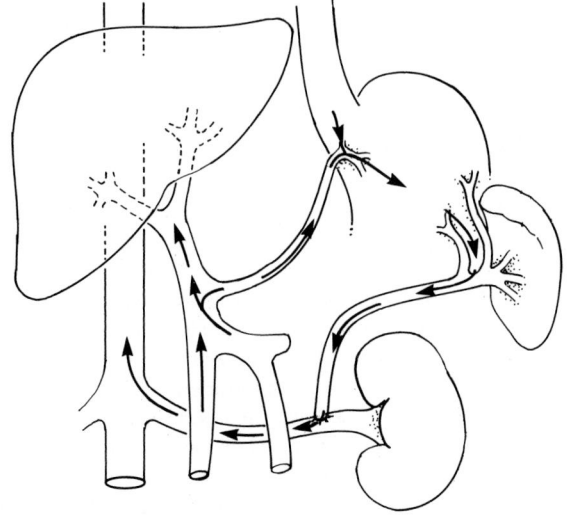

DISTAL END-TO-SIDE SPLENORENAL SHUNT

FIGURE 30–4. Illustration of the distal splenorenal shunt that was designed to prevent diversion of gut venous flow to the liver.

Mallory–Weiss Tear

Mallory–Weiss tears occur near the gastroesophageal junction in either gastric or esophageal mucosa (see ch 58). They are caused by retching, perhaps with forceful gastric mucosal prolapse as identified at endoscopy.[190] They account for 5% to 10% of UGI hemorrhages.[191] There is usually a history of vomiting foodstuffs prior to hematemesis, although the blood can occur with the first emesis.[192] Many patients with Mallory–Weiss tears have a history of alcohol intake.[193] The bleeding usually resolves with conservative management, although endoscopic therapy or intra-arterial vasopressin may be required. Rarely, patients with rebleeding or uncontrollable hemorrhage will require oversewing of the bleeding mucosa.

Esophagitis and Esophageal Ulcers

Esophagitis and esophageal ulcers account for approximately 8% of UGI hemorrhages (see ch 55). The primary etiology of these lesions is peptic reflux, but radiation, infectious esophagitis due to pathogens such as *Candida* or herpes, pill-induced damage, and sclerotherapy-induced ulcers can also cause these lesions. The presentation of bleeding esophageal lesions is similar to that of peptic ulcer disease. Persistent or recurrent bleeding should be treated aggressively with therapeutic endoscopic or angiographic techniques, because esophageal lesions are less amenable to surgery than peptic ulcer disease. When the ulcer is sclerotherapy-induced, one must be certain of the source of bleeding, because recurrent varices would be managed differently. Sucralfate has been suggested for treatment of these chemically induced ulcers,[194] although a controlled trial did not prove efficacy.[195]

Erosive Duodenitis

Hemorrhage from erosive duodenitis is closely related to duodenal ulcer bleeding but is usually less severe because the lesions are shallower and involve smaller vessels. It accounts for approximately 5% of UGI hemorrhages. It generally occurs in patients with a history of peptic ulcer disease or with similar risk factors. Bleeding from duodenitis is almost always self-limited, rarely requiring therapeutic endoscopic intervention.

Neoplasms

Neoplasms of the stomach, esophagus, or duodenum are uncommon causes (2%–4%) of UGI hemorrhage. Bleeding from these lesions is usually self limited, and treatment is ultimately in the hands of the oncologist or surgeon. If persistent or recurrent bleeding occurs in a patient unsuitable for surgical resection, endoscopic therapy or angiographic arterial embolization may be used.[196] Intra-arterial vasopressin is not usually effective because of the large size of the bleeding vessels.

Angiodysplasia

Vascular ectasias or angiodysplasia, which occurs less commonly in the stomach or duodenum than in the colon,[197] was the cause of UGI bleeding in 5% to 7% of patients (see ch 108).[18,198] Often found in advanced age, they have been associated with aortic valve disease,[199] chronic renal failure,[198] hereditary hemorrhagic telangiectasia or Osler-Weber-Rendu syndrome,[200] and prior radiation therapy.[201] The diagnosis is usually made endoscopically by visualization of small, punctate, bright red mucosal vascular lesions. Controlled studies of therapeutic alternatives are not available, but most clinicians would first attempt endoscopic coagulation techniques. These have been reported to be successful,[202] although they are associated with high rebleeding rates in patients with hereditary Osler-Weber-Rendu lesions.[203] When these vascular ectasias are associated with chronic renal failure and its attendant prolonged bleeding time due to platelet dysfunction, estrogen-progesterone therapy has been reported to be beneficial.[204,205] Recently, similar efficacy has been reported in patients with normal renal function and chronic GI blood loss from vascular ectasias.[206,207] This suggests that the abnormal platelet function present in renal failure may not be a prerequisite for estrogen-progesterone treatment. Controlled trials are needed to further assess this form of therapy.

An unusual variant of gastric vascular ectasias is the watermelon stomach.[208] The endoscopic appearance is a jagged column of vessels that run along the top of longitudinal rugal folds traversing the antrum and converging on the pylorus. This vascular aggregate resembles the stripes on a watermelon. Endoscopic biopsy or resected specimens show dilated mucosal capillaries with focal thrombosis and fibromuscular hyperplasia of vessels in the lamina propria.[209] It has been associated clinically with hypochlorhydria and occasionally with portal hypertension.[210] Antrectomy with

Billroth I anastomosis appears to be effective,[211] although oral corticosteroids have been reported to be successful in a poor surgical risk patient.[212] Endoscopic coagulation treatment with the YAG laser, Bicap, or heater probe may also be useful.[213]

Aorto-Enteric Fistula

Arterial-enteric fistulae usually involve the aorta but occasionally arise from branches of the celiac axis. The majority of aorto-enteric fistulae are secondary to prior aortic Dacron graft surgery,[214] although they may occur as primary fistulae due to atherosclerotic vessels or more rarely from mycotic aneurysms, tuberculosis, or syphilis.[215] Aorto-enteric fistulae almost always involve the third portion of the duodenum, although they may rupture into the jejunum, ileum, stomach, and colon. In patients with Dacron grafts, the fistula usually arises from the proximal portion of the graft and may be associated with false aneurysms. The classic clinical presentation is a "herald" bleed, which occurs and stops spontaneously hours or occasionally weeks before the exsanguinating hemorrhage. A high index of suspicion is necessary to make the diagnosis because the fistula is difficult to discern by radiography, endoscopy, and angiography. Whenever there is a prior history of aortic Dacron graft surgery in a patient presenting with GI hemorrhage, endoscopy should be performed to rule out other causes of bleeding, and the endoscopist should attempt to reach the third portion of the duodenum hoping to visualize the fistula.[216] If a fistula is not identified, it should still be the presumed source of bleeding, and the patient should have surgery. Arteriography is often not helpful and may delay surgery.

Hematobilia and Hemosuccus Pancreaticus

Hematobilia is defined as hemorrhage into the biliary tract from any cause. Hemorrhage traversing the pancreatic duct has been termed "hemosuccus pancreaticus," although it is often included with hematobilia because it exits the ampulla. Mortality from hemorrhage from both of these sites is significant (30%–50%). The most common cause of hematobilia is prior liver or biliary tree trauma, including prior percutaneous liver biopsy.[217] Extra- or intrahepatic aneurysms of the hepatic artery or its branches are often caused by the trauma and may communicate with the bile ducts. Less common causes of hematobilia are extra- or intrahepatic tumors and gallstones and cholecystitis.[218]

Hemosuccus pancreaticus represents bleeding from peripancreatic blood vessels into a pancreatic duct. Hemorrhage emanates from digested peripancreatic pseudoaneurysms or veins that rupture into a pseudocyst or from true aneurysms of the peripancreatic vessels that rupture into pancreatic parenchyma and ducts.[219] This usually occurs in patients with a history of chronic pancreatitis and pseudocysts. Diagnosis may be made at endoscopy with visualization of blood coming from the papilla, although it is easily missed when the bleeding has ceased. Angiography is indicated to define the bleeding site and may be used for treatment by em-

bolizing the vessel.[219–221] If embolotherapy is not successful, surgery may be required.

Dieulafoy's Disease

The Dieulafoy's lesion is defined as a ruptured thick-walled arterial vessel that is larger than other surrounding submucosal vessels with little or no associated ulceration.[222,223] The cause of bleeding is not thought to be a primary ulcerative process but rather pressure erosion of the overlying epithelium by this ectatic vessel.[224] The Dieulafoy's vessel occurs in the fundus and endoscopically appears as a round mucosal defect with a protruding artery at the base. It is an uncommon lesion, although it has been recognized more frequently because of greater use of endoscopy. Patients present with hematemesis and/or melena without any relevant history. Endoscopic injection therapy or electrocoagulation techniques have been reported to be successful in the cessation of bleeding in the majority of patients, although surgery is occasionally required.[225]

Factitious Bleeding or Bleeding From Non-GI Sources

Occasionally patients present with hematemesis or melena that does not originate from a GI source. Usually it is due to swallowed blood from epistaxis, hemoptysis, or oral lesions. These diagnoses are best determined by careful history and physical examination. Endoscopy to rule out GI sources may be required if the diagnosis remains uncertain. Rarely patients will present with factitious bleeding. They may bleed themselves by venopuncture and then swallow the blood prior to presentation. A high index of suspicion is necessary to make this diagnosis.

DIAGNOSTIC APPROACH TO UGI BLEEDING

There is controversy about whether all patients with upper GI bleeding should have a diagnostic examination. Those with self-limited minor bleeding and other more serious medical problems may not require endoscopy, because this has not been shown to alter prognosis.[226] However, in the majority of patients, even those with relatively minor bleeding, an accurate diagnosis or localization of the source is desirable to direct further patient management. In patients with significant bleeding, endoscopy may also be used for therapeutic maneuvers.

History and Physical Examination

As initial resuscitative measures are being implemented, a history and physical examination should be performed. It must be noted that even experienced gastroenterologists can guess the etiology of bleeding only 50% of the time after a careful history and physical examination. However, the history may raise specific diagnostic possibilities. Prior history of peptic disease or dyspeptic symptoms will suggest ulcer bleeding. Recent use of nonsteroidal anti-inflammatory drugs must always be determined. A history of alcohol or caustic substance ingestion is important to obtain. Prior history of cirrhosis or symptoms of cirrhosis such as ascites may suggest the need for urgent endoscopy to diagnose variceal bleeding. Other medical problems such as prior aortic graft surgery, coagulopathies, cancer, or recent nosebleeds may all suggest likely diagnoses.

Physical examination of the skin may provide diagnostic clues. Stigmata of cirrhosis, evidence of underlying malignancy (Kaposi's sarcoma), or hereditary vascular anomalies may be present. In addition, findings of lymphadenopathy or abdominal masses may suggest malignancy. Abdominal tenderness in the epigastrium is common in peptic disease. Hepatic or splenic enlargement may be present in liver disease or in certain malignant disorders. When patients present with upper GI bleeding, a rectal examination may indicate the magnitude of blood loss by demonstrating maroon or melenic stool in patients with severe bleeding or normal-colored stool in patients with minimal or recent bleeding.

Endoscopy

Barium contrast studies have been replaced by endoscopy for diagnosis of upper GI bleeding (see ch 111). The greater accuracy and therapeutic potential of endoscopy generally makes it the diagnostic procedure of choice.[227–229] Diagnostic endoscopy is viewed as a safe and simple procedure by both patient and physician, although morbidity rates of 1.0% and mortality rates of 0.1% have been reported. Endoscopy is contraindicated in uncooperative patients or in patients with suspected perforated viscus. Relative contraindications include compromised cardiopulmonary status or depressed level of consciousness. Endoscopy can locate precisely the site of bleeding when there is continued bleeding or when stigmata of bleeding persist. In patients with massive hemorrhage, the source of bleeding occasionally cannot be discerned by endoscopy. In patients whose bleeding has stopped and no stigmata of bleeding remain, a significant lesion seen on endoscopy (e.g., a clean ulcer base) is the presumed source. If either more than one lesion or no lesions are identified, no definitive diagnosis can be made, and these patients need to be restudied if they bleed again. It is important not to mislead those caring for the patient by overstating the certainty of the localization or diagnosis of the bleeding site.

The timing of the diagnostic endoscopy depends on the severity and suspected etiology of the hemorrhage. Patients who fail to stop bleeding with simple supportive care require urgent endoscopy to guide further therapeutic techniques. Also, patients with underlying cirrhosis should have endoscopy as close to the bleeding episode as possible, because these patients often have more than one source of potential hemorrhage and the diagnosis of bleeding varices will alter future approaches to treatment. For the majority of patients whose bleeding ceases, diagnostic endoscopy can be postponed for 24 hours without seriously altering diagnostic accuracy or clinical outcome.[230] In an uncomplicated patient who, along with the physician, is comfortable without a specific diagnosis, an empiric trial of treatment may be indicated. Barium x-ray may be used in this situation to rule out more serious or unexpected lesions, thereby avoiding the endoscopy altogether.

Radionuclide Scans

Localization of the site of gastrointestinal bleeding can be accomplished by scanning for extravasation of intravascular radiolabeled blood (see ch 121). Technetium-99 sulfur colloid scans are obtained shortly after injection. Technetium-99 pertechnetate–labeled red cells allow repeated scans over 24 to 36 hours after injection to detect intermittent bleeding. These techniques can reveal bleeding when the rate of blood loss is as low as 0.5 ml per minute and have no associated morbidity.[231] The major disadvantage of radionuclide scans is that they merely localize the bleeding to an area of the abdomen and do not diagnose the specific location or the responsible lesion. For this reason, radionuclide studies are often used to screen patients to determine which patients have sufficient ongoing bleeding to warrant angiography. In addition, they may allow more selective angiographic studies, thereby decreasing the dye load. Radionuclide scans are much more commonly used in the diagnosis of lower GI bleeding because the accuracy and therapeutic alternatives of upper endoscopy makes this the diagnostic method of choice in UGI bleeding, even in the rapidly bleeding patient. In the rare situation when massive hemorrhage makes endoscopy impossible, angiography should be obtained immediately and not delayed by prior radionuclide scans.

Angiography

Angiography is used in the diagnosis of acute upper GI bleeding only when endoscopy has failed (see ch 122). The bleeding must be arterial and at a rate of 0.5 to 0.6 ml per minute to detect extravasation. Angiography represents a therapeutic alternative for delivery of intra-arterial vasopressin in stress gastritis or for embolization of bleeding ulcers or neoplasms in inoperable patients. In addition, angiography may be used to diagnose difficult cases of recurrent GI bleeding from an unknown source. Angiographic demonstration of vascular ectasias may suggest the source of bleeding, although in patients who are not actively bleeding the diagnosis is uncertain, because these are common lesions. Angiography provides an accurate diagnosis in 50% to 75% of patients but is associated with a serious complication rate of about 2%.[232] Complications from angiography are related either to catheter placement (dissection, thrombosis, false aneurysm) or to the contrast material (allergic reactions, renal failure). When embolic occlusion of vessels with Gelfoam or autologous clot is used, the complication rate increases because of ischemic necrosis and perforation.[233]

TREATMENT OF UGI BLEEDING

Treatment of upper GI bleeding always begins with resuscitative measures. Once the patient is stable, two types of treatment are available: empiric and specific. The specific treatments depend on the diagnosis and the presence or absence of continued bleeding. For patients with severe bleeding, specific treatments include endoscopic or angiographic means of control or surgery. Empiric treatment is often initiated prior to diagnostic procedures, especially in the majority of patients whose bleeding stops.

Gastric Lavage

Gastric lavage with iced saline has been recommended as a method of treatment of upper GI bleeding.[234] Traditionally, this is performed through a nasogastric tube that has been placed to diagnose the location of bleeding. Cold solutions have a theoretical advantage of slowing blood flow. However, it can also be argued that ice water may impair coagulation factors, and certainly it increases discomfort by making the patient cold. Controlled trials have not shown any therapeutic benefit from cold lavage solutions.[235,236] Instillation of levarterenol for vasoconstriction has also been proposed, but this has not been shown to be superior to simple lavage.[237] Therefore, one should simply lavage with room-temperature tap water for the important task of monitoring the rapidity of bleeding. A large-bore orogastric tube should replace the diagnostic nasogastric tube when cleansing for subsequent endoscopy is needed. Aliquots of 100 to 500 ml of water are instilled and removed, preferably by gravity drainage to prevent extensive suction trauma.

Medical Therapy

Acid-reducing therapy is usually instituted in patients with upper GI bleeding even before a diagnosis is confirmed. Since acid is one of the important pathogenetic factors in peptic disease, antacids or H2 blockers are frequently used. Placebo-controlled trials have not been able to demonstrate either earlier cessation of bleeding, reduced rates of rebleeding, or decreased mortality with use of these agents. However, combining the results of the multiple studies suggests a positive therapeutic advantage for treatment.[42] Since it would take a trial of over 10,000 patients in order to demonstrate only a 20% decrease in deaths, it seems reasonable to continue this empiric treatment of upper GI bleeding inasmuch as the complication rate of acid-reducing therapy is extremely low and potential benefit exists. Whether use of agents capable of raising gastric pH to higher levels, such as a combination of H2 blocker and antacid or omeprazole, would be more effective is not known at this time.

Several other drug treatments have been studied. Intravenous somatostatin decreases acid secretion, splanchnic blood flow, and portal pressure, but the evidence for its efficacy in treatment of acute GI bleeding is not strong.[43] Tranexamic acid, an antifibrinolytic agent, has also been studied without very promising results.[44] Intravenous vasopressin is reportedly helpful in variceal hemorrhage, although even this is controversial. For other types of bleeding lesions, most experience with vasopressin is with intra-arterial delivery via an angiographically placed catheter.

Mucosal protective agents such as sucralfate or prostaglandins have not been well studied in bleeding patients but may be of similar benefit as acid-reducing therapy.

Surgical Therapy for UGI Bleeding

The indications for urgent surgery in UGI bleeding have remained essentially the same over the last 40 years except that now endoscopic therapy may be tried as a first approach. Patients who continue to bleed for more than 24 hours, require more than a 6- to 8-unit transfusion, or have recurrent bleeding despite endoscopic treatment require surgery. This decision may be delayed in patients who are very poor operative risks in whom angiographic treatment may be chosen,[238] or in specific diagnoses with known high surgical mortality rates, such as stress gastritis or acute variceal hemorrhage. If the patient is going to require surgery, promptness is desirable before the patient deteriorates.[239]

ACUTE LOWER GASTROINTESTINAL BLEEDING

Lower GI bleeding is defined as bleeding from below the ligament of Treitz. The average patient is older than those with upper GI bleeding. The mortality from acute lower GI bleeding has decreased in the last two decades.[240] This may be attributed to better localization and diagnosis of bleeding via colonoscopy and angiography, which in turn allows more selective surgical and angiographic treatment to be performed. Alternatively, this may be attributed to better resuscitative care and medical and surgical management. In the 1950s and 1960s, surgery for massive or recurrent lower GI bleeding usually involved segmental left colonic resections. This was based on the belief that most LGI bleeding originated in left colon diverticula. Postoperatively, recurrent bleeding was very frequent and mortality was high.[241] The superior techniques now available for localization of the bleeding site have increased the number of right colonic resections, and mortality rates of less than 5% are reported.[242]

ETIOLOGIES OF LOWER GI BLEEDING

The two major causes of acute lower GI bleeding are diverticulosis and angiodysplasia (Table 30-3). As is the case with upper GI bleeding, 80% of bleeding episodes resolve spontaneously. In the patients in whom bleeding ceases, ~25% have recurrent bleeding. In contrast to upper GI bleeding, most lower GI bleeding is slow and intermittent and does not require hospitalization. The most common causes of chronic lower GI bleeding are hemorrhoids and colonic neoplasia.

TABLE 30-3
Final Diagnoses of Major Lower GI Bleeding

DIAGNOSIS	% OF TOTAL DIAGNOSIS
Diverticulosis	43
Angiodysplasia	20
Undetermined	12
Neoplasia	9
Colitis	
Radiation	6
Ischemic	2
Ulcerative	1
Other	7

Modified from Boley SJ, DiBiase A, Brandt LJ, et al. Lower intestinal bleeding in the elderly. Am J Surg 1979;137:57.

Diverticular Bleeding

Diverticular bleeding occurs in only ~3% of patients with diverticulosis. However, it is the most common cause of major lower GI hemorrhage because of the high prevalence of diverticulosis in the Western world (see ch 82). Prior to widespread availability of colonoscopy and angiography, the true incidence of diverticular bleeding was overestimated because this diagnosis is so frequently made by barium enema. Later angiographic studies have demonstrated that despite the left-sided preponderance of diverticula, 70% of bleeding diverticula occur in the right colon.[243] Some of the decreased mortality from lower GI hemorrhage is likely due to better localization of the bleeding source, allowing directed surgical therapy and lower postsurgical rebleeding rates.

Diverticula are usually located in the colonic wall at the site of penetration of nutrient vessels. Bleeding presumably results from a colonic artery that penetrates into the dome of the diverticulum. The artery ruptures into the diverticular sac and causes copious bleeding. Clinical evidence of associated diverticulitis or inflammation is usually not present, so vessel rupture is thought to be due to pressure erosion.

Diverticular bleeding presents with acute, painless, maroon to bright red hematochezia, although melenic stools may occur. The degree of blood loss is often significant and may not be well tolerated in the elderly population at risk. Diverticulosis is not thought to be a cause of occult heme-positive stool or slow bleeding.[244] If the initial bout of diverticular bleeding ceases spontaneously, no further therapy is indicated, because bleeding does not recur in the majority of patients. In the 80% of patients in whom bleeding ceases, 75% will not have a recurrence and 25% will have repeated episodes of diverticular hemorrhage.[241]

In the 20% of patients with persistent hemorrhage from diverticulosis, angiography is useful for both diagnosis and treatment.[245-247] Selective catheterization with administration of intraarterial vasopressin successfully controls the bleeding in the majority of patients. Any patient who fails angiographic control of diverticular bleeding should have urgent surgery to remove the portion of the colon bearing the bleeding site. In the event of failure to localize the bleeding site, emergent subtotal colectomy should be performed.[248] Patients with recurrent diverticular bleeding should have elective surgery if the patient's general medical condition and anticipated life-span warrant such aggressive therapy.

Angiodysplasia

Vascular ectasias, or angiodysplasias, are common causes of both acute major lower GI hemorrhage and slow intermittent blood loss (see ch 108). Forty-six percent of 80 patients with LGI angiodysplasia presented with acute hemorrhage and 56% presented with chronic or occult blood loss.[249] Angiography in acute LGI bleeding shows 20% to 40% of the cases to be due to angiodysplasias.[250,251] The majority of these vascular ectasias are degenerative lesions associated with aging. Two thirds of patients with colonic angiodysplasia are over 70 years of age. They are quite different from the congenital vascular lesions that occur throughout the GI tract in various age groups. Angiodysplastic lesions are usually multiple, less than 5 mm in diameter, and involve primarily the cecum and right colon (Fig 30-5; Color Fig 2). The clinical association with aortic valve stenosis is recognized, but the reasons for this are uncertain.[252-254] Indeed, it has been reported that aortic valve replacement decreases bleeding frequency.[255,256] However, an analysis of these studies has questioned the validity of the association between angiodysplasia and aortic valve disease.[257]

The pathogenesis of angiodysplasias is unknown, but one theory is that repeated, partial intermittent obstruction of the submucosal veins where they pierce the muscle layers of the colon leads to dilatation and tortuosity of the veins.[258] Eventually, the entire arteriole–capillar–venular unit dilates, creating a small arteriovenous communication (Fig 30-6; Color Fig 3). The predilection of these degenerative lesions for the right colon may be due to the greater tension in the cecal wall compared with the rest of the colon. However, the reported decrease in bleeding from angiodysplasias after aortic valve replacement does not support this theory of pathogenesis.

The diagnosis of vascular ectasias can be made by either colonoscopy or angiography (see Figs 30-5 and 30-6; Color Figs 2 and 3). The diagnostic sensitivity of colonoscopy is ~80% with a 90% specificity.[249] The sensitivity of angiography using pathology as the gold standard is unknown, although it has been suggested that angiography misses the small vascular ectasias. The earliest angiographic sign is a densely opacified, dilated, tortuous, slowly emptying intramural vein. A vascular tuft represents a more advanced lesion, and an early filling vein reflects an arteriovenous communication and is a late sign.[259] Both diagnostic modalities frequently identify the lesions without demonstrating active bleeding. Because active bleeding is infrequently identified and because these lesions appear to be very common in the elderly without a significant blood loss history, definitive diagnosis is difficult. Nevertheless, if no other source of GI bleeding is identified in a patient with recurrent or persistent GI bleeding sufficient to require transfusions or cause significant anemia, the presence of angiodysplasia is an indication for treatment. For control of con-

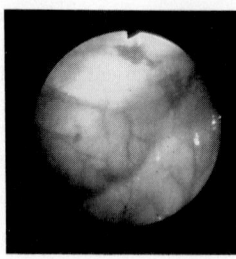 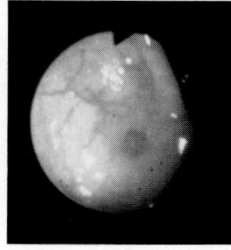

FIGURE 30–5. (See Color Fig 2). Two endoscopic pictures of angiodysplastic lesions in the right colon.

tinued gross hemorrhage, intra-arterial vasopressin has been very successful. In patients whose bleeding has ceased or slowed, endoscopic techniques of hemostasis may be tried.[260,261] When the lesions are too multiple or when recurrent bleeding occurs despite therapeutic colonoscopy, a hemicolectomy or colectomy is indicated depending on the localization of these lesions.

Neoplasms

Benign and malignant neoplasms of the colon are common lesions that, like diverticulosis and angiodysplasias, occur predominantly in the elderly (see ch 78 and ch 84). They rarely cause major hemorrhages but usually present with small intermittent bleeding or occult positive stools. The diagnosis is made by colonoscopy or barium enema, and treatment is by surgical or colonoscopic excision. Small-bowel tumors are rare but may be diagnosed by small-bowel x-ray or enteroclysis (see ch 70). Occasionally, angiography may be required to make the diagnosis. A history of

intermittent small-bowel obstruction is a clue to small-bowel tumors as the cause of LGI bleeding.

Perianal Disease

Hemorrhoids and anal fissures are probably the most common causes of minor intermittent lower GI bleeding (see ch 85). Only rarely is the amount of bleeding severe enough to cause iron-deficient anemia or acute and severe enough to require transfusions. Massive hemorrhage from simple hemorrhoids is very rare but may occur from rectal varices in patients with portal hypertension.[262] Bleeding usually comes from internal hemorrhoids and is painless. The characteristic clinical history is bright red blood on the toilet tissue or around the stool but not mixed in the stool. Bleeding often occurs with straining or passage of hard stool. A similar history is common in patients with bleeding from anal fissures, with the exception that anal fissures are often painful. Because rectal polyps and carcinomas may present with a similar bleeding history, patients should be evaluated with anoscopy and flexible sigmoidoscopy or with retroflexion of the flexible sigmoidoscope in the rectum in order to carefully visualize the proximal anal canal. Careful external examination of the external anal canal is also necessary. Perianal disease is treated with sitz baths, bulk-forming agents, avoidance of straining, and ointments or suppositories. It is unknown if actual therapeutic benefit is obtained with locally applied medications containing lubricants and hydrocortisone, but many patients report symptomatic relief. When bleeding or other symptoms continue to be troublesome, hemorrhoidal banding, coagulation techniques, or surgery may be indicated.[263]

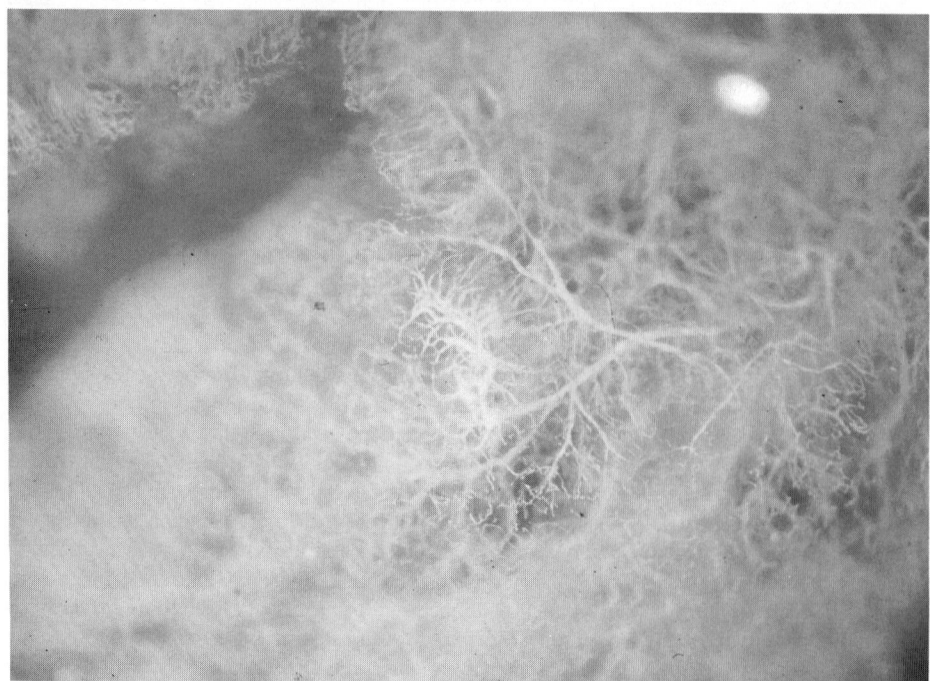

FIGURE 30–6. (See Color Fig 3) Acrylic cast of a surgical colonic specimen showing the tuft of dilated vessels in angiodysplasia.

Meckel's Diverticulum

Meckel's diverticulum is the most frequent congenital anomaly of the intestinal tract, with an incidence of 0.3% to 3.0% in autopsy reports.[264] It develops from incomplete obliteration of the vitelline duct, leaving an ileal diverticulum. Approximately 50% of these diverticula contain normal ileal mucosa, and the majority of the remaining 50% contain gastric mucosa or occasionally duodenal, colonic, and pancreatic ectopic mucosa. The gastric mucosa is capable of acid secretion that can result in ulceration of adjacent ileal mucosa (Fig 30-7; Color Fig 4). Most Meckel's diverticula remain asymptomatic and do not require surgical excision when discovered incidentally.[265] Bleeding, the most common complication, usually occurs in childhood, although rarely adults may present with it (Fig 30-7; Color Fig 4).[266] Patients present with painless bleeding that may be melenic or bright red, although classically it is described as "currant jelly" in appearance. Diagnosis can be made by radiolabeled technetium scanning, but false-neg-

ative scans are not uncommon and false-positive scans have also been reported.[267] It has been suggested that pentagastrin or cimetidine administration prior to the scan may improve sensitivity.[268,269] Barium filling of the diverticulum may occur, especially with an enteroclysis. Mesenteric angiography may demonstrate the site of bleeding. Surgical excision is the treatment of choice.

Inflammatory Bowel Disease

Bleeding from inflammatory bowel disease is usually small to moderate in quantity, but rarely it may be massive (see ch 77). It is not uncommon for patients to develop an iron-deficiency anemia, although transfusions are not often required. The blood is usually mixed in with the stool and is associated with other symptoms of the disease, such as diarrhea, tenesmus, and pain. The diagnosis and treatment of this bleeding depends on the management of the underlying disorder.

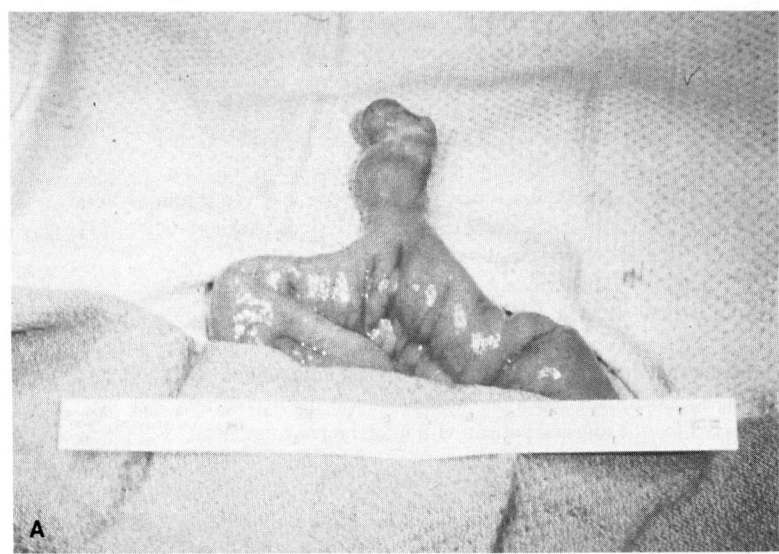

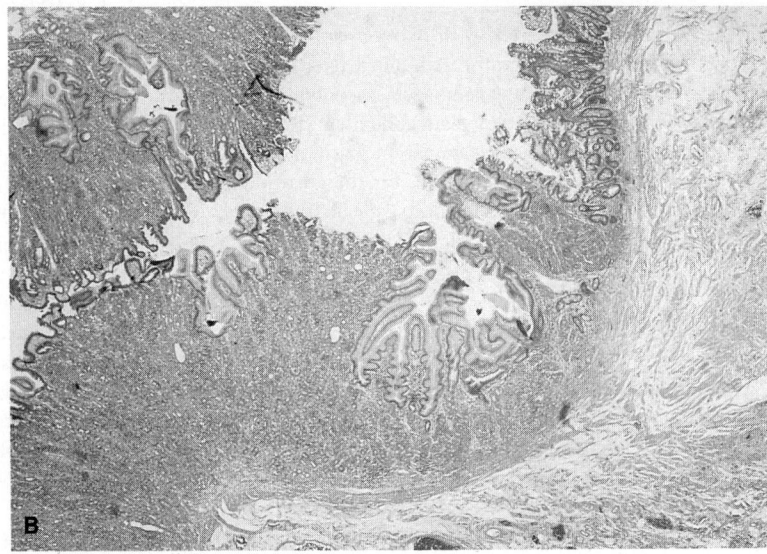

FIGURE 30-7. A, (See Color Fig 4) Operating picture of a gross specimen of a Meckel's diveticulum. **B,** Histologic slide from the same specimen showing gastric mucosa adjacent to ileal mucosa.

Colitis Due to Ischemia, Infections, or Radiation

Ischemic colitis is a common entity in the elderly population (see ch 109). It is usually due to "low-flow states" and small-vessel disease rather than large-vessel occlusion. Any segment of the colon may be involved, although the most common are the splenic flexure, descending, and sigmoid colon. The typical presentation is mild crampy abdominal pain localized to the lower left side followed within 24 hours by rectal bleeding or bloody diarrhea. The blood loss is characteristically minimal, although massive bleeding has rarely been described. Plain abdominal films may show the classic "thumbprinting" lesion of the colon. The diagnosis is best made by colonoscopy and biopsy. The majority of cases resolve spontaneously with observation and medical support. Surgery is reserved for the rare circumstance of clinical deterioration with fever and rising white blood cell count or persistent hemorrhage.

Infectious colitis due to *Campylobacter jejuni, Salmonella, Shigella,* invasive *Escherichia coli* or *E. coli* 0157, or *Clostridium difficile* often presents with bloody diarrhea. The degree of blood loss is rarely significant. The diagnosis is by sigmoidoscopy with biopsy and stool culture. Treatment is either not required or is determined by the specific pathogen.

Radiation-induced colitis is a chronic recurrent problem that may follow the radiation immediately or present several years later. Again, the blood loss is rarely massive but may cause iron deficiency because of the chronicity of the lesion. Diagnosis is made by the history of prior radiation with endoscopic biopsy confirmation. Medical treatment with bulk-forming agents or sulfasalazine may be tried, although efficacy is uncertain. Endoscopic coagulation treatment has been reported to be successful in decreasing transfusion requirements.[270] Surgical intervention is difficult because of the radiation damage to local tissue, and this is reserved for the unusual patient with intolerable symptoms.

Intussusception

Intussusception may present with maroon stools and is almost always accompanied by crampy abdominal pain. Uncommon in adults, it usually has a leading point such as a polyp or malignancy. Diagnosis may be suggested by plain abdominal films and a sausage-shaped mass on physical examination. Barium enema may be useful for diagnosis and, in children, for therapeutic reduction. Treatment of intussusception in adults is usually surgical.

Other Causes of Lower GI Bleeding

Several rare causes of lower Gl bleeding deserve brief mention. Ileal or colonic varices, which have a predilection for the area around ostomies,[271] may present with massive lower GI bleeding.[272] The diagnosis is often made by angiography, and treatment is portosystemic shunt surgery. Solitary colonic ulcer, which may occur in the rectum or in the cecum, is also a rare cause of lower Gl bleeding.[273,274] Aortoenteric fistulae, not associated with pros-

thetic grafts, have been described with ileum and colon. The diagnosis is usually made at angiography; the treatment is surgery.

DIAGNOSTIC APPROACH TO LGI BLEEDING

The diagnosis should be sought in all patients with lower Gl bleeding unless their overall prognosis is too poor to warrant further tests. In the majority of patients whose bleeding ceases spontaneously, an elective colonoscopy after routine preparation is indicated. Patients with continued bleeding require urgent diagnosis. If a perianal or rectal source is suspected, simple proctoscopy can be performed quickly and may provide the diagnosis. For most colonic bleeding, a more thorough examination will be required. If the bleeding is slow to moderate, rapid intestinal lavage via nasogastric intubation allows adequate preparation for urgent colonoscopy. For rapidly bleeding patients, the colonoscopic view may be obscured by blood so that the patient will require angiography. As with upper GI bleeding, most angiographers prefer prior radiolabeled nuclide scans to demonstrate active bleeding and to direct their examination. Prior to angiography, nasogastric lavage and even upper endoscopy should be considered to rule out an upper source of bleeding.

History and Physical Examination

A thorough history and physical examination often point to the correct diagnosis. For example, a prior diagnosis of hemorrhoids or inflammatory bowel disease is important. Symptoms that occur in association with bleeding, such as abdominal pain or diarrhea, suggest specific diagnoses. A recent history of anorexia or weight loss or an abdominal mass on physical examination may indicate underlying malignancy.

Colonoscopy

As in the upper Gl tract, colonoscopy has generally replaced barium enema for diagnostic evaluation of lower Gl bleeding (see ch 112). Several series have demonstrated the superior diagnostic sensitivity of colonoscopy even when compared to double-contrast barium enema.[275] In patients with lower Gl bleeding and normal barium enemas, 10% to 20% will have abnormal colonoscopies.[276] When lower Gl bleeding is the clinical indication for colonoscopy, the diagnostic yield is very high (40%–50%). In addition, if a barium enema is abnormal, a colonoscopy is still usually indicated for biopsy or therapeutic maneuvers. Therefore, when the indication for diagnostic study is Gl bleeding, a colonoscopy is usually indicated, regardless of the barium enema results. For these reasons, most clinicians favor colonoscopy as the primary examination. In the occasional patient in whom full colonoscopy is not technically feasible or when the colonoscopy is nondiagnostic, a barium enema is helpful.

Patients with rapid ongoing blood loss require either diagnostic angiography or urgent colonoscopy after purge. Although the traditional view is that colonoscopy in patients with severe hematochezia is impractical because of inadequate visualization, colonoscopy is feasible and useful after prior rapid cleansing.[277] Urgent colonoscopy preceded by upper endoscopy made a final diagnosis of colonic lesions in 74% of patients, UGI lesions in 11%, presumed small-bowel lesions in 9%, and no lesion site in 6% of 80 patients with ongoing hematochezia.[16] This diagnostic accuracy is similar or better than that of arteriography.

Angiography

In the rapidly bleeding patient, angiography offers both accurate diagnosis and therapy (see ch 122). There are advocates for an aggressive angiographic approach that includes pharmacologic techniques such as heparin or streptokinase to increase the possibility of demonstrating extravasation.[278] When dye extravasation is not demonstrated, angiography can lead to a presumptive diagnosis such as angiodysplasia. In addition, rare small-bowel lesions such as arteriovenous malformations or neoplasms may be demonstrated. Despite the diagnostic accuracy of both colonoscopy and angiography, the source of bleeding in many patients with a presumed lower GI source is not determined. This unfortunate, but not rare, group of patients often undergoes repeated studies.

TREATMENT OF LGI BLEEDING

Resuscitation of the patient must be the initial step in patient management. The majority of patients whose bleeding ceases will require elective treatment of the source of bleeding, depending on diagnosis. Urgent therapeutic maneuvers are indicated in patients requiring more than 3 units of red blood cell transfusion.[279]

Intra-arterial Vasopressin

Intra-arterial vasopressin is effective in controlling 90% of hemorrhages from both diverticula and angiodysplasia (see ch 123).[280] In patients with persistent bleeding, vasopressin should be infused at a rate of 0.2 U/min after selective catheterization of the bleeding vessels. Repeat contrast injection at 15 to 30 minutes should confirm cessation of hemorrhage. If hemorrhage is controlled, the vasopressin dose should be reduced to 0.1 U/min and maintained for about 12 hours. If the hemorrhage persists, the dose may be increased to 0.3 U/min. The complication rate of vasopressin infusion is 5% to 15% and includes its cardiovascular toxicity and the problems associated with an indwelling catheter.[281] Patients who fail vasopressin therapy will require surgery. Because 13% to 18% of patients receiving embolotherapy develop the serious complication of bowel infarction, with lesser degrees of ischemia being even more common, embolization techniques should be used as a last resort in patients who are poor surgical candidates. The elderly population that develops LGI bleeding may be at greater risk for ischemic complications from embolic therapy because of diffuse arteriosclerosis.

Therapeutic Colonoscopy

When bleeding has ceased or is very slow, electrocoagulation techniques may be used for angiodysplasia (see chs 107, 134). Heater probe, hot biopsy with monopolar coagulation, Bicap or multipolar coagulation, and neodymium-YAG laser have all been used successfully for these lesions. Rebleeding rates of 10% to 30% have been reported.[282] Options then include further endoscopic therapy or surgery. Occasionally, the lesions are too multiple to permit initial endoscopic therapy, and surgical excision is required. Complications from endoscopic therapy are uncommon but include induction of bleeding and perforation. A retrospective comparison of medical therapy, coagulation techniques, and surgery showed a significant decrease in transfusion requirement for all three types of management of angiodysplasia.[283] Specimen injection techniques have demonstrated incidental angiodysplastic lesions in up to 50% of surgically resected colons and autopsy specimens.[284] Therefore, it seems prudent to reserve endoscopic therapy for lesions causing significant blood loss or anemia.

Surgical Therapy for LGI Bleeding

As with UGI bleeding, surgery should not be postponed too long in the patient with persistent LGI bleeding because morbidity and mortality climb with delay. Prior surgical practice included left hemicolectomy for lower GI bleeding and was associated with high rebleeding rates. With the use of angiographic and colonoscopic diagnostic techniques, it has been shown that 70% to 80% of lower GI hemorrhage is from the right colon. This information has led to improved rebleeding rates for patients with lower GI bleeding. Surgical mortality in recent series is less than 5%.[285] For the difficult situation of recurrent bleeding without demonstration of bleeding site, a subtotal colectomy may be indicated in patients with a good overall prognosis.

BLEEDING FROM AN UNKNOWN SOURCE

There are always a few unfortunate patients with chronic bleeding or recurrent acute bleeding who elude diagnosis despite upper and lower GI x-rays, endoscopy, and angiography. It has been estimated that as many as 5% of patients will not have an identifiable source of bleeding despite extensive examination.[286] The etiology of GI bleeding in the majority of patients with bleeding from obscure origin is thought to be vascular ectasias.[287] This was determined in 80% of cases referred for small-bowel enteroscopy. Unfortunately, many of these lesions are too small to be detected by angiography and can be missed or not reached by endoscopy.[288] These are generally degenerative lesions that occur with aging. Rarely, arteriovenous malformations or vascular fragility syndromes may be associated with elastic tissue disorders such as pseudoxanthoma elasticum[289] and Ehlers–Danlos syndrome,[290] or with skin-associated vascular anomalies such as heredity hemorrhagic telangiectasia[291] or blue rubber bleb syndrome.[292]

The failure to make a diagnosis in some patients with chronic or recurrent bleeding is due to the relative inaccessibility of the small bowel. In young patients, a radionuclide scan for Meckel's diverticulum is valuable. The most useful approach toward identifying small-bowel sources of bleeding is by enteroclysis or small-bowel infusion x-ray (Fig 30-8). This requires intubation of the patient via the mouth with fluoroscopic positioning of the tip of the tube at the duodenojejunal junction. Barium is then rapidly injected to fill the small bowel. In addition, methylcellulose and water with or without parenteral glucagon are given to achieve a double-contrast effect.[293,294] If the small-bowel studies are also negative in patients bleeding from an unknown source and the blood loss can be offset with iron supplementation, no further evaluation may be necessary. If transfusions are required, however, visceral angiography or enteroscopy is indicated. Angiography in the patient who is not actively bleeding may reveal vascular anomalies or small-bowel tumors not identified by other tests.[295,296] Recently, small-bowel enteroscopy has been reported to be successful in 30% of patients with bleeding from obscure origin who have eluded all other diagnostic tests.[297] This is a tedious and time-consuming test for both patient and physician with three quarters of the patients having the ileum reached in an average intubation time of 6 hours. Other drawbacks include the lack of intervention capability, inability to completely visualize lumen (estimated at 50%–70%), and inavailability of this technique. Intraoperative transluminal endoscopic illumination has been useful in locating small-bowel angiodysplastic lesions.[298]

Endoscopic thermal ablation of angiodysplasia is recommended when the lesions are accessible. If this is unsuccessful or not feasible because of multiple lesions, surgical resection of the involved segments may be necessary. Perhaps a therapeutic trial of estrogen–progesterone therapy for the possible underlying diagnosis of vascular ectasias is worthwhile even in some patients without a definite diagnosis. Further study in this area is needed. Unfortunately, there are a few patients with bleeding from an unknown source who will defy diagnosis or be too ill for surgery and be relegated to receive transfusions as needed.

The reader is directed to Chapter 22, Gastrointestinal Blood Flow; Chapter 31, Approach to the Patient with Occult Gastrointestinal Bleeding; Chapter 44, Skin Lesions Associated with Gastrointestinal Diseases; Chapter 45, Approach to Gastrointestinal Problems in the Elderly; Chapter 55, Reflux Esophagitis; Chapter 58, Miscellaneous Diseases of the Esophagus; Chapter 61, Acid-Peptic Disorders; Chapter 62, Zollinger–Ellison Syndrome; Chapter 64, Surgery for Peptic Ulcer Disease; Chapter 70, Tumors and Other Neoplastic Diseases of the Small Intestine; Chapter 78, Colonic Polyps: Benign and Premalignant Neoplasms of the Colon; Chapter 82, Diverticulitis; Chapter 84, Malignant Tumors of the Colon; Chapter 108, Vascular Ectasias, Tumors, and Malformations; Chapter 109, Vascular Insufficiency; Chapter 111, Upper Gastrointestinal Endoscopy; Chapter 112, Colonoscopy and Flexible Sigmoidoscopy; Chapter 121, Gastrointestinal Radionuclide Imaging Procedures; Chapter 122, Angiography; Chapter 123, Interventional Radiology; Chapter 133, Sclerotherapy; and Chapter 134, Endoscopic Control of Nonvariceal Upper Gastrointestinal Hemorrhage.

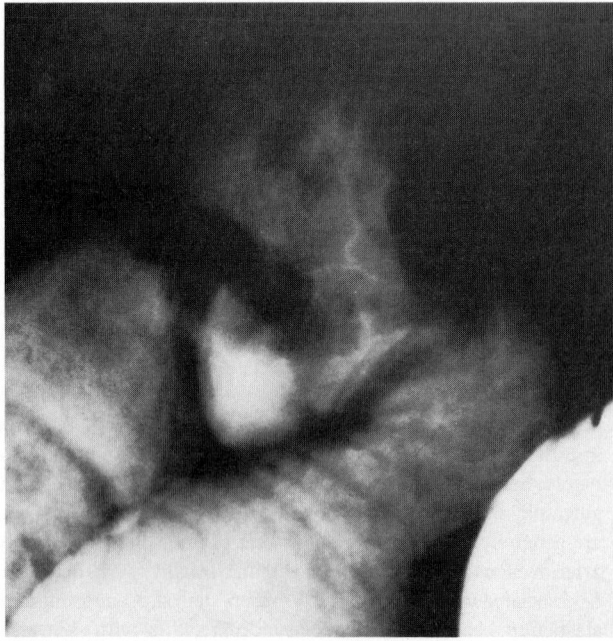

FIGURE 30–8. Enterocylsis demonstrating a small bowel tumor that had caused GI hemorrhage. It was missed on routine small bowel follow through.

REFERENCES

1. Cutler JA, Mendeloff AI. Upper gastrointestinal bleeding: Nature and magnitude of the problem in the U.S. Dig Dis Sci 1981;26:90s.
2. Shiller KFR, Truelove SC, Williams DG. Hematemesis and melena, with special reference to factors influencing the outcome. Br Med J 1970;2:7.
3. Hunt PS, Hansky J, Korman MG. Mortality in patients with haematemesis and melaena: A prospective study. Br Med J 1979;1:1238.
4. Kang JY, Piper DW. Improvement in mortality rates in bleeding peptic ulcer disease. Med J Aust 1980;1:213.
5. Wright HK. Massive colonic hemorrhage. Surg Clin North Am 1980;60:1297.
6. Peterson WL, Barnett CC, Smith HJ, et al. Routine early endoscopy in upper gastrointestinal tract bleeding. N Engl J Med 1981;304:925.
7. Morris DW, Levine GM, Soloway RD, et al. Prospective, randomized study of diagnosis and outcome in acute upper gastrointestinal bleeding: Endoscopy versus conventional radiography. Am J Dig Dis 1975;20:1103.
8. Conn HO. To scope or not to scope. N Engl J Med 1981;304:967.
9. Sander-Jensen K, Secher NH, Bie P, et al. Vagal slowing of the heart during hemorrhage: Observations from 20 consecutive hypotensive patients. Br Med J 1986;292:364.
10. Vladeck BC, Bassin R, Kark AE, et al. Rapid and slow hemorrhage in man: II. Sequential acid-base and oxygen transport responses. Am Surg 1971;173:331.
11. Boyan CP. Cold or warmed blood for massive transfusions. Am Surg 1964;160:282.
12. Silverstein FE, Gilbert DA, Tedesco FJ, et al. The national ASGE survey on upper gastrointestinal bleeding. II. Clinical prognostic factors. Gastrointest Endosc 1981;27:80.
13. Luke RG, Lees W, Rudick J. Appearances of the stools after the introduction of blood into the caecum. Gut 1964;5:77.
14. Stellato T, Rhodes RS, McDougal WS. Azotemia in upper gastrointestinal hemorrhage. Am J Gastroenterol 1980;73:486.
15. Layne EA, Mellow MH, Lipman TO. Insensitivity of guaiac slide

tests for detection of blood in gastric juice. Ann Intern Med 1981;94: 774.

16. Jensen DM, Machicado GA. Diagnosis and treatment of severe hematochezia. The role of urgent colonoscopy after purge. Gastroenterology 1988;95:1569.

17. Elashoff JD, Grossman MI. Trends in hospital admissions and death rates for peptic ulcer in the United States from 1970 to 1978. Gastroenterology 1980;78:280.

18. Fleischer D. Etiology and prevalence of severe persistent upper gastrointestinal bleeding. Gastroenterology 1983;84:538.

19. Thorne FL, Nyhus LM. Treatment of massive upper gastrointestinal bleeding. Am Surg 1965;31:413.

20. Graham DY, Smith JL. The course of patients after variceal hemorrhage. Gastroenterology 1981;80:800.

21. Silverstein FE, Gilbert DA, Tedesco FJ. The national ASGE survey on upper gastrointestinal bleeding. Gastrointest Endosc 1981;27:73.

22. Swain CP, Storey DW, Bown SG. Nature of the bleeding vessel in recurrently bleeding gastric ulcers. Gastroenterology 1986;90:595.

23. Wara P. Endoscopic prediction of major rebleeding—A prospective study of stigmata of hemorrhage in bleeding ulcer. Gastroenterology 1985;88:1209.

24. Griffiths WJ, Neumann DA, Welsh JD. The visible vessel as an indicator of uncontrolled or recurrent gastrointestinal hemorrhage. N Engl J Med 1979;300:1411.

25. Storey DW, Bown SG, Swain CP, et al. Endoscopic prediction of recurrent bleeding in peptic ulcers. N Engl J Med 1981;305:915.

26. Chang-Chien C, Wu C, Chen P, et al. Different implications of stigmata of recent hemorrhage in gastric and duodenal ulcers. Dig Dis Sci 1988;33:400.

27. Laine L. Multipolar electrocoagulation in the treatment of active upper gastrointestinal tract hemorrhage. N Engl J Med 1987;316: 1613.

28. Gregory PB, Knauer M, Fogel MR. Upper gastrointestinal bleeding. Accuracy of clinical diagnosis and prognosis. Dig Dis Sci 1981;26: 655.

29. Johnston SJ, Jones PF, Kyle J, et al. Epidemiology and course of gastrointestinal haemorrhage in Northeast Scotland. Br Med J 1973;29:655.

30. Lumsden K, MacLarnon JC, Dawson J. Giant duodenal ulcer. Gut 1970;11:592.

31. Cotton PB, Rosenberg MT, Waldram RPL, et al. Early endoscopy of oesophagus, stomach, and duodenal bulb in patients with haematemesis and melaena. Br Med J 1973;2:505.

32. Christensen A, Bousfield R, Christansen J. Incidence of perforated and bleeding peptic ulcers before and after the introduction of H2-receptor antagonists. Ann Surg 1988;207:4.

33. Jorde R, Burhol PG, Johnson JA. Peptic ulcer bleeding in patients with and without dyspepsia. Scand J Gastroenterol 1988;23:213.

34. Armstrong CP, Blower AL. Nonsteroidal antiinflammatory drugs and life threatening complications of peptic ulceration. Gut 1987;28: 527.

35. Swain CP, Salmon PR, Northfield PC. Does ulcer position influence presentation or prognosis of acute gastrointestinal bleeding? Gut 1986;27:A632.

36. LaBrooy SJ, Misiewicz JJ, Edwards J, et al. Controlled trial of cimetidine in upper gastrointestinal haemorrhage. Gut 1979;20:892.

37. Hoare AM, Bradby GVH, Hawkins CF, et al. Cimetidine in bleeding peptic ulcer. Lancet 1979;2:671.

38. Pickard RG, Sanderson I, South M, et al. Controlled trial of cimetidine in acute upper gastrointestinal bleeding. Br Med J 1979;1: 661.

39. Carstensen HE, Bulow S, Hansen OH, et al. Cimetidine for severe gastroduodenal hemorrhage; a randomized controlled trial. Scand J Gastroenterol 1980;15:103.

40. Zuckerman G, Welch R, Douglas A. Controlled trial of medical therapy for active upper gastrointestinal bleeding and prevention of rebleeding. Am J Med 1984;76:361.

41. Dawson J, Cockel R. Ranitidine in acute upper gastrointestinal haemorrhage. Br Med J 1982;285:476.

42. Collins R, Langman M. Treatment with histamine H2 antagonists in acute upper gastrointestinal hemorrhage. N Engl J Med 1985;131: 660.

43. Magnusson I, Ihre T, Johannson C, et al. Randomized double blind trial of somatostatin in the treatment of massive upper gastrointestinal haemorrhage. Gut 1985;26:221.

44. Lauritsen K, Laursen LS, Havelund T, et al. Controlled trial of arbaprostil in bleeding peptic ulcer. Br Med J 1985;291:1093.

45. Engvist A, Brostrom F, Feilitzen F, et al. Tranexamic acid in massive haemorrhage from the upper gastrointestinal tract: A double blind study. Scand J Gastroenterol 1979;14:839.

46. Barer D, Ogilvie A, Henry D, et al. Cimetidine and tranexamic acid in the treatment of acute upper gastrointestinal tract bleeding. N Engl J Med 1983;308:1571.

47. Hussey KP. Vasopressin therapy for upper gastrointestinal tract hemorrhage. Has its efficacy been proven? Arch Intern Med 1985;145: 1263.

48. Waltman AC, Greenfield AJ, Novelline RA, et al. Pyloroduodenal bleeding and intraarterial vasopressin: Clinical results. AJR Am J Roentgenol 1979;133:643.

49. Lieberman DA, Keller FS, Katon RM, et al. Arterial embolization for massive upper gastrointestinal tract bleeding in poor surgical candidates. Gastroenterology 1984;86:876.

50. Chen PC, Wu CS, Liau YU. Hemostatic effect of endoscopic local injection with hypertonic saline-epinephrine solution and pure ethanol for digestive tract bleeding. Gastrointest Endosc 1986;32: 319.

51. Panes J, Forne M, Marco C. Controlled trial of endoscopic sclerosis in bleeding peptic ulcers. Lancet 1987;1:1292.

52. Klein FA, Drueck C, Breuer RI, et al. Control of upper gastrointestinal bleeding with a microcrystalline collagen hemostat. Dig Dis Sci 1982;27:981.

53. Linsheer WG, Fazig TL. Control of upper gastrointestinal hemorrhage by endoscopic spraying of clotting factors. Gastroenterology 1979;77:642.

54. Peura DA, Johnson LF, Burkhalter EL. Use of tri fluoroisopropyl cyanoacrylate polymer (MBR 4197) in patients with bleeding peptic ulcers of the stomach and duodenum: A randomized controlled study. J Clin Gastroenterol 1982;4:325.

55. Protell RL, Gilbert DA, Silverstein FE, et al. Computer-assisted electrocoagulation: Bipolar vs monopolar in the treatment of experimental canine gastric ulcer bleeding. Gastroenterology 1981;80: 451.

56. O'Brien JD, Day SJ, Burnham WR. Controlled trial of small bipolar probe in bleeding peptic ulcers. Lancet 1986;1:464.

57. Fleischer D. Endoscopic therapy of upper gastrointestinal bleeding in humans. Gastroenterology 1986;90:217.

58. Rutgeerts P, Vantrappen G, Broeckaert L, et al. Controlled trial of YAG laser treatment of upper digestive hemorrhage. Gastroenterology 1982;83:410.

59. Fleischer D. The current status of gastrointestinal laser activity in the United States. Gastrointest Endosc 1982;28:157.

60. Green FW, Kaplan MM, Curtis LE, et al. Effect of acid and pepsin on blood coagulation and platelet aggregation. Gastroenterology 1978;74:38.

61. Berstad A, Holm HA, Kittang E. Experience with antipeptic agents. Scand J Gastroenterol 1979;14:121.

62. Berstad A. Management of acute upper gastrointestinal bleeding. Scand J Gastroenterol 1982;17:103.

63. Peterson WL, Richardson CT. Intravenous cimetidine or two regimens of ranitidine to reduce fasting gastric acidity. Ann Intern Med 1986;104:505.

64. Kernohan RM, Anderson JR, McKelvey STD, et al. A controlled trial of bipolar electrocoagulation in patients with upper gastrointestinal bleeding. Br J Surg 1984;71:889.

65. Elta GH, Appelman HD, Behler EM, et al. A study of the correlation between endoscopic and histologic diagnoses in gastroduodenitis. Am J Gastroenterol 1987;82:749.

66. Borch K, Jansson L, Sjodahl R, et al. Hemorrhagic gastritis. Incidence, etiological factors and prognosis. Acta Chir Scand 1987;154:211.

67. Graham DY, Smith JL. Aspirin and the stomach. Ann Intern Med 1986;104:390.

68. Silvoso GR, Ivey KJ, Butt JH, et al. Incidence of gastric lesions in patients with rheumatic disease on chronic aspirin therapy. Ann Intern Med 1979;91:517.

69. Cohen MM, McCready DR, Clark L, et al. Protection against aspirin-

induced antral and duodenal damage with enprostil. Gastroenterology 1985;88:382.

70. Lanza FL, Aspinall RL, Swabb EA, et al. Double-blind, placebo-controlled endoscopic comparison of the mucosal protective effects of misoprostol versus cimetidine on tolmetin-induced mucosal injury to the stomach and duodenum. Gastroenterology 1988;95:289.

71. Caldwell JR, Roth SH, Wu WC, et al. Sucralfate treatment of non-steroidal anti-inflammatory drug-induced gastrointestinal symptoms and mucosal damage. Am J Med 1987;83:74.

72. Hoftiezer JW, Silvoso GR, Burks M, et al. Comparison of the effects of regular and enteric coated aspirin on gastroduodenal mucosa of man. Lancet 1980;2:609.

73. Scheiman JM, Behler EM, Berardi RR, et al. Salicylsalicylic acid causes less gastroduodenal mucosal damage than enteric-coated aspirin. An endoscopic comparison. Dig Dis Sci 1989;34:229.

74. Wells JJ, Nostrant TT, Wilson JAP, et al. Gastroduodenal ulcerations in patients receiving selective hepatic artery infusion chemotherapy. Am J Gastroenterol 1985;80:425.

75. Chaudhury TK, Robert A. Prevention by mild irritants of gastric necrosis produced in rats by sodium taurocholate. Dig Dis Sci 1980;25:830.

76. Needham CD, Kyle J, Jones PF, et al. Aspirin and alcohol in gastrointestinal haemorrhage. Gut 1971;12:819.

77. Sarfeh IJ, Tarnawski A, Malki A, et al. Portal hypertension and gastric mucosal injury in rats. Effects of alcohol. Gastroenterology 1983;84:987.

78. Laine L, Weinstein WM. Histology of alcoholic hemorrhagic "gastritis": A prospective evaluation. Gastroenterology 1988;94:1254.

79. McCormack TT, Sims J, Eyre-Brook I, et al. Gastric lesions in portal hypertension: Inflammatory gastritis or congestive gastropathy? Gut 1985;26:1226.

80. VanVliet ACM, Tenkate FJW, Dees J, et al. Abnormal blood vessels of the prepyloric antrum in cirrhosis of the liver as a cause of chronic gastrointestinal bleeding. Endoscopy 1978;10:89.

81. Thomas E, Rosenthal WS, Rymer W, et al. Upper gastrointestinal hemorrhage in patients with alcoholic liver disease and esophageal varices. Am J Gastroenterol 1979;72:623.

82. Sarfeh IJ, Tabak C, Eugene J, et al. Clinical significance of erosive gastritis in patients with alcoholic liver disease and upper gastrointestinal hemorrhage. Ann Surg 1981;194:149.

83. Babb RR, Mitchell RL. Persistent hemorrhagic gastritis in a patient with portal hypertension and esophagogastric varices: The role of portal decompressive surgery. Am J Gastroenterol 1988;83:777.

84. Hosking SW, Kennedy HJ, Seddon I, et al. The role of propranolol in congestive gastropathy of portal hypertension. Hepatology 1987;7:437.

85. Skillman JJ, Silen W. Acute gastroduodenal "stress" ulceration: Barrier disruption of varied pathogenesis? Gastroenterology 1970;59:478.

86. Skillman JJ, Bushnell LS, Goldman H, et al. Respiratory failure, hypotension, sepsis and jaundice—A clinical syndrome associated with lethal hemorrhage from acute stress ulceration of the stomach. Am J Surg 1969;117:523.

87. Kamada T, Fusamoto H, Karuano S, et al. Acute gastroduodenal lesions in head injury. Am J Gastroenterol 1977;68:249.

88. Athanasoulis CA, Baum S, Waltman AC, et al. Control of acute mucosal hemorrhage. Intraarterial infusion of posterior pituitary extract. N Engl J Med 1974;290:597.

89. Semb BKH, Scjonsby H, Solhaug JH. Intravenous infusion of vasopressin in the treatment of bleeding from severe hemorrhagic gastritis. Acta Chir Scand 1983;149:579.

90. Hubert JP, Kierman PD, Welch JS, et al. The surgical management of bleeding stress ulcers. Ann Surg 1980;191:672.

91. Lucas CE, Sugawa C, Riddle J, et al. Natural history and surgical dilemma of "stress" gastric bleeding. Arch Surg 1971;102:266.

92. Hastings PR, Skillman JJ, Bushnell LS, et al. Antacid titration in the prevention of acute gastrointestinal bleeding. N Engl J Med 1978;298:1041.

93. Peura DA, Johnson LF. Cimetidine for prevention and treatment of gastroduodenal mucosal lesions in patients in an intensive care unit. Ann Intern Med 1985;103:173.

94. Borrero E, Bank S, Margolis I, et al. Comparison of antacid and

sucralfate in the prevention of gastrointestinal bleeding in patients who are critically ill. Am J Med 1985;79:62.

95. Priebe HJ, Skillman JJ, Bushnell LS, et al. Antacid versus cimetidine in preventing acute gastrointestinal bleeding. N Engl J Med 1980;302:426.

96. Ostro MJ, Russell JA, Soldin SJ, et al. Control of gastric pH with cimetidine boluses versus primed infusions. Gastroenterology 1985;89:532.

97. Shuman RB, Schuster DP, Zuckerman GR. Prophylactic therapy for stress ulcer bleeding: A reappraisal. Ann Intern Med 1987;106:562.

98. Tryba M, Zevounov F, Torok M, et al. Prevention of acute stress bleeding with sucralfate, antacids, or cimetidine. Am J Med 1986;79:55.

99. Driks MR, Craven DE, Celli BR, et al. Nosocomial pneumonia in intubated patients given sucralfate as compared with antacids or histamine type 2 blockers: The role of gastric colonization. N Engl J Med 1987;317:1376.

100. Infante-Rivard C, Esnaola S, Villeneuve JP. Role of endoscopic variceal sclerotherapy in the long term management of variceal bleeding: A meta-analysis. Gastroenterology 1989;96:1087.

101. Smith JL, Graham DY. Survival analysis of variceal hemorrhage: Does it matter when the meter is started? Hepatology 1988;8:193.

102. Snady H, Feinman L. Prediction of variceal hemorrhage: A prospective study. Am J Gastroenterol 1988;83:519.

103. Burroughs AK, D'iteygene F, McIntyre N. Pitfalls in studies of prophylactic therapy for variceal bleeding in cirrhotics. Hepatology 1986;6:1407.

104. Lebrec D, DeFleury P, Rueff B, et al. Portal hypertension, size of esophageal varices, and risk of gastrointestinal bleeding in alcoholic cirrhosis. Gastroenterology 1980;79:1139.

105. Bosch J, Bordas JM, Rigau J, et al. Noninvasive measurement of the pressure of esophageal varices using an endoscopic gauge: Comparison with measurements by variceal puncture in patients undergoing endoscopic sclerotherapy. Hepatology 1986;6:667.

106. Beppu K, Inokucki K, Koyanagi N, et al. Prediction of variceal hemorrhage by esophageal endoscopy. Gastrointest Endosc 1981;27:213.

107. Eckardt VF, Grace ND. Gastroesophageal reflux and bleeding esophageal varices. Gastroenterology 1979;76:39.

108. North Italian Endoscopic Club. Prediction of the first variceal hemorrhage in patients with cirrhosis of the liver and esophageal varices. N Engl J Med 1988;319:983.

109. Blackstone MO. Esophageal varices. In: Blackstone MO. Endoscopic interpretation. New York: Raven Press, 1984:66.

110. Foutch PG, Sullivan JA, Gaines JA, et al. Cutaneous vascular spiders in cirrhotic patients: Correlation with hemorrhage from esophageal varices. Am J Gastroenterol 1988;83:723.

111. Dagradi AE, Mehler R, Tan DTD, et al. Sources of upper gastrointestinal bleeding in patients with liver cirrhosis and large esophagogastric varices. Am J Gastroenterol 1970;54:458.

112. Conn HO, Ramsby GR, Storer EH, et al. Intraarterial vasopressin in the treatment of upper gastrointestinal hemorrhage: A prospective, controlled trial. Gastroenterology 1975;68:211.

113. Mallory A, Schaefer JW, Cohen JR, et al. Selective intraarterial vasopressin infusion for upper gastrointestinal tract hemorrhage. Arch Surg 1980;115:30.

114. Chojkier M, Groszmann RJ, Atterbury LE, et al. A controlled comparison of continuous intraarterial and intravenous infusions of vasopressin in hemorrhage from esophageal varices. Gastroenterology 1979;77:540.

115. Fogel MR, Knauer CM, Andres LL, et al. Continuous intravenous vasopressin in active upper gastrointestinal bleeding. Ann Intern Med 1982;96:565.

116. Conn HO. Vasopressin and nitroglycerin in the treatment of bleeding varices: The bottom line. Hepatology 1986;6:523.

117. Sirinek KR, Levine BA. High-dose vasopressin for acute variceal hemorrhage. Arch Surg 1988;123:876.

118. Tsai YU, Lay CS, Lai KH, et al. Controlled trial of vasopressin plus nitroglycerin vs. vasopressin alone in the treatment of bleeding esophageal varices. Hepatology 1986;6:406.

119. Gimson AES, Westaby D, Hegarty J, et al. A randomized trial of

vasopressin and vasopressin plus nitroglycerin in the control of acute variceal hemorrhage. Hepatology 1986;6:410.

120. Freeman JG, Lishman AH, Cobden I, et al. Controlled trial of ter-lipressin (glypressin) versus vasopressin in the early treatment of oesophageal varices. Lancet 1982;1:66.

121. Walker S, Stiehl A, Raedsch R, et al. Terlipressin in bleeding esophageal varices: A placebo controlled, double-blind study. Hepatology 1986;6:112.

122. Bosch J, Kravetz D, Rodes J. Effects of somatostatin on hepatic and systemic hemodynamics in patients with cirrhosis of the liver: Comparison with vasopressin. Gastroenterology 1981;80:518.

123. Kravetz D, Bosch J, Teres J, et al. Comparison of intravenous somatostatin and vasopressin infusions in treatment of acute variceal hemorrhage. Hepatology 1984;4:442.

124. Miskowiak J, Burcharth F, Jensen LI. Effect of lower oesophageal sphincter on oesophageal varices. Scand J Gastroenterol 1981;16: 957.

125. Hosking SW, Doss W, El-Zeiny H, et al. Pharmacological constriction of the lower oesophageal sphincter: A simple method of arresting variceal haemorrhage. Gut 1988;29:1098.

126. Crotty B, Wood LJ, Willett IR, et al. The management of acutely bleeding varices by injection sclerotherapy. Med J Aust 1986;145: 130.

127. Westaby D, Hayes PC, Gumson AES, et al. Injection sclerotherapy for active variceal bleeding: A controlled trial. Gut 1986;7:A1246.

128. Copenhagen Esophageal Varices Sclerotherapy Project. Sclerotherapy after first variceal hemorrhage in cirrhosis. A randomized multicenter trial. N Engl J Med 1984;311:1594.

129. Paquet KJ, Feussner H. Endoscopic sclerosis and esophageal balloon tamponade in acute hemorrhage from esophagogastric varices: A prospective controlled randomized trial. Hepatology 1985;5:580.

130. Panes J, Teres J, Bosch J, et al. Efficacy of balloon tamponade in treatment of bleeding gastric and esophageal varices. Dig Dis Sci 1988;33:454.

131. Feneyrou B, Hanana J, Davres JP, et al. Initial control of bleeding from esophageal varices with the Sengstaken-Blakemore tube. Am J Surg 1988;155:509.

132. Hunt PS, Korman MG, Hansky J, et al. An 8-year prospective experience with balloon tamponade in emergency control of bleeding esophageal varices. Dig Dis Sci 1982;27:413.

133. Teres J, Cecelia A, Bordas JM, et al. Esophageal tamponade for bleeding varices. Controlled trial between the Sengstaken–Blakemore tube and the Linton-Nachlas tube. Gastroenterology 1978;75:566.

134. Boyce MHW. Modification of the Sengstaken–Blakemore balloon tube. N Engl J Med 1962;267:195.

135. Chojkier M, Conn HO. Esophageal tamponade in the treatment of bleeding varices. A decadal progress report. Dig Dis Sci 1980;25: 267.

136. Mandelstam P, Zeppa R. Endotracheal intubation should precede esophagogastric balloon tamponade for control of variceal bleeding. J Clin Gastroenterol 1983;5:493.

137. Smith-Laing G, Scott J, Long RG, et al. Role of percutaneous transhepatic obliteration of varices in the management of hemorrhage from gastroesophageal varices. Gastroenterology 1981;80:1031.

138. Viamonte M, Pereiras R, Russell E, et al. Transhepatic obliteration of gastroesophageal varices: Results in acute and nonacute bleeders. AJR Am J Roentgenol 1977;129:237.

139. Bengmark S, Borjesson B, Hoevels J, et al. Obliteration of esophageal varices by PTP. Ann Surg 1979;190:549.

140. Malt RA, Abbolf WM, Warshaw AL, et al. Randomized trial of emergency mesocaval and portacaval shunts for bleeding esophageal varices. Am J Surg 1978;135:584.

141. Orloff MJ, Bell RH. Long-term survival after emergency portacaval shunting for bleeding varices in patients with alcoholic cirrhosis. Am J Surg 1986;151:176.

142. Terblanche J, Burroughs AK, Hobbs KEF. Controversies in the management of bleeding esophageal varices. N Engl J Med 1989;320: 1393.

143. Smith JL, Graham DY. Variceal hemorrhage: A critical evaluation of survival analysis. Gastroenterology 1982;82:968.

144. Terblanche J, Northover JMA, Bornman P, et al. A prospective controlled trial of sclerotherapy in the long term management of

patients after esophageal variceal bleeding. Surg Gynecol Obstet 1979;148:323.

145. Korula J, Balart LA, Radvan G, et al. A prospective randomized controlled trial of chronic esophageal variceal sclerotherapy. Hepatology 1985;5:584.

146. Cello JP, Grendell JH, Crass RA, et al. Endoscopic sclerotherapy versus portacaval shunt in patients with severe cirrhosis and variceal hemorrhage. N Engl J Med 1984;311:1589.

147. Schuman BM, Beckman JW, Tedesco FJ, et al. Complications of endoscopic injection sclerotherapy: A review. Am J Gastroenterol 1987;82:823.

148. Westaby D, MacDougall BRD, Williams R. Improved survival following injection sclerotherapy for esophageal varices: Final analysis of a controlled trial. Hepatology 1985;5:827.

149. Terblanche J, Kahn D, Campbell JA, et al. Failure of repeated injection sclerotherapy to improve long-term survival after oesophageal variceal bleeding. Lancet 1983;1:1328.

150. Larson AW, Cohen H, Zweiban B, et al. Acute esophageal variceal sclerotherapy. JAMA 1986;255:497.

151. Lebrec D, Pynard T, Hillon P, et al. Propranolol for prevention of recurrent gastrointestinal bleeding in patients with cirrhosis: A controlled study. N Engl J Med 1981;305:1371.

152. Lebrec D, Novel O, Corbic M, et al. Propranolol: A medical treatment for portal hypertension? Lancet 1980;2:180.

153. Garcia-Tsao G, Grace ND, Groszmann RJ, et al. Short-term effects of propranolol on portal venous pressure. Hepatology 1986;6:101.

154. Burroughs AK, Jenkins WJ, Scherlock S, et al. Controlled trial of propranolol for the prevention of recurrent variceal hemorrhage in patients with cirrhosis. N Engl J Med 1983;309:1539.

155. Villeneuve JP, Pomier-Layrangues G, Infante-Rivard C, et al. Propranolol for the prevention of recurrent variceal hemorrhage: A controlled trial. Hepatology 1986;6:1239.

156. Westaby D, Melia WM, MacDougall BRD, et al. β_1 selective adrenoreceptor blockade for the long term management of variceal bleeding. A prospective randomized trial to compare oral metoprolol with injection sclerotherapy in cirrhosis. Gut 1985;26:421.

157. Kroeger RJ, Groszmann RJ. Effect of selective blockade of β_2-adrenergic receptors on portal and systemic hemodynamics in a portal hypertensive rat model. Gastroenterology 1985;88:896.

158. Hillon P, Lebrec P, Munoz C, et al. Comparison of the effects of a cardioselective and a nonselective β-blockade on portal hypertension in patients with cirrhosis. Hepatology 1982;2:528.

159. Westaby D, Bihari DJ, Gimson AES, et al. Selective and nonselective beta receptor blockade in the reduction of portal pressure in patients with cirrhosis and portal hypertension. Gut 1984;25:121.

160. Malt RA. Portosystemic venous shunts. N Engl J Med 1976;295: 24,80.

161. Galambos JT, Warren WD, Rudman D, et al. Selective and total shunts in the treatment of bleeding varices. N Engl J Med 1976;295: 1089.

162. Langer B, Taylor BR, MacKenzie DR, et al. Further report of a prospective randomized trial comparing distal splenorenal shunt with end-to-side portacaval shunt. Gastroenterology 1985;88:424.

163. Reichle FA, Fahmy WF, Coolsorkhi M. Prospective comparative clinical trial with distal splenorenal and mesocaval shunts. Am J Surg 1979;137:13.

164. Fischer JE, Bower RH, Atamian S, et al. Comparison of distal and proximal splenorenal shunts. Ann Surg 1981;194:531.

165. Conn HO, Resnick RH, Grace ND, et al. Comparison of distal and proximal splenorenal shunt vs portal-systemic shunt: Current status of a controlled trial. Hepatology 1981;1:151.

166. Harley HAJ, Morgan T, Redker AG, et al. Results of a randomized trial of end-to-side portacaval shunt and distal splenorenal shunt in alcoholic liver disease and variceal bleeding. Gastroenterology 1986;91:802.

167. Rikkers LF. Portal hypertension. In: Moody FG, Carey LC, Jones RS, Kelly KA, Nahrwold DL, Skinner DB, eds. Surgical treatment of digestive disease. Chicago: Year Book Medical Publishers, 1986: 409.

168. Resnick RH, Iber FL, Ishihara AM, et al. A controlled study of the therapeutic portacaval shunt. Gastroenterology 1974;67:843.

169. Rueff B, Degos F, Degos JD, et al. A controlled study of therapeutic portacaval shunt in alcoholic cirrhosis. Lancet 1976;1:655.

170. Reynolds TB, Donovan AJ, Mikkelsen WP, et al. Results of a 12-year randomized trial of portacaval shunt in patients with alcoholic liver disease and bleeding varices. Gastroenterology 1981;80:1005.

171. Gouge TH, Ranson JHC. Esophageal transection and paraesophagogastric devascularization for bleeding esophageal varices. Am J Surg 1986;151:47.

172. Koyanagi N, Iso Y, Higashi H, et al. Recurrence of varices after oesophageal transection: Intra-operative and postoperative assessment by endoscopy. Br J Surg 1988;75:9.

173. Ono J, Katsuki T, Kodama Y. Combined therapy for esophageal varices: Sclerotherapy, embolization and splenopneumopexy. Surgery 1987;101:535.

174. Akita H, Sakoda K. Porto pulmonary shunt by splenopneumopexy as a surgical treatment of Budd-Chiari syndrome. Surgery 1980;87:85.

175. Resnick RH, Chalmers TC, Ishihara AM, et al. A controlled study of the prophylactic portacaval shunt. Ann Intern Med 1969;70:675.

176. Conn HO, Lindemuth WW, May CJ, et al. Prophylactic portacaval anastomosis. Medicine 1972;51:27.

177. Witzel L, Wolbergs E, Merki H, et al. Prophylactic endoscopic sclerotherapy of oesophageal varices. Lancet 1985;1:773.

178. Santangelo WC, Dueno MI, Estes BL, et al. Prophylactic sclerotherapy of large esophageal varices. N Engl J Med 1988;318:814.

179. Sauerbruch T, Wotzka R, Kopcke W, et al. Prophylactic sclerotherapy before the first episode of variceal hemorrhage in patients with cirrhosis. N Engl J Med 1988;319:8.

180. Pascal JP, Cales P, Multicenter Study Group. Propranolol in the prevention of first upper gastrointestinal tract hemorrhage in patients with cirrhosis of the liver and esophageal varices. N Engl J Med 1987;317:856.

181. Ideo G, Bellati G, Fesce E, et al. Nadolol can prevent the first gastrointestinal bleeding in cirrhotics: A prospective, randomized study. Hepatology 1988;8:6.

182. The Italian Multicenter Project for Propranolol in Prevention of Bleeding. Propranolol for prophylaxis of bleeding in cirrhotic patients with large varices: A multicenter randomized clinical trial. Hepatology 1988;8:1.

183. Hosking SW, Johnson AG. Gastric varices: A proposed classification leading to management. Br J Surg 1988;75:195.

184. Glynn MJ. Isolated splenic vein thrombosis. Arch Surg 1986;121:723.

185. Moossa AR, Gadd MA. Isolated splenic vein thrombosis. World J Surg 1985;9:384.

186. Keith RG, Mustard RA, Sarbil EA. Gastric variceal bleeding due to occlusion of splenic vein in pancreatic disease. Can J Surg 1982;25:301.

187. Sarin SK, Sachdeu G, Nanda R, et al. Endoscopic sclerotherapy in the treatment of gastric varices. Br J Surg 1988;75:747.

188. Yassin YM, Eita MS, Hussein A. Endoscopic sclerotherapy for bleeding gastric varices. Gut 1985;26:A1105.

189. Trudeau W, Prindiville T. Endoscopic injection sclerosis (EIS) of bleeding gastric varices. Gastroenterology 1983;84:1338A.

190. Shepard HA, Harvey J, Jackson A, et al. Recurrent retching with gastric mucosal prolapse. A proposed prolapse gastropathy syndrome. Dig Dis Sci 1984;29:121.

191. Knaver CM. Mallory-Weiss syndrome. Characterization of 75 Mallory-Weiss lacerations in 528 patients with upper gastrointestinal hemorrhage. Gastroenterology 1976;71:5.

192. Graham DY, Schwartz JT. The spectrum of the Mallory-Weiss tear. Medicine 1977;57:307.

193. Sugawa C, Benishek D, Walt AJ. Mallory-Weiss syndrome. A study of 224 patients. Am J Surg 1983;145:30.

194. Roark G. Treatment of postsclerotherapy esophageal ulcers with sucralfate. Gastrointest Endosc 1984;30:9.

195. Singal AK, Sarin SK, Misras P, et al. Ulceration after esophageal and gastric variceal sclerotherapy—Influence of sucralfate and other factors on healing. Endoscopy 1988;20:238.

196. Goldstein HM, Medellin H, Ben-Menachem Y, et al. Transcatheter arterial embolization in the management of bleeding in the cancer patient. Radiology 1975;115:603.

197. Meyer CT, Troncale FJ, Galloway S, et al. Arteriovenous malformations of the bowel: An analysis of 22 cases and a review of the literature. Medicine 1981;60:36.

198. Zuckerman GR, Cornette GL, Clouse RE, et al. Upper gastrointestinal bleeding in patients with chronic renal failure. Ann Intern Med 1985;102:588.

199. Weaver GA, Alpers HD, Davis JS, et al. Gastrointestinal angiodysplasia associated with aortic valve disease: Part of a spectrum of angiodysplasia of the gut. Gastroenterology 1979;77:1.

200. Vase P, Grove O. Gastrointestinal lesions in hereditary hemorrhagic telangiectasia. Gastroenterology 1986;91:1079.

201. Blackstone MO. Uncommon gastric appearances. In: Blackstone MO. Endoscopic interpretation. New York: Raven Press, 1984:195.

202. Marwick T, Kerlin P. Angiodysplasia of the upper gastrointestinal tract: Clinical spectrum in 41 cases. J Clin Gastroenterol 1986;8:404.

203. Rutgeerts P, VanGompel F, Geboes K, et al. Long term results of treatment of vascular malformations of the gastrointestinal tract by neodymium YAG laser photocoagulation. Gut 1985;26:586.

204. Livio M, Mannucci PM, Vigano G, et al. Conjugated estrogens for the management of bleeding associated with renal failure. N Engl J Med 1986;315:731.

205. Bronner MH, Pate MB, Cunningham JT, et al. Estrogen-progesterone therapy for bleeding gastrointestinal telangiectasias in chronic renal failure. Ann Intern Med 1986;105:371.

206. Granieri R, Mazzulla JP, Yarborough GW, et al. Estrogen-progesterone therapy for recurrent gastrointestinal bleeding secondary to gastrointestinal angiodysplasia. Am J Gastroenterol 1988;83:556.

207. Van Cutsem E, Rutgeerts P, Geboes K, et al. Treatment of bleeding gastrointestinal telangiectasias with estrogen-progesterone. Gastroenterology 1989;96:A523.

208. Rawlinson WD, Barr GD, Lin BPC. Antral vascular ectasia—The "watermelon" stomach. Med J Aust 1986;144:709.

209. Jabbari M, Cherry R, Lough JO, et al. Gastric antral vascular ectasia: The watermelon stomach. Gastroenterology 1984;87:1165.

210. Gilliam JH, Gersinger KR, Wu WC, et al. The "watermelon stomach." Morphologic diagnosis by endoscopy [Abstract]. Gastroenterology 1984;88:1394.

211. Wheeler MH, Smith DM, Cotton PB, et al. Abnormal blood vessels in the gastric antrum. A cause of upper gastrointestinal bleeding. Dig Dis Sci 1979;24:155.

212. Calam J, Walker RJ. Antral vascular lesion, achlorhydria and chronic gastrointestinal blood loss. Response to steroids. Dig Dis Sci 1980;25:236.

213. Petrini JL, Johnston JH. Heat probe treatment for antral vascular ectasia. Gastrointest Endosc 1989;35:324.

214. Champion MC, Sullivan SN, Coles JC, et al. Aortoenteric fistula. Ann Surg 1982;195:314.

215. Steffes BC, O'Leary JP. Primary aortoduodenal fistulas: A case report and review of the literature. Ann Surg 1980;46:121.

216. Connally JE, Kwaan JHM, McCart PM, et al. Aortoenteric fistula. Ann Surg 1981;194:402.

217. Larmi TK. Hemobilia associated with cholecystitis, postcholecystectomy conditions and trauma: Review of 12 cases. Ann Surg 1966;163:373.

218. Balldin G, Cronstedt J. Bleeding birth of a gallstone from a hanging papilla of Vater. Endoscopy 1983;15:36.

219. Steckman ML, Dooley MC, Jaques PF, et al. Major gastrointestinal hemorrhage from peripancreatic blood vessels in pancreatitis. Treatment by embolotherapy. Dig Dis Sci 1984;29:486.

220. Fagan EA, Allison DJ, Chadwick JS, et al. Treatment of haemobilia by selective arterial embolization. Gut 1980;21:541.

221. Wagner WH, Lundell CJ, Donovan AJ. Percutaneous angiographic embolization for hepatic arterial hemorrhage. Arch Surg 1985;120:1241.

222. Hoffmann J, Beck H, Jensen HE. Dieulafoy's lesion. Surg Gynecol Obstet 1984;159:537.

223. Mortensen NJ, Mountfond RA, Davies JD, et al. Dieulafoy's disease: A distinctive arteriovenous malformation causing massive gastric haemorrhage. Br J Surg 1983;70:76.

224. Juler GL, Labitzke HG, Lamb R, et al. The pathogenesis of Dieulafoy's gastric erosion. Am J Gastroenterol 1984;79:195.

225. Pointner R, Schwab G, Konigsrainer A, et al. Endoscopic treatment of Dieulafoy's disease. Gastroenterology 1988;94:563.

226. Graham DY. Limited value of early endoscopy in the management of acute upper gastrointestinal bleeding. Am J Surg 1980;140:284.

227. Dronfield MW, Langman MJS, Atkinson M, et al. Outcome of endoscopy and barium radiography for acute upper gastrointestinal bleeding: Controlled trial in 1037 patients. Br Med J 1982;284:545.

228. Keller RT, Logan GM. Comparison of emergent endoscopy and upper gastrointestinal series radiography in acute upper gastrointestinal haemorrhage. Gut 1976;17:180.

229. Morris DW, Levine GM, Soloway RD, et al. Prospective, randomized study of diagnosis and outcome in acute upper gastrointestinal bleeding: Endoscopy versus conventional radiography. Am J Dig Dis 1975;20;1103.

230. Leinicke JA, Schaffer RD, Hogan WJ, et al. Emergency endoscopy in acute upper GI bleeding (UGB): Does timing affect the significance of diagnostic yield? Gastrointest Endosc 1976;22:228.

231. Steer ML, Silen W. Diagnostic procedures in gastrointestinal hemorrhage. N Engl J Med 1983;309:646.

232. Keller FS, Rosch J. Value of angiography in diagnosis and therapy of acute upper gastrointestinal hemorrhage. Dig Dis Sci 1981;26:78s.

233. Twiford TW, Goldstein HM, Zornoza J. Transcatheter therapy of gastrointestinal arterial bleeding. Dig Dis 1978;23:1046.

234. Bryant LR, Mobin-Uddin K, Dillon ML, et al. Comparison of ice water with iced saline solution for gastric lavage in gastroduodenal hemorrhage. Am J Surg 1972;124:570.

235. Ponsky JL, Hoffman M, Swayngim DS. Saline irrigation in gastric hemorrhage: The effect of temperature. J Surg Res 1980;28:204.

236. Andrus CH, Ponsky JL. The effects of irrigant temperature in upper gastrointestinal hemorrhage: A requiem for iced saline lavage. Am J Gastroenterol 1987;82:1062.

237. Kiselow MC, Wagner M. Intragastric instillation of levarterenol. A method for control of upper gastrointestinal tract hemorrhage. Arch Surg 1973;107:387.

238. Lieberman DA, Keller FS, Katon RM, et al. Arterial embolization for massive upper gastrointestinal tract bleeding in poor surgical candidates. Gastroenterology 1984;86:876.

239. Morris DL, Hawker PC, Brearley S, et al. Optimal timing of operation for bleeding peptic ulcer: Prospective randomized trial. Br Med J 1984;288:1277.

240. Browder W, Cerise EJ, Litwin MS. Impact of emergency angiography in massive lower gastrointestinal bleeding. Ann Surg 1986;204:530.

241. McGuire HH, Hanes BW. Massive hemorrhage from diverticulosis of the colon. Ann Surg 1972;125:847.

242. Nath RL, Sequeira JC, Weitzman AF, et al. Lower gastrointestinal bleeding. Diagnostic approach and management conclusions. Am J Surg 1981;141:478.

243. Cassarella WJ, Kanter IE, Seaman WB. Right-sided colonic diverticula as a cause of acute rectal hemorrhage. N Engl J Med 1972;286:450.

244. Kewenter J, Hellzen-Ingemarsson A, Kewenter G, et al. Diverticular disease and minor rectal bleeding. Scand J Gastroenterol 1985;20:922.

245. Eisenberg H, Laufer I, Skillman JJ. Arteriographic diagnosis and management of suspected colonic diverticular hemorrhage. Gastroenterology 1973;64:1091.

246. Athanasoulis CA, Baum S, Rosch J, et al. Mesenteric arterial infusions of vasopressin for hemorrhage from colonic diverticula. Am J Surg 1975;129:212.

247. Bar AH, DeLaurentis DA, Parry CE, et al. Angiography in the management of massive lower gastrointestinal tract hemorrhage. Surg Gynecol Obstet 1980;150:226.

248. Drapanas T, Pennington G, Kappelman M, et al. Emergency subtotal colectomy: Preferred approach to management of massively bleeding diverticular disease. Ann Surg 1973;177:519.

249. Richter JM, Hedberg SE, Athanasoulis CA, et al. Angiodysplasia. Clinical presentation and colonoscopic diagnosis. Dig Dis Sci 1984;29:481.

250. Boley SJ, DiBiase A, Brandt LJ, et al. Lower intestinal bleeding in the elderly. Am J Surg 1979;137:57.

251. Wright HK, Pelliccia O, Higgins EF, et al. Controlled, semielective, segmental resection for massive colonic hemorrhage. Am J Surg 1980;139:535.

252. Rogers G. Endoscopic diagnosis and therapy of mucosal vascular abnormalities of the gastrointestinal tract occurring in elderly patients and associated with cardiac, vascular and pulmonary disease. Gastrointest Endosc 1980;26:134.

253. McNamara JJ, Austen WG. Gastrointestinal bleeding occurring in patients with acquired valvular heart disease. Arch Surg 1968;97:538.

254. Greenstein RJ, McElhinney AJ, Reuben D, et al. Colonic vascular ectasias and aortic stenosis: Coincidence or causal relationship? Am J Surg 1986;151:347.

255. Cappell MS, Lebwohl O. Cessation of recurrent bleeding from gastrointestinal angiodysplasias after aortic valve replacement. Ann Intern Med 1986;105:54.

256. Scheffer SM, Leatherman LL. Resolution of Heyd's syndrome of aortic stenosis and gastrointestinal bleeding after aortic valve replacement. Ann Thorac Surg 1986;42:477.

257. Imperiale TF, Ransohoff DF. Aortic stenosis, idiopathic gastrointestinal bleeding, and angiodysplasia: Is there an association? A methodologic critique of the literature. Gastroenterology 1988;95:1670.

258. Boley SJ, Sammartano R, Adams A, et al. On the nature and etiology of vascular ectasias of the colon. Gastroenterology 1977;72:650.

259. Boley SJ, Sammartano R, Brandt LJ. Vascular ectasias of the colon. Surg Gynecol Obstet 1979;149:353.

260. Howard OM, Buchanan JD, Hunt RH. Angiodysplasia of the colon. Lancet 1982;1:16.

261. Cello JP, Grendell JH. Endoscopic laser treatment for gastrointestinal vascular ectasias. Ann Intern Med 1986;104:352.

262. Hosking SW, Johnson AG. Bleeding anorectal varices: A misunderstood condition. Surgery 1988;104:70.

263. Buls JG, Goldberg SM. Modern management of hemorrhoids. Surg Clin North Am 1978;58:469.

264. Williams RS. Management of Meckel's diverticulum. Br J Surg 1981;68:477.

265. Soltero MJ, Bill AH. The natural history of Meckel's diverticulum and its relation to incidental removal. Am J Surg 1976;132:168.

266. Yamaguchi M, Takeuchi S, Awazu S. Meckel's diverticulum. Investigation of 600 patients in Japanese literature. Am J Surg 1978;136:247.

267. Stakianakis GN, Haase GM. Abdominal scintigraphy for ectopic gastric mucosa: A retrospective analysis of 143 studies. AJR Am J Roentgenol 1982;138:7.

268. Treves S, Grand RJ, Eraklis AJ. Pentagastrin stimulation of technetium-99 m uptake by ectopic gastric mucosa in a Meckel's diverticulum. Radiology 1978;128:711.

269. Baum S. Pertechnetate imaging following cimetidine administration in Meckel's diverticulum of the ileum. Am J Gastroenterol 1981;76:464.

270. Alexander TJ, Dwyer RM. Endoscopic Nd:Yag laser treatment of severe radiation injury of the lower gastrointestinal tract: Long-term follow-up. Gastrointest Endosc 1988;34:407.

271. Ricci RL, Lee KR, Greenberger NJ. Chronic gastrointestinal bleeding from ileal varices after total proctocolectomy for ulcerative colitis: Correction by mesocaval shunt. Gastroenterology 1980;78:1058.

272. Hamlyn AN, Morris JS, Lunzen MR, et al. Portal hypertension with varices in unusual sites. Lancet 1974;1:1531.

273. Levine DS. "Solitary" rectal ulcer syndrome. Gastroenterology 1987;92:243.

274. Sutherland DER, Chan FY, Fouceir E, et al. The bleeding cecal ulcer in transplant patients. Surgery 1979;86:386.

275. Aldridge MC, Sim AJW. Colonoscopy findings in symptomatic patients without x -ray evidence of colonic neoplasms. Lancet 1986;1:833.

276. Tedesco FJ, Waye JD, Raskin JB. Colonoscopic evaluation of rectal bleeding. A study of 304 patients. Ann Intern Med 1978;89:907.

277. Forde KA. Colonoscopy in acute rectal bleeding. Gastrointest Endosc 1981;27:219.

278. Koval G, Benner KG, Rosch J, et al. Aggressive angiographic diagnosis in acute lower gastrointestinal hemorrhage. Dig Dis Sci 1987;32:248.

279. Ramanath HK, Hinshaw JR. Management and mismanagement of bleeding colonic diverticula. Arch Surg 1971;103:311.

280. Waltman AC. Transcatheter embolization versus vasopressin infusion

for the control of arteriocapillary gastrointestinal bleeding. Cardiovasc Intervent Radiol 1980;3:289.

281. Uflacker R. Transcatheter embolization for treatment of acute lower gastrointestinal bleeding. Acta Radiol 1987;4:425.

282. Santos JCM, Apilli F, Guimaraes AS, et al. Angiodysplasia of the colon: Endoscopic diagnosis and treatment. Br J Surg 1988;75:256.

283. Hutcheon DF, Kablin J, Bulkley GB, et al. Effect of therapy on bleeding rates in gastrointestinal angiodysplasia. Am Surg 1987; 53:6.

284. Aldabagh SM, Trujillo YP, Taxy JB. Utility of specimen angiography in angiodysplasia of the colon. Gastroenterology 1986;91:725.

285. Welch CE, Athanasoulis CA, Galdabini JJ. Hemorrhage from the large bowel with special reference to angiodysplasia and diverticular disease. World J Surg 1978;2:73.

286. Thompson JN, Salen RR, Hemingway AP, et al. Specialist investigation of obscure gastrointestinal bleeding. Gut 1987;28:47.

287. Spechler SJ, Schummel EM. Gastrointestinal tract bleeding of unknown origin. Arch Intern Med 1982;142:236.

288. Duray PH, Marcal JM, LiVolsi VA, et al. Small intestinal angiodysplasia in the elderly. J Clin Gastroenterol 1984;6:311.

289. Strole WE. Case records of the Massachusetts General Hospital. N Engl J Med 1983;308:579.

290. Krane SM. Case records of the Massachusetts General Hospital. N Engl J Med 1979;300:129.

291. Smith CR, Bartholomew LG, Cain JC. Hereditary hemorrhagic telangiectasia and gastrointestinal hemorrhage. Gastroenterology 1963;44:1.

292. Baker AL, Kahn PC, Binder SC, et al. Gastrointestinal bleeding due to blue rubber bleb nevus syndrome. Gastroenterology 1971;61:530.

293. Maglinte DDT, Elmore MF, Chernish SM, et al. Enteroclysis in the diagnosis of chronic unexplained gastrointestinal bleeding. Dis Colon Rectum 1985;28:403.

294. Maglinte DDT, Hall R, Miller RE, et al. Detection of surgical lesions of the small bowel by enteroclysis. Am J Surg 1984;147:225.

295. Athow AC, Sheppard L, Subson DE. Selective visceral angiography for unexplained acute gastrointestinal bleeding in a distinct general hospital. Br J Surg 1985;72:120.

296. Best EB, Teaford AK, Rasler FH. Angiography in chronic recurrent gastrointestinal bleeding: A nine year study. Surg Clin North Am 1979;59:811.

297. Lewis BS, Waye JD. Chronic gastrointestinal bleeding of obscure origin: Role of small bowel enteroscopy. Gastroenterology 1988;94:1117.

298. Scott SD, Royle GT. Angiodysplasia of the small bowel; a brilliant technique for localizing the quiescent lesion. Postgrad Med J 1987;63:995.

31

Approach to the Patient with Occult Gastrointestinal Bleeding

DAVID A. AHLQUIST

By definition, occult gastrointestinal bleeding is hidden and not apparent on stool inspection. As with gross gastrointestinal bleeding (ch 30), occult bleeding may be either acute and self-limited or chronic, and its cause may either be known or remain obscure after diagnostic studies. However, unlike gross bleeding, which is overtly evidenced by melena or hematochezia, occult bleeding goes unnoticed unless detected by a test.

Occult gastrointestinal bleeding is exceedingly common. Abnormal fecal blood levels can be found in 1 of 20 adults on prevalence screens[1-5] but probably occur episodically in everyone through their lifetime. The causes of occult bleeding are protean and may occur at any anatomic level from the oropharynx to the rectum. Abnormal fecal blood levels often reflect trivial pathology but may herald a health-threatening benign or malignant lesion. As such, the clinician's judgment is challenged when he is faced with the finding of an abnormal fecal occult blood level.

The critical metabolic sequela of occult gastrointestinal bleeding is iron deficiency. The resulting morbidity from indolent fatigue and loss of productivity represents a major public health concern. In the United States alone, 20 million people are believed to be iron-deficient.[6] The global prevalence of iron deficiency is estimated at 15%, or a staggering total of 600 million people.[7] Iron deficiency is the most common cause of anemia worldwide and is usually due to chronic enteric blood loss, especially in men and postmenopausal women.[8,9] Because iron deficiency is common and treatable, recognition of its presence and association with gastrointestinal pathology is important.

In recent years, the most widespread application of fecal blood testing has been as a screening tool for colorectal cancer. Unfortunately, fecal blood is an inherently ambiguous marker for colorectal cancer because most abnormal fecal occult bleeding is due to other causes, and asymptomatic colorectal cancers often do not bleed. While it is hoped that such screening will eventuate in reduced cancer mortality, this common practice remains unproved and controversial.

PATHOPHYSIOLOGIC CONSIDERATIONS

Quantitative Relationships

Given a typical daily stool weight of 150 g (volume of 150 ml), an average circulating hemoglobin of 15 g/dl, and the known hemoglobin iron content of 0.34% by weight, the following equivalences can be calculated: volume of 2 ml fecal blood lost per day = concentration of 2 mg Hb/g of stool = total daily Hb loss of 300 mg = daily iron loss of 1 mg. A marked increase in stool volume or decrease in the circulating hemoglobin level would alter this equivalence accordingly.

Surprisingly large amounts of blood may be lost into the gastrointestinal lumen and yet remain occult. Ingestion of over 200 ml of blood is required to consistently produce melena in volunteers.[10] Bolus infusion of blood directly into the cecum must exceed 150 ml to routinely yield melena or hematochezia.[11,12] We have observed fecal hemoglobin concentrations of over 100 mg/g (equivalent to 100 ml/d blood loss or 10 g Hb/dl) in normal-appearing stools from patients with gastroduodenal bleeding (unreported data). Thus, hemoglobin concentrations of some stools may approach the hemoglobin concentration of circulating blood without being visibly apparent. Of incidental importance, the hemoglobin concentration of melena may surpass that of circulating blood by a factor of four or five, likely as a result of hemocon-

centration during colonic transit, because fecal hemoglobin concentrations of over 680 mg/g, or 68 g/dl, have been recorded.[13] In sharp contrast, as little as 1 or 2 ml of blood may be visible as a bright red streak on the stool surface from patients with anorectal lesions. Thus, depending on the rate of enteric bleeding, anatomic site of bleeding, enterocolic transit time, efficiency of luminal hemoglobin metabolism, and fecal mixing, the same amount of blood loss may be visually gross or occult.

NORMAL FECAL BLOOD LOSS

Fecal blood is not simply present or absent but ranges in a continuum from physiologic levels to pathologically elevated levels. Fecal blood levels quantified in groups of healthy volunteers by various investigators using the radiochromium[14-17] or heme-porphyrin[18,19] techniques have been strikingly similar. Reported mean fecal blood levels have been between 0.5 and 1.5 ml/d (0.5–1.5 mg Hb/g), with 90% to 95% of levels falling below 2 ml/day and 97% to 100% below 3 ml/day. Normal fecal blood losses do not appear to change with age or gender.[18]

Gastrointestinal Hemoglobin Metabolism

The metabolic fate of intraluminal hemoglobin depends in large part on the anatomic level and rate of bleeding. The variable degree of hemoglobin disassembly that occurs during transit dramatically impacts the measurement of fecal blood, because available fecal blood tests target different components of the hemoglobin molecule (Table 31-1). Accordingly, an appreciation of enterocolic hemoglobin metabolism helps to clarify test limitations and may be useful in selecting a test appropriate to the clinical indication.

HEME METABOLISM AND ABSORPTION

The heme moities of hemoglobin are cleaved from the globins primarily by pancreatic and intestinal proteases in the proximal small bowel and probably to a lesser extent by gastric pepsin.[20,21] A variable fraction of intraluminal heme is absorbed intact in the

TABLE 31-1
Effect of Gastrointestinal Bleeding Site on Metabolic Fate of Intraluminal Hemoglobin (Hb)

BLEEDING SITE	Hb INSULTS DURING LUMINAL TRANSIT	Hb COMPONENTS IN STOOL*		
		Globin	Heme	HDPs†
Upper gastrointestinal	Globin completely digested by gastric, enteric peptidases	0	+	+++
	Minimal heme absorption in duodenum and jejunum			
	Colonic flora convert heme to HDPs			
Distal ileum, proximal colon	Globin altered by peptidases of colonic flora	+	+	++
Rectosigmoid	Minimal alteration of Hb molecule	+++	+++	0/+

* *Immunochemical tests detect globin, guaiac tests react with intact heme, and the heme-porphyrin assay measures both heme and HDPs.*
† *HDPs, heme-derived porphyrins.*

proximal small intestine.[22,23] There is evidence that the mechanism of heme absorption is saturable. Fecal heme recovery is as low as 40% following ingestion of 5 to 10 ml of blood but increases to over 85% after ingestion of 15 ml or more of blood.[24,25] Binding of heme to the brush border, which may be facilitated by a specific receptor,[26] appears to be the rate-limiting step.[27,28] Once absorbed into epithelial cells, heme is initially compartmentalized into secondary lysosomes and eventually metabolized by microsomal heme oxidase to free iron and bilirubin, both of which rapidly enter the portal circulation.[22,29,30] The regulation of heme absorption remains ill-defined, but it is known that heme absorption may increase threefold in response to iron deficiency[31] and decrease following gastrectomy.[32]

Heme that escapes intestinal absorption enters the colon, where it is variably converted by bacteria to porphyrin and iron.[24,33] The fraction of heme converted to porphyrin varies from 1% to 99% of the total heme entering the colon[13,33] and is not detected by guaiac tests, which react only with intact heme. The fact that bacteria account for the conversion of heme to porphyrin is supported by observations that this heme-derived porphyrin fraction is absent in neonates prior to gut colonization,[34] is greater with proximal than distal colorectal bleeding,[18,33] and increases during fecal storage.[13]

GLOBIN METABOLISM

The globin chains of hemoglobin are digested by gastric pepsin and by pancreatic and intestinal proteases. Because immunoassays for hemoglobin are directed against antigenic sites on the globin chains, they are very insensitive for upper gastrointestinal bleeding. Immunoassays completely fail to detect ingested blood in quantities up to 100 ml.[27] Globin chains are also metabolized in the colon. This is probably due to bacteria, because bleeding from right-sided colon lesions is less likely to be detected by immunoassay than that from left-sided lesions,[35] and immunoreactivity is progressively lost during fecal storage (personal observations).

Iron Metabolism and Deficiency

Occult gastrointestinal bleeding may be compensated by increased iron absorption or mobilization of body iron stores, which, in turn, stimulates erythropoiesis. However, when iron loss from occult bleeding chronically exceeds intestinal iron absorption, iron stores are eventually depleted and iron deficiency with attendant anemia and other metabolic sequelae ensue. Thus, the time required to develop iron deficiency depends on the intestinal absorptive capacity for iron, the rate and chronicity of occult bleeding, and the size of body iron stores. Chapters 20 and 21 cover additional aspects of iron metabolism.

IRON ABSORPTION

Ordinarily, about 10% of dietary iron is absorbed. A daily adult Western diet typically contains 5 to 15 mg of elemental iron and 1 to 5 mg of heme-iron,[36] the latter primarily from myoglobin in meat. Intrinsic sources of iron are relatively small and originate from sloughed epithelial cells, which contain heme in cytochromes and catalase and traces of elemental iron bound in ferritin.[27] Heme-iron is preferentially absorbed and appears to provide 60% to 80% of the 1 to 2 mg of iron normally absorbed daily.[37] Both iron forms are absorbed primarily in the duodenum and proximal jejunum, although by different mechanisms. Dietary heme-iron is absorbed as described for hemoglobin-heme above. Elemental iron absorption occurs as an active process that is poorly characterized but regulated by numerous factors. Elemental iron absorption may be increased up to 10-fold by iron deficiency, anemia, hypoxia, liver disease, increased erythropoiesis, and elevated luminal iron concentration.[6,36,38] Its absorption is facilitated by reducing substances, such as ascorbate, by bile and pancreatic juice, by gastric acid, and possibly by a nonacidic gastric modulator.[6,39-42] Conversely, certain luminal substances, such as phytates in cereals, tannic acid in tea, oxalates, and desferrioxamine, chelate iron and impede its absorption.[36,38,43] Except for iron deficiency and anemia, the above factors do not influence the efficiency of heme-iron absorption.[20,31,43] Once absorbed, iron is either transported to hematopoietic or reticuloendothelial tissue by way of transferrin carriage or stored as ferritin in the epithelial cell.

Inadequate iron procurement results from either dietary deficiency or iron malabsorption. The former may occur in third-world countries, infants, some vegetarians, and derelicts.[6] General causes of malabsorption (ch 38 and 68 through 75) may eventuate in iron deficiency, which has been reported with achlorhydria and postgastrectomy states, celiac sprue, short bowel syndrome, Crohn's disease, lymphoma, radiation enteritis, amyloidosis, chronic mesenteric ischemia, and eosinophilic gastroenteritis.[6,32,33,44-46] Selective iron malabsorption rarely occurs as a result of an inherited defect of transferrin function in children[47] or as a result of an acquired autoimmunity to the transferrin receptor in adults.[48]

IRON LOSS

A physiologic mechanism to excrete excess iron does not exist. Under normal circumstances, absorption of dietary iron (average, 1 to 2 mg per day) equals or just exceeds iron loss through normal daily occult gastrointestinal bleeding (average 1 mg per day). Trace amounts of iron are also lost through cutaneous desquamation and intestinal epithelial sloughing.[27] Excessive iron loss by occult gastrointestinal bleeding, the most common cause of iron deficiency, is the most difficult to recognize clinically. Menorrhagia often contributes to iron deficiency in premenopausal women.[49] Although excessive bleeding can occur from the airway, urinary tract, or multiple phlebotomies, these are uncommon causes of iron deficiency and are clinically apparent.[6] As a general rule, occult gastrointestinal losses of 5 to 10 ml per day are required to overcome compensatory absorptive increases, in the absence of pharmacologic iron replacement, and lead to a negative iron balance.

IRON STORAGE

Most body iron is in metabolically active forms, with 65% to 70% in hemoglobin, about 4% in myoglobin, and less than 1% in various tissue enzymes.[6] Surplus iron is stored in a soluble complex with ferritin and in a particulate state as hemosiderin, especially in hepatocytes and in the reticuloendothelial cells of the liver, bone marrow, and spleen. Iron in these macromolecular storage forms accounts for the remaining 20% to 25% of total body iron.[6] The mechanism by which iron is mobilized from these stores is incompletely understood. A small amount of ferritin is present in plasma and correlates well with total body iron stores.[50]

METABOLIC CONSEQUENCES OF IRON DEFICIENCY

Iron is present in all mammalian cells and is of vital importance not only for oxygen transport and storage as hemoglobin but also for many nonhematologic functions. This ubiquitous metal is essential for nearly half of the enzymes of the Krebs and tricarboxylic acid cycles, for catecholamine metabolism, for DNA synthesis, and for several other cellular processes.[51] It is not surprising that the clinical and metabolic manifestations of iron deficiency are so generalized.

The fatigue associated with iron deficiency has traditionally been ascribed to the resultant anemia. Controlled studies of laborers in tropical countries with iron deficiency anemia primarily due to hookworm infestation have clearly shown that work productivity increases significantly with iron replacement and resolution of anemia.[52,53] However, such clinical studies do not distinguish the potential contribution of nonhematologic tissue iron depletion to the symptoms from that of anemia. Iron deficiency leads to decreased tissue myoglobin levels and to reduced activity in iron-requiring enzymes, including cytochrome oxidase, succinate dehydrogenase, xanthine oxidase, and others.[51] These tissue enzymes may be affected prior to the development of anemia, which is a relatively late stage of iron deficiency. Indeed, patients with proven iron deficiency by absent bone marrow stains but without anemia note a greater improvement in their fatigue with iron therapy than with placebo.[54] However, the strongest evidence that nonhemoglobin iron deficiency plays a role in muscle fatigue comes from a study comparing treadmill endurance in normal rats and in iron-deficient rats with hemoglobin levels adjusted to normal.[55] Running ability was markedly lower in iron-deficient animals (correlated with reduced tissue rates of oxidative phosphorylation) and normalized with iron therapy. Thus, the fatigue associated with iron deficiency is multifactorial and not due to anemia alone.

Numerous epithelial changes may accompany iron deficiency. While some, such as lingual atrophy and stomatitis, may occur with various nutrition deficiencies, others, like koilonychia and proximal esophageal webs, are more characteristic (see section on Clinical Manifestations). Achlorhydria may occur in over 40% of patients with iron deficiency.[56] Gastric hyposecretion resolves with iron replacement in some patients.[57] A spruelike small intestinal lesion may develop with associated malabsorption as the result of iron deficiency, and this may resolve histologically and clinically with iron repletion.[58] These gastric and small intestinal sequelae of iron deficiency can create a vicious cycle by further compromising iron absorption.

Iron deficiency has been causally linked to behavioral, immunologic, and growth disturbances.[51] Mental fatigue, cognitive impairment, and affective disturbances in children with iron de-

ficiency may resolve with iron therapy. Elevated levels of norepinephrine and decreased conversion of thyroxine to triiodothyronine reported in patients with iron deficiency may explain their irritability and cold intolerance. Iron appears to be important in cell-mediated immunity, and its deficiency may predispose the host to candidal and certain bacterial infections. Finally, slowed growth and delayed wound healing have been attributed to iron deficiency.

ETIOLOGY

Many of the lesions causing gross bleeding (ch 30) can ooze chronically and bleed occultly. Despite assumptions of the pre-endoscopic era, small diaphragmatic hernias and colonic diverticula probably do not produce occult bleeding.[18] The mechanism of occult gastrointestinal bleeding must involve a disruption of the epithelium and could be categorized as inflammatory, infectious, vascular, neoplastic, or traumatic. Much of our understanding of specific lesions responsible for occult bleeding has been inferred from gastrointestinal findings in patients with iron deficiency rather than from prospective studies using valid fecal assays. The prevalence of lesions responsible for occult bleeding varies depending on the age and geography of the population considered. For example, occult bleeding in infants most commonly arises from milk-induced enteritis,[59,60] but in the elderly it arises from peptic ulcer disease and neoplasms.[8,18,61,62] While rare in industrialized countries, intestinal helminth infestation is overwhelmingly the most common cause of harmful occult bleeding in tropical and subtropical countries.[63]

Although innumerable conditions can induce occult blood loss, this section will deal primarily with those causes of occult gastrointestinal bleeding which may present solely as iron deficiency or an abnormal fecal blood test result (Table 31-2).

Inflammatory Causes

ACID-PEPTIC DISEASE

In Western countries, erosions or ulceration of the esophagus, stomach, and duodenum are the most common gastrointestinal lesions associated with occult bleeding and iron deficiency (see ch 55, 61, and 62). Iron deficiency has been attributed to such acid-peptic disease in 30% to 70% of adult cases,[8,61,62,64] and patients often have no ulcer symptoms. Acid-peptic disease, particularly reflux esophagitis,[65] may also underlie iron deficiency in young children. Based on quantitative studies,[18] occult fecal blood levels are elevated in about two thirds of patients with peptic ulcers or erosions, and levels are significantly higher in those with associated anemia. It is not known whether occult blood levels are predictive of gross bleeding or other complications in patients with chronic peptic ulcers.

TABLE 31–2
Disorders That May Present as Occult Gastrointestinal Bleeding With or Without Iron Deficiency

Inflammatory Causes

Peptic esophagitis
Large hiatal hernia (Cameron erosions)
Crohn's disease
Chronic ulcerative colitis
Mild enterocolitis
Whipple's disease
Sprue
Eosinophilic gastroenteritis
Meckel's diverticulum
Solitary colon ulcer
Other

Infectious Causes

Hookworm
Strongyloidiasis
Ascariasis
Tuberculous enterocolitis
Amebiasis
Other

Vascular Causes

Angiodysplasia and vascular ectasias
Gastroesophageal varices and congestive
gastropathy
Hemangiomas
Blue rubber bleb nevus syndrome
Watermelon stomach
Other

Tumors and Neoplastic Causes

Primary gastrointestinal cancer at any site
Metastases to gastrointestinal tract
Large polyp at any site
Lymphoma
Leiomyoma
Leiomyosarcoma
Lipoma
Other

Drugs

Nonsteroidal anti-inflammatory drugs
Other

Extragastrointestinal Causes

Hemoptysis
Epistaxis
Oropharyngeal bleeding

Artifactual Causes

Hematuria
Menstrual bleeding
Nonspecific test positivity

Miscellaneous Causes

Long-distance running
Coagulopathies
Factitial

CAMERON EROSIONS

The association between large diaphragmatic hernias and iron deficiency anemia has long been known.[66] In up to 10% of iron-deficient patients, a large diaphragmatic hernia is found.[8,61] Furthermore, anemia is nearly 16 times more common in patients with large hernias than in those with none.[67] The chronic occult blood loss is due to characteristic longitudinal erosions, often called Cameron erosions (Fig 31-1), located in the gastric mucosa at the level of the diaphragm hiatus and felt to be secondary to mechanical trauma from breathing.[68] Hernias of the diaphragm are discussed elsewhere (ch 53).

MISCELLANEOUS ENTEROCOLITIDES

Many inflammatory conditions of the small and large intestines may bleed occultly (ch 70, 75, 77, 86, and 107). A heat-labile protein in bovine milk not uncommonly produces occult bleeding and iron deficiency in infants.[59] The secondary inflammatory reactions in the gastroduodenum, small intestine, and colon resolve when milk is stopped.[69,70] Meckel's diverticulum may be associated with both gross and occult bleeding in children and young adults.[60]

Crohn's disease and chronic ulcerative colitis can present with occult bleeding alone and together account for about 1% of iron deficiency in adults.[8,61] Occult blood loss with anemia may occur with celiac sprue, Whipple's disease, eosinophilic gastroenteritis, radiation enteritis, and solitary colon ulcer.

Infectious Causes

While occult bleeding may accompany many acute infectious enterocolitides (ch 68, 69, 83, and 103), it may be chronic and lead to iron deficiency from such conditions as gastrointestinal tuberculosis (ch 69), amebiasis (ch 104), and ascariasis (ch 105).

However, the most common infectious cause of chronic occult bleeding and, perhaps, the major single cause for iron deficiency anemia worldwide is hookworm.

HOOKWORM

Several hundred million people are infected with hookworm globally, and the prevalence in children and laborers in some countries

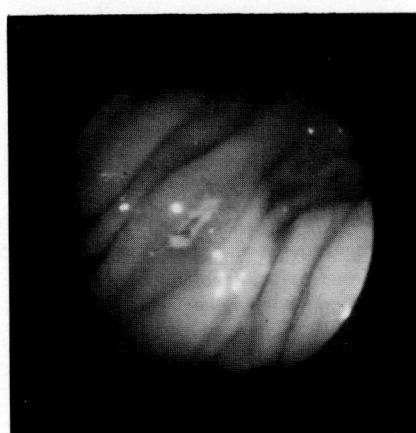

FIGURE 31–1. Cameron erosion. These characteristic longitudinal erosions accompany some large hiatal hernias, are located in the gastric mucosa at the level of the diaphragm, and commonly account for occult bleeding and iron deficiency. (Endophotograph contributed by Dr AJ Cameron, Mayo Clinic, Rochester, MN.)

exceeds 80%.[63] The major, and frequently only, manifestation is iron deficiency, which exacts an enormous socioeconomic toll in lost work productivity throughout the tropics and subtropics. The natural history is well established (ch 105). Daily occult fecal blood loss averages over 12 ml from most hosts, may exceed 100 ml, correlates with the hookworm burden, and drops precipitously following vermifuge.[63]

Vascular Causes

GASTROESOPHAGEAL VARICES

Varices are occasionally incriminated as the source of occult bleeding and have been reported in up to 3% of patients with iron deficiency.[8,67] Little is known about occult bleeding patterns from these lesions. Most patients with varices have normal fecal blood levels, but a few have levels over 100 mg Hb/g.[18] The attendant boggy and friable mucosa in the gastroduodenum, called congestive gastropathy,[71] may be responsible for some of the occult blood loss with portal hypertension.

VASCULAR MALFORMATIONS

Hereditary and acquired vascular malformations (ch 108) are an increasingly recognized source of occult gastrointestinal bleeding. Angiodysplasias are found in 0.4% to 6% of adults with iron deficiency anemia[8,61,64,70] and are common explanations for obscure occult bleeding. In a review of patients with transfusion-dependent anemia from vascular malformations, gastrointestinal bleeding remained occult in 43% of patients with acquired lesions and in 30% of patients with hereditary hemorrhagic telangiectasia.[72] Clinically significant occult bleeding has been described with other vascular lesions, including watermelon stomach,[73,74] postradiation telangiectasias,[75] and those associated with the blue rubber bleb

nevus syndrome,[76] scleroderma,[77] Turner's syndrome,[78] and Klippel–Trenaunay syndrome.[79]

Tumors and Neoplasms

Gastrointestinal tumors are second only to peptic disease as a cause for occult bleeding that leads to iron deficiency in adults in Western countries.[8,61,62,64] Because of the importance of fecal occult blood testing in the detection of colorectal adenocarcinoma and adenomas, these lesions will be discussed in detail below. Colorectal cancer is clearly the most common malignant lesion to cause occult bleeding in Western countries,[8,18,61] followed by primary cancers in the stomach, esophagus, and ampulla.[8,18,61,62,64] In some elderly populations with anemia, gastric cancer has been found at nearly the same frequency as has colorectal cancer.[62,80] Lymphoma, lipomas, leiomyoma, leiomyosarcoma, hamartomas, juvenile polyps, and metastatic lesions to the gut can also produce occult bleeding (see ch 57, 63, 70, 78, 79, 84, 90, and 96).

Drugs

Any ingestant that produces direct or indirect injury to the gastrointestinal tract may potentially cause abnormal occult bleeding. Ethanol may lead to hemorrhagic gastritis at high concentrations.[81] However, following ingestion of small to moderate amounts, ethanol does not appear to cause fecal blood level elevations,[82] and the contribution of social drinking to occult bleeding is probably minor. Anticoagulant use is associated with a higher incidence of positive fecal occult blood test results, but gastrointestinal disease is present in most patients with fecal blood elevations who are on anticoagulants.[83,84] Thus, anticoagulants may unmask bleeding from pre-existing lesions rather than produce bleeding per se. Certain antibiotics, potassium preparations, antimetabolites, and other drugs may cause occult bleeding secondary to caustic effects or epithelial sloughing, but few data are available. It is debatable whether steroids promote occult blood loss. Clearly, aspirin and related nonsteroidal anti-inflammatory drugs (NSAIDs) are responsible for most drug-induced occult gastrointestinal bleeding.

NONSTEROIDAL ANTI-INFLAMMATORY DRUGS

NSAIDs are among the most widely used prescription and nonprescription drugs worldwide. In the United States alone, over 30 billion tablets are consumed annually.[85] Except for acetaminophen and sodium salicylate, all NSAIDs may cause occult blood loss.[85,86] In sufficient quantities, NSAID ingestion may produce focal mucosal hemorrhages, erosions, or ulceration predominantly in the stomach in virtually anyone.[85,86] However, at usual therapeutic doses, some NSAIDs induce more occult bleeding than others.[87] These mucosal findings, often called NSAID gastropathy, result from inhibition of epithelial cyclooxygenase activity and consequent reduction in mucosoprotective prostaglandins.[88] A dose-response relationship exists between the amount of NSAID ingested and the degree of gastric mucosal injury or quantity of fecal blood loss in acute studies.[82,85,89] Approximately 70% of those taking therapeutic amounts of aspirin, two tablets q.i.d., will bleed occultly and average 2 to 5 ml of blood loss daily.[82,85] Individual susceptibility to NSAID injury varies, because some bleed more than 30 ml per day or develop anemia with a similar dose range of aspirin.[85] Of course, a large NSAID-induced ulcer may produce much higher levels of occult or gross fecal blood.

Long-Distance Running

Iron deficiency with or without anemia may develop in long-distance runners and may be associated with suboptimal performance.[90–92] Occult gastrointestinal bleeding appears to be a major cause. Based on quantitative studies,[93] fecal hemoglobin increased following a marathon event in 20 of 24 runners, peaking to an average of nearly 4 mg/g (4 ml blood loss/day) but to over 40 mg/g in some individuals. Furthermore, 8% to 23% of runners have been shown to have guaiac-positive stools after a marathon.[94] Although the mechanism of such occult bleeding is unknown, some have speculated that mesenteric ischemia or repetitive jarring trauma may be responsible. In elite class runners, both gastric and colonic erosions have been identified and have been shown to resolve with periods of running cessation.[95,96] Interestingly, occult bleeding is less likely to occur with other endurance activities, such as swimming or prolonged walking.[97]

Extragastrointestinal and Other Causes

Fecal occult blood levels may be elevated in patients who swallow blood arising from tracheobronchial, dental, otorhinolaryngologic, or factitial sources. Stools sampled from the toilet water may be contaminated if patients have hematuria or menstrual bleeding.[98]

Finally, numerous substances other than blood may react with guaiac and other tests to produce false-positive results (discussed below). This problem of test artifact might be called pseudo-occult bleeding.

CLINICAL MANIFESTATIONS

Occult gastrointestinal bleeding, in most cases, is clinically silent and unsuspected. However, characteristic symptoms and signs of iron deficiency may occur secondary to chronic occult blood loss from any cause. Also, there may be predominant manifestations of the underlying gastrointestinal disease responsible for occult bleeding.

Manifestations of Iron Deficiency

Fatigue, tachycardia, exertional dyspnea, and, when anemia co-exists, pallor are common concomitants of advanced iron defi-

ciency. Other less common but more specific overt sequelae of iron deficiency may be present.

PICA

Various types of pica, or compulsive eating behavior, are associated with iron deficiency, especially in women and children.[99] Pagophagia, or ice eating, is the most frequently recognized form of pica, and afflicted patients may consume up to 9 kg of ice daily.[99,100] Other variants of pica that have been described with iron deficiency include ingestion of soil or clay (geophagia), brittle or crunchy foods (gooberophagia), laundry starch, and chalk.[6,99] Surprisingly, such bizarre behavior resolves with iron repletion in nearly all cases.[99,100] When carefully sought, a mild degree of pica may accompany iron deficiency anemia in nearly 50% of patients.[99]

PHYSICAL FINDINGS

Specific physical findings may result from advanced depletion of tissue iron stores but are now uncommon in the United States. Papilledema, cranial nerve palsies, and retinal hemorrhages rarely occur with severe iron deficiency and resolve with iron repletion.[6] More characteristic are various epithelial abnormalities. Fingernails and toenails may become brittle, longitudinally furrowed, or spooned[101]—changes called koilonychia (Fig 31-2A). Glossitis (Fig 31-2B) may occur with erythema and loss of lingual papillae.[102] Scaling or fissuring of the lips, called cheilitis, and atrophic rhinitis may also result from iron deficiency.[103]

The association of postcricoid esophageal webs with iron deficiency has long been recognized as the Paterson-Kelly syndrome or the Plummer-Vinson syndrome.[104,105] These webs are eccentric, sometimes multiple, and are located in the proximal esophagus (Fig 31-2C). They are more common in women and may cause dysphagia. Although not pathognomonic for iron deficiency, these webs are more prevalent in patients with iron deficiency, often attended by other epithelial sequelae such as glossitis or achlorhydria, and may respond to iron therapy.[6,102,106] The premalignant potential of this lesion is controversial.[107]

Manifestations of Underlying Disease

In patients with occult gastrointestinal bleeding, clinical features of the underlying disease may be present and serve as clues to identification of the bleeding source. Just as the potential causes of occult bleeding are legion, so too are the possible symptoms and signs of these disorders. Cutaneous lesions associated with gastrointestinal disease are described in Chapter 44. Manifestations of specific etiologic disorders are covered in other chapters.

ASSESSMENT AND DIAGNOSTIC STRATEGIES

Occult gastrointestinal bleeding may be evidenced either indirectly by laboratory confirmation of iron deficiency or directly by mea-

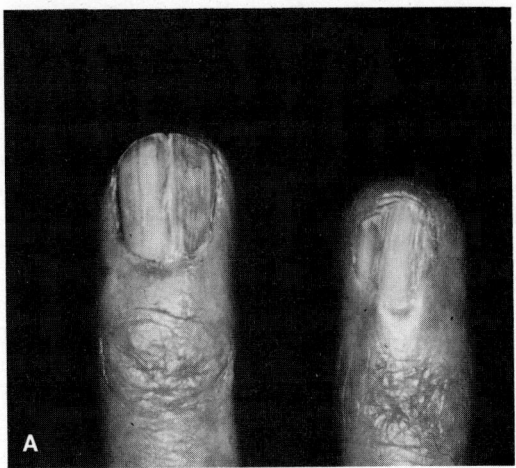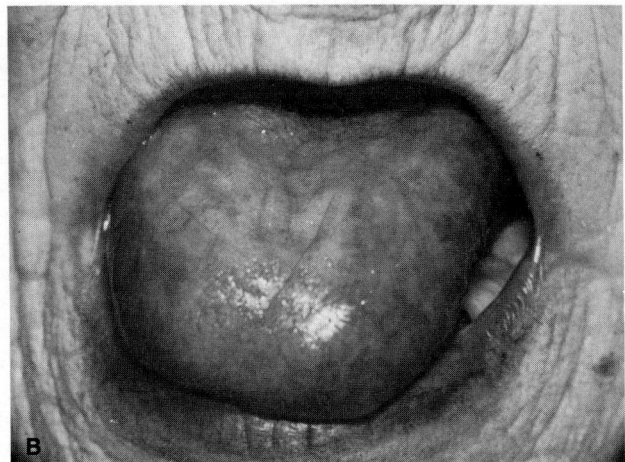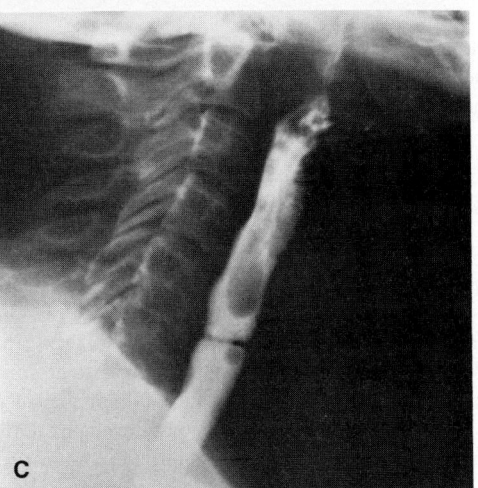

FIGURE 31–2. Epithelial changes associated with chronic iron deficiency include **A,** koilonychia; **B,** glossitis; and **C,** proximal esophageal webs.

surement of fecal blood. Neither approach is infallible, and they should be viewed as complementary. Iron deficiency would not be present if enteric blood loss were quantitatively minor or of inadequate duration. Fecal blood test results may be negative because of intermittent bleeding or because of deficiencies in the chemical performance of the tests themselves. Thus, it is important to appreciate the strengths and limitations of laboratory techniques used to establish occult bleeding. The subsequent gastrointestinal evaluation should be tailored to the clinical setting.

Tests for Iron Deficiency

The gold standard for iron deficiency is the absence of bone marrow hemosiderin by Prussian blue staining. However, bone marrow analysis is seldom required to document iron deficiency.

HEMATOLOGIC ASSESSMENT

Although hypochromic microcytic anemia is often the first clue to the presence of iron deficiency, it is a relatively late-stage manifestation of iron deficiency.[6] Hypochromic microcytic anemia may be determined by peripheral smear microscopy or by automated calculations revealing depressed mean corpuscular hemoglobin concentration and mean corpuscular volume. Anisocytosis, or variability in cell size, is also common with iron deficiency anemia and is reflected by elevation of another red cell index, called the red cell distribution width. Unfortunately, this characteristic profile on red cell indices appears to be present in only 50% to 70% of patients with iron deficiency anemia.[108] Furthermore, these red cell morphologic abnormalities are not specific for iron deficiency and may all occur with the anemia of chronic illness, thalassemia, and sideroblastic anemia.[6,108,109] Thus, the status of iron stores must also be evaluated to determine the etiology of hypochromic microcytic anemia.

CHEMICAL TESTS

Unlike iron deficiency, other causes of hypochromic microcytic anemia are associated with normal or increased tissue iron stores.[6,109] Although typically decreased with iron deficiency, serum iron levels and transferrin saturation correlate rather poorly with marrow iron stores, are influenced by many medical conditions, and therefore are suboptimal markers for iron deficiency.[6,108,109] Serum iron and transferrin saturation are also commonly low with the anemia of chronic illness, which is the most troublesome differential diagnosis.[6,108,109] In contrast, serum ferritin levels correlate well with tissue iron stores and better differentiate iron deficiency anemia from other anemias.[6,109] Serum ferritin levels often fall well before anemia develops. A low serum ferritin is pathognomonic for iron deficiency. However, inflammatory conditions, malignancy, and renal insufficiency can mildly elevate the serum ferritin and uncommonly cause a falsely normal serum level in the face of absent marrow iron stores.[6,108,109] Thus, iron deficiency anemia may occasionally present with normal serum ferritin levels, and a bone marrow study would be indicated if there were any question.

Fecal Blood Testing

A plethora of tests for the detection of fecal occult blood are commercially available, but there are four basic approaches, each with advantages and disadvantages.

GUAIAC (LEUCO-DYE) TESTS

Guaiac preparations have long been available to detect blood and remain the most widely used type of fecal blood test. Guaiac was first employed by Van Deen in 1864 to indicate fecal blood[110] and by Boas in 1901 as a means of detecting gastrointestinal malignancies.[111] However, the familiar guaiac-impregnated pad tests for colorectal cancer screening were not developed until 1967.[112]

Guaiac, a type of leuco-dye, is an impure, colorless compound that becomes colored in the presence of adequate concentrations of peroxidaselike substances, such as hemoglobin and hydrogen peroxide. Other leuco-dyes, such as benzidine, O-toluidine, and leuco-malachite green, have been used for occult blood detection. Unfortunately, this color reaction is not specific for blood. All leuco-dyes may react with nonhemoglobin peroxidases or with nonspecific oxidants in stool.

Currently marketed tests that are based on guaiac or other leuco-dyes include Hemoccult (SmithKline Diagnostics, Sunnyvale, CA), the most commonly used of these tests; HemoFec (Boehringer Mannheim, Mannheim, West Germany); Coloscreen (Helena Laboratories, Beaumont, TX); Colo-Rect (Roche Diagnostics, Nutley, NJ); Hema-Check (Miles Laboratories, Elkhart, IN); Quick-Cult (Laboratory Diagnostics, Morganville, NJ); Haemo-Screen (E. Merck Diagnostics, Darmstadt, West Germany); Early Detector (Warner-Lambert, Morris Plains, NJ); Seracult (Propper Manufacturing, Long Island, NY); and several new over-the-counter products. These leuco-dye pad tests are elegantly simple, inexpensive, highly portable, and require no sophisticated laboratory equipment. While most may be done at the bedside, one approach (EZ Detect, NMF Pharmaceuticals, Los Angeles, CA) employs a leuco-dye indicator placed into the toilet water.

The unpredictable reactivity of these qualitative tests confounds their clinical interpretation. There is no consistent fecal hemoglobin level above which guaiac tests become positive and below which they remain negative.[13,112–116] Guaiac tests may be positive in stools

with less than 1 mg hemoglobin/g[13] or remain negative in those with over 80 mg/g.[117] Fecal hemoglobin levels must exceed 10 mg/g (10 ml daily blood loss) before Hemoccult is positive at least half the time.[113–115]

Fecal hydration strongly influences guaiac reactivity. It is well known that Hemoccult sensitivity can be enhanced by wetting the fecal smear prior to addition of the peroxide catalyst.[118] Positive reactions can be induced in stools that are initially Hemoccult-negative simply by progressive aqueous dilution, even in stools with normal hemoglobin levels.[13] Most important, the native water content or consistency of individual stools varies widely and contributes significantly to variable Hemoccult reactivity (Fig 31-3). Wetter stools are more likely to be positive than are drier stools.[13,18]

Another major explanation for variability in guaiac test reactivity is the degradation by fecal flora of heme to porphyrin, which no longer possesses peroxidaselike activity. Enterocolic heme degradation accounts for the relative insensitivity of guaiac tests for occult bleeding arising from the right colon and more proximal gut[18,33,119] and for the inability of Hemoccult to detect fecal heme after ingestion of 15 to 30 ml of blood per day.[24,120] Conversion of heme to porphyrin continues during fecal storage and causes a corresponding fall in Hemoccult positivity.[13,121] This time-dependent heme degradation diminishes the validity of guaiac tests applied to mail-in stools. Thus, leuco-dye tests, which require intact heme for chemical detection, tend to underestimate enteric blood loss, especially with bleeding from proximal lesions or with stored specimens.

Several factors besides wet stools can produce chemical false-positive reactions. Certain fruits and vegetables have peroxidaselike activity, including radishes, turnips, cantaloupe, bean sprouts, cauliflower, broccoli, and grapes, and their removal from the diet reduces the rate of Hemoccult false-positives.[122,123] While some studies have shown that the rate of Hemoccult positivity may approach 60% following ingestion of therapeutic doses of iron,[124] others have observed much lower rates.[125] Other factors reported to cause a color reaction include cimetidine,[126] halogens,[127] and toilet bowl sanitizers.[128] Conversely, several substances or con-

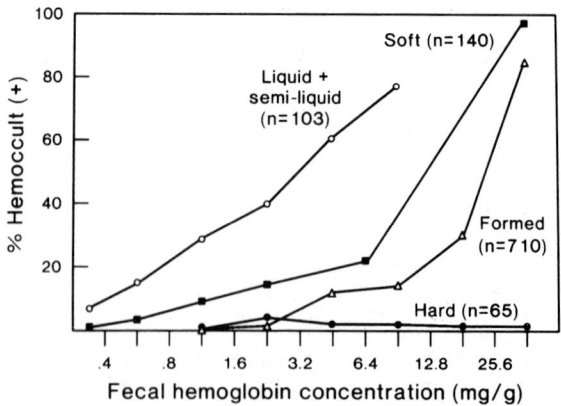

FIGURE 31–3. Effect of fecal hemoglobin concentration and stool consistency (native hydration) on guaiac test (Hemoccult) reactivity. The HemoQuant assay was used to quantify hemoglobin concentrations; its upper limit of normal is 2 mg/g. (Reproduced with permission from Ahlquist DA, McGill DB, Schwartz S. HemoQuant, a new quantitative assay for fecal hemoglobin, comparison with Hemoccult. Ann Intern Med 1984;101: 299.)

ditions may inhibit guaiac reactivity, in addition to dry stools and heme degradation, and produce false-negative reactions, including reducing substances such as ascorbic acid,[129] antacids,[130] heat, an acid *p*H, and defective reagents.[131]

Maneuvers to increase guaiac sensitivity, such as hydrating the smeared fecal aliquot prior to testing, often succeed at the expense of specificity.[118] Sensitivity can be enhanced without compromising specificity by first purifying fecal hemoglobin with the use of solvent extraction[132] or electrostatic filtration.[133] However, sensitivity cannot be restored if heme degradation to porphyrin has occurred.

IMMUNOCHEMICAL TESTS

Immunochemical detection of fecal blood has been studied for over a decade.[35,134–137] Antihemoglobin or antialbumin antibodies, used in these assays, do not react with nonhuman blood, diet peroxidases, or medications. Thus, they represent an advance in specificity over guaiac tests. A distinct practical advantage of immunochemical tests is the obviation of burdensome dietary preparations. Simple and relatively inexpensive smear punch-disc immunodiffusion techniques have been incorporated into commercially available tests, including HemeSelect (SmithKline Diagnostics, Sunnyvale, CA) and FECA-EIA (Lab Systems, Helsinki, Finland).

Metabolism of globin during enterocolic transit or storage compromises the immunologic measurement of fecal blood. Immunochemical tests may detect as little as 0.3 mg of blood added to a stool[134] but fail to detect fecal hemoglobin following ingestion of 20[35] to 100 ml[27] of blood. It is not surprising that immunochemical tests are much less likely to detect bleeding from proximal gut lesions than from distal lesions.[35] Some immunochemical approaches have been complicated by nonspecific positive reactions from certain fecal constituents,[134] and in some clinical studies false-positive rates have exceeded those of guaiac tests.[138] Thus, like guaiac tests, immunochemical tests are qualitative, variably sensitive, and influenced by the anatomic site of bleeding and by storage.

HEME-PORPHYRIN (HEMOQUANT) ASSAY

Quantitation of fecal blood levels provides the clinician with meaningful diagnostic information, because the predictive value of fecal blood elevation depends on the degree of elevation (Fig 31-4). A recently described assay,[13,24] called HemoQuant (Mayo Medical Laboratories, Rochester, MN; SmithKline BioSciences, Van Nuys, CA; Nichols Laboratory, Los Angeles, CA), offers certain advantages over other occult blood tests. It is quantitative, noninvasive, specific for heme, chemically sensitive, and suitable for automation. HemoQuant is based on the fluorimetric assay of heme and heme-derived porphyrin. Unlike guaiac and immunochemical tests, the HemoQuant test includes that important fraction of heme already degraded to porphyrin during fecal storage[18] or enterocolic transit.[13,18,24,33] Because of this feature, sensitivity for proximal gastrointestinal bleeding is higher with HemoQuant than with guaiac and immunochemical tests. HemoQuant may be affected by red meat but not by other dietary peroxidases, medications, or fecal contaminants.[13,18,24,25]

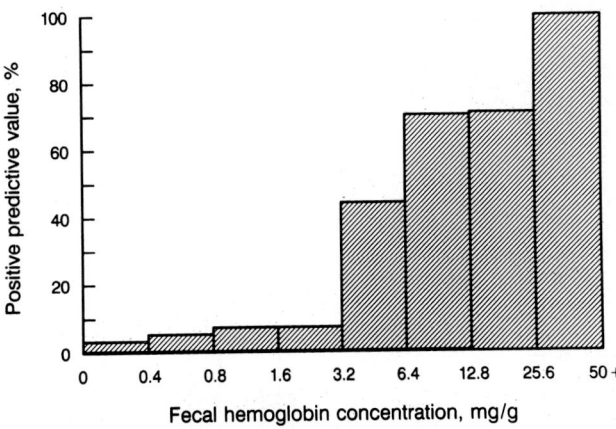

CG-12307ZX-4

FIGURE 31–4. Positive predictive value for hemorrhagic gastrointestinal lesions of fecal hemoglobin at varying concentrations. Based on data from 1000 patients tested by the HemoQuant assay prior to gastrointestinal studies. Hemorrhagic lesions included ulcers or erosions, vascular malformations, and malignancies.

HemoQuant results are calculated as hemoglobin-equivalents and reported as mg hemoglobin/g stool. Fecal hemoglobin concentrations from 0.01 to 500 mg/g are accurately measured without preliminary concentration or dilution of the specimens.[13,24] Values below 2 mg/g are considered normal.[18,19] HemoQuant has been validated by a greater than 99% recovery of blood added directly to stools,[13] by an 88% recovery of ingested blood,[24,25] and by a close correlation with other quantitative assays.[24] Because HemoQuant is currently performed for commercial use in a reference laboratory only, the inevitable 2- to 4-day delay in results is a distinct disincentive for many clinicians.

Because it quantifies fecal blood, HemoQuant has proved to be a useful research tool in studying patterns of occult gastrointestinal bleeding in health and disease (Fig 31-5).

RADIOLABELED ERYTHROCYTE TECHNIQUE

Fecal recovery of intravenously injected ^{51}Cr-labeled erythrocytes has been the accepted standard for quantifying enteric blood loss for over three decades.[14–17] Once chromium enters the gut lumen, its reabsorption is negligible, and therefore it has proved to be a valid quantitative marker for gastrointestinal bleeding. However, some have questioned its accuracy at very low levels of bleeding due to biliary excretion of free chromium.[139,140] The test is expensive, requires at least 3 full days of whole stool collections, and is obviously impractical for large-volume routine use. Slow enterocolic transit may cause falsely low results.[141]

SPECIMEN COLLECTION AND SAMPLING

Accurate fecal blood testing requires careful control of each step of the testing process. The technique to mobilize the stool for sampling has usually been ignored in commercial test kit instructions. A recent survey indicated that most patients sample their

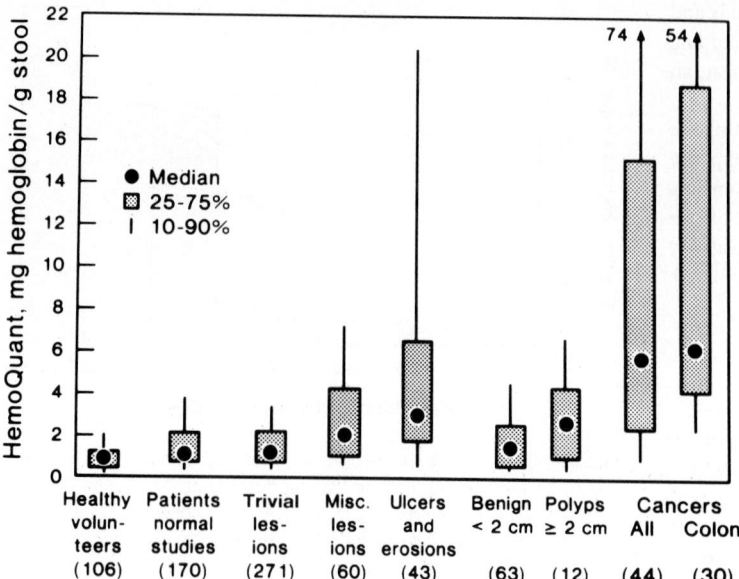

FIGURE 31–5. Fecal blood distribution in healthy volunteers and patients undergoing gastrointestinal evaluations. Data are based on a single HemoQuant measurement per subject. Minor lesions include diverticula, hemorrhoids, and small diaphragmatic hernias. Miscellaneous (Misc) lesions include large diaphragmatic hernias, varices, and vascular malformations. Reprinted with permission (From Ahlquist DA, McGill DB, Schwartz S. Fecal blood levels in health and disease—A study using HemoQuant. Reproduced by permission of The New England Journal of Medicine. 1985;312:422.)

stool specimen from within the toilet water.[128] Such a practice introduces potential measurement error due to leaching of blood from the stool into the toilet water[128] or to contamination by menstrual or urinary blood,[98] ascorbic acid and other urinary reducing substances,[127,129] and toilet bowl sanitizers.[128] Use of a disposal collection device prior to sampling may prevent these artifacts.[128]

Blood is nonuniformly distributed within the fecal specimen,[142] especially with bleeding from distal colorectal lesions (unpublished personal data). Testing of multiple aliquots or multiple stools will partially compensate for this nonuniformity.[19,143] The convention of testing two aliquots per stool to reduce sampling error, as originally suggested by Greegor,[112] has persisted in most testing programs.

Guaiac-based tests for the detection of blood in the toilet water or on stool wiped from the perineum after evacuation have been marketed to enhance patient compliance, but few published data are available. There is also a dearth of information on the value of the time-honored technique of guaiac testing stool obtained from a digital exam. One prospective study[144] showed that guaiac pad tests were more sensitive for colorectal cancer when performed by experienced technicians on stools sent to the laboratory than when performed by physicians on digital smears at the bedside.

TEST SELECTION

No single fecal blood test is appropriate for all applications. Until definitive comparative data are published, test selection should be guided by judicious consideration of test performance characteristics, availability, and cost (Table 31-3) relative to the clinical indication. For example, a simple, inexpensive, qualitative test may be preferred for large population screening. Immunochemical tests offer theoretic advantages for colorectal cancer screening because they are not affected by proximal gut bleeding and dietary preparations are unnecessary. In contrast, when evaluating iron deficiency or anemia, the heme-porphyrin assay may provide the

most useful information because it accurately quantifies luminal blood loss irrespective of the anatomic source. The radiolabeled erythrocyte technique yields the same quantitative information but is time-consuming, much more expensive, and logistically burdensome. Guaiac and immunochemical tests would appear less suitable because they are qualitative and insensitive for upper gastrointestinal bleeding. Future studies should be instructive in directing the clinical application of these and other newer approaches.

Patient Evaluation

In practice, abnormal occult gastrointestinal bleeding comes to the attention of clinicians when a positive fecal blood test result surfaces in patients undergoing colorectal cancer screening, when iron deficiency anemia is encountered, and, less commonly, when fecal blood tests are applied to investigate those presenting with gastrointestinal symptoms. The consequent diagnostic strategy should be individually tailored, but some general guidelines merit consideration.

ABNORMAL FECAL BLOOD TEST RESULTS IN AN ASYMPTOMATIC PATIENT WITHOUT ANEMIA

At present, this common situation occurs almost exclusively as the result of colorectal cancer screening, because there are very few other reasons to routinely check fecal occult blood levels. The major responsibility is to exclude colorectal cancer, although this finding can be expected in only 2% to 10% of cases overall.[1–5] Most agree that colonoscopy provides the most sensitive and specific approach to visualize the colorectum,[4,5,64,145,146] and some

TABLE 31–3
Comparative Features of Fecal Occult Blood Tests

	GUAIAC (LEUCO-DYE) TESTS	IMMUNOASSAYS	HEME-PORPHYRIN ASSAY	^{51}Cr-LABELED ERYTHROCYTE ASSAY
Quantitative	No	No	Yes	Yes
Chemical False-Positives				
Diet peroxidases	Yes	No	No	No
Animal Hb	Yes	No	Yes	No
Halogens	Yes	No	No	No
Toilet Sanitizers	Yes	No	No	No
Iron	Yes (?)	No	No	No
Wet stools	Yes	No	No	No
Chemical False-Negatives				
Ascorbic acid	Yes	No	No	No
Enterocolic Hb metabolism	Yes	Yes	No	No
Fecal storage	Yes	Yes	No	No
Dry stools	Yes	No	No	No
Sensitivity for Bleeding				
Upper GI source	Poor	Very poor	Good	Good
Proximal colon	Fair	Fair	Good	Good
Distal colon and rectum	Good	Good	Good	Good
Laboratory Required	No	Yes (small)	Yes	Yes
Assay time	5 min	1–24 hr	1 hr	≥72 hr
Cost to patient*	$5–7	$15–20	$20	$150–300

* Based on 1990 estimates

would argue that it is also the most cost-effective strategy.[146] However, the combination of double-contrast barium x-ray and proctosigmoidoscopy probably provides nearly the same sensitivity for cancer.[146] Because of technical limitations of both colonoscopy and colon x-ray, the two procedures are often complementary. Various mathematical models have been developed to optimize the cost-effectiveness of such a colorectal workup.[145,146]

Because of the relatively low point prevalence in most Western countries of malignancies proximal to the colon, physicians could justifiably stop their evaluation after colon studies in the absence of symptoms or anemia and repeat fecal blood testing in 6 to 12 months. However, a good case could be made for additionally checking a serum ferritin level, because this is inexpensive, introduces essentially no morbidity, and may indicate more significant chronic blood loss from an indolent proximal gastrointestinal lesion. If the ferritin were low, esophagogastroduodenoscopy would be the preferred next step, because the miss rate of barium x-ray of the stomach for peptic and other lesions is so high (see ch 61 and 111). If this were negative, a small-intestine x-ray would be appropriate. And if all gastrointestinal studies are nonrevealing, close hematologic follow-up would be in order. Finally, in populations with a high prevalence of gastric or esophageal cancer, it may be prudent to routinely extend the evaluation of an abnormal fecal blood test to the upper gut if colorectal studies are negative.

OCCULT BLEEDING IN THE ANEMIC PATIENT

Unless menorrhagia, chronic gross hematuria, or another source of extraintestinal blood loss is clinically apparent, most patients with iron deficiency anemia should undergo an aggressive gastrointestinal evaluation. Because a gastrointestinal lesion will be found in 66% to 97% of men and postmenopausal women with iron deficiency anemia,[8,61,62,64] it could be argued that fecal blood testing would be superfluous in these patients and that gastrointestinal studies should be done regardless of fecal blood test results. However, nutritional inadequacies, iron malabsorption, or extraintestinal bleeding may be contributing etiologic factors in some patient groups with iron deficiency anemia. As such, fecal blood testing would be indicated in those groups, including children, postgastrectomy patients, menstruating women, those with achlorhydria, the elderly, immigrants from underdeveloped countries, vegetarians, and patients with steatorrhea.

A practical schema for evaluating adults with iron deficiency anemia and occult gastrointestinal bleeding is shown in Figure 31-6. The large majority of lesions causing occult bleeding in anemic patients are demonstrated by routine endoscopic and radiographic procedures. Because further studies for more obscure bleeding sources are invasive, expensive, less revealing of lesions,

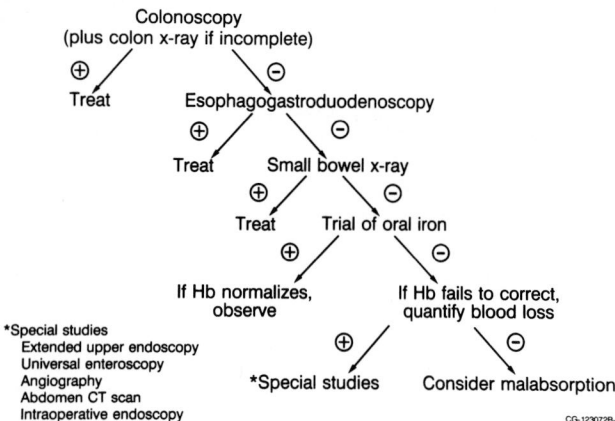

FIGURE 31–6. Diagnostic schema for adult patients with iron deficiency anemia and occult gastrointestinal bleeding.

and associated with more morbidity, it is often justifiable to observe a response to iron therapy and reconfirm fecal blood loss prior to embarking on these further studies. In patients who fail to respond to iron therapy and have continued enteric blood loss, special studies that may prove helpful include extended upper endoscopy,[147] universal enteroscopy,[148] angiography (ch 122), abdominal CT scan (ch 118), which may reveal intra-abdominal malignant disease or pancreaticobiliary pathology, or, in rare situations, surgical exploration and intra-operative endoscopy.[149] Radioisotope blood loss scans have no role in the evaluation of occult bleeding. Vascular malformations probably account for the majority of obscure causes of occult bleeding.[150]

OCCULT BLEEDING IN THE PATIENT WITH GASTROINTESTINAL SYMPTOMS

The sequence of diagnostic testing should be initially directed to the anatomic level from which the symptoms appear to arise. Some have suggested that a positive fecal blood test increases the likelihood that vague gastrointestinal symptoms are due to organic rather than functional disease.[151] Thus, clinical judgment is required to determine the extent of evaluation in such instances.

SCREENING FOR COLORECTAL NEOPLASIA

Fecal blood testing for the early detection of colorectal cancer is very widely practiced in Western countries.[152] In a multicenter North American survey, over 40% of nearly 11,000 respondents over the age of 50 years indicated that they had undergone fecal blood testing at least once prior to the study (unpublished personal data). Yet fecal blood screening is based not on established efficacy but on the assumptions that asymptomatic colorectal cancers bleed, that available tests will detect this bleeding, and that such detection will eventuate in reduced cancer mortality in the population screened. This section will deal only with fecal blood testing and

not with other approaches to the detection of colorectal neoplasia (see ch 78, 79, 84, 112, and 114).

Occult Bleeding Patterns of Colorectal Neoplasms

Fecal blood levels vary widely in patients with colorectal cancer, based on quantitative studies, and range from normal to markedly elevated.[18,19,113,118,142,153] Occult bleeding increases with surface ulceration[18,154] and with the size of colorectal neoplasms.[18,155,156] Of concern from a screening standpoint, fecal occult blood levels may be lower in patients with early-stage disease and asymptomatic disease compared with those with advanced-stage and symptomatic cancer.[156] Longitudinal observations in asymptomatic patients with colorectal cancer have shown that fecal blood levels are often below the detection threshold of guaiac tests and commonly within the normal range of quantitative tests (Fig 31-7).

Very little is known about the natural bleeding history of colorectal adenomas. It is well established that large polyps may bleed either occultly or grossly. Some reports of polyp bleeding rates have been based on patients who either presented with bleeding or had large polyps,[119] and such findings cannot be extrapolated to the general population. The fact that patients with small adenomas bleed more than those without adenomas is highly questionable. Most studies that have quantified bleeding from adenomas smaller than 2 cm have shown the distributions of fecal blood levels to be comparable to those in patients without adenomas.[18,118,153] Furthermore, only 3% to 4% of patients with endoscopically proven polyps were guaiac-positive in one prospective study,[157] a positivity rate no different from that of the general

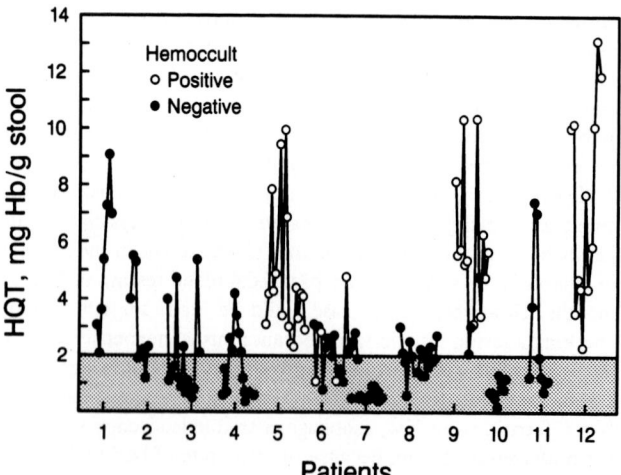

FIGURE 31–7. Occult blood levels in stools collected for 2 weeks from 12 patients with asymptomatic primary colorectal adenocarcinoma as determined by HemoQuant (HQT) and Hemoccult. The shaded zone below a HemoQuant level of 2 mg Hb/g stool represents the conventional normal range. (Reprinted with permission from Ahlquist DA, McGill DB, Fleming JL. Patterns of occult bleeding in asymptomatic colorectal cancer. Cancer 1989;63:1826.)

population. Guaiac positivity in screening trials has often been attributed to the finding of adenomas, despite the fact that most of those polyps have been diminutive and thus unlikely to bleed. Fecal blood appears to be a poor marker for adenomas, especially small ones.

Test Performance

VALIDITY

Validity is a function that combines sensitivity, specificity, and predictive value. The validity of a test must be high if the test is to perform effectively in the screening setting. Test validity varies with the techniques used and population studied. Sensitivity, or the detection rate, has ranged in patients with symptomatic colorectal cancer from 40% to 67% with guaiac,[18,135,152,155] from 85% to over 90% with immunochemical tests,[136,155] and from 56% to 97% with the heme-porphyrin test applied to a single stool.[18,156] Test sensitivity appears to be lower with asymptomatic colorectal cancers.[19] Multiple stool testing improves sensitivity.[19,143] In most prospective comparison studies, heme-porphyrin[18,19] and immunochemical tests[135,136,138] have proved more sensitive than guaiac in detecting colorectal cancer; however, few studies have compared sensitivity at matched specificity. Specificity, the rate of negative test results in those without cancer, has ranged from 90% to 98% with various test programs,[1–5,152] which translates to false-positive rates from 2% to 10%. Finally, the positive predictive value, or the probability that a positive test result will yield a colorectal cancer, is highly dependent on the cancer prevalence in the screened population. Population-based studies have, to date, been conducted primarily with guaiac, and positive predictive values have ranged from 2% to 18%.[1–5,152] Nevertheless, most causes of fecal blood elevation, however measured, are due to benign or trivial pathology.

COMPLIANCE

Screening effectiveness requires not only a high test validity but also a compliant patient population. Compliance rates have been as low as 19% in general populations to as high as 97% in carefully instructed outpatients using a stool collection device, but reported compliance rates generally average from 30% to 60% in population-based screening programs.[152] Compliance varies with socioeconomic and demographic factors and is highest when there has been an educational effort or a physician encounter.[158–160] Physician compliance in screening programs also varies.[152]

EFFECTIVENESS AND COST

Many uncontrolled studies have demonstrated that fecal blood screening will detect colorectal cancers at earlier than expected stages.[152] However, none of the ongoing controlled trials, some running for nearly 15 years, has yet demonstrated a significant reduction in mortality as a result of fecal blood screening.[1–5] Thus, the efficacy of this massive effort remains unproved. Several statistical models based on test performance assumptions have been developed to assess cost-effectiveness of screening.[152]

Some have argued that it is premature to evaluate cost-effectiveness until efficacy is established.[161] However, the cost of such screening is enormous.[162] The low unit price of a fecal blood test belies the true cost of screening. Because of the very expensive diagnostic studies done on the many patients with false-positive results, the total cost of fecal blood screening may approach that of performing a colon x-ray on all persons screened.[163]

Efficacy of cancer mortality reduction is largely dependent on test sensitivity, while screening cost is more a function of test specificity. Unfortunately, an increase in sensitivity usually results in a decreased specificity, and vice versa. Thus, maximal cost-effectiveness would be achieved by optimally balancing these test features.

Guidelines

HIGH-RISK PATIENTS

Patients with a strong family history of colorectal cancer, with chronic ulcerative colitis, with adenomatous polyposis, with a previous colorectal cancer, or with other criteria of high risk for colorectal cancer would be best served by having periodic structural studies such as colonoscopy or colon x-ray (see ch 84). Fecal blood screening is probably inappropriate in this group.

AVERAGE-RISK PATIENTS

Because sporadic colorectal cancer is so prevalent in Western countries, its incidence increases sharply after age 50, and its early detection confers a favorable prognosis, the American Cancer Society and National Cancer Institute currently recommend annual fecal blood testing in persons age 50 or older. No specific approach to fecal blood testing is advocated in these recommendations. The Preventive Task Forces in Canada and the United States, however, caution that these recommendations are based on expert opinion rather than established efficacy.[164] Thus, the controversy continues.

Most agree that population-based screening with fecal blood testing is not yet appropriate. However, in the absence of better surveillance measures, many physicians understandably use fecal blood tests for the case detection of colorectal cancer in their own patients. If fecal blood testing is to be practiced for cancer detection, clinicians should be aware of test limitations, understand the common causes of occult gastrointestinal bleeding, and follow a rational strategy in evaluating patients with elevated test results.

THERAPEUTIC CONSIDERATIONS

Treatment of abnormal occult gastrointestinal bleeding is dictated by the clinical setting. As above, the first step in management of newly discovered occult bleeding is to exclude a serious underlying lesion. In screen test–positive patients found to have normal structural colorectal studies, it is often appropriate to simply observe if iron stores are replete. However, if concomitant iron deficiency exists, then an aggressive search for the gastrointestinal bleeding source is warranted. Medical or extirpative therapy of the lesion may not only prevent lesion-specific morbidity or mortality but also definitively stop further iron loss. Whether the bleeding source is correctable or not, a cornerstone to treatment is the replenishment of iron stores. Some patients with chronically bleeding lesions, such as radiation enteritis or Cameron erosions,[68,75] may be appropriately managed with long-term iron replacement alone, because satisfactory medical cures are lacking and surgical approaches may be associated with unwanted morbidity. Uncommonly, blood transfusions are indicated initially in those with severe anemia and cardiovascular compromise.

Iron Therapy

Oral iron therapy with ferrous sulfate tablets is the preferred approach in the large majority with iron deficiency because it is cheap, effective, and usually well tolerated. More expensive oral preparations have included ferrous fumarate, ferrous gluconate, and those with added ascorbic acid or other absorption enhancers, but these preparations appear to offer no special advantages.[6] Dietary iron replacement is usually inefficient and unpractical. For example, it has been calculated that a daily consumption of 5 kg of red meat, the best dietary source, would be required to provide 60 mg of iron,[109] which is the amount contained in one 300-mg tablet of ferrous sulfate. An optimal adult dose of ferrous sulfate is 300 mg three times daily, because absorption is not appreciably increased with higher doses.[6] Although repletion of iron stores typically requires 3 to 6 months of oral therapy, a peak in reticulocytosis occurs after 7 to 10 days, epithelial abnormalities may resolve within weeks, and hemoglobin usually normalizes by 2 months.[6] Side effects from oral iron occur in 10% to 20% of patients, appear to be dose-related, are similar for the different preparations, and result in discontinuation of therapy in about 8%.[6,165,166] In a large prospective study,[165] side effects most commonly reported included constipation in 13%, diarrhea in 6%, heartburn or epigastric pain in 5%, and nausea in 4%.

Parenteral iron is indicated in patients who malabsorb or do not tolerate oral iron. It should be emphasized that oral iron is equally efficient in correcting iron deficiency anemia[166] and is safer in most cases. Because parenterally administered iron salts are toxic, iron must be injected in a complex. An iron dextran is available in the United States at a concentration containing 50 mg elemental iron per ml. A maximum daily dose of 5 ml can be given intramuscularly and 2 ml intravenously.

The number of injections required is determined by estimated total iron deficits but may average 7 to 10.[6] The iron dextran complex is taken up by reticuloendothelial tissues and slowly converted to bioavailable iron. Idiosyncratic reactions rarely occur, although cases of fatal anaphylaxis following either intramuscular or intravenous iron dextran have been reported.[6] About 10% of patients develop a serum sickness–like illness with fever, myalgias, arthralgias, lymphadenopathy, and urticaria.[6]

Because so many gastrointestinal disorders can present as, or be accompanied by, occult bleeding, most of the chapters in Parts II, III, and IV are pertinent to this chapter. Particularly important chapters for additional reading are Chapter 20, Vitamins and Minerals; Chapter 21, General Nutritional Principles; Chapter 28, Approach to the Patient with Dysphagia; Chapter 30, Approach to the Patient with Gross Gastrointestinal Bleeding; Chapter 38, Approach to the Patient with Diarrhea; Chapter 44, Skin Lesions Associated with Gastrointestinal Diseases; Chapter 48, Approach to the Patient Requiring Nutritional Supplementation; Chapter 53, Esophagus: Anatomy and Structural Anomalies; Chapter 55, Reflux Esophagitis; Chapter 57, Esophageal Tumors; Chapter 59, Stomach: Anatomy and Structural Anomalies; Chapter 61, Acid-Peptic Disorders; Chapter 62, Zollinger–Ellison Syndrome; Chapter 63, Tumors of the Stomach; Chapter 64, Surgery for Peptic Ulcer Disease; Chapter 68, Small Intestine: Infections with Common Bacterial and Viral Pathogens; Chapter 69, Chronic Infections of the Small Intestine; Chapter 70, Tumors and Other Neoplastic Diseases of the Small Intestine; Chapter 71, Celiac Disease; Chapter 72, Specific Mucosal Protein Deficiency States; Chapter 73, Bacterial Overgrowth; Chapter 74, Short Bowel Syndrome; Chapter 75, Miscellaneous Diseases of the Small Intestine; Chapter 77, Inflammatory Bowel Disease; Chapter 78, Colonic Polyps: Benign and Premalignant Neoplasms of the Colon; Chapter 79, Polyposis Syndromes; Chapter 82, Diverticulitis; Chapter 83, Bacterial Infections of the Colon; Chapter 84, Malignant Tumors of the Colon; Chapter 85, Anorectal Diseases; Chapter 86, Miscellaneous Inflammatory and Structural Disorders of the Colon; Chapter 104, Parasitic Diseases: Protozoa; Chapter 105, Parasitic Diseases: Helminths; Chapter 107, Gastrointestinal Manifestations of Immunologic Disorders; Chapter 108, Vascular Ectasias, Tumors, and Malformations; Chapter 109, Vascular Insufficiency; Chapter 110, General Considerations; Chapter 111, Upper Gastrointestinal Endoscopy; Chapter 112, Colonoscopy and Flexible Sigmoidoscopy; Chapter 113, Endoscopic Retrograde Cholangiopancreatography, Endoscopic Sphincterotomy and Stone Removal, Endoscopic Biliary and Pancreatic Drainage; Chapter 114, Contrast Radiology; Chapter 115, Cross-Sectional Anatomy; Chapter 116, Ultrasound; Chapter 117, Endoscopic Ultrasound; Chapter 118, Applications of Computed Tomography to the Gastrointestinal Tract; Chapter 119, Magnetic Resonance Imaging; Chapter 120, Positron Emission Tomography; Chapter 121, Gastrointestinal Radionuclide Imaging Procedures; Chapter 122, Angiography; and Chapter 123, Interventional Radiology.

REFERENCES

1. Kewenter J, Bjork S, Haglind E, et al. Screening and rescreening for colorectal cancer, a controlled trial of fecal occult blood testing in 27,700 subjects. Cancer 1988;62:645.
2. Hardcastle JD, Chamberlain J, Sheffield J, et al. Randomized, controlled trial of faecal occult blood screening for colorectal cancer. Lancet 1989;1:1160.
3. Kronborg O, Fenger C, Sondergaard K, et al. Initial mass screening for colorectal cancer with fecal occult blood test: A prospective randomized study at Funen in Denmark. Scand J Gastroenterol 1987;22:677.
4. Gilbertsen VA, McHugh R, Schuman LM, et al. The earlier detection of colorectal cancers: A preliminary report of the results of the Occult Blood Study. Cancer 1980;45:2899.
5. Winawer SJ, Andrews M, Miller CH, et al. Review of screening for colorectal cancer using fecal occult blood testing. In: Winawer SJ,

Schottenfeld D, Sherlock P, eds. Colorectal cancer: Prevention, epidemiology, and screening. New York: Raven Press, 1980:249.

6. Fairbanks VF, Beutler E. Erythrocyte disorders: Anemias related to disturbances of hemoglobin synthesis. In: Williams WJ, ed. Hematology. New York: McGraw-Hill, 1983:300.

7. DeMaeyer E, Adiels-Tegman M. The prevalence of anemia in the world. World Health Stat Q 1985;38:302.

8. Kerlin P, Reiner R, Davies M, et al. Iron deficiency anemia—A prospective study. Aust NZ J Med 1979;9:402.

9. Garby L. Iron deficiency: Definition and prevalence. Clin Haematol 1973;2:245.

10. Schiff L, Stevens RJ, Shapiro N, Goodman S. Observations on the oral administration of citrate blood in man. Am J Med Sci 1942;203:409.

11. Hilsman JH. The color of blood-containing feces following the instillation of citrated blood at various levels of the small intestine. Gastroenterology 1950;15:131.

12. Luke RG, Lees W, Rudick J. Appearances of the stools after the introduction of blood into the caecum. Gut 1964;5:77.

13. Ahlquist DA, McGill DB, Schwartz S, et al. HemoQuant, a new quantitative assay for fecal hemoglobin: Comparison with Hemoccult. Ann Intern Med 1984;101:297.

14. Ebaugh FG, Clermens T, Rodnan G, et al. Quantitative measurement of gastrointestinal blood loss. Am J Med 1958;25:169.

15. Owen CA Jr, Bollman JL, Grindlay JH. Radiochromium-labeled erythrocytes for the detection of gastrointestinal hemorrhage. J Lab Clin Med 1954;44:238.

16. Cameron AD. Gastrointestinal blood loss measured by radioactive chromium. Gut 1960;1:177.

17. Friedman BI. Radionuclide determination of gastrointestinal blood loss. Semin Nucl Med 1972;2:265.

18. Ahlquist DA, McGill DB, Schwartz S, et al. Fecal blood levels in health and disease: A study using HemoQuant. N Engl J Med 1985;312:1422.

19. Ahlquist DA, McGill DB, Fleming JL, et al. Patterns of occult bleeding in asymptomatic colorectal cancer. Cancer 1989;63:1826.

20. Wheby MS, Suttle GE, Ford KT. Intestinal absorption of hemoglobin iron. Gastroenterology 1970;58:647.

21. Conrad ME, Cortell S, Williams HL, et al. Polymerization and intraluminal factors in the absorption of hemoglobin-iron. J Lab Clin Med 1966;68:659.

22. Wyllie JC, Kaufman N. An electron microscopic study of heme uptake by rat duodenum. Lab Invest 1982;47:471.

23. Hallberg L, Bjorn-Rasmussen E, Howard L, et al. Dietary heme iron absorption. Scand J Gastroenterol 1979;14:769.

24. Schwartz S, Dahl J, Ellefson M, Ahlquist DA: The HemoQuant test: A specific and quantitative determination of heme (hemoglobin) in feces and other materials. Clin Chem 1983;29:2061.

25. Schwartz S, Ellefson M: Quantitative fecal recovery of ingested hemoglobin-heme in blood: Comparisons by HemoQuant assay with ingested meat and fish. Gastroenterology 1985;89:19.

26. Grasbeck R, Kouvonen I, Lundberg M, et al. An intestinal receptor for heme. Scand J Haematol 1979;23:5.

27. Young G, Rose IS, St John JB. Haem in the gut: Fate of haemoproteins and absorption of haem. J Gastroenterol Hepatol 1989;4:537.

28. Wheby MS, Spyker DA. Hemoglobin iron absorption kinetics in the iron-deficient dog. Am J Clin Nutr 1981;34:1686.

29. Raffin SB, Woo CH, Roost KT, et al. Intestinal absorption of heme iron: Heme cleavage by mucosal heme oxygenase. J Clin Invest 1974;54:1344.

30. Hartmann F, Bissell DM. Metabolism of heme and bilirubin in rat and human small intestinal mucosa. J Clin Invest 1982;70:23.

31. Hallberg L, Solvell L. Absorption of hemoglobin iron in man. Acta Med Scand 1967;181:335.

32. Baird IM, Wilson GM. The pathogenesis of anemia after partial gastrectomy; II. Iron absorption. Q J Med 1959;28:35.

33. Goldschmeidt M, Ahlquist DA, Wieand HS, et al. Measurement of degraded fecal hemoglobin-heme to estimate gastrointestinal site of occult bleeding: Appraisal of its clinical utility. Dig Dis Sci 1988;33:605.

34. Cifuentes PF, Engel RR, Ellefson M, et al. Quantitative determination of fecal blood by HemoQuant test in the newborn infant (abstr). Pediatr Res 1983;18:185A.

35. Adams EC, Layman KM. Immunochemical confirmation of gastrointestinal bleeding. Ann Clin Lab Sci 1974;4:343.

36. Rao BSN. Physiology of iron absorption and supplementation. Br Med Bull 1981;37:26.

37. Layrisse M. Model for measuring dietary absorption of heme iron. Am J Clin Nutr 1972;25:401.

38. Refsum SB, Schreiner BBI. Regulation of iron balance by absorption and excretion. Scand J Gastroenterol 1984;19:867.

39. Pollack S, Kaufman RM, Crosby WH. Iron absorption: Effects of sugars and reducing agents. Blood 1964;24:577.

40. Sorensen EW. Studies on iron absorption. VI. The effect of bile and pancreatin on the absorption of iron. Acta Med Scand 1967;181:707.

41. Jacobs A, Miles PM. Role of gastric secretion in iron absorption. Gut 1969;10:226.

42. Jacobs A, Rhodes J, Eakins JD. Gastric factors influencing iron absorption in anemic patients. Scand J Haematol 1967;4:105.

43. Hwang YF, Brown EB. Effect of deferoxamine on iron absorption. Lancet 1965;1:135.

44. Guiliani ER, Hagedorn AB, Owen CA, Scudamore HH. Anemia of non-tropical sprue studied with radioiron and radiochromium. J Nucl Med 1961;2:297.

45. Kalser MH, Roth JLA, Tumen H, Johnson TA. Relation of small bowel resection to nutrition in man. Gastroenterology 1960;38:605.

46. Greenberger NJ, Isselbacher KJ. Malabsorption following radiation injury to the GI tract. Am J Med 1964;36:450.

47. Goya N. A family of congenital atransferrinemia. Blood 1972;40:239.

48. Larrick W, Hyman ES. Acquired iron deficiency anemia caused by an antibody against transferrin receptor. N Engl J Med 1984;311:214.

49. Jacobs A, Butler EB. Menstrual blood loss in iron deficiency anemia. Lancet 1965;2:407.

50. Witte DL, Kraemer DF, Johnson DF, et al. Prediction of bone marrow iron findings from tests performed on peripheral blood. Am J Clin Pathol 1986;85:202.

51. Cooke JD, Lynch SR. The liabilities of iron deficiency. Blood 1986;68:803.

52. Basta SS, Soekirman MS, Karyadi D, Serinshaw NS. Iron deficiency anemia and the productivity of adult males in Indonesia. Am J Clin Nutr 1979;32:916.

53. Edgerton VT, Gardner GW, Ohira Y, et al. Iron-deficiency anemia and its effect on worker productivity and activity patterns. Br Med J 1979;2:1546.

54. Schoene RB, Escourrou P, Robertson HT, et al. Iron repletion decreases maximal exercise lactate concentrations in female athletes with minimal iron deficiency anemia. J Lab Clin Med 1983;102:306.

55. Finch CA, Miller LR, Inander AR, et al. Iron deficiency in the rat: Physiological and biochemical studies of muscle dysfunction. J Clin Invest 1976;58:447.

56. Jacobs A, Lawrie JH, Enwistle CC, Campbell H. Gastric acid secretion in chronic iron deficiency anemia. Lancet 1966;2:190.

57. Stone WD. Gastric secretory response to iron therapy. Gut 1968;9:99.

58. Guha DK, Walia BNS, Tandon BN, et al. Small bowel changes in iron-deficiency anemia of childhood. Arch Dis Child 1968;43:239.

59. Woodruff CW. Iron deficiency in infancy and childhood. Pediatr Clin North Am 1977;24:85.

60. Reeves JD, Vichinsky E, Addiego J, Lubin BH. Iron deficiency in health and disease. Adv Pediatr 1983;30:281.

61. Cook IJ, Pavli P, Riley JW, et al. Gastrointestinal investigation of iron deficiency anemia. Br Med J 1986;292:1380.

62. Calvey HD, Cestleden CM. Gastrointestinal investigations for anaemia in the elderly: A prospective study. Age Aging 1987;16:399.

63. Roche M, Layrisse M. The nature and causes of "hookworm anemia." Am J Trop Med Hyg 1966;15:1029.

64. Hershko C, Vitells A, Braverman Z. Causes of iron deficiency anemia in an adult inpatient population: Effect of diagnostic work-up on etiologic distribution. Blut 1984;49:347.

65. Euler AR, Ament ME. Gastroesophageal reflux in children: Clinical manifestations, diagnosis, pathophysiology, and therapy. Pediatr Ann 1976;5:678.

66. Segal HZ. Secondary anemia associated with diaphragmatic hernia. NY State J Med 1931;31:692.

67. Cameron AJ. Incidence of iron deficiency anemia in patients with large diaphragmatic hernia: A controlled study. Mayo Clinic Proc 1976;51:767.

68. Cameron AJ, Higgins JA. A lesion associated with large diaphragmatic hernia and chronic blood loss anemia. Gastroenterology 1986;91:338.

69. Coello-Ramirez P, Larrosa-Harro A. Gastrointestinal occult hemorrhage and gastroduodenitis in cow's milk protein intolerance. J Pediatr Gastroenterol Nutr 1984;3:215.

70. Savilalati E, Verkasalo M. Intestinal cow's milk allergy: Pathogenesis and clinical presentation. Clin Rev Allergy 1984;2:7.

71. McCormack TT, Sims J, Eyre-Brook I, et al. Gastric lesions in portal hypertension: Inflammatory gastritis or congestive gastropathy? Gut 1985;26:1226.

72. Gostout CJ, Bowyer BA, Ahlquist DA, et al. Mucosal vascular malformations of the gastrointestinal tract: Clinical observations and results of endoscopic neodymium:yttrium:aluminum-garnet laser therapy. Mayo Clin Proc 1988;63:993.

73. Gostout CJ, Ahlquist DA, Radford CM, et al. Endoscopic laser therapy for watermelon stomach. Gastroenterology 1989;96:1462.

74. Jabbari M, Cherry R, Lough JO, et al. Gastric antral vascular ectasia: The watermelon stomach. Gastroenterology 1984;87:1165.

75. Wellwood JM, Jackson BT. The intestinal complications of radiotherapy. Br J Surg 1973;60:814.

76. Belsheim MR, Sullivan SN. Blue rubber bleb nevus syndrome. Can J Surg 1980;23:274.

77. Holt JM, Wright R. Anemia due to the blood loss from the telangiectasias of scleroderma. Br Med J 1967;3:537.

78. Rosen KM, Sirota DK, Marinoff SC. Gastrointestinal bleeding in Turner's syndrome. Ann Intern Med 1967;67:145.

79. Schmitt B, Posselt HG, Waag KL, et al. Severe hemorrhage from intestinal hemangiomatosis in Klippel-Trenaunay syndrome: Pitfalls in diagnosis and management. J Pediatr Gastroenterol Nutr 1986;5:155.

80. Croker JR, Beynon G. Gastrointestinal bleeding–A major cause of iron deficiency in the elderly. Age Aging 1981;10:40.

81. Lee ER, Dagradi AE. Hemorrhagic erosive gastritis: A clinical study. Am J Gastroenterol 1975;65:201.

82. Fleming JL, Ahlquist DA, McGill DB, et al. Influence of aspirin and ethanol on fecal blood levels as determined by the HemoQuant assay. Mayo Clin Proc 1987;62:159.

83. Jaffin BW, Bliss CM, Larmont JT. Significance of occult gastrointestinal bleeding during anticoagulant therapy. Am J Med 1987;83:269.

84. Wilcox CM, Truss CD. Gastrointestinal bleeding in patients receiving long-term anticoagulant therapy. Am J Med 1988;84:683.

85. Ivey KJ. Gastrointestinal intolerance and bleeding with non-narcotic analgesics. Drugs 1986;32:71.

86. Graham DY, Smith SL. Gastroduodenal complications of chronic NSAID therapy. AM J Gastroenterol 1988;83:1081.

87. Carson JL, et al. The relative gastrointestinal toxicity of the NSAIDs. Arch Intern Med 1987;147:1054.

88. Schoen RT, Vender RJ. Mechanisms of non-steroidal anti-inflammatory drug-induced gastric damage. Am J Med 1989;86:449.

89. Loebl DH, Craig RM, Culic DD, et al. Gastrointestinal blood loss: Effect of aspirin, fenoprofen, and acetaminophen on rheumatoid arthritis as determined by sequential gastroscopy and radioactive fecal markers. JAMA 1977;237:976.

90. Brotherhood J, Brozovic B, Pugh LGC. Haematological status of middle and long-distance runners. Clin Sci Mol Med 1975;48:139.

91. Stewart GA, Steel JE, Toyne AH, Stewart MJ. Observations on the haematology and the iron and protein intake of Australian Olympic athletes. Med J Aust 1972;2:1339.

92. DeWijn JF, De Jongste JL, Mosterd W, Willebrand D. Hemoglobin, packed cell volume, serum iron and iron binding capacity of selected athletes during training. Nutr Metab 1971;13:129.

93. Stewart JG, Ahlquist DA, McGill DB, et al. Gastrointestinal blood loss and anemia in runners. Ann Intern Med 1984;100:843.

94. Fischer RL, McMahon LF, Ryan MJ, et al. Gastrointestinal bleeding in competitive runners. Dig Dis Sci 1986;31:1226.

95. Cooper BT, Douglas SA, Firth LA, et al. Erosive gastritis and gastrointestinal bleeding in a female runner. Gastroenterology 1987;92:2019.

96. Moses FM, Brewer TG, Peura DA. Running associated proximal hemorrhagic colitis. Ann Intern Med 1988;108:385.

97. Robertson JD, Marrghan RJ, Davidson RJL. Fecal blood loss in response to exercise. Br Med J 1987;295:303.

98. Dardick KR. Hematuria and false-positive tests for stool occult blood. Am Fam Physician 1984;29:201.

99. Crosby WH. Pica. JAMA 1976;235:2765.

100. Reynolds RD, Binder HJ, Miller MB, et al. Pagophagia and iron deficiency anemia. Ann Intern Med 1968;69:435.

101. Anderson NP. Syndrome of spoon nails, anemia, cheilitis, and dysphagia. Arch Dermatol 1938;37:816.

102. Baird IM. The tongue and oesophagus in iron-deficiency anemia and the effect of iron therapy. J Clin Pathol 1961;14:603.

103. Jacobs A, Cavill I. The oral lesions of iron deficiency anemia: Pyridoxine and riboflavin status. Br J Haematol 1968;14:291.

104. Hutten CF. Plummer Vinson syndrome. Br J Radiol 1956;29:81.

105. Jacobs A, Kilpatrick GS. The Paterson-Kelly syndrome. Br Med J 1964;2:79.

106. Khosla SN. Cricoid webs—Incidence and follow-up study in Indian patients. Postgrad Med J 1984;60:346.

107. Wynder EL, Hultberg S, Jacobsson F, Bross IJ. Environmental factors in cancer of the upper alimentary tract: A Swedish study with special reference to Plummer-Vinson (Paterson-Kelly) syndrome. Cancer 1957;10:470.,

108. Thompson WG, Meola T, Lipkin M, Freedman ML. Red cell distribution width, mean corpuscular volume, and transferrin saturation in the diagnosis of iron deficiency. Arch Intern Med 1988;148:2128.

109. Marcus DL, Freedman ML. Clinical disorders of iron metabolism in the elderly. Clin Geriatr Med 1985;1:729.

110. Van Deen J. Tincture gaujaci, und ein ozontrague, als reagens auf sehr geringe blutmengen, namentlich in medico-forensischen falen. Arch Holland Beitr Natura Heilk 1864;3:228.

111. Boas I. Uber okkulte magen blumtunge. Dtsch Med Wochenschr 1901;27:315.

112. Greegor DH. Occult blood testing for detection of asymptomatic colon cancer. Cancer 1971;28:131.

113. Doran J, Hardcastle JD. Bleeding patterns in colorectal cancer: The effect of aspirin and implications for faecal occult blood testing. Br J Surg 1982;69:711.

114. Ostrow JD, Mulvaeny CA, Hansell JR, et al. Sensitivity and reproducibility of chemical tests for fecal occult blood with an emphasis on false-positive reactions. Am J Dig Dis 1973;18:930.

115. Stroehlein JR, Fairbanks VG, McGill DS, et al. Hemoccult detection of fecal occult blood quantitated by radioassay. Am J Dig Dis 1976b;21:841.

116. Bassett ML, Goulston KJ. False positive and negative Hemoccult reactions on a normal diet and effect of diet restriction. Aust NZ J Med 1980;10:1.

117. Heinrich HCL. Letter: Occult blood tests. Lancet 1980;1:822.

118. Macrae FA, St John DJB. Relationship between patterns of bleeding and Hemoccult sensitivity in patients with colorectal cancers or adenomas. Gastroenterology 1982;82:891.

119. Herzog P, Holtermuller KH, Preiss J, et al. Fecal blood loss in patients with colonic polyps: A comparison of measurements with [51]chromium-labeled erythrocytes and with the Haemoccult test. Gastroenterology 1982;83:957.

120. Hunt RH. Evaluation of diagnostic techniques for colon cancer. Presented at the Second International Symposium on Colorectal Cancer. Washington, DC, 1981.

121. Stroehlein JR, Fairbanks VF, Go VL, et al. Hemocult stool tests: False-negative results due to storage of specimens. Mayo Clin Proc 1976a;51:548.

122. Illingworth DG. Influence of diet on occult blood tests. Gut 1965;6:595.

123. Macrae FA, St John DJB, Caligiore P, et al. Optimal dietary conditions for Hemoccult testing. Gastroenterology 1982;82:899.

124. Lifton LF, Kreiser J. False-positive stool occult blood tests caused by iron preparations. A controlled study and review of literature. Gastroenterology 1982;83:860.

125. Irons GV, Kirsner JB. Routine chemical tests of the stool for occult blood: An evaluation. Am J Med Sci 1965;249:247.

126. Schentag JJ. Letter: False positive "Hemoccult" reaction with cimetidine. N Engl J Med 1980;303:110.

127. Ahlquist DA, Schwartz S. Use of leuco-dyes in the quantitative colorimetric microdetermination of hemoglobin and other heme compounds. Clin Chem 1975;21:362.

128. Ahlquist DA, Schwartz S, Isaacson J, et al. A stool collection device: The first step in occult blood testing. Ann Intern Med 1988;108:609.

129. Jaffe RM, Kasten B, Young DS, et al. False-negative stool occult blood tests caused by ingestion of ascorbic acid (vitamin C). Ann Intern Med 1975;83:824.

130. Layne EA, Mellow MH, Lipman TO. Insensitivity of guaiac slide tests for detection of blood in gastric juice. Ann Intern Med 1981;94:774.

131. Markman HD. Letter: Errors in the guaiac test for occult blood. JAMA 1967;202:846.

132. Jaffe RM, Zierdt W. A new occult blood test not subject to false-negative results from reducing substances. J Lab Clin Med 1979;93:879.

133. Graham DY, Sackman JW, Wallis CH, et al. The Hemo-matic Analyzer: A new occult blood testing device. Am J Gastroenterol 1984;79:117.

134. Barrows GH, Burton RM, Jarrett DD, et al. Immunochemical detection of human blood in feces. Am J Clin Pathol 1978;69:342.

135. Songster CL, Barrows GH, Jarrett DD. Immunochemical detection of fecal occult blood—The fecal smear punch-disc test: A new non-invasive screening test for colorectal cancer. Cancer 1980;45:1099.

136. Yoshida Y, Saito H, Tsuchida S, et al. A simple sensitive immunologic fecal occult blood test suitable for mass screening for colorectal cancer (abstr). Gastroenterology 1986;90:1699.

137. Nakayama T, Yasuoka H, Kishino T, et al. Elisa for occult fecal albumin. Lancet 1987;1:1368.

138. Frommer DJ, Kapparisa A, Brown MK. Improved screening for colorectal cancer by immunochemical detection of occult blood. Br Med J 1988;296:1092.

139. Stephens FO, Lawrenson KB. The pathologic significance of occult blood in feces. Dis Colon Rectum 1970;13:425.

140. Stephens FO, Lawrenson KB. Cr^{51} excretion in bile. Lancet 1969;1:158.

141. Chafetz N, Taylor A, Schlief A, Verba J, Hooser CW. A potential error in the quantitation of fecal blood loss: Concise communication. J Nucl Med 1976;17:1053.

142. Rosenfield RE, Kochwa A, Kaczera A, et al. Non-uniform distribution of occult blood in feces. Am J Clin Pathol 1979;71:204.

143. Farrands PA, Hardcastle JD. Accuracy of occult blood tests over a six-day period. Clin Oncol 1983;9:217.

144. Hoffman A, Young Q, Bright-Asare P, et al. Early detection of bowel cancer at an urban public hospital: Demonstration project. CA 1983;33:344.

145. Brandeau ML, Eddy DM. The work-up of the asymptomatic patient with a positive fecal occult blood test. Med Decis Making 1987;7:32.

146. Barry MJ, Mulley AG, Richter JM. Effect of work-up strategy on the cost-effectiveness of fecal occult blood screening for colorectal cancer. Gastroenterology 1987;93:301.

147. Myers RT. Diagnosis and management of occult gastrointestinal bleeding: Visualization of the small bowel lumen by fiberoptic colonoscope. Am Surg 1976;42:92.

148. Lewis BS, Waye JD. Chronic gastrointestinal bleeding of obscure origin: Role of small bowel enteroscopy. Gastroenterology 1988;94:1117.

149. Bowden TA, Hooks VH, Mausberger AR. Intraoperative gastrointestinal endoscopy in the management of occult gastrointestinal bleeding. South Med J 1979;72:1532.

150. Spechler S, Schimmel E. Gastrointestinal tract bleeding of unknown origin. Arch Intern Med 1982;142:236.

151. Goulston K, Davidson P. Fecal occult blood testing in patients with colonic symptoms. Med J Aust 1980;2:667.

152. Simon JB. Occult blood screening for colorectal carcinoma: A critical review. Gastroenterology 1985;88:820.

153. Dybdahl JH, Daae LNW, Larsen S, et al. Occult faecal blood loss determined by a ^{51}Cr method and chemical tests in patients referred for colonoscopy. Scand J Gastroenterol 1984;19:245.

154. Griffith CDM, Turner DJ, Saunders JH. False-negative results of Hemoccult test in colorectal screening. Br Med J 1981;283:472.

155. Crowley ML, Freeman LD, Mottet MD, et al. Sensitivity of guaiac-impregnated cards for the detection of colorectal neoplasia. J Clin Gastroenterol 1983;5:127.

156. Ahlquist DA, Klee GG, McGill DB, Ellefson RD. Colorectal cancer detection in the practice setting: Impact of fecal blood testing. Arch Intern Med 1990;150:1041.

157. Demers RY, Stawick LE, Demers P. Relative sensitivity of the fecal occult blood test and flexible sigmoidoscopy in detecting polyps. Prev Med 1985;14:55.

158. Elwood TW, Erickson A, Liberman S. Comparative education approaches to screening for colorectal caner. Am J Public Health 1978;68:135.

159. Nichols S, Koch E, Lallermand RC, et al. Randomized trial of compliance with screening for colorectal cancer. Br Med J (Clin Res) 1986;293:107.

160. Morrow GR, Way J, Hoagland AC, et al. Patient compliance with self-directed Hemoccult testing. Prev Med 1982;11:512.

161. Frank JW. Occult blood screening for colorectal cancer: The yield and costs. Am J Prev Med 1985;1:18.

162. Clayman CG. Mass screening for colorectal cancer: Are we ready? JAMA 1989;261:609.

163. Neuhauser D. Letter: Cost effectiveness of screening for occult blood in the stool: Another look. N Engl J Med 1980;303:1306.

164. Knight KK, Fielding JE, Battista RN. Occult blood screening for colorectal cancer. JAMA 1989;261:586.

165. Hallberg L, Ryttinger L, Solvell L. Side-effects of oral iron therapy: A double-blind study of different iron components in tablet form. Acta Med Scand 1966;459:3.

166. McCurdy PR. Oral and parenteral iron therapy. JAMA 1965;191:155.

32

Approach to the Patient with Unexplained Weight Loss

DOUGLAS A. DROSSMAN

The evaluation of weight loss can be a challenge for the physician because: (1) the patient's concern may not reflect a true loss of weight, (2) the physician's concern may not be shared by the patient (e.g., patients with eating disorders), (3) the loss may not be clinically significant (e.g., from healthy dieting and exercise), (4) there may be multiple etiologies for the weight loss, (5) there may be a serious underlying disorder, which cannot be found, and (6) it may difficult to determine the relative roles of biologic and behavioral factors. As a result, the type and extent of diagnostic evaluation needed may be difficult to determine. The first part of this chapter presents a general approach to the evaluation of weight loss that considers these diagnostic difficulties. Part two focuses on evaluating and treating patients with eating disorders.

HUNGER AND SATIETY

While both *hunger* and *appetite* refer to the desire to eat, the determinants of hunger are usually attributed to physiologic mechanisms, while appetite is influenced by environmental and psychologic processes (aroma, appearance of food, mood, and so forth). *Satiety* refers to the gratification of hunger and appetite. *Anorexia* is a clinical symptom characterized by the absence of hunger or appetite. The experience of hunger and satiety appears to result from overlapping stimuli from the central nervous system (CNS) and gastrointestinal (GI) tract, which in the short-term affect food intake (by way of satiety) and in the long-term affect body weight. Both satiety and anorexia are determined by physiologic and psychologic processes.

The regulation of food intake has been attributed to certain physiologic constructs (e.g., the "set point" theory, which assumes that persons have a fixed reference point of body weight, and they return to this weight if they are over- or underfed).[1] It is proposed that GI, metabolic, and CNS stimuli affect, in an integrated fashion, peripheral and central receptors and, ultimately, the experience of hunger, satiety, and eating behavior.[2] Stimuli may include the thought and taste of food; concentrations of intestinal nutrients such as glucose, amino acids, and fatty acids; and gastric distention and emptying. In general, it is assumed that nutrients produced after food ingestion have an inhibitory affect on hunger. The hypothalamus appears to be the center for hunger (lateral nucleus)

and satiety (ventromedial nucleus), although the pathways and interactions of these areas are more complex than previously assumed.

In addition to nutrients, peptide hormones such as insulin and glucagon have been implicated in the modulation of food regulation by way of their effects on glucose metabolism.[2] Within the medial hypothalamus, norepinephrine stimulates the desire to eat by means of α_2-adrenergic receptors. Within the lateral hypothalamus, serotonin, dopaminergic, and β-adrenergic receptors mediate the inhibition of eating.[3] Agents that act on the opiate kappa receptor stimulate feeding,[4] and naloxone, an opiate antagonist, inhibits feeding in laboratory animals. Gamma-aminobutyric acid (GABA) and benzodiazepines also appear to play a role in food regulation, although their precise functions are not well established.[2]

Attention has been directed toward an additional peptide that may have primary effects on satiety.[5] Exogenous administration of cholecystokinin (CCK) and bombesin inhibit feeding activity in several animals.[6] These peptides, found in the GI tract and the CNS, may have origins and effects both centrally and peripherally. For example, CCK's effect on satiety by way of inhibition of gastric emptying[7] is blocked by vagotomy, suggesting a degree of CNS control.[8] CCK also appears to have independent effects on the hypothalamic satiety center and may play a role in the pathophysiology of the eating disorders. In one study, the postprandial serum level of CCK and the patient's satiety were found to be significantly less in bulimic patients.[9]

NAUSEA AND VOMITING

Nausea and vomiting are discussed in detail in Chapter 33. These symptoms may play an important role in weight loss, therefore, their mechanisms are briefly reviewed here also. *Nausea* is the unpleasant feeling that one is about to vomit. It is associated with anorexia and may represent the awareness of afferent stimuli to the medullary vomiting center. A variety of stimuli (e.g., labyrinthine, psychologic factors, bowel distention, peripheral pain) may produce nausea. The physiologic correlates of nausea include gastric hypomotility and increased parasympathetic tone, which precede and accompany retching and vomiting. *Retching* may occur without, or may precede vomiting. It is produced by forced re-

634

spiratory inspiration of the chest wall and diaphragm against a closed mouth and glottis, and forced spasmodic expiratory contractions of the abdominal musculature. During retching, the pyloris is closed and the antrum contracts while the fundus of the stomach relaxes. *Vomiting* or *emesis* occurs at a point when the esophageal sphincters and glottis open, and the cardia is forced into the thorax. The intrathoracic pressure effect is reversed, and gastric contents are forcefully expelled through the mouth.[10,11] It appears that retching is an attempt to inhibit vomiting; the glottis and respiratory muscles appear to counteract the abdominal efforts directed toward expulsion of gastric contents.

There appear to be two separate units in the medulla mediating the vomiting reflex: a vomiting center in the reticular formation, which receives visceral afferent impulses from the GI tract, and a chemoreceptor trigger zone in the area postrema in the floor of the fourth ventricle, which acts on the vomiting center.[12] Unlike the vomiting center, the chemoreceptor trigger zone responds to a variety chemical stimuli including the opiate drugs, ergot, cancer chemotherapy agents, cardiac glycosides, uremia, hypoxia, nicotine, and various enterotoxins. Dopamine receptors appear to mediate the vomiting response in the chemoreceptor trigger zone.[13] Therefore, dopamine agonists (e.g., apomorphine, bromocriptine; as well as possibly several other neuropeptides) cause vomiting, whereas dopamine antagonists (e.g., phenothiazines, metoclopramide) have antiemetic effects. The chemoreceptor trigger zone and the vomiting center have afferent neural connections not only from the GI tract (e.g., pharynx, mesenteric vasculature, and bile ducts) but also from corticobulbar areas that mediate smells, sights, and tastes. It, therefore, appears that the vomiting apparatus is responsive to a variety of GI and CNS inputs.

While the regulatory mechanisms for the GI symptoms (anorexia, nausea, vomiting) associated with weight loss are not fully established, one factor is evident: there is close interaction among the environment and CNS and GI function. These relationships support the validity of psychologic processes in initiating these symptoms.

INITIAL ASSESSMENT OF WEIGHT LOSS

Some general questions should be considered when seeing a patient presumed to have lost weight (Table 32-1):

TABLE 32–1
Initial Assessment of Weight Loss

1. What is normal variation in weight?
2. Has weight loss truly occurred?
3. Was it intentional?
4. What is the timeframe of the weight loss?
5. What are the biologic and behavioral determinants?
6. What are the contributing factors?
   a. Decreased intake
   b. Increased metabolic rate
   c. Incomplete absorption/digestion
   d. Increased catabolism or any combination?
7. Is further diagnostic assessment needed?

1. What is the Normal Variation in Weight?

As a result of normal deviations in intake and output of salt, water, and food, a person's weight fluctuates each day by as much as 1.5%. However, body weight tends to remain constant over long periods of time. Therefore, continued loss of greater than 5% of body weight (2–5 kg) is considered by most as a departure from normal and may require some investigation, although it may not necessarily reflect a clinically significant event.

2. Has Weight Loss Truly Occurred?

Most people weigh themselves periodically and can state their usual weight with reasonable accuracy, although large persons tend to underestimate[14] and small persons[14] and females[15] overestimate their weight. The recall of weight can also be inaccurate. Persons who lose weight slowly may not be aware of the change, and even diagnosis may affect recall of weight change. In one study of 105 patients, perceived weight loss was underestimated (by 1.8 kg) by patients with cancer, overestimated (by 1.7 kg) by patients with functional disorder, and accurate in patients with nonmalignant disease.[16] It can be assumed that up to half of patients who complain of significant weight loss will not have it documented by recorded values.[17,18] Therefore, the surest evidence of weight loss is comparison of current weight with previously recorded values. In the absence of this documentation, the physician must attempt to corroborate the patient's report by changes in clothing (e.g., belt) size or from family members.

3. Was it Intentional?

If weight loss is documented, it is helpful to know the contribution of dietary restriction, increased exercise, or other voluntary efforts. Particularly for the patient presumed to have an eating disorder, information from friends or family members of the person's eating behavior is needed.

4. What is the Timeframe of the Weight Loss?

In general, rapid weight loss is accompanied by physiologic effects (e.g., dehydration) and is often associated with signs of underlying disease and decline in everyday function. Conversely, patients losing weight over prolonged periods of time tend to adapt physiologically and psychologically. Even when malnourished, these patients may not be aware of the degree of weight change and may still function in their usual activities.

5. What are the Biologic and Behavioral Determinants?

Both biomedical and psychosocial etiologic factors must be assessed. It is *not* helpful to try to determine whether the cause is "organic *or* functional" because both are usually operative.

6. What are the Contributing Factors?[14]

Decreased intake is the most common contribution to weight loss and should always be considered. As shown in Table 32-2, the reasons for the decreased intake can be of diagnostic value. *Increased metabolic rate or a catabolic state* due to fever, tissue inflammation, cancer, hyperthyroidism, diabetes, and physical activity produces a modest amount of weight loss. Resting energy expenditure increases about 12% for each degree centigrade of temperature above normal. In a 70-kg person, physical activity equivalent to running 6 miles burns 2100 kJ. *Incomplete absorption or maldigestion* of nutrients either by mechanical obstruction or

TABLE 32-2
Causes of Decreased Food Intake

SYMPTOMS	POSSIBLE ETIOLOGIES
Loss of appetite with the thought, sight, or odor of food	Advanced malignancy
	Drugs
	Psychiatric (e.g., depression, psychosis)
	Alcohol/drug abuse
	ARC/AIDS
Abnormal taste (dysgeusia)	Drugs
	Psychiatric (e.g., depression, psychosis)
	Zinc deficiency
	B vitamin deficiency
	Sinusitis
Mechanical problems with swallowing, pain, or dyspnea limiting ingestion	Neurologic (bulbar) disturbance
	Oral/dental disease
	Esophageal stricture or motor disorder
	Severe cardiopulmonary disease
Abdominal pain with fear of eating (sitophobia)	Channel ulcer
	Partial intestinal obstruction
	Intestinal ischemia
	Pancreatitis
	Pancreatic cancer
	Cholecystitis, choledocholithiasis
	Psychiatric (e.g., conversion disorder)
	Irritable bowel syndrome
Lethargy, weakness	Severe malnutrition of any cause
	Neuromuscular disease
	Psychiatric (e.g., depression)
Overzealous dietary fads	
Conditioned aversion to foods when taken after a nauseating stimulus	Cancer chemotherapy Psychiatric
Infirmity or poverty	

Modified from Heizer WH. Weight loss. In Dornbrand L, Fletcher R, Hoole A, Pickard G, eds. Clinical problems in ambulatory care medicine. Boston: Little, Brown & Co, in press.

malabsorption due to GI disorders is detailed elsewhere (see ch 37, 38, 71 and 89).

7. Is Further Diagnostic Assessment Needed?
Finally, it should be determined if the weight loss might be explained by existing illnesses. If so, further diagnostic assessment may not be needed.

ETIOLOGIC CONSIDERATIONS

It may be assumed that a listing of etiologies causing weight loss would aid in the diagnostic plan. However, weight loss is only a clinical sign; the occurrence of other clinical findings establishes the diagnosis. Furthermore, weight loss is usually multifactorial, and the physician often needs to determine the relative contributions of several diagnoses. Finally, the distribution of etiologies for weight loss varies depending on the population; ambulatory patients seen in primary care have different etiologies than patients referred to a medical center.

Some general observations about etiology and the diagnostic approach can be made from two studies evaluating the etiologies of unexplained weight loss (Table 32-3). The studies were performed at referral centers: a California VA hospital[17] and an Israeli hospital[19]. In most cases, the causes, most often cancer or GI disease, were established initially or within a few months, and abnormal physical findings and laboratory studies were typically present on the first visit. Also, while GI disorders were frequent, the specific diagnoses varied between studies. The VA study patients had malabsorption, inflammatory bowel disease, diabetic enteropathy, and esophageal dysmotility; the Israeli study patients had peptic disease, bowel motility disorders, cholelithiasis, inflammatory bowel disease, hiatal hernia, and Zenker's diverticulum. So, while GI etiologies need to be considered as a cause for unexplained weight loss, prevalence studies do not help in planning the diagnostic evaluation. Finally, despite intensive investigations, about 25% of the patients remain undiagnosed, yet they seem to have a good long-term prognosis.

In these studies, there was a 10% prevalence of psychologic disorder, although it was not clear how systematically these diagnoses were considered. In two more recent studies, when psychologic diagnoses were pursued, the prevalences were much higher. Among 50 inpatients in Italy,[20] 42% had stress-related disorders, primarily depression; organic etiologies were found in an additional 34%. In an outpatient study of 105 patients in

TABLE 32-3
Etiologies for Unintentional Weight Loss at Referral Centers

DIAGNOSIS	CALIFORNIA VA HOSPITAL (n = 91)* (%)†	ISRAEL (n = 154)‡ (%)
Unknown	26	23
Neoplasia	19	36
GI disorders	14	17
Psychiatric	9	10
Cardiovascular	9	0
Alcohol	8	0
Pulmonary	6	0
Endocrine/metabolic	4	4
Infectious	3	4
Inflammatory	2	1
Renal	0	4
Miscellaneous	4	1

* Data from Martin KI, Sox HC Jr, Krupp JR. Involuntary weight loss: Diagnostic and prognostic significance. Ann Intern Med 1981;95:568.
† Some patients had more than one diagnosis.
‡ Data from Rabinowitz M, Pitlik SD, Leifer M, Garty M, Rosenfeld JB. Unintentional weight loss. A retrospective analysis of 154 cases. Arch Intern Med 1986;146:186.

France,[21] 60% were diagnosed to have primarily depression or other psychologic causes for the weight loss; gastroenterologic diagnoses were the next most common causes.

Three conclusions can be made from the data: (1) Most etiologies are established initially and with limited diagnostic evaluation. (2) If a diagnosis cannot be made, watchful waiting is reasonable, because the prognosis is good. (3) Greater efforts should be paid to establish psychologic etiologies.

CLINICAL ASSESSMENT

Historical Data

A well-organized medical interview (see ch 27) and the physical examination can help the physician determine the best diagnostic approach. The history can provide important etiologic clues.

GENERAL MEDICAL ETIOLOGIES

Certain medical disorders are characteristically associated with chronic weight loss. These include (1) *endocrine/metabolic disorders,* such as thyrotoxicosis, diabetes mellitus, and Addison's disease; (2) *chronic infections,* such as tuberculosis, fungal diseases, subacute bacterial endocarditis; (3) *occult malignancy,* such as GI cancers, lymphoma, gynecologic and renal tumors, and leukemia; and (4) *disorders of immunity,* such as acquired immunodeficiency syndrome (AIDS) or AIDS-related complex. In addition, physiologic changes in weight loss may occur in *elderly persons,* although pathologic etiologies are also common and are usually multidetermined.[18]

GASTROINTESTINAL ETIOLOGIES

Presumptive GI etiologies can be determined through the medical history. The *relation of symptom to meals* can provide information about the possible site of GI obstruction. GI obstruction is usually associated with worsening of symptoms (e.g., dysphagia, nausea, vomiting, abdominal pain) after eating. Depending on the volume of food consumed, symptoms can occur almost immediately (benign or malignant esophageal stricture, achalasia, rumination, psychiatric etiologies), 1 to 3 hours postprandially in gastric or high intestinal obstruction (e.g., pyloric channel ulcer, gastric motor emptying disorder, internal duodenal hernia), to several hours later with more distal lesions (e.g., Crohn's ileitis, colonic adenocarcinoma). Relief of symptoms with vomiting is also suggestive of an obstructing lesion, and the presence of abdominal distention and fecalent vomitus would indicate a more distal source. Pain arising from pancreatic or gallbladder disease may worsen after a meal because of induction of digestive enzyme production or gallbladder contraction, but this usually is not relieved by vomiting. *Weight loss associated with ingestion of normal or large quantities of food* may suggest malabsorption, hyperthyroidism, cancer, or diabetes mellitus. The production of *large volume, foul smelling and oily stools* suggests fat malabsorption due to pancreatic or intestinal disease. However, the discriminating value of these symptoms lessens over time as patients decrease their food intake to avoid pain (sitophobia) or diarrhea, or because of associated depressive symptoms.

BEHAVIORAL ETIOLOGIES

Weight loss due to behavioral factors is associated with decreased food intake and can be determined by the interview or, if needed, by psychologic testing or consultation. It is important to evaluate not only what is said, but how the patient behaves. For example, weight loss is "ego-syntonic" for patients with eating disorders (i.e., the motivation is to maintain the process). This is inferred when the patient acknowledges that it is *others* who believe she needs to gain weight ("My parents say I'm getting too thin"). These patients can also: (1) express reluctance to be weighed, (2) exercise vigorously, (3) eat low-calorie foods, or (4) overtly or covertly resist therapeutic efforts directed toward weight gain. The nonpsychiatrist can make a presumptive behavioral diagnosis based on certain features listed below (Table 32-4)[22,23] (see ch 27) and obtain psychiatric consultation for additional guidance.

The behavioral disorder most commonly associated with weight loss is *primary or secondary depression.* Typically, depression is associated with saddened affect, true anorexia, sleep disturbance, anhedonia, and a generalized sense of poor self-esteem. Patients with depression acknowledge a lack of interest and gratification in eating as well as a decreased appetite. Less commonly, patients may have loss of appetite and sometimes pain due to a *conversion disorder.* This disorder is associated with a symbolic association between food or eating and a psychologic conflict. For example, symptoms may result from the fantasied wish to rid the body of a forbidden thought (e.g., to get pregnant or to harm someone) or, in cases of unresolved grief, as a symbolic representation ("symptom model") of a deceased person who had similar symptoms. With conversion disorder, inquiry usually discloses an identifiable traumatic event that led to the onset of symptoms. These patients are not necessarily depressed, do not have body image disturbance, and may function normally except for circumscribed periods related to eating. Interestingly, patients with conversion disorder often have vomiting that is not associated with anorexia or nausea. Weight loss due to a *thought disorder,* such as schizophrenia or other psychosis, results from a more distorted alteration in perception or attitudes about food and eating. For example, the patient may believe that the food has been poisoned or that eating will cause the intestines to rot. These beliefs may be well circumscribed or may be part of more pervasive thought disturbances affecting daily function. Delusional thoughts can be elicited by asking the patient to describe his or her beliefs about the cause or meaning of the symptoms. Weight loss due to an *eating disorder (anorexia nervosa, bulimerexia, adult rumination syndrome)* is discussed in more detail later in this chapter. In brief, the eating disorders are distinguished from other behavioral disorders by the patient's intense drive to maintain thinness (dieting, exercise, self-induced vomiting, purging) in association with a body-image disturbance of being too fat. The fundamental psychologic problem is the need to maintain self-esteem through excess self-control of

TABLE 32–4
Behavioral Disorders Causing Weight Loss

FEATURE	ANOREXIA NERVOSA	CONVERSION	SCHIZOPHRENIA	DEPRESSION
Drive to be thin	Marked	None	None	None
Self-imposed starvation	Marked (fear of fatness)	None	Marked (delusional)	None
Body-image disturbance	Present	None	None	None
Appetite	Maintained	Variable	Maintained	True anorexia
Satiety	Early satiety	Variable	Variable	Variable
Food avoidance	Present	None	Present (delusional)	Loss of interest
Bulimia	30%–50%	Rare	Rare	Rare
Vomiting	Present (controls weight)	Present (symbolic)	Rare	Rare
Laxatives	Present	Rare	None	None
Activity	Increased	No change	No change	Reduced

Modified from Garfinkel DE, Kaplan AS, Garner DM, Darby PL. The differentiation of vomiting/weight loss as a conversion disorder from anorexia nervosa. Am J Psychiatry 1983;140:1019.

weight and body size. The patient does not experience true anorexia but, rather, struggles to stay thin despite the hunger.

Physical Findings

The physical findings of unexplained weight loss relate to the etiology of the weight loss and to the degree of malnutrition. A discussion of the physical effects of malnutrition can be found elsewhere (see ch 21).

Laboratory Assessment

Laboratory studies should be guided by the results of the history and physical examination. Table 32-5 lists the types of studies that can be obtained. The choice of studies must be individualized and determined by the data obtained from the history and physical examination.

APPROACH TO TREATMENT

In general, the treatment of weight loss must be directed at the underlying medical problem. Regardless of diagnosis, once the patient loses more than 15% of normal body weight, manifestations of malnutrition can develop (e.g., weakness, depressed immune function and susceptibility to infection, emotional changes of apathy and irritability), which may require nutritional supplementation. Several liquid diets are available that have the advantage of requiring no preparation and are nutritionally complete. However, many patients find them less palatable than food.

THE EATING DISORDERS

The eating disorders, anorexia nervosa, bulimia and rumination, are relatively common disorders, affecting about 5% to 10% of the young female population.[24,25] Gastroenterologists and primary care physicians usually see these patients at the time severe undernutrition or medical or psychologic complications develop. The diagnosis and treatment of patients with eating disorders require a recognition that these disorders result from a combination of biologic, psychologic, and social influences.[26]

ANOREXIA NERVOSA

ANOREXIA[27]
my face in the mirror
conjures the idle bone below,
sweet slow bloom,
yet still I am repelled
by its lewd fleshiness
at dinner the rage boils, a smoke
rising from the groaning plates
more obscene than any dream
my sister sits across the table
wrapped in private spite,
ready to thrust her spear
at any opening:
stop picking at your food—
if you can't eat all of it,
why eat at all, she says.
her words choke a thing in me
and my fork falls, lifeless.
mother, she doesn't like my boyfriend
she denounces him
for what she creates in me—
clean your plate, she says but
mother, she hasn't said I love you
to anyone in fifteen years.

TABLE 32-5
Diagnostic Studies for Evaluation of Weight Loss*

General

Chest x-ray, flat and upright of abdomen

Complete blood count, sedimentation rate

Glucose

Creatinine

Liver chemistry tests

Total protein, albumin

Immunoglobulins

Stool for occult blood X3

Urinalysis

TSH, T$_4$, T$_3$

PPD skin test

HIV assay

Malabsorption Suspected

Screening

Qualitative fecal fat (quantitative if possible)

Carotene

Prothrombin time

More Specific

D-xylose (intestinal)

Bentiromide (pancreatic)

Breath tests—Cholyl-^{14}C-glycine (bacterial overgrowth, ileal disease)

Small intestinal culture (bacterial overgrowth)

Schilling test (intestinal, pancreatic, bacterial overgrowth)

Most Specific

Small bowel biopsy (e.g., celiac sprue, giardiasis, Whipple's disease, amyloidosis, abetalipoproteinemia)

Endoscopic retrograde pancreatography (ERP)

Gastrointestinal Obstruction Suspected

Esophagogastroduodenoscopy

Upper GI/small intestinal series (or enteroclysis)

Colonoscopy

Occult Neoplasm Suspected (Rare)

CT scan of the abdomen

Abdominal/pelvic ultrasound

* Studies listed are guidelines to be selected on an individual basis. When in doubt, watchful waiting is recommended.

---

mother can't you find another way
to shrink me to something
you can embrace
I just want to be something
more than a child.

Peggy Hanson, M.D.

It is difficult to understand fully the experience of a person with anorexia nervosa. The fear of fatness and distortion of body image result in a variety of compulsive acts and rituals to lose weight. Underlying this "pursuit of thinness" are profound feelings of helplessness in what is perceived to be a controlling environment, and ineffectiveness in initiating actions of consequence. The anorectic person, never having developed a sense of autonomy, maintains the prospect that perfection is needed in order to be loved and accepted. Adolescence or other events that foster psychologic growth and individuation challenge these convictions and are particularly threatening to self-esteem. It is believed that the preanorectic person feels inadequate at these times and desperately attempts to control at least her body.[28] Dieting may be a visible accomplishment of the virtues of self-denial and mastery over bodily urges that enhance her feeling of control in other areas of her life.[29] The disorder can be characterized behaviorally by self-induced weight loss, psychologically by body-image and other perceptual disturbances, and biologically by physiologic alterations (e.g., amenorrhea) that result from nutritional depletion.

Epidemiology

Anorexia nervosa (DSM-IIIR 307.10) predominantly afflicts young, affluent, white females (95%) (Table 32-6), although the general clinical features in males are similar.[30] The incidence may be increasing.[31] In one community study, the number of new cases per year over a 10-year period rose from 0.35 per 100,000 to 0.64 per 100,000.[32] The disorder is associated with higher social class, occurring in up to 1 of every 250 adolescent students in private school and with a prevalence of 1%.[26]

Etiology And Pathogenesis— Putative Predisposing Factors

SOCIAL/CULTURAL FACTORS

The cultural ideal for women's bodies has shifted in the last century from that of plumpness (formerly representing wealth, abundance, maternalism, and fertility) to a slimmer female image (representing independence, assertiveness, and success). Thinner women are idealized and predominate on prime-time television and among beauty pageant contestants and high-fashion models.[31] Social pressures from peers, particularly during adolescence, seem to influence young women and girls to engage in anorectic behaviors. These factors are probably not sufficient for the disorder to develop but, in the predisposed person, may create the proper environment for its expression.

PSYCHOLOGIC FACTORS[26]

As previously noted, it is believed that anorectic persons have an incompletely developed personal identity and struggle to maintain a sense of control over their environment. Psychiatric interviews suggest that the patient develops within a family that values outward appearance, proper behavior, and achievement more than self-actualization. In response to parental expectations, the prean-

TABLE 32–6
Diagnostic Criteria for 307.10 Anorexia Nervosa

A. Refusal to maintain body weight over a minimal normal weight for age and height (e.g., weight loss leading to maintenance of body weight 15% below that expected) or failure to make expected weight gain during period of growth, leading to body weight 15% below that expected.
B. Intense fear of gaining weight or becoming fat, even though underweight.
C. Disturbance in the way in which one's body weight, size or shape is experienced (e.g., claiming to "feel fat" even when emaciated, or believes that one area of the body is "too fat" even when obviously underweight).
D. In females, absence of at least three consecutive menstrual cycles when otherwise expected to occur (primary or secondary amenorrhea; a woman is considered to have amenorrhea if her periods occur only following hormone [e.g., estrogen] administration).

From American Psychiatric Association. Eating disorders: 307.10 Anorexia nervosa. In: Diagnostic and statistical manual of mental disorders—DSM-III-R. Washington, DC: American Psychiatric Association, 1987:65.

orectic child learns to be hard working, eager to please, and attentive to family needs. In turn, the parents support and indulge in the behaviors of their child ("the best little girl in the world"). Therefore, these mutually reinforced actions produce interdependence among the family members (enmeshment). Because the high standards within the family are rarely achieved, the child obsessively struggles for parental approval.

It follows that "negative" childhood behaviors (e.g., assertiveness, rebellion) are not permitted. However, psychologists believe these behaviors to be necessary for the development of individual identity. As a result, the preanorectic child comes to rely on externally imposed ideal values to maintain self-esteem, but at the expense of autonomous development.

For reasons previously noted, it is not surprising that a distressing period for the preanorectic child occurs during or soon after puberty when physical, social, and psychologic events (menarche, growth spurt, school and adolescent peer pressure) encourage individuation and separation from the family. Over 80% of anorectic patients develop the disorder within 7 years of menarche.

Very recent data indicate that there is a high prevalence of sexual abuse among anorectic patients. In one study of 158 patients admitted to an eating disorder unit,[33] 50% of the anorectic and bulimic patients reported sexual abuse compared to 28% of the patients with other eating disorder diagnoses ($P < 0.01$). The relationship of this traumatic psychologic experience to the development or expression of anorexia nervosa requires further study.

BIOLOGIC FACTORS

It is likely, although unproven, that predisposing biologic factors increase susceptibility to developing anorexia nervosa. There is a 6% prevalence of anorexia nervosa in siblings, and in one study of twin pairs, 9 of 12 monozygotic and 1 of 14 dizygotic pairs were concordant for the disorder.[34] Family studies also show a co-association of anorexia nervosa and depressive disorder in first-degree relatives of anorectic patients.[35] These data suggest variable expressions of a common underlying disorder or of possibly two independent but linked disorders that, given the proper environmental stimulus (e.g., dieting, emotional stress), might manifest clinically as depression and anorexia nervosa.

Abnormalities in satiety, temperature regulation, and endocrine function suggest that a hypothalamic abnormality exists, although no specific lesion has been identified. It is more likely that the hypothalamus serves a modulating role. In the predisposed person, the biologic and psychosocial events around the time of adolescence may produce physiologic changes in neurotransmitter, endocrine, or immune function by way of the hypothalamus that lead to the characteristic behavioral effects. The biologic findings of anorexia nervosa appear to be homeostatic adaptations to starvation.

Clinical Manifestations

There are no characteristic pathologic or physiologic findings, and no consistent psychiatric diagnosis is found. However, the consistency of the behavioral and medical features supports the idea that anorexia nervosa is a distinct clinical entity.

PSYCHOLOGIC AND BEHAVIORAL FEATURES

Patients are not truly anorectic but *struggle against hunger* to achieve an unrealistic degree of weight loss. Interestingly, they are preoccupied with food and exhibit bizarre food preferences or elaborately prepare food for others. For most anorectics, weight loss is accomplished through dietary restriction and exercise (restrictor subgroup), although up to 50% also self-induce vomiting or take purgatives (bulimic subgroup).[36]

Anorectic persons exhibit *perceptual disturbances* in overestimating their body width and insisting they are too fat despite profound weight loss. Their assessment of the body habitus of others is not affected. Anorectic persons may also exhibit abnormalities in perceiving or reporting enteroceptive stimuli. They have altered satiety,[37] deny fatigue, and fail to recognize emotional states such as anger and depression.

Disturbances in mood are manifest primarily as depression. Several studies report major affective disorder to be present in about 50% of these patients.[35,38]

Defects in conceptual thought and abstract reasoning may also occur. Patients display a pervasive sense of ineffectiveness, feeling as if they are controlled by their environment. Failing to see the "grays" in life, patients also tend to view situations in extremes, interpreting events in a rigid and highly personalized form.

MEDICAL FEATURES

Most of the physical, metabolic, and endocrine abnormalities of anorexia nervosa are also seen in starvation secondary to other conditions. The severity of the findings correlates with the nutritional state.

The *physical signs* of anorexia nervosa include loss of subcutaneous fat and bony prominences. Secondary sexual features will be absent in the patient who develops anorexia nervosa before puberty. Core temperature, blood pressure, and pulse are decreased. Examination of the skin may reveal brittle hair and nails, decreased fat stores, acrocyanosis, and downy hair (lanugo).[39] There may also be a yellow discoloration of the skin (hypercarotenemia).

There are a variety of *endocrine abnormalities*.[26] Gonadal dysfunction for women presents as amenorrhea and in up to half occurs before weight loss occurs.[40] Male anorectic patients lose libido and are infertile. Patients have decreased follicle-stimulating (FSH) and luteinizing hormone (LH). They do not exhibit secretory bursts of LH throughout the day in response to endogenous luteinizing hormone releasing factor (LHRF), indicating an abnormality in hypothalamic regulation. This "immature" secretory pattern, characteristic of prepubertal girls, may result from the loss of a critical amount of body fat content or, as seen in female dancers and athletes,[41] from the physiologic effects of stress or exercise. Normal menses may reoccur with weight gain, when body fat content reaches 22%.

Patients may exhibit clinical features suggestive of hypothyroidism, such as decreased vital signs, dry skin, constipation, cold intolerance, and a delayed ankle jerk, although lethargy is not usually observed until severe malnutrition develops. Serum T_4 and TSH are low or normal, and there is a delayed TSH response to TRH.[42] T_3 levels tend to be low, with a corresponding increase in reverse T_3, the relatively inactive isomer of T_3. Under the stress of malnutrition, the liver preferentially deiodinates T_4 to rT_3. The clinical findings of mild hypothyroidism may arise from a decreased availability of the more active T_3 isomer, which preferentially binds to the thyroid receptor. However, free thyroxine tends to be normal. Clinically significant hypothyroidism does not occur, and treatment with exogenous thyroid is not indicated. These abnormalities reverse with weight gain.[42]

Anorectic patients usually have normal or slightly elevated plasma cortisol levels with decreased urinary levels of 17-hydroxycorticosteroids. This is due to a decrease in the metabolic clearance of cortisol from plasma with an increase in cortisol-binding capacity. The 24-hour cortisol production rate and basal ACTH secretion are normal. The response to ACTH stimulation may be increased, and the response to metyrapone stimulation is normal. Decreased libido and, in males, delayed virilization may be due to a shift of androgen metabolism from the 5α-reductase enzyme system (yielding testosterone and congeners) to the 5β-reductase system, producing the weaker androgen etiocholanolone.

Human growth hormone (HGH) levels are normal or slightly elevated. Concurrently, there is a decrease in somatomedin levels. This growth-promoting peptide is produced by the liver and other tissues under the influence of HGH. Somatomedin mediates the anabolic effects of HGH but not its lipolytic effects. Thus, anorectic patients and other malnourished persons maintain their adipose tissue breakdown (increased HGH) without growth effects.

Changes in *GI function* may underlie the common complaints of early satiety, bloating, vomiting, and constipation reported by these patients. There is physiologic evidence of gastric electrical dysrhythmias, impaired antral contraction, and delayed emptying of a solid meal.[43] Improvement in gastric emptying with domperidone[44,45] suggests that dysfunction of dopaminergic peptides or their receptors in the enteric nervous system (ENS) as well as the CNS may exist in anorexia nervosa.

Depletion of tissue protein stores secondary to malnutrition may explain some of the GI complications seen in these patients. Acute gastric or duodenal dilatation may result from rapid refeeding in the malnourished, protein-deficient patient.[46] Similarly, refeeding pancreatitis and diarrhea also occur.[26] The diarrhea may be due to diet-induced depletion of pancreatic and intestinal brush border enzymes. Elevations occur in serum amylase of salivary and pancreatic origin, and ultrasonography has shown decreased echogenicity of the pancreas, possibly due to atrophy.[47] These abnormalities revert to normal after refeeding.

Chronic constipation may result from decreased oral intake, decreased intestinal transit, laxative/diuretic abuse, or any combination. With the sudden development of constipation, the possibility of fecal impaction should be considered. Barium enema studies, with or without laxative abuse, may show a dilated, atonic, and ahaustral colon. Laxative abuse can be confirmed by the presence of melanosis coli or testing for phenolphthalein in the stool.

Patients exhibit *depressed cardiovascular function* with a decreased cardiac O_2 consumption, left ventricular wall thickness, cardiac chamber size, and blood pressure.[48] These are adaptive responses to malnutrition and decreased catecholamine levels. Electrocardiographic changes include bradycardia, decreased QRS amplitude, prolonged QT interval, nonspecific ST segment changes, and U waves. Patients may also develop arrhythmias (tachycardia, sinus arrest, and ectopic atrial, junctional or ventricular rhythms) and sudden death either due to the primary disorder or to metabolic disturbances secondary to purgation. Death from ipecac (emetine) cardiomyopathy has been reported.[49]

Laboratory findings include leukopenia and decreased white cell function, anemia and thrombocytopenia, and hypocomplementemia may occur. However, anorectic patients do not seem to have a greater susceptibility to infection. Biochemical findings include increases in gamma-glutamyltranspeptidase, lactate dehydrogenase, ALT, AST, and cholesterol, and decreases in serum proteins, albumin and globulins, and blood sugar.[50] In contrast, patients who are anorectic secondary to other diseases tend to have a more pronounced drop in albumin and increases in serum globulins. Steatosis or nonspecific periportal infiltrates appear to be the basis for the liver chemistry findings[46] and usually require no further evaluation. The elevated serum carotene and vitamin A levels are due either to an excess intake of dietary carotenoids or to an acquired defect in the utilization or metabolism of these compounds.

Diagnosis

It is difficult to know when the diagnosis should be made because social and cultural factors promote and maintain anorectic behaviors. Five percent of college women without weight loss display attitudes and behaviors consistent with the diagnosis.[51] Within some population groups (e.g., high-fashion models, ballerinas), low body weight is *de rigueur*,[52] and the associated anorectic behaviors are accepted. The diagnosis of anorexia nervosa should be considered when the person voluntarily withholds food in the face of hunger to achieve an unrealistic degree of weight loss and becomes psychosocially dysfunctional. Diagnosis is confirmed by identifying the described behavioral features and by excluding any treatable medical disorders.

Use of clinical criteria for anorexia nervosa as proposed by the American Psychiatric Association[53] (Table 32-6) is recommended. The differential diagnosis in a young population includes primary endocrine disorders (panhypopituitarism, Addison's disease, hyperthyroidism, diabetes mellitus), GI disease (Crohn's disease, celiac sprue), chronic infection (tuberculosis), neoplastic disorders (lymphoma), and, rarely, CNS disorders (hypothalamic tumor, vascular malformation).

Screening laboratory evaluation should include a CBC, sedimentation rate, electrolytes, blood urea nitrogen, liver chemistries, serum amylase, serum carotene, thyroid function studies, and possibly fasting cortisol level.[26] Particularly in the adolescent patient, or the older patient with recent weight loss, an assessment might also be done for Crohn's disease[54] (sigmoidoscopy/colonoscopy, small bowel series) and malabsorptive disorders (stool examination for fat and parasites, small bowel biopsy). A CT scan or specialized endocrine studies (e.g., TRH stimulation, ACTH stimulation) may be indicated if a CNS disorder or pituitary dysfunction is suspected.

All patients should receive a nutritional assessment to determine the severity of the malnutrition and to establish a baseline for follow-up. Height and weight are usually sufficient. Patients with marked weight loss should have other nutritional measures (serum transferrin, albumin, measurement of triceps skinfold thickness, skin test reactivity to *Candida* antigen) obtained to gauge progress in nutritional treatment. A Prognostic Nutritional Index,[55] which is predictive of perioperative morbidity, can be used as a quantitative measure of nutritional status for these patients.[26]

Treatment

The treatment of patients with anorexia nervosa involves nutritional restitution with alleviation of medical complications and modification of the psycho-environmental factors that promote anorectic behavior. No one treatment is superior, and a multidisciplinary approach involving medical, psychiatric/psychologic, and nutritional personnel is needed.[26]

While the gastroenterology consultant may play an important role in the initial evaluation and the treatment of complications, the primary care physician is responsible for the ongoing medical and nutritional care and the provision of psychologic support. This includes: (1) fostering a sense of autonomy in the patient by encouraging her to take personal responsibility in the treatment plan, (2) remaining objective, consistent, and honest so as to develop and maintain the patient's sense of trust, (3) working with the family in the treatment, and (4) serving as liaison and patient advocate with the various consultants and counselors. At times, when complications develop, or when the patient seeks out "the expert," the primary care physician's involvement may seem to lessen. Because maintaining a long-term physician–patient relationship is essential, the gastroenterology or nutritional consultant must actively involve the referring physician in long-term treatment decisions.

All anorectic patients require some *dietary management*, although nutritional supplementation is not needed unless the patient is at risk of medical complications. With mild degrees of weight loss (e.g., weight 80% of ideal or better), nutritional and psychologic counseling is sufficient. The physician's role includes personal support, education about adolescent body development and its relationship to diet, and scheduling of periodic visits to observe for clinical deterioration. With moderate malnutrition (weight 65% to 80% of ideal), nutritional supplements may be necessary, but hospitalization usually is not required. Oral replacement with a palatable, nutritionally complete formulation (e.g., Ensure Plus) may help, with the goal being intake of 1050 to 2100 J above daily energy requirement. In some cases, metoclopramide or bethanecol may be used to improve gastric emptying and the patient's tolerance of larger meals. With severe malnutrition (weight less than 65% of ideal), hospitalization with active involvement of the gastroenterologist and nutritional service is usually required. Oral replacement may be attempted, but if the patient is unable or unwilling to comply, tube feeding into the duodenum[56] and supplementation with prokinetic agents may be necessary. The patient can receive 1680 to 2520 J above daily caloric need, with the goal being no more than 1 to 2 kg weight gain per week.

If the patient is severely malnourished and tolerates a feeding tube poorly or refuses to eat, *parenteral nutrition* may be considered. The peripheral venous route is preferred because central hyperalimentation is more expensive and is associated with a greater frequency of complications. If a central venous route is chosen, it should be supervised by an experienced hyperalimentation team. Caloric delivery should begin with one half of the daily requirement, progressing to full requirement by day 3 or 4. Electrolytes, serum chemistries, and hepatic and renal function must be monitored.

The goal of enteral or parenteral supplementation is to get the patient slowly to a body weight out of the range of medical risk. Rapid refeeding produces excess water stores and edema, secondary metabolic disturbances, and possibly cardiac failure. Continued nutritional intervention beyond achieving a dry weight of 80% ideal is not recommended. These procedures are psychologically invasive and minimize the patient's involvement in treatment, thereby increasing anxiety and resistance. Furthermore, supplements interfere with appetite and with attempts to reestablish normal eating patterns.

No *pharmacologic agents* are of proven value. However, data suggesting a biologic relationship between eating disorders and affective disturbance (see Psychologic and Behavioral Features) provide a theoretical basis for the use of antidepressants in eating disorders, and recent clinical studies show some benefit, particularly for patients with bulimia.[57] Chlorpromazine, lithium carbonate, and cyproheptadine have been reported effective in small short-term inpatient treatment trials.[26] The use of pharmacologic agents should be ancillary to the long-term nutritional and behavioral approaches.

Psychotherapy is used to help the patient modify the aberrant eating behavior and to improve psychosocial function. Behavior modification is an effective means of achieving short-term weight gain. Family therapy offers the best potential for long-term benefit because treatment is directed toward modifying the family interactions that maintain the anorectic behavior. Insight therapy may occasionally help the motivated patient. Further discussion of psychotherapeutic treatment approaches can be found elsewhere.[58]

Prognosis

The short-term prognosis is generally favorable.[26] Over three fourths of patients attain a body weight above 75% of ideal. Menses resume in at least half. However, less than one third of patients resume normal eating patterns. The long-term prognosis is variable, and relapses requiring hospitalization occur in about half the patients. Mortality among hospitalized patients averages 6%, with the main causes of death being inanition and severe electrolyte disturbances; suicide occurs in 1%.

A recent analysis of the clinical and behavioral factors predicting long-term outcome (at 6.4 years) indicates that psychosocial factors play a more important role than clinical interventions, including psychotherapy.[59] The best predictors related to the degree of social integration (e.g., with father, spouse, children, friends, coworkers) that the patient achieved. Interestingly, the type of medical treatment, return to work, and a good relationship with a psychotherapist were not sufficient to ensure a positive prognosis. To quote the author: "If, because a patient's life is at stake, and tube feeding is required, it should be carried out. . . . The criterion for discharge is not the patient's weight, but rather the question whether she can convincingly name at least one or two persons who will accompany her into her future life and who will keep in touch with her. . . . In those cases where no positive social relationship exists, the fostering of such relations must be the first and foremost objective of follow-up outpatient therapy."[59]

BULIMIA NERVOSA

For me, binge eating is continuous eating lasting from 2 hours to 2 days. I will eat any kind of food, regardless of when I ate my last meal, how much I ate, etc. It's almost an unconscious act; sometimes I'm not even aware that I'm eating. Sometimes I can't remember what or when I ate. I only know that I've stuffed myself. At times I will "come to" in the middle of stuffing myself and then struggle with the decision to stop eating or finish.
Anonymous[26]

Bulimia, derived from the Greek word meaning "ox-eating," is a compulsive behavior characterized by episodes of overeating (binging) usually followed by acts to "undo" the threatened weight gain with self-induced vomiting, cathartic or diuretic abuse (purging), fasting or excessive physical activity. As shown in this poem by a woman with bulimia, the experience can be associated with a sense of both depersonalization and gratification. Bulimia defines a behavior that is also found in patients with anorexia nervosa. However, patients having the *syndrome* of bulimia nervosa (DSM-IIIR 307.51) are distinguished by their having normal body size (Table 32-7). While some argue that the two groups seem more alike than different,[60,61] bulimics tend to have less body image distortion, are more aware that their secret compulsive behaviors are aberrant, and may be more accepting of treatment.[26]

Epidemiology[26]

Bulimia was only first reported as a diagnostic entity in 1979,[62] yet its prevalence is high and the disorder has probably existed a long time. Binge eating at least once occurs in half of the population, and weekly binge eating is reported by up to 15%. Self-induced vomiting or laxative/diuretic abuse associated with binge eating occurs in up to 20% of college students, and 4% report this type of behavior at least weekly. Bulimia is almost exclusively diagnosed in young (< 30 years) women (> 95%). Most all bulimics carry on their activity secretly; less than one third have discussed their behavior with their physician, and in one survey only 2.5% were under medical care.

Etiology and Pathogenesis

Patients commonly report obesity during childhood or adolescence, and the onset of bulimia is associated with a conscious decision to diet. At some point, the patients lose control of their compulsion to eat large amounts of "forbidden foods" and do binge. Self-induced vomiting is discovered as a convenient method of reestablishing weight control. Thus, a binge–purge cycle becomes established.

As with anorexia nervosa, societal influences seem to play a prominent role in the desire to be thin. Also, there are historical and social precedents for self-induced vomiting. The ancient Ro-

---

TABLE 32-7
Diagnostic Criteria for 307.51 Bulimia Nervosa

A. Recurrent episodes of binge eating (rapid consumption of a large amount of food in a discrete period of time).
B. A feeling of lack of control over eating behavior during the eating binges.
C. The person regularly engages in either self-induced vomiting, use of laxatives or diuretics, strict dieting or fasting or rigorous exercise to prevent weight gain.
D. A minimum average of two binge eating episodes per week for at least 3 months.
E. Persistent overconcern with body shape and weight.

From American Psychiatric Association. Eating disorders: 307.51 Bulimia nervosa. In: Diagnostic and statistical manual of mental disorders—DSM-IIIR. Washington, DC: American Psychiatric Association, 1987:67.

mans ate lavishly and then induced vomiting at feasts. Socialites who must attend many dinner parties may induce vomiting. Bulimics report coming from families that emphasize hearty eating and where food is used to celebrate happy times and to console during sad times. For these patients, eating takes on greater meaning than simply to achieve nutritional benefit, and this may help explain the emotional and behavioral investment present around food and eating. Therefore, social mores may be important in the clinical expression of the disorder.

A role for CCK (a satiety-inducing nerve-gut peptide) as a biologic determinant of the disorder has been recently supported by a study showing that bulimic patients, when compared to normal controls, have a blunted meal-induced secretion of CCK.[9] Furthermore, the authors reported that these abnormalities improved when a small number of patients were treated with a tricyclic antidepressant. Further research is needed to confirm these findings.

Clinical Manifestations[26,46,63]

The characteristic behavioral feature is the *binge–purge cycle:* an eating compulsion with a failure to achieve or to respond to normal satiety. Typically, these episodes occur secretly and are often associated with feelings of frustration, loneliness, or the sight of tempting food items. Binges are usually planned, and the preparation is associated with anxiety and excitement. During the binge, high-calorie "junk" foods are pleasurably consumed. The binge is usually terminated when feelings of guilt or physical discomfort such as nausea, abdominal pain, or headache occur. At this point, the patient self-induces vomiting or takes cathartics or laxatives.

Bulimics generally look healthy, and their behaviors are often unnoticed by friends and family. They are usually more outgoing than their anorectic counterparts. Some patients exhibit impulsive or antisocial behaviors such as drug abuse, kleptomania, and sexual promiscuity. The patient who seeks help does so because of feelings of guilt, anxiety, or depression, or because she is no longer able to continue the habit and still function in daily activities. Therefore, physicians tend to see the "tip of the iceberg": bulimic patients who have become dysphoric or dysfunctional from their disorder.

The *medical findings* of bulimia are consequences of the vomiting and laxative abuse. The physical examination may reveal parotid or salivary gland swelling due to vomiting, nutritional disturbances, or alcoholism. The knuckles may be bruised from their rubbing against the upper incisors during the induction of vomiting. Pharyngitis, dental and gingival erosions result from reflux of gastric acid, and conjunctival hemorrhages may occur from retching.

Frequent vomiting may also be complicated by esophagitis, esophageal erosions or strictures, Boerhaave's syndrome, Mallory-Weiss tears, or aspiration pneumonitis. Electrolyte disturbances are common, affecting up to 50% of patients.[36] Hypokalemic, hypochloremic, metabolic alkalosis due to loss of H^+, Cl^-, and K^+ is the most common metabolic complication, and this may lead to cardiac arrhythmias or renal injury. Secondary metabolic disturbances may produce weakness, tetany, and seizures. Emetics, such as ipecac, may produce cardiac conduction defects and arrhythmias. Stimulant laxatives can produce a "cathartic colon" with degeneration of Auerbach's plexus.

The majority of patients are clinically depressed by the time of clinical presentation, and 5% have attempted suicide. As stated, bulimia may be a manifestation of an underlying depressive disorder because a large proportion of patients have first-degree relatives with major affective disorders.

Diagnosis

The diagnosis of bulimia is based on recognition of the binge eating pattern and the exclusion of other medical disease to explain the behavior. Diagnostic criteria are listed in Table 32-7. The differential diagnosis in this young and otherwise healthy population is limited and would include schizophrenia, use of oral contraceptives, seizures, and rare neurologic disorders (Klüver-Bucy syndrome: a disorder of bilateral temporal lobe damage associated with indiscriminate sexual behavior, excessive orality and placidity; Kleine-Levin syndrome: a sleep disorder associated with hypersomnia and overeating).

Treatment

The goal of treatment is to help the patient overcome the urge to overeat. Bulimic patients recognize their behaviors as maladaptive. Compared to anorectic patients, they are more aware of associated psychologic difficulties and are more willing to work with physicians and counselors in a treatment plan.

The current psychotherapeutic technique is cognitive-behavioral treatment: the patient identifies the abnormal behaviors and uses behavioral techniques to extinguish them, thereby accomplishing greater self-control. The treatment is safe and probably effective, at least in the short-term.

Antidepressants have been reported successful in decreasing the binge activity and increasing the patient's sense of well-being. They may be more effective for bulimic patients than for patients with anorexia nervosa.[57]

RUMINATION SYNDROME[64,65]

Rumination syndrome or merycism is an eating disorder in which the person repetitively regurgitates small amounts of food from the stomach, rechews the food, and reswallows it. The disorder has been recognized as a medical curiosity for over 300 years, and ruminators have been known for their tendencies to offer public performances.

Infants frequently ruminate, and the disorder is described among institutionalized adults and children with emotional and intellectual deficits. However, there is no characteristic psychologic profile or psychiatric diagnosis reported. There may be three subpopulations with the disorder: emotionally deprived or mentally retarded children and adults, persons in whom the behavior develops as a learned maladaptive habit worsening at times of stress, and persons in whom rumination is associated with bulimia. A familial association is reported, although the role for genetic factors in the pathogenesis is not established.

The prevalence of rumination in adults is unknown because, generally, physicians are unfamiliar with the clinical features. Patients who seek treatment report symptoms of weight loss, regurgitation, or vomiting, and may express concern of an underlying medical disorder. Parents may bring the adolescent child to the physician because of halitosis or dental problems.

Rumination in humans is not the same physiologic event as in ruminant animals because reverse peristalsis does not occur. X-ray and manometric studies indicate that an episode is initiated by a belch or swallow, at which time the lower esophageal sphincter pressure is lowered, creating a common channel between the stomach and esophagus. At the same time, diaphragmatic and rectus muscle contractions raise the intraabdominal pressure, thereby leading to regurgitation. When the upper esophageal sphincter is relaxed, food is ejected into the mouth where it is expectorated or reswallowed. The manometric pattern is considered characteristic.[65]

Diagnosis depends on identifying the typical clinical features in the absence of other organic or psychiatric disease. While characteristic physiologic findings exist, extensive testing is not needed. As with other functional disorders, an awareness of the condition and a complete history and physical examination may be all that is needed. In some cases, medical conditions such as esophageal stricture, reflux esophagitis, intestinal obstruction, or esophageal motor disorders (achalasia, diffuse esophageal spasm) need to be excluded by x-ray, video fluoroscopy, and manometry. Because the disorder appears to be a learned maladaptive habit, behavioral modification and biofeedback techniques are recommended as treatment approaches. Treatment may be difficult because the act is pleasurable to some, and these patients may not be as motivated.

The reader is directed to Chapter 17, Carbohydrate Assimilation; Chapter 18, Intestinal Lipid Absorption; Chapter 19, Protein Digestion and Assimilation; Chapter 20, Vitamins and Minerals; Chapter 21, General Nutritional Principles; Chapter 48, Approach to the Patient Requiring Nurtitional Supplementation; Chapter 50, Approach to the Patient with Drug or Alcohol Dependency; Chapter 57, Esophageal Tumors; Chapter 63, Tumors of the Stomach; Chapter 70, Tumors and Other Neoplastic Diseases of the Small Intestine; Chapter 71, Celiac Disease; Chapter 74, Short Bowel Syndrome; Chapter 84, Malignant Tumors of the Colon; Chapter 90, Pancreatic Adenocarcinoma; Chapter 109, Vascular Insufficiency; Chapter 130, Psychiatric Evaluation and Management in Gastrointestinal Illness; and the corresponding chapters in the Atlas.

REFERENCES

1. Mrosovsky N, Powley TL. Set points for body weight and fat. Behav Biol 1977;20:205.
2. Alpers DH, Rosenberg IH. Eating behavior and nutrient requirements. In: Sleisenger MH, Fordtran JS, eds. Gastrointestinal disease: Pathophysiology, diagnosis, management. Philadelphia: WB Saunders, 1989:1971.
3. Herzog DB, Copeland PM. Bulimia nervosa—Psyche and satiety. N Engl J Med 1988;319:716.
4. Morley JE, Levine AS. The central control of appetite. Lancet 1983;1:398.
5. Smith GP, Gibbs J. The effect of gut peptides on hunger, satiety, and food intake in humans. Ann NY Acad Sci 1987;499:132.
6. Smith GP. Satiety effect of gastrointestinal hormones. In: Beers RF Jr, Bassett EG, eds. Polypeptide hormones. New York: Raven Press, 1980:413.
7. Smith GP. The peripheral control of appetite. Lancet 1983;2:88.
8. Smith GP, Gibbs J. Gut peptides and postprandial satiety. Fed Proc 1984;43:2889.
9. Geracioti TD Jr, Liddle RA. Impaired cholecystokinin secretion in bulimia nervosa. N Engl J Med 1988;319:683.
10. Johnson HD, Laws JW. The cardia in swallowing, eructation, and vomiting. Lancet 1966;2:1268.
11. McCarthy LE, Borison HL, Spiegel PK, Friedlander RM. Vomiting: Radiographic and oscillographic correlates in the decerebrate cat. Gastroenterology 1974;67:1126.
12. Feldman M. Nausea and vomiting. In: Sleisenger MH, Fordtran JS, eds. Gastrointestinal disease: Pathophysiology, diagnosis, management. Philadelphia: WB Saunders, 1989:222.
13. Sourkes TL. Neural and neuroendocrine functions of dopamine. Psychoneuroendocrinology 1975;1:69.
14. Heizer WH. Weight loss. In: Dornbrand L, Fletcher R, Hoole A, Pickard G, eds. Clinical problems in ambulatory care medicine. Boston: Little, Brown & Co, 1990: in press.
15. Connor Greene PA. Gender differences in body weight perception and weight-loss strategies of college students. Women Health 1988;14:27.
16. Ramboer C, Verhamme M, Vermeire L. Patients' perception of involuntary weight loss: Implications of underestimation and overestimation. Br Med J [Clin Res] 1985;291:1091.
17. Marton KI, Sox HC Jr, Krupp JR. Involuntary weight loss: Diagnostic and prognostic significance. Ann Intern Med 1981;95:568.
18. Robbins LJ. Evaluation of weight loss in the elderly. Geriatrics 1989;44:31.
19. Rabinovitz M, Pitlik SD, Leifer M, Garty M, Rosenfeld JB. Unintentional weight loss. A retrospective analysis of 154 cases. Arch Intern Med 1986;146:186.
20. Huerta G, Viniegra L. Involuntary weight loss as a clinical problem. Rev Invest Clin 1989;41:5.
21. Leduc D, Rouge PE, Rousset H, Maitre A, Champay Hirsch AS. Clinical study of 105 cases of isolated weight loss in internal medicine. Rev Med Interne 1988;9:480.
22. Garfinkel PE, Garner DM, Kaplan AS, Rodin G, Kennedy S. Differential diagnosis of emotional disorders that cause weight loss. Can Med Assoc J 1983;129:939.
23. Garfinkel PE, Kaplan AS, Garner DM, Darby PL. The differentiation of vomiting/weight loss as a conversion disorder from anorexia nervosa. Am J Psychiatry 1983;140:1019.
24. Kurtzman FD, Yager J, Landsverk J, Wiesmeier E, Bodurka DC. Eating disorders among selected female student populations at UCLA. J Am Diet Assoc 1989;89:45.
25. Pope HG Jr, Hudson JI, Yurgelun-Todd D. Prevalence of anorexia nervosa and bulimia in three student populations. Int J Eating Disorders 1984;3:45.
26. Balaa MA, Drossman DA. Anorexia nervosa and bulimia: The eating disorders. Dis Mon 1985;31:1.
27. Hanson P. Anorexia. NC Med J 1989;50:500.
28. Bruch H. Eating disorders: Obesity, anorexia nervosa and the person within. New York: Basic Books, 1973:3.
29. Garfield PE. To fast or not to fast: Part I. The claim for fasting in the popular literature. Curr Concepts Nutr 1981;24:5.
30. Margo JL. Anorexia nervosa in males. A comparison with female patients. Br J Psychiatry 1987;151:80.
31. Garner DM, Garfinkel PE, Olmstead MP. An overview of sociocultural factors in the development of anorexia nervosa. In: Darby PL, Garfinkel PE, Garner DM, eds. Anorexia nervosa: Recent developments in research. New York: Alan R Liss, 1983:66.
32. Herzog DB, Copeland PM. Eating disorders. N Engl J Med 1985;313:295.
33. Hall RC, Tice L, Beresford TP, Wooley B, Hall AK. Sexual abuse in patients with anorexia nervosa and bulimia. Psychosomatics 1989;30:73.
34. Holland AG. Anorexia nervosa: A study of 34 twin pairs and one set of triplets. Br J Psychiatry 1984;145:414.

35. Lotstra F, Sevy S, Medlewicz J. Genetic and biological markers in psychosomatic research. Adv Psychosom Med 1987;17:252.
36. Halmi KA. Anorexia nervosa and bulimia. Annu Rev Med 1987;38: 373.
37. Owen WP, Halmi KA, Gibbs J, Smith GP. Satiety responses in eating disorders. J Psychiatr Res 1985;19:279.
38. Laessle RG, Kittl S, Fichter MM, Wittchen HU, Pirke KM. Major affective disorder in anorexia nervosa and bulimia. A descriptive diagnostic study. Br J Psychiatry 1987;151:785.
39. Gupta MA, Gupta AK, Haberman HF. Dermatologic signs in anorexia nervosa and bulimia nervosa. Arch Dermatol 1987;123:1386.
40. Halmi KA. Anorexia nervosa. Demographic and clinical features in 94 cases. Psychosom Med 1974;36:18.
41. Vigersky RA. Hypothalamic-pituitary functions in anorexia nervosa and simple weight loss. In: Goodstein EL, ed. Eating and weight disorders. New York: Springer, 1983:105.
42. Tamai H, Mori K, Matsubayashi S, et al. Hypothalamic-pituitary-thyroidal dysfunctions in anorexia nervosa. Psychother Psychosom 1986;46:127.
43. Abell TL, Malagelada JR, Lucas AR, et al. Gastric electromechanical and neurohormonal function in anorexia nervosa. Gastroenterology 1987;93:958.
44. Stacher G, Kiss A, Wiesnagrotzki S, Bergmann H, Hobart J, Schneider C. Oesophageal and gastric motility disorders in patients categorised as having primary anorexia nervosa. Gut 1986;27:1120.
45. Russell DM, Freedman ML, Feiglin DH, Jeejeeboy KN, Swinson RP, Garfinkel PE. Delayed gastric emptying and improvement with domperidone in a patient with anorexia nervosa. Am J Psychiatry 1983;140:1235.
46. Cuellar RE, Van Thiel DH. Gastrointestinal consequences of the eating disorders: Anorexia nervosa and bulimia. Am J Gastroenterol 1986;81:1113.
47. Cox KL, Cannon RA, Ament ME, Phillips HE, Schaffer CB. Biochemical and ultrasonic abnormalities of the pancreas in anorexia nervosa. Dig Dis Sci 1983;28:225.
48. Fohlin L, Freyschuss U, Bjarbe B. Function and dimensions of the circulatory system in anorexia nervosa. Acta Pediatr Scand 1978;67: 11.
49. Friedman EJ. Death from ipecac intoxication in a patient with anorexia nervosa. Am J Psychiatry 1984;141:702.
50. Umeki S. Biochemical abnormalities of the serum in anorexia nervosa. J Nerv Ment Dis 1988;176:503.
51. Button EJ, Whitehouse A. Subclinical anorexia nervosa. Psychol Med 1981;11:509.
52. Frisch RE, Wyshak G, Vincent L. Delayed menarche and amenorrhea in ballet dancers. N Engl J Med 1980;303:17.
53. American Psychiatric Association. Eating disorders: 307.10 Anorexia nervosa. In: Diagnostic and statistical manual of mental disorders—DSM-IIIR. Washington, DC: American Psychiatric Association, 1987:65.
54. Jenkins AP, Treasure J, Thompson RP. Crohn's disease presenting as anorexia nervosa. Br Med J [Clin Res] 1988;296:699.
55. Buzby GP, Mullen JL, Mathews DC. Prognostic nutritional index in gastrointestinal surgery. Am J Surg 1980;139:160.
56. Allison SP. How I feed patients enterally. Proc Nutr Soc 1986;45: 163.
57. Herzog DB, Brotman AW, Bradburn IS. Treating eating disorders with antidepressants. Aust Paediatr J 1988;24:169.
58. Crisp AH, Norton KR, Jurczak S, Bowyer C, Duncan S. A treatment approach to anorexia nervosa—25 years on. J Psychiatr Res 1985;19: 393.
59. Engel K. Prognostic factors in anorexia nervosa. Psychother Psychosom 1988;49:137.
60. Scott RL, Baroffio JR. An MMPI analysis of similarities and differences in three classifications of eating disorders: Anorexia nervosa, bulimia, and morbid obesity. J Clin Psych 1986;42:708.
61. Garner DM, Garfinkel PE, O'Shaughnessy M. The validity of the distinction between bulimia with and without anorexia nervosa. Am J Psychiatry 1985;142:581.
62. Russell G. Bulimia nervosa: An ominous variant of anorexia nervosa. Psychol Med 1979;9:429.
63. Harris RT. Bulimia and related serious eating disorders with medical complications. Ann Intern Med 1983;99:800.
64. Rumination. Lancet 1987;1:200.
65. Amarnath RP, Abell TL, Malagelada JT. The rumination syndrome in adults. A characteristic manometric pattern. Ann Intern Med 1986;105:513.
66. American Psychiatric Association. Eating disorders: 307.51 Bulimia nervosa. In: Diagnostic and statistical manual of mental disorders—DSM-IIIR. Washington, DC: American Psychiatric Association, 1987:67.

33

Approach to the Patient with Nausea and Vomiting

ANN OUYANG

Nausea and vomiting are symptoms that occur commonly throughout life. Nausea is a *sensation* that may or may not lead to vomiting. The pathways controlling the perception of nausea are poorly understood because the sensory nature of this problem makes it difficult to study in an animal model. It has been assumed that, in animals, the presence of many of the behavioral findings that are commonly associated with vomiting represent nausea when seen in the absence of the act of vomiting. Retching and vomiting are separate motor acts, each associated with a well-characterized group of motor activities that involves somatic muscle groups, including respiratory muscles (i.e., intercostal muscles and diaphragm), and muscle groups resulting in posturing as well as smooth muscle in the gastrointestinal (GI) tract and oropharynx.[1-4] Retching usually, but not invariably, culminates in vomiting. The symptoms of nausea and vomiting commonly occur together, although not always. The fact that a patient complains of both symptoms or of one alone may provide insight into the specific underlying disorder. Several other symptoms (regurgitation, anorexia, and early satiety) may be called vomiting or nausea by the patient. They suggest specific and different underlying problems, and the true complaint of the patient should be determined by a careful history. *Regurgitation,* the act by which food is brought back into the mouth without the constellation of motor and autonomic activity that characterizes vomiting, is a symptom of either free gastroesophageal reflux or an obstructed esophagus, whether obstructed mechanically by a stricture or tumor or physiologically, as in achalasia or diffuse esophageal spasm. *Anorexia* is the loss of appetite such that the patient does not even feel the urge to eat. It may or may not be associated with nausea. Patients with nausea, particularly if it is chronic, do not necessarily lose their appetite. *Early satiety* is often confused with anorexia. Specifically, early satiety is the feeling of being full after eating an unusually small quantity of food. The patient may have a normal desire for food prior to starting a meal. It is important to determine which symptom is being described by the patient during an evaluation.

PATHOPHYSIOLOGY OF NAUSEA AND VOMITING

Most research on the pathophysiology of vomiting has been conducted in animal models and should be applied to man with caution. There is marked species variation in the vomiting reflex. For example, no vomiting is seen in rodents with stimuli that induce vomiting in dogs.

Figure 33-1 is a schematic of the pathways involved in the vomiting response. In cats, two areas of the brain stem have been implicated in the vomiting reflex. Intravenously injected apomorphine results in vomiting, a response that is no longer present after ablation of either the vomiting center in the medulla or the area postrema in the floor of the fourth ventricle. The area postrema is called the chemoreceptor trigger zone (CTZ). Direct electrical stimulation does not result in vomiting, suggesting that it is important for detecting circulating emetic agents. The area postrema is a vascular body protruding into the floor of the fourth ventricle. It receives afferent input from the viscera by way of the vagus nerve. The main efferent path from the area postrema is to the nucleus tractus solitarius and to the parabranchial region. Despite the afferent vagal input, stimulation of the gut by agents such as copper sulfate, given orally, results in vomiting that is not abolished by ablation of the CTZ or area postrema, suggesting an alternate afferent pathway by way of the vagus and splanchnic nerves. Direct electrical stimulation of the parvicellular reticular formation (PCRF) or vomiting center in the brain stem will result in the motor acts of retching and vomiting, suggesting that it is the efferent arm of this reflex. Until recently, it has been accepted that this "vomiting center" is a discrete group of neurones that, when stimulated, initiate the prodromal responses and motor responses associated with vomiting and retching. The concept of a "center" was proposed as a result of the observation that there

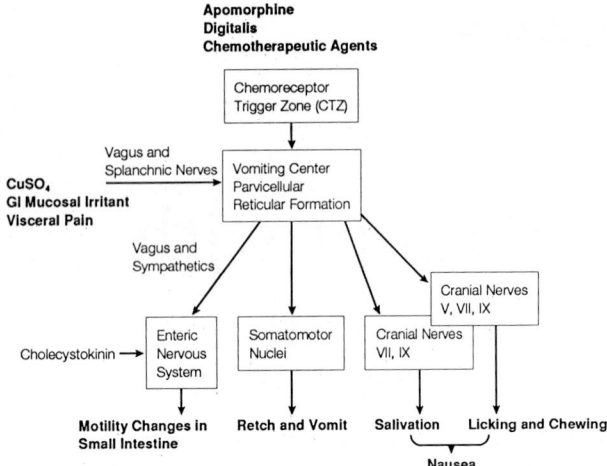

FIGURE 33–1. Relationships of the components of the vomiting center.

was a highly reproducible and complex set of motor and autonomic events associated with vomiting in response to a variety of stimuli, and that ablation of a specific area of the brain stem resulted in loss or reduced sensitivity to these emetic agents. This area of the brain stem was also closely related anatomically to the nuclei controlling a number of autonomic functions that are altered during retching and vomiting, such as salivation and respiration. However, the multiple components of the acts of retching and vomiting are not associated with each other in an all-or-none fashion. The concept of the "vomiting center" is therefore simplistic and probably applies to an area in the brain stem that coordinates the interaction of the several effector nuclei involved in the motor output resulting in vomiting and its associated actions.[5,6] This concept of a vomiting center does serve to outline the general sites of action of emetic agents. The complexity of the true system explains the difficulty in finding an antiemetic agent that is useful in all situations.

The act of vomiting is a highly integrated reflex that involves both the autonomic and somatic nervous systems. Profuse salivation, a major prodromal sign of vomiting, is seen prior to vomiting and is seen with nausea. The salivary glands are innervated by the facial and glossopharyngeal nerves whose cell bodies reside in the parvicellular reticular formation (PCRF or vomiting center). During nausea, tachycardia is prominent and may result from a generalized response to the stress of nausea or as part of the vomiting reflex. During retching, the changes in intrathoracic pressure may activate vagal efferents. Licking and rhythmic chewing are described during the pre-emetic phase, which has been assumed to be the animal equivalent of nausea and which results from the output of the trigeminal, facial, and hypoglossal nuclei. These nuclei appear to receive inputs from the PCRF. Nausea in man and the pre-emetic phase in animals do not inevitably result in vomiting, suggesting that these two phases can be linked but are not controlled by one set of neurones, as might be predicted from a true "center" model.

During retching, the mouth is closed and there is rhythmic, synchronous contraction of the diaphragm, abdominal muscles, and external intercostal muscles with a closed glottis.[2–4] This results in rapid decreases in intrathoracic pressure. The concurrent increases in intra-abdominal pressure result in movement of gastric contents into the esophagus. The gastric contents oscillate between the stomach and the esophagus, while the upper esophageal sphincter is closed between retches and is relaxed during retching. A characteristic posture is adopted.

During vomiting there is contraction of the abdominal rectus muscles and the external oblique muscles. As a result, both intrathoracic and intra-abdominal pressures are positive; the upper esophageal sphincter relaxes and the hiatal region of the diaphragm is inactive, in contrast to retching, resulting in the forceful ejection of intragastric contents through an open mouth and glottis.[7] Again, a characteristic posture is seen.

The gastrointestinal tract demonstrates a variety of changes during retching and vomiting. Acid secretion is decreased during nausea and vomiting. The significance of this event is uncertain. Complex motility changes in the stomach and small intestine have also been described. These changes can be seen both at the level of the membrane potential of the smooth muscle cell, as manifested by changes in the amplitude of slow waves, and at the level of the final event, patterns of contraction. (See ch 8 and 9 for a detailed description of the control of upper intestinal contractile events.) In cats given a number of emetic agents intracerebroventricularly, a characteristic myoelectric pattern preceded emesis.[8] This consisted of a dampening of slow wave amplitude, followed by an intense burst of spike potentials lasting several seconds, which appeared to migrate in an orad direction. This pattern started in the small intestine and could propagate over the proximal 50% of the intestine. Retching and vomiting began a few seconds after the spike burst reached the duodenal electrodes. This orally migrating spike burst was not essential for the development of vomiting in that atropine pretreatment blocked the spike pattern but retching and vomiting were still seen. Similar findings have been reported in dogs.[9] The gastrointestinal motor correlates of vomiting can occur without actual somatic motor acts of retching and vomiting, suggesting separate control pathways.[10] High doses of dopamine given intravenously in the dog induce retrograde duodenal contractions that move chyme back into the stomach. At the same time, gastric emptying is delayed.[11] Whether this peripheral dopaminergic effect is significant in vomiting is uncertain, because studies have suggested that the *peripheral* intestinal motor events seen with vomiting when induced by apomorphine, copper sulfate, or cholecystokinin in the conscious dog are not inhibited by any dopaminergic antagonists. In contrast, the effect of apomorphine, which acts by way of the chemoreceptor trigger zone, and the effect of copper sulfate, which acts at the vomiting center or parvicellular reticular formation, are blocked by D_2 dopaminergic antagonists.[9] Thus, although central stimulation of the vomiting center triggers both gastrointestinal motor events and somatomotor events leading to retching and vomiting, the peripheral pathways are different. These findings are supportive of the concept of a number of closely linked efferent nuclei constituting the vomiting center rather than a group of nuclei with a prepatterned all-or-none response. The findings in man are less well studied, but there is less evidence for reverse peristalsis occurring in the duodenum. Balloons in the duodenum were expelled into the stomach, but a simultaneous contraction in the proximal and distal duodenum was described.[12]

Thus, nausea and vomiting may result from a variety of factors that impact on the sensory pathways from the gut or by way of the circulation or central nervous system on the brain "centers" that integrate the motor pathways concerned with vomiting. The sites at which many a variety of emetic agents act in this pathway are shown in Figure 33-1.

CLINICAL APPROACH TO PATIENTS WITH NAUSEA AND VOMITING

History and Physical Examination

The most important aspects of the history in patients presenting with a complaint of "feeling sick" or being "sick" are the true nature of their symptoms and the duration and severity of symptoms. Patients presenting with anorexia have a differential diagnosis different from those presenting with nausea and vomiting. Regurgitation is often mistaken by the patient as vomiting, but a careful history should ascertain the true nature of the symptom. The differential diagnosis for regurgitation is, again, different from that for nausea and vomiting and includes disorders that cause anatomic or functional obstruction of the esophagus. These include a Zenker's diverticulum, an epiphrenic diverticulum, achalasia, diffuse esophageal spasm, and an esophageal stricture. In addition, free severe gastroesophageal reflux disease may result in regurgitation of food, although there is frequently a prominent postural component to the symptoms. These disorders are covered in detail in other chapters.

Nausea and vomiting are frequently, but not always, associated. Patients rarely present acutely with nausea without vomiting. More insidious nausea without vomiting is often seen and should raise the suspicion of gastroparesis, medication, or pregnancy. In a female of childbearing age, a pregnancy test should be performed before additional invasive tests are considered, particularly if they should involve radiation exposure.

When seeing a patient with true nausea and/or vomiting, one should first elicit whether the condition is acute or chronic. The differential diagnosis of acute nausea and vomiting is listed in Table 33-1, and the differential diagnosis of chronic nausea and vomiting is listed in Table 33-2. Acute nausea and vomiting without marked abdominal pain are usually associated with an infectious, toxic, or drug etiology. Head trauma and a raised intracranial pressure can also present with nausea and vomiting, but the associated injury is usually obvious to the patient. Similarly, an acute abdominal emergency associated with severe visceral pain may result in nausea and vomiting, but the pain becomes the major presenting symptom. The presence, therefore, of specific associated symptoms is very important when evaluating a patient with acute nausea and vomiting. These include abdominal pain, fever, diarrhea, vertigo, and the historical facts of whether family or friends have similar symptoms. Severe abdominal pain other than cramping pain associated with diarrhea should raise the suspicion of visceral

TABLE 33–1
Causes of Acute Nausea and Vomiting

1. Infectious
   Epidemic
     Norwalk agent, Hawaii agent
   Sporadic
     "food poisoning"
       Staphylococcus aureus toxin, *Bacillus cereus* toxin, *Clostridium perfringens* toxin
     Salmonella (nontyphoid)
   Hepatitis A or B
   In immunosuppressed host: gastric herpes simplex infection
   In bone marrow transplant: graft-versus-host disease
   Cutaneous herpes zoster infection
2. Drugs
   Chemotherapeutic agents
   Antibiotics (oral)
   Narcotics
   Cardiac glycosides
   Aminophylline
3. Visceral pain
   Peritonitis from any perforated viscus
   Small-bowel obstruction or pseudo-obstruction
     True mechanical obstruction
       Inguinal, femoral, obturator or incisional hernia
       Adhesions
       Volvulus
       Malrotation
       Internal hernia
       Crohn's disease
       Small intestinal tumor, intrinsic or serosal metastases
       Carcinoid tumor
       Meckel's diverticulum
       Intussusception
       Intestinal duplication
       Intestinal concretions from foreign bodies
       Gallstone ileus
       Parasitic infection: ascariasis
     Intestinal pseudo-obstruction (usually presents as chronic nausea and vomiting: see Table 33–2)
   Acute pancreatitis
   Acute cholecystitis
4. Central nervous system causes
   Vestibular disorders
     Motion sickness, labyrinthitis, migraine equivalent
   Central nervous system tumors or pseudotumors
   Meningitis
   Reye's syndrome
   Head injury
5. Others
   Ionizing radiation
   Radiation therapy

peritoneal irritation or acute mechanical obstruction. If obstruction is suspected, the quality of the vomitus may indicate if there is gastric outlet obstruction (partly digested food, no bile) or intestinal obstruction (bilious vomiting). Gastric outlet obstruction, even if acute, is not usually painful unless the patient has a gastric volvulus. Conversely, the site of mechanical obstruction causing chronic nausea and vomiting is usually gastric. Small-bowel mechanical obstruction is usually painful, with the vomiting often being preceded by severe colicky abdominal pain that may improve temporarily after vomiting.

TABLE 33–2

Differential Diagnosis in a Patient Complaining of Chronic Nausea and Vomiting

Disorders causing true nausea and/or vomiting
1. Gastric
   Causes of mechanical gastric outlet obstruction
      Chronic peptic ulcer disease
      Acute pyloric channel ulcer
      Gastric carcinoma
      Gastric lymphoma
      Duodenal carcinoma
      Pancreatic disease
      Crohn's disease
   Functional gastric outlet obstruction
      Gastroparesis: diabetes, scleroderma, metabolic, idiopathic
      Drug-induced
      Postviral
      Postgastric surgery
      Anorexia nervosa
2. Small intestine
   Mechanical obstruction: usually presents acutely or with intermittent acute symptoms (see Table 33–1)
   Motility disorder: intestinal pseudo-obstruction
      Scleroderma
      Diabetes
      Jejunal diverticulosis
      Amyloidosis
      Peritoneal studding with metastases
      Oat cell tumor of the lung with paraneoplastic neuropathy involving intestine
      Familial visceral myopathy
      Familial visceral neuropathy
      Hypothyroidism
3. Psychogenic
   Bulimia
   Psychogenic, not bulimic
4. Central nervous system
   Increased intracranial pressure secondary to tumor
   Pseudotumor
5. Drugs
   Narcotic
   Cardiac glycosides
   Theophylline derivatives
6. Pregnancy
   Nausea and vomiting of pregnancy
   Hyperemesis gravidarum
7. Metabolic/endocrine
   Hyperthyroidism
   Addison's disease
8. Other
   Idiopathic cyclic vomiting (motility disorder)

The timing of vomiting in relation to eating can also be a helpful clue in making the diagnosis. Regurgitation of undigested food, often when assuming a recumbent position, is suggestive of achalasia. Vomiting soon after eating can be seen in gastric ulcer disease, psychogenic disorders, and bulimia, while vomiting undigested food several hours after a meal suggests gastric outlet obstruction or gastroparesis. A previous history of peptic ulcer disease should be determined, because this is the most likely cause of gastric outlet obstruction. Patients with benign causes of gastric outlet obstruction may not lose much weight initially because they compensate for the food lost during vomiting. They are often hungry, while patients with malignant causes of gastric outlet obstruction often have significant anorexia, early satiety, and weight loss. Possible causes of nonobstructive gastroparesis, such as diabetes mellitus, should be determined. Drugs that may cause gastroparesis or vomiting from a central nervous system effect or by delaying gastric emptying should be considered.

Acute systemic symptoms such as fever or myalgia suggest a viral etiology. If the patient can give a history of eating food prepared by others, particularly if other people eating at the same function have similar symptoms, the possibility of ingesting a bacterial toxin should be considered. The presence of vertigo would suggest a labyrinthine problem, while a headache and stiff neck would raise the suspicion of meningitis.

In patients with chronic nausea and vomiting, associated headaches, a change in mental status, or any neurologic impairment should raise the suspicion of a central nervous system lesion. Projectile vomiting may also be seen, particularly if there is raised intracranial pressure. An inappropriate attitude to symptoms of vomiting and weight loss, particularly in a young woman, should suggest an eating disorder. Patients with bulimia may have calluses on the metacarpophalangeal joints from self-induction of vomiting.

In addition to obtaining a detailed history that can indicate the etiology of the problem, the severity of the condition should be determined based on physical findings of weight loss and dehydration and evidence of volume contraction by postural changes in the pulse or blood pressure. A number of features on the physical examination may be helpful when making a diagnosis. The abdomen should be examined for the presence of tenderness and auscultated to determine the presence or absence of a succussion splash and to determine the quality of bowel sounds. The hernial orifices should be examined carefully. The presence of occult blood in the stool should be determined. A detailed neurologic examination and funduscopic examination are necessary. The patient should be examined for postural hypotension. This is important in assessing the severity of the problem and in determining whether there is an autonomic neuropathy.

The choice of laboratory studies should be directed by the history and physical examination (see below). If mechanical obstruction is in the differential diagnosis based on the history and physical examination, an upright and supine abdominal x-ray should be taken. The upright film suggests the presence or absence of obstructed loops of bowel by the presence or absence of air-fluid levels, while the supine film allows an examination of the features of the obstructed loops that assist in determining the site of obstruction. The presence of metabolic abnormalities should be determined. These features provide an indication of the severity of the condition. Treatment depends on the etiology of the nausea and vomiting but can be considered as directed at two aspects of the patient's condition. Both the sequelae of nausea and vomiting, namely, the fluid and electrolyte disturbances, and the specific underlying etiology need to be addressed.

DIFFERENTIAL DIAGNOSIS AND DIAGNOSTIC STRATEGIES

Algorithms outlining the approach to patients with acute or chronic nausea and vomiting are shown in Figures 33-2 and 33-3. Details concerning the different diseases associated with this symptom complex are included below and in other chapters as indicated.

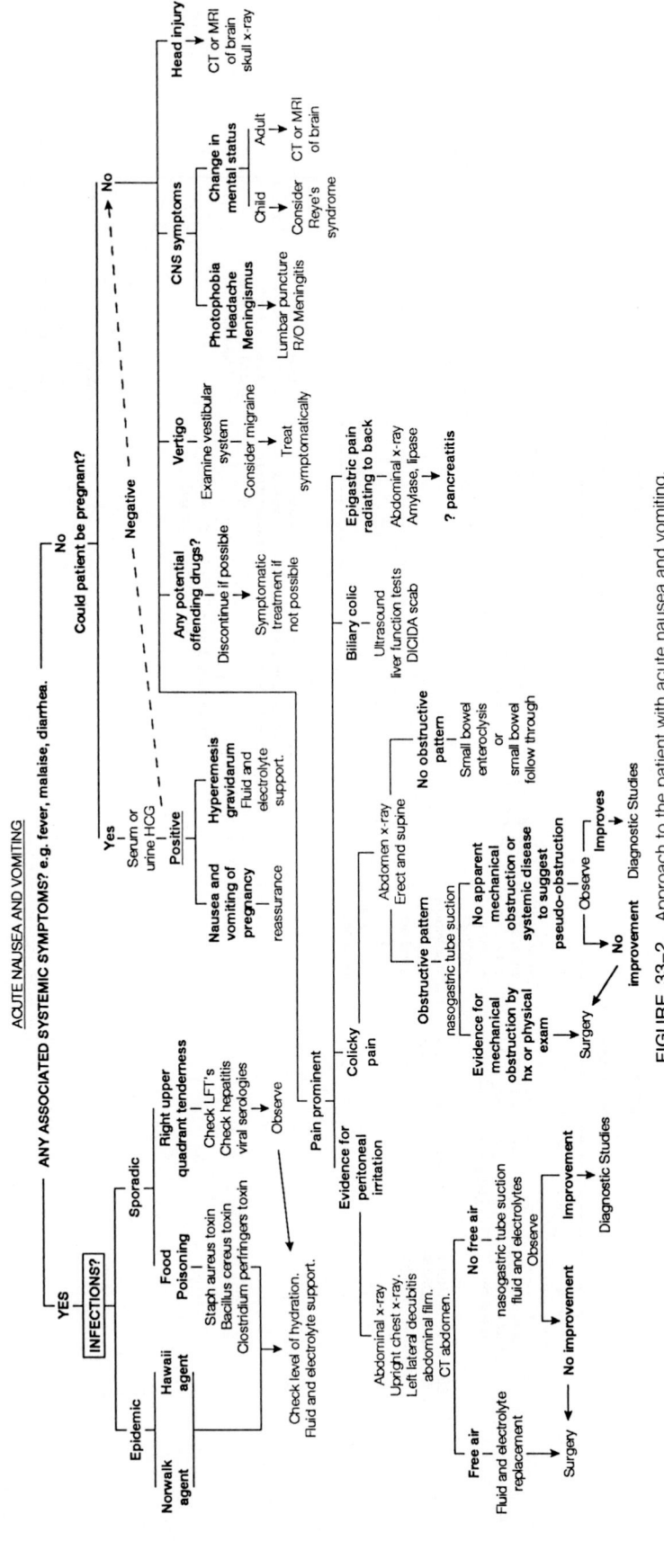

FIGURE 33–2. Approach to the patient with acute nausea and vomiting.

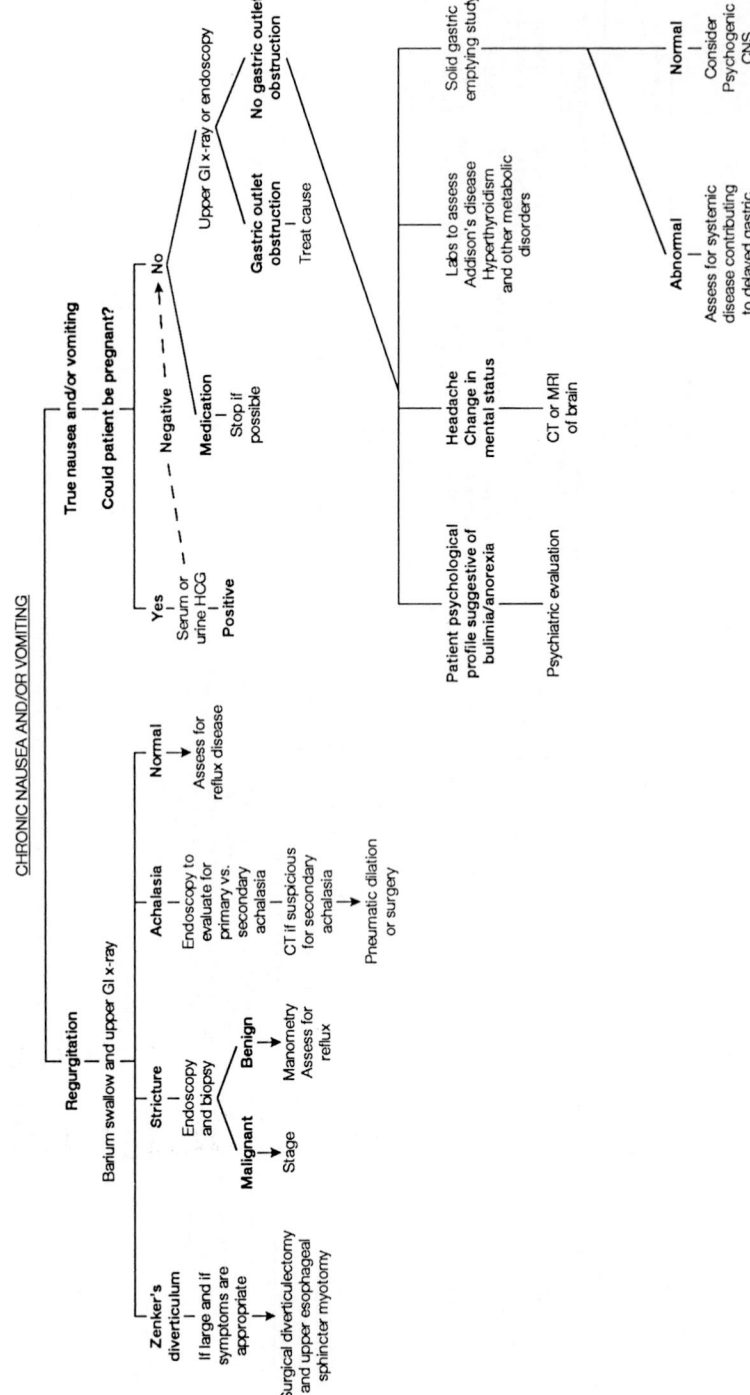

FIGURE 33–3. Approach to the patient with chronic nausea and vomiting.

Acute Nausea and Vomiting

INFECTIOUS

Symptoms of diarrhea, abdominal cramps, headache, and myalgia associated with nausea and vomiting are highly suggestive of viral gastroenteritis. These constitute a group of nonbacterial acute infectious gastroenteritis illnesses that have been labeled as a variety of syndromes: viral diarrhea, epidemic diarrhea and vomiting, winter vomiting disease, epidemic collapse, and epidemic nausea and vomiting. As a group, these illnesses account for the most frequent form of disease secondary to acute respiratory illnesses.[13] The Norwalk agent is associated with winter vomiting disease and is a 24-hour self-limited disease characterized by vomiting and nausea. It was described in an outbreak that affected 50% of students in an elementary school in Norwalk, Ohio.[14] During infections with the Norwalk agent, a parvoviruslike agent, jejunal biopsies demonstrate partial villous flattening, disorganization of the epithelial cells, vacuolization of the cytoplasm, and mononuclear infiltration of the lamina propria. These changes resolved with convalescence. Norwalk agent has also been implicated in gastroenteritis associated with the ingestion of raw clams and oysters.[15] Another parvoviruslike agent, the Hawaii agent, is also implicated as an infectious cause of acute nausea and vomiting. The pathophysiology of the nausea and vomiting is unknown, but there is evidence of impaired gastric motility in normals who ingested either agent. The degree of symptoms of nausea and vomiting did not correlate with the severity of gastric emptying, suggesting that this may be an association rather than the cause of nausea and vomiting.[16] Delayed gastric emptying has also been seen in patients with persistent nausea and vomiting long after the resolution of an acute viral syndrome.[17] Bacterial causes of acute nausea and vomiting are usually part of a syndrome associated with diarrhea and include infection with *Salmonella* (nontyphoid). Food poisoning with bacterial toxins is a common cause of the sudden onset of nausea and vomiting and, frequently, diarrhea. The enterotoxins of *Staphylococcus aureus, Clostridium perfringens,* and *Bacillus cereus* account for illness with an onset of a few hours to 24 hours after exposure. In most patients, a careful history and examination will determine the etiology of the acute infectious nausea and vomiting with or without diarrhea. Generally, these are acute self-limited disorders, and the patient should be treated symptomatically. With *Bacillus cereus* infection, diarrhea is prominent, and vomiting is seen in a minority of patients. Transmission of the disease to household contacts is uncommon.[18–20] Acute infectious hepatitis may present with nausea and vomiting before the right upper quadrant tenderness and icterus become apparent. In patients with acute hepatitis, the inability to eat and drink is one of the most common indications for admission. Usually these symptoms resolve as the patient becomes icteric.

A rare cause of nausea and vomiting is cutaneous herpes zoster infection. There is one report of transient symptoms associated with cutaneous findings and evidence of delayed gastric emptying.[21]

Nausea and vomiting are common after allogeneic bone marrow transplantation and may be associated with cytomegalovirus and/or herpes simplex virus infections of the gastrointestinal tract, or with graft-versus-host disease. A combination of endoscopic brushings, biopsies, and cultures may be necessary to identify the viral infections.[22]

DRUGS

Drugs associated with acute nausea and vomiting include chemotherapeutic agents, some of which cause nausea without vomiting, antibiotics such as erythromycin, opiates, and cardiac glycosides. The sites of action of drugs vary. Cardiac glycosides and chemotherapeutic agents act by way of the central nervous system. Studies in cats have demonstrated that, in cats, the emetic response to cisplatin was eliminated by ablation of the area postrema.[23] There is often a delay between administration of cytotoxic agents and the onset of nausea and vomiting.[24] The delay is variable depending on the cytotoxic agent, suggesting that these agents act indirectly rather than directly on the chemoreceptor trigger zone. The associated gastrointestinal side effects vary depending on the drug. For example, anorexia is prominent in patients receiving 6-mercaptopurine, vinblastine, and etoposide. Diarrhea may be seen with 5-fluorouracil. Vomiting is prominent with cisplatin, vinblastine, and etoposide and starts within a few hours of receiving dactinomycin, but it is not prominent in patients receiving 5-fluorouracil and is seen as a toxic manifestation of bleomycin. There is not much data to define the sites of action of the chemotherapeutic agents other than cisplatin, which has been suggested to act peripherally. There is also interspecies variability, which makes it difficult to extrapolate from animals to man. The delay seen frequently between the administration of the chemotherapeutic agent and the onset of vomiting has been taken to indicate an indirect action of the drug, resulting, perhaps, in the accumulation of an intermediate factor. One hypothesis is that cytotoxic drugs produce an emetic effect by inhibiting enzyme systems responsible for the rapid breakdown of neurotransmitters. This might result in an increased concentration of neurotransmitters in the vomiting pathway.[25] The efferent pathway that results in a combination of nausea, retching, and vomiting is probably complex and involves many neurotransmitters and interneurons. Such a complex circuit may explain the lack of uniformity of efficacy of most antiemetic agents for different cytotoxic agents. Narcotic analgesia can induce the sudden onset of nausea and vomiting, also probably by way of a central action. Most agents can be identified by the history. Any drugs that may be the offending agent and that can be either discontinued or replaced should be discontinued. If this is not possible, antiemetic agents as discussed below should be given.

VISCERAL PAIN

Acute visceral pain can induce nausea and vomiting and presumably affects visceral afferents. The prominence of pain usually indicates the source of the problem. The presence of peritonitis is suggested by abdominal rigidity and rebound tenderness, while an obstructive process is suggested by a history of waves of colicky pain separated by relatively pain-free periods. The differential diagnosis of an acute intestinal obstruction is outlined in Table 33-1. Any evidence for causes of obstruction, such as previous surgery predisposing to adhesions or previous medical conditions such as inflammatory bowel disease, should be determined. Physical examination should include specific examination of possible hernial orifices. An abdominal x-ray, upright and supine, should be performed to look for evidence of obstruction with air–fluid levels or for perforation with free air under the diaphragm. Treatment depends on the etiology of obstruction. Most causes of bowel obstruction can be managed only surgically. Partial obstruction due to adhesions may resolve with nasogastric suction, and small-bowel obstruction secondary to Crohn's disease may improve with medical therapy.

Severe epigastric pain radiating to the back and associated with nausea and vomiting is suggestive of acute pancreatitis. In addition to obtaining a serum amylase (and lipase if there is any question of the interpretation of the results), the patients should be assessed for the severity of the pancreatitis. The presence of an ileus should be determined both clinically and by abdominal x-ray. The severity of the pancreatitis should be determined by looking for signs associated with a worse prognosis. These include hypotension, a fall in hemoglobin, leukocytosis, an increase in blood urea nitrogen (BUN), hypoxia, hypocalcemia, hypoalbuminemia, renal dysfunction, and acidosis.[26,27]

Biliary colic is somewhat of a misnomer in that the pain is not colicky, as seen in intestinal obstruction, but tends to be constant, increasing in severity over hours, and often associated with nausea and vomiting, and then decreasing over a period of time. Because biliary colic is usually associated with a gallstone impacted in the cystic duct and not in the common bile duct, the liver function tests may be normal. If a stone is passed into the common bile duct, jaundice may be seen along with a transient cholestatic enzyme pattern. Acute cholecystitis is associated with more severe pain, a positive Murphy's sign, and sometimes fever. Imaging with a DICIDA scan (^{99m}Tc-labeled derivative of iminodiacetic acid) may help to determine the presence of acute cholecystitis. Although there are several causes of failure of the gallbladder to visualize on the DICIDA scan, in the appropriate clinical setting the study can be very helpful.[28]

VESTIBULAR DISORDERS

Vestibular disturbances may result in nausea and vomiting, usually associated with severe vertigo. Motion sickness has been examined experimentally in dogs, where it has been demonstrated that motion stimulates labyrinthine receptors. Labyrinthectomy or ablation of parts of the cerebellum abolish the vomiting induced by motion without affecting the responses to intravenously administered apomorphine or orally administered copper sulfate.[29] Labyrinthine stimulation can result in severe nausea and vomiting, usually associated with vertigo.

CENTRAL NERVOUS SYSTEM

Meningitis may present with nausea and vomiting but is usually associated with headache and photophobia and findings of men-

ingismus or stiff neck. In children who present with vomiting and who are unable to give a history, one should consider head trauma or meningitis. If meningitis is considered and there is no evidence for increased intracranial pressure, a spinal tap to examine the cerebrospinal fluid for cells and organisms and for culture should be obtained. Episodic vertigo, nausea, and vomiting can also be a rare presentation of a migraine equivalent.[30] Patients usually have either a personal or family history of more classical migraine symptoms.

REYE'S SYNDROME

Reye's syndrome, found exclusively in children, is characterized by encephalopathy and hepatomegaly with evidence of fatty degeneration of the viscera, including microvesicular fatty infiltration of the liver.[31] This syndrome, described initially in 1963, usually follows a prodromal illness, usually influenza or varicella.[32] Vomiting is a prominent feature of this syndrome, associated with variable changes in levels of consciousness, which can result in coma. Coma is associated with increased blood ammonia levels. Marked metabolic changes are seen with increases in serum free fatty acid concentrations and serum ammonia. Abnormalities in mitochondrial enzymes involved in the urea cycle and in enzymes associated with the citric acid cycle have been observed. Dicarboxylic acids in the urine and serum indicate mitochondrial injury. Some similarities in metabolic abnormalities are seen between Reye's syndrome and salicylate intoxication, and salicylates may serve as an additive factor in the pathogenesis of Reye's syndrome.[33–35] The management involves supportive care and monitoring of the intracerebral pressures. The incidence of Reye's syndrome as reported to the Centers for Disease Control (CDC) rose between its first description in 1963 to a peak of 555 reported cases in 1979–1980. Since then there has been a steady decline. An epidemiologic association has been described with aspirin use, and the decline in incidence of Reye's has been concurrent with a decrease in aspirin use in children with such prodromal symptoms. The true pathogenesis of Reye's is unknown, and studies are complicated by the lack of an animal model and the marked decrease in case occurrence.

Chronic Nausea and Vomiting

The causes of chronic nausea and vomiting are legion (Table 33-2). In addition to the obvious causes of nausea and vomiting, such as gastric outlet obstruction, are less well defined conditions. In such conditions, abnormalities in gastric or small intestinal physiology can be demonstrated, but the causal association of findings with the symptoms is less clear.

MECHANICAL GASTRIC OUTLET OBSTRUCTION

Any obstruction to the gastrointestinal tract can cause nausea and vomiting. Usually colonic obstruction presents as obstipation and pain rather than vomiting. Both gastric outlet obstruction and small intestinal obstruction present with vomiting. Small intestinal obstruction is associated with abdominal pain as a prominent accompanying symptom and usually presents acutely. Gastric outlet obstruction can be transient in the presence of pyloric channel ulcer or Crohn's disease, where medical therapy may decrease the edema and relieve the obstruction sufficiently to avoid immediate surgery, or it can be irreversible, as is seen with chronic peptic ulcer disease with scarring or carcinoma, in which case surgical bypass, pyloroplasty, or balloon dilatation will be required.[36–39] In addition to anatomic obstruction, functional disorders affecting gastric emptying are common. It is important to realize that if a patient is vomiting, and no obstructive lesions are found, both central nervous system causes and functional gastroparesis should be investigated.

FUNCTIONAL GASTRIC OUTLET OBSTRUCTION

Gastroparesis results from an impairment of the normal mechanism for gastric emptying. This will be described in detail in Chapter 60. Abnormalities in antral function, and therefore in solid gastric emptying, are seen most commonly. A radionuclide study to examine the emptying of solids is therefore more helpful than one to examine the emptying of liquids when abnormal gastric emptying is suspected. Gastroparesis is frequently seen in diabetes and is probably related to vagal neuropathy. Recordings of intragastric contractile activity have indicated a loss of phase 3 of the migrating myoelectric complex, which involves the antrum and small intestine. The finding of a similar loss in patients who have undergone surgical vagotomy suggests that the loss of phase 3 in patients with diabetic gastroparesis is due to an autonomic neuropathy.[40,41]

In scleroderma, the gastric emptying problems are usually seen in conjunction with involvement of other areas of the intestine. Nausea and vomiting may be minor compared with symptoms related to involvement of other areas of the gastrointestinal tract, including gastroesophageal reflux, intestinal overgrowth and malabsorption, pseudo-obstruction, and constipation.[42,43]

Idiopathic gastroparesis is the most common cause of delayed gastric emptying found on scintigraphic study. Studies of the electrical control of gastric antral contractions in some of these patients have suggested that abnormalities in the control activity are associated with episodic nausea and vomiting. Normally, in man, the antrum displays a three-cycle-per-minute slow wave activity. Although this is a property of the smooth muscle cell membrane, this activity can be recorded by way of surgically applied external serosal electrodes or by electrodes over the abdominal wall, the electrogastrogram.[44,45] In patients with nausea and evidence of delayed gastric emptying, changes in this three-cycle-per-minute activity have been recorded both directly from the antral muscle wall and by way of electrogastrograms. Such an increase in the rate of slow wave activity is called tachygastria and is discussed in greater detail in Chapters 8 and 60.

Drug-induced nausea and delayed gastric emptying are seen with many drugs, particularly narcotic agents. In addition, antacids have been reported to delay gastric emptying, as have histamine-H_2 receptor antagonists.[46–48] A delay in gastric emptying of liquids has been described with alcohol and a mixed meal.[49] These findings are not surprising, because pyloric sphincter responses to intraduodenal acid, amino acids, and fat have been described.[50–52] In addition, high concentrations of cholecystokinin receptors have been described in the rat pylorus.[53]

Any patient in whom gastric outlet obstruction is suspected should undergo visualization of the stomach, either by upper endoscopy or an upper GI barium study. If an anatomic obstruction is found, the patient should undergo endoscopy with biopsy of the obstructing lesion if it is anything other than clear chronic peptic ulcer disease. If no mucosal lesion is found, a computed tomography (CT) scan to visualize the thickness of the gastric antral wall and to image the pancreas is necessary. In some cases of lymphoma or submucosal infiltrative tumors, laparotomy and biopsy may be necessary. If no anatomic obstructing lesion is found, other causes of chronic nausea and vomiting should be considered. In patients with other systemic diseases that could explain the presence of gastroparesis, such as diabetes or scleroderma, the likelihood of gastroparesis is quite high, and an extensive search for more obscure causes, such as central nervous system causes, may not be necessary. If these conditions are not present, or if the patient is being considered for a prokinetic agent, a gastric emptying scan to confirm the delay in gastric emptying is useful. Because there is more often a problem with a delay in solid gastric emptying than with liquid emptying, an appropriately tagged solid should be used for the study. Often, technetium-labeled egg white is used. The only widely available prokinetic agent, metoclopramide, is associated with a significant likelihood of side effects, making a positive diagnosis of delayed gastric emptying important in the decision to use this agent (see below).

INTESTINAL PSEUDO-OBSTRUCTION

The definition of intestinal pseudo-obstruction is the presence of symptoms and findings consistent with acute intestinal obstruction in the absence of mechanical obstruction. Although the initial presentation of the patient may be acute, once a mechanical obstruction has been eliminated by a contrast study of the small and large intestine and a diagnosis of pseudo-obstruction has been made, the patients will often present with recurrent exacerbations. Intestinal pseudo-obstruction is frequently associated with an underlying systemic disorder (see Table 33-2). The focus of the evaluation should be directed at determining the presence of these associated systemic disorders. The specific studies are covered in other chapters.

EATING DISORDERS

In anorexia nervosa and bulimia, altered eating habits are prominent, although this may be hidden by the patient. Anorexia nervosa is an eating disorder in which the patient starves. The patient may occasionally have an eating binge and induce vomiting, but a decreased intake is the primary disorder. The patient, usually a young female, suffers from a markedly disturbed perception of body image. Bulimia is characterized by frequent binge eating and vomiting and may include surreptitious laxative and diuretic abuse. Metabolic disturbances are seen more commonly in bulimia because of the induced vomiting. In addition to psychologic abnormalities and interpersonal conflicts, abnormalities in gastric function have been described in anorexics—in particular, delayed gastric emptying and abnormal cholecystokinin levels have been described.[54] These eating disorders are covered in detail in Chapter 32.

CENTRAL NERVOUS SYSTEM DISORDERS

Nausea and vomiting may be a manifestation of increased intracranial pressure, seen with intracerebral tumors or pseudotumor cerebri. Increased intracranial pressure presents with headache, nausea, vomiting, mental changes, and disturbances in levels of consciousness. Initially, symptoms are most prominent in the morning. The additional neurologic deficits depend on the site of the lesion and the degree of local edema.[55,56] The diagnosis is made by either CT or magnetic resonance imaging (MRI) of the brain.

PREGNANCY

Nausea and vomiting are common in pregnancy, with 90% of women reporting nausea and/or vomiting.[57] About 86% complain of nausea, while far fewer complain of vomiting. The onset is often soon after the first missed period and may occur before pregnancy is diagnosed. Fifty percent of women have resolution of either symptom by the 15th week of gestation. Nausea and vomiting of pregnancy are not associated with any adverse outcome of the pregnancy. In a minority of cases, about 3.5 per 1000 deliveries, it is severe enough to cause fluid and electrolyte abnormalities or nutritional deficiencies, in which case it is called hyperemesis gravidarum. Like nausea and vomiting of pregnancy, it starts soon after the first missed period and often resolves during the third month. An increased incidence of hyperemesis gravidarum is reported with twins or with the presence of a hydatidiform mole. Although these conditions are associated with a higher than usual human chorionic gonadotropin (HCG) level, the level of HCG cannot predict the presence of hyperemesis gravidarum. Factors that may increase the risk of hyperemesis gravidarum are nulliparity and younger age. In one study, patients with hyperemesis had a higher serum estrogen level than control pregnant patients.[58] The role of psychologic abnormalities in hyperemesis gravidarum has received much attention. Researchers have demonstrated that patients with hyperemesis gravidarum often have a history of responding to emotional stress with vomiting, and the psychologic profile of patients suggests an increased prevalence of hysteria compared with control subjects.[59,60] There is no increase in fetal loss in these patients; however, in some studies, infants born to mothers with more impaired weight gain had lower birth weights than those born to mothers with greater weight gain.[61] Fluid and electrolyte replacement is important. Support psychotherapy is warranted based on studies suggesting that it is treatable by hypnosis.

PSYCHOGENIC VOMITING

Vomiting is seen in patients who do not necessarily fit the criteria of anorexia or bulimia. Psychogenic vomiting has been described in patients in whom psychiatric evaluation reveals significant life experiences that appear to be temporally related to the onset of vomiting. These include cohabitation with a person to whom they were antagonistic, parental loss at a young age, history of recurrent vomiting as children, and a family history of functional or persistent organic vomiting. In addition, some patients experienced abdominal pain as a prominent symptom.[62,63]

IDIOPATHIC CYCLIC VOMITING

Abnormalities of intestinal motor activity as evidenced by delayed gastric emptying or abnormal small intestinal motility have been described in patients with unexplained nausea and vomiting that present in a recurrent cyclic fashion. These abnormalities can be found even during asymptomatic periods. This cyclic vomiting is an unusual presentation (1% of patients with unexplained nausea and vomiting in a referral center) and is not associated with marked psychologic abnormalities, as tested by the Minnesota Multiphasic Personality Inventory (MMPI) test.[64]

CONSEQUENCES OF VOMITING

The medical consequences of vomiting result from decreased fluid intake, increased fluid loss, decreased nutrient intake, and loss of gastric and sometimes duodenal juices. Thus, volume depletion can be seen with its resultant metabolic alkalosis. In addition, a metabolic alkalosis can be seen with loss of hydrogen ion from the vomitus. Sodium depletion and potassium depletion occur from loss of the electrolytes in the vomitus. In addition, volume contraction results in an increased distal tubule Na^+/K^+ exchange, with loss of potassium by way of the renin angiotensin–aldosterone pathway. If the T_m for bicarbonate is exceeded, an obligatory loss of sodium will accompany the bicarbonate excretion from the kidneys, with increased sodium in the urine in the face of sodium depletion.

Clinically, the sudden increase in intrathoracic pressure may result in petechiae over the face and upper neck. Dental disease can result from chronic vomiting, and vomiting can be associated with a mucosal tear at the gastroesophageal junction with a resultant Mallory–Weiss tear and upper gastrointestinal bleeding. Rarely, a transmural tear of the esophagus with free perforation may be seen (Boerhaave's syndrome).

TREATMENT

The treatment of nausea and vomiting depends on the severity of the metabolic consequences of the condition and the underlying disorder. Treatment should include resuscitation of the patient and restoration of normal fluid and electrolyte balance as well as treatment of the underlying disorder if the condition is not a short-lived problem. Treatment of the various underlying disorders was discussed briefly earlier in this chapter and is discussed in detail in chapters covering each specific disorder. The symptomatic treatment of nausea and vomiting involves medications that act centrally and those which act on the gastrointestinal tract, the prokinetic agents (Table 33-3).

Centrally acting drugs include anticholinergics such as scopolamine, which has proved to be the most effective drug for motion sickness.[65,66] For other causes of nausea and vomiting, neuroleptic agents that act centrally have proved to provide symptomatic relief.[67]

The major psychoactive constituent of marijuana, delta-9-tetrahydrocannabinol (THC), was found to be an effective antiemetic agent in patients receiving cancer chemotherapy. The site of action of this antiemetic site was not clearly defined, although in animals it appeared to act primarily on the level of the reticular formation, thalamus, and cerebellum and also had an inhibitory effect on intestinal motility.[68,69] The interest in the clinical use of this agent has decreased with the development of the prokinetic agents.

TABLE 33–3
Antiemetic Agents[65–76]

Anticholinergic

Scopolamine

(Most effective drug for motion sickness)

Antihistamine (H₁-Receptor Antagonist)

Promethazine

Meclizine

Dimenhydrinate

(H$_1$-receptor antagonists are useful in the treatment of motion sickness and some causes of vestibular disturbances [e.g., Meniere's disease].)

Neuroleptic Agents (Includes Antipsychotic Agents)

Chlorpromazine

Perphenazine

Prochlorperazine

Promethazine

Thiethylperazine

Triflupromazine

Trimeprazine

(Phenothiazines may be helpful in a variety of conditions, including uremia, radiation sickness, drug-induced vomiting, and carcinomatosis. Dystonia can be a major side effect.)

Prokinetic Agents

Metoclopramide

Domperidone

Cisapride

(Useful in patients with chemotherapy-induced nausea and vomiting and in patients with functional gastroparesis or intestinal pseudo-obstruction.)

Δ-9-Tetracannabinoids

(Effective in patients with chemotherapy-induced nausea and vomiting but not currently used.)

Prokinetic agents are drugs that increase intestinal contractile force and accelerate intestinal transit. They have proved useful for both drug-induced nausea and vomiting in chemotherapy and intestinal motility disorders that result in gastroparesis or intestinal pseudo-obstruction. These agents include metoclopramide and two agents that are currently not available in the United States, domperidone and cisapride. The mechanism of action of these drugs is either to increase the effect of an agonist such as acetylcholine or to inhibit the effect of an inhibitory neurotransmitter such as dopamine.[70]

Metoclopramide (methoxy-2-chloro-5-procainamide) is related structurally to the antiarrhythmic agent procainamide. Its effects on the gastrointestinal tract are mediated by way of a central antidopamine effect, a peripheral antidopamine effect, and direct and indirect stimulation of cholinergic receptors.[71] It has been used to treat chemotherapy-associated nausea and vomiting and blocks emesis induced by apomorphine by way of antagonism of dopamine receptors in the vomiting center and chemoreceptor trigger zone.[72] In addition, it increases the rate of gastric emptying and may therefore also be useful in idiopathic gastroparesis or gastroparesis due to autonomic neuropathies. The major restriction to its use is the frequency of side effects related to its antidopaminergic properties. The incidence of side effects is as high as 10% to 20% in some studies.[71] Side effects range from central nervous system effects of mild anxiety, nervousness, and insomnia to more debilitating symptoms of marked anxiety and hallucinations and includes sleepiness, lethargy, and depression. Dystonic reactions are seen, often in younger patients, and parkinsonian reactions with tardive dyskinesia and akathisia may be seen in older patients.[71,73,74] Gynecomastia may be seen as a result of the peripheral antidopamine effects of metoclopramide, which increases the release of prolactin.[71] The neurologic side effects usually resolve on withdrawal of the drug.

The newer prokinetic agents have fewer central effects than metoclopramide. Domperidone has a specific antagonist effect on the inhibitory effects of dopamine on the upper gastrointestinal tract. It has limited ability to cross the blood–brain barrier and will probably be most useful for the treatment of gastroparesis. It has the same side effect of increasing prolactin levels as metoclopramide.[75] The latest prokinetic agent, cisapride, is a benzamide derivative that has no antidopaminergic effect and therefore does not have either the extrapyramidal side effects or increased prolactin levels that accompany metoclopramide and domperidone. It appears to act by way of indirect stimulation of cholinergic nerves.[70,76] Its usefulness should be similar to that of domperidone (i.e., mainly for gastrointestinal disorders associated with impaired gastric emptying and intestinal transit).

VOMITING IN CHILDREN

In the very young child, vomiting is a frequent symptom. The patient is unable to complain of nausea; thus, the differential diagnosis of a vomiting child includes causes of regurgitation. The differential diagnosis changes depending on the age of the child. In older children, the differential diagnosis is similar to that in adults, although peptic ulcer disease is less common and psychogenic vomiting may be more common. In infants, one needs to include congenital abnormalities that result in intestinal obstruction and metabolic disturbances. As in adults, acute obstruction distal to the duodenum, such as a malrotation, is usually associated with pain. Other causes of vomiting in infants may be pain-free. Regurgitation in infants is common and is often related to posture after feeding. If only small amounts of food are regurgitated and the infant is developing well, minor alterations in feeding habits and reassurance are usually sufficient. Most reflux symptoms resolve as the child develops, and only in cases where the infant is failing to thrive or is suffering from pulmonary problems should more extensive examination for gastroesophageal reflux be pursued. Esophageal strictures or, uncommonly, achalasia can also cause regurgitation that is usually severe enough to result in a barium study, which will delineate the problem. Gastric or pyloric channel ulcers, pyloric stenosis, and antral webs may cause postprandial vomiting in children.

Pyloric stenosis is found in 4 or 5 per 1000 live births and is found more frequently in males. The condition may be congenital but presents when the infant is between 2 and 6 weeks old. The vomiting is characteristically projectile and eventually follows all meals. On physical examination the infant is eager to feed, and peristaltic waves may be seen in the left upper quadrant. After feeding and vomiting, the pyloric stenotic lesion may be palpable as a small, firm mass often described as an "olive." Laboratory studies classically show a metabolic alkalosis secondary to the loss of gastric acid contents. An abdominal plain film shows a dilated air-filled stomach and a nondilated pyloric canal. Abdominal ultrasound may also be helpful. Contrast studies are not usually needed but may be helpful in less obvious cases.

Metabolic causes of vomiting in children include adrenal insufficiency, renal tubular acidosis, uremia, and hyperammonemia secondary to urea cycle enzyme deficiencies.

Central nervous system causes of vomiting include increased intracranial pressure from tumors that, as in adults, are often associated with morning vomiting. No preceding intra-abdominal discomfort is evident.

In toddlers, ingestion of drugs or chemical agents should always be considered when the child presents with acute vomiting, particularly if the parent cannot vouch for the child's activities.

In older children, although usually starting between the ages of 2 and 5, cyclic vomiting has been described. It is characterized by recurrent attacks of vomiting, fever, headaches, and abdominal pain. Vomiting has been described to occur as infrequently as once a month to as frequently as several times a day. Each episode may last a few hours to a few days. The etiology is unknown, and a form of seizure disorder and psychosocial stress have both been postulated.[77,78]

A child who is vomiting and has altered mental status following a prodromal viral illness should be considered to have Reye's syndrome even if there is no history of recent aspirin ingestion (see above and Fig 33-2).

The reader is directed to Chapter 8, The Physiology of Gastric Motility and Gastric Emptying; Chapter 32, Approach to the Patient with Unexplained Weight Loss; Chapter 37, Approach to the Patient with Ileus and Obstruction; and Chapter 60, Disorders of Gastric Emptying.

REFERENCES

1. Andrews PLR, Hawthorn J. The neurophysiology of vomiting. Baillieres Clin Gastroenterol 1988;2:141.
2. McCarthy LE, Borison HL. Respiratory mechanics of vomiting in decerebrate cats. Am J Physiol 1974;226:738.
3. McCarthy LE, Borison HL, Spiegel PK, et al. Vomiting: Radiographic and oscillographic correlates in the decerebrate cat. Gastroenterology 1974;67:1126.
4. Smith CC, Brizzee KR. Cineradiographic analysis of vomiting of the cat. Gastroenterology 1961;40:654.
5. Brizzee KR, Mehler WR. The central nervous connections involved in the vomiting reflex. In: Davis CJ, Lake-Bakaar GV, Grahame-Smith DG, eds. Nausea and vomiting: Mechanisms and treatment. Berlin: Springer-Verlag, 1986:31.
6. Mehler WR. Observations of the connectivity of the parvicellular reticular formation with respect to a vomiting center. Brain Behav Evol 1983;23:63.
7. Tan LK, Miller AD. Innervation of periesophageal region of cat's diaphragm: Implications for studies of control of vomiting. Neurosci Lett 1986;68:339.
8. Stewart JJ, Burks TF, Weisbrodt NW. Intestinal myoelectric activity after activation of central emetic mechanisms. Am J Physiol 1977;233:E131.
9. Lang IM, Marvig J. Functional localization of specific receptors mediating gastrointestinal motor correlates of vomiting. Am J Physiol 1989;256:G92.
10. Lang IM, Sarna SK, Condon RE. Gastrointestinal correlates of vomiting in the dog: Quantification and characterization as an independent phenomenon. Gastroenterology 1986;90:40.
11. Ehrlein HJ. Dopamine delays gastric emptying and induces retrograde power contraction with enterogastric reflux. Z Gastroenterol 1988:26:160.
12. Inglefinger FJ, Moss RE. The activity of the descending duodenum during nausea. Am J Physiol 1942;136:561.
13. Plotkin GR, Kluge RM, Waldman RH. Gastroenteritis: Etiology, pathophysiology, and clinical manifestations. Medicine 1979;58:95.
14. Adler JL, Zickl R. Winter vomiting disease. J Infect Dis 1969;119:668.
15. Morse DL, Guzewich JJ, Hanrahan HP, et al. Widespread outbreaks of clam-and oyster-associated gastroenteritis. N Engl J Med 1986;314:678.
16. Meeroff JC, Schriber DS, Trier JS, et al. Abnormal gastric motor function in viral gastroenteritis. Ann Intern Med 1980;92:370.
17. Rhoades JB, Robinson RG, McBride N. Sudden onset of slow gastric emptying of food. Gastroenterology 1979;77:569.
18. Terranova W, Blake PA. Bacillus cereus food poisoning. N Engl J Med 1978;298:143.
19. Melling J, Capel BJ, Turnbull PCB, et al. Identification of a novel enterotoxigenic activity associated with Bacillus cereus. J Clin Pathol 1976;29:938.
20. Turnbull PCB. Studies on the production of enterotoxins by Bacillus cereus. J Clin Pathol 1976;29:941.
21. Kebede D, Barthel JS, Singh A. Transient gastroparesis associated with cutaneous herpes zoster. Dig Dis Sci 1987;32:318.
22. Spencer GD, Hackman RC, McDonald GB, et al. A prospective study of unexplained nausea and vomiting after marrow transplantation. Transplantation 1986;42:602.
23. McCarthy LE, Borison HL. Cisplatin-induced vomiting eliminated by ablation of the area postrema in cats. Cancer Treat Rep 1984;68:401.
24. Calabresi P, Parks RE Jr. Chemotherapy of neoplastic diseases. In: Gilman AG, Goodman LG, Rall TW, et al, eds. The pharmacological basis of therapeutics, ed 7. New York: Macmillan, 1985:1240.
25. Edwards CM. Chemotherapy induced emesis. Mechanisms and treatment: A review. J R Soc Med 1988;81:658.
26. Ranson JHC, Rifkind KM, Turner JW. Prognostic signs and nonoperative peritoneal lavage in acute pancreatitis. Surg Gynecol Obstet 1976;143:209.
27. Ranson JHC, Pasternak BS. Statistical methods for quantifying the severity of clinical acute pancreatitis. J Surg Res 1977;22:79.

28. Mauro MA, McCartney WH, Melmed JR. Hepatobiliary scanning with ^{99m}Tc PIPIDA in acute cholecystitis. Radiology 1982;142:193.

29. Wang SC, Chinn HI. Experimental motion sickness in dogs. Importance of labyrinth and vestibular cerebellum. Am J Physiol 1956;185:617.

30. Harker LA, Rassekh C. Migraine equivalent as a cause of episodic vertigo. Laryngoscope 1988;98:160.

31. Heubi JE, Partin JC, Partin JS, et al. Reye's syndrome: Current concepts. Hepatology 1987;7:155.

32. Reye RDK, Morgan G, Baral J. Encephalopathy and fatty degeneration of the viscera: A disease entity in childhood. Lancet 1963;2:749.

33. Starko KM, Mullick FG. Hepatic and cerebral pathology findings in children with fatal salicylate intoxication: Further evidence for a causal relation between salicylate and Reye's syndrome. Lancet 1983;1:326.

34. You KS. Salicylate and mitochondrial injury in Reye's syndrome. Science 1983;221:163.

35. Martens ME, Lee CP. Reye's syndrome. Salicylates and mitochondrial function. Biochem Pharmacol 1984;33:2869.

36. Ellis H. Pyloric stenosis complicating duodenal ulceration. World J Surg 1987;11:315.

37. Lindor K, Ott BJ, Hughes RW Jr. Balloon dilatation of upper digestive tract strictures. Gastroenterology 1983;89:545.

38. Benjamin SB, Glass RL, Cattau EL Jr, et al. Preliminary experience with balloon dilation of the pylorus. Gastrointest Endosc 1984;30:93.

39. Schmudderich W. Through-the-scope balloon dilation of benign pyloric stenosis. Endoscopy 1989;21:7.

40. Malagelada J, Rees WDW, Mazotta LJ, et al. Gastric motor abnormalities in diabetic and postvagotomy gastroparesis: Effect of metoclopramide and bethanechol. Gastroenterology 1980;78:286.

41. Fox S, Behar J. Pathogenesis of diabetic gastroparesis: A pharmacologic study. Gastroenterology 1980;78:757.

42. Cohen S, Laufer I, Snape WJ Jr, Shiau Y-F, et al. The gastrointestinal manifestations of scleroderma: Pathogenesis and management. Gastroenterology 1980;79:155.

43. Greydanus MP, Camilleri M. Abnormal postcibal antral and small bowel motility due to neuropathy or myopathy in systemic sclerosis. Gastroenterology 1989;96:110.

44. Alvarez WC. The electrogastrogram and what it shows. JAMA 1922;78:1116.

45. Hamilton J, Bellahsene BE, Reichelderfer M, et al. Human electrogastrograms. Comparison of surface and mucosal recordings. Dig Dis Sci 1986;31:33.

46. Hurwitz A, Robinson RG, Vats TS, et al. Effect of antacids on gastric emptying. Gastroenterology 1976;71:268.

47. Scarpignato C, Beraccini G. Different effects of cimetidine and ranitidine on gastric emptying in rats and man. Agents Actions 1982;12:172.

48. Krzysztof J. Influence of oral cimetidine and ranitidine on gastric emptying in active duodenal ulcer. J Clin Gastroenterol 1988;10:143.

49. Barboriak JJ, Meade RC. Effect of alcohol on gastric emptying in man. Am J Clin Nutr 1970;23:1151.

50. Reynolds JC, Ouyang A, Cohen S. Evidence for an opiate-mediated pyloric sphincter reflex. Am J Physiol 1984;246:G130.

51. Reynolds JC, Ouyang A, Cohen S. Opiate nerves mediate feline pyloric response to intraduodenal amino acids. Am J Physiol 1985;248:G307.

52. White CM, Poxon V, Alexander-Williams J. Effect of nutrient liquids on human gastroduodenal motor activity. Gut 1983;24:1109.

53. Smith GT, Moran TH, Coyle JT, et al. Anatomic localization of cholecystokinin receptors to the pyloric sphincter. Am J Physiol 1984;246:R127.

54. Abell TL, Malagelada JR, Lucas AR, et al. Gastric electromechanical and neurohormonal function in anorexia nervosa. Gastroenterology 1987;93:958.

55. Pruitt A, Hochberg F. Neoplastic diseases of the central nervous system. In: Petersdorf RG, Adams RD, Braunwald E, et al, eds. Harrison's principles of internal medicine. New York: McGraw-Hill, 1987:1968.

56. Vakili ST, Muller J, Shidnia H, et al. Primary lymphoma of the central nervous system: A clinicopathologic analysis of 26 cases. J Surg Oncol 1986;33:95.

57. Tierson FD, Olsen CL, Hook EB. Nausea and vomiting of pregnancy and association with pregnancy outcome. Am J Obstet Gynecol 1986;155:1017.

58. Depue RH, Bernstein L, Ross RK, et al. Hyperemesis gravidarum in relation to estradiol levels, pregnancy outcome, and other maternal factors: A seroepidemiologic study. Am J Obstet Gynecol 1987;156:137.

59. Harvey WA, Sherfey MJ. Vomiting in pregnancy. A psychiatric study. Psychosom Med 1954;16:1.

60. Guze SB, DeLong WB, Majerus PW, et al. Association of clinical psychiatric disease with hyperemesis gravidarum. A three and a half year follow up study of 48 patients and 45 controls. N Engl J Med 1959;261:1363.

61. Gross S, Librach C, Cecutti A. Maternal weight loss associated with hyperemesis gravidarum: A predictor of fetal outcome. Am J Obstet Gynecol 1989;160:906.

62. Hill OW. Psychogenic vomiting. Gut 1968;9:348.

63. Cleghorn RA, Brown WT. Psychogenesis of vomiting. Can Psychiatr Assoc J 1964;9:299.

64. Abell TL, Kim CH, Malagelada J-R. Idiopathic cyclic nausea and vomiting—A disorder of gastrointestinal motility? Mayo Clin Proc 1988;53:1169.

65. Graybiel A, Wood CD, Knepton J, et al. Human assay of antimotion sickness drugs. Aviat Space Environ Med 1975;46:1107.

66. Wood CD. Antimotion drugs and antiemetic drugs. Drugs 1979;17:471.

67. Baldessarini RJ. Drugs and the treatment of psychiatric disorders. In: Goodman LG, Rall TW, Murad F, et al, eds. The pharmacological basis of therapeutics, ed 7. New York: Macmillan, 1985:387.

68. Vincent BJ, McQuiston DJ, Einhorn LH, Nagy CM, Brames MJ. Review of cannabinoids and their antiemetic effectiveness. Drugs 1983;25(Suppl 1):52.

69. Hollister LE. Health aspects of cannabis. Pharmacol Rev 1986;38:2.

70. Reynolds JC. Prokinetic agents: A key in the future of gastroenterology in motility disorders. Gastroenterol Clin North Am 1989;18:437.

71. Harrington PR, Hamilton CW, Brogden RN, et al. Metoclopramide. An updated review of its pharmacological properties and clinical use. Drugs 1983;25:451.

72. Albibi R, McCallum RW. Metoclopramide: Pharmacology and clinical application. Ann Intern Med 1983;98:86.

73. Bateman DN, Rawlins MD, Simpson JM. Extrapyramidal reactions with metoclopramide. Br Med J 1985;219:930.

74. Casteels-Van Daele M, Jaeke J, Van Der Scheuren P, et al. Dystonic reactions in children caused by metoclopramide. Arch Dis Child 1970;45:130.

75. Brogden RN, Carmine AA, Heel RC, et al. Domperidone: A review of its pharmacological activity, pharmacokinetics and therapeutic efficacy in the symptomatic treatment of chronic dyspepsia and as an antiemetic. Drugs 1982;24:360.

76. Van Neuten JM, Schuurkes JAJ. Pharmacodynamics of cisapride, a prokinetic agent with indirect cholinergic properties. Digestion 1986;34:137.

77. Mitchell WG, Greenwood RS, Messenheimer JA. Abdominal epilepsy: Cyclic vomiting as the major symptom of simple partial seizures. Arch Neurol 1983;40:251.

78. Reinhart JB, Evans SL, McFadden DL. Cyclic vomiting in children seen through the psychiatrist's eye. Pediatrics 1977;59:371.

34

Approach to the Patient with Abdominal Pain

KENNETH B. KLEIN
SHERMAN M. MELLINKOFF

Abdominal pain is an extremely common human experience.[1-3] It is the most frequent reason for patients to consult a gastroenterologist[4,5] and is a leading cause of disability and absence from work.[6] Abdominal pain is also costly. Investigations in response to a complaint of abdominal pain may be quite expensive, and the costs of inappropriate or delayed diagnosis and treatment may be considerable. Continuing care for a patient with chronic abdominal pain is extremely demanding of medical resources. Most important are the human costs; the suffering abdominal pain imposes on the patient, and often on the family, can be substantial.

Abdominal pain is an entirely subjective experience that cannot be accounted for simply by the location and extent of any tissue damage or disordered physiology. For example, one patient with a shallow duodenal ulcer crater may have severe epigastric pain, while another with profound hemorrhage from a penetrating ulcer may be asymptomatic. The pain experienced in association with similar lesions may vary greatly among patients not only in intensity but in location and character.[7] This variability may be accounted for only by considering pathophysiologic, neurophysiologic, and psychosocial mechanisms.

At the pathophysiologic level, the lesion's impact is influenced by such things as the nature and rate of progression of the noxious process, previous injury in the same location, and local motility patterns. Neuroanatomic and neurophysiologic determinants of abdominal pain include the nature of visceral sensory receptors, the organization of the pathways that pain information takes from the abdomen to the brain, and the wide range of modifying influences on the transmission and inhibition of pain messages at various levels of the nervous system. Finally, many psychosocial factors such as personality, family and cultural background, and the setting in which the pain occurs may profoundly affect the patient's subjective experience of abdominal pain.

The physician's major task in caring for patients with abdominal pain is to minimize suffering. In most cases of acute abdominal pain this is best achieved by making an expeditious diagnosis and then instituting appropriate, and usually curative, treatment. Especially with chronic abdominal pain, entirely eliminating the pain is not always possible. Thus, minimizing suffering often requires considerable attention to reducing the disruption the pain may cause in the patient's work, family, and personal life. Finally, minimizing suffering means minimizing potential morbidity—that resulting from delay in initiating specific therapy, from administering less than optimal therapy, and from performing inappropriate or unnecessary tests and procedures.

Expert diagnosis and treatment of patients with abdominal pain require knowledge of a number of areas in addition to the pathophysiology and natural history of the many conditions that may give rise to abdominal pain. Such areas include visceral neuroanatomy and neurophysiology, pain psychophysiology, and the mechanisms of action and effectiveness of a wide range of therapeutic options. The goal of this chapter is to provide the clinician with a broad-based background from which to draw in approaching patients with abdominal pain.

The first section will review the neuroanatomy and neurophysiology of abdominal pain. The focus will be how information from these fields may aid our understanding of many clinical facets of abdominal pain. The next section, on acute abdominal pain, will develop the principles of the previous section with an emphasis on expeditiously arriving at an accurate pathophysiologic diagnosis by means of a careful evaluation of clues from the history and physical examination. Last is a consideration of the three major classes of chronic abdominal pain: chronic intermittent abdominal pain, in which the focus is on arriving at a diagnosis, because specific therapy will usually follow; chronic unrelenting abdominal pain associated with an established cause, with emphasis on methods of minimizing the pain; and chronic intractable abdominal pain without a simple pathophysiologic explanation, in which a biopsychosocial approach is employed for understanding its complex pathogenesis and for optimal management.

NEUROANATOMY AND NEUROPHYSIOLOGY OF ABDOMINAL PAIN

Much more is known about "somatic" (especially cutaneous) pain than about abdominal visceral pain. Unfortunately, it is often inappropriate to make inferences from the first to the second because there are important neuroanatomic, functional, and clinical differences between skin and abdominal visceral nociception. The skin is much more densely innervated than the viscera. This presumably accounts for the fact that cutaneous pain is usually "bright" and precisely localized, whereas visceral pain tends to be ill-defined and poorly localized. Unlike skin pain, visceral pain may be referred to and result in hyperalgesia of areas remote from the site of pathology or injury. Stimuli affecting the skin may give rise to a wide variety of feelings, whereas the only consciously perceived sensation from most of the abdominal viscera is discomfort or pain. Pain arising from the skin always implies actual or potential tissue damage, whereas severe abdominal pain may result from stimuli (e.g., vigorous contraction of a hollow viscus) that don't threaten tissue integrity at all. The remainder of this section will suggest the anatomic and functional basis for these characteristics of abdominal pain.

Visceral Nerve Receptors That Mediate Abdominal Pain

A wide variety of destructive stimuli to the abdominal viscera cause no pain, and in fact often no conscious sensation whatsoever. For example, virtually all of the abdominal organs are insensitive to pinching, burning, stabbing, cutting, and electrical and thermal stimulation.[8-13] The same is true for acid and alkali when applied to normal gut mucosa.[8,11,13]

There are four general classes of stimuli that do result in abdominal pain. These are distention and contraction[8-10,14-17]; traction, compression, and torsion[9,10,14,17,18]; stretch[9,17-19]; and certain chemicals.[14,20,21] The abdominal visceral receptors mediating these responses are located within the walls of hollow organs, on serosal structures such as the visceral peritoneum and the capsule of solid organs, within the mesentery (especially associated with large mesenteric vessels and ligaments), and within the mucosa.[14,22-26] Receptors located in most of these sites appear to be "polymodal," that is, they respond to both mechanical and chemical stimuli.[25,27] However, mucosal receptors seem to respond primarily, if not exclusively, to chemicals.[18]

In terms of response to mechanical forces, best characterized are the "tension receptors," which are functionally, if not anatomically, in series with the smooth muscle of the wall of hollow organs.[14,26] They are located within the muscular layers as well as between the muscularis mucosa and the submucosa. Pain occurs whenever the smooth muscle in these locations undergoes a sufficient increase in tension. This commonly occurs when an organ is being stretched (e.g., gastric distention as a result of gastric outlet obstruction) or is forcefully contracting (e.g., the vigorous intestinal peristalsis that may occur proximal to an intussusception). These receptors will also be activated when the smooth muscle of an organ is isometrically contracting, that is, when the tension in the muscle cells increases but the organ doesn't change in diameter. Colonic contraction around an impaction and ampullary spasm around a stone are examples of isometric contraction. On the other hand, isotonic contraction or stretch, when the organ changes in diameter but there is no change in muscle tension (e.g., rectal accommodation to a fecal bolus), does not activate these tension receptors and is therefore not associated with pain.

The receptors in serosal and mesenteric structures respond most notably to stretch and torsion, respectively.[18] Stimulation of serosal receptors within the liver capsule presumably accounts for the pain experienced with hepatic distention in severe right-sided congestive heart failure. Similarly, mesenteric receptors are activated by a sigmoid volvulus or ovarian torsion.

Abdominal visceral receptors that initiate the transmission of pain information appear to respond to a wide variety of chemicals. Although a response may be elicited experimentally to chemicals such as KCl, HCl, and hypertonic saline,[14,24,27] of greater clinical interest is their activation by substances that are generated or released in the presence of inflammation, tissue necrosis, ischemia, and hypoxia. These include bradykinin, substance P, serotonin, histamine, and some of the prostaglandins.[14,21,24,27] Of these, bradykinin seems to be the most potent stimulus for pain.[24] Mesenteric insufficiency and inflammatory bowel disease probably cause pain through stimulation of these receptors. Chemically induced pain may result directly from chemical stimulation of the receptor. Recently, however, it has been suggested that such pain may be mediated through local smooth muscle contraction triggered by these chemicals.[22,24,28] Perhaps this indirect effect is one reason why it cannot be consistently demonstrated that applying acid to an ulcer crater is painful[29,30]; it could be that pain occurs only if local conditions favor smooth muscle contraction in response to the acid stimulus.

In many clinical situations it is likely that the subjective experience of abdominal pain is the result of multiple stimuli. Pancreatic cancer pain may result from a combination of serosal stretch, the compression of vessels and mesentery, and perhaps direct infiltration of nerves. Furthermore, the sensitivity of visceral receptors may be altered in certain settings. Pressure on, or chemicals applied to, the normal gastric mucosa usually causes no discomfort, but when the mucosa is inflamed, these same stimuli may be quite painful.[12,13]

Neuroanatomy of Abdominal Pain

Most abdominal visceral nerves play no role in pain perception. The walls of the gut, for example, house many sensory neurons whose cell bodies lie within the submucosal or myenteric plexuses. These nerves, which form part of the extensive enteric nervous system, are involved with the regulation of such activities as motility and secretion in response to local gut conditions. They do not project to the central nervous system (CNS) and are thought to have no role in nociception.[25] A second class of non-nociceptive abdominal nerves travel to the CNS along with the parasympathetic nerves, primarily the vagus. They transmit information concerning local osmolarity, pH, the concentration of nutrients, and the state of distention.[14,31] Little if any of this information reaches consciousness, and none is associated with pain.

Just as there are major differences in the types of stimuli that induce pain in the abdomen and the skin, there are major differences between the abdominal viscera and the skin in the nature of the afferent nerve fibers that do mediate pain. Associated with the skin are two separate types of nociceptive fibers: the myelinated, rapidly conducting A-delta fibers and the unmyelinated, slowly conducting c fibers. For the abdominal viscera, on the other hand, the great majority of afferent fibers, and virtually all the ones mediating nociception, are c fibers.[32]

The neuronal pathways that mediate abdominal pain sensation

involve three levels of neurons between the abdominal viscera and the cerebral cortex (Fig 34-1). First-order neurons travel from the viscera to the spinal cord, second-order neurons link the cord and the brain stem, and third-order neurons travel from the brain stem to higher levels of the brain. Virtually all nerve fibers that carry abdominal nociceptive information run wholly or almost wholly with the sympathetic nervous system (i.e., the thoracolumbar input).[25,26,32,33]

After leaving the viscus they innervate, the first-order nerves pass through the adjacent autonomic plexus. In general, the plexus appears as a web of nerve tissue associated with the major artery supplying the organ (e.g., the celiac, hepatic, superior mesenteric). These plexuses coalesce to form ganglia. From the ganglion, the afferent fibers then travel within the regional splanchnic nerve to the sympathetic chain, which runs parallel to the spinal cord on either side. From there they proceed to the spinal nerve by way of the white ramus communicans. Finally, they enter the spinal cord by way of dorsal and, which is unusual for afferent nerves,

possibly by way of ventral roots,[34] though this is controversial.[24] The cell bodies of these first-order neurons lie in the dorsal root ganglia. The neurons finally synapse in the dorsal horn of the spinal cord, predominantly in laminae I and V.[26,32,34,35] This is in contrast to "somatic" nerves, such as those from the skin, that synapse primarily in laminae II to IV, again highlighting the neuroanatomic differences between visceral and somatic pain.

The postsynaptic (second-order) neurons mediating abdominal visceral pain begin in the dorsal horn, cross the midline to the contralateral side, and then travel cephalad within the ventrolateral quadrant of the spinal cord. These neurons run in several ascending pathways, but mainly the spinothalamic tract, to synapse within a number of thalamic nuclei, and the spinoreticular tract, to synapse within reticular-formation nuclei of the pons and medulla.[26,34] Little is known about the pathways of the third-order nerves that transmit abdominal pain sensation, but by analogy to somatic pain pathways, they probably travel widely throughout the brain. Pain pathway projections from the spinothalamic tract travel primarily

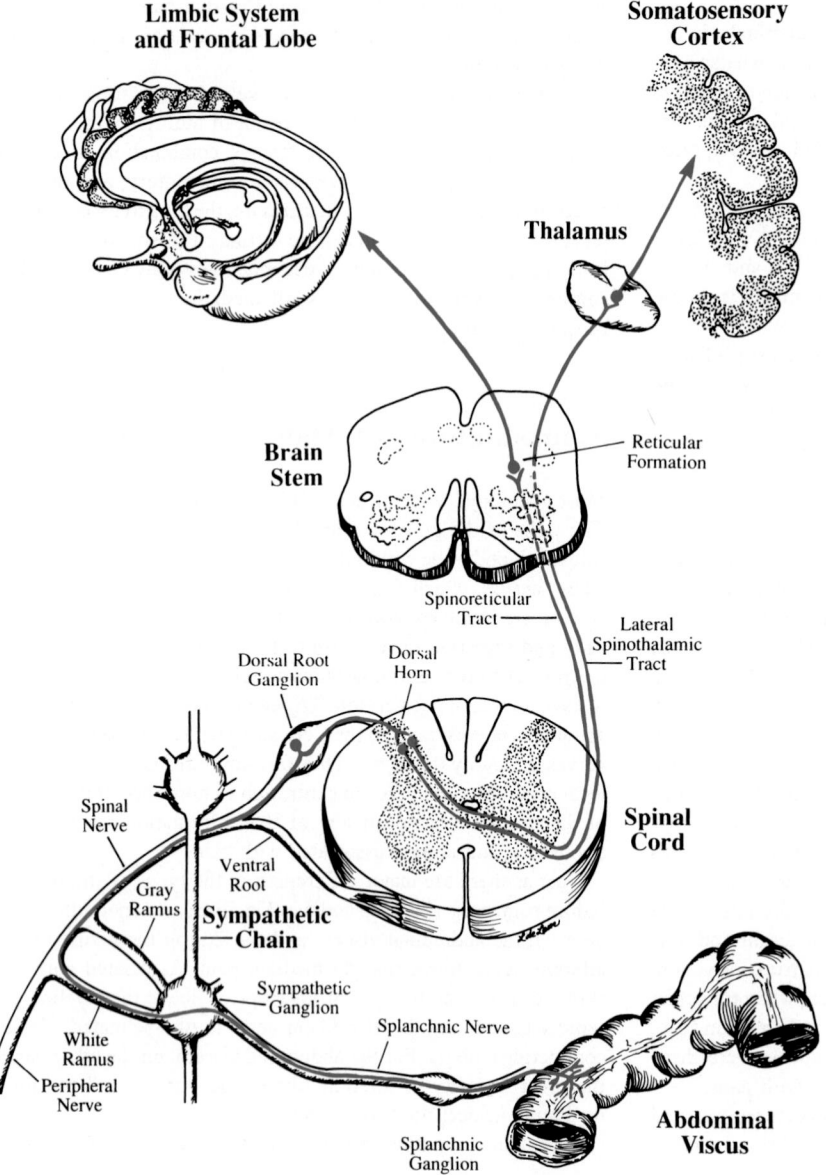

Limbic System and Frontal Lobe

Somatosensory Cortex

Thalamus

Brain Stem

Reticular Formation

Spinoreticular Tract

Lateral Spinothalamic Tract

Dorsal Root Ganglion

Dorsal Horn

Spinal Cord

Spinal Nerve

Ventral Root

Gray Ramus

Sympathetic Chain

Sympathetic Ganglion

Splanchnic Nerve

White Ramus

Peripheral Nerve

Splanchnic Ganglion

Abdominal Viscus

FIGURE 34–1. Neuronal pathways mediating abdominal visceral pain sensation. There are three orders of neurons mediating pain sensation. The first-order neuron travels from the abdominal viscus by way of the adjacent autonomic plexus to the regional splanchnic ganglion, then along the corresponding splanchnic nerve through a ganglion of the sympathetic chain, then by way of the white ramus communicans to the spinal nerve. From there it traverses the dorsal root (its cell body lies in the dorsal root ganglion) to enter the dorsal horn of the spinal cord, where it synapses predominantly within laminae I and V. The second-order neurons leave the dorsal horn, cross the midline, and ascend primarily in two tracts. The spinothalamic tract neurons travel through the brain stem to various nuclei within the thalamus, where they synapse with third-order neurons that go predominantly to the somatosensory cortex, mediating the sensory and discriminative aspects of pain. Spinoreticular tract neurons synapse within reticular formation nuclei located primarily in the pons and medulla. From there, third-order neurons travel predominantly to the limbic system and frontal cortex, mediating aspects of pain that have to do with feelings and actions, but also make connections within the thalamus and elsewhere.

to the somatosensory cortex, which seems to subserve the "sensory-discriminative" components of pain perception (that is, those concerned with the quality and localization of the pain). Third-order neurons synapsing with spinoreticular tract neurons seem to go predominantly to the limbic system and frontal cortex, subserving the "motivational-affective" aspects of pain perception (the aversive, unpleasant features).[36,37]

Functional Neuroanatomy and Neurophysiology

PAIN SIGNAL TRANSMISSION AND THE GATE CONTROL THEORY OF PAIN

Just how do the visceral afferent nerves of the abdomen transmit the information that is ultimately experienced as pain? Unlike the skin, where there are nerves that transmit pain information exclusively ("nociceptors"), it appears that there are few if any abdominal afferents solely concerned with nociception. With only rare possible exceptions,[38] afferent c fibers from the abdominal viscera grade their response to the strength of the stimulus through an "intensity coding" mechanism.[23,26,27] When a certain threshold is surpassed, the signal is interpreted as painful. However, although a certain level of stimulus intensity is necessary for the experience of abdominal pain, it is far from sufficient.[24,25] The "gate control theory of pain," proposed in 1965 by Melzack and Wall,[39] suggests

that whether the peripheral stimulus will be perceived as painful is influenced by interacting factors at the site of the stimulus, within the spinal cord, and in the brain.[40,41]

The focus of the gate control theory is the dorsal horn of the spinal cord (Fig 34-2). As discussed earlier, this is the site of the synapse between afferent neurons that carry sensory (especially nociceptive) information from the periphery and second-order neurons—in this context called "transmission cells" or "T-cells"—that relay signals to the brain stem and then ultimately to consciousness in the cortex. Two classes of peripheral neurons converge on the T-cell, one with large- and the other with small-diameter fibers. Both types of neurons directly stimulate the T-cell, thus tending to "open the gate" to pain signal transmission. Both also send branches to the substantia gelatinosa, located within the dorsal horn, where they synapse with inhibitory "interneurons." The large fibers *stimulate* the interneurons, which, when activated, tend to suppress T-cell firing (and thus "close the gate"), while the small fibers *inhibit* interneuron activity, creating the opposite effect. The balance of stimulatory and inhibitory inputs determines whether the T-cell will fire and thus transmit nociceptive information.

"Descending inhibitory systems" also provide input to the dorsal horn.[37,42,43] Neurons arising within the periaqueductal gray area of the midbrain, which are rich in enkephalins and opiate receptors, send projections to structures in the medulla, particularly the nucleus raphe magnus and the reticular formation. From there, fibers travel to the substantia gelatinosa, where a variety of neurotransmitters are released. These activate the inhibitory interneurons, decreasing the likelihood of rostral transmission of nociceptive information and thus the perception of pain. The endogenous opioids, especially the enkephalins, are key neurotransmitters of the descending inhibitory pathways. These pathways may also be stimulated by exogenous opioids, which is how these drugs are thought to work as analgesics.[42,44,45]

The descending inhibitory pathways are activated by a variety of immediate influences such as acute pain, stress, and the administration of placebos.[43] The degree to which these systems respond in various circumstances is determined by such complex factors as the setting in which the potentially painful event is occurring, previous pain experiences, and even personality characteristics and cultural background.[37,46] Descending inhibitory inputs to the dorsal horn have been specifically identified for abdominal visceral afferents.[47]

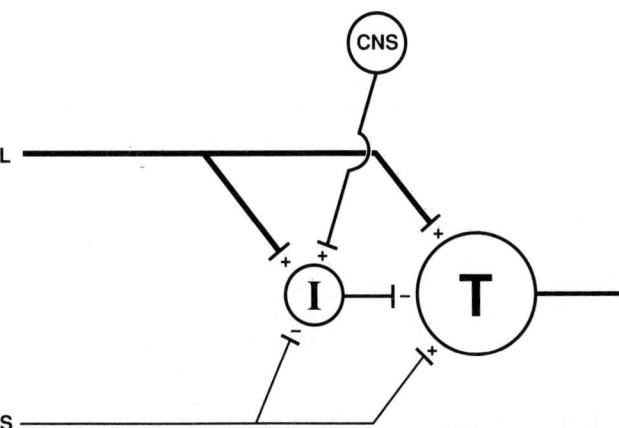

FIGURE 34-2. The gate control theory of pain. Sensory inputs from the periphery come to the dorsal horn of the spinal cord by way of large (*L*) and small (*S*) nerve fibers. Both fiber types synapse on the second-order ("transmission cell") neurons (*T*); when the T-cell neurons are activated, they communicate nociceptive information to the brain. The peripheral nerve fibers also synapse on interneurons (*I*) within the substantia gelatinosa of the dorsal horn that, when stimulated, *inhibit* T-cell firing. The large neurons stimulate and the small neurons inhibit these inhibitory interneurons, thus tending to prevent and promote, respectively, central transmission of incoming nociceptive signals. "Descending inhibitory systems" arising within the central nervous system (*CNS*), when activated by a variety of factors, also stimulate the interneuron to inhibit T-cell firing. The balance of these excitatory and inhibitory forces determines the degree to which nociceptive information is transmitted to the brain. (+ = excitatory signals; − = inhibitory signals)

LOCALIZATION OF ABDOMINAL PAIN

It is a common and sometimes frustrating clinical experience that patients find it difficult to precisely localize their abdominal pain. This imprecision was dramatically illustrated by a study in which various abdominal structures were distended by means of balloons.[15] Usually subjects were unable to distinguish any difference in pain location when the distal esophagus, biliary tree, and upper small intestine were distended.

Abdominal pain is so poorly localized in part because of the paucity of visceral afferent nerves. Indeed, the skin has a much greater density of afferents that conduct nociceptive information. Even at the levels where most of the incoming abdominal fibers enter, less than 10% of the total input to the spinal cord consists of such afferents; by far the predominant input is somatic nerves.[24,26,32] Furthermore, as opposed to the more tidy ordering of somatic afferents, one splanchnic nerve may carry fibers from several organs, and nerves from a single organ may enter the spinal cord by way of several spinal segments.

Although there is a relatively sparse input to the spinal cord from nerves that mediate abdominal pain, when a splanchnic nerve is stimulated, more than 50% of the second-order neurons at that level respond.[32] This characteristic, called "functional divergence," is probably another reason why abdominal pain is so diffusely experienced—a small number of abdominal afferent nerves stimulate a great number of spinothalamic tract neurons, precluding precise localization.[25] Another result of functional divergence is that abdominal visceral input that results in pain often also triggers a multitude of other, primarily autonomic, effects such as changes in muscle tone, pulse, blood pressure, and motor and secretory reflexes.[25,32]

The general region of the abdomen where pain is experienced is a reflection of the characteristics of the afferent nerves innervating the structure being stimulated. Most abdominal organs, including most of the gut, began embryologically as midline structures and therefore have bilaterally symmetric innervation.[10,17,24] And indeed, most digestive tract pain is midline pain.[10,15,17,48–53] Abdominal pain that is clearly lateralized is likely to be from the relatively few organs whose innervation is predominantly lateralized, such as the kidneys, ureters, and ovaries,[10,17,24] or from structures with somatic rather than visceral innervation, as will be discussed below. Some organs with bilateral innervation may have a predominance of one side over the other; this results in a tendency to pain perception away from the midline. Examples of such organs are the ascending and descending colon and the gallbladder.[24]

The spinal segments at which the afferent nerves from abdominal viscera enter the spinal cord determine the location within the abdomen where pain is experienced (Fig 34-3).[24] The embryologic origins of the abdominal viscera provide a general guideline as to the expected location (Table 34-1). Foregut structures (the distal esophagus, stomach, proximal duodenum, liver, biliary tree, and pancreas) are innervated by nerves that enter the spinal cord at the T5–T6 to T8–T9 level.[9,17,24,33] When these organs are artificially distended, the resultant pain tends to be in the midline, between the xiphoid and the umbilicus.[10,15,19,48,49,51,54] Similarly, clinical pain from foregut structures, such as the pain of peptic esophagitis and gastric ulcer, is usually felt in the epigastrium.

Organs arising from the midgut, including the small intestine, appendix, ascending colon, and the proximal two thirds of the transverse colon, are innervated by afferent nerves that enter the spinal cord roughly between T8–T11 and L1.[17,33,55] When these midgut organs are distended, pain is perceived in the periumbilical region.[10,16,24,48,51,52,54] This, not unexpectedly, is the same location as that for clinical pain involving these organs, for example, that of small-bowel obstruction and early appendicitis. Hindgut-derived organs, including the distal one third of the transverse colon, the descending colon, and the rectosigmoid, are innervated by spinal nerves T11 to L1.[17,33,55] Pain arising from experimental stimulation of these organs, and the corresponding clinical pain, is usually felt between the umbilicus and the pubis.[10,16,48,52]

Although these generalizations are clinically useful, it must be kept in mind that for a number of reasons, including variability of innervation, abdominal pain arising in a particular organ may be perceived by different patients in widely varying locations. This is true, for example, of the pain associated with cholecystitis.[56,57] Similarly, inflating a balloon in one location within the colon may result in pain in quite different parts of the abdomen in different subjects.[48,50,58,59]

Changes in the location of abdominal pain in the course of a developing illness are easier to understand if the basic principles of innervation of abdominal structures are remembered. Zollinger showed that distention of the biliary tree results in midline epigastric pain. When the parietal peritoneum overlying the gallbladder was stimulated, however, pain became sharply localized to the right upper quadrant.[19] This is because the parietal peritoneum is innervated by somatic rather than visceral nerves; somatic nerves provide much denser innervation, resulting in more precise localization of the tissue injury. Clinically, appendicitis usually presents with periumbilical pain, reflecting the midgut origins and bilaterally symmetric innervation of the appendix. The pain shifts to the right lower quadrant when appendiceal inflammation proceeds to the point where the parietal peritoneum is involved.[53]

REFERRED PAIN

One of the most characteristic features of abdominal pain is its propensity to be associated with pain at a site distant from the affected organ.[9,35,48,49,53,60–62] This is known as "referred pain." Re-

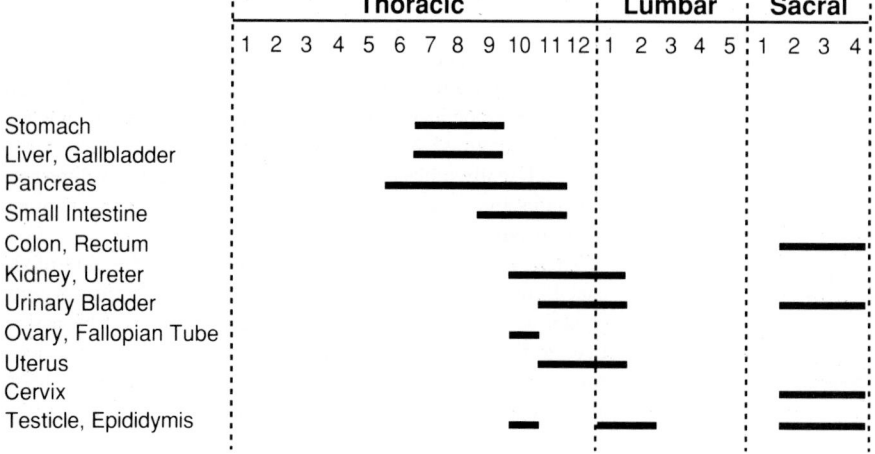

FIGURE 34–3. Relief of visceral abdominal pain by transection of spinal nerves. The bars indicate the spinal nerves that were sectioned to give relief of pain arising from the indicated visceral organs. (Modified from Jänig W, Morrison JFB. Functional properties of spinal visceral afferents supplying abdominal and pelvic organs, with special emphasis on visceral nociception. In: Cervero F, Morrison JFB, eds. Visceral sensation. Amsterdam: Elsevier, 1986:87.)

TABLE 34-1
General Rules of Abdominal Pain Localization

EMBRYOLOGIC ORIGIN	ADULT STRUCTURES	SPINAL SEGMENTS	CLINICAL PAIN LOCATION
Foregut	Distal esophagus, stomach prox. duodenum, liver, biliary tree, pancreas	T5–T6 to T8–T9	Between xiphoid and umbilicus
Midgut	Small intestine, appendix, ascending colon, proximal 2/3 of transverse colon	T8–T11 to L1	Periumbilical
Hindgut	Distal 1/3 of transverse colon, descending colon, rectosigmoid	T11–L1	Between umbilicus and pubis

ferred pain from an abdominal source is usually a deep, aching sensation that is perceived to be near the surface of the body.[9,63] Two associated features of referred pain are skin hyperalgesia[17,24,35,53,63,64] and increased muscle tone of the abdominal wall.[35,53,65]

In general, referred pain is associated with the cutaneous dermatomes whose afferent nerve roots enter the same levels of the spinal cord as those of the painful abdominal structure (Fig 34-4). Knowledge of the characteristic patterns of pain referral can be extremely helpful in making a diagnosis. For example, the biliary tree is innervated by visceral nerves that enter the spinal cord between T5 and T9. Thus, pain from a biliary tree lesion is referred to cutaneous dermatomes with T5 to T9 innervation, that is, the region of the back, right shoulder, and right scapula.[66]

What is the neuroanatomic basis for referred pain? A great deal of evidence in recent years has confirmed the "convergence–projection" theory (Fig 34-5). As mentioned previously, abdominal visceral afferent fibers terminate predominately in laminae I and V of the dorsal horn, thus flanking the sites where somatic nerves (i.e., nerves from skin, muscle, joints, and so forth) primarily terminate. Both sets of afferent inputs, however, activate the same spinothalamic tract neurons[26,67,68]; there are no separate pathways within the spinal cord for visceral and somatic pain.[35] Because somatic afferents are far more numerous and more commonly stimulated than abdominal visceral afferents, the brain tends to associate activation of the second-order neurons with a somatic source, even when it is due to abdominal visceral input.

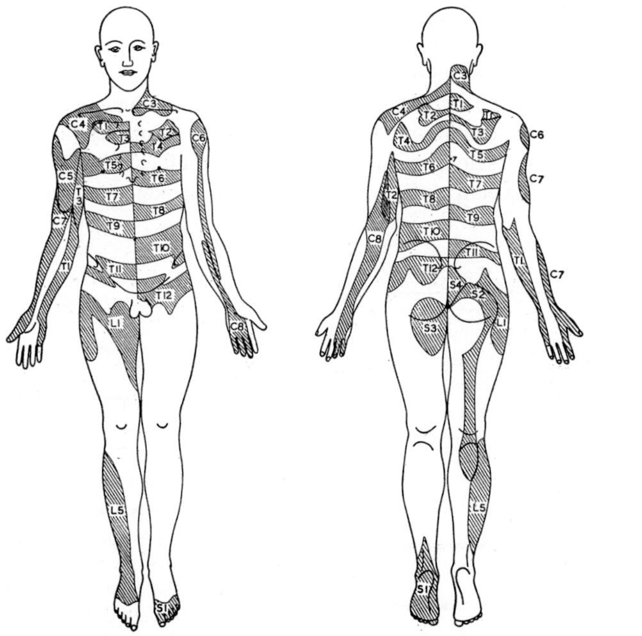

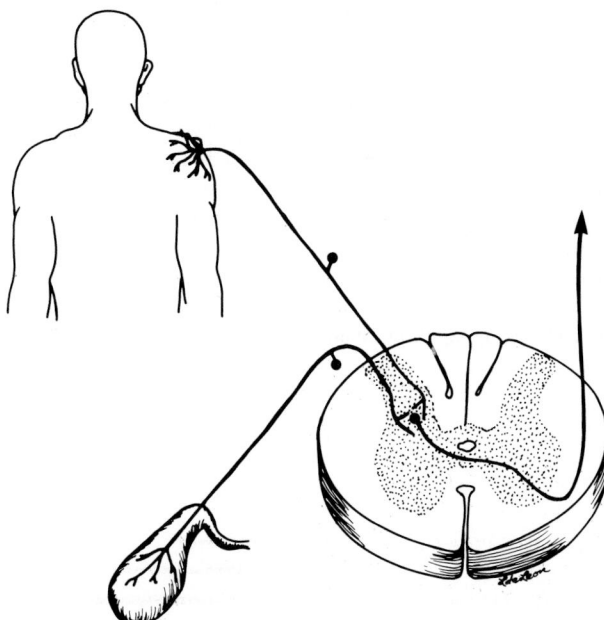

FIGURE 34-5. Neuroanatomic basis of referred pain. According to the "convergence–projection theory," afferent nociceptive signals from abdominal visceral structures synapse within the dorsal horn of the spinal cord with the second-order neurons that receive somatic (e.g., cutaneous) input from the same spinal level. Thus, a nociceptive signal from an abdominal organ triggers firing of the same second-order neurons that would respond if noxious input were received from the corresponding somatic structure. The resulting conscious perception of pain is referred to the somatic structure, because afferent signals from this source are received more commonly than are those from the viscera. Thus, the brain is "fooled" as to the true origin of the incoming signal.

FIGURE 34-4. Cutaneous dermatomes: Pattern of referral of pain from abdominal viscera. In general, pain is referred to the cutaneous dermatomes whose afferent nerves enter the same levels of the spinal cord as those of the affected abdominal organ. (From Lewis T. Pain. New York: Macmillan, 1942.)

The heightened skin sensitivity associated with referred pain is thought to occur as a result of the increased excitability of spinothalamic tract neurons that is caused by incoming abdominal visceral impulses. Thus, these neurons are primed for a relatively intense response to cutaneous input—even that triggered by skin stimulation that would not ordinarily be painful—entering the spinal cord at the same level.[35,63] The increased tone of abdominal muscles that may accompany visceral pain seems to be a result of facilitation of flexion reflexes[35,63,65] or a result of direct peritoneal irritation.[53,65] Figure 34-6 shows the spinal segmental distribution of cutaneous hyperalgesia associated with pain in various visceral organs. As can be seen by comparing Figures 34-6 and 34-3, there is a close correspondence between the segmental pattern of hyperalgesia and the spinal nerves that must be severed to give relief of abdominal pain arising from the same organs.

Neurophysiology of Chronic Abdominal Pain

Chronic pain may be due to ongoing peripheral pathology. However, even when it is intense and debilitating, some types of chronic pain may occur without any continued nociceptive input from the end-organ. This is probably true, for example, in many cases of chronic pancreatitis, where abdominal pain may persist long after significant pancreatic inflammation or even ductal distention has resolved. Indeed, severe chronic pain may be present without any identifiable inciting event.[45]

A variety of mechanisms may contribute to the establishment and maintenance of chronic abdominal pain states. Some involve neurons that are part of peripheral or central nociceptive circuits[45]: if there is selective damage to afferent large-diameter fibers or to fibers within the descending inhibitory pathways, inhibitory input to the spinal cord T cells will be reduced. The result would be that central transmission of nociceptive inputs would be facilitated. If such damage is sustained, chronic pain may develop.[45] Changes in the physiology of the c fibers, which convey nociceptive information from the abdominal viscera, may also promote chronic pain. When c fibers are repeatedly stimulated by processes such as acute tissue injury or changes in tissue composition, they may

begin to synthesize peptides rather than the amino acids that serve as neurotransmitters under usual circumstances. With more prolonged c-fiber stimulation, yet other neurotransmitters, whose identity is currently unknown, are synthesized. The release of these peptides and other "new" neurotransmitters tends to increase the sensitivity and excitability of the region of the dorsal horn in contact with the involved c fibers. The result is that there is a lowering of the threshold for transmission of nociceptive input from the structures that the c fibers innervate. In some cases such new patterns of neurotransmitter synthesis and release may become fixed, leading to the establishment of chronic pain, even after the original peripheral injury has resolved.[45]

An especially intriguing mechanism whereby chronic pain may develop involves the concept of a pain "memory trace." After acute pain has been experienced for more than several hours, there is evidence that a record of this pain is stored within the CNS.[45] Under certain circumstances, an acute noxious stimulus occurring within the same receptive field as that from which this memory trace arose will activate it, resulting in a recapitulation of the original pain.[69] Such pain may become self-sustaining if, for example, descending inhibitory pathways are compromised, allowing persistent firing of the memory trace.

The "central pattern generating mechanism" theory[40] suggests a means whereby these and other observations may be synthesized in a model to explain the occurrence of chronic pain without continued peripheral nociceptive input. Although originally proposed to account for the "phantom pain" sometimes experienced by paraplegic patients,[70] it is also useful in explaining some types of chronic abdominal pain. According to this theory, collections of neurons at various levels along the somatosensory pain projection systems from the dorsal horn to the cortex may develop abnormal firing patterns as a result of alterations in normal input, for example from reduced signals from damaged or severed afferent nociceptive fibers. Such abnormally functioning neurons may become stabilized (the "pattern generating mechanism") but might not result in nociceptive signals reaching consciousness unless they are triggered. Immediate triggers range from certain emotional states to acute visceral pathology. More long-term and continuous ("tonic") influences could cause self-perpetuating firing of these abnormal neurons, resulting in chronic pain.[40,45] Such influences may operate within the peripheral nervous system (e.g., a reduction in the ratio

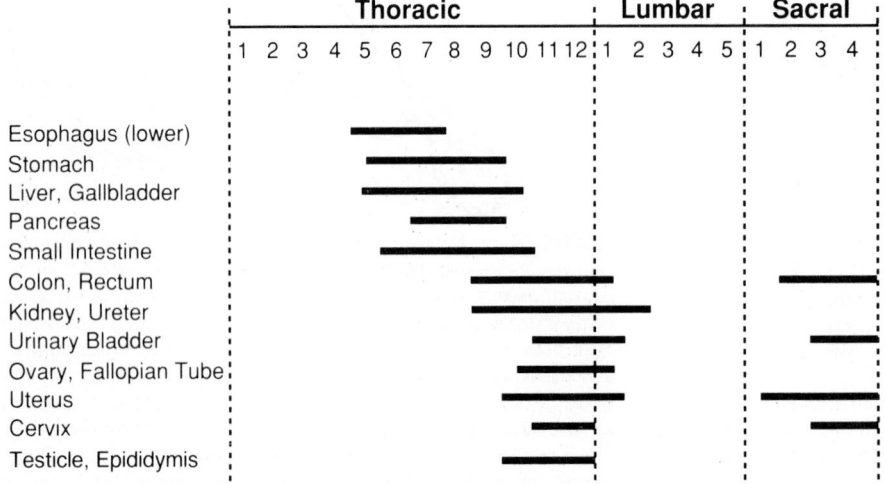

FIGURE 34–6. Segmental distribution of cutaneous hyperalgesia associated with pain in the abdominal viscera. The bars indicate the spinal levels of the cutaneous dermatomes where spontaneous or induced (by light stroking of the skin) hyperalgesia was experienced in patients who had abdominal pain arising in the indicated organs. (Modified from Jänig W, Morrison JFB. Functional properties of spinal visceral afferents supplying abdominal and pelvic organs, with special emphasis on visceral nociception. In: Cevero F, Morrison JFB, eds. Visceral sensation. Amsterdam: Elsevier, 1986:87.)

of large- to small-diameter nerve fiber afferent inputs to the dorsal horn) or the central nervous system (decreased descending inhibitory input, a particular cultural background, a personality disorder). Obviously, the detailed neurophysiology of such mechanisms is yet to be worked out, but they emphasize the point that complex interactions at various levels within the nervous system may result in chronic pain.

ACUTE ABDOMINAL PAIN

In caring for patients with acute abdominal pain, the central task is establishing an accurate diagnosis as quickly and efficiently as possible. This is because making a diagnosis almost always leads to specific therapy, such as surgery, drugs, or symptomatic treatment. The history and the physical examination are the keys to this process. They may point to the diagnosis in various ways: sometimes through anatomic, especially neuroanatomic, implications of readily obtained findings; sometimes through the pattern of the pain and the associated behavior of the patient; and sometimes through knowledge of the patient's social relationships or occupation.

History

LOCATION

The location where pain arising from various abdominal viscera is generally experienced was discussed in the section on neuroanatomy and neurophysiology. Table 34-1 and Figure 34-3 summarize this information. Likewise, Figures 34-4 and 34-6 together illustrate the expected pattern of referred pain from abdominal organs.

SUBJECTIVE CHARACTERIZATION

The subjective experience of pain is determined by a wide array of factors, including the setting in which the pain is occurring, the patient's past experience with various types of pain, personality, and culture. Trying to communicate an experience as private as abdominal pain can be a daunting task even in the best of circumstances. When the patient is actively in pain and is in an unfamiliar and sometimes threatening medical setting, his or her ability to meaningfully describe what he or she is feeling may be severely compromised. Thus, it is essential that the clinician be forbearing, generous, and respectful in hearing the patient's story. It is usually best to begin by listening without interrupting. The patient's original account and accompanying facial expressions often provide helpful leads to be followed later by specific questions.

In seeking to characterize the patient's pain, it is generally unwise to rely upon words or descriptions without careful clarification of their meaning. For example, the words "colic" or "cramps" may mean very different things to different people. To some people, "colic" merely means a severe pain, and a "cramp" is any pain localized to the belly. Such words may have rather different implications even for physicians: despite the usual meaning of "colic" as a paroxysmal pain that rises and falls in intensity, "biliary colic" quickly reaches maximal severity and varies little.[56] Renal colic more commonly tends to wax and wane,[56] while the "colic" associated with bowel obstruction is generally characterized by major fluctuations in pain intensity.

In actual practice there is tremendous variability in patients' characterizations of pain associated with the same pathologic process. For example, different patients have described the pain associated with their peptic ulcer disease as, among other things, aching, gnawing, sharp, burning, tearing, and squeezing.[7] Thus, it is usually best not to dismiss the possibility that a particular patient's abdominal pain is due to a specific condition simply because the pain description doesn't fit the classical teaching.

TEMPORAL CONSIDERATIONS

Causes of acute abdominal pain may often be differentiated by their tempo of onset and progression. Free rupture of a viscus or blood vessel into the peritoneal cavity, a dissecting aneurysm, or obstruction by a biliary or renal stone usually results in severe pain within seconds to minutes. Some inflammatory conditions such as pancreatitis and cholecystitis may take an hour or more to reach peak pain intensity, while with others such as appendicitis, diverticulitis, and bowel obstruction, the progression to maximal severity is generally slower yet. It may be helpful to ask approximately how much time elapsed between the first twinge of pain and the pain at its worst. Even if imprecise, the answer may still give more reliable information than asking simply whether the onset of the pain was "sudden" or "gradual." Another useful question is to ask what the patient was doing when the pain began. A patient with biliary colic may answer that question with astonishing precision ("I just opened the car door"). A patient with appendicitis is much more likely to set the onset of his pain as "sometime in the afternoon."

With some conditions, pain is characteristically present at certain times of the day. The pain of duodenal ulcer, for example, is particularly likely to awaken the patient at night[71] but is rarely present in the morning before breakfast. Mesenteric ischemia typically results in pain after meals.

The duration of the abdominal pain may help discriminate the underlying cause. An episode of uncomplicated biliary colic lasts for a few minutes up to an hour or two, then rapidly diminishes. On the other hand, with acute pancreatitis, the pain may be present for many hours or even days.

RELIEVING AND AGGRAVATING FACTORS

It is often helpful to ask the patient what makes his pain worse and what makes it better. Pain initiated by swallowing implicates the esophagus. If bowel movements relieve the pain, the colon is likely to be the source. Pain aggravated by any action that moves the peritoneum suggests peritonitis. Pain made worse by anger but not by laughter may arise from increased tension in smooth muscle or from ischemia, as in angina pectoris. Pain aggravated by fatigue but by no particular bodily movement is sometimes caused by musculoskeletal aches or by cancer.

With obstruction of a hollow viscus, the patient may move about, writhe, or change positions vainly seeking relief but without making the pain worse. On the other hand, with peritonitis, movement is likely to aggravate the pain, and the patient usually prefers to lie still, and even avoid coughing or deep breathing. Some retroperitoneal processes, for example a pancreatic cancer, are often aggravated by lying supine and relieved by sitting up or bending forward. In the supine position, the normal lumbar curve of the spine tightens the limited retroperitoneal space around the cancer; leaning forward tends to do the opposite as the curvature of the spine is reversed. Pain arising in the colon may give the patient the feeling that passing flatus or having a bowel movement would bring relief. Lesions in the small bowel may also make the patient feel that a bowel movement would relieve the pain, but usually the feeling is less urgent than with large-bowel disease.

Some kinds of abdominal pain, for example that of duodenal ulcer, may prompt the patient to eat. Other painful conditions, such as pancreatitis or appendicitis, tend to diminish or wholly abolish appetite or to be accompanied by nausea and vomiting.

In general, detailed consideration of what foods make the pain worse are unlikely to be helpful in diagnosis. To be sure, foods capable of delivering fermentable carbohydrate to the colon, such as beans and cabbage, are apt to result in increased colonic gas and may provoke symptoms. Similarly, patients may experience abdominal pain if they have lactase deficiency and consume milk products, or if they are especially susceptible to the effects of sorbitol or fructose.[72] However, commonly held beliefs about certain foods provoking abdominal pain in certain conditions have not been proved accurate. Fatty foods, for instance, do not cause pain in patients with biliary tree disease,[71,73] and spicy foods have not been shown to trigger peptic ulcer pain.

ATYPICAL PAIN

Usually, readily accessible characteristics of abdominal pain—its location, onset, periodicity, progression, and relieving and aggravating factors—suggest a diagnosis. Sometimes, however, abdominal pain seems baffling. The pain may be present all over the abdomen, or in various parts of it at different times, and may wax and wane in peculiar ways. There may not seem to be a relationship between the intensity or timing of the pain and any visceral function. Such pain may appear in sudden attacks or may come and go gradually over a period of hours or days. There may or may not be accompanying anorexia or vomiting, constipation, or, less often, diarrhea, but neither vomiting, bowel movement, eating, nor fasting seems to affect the pain very much. Pain with these characteristics should raise suspicion of an illness that afflicts the nerves of the abdominal viscera. Among these are acute intermittent porphyria, tabes dorsalis, and chronic poisoning with lead or arsenic. Black widow spider bite may also cause severe abdominal pain of this character. The family, social, or occupational histories may provide helpful clues in patients with this type of abdominal pain.

Mesenteric venous thrombosis (which may occur in women taking oral contraceptives) and mesenteric arterial thrombosis (in elderly patients) may result in severe abdominal pain that comes and goes capriciously for weeks and may be associated with no physical examination or laboratory findings until gangrene appears.

Perplexing abdominal pain is discussed further in the section on chronic intermittent abdominal pain.

Physical Examination

When the physician is consulted about acute abdominal pain, it is often most important to decide whether or not emergency surgery will be required. The medical history is frequently helpful, but physical examination is usually indispensable. It is most unwise to decide by telephone that a surgical abdomen is or is not present.

FACIAL EXPRESSION

The first—and often vital—part of the physical examination will already have begun while the history is being elicited: interpretation of the patient's facial expressions. Severe pain is almost always reflected in the face; even when the patient is describing severe pain that is no longer present, the intensity of the former feelings is evident. Especially characteristic of acute inflammatory processes within the abdomen, appendicitis in particular, is an expression that seems to reflect a combination of pain and nausea characterized by an aura of malaise and an upward curling of the upper lip.[74]

ABDOMINAL EXAMINATION

The critical signs of a surgical abdomen are generally those indicating peritonitis or bowel obstruction. These are described in some detail in the chapter on the acute abdomen (ch 36). It is important to remember that they should be sought before giving a narcotic, which can obscure the signs of peritonitis and cause or aggravate a paralytic ileus.

Eliciting the signs of peritoneal irritation is an art requiring practice and careful attention to the patient. Pain tends to cause apprehension, and so does the doctor who is perceived as hurried, insensitive, or rough. Without the patient's confidence and cooperation—as nearly as his condition permits—it is far more difficult to distinguish between tenderness caused by an inflamed peritoneum and guarding caused by the approach of the doctor's hand.

It is best to begin by simply observing the patient and then to proceed only as necessary to maneuvers likely to cause pain. In most kinds of peritonitis the patient will be least uncomfortable lying supine, sometimes with the knees drawn up, and avoiding movement that impinges upon the most tender area. Thus, cholecystitis or a pulmonary infarct impinging upon the supradiaphragmatic pleura may cause visible splinting of the muscles in the right upper quadrant and diminished respiratory excursion on the right. Sometimes a ruptured ectopic pregnancy—occasionally mittelschmerz with unusually profuse bleeding—will catch the patient between faintness and nausea if she sits up and aggravation of shoulder pain from irritation of the peritoneum under the left leaf of the diaphragm if she lies down. Acute osteomyelitis of the ilium, which can cause hip and lower abdominal pain, usually causes the patient to insist upon lying prone. The important thing about observation is to try to understand anatomically the patient's position and movements, whether voluntary or reflexive. If not precluded by obvious involuntary spasm, asking the supine patient to take a deep breath slowly may indicate which part of the peritoneum is inflamed. Pain associated by deep breathing may be much more marked after coughing.

Other means of finding peritoneal tenderness and comparing its severity in different locations include gentle percussion, steady pressure with the fingers, and sudden release of pressure. The latter may cause severe pain where the peritoneum is maximally inflamed and should not be undertaken when lesser maneuvers have suggested where the most marked peritonitis lies. Thus, with acute cholecystitis, gradual deep pressure in the left lower quadrant of the abdomen may cause little or no pain while sudden release of that pressure results in pain and muscle spasm in the right upper quadrant. Pain elicited by pressure over the inflamed peritoneum usually causes reflexive (involuntary) tightening or "guarding" of the overlying abdominal muscles. With severe, generalized peritonitis, the whole abdominal wall may be rigid. In contrast, pressure over an uninflamed cecum distended by gas may cause pain without involuntary guarding. Sometimes the distinction between voluntary and involuntary guarding is difficult. Occasionally an apprehensive patient without peritonitis will tighten his abdominal muscles as soon as they are touched by the palpating fingers, but no guarding is elicited by the pressure of a stethoscope. The latter is not feared because it appears that the doctor is listening, not directly palpating. Another way to look for peritoneal tenderness is to jar the patient's heel as he is lying supine with legs extended. This sudden blow may elicit pain in the abdomen where the peritoneum is inflamed but should not cause pain in the heel, where an apprehensive patient might expect it.

The stethoscope is often helpful in appraising the quality of peristalsis. In the presence of peritonitis, peristalsis may be absent or infrequent, depending upon the severity, extent, and duration of the inflammation. Hyperactive, nearly constant peristalsis all over the abdomen may be heard when irritation is present inside the intestine (as from a cathartic) but not in the peritoneum. Infrequent prolonged rushes of high-pitched or tinkling peristalsis may be heard over obstructed bowel or stomach. Because of their wide variability in normal people, the pattern of bowel sounds in general can be only suggestive or supportive of a distinct diagnosis, not definitive.

If surges of peristalsis are sufficiently powerful, and if the patient's abdominal wall is not too thick, the peristaltic wave may be visible, especially when light strikes the abdomen horizontally and the observer's eyes are at the level of the abdomen. Shadows accentuate the wavelike rise and fall of the abdominal wall. Similarly, lighted observation may also reveal a tightly distended gallbladder or some other abdominal mass.

OTHER EXAMINATIONS

Virtually any part of the physical examination may bear upon the evaluation of abdominal pain. Nonthrombocytopenic petechiae and purpura may accompany abdominal pain due to autoimmune reactions involving the intestine (Henoch–Schönlein purpura). Jaundice focuses attention on hemolysis, obstruction of the common bile duct, or liver disease; jaundice undetectable in artificial light may be clearly visible in sunlight. The irregular heartbeat of atrial fibrillation may be the clue to an intestinal or splenic thromboembolus. Congestive heart failure can cause right upper quadrant pain due to passive congestion of the liver. Diseases of organs near the abdomen, such as the lungs and spine, may cause abdominal pain; thus, these areas must be examined with care.

Rectal examination may be decisive in locating peritonitis that can be reached through the wall of the rectum. An inflamed appendix not detected convincingly by palpation of the right lower quadrant will sometimes be revealed by right-sided tenderness elicited through the rectal examination. In women, a pelvic examination may be most helpful in finding signs of peritonitis in the pelvic region.

With an inflamed retrocecal appendix, pain may be elicited only when the supine patient tries to raise his right leg without bending the knee. This "psoas sign" may also occur in the presence of inflammation overlying either psoas muscle. Similarly, if there is inflammation in the region of an obturator muscle, as may occasionally happen in appendicitis, pain may be produced not by abdominal pressure but rather by passive flexion of the hip 90° and then moving the knee to the limit of tolerance to the right or to the left. This is the so-called obturator sign.

OBSCURING FACTORS AND CONFUSING ISSUES

Every physician accumulates a list of confusing experiences. Perhaps the most common occur not with rare diseases but rather with common diseases in which the history or the physical signs are atypical. This is frequently the case with the elderly; fever may be absent or slight and signs of peritoneal irritation minimal in the presence of an inflamed viscus, such as with cholecystitis or appendicitis. Dementia at any age or other altered mental states may obscure the diagnosis by making both the history and physical examination problematic. Narcotics, alcohol, sedatives, cocaine, and adrenocorticosteroids may likewise interfere with expected observations. Steroids, for example, may prevent fever, cause euphoria, and suppress inflammation.

Peritonitis, readily detected by history and physical examination, is usually, but not always, an indication for surgery. Acute pancreatitis with peritonitis may require either medical or surgical treatment depending upon the circumstances. Very severe acute ulcerative colitis may cause inflammation from the mucosa through the colonic wall to the peritoneum. It may be very difficult to tell whether peritonitis is due to a ruptured colon—definitely an indication for surgery—or to the colitis, possibly an indication for surgery. A ruptured graafian follicle (mittelschmerz) may cause signs of peritoneal irritation but not require surgery. Familial Mediterranean fever (FMF) causes repeated, self-limited short attacks of sterile peritonitis and fever. If the peritonitis of FMF happens to be in the right lower quadrant, it can be mistaken for appendicitis, or if it is in the right upper quadrant, it can be mistaken for cholecystitis.

Acute obstruction of visceral arteries or veins, due to embolus, thrombosis, or dissecting aneurysm, may cause severe abdominal pain with no signs of peritonitis until a segment of gangrenous bowel is close to rupturing. Surgery is obviously preferable before the bowel ruptures, when peritoneal signs are absent.

Laboratory Examinations

Laboratory tests useful in the diagnosis of abdominal pain are discussed in detail in Part IV of this book, "Diagnostic and Therapeutic Modalities in Gastroenterology," as well as in the chapters concerned with specific disease entities that may give rise to abdominal pain. Some general principles regarding laboratory examinations are discussed in this chapter in the section on chronic intermittent abdominal pain.

CHRONIC ABDOMINAL PAIN

The pain pattern in patients with chronic abdominal pain may provide an important clue to the diagnosis. Pain that presents as discrete bouts, with the patient being entirely normal between attacks, may usually be explained by a discrete intermittent disorder of physiology. The etiology may be difficult to determine, but when it is, the condition may often be specifically treated. Examples of this sort of chronic abdominal pain include acute intermittent porphyria, internal hernias, endometriosis, and some cases of choledocholithiasis. Chronic abdominal pain that is present much or all of the time may also be associated with a clear pathophysiologic abnormality, such as chronic pancreatitis or metastatic colon cancer. In such cases the diagnosis is often obvious, but effective therapy may be quite difficult.

Other cases of chronic abdominal pain have no discrete pathophysiologic explanation. Such chronic abdominal pain may occur in bouts lasting for hours to days or weeks, and even between attacks there may be some residual discomfort. If the pain is primarily epigastric in location and "ulcerlike" in character, but no ulcer crater can be documented, it is called "nonulcer dyspepsia" (NUD) or "essential dyspepsia"[75,76] (see ch 61). If the abdominal pain is associated with abnormal bowel habits, perhaps bloating, and is otherwise undiagnosed, it may be considered to be a manifestation of the irritable bowel syndrome (IBS)[77-79] (see ch 80). Finally, undiagnosed chronic abdominal pain that is present most or all of the time for at least 6 months without features of nonulcer dyspepsia or irritable bowel syndrome may be termed "chronic intractable abdominal pain" (CIAP).

When a person experiences acute pain, the expectation is usually that the underlying process will resolve, either spontaneously or with specific treatment, and the pain will soon cease. With the prolonged suffering of chronic pain, however, many issues must be faced, including loss of autonomy, increased dependency, altered work and family roles, and a declining self-image.[80,81] Common psychologic responses to chronic pain include depression, anxiety, sleep disturbances, withdrawal, decreased activity, loss of libido, fatigue, and preoccupation with the pain.[80,82] Interestingly, there do not appear to be differences in psychologic responses in patients with and without a discrete, identifiable source of pain.[83-85] This seems to be true specifically in the case of abdominal pain.[86] How the patient deals with the many issues and emotions associated with chronic abdominal pain is determined in part by the complex interaction of the pain experience and the psychologic state, culture, and social and family circumstances.[46] Such factors are important to consider in both diagnosis and treatment of chronic abdominal pain, no matter what the underlying cause.

This section will discuss the three categories of chronic abdominal pain mentioned above: chronic intermittent abdominal pain, chronic unrelenting abdominal pain with an identifiable underlying cause, and chronic intractable abdominal pain without a discrete pathophysiologic basis. Issues of particular importance in caring for patients with each type of chronic abdominal pain syndrome will be emphasized; the reader should consult appropriate chapters for more encyclopedic information on specific entities.

Chronic Intermittent Abdominal Pain

DIAGNOSIS

A particularly difficult to diagnose type of chronic abdominal pain is that which is present for up to several hours, or at most several days, with the patient being entirely normal between attacks (Table 34–2). Indeed, such patients may be mistakenly dismissed as having a "functional" problem. It is vital to assiduously seek out the potential underlying etiology of this type of chronic abdominal pain, because, as with acute abdominal pain, specific (and often curative) treatment is usually available. This is best accomplished by means of a careful history, the elements of which were detailed in the section on acute abdominal pain. Here are highlighted historical considerations especially pertinent to patients with chronic intermittent abdominal pain.

History. Circumstances that trigger the abdominal pain often provide a clue to the diagnosis. Abdominal pain occurring at roughly monthly intervals suggests endometriosis. If pain follows the ingestion of drugs, one might think of acute intermittent porphyria (barbiturates) or pancreatitis (steroids, tetracyclines, or thiazide diuretics). If eating leads to abdominal pain, mesenteric ischemia and some varieties of chronic pancreatitis are possible explanations. Pain brought on when certain body positions are assumed raises the possibility of nerve root compression by a mass

TABLE 34–2

Some Causes of Chronic Intermittent Abdominal Pain

Physical	Neurologic
Ampullary stenosis	Abdominal epilepsy
Cholelithiasis	Diabetic radiculopathy
Intermittent intestinal obstruction	Nerve entrapment syndromes
Intussusception	Vertebral nerve root compression
Internal hernia	
	Miscellaneous
	Crohn's disease
Metabolic and/or genetic	Endometriosis
Acute intermittent porphyria	Heavy metal poisoning
Familial Mediterranean fever	Mesenteric ischemia
Familial pancreatitis	Ovulation ("mittelschmerz")

or as a result of a vertebral body fracture or a nerve entrapment syndrome.

Radiculopathy should be considered in a diabetic patient with intermittent abdominal pain, and Crohn's disease should be considered in a patient with a history of perianal pathology. Patients with FMF may have a history of arthritis or pleuritic pain.

Physical Examination. Jaundice associated with intermittent abdominal pain suggests choledocholithiasis or gallstone pancreatitis. Purpura or retinal cytoid bodies raise the possibility of an autoimmune process as the cause of the abdominal pain, such as periarteritis nodosa or systemic lupus erythematosus. Spasm and rigidity of the abdominal musculature may occur with heavy-metal poisoning. A distended abdomen, particularly if there is visible bowel peristalsis, could be the result of intermittent bowel obstruction. Some hernias may be detected by careful palpation. An asymmetry in sensation or strength could be caused by spinal nerve root compression, which in turn could be due to vertebral body collapse or impingement by a mass. An anal fissure would be characteristic of Crohn's disease.

Laboratory Examinations. In general, simple tests, especially if interpreted in light of the history and physical examination, will identify most discrete causes of chronic intermittent abdominal pain. Anemia is often present with ischemic colitis or lead poisoning, a high white blood cell (WBC) count may occur in FMF, and an elevated sedimentation rate may occur with an autoimmune process or FMF; all three might be present in patients with Crohn's disease. Elevated alkaline phosphatase and bilirubin are commonly present during symptomatic episodes of cholelithiasis, especially if they are prolonged, but sometimes an acute elevation of aminotransferases or amylase may be the only clue. Amylase, of course, is also elevated in pancreatitis, although its rise may not necessarily span the time of abdominal pain. Serum lead determination would rule out lead intoxication, and urine for porphobilinogen would rule out acute intermittent porphyria.

Abdominal radiographs—especially if taken with the patient in the upright position—may be very valuable when done during an acute attack of pain. Dilated loops of bowel would be suggestive of bowel obstruction due, for example, to an intermittently obstructing internal hernia or to intussusception. Sigmoidoscopy or barium enema could show evidence of ischemic colitis or endometriosis. Abdominal and pelvic ultrasonography or computed tomography (CT) scanning may reveal a variety of pancreatic or biliary tract lesions, intra-abdominal masses, or dilated bowel loops. Bones seen on various radiographic studies may show unexpected osteoporosis or vertebral body collapse.

TREATMENT

The treatment of patients with chronic intermittent abdominal pain associated with particular diagnoses is reviewed in the appropriate chapters of this book. The two following sections discuss general treatment approaches that may be relevant for some patients with chronic intermittent abdominal pain, especially when specific therapy is not available or not curative.

Chronic Unrelenting Abdominal Pain With an Identifiable Etiology

DIAGNOSIS

The cause of abdominal pain that is present much or all of the time for more than several months is often obvious. Weight loss suggests malignancy, depression, or chronic pancreatitis with pancreatic insufficiency. A history of pathologic fractures should make one think of metastatic malignancy or osteoporosis, and fever suggests an occult intraperitoneal abscess or certain autoimmune processes. If the patient has been a heavy alcohol consumer or has a family history of pancreatitis, chronic pancreatitis must be considered.

Physical examination may reveal jaundice, suggesting hepatic metastases, or pancreatic or biliary tree cancer. Fever may be present with some intra-abdominal malignancies (e.g., lymphoma). There may be an abdominal or pelvic mass suggestive of a visceral neoplasm. Ascites could be due to the intraperitoneal seeding of a malignancy or extensive liver replacement by metastatic tumor. Asymmetries of strength, sensation, or muscle mass could point to a nerve entrapment syndrome.

TREATMENT

The best symptomatic treatment for patients with chronic continuous abdominal pain for which there is usually no "curative" therapy is an individualized blend of therapeutic approaches. Most pertinent may be drugs and various nerve destruction and stimulation techniques, which are discussed here. Additional methods include relaxation therapies, hypnosis, various forms of psychologic support, and formally integrated treatment programs such as the pain clinic. These latter methods, along with a general approach to the patient, are discussed in the section on chronic intractable abdominal pain, but in many cases they are relevant to patients with chronic abdominal pain of known pathophysiologic origin.

Drugs. Drugs are probably the most commonly used form of therapy for treating pain. They are extremely effective in many types of acute pain. Unfortunately, pharmacologic agents have a more limited role in chronic pain.

Nonsteroidal Anti-Inflammatory Drugs (NSAIDs). Aspirin and the other NSAIDs are thought to act primarily at the site of tissue injury by blocking the enzyme cyclooxygenase, which in turn prevents the breakdown of tissue arachidonic acid to prostaglandins. As previously discussed, prostaglandins, which are produced in many types of injury, have an important role in directly and indirectly activating nociceptors. In many types of chronic abdominal pain there is no ongoing tissue damage or active inflammation; therefore, it is not surprising that these drugs may not be of benefit.

Opioids. By mimicking endogenous opioids (the enkephalins and endorphins), the opioid analgesics act within the midbrain, especially on the periaqueductal gray matter, to stimulate the descending inhibitory neurons that project to the dorsal horn.[87,88] Opioids probably work directly within the substantia gelatinosa as well, blocking incoming pain signals at the level of the spinal cord. Because the ultimate site of action of opioid analgesics is probably primarily within the spinal cord, they should inhibit chronic pain due to lesions that result in activation of peripheral nociceptors. On the other hand, opioids would be expected to be less effective in chronic abdominal pain where mechanisms giving rise to the pain are central to the spinal cord. Unfortunately, as discussed previously, even causes of chronic abdominal pain associated with clear peripheral lesions may develop a self-sustaining central component, making them less likely to be adequately treated by opioid analgesics.

Most clinicians feel comfortable prescribing narcotics to patients with abdominal pain associated with malignancy. Their use in nonmalignant chronic pain states (e.g., chronic pancreatitis) is controversial.[89] Clearly, no matter what the indication, narcotics are best administered within the context of an integrated treatment program with careful patient selection and frequent follow-up. In this setting, physical dependency and abuse are uncommon.[90,91] Patients are treated more effectively with opioids dosed at regular intervals than with opioids given on an "as needed" basis.[92] The "pain cocktail" has become popular because it allows flexible dosing as well as the incorporation of adjuvant drugs such as acetaminophen and antiemetics.[90] Such flexible dosing helps to minimize opioid side effects such as mental clouding, respiratory depression, nausea and vomiting, and constipation. Detailed discussions of treatment regimens for opioids are available.[90,92] Managing the opioid dependence of some patients with chronic abdominal pain on long-term narcotics can be a major problem; guidelines are available (also see ch 50).[93]

Antidepressants. Antidepressants, especially the tricyclics, are widely used in the treatment of chronic pain, both because such patients are commonly depressed and because these drugs may have intrinsic analgesic properties.[94–96] Their mechanism of analgesic action is not clear but may be due to their ability to inhibit serotonin reuptake within CNS neurons; serotonin is probably a neurotransmitter within the descending inhibitory pathways that terminate in the dorsal horn.[95,97] It would seem most reasonable to consider the use of antidepressants in patients with chronic abdominal pain when depression is prominent, or in situations where there seems to be an ongoing peripheral pathologic process whose nociceptive signals could be inhibited at the level of the spinal cord. It is important to consider potential side effects and drug interactions before prescribing these agents. Further information concerning the use of antidepressants in chronic pain is available.[98]

Anxiolytics. In the short term, anxiolytics may reduce the anxiety often present in patients with chronic abdominal pain, but they do not treat the pain per se. Long-term administration of benzodiazepine anxiolytics may lead to oversedation, cognitive impairments, or dependence and may result in a withdrawal syndrome on discontinuation.[99,100] As well, these drugs may actually worsen both depression and pain,[100] possibly by stimulating GABA production, which in turn depletes brain serotonin.[97] The nonbenzodiazepine anxiolytic buspirone works by a different mechanism of action and may have less abuse liability,[101] but there is not enough experience with the drug to judge whether it would be safe and effective in anxious patients with chronic abdominal pain.

Nerve Destruction and Stimulation Techniques

Chemical and Surgical Nerve Destruction. Chemical or surgical techniques that have been used to treat chronic abdominal pain by destroying the nociceptive pathways between the viscera and the brain include, going from the periphery centrally, celiac plexus blockade,[102,103] sympathectomy,[33,104] dorsal rhizotomy,[33,104] and cordotomy.[33,105,106] Celiac plexus blockade, by injection of nerve-destroying substances, has been widely used in chronic pancreatitis, where the results have been mixed,[107,108] and in pancreatic carcinoma, where the results have been more encouraging.[108,109] More central neurosurgical approaches (especially rhizotomy and cordotomy) are most appropriate in patients with a short life expectancy (no more than about 6 months), because serious complications, such as bowel and bladder dysfunction, dysesthesias, and even marked worsening of the pain, are not rare. Furthermore, even in initially successful procedures (roughly half the cases) the pain tends to recur.[33,104–106] This is probably true for several reasons. First, no matter what the inciting lesion, chronic abdominal pain may be sustained by pain-generating mechanisms that operate more centrally than even the high spinal cord. Second, after normal visceral inputs are severed, "denervation hypersensitivity" may occur,[104] which could also explain why pain, rather than being eliminated, sometimes becomes more intense after these procedures. Third, because of the plasticity of the nervous system, new neural connections may be formed after neurosurgery that ultimately result in new pain.[104]

Transcutaneous Electrical Nerve Stimulation. Transcutaneous electrical nerve stimulation (TENS) and dorsal column stimulation are attractive treatments for chronic pain because they are simple and devoid of significant side effects.[110–112] Theoretically, they work by selectively stimulating the large diameter peripheral nerves that have an inhibitory component to pain signal transmission within the dorsal horn (i.e., they help "close the gate").[104] Activation of endogenous opioids may also occur.[37] Thus, it is not surprising that they seem to be most effective in chronic pain states characterized by continuous nociceptive input from a peripheral site of pathology,[112] although even in these cases long-term success is difficult to demonstrate. Although there are several reports of apparent benefit in patients with chronic abdominal pain, the consensus seems to be that chronic abdominal pain of any etiology in general responds rather poorly to this technique.[110,112] Acupuncture may work in a similar fashion, or by stimulating specific inhibitory "trigger points,"[104] but again there is little encouraging information on its efficacy in chronic abdominal pain.

Chronic Intractable Abdominal Pain

CLINICAL FEATURES

Definition. Chronic intractable abdominal pain (CIAP), sometimes called "chronic idiopathic abdominal pain,"[113] "chronic undiagnosed abdominal pain,"[114] or "chronic functional abdominal pain,"[115] may be defined as abdominal pain that is present much or all of the time for at least 6 months for which no discrete pathophysiologic diagnosis is made after appropriate medical histories, physical examinations, and laboratory testing (Table 34-3).

What are the characteristic features of patients with CIAP? In most series, women account for 70% or more of the cases.[116-120] Many of these patients experienced abdominal pain as children, and relatives with a history of abdominal pain are common.[121] A history of childhood physical or sexual abuse is extremely frequent, probably having occurred in over half of such patients.[122] Typically there is a history of extensive diagnostic testing and previous abdominal or pelvic surgeries, usually with "negative" or nondefinitive findings.[118,119,123] Pain in locations other than the abdomen is frequent,[119,123-125] as are other somatic symptoms. The abdominal pain is often described in vague terms, sometimes in bizarre or idiosyncratic language. It is common for the onset of pain to follow the loss of a parent, spouse, or some other important figure and be worse on the anniversary of a loss.[119] Even so, these patients appear unable to acknowledge or understand that psychologic factors may trigger abdominal pain. Patients are often insistent that a serious problem is present and may frustrate their physician's attempts to care for them by abusive behavior and by demanding inappropriate diagnostic tests and procedures.

Patients with CIAP, like patients with many other sorts of chronic pain, are often globally disabled, with severely compromised work, family, and social functioning.[80,81] Also in common with patients with other types of chronic pain, patients with CIAP share many psychologic characteristics, including depression, anxiety, sleep disturbances, withdrawal, decreased activity, fatigue, loss of libido, and preoccupation with the pain.[80,82] Depression is especially frequent in patients with CIAP[116,118,119,121,126-128] and may be severe.

Characteristic Personality Features. Patients with certain chronic pain syndromes, including CIAP, have characteristic personality and behavioral features. These will be discussed in some detail, because they are of central importance in diagnosing and effectively treating these patients.

The literature concerning the relationship between personality and chronic pain is complex and may be confusing because of the very different orientations from which personality is discussed. Personality may be defined operationally, that is, by observable features. This approach, taken by the Diagnostic and Statistical Manual of the American Psychiatric Association (DSM-III-R),[129] has had considerable influence in describing personality types associated with chronic pain. Personality may also be characterized behaviorally as a set of responses to environmental contingencies. Finally, personality may be examined by use of an integrated approach that includes operational, behavioral, and psychodynamic perspectives.

The Somatoform Disorders. The DSM-III-R defines three personality subtypes among the somatoform disorders that are commonly associated with the experience of chronic pain. These are "hypochondriasis," "somatization disorder," and "somatoform pain disorder." Hypochondriasis is characterized by a preoccupation with bodily functions and sensations, usually within one organ system or body region, and an exaggerated concern by the patient for the presence of serious illness.[129] Hypochondriacs often go from doctor to doctor seeking reassurance that "nothing is wrong." Pain often becomes manifest in the course of this quest. Features of hypochondriasis are common in patients with CIAP.[119]

Patients with somatization disorder, formerly termed "hysteria," dramatically describe numerous physical symptoms, which are frequently exacerbated by stress.[129-131] Pain in general, and symptoms specifically referable to the gastrointestinal tract, are especially common. This personality type usually becomes manifest before age 20 and is seen almost exclusively in females. Because symptoms are maintained for many years, those with somatization

---

TABLE 34-3
Chronic Intractable Abdominal Pain: Diagnostic Criteria

Definition
1. Abdominal pain for > 6 months that is present much or all of the time
2. No evidence of a pathophysiologic abnormality that would explain the symptoms after investigations appropriate to findings on repeated histories and physical examinations

Highly characteristic features
A. Past history
   1. Childhood physical or sexual abuse
   2. Multiple procedures and/or surgeries, usually with negative results
   3. Multiple somatic complaints, including pain outside the abdomen
B. Abdominal pain features
   1. Does not vary in intensity, character, or location in response to physiologic states such as defecation, meals, and so forth, or does so in nonpredictable ways
   2. The description is dramatic and idiosyncratic
   3. May be triggered or exacerbated by psychologic factors
   4. Associated with major interferences with the patient's relationships and work
   5. Unresponsive to usual treatments
C. Psychologic features
   1. Depression, anxiety, and preoccupation with the pain
   2. Illness behavior
   3. "Pain-prone personality"
   4. High prevalence of DSM-III-R somatoform disorders[129] (e.g., hypochondriasis, somatization disorder, and somatoform pain disorder)

disorder, like hypochondriacal patients, are at high risk for inappropriate tests and procedures, including abdominal surgery. Somatization disorder is often seen in CIAP patients.[119,123,127]

Finally, somatoform pain disorder (formerly called "psychogenic pain disorder") is characterized by a preoccupation with pain for at least 6 months that does not have an identifiable "cause," or, if there is related pathology, the pain complaint seems out of proportion to the objective findings.[129,130] Usually the onset of pain is triggered by a stimulus that is related to a psychologic conflict, although such patients find it very difficult to consider their symptoms in psychologic terms; they deny current life problems or attribute them exclusively to their pain. A focus on the pain experience may enable the patient to avoid an unwelcome activity or get attention from others.

"Abnormal Illness Behavior." The behavioral psychology literature conceptualizes the "pain personality" as a set of behaviors that reinforce a chronic pain state.[132,133] According to this formulation, actions that are associated with diminution of pain, such as decreasing physical activity and taking medications, are called "avoidance behaviors." The resultant decrease in pain reinforces the continuation of these behaviors, even after the acute inciting event is resolved. At the same time, other behaviors (appearing uncomfortable and helpless, not reporting for work) may receive positive reinforcement, such as attention from family, avoidance of the stress of work and family responsibilities, and monetary compensation. Thus, there are a variety of factors in susceptible individuals that reinforce a set of behaviors that help to maintain the chronic pain state.[82] When these behaviors become a continual focus of concern, they are called "abnormal illness behavior" or "learned pain behavior."[130,134,135] It is common for patients with CIAP to exhibit such behavioral characteristics.

The Pain-Prone Personality. A constellation of personality characteristics with chronic pain as the most notable manifestation has been called the "pain-prone personality" by Engel[136] and the "pain-prone disorder" by Blumer and Heilbronn.[137] This formulation integrates behavioral and psychodynamic perspectives and includes elements of several DSM-III-R personality types, especially somatoform pain disorder. The experience of pain becomes a central feature in the lives of these people, leading to what has been termed a "pain career." They usually have a long history of numerous traumatic events, often beginning in childhood with exposure to violence, abuse, and rigid discipline. This results in poor self-esteem, because the vulnerable child cannot see these events as external and takes responsibility for their occurrence. For similar reasons, the patient carries a heavy burden of guilt; the experience of pain may serve as a means of atonement. Intolerance of success is common; pain may be a means of derailing threatened success. There is a great fear of loss of relationships; with such losses may come emotional or physical decompensation. Although professing strong independence and idealized interpersonal relationships, pain-prone patients tend to be passive, demanding, and critical of others. Finally, pain, which often occurs or worsens with an actual loss or threat of loss, serves to replace the loss itself. Thus, although maladaptive, the pain-prone patient's focus on pain allows him to avoid facing a number

of conflicts and tensions. Such a personality type has been repeatedly observed in patients with CIAP.[119,123]

No matter what the formulation or diagnosis, the personality disorders seen in many CIAP patients may have similar consequences, including "doctor shopping," proneness to surgery, inability to see aspects of their pain in psychologic terms, and reluctance to entertain the possibility that there may not be a discrete diagnosis or "explanation" for their pain. For all these reasons, it may be especially difficult for medical personnel to care for such patients.

EPIDEMIOLOGY AND PROGNOSIS

CIAP is not generally acknowledged as a distinct diagnostic entity. This is unfortunate, because more widespread recognition of the characteristic clinical features would aid in appropriate diagnosis and therapy of such patients and would help advance research into pathophysiology and treatment. No reliable information is available on its prevalence, but in one gastroenterology clinic referral practice patients with CIAP were as common as those with cholelithiasis and were seen substantially more frequently than patients with colon cancer or cirrhosis.[4] Whatever the prevalence, it is clear that patients with CIAP are heavy utilizers of medical resources.[118,119,123,128]

What is the outcome in patients with CIAP? Despite many inherent selection biases, published series are the best source for an answer. If not established initially, a discrete diagnosis is rarely made during follow-up.[117–119,125,138,139] Often, when a "cause" is discovered, it is not clear whether it is truly the source of the pain, is incidental, or even developed subsequent to the original complaint. It is unusual for the outcome to be reported after the presumed cause of pain is diagnosed and treated in these cases; clinical experience suggests that usually the pain remains, or pain becomes manifest elsewhere. Just as a discrete diagnosis rarely is made, it is unusual for patients with chronic abdominal pain to be substantially pain-free after one or more years.[86,117,119,125,140,141] This fact emphasizes the importance of focusing on adaptation to the pain rather than cure.

PATHOGENESIS

A "biopsychosocial" perspective[142,143] would seem to be the best way to frame the complex interaction of physiologic, historical, environmental, and psychologic factors whose final clinical expression is CIAP. Thus, rather than the more traditional view of illness causality, where a primary pathologic abnormality (e.g., intussusception) leads to physiologic consequences (bowel obstruction) resulting in clinical symptoms (abdominal pain, bloating, vomiting), the biopsychosocial model suggests that clinical states such as CIAP are multidetermined. Thus, the symptoms associated with CIAP are seen as the result of the interaction of many factors operating within and around the patient.

An example of a biopsychosocial approach to the understanding of the pathogenesis of CIAP is illustrated in Figure 34-7. It employs the "central pattern generating mechanism" theory proposed by Melzack and Loeser,[40,70] which was discussed earlier. Once ab-

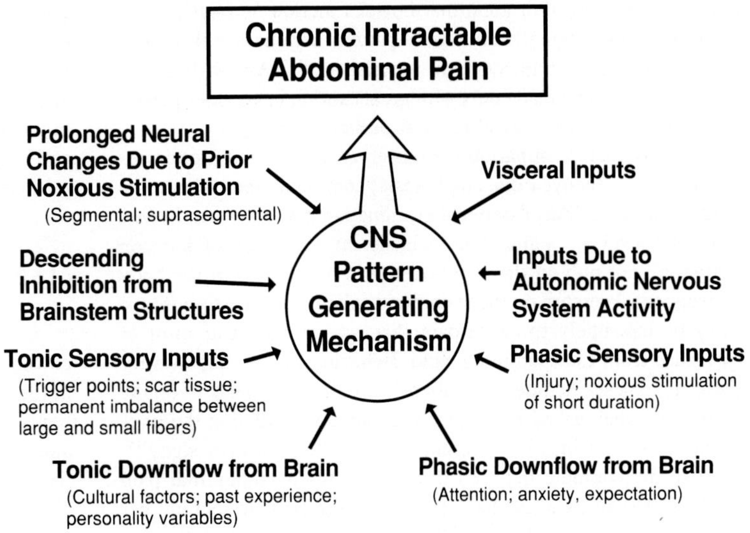

FIGURE 34–7. Model for the genesis of chronic intractable abdominal pain, based on the central pattern generating mechanism theory of Melzack and Loeser.[70] Groups of neurons along the somatosensory projection pathways from the dorsal horn to the cortex may develop abnormal firing patterns under certain circumstances—for example, when normal inputs from the abdominal viscera are reduced. This abnormal activity may become self-sustaining and then be triggered by a wide variety of influences, resulting in the conscious experience of abdominal pain. If triggers are repetitive or if inhibitory forces are compromised (e.g., defects in the descending inhibitory pathways), the pattern generating mechanism may become more or less continually activated, resulting in chronic abdominal pain. Note that although some of these influences originate within the periphery, many arise from within the CNS, indicating that chronic intractable abdominal pain may develop without ongoing nociceptive input from the abdominal viscera. (Modified, from Melzack R. Neurophysiological foundations of pain. In: Sternbach RA, ed. The psychology of pain, ed 2. New York: Raven Press, 1986:1.)

Chronic Intractable Abdominal Pain

CNS Pattern Generating Mechanism

Prolonged Neural Changes Due to Prior Noxious Stimulation (Segmental; suprasegmental)

Visceral Inputs

Descending Inhibition from Brainstem Structures

Inputs Due to Autonomic Nervous System Activity

Tonic Sensory Inputs (Trigger points; scar tissue; permanent imbalance between large and small fibers)

Phasic Sensory Inputs (Injury; noxious stimulation of short duration)

Tonic Downflow from Brain (Cultural factors; past experience; personality variables)

Phasic Downflow from Brain (Attention; anxiety, expectation)

normal firing patterns within neuronal pools along the pain projection pathways are established, they may be perpetuated or triggered as a result of some abnormality within the peripheral or central nervous system (e.g., defective descending inhibitory input), acute abdominal visceral disease or injury (viral gastroenteritis), emotional states (depression, stress), life experiences (childhood sexual abuse, loss of a spouse), or behavioral style (abnormal illness behavior). If the right circumstances are present, for instance if a certain personality disorder is present, these and other interacting factors could lead to self-sustaining abdominal pain. Though much more research is necessary to refine this model, there seems little doubt that an interaction of biology, psychology, and environment will ultimately explain the pathogenesis of CIAP.

Epidemiologic data support the concept that in addition to strictly biologic processes, psychosocial factors play a role in the genesis of many illnesses. By analogy with the irritable bowel syndrome, for instance, many people are likely to experience chronic abdominal pain but do not contact a physician because they do not see their symptoms as distressing enough to require medical attention.[3,144,145] An examination of the physiologic and psychologic differences between this population and patients with CIAP who are under medical care would be a fruitful area of study.

DIAGNOSIS

It is unusual to make a discrete pathophysiologic diagnosis in a patient with abdominal pain occurring much or all of the time for more than 6 to 9 months who has had appropriate evaluations.[117–120,138] In spite of this fact, some physicians may feel compelled to perform a series of ever more expensive and invasive tests in hopes of uncovering the elusive explanation for the patient's symptoms. This propensity may be reinforced by demands of the patient and the family, who express the opinion that if the physician would only do the right test, the cause of all the patient's troubles would be discovered. The resultant frenzied ordering of tests and procedures has been termed "furor medicus."[123] Such behavior may be harmful, because it reinforces the belief that there is indeed

a discrete cause of the pain that, if found, would be amenable to corrective treatment.

History and Physical Examination. There are a number of clinical features in patients with chronic abdominal pain that help identify a population likely to have CIAP. A key distinguishing characteristic is pain that is always or almost always present and is unchanging in character, intensity, and location.[118,120,121,123,127] When changes in the pain do occur, there seems to be no consistent pattern, or the pattern cannot be explained by known neuroanatomic pathways. This is in contrast to chronic abdominal pain associated with a specific diagnosis, which usually occurs with particular activities, positions, times of day, food or drug ingestions, or predictably accompanying symptoms in addition to the pain. Lack of weight loss in the absence of significant depression and lack of fever also favor a diagnosis of CIAP.[118,120,121,140] It is often stated that abdominal pain that awakens a patient from sleep is probably "organic." Indeed, such abdominal pain is somewhat more likely to awaken a patient, but "functional" pains may well do so too.[71,144,146] Therefore, nocturnal awakening with abdominal pain only weakly argues against a diagnosis of CIAP.

Compared with patients having a discrete etiologic diagnosis, patients with CIAP are more likely to have a history of other chronic pains and of psychopathology, to have had a friend or relative with abdominal pain, to worry about having cancer, to be burdened with guilt, to describe the pain in vague and bizarre terms, to have suffered abdominal pain and/or abuse as a child, and to be demanding and inappropriate in dealing with medical personnel.[119,122–125] In general, the presence of any of the personality characteristics associated with chronic pain, as discussed previously, favors a diagnosis of CIAP.

There is a potential overlap in clinical features with the irritable bowel syndrome and nonulcer dyspepsia, and indeed some patients with these entities with appropriate risk factors probably go on to develop CIAP. A main distinguishing feature is that abdominal pain in patients with CIAP is present much or all of the time, whereas that in patients with IBS or NUD is generally cyclical and is associated with abnormal bowel function and eating, respectively. Occasionally an elderly patient with an occult malignancy may present with some characteristics of CIAP—a diagnosis of CIAP should be made only with great caution in an older person who had not shown typical features earlier in life.

On physical examination there is an absence of autonomic activation (e.g., tachycardia, diaphoresis) commonly seen with acute abdominal pain. The abdominal examination may show tenderness but no "surgical" signs. The inconsistent elicitation of pain on palpation not only in the abdomen but in other parts of the body is frequent. Pressure on the abdomen applied with the stethoscope may be less likely to cause pain than an equivalent amount of pressure from the examining hand. Behavioral clues may be very helpful. These include the patient's circling her hand over the abdomen when asked to localize the pain and clutching the physician's arm during the examination. The "closed eyes sign,"[147] said to discriminate between discrete causes of abdominal pain and CIAP-like pain, is characterized by the patient keeping her eyes closed, often with a fixed "beatific smile," during abdominal palpation.

Laboratory Examinations. Tests to exclude other diagnoses in patients with possible CIAP must be individualized based on the patient's age, family and medical history, physical examination, and cost/benefit considerations. In general, though, simple laboratory tests will rule out most other causes of chronic abdominal pain. These may include complete blood count (CBC), sedimentation rate, chemistry screen, flat plate and upright abdominal radiographs, and sigmoidoscopy. When the history or physical examination suggests the possibility of a specific pathophysiologic abnormality, specialized tests must be pursued. Examples would include bowel contrast studies in a patient with a history compatible with intermittent or low-grade bowel obstruction, or endoscopic retrograde cholangiopancreatography (ERCP) in patients with gallstone disease or possible alcoholism.

Unless there is a specific indication for performing them, more complex diagnostic tests (e.g., ERCP) done for "screening" purposes in the patient with chronic abdominal pain of greater than 6 months' duration are unlikely to be helpful.[148,149] When abnormalities are identified in such circumstances, they are often minor and of questionable relevance to the patient's complaints (e.g., minimal changes in the secondary branches of the pancreatic duct) and may serve to divert the physician's attention from appropriate management.

MANAGEMENT

General Management Approach. Like most other chronic illnesses, CIAP has no cure. Nonetheless, when framed in the biopsychosocial perspective discussed above, caring for patients with CIAP may be very rewarding, leading to greater patient and physician satisfaction. Although patients with CIAP are unlikely to become entirely free of symptoms, they should be able to live a much fuller and more functional life. Unlike acute abdominal pain, which often has a single cause and is therefore responsive to a single treatment (e.g., drugs, surgery, or reassurance), CIAP is complex in its pathogenesis—again like many other chronic illnesses. Thus, optimal treatment must incorporate a number of therapeutic approaches (Table 34-4).

Establish Rapport and Trust. It is essential for the physician to establish a good working relationship with the patient. For example, patients with CIAP frequently infer that their pain is "all in their head." Acknowledging the reality of the pain and its resultant suffering is crucial. This should not be difficult except in rare cases when the patient is consciously malingering. Otherwise, because the complaint of pain reflects the patient's inner experience, it must be believed. To not do so, either by explicit statement or by behavior, rejects the patient's reality, which will interfere with the development of a mutually respectful and trusting relationship.

An important aspect of establishing rapport is scheduling brief, but frequent, visits. This serves several purposes. First, it dem-

---

TABLE 34-4

General Principles of Caring for Patients With Chronic Intractable Abdominal Pain

---

1. **Establish rapport and trust**
   a. Acknowledge the reality and pain of the patient's symptoms
   b. Convey a respectful and nonjudgmental attitude toward the patient
   c. Schedule brief but frequent visits
   d. Provide reassurance
2. **Set appropriate goals**
   a. Do not expect the patient to become "cured"
   b. Reduce impact of the illness on the patient's life
   c. Allow for setbacks without undue discouragement
3. **Shift emphasis from diagnosis to treatment**
4. **Focus on adjustment to illness rather than cure**
   a. Emphasize coping and adaptation ("wellness behaviors") rather than treatment of symptoms
   b. Orient treatment toward improvement in function, even in the face of continued pain
   c. Encourage the patient to take an active role in the treatment program
5. **Maintain a multidisciplinary orientation for referral and care**
   a. Consider specialized referrals for both diagnosis and treatment (psychiatry, psychology, neurology, pain clinic, and so forth)
   b. Take advantage of "ancillary" treatment modalities (physical therapy, relaxation training, job and family counseling, and so forth)

onstrates that the physician acknowledges the reality of the patient's illness and is committed to a treatment program. Second, the patient is reassured that the physician will be available and interested. Finally, it reduces the likelihood of unexpected "emergencies."

A frequent fear of patients and their families is that a serious underlying condition is being missed. The clinician, of course, can never absolutely guarantee that a disorder such as cancer does not exist, but he or she can provide reassurance that a considered review of existing data gives no reason for such a concern. Careful attention to new symptoms and signs in future visits will alert the physician to the possible need for further studies. Often, reassurance may be of more benefit to the family than to the patient, who may derive considerable benefit from maintaining the sick role.

Set Appropriate Goals. CIAP is a chronic, often lifelong, illness. Rather than striving for the patient to become totally asymptomatic, the goal should be to minimize the impact of the illness on the patient's life and to promote functioning that is as normal as possible. Such a goal allows for occasional periods of worsening of symptoms. When the physician communicates this expectation, such occurrences are less likely to be seen as major setbacks. Realistic treatment goals are important, even (and perhaps especially) when the patient does not share them. With achievable goals, the physician is more likely to be satisfied with the patient care plan because there will not be a setup for failure. The result will be a more effective therapeutic relationship.

Shift Emphasis From Diagnosis to Treatment. There is a tendency to emphasize diagnosis rather than management in patients with CIAP. As previously mentioned, a discrete diagnosis is not likely in a patient with abdominal pain of at least 6 months' duration who has had an adequate medical evaluation. Thus, expectations for ultimately finding a single etiology for the pain must be modest, and these must be clearly and convincingly communicated to the patient. A much more fruitful focus is on optimal treatment.

Focus on Adjustment to Illness Rather Than Cure. As stated, it is unlikely that a patient with CIAP will become pain-free. Thus, the physician must help the patient accept some degree of pain but minimize its impact on her life. In other words, the focus should be on restoration of more normal functioning despite the persistence of at least some pain, rather than attention to the pain itself. In behavioral terms this means attention to "well behaviors" rather than "sick behaviors."

Patients with CIAP, like chronic pain patients in general, are frequently characterized by passivity, which limits the fullness of their lives and puts inappropriate responsibility on the physician and the family. Patients must be encouraged to take an active role in their treatment. This might include the patient's making decisions about the administration of certain medications, planning a work and exercise schedule, and using self-hypnosis for relaxation. Such active participation improves the patient's self-esteem, which may result in improved functioning.

Maintain a Multidisciplinary Orientation for Consultation and Care. Because patients with CIAP exhibit an often complex blend of physical complaints and psychologic issues, a wide range of referral options should be considered. This provides for more comprehensive treatment and lessens the burden on the primary physician. Psychologic or psychiatric evaluation and possibly treatment are indicated when the clinician suspects that a major affective or personality disorder is present, needs advice in psychologic management, or feels uncomfortable with some aspect of the therapeutic relationship. Similarly, various forms of counseling (family, vocational, and so forth) may be appropriate if areas of the patient's life are identified that are significantly compromised because of the direct or indirect effects of the abdominal pain. Physical therapy and other specialized therapies such as biofeedback and relaxation should also be considered.

Over the last several decades, the integrated, multidisciplinary "pain clinic" has emerged as a popular way to treat patients with chronic pain of all types.[150,151] Usually one physician coordinates a treatment program that may incorporate many of the approaches mentioned previously. Referral of patients with CIAP to a pain clinic should be considered to help resolve any complex diagnostic issues as well as when the need is felt for a nonfragmented and comprehensive approach to the patient's care. A recent report suggests that some patients with chronic pain may achieve long-term benefit from participation in a pain clinic program.[152]

Specific Therapies. Drugs and neurostimulatory and destructive techniques have been discussed in the sections on other types of chronic abdominal pain. With the exception of antidepressants, they have a rather limited role in the treatment of patients with CIAP. Narcotics, in particular, are virtually never indicated in such patients—many patients with CIAP have become addicted to these drugs, considerably complicating their care.

Relaxation Training, Biofeedback, and Hypnosis. The premise behind procedures such as relaxation training and biofeedback is that altering physiologic states such as muscle tone or blood flow will control the physical factors that give rise to or help sustain the chronic pain.[153] Though they do not address the complex and multidetermined nature of CIAP, these techniques, as tools to promote well-being and a sense of control, could contribute an important element to an overall treatment program.

Although there are some enthusiastic proponents of hypnotherapy in the treatment of chronic pain,[154] the evidence that it is truly effective is limited.[155] Of interest are several studies suggesting that hypnosis may be effective for the chronic abdominal pain associated with the irritable bowel syndrome.[156,157] Whether this benefit would extend to patients with CIAP is speculative, but hypnosis is an attractive treatment option because it is safe, simple, and, like relaxation training, may serve to promote well-being. Furthermore, teaching the patient self-hypnosis may provide the patient with a sense of control. Like many behavioral therapies, success with hypnosis depends in large part on the patient's motivation.

Psychologic Therapies. Psychologically related treatments that have been employed in various chronic pain states include behavioral therapy, various "cognitive" therapies, and psychodynamic psychotherapy.

The goal of behavioral therapy is to reduce "chronic pain behaviors" by withdrawing their usual benefits and to reinforce "well behaviors" by rewarding them instead.[132,158,159] Behavior modification methods have been criticized for focusing on *behaviors* rather than the patient's pain *experience* and for ignoring the complex cognitive issues associated with most cases of chronic pain.[155] However, behavioral approaches have been widely used in the treatment of chronic pain, and there is good evidence that they may result in improvement in patients with a variety of chronic pain syndromes.[160]

Recently there has been a great deal of interest in "cognitive" treatments for chronic pain. The goal of cognitive therapy is to improve symptoms by modifying maladaptive thought processes, such as, "This pain means I am ill; therefore, I cannot continue to function."[161] The more comprehensive "cognitive-behavioral" methods combine cognitive interventions with behavioral components such as relaxation training or behavior modification through contingency management.[155,161] The assumption underlying these approaches is that the patient's attitudes, beliefs, and expectations can determine his emotional and behavioral reactions. In practice, cognitive-behavioral therapies teach pain control and promote "healthy behaviors" through increasing the patient's awareness of events or situations that tend to be associated with increased pain, in hopes that this awareness will lead to increased control over such occurrences. Other methods include reinterpreting and "relabeling" sensations normally regarded as painful, and imagery and relaxation exercises to lessen pain sensation in various situations. Though some studies based on these methods report striking success in patients with a variety of chronic pain states, a number of methodologic limitations moderate enthusiasm for this approach.[155,161]

More conventional psychotherapeutic approaches to chronic pain (e.g., psychodynamic psychotherapy) appear to have limited success in this population. Perhaps this is because patients whose chronic pain has a significant psychologic component in general lack insight into contributing psychologic issues and are resistant to exploring them.[119,134] There is, however, some evidence that patients with chronic abdominal pain associated with the irritable bowel syndrome may improve with psychotherapy[162]; there may be a subset of patients with CIAP who could also benefit from such an approach.

The reader is directed to Chapter 1, The Enteric Nervous System and Its Extrinsic Connections; Chapter 3, The Brain–Gut Axis; Chapter 25, Pharmacology of the Gastrointestinal Tract; Chapter 27, Psychosocial Factors in the Care of Patients with Gastrointestinal Disease; Chapter 29, Approach to the Patient with Chest Pain; Chapter 32, Approach to the Patient with Unexplained Weight Loss; Chapter 35, Approach to the Patient with Gas and Bloating; Chapter 36, Approach to the Patient with Acute Abdomen and Fever of Abdominal Origin; Chapter 50, Approach to the Patient with Drug or Alcohol Dependency; Chapter 61, Acid-Peptic Disorders; Chapter 80, Irritable Bowel Syndrome; Chapter 130, Psychiatric Evaluation and Management in Gastrointestinal Illness; and the corresponding chapters in the Atlas.

REFERENCES

1. Jones R, Lydeard S. Prevalence of symptoms of dyspepsia in the community. Br Med J 1989;298:30.
2. Jones R. Dyspeptic symptoms in the community. Gut 1989;30:893.
3. Sandler RS, Drossman DA, Nathan HP, McKee DC. Symptom complaints and health care seeking behavior in subjects with bowel dysfunction. Gastroenterology 1984;87:314.
4. Harvey RF, Salih SY, Read AE. Organic and functional disorders in 2000 gastroenterology outpatients. Lancet 1983;1:632.
5. Switz DM. What the gastroenterologist does all day: A survey of a state society's practice. Gastroenterology 1976;70:1048.
6. National Ambulatory Medical Care Survey, United States, 1985 (unpublished data).
7. Edwards FC, Coghill NF. Clinical manifestations in patients with chronic atrophic gastritis, gastric ulcer, and duodenal ulcer. Q J Med 1968;37:337.
8. Hertz AF. The sensibility of the alimentary canal in health and disease. Lancet 1911;1:1051.
9. Lewis T. Pain. New York: Macmillan, 1942.
10. Ray BS, Neill CL. Abdominal visceral sensation in man. Ann Surg 1947;126:709.
11. Nathan PW. Gastric sensation: Report of a case. Pain 1981;10:259.
12. Bentley FH. Observations on visceral pain. Ann Surg 1948;128:881.
13. Wolf S. Gastric sensibility. In: Wolf S, ed. The stomach. New York: Oxford University Press, 1965:88.
14. Leek BF. Abdominal visceral receptors. In: Neil E, ed. Enteroceptors. Handbook of sensory physiology, vol 3, part 1. New York: Springer-Verlag, 1972:113.
15. Chapman WP, Herrera R, Jones CM. A comparison of pain produced experimentally in lower esophagus, common bile duct, and upper small intestine with pain experienced by patients with diseases of biliary tract and pancreas. Surg Gynecol Obstet 1949;89:573.
16. Lipkin M, Sleisenger MH. Studies of visceral pain: Measurements of stimulus intensity and duration associated with the onset of pain in esophagus, ileum and colon. J Clin Invest 1958;37:28.
17. Almy TP. Basic considerations in the study of abdominal pain. In: Mellinkoff SM, ed. The differential diagnosis of abdominal pain. New York: McGraw-Hill, 1959:1.
18. Leek BF. Abdominal and pelvic visceral receptors. Br Med Bull 1977;33:163.
19. Zollinger R. Observations following distension of the gallbladder and common duct in man. Proc Soc Exp Biol Med 1933;30:1260.
20. Procacci P, Zoppi M, Maresca M. Clinical approach to visceral sensation. In: Cervero F, Morrison JFB, eds. Visceral sensation. Amsterdam: Elsevier, 1986:21.
21. Higashi H. Pharmacological aspects of visceral sensory receptors. In: Cervero F, Morrison JFB, eds. Visceral sensation. Amsterdam: Elsevier, 1986:149.
22. Morrison JFB. The afferent innervation of the gastrointestinal tract. In: Brooks FP, Evers PW, eds. Nerves and the gut. Thorofare, NJ: CB Slack, 1977:297.
23. Blumberg H, Haupt P, Janig W, Kohler W. Encoding of visceral noxious stimuli in the discharge patterns of visceral afferent fibres from the colon. Pflugers Archiv: Eur J Physiol 1983;398:33.
24. Jänig W, Morrison JFB. Functional properties of spinal visceral afferents supplying abdominal and pelvic organs, with special emphasis on visceral nociception. In: Cervero F, Morrison JFB, eds. Visceral sensation. New York: Elsevier, 1986:87.
25. Cervero F. Neurophysiology of gastrointestinal pain. Baillieres Clin Gastroenterol 1988;2:183.
26. Cervero F. Visceral nociception: Peripheral and central aspects of visceral nociceptive systems. Philos Trans R Soc Lond [Biol] 1985;308:325.
27. Haupt P, Jänig W, Kohler W. Response pattern of visceral afferent fibres, supplying the colon, upon chemical and mechanical stimuli. Pflugers Arch 1983;398:41.
28. Iggo A. Afferent C-fibres and visceral sensation. In: Cervero F, Morrison JFB, eds. Visceral sensation. Amsterdam: Elsevier, 1986:29.

29. Harrison A, Isenberg JI, Schapira M, Hagie L. Most patients with active symptomatic duodenal ulcers fail to develop ulcer-type pain in response to gastroduodenal acidification. J Clin Gastroenterol 1982;4:105.

30. Kang JY, Yap I, Guan R, Tay HH, Math MV. Acid induced duodenal ulcer pain: The influence of symptom status and the effect of an antispasmodic. Gut 1989;30:166.

31. Andrews PLR. Vagal afferent innervation of the gastrointestinal tract. In: Cervero F, Morrison JFB, eds. Visceral sensation. Amsterdam: Elsevier, 1986:65.

32. Cervero F, Tattersall JEH. Somatic and visceral sensory integration in the thoracic spinal cord. In: Cervero F, Morrison JFB, eds. Visceral sensation. New York: Elsevier, 1986:189.

33. White JC, Sweet WH. Pain in abdominal visceral disease. In: Pain and the neurosurgeon. Springfield, IL: Charles C Thomas, 1969: 560.

34. Willis WD Jr. Visceral inputs to sensory pathways in the spinal cord. In: Cervero F, Morrison JFB, eds. Visceral sensation. Amsterdam: Elsevier, 1986:207.

35. Fields HL. Pain from deep tissues and referred pain. In: Pain. New York: McGraw-Hill, 1987:79.

36. Fields HL. Pain pathways in the central nervous system. In: Pain. New York: McGraw-Hill, 1987:41.

37. Melzack R, Wall PD. Brain mechanisms. In: The challenge of pain, ed 2. London: Penguin Books, 1988:122.

38. Cervero F. Afferent activity evoked by natural stimulation of the biliary system in the ferret. Pain 1982;13:137.

39. Melzack R, Wall PD. Pain mechanisms: A new theory. Science 1965;150:971.

40. Melzack R. Neurophysiological foundations of pain. In: Sternbach RA, ed. The psychology of pain, ed 2. New York: Raven Press, 1986:1.

41. Melzack R, Wall P. The challenge of pain, ed 2. London: Penguin Books, 1988:1.

42. Frenk H, Cannon JT, Lewis JW, Liebeskind JC. Neural and neurochemical mechanisms of pain inhibition. In: Sternbach RA, ed. The psychology of pain, ed 2. New York: Raven Press, 1986:25.

43. Fields HL. Central nervous system mechanisms for control of pain transmission. In: Pain. New York: McGraw-Hill, 1987:99.

44. Fields HL. Neurophysiology of pain and pain modulation. Am J Med 1984;77(Suppl 3A):2.

45. Melzack R, Wall PD. Gate-control and other mechanisms. In: The challenge of pain, ed 2. London: Penguin Books, 1988:165.

46. Zborowski M. People in pain. San Francisco: Jossey-Bass, 1969.

47. Lumb BM. Brainstem control of visceral afferent pathways in the spinal cord. In: Cervero F, Morrison JFB, eds. Visceral sensation. Amsterdam: Elsevier, 1986:279.

48. Bloomfield AL, Polland WS. Experimental referred pain from the gastro-intestinal tract. Part II. Stomach, duodenum, and colon. J Clin Invest 1931;10:453.

49. Doran FSA. The sites to which pain is referred from the common bile-duct in man and its implication for the theory of referred pain. Br J Surg 1967;54:599.

50. Swarbrick ET, Hegarty JE, Bat L, Williams CB, Dawson AM. Site of pain from the irritable bowel. Lancet 1980;2:443.

51. Bentley FH, Smithwick RH. Visceral pain produced by balloon distension of the jejunum. Lancet 1940;2:389.

52. Jones CM, Pierce FD. The mechanism and reference of pain from the lower intestinal tract. Trans Assoc Am Physicians 1931;46:311.

53. Silen W. Cope's early diagnosis of the acute abdomen, ed 17. New York: Oxford University Press, 1987.

54. Brown FR. The problem of abdominal pain. With special reference to the localization of visceral pain. Br Med J 1942;1:543.

55. Currie DJ. Embryology and sensory innervation of the viscera. In: Abdominal pain. New York: McGraw-Hill, 1979:37.

56. French EB, Robb WAT. Biliary and renal colic. Br Med J 1963;2: 135.

57. Gaensler EA. Quantitative determination of the visceral pain threshold in man. J Clin Invest 1951;30:406.

58. Ritchie J. Pain from distension of the pelvic colon by inflating a balloon in the irritable colon syndrome. Gut 1973;14:125.

59. Moriarty KJ, Dawson AM. Functional abdominal pain: Further evidence that whole gut is affected. Br Med J 1982;284:1670.

60. Mellinkoff SM, ed. The differential diagnosis of abdominal pain. New York: McGraw-Hill, 1959.

61. Dworken HJ, Biel FJ, Machella TE. Supradiaphragmatic reference of pain from the colon. Gastroenterology 1952;22:222.

62. Ryle JA. Visceral pain and referred pain. Lancet 1926;1:895.

63. Cervero F. Mechanisms of visceral pain. In: Lipton S, Miles J, eds. Persistent pain: Modern methods of treatment, vol 4. London: Grune & Stratton, 1983:1.

64. Selzer M, Spencer WA. Interactions between visceral and cutaneous afferents in the spinal cord: Reciprocal primary afferent fiber depolarization. Brain Res 1969;14:349.

65. Richards V. An approach to surgical diseases of the abdomen and pelvis. In: Mellinkoff SM, ed. The differential diagnosis of abdominal pain. New York: McGraw-Hill, 1959:85.

66. Richards V. Other painful abdominal diseases requiring surgery. In: Mellinkoff SM, ed. The differential diagnosis of abdominal pain. New York: McGraw-Hill, 1959:173.

67. Selzer M, Spencer WA. Convergence of visceral and cutaneous afferent pathways in the lumbar spinal cord. Brain Res 1969;14:331.

68. Cervero F. Noxious intensities of visceral stimulation are required to activate viscero-somatic multireceptive neurons in the thoracic spinal cord of the cat. Brain Res 1982;240:350.

69. Hutchins HC, Reynolds OE. Experimental investigation of the referred pain of aerodontalgia. J Dent Res 1947;26:3.

70. Melzack R, Loeser JD. Phantom body pain in paraplegics: Evidence for a central "pattern generating mechanism" for pain. Pain 1978;4: 195.

71. Horrocks JC, De Dombal FT. Clinical presentation of patients with 'dyspepsia.' Detailed symptomatic study of 360 patients. Gut 1978;19: 19.

72. Rumessen JJ, Gudmand-Høyer E. Functional bowel disease: Malabsorption and abdominal distress after ingestion of fructose, sorbitol, and fructose–sorbitol mixtures. Gastroenterology 1988;95:694.

73. Price WH. Gall-bladder dyspepsia. Br Med J 1963;2:138.

74. Odom NJ. Facial expression in acute appendicitis. Ann R Coll Surg Engl 1982;64:260.

75. Talley NJ, Phillips SF. Non-ulcer dyspepsia: Potential causes and pathophysiology. Ann Intern Med 1988;108:865.

76. Gustavsson S, Bates S, Adami HO, Lööf L, Nyrén O. Dyspepsia. Definition and discussion of nomenclature. Scand J Gastroenterol 1985(Suppl);109:11.

77. Thompson WG. The irritable bowel. Gut 1984;25:305.

78. Thompson WG, Dotevall G, Drossman DA, Heaton KW, Kruis W. Irritable bowel syndrome: Guidelines for diagnosis. Gastroenterology Int 1989;2:92.

79. Drossman DA, Lowman BC. Irritable bowel syndrome: Epidemiology, diagnosis and treatment. Clin Gastroenterol 1985;14:559.

80. France RD, Krishnan KRR, Houpt JL, Maltbie AA. Personality and chronic pain. In: France RD, Krishnan KRR, eds. Chronic pain. Washington, DC: American Psychiatric Press, 1988:76.

81. Merskey H. Psychiatry and pain. In: Sternbach RA, ed. The psychology of pain, ed 2. New York: Raven Press, 1986:97.

82. Fields HL. The psychology of pain. In: Pain. New York: McGraw-Hill, 1987:171.

83. Reuler JB, Girard DE, Nardone DA. The chronic pain syndrome: Misconceptions and management. Ann Intern Med 1980;93:588.

84. Woodforde JM, Merskey H. Personality traits of patients with chronic pain. J Psychosom Res 1972;16:167.

85. Cox GB, Chapman CR, Black RG. The MMPI and chronic pain: The diagnosis of psychogenic pain. J Behav Med 1978;1:437.

86. Bleijenberg G, Fennis JFM. Anamnestic and psychological features in diagnosis and prognosis of functional abdominal complaints: A prospective study. Gut 1989;30:1076.

87. Melzack R, Wall PD. The search for drugs. In: The challenge of pain, ed 3. London: Penguin Books, 1983:197.

88. Fields HL. Analgesic drugs. In: Pain. New York: McGraw-Hill, 1987:251.

89. France RD, Urban BJ, Keefe FJ. Long-term use of narcotic analgesics in chronic pain. Soc Sci Med 1984;19:1379.

90. France RD, Krishnan KRR, Manepalli AN. Analgesics in chronic pain. In: France RD, Krishnan KRR, eds. Chronic pain. Washington, DC: American Psychiatric Press, 1988:414.

91. Portenoy RK, Foley KM. Chronic use of opioid analgesics in non-malignant pain: Report of 38 cases. Pain 1986;25:171.

92. McQuay HJ. Opioids in chronic pain. Br J Anaesth 1989;63:213.

93. France RD, Krishnan KRR. Management of opioid dependence. In: France RD, Krishnan KRR, eds. Chronic pain. Washington, DC: American Psychiatric Press, 1988:447.

94. Walsh TD. Antidepressants in chronic pain. Clin Neuropharmacol 1983;6:271.

95. Rosenblatt RM, Reich J, Dehring D. Tricyclic antidepressants in treatment of depression and chronic pain: Analysis of the supporting evidence. Anesth Analg 1984;63:1025.

96. Feinmann C. Pain relief by antidepressants: Possible modes of action. Pain 1985;23:1.

97. Hendler N. The anatomy and psychopharmacology of chronic pain. J Clin Psychiatry 1982;43(8)[Sec 2]:15.

98. France RD, Krishnan KRR. Psychotropic drugs in chronic pain. In: France RD, Krishnan KRR, eds. Chronic pain. Washington, DC: American Psychiatric Press, 1988:322.

99. Roy-Byrne PP, Hommer D. Benzodiazepine withdrawal: Overview and implications for the treatment of anxiety. Am J Med 1988;84:1041.

100. King SA, Strain JJ. Benzodiazepines and chronic pain. Pain 1990;41:3.

101. Buspirone—a radical advance in the treatment of anxiety? Lancet 1988;1:804.

102. Hanowell ST, Kennedy SF, MacNamara TE, Lees DE. Celiac plexus block: Diagnostic and therapeutic applications in abdominal pain. South Med J 1980;73:1330.

103. Owitz S, Koppolu S. Celiac plexus block: An overview. Mt Sinai J Med 1983;50:486.

104. Melzack R, Wall P. Sensory modulation of pain. In: The challenge of pain, ed 2. London: Penguin Books, 1988:214.

105. Mullan SF. Cordotomy and rhizotomy for pain. Clin Neurosurg 1983;31:344.

106. Jack TM, Lloyd JW. Long-term efficacy of surgical cordotomy in intractable non-malignant pain. Ann R Coll Surg Engl 1983;65:97.

107. Myhre J, Hilsted J, Tronier B, et al. Monitoring of celiac plexus block in chronic pancreatitis. Pain 1989;38:269.

108. Leung JWC, Bowen-Wright M, Aveling W, Shorvon PJ, Cotton PB. Coeliac plexus block for pain in pancreatic cancer and chronic pancreatitis. Br J Surg 1983;70:730.

109. Lebovits AH, Lefkowitz M. Pain management of pancreatic carcinoma: A review. Pain 1989;36:1.

110. Loeser JD, Black RG, Christman A. Relief of pain by transcutaneous stimulation. J Neurosurg 1975;42:308.

111. North RB. Neural stimulation techniques. In: Tollison CD, ed. Handbook of chronic pain management. Baltimore: Williams & Wilkins, 1989:136.

112. Long DM. Stimulation of the peripheral nervous system for pain control. Clin Neurosurg 1983;31:323.

113. Buccini RV, Drossman DA. Chronic idiopathic abdominal pain. Curr Concepts Gastroenterol 1987;12, 1:3-7,10.

114. Drossman DA. The patient with chronic undiagnosed abdominal pain. Hosp Pract [Off] 1986;21:22,24.

115. Drossman DA, Funch-Jensen P, Janssens J, Read NW, Talley NJ, Thompson WG. Identification of subgroups of functional gastrointestinal diseases. Gastroenterology Int 1990;December.

116. Kingham JGC, Dawson AM. Origin of chronic right upper quadrant pain. Gut 1985;26:783.

117. Sarfeh IJ. Abdominal pain of unknown etiology. Am J Surg 1976;133:22.

118. Devor D, Knauft RD. Exploratory laparotomy for abdominal pain of unknown etiology: Diagnosis, management, and follow-up of 40 cases. Arch Surg 1968;96:836.

119. Drossman DA. Patients with psychogenic abdominal pain: Six years' observation in the medical setting. Am J Psychiatry 1982;139:1549.

120. Rothman DL, Schwartz SI, Adams JT. Diagnostic laparotomy for fever or abdominal pain of unknown origin. Am J Surg 1977;133:273.

121. Hill OW, Blendis L. Physical and psychological evaluation of "non-organic" abdominal pain. Gut 1967;8:221.

122. Drossman DA, Leserman J, Nachman G, et al. Sexual and physical abuse among women with functional and organic gastrointestinal disorders. Ann Int Med, 1990;113:828.

123. DeVaul RA, Faillace LA. Persistent pain and illness insistence: A medical profile of proneness to surgery. Am J Surg 1978;135:828.

124. Eisendrath SJ, Way LW, Ostroff JW, Johanson CA. Identification of psychogenic abdominal pain. Psychosomatics 1986;27:705.

125. Sloth H, Jorgensen LS. Chronic non-organic upper abdominal pain: Diagnostic safety and prognosis of gastrointestinal and non-intestinal symptoms. A 5- to 7-year follow-up study. Scand J Gastroenterol 1988;23:1275.

126. Rose JDR, Troughton AH, Harvey JS, Smith PM. Depression and functional bowel disorders in gastrointestinal outpatients. Gut 1986;27:1025.

127. Gomez J, Dally P. Psychologically mediated abdominal pain in surgical and medical outpatient clinics. Br Med J 1977;1:1451.

128. Bouchier IAD, Mason CM. A study of patients with abdominal symptoms of undefined cause. Scott Med J 1979;24:199.

129. American Psychiatric Association. Diagnostic and statistical manual of mental disorders (DSM-III-R), ed 3. Washington, DC: American Psychiatric Association, 1987:1.

130. France RD, Krishnan KRR. Pain in psychiatric disorders. In: France RD, Krishnan KRR, eds. Chronic pain. Washington, DC: American Psychiatric Press, 1988:116.

131. Murphy M. Somatisation: Embodying the problem. Br Med J 1989;298:1331.

132. Fordyce WE. Learning processes in pain. In: Sternbach RA, ed. The psychology of pain, ed 2. New York: Raven Press, 1986:49.

133. Fordyce WE. Pain viewed as learned behavior. Adv Neurol 1974;4:415.

134. Pilowsky I, Chapman CR, Bonica JJ. Pain, depression, and illness behavior in a pain clinic population. Pain 1977;4:183.

135. Tyrer SP. Learned pain behaviour. Br Med J 1986;292:1.

136. Engel GL. "Psychogenic" pain and the pain-prone patient. Am J Med 1959;26:899.

137. Blumer D, Heilbronn M. Chronic pain as a variant of depressive disease: The pain-prone disorder. J Nerv Ment Dis 1982;170:381.

138. Woodhouse CJR, Bockner S. Chronic abdominal pain: A surgical or psychiatric symptom? Br J Surg 1979;66:348.

139. Svendsen JH, Munck LK, Andersen JR. Irritable bowel syndrome—Prognosis and diagnostic safety. A 5-year follow-up study. Scand J Gastroenterol 1985;20:415.

140. Waller SL, Misiewicz JJ. Prognosis in the irritable-bowel syndrome. Lancet 1969;2:753.

141. Talley NJ, McNeil D, Hayden A, Colreavy C, Piper DW. Prognosis of chronic unexplained dyspepsia. A prospective study of potential predictor variables in patients with endoscopically diagnosed nonulcer dyspepsia. Gastroenterology 1987;92:1060.

142. Engel GL. The need for a new medical model: A challenge for biomedicine. Science 1977;196:129.

143. Drossman DA. The physician and the patient: Review of the psychosocial gastrointestinal literature with an integrated approach to the patient. In: Sleisenger MH, Fordtran JS, eds. Gastrointestinal disease: Pathophysiology, diagnosis, management, ed 4. Philadelphia: WB Saunders, 1989:3.

144. Drossman DA, McKee DC, Sandler RS, et al. Psychosocial factors in the irritable bowel syndrome. A multivariate study of patients and nonpatients with irritable bowel syndrome. Gastroenterology 1988;95:701.

145. Whitehead WE, Bosmajian L, Zonderman AB, Costa PT Jr, Schuster MM. Symptoms of psychologic distress associated with irritable bowel syndrome. Comparison of community and medical clinic samples. Gastroenterology 1988;95:709.

146. Lawson MJ, Grant AK, Paull A, Read TR. Significance of nocturnal abdominal pain: A prospective study. Br Med J 1980;280:1302.

147. Gray DWR, Dixon JM, Collin J. The closed eyes sign: An aid to diagnosing non-specific abdominal pain. Br Med J 1988;297:837.

148. Bull J, Keeling PWN, Thompson RPH. Endoscopic retrograde cholangiopancreatography for unexplained upper abdominal pain. Br Med J 1980;1:764.

149. Ruddell WSJ, Lintott DJ, Axon ATR. The diagnostic yield of ERCP in the investigation of unexplained abdominal pain. Br J Surg 1983;70:74.
150. Loeser JD, Egan KJ. Managing the chronic pain patient. New York: Raven Press, 1989.
151. Melzack R, Wall PD. Pain clinics, hospices, and the challenge of needless pain. In: The challenge of pain, ed 2. London: Penguin Books, 1988:262.
152. Maruta T, Swanson DW, McHardy MJ. Three year follow-up of patients with chronic pain who were treated in a multidisciplinary pain management center. Pain 1990;41:47.
153. Turner JA, Chapman CR. Psychological interventions for chronic pain: A critical review I. Relaxation training and biofeedback. Pain 1982;12:1.
154. Hilgard ER. Hypnosis and pain. In: Sternbach RA, ed. The psychology of pain, ed 2. New York: Raven Press, 1986:197.
155. Turner JA, Chapman CR. Psychological interventions for chronic pain: A critical review II. Operant conditioning, hypnosis, and cognitive-behavioral therapy. Pain 1982;12:23.
156. Harvey RF, Hinton RA, Gunary RM, Barry RE. Individual and group hypnotherapy in treatment of refractory irritable bowel syndrome. Lancet 1989;1:424.
157. Whorwell PJ, Prior A, Faragher EB. Controlled trial of hypnotherapy in the treatment of severe refractory irritable-bowel syndrome. Lancet 1984;2:1232.
158. Fordyce WE. Treating chronic pain by contingency management. Adv Neurol 1974;4:583.
159. Gil KM, Ross SL, Keefe FJ. Behavioral treatment of chronic pain: Four pain management protocols. In: France RD, Krishnan KRR, eds. Chronic pain. Washington, DC: American Psychiatric Press, 1988:376.
160. Fordyce WE, Roberts AH, Sternbach RA. The behavioral management of chronic pain: A response to critics. Pain 1985;22:113.
161. Tan S-Y. Cognitive and cognitive-behavioral methods for pain control: A selective review. Pain 1982;12:201.
162. Svedlund J, Sjödin I, Ottosson J-O, Dotevall G. Controlled study of psychotherapy in irritable bowel syndrome. Lancet 1983;2:589.

35

Approach to the Patient with Gas and Bloating

JAY A. PERMAN
DAVID M. SALTZBERG

Excessive gas production is one of the most common gastrointestinal complaints for which patients seek physician advice. Patients may attribute abdominal cramps, bloating, chest pain, audible bowel sounds, nausea, anorexia, dyspepsia, belching, or flatulence to gaseousness.[1-5] Multiple terms have been applied to this constellation of complaints, including functional dyspepsia,[6,7] flatulent dyspepsia,[8-10] and functional bowel disease.[11,12]

Production of intestinal gas also forms the basis for the technique of breath analysis by which a variety of digestive functions and disease states can be detected and monitored noninvasively. In this chapter we review the physiology of intestinal gas production, clinical gas syndromes, and the evaluation and therapy of the gassy patient. A subsequent section reviews the clinical utility of breath analysis as a useful diagnostic technique.

COMPOSITION AND SOURCES OF INTESTINAL GAS

The principal gases demonstrable in flatus are nitrogen (N_2), oxygen (O_2), carbon dioxide (CO_2), hydrogen (H_2), and methane (CH_4) (Fig 35-1). Nitrogen is usually present in the highest concentrations, ranging as high as 90%.[13] These principal components of intestinal gas are present in the lumen in concentrations higher than those in blood, indicating that they could not have diffused from the bloodstream into the lumen. Likewise, H_2, CH_4, and CO_2 could not have been swallowed because they are not present in significant concentrations in the atmosphere. Rather, they are produced by processes in the intestinal lumen that are discussed in the following paragraphs.

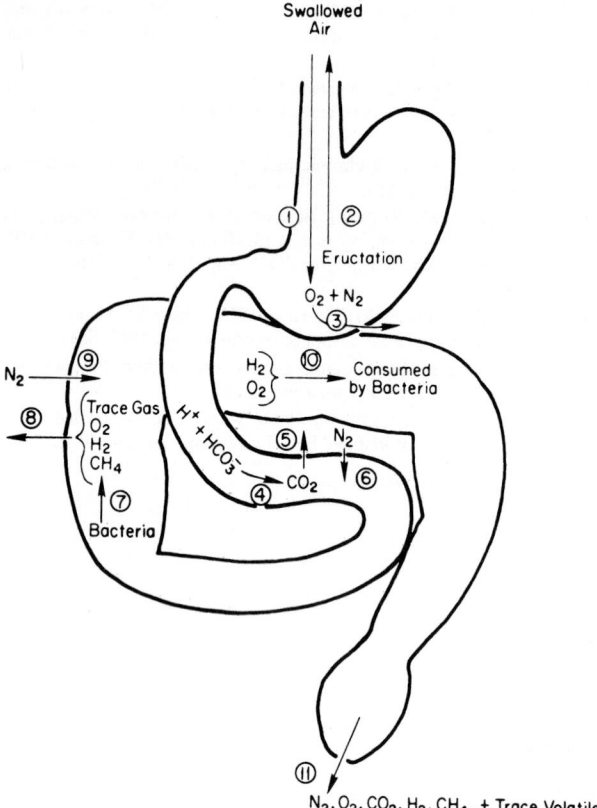

FIGURE 35–1. Mechanisms influencing rate of accumulation of gas in the gastrointestinal tract. Air is swallowed (1) and a sizable fraction is then eructated (2). The O_2 of gastric air diffuses into the blood draining the stomach. The reaction of H^+ and HCO_3^- yields CO_2 (4), which rapidly diffuses into the blood (5) while N_2 (6) diffuses into the lumen down a gradient established by the CO_2, H_2, and CH_4 (7), which diffuse into the blood perfusing the colon (8). Bacteria also consume O_2 and H_2 (9). N_2 diffuses into the colon (10) down a gradient established by bacterial production of CO_2, H_2, and CH_4. The net result of all these processes determines the composition and rate of passage of gas per rectum (11). (Reprinted with permission from Johnson LR, ed. Physiology of the gastrointestinal tract, Vol 2. New York: Raven Press, 1981:1314.)

Hydrogen (H_2)

Mammalian cells do not produce H_2, nor do newborns or germ-free rats.[14] H_2 production has been detected within 1 week of birth as bacterial colonization takes place and results chiefly from fermentation of dietary carbohydrates that escape absorption and enter the colon.[15] While ingested sugars, including nonabsorbable carbohydrates such as the oligosaccharides stachyose and raffinose, and incompletely absorbed sugars, such as dietary starches and fructose, are the principal substrates for H_2 production, in vitro studies using fecal homogenates indicate that glycoproteins are also substrates for H_2 production.[16] Thus, both exogenous and endogenous fermentable substrates may be metabolized to H_2 by fermentative processes present in the vast majority of individuals.

The quantity of carbohydrate available for fermentation in the colon rises under conditions of carbohydrate malabsorption, which may occur on a genetic basis, as in primary lactase deficiency, or secondary to intestinal injury. An increase in the rate and volume

of H_2 production following ingestion of a dietary sugar forms the basis for the H_2 breath test for carbohydrate malabsorption.[17] It has been established that virtually all H_2 production occurs in the large bowel. However, under conditions of bacterial overgrowth, the fermentative processes discussed previously may occur in the small bowel as well.[18]

Methane (CH_4)

As with H_2, methane is exclusively a product of bacterial metabolism. CH_4 is a volatile metabolite produced by highly anaerobic methanogenic bacteria, principally *Methanobrevibacter smithii*. A fraction of the CH_4 evolved is absorbed into the portal circulation and excreted in expired air, as with H_2. It is thus possible to detect luminal CH_4 production by measurement of the gas in expired air.[19] It has been estimated on the basis of several studies that 33% to 41% of healthy North American and European adults produce and excrete CH_4 in the breath.[19,20] A strong correlation has been reported between CH_4 excreter status of an individual and that of other members of his family. When both parents excrete CH_4, 92% of their children also excrete CH_4, and 84% of siblings of CH_4 excreters likewise excrete methane. While genetic factors may be an essential influence on CH_4 excreter status, Bond and colleagues could not demonstrate complete concordance in identical twins. Institutionalization is associated with a high frequency of CH_4 excretion in the mentally retarded, further supporting the role of environment in the development of CH_4 excreter status.[19]

Growth of methanogens and formation of CH_4 require substrate, principally carbohydrates and proteins. These substrates may be of dietary or exogenous origin, but dietary influences on CH_4 excretion have not been consistently demonstrated.[19–24] Methane excretion occurs in the fasted state and may result from metabolism of endogenous glycoproteins and proteins.[16]

Carbon Dioxide (CO_2)

Carbon dioxide may also be derived from bacterial fermentation of dietary substrates. A marked increase in flatus CO_2 per hour is passed in a diet containing beans compared with a bean-free diet.[25] Levitt has argued that an important source of CO_2 intraluminally may be that produced during neutralization of acid by bicarbonate secreted from the pancreas or intestine. Reaction of 1 mEq bicarbonate and 1 mEq acid results in liberation of 22.4 ml CO_2. Based on an average estimated daily secretion of acid of 100 mEq, neutralization of this acid by bicarbonate would result in production of over 2 L of CO_2.[26] Similarly, CO_2 may derive from the digestion of fat and protein. The lipolysis of triglyceride results in the production of fatty acids. Reaction of fatty acids with bicarbonate would in turn result in CO_2 production, as would the amino acids released by protein digestion reacting with bicarbonate. Thus, a meal of fat and protein could result in considerable production of CO_2. Because these sources of CO_2 are restricted to the upper small bowel, it is unlikely that significant amounts of CO_2 resulting from these sources would reach the colon. Rather, the bulk of this gas would be absorbed as it passed down the small bowel.

Oxygen and Nitrogen (O_2 and N_2)

These components of intestinal gas, which represent virtually all of atmospheric gas, are in large part derived from swallowed air. Nitrogen may diffuse into the bowel lumen from the blood, especially if the luminal concentration of nitrogen falls below that of the blood.

CLINICAL GAS SYNDROMES

Gas and Functional Abdominal Discomfort

The intestine of normal individuals generally contains less than 200 ml of gas, as measured by plethysmographic techniques,[27] and excretion of gas per rectum averages 600 ml per day in healthy subjects.[28] Evaluation of intestinal gas content in patients complaining of "gassiness" has revealed gut volumes no different from those of controls both in the fasting state[29,30] and following meals.[31] Using an argon washout technique, Levitt[32] demonstrated an average volume of intestinal gas of 176 ml in patients with chronic complaints of gaseousness compared with 199 ml for controls.[29] However, patients experienced marked abdominal discomfort with intestinal gas infusion, and several required discontinuation of the infusion because of severe pain. In contrast, healthy subjects tolerated infusion without difficulty. Significant reflux of gas from the small intestine into the stomach and prolonged transit times were detected in symptomatic individuals, confirming observations of other investigators.[2,9,33,34]

These findings suggest a heightened sensitivity to intestinal stretch and/or the presence of abnormal upper gastrointestinal motility in gassy patients rather than increased gas volume. Similar observations have been made in the irritable bowel syndrome.[35] Balloon distention of the rectum in patients with the irritable bowel syndrome will result in pain and spasm at considerably smaller volumes than in controls.[36,37] Recent studies of individuals with the irritable bowel syndrome have identified abnormal motility of the esophagus,[38,39] stomach,[7,40] colon,[37,41] and small intestine.[34,42] The disturbed motility patterns have correlated with the patient's typical abdominal symptoms,[43,44] suggesting generalized motor dysfunction.

Thus, patients with chronic vague, diffuse complaints and gaseousness may have a variant of the irritable bowel syndrome. Altered perception of gaseous distention or an exaggerated motor response to normal amounts of gas may explain their symptoms. Alternatively, the primary process may be a motor disorder, resulting in spasm with focal obstruction and secondary accumulation of localized areas of gas, such as in the splenic flexure syndrome.[45] Gastrointestinal gas is also involved in multiple other clinical syndromes, listed in Table 35-1, which will be discussed in the following sections.

TABLE 35-1
Clinical Gas Syndromes

Chronic belching/eructation
Aerophagia
Abdominal cramps and bloating
Hepatic/splenic flexure syndromes
Flatulence
Chronic carbohydrate malabsorption (lactose, sorbitol, fructose, starch)
Gas-bloat syndrome
Colonic explosion
Magenblase syndrome

Belching/Eructation

Belching may be defined as the retrograde passage of esophageal or gastric gas across the upper esophageal sphincter and out the oral cavity.[46,47] Technical advances in measurement of upper esophageal sphincter function have permitted better understanding of this process.[47] Belching is initiated by relaxation of the lower esophageal sphincter with formation of a common esophageal-gastric chamber of equal pressures. The upper sphincter next relaxes, allowing reflux of esophageal gas. The esophageal pressure is returned to normal only by a peristaltic contraction. No movement of the cricoid cartilage is detectable, as is seen with swallowing.

Involuntary belching following a meal is a normal phenomenon due to release of swallowed gas following distention of the stomach with food. Factors that decrease the lower esophageal sphincter tone, including such foods as onions, tomatoes, and mints, will facilitate belching.[48] The supine position allows the posteriorly placed gastroesophageal junction to be covered with fluid, inhibiting gas release.[2,5] A syndrome of postprandial epigastric fullness and bloating relieved by belching has been described as the Magenblase syndrome.[1] Accumulation of swallowed air throughout the day may lead to marked distention and may be exacerbated by food. Reflex release of this gas leads to resolution.

The bulk of upper gastrointestinal air accumulates secondary to aerophagia, or air swallowing. Large quantities of air may be swallowed while eating and particularly during drinking. Hypersalivation from gum chewing, smoking, or oral irritation will also lead to aerophagia. Anxious patients may unconsciously relax their upper esophageal sphincter, and the negative intrathoracic pressures generated during respiration will suck air into the esophagus.[1,2]

Chronic belching is not due to a pathologic organic process but is invariably a voluntary occurrence. These patients may be observed to swallow prior to each belch and have been shown with cineradiography to relax the upper sphincter, swallow, and then release the air from the esophagus before it reaches the stomach.[1,2,5] Commonly, they may have discomfort from a chronic disorder of the chest or upper abdomen, such as cholecystitis, peptic ulcer disease, or gastroesophageal reflux, and believe that it is relieved by belching. The patients are frequently anxious, and belching becomes habitual and is regarded as indicative of digestive problems.[1]

Inability to belch secondary to failure of the upper esophageal sphincter to relax in response to gaseous esophageal distention has been reported in a single patient. The patient had severe postprandial chest pain that was relieved only on expulsion of esophageal air back into the stomach. The sphincter relaxed appropriately with swallowing.[49] Inability to belch may also occur in patients following fundoplication for reflux esophagitis. This will be discussed in a later section.

Hepatic/Splenic Flexure Syndromes

These syndromes are believed to be caused by the trapping of gas at the colonic flexures with subsequent distention of the colon, resulting in upper abdominal discomfort.[45] Pain may be referred to the chest, shoulder, and neck because of diaphragmatic irritation and may simulate myocardial ischemia.[1] Most patients are constipated and have evidence of emotional disorders.[1,45] Symptoms are improved by defecation or enema during an attack. The involved flexure will appear distended with air on a plain radiograph of the abdomen. Machella and colleagues noted no lesions on barium enema in patients with the splenic flexure syndrome, but spasm was frequently identified.[45] Several patients had their pain reproduced by the barium enema or by distention of a balloon placed in the flexure. Although anatomic anomalies may contribute to air trapping, these syndromes likely represent motor disorders of the colon and should be regarded as variants of irritable bowel syndrome. Therapy directed at relieving constipation is usually effective.

Flatulence

Frequent passage of gas per rectum is a disturbing symptom for patients, but rarely is it an indicator of serious disease. Studies of healthy young men have found that flatus is passed an average of 14 times per day, with less than 25 considered normal.[50–52] Less than 100 ml of rectal gas per hour is usually passed in the basal state.[53] While gas in the upper gastrointestinal (GI) tract is composed of swallowed air and is largely nitrogen, reflecting its origin in ambient air,[54] flatus composition is in contrast determined largely by dietary intake of carbohydrates[2] and the metabolic activity of colonic flora.[55] Passage of carbohydrate or glycoprotein[56] into the cecum will lead to anaerobic bacterial fermentation with production of H_2,[57] CO_2,[58] and in some patients CH_4.[59] Arrival of carbohydrates into the colon may occur as a result of (1) malabsorption or maldigestion, (2) ingestion of nonabsorbable carbohydrates such as stachyose and raffinose in beans or legumes,[60–62] (3) consumption of poorly absorbed carbohydrates such as fructose[63,64] and sorbitol[65] in fruit, or (4) physiologic malabsorption of small quantities of dietary starches.[66,67] Endoscopic or radiologic evaluation of the colon is unwarranted in these patients.

The frequency and volume of flatus passed and the accompanying symptoms may be influenced by underlying disorders of motility or metabolism. The patient with irritable bowel syndrome and delayed colonic transit may produce more colonic gas because of prolonged bacterial exposure to carbohydrates.[68] The capacity of colonic bacteria to produce gas also varies among individuals[63,68–70] and may be altered by changes in colonic pH,[71] antibiotics,[72] or bowel cleansing.[73]

Although rarely done, analysis of flatus composition and volume may be helpful in identifying its cause and deciding on therapy. If the flatus is of low volume and predominantly nitrogen, the patient is likely to be a compulsive air swallower and in need of reassurance and therapy for anxiety. Gas composed primarily of H_2 and CO_2 suggests bacterial fermentation, and an evaluation for malabsorption together with dietary restriction of carbohydrates would be appropriate.[2]

Carbohydrate Malabsorption

Recent applications of hydrogen breath testing have provided evidence that malabsorption of small quantities of carbohydrates may result in chronic complaints of gas, abdominal pain, and flatulence.[74] Clinically inapparent malabsorption of lactose,[75] sorbitol,[65] fructose,[63,64] and starch[66,67] has been described. In susceptible individuals, gas released from bacterial fermentation of these sugars may result in an array of unexplained symptoms. Barr and colleagues examined children with chronic unexplained abdominal pain and documented that 40% malabsorbed lactose.[75] Lactose restriction resulted in resolution of the pain in 70%. Thus, subtle carbohydrate malabsorption may result in significant complaints of gas and bloating.

Levitt examined the absorption of a series of complex carbohydrates with H_2 breath testing in healthy subjects and found that up to 20% of an administered carbohydrate is not absorbed.[66] Only rice and gluten-free wheat were completely absorbed, while flour of whole wheat, oats, potatoes, and corn was partially malabsorbed.[66,67] In contrast, dietary fibers including cellulose, lignin, bran, and gums are inefficiently converted to gases by bacterial fermentation.[76–78] Hemicellulose and pectin fermentation result in more gas production but only about one third as much as lactulose on a weight basis.[79]

Fructose has been used increasingly as a sweetener, and oligosaccharides containing fructose are present in onions, asparagus, and wheat.[80] Symptomatic malabsorption with bloating, cramps, eructation, and flatulence has been described by several investigators. Ravich and colleagues noted that 50 g of fructose is malabsorbed by the majority of healthy individuals; volunteers consuming this dose generally developed cramps and diarrhea.[63] Rumessen found that 50% of patients with functional bowel disease malabsorbed 25 g of fructose and developed gastrointestinal distress.[74] Similar findings were noted with sorbitol, suggesting that sugar malabsorption was contributing to the clinical manifestations of their illness. Thus, a detailed dietary history should be taken in patients with apparently functional bowel disorders, and consideration should be given to the evaluation of problematic foods with H_2 breath testing.

Colonic Explosions

Colonic explosion with perforation due to ignition of H_2 and/or CH_4 during surgery,[81,82] sigmoidoscopy,[83] and colonoscopy[84] has been well documented. The flatus concentration of H_2 may reach 44%, and methane 30%, both of which are in the combustible range.[85,86] Cases have occurred in the setting of inadequate bowel preparation or in purging with mannitol or sorbitol, which may serve as a substrate for bacterial fermentation.[84] Use of the electrocautery[81,82] and polypectomy snares[84] has been associated with ignition of the high colonic gas concentration in these patients. Bowel cleansing with a liquid diet, enemas, and laxatives has been shown to effectively decrease colonic H_2 and CH_4 concentration to safe levels.[85] Although CO_2 infusion has been recommended into regions of polypectomy performance to clear combustible gases,[86] this is rarely done, and few colonic explosions have been noted in recent years.[84,87]

Gas-Bloat Syndrome

The Nissen fundoplication procedure for reflux esophagitis involves wrapping the fundus around the gastroesophageal junction. This results in a one-way valve that allows food and gas to enter the stomach but prevents most patients from belching or vomiting.[88] During the first few postoperative months, 25% to 50% of patients will have significant symptoms of bloating, upper abdominal cramping, and excessive flatus, known as the gas-bloat syndrome, due to gastric distention.[88–90] Difficulties with gastric emptying or partial small-bowel obstruction may exacerbate symptoms, and early postoperative gastric perforation due to severe distention has been described.[91] Most patients will improve slowly with time, and surgical revision is rarely required.[92]

Patients with total laryngectomies may also exhibit this syndrome when developing esophageal speech. They learn to relax the upper esophageal sphincter and swallow air that is then expelled through the mouth to form words. Excessive amounts of air may be passed into the upper gastrointestinal tract in this manner.[5]

CLINICAL ASSESSMENT

History and Physical Examination

Evaluation of the gaseous patient is summarized in Table 35-2. The patient presenting with complaints of excessive gas may have myriad symptoms, including abdominal pain in any quadrant, bloating, foul breath, anorexia, early satiety, nausea, belching, audible borborygmi, constipation, and flatulence. Although these symptoms are largely functional in nature, they overlap with those of more serious disorders, which need to be considered. Similar to the patient with irritable bowel syndrome, the patient with gas rarely wakens from sleep with abdominal distress, and symptoms are often relieved by a bowel movement.[93] Patients are frequently anxious and may have a history of psychiatric disorders. Medications that slow gut transit may also precipitate symptoms, especially narcotics, anticholinergics, and calcium channel antagonists.[94] A precise diet history is crucial, and a prospective diary

TABLE 35-2
Assessment of the Gaseous Patient

History

Dietary history—consumption of legumes, beans, apples, prunes, raisins, starch

Medications—narcotics, anticholinergics, calcium channel blockers

Surgery—abdominal surgery that may affect gastric motor function or predispose to mechanical obstruction

Psychiatric disturbances—anxiety, depression

Systemic disease—diabetes, muscular dystrophy, hypothyroidism, progressive systemic sclerosis

Physical Examination

Abdominal distention, ascites, peritonitis, weight loss

Lab

CBC, electrolytes, liver function tests

X-rays—flat and upright abdomen, barium enema, UGI series

Breath testing

Manometry—esophageal, gastric, rectal, intestinal

Nuclear studies—gastric emptying

---

may be of benefit to correlate specific foods with symptoms. Ingestion of legumes, beans, apples, prunes, raisins, and unrefined starches should be specifically addressed.[60,64,95] Consumption of diet foods, candy, and soda, which may result in the ingestion of large unappreciated quantities of sorbitol and fructose, should be considered.[63] Gum chewing, smoking, and chewing tobacco may result in significant air swallowing in the chronic belcher.[1,2] However, the presence of vomiting, fever, weight loss, nocturnal diarrhea, steatorrhea, or rectal bleeding suggests an organic origin, and an appropriate evaluation should be initiated.

Physical examination is generally unremarkable in patients with gaseousness. The patient should be observed for signs of weight loss, anxiety, hyperventilation, and air swallowing. The distended abdomen should be assessed for ascites by attempting to elicit shifting dullness and a fluid wave. A succussion splash should be listened for to exclude gastric outlet obstruction in distended patients. A tense or tender, diffusely tympanitic abdomen in a patient may suggest obstruction or peritonitis with ileus. Evidence of blood in the stool should prompt evaluation for colonic lesions.

Differential Diagnosis

The major etiologies to exclude are those which cause intestinal obstruction on either an anatomic or functional basis. In the patient with multiple previous operations, adhesions or internal hernias may lead to colicky abdominal pain and progressive distention and vomiting. Recurrent peptic ulcer disease may result in gastric outlet obstruction, while neoplastic disease of the stomach, small intestine, or colon must be considered in the elderly.

Many disorders associated with gaseous discomfort are attributable to altered gastrointestinal motility. Diabetes mellitus with autonomic neuropathy may result in impaired gastric emptying (gastroparesis) with upper abdominal pain, bloating, and early satiety.[96] Scleroderma may cause disturbed gastric emptying and small intestinal transit as a result of neuromuscular dysfunction.[97] The presence of Raynaud's syndrome may indicate an early case of scleroderma. Malabsorption and partial obstruction may result in bloating, pain, and flatulence. Neuromuscular disorders such as muscular dystrophy[98] and spinal cord injury may produce similar findings.[99] Idiopathic degeneration of intestinal muscle or ganglia may occur, resulting in intestinal distention and simulation of mechanical obstruction. These disorders are frequently familial and are known as intestinal pseudo-obstruction.[100] Abnormal thyroid function may affect gastrointestinal motility and should be considered in patients with abdominal distention and constipation.[69]

Motility disorders predispose the patient to stasis of intestinal contents, allowing proliferation of upper intestinal bacteria. This may result in bacterial overgrowth with metabolism of dietary constituents to gases by anaerobic bacteria in the upper GI tract.[101] This condition results in further gaseous distention.

Laboratory Testing and Radiologic Evaluation

Simple laboratory screens and abdominal x-rays are of assistance in excluding multiple diagnostic possibilities. Normal complete blood count, glucose, prothrombin time, albumin, protein, calcium, phosphate, and liver function tests are of help in excluding diabetes, malignancy, occult malabsorption, and cirrhosis.

Flat and upright radiographs of the abdomen may suggest intestinal obstruction, perforation, or ascites. Localized gas collections at the hepatic or splenic flexures may correlate with the patient's symptoms. No correlation between quantity of gas noted and the patient's complaints exists. If symptoms persist or abnormal findings are present, barium studies of the upper or lower GI tract may be of use to identify obstruction. Endoscopy should be reserved for confirmation of abnormal barium findings or evaluation of significant laboratory abnormalities such as anemia. Sonography may be useful to identify ascites as a cause of distention.

H_2 breath tests may be used to confirm a relationship between symptoms and individual foods. A rise in breath H_2, especially if associated with the onset of typical symptoms, strongly suggests the test carbohydrate as the causative agent.[74] In patients with suspected motility disorders, esophageal and/or rectal motility may provide a measure of smooth muscle function throughout the GI tract.[102] Gastric and small intestinal manometric and electrophysiologic studies are available in referral centers.[103] Nuclear studies may also be of assistance, particularly in the assessment of gastric emptying.[104]

THERAPY

Because symptoms of gaseousness seem to be due largely to an exaggerated response to intestinal gas and/or motility disorders, attempts should be made to decrease intestinal gas and to regulate bowel function (Table 35-3). Aerophagia may be controlled with

TABLE 35-3
Therapy of Gaseousness

Reduce Intestinal Gas

Control aerophagia
  Cease gum or candy chewing, smoking
  Improve oral hygiene
  Treat anxiety
Dietary restriction (as guided by H_2 breath tests)
  Legumes, beans, fruits, starches
Drug therapy
  Activated charcoal prior to meals
  ? simethicone

Regulate bowel function

Promote laxation
  Fluids, fiber, osmotic laxatives
Enhance gut motility
  Metoclopramide

changes of simple habits. Cessation of gum and candy chewing, as well as cessation of smoking and improved oral hygiene, will decrease air swallowing.[2] The chronic belcher may be aided by observation of himself in the mirror in order to note that each belch is preceded by a swallow that the patient can learn to control.[3] Reassurance and judicious use of anxiolytics will help many air swallowers. Belching commonly occurs in response to discomfort from gastroesophageal reflux, and patients with concomitant pyrosis may benefit from treatment with an H_2 blocker.

Patients with complaints of excessive flatus may require dietary alterations as directed by H_2 breath testing. Restriction of ingestion of legumes, beans, fruits, and complex carbohydrates may be required.[95] The possibility of bacterial overgrowth should be considered, especially if conditions predisposing to overgrowth exist. If bacterial overgrowth is documented, treatment with tetracycline or metronidazole for 2 weeks is usually effective.[105]

Several agents have been used to bind or alter intestinal gas. Activated charcoal appears to be effective in reducing breath H_2 and intestinal complaints caused by consumption of indigestible carbohydrates, particularly when the charcoal is administered prior to the meal.[106,107] The mechanism is uncertain, and in vitro studies have been unable to confirm binding of the charcoal to H_2 or carbohydrate substrates.[108] Simethicone alters the elasticity of mucus-coated bubbles, resulting in the bubbles being broken or coalescing.[109] Although simethicone is frequently used, there are limited data to support its effectiveness.[110,111]

Regulation of bowel function is an important aspect of the treatment of abdominal cramps, gas, and bloating. Many patients have delayed transit and are constipated. Treatment with increased dietary fiber and/or osmotic laxatives will promote more rapid transit and relieve constipation and functional obstruction. Fiber is inefficiently converted to gas and is thus an ideal agent.[78,79] Metoclopramide has also been demonstrated to significantly reduce gaseous complaints, probably by its action on gut motor activity.[112] However, its use should be limited to patients with documented dysmotility.

BREATH TESTS

Breath Hydrogen (H₂) Testing

Breath H_2 testing has been applied most frequently in the detection of carbohydrate maldigestion and malabsorption, bacterial overgrowth, mouth-to-cecum transit time measurements, and intestinal gas syndromes (Table 35-4).

PERFORMANCE

Breath hydrogen tests for the detection of monosaccharide or disaccharide malabsorption are generally performed by obtaining samples of expired air before and at 30-minute intervals for 3 hours following administration of aqueous sugar solutions that represent the test substrate.[113] More than 90% of malabsorbers will exhibit H_2 excretion curves consistent with a positive response by 2 hours following substrate ingestion. Detection of carbohydrate malabsorption following administration of a complex test meal (e.g., detection of lactose malabsorption after ingestion of milk or yogurt) requires a longer testing period to compensate for the slower gastric emptying induced by fat in the test meal.[114] Detection of starch malabsorption, especially in patients with cystic fibrosis, may require a monitoring period of 8 to 10 hours.[115,116]

SAMPLING

Original techniques for breath H_2 measurements were applicable only to the totally cooperative patient. These techniques required a closed continuous collection system in which the patient remained for hours. Using this method, total excretion of specific components of breath could be determined without concern for minute-to-minute variation in endogenous gas production. Because this methodology was complicated and unwieldy, interval sampling methods have been developed that are less precise than closed continuous collection systems but are certainly adequate for patient care and clinical research. A semiquantitative estimate of the total excretion of a gas component over time can be determined using interval sampling by assuming a constant output of respiratory gases. More specifically, the total amount of gas expired during a period of observation can be calculated, assuming there is a constant production per unit time of the specific components of breath being measured and taking the mean value of two sample points.[117] For most clinical applications, however, the concentration of the specific gas is sufficient, and calculation of the total quantity excreted is not required.

Application of breath tests in the pediatric population has required the development of well tolerated collecting systems that, in the case of infants and toddlers, do not require the child's active cooperation. Face masks are commonly used for collecting techniques in infants and children.[118] Much of this author's (JAP) work in patients of any age has utilized a simple nasal prong into which the patient breathes normally while the prong is held at the nose by either the patient himself or the examiner.[119] While watching the subject's breathing pattern, the examiner aspirates 3

TABLE 35–4
Frequently Applied Breath Tests

DETECTION OF	SUBSTRATE	COMPONENT OF EXPIRED AIR MEASURED
Carbohydrate maldigestion/malabsorption		
Lactase deficiency	Lactose	H_2
	^{14}C-lactose	$^{14}CO_2$
Sucrase–isomaltase deficiency	Sucrose	H_2
Glucose malabsorption	Glucose	H_2
Starch	Rice	H_2
Fat maldigestion/malabsorption	^{14}C- or ^{13}C-trioctanoin	$^{14/13}CO_2$
	^{14}C- or ^{13}C-tripalmitin	$^{14/13}CO_2$
	^{14}C- or ^{13}C-triolein	$^{14/13}CO_2$
	^{14}C- or ^{13}C-palmitic acid	$^{14/13}CO_2$
Bacterial overgrowth	^{14}C- or ^{13}C-glycocholate	$^{14/13}CO_2$
	Glucose	H_2
	Lactulose	H_2
	^{14}C-xylose	$^{14}CO_2$
Ileal dysfunction	^{14}C- or ^{13}C-glycocholate	$^{14/13}CO_2$
Mouth-to-cecum transit time	Lactulose	H_2
Intestinal gas syndromes	Foods	H_2
Hepatic function	^{14}C-aminopyrine	$^{14}CO_2$

to 5 ml in the latter half of expiration until a sample sufficient for analysis has been obtained. The nasal prong technique has been found to be well-tolerated by patients of all ages, and satisfactory samples have been obtained.

SUBSTRATE SELECTION

Breath hydrogen testing permits flexibility in substrate selection, substrate form, and dosage. The only rigid requirement is that the substrate be appropriate to the function one wishes to evaluate. Thus, detection of lactose malabsorption requires the administration of lactose as the test substrate. Conventionally, 2 g/kg lactose in a 20% solution is the test dose.[117] This dosage is adapted from the standard lactose tolerance test using blood glucose as the measured response. The osmolality of the solution may need to be modified in patients younger than 6 months of age. Should one wish to determine whether an individual malabsorbs a more physiologic dose, one could use lactose in a given serving of milk or yogurt as the test substrate.[114]

SAMPLE ANALYSIS

Hydrogen is usually measured by gas chromatography, and relatively inexpensive and dedicated instruments are available commercially for this purpose. Other methods for measuring breath hydrogen are available. These include electrochemical cells, helium ionization detectors, and reduction gas detectors.[118,119] Samples are conventionally collected in plastic syringes. Alternatively, samples may be collected in specialized collection bags and transferred to syringes for application directly to the sample loop of the instrument. There are no intermediate separation steps required prior to analyzing the sample.

SAMPLE STORAGE

Breath hydrogen methodology has been applied to outpatient and field studies because of its ease and simplicity and because samples can be stored in a variety of systems. Samples stored in the collection syringes themselves over an 8-hour period demonstrated no change in hydrogen concentration, but deterioration does occur over a period of days.[113] Sealing methods and refrigeration of samples appear to retard the deterioration in the sample if stored in a syringe over time. Specialized nonsterile vacutainers have been successfully used for storing and shipping samples, and these vacutainers have been demonstrated to be stable for periods exceeding 30 days.[113] Mylar bags are also available for prolonged sample storage.

INTERPRETATION OF DATA

A typical breath H_2 curve is shown in Figure 35-2. Results are most commonly expressed as the concentration of hydrogen excreted in parts per million (ppm) above baseline. Hydrogen concentrations tend to decline in the fasting state, and the baseline value can therefore be defined as the lowest value of hydrogen

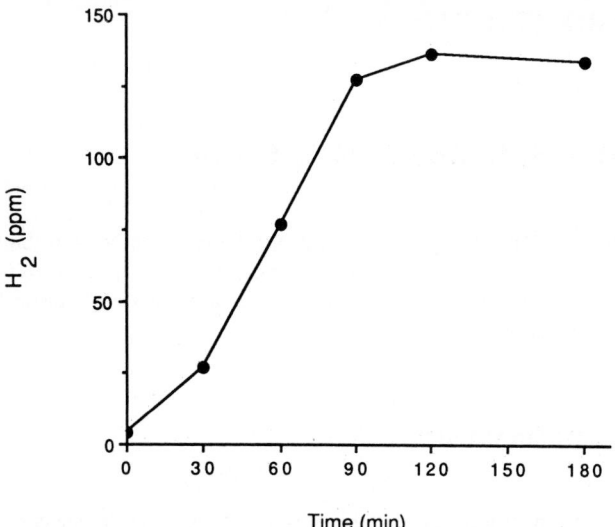

FIGURE 35-2. Breath H_2 curve after ingestion of lactose (2 g/kg in 20% solution) by a 15-year-old boy with a 2-year history of recurrent abdominal pain. A 10-ppm rise above the basal (lowest) value is consistent with lactose malabsorption.

obtained at any sampling time.[117] Parts per million above baseline, or delta ppm, is then calculated by subtraction of this value from the subsequent hydrogen concentrations. An increase in breath H_2 of more than 10 ppm above baseline completely discriminates biopsy-proven isolated lactase-insufficient subjects from lactase-sufficient subjects. An increase occurring later than 120 minutes after ingestion of substrate, more specifically at 180 minutes, suggests either normal mucosal function or partial or secondary lactase deficiency due to mucosal injury.[113] In practice, most clinicians prefer to use a rise of 20 ppm rather than 10 ppm above baseline or greater as the criterion for an unequivocally positive response, with rises of 10 to 20 ppm considered equivocal.

In addition, an early rise in H_2 concentration in the first 30 minutes following substrate ingestion may be consistent with small-bowel bacterial overgrowth, especially if accompanied by a subsequent second peak in expired H_2.[120] The latter is thought to be due to the bolus of the substrate reaching the colon. Unfortunately, the second peak does not commonly occur in practice, and one must therefore rely on either the early rise in breath hydrogen or the elevation of the fasting H_2 (discussed below) as an indictor of bacterial overgrowth. Kerlin and Wong have recently shown that a rise in breath H_2 following glucose is a reliable indirect test for bacterial overgrowth.[121]

Criteria for the interpretation of breath hydrogen tests in the detection of carbohydrate malabsorption may vary, but all are based on comparisons of H_2 concentrations in interval samples with a pretest value obtained after an overnight fast. The diagnostic significance of the fasting breath H_2 (FH_2) concentration itself has been examined. Values defined as greater than 42 ppm may indicate the presence of gastrointestinal stasis and bacterial overgrowth.[122] Because laboratories may vary, an elevated fasting hydrogen can probably be described more generically as that which exceeds two standard deviations beyond the mean fasting hydrogen for that laboratory. FH_2 is of use only if a red meat–rice meal with no other source of carbohydrate other than the rice is ingested the night before.[122,123]

CO_2 Breath Testing

Dodds was the first to recognize CO_2 measurements as a test of intestinal function. He was able to demonstrate a rise in breath CO_2 concentration after meals and to document postprandial changes in CO_2 excretion in disorders of malabsorption.[124] Because CO_2 is normally present in considerable quantities in expired air, breath tests dependent on changes in breath CO_2 concentration require labeled substrates. The radioactive ^{14}C isotope of carbon is most commonly used,[125] but nonradioactive ^{13}C has been used in children.[126] The labeled carbon is placed in a specific small-molecular-weight segment of the test substrate, which will be cleaved off by the enzymatic process being studied, yielding a moiety that is oxidized to CO_2 by mammalian enzymes or bacteria. The rate of labeled CO_2 excretion can be used as a measure of enzymatic activity.[127]

Tests are performed by administering a labeled substrate and having the subject exhale through a pipette at 15 to 30–minute intervals into a scintillation vial containing an alkaline binding compound and phenolphthalein.[128] CO_2 is bound in a stoichiometric fashion. When the compound is saturated, a carbonate is formed, resulting in a color change. Liquid scintillation counting is performed, and results are expressed as the ratio of $^{14}CO_2$ to total bound CO_2.[125] The dose of ^{14}C generally used is 10 μCi, which results in total body irradiation approximately equal to that of a chest x-ray.[129]

CO_2 breath testing has been used to evaluate fat absorption,[130-132] bacterial overgrowth,[133-137] bile acid absorption,[138-142] hepatic drug metabolism,[143-146] and carbohydrate absorption (see Table 35-4).[146] Labeled triglycerides have been investigated as an alternative to stool collection in assessing fat absorption. The appearance of $^{14}CO_2$ in the breath indicates intact digestive and absorptive processes permitting oxidation of fat to $^{14}CO_2$. These tests are helpful in identifying patients with lipolytic disorders, but there is great overlap between controls and patients with other causes of fat malabsorption, making the test less useful. Similarly, the rapid appearance of $^{14}CO_2$ has been used as a marker of intact function of cytochrome P-450 following the administration of microsomally metabolized aminopyrine. Decreased excretion has been found in severe alcoholic hepatitis[143] and cirrhosis[144,145] and with acetaminophen-induced injury and hepatic injury.[146]

Bacterial overgrowth syndromes have also been extensively evaluated with the aid of CO_2 breath testing. Metabolism of the labeled substrate by bacteria in the upper gastrointestinal tract results in the rapid release of large amounts of $^{14}CO_2$ compared with controls.[133] Glycine is cleaved from the conjugated bile acid cholylglycine by those anaerobic bacteria possessing deconjugase enzymes, with subsequent metabolism of labeled glycine to CO_2.[138,139] Although the test is sensitive, it lacks specificity, because ileal resection or dysfunction will result in malabsorption of the bile acid with rapid degradation by colonic bacteria.[140-142] ^{14}C-D-xylose appears to be a more specific substrate,[134] correlating well with jejunal culture in identifying clinical cases of bacterial overgrowth.[135] Even in the presence of extensive small-bowel disease, the small quantity of D-xylose administered is absorbed and excreted unmetabolized in the urine. Thus, $^{14}CO_2$ appearing in the breath within 30 to 60 minutes is invariably secondary to bacterial processes.[136,137]

The reader is directed to Chapter 17, Carbohydrate Assimilation; Chapter 26, The Gastrointestinal Microflora; Chapter 37, Approach to the Patient with Ileus and Obstruction; Chapter 38, Approach to the Patient with Diarrhea; Chapter 39, Approach to the Patient with Constipation; Chapter 60, Disorders of Gastric Emptying; Chapter 67, Dysmotility of the Small Intestine; Chapter 72, Specific Mucosal Protein Deficiency States; Chapter 73, Bacterial Overgrowth; Chapter 80, Irritable Bowel Syndrome; and Chapter 81, Motility Disorders of the Colon.

REFERENCES

1. Roth JLA. Gaseousness. In: Berk JE, ed. Gastroenterology. Philadelphia: WB Saunders, 1985:142.
2. Danhof IE. The clinical gas syndromes: A pathophysiologic approach. Ann NY Acad Sci 1968;150:127.
3. Levitt MD, Bond JH. Flatulence. Annu Rev Med 1980;31:127.
4. Altman DF. Downwing update—A discourse on matters gaseous. [Medical Staff Conference] West J Med 1986;145:502.
5. Maddock WG, Bell JL, Tremaine MJ. Gastrointestinal gas. Ann Surg 1949;130:512.
6. Rees WDW, Miller LF, Malagelada J-R. Dyspepsia, antral motor dysfunction and gastric stasis of solids. Gastroenterology 1980;78:360.
7. Camilleri M, Malagelada J-R, Kao PC, Zinsmeister AR. Gastric and autonomic responses to stress in functional dyspepsia. Dig Dis Sci 1986;31:1169.
8. Rhiad JA, Watson L. Gallstone dyspepsia. Br Med J 1968;1:32.
9. Johnson AG. Pyloric function and gall-stone dyspepsia. Br J Surg 1972;59:449.
10. Watson RGP, Love AHG. Gastric emptying in patients with a flatulent dyspepsia with and without gallbladder disease. Scand J Gastroenterol 1987;21:47.
11. Lenhard-Jones JE. Functional gastrointestinal disorders. N Engl J Med 1983;308:431.
12. Thompson WG, Heaton KW. Functional bowel disorders in apparently healthy people. Gastroenterology 1980;79:283.
13. Levitt MD. Volume and composition of human intestinal gas. N Engl J Med 1971;284:1394.
14. Engel RR, Levitt MD. Intestinal trace gas formation in newborns (abstr). San Francisco: American Pediatric Society and Society for Pediatric Research, 1970:266.
15. MacLean WC, Fink BB. Lactose malabsorption by premature infants: Magnitude and clinical significance. J Pediatr 1980;97:383.
16. Perman JA, Modler S. Glycoproteins as substrates for production of hydrogen and methane by colonic bacterial flora. Gastroenterology 1982;82:911.
17. Newcomer AD, McGill DB, Thomas PJ, Hofmann AF. Prospective comparison of indirect methods for detecting lactase deficiency. N Engl J Med 1975;293:1232.
18. Levitt MD. Production and excretion of hydrogen gas in man. N Engl J Med 1969;281:122.
19. Bond JH, Engel RR, Levitt MD. Factors influencing pulmonary methane excretion in man. An indirect method of studying *in situ* metabolism of the methane-producing colonic bacteria. J Exp Med 1971;133:572.
20. Pitt P, DeBruijn KM, Beeching MF, Goldberg E, Blendis LM. Studies on breath methane: The effect of ethnic origins and lactulose. Gut 1980;21:941.
21. Calloway DH. Respiratory hydrogen and methane as affected by consumption of gas forming food. Gastroenterology 1966;51:3383.
22. Tadesse K, Smith D, Eastwood MA. Breath hydrogen (H_2) and methane (CH_4) excretion patterns in normal man and in clinical practice. Q J Exp Med 1980;65:85.

23. Tadesse K, Eastwood MA. Metabolism of dietary fiber components in man assessed by breath hydrogen and methane. Br J Nutr 1978;40:393.

24. McKay LF, Brydon WG, Eastwood MA, Smith JH. The influence of pentose on breath methane. Am J Clin Nutr 1981;34:2728.

25. Steggerda FR. Gastrointestinal gas following food consumption. Ann NY Acad Sci 1968;150:57.

26. Levitt MD. Intestinal gas production. J Am Diet Assoc 1972;60:487.

27. Bedell GN, Marshall R, Dubois AB, Harris JH. Measurement of the volume of gas in the gastrointestinal tract. J Clin Invest 1956;35:336.

28. Kirk E. The quantity and composition of human colonic flatus. Gastroenterology 1949;12:782.

29. Lasser RB, Bond JH, Levitt MD. The role of intestinal gas in functional abdominal pain. N Engl J Med 1975;293:524.

30. Oppenheimer A. Gas in the bowels: Observations and experiment in man. Surg Gynecol Obstet 1940;70:105.

31. Lasser RB, Levitt MD, Bond JH. Studies of intestinal gas after ingestion of a standard meal. Gastroenterology 1976;70:906A.

32. Levitt MD. Volume and composition of human intestinal gas determined by means of an intestinal washout technique. N Engl J Med 1971;284:1396.

33. Capper WM, Butler TJ, Kilby JO, Gibson MJ. Gallstones, gastric secretion, and flatulent dyspepsia. Lancet 1967;1:413.

34. Cann PA, Read NW, Brown C, Hobson N, Holdsworth CD. Irritable bowel syndrome: Relationship of disorders in the transit of a single solid meal to symptom patterns. Gut 1983;24:405.

35. Schuster MM, Whitehead WE. Physiologic insights into irritable bowel syndrome. Clin Gastroenterol 1986;15:839.

36. Ritchie J. Pain from distention of the pelvic colon by inflating a balloon in the irritable colon syndrome. Gut 1973;14:125.

37. Whitehead WE, Engel BT, Schuster MM. Irritable bowel syndrome. Physiological differences between diarrhea-predominant and constipation-predominant patients. Dig Dis Sci 1980;25:404.

38. Whorwell PJ, Klouter C, Smith CL. Esophageal motility in irritable bowel syndrome. Br Med J 1981;282:1101.

39. Swarbrick ET, Hegarty JE, Bat I, Williams CB, Dawson AM. Site of pain from the irritable bowel syndrome. Lancet 1980;2:443.

40. Malagelada J-R, Standhellini V. Manometric evaluation of functional upper gut symptoms. Gastroenterology 1985;88:1223.

41. Snape WT, Carlson GT, Matarazzo SA, Cohen S. Evidence that abnormal myoelectric activity produces colonic motor dysfunction in the irritable bowel syndrome. Gastroenterology 1977;72:383.

42. Neilsen OH, Gjorup J, Christiansen FN. Gastric emptying rate and small bowel transit time in patients with irritable bowel syndrome determined with Tc-99–labeled pellets and scintigraphy. Dig Dis Sci 1986;31:1287.

43. Kellow JE, Phillips SF. Altered small bowel motility in irritable bowel syndrome is correlated with symptoms. Gastroenterology 1987;92:1885.

44. Kumar D, Wingate DL. The irritable bowel syndrome: A paroxysmal motor disorder. Lancet 1985;2:973.

45. Macella TE, Dworken HJ, Biel FJ. Observations on the splenic flexure syndrome. Ann Intern Med 1952;37:543.

46. McNally EF, Kelly JE, Inglefinger FJ. Mechanism of belching: Effects of gastric distention with air. Gastroenterology 1964;46:254.

47. Kahrilas PJ, Dodds WJ, Dent J, Wyman JB, Hogan WJ, Arndorfor RC. Upper esophageal sphincter function during belching. Gastroenterology 1986;91:133.

48. Castell DO. The lower esophageal sphincter. Ann Intern Med 1975;83:390.

49. Kahrilas PJ, Dodds WJ, Hogan WJ. Dysfunction of the belch reflex—A cause of incapaciting chest pain. Gastroenterology 1987;93:818.

50. Levitt MD, Lasser RB, Schwartz JS, Bond JH. Studies of a flatulent patient. N Engl J Med 1976;295:260.

51. Sutalff LO, Levitt MD. Follow-up of a flatulent patient. Dig Dis Sci 1979;26:652.

52. Steggerda FR. Gastrointestinal gas following food consumption. Ann NY Acad Sci 1968;150:57.

53. Kirk E. The quantity and composition of human colonic flatus. Gastroenterology 1949;12:782.

54. Levitt MD. Volume and composition of human intestinal gas. N Engl J Med 1971;284:1394.

55. Florent C, Flourie B, Leblond A, Rautureamu M, Bernier JJ, Rambaud JC. Influence of chronic lactulose ingestion on the colonic metabolism of lactulose in man (an in vivo study). J Clin Invest 1985;75:608.

56. Perman JA, Modler S. Glycoproteins as substrates for production of hydrogen and methane by colonic bacterial flora. Gastroenterology 1982;83:388.

57. Levitt MD. Production and excretion of hydrogen gas in man. N Engl J Med 1969;281:122.

58. Cummings JC. Fermentation in the human large intestine: Evidence and implications for health. Lancet 1983;1:1206.

59. McKay LF, Eastwood MA, Brydon WG. Methane excretion in man—A study of breath, flatus and feces. Gut 1985;26:69.

60. Wagner JR, Carcson JF, Becker R, Gumbann MR, Danhof IE. Comparative flatulence activity of beans and bean fractions for man and the rat. J Nutr 1977;107:680.

61. Saunders DR, Wiggins HS. Conservation of mannitol, lactulose and raffinose by the human colon. Am J Physiol 1981;241:G397.

62. Layer P, Carlson GL, DiMagno EP. Partially purified white bean amylase inhibitor reduces starch digestion in vitro and inactivates intraduodenal amylase in humans. Gastroenterology 1985;88:1895.

63. Ravich WJ, Bayless TM, Thomas M. Fructose: Incomplete intestinal absorption in humans. Gastroenterology 1983;84:26.

64. Kneepkens MF, Vonk RJ, Furnandes J. Incomplete intestinal absorption of fructose. Arch Dis Child 1984;59:735.

65. Hymas JS. Sorbitol intolerance: An unappreciated cause of functional gastrointestinal complaints. Gastroenterology 1983;84:30.

66. Anderson IH, Levine AS, Levitt MD. Incomplete absorption of the carbohydrate in all-purpose wheat flour. N Engl J Med 1981;304:891.

67. Levitt MD, Hirsh P, Fetzer CA, Sheahan M, Levine As. H_2 excretion after ingestion of complex carbohydrates. Gastroenterology 1987;92:383.

68. Saltzberg DM, Levine GM, Lubar C. Impact of age, sex, race and functional complaints on hydrogen (H_2) production. Dig Dis Sci 1988;33:308.

69. Shafer RB, Prentiss RA, Bond JH. Gastrointestinal transit in thyroid disease. Gastroenterology 1984;86:852.

70. Bjorneklett A, Jenessen E. Relationships between hydrogen (H_2) and methane (CH_4) production in man. Scand J Gastroenterol 1980;17:985.

71. Perman JA, Modler S, Olson AC. Role of pH in production of hydrogen from carbohydrates by colonic bacterial flora. J Clin Invest 1983;67:643.

72. Murphy EL, Calloway DH. The effect of antibiotic drugs on the volume and composition of intestinal gas from beans. Am J Dig Dis 1972;17:639.

73. Gilat T, Benhur H, Gelman-Malachin OE, Terdiman R, Peled Y. Alterations of the colonic flora and their effect on the hydrogen breath test. Gut 1978;19:602.

74. Rumessen JJ, Gudmand-Hoyer E. Functional bowel disease: Malabsorption and abdominal distress after ingestion of fructose, sorbitol and fructose–sorbitol mixtures. Gastroenterology 1988;95:696.

75. Barr RG, Levine MD, Watkins JB. Recurrent abdominal pain of childhood due to lactose intolerance. N Engl J Med 1979;300:1449.

76. Marthinsen D, Fleming SE. Excretion of breath and flatus gases by humans consuming high-fiber diets. J Nutr 1982;112:1133.

77. Hanson CF, Wintorfeldt EA. Dietary fiber effects on passage rate and breath hydrogen. Am J Clin Nutr 1985;42:44.

78. Bond JH, Levitt MD. Effect of dietary fiber on intestinal gas production and small bowel transit time in man. Am J Clin Nutr 1978;31:S169.

79. Tadesse K, Eastwood MA. Metabolism of dietary fiber components in man assessed by breath hydrogen and methane. Br J Nutr 1978;40:393.

80. Stone-Dorshow T, Levitt MD. Gaseous response to ingestion of a poorly absorbed fructo-oligosaccharide sweetener. Am J Clin Nutr 1987;46:61.

81. Becker GL. Prevention of gas explosions in the large bowel during electrosurgery. Surg Gynecol Obstet 1953;97:463.

82. Levy EI. Explosions during lower bowel electrosurgery. Am J Surg 1954;88:754.

83. Bond JH, Levy M, Levitt MD. Explosions of hydrogen gas in the colon during proctosigmoidoscopy. Gastrointest Endosc 1976;23:41.

84. Bigard MA, Gaucher P, Lassalle C. Fatal colonic explosion during colonoscopic polypectomy. Gastroenterology 1979;77:1307.

85. Bond JH, Levitt MD. Factors affecting the concentration of combustible gases in the colon during colonoscopy. Gastroenterology 1976;68:1445.

86. Woodward NW. Prevention of explosion while fulgurating polyps of the colon. Dis Colon Rectum 1961;4:32.

87. Ragins H, Shinya H, Wolfee WI. The explosive potential of colonic gas during colonoscopic electrosurgical polypectomy. Surg Gynecol Obstet 1974;138:554.

88. Hocking MP, Maher JW, Woodward ER. Definitive surgical therapy for incapacitating "gas-bloat" syndrome. Am Surg 1982;48:131.

89. Bushkin FL, Neustein CL, Parker TH, et al. Nissen fundoplication for reflux peptic esophagitis. Ann Surg 1977;185:672.

90. Walls ADF, Gonzales JG. The incidence of gas-bloat syndrome and dysphagia following fundoplication for hiatus hernia. J R Coll Surg Edinb 1977;22:391.

91. Harvey CF, McKelvey STD. Fundal perforation complicating the gas-bloat syndrome. J R Coll Surg Edinb 1986;31:183.

92. Rossetti M, Hell K. Fundoplication for the treatment of gastroesophageal reflux in hiatal hernia. World J Surg 1977;1:439.

93. Manning AP, Thompson WG, Heaton KW, Morris AF. Towards positive diagnosis of the irritable bowel. Br Med J 1978;2:653.

94. Lewis JG. Adverse reactions to calcium antagonists. Drugs 1983;25:196.

95. Hickey CA, Calloway DH, Murphy EL. Intestinal gas production following ingestion of fruits and fruit juices. Dig Dis Sci 1972;17:383.

96. Keshavarzian A, Iber FL, Vaeth J. Gastric emptying in patients with insulin-requiring diabetes mellitus. Am J Gastroenterol 1987;82:29.

97. Cohen S. The gastrointestinal manifestations of scleroderma: Pathogenesis and management. Gastroenterology 1980;79:155.

98. Leon SH, Schuffler MD, Kettler M, Rohrmann CA. Chronic intestinal pseudoobstruction as a complication of Duchenne's muscular dystrophy. Gastroenterology 1986;90:455.

99. Glick ME, Meshkinpour H, Haldeman S, Hoehler F, Downey H, Bradley WE. Colonic dysfunction in patients with thoracic spinal cord injury. Gastroenterology 1984;86:287.

100. Schuffler MD. Chronic intestinal pseudo-obstruction syndromes. Med Clin North Am 1981;65:1331.

101. Simon GL, Gorbach SL. Intestinal flora in health and disease. Gastroenterology 1984;86:174.

102. Sullivan MA, Snape WJ Jr, Matarazzo SA, et al. Gastrointestinal myoelectric activity in idiopathic intestinal pseudo-obstruction. N Engl J Med 1977;297:233.

103. Kim CH, Malagelada JR. Electrical activity of the stomach: Clinical implications. Mayo Clin Proc 1986;61:205.

104. Ricci DA, McCallum RW. Diagnosis and treatment of delayed gastric emptying. Adv Intern Med 1988;33:357.

105. King CE, Toskes PP. Small intestinal bacterial overgrowth. Gastroenterology 1979;76:1035.

106. Hall RG, Thompson H, Strother A. Effects of orally administered activated charcoal on intestinal gas. Am J Gastroenterol 1981;75:192.

107. Jain NK, Patel VP, Pitchumoni S. Activated charcoal, simethicone and intestinal gas: A double-blind study. Ann Intern Med 1986;105:61.

108. Potter T, Elcis C, Levitt M. Activated charcoal: In vivo and in vitro studies of effect on gas formation. Gastroenterology 1985;88:620.

109. Bernstein JE, Schwartz SR. An evaluation of the effectiveness of simethicone in acute upper gastrointestinal distress. Curr Ther Res 1974;16:617.

110. Lifschitz CH, Irving CS, O'Brian-Smith E. Effect of a simethicone-containing tablet on colonic gas elimination in breath. Dig Dis Sci 1985;30:426.

111. Bernstein JE, Kasich AM. A double-blind trial of simethicone in functional disease of the upper gastrointestinal tract. J Clin Pharmacol 1974;14:617.

112. Johnson AG. Controlled trial of metoclopramide in the treatment of flatulent dyspepsia. Br Med J 1971;2:25.

113. Perman JA, Barr RB, Watkins JB. Sucrose malabsorption in children; non-invasive diagnosis by interval breath hydrogen determination. J Pediatr 1978;93:17.

114. Solomons NW, Garcia-Ibanez R, Viteri FE. Reduced rates of breath hydrogen (H_2) excretion with lactose tolerance tests in young children using whole milk. Am J Clin Nutr 1979;32:783.

115. Kerlin P, Wong L, Harris B, Capra S. Rice flour, breath hydrogen and malabsorption. Gastroenterology 1984;87:578.

116. Perman JA, Rosenstein BJ. Carbohydrate digestion in cystic fibrosis (CF): Application of breath H_2 measurements. Pediatr Res 1986;20:246A.

117. Barr RG, Watkins JB, Perman JA. Mucosal function and breath hydrogen excretion: Comparative studies in the clinical evaluation of children with non-specific abdominal complaints. Pediatrics 1981;68:526.

118. Bartlett K, Dobson JV, Eastham E. A new method for the detection of hydrogen in breath and its application to acquired and inborn sugar malabsorption. Clin Chim Acta 1980;108:189.

119. Stevenson D, Cohen RS, Ostrander CR, Shahin SM, Kerner JA, Wetmore DL, Werner SB, Tomczyk M, Johnson JD. A sensitive analytical apparatus for measuring hydrogen production rates. II. Application to studies in human infants. J Pediatr Gastroenterol Nutr 1982;1:233.

120. Rhodes JM, Middleton P, Jewell DP. The lactulose hydrogen breath test as a diagnostic test for small-bowel bacterial overgrowth. Scand J Gastroenterol 1979;14:333.

121. Kerlin P, Wong L. Breath hydrogen testing in bacterial overgrowth of the small intestine. Gastroenterology 1988;95:982.

122. Perman JA, Modler S, Barr RG, Rosenthal P. Fasting breath hydrogen concentration: Normal values and clinical application. Gastroenterology 1984;87:1358.

123. Kotler DP, Holt PR, Rosensweig NS. Modification of the breath hydrogen test: Increased sensitivity for the detection of carbohydrate malabsorption. J Lab Clin Med 1982;100:798.

124. Dodds EC, Bennett TI. Variations in alveolar carbon dioxide pressure in relation to meals: A further study. J Physiol 1920;54:381.

125. King CE, Toskes PP. The use of breath tests in the study of malabsorption. Clin Gastroenterol 1983;12:591.

126. Watkins JB, Klein PD, Schoeller DA, Kirschner BS, Park R, Perman JA. Diagnosis and differentiation of fat malabsorption in children using ^{13}C-labeled lipids: Trioctanoin, triolein, and palmitic acid breath test. Gastroenterology 1982;82:911.

127. Reba RC, Salkeld J. In vitro studies of malabsorption and other GI disorders. Semin Nucl Med 1972;12:147.

128. Abt AF, Von Schching SL. Fat utilization test in disorders of fat metabolism. Bull Johns Hopkins Hosp 166;119:316.

129. King CE, Toskes PP, Guilarte TR, Brokeman VA, Fitzgerald L, Staley G. Safety of carbon-14 breath tests: Elimination and tissue retention studies of ^{14}C-D-xylose and ^{14}-cholyl glycine. Clin Res 1980;28:483.

130. Schwabe AD, Hepner GW. Breath tests for the detection of fat malabsorption. Gastroenterology 1979;76:216.

131. Newcomer AD, Hofmann AF, DiMagno EP, Thomas PJ, Carlson GL. Triolein breath test: A sensitive and specific test for fat malabsorption. Gastroenterology 1979;76:6.

132. Cole SG, Rossis S, Stern A, Hofmann AF. Cholesteryl octanoate breath test: Preliminary studies on a new noninvasive test of human pancreatic exocrine function. Gastroenterology 1987;93:1372.

133. King LE, Toskes PP, Spivey JC, Lorenz E, Welkos S. Detection of small intestinal bacterial overgrowth by means of a ^{14}C-D-xylose breath test. Gastroenterology 1979;77:75.

134. King CE, Toskes PP, Guilarte TR, Lorenz E, Welkos SL. Comparison on the gram d-^{14}C-xylose breath test to the ^{14}C bile acid breath test in patients with small intestine bacterial overgrowth. Dig Dis Sci 1980;25:53.

135. Tillman R, King CE, Toskes PP. Continued experience with the xylose breath test: Evidence that the small bowel culture as the gold standard for bacterial overgrowth may be tarnished. Gastroenterology 1981;80:1304.

136. Schneider A, Novis B, Chen V, Leichtman G. Value of the ^{14}C-D-xylose breath test in patients with intestinal bacterial overgrowth. Digestion 1985;32:86.

137. King CE, Toskes PP. Comparison of the 1-gram ^{14}C xylose, 10-

gram lactose-H_2 and 80-gram glucose-H_2 breath tests in patients with a small intestine bacterial overgrowth. Gastroenterology 1986;91:1447.

138. Fromm H, Hofmann AF. Breath test for altered bile-acid metabolism. Lancet 1971;2:621.

139. Sherr HP, Yasuhito S, Newman A, Banwell JG, Wagner HN, Hendrix JR. Detection of bacterial deconjugation of bile salts by a convenient breath analysis technic. N Engl J Med 1971;285:256.

140. Lauterburg DH, Newcomer AD, Hofmann AF. Clinical value of the bile acid breath test. Evaluation of the Mayo Clinic experience. Mayo Clin Proc 1978;53:227.

141. Farvivar S, Fromm H, Schindler D, McJunkin B, Schmidt FW. Tests of bile acid and vitamin B12 metabolism in ileal Crohn's disease. Am J Clin Pathol 1980;73:69.

142. Ferguson J, Walker K, Thomson ABR. Limitations in the use of

^{14}C-glyco cholate breath and stool bile determinations in patients with chronic diarrhea. J Clin Gastroenterol 1986;8:258.

143. Schneider JF, Baker AL, Haines NW, Hatfield G, Boyer JL. Aminopyrine N-demethylation: A prognostic test of liver. Gastroenterology 1980;79:1145.

144. Villeneuve JP, Infante-Rivard C, Ampelas M, Pomier-Layargues G, Huet PM, Marleau D. Prognostic value of the aminopyrine breath test in cirrhotic patients. Hepatology 1986;5:928.

145. Morelli A, Naroucci F, Pelli MA, Farroni F, Vedovelli A. The relationship between aminopyrine breath test and severity of liver disease in cirrhosis. Am J Gastroenterol 1981;76:110.

146. Sampors JB, Wright N, Lewis KO. Predicting outcome of paracetamol poisoning by using ^{14}C-aminopyrine breath test. Br Med J 1980;280:279.

36

Approach to the Patient with Acute Abdomen and Fever of Abdominal Origin

DAVID McFADDEN
MICHAEL J. ZINNER

THE ACUTE ABDOMEN

Introduction

The patient presenting with acute abdominal pain remains the last crucible of the physician's diagnostic and therapeutic abilities. The term *acute abdomen* refers to the sudden and unexpected onset of acute abdominal pain. As stated succinctly by Cope in 1921, the term *acute abdomen* should never be equated with the invariable need for operation.[1] The acute abdomen defines pain that has been present for less than 24 hours and may be associated with other symptoms such as nausea or vomiting, abdominal distention, diarrhea, constipation, and anorexia. The pain and associated symptoms can be caused by many intra-abdominal and extra-abdominal pro-

cesses, which may, in turn, present clinically in a variety of ways. The first tenet in managing patients with acute abdominal pain is a thorough attempt at diagnosis, using fundamentals of history taking and physical examination.[1-3] Accurate diagnosis of the acute abdomen depends on the physician's grasp of the anatomy and physiology of the abdominal viscera and extra-abdominal conditions that may simulate an acute abdomen. The purpose of this chapter is not to give a comprehensive treatise on the diagnosis and treatment of acute abdominal pain, but rather to provide a succinct review of the differential diagnoses, diagnostic tests, and therapeutic alternatives for the patient presenting with acute abdominal pain so that a prompt diagnosis and therapeutic plan may be formulated.

The second section of this chapter deals with the topic of fevers of abdominal origin. The biology, physiology, and treatment of peritonitis, intra-abdominal abscesses, and postoperative etiologies are described.

Embryologic and Anatomic Considerations

Because acute abdominal pain is capable of arising from almost any intra-abdominal or extra-abdominal structure, a brief review of the embryology and anatomy of the abdominal cavity follows.[4]

The gut tube comprises a foregut, midgut, and hindgut, each of which has its own blood supply and innervation and retains these relationships throughout development and into adulthood. The foregut extends from the oropharynx to the duodenum at the level of the entrance of the common bile duct.[5] It includes the pancreas, liver, biliary tree, and spleen. The midgut comprises the distal duodenum, jejunum, ileum, appendix, ascending colon, and proximal two thirds of the transverse colon. The hindgut consists of the distal one third of the transverse colon down to the cloacal bulge, which constitutes the point of contact between the surface ectoderm and endoderm of the cloaca.

The peritoneum constitutes a continuous visceral and parietal layer. Although both layers are mesodermally derived, they develop separately. Importantly, for diagnostic reasons, the nerve supply to each layer is separate. The visceral layer is supplied by autonomic nerves (sympathetic and parasympathetic), and the parietal peritoneum is supplied by somatic innervation (spinal nerves).[5] The pathways relaying the sensation of pain differ for each layer and in quality as well. Visceral pain is dull, crampy, or aching; parietal pain is sharp, severe, and persistent.

Normal embryologic development of abdominal viscera proceeds with bilateral midline autonomic innervation; therefore, visceral pain is usually felt in the abdominal midline. The position of pain in the midline is determined by the embryologic origin of the involved viscus. Epigastric pain is typical of foregut origin. Periumbilical midline pain signifies pain arising from the midgut. Hypogastric or lower abdominal midline pain indicates an origin from the hindgut structures. Pelvic pain is more typical of disease originating in structures derived from the cloaca.[5]

For abdominal pain to be recognized by the patient, nociceptors, or pain receptors, must be noxiously stimulated. Two types of neuronal fibers are involved. A-delta fibers are rapid transmitters and give rise to sharp, well-localized pain sensations. These fibers are distributed to muscle and skin and are involved with the somatic pain transmission through spinal nerves. C-fibers are slow transmitters and generate the sensation of dull, poorly localized pain that is more gradual in its onset and of longer duration. These fibers are located intramurally in hollow viscera and in the capsule of solid organs. They are also found in muscle, periosteum, and the parietal peritoneum. These fibers are predominantly involved in the visceral pain transmission through the autonomic nervous system.

Different neural pathways are responsible for pain mediation, depending on whether the source of the pain is the abdominal wall or intra-abdominal viscera. The anterior and lateral abdominal walls are supplied by nerves coming from spinal segments T7–L1.[5] The posterior abdominal wall is innervated from spinal segments L2–L5. Pain arising from the abdominal wall is relayed to the spinal cord through the spinal nerves. Because these pain fibers enter the spinal cord ipsilaterally from the focus of pain, it is perceived as originating from that side. Also, such pain localizes to the area of the abdomen from which it originates. In contrast, pain coming from intra-abdominal viscera is perceived to arise in the midline because sensory input from such viscera enters the spinal cord on both sides.

Abdominal pain can be divided into three categories: visceral, somatic, and referred.[5] The aforementioned intramural sensory receptors of the abdominal viscus are responsible for visceral pain. The major forces that produce this type of pain arise from geometric changes such as stretching or distention, resulting in increased wall tension of the particular viscus affected. Other factors believed to be responsible for development of visceral pain include inflammation and ischemia. Visceral pain almost always heralds intra-abdominal disease but does not necessitate surgical intervention. When visceral pain becomes supplanted by somatic pain, surgical intervention becomes a likely possibility.

Somatic or parietal pain arises from irritation of the parietal peritoneum. Mediated mainly by spinal nerve fibers that supply the abdominal wall, somatic pain is localized and is perceived as originating from one of the four quadrants of the abdominal wall. In contrast to visceral pain where geometric changes are responsible for the stimulation of nerve endings, somatic pain arises as a response to acute changes in pH or temperature as seen in bacterial or chemical inflammation.[6] In addition, somatic pain is felt in response to sudden increases in pressure as with a surgical incision. Somatic pain is perceived as sharp and pricking and is usually constant.

Referred pain is felt in an area of the body other than the site of its origin.[5] Referred pain usually arises from a deep structure, is superficial at its distant presenting location, and frequently is sharp and localized at the distant site. It occurs secondary to the existence of shared central pathways for afferent neurons arising from different sites. A classic example is the ruptured spleen that results in irritation of the left hemidiaphragm, which is innervated by cervical nerves.[3–5] In this setting, referred pain is perceived as arising in the left shoulder (Kehr's sign), also supplied by these nerve roots. A knowledge of referred pain and its patterns may be of diagnostic assistance when other evidence of disease is lacking or absent (Table 36-1).

Clinical Assessment of the Acute Abdomen

HISTORY

Sir Zachary Cope's treatise on the acute abdomen centers on early diagnosis.[1] No aspect of diagnosis is more important than a careful and thorough history. If possible, it is best to allow the patient to give his or her entire current history before asking specific questions. This should include a past medical history and information concerning associated illnesses. A history of prior similar symptoms is also sought as well as the presence of any prodromal symptoms.

The character and onset of the pain are particularly important (Fig 36-2). Colicky pain usually indicates some type of obstructive process and may be associated with intestinal obstruction, the passage of a ureteral calculus, or acute cholecystitis. It signifies hyperperistalsis of smooth muscle in an attempt to move fluid past an obstruction. Between colicky episodes, the pain lessens or disappears. During attacks, the pain is persistent and unrelenting. The pain seen with infectious processes such as appendicitis, di-

TABLE 36–1
Referred Pain Patterns

SITE	REFERRING VISCUS
Left shoulder	Left diaphragmatic irritation (spleen, subphrenic fluid or abscess) esophagus, heart
Right shoulder	Right diaphragmatic irritation Liver
Right subscapular	Biliary tree, liver
Epigastrium	Stomach, transverse colon
Right upper quadrant	Liver, biliary tree, pylorus, duodenum
Flank	Kidney, pancreas
Sacrum, lumbar area	Uterus, rectum
Hypogastrium	Colon, kidney
Groins, genitalia	Ureter, bladder
Umbilicus	Appendix, midgut

verticulitis, or intra-abdominal abscess is usually sustained and may increase in severity over time. Clues to the underlying cause of pain may be evidenced by the type of onset. Pancreatitis is usually gradual in onset and commonly follows an episode of alcoholic abuse. In contrast, a perforated hollow viscus such as a peptic ulcer or abdominal aortic aneurysm produces a sudden onset of pain that the patient may be able to time precisely. Pain location can also be helpful in establishing the underlying diagnosis (Fig

TABLE 36–2
Abdominal Pain Onset Patterns

I. *Sudden (Seconds)*
  A. Perforation or rupture of viscus/abscess/hematoma
     Peptic ulcer, abdominal aortic aneurysm, esophagus (Boerhaave's syndrome), ectopic pregnancy, spontaneous pneumothorax
  B. Infarction
     Gut, heart, lung
II. *Rapid (Minutes)*
  A. Colic syndromes
     Biliary, ureteral, small bowel obstruction (high)
  B. Inflammatory processes
     Pancreatitis, diverticulitis, peptic ulcer, appendicitis, cholecystitis, pneumonitis
  C. Ischemic processes
     Strangulation obstruction of intestine, mesenteric ischemia, torsion/volvulus
III. *Gradual (Hours)*
  A. Inflammatory processes
     Appendicitis, cholecystitis, pancreatitis, gastritis, lymphadenitis, inflammatory bowel disease, diverticulitis, salpingitis, cystitis, prostatitis, intra-abdominal abscess.
  B. Obstruction
     Distal small bowel or colon, urinary retention, incarcerated hernia, ectopic pregnancy
  C. Neoplastic
     Perforating or penetrating tumors (colon, stomach, small intestine)

36-1). This is especially true with somatic pain that results from an irritation of the parietal peritoneum.

Other factors must also be considered in evaluating the patient with acute abdominal pain. These include any previous history of intra-abdominal disease, previous abdominal surgery, and current medications. Familial or concomitant diseases in family members should also be elicited. Vomiting is a less specific diagnostic aid in evaluating the patient with acute abdomen. If vomiting is present, it is important to document the frequency and character of the vomitus as well as questions concerning the recent passage or urine, stool, or flatus. A woman's precise menstrual history should be obtained because this may be the sole clue to the presence of gynecologic pathology.

PHYSICAL EXAMINATION

The first and most important step in physical examination of the patient with acute abdominal pain is a careful observation of the patient's body habitus and facial expression. The patient's unwillingness to change postural positions may be evidence of an underlying peritonitis. Hip flexion with the knees drawn up to maintain comfort suggests tension on the abdominal wall and possible peritoneal irritation. Restriction of diaphragmatic excursion

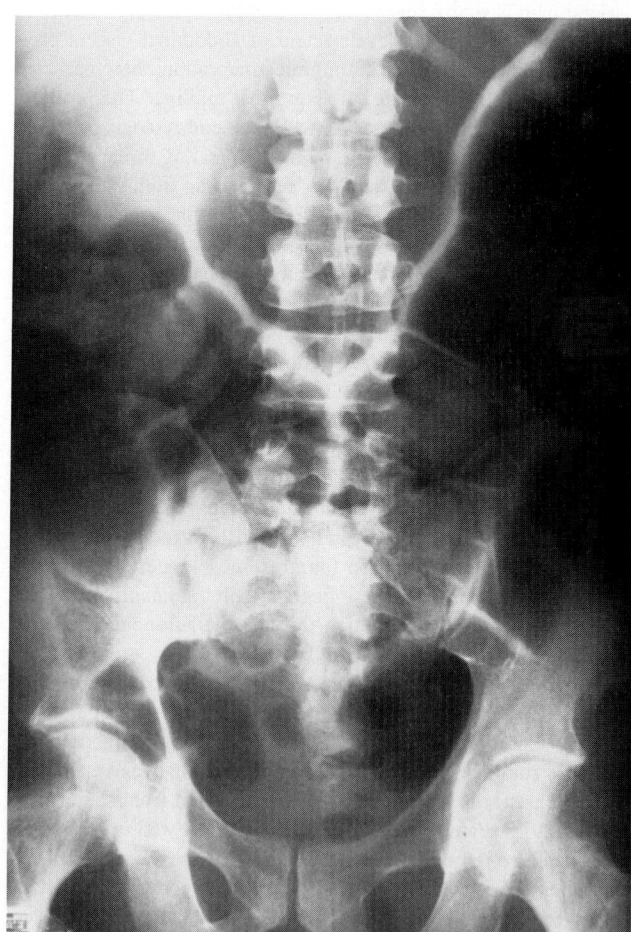

FIGURE 36–1. Emphysematous cholecystitis in an elderly diabetic patient. Gas is present within lumen and wall of gallbladder.

with respiration as noted by shallow breathing and the use of accessory respiratory muscles is also consistent with peritoneal irritation. In contrast, the presence of colicky pain is often manifested by intense movement in an effort to alleviate pain followed by quiescent periods between colicky attacks.

Inspection of the abdomen should also be performed to note any localized or generalized distention, hernial bulges, or areas of erythema or infection. After inspection, careful auscultation for bowel sounds must be performed. Many acute abdominal conditions lead to a partial or complete ileus with decreased or absent bowel sounds. Patients suffering bowel obstructions have hyperactive sounds usually occurring simultaneously with colicky pain. The presence of bruits should also be noted in the abdomen, flanks, and groins. A careful auscultation of the chest, particularly in the diaphragmatic area, should be performed to document diaphragmatic movement and to search for the possibility of basilar pneumonias that may simulate an acute abdomen. Gentle palpation of all quadrants of the abdomen should be performed after auscultation. Gentle, rather superficial, palpation should be initially performed proceeding from the least painful areas to the most painful areas as suggested from the patient's history. Peritoneal signs may be suspected by the findings on gentle palpation, but, after this, deeper palpation should also be attempted. Deeper palpation should identify localized or generalized peritonitis and may define any masses present. Classic rebound tenderness, as diagnosed by deep palpation followed by rapid release, should be discouraged because it may cause pain even in normal persons and is not reproducible. Percussion tenderness is a kinder and gentler way of eliciting peritoneal signs. A useful technique is to shake gently the patient's torso back and forth laterally by holding the hips or firmly striking the heel of the patient. This often causes a friction between inflamed peritoneal surfaces yielding specific somatic pain. Having the patient cough, laugh, or distend or maximally reduce his or her abdominal girth is often helpful in localizing specific peritoneal inflammations, especially in children. Other techniques, such as using a stethoscope to palpate and release, can be helpful. This is particularly true in the multiply-examined patient. A mandatory rectal and pelvic evaluation completes the physical examination.

Several signs usually associated with appendicitis have been described and may prove helpful in the diagnosis of the acute abdomen. The psoas sign is elicited by stretching the peritoneum over the psoas muscle by extension of the thigh at the hip. If inflammation involves either psoas sheath, as may occur with psoas abscess or pelvic or retrocecal appendix, pain is elicited by this maneuver. The obturator sign is performed by internally rotating the thigh with the knee flexed, thereby stretching the obturator fascia. Again, if inflammation is present that involves the obturator fascia, as may occur for appendicitis, obturator hernia, or pelvic abscess, pain is elicited by this maneuver. Hyperesthesia is uncommonly present but is defined as exquisitely sensitive skin, usually to gentle touch, in the dermatone corresponding to that supplied by the same nerve roots as an area of parietal peritoneum that is being irritated by an intra-abdominal inflammatory process. However, this is not a reliable sign.

LABORATORY EVALUATION

A number of laboratory tests may provide useful information in evaluating the patient with acute abdominal pain. A minimal evaluation consists of a complete blood count, urinalysis, serum amylase, and a beta human chorionic gonadotropin (HCG) test in females. A set of serum electrolytes, blood urea nitrogen, creatinine, and glucose may be useful in evaluating the patient's hydration status, renal function, and basic metabolic state. Liver function tests may be helpful in the patient with upper abdominal pain. A "shotgun" approach to the laboratory evaluation of the patient presenting with acute abdominal pain should be avoided. Laboratory investigations should not be performed unless their results could change the need for additional tests or therapy.

Four roentgenographic views of the chest and abdomen are mandatory in the patient with acute abdominal pain who does not have an obvious diagnosis. These films include a supine and erect plain film of the abdomen as well as an upright PA and lateral film of the chest. The upright abdominal film should be centered to include the diaphragms, permitting detection of free intraperitoneal air but also of air–fluid levels within the bowel that can be detected only on horizontal beam films (Fig. 36-2).[7] If patients are too sick or debilitated to stand, lateral decubitus films should be obtained. The left lateral decubitus view is best for detecting pneumoperitoneum, because free intraperitoneal air is more easily visualized between the liver and the right lateral abdominal wall.[8] It is worth noting that only 10% of patients with an acute abdomen exhibit abnormalities on screening radiographs.[9] Nevertheless, in the patient without a clear-cut diagnosis based on history, physical examination, and simple blood tests, we feel that such radiologic evaluation is indicated.[10]

Depending on the clinical, laboratory, or plain film findings, a contrast study with barium or water-soluble contrast agents may be required for more definitive diagnosis. If plain film suggests intestinal necrosis, toxic megacolon, or pneumoperitoneum, barium studies should be avoided because of the risk of extravasation of barium into the peritoneal cavity.[9,10]

More sophisticated radiologic studies may be needed in the evaluation of certain conditions. Abdominal ultrasound is a safe method of evaluating the biliary tree, the abdominal aorta, the

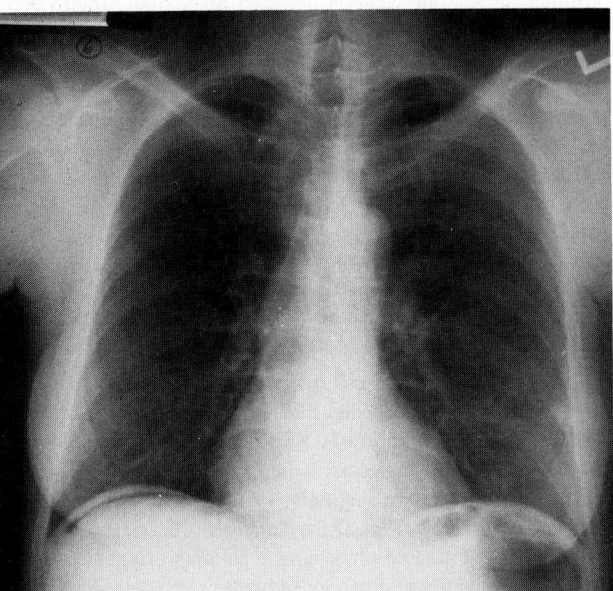

FIGURE 36-2. Upright chest radiograph of patient with perforated duodenal ulcer. Note small pneumoperitoneum on right side.

pancreas, or other inflammatory processes or fluid collections.[11,12] Computed tomography (CT) has proved itself in the diagnosis of many abdominal disorders, including the acute abdomen, and in many instances provides information superior to that of other more conventional studies.[13] Magnetic resonance imaging (MRI) does not have an established role in the diagnosis of acute abdominal disorders. Angiographic evaluation of the abdominal vessels can be both diagnostic and therapeutic in the treatment of patients with vascular disease of the abdomen presenting with acute abdominal pain. Various nuclear medicine studies are also useful in various clinical situations.

Causes of Acute Abdomen in Adults

APPENDICITIS

Appendicitis is a relatively modern term dating from 1886.[14] It is the wise physician who never places appendicitis lower than second on the list of differential diagnoses for the patient presenting with acute abdominal pain unless the physician performed a previous appendectomy on that patient. Appendicitis remains a significant cause of morbidity and mortality especially in the extreme age groups.[15]

As with any other medical condition, diagnosis begins with a complete history, physical examination, and appropriate laboratory tests. The history of a patient with appendicitis usually follows a distinct pattern: (1) pain in the abdomen, typically midabdominal, (2) onset of nausea and vomiting, (3) relocation or movement of the pain to the right lower quadrant, and (4) elevation of temperature.[14] Anorexia is an important sign in patients who do not complain of nausea or vomiting. Pain elicited in the right lower quadrant by bumping, coughing, or laughing may represent peritoneal irritation in that area.[16] A history of diarrhea does not rule out appendicitis but suggests the need for a stool Gram's stain and culture to look for leukocytes and organisms associated with gastroenteritis, such as *Salmonella, Campylobacter,* or *Shigella.*

The physical examination is most important in assessing the patient with suspected appendicitis. The decision to operate on a patient is based on clinical evidence of peritoneal inflammation rather than abnormal laboratory values or historic findings. If the patient has no evidence of peritoneal irritation despite an appropriate history and abnormal laboratory data, one may elect to observe the patient by carefully examining him or her at frequent intervals to check for the development of localized or diffuse tenderness. If signs of peritonitis are present, operative intervention is recommended, regardless of other findings.

The basic laboratory evaluation for a patient with suspected appendicitis includes a white blood cell count with differential urinalysis, and a serum beta-HCG if the patient is female. Rarely is an abdominal x-ray necessary if the physical examination, history, and laboratory data are suggestive or indicative of appendicitis. It may be useful, however, if the diagnosis is in question.[16] Some authors have advocated ultrasound evaluation of the right lower quadrant for evidence of periappendiceal fluid, edema, or abscess formation. Urinalysis is essential, but it must be remembered that several red cells or white cells may be seen per high power field secondary to the overlying inflammation caused by an inflamed organ, such as the appendix near the ureter. The diagnosis of appendicitis is most difficult in preschool children, young women from age 20 to 40, and elderly persons. Preschool children have a high rate of perforative appendicitis (up to 63%)[17] but, fortunately, have a very low mortality because of their general good health. Most authors advocate that any preschool child with unexplained abdominal pain be admitted to the hospital for serial examination and observation.[17,18] Young women who have regular menstrual cycles and present with right lower quadrant pain have the highest negative appendectomy rate (40%) of all patients explored for presumed appendicitis. Pelvic inflammatory disease is a common diagnosis in this group.[19] A recent prospective study found several criteria were to be useful in differentiating between pelvic inflammatory disease and appendicitis in young females. These include: (1) duration of symptoms, (2) the presence of nausea, vomiting, or both, (3) a history of venereal disease, (4) cervical motion tenderness on pelvic exam, (5) adnexal tenderness, and (6) isolated peritoneal signs on the right lower quadrant.[19] Using these simple physical and historic signs and symptoms, this group was able to reduce the negative laparotomy rate in young females to 15.4%. Laparoscopy has also been advocated by multiple authors[20,21] but usually requires a general anesthetic and is not universally accepted. We would not favor this approach in young females.

Elderly persons are at an increased risk from appendicitis because the illness is often recognized late. Perforation rates of 75% have been reported.[22] Elderly patients frequently have multiple underlying medical conditions, and death may result in as many as 24%.[22] Elderly patients are often difficult to diagnose because as many as one fourth do not have an elevation of temperature or white blood cell count.[16] Pain is generally the chief complaint in the majority of elderly patients. A high index of suspicion should be upheld for elderly patients presenting with abdominal pain.

Other diagnoses to be considered in the evaluation of right lower quadrant pain include ruptured ectopic pregnancy, ovarian cyst, mesenteric lymphadenitis, mittelschmerz, pelvic inflammatory disease, gastroenteritis, pyelonephritis, cecal diverticulitis, inflammatory bowel disease, and Meckel's diverticula. The overall mortality of appendectomy for appendicitis is less than one in a thousand but increases tenfold in the presence of free perforation. We and others feel no great shame in a negative appendectomy rate of 10% to 20% given the increased and striking mortality seen in patients who are allowed to perforate in hospital.[16,18,22] The management of patients with appendicitis is discussed in detail elsewhere.[23,24]

ACUTE CHOLECYSTITIS

Acute cholecystitis is a common cause of the acute abdomen in adults as documented by the approximately 100,000 cholecystectomies done in this country each year for acute cholecystitis.[25] Most cases of acute cholecystitis are secondary to gallstones obstructing the cystic duct with subsequent edema, inflammation, and frequently bacterial invasion. Acute acalculous cholecystitis accounts for approximately 5% of all cases of acute cholecystitis and generally presents in hospitalized patients.[26] Acalculus cholecystitis is rarely seen in patients presenting to hospital emergency rooms or outpatient clinics.

The usual clinical presentation of acute cholecystitis is in a middle-aged patient, approximately 80% of whom have had previous biliary colic. The pain of early acute cholecystitis is difficult to distinguish from that of biliary colic. However, once the pain of biliary colic has persisted beyond 6 hours or is associated with fever or leukocytosis, the diagnosis of acute cholecystitis should be entertained.[26] Pain is classically crampy but does not cease between cramps as in small bowel, large bowel, or ureteral colic.[27] Pain may radiate to the epigastrium and occasionally to the back. Nausea and vomiting are common, and fever is usually less than 101°F. Temperatures greater than this should raise the suspicion of local complications such as gangrene or perforation.

The classic physical findings are right upper quadrant tenderness, guarding, and a Murphy's sign (inspiratory arrest elicited when palpating the right upper quadrant while asking the patient to take a deep breath). Right upper quadrant tenderness may vary from extremely mild to right upper quadrant rigidity. A mass in the right upper quadrant is found in approximately 20% of cases and is generally related to a mass of omentum overlying the inflamed gallbladder.[25] Generalized peritonitis is rarely seen in acute cholecystitis unless gallbladder perforation has occurred.[28]

Laboratory findings in acute cholecystitis reflect the spectrum of the disease. A mild clinical presentation produces few abnormalities on routine laboratory investigations. A leukocytosis of between 12,000 and 15,000 cells/ml is common. Jaundice is occasionally present but mild with bilirubin levels less than 4 mg/dl.[25] This hyperbilirubinemia is usually due to local inflammation of the liver around an inflamed gallbladder rather than biliary obstruction. A bilirubin of greater than 4 mg/dl significantly increases the probability of common duct stones. The serum amylase concentration is frequently elevated despite an absence of clinical pancreatitis.[29] Thus, the differentiation between acute cholecystitis and acute pancreatitis may be difficult on clinical grounds. Although increases in hepatic transaminases are frequent in cases of acute cholecystitis, these abnormalities rarely exceed two to three times the normal levels.

Specific radiologic examinations are frequently obtained in patients with suspected acute cholecystitis. Plain abdominal films rarely confirm the diagnosis of acute cholecystitis. Radiopaque gallstones are seen in approximately 15% of patients with gallstones; however, their presence does not prove the diagnosis of acute cholecystitis. Infrequent signs specific to the diagnosis of acute cholecystitis on the plain abdominal film include air in the gallbladder, gallbladder wall, or occasionally the biliary tract itself. Today neither oral cholecystograms nor intravenous cholangiograms have any role in the diagnosis of acute cholecystitis.[30]

Ultrasonography is the most commonly used screening test for acute or chronic cholecystitis. This test combines noninvasiveness, safety, and a high degree of accuracy and is available in most hospitals. Ultrasound is also helpful for the additional data that may be obtained, such as the presence of liver masses, common duct dilatation or stones, pancreatitis, or abdominal fluid collections.[25] Ultrasonographic signs of acute cholecystitis include gallbladder dilatation, mural thickening, sludge in the gallbladder, and pericholecystic fluid collections.[31] Some radiologists have described the "ultrasonographic Murphy's sign" in which the ultrasonographer locates the most tender point on the patient's abdomen with the ultrasound probe and correlates it with the position of the gallbladder. Ultrasound is sensitive for the detection of gallstones, but its specificity for the detection of acute cholecystitis is considerably lower.

The recent development of a family of technetium-labeled compounds rapidly excreted by hepatocytes into the bile canaliculi has revolutionized the imaging of the biliary tract. After intravenous injection, flow is rapidly seen in the common bile duct and into the duodenum. Gallbladder filling with the isotope occurs rapidly, usually within 15 to 30 minutes.[25] The radionuclides are concentrated in the gallbladder over a period of 1 to 4 hours with a normal scan showing an initial rapid imaging of the liver followed by excretion into the common duct and concentration in the gallbladder.[32] Failure to visualize the gallbladder within 60 minutes is highly suspicious for cystic duct obstruction and acute cholecystitis. This test has the advantage of being a test of function rather than anatomy. Occasionally, normal gallbladders do not visualize within 1 hour; therefore, most examinations continue for up to 4 hours before concluding that the cystic duct is obstructed. False positives are occasionally seen in patients who are receiving total parenteral nutrition or who have undergone prolonged fasting, which result in gallbladder stasis and an inability to fill. Also, local inflammatory conditions in the right upper quadrant may decrease the technetium-labeled compound excreted by the liver or render the gallbladder stagnant, such as acute pancreatitis, acute hepatitis, and perforated peptic ulcer disease, accounting for a small number of false-positive studies. The sensitivity of nuclear medicine scanning in acute acalculus cholecystitis is good with more than 97% of patients with this condition showing no imaging of the gallbladder within 4 hours; however, its specificity is considerably lower.[32,33]

Although the standard treatment of acute cholecystitis is cholecystectomy, the initial approach to the patient centers on proper resuscitation and medical treatment. The management of patients with acute cholecystitis is discussed elsewhere[34–39] and in Chapter 94.

ACUTE PANCREATITIS

Acute pancreatitis poses many problems in differential diagnosis and treatment. Fortunately, the illness is usually mild and self-limited with a mortality of less than 5%. However, when the illness is severe and pancreatic injury is characterized by necrosis and hemorrhage, mortality varies between 15% and 100%.[40] In the United States, the major etiologies of acute pancreatitis are alcohol abuse (approximately 70%) or gallstones (approximately 15%). Other rarer causes of acute pancreatitis include hyperparathyroidism, pregnancy, hyperlipidemia, surgery, trauma, and shock.

The clinical presentation of acute pancreatitis varies. Abdominal pain can be very severe and may increase gradually for several hours before achieving maximum intensity. It may also develop suddenly, simulating an acute abdominal or vascular catastrophe.[41] Characteristically, once it begins, the pain persists for many hours and frequently for days. Abdominal pain that varies markedly in intensity or stops for periods of time is rarely pancreatitis.[40] Nausea and vomiting occur commonly and may persist as retching and dry heaves. Palpation of the upper abdomen frequently demonstrates guarding, but the abdomen is rarely as rigid as seen with the perforation of a hollow viscus. However, peritoneal signs may be present. Hypoactive bowel sounds are common, and the vital signs may demonstrate an elevated temperature and pulse with a corresponding decrease in blood pressure from relative hypovolemia.

An elevated serum amylase remains the *sine qua non* of the diagnosis of acute pancreatitis. Nevertheless, elevated serum amylase levels may be seen in other important abdominal conditions including perforated peptic ulcer, small bowel obstruction, ectopic pregnancy, and mesenteric ischemia.[42] In acute pancreatitis, serum amylase values rise within a few hours after the onset of symptoms and may return to normal within 72 hours. Up to 32% of patients presenting with acute alcoholic pancreatitis may have normal levels of serum amylase on admission.[43] In patients who present to a physician relatively late, a 2-hour sample of urine for urine amylase may be sent. The urinary amylase level may remain elevated for 5 to 7 days after the start of the attack.[43] Other blood tests that should be immediately sent from the patient suspected of having acute pancreatitis include hematocrit and white blood cell count, serum electrolytes, blood glucose, arterial blood gas, and serum calcium. Serum lipase concentrations are also elevated in patients with acute pancreatitis and may remain elevated longer than serum amylase levels. Unfortunately, lipase may also be elevated in patients with other serious abdominal illnesses.[43]

Several plain radiologic indicators of acute pancreatitis have been described, including the colon "cut-off" sign, and the sentinel loop.[44] Although these may be found retrospectively in up to 90% of patients presenting with acute pancreatitis, their findings are not diagnostic (Fig. 36-3). In an emergency, a water-soluble contrast upper gastrointestinal series may be helpful in differentiating between perforated peptic ulcer and acute pancreatitis if no pneumoperitoneum is seen on plain films.[41]

The treatment of acute pancreatitis is nonsurgical in most cases. The management of acute pancreatitis is discussed elsewhere[45-56] and in Chapter 88.

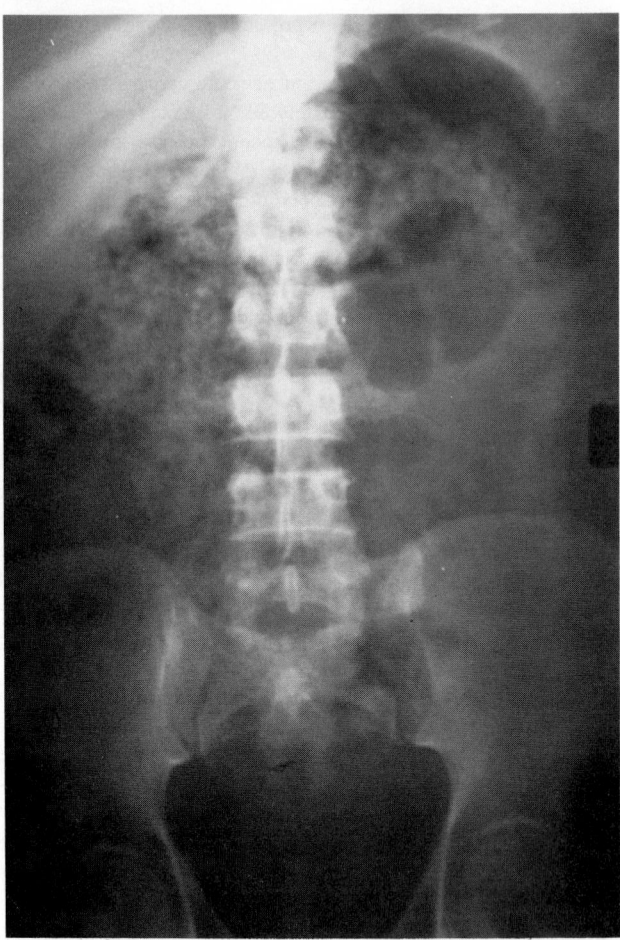

FIGURE 36–3. Plain radiograph of patient with pancreatic sepsis. Note generalized ileus pattern and retroperitoneal air bubbles.

DIVERTICULITIS

Acute colonic diverticulitis is a common cause of acute abdominal pain in the older population. Although colonic diverticulitis occurs in approximately 5% of the population, the prevalence of colonic diverticuli increases with age so that by the ninth decade it is present in approximately 70% of the population.[57,58] Although only 2% to 5% of patients admitted for diverticular disease are under the age of 40, diverticulitis in young patients is much more aggressive and requires surgery in as many as 88% of all cases.[59]

The sigmoid colon is the most commonly involved segment of bowel (90%) and is the only segment of bowel involved in 50% of patients.[57] Solitary right-sided, or cecal, diverticular disease constitutes only 0.1% to 2.5% of all cases. It is more common in Asian countries, especially Japan.[60] Interestingly, the average age of patients with right-sided diverticulitis is 10 to 15 years less than that of patients with left-sided disease.

The signs and symptoms of acute diverticulitis are protean and can involve multiple organ systems such as the colon, small intestine, and genitourinary organs. A history of previous episodes of diverticulitis or radiographic evidence of diverticulosis is helpful but rarely found. The classic picture of left lower quadrant abdominal pain, low grade fever, leukocytosis, nausea with occasional vomiting, and mild abdominal distention is not always present. The signs and symptoms depend on the degree and location of the inflammatory process. A palpable mass may be present in the left lower quadrant, but, in the absence of inflammation, it is not diagnostic of diverticulitis.[57]

The diagnosis of diverticulitis is a clinical one. Even so, the sensitivity and specificity of clinical decision making with diverticulitis is not perfect because one third of surgical specimens resected for diverticulitis show no evidence of inflammation. Laboratory evaluation may be misleading because 64% of patients presenting with complicated diverticular disease have a normal white cell count.[57,61] Plain roentgenograms of the abdomen or erect films of the chest rarely show pneumoperitoneum even in the presence of free diverticular perforation. Other more common but nonspecific findings noted on plain abdominal films may include an ileus pattern, a mass effect in the left lower quadrant, or evidence of partial or complete obstruction of the large or small bowel.[62] Acute endoscopic evaluation is generally not indicated in the patient with suspected diverticulitis. The sigmoidoscope cannot usually be passed beyond the rectosigmoid junction and is extremely uncomfortable. Also, perforation may occur because of the fixation that occurs secondary to the inflammatory reaction or the installation of air. However, we do recommend sigmoidoscopy after resolution of the edema and inflammation, usually within 1 to 2 weeks. At that time, endoscopy may be better tolerated and more informative, especially in excluding the diagnosis of carcinoma of the sigmoid colon.[57] As with sigmoidoscopy, we do not recommend barium enema examination in the acute phase of diverticular disease. There is a high risk of barium peritonitis should perforation exist or be caused by insufflation of barium. If a contrast study is deemed necessary because of diagnostic difficulties, a water-soluble contrast agent should be used. Elective barium enema examination may be performed at a later date after resolution of symptoms (Fig. 36-4).

CT scanning had been advocated as the radiographic procedure of choice in patients presenting with acute diverticulitis.[63,64] The most frequent findings described include localized thickening of the colonic wall and increased density in the periodic fat. We do not recommend routine CT scanning in all patients admitted with the diagnosis of diverticulitis but reserve it for patients with suspected complications or in whom the diagnosis is uncertain. The initial management of patients thought to have diverticulitis consists of bowel rest with or without nasogastric suction, intravenous fluids, and systemic parenteral antibodies.[57] Information regarding the management of patients with acute diverticulitis is presented in Chapter 82.

PERFORATED PEPTIC ULCER

Perforated peptic ulcer accounts for approximately 10% of all hospital admissions related to ulcer disease and occurs in 7 to 10

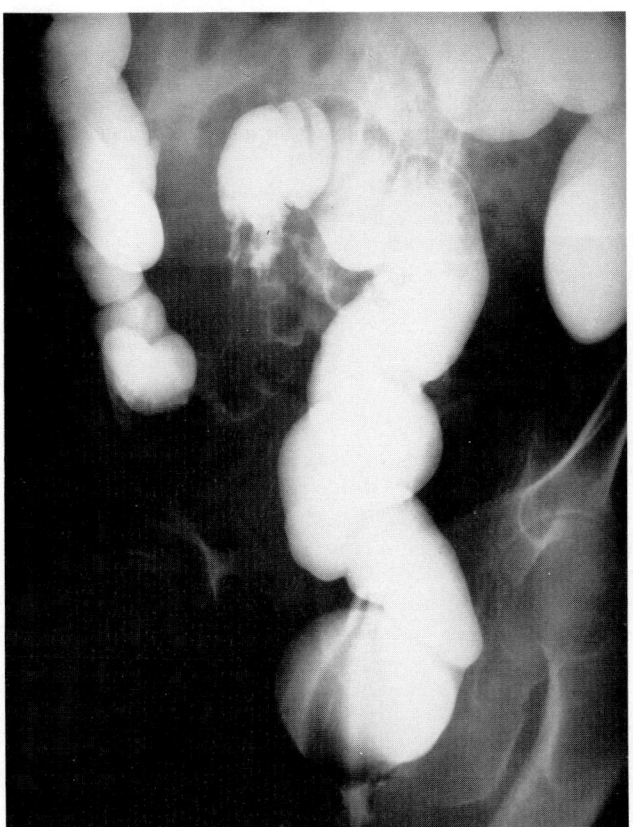

FIGURE 36–4. Barium enema demonstrating segment of sigmoid diverticulitis with intramural fistula.

patients per 100,000 per year.[65] Although this emergency can occur at any age, it is important to be prepared for its management in an increasingly older population.[66] The diagnosis of perforation is most often delayed in elderly patients admitted to the hospital for conditions other than a gastrointestinal problem, particularly neurologic problems. Left undiagnosed and untreated, these patients inevitably die from continued loss of intravascular fluid, hypotension, and sepsis.

The increased usage of nonsteroidal antiinflammatory drugs has led to the speculation that patients taking these drugs are at increased risk for the development of peptic ulcer. Studies report that between 16% and 80% of all patients presenting with perforated gastric or duodenal ulcers were taking nonsteroidal antiinflammatory drugs at the time of diagnosis. No prospective studies have proven this relationship. Perforation of duodenal ulcers occurs six to eight times more frequently than perforation of gastric ulcers.[67]

The sudden onset of severe epigastric pain that quickly spreads to involve the entire abdomen is the most common presentation of a perforated peptic ulcer. Patients can often state the exact time the pain began and usually seek medical attention within 6 to 12 hours. Evidence of peritonitis is overtly manifested by the appearance of an acutely ill patient who complains of severe pain and who avoids movement and examination because both exacerbate the pain. In elderly patients and in patients who are immunosuppressed, a benign pain pattern and a relative paucity of findings may deceive the patient and the physician, thereby delaying treatment for this abdominal catastrophe.[68]

The abdomen is usually rigid and diffusely tender to examination; occasionally, maximum tenderness is elicited in the epigastrium. The presence or absence of bowel sounds is of little help in the diagnosis. The extent to which the visceral and parietal peritoneum are exposed to gastroduodenal contents governs the severity of the peritonitis and the resultant loss of intravascular fluid. Patients when initially seen may have a deceptively normal pulse rate and blood pressure so that the severity of their condition may be underestimated. Eventually, however, the patient suffers hypovolemia and circulatory shock. The serum amylase concentration may increase to two to three times the normal value due to absorption of spilled salivary and pancreatic amylase into the peritoneal cavity.[65-67]

The diagnosis of perforated peptic ulcer is supported by the presence of pneumoperitoneum. This may be suspected on physical examination by the loss of liver dullness on percussion. It is confirmed by the demonstration of free intraperitoneal air on upright chest or left lateral decubitus x-ray. Pneumoperitoneum is demonstrated between 55% and 85% of the time in patients with perforated peptic ulcer.[69,70] If pneumoperitoneum is absent and the diagnosis of perforated ulcer is strongly suspected, we proceed with oral or nasogastric tube instillation of water-soluble contrast as an additional roentgenographic study.

The most commonly confused differential diagnoses include acute cholecystitis, acute pancreatitis, acute diverticulitis, and appendicitis. An ulcer that seals spontaneously after perforation or one that perforates and is contained within the lesser sac may complicate accurate diagnosis. Duodenal ulcers perforate through the anterior wall of the duodenal bulb into the free peritoneal cavity in 92% of cases.[65,71] However, giant (> 2 cm) duodenal ulcers are usually posterior and only 10% perforate.[72] Patients with giant duodenal ulcers almost always require gastric resection.

A small but important subset (approximately 10%) of patients with perforated duodenal ulcers may have simultaneous bleeding from a posterior "kissing ulcer." The surgeon must not overlook the second ulcer in these patients because a significant risk of postoperative gastrointestinal bleeding has been reported.[73] The patients diagnosed with acute perforated ulcer should be initially managed with intravenous fluid resuscitation, broad-spectrum antibiotic coverage, correction of metabolic abnormalities, and preparation for the operating room. A detailed discussion on the management of perforated peptic ulcer can be found elsewhere[74-78] and in Chapters 61 and 64.

BOWEL OBSTRUCTION

Small bowel obstruction accounts for approximately 20% of all acute surgical admissions and constitutes one of the most common indications for emergency surgical intervention.[79] Postoperative intra-abdominal adhesions account for the majority of small bowel obstructions (50%–70%), with hernias accounting for another one fourth.[80] Malignancy, intussusception, inflammatory bowel disease, and miscellaneous causes make up the remainder.

The classic clinical findings in patients with small bowel obstruction are abdominal pain, usually crampy in nature; vomiting; abdominal distention; and obstipation. Tachycardia, fever, and elevated white blood cell count are useful in determining the surgical urgency. However, these signs are not indicative of the presence or absence of gangrenous intestine, particularly in patients over the age of 50. Several studies have documented the lack of predictive ability of experienced surgeons in diagnosing strangulation obstruction preoperatively.[81,82]

Flat and upright chest and abdominal x-rays are the most helpful roentgenographic examinations in assessing small bowel obstruction and may also help in determining if the obstruction is complete or incomplete. The presence of air–fluid levels in the small bowel, usually in a stepladder pattern, associated with colicky abdominal pain and hyperperistaltic bowel sounds, is classic for bowel obstruction[83] (Fig 36-5). The onus on the physician is to determine whether this is small bowel or large bowel and whether nonoperative therapy is indicated versus urgent operation. If there is difficulty in determining whether large bowel or small bowel is involved, the use of a barium enema may help rule out an obstructing lesion in the colon.[84] We do not routinely recommend the use of barium upper gastrointestinal series in patients presenting with acute bowel obstruction.

Large bowel obstruction is most frequently caused by carcinoma, diverticulitis, and volvulus.[85] The pain of large bowel obstruction is usually less acute. Shock is unusual, except in some cases of volvulus or intussusception, and vomiting is a late symptom. Early abdominal distention is common in large bowel obstruction. The consequences of large bowel obstruction are influenced by the competency of the ileocecal valve.[86] If the valve is incompetent (as it is in approximately 15% to 20% of patients with colonic obstruction) and allows reflux into the small intestine, the patient's condition and the radiologic picture resemble those found in patients with partial small bowel obstruction. If the ileocecal valve is competent, a closed loop exists between the obstructing lesion and the ileocecal valve. Gangrene and perforation of the cecum as a result of severe distention may occur. Tenderness in the right lower quadrant in such a case usually suggests that this complication is imminent or has already occurred.

Plain abdominal x-rays may lead to the diagnosis of volvulus. However, when such a differentiation between large and small bowel obstruction is unclear or when suspected large bowel obstruction is present without the classic findings of a volvulus on plain x-rays, we recommend an emergency contrast enema as an early diagnostic test.[79]

Treatment of small and large bowel obstruction depends on the cause of the obstruction, and the interested reader is referred elsewhere.[81-90]

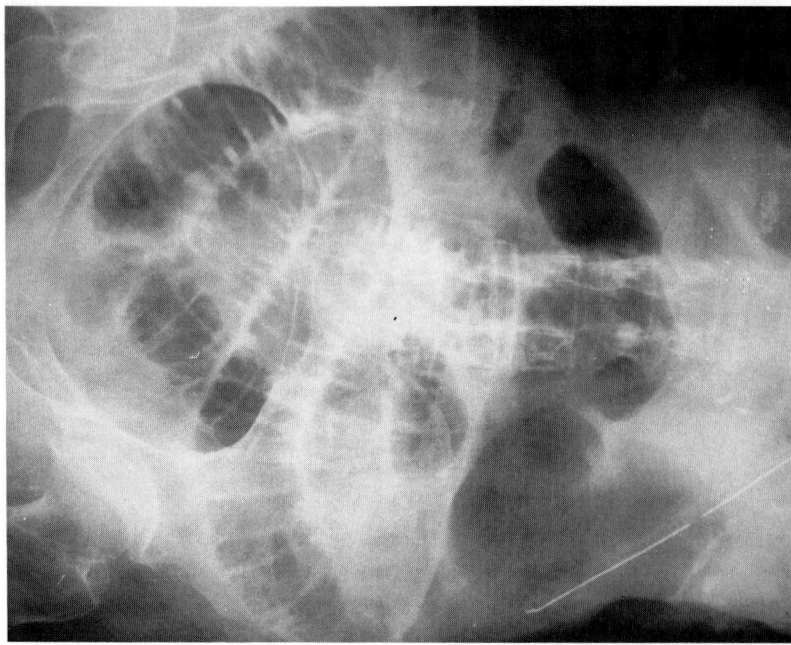

FIGURE 36–5. Small bowel obstruction in patient with incarcerated inguinal hernia.

MESENTERIC ISCHEMIA

Vascular disorders of the intestines are an unusual but extremely important cause of acute abdominal problems, accounting for only 0.4% of acute abdominal operations.[91] Acute abdominal vascular processes are usually catastrophic illnesses with extremely high mortality, therefore, prompt diagnosis and therapy are the only possibilities for improving prognosis. Acute ischemic syndromes of the abdominal viscera are the result of: embolic occlusions of visceral branches of the abdominal aorta; thrombotic occlusions of an atherosclerotic branch of the mesenteric arterial system; mesenteric venous thrombosis; or nonocclusive mesenteric ischemia (low-flow syndrome).[91,92] The usual consequence of any of these conditions is intestinal infarction with overall mortalities ranging from 40% to 70%.[91] The mortality of these conditions is directly related to the presence of gangrenous bowel and the frequent association with significant cardiovascular disease. Attempts should be made to differentiate among the causes of acute mesenteric ischemia because both treatment and prognoses differ.[92]

Nearly 70% of affected patients are over the age of 60, and about 90% report the acute onset of crampy abdominal pain, usually epigastric or periumbilical in location. The hallmark of this disease is pain out of proportion to physical findings.[92] Abdominal pain with subsequent spontaneous bowel evacuation in the absence of significant physical findings is frequently seen in early occlusive mesenteric ischemia.[92] In contrast, patients with nonocclusive mesenteric ischemia initially have pain in the absence of defecatory

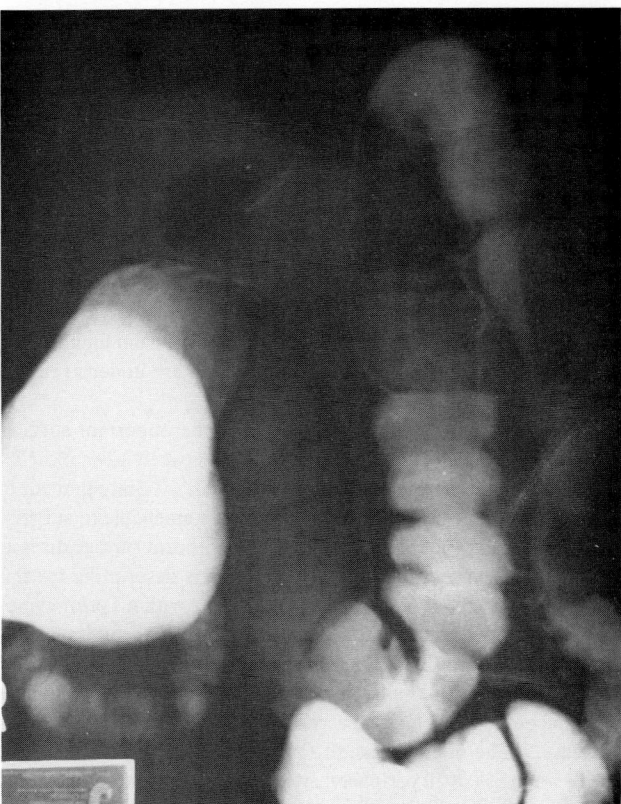

FIGURE 36–7. "Thumbprinting" of ischemic colitis. This phenomenon is occasionally seen on plain radiographs.

urge or evacuation.[93] Other clinical signs include vomiting, diarrhea, abdominal distention or tenderness, and melena. Bowel sounds range from an early hyperactivity to absent as transmural necrosis proceeds. Occult blood is a frequent but nonspecific finding in stool examination. A history of preexisting postprandial abdominal pain, "intestinal angina," is elicited in only about 10% of patients but is an important diagnostic aid.[92] Shock, secondary to volume depletion or perforative sepsis, is seen in one fourth of the patients on presentation.[94] Hemoconcentration and leukocytosis greater than 20,000/mm^3 are frequently seen, but no single test or combination of blood tests is diagnostic. Serum amylase is elevated in one third of patients with mesenteric ischemia.[92] Metabolic acidosis is a late, but significant finding in these patients. It cannot be overemphasized that acute, severe abdominal pain, especially in the elderly, in the absence of associated physical findings, is usually the earliest sign of mesenteric ischemia, and, at this stage, most patients have not progressed to intestinal infarction.[91] The development of abdominal or peritoneal signs implies infarction and significantly increases mortality.

Plain abdominal x-rays are rarely helpful, but a "gasless" abdomen has been described in association with mesenteric ischemia as a result of small bowel spasm with subsequent distention and ileus.[94] Portal venous gas is rare and considered a terminal finding (Fig. 36-6). Barium examinations may help in more chronic processes by revealing a thumbprinting pattern caused by submucosal hemorrhage or edema and superficial mucosal ulceration (Fig. 36-7).[92] If the diagnosis of acute mesenteric ischemia is suspected,

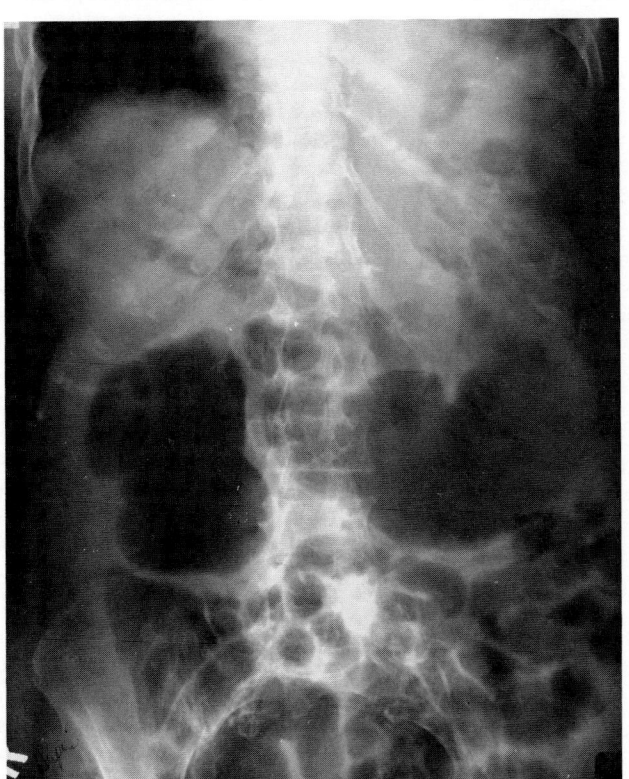

FIGURE 36–6. Portal venous gas in a patient with mesenteric infarction. Portal venous gas can usually be differentiated from biliary gas by its centrifugal spread toward liver boundaries.

many surgeons advocate rapid use of visceral arteriography. Arteriography may be helpful in differentiating the causes of intestinal ischemia. Acute thromboses usually involve the origin of any or all of the three main vessels, whereas embolic phenomena typically affect the superior mesenteric artery (SMA), usually several centimeters distal to its origin and often at the orifice of the middle colic artery.[92] Nonocclusive ischemic disease characteristically shows segmental mesenteric arterial constriction, often within associated proximal stenosis of the SMA. Both anterior, anteroposterior, and anterolateral arteriographic views are necessary to evaluate the arterial tree, and the selective infusion of vasodilating agents such as papaverine has been advocated to maintain intestinal perfusion while other resuscitative measures are undertaken and the surgical team is assembled.

Acute mesenteric arterial embolism is the important surgical cause of intestinal ischemia, constituting between 12% and 67% of all acute mesenteric vascular catastrophes.[92,95] Sixty percent of acute mesenteric arterial embolic events are amenable to surgery. Bergan's triad of acute abdominal pain, significant cardiac disease, and spontaneous gastrointestinal emptying is descriptive for this disorder.[96] Affected patients may be younger with no prior symptoms of intestinal angina. Important historic or concomitant findings include arrhythmias in 70% of patients, the majority of which are atrial tachyarrhythmias, recent myocardial infarctions, previous arterial emboli, rheumatic heart disease, and atherosclerotic heart disease.[92] The oblique takeoff for the SMA favors embolization with about 5% of all peripheral arterial emboli involving this vessel or a distal branch.[97] Emboli usually lodge several centimeters distal to the SMA origin, occluding the middle colic artery, right colic artery, ileocolic artery, or even smaller peripheral branches.

Acute mesenteric thrombosis of a previously atherosclerotic vessel is the most common cause of acute mesenteric ischemia. Various series report this entity as making up between 44% and 82% of all mesenteric ischemic disorders.[92] Most of these patients have had a significant gastrointestinal history. Between 50% and 70% have had in the previous year a significant history of weight loss, diarrhea, abdominal pain, or the diagnosis of an abdominal bruit. Many patients have had an unsuccessful investigation the preceding months for peptic ulcer or gallbladder disease, and many carry the label of having psychiatric or functional abdominal pain. The exact percentage of patients with intestinal angina who progress to frank bowel infarction is unknown.[92] Overall mortality of acute thromboses averages 80%, with most of these patients in some series undergoing either an "open and close" laparotomy because of extensive intestinal necrosis or heroic massive bowel resections.

Acute or subacute thrombosis of the mesenteric veins accounts for approximately 10% of all cases of mesenteric ischemia.[92] Although the majority of these patients lack predisposing conditions, associated disorders include peritonitis or abdominal inflammation, abdominal trauma, portal hypertension, intra-abdominal tumors, adhesions, volvulus, sickle-cell disease, polycythemia vera, coagulopathies, pregnancy, recent splenectomy, and the use of oral contraceptives. Over 40% of patients have had a previous vein thrombophlebitis of the lower extremity.[98] The reported age range is from 11 months to 89 years, but most series report an average age of only 47 years.[92]

Acute abdominal presentations of mesenteric venous thrombosis are unusual and usually represent primary thrombosis of the large mesenteric veins, although rarely are veins in the inferior mesenteric system involved. By the time of presentation, most patients have significant abdominal pain, tenderness, and distention. Laboratory investigations reveal a leukocytosis, hemoconcentration, and a copious bloody peritoneal transudate.[98] The entity of nonocclusive mesenteric ischemia is a diverse series of interrelated events that accounts for 20% to 50% of all mesenteric infarctions in which autopsy data are included. It involves the distribution of the SMA almost exclusively. These patients are usually hospitalized for other medical problems when this condition arises. The presence of abdominal pain and evidence of low cardiac output are the major diagnostic aids. Arteriography is useful in distinguishing this condition from occlusive mesenteric ischemia. In addition, careful angiography may reveal segmental spastic arterial constriction as well as a failure of visualization of mesenteric vascular arcades and intramural vessels.[99] The intraarterial infusion of vasodilators has been reported with some success during which aggressive attempts to increase cardiac output and restore intravascular volume are performed. Repeat angiography is performed after vasodilator therapy has begun to document improvement.

Unlike other types of acute mesenteric ischemia, immediate surgery is not indicated in nonocclusive ischemia. Furthermore, anesthesia and intraoperative manipulation decrease intestinal blood flow. Generally, 8 to 12 hours of observation of the patient while vasodilator therapy is administered and cardiac output restoration is attempted is the initial treatment of choice. After this, or sooner if evidence of infarcted bowel is present, laparotomy is performed in the majority of patients. A more detailed discussion on the management of mesenteric ischemia is presented in Chapter 109.

RUPTURED ABDOMINAL AORTIC ANEURYSMS

Rupture of an abdominal aortic aneurysm is the most urgent nontraumatic emergency faced by physicians and surgeons.[100,101] The mortality for ruptured aortic aneurysms is 100% without surgical treatment, therefore, it is imperative that emergency room physicians and surgeons are able to make the diagnosis and begin appropriate emergency care.[100]

Pain is the most common complaint of patients with ruptured aneurysms. The pain is usually of sudden onset in the midabdominal or paravertebral area. As the retroperitoneal hematoma enlarges, pain may be experienced in the flank, usually on the left side. Pressure on the ilioinguinal nerve may cause the pain to radiate to the inguinal area. The pain is frequently associated with diaphoresis, lightheadedness, and nausea, caused by the sudden hypotension.

The most important clinical finding, present in over 90% of patients, is a pulsatile, often tender, abdominal mass. On palpation, the mass may be more diffuse and difficult to define than an intact abdominal aneurysm. Shock, defined as a blood pressure of less than 100 mm Hg and a pulse greater than 100, is found in at least 60% of patients.[102]

Approximately three fourths of patients with a ruptured abdominal aortic aneurysm have the classic triad of abdominal pain, pulsatile mass, and hypotension.[100] The presence of these three signs and symptoms suffices to make the diagnosis of aneurysmal rupture, and other confirmatory tests are superfluous. Preparations for emergency surgery should begin immediately. Occasionally, the pain of ruptured aneurysm predominates in the flank, and the true diagnosis may be missed. Renal colic, diverticulitis, lumbosacral disk disease, perforated appendicitis, and duodenal ulcer are the diagnoses most often confused with ruptured abdominal aortic aneurysm.[100] In approximately 10% to 20% of patients, the diagnosis of aneurysmal rupture cannot be made solely on clinical grounds. In such patients, a pulsatile abdominal mass may not have been noticed because of the patient's obesity, the small size of the aneurysm, or an inadequate examination. When one or more of these components of the classic diagnostic triad are absent, objective laboratory tests may be necessary to suggest or confirm the diagnosis. It should be emphasized that, even in the patient who appears hemodynamically stable, a need for rapid diagnosis and expeditious surgery exists.

A complete blood count may be helpful in the diagnosis. A hematocrit value of less than 35% in a patient with a known or suspected aortic aneurysm correlates well with rupture.[103] Plain radiographs of the abdomen may be helpful when the diagnosis is in doubt. Eighty-five percent of abdominal aortic aneurysms have sufficient calcification to outline the dimension of the aorta on standard x-rays.[7] Lateral lumbar spine films are the most useful because the aortic outline may be demonstrated without obscuration by underlying vertebral bodies.[100] Although aortography allows the diagnosis of leaking abdominal aneurysm, its routine use is condemned. The time interval required to obtain aortography is potentially hazardous. Furthermore, there have been multiple reports of rupture precipitated by intraaortic injection of contrast media.[104] If the diagnosis of ruptured aneurysm is not made, the correct diagnosis may not be suspected until other studies are performed to evaluate the abdominal pain. Ureteral deviation on an intravenous pyelogram, or displacement of loops of colon by the retroperitoneal mass on barium enema may be the first clue in diagnosis (Fig. 36-8).[100]

Unlike most patients with abdominal surgical emergencies, patients with ruptured aortic aneurysms are best resuscitated in the operating room rather than the emergency area. Patients who survive ruptured aneurysms do so because of temporary tamponade of the bleeding by the intact retroperitoneum. If the tamponade effect is lost during the resuscitative effort and free rupture in the peritoneal cavity occurs, only expeditious laparotomy and aortic cross-clamping will save the patient's life. This maneuver should be performed in the emergency department. Any procedures likely to cause a Valsalva's maneuver, such as the placement of a urinary catheter or passage of a nasogastric tube, should be delayed because they may induce free rupture.

MISCELLANEOUS CAUSES

In addition to the above entities, acute abdominal catastrophies can result from a diverse set of disorders including toxic megacolon from inflammatory bowel disease and infectious colitides as well as ascending cholangitis. These problems are covered in detail in Chapters 77 and 95.

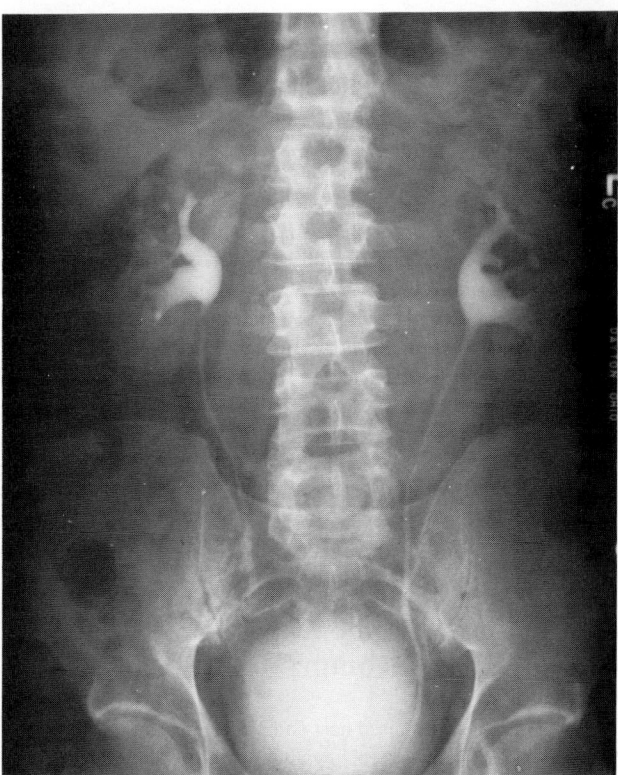

FIGURE 36–8. Intravenous pyelogram of patient with unsuspected leaking abdominal aortic aneurysm. Note bilateral deviation of ureters and calcific rim along left side of aneurysm.

The Acute Abdomen in Children

Evaluation of acute abdominal pain in children is a major challenge for both pediatricians and surgeons. Appendicitis remains one of the most difficult diagnoses in children, with reported perforation rates of up to 40%.[17,105] Unfortunately, delay in making the correct diagnosis appears to be the major factor contributing to the increased rate of appendiceal perforation in children.

As in adults, a careful clinical history and thorough physical examination are critical in the diagnostic evaluation of a child with acute abdomen.[106,107] The basic laboratory evaluation includes a complete blood count and urinalysis. A beta-HCG is recommended in all females over the age of 10. A normal white blood cell count and differential should not delay surgical exploration in the child with obvious localized right lower quadrant peritonitis. The urinalysis is very important in helping to differentiate urinary tract infections or renal calculus from acute appendicitis. A few (< 5) white blood cells or red blood cells are common in a child with an inflamed appendix lying near the ureter or bladder. We do not recommend routine radiologic evaluations of the child with obvious appendicitis. However, in the child with a puzzling presentation, a chest x-ray may be helpful to rule out pneumonia, and abdominal films may demonstrate intussusception, intestinal obstruction, volvulus, complicated Meckel's diverticulum, ruptured tumors, or other rare pathology.[105] Recent reports on the use of barium enema to help diagnose acute appendicitis have been contradictory.[107,108] We believe that barium enemas have occasional utility but should not be the basis for operating or not operating on a child with acute abdominal pain. Ultrasound imaging may be a useful adjunct in patients with an appendiceal abscess, but it has been of little help in the child with possible acute appendicitis.[12]

The other frequently mentioned diagnoses in the child presenting with abdominal pain are gastroenteritis, urinary tract infection, and mesenteric lymphadenitis. The differential diagnosis of these conditions is summarized in Table 36-1.

One of the most common causes of abdominal pain in infancy is intussusception. The classic picture of intussusception is a 3- to 18-month-old child with severe intermittent abdominal pain associated with "currant jelly" stools and a palpable midabdominal mass.[109] After surgical evaluation and intravenous fluids, a careful barium enema frequently reduces the idiopathic intussusception in this age group. Operative intervention is reserved for the infant with peritonitis or unsuccessful reduction or recurrence after barium enema.[110] Causes of abdominal pain in different age groups of children are listed in Table 36-3.

The Acute Abdomen in the Immunocompromised Patient

The immunocompromised host comprises a heterogeneous group that includes patients receiving allografts, chemotherapy for malignant disease, and steroids for autoimmune diseases, as well as patients with the acquired immunodeficiency syndrome (AIDS). Each of these groups has specific abdominal complications. The clinician should be familiar with each of the causes of the acute abdomen in each subset of immunocompromised hosts. The etiology of the acute abdomen in these patients may be divided into two broad categories: (1) disorders associated with immunocompromised states, such as neutropenic enterocolitis and cytomegalovirus (CMV) infection, and (2) processes that can occur in any patient regardless of host defenses, such as appendicitis, cholecystitis, or peptic ulcer disease.[111] Some general principles of the approach and management of immunocompromised patients with acute abdominal pain are addressed here.[111-113]

An aggressive diagnostic approach must be undertaken in evaluating immunocompromised patients with acute abdominal pain because these patients may have minimal systemic findings, covert abdominal signs, and suppressed laboratory findings. The immunocompromised host also is prone to some unusual problems such as pneumatosis intestinalis that may not require surgery but may mimic the presentation of more serious problems.[111] Other conditions with significant signs and symptoms not requiring surgical intervention include CMV infection, focal hepatic or splenic fungal disease, neutropenic enterocolitis, and Kaposi's sarcoma (Fig. 36-9). The diagnostic work-up should include the appropriate screening blood chemistry and hematologic evaluations as well as plain films of the chest and abdomen.

Polymicrobial sepsis in the immunocompromised host is one of the most reliable indicators of significant intra-abdominal pathology.[11] The search for intraperitoneal infection often requires the use of ultrasonography, CT scanning, or radioactive isotopic (WBC) scanning. Because negative results of any of these tests do not rule out an active process, diagnostic laparotomies are occasionally indicated for steady, undiagnosed abdominal pain or deteriorating clinical status. The decision must be balanced against postoperative mortality of between 20% and 50% in patients with severe immunosuppression.[113]

Preoperative preparation must be precise and compulsive in the immunocompromised patient. The usual resuscitative measures, including volume replacement and correction of electrolyte imbalances, must be performed as well as the institution of broad-

TABLE 36–3
Pediatric Acute Abdomen—Differential Diagnoses

INFANTS	CHILDREN	ADOLESCENTS
Intussusception	Meckel's diverticulitis	Pelvic inflammatory disease
Pyelonephritis	Pneumonitis	Mittelschmerz
Meckel's diverticulitis	Bacterial enterocolitis	Hematocolpos
Bacterial enterocolitis	Viral enteritis	Crohn's disease
Viral enteritis	Pancreatitis	Bacterial enterocolitis
Gastroesophageal reflux	Crohn's disease	Viral enteritis
Hypertrophic pyloric stenosis	Ruptured tumors	Peptic ulcer disease
Hirschsprung's disease	Pyelonephritis	Cholelithiasis
Strangulated hernia	Cystitis	Pancreatitis
Pneumonitis	Appendicitis	Pneumonia
Testicular torsion	Trauma (child abuse)	Ectopic pregnancy
Mesenteric cysts		Psychosomatic
Pancreatitis		Pregnancy
Ruptured tumors		Appendicitis
Appendicitis*		Trauma (child abuse)
Trauma (child abuse)*		

* Although on the bottom of the lists, these two etiologies must always be considered in any child.

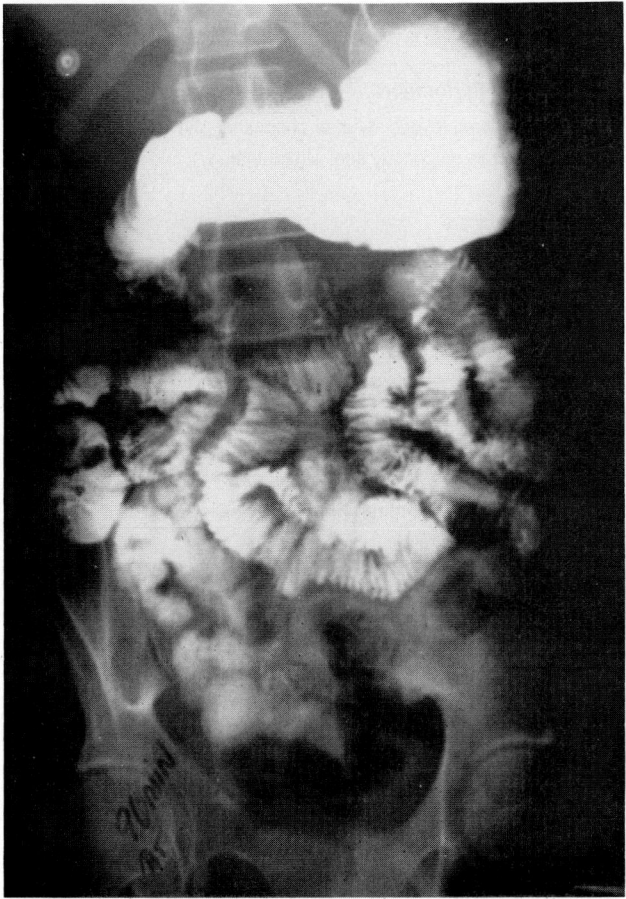

FIGURE 36–9. Diffuse involvement of upper gastrointestinal tract with Kaposi's sarcoma in a young man with acquired immunodefeciency syndrome.

spectrum antibiotic coverage. Acute adrenal deficiency must be avoided in patients previously receiving steroids. Clotting abnormalities must be corrected in patients with severe liver dysfunction or severe thrombocytopenia. Any indwelling catheters in these patients can be the source of fatal bacteremia, therefore, their indications should be precise. These catheters should always be removed as soon as possible postoperatively.

Specific intraoperative considerations must be kept in mind for these patients. In operations on the gut, stomas and mucous fistulas should be used preference to primary anastomoses.[111] Long periods of bowel dysfunction must be expected after abdominal surgery. Although any enterotomy may leak, we prefer gastrostomy and feeding jejunostomies for patients in whom a long recovery is expected. Specific abdominal processes for various immunocompromised hosts are outlined in Table 36-4.

The Acute Abdomen After Cardiovascular Surgery

Intra-abdominal complications or acute surgical abdomens after cardiac procedures occur in less than 1% of patients.[114-116] Despite the low incidence of these complications, they carry a mortality between 25% and 60%. These deaths represent 7% to 10% of the total mortality for cardiopulmonary bypass operations.

The most commonly reported intra-abdominal complication is gastrointestinal tract bleeding.[114-116] Causes of acute abdominal pain include intestinal ischemia, acute cholecystitis, acute pancreatitis, and acute colitis. The pathophysiology of intra-abdominal complications secondary to cardiovascular surgery is thought to be visceral hypoperfusion. Although suggested by some writers,[114] a statistical association between prolonged pump time and intraabdominal complications has not been reported. Other risk factors for the development of intra-abdominal complications include the need for an emergency cardiac operation, advanced age, the use of the intraaortic balloon pump, the use of vasopressor agents, valvular operations, and intraoperative hypotension.[114-116]

It should be noted that the etiologies of the acute surgical abdomen after cardiac surgery are not unusual abdominal disease processes. What has generally been reported are common general surgical problems that are seen in most every general surgical practice.[114] When caring for these patients, several factors should be remembered. Patients must undergo an aggressive although directed work-up to diagnose the abdominal process causing a suspected acute surgical abdomen. Surgery must be performed promptly when indicated. Abdominal surgery should be delayed only for prompt and aggressive resuscitation because the unnecessary delays are accompanied by unacceptable mortality.[115] Furthermore, it should be remembered that it is unacceptable to believe that these patients are too sick for surgery, because patients after cardiac revascularization are more suitable for abdominal surgery than before their cardiac surgery.

Gynecologic Causes of the Acute Abdomen

Acute abdominal emergencies of gynecologic origin usually occur in women of reproductive age, but occasionally are seen in newborn, adolescent, and postmenopausal patients. The most common and important conditions to be considered include pelvic inflammatory disease (PID) with or without abscess, ectopic pregnancy, hemorrhage from a functional ovarian cyst, and adnexal or ovarian torsion.[117]

PID must be considered in virtually every woman of reproductive age with lower abdominal pain. The clinician must be experienced in distinguishing those patients that require medical management from those that require operative intervention. Tuboovarian abscess (TOA) is a frequent complication in patients with acute salpingitis and is more likely when treatment has been delayed or there have been repeated episodes of acute salpingitis, or when an intrauterine device (IUD) is present. The abscess is usually polymicrobial including aerobes such as *Streptococcus*, *Escherichia coli*, and *Hemophilus influenzae*, as well as anaerobes such as *Peptococcus*, *Peptostreptococcus*, and *Bacteroides*.[118] Sexually transmitted organisms, such as gonococcus and *Chlamydia*, are usually not present within the abscess but may be cultured from the cervix in about one third of the cases.[117]

Pelvic examination usually reveals extreme pelvic tenderness with increased pain on cervical motion. Identification of a pelvic mass is difficult because pain tenderness often precludes an optimal examination. Abnormal findings on abdominal examination are

TABLE 36–4
Acute Abdominal Pain in the Immunocompromised Host

Cytomegaloviral Infection (CMV)	**Bowel Perforation**
Interstitial pneumonitis	Lymphoma (especially after chemotherapy)
Mononucleosis	Leukemia (especially after chemotherapy)
Cholecystitis	CMV
Hepatitis	Colon ulcers
Pancreatitis	Pseudomembranous colitis
Gastrointestinal ulceration	Kaposi's sarcoma
	Iatrogenic
Neutropenic Enterocolitis	Mycobacterial
Cholecystitis	
Campylobacter	**Acute Graft Versus Host Disease**
CMV	**Fecal Impaction**
Acalculous	**Pseudoacute Abdomen**
	Standard Abdominal Processes
Pancreatitis	Appendicitis
Steroid	Cholecystitis
Azothiaprine	Diverticulitis
Pentamidine	Peptic ulcer disease
CMV	Small bowel obstruction
	Pelvic inflammatory disease
Hepatitis	Urinary tract infection
A, B, C	Perirectal abscess
CMV	Lymphadenitis
Ebstein-Barr virus	
Hepatosplenic Abscess	
Candida	
Mycobacterial	
Splenic rupture	

largely confined to the lower abdomen and include signs of peritonitis and sometimes a tender, fluctuant mass.[119] Most often, the abnormalities are bilateral, but there may be unilateral accentuation. Careful examination usually demonstrates that the signs of peritonitis become more severe as the examining hand approaches the pelvic brim with maximal intensity deep in the pelvis, as demonstrated by rectal examination. When the intensity of peritonitis increases as the examiner moves away from the pelvic brim, especially on the right side, it is circumstantial evidence that the inflammatory process is coming from an intra-abdominal rather than a pelvic source.[19,117] Although classic bedside teaching is that PID and its associated TOA most commonly occur within 1 week of the beginning or end of a menstrual period, several studies have documented that this is not so.[120,121]

Ultrasonography has become the diagnostic tool of choice and provides information that may become extremely useful in the patient's management. If an abscess is present, ultrasonography usually shows a complex adnexal mass.[117] The onus lies on the surgeon or gynecologist to determine if the suspected tubo-ovarian abscess is confined to the pelvis or if there is evidence of rupture; the latter is a surgical emergency.[119]

For the patient with an unruptured TOA, the initial management is medical with antibiotics appropriate for a polymicrobial aerobic and anaerobic infection. In the absence of rupture or leakage, nonoperative management with appropriate antibiotics may be successful in 33% to 74% of cases. With leakage or rupture, surgical intervention should be carried out promptly.[117]

In the United States, approximately 1 out of every 200 diagnosed pregnancies is ectopic, and about 50,000 of such cases are reported each year.[117] Ectopic pregnancy continues to be a major cause of maternal death. Early diagnosis and surgical intervention require an awareness of the conditions and circumstances that increase the risk that a given pregnancy will be in an ectopic location. Although the overall risk is only 1 in 200 pregnancies, in selected groups of women the risk is increased 20- to 100-fold. Risk factors include prior salpingitis, prior tubal ligation, prior tubal repair, presence of an intrauterine device, and prior ectopic pregnancy.[117,122]

Pain is the most common symptom of ectopic pregnancy but can be extremely variable in degree or location. A history of some menstrual abnormality is invariably present, but its detection requires careful and detailed inquiries. Ammenorrhea, a delayed menstrual period, an abnormal period, and noncyclic bleeding are examples of typical menstrual abnormalities.[117] Subjective symptoms of pregnancy are present in less than half of patients.[117]

The physical examination is especially useful in making the diagnosis and distinguishing this condition from PID. Fever is generally absent, and the findings on pelvic examination are also highly variable. Diffuse pelvic tenderness and pain on cervical motion may suggest free blood within the pelvis. The acute rupture of a blood-filled fallopian tube or walled-off pelvic blood collection produces the classic picture of severe pelvic and abdominal pain, shoulder pain, urge to defecate, and syncope, even in the absence of hypovolemia.[117] Fortunately, severe hypovolemic shock associated with massive intraperitoneal hemorrhage is rare (less than 5%).[122,123] Other diagnostic aids include a positive urine or serum pregnancy test, culdocentesis or needle aspiration of the posterior cul-de-sac with withdrawal of at least 0.5 ml of nonclotting blood, ultrasound, and laparoscopy.

Although a spontaneous resolution of ectopic pregnancy is possible and may be even more frequent than suspected, the risk of intraperitoneal hemorrhage warrants early operative intervention in every patient. The choice of the best operative procedure requires consideration of the operative findings in the pelvis, the patient's general condition, and her desire for subsequent childbearing.[117]

Other gynecologic causes of acute abdominal pain include hemorrhage from a functional ovarian cyst, mittelschmerz disease, and adnexal torsion.

Urologic Causes of the Acute Abdomen

Fortunately, most acute urologic processes are distinguishable from nonurologic causes of the acute abdomen. Because genitourinary organs exhibit significant overlap of autonomic innervation with visceral structures, referred pain is common. Three primary urologic areas should be considered in the differential diagnosis of the patient with acute abdominal pain: renal and perirenal infections, obstructions of the ureter and renal pelvis, and acute intrascrotal events.[124–130]

Cystitis must be in the differential diagnosis for all patients presenting with acute lower abdominal pain. Urinalysis for suspected infected urine should be performed on all patients presenting with lower abdominal pain.[3] Uncomplicated pyelonephritis in otherwise healthy persons is usually not a difficult diagnosis. Patients classically present with urinary frequency, dysuria, flank pain, fever, chills, and leukocytosis.[124] Urinalysis is usually diagnostic, revealing pyuria, white blood cell casts, bacteriuria, and occasionally microscopic hematuria.

Two subgroups with pyelonephritis deserve special consideration with regard to their evaluation and management. The elderly patient is at increased risk for both infections of the urinary tract and bacteremic complications.[125] The second group that should be specially considered are patients who are diabetic. These patients are more prone to an unusual form of renal infection, commonly referred to as emphysematous pyelonephritis, which is associated with a mortality of approximately 40%.[126]

Renal and perirenal abscesses rarely present as acute abdominal pain. Unfortunately, urinalysis and urine culture are not consistently diagnostic in these patients. An intravenous urogram is normal in most cases but may reveal caliceal distortion and a mass effect. Symptoms are usually localized to the flank, and abdominal pain is the principal complaint in up to one half of patients.[124]

Acute ureteral or renal pelvic obstruction is the most common urologic problem confused with nonurologic causes of the acute abdomen. Urolithiasis is the most common cause of upper urinary obstruction.[124] The patient with upper urinary tract obstruction complains of pain that begins in the flank, courses laterally and anteriorly to the ipsilateral lower abdominal quadrant, and may radiate to the groin and genitalia. Rarely does acute renal obstruction present as severe, diffuse abdominal pain. Renal colic may appear very similar to the pain of leaking abdominal aneurysms, resulting in a misdiagnosis of one or the other.

Urinalysis in most patients with urinary calculi reveals gross or microscopic hematuria. Radiographic evaluation remains the cornerstone of diagnosis. A plain abdominal film is rarely sufficient.[7] Although the majority of urinary calculi are radiopaque, a 1- or 2-mm calculus may cause complete ureteral obstruction yet be very difficult to see on plain films of the abdomen. All patients with acceptable renal function should undergo intravenous pyelography at their initial presentation.[124] The treatment of such affected patients includes brisk hydration; the use of strong, parenteral narcotics for pain relief; and consideration of extracorporeal shock wave lithotripsy (ESWL), which has become the treatment of choice for upper ureteral and renal pelvic calculi that do not pass spontaneously.[127]

Nonsurgical Simulators of the Acute Abdomen

A number of diseases either do not need or possibly contraindicate operation yet may cause symptoms very suggestive of conditions for which operation is the best procedure.[131] In some cases, the symptoms arise from disease within the abdomen and, in other instances, the pain is referred to the abdomen from another part of the body. Table 36-5 lists a variety of nonsurgical and nonabdominal considerations that may simulate the acute abdominal pain seen by the examining physician. The reader is referred to several excellent reviews for more illumination on these points.[131,132]

FEVER OF ABDOMINAL ORIGIN

Introduction

Fever of abdominal origin usually results from infection of the abdominal cavity, which may be classified as monomicrobial or polymicrobial. Classic monomicrobial infections include biliary tract infections and spontaneous or primary peritonitis. Most cases of intra-abdominal sepsis are polymicrobial and include both aerobic and anaerobic bacteria derived from normal intestinal flora.[133] The problem in treating these infections is that complete bacteriologic data are not often available at the time that therapeutic decisions are required. Additionally, valid specimens other than blood cultures are difficult to obtain. Nevertheless, repeated studies have shown that the predominant isolates in abdominal infections are the coliforms and *Bacteroides* species.[133,134]

TABLE 36-5
Nonsurgical Simulators of the Acute Abdomen

Pulmonary

Pneumonia, pleurodynia (Bornholm's disease), pulmonary embolism, pneumothorax

Cardiac

Myocardial infarction, angina, congestive heart failure, pericarditis

Neurologic

Tabes dorsalis, herpes zoster, epilepsy

Urologic

Pyelonephritis, cystitis, prostatitis

Gynecologic

Pelvic inflammatory disease, Mittelschmerz, ovarian cysts

Metabolic/Toxic

Diabetes, uremia, lead poisoning, hyperlipidemia, hyperparathyroidism, Addison's disease, arachnoidism

Infectious

Viral gastroenteritis, typhoid, malaria, tuberculous peritonitis, food poisoning, spinal osteomyelitis, spontaneous bacterial peritonitis

Hematologic

Porphyria, leukemia, hemolytic crises, hemachromatosis

Miscellaneous

Periarteritis nodosa, familial mediterranean fever, drug addiction, psychiatric disorders

Causes of Fever of Abdominal Origin

PERITONITIS

Peritonitis is generally divided in two categories, spontaneous or primary peritonitis and secondary bacterial peritonitis. Spontaneous or primary peritonitis is a relatively common complication of ascites found primarily in children with nephrotic syndrome or patients with cirrhosis. The presumed mechanism is seeding of the ascitic fluid from a hematogenous source such as portal bacteremia, remote infection, or transient bacteremia.[135] Most adult cases are monomicrobial, usually *Escherichia coli,* although other organisms such as streptococci are common.[136] *Streptococcus pneumonia* is most commonly seen in children.[137] Anaerobic bacteria are distinctly unusual and suggest a secondary bacterial peritonitis. Although fever, abdominal pain, and tenderness do occur in most patients, symptoms are occasionally minimal and easily overlooked.[136] Nausea, vomiting, and diarrhea are common. In more than one third of patients, there are no symptoms or signs directly referable to the abdomen.[135] Indirect findings suggesting the presence of peritonitis include deterioration in hepatic or renal function, increasing encephalopathy, or temporary resistance to diuretics.[135] Diagnostic paracentesis is required in the patient with any of these features. In view of the high mortality of this condition

(48%–70%), early diagnosis and treatment are imperative. Because the results of bacterial culture are generally unavailable for 24 and 48 hours, reliance has to be placed on other characteristics of ascitic fluid infection.[135] Cloudy fluid is present in more than three quarters of patients with spontaneous bacterial peritonitis (SBP) and in one third of those with sterile ascites.[136] Gram's stain of a centrifuged deposit of ascitic fluid should be examined, although organisms are detected in less than one third of cases in which SBP is subsequently proven by bacterial culture.[137]

The most common way in which the diagnosis is established is measurement of the ascitic fluid white cell count. Sterile ascites normally contains less than 300 white blood cells/mm^3, most of which are lymphocytes, and less than 25% are polymorphonuclear cells (PMNs). Therefore, a diagnosis of SBP is considered probable when these values are exceeded. We feel the diagnosis must be based on the findings of greater than 250 PMNs/mm^3.

Antibiotic selection is best guided by culture results, but suggested regimens, while cultures are either pending or negative, include the use of third-generation cephalosporin or, alternatively, an aminoglycoside plus a broad-spectrum penicillin derivative.[133] Essentially, all antibiotics equilibrate into the peritoneum so that direct infusion into the abdominal cavity is unnecessary. A frequent problem with aminoglycosides is that these agents are distributed in free body water, which may be increased by several liters in patients with ascites.[133] Thus, therapeutic levels may be difficult to achieve and serum levels must be followed, and an alternative agent should be used when possible.

Secondary bacterial peritonitis implies the perforation or leakage from a hollow viscus within the abdominal cavity. The pathophysiology of ensuing complications depends on the nature of the insult, which may be chemical, as in gastric acid, or bacterial.[133] Secondary bacterial peritonitis usually involves fecal flora and includes an imposing array of bacteria. Fecal spillage or free perforation of the colon causes generalized peritonitis with large collections of fluid in the abdomen, hypotension, shock, and rapid death. Therapy is directed at stabilizing hemodynamic status, administration of appropriate antibiotics, and early surgical intervention. Localized peritonitis is far more subtle but may involve the same bacteria and is treated with the same antibiotics.[133,134]

Antibiotics should be started after the collection of at least two blood cultures and the institution of intravenous fluid support. Surgery is conducted as soon as the diagnosis is established and the patient is sufficiently stabilized. The major goals of surgery are to control the source of contamination.

Another specific infection seen in surgical patients is the peritonitis associated with ventriculoperitoneal shunts, such as LeVeen or Denver shunts, or peritoneal dialysis catheters. These infections represent complications of medical progress in which the major therapeutic dilemma is the decision to treat with locally or systemically administered antibiotics and the necessity to remove the foreign body.[138] The treatment is modified on the basis of clinical and laboratory findings. Most patients have abdominal pain or tenderness, cloudy ascitic or dialysate fluid with over 250 PMNs/ml and positive cultures on primary isolation plates.[133] Although all antibiotics penetrate into the peritoneal fluid, it is compelling to deliver these antibiotics locally in patients receiving peritoneal dialysis because the desired serum levels are more easily obtained by using dialysates containing the drug. The decision to remove the catheter is influenced by the necessity of the device and the response to treatment.[138,139]

Peritonitis complicating peritoneal dialysis usually involves gram-positive organisms. The commonly used drug for these infections is vancomycin because all gram-positive bacteria are sensitive as of this writing, and a single intravenous dose of 1 g provides a complete 7- to 14-day course in anuric patients.[140] Only 10% to 12% of patients require removal of their dialysis catheters. Indications for catheter removal include catheter malfunction with poor flow, refractory infection with persistently positive cultures after 5 to 7 days, or relapse when treatment is discontinued.[133]

Peritoneovenous shunts that become infected require antibiotics directly against the isolated organisms.[141] Most patients have a suboptimal response to therapy or relapse when antibiotics are discontinued. Thus, in contrast to infection with peritoneal dialysis catheters, definitive cure usually requires removal of the peritoneovenous shunts.

Candida peritonitis is a frequently recognized complication of peritoneal dialysis or intestinal surgery. Treatment with steroids and antibacterial agents are the contributing factors.[142] Although there usually is no evidence of disseminated candidiasis in these patients, the prognosis with this localized form remains poor.[133] The factors that influence the decision to treat *Candida* species recovered from peritoneal fluid are the reproducibility of culture results, semiquantitative assessment, cell count, and response to antibiotic.[133,134] Preferred criteria are repeatedly positive cultures, recovery on primary isolation plates to the exclusion of other organisms, and a polymorphonuclear cell count exceeding 250 cells/ml.[133] Most of these patients are febrile and fail to respond to additional bacterial agents. The preferred treatment is systemic amphotericin B.[142] The response is monitored by clinical signs such as decreasing fever, leukocytosis, and abdominal tenderness; peritoneal fluid cell counts; and follow-up cultures.[133] The addition of amphotericin B to the dialysate fluid has been attempted but is often precluded by the local pain stimulated by local administration.[143] Most dialysis patients fail to respond and require removal of their catheters.

Tuberculous peritonitis is based on the detection of mycobacteria on peritoneal biopsy or from any distant site in association with clinical evidence of chronic peritonitis.[144] Relative findings that are sufficient to initiate antitubercular treatment are mononuclear peritonitis preferably coupled with a peritoneal biopsy or pleural biopsy that shows granulomatous changes.[133,144]

INTRA-ABDOMINAL ABSCESSES

The clinical presentations of intra-abdominal abscesses and their diagnostic work-ups are covered in detail in Chapter 99. It is important to remember that all intra-abdominal abscesses require drainage with the exceptions of some amoebic liver abscesses, some hepatic abscesses, and about 70% of tubo-ovarian abscesses.[133] The usual mode of drainage is operative intervention, but an alternative is percutaneous drainage using ultrasound or CT guidance.[145] These techniques have the advantage of avoiding general anesthesia and postoperative complications. In most series, percutaneous drainage has been accomplished with reduced mortality, reduced recurrence rates, reduced hospital stays, and reduced costs when compared to the reported experience of surgery.[145-148] The factors that may influence the decision for percutaneous drainage are outlined in Table 36-6.

TABLE 36-6
Decision Tree: Intraabdominal Abscess

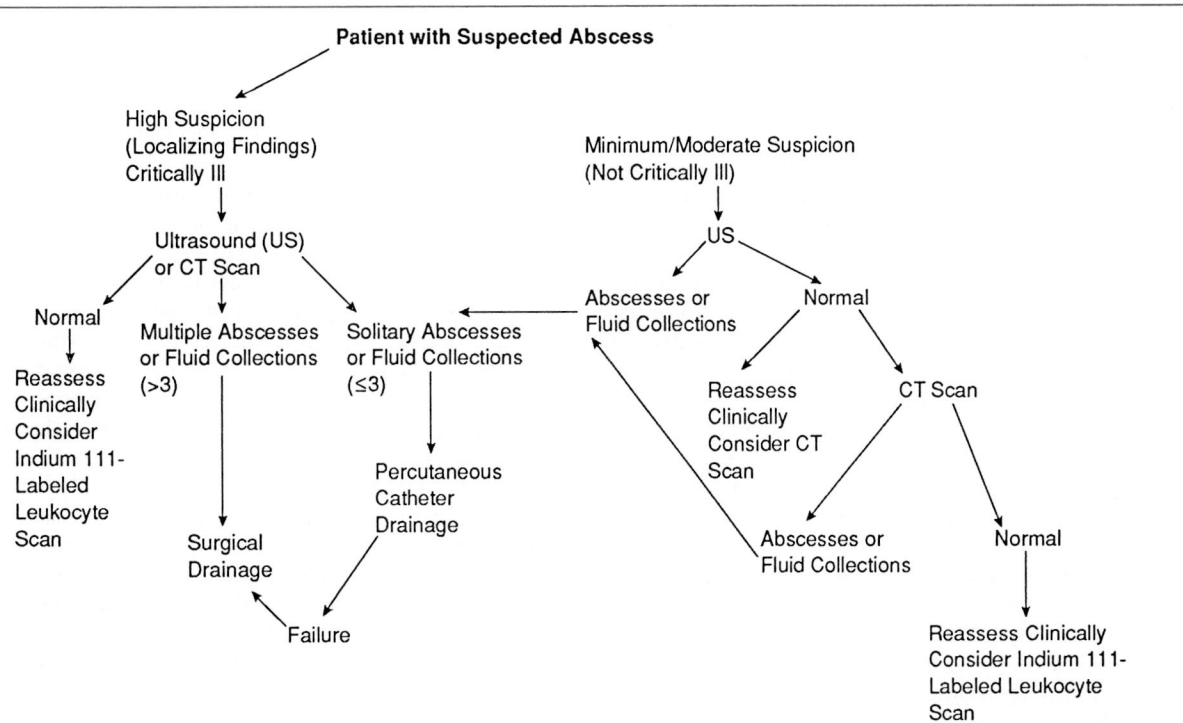

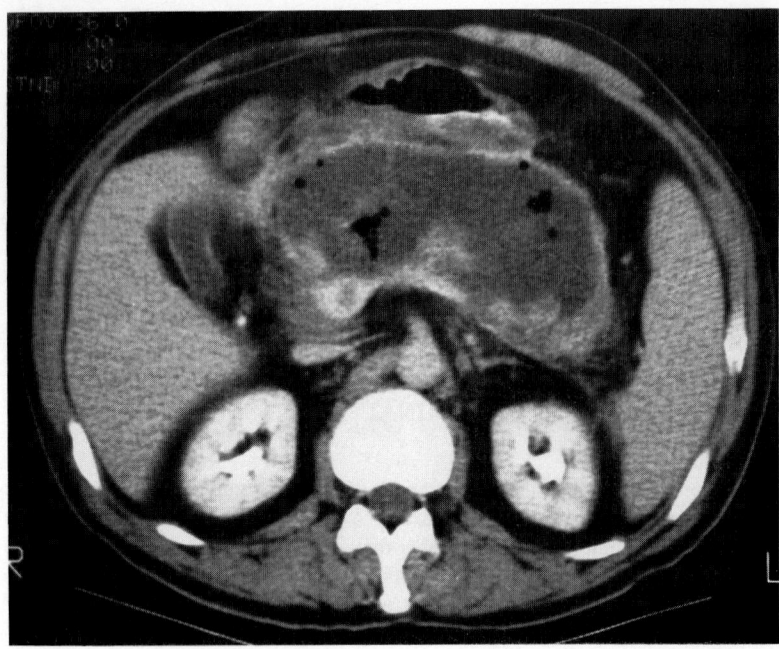

FIGURE 36–10. CT scan of pancreatic abscess. Gas bubbles in fluid collection are diagnostic.

Pancreatic abscesses generally occur after an acute attack of pancreatitis (Fig. 36-10). Pancreatic abscesses are invariably fatal if drainage is not performed.[54-56] The usual procedure is surgical debridement with external drainage. The most common pathogens recovered are the coliforms, with anaerobic bacteria being uncommon.[55] The recent use of CT scanning with percutaneous aspiration of suspicious peripancreatic fluid collections has led to an earlier diagnosis and improved prognosis of this life-threatening condition.[133]

Liver abscesses are classified by etiologies as pyogenic or amoebic, although about 4% of amoebic abscesses also harbor bacteria.[133] Preferred studies to distinguish these possibilities are the *Entamoeba histolytica* serology, blood cultures, and liver aspiration for microscopic examination and culture.[149] Amoebic abscesses are treated medically using metronidazole. Emetine or chloroquine are excellent drugs that may be used in patients who are unable to take metronidazole. Indications for percutaneous aspiration include facilitation of establishing the diagnosis, very large abscesses (> 10 cm), imminent rupture, failure to respond to appropriate medical therapy after 5 days, and left-sided amoebic abscesses because of their propensity for intramediastinal and retroperitoneal rupture.[149] Open drainage is reserved for patients who have failed to respond after 4 to 5 days of medical therapy and the abscesses are inaccessible to needle drainage.[150]

Three approaches are used in the management of the patient with a pyogenic liver abscess. The use of antibiotics alone is advocated by some but generally recommended only for patients who have multiple, widely distributed liver abscesses or a solitary abscess in which there is an impressive response to antibiotic treatment during diagnostic evaluation.[151] The use of antibiotics combined with surgical drainage is a time-honored approach advocated for solitary pyogenic liver abscesses although some authorities have recommended repeated percutaneous aspiration as an alternative to open surgical intervention.[133,151] Drains can be placed either by an operative approach or by percutaneous insertion using CT or ultrasound guidance. The predominant bacterial isolates are the coliform species, although anaerobic organisms are isolated from approximately one half of pyogenic liver abscesses.[150]

Splenic abscesses are most frequently secondary to staphylococcus, streptococcus, coliforms, and anaerobes. The usual definitive treatment is splenectomy, although recent reports have advocated percutaneous needle aspiration under ultrasound or CT guidance.[152]

FEVER ASSOCIATED WITH CROHN'S DISEASE

In addition to the common presenting symptoms of diarrhea, pain, and a palpable abdominal mass, fever can be seen in over 50% of patients with Crohn's disease. In cases that present with acute pain, fever, and surgical signs on abdominal examination, the patient may be mistakenly believed to have appendicitis (Fig. 36-11). However, most patients have more chronic courses with intermittent flares of pain, diarrhea, and fever. In most cases of Crohn's disease, the fever is relatively low grade with temperatures rarely exceeding 102°F. The presence of a temperature in excess of 102°F suggests the presence of a complication within the abdomen such as an abscess. This necessitates evaluation for an infectious source of fever in addition to the inflammatory process in active Crohn's. Another source of fever in Crohn's disease is the presence of active perianal disease. At least half of patients experience perianal complications during the course of their disease, which may be unrelated to the activity of the intra-abdominal process. Perianal or perirectal abscess formation may be associated with temperature elevations to 103°F, which require surgical drainage and parenteral antibiotic therapy. The evaluation and therapy of Crohn's disease and its complications are discussed in greater detail in Chapter 77.

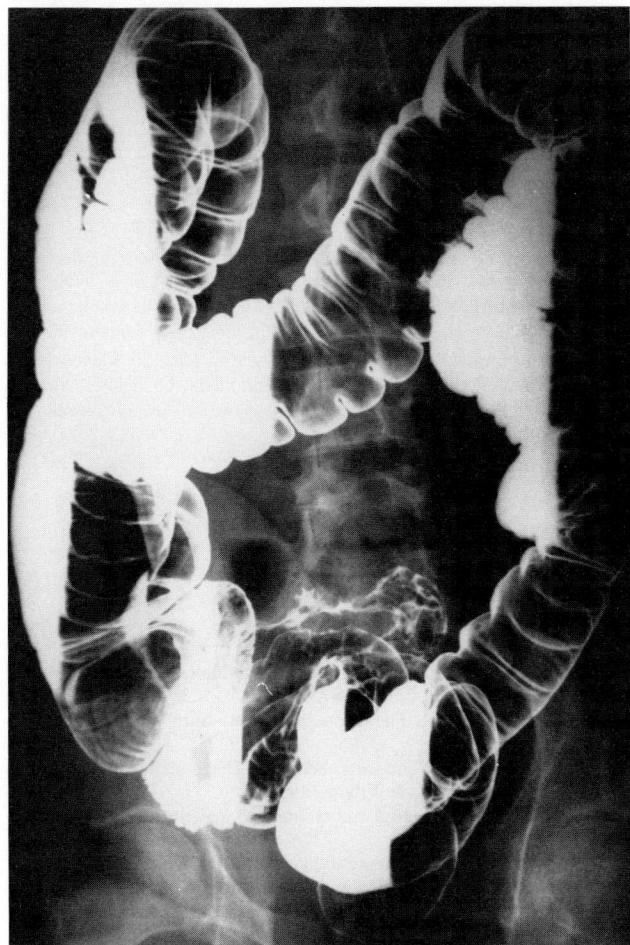

FIGURE 36–11. Crohn's disease of terminal ileum noted on barium enema examination in patient with suspected "chronic" appendicitis. Note stricture and mucosal blunting.

POSTOPERATIVE ABDOMINAL FEVERS

Postoperative fever is common, although its clinical significance is often unclear. Although a temperature elevation may herald a serious infection, in most cases, none is found.[153]

Postoperative fevers occur in 15% to 30% of patients subjected to laparotomy.[154] Most series report a 20% to 30% culture-proven infection for patients with postoperative fevers.[153] When approaching the patient with a postoperative fever, attention should be directed to infections related to the surgical procedure itself and other iatrogenic maneuvers that may alter host defenses.[155]

The timing of the onset of fever is a classic aid in determining the possible cause of these infections.[155] Temperature elevation in the first 48 hours after surgery is generally related to pulmonary atelectasis. In the next 24 to 48 hours, urinary tract infections become apparent. Under most conditions, wound infections do not cause fever until 3 to 5 days postoperatively, although streptococcal and clostridial wound infections may be seen as early as 24 hours after surgery.[153] Thrombophlebitis rarely occurs before the third postoperative day and usually does not become apparent until a week to 10 days after surgery. A mnemonic aid to assist in remembering the sequence of fever onset is wind (pulmonary), water (urinary), wound, and walking (phlebitis).[155]

In addition to the careful taking of the patient's history, the examination should be focused on the areas that are likely to represent sources of postoperative fevers. Wound and drain sites must be inspected carefully. The patient's urinary catheter should be examined for signs of urinary tract infection. Intravascular catheter sites are potential sources of serious infection even though evidence for inflammation at the catheter site is often minimal. Routine ordering of unnecessary laboratory tests is not cost effective, and one study concluded that routine evaluations of fever had no influence on the outcome in the majority of patients.[153] Additionally, the empiric use of antibiotics for treatment of postoperative fever is to be discouraged. Only when the established source of infection has been defined or strongly suspected should antibiotic coverage be provided.[153-155]

Abdominal sources of fever in the postoperative patient generally occur later (5–10 days postoperatively) than more common causes of postoperative fever. Wound infections may have extremely subtle clinical manifestations. All wounds require careful daily inspection for erythema, tenderness, edema, and warmth. If a wound infection is suspected, partly opening the wound under sterile conditions and probing it to examine the contents may prove diagnostic.[156] Most simple wound infections are treated by opening the wound and do not require the use of antibiotics. Wound infections are more likely to occur in patients who are immunocompromised from shock, malnutrition, malignancy, prior sepsis, or severe injury.[156]

Wound dehiscence usually declares itself between the fifth and seventh days postoperatively.[157] This is true for any wound, including intestinal anastomoses, in which the wound dehiscence produces an anastomotic leak.[155] Malnutrition, prior ongoing sepsis, cancer, diabetes, steroid use, and wound infection all increase the risk of wound dehiscence.[155,157] Wound dehiscence typically declares itself with a sudden gush of serosanguineous (salmon-colored) fluid that represents intra-abdominal or intrapleural contents that erupt from the wound. When possible, the best treatment for dehiscence is reclosure of the wound, however, if the patient is too ill, simple packing of the wound should be performed and the resulting hernia may be repaired at a later date.[157,158]

Intra-abdominal abscesses may also present during the late postoperative period. intra-abdominal abscesses most commonly follow operations that are associated with significant contamination of the abdominal cavity. They also are most likely to present in patients with severe immunosuppression (i.e., cancer, malnutrition, previous sepsis, trauma, chemotherapy, or diabetes).[133] intra-abdominal abscesses should be considered as a cause of fever in any patient who has undergone a major intra-abdominal procedure. Examination may reveal localized tenderness in the abdomen with physical findings consistent with local peritonitis, although, in most cases, the abdominal examination is unrevealing. CT scanning has proved to be the most useful diagnostic test in these situations, although reexploration of the abdomen has also had a high yield in patients with radiographically undiagnosed intra-abdominal abscesses.[159] Either percutaneous or surgical drainage of intra-abdominal abscesses is necessary.

Acalculus cholecystitis is an important cause of postoperative fever. With this disorder, fever is commonly associated with tenderness in the right upper quadrant and occasionally a palpable gallbladder.[26] The patient may also become jaundiced. Laboratory tests that may help confirm acalculus cholecystitis are ultrasonography, demonstrating an edematous gallbladder with sludge within its lumen, or a radioisotope scan, demonstrating nonvisualization of the gallbladder.[31,33] One must realize that false-positive radioisotope scans are common in the critically ill population with either other intra-abdominal processes or sepsis from other foci that may depress liver function.[26] The proper treatment for acalculus cholecystitis is cholecystectomy. On occasion, cholecystostomy, either in the operating room or by percutaneous approach, is adequate therapy.[160]

Critically ill surgical patients who have spent 7 or more days in the hospital are predisposed to infection from organisms that are generally considered of low virulence.[133] Risk factors include gastrointestinal operations, older age, prior bacterial sepsis, antibiotic administration, central venous catheter placement, respiratory therapy, and total parenteral nutrition.[135] When fever develops more than 7 days after surgery in patients with these risk factors, infections with fungi (particularly *Candida*), *Staphylococcus* epidermitis, enterococcus, *Serratia*, CMV, and *Legionella* should also be considered.[161]

FEVER ASSOCIATED WITH HALOTHANE HEPATITIS

Fever is the presenting symptom in three quarters of patients with acute hepatitis due to halothane anesthesia. Although halothane is the most common cause of anesthesia-induced hepatitis, other haloalkane anesthetics can also induce idiosyncratic hepatotoxicity. The risk factors for the development of halothane hepatitis include multiple exposures to the anesthetic (especially if the administrations are temporally close), obesity, female sex, and adulthood. Some studies have suggested that patients with allergies may be at increased risk, although this finding is not universally accepted. In general, fever with or without rash is the initial sign occurring 6 to 14 days after an initial exposure to halothane or as early as 1 day after multiple exposures. After 2 to 5 days of fever, jaundice with malaise, abdominal pain, and nausea may develop. In fulminant cases, coagulopathy and encephalopathy develop and may progress to death within 7 to 10 days. Laboratory tests reveal serum aminotransaminase levels greater than 10 times normal and a high bilirubin level. The alkaline phosphatase usually is elevated to a lesser extent. The onset of an elevated prothrombin time is an ominous finding and suggests a possible fulminant outcome. The mortality rate for halothane hepatitis is roughly 10% to 30% in recent series. In those persons who survive, complete recovery can be expected usually within 1 to 2 weeks. Only very rare cases of chronic liver disease secondary to halothane exposure have been described. In general, the therapy of halothane hepatitis involves the standard supportive care that would be given a person with severe viral hepatitis. In fulminant cases, orthotopic liver transplantation may represent the only viable option for saving the patient's life.

MISCELLANEOUS INTRA-ABDOMINAL SOURCES OF FEVER

It should not be forgotten that occult tumors may present as fevers. Twenty percent of fevers of unknown origin are secondary to cancers, either primary or metastatically involved in the abdomen.[162] Approximately 5% of fevers in patients with neoplasms

are related to the tumor. Most commonly implicated tumors are hypernephroma, liver tumors, and lymphomas. Rarely, carcinomas of the stomach, colon, and pancreas are cited.[162,163]

The reader is directed to Chapters 34, Approach to the Patient with Abdominal Pain; Chapter 61, Acid-Peptic Disorders; Chapter 64, Surgery for Peptic Ulcer Disease; Chapter 68, Small Intestine: Infections with Common Bacterial and Viral Pathogens; Chapter 77, Inflammatory Bowel Disease; Chapter 82, Diverticulitis; Chapter 83, Bacterial Infections of the Colon; Chapter 86, Miscellaneous Inflammatory and Structural Disorders of the Colon; Chapter 88, Acute Pancreatitis; Chapter 94, Gallstones; Chapter 95, Diseases of the Biliary Tree; Chapter 99, Intra-abdominal Abscesses and Fistulas; Chapter 100, Diseases of the Mesentery and Omentum; and Chapter 109, Vascular Insufficiency.

REFERENCES

1. Cope Z. Extract from the preface to the first edition. In: Silen W, ed. Cope's early diagnosis of the acute abdomen, ed 17. New York: Oxford University Press, 1987.
2. Williams LF, ed. The acute abdomen. Surg Clin North Am 1988;68(2):355.
3. Kirkpatrick JR, ed. The acute abdomen—Diagnosis and management. Baltimore: Williams & Wilkins, 1984.
4. Langman J, ed. Medical embryology, ed 2. Baltimore: Williams & Wilkins, 1969.
5. Myers SI, Miller TA. Acute abdominal pain: Physiology of the acute abdomen. In: Miller TA, Rowland B, eds. The physiologic basis of modern surgical care. St Louis: CV Mosby, 1988:525.
6. Kandel ER, Schwartz JH, eds. Principles of neuroscience, ed 2. New York: Elsevier, 1985:693.
7. Levine MS. Plain film diagnosis of the acute abdomen. Emerg Med Clin North Am 1985;3:541.
8. Eisenberg RL, Heineken P, Hedgcock MW, et al. Evaluation of plain abdominal radiographs in the diagnosis of abdominal pain. Ann Surg 1983;197:464.
9. Abrams HL. The over utilization of X-rays. N Engl J Med 1979;300: 1213.
10. Lee PWR. The plain X-ray in the acute abdomen: A surgeon's evaluation. Br J Surg 1976;63:763.
11. Doust BD, Thompson R. Ultrasonography of abdominal fluid collections. Gastrointest Radiol 1978;3:273.
12. Bagi P, Dueholm S. Nonoperative management of the ultrasonographically evaluated appendiceal mass. Surgery 1987;101:602.
13. Shaff MI, Tarr RW, Partain CL, et al. Computed tomography and magnetic resonance imaging of the acute abdomen. Surg Clin North Am 1988;68:233.
14. Cooperman M. Complications of appendectomy. Surg Clin North Am 1983;63:1233.
15. Williams GR. A history of appendicitis. Ann Surg 1983;197:495.
16. Dodson TF. Right lower quadrant pain: "Do I have appendicitis, Doctor?" In: Cutler BS, ed. Manual of clinical problems in surgery. Boston: Little, Brown & Co, 1984:149.
17. Bell MJ, Bower RJ, Ternberg JL. Appendectomy in childhood. Analysis of 105 negative explorations. Am J Surg 1982;144:335.
18. Elmore JR, Dibbins AW, Curci MR. The treatment of complicated appendicitis in children. Arch Surg 1987;122:424.
19. Bongard F, Lander DV, Lewis F. Differential diagnosis of appendicitis and pelvic inflammatory disease. Am J Surg 1985;150:90.
20. Robinson JA, Burch BH. An assessment of the value of the menstrual history in differentiating acute appendicitis from pelvic inflammatory disease. Surg Gynecol Obstet 1984;159:149.
21. Leape LL, Ramenofsky ML. Laparoscopy for questionable appendicitis. Can it reduce the negative appendectomy rate? Ann Surg 1980;191:410.

22. Peltokallio P, Tykka H. Evolution of the age distribution and mortality of acute appendicitis. Arch Surg 1981;116:153.
23. Puylaerr JBCM, Rutgers PH, Lalisang RI, et al. A prospective study of ultrasonography in the diagnosis of appendicitis. N Engl J Med 1987;317:666.
24. Skoubo-Kristensen E, Hvid I. The appendiceal mass. Ann Surg 1982;196:584.
25. Sharp K. Acute cholecystitis. Surg Clin North Am 1988;68:269.
26. Orlando R, Gleason E, Drezner AD. Acute acalculous cholecystitis in critically ill patients. Am J Surg 1983;145:472.
27. Patwardhan NA. Cholelithiasis and cholecystitis. In: Cutler BS, ed. Manual of clinical problems in surgery. Boston: Little, Brown & Co, 1984:61.
28. Friley M. Perforation of the gallbladder. Curr Surg 1972;29:377.
29. Koop H. Serum levels of pancreatic enzymes and their clinical significance. Clin Gastroenterol 1984;13:739.
30. Smith G, Bixler TJ, Sterioff S. Oral cholecystography in assessment of acute abdominal pain. Arch Surg 1980;115:642.
31. Cooperberg PL, Burhenne HJ. Real-time ultrasonography. Diagnostic technique of choice in calculous gallbladder disease. N Engl J Med 1980;302:1277.
32. Szlabick RE, Catto JA, Fink-Bennett D, et al. Hepatobiliary scanning in the diagnosis of acute cholecystitis. Arch Surg 1980;115:540.
33. Belsore JV. Acalculous cholecystitis. Contemp Surg 1983;22:90.
34. Pitt HA, Postier RG, Cameron JL. Biliary bacteria. Arch Surg 1982;117:445.
35. van der Linden W, Suneel H. Early versus delayed operation for acute cholecystitis: A controlled clinical trial. Am J Surg 1970;120:7.
36. McArthur P, Cuschieri A, Sells RA, et al. Controlled clinical trial comparing early with interval cholecystectomy for acute cholecystitis. Br J Surg 1978;62:850.
37. Gingrich RA, Awe WC, Boyden AM, et al. Cholecystostomy in acute cholecystitis: Factors influencing morbidity and mortality. Am J Surg 1968;116:310.
38. O'Connor MJ, Schwartz ML, McQuarrie DG, et al. Acute bacterial cholangitis. Arch Surg 1982;117:437.
39. Klimbera S, Hawkins I, Vogel SB. Percutaneous cholecystostomy for acute cholecystitis in high-risk patients. Am J Surg 1987;153:125.
40. Potts JR. Acute pancreatitis. Surg Clin North Am 1988;68:281.
41. Dodson TF. Surgical intervention in acute pancreatitis. In: Cutler BS, ed. Manual of clinical problems in surgery. Boston: Little, Brown & Co, 1984:67.
42. Geokas MC, Baltaxe HA, Banks PA, Silva J, Frey CF. Acute pancreatitis. Ann Intern Med 1985;103:86.
43. Moossa AR. Diagnostic tests and procedures in acute pancreatitis. N Engl J Med 1984;311:639.
44. Ranson JHC. Acute pancreatitis. Curr Probl Surg 1970;16:1.
45. Sarr MG, Santey H, Cameron JL. Prospective, randomized trial of nasogastric suction in patients with acute pancreatitis. Surgery 1986;100:500.
46. Finch WT, Sawyers JL, Schenker S. A prospective study to determine the efficacy of antibiotics in acute pancreatitis. Ann Surg 1976;183:667.
47. Ranson JHC. Acute pancreatitis: Pathogenesis, outcome, and treatment. Clin Gastroenterol 1984;13:843.
48. Martin JK, van Heerden JA, Bess MA. Surgical management of acute pancreatitis. Mayo Clin Proc 1984;59:259.
49. Rattner DW, Warshaw AL. Surgical intervention in acute pancreatitis. Crit Care Med 1988;16:89.
50. Kelley TR, Wagner DS. Gallstone pancreatitis: A prospective randomized of the timing of surgery. Surgery 1988;104:600.
51. Ranson JHC, Gliedman ML. Management of acute biliary pancreatitis. Contemp Surg 1986;29:93.
52. Frey CF. A strategy for the surgical management of gallstone pancreatitis. In: Beger HG, Buchler M, ed. Acute pancreatitis. Berlin: Springer-Verlag, 1987:242.
53. Hunt JL, Epharave K. Presentation of pancreatic pseudocysts: Implications for timing of surgical intervention. Am J Surg 1986;151:749.
54. Hiatt JR, Fink AS, King W, et al. Percutaneous aspiration of peripancreatic fluid collections: A safe method to detect infection. Surgery 1987;101:523.
55. Fink AS, Hiatt JR, Pitt HA, et al. Indolent presentation of pancreatic abscess. Arch Surg 1988;123:1067.
56. Bradley EL. Management of infected pancreatic necrosis by open drainage. Ann Surg 1987;206:542.
57. Chappuis CW, Cohn I. Acute colonic diverticulitis. Surg Clin North Am 1988;68:301.
58. Rodkey GV, Welch CE. Diverticulitis of the colon: Evolution in concept and therapy. Surg Clin North Am 1965;45:1231.
59. Freischlag J, Bennion RS, Thompson JE. Complications of diverticular disease of the colon in young people. Dis Colon Rectum 1986;29:639.
60. Hughes LE. Postmortem survey of diverticular disease of the colon. Gut 1969;10:336.
61. Kolvalcik PJ, Sustarik DL. Cecal diverticulitis. Am Surg 1981;47:72.
62. Roth SLA. Diagnosis and differential diagnosis of colonic diverticulitis. Postgrad Med 1976;60:95.
63. Labs JD, Sarr MG, Fishman EK, et al. Complications of acute diverticulitis of the colon: Improved early diagnosis with computerized tomography. Am J Surg 1988;155:331.
64. Hulnick DH, Megibow AJ, Balthazar ES, et al. Computed tomography in the evaluation of diverticulitis. Radiology 1984;152:491.
65. Jordan PH, Morrow C. Perforated peptic ulcer. Surg Clin North Am 1988;68:315.
66. Boey J, Lee NW, Wong J, et al. Perforation in acute duodenal ulcers. Surg Gynecol Obstet 1982;155:193.
67. Sawyers JL, Herrington LH, Mulherin JL, et al. Acute perforated duodenal ulcer. An evaluation of surgical management. Arch Surg 1975;110:527.
68. Collier DSS, Pain JA. Non-steroidal anti-inflammatory drugs and peptic ulcer perforation. Gut 1985;26:359.
69. Roh JJ, Thompson JS, Harned RK, et al. Value of pneumoperitoneum in the diagnosis of visceral perforation. Am J Surg 1983;146:830.
70. Madura MJ, Craig RM, Shields TW. Unusual causes of spontaneous pneumoperitoneum. Surg Gynecol Obstet 1982;154:417.
71. Maull KI, Reater DB. Pneumogastrography in the diagnosis of perforated peptic ulcer. Am J Surg 1984;148:340.
72. Morrow CE, Mulholland MW, Dunn DH, et al. Giant duodenal ulcer. Am J Surg 1982;144:330.
73. McGee GS, Sawyers JL. Perforated gastric ulcers. Arch Surg 1987;122:555.
74. Crofts TJ, Park KGM, Steele RJC, et al. A randomized trial of nonoperative treatment for perforated peptic ulcer. N Engl J Med 1989;320:970.
75. Hodnett RM, Gonzalez F, Lee WC, et al. The need for definitive therapy in the management of perforated gastric ulcers. Ann Surg 1989;209:36.
76. Griffin GE, Organ CH. The natural history of the perforated duodenal ulcer treated by suture plication. Ann Surg 1976;183:382.
77. Jordan PH. Proximal gastric vagotomy without drainage for treatment of perforated duodenal ulcers. Gastroenterology 1982;83:179.
78. Boey J, Lee NW, Koo J, et al. Immediate definite surgery for perforated duodenal ulcers. Am J Surg 1982;196:338.
79. Richards WO, Williams LF. Obstruction of the large and small intestine. Surg Clin North Am 1988;68:355.
80. Wangensteen OH. Historical aspects of the management of acute intestinal obstruction. Surgery 1969;65:363.
81. Sarr MG, Bulkley GB, Zuidema GD. Preoperative recognition of intestinal strangulation obstruction. Am J Surg 1983;145:175.
82. Silen W, Hein MF, Goldman L. Strangulation obstruction of the small intestine. Am J Surg 1962;85:121.
83. Bizer LS, Liebling RW, Delaney HM, et al. Small bowel obstruction. Surgery 1981;89:407.
84. Brolin RE, Krasna MD, Mast BA. Use of tubes and radiographs in the management of small bowel obstruction. Ann Surg 1987;206:126.
85. Dodson TF. Small bowel obstruction. In: Cutler BS, ed. Manual of clinical problems in surgery. Boston: Little, Brown & Co, 1984:123.
86. Kelley WE, Brown PW, Lawrence WL, et al. Penetrating, obstructing, and perforating carcinomas of the colon and rectum. Arch Surg 1981;116:381.
87. Bak MP, Bowel SJ. Sigmoid volvulus in elderly patients. Am J Surg 1986;151:71.

88. Bode WE, Beart RW, Spencer RJ, et al. Colonoscopic decompression for acute pseudo-obstruction of the colon. Am J Surg 1984;147:243.

89. Geelhoed GW. Colonic pseudo-obstruction in surgical patients. Am J Surg 1985;149:258.

90. Stewardson RH, Banbeck CT, Nyhus LM. Critical operative management of small bowel obstruction. Ann Surg 1978;187:189.

91. Williams LF. Mesenteric ischemia. Surg Clin North Am 1988;68:331.

92. McFadden DW, Zinner MJ. Intestinal circulation and vascular disorders. In: Miller TA, Rowland BJ, ed. Physiologic basis of modern surgical care. St Louis: CV Mosby, 1988:360.

93. Silva WE. Intestinal vascular disease. In: Cutler BS, ed. Manual of clinical problems in surgery. Boston: Little, Brown & Co, 1984:129.

94. Andersson R, Parsson H, Isaksson B, et al. Acute intestinal ischemia. Acta Chir Scand 1984;150:217.

95. Kaufman SL, Harrington DP, Siegelman SS. Superior mesenteric artery embolization: An angiographic emergency. Radiology 1979;124:625.

96. Bergan JJ. Revascularization in treatment of mesenteric infarction. Ann Surg 1975;187:430.

97. Rogers DM, Thompson JE, Garrett WV, et al. Mesenteric vascular problems. A 26-year experience. Ann Surg 1982;195:554.

98. Sack J, Aldrete JS. Primary mesenteric venous thrombosis. Surg Gynecol Obstet 1982;154:205.

99. Russ JE. Surgical therapy of non-occlusive mesenteric infarction. Am J Surg 1977;134:638.

100. Mannick JA, Whitlemore AO. Management of ruptured or symptomatic abdominal aortic aneurysms. Surg Clin North Am 1988;68:377.

101. Cutler BS. Ruptured abdominal aortic aneurysm. In: Cutler BS, ed. Manual of clinical problems in surgery. Boston: Little, Brown & Co, 1984:306.

102. Johnson G. Surgical management of suprarenal and infrarenal abdominal aortic aneurysm. Contemp Surg 1987;30:22.

103. Swanson RJ, Littooy FN, Hunt TK, et al. Laparotomy as a precipitating factor in the rupture of intra-abdominal aneurysms. Arch Surg 1980;115:299.

104. Youkey JR, Clagett GP, Rich NR, et al. Vascular trauma secondary to diagnostic and therapeutic procedures. Am J Surg 1983;146:788.

105. Neblett WW, Pietsch JB, Holcomb GW. Acute abdominal conditions in children and adolescents. Surg Clin North Am 1988;68:415.

106. Saebo A. The *Yersinia enterocolitica* infection in acute abdominal surgery. Ann Surg 1983;198:760.

107. Hatch EI. The acute abdomen in children. Pediatr Clin North Am 1985;32:1151.

108. Hatch EI, Naffis O, Chandler NW. Pitfalls in the use of barium enema in early appendicitis in children. J Pediatr Surg 1981;16:309.

109. Ein SH. Leading points in childhood intussusception. J Pediatr Surg 1976;11:209.

110. Wayne ER, Campbell JD, Koloske AM, et al. Intussusception in the older child. J Pediatr Surg 1976;11:789.

111. Nylander WA. The acute abdomen in the immunocompromised host. Surg Clin North Am 1988;68:457.

112. La Raja RD, Rothenberg RE, Odom JW, et al. The incidence of intra-abdominal surgery in acquired immunodeficiency syndrome: A statistical review of 904 patients. Surgery 1989;105:175.

113. Barone JE, Gingold BS, Nealon TF, et al. Abdominal pain in patients with acquired immune deficiency syndrome. Ann Surg 1986;204:619.

114. Leitman, IM, Paull DE, Barie PS, et al. Intra-abdominal complications of cardiopulmonary bypass operations. Surg Gynecol Obstet 1987;165:251.

115. Rosemurgy AS, McAllister E, Karl RC. The acute surgical abdomen after cardiac surgery involving extracorporeal circulation. Ann Surg 1988;207:323.

116. Lawhorne TW, Davis JL, Smith GW. General surgical complications after cardiac surgery. Am J Surg 1978;136:254.

117. Burnett LS. Gynecologic causes of the acute abdomen. Surg Clin North Am 1988;68:385.

118. Cilley RE, Colletti LM, Dent TL, et al. Management of common gynecologic problems encountered during abdominal exploration. Ann Surg 1987;53:617.

119. Kao MS. Unexpected gynecologic findings at laparotomy. Probl Gen Surg 1984;1:290.

120. Ginsberg K, Faro S. Management of pelvic inflammatory disease. Infections Surg 1987;6:562.

121. Eschenbach DA. Epidemiology and diagnosis of acute pelvic inflammatory disease. Obstet Gynecol 1980;55:1425.

122. Rubin GL, Peterson HB, Dorfman SF, et al. Ectopic pregnancy in the United States 1970–1978. JAMA 1983;249:1725.

123. Berkeley AS. Ectopic pregnancy: Update on diagnosis and surgical management. Infect Surg 1983;1:431.

124. Koch MO, McDougal WS. Urologic causes of the acute abdomen. Surg Clin North Am 1988;68:399.

125. Kunin CM. Urinary tract infections. Surg Clin North Am 1980;60:223.

126. Hawes S, Whigham T, Ehrmann S, et al. Emphysematous pyelonephritis. Infect Surg 1983;2:191.

127. Chaussy C, Schmiedt E, Jocham D, et al. First clinical experience with extracorporeally induced destruction of kidney stones by shock waves. J Urol 1982;127:417.

128. Nadel NS, Gitter MH, Hahn LC, et al. Preoperative diagnosis of testicular torsion. Urology 1973;1:478.

129. Levy BJ. The diagnosis of torsion of the testicle using the Doppler ultrasonic stethoscope. J Urol 1975;113:63.

130. Sufrin G. Acute epididymitis. Sex Transm Dis 1981;8:132.

131. Diseases which may simulate the acute abdomen. In: Silen W, ed. Cope's early diagnosis of the acute abdomen, ed 17. New York: Oxford University Press, 1987:271.

132. Gilmore OJA. Appendicitis and mimicking conditions. A prospective study. Lancet 1975;2:421.

133. Bartlett JG. Intra-abdominal sepsis. In: Bayless TM, ed. Current therapy in gastroenterology and liver disease—2. Toronto: BC Decker, 1986:270.

134. Lewis FR. Abdominal abscess—The role of the surgeon. In: Root RK, ed. New surgical and medical approaches in infectious diseases. New York: Churchill Livingstone, 1987:167.

135. Crossley IR, Williams R. Spontaneous bacterial peritonitis. Gut 1985;26:325.

136. Hallak A. Spontaneous bacterial peritonitis. Am J Gastroenterol 1989;84:345.

137. Conn HO. Bacterial peritonitis: Spontaneous or paracentetic? Gastroenterology 1979;77:1145.

138. Wormser GP, Hubbard RC. Peritonitis in cirrhotic patients with LeVeen shunts. Am J Med 1981;71:358.

139. Hubschmann OR, Counter RW. Gram-positive peritonitis in patients with infected ventriculoperitoneal shunts. Surg Gynecol Obstet 1979;149:69.

140. Fenton SS. Clinical aspects of peritonitis in patients on chronic ambulatory peritoneal dialysis. Peritoneal Dial Bull 1981¹:1.

141. Solomkin JS, Flohr AB, Quie PG, et al. The role of *Candida* in intraperitoneal infections. Surgery 1980;88:524.

142. Marsh PK, Tally FP, Kellum J, et al. *Candida* infections in surgical patients. Ann Surg 1983;198:42.

143. Smith JW. Synergism of amphotericin B with other antimicrobial agents. Ann Intern Med 1978;78:450.

144. Sherman S. Tuberculous enteritis and peritonitis. Arch Intern Med 1980;140:506.

145. Glick PL, Pellegrini CA, Stein S, et al. Abdominal abscess. A surgical strategy. Arch Surg 1983;118:646.

146. Aeder MI, Wellman JL, Haaga JR, et al. Role of surgical and percutaneous drainage in the treatment of abdominal abscesses. Arch Surg 1983;118:273.

147. Saini S, Kellum JM, O'Leary MP, et al. Improved localization and survival in patients with intra-abdominal abscesses. Am J Surg 1983;145:136.

148. Hinsdale JG, Jaffe BM. Re-operation for intra-abdominal sepsis. Ann Surg 1984;199:31.

149. Pitt HA. Liver abscess. In: Cameron JL, ed. Current surgical therapy—2. Toronto: BC Decker, 1986:153.

150. Basile JA, Klein SR, Worthen NJ, et al. Amebic liver abscess. The surgeon's role in management. Am J Surg 1983;146:67.

151. Miedema BW, Dineen P. The diagnosis and treatment of pyogenic liver abscess. Ann Surg 1984;200:328.

152. Sarr MG, Zuidema GD. Splenic abscess. Presentation, diagnosis, and treatment. Surgery 1983;92:480.
153. Yeung RSW, Buck JR, Filler RM. The significance of fever following operations in children. J Pediatr Surg 1982;17:347.
154. Freischlag J, Busuttil RW. The value of postoperative fever evaluation. Surgery 1983;94:358.
155. Gantz NM. Postoperative fever. In: Cutler BS, ed. Manual of clinical problems in surgery. Boston: Little, Brown & Co, 1984:26.
156. Olson M, O'Connor M, Schwartz ML. Surgical wound infections. Ann Surg 1984;199:253.
157. Poole GV. Mechanical factors in abdominal wound closure: The prevention of fascial dehiscence. Surgery 1985;97:631.
158. Richards PC, Balch CM. Abdominal wound closure. Ann Surg 1983;197:238.
159. Harbrecht PS, Garrison RN, Fry DE. Early urgent relaparotomy. Arch Surg 1984;119:369.
160. Flint LM. Early postoperative acute abdominal complications. Surg Clin North Am 1988;68:445.
161. Dunn DL, Simmons RL. Empiric therapy of peritonitis and intra-abdominal infection. Infect Surg 1983;5:466.
162. Musher DM. Fever of unknown origin. Diagnostic principles. Hosp Pract 1982;17:89.
163. Molavi A, Weinstein L. Persistent perplexing pyrexia. Med Clin North Am 1970;54:379.

37

Approach to the Patient with Ileus and Obstruction

ROBERT W. SUMMERS
CHARLES C. LU

TERMINOLOGY

Ileus refers to a state of inhibited motility in the gastrointestinal tract. The adjectives *paralytic* or *adynamic* are useful to emphasize the inhibition of propulsive activity. Perhaps the term *motor paralysis* or *paresis* might be a better term than ileus because such terms describe the physiologic malfunction more clearly; unfortunately neither enjoys wide usage.

Ileus is a pathophysiologic inhibition of motor activity. The term *functional obstruction* might be used but is confusing because the word "functional" often implies a psychological component, as in the "functional bowel disorder," and "obstruction" implies an anatomic impediment to flow. *Pseudo-obstruction* might also be used, but this term is often employed in the context of a chronic disorder. Sudden massive idiopathic dilatation of the colon is, however, sometimes called *acute colonic pseudo-obstruction* or Ogilvie's syndrome. *Toxic megacolon* is a special sort of ileus in which transmural inflammation produces atony of the muscle and at the same time the mucosal barrier is disrupted, resulting in systemic toxemia.

Ileus can clinically resemble mechanical obstruction. *Obstruction* implies blockage of the gut at one or more sites; the adjective *mechanical* emphasizes the anatomic nature of the problem. *Obturation* is a synonym that implies that the process is intraluminal. The obstruction is *complete* if there is complete inability of intestinal contents to pass through the digestive tract or *partial* if passage continues but is difficult. If obstruction is described as *simple*, the lumen is occluded only at one location. The term *closed loop obstruction* is used when the lumen is obliterated at two sites, and this situation is often accompanied by impairment of the blood supply. If the blood supply is inadequate to maintain the viability of the gut, the term *strangulated obstruction* is used.

PATHOPHYSIOLOGIC CONSIDERATIONS (FIG 37-1)

Changes in Blood Flow

Strangulation obstruction can result in severe impairment of blood flow and is a potentially lethal complication, requiring urgent rec-

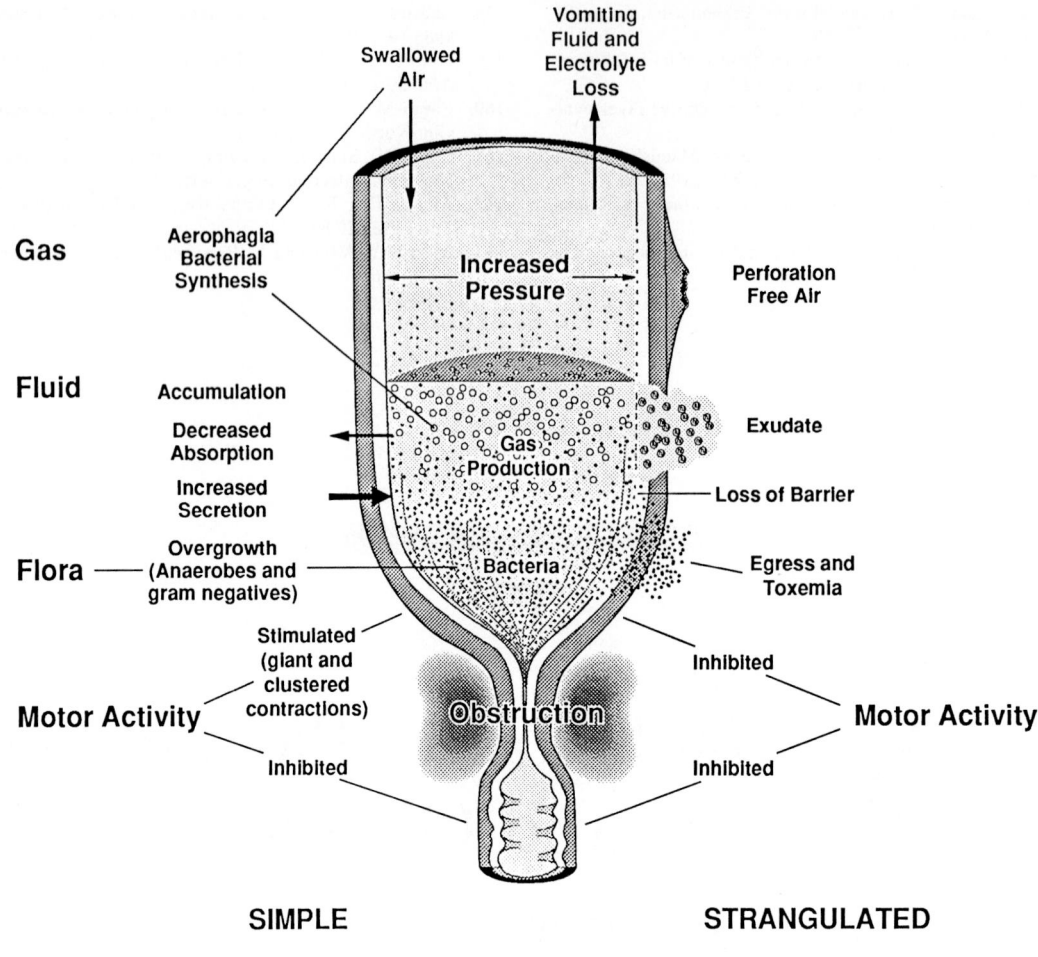

OBSTRUCTION

FIGURE 37–1. Pathophysiology of simple and strangulated obstructions.

ognition and management. Few studies in humans have been performed because of the invasive methods required to measure blood flow and the critical nature of the clinical problem. However, the major underlying threat to life in closed loop obstruction is impairment of blood flow in large vessels. The vascular supply of the bowel can be compromised through external compression of the bowel or its mesentery by adhesions, hernial orifices, tumors, torsion (volvulus), or intussusception. Although an increase in intraluminal pressure had been thought to cause local ischemia, this probably occurs only as a very late event except in closed loop obstruction. Pressures only reach 8 to 10 cm H_2O in simple obstruction and are not high enough to produce transmural ischemia.[1] Total mesenteric blood flow actually increases in experimentally induced simple obstruction, and an increase in muscle blood flow occurs during increased motor activity.[2] However, some shunting of blood from mucosa to the muscle does occur with increased intraluminal pressure, without any change in total blood flow.

The mucosa has the greatest metabolic need for blood and is the layer of the bowel that is most sensitive to ischemia. Within minutes after vascular occlusion, damage to the tips of the villi is manifest by sloughing of the epithelial cells.[3] If ischemia continues for 30 to 60 minutes, the villi are almost completely denuded and only the crypt epithelium is preserved.[4] The major early consequences of these changes are (1) impairment of the basic transport processes, (2) loss of the protective barrier to gut bacteria and their toxic products, and (3) exudation and hemorrhage into the lumen.

Failure to recognize and treat strangulation obstruction will inevitably lead to infarction, necrosis, and perforation of the bowel wall with peritonitis and/or sepsis and death. The mortality of obstruction complicated by transmural necrosis is commonly said to be 30%. Advanced sepsis can be associated with disseminated intravascular coagulation; however, the full-blown picture with prolonged prothrombin and partial thromboplastin times, thrombocytopenia, reduced fibrinogen, and increased fibrin degradation products is seldom encountered.

Ileus can be the result of arterial blockade from causes such as mesenteric vasculitis, atherosclerosis, or emboli. The converse is not the case; that is, ileus does not impair large arterial blood flow and the intraluminal pressures generated with ileus are not great enough to compromise mucosal blood flow.

Changes in Bowel Flora

The clinical picture in ileus and obstruction is affected by the bowel flora. Normally the flora of the stomach, jejunum, and proximal ileum are mainly gram-positive and facultative. Organisms are present in low concentrations (10^3 to 10^4 organisms per milliliter of fluid). Aerobic lactobacilli, streptococci, staphylococci, and fungi are most often cultured in this region, while anaerobes and coliforms are rare and in even lower concentrations.[5] The organisms in the colon are drastically different in numbers and kind. Approximately 10^9 to 12^{12} organisms per gram of feces exist in the colon, and they make up to 40% of the fecal dry weight. The vast majority (99%) are non-spore-forming anaerobic rods, including *Bacteroides* species, lactobacilli, and enterobacteria.[6] About 1% are aerobic gram-negative rods, mostly coliforms. Distal ileal flora represents a mixture of upper intestinal and colonic flora. The concentrations are commonly 10^6 to 10^7/mL.

Mechanisms regulating gut flora are complex but primarily involve gastric acidity and propulsive motility. Large numbers of bacteria are normally destroyed by the acid milieu in the stomach, but if the pH is high because of achlorhydria or antisecretory drugs, higher concentrations of organisms are found in the upper intestine.[7] Normal motility clears both nutrients and organisms from the intestine; but if propulsive activity is impaired, stasis and bacterial overgrowth occur. Within a few hours after complete obstruction, the contents of the proximal bowel become malodorous and feculent due to a marked increase in anaerobic organisms, especially *Bacteroides*.[8]

In partial obstruction (e.g., ileal strictures from Crohn's disease) or with impaired motility (e.g., diabetic autonomic neuropathy or scleroderma), intestinal stasis promotes bacterial overgrowth and malabsorption. Excessive luminal organisms cause mild mucosal injury, excessive gas formation, catabolism of nutrients with formation of short-chain fatty acids, and protein deprivation. Deconjugation of bile acids by bacteria causes impaired micelle formation and steatorrhea, and in some cases vitamin B_{12} deficiency develops from bacterial binding of the vitamin B_{12}–intrinsic factor complex.

The most serious consequence of increased luminal bacteria occurs in strangulation obstruction. The ischemia compromises the integrity of the bowel wall's defense barrier. The mucosa is especially susceptible to anoxia and necrosis, which leads to hemorrhage and increased permeability with transudation of toxic, infected intraluminal fluid across the bowel into the peritoneum and mesenteric circulation. This exudate is particularly lethal if clostridia and their exotoxins are present in the fluid.

Less is known about changes in bowel flora with ileus, but it is likely that qualitative and quantitative changes occur that are similar to that seen with mechanical obstruction. Bacterial overgrowth has been shown to occur with impaired propulsive motility and likely persists when it ceases.[9]

Changes in Bowel Contents

Normally, absorption and secretion of fluid and electrolytes take place in both the small and the large intestines. The duodenum and jejunum accomplish high-capacity absorption while the ileum and colon provide high efficiency. Following intestinal obstruction, fluid and electrolytes accumulate proximal to the obstructive site. Isotopic studies of water and electrolyte flux demonstrate both reduced net absorption during the first 12 hours after obstruction and increased secretion of water, sodium, and potassium.[10] As obstruction is prolonged, failure of absorption and enhanced secretion of water and electrolytes increase still further and net absorption becomes net secretion. Bacterial overgrowth may contribute to the enhanced secretion partly through the metabolism of ingested nutrients, but the exact mechanism is not known.[11] It is likely that neural reflexes contribute to secretion, activated by stretch receptors. In contrast, absorption of water and electrolytes continues in the obstructed colon, resulting in the conversion of the liquid ileal effluent to a solid fecal mass. Fluid and electrolyte fluxes with ileus have not been studied satisfactorily but probably are not greatly different from normal.

In addition to increased fluid in the bowel, intestinal gas contributes to the abdominal distention and the gas-filled loops routinely observed on plain abdominal radiographs. The origin of the gas is mainly from swallowed air in both ileus and obstruction. Gas does not accumulate to any degree if a cervical esophagostomy is performed in experimental obstruction, and analysis of the gas composition reveals high concentrations of nitrogen and low concentrations of carbon dioxide, hydrogen, and methane. The latter three gases are all products of bacterial fermentation, while nitrogen originates almost solely from swallowed air. If oral intake continues, as it does in partial obstruction, bacterial metabolism produces gas from ingested nutrients and contributes to distention and increased flatus.

Bowel distention can become severe and contribute significantly to the patient's discomfort. Abdominal pain is much more severe in obstruction than it is in ileus. Distention may also compromise respiration, especially in patients with cardiorespiratory problems, through impairment of diaphragmatic motion. Finally, the luminal sequestration of fluid and electrolytes, loss of absorptive capacity, and vomiting contribute to dehydration and circulatory insufficiency through fluid loss from the extracellular and intravascular compartments.

Changes in Motility (Fig 37-2)

Marked changes in motor activity occur in small intestinal and colonic obstruction. In experimental obstruction of the intestine, the aborad segment is inhibited almost immediately while a temporary increase in contractile activity occurs proximally.[12] This may represent enhancement of the so-called peristaltic reflex. The stimulus for the transient proximal hyperactivity is increase in wall tension. Accumulated fluid, gas, and nutrients raise intraluminal pressure, stimulating stretch receptors. The increased motor activity proximally is probably cholinergically mediated, as it is prevented by atropine.[13] With more prolonged obstruction, 1 minute or longer periods of quiescent motor activity are interspersed with intense regular spike bursts, some of which occur only at one recording site while others migrate aborally. Clustered contraction patterns are frequently seen in the normal fasting state but are

Fed-Normal   Fed-Mechanical Obstruction

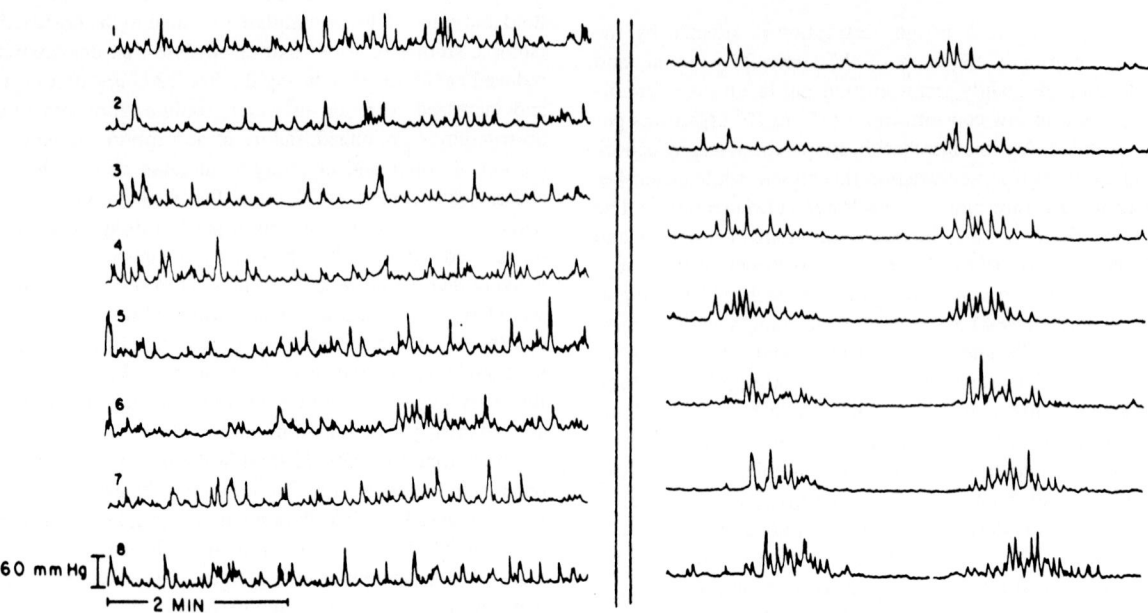

FIGURE 37–2. Comparison of motor activity in the normal and obstructed small intestine.

not normal after a meal. They likely represent the intermittent colic that patients having distention typically experience after eating. The same pattern can be detected by external recording of bowel sounds from patients with total or subtotal obstruction.[14] These migrating clustered contractions are typical of partial as well as complete obstruction after a meal, but they are not diagnostic because they occur in other conditions, including pseudo-obstruction.[15] If the obstruction is allowed to continue, the quiescent periods become progressively longer and motor activity is gradually reduced. This probably occurs through activation of inhibitory intestinointestinal reflexes.

Distal to intestinal obstruction, motor activity is markedly inhibited. In experimental obstruction, almost no contractile activity occurs in the segment of small bowel aborad to the obstruction throughout the period of obstruction. The mechanism of this inhibition is not established. It is not due to absence of intestinal contents because contractions do not increase when chyme is infused.[13] Although it has been suggested that the inhibition might be due to sympathetic reflexes, it is not reversed by α- or β-adrenergic antagonists, nor is it overcome by cholinergic agonists. It may be due to activity of the nonadrenergic, noncholinergic inhibitory nerves, but this is unproven.

Colonic obstruction is less well studied but also causes changes in motility, although they occur more slowly owing to the larger accommodative volume.[16,17] When the right colon is obstructed, both the segment proximal to the obstruction and the distal colon exhibit reduced contractions. However, when the left colon is obstructed, motor activity increases throughout the large bowel, exhibiting a pattern of clustered contractions similar to that seen in small bowel obstruction.

Mechanisms involved in adynamic ileus may be neurogenic, myogenic, or humoral. They may include either excessive inhibition or deficient excitation. Least is understood about the reflex mechanisms and muscle failure, while most is known about circulating substances because many are easily measurable. Any of the following may reduce or abolish motor activity: blood-borne toxins, drugs, circulating hormones, and abnormalities in mineral balance, acid–base balance, and oxygen supply.

Postoperative ileus has been studied more than some other causes of motor paralysis and may be a prototype for some of the other conditions. Following an operation, gastrointestinal motor failure ensues for several days; food and fluids are not tolerated, and no flatus or stool is passed per rectum. Studies of motor activity in animals have shown that contractions return first in the small intestine 3 to 6 hours after laparotomy, in the stomach after 24 hours and in the colon after several days.[18–20] Analogous human studies confirm that the colon is slowest to recover and that the right colon activity returns several days before the sigmoid colon.[21,22] Motility patterns do not return entirely to normal as soon as contractions return so that normal digestive function is delayed. The factors influencing the duration of ileus are varied. Manipulation of the abdominal organs delays return of function longer than a laparotomy alone. Chemical or physical irritants in the peritoneal cavity such as bile, blood, or talc delay recovery even longer. Bowel dilatation from gas and fluid accumulation activates visceral afferents and an inhibitory reflex arc.[23,24] Somatic inhibitory reflexes are activated at the beginning of a laparotomy when the parietal peritoneum is entered. In the postoperative period a low-grade sterile peritonitis may stimulate the same somatic inhibitory reflexes, augmented by opioid narcotics.

The mediators involved in postoperative ileus are unknown. Adrenergic inhibition has been believed to be the cause; however, it does not explain why the process lasts several days. Plasma concentrations of catecholamines are elevated after general anesthesia and laparotomy, but the benefit of adrenalectomy, demedullation, or adrenergic antagonists in reducing ileus is controversial.[18,25] Other experimental evidence supports the idea that propulsive contractions are inhibited by sympathetic nerves. The return of migrating motor complexes is more rapid if an operative splanchnicectomy is performed, and measurement of norepinephrine turnover confirms the stimulation of the sympathetic nervous system following a laparotomy and intestinal manipulation.[26,27] However, the use of epidural anesthesia (which blocks efferent sympathetic nerves) does not shorten ileus or the time of first passage of gas or feces. This suggests that mechanisms other than spinal reflexes play a major role in development and maintenance of postoperative ileus.[28]

Damage to cholinergic nerves from handling or hypoxemia could explain ileus,[29] but the activation of the nonadrenergic, noncholinergic inhibitory nerves may be more likely. However, until the neurotransmitter of these nerves is established or effective and specific antagonists can be found, it is not possible to test this hypothesis and the role of active reflex inhibition remains speculative.

Metabolic Consequences and Systemic Effects

One of the first systemic consequences of obstruction or ileus is fluid and electrolyte imbalance. With obstruction, the type of disturbance is largely dependent on the anatomic site of the block. With gastric outlet obstruction, repeated emesis of clear fluid high in hydrochloric acid and potassium chloride leads to metabolic alkalosis with hypokalemia and hypochloremia. With distal duodenal or proximal jejunal obstruction, alkaline biliary and pancreatic secretions are lost, producing metabolic acidosis. The volume of emesis is less with distal intestinal obstruction, but vomiting is less likely to decompress the bowel and thus the colicky pain and abdominal distention are more severe. Vomiting and dehydration are uncommon in colonic obstruction, but distention and pain may be intense. If the ileocecal valve is incompetent, colonic obstruction more closely resembles ileal obstruction, but if it is competent, gas accumulates rapidly from both swallowed air and bacterial fermentation. The pressure inside the colon may rise rapidly and cause rupture, most commonly in the cecum. The tensile strength of the cecum is relatively low, and the mucosal microcirculation is more tenuous than in the small bowel. By LaPlace's law the tension in the wall is greatest where the radius is the greatest. Thus emergent decompression of the colon is required when the diameter of the colon rapidly enlarges, risking perforation.

The same metabolic consequences may occur as a result of ileus, although in most situations ileus is caused by metabolic abnormalities. Vomiting, changes in flora, and alterations in absorption and secretion may produce a clinical situation identical to that seen in simple obstruction. Fortunately ischemic complications and sepsis are very uncommon.

With closed loop obstruction and strangulation, a systemic inflammatory response occurs as a result of the release of a wide range of substances from necrotic bowel. Cyclooxygenase and lipoxygenase metabolites, slow-reacting substance, and a variety of kinins, histamine and serotonin, lysosomal enzymes, and free radicals all likely play a role in the fever, leukocytosis, fluid shifts, and shock that may precede or coexist with the developing sepsis. Finally organ failure and death may ensue with one or more of the following: metabolic encephalopathy, acute renal insufficiency, hepatic failure, high-output shock and myocardial dysfunction, adult respiratory distress syndrome, or disseminated intravascular coagulation.

HISTORY

The clinical findings in ileus and obstruction depend on the anatomic site (Table 37-1). In performing the clinical evaluation, the physician should attempt to determine the anatomic site involved and ascertain the underlying cause. For management decisions it is important to know the duration of the process and especially whether complications such as peritonitis, perforation sepsis, or strangulation are present. The main signs and symptoms of obstruction are crampy spasmodic abdominal pain, vomiting, borborygmi, abdominal distention, and obstipation. These clinical features may develop slowly over months or years or acutely over a few hours.

If obstruction is incomplete or if only mild to moderate hypomotility exists, the patient may describe only intermittent crampy abdominal pain occurring after meals. The pain is located

TABLE 37-1
Clinical Features of Ileus and Obstruction Dependent on Anatomic Site

FEATURE	SITE OF OBSTRUCTION				
	Ileus	Gastric Outlet	Distal Duodenum	Jejunoileal	Colonic
Pain	Mild	Mild	Mild	Moderate	Severe
Distention	Moderate–severe	Mild	Mild	Moderate	Severe
Emesis					
Amount/frequency	Small/infrequent	Copious/frequent	Copious/frequent	Smaller/less frequent	Uncommon
Nature	Sour/bilious	Clear, sour, HCl & KCl	Bile-stained, bitter, NaCl and NaHCO₃	Malodorous, feculent	Variable
Acid–base problem	Variable	Metabolic alkalosis	Metabolic acidosis	Dehydration, hypotension	Usually not severe

in the mid and upper abdomen with small bowel obstruction and in the lower abdomen with left-sided colonic obstruction. Eating fiber-rich foods with undigestible components such as skins, seeds, nuts, and raw vegetables such as celery, cabbage, or water chestnuts may aggravate the symptoms of obstruction. If the patient eats a low-residue diet or avoids eating entirely, the symptoms may be reduced or avoided. As the obstruction becomes increasingly complete, the pain intensifies and comes in waves or spasms. This is true intestinal colic with severe crescendos of pain followed by waning intervals of rest in 3- to 10- minute cycles. With ileus, pain is much less intense and may only be sensed as a feeling of pressure or fullness. In more proximal obstruction, pain is relieved by vomiting. Bloating or abdominal distention may be experienced after a meal in association with waxing and waning pain, which may be described as dull, squeezing, and ill defined. Bowel sounds may be so loud that they are heard by others in the room (borborygmi). Patients may observe abdominal distention, which they may describe as a feeling that their clothing is tight or that they look pregnant.

As the situation becomes more advanced, nausea and vomiting are more frequent and more severe. If emesis appears and tastes like swallowed food or is clear, foamy tasteless fluid, the obstruction is probably above the lower esophageal sphincter. If the fluid or food is sour but not bile-stained or bitter, the obstruction is probably near the gastric outlet. Bitter bile-stained emesis suggests a proximal small bowel obstruction while malodorous feculent emesis suggests a distal small bowel obstruction or a colonic obstruction with an incompetent ileocecal valve. With complete obstruction and protracted vomiting, dehydration and orthostatic hypotension occur in association with reduced urine output. With complete bowel obstruction, patients develop obstipation and fail to pass flatus. Patients with fecal impaction may present with paradoxic diarrhea. In children, passage of bloody mucus often indicates intussusception ("red currant jelly").

In order to investigate the underlying causes of obstruction, inquiry should be made about the following: previous operations (adhesions), previous episodes of obstruction, bulges on the abdomen wall or in the groin (hernias), previous cancers or polyps, abdominal irradiation, inflammatory bowel disease, peptic ulcer, gallstone disease, pancreatitis, foreign body ingestion, or divertic-

ular disease. A psychiatric history and a family history of polyps or cancer may provide helpful clues to the underlying diagnosis.

Hypomotility and paralytic ileus are most often due to metabolic, electrolyte, and acid–base disorders; pharmacologic inhibition of motility; or primary or secondary neuropathies or myopathies. Careful drug, endocrine, and immunologic histories are important in discovering the underlying cause. One must be alert to thyroid and parathyroid disorders, diabetes mellitus, scleroderma, heavy metal poisoning, and porphyria.

The development of constant unremitting localized pain, fever, chills, and rigors and of a general sudden worsening of the clinical state suggest ischemia and infarction. However, waiting for such features to develop is poor clinical judgment. Strangulation and necrotic bowel may exist with none of these findings being present. A high index of suspicion and aggressive management are important practices to adopt if mortality is to be kept low. If the clinical condition changes and if any of these systemic symptoms appear, urgent steps must be taken to search for and treat potentially ischemic or necrotic bowel.

PHYSICAL EXAMINATION

Inspection

Observation of the patient's behavior during a bout of mechanical obstruction is critical in evaluation. A great deal of distress is apparent, manifest by a pained expression and active body language. The patient may be doubled over, holding the abdomen and writhing restlessly in bed, frequently changing position and vomiting or retching. Intervals of relief may occur during which the patient may lie still. With ileus, the pain is less severe in the face of moderate abdominal distention, but it is more steady and unrelenting and the patient usually lies quietly in bed.

The abdominal examination should always be begun by careful inspection. A number of dermatologic findings may provide clues to the underlying cause of the obstruction or ileus (Table 37-2).

TABLE 37–2
Cutaneous Findings That Are Clues to the Cause of Obstruction

PHYSICAL SIGNS	DIAGNOSIS
Abdominal scars	Adhesions
Pyoderma gangrenosum/erythema nodosum	Ulcerative colitis/Crohn's disease
Buccal, palmar, plantar pigmentation	Peutz-Jegher syndrome
Cullen's/Grey Turner's sign	Hemorrhagic pancreatitis
Cutaneous atrophy, hyperpigmentation	Chronic pancreatitis/abdominal radiation
Vesicles, bullae, scars, pigmentation	Porphyria
Neurofibromas	Von Recklinghausen's disease
Acanthosis nigricans	Gastrointestinal malignancies
Butterfly dermatitis	Lupus erythematosus
Atrophy/telangiectasia/variable pigmentation	Scleroderma/dermatomyositis

Abdominal distention is more typical of low intestinal and colonic obstruction. The greatest distention occurs with rectal cancer. Occasionally with obstruction, loops of bowel can be seen moving beneath the abdominal wall (visible peristalsis).

Palpation

It is mandatory to carefully palpate the umbilicus, the lower trunk, and both inguinal and femoral areas in every case of suspected obstruction in order to detect external hernias. Incarcerated femoral hernias are especially easy to overlook in the obese patient. Recognition of such hernias is important not only for diagnosis but also for treatment, since they can sometimes be manually reduced, relieving the obstruction and avoiding the hazards of strangulation. Careful palpation of the abdomen is also imperative to detect hepatosplenomegaly, liver masses, or other intra-abdominal masses suggesting malignant neoplasms. Tender lumps may suggest an abscess from Crohn's disease or diverticulitis, an intussusception, or an ischemic loop of bowel. Metastatic nodes in the umbilicus or inguinal region may also suggest colonic or other neoplasms. A careful rectal and pelvic examination should always be done to find rectal or vaginal tenderness or masses and fecal or barium impaction, although these may lie beyond the examining finger.

Percussion

Resonant percussion or tympany occurs in both ileus and obstruction because of entrapped intestinal or colonic gas. Shifting dullness or a "puddle sign" occurs when there is free abdominal fluid and might suggest associated malignant ascites or inflammation, as in complicated pancreatitis, bowel necrosis, or early tuberculous peritonitis.

Auscultation

Auscultation is important in distinguishing obstruction from ileus. In ileus, the bowel sounds are infrequent and hypoactive. The findings in obstruction are quite different, unless the obstruction is prolonged for several days or is complicated by ischemia and necrosis. Bowel sounds become louder, higher pitched, and hyperactive in obstruction. They have a musical, tinkling, or metallic quality and occur in clusters or rushes. These rushes often coincide with colic. In recent-onset proximal obstructions, they may occur every 3 to 5 minutes or up to 15 minutes if obstruction is in the distal bowel or if it is more prolonged or complicated by strangulation. This means that the examiner may need to listen for 10 to 15 minutes to hear the abnormal sounds. With ileus, the abdomen is almost completely silent. Rare low-pitched gurgles or weak tinkles are heard plus transmitted heart tones and moving water if the patient changes position. Shaking of the abdomen and pelvis while listening with a stethoscope several hours after a meal may reveal a "succussion splash." Although this splashing noise is most characteristic of gastric outlet obstruction, it may also occur in

intestinal or colonic obstruction or even in paralytic ileus when there are large volumes of gas and fluid in dilated loops of bowel.

Repeated abdominal examinations are essential because complications may develop with time and produce changing physical findings. If fevers, hypotension, rigors, or signs of sepsis develop, if bowel sounds disappear, or if signs of peritoneal irritation such as low-pitched rubs, muscle guarding, rigidity, or rebound tenderness intervene, the bowel is probably ischemic and rapid intervention is imperative. Ischemia may have developed before these signs appear, but when any one of them is detected it is an ominous finding that often signifies a life-threatening event.

DIFFERENTIAL DIAGNOSIS AND DIAGNOSTIC STRATEGIES

Causes of Mechanical Obstruction

The causes of mechanical obstruction are extremely varied and may be divided into (1) extrinsic lesions, (2) intrinsic lesions, and (3) intraluminal objects (Table 37-3). In adults, the most common causes of obstruction are adhesions and hernias in the small bowel and cancer in the colon. Frequently it is not possible to diagnose the cause of the obstruction preoperatively, but a careful history may allow one to make a diagnosis with a high degree of probability. This is important not only to satisfy intellectual curiosity but also as an aid in management decisions.

EXTRINSIC LESIONS

Extrinsic masses can compress the bowel or mesentery to cause obstruction. *Adhesions* are the most common cause of small intestinal obstruction in adults, but they uncommonly obstruct the colon. They most commonly occur after gynecologic procedures and operations on the small and large intestine and uncommonly occur following gastric and biliary procedures. Adhesions may occur from a few days to 10 or 20 years after an operation. They may occur without a history of an operation, most commonly following infection (peritonitis) or irradiation. Adhesive bands form and contract with time, entrapping a loop of bowel. They often cause a closed loop obstruction, commonly associated with strangulation. *Congenital bands* behave clinically in much the same way as adhesions, but they may occur in association with malrotation (Ladd's bands) or in the absence of any known cause.

Hernias may cause either simple obstruction or closed loop obstruction with or without strangulation as the blood supply is compromised by the hernial ring. A listing of the more common hernias is included in Table 37-4. *External hernias* protrude through the abdominal wall, are palpable as tender masses, and may be reducible. *Internal hernias* are not palpable and are usually identified at the time of operation. *Diaphragmatic hernias* rarely cause obstruction unless they are paraesophageal. Uncommon *pelvic hernias* may be palpable but require careful pelvic, rectal, and perineal examination and are usually only recognized at operation as the cause of bowel obstruction.

TABLE 37–3
Causes of Mechanical Obstruction

Extrinsic Lesions	Intrinsic Lesions
Extrinsic Lesions	**Intrinsic Lesions**
Adhesions and congenital bands	Benign and malignant neoplasms
Hernias	Adenocarcinomas
External hernias	Lymphoma, lymphosarcoma
Internal hernias	Carcinoid tumors
Diaphragmatic hernias	Inflammatory conditions
Pelvic hernias	Tuberculous enteritis, Crohn's disease
Volvulus	Ischemic stricture, KCl strictures
Gastric	Radiation injury, caustic ingestants
Mid gut	Eosinophilic gastroenteritis, ameboma
Cecal	Diverticulitis, pelvic inflammatory disease
Sigmoid	Intussusception
Extrinsic masses	Congenital defects
Benign or malignant tumors	Hypertrophic pyloric stenosis, annular pancreas
Abscesses	Intestinal atresia/agenesis
Aneurysms	Malrotation/volvulus
Hematomas	Intestinal duplication, mesenteric cysts
Endometriomas	Meckel's diverticulum
	Hirschsprung's disease
Intraluminal Objects	Hematoma
Meconium ileus	Abdominal trauma
Barium impaction	Thrombocytopenia
Fecal impaction	Henoch-Schönlein purpura
Gallstone ileus	
Gastric bezoars	
Foreign bodies	

A *volvulus* is an abnormal torsion of a segment of bowel, usually colon, producing a closed loop obstruction and occlusion of the blood supply. It involves the sigmoid colon in 70% to 80% of cases and the cecum in 10% to 20% of cases. Typically, pain comes on suddenly and is severe, followed rapidly by severe abdominal distention. A tender mass may be palpated, and characteristic abdominal plain radiographic findings are often present (Fig 37-3). Occasionally they may be reduced by barium enema or colonoscopy, but they are prone to recur. Volvulus of the small intestine occurs in newborns but is rare in adults. Volvulus of the stomach is often associated with large defects in the diaphragm, congenital malrotation, or large paraesophageal hernias.

INTRINSIC LESIONS

Tumors may narrow or obstruct the lumen or may be the leading point of an intussusception. *Neoplasms* causing obstruction may be benign or malignant, and if malignant they may be primary or metastatic. The most common primary malignant cause is adenocarcinoma of the colon.

Inflammatory or ischemic processes involving the bowel wall produce strictures, luminal narrowing, muscle dysfunction, and impaired transit. Blunt trauma to the abdomen may produce intramural hemorrhage and compromise of the lumen. *Hematomas* may also occur as a result of severe thrombocytopenia or clotting disorders without or with vascular fragility as in Henoch-Schönlein purpura.

Intussusception exists when a leading segment of bowel invaginates into an accepting segment. In infants this is usually idiopathic, but in older children and adults an intrinsic bowel lesion initiates the process. The inner advancing invaginated segment is called the *intussuscipiens*, while the outer accepting invaginating segment is termed the *intussusceptum*. Initially the inner walls become edematous because of lymphatic obstruction. As the process advances, venous obstruction, infarction, and necrosis follow.

A variety of *congenital anomalies* predisposes to intestinal obstruction, which usually but not always becomes evident in the newborn period. *Hypertrophic pyloric stenosis* may cause intractable vomiting in neonates. Congenital stenoses most often occur in the duodenum and are frequently associated with an *annular pancreas* or *aberrant pancreatic tissue* in the wall. *Atresias* and *agenesis* are also most common in the duodenum but may occur elsewhere in the small bowel, colon, or anus. The length of involvement may be merely a membrane, multiple short segments, or an extensive portion of the gut. If the endoderm fails to separate from the notochord early in gestation, the end result may be an obstruction from *intestinal duplication* or *mesenteric cyst*. A *Meckel's diverticulum* may be the cause of intussusception. *Malrotation, nonrotation, reverse rotation,* or errors in mesenteric fixation increase

TABLE 37-4
Common Hernias

External Hernias

Indirect inguinal—may incarcerate at internal or external ring

Femoral—adjacent to the femoral vein

Umbilical—with or without an omphalocele

Internal supravesical—through vesical fascia into space of Retzius

*Lateral ventral (Spigelian)—at junction of internal oblique muscle and rectus abdominis (usually tiny, causes intense localized tenderness)

Lumbar—between external oblique muscle and latissimus dorsi

Incisional—closely related to a scar

Internal Hernias

Paraduodenal

Transomental

Iliac fossa

Epiploic foramen

Transmesenteric

Diaphragmatic Hernias

*Sliding hiatal

Paraesophageal

Posterolateral diaphragmatic (Bochdalek's)

Anterior diaphragmatic (Morgagni)

Pelvic Hernias

Obturator—palpable on pelvic examination

Sciatic—palpable on rectal examination

Perineal—lateral to bulbocavernosus muscle or rectum

* *Uncommonly causes obstruction*

the risk of volvulus. Defects in migration of neural crest ganglion cells cause aganglionic segments of distal colon or rectum. Impaired motility in these segments produces megacolon, also known as *Hirschsprung's disease*.

INTRALUMINAL OBJECTS

In the newborn period, ultra-thick *meconium* may cause bowel obstruction or even perforation (the common term "meconium ileus" is a misnomer). This abnormal material is almost always due to underlying cystic fibrosis with its reduced secretion of proteolytic enzymes. An analogous situation is the development of *barium impaction* in adults. Excessive extraction of water from the barium occurs when there is prolonged colonic stasis. Often this is due to an underlying motility disorder such as scleroderma, chronic intestinal obstruction or colonic pseudo-obstruction.[30] *Fecal impaction* itself may also cause colonic obstruction. This may result from severe chronic constipation or from a variety of drugs such as the narcotics or antipsychotics, but it may also be due to an underlying colonic carcinoma or diverticulitis. Large gallstones occasionally erode through the gallbladder wall into the duodenum or more rarely into the colon or stomach. Some of these

stones are large enough to obstruct the bowel, most commonly in the distal ileum. This condition is misnamed "gallstone ileus" and may be suspected if dilated loops of bowel proximal to a small bowel obstruction are associated with air in the biliary tree from the cholecystoduodenal fistula. Finally, objects from the stomach may produce intestinal obstruction if they pass the pylorus or a gastrointestinal stoma. Such objects include gastric bezoars, ingested foreign bodies, or iatrogenically introduced bodies. Coins, bottles, gastric balloons, illicit drugs in condoms, Angelchick prostheses, and almost anything imaginable can be discovered in an obstructed intestine.

Causes of Adynamic Ileus

Just as mechanical obstruction always has an underlying cause, ileus is never primary, and a search for the cause is essential to achieve success in management. Because the clinical picture in ileus is so similar to that in mechanical obstruction, diagnostic considerations for both disorders must proceed concurrently. Long-standing or complicated mechanical obstruction may even terminate with ileus. The underlying causes of mechanical obstruction are overt, simple, anatomic, and almost always conclusively apparent. Conversely, the underlying mechanisms in acute motor paralysis are occult, complex, and rarely completely understood. Causes of adynamic ileus are outlined in Table 37-5. The conditions associated with ileus can often be defined, but a great deal is yet to be learned before mechanisms are understood and rational therapy can be applied. On the other hand, treatment is usually successful through management of the underlying causal condition.

The term *acute colonic pseudo-obstruction* implies that non-obstructive massive dilatation of the colon is temporary and reversible. Ogilvie described this dilatation in association with invasion and destruction of the celiac axis and semilunar ganglion by retroperitoneal malignancy.[31] He hypothesized that the cause was "sympathetic deprivation." The constellation of findings has been reported in association with a widely heterogeneous group of clinical disorders, and therefore a variety of causes are operative (Table 37-6).[32] The list is very similar to that compiled for ileus (see Table 37-5). Numerous mechanisms must be operative for such a range of associated conditions. Impaired motility and aerophagia play an important role, but which comes first and which dominates is uncertain. It is likely that the massive dilatation initiates autoinhibitory reflexes that perpetuate the problem.

Toxic megacolon occurs in severe inflammatory bowel disease and in other forms of colitis including bacillary or amebic dysentery. The exact pathogenesis remains an enigma, but it is likely that transmural inflammation adversely affects the muscle layer in some way. Inhibitory drugs such as anticholinergics, opiates, and antidiarrheals probably have an important deleterious effect and must be avoided or discontinued.

Other Considerations

Probably the catastrophic condition most easily confused with obstruction is mesenteric insufficiency. This is most commonly

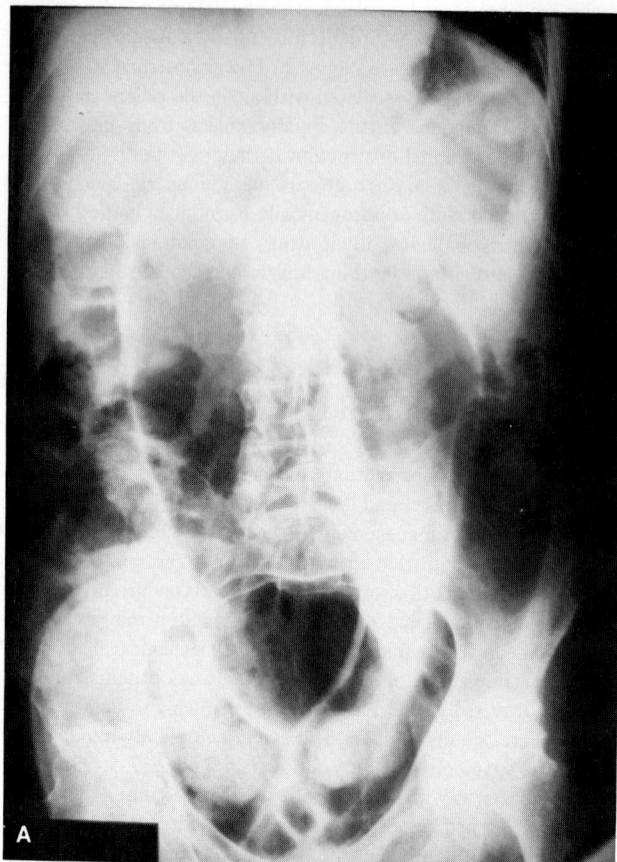
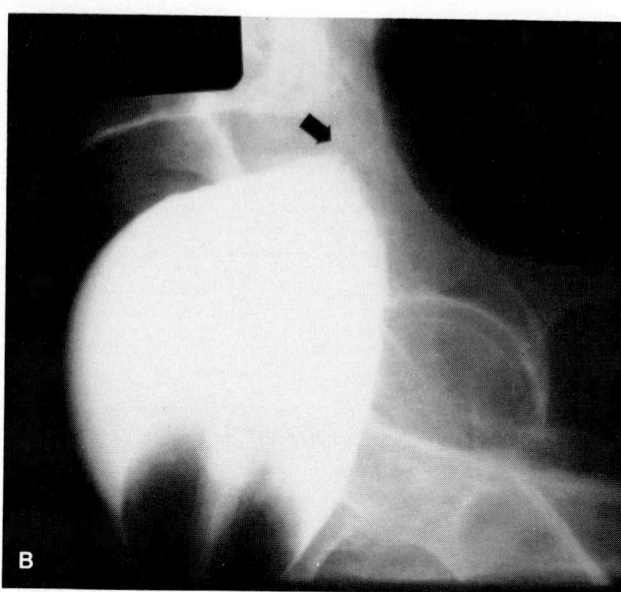

FIGURE 37–3. Plain abdominal x-ray showing colonic obstruction secondary to sigmoid volvulus.

caused by emboli, atherosclerotic plaques, low blood flow states, or dissecting abdominal aortic aneurysms. Patients may experience colicky abdominal pain following meals and later develop a picture more like ileus. If mesenteric insufficiency is suspected, an immediate angiogram is indicated to confirm the diagnosis. Other acute abdominal disorders with severe pain may also simulate obstruction or ileus or actually coexist with either of them. Therefore in planning the diagnostic strategy, it is necessary to consider the lists of differential diagnoses outlined in Tables 37-3 through 37-6. During the initial patient encounter, the studies marked by an asterisk in Table 37-7 should be obtained as quickly as possible in combination with a history and physical examination. Other listed studies will be included as suggested by the clinical examination and initial study results.

ASSESSMENT

Biochemical and Hematologic Tests

Laboratory studies have limited usefulness in the diagnosis of mechanical obstruction, but they may be important in adynamic ileus, and they are sometimes critical in the management of both of these problems (see Table 37-7). Early in the course of ob-

struction all of the results of the blood tests are usually normal. Except for laboratory indications of infection, inflammation, or tumors (e.g., abscesses, tuberculosis, eosinophilic gastroenteritis, Crohn's disease, carcinoid neoplasms, lymphomas, or adenocarcinomas), there are rare occasions when biochemical and hematologic tests aid in establishing the cause of mechanical obstruction. In contrast, because of the frequent metabolic abnormalities that cause or are associated with ileus, laboratory tests are essential in discovering the underlying cause of ileus and in determining its management. In more mild conditions, measurement of electrolytes, blood urea nitrogen, and creatinine is helpful in assessing fluid balance and the presence and severity of dehydration. As vomiting and dehydration are more prolonged, hemoconcentration increases and the hemoglobin, hematocrit, and serum albumin levels rise. Leukocytosis is common in infectious and inflammatory disorders. In more severe cases, the measurement of arterial blood gases is also necessary to assess acid–base balance. More proximal obstructions cause greater acid–base imbalance, while the more distal obstructions cause greater electrolyte disorders.

If the bowel is ischemic or infarcted, a variety of enzymes may "leak" across the intestine and/or be released into the circulation. Elevations in amylase, alkaline phosphatase, creatine phosphokinase, aspartate aminotransferase, alanine aminotransferase, and lactate dehydrogenase may all be encountered in ischemia or infarction with or without sepsis. It must be emphasized that their levels may also be normal and that no laboratory test is a reliable indicator of infarction. Any of these enzyme levels may be elevated

TABLE 37–5
Causes of Adynamic Ileus

INTRA-ABDOMINAL CAUSES	EXTRA-ABDOMINAL CAUSES
Reflex inhibition	Reflex inhibition
Laparotomy	Rib, spine, or pelvic fractures
Abdominal trauma	Myocardial infarction
Inflammatory conditions	Pneumonia/pulmonary embolus
Perforated viscous/penetrating wounds	Burns
Bile peritonitis	Black widow spider bites
Chemical peritonitis	Drug-induced
Intraperitoneal hemorrhage	Anticholinergic/ganglionic antagonists
Toxic megacolon	Opiates
Familial Mediterranean fever	Chemotherapeutic agents
Acute pancreatitis	Metabolic abnormalities
Celiac disease	Septicemia
Acute irradiation injury	Electrolyte imbalance
Abdominal irradiation	Heavy metal poisoning (lead, mercury)
Infectious processes	Porphyria
Bacterial peritonitis	Uremia
Appendicitis	Diabetic ketoacidosis
Cholecystitis	Sickle cell disease
Diverticulitis	
Ischemic processes	
Arterial insufficiency	
Venous thrombosis	
Mesenteric arteritis	
Strangulation obstruction	
Retroperitoneal processes	
Ureteropelvic stones	
Pyelonephritis	
Retroperitoneal hemorrhage	
Pheochromocytoma	

because of primary pancreatic or hepatic disease. Sepsis may contribute to most of the same abnormalities plus elevations in bilirubin and serum and urine phosphate. Most of the abnormalities show up very late in the course of the disease.[33–36] Gross or occult blood in the stool often occurs with cancer of the colon or infarction. Therefore even though abnormalities in laboratory tests may occur because of intestinal infarction, they are neither sensitive nor specific in this setting.

Radiologic Studies

PLAIN FILMS

When the clinical evaluation suggests either obstruction or ileus, radiographic examination is extremely helpful to confirm their presence, differentiate between the two disorders, localize the level of an obstruction, and contribute to an understanding of the underlying cause.[37] The first studies to be selected include posteroanterior and lateral chest films and upright and supine films of the abdomen without contrast media. The chest radiograph is important to detect pneumonia or other extra-abdominal processes as a cause of ileus, to evaluate cardiorespiratory status preoperatively, and to discover free air or other subdiaphragmatic abnormalities. If an upright chest film is not physically or technically possible, a cross-table lateral film of the abdomen with the left side down may demonstrate free peritoneal air. It is important to wait 5 to 10 minutes after assumption of this position to allow migration of small amounts of air to the paracolic gutter to the nondependent surface.

The abdominal films demonstrate the distribution of gas and fluid in the gastrointestinal tract. The jejunum lies in the left upper and central abdomen, the ileum lies in the right central and lower abdomen, while the colon occupies the flanks and right iliac fossa. Some radiologists recommend a prone abdominal view instead of or in addition to a supine view because it allows intestinal gas to fill the left colon and rectum, improving the assessment of colonic obstruction.[38]

Normally there is almost no air in the small intestine and only scattered gas bubbles and feces in the colon. In early or incomplete small bowel obstruction, gas and fluid begin to accumulate, causing the lumen to become dilated. Air, fluid, and feces persist in the colon, and it is difficult to determine the level of obstruction or

TABLE 37–6
Causes of Acute Colonic Pseudo-Obstruction

INTRA-ABDOMINAL CAUSES	EXTRA-ABDOMINAL CAUSES
Reflex inhibition	Reflex inhibition
Cholecystectomy	Craniotomy
Cesarean section	Coronary bypass
Renal transplantation	Open heart surgery
Urologic operations	Fractures
Trauma	Drug-induced
Inflammatory conditions	Phenothiazines
Acute cholecystitis	Tricyclic antidepressants
Acute pancreatitis	Laxative abuse
Inflammatory bowel disease	Chemotherapy
Acute irradiation injury	Metabolic abnormalities
Pelvic irradiation	Systemic infection
Infectious processes	Alcohol
Spontaneous bacterial peritonitis	Lead poisoning
Herpes zoster	Acute or chronic renal failure
Anorectal herpes simplex	Narcolepsy
Ischemic process	Chronic obstructive pulmonary disease
Inferior mesenteric insufficiency	
Retroperitoneal processes	
Malignancy	
Hematoma/hemorrhage	

Adapted from Anuras S, Shirazi S. Colonic pseudo-obstruction. Am J Gastroenterol 1984;79:525.

TABLE 37–7
Laboratory Tests That May Be Helpful in Evaluation and Treatment of Ileus and Obstruction

Gastrointestinal Tests

*Stool occult blood
*Plain upright/supine radiographs
Barium/liquid contrast radiographs
Endoscopy—upper and lower
Arteriography
Bile acid breath test
Quantitative intestinal fluid culture
Scintigraphic emptying and transit studies
Computed tomography
Manometry

Hematologic Tests

*Complete blood cell count
  Erythrocytes
  Hemoglobin/hematocrit
  Leukocytes
  Platelets
Iron/TIBC/ferritin
Blood culture
Clotting function
  Fibrinogen
  Prothrombin
  Partial thromboplastin
  Fibrin split products
Vitamin B_{12}, folate

Fluid/Electrolyte/Acid–Base Balance

*Serum concentrations
  Sodium
  Potassium
  Chloride
  Bicarbonate
*Blood gases
  Po_2
  Pco_2
  pH

Cardiorespiratory Tests

*Electrocardiogram
Central venous pressure
Pulmonary artery wedge pressure
*Chest radiograph
Pulmonary function studies
Sputum culture

Renal Tests

*Urinalysis
  Volume
  Sugar
  Electrolytes
  Osmolality
  Blood/bacteria
*Serum urea/creatinine
Urine culture
Intravenous pyelography
Ultrasonography

Hepatobiliary and Pancreatic Tests

*Bilirubin
*Alkaline phosphatase
*Transaminases
Lactate dehydrogenase
Creatine phosphokinase
*Cholesterol/triglycerides
*Serum/urine amylase
*Lipase
Endoscopic retrograde cholangiopancreatography
Ascitic fluid culture

Endocrine/Metabolic Tests

*Blood glucose
Thyroid function
Vanillylmandelic acid/catecholamines
*Calcium/magnesium/phosphate
Somatostatin
Blood alcohol
Toxins
Blood drug concentrations

* *Test indicated in essentially all patients with suspected ileus or obstruction.*

---

even to differentiate obstruction from a localized ileus without contrast media. With total luminal blockage, more gas and fluid accumulate proximal to the level of the obstruction and the lumen becomes widely dilated (often greater than 3.5 cm in the jejunum). The small intestinal valvulae conniventes produce markings across the entire luminal diameter (Fig 37-4). In the upright or decubitus position, multiple air-fluid levels occur with a "step-ladder" pattern (i.e. different levels in adjacent loops). Distal to the obstruction, the bowel, including the colon, empties and collapses within 12

to 24 hours. When air persists in the colon, its diameter is less than that of the small bowel.

With colonic obstruction, most or all of the air and fluid accumulate in the colon proximal to the obstruction if the ileocecal valve is competent. The haustra cause incomplete indentations in the contour of the wall, producing a scalloped effect. Distal to the obstruction the colon and rectum become free of gas and feces. If the ileocecal valve is incompetent or absent, gas and fluid will be seen throughout both the proximal colon and the small bowel

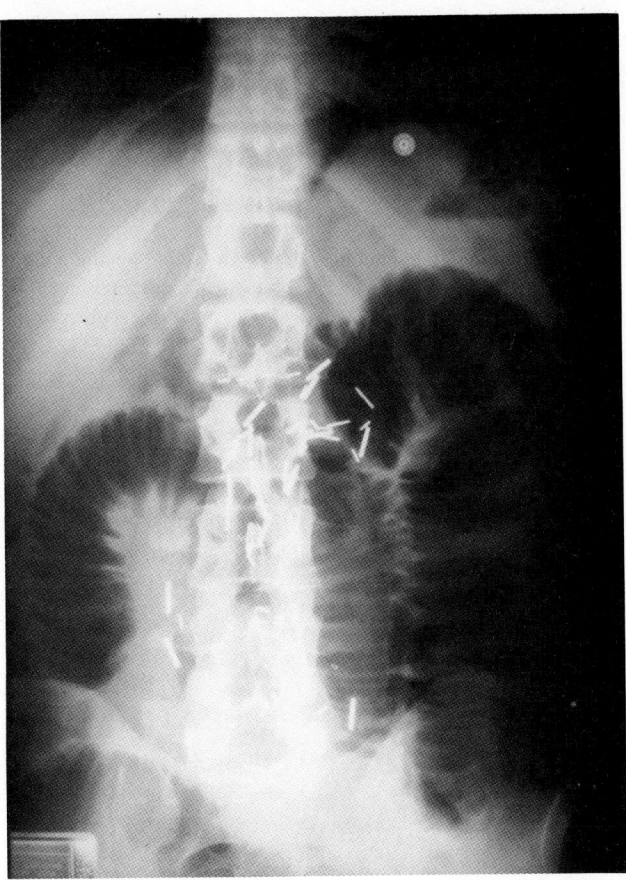

FIGURE 37–4. Plain abdominal x-ray showing multiple dilated loops of intestine indicating small bowel obstruction due to adhesions from previous surgery.

air-fluid levels tend to be longer and more pronounced. A "step-ladder" appearance can occur in either obstruction or ileus. However, if multiple air-fluid levels appear in a "string of beads" pattern, a high-grade partial or complete obstruction of small bowel is highly likely. This is caused by small air bubbles trapped in the superior recesses of splayed-out valvulae conniventes in an upright or decubitus position while the dilated loop is filled with large amounts of fluid. Supine films, on the other hand, may show little or no gas in the small intestine.

CONTRAST STUDIES

The differentiation of ileus from mechanical obstruction is not always possible with plain abdominal films, and the presence or absence of obstruction can only be determined by using contrast media. Barium provides better contrast and detail than water-soluble media, but it should not be used if there is any question of bowel viability or perforation. If there is any doubt about the site of obstruction, barium should not be given orally until colonic obstruction is excluded by barium enema or colonoscopy. If orally administered barium accumulates proximal to an obstruction in the colon, water continues to be extracted and the barium becomes inspissated and impacted. It can only be removed at the time of operation, which may be hazardous because of potential spillage. Barium should be used for retrograde studies but avoided if there is a possibility of perforation. Free barium within the peritoneal cavity creates an intense inflammatory reaction. It is acceptable to give barium orally or by intubation in small bowel obstruction

and the findings will resemble small bowel obstruction. Except with proximal colonic obstruction, the diameter of the transverse colon will be greater than that of the small bowel.

Early in the course of strangulation, no features clearly distinguish the radiologic findings from those of simple obstruction. When strangulation is far advanced, the necrotic bowel loses its mucosal contour and becomes splayed by edema, exhibiting a "thumb-printed" appearance. Air may be seen in the bowel wall, in branches of the portal venous system, or lying free within the peritoneal cavity, signifying perforation.

In ileus, gas and fluid accumulate differently throughout the gastrointestinal tract (Fig 37-5). Loops of mildly distended bowel may develop proximal or adjacent to an acute inflammatory process such as appendicitis or pancreatitis. These loops are involved by a localized ileus and are called "sentinel loops." If peritonitis co-exists with ileus, the bowel wall becomes thickened and the pro-peritoneal fat line becomes obscured. If ascites is present, it produces a "ground-glass" density throughout the abdomen. In acute colonic pseudo-obstruction, the entire colon becomes dilated, but the cecal diameter is usually the greatest.

In the differentiation between ileus and obstruction, the degree of intestinal distention, the amount of intraluminal fluid and gas, and the distribution pattern of air-fluid levels in upright or decubitus position are important features to compare. Obstruction usually causes more fluid and gas accumulation than ileus, and

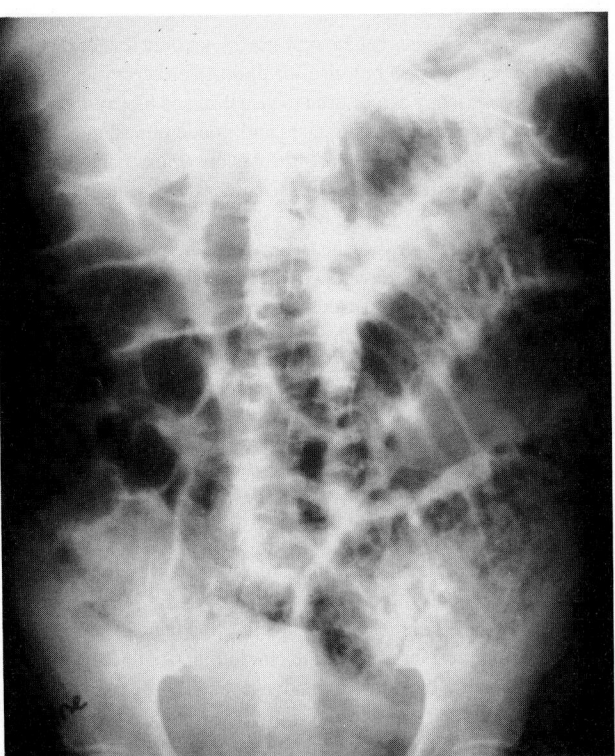

FIGURE 37–5. The small intestine is dilated and distended with gas and a small amount of air is also present in the colon. These findings are suggestive of ileus, in this situation due to jejunal ischemic necrosis.

after colonic obstruction is excluded. Net secretion keeps the barium in a liquid suspension, and it can be removed through an intraluminal tube. In small bowel obstruction, barium provides superior definition to water-soluble media, which is hyperosmolar and becomes diluted by secretion and mixing with intestinal contents, thus reducing contrast.

A nonionic contrast agent such as metrizamide (Amipaque) is isotonic with blood. Therefore, it is the contrast agent of choice whenever a water-soluble agent is needed. However, high cost at the present time limits its clinical application to neonates and young children.

OTHER IMAGING PROCEDURES

Angiography is sometimes useful in diagnosing abdominal tumors, but other modalities have now nearly replaced this method. It is most useful in some cases of mesenteric ischemia and infarction. Ultrasonography has a very limited role in both obstruction and ileus because the "gas blocking" from the dilated loops of bowel prevents imaging beyond the tissue–gas interface. Computed axial tomography may be helpful in establishing the diagnosis and should be used if the plain and contrast radiographs are inconclusive. It should be remembered, however, that establishing the diagnosis with certainty preoperatively is not always necessary. It may not even be desirable if a needed operation is delayed by waiting for the test.

Other Studies

Endoscopic techniques can be very useful not only for the diagnosis of ileus or obstruction but also for definitive therapy. Esophagogastroduodenoscopy can be used to visualize and biopsy obstructive lesions in the esophagus, stomach, and duodenum. Benign ulcers, strictures, and carcinomas are the lesions most commonly encountered. Sometimes edema or submucosal extension of the process may obscure the lesion, but in the majority of cases it can be seen and biopsied or brushed. In addition, pneumatic balloon catheters have been developed in graded sizes to accomplish brusque dilatation of obstructing lesions. Radial cuts can be made in narrow short strictures and membranes, and heater probes, bipolar cautery devices, and lasers can be used to rapidly heat and coagulate obstructing tumors. The necrotic tissue then sloughs and provides a larger opening in the lumen. A long fiberoptic enteroscope has been developed to examine the small bowel, but it is not yet widely available. In all endoscopic studies, especially upper gastrointestinal endoscopies, the use of carbon dioxide should be seriously considered for insufflation instead of air. Carbon dioxide is rapidly absorbed and can reduce excessive distention and pain proximal to the obstruction.

The same techniques are available for diagnosis and therapy in the rectum and large intestine (including the ileocecal valve). The instruments include the rigid sigmoidoscope, the flexible fiberoptic or video sigmoidoscope, and the fiberoptic or video colonoscope for visualization and biopsy of lesions, dilatation, and cauterization.

Intestinal or, to a lesser extent, colonic manometry is used to evaluate motor function. Experience with the technique is limited

in acute disorders, and it is more helpful in chronic disorders. Total contractile activity is reduced or absent in ileus. Abnormal contractile patterns may be present in obstruction. The typical pattern seen in small bowel obstruction after a meal is clustered contractions: brief regular contractions occurring at 5-second intervals and preceded and followed by quiescent periods lasting longer than a minute (see Fig 37-2). Giant, high-amplitude contractions may also occur, but they are not present in normal postprandial motility recordings. This pattern is not specific for obstruction because it has been reported in other conditions, including pseudo-obstruction. Fortunately ileus and mechanical obstruction can be distinguished using ordinary clinical techniques. At this time, manometry must be considered to be a research rather than a reliable clinical tool to definitively establish the cause of ileus or obstruction. Interesting findings have been reported, but caution is in order before using manometry to make important therapeutic decisions.

An abdominal paracentesis should be done in situations in which fluid is present and the cause of obstruction or ileus is not clear. The presence of blood, bile, amylase, proteins, leukocytes, bacteria, or malignant cells may be very helpful in therapeutic decisions.

THERAPEUTIC CONSIDERATIONS

Therapeutic Strategy

Following the initial evaluation and establishment of the presence of obstruction or ileus, fluid, electrolytes and acid–base resuscitation should begin. Adjustments in the composition and rate of administration are made as soon as the relevant laboratory tests become available. Decompression of the distended bowel is instituted at the same time via nasogastric aspiration. The next decision to be made is that of urgent operative therapy versus expectant operative therapy versus nonoperative therapy.

Acute complete bowel obstruction is a surgical emergency. The objective of treatment is to relieve the mechanical impediment to propulsion, and operative therapy is most often the means to that end. Ileus is managed by treating the underlying cause, and operative therapy should be avoided entirely unless some other intraabdominal catastrophe requires laparotomy. Close communication with a surgeon is essential in deciding the course of action.

Replacement of Fluids

Correction of fluid, electrolyte, and acid–base imbalance must be guided by the level and duration of obstruction and measurements of the hematocrit, serum sodium, potassium, chloride, bicarbonate, blood urea nitrogen, creatinine, and arterial blood gases and pH. Bedside estimates of dehydration are inaccurate, although orthostatic hypotension and tachycardia support the need to begin therapy. If severe hypovolemia exists, restoration of intravascular fluid volume should be monitored by urinary output, central venous pressure, and arterial blood pressure. If heart failure, chronic obstructive pulmonary disease, or renal failure is a concurrent problem, a Swan-Ganz catheter should be used to monitor left ventricular function.

Fluid replacement should be based on estimates of previous deficits, daily maintenance requirements, and current losses. Mild to moderately severe dehydration may vary from 4% to 8% of total body weight. Half of this deficit should be given during the first 24 hours and half during the second 24 hours. Maintenance requirements amount to an average of 1500 to 2000 mL in an afebrile 70-kg person having normal renal function. Continued losses through vomiting or nasogastric suction can be measured to allow calculation of total fluid replacement and caloric loss. A balanced salt solution, such as lactated Ringer's solution, should be used to correct the deficit.

With metabolic *alkalosis* from a gastric outlet obstruction, fluid replacement should begin with isotonic sodium chloride. As soon as adequate urine output is assured, potassium chloride should be given, because renal potassium loss is great in gastric outlet obstruction. The potassium loss can be measured in a 24-hour urine sample. Hydrochloric acid can be given intravenously, but it is rarely needed. In metabolic *acidosis*, 2 mM sodium bicarbonate or one-sixth molar sodium lactate should be given. Large amounts of sodium bicarbonate given as ampules of 44.6 mM may produce intracellular volume depletion. If correction of acidosis with sodium bicarbonate is too rapid, cerebrospinal fluid pH may fall rapidly and worsen neurologic symptoms. Overcorrection of arterial pH above 7.4 shifts the hemoglobin dissociation curve to the left and reduces delivery of oxygen to the tissue by increasing the affinity of hemoglobin for oxygen. Slower restoration of pH to 7.4 may be desirable, and if there is no liver dysfunction, sodium lactate may be preferred over sodium bicarbonate. The following is a rough calculation for net bicarbonate deficit due to gastrointestinal loss:

$$(24 \text{ mEq/L} - \text{measured plasma } [HCO_3^-])$$

$$\times \ 0.6 \text{ body weight (kg)}$$

Bicarbonate should be given if the arterial pH is less than 7.1. Half of the calculated deficit should be given to raise the plasma bicarbonate concentration to 16 mEq/L over 12 to 24 hours.

Decompression of the Bowel

There is value in reducing gaseous distention. It is distressing for the patient because it causes pain and respiratory embarrassment. Distention also causes nausea and vomiting and may result in aspiration, particularly during induction of anesthesia. Nasogastric suction is appropriate in both obstruction and ileus, but the use of long indwelling intestinal tubes such as the Cantor tube or Miller-Abbott tube is controversial and not routinely recommended.[39] The long tubes are difficult and sometimes impossible to pass into the intestine. They have balloons that may expand to dangerous volumes during passage, and they are probably no more effective in reducing distention than a nasogastric tube. They may be tried if strangulation is unlikely, if nasogastric suction is ineffective, or if long-term nonoperative therapy is planned. If nothing is allowed by mouth for several days, some provision must be made for nutrition.

Principles of Surgical Treatment

As a general rule, acute complete mechanical obstruction of the small intestine should be relieved as soon as preoperative resuscitation is adequate and nasogastric decompression is established. In the presence of complete obstruction, strangulation cannot be excluded by clinical criteria and delay in operation may be fatal.[40] The reason for urgency is that the mortality associated with ischemic bowel complicating obstruction is high, and this problem can be detected with certainty only at operation. Thus an operation provides the ultimate procedure to detect strangulation and to accomplish definitive treatment. Antibiotics are almost always given prophylactically because an enterotomy in an unprepared bowel has a high incidence of wound infection and sepsis is a frequent complication whenever blood flow is compromised. Coverage must be provided for anaerobes and gram-negative organisms.

When strangulation is encountered from any cause, the grossly necrotic bowel is resected and the viability of the adjacent bowel must be assessed. This is difficult if not impossible on the basis of gross observation of the tissue. Two important new intraoperative aids in improving the accuracy include Doppler ultrasonography and fluoroscein dye injection. After restoring mesenteric circulation, a hand-held Doppler probe sends and receives the sound waves to assess blood flow.[41] The technique is easy to perform and has been shown to determine viability accurately as confirmed by a second-look operation.[42] Intravenous fluoroscein can be quantitatively detected in the bowel through the use of a perfusion fluorimeter. This method is also highly accurate and useful in determining viability, especially in longer segments.[43,44] Nonperfused segments are resected followed by an end-to-end anastomosis. Primary neoplasms of the small intestine are rare but require adequate resection with lymph node dissection when the lesion is malignant.

In partial small bowel obstruction immediate operative therapy is not usually necessary. There is time to establish the severity and underlying cause with the relevant diagnostic tests. If the patient continues to pass stool and flatus and if air persists in the colon, strangulation is unlikely and expectant therapy is usually appropriate. If any worrisome signs should arise such as fever, rebound tenderness, leukocytosis, or unexplained hyperamylasemia, laparotomy is indicated. If and when total obstruction develops, immediate laparotomy must be considered. If an external hernia can be found, gentle attempts should be made to reduce it, avoiding excessive force and watching for evidence of infarction or perforation after successful reduction.

Immediate operation is also usually not indicated if the patient has had a history of multiple previous episodes of bowel obstruction, multiple abdominal operations with extensive adhesions, extensive abdominal radiation therapy, bacterial peritonitis, Crohn's disease, or carcinomatosis with widespread metastases. In these situations, strangulation is less likely due to fixation of the bowel. Operative procedures in this setting are exceedingly difficult owing to dense adhesions, increasing the risk of inadvertent enterotomies that risk wound contamination, infection, and postoperative intestinal fistulas. If the condition persists for 2 days or clinical deterioration ensues, an operation should be performed.[45] If it resolves, the patient may be followed. If nonoperative therapy is chosen and decompression does not produce marked clinical improvement and resolution of bowel distention in 24 to 48 hours, successful nonoperative therapy is unlikely and surgical intervention is indicated.[39,45] If signs of bowel infarction do appear at any time, abdominal exploration is urgently indicated. It should be stressed that immediate operation versus tube decompression and close observation for 48 hours in the treatment of small bowel obstruction remains controversial. The mortality with ischemic bowel is about 30%, and the high risk of this potential complication plus the difficulty in prompt detection supports early operative therapy as the more prudent plan in most settings.

In obstruction of the colon, the principles of correcting dehydration and electrolyte balance, decompressing the bowel, and administering antibiotics before operation also apply. Nasogastric suction may or may not be effective in reducing the distention. The two most common obstructing colonic lesions are diverticulitis and colon carcinoma. The two may be difficult or impossible to distinguish on clinical or radiologic grounds, and they may coexist. If there is any doubt about the diagnosis of diverticular disease after radiologic or endoscopic studies, a resection should be done. Sometimes the cancer is apparent only after careful histologic examination. If the problem presents as an acute obstruction, proper bowel cleansing is often not possible. A two-stage operation consisting of resection and diversion followed by reanastomosis at a later date is necessary because primary anastomoses have a high rate of anastomotic leaks, wound contamination, and abscess formation. The management problems with diverticular disease are very similar to those with cancer. If there is a perforation and abscess, the diseased bowel is often resected and the proximal segment temporarily diverted.[46]

Nonoperative therapy may be possible in a number of situations. Frequently volvulus of the sigmoid colon and less often the cecum can be reduced by aspirating the gas with a colonoscopically placed tube. Another technique that may be tried in sequence is to exert gentle hydrostatic pressure with a barium enema or other rectally introduced contrast medium. The risk of perforation or necrosis cannot be ignored using either of these procedures. If they are successful, frequent examinations should continue for several days to watch for signs of infarction. Because there is a tendency for recurrence with both cecal and sigmoid volvulus, elective repair is usually advisable. Resection rather than fixation is indicated if there is evidence of ischemia, and some recommend it in all cases.[47] Adhesions or radiation-induced strictures are uncommon causes of obstruction in the colon. Endoscopic treatment with hydrostatic or pneumatic balloons can sometimes relieve the obstruction, obviating the need for emergency surgery in some cases, although recurrences demand definitive surgical therapy.[48]

Palliative relief of obstruction can sometimes be accomplished in inoperable cancer through the use of laser coagulation.[49,50] The neodymium-YAG laser is directed at the lesion under endoscopic guidance. The tumor is partially vaporized and coagulated; the necrotic tissue sloughs, and the lumen is restored. Although perforation is a risk, this procedure may be preferable to surgical therapy in elderly patients with other serious medical problems.

The therapy for ileus is primarily directed toward treatment of the underlying or associated disease. Sometimes that is not apparent and the ileus resolves spontaneously. Supportive care and the resolution of the associated condition is accompanied by return of intestinal or colonic motor activity. Drugs inhibitory to motility should be withdrawn if at all possible. In most cases,

however, thorough search for the underlying cause is the key to successful management. In the postoperative period temporary ileus is expected. The use of sympathetic antagonists or cholinergic agonists is not helpful. The use of the newer prokinetic drugs such as metoclopramide or domperidone have not been fully evaluated. Withdrawal of any drugs that inhibit motility, especially narcotics, is of benefit. If evidence of obstruction appears after the ileus has resolved and the patient has begun oral intake, then a new mechanical obstruction must be suspected and proper steps must be initiated to document and treat the problem, including a repeat laparotomy if necessary.[51]

In acute colonic pseudo-obstruction, fluids and electrolyte imbalance must be corrected; nothing is allowed by mouth and nasogastric suction is instituted. The patient must be examined frequently to assess abdominal girth, tenderness, and signs of peritoneal irritation or sepsis. As in intestinal ileus, treatment must be directed toward any underlying cause such as sepsis and inhibitory drugs should be withdrawn. Gentle enemas may aid in evacuation of the distal bowel, but the use of prokinetic (motor stimulating) drugs has been disappointing. Plain abdominal radiographs should be obtained regularly to determine changes in colonic diameter. If the condition can be anticipated or recognized early, it is likely that massive dilatation can be prevented with supportive care. Although 12 cm is often stated to be the upper limit of colonic diameter to continue medical management, a rapidly expanding colonic diameter is better evidence of impending perforation and a more important indicator of risk than a single numeric value. Furthermore, the risk of perforation appears to correlate better with the duration of dilatation than with the diameter.[52] If an ominous degree of dilatation appears, some method of rapid decompression must be instituted because perforation, massive peritoneal soilage, and fatal sepsis may be the result. A surgical cecostomy has been the standard therapy and may still be indicated in some cases. More recently, colonoscopic deflation has been enthusiastically recommended with a high success rate from 75% to 100%.[53,54] The use of carbon dioxide insufflation and a large-bore catheter taped alongside the colonoscope may facilitate the procedure. However, new information is altering the approach to the problem. Acute colonic pseudo-obstruction may not be as hazardous as previously thought; colonoscopy has its own inherent risk of perforation, especially in a poorly prepared colon, and the dilatation often resolves spontaneously with conservative, nonendoscopic, and nonsurgical treatment (86%).[55] Therefore, present information supports initial conservative therapy of acute colonic pseudo-obstruction, but careful clinical monitoring continues to be mandatory because perforation remains a disastrous complication. If the problem is unresponsive or worsens, then colonoscopic deflation should be attempted, followed by operative cecostomy in the event of failure.

The reader is directed to Chapter 34, Approach to the Patient with Abdominal Pain; Chapter 36, Approach to the Patient with Acute Abdomen and Fever of Abdominal Origin; Chapter 67, Dysmotility of the Small Intestine; Chapter 73, Bacterial Overgrowth; and Chapter 81, Motility Disorders of the Colon.

REFERENCES

1. Shikata CI, Shida T, Amino K, et al. Experimental studies on the hemodynamics of the small intestine following increased intraluminal pressure. Surg Gynecol Obstet 1983;156:155.
2. Papanicolaou G, Nikas D, Ahn YK, et al. Regional blood flow and water content of the obstructed small intestine. Arch Surg 1985;20:926.
3. Wagner R, Gabbert H, Höhn P. The mechanism of epithelial shedding after ischemic damage to the small intestinal mucosa: a light and electron microscopic investigation. Virchows Arch (Cell Pathol) 1979;30:25.
4. Robinson JWL, Mirkovitch V. The recovery of function and microcirculation in small intestinal loops. Gut 1972;13:784.
5. Gorbach SL. Intestinal microflora. Gastroenterology 1971;60:1110.
6. Hill MJ, Drasar BS. The normal colonic bacterial flora. Gut 1975;16:318.
7. Giannella RA, Broitman SA, Zamcheck N. Gastric acid barrier to ingested microorganisms in man: studies in vivo and in vitro. Gut 1972;13:251.
8. Sykes PA, Boulter KH, Schofield PF. The microflora of the obstructed bowel. Br J Surg 1976;63:721.
9. Van Trappen G, Janssens J, Hellemans J, et al: The interdigestive motor complex of normal subjects and patients with bacterial overgrowth of the small intestine. J Clin Invest 1977;59:1158.
10. Shields R. The absorption and secretion of fluid and electrolytes by the obstructed bowel. Br J Surg 1965;52:774.
11. Heneghan JB, Robinson JWL, Menge H, et al. Intestinal obstruction in germ-free dogs. Eur J Clin Invest 1981;11:285.
12. Summers RW, Yanda R, Prihoda M, et al. Acute intestinal obstruction: an electromyographic study in dogs. Gastroenterology 1983;85:1301.
13. Prihoda J, Flatt A, Summers RW. Mechanisms of motility changes during acute intestinal pseudo-obstruction. Am J Physiol 1984;247(Gastrointest Liver Physiol 10):G37.
14. Arnbjornsson E. Normal and pathological bowel sound patterns. Ann Chir Gynaecol 1986;75:314.
15. Summers RW, Anuras S, Green J. Jejunal manometry patterns in health: partial intestinal obstruction and pseudo-obstruction. Gastroenterology 1983;85:1290.
16. Coxon JE, Dickson C, Taylor I. Changes in colonic motility during the development of chronic large bowel obstruction. Br J Surg 1985
17. Fraser ID, Condon RE, Schulte WJ, et al. Intestinal motility in experimental large bowel obstruction. Surgery 1980;87:677.
18. Smith J, Kelly KA, Weinshilboum RM. Pathophysiology of postoperative ileus. Arch Surg 1977;112:203.
19. Woods JH, Erickson LW, Condon RE, et al. Postoperative ileus: a colonic problem? Surgery 1978;84:527.
20. Bueno L, Fioramonti J, Ruckebusch Y. Postoperative intestinal motility in dogs and sheep. Dig Dis Sci 1978;23:682.
21. Wilson, JP. Postoperative motility of the large intestine in man. Gut 1975;16:689.
22. Condon RE, Cowles VE, Schulte WJ, et al. Resolution of postoperative ileus in humans. Ann Surg 1986;203:574.
23. Jahnberg T, Abrahamsson H, Jansson G, et al. Vagal gastric relaxation in the dog. Scand J Gastroenterol 1977;12:221.
24. Abrahamsson H, Glise H, Glise K. Reflux suppression of gastric motility during laparotomy and gastroduodenal nociceptive stimulation. Scand J Gastroenterol 1979;14:101.
25. Dubois A, Henry DP, Kopin IJ. Plasma catecholamine and postoperative gastrointestinal propulsion in the rat. Gastroenterology 1975;68:466.
26. Dubois A, Weise VK, Kopin IJ. Postoperative ileus in the rat; physiopathology, etiology and treatment. Ann Surg 1973;178:781.
27. Dubois A, Kopin IJ, Pettigrew K, et al. Chemical and histochemical studies of postoperative sympathetic activity in the digestive tract. Gastroenterology 1974;66:403.
28. Wallin G, Cassuto J, Hogstrom S, et al. Failure of epidural anesthesia to prevent postoperative paralytic ileus. Anesthesiology 1986;65:292.
29. Malone PC. The physiology of intestinal oxygenation and the pathophysiology of intestinal ileus. Med Hypotheses 1987;22:111.
30. Thompson MA, Summers R. Barium impaction as a complication of gastrointestinal scleroderma. JAMA 1976;235:1715.
31. Ogilvie H. Large intestine colic due to sympathetic deprivation: a new clinical syndrome. Br Med J 1948;2:671.
32. Anuras S, Shirazi S. Colonic pseudo-obstruction. Am J Gastroenterol 1984;79:525.
33. Graeber GM, O'Niell JF, Wolf RE, et al. Elevated levels of peripheral serum creatine phosphokinase with strangulated small bowel obstruction. Arch Surg 1983;118:837.
34. Sachs SM, Morton JH, Schwartz SI. Acute mesenteric ischemia. Surg 1982;92:646.
35. Lamar W, Woodward L, Statland BE. Clinical implications of creatine kinase-BB isoenzymes. N Engl J Med 1978;299:234.
36. Jamieson WG, Taylor BM, Troster M. The significance of urine phosphate measurements in the early diagnosis of intestinal infarction. Surg Gynecol Obstet 1979;148:334.
37. Gonzalez R, Siskind BN, Burrell MI. The role of radiology in the evaluation of intestinal obstruction. In: Fielding LP, Welch JP, Moore FD, eds. Intestinal obstruction. Edinburgh: Churchill Livingstone, 1982:28.
38. Buckell NA, Williams GT, Bartram CT, et al. Depth of ulceration in acute colitis: correlation with outcome and radiologic features. Gastroenterology 1980;79:19.
39. Brolin RE. The role of gastrointestinal tube decompression in the treatment of mechanical intestinal obstruction. Am Surgeon 1983;49:131.
40. Sarr MG, Bulkley GB, Zuidema GD. Preoperative recognition of intestinal strangulation obstruction: prospective evaluation of diagnostic capability. Am J Surg 1983;145:176.
41. Cooperman M, Martin EW, Carey LC. Evaluation of ischemic intestine by Doppler ultrasound. Am J Surg 1980;139:73.
42. O'Donnell JA, Hobson RWW. Operative confirmation of Doppler ultrasound in evaluation of intestinal ischemia. Surgery 1980;87:109.
43. Carter MS, Fantine GA, Sammurtano RJ, et al. Quantitative and qualitative fluorescein fluorescence in determining intestinal viability. Am J Surg 1984;147:117.
44. Bulkley GB, Zuidema GD, Hamilton SR, et al. Intraoperative determination of small intestinal viability following ischemic injury. Ann Surg 1981;193:628.
45. Brolin R, Crasna M, Mast B. Use of tubes and radiographs in the management of small bowel obstruction. Ann Surg 1987;206:126.
46. Krukowski Z, Matheson N. Emergency surgery for diverticular disease complicated by generalized and fecal peritonitis: a review. Br J Surg 1984;71:921.
47. Tejler G, Jiborn H. Volvulus of the cecum: report of 26 cases and review of the literature. Dis Colon Rectum 1988;31:445.
48. Siegel J, Yalto R. Hydrostatic balloon catheters: a new dimension of therapeutic endoscopy. Endoscopy 1984;16:231.
49. Eckhauser M. Endoscopic laser vaporization of obstructing left colonic cancer to avoid decompressive colostomy. Gastrointest Endosc 1987;33:105.
50. Kreifhaber P, Huber F, Kreifhaber K. Palliative and preoperative endoscopic neodymium-YAG laser treatment of colorectal cancer. Endoscopy 1987;19:43.
51. Steward R, Page C, Brender J, et al. The incidence and risk of early postoperative small bowel obstruction. Am J Surg 1987;154:643.
52. Johnson CD, Rice RP, Kelvin FM, et al. The radiographic evaluation of gross cecal distension. AJR 1985;145:1211.
53. Strodel WE, Nostrant TT, Eckhauser FE, et al. Therapeutic and diagnostic colonoscopy in nonobstructive colonic dilatation. Ann Surg 1983;197:416.
54. Bode WE, Beart RW: Colonoscopic decompression for acute pseudo-obstruction of the colon. Am J Surg 1984;147:243.
55. Sloyer AF, Panella VS, Demas BE. Ogilvie's syndrome: successful management without colonoscopy. Dig Dis Sci 1988;33:1391.

38

Approach to the Patient with Diarrhea

DON W. POWELL

No group of diseases contrasts better the differences in health care problems faced by developed nations and developing nations than do the diarrheal disorders. In developed nations, diarrheal disorders are primarily of economic significance, accounting for loss of time and productivity from work. In 1980, one could estimate hospitalization costs in the United States of some $2 billion yearly to diagnose and treat acute and chronic diarrhea.[1] In addition, in that same year, neonatal infectious diarrhea in livestock (due to the same diseases that affect man) cost the United States an additional $1 billion.[2] Using a different approach that included outpatient costs and loss of time from work, Garthright and colleagues estimated a cost of $23 billion per year, or $106 per person, in the United States for acute infectious diarrheas.[3] That is not to say that diarrhea is not a cause of death in industrialized nations; it certainly is (see below), and the magnitude of this statistic may be underestimated. However, there is little question that diarrheal diseases are among the leading causes of death and morbidity in the Third World, accounting for 5 to 8 million deaths per year in infants and small children.[4–8]

In both primitive and sophisticated cultures, diarrhea is thought to be a consequence of the ingestion of tainted or unsavory (e.g., "rich" or fatty) food, but it may also have sociologic or moral connotations (e.g., to result from some supernatural cause such as "evil eye," which is known as *mal de ojo* in Central American cultures, *quebranto* in Brazil, *eshwaha* in Sri Lanka, and *nazar* in Pakistan).[9–11] The experienced clinician cannot help but wonder if some of these mystical concerns may also carry over into the cultures of developed nations, because even here diarrhea seems to cause emotional distress far in excess of the physical symptoms that accompany it. Perhaps in Western cultures, Freudian issues involving toilet training are operative.

To the gastroenterologist, diarrhea has special significance as one of the "big three" symptoms of gastrointestinal disease: abdominal pain, nausea/vomiting, and diarrhea. To care for patients well, the physician must understand the pathophysiology of this common symptom and know its many causes.

This chapter will attempt to define, classify, and explain general concepts of the pathophysiology of diarrhea and summarize the epidemiology, clinical presentation, diagnostic evaluation, and therapy of acute diarrhea and of an entirely different group of illnesses that make up chronic diarrhea. This chapter is meant to be considered in conjunction with the information presented in Parts I, II, III, and IV of this book. References to and specific details about the many diseases can be found in those chapters.

DEFINITION

As far as the patient is concerned, diarrhea is best defined as it was by Doctors Roux and Ryle at the turn of the century[12]: "The too rapid evacuation of too fluid stools." Although normal stooling frequency ranges from three times a week to three times a day, the individual patient may report any departure from his or her own standard of frequency or fluidity, as well as stools that cause urgency or abdominal discomfort, as diarrhea.[13,14] Such a definition is "too loose" (sic) for the scientific physician or clinical investigator who prefers to define diarrhea as a physical sign (24-hour excretion weight or volume) rather than as a symptom. Healthy children and adults have daily stool weights of less than 200 g,[15–17] and infants have a daily stool weight of less than 10 g/kg.[18] Stool weights in excess of this are considered as diarrhea by the physician, and because stool varies from 60% to 85% water,[19,20] this definition implies that diarrhea is a disease of intestinal water and electrolyte transport.

Diarrhea should be distinguished from two other symptom complexes often confused by patients: (1) "Pseudodiarrhea" is an increased frequency of defecation with either no change in consistency or a 24-hour stool output below 200 g. Such a stooling pattern often accompanies motility disorders or anorectal disease. It is a common symptom in proctitis of any cause and in the irritable bowel syndrome. (2) Incontinence, which is defined as the involuntary release of rectal contents, is a relatively common but under-reported condition.[21] Although incontinence may be more common when stool is liquid, it is more often due to abnormal neuromuscular function and occurs as a result of neurologic disease (afferent abnormalities of sensation or efferent motor abnormalities) or pelvic problems (trauma to or disease of the sphincter or pelvic muscles).[22] Both pseudodiarrhea and incontinence may be accompanied by urgency and abdominal discomfort.

The factors, aside from water content, governing normal stool weight are not completely understood, but certainly fiber content and bacterial mass are important. One half of the dry weight of stool is due to bacterial cell bodies.[23] Increasing fiber (wheat bran) ingestion from 10 to 26 g per day increases average stool weight from 100 g per day to 149 g per day and increases stool frequency from <1 to nearly 2 times per day.[16,17] The weight of women's stool is less than that of men by one half.[17] This may reflect differences in dietary fiber intake, although hormonal factors have also been implicated. There is some controversy as to whether the ovarian cycles do[17] or do not[24] influence stool weight and consistency. There is reason to believe that both exercise[25] and stress[26] might influence stool weight in that both have been shown to decrease fluid and electrolyte absorption of human jejunum by 50% or greater. Whether the colon can subsequently compensate for these small-bowel changes is unclear. Even personality factors correlate with stool weight.[16] Lastly, intraluminal bile acid content might influence stool weight. The ingestion of cholestyramine[27] or aluminum hydroxide,[28,29] potent bile acid–binding substances, induces constipation. The factors causing abnormal stool weight are now more completely defined and, as described below, result in either a failure of intestinal solute and fluid absorption or actual solute and fluid secretion.

PATHOPHYSIOLOGY AND CLASSIFICATION

There are many ways to classify diarrhea, and each classification permits informative insights into the pathophysiology of this symptom complex. Because no single classification does complete justice to this complicated entity, several classifications are considered below with the idea that in their sum they allow a better definition and understanding of this complex and multifactorial condition.

A Condition of Abnormal Motor Function

In the early part of this century, diarrhea was thought to be due predominantly to abnormal gastrointestinal muscle contraction. Beginning in the 1950s with an increasing number of studies of intestinal water and electrolyte transport in both health and disease, the role of motor activity was relegated more to that of a secondary cause. Certainly the role of gastrointestinal motility in diarrhea was not then, nor is now, completely understood (ch 9 and 10). Suffice it to say that the movement of fluid down the gastrointestinal tract is not a passive phenomenon, nor is defecation; both require muscle contraction. Furthermore, most of the diarrheal conditions that have been studied, both natural and experimental, have been shown to alter *both* intestinal fluid and electrolyte transport as well as smooth muscle function, often with the induction of propagative forms of intestinal motility.[30] What is less clear is whether there is a diarrhea that is caused specifically and only by abnormal motor function—so-called *diarrhée motrice*, as this condition has been labeled by Read.[30] Perhaps the "pseudo-diarrhea" of anorectal disease and rapid small intestinal transit with carbohydrate wastage (see below) are examples of motor diarrhea. Most, however, would agree with the concept of the "diarrhea spiral" (Fig 38-1).

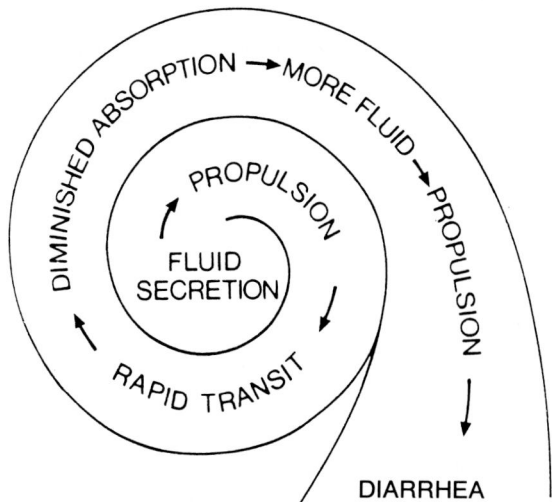

FIGURE 38-1. The diarrhea spiral. Increased intraluminal fluid as the result of abnormalities in intestinal fluid and electrolyte transport initiate propulsive activity both by reflex and as a result of the same pathophysiologic processes that disturbed epithelial function. Rapid transit follows with decreased contact time (and perhaps also diminished surface area). This causes diminished absorption, more intraluminal fluid, more propulsion, and finally diarrhea. (Read NW. Diarrhée motrice. Clin Gastroenterol 1986;15:657.)

A Condition of Abnormal Fluid and Electrolyte Transport

ABNORMAL ABSORPTION

Between 1950 and 1965, physiologists defined the basic concept of the sodium gradient hypothesis and solute-driven water absorption (ch 14).[31–33] These investigators showed that the low intracellular Na concentration, brought about by the basolateral membrane–located Na pump (NaK ATPase), provided the energy for the absorption of Na and the cotransport of nutrients such as glucose and amino acids. They also demonstrated that the transport of water from lumen to blood resulted from an increased osmolality in the intercellular space due to Na and solute absorption. Triple-lumen tube perfusion studies in humans defined the fluid and electrolyte loads and absorptive capacities of the human small intestine and colon.[19,20]

As shown in Table 38-1, entering the duodenum each 24 hours is 8 to 10 L of fluid containing 800 mmol Na, 700 mmol Cl, and 100 mmol K. Two liters of this duodenal load are derived from the diet; the remainder comes from secretions of the salivary glands, stomach, liver, pancreas, and the duodenum itself. The small intestine normally absorbs all but 1.5 L of this fluid, and this is the volume characteristically presented to the colon for absorption. The colon, in turn, absorbs all but approximately 100 ml of this fluid, which contains 3, 8, and 2 mmol of Na, K, and Cl, respectively. Although the maximum absorptive capacity of the small intestine remains undefined, it has been shown that the capacity of the normal adult human colon is 4 to 5 L per 24 hours. Diarrhea, therefore, can be viewed as either small intestinal or colonic in origin. If the small intestine is deranged by disease or pharmacologic agents such that its absorptive capacity is reduced by 50%,

TABLE 38–1
The Organ Physiology of Human Intestinal Water and Solute Transport

	WATER (ml/24 h)	Na$^+$ (mmol/24 h)	K$^+$ (mmol/24 h)	Cl$^-$ (mmol/24 h)
Entering duodenum (diet plus endogenous secretions)	8000–10,000	800	100	700
Entering colon	1500	200	10	100
Stool	100	3	8	2

the volume of fluid presented to the normal colon will exceed its absorptive capacity of ∼4 L. A stool excretion greater than 200 g (over ∼200 ml) would result; by definition, this is diarrhea. Alternatively, if the colon is deranged so that it cannot absorb even the 1.5 L presented to it by the normal small intestine, then diarrhea would result with stool volumes greater than ∼200 ml. This excess fluid excretion may come about because of the failure of absorption of Na and H$_2$O as the result of either a deranged epithelial transport mechanism or the presence of nonabsorbable solutes in the intestinal lumen.

ABNORMAL SECRETION

Investigations in the decade following 1965 rediscovered and documented the ability of the intestine to secrete as well as absorb fluid and electrolytes.[31–33] The revolutionary discovery by Michael Field in 1968 of the role of intracellular cyclic nucleotides in initiating intestinal Cl and H$_2$O secretion led to an entirely new concept of diarrhea. The subsequent discoveries that neurotransmitters, hormones, bacterial enterotoxins, and cathartics all stimulated intestinal Cl and water secretion by way of changes in intracellular cyclic AMP, cyclic GMP, or ionized Ca^{2+} further developed this concept (ch 14). Thus, a new transport abnormality, intestinal secretion, was added to abnormal absorption as a pathophysiologic mechanism of diarrhea (Table 38-2).

Although initially it was thought that bacterial enterotoxins increased intracellular messengers by way of a direct effect on enterocyte receptors, studies by Lundgren and his co-investigators demonstrated that at least 50% of the intestinal secretion initiated by bacterial enterotoxins in vivo comes about from stimulation of receptors on enterochromaffin cells. These endocrine cells release hormones that activate the enteric nervous system, releasing neurotransmitters that secondarily stimulate the enterocyte.[34]

The most recent addition to our knowledge of the physiology of intestinal secretion has been the realization that inflammatory mediators released from immune cells (mucosal mast cells and resident phagocytes such as eosinophils, macrophages, and neutrophils) and mesenchymal cells (fibroblasts, endothelium, and smooth muscle) in the lamina propria and submucosa are also capable of initiating intestinal secretion.[35] Adenosine, histamine, serotonin, hydrogen peroxide, platelet activating factor, leukotrienes, and prostaglandins released by mast cells, activated phagocytes, or mesenchymal cells may directly stimulate the en-

TABLE 38–2
Stool Osmotic Gap as a Guide to the Pathophysiology of Diarrhea

Stool osmolality or 290 mosm/kg H$_2$O − 2 [Na + K] mmol/L	=	Stool osmotic gap
Stool [Na] > 90 mmol/L and Osmotic gap < 50 mosm/kg H$_2$O	=	Secretory diarrhea; rarely, osmotic diarrhea due to Na$_2$SO$_4$ or Na$_2$PO$_4$ ingestion*
Stool [Na] < 60 mmol/L and Osmotic gap > 100 mosm/kg H$_2$O	=	Osmotic diarrhea; if stool volume does not return to normal on fast, suspect surreptitious Mg ingestion†
Stool [Na] > 150 mmol/L and Stool osmolality > 375–400 mosm/Kg H$_2$O	=	Suspect contamination of specimen with concentrated urine
Stool osmolality < 200–250 mosm/Kg H$_2$O	=	Suspect contamination of specimen with dilute urine or water

* *Normal stool SO$_4$ and PO$_4$ is usually < 5 mmol; exact values not established.*
† *Normal stool Mg on regular diet is 20–50 mmol/L; on fast, the concentration should be less than 10 mmol/L. Exact values not well established.*

terocyte or may initiate intestinal secretion by releasing prostaglandins from other immune and mesenchymal cells in the subepithelial layers of the bowel. These mediators may also activate the enteric nervous system. Thus, the diarrhea of intestinal anaphylaxis or inflammation, which had heretofore been ascribed to deranged Na, nutrient, and H_2O absorption or to exudation of plasma from denuded intestinal blood vessels, may also be due in part to active intestinal electrolyte and H_2O secretion.

These studies of electrolyte and water secretion also revealed that the intracellular messengers have an effect on absorption as well as secretion. In addition to stimulating electrogenic Cl (and perhaps HCO_3) secretion from the crypt cells of the small intestine and colon, these messengers also inhibit electrically neutral NaCl absorption from the villus cells of the small intestine and surface cells of the colon. Because the direction of net fluid movement is in response to the net direction of solute movement, a submaximal secretory stimulus will give the appearance of an inhibition of absorption rather than stimulated secretion (Fig 38-2).

Malabsorption (Osmotic) Versus Secretory (Electrolyte Transport) Diarrhea

The increased understanding of intestinal water and electrolyte transport and how Na and Cl absorption and secretion are altered by increased intracellular levels of cyclic nucleotides or Ca^{2+} led to the idea that there were two general categories of diarrheal pathophysiology—malabsorption and secretion—although, as noted above, the latter could not be clearly separated from conditions where there was inhibition of absorption rather than frank secretion. From an understanding of the physiology it should be possible to distinguish between these two kinds of diarrhea: (1) by the responses to feeding and to fast and (2) by measurements of stool osmolality and electrolytes. To understand these principles, we must consider how a normal intestine alters interluminal ionic concentrations and osmolality and subsequently how these parameters are altered by secretory agonists or by the presence of nonabsorbable (osmotic) solutes.

NORMAL PHYSIOLOGY

The magnitude of fluid flows as well as the ionic concentration and osmolality of the fluid at different points in the gastrointestinal tract give insight into the organ physiology of intestinal electrolyte and water transport. The fasting intestinal flow rate in healthy humans averages approximately 2.5 ml per minute in the upper jejunum and 0.4 to 0.9 ml per minute across the ileocecal valve.[36] Following meals, flow rates in the upper jejunum depend on the rate of gastric emptying, the rates of pancreatic and biliary secretion, and also the osmolality of the ingested meal. Rates may approximate 20 to 50 ml per minute in the upper jejunum and 5 to 10 ml per minute across the ileocecal valve. Nonetheless, regardless of whether a subject ingests a hypotonic meal (e.g., a steak meal with an osmolality of 230 mosm/kg H_2O) or a hypertonic meal (e.g., a milk and doughnut meal with an osmolality of 630 mosm/kg H_2O), the very permeable duodenum allows the movement of

water and electrolytes into or out of the lumen such that the meal is approximately isotonic by the time it reaches the proximal jejunum (Fig 38-3). At this point it will have an electrolyte content essentially that of plasma (Fig 38-4). Furthermore, the volume of this meal is augmented by gastric, pancreatic, biliary, and duodenal secretions such that the 313-ml milk and doughnut meal expands to 1200 ml and the 645-ml steak meal approaches 2000 ml by distal duodenum or proximal jejunum.[37] However, the high-carbohydrate hypertonic meal is handled differently from the high-protein hypotonic meal. The rapid digestion of starches and lactose into osmotically active sugars presents a larger osmotic load to the proximal small bowel, and considerable amounts of fluid must passively enter to equilibrate the osmolalities and electrolyte contents. After ingesting this meal, it may be midjejunum before efficient absorption of the fluid and electrolytes begins. In contrast, after ingesting the hypotonic steak meal, absorption begins virtually in the duodenum (see Fig 38-3). In either case, as the chyme moves toward the colon, the electrolyte concentrations in the luminal fluid remain approximately those of plasma, except for Cl, which is reduced to concentrations of 60 to 70 mmol/L, and HCO_3, which is increased to a similar concentration as the result of the Cl and HCO_3 transport mechanisms residing in the small intestine (see Fig 38-4). In the colon, the amiloride-sensitive Na channel and the low epithelial permeability allow this segment to extract Na and fluid very efficiently from the contents.[37] As a result, the Na content of stool drops to approximately 30 mmol/L, and poorly absorbed divalent cations such as Mg^{2+} and Ca^{2+} are concentrated to values of 5 to 100 mmol/L, depending on diet (Fig 38-5). Potassium values increase from 5 to 10 mmol/L in the small bowel to 75 mmol/L in stool as the result of both the lumen negative electrical potential difference, which favors the movement of cations from blood to lumen, and the active K^+ secretory mechanisms present in the colon. The anion concentrations in the intestinal lumen change drastically in the colon. Bacterial degradation of carbohydrate (unabsorbed starches, sugars, and fiber) creates short-chain fatty acids (at colonic pH these are present as organic anions, mainly acetate, propionate, and butyrate) that attain concentrations of 80 to 180 mmol/L.[38] Depending on the concentrations and quantities of organic anions created, stool pH may drop to 4 or lower. Even though colonic bacteria degrade carbohydrates and increase the concentration of organic anions (and therefore the number of osmotically active particles), the osmolality of stool, if measured as soon as it is passed, is approximately that of plasma—280 to 310 mosm.[39,40] If stool osmolality is measured hours to days after passage, even if it has been stored in deep freeze, the osmolality may increase to greater than 350 mosm because of continued bacterial degradation of carbohydrate in the collecting container.

PATHOPHYSIOLOGY OF OSMOTIC (MALABSORPTIVE) DIARRHEA

Contrast the events above with what transpires when a lactase-deficient subject ingests a lactose test meal[41,42] or when the normal subject ingests a nonabsorbable solute such as polyethylene glycol (PEG).[39] Although the same dilution of the meal occurs in the duodenum (Fig 38-6), the lactase-deficient subject is unable to reabsorb the fluid because the lactose is not metabolized to glucose and galactose, which are substrates for the normal Na-coupled

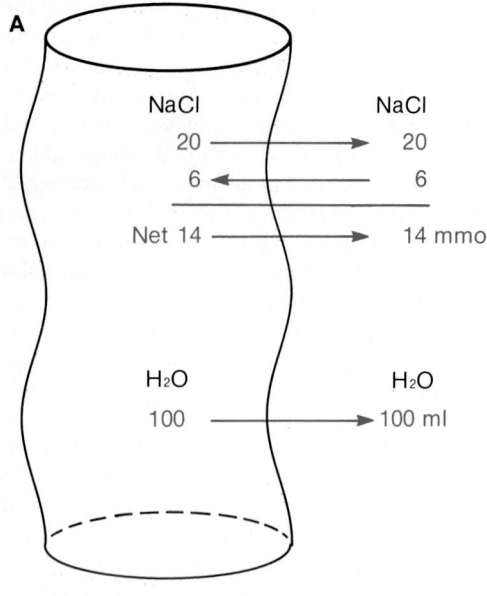

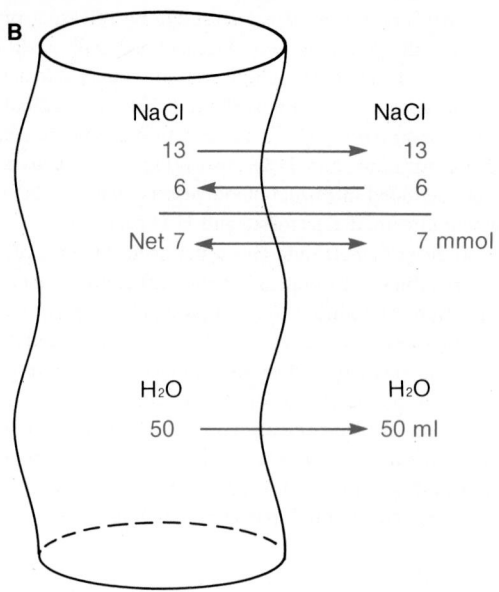

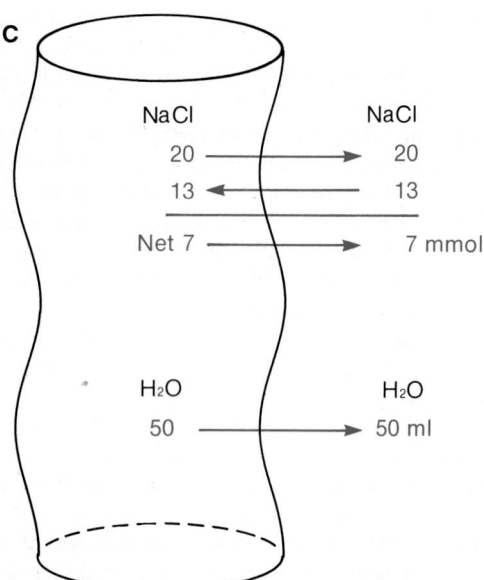

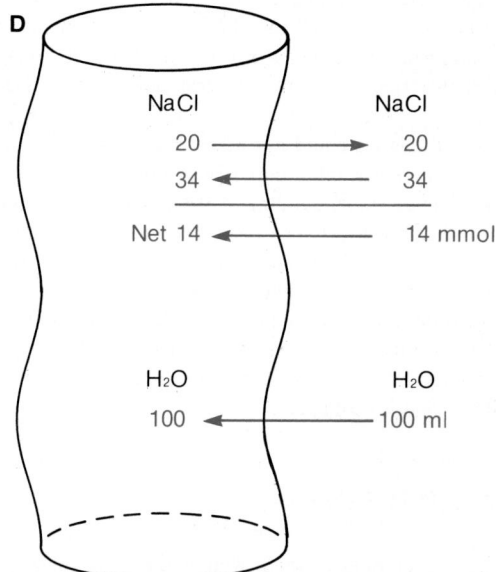

FIGURE 38–2. Theoretic changes in the intraluminal fluid volume in response to changes in electrolyte transport. **A,** In the control state, Na and Cl absorption of 20 mmol by the villus epithelium of the small intestine or the surface epithelium of the colon is offset by NaCl secretion of 6 mmol. Thus, there is net transport of 14 mmol from lumen to blood. This results in a net movement of 100 ml of fluid from lumen to blood. **B,** If some disease process reduces NaCl absorption from 20 to 13 mmol without changing crypt secretion, the amount of NaCl absorbed is reduced by 50% (to 7 mmol). Fluid absorption would also be reduced by 50% to 50 ml. **C,** If NaCl absorption is unaffected and yet some process stimulated NaCl secretion from the crypt from 6 to 13 mmol, the result is only 7 mmol of NaCl and only 50 ml of H_2O absorbed. The net result appears to be identical to the example in **B,** but the process causing this is quite different. **D,** If NaCl absorption remains at control values of 20 mmol and yet secretion increases to 34 mmol, there would be a net movement of 14 mmol NaCl from the blood into the lumen and a corresponding secretion of 100 ml fluid. Obviously, some combination of reduced NaCl absorption and stimulated NaCl secretion could also result in a similar amount of fluid secretion.

sugar absorptive mechanisms of the small intestine. Similarly, ingested PEG would result in fluid entry into the small bowel, rendering the intraluminal solutions isosmotic with plasma. Intraluminal Na concentrations drop below 80 mmol/L, and the permeable jejunum cannot absorb Na against such a steep lumen-to-plasma gradient. What happens to the chyme when it reaches

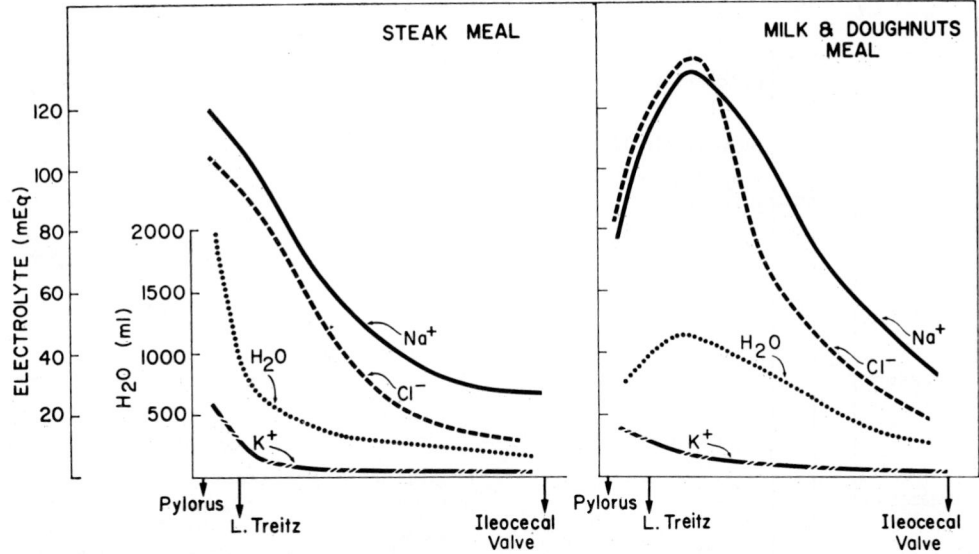

FIGURE 38–3. Intraluminal volumes and electrolyte content in the human small intestine following a hypotonic (steak) meal and a hypertonic (milk and doughnut) meal. (Fordtran JS. Speculations on the pathogenesis of diarrhea. Fed Proc 1967;26:1405; Fordtran JS, Locklear TW. Ionic constituents and osmolality of gastric and small intestinal fluids after eating. Am J Dig Dis 1966;11:503.)

the colon depends on the nature of the unabsorbed solute. If the solute is nonmetabolizable (i.e., PEG or Mg citrate), some Na and H_2O may be absorbed by the colon (which is less permeable and can concentrate Na from luminal concentrations below 30 mmol/L), resulting in a linear relationship between the ingested osmotic load of PEG and stool water output (stool weight) (Fig 38–7). If the unabsorbed solute is a carbohydrate that can be me-

tabolized by colonic bacteria (e.g., lactulose or lactose), it has three effects on stool weight: (1) One mole of disaccharide is metabolized to 3.7 mol of short-chain fatty acids (organic anion), thus nearly quadrupling the number of osmotically active particles in the colon. This increases the solute load, promoting the movement of more fluid into the colon. (2) The organic anions obligate retention of inorganic cations, further increasing the osmotic load

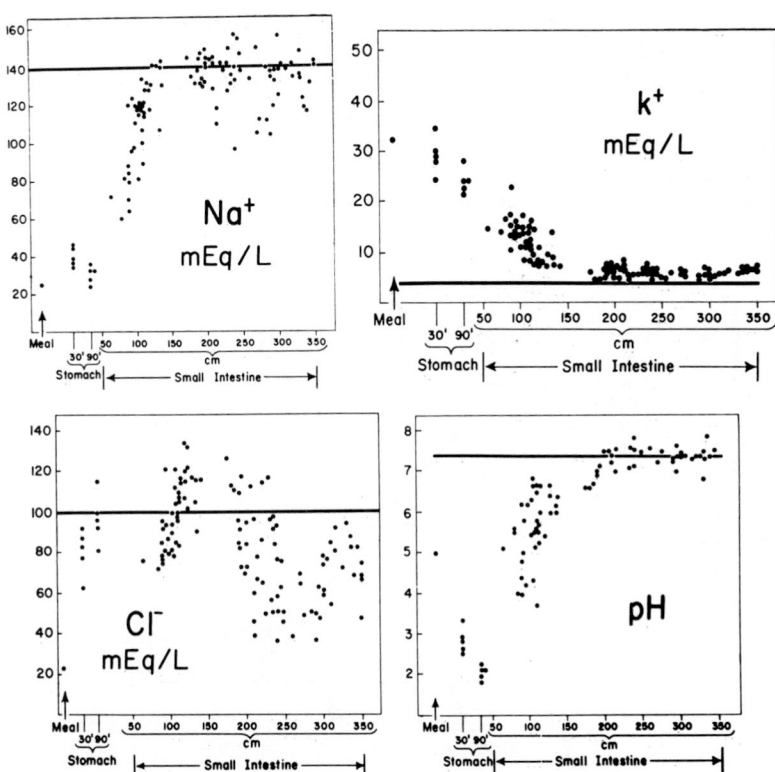

FIGURE 38–4. Na, K, and Cl concentrations and *p*H values in human gastric and small intestinal fluid following steak meal. The horizontal line in each figure indicates normal plasma concentrations or pH. (Fordtran JS. Speculations on the pathogenesis of diarrhea. Fed Proc 1967;26:1405.)

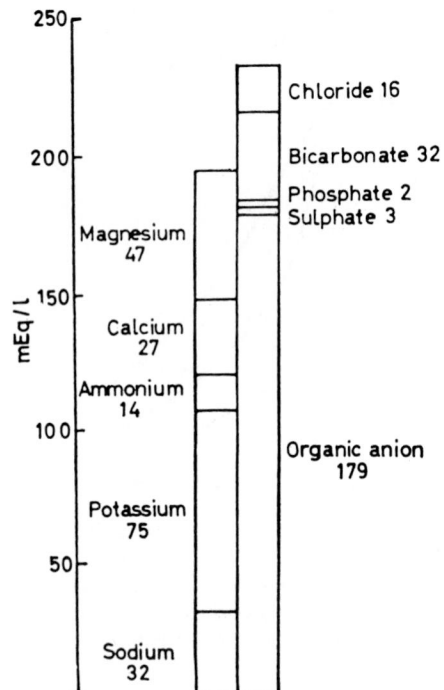

FIGURE 38-5. Human stool electrolyte concentrations obtained by fecal dialysis. (Wrong O, Metcalfe-Gibson A, Morrison BIR, Ng ST, Howard AV. *In vivo* dialysis of faeces as a method of stool analysis. Clin Sci 1965;28: 357.)

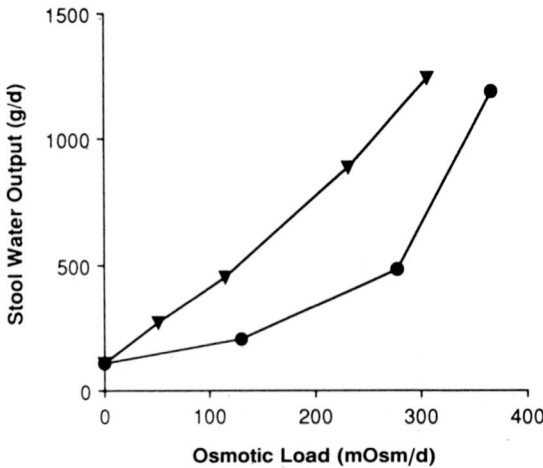

FIGURE 38-7. The effect of ingested osmotic load of polyethylene glycol (PEG) (triangles) and lactulose (circles) on 24-hr stool water output (see text). (Hammer HF, Santa Ana CA, Schiller LR, Fordtran JS. Studies of osmotic diarrhea induced in normal subjects by ingestion of polyethylene glycol and lactulose. J Clin Invest 1989;84:1056.)

(and thus the fluid) in the colon. (3) Because some of the organic anions are absorbed, fluid is absorbed as it traverses the colon. The net result of these three effects is also shown in Figure 38-7. At lower ingested osmotic loads, the stool weight is less when the ingested solute is lactulose or lactose. This is due to metabolism of carbohydrate by the colonic flora and the absorption of the resulting organic anions. When the capacity of the colonic flora to metabolize the carbohydrate is exceeded, the unabsorbed carbohydrate, the organic anions with their obligate cations, and fluid are retained in the colon. Stool weight then may increase at a rate (slope of the line) that exceeds that seen with PEG ingestion.

Because PEG is not metabolized by the bacteria, it exerts its full osmotic effect in proportion to the amount ingested.

With either unabsorbable solute (e.g., Mg or PEG) or unabsorbed carbohydrate (e.g., lactulose or, in some individuals, lactose) ingestion, a considerable amount of the osmolality of stool is due to the nonabsorbed solute, so that there is an osmotic gap between stool osmolality and the sum of the inorganic ions in the stool (Table 38-2). In practice, one need not measure stool osmolality, which may be falsely altered by bacterial degradation of carbohydrate after the stool is passed, but may simply use plasma osmolality (290 mosm/kg H_2O) as the proper number, because newly passed stool is essentially osmotic with plasma. Furthermore, only Na and K must be measured in the stool and then multiplied by 2 in order to account for the obligate (mainly organic) anions in the stool. The difference between stool osmolality (or 290 mosm) and 2 × [Na + K] concentrations normally should be less than 100. The 100 value (osmotic gap) takes into account unabsorbed divalent cations (Ca^{2+} and Mg^{2+}) and ammonium and their obligate

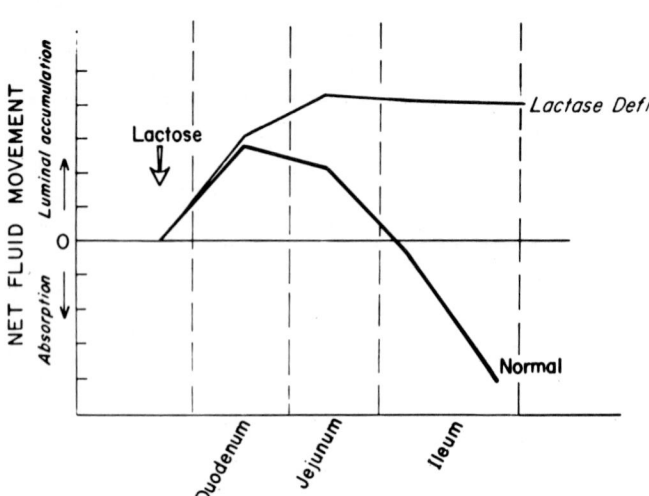

FIGURE 38-6. Changes in fluid absorption and secretion in the small intestine of normal and lactase-deficient subjects following a lactose meal of 50 g/m² body surface area in 400 ml of distilled water. (Binder HJ, Bayless TM, Whiting DS. Pathophysiology of diarrhea. Unit VIIB. In: Timonium, MD: The Undergraduate Teaching Project in Gastroenterology Liver Disease. American Gastroenterological Association, 1979. Data from Christopher NL, Bayless TM. Role of the small bowel and colon in lactose-induced diarrhea. Gastroenterology 1971;60:845.)

anions. Furthermore, because it is the *ingestion* of nonabsorbable (or nonabsorbed) solutes that causes the osmotic gap and the diarrhea, the diarrhea should disappear when the patient fasts, and stool weights should return to values less than 200 g/24 h.

The osmotic effect of a solute is governed by the number of molecules present in a given volume of solution and their inability to passively move across the epithelium by which they are confined. Therefore, water-soluble, low-molecular-weight solutes such as sugars and amino acids will exert more significant osmotic effects than will high-molecular-weight polymers of carbohydrate (starches or dextrans) or amino acids (proteins) or cell membrane-soluble lipids. Osmotic diarrheas are due to increased intraluminal fluid secondary to water movement into the bowel as a result of unabsorbed osmotic solutes in the lumen. These osmotic solutes can be derived from either exogenous (ingested) or endogenous sources or because of congenital or acquired malabsorptive disease. The causes are listed in Table 38-3 and are discussed in more detail in the sections on acute and chronic diarrhea.

PATHOPHYSIOLOGY OF SECRETORY (DERANGED ELECTROLYTE TRANSPORT) DIARRHEAS

In secretory diarrheas, particularly in the fasting state, the major solutes in the lumen are Na, K, Cl, and HCO_3. It is the failure to absorb these electrolytes and/or their active secretion that determines the amount of fluid entering or leaving the colon. Therefore, in secretory diarrheas, twice the Na + K concentrations will approximate stool osmolality. Furthermore, unless the secretory stimulus is something that is being ingested, the diarrhea and stool weight should be only minimally or moderately reduced when the patient fasts; thus, stool weight will remain above 200 g/24 h.

There are many conceptual and practical problems encountered in using the response to fasting and feeding and measurements of stool osmotic gap.[43,44] First, in some diseases the ingestion of a drug and/or the act of feeding itself seems to initiate the secretory phenomenon. Under these circumstances, the fasting stool may return to normal, and yet the pathophysiology is that of a secretory diarrhea. Examples are the patients who factitiously ingest laxatives and patients with microscopic (lymphocytic) and/or collagenous colitis. Second, the stool specimen may be accidentally contaminated with urine or purposefully diluted with water. Third, there may be malabsorptive diseases that also have a secretory component. For example, in celiac sprue there is secretion by the small intestine, and malabsorbed fat may also initiate active secretion in the colon. Similarly, in viral diarrhea there may be simultaneous secretion by the hyperplastic crypts and malabsorption by the damaged villus epithelium. Thus, the use of stool response to fasting and feeding and the measurements of stool electrolyte for calculation for osmotic gap are useful guidelines only for the classification of diarrhea. In general, if stool Na concentrations are greater than 90 mmol/L and the osmotic gap is less than 50, then a secretory diarrhea is present (Table 38-2). Conversely, if stool Na is less than 60 mmol/L and the osmotic gap is greater than 100, then it is likely to be an osmotic form of diarrhea. Stools with Na concentration between 60 and 90 mmol/L and calculated osmotic gaps between 50 and 100 can be due to either secretory or malabsorptive abnormalities or to diseases that have as their pathophysiologic basis some element of both secretion and malabsorption.[40,42,43]

TABLE 38–3
Classification of Osmotic (Malabsorptive) Diarrhea

I. Exogenous
- A. Laxatives:
  Polyethylene glycol/saline (Golytely), $Mg(OH)_2$ (Milk of Magnesia), $MgSO_4$ (Epsom salts), Na_2SO_4 (Glauber's or Calsbad salt), Na_2PO_4 (neutral phosphate)
- B. Antacids:
  Those containing MgO or $Mg(OH)_2$
- C. Dietetic foods, candy or chewing gum, and elixirs:
  Those containing sorbitol, mannitol, or xylitol
- D. Miscellaneous drugs:
  Chronic ingestion of colchicine, cholestyramine, neomycin, para-aminosalicylic acid, lactulose

II. Endogenous
- A. Congenital:
  (Specific malabsorptive diseases)
  Disaccharidase deficiencies (lactase, sucrase–isomaltase, trehalase)
  Glucose–galactose or fructose malabsorption
  (Generalized malabsorptive diseases)
  Abetalipoproteinemia and hypobetalipoproteinemia
  Congenital lymphangiectasia, microvillus inclusion disease
  Enterokinase deficiency
  Pancreatic insufficiency (cystic fibrosis or Shwachman's syndrome)
- B. Acquired:
  (Specific malabsorptive diseases)
  Postenteritis disaccharidase deficiency
  (Generalized malabsorptive diseases)
  Pancreatic insufficiency (alcohol), bacterial overgrowth, celiac sprue, rotavirus enteritis, parasitic diseases (*Giardia*, coccidiosis), metabolic diseases (thyrotoxicosis, adrenal insufficiency), inflammatory disease (eosinophilic enteritis, mastocytosis), protein–calorie malnutrition, short-bowel syndrome, jejunoileal bypass

Secretory diarrheas are due to specific alterations in the mechanisms of water and electrolyte transport, usually secondary to stimulation of intestinal Cl and HCO_3 secretion and inhibition of Na and Cl absorption, by agents that increase the intracellular messengers responsible for these events (cyclic nucleotides and ionized Ca^{2+}).[31-35] The correlations between enterotoxins or laxatives and intracellular messengers are described in more detail in Chapter 14. As is the case with osmotic causes of diarrhea, these secretory stimuli may be of exogenous origin or they may be endogenous (Table 38-4).

Endogenous detergents that produce secretory diarrhea include dihydroxy bile acids[45,46] and long-chain fatty acids,[47,48] particularly if they have been hydroxylated by intestinal microflora.[49] The detergent "stool softener" dioctyl sodium sulfosuccinate[50] and the cathartic ricinoleic acid (castor oil)[51] are secretagogues also. These agents change intracellular cyclic AMP and Ca^{2+} and alter epithelial tight junctional permeability, but the exact mechanism of diarrhea with such detergents remains unclear. The important concept here is that these "malabsorbed" endogenous detergents may lend an element of secretory diarrhea to otherwise malabsorptive diseases.

Diarrheas Due to Brush Border or Enterocyte Damage/Death With Inflammation

Recently it has become more clear that every diarrhea cannot be easily classified as malabsorptive or secretory. There is also a large group of diarrheas characterized by enterocyte damage/death with minimal to severe inflammation in which both malabsorption and secretion occur.

The histologic response to enterocyte damage and death is different in the small intestine and in the colon, although functionally the processes are probably the same (ch 126). In the small intestine, both the microvilli of the enterocyte and the villi become initially shorter and broader and then disappear completely, while at the same time there is a compensatory hyperplasia of the crypts as they respond to signals that cause the stem cells to divide and the new enterocytes to migrate up the crypts in an attempt to repopulate the villus.[52] The histologic response of the colon to epithelium cell death is one of attenuated surface cells but hyperplastic irregular regenerative crypts.[53] The result of these events is the presence of immature cells on rudimentary, or nonexistent, villi of the small intestine and on the surface of the colon. These immature "absorptive" cells have poor disaccharidase and peptide hydrolase activity, reduced or absent Na-coupled sugar or amino acid transport mechanisms, and reduced or absent NaCl absorptive transporters. Conversely, the crypt cells and the new, immature villus or surface cells maintain their ability to secrete Cl (and perhaps HCO_3). A well-studied example of this phenomenon is experimental viral enteritis in which such transport abnormalities have been documented by Hamilton and his cohorts.[54-61]

The lamina propria of damaged small intestine or colon reveals varying degrees of either chronic (lymphocyte and plasma cell) or acute (mast cell, macrophage, eosinophil, and neutrophil) inflammatory infiltrate. These inflammatory cells respond either to various soluble mediators of inflammation or, as part of the process

TABLE 38-4
Classification of Secretory (Deranged Electrolyte Transport) Diarrhea

I. Exogenous
  A. Laxatives:
    Phenolphthalein, anthraquinones, bisacodyl, oxyphenisatin, senna, aloe, ricinoleic acid (castor oil), dioctyl sodium sulfosuccinate
  B. Medications:
    Diuretics (furosemide, thiazides); asthma medication (theophylline)
    Cholinergic drugs—glaucoma eye drops and bladder stimulants (acetylcholine analogues or mimetics); myesthenia gravis medication (cholinesterase inhibitors); cardiac drug (quinidine and quinine); gout medication (colchicine)
    Prostaglandins (misoprostol); di-5-aminosalicylic acid (azodisalicylate); gold (may also cause colitis)
  C. Toxins:
    Metals (arsenic), plant (mushroom, e.g., Amanita phalloides), organophosphates (insecticides and nerve poisons), seafood toxins (ciguatera, scombroid poisoning, paralytic or neurotoxic shellfish poisoning), coffee, tea, or cola (caffeine and other methylxanthines), ethanol.
  D. Bacterial toxin:
    Staphylococcus aureus, Clostridium perfringens and *botulinum, Bacillus cereus*
  E. Gut allergy without histologic change
II. Endogenous
  A. Congenital:
    Microvillus inclusion disease
    Congenital chloridorrhea (absence of Cl:HCO_3 exchanger)
    Congenital Na diarrhea (absence of Na:H exchanger)
  B. Bacterial enterotoxins:
    Vibrio cholera, toxigenic E. coli (LT and ST), *Campylobacter jejuni, Yersinia enterocolitica, Klebsiella pneumoniae, Clostridium difficile, S. aureus* (toxic shock syndrome)
  C. Endogenous laxatives:
    Dihydroxy bile acids and long-chain fatty acids, especially hydroxylated ones
  D. Hormone-producing tumors:
    Pancreatic cholera syndrome and ganglioneuromas (VIP), medullary carcinoma of thyroid (calcitonin and prostaglandins), mastocytosis (histimine), villous adenoma (secretagogue unknown)

of phagocytosis, by secreting inflammatory mediators such as his-tamine, serotonin, adenosine, cytokines, platelet activating factor, and eicosanoids (prostaglandins and leukotrienes), which are po-tent stimulants of intestinal secretion.[35,62] Depending on the cause and intensity of the inflammation, white blood cells (lymphocytes, eosinophils, or neutrophils) may invade the epithelium and reside between the enterocytes. If the neutrophils cross the epithelium of the colon, they present as the classic crypt abscess, which can be seen in both infectious enteritis and inflammatory bowel disease. If the inflammation is severe enough, there will be frank ulceration ranging from a simple loss of the surface epithelium with an intact basement membrane to ulcerations extending into the lamina pro-pria or deeper.

The mechanisms of brush border damage or cell death with ulceration may be quite different in different diseases. Based on current knowledge, there seem to be two general mechanisms: (1) direct damage/death by luminal or invading microorganisms or parasites[63] or (2) immunologic damage/death due to complement attack[64,65] or T lymphocyte–mediated death[66,67] or damage/death secondary to products (proteases and oxidants) secreted by mast cells[35,68] and phagocytes (Fig 38-8).[35,69] If the primary event is autoimmunity with complement-mediated or cytotoxic T-cell killing of enterocytes, then the inflammatory response would be secondary to the cell death. Conversely, if the primary event is uncontrolled acute inflammation, the enterocyte death may be secondary to products (oxidants and proteases) of phagocyte and mast cell degranulation. In this case, the enterocyte cell death is an example of an innocent bystander event. With either mechanism, the damage to the absorptive epithelium and/or the presence of immature cells with poor absorptive capabilities now populating the previously damaged absorptive surface results in malabsorption of ions and nutrients. At the same time, the release of inflammatory mediators from the inflammatory cells of the lamina propria stim-ulates secretion from the remaining crypt and immature villus/surface cells.[35,62] Immune-mediated vascular damage may cause protein to leak from capillaries. If severe ulceration has occurred, exudation from capillaries and lymphatics may contribute to the diarrhea. Release of interleukin-1 and tumor necrosis factor may also account for some of the systemic effects of severe inflammation as well as the glucocorticoid stress response (Fig 38-9).

In both the small intestine and colon there are four general categories of enterocyte damage/death and inflammation: infection, hypersensitivity, cytostatic (anticancer) agents, and idiopathic (? autoimmune) diseases (Table 38-5).

ACUTE DIARRHEAS

Definition and Classification

Acute diarrheas are those defined as being less than 2 to 3 weeks in duration. They may be due to ingested drugs or toxins or may occur in particular environmental circumstances, such as hospi-talization or marathon races (runner's diarrhea). However, the most common acute diarrheas are those due to infectious agents.

Infectious Diarrheas

EPIDEMIOLOGY

Acute infectious diarrhea accounts for more than 4 million deaths each year in children less than 5 years of age.[3–8] These figures add up to 10,000 children per day or 7 deaths per minute. It is also the major cause of protein–calorie malnutrition in the world. These deaths occur overwhelmingly in developing nations, where two thirds of the world's population live in areas where there is extreme poverty, rapid urbanization, crowded substandard housing with inadequate sewage disposal and inadequate water supplies, insuf-ficient food with lack of refrigeration, poor education (particularly in regard to personal hygiene), and a fundamental lack of access to health care.[7,8] In the Third World, children have 50 to 60 days of diarrhea per year, and approximately 10% of the episodes result in dehydration requiring therapy.[7,8]

Deaths occur in the United States as well, and they occur dis-proportionately among the black population and in the southern part of the United States. As in the undeveloped countries, the major cause seems to be poverty and lack of education, and not some inordinate racial susceptibility. In the United States, diarrhea is listed as the principal cause of death in over 500 children each year.[70] Fifty to 100 of these deaths will be due to rotavirus.[71] No doubt these reported rates in the United States are an underes-timate.

In the United States there is also a significant incidence of diarrhea that is less likely to cause death but causes considerable economic loss. Children have approximately two episodes per year, and among all of the population in the United States, the illness is frequent and severe enough to result in 250,000 hospital ad-missions, 7.9 million visits to physicians, and 48 million episodes that last at least 1 full day, causing restricted activity.[3,6] With improvement in sanitation and education in the United States, rates for certain infectious etiologies of diarrhea have declined. For example, the detection rate of *Entamoeba histolytica* cysts has declined from approximately 10% 40 years ago to less than 1% in 1976.[71] However, in those diseases in which person-to-person contact is a method of transmission (e.g., rotavirus) or in which the reservoirs of organisms are in domestic food animals (e.g., *Salmonella* or *Campylobacter*), the incidences remain constant or have increased.[71,72] In fact, cases of salmonellosis have doubled over the past 10 years, perhaps as the result of both mass production and distribution of food products and increased reporting. Sal-monellosis yearly may account for over 40,000 reported cases, 500 deaths, and financial costs of over $50,000,000.[72] The incidence of antibiotic-resistant *Salmonella* is also increasing, probably be-cause of increased use of antibiotic therapy in humans and because antibiotics are added to animal feed to treat diseases and to enhance growth.[73]

HISTORY

Infectious diarrhea can be suspected by knowledge of the routes of infection, by recognition of high-risk groups, and by an un-derstanding of the pathophysiology of infections.

Except for certain parasites that have the ability to enter humans by boring through the skin (ch 105), most infectious diarrheas are

I. DIRECT CELL DAMAGE DEATH

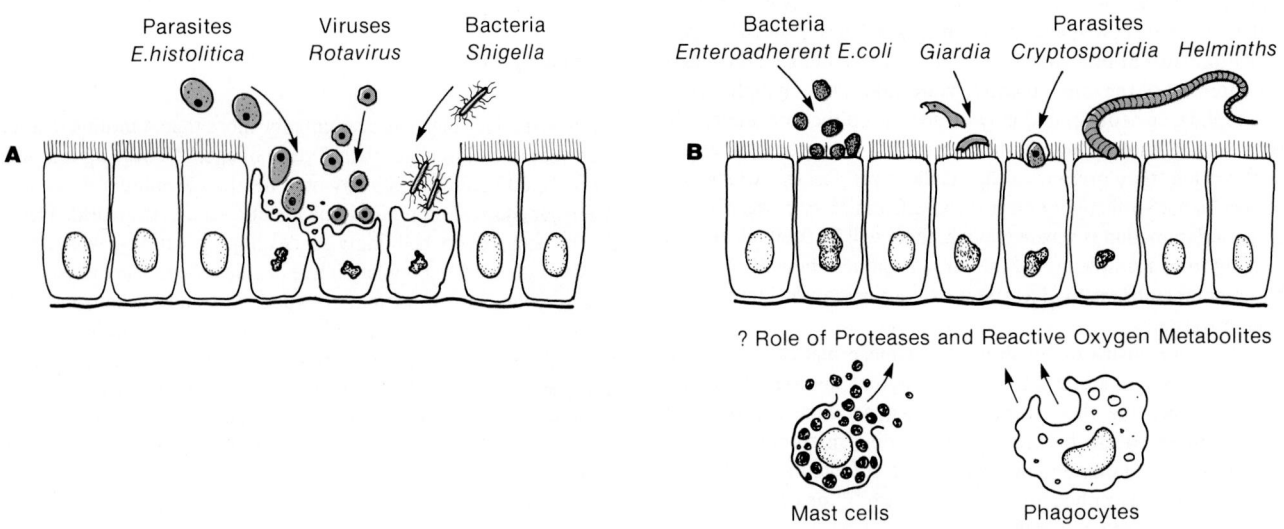

II. IMMUNE SYSTEM-MEDIATED CELL DAMAGE/DEATH

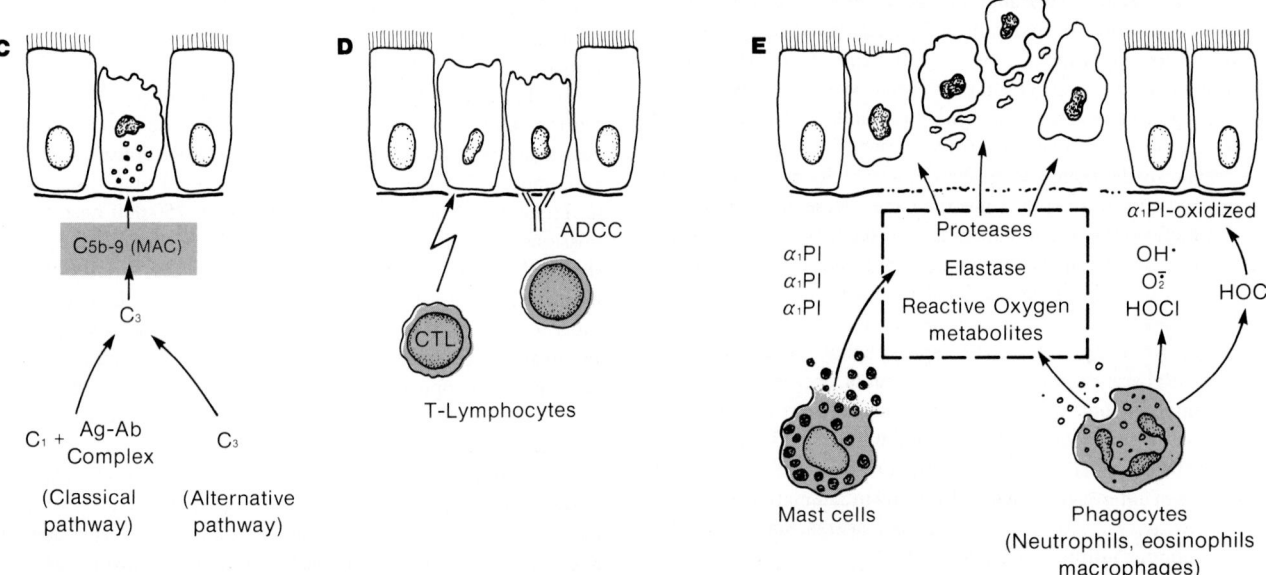

FIGURE 38–8. Proposed mechanism of enterocyte damage and death. I. Direct damage as a result of (**A**) enterocyte penetration and (**B**) secretion of toxic products by adherent bacteria or parasites. There may be a role for immune cell products in the damage also (see II **E**). II. Indirect (immune system–mediated) damage/death as a result of (**C**) complement membrane–attack complex (MAC), (**D**) cytotoxic T-lymphocyte (CTL) or antibody- dependent cellular cytotoxicity (ADCC) by T-lymphocytes, or (**E**) mast cell or phagocyte protease (elastase) secretion. These proteases are normally inhibited by plasma α_1-antiproteases that are inactivated by hypochlorous acid (HOCl). HOCl is formed from Cl and H_2O_2 in the presence of myelo- peroxidase. H_2O_2 and myeloperoxidase are both secreted by neutrophils.

acquired by the oral ingestion of stool (Table 38-6).[8,71,74] An exception may be the vibrios, which have brackish water as their natural habitat. Fecal–oral transmission can come by way of water or food. Water systems might be contaminated by human waste as the result of poor sewage systems, or by either wild or domestic animal feces if the water is not properly purified. Beef, pork, or poultry may be the source of infection if it is poorly cooked, but more often in developed nations infection comes from contamination of food-preparing surfaces with organisms present in these meats.[75] The organisms then are spread to uncooked food, such as salads, that is prepared on these same surfaces. Food-borne diarrhea also comes from minute inoculation of certain foods that then proliferates because the food is either poorly refrigerated or inadequately heated prior to serving. This occurs at picnics, banquets, or restaurants.

Person-to-person transmission (Table 38-6) can occur through aerosolization (rotavirus), through contamination of hands (*Clostridium difficile*), or through contamination of fomites.[76,77] Spread

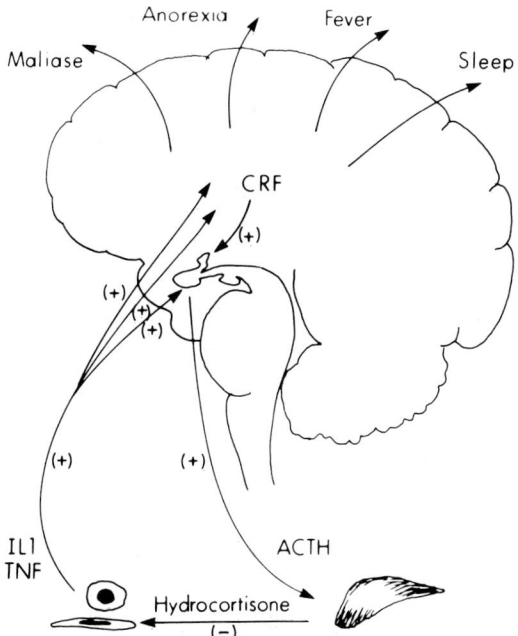

FIGURE 38–9. The systemic manifestations of severe intestinal inflammation are due primarily to release of interleukin-1 (IL1) and tumor necrosis factor (TNF)$_2$, which have effects in the central nervous system, as shown. These agents also stimulate the pituitary–adrenal axis and initiate the glucocorticoid stress response. Glucocorticoids through a negative feedback action down-regulate the inflammatory cells in the lamina propria, thus decreasing IL1 and TNF release.

also comes from sexual activity, particularly oral–genital or oral–anal contact.

There are certain high-risk groups in which infectious diarrheas occur (Table 38-7). The most obvious are travelers to or those

recently coming from developing nations. Traveler's diarrhea is considered in depth in Chapter 68. In addition, vacationers in the United States, especially campers who have been ingesting ground water, are at risk.

There are certain unusual foods that represent risk above normal (Table 38-6). Approximately 8% of the people ingesting shellfish from federally approved but close-in shellfish beds will have diarrhea. The rate is 4% when shellfish come from pristine beds[78] (and Weber D. Personal communication). Deep-sea fish and shellfish also cause diarrhea by way of toxigenic mechanisms (see ch 68 for discussion of scombroid, ciguatera, and the paralytic/neurotoxic food poisonings).

Homosexuals (gay bowel syndrome), prostitutes, and intravenous drug users are apt to develop infectious diarrhea through the oral–fecal route or because they have AIDS. The incidence of infectious diarrhea among homosexuals without AIDS has markedly decreased as a result of the AIDS threat, most assuredly because of a decrease in promiscuity and the practice of "safe sex." However, the decline in this particular risk group has been more than offset by the high incidence and seriousness of enteric infections in AIDS. Gay bowel syndrome is detailed in Chapter 83, and AIDS diarrhea is covered in Chapter 103.

In this country, daycare diarrhea represents the equivalent of Third World diarrhea. The number of children in the United States currently attending daycare is probably 6.3 million or more. Diarrhea is extremely prevalent in both endemic and outbreak form and usually involves those organisms which colonize at a low inoculum dose (*Shigella, Giardia, Cryptosporidium*) or those which are spread easily (rotavirus).[77,79,80] However, any organism can be isolated in outbreaks of daycare diarrhea, including *C. difficile* and *Salmonella*. The mechanism of transmission in daycare centers is person-to-person by way of fecal contamination of hands and fomites (toys, surfaces in diaper changing areas, bathroom tap and flush handles, and so forth). Not only does daycare represent an

TABLE 38–5
Classification of Diarrheas Due to Brush Border or Enterocyte Damage/Death With Inflammation

I. With minimal to moderate inflammation
  A. Infections:
    Bacteria (enteroadherent or enteropathogenic *E. coli*)
    Viruses (rotavirus and Norwalk agent, HIV)
    Parasites (*Giardia, Cryptosporidium, Isospora, Ascaris, Trichinella*)
    Mixed organisms (tropical sprue, bacterial overgrowth)
  B. Cytostatic (anticancer) agents:
    Chemotherapy (mucositis)
    Radiation therapy (acute or chronic radiation enteritis, radiation sickness)
  C. Hypersensitivity:
    Nematode infestation, ?food allergy
  D. Idiopathic or autoimmune:
    Microscopic (lymphocytic) and collagenous colitis, Canada–Cronkhite syndrome, graft-versus-host disease

II. With moderate–severe inflammation ± ulceration
  A. Infections:
    Destruction of enterocytes (*Shigella*, enteroinvasive *E. coli, Entamoeba histolytica,* hookworm)
    Penetration of mucosa (*Salmonella, Campylobacter jejuni, Yersinia enterocolitica, Mycobacterium avium-intracellulare,* Whipple's disease)
  B. Hypersensitivity:
    Celiac sprue, milk or soybean protein hypersensitivity, eosinophilic gastroenteritis, nematode infestation (reinfection)
    Drug-induced colitis (gold, methyldopa)
  C. Idiopathic or autoimmune:
    Ulcerative colitis/proctitis, Crohn's disease, lymphoma

TABLE 38–6
Fecal–Oral Spread of Infectious Diarrhea

VEHICLE	MAJOR PATHOGENS		
	Bacteria	Viruses	Parasites
Water and raw vegetables or fruits washed in such water	V, cholerae, *Aeromonas*, ?*E. coli* of all types	Norwalk agent	*Giardia*, cryptosporidiosis, *E. histolytica*, *Isospora*
Food: poultry, beef, pork, as well as eggs and dairy products	*Campylobacter, Salmonella, E. coli, Yersinia, Aeronomas, Shigella* (in tropics)	Norwalk agent	Cryptosporidiosis, *E. histolytica*, *Isospora*, tapeworms (beef and pork), *Echinococcus*
Seafood and shellfish	*V. cholerae, V. parahaemolyticus,* and *V. vulnificus, Aeromonas, Plesiomonas, Salmonella, Shigella*	Norwalk agent, hepatitis A, B, C	Fish tapeworm, anisakiasis
	Food poisonings–scombroid, ciguatera, paralytic and neurotoxin diseases		
Ethnic and specific foods:			
Fried rice	*B. Cereus* food poisoning		
Suchi		Fish food poisonings	Anisakiasis, fish tapeworm
Gefilte fish			
Fast-food hamburger	Hemorrhagic *E. coli, Salmonella,*		
Raw-egg milk shake, eggs	*Staphylococcus*, food poisoning, clostridial food poisoning		
Potato salad and cream pie			
Home-canned food			
Person-to-person	*Shigella, C. difficile*	Rotavirus	*Giardia*, cryptosporidiosis
Animal-to-person	*Campylobacter*	Cryptosporidiosis	
Pets or livestock (children, veterinarians, farm workers)			
Sexual contact:	Almost all bacteria, viruses and parasites, but especially:		
	Salmonella, Shigella, Campylobacter Gonorrhea, Syphilis	CMV, herpes	*Giardia, E. histolytica*, cryptosporidiosis

important source of infection for the children housed there, but because the secondary attack rate ranges between 10% and 20%, daycare represents an important source of infection for parents and siblings as well.[77–80]

Hospitals, mental institutions, and nursing homes represent high-risk areas for the easily transmitted organism. This is discussed in detail below.

CORRELATION OF SIGNS AND SYMPTOMS WITH PATHOPHYSIOLOGY

Patients with infectious diarrhea complain of nausea, vomiting, and abdominal pain and have either watery, malabsorptive, or bloody diarrhea and fever. The type of symptoms can be related to the segment of intestine that the organisms infect (i.e., small intestine, which tends to give a watery diarrheal disease, or large intestine, which tends to cause bloody diarrhea). However, the considerable overlap among the diseases often makes this classification less useful. Although the various organisms discussed here and in Chapters 68, 69, 83, 104, and 105 can present with any combination of these signs and symptoms, there are certain patterns that tend to occur characteristically (Table 38-8).

The diseases that have a toxin pathogenesis—either a preformed toxin or enterotoxin production after adherence (colonization)—have nausea and vomiting as a prominent symptom, and rarely is there high fever. The food poisonings due to preformed toxins frequently cause vomiting within 4 hours of ingesting the food, and this can be a useful clue to the diagnosis.[75,81]

Patients ingesting toxins or those with toxigenic infection complain of abdominal pain that is generally mild, diffuse, and crampy and that is often due to the high volumes of secreted fluid and the resulting stimulation of peristalsis. Parasites that do not invade (e.g., *Giardia*, cryptosporidiosis, and the helminths) produce only moderate abdominal discomfort.[82,83] The invasive bacteria[84–87] (category III of Table 38-8) and the organisms that produce local cytotoxins, such as *C. difficile*[88] and enterohemorrhagic *Escherichia coli*,[89] cause severe inflammation, severe abdominal pain, and, with the exception of the cytotoxin producers, usually high fever. Yersinosis is often relegated to the terminal ileum and cecum and presents with right lower quadrant pain and tenderness, suggesting appendicitis.[87,90,91] The localized right lower quadrant tenderness of yersinosis and the severe peritoneal signs seen with *C. difficile* enterocolitis or enterohemorrhagic *E. coli* colitis can raise the question of surgically urgent disease, and many such patients have been operated on in error.

TABLE 38–7
High-Risk Groups for Infectious Diarrhea

Recent travel

Developing nations
Peace Corps workers
Campers (ground water)

Unusual food

Seafood and shellfish, especially raw
Restaurants and fast-food houses
Banquets and picnics

Homosexuals, prostitutes, and I.V. drug users

"Gay bowel syndrome"
AIDS

Daycare

Children
Secondary contacts (family members)

Institutions

Mental institutions
Nursing homes
Hospitals

Toxin-producing organisms,[75,81,82] the invasive organisms that cause minimal inflammation (e.g., enteric viruses),[92] and those organisms which adhere, infect, or colonize but do not destroy the epithelium (enteropathogenic or enteroadherent *E. coli*[81] and both protozoan and helminth parasites)[82,83] cause watery diarrhea. The organisms that produce enterotoxins *and* invade (*Campylobacter, Aeromonas, Shigella, Vibrio parahaemolyticus,* and *V. fulnificus*) initially cause a watery diarrhea that is followed within hours or days by bloody diarrhea as the additional component of inflammation develops after the organism has penetrated and multiplied.[84–87,93] Organisms that simply penetrate and multiply may or may not cause bloody diarrhea depending on the degree of inflammation and mucosal destruction that ensues (e.g., *Salmonella* may or may not cause bloody diarrhea; *Mycobacterium avium-intracellulare* does not). Fecal leukocytes may or may not be present. The diarrheas due to the cytotoxin-producing organisms *C. difficile* and enterohemorrhagic *E. coli* present with watery diarrhea that either rarely (*C. difficile*) or always and rapidly (enterohemorrhagic *E. coli*) changes to a bloody diarrhea.[88,89]

SYSTEMIC SYMPTOMS WITH INFECTIOUS DIARRHEAL DISEASES

Certain enteric infections are accompanied by systemic symptoms that may be clues to their diagnosis. The hemolytic uremic syndrome that is characterized by acute hemolytic anemia, renal failure with uremia, and disseminated intravascular coagulation occurs

TABLE 38–8
Correlations Between Pathophysiology and Symptoms of Infectious Diarrhea

PATHOPHYSIOLOGY	MICROORGANISMS	SYMPTOMS
I. Preformed toxins (food poisonings)	*B. cereus, S. aureus, C. perfringens, C. botulinum*	Nausea, vomiting, watery diarrhea, low-grade fever, mild–moderate pain
II. Enterotoxin production Adherent organisms:	*V. cholerae,* enterotoxigenic *E. coli, K. pneumoniae*	Watery diarrhea; may contain mucus (i.e., "rice water" stool), low-grade fever, mild–moderate pain
Invading organisms:	*Campylobacter, Aeromonas, Shigella,* noncholera *Vibrio*	Initially watery diarrhea, then bloody; high fever, severe pain
III. Invasive organisms Enterocyte invasion and destruction (Minimal inflammation):	Rotavirus, Norwalk agent	Watery diarrhea and malabsorption, high fever, moderate pain
(Severe inflammation):	*Shigella,* enteroinvasive *E. coli, E. histolytica*	Bloody diarrhea, high fever, severe pain
Mucosal penetration with multiplication in lamina propria and inflammation:	*Campylobacter, Salmonella, Aeromonas,* ?*Plesiomonas, Yersinia, V. parahemolyticus* and *fulnificus, Mycobacterium avium-intracellulare* and *tuberculosis, Histoplasmosis*	Either watery or bloody diarrhea depending on degree of mucosal destruction, high fever, severe pain
IV. Attachment or colonization Local cytotoxin and inflammation: Adherent:	Enteropathogenic (enteroadherent) *E. coli, Giardia,* cryptosporidiosis, helminths	Watery diarrhea, low–moderate fever, moderate–severe pain
Cytotoxic:	*C. difficile*	Usually watery diarrhea, occasionally bloody diarrhea, low–moderate fever, severe pain
	Enterohemorrhagic *E. coli*	Watery diarrhea for short time, then bloody diarrhea; low–moderate fever, severe pain
V. Systemic infection:	Hepatitis, listeriosis, legionellosis, Rocky Mountain spotted fever, psittacosis, otitis media in infants, toxic shock syndrome (*S. aureus*), measles	Watery diarrhea may be initially a part of disease or it may accompany disease, clinical manifestations are overwhelmingly those of the organs and tissues primarily involved by the organisms

with both shigellosis[84] and infection with enterohemorrhagic *E. coli.*[89] This serious and often fatal complication develops most commonly in the very young and the very old (inhabitants of nursing homes). Reiter's syndrome (arthritis, urethritis, and conjunctivitis) occurs following infection with *Salmonella, Shigella, Campylobacter,* and *Yersinia.*[84-87,91] Thyroiditis, pericarditis, and glomerulonephritis may also occur in yersinosis.[87]

Differential Diagnosis

The differential diagnosis of *acute watery diarrhea* includes the foods, drugs, and medications listed in Tables 38-3 and 38-4. Although the drugs and medications listed in these tables are the most common culprits, any medication can cause diarrhea, and therefore the medication history should be considered seriously. Toxin ingestion from either the environment (organophosphate insecticides)[94] or food (mushroom,[95-97] seafood [see ch 68], caffeine, and carbohydrate-containing drinks) should be apparent from the patient's history. This may not be true for chronic arsenic poisoning, which may present initially as a watery, then as a bloody, diarrhea.[98,99] In the southern United States, arsenic usually is administered by a third party (usually spouses) as an attempted homicide. Such toxins can be recognized by the accompanying systemic symptoms (e.g., cardiovascular collapse in arsenic intoxication or the muscarinic signs of organophosphate intoxication and mushroom poisoning—the latter accompanied by hepatotoxicity).

The differential diagnosis of *acute bloody diarrhea* includes superior mesenteric arterial or venous thrombosis or ischemic colitis (ch 109), inflammatory bowel disease (ch 77), and drug-induced colitis (ch 86). Although age and the presence of other manifestations of atherosclerosis may suggest mesenteric vascular insufficiency or ischemic colitis, older people may also have more severe clinical manifestations with invasive infectious agents as well. Enterohemorrhagic *E. coli* can mimic ischemic colitis with submucosal hemorrhage presenting as thumb-printing on flat plate of the abdomen. Ulcerative proctitis/colitis and Crohn's disease can present with an acute course that suggests infectious enterocolitis. It is important to remember that the colonoscopic and radiographic appearance of the various invasive enteritides can mimic almost identically inflammatory bowel disease (IBD). At their various stages, shigellosis, salmonellosis, campylobacteriosis, yersinosis, and amebiasis can present as either aphthouslike ulcers or segmental colitis or pancolitis. There are histologic hallmarks that differentiate IBD from infectious diarrheas. *Clostridium difficile* may have the classic pseudomembranous enterocolitis appearance by x-ray or endoscopy, but on occasion the pseudomembrane is not present (particularly in pancytopenic cancer chemotherapy patients), and then the disease looks more like IBD. On rare occasions, the opposite mistake is made, and blood-filled macrophages in the stool of a patient with ulcerative colitis are mistaken as blood-filled trophozoites of amebiasis, or chronic ischemic colitis masquerades as pseudomembranous colitis. Furthermore, the colonic mucosa inflamed with ulcerative colitis appears to be more susceptible to colonization by pathogenic enteric bacteria, and *Salmonella, Campylobacter,* or *C. difficile* infection may accompany IBD and complicate the diagnosis and treatment. Drugs that may induce a colitis indistinguishable from ulcerative

colitis include gold (rheumatoid arthritis) and methyldopa (hypertension).

LABORATORY DIAGNOSIS OF ACUTE DIARRHEA

The diagnosis and treatment of the infectious diarrheas are complicated by the fact that these diseases are common and by the cost of both making the diagnosis and delivering specific (antibiotic) therapy, especially when the disease is usually mild and self-limited. It has been shown that the high cost of a single positive stool culture ($1200), if all frequent and important bacterial causes are not sought and if there is no discrimination as to which stools are cultured, can be reduced to $30 per culture if *Campylobacter* is looked for in addition to *Salmonella* and *Shigella* and if only liquid stools are cultured.[100] Furthermore, antibiotic therapy may prolong carriage rate for the infectious organism without altering the clinical course of the disease, and motility-altering drugs may even worsen the infection. Therefore, the questions revolve around who should undergo a diagnostic evaluation, who should be treated and when should they be treated, and whether treatment should consist of only symptomatic therapy or symptomatic therapy plus specific antibiotics.

An algorithm for the approach to acute diarrhea is shown in Figure 38-10. The key to this approach is the use of discriminating symptoms to determine when fecal specimens should be sent for laboratory diagnosis.[101] It is important to remember that certain organisms that can cause either watery or bloody diarrhea are not routinely sought by most clinical microbiology laboratories. For example, certain causes of bloody diarrhea, such as *Yersinia, Plesiomonas,* and enterohemorrhagic *E. coli,* may require specific special culture techniques or can be identified only with type-specific antisera.[102] Similarly, the watery diarrheas caused by *Aeromonas, Cryptosporidium,* and non-cholera *Vibrio* may require special laboratory attention.[102-104] The enteropathogenic and enteroadherent *E. coli* are diagnosed only by specific methods. Most labs have the ability to recognize or serotype for the 0157:H7 enterohemorrhagic strain.[81,89] The diagnosis of enterotoxigenic *E. coli* and enteroinvasive *E. coli* requires biologic intestinal loop or conjunctival invasion assays.[81] The enteroadherent bacteria are perhaps best diagnosed by biopsy. In addition, certain parasites (*Giardia* and *Strongyloides*) may be difficult to detect in stool and could best be diagnosed by duodenal aspiration, by string test (*Giardia*), or by intestinal biopsy.[82] Therefore, the physician may need to communicate his presumptive diagnosis to the laboratory, if warranted by history or epidemiologic evidence. Lastly, it must be remembered that anywhere between 20% and 40% of all acute infectious diarrheas will remain undiagnosed even with the application of all laboratory techniques.

TREATMENT OF ACUTE DIARRHEA

The treatment of diarrhea can be divided into symptomatic (fluid replacement and antidiarrheal) therapy and specific, antimicrobial therapy.[103-106] Death in most instances of acute diarrhea is due to dehydration. Therefore, a cardinal principle of the management of any diarrhea is attention to and replacement of fluid and electrolyte deficits. Severely dehydrated individuals, particularly those

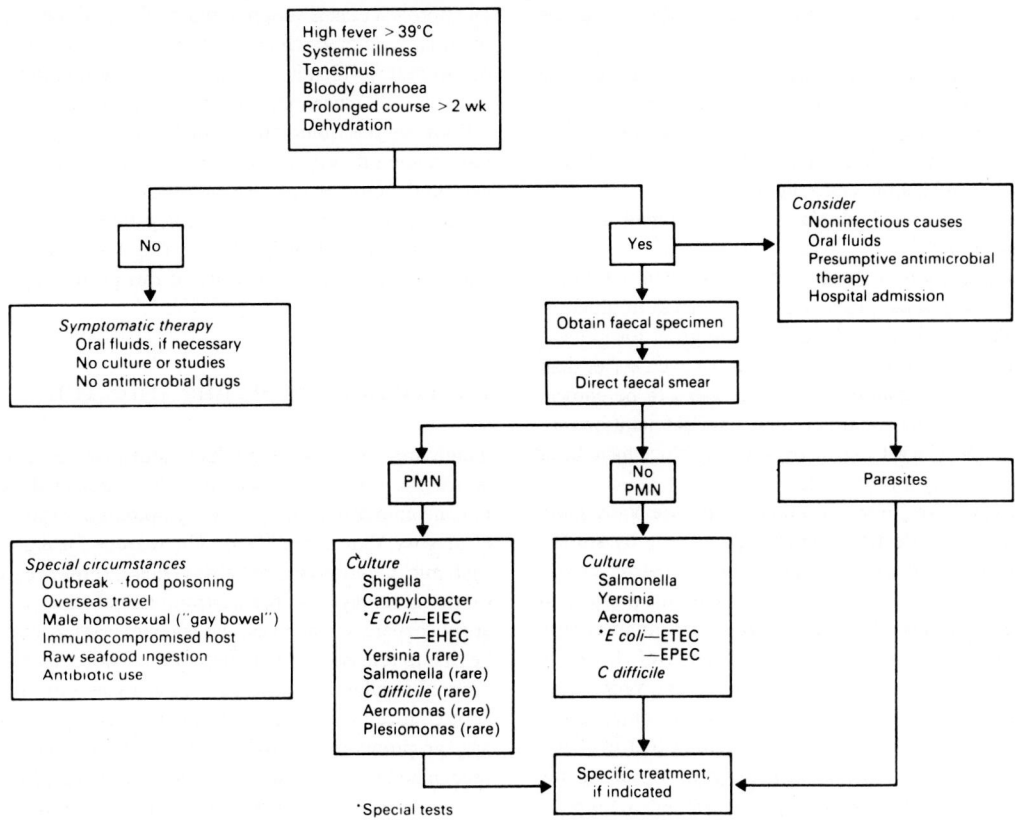

FIGURE 38–10. Algorithm for the diagnostic approach to acute diarrhea. (Gorbach SL. Bacterial diarrhoea and its treatment. Lancet 1987;2:1378.)

with altered mental status, should be rehydrated with intravenous Ringer's lactate or saline solutions to which additional K and NaHCO$_3$ may be added as necessary.[107] Alert patients should be given oral replacement solutions (ORS) (Table 38-9). Experience

in the developing nations has demonstrated the efficacy of ORS in most causes of severe dehydrating diarrhea.[108] Their use in developed nations has lagged behind, and this may in part account for some of the morbidity and mortality still experienced in the

TABLE 38–9
Composition of Oral Replacement Solutions for the Treatment of Diarrhea

SOLUTION	Na mmol/L	K mmol/L	Cl mmol/L	CITRATE mmol/L	GLUCOSE† mmol/L
WHO solution	90	20	80	30	111 (20)
Pedialyte RS	75	20	65	30	139 (25)
Pedialyte	45	20	35	30	139 (25)
Resol	50	20	50	34	111 (20)
Lytren	50	25	45	30	111 (20)
Infalyte	50	20	40	30*	111 (20)
Gatorade	23.5	<1	17	—	(40)
Coca-Cola	1.6	<1	—	13.4*	(100)
Apple juice	<1	25	—	—	(120)
Orange juice	<1	50	—	50	(120)

* Bicarbonate concentration rather than citrate.
† Figures in parentheses represent grams of carbohydrate.
See reference 106 for the names and composition of solutions available in the United Kingdom.
(Modified from Di John D, Levine MM. Treatment of diarrhea. Infect Dis Clin North Am 1988;2:719.)

United States.[109] In mild to moderate dehydration, ORS can be given to infants and children in volumes of 50 to 100 ml per kg over 4 to 6 hours, whereas adults may need to drink up to 1000 ml per hour.[107] Once the patient is rehydrated, 100 to 200 ml per kg can be given every 24 hours until the diarrhea ceases. The World Health Organization (WHO) solution is endorsed for use in both rehydration and maintenance therapy worldwide, although some are concerned that the high Na content (90 mmol/L) may lead to hypernatremia.[105,106]

Recently, investigation of these solutions has centered on increasing their efficacy. The addition of amino acids to glucose-based ORS or the substitution of rice or grain gruel for glucose suggests that such "super ORS" solutions may be even better than the conventional WHO solution.[110] This remains to be shown. Clearly, the WHO solution and the commercial ORS solutions are superior to Gatorade, Coca-Cola, or fruit juices, which have been frequently used for rehydration in this country.

Bismuth subsalicylate (Pepto-Bismol) is safe (see below) and efficacious in bacterial infectious diarrheas, as shown by studies of traveler's diarrhea.[111] It may not have antidiarrheal activity in viral diarrhea,[112] raising the question whether its main effect in travelers diarrhea is through its antibacterial or anti-inflammatory action or perhaps because its clay vehicle is capable of absorbing enterotoxins.[113] Kaolin–pectin preparations are not very effective.[114] Because of the possibility of worsening the colonization or invasion of the organism by paralyzing intestinal motility, and evidence that the use of motility-altering drugs may prolong microorganism excretion time, neither opiates nor anticholinergic drugs are recommended for infectious diarrheas. However, it has been shown that loperamide can be both useful and safe in traveler's diarrhea, provided it is not given to patients who have high fever or those with blood or pus in the stool.[115] The anxiolytics and antiemetics that decrease sensory perception may make symptoms more tolerable and generally are safe.

Antibiotic therapy in the infectious diarrheas is controversial (see ch 68, 83, 104, and 105). Those with mild disease or those who are clearly improving probably do not need antibiotic treatment. There are certain infectious diarrheas in which treatment is recommended: *shigellosis, cholera, traveler's diarrhea, pseudomembranous enterocolitis,* and the *parasitic diseases.* There are other diarrheas in which treatment is not indicated, primarily because there is no effective therapy (e.g., viral diarrhea and cryptosporidiosis). There are several diseases where the indications are less clear but treatment is usually recommended (i.e., infection with the noncholera vibrios, prolonged or protracted infection with *Yersinia,* early in the course of campylobacteriosis, and nursery outbreaks of enteropathogenic *E. coli* diarrhea). Regardless of the cause of infectious diarrhea, patients should be treated if they are debilitated with malignancy, are immunosuppressed, have an abnormal cardiovascular system or valvular, vascular, or orthopedic prostheses, have hemolytic anemia (especially when salmonellosis is involved), or are extremely young or old. Treatment is also advised for those with prolonged symptoms and those who relapse. These guidelines were developed for patients with salmonellosis,[101] but they are useful guidelines for all infectious diarrheas.

Chapters 68, 69, 83, 103, 104, and 105 outline the antimicrobials of choice for the various infections. However, usually it will be 3 to 5 days after obtaining stools before specific organisms can be grown and identified. Although there is no clear evidence that early treatment will alter the course of an infectious diarrhea, such

an approach makes common sense. The antibiotics to use, if treatment is warranted while awaiting specific diagnosis, are trimethoprim-sulfa, which is at least second-line therapy for most of the infectious diarrheas except for *Campylobacter, C. difficile,* and the vibrios, or the quinolones (norfloxacin or ciprofloxacin), which have some efficacy against these other organisms as well. If the symptom complex suggests giardiasis, a course of metronidazole might be given even if stools are negative for cysts, although duodenal aspiration/biopsy or the string test might be indicated to clarify the presence or absence of this protozoa.[82]

Diarrhea in Systemic Infection

There are several systemic infectious diseases in which diarrhea is often a prominent symptom either early in the clinical course or concomitantly with the other symptoms as the disease progresses (Category V in Table 38-8). The reasons for diarrhea with these systemic infections are not always clear. It may represent invasion of the enterocyte or the gastrointestinal mucosa as a portal of entry (hepatitis, listeriosis, and legionellosis). Alternatively, it may be due to release of inflammatory mediators, such as the interleukins or bradykinin, in severe systemic diseases like Rocky Mountain spotted fever or psittacosis. Nausea, vomiting, and severe diarrhea are symptoms in the toxic shock syndrome. This disease can be recognized by its occurrence in menstruating young females who use tampons and by the accompanying symptoms of skin rash with desquamation and hypotension.

Prolonged Infectious Diarrhea

POSTINFECTIOUS MALABSORPTION

There are a number of syndromes where infectious watery or bloody diarrheas seem to persist[116] or else change to malabsorptive diarrheas.[117] Infants with severe infectious diarrhea may become severely malnourished and then develop disaccharidase deficiency or what appears to be a chronic malabsorptive disease. The resulting protein deficits may cause poor repair, but the role of bacterial overgrowth and the possibility of unidentified, persistent infection remain to be clarified in this syndrome. These infants can be managed with total parenteral and then enteral nutrition.[118] Many will recover normal intestinal function with time.

PROTRACTED INFECTION

A form of protracted diarrhea has been seen in travelers, and undiagnosed chronic infections or nonspecific bacterial overgrowth has been postulated.[119] Such a pathophysiologic mechanism is similar to that proposed for tropical sprue (ch 69). Thus, where *protracted travelers diarrhea* ends and *tropical sprue* begins may be a matter of small-bowel histology. Hard-to-diagnose organisms that are known to cause protracted or prolonged diarrheas include enteropathogenic (enteroadherent) *E. coli, Giardia* and *Amoeba,* and cryptosporidiosis. *Aeromonas*[120] and *Yersinia enterocolitica*[87] can both present with a chronic watery diarrheal syndrome or as a colitis. *C. difficile* is a disease that often is difficult to clear, and as many as four to five relapses have been observed. Patients with chronic diarrheas should have these diseases ruled out.

RAW MILK DIARRHEA

Prolonged diarrhea may be due to organisms that have not yet been identified. An example of this may be raw milk diarrhea, which was reported in outbreak form in Minnesota.[121] These patients developed chronic watery diarrhea with weight loss that often lasted 18 months and was labeled frequently as irritable bowel syndrome. It has also been reported in other states associated with raw milk ingestion,[122] and a disease of similar clinical manifestations, without raw milk ingestion, has been recorded.[123] This just points out that there are still unidentified organisms that can cause both acute and chronic diarrheas.

Hospital- and Health Care Facility-Acquired Diarrhea

The incidence of diarrhea is extremely high among hospitalized patients and those residing in chronic care facilities for the retarded/mentally disturbed or for the elderly. Often this is a hidden problem, known only by the nurse's aide who changes the bed sheets. In the intensive care setting it occurs in 30% to 50% of patients, and in chronic care facilities over one third of patients will have a significant diarrheal illness each year.[6,124–126] This is a multifactorial condition and, no doubt, all of the factors are not yet understood. Recognized causes include fecal impaction, nosocomial gastrointestinal infections, diarrheogenic drugs, enteral feeding, and anticancer therapy.

FECAL IMPACTION

Clinical lore has it that the most common cause of diarrhea in hospitalized or institutionalized patients is a fecal impaction. Such paradoxical diarrhea and incontinence appear to be most common in patients with dementia or psychosis.[127,128] While the validity of this clinical impression remains uncertain, the need to perform a rectal examination and perhaps a flat and upright abdominal x-ray in such patients can certainly be recommended, if for no other reason than because important findings can ensue from such an exam. A gentle rectal examination can be well tolerated and safe even in a coronary care unit.

DRUGS

In a given patient, any of his or her medications may be initiating diarrhea. There are, however, certain medications that are more apt to cause diarrhea than others (Tables 38-3 and 38-4). A proportion of antibiotic-induced diarrhea is due to *C. difficile* infection. Whether non-*difficile* antibiotic-induced diarrhea is due to a nonspecific change in flora, a chemical effect of the antibiotic, or

overgrowth of some other enterotoxin-producing microorganism remains to be determined.

ELIXIR DIARRHEA

Drugs such as theophylline or KCl made up in liquid formulations (elixirs) may cause diarrhea because of the high content of sorbitol used to sweeten the elixir.[129,130] This is the iatrogenic equivalent of "chewing gum diarrhea" (see below).

ENTERAL FEEDING

An important but poorly understood cause of diarrhea is tube feeding, particularly in the critically ill patient.[6,124–126,129–135] Up to 25% to 35% of patients on tube feeding will develop diarrhea. Various pathophysiologic factors are hypothesized: (1) bacterial contamination of the enteral formula, particularly as it warms to room temperature, allowing proliferation of a bacteria as the feeding is slowly infused, (2) the administration of hypertonic solutions that cause diarrhea by inducing a form of "dumping syndrome," (3) the administration of lactose-containing formulas to lactase-deficient subjects, (4) the administration of sorbitol-containing elixirs, (5) the administration of low-Na formulas that result in considerable blood-to-lumen Na diffusion in addition to fluid movement if the formula is hypertonic as well, and (6) the presence of hypoalbuminemia in malnourished patients, which alters the oncotic or Starling forces in the gut capillaries, thus preventing absorption or inducing secretion. Although there are experimental studies that support all of the possibilities above, the administration of tube feeding to otherwise normal patients is usually not accompanied by diarrhea,[136–138] and the presence of hypoalbuminemia does not always correlate with the presence of diarrhea.[138] Furthermore, a closely monitored and controlled study comparing elemental (osmolality 690 mosm/kg) with polymeric (395 mosm/kg) diets has shown no difference in the incidence of diarrhea (24%–31%) in such patients.[139] It is tempting, therefore, to consider the possibility of physiologic abnormalities in these critically ill patients, which, under the setting of enteral feeding, lead to either inhibited Na and water absorption or stimulated Cl and water secretion. While studies have shown essentially normal fat absorption in the debilitated and elderly,[140] there are few studies of water and electrolyte transport in such patients.

NOSOCOMIAL DIARRHEA

Mental institutions have high incidences of shigellosis[84] and diseases caused by protozoan parasites (*E. histolytica* and *Giardia*)[82] and the helminths.[141] Infectious diarrhea is common in hospitals, accounting for over 20% of nosocomial infections and being second only to respiratory infections on pediatric wards.[6,142] The rates are particularly high in intensive care settings, where 8 cases per 100 admissions exceed the rates of even pediatric wards by a factor of 4.[6,142] In the ICU setting, the role of tube feeding as a source of infection and H$_2$ blockers, which eradicate the gastric acid barrier, has been postulated. Although in years past the most common cause was infection with *Salmonella* species,[142] since 1980 *C. difficile* accounts for over 50%[143] and *Salmonella* only 12% of cases.[144]

In fact, the likelihood of a nosocomial infection due to *Salmonella* or *Shigella* in the tertiary, big city hospital is so rare that routine cultures for *Salmonella* and *Shigella* and ova/parasite exams are not cost-effective if diarrhea begins after hospital admission.[145] Immunosuppressed patients are another important group susceptible to nosocomial diarrhea. Viral infections (rotavirus, adenovirus, and Coxsackie) may be an important cause of nosocomial infectious diarrheas in bone marrow transplant units, where they cause increased mortality.[146] These causes must be differentiated from the diarrhea of graft-versus-host disease.

Outbreaks of hemorrhagic *E. coli* infections and *C. difficile* have been recognized in nursing homes.[93,143] *Clostridium difficile* cytotoxin may be found in the stool of a quarter of these elderly patients, and one third of these may have diarrhea.[143] There is a distinct possibility that some of the strokes, injuries from falls, and even myocardial infarctions occurring in nursing home settings could be due to the hypovolemia and toxic state induced by these nosocomial diarrheas. Hand washing and use of gloves by health care personnel may reduce the incidence of *C. difficile* diarrhea.[147,148]

Hospital-acquired diarrheas may be a causative factor in other nosocomial hospital infections (i.e., of the urinary tract).[142] Thus, the impact of nosocomial diarrhea on the duration and cost of hospitalization and on morbidity is probably substantial.

ACUTE DIARRHEA CONCOMITANT WITH CANCER TREATMENT

The incidence of acute, mild diarrhea with chemotherapy or radiation therapy is quite high, approaching 100% with some agents or regimens. Radiation therapy causes chronic diarrhea as well, and this is discussed later. Nausea, vomiting, and diarrhea are dose- and agent-related phenomena; induced diarrhea requires a greater amount of radiation,[149,150] and diarrhea occurs usually with specific forms of chemotherapy.[151] The nausea and vomiting may well be due to circulating chemicals (beta-endorphins, histamine, prostaglandins, and endotoxin) or to the central nervous system (CNS) effect of the agent itself. The diarrhea appears to require changes in intestinal morphology. The stem cell for enterocytes, which resides in the crypt, is among the cells more sensitive to the effects of cytotoxic drugs and irradiation. With significant doses of either form of cytotoxic therapy there is disintegration of the crypt epithelium, decreases in mitoses, decreases in digestive brush border enzymes, and often the development of villus atrophy.[152-154] With recovery from the acute injury, crypt hyperplasia may develop. A significant inflammatory infiltrate develops in the lamina propria, and if the doses are high enough or continued for long enough, there will be ulceration of the epithelium. These changes are similar to those described for rotavirus (see above), and abnormalities of motility and water and electrolyte transport also occur.[155,156] The chemotherapeutic agents most likely to cause severe diarrhea are amsacrine, azacitidine, cytosine arabinoside, actinomycin D, daunorubicin, doxorubicin, floxuridine, 5-fluorouracil, 6-mercaptopurine, methotrexate, and Mithracin.[151] The combination of 5-fluorouracil plus leucovorin causes a severe watery diarrhea.[157] It has been recognized recently that the incidence of diarrhea with interleukin-2 therapy approaches 80%.[158]

Radiation may induce diarrhea either through damage to segments of bowel during pelvic irradiation or through damage to the entire bowel when total body radiation is received.[150,159,160] Total body radiation at low doses (1.5 Gy) causes only nausea and vomiting. Either watery or bloody diarrhea ensues at total body doses greater than 6 Gy,[150] and pelvic irradiation over 4 weeks with doses of 3 to 4 Gy may also cause diarrhea.[160] Current treatment for both chemotherapy and radiation-induced diarrhea is symptomatic and includes antimotility drugs and cyclooxygenase blockers.

Runner's Diarrhea

Gastrointestinal disturbances including anorexia, heartburn, nausea, vomiting, cramps, urgency, and diarrhea are quite common in those who exercise vigorously, particularly marathon runners and triathletes.[161] Diarrhea may occur in 10% to 25% and is particularly common (40%-70%) in women runners. "Runner's trots" usually is a watery diarrhea that is self-limiting. The mechanisms operative in runner's diarrhea are unclear but may involve release of gastrointestinal hormones such as gastrin, motilin, or vasoactive intestinal polypeptide (VIP)[162] or release of inflammatory mediators such as prostaglandins.[163] A role for ischemia has been postulated because of the occurrence of ischemia colitis in marathon runners.[164] Many treatment regimens have been used, but none has been studied. Because there is already a delayed transit time with exercise,[165] antimotility drugs may not help. Nevertheless, they might be tried. Nonsteroidal anti-inflammatory agents are taken by many runners, but it is not clear whether they help in this condition.

CHRONIC DIARRHEA

Definition and Classification

Chronic diarrheas are those of at least 3 to 6 weeks' duration, and they fall into three categories broadly based on pathophysiologic mechanisms—osmotic diarrhea (Table 38-3), deranged electrolyte transport diarrhea (Table 38-4), or enterocyte damage/death with inflammation (Table 38-5)—that correspond basically to malabsorptive, secretory, and inflammatory diarrheas, respectively. It would be convenient clinically if the character of the stool that results from a specific pathophysiology correlated as well (i.e., steatorrhea with all cases of malabsorption, watery stool only with secretory diarrheas, or bloody stool with inflammation). Unfortunately, this is not the case. Carbohydrate malabsorption causes a watery diarrhea, as does inflammation that is not severe enough to cause ulceration and blood vessel abnormalities. Inflammation may also cause malabsorption (e.g., eosinophilic gastroenteritis or mastocytosis). Similarly, diseases whose hallmark is intestinal malabsorption may actually have impressive inflammation (e.g., celiac sprue),[166] and malabsorptive diseases often have an element of intestinal secretion.[167] Nonetheless, for clinical purposes it is reasonable to initially classify diarrheas as either steatorrhea, watery diarrhea, or inflammatory diarrhea, realizing that these categories are mixed with regard to pathophysiology. Such a categorization directs the physician to certain diagnostic algorithms.

Epidemiology

It is impossible to arrive at exact figures for the incidence or prevalence of chronic diarrhea because of the many causes and because epidemiologists have not performed the appropriate population studies. Specific prevalence and incidence figures for the major diarrheal diseases can be obtained in the chapters on those specific entities. Suffice it to say it is a symptom present in probably 30% of patients coming to the gastroenterologist.

STEATORRHEA (GENERALIZED MALABSORPTIVE DISEASES)

Although the three major nutrients—fat, carbohydrate, and protein—may all be malabsorbed, we generally recognize clinical symptoms because of the malabsorption of either carbohydrate or fat. Protein or amino acid malabsorption (azotorrhea) occurs but is not clinically recognized unless it is severe enough to cause malnutrition or unless specific amino acid transport defects cause congenital systemic disease (see ch 19 and 72). Malabsorption of electrolytes and water is also part of the pathophysiology of malabsorptive diarrheas. The gut's limited ability to absorb high concentrations of divalent ions (i.e., mg, SO_4, and PO_4) results in clinically evident diarrhea when these ions are ingested in excess. Clinically, the generalized malabsorptive diseases present as steatorrhea.

Fat absorption is discussed in Chapter 18. Based on the normal physiology of absorption, fat malabsorption can be divided into three broad categories: (1) intraluminal maldigestion, (2) mucosal malabsorption, and (3) postmucosal malabsorption due to lymphatic obstruction. The diseases listed in Table 38-3 can be allocated to one or more of these three general categories.

Intraluminal Maldigestion

CHRONIC LIVER DISEASE AND BILE DUCT OBSTRUCTION

Because bile duct obstruction from cancer of the head of the pancreas can cause steatorrhea, presumably through both pancreatic and bile salt insufficiency, it is natural to assume that the 25% to 100% incidence of mild steatorrhea in patients with cirrhosis is also due to inadequate micelle formation from bile salt insufficiency.[168] However, secondary factors, including malnutrition, portal hypertension, bacterial overgrowth, and drugs (e.g., neomycin), may also play a role. In both cancer of the pancreas and severe liver disease, diarrhea is not usually a significant clinical problem; the fat malabsorption is usually mild. Certainly the weight loss in these two conditions is multifactorial.

BACTERIAL OVERGROWTH

Stasis syndromes cause steatorrhea as well as an inflammatory and secretory form of diarrhea.[169] Steatorrhea is due to deconjugation of bile salts, causing poor micelle formation. However, brush border injury, mucosal inflammation, hydroxylation of fat with resulting fatty acid diarrhea, and changes in intestinal motility all play a role in this disease as well (see ch 73).

PANCREATIC EXOCRINE INSUFFICIENCY

Chronic pancreatitis may cause weight loss because of anorexia or because of fear that eating will cause pain by aggravating pancreatitis. When at least 90% of the secretory capacity of the pancreas is lost, *chronic pancreatic exocrine insufficiency* supervenes, and malabsorption leads to continued weight loss, in spite of a good-to-excellent appetite (see ch 89). Up to 70% of patients with pancreatic calcification have chronic pancreatitis severe enough to cause malabsorption.

Cystic fibrosis is a childhood equivalent of chronic pancreatic insufficiency, but the weight loss in this disease is probably due as much to the anorexia of chronic infection[170] as to the malabsorption induced by pancreatic enzyme and bile acid deficiencies.[171]

Somatostatinoma is a rare pancreatic islet tumor with highly variable symptoms but may present with gallstones, diabetes, and diarrhea.[172] However, it is the one neuroendocrine tumor in which the diarrhea is due to steatorrhea rather than intestinal secretion. Presumably, the steatorrhea is secondary to inhibition of pancreatic secretion.

Mucosal Malabsorption

DRUGS

The chronic ingestion of *drugs* such as colchicine,[173] cholestyramine,[174] neomycin,[175] or para-aminosalicylic acid (PAS)[176] induces steatorrhea either by enterocyte damage or, in the case of cholestyramine, by binding bile acids.

INFECTIOUS DISEASES

Parasites may cause malabsorption, particularly the protozoa *Giardia* and *Isospora*[177-179] and the helminth *Strongyloides,*[180] through brush border damage. Because these are treatable diseases, they must be sought and rigorously excluded by stool exam or small intestinal biopsy. *Mycobacterium avium-intracellulare* also causes malabsorption; unfortunately, it responds poorly to treatment (see ch 103).

IMMUNE SYSTEM DISEASES

There are several inflammatory diseases, including *systemic mastocytosis*[181] and *eosinophilic gastroenteritis,*[182] in which gross distortion of the mucosa is associated with fat malabsorption. On occasion, the steatorrhea may be profound, and the patients thus present with a "spruelike" syndrome. In other patients, the watery diarrhea, systemic flushing, abdominal pain, tachycardia, and protein-losing enteropathy overshadow the steatorrhea (see below).

TROPICAL SPRUE

This disease of unknown etiology affects those in certain tropical parts of the world, including the Indian subcontinent and Asia, the West Indies, northern South America, and parts of Central America and central and southern Africa (see ch 69). It can occur in visitors residing in these areas for as short a time as 1 to 3 months. Its acute onset suggests an infectious origin, and an unknown infection either persists or leads to brush border damage and bacterial overgrowth with perpetuation of the disease. Small-bowel histology may show minimal villus blunting and inflammatory infiltrate or may reveal severe villus atrophy and crypt hyperplasia. If the patient is removed from the tropical areas and the mucosal change is mild, the disease may remit spontaneously.[183] A combination of tetracycline and folic acid is effective therapy.

CELIAC SPRUE

This disease, also called nontropical sprue, celiac disease, and gluten-sensitive enteropathy, is the prototype mucosal malabsorptive disease (see ch 71). Although it presents classically with the signs and symptoms of malabsorption (Table 38-10), it may have occult presentations as well. It presents as a failure to thrive in the very young[184] with muscle wasting, abdominal distention, and irritability ("the clinging child"). It may become asymptomatic during adolescence and then present during this period as unexplained iron deficiency anemia, growth retardation, or anorexia to the point of suggesting an eating disorder, or the development of recurrent mouth ulcerations (aphthous ulcers) and diarrhea in the young adult may suggest inflammatory bowel disease.[185-187] (The term *sprue* comes from the Dutch "spruw," which means thrush, in recognition of the frequent oral aphthae).[185] In later life it may present with insidious nutritional deficiencies, including infertility and neuromuscular and skeletal disease.[188-190]

DERMATITIS HERPETIFORMIS

This form of skin disease is associated with celiaclike intestinal morphology in 70% to 80% of cases.[191] The blistering skin disease,

TABLE 38-10

Comparison of Clinical Features of Malabsorption Due to Mucosal Disease (Celiac Sprue) With Impaired Intraluminal Digestion (Chronic Pancreatic Insufficiency)

CLINICAL MANIFESTATIONS	CELIAC SPRUE	PANCREATIC INSUFFICIENCY
Symptom/sign		
Sex	F > M (2:1)	M > F (3:1)
Age of onset	<3; 20–40	30–60
Diarrhea (%)	70–90	70–90
Weight loss (%)	60–90	90
Flatulence & bloating (%)	40	0
Weakness & lethargy (%)	95	4
Anorexia (%)	30–50	0
Oral aphthous ulcers, recurrent (%)	60	0
Severe abdominal pain (%)	0	64
Increased appetite (%)	15	70
Oil separates from stool (%)	0	57
Extraintestinal symptoms		
Tetany, bone pain, hemorrhagic diathesis, edema or ascites, nocturnal polyuria (%)	20–50	0–10
Lab tests		
Stool fat, g/24 h	25 (range, 3.5–87)	48 (range, 8–180)
Stool fat concentration, g/100 g stool (%)	<9.5	>9.5
Total serum protein < 6 g/dL (%)	71	14
Anemia (%)	21	0

(Modified from Evans WB, Wollaeger EE. Incidence and severity of nutritional deficiency states in chronic exocrine pancreatic insufficiency: Comparison with nontropical sprue. Am J Dig Dis 1966;11:594; Bo-Linn GW, Fordtran JS. Fecal fat concentration in patients with steatorrhea. Gastroenterology 1984;87:319.)

which is characterized by IgA deposits in the dermal papilla, usually responds to dapsone, while the mucosal lesion responds to gluten-free diet. The diet also seems to have a beneficial effect on the skin lesion, and about 50% of patients will be able to stop dapsone medication.

WHIPPLE'S DISEASE

This is a systemic infectious disease classically involving the intestine of middle-aged males (M:F ratio is 5:1). The peak incidence occurs at ages 40 to 50, but it is reported in infants and in octogenarians. It presents with all of the signs and symptoms of severe mucosal disease (Table 38-10) but has some additional characteristics: arthralgias in 65%, chills and fever in up to 40%, hypotension (blood pressure < 110/60) in 70%, lymphadenopathy in over 50%, and, most important, involvement of the central nervous system in a plethora of ways.[192] This disease is discussed in more detail in Chapter 75.

ABETALIPOPROTEINEMIA

This is a rare defect in chylomicron formation (absence of Apo B) that presents in children as steatorrhea, acanthocytic red cells, ataxia, and retinitis pigmentosa (see ch 18 and 72). A variant, chylomicron retention disease, has been reported. Patients with Tangier disease (absence of Apo AI and Apo II) have yellow-orange streaks and spots in the tonsils and colonic mucosa. They may have diarrhea but not steatorrhea.

Postmucosal Obstruction

INTESTINAL LYMPHANGIECTASIA

This is either a congenital or acquired (post-traumatic, lymphoma, carcinomas, and Whipple's) disease that causes protein-losing enteropathy with significant steatorrhea.[193-195] It is the classic form of postmucosal obstruction malabsorption. The unique pathophysiology (malabsorption of fat with loss of protein and lymphocytes, but normal absorption of carbohydrates) relates to the obstructed lymphatics channels, which are the route of absorption for fat and for the recovery of lymphocyte and protein-laden lymph. The absorption of carbohydrates and amino acids takes place by way of the portal circulation and remains unaffected.

Mixed Causes of Steatorrhea

SHORT-BOWEL SYNDROME

Extensive intestinal resection represents another complicated, multifactorial form of steatorrhea resulting from the lack of sufficient absorptive surface, decreased transit time, and diminished

bile salt pool (see ch 74). The diarrhea is heightened by the osmotic effect of nonabsorbed solutes, by gastric hypersecretion, perhaps by bacterial overgrowth, and conceivably even by intestinal secretion.

METABOLIC DISEASES

Diseases such as *thyrotoxicosis*,[196] *adrenal insufficiency*,[197] and *protein–calorie malnutrition*[198,199] may result in malabsorption through different mechanisms. Thyrotoxicosis may simply shorten transit time so as to disturb the intraluminal phase of the fat absorption. Adrenal insufficiency appears to generally disturb intraluminal and mucosal absorption, as does protein–calorie malnutrition, which also causes a villus atrophy. As is the case with *liver disease*,[168] the clinical picture usually overshadows the diarrhea and malabsorption, and certainly the weight loss in these conditions is only partly due to the malabsorption.

History and Physical Examination in Malabsorption

The signs and symptoms of generalized malabsorption are outlined in Table 38-11, along with the responsible pathophysiologic mechanisms and the expected laboratory test abnormalities.[200] Mild degrees of malabsorption may be entirely asymptomatic and may not result in the classic gastrointestinal manifestations of flatulence, bulky or greasy foul-smelling stools, and weight loss. In fact, the mild steatorrhea of common bile duct obstruction, chronic liver disease, early pancreatic insufficiency, and even mild celiac disease may be undetected by the patient. For these reasons, malabsorption sometimes presents as an aberration of one of the other body systems: anemias, hemorrhagic diathesis, osteopenic bone disease, tetany, amenorrhea, or infertility. The skin, mucous membrane, and visual and peripheral nervous system manifestations of essential nutrient malabsorption may occur also.

There are certain clues to help differentiate clinically severe mucosal disease, as manifested by celiac sprue or Whipple's disease, from the malabsorption due to exocrine pancreatic insufficiency (Table 38-11). Although sex and age may be helpful, they are not nearly as discriminating between mucosal and pancreatic disease as are the anorexia, lethargy, and malaise of intestinal mucosal disease. Most likely these symptoms are due to activation of the increased number of lamina propria inflammatory cells with release of inflammatory mediators, particularly cytokines (see Fig 38-9). The systemic manifestations of malabsorption with mucosal disease are usually more severe than those of pancreatic insufficiency, and therefore extraintestinal symptoms are more common. Repeated bouts of pancreatitis in patients with pancreatic insufficiency, however, can cause severe abdominal pain, and this may be a useful clue to this diagnosis.

The character of the stool may be a useful differentiating symptom. The fat content (%) of the stool in pancreatic insufficiency is considerably higher than in mucosal disease.[201] At body temperature, the fat may be present as oil, and the oil may separate from the stool, manifesting as oily seepage from the anus or as oil droplets floating in the toilet bowl after passage of the steatorrheic

TABLE 38-11
Correlation of Clinical Manifestations, Pathophysiology, and Laboratory Findings in Malabsorptive Processes

SIGNS AND SYMPTOMS	PATHOPHYSIOLOGIC MECHANISM	LABORATORY ABNORMALITIES
Gastrointestinal		
Diarrhea	Malabsorption of fat, CHO, and protein Increased secretion due to crypt hyperplasia, inflammatory mediators, bile and fatty acids	Stool weights > 200 g Stool weight ↓ to normal with fast Stool osmotic gap > 100 mosm/kg H_2O [Na] < 60 mmol/L
Weight loss	Nutrient malabsorption, anorexia in mucosal diseases	Increased stool fat, decreased serum proteins
Flatulence, borborygmus, abdominal distention, foul-smelling stools	Bacterial fermentation of malabsorbed carbohydrates and proteins	Increased flatus production
Bulky, greasy stools	Fat malabsorption	Increased stool fat, low serum carotene
Abdominal pain	If severe, due to chronic pancreatitis If mild, distention of bowel and inflammation	
Hematopoietic		
Anemia	Fe, pyridoxine, folate, and B_{12} deficiency	Microcytic, macrocytic, or dimorphic anemia
Hemorrhagic diathesis	Vitamin K deficiency	Prolonged prothrombin time
Musculoskeletal		
Bone pain (osteopenic bone disease)	Ca, Vitamin D, and protein malabsorption	Hypocalcemia, hypophosphatemia, increased serum alkaline phosphatase
Tetany	Ca, Mg, Vitamin D malabsorption	Above plus hypomagnesemia
Endocrine		
Amenorrhea, infertility, impotence	Malabsorption with protein–caloric malnutrition	Low serum proteins; may have abnormalities in gonadotropin secretion
Secondary hyperparathyroidism	Probably Vitamin D and Ca deficiency	Increased alkaline phosphatase, increased serum PTH
Skin and mucous membranes		
Cheilosis, glossitis, stomatitis,	Iron, riboflavin, niacin, folate, and B_{12} deficiency	Low serum Fe, folate, B_{12}
Purpura	Vitamin K deficiency	Prolonged prothrombin time
Follicular hyperkeratosis	Vitamin A deficiency	Low serum carotene
Scaly dermatitis or acrodermatitis	Zinc and essential fatty acid deficiency	Low serum or urinary Zn
Hyperpigmented dermatitis	Niacin deficiency	
Edema and/or ascites	Protein malabsorption	Low serum albumin
Nervous system		
Xerophthalmia and night blindness	Vitamin A deficiency	Decreased serum carotene
Peripheral neuropathy	Vitamin B, thiamine deficiency	Decreased serum B_{12}

(Modified from Trier JS. Intestinal malabsorption: Differentiation of cause. Hosp Pract 1988; 23:195.)

stool. Patients with pancreatic insufficiency rarely have flatulence and bloating, perhaps because salivary or gastric amylase ameliorates somewhat the carbohydrate malabsorption. Stools tend to float in malabsorptive diseases as a result of the gas content, which is due to carbohydrate malabsorption and not fat malabsorption.[202] Total serum protein concentrations are usually lower in intestinal mucosal diseases, most likely because of concomitant protein-losing enteropathy, and anemia is more common because of both iron and folate malabsorption.

Laboratory Diagnosis of Steatorrhea (Malabsorptive Syndromes)

There are numerous laboratory tests (Table 38-12) directed at establishing the presence of steatorrhea and whether that steatorrhea comes from intestinal mucosal disease, lymphatic obstruction, or impaired intraluminal digestion. There are also therapeutic trials of varying philosophic acceptance: pancreatic enzyme ad-

TABLE 38–12

Comparison of Laboratory Results in the Three Types of Malabsorption: Musocal Disease, Impaired Intraluminal Digestion, and Postmucosal (Lymphatic) Obstruction

TEST	MUCOSAL DISEASE	IMPAIRED LUMINAL DIGESTION		LYMPHATIC OBSTRUCTION
		Pancreatic Disease	Bacterial Overgrowth	
Stool fat	↑↑	↑↑↑	↑	↑↑
Intestinal biopsy	Abnormal	Normal	Mildly abnormal	Usually abnormal
Screening (blood) tests of malabsorption				
Prothrombin time	May be ↓	May be ↓	May be ↓	May be ↓
Serum carotene	↓	↓	May be ↓	↓
Serum cholesterol	↓	↓	↓	↓
Serum albumin	↓	Normal	May be ↓	↓
Serum Fe	↓	Normal	Normal	Normal
Serum folate	↓	Normal	Normal	Normal
Serum B$_{12}$	Normal	Normal	May be ↓	Normal
Specific malabsorption tests				
^{14}C-triolein breath test	↓	↓	↓	↓
D-xylose absorption	↓	Normal	May be ↓	Normal
Schilling test	Normal	↓	↓	Normal
Breath tests (H$_2$, ^{14}C-xylose, or ^{14}C-cholylglycine)	Norm or abn	Normal	Abnormal	Normal
Bentiromide test	Normal or ↓	Normal or ↓	Normal or ?	Normal

(Modified from Trier JS. Intestinal malabsorption: Differentiation of cause. Hosp Pract 1988;23:195.)

ministration to diagnose pancreatic insufficiency, and antibiotic administration (tetracycline) coupled with the Schilling test to prove bacterial overgrowth. To diagnose the cause of steatorrhea, one should use the most specific, the least expensive, and the least invasive tests as dictated by clinical history and physical examination.

SCREENING TESTS

Blood tests that may be important clues to the presence of significant malabsorption include a complete blood count, prothrombin time, serum protein determination, and alkaline phosphatase. These may signal the presence of iron, folate, Vitamin B$_{12}$, Vitamin K, or severe Vitamin D malabsorption (osteomalacia is accompanied by an increased alkaline phosphatase). Serum carotene, cholesterol, albumin, serum iron, folate, and B$_{12}$ determination give additional clues to the presence of malabsorption, and these usually point to intestinal mucosal disease. Serum carotene may be low simply from poor intake, but not usually less than 50 μg/dL, as is commonly seen in severe malabsorption.

One should seriously consider early on sending stools for ova and parasite prior to beginning 24-hour stool collections or ob-taining barium x-rays, although this is not always cost-effective. The presence of barium interferes with the ability to find ova or parasites, even for 1 to 3 weeks after the procedure. Most important, before ordering any stool test, *look at the stool.* Although the stool in severe protein-losing enteropathy may, on occasion, be mistaken for the greasy, bulky, puttylike, foul-smelling stool of steatorrhea, the stool of neither of these types of diarrhea will be mistaken for watery or bloody diarrhea.

FECAL FAT TESTS

The usual intake of fat in the typical American diet is 100 to 150 g/day, mostly as triglycerides (ch 18). Previously it was thought that 93% to 97% of this fat was absorbed and that this percentage capability extended up to an intake of 200 g/day.[203] This relationship was recognized not to hold for neonates, whose stool fat may normally exceed 10% of intake.[18] Recently it has become clear that the normal coefficient of absorption of dietary triglycerides is 99%, while that for phospholipid of endogenous sources (bile, sloughed enterocytes, and bacteria) is 90% or better. Thus, 5 to 6 g of normal fecal fat is unabsorbed phospholipid from the 40- to 50-g endogenous pool.[204] Nonetheless, when total stool fat exceeds the normal 6 g/24 h (or triglyceride content exceeds 1 g/24 h), this can be detected by a simple *qualitative fecal fat determination* with an impressive degree (~90%) of sensitivity and specificity.[205-208] To perform the qualitative stool fat exam, stool is mixed with water and alcohol and heated, and then Sudan 3 or 4 stain is added. This will stain neutral fat (triglycerides) but will not stain fatty acid soaps. The latter can be dissociated by mixing glacial acetic acid and Sudan stain with the stool and heating it to boiling. The slide must be viewed while it is warm, because fatty acids and cholesterol will crystalize with cooling. A positive test is recorded when there are more than 100 orange-red globules of fat at least 6 to 75 μm in diameter (bigger than red blood cells) per medium power (40×) field. There is a positive correlation between the number of droplets and the fat content of the stool and a less clear relationship between the size of the droplets and the fat content.[208] The test loses some sensitivity with mild steatorrhea (fecal fat in the 6–10 g/24 h range). There are also false-negatives when fat intake is inadequate; therefore, it is wise to ensure that the patient is ingesting a normal diet (at least 100 g fat/24 h). False-positives can occur when mineral oil laxatives or rectal suppositories (cocoa butter) are given to the patient prior to stool collection. Obviously, the accuracy of the test depends also on the experience of the laboratory personnel.

The *quantitative fecal fat determination* is the gold standard with which all malabsorption tests are compared. Homogenized stool specimens are analyzed by the technics of Van de Kamer,[209] which involve the saponification of wet feces with alcohol and sodium hydroxide, liberation of the fatty acids with HCl, extraction with petroleum ether, and then titration of the fatty acids. The major problem with the quantitative fecal fat analysis is being sure that an adequate stool specimen has been collected. Because a patient's bowel movements might vary from day to day, the latter is possible only with a 72-hour collection. Even so, in 3 days less than 50% of patients will pass over 90% of ingested stool markers.[210] Furthermore, because phospholipids and cholesterol are derived primarily from endogenous sources, while triglyceride is the primary dietary fat, the Van de Kamer method with its 5 to 6 g/24 h upper limit of normal is actually not measuring just unabsorbed dietary fat. One could argue, therefore, that the alcohol part of the quantitative fecal fat test (Sudan stain) is more specific for detecting abnormalities of dietary fat absorption. This presupposes, however, that this basically qualitative test can be read quantitatively and uniformly. Therefore, the 3-day fecal quantitative fat determination remains the single best test for detection of steatorrhea. It is possible for patients to obtain the 3-day collection on an outpatient basis by providing them with a weighed paint can and toilet bowel inserts to separate stool from urine, and by having them purchase an inexpensive Styrofoam ice chest to keep the specimen on ice during the 3-day collection period.

Although stool fat excretion for 24 hours may be the same for mucosal and pancreatic disease, mucosal disease generally causes more water malabsorption or outright secretion.[201] The result is stool fat that is excessive but is diluted by the excess fluid. Consequently, the stool fat concentration (grams fat/100 g wet stool weight) is usually less than 9.5% in mucosal diseases such as celiac sprue and greater than 9.5% in chronic pancreatic insufficiency (Fig 38-11).

SMALL INTESTINAL BIOPSY

Once significant steatorrhea has been documented by either the qualitative or quantitative fecal fat determination, small intestinal biopsy is probably the most cost-effective way to determine whether the steatorrhea is due to intestinal disease or impaired luminal digestion. Small-bowel biopsy instruments such as the Rubin–Quentin multipurpose tube, the Crosby–Kugler capsule, or the Carey capsule are useful for distal duodenal biopsy, as is the hydraulic Rubin–Quentin tube that allows one to make several biopsies over a more extensive length of jejunum. The capsule technique is frequently used in infants because of its safety and the ease of passing this orally to the suckling child.[211] However, in adults, upper intestinal endoscopy with forceps biopsy of the

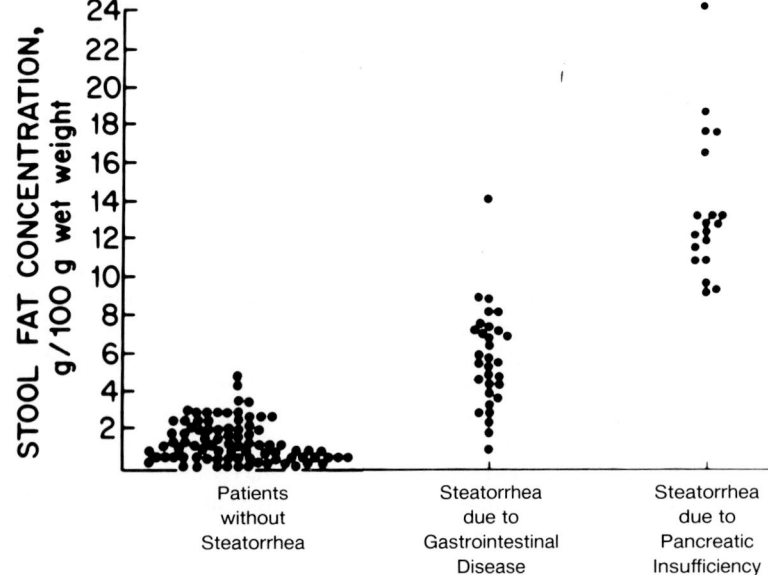

FIGURE 38-11. Stool fat concentrations in patients with intestinal mucosal disease and pancreatic insufficiency are compared with those in patients without steatorrhea. Steatorrhea due to pancreatic insufficiency is usually >9.5% (g fat/g weight of stool). (Bo-Linn GW, Fordtran JS. Fecal fat concentration in patients with steatorrhea. Gastroenterology 1984;87:319.)

duodenum has, for all intents and purposes, supplanted the use of these biopsy tubes (see ch 126). Endoscopy may also be diagnostic in celiac sprue because of the characteristic gross appearance of the duodenum (scalloped valvulae conniventes).[212]

There are a few diseases in which small-bowel biopsy is diagnostic (Table 38-13). Diseases that have a patchy distribution within the gastrointestinal tract might not be picked up on small-bowel biopsies obtained at endoscopy or, for that matter, even with single small intestinal capsule biopsies. Miscellaneous lesions not included in Table 38-13 that might be discovered with small-bowel biopsy include benign lymphoid hyperplasia, allergic enteropathies such as milk or soy protein hypersensitivity, lipid storage diseases such as Fabry's or Niemann-Pick disease, histoplasmosis, capillariasis, cytomegalovirus enteritis, schistosomiasis, and Waldenström's macroglobulinemia.[52,213]

Malabsorption Tests

D-XYLOSE ABSORPTION TEST

D-xylose is a five-carbon sugar that is incompletely absorbed in the duodenum and jejunum by both Na-dependent transcellular and passive paracellular mechanisms. Xylose is not completely metabolized, and therefore its excretion into urine or its concentrations in blood following ingestion of a standardized dose has been used for over 30 years as a small intestinal absorption test.[214] After an overnight fast, either 5 or 25 g is given orally, and the patient is encouraged to drink fluids in order to maintain a good urinary output. The large dose may cause nausea and vomiting or

TABLE 38-13
Diagnostic Reliability of Peroral Small Intestinal Biopsy

Diagnostic histology; diffuse lesions; should be present on endoscopic biopsy

Whipple's disease	PAS-positive lamina propria macrophages
Mycobacterium avium-intracellulare	Acid-fast lamina propria macrophages
Abetalipoproteinemia	Vacuolated, lipid-laden enterocytes with normal architecture
Agammaglobulinemia	Spruelike histology with *Giardia*

Abnormal, but not diagnostic, histology; diffuse lesions; should be present on endoscopic biopsy

Celiac, refractory, and tropical sprue	Varying degrees of villus atrophy and crypt hyperplasia with lamina propria inflammation
Viral enteritis	Same as mild–moderate sprue
Bacterial overgrowth	Same as mild–moderate sprue
Severe, prolonged folate and B_{12} deficiency	Same as sprue, reduced mitoses in crypts

Diagnostic histology; patchy distribution; therefore may be missed on endoscopic biopsy

Lymphoma	Villi widened and lamina propria filled with malignant lymphoma cells
Lymphangiectasia	Dilated lymphatics in lamina propria and submucosa
Eosinophilic enteritis	Lamina propria infiltrated with eosinophils and neutrophils; musoca normal to flat
Mastocytosis	Lamina propria infiltrated with mast cells, eosinophils and neutrophils; mucosa normal to flat
Amyloidosis	Amyloid in lamina propria and submucosa with Congo red stain; normal mucosa and architecture
Crohn's disease	Varying inflammation and ulceration with subepithelial granulomas
Giardiasis, Coccidia, strongyloidiasis	Mucosa normal to flat with *Giardia*, *Cryptosporidium* or *Strongyloides* on surfaces of villi or crypts; *Eimeria*, *Isospora* or Microsporidia within enterocytes

Abnormal but not diagnostic; patchy distribution; may be missed on endoscopic biopsy

Acute radiation enteritis, enteropathy of dermatitis herpetiformis	Spruelike lesion of varying severity

(Modified from Trier JS. Intestinal malabsorption: Differentiation of cause. Hosp Pract 1988;23:195; Trier JS. Diagnostic value of peroral biopsy of the proximal small intestine. N Engl J Med 1971;285:1470.)

a "dumpinglike" syndrome with diarrhea and side effects that may invalidate the test. Hepatic metabolism or excretion into the bowel accounts for a loss of about 35% of ingested dose, and approximately 25% of the administered dose is excreted in the urine. Patients with normal renal function will, therefore, excrete more than 4 g after a 25-g dose. The test has poor sensitivity in mild mucosal disease, although this can be increased by obtaining blood values following the oral dose. A blood level of greater than 25 mg/dL 1 hr following the 25-g dose, or greater than 20 mg/dL 1 hr after the 5-g dose, can be expected. Because the test depends on normal renal function, it is less useful in elderly patients in whom glomerular filtration rate (GFR) is reduced or in patients with known renal disease. Because it can be distributed into sequestered fluids, it is less useful in patients with ascites. Indeed, increased portal pressure alone has been shown to decrease xylose absorption. Furthermore, nonsteroidal anti-inflammatory drugs impair either absorption or urinary excretion. It has therefore lost diagnostic favor in the adult population, in whom the easy endoscopic small-bowel biopsy, with its increased sensitivity, has largely supplanted the d-xylose test. It should still be considered in those mucosal diseases in which a patchy distribution of the histologic lesion may invalidate the endoscopic biopsy (Table 38-13). It is, however, still used in the pediatric evaluation of mucosal malabsorption and can be used to follow the response to gluten-free diet.[214]

^{14}C-TRIOLEIN BREATH TEST

Following enzymatic hydrolysis by pancreatic proteins and micelle formation with bile salts, triglycerides are absorbed within the first 150 cm of jejunum. If a triglyceride such as triolein, labeled with ^{14}C at the carboxyl groups, is given with 20 to 30 g of non-labeled triolein (to promote biliary emptying), it should be efficiently absorbed, should be essentially completely metabolized to CO_2 and water, and the $^{14}CO_2$ should appear in the breath. This forms the basis for the ^{14}C-triolein breath test.[215–218] The CO_2 is collected by having the patient breathe for 60 to 90 seconds into a trap containing 1 to 2 mmol/L hyamine hydroxide and phenolphthalein. When the CO_2 has been converted to HCO_3 and carbonic acid, the reagents change color and a known molar quantity of CO_2 is quantitated in a β-scintillation counter. In patients with impaired fat absorption there is a reduction in the $^{14}CO_2$ excreted. Either cumulative or peak values provide discrimination, with 85% to 95% sensitivity and specificity. False-positives are obtained if there is poor gastric emptying (such as in diabetes and following gastric surgery), if there are conditions that lead to dilution of $^{14}CO_2$ (such as obesity, hyperlipidemia, and ascites), in impaired metabolism (such as severe liver disease), and when there is CO_2 retention (such as in chronic lung disease). False-negatives (increased CO_2 production) can be seen (theoretically, at least) in fever, starvation, and hyperthyroidism. The amount of radioactivity is approximately the same as in a chest film and is confined almost exclusively to the lungs. The major disadvantages of the test are the false-positives in healthy individuals (20% in irritable bowel syndrome) and the false-negatives in patients with mild degrees of fat malabsorption.

Pancreatic Function Tests

BENTIROMIDE TEST

Pancreatic chymotrypsin will cleave free para-aminobenzoic acid (PABA) from the synthetic peptide N-benzoyl-L-tyrosyl-para-aminobenzoic acid (bentiromide). If 500 to 1000 mg are administered orally and normal pancreatic chymotrypsin is present, the free PABA should be absorbed, conjugated in the liver, and excreted in the urine. With severe pancreatic insufficiency, less than 57% of the PABA is excreted in 6 hours.[219,220] Unfortunately, severe intestinal mucosal disease, renal disease, diabetes, and severe liver disease all diminish PABA absorption or excretion in the absence of pancreatic insufficiency, and the test is not very sensitive in those with mild pancreatic insufficiency. Furthermore, several ingested substances, including medications (acetaminophen, benzocaine, Xylocaine, lidocaine, procaine, sulfa-containing antibiotics, chloramphenicol, chlorthiazide, furosemide) as well as certain foods (prunes and cranberries), interfere with the laboratory determination.[221] Recent attempts to increase the sensitivity of the test by obtaining plasma values[222] or by administering PAS[223] suggest that the test can be made more accurate and sensitive. Certainly, the test is not sufficiently sensitive or specific to end the search for a better pancreatic function test.

PANCREATIC STIMULATION TESTS

Following duodenal intubation with a double-lumen tube (one lumen having an aspiration port to remove contaminating gastric juice), the pancreas can be stimulated either with the intravenous secretin or cholecystokinin or by an intragastric liquid meal containing fat, protein, and carbohydrates (Lundh meal).[224,225] Pancreatic juice is aspirated from the duodenal port, and the serially collected samples are analyzed for volume, HCO_3 concentration, and, in some laboratories, pancreatic enzymes (lipase, colipase, trypsin, or chymotrypsin). A HCO_3 concentration less than 90 mmol/L suggests chronic pancreatitis, and in research laboratories there are normal values for specific pancreatic enzyme concentration or output. Although the test may be accurate and sensitive, it requires intestinal intubation and is time-consuming. Therefore, this test is not uniformly available in all medical centers.

SCHILLING TEST

Vitamin B_{12}(cobalamin) will not be absorbed unless it is bound to intrinsic factor, and intrinsic factor cannot bind if salivary and gastric R-proteins are not degraded by the pancreatic proteolytic activity in the upper small intestine. Thus, approximately 50% of patients with severe pancreatic insufficiency will have impaired Vitamin B_{12} absorption when measured with the Schilling test. Obviously, this is not very specific because of diminished B_{12} absorption in patients with pernicious anemia, bacterial overgrowth, severe mucosal intestinal disease, or extensive ileal disease/resection. A variant of this test involves the dual labeling of cobalamin with different isotopes: (^{58}CO)-cobalamin bound to hog R-protein is mixed with (^{57}CO)-cobalamin bound to intrinsic factor.[226,227] In pancreatic insufficiency, the R-factor–bound cobalamin is not absorbed because of the absence of pancreatic proteases, whereas the (^{57}CO)-cobalamin that is bound to intrinsic factor will be normally absorbed. The urinary ratio of ^{58}CO/^{57}CO can then discriminate between normal and pancreatic insufficiency, with an excretion ratio normally being greater than 0.7.

Tests For Bacterial Overgrowth

DUODENAL INTUBATION WITH QUANTITATIVE BACTERIAL CULTURE

The duodenum and upper jejunum can be intubated either with passage of a small intestinal tube under fluoroscopic control or by way of a tube passed through the endoscope, and fluid can be aspirated from the upper intestine, or nonbacteriostatic saline can be flushed through the tube and then aspirated for aerobic and anaerobic culture.[228] The growth of more than 10^5 bacterial colonies per milliliter suggests bacterial overgrowth. Care should be taken to collect samples anaerobically, and they should be plated for aerobic and anaerobic cultures immediately. The test has not been standardized, and contamination with oropharyngeal bacteria can be a problem.

BREATH TEST

The *breath hydrogen test* (see below and Fig. 38-12) can be used to diagnose bacterial overgrowth and has a sensitivity of over 90% and a specificity of 78%[229] when breath H_2 increases are found *within the first 2 hours* of either glucose or rice flour ingestion (see ch 35 and 73). The combination of a high fasting breath hydrogen excretion and a diagnostic increase in breath hydrogen after glucose will be present in approximately half of the patients with bacterial overgrowth.[230]

The ^{14}C-D-xylose breath test is said to be more specific for bacterial overgrowth, with 85% of patients having an increase exhaled $^{14}CO_2$ within 60 minutes of ingesting 1 g of ^{14}C-D-xylose.[231,232] Because most of the ^{14}C-labeled xylose is absorbed in the small intestine, less reaches the colon, where it can be metabolized to CO_2 by bacteria, falsely increasing excretion. Although the test can be complicated by delayed gastric emptying, the champions of the test claim near 100% specificity and sensitivity and an even greater reproducibility than that found in duodenal intubation with culture. This test is not available in many laboratories.

The *cholyl-^{14}C-glycine breath test* is based on the rationale that conjugated (glycine or taurine) bile acids are reabsorbed passively throughout the jejunum and actively absorbed in the terminal ileum.[233,234] Bacterial overgrowth will hydrolyze the peptide bond, releasing the ^{14}C-labeled glycine, which is then absorbed, metabolized as CO_2, and exhaled in expired air. Unfortunately, the test is not specific, and it will show similar results in patients with terminal ileal disease/resection and may be misleading in severe mucosal disease.

Radiologic Tests For Malabsorption

Radiology should be viewed as an adjunct to the diagnosis of malabsorption and not a primary test. A flat plate of the abdomen demonstrating pancreatic calcification, pancreatic ultrasound, computed tomography, and endoscopic retrograde cholangiopancreatography (ERCP) can be used to confirm the presence of pancreatic disease as a cause of malabsorption. Small intestinal disease can also be revealed by barium contrast radiographs,[235] either an upper GI series with small intestinal follow-through or an enteroclysis examination (see ch 114). Previous gastric surgery, gastrocolic fistulae, blind loops from previous intestinal anastomoses, small intestinal strictures, multiple jejunal diverticuli, and abnormal intestinal motility that could lead to bacterial overgrowth might be demonstrated. Certain diseases may present radiographically as uniform thickening of the valvulae conniventes (e.g., amyloidosis, lymphoma, Whipple's disease); uniform or patchy diseases such as lymphoma or lymphangiectasia might also be seen. Patients with sprue show dilatation of the small intestine with little mucosal abnormality. Segmentation of the barium column also occurs in sprue or in any of the malabsorptive or severe secretory diarrheas if there is sufficient intraluminal fluid to cause precipitation or flocculation of the barium.

WATERY DIARRHEA

Watery diarrheas can result from either malabsorption, inflammation, or intestinal secretion. The malabsorption of carbohydrate or the malabsorption of some secretagogues (such as bile acids or long-chain fatty acids) that stimulate colonic water and electrolyte secretion results in diarrheas that disappear on fast. Postvagotomy diarrhea, which is initiated by eating, disappears on fast also. In contrast, the secretory diarrheas due to neuroendocrine tumors may diminish slightly but do not return to normal when the patient is fasting. This maneuver, together with measurements of the stool osmotic gap, can be useful in diagnosing these various conditions.

Watery Diarrheas That Respond to Fast

CARBOHYDRATE MALABSORPTION

Carbohydrate malabsorption may be either specific or generalized (Table 38-3). Diarrhea can result from the chronic ingestion of dietetic foods, candy, chewing gum, or medication elixirs that are sweetened with unabsorbable carbohydrates such as sorbitol (chewing gum and elixir diarrhea).[129,236,237] Sorbitol (and fructose) is also present in pears, prunes, peaches, and apple juice,[237] and excessive ingestion of these results in diarrhea as well. Chronic drug ingestion of the types that cause malabsorption of fat (see above) also causes carbohydrate malabsorption.[238]

Congenital absence of enterocyte brush border carbohydrate hydrolases and transport proteins may cause diarrhea[238] (e.g., *glucose-galactose malabsorption* and the various *disaccharidase deficiencies:* lactase, sucrase-isomaltase, and trehalase). These are discussed in more detail in Chapter 72. Lactose intolerance usually presents in childhood or adolescence,[239–241] but it may not be recognized in adults.[242] For this reason, unexplained watery diarrhea, especially when accompanied by abdominal cramps, bloating, and flatus, should be considered as possibly due to *lactase deficiency,* even if it occurs in people not considered to be among the high-risk groups[239] (i.e., Orientals and native American Indians [90% prevalence of lactase deficiency] or American blacks, Jews, Hispanics, and Southern Europeans [60%–70% prevalence]). A 10% to 15% prevalence of lactase deficiency can be expected in Northern or Western Europeans and their American descendants. Either trial of a lactose-free diet, breath hydrogen test, or lactose absorption test may be diagnostic. Disaccharidase deficiency can occur secondarily as well following a variety of intestinal insults and can last for months.[238]

A certain amount of carbohydrate normally is unabsorbed. As much as 50 g of a normal 200-g carbohydrate diet may be "wasted" by the normal small intestine and pass into the colon where it is metabolized by colonic flora.[243,244] Fructose may be malabsorbed when ingested in high concentrations, particularly when ingested alone and not as a component of sucrose.[245–247] *Toddler's diarrhea* in children may be secondary to drinking large amounts of fructose-containing fruit juice,[248] and colic in infants has been proposed to be due to carbohydrate malabsorption.[249] An occasional adult diarrhea also appears to be due to ingestion of large volumes of fruit juice or soft drinks that are sweetened with fructose-containing corn syrup. Diets high in carbohydrate and low in fat might be particularly apt to cause this kind of diarrhea because the low fat content would allow rapid gastric emptying and rapid small intestinal motility. Some of these children with toddler's diarrhea are suspected of having a primary intestinal motility abnormality in which the migrating motor complex (MMC) is not disrupted by eating.[250] Continuation of the propagative motility pattern characteristic of the MMC might worsen carbohydrate malabsorption and result in an osmotic form of diarrhea.

Kellow and colleagues[251] have reported similar abnormalities of the MMC in patients with the painless diarrhea variant of irritable bowel syndrome, while others have shown a rapid orocecal transit time in these patients.[252–256] The question has also been posed whether carbohydrate wastage may be part of the pathophysiology of diarrhea in other diseases such as thyrotoxicosis[257] and even ulcerative colitis[258] where a rapid transit time has been recorded. Because carbohydrate is metabolized to H_2 and CO_2 by colonic bacteria, the symptoms of excess flatus, abdominal bloating, and cramping abdominal pain may be important clues to the diagnosis of carbohydrate malabsorption.

BILE ACID DIARRHEA

Three types of bile acid–induced diarrhea are proposed: type 1, which is due to severe disease, resection, or bypass of the distal ileum; type 2, or primary bile acid malabsorption; and type 3, where bile acid malabsorption follows upper abdominal surgery, either truncal vagotomy or cholecystectomy.

There is little question that type 1 bile acid diarrhea exists.[259,260] *Ileal disease, resection,* and *bypass* (e.g., in Crohn's disease or postoperative adhesions) allow dihydroxy bile salts to escape absorption. If concentrations above 2 mmol are attained in the colon, diarrhea will ensue.[45,46] The exact mechanisms of this diarrhea have not been entirely defined (see ch 14), although pathophysiologically it is a secretory diarrhea. Fasting prevents gallbladder contraction so that large boluses of bile do not enter the intestine. Therefore, type 1 bile acid diarrhea commonly disappears on fast. This form of diarrhea can be recognized by the history of previous ileal surgery or the presence of ileal disease. Bile acid diarrhea must be differentiated from fatty acid diarrhea, which occurs when ileal disease or resection involves such a large segment of ileum (>100 cm) that hepatic synthesis cannot maintain an adequate intraluminal bile salt pool.[260,261] Under these circumstances, steatorrhea ensues, and fatty acid–induced intestinal secretion complicates the picture. It is important to differentiate these two related syndromes because bile acid diarrhea will respond to bile salt binders such as cholestyramine, whereas the diarrhea of fatty acid malabsorption will not and may worsen with such therapy. Fatty acid diarrhea requires a low-fat diet that is supplemented with medium-chain triglycerides to prevent severe weight loss.

Postcholecystectomy diarrhea, one of the proposed type 3 bile acid malabsorption syndromes, is recognized, and a measured increase in fecal bile acids in these patients suggests this as the pathogenesis.[262,263] Why interruption of gallbladder storage would lead to increased bile acid wastage is unclear. Although many patients respond to cholestyramine, some do not, raising the question whether there are other pathophysiologic mechanisms involved in this form of diarrhea.[263]

POSTVAGOTOMY DIARRHEA

Truncal vagotomy combined with some type of drainage procedure is the most common operation for peptic ulcer disease. It is accompanied by diarrhea in 20% to 30% of patients, and this diarrhea may be severe enough to cause 5% to 10% to seek medical care.[264–267] Because the incidence of diarrhea is much less following selective or superselective vagotomy, a vagus-mediated discoordination of gastric motility, intestinal secretion, or intestinal absorption may be involved, although the exact pathophysiology is unknown.[267,268] Various theories of pathogenesis have been proposed, including disordered gastric emptying with presentation of hyperosmolar loads to the proximal intestine, thus releasing kinins and other secretory agents; rapid small intestinal transit that could cause carbohydrate wastage; or rapid transit that might increase bile acid or fatty acid concentrations reaching the colon.[264–268] The idea that bile acids play an important role in the diarrhea accounts for its classification as a type of bile acid diarrhea. The treatment for this condition, in the absence of a clear understanding of the pathophysiology, is not always rewarding. Cholestyramine (occasionally) and motility-altering drugs (opiates and anticholinergics) will benefit some patients.[269]

Watery Diarrheas That May or May Not Respond to Fast (Diarrheas of Mixed or Uncertain Pathophysiology)

TYPE 2 BILE ACID DIARRHEA

Type 2 bile acid diarrhea, or *primary bile acid malabsorption,* may be congenital or acquired. It has been proposed as the cause of chronic unexplained diarrheas. The acquired variety was first described by Thaysen and Pedersen in Denmark as a disease of excess bile acid loss responsive to cholestyramine but not associated with other types of ileal dysfunction.[270] It was suggested that there might be an ileal absence of bile acid receptors or transport proteins (see ch 72) similar to the cases of congenital type 2 bile acid diarrhea that have been reported.[271,272] A similar group of patients from Yugoslavia was reported who had documented bile acid malabsorption but also had features suggestive of an autoimmune disease and displayed histologic abnormalities of the terminal ileum, which included subtotal villus atrophy and crypt hyperplasia.[273] It is unclear whether this disease exists in the United States. A well-studied group of such patients in Texas had documented bile acid malabsorption, normal stool fat excretion, and a Shilling test that was normal, but the B_{12} absorption correlated well with the half-time of C^{14}-labeled bile acid retention.[274,275] These findings suggested some subtle abnormality of the terminal ileum (ileal biopsies were not done), or else some abnormality of motility that interferes with both B_{12} and bile acid absorption. Of significance, however, is that the diarrhea of these patients did not respond to cholestyramine. Thus, there appears to be a form of idiopathic diarrhea in which bile acids are malabsorbed but the diarrhea does not appear to be due to the bile acids. This syndrome needs further study.

IRRITABLE BOWEL SYNDROME

Among patients defined as having irritable bowel syndrome (IBS), a small percent (~25%) have a predominant symptom complex of painless diarrhea. As time goes on, the size of this category of IBS becomes smaller and smaller as new organic conditions are discovered. The first major group removed from this category consisted of those adults found to have occult lactose intolerance. More recently, the discovery of collagenous or microscopic/lymphocytic colitis has depleted this category even further. Now it has been suggested, as noted above, that many of these patients may turn out to have a motility disorder that leads to a form of carbohydrate-wasting diarrhea or even primary bile acid malabsorption (type 2). Furthermore, a certain percentage of patients can be shown to malabsorb fructose or sorbitol, suggesting another form of carbohydrate-wasting diarrhea in certain patients who are labeled as having IBS. Food hypersensitivities have been suggested as the etiology of IBS diarrhea (see below), and the documentation by history of food intolerance[276–278] has been given even more credibility by the objective findings of increased prostaglandin E_2 content in the stool and jejunal fluid of such patients.[276,279] Such increases in prostaglandin production would be expected as a result

of a gut hypersensitivity reaction to some ingested antigen. Lastly, patients with raw milk diarrhea (see above), most likely an infectious diarrhea of unknown etiology, also have a symptom complex compatible with the diarrhea of IBS. All of these examples should give the clinician pause before he attributes the painless diarrhea variant of IBS to any psychosocial etiologies, particularly in males in whom IBS is rare in the first place. Perhaps such patients are better labeled as having idiopathic chronic diarrhea.

FOOD ALLERGY

Although dietary hypersensitivity is clearly recognized in infants and adults (particularly to milk or soybean protein; see below) and systemic anaphylaxis has long been recognized with seafood ingestion, diarrhea as a result of food allergy without significant histologic hallmarks in the intestine remains an area of controversy that needs better definition (see ch 107). Commonly suspected allergies include milk, eggs, seafood, nuts, artificial flavors, and food coloring. Although such patients may have enhanced release of histamine from peripheral blood basophils,[280] serum markers for gut mucosal mast cell degranulation are needed to better determine if gut-related food allergy type 1 hypersensitivity does exist and how often it causes symptoms.

MICROSCOPIC (LYMPHOCYTIC) AND COLLAGENOUS COLITIS

These two diseases may be the same or variants of the same disease.[281–283] However, microscopic/lymphocytic colitis seems to be equally prevalent in males and females, while collagenous colitis occurs predominantly in females (10 to 1) who are usually, but not always, middle-aged to elderly.[283] This disease could be categorized under either inflammatory diarrhea or secretory diarrhea because intraepithelial lymphocytes, lamina propria inflammation (lymphocytes), and intestinal secretion are the hallmarks of the disease.[283–285] However, in many cases the secretory process is mild, and diarrhea stool volumes may return to normal with fasting.[286] Other patients with more severe diarrhea will continue to have elevated stool volumes on fast. A few appear to have small-bowel villus atrophy and may even present with malabsorption.[287] Increased luminal prostaglandin levels suggest that this inflammatory mediator is being released by the subepithelial immune cells and is causing the diarrhea in this disease. It is intriguing to consider whether food hypersensitivity or bile may be the trigger for such prostaglandin release.

Watery Diarrheas That Do Not Respond to Fast (True Secretory Diarrheas)

CARCINOID SYNDROME

Patients with metastatic carcinoid tumors of the gastrointestinal tract, and rarely primary nonmetastatic carcinoid tumors of the bronchial epithelium, produce a syndrome that includes watery diarrhea, cramping abdominal pain with borborygmus, episodic flushing, skin changes including telangiectasia, cyanosis, and pellagralike skin lesions, bronchospasm with asthma attacks and dyspnea, and cardiac murmurs usually due to right-sided valvular lesions.[288-290] The symptoms are due to secretion of serotonin, histamine, catecholamines, kinins, prostaglandin, and tachykinins (e.g., substance P) by the tumor mass. All of these agents, excluding catecholamines, are potent intestinal secretagogues (see ch 14). Up to one third of these patients will not report flushing episodes, and the pellagralike skin changes and heart murmurs may take some time to develop to clinical appearance. Therefore, this disease should be considered when one is faced with secretory diarrheas.

GASTRINOMA

Although 90% of patients with Zollinger–Ellison syndrome will develop peptic ulcers at some time during the course of their disease, diarrhea also occurs in up to one third of patients and may precede the ulcer symptoms; furthermore, in 10% of patients diarrhea may be the major pathophysiologic manifestation of the disease.[291-295] The diarrhea is not classically a secretory diarrhea. It is due in part to high volumes of HCl secretion, because it can be reduced by nasogastric aspiration. Maldigestion of fat due to inactivation of the pancreatic lipase and precipitation of bile acids by the low pH may also play a role. Because Zollinger–Ellison syndrome is the most common of the neuroendocrine tumors, it must be ruled out as a cause of secretory diarrhea.

VIPOMA OR WATERY DIARRHEA–HYPOKALEMIA–ACHLORHYDRIA (WDHA) SYNDROME

Non-beta cell pancreatic adenomas secrete a host of peptides, including vasoactive intestinal polypeptide (VIP), pancreatic polypeptide (PP), peptide histidine isoleucine (PHI), and occasionally secretin, gastrin inhibitory polypeptide (GIP), neurotensin, calcitonin, and prostaglandins.[288,289,291-297] Of these, only VIP has been found to be elevated in virtually all patients with WDHA syndrome, and because infusions of this hormone can produce all of the symptoms, it therefore seems likely to be the primary mediator of this disease. Thus, vipoma seems to be a reasonable and perhaps a more descriptive name than pancreatic cholera or WDHA syndrome. Patients with this tumor have secretory diarrhea, with 70% of patients having more than 3 L of stool per day and virtually all having more than 700 ml per day. Diarrheas of 10 to 20 L/24 h have been reported. With high levels of circulating VIP, all segments of the intestine may secrete Na, K, Cl, and HCO_3, as well as H_2O, thus accounting for the dehydration, hypokalemia, and acidosis that may accompany this disease.[298] Abdominal pain is not an important symptom of this disease, and as many as 20% of patients will exhibit flushing. These skin manifestations, as well as hypercalcemia (without hyperparathyroidism) in over 70% of patients, are probably due to the tumor release of neuroendocrine products. Other features of the syndrome include achlorhydria,

hypokalemia, hypomagnesemia, enlarged gallbladder, hypokalemic myopathy or nephropathy, flushing, hyperglycemia, and lacrimal gland hypersecretion (tearing).

In the pediatric age group, vipomas may present as neurocrest (sympathetic chain) tumors—ganglioneuromas, neuroblastomas, neurofibromas, and pheochromocytomas. Some of these tumors will secrete VIP and produce secretory diarrheas that resolve when the tumor is removed.[299-301]

Occasional patients will have pancreatic islet tumors and watery diarrhea with normal VIP levels, suggesting the secretion of some other peptide. Pancreatic polypeptide, neurotensin, calcitonin, and prostaglandins are all candidate hormones.[288,289]

MEDULLARY CARCINOMA OF THE THYROID

Medullary carcinoma of the thyroid may present in sporadic form or in 25% to 50% of patients it may present as part of the multiple endocrine neoplasia (MEN IIa) syndrome with pheochromocytomas and hyperparathyroidism.[288,289] Watery (secretory) diarrhea is a prominent part of the syndrome, and it is thought to be due to the secretion of calcitonin by the tumor.[302-304] However, these tumors also secrete prostaglandins, VIP, substance P, and rarely serotonin or kallikrein (which activates bradykinin). Although studies in some patients have shown small intestinal secretion,[303] others have shown severely shortened colonic transit time.[304] Therefore, the pathophysiology in this disease may not always be a straightforward secretory one. Usually by the time watery diarrhea occurs (30% of cases) it indicates metastasis with poor prognosis.

GLUCAGONOMA

Patients with glucagon-secreting pancreatic islet tumors present with diabetes, a form of eczematous skin rash called migratory necrolytic erythema, and occasionally mild diarrhea, psychiatric or neurologic aberrations, and thromboembolic propensities.[289,305] The cause of the diarrhea in these patients is unclear.

VILLOUS ADENOMAS

Villous adenomas of the rectum or rectosigmoid may cause a secretory form of diarrhea with K loss.[306-309] Diarrhea in the range of 500 to 3000 ml/24 h has been recorded. Tumors that are capable of causing such secretory diarrhea are usually large—more than 3 to 4 cm in diameter and often as large as 10 to 12 cm. While the cause of the secretion may be intrinsic to the nature of this neoplastic epithelium, secretagogues have been extracted from such tumors,[310] and high levels of prostaglandins have been found in both the tumor and rectal effluent of such patients.[311] Indeed, the reduction in diarrhea in some patients by indomethacin administration suggests that prostaglandins may play some role in the pathophysiology of diarrhea observed with these tumors.[311]

SYSTEMIC MASTOCYTOSIS

When mast cell proliferation is limited to the skin, it is termed urticaria pigmentosa. When it involves the bones, liver, spleen, lymph nodes, and gastrointestinal tract, it is known as systemic mastocytosis. The diarrhea of systemic mastocytosis may be continuous and accompanied by steatorrhea[181]; in these cases, the infiltration of the mucosa and the resulting villus atrophy cause a malabsorptive syndrome (see above). However, the diarrhea may be intermittent and may be associated with flushing, tachycardia, hypotension, and occasionally headache, cognitive disorders, nausea and vomiting, peptic ulcers, syncope, itching, and urticaria, which may be provoked by alcohol ingestion.[289] Under those circumstances, histamine, or other mast cell mediators, may well be the secretagogue responsible, by virtue of either stimulating gastric acid secretion (much as in Zollinger–Ellison syndrome) or having a secretory effect on the intestine. A rare patient's diarrhea will improve with cyclooxygenase blockade, suggesting a role for high circulating prostaglandins as a cause of the diarrhea as well.[312] Blockade of mast cell degranulation with disodium cromoglycate may reduce all these symptoms and diarrhea but not the steatorrhea.[313]

FACTITIOUS DIARRHEA

Approximately 15% of patients referred to secondary or tertiary centers for diarrhea,[314] and 25% of patients with proven secretory diarrheas,[315-318] will turn out to be surreptitiously ingesting either laxatives or diuretics. These patients present with severe chronic watery diarrhea, often with abdominal pain, weight loss, nausea and vomiting, and sometimes with myopathy and hypokalemia. Occasionally they will have severe protein-losing enteropathy as well. They have 10 to 20 bowel movements per day with 24-hour stool volumes in the range of 300 to 3000 ml and may have nocturnal diarrhea as well. The most common drugs ingested are diphenolic laxatives (in the country, phenolphthalein) and anthraquinones, which include senna, cascara, aloe, rhubarb, frangula, and danthron, agents that cause intestinal secretion.[319,320] However, osmotic laxatives such as Na_2SO_4, Na_2PO_4, $MgSO_4$, and Mg citrate are occasionally used. In the absence of a readily available assay for one of the more common laxatives, dioctyl sodium sulfosuccinate (the docusate salts), we are uncertain of its frequency in this syndrome. Rare patients will ingest large quantities of diuretics. The reason these patients, over 90% of whom are women, ingest these drugs to the point of requiring hospitalization and medical evaluation is unclear. There appear to be two different clinical syndromes[289,321]: (1) Women under 30 in whom some elements of eating disorders, such as anorexia nervosa and bulimia, appear to be part of the psychic abnormality. Whether this is indeed part of the eating disorder or whether the use of laxatives was learned only in an earlier eating disorder is uncertain. (2) The other group consists of middle-aged to elderly women who often have histories of extensive medical care and who seem to gain some kind of secondary benefit from the sick role and the personal attention they receive with hospitalization and diagnostic evaluation. Many of these patients are health care workers (e.g., nurse's aides), and this is particularly true in the rare males that present with this

syndrome. Upon confrontation, these patients will sometimes deny the drug ingestion and will leave the physician's care. Others will admit the aberrant behavior and can be helped with psychiatric care. When laxatives are discontinued, these patients will develop edema as a result of secondary hyperaldosteronism, but it will subside spontaneously within 1 to 2 months if left untreated.

This syndrome also exists in pediatrics, where it has been called Münchausen's syndrome by proxy or Polle's syndrome.[322-325] (Polle was Baron von Münchausen's son who died at an early age of unknown causes). In these circumstances it is a form of child abuse where the guilty parent, usually the mother, again derives some kind of secondary gain from the extensive hospitalizations and evaluations of the child.

The frequency of this factitious disorder as a cause of severe diarrhea is high enough to warrant laxative screening to rule out this syndrome prior to initiating extensive medical evaluation for the other causes of diarrhea.

CHRONIC IDIOPATHIC DIARRHEA AND PSEUDOPANCREATIC CHOLERA SYNDROME

Patients in whom extensive evaluation for a cause of apparent secretory diarrhea is negative, including a search for hormone-secreting tumors and laxative and drug ingestion, are labeled as either chronic idiopathic diarrhea or pseudopancreatic cholera syndrome, depending on whether the fasting stool volumes are greater than or less than 700 ml/24 h.[286,316,321] Some of these patients may have microscopic/lymphocytic colitis or may be patients with the type 2 bile acid diarrhea variant (see above). Others could be ingesting laxatives or drugs for which assays are not readily available. It is important to remember that these patients, in whom no diagnosis can be made, are more common than are patients with neuroendocrine secretory tumors. Once factitious drug ingestion can be ruled out as best as possible, they deserve thorough evaluation. If no diagnosis is revealed, symptomatic therapy with bile salt-binding drugs, opiates, and anticholinergic medications might be tried.

DIABETIC DIARRHEA

Young to middle-aged people whose diabetes has been poorly controlled for over 5 years, particularly males ages 20 to 40, may have a profuse watery, urgent diarrhea often occurring at night with incontinence.[326-328] These patients usually have severe neuropathy and often have both nephropathy and retinopathy. An occasional patient will have exocrine pancreatic insufficiency or bacterial overgrowth secondary to the motility disturbances of the autonomic neuropathy, and even more rarely a diabetic with diarrhea will have concomitant celiac disease. In these patients, steatorrhea with resulting fatty acid-induced colonic secretion may be the cause of the diarrhea, and they may respond to specific treatment for these forms of malabsorption. Unfortunately, the majority of diabetic patients with severe diarrhea do not have steatorrhea, and the cause of their diarrheal condition is unknown. A series of experiments by Chang and colleagues in animals given diabetes by streptozocin administration suggests that diabetes induces specific sympathetic denervation of the bowel.[329-331] This leaves unopposed cholinergic tone, which impairs fluid and electrolyte absorption or actually stimulates frank intestinal secretion. It is on this basis that clonidine, a specific α2-adrenergic agent, has been recommended as a treatment for diabetic diarrhea.[331] Indeed, responses can be demonstrated, although it is uncertain whether these are nonspecific antisecretory responses compatible with α2-adrenergic agents or whether they are more specific with regard to the pathophysiology of diarrhea in diabetes. These patients with neuropathy frequently have impaired anal sphincter function, and this is a part of their incontinence.[332] Two possible causes of diarrhea in these patients that deserve more evaluation are (1) increases in systemic levels of kinins and (2) diffusion of glucose from blood to colonic lumen (secondary to nocturnal hyperglycemia) with the induction of a "carbohydrate" form of osmotic diarrhea.

ALCOHOLIC DIARRHEA

Binge drinking of alcohol (as the reader may recognize) will cause a brief episode of diarrhea that usually lasts less than 1 day. This may result from acute damage to both the microvasculature and the epithelium, as shown by infusing experimental animals with concentrations of ethanol equivalent to that obtained with moderate drinking.[333-337] These histologic changes are accompanied by alterations in H_2O, electrolyte, and nutrient absorption. The microvascular changes appear to be due to the release of inflammatory mediators from mast cells and phagocytes and are prevented by pretreatment with prostaglandins, but such treatment does not prevent the changes in intestinal absorption.[338] Thus, it remains unknown whether the epithelial damage is due to the direct effects of alcohol or whether release of other mediators, not prevented by prostaglandin treatment, are involved.

Chronic alcoholics often have a severe watery diarrhea that persists for days or even weeks following hospitalization. Chronic changes in intestinal histology can be demonstrated with prolonged alcohol ingestion in animals.[333-337] Additional abnormalities described in alcoholics include more rapid oral–cecal transit, decreased intestinal disaccharidases, decreased bile secretion (particularly in those with cirrhosis), and decreased pancreatic secretion.[321] Because many of these patients are either folate-, B_{12}- or protein-malnourished, these deficiencies may also play a role.[335] With abstinence, renourishment, and replacement of vitamin deficiencies, most patients' diarrhea will slowly improve.

Congenital Secretory Diarrheas

Five causes of congenital diarrhea have been proposed: (1) a congenital short bowel syndrome,[339] (2) a primary form of ileal dysfunction with bile acid malabsorption,[271,272] (3) congenital chloridorrhea,[340,341] (4) congenital Na diarrhea,[342,343] and (5) microvillus inclusion disease.[344,345] The latter three autosomal recessive disorders present with severe secretory diarrheas. *Congenital chloridorrhea* and *congenital Na diarrhea* are discussed in Chapter 72. In contrast to congenital diarrheas 1 through 4 listed above, in which the mother commonly presents with hydramnios, *microvillus*

inclusion disease presents soon after birth with severe watery diarrhea that involves all segments of the intestine.[344] The volumes of diarrhea in these infants are tantamount to diarrheas of 9 to 10 L/24 h in adults. Biopsies in this disease show a flat mucosa in which enteroendocrine cells and goblet cells are normal, but enterocytes show absent or markedly shortened microvilli and intracellular vesicular bodies that appear to be the brush border structures that are not expressed on the apical surface. Electrolyte studies in this disease show the intestine to be in a secretory state, although there is some rudimentary absorption of glucose.[345] These patients must be managed with parenteral nutrition if they are to live past infancy.

History and Physical Examination in Watery Diarrhea

Certain clues as to etiology can be determined from age, sex, and history. Age is the least helpful (save the congenital syndromes of infancy) because watery diarrheal syndromes can occur in both children and adults. Villous adenomas are diseases of adulthood, as is carcinoid syndrome. However, vipomas can occur in children, as do the factitious diarrheas. Middle-aged and older females are more apt to have collagenous colitis and some form of factitious diarrhea, whereas younger females may have irritable bowel syndrome disease or the bulimic-type factitious diarrhea. Previous operations are important events because of the possibility of postvagotomy diarrhea or ileal resection with type 1 bile acid diarrhea. The absence of nocturnal diarrhea, incontinence, or a history of hypokalemia is more compatible with the mild diarrheas that are due to carbohydrate malabsorption, IBS, type 2 bile acid diarrhea, and collagenous colitis. These diarrheas often respond (at least partially) to fast. Conversely, a history of 10 to 20 bowel movements per day, particularly nocturnal bowel movements with incontinence, should suggest the secretory diarrheas, as should documented electrolyte abnormalities (hypokalemia and acidosis) or dehydration, particularly when accompanied by systemic symptoms such as flushing. The presence of long-standing diabetes or alcoholism obviously is necessary for a diagnosis of these forms of diarrhea. Weight loss is not usually part of most of the watery diarrheas, except for advanced neuroendocrine tumors and mastocytosis.

Physical examination is helpful only when the cutaneous flushing of the neuroendocrine tumors and systemic mastocytosis is evident, or when there is the dermatographism of systemic mastocytosis. The concomitant presence of peptic ulcer should suggest gastrinoma or systemic mastocytosis. Scars from previous surgery raise the question of postvagotomy diarrhea or terminal ileal resection. Autonomic dysfunction (postural hypotension, impotence, gustatory sweating) is almost invariably present in diabetic diarrhea.

Laboratory Diagnosis of Mild Watery Diarrheas That Respond to Fast

Patients with irritable bowel syndrome, food allergy, postvagotomy diarrhea, microscopic/lymphocytic and collagenous colitis, various forms of carboyhdrate malabsorption, and types 1 and 3 bile acid have mild diarrhea by history, usually with no nocturnal comonment. The diarrhea usually responds to fast with a reduction in stool volume from values less than 100 g to below 200 g/24 h. Occasional diarrheas of collagenous colitis and type 2 bile acid diarrhea may not respond to fast. If carbohydrate malabsorption is present, the stool osmotic gap is usually greater than 100 mOsm. The response to fast, to carbohydrate restriction, conceivably to elimination diets for food allergy, and to cholestyramine administration will differentiate many of these forms of watery diarrheas from the more severe secretory diarrheas.

In those individuals in whom therapeutic trial of carbohydrate restricted free diet is inconclusive, either breath hydrogen testing or lactose tolerance testing may be indicated.[346] Because hydrogen is produced only by bacterial fermentation of carbohydrates, increased breath hydrogen excretion following a carbohydrate challenge can be used to uncover disaccharidase deficiency, small intestinal bacterial overgrowth, even excess carbohydrate wastes that might occur with motility disorders (see above). Patients with small intestinal mucosal disease and pancreatic exocrine insufficiency may also have mild carbohydrate malabsorption. Bacterial overgrowth may cause a peak of increased hydrogen production within 2 hours of giving a carbohydrate meal. In disaccharidase deficiency, small intestinal mucosal disease, or pancreatic insufficiency, the peak in hydrogen may come later, between 3 and 6 hours after ingestion[347] (Fig. 38-12). The increase in hydrogen excretion by patients with pancreatic insufficiency can be reduced by concomitant administration of pancreatic enzymes. Therefore, depending on what kind of carbohydrate malabsorption is sought, an oral dose of lactose (g/kg body weight), glucose (50 g), lactulose (10 g), or rice flour (100 g) may be given after an overnight fast and measurement of baseline breath hydrogen values. The test needs to be standardized for each carbohydrate, but in general, a rise of over 20 ppm in exhaled hydrogen within the first 3 to 6 hours of ingestion is diagnostic. Breath hydrogen tests may not correlate with either stool weight or stool fat, even in the presence of significant intestinal mucosal disease, because significant colonic salvage of the nonabsorbed carbohydrate may occur and diarrhea may not be precipitated. Furthermore, the breath hydrogen test measures only carbohydrate malabsorption. This test is useful in children because it is simple and does not involve administration of radioisotopes. Because of the greater absorption of rice flour than other natural carbohydrates, it has been proposed that this be the only complex carbohydrate in the diet for 24 hours prior to hydrogen breath testing in order to lower baseline (fasting) H_2 excretion.

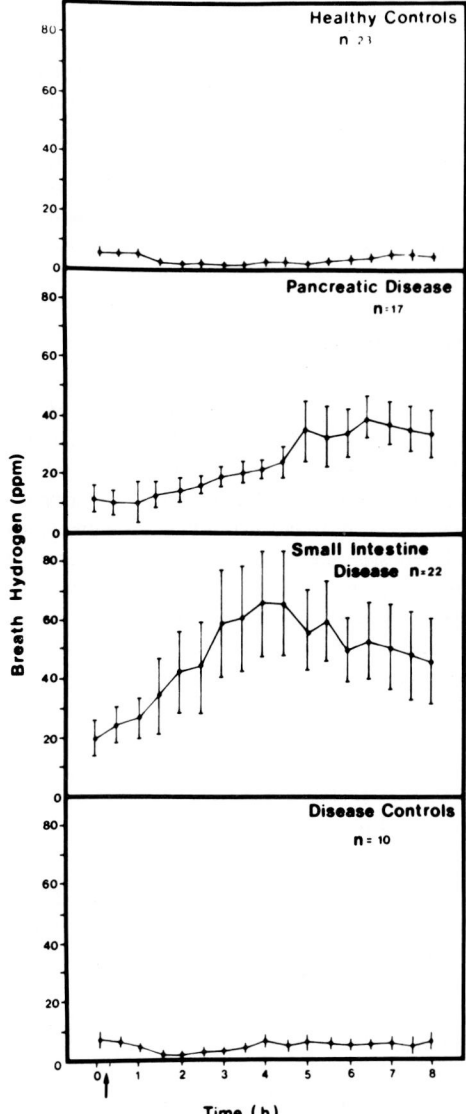

FIGURE 38–12. Breath H_2 production following ingestion of 100 g of rice carbohydrate. Healthy and disease controls are compared with patients with pancreatic insufficiency and intestinal mucosal disease. The increased H_2 produced in patients with pancreatic insufficiency was corrected by addition of pancreatic extract to the rice pancake test meal. (Kerlin P, Wong L, Harris B, Capra S. Rice flour, breath hydrogen, and malabsorption. Gastroenterology 1984;87:578.)

LACTOSE TOLERANCE TEST

To detect either congenital or acquired lactase deficiency, 50 g of lactose is administered and plasma glucose is measured at 1 and 2 hours. A plasma glucose increase of more than 20 mg/dL is a normal response.[242] Patients who lack lactase and, therefore, the ability to split lactose into glucose and galactose will have little increase in plasma glucose. This test does not have good sensitivity and may miss patients with biopsy-proven lactase deficiency, even though they may have symptoms upon the lactose administration.

This test has largely fallen out of favor because of the more sensitive and simple breath hydrogen lactose test.

CHOLYL-^{14}C-GLYCINE BREATH TEST

This test can be used to identify impaired ileal absorption of bile acids, although it is neither specific nor sensitive.[233] The measurement of cholyl-^{14}C-glycine excreted in the stool may increase the sensitivity but adds to the difficulty of performing the test.

⁷⁵SeHCAT TEST

Selenahomotaurocholic acid is an analogue of taurocholic acid and thus has a similar enterohepatic circulation. When radioactively labeled with ^{75}Se, it can be given orally and the patient can be scanned with the gamma camera; those who retain less than 34% of the administered dose after 3 days are considered to have increased bile acid loss.[348] This test is currently available only in research laboratories.

COLONOSCOPY WITH BIOPSY

Patients with mild diarrhea with variable response to fast, but no osmotic gap, should undergo colonic and possibly terminal ileal biopsy if history does not reveal exogenous cause and therapeutic trials have not been helpful. Microscopic/lymphocytic and collagenous colitis may be found on histologic examination of colonic (not rectal) biopsies and type 2 bile acid diarrhea (if it exists) on terminal ileal biopsies. Early in the course of even secretory states, diarrhea volumes may be low, and there may be some significant response to fast. Therefore, in the case of negative evaluations, the true secretory diarrheas must be sought (see below).

Laboratory Diagnosis of Severe Diarrheas That Do Not Respond to Fast

Patients with a history of 10 to 20 bowel movements/24 h, nocturnal diarrhea with incontinence, and 24-hour stool volumes on fast more than 200 g (usually more than 700 g) are apt to have one of the true secretory diarrheas. The aim of the evaluation is to obtain evidence for a severe form of microscopic/lymphocytic and collagenous colitis, for factitious diarrhea, or for the presence of one of the neuroendocrine tumors or systematic mastocytosis, and, following a negative evaluation, to assign the label of chronic idiopathic diarrhea or pseudopancreatic cholera syndrome.

CATHARTIC SCREEN

Because of the cost of an extensive evaluation and the frequency of factitious diarrhea, it is wise to undertake a cathartic screen as the initial evaluation of secretory diarrhea. Phenolphthalein, if recently ingested, can be detected "at the bedside" by alkalinizing the stool with either NaOH or KOH, which will cause a pink to purple color.[315,321] The other diphenolic laxatives (bisacodyl and oxyphenisatin), the anthraquinones, and castor oil can be detected only by chemical analysis of urine or stool. Cathartic screens are available from commercial laboratories, although the docusate salts (dioctyl sodium sulfosuccinate), which are present in many of the over-the-counter cathartics, are not part of these screens. Stool SO_4, PO_4, and Mg analysis will detect those factitious diarrheas due to osmotic cathartics. It should be remembered that Na_2SO_4 and Na_2PO_4 will not cause an osmotic gap (Table 38-2). Although

there is controversy regarding the ethicality and legality of a room search for laxatives and diuretics, most feel it is warranted because of the expense and risk to the patient of the extensive evaluation. Certainly a room search can be a test with the highest diagnostic yield for surreptitious laxative abuse.[314-318]

BLOOD AND URINE HORMONE LEVELS

If a true secretory diarrhea is demonstrated, blood levels of serotonin or urinary 5-hydroxyindole acetic acid (5-HIAA) and serum levels for gastrin, VIP, PP, and PHI may be obtained through commercial or research laboratories.[289,297] The diagnosis of patients with glucagonoma, somatostatinoma, and systemic mastocytosis will be aided by research laboratories that are capable of measuring blood or urinary levels of glucagon, somatostatin, histamine, and prostaglandins.

ENDOSCOPY AND CONTRAST X-RAYS

Patients with true secretory diarrheas or severe nonosmotic watery diarrheas should have colonoscopy to rule out villous adenomas of the rectosigmoid and biopsy to rule out microscopic or collagenous colitis or mastocytosis. Colonoscopy may also reveal melanosis coli secondary to chronic anthracene laxative use, and this can be confirmed by biopsy. Melanosis coli can develop as early as 4 months after beginning such laxatives and may require a year after discontinuance to resolve.[349]

Contrast x-rays have little role in the diagnosis of watery diarrheas, although an ahaustral colon with focal areas of spasm ("pseudostrictures") may suggest chronic laxative abuse (the cathartic colon—see ch 86).[350]

INFLAMMATORY DIARRHEAS

Although the inflammatory diarrheas are actually often due to intestinal secretion or to malabsorption, clinically it is useful to separate these from other diarrheas because they can be suspected, and therefore diagnosed, by certain hallmarks: the presence of fever, particularly when accompanied by localized abdominal tenderness; the presence of blood or leukocytes (neutrophils or eosinophils) in the stool; the presence of severe hypoalbuminemia and hypoglobulinemia with the demonstration of protein-losing enteropathy; and the presence of characteristic lesions on biopsy. The common inflammatory diarrheas are inflammatory bowel disease, eosinophilic gastroenteritis, allergic enteropathy, and chronic radiation enteritis.

Inflammatory Bowel Disease

Patients with inflammatory bowel disease (IBD), either Crohn's disease of the small or large intestine or ulcerative colitis, have diarrhea usually less than 1 L/24 h that frequently, but not always, improves with fast. Decreased Na, Cl, and H_2O absorption or frank secretion can be demonstrated in both the small intestine and colon of patients with IBD.[351-356] Interestingly, patients with severe ulcerative colitis may have water and electrolyte secretion in the unaffected small intestine, suggesting the presence of circulating secretagogues when the colon is severely inflamed.[354] The abnormalities of transport are due to the presence of locally released secretagogues, such as histamine, prostaglandins, and leukotrienes; platelet-activating factor; and cytokines (interleukins) from mast cells, phagocytes, and mesenchymal cells.[355-361] While these mediators may directly affect the epithelium, they also stimulate the enteric nervous system, and increased concentrations of secretory neurotransmitters such as VIP are also found in the tissues of patients with IBD.[362,363] The abnormalities of electrolyte transport brought about by these secretagogues are further enhanced by a damaged absorptive surface epithelium and, indeed, even denuded mucosa with leakage of plasma or blood into the lumen.

Effective treatment of IBD with sulfasalazine, 5-aminosalicylic acid, or steroids is accompanied by reductions in the levels of inflammatory mediators and improved histology. It is therefore not surprising that effective treatment is accompanied also by reduction in diarrhea (see below).

Eosinophilic Gastroenteritis

Infiltration of the gastrointestinal tract with eosinophils is a recognized clinical entity accompanied by diarrhea.[182,364,365] Diarrhea occurs in 30% to 60% of patients with eosinophilic enteritis regardless of whether the eosinophils are infiltrating the mucosa, the muscle, or the serosal layers of the gut.[365] The disease may involve the entire gastrointestinal tract from esophagus to anus, or it may be isolated to the colon. Abdominal pain, nausea, vomiting, and weight loss are other prominent symptoms of this disease, which occurs in both adults and children. Steatorrhea and protein-losing enteropathy are present in 10% to 30% of these patients, and 75% will have peripheral eosinophilia. A small group of patients with peripheral eosinophilia but no evidence of gastrointestinal infiltration appear to have symptoms similar to those with gastrointestinal involvement.[365] The etiology of this disease is unknown, but approximately 50% have atopic (allergic) histories. Food allergy is suspected in these patients, but elimination diets are only occasionally successful. Steroids remain the mainstay of therapy.

Milk and Soy Protein Allergy

Intolerance to cow's milk and soy protein is a well-established cause of enterocolitis in infants.[366-369] The disease involves both the small intestine and the colon and may present within the first 6 months of life with either acute or gradual onset of vomiting and diarrhea, occasionally with bloody stools due to an ulcerative proctocolitis. Approximately 50% of the patients who are allergic to one of these proteins will be allergic to the other. Small intestinal

and rectal biopsies after protein challenge will show abnormalities ranging from inflammatory infiltrate to sloughing of the epithelium.

Protein-Losing Enteropathy

Severe protein loss by the gastrointestinal tract occurs in a variety of disease states[370-373]: infection (*C. difficile* enterocolitis, viral gastroenteritis, parasite infestation, bacterial overgrowth, Whipple's disease), diseases with mucosal erosion or ulcerations (gastritis, gastric cancer, and inflammatory bowel disease), diseases marked by lymphatic obstruction (congenital intestinal lymphangiectasia, lymphoma, or mesenteric tuberculosis), mucosal diseases without ulcerations (Ménétrier's disease, sprue, and eosinophilic gastroenteritis), and immune diseases (systemic lupus erythematosus or food allergies, primarily to milk). While the protein loss due to ulceration with denudation of mucosal capillaries and lymphatics and that due to obstructed lymphatics are easy to comprehend, our recent understanding of immune vascular injury in other sites (lung, kidney, and so forth) allows a better appreciation of this phenomenon in the gastrointestinal tract.

Chronic Radiation Enterocolitis

Although acute radiation diarrhea is common (see above), patients receiving pelvic radiation for malignancies of the female urogenital tract or the male prostate may develop chronic radiation enterocolitis 6 to 12 months following total doses of radiation greater than 4 to 6 Gy.[158,374-378] The terminal ileum, cecum, and the rectosigmoid are the segments usually involved because they are fixed in the pelvis and therefore may receive the full brunt of the weekly radiation dosages. The histology is one of endarteritis, occasionally with lymphangiectasia, partial villous atrophy, fibrosis, and strictures. With time, severely bleeding telangiectasia develops in the rectum of many patients.[377] The diarrhea may be due to bile acid malabsorption when the ileum is involved, to bacterial overgrowth if small intestinal strictures occur, or to the chronic inflammation of the small intestine and colon.[376,378,379] Anti-inflammatory drugs such as sulfasalazine and corticosteroids have been tried with little success; occasionally cholestyramine and nonsteroidal anti-inflammatory drugs may help, as do nonspecific antidiarrheal medications. The bleeding rectal telangiectasia may respond to laser ablation.

Miscellaneous Diseases

Several diseases whose histology is chronic inflammation of the lamina propria and submucosa present with acute, subacute, or chronic diarrhea. Although *acute mesenteric arterial/venous thrombosis* presents as an acute bloody diarrhea, *chronic mesenteric vascular ischemia* may present as watery diarrhea with spotty inflammation that can mislead the physician to think of inflammatory bowel disease (see ch 109). Chronic infections including gastrointestinal *tuberculosis* and *histoplasmosis* present with diarrhea that may be bloody or may have characteristics of a secretory process.[380,381] Immunologic diseases such as *Behçet's syndrome* have diarrhea as a frequent component.[382] Diarrhea is the hallmark of acute *graft-versus-host disease* following allogeneic bone marrow transplantation.[383,384] The triad of dermatitis, hepatic cholestasis, and enteritis with diarrhea define this disease, and the volume of diarrhea has even been proposed as part of clinical staging. The *Cronkhite–Canada syndrome,* usually listed under the polyposes because of the characteristic retention polyps, has most of the hallmarks of an immune disorder, and severe gastrointestinal protein loss and diarrhea are present.[385–387]

History and Physical Examination in Inflammatory Diarrheas

The important clinical manifestations of inflammatory diarrheas are the signs and symptoms of inflammation and the effects of severe chronic protein loss. Fever with acute or chronic abdominal pain, particularly if it is localized to either right or left lower quadrants, may be an important clue to IBD ileitis or colitis. Eosinophilic, allergic, and immunologic enteritis usually cause diffuse pain and tenderness. Severe protein-losing enteropathy is manifested either as peripheral edema, ascites, or even anasarca. Diarrhea in these inflammatory diseases may be meager (i.e., the pseudodiarrhea of proctitis) or it may be a fairly severe. Exsanguinating hemorrhage can occur, as in fulminant colitis, or moderately severe secretory watery-type diarrhea, as in graft-versus-host disease.

Systemic manifestations of inflammatory disease may be prominent in these patients. These include polymigratory arthritis, uveitis, and various dermatitides, including erythema nodosum, pyoderma gangrenosum, and the palpable purpura of vasculitis. As is the case with the mucosal malabsorptive disease with severe subepithelial inflammation, anorexia can be an important cause of the weight loss.

LABORATORY DIAGNOSIS IN INFLAMMATORY DIARRHEAS

Peripheral blood findings of leukocytosis, eosinophilia, elevated sedimentation rate, hypoalbuminemia, and/or low total serum proteins suggest the presence of inflammation, hypersensitivity, and/or severe protein-losing enteropathy. Low serum proteins and/or anasarca in the absence of nephrotic syndrome should always alert one to the possibility of protein-losing enteropathy.

TABLE 38–14
Antidiarrheal Agents for Mild–Moderate Diarrheas

DRUG	MECHANISM OF ACTION IN HUMANS	SIDE EFFECTS
Bismuth subsalicylate	Anti-inflammatory, but not anticyclooxygenase; mechanism not known, has bacteriocidal activity. Suspended in clay that might bind enterotoxins.	Salicylate toxicity, encephalopathy in high doses or with impaired renal function, black stools confused with melena
Opiates Paregoric Deodorized tincture of opium Codeine Diphenoxylate with atropine* Loperamide†	Alters motility, dilatation, and decreased peristalsis of small bowel, ?nonpropulsive contractions of distal colon; increased anal sphincter tone	May enhance bacterial invasion, may precipicate toxic megacolon, may prolong excretion of pathogens, CNS and respiratory depression, delayed gastric emptying, addiction potential
Anticholinergics Atropine Hyoscyamine Synthetic drugs	Alters motility, dilatation of both small and large intestine	Same as above plus atropine toxicity but minus addiction and CNS/respiratory depression
Cholestyramine	Binds bile acids	Binds medications and vitamins, steatorrhea with high doses
Bulk-forming agents Psyllium Methylcellulose	Hydroscopic, partially nonabsorbed bulk added to stool Alters bacterial cell mass	Bloating and flatus, intestinal obstruction behind pre-existing strictures

* *Atropine toxicity, especially tachycardia, occurs with overdose*
† *Poor passage of blood–brain barrier and good first-pass hepatic metabolism make this opiate the one with the fewest side effects*

Stool volumes may vary with variable osmotic gap and with a variable response to fasting. The hallmark of the inflammatory diarrheas, however, is the presence of blood, either gross or occult, and leukocytes in the stool. Stool exam for leukocytes should use methylene blue stain and not Gram stain for best results.[388] Upper gastrointestinal endoscopy or colonoscopy may allow diagnostic biopsies. Contrast x-rays are useful for defining the extent of small intestinal involvement.

SPECIAL LABORATORY TESTS

Indium-labeled white blood cell scans may be useful in detecting bowel inflammation not evident by endoscopy or conventional barium contrast radiography (see ch 114). In specific research laboratories, stool excretion of [11]In-labeled white cells can be used as a quantitative index of fecal white cell loss.[389]

The most sensitive test for this group of inflammatory diarrheas is measurement of intestinal protein loss. Until recently, this was accomplished by measuring 24-hour stool excretion or clearance (24-hour stool excretion divided by mean serum activity just as creatinine clearance is performed) of ^{51}Cr-labeled albumin.[390] Endogenous labeling of albumin can be accomplished by injecting 50 μci of [51]CrCl$_3$ 2 days before collecting 24- to 72-hour stool collections. A sample of blood is drawn during the stool collection to determine serum activity in order to calculate clearance.

More recently, the clearance of native endogenous proteins, particularly alpha$_1$-antitrypsin (α_1-AT), has proved to be as sensitive as ^{51}Cr-labeled protein clearance and avoids the administration of radioactive material.[389,391,392] The principle of the clearance studies is the same as with radioactive albumin. α_1-AT is measured in serum and stool either by radial immunodiffusion or with laser nephelometry with monospecific antisera. Stool determination requires an aliquot of lyophilized stool to be extracted with saline. This test at present requires laboratory expertise and is not uniformly available.

ANTIDIARRHEAL THERAPY

Antidiarrheal agents can be divided into two categories: agents useful for mild to moderate diarrheas (Table 38-14) and those helpful in secretory and other severe diarrheas (Table 38-15). A major drawback of current antidiarrheal drugs is that they have

TABLE 38–15
Agents Helpful in Secretory and Other Severe Diarrheas

DRUG	MECHANISM IN HUMAN	SIDE EFFECTS	DISEASES USEFUL
Octreotide	Suppresses hormone secretion from neuroendocrine cells, mild antisecretory effect, alters motility (dilatation and decreased peristalis)	Suppresses pancreatic secretion (steatorrhea), delays gallbladder emptying (cholelithiasis), suppresses insulin secretion (hyperglycemia)	Carcinoid syndrome, vipoma and other neuroendocrine tumors, unexplained secretory diarrhea; occasionally helpful in short bowel syndrome
Clonidine	α_2-adrenergic agonist, mild antisecretory effect, alters motility	Postural hypotension, depression, rebound hypertension when discontinued	Diabetic diarrhea, diarrhea of opiate withdrawal, unexplained secretory diarrhea
Phenothiazines	Calmodulin inhibition, mild antisecretory effect, alters motility (as above)	Postural hypotension, depression, tardive dyskinesia diarrhea	Vipomas and other neuroendocrine tumors, unexplained secretory
Calcium channel blockers	Mild antisecretory effect, alters motility (as above)	Postural hypotension, cardiac effects	Neuroendocrine tumors, unexplained secretory diarrheas
H, K, ATPase inhibitors and H$_2$ antagonist	↓ Gastric secretion	Encephalopathy, bone marrow toxicity, antiandrogen (cimetidine)	Zollinger–Ellison syndrome, systemic mastocytosis
H$_1$ antagonist	↓ Intestinal secretion	Bone marrow toxicity	Systemic mastocytosis
Serotonin antagonist Methysergide Ketanserin Cyproheptadine	↓ Intestinal secretion Alters motility (as above), ↓ flushing	Tardive dyskinesia	Carcinoid syndrome
Indomethacin	Inhibits prostaglandin synthesis and secretion, mild proabsorptive effect	Gastric ulceration	Medullary carcinoma of thyroid, villous adenoma, AIDS enteropathy, rare neuroendocrine tumor
Glucocorticoids	Anti-inflammatory, proabsorptive	Cushing's syndrome	Inflammatory bowel disease

Isolated case reports indicate antisecretory activity of bromocriptine, lithium carbonate, nicotinic acid, and berberine.

only mild proabsorptive or antisecretory action. Although studies in experimental animals, particularly in vitro, suggest that many of the current agents listed in Tables 38-14 and 38-15 have proabsorptive or antisecretory activity,[393–395] when studied in man most of these agents are lacking this effect, or else it is minimal.[396–399] Most of the current antidiarrheal agents in Table 38-14 and many in Table 38-15 have their activity by altering the intestinal motility. Loperamide, clonidine, phenothiazines, and somatostatin have mild antisecretory activity but also cause dilatation of the small intestine and colon and decrease peristalsis,[395,400–402] while the opiates also cause disordered contractions of the distal large bowel and increased anal sphincter tone.[403–405] The sum of these effects is to trap fluid within the intestine, put it in contact with the mucosa for a greater period of time, and thus eventually allow more complete absorption. Therefore, these drugs may be useful in mild diarrheas, but they can be potentially harmful in severe diarrheas if one is relying on stool output as a gauge for replacing fluid losses. Furthermore, the antimotility effects are not desired if the diarrhea is due to microbiologic organisms because stasis may enhance their invasion and also delay subsequent clearance of the microorganisms from the bowel, thus increasing carriage time. Also, clinical evidence suggests that such drugs are dangerous in severe inflammatory bowel disease, where they may be a precipitating factor in toxic megacolon. Therefore, their use must be tempered.

When faced with a severe secretory diarrhea, the use of drugs with serious side effects (Table 38-15) can be justified for the diarrheas of carcinoid syndrome, neuroendocrine tumors, diabetic diarrhea, and secretory diarrheas of cholera. The somatostatin analogue octreotide appears to have its major antisecretory effect in carcinoid syndrome and in some other neuroendocrine tumors because it inhibits hormone secretion by the tumor.[402,406–412] It may also, therefore, prevent some of the other clinical manifestations of hormone release (e.g., flushing, tachycardia, and skin rash). Unfortunately, patients with large tumor burdens may escape from the drug, and then their management may require debulking surgery and/or agents such as phenothiazines or calcium channel blockers, which have serious side effects. Octreotide may be of limited usefulness in short-bowel syndrome.[405,406]

Although clonidine is very useful in the diarrhea of opiate withdrawal and sometimes in patients with diabetic diarrhea, particularly those who already have severe postural hypotension that cannot be made much worse by the agent, side effects such as this become a limiting factor.[331] Lithium carbonate, bromocriptine, nicotinic acid, and the Indian drug berberine have all been reported to be useful in certain secretory diarrheas.[393,394] However, these reports are largely anecdotal, and these drugs are not well studied as antisecretory agents.

Indomethacin, a cyclooxygenase blocker that inhibits prostaglandin production, may be useful in radiation enteritis, occasional infectious diarrheas, neuroendocrine tumors, villous adenomas, AIDS enteropathy, and occasional patients with irritable bowel (? food allergy) diarrhea (see text above), but it is not useful in IBD. In IBD, glucocorticoids have an effect within 72 hours on *both* prostaglandin and leukotriene production[413] and can be shown to have a proabsorptive effect on the intestine within 5 hours of administration.[414,415] Thus, in IBD, steroids are both anti-inflammatory and antidiarrheal.

The reader is directed to Chapter 1, The Enteric Nervous System and Its Extrinsic Connections; Chapter 2, Gastrointestinal Hormones; Chapter 3, The Brain–Gut Axis; Chapter 4, Smooth Muscle of the Gut; Chapter 5, The Immune System; Chapter 9, Motility of the Small Intestine; Chapter 10, The Motor Function of the Colon; Chapter 14, Secretion and Absorption: Small Intestine and Colon; Chapter 17, Carbohydrate Assimilation; Chapter 18, Intestinal Lipid Absorption; Chapter 19, Protein Digestion and Assimilation; Chapter 26, The Gastrointestinal Microflora; Chapter 31, Approach to the Patient with Occult Gastrointestinal Bleeding; Chapter 34, Approach to the Patient with Abdominal Pain; Chapter 39, Approach to the Patient with Constipation; Chapter 43, Approach to the Patient with Ascites; Chapter 44, Skin Lesions Associated with Gastrointestinal Diseases; Chapter 45, Approach to Gastrointestinal Problems in the Elderly; Chapter 46, Approach to Gastrointestinal Problems in the Immunocompromised Patient; Chapter 51, Advice to Travelers; Chapter 52, Public Health for Medical Staff; Chapter 62, Zollinger–Ellison Syndrome; Chapter 64, Surgery for Peptic Ulcer Disease; Chapter 66, Small Intestine: Anatomy and Structural Anomalies; Chapter 67, Dysmotility of the Small Intestine; Chapter 68, Small Intestine: Infections with Common Bacterial and Viral Pathogens; Chapter 69, Chronic Infections of the Small Intestine; Chapter 70, Tumors and Other Neoplastic Diseases of the Small Intestine; Chapter 71, Celiac Disease; Chapter 72, Specific Mucosal Protein Deficiency States; Chapter 73, Bacterial Overgrowth; Chapter 74, Short Bowel Syndrome; Chapter 75, Miscellaneous Diseases of the Small Intestine; Chapter 76, Colon: Anatomy and Structural Anomalies; Chapter 77, Inflammatory Bowel Disease; Chapter 78, Colonic Polyps: Benign and Premalignant Neoplasms of the Colon; Chapter 79, Polyposis Syndromes; Chapter 80, Irritable Bowel Syndrome; Chapter 81, Motility Disorders of the Colon; Chapter 82, Diverticulitis; Chapter 83, Bacterial Infections of the Colon; Chapter 84, Malignant Tumors of the Colon; Chapter 85, Anorectal Diseases; Chapter 86, Miscellaneous Inflammatory and Structural Disorders of the Colon; Chapter 89, Chronic Pancreatitis; Chapter 90, Pancreatic Adenocarcinoma; Chapter 91, Endocrine Neoplasms of the Pancreas; Chapter 103, Gastrointestinal Complications of the Acquired Immunodeficiency Syndrome; Chapter 104, Parasitic Diseases: Protozoa; Chapter 105, Parasitic Diseases: Helminths; Chapter 106, Gastrointestinal Manifestations of Systemic Diseases; Chapter 107, Gastrointestinal Manifestations of Immunologic Disorders; Chapter 108, Vascular Ectasias, Tumors, and Malformations; Chapter 109, Vascular Insufficiency; Chapter 111, Upper Gastrointestinal Endoscopy; Chapter 112, Colonoscopy and Flexible Sigmoidoscopy; Chapter 113, Endoscopic Retrograde Cholangiopancreatography, Endoscopic Sphincterotomy and Stone Removal, Endoscopic Biliary and Pancreatic Drainage; Chapter 114, Contrast Radiology; Chapter 126, Endoscopic Mucosal Biopsy; Chapter 127, Microbiologic Studies; Chapter 129, Tests of Gastric and Exocrine Pancreatic Function and Absorption; and Chapter 138, Applications of New Technology in Tissue Examination.

REFERENCES

1. U.S. National Commission on Digestive Diseases. Digestive Diseases: Neglected problems–exciting opportunities. Washington, D.C.: U.S. Department of Health Education and Welfare, Public Health Service, National Institutes of Health, 1979.

2. Annual Report of the Animal Health Scientific Research Advisory Board of the USDA, 1980.

3. Garthright WE, Archer DL, Kvenberg JE. Estimates of incidence and costs of intestinal infectious diseases in the United States. Public Health Rep 1988;103:107.

4. Rohde JE, Northrup RS. Taking science where the diarrhea is. In: Elliott K, Knight J, eds. Acute diarrhoea in childhood. Amsterdam: Elsevier-Excerpta Medica-North Holland, 1990:338.

5. Snyder JD, Merson MH. The magnitude of the global problem of acute diarrhoeal disease: A review of active surveillance data. Bull WORLD Health Organ 1982;60:605.

6. Guerrant RL, Hughes JM, Lima NL, Crane J. Diarrhea in developed and developing countries: Magnitude, special settings, and etiologies. Rev Infect Dis 1990;12(Suppl 1):S41.

7. Gold R. Overview of the worldwide problem of diarrhoea. Drugs 1988;36:1.

8. Levine MM, Losonsky G, Herrington D, Kaper JB, Tacket C, Rennels MB, Morris JG. Pediatric diarrhea: The challenge of prevention. Pediatr Infect Dis J 1986;5:S29.

9. Weiss MG. Cultural models of diarrheal illness: Conceptual framework and review. Soc Sci Med 1988;27:5.

10. Nichter M. From *Aralu* to ORS: Sinhalese perceptions of digestion, diarrhea, and dehydration. Soc Sci Med 1988;27:39.

11. Mull JD, Mull DS. Mothers' concepts of childhood diarrhea in rural Pakistan: What ORT program planners should know. Soc Sci Med 1988;27:53.

12. Ryle JA. An address on chronic diarrhea. Lancet 1924;2:101.

13. Drossman DA, Sandler RS, McKee DC, Lovitz AJ. Bowel patterns among subjects not seeking health care: Use of a questionnaire to identify a population with bowel dysfunction. Gastroenterology 1982;83:529.

14. Sandler RS, Drossman DA. Bowel habits in young adults not seeking health care. Dig Dis Sci 1987;32:841.

15. Goy JAE, Eastwood MA, Mitchell WD, Pritchard JL, Smith AN. Fecal characteristics contrasted in the irritable bowel syndrome and diverticular disease. Am J Clin Nutr 1976;29:1480.

16. Tucker DM, Sandstead HH, Logan GM Jr, Klevay LM, Mahalko J, Johnson LK, Inman L, Inglett GE. Dietary fiber and personality factors as determinants of stool output. Gastroenterology 1981;81:879.

17. Davies GJ, Crowder M, Reid B, Dickerson JWT. Bowel function measurements of individuals with different eating patterns. Gut 1986;27:164.

18. Rhoads JM, Powell DW. Diarrhea. In: Walker WA, Durie PR, Hamilton JR, Walker-Smith JA, Watkins JB, eds. Pediatric gastrointestinal disease. Ontario: BC Decker, 1990.

19. Fordtran JS. Speculations on the pathogenesis of diarrhea. Fed Proc 1967;26:1405.

20. Phillips SF. Diarrhea: A current view of the pathophysiology. Gastroenterology 1972;63:495.

21. Leigh RJ, Turnberg LA. Fecal incontinence: The unvoiced symptom. Lancet 1982;1:1349.

22. Schiller LR. Faecal incontinence. Clin Gastroenterol 1986;15:687.

23. Cummings JH. Short chain fatty acids in the human colon. Gut 1981;22:763.

24. Kamm MA, Farthing MJG, Lennard-Jones JE. Bowel function and transit rate during the menstrual cycle. Gut 1989;30:605.

25. Barclay GR, Turnberg LA. Effect of moderate exercise on salt and water transport in the human jejunum. Gut 1988;29:816.

26. Barclay GR, Turnberg LA. Effect of psychological stress on salt and water transport in the human jejunum. Gastroenterology 1987;93:91.

27. Hofmann AF, Poley JR. Cholestyramine treatment of diarrhea associated with ileal resection. N Engl J Med 1969;281:397.

28. Clain JE, Malagelada JR, Chadwick VS, Hofmann AF. Binding properties in vitro of antacids for conjugated bile acids. Gastroenterology 1977;73:556.

29. Sali A, Murray WR, MacKay C. Aluminum hydroxide in bile-salt diarrhea. Lancet 1977;2:1051.

30. Read NW. Diarrhée motrice. Clin Gastroenterol 1986;15:657.

31. Powell DW. Intestinal water and electrolyte transport. In: Johnson LR, ed. Physiology of the gastrointestinal tract. New York: Raven Press, 1987:1267.

32. Field M, Rao MC, Chang EB. Intestinal electrolyte transport and diarrheal disease (Part One). N Engl J Med 1989;321:800.

33. Fondacaro JD. Intestinal ion transport and diarrheal disease. Am J Physiol (Gastrointest Liver Physiol 13) 1986;250:G1.

34. Lundgren O, Svanvik J, Jivegård L. Enteric nervous system: I. Physiology and pathophysiology of the intestinal tract. Dig Dis Sci 1989;34:264.

35. Powell DW. The immunophysiology of intestinal electrolyte transport. In: Field M, Frizzel R, eds. Handbook of physiology: The gastrointestinal system, Vol 4. Intestinal absorption and secretion. Bethesda, MD: American Physiological Society, 1991:591.

36. Phillips S, Giller J. The contributions of the colon to electrolyte and water conservation in man. J Lab Clin Med 1973;81:733.

37. Fordtran JS, Locklear TW. Ionic constituents and osmolality of gastric and small intestinal fluids after eating. Am J Dig Dis 1966;11:503.

38. Wrong O, Metcalfe-Gibson A, Morrison BIR, Ng ST, Howard AV. *In vivo* dialysis of faeces as a method of stool analysis. Clin Sci 1965;28:357.

39. Hammer HF, Santa Ana CA, Schiller LR, Fordtran JS. Studies of osmotic diarrhea induced in normal subjects by ingestion of polyethylene glycol and lactulose. J Clin Invest 1989;84:1056.

40. Shiau YF, Feldman GM, Resnick MA, Coff PM. Stool electrolyte and osmolality measurements in the evaluation of diarrheal disorders. Ann Intern Med 1985;102:773.

41. Christopher NL, Bayless TM. Role of the small bowel and colon in lactose-induced diarrhea. Gastroenterology 1971;60:845.

42. Binder HJ, Bayless TM, Whiting DS. Pathophysiology of diarrhea. Unit VIIB. In: Timonium, MD: The Undergraduate Teaching Project in Gastroenterology Liver Disease. American Gastroenterological Association: Distributed by Milner Fenwick, 1979.

43. Ladefoged K, Schaffalitzky De Muckadell OB, Jarnum S. Faecal osmolality and electrolyte concentrations in chronic diarrhoea: Do they provide diagnostic clues? Scand J Gastroenterol 1987;22:813.

44. Molla AM, Rahman M, Sarker SA, Sack DA, Molla A. Stool electrolyte content and purging rates in diarrhea caused by rotavirus, enterotoxigenic *E. coli* and *V. cholerae* in children. J Pediatr 1981;98:835.

45. Mekhjian HS, Phillips SF, Hofmann AF. Colonic secretion of water and electrolytes induced by bile acids: Perfusion studies in man. J Clin Invest 1971;50:1569.

46. Binder HJ, Rawlins CL. Effect of conjugated dihydroxy bile salts on electrolyte transport in rat colon. J Clin Invest 1973;52:1460.

47. Ammon HV, Phillips SF. Inhibition of colonic water and electrolyte absorption by fatty acids in man. Gastroenterology 1973;65:744.

48. Bright-Asare P, Binder HJ. Stimulation of colonic secretion of water and electrolytes by hydroxy fatty acids. Gastroenterology 1973;64:81.

49. Wiggins HS, Cummings JH, Pearson JR. Hydroxystearic acid and diarrhoea following ileal resection. Gut 1974;15:392.

50. Donowitz M, Binder HJ. Effect of dioctyl sodium sulfosuccinate on colonic fluid and electrolyte movement. Gastroenterology 1975;69:941.

51. Gaginella TS, Chadwick VS, Debongnie JC, Lewis JC, Phillips SF. Perfusion of rabbit colon with ricinoleic acid: Dose-related mucosal injury, fluid secretion, and increased permeability. Gastroenterology 1977;73:95.

52. Perera DR, Weinstein WM, Rubin CE. Symposium of pathology on the gastrointestinal tract—Part II: Small intestinal biopsy. Hum Pathol 1975;6:456.

53. Riddell RH. Pathology of idiopathic inflammatory bowel disease. In: Kirsner JB, Shorter RG, eds. Inflammatory bowel disease. Philadelphia: Lea & Febiger, 1988:329.

54. Butler DG, Gall DG, Kelly MN, Hamilton JR. Transmissible gastroenteritis. Mechanisms responsible for diarrhea in an acute viral enteritis in piglets. J Clin Invest 1974;53:1335.

55. McClung HJ, Butler DG, Kerzner G, Gall DG, Hamilton JR. Transmissible gastroenteritis: Mucosal ion transport in acute viral enteritis. Gastroenterology 1976;70:1091.

56. Kerzner B, Kelly MH, Gall DG, Butler DG, Hamilton JR. Transmissible gastroenteritis: Sodium transport and the intestinal epithelium during the course of viral enteritis. Gastroenterology 1977;72:457.

57. Gall DG, Chapman D, Kelly M, Hamilton JR. Na$^+$ transport in jejunal crypt cells. Gastroenterology 1977;72:452.

58. Shepherd RW, Gall DG, Butler DG, Hamilton JR. Determinants of diarrhea in viral enteritis. The role of ion transport and epithelial changes in the ileum in transmissible gastroenteritis in piglets. Gastroenterology 1979;76:20.

59. Keljo DJ, MacLeod RJ, Perdue MH, Butler DG, Hamilton JR. D-glucose transport in piglet jejunal brush-border membranes: Insights from a disease model. Am J Physiol (Gastrointest Liver Physiol 12) 1985;249:G751.

60. MacLeod RJ, Hamilton R. Absence of a cAMP-mediated antiabsorptive effect in an undifferentiated jejunal epithelium. Am J Physiol (Gastrointest Liver Physiol 15) 1987;252:G776.

61. Rhoads JM, MacLeod RJ, Hamilton JR. Alanine enhances jejunal sodium absorption in the presence of glucose: Studies in piglet viral diarrhea. Pediatr Res 1986;20:879.

62. Sartor RB, Powell DW. Mechanisms of diarrhea in intestinal inflammation and hypersensitivity: Immune system modulation of intestinal transport. In: Field M, ed. Diarrheal diseases. New York: Elsevier 1991, (In Press)

63. Levine MM, Kaper JB, Black RE, Clements ML. New knowledge on pathogenesis of bacterial enteric infections as applied to vaccine development. Microbiol Rev 1983;47:510.

64. Frank MM. Complement in the pathophysiology of human disease. N Engl J Med 1987;316:1525.

65. Müller-Eberhard HJ. Molecular organization and function of the complement system. Annu Rev Biochem 1988;57:321.

66. Shanahan F. Pathogenesis of inflammatory bowel disease. Autoimmunity forum. Gastroenterology 1989;1:2.

67. Shanahan F, Leman B, Deem R, Targan S. In vivo primed cytotoxic T cells in inflammatory bowel disease. In: MacDermott RP, ed. Inflammatory bowel disease: Current status and future approach. New York: Elsevier, 1988:101.

68. Patrick MK, Dunn IJ, Buret A, Miller HRP, Huntley JF, Gibson S, Gall DG. Mast cell protease release and mucosal ultrastructure during intestinal anaphylaxis in the rat. Gastroenterology 1988;94:1.

69. Weiss SJ. Tissue destruction by neutrophils. N Engl J Med 1989;320:365.

70. Ho MS, Glass RI, Pinsky PF, Young-Okoh N, Sappenfield WM, Buehler JW, Gunter N, Anderson LJ. Diarrheal deaths in American children: Are they preventable? JAMA 1988;260:3281.

71. Cohen ML. The epidemiology of diarrheal disease in the United States. Infect Dis Clin North Am 1988;2:557.

72. Goldberg MB, Rubin RH. The spectrum of salmonella infection. Infect Dis Clin North Am 1988;2:571.

73. Cohen ML, Tauxe RV. Drug-resistant *Salmonella* in the United States: An epidemiologic perspective. Science 1986;234:964.

74. Fekety R. Recent advances in management of bacterial diarrhea. Rev Infect Dis 1983;5:246.

75. Snydman DR. Bacterial food poisoning. In: Gorbach SL, ed. Infectious diarrhea. Boston: Blackwell, 1986:201.

76. McFarland LV, Mulligan ME, Kwok RYY, Stamm WE. Nosocomial acquisition of *Clostridium difficile* infection. N Engl J Med 1989;320:204.

77. Ekanem EE, DuPont HL, Pickering LK, Selwyn BJ, Hawkins CM. Transmission dynamics of enteric bacteria in day-care centers. Am J Epidemiol 1983;118:562.

78. Dupont HL. Consumption of raw shellfish—Is the risk now unacceptable? N Engl J Med 1986;314:707.

79. Pickering LK, Woodward WE. Diarrhea in day care centers. Pediatr Infect Dis J 1982;1:47.

80. Kim K, DuPont HL, Pickering LK. Outbreaks of diarrhea associated with *Clostridium difficile* and its toxin in day-care centers: Evidence of person-to-person spread. J Pediatr 1983;102:376.

81. Mathewson JJ, DuPont HL. *Escherichia coli.* In: Gorbach SL, ed. Infectious diarrhea. Boston: Blackwell, 1986:85.

82. Wolfe MS. Parasites. In: Gorbach SL, ed. Infectious diarrhea. Boston: Blackwell, 1986:141.

83. Jokipii L, Jokipii AMM. Timing of symptoms and oocyst excretion in human cryptosporidiosis. N Engl J Med 1986;315:1643.

84. Keusch GT. *Shigella.* In: Gorbach SL, ed. Infectious diarrhea. Boston: Blackwell, 1986:31.

85. Hornick RB. *Salmonella.* In: Gorbach SL, ed. Infectious diarrhea. Boston: Blackwell, 1986:17.

86. Cover TL, Blaser MJ. The pathobiology of *Campylobacter* infections in humans. Annu Rev Med 1989;40:269.

87. Cover TL, Aber RC. *Yersinia enterocolitica.* N Engl J Med 1989;321:16.

88. Bartlett JG. *Clostridium difficile:* Pseudomembranous colitis and antibiotic-associated diarrhea. In: Gorbach SL, ed. Infectious diarrhea. Boston: Blackwell, 1986:157.

89. Riley LW. The epidemiologic, clinical, and microbiologic features of hemorrhagic colitis. Annu Rev Microbiol 1987;41:383.

90. Attwood SEA, Cafferkey MT, West AB, Healy E, Mealy K, Buckley TF, Boyle N, Keane FBV. *Yersinia* infection and acute abdominal pain. Lancet 1987;1:529.

91. Vantrappen G, Agg HO, Ponette E, Geboes K, Bertrand P. *Yersinia* enteritis and enterocolitis: Gastroenterological aspects. Gastroenterology 1977;72:220.

92. Dascal A, Blacklow NR. Viral diarrhea. In: Grobach SL, ed. Infectious diarrhea. Boston: Blackwell, 1986:125.

93. Holmberg SD. *Vibrios* and *Aeromonas.* Infect Dis Clin North Am 1988;2:655.

94. Risher JF, Mink FL, Stara JF. The toxicologic effects of the carbamate insecticide aldicarb in mammals: A review. Environ Health Perspect 1987;72:267.

95. McClain JL, Hause DW, Clark MA. Amanita phalloides mushroom poisoning: A cluster of four fatalities. J Forensic Sci 1989;34:83.

96. French AL, Garrettson LK. Poisoning with the North American jack o'lantern mushroom, *Omphalotus illudens.* J Toxicol Clin Toxicol 1988;26:81.

97. Stallard D. Muscarinic poisoning from medications and mushrooms: A puzzling symptom complex. Postgrad Med 1989;85:341.

98. Massey EW, Wold D, Heyman A. Arsenic: Homicidal intoxication. South Med J 1984;77:848.

99. Schoolmeester WL, White DR. Arsenic poisoning. South Med J 1980;73:198.

100. Guerrant RL, Sheilds DS, Thorson SM, Schorling JB, Gröschel DHM. Evaluation and diagnosis of acute infectious diarrhea. Am J Med 1985;78(Suppl 6B):91.

101. Gorbach SL. Bacterial diarrhoea and its treatment. Lancet 1987;2:1378.

102. Thorne GM. Diagnosis of infectious diarrheal diseases. Infect Dis Clin North Am 1988;2:747.

103. Gertler S, Pressman J, Cartwright C, Dharmsathaphorn K. Management of acute diarrhea. J Clin Gastroenterol 1983;5:523.

104. Banwell JG. Nonspecific therapy. In: Gorbach SL, ed. Infectious diarrhea. Boston: Blackwell, 1986:219.

105. Di John D, Levine MM. Treatment of diarrhea. Infect Dis Clin North Am 1988;2:719.

106. Elliott EJ, Cunha-Ferreira R, Walker-Smith JA, Farthing MJG. Sodium content of oral rehydration solutions: A reappraisal. Gut 1989;30:1610.

107. Carpenter CCJ. Fluid and electrolyte therapy. In: Gorbach SL, ed. Infectious diarrhea. Boston: Blackwell, 1986:237.

108. Pizarro D. Oral rehydration in infants in developing countries. Drugs 1988;36:39.

109. Mackenzie A, Barnes G. Oral rehydration in infantile diarrhoea in the developed world. Drugs 1988;36:48.

110. Carpenter CCJ, Greenough WB, Pierce NF. Oral-rehydration therapy—The role of polymeric substrates. N Engl J Med 1988;319:1346.

111. DuPont HL, Sullivan P, Pickering LK, Haynes G, Ackerman PB. Symptomatic treatment of diarrhea with bismuth subsalicylate among students attending a Mexican university. Gastroenterology 1977;73:715.

112. Steinhoff MC, Douglas RG Jr, Greenberg HB, Callahan DR. Bismuth subsalicylate therapy of viral gastroenteritis. Gastroenterology 1980;78:1495.

113. Graham DY, Estes MK, Gentry LO. Double-blind comparison of

bismuth subsalicylate and placebo in the prevention and treatment of enterotoxigenic *Escherichia coli*-induced diarrhea in volunteers. Gastroenterology 1983;85:1017.

114. Portnoy BL, DuPont HL, Pruitt D, Abdo JA, Rodriguez JT. Antidiarrheal agents in the treatment of acute diarrhea in children. JAMA 1976;236:844.

115. Johnson PC, Ericsson CD, DuPont HL, Morgan DR, Bitsura JAM, Wood LV. Comparison of loperamide with bismuth subsalicylate for the treatment of acute travelers' diarrhea. JAMA 1986;255:757.

116. Blaser MJ. Infectious diarrheas: Acute, chronic, and iatrogenic. Ann Intern Med 1986;105:785.

117. WHO. Persistent diarrhoea in children in developing countries: Report of a WHO meeting. Geneva 14–17 December 1987. Geneva: WHO Diarrhoeal Diseases Control Programme, 1988.

118. Young R, Allely C, Kaufman SS. Nutrition support of intractable diarrhea: A case report and literature review. Nutr Clin Pract 1989;4:19.

119. Giannella RA. Chronic diarrhea in travelers: Diagnostic and therapeutic considerations. Rev Infect Dis 1986;8(Suppl 2):S223.

120. Willoughby JMT, Rahman AFMS, Gregory MM. Chronic colitis after *Aeromonas* infection. Gut 1989;30:686.

121. Osterholm MT, MacDonald KL, White KE, Wells JG, Spika JS, Potter ME, Forfang JC, Sorenson RM, Milloy PT, Blake PA. An outbreak of a newly recognized chronic diarrhea syndrome associated with raw milk consumption. JAMA 1986;256:484.

122. Blaser MJ. Brainerd diarrhea: A newly recognized raw milk–associated enteropathy. JAMA 1986;256:510.

123. Martin DL, Hoberman LJ. A point source outbreak of chronic diarrhea in Texas: No known exposure to raw milk. JAMA 1986;256:496.

124. Kelly TWJ, Patrick MR, Hillman KM. Study of diarrhea in critically ill patients. Crit Care Med 1983;11:7.

125. Gottschlich MM, Warden GD, Michel MA, Havens P, Kopcha R, Jenkins M, Alexander JW. Diarrhea in tube-fed burn patients: Incidence, etiology, nutritional impact, and prevention. J Parenter Enteral Nutr 1988;12:338.

126. Brinson RR, Kolts BE. Hypoalbuminemia as an indicator of diarrheal incidence in critically ill patients. Crit Care Med 1987;15:506.

127. Wrenn K. Fecal impaction. N Engl J Med 1989;321:658.

128. Read NW, Abouzekry L. Why do patients with faecal impaction have faecal incontinence? Gut 1986;27:283.

129. Edes TE, Walk BE, Austin JL. Diarrhea in tube-fed patients: Feeding formula not necessarily the cause. Am J Med 1990;88:91.

130. Heimburger DC. Diarrhea with enteral feeding: Will the real cause please stand up? Am J Med 1990;88:89.

131. Silk DBA. Towards the optimization of enteral nutrition. Clin Nutr 1987;6:61.

132. Breach CL, Saldanha LG. Tube feeding complications, Part I: Gastrointestinal. Nutritional Support Services 1988;8:15.

133. Silk DBA, Payne-James J. Letter: Gastrointestinal complications? Nutritional Support Services 1988;8:5.

134. Keohane PP, Attrill H, Love M, Frost P, Silk DBA. Relation between osmolality of diet and gastrointestinal side effects in enteral nutrition. Br Med J 1984;288:678.

135. Halperin ML, Wolman ST, Greenberg GR. Paracellular recirculation of sodium is essential to support nutrient absorption in the gastrointestinal tract: An hypothesis. Clin Invest Med 1986;9:209.

136. Spiller RC, Jones BJM, Silk DBA. Jejunal water and electrolyte absorption from two proprietary enteral feeds in man: Importance of sodium content. Gut 1987;28:681.

137. Zarling EJ, Parmar JR, Mobarhan S, Clapper M. Effect of enteral formula infusion rate, osmolality, and chemical composition upon clinical tolerance and carbohydrate absorption in normal subjects. J Parenter Enteral Nutr 1986;10:588.

138. Pesola GE, Hogg JE, Yonnios T, McConnell RE, Carlon GC. Isotonic nasogastric tube feedings: Do they cause diarrhea? Crit Care Med 1989;17:1151.

139. Jones BJM, Lees R, Andrews J, Frost P, Silk DBA. Comparison of an elemental and polymeric enteral diet in patients with normal gastrointestinal function. Gut 1983;24:78.

140. Simko V, Michael S. Absorptive capacity for dietary fat in elderly patients with debilitating disorders. Arch Intern Med 1989;149:557.

141. Braun TI, Fekete T, Lynch A. Strongyloidiasis in an institution for mentally retarded adults. Arch Intern Med 1988;148:634.

142. Lima NL, Guerrant RL, Kaiser DL, Germanson T, Farr BM. A retrospective cohort study of nosocomial diarrhea as a risk factor for nosocomial infection. J Infect Dis 1990;161:948.

143. Bender BS, Laughon BE, Gaydos C, Forman MS, Bennett R, Greenough WB, Sears SD, Bartlett JG. Is *Clostridium difficile* endemic in chronic-care facilities? Lancet 1986;2:11.

144. Hughes JM, Jarvis WR. Nosocomial gastrointestinal infections. In: Wenzel RP, ed. Prevention and control of nosocomial infections. Baltimore: Williams & Wilkins, 1987:405.

145. Siegel DL, Edelstein PH, Nachamkin I. Inappropriate testing for diarrheal diseases in the hospital. JAMA 1990;263:979.

146. Yolken RH, Bishop CA, Townsend RT, Bolyard EA, Barlett J, Santos GW, Saral R. Infectious gastroenteritis in bone-marrow-transplant recipients. N Engl J Med 1982;306:1009.

147. Johnson S, Gerding DN, Olson MM, Weiler MD, Hughes RA, Clabots CR, Peterson LR. Prospective, controlled study of vinyl glove use to interrupt *Clostridium difficile* nosocomial transmission. Am J Med 1990;88:137.

148. Nolan NPM, Kelly CP, Humphreys JFH, Cooney C, O'Connor R, Walsh TN, Weir DG, O'Briain DS. An epidemic of pseudomembranous colitis: Importance of person to person spread. Gut 1987;28:1467.

149. Mitchell EP, Schein PS. Gastrointestinal toxicity of chemotherapeutic agents. Semin Oncol 1982;9:52.

150. Dubois A, Walker RI. Prospects for management of gastrointestinal injury associated with the acute radiation syndrome. Gastroenterology 1988;95:500.

151. Longo DL. Principles of cancer treatment. In: Kelly WV, ed. Textbook of internal medicine. Philadelphia: JB Lippincott, 1989:1214.

152. Kralovánszky J, Prajda N. Biochemical changes of intestinal epithelial cells induced by cytostatic agents in rats. Arch Toxicol 1985;Suppl 8:94.

153. Baskerville A, Batter-Hatton D. Intestinal lesions induced experimentally by methotrexate. Br J Exp Pathol 1977;58:663.

154. Trier JS, Browning TJ. Morphologic response of the mucosa of human small intestine to X-ray exposure. J Clin Invest 1966;45:194.

155. Curran PF, Webster EW, Hovsepian JA. The effect of X-irradiation on sodium and water transport in rat ileum. Radiat Res 1960;13:369.

156. Gunter-Smith PJ. Gamma radiation affects active electrolyte transport by rabbit ileum: Basal Na and Cl transport. Am J Physiol 1986;250(Gastrointest Liver Physiol 13):G540.

157. Grem JL, Shoemaker DD, Petrelli NJ, Douglass HO Jr. Severe and fatal toxic effects observed in treatment with high- and low-dose leucovorin plus 5-fluorouracil for colorectal carcinoma. Cancer Treat Rep 1987;71:1122.

158. Rosenberg SA, Lotze MT, Mulé JJ. New approaches to the immunotherapy of cancer using interleukin-2. Ann Intern Med 1988;108:853.

159. Gelfand MD, Tepper M, Katz LA, Binder HJ, Yesner R, Floch MH. Acute irradiation proctitis in man: Development of eosinophilic crypt abscesses. Gastroenterology 1968;54:401.

160. Editorial: Radiation-induced proctosigmoiditis. Lancet 1983;1:1082.

161. Riddoch C, Trinick T. Gastrointestinal disturbances in marathon runners. Br J Sports Med 1988;22:71.

162. Sullivan SN, Champion MC, Christofides ND, Adrian TE, Bloom SR. Gastrointestinal regulatory peptide responses in long-distance runners. Physician and Sports Medicine 1984;12:77.

163. Demers LM, Harrison TS, Halbert DR, Santen RJ. Effect of prolonged exercise on plasma prostaglandin levels. Prostagland Med 1981;6:413.

164. Heer M, Repond F, Hany A, Sulser H, Kehl O, Jäger K. Acute ischaemic colitis in a female long distance runner. Gut 1987;28:896.

165. Meshkinpour H, Kemp C, Fairshter R. Effect of aerobic exercise on mouth-to-cecum transit time. Gastroenterology 1989;96:938.

166. Marsh MN, Hinde J. Inflammatory component of celiac sprue mucosa. I. Mast cells, basophils, and eosinophils. Gastroenterology 1985;89:92.

167. Fordtran JS, Rector FC, Locklear TW, Ewton MF. Water and solute

movement in the small intestine of patients with sprue. J Clin Invest 1967;46:287.

168. Losowsky MS, Walker BE. Liver disease and malabsorption. Gastroenterology 1969;56:589.

169. Mathias JR, Clench MH. Review: Pathophysiology of diarrhea caused by bacterial overgrowth of the small intestine. Am J Med Sci 1985;289:243.

170. Zentler-Munro PL. Cystic fibrosis—A gastroenterological cornucopia. Gut 1987;28:1531.

171. Weizman Z, Durie PR, Kopelman HR, Vesely SM, Forstner GG. Bile acid secretion in cystic fibrosis: Evidence for a defect unrelated to fat malabsorption. Gut 1986;27:1043.

172. Krejs GJ, Orci L, Conlon JM, et al. Somatostatinoma syndrome: Biochemical, morphologic and clinical features. N Engl J Med 1979;301:285.

173. Race TF, Paes IC, Faloon WW. Intestinal malabsorption induced by oral colchicine. Comparison with neomycin and cathartic agents. Am J Med Sci 1970;259:32.

174. West RJ, Lloyd JK. The effect of cholestyramine on intestinal absorption. Gut 1975;16:93.

175. Rogers AI, Vloedman DA, Bloom EC, Kalser MH. Neomycin-induced steatorrhea. JAMA 1966;197:185.

176. Halsted CH, McIntyre PA. Intestinal malabsorption caused by aminosalicylic acid therapy. Arch Intern Med 1972;130:935.

177. Hoskins LC, Winawer SJ, Broitman SA, Gottlieb LS, Zamcheck N. Clinical giardiasis and intestinal malabsorption. Gastroenterology 1967;53:265.

178. Brandborg LL, Goldberg SB, Breidenbach WC. Human coccidiosis—A possible cause of malabsorption. N Engl J Med 1970;283:1306.

179. Kotcher E, Miranda M, Esquivel R, Peña-Chavarría A, Donohugh DL, Baldizón C, Acosta A, Apuy JL. Intestinal malabsorption and helminthic and protozoan infections of the small intestine. Gastroenterology 1966;50:366.

180. Milner PF, Irvine RA, Barton CJ, Bras G, Richards R. Intestinal malabsorption in *Strongyloides stercoralis* infestation. Gut 1966;6:574.

181. Broitman SA, McCray RS, May JC, Deren JJ, Ackroyd F, Gottlieb LS, McDermott W, Zamcheck N. Mastocytosis and intestinal malabsorption. Am J Med 1970;48:382.

182. Leinbach GE, Rubin CE. Eosinophilic gastroenteritis: A simple reaction to food allergens? Gastroenterology 1970;59:874.

183. Lindenbaum J, Gerson CD, Kent TH. Recovery of small-intestinal structure and function after residence in the tropics. I. Studies in Peace Corps volunteers. Ann Intern Med 1971;74:218.

184. Hamilton JR, Lynch MJ, Reilly BJ. Active coeliac disease in childhood: Clinical and laboratory findings of forty-two cases. Q J Med 1969;38:135.

185. Westergaard H. Southwestern Internal Medicine Conference: The sprue syndromes. Am J Med Sci 1985;290:249.

186. Evans WB, Wollaeger EE. Incidence and severity of nutritional deficiency states in chronic exocrine pancreatic insufficiency: Comparison with nontropical sprue. Am J Dig Dis 1966;11:594.

187. Mann JG, Brown WR, Kern F Jr. The subtle and variable clinical expressions of gluten-induced enteropathy (adult celiac disease, nontropical sprue): An analysis of twenty-one consecutive cases. Am J Med 1970;48:357.

188. Wilson C, Eade OE, Elstein M, Wright R. Subclinical coeliac disease and infertility. Br Med J 1976;2:215.

189. Ross JR, Gibb SP, Hoffman DE, Clerkin EP, Dotter WE, Hurxthal LM. Gluten enteropathy and skeletal disease. JAMA 1966;196:270.

190. Cooke WT, Smith WT. Neurological disorders associated with adult coeliac disease. Brain 1966;89:683.

191. Gawkrodger DJ, Blackwell JN, Gilmour HM, Rifkind EA, Heading RC, Barnetson R StC. Dermatitis herpetiformis: Diagnosis, diet and demography. Gut 1984;25:151.

192. Feldman M. Southern Internal Medicine Conference: Whipple's disease. Am J Med Sci 1986;291:56.

193. Waldmann TA, Steinfeld JL, Dutcher TF, Davidson JD, Gordon RS Jr. The role of the gastrointestinal system in "idiopathic hypoproteinemia." Gastroenterology 1961;41:197.

194. Mistilis SP, Skyring AP. Intestinal lymphangiectasia. Am J Med 1966;40:634.

195. Asakura H, Tsuchiya M, Katoh S, Kobayashi K, Yonei Y, Yoshida T, Hamada Y, Miura S, Morita A, Kuramochi S, Teramoto T. Pathological findings of lymphangiectasia of the large intestine in a patient with protein-losing enteropathy. Gastroenterology 1986;91:719.

196. Miller LJ, Gorman CA, Go VLW. Gut–thyroid interrelationships. Gastroenterology 1978;75:901.

197. Rodgers JB, Riley EM, Drummey GD, Isselbacher KJ. Lipid absorption in adrenalectomized rats: The role of altered enzyme activity in the intestinal mucosa. Gastroenterology 1967;53:547.

198. James WPT. Intestinal absorption in protein-calorie malnutrition. Lancet 1968;1:333.

199. Stanfield JP, Hutt MSR, Tunnicliffe R. Intestinal biopsy in kwashiorkor. Lancet 1965;2:519.

200. Trier JS. Intestinal malabsorption: Differentiation of cause. Hosp Pract 1988;23:195.

201. Bo-Linn GW, Fordtran JS. Fecal fat concentration in patients with steatorrhea. Gastroenterology 1984;87:319.

202. Levitt MD, Duane WC. Floating stools—Flatus versus fat. N Engl J Med 1972;286:973.

203. Wiggins HS, Howell KE, Kellock TD, Stalder J. The origin of faecal fat. Gut 1969;10:400.

204. Khouri MR, Huang G, Shiau YF. Sudan stain of fecal fat: New insight into an old test. Gastroenterology 1989;96:421.

205. Drummey GD, Benson JA Jr, Jones CM. Microscopical examination of the stool for steatorrhea. N Engl J Med 1961;264:85.

206. Ghosh SK, Littlewood JM, Goddard D, Steel AE. Stool microscopy in screening for steatorrhoea. J Clin Pathol 1977;30:749.

207. Rosenberg IH, Sitrin MD. Screening for fat malabsorption. Ann Intern Med 1981;95:776.

208. Simko V. Fecal fat microscopy: Acceptable predictive value in screening for steatorrhea. Am J Gastroenterol 1981;75:204.

209. Van de Kamer JH, Ten Bokkel Huinink H, Weyers HA. Rapid method for the determination of fat in feces. J Biol Chem 1949;177:347.

210. Ditchburn RK, Smith AH, Hayter CJ. Use of unabsorbed radioactive marker substances in a re-assessment of the radioactive triolein test of fat absorption. J Clin Pathol 1971;24:506.

211. Greene HL, Rosensweig NS, Lufkin EG, Hagler L, Gozansky D, Taunton OD, Herman RH. Biopsy of the small intestine with the Crosby–Kugler capsule: Experience in 3,866 peroral biopsies in children and adults. Am J Dig Dis 1974;19:189.

212. Jabbari M, Wild G, Goresky CA, Daly DS, Lough JO, Cleland DP, Kinnear DG. Scalloped valvulae conniventes: An endoscopic marker of celiac sprue. Gastroenterology 1988;95:1518.

213. Trier JS. Diagnostic value of peroral biopsy of the proximal small intestine. N Engl J Med 1971;285:1470.

214. Craig RM, Atkinson AJ Jr. D-xylose testing: A review. Gastroenterology 1988;95:223.

215. Newcomer AD, Hofmann AF, DiMagno EP, Thomas PJ, Carlson GL. Triolein breath test: A sensitive and specific test for fat malabsorption. Gastroenterology 1979;76:6.

216. West PS, Levin GE, Griffin GE, Maxwell JD. Comparison of simple screening tests for fat malabsorption. Br Med J 1981;282:1501.

217. Mylvaganam K, Hudson PR, Ross A, Williams CP. ^{14}C triolein breath test: A routine test in the gastroenterology clinic? Gut 1986;27:1347.

218. Turner JM, Lawrence S, Fellows IW, Johnson I, Hill PG, Holmes GKT. [^{14}C]-triolein absorption: A useful test in the diagnosis of malabsorption. Gut 1987;28:694.

219. Arvanitakis C, Greenberger NJ. Diagnosis of pancreatic disease by a synthetic peptide: A new test of exocrine pancreatic function. Lancet 1976;1:663.

220. Mee AS, Girdwood AH, Walker E, Gilinsky NH, Kottler RE, Marks IN. Comparison of the oral (PABA) pancreatic function test, the secretin-pancreozymin test and endoscopic retrograde pancreatography in chronic alcohol induced pancreatitis. Gut 1985;26:1257.

221. Heyman MB. The bentiromide test: How good is it? Gastroenterology 1985;89:685.

222. Weizman ZE, Forstner GG, Gaskin KJ, Kopelman H, Wong S, Durie PR. Bentiromide test for assessing pancreatic dysfunction using analysis of para-aminobenzoic acid in plasma and urine: Studies

in cystic fibrosis and Shwachman's syndrome. Gastroenterology 1985;89:596.

223. Hoek FJ, Van den Bergh FAJTM, Elhorst JTK, Meijer JL, Timmer E, Tytgat GNJ. Improved specificity of the PABA test with p-aminosalicylic acid (PAS). Gut 1987;28:468.

224. Orlando R. Secretin test. In: Drossman DA, ed. Manual of gastroenterologic procedures, ed 2. New York: Raven Press, 1987:66.

225. Arvanitakis C, Cooke AR. Diagnostic tests of exocrine pancreatic function and disease. Gastroenterology 1978;74:932.

226. Brugge WR, Goff JS, Allen NC, Podell ER, Allen RH. Development of a dual label Schilling test for pancreatic exocrine function based on the differential absorption of cobalamin bound to intrinsic factor and R protein. Gastroenterology 1980;78:937.

227. Chen W-L, Morishita R, Eguchi T, Kawai T, Sakai M, Tateishi H, Uchino H. Clinical usefulness of dual-label Schilling test for pancreatic exocrine function. Gastroenterology 1989;96:1337.

228. Isaacs PET, Kim YS. The contaminated small bowel syndrome. Am J Med 1979;67:1049.

229. Kerlin P, Wong L. Breath hydrogen testing in bacterial overgrowth of the small intestine. Gastroenterology 1988;95:982.

230. Perman JA, Modler S, Barr RG, Rosenthal P. Fasting breath hydrogen concentration: Normal values and clinical application. Gastroenterology 1984;87:1358.

231. King CE, Toskes PP, Spivey JC, Lorenz E, Welkos SL. Detection of small intestine bacterial overgrowth by means of a ^{14}C-d-xylose breath test. Gastroenterology 1979;77:75.

232. King CE, Toskes PP, Guilarte TR, Lorenz E, Welkos SL. Comparison of the one-gram d-(^{14}C) xylose breath test to the (^{14}C) bile acid breath test in patients with small-intestine bacterial overgrowth. Dig Dis Sci 1980;25:53.

233. Fromm H, Hofmann AF. Breath test for altered bile–acid metabolism. Lancet 1971;2:621.

234. Farivar S, Fromm H, Schindler D, Schmidt FW. Sensitivity of bile acid breath test in the diagnosis of bacterial overgrowth in the small intestine with and without the stagnant (blind) loop syndrome. Dig Dis Sci 1979;24:33.

235. Swischuk LE, Welsh JD. Roentgenographic mucosal patterns in the "malabsorption syndrome": A scheme of diagnosis. Am J Dig Dis 1968;13:59.

236. Gryboski JD. Diarrhea from dietetic candies. N Engl J Med 1966;29:718.

237. Hyams JS. Sorbitol intolerance: An unappreciated cause of functional gastrointestinal complaints. Gastroenterology 1983;84:30.

238. Caspary WF. Diarrhoea associated with carbohydrate malabsorption. Clin Gastroenterol 1986;15:631.

239. Bayless TM. Lactase deficiency and intolerance to milk. Viewpoints on Digestive Diseases 1971;3:1.

240. Bayless TM, Rothfeld B, Massa C, Wise L, Paige D, Bedine MS. Lactose and milk intolerance: Clinical implications. N Engl J Med 1975;292:1156.

241. Barr RG, Levine MD, Watkins JB. Recurrent abdominal pain of childhood due to lactose intolerance: A prospective study. N Engl J Med 1979;300:1449.

242. DiPalma JA, Narvaez RM. Prediction of lactose malabsorption in referral patients. Dig Dis Sci 1988;33:303.

243. Bond JH, Currier BE, Buchwald H, Levitt MD. Colonic conservation of malabsorbed carbohydrate. Gastroenterology 1980;78:444.

244. Stephen AM, Haddad AC, Phillips SF. Passage of carbohydrate into the colon: Direct measurements in humans. Gastroenterology 1983;85:589.

245. Rumessen JJ, Gudmand-Høyer E. Absorption capacity of fructose in healthy adults. Comparison with sucrose and its constituent monosaccharides. Gut 1986;27:1161.

246. Rumessen JJ, Gudmand-Høyer E. Functional bowel disease: Malabsorption and abdominal distress after ingestion of fructose, sorbitol and fructose-sorbitol mixtures. Gastroenterology 1988;95:694.

247. Andersson DEH, Nygren A. Four cases of long-standing diarrhoea and colic pains cured by fructose-free diet—A pathogenic discussion. Acta Med Scand 1978;203:87.

248. Andres JM. Advances in understanding the pathogenesis of persistent diarrhea in young children. Adv Pediatr 1988;35:483.

249. Woolridge MW, Fisher C. Colic, "overfeeding," and symptoms of lactose malabsorption in the breast-fed baby: A possible artifact of feed management? Lancet 1988;2:382.

250. Fenton TR, Harries JT, Milla PJ. Disordered small intestinal motility: A rational basis for toddlers' diarrhoea. Gut 1983;24:897.

251. Kellow JE, Phillips SF. Altered small bowel motility in irritable bowel syndrome is correlated with symptoms. Gastroenterology 1987;92:1885.

252. Gilmore IT. Orocaecal transit time in health and disease. Gut 1990;31:250.

253. Corbett CL, Thomas S, Read NW, Hobson N, Bergman I, Holdsworth CD. Electrochemical detector for breath hydrogen determination: Measurement of small bowel transit time in normal subjects and patients with the irritable bowel syndrome. Gut 1981;22:836.

254. Cann PA, Read NW, Brown C, Hobson N, Holdsworth CD. Irritable bowel syndrome: Relationship of disorders in the transit of a single solid meal to symptom patterns. Gut 1983;24:405.

255. Read NW, Miles CA, Fisher D, Holgate AM, Kime ND, Mitchell MA, Reeve AM, Roche TB, Walker M. Transit of a meal through the stomach, small intestine, and colon in normal subjects and its role in the pathogenesis of diarrhea. Gastroenterology 1980;79:1276.

256. Read NW. Small bowel transit time of food in man: Measurement, regulation and possible importance. Scand J Gastroenterol 1984(Suppl);96:77.

257. Tobin MV, Fisken RA, Diggory RT, Morris AI, Gilmore IT. Orocaecal transit time in health and in thyroid disease. Gut 1989;30:26.

258. Rao SSC, Read NW, Holdsworth CD. Is the diarrhoea in ulcerative colitis related to impaired colonic salvage of carbohydrate? Gut 1987;28:1090.

259. Hofmann AF. Bile acid malabsorption caused by ileal resection. Arch Intern Med 1972;130:597.

260. Hofmann AF, Poley JR. Role of bile acid malabsorption in pathogenesis of diarrhea and steatorrhea in patients with ileal resection. Gastroenterology 1972;62:918.

261. Hardison WGM, Rosenberg IH. Bile-salt deficiency in the steatorrhea following resection of the ileum and proximal colon. N Engl J Med 1967;277:337.

262. Hutcheon DF, Bayless TM, Gadacz TR. Postcholecystectomy diarrhea. JAMA 1979;241:823.

263. Fromm H, Tunuguntla AK, Malavolti M, Sherman C, Ceryak S. Absence of a significant role of bile acids in diarrhea of a heterogenous group of postcholecystectomy patients. Dig Dis Sci 1987;32:33.

264. Raimes SA, Smirniotis V, Wheldon EJ, Venables CW, Johnston IDA. Postvagotomy diarrhea put into perspective. Lancet 1986;2:851.

265. Cuschieri A. Postvagotomy diarrhoea: Is there a place for surgical management? Gut 1990;31:245.

266. Browning GG, Buchan KA, MacKay C. Clinical and laboratory study of postvagotomy diarrhoea. Gut 1974;15:644.

267. Ladas SD, Isaacs PET, Quereshi Y, Sladen G. Role of the small intestine in postvagotomy diarrhea. Gastroenterology 1983;85:1088.

268. Doty JE, Meyer JH. Vagotomy and antrectomy impairs canine fat absorption from solid but not liquid dietary sources. Gastroenterology 1988;94:50.

269. O'Brien JD, Thompson DG, McIntyre A, Burnham WR, Walker E. Effect of codeine and loperamide on upper intestinal transit and absorption in normal subjects and patients with postvagotomy diarrhoea. Gut 1988;29:312.

270. Thaysen EH, Pedersen L. Idiopathic bile acid catharsis. Gut 1976;17:965.

271. Balistreri WF, Partin JC, Schubert WK. Bile acid malabsorption— A consequence of terminal ileal dysfunction in protracted diarrhea of infancy. J Pediatr 1977;89:21.

272. Heubi JE, Balistreri WF, Fondacaro JD, Partin JC, Schubert WK. Primary bile salt malabsorption: Defective in vitro active bile acid transport. Gastroenterology 1982;83:804.

273. Popović OS, Kostić KM, Milović VB, Milutinović-Djurić S, Miletić VD, Šešić L, Djordjević M, Bulajić M, Bojić P, Rubinić M, Borisavljević N. Primary bile acid malabsorption: Histologic and immunologic study in three patients. Gastroenterology 1987;92:1851.

274. Schiller LR, Hogan RB, Morawski SG, Santa Ana CA, Bern MJ, Norgaard RP, Bo-Linn GW, Fordtran JS. Studies of the prevalence and significance of radiolabeled bile acid malabsorption in a group

of patients with idiopathic chronic diarrhea. Gastroenterology 1987;92:151.

275. Schiller LR, Bilhartz LE, Santa Ana CA, Fordtran JS. Comparison of endogenous and radiolabeled bile acid excretion in patients with idiopathic chronic diarrhea. Gastroenterology 1990;98:1036.

276. Alun Jones V, McLaughlan P, Shorthouse M, Workman E, Hunter JO. Food intolerance: A major factor in the pathogenesis of irritable bowel syndrome. Lancet 1982;2:1115.

277. Nanda R, James R, Smith H, Dudley CRK, Jewell DP. Food intolerance and the irritable bowel syndrome. Gut 1989;30:1099.

278. Bentley SJ, Pearson DJ, Rix KJB. Food hypersensitivity in irritable bowel syndrome. Lancet 1983;2:295.

279. Bukhave K, Rask-Madsen J. Prostaglandin E_2 in jejunal fluids and its potential diagnostic value for selecting patients with indomethacin-sensitive diarrhoea. Eur J Clin Invest 1981;11:191.

280. Sampson HA, Broadbent KR, Bernhisel-Broadbent J. Spontaneous release of histamine from basophils and histamine-releasing factor in patients with atopic dermatitis and food hypersensitivity. N Engl J Med 1989;321:228.

281. Hwang WS, Kelly JK, Shaffer EA, Hershfield NB. Collagenous colitis: A disease of pericryptal fibroblast sheath? J Pathol 1986;149:33.

282. Rams H, Rogers AI, Ghandur-Mnaymneh L. Collagenous colitis. Ann Intern Med 1987;106:108.

283. Lazenby AJ, Yardley JH, Giardiello FM, Jessurun J, Bayless TM. Lymphocytic ("microscopic") colitis: A comparative histopathologic study with particular reference to collagenous colitis. Hum Pathol 1989;20:784.

284. Baum CA, Bhatia P, Miner PB Jr. Increased colonic mucosal mast cells associated with severe watery diarrhea and microscopic colitis. Dig Dis Sci 1989;34:1462.

285. Rask-Madsen J, Grove O, Hansen MGJ, Bukhave K, Henrik-Nielsen R. Colonic transport of water and electrolytes in a patient with secretory diarrhea due to collagenous colitis. Dig Dis Sci 1983;28:1141.

286. Fordtran JS, Santa Ana CA, Morawski SG, Bo-Linn GW, Schiller LR. Pathophysiology of chronic diarrhoea: Insights derived from intestinal perfusion studies in 31 patients. Clin Gastroenterol 1986;15:447.

287. Hamilton I, Sanders S, Hopwood D, Boucchier IAD. Collagenous colitis associated with small intestinal villous atrophy. Gut 1986;27:1394.

288. Weil C. Gastroenteropancreatic endocrine tumors. Klin Wochenschr 1985;63:433.

289. Rambaud J-C, Hautefeuille M, Ruskoné A, Jacquenod P. Diarrhoea due to circulating agents. Clin Gastroenterol 1986;15:603.

290. Donowitz M, Binder HJ. Jejunal fluid and electrolyte secretion in carcinoid syndrome. Dig Dis 1975;20:1115.

291. Kingham JG, Levison DA, Fairclough PD. Diarrhoea and reversible enteropathy in Zollinger–Ellison syndrome. Lancet 1981;2:610.

292. Rambaud JC, Modigliani R, Emonts P, Matuchansky C, Vidon N, Besterman H, Bernier J-J. Fluid secretion in the duodenum and intestinal handling of water and electrolytes in Zollinger–Ellison syndrome. Dig Dis 1978;23:1089.

293. Fang M, Ginsberg AL, Glassman L, McCarthy DM, Cohen P, Geelhoed GW, Dobbins WO. Zollinger–Ellison syndrome with diarrhea as the predominant clinical feature. Gastroenterology 1979;76:378.

294. Carney JA, Hayles AB. Alimentary tract manifestations of multiple endocrine neoplasia, type 2b. Mayo Clin Proc 1977;52:543.

295. McGill DB, Miller LJ, Carney JA, Phillips SF, Go VLW, Schutt AJ. Hormonal diarrhea due to pancreatic tumor. Gastroenterology 1980;79:571.

296. Friesen SR. Tumors of the endocrine pancreas. N Engl J Med 1982;306:580.

297. Krejs GJ. VIPoma syndrome. Am J Med 1987;82(Suppl 15B):37.

298. Rood RP, DeLellis RA, Dayal Y, Donowitz M. Pancreatic cholera syndrome due to a vasoactive intestinal polypeptide–producing tumor: Further insights into the pathophysiology. Gastroenterology 1988;94:813.

299. Green M, Cooke RE, Lattanzi W. Occurrence of chronic diarrhea in three patients with ganglioneuromas. Pediatrics 1959;23:951.

300. Stickler GB, Hallenbeck GA, Flock EV, Rosevear JW. Catechol-amines and diarrhea in ganglioneuroblastoma. Am J Dis Child 1962;104:598.

301. Carney JA, Go VLW, Sizemore GW, Hayles AB. Alimentary-tract ganglioneuromatosis: A major component of the syndrome of multiple endocrine neoplasia, type 2b. N Engl J Med 1976;295:1287.

302. Bernier JJ, Rambaud JC, Cattan D, Prost A. Diarrhoea associated with medullary carcinoma of the thyroid. Gut 1969;10:980.

303. Isaacs P, Whittaker SM, Turnberg LA. Diarrhea associated with medullary carcinoma of the thyroid: Studies of intestinal function in a patient. Gastroenterology 1974;67:521.

304. Rambaud JC, Jian R, Flourié RJB, Hautefeuille M, Salmeron M, Thuillier F, Ruskoné A, Florent C, Chaoui F, Bernier J-J. Pathophysiology study of diarrhoea in a patient with medullary thyroid carcinoma. Evidence against a secretory mechanism and for the role of shortened colonic transit time. Gut 1988;29:537.

305. Leichter SB. Clinical and metabolic aspects of glucagonoma. Medicine 1980;59:100.

306. Duthie HL, Atwell JD. The absorption of water, sodium, and potassium in the large intestine with particular reference to the effects of villous papillomas. Gut 1963;4:373.

307. Solomon SS, Moran JM, Nabseth DC. Villous adenoma of recto-sigmoid accompanied by electrolyte depletion. JAMA 1965;194:5.

308. Shields R. Absorption and secretion of electrolytes and water by the human colon, with particular reference to benign adenoma and papilloma. Br J Surg 1966;53:893.

309. Lee RO, Keown D. Villous tumours of the rectum associated with severe fluid and electrolyte disturbance. Br J Surg 1970;57:197.

310. DaCruz GMG, Gardner JD, Peskin GW. Mechanism of diarrhea of villous adenomas. Am J Surg 1968;115:203.

311. Steven K, Lange P, Bukhave K, Rask-Madsen J. Prostaglandin E_2-mediated secretory diarrhea in villous adenoma of rectum: Effect of treatment with indomethacin. Gastroenterology 1981;80:1562.

312. Roberts LJ II, Sweetman BJ, Lewis RA, Austen KF, Oates JA. Increased production of prostaglandin D_2 in patients with systemic mastocytosis. N Engl J Med 1980;303:1400.

313. Soter NA, Austen KF, Wasserman SI. Oral disodium cromoglycate in the treatment of systemic mastocytosis. N Engl J Med 1979;301:465.

314. Bytzer P, Stokholm M, Andersen I, Klitgaard NA, Schaffalitzky de Muckadell OB. Prevalence of surreptitious laxative abuse in patients with diarrhoea of uncertain origin: A cost benefit analysis of a screening procedure. Gut 1989;30:1379.

315. Ewe K, Karbach U. Factitious diarrhoea. Clin Gastroenterol 1986;15:723.

316. Read NW, Krejs GJ, Read MG, Santa Ana CA, Morawski SG, Fordtran JS. Chronic diarrhea of unknown origin. Gastroenterology 1980;78:264.

317. Krejs GJ, Walsh JH, Morawski SG, Fordtran JS. Intractable diarrhea: Intestinal perfusion studies and plasma VIP concentrations in patients with pancreatic cholera syndrome and surreptitious ingestion of laxatives and diuretics. Am J Dig Dis 1977;22:280.

318. Morris AI, Turnberg LA. Surreptitious laxative abuse. Gastroenterology 1979;77:780.

319. Binder HJ. Pharmacology of laxatives. Annu Rev Pharmacol Toxicol 1977;17:355.

320. Sekas G. The use and abuse of laxatives: Recognizing the abusive patient. Practical Gastroenterology 1987;11:33.

321. Fine KD, Krejs GJ, Fordtran JS. Diarrhea. In: Sleisenger MH, Fordtran JS, eds. Gastrointestinal disease: Pathophysiology, diagnosis, management, ed 4. Philadelphia: WB Saunders, 1989:290.

322. Burman D, Stevens D. Münchausen family. Lancet 1977;2:456.

323. Chan AA, Salcedo JR, Atkins DM, Ruley EJ. Münchausen syndrome by proxy: A review and case study. J Pediatr Psychol 1986;11:1.

324. DeVore CD, Ulshen MH, Cross RE. Phenolphthalein laxatives and factitious diarrhea. Clin Pediatr 1982;21:573.

325. Rosenberg DA. Web of deceit: A literature review of Munchausen syndrome by proxy. Child Abuse Negl 1987;11:547.

326. Katz LA, Spiro HM. Gastrointestinal manifestations of diabetes. N Engl J Med 1966;275:1350.

327. Goldstein F, Wirts CW, Kowlessar OD. Diabetic diarrhea and steatorrhea: Microbiologic and clinical observations. Ann Intern Med 1970;72:215.

328. Scarpello JHB, Sladen GE. Progress report: Diabetes and the gut. Gut 1978;19:1153.

329. Chang EB, Bergenstal RM, Field M. Diarrhea in streptozocin-treated rats: Loss of adrenergic regulation of intestinal fluid and electrolyte transport. J Clin Invest 1985;75:1.

330. Chang EB, Fedorak RN, Field M. Experimental diabetic diarrhea in rats. Gastroenterology 1986;91:564.

331. Fedorak RN, Field M, Chang EB. Treatment of diabetic diarrhea with clonidine. Ann Intern Med 1985;102:197.

332. Schiller LR, Santa Ana CA, Schmulen AC, Hendler RS, Harford WV, Fordtran JS. Pathogenesis of fecal incontinence in diabetes mellitus: Evidence of internal-anal-sphincter dysfunction. N Engl J Med 1982;307:1666.

333. Rubin E, Rybak BJ, Lindenbaum J, Gerson CD, Walker G, Lieber CS. Ultrastructural changes in the small intestine induced by ethanol. Gastroenterology 1972;63:801.

334. Kvietys PR, Patterson WG, Russell JM, Barrowman JA, Granger DN. Role of the microcirculation in ethanol-induced mucosal injury in the dog. Gastroenterology 1984;87:562.

335. Hermos JA, Adams WH, Liu YK, Sullivan LW, Trier JS. Mucosa of the small intestine in folate-deficient alcoholics. Ann Intern Med 1972;76:957.

336. Ray M, Dinda PK, Beck IT. Mechanism of ethanol-induced jejunal microvascular and morphologic changes in the dog. Gastroenterology 1989;96:345.

337. Colombel JF, Hällgren R, Venge P, Mesnard B, Rambaud JC. Neutrophil and eosinophil involvement of the small bowel affected by chronic alcoholism. Gut 1988;29:1656.

338. Leddin DJ, Ray M, Dinda PK, Prokopiw I, Beck IT. 16, 16-dimethyl prostaglandin E$_2$ alleviates jejunal microvascular effects of ethanol but not the ethanol-induced inhibition of water, sodium, and glucose absorption. Gastroenterology 1988;94:726.

339. Hamilton JR, Reilly BJ, Morecki R. Short small intestine associated with malrotation: A newly described congenital cause of intestinal malabsorption. Gastroenterology 1969;56:124.

340. Turnberg LA. Abnormalities in intestinal electrolyte transport in congenital chloridorrhoea. Gut 1971;12:544.

341. Holmberg C. Congenital chloride diarrhoea. Clin Gastroenterol 1986;15:583.

342. Holmberg C, Perheentupa J. Congenital Na$^+$ diarrhea: A new type of secretory diarrhea. J Pediatr 1985;106:56.

343. Booth IW, Murer H, Milla PJ, Stange G, Fenton TR. Defective jejunal brush-border Na$^+$/H$^+$ exchange: A cause of congenital secretory diarrhoea. Lancet 1985;1:1066.

344. Cutz E, Rhoads JM, Drumm B, Sherman PM, Durie PR, Forstner GG. Microvillus inclusion disease: An inherited defect of brush-border assembly and differentiation. N Engl J Med 1989;320:646.

345. Rhoads JM, Vogler RC, Lacey SR, Reddick RL, Keku EO, Azizkhan RG, Berschneider HM. Microvillus inclusion disease: In vitro jejunal electrolyte transport. (In press)

346. Newcomer AD, McGill DB, Thomas PJ, Hofmann AF. Prospective comparison of indirect methods for detecting lactase deficiency. N Engl J Med 1975;293:1232.

347. Kerlin P, Wong L, Harris B, Capra S. Rice flour, breath hydrogen, and malabsorption. Gastroenterology 1984;87:578.

348. Sciarretta G, Vicini G, Fagioli G, Verri A, Ginevra A, Malaguti P. Use of 23-selena-25-homocholyltaurine to detect bile acid malabsorption in patients with ileal dysfunction or diarrhea. Gastroenterology 1986;91:1.

349. Wittoesch JH, Jackman RJ, McDonald JR. Melanosis coli: General review and a study of 887 cases. Dis Colon Rectum 1958;1:172.

350. Plum GE, Weber HM, Sauer WG. Prolonged cathartic abuse resulting in roentgen evidence suggestive of enterocolitis. Am J Roentgenol 1960;83:919.

351. Head LH, Heaton JW Jr, Kivel RM. Absorption of water and electrolytes in Crohn's disease of the colon. Gastroenterology 1969;56:571.

352. Archampong EQ, Harris J, Clark CG. The absorption and secretion of water and electrolytes across the healthy and the diseased human colonic mucosa measured *in vitro*. Gut 1972;13:880.

353. Edmonds CJ, Pilcher D. Electrical potential difference and sodium and potassium fluxes across rectal mucosa in ulcerative colitis. Gut 1973;14:784.

354. Binder HJ, Ptak T. Jejunal absorption of water and electrolytes in inflammatory bowel disease. J Lab Clin Med 1970;76:915.

355. Knutson L, Ahrenstedt Ö, Odlind B, Hällgren R. The jejunal secretion of histamine is increased in active Crohn's disease. Gastroenterology 1990;98:849.

356. Rask-Madsen J. Eicosanoids and their role in the pathogenesis of diarrhoeal diseases. Clin Gastroenterol 1986;15:545.

357. Zifroni A, Treves AJ, Sachar DB, Rachmilewitz D. Prostanoid synthesis by cultured intestinal epithelial and mononuclear cells in inflammatory bowel disease. Gut 1983;24:659.

358. Lauritsen K, Laursen LS, Bukhave K, Rask-Madsen J. *In vivo* profiles of eicosanoids in ulcerative colitis, Crohn's colitis, and *Clostridium difficile* colitis. Gastroenterology 1988;95:11.

359. Sharon P, Stenson WF. Enhanced synthesis of leukotriene B$_4$ by colonic mucosa in inflammatory bowel disease. Gastroenterology 1984;86:453.

360. Eliakim R, Karmeli F, Razin E, Rachmilewitz D. Role of platelet-activating factor for ulcerative colitis: Enhanced production during active disease and inhibition by sulfasalazine and prednisolone. Gastroenterology 1988;95:1167.

361. Sartor RB, Chapman EJ, Schwab JH. Increased interleukin 1b concentrations in resected inflammatory bowel disease (IBD) tissue. Gastroenterology 1988;94:A399.

362. O'Morain C, Bishop AE, McGregor GP, Levi AJ, Bloom SR, Polak JM, Peters TJ. Vasoactive intestinal peptide concentrations and immunocytochemical studies in rectal biopsies from patients with inflammatory bowel disease. Gut 1984;25:57.

363. Duffy LC, Zielezny MA, Riepenhoff-Talty M, Byers TE, Marshall J, Weiser MM, Graham S, Ogra PL. Vasoactive intestinal peptide as a laboratory supplement to clinical activity index in inflammatory bowel disease. Dig Dis Sci 1989;34:1528.

364. Cello JP. Eosinophilic gastroenteritis—A complex disease entity. Am J Med 1979;67:1097.

365. Talley NJ, Shorter RG, Phillips SF, Zinsmeister AR. Eosinophilic gastroenteritis: A clinicopathological study of patients with disease of the mucosa, muscle layer, and subserosal tissues. Gut 1990;31:54.

366. Gryboski JD. Gastrointestinal milk allergy in infants. Pediatrics 1967;40:354.

367. Powell GK. Milk- and soy-induced enterocolitis of infancy: Clinical features and standardization of challenge. J Pediatr 1978;93:553.

368. Whitington PF, Gibson R. Soy protein intolerance: Four patients with concomitant cow's milk intolerance. Pediatrics 1977;59:730.

369. Van Sickle GJ, Powell GK, McDonald PJ, Goldblum RM. Milk- and soy protein–induced enterocolitis: Evidence for lymphocyte sensitization to specific food proteins. Gastroenterology 1985;88:1915.

370. Waldmann TA. Protein-losing enteropathy. Gastroenterology 1966;50:422.

371. Waldmann TA, Wochner RD, Laster L, Gordon RS Jr. Allergic gastroenteropathy. N Engl J Med 1967;276:761.

372. Greenberger NJ, Tennenbaum JI, Ruppert RD. Protein-losing enteropathy associated with gastrointestinal allergy. Am J Med 1967;43:777.

373. Monballyu J, Hauglustaine D, Geboes K, Desmet V, Michielsen P. Protein-losing enteropathy in systemic lupus erythematosus. Digestion 1985;31:243.

374. Lantz B, Einhorn N. Intestinal damage and malabsorption after treatment for cervical carcinoma. Acta Radiol Oncol 1984;23:33.

375. Newman A, Katsaris J, Blendis LM, Charlesworth M, Walter LH. Small-intestinal injury in women who have had pelvic radiotherapy. Lancet 1973;2:1471.

376. Schuster JJ, Stryker JA, Demers LM, Mortel R. Absence of bile acid malabsorption as a late effect of pelvic irradiation. Int J Radiat Oncol Biol Phys 1986;12:1605.

377. Ahlquist DA, Gostout CJ, Viggiano TR, Pemberton JH. Laser therapy for severe radiation-induced rectal bleeding. Mayo Clin Proc 1986;61:927.

378. DeCosse JJ, Rhodes RS, Wentz WB, Reagan JW, Dworken HJ, Holden WD. The natural history and management of radiation induced injury of the gastrointestinal tract. Ann Surg 1969;170:369.

379. Tankel HI, Clark DH, Lee FD. Radiation enteritis with malabsorption. Gut 1965;6:560.

380. Davis GR, Corbett DB, Krejs GJ. Ileal chloride secretion as a cause of secretory diarrhea in a patient with primary intestinal tuberculosis. Gastroenterology 1979;76:829.

381. Cappell MS, Mandell W, Grimes MM, Neu HC. Gastrointestinal histoplasmosis. Dig Dis Sci 1988;33:353.

382. O'Duffy JD. Behçet's syndrome. N Engl J Med 1990;322:326.

383. Shulman HM, Sullivan KM. Graft-versus-host disease: Allo- and autoimmunity after bone marrow transplantation. In: Cruse J, Lewis RE Jr, eds. Concepts in immunopathology: Cellular aspects of autoimmunity, Vol 6. Basel: Karger, 1988:141.

384. Martin PJ. Pharmacologic approaches for prevention and treatment of acute graft-versus-host disease. Clinical Aspects of Autoimmunity 1990;4:8.

385. Cronkhite LW, Canada WJ. Generalized gastrointestinal polyposis: An unusual syndrome of polyposis, pigmentation, alopecia and onychotrophia. N Engl J Med 1955;252:1011.

386. Daniel ES, Ludwig SL, Lewin KJ, et al. The Cronkhite Canada syndrome: An analysis of clinical and pathologic features and therapy in 55 patients. Medicine 1982;61:293.

387. Burke AP, Sobin LH. The pathology of Cronkhite–Canada polyps: A comparison to juvenile polyposis. Am J Surg Pathol 1989;13:940.

388. Harris JC, Dupont HL, Hornick RB. Fecal leukocytes in diarrheal illness. Ann Intern Med 1972;76:697.

389. Fischbach W, Becker W, Mössner J, Koch W, Reiners C. Faecal alpha-1-antitrypsin and excretion of ^{111}indium granulocytes in assessment of disease activity in chronic inflammatory bowel diseases. Gut 1987;28:386.

390. Crossley JR, Elliott RB. Simple method for diagnosing protein-losing enteropathies. Br Med J 1977;1:428.

391. Florent C, L'Hirondel C, Desmazures C, Aymes C, Bernier JJ. Intestinal clearance of α_1-antitrypsin: A sensitive method for the detection of protein-losing enteropathy. Gastroenterology 1981;81:777.

392. Karbach U, Ewe K, Bodenstein H. Alpha$_1$-antitrypsin, a reliable endogenous marker for intestinal protein loss and its application in patients with Crohn's disease. Gut 1983;24:718.

393. Powell DW, Field M. Pharmacological approaches to treatment of secretory diarrhea. In: Field M, Fordtran JS, Schultz SG, eds. Secretory diarrhea. Bethesda, MD: American Physiological Society, 1980:187.

394. Powell DW. Mechanisms of antisecretory agents and prospects for novel drugs. In: Holmgren J, Lindberg A, Möllby R, eds. Development of vaccines and drugs against diarrhea. Lund, Sweden: Studentlitteratur, 1986:257.

395. Dharmsathaphorn K. α_2-Adrenergic agonists: A newer class of antidiarrheal drugs. Gastroenterology 1986;91:769.

396. Krejs GJ, Browne R, Raskin P. Effect of intravenous somatostatin on jejunal absorption of glucose, amino acids, water and electrolytes. Gastroenterology 1980;78:26.

397. Hughes S, Higgs NB, Turnberg LA. Loperamide has antisecretory activity in the human jejunum in vivo. Gut 1984;25:931.

398. Molla AM, Gyr K, Bardhan PK, Molla A. Effect of intravenous somatostatin on stool output in diarrhea due to *Vibrio cholerae*. Gastroenterology 1984;87:845.

399. Rabbani GH, Butler T, Patte D, Abud RL. Clinical trial of clonidine hydrochloride as an antisecretory agent in cholera. Gastroenterology 1989;97:321.

400. Schiller LR, Santa Ana CA, Morawski SG, Fordtran JS. Mechanism of the antidiarrheal effect of loperamide. Gastroenterology 1984;86:1475.

401. Schiller LR, Santa Ana CA, Morawski SG, Fordtran JS. Studies of the antidiarrheal action of clonidine: Effects on motility and intestinal absorption. Gastroenterology 1985;89:982.

402. Ruskoné A, René E, Chayvialle JA, Bonin N, Pignal F, Kremer M, Bonfils S, Rambaud JC. Effect of somatostatin on diarrhea and on small intestinal water and electrolyte transport in a patient with pancreatic cholera. Dig Dis Sci 1982;27:459.

403. Frantzides CT, Condon RE, Schulte WJ, Cowles V. Effects of morphine on colonic myoelectric and motor activity in subhuman primates. Am J Physiol 1990;258(Gastrointest Liver Physiol 21):G247.

404. Sarna SK, Otterson MF. Small intestinal amyogenesis and dysmyogenesis induced by morphine and loperamide. Am J Physiol 1990;258(Gastrointest Liver Physiol 21):G282.

405. Read M, Read NW, Barber DC, Duthie HL. Effects of loperamide on anal sphincter function in patients complaining of chronic diarrhea with fecal incontinence and urgency. Dig Dis Sci 1982;27:807.

406. Davis GR, Camp RC, Raskin P, Krejs GJ. Effect of somatostatin infusion on jejunal water and electrolyte transport in a patient with secretory diarrhea due to malignant carcinoid syndrome. Gastroenterology 1980;78:346.

407. Kvols LK, Moertel CG, O'Connell MJ, Schutt AJ, Rubin J, Hahn RG. Treatment of the malignant carcinoid syndrome: Evaluation of a long-acting somatostatin analogue. N Engl J Med 1986;315:663.

408. Ch'ng JLC, Anderson JV, Williams SJ, Carr DH, Bloom SR. Remission of symptoms during long term treatment of metastatic pancreatic endocrine tumours with long acting somatostatin analogue. Br Med J 1986;292:981.

409. Maton PN, O'Dorisio TM, Howe BA, McArthur KE, Howard JM, Cherner JA, Malarkey TB, Collen MJ, Gardner JD, Jensen RT. Effect of a long-acting somatostatin analogue (SMS 201-995) in a patient with pancreatic cholera. N Engl J Med 1985;312:17.

410. Gorden P, Comi RJ, Maton PN, Go VLW. NIH Conference: Somatostatin and somatostatin analogue (SMS 201-995) in treatment of hormone-secreting tumors of the pituitary and gastrointestinal tract and non-neoplastic diseases of the gut. Ann Intern Med 1989;110:35.

411. Dharmsathaphorn K, Gorelick FS, Sherwin RS, Cataland S, Dobbins JW. Somatostatin decreases diarrhea in patients with the short-bowel syndrome. J Clin Gastroenterol 1982;4:521.

412. Nightingale JMD, Walker ER, Burnham WR, Farthing MJG, Lennard-Jones JE. Octreotide (a somatostatin analogue) improves quality of life in some patients with a short intestine. Aliment Pharmacol Therap 1989;3:367.

413. Lauritsen K, Laursen LS, Bukhave K, Rask-Madsen J. In vivo effects of orally administered prednisolone on prostaglandin and leucotriene production in ulcerative colitis. Gut 1987;28:1095.

414. Sandle GI, Hayslett JP, Binder HJ. Effect of glucocorticoids on rectal transport in normal subjects and patients with ulcerative colitis. Gut 1986;27:309.

415. Sandle GI, McGlone F. Acute effects of dexamethasone on cation transport in colonic epithelium. Gut 1987;28:701.

39

Approach to the Patient with Constipation

ARNOLD WALD

DEFINITIONS

Although constipation is a common gastrointestinal complaint in clinical practice, some uncertainty exists as to the precise definition of the term. In part, this derives from the fact that constipation is a symptom rather than a disease and, as such, represents a subjective interpretation of a real or imaginary somatic disturbance by the patient. Individuals complain of constipation if they think that they defecate too infrequently or with too much effort, if their stools are too hard or too small, if defecation is painful, or if they have a sense of incomplete evacuation. This lack of objectivity has contributed to the controversy concerning the incidence, pathogenesis, and treatment of constipation and defecation disorders. Furthermore, the availability of over-the-counter laxatives and other evacuation aids adds to the complexity of managing patients with bowel complaints. Chronic and often inappropriate use of laxatives may result in laxative dependence, produce damage to the bowel, and lead to problems where none previously existed.

Although no single definition is applicable to all constipated individuals, it is useful to review the most common ones in order to provide guidelines for clinical practice. *Bowel frequency* has received much attention because it lends itself to quantification and is a convenient measurement to use when evaluating patients or surveying large populations. Because a number of population surveys have found that the vast majority of people consuming a western diet defecate at least three times per week,[1–3] constipation has been defined as a frequency of defecation of twice weekly or less. Recent smaller surveys suggest that the lower limit of normal is five times per week, varying according to sex and race[4,5]; however, this has not been widely adopted as the standard. Furthermore, frequency alone may not be a sufficient criterion to use because many constipated patients complain of excessive straining at defecation, with or without hard stools, although frequency of defecation is within the normal range. *Difficulty during defecation* is highly subjective and difficult to quantify. Attempts to do so have been reported with the use of expulsion of water-filled balloons, solid spheres of different volumes,[6,7] and synthetic stool with the use of radiologic or scintigraphic techniques.[8,9] These techniques have methodologic shortcomings and cannot be used for large population surveys because of their invasive nature and/or exposure to radioactivity. Even more problematic are measurements of *stool weight* and *consistency*. Normal stool weight ranges widely among individuals, with considerable day-to-day variability[1,10]; measurement of stool consistency is unpleasant to perform and difficult to quantify.[11] Other definitions of constipation are entirely subjective. For clinical purposes, one should use a combination of subjective and objective criteria as a starting point in assessing such complaints. These include a frequency of defecation less than three times weekly alone or in conjunction with other subjective complaints, especially if there has also been a distinct change in regular bowel habits.[3]

SOCIOECONOMIC AND MEDICAL CONSEQUENCES

The costs of constipation are considerable. In the United States, 368 million dollars were spent for laxatives in 1982[12]; many are used unnecessarily, and some may be harmful. No data exist regarding additional costs generated as a result of medical evaluations, diagnostic studies, surgery, and absences from work relating to constipation.

Management of problems secondary to constipation adds to the economic burden of this condition. For example, chronic constipation may be associated with urinary tract infections,[13,14] and in children it may be associated with enuresis and vesicoureteral reflux as well as fecal soiling.[15] These conditions frequently improve or disappear with treatment of constipation.

Fecal impaction consequent to constipation is the most frequent cause of fecal soiling in the institutionalized elderly. Together with urinary incontinence, it is a contributing factor in the removal of elderly individuals from their homes. Chronic constipation may also lead to perineal descent, pudendal nerve damage, and fecal incontinence in middle-aged and older women.[16,17] In more advanced cases, rectal prolapse may result.

In young women, chronic severe constipation is associated with an increased incidence of unnecessary surgery, particularly appendectomy, hysterectomy, and ovarian cystectomy.[18] The reasons for this are unknown. In older individuals, dilated loops of colon may result in volvulus or ischemic colitis. Stercorous ulcers with bleeding or perforation are a hazard in patients with fecal impaction.[19] Finally, there is some evidence that links constipation with colon and rectal cancer in women.[20]

PATHOPHYSIOLOGIC CONSIDERATIONS

Constipation may be conceptually regarded as disordered movement through the colon and/or anorectum because, with few exceptions, transit through the more proximal regions of the gastrointestinal tract are normal. From a pathophysiologic viewpoint, impairment of large intestinal transit can occur because of a primary motor disorder, in association with a large number of diseases, or as a side effect of many drugs (Tables 39-1 and 39-2). Diseases associated with constipation include metabolic and endocrine disorders and those neurogenic disorders which affect the gastrointestinal tract.

Chronic illnesses often lead to both physical and mental impairments that can produce or exaggerate constipation. This may be further exacerbated by inactivity or physical immobility that can lead to fecal retention. A bedridden patient may be unable to respond to defecatory signals because of inadequate toileting arrangements; as a result, fecal retention may lead to megarectum,

TABLE 39–1
Secondary Causes of Functional Constipation

Metabolic and Endocrine Disorders

Diabetes mellitus
Hypothyroidism
Hypercalcemia, hypokalemia
Pregnancy
Porphyria
Panhypopituitarism
Pheochromocytoma
Glucagonoma

Neurogenic Disorders

Peripheral

Hirschsprung's disease
Chagas' disease
Neurofibromatosis
Ganglioneuromatosis
Autonomic neuropathy
Hypoganglionosis
Intestinal pseudo-obstruction (myopathy, neuropathy)

Central

Multiple sclerosis
Spinal cord lesions
Parkinson's disease
Shy-Drager syndrome
Trauma to nervi erigentes
Cerebrovascular accidents

Collagen vascular and muscle disorders

Systemic sclerosis
Amyloidosis
Dermatomyositis
Myotonic dystrophy

TABLE 39–2
Drugs Associated with Constipation

Analgesics

Anticholinergics

Antispasmodics
Antidepressants
Antipsychotics
Antiparkinsonian drugs

Cation-containing agents

Iron supplements
Aluminum (antacids, sucralfate)
Calcium (antacids, supplements)
Barium sulfate
Metallic intoxication (arsenic, lead, mercury)

Neutrally active agents

Opiates
Antihypertensives
Ganglionic blockers
Vinca alkaloids
Anticonvulsants
Calcium channel blockers

diminished rectal sensation, and fecal impaction. Other factors that may contribute to constipation in the bedridden patient include underlying illness, medications, or dietary inadequacies. Generalized weakness or striated muscle diseases, such as dermatomyositis, may result in significant constipation due to poor expulsion efforts.[31]

Metabolic and Endocrine Disorders

The most common of the endocrine disorders that cause constipation are diabetes mellitus and hypothyroidism. Constipation was reported by 60% of an unselected clinic population of diabetics.[21] While constipation may occasionally be severe, in our experience symptoms tend to be mild and responsive to relatively simple measures. Constipation associated with hypothyroidism is also usually mild and improves with thyroid replacement therapy but can present with life-threatening megacolon in patients with myxedema.[22] Constipation is said to be common during pregnancy,[23] and some women report that they are constipated immediately prior to menstruation.[24] Alterations of progesterone and estrogen may be responsible, because pregnancy is also associated with decreased lower esophageal sphincter pressures,[25] delayed orocecal transit times,[26] and increased gallbladder volume.[27] Similar changes in orocecal and gallbladder function have been documented during the luteal phase of the menstrual cycle.[28] Although delayed colonic transit has also been reported during the luteal phase,[29] a recent study failed to substantiate such changes in a nonconstipated population.[30] Other less common endocrinopathies that cause constipation are listed in Table 39-1.

Neurogenic Disorders

Because colonic and anorectal motor functions are coordinated by both the enteric nerves and the extrinsic innervation of the sympathetic and parasympathetic nerves (ch 10), it is not surprising that diseases of the central and peripheral nervous systems are often associated with constipation (Table 39-1).

DISORDERS OF EXTRINSIC INNERVATION

The distal colon is supplied by parasympathetic innervation derived from the sacral nerves that pass through the pelvis as the nervi erigentes and enter the bowel wall in the lower part of the rectum.[32] Transection of these nerves or lesions in the sacral cauda equina may produce constipation associated with hypomotility, colonic dilatation, decreased rectal tone and sensation, stasis of the distal colon, and impaired defecation.[33,34] Similar findings occur in patients with injury to the lumbosacral spine,[35] in patients with meningomyelocele,[36] and following low spinal anesthesia.[37] Constipation may also occur with high spinal cord damage, but in these patients colonic reflexes are intact and defecation can often be triggered by digital stimulation of the anal canal.[38] Although the motor response of the sigmoid colon after a meal is reduced following high spinal injuries, responses to pharmacologic stimuli are normal.[39] In contrast to low spinal cord lesions, anal sphincter pressures are normal, but rectal sensation may be impaired and rectal compliance is reduced in patients with high spinal injuries.[39,40]

The prevalence of constipation in multiple sclerosis is high and is strongly associated with neurogenic dysfunction of other organ systems.[41] Constipation in these patients may be exacerbated by physical inactivity or use of medications with constipating side effects. Severely disabled and constipated patients with multiple sclerosis demonstrate absent colonic motor responses after eating a meal and high pressure/volume colonmetrograms that probably result from interruption of normal cortical inhibition of colonic motor activity.[42] Others have found prolonged colonic transit and anorectal changes suggestive of rectosphincteric dyssynergia (see below) leading to poor rectal evacuation.[43] Whether these findings apply to most multiple sclerosis patients with bowel dysfunction is unknown.

DISORDERS OF THE ENTERIC NERVOUS SYSTEM

Hirschsprung's Disease. The classic form of this disorder is characterized by obstipation from birth and colonic dilatation proximal to a contracted nonpropulsive segment of distal bowel. Rectal examination reveals an empty rectal vault, but the abdomen is markedly distended by a colon filled with stool. Barium enema discloses the characteristic findings in the distal colon and rectum.

In contrast to normal individuals, the internal anal sphincter does not relax following rectal distention[44] and, indeed, often contracts. The absence of this rectosphincteric inhibitory reflex is universal in Hirschsprung's disease,[45] reflecting the absence of intramural ganglion cells of both the submucosal and myenteric plexuses; this results from a developmental arrest of caudal mi-

gration of neural crest cells from the notochord during embryonic development. Characteristic histochemical findings include increased acetylcholinesterase and catecholamine activity.[46,47] In addition, neurons containing hydroxytryptamine are absent,[48] and there is a depletion of inhibitory neurotransmitters such as substance P and vasoactive intestinal polypeptide.[49,50]

The demonstration by manometry of the rectosphincteric inhibitory reflex excludes Hirschsprung's disease from diagnostic consideration. However, except in the ultrashort-segment variant of the disease, *rectal biopsies to document the absence of neurons must be obtained to confirm the diagnosis.* Tissue specimens may be obtained by suction biopsy techniques or by a full-thickness biopsy of the rectal wall. In addition to absent neurons, increased acetylcholinesterase staining can also be useful to establish the diagnosis.[46] Although most patients with Hirschsprung's disease are diagnosed by 6 months of age, some patients have a clinically milder disease, and the diagnosis may be delayed well into adulthood.[51,52] Some of these patients have a very short aganglionic segment, so that in contrast to the classical form of the disease, stool may be present in the rectum and fecal incontinence may occur. In such patients, the barium enema does not demonstrate a narrow segment; however, the rectosphincteric inhibitory reflex is absent because the internal anal sphincter is invariably denervated.[45] Although one might expect that clinical severity increases with the length of the aganglionic segment, in fact the clinical course correlates poorly with this parameter.

Some investigators have postulated the existence of ultrashort-segment Hirschsprung's disease in which the disease is limited to the anal canal.[20] Because this area normally contains no ganglia, the rectal biopsy will not be useful and barium studies are normal. Thus, diagnosis rests entirely upon the manometric demonstration of an absent rectosphincteric inhibitory reflex. However, care must be taken because the most common reasons for failure to elicit internal sphincter relaxation are technical ones. The recording instrument must be calibrated correctly, settings must be of adequate sensitivity, the probe must be properly positioned, and balloon inflation of the rectum must be of sufficient volume, particularly in patients with megarectum. In addition, the rectum should be emptied prior to manometry because relaxation may not be elicited if the rectum is filled with stool. Finally, there often is no inhibitory reflex in premature or low-birth-weight neonates in whom the reflex may take up to 2 weeks to appear.[53]

Other Peripheral Neurologic Diseases. Constipation has been reported in patients with both decreased[54] and increased[55] numbers of ganglion cells in the colon, although it should be emphasized that quantification of ganglion cells in biopsy specimens is difficult.[20] There have also been reported cases of "zonal colonic aganglionosis" in which discrete areas of the colon are devoid of enteric neurons.[56] The etiology of these disorders may be congenital or acquired secondary to a vascular accident.

Abnormal-appearing enteric neurons in the large intestine have been described as a paraneoplastic phenomenon in patients with generalized intestinal pseudo-obstruction and in patients with severe chronic constipation associated with slow transit (see below). The role of chronic laxative use in producing damage to the enteric neurons is uncertain in such patients.[57,58] Diagnosis requires special staining and labor-intensive quantification of neurogenic elements of colon specimens[59]; it is also potentially susceptible to interpretive bias.

Primary autonomic neuropathy may be associated with bladder dysfunction and constipation,[60] and secondary autonomic dysfunction is believed to underlie constipation in patients with diabetes mellitus.[21] Diabetic patients with constipation may have delayed or absent[61] increases in colonic motor function following a meal.

Idiopathic Constipation

The vast majority of constipated patients have no obvious cause to explain their symptoms but are presumed to have an underlying disorder of colonic or anorectal motor function. The precise categorization of distinct subtypes of idiopathic constipation is somewhat difficult because of variable definitions and methodology. However, it is possible to attempt to categorize patients with idiopathic constipation into several broad groups based upon age of presentation, symptoms and duration of complaint, studies of colonic transit and anorectal sensorimotor function, and, in some instances, psychologic profiles.

Idiopathic Childhood Constipation.

Chronic constipation in childhood is undoubtedly multifactorial in origin and involves both psychologic and physiologic factors.[62] Although severe behavioral problems may be important and should be identified, idiopathic constipation in children is *not* synonymous with psychogenic constipation; indeed, behavioral abnormalities are usually mild in the majority of affected children and may be secondary to bowel dysfunction.[63,64]

Constipation in children is frequently associated with fecal impaction and dilatation of the rectum and sigmoid colon.[65] Many children have slow colonic transit, usually localized to the distal colon and rectum,[66] which suggests either voluntary withholding behavior or abnormal anorectal function. Many constipated children complain that they do not sense an urge to defecate. Although it is commonly believed that rectal sensation is impaired, demonstration of rectal sensory impairment has been inconsistent.[67–69] In one report, impaired perception of sustained distention of a rectal balloon persisted for as long as 3 years in five of eight children who had been successfully treated.[70] If confirmed, such findings could, in part, explain the high frequency of clinical relapse in successfully treated children. However, another study found that rectal sensory impairment had little effect on therapeutic outcome.[59]

Studies of anal sphincter pressures have also been contradictory; resting anal canal tone has been reported to be increased,[67,71,72] decreased,[73] or similar[69] compared to that of nonconstipated children. Relaxation of the internal anal sphincter is usually normal,[69] and its absence suggests short-segment Hirschsprung's disease. Finally, up to 63% of constipated children with fecal soiling fail to relax the puborectalis and external sphincter muscles when asked to defecate,[69,74] a phenomenon that has been termed *rectosphincteric dyssynergia*. This may be a learned behavior acquired at an earlier age when attempts to evacuate a large fecal bolus were associated with discomfort or an anal fissure (see below). It is hypothesized that rectosphincteric dyssynergia may lead to further retention of stool, which continues the vicious cycle of events. However, the contribution of this finding to the pathogenesis and/or maintenance of constipation in children has not been defined.

Severe Constipation in Young to Middle-Aged Adults.

Chronic constipation in this age group is predominantly confined to women. Abdominal pain is uncommon and megacolon is rare. Patients may complain of infrequent defecation, excessive straining when defecating, or both, and often fail to improve with fiber supplements or mild laxatives. Many report symptoms beginning in childhood or adolescence. There are several subtypes within this group of patients who, despite similarities with respect to their clinical pictures, may be distinguished by studies of bowel function and psychologic profiles.

Approximately 30% of patients who consult for complaints of infrequent defecation and who are unresponsive to therapeutic intervention have normal colonic transit.[75] Patients with normal transit constipation may consciously or unconsciously deny that they defecate and often exhibit evidence of increased psychosocial distress.[76] Because these patients do not complain of abdominal pain, they cannot be diagnosed as having irritable bowel syndrome, but the psychologic profiles of these two groups are similar.[76,77] Some patients with normal transit constipation demonstrate abnormalities of anorectal sensory and motor function that are indistinguishable from those in patients with slow transit constipation (see below); the relationship of these findings to the patients' complaints is unclear.

The remaining 70% of patients with severe constipation characterized mainly by infrequent defecation exhibit slow colonic transit. The majority have "colonic inertia," which may be defined simply as the delayed passage of radiopaque markers through the proximal colon (Fig 39-1). Unlike patients with normal colonic transit, those with slow transit have significantly lower psychologic distress scores, which are similar to those of nonconstipated patients with other gastrointestinal disorders.[77]

Controversy exists concerning the validity of the concept of colonic inertia. Some investigators[38] have argued that colonic transit can vary considerably in the same subject on different days and is affected by diet and the menstrual cycle (potentially important in young women). Furthermore, criteria for colonic inertia are imprecise, because colonic stasis could occur as a result of decreased propulsion (hypomotility) or increased distal motility and retropulsion (hypermotility) of markers. Our experience suggests that the menstrual cycle affects colonic transit of markers minimally, if at all,[30] and that significantly slow colonic transit is sufficiently reproducible for clinical purposes. However, one should reserve the term *colonic inertia* for cases in which transit in the proximal colon is delayed without evidence of retropulsion of markers from the left colon; the use of differently shaped markers and shorter sampling intervals may be helpful. Perhaps colonic scintigraphy to measure transit in these patients may help to clarify terminology and pathophysiology.[78]

It is not entirely clear which pathophysiologic mechanisms are important in patients with colonic inertia. At rest, colonic motility appears to be similar to that of normal controls,[79–81] but several studies have demonstrated no increase of motor activity after meals[82] or following the administration of bisacodyl.[79,80] Such findings suggest that abnormalities of the enteric nerve plexus may exist, and, indeed, a number of histologic abnormalities have been demonstrated in resected colon specimens from such patients.[83] These include decreased numbers of neurons and axons as well as nuclear abnormalities in the ganglia. The frequent use of laxatives by constipated patients potentially confounds the interpretation of the origin of such changes.

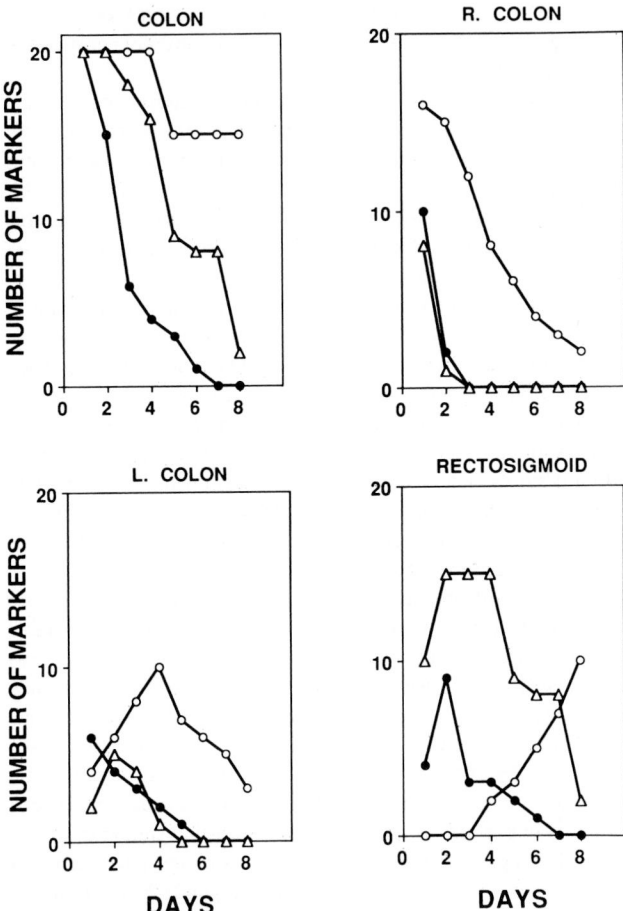

FIGURE 39–1. Characteristic transit patterns of 20 radiopaque markers through the colon during an 8-day period in three groups of constipated patients. With normal transit, (– ● –), there is rapid disappearance of markers from the colon. In colonic inertia (– ○ –), there is prolonged transit through the right and left colon segments with delayed appearance in the rectosigmoid colon. In outlet obstruction (– △ –), transit is normal in the right and left colons, but stagnation occurs in the rectosigmoid colon. (Redrawn from Wald A. Colonic transit and anorectal manometry in chronic idiopathic constipation. Arch Intern Med 1986;146:1713.)

Patients with severe colonic inertia frequently have symptoms and abnormalities in other areas. These include esophageal dysmotility,[81] delayed transit through the small intestine,[85] and a high incidence of bladder dysfunction and urinary symptoms.[14,84] While such disturbances suggest possible neurogenic dysfunction, the precise mechanisms of colonic disturbances remain to be defined.

The term *outlet obstruction*[86] has been used to designate a form of idiopathic slow transit constipation in which markers progress normally through the proximal colon but stagnate in the rectum (Fig 39-1). This pattern is not specific and may be seen in children with Hirschsprung's disease or idiopathic constipation, in the nonambulatory or infirm elderly with fecal impaction,[87] in patients with megarectum,[88] and in young and middle-aged adults with idiopathic slow transit constipation who demonstrate abnormal responses of the pelvic floor muscles during defecation.[89] This recently described entity provides another plausible mechanism by which constipation may be produced or exacerbated.

Normally, defecation involves the coordinated relaxation of the puborectalis and external anal sphincter muscles together with increased intra-abdominal pressure and inhibition of colonic segmenting activity, which propels stool toward the rectum. In patients with rectosphincteric dyssynergia (anismus), ineffective defecation appears to be associated with failure to relax, or inappropriate contraction of, the puborectalis and external anal sphincter muscles.[69,74,89,90] This narrows the anorectal angle and increases the pressures of the anal canal so that evacuation is less effective. Such patients also have difficulty in expelling spheres, water-filled balloons, or artificial stool from the rectum, in comparison to most nonconstipated subjects.[74,89,91] Because relaxation of these muscles involves cortical inhibition of the spinal reflex during defecation, this pattern may represent a conscious or unconscious act. It can be modified, as has been demonstrated by studies in which biofeedback has normalized defecation patterns in both children and adults with this abnormality.[92-94]

The pathogenesis of rectosphincteric dyssynergia is not completely understood but is probably multifactorial. Because it can often be modified with operant conditioning training, it is probably an acquired learned dysfunction rather than an organic or neurogenic disease. Recent studies indicate that rectosphincteric dysfunction occurs in constipated patients with normal as well as slow transit and can occur in patients with colonic inertia as well as in those with outlet obstruction.[38]

The presence of rectosphincteric dyssynergia can be established in various ways, ranging from simple to sophisticated. During the rectal exam, the contraction of the puborectalis and external anal sphincter muscles can be felt when the patient is asked to strain. During anorectal manometry, when the patient is asked to expel the manometer, the characteristic normal pattern is one in which intrarectal pressure increases and external sphincter pressure decreases; in anismus, external pressure increases during attempted expulsion of the manometer. This can also be demonstrated with electromyographic recordings of either or both muscles; normally, electromyographic activity is inhibited during defecation, but it increases sharply with rectosphincteric dyssynergia. Finally, one can use defecography to radiographically evaluate the expulsion of thickened barium from the rectum.[8,95-97] In rectosphincteric dyssynergia, the anorectal angle either does not widen or actually narrows during attempts to expel the barium so that little or no expulsion occurs.[20,98] In our experience, there is agreement on the diagnosis of rectosphincteric dyssynergia between manometry and defecography in approximately 67% of cases.[99]

Irritable Bowel Syndrome. Constipation in patients with irritable bowel syndrome is most commonly seen in young to middle-aged adults and is more common in women than men. It is distinguished clinically by the presence of abdominal pain, especially in the lower abdomen, and by the passage of small, hard stools, often with a sense of incomplete evacuation and excessive straining. Not uncommonly, patients also complain of abdominal bloating, flatulence, and upper gastrointestinal as well as nongastrointestinal symptoms.[100] These include heartburn, dysphagia, nausea, genitourinary complaints, back pain, and, in women, dyspareunia. Patients with irritable bowel syndrome frequently demonstrate evidence of increased psychosocial distress.[76]

Colonic transit times in these patients are often normal or only modestly slowed.[101] A number of suggestive findings on colonic radiographs and patterns of colonic dysmotility have been described. These changes are more fully described in Chapters 80 and 81.

Constipation in the Elderly. Most elderly individuals with chronic constipation had this complaint when they were younger. Others develop constipation due to colonic or systemic disorders or as a side effect of medications (Table 39-2). There are few data to suggest that aging significantly affects colonic motor function or that healthy elderly subjects have a higher incidence of constipation than do younger individuals.[1,102] However, fecal impaction is a significant problem in elderly individuals who are institutionalized.[103] Mental confusion, immobility, or inadequate toilet arrangements may cause such persons to ignore or not act upon the urge to defecate so that the fecal bolus becomes too large or uncomfortable to pass. The development of megarectum often leads to blunting of rectal and anal sensation, which persists even after disimpaction.[87] This predisposes such patients to reaccumulation of feces unless scrupulous toileting programs or periodic evacuation is instituted. Fecal impaction is the most common cause of spurious diarrhea and of fecal incontinence in the institutionalized elderly.[104]

Megarectum and Megacolon. While only a small percentage of patients with constipation have megacolon or megarectum, most patients with a dilated colon or rectum have constipation or defecatory difficulties. In addition, megarectum and megacolon may occur together, or each may be present in the absence of the other.[38,105] Although radiographic criteria exist to diagnose these entities,[106] radiologic assessment does not always correlate with manometric evaluation of rectal elasticity.[65]

Idiopathic megacolon may be divided into *primary (congenital) megacolon* and *secondary (acquired) disease*. Primary megacolon is thought to be associated with neurogenic dysfunction, although histologic changes may not be evident without specialized neurohistologic staining.[59] In contrast, secondary megacolon and megarectum often develop later in life and may occur in response to chronic fecal retention. These patients have increased rectal compliance and elasticity, blunted rectal sensation, an increased threshold and decreased depth of internal anal sphincter relaxation.[88] To avoid misdiagnosing Hirschsprung's disease by anorectal manometry, effective rectal cleansing and larger volumes of rectal distention are often necessary to induce internal anal sphincter relaxation in these patients.

Megarectum is generally associated with fecal impaction and soiling, which often occurs in children and in the physically and mentally impaired elderly.[107] In addition, megarectum can occur in Hirschsprung's disease, meningomyelocele, and other lesions of the lumbosacral cord, and in patients with poor toileting routines. Presumably, the sensory and motor abnormalities associated with megarectum are reversible with appropriate therapy in many patients, but this has not been established in the elderly, and abnormalities may persist long after successful treatment in children.[70]

diagnostic studies and treatment. This information should be obtained with knowledge of the many potential causes of constipation previously detailed.

A critical question concerns the onset and duration of the complaint. Constipation that is present from birth or the neonatal period is most certainly congenital in origin, whereas onset in later life suggests an acquired disorder. A recent change in bowel habit demands a workup for organic disorders, especially in adults, whereas complaints of several years' duration or longer are more likely due to functional disorders.

Next, establishing the nature of the symptoms is important in suggesting various categories of bowel dysfunction and addressing the specific concerns of the patient. Inquiry concerning frequency of defecation and defecatory difficulties such as excessive straining, discomfort, or sense of incomplete evacuation of the rectum may help to identify specific areas of concern. A complaint of small or hard stools is subjective; it may be helpful to ask the patient to draw a typical stool and an "ideal" one in order to determine if misperceptions or unrealistic expectations exist. The presence of pain or bleeding with defecation should be noted.

A history of abdominal pain or bloating in association with constipation leads to consideration of the diagnosis of irritable bowel syndrome. Upper gastrointestinal symptoms such as dysphagia, heartburn, early satiety, or vomiting also suggest irritable bowel syndrome or a more diffuse disorder of gastrointestinal function. Genitourinary symptoms, while not specific for constipation of any etiology, may also suggest a central or peripheral neurogenic disorder. Inquiry concerning laxative use and its duration is important, as are questions concerning similar gastrointestinal complaints in other family members and parental views on laxatives and bowel habits. Finally, a gentle but careful assessment for evidence of affective disorders, dysphoria, emotional distresses (such as litigation or psychologic counseling), and the use of mood-altering drugs will help to establish potential contributing factors to subjective complaints in the patient. Questionnaires such as the Hopkins Symptom Checklist[108] can be helpful in this regard; it takes less than 15 minutes to complete, is acceptable to most patients, and reveals a high incidence of psychologic distress in a number of subgroups of idiopathic constipation.[77] It correlates quite well with the Minnesota Multiphasic Personality Inventory (MMPI), which is far too time-consuming to administer and score for routine use in clinical practice. These instruments should be used as an adjunct to careful history taking and not substitute for it. In children, inquiry should be made concerning nightmares, enuresis, school performance, and intrafamilial tensions. In addition, a history of bowel disturbances in the family should be elicited because there is an increased incidence of constipation and defecatory difficulties in one or both parents of children with encopresis.[109]

EVALUATION OF CONSTIPATION

History

Evaluating complaints of constipation involves a careful delineation of its duration and characteristics and a review of any previous

Physical Examination

Physical examination includes a search for evidence of nongastrointestinal diseases that may cause or exacerbate constipation. Particular attention should be given to a careful neurologic examination, including an assessment of autonomic function, and abdominal palpation for evidence of bowel distention, retained stool, or prior surgical procedures.

Anorectal and perineal examinations should search for perineal disease or deformity, abnormal location of the anal orifice, atrophy of the gluteal muscles, and rectal prolapse. Digital exam will elicit the pain of an anal fissure, detect a fixed stenosis of the anal canal, assess tone and strength of the anal canal at rest and with squeeze, or detect the presence of a rectal mass or fecal impaction. When the patient strains, one should evaluate for the presence of rectosphincteric dyssynergia, or a rectocele bulging anteriorly into the vagina, and one should also look for perineal descent or rectal prolapse. Gaping of the anal canal when the examiner pulls the puborectalis muscle posteriorly or immediately upon withdrawing the finger from the anal canal suggests denervation of the external anal sphincter. Perineal sensation should be assessed, and reflex contraction of the anal canal following pinprick of the perianal area ("anal wink") also can be used to test neurologic function of the perineal areas.

Studies of Colorectal Structure

These studies are important in order to exclude organic disease. However, they provide little, if any, useful information about colonic and anorectal function and are generally overused in patients with long-standing symptoms.

Flexible sigmoidoscopy is a technique to assess bowel mucosa and intraluminal characteristics. It will identify lesions that narrow or occlude the bowel and will detect melanosis coli, a brown-black discoloration of the bowel mucosa that is produced by lipofuscin deposits in the lamina propria with chronic use of anthraquinone laxatives.[110] Flexible sigmoidoscopy can also be used to estimate bowel diameter and will detect the featureless characteristics of the distal bowel in many patients with laxative abuse ("cathartic colon").

When patients complain of constipation of short duration or a recent change in bowel habit, *barium radiographs* are an important complement to sigmoidoscopy in detecting organic causes and are also useful to diagnose megacolon and megarectum. Contrary to studies that have found a poor relationship between rectal size on radiography and rectal elastic properties,[65] we and others have found reasonably good correlation between these two parameters.[88,99] However, barium enema provides limited information about colonic transit and motor function in most patients with chronic constipation.[111] On balance, studies of anorectal manometry and compliance provide more useful measurements of anorectal function than do barium studies in patients with functional constipation.

Barium radiographs will show the characteristic denervated bowel segment with proximal dilatation of the colon in classical Hirschsprung's disease and should be obtained if this disorder is suspected. In such circumstances, bowel cleansing should *not* be ordered so that the characteristic changes will be accentuated. It is also important to remember that complete filling of the colon is not necessary for diagnosis of this disorder. Plain films of the abdomen can be useful in the evaluation and treatment of chronic constipation. They can detect significant stool retention in the pelvic colon or throughout the entire colon, can suggest the diagnosis of megacolon, and can be used to monitor the adequacy of bowel cleansing of patients with fecal retention if there is uncertainty on physical examination.

Rectal biopsies are useful only in patients with suspected Hirschsprung's disease. Suction biopsies should be obtained at least 3 cm above the distal portion of the internal anal sphincter in order to exclude the disease. For other patients with constipation, rectal and colonic biopsies with the use of endoscopic forceps are too superficial to be of clinical utility.

Studies of Colonic and Anorectal Function

These tests are generally reserved for patients with severe idiopathic constipation who fail to respond to relatively simple therapeutic measures (see below). They are also useful in defining the patterns of bowel function in various subgroups of patients with constipation in order to identify potentially useful therapeutic strategies.

Colonic Transit Studies. This test is most useful when evaluating a patient with severe constipation whose major complaint is that of infrequent defecation. Although the methods vary somewhat, the principle of the test is the same. The subject ingests a high-fiber diet (20–30 g/day) while abstaining from the use of laxatives, enemas, and medications that may affect bowel function. Radiopaque markers are ingested, and their transit through the colon is monitored by abdominal radiographs until at least 80% have passed or a defined period of time has elapsed (usually 6–8 days). Transit is then correlated with bowel habit before and during the test.

The original technique described by Arhan and colleagues[112] involves the ingestion of 20 radiopaque markers cut from a No. 16 Fr radiopaque Levin tube. Abdominal radiographs are obtained at 24-hour intervals; markers are counted in the right, left, and rectosigmoid colons, as defined by certain anatomic landmarks, and can be followed as they move distally until expelled. The markers in each segment each day are totaled and multiplied by a factor of 1.2 to obtain segmental and total transit times.

Recently, the technique has been modified in order to reduce exposure to radioactivity and the number of patient visits to the radiology suite. Daily doses of markers are given for 2[30] or 3[113,114] days, each dose of marker being a different shape. Thus, radiographs may be obtained at 2- or 3-day intervals, respectively. Using fast-film techniques with up to 110 keV, radiation exposure can be significantly reduced while sufficient detail is obtained to identify the markers and the anatomic landmarks.

Notwithstanding differences in patients with respect to national origin, diet, and other factors that might affect colonic transit, studies of normal subjects on diets containing 20 to 30 g of fiber/day indicate a range of normal (Table 39-3). The original studies seem to have overestimated the normal range; the upper limit of normal for most adults is approximately 70 hours.[30,113,114] Although transit times differ between men and women, these differences appear to be inconsequential for clinical purposes. In addition, there are no important differences between the two phases of the menstrual cycle,[30] an important consideration because women are most commonly evaluated for severe constipation.

Keeping in mind the possible limitations of the test,[38] we have found it to be a most helpful instrument when evaluating patients with severe intractable constipation and one that has prognostic and therapeutic implications as well. Patients with normal colonic

TABLE 39–3
Segmental and Total Colonic Transit Times* in Normal Subjects

STUDY (REF.)	NUMBER	RIGHT COLON	LEFT COLON	RECTOSIGMOID	TOTAL COLONIC	DAILY FIBER INTAKE
Chaussade (113)	22	24	30	44	67	20 g
Hinds (30)	36	20	27	37	70	20–25 g
Metcalf (114)	73	30	35	31	71	15–25 g
Arhan (112)	38	38	37	34	93	0.2 g/kg
Verduron (88)	11	18	13	20	34	30 g

* Hr; mean + 2 S.D.

transit who complain predominantly of infrequent defecation may consciously or unconsciously misrepresent or misperceive bowel habit and, as a group, exhibit higher levels of psychologic distress than do patients with slow-transit constipation.[77] In contrast, patients with painless constipation and slow colonic transit have less psychologic dysfunction.[77] Patients with the pattern of colonic inertia often do not respond to therapeutic intervention.[75] At the risk of being too simplistic, it may be hypothesized that patients with slow transit have a physiologic basis to their symptoms, in contrast to those with normal transit who may have a significant psychologic or behavioral component to their complaints.

An interesting method that measures colonic transit by scintigraphy has been recently introduced.[78] This technique involves placement of a radioisotope into the cecum through a nasointestinal tube followed by nuclear imaging at various intervals. Although it appears promising as an investigational tool, it provides no more clinical information than does the conventional marker study. In addition, the invasiveness of the procedure and the need for nuclear medicine facilities are likely to limit its clinical utility.

Finally, one can assess bowel transit by collecting stools after the administration of radiopaque markers (x-ray the stools) or liquid markers that are nonabsorbable (inspection of the stools). These are somewhat unpleasant for both patients and technicians and can quantitate only total gastrointestinal transit rather than provide an assessment of segmental colonic transit. Consequently, they are less useful and not widely performed.

Anorectal Manometry. Anorectal motility studies may provide useful information in many patients with severe constipation. The most useful parameters are rectal sensation, viscoelasticity, relaxation of the internal anal sphincter, and defecatory patterns produced upon attempted expulsion of the apparatus.

Satisfactory measurements of anal sphincter responses can be obtained with open-tipped perfused catheters, direct on-line pressure transducers, or air-filled balloons of various sizes and configurations. If rectal sensation is impaired, as it is in many patients with severe constipation, it is helpful to know whether it is associated with increased rectal compliance or megarectum. Compliance can be measured by sequentially inflating a balloon placed in the rectum and measuring pressures at each level of distention. Pressures should be corrected by subtracting those obtained by inflation outside the patient. One should note the volume at which the first urge to expel the balloon occurs and also the symptoms elicited with increasing inflation of the balloon. Patients with constipation associated with irritable bowel syndrome often have low compliance and tolerate distention poorly, in striking contrast to

patients with megarectum.[88] The absence of internal anal sphincter relaxation strongly suggests Hirschsprung's disease; in the presence of megarectum, it is important to use larger volumes of rectal distention and to evacuate the rectum to avoid an inappropriate diagnosis of aganglionosis.

We have found that the triple balloon manometer is a satisfactory instrument to assess anorectal patterns during attempted expulsion. Pressures recorded by the rectal balloon give some indication of intra-abdominal pressures generated during expulsion, while pressure recordings of the external balloon indicate relaxation or inappropriate contraction of the external anal sphincter and/or gluteal muscles.[69] Manometry can be supplemented by electromyogram (EMG) studies with the use of concentric needle recordings of the external anal sphincter or by electrodes on the surface of an anal plug. Electromyogram recordings of the anal sphincters with the use of surface electrodes are difficult to perform and interpret; recordings with surface electrodes may reflect activity of the gluteal muscles as well.

Studies of Defecation. Defecation can be evaluated by both radiographic and nonradiographic techniques and may be especially useful in patients who complain of excessive straining during defecation or who employ digital manipulation to facilitate evacuation. These tests vary in their complexity and the information provided, and each has potential limitations.

Defecography is a technique in which barium thickened to a consistency that approximates stool is introduced into the rectum. Evacuation of the barium is monitored by fluoroscopy and videotape while the patient sits on a specially constructed commode. Assessment of the anorectal structures, including the anorectal angle, are obtained at rest and during defecation; also, anatomic abnormalities such as rectoceles and intussusceptions that are not observed at rest may be apparent during defecation. However, emptying is semiquantitative, subjective, and liable to bias. It is probable that many patients feel embarrassed by the nature and setting of the procedure; such inhibitions can potentially result in an abnormal study. Recent studies indicate that anatomic abnormalities such as rectocele and intussusception are not uncommon in normal volunteers without constipation.[96,115] Therefore, caution should be taken when interpreting defecography, and more experience with this technique is needed, in both normal subjects and constipated patients, before definitive decisions can be made on the basis of radiographic findings.

Similar anatomic information can be obtained with balloon topography[116] or simple proctography with ordinary barium and a chain to outline the anal canal.[117] These tests provide no information about the completeness of defecation. Scintigraphic techniques using radioisotope-labeled artificial stool can provide quantitative information concerning rectal emptying but provide little or no anatomic information.[9] Expulsion of water-filled balloons or solid spheres of different sizes and volumes[118] provides some information about expulsion but no information about anatomic changes or relationships in the anorectum.

DIAGNOSTIC STRATEGIES

Most chronically constipated patients do not require extensive diagnostic studies beyond a careful history and physical examination and the appropriate exclusion of systemic or gastrointestinal causes for their complaints. Functional evaluation of the colon and anorectum should generally be reserved for those who fail to respond to initial simple therapy and express continued dissatisfaction with their bowel habit. Complaints exceeding 6 months' duration may be a reasonable definition of chronicity. Most patients with constipation-predominant irritable bowel syndrome do not require extensive diagnostic testing and rarely complain of persistent constipation beyond 3 to 6 months' duration.

The functional evaluation of chronic severe constipation begins with carefully defining the complaint and choosing studies that are most likely to yield diagnostic information concerning that complaint (Fig 39-2). For example, it does not seem important to measure colonic transit if a patient defecates several times per day but does so only with excessive straining and/or digital manipulation. Likewise, performing anorectal manometry adds little

to the evaluation of a patient who claims to have a bowel movement once every 8 days but has normal colonic transit. However, it may provide useful information if colonic transit is prolonged.

For the patient with infrequent defecation who fails to respond to initial therapy, measurement of colonic transit time is the single most useful diagnostic study to obtain. In my experience, a normal study eliminates the need for further diagnostic tests of gastrointestinal function and may serve to reassure both physician and patient that colorectal function is not seriously impaired. In contrast, significant slowing of colonic transit serves to corroborate the complaint on physiologic grounds and suggests the need for additional studies to further characterize various aspects of gastrointestinal motor function (Fig 39-2).

Patients with *colonic inertia* generally have persistent complaints and respond poorly to medical therapy.[75] Anorectal manometry should be performed to characterize sensorimotor function of the bowel such as rectal sensation and viscoelasticity. Appropriate studies of upper gastrointestinal motor function should be obtained to look for evidence of gastrointestinal pseudo-obstruction (ch 67), because such information may have both prognostic and therapeutic implications (see below). In contrast, the pattern of *outlet dysfunction* suggests a more localized problem of the anorectum that can be further characterized by anorectal manometry, defecography, and a search for anatomic or functional abnormalities. The finding of normal anorectal function in a patient with outlet obstruction may suggest possible withholding behavior and is common in children.

For the patient who complains of *excessive defecatory straining* in the absence of an organic cause, studies of colonic transit appear to have little or no utility. However, studies of anorectal function

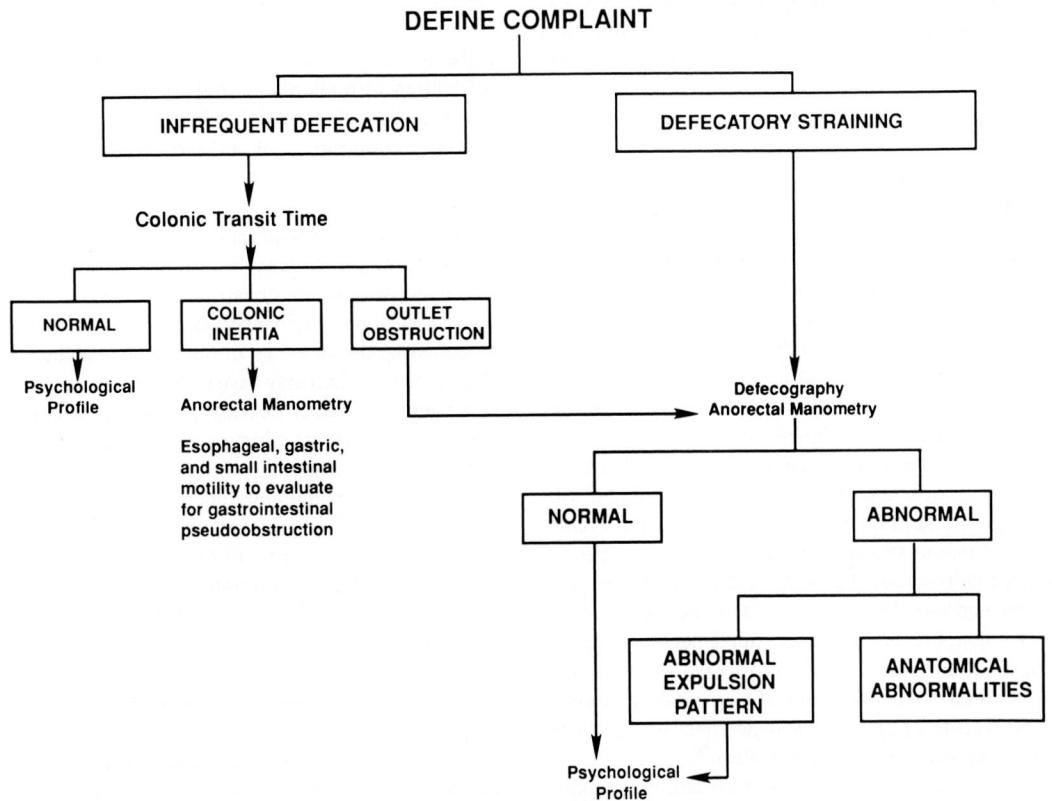

FIGURE 39–2. Suggested algorithm for the evaluation of a patient with severe constipation who has not responded to simple dietary measures.

may be helpful. Normal anorectal motility and defecography may help to reassure patients that there is nothing seriously wrong from a functional standpoint; many of these patients exhibit high levels of psychologic distress similar to patients with normal transit constipation.[119] The importance of anatomic abnormalities and rectosphincteric dyssynergia as seen by defecography in such patients remains to be established.

TREATMENT CONSIDERATIONS

Much has been written about the treatment of constipation. There is general agreement that selecting therapeutic strategies requires understanding of the "whole patient," that fiber supplements should be added to the diet, that establishing proper toileting arrangements can be helpful to certain patients, and that chronic use of "harsh laxatives" should be avoided if possible. Moreover, treatment should be individualized, taking into consideration the age of the patient, duration and severity of constipation, potential contributing factors, and the patient's concerns and expectations. While all of this is reasonable, it should be stated that there is often little objective evidence to support such approaches, in part because of the paucity of controlled trials and the heterogeneity of the population who consult for constipation. In addition, short-term results do not always reflect long-term outcome, and there is probably a significant placebo component to most of the therapeutic approaches currently in vogue. Broadly speaking, *nonsurgical treatment* can be separated into several categories: (1) *dietary approaches* such as fiber supplementation, (2) *behavioral approaches* such as habit training, contingency management, and biofeedback, and (3) *pharmacologic approaches*. In selected patients with severe constipation, surgery has a definite role when abnormal bowel function can be ameliorated by operative intervention.

Dietary Approaches

Dietary adjustments are the first line of intervention for most adults with constipation. Inadequate intake of dietary fiber is widely believed to contribute to constipation in industrialized nations, because high fiber consumption in other parts of the world is generally associated with the daily passage of several bowel movements of considerable volume.[120] Indeed, increases in dietary fiber by nonconstipated persons increase stool weight and frequency of defecation and decrease gastrointestinal transit times.[121] With few exceptions, dietary approaches are not often used in children with constipation because other factors are believed to be important.

Although constipation appears to result from dietary fiber inadequacy in some individuals, there is no evidence that most constipated patients consume less fiber than do nonconstipated individuals.[38] This is not to say that fiber supplementation should not be attempted. Many constipated individuals do respond to increases in fiber intake to between 20 and 30 g per day, although whether this represents a purely physiologic effect or is, at least in part, a placebo response is not entirely clear.[20]

Fiber components are not equivalent in their ability to modify stool characteristics and bowel habit. For example, wheat bran is most effective in increasing stool weight, followed by fruits and vegetables, oats, mucilages, corn, cellulose, soya, and pectin.[121,122] In animal studies, wheat bran accelerated colonic transit, whereas cellulose produced no change compared with fiber-free controls; pectin, sugar, and oat brans had more variable effects on different regions of the colon.[123] The "bulking" effect of fiber is also not so much related to water retention capabilities or to mechanical factors as to colonic microbial ecology and interaction with intraluminal contents (Fig 39-3). Thus, fiber may serve as a substrate for colonic bacteria that increases stool bulk by proliferation of bacteria and production of gases that are trapped in the stool.[121,122,124] Microbial breakdown products such as short-chain fatty acids may also stimulate colonic motility.[122] The net effect is increased stool bulk and shortened colonic transit in many individuals.

It is not unreasonable to recommend a high-fiber diet in all ambulatory adult patients who have constipation without megacolon (Table 39-4). It will be of greatest help in those with low fiber intake and for patients with constipation-predominant irritable bowel syndrome in whom fiber intake should be increased gradually to avoid undue cramping and bloating. If there is a fecal impaction, this should be removed before initiating fiber supplementation. Patients with obstructive lesions anywhere in the gastrointestinal tract should not be given fiber supplements. Fiber is not indicated in patients with megacolon or megarectum, especially if such patients are confined to bed, are demented, or have neurogenic constipation. Such patients are better managed by reducing colonic contents and periodic timed evacuation.

Behavioral Approaches

Habit training and contingency management are often employed in children with idiopathic constipation with or without soiling.[62] The goal of such approaches is to achieve regular evacuation to prevent buildup of stool and fecal soiling. They may also play a role in patients with neurogenic constipation with or without soiling.

An important principle is that before embarking on a behavioral approach, the patient must be disimpacted and the colon evacuated effectively with saline or tap water enemas. This can be accomplished with twice-daily enemas for 3 days and can be monitored by palpating the abdomen or obtaining an abdominal radiograph. Occasionally, a child may have to be hospitalized if cleansing cannot be achieved at home. Recently, colonic evacuation has been accomplished by having constipated children drink a balanced electrolyte solution containing polyethylene glycol 3350 (GoLYTELY; COLYTE) in amounts totaling 5 to 19 L.[125]

After bowel cleansing, light mineral oil in doses of 5 to 15 ml/kg/day or lactulose 15 to 30 ml/day is given to produce at least one stool per day. In addition, the child is instructed to use the bathroom after breakfast or dinner to take advantage of meal-stimulated increases in colonic motility. If no bowel movement is produced after breakfast, attempts are made after dinner as well. A contingency plan is that failure to defecate after 2 days results in a cleansing enema to prevent recurrence of fecal impaction. Once postprandial defecation occurs regularly for 2 to 3 months, weaning from the mineral oil or lactulose is attempted gradually. Positive reinforcement is given for successful toileting and pun-

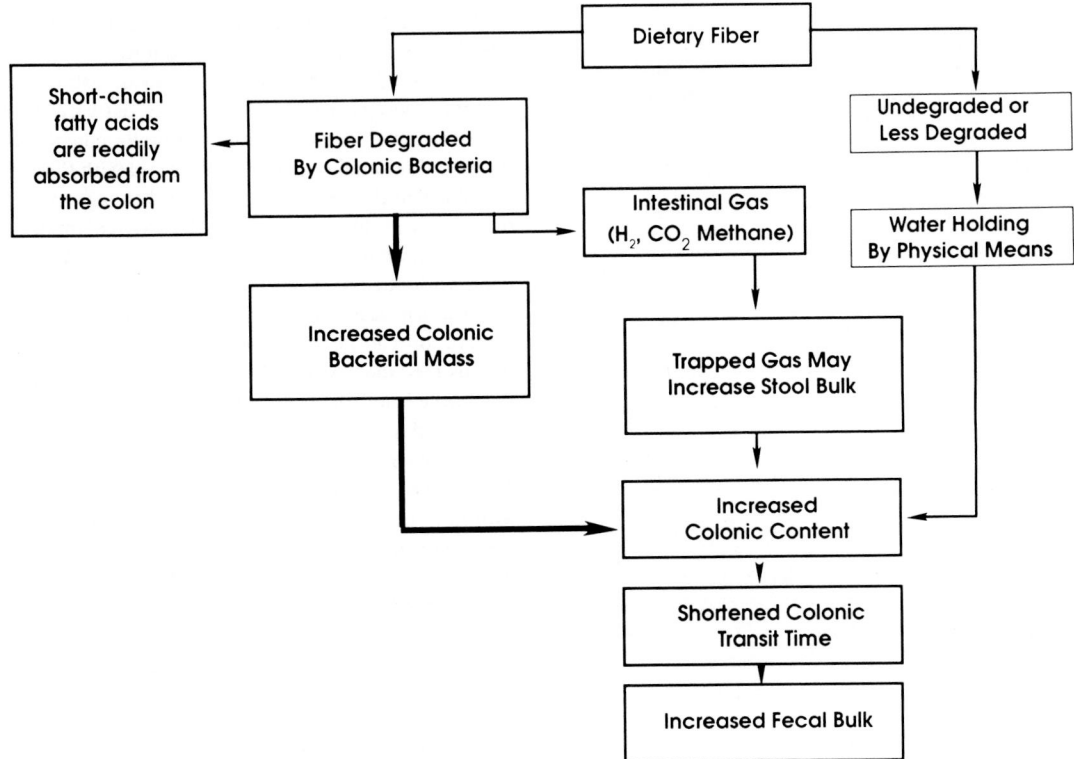

FIGURE 39–3. Mechanisms by which dietary fiber increases fecal bulk. (From Yang P, Banwell JG. Dietary fiber: Its role in the pathogenesis and treatment of constipation. Pract Gastroenterol 1986;10:28.)

ishment for failure is prohibited. Contact with the child and at least one parent should be maintained regularly.

These types of behavioral approaches to idiopathic constipation in children have achieved success rates of up to 78%,[64,126,127] although relapses are not uncommon.[64,128] The relative importance of each aspect of such strategies is unknown because no component analysis has been reported.[62] Treatment failures have been traditionally attributed to patient and family behavioral disturbances and noncompliance, but underlying disturbances of bowel function have also been hypothesized to play a role in some children.[67–74] In a small study, children with rectosphincteric dyssynergia did not respond to mineral oil and bowel retraining as well as did children with normal rectal expulsion patterns.[94]

Another behavioral approach is the use of *biofeedback* to correct inappropriate contraction of the pelvic floor muscles and external anal sphincter during defecation. Studies have employed EMG recordings with the use of anal plugs[93] or anorectal manometers to monitor external anal sphincter pressures during attempted expulsion of the apparatus.[92,94] The patient watches the recordings of EMG or pressure responses and is told to modify inappropriate responses through trial and error efforts. In a recent study, six of nine children with constipation and soiling associated with rectosphincteric dyssynergia were markedly improved 12 months after receiving biofeedback compared with only three of nine children receiving conventional therapy.[94] Biofeedback seemed to be somewhat specific because only 40% of children with normal defecation patterns were improved 12 months after biofeedback, but clearly factors other than normalizing expulsion patterns played a role in treating these children. Similar improvement has been reported in constipated adults receiving biofeedback for rectosphincteric

dyssynergia, but these studies are small and uncontrolled.[92,93] Biofeedback warrants further evaluation in such patients and may prove helpful to some. It will also be important to assess behavioral parameters in future studies because some reports suggest that biofeedback has a higher failure rate in patients with psychosocial distress.[129]

Despite the widespread belief that childhood encopresis is secondary to behavioral disturbances, the importance of behavioral factors is uncertain. Most of the controversy centers around differences in the reported frequency and severity of behavioral disorders in encopretic children and whether they precede soiling or occur as a result of the underlying bowel dysfunction. Inconsistencies among various studies may be due to differences in study populations; children with encopresis who were evaluated in psychiatric settings exhibited significant psychologic dysfunction, whereas those referred to medical settings were less likely to do so. Several studies have reported only mild behavioral dysfunction and unremarkable toilet experiences in encopretic children treated in medical settings.[63,126,130] In contrast, others have reported more anxiety, less tolerance for demands, more submission in the face of peer aggression, less control of aggressive impulses, and more academic difficulties among encopretic children than among matched controls. Landman and colleagues,[131] using a measure of locus of control (the extent to which one perceives that an event is contingent upon one's own behavior), found that children with encopresis tended to feel less in control of positive life events and had lower self-esteem than children with other chronic illnesses such as recurrent abdominal pain, enuresis, or headache. Although others have made similar observations, they concluded that such personality characteristics developed because of negative experi-

TABLE 39–4
Food Sources of Dietary Fiber

	AMOUNT OF SERVING (g)	AMOUNT/100 g OF FOOD
Breakfast Cereals		
All-Bran	9.9	26.70
Cornflakes	2.8	11.00
Rice Krispies	1.4	4.51
Shredded Wheat	3.0	12.31
Special K	1.7	5.41
Breads		
White bread	0.8	2.71
Whole wheat	2.4	8.51
Fruits		
Apple	3.2	1.41
Banana	5.9	1.71
Peach	2.1	2.38
Pear	3.1	2.41
Strawberry	3.3	2.12
Nuts		
Brazil	5.4	7.71
Peanut	5.7	9.31
Peanut butter	2.1	7.51
Vegetables		
Broccoli	5.6	4.11
Cabbage	1.9	2.81
Cauliflower	2.5	1.81
Lettuce	0.8	1.51
Carrot	3.7	3.20
Baked beans	18.6	7.31
Peas	11.3	6.31
Tomato	3.0	1.41

(Yang P, Banwell JG. Dietary fiber: Its role in the pathogenesis and treatment of constipation. Pract Gastroenterol 1986; 10:28.)

ences associated with soiling.[132,133] Consistent with this interpretation, Levine and Bakow[64] found that successfully treated encopretic children became better adjusted and exhibited no evidence of symptom substitution as long as 3 years after therapy. These observations imply that one consequence of fecal soiling is the development of poor coping skills, low self-esteem, and passivity, which are potentially reversible with successful therapy.

Pharmacologic Therapy

The use of laxatives is deeply rooted in medical and social traditions,[134] and vast amounts are consumed in the western world,[12] especially by elderly persons.[1,105] Laxatives are classified into five groups on the basis of their presumed mode of action (Table 39-

5). Except for the bulk laxatives, routine use of these agents over long periods of time should be discouraged.

The *bulk-forming laxatives* consist of natural (psyllium) or synthetic polysaccharides or cellulose derivatives that act in a manner similar to that of fiber naturally contained in the diet. Because fluid intake should be increased with these preparations, caution should be exercised in using these agents in patients who require severe fluid restriction. "Sugar-free" bulk laxatives may contain aspartame (NutraSweet) and are contraindicated in patients with phenylketonuria.

Emollient laxatives consist of mineral oil and docusate salts. Mineral oil can be given orally or by enema; it penetrates and softens the stool. Although some orally administered mineral oil is absorbed and deposited in the liver, spleen, and mesenteric lymph nodes,[135] there are no described harmful effects. Because mineral oil may decrease the absorption of fat-soluble Vitamins A, D, and K, it should be administered between meals. Aspiration with lipid pneumonia is well described; therefore, mineral oil is contraindicated in patients with esophageal dysmotility or dysphagia and in elderly or debilitated patients and should not be given at bedtime.

Docusate salts are anionic surfactants that lower the surface tension of stool to allow mixing of aqueous and fatty substances. This softens stool to permit easier defecation. They also stimulate intestinal fluid and electrolyte secretion by increasing mucosal cyclic-AMP.[136] Although not absorbed, they alter intestinal mucosal permeability and increase the absorption of other laxatives, such as mineral oil, phenolphthalein, and danthron.[12] Recent placebo-controlled studies failed to demonstrate changes in stool water content, stool weight, frequency of defecation, or colonic transit times when docusates were given in currently recommended doses, suggesting that any therapeutic benefit from these agents may be secondary to a placebo effect.[137]

Hyperosmolar agents include mixed electrolyte solutions containing polyethylene glycol and nonabsorbable sugars such as lactulose and sorbitol. Sorbitol and lactulose are degraded by colonic bacteria to low-molecular-weight acids that increase stool acidity and osmolarity. Doses should be adjusted to reduce side effects and modulate defecation. Sorbitol and glycerin are given intrarectally and may produce rectal irritation. Polyethylene glycol solutions are most often given for bowel cleansing prior to colonoscopy or to instituting bowel programs. There have been recent anecdotal reports of using 8 to 24 oz daily to treat intractable constipation.

Saline laxatives contain relatively nonabsorbable cations and anions that exert an osmotic effect to increase intraluminal water content. Magnesium may also stimulate the release of cholecystokinin to increase intestinal motor activity.[138] Because an appreciable amount of magnesium may be absorbed, it should be avoided in patients with renal insufficiency because of the danger of magnesium toxicity.[139] Other side effects include hypocalcemia in children[12] and mineral imbalances. Saline laxatives can also be administered by enemas or suppositories.

Stimulant laxatives consist of castor oil, anthraquinones (cascara sagrada, senna, casanthranol, and danthron), and diphenylmethanes (phenolphthalein and bisacodyl) (Table 39-6). Castor oil is hydrolyzed by intestinal lipases to ricinoleic acid, which stimulates intestinal secretion, decreases glucose absorption, and increases intestinal motility.[140]

The anthraquinone laxatives increase fluid and electrolyte accumulation in the distal ileum and colon through incompletely

TABLE 39–5
Laxatives

LAXATIVE	USUAL ADULT DOSE	ONSET OF ACTION	SIDE EFFECTS
Bulk-Forming Laxatives			
Natural (psyllium)	7 g P.O.	12–72 hrs	Impaction above strictures
Synthetic (methylcellulose)	4–6 g P.O.	12–72 hrs	Fluid overload
Emollient Laxatives			
Docusate salts	50–500 mg P.O.	24–72 hrs	Skin rashes
Mineral oil	15–45 ml P.O.	6–8 hrs	Decreased absorption of vitamins
			Lipid pneumonia
			Decreased absorption of Coumadin, oral contraceptives
Hyperosmolar Laxatives			
Polyethylene glycol	3–22 L P.O.	1 hr	Abdominal bloating
Lactulose	15–60 ml P.O.	24–48 hrs	Abdominal bloating
Sorbitol	120 ml of 25% soln P.O.	24–48 hrs	Abdominal bloating
Glycerine	3 g suppository	15–60 min	Rectal irritation
	5–15 ml enema	15–30 min	Rectal irritation
Saline Laxatives			
Magnesium sulfate	15 g P.O.	0.5–3 hrs	Magnesium toxicity (with renal insufficiency)
Magnesium phosphate	10 gm P.O.	0.5–3 hrs	
Magnesium citrate	200 ml P.O.	0.5–3 hrs	
Stimulant Laxatives			
Castor oil	15–60 ml P.O.	2–6 hrs	Nutrient malabsorption
Diphenylmethanes			
Phenolphthalein	60–100 mg P.O.	6–8 hrs	Skin rashes
Bisacodyl	30 mg P.O.	6–10 hrs	Gastric irritation
	10 mg P.R.	0.25–1 hrs	Rectal stimulation
Anthraquinones			
Cascara sagrada	1 ml P.O.	6–12 hrs	Melanosis coli
Senna	2 ml P.O.	6–12 hrs	Degeneration of Meissner's and Auerbach's plexuses
Aloe (casanthrol)	250 mg P.O.	6–12 hrs	
Danthron	75–150 mg P.O.	6–12 hrs	Hepatotoxicity (with docusate)

(Sekas G. The use and abuse of laxatives. Pract Gastroenterol 1987;11:33.)

understood actions.[12] All are absorbed from the small intestine to some extent (especially danthron) and are metabolized by the liver. Anthraquinones are converted to a pharmacologically active state when they come in contact with intestinal microorganisms. Pathologic changes in the colon produced by chronic anthraquinone use include melanosis coli, a benign and reversible condition, and perhaps smooth muscle atrophy and damage to the myenteric plexus.[58] Danthron may cause hepatotoxicity similar to chronic active hepatitis when given together with docusate.[20]

Approximately 15% of phenolphthalein is absorbed from the small intestine and undergoes an enterohepatic circulation, which explains its often long duration of action. It acts directly to stim-ulate colonic motor activity and inhibits glucose and sodium absorption to increase intraluminal fluid content. Side effects include fixed-drug skin eruptions, erythema multiforme, and photosensitive bullous skin lesions.[141] Fatalities have been reported in allergic individuals who were rechallenged with the drug.[134]

Bisacodyl is structurally similar to phenolphthalein and exhibits similar actions on small intestinal fluid accumulation and colonic motor activity. Because the drug is a gastric irritant, tablets are enteric coated and should not be broken or chewed.[134]

The use of drugs to enhance colonic transit by increasing propulsive motor activity has been hampered somewhat by our limited knowledge of the control of various aspects of colonic motility

TABLE 39–6
Composition of Commonly Used Laxatives

BRAND	ALOE	BISACODYL	CASCARA	DANTHRON	DOCUSATE	MINERAL OIL	PHENOLPHTHALEIN	SENNA
Agoral							×	
Black–Draught	×						×	
Carter's Little Pills					×			×
Colace					×			×
Correctol					×		×	
Dialose					×			
Doxidan				×	×			
Ducolax		×						
Evac-U-Gen							×	
Ex-Lax							×	
Extra Gentle Ex-Lax					×		×	
Feen-a-Mint					×		×	
Haley's MO						×		
Modane				×				
Modane Plus				×	×			
Nature's Remedy	×		×					
Peri-Colac			×		×			
Petrogalar						×		
Senokot								×
Surfak					×			
Unilax				×	×			
X-Prep								×
Yellowlax							×	

(Sekas G. The use and abuse of laxatives. Pract Gastroenterol 1987;11:33.)

(see ch 10) and the pathophysiology of severe idiopathic constipation. *Cholinergic agents* such as bethanechol have been used with little success and exhibit moderate side effects in patients with colonic inertia.[75] *Cholinesterase inhibitors* such as neostigmine may have fewer side effects, but there is no evidence of increased efficacy.[39]

Prokinetic agents represent a new class of drugs that stimulate gastrointestinal motor activity to enhance transit of intraluminal contents. Metoclopramide has been used to treat upper gastrointestinal motor disorders but exerts little effect on colonic motility and is not effective in constipated patients.[142] Cisapride is a newer prokinetic agent that appears to enhance transit through the proximal colon in man[143] and has been shown to stimulate distal colonic motility and improve rectal sensation in chronically constipated patients.[144] Although some studies suggest that clinical improvement occurs with the drug,[145] others report highly variable and often disappointing results in patients with severe idiopathic constipation.

It has been hypothesized that motility disorders leading to chronic constipation are caused by excessive endogenous opioids. Several patients with severe constipation have been treated successfully with intravenous naloxone, an opioid receptor antagonist.[146] With use of scintigraphic techniques, naloxone accelerates transit in various parts of the colon in normal volunteers.[147] Preliminary studies suggest that oral naloxone may increase stool volumes in elderly constipated individuals when compared with placebo.[148] Further studies are required to assess the role of this class of agents.

Surgical Treatment

With several important exceptions, the indications for surgical intervention in managing patients with chronic constipation are somewhat controversial. The generally agreed upon indications and contraindications for surgery are discussed below.

Hirschsprung's Disease. Surgery is the treatment of choice for all forms of this disease but will vary according to the length of the aganglionic segment. In patients with short-segment or ultrashort-segment disease, anal myotomy, in which the internal sphincter and a varying length of rectal smooth muscle are incised, can be extremely beneficial.[149,150] In the classic form of the disease, more extensive procedures are used to overcome the obstructing effect of the aganglionic segment. These approaches consist of removing the segment, as in the Swenson operation,[151] or bypassing it, as in the Duhamel operation,[152] or the endorectal pull-through techniques of Soave[153] and Boley.[154] The choice of surgical technique depends upon the surgeon, but excellent results have been reported for all of them.[155,156] For good results to be obtained, thorough cleansing of the colon prior to surgery is mandatory.[150]

Colonic Inertia. In selected patients with colonic inertia, subtotal colectomy with ileorectal anastomosis can be dramatically beneficial in ameliorating incapacitating symptoms that are unresponsive to medical management.[157–159] It is now abundantly clear that limited resection of the colon produces unsatisfactory results and a high rate of anastomotic leaks.[157] *Before surgery is undertaken, it is important to document that the disorder is confined to the large intestine by performing radiologic and/or manometric studies to establish normal esophageal, gastric, and small-intestine motor function.* Nevertheless, in one study, abnormal gastroduodenal manometry did not necessarily predict failure of colectomy,[160] and normal studies do not guarantee success. Patients who have evidence of a more extensive dysmotility disorder can be anticipated to have less satisfactory results,[161] and such procedures should be done only if colonic distention is life-threatening or severely incapacitating.

Rectocele. Surgical therapy consists of reducing or eliminating the pouch with posterior culporrhaphy. Because rectoceles are commonly seen in nonconstipated persons, care must be taken before attributing defecatory difficulties to this entity. Ideally, one should observe improved rectal evacuation after the patient exerts finger pressure on the posterior wall of the vagina during defecography. Rectocele repairs frequently do not alleviate symptoms of difficult defecation.

Rectal Intussusception and Prolapse. Surgical therapy consists of various resuspension procedures such as the Ripstein procedure,[162] the Thiersch operation,[150] the Ivalon sponge wrap,[163] and abdominal rectopexy with sigmoid resection.[150] However, most patients who undergo surgery experience no improvement in their defecatory difficulties.[164] As with rectoceles, rectal intussusceptions are not uncommon in nonconstipated individuals, and their presence in constipated patients should not imply causation.

Rectosphincteric Dyssynergia. *Surgery for this disorder is contraindicated* because patients receive no benefits from posterior division of the puborectalis muscle and fecal incontinence commonly occurs after surgery.[165]

The reader is directed to Chapter 10, The Motor Function of the Colon; Chapter 67, Dysmotility of the Small Intestine; Chapter 80, Irritable Bowel Syndrome; Chapter 81, Motility Disorders of the Colon; Chapter 82, Diverticulitis; and Chapter 85, Anorectal Diseases.

REFERENCES

1. Connell AM, Hilton C, Irvine G, Lennard-Jones JE, Miscewicz JJ. Variation in bowel habit in two population samples. Br Med J 1965;2:1095.

2. Drossman DA, Sandler RS, Mekel DC, Lovitz AJ. Bowel patterns among subjects not seeking health care. Gastroenterology 1982;83:529.

3. Schuster MM. Evaluation and treatment of constipation: The need for hard data about hard stools. Pract Gastroenterol 1986;10:15.

4. Martelli H, Devroede G, Arhan P, Duguay C, Dornic C, Faverdin C. Some parameters of large bowel function in normal man. Gastroenterology 1978;75:612.

5. Sandler RS, Drossman DA. Bowel habits in apparently healthy young adults. Dig Dis Sci 1987;32:841.

6. Bannister JJ, Gibbons CP, Trowbridge EA, Read NW. Experimental support for a simple model of defecation. Gut 1985;26:A1131.

7. Barnes PRH, Lennard-Jones JE. Balloon expulsion from the rectum in constipation of different types. Gut 1985;26:1049.

8. Mahieu P, Pringot J, Bodart P. Defecography I. Description of a new procedure and results in normal patients. Gastrointest Radiol 1984;9:247.

9. O'Connell JP, Kelly KA, Brown ML. Scintigraphic assessment of neorectal motor function. J Nucl Med 1986;27:460.

10. Rendtorff RC, Kashgarian M. Stool patterns of healthy adult males. Dis Colon Rectum 1967;10:222.

11. Exton-Smith AN, Bendall MJ, Kent F. A new technique for measuring the consistency of feces: A report on its application to the assessment of Senokot therapy in the elderly. Age Ageing 1975;4:58.

12. Tedesco FJ, DiPiro JT. Laxative use in constipation. Am J Gastroenterol 1985;80:303.

13. Neumann PZ, deDomenico IJ, Nogrady MB. Constipation and urinary tract infection. Pediatrics 1973;52:241.

14. Bannister JJ, Lawrence WT, Smith A, Thomas DG, Read NW. Urological abnormalities in young women with severe constipation. Gut 1988;29:17.

15. Levine MD. Children with encopresis: A descriptive analysis. Pediatrics 1975;56:412.

16. Kiff ES, Barnes PRH, Swash M. Evidence of pudendal neuropathy in patients with perineal descent and chronic constipation. Gut 1984;25:1279.

17. Snooks SJ, Barnes PRH, Swash M, Henry MM. Damage to the innervation of the pelvic floor musculature in chronic constipation. Gastroenterology 1985;89:977.

18. Preston DM, Lennard-Jones JE. Severe chronic constipation in young women: Idiopathic slow transit constipation. Gut 1986;27:41.

19. Gekas P, Schuster MM. Stercoral perforation of the colon: Case report and review of the literature. Gastroenterology 1981;80:1054.

20. Devroede G. Constipation. In: Sleisenger MH, Fordtran JS, eds. Gastrointestinal disease: Pathophysiology, diagnosis and management, ed 4. Philadelphia: WB Saunders, 1989:331.

21. Feldman M, Schiller LR. Disorders of gastrointestinal motility associated with diabetes mellitus. Ann Intern Med 1983;98:378.

22. Solano FX, Starling RC, Levey GS. Myxedema megacolon. Arch Intern Med 1985;145:231.

23. Anderson AS. Constipation during pregnancy. Incidence and methods used in its treatment in a group of Cambridgeshire women. J Health Visitor 1984;57:363.

24. Rees DW, Rhodes J. Altered bowel habit and menstruation. Lancet 1975;2:475.

25. Dodds WJ, Dent J, Hogan WJ. Pregnancy and the lower esophageal sphincter. Gastroenterology 1978;74:1334.

26. Wald A, Van Thiel DH, Hoechstetter L, et al. Effect of pregnancy on gastrointestinal transit. Dig Dis Sci 1982;26:1015.

27. Everson GT, McKinley C, Lawson M, Johnson M, Kern F. Gallbladder function in the human female: Effect of the ovulatory cycle, pregnancy and contraceptive steroids. Gastroenterology 1982;82:711.

28. Wald A, Van Thiel DH, Hoechstetter L, et al. Gastrointestinal transit: The effect of the menstrual cycle. Gastroenterology 1981;80:1497.

29. Davies GJ, Crowder M, Reid B, Dickerson JWT. Bowel function measurements of individuals with different eating patterns. Gut 1986;27:164.

30. Hinds JP, Stoney B, Wald A. Does gender or the menstrual cycle affect colonic transit? Am J Gastroenterol 1989;84:123.

31. Swenson WM, Witkowski LJ, Roskelly RC. Total colectomy for dermatomyositis. Am J Surg 1968;11:405.

32. Fukari K, Fukada H. The intramural pelvic nerves in the colon of dogs. J Physiol 1984;354:89.

33. Gunterberg B, Kewenter J, Peterson I, Steiner B. Anorectal function after major resections of the sacrum with bilateral or unilateral sacrifice of sacral nerves. Br J Surg 1976;63:546.

34. Devroede G, Lamarche J. Functional importance of extrinsic parasympathetic innervation to the distal colon and rectum in man. Gastroenterology 1974;66:273.

35. Devroede G, Arhan P, Duguay C, et al. Traumatic constipation. Gastroenterology 1979;77:1258.

36. Arhan P, Faverdin C, Thouvenot J. Anorectal motility in sick children. Scand J Gastroenterol 1972;7:309.

37. Freckner B, Ihre T. Influence of autonomic nerves on the internal anal sphincter in man. Gut 1976;17:306.

38. Read NW, Times JM. Defecation and the pathophysiology of constipation. Clin Gastroenterol 1986;15:937.

39. Glick ME, Meshkinpour H, Haldeman S, et al. Colonic dysfunction in patients with thoracic spinal cord injury. Gastroenterology 1984;86:287.

40. Freckner B. Function of the anal sphincter in spinal man. Gut 1975;16:638.

41. Hinds JP, Wald A. Colonic and anorectal dysfunction associated with multiple sclerosis. Am J Gastroenterol 1989;84:587.

42. Glick ME, Meshkinpour H, Haldeman S, Bhatia NN, Bradley WE. Colonic dysfunction in multiple sclerosis. Gastroenterology 1982;83:1002.

43. Weber J, Grise P, Roquebert M, et al. Radiopaque markers transit and anorectal manometry in 16 patients with multiple sclerosis and urinary bladder dysfunction. Dis Colon Rectum 1987;30:95.

44. Tobon F, Reid NCRW, Talbert JL, et al. A nonsurgical diagnostic test for Hirschsprung's disease. N Engl J Med 1968;278:188.

45. Schuster MM. The riddle of the sphincters. Gastroenterology 1975;69:249.

46. Boston VE, Dale G, Riley KWA. Diagnosis of Hirschsprung's disease by quantitative biochemical assay of acetylcholinesterase in rectal tissue. Lancet 1975;2:951.

47. Garrett JR, Howard ER, Nixon HH. Autonomic nerves in rectum and colon in Hirschsprung's disease. A cholinesterase and catecholamine histochemical study. Arch Dis Child 1969;44:406.

48. Rogawski MA, Goodrich JT, Gershon MD, Touloukian RJ. Hirschsprung's disease: Absence of serotonergic neurons in the aganglionic colon. J Pediatr Surg 1978;13:608.

49. Freund HR, Humphrey CJ, Fischer JE. Reduced tissue content of vasoactive intestinal peptide in aganglionic colon of Hirschsprung's disease. Am J Surg 1981;141:243.

50. Tafuri WL, Maria TA, Pitella JEH, et al. An electron microscope study of the Auerbach's plexus and determination of substance P of the colon in Hirschsprung's disease. Virchows Arch [A] 1974;362:41.

51. Fairgrieve J. Hirschsprung's disease in the adult. Br J Surg 1963;50:506.

52. Metzger PP, Alvear DT, Arnold GC, Stoner RR. Hirschsprung's disease in adults: Report of a case and review of the literature. Dis Colon Rectum 1978;21:113.

53. Morikawa P, Donahoe PD, Hendren WH. Manometry and histochemistry in the diagnosis of Hirschsprung's disease. Pediatrics 1979;63:865.

54. Howard ER, Garrett JR, Kidd A. Constipation and congenital disorders of the myenteric plexus. J R Soc Med 1984;77(Suppl 3):13.

55. Aidan Carney J, Go VLM, Sizemore GW, Hayles AB. Alimentary tract ganglioneuromatosis. A major complication of the syndrome of multiple endocrine neoplasia type 2B. N Engl J Med 1976;295:1287.

56. MacIver AG, Whitehead R. Zonal colonic aganglionosis: A variant of Hirschsprung's disease. Arch Dis Child 1972;47:233.

57. Smith B. Effect of irritant purgatives on the myenteric plexus in man and mouse. Gut 1968;9:139.

58. Smith B. Pathologic changes in the colon produced by anthraquinone purgatives. Dis Colon Rectum 1973;16:455.

59. Schuffler MD, Jonak Z. Chronic idiopathic intestinal pseudoobstruction caused by a degenerative disorder of the myenteric plexus: The use of Smith's method to define the neuropathology. Gastroenterology 1982;82:476.

60. Caronna JJ, Plum F. Cerebrovascular regulation in preganglionic and postganglionic autonomic insufficiency. Stroke 1973;4:12.

61. Battle WM, Snape WJ, Alair A, Cohen S, Braunstein S. Colonic dysfunction in diabetes mellitus. Gastroenterology 1980;79:1217.

62. Wald A, Handen BL. Behavioral aspects of disorders of defecation and fecal continence. Ann Behav Med 1987;9:19.

63. Gabel S, Hegedus AM, Wald A, Chandra R, Chiponis D. Prevalence of behavior problems and mental health utilization among encopretic children: Implications for behavioral pediatrics. Dev Behav Pediatr 1986;7:111.

64. Levine MD, Bakow H. Children with encopresis: A study of treatment outcome. Pediatrics 1976;58:845.

65. Meunier P, Louis D, deBeaujeu MJ. Physiologic investigation of primary colonic constipation in children. Comparison with the barium enema study. Gastroenterology 1984;87:1351.

66. Corazzari E, Cucchiara S, Staiano A, et al. Gastrointestinal transit time, frequency of defecation, and anorectal manometry in healthy and constipated children. J Pediatr 1985;106:379.

67. Meunier P, Marechal JM, deBeaujeu MJ. Rectoanal pressures and rectal sensitivity studies in chronic childhood constipation. Gastroenterology 1979;77:330.

68. Loening-Baucke V. Sensitivity of the sigmoid colon and rectum in children treated for chronic constipation. J Pediatr Gastroenterol Nutr 1984;3:454.

69. Wald A, Chandra R, Chiponis D, Gabel S. Anorectal function and continence mechanisms in childhood encopresis. J Pediatr Gastroenterol Nutr 1986;5:346.

70. Loening-Baucke VA. Factors responsible for persistence of childhood constipation. J Pediatr Gastroenterol Nutr 1987;6:915.

71. Molnar D, Taitz LS, Urwin OM, Wales JKH. Anorectal manometry results in defecation disorders. Arch Dis Child 1983;58:257.

72. Arhan P, Devroede G, Jehannin B, et al. Idiopathic disorders of fecal continence in children. Pediatrics 1983;71:774.

73. Loening-Baucke VA, Younoszai MK. Effect of treatment on rectal and sigmoid motility in chronically constipated children. Pediatrics 1984;73:199.

74. Loening-Baucke V, Cruikshank B, Savage C. Defecation dynamics and behavior profiles in encopretic children. Pediatrics 1987;80:672.

75. Wald A. Colonic transit and anorectal manometry in chronic idiopathic constipation. Arch Intern Med 1986;146:1713.

76. Whitehead WE, Engel BT, Schuster MM. Irritable bowel syndrome. Physiological and psychological differences between diarrhea-predominant and constipation-predominant patients. Dig Dis Sci 1980;25:404.

77. Wald A, Stoney B, Hinds JP. Psychological profiles in patients with constipation associated with normal and slow colonic transit. Gastroenterology 1988;95:892.

78. Krevsky B, Malmud LS, D'Ercole F, et al. Colonic transit scintigraphy. A physiologic approach to the measurement of colonic transit in humans. Gastroenterology 1986;91:1102.

79. Preston DM, Lennard-Jones JE. Pelvic motility and response to intraluminal bisacodyl in slow-transit constipation. Dig Dis Sci 1985;30:289.

80. Shouler P, Keighley MRB. Changes in colorectal function in severe idiopathic chronic constipation. Gastroenterology 1986;90:414.

81. Waldron D, Bowes KL, Kingma YJ, Cote KR. Colonic and anorectal motility in young women with severe idiopathic constipation. Gastroenterology 1988;95:1388.

82. Meunier P, Rochas A, Lambert R. Motor activity of the sigmoid colon in chronic constipation: Comparative study with normal subjects. Gut 1979;20:1095.

83. Krishnamurthy S, Schuffler MD, Rohrmann CA, Pope CE. Severe idiopathic constipation is associated with a distinctive abnormality of the colonic myenteric plexus. Gastroenterology 1985;88:26.

84. Watier A, Devroede G, Duranceau A, et al. Constipation with colonic inertia. A manifestation of systemic disease? Dig Dis Sci 1983;28:1025.

85. Bannister JJ, Timms JM, Barfield L, Read NW. Physiologic studies in young women with chronic constipation. Int J Colorectal Dis 1986;1(3):175.

86. Martelli H, Devroede G, Arhan P, Duguay C. Mechanisms of idiopathic constipation: Outlet obstruction. Gastroenterology 1978;75:623.

87. Read NW, Abouzekry L, Read MG, et al. Anorectal function in elderly patients with fecal impaction. Gastroenterology 1985;89:959.

88. Verduron A, Devroede G, Bouchoucha M, et al. Megarectum. Dig Dis Sci 1988;33:1164.

89. Preston DM, Lennard-Jones JE. Anismus in chronic constipation. Dig Dis Sci 1985;30:413.

90. Read NW, Timms JM, Barfield LJ, et al. Impairment of defecation in young women with severe constipation. Gastroenterology 1986;90:53.

91. Turnbull GK, Lennard-Jones JE, Bartram CI. Failure of rectal expulsion as a cause of constipation: Why fibre and laxatives sometimes fail. Lancet 1986;1:767.

92. Van Ball JG, Leguit P, Brummelkamp WH. Relaxation biofeedback conditioning as treatment of a disturbed defecation reflex: Report of a case. Dis Colon Rectum 1984;27:187.

93. Bleijenberg G, Kuijpers HC. Treatment of the spastic pelvic floor syndrome with biofeedback. Dis Colon Rectum 1987;30:108.

94. Wald A, Chandra R, Gabel S, Chiponis D. Evaluation of biofeedback in childhood encopresis. J Pediatr Gastroenterol Nutr 1987;6:554.

95. Ekberg O, Nyslander G, Fork F-T. Defecography. Radiology 1985;155:45.

96. Bartram CI, Turnbull GK, Lennard-Jones JE. Evacuation proctography: An investigation of rectal expulsion in 20 subjects without defecatory disturbance. Gastrointest Radiol 1988;13:72.

97. Turnbull GK, Bartram CI, Lennard-Jones JE. Radiologic studies of rectal evacuation in adults with idiopathic constipation. Dis Colon Rectum 1988;31:190.

98. Mahieu P, Pringot J, Bodart P. Defecography. II. Contribution to the diagnosis of defecation disorders. Gastrointest Radiol 1984;9:253.

99. Wald A, Friemanis M, Stoney B, Hinds JP. Anorectal manometry and defecography in severe idiopathic constipation. Gastroenterology 1988;95:892.

100. Whorwell PJ, McCallum M, Creed FM, Roberts CT. Non-colonic features of irritable bowel syndrome. Gut 1986;27:37.

101. Cann PA, Read NW, Brown C, Hobson N, Holdsworth CD. The irritable bowel syndrome (IBS) relationship of disorders in the transit of a single solid meal to symptom patterns. Gut 1983 1983;24:405.

102. Milne JS, Williamson J. Bowel habit in older people. Gerontologia Clinica 1972;14:55.

103. Wilkins EG. Constipation in the elderly. Postgrad Med J 1968;44:728.

104. Brocklehurst JC. Colonic disease in the elderly. Clin Gastroenterol 1985;14:725.

105. Barnes PRH, Lennard-Jones JE, Hawley PR, Todd IP. Hirschsprung's disease and idiopathic megacolon in adults and adolescents. Gut 1986;27:534.

106. Preston DM, Lennard-Jones JE, Thomas BM. Towards a radiologic definition of idiopathic megacolon. Gastrointest Radiol 1985;10:167.

107. Brocklehurst JC, Khan MY. A study of fecal stasis in old age and the use of Dorbanex in its prevention. Gerontologia Clinica 1969;11:293.

108. Derogatis LR. The SCL-90-R. Administration, scoring and procedure manual II. Towson, MD: Clinical Psychometric Research, 1983.

109. Bellman MM. Studies on encopresis. Acta Pediatr Scand 1966;56(Suppl 170):1.

110. Wittoesch JH, Jackman RJ, McDonald JR. Melanosis coli: General review and a study of 887 cases. Dis Colon Rectum 1958;1:172.

111. Patriquin H, Martelli H, Devroede G. Barium enema in chronic constipation: Is it meaningful? Gastroenterology 1978;75:619.

112. Arhan P, Devroede G, Jehannin B, et al. Segmental colonic transit time. Dis Colon Rectum 1981;24:625.

113. Chaussade S, Roche H, Khyardi A, Conturier D, Guerre J. A new method for measuring colonic transit time. Description and validation. Gastroenterol Clin Biol 1986;10:385.

114. Metcalf AM, Phillips SF, Zinsmeister AR, MacCarty RL, Beart RW, Wolff BG. Simplified assessment of segmental colon transit. Gastroenterology 1987;92:40.

115. Shorvon PJ, McHugh F, Somers S, Stevenson GW. Defecographic findings in young healthy volunteers. Gut 1987;28:A1361.

116. Lahr CJ, Rothenberger DA, Jensen LL, Goldberg SM. Balloon topography. A simple method of evaluating anal function. Dis Colon Rectum 1986;29:1.

117. Bartolo DC, Read NW, Jarratt JA, Read MG, Donnelly TC, Johnson AG. Differences in anal sphincter function and clinical presentation in patients with pelvic floor descent. Gastroenterology 1983;85:68.

118. Barnes PRH, Lennard-Jones JE. Balloon expulsion from the rectum in constipation of different types. Gut 1985;26:1049.

119. Caruana BJ, Hinds JP, Friemanis M, Wald A. Psychological and physiological characteristics of patients with defecation difficulties. Gastroenterology 1989;97:932.

120. Burkitt DP, Walker ARP, Painter NS. Effect of dietary fibre on stool and transit times and its role in the causation of disease. Lancet 1972;2:1408.

121. Cummings JH. Constipation, dietary fibre and the control of large bowel function. Postgrad Med J 1983;1:1206.

122. Yang P, Banwell JG. Dietary fiber: Its role in the pathogenesis and treatment of constipation. Pract Gastroenterol 1986;10:28.

123. Lupton JR, Meacher MM. Radiographic analysis of the effect of dietary fibers on rat colonic transit time. Am J Physiol 1988;255:G633.

124. Wolin MJ. Fermentation in the rumen and human large intestine. Science 1981;213:1463.

125. Ingebo KB, Heyman MB. Polyethylene glycol-electrolyte solution for intestinal clearance in children with refractory encopresis. Am J Dis Child 1988;142:340.

126. Lowery SP, Srour JW, Whitehead WE, et al. Habit training as treatment of encopresis secondary to chronic constipation. J Pediatr Gastroenterol Nutr 1985;4:397.

127. Christopherson ER, Rainey SK. Management of encopresis through a pediatric outpatient clinic. J Pediatr Psychol 1976;4:38.

128. Abrahamian FP, Lloyd-Still JD. Chronic constipation in childhood: A longitudinal study of 186 patients. J Pediatr Gastroenterol Nutr 1984;3:460.

129. Ford MR. Interpersonal stress and style as predictors of biofeedback/relaxation training outcome: Preliminary findings. Biofeedback Self Regul 1985;10:223.

130. Wolters WHG, Wauters EAK. A study of somatopsychic vulnerability in encopretic children. Psychother Psychosom 1975;26:37.

131. Landman GB, Rappaport L, Fenton T, Levine M. Locus of control and self-esteem in children with encopresis. Dev Behav Pediatr 1986;7:111.

132. Hoag JM, Norriss NG, Himeno ET, Jacobs J. The encopretic child and his family. J Am Acad Child Psychiatry 1971;10:242.

133. Bemporad JR, Kresch RA, Asnes R, Wilson A. Chronic neurotic encopresis as a paradigm of a multifactorial psychotic disorder. J Nerv Ment Dis 1978;166:472.

134. Sekas G. The use and abuse of laxatives. Pract Gastroenterol 1987;11:33.

135. Stryker WA. Absorption of liquid-petrolatum ("mineral oil") from the intestine: A histological and chemical study. Arch Pathol 1941;31:670.

136. Donowitz M, Binder HJ. Effect of dioctyl sodium sulfosuccinate on colonic fluid and electrolyte movement. Gastroenterology 1975;69:941.

137. Chapman RW, Sillery J, Fontana DD, Matthys C, Saunders DR. Effect of oral dioctyl sodium sulfosuccinate on intake–output studies of human small and large intestine. Gastroenterology 1985;89:489.

138. Donowitz M. Current concepts of laxative action: Mechanisms by which laxatives increase stool water. Clin Gastroenterol 1979;1:77.

139. Pietrusko RG. Use and abuse of laxatives. Am J Hosp Pharm 1977;34:291.

140. Ammon HV, Phillips SF. Inhibition of colonic water and electrolyte absorption by fatty acids in man. Gastroenterology 1973;65:744.

141. Wyatt E, Greaves M, Sondergard J. Fixed drug eruption (phenolphthalein). Arch Dermatol 1972;106:671.

142. Reynolds JC. Chronic severe constipation. In: Cohen S, Soloway RD, eds. Functional disorders of the gastrointestinal tract. New York: Churchill Livingstone, 1987:95.

143. Krevsky B, Malmud L, Mauer A, et al. The effect of cisapride on colonic transit. Alimentary Pharmacol Ther 1987;1:293.

144. Reboa G, Arnulfo G, Frascio M, DiSomma C, Pitto G, Berti-Riboli E. Colon motility and coloanal reflexes in chronic idiopathic constipation. Effects of a novel enterokinetic agent cisapride. Eur J Clin Pharmacol 1984;26:745.

145. Müller-Cissner JA, Bavarian Constipation Study Group. Treatment

of chronic constipation with cisapride and placebo. Gut 1987;28:1033.

146. Kreek MJ, Schaffer RA, Hahn EF, Fishman J. Naloxone, a specific opioid antagonist, reverses chronic idiopathic constipation. Lancet 1983;1;261.

147. Kaufman PN, Krevsky B, Malmud LS, et al. Role of opiate receptors in the regulation of colonic transit. Gastroenterology 1988;94:1351.

148. Kreek MJ, Paris P, Bartol MA, Mueller D. Effects of short-term oral administration of the specific opioid antagonist naloxone on fecal evacuation in geriatric patients. Gastroenterology 1984;86:1144.

149. Lynn HB, van Heerden JA. Rectal myectomy in Hirschsprung's disease. Arch Surg 1975;110:991.

150. Poisson J, Devroede G. Severe chronic constipation as a surgical disease. Surg Clin North Am 1983;63:193.

151. Swenson O. A new surgical treatment for Hirschsprung's disease. Surgery 1950;28:371.

152. Duhamel B. New operation for treatment of Hirschsprung's disease. Arch Dis Child 1960;35:38.

153. Soave F. Hirschsprung's disease: A new surgical technique. Arch Dis Child 1964;39:116.

154. Boley SJ. An endorectal pull-through operation with primary anastomosis for Hirschsprung's disease. Surg Gynecol Obstet 1968;127:353.

155. Nixon HH. Hirschsprung's disease: Progress in management and diagnostics. World J Surg 1985;9:189.

156. Martin LW, Torres AM. Hirschsprung's disease. Surg Clin North Am 1985;65:1171.

157. Preston DM, Hawley PR, Lennard-Jones JE, Todd IP. Results of colectomy for severe idiopathic constipation in women (Arbuthnot Lane's disease). Br J Surg 1984;71:547.

158. Roe AM, Bartolo DC, Mortensen NJ McC. Diagnosis and surgical management of intractable constipation. Br J Surg 1986;73:854.

159. Loening-Baucke VA, Anuras S, Mitros FA. Changes in colorectal function in patients with chronic colonic pseudoobstruction. Dig Dis Sci 1987;32:1104.

160. Howard RJ, Davis RH, Clench MH, Mathias JR. Subtotal colectomy as a therapeutic consideration in patients with chronic constipation refractory to medical therapy. Gastroenterology 1985;88:1423.

161. Belliveau P, Goldberg SM, Rothenberger DA, et al. Idiopathic acquired megacolon: The value of subtotal colectomy. Dis Colon Rectum 1982;25:118.

162. Ripstein CB. Definitive corrective surgery. Dis Colon Rectum 1972;15:334.

163. Wells C. New operation for rectal prolapse. Proc R Soc Med 1959;52:602.

164. Ihre T, Seligson V. Intussusception of the rectum-internal procidentia: Treatment and results in 90 patients. Dis Colon Rectum 1975;18:391.

165. Barnes PRH, Hawley PR, Preston DM, Lennard-Jones JE. Experience of posterior division of the puborectalis muscle in the management of chronic constipation. Br J Surg 1985;72:475.

40

Approach to the Patient with Ileostomy and Ileal Pouch

KEITH A. KELLY

This chapter will deal with ileostomies, both standard and continent, and with ileal pouches used as reservoirs to replace an excised colorectum. The ileal pouch in particular will be emphasized, because when it is anastomosed to the anal canal, it restores transanal defecation, maintains reasonable fecal continence, and obviates a permanent abdominal ileostomy.

The positions taken in this chapter are based on a large experience with these operations at the Mayo Clinic over the past 20 years as cited in a series of reports.[1-44] The data of others are also used.[45-64]

STANDARD END ILEOSTOMY

Proctocolectomy with end ileostomy (Brooke ileostomy) is the standard procedure for patients who require excision of the entire colon and rectum for ulcerative colitis, familial adenomatous polyposis, or multiple colonic malignancies. The ileostomy is made from the terminal ileum and is positioned in the right lower quadrant of the abdomen. The patient's fecal effluent discharges through the stoma and is collected by an external appliance that the patient wears continuously, day and night. These ileostomies, when properly constructed and managed, have proved remarkably safe and trouble-free.

Rationale

The rationale is that excision of the entire large intestine will cure the patient of his colorectal disease, while the establishment of the Brooke ileostomy will afford a satisfactory life-style.

Type of Patient

The operation can be done for patients of any age or sex who require excision of the large intestine. Because of the advent of continence-preserving operations, however, the operation is used today mainly in older patients or in obese patients who are not candidates for the continence-preserving procedures.

Preoperative Preparation

The nutritional status of the patient is stabilized before operation. This sometimes, but not often, requires parenteral supplementation. Anemia is treated by blood transfusion. For patients who currently receive or who recently completed steroid therapy, additional steroid (usually 100 mg of hydrocortisone intravenously every 8 hours) is given to ensure adequate supply during the operative stress. The bowels are cleansed with laxatives and enemas for 2 days prior to operation. Alternatively, 4 L of an electrolyte solution can be given by mouth the night before operation to wash out the gastrointestinal tract. Diet is restricted to clear liquids the day before operation. The growth of enteric bacteria is suppressed by giving neomycin, 0.5 g every 4 hours, and tetracycline, erythromycin, or metronidazole, 250 mg every 4 hours, for 1 day prior to operation. Cefazolin, 0.5 g, is given intravenously just prior to the operation and is continued every 8 hours for two more doses.

At a preoperative interview, the exact description of the procedure and an understanding of the new anatomy produced by the operation are thoroughly discussed with the patient. The patient must understand that the ileostomy provides a permanent abdominal stoma and that an appliance must be worn continuously to collect the fecal effluent. A visit with a person who has made a successful adjustment to an ileostomy is also most helpful. The old patient can frequently dispel the new patient's fears and misconceptions about the operation.

In addition, before operation, an appropriate site should be selected for the ileostomy by actually positioning an appliance on the patient's abdomen. The site is usually just lateral to and inferior to the umbilicus, midway between the midline and the right anterior iliac spine. This position allows the patient to bend and move the body in all directions without dislodging the appliance. The site selected should also be free of abdominal skin folds, creases, and scars that might hinder effective sealing of the appliance to the skin. The assistance of a competent stomal therapist is invaluable.

Technique

The patient is placed in a modified lithotomy position to allow the surgeon access to both the abdomen and the perineum. A catheter is inserted into the urinary bladder for continuous drainage, and the skin is prepared with a dilute solution of povidone-iodine (Betadine) or another suitable antiseptic.

Through a vertical midline abdominal incision, a thorough inspection of the abdominal content is made to confirm the presence or absence of disease. The diseased large intestine is then excised, making every effort to preserve as much of the small intestine as possible. Usually, all but a centimeter or two of terminal ileum can be saved. The surgeon should also carefully preserve the greater omentum and the mesentery of the small intestine and of the right colon. The latter is used in closing the peritoneal space lateral to the terminal ileum.

The terminal ileum is next prepared for construction of the stoma by dividing its secondary and tertiary vascular arcades while preserving its marginal artery and vein. This "trimming down" of the mesentery allows the bowel to be more easily turned inside out later during construction of the stoma.

The surgeon then moves to the cutaneous surface of the right lower abdomen to begin the construction of the stoma. The abdominal skin at the exact center of the site selected for the ileostomy is grasped with a clamp and elevated into the operative field. With use of a knife passed in the plane parallel to the surface of the abdomen, a circular defect approximately 2 cm in diameter is created in the skin. A 1-cm circle of the anterior rectus sheath is then excised, and the dissection is continued posteriorly through the rectus muscle and into the abdominal cavity. The surgeon should assure himself that the defect created in the abdominal wall will easily admit the index and middle fingers simultaneously, a defect with a diameter of about 4 cm. Smaller defects may narrow and obstruct the terminal ileum, while larger defects may predispose to parastomal hernia.

A noncrushing clamp is then passed from the exterior through the defect and into the abdominal cavity. The distal cut end of the ileum is grasped in the blades of the clamp, and the ileum is brought through the anterior abdominal wall to the skin surface. The ileum should project above the skin surface for a distance of about 5 cm. The ileum is then anchored to the abdominal wall from the peritoneal side using three interrupted 4-0 Dacron sutures. These sutures approximate the seromuscular layer of the ileum to the endoabdominal fascia at the site of exit of the ileum from the abdomen. This prevents prolapse or retraction of the stoma and peristomal hernia in the postoperative period.

Next, the space lateral to the terminal ileum is closed by approximating the ileal mesentery to the retroperitoneum and to the right lateral parietal peritoneum with use of a continuous 3-0 absorbable suture. This maneuver prevents later internal herniation and obstruction of more proximal small intestine at this site.

The stoma is then constructed by turning the terminal ileum inside out so that its mucosal surface is exposed and its serosal surface is covered and protected by the eversion (Fig 40-1). Because 5 cm of terminal ileum has been pulled through to the exterior from the abdomen, when the terminal ileum is turned inside out, a stoma 2.5 cm in length results. A stoma of this length projects well into an ileostomy bag. Leakage and slippage of the bag are

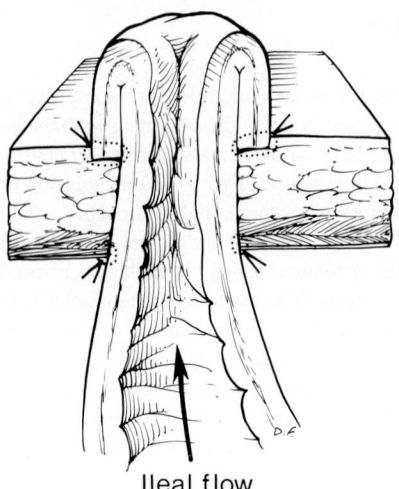

Ileal flow

FIGURE 40–1. Diagram of Brooke ileostomy.

minimized. Yet the stoma is not long enough to be excessively bulky or physically unattractive. The distal cut edge of the everted ileum is sewn to the dermis at the site of the stoma with eight interrupted absorbable sutures. Some of these sutures also include the seromuscular layer of the inner wall of the ileum at the skin level. The stoma should be bright red at the completion of its construction. This assures the surgeon that its blood supply is satisfactory.

An alternative method is to construct a loop ileostomy instead of a Brooke or end ileostomy. In this technique, the distal cut end of the ileum is closed, and a loop of ileum is brought to the surface 5 cm to 10 cm proximal to the closure (Fig 40-2). An external rod passed beneath the loop supports the loop at skin level in the postoperative period and prevents retraction of the stoma. This has an advantage in obese subjects in whom the ileostomy is especially likely to retract. A semicircular incision is made into the distal arm of the ileal loop at the level of the skin. The distal cut edge of the incision is sewn to the adjacent dermis. The proximal

cut edge is everted back over the proximal arm of the loop and sewn to the skin edge near the proximal arm. The final result is a stoma not dissimilar in appearance and function to a Brooke ileostomy.

After construction of the ileostomy, the abdomen is irrigated with an isotonic saline solution to remove blood, necrotic tissue, enteric content, and other debris that may remain after the intra-abdominal dissection. The abdominal incision is closed with absorbable sutures. We place a subcuticular catheter in the wound for suction and irrigation with antibiotics in the postoperative period.[3] This technique has reduced our incidence of wound infection to approximately 1% of operated patients. After the wound is closed, an ileostomy appliance is applied immediately to cover the stoma. The appliance protects the skin from irritation by ileal content discharged in the postoperative period.

The rectum and anus are excised in the intersphincteric plane[48] or the submucosal plane. The anal canal is closed primarily, by approximating the tunica muscularis of the distal rectum to itself with 2-0 absorbable sutures. A 5-mm suction-catheter is placed into the depths of the pelvis transabdominally and brought to the surface through a stab wound in the left flank. An alternative technique is to insert a double-lumen catheter into the perineal wound. One arm of the drain is irrigated with 154 mmol NaCl, 50 ml/hr, in the postoperative period, while suction is applied to the other arm. Such a technique removes blood, serum, necrotic debris, and intestinal content from the wound and minimizes the possibility of wound infection.[2]

Postoperative Care

Postoperatively, the patient is given nothing by mouth and is nourished by intravenous fluid and electrolyte solutions. The stomach is aspirated by way of a nasogastric tube. The urinary catheter is left in place, and the patient is ambulated beginning the day after operation.

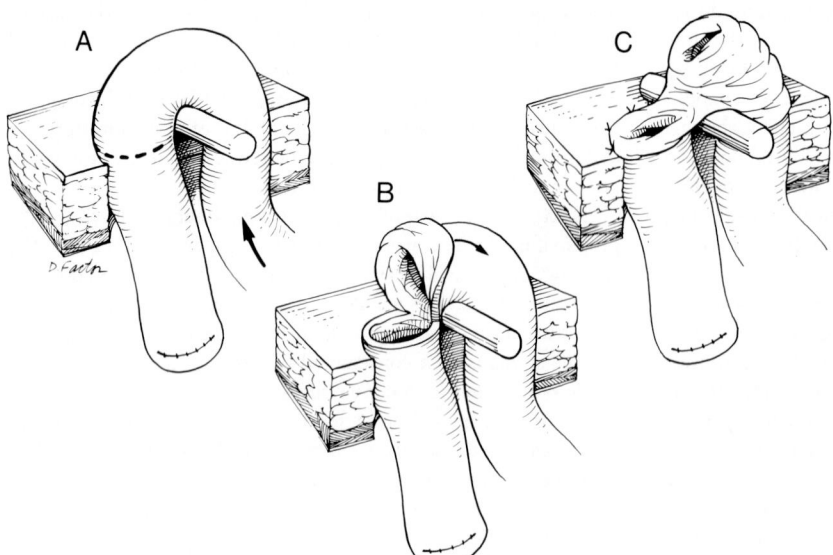

FIGURE 40–2. Construction of loop ileostomy. **A,** Loop of terminal ileum brought to surface and supported by rod. **B,** Ileum incised and proximal lip folded over. **C,** Completed stoma.

The ileostomy often begins discharging content on about the third postoperative day, at which time the nasogastric tube can be removed. The urinary catheter and pelvic drain are usually removed about the fifth day. At this time the patient is ready to begin taking oral feedings. We begin with a liquid diet, gradually increasing the solid content, so that by the seventh day the patient is usually taking a low-fiber solid diet. At this point, the patient is ready to learn self-care of the ileostomy, assisted by the stomal therapist.

Ileostomy output should be carefully monitored in the early postoperative period to ensure that the patient does not have excessive losses. The output from a healthy ileostomy is about 600 ml/day. If volumes greater than 1 L/day are passed, the patient may need intravenous supplementation of the oral intake to ensure that water and electrolyte depletion do not result.

The patient is usually ready for hospital discharge on approximately the tenth day after operation. After discharge, we encourage patients to eat all types of food but caution them to masticate thoroughly indigestible fiber. Undispersed fiber may obstruct an ileostomy. Food such as mushrooms, raw vegetables, and nuts are of particular concern. Patients generally require no long-term medications. In particular, Vitamin B_{12} usually is not needed, provided not more than a few centimeters of terminal ileum have been resected.

Patients must care properly for their stoma to protect the skin from the ileostomy content. The skin becomes irritated, and peristomal dermatitis will develop if the content gets on it. This problem can usually be prevented by proper stoma care.

Patients generally return to an active physical life after operation and resume their previous work. They can pursue sports such as tennis, swimming, and golf. An active sex life and pregnancy are not contraindications. Most patients adjust well to the presence of the stoma and report a satisfactory quality of life.

Complications

Complications from the operation are infrequent. Infection, abscess, and bleeding may occur in the early postoperative period, but they are usually prevented by careful attention to preoperative preparation and operative detail. Stomal obstruction, diarrhea, retraction of the stoma, prolapse of the stoma, and peristomal hernia may appear in the later postoperative period, but they are also rare (5% of patients or fewer) when the techniques described above are employed. Should they occur, revision of the stoma is often required. Urinary and sexual dysfunction may be long-term sequelae when nerves to these organs are damaged by the operative dissection. These complications are minimized when the excision of the rectum and anus is done in the intersphincteric or submucosal plane close to the anorectal lumen and away from the nerves.[48]

Patients with Brooke ileostomies are susceptible to two long-term metabolic complications: urinary stones and gallstones. In regard to urinary stones, these patients are in a state of chronic water and sodium loss. In health, the colon ordinarily absorbs water and electrolytes. Removal of the colon leads to a greater loss of water, sodium, chloride, potassium, and bicarbonate through the stoma than that occurring with normal defecation. Mild chronic dehydration and slight acidosis develop.[53] The ensuing low output

of acidic urine may lead to precipitation of uric acid stones in the urinary tract. To prevent this, the patients should be encouraged to drink adequate amounts of fluids. The taking of an alkali may also be indicated.

With regard to gallstones, the loss of bile salts through the stoma in patients who have had extensive resection of the ileum during the colectomy may deplete the bile salt pool and make patients susceptible to the formation of gallstones. No adequate form of prophylaxis has proved efficacious to date, but oral ingestion of a bile salt, such as ursodeoxycholic acid, might be considered. Should gallstones develop, cholecystectomy may be indicated. In contrast to ileostomy patients who have had ileal resection, those without ileal resection and with no ileal disease may be no more likely to form gallstones than a healthy control population.

Outcome

Patients are restored to good health. While the Brooke stoma is incontinent and requires the patients to wear an appliance day and night to collect the outflow from the enteric tract, these ileostomies are compatible with a satisfactory life-style over the long term. Nonetheless, patients and physicians have been reluctant to accept this operation, which, until recent years, was their only alternative. As a consequence, operation was often delayed or even postponed indefinitely despite strong indications for surgical therapy. Reluctance has arisen because of the fear of ileostomy and its physical, social, and psychologic consequences.

The Brooke ileostomy does leave the patient with complete fecal incontinence. An appliance must be worn day and night to collect the output from the stoma. The appliances are unsightly, uncomfortable, and somewhat odoriferous. Noises may issue from the stoma during times of fecal discharge, causing embarrassment to the patient. There is also the ever-present danger of leakage of stool or gas at the site of attachment of the appliance to the skin. The peristomal skin may become irritated.[1] Because of all of these factors, patients experience mild to moderate (15% of patients) or severe (9% of patients) restrictions of their activities (Table 40-1). In addition, the appliances are expensive. Patients estimate the cost of maintaining the appliance and servicing the ileostomy to be in the neighborhood of $500 per year. Thus, alternatives to an incontinent Brooke ileostomy are welcome. In our own series, 40% of patients with a Brooke ileostomy would like a change if one were available.[41]

Today, alternative operations are available that allow the disease to be removed and yet preserve fecal continence and avoid ileostomy. The newer operative approaches include the ileal pouch-anal anastomosis and the continent ileostomy (Kock pouch).

THE ILEAL POUCH–ANAL ANASTOMOSIS

The ileal pouch–anal anastomosis is currently being used with increasing frequency in the surgical management of chronic ulcerative colitis and familial adenomatous polyposis.

TABLE 40-1
Effect of Abdominal Ileostomy on Daily Activity in 685 Patients

ACTIVITY	% OF PATIENTS WITH			
	Moderate–Severe Restriction	Mild Restriction	No Restriction	Improvement Over Preoperative Status
Social life	7	14	51	28
Sports	17	26	42	15
Work at home	4	8	68	20
Recreation	8	21	48	23
Family relationships	3	5	68	24
Sex	14	15	56	15
Travel	8	18	48	26
Mean ± SEM, all categories	9 ± 2	15 ± 3	54 ± 4	22 ± 2

Rationale

The rationale is that the ileal pouch–anal operation, when combined with colectomy and rectal mucosal stripping, excises the entire colorectal disease in ulcerative colitis and polyposis coli and yet preserves transanal defecation and reasonable fecal continence. A permanent abdominal ileostomy is avoided. Because the rectal mucosal stripping is done endorectally, the nerves to the anal canal, urinary bladder, and genitalia are unlikely to be disturbed during the operation; thus, postoperative anal, urinary, and sexual dysfunction should be rare. Moreover, no perineal wound is made with this procedure, a wound that is sometimes difficult to heal.

Type of Patient

Patients with chronic ulcerative colitis, familial adenomatous polyposis of the colorectum, or multiple colorectal carcinomas are candidates for the operation, but those with Crohn's disease are not (Table 40-2). Crohn's disease may involve the small intestine as well as the large intestine. The risk of recurrence of Crohn's disease in the newly constructed pouch and the adverse sequelae

TABLE 40-2
Indications and Contraindications for Ileal Pouch–Anal Anastomosis

Indications	Relative Contraindications
Chronic ulcerative colitis	Massive obesity
Familial adenomatous polyposis	Emergency operation
Multiple colorectal malignancies	Inanition
	Use of steroid medication
Contraindications	Indeterminate colitis
Crohn's disease	
Cancer of the distal rectum	
Poor anal sphincter function	
Anal sphincter excised	
Age >65 years	

that might ensue argue against the use of the operation for this condition.

In contrast to Crohn's patients, patients with indeterminate colitis are candidates for the ileal pouch procedure. In these patients, in spite of historic, physical, endoscopic, radiologic, or pathologic examination, the exact diagnosis, colitis versus Crohn's, is not clear. The ileal pouch–anal operation in 25 such patients done at Mayo has been followed by results similar to those obtained in patients with clear-cut ulcerative colitis.[44] Crohn's disease has appeared in only 2 of these 25 patients to date over a 3-year follow-up. Rectal–vaginal fistula, however, is an indicator of a poor prognosis in patients with indeterminate colitis. Patients in our series with such a fistula often developed a recurrent fistula after the pouch procedure.

The ileal pouch–anal operation can also be done in patients with colitis and polyposis who have developed cancer in the colon or proximal rectum, provided the cancer and the adjacent lymph nodes to which it might have spread can be completely excised during the colectomy. Among 17 patients with cancer complicating ulcerative colitis and polyposis coli, the functional results of the operation were as good as in those in patients who had no cancer, and the recurrent cancer rate was comparable to that found among patients with similar malignancies that were treated by conventional operative techniques.[32] When cancer involves the mid or distal rectum, however, proctectomy must usually be done to ensure complete removal of the primary tumor. With proctectomy, ileal pouch–anal anastomosis is no longer possible. In patients with widespread metastatic malignancy, excision of the segment of bowel containing the primary tumor and reanastomosis seem preferable to performing the more extensive proctocolectomy and ileoanal anastomosis.

The operation should not be done as an emergency to treat an acute complication of colitis or polyposis, with one exception. The exception is patients who are exsanguinating from severe and unremitting hemorrhage of their rectal mucosa. In this situation, the rectal mucosa must be removed in order to control the hemorrhage. The ileal pouch and the pouch–anal anastomosis must then be made at the emergent operation to preserve the transanal route of defecation. In other emergencies, however, such as acute severe colitis, toxic megacolon, colonic perforation with peritonitis, and acute colonic obstruction, the colon should be removed, the rectum closed at its proximal end, and a Brooke ileostomy established.

The ileal pouch–anal procedure can then be accomplished during a second operation 6 to 12 months later.

Children, young adults, and middle-age adults up to the age of 65 years are candidates for the operation. They have sufficient anal sphincter strength to prevent fecal leakage after operation. Beyond age 65, anal sphincter strength begins to decline and might reach levels insufficient to maintain satisfactory continence after an ileal pouch–anal operation. We have not performed the operation on patients over the age of 65.

Inanition, weight loss, systemic steroids, and previous colonic operations are only relative contraindications to the operation, but loss of or severe damage to the anal sphincter by operation or disease is a contraindication. Obese patients are less likely to be able to undergo the procedure. The presence of excess fat in the ileal mesentery of obese subjects sometimes prevents the ileal pouch from reaching inferiorly far enough to meet the dentate line for the anastomosis. Obese subjects should be counseled to lose weight prior to operation. Another option is to perform colectomy, ileostomy, and retention of the rectum, withdraw steroids, have the patient lose weight, and then carry out the mucosal rectectomy and ileal pouch–anal operation at a second procedure.

Technique

EXTENT OF RESECTION

A major goal of the operation is removal of all diseased tissue, which means complete excision of all colonic and rectal mucosa.

This is accomplished by resection of the cecum, the colon (including the ileocolic valve), the proximal and midrectum, and the mucosa of the distal rectum down to the dentate line. The ileum should be preserved, even if it is involved with "backwash ileitis." We found that a pouch made from an ileum involved with backwash ileitis heals as well as a pouch made from uninvolved ileum.[26] Backwash ileitis also did not predispose the patient to a greater risk of nonspecific "pouchitis" in the postoperative period.

The colon should be removed, but the greater omentum should be preserved. The ileum is divided just proximal to the ileocolic valve. The rectum is mobilized by dividing and ligating its vasculature close to the bowel wall and away from the presacral neural plexuses and the innervation to the anal sphincter, bladder, and genitalia. Division of the fascia of Denonvilliers allows entrance into the avascular plane just anterior to the rectum to allow separation of the rectum from the prostate gland, seminal vesicles, and urethra in the male. Entrance into a similar plane in the female prevents injury to the vagina.

The length of the distal rectal mucosal stripping has shortened in recent years. Martin and colleagues[49] and others[56] advised a 10-cm to 15-cm length of stripping mostly accomplished by way of the abdominal route, but most surgeons today perform a 3-cm to 5-cm stripping by way of the perineal, transanal approach. The short length and perineal approach facilitate the operation while preserving the anal sphincteric mechanism satisfactorily. The anal sphincter has a length of 3 cm to 4 cm, only 1 cm to 2 cm of which are proximal to the dentate line. The short stripping preserves the muscle and innervation of the anal sphincter adequately.[8]

The anal canal is dilated to a diameter of 3 cm, not larger, and the dissection is begun endoluminally at the dentate line and extended proximally (Fig 40-3). A dilute solution of epinephrine (1/100,000) injected into the submucosa elevates the mucosa away

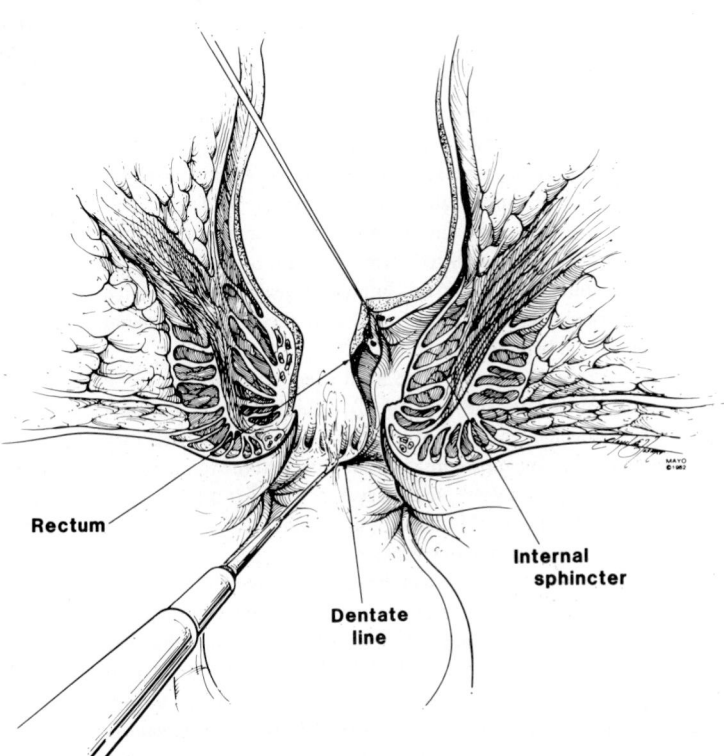

FIGURE 40–3. Technique of distal rectal mucosal stripping. (Reprinted, with permission, from Kelly KA. Ileal pouch–anal anastomosis: A critical look. In: Tytgat, G, van Blankenstein M, eds. Current Topics in Gastroenterology and Hepatology. Stuttgart, West Germany: Georg Thieme Verlag, 1990.)

from the underlying tunica muscularis and decreases bleeding, as does the use of cautery dissection. Once the distal 2 cm to 3 cm of rectal mucosa have been freed, eversion of the midrectum through the anus and onto the surface of the perineum facilitates the removal of the more proximal portion of the distal rectal mucosa.[14] Everting the rectum onto the perineum does not injure the anal sphincter or the perineal nerves more than does the pure endoluminal approach. Anal sphincteric, urinary, and sexual function with the eversion technique are excellent and similar to those obtained with the noneversion technique.[16] The distal rectal mucosa is freed to a level 5 cm proximal to the dentate line, where the bowel is then transected and more orad portions of full-thickness rectum are removed.

An alternative approach being used with increasing frequency today employs *no* distal rectal mucosal stripping.[57,58,61,62] The distal rectal wall is thoroughly mobilized from the abdominal route, after which the distal rectum is stapled transversely and divided at a site 1 cm to 2 cm above the dentate line. The rationale of this approach is that the distal 1 cm to 2 cm of rectum are lined not by columnar mucosa but by "transitional" mucosa, which may not be involved in colitis or polyposis. Preservation of the entire thickness of the distal rectal wall, including its transitional mucosa, facilitates the operation, preserves anal canal sensation, and may improve postoperative continence. The ileal pouch can be stapled to the distal rectal stump with a circular stapler.

While this approach appears attractive, we have found that the distal 1 to 2 cm of rectal mucosa in many of our patients are involved in the colitis or polyposis, just as is the more proximal mucosa. Leaving this mucosa behind commits the patient to the need for continued surveillance and the risk of continuing inflammation and possible neoplastic transformation. We advise the complete excision of all diseased mucosa, including the transitional mucosa.

CONSTRUCTION OF ILEAL POUCH

With excision of all diseased colorectum complete, construction of the ileal pouch is next addressed. A pouch should be made (Fig 40-4). Early experience with straight ileoanal anastomosis without an ileal pouch was unfavorable. Patients experienced stool frequencies of 10 to 20 stools/day and not infrequent incontinence.[11] The capacity of the unmodified terminal ileum to store the fecal content and defer defecation was limited, at least in our practice in adult patients. Others have found that the straight ileoanal anastomosis is satisfactory in children.[64]

Several types of pouches have been used, and all seem to be satisfactory. We prefer the "J-shaped" pouch because of the simplicity of its design, the ease of its construction, the satisfactory volume that it holds (approximately 300 ml), and the rapid, spontaneous, and near complete voluntary evacuation it affords. The "S-shaped" pouch and "H-shaped" pouch are also satisfactory, providing the efferent outflow limbs are not longer than 1 cm to 2 cm.[51,52] The "W-shaped" pouch has an attractive globular configuration that sits deep in the pelvis just above the levator ani.[55,64] It allows slightly more length to reach to the dentate line than the J-shaped pouch because the bend of the first loop of bowel used to make the "W" pouch, the site of anastomosis, is only 8 cm from the terminal cut end of the ileum. In the "J" pouch, the bend is 15 cm from the terminal cut end. Thus, the "W" pouch is useful

in obese, stocky patients with a short ileal mesentery. We have found the "W" pouch to have a slightly larger capacity and a slightly better compliance than the "J" pouch, perhaps because of its slightly larger size. (Johnson G, Pemberton JH, Kelly KA. Unpublished observations.) Nonetheless, all of the pouches provide a capacity similar to that of the rectum in health (approximately 300 ml), have similar distensibility (approximately 15 ml/mm Hg), and evacuate satisfactorily (65%–85% of content evacuated in 15–30 seconds).

The ileal mesentery is thoroughly mobilized up to the level of the pancreas. Division of a major ileal vascular arcade is usually required to allow the ileum to reach to the dentate line. Either the ileocolic vascular pedicle or the distal superior mesenteric vessels should be divided. Temporary occlusion with a "bulldog" vascular clamp prior to division allows the surgeon to be certain that vascular perfusion of the terminal ileum after division will be satisfactory.

The pouch is made from the distal 30 cm to 35 cm of ileum. Construction can be done with either absorbable sutures (2-0 chromic or polyglycolic acid) or staples. I prefer sutures because they offer a more water-tight closure, control bleeding from the cut edges better, and allow the surgeon to "sculpt" the pouch more exactly. Also, sutures are cheaper than staples. The advantage of staples is that they may shorten the time required for construction of the pouch.

POUCH–ANAL ANASTOMOSIS

The newly constructed pouch is advanced endorectally to the dentate line. The most dependent portion of the pouch is opened and the full thickness of ileal pouch wall is sewn to the anal canal at the dentate line (Fig 40-5). The 2-0 and 3-0 absorbable sutures include the cut edge of the pouch on one side and the anal sphincter and the anal mucosa at the dentate line on the other side. The anastomosis should ideally be under no tension, have good blood supply, and allow accurate mucosa-to-mucosa approximation.

Some surgeons have used a circular stapler to accomplish the anastomosis, but we have not, believing that the stapler may damage the anal sphincter by crushing it and excising a portion of it. The stapler can be used when the surgeon elects an ileal pouch–*distal rectal* anastomosis, as described above. In this instance, the anal sphincter would likely not be damaged by the stapler, and the stapler usually accomplishes a leak-free anastomosis with a satisfactory lumen.[49,53,56,57]

TEMPORARY ILEOSTOMY

A temporary diverting loop ileostomy should be employed in most patients.[22] The ileostomy allows the ileal pouch–anal anastomosis to heal prior to being stressed by the fecal stream passing over it. Even with a diverting ileostomy, about 5% of the pouch-anal anastomoses will show sinuses from lack of complete healing when the anastomoses are checked for healing 2 months after their construction.

We employ a loop ileostomy, as described earlier, positioning the afferent or proximal limb at five o'clock and the efferent or distal limb at 11 o'clock on the anterior frontal view. The efferent limb is not transected distal to the stoma, as it is in end ileostomy

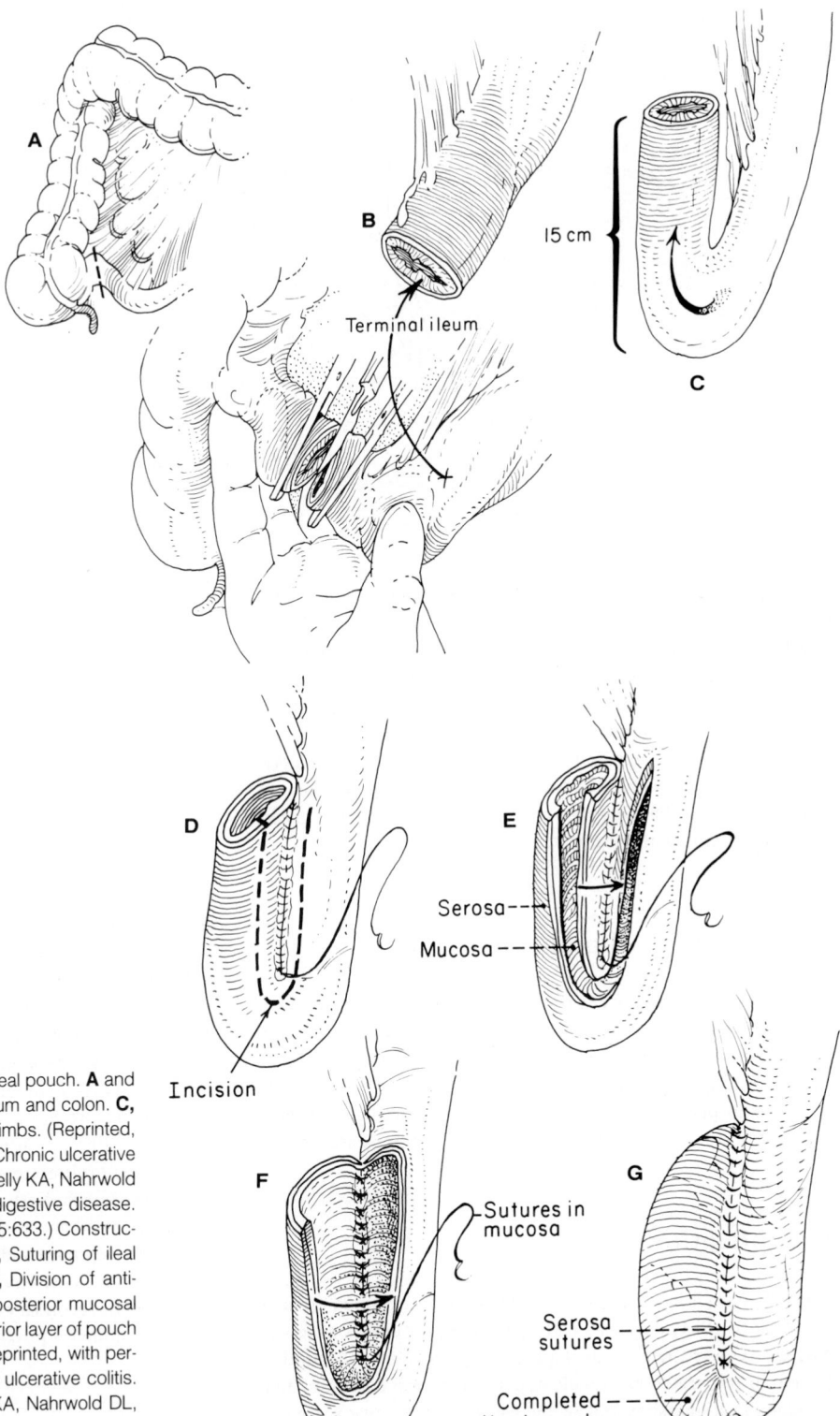

FIGURE 40–4. Construction of J-shaped ileal pouch. **A** and **B,** Division of terminal ileum, removal of cecum and colon. **C,** Fashioning ileum into a J shape with 15-cm limbs. (Reprinted, with permission, from Kelly KA, Dozois RR. Chronic ulcerative colitis. In: Moody FG, Carey LC, Jones RS, Kelly KA, Nahrwold DL, Skinner DB, eds. Surgical treatment of digestive disease. Chicago: Year Book Medical Publishers, 1985:633.) Construction of J-shaped ileal pouch (continued). **D,** Suturing of ileal limbs with 2-0 absorbable suture. **D** and **E,** Division of antimesenteric border of ileum. **F,** Suturing of posterior mucosal layer of pouch. **G,** Completed closure of anterior layer of pouch with two rows of 2-0 absorbable sutures. (Reprinted, with permission, from Kelly KA, Dozois RR. Chronic ulcerative colitis. In: Moody FG, Carey LC, Jones RS, Kelly KA, Nahrwold DL, Skinner DB, eds. Surgical treatment of digestive disease. Chicago: Year Book Medical Publishers, 1985:633.)

with proctocolectomy. Ileal continuity between the stoma and the pouch is maintained. The afferent limb is splinted with a Foley catheter (No. 16 French) during the first postoperative week to combat the tendency of this limb to form a volvulus around the stoma.

The ileostomy is closed at a second operation 2 months later, providing radiologic assessment shows complete healing of the pouch and anastomosis with no evidence of leak, fistula, or abscess. Should a leak be present when the anastomosis is assessed at 2 months, the ileostomy should not be closed. A 2-month to 6-

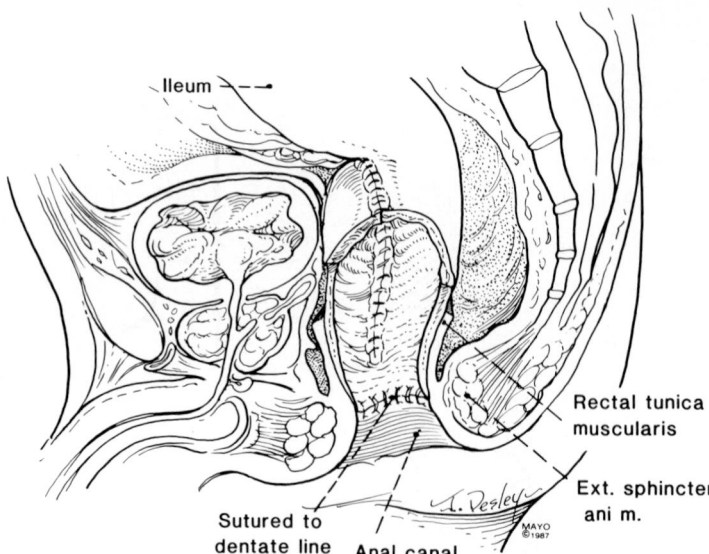

Ileum

Rectal tunica
muscularis

Ext. sphincter
ani m.

Sutured to
dentate line   Anal canal

FIGURE 40–5. Diagram of endorectal, ileal pouch–anal anastomosis. (Modified from Taylor BM, Beart RW Jr, Dozois RR, et al. Straight ileoanal anastomosis vs ileal pouch–anal anastomosis after colectomy and mucosal proctectomy. Arch Surg 1983;118:696.)

month additional period of waiting will usually allow healing, after which the closure can be done. The closure is accomplished without bowel resection through a transverse peristomal incision; the original, main midline incision need not be reopened.

Young patients (≤30 years of age) with minimal or no inflammation of their rectal mucosa, in good general health, and not on steroids, in whom a clean, tension-free, technically excellent anastomosis is made, may not require the protective loop ileostomy.[20] Patients with familial polyposis are more likely to be in this group than are patients with ulcerative colitis.[43]

Postoperative Management

Once intestinal continuity is re-established, the patients follow a fiber-free diet for 1 month and take loperamide HCl as needed to decrease stool frequency and enhance intestinal absorption. Fiber should then be introduced and encouraged. The patients should be urged to participate freely in social, domestic, occupational, sporting, and sexual activities as appropriate to their status in life.

Complications

The operation is safe. Among over 950 patients operated upon at Mayo since 1981, only two early postoperative deaths have occurred.[43] One patient died of pulmonary embolus and another patient of perforated gastric ulcer, peritonitis, and enteric fistula.

Complications appeared in the early postoperative period in 46% of patients. Intestinal obstruction was the most common complication (20% incidence). About one half of the patients developing it required operative relief. Abdominal and pelvic infection, which occurred in about 10% of our first 200 patients, developed in less than 5% of our last 200 patients. With infection, long-term results are poor. Sepsis led to pouch removal in 23 of the 48 colitis patients in whom removal was necessary.

Outcome

OVERALL DIGESTIVE FUNCTION

Overall digestive function returns to near normal status after ileostomy closure. Gastric emptying is unaltered, but transit through the small intestine is slowed, perhaps to compensate for loss of the large intestine.[36] Absorption of foodstuffs, vitamins, minerals, and bile salts is unimpaired. Few secondary bile acids are present, but the pool of primary bile salt acids is of sufficient size to allow complete digestion and absorption of fat and fat-soluble vitamins. Vitamin B_{12} is absorbed by the ileum and ileal pouch; deficiencies of Vitamin B_{12} have not appeared in the patients. Water absorption is satisfactory; the ratio of total body water to fat-free body mass is unaltered.[63] Urine output tends to be low, however, and the urine contains less sodium and is more acidic than that from healthy controls. Short-chain fatty acids are present in the fecal discharge, but they are present in concentrations smaller than those found in health.[38] Enteric output averages about 650 ml/day.

Bacteria proliferate in the pouch and in the small bowel proximal to the pouch. Both aerobic and anaerobic bacteria are present in greater numbers in the pouch and jejunum of pouch patients than in the jejunum and terminal ileum of patients with conventional Brooke ileostomy.[23] The bacterial overgrowth in pouch patients may be secondary to stasis in the pouch and may slow transit in the jejunoileum proximal to the pouch.

ANAL FUNCTION

The resting pressure of the anal sphincter is initially decreased about 10% from that of healthy controls, but the pressure returns to the control level after 6 months to 1 year.[31,56] The magnitude of the resting pressure (about 50 mm Hg) is similar during the day while fasting or after feeding and at night during sleep. Episodic decreases in pressure of 10 mm Hg to 30 mm Hg do occur at night during REM sleep, however, as they do in healthy controls.[40] Such episodes likely predispose the patients to nocturnal fecal leakage during REM sleep. Anal squeeze pressure, however, is greater than that of controls. Anal slow waves (the small, slow phasic changes in pressure that are superimposed on the baseline pressure) oscillate at a slower frequency and with a larger amplitude after operation.[31] The physiologic consequences of the changes in anal slow waves are unknown.

Sensation in the anal canal remains intact; the patients can distinguish gas, liquid, and solid enteric content as it enters the anal canal.[18] The rectal–anal inhibitory reflex is often lost, but this does not seem to influence continence.[8] The rectal–anal angle is preserved, although descent of the angle on straining may be limited.[33]

POUCH FUNCTION

The ileal pouch accommodates distention well. The distensibility of the pouch (15 ml/mm Hg) is similar to that of the healthy rectum, as is the maximum tolerable capacity (approximately 300 ml). Large phasic contractions appear in the pouch on distention, but not in the healthy rectum. The call to stool ensues when mean intraluminal pressure in the pouch reaches about 27 mm Hg[64] and when the large pouch contractions become frequent and reach amplitudes similar to mean anal sphincteric pressure.[19,28] Evacuation occurs voluntarily, rapidly (11 ml/second), and nearly completely (approximately 80% of pouch content emptied). The size of the average bowel movement is about 100 g.[27]

GENITOURINARY FUNCTION

Urinary function, beyond the first week or two after operation, is clinically unaltered. Postoperative sexual function has also been unaffected in some series,[56] but in our Mayo series 2% of male patients were impotent and 2% had retrograde ejaculation.[43] Postoperative sexual dysfunction was more common in older men than in younger men.[27] Among females, temporary dyspareunia occurred after operation in 7% of patients (Table 40-3).

Pregnancy is a viable option for women. Among 20 ileal pouch patients who became pregnant in the Mayo series, all delivered healthy infants. Eleven patients were delivered vaginally and nine by cesarean section. Pouch–anal function during and after pregnancy remained essentially unchanged from prepregnancy status regardless of the method of delivery.[39]

CLINICAL FUNCTION

Stool frequency remains steady at six small, soft bowel movements/day and one movement/night when patients are assessed from 6 months after operation up to 4 years after operation. Stool continence is perfect in 75% of patients during the day and 50% of patients at night. Mild fecal spotting (3-cm spot on underclothes

TABLE 40-3
Outcome of Ileal Pouch–Anal Anastomosis in 790 Patients

CATEGORY	STOOLING FREQUENCY (NO./DAY)	NOCTURNAL FECAL SPOTTING (% OF PATIENTS)	SEXUAL DYSFUNCTION (% OF PATIENTS)
Gender			
Men	6	44	2
Women	6	56*	7
Age			
<50 years	6	40	—
>50 years	8*	40	—†
Disease			
Colitis	6	40	8
Polyposis	4*	26*	5

* $P < 0.05$ compared to value just above.
† Greater in older subjects; see text.

two times/week) occurred in 23% of the patients during the day and 48% of the patients at night at 6 months. Continence improved by 4 years after operation, when 75% of patients were perfect at night. Only 2% of patients have gross fecal leakage; they usually end up with re-establishment of an abdominal ileostomy. The overall failure rate is 5% (i.e., abdominal stoma re-established, pouch excised), but the incidence of failure in recent years is about 2% to 3%.

Older patients have more bowel movements per day than younger patients but have a similar incidence of fecal spotting (Table 40-3). Women have more spotting than men. Patients with familial polyposis have less postoperative sepsis (none), fewer bowel movements (4.5/day), better nocturnal continence (26% with spotting), and fewer pouch excisions (none) than patients with colitis (6% sepsis, 5.8 stools/day, 40% nocturnal spotting, 5% pouch excisions).[43]

Nonspecific pouchitis has appeared symptomatically in 22% of colitis patients on mean follow-up of 4 years but in only 7% of polyposis patients. The pouchitis is heralded by the onset of watery diarrhea, sometimes with small amounts of blood, low-grade fever, malaise, pelvic pain, and systemic symptoms, such as arthralgias and uveitis. Endoscopic inspection of the pouch in such patients usually shows mucosal edema, hyperemia, punctate ulcerations, and friability. Biopsy shows acute and chronic inflammation, although the findings may be discontinuous. Also, sometimes inflammation is found in the absence of symptoms.

Bacterial overgrowth of anaerobic organisms in the pouch and in the bowel proximal to the pouch seems to have a role in the pathogenesis of pouchitis, because the clinical symptoms diminish markedly when the patients are treated with metronidazole.[23] Also, subsidence of histologic changes with therapy is often, but not necessarily, found. Most patients have one or only a few attacks, while others have persistent and recurring attacks that require long-term maintenance therapy with metronidazole or anti-inflammatory agents.

While bacteria or their toxins may have a role in the pathogenesis, other factors must be operative as well. Patients with polyposis have bacterial overgrowth in the pouch, but they have a lower incidence of pouchitis than patients with colitis. No specific bacterial pathogens have been identified. A systemic response may occur with the pouchitis. The systemic symptoms with pouchitis are oftentimes similar to those that occurred with the colitis before operation. (Lolmuller JL, Dozois RR, Wolff BG. Unpublished observations.) While anastomotic stricture and stasis in a large pouch that empties poorly can lead to pouchitis, these factors are not usually operative in most patients.

The quality of life has been excellent, with 75% to 90% of patients experiencing improved or satisfactory social, sexual, sporting, occupational, and domestic performance. Only 6% would desire a change in their postoperative status if one were available, in contrast to 40% of Brooke ileostomy patients who would like a change.[41]

To summarize, the ileal pouch–anal operation, when combined with colectomy and rectal mucosal stripping, eliminates the colorectal disease in ulcerative colitis and familial adenomatous polyposis while maintaining transanal voluntary defecation and reasonable fecal continence. A permanent abdominal ileostomy is avoided. After operation, the patients return to good health and a quality of life not dissimilar from that enjoyed by those in health. The main postoperative drawbacks, intestinal obstruction and nonspecific inflammation in the ileal pouch, are usually managed satisfactorily with medical and surgical therapy.

THE CONTINENT ILEOSTOMY (KOCK POUCH)

The continent ileostomy or Kock pouch consists of three parts: a reservoir or pouch made of distal ileum, a valve made of terminal ileum interposed between the pouch and the exterior, and an efferent ileal limb leading from the valve to the stoma. For patients who require an ileostomy, the Kock pouch provides fecal continence and eliminates the need for an ileostomy appliance.[4,47,59,60] Because of this, the stoma can be fashioned flush with the skin and placed nearer the pubis to make it less conspicuous.

Rationale

The rationale behind the procedure is that the pouch collects and holds fecal content until it is emptied by passing a catheter through the stoma and valve into the pouch. The content then drains through the catheter directly into the toilet bowl, after which the catheter is removed. The catheter is rinsed after its use and placed in a purse to be carried in the patient's pocket during the day. A small dressing is placed over the stoma after drainage to prevent mucus secreted by the surface epithelium of the ileum from soiling the clothes. In between intubations, no gas or stool leaks, so no ileal appliance need be worn. The patient has complete control over fecal discharge.

Type of Patient

This operation is suitable for young or middle-aged adults who already have an incontinent Brooke ileostomy after proctectomy or who require proctocolectomy but wish to avoid the drawbacks of an ileoanal anastomosis. Patients must have sufficient understanding, intelligence, and physical capabilities to deal with catheterization and care of the pouch. Thus, children or patients over 70 years of age are often not candidates. Also, construction of a Kock pouch is difficult in obese patients.

Technique

The operation is done in one stage and is performed with the patient in the modified lithotomy position. The proctocolectomy is accomplished, after which the pouch is fashioned from the terminal 45 cm of ileum (Figs 40-6). The anterior and posterior walls of the pouch are constructed with two layers of continuous 2-0 absorbable suture. The terminal ileum is intussuscepted into the newly formed pouch for a distance of 5 cm to form the valve. The serosal surface of the intussuscepted ileum is scarified with cautery prior to the intussusception, the adjacent mesentery is stripped of its peritoneal coat, and a window is made in the mesentery adjacent to the intussuscepted bowel to encourage adhesions and to discourage disintussusception. The intussuscepted ileum is anchored in place with four cartridges of stainless steel staples or with sutures. Additional sutures of 4-0 Dacron are placed at the exit of the efferent limb from the pouch to further anchor the valve in place. We have not used fascia lata or plastic mesh to enhance fixation of the valve because of the risk of infection and fistula. The efferent ileal limb leading to the stoma is made as short as possible, and the stoma is placed just above the hairline in the right lower quadrant. The pouch is sewn to the anterior abdominal wall just beneath the stoma, again with interrupted 4-0 Dacron sutures. The ileostomy is made flush with the skin. The space lateral to the pouch is closed by approximating the ileal mesentery to the parietal peritoneum of the right lower quadrant of the abdomen. This obviates volvulus of the pouch and peripouch herniation of the more proximal small intestine.

Postoperative Care

The pouch is intubated and drained continuously for the first postoperative month to ensure that it and the valve remain in the appropriate position while the fibrous tissue of healing fixes the structures in place. The tube is then removed, and the patient begins intermittent intubation of the pouch. At first, the intubations are done every 2 hours during the day, and the catheter is left in place continuously overnight. The interval between intubations is increased gradually so that after the second month the patient is intubating the pouch four times a day, but not at night. Patients require no medication and can eat a general diet provided that they masticate thoroughly. Poorly masticated, indigestible materials, such as mushrooms, kernels of corn, string beans, and cab-

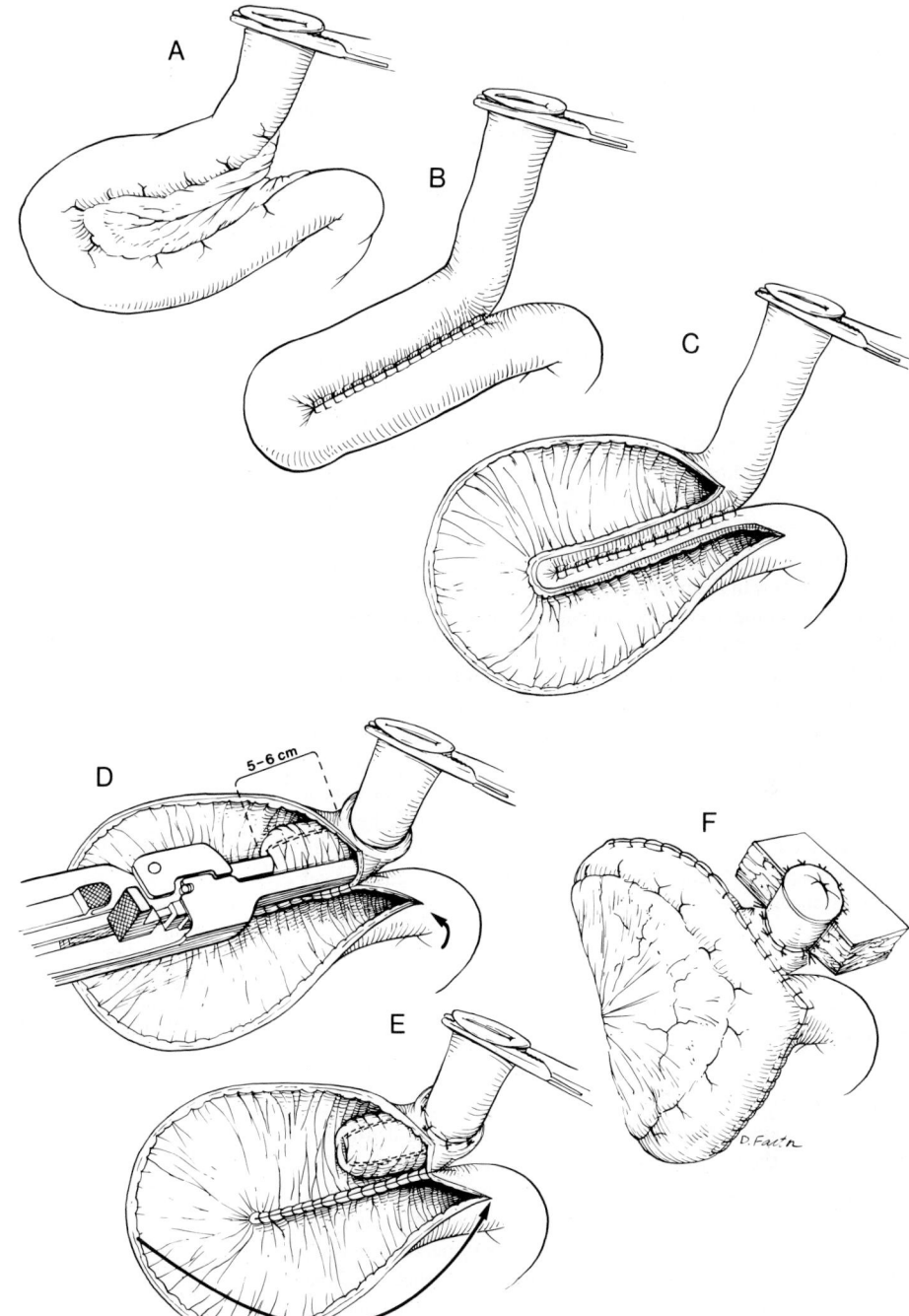

FIGURE 40–6. Construction of continent ileal pouch (Kock pouch). **A,** Terminal 45 cm of ileum positioned to form pouch. **B,** 15-cm limbs approximated with 2-0 continuous catgut. **C,** Incision made into antimesenteric border of limbs. Construction of continent ileal pouch (continued). **D,** Terminal ileum intussuscepted into newly forming pouch and anchored with staples. **E,** Anterior wall of pouch formed by folding over the ileum. **F,** Completed pouch with short efferent limb and skin-flush stoma.

bage, may plug the catheter during intubations and interfere with emptying. The patients should irrigate the pouch free of debris at least once a day with warm water or a saline solution.

Complications

The immediate postoperative complications (e.g., intestinal obstruction and sepsis) and the long-term complications (e.g., gall-

stones and urinary stones) are similar to those of other types of ileostomy. In addition, complications specific to the procedure may occur: slippage of the valve, valve prolapse, stomal stenosis, and pouch-related diarrhea.

Slippage of the valve occurs because the intussuscepted terminal ileum used to make the valve sometimes reduces partially, resulting in a tortuous tract leading from the pouch to the exterior. The patient then has two problems: difficulty intubating the pouch and leakage of content from the pouch. Reoperation is usually required, at which time the valve must be replaced within the pouch and

TABLE 40–4
Outcome of Ileostomy and Ileal Pouch Operations

PROCEDURE	FECAL CONTINENCE PRESERVED	STOMA PRESENT	INTUBATIONS REQUIRED	DISADVANTAGES
Brooke ileostomy	No	Yes	No	Ileostomy bag required
Ileal pouch–anal anastomosis	Yes	No	No	Occasional fecal leakage, pouchitis
Continent ileostomy (Kock pouch)	Yes	Yes	Yes	Valve malfunction, pouchitis

reanchored with stainless steel staples and sutures. Reoperation is necessary today in about 15% of patients and is usually successful.[4] However, reoperation does not guarantee that the valve will function perfectly henceforth. A second reoperation may be required in an additional 15% to 20% of patients.

Prolapse of the valve through the stoma to the exterior can also occur. Again, reoperation is required, replacing the valve into the pouch, reanchoring it in place, and narrowing the opening in the abdominal wall through which the prolapse has occurred. Stenosis of the stoma, a complication usually related to ischemia of the stoma, can usually be managed by a local operation, during which the stoma is excised, the efferent ileum mobilized, and a new stoma made at the same site.

Diarrhea, which occurs in about one third of patients over the long term, likely results from "pouchitis" that may be caused by bacterial overgrowth in the pouch, just as in the ileal pouch–anal operation. The diarrhea, when symptomatic, can usually be managed satisfactorily with antibiotics, such as metronidazole, 250 mg q.i.d. Other possible causes of diarrhea, such as partial small bowel obstruction and lactase deficiency, may be responsible and require correction.

Outcome

The procedure does achieve its objective of providing complete control over fecal discharge. The patients do have an ileostomy, however, and they must intubate the ileal pouch to empty it. The physiology and bacteriology of the Kock pouch are similar to those of the ileal pouch used in the ileal–anal operation. A greater dilatation of the Kock pouch occurs in the postoperative period, however, likely because of the more complete obstruction of the outflow of gas and stool occasioned by the valve of the pouch as opposed to the natural anal sphincter of the ileal–anal anastomosis. The pouch retains the absorptive and motor functions of the ileum in health, but the capacity of the pouch is much greater than that of the unoperated terminal ileum.

CHOICE OF OPERATION

Nonobese patients who are less than 65 years of age, who have a competent anal sphincter, and who require operation for chronic ulcerative colitis and polyposis coli usually choose the ileal pouch–anal anastomosis. The major advantages of this operation include total excision of the disease, avoidance of a permanent ileostomy,

maintenance of transanal fecal flow, and reasonable fecal continence (Table 40-4). Obese patients and older patients usually require proctocolectomy and a Brooke ileostomy. The continent ileal pouch of Kock is used mainly for patients who already have had their rectum excised and who have an incontinent Brooke ileostomy.

> The reader is directed to Chapter 14, Secretion and Absorption: Small Intestine and Colon; Chapter 38, Approach to the Patient with Diarrhea; and Chapter 77, Inflammatory Bowel Disease.

REFERENCES

1. Roy PH, Sauer WG, Beahrs OH, et al. Experience with ileostomies: Evaluation of long-term rehabilitation in 497 patients. Am J Surg 1970;119:77.
2. Schwab PM, Kelly KA. Primary closure of the perineal wound after proctectomy: A new technique. Mayo Clin Proc 1974;49:176.
3. McIlrath DC, van Heerden JA, Edis AJ, et al. Closure of abdominal incisions with subcutaneous catheters. Surgery 1976;80:411.
4. Dozois RR, Kelly KA, Ilstrup D, et al. Factors affecting revision rate after continent ileostomy. Arch Surg 1981;116:610.
5. Telander RL, Perrault J. Colectomy with rectal mucosectomy and ileo-anal anastomosis in young patients. Arch Surg 1981;116:623.
6. Beart RW Jr, Dozois RR, Kelly KA. Ileoanal anastomosis in the adult. Surg Gynecol Obstet 1982;154:826.
7. Heppell J, Kelly KA, Phillips SF, et al. Physiologic aspects of continence after colectomy, mucosal proctectomy, and endorectal ileo-anal anastomosis. Ann Surg 1982;195:435.
8. Heppell J, Pemberton JH, Kelly KA, Phillips SF. Ileal motility after endorectal ileo-anal anastomosis. Surg Gastroenterol 1982;1:123.
9. Heppell J, Taylor BM, Beart RW Jr, et al. Predicting outcome after endorectal ileoanal anastomosis. Can J Surg 1983;26:132.
10. Taylor BM, Beart RW Jr, Dozois RR, et al. Straight ileoanal anastomosis vs ileal pouch-anal anastomosis after colectomy and mucosal proctectomy. Arch Surg 1983;118:696.
11. Taylor BM, Cranley B, Kelly KA, et al. A clinico-physiological comparison of ileal pouch–anal and straight ileoanal anastomoses. Ann Surg 1983;198:462.
12. Taylor BM, Beart RW Jr, Dozois RR, et al. The endorectal ileal pouch–anal anastomosis: Current clinical results. Dis Colon Rectum 1984;27:347.
13. Pemberton JH, Phillips SF, Dozois RR, et al. Conventional ileostomy—Current clinical results. In: Dozois RR, ed. Alternatives to conventional ileostomy. Chicago: Year Book Medical Publishers, 1985:40.
14. Kelly KA. Ileal pouch–anal anastomosis after proctocolectomy. Surg Rounds 1985;8:48.

15. Stryker SJ, Borody TJ, Phillips SF, et al. Motility of the small intestine after proctocolectomy and ileal pouch–anal anastomosis. Ann Surg 1985;201:351.

16. Stryker SJ, Daube JR, Kelly KA, et al. Anal sphincter electromyography after colectomy, mucosal rectectomy, and ileoanal anastomosis. Arch Surg 1985;120:713.

17. Metcalf AM, Dozois RR, Kelly KA, et al. Ileal "J" pouch–anal anastomosis: Clinical outcome. Ann Surg 1985;202:735.

18. Beart RW Jr, Dozois RR, Wolff BG, Pemberton JH. Mechanisms of rectal continence. Lessons from the ileoanal procedure. Am J Surg 1985;149:31.

19. Stryker SJ, Kelly KA, Phillips SF, et al. Anal and neorectal function after ileal pouch–anal anastomosis. Ann Surg 1986;203:55.

20. Metcalf AM, Dozois RR, Kelly KA, Wolff BG. Ileal pouch–anal anastomosis without temporary, diverting ileostomy. Dis Colon Rectum 1986;29:33.

21. O'Connell PR, Kelly KA, Brown ML. Scintigraphic assessment of neorectal motor function. J Nucl Med 1986;27:460.

22. Metcalf AM, Dozois RR, Beart RW Jr, et al. Temporary ileostomy for ileal pouch–anal anastomosis: Functions and complications. Dis Colon Rectum 1986;29:300.

23. O'Connell PR, Rankin DR, Weiland LH, Kelly KA. Enteric bacteriology, absorption, morphology and emptying after ileal pouch–anal anastomosis. Br J Surg 1986;73:909.

24. Metcalf AM, Dozois RR, Kelly KA. Sexual function in women after proctocolectomy. Ann Surg 1986;204:624.

25. O'Connell PR, Pemberton JH, Brown ML, Kelly KA. Determinants of stool frequency after ileal pouch–anal anastomosis. Am J Surg 1987;153:157.

26. Gustavsson S, Weiland LH, Kelly KA. Relationship of backwash ileitis to ileal pouchitis after ileal pouch–anal anastomosis. Dis Colon Rectum 1987;30:25.

27. Pemberton JH, Kelly KA, Beart RW Jr, et al. Ileal pouch–anal anastomosis for chronic ulcerative colitis: Long-term results. Ann Surg 1987;206:504.

28. O'Connell PR, Pemberton JH, Kelly KA. Motor function of the ileal J pouch and its relation to clinical outcome after ileal pouch–anal anastomosis. World J Surg 1987;11:735.

29. O'Connell PR, Pemberton JH, Weiland LH, et al. Does rectal mucosa regenerate after ileoanal anastomosis? Dis Colon Rectum 1987;30:1.

30. Dozois RR. Pelvic and perianastomotic complications after ileal pouch–anal anastomosis. Perspectives in Colon and Rectal Surgery 1988;1:113.

31. O'Connell PR, Stryker SJ, Metcalf AM, et al. Anal canal pressure and motility after ileoanal anastomosis. Surg Gynecol Obstet 1988;166:47.

32. Taylor BA, Wolff BG, Dozois RR, et al. Ileal pouch–anal anastomosis for chronic ulcerative colitis and familial polyposis coli complicated by adenocarcinoma. Dis Colon Rectum 1988;31:358.

33. Barkel DC, Pemberton JH, Pezim ME, et al. Scintigraphic assessment of the anorectal angle in health and after ileal pouch–anal anastomosis. Ann Surg 1988;208:42.

34. Scott NA, Dozois RR, Beart RW Jr, et al. Postoperative intra-abdominal and pelvic sepsis complicating ileal pouch–anal anastomosis. Int J Colorectal Dis 1988;3:149.

35. Francois Y, Dozois RR, Kelly KA, et al. Small intestinal obstruction complicating ileal pouch–anal anastomosis. Ann Surg 1989;209:46.

36. Soper NJ, Orkin BA, Kelly KA, et al. Gastrointestinal transit after proctocolectomy with ileal pouch–anal anastomosis or ileostomy. J Surg Res 1989;46:300.

37. Ambroze WL, Bell AM, Pemberton JH, et al. The effect of stool consistency on rectal and neorectal emptying. Gastroenterology 1989;96:A11.

38. Ambroze WL, Pemberton JH, Bell AM, et al. Fecal short chain fatty acids after ileal pouch–anal anastomosis. Gastroenterology 1989;96:A11.

39. Nelson H, Dozois RR, Kelly KA, et al. The effect of pregnancy and delivery on the ileal pouch–anal anastomosis functions. Dis Colon Rectum 1989;32:384.

40. Orkin BA, Kelly KA, Dent J. Influence of sleep on anal canal resting pressure. Gastroenterology 1989;96:A378.

41. Pemberton JH, Phillips SF, Ready RR, et al. Quality of life after Brooke ileostomy and ileal pouch–anal anastomosis: Comparison of performance status. Ann Surg 1989;209:620.

42. Scott NA, Barkel DC, Wolff BG, et al. Anal and ileal pouch manometric measurements before ileostomy closure are related to functional outcome after ileostomy closure. Br J Surg 1989;76:613.

43. Dozois RR, Kelly KA, Welling DR, et al. Ileal pouch–anal anastomosis: Comparison of results in familial adenomatous polyposis and chronic ulcerative colitis. Ann Surg 1989;210:268.

44. Pezim ME, Pemberton JH, Beart RW Jr, et al. Outcome of "indeterminate" colitis following ileal pouch–anal anastomosis. Dis Colon Rectum 1989;32:653.

45. Brooke BN. The management of an ileostomy including its complications. Lancet 1952;2:102.

46. Turnbull RB Jr. Management of ileostomy. Am J Surg 1953;86:617.

47. Kock NG. A new look at ileostomy. Surg Annu 1976;8:241.

48. Lyttle JA, Parks AG. Intersphincteric excision of the rectum. Br J Surg 1977;64:413.

49. Martin LW, LeCoultre C, Shubert WK. Total colectomy and mucosal proctectomy with preservation of continence in ulcerative colitis. Ann Surg 1977;186:477.

50. Utsunomiya J, Iwama T, Imago M, et al. Total colectomy, mucosal proctectomy and ileoanal anastomosis. Dis Colon Rectum 1980;23:459.

51. Parks AG, Nicholls RJ, Belliveau P. Proctocolectomy with ileal reservoir and anal anastomosis. Br J Surg 1980;67:533.

52. Fonkalsrud EW. Endorectal pull-through with ileal reservoir for ulcerative colitis and polyposis. Am J Surg 1982;144:81.

53. Kennedy HJ, Al-Dujaili EAS, Edwards CRW, et al. Water and electrolyte balance in subjects with a permanent ileostomy. Gut 1983;24:702.

54. Coran AG, Sarahan TM, Dent TL, et al. The endorectal pullthrough for the management of ulcerative colitis in children and adults. Ann Surg 1983;197:99.

55. Nicholls RJ, Pezim ME. Restorative proctocolectomy with ileal reservoir for ulcerative colitis and familial adenomatous polyposis: A comparison of three reservoir designs. Br J Surg 1985;72:470.

56. Becker JM, Raymond JL. Ileal pouch–anal anastomosis: A single surgeon's experience with 100 consecutive cases. Ann Surg 1986;204:375.

57. Heald RJ, Allen DR. Stapled ileo-anal anastomosis: A technique to avoid mucosal proctectomy in the ileal pouch operation. Br J Surg 1986;73:571.

58. Johnston D, Holdsworth PJ, Nasmyth DG, et al. Preservation of the entire anal canal in conservative proctocolectomy for ulcerative colitis: A pilot study comparing end-to-end ileo-anal anastomosis without mucosal resection with mucosal proctectomy and endo-anal anastomosis. Br J Surg 1987;74:940.

59. Myrvold HE. The continent ileostomy. World J Surg 1987;11:735.

60. Fazio VW, Church JM. Complications and function of the continent ileostomy of the Cleveland Clinic. World J Surg 1988;12:148.

61. Brough WA, Schofield PF. An improved technique of J pouch construction and ileoanal anastomosis. Br J Surg 1989;76:350.

62. Williams NS. Stapling technique for pouch–anal anastomosis without the need for purse-string sutures. Br J Surg 1989;76:348.

63. Christie PM, Knight GS, Hill GL. Metabolism of body water and electrolytes after surgery for ulcerative colitis: Brooke ileostomy versus J pouch. Aust N Z J Surg 1989;59:268.

64. Harms BA, Pahl AC, Starling JR. Comparison of clinical and compliance characteristics between "S" and "W" ileal reservoirs. Am J Surg 1990;159:34.

41

Approach to the Patient with Jaundice

PETER G. TRABER
JORGE J. GUMUCIO

Jaundice (or icterus) is yellow pigmentation of the sclerae, skin, and mucous membranes that occurs as a result of tissue deposition of excess levels of serum bilirubin. Many important clinical disorders present with jaundice, and its presence centers attention on the liver, biliary tree, and pancreas. Hyperbilirubinemia becomes clinically manifest as jaundice when the serum bilirubin is between 2 and 4 mg/dl (34–68 μmole/liter); the level of detection will vary depending on natural skin coloration, the type of light in which the patient is examined (i.e., natural versus fluorescent), and the rapidity of the rise in serum bilirubin. The bilirubin pigment is most intense in tissues that contain large amounts of elastin, such as the sclerae, because bilirubin avidly binds to this extracellular matrix protein. Detection of minimal elevations in serum bilirubin may be first detected in the frenulum of the tongue. Yellow discoloration of skin can also occur from massive ingestion of carotene- or lycopene-containing vegetables, the antimalarial drug quinacrine, uremia, and exposure to dinitrophenol or picric acid; these can easily be distinguished from jaundice by determination of the serum bilirubin and the lack of scleral icterus.

The evaluation of jaundice requires a thorough understanding of the differential diagnosis of hyperbilirubinemia as well as the differential diagnoses of hepatocellular disease and cholestasis. In this chapter, bilirubin metabolism will be reviewed and the causes of hyperbilirubinemia will be presented based on abnormalities in the formation, metabolism, or excretion of this bile pigment. Hyperbilirubinemia in adults is most often associated with diffuse dysfunction or necrosis of hepatocytes or with a cholestatic syndrome. The hepatic disorders that cause hepatocellular necrosis or dysfunction resulting in jaundice include virtually every liver disease and, therefore, will not be discussed in detail.

Cholestasis is a syndrome of characteristic serum biochemical and hepatic morphologic findings that result from impaired bile formation or bile flow and may be caused by diseases that affect hepatocytes, the biliary system, or the pancreas. The etiologic classification of cholestasis has, in previous discussions of this syndrome, been subdivided into "medical" and "surgical" causes of jaundice as related to the form of therapy required. In the era of modern gastroenterologic and surgical practice, the distinction between "medical" and "surgical" jaundice has blurred. For in-stance, classical "surgical" etiologies, such as choledocholithiasis, are now amenable to "medical" therapy, such as endoscopic retrograde cholangiography with sphincterotomy and stone extraction or biliary lithotripsy. Therefore, it is more useful to subdivide cholestasis into intrahepatic and extrahepatic (biliary) causes without reference to the required therapy.

The diagnostic approach to the patient with jaundice will be discussed by reviewing important aspects of the history, physical examination, and routine laboratory tests. From this evaluation the type of hyperbilirubinemia can be discerned and, if due to hepatobiliary disease, the disease process can be classified as primarily hepatocellular or cholestatic. In addition, from these routine examinations, the site of the pathologic process in many cholestatic patients can be ascertained and can, therefore, guide the use of other diagnostic modalities. Strategies for the use of specialized diagnostic tests will be presented so that a logical and cost-effective evaluation can be designed for the individual patient.

BILIRUBIN METABOLISM

Bilirubin is a yellow tetrapyrrole compound that is, essentially, a waste product of heme metabolism (Fig 41-1).[1-3] Recently, it has been suggested that bilirubin may function as an antioxidant and, therefore, may perform a physiologic function.[4] The bilirubin molecule is configured such that internal hydrogen bonds expose hydrophobic groups on the exterior of the molecule; the result is that bilirubin is highly lipid soluble.[5] Because of its hydrophobicity, bilirubin is solubilized in bile by micelles and in serum by binding to serum proteins such as albumin.[5] Investigation of the production and excretion of bilirubin has been a difficult challenge because of the molecule's hydrophobicity, its instability in aqueous solution, and its sensitivity to oxidation when exposed to light.[5] The metabolic pathway outlined below represents the work of many investigators and has been summarized in an excellent monograph.[1] Bilirubin metabolic pathways are summarized in Figure 41-2.

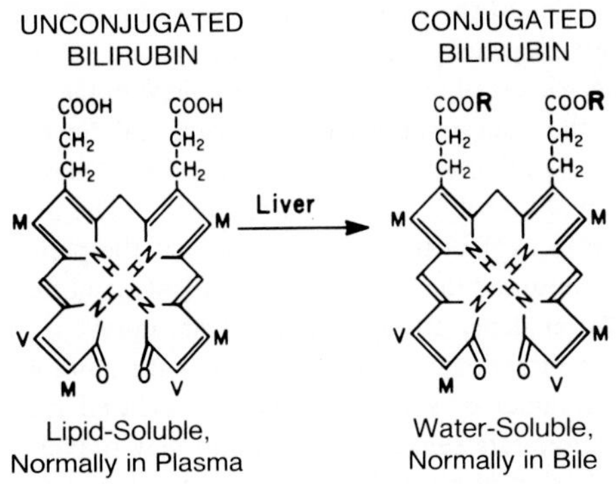

UNCONJUGATED
BILIRUBIN

CONJUGATED
BILIRUBIN

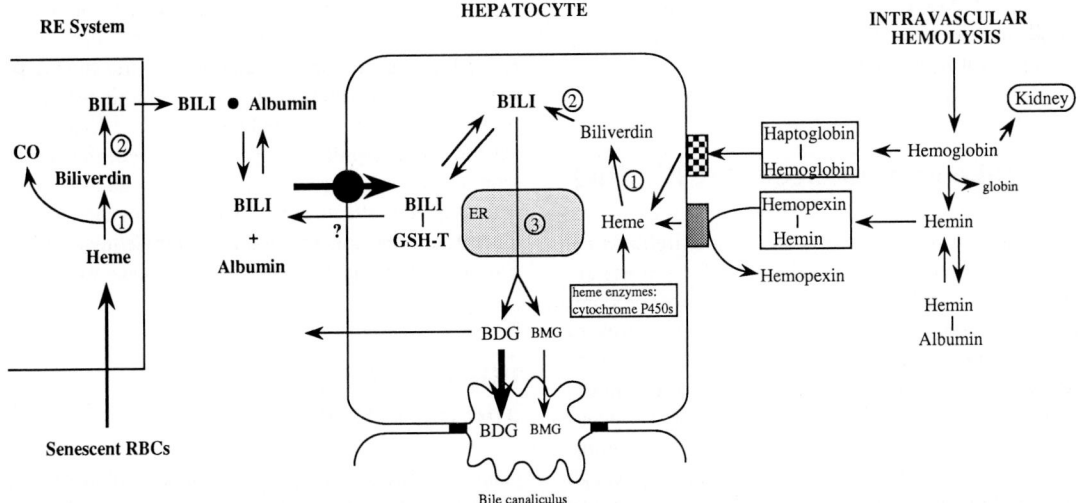

Lipid-Soluble,
Normally in Plasma

Water-Soluble,
Normally in Bile

FIGURE 41–1. Chemical structures of unconjugated and conjugated bilirubin (*M,* methyl; *V,* vinyl; *R,* conjugated group that may be glucuronic acid, glucose, or xylose). (From Ostrow JD. Bile pigments and jaundice: molecular, metabolic and medical aspects. New York: Marcel Dekker, 1986.)

Bilirubin Production

The source of the heme that is converted to bilirubin has been studied in vivo by labeling of the heme pool with ^{14}C aminolevulinic acid in both animals and humans.[6–8] The major peak of radiolabeled bilirubin, in humans, occurs at approximately 120 days following the injection of the label.[8] The average life span of a red blood cell is 120 days, and, therefore, the timing of this peak of labeled bilirubin suggested that the majority of bilirubin production results from the breakdown of senescent red blood cells and hemoglobin catabolism.[8] Indeed, it has been confirmed in numerous studies that hemoglobin is the source for approximately 80% of bilirubin in animals and man.[2,3,8] There is also an early peak of labeled bilirubin that is detected within 72 hours following labeling of the heme pool; this can constitute up to 26% of bilirubin production in humans.[6] This "early peak" bilirubin actually has two components. The initial bilirubin production results from turnover of the hepatic free heme pool and the catabolism of heme-containing enzymes in liver, predominantly the cytochrome P450. The later component of "early peak" bilirubin results from intramarrow breakdown of red blood cells, or ineffective erythropoiesis, and a small fraction results from the breakdown of renal heme.[6] Myoglobin, another major heme-containing protein, has a very slow turnover rate, and the contribution to the bilirubin load by its catabolism appears to be insignificant.[6]

Senescent red blood cells are phagocytized by reticuloendothelial cells located predominantly in spleen, liver (Kupffer cells) and, to a more limited extent, bone marrow. In addition to the phagocytosis of senescent blood cells, hemoglobin-derived heme

FIGURE 41–2. Pathways of bilirubin metabolism. The breakdown of senescent red blood cells in reticuloendothelial (RE) cells located in spleen, liver, and bone marrow (RE system) contributes approximately 80% of the total daily bilirubin load. The remaining 20% of bilirubin is derived from heme that results primarily from metabolism of heme-containing enzymes, and a small fraction comes from intravascular hemolysis or ineffective erythropoesis. In hemolytic states, the load of hemolytic heme can be dramatically increased. In this situation, hemoglobin binds to haptoglobin and is taken up by hepatocytes by a receptor-mediated process; a proportion of hemoglobin is oxidized to hemin and globin, and the hemin is bound to hemopexin with subsequent uptake by the liver. In addition, a significant proportion of intravascular hemoglobin may be metabolized by the renal cortex in hemolytic anemias. In either the RE system macrophages or in the hepatocyte, heme is oxidized to biliverdin by heme oxygenase (1) with the production of stoichiometric amounts of carbon monoxide. The biliverdin is converted to bilirubin by biliverdin reductase (2), which requires NADPH or NADH for activity. Bilirubin is transported in the serum reversibly and is noncovalently bound to albumin. At the hepatocellular sinusoidal membrane, bilirubin that dissociates from albumin is available for transport across the membrane by a specific transport protein. The bilirubin that is taken up can flow back into sinusoidal blood, but the mechanism is unknown. In the cytoplasm, bilirubin reversibly binds to glutathione S-transferase B (formerly called ligandin [*GSH-T* in figure]); this binding effectively traps bilirubin in the hepatocyte cytosolic compartment. Bilirubin is conjugated in the endoplasmic reticulum (ER) by UDP-glucuronosyltransferase (3). The bilirubin conjugates, *BDG* (bilirubin diglucuronide) and *BMG* (bilirubin monoglucuronide), are transported across the canalicular membrane and into bile. There may be reflux of some of the conjugated bilirubin into the sinusoidal blood by unknown mechanisms; although this is a small amount in normal subjects, there is a large reflux in liver diseases.

may be available for metabolism to bilirubin as a result of ineffective erythropoiesis or intravascular hemolysis. Ineffective erythropoiesis refers to the destruction of nascent red blood cells in the bone marrow before they are able to enter the circulation. Under normal circumstances, ineffective erythropoiesis accounts for less than 3% of bilirubin production,[6] but this may be greatly increased in certain pathologic processes such as pernicious anemia. Intravascular hemolysis ordinarily accounts for an even smaller fraction of total bilirubin production but can become the predominant source in certain hemolytic disorders. Hemoglobin and heme that are released into the serum as a result of hemolysis are bound to haptoglobin and to hemopexin, respectively, and the complexes bind to specific hepatic receptors; uptake and subsequent metabolism in hepatocytes follow.[6]

The first step in the metabolism of heme (iron-protoporphyrin IX-α is the specific stereoisomer produced in mammals) is catalyzed by heme oxygenase, a microsomal enzyme present in high concentrations in splenic macrophages, Kupffer cells, and bone marrow macrophages.[1,3,6] In hemolytic states, heme oxygenase can be induced to high levels in renal tubular cells as well.[6] The cleavage of the heme ring by heme oxygenase releases iron and generates one molecule of carbon monoxide and biliverdin IX-α. The carbon monoxide is excreted via the lungs; exhaled carbon monoxide is a sensitive measure of heme catabolism, but this test is available only in research centers.[2,3,6] Biliverdin IX-α is converted to bilirubin IX-α by biliverdin reductase, a cytosolic enzyme, in a reaction that requires NADPH as a cofactor.[6] The conversion of biliverdin to bilirubin is quite efficient, and, therefore, virtually no biliverdin is present in serum or bile.[6]

Hepatic Uptake and Intracellular Binding

Following generation in reticuloendothelial cells, bilirubin is released into the circulation (the mechanisms of this process are unknown), where it is tightly bound to serum proteins, predominantly albumin.[9] Binding of bilirubin to albumin helps to prevent its toxic effects on the immature brain.[10,11] Drugs that compete with bilirubin for binding sites on albumin, such as sulfonamides and anti-inflammatory drugs, increase the free bilirubin concentration and increase toxicity of bilirubin in infants.[10,11] Albumin-bound bilirubin is accessible for uptake into hepatocytes through the fenestrated endothelial cells that line the hepatic sinusoids; the fenestrae allow large protein molecules to pass into the space of Disse and interact with the hepatocyte basolateral membrane.[12]

Bilirubin is transported across the hepatocyte basolateral membrane by a saturable, carrier-mediated transport process that is distinct from the carrier involved in bile acid transport.[12] This transport process is bidirectional, and, therefore, intracellular bilirubin can also be transported back into the sinusoidal space.[12] It appears that the membrane transporter is a dimer of approximately 105,000 dalton molecular weight that can be dissociated into two 55,000 molecular weight proteins.[13,14] The polypeptide monomers bind sulfobromophthalein (BSP) and bilirubin, but not bile acids, and antibodies to these monomers stain both basolateral and canalicular membrane domains of hepatocytes, but not other parenchymal cells.[14] In addition, antibodies to this membrane protein inhibit uptake of BSP into isolated rat hepatocytes.[15] Further

characterization of the transporter must await purification of the protein to homogeneity, protein sequencing, and cDNA cloning.

The mechanism of interaction of bilirubin with the extracellular domain of the transport protein is controversial. Several investigators proposed that uptake of bilirubin and BSP may depend on the fraction of bilirubin bound to albumin.[16–19] The hypothesized mechanism to explain this phenomenon was the presence of an albumin receptor on the hepatocyte sinusoidal membrane.[19] However, recent evidence strongly suggests that uptake is dependent on the "free" fraction,[12,20,21] and this is now the more widely held theory. A number of studies in isolated perfused rat liver and analbuminemic rats suggest that albumin may prevent the nonspecific diffusion of bilirubin into tissues but is not required for hepatic uptake.[2] The effects of binding of organic anions (i.e., BSP) to albumin have been studied in the isolated perfused rat liver. Albumin binding serves the purpose of distributing BSP throughout hepatocytes of the liver acinus.[2,12,22–24] Although similar studies have not been performed with bilirubin, the principal findings may pertain to bilirubin as well. In the absence of albumin, BSP concentrates in the few hepatocytes located in the periportal area, the cells first exposed to the incoming load.[23] This may result in the attainment of high and potentially toxic concentrations of organic anions in these cells. Binding to albumin, by distributing the incoming concentration into hepatocytes throughout the acinus, avoids this possible overload of a few hepatocytes.

Following uptake, bilirubin is bound by intracellular proteins, a process that may trap bilirubin in the intracellular compartment and prevent reflux into the sinusoidal blood.[2,12] The major bilirubin-binding protein is glutathione S-transferase B (ligandin), with smaller contributions by other glutathione S-transferases and by the liver fatty acid–binding protein.[2,12] Increases in the concentration of ligandin in the rat liver reduce the efflux of bilirubin from hepatocytes into the sinusoid, but the rate of uptake of bilirubin is not affected by changes in ligandin concentration.[25] Therefore, the concentration of intracellular bilirubin-binding proteins influences the net bilirubin uptake by hepatocytes.[25]

Bilirubin Conjugation and Secretion Into Bile

Conversion of bilirubin to glucuronides is obligatory for excretion of bilirubin from hepatocytes into bile canaliculi.[2,3,26] UDP-glucuronic acid is added to the propionic side chains of bilirubin by esterification catalyzed by bilirubin UDP-glucuronosyltransferase.[27] This enzyme is a member of a family of glucuronosyltransferases that are located in the smooth and rough endoplasmic reticulum of hepatocytes.[26] Since there are two propionic side chains on each bilirubin molecule, glucuronic acid may be conjugated to one or both of the propionic acids; 80% of bilirubin in bile is in the form of bilirubin diglucuronide.[2,26] Trace amounts of other sugar conjugates such as bilirubin glucoside and xyloside are also found in human bile.[26]

Current theory maintains that conjugated bilirubin is secreted into bile via a carrier-mediated transport process to transport bilirubin conjugates against a concentration gradient.[27] Although there is considerable evidence to support this hypothesis, definitive measurements of bile pigment concentration in canaliculi and other technical considerations have made this theory difficult to rigorously substantiate.[27] In studies of bilirubin clearance in vivo and in the isolated perfused rat liver, secretion of conjugated bilirubin across the canalicular membrane appears to be the rate-limiting step in the transport of bilirubin into bile.[27] Therefore, in hepatocellular disease, bilirubin secretion is relatively more impaired than are uptake and conjugation, and conjugated bilirubin accumulates intracellularly, is secreted back into sinusoids, and its levels increase in blood.

Metabolism Within the Gastrointestinal Lumen and Extrahepatic Excretion

Bilirubin glucuronides traverse most of the length of the small intestine without undergoing absorption or metabolism.[28] In this way, conjugation of bilirubin may be viewed as a mechanism designed to prevent bilirubin re-entry into the systemic circulation. In the distal ileum and colon, bilirubin glucuronides are subjected to metabolism by bacteria.[28] Bacteria act on bilirubin glucuronides to remove the sugar conjugate by the action of β-glucuronidase and, subsequently, to convert bilirubin to a series of colorless compounds called urobilinogens. Both unconjugated bilirubin and urobilinogens are absorbed by the distal small intestine and colon and undergo enterohepatic circulation with the majority excreted into bile; a small fraction of urobilinogen is excreted into urine.[28] Urobilinogens, in addition, can be further metabolized to urobilin and other compounds that are excreted in stool and provide some of the pigmentation characteristic of feces.[28] Measurement of urobilinogens in urine has been used as an indication of the bilirubin load excreted into the gastrointestinal tract. In disease states in which the production of bilirubin is increased, such as hemolytic anemia, urinary urobilinogen may be increased, and conversely, in biliary obstruction, urinary urobilinogen may be very low. This measurement plays a minor role in the evaluation of a jaundiced patient because it does not sufficiently discriminate between overproduction of bilirubin and cholestatic states.

Conjugated bilirubin is more water-soluble than unconjugated bilirubin and is not highly protein-bound; therefore, it is excreted into urine.[28] Conjugated bilirubin is filtered at the glomerulus, and the majority is then reabsorbed by the proximal tubules; only a small fraction is excreted in the urine. Unconjugated bilirubin is tightly bound to serum proteins and is thus not filtered at the glomerulus, and none is detected in urine. Therefore, the presence or absence of bilirubin in the urine may be an early clinical clue to the nature of the hyperbilirubinemia. Unconjugated hyperbilirubinemia will not lead to bile pigment in urine, whereas bilirubin may be detected in the urine in conjugated hyperbilirubinemia. The detection of bilirubin in the urine in conjugated hyperbilirubinemia depends on the stage of the liver disease. Early in the course of viral hepatitis, bilirubin may be detected in the urine before jaundice is evident, whereas later in the disease process, urinary bilirubin may be absent in the presence of overt jaundice. This phenomenon may be due to the accumulation of bilirubin–albumin over the course of the hepatitis. Thus, the absence of bilirubin in the urine does not exclude conjugated hyperbilirubinemia in a jaundiced patient.

DIFFERENTIAL DIAGNOSIS OF HYPERBILIRUBINEMIA

Measurement of Serum Bilirubin

The level of serum bilirubin in 95% of normal adults ($+2$ S.D. from mean) is 3 to 15 μmole/liter (0.2–0.9 mg/dl), and approximately 96% of the total bilirubin is present as unconjugated bilirubin IX-alpha.[29] The remaining fraction of total bilirubin, approximately 4%, is in the form of mono- and diester conjugates as demonstrated by a sensitive liquid chromatographic technique.[29] In jaundiced patients there may be small amounts of bilirubin IX-alpha isomers that form as a result of photoreactions in skin as well as bilirubin covalently bound to serum proteins.[29] In patients with conjugated hyperbilirubinemia, up to 60% of the serum bilirubin may be covalently bound to serum proteins, primarily albumin; of the bilirubin conjugates, only bilirubin glucuronides are involved in this reaction.[29] Therefore, in those patients with significant amounts of bilirubin–albumin (also called delta bilirubin and bil-alb) in serum, the half-life of the serum bilirubin will be the same as albumin, approximately 12 to 14 days. This may account for the persistence of jaundice after the relief of a biliary obstruction.

Knowledge of how serum bilirubin is measured is necessary to properly evaluate bilirubin levels. The most common method employed in clinical laboratories uses spectrophotometric quantitation of azo derivatives of bilirubin (van den Bergh reaction or variations of this original method).[29] Diazotized aromatic amines cleave the bilirubin molecule into two identical molecules bound to the azo compound that are detected spectrophotometrically and differentiated from other serum components. If the reaction is performed in acidic aqueous media (the "direct reaction") conjugated bilirubin, both free and bilirubin conjugates that are covalently bound to albumin will react with the azo compound; this is referred to as direct-reacting bilirubin. An accelerator compound, such as alcohol, is then added, which promotes the cleavage of unconjugated bilirubin by the azo compound, thus yielding a measurement of total serum bilirubin. The "indirect" fraction, or unconjugated bilirubin, is calculated from the difference between total and direct bilirubin. However, this method does not accurately reflect the true concentration of either unconjugated or conjugated bilirubin. The direct measurement also detects other bilirubin isomers present in small amounts and, importantly, a small fraction of unconjugated bilirubin.[29] Therefore, this method overestimates the amount of conjugated bilirubin in serum, and some commercial assays may detect as much as 50% direct-reacting bilirubin in normal individuals (as stated above, only 4% is conjugated when accurate chromatographic assays are used).

Based on data accumulated using the most reproducible commercial diazo assays, normal individuals' serum may contain up to 0.3 mg/dl or 30% of direct-reacting bilirubin; therefore, values greater than these indicate the presence of conjugated hyperbilirubinemia. It should be noted, however, that in most cases of conjugated hyperbilirubinemia the direct fraction will be in excess of 70% to 80%. In adults, the measurement of direct and indirect fractions of bilirubin is useful only when total serum bilirubin is less than 5 to 6 mg/dl. Disorders that result in unconjugated hyperbilirubinemia (see next section) do not in and of themselves lead to bilirubins above this level.

Several more accurate methods for the quantitation of bilirubins have been developed that may be adapted for routine clinical use in the future. In one method, bilirubin conjugates are converted to mono and dimethyl esters, and the unconjugated and esterified bilirubins are extracted using methanol. The extracted products can be quantitatively analyzed using either high-pressure liquid chromatography or thin-layer chromatography. Protein-conjugated bilirubins can be quantitated by first extracting proteins using an alkaline/methanol extraction procedure. Although this method is time consuming, the recently developed Kodak Ektachem system is able to rapidly determine protein-bound bilirubin and total bilirubin and is now in use in some hospitals.

Causes of Hyperbilirubinemia

UNCONJUGATED HYPERBILIRUBINEMIA

Elevation of unconjugated bilirubin can be due to an overproduction of bilirubin, impaired delivery of bilirubin to the liver, or impaired hepatic uptake of bilirubin, or it can occur as a result of a hereditary defect in the metabolism of unconjugated bilirubin (Table 41-1).[30]

Increased production of bilirubin can occur when there is a high rate of heme turnover, as in hemolytic disorders, which can be classified as either inherited or acquired.[31] Inherited hemolytic disorders include: (1) erythrocyte membrane defects such as spherocytosis, elliptocytosis, and abetalipoproteinemia, (2) glycolytic or pentose phosphate enzyme deficiencies such as pyruvate kinase or glucose-6-phosphate dehydrogenase deficiency, and (3) defects in globin structure or synthesis such as sickle cell anemia and thalassemia. Adults with hereditary spherocytosis have mild hyperbilirubinemia, and 50% have a history of marked jaundice as an infant.[32] Under stable, steady-state conditions, serum bilirubin levels in patients with hemolysis do not exceed 4 to 5 mg/

dl, because this reflects the maximum rate of production.[30,31] However, in acute hemolysis or in the presence of renal or hepatobiliary disease, hemolytic disease can result in much greater levels of serum bilirubin. For example, patients with sickle cell anemia may have marked hyperbilirubinemia due to the coexistence of massive, acute hemolysis, liver disease (transfusion-related hepatitis or choledocholithiasis), and renal insufficiency. It is of particular importance to consider cholelithiasis in patients with long-standing hemolytic disease because there is a high incidence of calcium bilirubinate stones (pigment stones) in these conditions.[33,34]

Acquired hemolytic disorders include: (1) immune-mediated hemolytic anemia due to incompatible blood transfusions, autoimmune antibodies associated with drug reactions or malignant disease, cold hemagglutinin disease or paroxysmal cold hemoglobinuria, (2) microangioplastic hemolytic anemia associated with prosthetic heart valves, disseminated intravascular coagulation, and hemolytic-uremic syndrome, (3) direct red cell injury due to chemicals, venoms, thermal injury, or physical damage as in hemodialysis, (4) paroxysmal nocturnal hemoglobinuria, and (5) metabolic derangements such as hypophosphatemia.

Ineffective erythropoiesis, the destruction of red blood cells before release from the bone marrow, can also markedly increase the bilirubin load and lead to mild degrees of jaundice.[30] Diseases that cause ineffective erythropoiesis include pernicious anemia, severe iron deficiency anemia, sideroblastic anemia, folate deficiency, erythropoietic porphyria, and lead poisoning.

Extravasation of blood into extravascular spaces, as occurs with hematomas following femur fractures or retroperitoneal bleeding, can lead to a large bilirubin load when the sequestered hemoglobin is reabsorbed. Impaired bilirubin uptake as caused by certain drugs, notably rifampicin, and impaired delivery of bilirubin to the liver, as may occur with portal systemic shunting in cirrhosis or following portacaval shunt, may also lead to mild unconjugated hyperbilirubinemia.[1] In addition, some patients with congestive heart failure may have predominantly unconjugated hyperbilirubinemia.[1]

Hereditary unconjugated hyperbilirubinemias include Crigler-Najjar syndrome and Gilbert's sydrome, which will be discussed below.

CONJUGATED HYPERBILIRUBINEMIA

Conjugated hyperbilirubinemia can be caused by hereditary syndromes (Dubin-Johnson and Rotor's syndromes), diseases causing diffuse necrosis or dysfunction of hepatocytes, familial and acquired cholestatic syndromes, and diseases that cause infiltration of the liver parenchyma, such as amyloidosis or carcinoma (Table 41-1).

Hereditary Hyperbilirubinemia

Hereditary syndromes of hyperbilirubinemia are discussed here primarily to emphasize the diseases that are important to be aware of in the evaluation of adult patients with jaundice. Complete reviews on the pathogenesis, genetics, and clinical manifestations of each of these syndromes can be found elsewhere.[3,35,36]

Unconjugated, nonhemolytic hyperbilirubinemia can be caused

TABLE 41-1
Differential Diagnosis of Hyperbilirubinemia

I. Unconjugated hyperbilirubinemia
  A. Overproduction of bilirubin
    1. Red blood cell destruction
      a) Inherited hemolytic anemia
      b) Acquired hemolytic anemia
    2. Ineffective erythropoiesis
    3. Red blood cell extravasation
  B. Impaired hepatic uptake of bilirubin
  C. Impaired delivery of bilirubin to the liver
  D. Hereditary unconjugated hyperbilirubinemias
    1. Crigler-Najjar syndromes I and II
    2. Gilbert's syndrome
II. Conjugated hyperbilirubinemias
  A. Hereditary syndromes
    1. Rotor's syndrome
    2. Dubin-Johnson syndrome
  B. Diffuse hepatocellular disease
  C. Cholestatic syndromes
  D. Infiltrative liver disease

by three well-characterized hereditary syndromes—Crigler-Najjar syndrome, types I and II, and Gilbert's syndrome. In each of these syndromes a deficiency of bilirubin UDP-glucuronosyltransferase is the underlying defect in bilirubin metabolism. Patients with Crigler-Najjar syndrome type I have total absence of UDP-glucuronosyltransferase and markedly elevated bilirubins (>20 mg/dl). Patients develop kernicterus in infancy, and this disease is uniformly fatal with only a few patients reaching adolescence. In Crigler-Najjar syndrome type II there is a partial, yet severe, deficiency of the enzyme, bilirubins are < 20 mg/dl, kernicterus can be prevented, and the prognosis for these patients is good. Although Crigler-Najjar syndromes are rare and present in infancy, Gilbert's syndrome is common and often presents in early adulthood. In Gilbert's syndrome there is mild deficiency of bilirubin UDP-glucuronosyltransferase; however, this group of patients appears to be heterogeneous and there are defects in the uptake of BSP and/or a mild decrease in red blood cell survival in some subsets of patients.[35] The result of these defects is a mild unconjugated hyperbilirubinemia (1–6 mg/dl) in the absence of overt hemolytic states and in the absence of liver disease. There tend to be exacerbations of the jaundice during periods of fasting and stress and in association with febrile illnesses. The condition is completely benign, causes no symptoms, and the only required therapy is calm reassurance to the patient that the hyperbilirubinemia is not due to a serious disease. Hemolytic anemia and liver disease must be excluded when the patient initially presents; the absence of liver disease is best confirmed by demonstration of a normal fasting serum bile acid level and normal transaminases in the presence of an elevated bilirubin. A liver biopsy is not required.

Conjugated hyperbilirubinemia can be caused by two well-described, but rare, hereditary disorders: the Dubin-Johnson syndrome and Rotor's syndrome. Dubin-Johnson syndrome is caused by a defect in the transport of organic anions across the canalicular membrane into the canalicular space and is characterized by mild conjugated hyperbilirubinemia (2–6 mg/dl) and brown-black pigmentation of the liver. Patients present before the age of 20, and the disorder runs a benign course. The defect extends to the excretion of radiographic and radioscintigraphic agents; thus, there is nonvisualization of the biliary tree and gallbladder on oral cholecystography or hepatobiliary scintigraphy. Rotor's syndrome is also characterized by a mild conjugated hyperbilirubinemia, usually presenting in the second decade of life, that is probably due to a markedly reduced storage capacity of the hepatocyte for bilirubin; liver histology and excretion of radiographic compounds are normal.

ETIOLOGIES OF ACQUIRED CONJUGATED HYPERBILIRUBINEMIA

Diffuse Hepatocellular Disease

Virtually all diffuse hepatocellular diseases can present with jaundice; the clinical manifestations differ depending on the specific etiology and on whether the process is acute or chronic (Table 41-2). An exhaustive discussion of the many etiologies is beyond the scope of this chapter; details of acute and chronic hepatocellular disease can be found in textbooks of hepatology. Many acute dis-

TABLE 41-2
Diffuse Hepatocellular Disease

Acute Injury	Chronic Injury
Viral hepatitis	Chronic hepatitis
Drug toxicity	Cirrhosis
Alcohol-related disease	Metabolic disorders

eases directly damage the hepatocyte by affecting vital metabolic functions, by damaging organelles such as mitochondria or lysosomes, or by damaging the plasma membrane. The clinical presentation varies widely depending on the specific etiology and the severity of the damage to hepatocytes. The serum enzyme pattern of acute hepatocellular disease is characterized by marked elevation of aminotransferases (AST [aspartate aminotransferase] and ALT [alanine aminotransferase]), usually greater than fivefold, and a mild elevation of alkaline phosphatase (two- to threefold increase). Depending on the severity of the process, the serum prothrombin time may be prolonged on the basis of decreased synthesis of coagulation factors, and serum glucose may be low secondary to impaired gluconeogenesis. The major etiologies of acute hepatocellular disease include the viral hepatitides, drug toxicity (predictable toxins such as acetaminophen and many drugs that can cause idiosyncratic toxicity), and alcohol-related disease. Alcoholic hepatitis may be distinguished from acute viral hepatitis based on the pattern of serum transaminases. In alcoholic hepatitis, the transaminases are usually less than 300 IU/liter and the ratio of AST/ALT is usually greater than 2, whereas in acute viral hepatitis the transaminases are usually greater than 300 IU/liter and the AST/ALT ratio is usually less than or equal to 1 (see ch 42).

Chronic, diffuse hepatocellular disease results from the combination of direct damage to hepatocytes and alterations in the architecture of the liver due to fibrosis. Serum enzyme analysis is of little use in discerning the etiology of chronic hepatocellular disease. The etiologies include chronic hepatitis, cirrhosis, and miscellaneous metabolic disorders. Chronic hepatitis may be due to autoimmune immunologic damage ("lupoid" or autoimmune chronic hepatitis), chronic viral infection with either hepatitis B or C virus or combined hepatitis B and D infection, or chronic ingestion of certain drugs (oxyphenisatin, nitrofurantoin, methyldopa, isoniazid). The most common etiologies of cirrhosis include alcoholic cirrhosis, postviral hepatitic and cryptogenic; less common etiologies that should be considered include hemochromatosis, Wilson's disease, and alpha-1 antitrypsin deficiency. The degree of jaundice in cirrhotic patients depends primarily on the activity of ongoing damage to hepatocytes by the underlying etiology. Many patients with inactive cirrhosis will have normal or minimally elevated bilirubins. The approach to the laboratory diagnosis of these disorders can be found in Chapter 42.

Cholestatic Syndromes

Cholestasis, or bile secretory failure, is a term that means different things to various people. From the clinical standpoint, cholestasis is a syndrome that may present with or without jaundice, sometimes accompanied by pruritus, and usually presents with significant elevations of alkaline phosphatases or serum leucine aminopeptidases, variable levels of transaminases, and elevation of the serum concentration of bile acids.[37,38] Pruritus was previously attributed to the accumulation of bile salts in the blood and subsequently in the subcutaneous tissues; however, there is very poor correlation of symptoms with serum bile acid levels, and pruritus is probably due to the accumulation of unknown cholephilic pruritigens. On biopsy, cholestasis of some duration will present to the pathologist as bile pigment deposits either in hepatocytes, in bile ducts, or in both. Basically, the morphologic and clinical abnormalities observed in cholestasis result from an impairment in bile secretion. Solutes that are normally secreted into bile are now retained in hepatic cells. The increased concentration of solutes intracellularly alters cellular function. For instance, the increased intracellular concentration of bile salts stimulates the synthesis of alkaline phosphatase.[39] Subsequent increments in the intracellular concentrations of bile acids may result in cellular damage. As a result of increased permeability of membranes and increased intracellular concentration, solutes reflux into sinusoids. At that point, other processes such as uptake may be impaired, although the initial pathophysiologic event leading to cholestasis may have been at the canalicular level. This limits the interpretation of studies attempting to elucidate the initial events resulting in cholestasis. It is difficult at times to differentiate what is cause and what is effect. Regardless, the result will be an increased concentration in blood of solutes that are normally secreted into bile. One class of solutes that is most sensitive as an indicator of cholestasis is the bile acids. The concentration of bile acids in serum is always elevated in cholestasis, even at times when bilirubin concentration is normal or barely increased. Serum bile acid levels are elevated in most moderately severe liver diseases, and therefore one cannot differentiate cholestatic from diffuse hepatocellular disease. This cascade of pathophysiologic events occurs whether the impairment to bile secretion (i.e., the cause of cholestasis) is in hepatic cells or in the biliary tree (mechanical obstruction). For this reason, it is not possible to differentiate intrahepatic from extrahepatic cholestasis on the basis of the chemical abnormalities found in blood. Clinical assessment in conjunction with specialized tests will play a fundamental role in this differential diagnosis.

INTRAHEPATIC CHOLESTASIS

Diseases that usually cause a clinical and pathologic picture of diffuse hepatocellular injury can, on occasion, present with primarily a cholestatic spectrum of findings (Table 41-3). The majority of cases of viral hepatitis lack the typical clinical and laboratory findings of cholestasis, although liver biopsies may show histologic evidence of cholestasis (bile plugs) in some patients with typical acute hepatitis. Rarely, a clinical variant of acute hepatitis, cholestatic viral hepatitis, may present with findings similar to those of extrahepatic biliary obstruction, with jaundice, fever, weight loss pruritus, elevated alkaline phosphatase, and elevated cholesterol.[40–43] The jaundice can be prolonged, lasting 2 to 8 months, and has been shown to be associated with hepatitis A infection[43]; however, other viral agents may also cause this syndrome.

Severe fatty infiltration of the liver associated with alcohol abuse can present with hepatomegaly, jaundice, fever (in 50%),

TABLE 41-3
Causes of Intrahepatic Cholestasis

Hepatocellular Disease

Viral hepatitis
Alcoholic liver disease

Hepatotoxicity Due to Drugs and Environmental Toxins

Canalicular cholestasis
Hepatocanalicular cholestasis
Cholangiolar cholestasis
Cholangiodestructive cholestais

Familial

Idiopathic cholestasis of pregnancy
Idiopathic benign recurrent cholestasis
Familial intrahepatic cholestasis

Immunologic Liver Disease

Primary biliary cirrhosis
Intrahepatic primary sclerosing cholangitis

Cystic Liver Diseases

Extrahepatic Bacterial Infections

Parenteral Hyperalimentation

Distant Effects of Malignancies

and a cholestatic pattern of liver enzyme abnormalities with markedly elevated alkaline phosphatase, mildly elevated transaminases, and elevated cholesterol.[44] Alcoholic hepatitis, with or without evidence of cirrhosis or fatty infiltration, can also present with these clinical findings.[45] Primary biliary cirrhosis, a chronic disease characterized by progressive destruction of intrahepatic bile ducts, usually presents with pruritus and malaise with elevated alkaline phosphatase and not with jaundice.[46]

Drug-induced cholestasis can be categorized by the type of histologic lesion caused by the offending agent.[47] *Canalicular cholestasis* is characterized by bilirubin casts in canaliculi without parenchymal inflammation; the agents primarily responsible for this lesion are C-17 alkylated anabolic and contraceptive steroids[47] such as norethandrolone and ethinyl estradiol.[48] On occasion, non–C-17 substituted steroids such as testosterone may cause cholestatic jaundice.[49] In *hepatocanalicular cholestasis* there is mild parenchymal damage in addition to cholestasis; this form of damage is classically caused by chlorpromazine (also, rarely, with haloperidol) as well as by erythromycin estolate and organic arsenicals.[47] Numerous other drugs may, on occasion, cause this type of injury, including captopril,[50] semisynthetic penicillins,[51] carbamazepine,[52] nonsteroidal anti-inflammatory drugs (naproxen,[53] indomethacin,[54] phenylbutazone,[55] sulindac[56]), sulfasalazine,[57] gold therapy,[47] antithyroid drugs (carbimazole),[47] oral hypoglycemics,[47] thiabendazole,[58] and nitrofurantoin.[47] A new type of cholestatic drug injury, called *cholangiolar cholestasis*, was identified as resulting from benoxaprofen hepatotoxicity.[47] This injury was characterized by the presence of a bile-stained precipitate in cholangioles, occurred predominantly in elderly women, and had a high case mortality rate, which is unusual in typical cholestatic drug injury.[59] Destruction of cholangioles and larger bile ducts as a result of toxic injury has been called *cholangiodestructive cholestasis* and is caused by exposure to environmental and industrial toxicants such as aniline oil,[60] paraquat,[61] and 4,4'-diaminodiphenylmethane (Epping jaundice).[62]

Cholestatic syndromes that appear to have a familial association include idiopathic cholestasis of pregnancy[63–65] and idiopathic benign recurrent cholestasis,[66] which are generally benign conditions that do not lead to chronic liver disease. Familial intrahepatic cholestasis, including Alagille syndrome, Byler syndrome, and nonsyndromic ductal hypoplasia, is usually identified in infancy or early childhood and leads to progressive liver failure.[67] Intrahepatic cholestasis is the hallmark of primary biliary cirrhosis and, on occasion, can occur with primary sclerosing cholangitis when only intrahepatic ducts are involved. Of the congenital cystic diseases of the liver, generally only multiple cystic dilation of the intrahepatic bile ducts, or Caroli's disease, causes cholestasis, although polycystic disease on occasion may present with jaundice if a large cyst compresses the extrahepatic biliary tree. The major acquired cystic disease of the liver that may present with jaundice in a small number of patients is infestation with several species of *Echinococcus* (hydatid cysts).

Extrahepatic bacterial infections, both bacteremic and nonbacteremic, are important causes of intrahepatic cholestasis that, if missed in the clinical investigation, can delay appropriate therapy.[68–71] Jaundice in adults has usually been associated with infection with gram-negative organisms,[70] although gram-positive organisms can cause the same syndrome.[70] The usual sites of infection include diverticulitis, appendiceal abscess, pelvic infection and abscess, pyelonephritis, cholecystitis, endocarditis, and pneumonia (usually lobar pneumonia with *Streptococcus pneumoniae*).[70] The pathophysiology of cholestasis caused by bacterial infections is unclear; however, circulating endotoxin probably plays a significant role.[70,72]

Total parenteral nutrition can cause several hepatic abnormalities, including fatty liver, cholestasis, portal inflammation, gallstone formation, and, rarely, following long-term administration, steatonecrosis and micronodular cirrhosis.[73] The cholestasis associated with parenteral nutrition usually occurs after 3 to 4 weeks of administration and resolves upon discontinuing infusions; the pathogenesis is unknown.

Jaundice and cholestasis occur in approximately 13% of patients with Hodgkin's disease at the initial presentation of the illness; by the time of death, jaundice is present in up to 75% of patients. At presentation, 7% of patients have malignant hepatic involvement (stage IV disease) with destruction of portal areas with a lymphocytic and an immature mesenchymal cell infiltrate; obstruction of extrahepatic ducts by mass lesions is much less common. On occasion, Hodgkin's disease[74,75] may cause a bland intrahepatic cholestasis that may be present well before the appearance of the overt disease. Hypernephromas have been associated with hepatocellular dysfunction, which has been termed the "nephrogenic hepatic dysfunction syndrome." In this syndrome, patients with nonmetastatic hypernephromas have fever, weight loss, hepatomegaly, splenomegaly, and abnormal liver enzymes, including elevation of alkaline phosphatase (up to fivefold increase) as well as gamma glutamyl transpeptidase and 5' nucleotidase. Hyperbilirubinemia and jaundice are uncommon but have been reported to occur in 10% of individuals with this syndrome.

EXTRAHEPATIC CHOLESTASIS

The many etiologies of extrahepatic cholestasis or obstruction are best categorized by anatomic location of the pathologic process (Table 41-4). The most common biliary etiology, by far, is choledocholithiasis, with less common causes including primary sclerosing cholangitis, cholangiocarcinoma (many occur as a complication of long-standing sclerosing cholangitis[76]), and benign biliary stricture due to operative trauma.[77] In choledocholithiasis, the bilirubin level is generally 2 to 5 mg/dl and rarely is greater than 12 mg/dl,[78] pain and fever are often present, the jaundice is transient or of short duration, and the patient may have a history of biliary colic. However, at times the history of jaundice may be of longer duration and pain may be a less prominant complaint; the long duration of obstruction in these patients may lead to biliary cirrhosis. Some patients with choledocholithiasis may present with bacterial cholangitis associated with jaundice, high fever, chills, right upper quadrant pain, and, in the most severe cases, hypotension and septic shock.

Primary sclerosing cholangitis may occur as an isolated disease process or, in 50% of cases, in association with inflammatory bowel disease, mostly ulcerative colitis.[76] An anatomic picture similar to that of primary sclerosing cholangitis, including multiple bile duct strictures with intervening dilated ducts, can occur as a result of administration of chemotherapeutic agents via the hepatic artery.[79,80] Cholangiocarcinoma is often detected late, because the common bile duct must be nearly completely occluded before jaundice develops. When the tumor is located at the bifurcation of the right and left common hepatic bile ducts, one of the ducts can be completely occluded without causing jaundice; the patient develops jaundice only when the second duct is occluded. Miscellaneous and uncommon causes of biliary obstruction include hemobilia,[81] Caroli's disease when involving the common bile duct,[81,82] choledochal cyst,[81] adenomyoma of the bile duct,[83] rupture of a hydatid cyst into the common bile duct,[84] metastatic carcinoma,[85,86] lymphoma involving the hilum of the liver or bile duct,[87] biliary ectasia due to Marfan's syndrome,[88] and parasitic infestation of the biliary tree.[89] Infestation of the bile and pancreatic duct with *Ascaris lumbricoides* can cause biliary colic (jaundice less common), and pyogenic cholangitis and pancreatitis should be

TABLE 41-4
Causes of Extrahepatic Cholestasis

Biliary Disease

Choledocholithiasis

Cholangiocarcinoma

Benign biliary stricture

Primary sclerosing cholangitis

Miscellaneous

Pancreatic Disease

Carcinoma

Acute pancreatitis

Chronic Pancreatitis

Retroperitoneal and Duodenal Disease

considered in patients from endemic areas, such as India, Southeast Asia, and South America.[90] Liver fluke disease (distomiasis) can lead to biliary obstruction and jaundice.[89] One of the more important liver flukes is *Clonorchis sinensis,* which is common in Southeast Asia, is acquired by ingesting raw fish, and can, in severe infestations, cause jaundice and recurrent cholangitis.[89] The increasing popularity of eating raw fish in the U.S. (i.e., sushi and sashimi) has led to reports of unusual parasitic disease[91] and should alert the clinician to potential liver fluke infection.

Pancreatic etiologies of common bile duct obstruction include carcinomas and complications of acute and chronic pancreatitis. Carcinoma of the head of the pancreas is an important and common cause of common bile duct obstruction. These patients may have a longer duration of steady jaundice, weight loss, symptoms of malabsorption, and higher levels of bilirubin than patients with choledocholithiasis, many in excess of 15 mg/dl.[78] Fever from cholangitis is not as common in malignant strictures as in choledocholithiasis or postsurgical benign strictures. Swelling of the pancreatic head in acute pancreatitis may cause partial obstruction of the common bile duct but rarely causes jaundice[81]; when jaundice is present it is imperative to determine if a gallstone is impacted in the distal common bile duct and is responsible for the acute pancreatitis. Chronic pancreatitis may cause partial or total distal common bile duct obstruction from fibrotic narrowing of the intrahepatic portion of the duct or by compression from a pseudocyst.[92,93]

Rarely, distal common bile duct obstruction may be caused by disease in the duodenum or retroperitoneum, including ampullary carcinoma, duodenal Crohn's disease,[94] duodenal eosinophilic enteritis,[95] duodenal diverticulum,[81] hepatic artery aneurysm,[96] and blunt abdominal trauma with retroperitoneal bleeding or intramural duodenal hemorrhage.

Infiltrative Liver Disease

Infiltrative diseases of the liver include systemic amyloidosis, granulomatous hepatitis, primary and metastatic carcinoma, and hematologic malignancies (Table 41-5). Although these diseases are relatively uncommon causes of jaundice, they are frequently found in association with an increase in serum alkaline phosphatase

TABLE 41-5
Infiltrative Liver Disease

Systemic Amyloidosis

Granulomatous Hepatitis

Infections
Drug toxicity
Malignancies
Sarcoidosis
Other disorders

Primary and Metastatic Carcinomas

Hematologic Malignancies

activity. Amyloidosis of the liver, which usually presents with minimal clinical or laboratory abnormalities referable to the liver, has been reported to cause severe cholestasis with marked hyperbilirubinemia; histopathology often demonstrates massive infiltration of amyloid within the parenchyma[97,98] and, in one case, massive infiltration in the portal tracts alone.[99] There are many etiologies of granulomatous liver disease, including infections (bacterial—tuberculosis, leprosy, and brucellosis; mycotic—histoplasmosis, coccidiomycosis; parasitic—schistosomiasis and toxocariasis; viral—mononucleosis, cytomegalovirus [CMV], psittacosis; rickettsia; spirochetal—syphilis), reactions to drugs and foreign substances (most frequent agents—beryllium, allopurinol, sulfonamides, phenylbutazone, chlorpropamide, quinidine), and many miscellaneous disorders (sarcoidosis, primary biliary cirrhosis, Crohn's disease, lymphomas). Although alkaline phosphatase is elevated in the majority of patients and serum bilirubin is slightly elevated in a significant minority of patients, overt jaundice is uncommon in granulomatous hepatitis. When jaundice is present, the most likely etiology is either tuberculosis or sarcoidosis; on rare occasions the jaundice may be profound in sarcoidosis. Primary and metastatic carcinoma may on occasion present with cholestatic jaundice; this usually occurs in patients with a large hepatic tumor load. Hematologic malignancies or disorders that may infiltrate the liver and rarely cause jaundice include Hodgkin's disease (discussed above), non-Hodgkin's lymphoma (25% with liver involvement at initial diagnosis), multiple myeloma, and myeloid metaplasia.

The Postsurgical and Critically Ill Patient

The evaluation of jaundice in complicated postoperative patients or in critically ill patients in the intensive care unit is a challenging task. These patients may have combined effects of increased production of bilirubin, impaired hepatocellular function, total parenteral nutrition, sepsis, and, in some cases, extrahepatic biliary obstruction.[100-103] Increased bilirubin production may occur from rapid destruction of transfused blood (20% of administered blood cells stored for 21 days is destroyed within 24 hours), immunologic destruction of mismatched red cell transfusions, breakdown of endogenous blood cells because of damage to cell membrane from cell-savers, reabsorption of blood from hematomas, and intravascular destruction of red cells by artificial heart valves. Massive hemolysis can occur from infections of devascularized or necrotic tissues by *Clostridium welchii.* Hemolysis as a result of stress or drugs may also occur in patients with G-6PD deficiency, which is present in approximately 10% of American blacks.

Hepatocellular dysfunction can result from a variety of insults to the liver, including hypotension and hypoxia resulting in ischemic hepatitis, systemic bacterial infections, hepatotoxicity from anesthetic agents or other drugs, or viral hepatitis. Pre-existing congestive hepatopathy as a result of right heart failure may impair the liver's ability to handle an increased bilirubin load and may partially explain the high incidence of postoperative jaundice following cardiac surgery.[104] Prolonged parenteral alimentation, which is often required in seriously ill patients, may produce cholestasis. Renal failure may contribute to the degree of jaundice because of decreased clearance of conjugated bilirubin. Extrahepatic biliary obstruction is uncommon and should be considered primarily in patients who are recovering from biliary surgery. A very important etiology to consider for jaundice in seriously ill patients is acute acalculous cholecystitis[105]; this condition can be difficult to diagnose and, if left untreated, is virtually always fatal. Although approximately 50% of these patients may have hyperbilirubinemia,[105] the degree of jaundice is usually not marked unless there are other underlying liver abnormalities.

In some patients a syndrome of benign postoperative cholestatic jaundice has been described in which hyperbilirubinemia is noted on the first or second postoperative day and disappears by day 14 to 18.[106] The majority of these patients experienced an episode of decreased hepatic perfusion or congestive heart failure or had long, difficult operative procedures in combination with an increased bilirubin load (hematomas and/or blood transfusions).[106,107]

The Immunocompromised Patient

Individuals who are infected with the human immunodeficiency virus I (HIV-1) resulting in the acquired immunodeficiency syndrome (AIDS) may develop hepatobiliary complications that are unique to these patients.[108–110] Many patients with AIDS are homosexual males or use intravenous drugs, and, because of exposure, in some series up to 95% of patients have active or remote hepatitis B infection.[108] However, the prevalence of chronic active hepatitis secondary to hepatitis B or superinfection with hepatitis D does not seem to be greater in patients with AIDS than in the general, nonimmunosuppressed population.[108]

Evidence of hepatobiliary disease is quite common in AIDS, with hepatomegaly detected in 60% to 73%, elevated liver enzymes in 66%, and histologic abnormalities in 85% of patients.[108] The liver disease is usually mild and does not cause morbidity or clinical jaundice. Hepatic granulomatous disease is common and may be caused by infection with *Mycobacterium avium-intracellulare* or tuberculosis, *Cryptococcus neoformans*, *Histoplasma capsulatum*, *Coccidioides immitis,* or *Candida albicans*.[108–110] Hepatic infection with cytomegalovirus is common and is usually associated with widespread systemic infection with the virus. Patients with AIDS are frequently on multiple medications, in particular sulfonamides for *Pneumocystis carinii* pneumonia, that may cause hepatic granulomatous disease or other forms of hepatotoxicity.[108–110] The most common malignancies involving the liver are Kaposi's sarcoma and lymphoma[108]; a primary bile duct lymphoma may cause extrahepatic biliary obstruction.[111]

Unusual biliary tract infections may occur and produce a clinical and laboratory picture of cholestasis,[108,109,112–115] although jaundice is uncommon. Acalculous cholecystitis may be caused by infections with cytomegalovirus, *Cryptosporidium*, or, rarely, *Campylobacter fetus*. Obstruction of both intrahepatic and extrahepatic bile ducts may occur as a result of infection of the biliary tree with cytomegalovirus and/or *Cryptosporidium*.[108,113–115] The clinical and radiographic findings are similar to those of sclerosing cholangitis and/or papillary stenosis.[108,115] In patients with papillary stenosis, endoscopic sphincterotomy has been found to improve symptoms and reverse the cholestatic laboratory picture.[115]

CLINICAL EVALUATION OF THE JAUNDICED PATIENT

History

Symptoms that the patient relates at the time of presentation with jaundice may be helpful in suggesting certain etiologies for jaundice. Dark or "tea-colored" urine indicates the presence of conjugated hyperbilirubinemia associated with hepatocellular or cholestatic disease. Pruritus is associated with cholestasis and occasionally with hepatocellular disease but is absent in unconjugated hyperbilirubinemias. However, the presence or absence of pruritus is of little use in differentiating intrahepatic from extrahepatic cholestasis. Abdominal pain in the right upper quadrant and fever are usually associated with extrahepatic biliary obstruction secondary to choledocholithiasis or biliary stricture, which may be complicated by cholangitis; shaking chills suggest bacteremia. However, drug-induced or viral hepatitis and alcoholic liver disease may also present with abdominal pain and fever (in the absence of rigors) and can be indistinguishable from choledocholithiasis. Constant abdominal pain that radiates through to the midback and is partially relieved by bending forward is more characteristic of pancreatic carcinoma that has locally invaded the retroperitoneum. Pancreatic carcinoma that causes jaundice by obstructing the distal common bile duct may be contained in the pancreatic head and may, therefore, not cause pain. Most of the icteric syndromes are associated with constitutional symptoms of anorexia, nausea, malaise, and fatigue and are of little use in differential diagnosis.

The history of the onset and duration of the symptoms is more informative in narrowing the differential diagnosis than the symptoms at the time of presentation. Recent and sudden onset of abdominal pain associated with fever is highly suggestive of choledocholithiasis; previous episodes of biliary colic provides additional confirmation of this impression. A family history of gallstones or ethnic predisposition may indicate the patient's risk for the development of cholelithiasis. A sustained period of icterus lasting several weeks associated with weight loss, depression, and malabsorption is more consistent with pancreatic carcinoma. Viral hepatitides are frequently associated with prodromal symptoms. Malaise, fever, joint pains, and a skin rash may be present for several weeks before the onset of jaundice associated with hepatitis B. A shorter prodromal period is more common with hepatitis A infection consisting of acute gastrointestinal or upper respiratory tract symptoms. If viral hepatitis is suspected, information concerning predisposing factors should be sought, including travel history, blood product transfusions, intravenous drug use, tattoo exposure, sexual preference and contacts, exposures to jaundiced individuals, and potential contact with infected food products.

Review of symptoms related to other organs may suggest that certain etiologies for jaundice are more likely. History of chronic intermittent bloody diarrhea may indicate inflammatory bowel disease, in particular ulcerative colitis, and should prompt the clinician to consider sclerosing cholangitis. Diarrhea may precede the development of sclerosing cholangitis by years and be quiescent when the patient presents with jaundice, or, conversely, sclerosing cholangitis may be the first manifestation of ulcerative colitis.

Primary biliary cirrhosis may be associated with other autoimmune disorders, such as Sjögren's syndrome and thyroiditis. Chronic cough, dysphagia, early satiety, change in bowel habits, or skin lesions may indicate a malignancy in another organ that may be metastatic to the hepatobiliary system. Secondary amenorrhea and decreased libido in women and impotence or decreased libido in men may be indicative of chronic liver disease. Risk factors for the development of gallstones should be assessed, including female sex, ethnic background (Pima Indians, Mexican Americans), obesity, ileal disease (i.e., Crohn's disease), chronic hemolysis, and cirrhosis.

The history of drug and alcohol intake is an essential aspect of the investigation that must be performed thoroughly. Some patients may not tell the physician that they are taking certain medications because they are over-the-counter preparations or not prescribed for a medical illness. However, a number of these drugs can cause hepatocellular and cholestatic disease, including nonsteroidal anti-inflammatory drugs and oral contraceptives. In addition, patients should be asked about illicit drug use, including the use of anabolic steroids by athletes. The patient should be asked if he takes any "health food" preparations that may contain hepatotoxins, such as Vitamin A or pyrrolizidine alkaloids (Jamaican bush tea), which may cause hepatic veno-occlusive disease. The patient should be questioned in depth concerning alcohol intake; corroborate the history with a family member, if possible. Finally, a careful occupational history may reveal potential exposure to hepatotoxic industrial compounds. A family or previous personal history of jaundice or liver disease may suggest inherited disease such as Gilbert's syndrome, cholestasis of pregnancy, benign intrahepatic cholestasis, or pancreatic disease (hyperlipidemia or familial pancreatitis).

Physical Examination

The general physical examination may reveal evidence of cachexia, malnutrition, weight loss, or temporal wasting and may suggest the presence of malignancy. Often the general appearance and vitality of the patient give the clinician a sense of whether benign or malignant disease may be the underlying etiology of jaundice. Evidence of an epigastric mass or lymphadenopathy may further indicate intra-abdominal malignancy. Skin rash may be associated with hepatitis B infection; pyoderma gangrenosum or erythema nodosum may complicate inflammatory bowel disease and may suggest the possibility of sclerosing cholangitis. Physical findings of chronic liver disease include spider angiomata, body hair pattern, parotid gland enlargement, gynecomastia, palmar erythema, or testicular atrophy. Inspection of the abdomen in cirrhotic patients may reveal collateral vessels on the abdominal wall.

The presence of a dilated, palpable gallbladder suggests a malignant obstruction of the common bile duct. This occurs because the obstruction in malignancy is often complete and the gallbladder is free of disease and is thus able to distend. In contrast, in choledocholithiasis the obstruction is often partial or intermittent and the gallbladder is nondistensible because of fibrosis secondary to cholelithiasis. However, the presence of a palpable distended gallbladder is present in only 25% of patients with malignant obstruction of the common bile duct.[84] The presence of right upper quadrant tenderness with splinting of inspiratory movement while palpating this area (Murphy's sign) suggests cholecystitis or cholangitis.

Palpation of the liver may yield important information and should be performed carefully in every patient.[116] The normal liver is soft with a sharp, smooth edge and will be palpable just below the right costal margin upon deep inspiration. A firm liver suggests the presence of cirrhosis, and an irregular edge may be palpable, particularly in macronodular cirrhosis; in addition, the left lobe of the liver may be prominent. Splenomegaly with a firm liver provides further evidence of cirrhosis with portal hypertension. A very hard liver in the presence of large nodules suggests primary or metastatic hepatic malignancy. The liver is frequently tender and somewhat enlarged in hepatitis and may be very large (4–5 cm below the costal margin) in fatty liver, amyloidosis, or congestive heart failure. When extrahepatic biliary obstruction has been present long enough to cause dilation of intrahepatic bile ducts, there is usually hepatomegaly with a rounded, smooth edge; however, if secondary biliary cirrhosis is present, the edge will be firm.

The presence of ascites may be associated with cirrhosis, metastatic disease to the peritoneum, obstruction of lymphatics from tumor or lymphoma resulting in chylous ascites, or pancreatic disease with ruptured pseudocyst or pancreatic fistula.

Routine Laboratory Tests

Hematologic tests such as the complete blood count, red cell indices, reticulocyte count, and examination of a peripheral blood smear may alert one to the possibility of hemolysis or ineffective erythropoiesis. The most important laboratory tests are the transaminases, which are elevated primarily in hepatocellular necrosis, and alkaline phosphatase, 5' nucleotidase, and leucine aminopeptidase, which are canalicular enzymes and are elevated primarily in cholestasis (the origin of these enzymes and their interpretation are discussed in Chapter 42). Analysis of the pattern of transaminase and alkaline phosphatase elevation in patients with jaundice allows the categorization of disease into hepatocellular or cholestatic. Elevation of serum transaminases to greater than fivefold normal values with a mild elevation in alkaline phosphatase (two- to threefold) is characteristic of diffuse hepatocellular diseases such as viral hepatitis. Marked elevation of alkaline phosphatase levels (greater than three- to fivefold) with or without mild increases in serum transaminases (less than three- to fivefold) suggests the presence of a cholestatic process. However, the differentiation of intrahepatic from extrahepatic biliary obstruction cannot be made by analysis of laboratory tests alone. Soon after an acute obstruction of the biliary tree, as in choledocholithiasis, there may be a transient, marked elevation of transaminases that rapidly decreases over 24 to 72 hours.[117]

DIAGNOSTIC EVALUATION: ESTABLISHING THE SITE OF HEPATOBILIARY OBSTRUCTION

When the initial clinical evaluation suggests cholestasis, the main emphasis of the diagnostic evaluation is directed toward establishing whether the cholestatic syndrome is due to an intrahepatic or an extrahepatic cause and determining the specific disorder responsible for the cholestasis.

Extensive published information on widely used diagnostic tests, including ultrasonography (US), computerized tomography (CT), hepatobiliary scintigraphy (HS), percutaneous transhepatic cholangiography (PTC), and endoscopic retrograde cholangiopancreatography (ERCP), allows one to predict the utility of each test in establishing the presence and the site of cholestasis. Oral cholecystography and intravenous cholangiography will not be discussed because they are of little use in the evaluation of jaundice. The principles of selection and interpretation of diagnostic tests will be reviewed and then applied to the selection of diagnostic tests in the evaluation of jaundice.

The usefulness of diagnostic tests can be defined by the sensitivity and specificity of the tests and by the complementary measures of the percentage of false-negative and false-positive results.[118,119] The sensitivity of a test is the likelihood of a positive result in patients known to have the disease (in this case, extrahepatic cholestasis). Mathematically, this relationship is expressed as the number of patients with the disease who have a positive test (true positives) divided by the total number of patients with the disease. The false-negative rate for the test is 1 − sensitivity. The specificity of a test is the likelihood of a negative result in patients known to be free of the disease or the number of true negatives divided by the total number of patients without the disease. Finally, the false-positive rate is dependent on the specificity of the test, or 1 − specificity. It should be emphasized that these parameters for any given test apply only if the tests are performed and analyzed in the same manner as when the measurements were made. Hence, if there are advances in technology or differences in operator training, the sensitivity or specificity of a test may be altered.

In order to interpret the results of a positive or negative test result, in addition to the sensitivity and specificity of the test, one must have information on the prevalence of the disease in the tested population, or the pretest probability of disease.[118,119] For the evaluation of the jaundiced patient, the routine clinical examination is reasonably accurate in determining the probability of extrahepatic or intrahepatic biliary obstruction and plays a central role in the strategies for evaluation as described by many authors.[120–129] Although principles of diagnostic testing are useful, the selection of diagnostic strategies for individual patients must be based on many criteria that defy strict mathematical considerations. In fact, a computer simulation of multiple diagnostic strategies using decision analysis determined that there was little difference between several common diagnostic strategies.[130] Therefore, a rigid algorithm for the use of diagnostic tests will be avoided. The characteristics of the pertinent tests will be presented followed by an overall diagnostic strategy. For a more in-depth analysis of diagnostic tests, the reader is referred to a review by Lumeng and O'Connor.[128]

Noninvasive Tests

CLINICAL EXAMINATION

The routine history, physical examination, and laboratory evaluation in jaundiced patients have been shown to be quite accurate in defining whether cholestasis is due to an intrahepatic or an extrahepatic cause.[121,124,128] The accuracy of the clinical examination for the detection of extrahepatic biliary obstruction in various studies has ranged from 69% to 90%. In a direct comparison of the clinical examination with noninvasive diagnostic tests, the clinical examination was found to be more sensitive than US, CT, or HS alone and had an overall greater accuracy as well.[124] In this study, patients were excluded if they had obvious hepatitis, metastatic disease, or cirrhosis that was previously known to be complicated by cholestasis[124]; therefore, the patient population included patients with cholestasis of undetermined etiology similar to that seen in practice. Fifty consecutive patients were prospectively evaluated by three gastroenterologists and noninvasive diagnostic tests including US, CT, and HS; the diagnostic studies were read by observers who were unaware of clinical information or laboratory tests. All patients had confirmed diagnoses by invasive techniques such as surgery, ERCP, PTC, or autopsy. The clinical examination alone was found to be 95% sensitive and 76% specific in diagnosing the presence of extrahepatic cholestasis in this group of patients. The sensitivity of each of the noninvasive tests was lower, although the specificities were greater than those of the clinical examination. These data should not be interpreted as indicating that clinical evaluation alone is sufficient in the evaluation of patients with jaundice. The majority of individual patients require further noninvasive and invasive diagnostic testing to confirm the presence of extrahepatic obstruction and to identify the site of cholestasis as well as the specific etiology. Rather, these studies underscore the importance of a careful clinical examination of the jaundiced patient for determining the pretest probability of disease and for guiding the subsequent diagnostic evaluation. In addition, the interpretation of results of diagnostic tests may rely heavily on the clinical assessment.

ULTRASONOGRAPHY

Examination of the liver, biliary tree, and pancreas by US is in widespread clinical use and has been advocated by many authors as the initial diagnostic test in the evaluation of jaundice. Initially, gray-scale, static ultrasound technology was capable of imaging only a single-tissue plane, and, consequently, multiple images had to be visually pieced together in order to evaluate contiguous structures. This made the success of the technique dependent on the skill and, more important, the persistence of the operator. With the advent of dynamic ultrasound imaging technology, the operator was provided a two-dimensional image of the tissue that changed in "real time" with the movement of the transducer on the surface of the patient's abdomen. This technology is now available to virtually all clinical radiology departments and provides for a more accurate and rapid diagnostic procedure.

Many studies have reported on the use of ultrasound in the evaluation of jaundice.[131–140] The sensitivity of ultrasound for the diagnosis of extrahepatic biliary obstruction in these studies has ranged from 88% to 98% and the specificity from 86% to 100%. In general, the specificity of ultrasound in the diagnosis of extrahepatic biliary obstruction has been shown to be greater than its sensitivity. In cases where the serum bilirubin is moderately to markedly elevated, the sensitivity approaches 100%, but in cases where the biliary obstruction is acute, partial, or intermittent, the sensitivity is lower. Although quite sensitive for the detection of cholelithiasis, US is not a sensitive modality for the detection of stones in the gallbladder neck/cystic duct or in the common bile duct, with sensitivities in the range of 25% to 55%.[128,141,142] Following cholecystectomy, the diameter of the common bile duct may be larger than normal, and, therefore, this has to be taken into consideration when interpreting US in these patients. US, for safety reasons, is the most acceptable procedure in the pregnant patient with jaundice and, in addition to detecting cholelithiasis and biliary dilatation, may be useful in the diagnosis of fatty liver of pregnancy.[143]

The diagnostic usefulness of ultrasound in localizing the site of obstruction in the jaundiced patient is based on the detection of a dilated biliary system or on the identification of a mass lesion in the liver, biliary tract, pancreas, duodenum, or retroperitoneum. Therefore, in cases where a mass lesion is small and thus not identified, or when the biliary system is not dilated (i.e., sclerosing cholangitis or acute obstruction from a gallstone), the ultrasound may not correctly identify the site of cholestasis as extrahepatic. Patient factors that may lead to a nondiagnostic ultrasound include marked obesity, distortion of the normal anatomy secondary to surgery, and the presence of intestinal gas that lies in the path between the ultrasound transducer and the organ of interest, usually the distal common bile duct and pancreas. Imaging of the pancreas with ultrasound is technically inadequate in approximately 14% of examinations, even with experienced operators.[144,145]

COMPUTERIZED TOMOGRAPHY

Computerized tomography produces a cross-sectional image of the abdominal contents with high resolution. The principle of using CT in the detection of extrahepatic biliary obstruction is similar to that of ultrasound (i.e., identification of dilation of bile ducts and/or demonstration of a mass lesion that is obstructing the biliary tree). CT has been shown, in most studies, to be as sensitive and specific as US in the diagnosis of extrahepatic biliary obstruction.[124,128,130,138,139,146,147] However, CT has several advantages over US in imaging the distal common bile duct (CBD) and pancreas and has been shown to be much more accurate than US in the diagnosis of pancreatic carcinoma.[144,145,148] In one prospective study CT had a sensitivity of 87% in detecting a pancreatic lesion, whereas ultrasound had a sensitivity of only 69%.[144] These differences are probably due to the fact that bowel gas and obesity do not obscure the view of the pancreas with CT as is often the case with US. CT is accurate in delineating the level of the obstruction,[149] more accurate than ultrasound in detecting common bile duct stones,[128,150,151] may be helpful in diagnosing sclerosing cholangitis when there is no generalized biliary dilation,[152] and may detect duodenal malignancy.[153]

Although US and CT have been of equivalent efficacy in most comparative studies, US has been chosen as the initial test in the evaluation of jaundice by most authors. This is because US is, in general, more available, less expensive, takes less time to perform an adequate test, and lacks the radiation exposure of CT. However, these two modalities should be considered equivalent for the identification of extrahepatic biliary obstruction and complementary for determining the specific etiology of obstruction. When pancreatic malignancy is the most likely diagnosis, CT should be the initial test, because this is the most efficient way of confirming the diagnosis and evaluating the extent of local or intra-abdominal spread of malignancy.[148,154]

HEPATOBILIARY SCINTIGRAPHY

Hepatobiliary scintigraphy evaluates the capacity of the liver to secrete an organic anion and, by extension, bile into the intestinal tract. Therefore, the impaired physiologic function in cholestasis can be directly assessed rather than the anatomic consequences of extrahepatic biliary obstruction, which are detected by US and CT. In HS, a radiolabeled organic anion is taken up by hepatocytes and excreted into the canaliculus and biliary tree. The time course of radionuclide excretion into the duodenum as well as anatomic information from the image can be used to determine the presence of both partial and complete biliary obstruction.

The most effective biliary imaging agents are N-substituted iminodiacetic acid (IDA) compounds that have been complexed to ^{99m}Tc.[155-158] These compounds circulate bound to albumin and appear to be handled as organic anions by hepatocytes; uptake is competitively inhibited by BSP, bilirubin, and taurocholate. Therefore, these imaging agents may be transported by both bilirubin and bile acid membrane transport proteins. DISIDA (o-diisopropyl IDA), PIPIDA (p-isopropyl IDA), and BIDA (p-n butyl IDA) effectively compete with endogenous anions and are often able to be secreted into the biliary tree in high enough concentrations for imaging even when bilirubin is elevated. The newly approved agent mebrofenin (m-bromo-o, p-trimethyl IDA) appears to be superior to these agents in hepatic uptake and biliary excretion and may further improve the quality of images in patients with hyperbilirubinemia[153]; however, clinical trials will be required to determine whether this agent will improve the usefulness of HS.

Hepatobiliary scintigraphy is a sensitive test for the detection of complete biliary obstruction, but the specificity and predictive value of a positive test are lower.[159-164] In one study of 60 scans that demonstrated a pattern consistent with complete biliary obstruction, 19 were found to be false-positives and due to severe hepatocellular disease,[14] liver metastases,[4] or portal venous thrombosis.[1,159] False-positive results have also been frequently reported in patients with cholestatic drug toxicity[160,164] and occasionally in alcoholic hepatitis.[160] Several studies have indicated that HS is able to detect partial bile duct obstruction when the bilirubin is only mildly elevated or in the absence of jaundice and may be better than US in these patients.[165,166] It has been proposed that the combination of HS with US may have a diagnostic accuracy greater than when either test is used alone.[166]

Some have proposed that HS be used as a screening test in jaundiced patients[153]; however, it has not been employed by most clinicians in the initial evaluation of jaundice. The major reasons for this are a lack of precise anatomic information provided by the images and the high number of false-positive tests in patients with hepatocellular disease such as cholestatic drug toxicity. When compared to US in the evaluation of jaundiced patients presenting to a general hospital, HS was of little use in determining the site of cholestasis.[162] In a prospective study, HS was compared to US and CT in the evaluation of 56 patients who ultimately had a definitive diagnosis made by biopsy, surgery, or clinical course.[164] US and CT were equally useful, but HS could not be recommended in the evaluation of jaundice primarily because of the large number of false-positive tests in patients with intrahepatic cholestasis.[164] In another prospective study comparing the effectiveness of non-invasive tests in jaundiced patients, HS was found to have an overall accuracy of only 68%.[124]

HS may be indicated in the evaluation of certain nonicteric conditions such as acute cholecystitis[155,167] and in the detection of postoperative or post-traumatic biliary leaks.[168] However, at the present time the inclusion of HS as a screening modality in the evaluation of jaundice is not warranted.

Invasive Tests

PERCUTANEOUS CHOLANGIOGRAPHY

In this procedure, a long, 22-gauge needle (Chiba-type or "skinny" needle) is introduced into the liver and withdrawn while injecting radiocontrast dye until the dye enters the biliary tree.[169–172] The biliary tree may then be filled with contrast through the needle itself, or, as is more often done, a catheter may be placed over the needle and threaded into the biliary tree. Because the "skinny" needle is relatively atraumatic to the liver capsule and parenchyma, multiple passes can be made without increasing the risk of complication.[172] The success rate of bile duct opacification using multiple passes, if necessary, is approximately 70% when the bile ducts are not dilated and approaches 100% when the ducts are dilated.[172] The accuracy of PTC for defining the level of obstruction and the specific lesion responsible for the obstruction is 89% to 95% and 75% to 90%, respectively.[169–172] Difficulties in interpretation may occur when there is poor mixing of contrast with CBD bile or when the lesion is in the distal CBD. Samples of brushings or aspirates of bile may be examined by cytology and prove useful in the diagnosis of malignant disease. In addition to the diagnostic utility of PTC, there are multiple techniques for therapy via the percutaneous catheter, such as balloon dilation of strictures,[173] stent placement (internal and external draining),[174,175] and stone removal.[176]

The rate of major complications with PTC is approximately 5%, and the most serious and frequent complications include bile peritonitis, bleeding, and sepsis, each of which may result in death[172]; the overall mortality is 0.2% to 1.0%.[128] Prophylaxis with antibiotics that cover typical organisms known to infect the obstructed biliary tract may decrease the incidence of septicemia.[172] The use of this test in evaluation of the jaundiced patient will be discussed below.

ENDOSCOPIC RETROGRADE CHOLANGIOPANCREATOGRAPHY

This examination is performed by inserting a catheter into the distal CBD via a side-viewing endoscope and injecting radiocontrast dye into the CBD and pancreatic duct. The advantages of ERCP over PTC include examination of the stomach and duodenum, which may detect other disease; evaluation of the pancreatic duct, which is not seen on PTC; and direct visualization of the papilla of Vater, which can be biopsied in the case of suspected ampullary carcinoma. In addition, ERCP is minimally invasive. Also, many therapeutic maneuvers can be attempted via the endoscope, including biliary stent placement, nasobiliary drainage, papillotomy or sphincterotomy, stone extraction, and stricture dilation.[177–184] Recently, intracavitary radiation therapy has been performed for palliation of malignant obstruction of the biliary tree by placing the radiation source in the bile duct endoscopically.[185] Disadvantages, as compared with PTC, include the greater expense of the procedure and the fact that it is technically more difficult to perform, thus requiring more operator training.

The success rate of performing a technically adequate ERCP is approximately 90%. The overall major complication rate for ERCP is 1.9% to 2.8%, as reported from a review of the literature by Lumeng and O'Connor.[128] The most important complications are pancreatitis, cholangitis, pancreatic abscess, drug reactions, and pulmonary aspiration.[186] The mortality rate of 0.1% is somewhat lower than that for PTC, but, as has been pointed out,[128] the local expertise and experience with both of these techniques may vary significantly.

LIVER BIOPSY

Liver biopsies can generally be performed safely in jaundiced patients, even in the presence of extrahepatic biliary obstruction, if the prothrombin time is less than 3 seconds prolonged and the platelet count is greater than 80,000 per microliter. However, histologic examination of the liver is seldom of help in distinguishing intrahepatic from extrahepatic cholestasis. Some histologic findings are highly suggestive of extrahepatic biliary obstruction, such as bile lakes and extravasates and bile infarcts, and others are moderately suggestive, such as portal tract edema, bile ductular proliferation, and a neutrophilic portal infiltrate. However, the frequency and specificity of these findings do not warrant the routine use of liver biopsy in cholestasis. Liver biopsy should be reserved for the evaluation of patients with presumed diffuse hepatocellular disease or in those patients with probable intrahepatic cholestasis from an obscure etiology.

Diagnostic Strategy

The proper sequence of noninvasive and invasive diagnostic testing in the evaluation of jaundice has been the subject of numerous articles and textbook chapters. Most of these authors have used a generalized algorithm to guide the clinician through the diagnostic evaluation using noninvasive tests to determine the choice of more invasive tests; the aim is to provide a definitive diagnosis to direct therapy. Most of these algorithms are based on a thorough analysis of the diagnostic modalities available and provide a good framework upon which to build a logical diagnostic strategy. However, the uninitiated clinician may interpret these algorithms in a rigid fashion and forget that the focus of the evaluation is the individual patient. Therefore, the approach outlined here uses the clinical evaluation of the patient as the focus of the diagnostic evaluation, and noninvasive and invasive tests are chosen based on the unique attributes of the individual tests.

With knowledge of the history, physical examination, and routine laboratory tests, the clinician should be able to categorize patients with cholestasis into several broad groups: (1) those patients with a very low likelihood of extrahepatic obstruction, (2) those patients in whom extrahepatic obstruction is possible, but the clinician does not have a high degree of certainty, and (3) those patients with a high likelihood of extrahepatic obstruction.

Noninvasive diagnostic tests in patients who have a low likelihood of extrahepatic obstruction (i.e., <10%) would be expected to have a low probability of changing the clinical impression. For example, if US is performed on a group of patients with a 10% prevalence of extrahepatic biliary obstruction and the sensitivity and specificity of ultrasound are both estimated to be 90% (this example could be extended to CT as well), the predictive value of a positive test as being indicative of biliary obstruction would only be 50%. On the other hand, the predictive value of a negative test as indicative of the absence of biliary obstruction would be 98.7%. Therefore, it is unlikely that the ultrasound examination would compel the physician to change the clinical impression or management in this group of patients.

In practice, the clinician may have this degree of certainty only in ascertaining the absence of extrabiliary obstruction in selected patients. Young patients with viral hepatitis, patients with drug-induced cholestasis, and patients with alcoholic liver disease may have a clinical presentation that allows one to predict a very low likelihood of biliary obstruction. In these patients it is not necessary to obtain initially a noninvasive test such as US or CT. For instance, a 17-year-old college student develops jaundice after returning from vacation on a Caribbean island. For one week prior to noticing yellow eyes and dark urine, she complained of malaise, a sore throat, and a nonproductive cough. Her companion on the trip has similar symptoms but is not jaundiced. Physical examination reveals only a mildly tender liver edge. Laboratory studies showed a bilirubin of 5.0 mg/dl with 50% of the total as direct bilirubin, aspartate aminotransferase was 980 IU/liter (normal, <50 IU/liter), and there was a normal alkaline phosphatase. The most likely diagnosis is hepatitis A, and the initial diagnostic test should be hepatitis viral serologies. In this case, hepatitis A IgM antibody was positive, and an ultrasound was not indicated. In patients with a low likelihood of extrahepatic obstruction, if the clinical course is atypical for the presumed diagnosis or if new signs or symptoms develop, US or CT would be indicated. Unless the new symptoms indicate the need for CT, the preferred test in this situation would be US. Finally, if special diagnostic tests do not yield a diagnosis or if jaundice persists in the absence of dilated bile ducts on US, a liver biopsy should be performed.

If the clinical examination indicates that obstructive cholestasis is possible, but the likelihood is not high, further noninvasive diagnostic tests are indicated. It is in this situation that the result of diagnostic testing is most likely to alter the clinical impression and, thus, the subsequent diagnostic and therapeutic management.[118] In extending the example of US as illustrated above, if the prevalence of biliary obstruction in this clinical situation was estimated to be 50%, the predictive value of a positive scan as being indicative of biliary obstruction would be 90%; therefore, the degree of certainty of the clinician regarding the presence of obstruction was raised from 50% to 90%. In addition, the predictive value of a negative test as being indicative of the absence of obstruction would also be 90%. Either US or CT could be chosen as the initial noninvasive test in these patients; however, the greater availability, lack of a requirement for intravenous contrast, lack of radiation exposure, and lower cost of ultrasonography makes this the preferred initial test. If the US does not demonstrate evidence for obstruction, the clinician may elect a period of observation before proceeding with further evaluation or may perform a liver biopsy. If US demonstrates ductal dilation but the etiology of the obstruction is unclear, or if the obstruction is located in the distal CBD or pancreas, CT may be helpful and should be considered complementary to US. However, the practice of obtaining multiple noninvasive tests, in general, should be avoided. The choice of invasive tests will be discussed below.

In patients in whom the likelihood of extrahepatic obstruction is high as indicated by the clinical evaluation, a normal noninvasive test should not dissuade one from further evaluation of the patient. To extend our example of an idealized patient population to this clinical situation, if the prevalence of extrahepatic obstruction is estimated to be 90%, the predictive value of a negative US would be 50%, much less than the clinical estimate of biliary obstruction; in most instances the clinician, appropriately, would ignore this test result. The predictive value of a positive test in indicating the presence of biliary obstruction would be 98.7%, not much greater than the clinical impression.

We feel that CT, rather than US, is the best initial test in these patients because CT provides more information as to the etiology of the obstruction and the specific level of obstruction and provides better imaging of the distal CBD and the pancreas, common areas of extrahepatic obstruction. If a pancreatic mass is identified on CT, it may be immediately aspirated via a thin needle to rapidly obtain a tissue diagnosis. Many patients with a high likelihood of extrahepatic obstruction who have US as the initial test also have a CT to evaluate the US abnormalities, and therefore the noninvasive testing is needlessly expensive and the added time delays obtaining a definitive diagnosis.

An example of a patient who has a high likelihood of extrahepatic obstruction would be a 65-year-old man who has had epigastric pain for about 4 months. The pain is constant and interferes with sleep. His appetite is poor and he has noted the loss of about 35 pounds during this interval. About a month ago he noticed dark urine and light-colored stools followed a few days later by jaundice. About 2 weeks ago, pruritus appeared. On physical examination there is loss of fat and muscular mass and jaundice. On abdominal palpation there is the sensation of fullness in the epigastrium. Complete blood count reveals a slight normocytic, normochromic anemia. Bilirubin is 17 mg/dl, ALT is two times normal, and AST is 2.5 times normal values. Alkaline phosphatase is five times normal values. An abdominal CT reveals a mass in the head of the pancreas, which on aspiration by thin needle reveals an adenocarcinoma of the pancreas.

Most authors have indicated that the choice of PTC versus ERCP for the invasive evaluation of biliary obstruction should be guided by the presence or absence of a dilated biliary system as shown by noninvasive testing. However, we, and others,[187] feel that ERCP should be the invasive test of choice in the majority of patients; this will depend, of course, on the local expertise in this procedure. ERCP has the following advantages: it does not require puncture of the skin and liver capsule, it has fewer severe complications than PTC, and it evaluates the areas most often affected in obstructive jaundice (distal CBD and pancreas) better than PTC. In addition, specific therapeutic measures may be implemented at the time of ERCP, such as sphincterotomy, CBD stone extraction, or stent placement. Stone extraction and stent placement can be done by PTC, but larger catheters must be placed into the liver, and, in most cases, the patient is left with an external biliary drain, at least temporarily. It is prudent, therefore, to attempt biliary therapeutic maneuvers via the endoscope before resorting to the percutaneous approach. If ERCP is unsuccessful or if additional information is required from portions of the biliary tree not visualized well by the procedure, PTC may be performed.

There are certain patients in whom the evaluation of the cause of jaundice becomes an urgent process. This may occur in patients in whom one suspects that the cause of jaundice may be extrahepatic but who present with rapidly progressive fever, leukocytosis with a shift to the left, and at times with mental alterations or hypotension. In these cases, cholangitis should be suspected and the diagnostic evaluation must be performed without delay. In mild to moderate cases of cholangitis, antibiotic therapy may improve the clinical situation within 6 to 12 hours of initiating therapy. However, the patient with evidence of severe sepsis or shock should either be taken to surgery promptly or undergo emergent ERCP to drain and decompress the bile ducts; antibiotics must be administered concomitantly. In more stable patients who may require surgery, an abdominal US showing dilated bile ducts may be all that is needed, and this is preferred over CT because it can usually be obtained more rapidly. However, common duct obstruction and cholangitis may be present in the absence of ductal dilation, and a normal exam should not delay surgery or ERCP in the seriously ill patient.

The reader is directed to Chapter 16, Bile Secretion; Chapter 42, Approach to the Patient with Abnormal Liver Chemistries; Chapter 93, Gallbladder and Biliary Tree: Anatomy and Structural Anomalies; Chapter 95, Diseases of the Biliary Tree; Chapter 113, Endoscopic Retrograde Cholangiopancreatography, Endoscopic Sphincterotomy and Stone Removal, Endoscopic Biliary and Pancreatic Drainage; and Chapter 136, Mechanical and Chemical Management of Gallstones.

REFERENCES

1. Ostrow JD, ed. Bile pigments and jaundice: Molecular, metabolic and medical aspects. New York: Marcel Dekker, 1986.
2. Chowdhury JR, Wolkoff AW, Arias IM. Heme and bile pigment metabolism. In: Arias IM, Jakoliz WB, Popper H, Schachter D, Shafritz DA, eds. The liver: Biology and pathology. New York: Raven Press, 1988:419.
3. Blanckaert N, Schmid R. Physiology and pathophysiology of bilirubin metabolism. In: Zakim D, Boyer TA, eds. Hepatology: A textbook of liver disease. Philadelphia: WB Saunders, 1982:246.
4. Stocker R, Yamamoto Y, McDonagh AF, et al. Bilirubin is an antioxidant of possible biological significance. Science 1987;235:1043.
5. Carey MC, Spinak W. Physical chemistry of bile pigments and porphyrins with particular reference to bile. In: Ostrow JD, ed. Bile pigments and jaundice: Molecular, metabolic and medical aspects. New York: Marcel Dekker, 1986:81.
6. Bissell DM. Heme catabolism and bilirubin formation. In: Ostrow JD, ed. Bile pigments and jaundice: Molecular, metabolic and medical aspects. New York: Marcel Dekker, 1986:133.
7. Robinson SH, Tsong M, Brown BW, Schmidt R. The sources of bile pigment in the rat: Studies of the 'early-labeled' fraction. J Clin Invest 1966;45:1569.
8. Berk PD, Howe RB, Bloomer JR, Berlin NI. Studies of bilirubin kinetics in normal adults. J Clin Invest 1969;48:2176.
9. Brodersen R. Aqueous solubility, albumin binding, and tissue distribution of bilirubin. In: Ostrow JD, ed. Bile pigments and jaundice: Molecular, metabolic and medical aspects. New York: Marcel Dekker, 1986:157.
10. Kwang-Sun L, Gartner LM. Fetal bilirubin metabolism and neonatal jaundice. In: Ostrow JD, ed. Bile pigments and jaundice: Molecular, metabolic and medical aspects. New York: Marcel Dekker, 1986:373.
11. Schenker S, Hoyumpa AM, McCandless DW. Bilirubin toxicity to the brain (kernicterus) and other tissues. In: Ostrow JD, ed. Bile pigments and jaundice: Molecular, metabolic and medical aspects. New York: Marcel Dekker, 1986:395.
12. Goresky CA. Hepatic uptake of bile pigments. In: Ostrow JD, ed. Bile pigments and jaundice: Molecular, metabolic and medical aspects. New York: Marcel Dekker, 1986:183.
13. Wolkoff AW, Chung CT. Identification, purification, and partial characterization of an organic anion binding protein from rat liver cell plasma membrane. J Clin Invest 1980;65:1152.
14. Stremmel W, Gerber MA, Glezerov V, et al. Physiochemical and immunohistological studies of a sulfobromophthalein- and bilirubin-binding protein from rat liver plasma membranes. J Clin Invest 1983;71:1796.
15. Stremmel W, Berk P. Hepatocellular uptake of sulfobromophthalein and bilirubin is selectively inhibited by an antibody to the liver plasma membrane sulfobromophthalein/bilirubin binding protein. J Clin Invest 1986;78:822.
16. Forker EL, Luxon BA. Albumin helps mediate removal of taurocholate by rat liver. J Clin Invest 1981;67:1517.
17. Forker EL, Luxon BA. Hepatic transport kinetics and plasma disappearance curves: Distributed modeling versus conventional approach. Am J Physiol 1978;235:648.
18. Weisiger RA, Gollan J, Ockner R. The role of albumin in hepatic uptake process. In: Popper H, Schaffner F, eds. Progress in liver disease. New York: Grune & Stratton, 1982:71.
19. Ockner R, Weisiger RA, Gollan J. Hepatic uptake of albumin-bound substances: Albumin receptor concept. Am J Physiol 1983;245:G13.
20. Weisiger RA. Dissociation from albumin: A potentially rate-limiting step in the clearance of substances by the liver. Proc Natl Acad Sci USA 1985;82:1563.
21. Weisiger RA, Ma WL. Uptake of oleate from albumin solutions by rat liver. Failure to detect catalysis of the dissociation of oleate from albumin by an albumin receptor. J Clin Invest 1987;79:1070.
22. Traber PG, Chianale J, Gumucio JJ. Physiologic significance and regulation of hepatocellular heterogeneity. Gastroenterology 1988;95:1130.
23. Gumucio DL, Gumucio JJ, Wilson JAP, et al. Albumin influences sulfobromophthalein transport by hepatocytes of each acinar zone. Am J Physiol 1984;246:G86.
24. Gumucio JJ, Miller DL. Functional implications of liver cell heterogeneity. Gastroenterology 1981;80:393.
25. Wolkoff AW, Goresky CA, Sellin J, et al. Role of ligandin in transfer of bilirubin from plasma to liver. Am J Physiol 1979;236:E638.
26. Hauser SC, Gollan JL. Hepatic UDP glucuronosyltransferases and the conjugation of bilirubin. In: Ostrow JD, ed. Bile Pigments and Jaundice: Molecular, Metabolic and Medical Aspects. New York: Marcel Dekker, 1986:211.
27. Scharschmidt BF. Biliary secretion of bile pigments. In: Ostrow JD, ed. Bile pigments and jaundice: Molecular, metabolic and medical aspects. New York: Marcel Dekker, 1986:243.
28. Billing BH. Intestinal and renal metabolism of bilirubin including enterohepatic circulation. In: Ostrow JD, ed. Bile pigments and jaundice: Molecular, metabolic and medical aspects. New York: Marcel Dekker, 1986:255.
29. Blanckaert N, Heirwegh KPM. Analysis and preparation of bilirubins and biliverdins. In: Ostrow JD, ed. Bile pigments and jaundice: Molecular, metabolic and medical aspects. New York: Marcel Dekker, 1986:31.
30. Powell LW. Clinical aspects of unconjugated hyperbilirubinemia. Semin Hematol 1972;9:91.

31. Wintobe MM, ed. Clinical hematology. Philadelphia: Lea & Febiger, 1981:734.

32. MacKinney AA, Morton NE, Kosower NS, Schilling RF. Ascertaining genetic carriers of hereditary spherocytosis by statistical analysis of multiple laboratory tests. J Clin Invest 1962;41:554.

33. Bates GC, Brown CH. Incidence of gallbladder disease in chronic hemolytic anemia (spherocytosis). Gastroenterology 1952;21:104.

34. Jordan RA. Cholelithiasis in sickle cell disease. Gastroenterology 1957;33:952.

35. Berk PD, Isola LM, Jones EA. Specific defects in hepatic storage and clearance of bilirubin. In: Ostrow JD, ed. Bile pigments and jaundice: Molecular, metabolic and medical aspects. New York: Marcel Dekker, 1986:279.

36. Chowdhury JR, Arias IM. Disorders of bilirubin conjugation. In: Ostrow JD, ed. Bile pigments and jaundice: Molecular, metabolic and medical aspects. New York: Marcel Dekker, 1986:317.

37. Duffy MC, Boyer JL. Pathophysiology of intrahepatic cholestasis and biliary obstruction. In: Ostrow JD, ed. Bile pigments and jaundice: Molecular, metabolic and medical aspects. New York: Marcel Dekker, 1986:333.

38. Moseley RH. Mechanism of bile formation and cholestasis: Clinical significance of recent experimental work. Am J Gastroenterol 1986;81:731.

39. Hatoff DE, Hardison WGM. Induced synthesis of alkaline phosphatase by bile acids in rat liver cell culture. Gastroenterology 1979;77:1062.

40. Eliakim M, Rachmilewitz M. Cholangiolitic manifestations in virus hepatitis. Gastroenterology 1956;31:369.

41. Shaldon S, Sherlock S. Virus hepatitis with features of prolonged bile retention. Br Med J 1957;2:734.

42. Morrow RH Jr, Smetana HF, Sai FT, Edgcomb JH. Unusual features of viral hepatitis in Accra, Ghana. Ann Intern Med 1968;68:1250.

43. Gordon SC, Reddy KR, Schiff L, Schiff ER. Prolonged intrahepatic cholestasis secondary to acute hepatitis A. Ann Intern Med 1984;101:635.

44. Ballard H, Bernstein M, Farrar JT. Fatty liver presenting as obstructive jaundice. Am J Med 1961;30:196.

45. Perrillo RP, Griffin R, DeSchryver-Kecskemeti K, Lander JJ, Zuckerman GR. Alcoholic liver disease presenting with marked elevation of serum alkaline phosphatase. Dig Dis Sci 1978;23:1061.

46. Kaplan MM. Primary biliary cirrhosis. N Engl J Med 1987;316:521.

47. Zimmerman HJ, Maddrey WC. Toxic and drug-induced hepatitis. In: Schiff L, Schiff ER, eds. Diseases of the liver. Philadelphia: JB Lippincott, 1987:591.

48. Lieberman DA, Keeffe EM, Stenzel P. Severe and prolonged oral contraceptive jaundice. J Clin Gastroenterol 1984;6:145.

49. Lucey MR, Moseley RH. Severe cholestasis associated with methyltestosterone: A case report. Am J Gastroenterol 1987;82:461.

50. Rahmat J, Gelfand RL, Gelfand MC, Winchester JF, Schreiner GE, Zimmerman HJ. Captopril-associated cholestatic jaundice. Ann Intern Med 1985;102:56.

51. Konikoff F, Alcalay J, Halevy J. Cloxacillin-induced cholestatic jaundice. Am J Gastroenterol 1986;81:1082.

52. Ramsay ID. Carbamazepine-induced jaundice. Br Med J 1967;4:155.

53. Vitorino RMM, Silveira JCB, Baptista A, De Moura MC. Jaundice associated with naproxen. Postgrad Med J 1980;56:368.

54. Cappell MS, Kozicky O, Competiello LS. Indomethacin-associated cholestasis. J Clin Gastroenterol 1988;10(4):445.

55. Benjamin SB. Phenylbutazine liver injury: A clinicopathological survey of 23 cases and review of the literature. Hepatology 1988;1:255.

56. Whittaker SJ, Amar JN, Wanless IR, Heathcote J. Sulindac hepatotoxicity. Gut 1982;23:875.

57. Mitrane MP, Singh A, Seibold JR. Cholestasis and fatal agranulocytosis complicating sulfasalazine therapy. J Rheumatol 1986;13:969.

58. Rex D, Lumeng L, Eble J, Rex L. Intrahepatic cholestasis and sicca complex after thiabendazole. Gastroenterology 1983;85:718.

59. Taggart HM, Alderdice JM. Fatal cholestatic jaundice in elderly patients taking benoxaprofen. Br Med J 1982;284:1372.

60. Solis-Herruzo JA, Castellano G, Colina F, Morillas JD, Munoz-Yague MT, Coca MC, Jelavic D. Hepatic injury in the toxic epidemic syndrome caused by ingestion of adulterated cooking oil (Spain, 1981). Hepatology 1984;4:131.

61. Mullick FG, Ishak KG, Mahabir R, Stromeyer FW. Hepatic injury associated with paraquat toxicity in humans. Liver 1981;1:209.

62. Kopelman H, Scheuer PJ, Williams R. The liver lesion of the Epping jaundice. Q J Med 1966;140:553.

63. Reyes H. The enigma of intrahepatic cholestasis of pregnancy: Lessons from Chile. Hepatology 1982;2:87.

64. Holzbach RT, Sanders JH. Recurrent intrahepatic cholestasis of pregnancy. JAMA 1965;193:204.

65. Frezza M, Pozzato G, Chiesa L, Stramentinoli G, Di Padova C. Reversal of intrahepatic cholestasis of pregnancy in women after high dose S-adenosyl-L-methionine administration. Hepatology 1984;4:274.

66. Pagter AGF, van Berge Henegouwen GP, Ten Bokkel Huinink JA, Brandt K-H. Familial benign recurrent intrahepatic cholestasis. Gastroenterology 1976;71:202.

67. LaBrecque DR, Mitros FA, Nathan RJ, Romanchuk KG, Judisch GF, El-Khoury GH. Four generations of arteriohepatic dysplasia. Hepatology 1982;2:467.

68. Fahrlander H, Huber F, Gloor F. Intrahepatic retention of bile in severe bacterial infections. Gastroenterology 1964;47:590.

69. Vermillion SE, Gregg JA, Baggenstoss AH, Bartholomew LG. Jaundice associated with bacteremia. Arch Intern Med 1969;124:611.

70. Zimmerman HJ, Fang M, Utili R, Seeff LB, Hoofnagle J. Jaundice due to bacterial infection. Gastroenterology 1979;77:362.

71. Paton A. Sepsis and cholestasis. Br Med J 1984;289:857.

72. Utili R, Abernathy CO, Zimmerman HJ. Inhibition of Na+, K+-adenosinetriphosphatase by endotoxin: A possible mechanism for endotoxin-induced cholestasis. J Infect Dis 1977;136:583.

73. Baker AL, Rosenberg IR. Hepatic complications of total parenteral nutrition. Am J Med 1987;82:489.

74. Perea DR, Greene MC, Fenster LF. Cholestasis associated with extrabiliary Hodgkin's disease. Gastroenterology 1974;67:680.

75. Piken EP, Abraham GE, Hepner GW. Investigation of a patient with Hodgkin's disease and cholestasis. Gastroenterology 1979;77:145.

76. Lefkowitch JH, Martin EC. Primary sclerosing cholangitis. In: Popper H, Schaffner F, eds. Progress in liver diseases. New York: Grune & Stratton, 1986:557.

77. Genest JF, Namas E, Grundfest-Broniatowski S, et al. Benign biliary structures: An analytic review (1970–1984). Surgery 1986;99:409.

78. Pellegrini CA, Thomas MJ, Way LW. Bilirubin and alkaline phosphatase valves before and after surgery for biliary observation. Am J Surg 1982;143:67.

79. Zimmerman HJ. Hepatologic effects of oncotherapeutic agents. In: Popper H, Schaffner F, eds. Progress in liver diseases. New York: Grune & Stratton, 1986:621.

80. Anderson SD, Holley HC, Berland LL, et al. Causes of jaundice during hepatic artery infusion chemotherapy. Radiology 1986;161:439.

81. Way LW, Sleisenger MH. Biliary obstruction, cholangitis, and choledocholithiasis. In: Sleisenger MH, Fordtran JS, eds. Gastrointestinal diseases. Philadelphia: WB Saunders, 1989:1714.

82. Nichols T, Craig RM. Caroli's disease: Clinical presentation simulating carcinoma of the pancreas. Am J Gastroenterol 1979;72:79.

83. Cook DJ, Salena BJ, Vincic LM. Adenomyoma of the common bile duct. Am J Gastroenterol 1988;83:432.

84. Shemesh E, Klein E, Abramowich D, Pines A. Common bile duct obstruction caused by hydatid daughter cysts—Management by endoscopic retrograde sphincterotomy. Am J Gastroenterol 1986;81:280.

85. Sung MW, Bruckner HW, Szabo S, Miltz HA. Extrahepatic obstructive jaundice due to colorectal cancer. Am J Gastroenterol 1988;83:267.

86. Johnson DH, Hainsworth JD, Greco FA. Extrahepatic biliary obstruction caused by small-cell lung cancer. Ann Intern Med 1985;102:487.

87. Radhakrishnan S, Nakib BA, Liddawi HA, Ruwaih AA. Primary gastrointestinal lymphoma complicated by common bile duct obstruction: Report of two cases. Am J Gastroenterol 1986;81:691.

88. Merza AP, Raiser MW. Biliary tract manifestations of the Marfan syndrome. Am J Gastroenterol 1987;82:779.
89. Marcial MA, Marcial-Rojas RA. Parasitic diseases of the liver. In: Schiff L, Schiff ER, eds. Diseases of the liver. Philadelphia: JB Lippincott, 1987:1171.
90. Khuroo MS, Zargar SA. Biliary ascariasis: A common cause of biliary and pancreatic disease in an endemic area. Gastroenterology 1985;88:418.
91. Wittner M, Turner JW, Jacquette G, et al. Eustrongylidiasis—A parasitic infection acquired by eating sushi. New Engl J Med 1989, 320:1124.
92. Littenberg G, Afroudakis A, Kaplowitz N. Common bile duct stenosis from chronic pancreatitis: A clinical and pathologic spectrum. Medicine 1979;58:385.
93. Cooperman AM. Chronic pancreatitis. Surg Clin North Am 1981;61:71.
94. Fontch PG, Ferguson DR. Duodenal Crohn's disease complicated by common bile duct obstruction: Report of a case and review of the literature. Am J Gastroenterol 1984;79:520.
95. Rumane MC, Lieberman DA. Eosinophilic gastroenteritis presenting with biliary and duodenal obstruction. Am J Gastroenterol 1987;82:775.
96. Zacharz K, Geier S, Pellecchia C, Irwin G. Jaundice secondary to hepatic artery aneurysm: Radiological appearance and clinical features. Am J Gastroenterol 1986;81:295.
97. Levy M, Fryd DH, Eliakim M. Intrahepatic destructive jaundice due to amyloidosis of the liver: A case report and review of the literature. Gastroenterology 1971;61:234.
98. Rubinow A, Koff RS, Cohen AS. Severe intrahepatic cholestasis in primary amyloidosis: A report of four cases and review of the literature. Am J Med 1978;64:937.
99. Hoffman MS, Stein BE, Davidian MM, Rosenthal WS. Hepatic amyloidosis presenting as severe intrahepatic cholestasis: A case report and review of the literature. Am J Gastroenterol 1988;83:783.
100. Morgenstern L. Postoperative jaundice. Am J Surg 1974;128:255.
101. LaMont JT, Isselbacher KJ. Postoperative jaundice. N Engl J Med 1973;288:305.
102. Nunes G, Blaisdell FW, Margaretten W. Mechanism of hepatic dysfunction following shock and trauma. Arch Surg 1970;100:546.
103. Boekhorst T, Ureus M, Doesburg W, et al. Etiologic factors of jaundice in severely ill patients. J Hepatol 1988;7:111.
104. Chu C-M, Chang C-H, Liaw Y-F, Hsieh M-J. Jaundice after open heart surgery: A prospective study. Thorax 1984;39:52.
105. Orlando R III, Gleason E, Drezner AD. Acute acalculous cholecystitis in the critically ill patient. Am J Surg 1983;145:472.
106. Schmid M, Hefti ML, Gattiker R, Kistler HJ, Senning A. Benign postoperative intrahepatic cholestasis. N Engl J Med 1965;272:545.
107. Kantrowitz PA, Jones WA, Greenberger NJ, Isselbacher KJ. Severe postoperative hyperbilirubinemia simulating obstructive jaundice. N Engl J Med 1967;11:276.
108. Schneiderman DJ. Hepatobiliary abnormalities of AIDS. Gastroenterol Clin North Am 1988;17:615.
109. Lebovics E, Dworkin BM, Heier SK, Rosenthal WS. The hepatobiliary manifestations of human immunodeficiency virus infection. Am J Gastroenterol 1988;83:1.
110. Schneiderman DJ, Arenson DM, Cello JP, Margaretten W, Weber TE. Hepatic disease in patients with the acquired immune deficiency syndrome (AIDS). Hepatology 1987;7:925.
111. Kaplan LD, Kahn J, Jacobson M, Bottles K, Cello J. Primary bile duct lymphoma in the acquired immunodeficiency syndrome (AIDS). Ann Intern Med 1989;110:161.
112. Kavin H, Jonas RB, Chowdhury L, Kabins S. Acalculous cholecystitis and cytomegalovirus infection in the acquired immunodeficiency syndrome. Ann Intern Med 1986;104:53.
113. Agha FP, Nostrant TT, Abrams GD, Mazanec M, Van Moll L, Gumucio JJ. Cytomegalovirus cholangitis in a homosexual man with acquired immune deficiency syndrome. Am J Gastroenterol 1986;81:1068.
114. Jacobson MA, Cello JP, Sande MA. Cholestasis and disseminated cytomegalovirus disease in patients with the acquired immunodeficiency syndrome. Am J Med 1988;84:218.
115. Dolmatch BL, Laing FC, Federle MP, Jeffrey RB, Cello J. AIDS-related cholangitis: Radiographic findings in nine patients. Radiology 1987;163:313.
116. Schiff L. Jaundice: A clinical approach. In: Schiff L, Schiff ER, eds. Diseases of the liver. Philadelphia: JB Lippincott, 1987:209.
117. Fortson WC, Tedesco FJ, Starnes EC, Shaw CT. Marked elevation of serum transaminase activity associated with extrahepatic biliary tract disease. J Clin Invest 1985;7(6):502.
118. Griner PF, Mazewski RJ, Mushlin AI, Greenland P. Selection and interpretations of diagnostic tests and procedures. Ann Intern Med 1981;94:553.
119. Pauker SG, Eckman MH. Principles of diagnostic testing. In: Kelley WN, ed. Textbook of internal medicine. Philadelphia: JB Lippincott, 1989:16.
120. Martin WB, Apostolakos PC. Clinical versus actuarial prediction in the differential diagnosis of jaundice. Am J Med Sci 1960;240:571.
121. Schenker S, Balint J, Schiff L. Differential diagnosis of jaundice: Report of a prospective study of 61 proved cases. Am J Dig Dis 1962;7:449.
122. Malchow-Moller A, Matzen P, Bjerregaard B, Hilden J, Holst-Christensen J, Staehr Johansen T, Altman L, Thomsen C, Juhl E. Causes and characteristics of 500 consecutive cases of jaundice. Scand J Gastroenterol 1981;16:1.
123. Stern B, Knill-Jones RP, Williams R. Use of computer program for diagnosing jaundice in district hospitals and specialized liver unit. Br Med J 1975;2:659.
124. O'Connor KW, Snodgrass PJ, Swonder JE, Mahoney S, Burt R, Cockerrill EDM, Lumeng L. A blinded prospective study comparing four current noninvasive approaches in the differential diagnosis of medical versus surgical jaundice. Gastroenterology 1983;84:1498.
125. Scharschmidt BF, Goldberg HI, Schmid R. Approach to the patient with cholestatic jaundice. Med Intel 1983;308:1515.
126. Vennes JA, Bond JH. Approach to the jaundiced patient. Gastroenterology 1983;84:1615.
127. Saint-Marc Girardin M-F, Le Minor M, Alperovitch A, Roudot-Thoraval F, Metreau J-M, Dhumeaux D. Computer-aided selection of diagnostic tests in jaundiced patients. Gut 1985;26:961.
128. Lumeng L, O'Connor KW. Differential diagnosis of jaundice. In: Ostrow JD, ed. Bile pigments and jaundice: Molecular, metabolic and medical aspects. New York: Marcel Dekker, 1986:475.
129. Lindberg G, Nilsson LH, Thulin L. Decision theory as an aid in the diagnosis of cholestatic jaundice. Acta Chir Scand 1983;149:521.
130. Richter JM, Silverstein MD, Schapiro R. Suspected obstructive jaundice: A decision analysis of diagnostic strategies. Ann Intern Med 1983;99:46.
131. Wheeler PG, Theodossi A, Pickford R, Laws J, Knill-Jones RP, Williams R. Non-invasive techniques in the diagnosis of jaundice—ultrasound and computer. Gut 1979;20:196.
132. Vicary FR, Cusick G, Shirley IM, Blackwell RJ. Ultrasound and jaundice. Gut 1977;18:161.
133. Vallon AG, Lees WR, Cotton PB. Grey-scale ultrasonography in cholestatic jaundice. Gut 1979;20:51.
134. Taylor KJW, Rosenfield AT, Spiro HM. Diagnostic accuracy of gray scale ultrasonography for the jaundiced patient. Arch Intern Med 1979;139:60.
135. Taylor KJW, Rosenfield AT. Grey-scale ultrasonography in the differential diagnosis of jaundice. Arch Surg 1977;112:820.
136. Malini S, Sabel J. Ultrasonography in obstructive jaundice. Radiology 1977;123:429.
137. Bolondi L, Gandolfi L, Rossi A, Caletti GC, Fontana G, Labo G. Ultrasound in the diagnosis of cholestatic jaundice. Am J Gastroenterol 1979;71:168.
138. Haubek A, Pedersen JH, Burcharth F, Gammelgaard J, Hancke S, Willumsen L. Dynamic sonography in the evaluation of jaundice. Am J Roentgenology 1981;136:1071.
139. Morris AI, Fawcitt RA, Wood R, Forbes WSC, Isherwood I, Marsh MN. Computed tomography, ultrasound, and cholestatic jaundice. Gut 1978;19:685.
140. Cotton PB, Denyer ME, Kreel L, Husband J, Meire HB, Lees W. Comparative clinical impact of endoscopic pancreatography, grey-scale ultrasonography, and computer tomography (EMI scanning) in pancreatic disease: Preliminary report. Gut 1978;19:679.
141. Gross BH, Harter LP, Gore RM, Callen PW, Filly RA, Shapiro HA, Goldberg HI. Ultrasonic evaluation of common bile duct stones:

Prospective comparison with endoscopic retrograde cholangiopancreatography. Radiology 1983;146:471.

142. Laing FC, Jeffrey RB Jr. Choledocholithiasis and cystic duct obstruction: Difficult ultrasonographic diagnosis. Radiology 1983;146:475.

143. Campillo B, Bernuau J, Witz M-O, Lorphelin J-M, Degott C, Rueff B, Benhamou J-P. Ultrasonography in acute fatty liver of pregnancy. Ann Intern Med 1986;105:383.

144. Hessel SJ, Siegelman SS, McNeil BJ, Sanders R, Adams DF, Alderson PO, Finberg HJ, Abrams HL. A prospective evaluation of computed tomography and ultrasound of the pancreas. Radiology 1982;143:129.

145. Kamin PD, Bernardino ME, Wallace S, Jing B-S. Comparison of ultrasound and computed tomography in the detection of pancreatic malignancy. Cancer 1980;46:2410.

146. Pedrosa CS, Casanova R, Rodriguez R. Computed tomography in obstructive jaundice. Radiology 1981;139:627.

147. Pedrosa CS, Casanova R, Lezana AH, Fernandez MC. Computed tomography in obstructive jaundice. Radiology 1981;139:635.

148. Van Dyke JA, Stanley RJ, Berland LL. Pancreatic imaging. Ann Intern Med 1985;102:212.

149. Reiman TH, Balfe DM, Weyman PJ. Suprapancreatic biliary obstruction: CT evaluation. Radiology 1987;163:49.

150. Barakos JA, Ralls PW, Lapin SA, Johnson MB, Radin DR, Colletti PM, Boswell WD Jr, Halls JM. Cholelithiasis: Evaluation with CT. Radiology 1987;162:415.

151. Baron RL. Common bile duct stones: Reassessment of criteria for CT diagnosis. Radiology 1987;162:419.

152. Teefey SA, Baron RL, Rohrmann CA, Shuman WP, Freeny PC. Sclerosing cholangitis: CT findings. Radiology 1988;169:635.

153. Farah MC, Jafri SZH, Schwab RE, Mezwa DG, Francis IR, Noujaim S, Kim C. Duodenal neoplasms: Role of CT. Radiology 1987;162:839.

154. Freeny PC, Marks WM, Ryan JA, Traverso LW. Pancreatic ductal adenocarcinoma: Diagnosis and staging with dynamic CT. Radiology 1988;166:125.

155. Krishnamurthy S, Krishnamurthy GT. Technetium-99m-iminodiacetic acid organic anions: Review of biokinetics and clinical application in hepatology. Hepatology 1989;9:139.

156. Chervu LR, Nunn AD, Loberg MD. Radiopharmaceuticals for hepatobiliary imaging. Semin Nucl Med 1982;8:5.

157. Klingensmith WC III, Fritzberg AR, Spitzer VM, Kuni CC, Shanahan WSM. Clinical comparison of diisopropyl-IDA Tc 99m and diethyl-IDA Tc 99m for evaluation of the hepatobiliary system. Radiology 1981;140:791.

158. Rosenthall L. Cholescintigraphy in the presence of jaundice utilizing Tc-IDA. Semin Nucl Med 1982;8:53.

159. Egbert RN, Braunstein P, Lyons KP, Miller DR. Total bile duct obstruction: Prompt diagnosis by hepatobiliary imaging. Arch Surg 1983;118:709.

160. Lee AW, Ram MD, Shis W-J, Murphy K. Technetium-99m BIDA biliary scintigraphy in the evaluation of the jaundiced patient. J Nucl Med 1986;27:1407.

161. Lecklitner ML, Austin AR, Benedetto AR, Growcock GW. Positive predictive value of cholescintigraphy in common bile duct obstruction. J Nucl Med 1986;27:1403.

162. Scott BB, Evans JA, Unsworth J. The initial investigation of jaundice in a district general hospital: A study of ultrasonography and hepatobiliary scintigraphy. Br J Radiol 1980;53:557.

163. Krishnamurthy GT, Lieberman DA, Brar HS. Detection, localization, and quantitation of degree of common bile duct obstruction by scintigraphy. J Nucl Med 1985;26:726.

164. Matzen P, Malchow-Moller A, Brun B, Gronvall S, Haubek A, Henriksen JH, Laursen K, Lejerstofte J, Stage P, Winkler K, Juhl E. Ultrasonography, computed tomography and cholescintigraphy in suspected obstructive jaundice—A prospective comparative study. Gastroenterology 1983;84:1492.

165. Zeman RK, Lee C, Jaffe MH, Burrell MI. Hepatobiliary scintigraphy and sonography in early biliary obstruction. Radiology 1984;153:793.

166. Lieberman DA, Krishnamurthy GT. Intrahepatic versus extrahepatic cholestasis. Gastroenterology 1986;90:734.

167. Freitas JE. Cholescintigraphy in acute and chronic cholecystitis. Semin Nucl Med 1982;8:18.

168. Weissmann HS, Gliedman ML, Wilk PJ, Sugarman LA, Badia J, Guglielmo K, Freeman LM. Evaluation of the postoperative patient with 99mTc-IDA cholescintigraphy. Semin Nucl Med 1982;8:27.

169. Burcharth F, Nielbo N. Percutaneous transhepatic cholangiography with selective catheterization of the common bile duct. AJR Am J Roentgenol 1976;127:409.

170. Ferrucci JT, Wittenberg J. Refinements in Chiba needle transhepatic cholangiography. AJR Am J Roentgenol 1977;129:11.

171. Juttner H-U, Redeker AG. Fine needle transhepatic cholangiography. Am J Gastroenterol 1981;75:454.

172. Mueller PR, vanSonnenberg E, Simeone JF. Fine-needle transhepatic cholangiography. Ann Intern Med 1982;97:567.

173. Moore AV, Illescas FF, Mills SR, Wertman DE, Heaston DK, Newman GE, Zuger JH, Salmon RB, Dunnick NR. Percutaneous dilation of benign biliary strictures. Radiology 1987;163:625.

174. Nilsson U, Evander A, Ihse I, Lunderquist A, Mocibob A. Percutaneous transhepatic cholangiography and drainage. Acta Radiol 1983;24:433.

175. Nakayama T, Ikeda A, Okuda K. Percutaneous transhepatic drainage of the biliary tract. Gastroenterology 1978;74:554.

176. Park JH, Choi BI, Han MC, Sung KB, Choo IW, Kim C-W. Percutaneous removal of residual intrahepatic stones. Radiology 1987;163:619.

177. Cotton PB. Progress report: ERCP. Gut 1977;18:316.

178. Dowsett JF, Vaira D, Polydorou A, Russell ROG, Salmon PR. Interventional endoscopy in the pancreatobiliary tree. Am J Gastroenterol 1988;83:1328.

179. Kozarek RA. Direct cholangioscopy and pancreatoscopy at time of endoscopic retrograde cholangiopancreatography. Am J Gastroenterol 1988;83:55.

180. Brandabur JJ, Kozarek RA, Ball TJ, Hofer BO, Ryan JA, Traverso LW, Freeny PC, Lewis GP. Nonoperative versus operative treatment of obstructive jaundice in pancreatic cancer: Cost and survival analysis. Am J Gastroenterol 1988;83:1132.

181. Siegel JH, Snady H. The significance of endoscopically placed prostheses in the management of biliary obstruction due to carcinoma of the pancreas: Results of nonoperative decompression in 277 patients. Am J Gastroenterol 1986;81:634.

182. Siegel JH, Tone P, Menikeim D. Gallstone pancreatitis: Pathogenesis and clinical forms—The emerging role of endoscopic management. Am J Gastroenterol 1986;81:774.

183. Williams HJ Jr, Bender CE, May GR. Benign postoperative biliary strictures: Dilation with fluoroscopic guidance. Radiology 1987;163:629.

184. Huibregtse K, Katon RM, Coene PP, Tytgat GNJ. Endoscopic palliative treatment in pancreatic cancer. Gastrointest Endo 1986;32:334.

185. Siegel JH, Lichtenstein JL, Pullano WE, Ramsey WH, Rosenbaum A, Halpern G, Nonkin R, Jacob H. Treatment of malignant biliary obstruction by endoscopic implantation of iridium 192 using a new double lumen endoprosthesis. Gastrointest Endo 1988;34:301.

186. Bilbao MK, Dotter CT, Lee TG, Katon RM. Complications of endoscopic retrograde cholangiopancreatography (ERCP). Gastroenterology 1976;70:314.

187. Summerfield JA. Biliary obstruction is best managed by endoscopists. Gut 1988;29:741.

42

Approach to the Patient with Abnormal Liver Chemistries

RICHARD H. MOSELEY

The approach to the patient with abnormal liver chemistries is not governed by any well-defined diagnostic algorithms. Instead, a systematic approach to patients with suspected underlying liver disease involves, first, a thorough understanding of the diverse panel of available measurements of liver function and serum markers of hepatobiliary disease. From this panel, a group of indices most appropriate to the particular clinical problem is then selected. A single test is rarely sufficient in the approach to most clinical problems. The selection process is, however, facilitated by several distinct patterns of hepatocellular injury. Because diagnostic tests are imperfect, they are usually discussed in terms that allow assessment of their diagnostic value. The sensitivity of a test is defined as the likelihood of an abnormal test result in patients known to have a disease, and specificity is the likelihood of a normal test result in patients known to be free of the disease. The false-positive rate is the likelihood of an abnormal test result in patients without the disease (1 − specificity), and the false-negative rate is the likelihood of a normal test result in patients known to have the disease (1 − sensitivity). Thus, sensitivity and the false-negative rate evaluate a diagnostic test in patients with disease, and specificity and the false-positive rate evaluate a test in patients without disease.[1] This chapter consists of a discussion of representative and commonly used tests and offers guidelines in the interpretation of results.

CLINICAL EVALUATION

As in most disease states, an accurate history is critical in the approach to the patient with laboratory evidence of liver disease. Although systemic symptoms of liver disease, such as anorexia, weight loss, chills and fever, nausea, and vomiting are nonspecific and typically of little help in the differential diagnosis, valuable information can be elicited by questions regarding family history, drug use (prescription as well as over-the-counter medications), alcohol consumption and illicit substance use/abuse, exposure history, sexual and menstrual history, occupational and/or environmental history, travel history, and past surgical (including, if available, anesthesia records) and transfusion history.

A family history of jaundice may be present in hereditary hemolytic states, such as hereditary spherocytosis, in Gilbert's syndrome, in Dubin-Johnson and Rotor's syndrome, and in benign idiopathic recurrent cholestasis. Familial forms of intrahepatic cholestasis, such as arteriohepatic dysplasia (Alagille's syndrome), have been well described. Hemochromatosis, Wilson's disease (hepatolenticular degeneration), and alpha$_1$-antitrypsin deficiency are examples of liver diseases transmitted by an autosomal recessive mode of inheritance, and genetic factors may play a role in other hepatobiliary disorders, such as primary sclerosing cholangitis and autoimmune chronic active hepatitis.

Given the relatively nonspecific presentation of drug-induced liver disease, drug-related hepatic injury may not be immediately suspected in a patient with impaired liver function. Difficulties in diagnosis are compounded by the unknown hepatotoxicity of newly introduced agents. Nevertheless, the possibility of drug-induced liver injury should be considered in all patients with a seemingly nonspecific change or worsening of liver chemistries, and such considerations are aided by a complete drug history. Alcohol and nonprescription medication use is an important part of this inquiry. Alcohol intake should be quantified and expressed, when possible, in terms of grams per day of alcohol (daily consumption, converted to milliliters, is multiplied by the percentage of the form of alcohol ingested and by 0.78). A threshold for the development of cirrhosis of 160 g/day for 15 years has been described in male alcoholics,[2] and it is likely that a lower threshold exists in women.[3] Alcoholic patients presenting with jaundice and profoundly abnormal serum transaminase levels should always be questioned regarding the use of acetaminophen. A high incidence of aspirin-induced hepatotoxicity has been observed in patients with rheumatic diseases, including juvenile rheumatoid arthritis and systemic lupus erythematosus, that appears to correlate with serum salicylate levels.[4] Hypervitaminosis A is a well-recognized clinical syndrome associated with hepatic injury, intracranial hypertension, and desquamative dermatitis.[5] Although most cases of hepatic injury from vitamin A have occurred with massive long-term intake, toxicity may be potentiated by ethanol,[6] severe hypertriglyceridemia,[7] and renal failure.[8]

Viral hepatitis should be suspected in patients with abnormal liver chemistries and a history of exposure to and/or contact with jaundiced individuals, syringes and/or needles (including tattoo paraphernalia), or blood and blood products. A history of recent ingestion of raw oysters or steamed clams should suggest hepatitis A infection, although specific risk factors that have been associated with hepatitis A within the United States also include homosexual contact[9] and contact with children attending daycare centers.[10] In contrast to the well-recognized problem of nosocomial hepatitis B, nosocomial outbreaks of hepatitis A have, until recently, received little attention.[11] Questions directed at determining the source of water for patients are occasionally relevant, because private water supplies contaminated with sewage have been frequently implicated in outbreaks of hepatitis A. The development of abnormal liver chemistries in the "healthy" hepatitis B carrier warrants strong consideration of superinfection with hepatitis delta virus. Recent travel to areas endemic for viral hepatitis should be noted; waterborne outbreaks of non-A, non-B hepatitis have been clearly documented in Southeast Asia and the Indian subcontinent. Abnormalities in smell (dysosmia) and taste (dysgeusia) may be noted by patients afflicted with viral hepatitis. Arthritis, abrupt in onset and with a strong predilection for proximal interphalangeal joints, has been noted during the prodromal phase in approximately 20% of patients with hepatitis B.[12]

Sexually transmitted diseases are an important cause of abnormal liver chemistries, and a sexual history should be included in the evaluation of such patients. Efforts to obtain accurate historical information are usually compromised by apprehension felt on the part of the interviewer rather than the patient. Relevant historical elements include information regarding whether or not the patient is currently sexually active, the number of sexual partners the patient has had in the preceding 6 months (the average incubation period of hepatitis B is from 6 to 12 weeks), whether the patient's sexual partners are of the same or different sex, whether the patient has been recently exposed to a new sexual partner, and the sites of sexual exposure. A sexual history in the female patient should always include information on contraceptive use. A menstrual history may reveal the presence of secondary amenorrhea, a frequent complication of chronic liver disease.

Although the use of hepatotoxins such as carbon tetrachloride, chloroform, and trinitrotoluene has diminished, liver injury associated with accidental and occupational exposure to workplace chemicals remains a significant problem.[13] Although an itemized list is beyond the scope of this text, exposure to industrial and environmental hepatotoxins such as trichlorethylene (a commonly used solvent in dry cleaning that can cause an acute centrilobular hepatitis)[14] and vinyl chloride (used in the plastics industry and associated with the occurrence of hepatic angiosarcomas)[15] may be elicited by a thorough occupational history. Arsenic, used in insecticide sprays by vineyard workers, has been implicated in a spectrum of chronic liver disease, including noncirrhotic portal hypertension[16] and hepatic angiosarcoma.[17] Occupational exposure to 2-nitropropane in industrial construction, highway maintenance, ship building, and plastic production has resulted in fulminant hepatic failure.[18] Although more commonly observed as a complication of high-dose antineoplastic chemotherapy, particularly in the setting of bone marrow transplantation,[19] hepatic veno-occlusive disease due to poisoning with pyrrolizidine alkaloids present in herbal teas has been reported in this country.[20]

The liver may be a target organ in a vast array of systemic disorders. In particular, but by no means exclusively, the presence of coexistent cardiac, pancreatic, and inflammatory bowel disease should be considered in the evaluation of any patient with abnormal liver chemistries. Right-sided congestive heart failure, hypotension, and shock are well-recognized causes of abnormal liver chemistries.

Prolongation of the prothrombin time, often disproportionate to other signs of liver dysfunction, is the most frequent abnormality in patients with congestive heart failure, although elevations in serum bilirubin (primarily of the unconjugated form and rarely greater than 3 mg/dl) and serum transaminases can also occur.[21] Clinically inapparent left-sided heart failure may present with a picture like that of acute or chronic hepatitis.[22] Hemochromatosis, in turn, may present as a congestive cardiomyopathy,[23] in addition to hypogonadism, arthropathy, diabetes, and hyperpigmentation. Distal common bile duct stenosis is a well-described complication of chronic alcoholic pancreatitis to be considered in the setting of anicteric alkaline phosphatase elevations of a persistent nature.[24,25] The biliary tree may be similarly affected in cystic fibrosis.[26] Hepatobiliary manifestations of inflammatory bowel disease of clinical import occur in up to 10% of patients.[27] Hematologic disorders, such as polycythemia rubra vera, myeloproliferative disorders, and paroxysmal nocturnal hemoglobinuria may predispose to hepatic vein thrombosis. Hemoglobinopathies, such as sickle cell anemia and thalassemia, have been implicated as risk factors for pigment stone formation, and for sickle cell disease, a spectrum of morphologic and clinical features of hepatic dysfunction has been described, including unexplained hepatic necrosis, portal fibrosis, regenerative nodules, and cirrhosis.[28] Bacteremia, particularly with gram-negative organisms and *Staphylococcus aureus,* should be considered in any ill individual with disproportionate elevations of direct and total serum bilirubin values in comparison to levels of alkaline phosphatase and aspartate aminotransferase.[29] Bilirubin elevations may become manifest prior to the clinical recognition of infection, and persistent or progressive hyperbilirubinemia despite anti-infective therapy portends a poor prognosis and may warrant institution of additional therapeutic agents.[30] Leptospirosis should be regarded with a high index of suspicion in the febrile patient with both hepatic and renal abnormalities and a history of potential contact with animal urine or water. Renal cell carcinoma may present with abnormalities in liver chemistries, primarily elevated alkaline phosphatase levels, in the absence of hepatic metastases (nephrogenic hepatic dysfunction syndrome).[31] Liver diseases peculiar to the gravid female include intrahepatic cholestasis of pregnancy, toxemia, and acute fatty liver of pregnancy, although viral hepatitis is the most common cause of jaundice during pregnancy.[32]

Fatty liver, or hepatic steatosis, should be considered in the obese patient presenting with abnormal liver chemistries. Mild degrees of fatty infiltration have been observed in approximately 50% of obese and in 60% to 100% of morbidly obese (>45 kg overweight) individuals, manifesting biochemically as mild elevations of serum transaminases and alkaline phosphatase.[33] Furthermore, a form of nonalcoholic liver disease resembling alcoholic hepatitis and cirrhosis has been described predominantly in middle-aged obese women with diabetes mellitus and/or hyperlipidemia.[34] Obesity appears to be the major factor in the fatty infiltration observed in adult-onset diabetes mellitus.[33]

The nature of, and indications for, previous abdominal surgical procedures should be fully ascertained. Information, if available, concerning the gross appearance of the liver at the time of operation may prove valuable. In the postoperative patient, surgical and anesthesia records should be carefully reviewed for the inhalational agent administered, the presence and duration of intraoperative hypotension, and the amount of blood product support required.

Hepatic injury has been observed with most of the halogen-substituted inhalation anesthetics (e.g., halothane, methoxyflurane, and enflurane), initially presenting with fever, followed by the appearance of jaundice, with or without eosinophilia, after a latent period of several days.[35] Transfusions, particularly of stored blood, can be a factor in the development of postoperative jaundice. Progressive liver disease, including cirrhosis, has been described as a late complication of jejunoileal bypass surgery.[36] Biliary strictures, retained and recurrent stones, or papillary stenosis should be considered in the diagnosis of the postcholecystectomy patient with abnormal liver chemistries.

Generalized pruritus may be a presenting symptom in patients with liver disease, particularly cholestatic syndromes. The exact mechanism responsible for this often disabling symptom is unclear. Despite the frequent response to oral cholestyramine, a bile acid-binding agent, there is no apparent correlation between either serum or tissue levels of bile acids and the degree of pruritus.[37] Clinical experience suggests that pruritus in the jaundiced patient is frequently nocturnal and most pronounced on the palms and soles.

The presence, or absence, and character of abdominal pain may provide some clues in the approach to establishing an etiology to abnormal liver chemistries. In contrast to the intense and rapidly developing right upper quadrant abdominal pain of acute extrahepatic obstruction, such as occurs in choledocholithiasis, the pain associated with acute viral hepatitis can be best described as a heavy or dragging sensation. Pain from primary and metastatic tumors of the liver may be distinguished by its dull or boring character, although hemorrhage into the tumor may result in the sudden onset of severe pain.

Physical findings of some discriminative value in the patient with abnormal liver chemistries include stigmata of chronic liver disease (e.g., spider angiomata, palmar erythema, parotid gland enlargement, gynecomastia, Dupuytren's contracture, and testicular atrophy), hepatomegaly and liver consistency, splenomegaly, gallbladder distention, and abdominal tenderness. However, poor interobserver agreement for several of these clinical signs has been reported,[38] and for other signs, such as Dupuytren's contracture, the correlation with chronic liver disease is poor.[39] Although the degree of hepatomegaly can be quite variable in all forms of hepatobiliary disease, a liver span greater than 15 cm is more often associated with passive congestion from right-sided heart failure or neoplastic and infiltrative processes (e.g., amyloidosis, myeloproliferative disorders, hepatic steatosis, and the glycogen and lipid-storage disorders).[40] A pulsatile liver may be encountered in tricuspid insufficiency. A hepatic bruit or friction rub should alert the examiner to the possibility of an underlying hepatocellular carcinoma; alternatively, a friction rub may occur with a hepatic abscess or in acute cholecystitis.[41] The presence of sunflower cataracts and Kayser-Fleischer rings, golden brown or greenish discoloration of Descemet's membrane in the limbic region of the cornea, initially appearing at the superior corneal quadrant, should be sought with either the unaided eye or with slit-lamp ophthalmoscopy, even if the latter is no longer considered pathognomonic for Wilson's disease.[42] Conjuctival suffusion, with or without hemorrhage, should suggest leptospirosis. Murphy's sign, or inspiratory arrest during deep palpation of the right upper quadrant, is highly suggestive of acute cholecystitis. Punch or fist percussion tenderness can also be elicited in acute cholecystitis (and in acute

hepatocellular injury) and may help to differentiate hepatobiliary from pleural-based pain. A distended gallbladder, detected by either inspection or palpation, may be a presentation of malignant obstruction of the common bile duct (Courvoisier's sign).

Jaundice, manifested by yellow pigmentation of the skin, mucous membranes, and sclerae, typically requires a serum bilirubin concentration of greater than 3 mg/dl for detection. Artificial light makes detection at low levels more difficult. Ingestion of foods rich in carotene (such as carrots) and lycopene (such as tomato juice), of drugs such as quinacrine and busulfan, or of toxins, such as picric acid, may result in similar skin discoloration that is readily distinguished from jaundice by the absence of scleral icterus.

In addition to jaundice and excoriations resulting from pruritus, skin manifestations of potential aid in the differential diagnosis of patients with abnormal liver chemistries include the hyperpigmentation associated with primary biliary cirrhosis and hemochromatosis, xanthomas and xanthelasmas present in chronic cholestasis, and the hypertrichosis of periorbital and malar regions and eczematoid dermatitis of sun-exposed areas in porphyria cutanea tarda. A high frequency of ichthyosislike states and koilonychia has also been reported in hemochromatosis,[43] and lichen planus has been associated with autoimmune chronic active hepatitis[44] and primary biliary cirrhosis.[45]

HEPATIC FUNCTION TESTS

Laboratory determinations that reflect hepatic disease are collectively called "liver function tests." However, only some are true measurements of hepatic function, and the use of this descriptive term should be discouraged. Tests that examine the ability of the liver to excrete substances, particularly organic anions, into bile fall within this strict definition, as do laboratory assessments of the synthetic and metabolic capacity of the liver.

Bilirubin

Tests of bilirubin metabolism are important in the assessment of hepatic function, because bilirubin is an endogenous organic anion, derived primarily from the degradation of hemoglobin from senescent erythroid cells. Photometric determination of the azo derivatives obtained by reaction of plasma with the diazonium ion of sulfanilic acid (the diazo, or van den Bergh, reaction) separates bilirubin into two fractions, a water-soluble direct-reacting conjugated form and a lipid-soluble indirect-reacting form representing unconjugated bilirubin. Normal plasma total bilirubin concentrations in males are significantly higher than in females, and virtually all the bilirubin normally present in serum is the unconjugated fraction. Hyperbilirubinemia, clinically manifested as jaundice, can accordingly be classified as either predominantly unconjugated or predominantly conjugated, simply by subtracting direct from total serum bilirubin to estimate indirect, or unconjugated, bilirubin. Increased production of bilirubin, impaired transport into hepatocytes, and defective bilirubin conjugation within the hepatocyte characterize disorders associated with unconjugated hyperbilirubinemia. Up to 85% of total serum bilirubin is the unconjugated form in these disease states.[40] Besides the rate of hemolysis, the ability of the liver to conjugate bilirubin determines the degree of unconjugated hyperbilirubinemia observed. Even in severe hemolytic disorders, total serum bilirubin rarely exceeds 5 mg/dl in the presence of normal hepatic function.[40] Unconjugated hyperbilirubinemia may also be observed in disease states that interfere with the delivery of bilirubin to the liver, such as congestive heart failure, or in the presence of portosystemic shunts. In contrast, in disorders with impaired intrahepatic excretion of bilirubin, the rate-limiting step in overall bilirubin metabolism, and in extrahepatic obstruction, a conjugated hyperbilirubinemia is observed. In these settings, typically greater than 50% of the serum bilirubin is in the direct-reacting form.[40]

A directly reacting fraction of bilirubin that is apparently covalently bound to albumin (albumin-bound bilirubin or delta bilirubin) has also been recently identified.[46] It represents a significant fraction of total bilirubin in patients with both hepatocellular and cholestatic forms of jaundice when hepatic excretion of conjugated bilirubin is impaired, but it is not present in disorders associated with a predominant unconjugated hyperbilirubinemia. During recovery from jaundice, albumin-bound bilirubin tends to persist in plasma because the albumin–bilirubin complex is minimally filtered by the kidney.[46] This provides an explanation for the slow resolution of jaundice in convalescent patients with otherwise apparently normal liver function.

Urine bilirubin is invariably conjugated bilirubin and thus is encountered only in conditions in which serum levels of direct or conjugated bilirubin are elevated. The tea-colored appearance of urine caused by the presence of bilirubin must be differentiated from similar discoloration by hemoglobinuria and myoglobinuria. Prolonged storage before testing may produce false-negative results; phenothiazine administration may cause false-positive findings.[40] Bilirubinuria may precede the clinical appearance of jaundice, largely because of the low (<1.0 mg/dl) renal threshold for conjugated bilirubin.

Conjugated bilirubin excreted in bile is acted upon by intestinal bacteria to form urobilinogen. Unlike conjugated bilirubin, urobilinogen may undergo an enterohepatic circulation. Urobilinogen not excreted into bile is filtered at the glomerulus, accounting for its presence, in minimal amounts (<4 mg/day), in urine. Although rarely performed, urinary urobilinogen can be elevated in disorders of bilirubin overproduction, such as hemolytic states, and decreased in extrahepatic obstruction when conjugated bilirubin is prevented from reaching the gut. Impaired hepatobiliary excretion of urobilinogen in disorders characterized by hepatocellular dysfunction results in mild elevations in urinary urobilinogen. Similarly, variations from normal fecal urobilinogen output, typically ranging from 50 to 280 mg/day, can be assessed. Antibiotic suppression of intestinal bacterial flora and impaired bilirubin excretion decrease fecal output, whereas output is increased with hemolysis.

Serum Bile Acids

Two primary bile acids, cholic and chenodeoxycholic acid, are synthesized in the liver from cholesterol and converted by intestinal bacteria to the secondary bile acids, deoxycholic and lithocholic acid. Chenodeoxycholate can also be transformed into the tertiary

bile acid, ursodeoxycholate. Serum bile acid determination in the assessment of patients with liver disease has been recently advocated. Although almost always elevated in moderate-to-severe liver disease, poor diagnostic sensitivity in patients with mild liver disease has prevented widespread application.[47] The finding of normal fasting levels of cholic acid conjugates may, however, be helpful in supporting a diagnosis of Gilbert's syndrome in patients with unconjugated hyperbilirubinemia.[48] Higher sensitivity of serum bile acid levels as compared with conventional tests has also been demonstrated in the detection of patients with cirrhosis,[49] reflecting decreased first-pass elimination due to portosystemic shunting.[50] Elevated serum levels of bile acids in these patients may have, in addition, prognostic implications.[51] It should be recognized that the increase in serum bile acids that uniformly occurs as a result of diminished hepatic uptake or biliary excretion may be absent in patients with coexisting ileal disease that interferes with the intestinal phase of the enterohepatic circulation of bile acids. Conversely, small intestinal bacterial overgrowth may elevate serum bile acid levels.[52] Furthermore, serum bile acid determination was demonstrated to be of no value in assessing the patency of surgical portosystemic shunts.[53]

Dye Tests

Sulfobromophthalein (BSP) is a cholephilic organic anion previously used to assess hepatic function. The only current clinical application of the BSP plasma disappearance test is in the diagnosis of the inherited conjugated hyperbilirubinemic states, Dubin-Johnson syndrome, and Rotor's syndrome. In the former, BSP retention in plasma is normal (5% retention) or only slightly elevated at 45 minutes, but there is a characteristic rise in plasma BSP levels at approximately 90 minutes, whereas in Rotor's syndrome a 30% to 50% retention of the injected dose is observed at 45 minutes without a secondary elevation at 90 minutes.[54] Anaphylactic reactions have been reported following BSP injections, largely limiting studies of BSP uptake and biliary excretion to research settings.

Indocyanine green (ICG) is a less toxic dye, with hepatic uptake and excretion characteristics similar to those of BSP. However, because of greater hepatic clearance, ICG appears to be a less sensitive indicator of mild hepatic dysfunction than BSP.[55] Negligible removal by extrahepatic tissues makes ICG an ideal indicator of hepatic blood flow.[56]

Clotting Factors

Liver disease is a frequent cause of impaired coagulation. Normal serum activities of the vitamin K–dependent coagulation-factor proenzymes (Factors II, VII, IX, and X), as assessed by the one-stage prothrombin time, depend upon both intact hepatic synthesis and adequate intestinal absorption of lipid-soluble vitamin K. Vitamin K is required for the post-translational formation of γ-carboxyglutamyl residues that are essential for physiologic activation of the factors.[57] Prolonged prothrombin times can, therefore, be observed in both hepatocellular disorders that impair hepatic synthetic function, such as hepatitis and cirrhosis, and cholestatic syndromes that interfere with lipid absorption. Hepatocellular injury can be differentiated from cholestatic causes of prothrombin time prolongation by the parenteral administration of vitamin K.[58] Intact hepatic function is established by a greater than 30% improvement in the prothrombin time within 24 hours of administration. It should be recognized that a prolonged prothrombin time may occur in the absence of liver disease, such as in dietary deficiency of vitamin K, consumption coagulopathies, anticoagulant and antibiotic use, and steatorrhea. Correction of the abnormal prothrombin time by parenteral vitamin K will also be observed in these conditions. Prolongation of prothrombin time in acute hepatocellular injury signifies severe hepatocellular necrosis, may antedate other manifestations of hepatic failure, and is associated with a worse prognosis.[59] Similarly, in chronic liver disease, a prolonged prothrombin time carries a poor long-term prognosis.[60] Plasma concentrations of individual proteins may be useful clinical guides; in view of its short half-life, Factor VII is considered the best index of severity of liver disease and of prognosis.[61] A characteristic pattern of hemostatic abnormalities occurs in patients with severe liver dysfunction consisting of a low plasma fibrinogen level, a prolonged prothrombin time, and a normal or prolonged partial thromboplastin time. A hepatoma-associated dysfibrinogen, similar to fetal fibrinogen, has been described that produces prolonged prothrombin, thrombin, and reptilase times and inhibition of normal plasma coagulation.[62]

Albumin

Albumin is quantitatively the most important of a number of plasma proteins formed in the liver. Accordingly, measurement of total concentration of serum albumin is a useful test of hepatic synthetic function. The relatively long half-life of serum albumin (20 days) makes the serum albumin level a better index of severity and prognosis in patients with chronic liver disease than in patients with acute hepatic injury, where levels are usually normal or only minimally depressed.[55] Nutritional factors, namely, the availability of amino acids, are critical determinants of the rate of albumin synthesis.[63] Moreover, alterations in serum albumin levels may reflect not only disturbances in synthesis but also changes in the rate of catabolism, dilution by expanded plasma volume, as seen in cirrhosis, and/or enhanced loss via the gastrointestinal tract or kidneys. The shorter half-life of prealbumin (1.9 days), a glycoprotein synthesized by the liver with a faster electrophoretic migration relative to albumin, was exploited to demonstrate that serum prealbumin levels may be a sensitive index of liver function following acetaminophen overdose.[64] Serum prealbumin was also found to be useful in monitoring patients with α_1-antitrypsin deficiency.[65]

Immunoglobulins

Although measurement of serum globulins does not fulfill the operational definition of a liver function test, the hypergammaglobulinemia that is commonly observed in patients with liver disease indirectly represents functional impairment of the reticuloendothelial cells of the hepatic sinusoids.[55] Nondiagnostic im-

munoglobulin abnormalities can be detected in most acute and chronic forms of liver disease, with drug-induced and extrahepatic cholestasis being notable exceptions. Although there is considerable overlap, hypergammaglobulinemia above 3.0 g/dl in a patient with chronic hepatitis is more consistent with autoimmune liver disease than viral hepatitis. Rarely, the hypergammaglobulinemia in autoimmune hepatitis may be so pronounced that it causes the hyperviscosity syndrome.[66] A predominant rise in the IgA fraction is observed in hypergammaglobulinemia associated with alcoholic cirrhosis, whereas a disproportionate elevation of IgM is a feature that differentiates primary biliary cirrhosis from other liver diseases, specifically chronic active hepatitis, that are associated with prominent hypergammaglobulinemia.[67] However, a specific diagnosis is rarely established by quantitative determinations of immunoglobulins. Demonstrating hyperglobulinemia on serum protein electrophoresis is a clue to the presence of chronic liver disease.[55] Conversely, hypoglobulinemia should suggest a protein-losing enteropathy.

Lipoproteins

The pivotal role the liver plays in normal lipoprotein and cholesterol metabolism is reflected in the characteristic finding of abnormal lipoproteins and mild hypertriglyceridemia in acute forms of hepatocellular injury. Decreases in hepatic lecithin:cholesterol acyltransferase (LCAT) activity appear to account for the absence of alpha and pre-beta bands on lipoprotein electrophoresis commonly associated with acute viral hepatitis and alcoholic hepatitis.[68] Alterations in hepatic triglyceride lipase activity may result in the characteristic elevation in low-density lipoprotein triglyceride that, in turn, gives rise to the broad beta electrophoretic band observed in these disorders.[69] Abnormalities in serum lipoproteins in chronic forms of liver disease are a reflection of the degree of ongoing liver injury.[55] Target and spur cell formation in chronic liver disease may result from enhanced incorporation of cholesterol into the erythrocyte plasma membrane.[70] Lipoprotein alterations in cholestatic disorders are discussed below.

Tests of Hepatic Metabolism

Drug metabolism is another critical hepatic function, and liver disease is frequently associated with impaired drug metabolism. The most widely performed tests of hepatic metabolic capacity are antipyrine clearance determination and the aminopyrine demethylation breath test. Antipyrine is a minor analgesic that, on the basis of rapid and complete absorption from the gastrointestinal tract, distribution in total body water, and minimal nonhepatic elimination, would seem to qualify as an ideal probe for studies of hepatic drug metabolism. Impaired antipyrine metabolism by the cytochrome P-450 oxidase system, however, appears to be more a reflection of chronic active liver disease, the extent of impairment correlating well with serum albumin and prothrombin time determinations, and the degree of necrosis and inflammation on liver biopsy.[71] Little or no impairment in antipyrine metabolism is observed in patients with acute hepatitis or well-compensated cirrhosis.[72] The aminopyrine breath test avoids the need for multiple blood determinations. ^{14}C-aminopyrine is demethylated, via a ^{14}C-formaldehyde intermediate, to [14]CO$_2$, which is measured in expired air. Single-sample, 2-hour breath [14]CO$_2$ determinations are significantly decreased (expressed as a percentage of the administered dose) in patients with both acute and chronic hepatocellular injury but are normal or minimally decreased in patients with intrahepatic and extrahepatic cholestasis without hepatocellular injury.[73] The aminopyrine breath test has also been used as a prognostic test in patients with alcoholic hepatitis, a value of >1% of the administered dose correlating with improved 3-week survival.[74] Overall, while these quantitative tests may be noninvasive predictors of hepatic histology, difficulties with interindividual differences in the metabolism of a single drug and intraindividual differences in the metabolism of different drugs make interpretation difficult, and it is unlikely that these tests will supplant percutaneous liver biopsy, for example, in the diagnostic approach to the patient with liver disease.

There is increasing evidence to suggest that susceptibility of individuals to hepatotoxic drug reactions or disease states is related to a genetically determined capacity for oxidative metabolism.[75] In this regard, it is important to note the recent development of noninvasive tests that identify significant interpatient differences in hepatic concentrations and activities of certain forms of the cytochromes P-450 that underlie this polymorphism in oxidative drug metabolism.[76,77] The high incidence of impaired sulfoxidation in patients with primary biliary cirrhosis[78] and in patients with chlorpromazine-induced hepatotoxicity[79] may be a pathophysiologic manifestation of this polymorphism.

SERUM MARKERS OF HEPATOBILIARY DYSFUNCTION

As discussed above, routine biochemical laboratory tests are not true indices of hepatic function. Instead, they serve as markers of hepatobiliary dysfunction resulting from either hepatocellular necrosis, cholestasis, or infiltrative processes.

Aminotransferases (Transaminases)

Aspartate aminotransferase (AST; SGOT) and alanine aminotransferase (ALT; SGPT) are important markers of hepatocellular injury. While AST can be found in various tissues, notably cardiac and skeletal muscle, kidney, and brain, ALT is limited primarily to the liver. Within the liver cell, AST is present in two isozymic forms in mitochondria and the cytosol,[80] and ALT is localized to the cytosol. In normal serum, most of the AST activity is accounted for by the cytosolic isoenzyme.[81] Given the tissue distribution of these two enzymes, elevations of serum ALT are a more specific reflection of hepatocellular disease than are serum AST levels. Following acute myocardial infarction, serum AST levels are elevated more frequently than are ALT levels; furthermore, elevations in ALT levels that occur in this setting are commonly the result of hepatic ischemia brought on by extensive myocardial injury, congestive heart failure, or cardiogenic shock.[82] The highest serum elevations of both enzymes are seen in patients with viral, toxin-induced, and ischemic hepatitis, whereas smaller (<300 IU)

elevations relative to the degree of histologic necrosis are usually encountered in alcoholic hepatitis.[82] The AST/ALT ratio in serum is also regarded as a useful indicator of alcoholic liver disease, with a ratio greater than 2 being highly suggestive of alcohol-induced hepatic injury.[83] In contrast, in patients with acute and chronic viral hepatitis (and extrahepatic biliary obstruction), an AST/ALT ratio of less than 1.0 is typically observed, although a correlation between an AST/ALT ratio greater than 1.0 and the presence of underlying cirrhosis has been recently described in patients with chronic hepatitis B infection.[84] Thus, not only should an AST/ALT ratio of greater than 1.0 in the setting of nonalcoholic chronic liver disease raise suspicion regarding underlying cirrhosis, but also in the presence of cirrhosis the AST/ALT ratio may be less useful in differentiating alcoholic from nonalcoholic forms of liver disease. Several mechanisms have been proposed for the disproportionate elevation of serum AST levels in alcoholic liver disease. Hepatic ALT activity in alcoholic liver disease is diminished to a greater extent than hepatic AST activity.[85] Pyridoxal 5'-phosphate is necessary for the activity of both aminotransferases, and there may be enhanced sensitivity of hepatic ALT to alcohol-induced pyridoxine deficiency.[86] Preferential alcohol-induced injury to mitochondria enriched in AST is an alternative hypothesis (see below). Impaired plasma clearance of AST by sinusoidal cells[87] may play a role in the relative increase in serum AST levels observed in cirrhosis.[84]

Although these indices of hepatocellular injury are not predictive of histologic findings, serial determinations of serum AST and ALT levels may reflect the extent of hepatocellular injury and are useful in following the progression of liver disease. However, decreases in AST and ALT levels in serum may be either a sign of recovery from an acute injury or, particularly in the case of fulminant hepatic failure, an indication of limited hepatic reserve following overwhelming hepatocyte necrosis. In addition, falsely low serum AST levels, corrected by dialysis, have been reported in patients with uremia.[88] False elevations of AST have been observed in patients receiving para-aminosalicylic acid and erythromycin, and AST may rarely exist as a macroenzyme by forming a complex with immunoglobulin, leading to an otherwise unexplained elevation in serum AST activity.[89]

Serum levels of the mitochondrial isoenzyme of aspartate aminotransferase (mAST) and the ratio of mAST to total AST have been reported to be specific and sensitive markers of chronic alcoholism.[90] At present, until these and other new markers of alcohol abuse are better evaluated, γ-glutamyl transpeptidase determination, in combination with mean corpuscular volume and serum AST levels, remains the recommended biochemical indicator of recent alcohol abuse.[91]

Other Enzyme Markers of Hepatocellular Injury

Within the liver, the mitochondrial enzyme, glutamate dehydrogenase (GDH), is preferentially localized in centrizonal hepatocytes. The observation that alcohol exerts a toxic effect predominantly on mitochondria in centrizonal hepatocytes may account for the finding, in a large series of alcoholic patients, that serum GDH determination was more useful than serum AST levels in diagnosing patients with histologically documented alcoholic hepatitis.[92] Serum GDH levels have also been reported to be increased in the congestive hepatopathy observed in acute right-sided heart failure.[92] However, the specificity of GDH as a marker of pericentral hepatocellular necrosis in alcoholic liver disease is open to question,[93] and to date, serum GDH determinations have not received widespread application. Preliminary evidence suggests that levels of serum alcohol dehydrogenase, another enzyme distributed predominantly in hepatocytes in zone 3 of the hepatic acinus, may be useful in differentiating ischemic hepatitis, associated with centrilobular necrosis, from other forms of acute hepatitis.[94] The activities of sorbitol dehydrogenase,[95] isocitrate dehydrogenase,[96] and ornithine carbamyltransferase[97] parallel those of the aminotransferases. While all have high specificity for disorders associated with hepatocellular injury, lower sensitivity compared with aminotransferase determinations has limited their clinical use.

Alkaline Phosphatase

In the liver, alkaline phosphatase appears to be an integral enzyme of the exterior surface of the bile canalicular membrane.[98] While hepatocellular injury invariably results in increases in serum aminotransferase activity, significant (fourfold or greater) elevations of serum alkaline phosphatase activity are typically observed in patients with cholestatic syndromes. Lesser increases in serum alkaline phosphatase levels lack specificity and may be present in all forms of liver disease. The major mechanism underlying these elevations is increased synthesis, via enhanced mRNA translation,[99] of hepatic alkaline phosphatase rather than impaired biliary secretion of the enzyme. The mechanism(s) by which increased hepatic alkaline phosphatase activity leads to elevations in serum activity is less clear. Alkaline phosphatase contained within the bile canalicular membrane may be solubilized by bile acids that accumulate during cholestasis that, in turn, alter the permeability characteristics of the intercellular tight junctions.[100] Alternatively, the distribution of hepatic alkaline phosphatase activity may be altered, again by the high intrahepatic concentrations of bile acids in patients with cholestasis, so that it is found in all domains of the hepatocyte plasma membrane and enters serum directly from the plasma membrane.[100]

Alkaline phosphatase activity can also be demonstrated in bone, placenta, intestine, kidney, and leukocytes. Liver and bone represent the predominant source of serum alkaline phosphatase activity in normal subjects, with less than 20% derived from the intestine. Elevations of the intestinal isoenzyme occur in chronic renal failure, in individuals secreting the ABH red blood cell antigen, and in those of B and O blood groups.[101] In pregnancy, a substantial fraction may be derived from the placenta. Low levels of serum alkaline phosphatase have received comparatively less attention but may be encountered in hypothyroidism, pernicious anemia, zinc deficiency, and congenital hypophosphatasia. Recently, decreased serum alkaline phosphatase levels were observed in acute hemolytic anemia complicating Wilson's disease.[102] Benign familial elevation of serum alkaline phosphatase in a pattern suggesting autosomal-dominant inheritance has been reported.[103] Ectopic production of an alkaline phosphatase isoenzyme (Regan isoenzyme) occurs in patients with cancer, and elevations in serum alkaline phosphatase levels may, therefore, be observed in the absence of bony or hepatic metastasis.[104] Similarly, patients with stage I and II Hodgkin's disease, osteomyelitis, and congestive heart failure have been found to have marked elevations in serum alkaline phosphatase levels in the absence of hepatic involvement.[105]

Other Enzyme Markers of Cholestasis

Although the alkaline phosphatase isoenzymes exhibit different susceptibility to heat inactivation, and separation is possible with polyacrylamide gel electrophoresis,[106] alternative approaches are used in clinical practice. Serum gamma-glutamyl transferase or transpeptidase (GGTP) determination establishes the hepatic origin of an elevated alkaline phosphatase by virtue of its localization within the hepatobiliary tree, as well as kidney, pancreas, and intestine. Alcohol, presumably via enzyme induction, will result in elevated serum enzyme levels, and this finding has been invoked as a sensitive marker of chronic alcohol consumption that occurs independently of any liver damage.[107] However, sensitivity varies from 30% to 80%, depending on the population studied,[91] and elevated serum GGTP levels are also encountered in pancreatic disorders, myocardial infarction, uremia, chronic obstructive pulmonary disease, rheumatoid arthritis, diabetes mellitus, and in patients using microsomal enzyme-inducing drugs such as anticonvulsants and warfarin.

Determination of serum 5'-nucleotidase (5'-NT) and/or leucine amino peptidase (LAP) levels fulfills a role similar to that of serum GGTP determination. Despite their presence in a wide variety of other body tissues, elevated enzyme levels in the nonpregnant patient are specific for hepatobiliary disease and correlate well with elevated alkaline phosphatase levels of hepatic origin. Serum leucine aminopeptidase levels are elevated in pregnancy,[108] and conflicting data exist concerning 5'-nucleotidase levels in pregnancy. In patients with cancer, elevated 5'-nucleotidase levels are a sensitive marker in the diagnosis of metastatic disease to the liver.[109] Of significant note, a normal 5'-nucleotidase level does not necessarily exclude liver disease in the setting of an elevated alkaline phosphatase, because these enzyme markers may not increase in parallel in early or mild hepatic injury.[110]

Lactate Dehydrogenase

Although commonly available, measurement of total serum lactate dehydrogenase (LDH) has limited diagnostic specificity for hepatocellular disease, and fractionation of LDH to determine levels of the isoenzyme of hepatic origin (LDH-5) is rarely indicated. Moderate elevations of LDH are frequently encountered in hepatocellular disorders such as viral hepatitis and cirrhosis and are less common in cholestatic disorders.

DISEASE-SPECIFIC MARKERS

The laboratory tests outlined above alert the physician to the presence of hepatobiliary disease. In the section that follows, additional markers of specific disorders are discussed.

Viral Serology

Diagnosis of acute hepatitis A is based on serologic detection of hepatitis A virus–specific IgM antibody (IgM anti-HAV). Seropositivity first becomes detectable at the onset of clinical illness and is invariably present at the onset of jaundice. This serologic marker typically persists for 120 days, far exceeding both clinical and biochemical resolution of illness, and prolonged periods of seropositivity of greater than 200 days have been observed.[111] Nevertheless, it is best regarded as a marker of acute or recent hepatitis A viral infection. In contrast, IgG anti-HAV is present primarily in convalescent sera and persists for long periods following infection, perhaps for life.

A number of serologic tests are available to establish a diagnosis of hepatitis B viral infection. Hepatitis B surface antigen (HB_sAg) is the first marker detectable in serum, preceding elevations in serum aminotransferases as well as the onset of symptoms. HB_s antigenemia typically lasts for 1 to 2 months in self-limited infections. The titer of HB_sAg, although not routinely reported, appears to be inversely related to the degree of hepatic inflammation. Persistence of HB_sAg beyond 20 weeks is associated with a chronic carrier state, although it should be recognized that persistence of the hepatitis B virus may occur in the absence of any conventional serologic marker.[112]

Antibody to core antigen (anti-HB_c) is detected in serum approximately 2 weeks after the appearance of HB_sAg; typically, a "window" or lag period then occurs before the appearance of specific antibody to HB_sAg (anti-HB_s). During this period, and in the 10% of patients who do not manifest detectable levels of HB_sAg, anti-HB_c may be the only detectable serologic marker of recent infection with hepatitis B virus. The highest titers of anti-HB_c occur in patients with the longest periods of HB_sAg positivity. Antibody to the core antigen of HBV of the IgM class (IgM anti-HB_c) is the most sensitive marker of acute hepatitis B.[113] The specificity of IgM anti-HB_c as a test, however, is lessened by the persistence, at low levels, of IgM anti-HB_c in some patients with chronic active hepatitis B.[114]

At present, the commercially available serologic tests for the detection of the agent(s) responsible for non-A, non-B hepatitis detects antibody about 6 months after infection. Acute diagnosis of this disorder currently relies on the serologic exclusion of hepatitis A virus, hepatitis B virus, and other occasionally observed hepatotrophic viruses such as cytomegalovirus, herpes simplex and Epstein–Barr virus. Using these diagnostic criteria, studies have demonstrated that levels of serum alanine aminotransferase (ALT) greater than 300 IU/liter in anicteric patients with non-A, non-B hepatitis are associated with the development of chronic forms of hepatitis.[115] In addition, a relationship between elevated alanine aminotransferase levels[116] and/or antibody to hepatitis B core antigen[117,118] in donor blood and the incidence of non-A, non-B hepatitis in recipients of such blood has been established. The recent development of a specific assay for antibodies to a major etiologic virus of post-transfusional hepatitis will, undoubtedly, provide an important clinical diagnostic tool.[119]

Immunologic Tests

Immunologic abnormalities occur in a wide spectrum of liver diseases. The antinuclear antibody (ANA) reaction in autoimmune chronic active hepatitis is of the homogenous pattern by immunofluorescence, and a titer of >1:160 is usually required for diagnosis. Antibodies to double-stranded (native) DNA occur in more than 40% of patients with autoimmune hepatitis.[120] However, these antibodies are also present in similar percentages of patients with acute and chronic hepatitis B, suggesting that they represent a response to DNA released from hepatocyte necrosis.[121] Antimitochondrial antibodies (AMA), although apparently playing no role in the pathogenesis of the disease, are present in over 90% of patients with primary biliary cirrhosis (PBC) and in about 25% of patients with chronic active hepatitis and drug-induced liver injury.[122,123] In fact, an antimitochondrial antibody titer of greater than 1:40, even in the absence of serum alkaline phosphatase elevation or symptoms, may be strongly suggestive of primary biliary cirrhosis.[124] Four major mitochondrial antigens related to PBC have been described: M2 antigen on the inner mitochondrial membrane, recently identified as the dihydrolipoamide acyltransferase of the branched-chain α-keto acid dehydrogenase complex[125]; and M4, M8, and M9 antigen on the outer mitochondrial membrane. The specific profile of antibodies to these antigens in patients may have clinical and prognostic importance.[126] Antibodies to the soluble Ro antigen,[127] frequently present in patients with Sjögren's syndrome and systemic lupus erythematosus, and anticentromere antibodies[128] have also been identified in patients with primary biliary cirrhosis, particularly those with extrahepatic autoimmune disorders such as sicca syndrome and the CREST (calcinosis, Raynaud's phenomenon, esophageal dysmotility, sclerodactyly, telangiectasia) syndrome, respectively.

Smooth muscle antibodies, reactive to S actin, may be detected in up to 70% of patients with autoimmune chronic active hepatitis, in approximately 50% of patients with PBC, and occasionally in patients with acute viral hepatitis.[129] The presence of antiliver/kidney microsomal antibodies (anti-LKM_1) and absent or low titer antiactin or antinuclear antibodies serve to segregate patients with idiopathic autoimmune chronic active hepatitis into a subset characterized by a more aggressive course and a young female predominance.[130] The antigen to which anti-LKM_1 is directed has been recently identified as the polymorphic cytochrome P-450 isozyme, P-450db1.[131] Similarly, anti-LKM_2 antibodies directed against cytochrome P-450-8 have been described in patients with hepatitis and concomitant administration of the diuretic tienilic acid (ticrynafen).[132]

Human leukocyte antigens (HLA) have been associated with a wide spectrum of liver diseases. Specifically, HLA-B8 and DRw3 have been associated with autoimmune chronic active hepatitis,[133] and HLA-A3 and B14[134] with hemochromatosis. However, the increased frequencies of these HLA-haplotypes are neither absolute nor diagnostic. Thus, while HLA typing provides information on gene frequencies, it is neither routinely performed nor recommended. In hemochromatosis, the greater expense of HLA typing compared with tests of iron stores can be justified, however, in the management of young siblings of abnormal homozygotes, who on initial evaluation may have normal body iron stores.[135]

Ceruloplasmin

Determination of the serum concentration of ceruloplasmin, a copper transport protein in plasma, is particularly useful in the diagnosis of Wilson's disease. Although not directly involved in the pathogenesis of this autosomal recessively inherited copper storage disorder, low levels of ceruloplasmin (<20 mg/dl) are found in approximately 90% of homozygotes and in about 10% of heterozygotes. In contrast to Wilson's disease, serum ceruloplasmin is typically elevated in primary biliary cirrhosis, another disorder associated with increased hepatic copper concentrations.[136] Increased serum levels in this disorder and other forms of liver disease reflect the role of ceruloplasmin as a nonspecific acute-phase reactant. Accordingly, normal values may occasionally be observed during the chronic active hepatitis phase of Wilson's disease.[137] Pregnancy and exogenous estrogen administration may also lead to elevated values for this protein.[138,139] Likewise, hypoceruloplasminemia may result from the diminution in hepatic synthetic function observed in non-Wilsonian fulminant hepatic injury[140] and chronic hepatitis,[141] and less commonly in severe malnutrition, other protein-losing states, and Menkes' syndrome.[138] A high incidence of low ceruloplasmin levels has been described in otherwise healthy members of a pedigree and has been termed hereditary hypoceruloplasminemia to distinguish this benign disorder from Wilson's disease.[142]

Iron Storage Parameters

Measurements of serum iron level and total iron-binding capacity (or transferrin) are useful in the diagnosis of the hepatic iron overload state, hemochromatosis. Transferrin is normally 20% to 45% saturated, and both serum iron level and percent saturation of transferrin are elevated early in the course of this disorder. However, these tests have a relatively low degree of specificity in patients with liver disease; increased serum iron levels, with normal transferrin saturation, are commonly observed in patients with alcohol-induced liver injury.[143] Acute elevations in serum iron levels have also been observed in acute viral hepatitis.[144] Assays of serum ferritin may more closely estimate hepatic and total body iron stores,[143,145] and elevated serum ferritin levels are commonly observed early in the course of hemochromatosis, even before there is any histologic evidence of liver injury.[146] Ascorbic acid deficiency in patients with iron overload may lead to inappropriately low serum ferritin levels,[147] and several families have been described in which asymptomatic relatives of patients with idiopathic hemochromatosis had normal serum ferritin levels despite evidence of moderate hepatic iron overload.[148] Because serum ferritin is an acute-phase reactant, other forms of hepatocellular necrosis and systemic infection can be associated with elevated serum ferritin levels disproportionate to body iron stores.[149] For this reason, quantitative determination of tissue iron concentration on liver biopsy remains the definitive test for the diagnosis of hemochromatosis.

Alpha-Fetoprotein

A sensitive radioimmunoassay for alpha-fetoprotein (AFP), a major serum protein during fetal life, has been employed in the screening for primary hepatocellular carcinoma. While 70% to 90% of patients with hepatocellular carcinoma will have elevations in serum α-fetoprotein, significant elevations are also observed in patients with germ-cell tumors, other gastrointestinal malignancies,

and non-neoplastic hepatic disorders such as chronic active hepatitis, viral and alcoholic hepatitis, and primary biliary cirrhosis.[150] To enhance the specificity of this test in the diagnosis of hepatocellular carcinoma, concentrations exceeding 400 ng per milliliter have been generally cited,[151] although this arbitrary cutoff may exclude up to one third of patients with biopsy-proven hepatocellular carcinoma. A recently developed monoclonal radioimmunoassay may improve the specificity of AFP screening.[152] In addition, although presently not widely available, assays for des-γ-carboxy prothrombin, an abnormal prothrombin, may become useful in the detection of primary hepatocellular carcinoma.[153,154] Serum complement levels, typically depressed in cirrhosis, are elevated in patients with well-differentiated hepatocellular carcinoma,[155] although a role of this test in the early detection of hepatocellular carcinoma remains to be established.

Alpha$_1$-Antitrypsin

Alpha$_1$-antitrypsin is a 52-kd glycoprotein synthesized in the liver and, to a lesser extent, in monocytes and macrophages,[156] that migrates in the alpha$_1$-globulin fraction on serum protein electrophoresis. Normal serum levels (which range from 150 to 350 mg/dl) may increase postoperatively and in association with inflammation, malignancy, pregnancy, or estrogen therapy. The principal function of this protein is the inhibition of leukocyte elastase. The single gene coding for the synthesis of alpha$_1$-antitrypsin is contained within a 10-Kb segment of five exons on chromosome 14.[157] More than 25 codominantly expressed alleles have been described at this locus, and the normal phenotype for the protease inhibitor (Pi) system has been designated Pi MM by electrophoretic mobility. Individuals homozygous for the electrophoretically slowest of the genetic variants of this protein, designated Pi ZZ, exhibit markedly decreased serum alpha$_1$-antitrypsin levels and are predisposed to the early onset of chronic active hepatitis and cryptogenic cirrhosis.[158] Heterozygotes (Pi MZ) demonstrate serum levels that are 50% to 60% of normal values.[159] The inability of the hepatocyte to process and secrete the Z protein, which differs from the normal M protein by a single amino acid substitution,[160] results in the characteristic presence of periodic acid-Schiff (PAS)–positive diastase-resistant globules in periportal hepatocytes on percutaneous liver biopsy. The diagnosis of alpha$_1$-antitrypsin deficiency should be entertained in a patient with a hepatocellular injury pattern to liver chemistry abnormalities when an absent alpha$_1$-globulin peak is observed on serum electrophoresis and confirmed by serum antitrypsin activity determination and genetic Pi typing.

Serum Ammonia

Urea formation in the liver, via the Krebs-Henseleit cycle, is required for the disposal of the toxic product of nitrogen metabolism, ammonia. Thus, elevated serum ammonia levels are frequently observed in both acute and chronic forms of liver disease. Striking elevations in fulminant hepatic failure are the result of impaired conversion of ammonia to urea in the setting of severe hepatocellular necrosis, whereas the hyperammonemia present in patients with cirrhosis and portal hypertension primarily reflects portosystemic shunting of ammonia derived from colonic bacteria.[161] Additional factors that influence the level of serum ammonia in patients with cirrhosis include: (1) intestinal production of ammonia by bacterial deamination of blood or dietary protein, (2) renal production of ammonia by glutaminase in response to metabolic alkalosis and/or hypokalemia, (3) intestinal production of ammonia from urea by urease-forming bacteria in the setting of diminished renal function, and (4) hepatic production of ammonia from amino acids in response to increased glucagon secretion.[162] Although routinely determined in patients with suspected hepatic encephalopathy and used as an index of the success of therapy, serum ammonia levels only roughly correlate with the degree of encephalopathy.[162] Hyperammonemia and encephalopathy in the absence of liver disease have been reported in patients with urea cycle enzyme deficiencies, following ureterosigmoidostomy, and in a patient with a neurogenic bladder infected with urease-producing bacteria.[163] Thus, serum ammonia determination, most accurately measured on arterial blood, is best regarded merely as an aid in the differential diagnosis of encephalopathy.

Additional abnormalities that can be observed in hepatic encephalopathy include decreased serum levels of branched-chain amino acids and elevated serum levels of aromatic amino acids, methanethiol, and short-chain fatty acids.[162] This serum amino acid profile contrasts with that observed in severe autoimmune hepatitis, in which both aromatic and branched-chain amino acid levels are increased and do not distinguish patients with and without clinical manifestations of hepatic encephalopathy.[164]

Thyroid Function Tests

Acute hepatocellular injury is associated with elevated serum levels of T_4 and increased circulating concentrations of TBG[165,166] without clinical signs of hyperthyroidism. A significant correlation exists between serum TBG levels and AST levels, consistent with increased release of TBG from damaged hepatocytes.[165] Decreased extrathyroidal conversion of T_4 to T_3 in chronic liver disease results in the characteristic finding of low serum levels of T_3.[167] In contrast, reverse T_3 levels are elevated in patients with chronic liver disease, owing to a reduced activity of 5'-monodeiodinase.[168] The levels of rT_3 have prognostic significance for patients awaiting orthotopic liver transplantation and for patients recovering from alcoholic hepatitis.[169,170] Increased levels of TBG and, consequently, T_4 are found in patients with hepatocellular carcinoma, and serial monitoring of these levels may assist in the identification of cirrhotic patients who have undergone malignant transformation.[171] Hypothyroidism may be a presenting manifestation of primary biliary cirrhosis.[172]

Vitamins

The liver is the principal storage site for vitamin B_{12}. Increases in serum vitamin B_{12} levels in patients with acute hepatocellular injury, particularly viral hepatitis, reflect release from necrotic hepatocytes.[173] Similar elevations may be observed in patients with cirrhosis.[173] Elevated levels of serum vitamin B_{12} have been observed in patients with hepatic abscesses and portal pyophlebitis and thus may be used to differentiate jaundice due to intrahepatic infection from jaundice resulting from systemic bacterial infection.[174] However, this test has not received widespread use in the diagnostic approach to patients with liver disease. In acute viral hepatitis and cirrhosis, serum vitamin A levels are decreased,[175] but to date, the value in determining levels is restricted to studies of abnormal dark adaptation.

Lipoprotein-X

An abnormal lipoprotein, referred to as lipoprotein-X, is characteristically detectable in cholestatic syndromes.[176] This lipoprotein has beta mobility on electrophoresis and is composed primarily of unesterified cholesterol, phospholipid, and albumin, in characteristic biconcave discs on electron microscopy.[177] Unfortunately, despite initial reports to the contrary,[178] lipoprotein-X determinations are of limited value in distinguishing intra- from extrahepatic cholestasis, although they are helpful in differentiating cholestasis from hepatocellular injury.[179]

Percutaneous Liver Biopsy

Unlike most of the laboratory tests discussed above, a predictive value cannot be assigned to a specific morphologic feature observed with a percutaneous liver biopsy. Yet liver biopsy can be extremely useful in the diagnostic approach to the patient with abnormal liver chemistries. Proper biopsy interpretation is assisted by the availability of all clinical, biochemical, immunologic, and radiographic data in order to correlate histologic features with an etiologic diagnosis. As a general rule, direct forms of liver injury tend to cause predominant centrizonal necrosis, immunologically mediated forms of hepatocyte injury are localized to the periportal regions, and cholestatic liver injury can be recognized by the accumulation of canalicular bile and feathery degeneration of hepatocytes in the absence of a significant inflammatory infiltrate. Major applications of liver biopsy, other than in the evaluation of a patient with persistently abnormal liver chemistries, include establishing the diagnosis in patients with: (1) unexplained hepatomegaly; (2) suspected systemic disease, such as tuberculosis, sarcoidosis, or fever of unknown origin[180]; and (3) suspected primary or metastatic carcinoma. Contraindications to needle biopsy of the liver include: (1) uncooperative or unstable patient, (2) impaired coagulation, (3) ascites, (4) right-sided empyema, and (5) suspected hemangioma or echinococcal cyst.

GENERAL APPROACH

An extensive number of tests has been described in the preceding pages and other chapters. Initially, nonhepatic causes for any observed abnormalities must be considered (Table 42-1). The dilemma then faced is in selecting a proper diagnostic approach to the patient with suspected liver disease. Liver disease can be classified into four major types, namely, cholestatic, hepatocellular, and immunologic forms of injury, and infiltrative processes. Depending on the target of the immune response, immunologic injury will result in either a cholestatic picture (when the bile ducts are

TABLE 42–1
Nonhepatic Causes for Abnormal Liver Chemistries

TEST	NONHEPATIC CAUSES	DISCRIMINATING TESTS
Albumin	Protein-losing enteropathy	Serum globulins, α_1-antitrypsin clearance
	Nephrotic syndrome	Urinalysis, 24-hr urinary protein
	Malnutrition	Clinical setting
	Congestive heart failure	Clinical setting
Alkaline phosphatase (AP)	Bone disease	GGTP, LAP, 5'NT
	Pregnancy	GGTP, 5'NT
	Malignancy	AP electrophoresis
Serum AST	Myocardial infarction	MB-CPK
	Muscle disorders	Creatine kinase
Bilirubin	Hemolysis	Reticulocyte count, peripheral smear, urine bilirubin
	Sepsis	Clinical setting, cultures
	Ineffective Erythropoiesis	Peripheral smear, urine bilirubin, Hgb electrophoresis, bone marrow examination
	"Shunt" hyperbilirubinemia	Clinical setting
GGTP	Alcohol, drugs	History
Ferritin	Systemic disease, chronic inflammation	Clinical setting
Prothrombin time	Dietary deficiency of vitamin K, antibiotic and anticoagulant use, steatorrhea	Response to vitamin K, clinical setting

preferentially involved, as in primary biliary cirrhosis) or a hepatocellular form of injury (when the primary insult is to the hepatocyte membrane, as in viral and autoimmune hepatitis). Cholestasis can be further categorized as either a functional defect in bile formation at the level of the hepatocyte (intrahepatic cholestasis) or a structural impairment in bile secretion and flow (extrahepatic cholestasis). Evaluation is aided by the presence of these relatively discrete patterns of liver injury and tests of discriminative value in the detection of these patterns. Routinely, the results of the following tests should be determined in all patients with suspected liver disease before disease-specific markers are sought:

1. Serum aminotransferase (AST;SGOT and ALT;SGPT) activity
2. Serum alkaline phosphatase
3. Serum total and direct bilirubin
4. Serum total protein, with albumin and globulin fractionation
5. Prothrombin time

A pattern of typical abnormalities that are seen in the various forms of hepatobiliary injury emerges from this battery of tests, as outlined in Table 42-2. Additional diagnostic information may be provided by the disease-specific markers, as listed in Table 42-3. Further laboratory evaluation of any patient with evidence of chronic (>6 months) hepatitis should, at the minimum, include:

1. Serum protein electrophoresis
2. Serum ferritin
3. Antinuclear antibody
4. Serum ceruloplasmin
5. Hepatitis B viral serology

TABLE 42–2
Routine Biochemical Tests in the Patient With Idealized Hepatobiliary Disease

TEST	HEPATOCELLULAR NECROSIS	CHOLESTASIS	INFILTRATIVE PROCESS
Aminotransferase	++ – +++	0 – +	0 – +
Alkaline phosphatase	0 – +	++ – +++	++ – +++
Total/direct bilirubin	0 – +++	0 – +++	0 – +
Prothrombin time	Prolonged	Prolonged; responsive to Vit. K	Normal
Albumin	Decreased in chronic disorders	Normal	Normal

0, normal; + to +++, degrees of abnormality.

TABLE 42–3
Diagnosis of Selected Hepatobiliary Disorders

FORM OF LIVER INJURY	SUPPORTING LABORATORY DATA	ROLE OF LIVER BIOPSY
Hepatocellular		
Viral hepatitis	Viral serology	Rarely required
Drug-induced hepatitis	Eosinophil count	Rarely diagnostic
Autoimmune chronic active hepatitis	Immunoelectrophoresis	Usually required
	Antinuclear antibody	
	Anti–smooth muscle antibody	
Wilson's disease	Serum ceruloplasmin	Essential
Hemochromatosis	Serum iron/TIBC	Essential
	Serum ferritin	
Alpha1-antitrypsin (AAT) deficiency	Protein electrophoresis	Usually required
	Serum AAT level	
	Pi typing	
Cholestatic		
Primary biliary cirrhosis	Antimitochondrial antibody	Essential
	Immunoelectrophoresis	
Infiltrative		
Hepatocellular carcinoma	Alpha-fetoprotein	Essential

The differential diagnosis of a patient with abnormal liver chemistries consistent with cholestatic injury (i.e., elevations of serum alkaline phosphatase and bilirubin levels, with or without moderate elevations of serum aminotransferase levels) represents a formidable clinical challenge. Hyperbilirubinemia resulting from extrahepatic biliary obstruction, in contrast to that observed in acute and chronic forms of hepatocellular injury, over time tends to level off and rarely exceeds levels of 35 mg/dl in the absence of oliguria and/or hemolysis. The mechanism for this plateau effect appears to be related to altered bilirubin metabolism, including enhanced renal excretion of conjugated bilirubin. In addition, a daily increase of 1.5 mg/dl in total serum bilirubin is characteristic of extrahepatic biliary obstruction.[181] Nevertheless, none of the routine biochemical laboratory tests can reliably distinguish intrahepatic cholestasis from extrahepatic biliary obstruction. Furthermore, it should be recognized that within 24 to 48 hours of acute extrahepatic obstruction, profound elevations in serum ALT and AST levels may be observed, followed by a rapid decline.[182,183]

Although there are no symptoms or signs that are pathognomonic for intra- or extrahepatic forms of cholestasis, a history of previous biliary tract surgery, the presence of abdominal pain or significant weight loss, palpable gallbladder or abdominal mass, fever or other signs of cholangitis, and an elevated serum amylase should point to an extrahepatic cause such as choledocholithiasis, pancreatitis, cholangiocarcinoma, or carcinoma of the pancreas. Partial obstruction and obstruction involving only a portion of the intrahepatic biliary tree may result in an elevated serum alkaline phosphatase level in the absence of hyperbilirubinemia. Conversely, a normal alkaline phosphatase level in a jaundiced patient strongly rules against the presence of extrahepatic biliary obstruction.[40] Fever and right upper quadrant abdominal pain may occur in drug-induced cholestasis and lead to confusion if a detailed drug history is not available. A cholestatic biochemical profile with fluctuating levels of serum alkaline phosphatase in a patient with inflammatory bowel disease should suggest primary sclerosing cholangitis. Marked cholangiographic changes in the presence of advanced histologic stage may, however, occur without a concomitant increase in serum alkaline phosphatase activity.[184]

Thus, additional laboratory tests, even liver biopsy, may not further differentiate between intrahepatic and extrahepatic cholestasis. Moreover, in drug-induced cholestasis, discontinuation of the offending drug, one of the more common causes of intrahepatic cholestasis, may not be immediately followed by resolution of the cholestatic picture. As discussed in greater detail in other chapters, the most direct approach to the differential diagnosis of cholestatic injury is the use of abdominal ultrasonography to assess bile duct size, followed, if biliary dilatation is present, by endoscopic retrograde cholangiopancreatography (ERCP) or percutaneous transhepatic cholangiography (PTC). Biliary tract obstruction of short duration may not be accompanied by detectable dilatation of the bile ducts, and in cases where there is a strong clinical suspicion of an extrahepatic cause of cholestasis, ERCP or PTC may be indicated even in the presence of a normal ultrasonographic examination.[185]

While other features, such as serum bilirubin levels and prolongation of the prothrombin time, may vary and correlate with the severity of the injury, elevated serum aminotransferases are characteristically associated with hepatocellular forms of injury and reflect release of intracellular enzymes from hepatocytes undergoing necrosis. As a general rule, aminotransferase levels greater than 400 units are indicative of hepatocellular injury. In contrast, milder degrees of serum aminotransferase elevation (<300 units) are of little diagnostic benefit, because they are observed in cholestatic disorders as frequently as in acute and chronic hepatocellular disease. Establishing the cause of hepatocellular necrosis usually requires more information than routine laboratory results provide.

As discussed previously, the nature and degree of aminotransferase elevation may be helpful in distinguishing between alcoholic hepatitis and ischemic, viral-induced, or drug-induced hepatitis. Leukocytosis can be a prominent feature associated with alcoholic hepatitis. Ischemic liver injury is, at times, indistinguishable from acute viral hepatitis. A disproportionate and marked elevation in serum transaminases in the setting of generalized malaise, anorexia, jaundice, and tender hepatomegaly characterize both disorders. However, measures to improve hepatic blood flow (e.g., correction of hypotension or congestive heart failure) are accompanied by a more rapid fall in serum aminotransferase levels than is observed in the course of acute viral hepatitis.[186] Normal values are occasionally found within 48 to 72 hours in cases of ischemic hepatitis. Features suggestive of drug-related hepatotoxicity include a history of recent institution of therapy and indirect evidence of a hypersensitivity reaction, such as rash, arthralgia, and eosinophilia. Profoundly abnormal aminotransferase activities, with preservation of an elevated SGOT/SGPT ratio, are observed in alcoholic patients with acetaminophen hepatotoxicity,[187] and a positive response to questions regarding the use of acetaminophen mandates measurement of the blood level of acetaminophen. A high index of suspicion is required in the diagnosis of Wilson's disease, and ceruloplasmin levels should be routinely determined in patients below the age of 35 years with a pattern of abnormalities (variable elevations in serum aminotransferases in the presence of mild hyperbilirubinemia and hypoalbuminemia) suggesting HB_sAg-negative chronic active hepatitis, autoimmune chronic active hepatitis, or cryptogenic cirrhosis. Although a reduced serum ceruloplasmin level may be observed in other disorders, as discussed above, its presence in an asymptomatic individual with elevated serum aminotransferase levels is highly suggestive of Wilson's disease.

Isolated elevation of serum alkaline phosphatase, confirmed by serum leucine aminopeptidase, 5'-nucleotidase, or GGTP to be of hepatic origin, is strongly suggestive of an infiltrative process, whether a localized (i.e, primary biliary cirrhosis) or systemic granulomatous disease, such as sarcoidosis, miliary tuberculosis, coccidiomycosis, histoplasmosis, brucellosis, Q fever, or a drug reaction (e.g., allopurinol, quinidine), or, alternatively, the first indication of metastatic carcinoma to the liver. A greater than threefold elevation in serum alkaline phosphatase levels in patients with cirrhosis should raise concern for the development of hepatocellular carcinoma.[188] The triad of an elevated serum alkaline phosphatase level, detectable titers of antimitochondrial antibody, and an elevated serum IgM level in a middle-aged woman is of considerable discriminative value in the diagnosis of primary biliary cirrhosis. Alternatively, in a patient with a history of malignancy, particularly of the breast or colon, the presence of an elevated serum alkaline phosphatase warrants an evaluation for metastases. The absence of diagnostic findings on abdominal ultrasound, computerized axial tomography of the abdomen, technetium sulfur colloid nuclear imaging, and invasive tests such as endoscopic retrograde cholangiopancreatography, represents one of the major indications for percutaneous and/or laparoscopic liver biopsy.

The extent of hepatic dysfunction in any form of injury is routinely assessed by the prothrombin time and serum albumin concentration. Prolongation of the prothrombin time without improvement by parenteral vitamin K administration and serum albumin concentration below 3 g/dl both reflect the prognosis and severity of underlying liver disease.

Recent studies have addressed the issue of evaluating asymptomatic patients with moderate elevations in serum aminotransferase levels.[189,190] Apart from determinations of ferritin, ceruloplasmin, alpha$_1$-antitrypsin, and markers for hepatitis B virus, blood tests had little discriminative value. A high incidence of obesity and regular alcohol use was demonstrated in these patients. Fatty infiltration, consequently, was the most common finding on liver biopsy; however, histologic findings of chronic persistent or active hepatitis in 20% of patients in one study[189] lent support for the use of percutaneous liver biopsy in the diagnostic approach to patients with persistently elevated levels of serum aminotransferases. Furthermore, examination of a highly select population of individuals with unexplained chronic serum ALT elevations, in whom viral-, alcohol-, or drug-related disease was excluded, demonstrated histologic features of chronic active hepatitis, including cirrhosis, in more than two thirds of patients.[191] Steatohepatitis was the most frequent alternative diagnosis, with clinical and laboratory findings, including seropositivity for antinuclear antibodies, indistinguishable from those of patients with chronic active hepatitis.[191]

The significance of hepatic abnormalities has been examined in several other clinical situations. In the acquired immunodeficiency syndrome (AIDS), mild to moderate increases in serum aminotransferase activities (range, 40–605 IU/liter; mean, 172 IU/liter) are observed in 70% of patients, with higher elevations noted in populations referred for liver biopsy.[192] Increases in alkaline phosphatase levels (range, 200–270 IU/liter) were present in a slightly smaller percentage of patients, and jaundice was present in only 15% of patients.[192] Macrosteatosis and nonspecific portal inflammation were the most common histologic abnormalities,[193,194] and, in general, the information provided by liver biopsy had little effect on therapy or survival.[194] An exception to an otherwise noninvasive approach to abnormal liver chemistries in patients with AIDS, however, is endoscopic sphincterotomy in the setting of clinical, biochemical, and radiologic features of papillary stenosis and sclerosing cholangitis.[195]

Multitransfused hemophiliacs have a high incidence of asymptomatic abnormalities in liver chemistries, and liver biopsies demonstrate a wide histologic spectrum of liver disease, ranging from mild chronic persistent hepatitis to chronic active hepatitis and cirrhosis.[196] As with other forms of chronic liver injury, there is a poor correlation with serum transaminase levels and histology.[197] Given the limitations of liver biopsy in this population, however, noninvasive determinations of underlying liver dysfunction have been sought, including serum procollagen III peptide[198] and serum γ-globulin levels.[199]

Elevated serum transaminase levels occurring during therapy for acute lymphoplastic leukemia have been recently associated with a pattern more consistent with non-A, non-B hepatitis than with chemotherapy-induced hepatotoxicity.[200] In contrast, the presence of an elevated alkaline phosphatase level and a persistent fever, often coupled with abdominal pain, in a neutropenic patient should suggest focal hepatosplenic candidiasis.[201]

In conclusion, it is worthwhile to reiterate that the diagnostic tests discussed above suggest but rarely provide a specific diagnosis in a patient with suspected liver disease. Nevertheless, information obtained from these tests should facilitate the efficient and proper use of other noninvasive and invasive tests such as ultrasonography, computed tomography, radionuclide hepatobiliary scanning, PTC, ERCP, and laparoscopy.

The reader is directed to Chapter 16, Bile Secretion; Chapter 41, Approach to the Patient with Jaundice; Chapter 93, Gallbladder and Biliary Tree: Anatomy and Structural Anomalies; Chapter 94, Gallstones; Chapter 95, Diseases of the Biliary Tree; Chapter 113, Endoscopic Retrograde Cholangiopancreatography, Endoscopic Sphincterotomy and Stone Removal, Endoscopic Biliary and Pancreatic Drainage; and Chapter 116, Ultrasound.

REFERENCES

1. Pauker SG, Eckman MH. Principles of diagnostic testing. In: Kelley WN, ed. Textbook of internal medicine. Philadelphia: JB Lippincott, 1989:16.
2. Lelbach WK. Organic pathology related to volume and pattern of alcohol use. In: Gibbins RJ, Israel Y, Kalant H, Popham RE, Schmidt W, Smart RG, eds. Research advances in alcohol and drug problems. New York: John Wiley & Sons, 1974:93.
3. Saunders JB, Davis M, Williams R. Do women develop alcoholic liver disease more readily than men? Br Med J 1981;282:1140.
4. Zimmerman HJ. Effects of aspirin and acetaminophen on the liver. Arch Intern Med 1981;141:333.
5. Leo MA, Lieber CS. Hypervitaminosis A: A liver lover's lament. Hepatology 1988;8:412.
6. Worner TM, Gordon GG, Leo MA, et al. Vitamin A treatment of sexual dysfunction in male alcoholics. Am J Clin Nutr 1988;48:1431.
7. Ellis JK, Russell RM, Makrauer FL, et al. Increased risk for vitamin A toxicity in severe hypertriglyceridemia. Ann Intern Med 1986;105:877.
8. Schmunes E. Hypervitaminosis A in a patient with alopecia receiving renal dialysis. Arch Dermatol 1979;115:882.
9. Corey L, Holmes KK. Sexual transmission of hepatitis A in homosexual men: Incidence and mechanism. N Engl J Med 1980;302:435.
10. Hadler SC, Webster HM, Erben JJ, et al. Hepatitis A in day-care centers: A community-wide assessment. N Engl J Med 1980;302:1222.
11. Goodman RA. Nosocomial hepatitis A. Ann Intern Med 1985;103:452.
12. Inman RD. Rheumatic manifestations of hepatitis B virus infection. Semin Arthritis Rheum 1982;11:406.
13. Sotaniemi EA, Sutinen S, Sutinen S, et al. Liver injury in subjects occupationally exposed to chemicals in low doses. Acta Med Scand 1982;212:207.
14. Baerg RD, Kimberg DV. Centrilobular hepatic necrosis and acute renal failure in "solvent sniffers." Ann Intern Med 1970;73:713.
15. Dannaher CL, Tamburro CH, Yam LT. Occupational carcinogenesis: The Louisville experience with vinyl-chloride–associated hepatic angiosarcoma. Am J Med 1981;70:279.
16. Morris JS, Schmid M, Newman S, et al. Arsenic and noncirrhotic portal hypertension. Gastroenterology 1974;64:86.
17. Regelson W, Kim U, Ospina J, et al. Hemangioendothelial sarcoma of liver from chronic arsenic intoxication by Fowler's solution. Cancer 1968;21:514.
18. Harrison R, Letz G, Pasternak G, et al. Fulminant hepatic failure after occupational exposure to 2-nitropropane. Ann Intern Med 1987;107:466.
19. Rollins BJ. Hepatic veno-occlusive disease. Am J Med 1986;81:297.
20. Stillman AE, Huxtable R, Consroe P, et al. Hepatic veno-occlusive disease due to pyrrolizidine (Senecio) poisoning in Arizona. Gastroenterology 1977;73:349.
21. Ware AJ. The liver when the heart fails. Gastroenterology 1978;74:627.
22. Cohen JA, Kaplan MM. Left-sided heart failure presenting as hepatitis. Gastroenterology 1978;74:583.
23. Skinner C, Denmure ACF. Hemochromatosis presenting as congestive cardiomyopathy associated with hemochromatosis. N Engl J Med 1972;287:866.
24. Littenberg G, Afroudakis A, Kaplowitz N. Common bile duct stenosis from chronic pancreatitis: A clinical and pathologic spectrum. Medicine 1979;58:385.
25. Petrozza JA, Dutta SK, Latham PS, et al. Prevalence and natural history of distal common bile duct stenosis in alcoholic pancreatitis. Dig Dis Sci 1984;29:890.
26. Gaskin KJ, Waters DLM, Howman-Giles R, et al. Liver disease and common-bile-duct stenosis in cystic fibrosis. N Engl J Med 1988;318:340.
27. Danzi JT. Extraintestinal manifestations of idiopathic inflammatory bowel disease. Arch Intern Med 1988;148:297.
28. Bauer TW, Moore GW, Hutchins GM. The liver in sickle cell disease: A clinicopathologic study of 70 patients. Am J Med 1980;69:833.
29. Franson TR, Hierholzer WJ, LaBrecque DR. Frequency and characteristics of hyperbilirubinemia associated with bacteremia. Rev Infect Dis 1985;7:1.
30. Franson TR, LaBrecque DR, Buggy BP, et al. Serial bilirubin determinations as a prognostic marker in clinical infections. Am J Med Sci 1989;297:149.
31. Strickland RC, Schenker S. The nephrogenic hepatic dysfunction syndrome: A review. Dig Dis 1977;22:49.
32. Steven MM. Pregnancy and liver disease. Gut 1981;22:592.
33. Alpers DH, Sabesin SM. Fatty liver: Biochemical and clinical aspects. In: Schiff L, Schiff ER, eds. Diseases of the liver. Philadelphia: JB Lippincott, 1987:949.
34. Ludwig J, Viggiano TR, McGill DB, et al. Nonalcoholic steatohepatitis: Mayo Clinic experiences with a hitherto unnamed disease. Mayo Clin Proc 1980;55:434.
35. Lewis JH, Zimmerman HJ, Ishak KG, et al. Enflurane hepatotoxicity: A clinicopathologic study of 24 cases. Ann Intern Med 1983;98:984.
36. Hocking MP, Duerson MC, O'Leary JP, et al. Jejunoileal bypass for morbid obesity: Late follow-up in 100 cases. N Engl J Med 1983;308:995.
37. Freedman MR, Holzbach RT, Ferguson DR. Pruritus in cholestasis: No direct causative role for bile acid retention. Am J Med 1981;70:1011.
38. Espinoza P, Ducot B, Pelletier G, et al. Interobserver agreement in the physical diagnosis of alcoholic liver disease. Dig Dis Sci 1987;32:244.
39. Attali P, Ink O, Pelletier G, et al. Dupuytren's contracture, alcohol consumption, and chronic liver disease. Arch Intern Med 1987;147:1065.
40. Lumeng L, O'Connor KW. Differential diagnosis of jaundice. In: Ostrow JD, ed. Bilirubin, bile pigments and jaundice. New York: Marcel Dekker, 1986:475.
41. Nicholas GG, Williams E. Friction rub in acute cholecystitis: An unusual finding. JAMA 1971;218:1945.
42. Frommer D, Morris J, Sherlock S, et al. Kayser-Fleischer–like rings in patients without Wilson's disease. Gastroenterology 1977;72:1331.
43. Chevrant-Breton J, Simon M, Bourel M, et al. Cutaneous manifestations of idiopathic hemochromatosis. Arch Dermatol 1977;113:161.
44. Rebora A. Lichen planus and the liver [Letter]. Lancet 1981;2:805.
45. Graham-Brown RAC, Sarkany I, Sherlock S. Lichen planus and primary biliary cirrhosis. Br J Dermatol 1982;106:699.
46. Weiss JS, Gautam A, Lauff JJ, et al. The clinical importance of a protein-bound fraction of serum bilirubin in patients with hyperbilirubinemia. N Engl J Med 1983;309:147.
47. Ferraris R, Colombatti G, Fiorentini MT, et al. Diagnostic value of serum bile acids and routine liver function tests in hepatobiliary diseases: Sensitivity, specificity, and predictive value. Dig Dis Sci 1983;28:129.
48. Vierling JM, Berk PD, Hofmann A, et al. Normal fasting-state levels

of serum cholyl–conjugated bile acids in Gilbert's syndrome: An aid to the diagnosis. Hepatology 1982;2:340.

49. Festi D, Labate AMM, Roda A, et al. Diagnostic effectiveness of serum bile acids in liver diseases as evaluated by multivariate statistical methods. Hepatology 1983;3:707.

50. Ohkubo H, Okuda K, Iida S, et al. Role of portal and splenic vein shunts and impaired hepatic extraction in the elevated serum bile acids in liver cirrhosis. Gastroenterology 1984;86:514.

51. Mannes GA, Thieme C, Stellaard F, et al. Prognostic significance of serum bile acids in cirrhosis. Hepatology 1986;6:50.

52. Setchell KDR, Harrison DL, Gilbert JM, et al. Serum unconjugated bile acids: Qualitative and quantitative profiles in ileal resection and bacterial overgrowth. Clin Chim Acta 1985;152:297.

53. Tabibian N, Reynolds TB. Serum bile acid determination for assessing patency of portosystemic shunts: Lack of value. Arch Intern Med 1987;147:911.

54. Wolpert E, Pascasio FM, Wolkoff AW, et al. Abnormal sulfobromophthalein metabolism in Rotor's syndrome and obligate heterozygotes. N Engl J Med 1977;296:1099.

55. Kaplowitz N, Eberle D, Yamada T. Biochemical tests for liver disease. In: Zakim D, Boyer TD, eds. Hepatology: A textbook of liver disease. Philadelphia: WB Saunders, 1982:583.

56. Groszmann RJ. The measurement of liver blood flow using clearance techniques. Hepatology 1983;3:1039.

57. Friedman PA. Vitamin K–dependent proteins. N Engl J Med 1984;310:1458.

58. Lord JW, Andrus WW. Differentiation of intrahepatic and extrahepatic jaundice: Response of the plasma prothrombin to intramuscular injection of menadione (2-methyl-1,4-naphthaquinone) as a diagnostic aid. Arch Intern Med 1941;68:199.

59. Clarke R, Rake MO, Flute PT, et al. Coagulation abnormalities in acute liver failure: Pathogenetic and therapeutic implications. Scand J Gastroenterol 1973;8(19):63.

60. Christensen E, Schlichting P, Andersen PK, et al. Updating prognosis and therapeutic effect evaluation in cirrhosis with Cox's multiple regression model for time-dependent variables. Scand J Gastroenterol 1986;21:163.

61. Kelly DA, Summerfield JA. Hemostasis in liver disease. Semin Liver Dis 1987;7:182.

62. Gralnick HR, Givelber H, Abrams E. Dysfibrinogenemia associated with hepatoma: Increased carbohydrate content of the fibrinogen molecule. N Engl J Med 1978;299:221.

63. Rothschild MA, Oratz M, Schreiber SS. Alcohol, amino acids, and albumin synthesis. Gastroenterology 1974;67:1200.

64. Hutchinson DR, Smith MG, Parke DV. Prealbumin as an index of liver function after acute paracetamol poisoning. Lancet 1980;ii: 121.

65. Cox DW, Smyth S. Risk for liver disease in adults with alpha₁-antitrypsin deficiency. Am J Med 1983;74:221.

66. Lee WM, Lebwohl O, Chien S. Hyperviscosity syndrome attributable to hyperglobulinemia in chronic active hepatitis. Gastroenterology 1978;74:918.

67. Feizi T. Immunoglobulins in chronic liver disease. Gut 1968;9:193.

68. Day RC, Harry DS, Owen JS, et al. Plasma lecithin cholesterol-acyltransferase activity and the lipoprotein abnormalities of parenchymal liver disease. Clin Sci Mol Med 1978;54:36.

69. Muller PR, Fellin R, Lambrecht J, et al. Hypertriglyceridemia secondary to liver disease. Eur J Clin Invest 1974;4:419.

70. Cooper RA. Hemolytic syndromes and red cell membrane abnormalities in liver disease. Semin Hematol 1980;17:103.

71. Branch RA, Herbert CM, Read AE. Determinants of serum antipyrine half-lives in patients with liver disease. Gut 1973;14:569.

72. Branch RA, Herbert CM, Read AE. Determinants of serum antipyrine half-lives in patients with liver disease. Gut 1973;14:569.

73. Hepner GW, Vesell EJ. Quantitative assessment of hepatic function by breath analysis after oral administration of [¹⁴C]aminopyrine. Ann Intern Med 1975;83:632.

74. Schneider JF, Baker AL, Haines NW, et al. Aminopyrine N-demethylation: A prognostic test of liver function in patients with alcoholic liver disease. Gastroenterology 1980;79:1145.

75. Jacqz E, Hall SD, Branch RA. Genetically determined polymorphisms in drug oxidation. Hepatology 1986;6:1020.

76. Mahgoub A, Idle JR, Lancaster R, et al. Polymorphic hydroxylation of debrisoquine in man. Lancet 1977;2:584.

77. Watkins PB, Murray SA, Winkelman LG, et al. Erythromycin breath test as an assay of glucocorticoid-inducible liver cytochromes P-450: Studies in rats and patients. J Clin Invest 1989;83:688.

78. Watson RGP, Olomu A, Clements D, et al. A proposed mechanism for chlorpromazine jaundice–defective hepatic sulphoxidation combined with rapid hydroxylation. J Hepatol 1988;7:72.

79. Olomu AB, Vickers CR, Waring RH, et al. High incidence of poor sulfoxidation in patients with primary biliary cirrhosis. N Engl J Med 1988;318:1089.

80. Morino Y, Kagamiyama H, Wada H. Immunochemical distinction between glutamic-oxaloacetic transaminase from the soluble and mitochondrial fractions of mammalian tissues. J Biol Chem 1964;239: 943.

81. Boyde TRC, Latner AL. Starch gel electrophoresis of transaminase in human tissue extracts and serum. Biochem J 1961;82:52.

82. Reichling JJ, Kaplan MM. Clinical use of serum enzymes in liver disease. Dig Dis Sci 1988;33:1601.

83. Cohen JA, Kaplan MM. The SGOT/SGPT ratio—An indicator of alcoholic liver disease. Dig Dis Sci 1979;24:835.

84. William ALB, Hoofnagle JH. Ratio of serum aspartate to alanine aminotransferase in chronic hepatitis: Relationship to cirrhosis. Gastroenterology 1988;95:734.

85. Matloff DS, Selinger MJ, Kaplan MM. Hepatic transaminase activity in alcoholic liver disease. Gastroenterology 1980;78:1389.

86. Diehl AM, Potter J, Boitnott J, et al. Relationship between pyridoxal 5′phosphate deficiency and aminotransferase levels in alcoholic hepatitis. Gastroenterology 1984;86:632.

87. Kamimoto Y, Horiuchi S, Tanase S, et al. Plasma clearance of intravenously injected aspartate aminotransferase isozymes: Evidence for preferential uptake by sinusoidal liver cells. Hepatology 1985;5: 367.

88. Cohen GA, Goffinet JA, Donabedian RK, et al. Observations on decreased serum glutamine oxaloacetic transaminase (SGOT) activity in azotemic patients. Ann Intern Med 1976;84:275.

89. Litin SC, O'Brien JF, Pruett S, et al. Macroenzyme as a cause of unexplained elevation of aspartate aminotransferase. Mayo Clin Proc 1987;62:681.

90. Nalpas B, Vassault A, Charpin S, et al. Serum mitochondrial aspartate aminotransferase as a marker of chronic alcoholism: Diagnostic value and interpretation in a liver unit. Hepatology 1986;6:608.

91. Lumeng L. New diagnostic markers of alcohol abuse. Hepatology 1986;4:742.

92. Waes LV, Lieber CS. Glutamate dehydrogenase: A reliable marker of liver cell necrosis in the alcoholic. Br Med J 1977;2:1508.

93. Jenkins WJ, Rosalki SB, Foo Y, et al. Serum glutamate dehydrogenase is not a reliable marker of liver cell necrosis in alcoholics. J Clin Pathol 1982;35:207.

94. Kato S, Ishii H, Kano S, et al. Alcohol dehydrogenase: A new sensitive indicator of hepatic damage due to cardiorespiratory failure [Abstract]. Gastroenterology 1985;88:1438.

95. DeRitis F, Giusti G, Piccinino F, et al. Biochemical lab tests in viral hepatitis and other hepatic diseases. Bull WORLD Health Organ 1965;32:59.

96. Okumura M, Spellberg MA. Serum isocitric dehydrogenase activity in the differential diagnosis of liver disease. Gastroenterology 1960;39:305.

97. Reichard H. Ornithine carbamyl transferase activity in human serum in diseases of the liver and biliary system. J Lab Clin Med 1961;57: 78.

98. Blitzer BL, Boyer JL. Cytochemical localization of Na⁺,K⁺-ATPase in the rat hepatocyte. J Clin Invest 1978;62:1104.

99. Seetharam S, Sussman NL, Komoda T, et al. The mechanism of elevated alkaline phosphatase activity after bile duct ligation in the rat. Hepatology 1986;6:374.

100. Kaplan MM. Serum alkaline phosphatase—Another piece is added to the puzzle. Hepatology 1986;6:526.

101. Robinson JC, Goldsmith LA. Genetically determined variants of serum alkaline phosphatase: A review. Vox Sang 1967;13:289.

102. Shaver WA, Bhatt H, Combes B. Low serum alkaline phosphatase activity in Wilson's disease. Hepatology 1986;6:859.

103. Wilson JW. Inherited elevation of alkaline phosphatase activity in the absence of disease. N Engl J Med 1979;301:983.

104. Stolbach LL, Krant MJ, Fishman WH. Ectopic production of an alkaline phosphatase isoenzyme in patients with cancer. N Engl J Med 1969;281:757.

105. Brensilver HL, Kaplan MM. Significance of elevated liver alkaline phosphatase in serum. Gastroenterology 1975;68:1556.

106. Kaplan MM, Rogers L. Separation of human serum alkaline phosphatase isoenzymes by polyacrylamide gel electrophoresis. Lancet 1969;ii:1029.

107. Kristenson H, Trell E, Eriksson S, et al. Serum gamma-glutamyl-transferase in alcoholism. Lancet 1977;1:609.

108. Bressler R, Forsyth BR. Serum leucine aminopeptidase activity in normal pregnancy and in patients with hydatidiform mole. N Engl J Med 1959;261:746.

109. Kim NK, Yasmineh WG, Freier EF, et al. Value of alkaline phosphatase, 5′-nucleotidase, γ-glutamyl-transferase and glutamate dehydrogenase activity measurements (single and combined) in serum in diagnosis of metastasis to the liver. Clin Chem 1977;23:2034.

110. Connell MD, Dinwoodie AJ. Diagnostic use of serum alkaline phosphatase isoenzymes and 5′-nucleotidase. Clin Chim Acta 1970;30:235.

111. Kao HW, Aschcavai M, Redeker AG. The persistence of hepatitis A IgM antibody after acute clinical hepatitis A. Hepatology 1984;4:933.

112. Brechot C, Degos F, Lugassy C, et al. Hepatitis B virus DNA in patients with chronic liver disease and negative tests for hepatitis B surface antigen. N Engl J Med 1985;312:270.

113. Lemon SM, Gates NL, Simms TE, et al. IgM antibody to hepatitis B core antigen as a diagnostic parameter of acute infection with hepatitis B virus. J Infect Dis 1981;143:803.

114. Banninger P, Altorfer J, Frosner GG, et al. Prevalence and significance of anti-HB$_c$ IgM (radioimmunoassay) in acute and chronic hepatitis B and in blood donors. Hepatology 1983;3:337.

115. Berman M, Alter HJ, Ishak KG, et al. The chronic sequelae of non-A, non-B hepatitis. Ann Intern Med 1979;91:1.

116. Aach RD, Szmuness W, Mosley JW, et al. Serum alanine aminotransferase of donors in relation to the risk of non-A, non-B hepatitis in recipients: The Transfusion-Transmitted Viruses Study. N Engl J Med 1981;304:989.

117. Stevens CE, Aach RD, Hollinger B, et al. Hepatitis B virus antibody in blood donors and the occurrence of non-A, non-B hepatitis in transfusion recipients: An analysis of the Transfusion-Transmitted Viruses Study. Ann Intern Med 1984;101:733.

118. Koziol DE, Holland PV, Alling DW, et al. Antibody to hepatitis B core antigen as a paradoxical marker for non-A, non-B hepatitis agents in donated blood. Ann Intern Med 1986;104:488.

119. Kuo G, Choo Q-L, Alter HJ, et al. An assay for circulating antibodies to a major etiologic virus of human non-A, non-B hepatitis. Science 1989;244:362.

120. Davis P, Read AE. Antibodies to double-stranded (native) DNA in active chronic hepatitis. Gut 1975;16:413.

121. Jain S, Markham R, Thomas HC, et al. Double-stranded DNA-binding capacity in serum in acute and chronic liver disease. Clin Exp Immunol 1976;26:35.

122. Doniach D, Roitt IM, Walker JG, et al. Tissue antibodies in primary biliary cirrhosis, active chronic (lupoid) hepatitis, cryptogenic cirrhosis and other liver diseases and their clinical implications. Clin Exp Immunol 1966;1:237.

123. Klatskin G, Kantor FS. Mitochondrial antibody in primary biliary cirrhosis and other diseases. Ann Intern Med 1972;77:533.

124. Mitchison HC, Bassendine MF, Hendrick A, et al. Positive antimitochondrial antibody but normal alkaline phosphatase: Is this primary biliary cirrhosis? Hepatology 1986;6:1279.

125. Surh CD, Danner DJ, Ahmed A, et al. Reactivity of primary biliary cirrhosis sera with a human fetal liver cDNA clone of branched-chain α-keto acid dehydrogenase dihydrolipoamide acyltransferase, the 52kD mitochondrial autoantigen. Hepatology 1989;9:63.

126. Weber P, Brenner J, Stechemesser E, et al. Characterization and clinical relevance of a new complement-fixing antibody—anti-M8—in patients with primary biliary cirrhosis. Hepatology 1986;6:553.

127. Penner E. Demonstration of immune complexes containing the ribonucleoprotein antigen Ro in primary biliary cirrhosis. Gastroenterology 1986;90:724.

128. Bernstein RM, Callender ME, Neuberger JM, et al. Anticentromere antibody in primary biliary cirrhosis. Ann Rheum Dis 1982;41:612.

129. Whittingham S, Irwin J, MacKay DR, et al. Smooth muscle autoantibody in "autoimmune" hepatitis. Gastroenterology 1966;51:499.

130. Homberg J-C, Abuaf N, Bernard O, et al. Chronic active hepatitis associated with antiliver/kidney microsome antibody type 1: A second type of "autoimmune" hepatitis. Hepatology 1987;7:1333.

131. Zanger UM, Hauri H-P, Loeper J, et al. Antibodies against human cytochrome P-450db1 in autoimmune hepatitis type II. Proc Natl Acad Sci USA 1988;85:8256.

132. Beaune P, Dansette PM, Mansuy D, et al. Human anti-endoplasmic reticulum autoantibodies appearing in a drug-induced hepatitis are directed against a human liver cytochrome P-450 that hydroxylates the drug. Proc Natl Acad Sci USA 1987;84:551.

133. MacKay DR. Genetic aspects of immunologically mediated liver disease. Semin Liver Dis 1984;4:13.

134. Simon M, Fauchet R, Hespel JP, et al. Idiopathic hemochromatosis: A study of biochemical expression in 247 heterozygous members of 63 families—Evidence for a single major HLA-linked gene. Gastroenterology 1980;78:703.

135. Edwards CQ. Early detection of hereditary hemochromatosis. Ann Intern Med 1984;101:707.

136. Kaplan MM. Primary biliary cirrhosis. N Engl J Med 1987;316:521.

137. Scott J, Gollan JL, Samourian S, et al. Wilson's disease, presenting as chronic active hepatitis. Gastroenterology 1978;74:645.

138. Scheinberg IH, Sternlieb I. Wilson's disease. Philadelphia: WB Saunders, 1984.

139. German JL, Bearn AG. Effect of estrogens on copper metabolism in Wilson's disease. J Clin Invest 1961;40:445.

140. McCullough AJ, Fleming CR, Thistle JL, et al. Diagnosis of Wilson's disease presenting as fulminant hepatic failure. Gastroenterology 1983;84:161.

141. Spechler SJ, Koff RS. Wilson's disease: Diagnostic difficulties in the patient with chronic hepatitis and hypoceruloplasminemia. Gastroenterology 1980;78:803.

142. Edwards CQ, Williams DM, Cartwright GE. Hereditary hypoceruloplasminemia. Clin Genet 1979;15:311.

143. Brissot P, Bourel M, Herry D, et al. Assessment of liver iron content in 271 patients: A reevaluation of direct and indirect methods. Gastroenterology 1981;80:557.

144. Turnberg LA. Iron absorption in acute hepatitis. Am J Dig Dis 1966;11:20.

145. Powell LW, Halliday JW, Cowlishaw JL. Relationship between serum ferritin and total body iron stores in idiopathic hemochromatosis. Gut 1978;19:583.

146. Halliday JW, Russo AM, Cowlishaw JL, et al. Serum ferritin in the diagnosis of hemochromatosis. Lancet 1977;2:621.

147. Chapman RW, Hussain MAM, Gorman A, et al. Effect of ascorbic acid deficiency on serum ferritin concentration in patients with β-thalassaemia major and iron overload. J Clin Pathol 1982;35:487.

148. Wands JR, Rowe JA, Mezey SE, et al. Normal serum ferritin concentrations in precirrhotic hemochromatosis. N Engl J Med 1976;294:302.

149. Prieto J, Barry M, Sherlock S. Serum ferritin in patients with iron overload and with acute and chronic liver diseases. Gastroenterology 1975;68:525.

150. Bloomer JR, Waldmann TA, McIntre KR, et al. α-Fetoprotein in nonneoplastic hepatic disorders. JAMA 1975;233:38.

151. Chen D-S, Sung J-L. Serum alphafetoprotein in hepatocellular carcinoma. Cancer 1977;40:779.

152. Bellet DH, Wands JR, Isselbacher KJ, et al. Serum α-fetoprotein levels in human disease: Perspective from a highly specific monoclonal radioimmunoassay. Proc Natl Acad Sci USA 1984;81:3869.

153. Liebman HA, Furie BC, Tong MJ, et al. Des-γ-carboxy (abnormal) prothrombin as a serum marker of primary hepatocellular carcinoma. N Engl J Med 1984;310:1427.

154. Soulier J-P, Gozin D, Lefrere J-J. A new method to assay des-γ-carboxyprothrombin: Results obtained in 75 cases of hepatocellular carcinoma. Gastroenterology 1986;91:1258.

155. Chang W-Y, Chuang W-L. Complements as new diagnostic tools of hepatocellular carcinoma in cirrhotic patients. Cancer 1988;62:227.

156. Perlmutter DH, Cole FS, Kilbridge P, et al. Expression of the α_1-proteinase inhibitor gene in human monocytes and macrophages. Proc Natl Acad Sci USA 1985;82:795.

157. Darlington GJ, Astrin KH, Muirhead SP, et al. Assignment of human α_1-antitrypsin to chromosome 14 by somatic cell hybrid analysis. Proc Natl Acad Sci USA 1982;79:870.

158. Berg NO, Eriksson S. Liver disease in adults with alpha$_1$-antitrypsin deficiency. N Engl J Med 1972;287:1264.

159. Eriksson S, Carlson J, Velez R. Risk of cirrhosis and primary liver cancer in alpha$_1$-antitrypsin deficiency. N Engl J Med 1986;314:736.

160. Brantly M, Nukiwa T, Crystal RG. Molecular basis of alpha$_1$-antitrypsin deficiency. Am J Med 1988;84(6A):13.

161. Black M. Hepatic detoxication of endogenously produced toxins and their importance for the pathogenesis of hepatic encephalopathy. In: Zakim D, Boyer TD, eds. Hepatology: A textbook of liver disease. Philadelphia: WB Saunders, 1982:397.

162. Fraser CL, Arieff AI. Hepatic encephalopathy. N Engl J Med 1985;313:865.

163. Drayna CJ, Titcomb CP, Varma RR, et al. Hyperammonemic encephalopathy caused by infection in a neurogenic bladder. N Engl J Med 1981;304:766.

164. McCullough AJ, Czaja AJ, Jones JD, et al. The nature and prognostic significance of serial amino acid determinations in severe chronic active liver disease. Gastroenterology 1981;81:645.

165. Gardner DF, Carithers RL, Utiger RD. Thyroid function tests in patients with acute and resolved hepatitis B virus infection. Ann Intern Med 1982;96:450.

166. Ross DS, Daniels GH, Dienstag JL, et al. Elevated thyroxine levels due to increased thyroxine binding globulin in acute hepatitis. Am J Med 1983;74:564.

167. Nomura S, Pittmen CS, Chambers JB, et al. Reduced peripheral conversion of thyroxine to triiodothyronine in patients with hepatic cirrhosis. J Clin Invest 1975;56:643.

168. Chopra IJ, Solomon DH, Hepner GW, et al. Misleading low free thyroxine index and usefulness of reverse triiodothyronine measurement in nonthyroidal illnesses. Ann Intern Med 1979;90:905.

169. Van Thiel DH, Udani M, Schade RR, et al. Prognostic value of thyroid hormone levels in patients evaluated for liver transplantation. Hepatology 1985;5:862.

170. Walfish PG, Orrego H, Israel Y, et al. Serum triiodothyronine and other clinical and laboratory indices of alcoholic liver disease. Ann Intern Med 1979;91:13.

171. Gershengorn MC, Larsen PR, Robbins J. Radioimmunoassay for serum thyroxine-binding globulin: Results in normal subjects and in patients with hepatocellular carcinoma. J Clin Endocrinol Metab 1976;42:907.

172. Elta GH, Sepersky RA, Goldberg MJ, et al. Increased incidence of hypothyroidism in primary biliary cirrhosis. Dig Dis Sci 1983;28:971.

173. Zimmerman HJ. Function and integrity of the liver. In: Henry JB, ed. Clinical diagnosis and management by laboratory methods. Philadelphia: WB Saunders, 1984:217.

174. Neale G, Caughey DE, Mollin DE, et al. Effects of intrahepatic and extrahepatic infection on liver function. Br Med J 1966;1:382.

175. Smith FR, Goodman DW. The effects of diseases of the liver, thyroid, and kidneys on the transport of vitamin A in human plasma. J Clin Invest 1971;50:2426.

176. Seidel D, Alaupovic P, Furman RH. A lipoprotein characterizing obstructive jaundice. I. Method for quantitative separation and identification of lipoproteins in jaundiced subjects. J Clin Invest 1969;48:1211.

177. Hamilton RL, Havel RJ, Kane JP, et al. Cholestasis: Lamellar structure of the abnormal human serum lipoprotein. Science 1971;172:475.

178. Magnani HN, Alaupovic P. Utilization of the quantitative assay of lipoprotein X in the differential diagnosis of extrahepatic obstructive jaundice and intrahepatic disease. Gastroenterology 1976;71:87.

179. Simon JB, Poon RWM. Lipoprotein-X levels in extrahepatic versus intrahepatic cholestasis. Gastroenterology 1978;75:177.

180. Mitchell DP, Hanes TE, Hoyumpa AM, et al. Fever of unknown origin: Assessment of the value of percutaneous liver biopsy. Arch Intern Med 1977;137:1001.

181. Schiff L. Jaundice: A clinical approach. In: Schiff L, Schiff ER, eds. Diseases of the liver. ed 6. Philadelphia: JB Lippincott, 1987:209.

182. Ginsberg AL. Very high levels of SGOT and LDH in patients with extrahepatic biliary tract obstruction. Am J Dig Dis 1970;15:803.

183. Patwardhan RV, Smith OJ, Farmelant MH. Serum transaminase levels and cholescintigraphic abnormalities in acute biliary tract obstruction. Arch Intern Med 1987;147:1249.

184. Balasubramaniam K, Wiesner RH, LaRusso NF. Primary sclerosing cholangitis with normal serum alkaline phosphatase activity. Gastroenterology 1988;95:1395.

185. Scharschmidt BF, Goldberg HI, Schmid R. Approach to the patient with cholestatic jaundice. N Engl J Med 1983;308:1515.

186. Bynum TE, Boitnott JK, Maddrey WC. Ischemic hepatitis. Dig Dis Sci 1979;24:129.

187. Himmelstein DU, Woolhandler SJ, Adler RD. Elevated SGOT/SGPT ratio in alcoholic patients with acetaminophen hepatoxicity. Am J Gastroenterol 1984;79:718.

188. San Jose D, Cady A, West M, et al. Primary carcinoma of the liver: Analysis of clinical and biochemical features of 80 cases. Am J Dig Dis 1965;10:657.

189. Hultcrantz R, Glaumann H, Lindberg G, et al. Liver investigation in 149 asymptomatic patients with moderately elevated activities of serum aminotransferases. Scand J Gastroenterol 1986;21:109.

190. Friedman LS, Dienstag JL, Watkins E, et al. Evaluation of blood donors with elevated serum alanine aminotransferase levels. Ann Intern Med 1987;107:137.

191. Hay JE, Czaja AJ, Rakela J, et al. The nature of unexplained chronic aminotransferase elevations of a mild to moderate degree in asymptomatic patients. Hepatology 1989;9:193.

192. Palmer M, Braly LF, Schaffner F. The liver in acquired immune deficiency disease. Semin Liver Dis 1987;7:192.

193. Lebovics E, Thung JN, Schaffner F, et al. The liver in the acquired immunodeficiency syndrome: A clinical and histologic study. Hepatology 1985;5:293.

194. Schneiderman DJ, Arenson DM, Cello JP, et al. Hepatic disease in patients with the acquired immune deficiency syndrome (AIDS). Hepatology 1987;7:925.

195. Schneiderman DJ, Cello JP, Laing FC. Papillary stenosis and sclerosing cholangitis in the acquired immunodeficiency syndrome. Ann Intern Med 1987;106:546.

196. Bianchi L, Desmet VJ, Popper H, et al. Histologic patterns of liver disease in hemophiliacs, with special reference to morphologic characteristics of non-A, non-B hepatitis. Semin Liver Dis 1987;7:203.

197. Spero JA, Lewis JH, Van Thiel DH, et al. Asymptomatic structural liver disease in hemophilia. N Engl J Med 1978;298:1373.

198. Miller EJ, Lee CA, Karayiannis P, et al. Non-invasive investigation of liver disease in haemophilic patients. J Clin Pathol 1988;41:1039.

199. Hay CRM, Preston FE, Triger DR, et al. Predictive markers of chronic liver disease in hemophiliacs. Blood 1987;69:1595.

200. Hetherington ML, Buchanan GR. Elevated serum transaminase values during therapy for acute lymphoblastic leukemia correlate with prior blood transfusions. Cancer 1988;62:1614.

201. Thaler M, Pastakia B, Shawker TH, et al. Hepatic candidiasis in cancer patients: The evolving picture of the syndrome. Ann Intern Med 1988;108:88.

43

Approach to the Patient with Ascites

BRUCE A. RUNYON
TELFER B. REYNOLDS

When the liver is full of fluid and this overflows into the peritoneal cavity, so that the belly becomes full of water, death follows.

Hippocrates, ca. 400 B.C.

The word "ascites" is of Greek derivation (askos) and means bag or sack. The word is singular and is used to refer to the condition of pathologic fluid accumulation within the abdominal cavity. The fluid that accumulates is referred to as ascitic fluid. Hippocrates is said to have been the first to note the association of liver disease and fluid overload. Sydenham noted that alcoholics were predisposed to this condition.

This chapter will deal with all aspects of ascites, but the authors will focus on (1) the most common causes of ascites, (2) the most common complications of ascites, and (3) the most treatable (or even curable) causes and complications of ascites. Some misconceptions have developed regarding diagnosis and treatment of ascites, based in part on assumptions, anecdotes, and extrapolations from other body fluids. This chapter attempts to provide *data-supported* concepts about ascites. Chapter 124, Paracentesis and Ascitic Fluid Analysis, was written in conjunction with this chapter and should be read concomitantly.

CAUSES OF ASCITES AND MECHANISMS OF ASCITES FORMATION

Table 43-1 lists the causes of ascites formation in a prospective series of 1196 paracenteses performed in 576 patients between 1982 and 1988 on the general medical and gastroenterology/hepatology wards of three academic institutions (Runyon BA. Unpublished observations). Cirrhosis and alcoholic hepatitis cause the vast majority of ascites in these settings; only 18.6% of patients had a cause other than chronic parenchymal liver disease. The causes of ascites would be distributed differently if the patients had been accessed from oncology, cardiology, or pediatric wards. The current causes of ascites also differ markedly from those

of a series of 5000 cases collected at the turn of the century[1] (Fig 43-1).

Mechanisms of Ascites Formation in Liver Disease

The fundamental forces postulated by Starling to control the distribution of extracellular fluid between the intravascular and interstitial compartments are hydrostatic and oncotic pressures. The presence of ascites implies an imbalance of these forces in the peritoneal cavity, a localized disruption in the integrity of the vascular wall barrier, or a leakage of extraneous fluid into the peritoneal cavity. In liver disease with ascites, there is invariably a rise in pressure in the portal venous bed and often a decrease in vascular oncotic pressure because of decreased serum albumin. Of these two factors, portal hypertension is much more important in the genesis of ascites than is hypoalbuminemia; patients with liver disease frequently have low serum albumin without ascites, whereas patients with ascites due to liver disease are never without portal hypertension. There have been efforts to develop an "ascites threshold index" to predict what combinations of portal hypertension and hypoalbuminemia are likely to result in ascites,[2] but such formulations have not been used much in practice.

As a result of both clinical and experimental observations, it is generally agreed that the most important site of ascites formation is the liver itself rather than the mesenteric and intestinal capillaries of the portal venous bed. For example, experimental ascites is easily created by hepatic venous constriction but only with difficulty (plasmapheresis is required) by portal vein constriction.[3] After experimental hepatic venous constriction, it can be shown, either by transposing the liver into the right pleural cavity or by wrapping it in cellophane, that most of the ascites forms from the

TABLE 43–1

CAUSE	NUMBER	(% OF TOTAL)
Chronic parenchymal liver disease (cirrhosis and alcoholic hepatitis)	469	81.4
Malignancy	57	10.0
Heart failure	17	3.0
Tuberculosis	10	1.7
Nephrogenous ("dialysis ascites")	6	1.0
Pancreatic	5	0.9
Fulminant hepatic failure	4	0.7
Biliary	3	0.5
Lymphatic tear	2	0.3
Chlamydia	2	0.3
Nephrotic syndrome	1	0.2

* Of these 576, 10 (1.7%) were chylous, including the two surgical lymphatic tear cases, three patients with lymphoma, and five patients with "cirrhotic chylous ascites."

† Of these 576, 25 (4.3%) patients had "mixed" ascites (i.e., two causes of ascites—e.g., cirrhosis and peritoneal carcinomatosis).

‡ (Runyon BA. Unpublished observations.)

liver.[3] The normal endothelium of the hepatic sinusoids is markedly fenestrated in order to permit easy entry of plasma into the space of Disse for interaction with the microvilli of the hepatocytes.[4] It is easy to envision a marked increase in hepatic interstitial fluid formation through this fenestrated endothelium as a consequence of increased sinusoidal hydrostatic pressure. Normally, the excess fluid is returned to the circulation by the hepatic lymphatics, which empty ultimately into the thoracic duct. There is ample evidence that the hepatic lymphatics are distended in patients with portal hypertension and that thoracic duct lymph flow is markedly increased.[5] When the capacity of the hepatic lymphatics is exceeded, then hepatic interstitial fluid enters the peritoneal cavity as ascites. No doubt the intestinal and mesenteric capillaries contribute in some degree to ascites formation, because patients with extrahepatic portal vein occlusion sometimes do develop ascites after variceal hemorrhage, and fluid and blood replacement lowers plasma oncotic pressure. Similarly, in experimental portal vein occlusion in dogs, ascites will appear after plasmapheresis.[6]

The imbalance in hydrostatic and oncotic pressures that creates ascites is rapidly restored to equilibrium by the small rise in plasma oncotic pressure and fall in portal pressure that result from the decrease in plasma volume that accompanies ascites formation. Progression of ascites, as seen in patients with liver disease, requires a positive sodium and water balance with return of plasma volume, portal pressure, and plasma oncotic pressure to their original values. This leads, in turn, to more ascites formation. Ascites formation and reabsorption remain in balance in the absence of sodium ingestion, whereas ascites increases in a quantitatively predictable fashion when there is intake of sodium. Most patients with ascites have avid renal sodium retention with 24-hour urinary sodium excretion of less than 10 mEq irrespective of sodium intake. The concentration of sodium in ascitic fluid is, because of the Gibbs-Donnan equilibrium, 95% of the serum sodium concentration. A positive balance of 120 to 125 mEq of sodium will, therefore,

result in a 1-kg weight gain. Accurate measurement of daily weight and 24-hour urinary sodium content allows a fairly precise calculation of dietary sodium intake. This is often of practical value in explaining why patients are not responding optimally to diuretic therapy. In practice, it is wise to concomitantly measure 24-hour urinary creatinine content to help assess the completeness of the 24-hour urine collection. Creatinine formation is below normal in most patients with chronic liver disease, ranging from 15 to 20 mg/kg body weight in males and 10 to 15 mg/kg in females. Osmotic diarrhea, as from lactulose administration, contains moderate amounts of sodium, which can confuse sodium balance calculation.

PATHOGENESIS OF RENAL SODIUM RETENTION

The traditional explanation for renal sodium retention in the ascites of liver disease has been called the "underfill" theory. At the point in time when ascites formation begins, there is a small contraction in the size of the intravascular fluid compartment, which results in a small rise in plasma oncotic pressure and a small fall in portal pressure so as to create a new balance between the intravascular and ascitic compartments. The circulatory volume sensors are activated by the fall in plasma volume, leading to both proximal and distal renal tubular sodium and water retention. Plasma volume and plasma oncotic pressure then return toward their original values. However, the activated volume sensors are not turned off by the sodium and water retention because further ascites formation prevents return of plasma volume to a normal level. This concept of the pathogenesis of renal sodium retention in cirrhotic patients with ascites is supported by the finding of increased levels of the various hormones that are stimulated by hypovolemia: vasopressin, noradrenaline, renin, angiotensin, and aldosterone. In support of

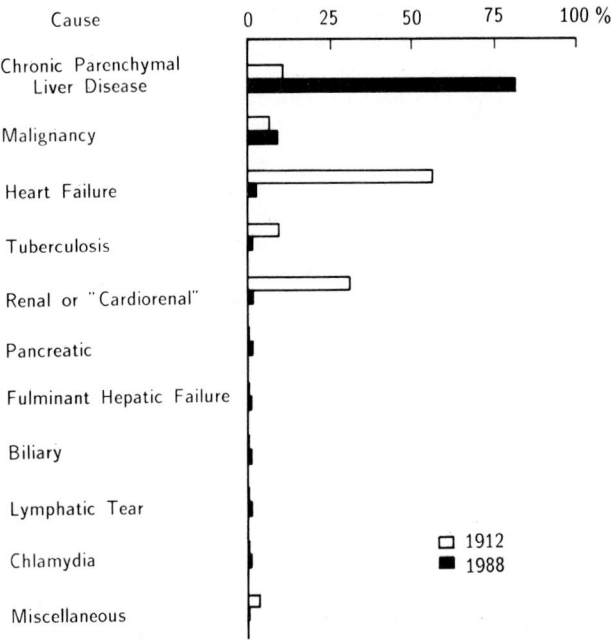

FIGURE 43–1. A comparison of cause of ascites formation in 1912 vs 1988.

the "underfill" theory, head-out water immersion often causes natriuresis in ascitic patients, presumably by increasing central blood volume,[7] and peritoneovenous shunt placement either causes natriuresis or enhances the natriuretic action of diuretics, presumably because of volume expansion.[8]

An alternative view is called the "overflow" theory. This was proposed by Lieberman in 1970 as a result of extensive studies in patients with liver disease showing consistently high plasma volumes in ascitic patients as compared with normal subjects and no difference in mean levels between ascitic and nonascitic patients with liver disease.[9] Lieberman postulated that some as-yet-unknown stimulus for renal sodium retention developed in patients with liver disease and that a primary increase in plasma volume together with portal hypertension resulted in ascites formation. Experimental support for this theory came from studies in dogs by Levy and co-workers[10] and in rats by Lopez-Novoa and colleagues,[11] who showed that nitrosamine-induced liver disease and carbon tetrachloride–induced liver disease, respectively, caused renal sodium retention that was demonstrable prior to the appearance of ascites.

It is unlikely that the high values for total plasma volume found by Lieberman and colleagues[9] and by others[12] in patients with ascites are artifacts of experimental study techniques (e.g., leakage of the radioiodinated human serum albumin marker from the plasma). However, "effective plasma volume" could still be subnormal, with high total plasma volume measurements accounted for by distention of the portal venous bed, portal venous collaterals, and hepatic lymphatics. Recently, Schrier and an international group have emphasized the evidence for increased vascular capacitance in the peripheral circulation in cirrhotic patients due to venous and arteriolar–capillary dilatation of uncertain cause.[13] Low peripheral vascular resistance and high cardiac outputs are commonly seen in this setting. Expansion of the plasma volume to fill this space could help account for sodium retention, measured plasma volume increase, and activation of pressor hormone systems prior to ascites formation. When the pressure threshold for ascites formation is exceeded, the "effective plasma volume" is further decreased in relation to the vascular capacity, and sodium retention is further increased.

Plasma levels of atrial natriuretic factor, a natriuretic peptide released from the atria in response to increased stretch and/or pressure, should be helpful in evaluating central blood volume. Reported values in patients with portal hypertension–induced ascites vary from laboratory to laboratory but tend to be on the high side of normal.[14] This provides no support for the "underfill" theory. However, the more important baroreceptors that are activated in ascitic patients may be in the territory of the arterial circulation.

EFFECTOR MECHANISMS FOR SODIUM RETENTION

Avid renal sodium retention is evident in most patients with chronic liver disease and ascites. Twenty-four-hour urinary sodium excretion is usually less than 20 mEq and often less than 1 mEq. Values over 20 mEq/24 hours, if not due to diuretic administration, suggest a relatively mild tendency to ascites formation or the onset of spontaneous diuresis, as in a patient with alcoholic liver disease who is improving with hospitalization. The renal sodium retention

is clearly due to increased tubular sodium reabsorption. Efforts to quantitate proximal and distal tubular sodium reabsorption rely of necessity on such indirect techniques as lithium clearance and measurement of free water clearance during hypotonic diuresis and are relatively imprecise. Almost certainly, both proximal and distal tubular sodium reabsorption are increased in patients who are forming ascites.

Atrial natriuretic factor seems not to play an important role in the sodium retention of liver disease, because values on the high side of normal are generally reported in ascitic patients and administration of a purified preparation intravenously does not cause much natriuresis.[15]

The renin–angiotensin–aldosterone system is activated in most patients with ascites. The finding of normal aldosterone levels in a proportion of patients with avid sodium retention suggests an increased tubular sensitivity to the action of aldosterone.[16]

Ascites Formation in Other Diseases

"MIXED" ASCITES

Approximately 5% of patients with ascites will have underlying cirrhosis as well as a second cause for ascites formation (e.g., tuberculosis or peritoneal carcinomatosis) (Table 43-1). This type of ascites is called "mixed." Therefore, when faced with a patient who has obvious liver disease and ascites, the astute clinician will not assume that the patient has *only* liver disease as the cause of ascites formation. Such an assumption could lead to a missed diagnosis of a curable, but potentially fatal, disease, such as tuberculous peritonitis. Interpretation of ascitic fluid analysis is difficult in patients with mixed ascites but critical to appropriate diagnosis (see ch 124).

MALIGNANCY

Fortunately, cancer is an uncommon cause of ascites formation. Unfortunately, most patients with malignancy-related ascites survive only a few weeks after onset of fluid retention.[17] In fact, if there is a delay in diagnosis because of confusion about how to diagnose malignancy-related ascites, many of these patients will die during the hospitalization in which the diagnosis is made. The physician's goal in treating this subgroup of ascites patients should be to do no harm and to maximize the time that the patient can spend out of the hospital. Exceptions to this very short life expectancy are the patients with ovarian carcinoma and lymphoma, who may respond to debulking surgery and chemotherapy, respectively. Contrary to popular belief, not all malignancy-related ascites is due to peritoneal carcinomatosis; the characteristics of the ascitic fluid and the treatments vary depending on the pathophysiology of ascites formation (Table 43-2)[17] (see also ch 124).

The mechanism of ascites formation in patients with malignant ascites depends on the location of the tumor. Although the data are not definitive, peritoneal carcinomatosis appears to cause ascites formation by "exudation" of proteinaceous fluid by tumor cells lining the peritoneum and entry of extracellular fluid into the peritoneal cavity for re-establishment of oncotic balance.[18] There

TABLE 43–2
Subtypes of Malignancy-Related Ascites and Their Prevalence

SUBTYPE	PREVALENCE (%)
Peritoneal carcinomatosis alone	53.3
Massive liver metastases alone	13.3
Peritoneal carcinomatosis *and* massive liver metastases	13.3
Hepatocellular carcinoma with portal hypertension	13.3
Malignant chylous ascites	6.7

Runyon BA, Hoefs JC, Morgan TR. Ascitic fluid analysis in malignancy-related ascites. Hepatology 1988;81:1104.

is very little information available regarding the cause of ascites formation in patients with massive liver metastases.[17–19] Presumably, occlusion of portal veins with tumor emboli leads to portal hypertension; then ascites forms as it does in patients with parenchymal liver disease and portal hypertension.[17] In the U.S., most patients with hepatocellular carcinoma have underlying portal hypertension; some of these patients do not develop fluid retention until the tumor becomes relatively large and replaces a significant percentage of the liver parenchyma. Alternatively, tumor-induced portal vein thrombosis may contribute to the patient's portal hypertension and predispose to fluid retention. Patients with hepatitis B viral cirrhosis may have no symptoms of liver disease during their entire lives until they develop ascites due to carcinoma. Chylous ascites due to malignancy appears to be caused by lymph node involvement by tumor and rupture of chyle-containing lymphatics.

TUBERCULOUS PERITONITIS

In the U.S., tuberculous peritonitis is essentially a disease of Asian and Mexican/Central American immigrants to the West Coast and of poor blacks on the East Coast. It is a rare disease. Despite the fact that the University of Southern California Liver Unit receives most of its ascites patients from a 1200-bed general hospital that houses these very subgroups of immigrants, only about six cases of tuberculous peritonitis are diagnosed per year (Runyon BA. Unpublished observations)! Half of these patients were found to have underlying cirrhosis, usually alcoholic in etiology. The presence of two causes of ascites formation (i.e., "mixed ascites") complicates diagnosis and treatment (see ch 124). Although patients with liver disease are not unusually prone to the hepatotoxicity of antituberculous therapy, their tolerance of drug toxicity is much poorer than that of patients with normal livers.

As in peritoneal carcinomatosis, tuberculous peritonitis probably causes ascites formation because of "exudation" of proteinaceous fluid by tubercles lining the peritoneum and entry of extracellular fluid into the peritoneal cavity for re-establishment of oncotic balance. At peritoneoscopy, the diffuse studding of the peritoneum by these lesions substantiates the plausibility of this mode of pathogenesis. Presumably, *Coccidioides* (a very rare form of inflammatory ascites) results in ascites formation by the same mechanism as tuberculosis.

HEART FAILURE

Apparently, the improved treatment of heart failure and the decreasing prevalence of heart disease have led to its decline as a cause of ascites formation. Ascites is currently an uncommon complication of heart disease.[20] The forms of heart failure recently reported to be complicated by ascites are listed in Table 43-3.[20]

Ascites forms in high-output and low-output heart failure. In the former situation, decreased peripheral resistance appears to initiate salt and water retention, whereas in the latter condition a diminished cardiac output is the first event.[13] Both of these initial events lead to a decreased "effective arterial blood volume" and subsequent activation of the vasopressin, renin–aldosterone, and sympathetic nervous systems. In turn, there is renal vasoconstriction and sodium and water retention.[13] Fluid then weeps from the congested hepatic sinusoids as lymph, just as in cirrhotic ascites.

It is unlikely that the perivenular fibrosis of chronic hepatic congestion (often referred to as "cardiac cirrhosis," although it is not true cirrhosis) plays an important role in fluid retention. Hepatic vein catheterization of a number of patients with cardiac ascites showed no evidence for vascular obstruction in the liver (Reynolds TB. Unpublished observations). Wedge vein pressures were high, but no higher than free hepatic vein pressures, and there was no abrupt fall in pressure as the catheter was withdrawn from a wedged to a free position in the hepatic vein.

PANCREATIC ASCITES

This rare form of ascites develops as part of severe acute (even hemorrhagic) pancreatitis, or as a result of pancreatic duct rupture or leakage from a pseudocyst as a complication of chronic pancreatitis. Patients with this form of ascites may also have underlying cirrhosis. Pancreatic ascites may occasionally be complicated by bacterial infection. Pleural effusions (left-sided usually) may be associated.

Ascites forms in this situation by leakage of pancreatic juice into the peritoneal cavity and/or by a "chemical burn" of the peritoneum. Extracellular fluid then enters to re-establish oncotic equilibrium. The ascitic fluid retains the unique characteristics of the source fluid (e.g., high amylase concentration), modified to some degree by the added extracellular fluid.

TABLE 43–3
Cause (and Prevalence of the Cause) of Cardiac Ascites

CAUSE	PREVALENCE (%)
Ischemia/aneurysm	31
Cardiomyopathy	23
Valvular heart disease	23
Restrictive lung disease	15
Constrictive pericarditis	8

Runyon BA. Cardiac ascites: A characterization. J Clin Gastroenterol 1988;10:410.

FULMINANT HEPATIC FAILURE

Ascites regularly develops along with hepatic coma as a manifestation of acute liver failure in viral hepatitis. However, because fulminant liver failure is quite uncommon, the total number of ascites patients who have acute liver failure is quite small. The ~80% mortality in patients with ascites due to acute hepatic failure (unless liver transplantation is performed) is much worse than that observed in patients with ascites due to chronic liver disease.

The ascites that forms in this setting has a high ($\geq$1.1 g/dl) serum-ascites albumin concentration gradient, indicating portal hypertension (Runyon BA. Unpublished observations). Ascites thus presumably forms in fulminant hepatic failure by mechanisms similar to those in ascites that forms in parenchymal liver disease.

BILIARY ASCITES

Bile can accumulate in the peritoneal cavity when the gallbladder, bile ducts, or gut rupture, or it can develop after biliary surgery. This is an uncommon form of ascites. Biliary ascites is most commonly due to rupture of the gallbladder—usually a complication of gangrene of the gallbladder in elderly men.[21]

The pathogenesis of ascites formation is similar to that of all forms of "extraneous fluids" that leak into the peritoneal cavity, as in pancreatic ascites.

LYMPHATIC TEAR

After extensive retroperitoneal dissection, as in distal splenorenal shunt or radical pelvic lymphadenectomy for testicular carcinoma, lymphatics may be transected and leak lymph for variable periods of time.[22] The leak may be chylous at first and then clarify. Usually this leakage is transient, but on occasion repeated therapeutic paracentesis (to relieve shortness of breath and distension-related pain) may cause massive protein depletion necessitating intervention, such as peritoneovenous shunt placement or reoperation and attempted ligation of the leak.[22]

The formation of ascites in this condition is similar to that of malignant chylous ascites (i.e., lymphatic leak). The presence or absence of chyle in the ascitic fluid depends on where the tear is in the lymphatic system—in chyle-containing channels or not. Patients with ascites due to lymphatic leak seem to have much more of a hypovolemia response to paracentesis than patients with other forms of ascites.

CHLAMYDIA PERITONITIS

In sexually active, otherwise healthy young women with fever and inflammatory ascites, chlamydial infection must be very high in the differential diagnosis. In recent years, *Chlamydia* apparently caused more Fitz-Hugh-Curtis syndrome than did the gonococcus.[23] This is one of the few curable causes of ascites formation. The pathogenesis of ascites formation is probably similar to that of tuberculous peritonitis.

NEPHROGENOUS (DIALYSIS) ASCITES

This poorly understood form of fluid overload develops in patients on hemodialysis.[24] On careful evaluation, many of these patients are found to have underlying chronic liver disease, which may be the reason that they develop fluid overload more readily than dialysis patients without liver disease. Evaluation of patients with nephrogenous ascites might include peritoneoscopy, which will assist with the differential diagnosis and confirm or rule out tuberculosis and cirrhosis.[24] The proper treatment of this condition is uncertain, and prognosis is poor.[24] This is one of the most poorly understood forms of ascites, and its pathogenesis is equally obscure.

NEPHROTIC SYNDROME

Although nephrotic syndrome is always listed as a cause of ascites as if it were quite common, in fact it is quite rare in adults. Only one patient was found among 576 ascites patients (Table 43-1).

It is postulated that in nephrotic syndrome loss of protein (in particular albumin) in the urine leads to decreased effective arterial blood volume, activated vasopressin, renin-aldosterone, and sympathetic nervous systems, with resulting renal sodium and water retention.[13]

CONTINUOUS AMBULATORY PERITONEAL DIALYSIS (CAPD) FLUID

This iatrogenic form of ascites is usually under the management of nephrologists. The major problem is infection, which occurs virtually once for every patient-year of treatment.[25] This form of infection is somewhat analogous to spontaneous peritonitis except that *Staphylococcus epidermidis* causes many cases of CAPD fluid infection but does not cause spontaneous bacterial peritonitis (SBP).[25]

"URINE" ASCITES

Urine may accumulate in the peritoneal cavity as a result of trauma or as a complication of renal transplantation or in the newborn.[26] Gastroenterologist/hepatologists are unlikely to be involved with the care of these patients.

CONNECTIVE TISSUE DISEASES

Serositis with ascites formation may complicate systemic lupus erythematosis.[27] This form of ascites has been reported to respond to steroid therapy.[27]

Pathogenesis presumably involves inflammation of the peritoneum with resultant exudation of proteinaceous fluid into the cavity.

OVARIAN DISEASE

In recent years, most ascites that is caused by ovarian disease is peritoneal carcinomatosis.[17] Meigs' syndrome (ascites and pleural effusion caused by benign ovarian neoplasms) is no longer a common cause of ascites formation (Table 43-1).

MYXEDEMA ASCITES

Ascites in patients with myxedema appears to be cardiac ascites, related to the subtle heart failure that these patients develop.[28] This ascitic fluid is high in protein and has a high albumin gradient—similar to cardiac ascites.[20,29] Treatment of the thyroid insufficiency cures the fluid retention.

BUDD-CHIARI SYNDROME

Patients with either acute or chronic Budd-Chiari syndrome frequently develop ascites because of portal hypertension and venous outflow obstruction. The protein concentration of this fluid is variable but the albumin gradient is high.

EVALUATION OF PATIENTS WITH ASCITES

History

Most ascites is due to liver disease and most liver disease in the U.S. is caused by alcohol; therefore, most patients with ascites are alcoholics. Ascites frequently develops as a part of the symptom complex of the patient's first decompensation of alcoholic liver disease—either alcoholic hepatitis or cirrhosis or both. Patients often state that the increasing abdominal girth has been noted for only a short time, but the laxity of the abdominal wall and the severity of the liver disease belie their chronology. Patients with alcoholic liver disease who intermittently cease or reduce alcohol consumption may be troubled by ascites in a cyclic fashion. The cycles of ascites/no ascites may be separated by many years and tend to parallel their alcohol consumption (Runyon BA. Unpublished observations). In contrast, patients who develop ascites with nonalcoholic liver disease tend to be persistently troubled by ascites after its onset, probably because of the late stage at which ascites forms and the lack of effective therapy (short of liver transplantation) for nonalcoholic liver disease. Patients who present with cirrhotic ascites often have a past medical history of liver disease including gastrointestinal bleeding and hepatic encephalopathy. When the patient has a very long history of stable cirrhosis and then develops ascites, the possibility of superimposed hepatocellular carcinoma should be considered. Patients with ascites should be questioned about other risk factors for liver disease (e.g., intravenous drug use, transfusions, acupuncture, tattoos, origination from an endemic area for hepatitis, and so forth).

Patients who have a history of cancer and develop ascites should be suspected of having a form of malignant ascites. Similarly, patients who have no risk factors for liver disease and who lose a significant amount of weight during ascites formation may harbor a neoplasm. Also, malignancy-related ascites is frequently painful, whereas cirrhotic ascites is usually not associated with pain in the absence of peritonitis or alcoholic hepatitis.

Patients with cardiac ascites often have a past history of heart disease.[20] Some alcoholics who develop ascites have alcoholic cardiomyopathy rather than liver disease.

Tuberculous peritonitis is usually manifested by fever and some abdominal discomfort. Half of patients with tuberculous peritonitis have underlying cirrhosis.

Patients who develop ascites in the setting of known diabetes and/or nephrotic syndrome should be suspected of having nephrotic ascites; these patients have anasarca. Ascites due to nephrotic syndrome in adults is very rare. Ascites developing in a patient with lethargy, cold intolerance, change in the skin and voice, and so forth, should be considered as possibly due to myxedema. Connective tissue diseases may be complicated by ascites as a manifestation of serositis.[27]

Physical Examination

Not all patients who complain of rapidly increasing abdominal girth have ascites. Some will simply have gaseous distention, and others may have the massive hepatomegaly of alcoholic hepatitis without fluid retention. Some female patients will have ovarian tumors without free fluid. Percussion of the flanks will rapidly determine which patients have ascites. If an experienced examiner detects no flank dullness, there is little or no ascites present (90% accuracy).[30] If flank dullness is detected, the patient should be rolled into a partial decubitus position to determine if the air-fluid interface shifts. The minimal volume of ascites detected by shifting dullness is said to be 1500 ml. The fluid wave has not been found to be of much value in detection of ascites; two examiners are required and, in general, very large volume obvious ascites is required before the fluid wave is present.[30] The puddle sign can detect as little as 120 ml of fluid, but many feeble patients cannot cooperate in the performance of this test (which requires the patient to maintain a hands-knees position for several minutes). Flank dullness was found to be a more helpful test than the puddle sign in a prospective study.[30]

The presence of blotchy palmar erythema (especially if the erythema extends onto the dorsum of the fingers) and/or large three-dimensional pulsatile vascular spiders are very suggestive of the presence of significant liver disease. Similarly, the presence of pathologically large abdominal wall collateral veins suggests that portal hypertension is present. The presence of large veins on the flanks and back of the patient suggests inferior vena cava block as in a web lesion or malignant obstruction. A firm nodule in the umbilicus, the Sister Mary Joseph nodule, is not common but is very suggestive of peritoneal carcinomatosis—most frequently from a gastric primary. A pathologic left-sided supraclavicular node (Virchow's node) suggests the presence of cancer in the upper abdomen. The neck veins of ascites patients should *always be examined* for distention in pursuit of a cardiac origin of ascites. Surprisingly, not all patients with cardiac ascites have peripheral edema. When cirrhotics have peripheral edema, it is usually in the lower extremities only. Nephrotics and patients with cardiac failure may have anasarca.

Ascites may be semiquantitated by use of the following system:

1+ detectable only by careful examination
2+ easily detected but of relatively small volume
3+ obvious ascites but not tense
4+ tense ascites.

This system works relatively well for patients with chronic ascites, but patients with fulminant hepatic failure or postoperative chylous ascites may have a tense abdomen without a large volume of fluid.

Differential Diagnosis by Ascitic Fluid Analysis

The details of paracentesis indications and technique, ascitic fluid analysis, and diagnosis by ascitic fluid analysis are provided in Chapter 124. Diagnostic paracentesis should be performed as a routine part of the evaluation of "new onset" ascites and should be repeated as part of the admission physical examination of patients hospitalized with ascites. Ascitic fluid infection is very common, frequently manifested by minimal symptoms, and under-diagnosed unless routine paracentesis is performed. Use of new

culture techniques and a new method of classification of ascites (albumin gradient rather than exudate/transudate) are detailed in Chapter 124.

Radiologic Assessment

Although many physicians order radiologic tests in the initial evaluation of the ascites patient, performing an abdominal paracentesis with appropriate testing of the fluid is probably a much more cost-effective approach. Usually the ascitic fluid analysis, in addition to the history and physical examination, provides a diagnosis. On occasion, performance of some radiologic tests may be of value. In the patient with infected ascites, if the initial ascitic fluid analysis meets criteria for gut perforation (Fig 43-2 and ch 124), and especially if large numbers of different bacteria are noted on Gram stain, emergency plain and upright abdominal films should be obtained to determine if free air is present. If there is free air, the patient probably needs laparotomy. If no free air is present, emergency water-soluble gut contrast studies should be performed. If the patient is young, a water-soluble upper gastrointestinal contrast study should be performed first, with a search for extravasation from a perforated duodenal ulcer. If the patient is elderly, a water-soluble contrast enema should be performed first, with a search for extravasation from a perforated colonic diverticulum. If extravasation is found, emergency surgical intervention should take place. The plain abdominal film may also be of value on rare occasions in detecting calcification of metastatic colonic carcinoma or ovarian neoplasms.

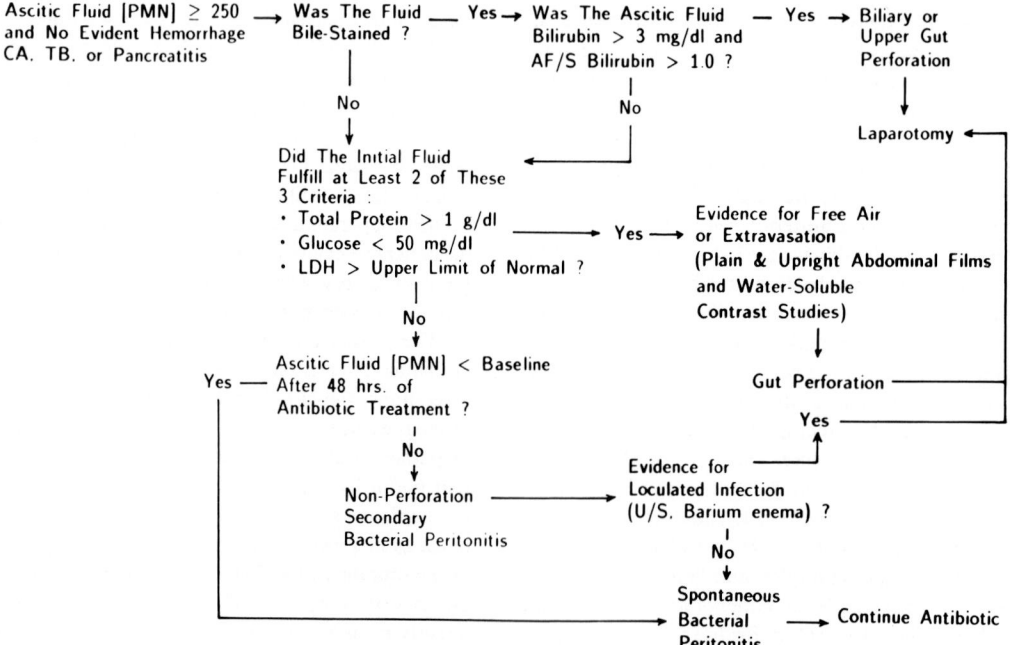

FIGURE 43–2. Algorithm for differentiating spontaneous from secondary bacterial peritonitis. *PMN*, polymorphonuclear leukocyte; *CA*, peritoneal carcinomatosis; *TB*, tuberculosis; *AF/S*, ascitic fluid/serum; *LDH*, lactate dehydrogenase; *U/S*, ultrasound.

Abdominal ultrasound may be of value in differentiating obesity from ascites or in detecting small-volume ascites. In the patient with ascites and multiple abdominal scars, ultrasound may be of value in determining where to safely insert the paracentesis needle.[31] Ultrasound may detect ovarian or pancreatic or mesenteric masses in the patient whose ascitic fluid analysis suggests peritoneal carcinomatosis. Computed tomographic studies may complement ultrasound and may be of additional value in detecting the increased density of the liver compared with the spleen in hemochromatosis. Imaging studies may be of value in detecting thrombosis of the hepatic or portal veins or of the inferior vena cava (e.g., Doppler ultrasound may confirm occluded or turbulent flow in the setting of thrombosis). The liver-spleen scan may be of some value in the evaluation of the ascites patient. The amount of colloid shift (i.e., redistribution of radionuclide from liver to spleen and bone marrow) is greatest in alcoholic liver disease but less abnormal or even normal in nonalcoholic liver disease. A normal liver–spleen scan excludes alcoholic liver disease as the cause of ascites formation.

COMPLICATIONS OF ASCITES

Infection

SPONTANEOUS BACTERIAL PERITONITIS

Ascitic fluid infection can be classified into five categories (Table 43-4). An abdominal paracentesis must be performed before a diagnosis of ascitic fluid infection can be made. Simply culturing blood and making a clinical diagnosis is not adequate. The prototype form of ascitic fluid infection is spontaneous bacterial peritonitis (SBP). This subtype is defined as ascitic fluid infection in which there is a positive ascitic fluid culture (essentially always pure growth of a single organism) and an elevated ascitic fluid absolute polymorphonuclear leukocyte (PMN) count (i.e., ≥250 cells/mm³) without an evident intra-abdominal source of infection that requires surgical treatment.

TABLE 43–4
Classification of Infected Ascites

CATEGORY	ASCITIC FLUID ANALYSIS
Spontaneous bacterial peritonitis	PMN ≥ 250/mm³, single organism
Culture-negative neutrocytic ascites	PMN ≥ 500/mm³, negative culture
Secondary bacterial peritonitis	PMN ≥ 250/mm³, usually multiple organisms
Monomicrobial bacterascites	PMN < 250/mm³, single organism
Polymicrobial bacterascites	PMN < 250/mm³, multiple organisms

Setting. For all practical purposes, SBP occurs only in the setting of liver disease—usually severe liver disease.[32,33] Ninety-five percent of patients with SBP have an elevated serum bilirubin, 81% are clinically jaundiced, and 98% have an abnormal prothrombin time.[34] Usually radionuclide liver–spleen scan demonstrates marked colloid redistribution.[34] The liver disease may be acute, as in fulminant hepatic failure; subacute, as in alcoholic hepatitis; or chronic, as in alcoholic cirrhosis. SBP is most common in alcoholic cirrhosis, but that is probably because alcoholic cirrhosis is the most common cause of ascites formation in this country. All forms of cirrhosis have been reported to be complicated by this infection. Ascites is a prerequisite to development of SBP, but the fluid may not always be clinically detectable. It is unlikely that SBP precedes ascites formation. Usually this infection develops in the patient at the time of his largest ascites volume. Nephrotic ascites was complicated regularly by SBP in the preantibiotic era, but the use of diuretics and antibiotics has made SBP uncommon in this setting currently. Cardiac ascites rarely is complicated by SBP, and patients with peritoneal carcinomatosis virtually never develop spontaneous peritonitis.[32,33] About half of SBP episodes are detected at the time of admission to the hospital; the remainder develop after admission.[34]

Pathogenesis. Recently, the pathogenesis of SBP has become more clear. There are several lines of evidence suggesting that this infection is probably the result of colonization of susceptible ascites as a result of spontaneous bacteremia (Fig 43-3). Bacteremia is common in patients with severe liver disease.[35] Fifty percent of patients with SBP have bacteremia documented at the time of diagnosis of peritoneal infection.[34] Cirrhotics with ascites usually have serum complement deficiency.[36] Neutrophil and reticuloendothelial system dysfunction are also common in cirrhosis.[37,38] Such abnormalities in host defense against infection would be expected to lead to frequent and prolonged bacteremia. Cirrhotic rats with ascites uniformly develop bacteremia after exposure to pneumococci and have more prolonged bacteremia and more fatalities compared with cirrhotic rats without ascites and compared with normal rats.[39] Although direct transmural migration of bacteria from the gut into ascites has been postulated as a route of colonization of ascitic fluid, this has been documented only in the setting of loss of mucosal integrity and/or irritation of the visceral peritoneum (in an animal model).[40,41] If organisms could easily traverse the gut wall, polymicrobial infections would be the rule rather than the exception. Also, the flora of the gut differ from the flora of SBP—anaerobes and enterococci predominate in the former, and *Escherichia coli, Klebsiella pneumoniae,* and the pneumococcus are the most common isolates in the latter.[34] In contrast to the flora of the gut, the flora of spontaneous bacteremia is similar to that of SBP and is also monomicrobial.

The protein concentration does not change with development of spontaneous infection.[42] Low protein ascites (e.g., <1 g/dl) has been shown to be particularly prone to SBP.[43] The opsonic activity (endogenous antimicrobial activity) of human ascitic fluid correlates directly with the fluid's protein concentration.[36] Patients with deficient ascitic fluid opsonic activity have been shown to be predisposed to SBP.[44]

In summary, ascitic fluid that is deficient in antimicrobial properties is the fertile soil in which SBP develops. Perhaps bacteremia is the seed that results in SBP when it occurs in the setting of fertile soil.

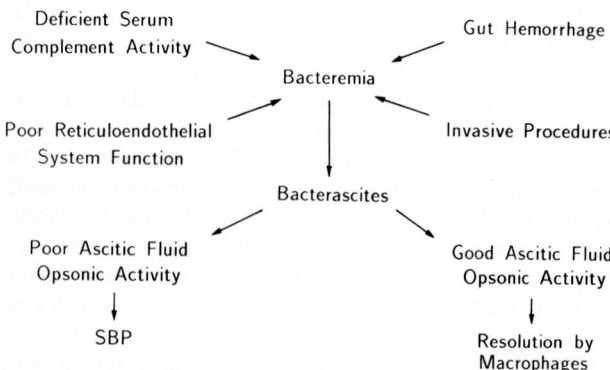

FIGURE 43–3. Proposed pathogenesis of spontaneous bacterial peritonitis (SBP).

Signs and Symptoms. Only two thirds of patients with SBP will have signs or symptoms of infection.[45] The most common signs and symptoms that were reported in series prior to 1985 are found in Table 43-5.[34] More recently it has become evident that the clinical manifestations of this infection are more subtle and the overall percentage of asymptomatic patients with SBP is increasing; the percentage of patients with rebound tenderness at the time of diagnosis now approaches zero (Runyon BA. Unpublished observations).

Prevalence. When abdominal paracentesis is performed routinely in patients with ascites on admission to the hospital (whether or not they have symptoms of infection), 10% to 27% are found to have SBP or a variant thereof.[43,44] Twelve to fifteen percent of hospitalized cirrhotics with ascites will be found to have SBP, as specifically defined, on hospital admission.[44,45] In contrast to the older retrospective studies that reported high rates of complications of paracentesis, recent prospective studies have demonstrated a complication rate of less than 1% in patients with ascites.[31,46] If the physician waits until the patient has convincing signs and symptoms of infection before performing a paracentesis, the infection is likely to be very advanced by the time the diagnosis is made. There have been no reported survivors of SBP when the

diagnosis is made after the creatinine has risen above 4 mg/dl. In order to maximize survival, it is important to perform paracentesis on hospital admission so that infection can be diagnosed and treated early. In addition, paracentesis should be repeated during hospitalization if any deterioration occurs—including pain, fever, mental status change, renal failure, acidosis, peripheral leukocytosis, or gastrointestinal bleeding.

There are no data on the frequency of SBP in outpatients. Fatal infection may be a common cause of death of cirrhotics who die at home.

Flora. As of 1985, 77% of SBP was caused by *E. coli*, streptococci (mostly pneumococci), and *Klebsiella* (Table 43-6).[34] Anaerobes cause ~approximately 1% of SBP.[47] Many reported cases of anaerobic SBP are polymicrobial and probably represent misdiagnosed secondary peritonitis. Presumably the infrequency of anaerobic SBP is due to the relatively high pO_2 of ascites—approaching that of arterial blood.[48] The prevalence of pneumococcal SBP appears to be increasing as ascitic fluid culture methods improve; as of 1988, 25% of SBP was caused by this organism, compared with an aggregate average of 8% in seven older series (Table 43-6).[49] Fungi do not cause SBP; fungal infection of ascitic fluid occurs only in the setting of secondary peritonitis.

Bacterial Infections Involving Sites Other than Ascites. Cirrhotics are unusually prone to bacterial infections because of multiple defects in immune defense (see Pathogenesis, above). This concept is only beginning to be widely appreciated, and the data substantiating it have only been published relatively recently. In a prospective study performed in Barcelona, 46% of 187 consecutive cirrhotics had bacterial infection of various types ranging from asymptomatic urinary tract infections to fatal sepsis at the time of admission to the hospital, or developed infection during hospitalization.[50] Thirty-five percent of 87 women with primary biliary cirrhosis developed bacteriuria (70% *E. coli*, 7% *Klebsiella*, 6% streptococcal) during a 12-month period.[51] Perhaps it is this high frequency of colonization of cirrhotics with bacteria and the inability of these immunocompromised patients to localize

TABLE 43-5
Signs and Symptoms in Patients with SBP

MANIFESTATION	FREQUENCY (%)
Fever	67
Abdominal pain	60
Abdominal tenderness	50
Rebound tenderness	42
Confusion	57
Diarrhea	34
Hypoactive bowel sounds	42
Hypotension	27
Hypothermia	11
Jaundice	81

Hoefs JC, Runyon BA. Spontaneous bacterial peritonitis. Dis Mon 1985;31:1.

TABLE 43-6
Flora of SBP

ORGANISM	%
Escherichia coli	43
Klebsiella pneumoniae	8
Streptococcus pneumoniae	8
Alpha-hemolytic streptococcus	5
Group D streptococcus	5
Unclassified streptococcus	4
Beta-hemolytic streptococcus	4
Beta-hemolytic streptococcus	4
Miscellaneous *Enterobacteriaceae*	3
Pseudomonas	2
Staphylococcus aureus	2
Miscellaneous	16

Hoefs JC, Runyon BA. Spontaneous bacterial peritonitis. Dis Mon 1985;31:1.

infection that lead to bacteremia and colonization of ascites. The flora of urinary tract infections in biliary cirrhosis patients is very reminiscent of the flora of SBP!

Risk Factors. The low-protein (opsonin-deficient) ascitic fluid risk factor has already been mentioned. The colloid redistribution of the liver–spleen scan is indicative of these patients' inability to rapidly remove particulate matter (e.g., bacteria) from the blood; this phenomenon would be expected to result in frequent and prolonged bacteremia.[50] Marked colloid redistribution appears to be a risk factor for SBP and spontaneous bacteremia.[50]

Some physicians are of the opinion that paracentesis itself poses a significant risk of causing ascitic fluid infection. This theoretic risk was not substantiated in the only published prospective study of paracentesis complications; in fact, no instances of needle-induced ascitic fluid infection were reported.[31] Furthermore, SBP was statistically more likely to be diagnosed at the time of the first paracentesis compared with subsequent taps. The most likely setting in which to expect iatrogenic peritonitis is when the paracentesis needle enters the bowel inadvertently during attempted paracentesis. Fortunately, this is very unusual (see Polymicrobial Bacterascites, below); only 10 cases were found among 1578 paracenteses in a retrospective study[52] and 1 case among 1196 paracenteses in a prospective study (Runyon BA. Unpublished observations).

Gastrointestinal hemorrhage has been linked to the development of spontaneous bacteremia and SBP.[53] The mechanism of this predisposition is not entirely clear. Experimental animals have prolonged bacteremia when inoculated with bacteria at the time of blood-letting, suggesting an acute deterioration in reticuloendothelial system function due to hemorrhage. In addition, invasive procedures performed in relation to gastrointestinal bleeding (e.g., endoscopy, intravascular catheter placement) may also predispose to bacteremia.

Even simple, seemingly innocuous procedures such as bladder catheter insertion in the setting of a bladder infection may cause bacteremia. Certainly, leaving a catheter in place for several days guarantees cystitis; urosepsis frequently follows in cirrhotics because of their inability to localize infections. For these reasons, bladder catheters are rarely used on the University of Southern California Liver Unit Ward.

Diagnosis. By definition, a positive ascitic fluid culture and an ascitic fluid PMN count of ≥250 cells/mm³ are required before a diagnosis of SBP is made. Empiric treatment is recommended based on the PMN count alone, before the culture result is available (see Treatment, below). A clinical diagnosis of ascitic fluid infection is not adequate; a paracentesis must be performed. Essentially no abnormalities in coagulation parameters preclude paracentesis[31] (see ch 124). A high index of suspicion of SBP and a low threshold for performing a paracentesis are required for early diagnosis of this infection.

Survival. In spite of treatment, 48% to 95% of patients with SBP die during the hospitalization in which the diagnosis is made.[45,54-56] The mean weighted mortality in the seven largest series as of 1985 was 78%.[34] The most recent series report the lowest mortality.[57] This is probably a reflection of earlier detection of infection in recent years as well as avoidance of nephrotoxic antibiotics in recent years. Many patients are cured of their in-

fection and yet die of liver and/or renal failure or gastrointestinal bleeding. In the older series, about half of SBP patients died of the infection despite antibiotic treatment; now, less than 5% of patients should die of infection if timely and appropriate antibiotics are used (see Treatment, below).

Treatment. Patients with ascitic fluid PMN counts of ≥250 cells/mm³ in a clinical setting compatible with SBP should be treated empirically with antibiotics. Patients with hemorrhage into ascites, peritoneal carcinomatosis, pancreatic ascites, or tuberculous peritonitis may have an elevated PMN count that is not related to SBP. They do not require empiric treatment. However, if the situation is initially unclear, treatment should be given until the diagnosis is clarified. Usually patients with uninfected neutrocytic ascitic fluid (except those with hemorrhage) have a predominance of lymphocytes in their ascitic fluid differential; this helps distinguish them from patients with SBP, in which PMNs predominate. Patients with bloody ascites should have a "corrected" PMN count calculated—one PMN is subtracted from the total absolute PMN count for every 250 red blood cells (RBCs). Such corrections of the PMN count may result in a negative number (i.e., less than zero). Patients with bloody ascites do not need antibiotics unless their corrected PMN count is ≥250 cells/mm³.

The ascitic fluid Gram stain is not of much value in the choice of empiric antibiotic. Only ~about 10% of Gram stains demonstrate organisms in early detected SBP, presumably because the median colony count is only one organism per milliliter of ascitic fluid in SBP.[49] In addition, in view of the potential for rapid death from this infection, it is difficult to justify "betting the patient's life" by narrowing the antibiotic spectrum of coverage based on the results of the Gram stain. Patients with suspected SBP require broad-spectrum therapy until the results of susceptibility testing are available. The recommendation for choice of empiric treatment has changed over the years. In 1971, the combination of a first-generation cephalosporin and kanamycin was recommended; in 1978, the combination of ampicillin and gentamicin was promoted.[56,58] Neither of these recommendations was based on susceptibility testing or efficacy data! Now we know that gentamicin has an unpredictable volume of distribution in patients with ascites and that the serum creatinine (and even the creatinine clearance) is a poor index of the glomerular filtration rate in ascites patients.[59,60] Therefore, it is very difficult to give appropriate loading or maintenance doses of gentamicin in these patients. If one chooses to use these drugs, a "stat" ascitic fluid and serum level should be obtained after each dose so that adequate but nontoxic levels are achieved and maintained; this is extremely cumbersome. Even if overdosing is avoided, up to 73% of cirrhotics develop nephrotoxicity.[61-63] Because of the difficulties in dosing and the apparent nephrotoxicity of aminoglycosides, their use was simultaneously abandoned in the treatment of cirrhotics in the early 1980s in many liver units around the world.

Aztreonam is a new monobactam that has been used in SBP; unfortunately, it's gram-positive coverage is negligible. Aztreonam treatment of SBP has been reported to result in an unacceptable 19% rate of superinfection.[64] Nearly 100% of SBP flora are sensitive to a third-generation cephalosporin or chloramphenicol.[34] Unfortunately, chloramphenicol is not a bactericidal drug for gram-negative bacteria; fatal recurrences are common just as in gram-negative meningitis treated with chloramphenicol.[65] The first- and second-generation cephalosporins lack the spectrum of coverage required for empiric treatment of this infection; organisms that are resistant to the empiric antibiotic may cause the patient's death before the susceptibility testing results are available. Cefotaxime, a third-generation cephalosporin, has been shown to be superior to ampicillin plus tobramycin in a controlled trial.[66] This drug covered 98% of the flora (including the pneumococcus), was more efficacious, and did not result in superinfection or nephrotoxicity.[66] This drug or a similar third-generation cephalosporin probably is the treatment of choice of suspected SBP. For cefotaxime, 2 g intravenously every 8 hours is more than adequate therapy. When susceptibility testing results are available, a drug with a more narrow spectrum can usually be substituted. Pneumococci will be sensitive to penicillin, and most *E. coli* species will be sensitive to ampicillin. Optimal duration of therapy is unclear. Most infectious disease experts treat life-threatening infections with 10 to 14 days of therapy; however, in SBP there are no data to support this duration of treatment. The ascitic fluid culture becomes negative after one dose of cefotaxime in 86% of patients.[67] The ascitic fluid PMN count, in general, drops exponentially after treatment is started such that the PMN count after 48 hours of therapy is always less than the pretreatment value in SBP treated with appropriate antibiotics.[67,68] Prolonged therapy is probably not necessary. Continuation of treatment until the PMN count normalizes has been reported to be efficacious.[69] A randomized controlled trial of short versus long duration of treatment is under way.

Recurrence. All series of patients with SBP report recurrences, although the older series did not report a high rate, in part because few patients survived the first episode. A prospective study reported in 1988 from Barcelona documents a 69% recurrence rate at 1 year.[57] An ascitic fluid protein concentration of <1.0 g/dl was the best predictor of recurrence. This impressive recurrence rate raises the question of antibiotic prophylaxis. This question warrants further study. Also, in view of the impressive recurrence rate, patients who survive SBP and are otherwise candidates for liver transplantation should be considered high priority for transplantation before a fatal recurrence of SBP occurs.

MONOMICROBIAL BACTERASCITES

The criteria for a diagnosis of monomicrobial bacterascites include a positive ascitic fluid culture for a single organism *and* an ascitic fluid PMN count of <250 cells/mm³.[70] The adjective "monomicrobial" is used to distinguish this variant of ascitic fluid infection from polymicrobial bacterascites (see below). In the older literature of SBP, this condition was either grouped with SBP or called asymptomatic bacterascites.[56] However, many patients with bacterascites have symptoms; therefore, the modifier asymptomatic does not seem appropriate. It does appear appropriate to distinguish this infection from SBP because of the absence of a PMN response in this condition. Monomicrobial bacterascites is to SBP as bacteriuria is to cystitis. Investigating the absence of PMNs in this variant of ascitic fluid infection may shed more light on the pathogenesis and natural history of ascitic fluid infection.

There is much less information available regarding monomicrobial bacterascites than there is for SBP.[70] However, the patients at risk for this variant of ascitic fluid infection appear to be the same patients that are at risk for SBP—the patients with severe acute and/or chronic liver disease and ascites. In fact, patients

who survive SBP may develop monomicrobial bacterascites and vice versa.[70]

It seems likely that the organisms of monomicrobial bacterascites reach ascites by the same route they use in SBP. Why does the host fail to mount a PMN response to the bacterial invasion? In fact, PMNs do enter the ascites in about half of the episodes, in which case monomicrobial bacterascites is simply early-detected SBP.[70] In the remaining half, the explanation is less clear. Lack of chemotactic factors (e.g., the complement fragment C5a) does not appear to be the explanation; ascitic fluid levels of C5a, one of the most important chemotactic factors, in monomicrobial bacterascites are not lower than in SBP.[71]

One possible explanation is that colonization of ascitic fluid might be very common, just as bacteremia is common even in normal hosts. The outcome of the bacterascites or bacteremia depends on the immune defenses of the host. Good immune defenses might eradicate the colonization without the host developing symptoms and without need for PMNs to enter the peritoneal cavity (i.e., peritoneal macrophages might kill the opsonized bacteria). Alternatively if defenses are weak, the bacteria may not be opsonized, and therefore they may not even be recognized as foreign matter. A third possibility is that peritoneal macrophages might not eradicate the organisms, and PMNs are called to the scene. SBP occurs and the patient will probably die without antibiotic treatment. Occasionally the patient dies of infection even before PMNs are recruited into the peritoneal cavity.

One series of bacterascites reported a predominance of gram-positive organisms,[45] whereas another series reported flora similar to that of SBP.[70] Gram-negative organisms do not colonize the skin and must be interpreted as pathogens, whereas gram-positives are routine skin flora and must be considered contaminants in the absence of a PMN response. *Staphylococcus epidermidis* cannot be interpreted as a pathogen in ascitic fluid unless a foreign body (e.g., peritoneovenous shunt) is present. Alpha-hemolytic streptococcus and *Staphylococcus aureus* also should be considered skin contaminants, unless there is a PMN response. Failure to use sterile technique when performing a paracentesis or failure to sterilize the blood culture bottle tops with iodine before inoculation will increase the presence of contaminants in the cultures.

Because of the mortality (22%–43%) associated with monomicrobial bacterascites, treatment appears to be warranted in many patients.[45,70] Even though the PMN count is not elevated, it is reasonable to use empiric antibiotics (e.g., cefotaxime 2 g I.V. every 8 hours) for patients with cirrhotic ascites who have *convincing signs or symptoms of infection* regardless of the PMN count in ascitic fluid. Empiric treatment can be discontinued after only 2 to 3 days if the culture remains negative. For patients who have asymptomatic monomicrobial bacterascites, paracentesis should be repeated for cell count and culture. If the PMN count has risen above 250/mm³, treatment should be started. Patients who have developed no PMN response or clinical evidence of infection do not require treatment. These are the patients who have probably eradicated the colonization by their own immune defenses.

CULTURE-NEGATIVE NEUTROCYTIC ASCITES (CNNA)

This diagnosis is made when (1) the ascitic fluid culture grows no bacteria, (2) the ascitic fluid PMN count is ≥500 cells/mm³,

(3) no antibiotics have been given (even a single dose usually makes the culture negative), and (4) there is no other explanation for an elevated PMN count (e.g., hemorrhage into ascites, peritoneal carcinomatosis, tuberculosis, or pancreatitis).[72] Patients who have negative cultures and PMN counts between 250 and 500/mm[3] are currently the subject of investigation.

This variant of ascitic fluid infection also occurs predominantly in the ascites patient with severe liver disease. The clinical signs, symptoms, course, and mortality are not different from those of SBP.[72] Approximately one third of these patients will have bacteremia at the time of their ascitic fluid infection. In 7% to 58% of neutrocytic ascites, the ability to grow organisms depends on the culture technique.[49,73] Thus, one explanation for the negative culture is inadequate culture technique.[49,73] In hospitals that use the older "conventional" culture method, negative cultures of infected ascites are common (see ch 124, Paracentesis and Ascitic Fluid Analysis). Patients who have CNNA despite good culture technique, in general, have spontaneously resolving SBP. This does not occur very often but is a real phenomenon.

One does not know the culture is destined to be "no growth" when initially faced with a patient with this variant of ascitic fluid infection. Therefore, empiric treatment should be given. When the preliminary report demonstrates no growth, it is helpful to repeat the paracentesis to assess the response of the PMN count to therapy. A decline in PMN count confirms a response to treatment and probably warrants a few more days of therapy. A stable PMN count, especially if there is not a predominance of PMNs, indicates that a nonbacterial (or mycobacterial) cause of the neutrocytosis is present. Cytology and culture for tuberculosis may be appropriate. Because improper culture techniques result in negative cultures, one of the most important methods to reduce the prevalence of CNNA in a hospital that is still using the conventional method of culture is to convince the microbiology lab to convert to the optimal method of culture.[49]

SECONDARY BACTERIAL PERITONITIS

This important variant of ascitic fluid infection is diagnosed when (1) the ascitic fluid culture is positive (usually for multiple organisms), (2) the PMN count is ≥250 cells/mm[3], and (3) there is an identified intra-abdominal primary source of infection (e.g., perforated gut, perinephric abscess).[67,74] The obvious importance of distinguishing this variant from SBP is that secondary peritonitis is usually treated with antibiotics *and* surgery, whereas SBP is essentially always treated with antibiotics *only*.[67] Performing a laparotomy in SBP or treating secondary peritonitis only with antibiotics usually results in the death of the patient.

Secondary bacterial infection of ascitic fluid can occur in any patient with ascites, even patients with noncirrhotic ascites.[75] Host defenses have little bearing on outcome when the gut perforates into ascitic fluid; the patient will die without surgical intervention. Secondary peritonitis should be *considered* in any ascites patient with peritonitis. However, because of the rarity of SBP in peritoneal carcinomatosis or cardiac ascites, a surgical source of peritonitis should be *presumed* in these conditions until proved otherwise.

The mechanism of ascitic fluid infection when the gut perforates into the ascitic fluid is no mystery. In the setting of a perinephric abscess or nonperforated inflamed appendix, bacteria presumably cross damaged tissue planes to enter the fluid.

Surprisingly, even with free perforation of the colon into ascitic fluid, patients do not develop a classic surgical abdomen.[75] Peritoneal signs require contact of inflamed visceral and parietal peritoneal surfaces. This does not happen when a large volume of fluid is present. Therefore, clinical signs and symptoms do not separate patients with secondary peritonitis from those with SBP.[75]

This variant of ascitic fluid infection is uncommon; only 2% of cirrhotic ascites patients have this at the time of admission to the hospital.[45] About 15% of patients who have symptoms initially resembling SBP will be shown to have secondary peritonitis; too often this diagnosis is made at autopsy.[34]

Gut perforation can be suspected and pursued if ascitic fluid analysis meets two of the following three criteria (Fig 43-2): total protein > 1 g/dl, glucose < 50 mg/dl, and LDH > 225 mU/ml (or more than the upper limit of normal for serum).[67,75] All ascitic fluids culture multiple organisms in the setting of a perforated viscus except for gallbladder rupture.[67] If multiple organisms and PMNs are seen on Gram stain, the likelihood of perforation is very high. Brown ascitic fluid with a bilirubin concentration of more than 6 mg/dl and greater than the serum level is indicative of biliary or gut (especially upper gut) perforation into ascites.[21] The initial ascitic fluid analysis is very helpful in delineating which patients are likely to have ruptured gut; these patients need an emergent radiologic evaluation (i.e., within minutes) to confirm and localize the site of rupture. Older patients should have a water-soluble contrast enema first to rule out perforated colonic diverticulum; younger patients, who are more likely to have a perforated duodenal ulcer, should have a water-soluble upper gastrointestinal contrast study first.[67] If perforation is documented, emergency intervention is mandatory to maximize survival; survivors have been reported.[67]

Patients with nonperforation secondary peritonitis tend *not* to have a diagnostic *initial* ascitic fluid analysis.[67,75] Fortunately, it is less urgent to make the diagnosis of secondary peritonitis in nonperforation peritonitis than it is in perforation peritonitis. Therefore, there may be time to evaluate the response of the ascitic fluid culture and PMN count to treatment. These parameters have been shown to be helpful in distinguishing secondary from spontaneous peritonitis.[67,75] The best time to perform a single repeat paracentesis to assess response is after 48 hours of treatment.[67] At 48 hours, essentially every SBP patient who has been treated with an appropriate antibiotic will have a PMN count lower than the pretreatment value, and the culture will be negative; in contrast, the culture remains positive and the PMN count rises in secondary peritonitis.[67,75]

Early diagnosis and surgical intervention reduce the mortality of secondary peritonitis into the same range as that of SBP (~50%).[67] Without surgical intervention, mortality approaches 100%. Patients suspected of having secondary peritonitis require broader spectrum empiric antibiotic coverage than those with SBP, in addition to an emergency evaluation to assess the need for surgical intervention (see above). Cefotaxime plus metronidazole provide excellent initial empiric therapy of suspected secondary peritonitis while the radiologic workup is being done.[67]

POLYMICROBIAL BACTERASCITES

This variant of ascitic fluid infection is diagnosed when (1) multiple organisms are cultured from ascitic fluid and (2) the PMN count is <250 cells/mm³.[52] This diagnosis should be suspected when (1) the paracentesis is difficult because of ileus or a traumatic tap, (2) stool and/or air is aspirated into the paracentesis syringe, or (3) multiple organisms but no PMNs are seen on Gram stain. Polymicrobial bacterascites is essentially diagnostic of inadvertent gut perforation by the paracentesis needle.[52] Fortunately, this variant of ascitic fluid infection is the rarest; only 10 cases (0.6%) were found among 1578 taps in a retrospective study,[52] and one case (0.08%) was found among 1196 taps in a prospective study (Runyon BA. Unpublished observations).

Surprisingly, needle perforation of the bowel is relatively well tolerated. Only 18% (2/11) of patients with needle perforation of the gut into ascitic fluid developed peritonitis; only 0.07% (2/2774) of paracenteses caused peritonitis.[52] Neither of these two patients required laparotomy, and none died because of the paracentesis-related peritonitis.[52] If needles larger than 22 gauge had been used, the results may have been different.

It appears that patients with low-protein ascitic fluid are at most risk of developing a PMN response and clinical peritonitis related to needle perforation of the gut.[52] Most of the patients with high-protein ascites (e.g., >1 g/dl) did not even receive antibiotics and yet did well. However, most physicians would probably feel uncomfortable withholding antibiotic treatment if needle perforation is suspected. If a decision to treat is made, anaerobic coverage should be included (e.g., cefotaxime and metronidazole). If a decision not to treat is made, follow-up paracentesis is helpful in following the PMN count and culture. If the number of organisms does not decrease and/or a PMN response occurs, antibiotic treatment should be initiated.

Figure 43-4 summarizes the approach to the patient with ascites. On admission to the hospital, all patients with ascites should have a paracentesis performed even if they have no signs or symptoms of infection and even if they have been tapped multiple times in the past. A PMN count and culture should be performed as a minimum ascitic fluid analysis. Ascitic fluid should be inoculated into blood culture bottles.[49] Blood cultures should be obtained (prior to antibiotics) if the patient appears ill, even if he is not febrile. Cirrhotic patients may respond to infection with hypothermia or hypotension rather than fever. If the initial fluid is neutrocytic and fulfills the criteria for perforation peritonitis, an emergency plain film, upright abdominal film, and water-soluble gut contrast studies should be performed. Emergency surgery is indicated if a surgically treated source of infection is identified.

Tense Ascites

Some patients ignore their growing abdomens and do not seek medical attention until they can no longer breathe comfortably because of the pressure the fluid exerts on the diaphragm. In this setting, the abdominal skin is usually stretched and glistening. This condition is called tense ascites. The volume of fluid required before "tenseness" occurs is highly variable. Some patients get tense ascites with 2 liters, while others are not tense with 20 liters of abdominal fluid. The rapid accumulation of fluid does not give the abdominal wall time to stretch; these patients have small-volume tense ascites. Truly tense ascites requires urgent treatment—therapeutic paracentesis. Tense ascites can be drained (even 20 or more liters) without untoward hemodynamic effect.[76-79]

However, in general, only 5 to 10 liters are removed. Although discarding all of the fluid obtained from patients who have difficulty synthesizing protein may be problematic, therapeutic paracentesis of cirrhotic ascites is less problematic than the textbooks of medicine would lead the reader to believe. The myth of the paracentesis-related hemodynamic disasters was based on observations in small numbers of patients—probably coincidences.[78] In fact, staged paracentesis of liter aliquots (up to 7 liters) of tense ascites resulted in incremental increases in cardiac output and stroke volume in one study.[79]

Patients who develop tense ascites are frequently the least compliant and/or the most refractory to conventional therapy. Careful attention should be given to the education of these patients regarding the chronicity of their disease as well as diet and diuretic therapy.

Abdominal Wall Hernias

Abdominal wall hernias (umbilical and inguinal) are common in patients with ascites and may cause serious complications (see Atlas). Unfortunately, there is little published information available about them. In one study, 17% of cirrhotics with ascites were found to have umbilical hernias on admission.[80] During follow-up, 14% of these patients' hernias became incarcerated, 35% developed skin ulceration, and 7% ruptured.[80]

Based on the above data, surgical treatment should be considered electively in all patients with hernias and ascites, because more than half will ultimately need surgery for a complication. Ascites should be medically removed preoperatively, because the hernia recurs in 73% of patients who have ascites at the time of hernia repair but only in 14% of patients who have no ascites at the time of repair.[81] If skin ulceration develops, surgery should be performed semiemergently. Emergent surgery should be performed for incarceration or rupture.[82] Rupture (i.e., Flood's syndrome) is the most feared complication of the umbilical hernia. The mortality of this complication is 11% to 43% overall, and 100% if the preoperative serum bilirubin is >2 mg/dl or the prothrombin time is prolonged more than 2.5 seconds.[82] A ruptured umbilical hernia requires emergent surgical repair, and this can usually be performed under local anesthesia.[82]

Hepatic Hydrothorax

Pleural effusions are not uncommon in patients with cirrhotic ascites. They are usually unilateral and right sided but occasionally may be bilateral with the right side predominating. Only rarely is there a unilateral left-sided effusion; tuberculosis is more common in left-sided effusions.[83] The volume of effusion varies widely. Small to moderate–sized collections probably form as a poorly understood reaction to the presence of the ascites. When the effusion is large and obscures most of the right lung, it is referred to as hepatic hydrothorax. This is thought to be due to a congenital weakness in the membranous portion of the right diaphragm, which ruptures because of the elevated intra-abdominal pressure associated with ascites.[84] Occasionally this results in sudden shortness of breath associated with decompression of the abdomen. On rare occasions no ascites is detected in the face of a huge pleural effusion—most likely this is due to a one-way valve mechanism in the diaphragm.[85]

The main symptom associated with hepatic hydrothorax is shortness of breath. Infection of this fluid is rare. When it does occur, it is usually a result of SBP.

Usually the fluid resembles ascites, but the analysis is not identical to that of the ascitic fluid because the pleural fluid is in a system with pressures different from those in the portal bed. The pleural fluid protein is usually 0.75 to 1.0 g/dl higher than that of ascitic fluid from the same patient.[84]

Treatment of hepatic hydrothorax is usually more difficult than expected. This complication tends to occur in patients who are the least compliant and/or the most refractory. Patients with hepatic hydrothorax were excluded from the Veterans Administration Cooperative LeVeen Shunt Study because it was recognized that they represent a difficult subgroup of ascites patients to treat. Some authors have recommended tetracycline sclerosis using a chest tube. However, chest tube insertion with suction has been reported to lead to serious fluid and protein depletion and death in two patients.[86] Once a chest tube is inserted, too often it becomes very difficult to remove it. Clamping the tube may cause fluid to leak around the tube's insertion site. Peritoneovenous shunt can be considered in the patient with large-volume ascites, but it is frequently accompanied by perioperative complications and shunt failure (see below). Direct surgical repair of the defect can be considered, but too often these patients are not good operative candidates. Sodium restriction and diuretics are probably the best and safest form of therapy of hepatic hydrothorax; this approach is the treatment used at the USC Liver Unit and is usually successful (Reynolds TB, Runyon BA. Unpublished observations).

TREATMENT OF ASCITES

Not all forms of ascites respond to the same treatment (see Fig 43-4). Therefore, the correct diagnosis of the cause of ascites formation is important. The diagnosis is usually apparent based on the history, physical examination, and ascitic fluid analysis (see ch 124).

Nonportal Hypertension–Related (Low-Albumin Gradient) Ascites

The prototype (and the most common form) of low-albumin gradient ascites is peritoneal carcinomatosis. Peripheral edema in these patients responds to diuretics, but the ascites usually does not respond to diuretics; edema-free patients treated with diuretics lose only intravascular volume without loss of ascites.[87] The mainstay of treatment of peritoneal carcinomatosis is therapeutic paracentesis.[76,77] Except for patients with ovarian carcinoma, patients with peritoneal carcinomatosis live only a matter of weeks; therefore, the total number of taps required to minimize symptoms is not great. Patients with ovarian malignancy may have a good response to debulking and chemotherapy. Experimental treatments of peritoneal carcinomatosis include intraperitoneal installation

of a streptococcal antigen OK-432[88] or melphalan.[89] Peritoneovenous shunts are said to be effective in malignant ascites and less morbid than in cirrhotic ascites[90]; however, in view of the very short life expectancy of these patients, a hospitalization for installation of a shunt may not be appropriate.

Nephrotic ascites is a rare form of ascites (0.2% of ascites overall), and it is also notable in that it is perhaps the only form of nonportal hypertension–related ascites that does respond to salt restriction and diuretics.

Tuberculous peritonitis requires antituberculous therapy; there is no point in using diuretics unless the patient has concomitant portal hypertension from cirrhosis. Pancreatic ascites may resolve spontaneously, but if caused by a duct leak they may require endoscopic stenting or operative intervention. A postoperative lymphatic leak may also resolve spontaneously but on occasion may require surgical intervention or peritoneovenous shunting.[22] *Chlamydia* peritonitis is cured by tetracycline therapy.[23] "Nephrogenous" ascites (dialysis ascites) (see ch 124) may respond to vigorous dialysis.[24]

Portal Hypertension–Related Ascites

TREAT THE UNDERLYING LIVER DISEASE

The first step in treating portal hypertension–related ascites (in the majority of cases this is cirrhotic ascites) is to treat the underlying liver disease. In most patients in the U.S., where the majority of liver disease is due to ethanol, this requires convincing the patient to stop drinking alcohol. With time and healing of alcoholic hepatitis, the ascites may resolve or at least convert from "refractory to medical therapy" to "nonrefractory to medical therapy." Patients with autoimmune chronic active hepatitis, iron-storage disease, or Wilson's disease should receive the specific therapy for those diseases; this may improve their overall liver function and increase ease of management of their ascites.

DETERMINE THE PRECIPITATING CAUSE OF ASCITES FORMATION

In the initial management of ascites, it is also of value to determine the precipitating cause of ascites formation. Frequently, ascites accumulates during an episode of dietary indiscretion or discontinuation of diuretics; the patient may decide that soup or whole milk is exactly what he thinks he needs and may consume large amounts of these high-salt foods. Education regarding these matters may help prevent future hospitalizations.

URINARY SODIUM

Twenty-four-hour urinary sodium measurements are useful in patients with portal hypertension–related ascites, in both assessing the need for diuretic therapy and monitoring its progress. Most patients retain sodium avidly and have less than 10 mEq in the 24-hour urine. They cannot be managed successfully with dietary sodium restriction alone and will need diuretic therapy or inter-

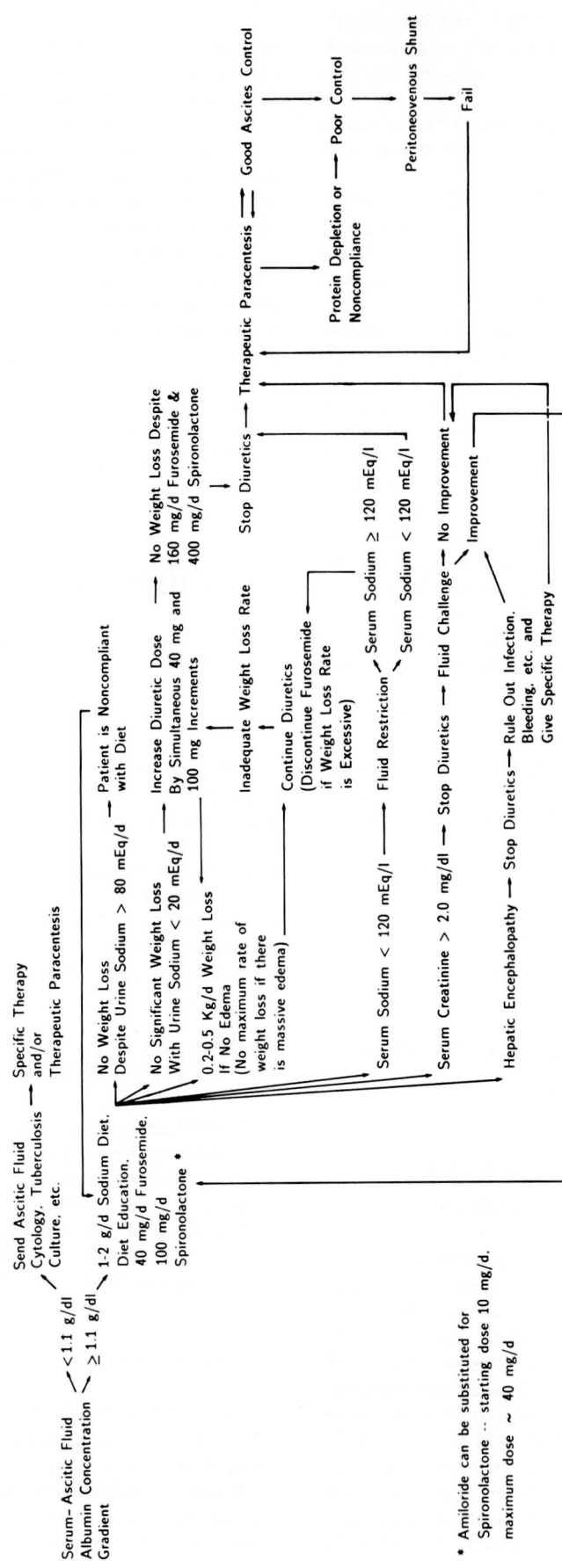

FIGURE 43–4. Algorithm for treatment of ascites.

mittent paracentesis. Those with <5 mEq/24 hours will need relatively high doses of diuretics and will not usually respond to the normal starting regimen of 100 mg of spironolactone and 40 mg of furosemide daily. More than 25 mEq of sodium in the initial 24-hour urine, if not due to recently administered diuretics, may be a sign of spontaneous natriuresis due to improvement in liver disease; such patients might be managed with dietary sodium restriction alone.[91] Since there is little circadian variation in urinary sodium concentration in patients with avid sodium retention, a "spot" urinary sodium concentration is a satisfactory substitute for a 24-hour collection for baseline assessment in most cases.

If diuretic therapy is not progressing satisfactorily, this can be due to inadequate natriuresis or to failure to properly restrict sodium intake, or both; monitoring 24-hour urinary sodium excretion and daily weight will usually clarify the problem. As mentioned earlier, the adequacy of 24-hour collections must be monitored by measurement of creatinine excretion.

DIET

In portal hypertension–related ascites, weight change is directly and predictably related to sodium balance. Dietary sodium restriction is, therefore, essential and should begin immediately. The patient and cook (if different from the patient) should be educated by an enthusiastic dietician. The more contact the dietician has with the patient and cook, the better. One patient–dietician encounter is not enough. Although a 500 mg (22 mEq)/day sodium diet is quite feasible in a hospital setting, it is an unrealistic goal for most outpatients. The advantage of such a diet while in hospital is a more negative sodium balance and more rapid loss of ascites. On the other hand, the advantage of a less restricted, 2 g (88 mEq)/day hospital diet is the opportunity to establish a diuretic regimen that will continue to be effective in the patient's home environment.

NO INDISCRIMINATE FLUID RESTRICTION

An indiscriminate fluid restriction is inappropriate. At the USC Liver Unit we do not restrict fluid in patients unless their serum sodium drops below 120 mEq/liter. Cirrhotics do not have symptoms from hyponatremia until the sodium is well below this level, unless the decline in sodium is very rapid—for example, related to use of hydrochlorothiazide. To fluid-restrict everyone serves only to alienate patients, nurses, and dieticians. There is no evidence that fluid restriction speeds diuresis. It is the sodium restriction that is important.

DIURETICS

If single-agent diuretic therapy is planned, spironolactone or amiloride is the best choice—starting with a minimum of 100 mg/day or 10 to 20 mg/day, respectively. Amiloride is more expensive but does not cause gynecomastia, as spironolactone occasionally does. Spironolactone is the mainstay of treatment of cirrhotic ascites. It is effective in 95% of patients as a single agent, compared with the 58% efficacy of furosemide alone.[92] The half-life of spironolactone is approximately 24 hours; it makes no sense to dose

the drug multiple times per day. Single daily doses of pills are most appropriate and enhance compliance—100-mg spironolactone pills are available. In general, spironolactone and furosemide are used together, starting with 100 mg/day spironolactone and 40 mg/day furosemide, then increasing each drug simultaneously as needed. If weight loss or urine sodium is inadequate, diuretics are increased up to a "ceiling" dose of 160 mg/day furosemide and 400 mg/day spironolactone. If diuresis is inadequate on these doses, one can add 25 to 50 mg hydrochlorothiazide or 5 mg of metolazone, but too often these three-drug combinations cause a massive urine sodium loss with profound hyponatremia, and diuretics must be stopped. Also, this "triple therapy" is probably too potent for outpatients. The ratio of spironolactone and furosemide can be adjusted to correct serum potassium problems. Combined with a 1000-mg sodium diet, this regimen will achieve successful diuresis in 93% of cirrhotics. There are very few reports regarding use of intravenous diuretics in these patients. If rapid weight loss is desired, therapeutic paracenteses should be done[46] (see below). For patients who have massive edema, there is no limit to the daily weight loss; once the edema has resolved, 0.5 kg/24 hours is probably a reasonable maximum.[93] If patients develop encephalopathy, serum sodium <120 mEq/liter despite fluid restriction, or serum creatinine >2.0 mg/dl, diuretics are usually stopped and the situation is reassessed. Potassium abnormalities are almost never prohibitive because of the ability to adjust the ratio of the diuretics. Many of the patients who develop serious complications of diuretic treatment will fail diuretic treatment and require second-line therapy. Prostaglandin inhibitors (e.g., nonsteroidal anti-inflammatory drugs) should not be used in patients with ascites because they curtail diuresis, may promote renal failure, and commonly cause gastrointestinal bleeding.[94] Complete removal of ascites may not be readily obtainable.[95] However, theoretically, the concentration of ascitic fluid through diuresis increases the fluid's opsonic activity 10-fold and may be of value in attempting to prevent SBP.[96]

REFRACTORY ASCITES

Patients who fail inpatient diuretic treatment (minimal to no weight loss or development of complications of diuretics) are treated with second-line therapy (i.e., therapeutic paracenteses)—first as inpatients and then as outpatients (see Fig 43-4, Therapeutic Paracentesis below, and ch 124).

PORTACAVAL SHUNT

In the 1960s, portacaval shunts were used for treatment of ascites, but operative complications, in particular portosystemic encephalopathy, led to an abandonment of this practice.[97]

RHODIASCIT ("PARIS PUMP")

In the 1970s, a device was used in Europe in the treatment of cirrhotic ascites that ultrafiltered the fluid after it was removed from the abdomen and then reinfused it intravenously.[98] Unfortunately, complications such as disseminated intravascular coagulation were common, and this form of treatment has been used very rarely in the U.S.

THERAPEUTIC PARACENTESIS

(See also ch 124 for details of use of albumin, and so forth.) From the time of the first recorded treatment of ascites until the late 1940s, therapeutic paracentesis was essentially the only available therapy. In the early 1950s, diuretics became available coincidently with reports of serious complications of therapeutic paracentesis in a small number of patients.[78] This resulted in therapeutic paracentesis being discarded as a viable treatment modality by many physicians in the 1950s without a "fair trial." In the 1980s, at least in part because of dissatisfaction with (1) the prolonged hospitalizations required for complete removal of ascites through use of diuretics and (2) dissatisfaction with peritoneovenous shunts, interest in therapeutic paracentesis resurged. Physicians who cared for ascites patients before 1950 remember that these patients tolerated outpatient "total paracentesis" with use of large trocars. Large volumes of fluid were removed in a matter of minutes, usually without incident. In the 1980s, some very well-designed and well-executed studies of large-volume (5 liter) paracentesis were reported from Barcelona, Spain, and from Los Angeles.[46,99,100] Patients were treated with (1) daily paracenteses followed by colloid infusion or (2) single paracentesis without intravenous colloid infusion.[46,99,100] Much to the surprise of many physicians, the patients tolerated these large-volume taps very well! In fact, if relatively small changes in electrolytes and serum creatinine are considered complications of therapy, daily therapeutic paracentesis was found to be safer than diuresis in the randomized controlled trial performed in Barcelona![46] If the goal of treatment is to achieve "dryness" of the abdomen while the patient is still in the hospital, taps are also faster than diuresis.[46] The authors of this study have concluded that therapeutic paracentesis is first-line therapy of patients with tense cirrhotic ascites. But not all physicians agree with this recommendation; in view of the ease and efficacy of diuretic therapy in >90% of patients, paracentesis should probably be reserved for treatment of tense ascites and ascites that is refractory to diuretic therapy. Also, therapeutic paracentesis lacks the ascitic fluid opsonin-conserving advantage of diuresis; theoretically, depletion of opsonins by paracentesis could predispose to spontaneous bacterial peritonitis.[101]

PERITONEOVENOUS SHUNTS

In the mid 1970s, the peritoneovenous shunt was promoted as a new "physiologic" treatment in the management of ascites.[102] It was initially unclear to some investigators whether this new tool should be used for initial therapy or should be reserved only for treatment of patients refractory to diuretics. Reports of complications of shunt insertion and shunt failure rapidly sobered the enthusiasm for this treatment and have removed it from first-line therapy of cirrhotic ascites. Reported complications include "recovery room pulmonary edema" (flow through a shunt exceeds 100 ml/min), variceal hemorrhage (from fluid overload), disseminated intravascular coagulation (DIC), thromboembolic phenomena including superior vena cava thrombosis, pseudocyst formation, and peritoneal fibrosis.[103] Unfortunately, shunt failure due

to thrombosis continues to be a serious problem. Most shunts clot in less than a year's time. "Second-generation" shunts (e.g., Denver shunts) have not reduced the shunt-failure rate due to thrombosis.[104] Finally, the Veterans Administration Cooperative Study of the peritoneovenous shunt enrolled ~3000 alcoholic cirrhotic ascites patients and randomized only those who were refractory to diuretic therapy to either continued diuretic therapy plus therapeutic paracentesis or peritoneovenous shunt (including use of Denver shunts in patients who clotted LeVeen shunts).[105] This study documented (1) no improved survival in shunted patients compared with medically treated patients, (2) excessive infections in shunted patients, (3) continued need for sodium restriction and diuretics despite a functional shunt, (4) excessive shunt failure, and (5) most important, *only 10% failure of diuretic therapy*.[105] Removal of most of the ascitic fluid intraoperatively prior to shunt insertion, with use of perioperative antiplatelet therapy, has reduced the incidence of DIC, and replacement of ascites with saline and administration of intraoperative intravenous furosemide have decreased the incidence of pulmonary edema.[106] At the present time, peritoneovenous shunting is reserved for the very small group of patients who fail both diuretic *and* paracentesis therapy. This does not happen very often—only when patients cannot or will not return for outpatient paracentesis.

EXTRACORPOREAL ULTRAFILTRATION AND PERITONEAL REINFUSION OF CIRRHOTIC ASCITES

Recently, a few patients with refractory ascites have been treated with a technique somewhat similar to the Paris pump, except that the concentrated ascitic fluid is reinfused into the abdomen rather than into the veins.[107] This route of reinfusion apparently avoids the complications associated with intravenous infusion, is rapid, conserves ascitic fluid protein, and may hold great promise for future treatment of ascites if controlled trials demonstrate efficacy.[108]

The reader is directed to Chapter 16, Bile Secretion; Chapter 26, The Gastrointestinal Microflora; Chapter 41, Approach to the Patient with Jaundice; Chapter 42, Approach to the Patient with Abnormal Liver Chemistries; Chapter 50, Approach to the Patient with Drug or Alcohol Dependency; Chapter 88, Acute Pancreatitis; Chapter 89, Chronic Pancreatitis; Chapter 101, Diseases of the Peritoneum; Chapter 124, Paracentesis and Ascitic Fluid Analysis; and Chapter 127, Microbiologic Studies.

REFERENCES

1. Cabot RC. The causes of ascites: A study of 5000 cases. Am J Med Sci 1912;143:1.
2. Atkinson M, Losowsky MS. The mechanism of ascites formation in chronic liver disease. Q J Med 1961;30:153.
3. Freeman S. Symposium on gastrointestinal diseases: Recent progress in physiology and biochemistry of liver. Med Clin North Am 1953;37:109.

4. Kessel RG, Kardon RH. Tissues and organs: A text-atlas of scanning electron microscopy. San Francisco, WH Freeman and Co, 1979.

5. Baggenstoss AH, Cain JC. The hepatic hylar lymphatics of man. N Engl J Med 1957;256:531.

6. Volwiler W, Grindlay JH, Bollman JL. Symposium on liver disease: Relation of portal vein pressure to formation of ascites—Experimental study. Gastroenterology 1950;14:40.

7. Epstein M. Deranged sodium homeostasis in cirrhosis. Gastroenterology 1979;76:622.

8. Blendis LM, Greig PD, Langer B, et al. The renal and hemodynamic effects of the peritoneovenous shunt for intractable hepatic ascites. Gastroenterology 1979;77:250.

9. Lieberman FL, Denison EK, Reynolds TB. The relationship of plasma volume, portal hypertension, ascites, and renal sodium retention in cirrhosis: The overflow theory of ascites formation. Ann NY Acad Sci 1970;170:202.

10. Levy M. Sodium retention and ascites formation in dogs with experimental portal cirrhosis. Am J Physiol 1977;233:F572.

11. Lopez-Novoa JM, Rengel MA, Hernando H. Dynamics of ascites formation in rats with experimental cirrhosis. Am J Physiol 1980;238:F353.

12. Murray JF, Dawson Am, Sherlock S. Circulatory changes in chronic liver disease. Am J Med 1958;24:358.

13. Schrier RW, Arroyo V, Bernardi M, et al. Peripheral arterial vasodilation hypothesis: A proposal for the initiation of renal sodium and water retention in cirrhosis. Hepatology 1988;8:1151.

14. Gines P, Jimenez W, Arroyo V, et al. Atrial natriuretic factor in cirrhosis with ascites: Plasma levels, cardiac release and splanchnic extraction. Hepatology 1988;8:636.

15. Laffi G, Tinzani M, Meacci E, et al. Renal hemodynamic and natriuretic effect of human atrial natriuretic factor infusion in cirrhosis with ascites. Gastroenterology 1989;96:167.

16. Wilkinson SP, Williams R: Renin–angiotensin–aldosterone system in cirrhosis. Gut 1980;21:545.

17. Runyon BA, Hoefs JC, Morgan TR. Ascitic fluid analysis in malignancy-related ascites. Hepatology 1988;8:1104.

18. Pockros PJ, Woods S. Malignant ascites from peritoneal carcinomatosis is immobile in comparison to cirrhotic ascites [Abstract]. Hepatology 1988;8:1450.

19. Greenway B, Johnson PJ, Williams R. Control of malignant ascites with spironolactone. Br J Surg 1982;69:441

20. Runyon BA. Cardiac ascites: A characterization. J Clin Gastroenterol 1988;10:410.

21. Runyon BA. Ascitic fluid bilirubin concentration as a key to the diagnosis of choleperitoneum. J Clin Gastroenterol 1987;9:543.

22. Miedema EB, Bissada NK, Finkbeiner AE, et al. Chylous ascites complicating retroperitoneal lymphadenectomy for testis tumors: Management with peritoneovenous shunting. J Urology 1978;120:377.

23. Muller-Schoop JW, Wang SP, Munzinger J, et al. Chlamydia trachomatosis as possible cause of peritonitis and perihepatitis in young women. Br Med J 1978;1:1022.

24. Mauk PM, Schwartz JT, Lowe JE, et al. Diagnosis and course of nephrogenic ascites. Arch Intern Med 1988;148:1577.

25. Rubin J, Rogers WA, Taylor HM, et al. Peritonitis during continuous ambulatory peritoneal dialysis. Ann Intern Med 1980;92:7.

26. Baghdassarian OM, Koehler PR, Schultze G. Massive neonatal ascites. Radiology 1961;76:586.

27. Wilkins KW, Hoffman GS. Massive ascites in systemic lupus erythematosus. J Rheumatol 1985;12:571.

28. Baker A, Kaplan M. Central congestive fibrosis of the liver in myxedema. Ann Intern Med 1972;77:927.

29. Mauer K, Manzione NC. Usefulness of the serum-ascites albumin gradient in separating transudative from exudative ascites: Another look. Dig Dis Sci 1988;33:1208.

30. Cattau EL, Benjamin SB, Knuff TE, et al. The accuracy of the physical exam in the diagnosis of suspected ascites. JAMA 1982;247:1164.

31. Runyon BA. Paracentesis of ascitic fluid: A safe procedure. Arch Intern Med 1986;146:2259.

32. Runyon BA. Spontaneous bacterial peritonitis associated with cardiac ascites. Am J Gastroenterol 1984;79:796.

33. Kurtz RC, Bronzo RL. Does spontaneous bacterial peritonitis occur in malignant ascites? Am J Gastroenterol 1982;77:146.

34. Hoefs JC, Runyon BA. Spontaneous bacterial peritonitis. Dis Mon 1985;31:1.

35. Graudal N, Milman N, Kirkegaard E, et al. Bacteremia in cirrhosis of the liver. Liver 1986;6:297.

36. Runyon BA, Morrissey R, Hoefs JC, Wyle F. Opsonic activity of human ascitic fluid: A potentially important protective mechanism against spontaneous bacterial peritonitis. Hepatology 1985;5:634.

37. Rajkovic IA, Williams R. Abnormalities of neutrophil phagocytosis, intracellular killing, and metabolic activity in alcoholic cirrhosis and hepatitis. Hepatology 1986;6:252.

38. Rimola A, Soto R, Bory F, et al. Reticuloendothelial system phagocytic activity in cirrhosis and its relation to bacterial infections and prognosis. Hepatology 1984;4:53.

39. Mellencamp MA, Preheim LC. Effect of cirrhosis on bacteremia and capsular antigenemia during experimental pneumococcal pneumonia [Abstract]. Proceedings of the 26th Interscience Congress on Antimicrobial Agents and Chemotherapy, Washington, DC, 1986:293.

40. Runyon BA. Fatal bacterial peritonitis secondary to nonobstructive colonic dilatation (Ogilvie's syndrome) in cirrhotic ascites. J Clin Gastroenterol 1986;8:687.

41. Schweinberg FB, Seligman AM, Fine J. Transmural migration of intestinal bacteria: A study based on the use of radioactive *Escherichia coli*. N Engl J Med 1950;242:47.

42. Runyon BA, Hoefs JC. Ascitic fluid analysis before, during, and after spontaneous bacterial peritonitis. Hepatology 1985;5:257.

43. Runyon BA. Low-protein-concentration ascitic fluid is predisposed to spontaneous bacterial peritonitis. Gastroenterology 1986;91:1343.

44. Runyon BA. Patients with deficient ascitic fluid opsonic activity are predisposed to spontaneous bacterial peritonitis. Hepatology 1988;8:632.

45. Pinzello G, Simonetti RG, Craxi A, et al. Spontaneous bacterial peritonitis: A prospective investigation in predominantly nonalcoholic cirrhotic patients. Hepatology 1983;3:545.

46. Gines P, Arroyo V, Quintero E, et al. Comparison of paracentesis and diuretics in the treatment of cirrhotics with tense ascites: Results of a randomized study. Gastroenterology 1987;93:234.

47. Targan SR, Chow AW, Guze LB. Role of anaerobic bacteria in spontaneous peritonitis of cirrhosis. Am J Med 1977;62:397.

48. Sheckman P, Onderdonk AB, Bartlett JG. Anaerobes in spontaneous peritonitis. Lancet 1977;2:1223.

49. Runyon BA, Canawati HN, Akriviadis EA. Optimization of ascitic fluid culture technique. Gastroenterology 1988;95:1351.

50. Rimola A, Soto R, Borg F, et al. Reticuloendothelial system phagocytic activity in cirrhosis and its relation to bacterial infections and prognosis. Hepatology 1984;4:53.

51. Burroughs AK, Rosenstein IJ, Epstein O, et al. Bacteriuria and primary biliary cirrhosis. Gut 1984;25:133.

52. Runyon BA, Canawati HN, Hoefs JC. Polymicrobial bacterascites: A unique entity in the spectrum of infected ascitic fluid. Arch Intern Med 1986;146:2173.

53. Rimola A, Bory F, Teres J, et al. Oral, nonabsorbable antibiotics prevent infection in cirrhotics with gastrointestinal hemorrhage. Hepatology 1985;5:463.

54. Correia JP, Conn HO. Spontaneous bacterial peritonitis in cirrhosis: Endemic or epidemic. Med Clin North Am 1975;59:963.

55. Hoefs JC, Canawati HN, Sapico FL, et al. Spontaneous bacterial peritonitis. Hepatology 1982;2:399.

56. Conn HO, Fessel JM. Spontaneous bacterial peritonitis in cirrhosis: Variations on a theme. Medicine 1971;50:161.

57. Tito L, Rimola A, Gines P, et al. Recurrence of spontaneous bacterial peritonitis in cirrhosis: Frequency and predictive factors. Hepatology 1988;8:27.

58. Weinstein MP, Iannini PB, Stratton CW, et al. Spontaneous bacterial peritonitis: A review of 28 cases with emphasis on improved survival and factors influencing prognosis. Am J Med 1978;64:592.

59. Gill MA, Kern JW. Altered gentamicin distribution in ascitic patients. Am J Hosp Pharm 1979;36:1704.

60. Papadakis MA, Arieff AI. Unpredictability of clinical evaluation of renal function in cirrhosis: Prospective study. Am J Med 1987;82:945.

61. Cabrera J, Arroyo V, Ballesta AM, et al. Aminoglycoside nephrotoxicity in cirrhosis. Gastroenterology 1982;82:97.
62. Moore RD, Smith CR, Lipsky JJ, et al. Risk factors for nephrotoxicity in patients treated with aminoglycosides. Ann Intern Med 1984;100:352.
63. Moore RD, Smith CR, Lietman PS. Increased risk of renal dysfunction due to interaction of liver disease and aminoglycosides. Am J Med 1986;80:1093.
64. Ariza J, Gudiol F, Dolz C, et al. Evaluation of aztreonam in the treatment of spontaneous bacterial peritonitis in patients with cirrhosis. Hepatology 1986;6:906.
65. Cherubin CE, Marr JS, Sierra MF, et al. Listeria and gram-negative bacillary meningitis. Am J Med 1981;71:199.
66. Felisart J, Rimola A, Arroyo V, et al. Randomized comparative study of efficacy and nephrotoxicity of ampicillin plus tobramycin versus cefotaxime in cirrhotics with severe infections. Hepatology 1985;5:457.
67. Akriviadis EA, Runyon BA. The value of an algorithm in differentiating spontaneous from secondary bacterial peritonitis. Gastroenterology 1990;98:127.
68. Runyon BA, Hoefs JC. Spontaneous vs secondary bacterial peritonitis: Differentiation by response of ascitic fluid neutrophil count to antimicrobial therapy. Arch Intern Med 1986;146:1563.
69. Fong TL, Akriviadis E, Runyon BA, Reynolds TB. Polymorphonuclear cell count response and duration of antibiotic therapy in spontaneous bacterial peritonitis. Hepatology 1989;9:423.
70. Runyon BA. Monomicrobial bacterascites: A potentially lethal variant of spontaneous bacterial peritonitis [Abstract]. Hepatology 1986;6:1140.
71. Runyon BA. The lack of ascitic fluid neutrocytosis in monomicrobial bacterascites is not due to ascitic fluid C5a deficiency [Abstract]. Hepatology 1987;7:1055.
72. Runyon BA, Hoefs JC. Culture-negative neutrocytic ascites: A variant of spontaneous bacterial peritonitis. Hepatology 1984;4:1209.
73. Runyon BA, Umland ET, Merlin T. Inoculation of blood culture bottle with ascitic fluid: Improved detection of spontaneous bacterial peritonitis. Arch Intern Med 1987;147:73.
74. Runyon BA. Spontaneous bacterial peritonitis: An explosion of information. Hepatology 1988;8:171.
75. Runyon BA, Hoefs JC. Ascitic fluid analysis in the differentiation of spontaneous bacterial peritonitis from gastrointestinal tract perforation into ascitic fluid. Hepatology 1984;4:447.
76. Cruikshank DP, Buchsbaum HJ. Effects of rapid paracentesis. JAMA 1973;225:1361.
77. Halpin TF, McCann TO. Dynamics of body fluids following the rapid removal of large volumes of ascites. Am J Obstet Gynecol 1971;110:103.
78. Reynolds TB. Therapeutic paracentesis: Have we come full circle? Gastroenterology 1987;93:386.
79. Guazzi M, Polese A, Magrini F, et al. Negative influences of ascites on the cardiac function of cirrhotic patients. Am J Med 1975;59:165.
80. Belghiti J, Rueff B, Fekete F. Umbilical hernia in cirrhotic patients with ascites [Abstract]. Gastroenterology 1983;84:1363.
81. Runyon BA, Juler GL. Natural history of umbilical hernias in patients with and without ascites. Am J Gastroenterol 1985;80:38.
82. Lemmer JH, Strodel WE, Knol JA. Management of spontaneous umbilical hernia disruption in the cirrhotic patient. Ann Surg 1983;198:30.
83. Mirouze D, Juttner HU, Reynolds TB. Left pleural effusion in patients with chronic liver disease and ascites: Prospective study of 22 cases. Dig Dis Sci 1981;26:984.
84. Lieberman FL, Hidemura R, Peters RL, Reynolds TB. Pathogenesis and treatment of hydrothorax complicating cirrhosis with ascites. Ann Intern Med 1966;64:341.
85. Rubinstein D, McInnes IA, Dudley FJ. Hepatic hydrothorax in the absence of clinical ascites: Diagnosis and management. Gastroenterology 1985;88:188.
86. Runyon BA, Greenblatt M, Ming RHC. Hepatic hydrothorax is a relative contraindication to chest tube insertion. Am J Gastroenterol 1986;81:566.
87. Pockros PJ, Woods S. Malignant ascites from peritoneal carcinomatosis is immobile in comparison to cirrhotic ascites. Hepatology 1988;8:1450.
88. Torisu M, Katano M, Kimura Y, et al. New approach to management of malignant ascites. Surgery 1983;93:357.
89. Howell SB, Pfeifle CE, Olshen RA. Intraperitoneal chemotherapy with melphalan. Ann Intern Med 1984;101:14.
90. Helzberg JH, Greenberger NJ. Peritoneovenous shunt in malignant ascites. Dig Dis Sci 1985;30:1104.
91. Strauss E, DeSa MDFG, Lacet CMC, et al. Standardization of a therapeutic approach for ascites due to chronic liver disease: A prospective study of 100 cases. Hepatology 1987;7:409.
92. Perez-Ayuso RM, Arroyo V, Planas R, et al. Randomized comparative study of efficacy of furosemide vs. spironolactone in nonazotemic cirrhosis with ascites. Gastroenterology 1983;84:961.
93. Pockros PJ, Reynolds TB. Rapid diuresis in patients with ascites from chronic liver disease: The importance of peripheral edema. Gastroenterology 1986;90:1827.
94. Mirouze D, Zipser RD, Reynolds TB. Effect of inhibitors of prostaglandin synthesis on induced diuresis in cirrhosis. Hepatology 1983;3:50.
95. Reynolds TB, Lieberman FL, Goodman AR. Advantages of treatment of ascites without sodium restriction and without complete removal of excess fluid. Gut 1979;19:549.
96. Runyon BA, Van Epps DE. Diuresis of cirrhotic ascites increases its opsonic activity and may help prevent spontaneous bacterial peritonitis. Hepatology 1986;6:396.
97. Franco D, Vons C, Traynor O, et al. Should portosystemic shunt be reconsidered in the treatment of intractable ascites in cirrhosis? Arch Surg 1988;123:987.
98. Parbhoo SP, Ajdukiewicz A, Sherlock S. Treatment of ascites by continuous ultrafiltration and reinfusion of protein concentrate. Lancet 1974.949.
99. Kao HW, Rakov NE, Savage E, et al. The effect of large volume paracentesis on plasma volume—A cause of hypovolemia? Hepatology 1985;5:403.
100. Pinto PC, Amerian J, Reynolds TB. Large-volume paracentesis in nonedematous patients with tense ascites: Its effect on intravascular volume. Hepatology 1988;8:207.
101. Runyon BA, Antillon MR, Montano AA. Effect of diuresis versus therapeutic paracentesis on ascitic fluid opsonic activity and serum complement. Gastroenterology 1989;97:158.
102. LeVeen HH, Christoudias G, Ip M, et al. Peritoneo-venous shunting for ascites. Ann Surg 1974;180:580.
103. Norfray JF, Henry HM, Givens JD, et al. Abdominal complications from peritoneal shunts. Gastroenterology 1979;77:337.
104. Fulenwider JT, Galambos JD, Smith RB, et al. LeVeen vs. Denver peritoneovenous shunts for intractable ascites of cirrhosis. Arch Surg 1986;121:351.
105. Stanley MM, Ochi S, Lee KK, et al. Peritoneovenous shunting as compared with medical treatment in patients with alcoholic cirrhosis and massive ascites. N Engl J Med 1989;321:1632.
106. Salem HH, Dudley FJ, Merrett A, et al. Coagulopathy of peritoneovenous shunts: Studies on the pathogenic role of ascitic fluid collagen and value of antiplatelet therapy. Gut 1983;24:412.
107. Lai KN, Leung JWC, Vallance-Owen J. Dialytic ultrafiltration by hemofilter in the treatment of patients with refractory ascites and renal insufficiency. Am J Gastroenterol 1987;82:665.
108. Runyon BA. Ultrafiltration and peritoneal reinfusion of ascitic fluid. Hepatology 1987;7:415.

44

Skin Lesions Associated with Gastrointestinal Diseases

ELIZABETH F. SHERERTZ
JOSEPH L. JORIZZO

There are many diseases that can involve both the skin and gastrointestinal (GI) tract. Primary disorders of the gut such as inflammatory bowel disease can initially manifest in the skin, and primary skin disorders such as pemphigus vulgaris may present with mucosal lesions. It is important that specialists in both disciplines be aware of how cutaneous lesions may be reflective of gastrointestinal diseases. This chapter reviews the skin lesions that may be associated with specific gastrointestinal-presenting complaints or known pathology. Once a dermatologic lesion or diagnosis is suspected, dermatologic consultation is suggested to assist in diagnosis and management.

INFLAMMATORY BOWEL DISEASE

Chronic nonspecific ulcerative colitis and Crohn's disease, though of unknown etiology, are associated with a host of immunologic abnormalities. Although the role of circulating immune complexes in producing extraintestinal manifestations has been debated (see ch 5, 77, and 107), it is not surprising that a number of reactive inflammatory vascular dermatoses occur in patients with these diseases. We will emphasize dermatoses reported in patients with inflammatory bowel disease.

Erythema—Generalized, Localized, and Annular

The concept of reactive inflammatory vascular dermatoses implies a spectrum of inflammatory blood vessel reactions that occur in association with internal disease.[1] The type of cutaneous lesion ranges from erythema (macular blanchable lesions characterized histologically by simple vasodilation and mild inflammation), through urticarial lesions (raised, peau d'orange lesions with vasodilation, and extravasation of edema fluid), through erythema multiforme (target lesions with purpura that results from extravasation of erythrocytes), to vasculitis (palpable purpuric lesions with histologic leukocytoclasis and fibrinoid necrosis of blood ves-

sel walls). A summary of various types of reactive erythema that may present in patients with GI disease is shown in Table 44-1.

Urticaria and Angioedema

Urticaria is a cutaneous vascular reaction characterized by dermal edema and erythema in which, by definition, individual lesions resolve within 24 hours.[1] Similar lesions occurring in a deep dermal or subcutaneous location are called *angioedema*. These are common conditions affecting up to 20% of people at least once in their lifetime, especially young adults. Urticaria has been well described in patients with inflammatory bowel disease[2]; usually it is drug-induced or due to some cause other than bowel disease. Hereditary or acquired C1 esterase deficiency is associated more with angioedema than urticaria; abdominal pain due to mucosal edema may occur. Chronic urticaria affects primarily middle-aged women and is characterized by the occurrence of daily hives (individual lesions still resolve within 24 hours) for more than 6 weeks. Individual lesions of urticarial vasculitis or a syndrome of urticarial lesions occurring in the setting of a serum sickness–like illness last for more than 24 hours, occur by a different mechanism, and are not, by definition, true urticaria. A skin biopsy should be performed on urticarial lesions that last for more than 24 hours to exclude vasculitis.

The cause of urticaria in an individual patient may be extremely difficult to establish, especially if the patient has chronic urticaria. Several practical approaches have been published.[3] Treatment of urticaria consists of an attempt to both eliminate the cause and relieve signs and symptoms with around-the-clock antihistamine therapy.

Erythema Multiforme

Erythema multiforme is an acute, self-limited, mucocutaneous syndrome characterized by targetoid cutaneous lesions that may be accompanied by serum sickness–like signs and symptoms (e.g., fever, arthralgias).[4] Erythema multiforme minor refers to patients

TABLE 44–1
Erythematous Eruptions in Patients with Gastrointestinal Disease

CLINICAL PATTERN	COMMON ASSOCIATIONS
Generalized Erythema Morbilliform (macules and papules) Scarlatiniform (confluent)	Drug or transfusion reaction; viral exanthem
Palmar Erythema	Nonspecific: oral contraceptive therapy, pregnancy, chronic liver disease, collagen–vascular diseases
Annular Erythema Erythema chronicum migrans single lesion, expanding, ? tick bite	Lyme disease
Erythema annulare centrifugum: multiple lesions, central clearing with rim of scale	Underlying infection; inflammatory disease
Erythema gyratum repens: malignancy, rare, "wood grain" pattern	Occult carcinoma: lung, stomach, esophagus
Urticaria Transient red wheals	Drug, food hypersensitivity; underlying infection; collagen–vascular disease
Erythema Multiforme (EM) EM minor—"target" lesions EM major—mucous membrane	Drug reaction; infections: *Mycoplasma,* herpes simplex, other; underlying inflammatory disease
Erythema Nodosum Tender red nodules on legs and elsewhere	Underlying inflammatory disease (e.g., bowel disease, sarcoid); drug reaction
Localized Erythema Patient with inflammatory bowel disease	Contact dermatitis Cutaneous granulomatous disease (Crohn's)

with a finite number of acrally located typical target lesions who, in general, lack mucosal lesions and other symptoms. Erythema multiforme major refers to patients with more severe disease and mucosal lesions.[4] Stevens–Johnson syndrome is used to describe patients with erythema multiforme who have significant mucosal involvement. Patients with toxic epidermal necrolysis (TEN), which may overlap with severe Stevens–Johnson syndrome, have a burnlike appearance. TEN is usually drug-induced and may be associated with a 30% mortality.

Well-documented causes of acute erythema multiforme include drugs (e.g., sulfonamides, phenytoin, and penicillin), herpes simplex, *Mycoplasma* infections, and other infections (e.g., tuberculosis), as well as a host of underlying diseases.[4] Typical erythema multiforme has been described in patients with inflammatory bowel disease.[2] Complications of erythema multiforme major may affect the gastrointestinal tract and may be severe in TEN. Esophagitis and esophageal stricture have been reported. There is considerable evidence that most cases of recurrent erythema multiforme are induced by recurrent herpes simplex infections.[4]

There is no therapy for erythema multiforme that has been assessed in a double-blind trial. Systemic corticosteroids are often prescribed for adults with erythema multiforme major in whom infection has been excluded. Ophthalmologic consultation for eye involvement and aggressive topical care are required to prevent secondary infection.

Erythema Nodosum

Erythema nodosum is characterized by the occurrence of tender, nonulcerative nodules most often on the legs resulting from inflammation in the subcutaneous fat (Fig 44-1; Color Fig 5). Usually these nodules last from 3 to 6 weeks and affect the anterior lower legs in a symmetrical distribution. Patients may have associated signs and symptoms including fever, malaise, arthritis, and arthralgias.[5]

Erythema nodosum has been well established as an extraintestinal manifestation of ulcerative colitis, Crohn's disease, and infectious colitis, such as from *Yersinia enterocolitica.*[5] The incidence of erythema nodosum in patients with ulcerative colitis was 7% in one large series, but the incidence in Crohn's disease is lower.[5] Other well-documented conditions associated with erythema nodosum include drugs (e.g., estrogen, sulfonamides, phenacetin), infections (e.g., bacterial, viral, fungal, chlamydial, acid-fast, spirochetal), malignancy, and other diseases, including Behçet's disease and sarcoidosis.[5] An immune complex–mediated mechanism

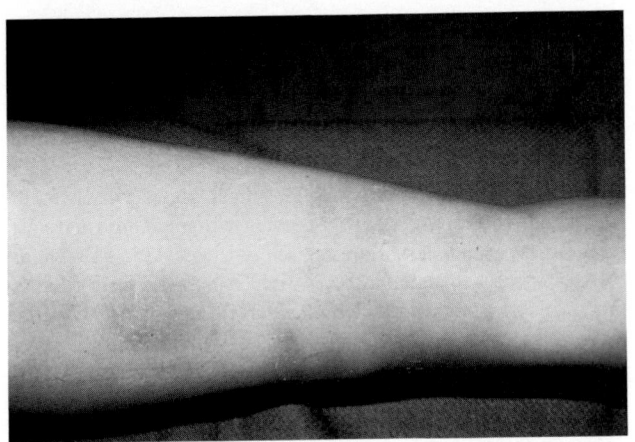

FIGURE 44–1. (See Color Fig 5) Erythema nodosum. These tender nodules occurred in association with ulcerative colitis.

affecting vessels in the septal panniculus has been proposed, although the exact pathogenesis of erythema nodosum remains unknown.

Treatment of erythema nodosum in patients with inflammatory bowel disease is directed at the underlying disease. Nonsteroidal anti-inflammatory drugs or even acetaminophen may alleviate the systemic symptoms.

Necrotizing Vasculitis

Leukocytoclastic vasculitis has been used to describe a form of vasculitis affecting postcapillary venules. We prefer to use that designation as a histopathologic description[6]: endothelial swelling, neutrophilic invasion of blood vessel walls, leukocytoclasia (karyorrhexis of nuclei of neutrophils), extravasation of erythrocytes, and fibrinoid necrosis of blood vessel walls. We prefer the name necrotizing venulitis for this disease process (other designations include Henoch-Schönlein purpura, which is actually a subgroup with IgA-containing immune complexes, allergic angiitis, hypersensitivity angiitis). Larger vessel involvement characterizes polyarteritis nodosa, granulomatous vasculitis (e.g., Wegener's and Churg-Strauss), and giant-cell arteritis. Palpable purpura on dependent sites is the typical cutaneous lesion of necrotizing venulitis.

Necrotizing venulitis has been proposed as a cutaneous model for circulating immune complex (CIC)–mediated vessel damage.[6] CICs deposit in postcapillary venules as a result of triggering factors (especially vasoactive amines). Complement is activated, and complement components (C5a) attract neutrophils, which then release their lysosomal enzymes and other products that mediate innocent bystander fibrinoid necrosis of blood vessel walls. Other organs besides skin (central and peripheral nervous system, synovium, pleura, pericardium, gastrointestinal tract, and kidney[6]) may act as filters for complexes with the similar end result of necrotizing lesions.

As many as 39% to 61% of patients with necrotizing venulitis do not have a precipitating cause that can be identified. Drugs, infections (e.g., hepatitis B, streptococcus), and diseases associated with immune complexes (e.g., collagen vascular diseases, cancers, and chronic active hepatitis) account for most of the identified

associations with necrotizing venulitis. Crohn's disease[7] and ulcerative colitis[8] have both been clearly described in association with necrotizing venulitis and occasionally with granulomatous vasculitis.[9]

Prognosis in all forms of vasculitis depends on the internal organ involvement. Treatment in a patient with vasculitis and inflammatory bowel disease would be directed at the underlying disease. Severe vasculitis might require acute therapy with plasmapheresis and/or high-dose therapy with systemic corticosteroids. Azathioprine or, for larger vessel vasculitis, cyclophosphamide may be important adjuvant therapies. Oral colchicine or sulfone drugs (e.g., dapsone) may be used for primarily cutaneous vasculitis.[6]

Pyoderma Gangrenosum

Pyoderma gangrenosum is a misleading designation for an ulcerating cutaneous disease of unknown cause. Typically fully evolved lesions have a dusky purple, undermined border and heal with cribriform scarring (Fig 44-2; Color Fig 6).[6] Lesions may demonstrate the pathergy phenomenon: the rapid extension of the lesion after trauma.

The diagnosis of pyoderma gangrenosum is a clinical diagnosis of exclusion. Bacterial, fungal, mycobacterial, and other infections, and vasculitis, squamous cell carcinoma, iododerma, bromoderma, and factitial disease must be excluded histologically with appropriate special stains and cultures. Controversy exists as to the exact histology of pyoderma gangrenosum, perhaps because older and/or partially treated lesions are often biopsied.[6] The pathogenesis of pyoderma gangrenosum remains unknown. Theories range from a forme fruste of vasculitis to a cell-mediated reactive process.[6]

More than 50% of patients with typical pyoderma gangrenosum do not have an associated disease. *The association with inflammatory bowel disease, however, is one of the best known associations and should be considered and excluded in every patient with pyoderma gangrenosum.*[10] Other associated conditions include chronic active and chronic persistent hepatitis, polyarthritis including rheumatoid arthritis, and myeloproliferative disorders.

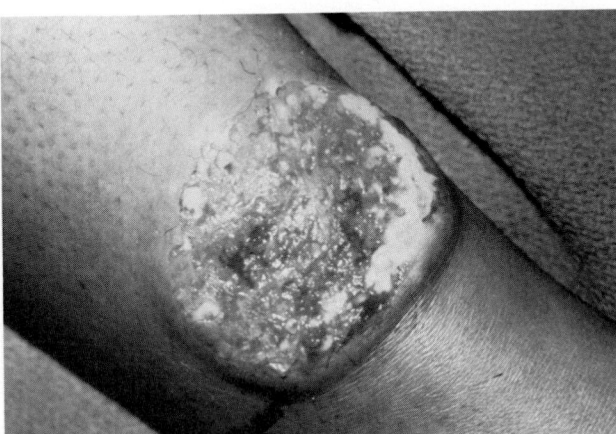

FIGURE 44–2. (See Color Fig 6) Pyoderma gangrenosum in a patient with Crohn's disease.

Aggressive therapy is often required because the disease can spread rapidly and predispose to sepsis or inanition and even death. Systemic corticosteroids in high doses, immunosuppressive agents, and sulfones are the mainstays of treatment.

Oral Manifestations

As many as 30% of patients with ulcerative colitis may have oral lesions including aphthae and angular stomatitis.[2] Specific lesions (i.e., granulomatous) of Crohn's disease may affect the mouth and lips more rarely. The lip lesions may cause confusion with Melkersson-Rosenthal syndrome, a condition in which granulomatous cheilitis can occur in association with facial nerve palsy. Granulomatous oral lesions may show a cobblestone pattern or may be nodular.[11]

Aphthae (canker sores) are nonspecific mucosal lesions that may be the most common oral lesions in patients with inflammatory bowel disease (Fig 44-3; Color Fig 7). Simple aphthae occur in up to 25% of normal individuals. Patients with numerous, almost constant, oral aphthae (complex aphthosis) should be evaluated to exclude inflammatory bowel disease.[12] This issue is discussed further under Behçet's Disease.

Angular cheilitis (perlèche and angular stomatitis) may occur as a manifestation of nutritional deficiency or more commonly as a manifestation of oral candidiasis. Pyostomatitis vegetans is a papular eruption of the oral mucosa that produces a cobblestone and eroded appearance. This distinctive oral disease is associated with Crohn's disease or ulcerative colitis in most patients.[13]

Miscellaneous Skin Lesions in Inflammatory Bowel Disease

Although certain reactive dermatoses occur more commonly in patients with inflammatory bowel disease, and are therefore of greatest relevance to physicians treating patients with diseases of the gastrointestinal tract, many reports exist of single case associations of a given dermatosis with Crohn's disease or ulcerative colitis. Metastatic Crohn's disease, which is the occurrence of

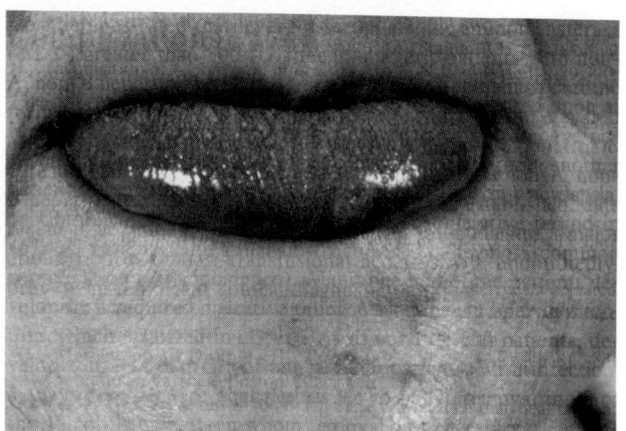

FIGURE 44-3. (See Color Fig 7) Aphthous ulcer involving the tongue in a patient with Behçet's disease.

TABLE 44-2

Some Cutaneous Associations of Crohn's Disease and Ulcerative Colitis

Erythemas (including annular erythemas)
Urticaria
Erythema nodosum
Necrotizing venulitis
Larger vessel necrotizing vasculitis
Pustular vasculitis
Pyoderma gangrenosum
Oral lesions
    Specific granulomas (Crohn's disease only)
    Aphthosis
    Angular cheilitis
    Pyostomatitis vegetans
Metastatic Crohn's disease
Finger clubbing
Acquired acrodermatitis enteropathica (zinc deficiency)
Striae
Epidermolysis bullosa acquisita
Psoriasis
Exfoliative erythroderma
Vitiligo
Lichen nitidus
Lichen planus

noncaseating granulomatous skin lesions remote from the gastrointestinal tract in patients with Crohn's disease, has been well described at a host of cutaneous sites.[14] Lesions are usually ulcers, papules, or nodules. Pustular vasculitis, which can occur with inflammatory bowel bypass syndrome, is discussed under jejunoileal bypass syndrome. Details of other less common associations can be sought in review articles[2,7] and in classic reports of large patient surveys.[15,16] Table 44-2 provides an overview.

RHEUMATOLOGIC DISEASE

Rheumatoid Arthritis and Systemic Lupus Erythematosus (SLE)

A review of skin manifestations of rheumatoid arthritis and SLE is beyond the scope of this review. Gastrointestinal involvement is usually related to vasculitis and is similar to that described above. See Chapters 47 and 106 for the gastrointestinal manifestations of rheumatic diseases.

Dermatomyositis

Dermatomyositis is an idiopathic inflammatory disorder that affects primarily skin and muscle and may manifest gastrointestinal symptoms (see ch 106). The cutaneous lesions are a violaceous poikiloderma (i.e., hyper- and hypopigmentation, telangiectasia, and epidermal atrophy) that occurs over the eyes ("heliotrope sign"), knuckles (Gottron's sign), and extensor surfaces. There is a photosensitivity component to the eruption. Periungual telangiectasia and cuticular dystrophy are also typical. As many as 25% of patients with primary idiopathic polymyositis may have dysphagia due to involvement of striated muscles of the pharynx and esophagus.[17] This may also occur with dermatomyositis. When dermatomyositis or polymyositis occurs as a paraneoplastic syndrome in adults, malignancy of the gastrointestinal tract is one of the most common culprits. *The evaluation of the adult patient with dermatomyositis or polymyositis should include an evaluation for occult malignancy.* Studies have suggested a complete history, physical examination, breast and pelvic examination in women, prostate examination in men, rectal examination, and screening laboratory tests as well as a chest x-ray. Pap smear and mammography are added for female patients.[18]

Scleroderma

Scleroderma is a cutaneous or multisystem disease of unknown etiology. A localized cutaneous form (morphea) is characterized by plaque, gyrate, generalized, or linear dermal sclerosis. The systemic form occurs as a CREST (calcinosis, Raynaud's phenomenon, esophageal dysmotility, sclerodactyly, and telangiectasia) variant or as progressive systemic sclerosis. These variants can be considered as overlapping ends of a continuum.[19]

The majority of patients with systemic scleroderma have the CREST variant. Although patients with CREST can become critically ill with any of the varied manifestations of systemic scleroderma, they generally are middle-aged or older women who have a chronic course and die with, not from, their disease. Calcium deposits occur primarily over joints late in the disease. Raynaud's phenomenon is associated with sequelae of this vasospasm that varies from "rat bite" trophic lesions on the fingertips to multiple sites of peripheral gangrene. Esophageal reflux should be treated to reduce esophageal fibrosis. Sclerosis occurs acrally, periorally, and can affect the trunk. A "salt and pepper" postinflammatory pigment change is particularly noticeable over sclerotic areas in darker-skinned patients. Telangiectasias are described as being "boxlike" or "matlike" and occur on the hands, face, and oral mucosa as well as on other sites.

The progressive systemic sclerosis type of systemic scleroderma occurs with an explosive onset. The dermal sclerosis is dramatic and is often truncal in onset with spread to the face and extremities. Postinflammatory pigment change is common, but CREST features are often absent or present to a lesser degree. The systemic and gastrointestinal features of scleroderma are discussed in Chapters 54, 67, 81, and 106.

Behçet's Disease

Behçet's disease is a complex multisystem disease first described by and named after a Turkish dermatologist.[6] Because there is no pathognomonic laboratory test for the diagnosis, several sets of diagnostic criteria have been proposed, including the modified O'Duffy criteria. Patients without inflammatory bowel disease or collagen vascular disease must have oral aphthosis (canker sores) plus at least two of the following: genital aphthae, synovitis, posterior uveitis, cutaneous pustular vasculitis, and meningoencephalitis.[20,21] The exclusion of patients with inflammatory bowel disease is crucial because patients with bowel disease may have recurrent aphthosis and (especially in patients with HLA-B27) may have an enteropathic arthritis syndrome. These patients are best considered as having the Reiter's disease/HLA-B27 spectrum of diseases rather than Behçet's disease.[22]

The oral lesions in Behçet's disease are aphthae, which can easily be distinguished from the psoriasiform oral lesions of Reiter's disease.[22] Genital aphthae resemble oral aphthae (Fig 44-4; Color Fig 8). Recurrent herpes simplex must be excluded by culture and/or by immunoperoxidase study of biopsy material. Cutaneous pustular vasculitis lesions show either leukocytoclastic vasculitis or a neutrophilic vascular reaction histologically.[23] Erythema nodosum–like lesions have also been described, as have pyoderma gangrenosum–like lesions.

A number of ocular changes have been described in these patients, although only posterior uveitis (i.e., retinal vasculitis) is an accepted diagnostic criterion. The synovitis produces an asymmetric, migratory, nonerosive, oligoarthritis. A host of diffuse or focal, central or peripheral neurologic manifestations have been reported, but only meningoencephalitis is a diagnostic criterion. Vascular involvement such as aneurysms, arterial occlusions, venous occlusions, and varices may occur, and they can prove fatal. The principal gastrointestinal manifestations are aphthae, which can occur at any gastrointestinal site (note that inflammatory bowel disease–like changes have been described, but these may be HLA-B27–positive patients with a Reiter's-like illness and aphthae).

Bowel-Associated Dermatosis– Arthritis Syndrome

Approximately 20% of patients develop a characteristic syndrome after jejunoileal bypass surgery[24] that includes pustular vasculitic cutaneous lesions, arthritis, and serum sickness–like features. Clinically and histopathologically, the skin lesions resemble the pustular vasculitis lesions seen in Behçet's disease. We expanded

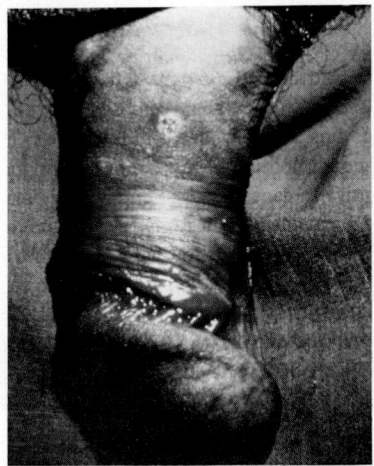

FIGURE 44–4. (See Color Fig 8) Behçet's disease. Note the early genital aphtha showing features of pustular vasculitis.

the concept to include patients who have not had bypass surgery but who had either inflammatory bowel disease or the occurrence of a blind loop after Billroth II surgery.[25]

The cutaneous lesions occur in crops with each episode lasting from 1 to 2 weeks and occurring at one to several-month intervals (Fig 44-5; Color Fig 9). Erythema nodosum–like lesions may occur. Fever, myalgias, chills, flulike symptoms, gastrointestinal upset, and arthralgias or nonerosive arthritis are often associated. Circulating immune complexes, perhaps containing bacterial peptidoglycans as antigens, have been postulated to mediate this syndrome.[24] Serum enhancement of neutrophil migration may also mediate the neutrophilic cutaneous lesions.[26]

The bowel bypass syndrome can be cured by restoration of normal bowel anatomy (see ch 74). Treatment of the underlying disease is necessary to control the syndrome when it occurs in patients with inflammatory bowel disease. Systemic antibiotic therapy with metronidazole, tetracycline, or erythromycin has proved beneficial in controlling cutaneous and systemic manifestations of this syndrome. It is unclear whether the effect is on reducing bacterial overgrowth or whether there is a more direct effect (e.g., on neutrophil function). Systemic corticosteroid therapy and oral dapsone are also effective therapies.[6]

Amyloidosis

Amyloidosis is a designation for a group of syndromes characterized by the extracellular deposition of an abnormal protein with certain staining properties and electron microscope features. Primary (AL) amyloidosis, also called light chain derived systemic amyloidosis,[27] often occurs in patients with multiple myeloma. Macroglossia occurs, as do specific dermal infiltrates presenting as cutaneous papules, plaques, and nodules with "pinch purpura" (Fig 44-6; Color Fig 10). Patients with primary (AL) amyloid have frequent gastrointestinal infiltrates as well as cardiac, renal, and other multisystem involvement. Skin biopsy of a cutaneous lesion in primary (AL) amyloid is virtually diagnostic of the disease.

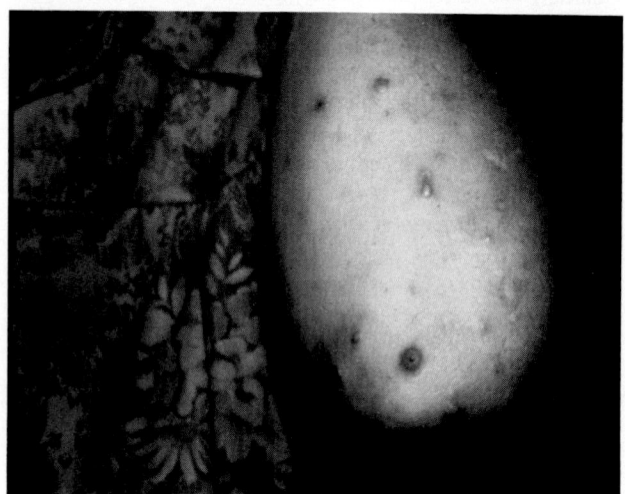

FIGURE 44–5. (See Color Fig 9) Bowel-associated dermatosis–arthritis syndrome. Pustular vasculitis lesions in a patient with a blind loop after Billroth II surgery.

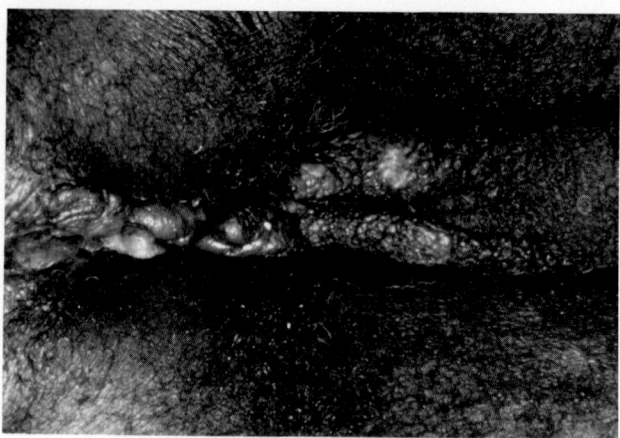

FIGURE 44–6. (See Color Fig 10) Amyloidosis. Note the perirectal amyloid nodules in this patient with multiple myeloma.

Patients with secondary (AA) amyloidosis do not have cutaneous involvement.[28] This pattern is associated with underlying disease such as chronic inflammatory bowel disease, tuberculosis, leprosy, chronic osteomyelitis, familial Mediterranean fever, or other diseases. Biopsy of normal skin may reveal amyloid deposits in less than one third of patients, whereas small bowel or colonic mucosal biopsies are positive in over 75% to 85% of patients.

SKIN DISEASE AND GI BLEEDING

Vascular Abnormalities

OSLER-WEBER-RENDU DISEASE (HEREDITARY HEMORRHAGIC TELANGIECTASIA)

This autosomal dominant trait is characterized by telangiectasias, aneurysms, and arteriovenous malformations that can affect mucocutaneous areas as well as internal organs.[29] The mucocutaneous hallmark for the syndrome is 1- to 3-mm telangiectatic mats resembling those seen in patients with scleroderma (Fig 44-7; Color Fig 11). These lesions may affect the lips and tongue, face, hands, chest, and feet[29] (ch 108).

Patients become symptomatic in childhood with epistaxis (80% of patients) and as adults with gastrointestinal hemorrhage.[29] Gastrointestinal bleeding may come from telangiectasias, aneurysms, or arteriovenous malformations and may require endoscopy for diagnosis because they are not detectable radiographically. Vascular abnormalities such as arteriovenous fistulae may also affect the liver, lungs, central nervous system, and retina (telangiectasias). Treatment has been reviewed in Chapter 108.

BLUE RUBBER BLEB NEVUS SYNDROME

Blue rubber bleb nevus syndrome is a rare autosomal dominant condition first described in the last century but named in 1958.[30]

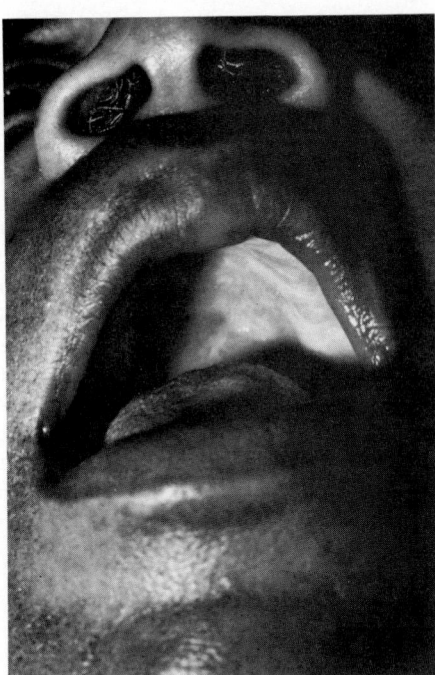

FIGURE 44–7. (See Color Fig 11) Typical telangiectasia of Osler-Weber-Rendu disease.

The cutaneous lesions are blue-colored, subcutaneous, rubbery, compressible, sometimes painful nodular vascular malformations that may be up to 10 cm in diameter. These vascular malformations are not true hemangiomas. They occur in the small intestine or colon but have also been reported to occur in the oropharynx, nasopharynx, esophagus, stomach, peritoneal cavity, mesentery, liver, lung, glans penis, eye, and central nervous system.[31] Gastrointestinal bleeding and intussusception may occur (ch 108).

KAPOSI'S SARCOMA

Most recent publications regarding Kaposi's sarcoma have focused on the epidemic form of the disease, which is associated with acquired immunodeficiency syndrome (AIDS)[32] (see ch 103). An endemic form has been long recognized in Africa, and the third variant is the classical type, which occurs primarily in individuals of Mediterranean ancestry.

The tumor in all groups is derived from proliferating endothelial cells, which are supported by the presence of Factor VIII–related antigen and other endothelium-associated antigens in the atypical cells. The cutaneous lesions vary from reddish purple macules to large vascular tumors. In the slowly progressive classical form of the disease, lesions begin on the feet or lower legs of the affected patients (who are typically elderly men) and extend proximally, becoming associated with severe peripheral edema. The most common site of internal involvement, but usually not a prominent feature, is the gastrointestinal tract. The small intestine, stomach, esophagus, and colon are the sites affected in order of decreasing frequency of involvement.[33] Extensive hemorrhage or partial bowel obstruction can occur. Other organs that may be affected include lymph nodes, larynx, spleen, liver, lungs, and other organs. The majority of the patients with the classical form of the disease die

with, and not from, their disease. In contrast, the Kaposi's sarcoma associated with AIDS is far more aggressive clinically (see ch 103). Gastrointestinal involvement in Kaposi's sarcoma occurring in the setting of immunosuppression associated with AIDS can be prominent and widespread.

Treatment may not be required for the patient with classic Kaposi's sarcoma that is localized. Local radiation therapy and intralesional chemotherapy (e.g., vinblastine) are commonly used therapies for more severe localized classical disease. Kaposi's sarcoma in AIDS patients has proved to be extremely refractory to therapy.

MALIGNANT ATROPHIC PAPULOSIS (DEGOS' DISEASE)

Malignant atrophic papulosis (Degos' disease) is a very rare, idiopathic, usually lethal disease with characteristic lesions that affect the skin, gastrointestinal tract, and central nervous system.[34] The cutaneous lesions are discrete, painless papules with umbilicated porcelain-white centers surrounded by telangiectatic rims. Histologically these lesions reveal an atrophic epidermis with a wedge-shaped dermal scar that is broader at the top than at the bottom.[35]

It is believed that most patients eventually develop visceral involvement. Gastrointestinal involvement may lead to massive gastrointestinal bleeding and to death (ch 108). The histopathology of gastrointestinal and central nervous system lesions is similar to that of cutaneous lesions. Current evidence is against an immunopathogenesis of this disease.[35] An endothelial defect with a secondary coagulation abnormality may be involved. There is no effective therapy. Patients who develop visceral involvement often have a fatal outcome.

Diseases of Connective Tissue

PSEUDOXANTHOMA ELASTICUM

Pseudoxanthoma elasticum (PXE) is a genetic disorder characterized by cutaneous and visceral manifestations that result from alterations to elastic fibers. Four genetic subtypes have been described, which include both autosomal recessive and dominant inheritance.[36] These types may have a variety of ocular, cardiovascular, and gastrointestinal manifestations.

The cutaneous lesions consist of yellow papules and plaques that produce a "chicken skin" appearance (Fig 44-8; Color Fig 12). These lesions begin early in life and may progress. They affect the neck, axillae, and possibly other flexures. The buccal mucosa may be affected. Histologically, lesions show calcification of mid-dermal elastic fibers. Angioid streaks are the characteristic retinal finding in patients affected with PXE but are not specific. The entire cardiovascular system is at risk for vascular calcification.

Gastrointestinal involvement may present with upper or lower gastrointestinal hemorrhage (ch 108). Endoscopy reveals the characteristic yellow cobblestone changes in the bowel. Bleeding is usually recurrent. The pathogenesis remains unknown. The treatment is aimed at complications, but no therapy exists to alter

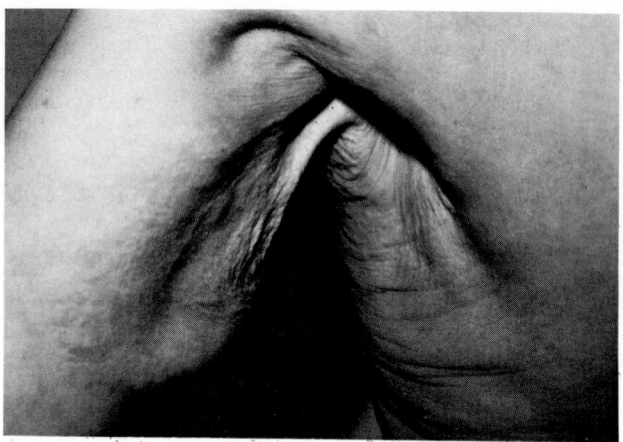

FIGURE 44–8. (See Color Fig 12) Pseudoxanthoma elasticum. Note the "chicken skin" appearance of the axillary skin.

the connective tissue abnormality. Prognosis depends on the subtype of disease.

EHLERS-DANLOS SYNDROME

Ehlers-Danlos syndrome is a heterogenous group of genetically inherited syndromes characterized by defective collagen. More than 10 distinct subtypes exist with various autosomal or X-linked inheritance patterns and with diverse abnormalities of collagen production ranging from lysyl oxidase deficiency to crosslinking abnormalities.[37]

The skin may be both hyperextensible and fragile. Wound healing is delayed and may produce "cigarette paper"–thin scars or "fish mouth" scars as well as pseudotumors over joints. Purpura due to easy bruising is a prominent feature in some subtypes of Ehlers-Danlos syndrome. Hyperextensibility of joints is a prominent feature of Ehlers-Danlos syndrome.

Visceral involvement is varied. Ocular and dental abnormalities are common. Large arteries may be affected by abnormal collagen, and rupture may occur, especially during pregnancy. Gastrointestinal perforation is prevalent in patients with type IV Ehlers-Danlos syndrome who have defective type III collagen and translucent skin with numerous ecchymoses. In addition to bowel perforation and gastrointestinal bleeding, these patients have a predisposition toward rupture of blood vessels, and therefore the prognosis is particularly grave[38] (ch 108).

CUTIS LAXA (GENERALIZED ELASTOLYSIS)

Cutis laxa is a heterogeneous group of disorders characterized by abnormalities primarily of elastic fibers. Various forms of autosomal and X-linked inheritance have been described, and an acquired form exists.[39] The skin appears to be "too large for the body." It sags and has a wrinkled, aged appearance. Gastrointestinal diverticula and hernias occur.[39] The genitourinary tract may also be affected. Progressive pulmonary involvement may lead to chronic obstructive pulmonary disease and cor pulmonale.

Typical "corkscrew" blood vessels are seen on arteriography. Various abnormalities, including deficient copper metabolism and reduced lysyl oxidase activity, have been described. Collagen fibers as well as elastic fibers may be abnormal. Pulmonary disease is not a rare cause of premature death in these patients.

NEUROFIBROMATOSIS (VON RECKLINGHAUSEN'S DISEASE)

A detailed discussion of neurofibromatosis is clearly beyond the scope of this chapter. This condition is inherited in an autosomal dominant fashion. Cutaneous features such as café-au-lait macules, axillary freckles, and cutaneous neurofibromas are hallmarks of this disease. Neurofibromas may occur throughout the gastrointestinal tract, and they affect 25% of patients.[40] The tongue, gallbladder, stomach, and jejunum are more commonly affected than the esophagus or colon. Ulceration, bleeding, volvulus, obstruction, perforation, and intussusception may occur. Malignant transformation of neurofibromas in the gut is not common, but it is well reported. Surgery is often required for symptomatic gastrointestinal involvement.

SYNDROMES ASSOCIATED WITH GASTROINTESTINAL POLYPS

Gardner's Syndrome (Familial Adenomatous Polyposis)

In 1953, Gardner refined his description of a dominantly inherited triad of osteomas, epidermoid cysts, and colorectal polyposis that predisposed to colonic adenocarcinoma.[41] Gardner's syndrome may occur as part of a spectrum that includes familial polyposis coli (no extracolonic lesions), Gardner's syndrome, and Turcot syndrome (features of Gardner's syndrome plus central nervous system neoplasms)[42] (see ch 79).

Patients with Gardner's syndrome develop multiple epidermoid cysts in their early teenage years. They occur in a generalized distribution especially on the scalp, face, and extremities[43] (Fig 44-9; Color Fig 13). Desmoid tumors, which represent locally aggressive but nonmetastasizing tumors of fibrous tissue, are associated with the syndrome and often affect the abdominal wall. Osteomas are benign osseous tumors that affect membranous bone. These lesions are often detectable by x-rays of the mandible or maxilla. Additional features that may be seen in a smaller number of patients with Gardner's syndrome include: dental abnormalities (congenitally absent teeth, extra teeth, and other developmental abnormalities of dentition), retinal abnormalities (pigmented truncal lesions), endocrine tumors (e.g., thyroid carcinoma), and hepatoblastoma.[44] When a diagnosis of Gardner's syndrome is suspected, ophthalmologic consultation, bone x-rays (including jaw x-rays), and endoscopy, sigmoidoscopy, and colonoscopy are required. Even after prophylactic colectomy, the rectal mucosal remnant, stomach, and duodenum must be monitored regularly.

Peutz–Jeghers Syndrome

Peutz and later Jeghers described a condition with an autosomal dominant inheritance pattern characterized by small intestinal ha-

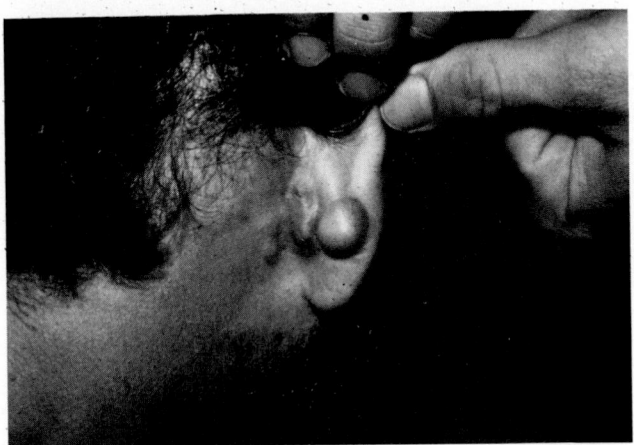

FIGURE 44-9. (See Color Fig 13) Gardner's syndrome. Note the typical epidermal inclusion cyst. This patient had multiple other cystic nodules, particularly on the scalp.

martomatous polyps and hyperpigmented macules of the lips.[45] Although most polyps occur in the jejunum, they also occur in the ileum, stomach, duodenum, and colon (ch 79). Lesions are present in childhood and may predispose to intussusception or to gastrointestinal bleeding.

The melanotic macules of Peutz-Jeghers syndrome begin in infancy. They affect the lips most commonly but may also affect the palms, soles, digits, periorbital skin, anus, and buccal mucosa. They histologically resemble ephelides (freckles). All except the buccal lesions fade with age.[46]

There is debate about the risk of gastrointestinal malignancy in patients with Peutz–Jeghers syndrome. Unusual bowel, ovarian, cervical, and testicular tumors, as well as breast cancers, have been reported in these patients.

Cronkhite-Canada Syndrome

The Cronkhite-Canada syndrome is a sporadically occurring disorder. Affected adults may develop the tetrad of cutaneous hyperpigmentation, alopecia, onychodystrophy, and intestinal polyposis.[47] The gastrointestinal signs and symptoms (e.g., diarrhea, abdominal pain, weight loss, and anorexia) often precede the onset of the hair, nail, and cutaneous manifestations by several months (see ch 79).

The predominating cutaneous lesions are macular hyperpigmented macules that coalesce to form plaques that are distributed primarily on the upper extremities but that may occur on most cutaneous sites.[44] Vitiligo occasionally may occur. Onycholysis, onychoschizia, and/or onychomadesis may affect all 20 nails. Widespread alopecia is nonscarring and may resemble alopecia areata.[44] The tongue may be fissured.

Cowden's Disease

Cowden's disease, also called multiple hamartoma syndrome, is inherited in an autosomal dominant fashion. Mucocutaneous markers for the syndrome include facial and oral mucosal papules

that histologically represent tricholemmomas (benign hair-derived tumors).[48] The oral lesions produce a cobblestone appearance. A "scrotal tongue" is often associated. Acral keratoses resemble acrokeratosis verruciformis.[44] Patients may also have lipomas, hemangiomas, neuromas, and café-au-lait macules.

Gastrointestinal hamartomatous polyps occur throughout the gastrointestinal tract, with the majority affecting the rectum and sigmoid colon. The polyps are not premalignant; however, up to one third of patients with Cowden's disease develop a malignancy, usually of breast or thyroid.[48]

Muir-Torre Syndrome

Muir and Torre each reported the association of sebaceous neoplasms and multiple visceral carcinomas.[49,50] The inheritance pattern is autosomal dominant. Cutaneous markers for the syndrome include sebaceous neoplasms (hyperplasia, adenoma, epithelioma, and carcinoma), basal cell carcinomas, and keratoacanthomas.[44]

Adenomatous colonic polyps are not a universal feature of the syndrome, but up to one half or more of these patients do have polyps. Malignancies that occur with the syndrome are usually colonic adenocarcinomas. Urogenital, hematologic, breast, and other malignancies may occur.[51] Patients should be screened for colonic polyps. If these are present, the patients must be screened frequently for colonic carcinoma and other malignancies.

Acrochordons and Colonic Polyps

In 1982, Klein and associates reported an increased incidence of acrochordons (skin tags) in patients with acromegaly observed for colonic polyps.[52] This same investigative group, after studying additional patients, reported that patients with more than six acrochordons might be targeted for evaluation for colonic polyps.[53] Several subsequent studies in patients who were referred for colonoscopy confirmed the correlation between acrochordons and colonic polyps. A prospective study in patients with no bowel disease also gave similar results.[54] In a recent autopsy study in which colonic polyps were assessed histologically, no correlation was noted between acrochordons and colonic polyps.[55] Obviously, additional prospective studies are required.

CUTANEOUS SIGNS OF GASTROINTESTINAL MALIGNANCY

Metastases and Direct Extension

Metastatic nodules of gastrointestinal adenocarcinoma are usually firm, pink dermal to subcutaneous masses and are most likely to occur on the abdomen or pelvic area. The primary lesion has usually already been diagnosed when metastases develop. The clinical presentation of an indurated nodule of the umbilicus, the so-called Sister Mary Joseph's nodule, may be the initial presentation of an underlying (usually advanced) abdominal malignancy, most commonly adenocarcinoma of the stomach or large bowel. Biopsy of such a lesion helps to diagnose the primary site in less than 50%.[56] Rarely, direct involvement of the lymphatics in the abdominal or thigh region draining a primary site can lead to extensive dermal infiltration, presenting as a sclerotic plaque. Occasionally, such a plaque can be quite erythematous and mimic cellulitis (carcinoma erysipeloides).

Cutaneous Lesions That Should Raise Suspicion of Possible Gastrointestinal Malignancy

Extramammary Paget's disease is a rare dermatosis of insidious onset, presenting as an erythematous scaling or lichenified patch, often with surface erosion or crusting. The site has usually been treated with topical corticosteroids and/or antifungals without response, and the diagnosis is made by clinical suspicion and skin biopsy. Extramammary Paget's disease is considered to be a cutaneous adenocarcinoma, probably of apocrine gland origin.[57] When it occurs in the perianal area, it should raise suspicion of a possible underlying rectal or cloacogenic carcinoma[58] (see ch 85). The frequency of underlying visceral carcinoma is reportedly up to 86%, though a more recent review showed that only 25% of perianal Paget's disease cases had a concurrent carcinoma of rectal origin.[58] Treatment of the Paget's disease is usually surgery (Mohs micrographic or wide excision) or radiation therapy. Frequent recurrences in the skin occur after either technique.

Acanthosis nigricans presents as a smooth, thickened, and dark appearance to the skin in body fold areas, most often in the axilla and around the neck (Fig 44-10; Color Fig 14). When more extensive, it may lead to a striking appearance, with thickening of the palms and soles and oral lesions of hyperkeratosis. Acrochordons (or skin tags) may also occur in affected sites. This clinical presentation is nonspecific and is most often seen without malignancy in obese patients in certain insulin-resistant diabetes syndromes, as a familial trait, and with certain medications.

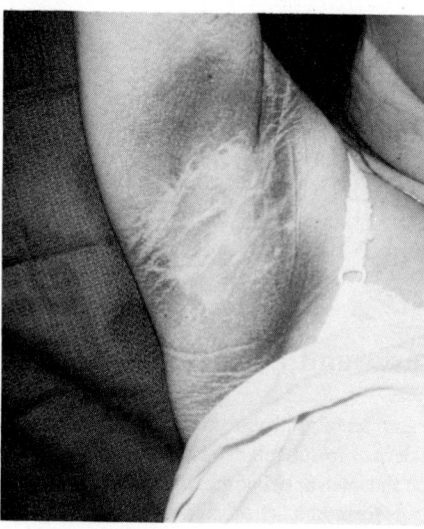

FIGURE 44–10. (See Color Fig 14) Acanthosis nigricans in a nonobese adult patient.

Suspicion for malignancy-associated acanthosis nigricans should arise when it occurs with recent onset in a nonobese patient who does not have diabetes. Biopsy of the skin is not helpful. Attention should be focused on the possibility of gastric adenocarcinoma, although other intra-abdominal and pelvic sites should also be evaluated for possible malignancy.[59,60] The malignancy appears concomitantly in 61% of patients, but in almost 20% the acanthosis nigricans may precede the diagnosable tumor by years. In these patients, frequent surveillance is necessary. In a patient known to have had an abdominal adenocarcinoma who then develops acanthosis nigricans, a vigorous search for recurrence or metastatic disease should be undertaken. The mechanism of malignant acanthosis nigricans is thought to be related to peptide growth factors released by the tumor.[61] Remission of the skin lesions occurs with removal of the tumor. There is not a good dermatologic/cosmetic treatment for acanthosis nigricans.

Keratoderma of the palms and soles (tylosis) is a nonspecific presentation of diffuse or punctate yellow hyperkeratosis of the palmar and plantar surfaces. There are multiple causes, and it is only in patients with long-standing skin lesions and a family history of cancer that the question of gastrointestinal malignancy should be raised. The strongest association has been with esophageal squamous cell carcinoma, and it may occur in an autosomal dominant pattern with up to 95% of family members developing esophageal carcinoma by age 65 (the Howell-Evans Syndrome)[62] (ch 57). In such kindreds, regular evaluations with barium swallow and esophagoscopy are warranted.[63] Other kindreds have been described with punctate keratodermas and carcinoma of the colon or pancreas. There are individual case reports of tylosis occurring in association with esophageal or bronchial carcinoma without a family history. In most of those cases, the palmar–plantar thickening was of recent onset without any other skin disease. The diagnosis of malignancy was usually apparent at the time of initial presentation and evaluation.

Generalized erythroderma is a nonspecific cutaneous reaction pattern with a large differential diagnosis of possible causes, including primary skin diseases, adverse drug reaction, or internal malignancy (especially lymphoma). The possibility of esophageal or other occult carcinoma should be raised in an erythrodermic patient with compatible symptoms.[64] *Hypertrichosis lanuginosa acquisita* refers to the sudden development of diffuse, fine, downy hair on the face and trunk. It is extremely rare but is strongly associated with internal malignancy. It has been seen most often with carcinoma of the lung or colon, but other gastrointestinal malignancy, including involvement of the pancreas and gallbladder, has been seen in such patients.[65]

Dyskeratosis congenita is a rare congenital, usually X-linked, genetic disorder with prominent mucocutaneous features. Reticulate skin pigmentation, dystrophic nails, and mucous membrane leukoplakia are hallmarks of the syndrome. Onset of skin lesions occurs in childhood, and patients often develop pancytopenia, which occasionally is a Fanconi-type anemia. Carcinoma may develop in areas of mucosal leukoplakia.[66]

Patients with the *Paterson-Brown-Kelly-Plummer-Vinson syndrome* present with mucocutaneous findings of brittle, spoon-shaped (koilonychia) nails, atrophic tongue, and angular stomatitis (ch 53). Dysphagia and iron deficiency complete the syndrome, with a carcinoma of the postcricoid area of the esophagus occasionally occurring in long-standing cases.[67]

Flushing episodes may be the presenting sign of *carcinoid syn-*

drome, which has been seen primarily with carcinoid tumors of the small intestine and liver metastases. The flushing is a bright red color on the face and upper chest, occasionally involving the entire trunk and extremities. Each episode lasts from 10 to 30 minutes, and after repeated episodes, permanent rosacealike telangiectasia and edema develop. Episodes may be provoked by food intake, alcohol, and emotional stress, among other factors. The mechanism of the flushing is related to contributions by various vasoactive and neuropeptides, as discussed in more detail in Chapter 70. The best current treatment for carcinoid flush is somatostatin analogue, which is effective in up to 90% of cases.[68] Similar flushing episodes can occur in patients with multiple endocrine neoplasia. Pellagralike skin lesions or cutaneous metastases have rarely been reported in patients with carcinoid tumors.

Necrolytic migratory erythema is the specific descriptive term for the cutaneous lesions of the glucagonoma syndrome, which occurs with a glucagon-secreting islet cell tumor of the pancreas (ch 91). The cutaneous eruption typically affects perioral, lower abdominal, and perineal sites with a configurative erythema, erosions, and superficial necrosis and scale. The clinical resemblance to zinc deficiency is notable. Patients often have angular cheilitis and a red, swollen tongue. Clinical presentation is more important than skin biopsy in making the diagnosis.[69] Skin lesions may respond to intravenous supplementation of amino acids, somatostatin or its analogue, or treatment of the underlying tumor.[70,71] Necrolytic migratory erythema has occasionally been reported in the absence of a pancreatic tumor, but a vigorous search for a tumor is needed when typical skin lesions occur in a patient with other suggestive symptoms, such as glucose intolerance, weight loss, psychologic changes, and/or anemia.

BULLOUS DISEASES OF THE SKIN THAT CAN DIRECTLY AFFECT THE GASTROINTESTINAL TRACT

Epidermolysis Bullosa (EB)

Epidermolysis bullosa is a spectrum of inherited mechanobullous diseases in which blisters occur spontaneously or at sites of friction or trauma. Classification of clinical subtypes of EB has been based on inheritance patterns and presence or absence of scarring, and more recently it has been based upon the electron microscopically determined level of the blistering. Both dominant and recessive forms of dystrophic EB occur. Onset of skin lesions occurs at birth or shortly after, and a dermatologic diagnosis of EB will usually have been made before a patient presents to a gastroenterologist. Rarely, pyloric atresia has been found in infants with junctional or recessive dystrophic EB, apparently resulting from mucosal blistering and scarring in utero. The major sites of gastrointestinal involvement, most often occurring in the recessive dystrophic form, are the oral cavity, esophagus, and anal areas[72,73] (see ch 58). In the mouth, recurring blisters lead to scarring and smooth tongue surface, restricted tongue movement, and restricted oral opening. Ability to chew, swallow, and speak is compromised. Patients with the scarring forms of EB may have dysplastic teeth and poor enamel.

Esophageal lesions may become symptomatic anytime in the first three decades of life. Dysphagia is the most common symptom and may reflect the presence of esophageal bullae or weblike scarring, which cause partial or total obstruction. Most such lesions occur in the cervical esophagus near the cricopharyngeal area. Anal involvement, with bullae and subsequent scarring, may lead to constipation. Lesions in this location are also prone to severe secondary infection. Nutritional deficiency is common in severe EB. The gastrointestinal aspects of this disease are covered more completely in Chapter 58.

Epidermolysis bullosa acquisita is an uncommon late-onset blistering disease associated with skin blistering and scarring at trauma sites.[74] It has a distinct immunohistologic pattern on immunofluorescence microscopy of skin biopsy tissue. There is no family history of EB in these patients. EB acquisita has been occasionally reported to cause extensive, scarring oral and esophageal lesions. It has occurred in association with inflammatory bowel disease.

Pemphigus Vulgaris

Pemphigus vulgaris is an immunologic blistering disease that commonly presents with oral erosions prior to the onset of cutaneous lesions. Skin or mucosal biopsy findings of an acantholytic blister and direct and indirect immunofluorescence microscopic evidence of IgG in the intraepidermal space confirm the diagnosis. Symptomatic esophageal involvement is rare.[75] Epigastric pain in a pemphigus patient being treated with systemic corticosteroids should raise the possibility of esophageal lesions, and endoscopy is indicated. Pemphigus involving the lower gastrointestinal tract can present with hemorrhage.[76]

Bullous Pemphigoid

Bullous pemphigoid is another immunologic blistering disease in which older patients present with tense bullae. Biopsied lesion skin shows a subepidermal blister, and IgG is found in the basement membrane zone in a linear pattern on direct and indirect immunofluorescence microscopy. Mucosal involvement is less common in bullous pemphigoid than in pemphigus, occurring in the mouth in about one third of pemphigoid patients. Esophageal or anal lesions rarely occur in patients with bullous pemphigoid, or in the variant known as cicatricial (mucous membrane) pemphigoid.[77] There have been case reports of bullous pemphigoid occurring coincident with gastrointestinal malignancy, particularly carcinoma of the colon.

Toxic Epidermal Necrolysis

Toxic epidermal necrolysis (TEN) is a severe mucocutaneous reaction most frequently associated with a drug reaction. It is sometimes considered to be the most severe expression of erythema multiforme. Patients with TEN present with a rapidly progressing toxic erythema that develops large bullae and widespread epidermal erosions. Gastrointestinal tract involvement can occur at any level, and the patient with this involvement most often presents with hemorrhage. Treatment is supportive with burn unit management for severe cases. Mortality is high (25%–50%) in drug-induced cases.

SKIN CONDITIONS ASSOCIATED WITH ABDOMINAL PAIN

Porphyrias

Variegate porphyria is the most likely porphyria in which patients present with skin lesions and episodic abdominal pain. The typical skin lesions (the same as are seen in porphyria cutanea tarda) are noninflamed blisters and erosions at sun-exposed sites, particularly the backs of the hands. Scarring with milia formation, hyperpigmentation, facial hypertrichosis, and sclerosis may occur. Photoprotection is of minimal benefit because the patients are exquisitely sensitive to light, and avoidance of inducing drugs is important. Hereditary coproporphyria is even more rare but may also have photosensitivity as a component.

Fabry's Disease

The skin lesions in *Fabry's disease*, a rare lysosomal storage disease, are punctate, 1-mm, red to blue angiokeratomas that do not blanch. They are most densely distributed from the mid-abdomen to the knees. Lesions have their onset from childhood to adolescence. Decreased or absent sweating may also occur. The gastrointestinal manifestations of this disease are covered in Chapter 106.

Mastocytosis

This is an uncommon disorder of mast cell proliferation. The most common skin lesions are *urticaria pigmentosa*, with childhood onset. These are usually reddish brown macules, but solitary nodules may occur. Upon stroking, these lesions typically itch, and a raised wheal or vesicle occurs (Darier's sign). Much less common is a telangiectatic variant or an erythroderma that occurs as adult forms. Skin biopsy confirms the increased numbers of mast cells in the dermis. Cutaneous symptoms may be controlled with antihistamines. Topical cromolyn and systemic psoralen in combination with ultraviolet A irradiation (PUVA) have been reported to be helpful in some patients. The gastrointestinal manifestations of mastocytosis are discussed in Chapter 106.[78]

Herpes Zoster

Dermatomal involvement of *herpes zoster* T_7–L_1 may cause abdominal pain prior to the onset of typical grouped vesicular lesions. Involvement of sacral nerve roots can produce constipation and pain with defecation.[79] Postherpetic neuralgia can cause persistent, recurrent pain in the involved dermatome.

PANCREATIC DISEASE

There are several cutaneous lesions that raise consideration of underlying pancreatic disease. Periumbilical purpura *(Cullen's sign)* and left flank purpura *(Grey Turner's sign)* are caused by dissection of blood along fascial planes from retroperitoneal bleeding of acute hemorrhagic pancreatitis. The abdominal symptoms predominate in this situation. Cutaneous metastases from pancreatic carcinoma are rare.

Presentation of tender, red subcutaneous nodules occurring most commonly on the pretibial region of the extremities, but which may occur at any site, should raise the diagnostic possibility of *panniculitis* (Fig 44-11; Color Fig 15). The clinical picture is often nonspecific, and the clinical assessment to determine the type of panniculitis may be difficult. *Pancreatic fat necrosis* may feel fluctuant, but lesions rarely ulcerate or discharge fluid.[80] Arthralgias and abdominal pain are frequent accompanying symptoms. Excisional (not punch) biopsy is indicated to confirm the diagnosis of panniculitis. The clinical differential diagnosis includes *superficial migratory thrombophlebitis*, which may be seen with pancreatic, gastric, or other cancers, Behçet's disease, and in some other settings. Pancreatic fat necrosis may be seen as the presenting sign in 22% of patients with pancreatitis, or in up to 65% of patients with pancreatic carcinoma. It has also been reported to occur in asymptomatic drug-induced pancreatitis.

The eruption of multiple yellow-red papules, predominating over extensor surfaces or buttock, suggests a diagnosis of *eruptive xanthomatosis*. These lesions occur in the presence of hypertriglyceridemia and may develop in a patient with pancreatitis, particularly in the setting of diabetes mellitus. Type IV or V hyperlipoproteinemia patterns are most often seen with the eruptive type of xanthomas. Lesions resolve as serum lipids return to normal.

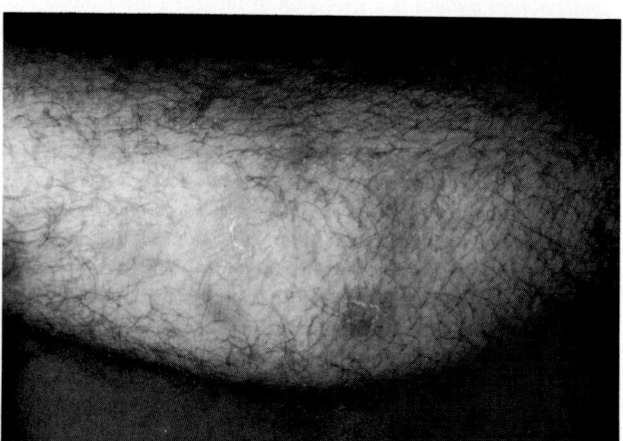

FIGURE 44–11. (See Color Fig 15) Panniculitis presenting as tender erythematous nodules in a patient with pancreatitis.

DERMATOLOGIC DISORDERS ASSOCIATED WITH MALABSORPTION

Dermatitis herpetiformis (DH) is an uncommon blistering disease characterized by intense pruritus and multiple grouped small vesicles distributed symmetrically over the body (Fig 44-12; Color Fig 16). Scalp and extensor surfaces are prominently involved, and the itching and excoriation may be so severe that intact blisters are not prominent. Diagnosis is made by skin biopsy, which shows a subepidermal blister with a neutrophilic infiltrate of the dermal papillae. Direct immunofluorescence of perilesional skin confirms the diagnosis of DH with the demonstration of IgA at the dermal-epidermal junction and/or within the dermal papillae.[81]

Gastrointestinal manifestations may not be clinically prominent in patients with DH who initially present to a dermatologist. Nevertheless, almost all DH patients will have some degree of demonstrable pathology related to gluten sensitivity in their small intestine. The characteristic changes include a mixed lymphocyte-plasma cell infiltrate and villous atrophy (see ch 71). Deposits of IgA can be found in the proximal jejunum in patients with DH before gluten-free diet manipulation.[82] Steatorrhea is observed in 20% to 30% of patients, usually associated with abnormal D-xylose absorption. Anemia may occur secondary to malabsorption (folate, iron), even before dapsone therapy. Even in the absence of GI symptoms, strict observance of a gluten-free diet will lead to improvement of the skin disease and will minimize the need for medication.[83,84] The improvement may take 6 months to 2 years of careful diet restriction, which is extremely difficult for most patients. Gluten challenge leads to flare of the skin lesions in patients previously controlled by diet. Thus, there is convincing evidence that dietary gluten plays a role in the pathogenesis of DH.

Therapy of DH is with one of the sulfones, usually diaminodiphenyl sulfone (dapsone), or with sulfapyridine. Prompt (within hours to a few days) relief of symptoms and halting of lesion formation is a hallmark of DH treatment with one of these agents. Oral dapsone is often started at a dose of 100 to 200 mg daily in adults and is titrated according to the clinical response and with the goal of minimizing side effects.

Malabsorption can occur with other skin diseases. Patients with extensive inflammatory skin disease, such as exfoliative erythroderma or atopic eczema, develop secondary malabsorption, termed *dermatopathic enteropathy*.[85] This is usually manifested as mild steatorrhea and is often asymptomatic, with prompt resolution with therapy of the skin disease. The mechanism is unclear but does not appear to be due to gluten sensitivity. Malabsorption can also occur as a result of abnormal motility or vascular compromise in systemic sclerosis and systemic vasculitides that may also affect the skin.

Skin manifestations of chronic malabsorption are largely nonspecific and reflect altered nutritional status. Dry skin, which may become inflamed (eczematous) or thick-scaled (ichthyotic), is common. Hyperpigmentation, slow hair and nail growth, and loss of skin elasticity also occur. There may be more specific skin changes with loss of certain nutrients, such as zinc deficiency (acrodermatitis enteropathica) or essential fatty acid deficiency, discussed below.

NUTRITIONAL DISORDERS

Although classically the cutaneous manifestations of nutritional deficiency have been separated with regard to specific nutrients, there is usually considerable overlap, and many of the skin signs are nonspecific.[86] This should be kept in mind when evaluating a patient with probable malnutrition due to inadequate or improper dietary intake, or GI disease that may lead to inadequate absorption of nutrients. See Chapters 17 to 21 and 48 for further information.

Protein Malnutrition

The terms marasmus (total starvation) and kwashiorkor (carbohydrate excess with protein deficiency) are often used. Marasmus in this country is usually limited to severely ill patients, and such patients have dry, loose skin, loss of subcutaneous fat, and thin, slowly growing hair. There may be prominent facial lanugo hair and hyperkeratosis around hair follicles. Absence of edema separates marasmus from kwashiorkor in most clinical descriptions. In kwashiorkor there may be hypo- and hyperpigmented scaling patches with peeling of the epidermis over edematous sites, joints, and flexural areas ("flaky paint"). Purpura may also occur, which results in mixed coloration. The hair may demonstrate alternative bands of dark and light pigmentation that correlate with episodes of inadequate protein intake ("flag sign"). Zinc and vitamin deficiency usually accompany these malnutrition states and undoubtedly contribute to the cutaneous findings.[87]

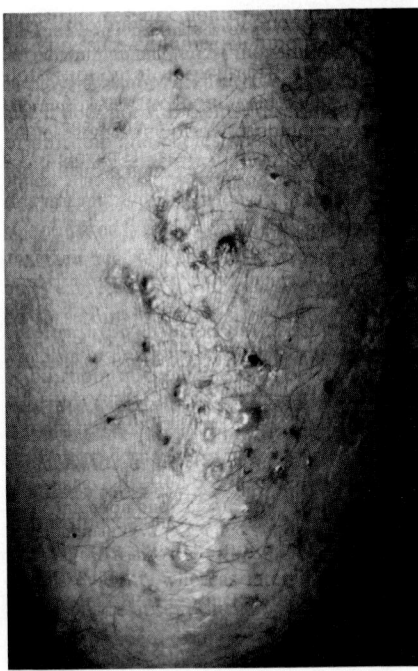

FIGURE 44–12. (See Color Fig 16) Dermatitis herpetiformis. Both elbows were involved. Note intact vesicles and multiple crusted (excoriated) lesions.

Essential Fatty Acid Deficiency

Essential fatty acid deficiency (EFAD) can occur in patients with fat malabsorption, in patients who have had partial bowel resection, or in patients who have been receiving fat-free parenteral nutrition. It has been less common since parenteral lipid supplement has been in routine use.[88]

Cutaneous lesions are typically diffusely distributed, erythematous scaling patches. There may be alopecia and traumatic purpura. The lesions do not develop for several weeks after there is biochemical evidence of EFAD. Linoleic acid is the major fatty acid involved, and there is direct evidence of its role in the repair of the skin lesions. Older studies suggested that topical application of linoleic acid, as sunflower or safflower oil, could correct the total deficiency, but more recent evidence stresses the importance of systemic replacement.

Vitamin Deficiencies

Vitamin A deficiency may occur with fat malabsorption or liver disease. The classic change is that of multiple keratotic follicular papules over the extremities (phrynoderma), usually with generalized dry skin. Keratinizing metaplasia may occur on mucosal surfaces. Skin improvement occurs slowly with replacement therapy. More common clinically is a syndrome of Vitamin A excess, especially with the use of synthetic retinoids but also seen with excess supplemental Vitamin A intake. Alopecia, fine erythematous scaling (sunburn appearance), cheilitis, skin fragility, and brittle nails are common. These problems slowly resolve when the excess is corrected.

There are many similarities in the cutaneous manifestations of deficiency of the *B vitamins* riboflavin, pyridoxine, and niacin. A seborrheic dermatitis appearance over the face, prominent involvement of the perioral and groin areas, and a smooth tongue are common features. In *pellagra* (niacin deficiency) there may be painful erosive and pigmented scaling patches, especially in sun-exposed sites. Occurrence on the upper chest is termed "Casal's necklace." Pellagra still occurs in those with inadequate intake (e.g., alcoholics, elderly) and in patients with gastric or small bowel disease leading to impaired absorption. It can rarely occur in patients with carcinoid, or in patients who are receiving therapy with isoniazid, 6-mercaptopurine, or 5-fluorouracil. Skin lesions respond dramatically to niacin replacement therapy.

Vitamin B_{12} deficiency certainly is a consideration in some patients with underlying gastrointestinal diseases, but cutaneous manifestations are uncommon. Generalized hyperpigmentation, which may specifically involve palms, soles, and nails, may occur. Onset of white hair, alopecia areata, or vitiligo may occur in association with pernicious anemia. Folic acid deficiency may present as an unusual "lemon" yellow color to the skin.

Vitamin C deficiency still occurs fairly often, especially in the elderly or in alcoholics who have inadequate dietary intake. Purpura and petechia, perifollicular hemorrhage with "corkscrew" hairs, and gingival erosions around teeth are the prominent features. Mucosal lesions respond first to replacement of Vitamin C, followed by slower resolution of purpura.

The skin is important in provitamin D_3 synthesis, which occurs in the epidermis in the presence of ultraviolet B radiation. Vitamin D deficiency does not have prominent cutaneous features. Vitamin K deficiency leads indirectly to purpura. Local injection of Vitamin K can lead to local eczematous reactions at the injection site, or rarely to the development of sclerotic morphealike plaques.

Zinc Deficiency

Zinc deficiency, acrodermatitis enteropathica, may be genetic or acquired.[89] The cutaneous manifestations are acrally distributed (hands, face, feet, anogenital region) and are typically erythematous, scaling, vesiculopustular, or eroded plaques. There may be alopecia, impaired wound healing, and stomatitis. Secondary candidal infection is common and should also be treated. Zinc replacement, pancreatic enzyme supplementation, and 8-hydroxy quinoline have been used in the therapy of acrodermatitis enteropathica.

TABLE 44–3

Perineal Skin Lesions (Practical List of Common Causes)

Erythema With Scale or Maceration

Contact dermatitis

Seborrheic dermatitis

Psoriasis

Candidiasis

Dermatophytosis

Secondary syphilis

Extramammary Paget's disease

Nutritional deficiencies

Bowen's disease

Vesicles, Erosions, Ulcers

Herpes simplex

Herpes zoster

Impetigo (streptococcal, staphylococcal)

Syphilis (primary or secondary)

Chancroid

Deep fungal, acid-fast bacilli, protozoal

Bullous pemphigoid

Pemphigus

Ecthyma

Nodules, Tumors, Ulceration

Condyloma acuminata (i.e., warts)

Hidradenitis suppurativa

Squamous or basal cell carcinoma

Crohn's disease

Carcinoma—metastatic or direct extension

Kaposi's sarcoma

Granulomatous herpes simplex

Other Nutritional Disorders

Glucagonoma syndrome, as discussed earlier, may have amino acid deficiency as a contributing factor in the development of skin lesions. Biotin deficiency leads to xerosis with an erosive perioral and intertriginous eruption and alopecia. Copper deficiency (Menkes' syndrome) has as its cutaneous manifestation pale, twisted hair (pili torti) and pale skin.

PERINEAL SKIN LESIONS

There are several skin lesions that occur in the perianal or perineal areas that may be encountered in the course of examination or endoscopy procedure (Table 44-3) (see also ch 85). Vesicles or erosions on an erythematous base should suggest herpetic lesions. *Herpes simplex* is often recurrent in this site, and in immunocompromised patients lesions may be persistent crusted erosions or ulcers. *Herpes zoster* usually presents acutely as dermatomal grouping of vesicles. Perianal ulcers and erosions may also occur in Crohn's disease, amebiasis, and in primary or secondary syphilis or in nontreponemal venereal disease.

Flesh-colored pedunculated papules in the perineal area are often *condyloma acuminatum* (venereal warts). Lesions, if they are few in number, usually respond well to therapy with cryosurgery, electrofulguration, or surgical or laser excision, or to topical podophyllin application. Refractory lesions may respond to intralesional or systemic interferon.

Erythema with scaling or maceration in the gluteal fold and perianal area raises the major considerations of *candidal infection, psoriasis, or seborrheic dermatitis;* irritant *contact dermatitis* (from fecal soiling); or bacterial (streptococcal/staphylococcal) *impetigo.* Clinical presentation, potassium hydroxide preparation of skin scrapings, and culture are helpful in differentiating these diagnoses. If lesions don't respond to appropriate therapy for one of these diagnoses, biopsy may be indicated to rule out *extramammary Paget's disease.*

TABLE 44–4
Dermatologic Side Effects of GI Medications

Antacids	**Clonidine**	**Metronidazole**	**Corticosteroids**
Exanthem	Exanthem	Exanthem*	Acanthosis nigricans
Fixed drug	Eczematous	Urticaria	Acne*
	Contact dermatitis (transdermal)*	Fixed drug	Hypertrichosis*
Bisacodyl	Exacerbates psoriasis		Striae
Fixed drug	Pemphigoid	**Ranitidine**	Purpura*
		Exanthem*	Panniculitis
Carbenoxylone	**Loperamide HCl**	Urticaria	Secondary skin infections
Exanthem	Urticaria	Gynecomastia	Vasculitis
Fixed drug	Exanthem	Vasculitis	
Bullous eruption	Erythema nodosum		**Cyanocobalamin**
		Sulfasalazine	Acne
Chenodeoxycholic Acid	**6-Mercaptopurine**	Alopecia	Eczematous
Xerosis	Alopecia	Exanthem*	
	Exanthem	Eczematous	**Domperidone**
Cholestyramine		Erythema multiforme	Lupus erythematosus
Exanthem	**Methotrexate**	Mononucleosislike	
	Alopecia*	Raynaud's	**Vitamin K**
Cimetidine	Exanthem	Toxic epidermal necrolysis	Eczematous
Alopecia	Photosensitivity*		Sclerotic plaque (injection site)
Exanthem	Oral ulceration	**Tetracyclines**	
Xerosis		Acnelike	
Exfoliative dermatitis	**Metoclopramide**	Phototoxicity*	
Exacerbates psoriasis	Exanthem	Lichenoid	
Erythema multiforme	Urticaria	Fixed drug	
Gynecomastia			
Purpura			
Urticaria			
Vasculitis			
Lupus erythematosus			
Erythema annulare centrifugum			

* *Common*

Idiopathic pruritus ani is a diagnosis that should be made only after a primary dermatosis, such as those listed above, has been ruled out. It is a common complaint, particularly in middle-aged males, and psychologic factors are stressed in some reviews.[90,91] The key to effective therapy of pruritus ani is eliminating underlying triggering factors, including infections, irritants, allergies, and abnormal anorectal pathology (e.g., rectal fissures or prolapse). Careful cleaning measures, dietary changes, and treatments ranging from topical corticosteroids to intralesional steroids or cryosurgery have been used successfully in different series. Treatment is most successful when the symptoms have been present for less than 2 years.

COMPLICATIONS OF MEDICATIONS

Dermatologic Side Effects of Medications Commonly Used in Gastroenterology

Some of the dermatologic side effects that have been reported in association with GI medications are noted in Table 44-4.[92] In general, onset of a drug eruption is correlated with recent institution of a medication. However, some reactions, such as xerosis or lupuslike reactions, may take longer (months) to develop. Skin biopsy will help confirm the type of cutaneous reaction but will not specify the medication involved. Skin testing, to predict or confirm drug allergy, is not routine. Desensitization has been successful for some medications, such as sulfasalazine.[93]

Gastrointestinal Side Effects of Dermatologic Therapy

Therapeutic modalities used in dermatology include topical and systemic agents ranging from corticosteroids to antibiotics and chemotherapeutic agents. Several specific drugs used primarily in dermatology are notable in their potential GI side effects. Topical clindamycin, used for treatment of acne vulgaris, has been rarely associated with *Clostridium difficile* toxin-positive pseudomembranous colitis.[94] Systemic retinoids have seen increasing dermatologic indications. Isotretinoin, used for severe cystic acne, has been temporally associated with inflammatory bowel disease onset or flare.[95] However, this drug has been used without adverse GI effects in some patients known to have pre-existent bowel disease. Dapsone, used for dermatitis herpetiformis and some other inflammatory dermatoses, has been occasionally associated with a mononucleosislike syndrome and with hepatitis, which is usually reversible when treatment is stopped.

The reader is directed to Chapter 5, The Immune System; Chapter 20, Vitamins and Minerals; Chapter 21, General Nutritional Principles; Chapter 30, Approach to the Patient with Gross Gastrointestinal Bleeding; Chapter 31, Approach to the Patient with Occult Gastrointestinal Bleeding; Chapter 38, Approach to the Patient with Diarrhea; Chapter 47, Approach to Gastrointestinal Problems Associated with Common Clinical Conditions; Chapter 48, Approach to the Patient Requiring Nutritional Supplementation; Chapter 53, Esophagus: Anatomy and Structural Anomalies; Chapter 54, Motility Disorders of the Esophagus; Chapter 57, Esophageal Tumors; Chapter 58, Miscellaneous Diseases of the Esophagus; Chapter 63, Tumors of the Stomach; Chapter 70, Tumors and Other Neoplastic Diseases of the Small Intestine; Chapter 71, Celiac Disease; Chapter 74, Short Bowel Syndrome; Chapter 77, Inflammatory Bowel Disease; Chapter 79, Polyposis Syndrome; Chapter 84, Malignant Tumors of the Colon; Chapter 85, Anorectal Diseases; Chapter 88, Acute Pancreatitis; Chapter 91, Endocrine Neoplasms of the Pancreas; Chapter 103, Gastrointestinal Complications of the Acquired Immunodeficiency Syndrome; Chapter 106, Gastrointestinal Manifestations of Systemic Disease; Chapter 107, Gastrointestinal Manifestations of Immunologic Disorders; and Chapter 108, Vascular Ectasias, Tumors, and Malformations.

REFERENCES

1. Jorizzo JL. Classification of urticaria and the reactive inflammatory vascular dermatoses. Dermatol Clin 1985;3:3.
2. Basler RSW, Dubin HV. Ulcerative colitis and the skin. Arch Dermatol 1976;112:531.
3. Archer ME, Jorizzo JL. Chronic urticaria. In: Taylor RB, ed. Difficult diagnosis. Philadelphia: WB Saunders, 1985:531.
4. Huff JC, Weston WL, Tonnesen MG. Erythema multiforme: A critical review of characteristics, diagnostic criteria and causes. J Am Acad Dermatol 1983;8:763.
5. White JW. Erythema nodosum. Derm Clin 1985;3:119.
6. Jorizzo JL, Solomon AR, Zanolli MD, Leshin B. Neutrophilic vascular reactions. J Am Acad Dermatol 1988;19:983.
7. Burgdorf W. Cutaneous manifestations of Crohn's disease. J Am Acad Dermatol 1981;5:689.
8. Speiser JC, Moore TL, Zuckner J. Ulcerative colitis with arthritis and vasculitis. Clin Rheumatol 1985;4:343.
9. Chalvardjian A, Nethercott JR. Cutaneous granulomatous vasculitis associated with Crohn's disease. Cutis 1982;30:645.
10. Holt PJA, Davis MG, Scunderski, NG. Pyoderma gangrenosum. Medicine 1980;59:114.
11. Frankel DH, .Mostofi RS, Lorincz AL. Oral Crohn's disease: Report of two cases in brothers with metallic dysgnosia and a review of the literature. J Am Acad Dermatol 1985;12:260.
12. Schreiner DT, Jorizzo JL. Behçet's disease and complex aphthosis. Dermatol Clin 1987;5:769.
13. Van Hale HM, Rogers RS, Zone JJ, Greippo PR. Pyostomatitis vegetans: A reactive mucosal marker in inflammatory disease of gut. Arch Dermatol 1985;121:94.
14. Lebwohl M, Fleischmajer R, Janowitz H, et al. Metastatic Crohn's disease. J Am Acad Dermatol 1984;10:33.
15. Sloan WP Jr, Bargen JA, Gage RP. Life histories of patients with chronic ulcerative colitis: A review of 2000 cases. Gastroenterology 1950;16:25.
16. Greenstein AJ, Janowitz HD, Sachar DB. The extraintestinal com-

plications of Crohn's disease and ulcerative colitis: A study of 700 patients. Medicine 1976;55:401.

17. Bohan A, Peter JB, Bowman RL, et al. A computer-assisted analysis of 153 patients with polymyositis and dermatomyositis. Medicine 1977;56:255.

18. Callen JP, Hyla JF, Boles GG, et al. The relationship of dermatomyositis and polymyositis to internal malignancy. Arch Dermatol 1980;116:295.

19. Rodnan GP, Medsger JA, Buckingham RB. Progressive systemic sclerosis—CREST syndrome: Observations on natural history and late complication in 90 patients. Arthritis Rheum 1975;18:423.

20. O'Duffy JD, Carney JA, Deodhar S. Behçet's disease: Report of 10 cases, 3 with new manifestations. Ann Intern Med 1971;75:561.

21. Jorizzo JL, Hudson RD, Schmalstieg FC, et al. Behçet's syndrome: Immune regulation, circulating immune complexes, neutrophil migration, and colchicine therapy. J Am Acad Dermatol 1984;10:205.

22. Jorizzo JL. Behçet's disease: An update based on the 1985 international conference based in London. Arch Dermatol 1986;122:556.

23. Jorizzo JL, Solomon AR, Cavallo T. Behçet's syndrome: Immunopathologic and histopathologic assessment of pathergy lesions is useful in diagnosis and follow up. Arch Pathol Lab Med 1985;109:747.

24. Ely PH. The bowel bypass syndrome: A response to bacterial peptidoglycans. J Am Acad Dermatol 1980;2:473.

25. Jorizzo JL, Apisarnthanarax P, Subrt P, et al. Bowel bypass syndrome without bowel bypass: Bowel-associated dermatosis-arthritis syndrome. Arch Intern Med 1983;143:457.

26. Jorizzo JL, Schmalstieg PC, Dinehart SM, et al. Bowel-associated dermatosis-arthritis syndrome: Immune complex–mediated vessel damage and increased neutrophil migration. Arch Intern Med 1984;144:738.

27. Kyle RA, Greippo PR, Garton JP, Gertz MA: Primary systemic amyloidosis. Am J Med 1985;79:708.

28. Breathnach SM, Black MM: Systemic amyloidosis and the skin: A review with special emphasis on clinical features and therapy. Clin Exp Dermatol 1979,4:517.

29. Peery WH. Clinical spectrum of hereditary hemorrhagic telangiectasis (Osler–Weber–Rendu disease). Am J Med 1987;82:989.

30. Bean WB. Blue rubber bleb nevi of the skin and gastrointestinal tract. In: Vascular spiders and related lesions of the skin. Springfield, Illinois: Charles C Thomas, 1958:178.

31. Sander KS, Cohen H, Radin R, et al. Blue rubber bleb nevus syndrome presenting with recurrences. Dig Dis Sci 1987;32:214.

32. Friedman-Kien AE, Laubenstein LJ, Rubenstein P, et al. Disseminated Kaposi's sarcoma in gay men. Ann Intern Med 1982;96:693.

33. Reed WB, Karmath HM, Weiss L. Kaposi sarcoma, with emphasis on the internal manifestations. Arch Dermatol 1974;110:115.

34. Degos R. Malignant atrophic papulosis. Br J Dermatol 1979;100:21.

35. Tribble K, Archer ME, Jorizzo JL, et al. Malignant atrophic papulosis: Absence of circulating immune complexes or vasculitis. J Am Acad Dermatol 1986;15:365.

36. Pope FM. Historical evidence for the genetic heterogeneity of pseudoxanthoma elasticum. Br J Dermatol 1975;92:493.

37. Uitto J, Shamban A. Heritable skin diseases with molecular defect in collagen or elastin. Dermatol Clin 1987;5:63.

38. Pope FM, Marin GR, Lichtenstein JR, et al. Patients with Ehlers–Danlos syndrome. Proc Natl Acad Sci USA 1975;72:1314.

39. Beighton P. The dominant and recessive forms of cutis laxa. J Med Genet 1972;9:216.

40. Davis GB, Berk RW. Intestinal neurofibroma in von Recklinghausen's disease. Am J Gastroenterol 1973;60:410.

41. Gardner EJ, Richards RC. Multiple cutaneous and subcutaneous lesions occurring simultaneously with hereditary polyposis and osteomatosis. Am J Hum Genet 1953;5:137.

42. Bussey HJR, Veale AMO, Morson BC. Genetics of gastrointestinal polyposis. Gastroenterology 1978;74:1325.

43. Weary PE, Linthicum A, Cawley EP, et al. Gardner's syndrome: A family group study and review. Arch Dermatol 1964;90:20.

44. Finan MC, Ray MK. Gastrointestinal polyposis syndrome. Dermatol Clin 1989;7:419.

45. Jeghers H, McKusick BA, Katz KH. Generalized intestinal polyposis and melanin spots of the oral mucosa, lips, and digits. N Engl J Med 1949;241:993 and 1031.

46. Hood AB, Krush AJ. Clinical and dermatologic aspects of the hereditary intestinal polyposes. Dis Colon Rectum 1983;26:546.

47. Daniel ES, Ludwig SL, Lewink J, et al. The Cronkhite–Canada syndrome: An analysis of clinical and pathological features and therapy. Medicine (Baltimore) 1982;61:293.

48. Salem OS, Steck WB. Cowden's disease (multiple hamartoma and neoplasia syndrome): A case report and review of the English literature. J Am Acad Dermatol 1983;8:686.

49. Muir EG, Bell AJY, Barlow KA. Multiple primary carcinomata of the colon, duodenum, and larynx associated with kerato-acanthoma of the face. Br J Surg 1967;54:191.

50. Torre D. Multiple sebaceous tumors. Arch Dermatol 1968;98:549.

51. Finan MC, Connolly SM. Sebaceous gland tumors and systemic disease: A clinico pathologic analysis. Medicine (Baltimore) 1984;63:232.

52. Klein J, Parbeen G, Gavaler JS, et al. Colonic polyps in patients with acromegaly. Ann Intern Med 1982;97:27.

53. Leavitt J, Klein J, Kendricks F, et al. Skin tags: A cutaneous marker for colonic polyps. Ann Intern Med 1983;98:92.

54. Chobanian S, Van Ness M, Winters C, et al. Skin tags as a marker for adenomatous polyps of the colon. Ann Intern Med 1985;103:892.

55. Dalton ADA, Coghill SB. No association between skin tags and colorectal adenomas. Lancet 1985;1:1332.

56. Powell FC, Cooper AJ, Massa MC, Goellner JR, Su WPD. Sister Mary Joseph's nodule: A clinical and histological study. J Am Acad Dermatol 1984;10:610.

57. Merot Y, Mazoujian G, Pinkus G, Momtaz TK, Murphy GF. Extramammary Paget's disease of the perianal and perineal regions: Evidence of apocrine derivation. Arch Dermatol 1985;121:750.

58. Chanda JL. Extramammary Paget's disease: Prognosis and relationship to internal malignancy. J Am Acad Dermatol 1985;13:1009.

59. Curth HO, Hilberg AW, Machacek GF. The site and histology of the cancer associated with malignant acanthosis nigricans. Cancer 1962;15:364.

60. Brown J, Winkelmann RK. Acanthosis nigricans: A study of 90 cases. Medicine 1968;47:33.

61. Ellis DL, Kafka SP, Chow JC, et al. Melanoma, growth factors, acanthosis nigricans, the sign of Leser–Trélat, and multiple acrochordons: A possible role for alpha-transforming growth factor in cutaneous paraneoplastic syndromes. N Engl J Med 1987;317:1582.

62. Harper PS, Harper RMJ, Howell-Evans AW. Carcinoma of the esophagus with tylosis. Q J Med 1970;39:317.

63. Bennion SD, Patterson JW. Keratosis punctata palmaris et plantaris and adenocarcinoma of the colon. J Am Acad Dermatol 1984;10:587.

64. Deffer TA, Overton-Keary PP, Goetle DK. Erythroderma secondary to esophageal carcinoma. J Am Acad Dermatol 1985;13:311.

65. Jemec GBE. Hypertrichosis lanuginosa acquisita. Arch Dermatol 1986;122:805.

66. Sirinavin C, Trowbridge AA. Dyskeratosis Congenita: Clinical features and genetic aspects: Report of a family and review of the literature. J Med Genet 1975;12:339.

67. Schetman D. The Plummer–Vinson syndrome. Arch Dermatol 1972;105:720.

68. Gorden P, Comi RJ, Maton PN, Go VL. NIH conference. Somatostatin and somatostatin analogue (SMS 201-995) in treatment of hormone-secreting tumors of the pituitary and gastrointestinal tract and non-neoplastic diseases of the gut. Ann Intern Med 1989;110:35.

69. Vanderstein PR, Scheithauer BW. Glucagonoma syndrome. J Am Acad Dermatol 1985;12:1032.

70. Norton JA, Kahn CR, Schiebinger R, Gorschboth C, Brennan MF. Amino acid deficiency and the skin rash associated with glucagonoma. Ann Intern Med 1979;91:213.

71. Schmid R, Allescher HD, Schepp W, Holscher A, Siewert R, Schuszdziarra V, Classen M. Effect of somatostatin on skin lesions and concentration of plasma amino acids in a patient with glucagonoma-syndrome. Hepatogastroenterology 1988;35:34.

72. Nowak AJ. Oropharyngeal lesions and their management in epidermolysis bullosa. Arch Dermatol 1988;124:742.

73. Gryboski JD, Touloukian R, Campanella RA. Gastrointestinal manifestations of epidermolysis bullosa in children. Arch Dermatol 1988;124:746.
74. Gammon WR, Briggaman RA, Woodley DT, Heald PW, Wheeler CE. Epidermolysis bullosa acquisita—A pemphigoid-like disease. J Am Acad Dermatol 1984;11:820.
75. Eliakim R, Goldin E, Livshin R, Okon E. Esophageal involvement in pemphigus vulgaris. Am J Gastroenterol 1988;83:155.
76. Ashworth J, Cox NH, Pickard WR, MacKay C, Roberts DT. Death in pemphigus vulgaris caused by lower gastrointestinal hemorrhage. J Am Acad Dermatol 1987;16:394.
77. Bernard P, Souyri N, Pillegand B, Bonnetblanc JM. Immunofluorescent studies of gastrointestinal tract mucosa in bullous pemphigoid. Arch Dermatol 1986;122:137.
78. Cherner JA, Jensen RT, Dubois A, O Dorisio TM, Gardner JD, Metcalfe DD. Gastrointestinal dysfunction in systemic mastocytosis. A prospective study. Gastroenterology 1988;95:657.
79. Jellinek EH, Tulloch WS. Herpes zoster with dysfunction of bladder and anus. Lancet 1976;2:1219.
80. Hughes PS, Apisarnthanarax, Mullins JF. Subcutaneous fat necrosis associated with pancreatic disease. Arch Dermatol 1975;111:506.
81. Katz SI, Hall RP, Lawley TJ, Strober W. Dermatitis herpetiformis: The skin and the gut. Ann Intern Med 198;93:857.
82. Karpati S, Kosnai I, Torok E, Kovacs JB. Immunoglobulin A deposition in jejunal mucosa of children with dermatitis herpetiformis. J Invest Dermatol 1988;91:336.
83. Reunala T, Blomqvist K, Tarpila S, et al. Gluten-free diet in dermatitis herpetiformis. I. Clinical response of skin lesions in 81 patients. Br J Dermatol 1977;97:473.
84. Leonard J, Haffenden G, Tucker W, Unsworth J, et al. Gluten challenge in dermatitis herpetiformis. N Engl J Med 1983;308:816.
85. Marks J, Shuster S. Small intestinal mucosal abnormalities in various skin diseases—Fact or fancy. Gut 1970;11:281.
86. Miller SJ. Nutritional deficiency and the skin. J Am Acad Dermatol 1989;21:1.
87. McLaren DS. Cutaneous changes in nutritional disorders. In: Fitzpatrick TB, Eisen AZ, Wolff K, et al, eds. Dermatology in general medicine. 3rd ed. New York: McGraw-Hill, 1987:1601.
88. Sherertz EF. The skin in essential fatty acid deficiency. In: Roe DA, ed. Nutrition and the skin. New York: Alan R Liss, Inc, 1986:117.
89. Neldner KH. Acrodermatitis enteropathica and other zinc-deficiency disorders. In: Fitzpatrick TB, Eisen AZ, Wolff K, et al, eds. Dermatology in general medicine. 3rd ed. New York, McGraw-Hill, 1987: 1613.
90. Hanno R, Murphy P. Pruritus ani: Classification and management. Dermatol Clin 1987;5:811.
91. Smith LE, Henrichs D, McCullah RD. Prospective studies on the etiology and treatment of pruritus ani. Dis Colon Rectum 1982;25: 358.
92. Bruinsma W. A guide to drug eruptions. 4th ed. Norwood, New Jersey: American Overseas Book Co, 1987.
93. Purdy BH, Philips DM, Summers RW. Desensitization for sulfasalazine skin rash. Ann Intern Med 1984;100:512.
94. Parry MF, Rha C-K. Pseudomembranous colitis caused by topical clindamycin phosphate. Arch Dermatol 1986;122:583.
95. Schleicher SM. Oral isotretinoin and inflammatory bowel disease. J Am Acad Dermatol 1985;13:834.

45

Approach to Gastrointestinal Problems in the Elderly

PETER R. HOLT

Gastroenterology, in contrast to cardiology and neurology, has been thought of as a specialty that deals more with diseases of the young than of the old. As a result, little attention has been paid to disorders of the elderly and solid, well-researched information generally is unavailable. Because many baseline physiologic gastrointestinal functions that have been studied are not affected by aging, many would argue that it has been unnecessary to consider the needs of the elderly patient in a gastroenterology practice.

However, a number of factors would lead one strongly to reject this prejudice.

First, the numbers of the elderly are increasing steadily. By the year 2025, those persons older than age 65 will represent more than 750 million in the world. Furthermore, several gastrointestinal disorders contribute to morbidity and mortality in advanced age. For example, the incidence of cancer of the colon continues to increase to the age of 85,[1] and over three-fourths of the deaths from peptic disease in the United States occur in persons older than 65.[2]

ALTERED PHYSIOLOGY

When disorders occur in the elderly, it is most important to separate age-related physiologic events from problems that are the consequence of disease. A common error when managing an elderly patient with a gastrointestinal symptom is to ascribe the complaint to the "aging process."[3] Thus, it is necessary to recognize the range of changes that lie within an age-dependent effect. One also should ask what pathologic problems occur generally in the elderly and how they may affect the gastrointestinal tract. For example, vascular atheromatous changes are almost universal in the elderly. Because the splanchnic circulation receives the largest fraction of cardiac output and has the lowest vascular resistance, a reduction in blood flow potentially can render the gastrointestinal mucosa susceptible to anoxic damage, particularly during low flow states such as hypotension and congestive heart failure. However, except following acute mesenteric arterial embolism or arterial or venous thrombosis, which may lead to gangrene of the mucosa, other changes (e.g., such as abdominal angina and anoxic strictures of the small and large bowel) are extremely rare.[4]

Age-associated degeneration of connective and neuronal tissues is common and, in the gastrointestinal tract, may contribute to diverticulosis or enteric nerve changes.[5] Changes in gastrointestinal epithelial cell production and modulation also occur. Recent evidence indicates that small and large intestinal epithelial cell production actually may increase both in experimental animals[6,7] and in humans,[8] and adaptive controls of proliferation are deranged in small intestine.[9] In the stomach, atrophic gastritis results from increased, and not reduced, cell production.[10]

Changes in gastrointestinal hormone action could result from reduction in hormone synthesis, reduced tissue release of the hormone or altered intravascular distribution, or changes in degradation rate or in destruction of the hormone (Table 45-1). Most hormone changes occurring in advanced age have been described at the end-organ cellular level.[11] Hormone receptor density or

TABLE 45-2
Drugs Whose Absorption Is Decreased by Antacids

Antibiotics
  Tetracycline, ketoconazole
  Fluoroquinolones
H_2 receptor antagonists
Digoxin
Phenothiazines
Isoniazid
Iron preparations

affinity may be less than in younger persons and post-receptor signal transduction or signal responses are commonly altered as a physiologic consequence of age.[12] In older humans, serum gastrin concentration may be increased because achlorhydria is present[13]; in the rat, no changes have been found.[14] Serum concentrations of pancreatic polypeptide,[15] of cholecystokinin,[16] and of motilin[17] are higher in the elderly than in the young. Reduced cholecystokinin receptor number or affinity has been found,[16] which may represent a desensitization phenomenon. The clinical consequences of these changes in gastrointestinal hormone levels or in receptors have not been elucidated.

Gastrointestinal immune responses also may be impaired. Aging generally leads to a decline in the functional capability of both helper and killer T cells, only subtle changes in B cell function, and little or no loss in antigen presenting cell function.[18] Circulating lymphocytes may be functionally more diverse and consist of a greater mosaic of responsive and nonresponsive cells,[19] but all of these changes have little clinical and functional impact.

Studies of age-related changes in the gut-associated lymphoid system have been sparse. Peyer's patches and mesenteric lymph node lymphocyte number and T cell–dependent mitogen responsiveness are reduced in senescent mice. However, gut secretion of IgA remains unaltered, suggesting that this mucosal associated host defense may be well maintained.[20] Reduction in transhepatic transport of dimeric immunoglobulin A into bile, described in aging rats, has not been confirmed in humans.

PHARMACOLOGIC CHANGES

The elderly consume the greatest number of drugs, take multiple medications most frequently, spend the greatest amount of money on medications, and have the highest incidence of drug reactions, yet our knowledge of pharmacologic changes in the elderly is relatively rudimentary and the application of this knowledge in practice is almost nonexistent.[21] Classic gastrointestinal drugs are quite frequently used by the elderly (see Table 45-1)[22,23] and cause one-fourth of the drug reactions.[24] Medications prescribed for gastrointestinal disorders can induce gastrointestinal side effects and alter the availability of distribution of these drugs or of other medications.[25] For example, antacids impair the absorption of many agents commonly used to treat the elderly (Table 45-2).

Changes in pharmacodynamics and pharmacokinetics can occur as a function of age.[26] Differences in pharmacodynamics (i.e., dif-

TABLE 45-1
Prevalence of Ingestion of Selected Drugs in the Elderly

CLASS OF DRUG	UNITED STATES (%)	UNITED KINGDOM (%)
Antibiotics	70	11.5
Psychotropics	35	50
Cardiotonics and antihypertensives	50	60
Antacids	15	2.5
Hematinics		13
Laxatives	11	7
Antiulcer drugs	6	

Abstracted from Holt PR. Gastrointestinal drugs in the elderly. Am J Gastroenterol 1986;81:403.

ferences in effective action at the end organ from the same drug concentration) occur quite uncommonly. Psychotropics, such as diazepam, nitrazepam, or chlordiazepoxide, have greater pharmacodynamic effects in the elderly, whereas β-adrenergic agonists and antagonists, such as propranolol and isoproterenol, have lesser effects. Pharmacokinetic differences are common and result from changes in drug disposition because of altered drug absorption, drug distribution, drug metabolism, or drug excretion. There is no evidence that absorptive capacity for drugs is reduced, although peak absorption may be slightly delayed.[27] The most common reason for altered clearances is a change in drug distribution because body weight falls and body composition changes. In the elderly, lean body mass and total body water decline and adipose tissue mass increases in relationship to total body weight. Fat represents an average of 36% of body weight in elderly men and 48% in elderly women, but only 18% in young men and 30% in young women.[26] Thus, the distribution of lipid-soluble drugs increases and that of water-soluble drugs decreases. However, such differences in body composition vary for individual subjects and may not hold for an active octogenarian.

Reduced renal function principally alters the excretion of water-soluble drugs. Inulin and creatinine clearances fall progressively after the age of 60[28] and are reduced by about one-third by age 80 from levels at age 20 to 30. The net effect of such reduced creatinine clearance for most drugs is quite small. Hepatic drug clearance also may be lower in the elderly because of reduced hepatic blood flow,[29] due to lower cardiac output and hepatic mass.[30] Such changes in liver blood flow may alter the distribution of drugs that are rapidly cleared by the liver, that is, have a considerable "first pass" effect, such as lidocaine and propranolol. Unfortunately, the clearance rates of agents such as propranolol are not predictable and considerable variation in clearance between individual patients is seen.[31] Changes in hepatic drug metabolism also can affect drug clearance. Phase 1 oxidative reactions are consistently reduced in rodents[32] but are only modestly altered in humans,[33] leading to lower drug clearance and higher steady-state plasma concentrations only after multiple doses of agents such as diazepam, theophylline, and antipyrine. However, phase 2 reactions, including glucuoronidation and acetylation, are affected minimally, if at all, as a function of age.[34]

Clinical Manifestations

Overall, clinical disorders may differ in the elderly for a number of reasons:

1. Diseases may occur only or principally in the old (e.g. pernicious anemia). The majority of gastrointestinal diseases that occur in the young also can occur in an older patient for the first time. Even celiac sprue (gluten-induced enteropathy) may present initially in the very old.[35]
2. Manifestations may differ in the old from those in the young. For example, colonic Crohn's disease more often affects the distal colon in the old but affects the proximal colonic segments in the young.[36]
3. The course of a disease may differ in the older patient (e.g., there may be fewer relapses from Crohn's disease in older than in younger patients).

4. Therapy for a disease may need to be altered (e.g., corticosteroids have serious side effects in older patients, so must be used sparingly for the treatment of inflammatory bowel disease).

Symptoms and signs of gastrointestinal disease may differ. This fact is recognized by physicians less commonly than is their belief that laboratory data can be "more abnormal" in the old than in the young. The clinical features of diseases in the elderly also may be altered because of central nervous system disease or depression or the patient may have a profound fear of complex medical care. There also are prejudices in the diagnostic evaluation of elderly patients with gastrointestinal disease, and management strategies must be carefully evaluated.

Acute abdominal pain appears to be muted with age, perhaps because endogenous opiate secretion is increased, nerve conduction falls, or the patient may be depressed.[37] The causes of acute abdominal pain in older persons also differ. Based on a multicenter review of more than 2400 patients over the age of 50, cholecystitis was found to be the cause in about 20%, appendicitis in 15%, intestinal obstruction in 12.3%, and cancer in 4%.[38] In younger patients, cholecystitis was the cause in only 6% and cancer in less than 1%. Cancer was found in no less than one-fourth of these emergency patients over age 70 with acute abdominal pain. The initial diagnostic impression in older patients with acute abdominal pain is wrong in up to two-thirds of patients.[39] Acute appendicitis often may be present, but with few overt abdominal signs[40,41] and more progression to gangrene and perforation.[42] Pain localization often is atypical in the over-60 age group (Table 45-3). Anorexia frequently results from impaired gastric emptying due to concomitant drug ingestion or from central effects of medications or depression.

Physical signs also are often altered in the elderly patient. The dramatic abdominal manifestations of an acute perforated viscus can be muted in the old.[37,43] One reason is that the chemical peritonitis induced by gastric hydrogen ions may be absent if the patient has hypochlorhydria. Sensory perception may be impaired, resulting in less abdominal tenderness, and drugs such as psychotropic agents also may alter the clinical features of the primary gastrointestinal disease. Laboratory data generally should not be considered any differently in an older patient than in the younger patient. The majority of tests are normal in the elderly (e.g., hemoglobin levels do not fall with age).[44,45] One clinical error in

TABLE 45-3
Pain in Acute Appendicitis

PAIN SITE	PERCENTAGE OF PATIENTS*	
	Age < 50 Years (2250)	Age > 60 Years (283)
Mid abdomen radiating to right iliac fossa	63%	41%
Right iliac fossa	34%	38%
Atypical pain distribution	3%	21%

* Number of patients shown in parentheses.
Modified from Arnbjornsson E. Recognizing appendicitis in the elderly. Geriatr Med Today 1984;3:72.

managing older patients with gastrointestinal disease is that diagnostic procedures are delayed or omitted. Rectal examination, sigmoidoscopy, and colonoscopy should be performed for the same indications in the old as in the young, particularly because the incidence of colon cancer in the United States increases progressively to the age of 85.[1] Patients generally prefer colonoscopy to double-contrast barium meals,[46] and the yield and value of this procedure in the elderly have been well justified.[47] For the diagnosis of upper gastrointestinal diseases, flexible esophagogastroduodenoscopy is accurate[48] and is done with no more risk in the old than in the young. Endoscopic complications most commonly occur from the sedating medication; with experience, sedation and analgesia can be much reduced in the old.[49] Upper gastrointestinal endoscopy is dangerous only with significant concomitant cardiorespiratory disease.

A difficult clinical problem is the approach to acute gastrointestinal bleeding in the elderly in whom mortality rates are high. The sources of upper gastrointestinal bleeding do not differ greatly with age. Peptic ulceration is commonly found,[50] esophageal bleeding is frequent,[49,51] but the incidence of hemorrhagic gastritis is relatively low.[52] In the past, lower gastrointestinal tract bleeding in the old usually was ascribed to neoplasms or diverticulitis and, more recently, to diverticulosis. Now the colonic vascular ectasias or angiodysplasia is considered more important than diverticulosis as a cause of lower gastrointestinal bleeding.[53] More prospective studies of the causes of upper and lower gastrointestinal tract bleeding in the elderly are needed.

Therapeutic approaches may need to be altered in older persons. Drugs excreted primarily by the kidney may need altered dosing. More or fewer side effects may occur. Corticosteroid therapy, for example, is more harmful in older persons because calcium is depleted from already osteopenic bones or cataract formation is accentuated. However, it is crucial to avoid the clinical trap of undertreating an older patient.[54] Previously, abdominal surgery often was avoided in the old; now it is recognized that patient risk reflects associated diseases and not age alone.[55] Severe cardiovascular and respiratory disease increases risk from abdominal surgery at any age. The spry, well, elderly individual can tolerate abdominal surgery, including colon resection for carcinoma, without significantly greater mortality or morbidity than the young[56] and usually can return to an active high quality of life.[57]

DISORDERS OF SWALLOWING AND FOOD INGESTION (SEE ALSO CH 28)

Disorders of swallowing and reduced food intake are among the most common problems facing clinicians who look after the health of older patients. Most symptoms occur from anorexia or during the pre-esophageal initiation of swallowing and not at the level of the esophagus. Reduced food intake often causes malnutrition in the elderly and can occur for many reasons. "Forgetting to eat" commonly is due to diseases of the brain, but the physician must consider the possible role of iatrogenic or drug-induced depression. Social influences, such as isolation and physical handicaps, can interfere with the patient's ability to prepare food. Food intake also can fall as a result of changes in taste or smell, from dental problems, or from swallowing disorders.

Disorders of Swallowing

Dysphagia may be oropharyngeal (pre-esophageal) or esophageal. Oropharyngeal dysphagia usually affects the patient's ability to swallow liquids, and esophageal dysphagia primarily alters the swallowing of solid foods. Few reproducible age-dependent physiologic changes occur in the pharynx and esophagus. Thinning of the tongue involves mucosa and muscle. The muscles of the mouth and pharynx are weaker in older subjects, resulting in altered masticatory muscle function.[58] Muscle contraction discoordination also can occur as a function of age, most commonly from disturbances in control originating in the extrapyramidal system, mainly in the basal ganglia,[59] and can be seen as an early feature of Parkinson's disease. Altered pharyngeal sensation and proprioception can result in changes in taste acuity and in differences in discrimination of the size of a food bolus in the pharynx.[58] As a result of all of these changes in the elderly, mastication tends to be slowed, tongue function is impaired (which can result in increased food spills), and swallowing takes longer. Drooling is a frequent, annoying, and embarrassing problem that can result from altered lip closure—a problem that dentists may help to improve.[60]

Generally, it has been held that salivary flow falls as a physiologic function of age because of a reduction in salivary gland cell mass and function. Recent studies demonstrate that salivary flow remains normal[61] so that medications or disease of the salivary glands are responsible for reduced salivary flow.

Disorders of taste acuity can reduce food intake.[62] In the absence of smoking, tests of taste sensitivity for bitter and sour have not shown consistent reduction with age.[63] However, the threshold for the detection of electrical stimuli is increased in the old, who also may lose the capacity to accurately identify blended foods. Changes in taste acuity are explained in a number of ways. The number of taste buds and papillae decreases with age,[64,65] increased salivary sodium secretion may lower the taste sensitivity to salt,[66] and lesions of the neural pathway for taste perception, especially the fifth, seventh, ninth, and tenth cranial nerves, also may contribute. Some have suggested that zinc deficiency might impair taste perception in the elderly, but plasma zinc levels usually are normal and do not correlate with altered taste acuity[67] and zinc supplementation does not improve taste acuity.[68] Taste disturbances more commonly occur from drugs taken to treat concomitant diseases in the patient.[69] Furthermore, the elderly often require dentures, and diminished taste often occurs following denture fitting. Oral hygiene also plays a role in taste, and regular professional hygiene care is undertaken less commonly in the elderly. The sense of smell is important in taste perception, and considerable impairment in this sense has been demonstrated in subjects over age 70.[70] All these factors can result in reduced food intake and nutrient depletion.

Physiologic Changes in the Esophagus

Although radiologic changes, described as "corkscrew esophagus" or presbyesophagus and consisting of tertiary contractions, have been shown to occur more commonly in the elderly,[71] these radiologic changes presently have no known pathophysiologic consequence.[72] Some have suggested that impaired peristalsis[73] or aperistalsis can occur in the very old (achalasia of the elderly),[74] but these patients have normal or low baseline pressures of the lower esophageal sphincter, a fact that distinguishes them from patients with classic achalasia of the esophagus.[75] The resting pressure in the lower esophageal sphincter does not change with age. When motility changes have been demonstrated in octogenarians, these have occurred in patients with concomitant diseases that can induce esophageal motor disturbances.[72] Unfortunately, direct measures of the transit of a bolus of different sizes in older subjects have not been performed.

Diseases of the Esophagus

Pharyngeal (Zenker's) diverticulum occurs most commonly in the elderly and consists of a herniation of the pharyngeal mucosa through the posterior pharyngeal wall between the oblique fibers of the inferior constrictor muscles and the transverse muscles of the cricopharyngeus. Premature closure of the cricopharyngeal muscle may generate higher than normal pharyngeal pressure. Zenker's diverticulum presents as dysphagia, regurgitation and pulmonary aspiration, or a mass in the neck. The diagnosis is readily made radiographically, using anteroposterior and lateral views of the lower pharynx. Endoscopy must be performed with great care to avoid perforation. Treatment of Zenker's diverticulum should include evaluation and treatment of cricopharyngeal function and surgical management of the primary diverticulum.[76] Endoscopic resection of the wall of the diverticulum has been advocated for elderly patients at high risk for surgical intervention or for recurrence after surgical treatment.[77]

Cricopharyngeal achalasia (i.e., abnormal or delayed relaxation of the upper esophageal sphincter without Zenker's diverticulum) also is found in the elderly.[78] A prominent posterior cricopharyngeal bar may be seen at barium swallow whether or not dysphagia is present.

Clinical reports and experimental studies show that pills can lodge in the esophagus and produce serious esophageal injury.[79,80] Drug-induced esophageal injury formerly was believed to occur only when large numbers of drugs were taken in suicide attempts or when underlying esophageal pathology was present. Pre-existing esophageal compression (e.g., due to valvular heart disease) can impair oropharyngeal transit and increase the chance of pill-induced esophageal injury, but most patients have no overt changes in esophageal anatomy or in function. Factors that can increase esophageal injury include the position of the patient on swallowing, the density, size, shape, and chemical composition of the medication,[81] and the volume of the fluid chaser taken with the medicine. Older patients who take medications before retiring are at particular risk since salivation and swallowing are less during sleep. Esophageal injury occurs with drugs (Table 45-4) that dissolve rapidly, resulting in high drug concentrations and an excessive pH that also may cause contact ulceration of the buccal mucosa.[82] Retention of pills occurs usually in the distal esophagus,[83] but pill-induced esophageal damage may be found higher.[81] Whether the changes in esophageal contractions that are found in the over-70 age group may enhance the frequency of pill esophagitis still is not completely clear. The management of pill esophagitis is discussed in Chapter 58.

TABLE 45-4
Drugs Associated With Esophageal Injury

Doxycycline hydrate

Tetracycline hydrochloride

Clindamycin

Emepromium bromide

Potassium chloride

Ferrous sulfate or succinate

Alprenolol chloride

Quinidine

Acetylsalicylic acid

Sustained-release theophylline

Modified from Carlborg B, Densert O. Esophageal lesions caused by orally administered drugs: an experimental study in the cat. Eur Surg Res 1980;12:270; and Kirkendall JW, Friedman AC, Oyewole MA, et al. Pill-induced esophageal injury: case reports and review of the medical literature. Dig Dis Sci 1983;28:174.

Carcinoma of the esophagus increases in frequency with advanced age with a peak frequency at 80 years of age. Esophageal carcinoma may be associated with alcoholism, Barrett's esophagus, reflux esophagitis, lye strictures, and achalasia.

PEPTIC DISEASE AND DISORDERS OF THE STOMACH (SEE ALSO CH 61)

The incidence of peptic ulcer disease and its complications in the elderly is rising throughout the world. In the United States, 80% of peptic ulcer-related deaths in 1984 occurred in the over-65 age group.[2] Surgery for the complications of peptic ulcer disease occurs mostly in the elderly.[84] Furthermore, the sex ratio for peptic disease also has changed. Whereas peptic ulcers occurred over twofold more commonly in men in 1965,[85] gastric ulcer in 1982 occurred with equal frequency in the two sexes, and disease in elderly women is particularly common.

Several factors may be important for greater peptic ulcer incidence in the elderly. The increase in life expectancy and in the numbers of the elderly is one factor. Clinical practitioners may be more aware of ulcer disease in the elderly, and fewer diagnostic errors may be made with the more extensive use of endoscopy. Smoking and poor nutrition also may contribute.[86] The increasing use of nonsteroidal anti-inflammatory drugs (NSAIDs) appears to be an important risk factor.[87,88] Finally, epidemiologic trends would suggest that cohort factors also may play a role.[89]

Changes in Gastric Physiology With Age

Gastric acid secretion probably does not change as a function of age. Approximately 75% of older, healthy persons retain gastric hydrogen ion secretion at rates similar to the young.[90] Only about 25% show acid hyposecretion, which is not due to an age-related change in the parietal cell but to the presence of atrophic gastritis.[91] There presently is no evidence for a decline in mucus gel strength with increasing age.[92] The gastric acid–secreting area in patients with duodenal ulcer disease older than the age of 60 does not differ significantly from that in the under-40 age group.[93] Therefore, therapeutic approaches that rely on reducing gastric acid secretion should aim to attain similar concentrations of drugs at the parietal cell in elderly and younger patients. The relative efficacy of the H_2 blockers in reducing acid secretion at differing ages is not clear. One study demonstrated no difference in the 24-hour gastric pH profile of young and elderly healthy volunteers and similar responses to cimetidine.[94] Intrinsic factor secretion usually is maintained into advanced age except in the presence of atrophic gastritis. Even when gastric atrophy develops, intrinsic factor secretion is retained longer than either acid or pepsin secretion. Gastric emptying rate for solids in healthy, elderly volunteers is unaltered,[95] although that for fluids may be prolonged.[96]

The symptoms associated with peptic ulcer disease in the elderly are more variable and subtle than in the young so that greater awareness of the disease is needed. Classic burning epigastric pain, temporal features related to food intake, and radiation of ulcer pain frequently are distorted or not present. The patient may complain of vague discomfort that is poorly localized and radiates inconsistently.[97] Precordial chest pain frequently may mimic angina and can cause clinical confusion. Anorexia and vague postprandial discomfort may be the sole presenting symptoms, and weight loss may be profound. In the older patient, active peptic ulcer disease frequently either is asymptomatic or painless. No abdominal pain was found in one-third of peptic ulcer patients admitted to a British hospital.[98] Thus, the "older" patient often has a complication as the initial presentation of a peptic ulcer. Because clinical features of complications also are muted, delayed diagnosis and increased morbidity and mortality result (Table 45-5).

The clinical features of a gastric ulcer in older patients can be quite bizarre[43] and frequently are characterized by severe weight loss and vague abdominal discomfort. The gastric ulcer has a more proximal location, often near the cardia.[99] The intrathoracic gastric ulcer, located in a hiatus hernia, may cause very atypical chest pain. Giant gastric ulcers (ulcers larger than 2.5 cm in diameter) occur more frequently in older patients and are difficult to differentiate from carcinoma. Fiberoptic endoscopy is the diagnostic modality of choice because the older patient must be investigated

intensively and the procedure is safe and has a greater sensitivity and specificity than the double contrast barium meal.[100]

Peptic ulcer complications are common, and the overall outcome is correlated with patient age. Over one-third of patients with peptic ulcer complications older than age 80 die.[101] Most acute upper gastrointestinal tract bleeding stops spontaneously, and there is no evidence that elderly patients bleed more severely or less often stop bleeding spontaneously than younger subjects; however, rigorous studies have not been performed. Rebleeding may occur more frequently in elderly patients.[102,103] The blood urea nitrogen level may rise more steeply in the bleeding elderly patient, hypotension may be more severe in the presence of concomitant antihypertensive therapy, and intravenous fluid replacement is tolerated less well. The mortality rate for acute peptic ulcer perforation is high[101] and is directly related to the presence of concomitant illnesses[104] and the speed with which a diagnosis is made and surgical intervention is possible.

Management

Antacids, the previous mainstay of peptic ulcer treatment, are not tolerated well in the older patient, even though the elderly consume large quantities of over-the-counter soluble and nonabsorbable antacids,[105,106] usually to reduce defecatory symptoms and not to relieve peptic pain. Diarrhea and colonic symptoms often accompany antacid use, and prolonged antacids may result in severe bone changes.[107] Sucralfate, a nonabsorbable complex of sulfated sucrose and aluminum hydroxide, has been advocated as particularly useful in the treatment of peptic disease in the elderly. However, constipation occurs frequently in all age groups and this symptom is particularly troublesome to the elderly. Furthermore, the pills are very large and are difficult to swallow. Increased aluminum absorption occurs and may be a potential hazard for encephalopathy in the older patients with renal insufficiency. The older patient with peptic ulcer disease can be treated with standard H_2 blocker therapy as easily as the young. Most experience is with cimetidine and ranitidine; both agents are effective, and peptic ulcer healing occurs as rapidly in the elderly as in the young. Despite much clinical prejudice, there also is no evidence that complications from the H_2 blockers differ with age, particularly in ambulatory patients. Suggestions that cimetidine administration causes more complications in older patients probably result from the fact that this agent has been in use for a longer period than the newer H_2 blockers. Although cimetidine alters P450-associated hepatic enzymes in vitro, clinical problems associated with the use of this H_2 blocking drug are very uncommon. Indeed, increasing evidence has demonstrated that drug-drug interaction with the most studied H_2 blockers, cimetidine and ranitidine, occur with about the same frequency.

When surgery becomes necessary, several issues become evident. Because emergency surgery is particularly hazardous in the old, elective surgery is indicated whenever possible. Thus, predicting ulcer severity is crucial. Surgical mortality or morbidity is related to the number and severity of other diseases present in the patient. Lung disease increases morbidity owing to frequent postoperative complications.[104,108] Rapid postsurgical ambulation has reduced the incidence of pulmonary emboli. Long-term post-

TABLE 45-5

Factors Contributing to Delayed Therapy for Peptic Ulcer Complications in the Elderly

Perforation associated with less pain
   Hypochlorhydria abolishes early chemical peritonitis
   Pain perception reduced due to
      CNS disease
      Endogenous opioids
      Psychotropic medication and nonsteroidal anti-inflammatory drugs
      Depression
Decreased vomiting from gastric outlet obstruction
Physical signs of perforation muted and laboratory data less pronounced
Fear of complex medical care and its cost
Physician misinformation and attitudes

gastrectomy problems, such as diarrhea, are difficult to handle by the elderly.

The increasing problem of peptic ulcer disease in elderly patients relates in part to their frequent use of NSAIDs.[89,109] Epidemiologic evidence from Europe, and recently from the United States,[88] shows a direct relationship between NSAID use and mortality or complications from peptic ulcer disease. However, there is no evidence that the elderly intrinsically are more susceptible to NSAID-induced peptic disease than younger patients, but only that they use more of these agents. Elderly patients with bleeding ulcers use nonaspirin NSAID three to four times more often than hospitalized and community controls.[87] Sixty percent of older patients with major peptic complications were taking NSAIDs.[101] However, these serious ulcer complications only occur once in 6000 NSAID prescriptions[110] even if gastric erosions are common. Concomitant NSAID use complicates the recognition and evaluation of peptic ulcer disease in the old. Diagnosis is delayed because ulcer patients frequently are asymptomatic and initially present with complications. NSAID-associated peptic ulcers also present more commonly as anemia than as pain.[111]

Treatment of NSAID-associated ulcers also differs. If the NSAID can be stopped, healing of gastric and duodenal ulcers occurs rapidly at any age. A full-dose course of H_2 blocker therapy (i.e., 6 weeks for duodenal ulcer disease and 8 to 12 weeks for a gastric ulcer) is recommended and 70% to 90% heal.[112,113] If NSAID therapy is not restarted, maintenance therapy to prevent ulcer recurrence is unnecessary. If the NSAID therapy is continued, 70% to 90% of duodenal and gastric ulcers can heal with effective H_2 blocker therapy in 8 to 12 weeks.[113] H_2 blocker treatment can prevent recurrence, but the role of prophylactic therapy presently is unclear. Initial studies have shown that misoprostol produces significant dose-dependent protection from gastric ulcer disease during NSAID use for a 2- to 3-week period but does not protect against duodenal ulcers.[114] Misoprostol probably also will be useful in the management of patients with active peptic ulcer disease associated with NSAID therapy.

Hypochlorhydria

Hypochlorhydria, due to chronic atrophic gastritis, occurs most commonly in the elderly. Using the criteria of serum pepsinogen

TABLE 45–6
Course of Gastritis in the Elderly*

CHANGE	BODY MUCOSA		ANTRAL MUCOSA	
	No. Patients	%	No. Patients	%
Progression	19	18	11	10
Regression	10	9	23	22
No change	79	73	71	68
Total	108	100	105	100

* Changes in the degree of gastritis in 10 years of follow-up.
Adapted from Ihamaki T, Kekki M, Sippen P, Siurala M. The sequelae and course of chronic gastritis during a 30- to 34-year bioptic follow-up study. Scand J Gastroenterol 1985;20:485.

TABLE 45–7
Impaired Nutrient Absorption With Achlorhydria

Hematinics
  Inorganic iron[128]
  Nonheme food iron[129]
  Food bound vitamin B_{12}[132,133]
  Folic acid[136]
Calcium carbonate[138]
Vitamin B_6[137]
Macronutrients if bacterial overgrowth occurs

I and II concentrations,[115] 31.5% of free-living, healthy persons aged 60 to 99 years were found to have some degree of atrophic gastritis.[91] In Scandinavia, up to two-thirds of severely hypochlorhydric older subjects were found to have pernicious anemia. The development of gastritis has been evaluated over a 30-year period[116] and mucosal inflammation progressed in half the cases (and regressed in 11%), but little progression was seen in the elderly (Table 45-6). No subject over age 60 with a normal gastric mucosa or superficial gastritis showed atrophic gastritis 10 years later. Gastric polyps develop in atrophic gastritis patients, but the long-term gastric cancer risk is only three to four times that of the population at large.[117] The risk of developing gastric cancer with achlorhydria is low[118] even if pernicious anemia with gastric mucosal dysplasia is present.[119,120]

A low intragastric pH is a major defense mechanism for the gut, and bacteria introduced into the stomach usually are destroyed within 15 minutes at a pH of 3.0 or below.[121] Gastric hypochlorhydria increases the pH of the proximal intestine[122] and predisposes to infection with typhoid and nontyphoid salmonellosis, cholera, giardiasis[123] and, perhaps, *Clostridium difficile* infection, leading to pseudomembranous colitis.[124] The relevance of these observations to the management of the elderly is not clear. Severe illness from salmonellosis is encountered more frequently with hypochlorhydria,[125] and *C. difficile* may be endemic in chronic care facilities.[126] It is conceivable that *Campylobacter pylori* infection of the stomach increases the risk of achlorhydria because epidemic hypochlorhydria occurs with this organism[127] and the prevalence of gastric *C. pylori* infection increases steadily with age.[128] Atrophic gastritis also occurs much more commonly in the elderly, and it is possible that *C. pylori* infection may be responsible.[129]

Malabsorption of several nutrients can occur with hypochlorhydria[130] (Table 45-7). For example, hydrochloric acid increases the absorption of ferric iron[131] and nonheme food iron[132] in achlorhydric subjects. Iron deficiency also occurs in treated pernicious anemia patients.[133] Food-bound vitamin B_{12} absorption falls with spontaneous[134] or drug-induced[135,136] hypochlorhydria. The potential role of food-bound vitamin B_{12} malabsorption in reducing serum vitamin B_{12} levels in healthy, elderly subjects presently is unclear.

Raising intraluminal pH reduces folic acid absorption[137] and feeding hydrochloric acid normalizes absorption in elderly subjects with achlorhydria.[138] However, such achlorhydric, atrophic gastritis patients may have higher than normal serum folate levels. The excessive numbers of bacteria in the proximal intestine lumen in these subjects produce enough folate to more than compensate for the dietary folate malabsorption. Vitamin B_6[139] and calcium carbonate[140] absorption also can fall in the absence of gastric hydrochloric acid. The absorption of trace metals such as copper also may be less.[141] The increase in gastrointestinal organisms also potentially produces malabsorption of dietary nutrients.

INTESTINAL ABSORPTION AND DISORDERS OF MALABSORPTION (SEE ALSO CH 38)

Physiologic Considerations

Intestinal absorption overall does not fall with age even if modest changes in digestive enzyme secretion and specific nutrient absorption can be detected. The anatomy of the human proximal intestinal epithelium in healthy elderly volunteers does not differ from the young.[142] Therefore, changes in villus architecture in the upper intestine of an elderly patient indicate gut disease and do not reflect the aging process. Pancreatic volume may diminish in the elderly,[143] although this is not universally found.[144] Dilatation of interlobular and intralobular ducts[145] may complicate interpretation of radiographs during endoscopic retrograde cholangiopancreatography. Fibrotic changes in the pancreas have been described at autopsy, although these may reflect nutritional factors and not aging.

There is little evidence for a reduction in basal or stimulated exocrine pancreatic secretion simply resulting from age and unassociated with disease, undernutrition, or medications. Enzyme secretion from the salivary glands, complementary organs, does not fall because of advanced age.[62] Although controversial,[146] a comparison of 61- to 78-year olds with younger controls showed no age-related differences in pancreatic trypsin, chymotrypsin, or lipase secretion following maximum doses of secretin and cerulein.[147-149] Because only 10% to 20% of maximal pancreatic enzyme output is needed for normal digestive capacity, modest changes in the pancreas are not likely to be functionally important.

There also is little evidence for any general age-associated changes in intestinal absorption. Human fecal fat excretion is no greater in the elderly than in the young with a diet containing approximately 100 g of fat per day.[150] One fragmentary study suggests that fecal fat excretion increases modestly if the dietary load of fat is increased.[151] However, undernourished elderly patients have been given up to 400 g of fat in a formula without inducing steatorrhea.[152] Earlier studies found lower chylomicron responses to standard meals,[153] but this method of evaluating lipid absorption depends on the production and turnover rate of intestinal lipoproteins and is indirect and inaccurate. Because of the simplicity of measuring xylose in the blood and urine, many xylose tolerance studies have been reported. Reduced urinary xylose excretion after standard oral xylose loads in older patients initially was misinterpreted as representing impaired absorption instead of reflecting changes in renal function, which occur so frequently in the healthy elderly.[154] More sophisticated studies, using combinations of oral and intravenous xylose, suggest that xylose absorption capacity does not fall significantly in healthy elderly subjects before the age of 80 but after this age they may be modestly reduced.[155] A reduction in carbohydrate absorptive capacity in

healthy, elderly volunteers has been detected when breath hydrogen excretion tests were used.[156]

Human calcium absorption falls in elderly men and women[157,158] because renal production of 1,25-hydroxycholecalciferol is reduced, lowering serum concentrations,[159] or the intestinal responsiveness to the circulating dihydroxycholecalciferol hormone is impaired.[160] Whether reduced calcium absorption contributes to senile osteoporosis is unclear. Some have recommended that dietary calcium intake should be higher in the elderly than in the young[161] or that supplemental vitamin D compound should be administered in order to reduce the bone calcium loss.[162] A contributing intestinal factor to lower total-body calcium is lactose intolerance as a consequence of intestinal mucosal lactase deficiency, which can lead to reduced dietary milk and dairy product ingestion. Finally, malabsorption of food-based vitamin B_{12} may occur in hypochlorhydric elderly subjects, resulting in inapparent vitamin B_{12} depletion.[163] The weight of these physiologic data suggests that, when malabsorption is detected in older persons, it is caused by disease and not by the effects of aging.

Clinical Malabsorption Syndromes

What are the diseases of malabsorption that occur in the elderly? The spectrum of diagnoses found in patients over the age of 65, referred to a specialist-consultant service in London, demonstrated that as many as 44% of patients had pancreatic disease and 25% had celiac sprue.[164] Thirty percent of nursing home residents showed "malabsorption," of whom two-thirds were anemic,[165] and these patients demonstrated multiple intestinal diverticula, had undergone gastrectomy or had a "malabsorption" pattern evident radiographically. Pancreatic insufficiency, small bowel diverticulosis, gastrectomy surgery, celiac sprue, intestinal strictures, or changes in bowel motility were found in another study of the elderly.[166] As many as 22% of patients with clear evidence of malabsorption had an anatomically normal small bowel.

These surveys of malabsorption in elderly patients indicate that pancreatic insufficiency is often present in the absence of a previous history. In one study, three-fourths of patients with chronic pancreatitis of unknown etiology were elderly[167] and vascular insufficiency was stated to be responsible.[168] Pancreatic calcification and exocrine failure of unknown etiology also occur in elderly Japanese.[169] Sarles and his group believe that chronic primary inflammatory pancreatitis—a condition characterized by mild recurrent abdominal pain, hypergammaglobulinemia leading to weight loss, pancreatic calcification, and recurrent fever—occurs in elderly women.[146] Because the pancreatic reserve for enzyme secretion is so large, the manifestations of malabsorption due to modest pancreatic enzyme deficiency are so subtle, and pancreatic insufficiency is so difficult to diagnose without complex and invasive diagnostic tests, the true extent of pancreatic insufficiency in the old is unknown.

The prevalence of celiac (nontropical) sprue in older patients is much greater than once was believed (see also ch. 71). Recent reports show that between one-fourth and one-third of newly diagnosed patients with sprue are older than 60.[35,170-172] Previously diagnosed sprue patients also are growing older,[173] and the need for surveillance of these patients is not known. Studies of younger celiac patients who have been treated with a "gluten-free diet" for a prolonged period have shown that intestinal architecture usually is distorted[174] and that modest malabsorption may be present.[175] Reduced serum folate levels suggest the presence of subclinical malabsorption.[176] It seems prudent to reevaluate the nutritional state and intestinal structure of older patients with a history of sprue at a younger age.

The clinical presentation of sprue in elderly patients differs considerably from that in the young. Only 25% of newly diagnosed sprue patients have diarrhea and weight loss as a principal feature.[35] Many older patients present with vague symptoms of dyspepsia and ill health. An unexpected hematologic finding in older patients, such as a low serum folate concentration, should suggest the possibility of sprue.[173,177] More elderly than younger patients appear to have clinical syndromes that result from micronutrient malabsorption, such as unusually severe osteopenia and osteomalacia, or a bleeding disorder due to hypoprothrombinemia. The frequency of making a diagnosis of sprue in the elderly is directly related to how often intestinal biopsies are performed.[35,178] Overall, elderly patients with malabsorption of any cause have clinical presentations that are much more subtle than those seen in the young. It is also possible that celiac disease behaves differently in the elderly. Lymphoma of the small intestine may be particularly common when celiac disease appears late in life.[179] The recorded incidence of differing malignancies among patients with sprue ranges from 11% to 14% and appears to increase the longer the duration of clinical follow-up. In addition to an increased incidence of malignancies, elderly patients with the histologic features of sprue may develop diffuse intestinal ulceration, which may be difficult to distinguish from classic celiac disease.[180] Ulceration can appear as a complication of untreated celiac disease that does not resolve even when patients are managed with a strict gluten-free diet. Splenic atrophy, associated with cavitation of mesenteric lymph nodes and accompanied by atrophy of the upper intestinal mucosa, occurs in older patients and occasionally responds to a gluten-free diet. Rarely, an elderly patient with celiac sprue will develop subacute intestinal pseudo-obstruction.[181] Older patients with sprue require intensive dietary training sessions to adjust to a gluten-free diet and need very close supervision to reduce the prevalence of micronutrient deficiencies.

Chronic intestinal vascular disease, causing abdominal pain and/or malabsorption, occurs rarely in the elderly. A syndrome of abdominal pain and malabsorption in association with vascular occlusion of mesenteric arteries, reversed after vascular surgery, has been reported in a few patients.[182] However, only one-fourth of patients with a diagnosis of possible chronic intestinal arterial occlusion were found to have potential clinical problems associated with vascular disease.[4] Symptoms were not related to the extent of mesenteric arterial occlusion determined radiographically. Only 2% were found to have steatorrhea and 2% had evidence of exudative enteropathy. Overall, one must conclude that vascular disease very rarely causes an overt clinical syndrome of malabsorption.

Bacterial Overgrowth Syndromes

Bacterial overgrowth syndrome can occur in elderly patients who are suspected of having malabsorption (see ch 73). Some have evidence of anatomic changes in the proximal small intestine, resulting in stasis of intestinal contents, such as small intestinal strictures, partial intestinal obstruction from Crohn's disease, postgastrectomy states, or multiple upper intestinal diverticulosis. The prevalence of upper intestinal diverticulosis increases greatly in the elderly.[183] In the duodenum, single very large diverticula may be present. Multiple diverticula also are present in the remaining small bowel and particularly in the upper jejunum. Small bowel diverticula occasionally may produce overt gastrointestinal symptoms because of local complications such as diverticular perforation, hemorrhage, enterolith formation, or entrapment. More commonly, the symptoms are due to intestinal bacterial overgrowth, so that only vitamin B_{12} malabsorption with anemia or hypoalbuminemia may be present.[184,185] However, most multiple intestinal diverticulosis does not result in symptoms or in bacterial overgrowth.[186]

A unique syndrome that appears to be restricted to the elderly is bacterial overgrowth without the presence of anatomic abnormality that should cause upper intestinal stasis. This usually is diagnosed by ^{14}C-cholylglycine breath testing, and treatment with antibiotics often results in clinical improvement.[187] Some patients with bacterial overgrowth have shown vitamin B_{12} deficiency.[166]

Thus, a proportion of older persons without gastrointestinal symptoms, but with clinical features indicating impaired nutrition, may have evidence of intestinal bacterial overgrowth. The frequency of bacterial overgrowth, demonstrated by the ^{14}C-cholylglycine breath test in the general population of the elderly, is uncertain. How frequently bacterial overgrowth is associated with evidence of nutritional deficits also is unknown. Further studies to elucidate the frequency and importance of such upper intestinal bacterial overgrowth in elderly patients are needed.

What may be the mechanism for such bacterial overgrowth in the absence of upper intestinal anatomic changes? The elderly patient may be achlorhydric or show modest changes in gut motility that alter the strength of postprandial intestinal contractions, but the available data on intestinal motility in patients with bacterial overgrowth are insufficient to permit conclusions. Intestinal factors that interfere with bacterial growth, such as lysozyme and immunoglobulin A secretion, also may play a role in such patients with intestinal bacterial overgrowth.

CONSTIPATION (SEE ALSO CH 39)

Most healthy, elderly patients living at home have normal bowel function[188] even though they commonly describe constipation.[189]

TABLE 45–8
Organic Causes of Constipation in the Elderly

MECHANISM	EXAMPLES
Obstruction	Tumors
Neuromuscular disorders	Parkinsonism
	Laxative colon
Endocrine disorders	Hypothyroidism
	Hypoparathyroidism
	Diabetes mellitus
Depression	

Normal bowel habits are found far less commonly in patients living in nursing homes or in chronic care hospitals.[190] Constipation frequently is defined by the elderly as painful, difficult, or incomplete evacuation and not by the number of bowel movements,[191] and antacids[105,106] or cathartics are used chronically for relief. Older persons who complain of constipation or alternating constipation and diarrhea often have had these symptoms for many years. The problem may simply become more evident in an older retired person who has more time to dwell on his infirmities. Indeed, when an elderly person develops constipation for the first time later in adult life, a careful evaluation to exclude systemic or obstructing disorders is mandatory (Table 45-8).

Physiologic Changes

Bowel transit, measured with radiopaque markers, does not differ between healthy younger and older subjects.[192] However, some delay in the rectal evacuation is found in many elderly patients who complain of constipation. Intestinal transit time also does not differ in constipated and nonconstipated geriatric patients.[193] Asymptomatic older volunteers also have normal small bowel transit time,[194] but this is delayed in elderly nursing home patients with a long history of bowel disturbances.[195] A common cause of altered gastrointestinal transit time and constipation is concomitant drug ingestion, which may be responsible for prolonged transit time in Parkinson's syndrome.[196]

Although colonic transit to the rectum may be normal, some elderly persons then cannot evacuate easily. A reduction in rectal wall elasticity can result in an increase in maximal tolerable volume and a relatively high rectal pressure.[197] Rectal sensitivity to distention may be less in constipated than in nonconstipated older patients.[198] The rectum may need to be distended with a larger volume of fluid in older patients who have had fecal impaction before the presence of a rectal balloon, pain, and the desire to defecate are perceived and before rectal contractions occur.[199] Rectal pressures also may be lower in such patients than in the young. These data imply that fecal impaction is related to a blunting in rectal sensation and suggest that neuropathic damage is present. Abnormalities of colonic ganglia cells also occur.[200]

Clinical Complications

The colon of elderly patients with chronic constipation may become massively dilated. This condition of "megacolon" usually is thought to represent an atonic colon that develops after prolonged disregard of the urge to defecate. It is particularly common in patients in chronic care nursing facilities with psychiatric disorders who are taking psychotropic medications, in patients with Parkinson's disease, and in patients with organic mental syndromes.[201] The elderly also are particularly predisposed to develop cecal volvulus.[202] Three clinical syndromes of cecal volvulus have been described: (1) an acute, fulminating type associated with gangrene and a high mortality; (2) an acute obstructing type presenting with pain and distention; and (3) a chronic recurring type featuring colicky abdominal pain. Acute fulminating volvulus usually presents as acute abdominal pain of less than 24 hours' duration and evidence of imminent perforation. In some patients, pain may last as long as a week or a history of recurrent chronic abdominal pain of many months duration can be obtained. Abdominal radiographs usually show small and large bowel obstruction. Classic radiologic features of cecal volvulus are found in less than one-half of the patients.[203] Sigmoid volvulus also may have an acute fulminating presentation owing to early occlusion of mesenteric vessels or subacute clinical features characterized by gradual progression of colicky abdominal pain and distention.[204] This diagnosis can only be made if the physician maintains a high index of suspicion, particularly in elderly, institutionalized patients who may have organic mental syndromes and depression and may not report accurately the development of chronic abdominal pain or even an acute abdominal catastrophe.

Surgical intervention remains the standard treatment of patients with colonic volvulus. When peritoneal signs are present, immediate laparotomy and colonic resection are needed. However, preoperative patient management with gastrointestinal suction and intravenous fluid replenishment[205] now can be complemented by colonoscopy, which is used to decompress colonic distention[206] as an interim approach in a patient whose clinical condition does not warrant emergency surgery. Some authors have suggested that colonoscopic decompression may be a definitive treatment, but long-term results have not been reported. Because a cecal volvulus tends to be recurrent and surgical resection is curative,[207] the principal role of successful colonoscopic decompression is to convert an acute emergency into more elective colon surgery.[208]

The management of constipation in the elderly must take into account contributing factors that might be present (Table 45-9). Initially, increasing fiber intake by providing unprocessed bran or cereals high in bran can be effective.[209,210] Fluid supplementation, particularly in incontinent patients, is important. Lactulose syrup can be used to treat chronic constipation in the elderly and may be helpful as long as it is introduced slowly and does not increase bloating.[211] Osmotic and irritant cathartics must be introduced carefully to avoid habituation. When simple measures do not work, then pelvic floor incoordination should be sought.

Fecal incontinence is one of the most common and disabling gastrointestinal symptoms that occur in the elderly. The majority of older patients who have diarrhea have some fecal incontinence whether the diarrhea is due to the irritable bowel syndrome or to inflammatory bowel disease,[212] and many patients do not admit to this symptom unless asked directly. In nursing homes, incontinence is common in the bedridden. Incontinence may follow rectal prolapse, perhaps due to denervation of the muscles of the anorectal sling and changes in anal sphincter tone.[213] Surgical reconstruction of the anorectal angle can be an effective treatment.[214]

TABLE 45-9
Contributory Factors to Constipation in the Elderly

Decreased food intake

Decreased fluid intake

Lack of bulk in the diet

Abuse of laxatives

Decreased defecatory sensation

Medications including sedatives, tranquilizers, antihypertensive and ganglion-blocking agents, narcotics, and calcium-containing antacids

Tests of motor function in patients with idiopathic fecal incontinence may show pelvic floor motor neuropathy.[215] External anal sphincter fiber density also may be significantly increased.[215] In fact, many patients with fecal incontinence have a background of fecal impaction and they may present clinically with so-called overflow incontinence, probably due to an obtuse anorectal angle and low anal pressures.[216] In some persons, relative ischemia of the rectum may be responsible.[217] Biofeedback retraining of the external anal sphincter, initially used to treat incontinent children and young patients with spinal cord injuries, now has been successfully appled in a limited manner to the treatment of fecal incontinence in the elderly.[218] Unfortunately, the technique is operator intensive and cannot be applied to the very common problem of fecal incontinence in the bed-bound elderly.

DIARRHEA

Diarrhea is not recognized as a common gastrointestinal problem in the elderly. Diarrhea, due to the irritable bowel syndrome or Crohn's disease, may have been present for many years; however, diarrhea also may occur as a new symptom in the older age group. It may result as a medication side effect or may occur from cathartic abuse. In nursing homes, diarrhea frequently is due to fecal impaction, but intestinal infection with hemorrhagic *Escherichia coli* or with *Clostridium difficile*[126] may be responsible. *C. difficile* infection may cause sufficient protein-losing enteropathy to produce hypoalbuminemia.[219]

INFLAMMATORY BOWEL DISEASE (SEE ALSO CH 77)

Inflammatory bowel disease is more common in the elderly than generally is recognized. Epidemiologic studies of Mendeloff and co-workers from the United States demonstrate a peak incidence of ulcerative colitis between the ages of 20 and 29 and another peak over the age of 70[220] and a trimodal distribution in Crohn's disease. In other parts of the world, a secondary peak of Crohn's disease occurred at around age 70.[221-223] Two-thirds of older patients with Crohn's disease are women who show predominantly colonic involvement,[224] often left-sided segmental colitis with a distribution similar to that found in diverticular disease. Some have suggested that the majority of elderly patients who are diagnosed as having inflammatory bowel disease involving the colon might be suffering from obliterative mesenteric vascular disease,[225,226] but this view is not widely accepted. On the other hand, many of the radiologic and pathologic criteria that are considered characteristic of ulcerative, granulomatous and ischemic colitis do not readily permit clear separation of these diseases in the colon[227] (Table 45-10).

In general, the manifestations of ulcerative colitis in older patients do not differ from those encountered in younger persons. Ulcerative colitis restricted to the rectum and sigmoid colon occurs more commonly in the older age group, and many elderly patients

TABLE 45-10

Clinical, Histologic, and Radiologic Features Characteristic of Inflammatory Bowel Disease or Ischemic Disease in the Elderly

Ulcerative Colitis

Universal colonic involvement or toxic megacolon

Extraintestinal manifestation (e.g., pyoderma)

Pseudopolyposis

Inflammatory reaction limited to the mucosa

Numerous crypt abscesses separated from ulcers

Crohn's Disease

Small bowel involvement, fistula formation, and perianal disease

Skip lesions, cobblestoning

Intestinal obstruction

Extraintestinal manifestation (e.g., ankylosing spondylitis)

Noncaseating granulomas, fissuring

Ischemic Disease

Transmucosal polymorphonuclear cell infiltration

Concurrent extraintestinal ischemic disease or precipitating cardiovascular event

Submucosal hemorrhage or necrosis

Rapid resolution without recurrence (in absence of anti-inflammatory treatment) and thumbprinting that reverses to normal

Segmental colitis proximal to tumor

Hemosiderin-laden macrophages

Major intravascular fibrin-platelet thrombi

with Crohn's disease showed inflammatory changes that are confined to this area of the bowel.[36,228,229] Previous suggestions that elderly patients with inflammatory bowel disease had a worse prognosis[230] have been discounted by a large study, showing that most older patients with ulcerative colitis were symptom-free 1 year after the initial attack.[231] Surgery appears to be necessary in fewer older patients and total colonic involvement with ulcerative colitis occurs in only 12.3% of the over-60 age group compared with 26.5% of those younger than 60. The mortality rate is modestly increased (2.4% vs. 1% in ulcerative colitis) in those older than age 60. Colonic disease occurs more commonly in older Crohn's patients. These data clearly demonstrate major differences in the results of recently treated patients compared with those managed 2 decades ago.

The differential diagnosis of an older patient with possible inflammatory bowel disease is complicated. Crohn's disease involving the distal small bowel may be lymphoma or carcinoma. Such patients often present clinically with abdominal pain, weight loss, anemia, and hypoalbuminemia, so that most physicians will seek the presence of carcinomatosis.

The differential diagnosis of colonic inflammatory bowel disease is even more difficult and includes colonic ischemic bowel disease and diverticulitis. The former closely mimics Crohn's disease because pseudopolyps, crypt abscesses, and strictures can occur and even the histology may be indistinguishable (see Table 45-10).[232] If abdominal radiography shows classic "thumbprinting," indicative of localized intramural bleeding and edema, acute mesenteric vascular disease usually is responsible. Barium enema may show segmental involvement with ulceration or stricture formation. In some patients, the radiograph will show the appearance of toxic megacolon.[233] Characteristically, the radiologic features change quite rapidly after the initial attack of ischemic disease, whereas the findings in inflammatory bowel disease do not alter quickly. Fiberendoscopic examination also is difficult. Ischemic disease usually is localized and not diffuse and does not involve the rectum. Strictures may occur both in Crohn's disease and in vascular disease with overlying inflamed-appearing mucosa. Pseudopolyps may be seen in both disorders. Histologic examination is helpful if the characteristic granulomas of Crohn's disease are seen or if mucosal necrosis is associated with evidence of recent submucosal hemorrhage, hemosiderin-laden macrophages, and the presence of extensive intravascular fibrin in ischemic disease.[232] Histologic evidence of cecal involvement has been noted in approximately 60% of patients with primarily ileal Crohn's disease.

Another important differential diagnosis is between segmental colonic inflammatory bowel disease and diverticulitis. Thirty to 50% of elderly patients with Crohn's disease involving the colon also may have diverticular disease[234] and the diagnosis may not be made prior to surgery. Patients with both conditions have pain, diarrhea, internal fistulae, and an abdominal mass so that symptoms and complications of Crohn's disease may be ascribed to diverticulitis.[235,236] The presence of blood in the stools is more suggestive of Crohn's disease, particularly when small amounts are passed persistently. On physical examination, the presence of anal lesions, rectovaginal fistulae, and extraintestinal complications, such as erythema nodosum, pyoderma gangrenosa, finger clubbing, or arthritis, all suggest Crohn's disease. If sigmoidoscopy discloses proctitis, then inflammatory bowel disease usually is present and diverticulitis is unlikely, although, occasionally, some involvement of the rectal mucosa may occur with extensive diverticular inflammation. Radiologic differences in inflammatory bowel disease include involvement of the rectum and ulcerating lesions of a long segment of involved bowel.[237]

When acute colonic distention occurs in an elderly patient, this also poses important problems in differential diagnosis. Massive colonic distention (megacolon) in the elderly usually is due to paralytic colonic ileus, but the differential diagnosis includes acute infectious colitis, inflammatory bowel disease, and ischemic colitis with full-thickness colonic infarction. Angiography plays only a minor role in differential diagnosis, because many patients with documented ischemic colitis have normal visceral angiography and many others, without ischemic colonic disease, have obliteration of two or three vessels.[238]

Most complications described in younger patients with inflammatory bowel disease also can occur in the older age group. Systemic complications occur less frequently in the elderly,[239] which may permit more restrictive forms of surgical therapy to be performed. In addition, the long-term prognosis for inflammatory bowel disease in older patients may be different from that found in the young. One reason for a high mortality in the first attack of inflammatory bowel disease in the elderly in early reports is that the correct diagnosis was greatly delayed and, when surgery was performed, it was often done as an emergency and was associated with a high mortality. Older patients who survive the first attack of inflammatory bowel disease or who have early surgery for the disease appear to do better than younger patients.[231]

Because long-standing inflammatory bowel disease is accompanied by an increased risk of cancer and colon cancer increases in prevalence with age,[1] it is appropriate to ask whether the coincidence of ulcerative colitis or Crohn's disease with advancing age may interact to greatly increase the chance of cancer formation. There are no data available that have separated the possible effects of the age of the patient from the length of time that he has suffered from the disease before the development of the cancer. The original hypothesis that colon cancer and ulcerative colitis develop most commonly when the disease started in childhood has been discounted. Cancer risk in ulcerative colitis is greater with generalized colonic involvement and increases in parallel with the length of time that the patient has had the disease after the first decade.[240] In Crohn's disease, cancer begins to occur after 20 years of active Crohn's disease. The relative efficacy of medical therapy in treating inflammatory bowel disease has permitted more patients with ongoing chronic, nonspecific inflammatory bowel disease to reach an older age.

There are several important medical therapeutic considerations when treating an older patient with inflammatory bowel disease. Some drugs used in treating younger patients must be handled more carefully in the elderly. It is important for the physician to evaluate each modality of treatment separately in order to avoid falling into the trap of undertreating the old. Opiate-containing drugs should be used with great care in treating diarrhea in older patients. They may be relatively ineffective because the elderly have higher endogenous serum opioid concentrations than the young. In addition, the elderly must not be oversedated in order to avoid unsteadiness and consequent falls. Loperamide may have fewer central effects and therefore be tolerated more easily. Anticholinergics should be used as little as possible to avoid potential cardiac complications, mental changes, and excessive gastrointestinal hypomotility.

Sulfasalazine and the newer 5-aminosalicylic acid agents generally are tolerated well. Metronidazole can interfere with the oxidation of warfarin and thus might induce excessive anticoagulation during concomitant metronidazole and warfarin treatment. Monitoring of plasma prothrombin levels is recommended under these circumstances. Immunosuppressive agents, such as azathioprine and 6-mercaptopurine, also appear to be tolerated well in the elderly patient. Corticosteroids have a higher risk of complications. Osteopenia appears to be greatly exacerbated during chronic corticosteroid therapy and may result in vertebral compression and bone fractures. Hyperglycemia is more prominent and eye changes may be accelerated, resulting in posterior subcapsular cataracts and an increase in intraocular pressure. The behavioral changes that may accompany corticosteroid therapy may be difficult to diagnose in the elderly and may be confused with the manifestations of cerebrovascular disease.

No studies have specifically described an optimal approach to surgical treatment of inflammatory bowel disease in the elderly. When surgery for extensive colonic disease is necessary, sphincter-saving operations should be performed whenever possible. However, it is my impression that elderly patients tolerate colectomy and ileostomy better than the passage of many loose bowel movements per day through a preserved rectum. Unfortunately, the older patient with major cerebrovascular disease and dementia cannot manage either type of surgery and becomes bed-bound in a nursing home after such operations.

HEPATIC AND BILIARY DISEASE

Hepatic Disease

Liver structure and function change remarkably little with age, which led to the important decision to increase the age of persons willing to donate livers potentially useful for hepatic transplantation from 45 to older than 55 years. Liver weight falls in advanced age, in part as a function of a lower lean body mass and in part in proportion to a reduced blood supply.[30] Liver size demonstrates more variation in the elderly than in the young. Minor morphologic changes have been described,[241] and the rate of hepatic regeneration may be slightly delayed,[242] but regeneration, in the end, is as complete as in the young. No distinctive differences in liver function tests are found in the elderly. The use of three liver function tests was determined prospectively in 523 unselected geriatric patients.[243] Some abnormalities were found in 27%, which were clinically helpful in half of the cases. An elevated serum alkaline phosphatase concentration was due to bone disease, including osteomalacia in 50% and liver disease in 25%, and no diagnosis was established in only 25% of patients. An unexpected elevation of serum bilirubin concentration usually indicates the presence of congestive cardiac failure and increases in serum aspartate aminotransferase with changes in serum alkaline phosphatase and bilirubin values suggest hepatocellular damage. Thus, abnormalities in liver function tests in older patients are due to hepatic or systemic disease and not to the aging process.[244]

The clinical course of liver disease in the majority of elderly patients does not differ from that in the young. Hepatitis may be milder in the elderly,[245] but, when complications occur, they may have more severe results.[246] Hepatic transplantation is being performed more commonly in older patients with little more mortality from the surgery than in the young and with a similar postoperative course.[247]

Biliary Tract Disease (see also ch 95)

The prevalence of gallstones rises steadily with age. Approximately 35% of persons older than age 80 have stones, reflecting changes in biliary bile salt and lipid composition, bile salt turnover, or changes in gallbladder contraction. Secondary bile acids are increased and higher cholic acid fractional turnover rates are found.[248] The elderly have higher fecal concentrations of lithocholic and deoxycholic acids without changes in gastrointestinal transit rates.[249] The lithogenic index and the concentration of biliary cholesterol may be increased, suggesting that canalicular secretion of cholesterol increases with age.[250] Gallbladder contractions also may be less responsive to cholecystokinin in the elderly.[16]

Juxtapapillary duodenal diverticula are most common in the elderly. Up to 65% to 85% of these patients have gallstones,[251] and biliary cannulation frequently demonstrates choledocholithiasis.[252] Postcholecystectomy stones also are common, pigment stones may predominate,[253] and sphincter motor activity may be less.[254]

The most common presentation of gallstone disease in the elderly is acute cholecystitis and cholangitis. Cholecystitis may present as a nonspecific clinical picture[251] or even with vague mental or physical disability.[255] Biliary tract infection may have a clinical picture of hypotension secondary to gram-negative bacterial shock. Acalculous cholecystitis also occurs frequently, is clinically difficult to diagnose, and is associated with a greater morbidity and mortality than calculous cholecystitis.[256] Empyema of the gallbladder may occur more commonly in the old and has a very high mortality. Even empyema may be painless or the pain may be tolerated for a surprisingly long time before hospital admission is sought by elderly patients.[257]

Cholelithiasis may present clinically with acute pancreatitis in the elderly. In 1959, gallstone-associated pancreatitis had a mortality rate of 40% in patients more than 75 years of age,[258] but now is much less.[259] The usual scoring systems used to predict pancreatitis severity[260,261] are less accurate in those older than age 75 than in younger patients.[262]

Obstructive jaundice from choledocholithiasis occurs commonly in the elderly patient[263] and may present a difficult clinical differential diagnosis because obstructing carcinomas of the pancreas and biliary tree are far more common in this age group. However, the clinical picture of obstructive jaundice does not differ from that seen in younger patients and the approach to diagnosis is identical.

The most important diagnostic procedure that should be performed in a patient with the least suspicion of acute biliary infection is a blood culture.[264] Much of the mortality from this disease in the elderly results from the presence of unrecognized subclinical infection, and bacteremia may be the only sign of cholangitis.[265] The detection of gallstones is of little help because asymptomatic stones are so frequently found. Ultrasonography can readily demonstrate bile duct dilatation and may be useful in detecting localized abscesses around the gallbladder.[266] The diagnosis of biliary tract disease affecting the bile duct most readily is made by endoscopic retrograde cholangiography.

There is no evidence that asymptomatic gallstones should be treated in the elderly, because complications occur very uncommonly.[267,268] Moreover, the previously held suggestion that patients with diabetes mellitus found to have asymptomatic gallstones require cholecystectomy has been discounted.[269] On the other hand, the therapeutic options for the management of gallstone disease have greatly expanded and can be combined in treating elderly patients with biliary tract disease. Lithotripsy, combined with stone dissolution therapy, is being performed in patients with modestly symptomatic gallstones (see ch 136). Direct instillation of methyl tert-butyl ether into the gallbladder for gallstone dissolution also is used.[270] Oral gallstone dissolution therapy by itself has not proven as effective as was once hoped. The precise role of these therapies in elderly patients with gallstones, as well as their side effects, has not been established.

Surgery for biliary tract disease is the most common form of abdominal surgery performed in the elderly. However, the complications of gallbladder surgery, particularly when performed as an emergency, are considerable in the frail elderly.[271] Mortality rates of 10% to 20% and morbidity rates of 30% to 40% commonly have been reported.[272] The mortality of elective biliary tract surgery is only in the range of 1% to 3% with a morbidity rate of 10% to 20%.[273-275]

The use of transduodenal retrograde endoscopic cholangiography and endoscopic drainage and sphincterotomy is a major advance in the management of elderly patients with acute cholangitis. Because the systemic consequences of biliary tract infection are the greatest hazard for the older patient, drainage of the biliary tree by sphincterotomy or transnasal drainage has reduced mortality and morbidity in acute cholecystitis and cholangitis.[276,277] Even if definitive treatment by sphincterotomy is not possible at the time of the acute attack of cholangitis, decompression permits subsequent definitive endoscopic or surgical treatment for most patients.[263] There is no evidence that the risks of endoscopic treatment of gallstones increase with age.

A novel use of endoscopic sphincterotomy has been in the treatment of elderly patients with symptoms from gallstone disease without surgical removal of the gallbladder. Endoscopic sphincterotomy reduces the symptoms and complications in such patients. Fibrosis and restenosis of the sphincter occur quite uncommonly,[263,278] and the risk of developing cholecystitis following endoscopic sphincterotomy in the presence of stones in the gallbladder is less than 15%.[277] The advantages and disadvantages of sphincterotomy compared with surgical exploration have been demonstrated, but direct comparison is difficult, because the groups inevitably are not perfectly comparable.[279]

> The reader is directed to Chapter 54, Motility Disorders of the Esophagus; Chapter 77, Inflammatory Bowel Disease; Chapter 78, Colonic Polyps: Benign and Premalignant Neoplasms of the Colon; Chapter 82, Diverticulitis; Chapter 84, Malignant Tumors of the Colon; and Chapter 94, Gallstones.

REFERENCES

1. Cutler SJ, Young JL. Third national cancer survey. NCI Monographs, 1975; DHEW publication nos. 785, 786, and 787.
2. World Health Organization. World health statistics annual of 1986. Geneva: World Health Organization, 1987.
3. Brody JA, Schneider EL. Diseases and disorders of aging: an hypothesis. J Chron Dis 1986;39:871.
4. Marston A, Clarke JMF, Garcia JG, Miller AL. Intestinal function and intestinal blood supply: a 20-year surgical study. Gut 1985;26:656.
5. Almy T. Factors leading to digestive disorders in the elderly. Bull NY Acad Med 1981;57:709.
6. Holt PR, Yeh KY. Colonic proliferation is increased in senescent rats. Gastroenterology 1988;95:1556.
7. Holt PR, Yeh KY. Small intestinal crypt cell proliferation rates are increased in senescent rats. J Gerontol 1989;44:B9.
8. Roncucci L, Ponz de Leon M, Scalmati A, et al. The influence of age on colonic epithelial cell proliferation. Cancer 1988;62:1973.
9. Holt PR, Yeh K-Y, Kotler DP. Altered controls of proliferation in small intestine of the senescent rat. Proc Natl Acad Sci USA 1988;85:2771.
10. Lipkin M, Correa P, Mikol YB, et al. Proliferative and antigenic modifications in human epithelial cells in chronic atrophic gastritis. J NCI 1985;75:613.
11. Roth GS. Effects of aging on mechanisms of alpha-adrenergic and dopaminergic action. Fed Proc 1986;45:60.
12. Wang SY, Halban PA, Rowe JW. Effects of aging on insulin synthesis and secretion. J Clin Invest 1988;81:176.
13. Trudeau WL, McGuigan JE. Serum gastrin levels in patients with peptic ulcer disease. Gastroenterology 1970;59:6.
14. Holt PR, Yeh K-Y. Aging and gastrin production: changes in serum and antral gastrin concentrations in the rat. J Gerontol 1989;44:M62.
15. Rayford PL, Texter EC Jr. Brain–gut peptides. In: Texter EC Jr, ed. The aging gut: pathophysiology, diagnosis and management. New York: Masson Publishing USA, 1983:173.
16. Khalil T, Walker JP, Wiener I, et al. Effect of aging on gallbladder contraction and release of cholecystokinin-33 in humans. Surgery 1985;98:423.
17. Bonora G, Vezzadini P, Frada G, et al. Interdigestive plasma motilin concentrations in aged adults. J Gerontol 1986;41:723.
18. Goidl EA. Aging and the immune response: cellular and humoral aspects. New York: Marcel Dekker, 1987.
19. Fulop T, Foris G, Worum I, et al. Age-related variations of some polymorphonuclear leukocyte functions. Mech Ageing Dev 1985;29:1.
20. Kawanishi H, Kiely J. Immune-related alterations in aged gut-associated lymphoid tissues in mice. Dig Dis Sci 1989;34:175.
21. Ouslander JG. Drug therapy in the elderly. Ann Intern Med 1981;95:711.
22. Lamy PP. Prescribing for the elderly. Littleton, MA: PSG Publishing Co, 1980.
23. Williamson J, Chopin JM. Adverse reactions to prescribed drugs in the elderly: a multicentre investigation. Age Ageing 1980;9:73.
24. Lakemedels Biverknings Kommitten. Report, January 1985. Uppsala, Sweden: National Board of Health and Welfare, 1985.
25. Holt PR. Gastrointestinal drugs in the elderly. Am J Gastroenterol 1986;81:403.
26. Greenblatt DJ, Sellers EM, Shader RI. Drug disposition in old age. N Engl J Med 1982;306:1081.
27. Weiner R, Dietze F, Laue R. Age-dependent alterations of intestinal absorption: II. A clinical study using a modified D-xylose absorption test. Arch Gerontol Geriatr 1984;3:97.
28. Rowe SE, Andres R, Tobin JD, et al. The effect of age on creatinine clearance in man: a cross-sectional and longitudinal study. J Gerontol 1976;31:155.
29. Sherlock S, Bearn AG, Billing BH, Patterson JGS. Splanchnic blood flow in man by the bromsulfalein method: the relation of peripheral plasma bromsulfalein level to the calculated flow. J Lab Clin Med 1950;35:923.
30. Wynne HA, Cope LH, Mutch E, et al. The effect of age upon liver volume and apparent liver blood flow in healthy man. Hepatology 1989;9:297.
31. Klotz U, Wilkenson GR. Hepatic elimination of drugs in the elderly. In: Kitani K, ed. The liver and aging. Amsterdam: Elsevier North-Holland, 1978:367.
32. Schmucker DL, Vessey DA, Wang RK, Maloney AG. Does aging compromise hepatic microsomal mono-oxygenase activity? In: Bianchi L, Holt P, James OFW, Butler RN, eds. Aging in liver and gastro-intestinal tract. Lancaster, UK: MTP Press, 1988:241.
33. James O, Rawoins M, Woodhouse K. Lack of aging effect on human microsomal monooxygenase enzyme activities and on inactivation pathways for reactive metabolic intermediates. In: Kitani K, ed: The liver and aging. Amsterdam: Elsevier North-Holland, 1982:395.
34. Fevery J. Class II reactions in aging. In: Bianchi L, Holt P, James OFW, Butler RN, eds. Aging in liver and gastro-intestinal tract. Lancaster, UK: MTP Press, 1988:267.
35. Swinson CM, Levi AJ. Is coeliac disease underdiagnosed? Br Med J 1980;281:1258.
36. Carr N, Schofield PF. Inflammatory bowel disease in the older patient. Br J Surg 1982;69:223.
37. Philips SL, Burns GP. Acute abdominal disease in the aged. Med Clin North Am 1988;72:1213.
38. Telfer S, Fenyo G, Holt PR, de Dombal FT. Acute abdominal pain in patients over 50 years of age. Scand J Gastroenterol 1988;23:47.
39. Oliver N. Abdominal pain in the elderly. Aust Fam Physician 1984;13:402.
40. Hangos G, Thurzo R. Appendicitis in the aged. Gerontol Clin 1961;3:55.
41. Arnbjornsson E. Recognizing appendicitis in the elderly. Geriatr Med Today 1984;3:72.
42. Arnbjornsson E, Adren-Sandberg A, Bengmark S. Appendicectomy

in the elderly: incidence and operative findings. Ann Chir Gynaecol 1983;72:223.

43. Narayanan M, Steinheber FU. The changing face of peptic ulcer in the elderly. Med Clin North Am 1976;60:1159.
44. Freedman ML, Marcus DL. Anemia and the elderly: is it physiology or pathology? Am J Med Sci 1980;280:81.
45. Zauber NP, Zauber AG. Hematologic data of healthy very old people. JAMA 1987;257:2181.
46. Lindsay DC, Freeman JG, Cobden I, Record CO. Should colonoscopy be the first investigation for colonic disease? Br Med J 1988;296:167.
47. Cobden I. Colonoscopy in the elderly patient. Geriatr Med Today 1988;7:32.
48. Lockhart SP, Schofield PM, Gribble RJN, Baron JH. Upper gastrointestinal endoscopy in the elderly. Br Med J 1985;290:283.
49. Cooper BT, Neuman CS. Upper gastrointestinal endoscopy in patients aged 80 years or more. Age Ageing 1986;15:343.
50. Cooper BT, Weston CFM, Neumann CS. Acute upper gastrointestinal hemorrhage. Q J Med 1988;69:765.
51. Booker JA. Haematemesis and melaena in the elderly. Age Ageing 1983;12:49.
52. Antler AS, Pitchumoni CS, Thomas E, et al. Gastrointestinal bleeding in the elderly: morbidity, mortality and cause. Am J Surg 1981;142:271.
53. Boley SJ, DiBiase A, Brandt LJ, Sammartano RJ. Lower intestinal bleeding in the elderly. Am J Surg 1979;137:57.
54. Wetle T. Age as a risk factor for inadequate treatment. JAMA 1987;258:516.
55. Djokovic JL, Hedley-Whyte J. Prediction of outcome of surgery and anesthesia in patients over 80. JAMA 1979;242:2301.
56. Seymour DG, Pringle R. Postoperative complications in the elderly surgical patient. Gerontology 1983;29:262.
57. Pedersen BV, Hougen HP, Kjaergaard J. A follow-up study of octogenarians after major gastrointestinal surgery. Danish Med Bull 1981;28:204.
58. Feldman RS, Kapus KK, Alman JE, Chauncey HH. Aging and mastication: changes in performance and in the swallowing threshold with natural dentition. J Am Geriatr Soc 1980;28:97.
59. Baum BJ, Bodner L. Aging and oral motor function: evidence for altered performance among older persons. J Dent Res 1983;61:2.
60. Baum BJ. Current research on aging and oral health. Spec Care Dent 1981;1:105.
61. Baum BJ. Evaluation of stimulated parotid saliva flow rate in different age groups. J Dent Res 1981;60:1292.
62. Schiffman SS. Food recognition by the elderly. J Gerontol 1977;32:586.
63. Weiffenbach JM, Baum BJ, Burghauser R. Taste thresholds: quality, specific variation with human aging. J Gerontol 1982;37:372.
64. Grzegorcizyk PB, Jones SW, Mistretta CM. Age-related differences in salt taste acuity. J Gerontol 1979;34:834.
65. Arey LB, Tremaine MJ, Monzingo FL. The numerical and topographical relations of taste buds to human circumvallate papillae throughout the life span. Anat Rec 1936;64:9.
66. Mochizuki Y. Studies on the papilla foliata of Japanese. Okajimas Folia Ana Jpn 1939;18:337.
67. Bales CW, Stinman LC, Freeland-Graves JH, et al. The effect of age on plasma zinc uptake and taste acuity. Am J Clin Nutr 1986;44:664.
68. Greger Jl, Geissler AH. Effect of zinc supplementation on taste acuity of the aged. Am J Clin Nutr 1978;31:633.
69. Schiffman SS. Taste and smell in disease: I and II. N Engl J Med 1983;308:1275, 1337.
70. Doty RL, Shaman P, Applebaum SL, et al. Smell identification ability: changes with age. Science 1984;226:1441.
71. Zboralske FF, Amberg JR, Soergel KH. Presbyesophagus: cineradiographic manifestations. Radiology 1964;82:463.
72. Hollis JB, Castell DO. Esophageal function in elderly man: a new look at "presbyesophagus." Ann Intern Med 1974;80:371.
73. Khan TA, Shragge BW, Crispin JS, Lind JF. Esophageal motility in the elderly. Am J Dig Dis 1977;22:1049.
74. Piaget F, Fouillet J. Le pharynx et l'oesophage seniles. J Med Lyon, 1959;40:951.
75. Reynolds JC, Ouyang A, Cohen S. Recent advances in Dx and Rx of esophageal disease. Geriatrics 1982;37:91.
76. Karamchandani MC, Neal HS. Zenker's diverticulum. Geriatr Med Today 1986;5:20.
77. White IL. Severe complication of a Zenker's diverticulum with endoscopic diverticulotomy rescue. Laryngoscope 1981;91:708.
78. Ekberg O, Wahlgre L. Dysfunction of pharyngeal swallowing: a cineradiographic investigation in 854 dysphagial patients. Acta Radiol [Diagn] 1985;26:389.
79. Bonavina L, DeMeester TR, McChesney L, et al. Drug-induced esophageal strictures. Ann Surg 1987;206:173.
80. Carlborg B, Densert O. Esophageal lesions caused by orally administered drugs: an experimental study in the cat. Eur Surg Res 1980;12:270.
81. Kirkendall JW, Friedman AC, Oyewole MA, et al. Pill-induced esophageal injury: case reports and review of the medical literature. Dig Dis Sci 1983;28:174.
82. Walts DC, Giddens JD, Johnson LF, et al. Localized proximal esophagitis secondary to ascorbic acid ingestion and esophageal motor disorder. Gastroenterology 1976;70:766.
83. Evans KT, Roberts GM. Where do all the tablets go? Lancet 1976;2:1237.
84. Walt R, Katschinski B, Logan R, et al. Rising frequency of ulcer perforation in elderly people in the United Kingdom. Lancet 1986;1:489.
85. Kurata JH, Haile BM, Elashoff JD. Sex differences in peptic ulcer disease. Gastroenterology 1985;88:96.
86. Myren J. The natural history of peptic ulcer—views in the 1980s. Scand J Gastroenterol 1983;18:993.
87. Somerville K, Faulkner G, Langmen M. Nonsteroidal anti-inflammatory drugs and bleeding peptic ulcer. Lancet 1986;1:462.
88. Griffin MK, Ray WA, Schaffner W. Nonsteroidal anti-inflammatory drug use and death from peptic ulcer in elderly persons. Ann Intern Med 1988;109:359.
89. Langman MJS. What is happening to peptic ulcer? Br Med J 1982;284:1063.
90. Kekki M, Sipponen P, Siurala M. Age behavior of gastric acid secretion in males and females with a normal antral and body mucosa. Scand J Gastroenterol 1983;18:1009.
91. Krasinski SD, Russell RM, Samloff IM, et al. Fundic atrophic gastritis in an elderly population. J Am Geriatr Soc 1986;34:800.
92. Allen A, Pearson JP, Blackburn A, et al. Pepsins and the mucus barrier in peptic ulcer disease. Scand J Gastroenterol 1988;23(suppl 146):50.
93. Tatsuta M, Ikuda S. Age-related changes in the acid-secreting area in patients with duodenal ulcer. Endoscopy 1983;15:243.
94. Frank W, Braverman A, Palmer R, et al. Comparison of the pharmacodynamics of cimetidine in an elderly population [Abstract]. Gastroenterology 1987;92:1395.
95. Kupfer RM, Heppell M, Haggith JW, Bateman DN. Gastric emptying and small-bowel transit rate in the elderly. J Am Geriatr Soc 1985;33:340.
96. Moore JG, Tweedy L, Christian PE, Datz FL. Effect of age on gastric emptying of liquid-solid meals in man. Dig Dis Sci 1983;28:340.
97. Gilinsky NH. Peptic ulcer disease in the elderly. Scand J Gastroenterol 1988;23(suppl 146):191.
98. Clinch D, Banerjee AK, Ostick G. Absence of abdominal pain in elderly patients with peptic ulcer. Age Ageing 1984;13:120.
99. Amberg JR, Aboralske FF. Gastric ulcers after 70. AJR 966;96:393.
100. Colin-Jones DG. Endoscopy or radiology for upper gastrointestinal symptoms? Lancet 1986;1:1022.
101. Armstrong CP, Blower AL. Nonsteroidal anti-inflammatory drugs and life-threatening complications of peptic ulceration. Gut 1987;28:527.
102. Permutt RP, Cello JP. Duodenal ulcer disease in the hospitalized elderly patient. Dig Dis Sci 1982;27:1.
103. Brearley S, Hawker PC, Morris DL, et al. Selection of patients for surgery following peptic ulcer hemorrhage. Br J Surg 1987;74:893.
104. Boey J, Wong J. Perforated duodenal ulcer. World J Surg 1987;11:319.
105. Stewart RB, Hale WE, Marks RG. Antacid use in an ambulatory elderly population. Dig Dis Sci 1983;28:1062.

106. Dunnell K, Cartwright A. Medicine takers, prescribers and hoarders. Boston: Routledge and Kegan, 1972:107.

107. Walan A. Antacids: metabolic side-effects and interactions. Scand J Gastroenterol 1982;25:63.

108. Brooks JR, Eraklis AJ. Factors affecting the mortality from peptic ulcer. N Engl J Med 1964;271:803.

109. Guess HA, West R, Strand LM, et al. Fatal upper gastrointestinal hemorrhage or perforation among users and nonusers of nonsteroidal anti-inflammatory drugs in Saskatchewan, Canada, 1983. J Clin Epidemiol 1988;41:35.

110. Langman MJ. Anti-inflammatory drug intake and the risk of ulcer complications. Med Toxicol 1986;1(suppl 1):34.

111. Collins AJ, Davies J, Dixon SA. Contrasting presentation and findings between patients with rheumatic complaints taking nonsteroidal and anti-inflammatory drugs and a general population referred for endoscopy. Br J Rheumatol 1986;25:50.

112. LoIudice TA, Saleem T, Land JA. Cimetidine in the treatment of gastric ulcer induced by steroidal and nonsteroidal anti-inflammatory agents. Am J Gastroenterol 1981;75:104.

113. Davies J, Collins AJ, Dixon AStJ. The influence of cimetidine on peptic ulcer in patients with arthritis taking anti-inflammatory drugs. Br J Rheumatol 1986;25:54.

114. Graham DY, Agrawal NM, Roth SH. Prevention of NSAID-induced gastric ulcer with misoprostol: multicentre double-blind, placebo-controlled trial. Lancet 1988;2:1277.

115. Samloff IM, Varis K, Khamaki T, et al. Relationships among serum pepsinogen I, serum pepsinogen II and gastric mucosal histology. Gastroenterology 1982;82:204.

116. Ihamaki T, Kekki M, Sipponen P, Siurala M. The sequelae and course of chronic gastritis during a 30- to 34-year bioptic follow-up study. Scand J Gastroenterol 1985;20:485.

117. Sipponen P, Kekki M, Haapakoski J, et al. Gastric cancer risk in chronic atrophic gastritis: statistical calculations of cross-sectional data. Int J Cancer 1985;35:173.

118. Svendsen JH, Dahl C, Svendsen LB, Christiansen PM. Gastric cancer risk in achlorhydric patients: a long-term follow-up study. Scand J Gastroenterol 1986;21:16.

119. Schafer LW, Larson DE, Melton LJ III, Higgins JA, Zinsmeister AR. Risk of development of gastric carcinoma in patients with pernicious anemia: a population-based study in Rochester, Minnesota. Mayo Clin Proc 1985;60:444.

120. Borch K, Renvall H, Liedberg G. Gastric endocrine cell hyperplasia and carcinoid tumors in pernicious anemia. Gastroenterology 1985;88:638.

121. Howden CW, Hunt RH. Relationship between gastric secretion and infection. Gut 1987;28:96.

122. Benn A, Cooke WT. Intraluminal pH of duodenum and jejunum in fasting subjects with normal and abnormal gastric or pancreatic function.

123. Gianella RA, Broitman SA, Zamcheck N. Influence of gastric acidity on bacterial and parasitic enteric infections. Ann Intern Med 1973;78:271.

124. Gurian L, Ward TT, Katon RM. Possible foodborne transmission in a case of pseudomembranous colitis due to *Clostridium difficile:* influence of gastrointestinal secretions on *Clostridium difficile* infection. Gastroenterology 1982;83:465.

125. Holt P. Severe *Salmonella* infection in patients with reduced gastric acidity. Practitioner 1985;229:1027.

126. Bender BS, Laughon BE, Gaydos C, et al. Is *Clostridium difficile* endemic in chronic-care facilities? Lancet 1986;2:11.

127. Morris A, Nicholson G. Ingestion of *Campylobacter pyloridis* causes gastritis and raised fasting pH. Am J Gastroenterol 1987;82:192.

128. Jones DM, Eldridge J, Fox AJ, et al. Antibody to the gastric *Campylobacter*-like organism *(Campylobacter pyloridis)*—clinical correlations and distribution in the normal population. J Med Microbiol 1986;22:57.

129. Faisal MKA, Russell RM, Samloff IM, Holt PR. Helicobacter Pylori infection and atrophic gastritis in the elderly (letter). Gastroenterology 1990;99:154.

130. Kassarjian Z, Russell RM. Hypochlorhydria: a factor in nutrition. In: Olson RE, ed. Annual review of nutrition 1989;9:271.

131. Jacobs P, Bothwell TH, Charlton RW. Role of hydrochloric acid in iron absorption. J Appl Physiol 1964;19:187.

132. Bezwoda W, Charlton R, Bothwell T, et al. The importance of gastric hydrochloric acid in the absorption of nonheme food iron. J Lab Clin Med 1978;92:108.

133. Carmel R, Weiner JM, Johnson CS. Iron deficiency occurs frequently in patients with pernicious anemia. JAMA 1987;257:1081.

134. Axon ATR. Potential hazards of hypochlorhydria in the treatment of peptic ulcer. Scand J Gastroenterol 1986;21:17.

135. Salom IL, Silvis SE, Doscherolmen A. Effect of cimetidine on the absorption of vitamin B-12. Scand J Gastroenterol 1982;17:129.

136. Belaiche J, Cattan D, Zittoun J, et al. Effect of ranitidine on cobalamin absorption. Dig Dis Sci 1983;28:667.

137. MacKenzie JF, Russell RI. The effect of pH on folic acid absorption in man. Clin Sci Mol Med 1976;51:363.

138. Russell RM, Krasinski SD, Samloff IM, et al. Folic acid malabsorption in atrophic gastritis: possible compensation by bacterial folate synthesis. Gastroenterology 1986;91:1476.

139. Middleton HM III. Intestinal hydrolysis of pyridoxal 5'-phosphate in vitro and in vivo in the rat: effect of protein binding and pH. Gastroenterology 1986;91:343.

140. Recker RR. Calcium absorption and achlorhydria. N Engl J Med 1985;313:70.

141. Holt PR, Rosenberg IH, Russell RM. Causes and consequences of hypochlorhydria in the elderly. Dig Dis Sci 1989;34:933.

142. Corazza GR, Frazzoni M, Gatto MRA, Gasbarrini G. Ageing and small bowel mucosa: a morphometric study. Gerontology 1986;32:60.

143. Andrew W. Cellular changes with age. Springfield, IL: Charles C Thomas, 1952.

144. Calloway NO, Foley CF, Langerbloom P. Uncertainties in geriatric data: II. Organ size. J Am Geriatr Soc 1965;13:20.

145. Kreel L, Sandin B. Changes in pancreatic morphology associated with aging. Gut 1973;14:962.

146. Laugier R, Sarles H. The pancreas. In: James OFW, ed. Clinics in gastroenterology. London: WB Saunders, 1985:749.

147. Gullo L, Priori P, Daniele C, et al. Exocrine pancreatic function in the elderly. Gerontology 1983;29:407.

148. Gullo L, Ventrucci M, Naldoni P, Pezzilli R. Aging and the exocrine pancreatic function. J Am Geriatr Soc 1986;34:790.

149. Dreiling DA, Triebling AT, Koiller M. The effect of age on human exocrine pancreatic secretion. Mt Sinai J Med 1985;52:336.

150. Arora S, Kassarjian Z, Krasinski SD, et al. Effect of age on tests of intestinal and hepatic function in healthy humans. Gastroenterology 1989;96:1560.

151. Weiner I, Hambraeus L. Digestive capacity of elderly people. In: Carlson LA, ed. Nutrition and old age. Uppsala, Sweden: Almquist and Wiksell, 1972:55.

152. Simko V, Shoukry M. Absorptive capacity for dietary fat in elderly patients with debilitating disorders. Arch Intern Med 1989;149:557.

153. Webster SGP, Wilkinson EM, Gowland E. A comparison of fat absorption in young and old subjects. Age Ageing 1977;6:113.

154. Kendall MJ. The influence of age on the xylose absorption test. Gut 1970;11:498.

155. Webster SGP, Leeming JT. Assessment of small bowel function in the elderly using a modified xylose tolerance test. Gut 1975;16:109.

156. Feibusch JM, Holt PR. Impaired absorptive capacity for carbohydrate in the aging human. Dig Dis Sci 1982;27:1095.

157. Avioli LV, McDonald JE, Lee SW. The influence of age on the intestinal absorption of ^{47}Ca absorption in postmenopausal osteoporosis. J Clin Invest 1965;44:1960.

158. Bullamore JR, Wilkinson R, Gallagher BE, et al. Effect of age on calcium absorption. Lancet 1970;2:535.

159. Barragary JM, France MKW, Corless D, et al. Intestinal cholecalciferol absorption in the elderly and in younger adults. Clin Sci Mol Med 1978;55:213.

160. Armbrecht HJ, Zenser TV, Bruns MEH, Davis BB. Effect of age on intestinal calcium absorption and adaptation to dietary calcium. Am J Physiol 1979;236:E769.

161. Nordin C, Morris HA. The calcium deficiency model for osteoporosis. Nutr Rev 1989;47:65.

162. Nordin BEC, Baker MR, Horsman A, Peacock M. A prospective trial of the effect of vitamin D supplementation on metacarpal bone loss in elderly women. Am J Clin Nutr 1985;42:470.

163. Carmel R, Sinow RM, Siegel ME, Samloff IM. Food cobalamin

malabsorption occurs frequently in patients with unexplained low serum cobalamin levels. Arch Intern Med 1988;148:1715.

164. Price HL, Gazzard BG, Dawson AM. Steatorrhoea in the elderly. Br Med J 1977;1:1582.

165. Montgomery RD, Haeney MR, Ross IN, et al. The ageing gut: a study of intestinal absorption in relation to nutrition in the elderly. Q J Med 1978;186:197.

166. Montgomery RD, Haboubi NY, Mike NH, et al. Causes of malabsorption in the elderly. Age Ageing 1986;15:235.

167. Ammann R, Sulser H. Die "senile" chronische Pankreatitis—eine neue nosologische Eiheit? Schweiz Med Wochenschr 1976;106:429.

168. Ammann R. Zur vaskularen Genese der chronischen Pankreatitis. Dtsch Med Wochenschr 1976;101:867.

169. Nagai H, Ohtsubo K. Pancreatic lithiasis in the aged. Gastroenterology 1984;86:331.

170. Logan RFA, Rifkind EA, Busuttil A, et al. Prevalence and "incidence" of celiac disease in Edinburgh and the Lothian region of Scotland. Gastroenterology 1986;90:334.

171. Campbell CB, Roberts RM, Cowen AE. The changing clinical presentation of coeliac disease in adults. Med J Aust 1977;1:89.

172. Kirby J, Fielding JF. Very adult coeliac disease! The need for jejunal biopsy in the middle aged and elderly. Irish Med J 1984;77:35.

173. Hallert C, Gotthard R, Norrby K, Walan A. On the prevalence of adult coeliac disease in Sweden. Scand J Gastroenterol 1981;16:257.

174. Kumar PJ, Walker-Smith J, Milla P, et al. The teenage coeliac: follow-up study of 102 patients. Arch Dis Child 1988;63:916.

175. Growing up with coeliac disease [Editorial]. Lancet 1988;2:1231.

176. Weir DG, Hourihane DO'B. Coeliac disease during the teenage period: the value of serial serum folate estimations. Gut 1974;15:450.

177. Pare P, Douville P, Caron D, Lagace R. Adult celiac sprue: changes in the pattern of clinical recognition. J Clin Gastroenterol 1988;10:395.

178. Gillberg R, Dotevall G, Kastrup W, et al. Conventional malabsorption tests: do they detect the adult patient with villous atrophy? Scand J Clin Lab Invest 1984;44:91.

179. Swinson CM, Clavin G, Coles EC, Booth CC. Coeliac disease and malignancy. Lancet 1983;1:111.

180. Robertson DAF, Dison MF, Scott BB, et al. Small intestinal ulceration: diagnostic difficulties in relation to coeliac disease. Gut 1983;24:565.

181. Dawson DJ, Sciberras CM, Whitwell H. Coeliac disease presenting with intestinal pseudo-obstruction. Gut 1984;25:1003.

182. Shaw RS, Maynard EP III. Acute and chronic thrombosis of the mesenteric arteries associated with malabsorption: a report of 2 cases successfully treated by thromboendarterectomy. N Engl J Med 1958;258:874.

183. Osnes M, Lotveit T, Larsen S, Aune S. Duodenal diverticula and their relationship to age, sex and biliary calculi. Scand J Gastroenterol 1981;16:103.

184. King CE, Toskes PA. Small intestinal bacterial overgrowth. Gastroenterology 1979;76:1035.

185. Clark ANG. Deficiency states in duodenal diverticular disease. Age Ageing 1972;1:14.

186. Pearce VR. The importance of duodenal diverticula in the elderly. Postgrad Med J 1980;56:777.

187. Roberts SH, James OFW, Jarvis EH. Bacterial overgrowth syndrome without "blind loop": a cause for malnutrition in the elderly. Lancet 1977;2:1193.

188. Connell AM, Hilton C, Irvine G, et al. Variation of bowel habit in two population samples. Br Med J 1965;2:1095.

189. Sonnenberg A, Koch TR. Physician visits in the United States for constipation: 1958 to 1986. Dig Dis Sci 1989;34:606.

190. Wigzell FW. The health of nonagenarians. Gerontology 1969;11:137.

191. Whitehead WE, Heller B, Schuster MM. Constipation, laxative use and incontinence in elderly people: community survey. Gastroenterology 1987;92:1693.

192. Eastwood HDH. Bowel transit studies in the elderly: radio-opaque markers in the investigation of constipation. Gerontol Clin 1972;14:154.

193. Wilkersson W, Andersson H, Bosaeus I, Falkheden T. Intestinal transit time in constipated and non-constipated geriatric patients. Scand J Gastroenterol 1983;18:593.

194. Kupfer RM, Heppell M, Haggith JW, Bateman DN. Gastric emptying and small-bowel transit rate in the elderly. J Am Geriatr Soc 1985;33:340.

195. Piccione PR, Kreek MJ, O'Bryan L, et al. Oro-cecal transit time correlated with symptoms of gastrointestinal dysmotility in geriatric facility residents [Abstract]. Gastroenterology 1987;92:1576.

196. Haboubi NY, Hudson P, Rahman Q, et al. Small-intestinal transit time in the elderly. Lancet 1988;1:933.

197. Ihre T. Studies on anal function in continent and incontinent patients. Scand J Gastroenterol 1974;9:5.

198. Newman HF, Freeman J. Physiologic factors affecting defecatory sensation: relation to aging. J Am Geriatr Soc 1974;22:553.

199. Read NW, Abouzedry L, Read MG, et al. Anorectal function in elderly patients with fecal impaction. Gastroenterology 1985;89:959.

200. Krishnamurthy S, Schuffler MD, Pope CC, Rohrmann CA. Severe idiopathic constipation is caused by distinct abnormality of the colonic myenteric plexus. In: Roman C, ed. Gastrointestinal motility. Lancaster, England: MTP Press, 1984;467.

201. Lane RHS, Todd IP. Idiopathic megacolon: a review of 42 cases. Br J Surg 1977;64:305.

202. Ballantyne GH. Review of sigmoid volvulus: clinical patterns and pathogenesis. Dis Colon Rectum 1982;25:823.

203. Anderson JR, Lee D. Acute caecal volvulus. Br J Surg 1980;67:39.

204. Petros JG, Bradley TM. Sigmoid volvulus: review of its incidence, etiology and management. Pract Gastroenterol 1988;12:62.

205. String ST, DeCosse JJ. Sigmoid volvulus: an examination of the mortality. Am J Surg 1971;121:293.

206. Staling JR. Initial treatment of sigmoid volvulus by colonoscopy. Ann Surg 1979;190:1.

207. Melchoir E. Volvulus of the cecum: appeal for primary resection with report of 6 cases. Surg 1949;25:251.

208. Bak MD, Boley SJ. Sigmoid volvulus in elderly patients. Am J Surg 1986;151:71.

209. Sandman PO, Adolfsson R, Hallsmans G, et al. Treatment of constipation with high-bran bread in long-term care of severely demented elderly patients. J Am Geriatr Soc 1983;5:289.

210. Smith RG, Rowe MJ, Smith AN, et al. A study of bulking agents in elderly patients. Age Ageing 1980;9:267.

211. Wesselium DE, Casparis A, Braadbaart S, et al. Treatment of chronic constipation with lactulose syrup: results of a double-blind study. Gut 1968;9:84.

212. Leigh RJ, Turnberg LA. Faecal incontinence: the unvoiced symptom. Lancet 1982;1:1349.

213. Parks AG, Swash M, Urich H. Sphincter denervation in anorectal incontinence and rectal prolapse. Gut 1977;18:656.

214. Parks AG. Anorectal incontinence. Proc R Soc Med 1975;68:681.

215. Rogers J, Henry MM, Misiewicz JJ. Combined sensory and motor deficit in primary neuropathic faecal incontinence. Gut 1988;29:5.

216. Read NW, Abouzekry L. Why do patients with faecal impaction have faecal incontinence? Gut 1986;27:283.

217. Devroede G, Vobecky S, Masse S, et al. Ischemic fecal incontinence and rectal angina. Gastroenterology 1982;83:970.

218. Wald A. Biofeedback therapy for fecal incontinence. Ann Intern Med 1981;95:146.

219. Rybold AH, Laughon BE, Greenough WB III, et al. Protein-losing enteropathy associated with *Clostridium difficile* infection. Lancet 1989;1:1353.

220. Garland CF, Lilienfeld AM, Mendeloff AT, et al. Incidence of rates of ulcerative colitis and Crohn's disease in fifteen areas of the United States. Gastroenterology 1981;81:1115.

221. Kyle J. An epidemiological study of Crohn's disease in Northeast Scotland. Gastroenterology 1971;61:826.

222. Norlen BJ, Krause U, Bergman L. An epidemiological study of Crohn's disease. Scand J Gastroenterol 1970;5:385.

223. Fahrlander H, Baerlocher C. Clinical features and epidemiological data on Crohn's disease in the Basle area. Scand J Gastroenterol 1971;6:657.

224. Lee FI, Giaffer M. Crohn's disease of late onset in Blackpool. Postgrad Med J 1987;63:471.

225. Rogers BHG, Clark LM, Kirsner JB. The epidemiological and demographic characteristics of IBD: an analysis of a computerized file of 1400 patients. J Chronic Dis 1971;23:743.

226. Brandt LJ, Boley SJ, Mitsudo S. Clinical characteristics and natural history of colitis in the elderly. Am J Gastroenterol 1982;77:382.

227. Margulis AR, Goldberg HI, Lawson TL, et al. The overlapping spectrum of ulcerative and granulomatous colitis: a roentgenographic-pathologic study. Am J Radiol 1971;113:325.

228. Williams NS, Macfie J, Celestin LR. Anorectal Crohn's disease. Br J Surg 1979;66:743.

229. Fabricius P, Gyde SN, Shoulder P, et al. Crohn's disease in the elderly. Gut 1985;26:461.

230. Watts JM, de Dombal FT, Watkinson G, Goligher JC. Early course of ulcerative colitis. Gut 1966;7:16.

231. Softley A, Myren J, Clamp SE, et al. Inflammatory bowel disease in the elderly patient. Scand J Gastroenterol 1988;23(suppl 144):27.

232. Brandt L, Boley S, Goldberg L, et al. Colitis in the elderly: a reappraisal. Am J Gastroenterol 1981;76:239.

233. Margolis IB, Faro RS, Howells EM, Organ CH. Megacolon in the elderly: ischemic or inflammatory? Ann Surg 1979;190:40.

234. Meyers MA, Alonso DR, Morson BC, Bartram C. Pathogenesis of diverticulitis complicating granulomatous colitis. Gastroenterology 1978;74:24.

235. Kratzer GL, Onsanit T. Diverticulitis in the elderly. J Am Geriatr Soc 1973;21:25.

236. Marshak RH, Janowitz HD, Present DH. Granulomatous colitis in association with diverticula. N Engl J Med 1970;283:1080.

237. Marshak RH, Lindner AE, Pochaczevsky R, et al. Longitudinal sinus tracts in granulomatous colitis and diverticulitis. Semin Roentgenol 1976;11:101.

238. Marston A, Pheils MKT, Thomas ML, Morson BC. Ischemic colitis. Gut 1966;7:1.

239. Rusch V, Simonowitz DA. Crohn's disease in the older patient. Surg Gynecol Obstet 1980;150:184.

240. Greenstein AJ, Sachar DB. Cancer in inflammatory bowel disease. Surv Dig Dis 1983;1:8.

241. David H. The hepatocyte: development, differentiation, and ageing. Jena, East Germany: VEB Gustav Fischer Verlag, 1985.

242. Schapiro H, Hotta SS, Outten WE, et al. The effect of aging on rat regeneration. Experientia 1982;38:1075.

243. Lubin JR, Millward BA, Coles JA, Croker JR. Value of profiling liver function in the elderly. Postgrad Med J 1982;49:763.

244. Kampmann JP, Sinding J, Jorgensen IM. Effect of age on liver function. Geriatrics 1975;30:91.

245. Zauli D, Crespi C, Fusconi M, et al. Different course of acute hepatitis B in elderly adults. J Gerontol 1985;40:415.

246. Gibinski K, Fojit E, Suchan S. Hepatitis in the aged. Digestion 1973;8:254.

247. Regt RH de, Minkoff HL, Feldman J, Starzl RH. Liver transplantation in older patients. N Engl J Med 1987;316:484.

248. Werf SDJ van der, Huijbregts AWM, Lamers HLM, et al. Age-dependent differences in human bile acid metabolism and 7-alpha-dehydroxylation. Eur J Clin Invest 1981;11:425.

249. Negengast FM, Hectors M, Werf SDJ, Tongeren JHM van. Age-dependent differences in secondary bile acid concentration in human feces [Abstract]. Gastroenterology 1985;88:1514.

250. Spellman SJ, Shaffer EA, Rosenthall L. Gallbladder emptying in response to cholecystokinin: a cholescintigraphic study. Gastroenterology 1979;77:115.

251. Croker JR. Biliary tract disease in the elderly. Clin Gastroenterol 1985;14:773.

252. Kennedy RH, Thompson MH. Are duodenal diverticula associated with choledocholithiasis? Gut 1988;29:1003.

253. Lotveit T, Osnes M, Larsen S. Recurrent biliary calculi: duodenal diverticula as a predisposing factor. Ann Surg 1982;196:30.

254. Viceconte G, Viceconte GW, Bogliolo G. Endoscopic manometry of the sphincter of Oddi in patients with and without juxtapapillary duodenal diverticula. Scand J Gastroenterol 1984;19:329.

255. Cobden I, Lendrum R, Venables CW, James OFW. Gallstones presenting as mental and physical disability in the elderly. Lancet 1984;1:1062.

256. Williamson RCN. Acalculous disease of the gallbladder. Gut 1988;29:860.

257. Thornton JR, Heaton KW, Espiner HJ, Eltringham WK. Empyema of the gallbladder—reappraisal of a neglected disease. Gut 1983;24:1183.

258. Pollack AV. Acute pancreatitis. Br Med J 1959;1:6.

259. Fan ST. Causes and prognosis of acute pancreatitis in the geriatric patient. Geriatr Med Today 1989;8:46.

260. Ranson JHC, Rifkind KM, Turner JW. Prognostic signs and nonoperative peritoneal lavage in acute pancreatitis. Surg Gynecol Obstet 1976;143:209.

261. Corfield AP, Williamson RCN, McMahon MJ, et al. Prediction of severity in acute pancreatitis: prospective comparison of 3 prognostic indices. Lancet 1985;88:403.

262. Lau WY, Yip WC, Poon GP, Wong KK. Optimal irrigation pressure in operative choledochoscopy. Aust NZ J Surg 1988;58:717.

263. Mee AS, Vallon AG, Croker JR, Cotton PB. Non-operative removal of bile duct stones by duodenoscopic sphincterotomy in the elderly. Br Med J 1981;283:521.

264. Madden JW, Croker JR, Beynon GPJ. Septicaemia in the elderly. Postgrad Med J 1981;57:502.

265. Esposito AL, Gleckman RA, Cram S, et al. Community acquired bacteremia in the elderly: analysis of 100 consecutive episodes. J Am Geriatr Soc 1980;28:315.

266. Taylor KJW, Rosenfield AT, Spiro HM. Diagnostic accuracy of gray-scale ultrasonography for the jaundiced patient. Arch Intern Med 1979;139:60.

267. Wenckert A, Robertson B. The natural course of gallstone disease. Gastroenterology 1966;50:376.

268. Gracie WS, Ransohoff DF. The natural history of silent gallstones. N Engl J Med 1982;307:798.

269. Ransohoff DF, Miller GL, Forsythe SB, Hermann RE. Outcome of acute cholecystitis in patients with diabetes mellitus. Ann Intern Med 1987;106:829.

270. Thistle JL, May GR, Bender CE, et al. Dissolution of cholesterol gallbladder stones by methyl tert-butyl ether administered by percutaneous transhepatic catheter. N Engl J Med 1989;320:633.

271. McSherry CK, Glenn F. The incidence and causes of death following surgery for non-malignant biliary tract disease. Ann Surg 1980;191:271.

272. Williamson BWA, Simpson CJ, McLatchie G, et al. Prospective randomised trial of early versus delayed surgery for acute biliary tract disease. Gut 1984;25:A1140.

273. Sullivan DM, Hood TR, Griffen WO. Biliary tract surgery in the elderly. Am J Surg 1982;143:218.

274. Houghton PJW, Donaldson LA. Elective biliary surgery—a safe procedure. Geriatr Med 1983;13:814.

275. Reiss R, Hoffman S, Deutsch AA. Cholecystectomy in patients above 70: review of 153 cases. Mt Sinai J Med 1982;49:71.

276. Leese T, Neoptolemos JP, Baker AR, Carr-Locke DL. Management of acute cholangitis and the impact of endoscopic sphincterotomy. Br J Surg 1986;73:988.

277. Escourrou J, Cordova JA, Lazorthes F, et al. Early and late complications after endoscopic sphincterotomy for biliary lithiasis, with and without the gallbladder in situ. Gut 1984;25:598.

278. Davidson BR, Neoptolemos JP, Carr-Locke DL. Endoscopic sphincterotomy for common bile duct calculi in patients with gallbladder in situ considered unfit for surgery. Gut 1988;29:114.

279. Cotton PB. Endoscopic management of bile duct stones (apples and oranges). Gut 1984;25:587.

46

Approach to Gastrointestinal Problems in the Immunocompromised Patient

GEORGE B. McDONALD
GEORGIA M. REES

The term *immunocompromised* is a broad one encompassing both elderly patients who have mild defects in lymphocyte function and marrow transplant patients whose immune defenses have been ablated. One can categorize immune defects as those involving granulocytes, the cellular immune system, and the humoral (antibody) immune system, since each is followed by its own spectrum of infections.[1,2] The normal intestinal tract has several additional nonimmune defenses against infection, for example, gastric acidity, the epithelial barrier, and motility, which prevents stasis of intestinal contents.[3,4] Disruption of these barriers to luminal organisms may not lead to systemic infection if the immune system is intact. However, if mucosal disruption occurs in patients with disordered immunity, particularly if granulocyte function is impaired, septicemia is likely.

The approach to gastrointestinal problems in an immunocompromised patient is made easier if the physician understands the nature of the immunodeficiency, or at least its medical name. Knowing which infections are common to which immunodeficiency disorders is quite useful in directing diagnosis and therapy.[5–8] The first section of this chapter is disease oriented, covering immunodeficiency diseases and their gastrointestinal manifestations. The second section is a problem-oriented approach to infection in the compromised patient, which emphasizes presenting signs and symptoms. The third section is a summary of prophylaxis and treatment of intestinal infections in the compromised host.

DISEASES WITH DISORDERED IMMUNITY: INTESTINAL AND LIVER COMPLICATIONS

Cancer and Its Treatment

The prevalence of intestinal involvement with malignant cells in both leukemia and lymphoma is high.[9,10] The consequences are bleeding, obstruction, perforation, and septicemia. Bleeding is most common after chemotherapy has caused lysis of malignant cells and suppression of platelet production.[9,11] Perforation is most common after treatment of lymphoma with gastric involvement but can occur at any site in the intestine, even in areas free of tumor.[12–15] Resection of transmural lymphomas reduces the chance of perforation and bleeding caused by cytotoxic therapy.[12] Malignant lymphoid cells may also involve the liver, spleen, pancreas, and retroperitoneum. In addition, malignant diseases derived from marrow and lymph node cells are commonly associated with disordered immunity, which may be manifest as intestinal and liver infections even before chemotherapy or radiation therapy ablates the immune system further. Septicemia, particularly with gut-derived fungal and clostridial organisms, is one manifestation of this immunodeficiency. *Clostridium septicum* causes both septicemia and typhlitis in these patients.[16–18]

Fungal and cytomegalovirus (CMV) infections cause both bleeding and perforation in patients with leukemia and lymphoma.[19,20] Surgical decision making in these patients is not necessarily dependent on defining the cause of intestinal ulceration, since this is usually apparent only in the resected specimen.[21]

In contrast, solid tumors themselves seldom give rise to profound immunodeficiency, aside from that seen in malnourished patients and after surgical trauma. Infectious processes that occur in the intestine and biliary system of patients with solid tumors are related to obstruction and local destruction of mucosa by tumor tissue. For example, fungal plaques are common in the esophagus obstructed by a carcinoma; bacterial overgrowth occurs with small bowel obstruction; diffuse colitis has been described above a high-grade colonic obstruction; and cholangitis occurs behind a partially obstructed biliary system. High-grade obstruction of the colon may lead to cecal perforation and peritonitis, and a necrotic tumor or metastasis to the intestine may perforate as well. Septicemia with two unusual organisms has been described in association with colon cancer. *C. septicum* is not found in the fecal flora normally but may be rarely seen in the bloodstream, in the stool, and at sites of distant infection in patients with colon cancer.[16,17] *Streptococcus bovis* septicemia has been described in similar patients.[22]

Cancer chemotherapy has profound effects on both lymphoid cells and granulocytes but, with some exceptions, minimal toxicity to the intestine. Granulocytopenia is a major risk factor for disseminated fungal and bacterial disease, often derived from the intestinal microbial flora.[23] Prolonged depression of lymphocyte function leads to reactivation of latent viruses (especially herpesviruses) and parasites (e.g., *Strongyloides*) and makes the patient more susceptible to viruses and parasites acquired from the environment.[23] Most multidrug chemotherapy regimens in common use do not cause significant mucosal, pancreatic, or liver injury.[24-26] There are some exceptions: sequential regimens that include cytarbine, chemotherapy with 5-fluorouracil and citrovorum factor, and concurrent use of chemotherapy with radiation may cause extensive mucosal necrosis.[27-29] Some agents cause oropharyngeal and esophageal mucositis and increase the damage that radiation therapy does to the esophagus when both are given concurrently. These drugs include doxorubicin, dactinomycin, bleomycin, cytarabine, fluorouracil, methotrexate, cyclophosphamide, etoposide, and cisplatin.[26,30,31] *Vinca* alkaloids are potentially neurotoxic and may cause dysphagia and colonic pseudo-obstruction, particularly in older patients.[32] Necrosis of the gastroduodenal mucosa has been described as a complication of intra-arterial chemotherapy delivered via the hepatic artery.[33] Drugs that have been reported to cause pancreatitis include L-asparaginase, azathioprine, 6-mercaptopurine, prednisone, and some combination chemotherapy regimens.[26] Pancreatitis has also occurred during estrogen treatment of metastatic prostate carcinoma.

Serious liver toxicity can occur after some high-dose chemotherapy regimens, particularly chemoradiation regimens used to prepare patients for marrow transplantation.[34-37] The site of injury is primarily hepatic venules, which become occluded, giving rise to hepatomegaly, necrosis of hepatocytes in zone 3 of the liver acinus, renal sodium retention, ascites, and weight gain (venoocclusive disease of the liver).[34-36] Veno-occlusive disease has also been described in patients on chronic therapy with 6-thioguanine and azathioprine.[26,34] Some agents (mithramycin, L-asparaginase, high-dose methotrexate) cause hepatocellular necrosis, which is usually transient.[26] Fatty liver has been described after therapy with L-asparaginase, dactinomycin, mitomycin-C, bleomycin, and methotrexate.[26] Cholestatic liver injury is an unusual manifestation of azathioprine, 6-mercaptopurine, busulfan, and amsacrine therapy.[26] Peliosis hepatis has occurred after therapy with hydroxyurea, azathioprine, 6-thioguanine, and androgen therapy.[26,38]

Cancer chemotherapy may affect the gastrointestinal tract in other ways as well. Vigorous retching and vomiting may lead to Mallory-Weiss tears, intramural hematomas of the esophagus, and esophageal perforation, as well as traumatize the gastric mucosa in the body of the stomach, which prolapses into the esophagus during emesis.[39,40] Bleeding and hematoma formation are more extensive in patients with platelet counts below $50,000/mm^3$. Hematomas may also occur in the small intestine, mesentery, and retroperitoneum and into the abdominal wall.[40,41] Rarely, chemotherapy will result in dissolution of a solid tumor or metastasis involving the esophagus or intestine. This leads to either perforation (with transmural tumors) or extensive ulcerations that bleed.[11-14]

In the cancer patient, endocrine and metabolic problems may have prominent gastrointestinal effects.[42] Hypercalcemia causes acid hypersecretion and anorexia and may be associated with pancreatitis. Hypophosphatemia leads to anorexia, nausea, and vomiting. Adrenal insufficiency, in the setting of disseminated tumor, sepsis, or coagulopathy, may cause severe abdominal pain, nausea, and vomiting. Hypothyroidism may be the result of radiation therapy or tumor infiltration of the thyroid gland; gastrointestinal manifestations include constipation and intestinal pseudo-obstruction.

Organ Transplantation

Transplantation of solid organs (kidney, liver, heart, lung) is frequently associated with intestinal and liver complications. Some of these complications are related to immunosuppressive drug therapy itself, but most are caused by infectious processes. Marrow transplantation has drug toxicity and infections in common with solid organ transplantation but in addition is frequently complicated by intestinal and liver disease caused by chemoradiation therapy and graft-versus-host disease.

RENAL TRANSPLANTATION

Patients with renal grafts receiving life-long therapy with immunosuppressive drugs have many gastrointestinal problems. However, in the event of a life-threatening infection or drug toxicity, immunosuppressive drugs can be stopped, the graft sacrificed, and uremia treated by dialysis. This option is not usually available to heart, lung, liver, or marrow recipients.

In the first month post transplant, preexisting viral hepatitis, tuberculosis, inapparent bacterial infection, and strongyloidiasis may become apparent. These unusual infections occur in patients with renal failure because of the effects of uremic toxins on host defenses.[43] Particular attention should be paid to screening graft recipients for *Strongyloides* before transplantation, since disseminated strongyloidiasis is frequently fatal.[44,45]

The most vulnerable period for infections is from 1 to 6 months post transplant.[5,46] Infection caused by herpesviruses and hepatitis viruses are frequent. The peak time for CMV infection is 6 to 8 weeks post transplant, with the insidious onset of malaise, myalgias, fever, anorexia, and occasionally a cough. About a third of patients have elevated levels of transaminase enzymes, without significant liver dysfunction. Intestinal bleeding from CMV ulceration, particularly in the right colon, can be a major problem. Herpes simplex virus (HSV) infections occur in about half of patients, affecting the mouth and nose primarily but also the esophagus, liver, and perianal areas.[5,47] HSV enteritis is rare. Varicella zoster virus (VZV) may involve the esophagus and liver in patients with disseminated disease.[5,46]

Liver disease is a major cause of morbidity after renal transplantation and the most common cause of death in graft recipients who have survived 5 years beyond transplantation.[48] Much of this morbidity is due to progressive chronic hepatitis, which is largely viral in nature, although immunosuppressive drugs may also contribute to chronic liver disease. The prevalence of chronic hepatitis B and of hepatitis C is high in candidates for renal transplantation, since most have been exposed to these viruses from hemodialysis and blood transfusions. In the first few years post transplant, patients with chronic hepatitis continue to have smouldering disease but otherwise have graft and patient survival comparable to patients without hepatitis.[49] In the ensuing years, however, progressive liver dysfunction becomes a major cause of morbidity. Cirrhosis, extrahepatic sepsis, and hepatomas are causes of death.[48,50] Although much attention has been directed at hepatitis B virus, there is evidence that the prevalence of chronic hepatitis in renal graft recipients is the same in both hepatitis B–positive and hepatitis B–negative renal graft recipients.[5] Hepatitis C virus and other non-A, non-B transfusion-borne hepatitis viruses appear to be the most important cause of chronic hepatitis post transplant.[5,51]

Renal transplant recipients appear to have more colonic problems than other organ transplant recipients, beyond the infectious colitis common to immunosuppressed patients. These problems include perforation, bleeding, and severe colitis. Diverticular perforation and pericolic abscess are particularly common, since long-term use of constipating phosphate-building antacids before transplantation appears to lead to sigmoid diverticula.[5,46] Perforations in both gastroduodenal and colonic areas have been attributed to corticosteroid therapy and to CMV infection.[19,52] Severe colitis has been described in 1% to 2% of renal transplant patients.[53] While infections due to CMV, *Clostridium difficile*, and enteric pathogens can cause colitis, these organisms are not usually found. Instead, intestinal ischemia, related to postsurgical changes in mesenteric flow or blood volume shifts after dialysis, has been invoked. Recent papers have also implicated polystyrene (Kayexalate)-sorbitol enemas (particularly the sorbitol component) in causing epithelial necrosis.[54,55]

Acalculous cholecystitis and pancreatitis are also causes of abdominal pain in renal transplant patients. These problems can be infectious (e.g., CMV) or related to drug toxicity, since cyclosporine, azathioprine, and prednisone have been implicated in biliary/pancreatic disease in these patients. Patients may develop abdominal pain as a manifestation of adrenal insufficiency if corticosteroid coverage is inadequate. "Peptic" ulcer disease may be more frequent in renal transplant patients than in a control population, but these ulcers may have CMV in their base.[56,57] Poor ulcer healing can be a consequence of CMV infection, particularly in patients who must maintain a high level of immunosuppression. The role of antiviral therapy in this setting has not been examined.

Infection with Epstein-Barr virus, usually reactivated from latency by immunosuppression, is also common in these patients. There are two sorts of presentations: one in younger patients with fever, pharyngitis, and enlarged nodes in the early post-transplant period and the other in older patients with an infiltrative lymphomatous process involving the viscera and central nervous system.[46,58] Intra-abdominal manifestations include infiltration of the stomach, small intestine, and liver with transformed lymphocytes. Abdominal pain, obstruction, anorexia, jaundice, and bleeding are common presenting features. The incidence of other kinds of tumors, particularly epithelial malignancy, is also increased in patients on chronic immunosuppressive therapy.[59]

Because immunosuppression masks the usual signs of intra-abdominal infection, an aggressive diagnostic approach, using barium enemas, Gastrografin upper intestinal studies, and ultrasound or computed tomography is recommended when renal transplant patients present with abdominal complaints.[46]

LIVER TRANSPLANTATION

The transplanted liver and its vascular and biliary anastomoses are at the center of most problems after liver transplantation. These topics are beyond the scope of this chapter. Nonhepatic gastrointestinal complications are usually due to infections, the effects of drug therapy, and vascular complications.

In the perioperative period, intestinal problems that may arise include variceal bleeding, colonic trauma, portal thrombosis with intestinal ischemia, pancreatitis, and intestinal overgrowth with Enterobacteriaceae and fungi. Although most early sepsis is related to hepatobiliary infection, the organisms are derived from these resident intestinal flora. The problem of systemic bacterial and fungal infection is multifactorial. Many candidates for liver transplantation exhibit diminished reticuloendothelial clearing of bacteria.[60] Transient leukopenia may result from large-volume transfusions during surgery. Other immunosuppressive factors (e.g., drugs, malnutrition, surgical trauma) contribute as well. The Pittsburgh group has reported a 50% incidence of gram-negative and fungal infections in liver graft recipients on cyclosporine and prednisone.[61,62] Oropharyngeal and selective bowel decontamination and prophylactic systemic antibiotics for 2 perioperative days reduced colonization with Enterobacteriaceae and *Candida* organisms as well as infections with these organisms.[63] Others prefer to preserve the colonization resistance provided by endogenous flora by avoiding preoperative antibiotics but giving perioperative antibiotics for 2 days.[64] At a minimum, antifungal prophylaxis seems indicated, given the high (> 50%) mortality associated with significant fungal infections after transplantation.[61]

Colonic perforations, enteric fistulae, and intra-abdominal abscesses have been described in the early transplant period.[65] Perforations are due to transmural injury caused by either surgical trauma or mucosal infection. Intestinal bleeding in the perioperative period can be variceal or from stress ulcers, ischemia, surgical anastomoses, and infectious ulcers (e.g., *Candida*, *Aspergillus*).[66]

Intestinal problems after operative recovery are similar to those after renal transplantation, since immunosuppressive therapy and herpesvirus infections are common to both groups of patients. Intra-abdominal infection may become recognizable weeks after operation, but herpesviruses, particularly CMV, are the most problematic pathogens.[67] In most liver transplant centers, it is not yet practical to screen the donor liver and transfused blood products for antibodies to CMV. As a result, most liver graft recipients are at risk for either primary or reactivation infection. Intestinal manifestations include persistent nausea and vomiting, bleeding, dysphagia, abdominal pain, and diarrhea.[67] Bleeding may result from cytomegaloviral ulcers throughout the intestinal tract.[66,67] The liver is frequently infected as well, but clinical liver disease is usually mild. Ganciclovir therapy has been reported to be effective in uncontrolled studies,[68,69] but return of immune function may be equally important.

Epstein-Barr virus infections and related lymphoproliferative syndromes may occur in chronically immunosuppressed liver graft recipients.[70]

CARDIAC TRANSPLANTATION

Heart and heart-lung recipients are as vulnerable to postoperative bacterial and fungal infections as recipients of other organs. However, intra-abdominal catastrophes are less common in the perioperative period than in renal and liver transplant recipients. Bacterial infection is the leading cause of death in the postoperative period, since the level of immunosuppression must be maintained at a high level.[71] While many of these infections are wound and intravenous-access related, the high prevalence of Enterobacteriaceae and gram-positive bacteria of intestinal origin suggest a breakdown of colonization resistance and mucosal barriers to infection.[72,73] Disseminated fungal infection in cardiac transplant patients is less common than bacteremia. Some success in treating visceral fungal infection has been reported, perhaps because of preserved granulocyte function.[73] Intestinal ischemia may result from poor cardiac output, particularly in patients with atherosclerotic disease of the mesenteric arteries. Ischemic hepatitis may be difficult to differentiate from other causes of hepatocellular injury (e.g., drugs, infection).

The major intestinal complications of cardiac transplantation are due to herpesviruses, since immunosuppressive therapy often cannot be diminished without cardiac rejection. As in other transplant settings, there is a latency before clinical disease caused by herpesviruses appears, usually 1 to 3 months after surgery. CMV causes disease in about 75% of cardiac graft recipients, some of whom are CMV seropositive before transplantation.[72,74] Others acquire the virus by blood product transfusion and from the donor heart itself. The clinical presentation is similar to that after other organ transplants: fever, malaise, myalgias, anorexia, and atypical lymphocytosis in most patients and organ damage in some. Intestinal manifestations of CMV infection are ulcerations of the esophagus, stomach, and intestine, usually discovered because of bleeding, pain, vomiting, or dysphagia.[73,75] Again, "peptic" ulcers in this patient population are as likely to be caused by CMV infection as by corticosteroids or gastric juice.[75] Bleeding can be a major problem when CMV infection has also caused thrombocytopenia. CMV hepatitis may be more severe after primary CMV infection, as compared with reactivation.[76]

HSV, VZV, and Epstein-Barr virus (EBV) cause the same spectrum of problems in cardiac transplant patients as discussed earlier.[73] The most serious complication is EBV-related lymphoproliferative disease.[70]

Surgical diseases in the abdomen (ulcer disease, cholecystitis, diverticulitis, pancreatitis) may be difficult to recognize in the heart transplant patient because of an impaired inflammatory response.[77] A high index of suspicion and an aggressive diagnostic approach are necessary to prevent unnecessary deaths.[78]

BONE MARROW TRANSPLANTATION

Although marrow graft recipients are prone to many of the same infections as solid-organ recipients, intestinal and liver complications caused by noninfectious processes make the approach to gastrointestinal problems quite different.[40] Candidates for marrow grafting usually have either hematologic malignancy or aplastic anemia, and they may have gastrointestinal diseases that would jeopardize a successful transplant. These include ulcerations caused by herpesviruses and fungi, parasite infestation, perianal bacterial infection, and liver disease (e.g., hepatitis C, fungal abscess, and hepatitis B). These problems must be addressed before transplantation, since the doses of chemotherapy or chemoradiotherapy used to ablate the host's residual marrow (and cancer cells, if present) cause profound depression of leukocytes and platelets for several weeks, until the donor marrow becomes established in the host. During this time, bacterial and fungal infections, many derived from the intestinal flora, are common.[79] Radiation therapy also damages the esophagus, intestinal mucosa, and the liver. Oropharyngeal mucositis may extend into the esophagus, causing dys-

phagia and painful swallowing. Intestinal damage is usually self-limited with regeneration of crypt epithelium by 3 weeks post transplant.[80] Liver toxicity is common, affecting up to 50% of patients conditioned with total-body irradiation and chemotherapy (usually cyclophosphamide) and leading to liver failure in a third of those affected.[35,36] This process, called veno-occlusive disease of the liver, is characterized by hepatomegaly, jaundice, weight gain, encephalopathy, and ascites, resulting from occlusion of terminal hepatic venules and damage to hepatocytes in zone 3 of the liver acinus.[35] Several risk factors for veno-occlusive disease have been identified: higher doses of chemotherapy or irradiation; hepatitis at the time of conditioning therapy; older age; and possibly estrogen-progestogen and cyclosporine therapy.[35,36,81] Veno-occlusive disease becomes apparent in the first several weeks after transplantation, but it must be differentiated from hepatic fungal infiltration, congestive heart failure, septicemia, drug toxicity, and graft-versus-host disease.[82]

A common noninfectious cause of intestinal and liver dysfunction is graft-versus-host disease (GVHD), an immunologic disorder that results from donor lymphoid cells reacting against host tissues (see also ch 107). Acute GVHD usually has its onset around day 20 post transplant but can occur earlier when prophylactic medications (e.g., methotrexate, cyclosporine) are not given. Intestinal manifestations of acute GVHD include protracted nausea and vomiting, profuse watery diarrhea with protein loss, abdominal pain, bleeding, and ileus.[83–86] Liver abnormalities include cholestasis and mild hepatocellular necrosis, with progressive jaundice in severe cases.[87,88] The diagnosis of acute GVHD can usually be made on clinical grounds and confirmed by biopsy of target organs. The differential diagnosis is usually between GVHD and infection, but it is also common to find both processes coexisting in the same patient. In most patients, the "immunologic hostilities" of acute GVHD cease after day 100, although some patients have unresolved acute GVHD beyond this time.

The syndrome of chronic GVHD occurs 3 to 9 months after transplantation. Intestinal problems include esophageal desquamation and stricture formation, bacterial overgrowth in the small intestine, and chronic cholestatic liver disease.[83,87–89]

Drug toxicity is another noninfectious cause of intestinal and liver disease in marrow graft recipients.[83,87] Total parenteral nutrition may cause liver injury and frequently leads to gallbladder sludge formation, which can cause symptoms. Antibiotic use is ubiquitous in the post-transplant period; suppression of anaerobic intestinal flora and colonization with fungi and Enterobacericeae is common. *Clostridium difficile* colitis may not be as readily recognized in these patients as in nontransplant patients, since pseudomembranes are absent in granulocytopenic patients. Other antibiotic complications are liver injury (sulfa-containing antibiotics, ketoconazole, some third-generation penicillins), pill esophagitis (clindamycin, tetracyclines), and nausea, vomiting, and anorexia (amphotericin, sulfa-containing drugs, oral nonabsorbable antibiotics). Immunosuppressive drugs, such as cyclosporine and azathioprine, in addition to predisposing to infection, may have direct toxicity to the liver, biliary system, and pancreas.

Infection remains a major impediment to survival after marrow transplantation.[79] When compared with patients who receive solid organ transplants, marrow transplant patients have more profound granulocytopenia and more deficient cell-mediated immunity and may require life-long immunosuppression because of GVHD. Successfully engrafted long-term survivors, however, may regain complete immune function and live normal lives without immunosuppressive therapy.

Infections during the period of granulocytopenia (before day 20 to 30) are usually fungal or bacterial, but viral and parasitic diseases present during conditioning therapy may become widespread during this time. Problems caused by fungal infection include esophagitis, invasive enteritis, colonization, portal fungemia of yeast forms from the small intestine, bleeding ulcers, and hepatobiliary disease.[79,83] Bacterial infections are frequently due to the resident oropharyngeal and intestinal flora and occasionally to clostridial organisms (*C. difficile, C. septicum*). Specific infections include bacterial esophagitis, phlegmonous gastritis, translocation of enteric bacteria into mesenteric tissue, *Pseudomonas* vasculitis, perianal cellulitis, typhlitis, and *C. difficile* colitis.[83] Bacterial liver abscess is unusual, but the hepatic effects of bacterial sepsis are common. HSV may cause necrotizing esophagitis or, rarely, fulminant hepatitis in this early post-transplant period. However, most HSV-seropositive patients now receive prophylactic acyclovir until engraftment.

After engraftment, viral infections of the intestine and liver begin to make their appearance. Currently most of the herpesvirus infections after marrow transplantation arise from latency, since most units screen blood products given to CMV-seronegative recipients and give prophylactic antiviral agents to seropositive patients.[90] CMV is the most problematic of the herpesviruses, with infection usually presenting as nausea and vomiting from day 40 to 60 after transplant.[84,91] Esophageal ulcers are the most frequent endoscopic finding. CMV may also be recovered from ulcerations throughout the intestine. CMV may also be associated with pancreatitis and infiltration of neural elements in the intestine. Serious liver disease caused by CMV is rare; the usual picture is that of a mild hepatitis with microabscesses, particularly in patients with CMV viremia and pneumonia.[92] HSV causes esophageal ulcerations, perianal disease, and rarely enteritis and hepatitis. Early diagnosis of HSV infection is critical, since acyclovir is effective therapy. VZV may cause esophagitis, fulminant hepatitis, and intestinal pseudo-obstruction because of neural involvement. VZV visceral infection may present before typical zoster skin lesions. Adenovirus usually causes a mild to moderately severe diarrheal illness, but severe disseminated disease, with fulminant hepatitis and necrotizing enteritis, has been reported.[93] Rotavirus causes mild to moderate enteritis but is usually self-limited. EBV–associated lymphoproliferative syndrome has been described in highly immunosuppressed marrow graft recipients with acute GVHD. The disease develops rapidly in these patients, infiltrating the stomach, intestine, mesentary, liver, and spleen.[94,95]

Hepatitis viruses, while highly prevalent in patients who have been multiply transfused before transplantation, are not usually a cause of serious liver disease in the early post-transplant period. Hepatitis predisposes patients to veno-occlusive disease of the liver, however.[35,36,81] Hepatitis C has some histologic features in common with acute GVHD and may present diagnostic problems after day 50 to 75.[88] Hepatitis B virus may replicate in the liver during prolonged immunosuppression and may rarely result in fulminant hepatic failure when the donor lymphoid system becomes functional.[96]

Parasitic diseases are unusual unless parasites go undetected in pretransplant screening. When patients are discharged to a less-controlled environment, they may acquire parasites such as *Giardia*

lamblia and *Cryptosporidium*, particularly from infected children and drinking water.[97,98]

Intestinal complications after day 100 are far less common but may be as serious. Chronic GVHD may cause intractable esophageal disease if not diagnosed and treated promptly.[89] Liver involvement with chronic GVHD may lead to cirrhosis, although in the reported cases, hepatitis C virus infection cannot be excluded.[99] Small intestinal bacterial and fungal overgrowth occurs in IgA-deficient patients with chronic GVHD. Secondary malignancy, mostly lymphomas, has been described in long-term survivors of marrow transplantation.[100]

Chronic Immunosuppressive Drug Therapy

Drugs that suppress the immune response are commonly used to treat allograft rejection, rheumatologic disorders, vasculitis, inflammatory bowel diseases, chronic liver diseases, obstructive pulmonary diseases, and a variety of other disorders characterized by excessive immune reactivity. The drugs most commonly used for this purpose are corticosteroids, cytotoxic drugs, cyclosporine, and antibodies to lymphocytes. These drugs are nonspecific in their effects and may depress not only excessive immune reactivity but also normal host defense mechanisms, thus predisposing to infection. The types of infections differ according to the immune cells being suppressed.

CORTICOSTEROIDS

In humans, corticosteroids exert their immunosuppressive effects by altering the circulation of leukocytes, the function of leukocytes, and the release of soluble mediators of inflammation.[101] Granulocyte migration to sites of infection is depressed by high-dose corticosteroid therapy. Infections with pyogenic bacteria (staphylococci, Enterobacteriaceae) and *Candida* species are the usual consequences. Eosinophils are markedly depleted by corticosteroid therapy, resulting in an increased susceptibility to such parasites as *Strongyloides, Toxoplasma*, and malarial organisms. Corticosteroids have profound effects on the monocyte-macrophage system and on T lymphocytes, which become redistributed in the body.[102] Activation of facultative intracellular organisms such as mycobacteria and latent viruses are consequences of corticosteroid therapy in patients harboring these organisms.

These effects of glucocorticoid therapy on the immune system are dependent on both the dosage level and the interval between doses. Prednisone in excess of 5 mg/d has some immunosuppressive effect, and marked effects are seen at doses of 40 to 60 mg/d. However, similar doses of corticosteroids, when given on an alternate-day basis do not result in significant immunosuppression and are not associated with an increased frequency of infection.[103]

CYTOTOXIC DRUGS

Patients with cancer who are treated with high doses of cytotoxic drugs such as cyclophosphamide, chlorambucil, azathioprine, and methotrexate develop profound immunosuppression. These drugs, which destroy immunocompetent cells or block their proliferation, can be given in lower doses to suppress an aberrant immune response while sparing host defense mechanisms.[101] When used to treat such conditions as Wegener's granulomatosis or necrotizing vasculitis, doses of the alkylating agents cyclophosphamide and chlorambucil are titrated to achieve total leukocyte counts in the $3000/\mu$L to $4000/\mu$L range, which suppress B- and T-lymphocyte responses.[101,104] The purine analogues azathioprine and 6-mercaptopurine destroy proliferating lymphocytes and deplete B- and T-lymphocytes.[101] Dose-limiting toxicity is marrow depression, particularly of leukocytes. Opportunistic infections can be seen with both alkylating agents and purine analogues in the absence of leukopenia, probably because these drugs affect monocyte-macrophage functions.[101] More serious infections occur when granulocyte counts fall below targeted levels. These drugs may also affect the gastrointestinal system directly, since hepatic toxicity (cholestasis, veno-occlusive disease), pancreatitis, and lymphoid malignancies occur in patients on chronic therapy with these agents.

The folate antagonist methotrexate is now used to treat rheumatologic disorders, inflammatory bowel disease, asthma, psoriasis, and other nonmalignant conditions. Although methotrexate affects granulocyte function and suppresses antibody responses,[105] opportunistic infections are unusual during treatment with low-dose pulse therapy with methotrexate. However, reactivation of latent viral infection has been reported.

CYCLOSPORINE

Cyclosporine is a cyclic peptide that inhibits certain humoral and cell-mediated responses without affecting marrow function or granulocytes.[106] With these properties, the drug found an immediate application in inhibiting allograft rejection in recipients of solid organ transplants and GVHD in marrow graft recipients. Since granulocytes and macrophages are relatively unaffected by cyclosporine, bacterial and fungal infections are not as common in patients who are treated with cyclosporine/prednisone as in those receiving azathioprine/prednisone, for example. However, reactivation of latent virus infection in cyclosporine-treated patients is a problem, since EBV and CMV may cause serious disease. Lymphoproliferative disorders are seen in organ transplant recipients on chronic cyclosporine/prednisone immunosuppression.[58,70] As cyclosporine becomes more widely used to treat inflammatory diseases other than allograft rejection, these viral diseases must be kept in mind, along with other side effects such as hepatic, renal, metabolic, and neurologic toxicity.[106]

ANTILYMPHOCYTE ANTIBODIES

Antibodies against immune cells can be infused intravenously into patients, destroying targeted lymphocytes by removing them in the reticuloendothelial system. Antilymphocyte serum and antithymocyte globulin are polyclonal antibodies that are relatively nonselective in their reactivity against T lymphocytes and some cells other than T lymphocytes.[107] These preparations have been used primarily in the organ transplant setting, but they have also been applied to autoimmune diseases and aplastic anemia. Recent developments in monoclonal antibody technology have led to more specific targeting of T-lymphocyte subsets. Antilymphocyte monoclonal antibody therapy has been applied to allograft rejection, certain lymphoid malignancies, and GVHD.[108,109] With both polyclonal and monoclonal antibody therapy, there is an increase in the activation of latent viral infections, particularly infection with CMV and EBV.[95,110,111]

Congenital Immunodeficiency Syndromes

The congenital immunodeficiency syndromes that affect the intestinal tract and the liver are described in chapter 107. The range of infections seen with these syndromes is wide, since there may be defects in antibody production, phagocytosis, lymphocyte function, and combinations of these.

DECREASED ANTIBODY PRODUCTION

Since immunoglobulins are important in opsonizing microbial organisms, patients with immunoglobulin deficiency tend to become infected with encapsulated bacteria, enteric pathogens, protozoa, and *Mycoplasma*. Named syndromes include Bruton's X-linked agammaglobulinemia, common variable hypogammaglobulinemia, and selective IgA deficiency. Patients with common variable hypogammaglobulinemia usually present with recurrent sinopulmonary infections but may have giardiasis, abnormal small intestinal villous architecture, nodular lymphoid hyperplasia, and bacterial overgrowth.[112] Achlorhydria is a feature of most immunoglobulin deficiency syndromes; the pathogenesis is not known, but *Helicobacter pylori* gastritis may be prevalent in these patients. Achlorhydria and deficient luminal immunoglobulin predispose to chronic infection with organisms such as *Salmonella*, *Shigella*, and *Campylobacter*. Persistence of disease with these organisms is seen in patients with the acquired immunodeficiency syndrome (AIDS) as well. Common variable hypogammaglobulinemia also predisposes patients to gastric adenocarcinoma and lymphoma.[113] Selective IgA deficiency, while the most common immunodeficiency state, is usually asymptomatic. There are a number of diseases that appear to be more common in patients with IgA deficiency than in the general population. These include achlorhydria and pernicious anemia, celiac sprue, inflammatory bowel disease, primary biliary cirrhosis, allergic disorders, autoimmune diseases, and malignancy.[114,115]

PHAGOCYTIC DEFECTS

Blood granulocyte counts under $500/\mu$L and defective granulocytes predispose to infections. Although granulocytopenia is most common with aplasia, with leukemia, and after chemotherapy, unusual congenital syndromes may also predispose patients to infections caused by staphylococci, gram-negative bacilli, and *Candida* organisms. Named syndromes include cyclic neutropenia, Chédiak-Higashi syndrome, and chronic granulomatous disease.[116,117]

DEFECTS IN CELLULAR IMMUNITY

Some organisms tend to persist intracellularly and are not readily killed by antibody/granulocyte defenses. These organisms include viruses, mycobacteria, and some fungi. These organisms are either eliminated or held in a latent state by monocyte/macrophages and lymphocytes. Isolated defects in T lymphocytes, as seen in the congenital disorders thymic-parathyroid hypoplasia (DiGeorge's syndrome) and thymic dysplasia (Nezelof's syndrome) commonly lead to skin and esophageal candidiasis, hepatitis, tuberculosis, and central nervous system infections.[118] Combined B-lymphocyte and T-lymphocyte defects, as in the Wiskott-Aldrich syndrome, ataxia-telangectasia, and severe combined immunodeficiency, lead to more severe infections. These include disseminated skin infections with staphylococci and herpesviruses, sinopulmonary infections, bacteremias and abscesses, and visceral herpesvirus infections.[119] Chronic mucocutaneous candidiasis is unusual, in that *Candida* infections are limited to the skin, nails, oropharynx, and esophagus. Bacterial, viral, and visceral fungal infections are not usually seen.[120]

Infections Leading to Immunodeficiency

Thus far in this chapter we have emphasized immunodeficiency leading to infection. There are examples of the reverse, that is, infection interfering with normal immunologic functions. Human immunodeficiency virus (HIV) infection is the most florid example of this type of acquired immunodeficiency (see ch 107). Nonspecific immunosuppression occurs after many other viral infections, probably because the viruses inhabit lymphoid or marrow progenitor cells. Examples are measles virus, rubella virus, HSV, and CMV.[121] CMV infections in transplant recipients and patients with AIDS may lead to granulocytopenia as well as to decreased lymphocyte and macrophage function, thus predisposing these patients to infections with yet other organisms.[122] EBV infections may rarely cause severe immunodeficiency in patients who had apparently normal immune responses before EBV infection. The resulting immunodeficiency disorders include mononucleosis with hepatic failure, aplastic anemia, agammaglobulinemia, and B-lymphocyte lymphomas.[1] When patients already receiving immunosuppressive therapy develop EBV infections, B-lymphocyte proliferation may cause a fatal lymphoma-like illness. Hepatitis viruses (particularly hepatitis C virus) may rarely cause aplastic anemia, and there is clinical evidence for an immunosuppressive effect of chronic hepatitis C virus infection in renal transplant patients, who may require fewer immunosuppressive drugs than renal graft recipients without hepatitis.[5]

Parasitic diseases also alter immune responses in their host. This phenomenon has been best studied in patients with helminth infections, particularly schistosomiasis and filariasis. After a prompt T-lymphocyte response to acute parasitic infection, the chronic stages of these diseases are characterized by depressed lymphocyte proliferation, lymphokine production, and circulating antibody levels.[123] Treatment reverses the immunosuppression, which is generally restricted to responses induced by parasite antigens. Some protozoal infections (e.g., kala-azar, leishmaniasis, Chagas' disease) also lead to suppression of specific cell-mediated immune responses to parasite antigens, but these patients do not appear to be more susceptible to other infections.[123]

Other Medical and Surgical Diseases With Immunodeficiency

OLD AGE

Infections in the elderly, while closely related to other diseases of aging, are also tied to the immunodeficiency that accompanies the aging process.[124] Infectious consequences of obstructing cancers, perforated bowel, and biliary stones are discussed elsewhere in this text. Recognition of these infections may be delayed, since fever, leukocytosis, and localized signs may be absent.[125] Instead, nonspecific lethargy and vague abdominal complaints may be the presenting symptoms.[126]

Infectious esophagitis in otherwise healthy elderly patients is usually caused by either *Candida albicans* or HSV. Enteric bacterial pathogens (especially *Salmonella*) may cause a more serious illness in the elderly than in younger patients.[127] Other enteric infections, often acquired in nursing home environments, include fungal overgrowth (*Candida*), viral enteritis (rotavirus, Norwalk agent), parasitic disease (*Giardia*, *Cryptosporidium*) and, rarely, verotoxin-producing *Escherichia coli*.[127–129]

New cases of tuberculosis are discovered more frequently in the elderly, especially in nursing home environments.[126,130] Most cases represent reactivation of pulmonary disease, but late generalized tuberculosis occurs as well. Hepatic involvement in generalized disease is common, but the presenting symptoms of fever, weakness, and anorexia are nonspecific.[130]

Obscure fever in the elderly is usually caused by neoplasm, connective tissue disorders, or infections.[131] Most of these infections are related to common intra-abdominal disorders such as appendicitis, perforation, and biliary sepsis.[131]

DIABETES MELLITUS

Patients with diabetes are susceptible to a variety of infections, which tend to be more severe than in nondiabetic patients. Immunologic abnormalities in poorly controlled diabetics appear to be secondary to alterations in the metabolic milieu, since metabolically well-controlled diabetics do not exhibit these abnormalities.[132] Diabetic patients have normal serum immunoglobulin and complement levels and respond appropriately to immunization. Cell-mediated immunity, however, is abnormal in patients with poor metabolic control. These abnormalities include decreased lymphocyte responsiveness to stimulation and defective suppressor T-lymphocyte activity. In vivo T-lymphocyte–mediated immunity has not been well studied in human diabetic patients, but numerous defects have been noted in diabetic animals. Granulocyte function is clearly affected by hyperglycemia, which causes decreased phagocytic activity, intracellular killing, and adherence.[132]

When diabetic patients develop diverticulitis, cholecystitis, or other infections caused by the intestinal flora, the resulting infection is more difficult to control. However, some primary infections of the intestine occur more frequently in diabetics: fungal esophagitis, parasitic infection, and intestinal overgrowth syndromes are the most common examples. Bacterial "translocation" from the colonic lumen to draining mesenteric nodes may also be more common in diabetic patients who have other risk factors for septicemia (e.g., trauma, burns, shock).[16,132]

PROTEIN-LOSING SYNDROMES (PROTEINURIA, ENTEROPATHY)

Significant amounts of serum immunoglobulin can be lost by patients with nephrotic syndrome and protein-losing enteropathy. In the case of nephrotic syndrome, the losses are mostly in the IgG class. Even though hypogammaglobulinemia may develop with these diseases, there appears to be sufficient remaining humoral immunity to avoid infection.[1] In contrast, when lymphocytes and immunoglobulins are lost, as is the case with intestinal lymphangiectasias, clinically significant immunodeficiency may develop.[1,133] Depletion of circulating lymphocytes leads to a high incidence of tuberculosis, fungal infections, and lymphoid malignancies. These abnormalities are reversible if the intestinal losses cease, as in a patient with constrictive pericarditis and intestinal lymphangiectasia who was cured by pericardiectomy.[134]

MALNUTRITION

Common infections are more morbid when they occur in malnourished patients, who may also be prone to infection with opportunistic organisms such as rotavirus, herpesviruses, fungi, intestinal parasites, and diarrhea-causing bacteria.[135] Defining the causes and nature of immunodeficiency in malnourished humans has proved difficult, since both macronutrient and micronutrient deficiences usually coexist in severely malnourished patients.[136] Much of the literature in this field is derived from controlled animal experiments.

In severe protein-energy malnutrition there is lymphoid depletion throughout the body. In the intestine, lymphoid aggregates, lamina propria plasma cells, and intraepithelial lymphocytes are reduced in number. Secretory IgA levels are low, and mucosal IgA response to viral vaccines is reduced. There are profound decreases in CD4 cells and moderately decreased CD8 cells.[137] Chemotactic migration of granulocytes is slower than normal, and intracellular microbe killing is defective. The opsonizing activity of plasma is also reduced since proteins with short half-lives (such as fibronectin) are closely linked to nutritional status.[138]

Deficiency of micronutrients, particularly zinc, folate, pyridoxine, and vitamin A, also affects cell-mediated immunity.[139] Zinc deficiency occurs as a genetic disease (acrodermatitis enteropathica) and as an element of pan-undernutrition; supplements of zinc reverse the immune abnormalities within weeks.[139] Zinc-deficient patients are susceptible to infections with *Salmonella*, coxsackievirus, and *Listeria*. Folate deficiency is common among malnourished patients, particularly among alcoholics and other hospitalized patients. Folate deficiency causes defects in granulocyte function as well as T-lymphocyte dysfunction.[140]

SURGICAL DISEASES

Surgical problems in immunodeficient patients are well recognized as being difficult to recognize and treat. Less well appreciated is the fact that previously healthy persons who develop acute surgical problems (e.g., trauma, burns, shock, sepsis, bleeding requiring transfusion) may develop defects in immune defenses and become secondarily infected. The intestinal tract is the source of most of the organisms causing such infections; the mechanisms by which these infections develop are the subject of much recent research.[141] The intestinal barrier to organisms and their toxins becomes "leaky" during many critical illnesses, especially when nutrients are supplied intravenously, rather than by the enteral route. Glutamine supplementation as well as enteral calories help preserve intestinal integrity.[141,142] Cell-mediated immunity plays a back-up role in preventing movement of organisms into the tissues.[143]

The phenomenon of bacterial translocation, by which organisms migrate through grossly intact mucosa into submucosal tissue, lymph nodes, and draining veins, has been studied in animal models. There appear to be several mechanisms for this process, including increased "permeability" of paracellular routes as well as increased numbers of aerobic organisms within the intestine. There is evidence that bacterial translocation occurs in humans with extensive burns, trauma, multiorgan failure, inflammatory bowel disease, and intestinal obstruction.[144-147] Furthermore, bacterial endotoxins appear to translocate during critical illness.[141] The inference has been made that these translocation phenomena are linked to infections in the liver, lungs, and spleen caused by enteric organisms and to the morbidity caused by endotoxemia. Proof of this linkage is lacking, but experiments in animals show that while translocation of bacteria in immunologically intact animals may not cause death, translocation in animals with defective immunity is lethal. These surgical studies form the basis for intestinal decontamination in many seriously ill patients, not just those with known immunodeficiency states.[148-150]

Other risk factors for immunosuppression in the surgical patient are malnutrition and blood transfusions. In several clinical series (involving surgical patients with colon cancer, Crohn's disease, abdominal trauma, and burns), blood transfusions have been identified as a risk factor for perioperative infection.[151] The mechanism for this putative immunomodulatory effect is not known. Transfusions may also transmit viruses (e.g., CMV and EBV) capable of causing immunosuppression.[152]

LIVER DISEASE

Infections are a significant cause of morbidity in fulminant hepatic failure.[153] When surveillance cultures are done routinely, 90% of these patients have evidence of infection.[154] Defects in the hepatic synthesis of proteins that enhance clearance of bacteria (e.g., fibronectin and other opsonins) and in macrophage and granulocyte function have been noted in hepatic failure.[155,156] Patients with chronic liver disease have decreased clearance of circulating bacteria, which is the probable explanation for spontaneous soft tissue infections and peritonitis in patients with cirrhosis.[60] Chronic alcoholics with cirrhosis have additional immune defects caused by the acute effects of ethanol.[157]

Patients with liver disease also demonstrate defects in cellular immunity, but the clinical consequences are not as apparent as with defects in bacterial clearance. In an animal model of liver dysfunction, a chain of events occurs that adversely affect these animals: bile duct obstruction leads to suppression of lymphocyte response to mitogens, probably via the absorption of intestinal endotoxin.[158,159] Endotoxemia also causes cytokine release (notably tumor necrosis factor), which in turn increases intestinal permeability to bacteria.[159] In seriously ill patients, liver dysfunction may lead to morbidity by similar mechanisms.

UREMIA

Infection is a major cause of morbidity in patients with renal failure, including those on chronic hemodialysis.[43,160] Defects in lymphocyte, granulocyte, and macrophage function have been described in these patients.[160-162] These defects are caused in large part by toxins, since improvements can be noted in vitro when uremic plasma is removed and occasionally by hemodialysis.[160] There are other potential causes for immunosuppression in uremic patients: malnutrition, micronutrient deficiency, chronic liver disease, high levels of endogenous glucocorticoids, and the mechanical effects of dialysis membranes on complement and granulocytes.[43,162] The result is a high prevalence of bacterial and fungal infections, poor response to vaccinations, and progressive chronic viral hepatitis in many patients.

GASTROINTESTINAL AND LIVER PROBLEMS IN THE IMMUNOCOMPROMISED PATIENT

Heartburn, Odynophagia, and Dysphagia

INFECTIOUS CAUSES

When symptoms of heartburn or painful swallowing appear suddenly in a patient with profound granulocytopenia (e.g., following chemotherapy) or with major abnormalities of T-lymphocyte function (e.g., HIV infection), an esophageal infection is likely. The organisms responsible are fungi, viruses, and bacteria, but infections due to multiple types of organisms are common in severely compromised patients.[163,164] Superficial brushings of infected lesions may yield fungal elements but may miss underlying cells infected by viruses. In contrast, less compromised patients may present with indolent esophageal infections by complaining of heartburn and dysphagia. This presentation can be seen in diabetic, corticosteroid-treated, or malnourished elderly patients as well as those with congenital disorders such as mucocutaneous candidiasis.[120,165] These patients rarely have deep fungal infections involving the spleen or liver, probably because of adequate granulocyte function. *Candida albicans* is the most common fungal organism causing esophagitis, but other *Candida* species and other fungi may be found in severely compromised patients.[165] The diagnosis of acute fungal esophagitis usually requires endoscopic brushings and biopsies, but esophageal symptoms in a patient with oral thrush may be adequate to prompt empiric treatment.

Three members of the herpesvirus family (HSV, VZV, and CMV) cause acute ulcerative esophagitis in the immunosuppressed patient. HSV and rarely VZV may also affect the normal host. For immunosuppressed patients the major risk factor for infections with these viruses is prior exposure, best demonstrated by seropositivity to the virus. CMV may also be transmitted by blood product transfusion, since latent virus is contained in leukocytes from CMV-seropositive blood donors. If immunosuppressed patients who are seronegative for CMV receive only CMV-seronegative blood products, they are unlikely to develop CMV infection.[166] The presentation of viral esophagitis is variable: some patients complain of excruciating retrosternal pain, and others present with nausea, anorexia, mild heartburn, or bleeding.[84,163,167] HSV first causes small vesicles in the esophagus identical to those in oral or nasal epithelium. Squamous cells in the center of the vesicles are infected with HSV, but when these cells are shed to form an ulcer, the centers are usually devoid of virus.[84,168] CMV does not infect squamous epithelium in the esophagus but, rather, subepithelial endothelial cells and fibroblasts.[84,163] Persistent anorexia, nausea, and vomiting are the most common presenting symptoms of CMV esophagitis in transplant patients.[84] Ulcers caused by CMV are shallow with slightly reddened, raised edges and may be very large.[169] Endoscopic brushings are seldom positive, since submucosal tissue at the base of ulcers must be sampled to find infected cells. Superinfection of these large ulcers by fungi and bacteria is common. Reflux of acid-peptic juice also contributes to the persistence of large ulcers, especially in patients with gastric stasis, vomiting caused by chemotherapy drugs, and poor salivary flow. Esophageal symptoms can be lessened by treating acid-peptic reflux vigorously.[91] VZV may cause both typical vesicles and necrotizing panesophagitis in severely immunodeficient patients, but there are usually other organs involved. VZV infects squamous epithelium and can be differentiated from HSV by immunohistologic staining.

Oropharyngeal bacteria, both gram-negative and gram-positive, may cause esophageal necrosis in patients who lack granulocytes.[163,170] Esophageal symptoms, fever, and bacteremia are the usual presenting symptoms. The diagnosis is difficult, since bacteria are not well seen in routine histologic stains. Bacterial esophagitis occurs in 10% to 20% of symptomatic patients in cancer center populations.[163,170]

Cryptosporidium and *Pneumocystis carinii* have been found in inflammatory esophagitis from patients with AIDS, but it is unclear whether these organisims are primary pathogens.

NONINFECTIOUS CAUSES

Patients receiving mediastinal radiation therapy commonly experience heartburn and dysphagia when the dose exceeds 30 Gy (3000 rad), but more severe and protracted esophagitis occurs with doses over 50 Gy.[171] Concomitant chemotherapy with doxorubicin, bleomycin, dactinomycin, cyclophosphamide, fluorouracil, etoposide, methotrexate, and cisplatin potentiate radiation effects.[26,31] Chemotherapy alone is an uncommon cause of esophagitis, but the oropharyngeal mucositis caused by some drugs may cause severe pain on swallowing. Retching after chemotherapy may cause retrosternal pain and dysphagia because of an intramural esophageal hematoma or even perforation.[39] Dysphagia due to motor abnormalities has been described as a complication of therapy with *Vinca* alkaloid chemotherapy, which is neurotoxic.[172] Carcinomas involving the esophageal wall transmurally may respond to effective radiation therapy by leading to fistulas and perforation. Cancers near the esophagus may compress its lumen, and remote cancers may rarely metastasize to the esophageal wall. Lymphoma and Kaposi's sarcoma in patients with AIDS can involve the esophagus concurrently with viral and esophageal infection.[173] Certain pills cause severe mucosal injury in the esophagus, notably antibiotics, iron and potassium tablets, and nonsteroidal anti-inflammatory drugs.[174]

Medical illness for which immunosuppressive drug therapy is commonly given may involve the esophagus. Examples are collagen vascular diseases, bullous skin diseases, and inflammatory processes such as Crohn's disease, sarcoidosis, Behçet's disease, and chronic GVHD following allogeneic marrow transplantation. Esophageal symptoms in patients such as these may be due to infection, the disease itself, or both.

Anorexia, Nausea, and Vomiting

INFECTIOUS CAUSES

Herpesvirus infections of the esophagus, stomach, or intestine commonly cause nausea in addition to more organ-specific symptoms such as painful swallowing or diarrhea. In a prospective study of 50 marrow transplant patients with unexplained nausea and vomiting, 23 patients had herpesvirus infection, usually in the esophagus.[84] CMV was the most common isolate, but HSV and VZV esophagitis cause nausea as well. When liver, kidney, and heart transplant patients are evaluated for either painful swallowing or nonspecific symptoms such as nausea or dyspepsia, a similar spectrum of viral infections is found.[5,67,72–75] VZV and CMV infections may also involve visceral neural elements to produce a pseudo-obstruction picture with distention and vomiting. Herpesvirus infections are common in other diseases with protracted T-lymphocyte dysfunction, such as AIDS, leukemia, lymphoma, and some immunodeficiency syndromes. Immunosuppressed patients may also develop gastric ulcers caused by CMV that fail to heal on acid-reducing medications.[56,57,75]

Anorexia may be a prominent symptom of intestinal parasitic infection, especially with *Giardia lamblia* and *Cryptosporidium*.[97,98] The latter organism may be widespread in patients with AIDS, involving the biliary ducts and esophagus.

Unrecognized bacterial infections cause anorexia and debility. In the immunocompromised patient with an abnormal granulocyte and macrophage responses to infection, typical signs and symptoms may be absent. Examples are *Clostridium difficile* colitis, bacterial liver abscess, perforated bowel, perianal cellulitis, appendicitis, cholecystitis, and visceral mycobacterial infections. Surgeons working in organ-transplant units have documented the difficulties of recognizing intra-abdominal infection in these patients.[46,65,66,77,78]

Central nervous system infections are another cause of nausea and vomiting in the immunosuppressed patient. Other signs and symptoms are usually present, however. For example, patients with AIDS who developed meningeal cryptococcosis had fever, headache, and malaise, but nausea or vomiting was present in 42% of patients.[175] CNS infections in the compromised host have been reviewed recently.[176]

NONINFECTIOUS CAUSES

Adverse drug reactions are a common noninfectious cause of anorexia, nausea, and vomiting. Some examples are nausea caused by chemotherapy agents, immunosuppressive drugs (such as methotrexate, cyclosporine, and azathioprine), and antibiotics (particularly trimethoprim-sulfamethoxazole). Terminal cancer patients frequently have nausea and vomiting partially caused by tumor necrosis factor, partly by obstruction, and partly by medication side effects.[177] In some cases, a search for treatable causes of anorexia should be undertaken even when the underlying disease will have a fatal outcome. Relief of nausea and vomiting is a worthy goal in a dying patient, if diagnosis and treatment can be done expeditiously.

Diarrhea

INFECTIOUS CAUSES

The differential diagnosis of diarrhea in the compromised host encompasses the same pathogens as in the normal host, as well as some that are very uncommon under ordinary circumstances. In addition, the usual pathogens often present with a more severe or more chronic course.

As in the normal host, a stool culture should be obtained to look for bacterial pathogens including *Salmonella*, *Shigella*, *Campylobacter*, and *Clostridium difficile*. Blood cultures for *Salmonella* and *Shigella* are positive more often in compromised patients than in sporadic cases.[178] While *Campylobacter* causes acute self-limited diarrhea in the normal host, it is a common cause of chronic bloody diarrhea and fever in patients with congenital hypogammaglobulinemia or AIDS (see ch 103).[179] Diarrhea, often bloody, is seen with neutropenic enterocolitis (typhlitis), frequently associated with *C. septicum* infection.[18,180–182] *Aeromonas* species have been recently implicated in diarrheal illness in both normal patients with community-acquired diarrhea and immunosuppressed patients.[183,184] Selective culture media are needed to isolate this anaerobic gram-negative rod, which can be effectively treated in the suppressed host.[185] Mycobacterial species may cause diarrhea, particularly in patients with AIDS (see ch 103 for a discussion of *M. avium-intracellulare* infection of the small intestine). Nonpathogenic organisms that colonize the small intestine in patients with immunologlobulin deficiency cause "stasis syndrome," which leads to mucosal dysfunction, malabsorption, and diarrhea.

Bacterial infections not obviously involving the intestine may cause diarrhea. For example, immunosuppressed patients are at risk for *Legionella* pneumonia. Diarrhea is a frequent symptom with this infection and occasionally is profuse.[186] Both *L. pneumophilia* and other *Legionella* species may cause diarrhea.[187] Toxic shock syndrome associated with *Staphylococcus aureus* infection may also have a diarrheal component.

In the minimally compromised patient, fungal overgrowth (usually *Candida albicans*) can be a cause of watery diarrhea.[129,188] Microscopy of stool specimens is a useful way of screening for this, but cultures are not, since some fungi are part of the normal flora. More severely compromised patients, especially those with prolonged granulocytopenia, may present with diarrhea due to mucosally invasive fungal infection.[20,83,94,189,190]

Parasitic infections are also common in the immunocompromised host. *Giardia lamblia* is a prominent pathogen in common variable hypogammaglobulinemia but is also seen in X-linked immunodeficiency, IgA deficiency, and AIDS.[191,192] *Cryptosporidium* is a coccidial protozoan that causes an acute self-limited diarrheal illness in normal hosts but can cause chronic diarrhea in the setting of T-lymphocyte dysfunction or hypogammaglobulinemia.[193] Diagnosis is usually made by performing a modified Ziehl-Nielson stain on the stool. A related pathogen is *Isospora belli*, which causes chronic diarrhea and weight loss in up to 15% of Haitian AIDS patients but is rarely seen in the United States.[194] *Isospora* responds to treatment but tends to recur. An important parasite pathogen in patients with AIDS, *Microsporidium*, is discussed in chapter 103. *Strongyloides stercoralis* enteritis may exacerbate during immunosuppressive therapy, causing diarrhea.[44,45] It is especially important to make this diagnosis before disseminated strongyloidiasis (hyperinfection) develops, since this complication is frequently fatal.[45] *Strongyloides* hyperinfection syndrome, however, appears to be rare in both patients with AIDS and marrow graft recipients.[195] *Blastocystis hominis* and *Enteromonas hominis*, long believed to be innocuous commensal parasites, have been blamed for persistent diarrhea in some immunodeficient patients.[196,197]

Viral infections can also result in severe or chronic diarrhea in the compromised host. In the setting of T-lymphocyte dysfunction, either congenital or acquired (as in the post-transplant setting), rotavirus has been shown to cause protracted diarrhea and malabsorption.[198–200] Persistent viral shedding was documented in one case for more than 450 days. Diagnosis is made by specific immunoassay of stool. Similar symptoms may result from coxsackievirus and adenovirus infections and probably from a host of other viruses that we are unable to detect in the clinical laboratory.[201–204] A more severe, necrotizing enteritis has been described in marrow transplant patients infected with adenovirus and HSV.[93,94]

CMV enteritis occurs commonly in patients with AIDS, transplant recipients, and patients with leukemia and lymphoma who receive chemotherapy.[67–69,74,84,91,94,205,206] It is less common in common variable hypogammaglobulinemia and other congenital syndromes. Sporadic cases have been described in patients without obvious immunodeficiency, suggesting a higher overall prevalence than we now recognize.[207] There are two sorts of diarrheal illness caused by CMV: one a profuse watery diarrhea with protein loss and the other an inflammatory colitis with diarrhea, bleeding, and pain. CMV enteritis does not always result in diarrhea, however, since infection can be focal, leading to nausea, vomiting, bleeding, and perforation. High-volume diarrhea and protein-losing enteropathy are due to diffuse small intestinal involvement.[208–210] Colonic involvement can range from small superficial erosions to severe hemorrhagic colitis with deep ulcerations, which can ultimately perforate.[68,69,211] Patients with CMV colitis are often febrile and have abdominal distention.[206] Although CMV may rarely be isolated on viral culture of stool, the diagnosis is more apt to be obtained with examination of biopsy specimens from involved tissue. Diagnostic tests that should be performed on biopsy specimens include centrifugation viral culture, routine histology, and specific immunohistochemical stains.[67,84,91,94,212]

NONINFECTIOUS CAUSES

While a specific infectious cause must always be sought, immunocompromised patients also have a higher incidence of certain noninfectious types of diarrhea. For example, nodular lymphoid hyperplasia and jejunal villous atrophy are seen in a significant number of patients with common variable hypogammaglobulinemia and can result in malabsorption and diarrhea.[112,213] Achlorhydria and intestinal bacterial overgrowth are also seen more frequently in patients with immunologic defects, including HIV infection.[112,114] Patients who are immunocompromised as a result of treatment for malignancy can have diarrhea as a result of drug or radiation injury to the bowel.

Abdominal Pain

The initial approach to pain in an immunosuppressed patient must be tempered by the knowledge that intra-abdominal catastrophes may occur without extreme signs and symptoms and that the time from presentation to death can be very short. This is particularly true in granulocytopenic patients and in those on chronic immunosuppressive drugs. Physicians experienced in the care of such patients have a sense of urgency in assessing abdominal pain.

Intestinal perforation and intra-abdominal abscess formation must be found early if the patient is to survive. Perforation is most common in the gastroduodenal region and the colon but can occur at any site in the intestine, particularly in patients with lymphoma involving the intestine.[14,15,21] Frequent abdominal examinations, radiographs, and contrast studies may be necessary to discern that a perforation has occurred and to locate the site. Causes of perforation include CMV infection, fungal infiltration, necrosis of transmural tumors, trauma, and diverticula.[12–15,21,52,211] Diverticular perforation seems to be particularly common in renal transplant patients.[46]

CMV and VZV can also involve neural plexi causing ileus and abdominal distention.[214] Severe abdominal pain is often the first manifestation of disseminated VZV infection, which may also progress to fulminant hepatitis. Early recognition and institution of acyclovir therapy may result in improved survival.[215,216]

Other focal infections of the intestinal tract that can present with abdominal pain include phlegmonous gastritis, appendicitis, and typhlitis (neutropenic enterocolitis). Phlegmonous gastritis, a bacterial infection of the gastric mucosa caused by organisms from the oral flora, has been described in patients with diabetes, alcoholism, AIDS, and following marrow transplantation.[217,218] Appendicitis occurs as commonly in children and adolescents with leukemia as it does in the general population. Most immunosuppressed patients with appendicitis have right lower quadrant pain, but in some the usual presentation is masked by corticosteroids and the lack of granulocytes.[219,220] Differentiating appendicitis from typhlitis can be difficult when imaging tests (computed tomography and ultrasound) are equivocal. Surgical exploration is recommended by most authorities, since mortality from a perforated appendix managed without operation is very high.[221,222] One surgical series of leukemic children with right lower quadrant pain found that half had appendicitis and half had typhlitis.[220] Typhlitis is a localized infection of the cecum and right colon that was first described in children with granulocytopenia and acute leukemia.[223] It is also seen in other diseases with granulocytopenia, after chemotherapy, after marrow grafting, and in patients with aplastic anemia, myeloma, and cyclic neutropenia.[180-182] Typhlitis has been rare after solid organ transplantation and in patients with AIDS, probably because of preserved granulocyte function. Patients present with nausea, vomiting, right-sided abdominal pain, fever and shock due to polymicrobial sepsis, and bloody diarrhea.[16,182,222,223] *Clostridium septicum* is the most frequently isolated organism associated with this condition.[16,18,181,182] Imaging studies help to confirm the diagnosis by demonstrating cecal wall edema.[224,225] The diagnosis is primarily a clinical one, however, and should lead to prompt empiric use of antibiotics and surgical consultation. There are other inflammatory diseases of the right colon that do not have the same poor prognosis as the typhlitis syndrome just described. These include *C. difficile* colitis, CMV ulcerations, fungal infiltrations, and acute GVHD in marrow graft recipients.

Biliary colic, cholecystitis, and gallbladder perforation can also be seen in suppressed hosts. Although immunocompromised patients may have pain related to stones or gallbladder sludge (particularly in patients on parenteral nutrition), they are also susceptible to unusual infections involving the biliary tree, most notably *Cryptosporidium* and CMV in patients with AIDS (see ch 103) Recognition of cholecystitis in a transplant patient on high-dose immunosuppressive therapy is difficult.

There is a higher incidence of lymphoproliferative disease in patients with immunodeficiency, especially in AIDS patients and solid-organ and marrow transplant recipients on immunosuppressive therapy.[1,46,58,70,94,95] Lymphoid infiltrates may involve the liver or bowel and present as abdominal pain, ileus, and bleeding. Recent studies have shown EBV transcripts to be present both in lymphoproliferative disease and in some lymphomas.[58,95]

Patients who are granulocytopenic because of treatment for malignancy may have abdominal pain related to that therapy and not necessarily to granulocytopenia. High-dose chemotherapy (particularly with regimens using cytarabine and 5-fluorouracil/citrovorum factor) and radiation therapy can injure the gut, causing crampy abdominal pain and diarrhea.[27-29, 171] This can rarely progress to mucosal necrosis with peritoneal signs. Certain chemotherapeutic agents may cause pancreatitis, particularly L-asparaginase and high-dose cytarabine.[26] Narcotics and antiemetics with anticholinergic properties are often used in these patients and can lead to ileus and painful bowel distention. Intra-arterial chemotherapy, usually given for hepatic metastases, may cause gastrointestinal mucosal necrosis.[33] Intraperitoneal therapy can cause a chemical peritonitis, may lead to infection or trauma from the catheter used, and may cause adhesions.[222]

Patients who are thrombocytopenic may have abdominal pain as a result of bleeding into the retroperitoneum, bowel wall, or abdominal wall. Hematomas within the sheath of the rectus abdominis cause sudden severe abdominal pain, which is frequently mistaken for intra-abdominal disease.[41] Diagnosis is made by ultrasound or computed tomography. Hematomas within the gut wall may occur at the site of a previous biopsy or at the site of an ulcer.[40,84] These cause abdominal pain and intestinal obstruction.

Management of intramural hematomas depends on the clinical situation. If blood loss is large and continuing, or if complete intestinal obstruction is present, surgical intervention is required. Many of these cases, however, can be managed conservatively with platelet support, parenteral nutrition, and observation.

In the early post–marrow transplant setting, abdominal pain can be caused by hepatic engorgement secondary to veno-occlusive disease of the liver.[35,36,81] GVHD can occur at any time after the bone marrow engrafts; gut involvement characteristically is associated with crampy abdominal pain and diarrhea.[80,83,85] These patients usually have evidence of GVHD of skin and liver. Diagnosis of intestinal GVHD can be confirmed by rectal, gastric, or duodenal biopsy if the platelet count can be supported at greater than $60,000/mm^3$.[80,83-86]

Perianal Pain

Perianal pain in a granulocytopenic patient is due to bacterial infection of perianal tissues until proven otherwise. This can be a difficult problem to recognize, since there may be little in the way of pus but instead only a painful cellulitis. These infections are usually polymicrobial, arising from either anal crypts or from tears in the anal canal.[226,227] Extensive supralevator and intersphincteric abscesses may also occur without being apparent on external examination. Digital rectal examination can be useful, but at the risk of precipitating bacteremia. Computed tomography of the pelvis gives a clear view of the anatomy involved if there is a true abscess.[228] A recent report from the National Cancer Institute places the controversy of surgical versus medical management into perspective.[227] Fifty-seven episodes of anorectal infection occurring in patients with prolonged neutropenia were reviewed. Most infections were due to multiple organisms, both aerobes and anaerobes. When antibiotics covering both types of organisms were given, there was control of infection in 15 of 17 patients, most of whom did not have evidence for extensive soft tissue destruction. Surgery plus antibiotic coverage was successful in 19 of 26 patients, many with obvious fluctuance, necrosis, or ongoing sepsis.[227] Seven patients died as a result of anorectal infection. Because of the lethal nature of uncontrolled anorectal infections in granulocytopenic patients, aggressive surgical approaches may be necessary in patients with tissue necrosis, even if such surgery carries the risk of poor wound healing and the spread of infection.[226,229,230] Early treatment of perianal cellulitis with proper antibiotics and the empiric treatment of fever in these patients probably accounts for fewer patients requiring surgical debridement than in the past.[227,231]

HSV causes painful chronic mucocutaneous ulcerations in patients with immunodeficiency syndromes, especially those with T-lymphocyte defects.[232-234] In the perianal area, the appearance is of multiple superficial ulcers with raised borders. When these ulcers coalesce and become macerated and secondarily infected, it is often difficult to identify them as viral.[232] In contrast to decubiti, HSV perianal ulcers are painful, have scalloped borders, and occur away from pressure points. The diagnosis is best made by scraping friable border areas and by rectal swabs, for viral cultures, immunocytology, or Tzanck smears. Acyclovir treatment is effective, but secondary bacterial or fungal infection may delay healing.[235] Recurrence is common unless immunosuppressive therapy can be decreased.[234]

Case reports of unusual anorectal infections include a patient with Job's syndrome (hyperimmunoglobulinemia E with recurrent infection) who had a chronic perianal abscess and colonic inflammation due to *Cryptococcus*.[236] Patients with AIDS may present with painful anorectal lesions caused by common venereal pathogens[237,238] as well as unusual diseases such as tuberculosis, Kaposi's sarcoma, cloacogenic carcinoma, squamous cell carcinoma, and lymphoma.[239-241] Papillomavirus infection and anal warts may be precursors of anal neoplasms in patients with AIDS.[242] These AIDS-related infections are discussed in chapter 103.

Gastrointestinal Bleeding

There are two categories of immunosuppressed patients with gastrointestinal bleeding: those with normal platelet and coagulation function and those with disordered hemostasis. In the latter group, even the most insignificant erosion can lead to continuous bleeding.

INFECTIOUS CAUSES

Viral ulcerations are the most common cause of bleeding in transplant patients as well as in those with prolonged T-lymphocyte immunodeficiency. They are less common during transient drops in leukocyte counts following chemotherapy for solid tumors. HSV may present as bleeding from esophageal lesions without symptoms referable to the esophagus.[84,163,167] The bleeding is more likely to be a slow ooze from coalescent herpetic ulcers rather than a spurting vessel. It is useful to brush the edges of these ulcers to make a diagnosis, but if the appearance suggests HSV infection, a course of acyclovir should be started empirically. Restoration of platelet and coagulation factors, protection of the ulcerated esophagus from acid-peptic reflux, and acyclovir are successful in controlling bleeding herpetic ulcers. HSV causes gastric and intestinal necrosis only rarely, usually in patients on high-dose immunosuppressive therapy.[94]

CMV causes ulcerations throughout the intestinal tract. Those in the esophagus are usually shallow, but those in the gastroduodenal, small intestinal, and colonic mucosa are deeper and capable of eroding into large vessels.[68,69,211,243-245] CMV may also cause diffuse gastritis or enteritis similar to inflammatory bowel disease.[67,74,84,91,94] In the gastroduodenal area, ulcers that appear to be typical peptic lesions may harbor CMV in the ulcer base and may fail to heal on standard ulcer therapy.[56,57,75] Identification of CMV as a cause of ulceration is very difficult when the ulcer is actually bleeding, since one is reluctant to biopsy the ulcer base where CMV-laden cells are usually found. When ulcers are in the midgut, radionuclide red cell or blood pool scans can localize the bleeding site, allowing angiographic control or surgical resection.[246,247] Endoscopic hemostasis of bleeding CMV ulcers can occasionally be achieved, but this is not a long-term solution since the infection remains long after a coagulation eschar has sloughed. There is little experience with antiviral therapy (ganciclovir or foscarnet) specifically for bleeding CMV lesions, although these drugs do have a significant antiviral effect in the intestine.[68,69,91,206]

Other viral infections may also cause bleeding, but these are far less common. VZV causes esophagitis similar to HSV, but not intestinal mucosal necrosis. EBV does not cause direct ulceration, but in immunosuppressed transplant patients (bone marrow, renal, cardiac, liver) it may lead to a lymphoma-like immunoproliferative disorder.[58,70,95] In the intestine, this disease presents as large submucosal nodules as well as diffuse mucosal infiltration with immunoblasts.[94] These areas commonly ulcerate and bleed. Adenovirus has been reported to cause extensive intestinal necrosis as well as fulminant hepatitis in immunosuppressed patients.[93] No therapy is effective. Other enteric viruses (e.g., rotavirus) are unusual causes of bleeding unless patients are severely thrombocytopenic.

Fungal plaques are frequently found at autopsy in the esophagus and intestine in a cancer center population but are uncommon causes of serious bleeding.[20] Exceptions are patients with prolonged granulocytopenia in whom deeper penetration of fungi can erode into large submucosal blood vessels, leading to massive bleeding.[83,94,189,248,249] Most fungal plaques are due to *Candida albicans*, but there is some evidence that other fungi (particularly *Aspergillus*) and other *Candida* species (such as *C. tropicalis* and *C. glabrata*) are more common causes of invasive ulceration. It should be noted that while *Candida* "colonization" of gastroduodenal peptic ulcers in normal hosts does not apparently alter their response to therapy, this may not be true in the granulocytopenic patient.

Any bacterial or parasitic infection capable of causing dysentery in a normal host will certainly do so in an immunosuppressed one. Thus bloody, high-volume diarrhea should prompt bacterial cultures as well as an examination for *E. histolytica*, if history and geography suggest this possibility. Pseudomembranous colitis due to *Clostridium difficile* may also present as bleeding, especially in patients with a low platelet count. In granulocytopenic patients, typical pseudomembranes may be absent but the colonic mucosa will be ulcerated and friable. Bloody diarrhea also occurs with typhlitis (*C. septicum* infection), especially if platelet counts are low.

NONINFECTIOUS CAUSES

Several noninfectious causes of serious bleeding must also be considered, especially in patients with low platelet counts. Patients receiving chemotherapy may traumatize their esophagus and stomach by retching, and if hemostasis is not normal, massive bleeding may result from Mallory-Weiss tears, ecchymoses in the upper body of the stomach, and intramural hematomas in the esophagus.[39,40] If a patient is receiving high-dose chemotherapy or radiation therapy for a tumor involving the wall of the intestinal tract, especially lymphoma or chloroma, tumor lysis may lead to a large area of ulceration or perforation at the site of the tumor.[11-14] High-dose chemotherapy regimens, especially those using cytarabine in combination with other agents and using 5-fluorouracil/citrovorum factor protocols, may cause intestinal mucosal necrosis and bleeding.[27-29] Fortunately, most combination chemotherapy regimens in current use do not cause this type of necrosis unless the drugs are infused intra-arterially. Hepatic artery infusions of chemotherapeutic agents may cause necrosis of duodenal and gastric mucosa.[33] In allogeneic marrow transplant patients, GVHD involving the intestine is a common cause of bleeding.[83-86,94] Viral and fungal superinfections as well as EBV lymphoproliferative lesions may coexist with GVHD.[83,94] In renal transplant patients, intestinal ischemia, with mucosal necrosis and bleeding, may occur in the perioperative period; severe colitis has also been described after Kayexalate-Sorbitol enemas.[53-55] Endoscopic biopsy sites and surgical anastomoses may bleed because of poor tissue repair in patients who are cachectic and in those who have received high-dose chemotherapy or irradiation to the intestine. Separating these noninfectious causes of bleeding from treatable infectious causes may be difficult, with the infections often becoming apparent only at surgery or autopsy. Patient outcome depends more on the reversibility of the primary illness than on the identification of preterminal infectious complications. It is unreasonable to recommend extensive, invasive studies to identify a bleeding site in a patient whose likelihood of survival is small.

Hepatobiliary Disease

Liver disease in the immunocompromised host can be caused by the same processes as in the normal host. There are a number of unusual pathogens, however, which are only seen in this setting and may respond to appropriate therapy if they are thought of and recognized.

INFECTIOUS CAUSES

Several viruses cause fulminant hepatic failure in immunosuppressed hosts. Death from massive hepatocyte necrosis may occur within days of the onset of illness. The most important viruses in this regard are HSV and VZV because they are sensitive to acyclovir therapy and thus potentially treatable.[47,250-253] In a compromised host with rapidly rising serum levels of hepatocellular enzymes, one should proceed promptly to liver biopsy for viral culture and immunohistology to identify the virus.[251-254] Transvenous liver biopsy may be an alternative to percutaneous biopsy when platelet counts are low. If a biopsy cannot be done safely, the empiric administration of acyclovir should be considered. Other viruses that cause massive hepatocellular necrosis in this setting include adenovirus, echovirus, and hepatitis B virus.[93,96,254-259] Fulminant hepatitis B differs from hepatitis caused by the other viruses mentioned previously in that hepatocyte destruction is caused not by hepatitis B virus but by a revived immune system. Hepatitis B virus replicates in the liver during immune suppression. When cancer chemotherapy ceases, or when doses of chronic immunosuppressive drugs are lowered, or when a marrow graft matures, there may be immune-mediated hepatocyte necrosis.[96,256-259] Fortunately, this is not common.

However, chronic viral hepatitis is very common in immunosuppressed patients, especially those who have received blood products. There is a problem in recognizing viral infection in these patients, since standard serologic tests may not be reliable. For example, hepatitis B virus can be demonstrated in the liver of seronegative children with leukemia.[260,261] A recent study of hepatitis B seronegative cancer patients showed that 12% had hepatitis B DNA in their serum.[262] The sensitivity of antibody tests to hepatitis C and D virus has not been examined in the compromised host. Chronic hepatitis is likely to occur in patients with chronic

renal failure on hemodialysis, organ transplant recipients, and patients with hematologic malignancies and aplastic anemia since these patients are often multiply transfused.[263] Hepatitis B and C tend to have a different clinical course in this population, probably because of the importance of the host immune response in the immunopathogenesis of liver necrosis. Patients with immature or impaired immune systems who are infected with the hepatitis B virus tend to have a higher level of virus replication within the liver but fewer acute symptoms, and tend to go on to the chronic carrier state rather than having an acute self-limited hepatitis.[264,265] The new onset of immunosuppression in a patient previously infected with hepatitis B can allow a marked rise in the level of viremia and may occasionally result in the re-expression of hepatitis B surface antigen (HbsAg) in a patient who was previously HBsAg negative and HBsAb positive.[257] In patients who remain immunocompromised, the clinical course can be quite variable. On initial liver biopsy one can find histology ranging from chronic persistent to chronic lobular to chronic active hepatitis; however, even the forms of hepatitis that are ordinarily nonprogressive in the normal host can progress in this group of patients to chronic active hepatitis or cirrhosis.[48-50,266,267]

Hepatitis C has become the more prominent cause of chronic liver disease in the immunosuppressed population as testing for the hepatitis B virus has become more sensitive, allowing more accurate screening of blood products. This form of hepatitis has also been well studied in the renal transplant population, which can probably serve as a model for other types of cellular immunodeficiency.[5,263] Chronic hepatitis has been found to develop in over 90% of renal transplant recipients who develop acute Hepatitis C during their first year post transplant and in 64% of those infected after that.[51] Those with hepatitis had a significantly higher mortality (45% versus 16% in those without hepatitis). Early on this mortality is due largely to extrahepatic sepsis, suggesting that the hepatitis itself may cause further immunosuppression. Over 5 to 10 years these patients also go on to develop progressive liver disease with cirrhosis.[263]

In marrow transplant patients with disseminated CMV infection, a diffuse hepatitis with microabscesses has been described but serious liver dysfunction is uncommon.[92] Hepatitis due to CMV is of particular concern in the liver transplant recipient.[268,269] The patient with CMV hepatitis presents with fever, jaundice, and elevated liver enzymes, all of which are also characteristic of acute rejection. Liver biopsy is necessary to distinguish the two since the treatment for CMV is to reduce the level of immunosuppression whereas the treatment for organ rejection is obviously an increase in immunosuppressive therapy. Ganciclovir therapy may also be effective in this setting.[68,69] Both CMV and EBV can occasionally produce long-standing elevations in serum hepatocellular enzyme levels in other types of immunocompromised hosts. The EBV-induced lymphoproliferative disorder can also involve the liver.[87,95]

In the patient who presents with liver function abnormalities that are primarily cholestatic, one must consider both biliary tract disease as well as infiltrative disease of the liver parenchyma. The most common infiltrative infectious processes in the liver producing elevated alkaline phosphatase and fever in immunocompromised patients are *Mycobacterium avium-intracellulare* (see ch 103) and hepatic candidiasis. Involvement of the liver with *Candida* can be part of an obviously disseminated infection, or the process can be localized to the liver. The triad of fever, right upper quadrant tenderness, and elevated alkaline phosphatase concentration in a granulocytopenic host should suggest the diagnosis of hepatic candidiasis.[87,270,271] The diagnosis is strongly supported by the finding of small nonenhancing lesions in the liver on abdominal computed tomography.[272,273] The diagnosis should be confirmed by ultrasound-directed needle aspiration, with culture and histologic examination of the biopsy material to ascertain the specific pathogen and its antibiotic sensitivity. Occasionally fungal microabscesses are seen at laparoscopy or on liver biopsy in a patient in whom no computed tomographic abnormalities were seen.[274] Presumably, these patients are those with early involvement. Other *Candida* species and other fungi (*Aspergillus, Trichosporon, Cryptococcus, Coccidioides, Histoplasma, Mucor*) may infect the liver.[275–279] Hepatic infection with *Aspergillus* and *Mucor* may present as Budd-Chiari syndrome because of the propensity of these organisms for vascular invasion.[276,278] *Pneumocystis carinii,* an organism recently reclassified as a fungus, may be widely disseminated in patients with AIDS, presenting as diffuse hepatic and visceral involvement.[280,281] *Toxoplasma gondii* may also involve the liver and other viscera. Other presentations of far advanced fungal diseases include large abscesses and cystic lesions and massed fungi in bile ducts.

Biliary infection is a common problem in patients with AIDS, due to infection with CMV and *Cryptosporidium* (see ch 103). These same organisms cause cholecystitis and cholangitis in congenital immunodeficiency syndromes and marrow graft recipients.[282,283]

Bacterial infections of the liver and biliary system are unusual in patients wtih disorders of cell-mediated immunity but are frequent in patients with biliary obstruction, intra-abdominal sepsis, granulocytopenia, and congenital disorders of granulocyte function. Even more common are the hepatic effects of remote bacterial infection, which may cause cholestatic jaundice and rises in serum alkaline phosphatase concentrations.[284–286] Unusual bacterial infections may also involve the liver when immune surveillance is defective. For example, granulomatous hepatitis in an adult marrow transplant patient was caused by the mycobacterium bacille Calmette-Guérin (BCG), given years earlier as a vaccine.[287]

NONINFECTIOUS CAUSES

Drug-induced liver disease must be considered in those patients who are immunocompromised on the basis of malignancy, since they are likely to be treated with chemotherapy that is hepatotoxic.[26,34–38]

Many immunosuppressed patients are treated with other drugs that are hepatotoxic. These include antibiotics (especially trimethorprim-sulfamethoxazole and third-generation penicillins, to a lesser extent), antifungal agents (ketoconazole, fluconazole, itraconazole), and immunosuppressive drugs (cyclosporine, methotrexate, azathioprine, prednisone).[87] Total parenteral nutrition may also cause liver dysfunction, especially in patients who are septic.[87,288]

Two conditions commonly seen in the bone marrow transplant setting are hepatic veno-occlusive disease and GVHD involving the liver. Veno-occlusive disease is a severe form of hepatotoxicity due to conditioning total-body irradiation and chemotherapy that precede the transplant.[34–37] GVHD is an immunologic disorder that affects bile ducts in the liver, usually in patients with evidence of GVHD in other organ systems, such as the skin and intestine.[87–88]

Idiopathic hyperammonemia, with coma, cerebral edema, and death, has been described in marrow transplant patients and after high-dose chemotherapy regimens.[289] Although overt liver dysfunction is not a feature of this syndrome, the inability to metabolize ammonia suggests a defect in hepatic enzyme systems. Sodium benzoate may be a useful therapy for hyperammonemia in these patients.

Fever

This section is not a comprehensive review of intestinal and hepatic causes of fever but rather a reminder of subtle disorders that may cause fever without organ-specific signs or symptoms. A common example is fungal liver disease, which frequently presents as fever unresponsive to empiric antibiotic therapy. A liver studded with miliary fungal lesions may not be tender until the lesions grow, may not lead to fungemia, and often appears normal by computed tomography or ultrasound because the size of individual lesions is below the sensitivity of imaging modalities.[271,274] Clues to the presence of hepatic fungus in a granulocytopenic patient can often be found in the mouth (oral thrush) or intestinal tract (fungal colonization on stool cultures), since the portal of entry for fungi is usually the intestine. Yeast forms of *Candida* transverse the normal small intestine into the portal circulation by a poorly understood process called persorption. This was conclusively demonstrated by an investigator who swallowed a *Candida* yeast broth, with subsequent fungemia and funguria.[290]

Mycobacterial infections of the liver and intestine are most commonly caused by *M. tuberculosis, M. avium-intracellulare,* and, in some Third World countries, *M. bovis. M. tuberculosis* infection of the liver and peritoneum was a well-recognized cause of fever of unknown origin before the advent of AIDS and aggressive chemotherapy regimens. Infection with this organism can be confined to the abdominal viscera, without typical chest radiographic abnormalities. *M. avium-intracellulare* infection of the intestine and liver occurs mostly in patients with AIDS (see ch 103). Severe, prolonged immunosuppression may lead to reactivation of latent mycobacteria.[287]

Esophageal infections caused by virus and fungi may be completely silent except for fever.[84,163] The ulcerated esophagus can be a portal of entry for bacteria, as illustrated by the case of an elderly man with recurrent fever whose distal esophagus allowed entry of both bacteria and particulate material.[291] Bacterial esophagitis in immunosuppressed patients usually occurs as a superinfection of already ulcerated epithelium and is commonly accompanied by fever.[163,170,291]

There are two types of bacterial infections of the stomach that present as fever. Phlegmonous gastritis is a suppurative infection of the mucosa and submucosa caused by polymicrobial flora from the oropharynx. Most reported cases have not been in severely immunosuppressed patients but rather in alcoholics and malnourished patients.[217,218] Abdominal pain develops as the pyogenic process progresses. *Pseudomonas* vasculitis is a blood-borne infection in which the blood vessels of the viscera become infected with bacteria.[292] An unremitting febrile illness with signs of septicemia may obscure the intra-abdominal/intravascular focus of infection.

When patients with parasitic diseases of the intestine become immunosuppressed, or when suppressed patients ingest parasites, intestinal symptoms are usually manifest, along with fever at times. One prominent exception is in patients with disseminated strongyloidiasis, in which extraintestinal symptoms, including fever, sepsis, and shock are prominent in the immunosuppressed patient.[45] *Entamoeba histolytica* may cause fulminant colitis and liver abscess when amebic dysentery is mistaken for ulcerative colitis and treated with corticosteroids. Recurrent fever due to bacteremia from organisms derived from the intestine is seen in patients with immunoglobulin deficiency and with AIDS. These organisms are normally intestinal pathogens, such as *Campylobacter fetus*, *Salmonella*, and *Shigella*, but the intestinal manifestations may not be prominent.[178,179,192] In other immunosuppressed patients, a similar phenomenon occurs, but the organisms are part of the usual intestinal flora. This phenomenon is called "translocation," in which luminal organisms gain access to lymphatic tissue and the portal circulation via an anatomically intact mucosa. Translocation is best defined in animal models of trauma and endotoxic shock and probably occurs in the analogous human conditions.[144-147] Translocation also occurs in immunosuppressed patients whose intestinal flora has been altered by antibiotic use, thus removing "colonization resistance." Aerobic organisms then proliferate instead of the usually dominant anaerobes.[293] Translocation of these aerobic organisms to adjacent tissues certainly occurs through mucosa damaged by chemotherapy or other infections, and possibly through normal mucosa as well.[294] A similar phenomenon occurs rarely in patients with colonic adenocarcinoma, in whom fever and bacteremia may occur spontaneously, without evidence of gross perforation of the bowel. The organisms most commonly isolated are clostridial species (especially *C. septicum*) and *Streptococcus bovis*.[16,22] *Clostridium* species are also responsible for other febrile illnesses seen regularly in hospitals that provide care for patients with cancer. These illnesses include typhlitis, an edematous process involving the cecum in granulocytopenic patients, associated with polymicrobial sepsis with colonic organisms; pseudomembranous colitis, caused by *C. difficile*; and biliary infections with gas-forming clostridia. There may be evidence of remote foci of clostridial infection.[16] Perianal bacterial infections in granulocytopenic patients commonly lead to fever but usually have local pain (albeit without much fluctuance). Intraabdominal abscesses from intestinal perforation may be difficult to recognize in immunosuppressed patients because of a paucity of clinical findings other than fever.[78]

COMMENTS ON TREATMENT OF INTESTINAL AND LIVER INFECTIONS IN THE IMMUNOCOMPROMISED HOST

Prophylaxis of Intestinally Derived Infections and Infections Involving the Intestine and Liver

The gastrointestinal tract is the origin of many of the bacteria, fungi, and parasites that are problematic in immunosuppressed patients. The development of viral infection is more complex, since viruses may be acquired from the environment, from blood-product transfusion, and from transplanted tissue but may also be activated from latency when immune surveillance is compromised. A large body of literature attests to efforts to prevent infection either by denying organisms access to the suppressed patient, by manipulating the patient's resident flora, or by giving antimicrobial drugs to prevent clinical illness.

PREVENTING NEW ORGANISMS FROM REACHING OR INFECTING THE PATIENT (SEE ALSO CH 52)

The air we breathe and the food we eat contain organisms that ordinarily do us no harm. Normal humans may even ingest small inocula of pathogenic organisms such as *Salmonella* without clinical illness, probably due to such defenses as gastric acidity and local mucosal immunity.[295] However, patients without granulocytes, without the "colonization resistance" of the normal intestinal flora, and without an intact mucosal barrier may be jeopardized by the organisms in normal food. *Escherichia coli*, *Klebsiella*, *Proteus*, *Serratia*, *Candida*, and *Aspergillus* organisms, for example, are commonly found on vegetables and fruits.[296] Prepared foods such as unpasteurized juices, snacks, and sandwiches have a similar range of organisms that may colonize the intestine and cause clinical illness.[297] Most oncology and marrow transplant units employ low microbial diets, eschewing contaminated items such as raw vegetables, salads, natural cheeses, cold soups from fresh vegetables, poorly cooked meat or fish salads, whipped cream, and uncooked spices.[298] Even bottled water and pasteurized milk may be contaminated. Sterile diets can be achieved, but evidence that they reduce clinical illness is lacking. Such measures as positive air pressure rooms, filtration of air, and cleaning of room surfaces are additional measures to protect vulnerable patients. Hospital-acquired organisms may be pathogens (e.g., *C. difficile*) but may also be normal organisms that acquire resistance to antibiotics.[150] Such organisms are difficult to eradicate once they have colonized and difficult to treat once they cause illness.

Physicians and nurses can be unwitting vectors of these organisms, but hospital-acquired organisms on hands can be eliminated by scrupulous hand washing. Endoscopists may transmit organisms from contaminated instruments such as endoscopes, brushes, and biopsy instruments. Cold disinfection procedures using glutaraldehyde are effective in removing organisms from the surface of endoscopes but not from the interstices of these instruments or the coiled wires of biopsy forceps.[299] Glutaraldehyde activity and contact time must be rigidly controlled to ensure that an instrument is adequately decontaminated; many prefer to gas-sterilize their instruments after thorough cleansing to ensure that a granulocytopenic patient does not become infected by a contaminated instrument.[40] It is more difficult to deal with bacteremia that occurs as a result of intestinal endoscopy. Immunologically normal patients may rarely develop bacteremia during upper endoscopy, colonoscopy, and esophageal dilation, but this is transient and seldom causes clinical illness.[300,301] The bacteria in these cases are usually derived from the patient's endogenous flora. However, a recent study of marrow transplant patients undergoing endoscopy revealed that 8 of 46 patients undergoing upper endoscopy with a gas-sterilized instrument developed clinically obvious bacteremia.[302] This was significantly more common among patients on high-dose prednisone therapy. What is transient bacteremia in a normal host may not be innocuous in an immunosuppressed one. There may be a role for antibiotic prophylaxis before endoscopy in this type of patient.

Prevention of newly acquired viral infections requires limiting patient exposure to viruses carried by other persons, including nurses, physicians, family members, and visitors, and careful transfusion practices. Viruses such as VZV, HSV, adenovirus, and enteroviruses may cause self-limited illness in a normal host, but immunosuppressed patients may develop severe visceral infections that can be fatal or may have a prolonged illness because a virus cannot be eliminated.[79,93,203,215] Obviously infected staff and visitors should not have close contact with a suppressed patient. Careful transfusion practices are necessary to prevent serious viral infections acquired from blood products.[152] Blood banks screen donor blood for hepatitis viruses A, B, and C, and for HIV. However, CMV remains a problem, since a high percentage of donor blood in many parts of the world is seropositive. CMV-seropositive patients harbor latent virus in leukocytes as well as in other cells. When CMV-bearing leukocytes are transfused in blood products, even normal recipients (such as cardiac bypass patients) may develop a clinical illness caused by CMV. When CMV is transmitted to transplant recipients in this way, potentially fatal pneumonia, intestinal infection, and pancreatitis may ensue.[5,79] The role of CMV in causing fever and debility in granulocytopenic cancer patients is apparently greater than first thought. A recent prospective study found that 39% of such patients had CMV disease, including CMV enteritis.[303] Better methods for diagnosis of CMV infection, such as centrifugation viral culture and molecular histochemistry of tissue specimens, should clarify the role of CMV in other groups of patients as well. In the marrow transplant setting, there is clear evidence that transfusing only CMV-seronegative blood products into CMV-seronegative patients reduces the incidence of CMV disease.[166] Ideally, this strategy should be applied to any immunosuppressed patient who needs blood products, but the supply of CMV seronegative blood is limited, especially in geographic areas where most of the populace is seropositive. A promising recent development in this area is filtration to remove leukocytes from banked blood.[304] Since leukocytes are the primary carriers of latent CMV in transfused blood, one would expect that leukofiltered blood products would lower the incidence of CMV disease in seronegative recipients. Preliminary studies are encouraging.[304] Although other organisms, such as *Salmonella* species, *Yersinia enterocolitica*, some parasites, and other blood-borne viruses can be transferred via blood products, cases involving such organisms are unusual.

PROPHYLACTIC ANTIBACTERIAL DRUG THERAPY

It is clear that the gastrointestinal tract is a major reservoir for organisms that cause systemic infection in granulocytopenic patients. Evidence is also accumulating that the intestinal flora may play a role in causing bloodstream infections in situations such as trauma, burns, and shock.[141] There have been several approaches to suppressing the bacterial flora of the intestine in patients at risk.

Total intestinal decontamination regimens employ a combination of poorly absorbed oral antibiotics along with low microbial or sterile diets.[305] Examples are gentamicin/vancomycin/nystatin, gentamicin/vancomycin/polymyxin/nystatin, and polymyxin/neomycin/nalidixic acid regimens. While these regimens are capable of achieving gut sterilization, in practice they seldom accomplish this because of poor patient compliance and the acquisition of antibiotic-resistant gram-negative bacilli.[306] These regimens are costly and unpopular with patients, but when patient compliance is good they appear to reduce the incidence of bacterial sepsis compared with nontreated controls.[307] These regimens should be reserved for patients who will be profoundly granulocytopenic for longer than just a few days, particularly if the intestinal mucosal barrier is disrupted. Surveillance cultures should be done regularly to detect the appearance of resistant organisms.[293,308]

Selective suppression of intestinally derived aerobic bacteria is more practical, better tolerated, and widely used than total decontamination. The theory is to allow the anaerobic bacterial flora of the colon to maintain their resistance to colonization by new organisms while suppressing the aerobic organisms (particularly Enterobacteriaceae) that cause most of the clinical infections.[305,309] Trimethoprim-sulfamethoxazole and quinolone antibiotics (ciprofloxacin and norfloxacin) are in current use, since controlled trials have shown them to be beneficial in reducing bacterial infections, especially those due to gram-negative bacilli.[310-312] It is important to point out that beneficial results are reported in trials in which patients were especially at risk for bacteremia because of profound, prolonged granulocytopenia. Oral antifungal therapy needs to be given with these antibiotics because of a high incidence of fungal colonization and infection when they are not given.[305,310] Trimethoprim-sulfamethoxazole may have several toxic reactions that limit its usefulness, among them rashes, nausea, liver dysfunction, and marrow suppression.

Another sort of selective antimicrobial prophylaxis involves the use of systemic antibiotics, usually in combination with oral antibiotics and antifungal drugs.[148,305] Prophylactic systemic antibiotics are aimed not only at organisms that appear in the bloodstream but also at aerobic gram-negative bacteria that colonize the oropharynx, upper airway, stomach, and colon of seriously ill patients.[148-150] These regimens have been applied to both severely immunosuppressed granulocytopenic patients as well as to medical-surgical patients in an intensive care unit setting.[148,313,314] In comparison to control groups, patients receiving prophylactic systemic antibiotics exhibit a lower incidence of infection and colonization with gram-negative bacteria. In the intensive care unit setting, the positive effect is mostly on the incidence of pulmonary infections.[148] It is more difficult to demonstrate improvement in survival with this prophylaxis, and such regimens require rigorous microbiologic surveillance to detect resistant strains.

Another prophylactic antimicrobial strategy is directed at organisms that are colonizing the intestinal tract but that are not yet causing clinical disease.[150] These organisms are detected by surveillance culture. This strategy is based on the observation that the majority of episodes of bacteremia in granulocytopenic patients are preceded by positive cultures from the intestinal tract with the same organism.[293] This applies not only to Enterobacteriaceae but to gram-positive organisms such as *S. epidermidis* and to *Candida* species. However, not all colonized patients develop infection, and enthusiasm for surveillance culture-directed therapy must be tempered by the costs of this approach as well as the lack of a clear effect on survival in granulocytopenic patients. It may be useful in controlling nosocomial colonization with resistant organisms in an intensive care unit setting.[150]

PROPHYLACTIC ANTIFUNGAL DRUG THERAPY

Oral and intestinal mucosal fungal infections are prevalent in general medical patients, many with subtle defects in cell-mediated immunity and many on antibiotics. As troublesome as these infections are, they are uncommon causes of mortality, as long as granulocyte function is preserved. In granulocytopenic patients, these mucosal fungal infections are more common, more extensive, more difficult to eradicate, and more likely to lead to fatal fungemia and fungal liver abscesses. Transintestinal passage of yeast forms of *Candida* species occurs through the normal human intestine, seeding the portal circulation and liver with fungi.[290] For this reason, prophylaxis of mucosal fungal infections takes on special importance in patients with prolonged granulocytopenia.

Candida species can be cultured from the normal intestinal tract, from mouth to anus, and have proven difficult to eradicate completely.[165] Part of the difficulty lies in the innate hardiness of fungi, but part lies with poor patient compliance with antifungal regimens. There are three sorts of prophylactic regimens: one employs oral nonabsorbable drugs, another uses oral absorbable drugs, and another uses intravenous antifungal agents.[305] As one moves from oral to parenteral prophylaxis there is increased patient compliance, cost, toxicity, and probably efficacy. The more complex regimens should be reserved for patients at highest risk for systemic fungal infection—those with prolonged granulocytopenia who are receiving antibiotics that alter the natural resistance to fungal colonization.

Commonly used oral nonabsorbable antifungal drugs include nystatin, amphotericin, and clotrimazole. Although these drugs are capable of suppressing fungi in the intestinal tract of hospitalized patients, this suppression is only partial. Studies of patients receiving chemotherapy for leukemia without antibiotic prophylaxis show that nystatin reduces colonization with fungi but not disseminated disease.[315] A stronger case can be made for use of these drugs in combination with oral antibiotic prophylaxis. Several studies have shown a decrease in fungal infections when nystatin or amphotericin is combined with oral antibiotics.[305,310,316] If regimens that attempt total suppression of bacterial flora are used, a yeast-free external environment may be necessary in addition to oral antifungal drugs.[317] Oral amphotericin has several theoretical advantages over oral nystatin: 12×10^6 IU of nystatin is needed to achieve adequate fecal concentrations, compared with 1 to 2 g of oral amphotericin.[318,319] Most *Candida* species are more sensitive to amphotericin than to nystatin.

Oral prophylaxis with azole antifungal agents (miconazole, ketoconazole, itraconazole, fluconazole) has the theoretic advantage of a systemic effect, since these drugs are absorbed by the intestine. These drugs do not affect colonization with *Candida*, but minor fungal infections are less frequent with imidazole prophylaxis when compared with placebo.[320–322] Most studies have not shown an advantage for oral imidazole drugs over oral nystatin or amphotericin in preventing major fungal infections, and in several studies, prophylactic azole therapy has led to colonization and infection with resistant fungi, notably *Aspergillus* species and *Candida* species other than *C. albicans*.[323,324]

Prophylaxis with intravenous antifungal agents (amphotericin and miconazole) is a logical step, given the morbidity of deep fungal infections and the problems with oral antifungal prophylaxis. Studies in granulocytopenic, febrile patients in whom fungal sepsis is suspected, can more appropriately be called empiric antifungal treatment. Positive results have been reported with both intravenous miconazole and amphotericin, but both negative results and toxicity have been noted in other randomized trials.[305,325–328]

PROPHYLACTIC ANTIVIRAL DRUG THERAPY

Exogenous viral infection is best prevented by limiting exposure to viruses, as outlined previously. Postexposure immunoglobulin prophylaxis is available for VZV (VZ immune globulin), hepatitis B (HB immune globulin), and hepatitis A (pooled immunoglobulin preparations). With the advent of effective antiviral drug therapy, prophylaxis against latent herpesviruses is now possible. Acyclovir prophylaxis for HSV and VZV infections is very effective and should be given to seropositive patients who are at risk for serious infections caused by these viruses.[329,330] Prophylactic acyclovir is given as 800 mg orally twice daily or 250 mg/m^2 intravenously every 12 hours. Acyclovir appears to partially protect against CMV infection in transplant recipients.[90] Ganciclovir therapy for CMV excretion, started before the onset of CMV disease, is the most effective way of preventing CMV pneumonia and enteritis in marrow transplant patients. Current trials examine the prophylactic effect of ganciclovir and foscarnet in CMV-seropositive immunosuppressed patients who are not yet excreting virus.

Treatment of Specific Infections in the Immunocompromised Patient

BACTERIAL INFECTIONS

Bacterial Esophagitis and Phlegmonous Gastritis. These infections are most commonly polymicrobial, owing to organisms that colonize the oropharynx, that is, streptococci, gram-negative bacilli, and anaerobic species.[170,331] In hospitalized patients, the stomach and esophagus may become colonized with Enterobacteriaceae as well.[148,149] Therapy for bacterial esophagitis and gastritis should be directed by the level of granulocyte function. Granulocytopenic patients should be treated with an antibiotic that covers Enterobacteriaceae as well as streptococci. Piperacillin or cefoxitin or imipenem/cilastin or ticarcillin/clavulamate, plus or minus an aminoglycoside, are suitable. In less-suppressed patients, penicillin, clindamycin, or cefoxitin will suffice, since most of infecting organisms are sensitive to penicillin.[331] Coexisting viral and fungal infections require treatment as well.

***Pseudomonas* Infections.** Although *Pseudomonas aeruginosa* can occasionally be cultured from ulcerations throughout the intestinal tract of granulocytopenic patients, sometimes in pure culture, its role as a primary pathogen is less clear.[332] When *Pseudomonas* organisms invade the submucosa or "translocate" into mesenteric tissues, the treatment imperative is obvious. *Pseudomonas* vasculitis may also involve the intestinal blood vessels without causing overlying ulceration.[292] Treatment requires an aminoglycoside plus a β-lactam antibiotic active against *Pseudomonas*, for example, tobramycin or gentamicin plus ticarcillin or carbenicillin or azlocillin or mezlocillin or piperacillin.[332]

Clostridium difficile Colitis.

The treatment of *C. difficile* colitis in granulocytopenic and other immunosuppressed patients is the same as in "normal" patients (see ch 83). Patients on oncology wards have a high rate of carriage of *C. difficile*, and colitis can occur without prior antibiotic use.[333–335] One recent study has demonstrated that a combination of environmental decontamination and vancomycin treatment of *C. difficile* carriers prevented colonization of hospitalized patients with leukemia.[336] Others have been less successful with a program of decontamination.[337]

Clostridium septicum Infections (Typhlitis/Neutropenic Enterocolitis and Septicemia Associated With Colon Cancer).

C. septicum is not normally found among fecal flora but has been associated with two clinical syndromes. The most common is typhlitis or inflammation of the cecum and ascending colon. Because this usually occurs in patients with profound granulocytopenia, mortality is high. Therapy is directed at both the putative causal organism (*C. septicum*) and at the polymicrobial colonic flora that may cause septic shock. *C. septicum* is sensitive to penicillin G (10 to 12 million units daily); alternative medications include cephalosporins, imipenen, clindamycin, and metronidazole.[16] There is variability in sensitivity of different *C. septicum* isolates. However, in an acutely ill, granulocytopenic patient, antibiotic coverage must be started empirically and must cover a wide range of enteric organisms. There is controversy about the role of surgery in managing patients with suspected typhlitis, since cases appear sporadically and only severe cases are reported. A plea can be made for a conservative approach (antibiotics and fluid resuscitation) if the patient's condition is not deteriorating, especially when granulocyte counts are rising.[338] When the patient's condition is unstable, particularly when there is no expectation for return of granulocyte function, surgical exploration is indicated.[182,222,223] Most surgeons resect the involved right colon.

The other syndrome associated with *C. septicum* is septicemia with tissue necrosis at distant sites. Although the source of the organism is invariably the colon, abdominal symptoms may be absent.[16] This is most commonly seen in patients with colorectal cancer and leukemia, in whom the portal of entry is believed to be malignant tissue.[16,17] Penicillin therapy should be instituted promptly. Resection of diseased colon may be necessary.[17]

Perianal Infections.

Anorectal infections caused by multiple enteric organisms (both aerobic and anaerobic) should be treated with a combination of antibiotics in the granulocytopenic patient. The National Cancer Institute suggests a third-generation cephalosporin, such as ceftazidime, plus an antibiotic active against anerobes, such as clindamycin.[227] An alternative regimen includes an extended-spectrum penicillin like piperacillin plus an aminoglycoside plus clindamycin. If cellulitis progresses, vancomycin can be added for better coverage against enterococci.[227] If a closed-space infection is being reinfected with luminal organisms, there may be a role for luminally active, nonabsorbable antibiotics, as well as systemic antibiotics.[231] However, an aggressive surgical

approach may be necessary if there is ongoing sepsis or tissue necrosis.[226,229,230]

Infection Caused by Enteric Bacterial Pathogens.

The treatment of patients infected with *Salmonella*, *Shigella*, *Campylobacter*, *Yersinia*, *Aeromonas*, and pathogenic *E. coli* is covered in Chapters 68 and 83. While normal hosts may have self-limited infections with these organisms, immunocompromised hosts are more frequently bacteremic and are more likely to become chronically infected.[178,179,192] Management of recurrent bacteremia and chronic diarrhea in patients with AIDS is covered in Chapter 103 and applies equally well to patients with congenital immunodeficiency. Breakthrough bacteremia and the need for extended courses of therapy remain problems with standard therapy (ampicillin, trimethoprim-sulfamethoxazole and chloramphenicol).[178] Ciprofloxacin effectively suppresses recurrent *Salmonella* bacteremia when given at a dose of 750 mg twice daily.[339]

FUNGAL INFECTIONS

Mucosal Fungal Infections.

Esophageal and enteric *Candida* infections involving the mucosa can be treated with luminal agents alone if the patient has intact granulocyte defenses and some degree of cellular immunity. The same drugs can be given for diarrhea associated with *Candida* overgrowth and for colonization with fungi. Available drugs include nystatin suspension (1 to 3 million units by mouth every 6 hours), clotrimazole (100 mg tablets, to be sucked every 6 hours), amphotericin (250 mg four times daily), or ketoconazole (200 mg tablets orally, once or twice daily). These drugs are not as effective in patients with defects in cellular immunity, such as in patients with AIDS and mucocutaneous candidiasis. Fluconazole (100 mg orally once daily) appears to be superior to ketoconazole in treating *Candida* esophagitis in these patients.[340]

A different approach must be taken for seemingly superficial mucosal infections caused by *Candida* in a patient with granulocytopenia. Even if the patient is afebrile and shows no signs of fungemia or disseminated candidiasis, a systemic antifungal drug should be given because of the propensity of yeast forms to seed the portal circulation. Amphotericin (0.3 to 0.5 mg/kg/d intravenously), ketoconazole (400 mg orally, once daily), and fluconazole (200 mg orally, once daily) are effective and may be needed for only 4 to 7 days. If a granulocytopenic patient with mucosal candidiasis exhibits clinical signs or symptoms of fungemia or invasive disease, higher doses of amphotericin should be given (0.5 to 1.0 mg/kg/d intravenously for 7 to 10 days). This holds for cases in which invasive disease cannot be proved by diagnostic imaging tests, since these tests are too insensitive to detect microscopic foci of infection.[274]

Fungal organisms other than *C. albicans* may be found in the compromised patient. These include other *Candida* species (especially *C. tropicalis* and *C. glabrata*), *Aspergillus*, *Mucor*, *Blastomyces*, *Cryptococcus*, *Pneumocystis carinii*, and *Histoplasma*, as well as plant fungi. These unusual fungi are more likely to be resistant to standard antifungal therapy.

Invasive Fungal Infections.

Transmural infiltration of the intestine, hepatic abscesses, peritonitis, and biliary fungal infection require treatment with high-dose amphotericin (0.5 to

1.0 mg/kg/d, often for prolonged courses of treatment). In the granulocytopenic patient with such infections, the prognosis is poor even with treatment unless patients regain granulocyte function. This can occasionally be accomplished by stopping immunosuppressive drug therapy, by successful treatment of leukemia, and by restoration of marrow granulocyte production with colony-stimulating factors. Other approaches include combinations of antifungal drugs (amphotericin with 5-flucytosine or rifampin),[341] liposomal amphotericin,[342] and newer azole derivatives (itraconazole, fluconazole).[343-345]

VIRAL INFECTIONS

Herpes Simplex Virus. Prophylaxis with acyclovir has almost eliminated esophageal, intestinal, and hepatic HSV infections in transplant units.[329] Higher doses are used to treat HSV esophagitis, enteritis, perianal ulceration, and hepatitis, that is, 250 mg/m^2 intravenously every 8 hours, or 400 mg orally, five times daily.[346,347] Esophageal symptoms resolve promptly, particularly if acid-peptic reflux is controlled as well. Failure to respond suggests a co-existing infection (bacterial, fungal, CMV) or rarely acyclovir-resistant HSV.[348,349] Foscarnet therapy has been reported to be effective in treating HSV resistant to acyclovir.[348,350] Another approach is to give continuous-infusion, high-dose acyclovir.[351]

Varicella Zoster Virus. Treatment of VZV esophagitis or hepatitis is with acyclovir 500 mg/m^2 intravenously every 8 hours.[215,216] Treatment response is less predictable than with HSV infection. In addition, acyclovir-resistant strains of VZV have been reported.[352]

Cytomegalovirus. Successful treatment of CMV esophagitis, enteritis, and hepatobiliary CMV infection with ganciclovir (5 mg/kg intravenously, every 12 hours) has been reported in several uncontrolled series, mostly in patients with AIDS.[68,69,205] A randomized trial of two weeks of ganciclovir therapy for CMV enteric infection in marrow transplant patients showed a significant effect on viral replication but no change in symptoms or endoscopic appearance.[91] Longer courses of therapy combined with intravenous immunoglobulin may be required for these patients. Because relapse of CMV infection is common after ganciclovir is stopped, maintenance therapy may be needed during prolonged immunosuppression. Experience with foscarnet in the treatment of CMV enteritis is limited.[353]

Rotavirus. There is no antiviral drug therapy for rotavirus enteritis. Ingestion of bovine colostrum containing antibodies to human rotavirus prevents disease in normal children.[354] There is little clinical experience with this form of therapy in immunodeficient patients or in those with established rotavirus infection.

PARASITIC INFECTIONS

Giardia lamblia. It is not more difficult to treat giardiasis in immunodeficient patients than in normal hosts, as shown in studies of patients with immunoglobulin deficiency and AIDS.[98,192,355,356] Quinacrine, metronidazole, tinidazole, and furazolidone are effective drugs when taken according to directions,

giving cure rates around 90%.[191] Metronidazole (and tinidazole, which is not currently available in the United States) is effective as a single dose of 1.5 to 2 g, which increases compliance in comparison to the usual dose of 5 mg/kg in three divided daily doses for 5 days. Quinacrine is probably more effective than imidazole drugs but also more poorly tolerated. Doses are 100 mg three times a day for 5 days for adults or 2 mg/kg in three divided doses daily for 5 days for children. Furazolidone may be an alternative, especially for children, since it is available as a palatable suspension. However, more than 10% of patients experience treatment failure and require repeated drug courses.[357] Some of these cases represent poor drug compliance and reinfection. Failure of symptoms to respond to treatment may also be due to co-existing pathogens, a common problem in patients with AIDS.[192] Bacterial overgrowth in the small intestine has also been described in association with giardiasis.[358]

Cryptosporidium. There are no established drugs for treatment of intestinal cryptosporidiasis in immunodeficient patients. Over 70 drugs have been tested, and only one has been reported to be effective.[193] Spiramycin (at 3 g/d orally) has been reported to be useful in treating *Cryptosporidium*-associated diarrhea in AIDS patients.[359,360] Others have not found spiramycin to be of value.[193] However, restoring immune competence does allow infected patients to shed this parasite. This is most readily done by discontinuing immunosuppressive drugs, as illustrated by several case reports.[361-363] Treatment of HIV infection with zidovudine (azathimodine, or AZT) has also been reported to result in clearance of the parasite.[360] The somatostatin analogue octreotide and opiates have been reported to lower diarrheal volume in AIDS patients.[360,364] Oral bovine colostrum (containing anti-*Cryptosporidium* antibodies) has been used with variable results.[365,366] Colostrum plus zidovudine had dramatic results in one AIDS patient, who apparently cleared the parasite.[367]

Entamoeba histolytica (Amebiasis). Immunosuppressed patients who are asymptomatic carriers of *E. histolytica* should be treated with a poorly absorbed luminal agent in order to prevent invasive disease. Available drugs include diloxanide furoate (500 mg three times a day for 10 days); paromomycin (30 mg/kg/d in three divided doses for 5 to 10 days); iodoquinol (650 mg three times a day for 20 days); and metronidazole (750 mg three times a day for 10 days).[368]

Patients with invasive disease (colitis, liver abscess) require treatment that eradicates luminal as well as tissue-invasive organisms. Metronidazole (750 mg orally or intravenously three times a day for 5 to 10 days) plus one of the nonabsorbable drugs mentioned previously is the treatment of choice. Amebic liver abscesses that do not respond to metronidazole are treated with dehydroemetine, 1 to 1.5 mg/kg/d intramuscularly for 5 days, plus chloroquine (base) 600 mg orally daily for 2 days, followed by 300 mg orally daily for 2 to 3 weeks.[369] Rarely, needle or surgical drainage will be required.

Strongyloides stercoralis (Strongyloidiasis). Patients with normal immune defenses who have *Strongyloides* infection should be treated whether symptomatic or not. This is especially important if the patient is to receive immunosuppressive chemotherapy, which may lead to disseminated disease.[45] Thiabendazole, 50 mg/kg/d (maximum 3 g) orally in two divided doses for 2 days, is successful 70% to 80% of the time, but proving that parasites have been eliminated can be difficult.[45] Repeated stool specimen examinations and intestinal biopsies and aspirates may be required. Decreases in serologic titers and eosinophil counts correlate with successful treatment.[370] In the immunosuppressed host, thiabendazole is again the drug of choice for intestinal strongyloidiasis, but a longer duration of therapy (5 to 7 days) may be required.[45] However, toxicity is more common with prolonged treatment. Toxic effects include vomiting, anorexia, and neurologic abnormalities, such as lethargy, hallucinations, dysphoria, and convulsions.[371] An alternative to thiabendazole is mebendazole, which is active primarily in the intestinal lumen. Doses range from 100 to 300 mg twice daily for 3 to 8 days to 500 mg daily for 21 days.[45]

Treatment of disseminated strongyloidiasis (hyperinfection syndrome) is less successful, with mortality of 30% to 40% even with therapy. Thiabendazole in the doses listed above should be given for 5 to 7 days or until clearance of parasites from stool and sputum.[45] Gram-negative sepsis frequently accompanies disseminated strongyloidiasis and must be treated. Immunosuppressive drugs should be discontinued if at all possible.

***Toxoplasma gondii* (Toxoplasmosis).** Therapy for toxoplasmosis in the immunosuppressed patient is indicated when there is either histologic evidence of infection or a strong clinical suspicion of neurologic or cardiac involvement. Treatment duration is usually 4 to 6 weeks after resolution of all signs and symptoms and even longer in patients whose immune response remains impaired.[372] The drugs of choice are pyrimethamine (200 mg/d loading dose, then 50 to 75 mg/d for several weeks, then 25-50 mg/d maintenance) plus sulfadiazine (6 to 8 g/d in four divided doses for an adult, or 100 mg/kg/d in four to six divided doses for a child).[372] Concomitant folinic acid (leucovorin) therapy may prevent marrow depression caused by pyrimethamine.

***Blastocystis hominis* and *Enteromonas hominis*.** These parasites may require treatment in the immunocompromised patient with prolonged diarrhea and no other causes that are obvious. Metronidazole and ketoconazole have been reported to be effective, but many patients so treated have been co-infected with other parasites.[196,197,373,374]

***Isospora belli*.** Unlike cryptosporidiasis, infection with this coccidial parasite responds to therapy with trimethoprim-sulfamethoxazole (given for 4 weeks), albeit with a high prevalence of side effects.[375,376] Pyrimethamine (50 to 75 mg/d) with folinic acid (10 mg/d) is an alternative drug.[377]

The reader is directed to Chapter 83, Bacterial Infections of the Colon; Chapter 103, Gastrointestinal Complications of the Acquired Immunodeficiency Syndrome; Chapter 104, Parasitic Diseases: Protozoa; Chapter 105, Parasitic Diseases: Helminths; Chapter 107, Gastrointestinal Manifestations of Immunologic Disorders; and Chapter 127, Microbiologic Studies.

REFERENCES

1. Waldmann TA. Immunodeficiency diseases: Primary and acquired. In: Samter M, Talmage DW, Frank M, Austen KF, eds. Immunological diseases, ed 4. Boston: Little, Brown, 1988:411.
2. Brown EJ, Joiner KA. Mechanisms of host resistance to infection. In: Samter M, Talmage DW, Frank M, Austen KF, eds. Immunological diseases, ed 4. Boston: Little, Brown, 1988:715.
3. Strober W, Brown WR. The mucosal immune system. In: Samter M, Talmage DW, Frank M, Austen KF, eds. Immunological diseases, ed 4. Boston: Little, Brown, 1988:79.
4. Van der Meer JWM. Defects in host-defense mechanisms. In: Rubin RH, Young LS, eds. Clinical approach to infection in the compromised host, ed 2. New York: Plenum Publishing, 1988:41.
5. Rubin RH. Infection in the renal and liver transplant patient. In: Rubin RH, Young LS, eds. Clinical approach to infection in the compromised host, ed 2. New York: Plenum Publishing, 1988:557.
6. Parrillo JE, Masur H. The critically ill immunosuppressed patient. Diagnosis and management. Rockville, MD: Aspen Publishers, 1987.
7. Ho M, Dummer JS. Risk factors and approaches to infections in transplant recipients. In: Mandell GL, Douglas RG, Bennett JE, eds. Principles and practice of infectious diseases, ed 3. New York: Churchill Livingstone, 1990:2284.
8. Stiehm ER, ed. Immunologic disorders in infants and children, ed 3. Philadelphia: WB Saunders, 1989.
9. Hermann R, Panahon AM, Barcos MP, et al. Gastrointestinal involvement in non-Hodgkin's lymphoma. Cancer 1980;46:215.
10. Prolla JC, Mirsner JB. The gastrointestinal lesions and complications of the leukemias. Ann Intern Med 1964;61:1084.
11. Fleming ID, Mitchell S, Dilawari RA. The role of surgery in the management of gastric lymphoma. Cancer 1982;49:1135.
12. List AF, Greer JP, Cousar JC, et al. Non-Hodgkin's lymphoma of the gastrointestinal tract: An analysis of clinical and pathologic features affecting outcome. J Clin Oncol 1988;6:1125.
13. Mittal B, Wasserman TH, Griffith RC. Non-Hodgkin's lymphoma of the stomach. Am J Gastroenterol 1983;78:780.
14. Ferrara JJ, Martin EW, Carey LC. Morbidity of emergency operations in patients with metastatic cancer receiving chemotherapy. Surgery 1982;92:605.
15. Hande HR, Fisher RI, Devita VT, et al. Diffuse histiocytic lymphoma involving the gastrointestinal tract. Cancer 1978;41:1984.
16. Kornbluth AA, Danzig JB, Bernstein LH. *Clostridium septicum* infection and associated malignancy. Report of 2 cases and review of the literature. Medicine 1989;68:30.
17. Katlic MR, Derkac WM, Coleman WS. *Clostridium septicum* infection and malignancy. Ann Surg 1980;193:361.
18. Editorial. *Clostridium septicum* and neutropenic enterocolitis. Lancet 1987;2:608.
19. Hirsch MS. Herpes group virus infections in the compromised host. In: Rubin RH, Young LS, eds. Clinical approach to infection in the compromised host, ed 2. New York: Plenum Publishing, 1988:347.
20. Eras P, Goldstein MJ, Sherlock P. Candida infection of the gastrointestinal tract. Medicine 1972;51:367.
21. Kemeny MM, Brennan MF. The surgical complications of chemotherapy in the cancer patient. Curr Probl Surg 1987;24:607.
22. Klein RS, Catalano MT, Edberg SC, et al. *Streptococcus bovis* septicemia and carcinoma of the colon. Ann Intern Med 1979;91:560.
23. Schimpff SC. Infections in the compromised host—An overview. In: Mandell GL, Douglas RG, Bennett JE, eds. Principles and practice of infectious diseases. New York: Churchill Livingstone, 1990:2258.
24. Shaw MT, Spector MH, Ladman AJ. Effects of cancer, radiotherapy and cytotoxic drugs on intestinal structure and function. Cancer Treat Rev 1979;6:141.
25. Smith FP, Kisner DL, Widerlite L, et al. Chemotherapeutic alteration of small intestinal morphology and function: A progress report. J Clin Gastroenterol 1979;1:203.
26. McDonald GB, Tirumali N. Intestinal and liver toxicity of antineoplastic drugs. West J Med 1984;140:250.
27. Slavin RE, Dias MA, Saral R. Cytosine arabinoside–induced gastrointestinal toxic alterations in sequential chemotherapeutic pro-

tocols—A clinical-pathologic study of 33 patients. Cancer 1978;42: 1747.

28. Petrelli N, Douglass HO, Herrera L, et al. The modulation of fluorouracil with leucovorin in metastatic colorectal carcinoma: A prospective randomized phase III trial. J Clin Oncol 1989;7:1419.

29. Phillips TL, Fu KK. The interaction of drug and radiation effects on normal tissues. Int J Radiat Oncol Biol Phys 1978;4:59.

30. Greco FA, Brereton MD, Kent H, et al. Adriamycin and enhanced radiation reaction in normal esophagus and skin. Ann Intern Med 1978;85:294.

31. Umsawasdi T, Valdivieso M, Barkley HT, et al. Esophageal complications from combined chemoradiotherapy (cyclophosphamide + Adriamycin + cisplatin + XRT) in the treatment of non–small cell lung cancer. Int J Radiat Oncol Biol Phys 1985;11:511.

32. Sandler SG, Tobin W, Henderson ES. Vincristine-induced neuropathy—A clinical study of 50 leukemia patients. Neurology 1969;19: 367.

33. Shike M, Gillin JS, Kemeny N, et al. Severe gastroduodenal ulcerations complicating hepatic artery infusion chemotherapy for metastatic colon cancer. Am J Gastroenterol 1986;81:176.

34. Rollins BJ. Hepatic veno-occlusive disease. Am J Med 1986;81:297.

35. McDonald GB, Sharma P, Matthews DE, et al. Venocclusive disease of the liver after bone marrow transplantation: Diagnosis, incidence, and predisposing factors. Hepatology 1984;4:116.

36. Jones RJ, Lee KSK, Beschorner WE, et al. Venoocclusive disease of the liver following bone marrow transplantation. Transplantation 1987;44:778.

37. Perry MC. Hepatotoxicity of chemotherapeutic agents. Semin Oncol 1982;9:65.

38. Larrey D, Freneaux E, Berson A, et al. Peliosis hepatis induced by 6-thioguanine administration. Gut 1988;29:1265.

39. Shay SS, Berendson RA, Johnson LF. Esophageal hematoma: Four new cases, a review, and proposed etiology. Dig Dis Sci 1981;26: 1019.

40. Wolford JL, McDonald GB. A problem-oriented approach to intestinal and liver disease after marrow transplantation. J Clin Gastroenterol 1988;10:419.

41. Titone C, Lipsius M, Krakauer JS. "Spontaneous" hematoma of the rectus abdominis muscle: Critical review of 50 cases with emphasis on early diagnosis and treatment. Surgery 1972;72:568.

42. Zaloga GP, Chernow B. Endocrine and metabolic problems in the critically ill immunocompromised patient. In: Parrillo JE, Masur H, eds. The critically ill immunosuppressed patient. Diagnosis and management. Rockville, MD: Aspen Publishers, 1987:155.

43. Tolkoff-Rubin NE, Rubin RH. Uremia and host defenses. N Engl J Med 1990;332:770.

44. Morgan JS, Schaffner W, Stone WJ. Opportunistic strongyloidiasis in renal transplant recipients. Transplantation 1986;42:518.

45. Genta RM, Walzer PD. Strongyloidiasis. In: Walzer PD, Genta RM, eds. Parasitic infections in the compromised host. New York: Marcel Dekker, 1989:463.

46. Auchincloss H, Rubin RH. Clinical management of the critically ill renal transplant patient. In: Parrillo JE, Masur H, eds. The critically ill immunosuppressed patient. Diagnosis and management. Rockville, MD: Aspen Publishers, 1987:347.

47. Taylor RJ, Saul SH, Dowling JN, et al. Primary disseminated herpes simplex virus infection with fulminant hepatitis following renal transplantation. Arch Intern Med 1981;141:1519.

48. Weir MR, Kirkamn RL, Strom TB, Tilney NC. Liver disease in recipients of long-functioning renal allografts. Kidney Int 1985;28: 839.

49. Dusheiko G, Song E, Bowyer S, et al. Natural history of hepatitis B virus infection in renal transplant recipients—Fifteen year follow-up. Hepatology 1983;3:330.

50. Parfrey PS, Forges RD, Hutchinson TA, et al. The clinical and pathological course of hepatitis B liver disease in renal transplant recipients. Transplantation 1984;37:461.

51. LaQuaglia MR, Tolkoff-Rubin NE, Dienstag JL, et al. Impact of hepatitis on renal transplantation. Transplantation 1981;32:504.

52. Warshaw AL, Welch JP, Ottinger LW. Acute perforation of the colon associated with chronic corticosteroid therapy. Am J Surg 1976;131:442.

53. Flanigan RC, Reckard CR, Lucas BA. Colonic complications of renal transplantation. J Urol 1988;139:503.

54. Lillemoe KD, Romolo JL, Hamilton SR, et al. Intestinal necrosis due to sodium polystyrene (Kayexalate) in sorbitol enemas: Clinical and experimental support for the hypothesis. Surgery 1987;101:266.

55. Wooton FT, Rhodes DF, Lee WM, Fitts CT. Colonic necrosis with Kayexalate-sorbitol enemas after renal transplantation. Ann Intern Med 1989;111:947.

56. Feduska NJ, Amend WJC, Vincenti F, et al. Peptic ulcer disease in kidney transplant recipients. Am J Surg 1984;148:51.

57. Cohen EB, Komorowski RA, Kauffman HM, Adams M. Unexpectedly high incidence of cytomegalovirus infection in apparent peptic ulcers in renal transplant recipients. Surgery 1985;97:606.

58. Hanto D, Frizzera G, Gajl-Peczalska K, et al. Epstein–Barr virus–induced B-cell lymphoma after renal transplantation. N Engl J Med 1982;306:913.

59. Penn I. Tumor incidence in human allograft recipients. Transplant Proc 1979;11:1047.

60. Rimola A, Soto R, Bory F, et al. Reticuloendothelial system phagocytic activity in cirrhosis and its relation to bacterial infections and prognosis. Hepatology 1984;4:53.

61. Wajsczcuk CP, Dummer JS, Ho M, et al. Fungal infection in liver transplant recipients. Transplantation 1985;40:347.

62. Dummer JS, Hardy A, Poorsattar A, Ho M. Early infections in kidney, heart, and liver transplant recipients on cyclosporine. Transplantation 1983;36:259.

63. Wiesner RH, Hermans P, Rakela J, Perkins J, Washington J, Di Cecco S, Krum RAF. Selective bowel decontamination to prevent gram-negative bacterial and fungal infection following orthotopic liver transplantation. Transplant Proc 1987;19:2420.

64. Carithers RL, Fairman RP, Mendez-Picon G, Posner MP, Mills AS, Friedenberg KT. Postoperative care. In: Maddrey WC, ed. Transplantation of the liver. New York: Elsevier, 1988:111.

65. Koep LJ, Peters TG, Starzl TE. Major colonic complications of hepatic transplantation. Dis Colon Rectum 1979;22:218.

66. Koep LJ, Starzl TE, Weil R. Gastrointestinal complications of hepatic transplantation. Transplant Proc 1979;11:257.

67. Alexander JA, Cueller RE, Fadden RJ, et al. Cytomegalovirus infection of the upper gastrointestinal tract before and after liver transplantation. Transplantation 1988;46:378.

68. Harbison MA, De Girolami PC, Jenkins RL, Hammer SM. Ganciclovir therapy of severe cytomegalovirus infections in solid-organ transplant recipients. Transplantation 1988;46:82.

69. Erice A, Jordan MC, Chace BA, Fletcher C, Chinnock BJ, Balfour HH. Ganciclovir treatment of cytomegalovirus disease in transplant recipients and other immunocompromised hosts. JAMA 1987;257: 3082.

70. Starzl TE, Porter KA, Inatsuki S, et al. Reversibility of lymphomas and lymphoproliferative lesions developing under cyclosporin-steroid therapy. Lancet 1984;1:583.

71. Pennock JL, Oyer PE, Reitz BA, et al. Cardiac transplantation in perspective for the future. Survival, complications, rehabilitation and cost. J Thorac Cardiovasc Surg 1982;83:168.

72. Hofflin JM, Potasman I, Baldwin JC, et al. Infectious complications in heart transplant patients receiving cyclosporine and corticosteroids. Ann Intern Med 1987;106:209.

73. Gentry LO, Zaluff B. Infection in the cardiac transplant patient. In: Rubin RH, Young LS, eds. Clinical approach to infection in the compromised host, ed 2. New York: Plenum Publishing, 1988:623.

74. Dummer JS, White LT, Ho M, et al. Morbidity of cytomegalovirus infection in recipients of heart or heart-lung transplants who received cyclosporine. J Infect Dis 1985;152:1182.

75. Johnson R, Peitzman AB, Webster MW, et al. Upper gastrointestinal endoscopy after cardiac transplantation. Surgery 1988;103:300.

76. Pollard RB, Rand KH, Merigan TC. Cell-mediated immunity to cytomegalovirus infection in normal subjects and cardiac transplant patients. J Infect Dis 1978;137:541.

77. Steed DL, Brown B, Reilly JJ, et al. General surgical complications in heart and heart-lung transplantation. Surgery 1985;98:739.

78. Cosimi AB. Surgical aspects of infection in the compromised host. In: Rubin RH, Young LS, eds. Clinical approach to infection in the compromised host, ed 2. New York: Plenum Publishing, 1988:649.

79. Meyers JD, Thomas ED. Infection complicating bone marrow transplantation in the compromised host. In: Rubin RH, Young LS, eds. Clinical approach to infection in the compromised host, ed 2. New York: Plenum Publishing, 1988:525.

80. Epstein RJ, McDonald GB, Sale GE, Shulman HM, Thomas ED. The diagnostic accuracy of the rectal biopsy in acute graft-versus-host disease: A prospective study of thirteen patients. Gastroenterology 1980;78:764.

81. Ganem G, Saint-Marc Girardin M-F, Kuentz M, et al. Venocclusive disease of the liver after allogeneic bone marrow transplantation in man. Int J Radiat Oncol Biol Phys 1988;14:879.

82. McDonald GB, Sharma P, Matthews DE, et al. The clinical course of 53 patients with venocclusive disease of the liver after marrow transplantation. Transplantation 1985;39:603.

83. McDonald GB, Shulman HM, Sullivan KM, Spencer GD. Intestinal and hepatic complications of human bone marrow transplantation. Gastroenterology 1986;90:460,770.

84. Spencer GD, Hackman RC, McDonald GB, et al. A prospective study of unexplained nausea and vomiting after marrow transplantation. Transplantation 1986;42:602.

85. Weisdorf SA, Salati LM, Longsdorf JA, et al. Graft-versus-host disease of the intestine: A protein-losing enteropathy characterized by fecal alpha-1-antitrypsin. Gastroenterology 1983;85:1076.

86. Snover DC, Weisdorf SA, Vercellotti GM, et al. A histopathologic study of gastric and small intestine graft-versus-host disease following allogeneic bone marrow transplantation. Hum Pathol 1985;16:387.

87. McDonald GB, Shulman HM, Wolford JL, Spencer GD. Liver disease after human marrow transplantation. Semin Liver Dis 1987;7:210.

88. Shulman HM, Sharma P, Amose D, et al. A coded histologic study of hepatic graft-versus-host disease after human bone marrow transplantation. Hepatology 1988;8:463.

89. McDonald GB, Sullivan KM, Schuffler MD, et al. Esophageal abnormalities in chronic graft-versus-host disease in humans. Gastroenterology 1981;80:914.

90. Meyers JD, Reed EC, Shepp DH, et al. Acyclovir for prevention of cytomegalovirus infection and disease after allogeneic marrow transplantation. N Engl J Med 1988;318:70.

91. Reed EC, Wolford JL, Kopecky KJ, et al. Ganciclovir for the treatment of cytomegalovirus gastroenteritis in marrow transplant patients. A randomized placebo-controlled trial. Ann Intern Med 1990;112:505.

92. Rees GM, Sarmiento JI, Myerson D, et al. Cytomegalovirus hepatitis in marrow transplant patients: Clinical, histologic and histochemical analysis. Gastroenterology 1990;98:A470.

93. Shields AF, Hackman RC, Fife KH, et al. Adenovirus infections in patients undergoing bone marrow transplantation. N Engl J Med 1985;312:529.

94. Spencer GD, Shulman HM, Myerson D, et al. Diffuse intestinal ulceration after marrow transplantation: A clinical-pathological study of 13 patients. Human Pathology 1986;17:621.

95. Zutter MM, Martin PJ, Sale GE, Shulman HM, et al. Epstein-Barr virus lymphoproliferation after bone marrow transplantation. Blood 1988;72:520.

96. Pariente EA, Goudeau A, DuBois F, et al. Fulminant hepatitis due to reactivation of chronic hepatitis B virus infection after allogeneic bone marrow transplantation. Dig Dis Sci 1988;33:1185.

97. Collier AC, Miller RA, Myers JD. Cryptosporidiosis after marrow transplantation: Person-to-person transmission and treatment with spiramycin. Ann Intern Med 1984;101:205.

98. Bromiker R, Korman SH, Or R, et al. Severe giardiasis in two patients undergoing bone marrow transplantation. Bone Marrow Transplant 1989;4:701.

99. Stechschulte DJ, Fishback JL, Emani A, Bhatia P. Secondary biliary cirrhosis as a consequence of graft-versus-host disease. Gastroenterology 1990;98:223.

100. Witherspoon RP, Fisher LD, Schoch G, et al. Secondary cancers after bone marrow transplantation for leukemia or aplastic anemia. N Engl J Med 1989;321:784.

101. Katz P, Fauci AS. Immunosuppressives and immunoadjuvants. In: Samter M, Talmage DW, Frank MM, Austen KF, Claman HN, eds. Immunological diseases, ed 4. Boston: Little, Brown, 1988:675.

102. Cupps TR, Fauci AS. Corticosteroid-mediated immunoregulation in man. Immunol Rev 1982;65:134.

103. Dale DC, Fauci AS, Wolff SM. Alternate-day prednisone: Leukocyte kinetics and susceptibility to infections. N Engl J Med 1974;291:1154.

104. Gershwin ME, Goetzl EJ, Steinberg AD. Cyclophosphamide use in practice. Ann Intern Med 1974;80:531.

105. Mitchell MS, Wade ME, DeConti RC, et al. Immunosuppressive effects of cytosine arabinoside and methotrexate in man. Ann Intern Med 1969;70:535.

106. Kahan BD. Cyclosporine. N Engl J Med 1989;321:1725.

107. Heyworth MF. Clinical experience with antilymphocyte serum. Immunol Rev 1982;65:79.

108. Ortho Multicenter Transplant Study Group. A randomized clinical trial of OKT3 monoclonal antibody for acute rejection of cadaveric renal transplants. N Engl J Med 1985;313:337.

109. Miller RA, Maloney DG, Warnke R, Levy R. Treatment of B-cell lymphoma with monoclonal anti-idiotype antibody. N Engl J Med 1982;306:517.

110. Rubin RH, Cosimi AB, Hirsch MD, et al. Effects of antithymocyte globulin on cytomegalovirus infection in renal transplant recipients. Transplantation 1981;31:143.

111. Metselaar HJ, Weimar W. Cytomegalovirus infection and renal transplantation. J Antimicrob Chemother 1989;23(Suppl E):37.

112. Sperber KE, Mayer L. Gastrointestinal manifestations of common variable immunodeficiency. Immunol Allergy Clin North Am 1988;8:423.

113. Kinlen LJ, Webster AD, Bird AG, et al. Prospective study of cancer with hypogammaglobulinemia. Lancet 1985;1:263.

114. Burks AW, Steel AW. Selective IgA deficiency. Ann Allergy 1986;57:3.

115. Cunningham-Rundles C, Pudifin DJ, Armstrong D, Good RA. Selective IgA deficiency and neoplasia. Vox Sang 1980;38:61.

116. Mills EL, Quie PG. Congenital disorders of the functions of polymorphonuclear neutrophils. Rev Infect Dis 1980;2:505.

117. Wright DG, Dale DC, Fauci AS, Wolff SM. Human cyclic neutropenia: Clinical review and long-term follow-up of patients. Medicine 1981;60:1.

118. Ament ME. Gastrointestinal manifestations of immunodeficiency diseases in infants, children and adults. In: Targan S, Shanahan F, eds. Immunology and immunopathology of the liver and gastrointestinal tract. New York: Igaku-Shoin, 1989:335.

119. Ammann AJ, Hong R. Disorders of the T-cell system. In: Shiehm ER, ed. Immunologic disorders in infants and children, ed 3. Philadelphia: WB Saunders, 1989:257.

120. Rohrmann CA, Kidd R. Chronic mucocutaneous candidiasis: Radiologic abnormalities in the esophagus. Am J Roentgenol 1978;130:473.

121. Greene MI, Fields BN. Host response to viruses. In: Samter M, Talmage DW, Frank MM, et al, eds. Immunological diseases, ed 4. Boston: Little, Brown, 1988:899.

122. Rakusan TA, Juneja HS, Fleischmann WR. Inhibition of hemopoietic colony formation by human cytomegalovirus in vitro. J Infect Dis 1989;159;127.

123. Sher A, Ottesen E. Immunoparasitology. In: Samter M, Talmage DW, Frank MM, eds. Immunological diseases, ed 4. Boston: Little, Brown, 1988:923.

124. Saltzman RL, Peterson PK. Immunodeficiency of the elderly. Rev Infect Dis 1987;9:1127.

125. Gleckman RA, Gantz NM. Infections in the elderly. Boston: Little, Brown, 1983.

126. Breitenbucher RB, Peterson PK. Infections in the elderly. In: Mandell GL, Douglas RG, Bennett JE, eds. Principles and practice of infectious diseases. New York: Churchill Livingstone, 1990:2315.

127. Gleckman R, Hibert D. Afebrile bacteremia: A phenomenon in geriatric patients. JAMA 1982;248:1478.

128. Ryan CA, Tauxe RV, Hosek GW, et al. *Escherichia coli* 0157:H7 diarrhea in a nursing home: Clinical, epidemiological, and pathological findings. J Infect Dis 1986;154:631.

129. Kane JG, Chretin JH, Garagusi VF. Diarrhoea caused by *Candida*. Lancet 1976;1:335.

130. Nagami PH, Yoshikawa TT. Tuberculosis in the geriatric patient. J Am Geriatr Soc 1983;31:356.

131. Esposito AL, Gleckman RA. Fever of unknown origin in the elderly. J Am Geriatr Soc 1978;26:498.

132. Handwerger BS. The immunology of diabetes mellitus. In: Samter M, Talmage DW, Frank MD, eds. Immunological diseases, ed 4. Boston: Little, Brown, 1988:1765.

133. Strober W, Wochner RD, Carbone PP, Waldmann TA. Intestinal lymphangiectasia: A protein-losing enteropathy with hypogamma-globulinemia, lymphocytopenia, and impaired homograft rejection. J Clin Invest 1967;46:1643.

134. Nelson DL, Blaese RM, Strober W, et al. Constrictive pericarditis, intestinal lymphangiectasia, and reversible immunologic deficiency. J Pediatr 1975;86:548.

135. Chandra RK. Nutrition, immunity, and infection: Present knowledge and future directions. Lancet 1983;1:688.

136. Garre MA, Boles JM, Youinou PY. Current concepts in immune derangement due to undernutrition. J Parenter Enteral Nutr 1987;11:309.

137. Chandra RK, Gupta S, Singh H. Inducer and suppressor T-cell subsets in protein-energy malnutrition: Analysis by monoclonal antibodies. Nutr Res 1982;2:21.

138. Scott RL, Solmer PR, MacDonald MG. The effect of starvation and repletion on plasma fibronectin in man. JAMA 1982;248:2025.

139. Chandra RK, Dayton DH. Trace element regulation of immunity and infection. Nutr Res 1982;2:721.

140. Youinou PY, Garre M, Menez JF, et al. Folic acid deficiency and neutrophil dysfunction. Am J Med 1982;73:652.

141. Wilmore DW, Smith RJ, O'Dwyer ST, et al. The gut: A central organ after surgical stress. Surgery 1988;104:917.

142. Hwang TL, O'Dwyer ST, Smith RJ, Wilmore DW. Preservation of the small bowel mucosa using glutamine enriched parenteral nutrition. Surg Forum 1986;37:56.

143. Maddaus MA, Wells CL, Simmons RL. Role of cell-mediated immunity in preventing the translocation of intestinal bacteria. Surg Forum 1986;37:107.

144. Carrico CJ, Meakins JL, Marshall JC, et al. Multiple-organ-failure syndrome. Arch Surg 1986;121:196.

145. Border JR, Hassett S, La Duca J, et al. The gut origin of septic states in blunt multiple trauma (ISS + 40) in the ICU. Ann Surg 1987;206:427.

146. Jarrett F, Balish E, Moylan JA, Ellerbe S. Clinical experience with prophylactic antibiotic bowel suppression in burn patients. Surgery 1978;83:523.

147. Deitch EA. Simple intestinal obstruction causes bacterial translocation in man. Arch Surg 1989;124:699.

148. Ledingham IM, Alcock SR, Eastway AT, et al. Triple regimen of selective decontamination of the digestive tract, systemic cefotaxime, and microbiological surveillance for prevention of acquired infection in intensive care. Lancet 1988;1:875.

149. Flynn DM, Weinstein RA, Nathan C, et al. Patients' endogenous flora as the source of "nosocomial" Enterobacter in cardiac surgery. J Infect Dis 1987;156:363.

150. Brun-Buisson C, Legrand P, Rauss A, et al. Intestinal decontamination for control of nosocomial multiresistant gram-negative bacilli. Study of an outbreak in an intensive care unit. Ann Intern Med 1989;110:873.

151. Waymack JP. The effect of blood transfusions on resistance to bacterial infections. Transplant Proc 1988;20:1105.

152. Rubin RH, Tolkoff-Rubin NE. Post-transfusion viral infections. Transplant Proc 1988;20:1112.

153. Larcher VF, Wyke RJ, Mowat AP, et al. Bacterial and fungal infection in children with fulminant hepatic failure: Possible role of opsonisation and complement deficiency. Gut 1982;23:1037.

154. Rolando N, Harvey F, Brahnn J, et al. Prospective study of bacterial infection in acute liver failure: An analysis of fifty patients. Hepatology 1990;11:49.

155. Imawari M, Hughes RD, Gove CD, et al. Fibronectin and Kupffer cell function in fulminant hepatic failure. Dig Dis Sci 1985;30:1028.

156. Wyke RJ, Jousif-Kadaru AGM, Rajkovic IA, et al. Serum stimulatory activity and polymorphonuclear leukocyte movement in patients with fulminant hepatic failure. Clin Exp Immunol 1982;50:442.

157. MacGregor RR. Alcohol and immune defense. JAMA 1986;256:1474.

158. Roughneen PT, Gouma DJ, Kulkarni AD, et al. Specific cell-mediated immunity in experimental biliary obstruction and its reversibility by internal biliary drainage. J Surg Res 1986;41:113.

159. Greve JW, Gouma DJ, Soeters PB, Buurman WA. Suppression of cellular immunity in obstructive jaundice is caused by endotoxins: A study with germ-free rats. Gastroenterology 1990;98:478.

160. Goldblum SE, Reed WP. Host defenses and immunologic alterations associated with chronic hemodialysis. Ann Intern Med 1980;93:597.

161. Goldblum SE, Van Epps DE, Reed WP. Serum inhibitor of C5 fragment-mediated polymorphonuclear leukocyte chemotaxis associated with chronic hemodialysis. J Clin Invest 1979;64:255.

162. Ruiz P, Gomez F, Schreiber AD. Impaired function of macrophage Fcq receptors in end-stage renal disease. N Engl J Med 1990;322:717.

163. McDonald GB, Sharma P, Hackman RC, et al. Esophageal infections in immunosuppressed patients after marrow transplantation. Gastroenterology 1985;88:1111.

164. Wheeler RR, Peacock JE, Cruz JM, Richter JE. Esophagitis in the immunocompromised host: Role of esophagoscopy in diagnosis. Rev Infect Dis 1987;9:88.

165. Trier JS, Bjorkman DJ. Esophageal, gastric, and intestinal candidiasis. Am J Med 1984;77:39.

166. Meyers JD. Prevention of cytomegalovirus infection after marrow transplantation. Rev Infect Dis 1989;11(Suppl 7):S1691.

167. Rattner HM, Cooper DJ, Zaman MB. Severe bleeding from herpes esophagitis. Am J Gastroenterol 1985;80:523.

168. Buss DH, Scharyj M. Herpesvirus infection of the esophagus and other visceral organs in adults. Incidence and clinical significance. Am J Med 1979;66:457.

169. St. Onge G, Bezahler GH. Giant esophageal ulcer associated with cytomegalovirus. Gastroenterology 1982;83:127.

170. Walsh TJ, Belitsos NJ, Hamilton SR. Bacterial esophagitis in immunocompromised patients. Arch Intern Med 1986;146:1345.

171. Novak JM, Collins JT, Donowitz M, et al. Effects of radiation on the human gastrointestinal tract. J Clin Gastroenterol 1979;1:9.

172. Chisholm RC, Curry SB. Vincristine-induced dysphagia. South Med J 1978;71:1364.

173. Pass HI, Potter DA, Macher AM, et al. Thoracic manifestations of the acquired immune deficiency syndrome. J Thorac Cardiovasc Surg 1984;88:654.

174. Bott S, Prakash C, McCallum RW. Medication-induced esophageal injury: Survey of the literature. Am J Gastroenterol 1987;82:758.

175. Chuck SL, Sande MA. Infections with Cryptococcus neoformans in the acquired immunodeficiency syndrome. N Engl J Med 1989;321:794.

176. Armstrong D, Polsby B. Central nervous system infections in the compromised host. In: Rubin RJ, Young LS. Clinical approach to infection in the compromised host, ed 2. New York: Plenum Publishing, 1988:165.

177. Reuben DB, Mor V. Nausea and vomiting in terminal cancer patients. Arch Intern Med 1986;146:2021.

178. Sperber SJ, Schleupner CJ. Salmonellosis during infection with human immunodeficiency virus. Rev Infect Dis 1987;9:925.

179. Perlman DM, Ampel NM, Schifman RB, et al. Persistent Campylobacter jejuni infections in patients infected with the human immunodeficiency virus (HIV). Ann Intern Med 1988;108:540.

180. Rifkin GD. Neutropenic enterocolitis and Clostridium septicum infection in patients with agranulocytosis. Arch Intern Med 1980;140:834.

181. Hopkins DG, Kushner JP. Clostridial species in the pathogenesis of necrotizing enterocolitis in patients with neutropenia. Am J Hematol 1983;4:289.

182. Alt BA, Glass NR, Sollinger H. Neutropenic enterocolitis in adults. Review of the literature and assessment of surgical intervention. Am J Hematol 1983;4:289.

183. Gracey M, Burke V, Robinson J. Aeromonas associated gastroenteritis. Lancet 1987;2:1304.

184. Golik A, Modai D, Gluskin I, et al. Aeromonas in adult diarrhea: An enteropathogen or an innocent bystander? J Clin Gastroenterol 1990;12:148.

185. Liao W-C, Cappell MS. Treatment with ciprofloxacin of Aeromonas hydrophilia associated colitis in a male with antibodies to the human immunodeficiency virus. J Clin Gastroenterol 1989;11:552.

186. Foltzer MA, Reese RE. Massive diarrhea in *Legionella micdadei* pneumonia. J Clin Gastroenterol 1985;7:525.
187. Fang D-G, Ju V, Vickers RM. Disease due to the *Legionellaceae* (other than *Legionella pneumophila*). Historical, microbiological, clinical, and epidemiological review. Medicine 1989;68:116.
188. Strober W, Krakauer R, Klaeveman HL, et al. Secretory component deficiency: A disorder of the IgA immune system. N Engl J Med 1976;294:351.
189. Myerowitz RL, Pazin GJ, Allen CM. Disseminated candidiasis. Changes in incidence, underlying diseases, and pathology. Am J Clin Pathol 1977;68:29.
190. Young RC, Bennett JE, Geelhoed GW, et al. Fungemia with compromised host resistance: A study of 70 cases. Ann Intern Med 1974;80:605.
191. Smith PD. *Giardia lamblia.* In: Walzer PD, Genta RM, eds. Parasitic infections in the compromised host. New York: Marcel Dekker, 1989:343.
192. Smith PD, Lane HC, Gill VJ, Manischewicz J, Quinnan GV, Fauci AS, Masur H. Intestinal infections in the acquired immunodeficiency syndrome: Etiology and response to therapy. Ann Intern Med 1988;108:328.
193. Current WL. *Cryptosporidium* spp. In: Walzer PD, Genta RM, eds. Parasitic infections in the compromised host. New York: Marcel Dekker, 1989:281.
194. DeHovitz JA, Pape JW, Boncy M, Johnson WD. Clinical manifestations and therapy of *Isospora belli* infection in patients with the acquired immunodeficiency syndrome. N Engl J Med 1986;315:87.
195. Neto VA, Pasternak J, Moreira AAB, et al. *Strongyloides stercoralis* hyperinfection in the acquired immunodeficiency syndrome. Am J Med 1989;87:602.
196. Babb RR, Wagener S. *Blastocystis hominis*—A potential intestinal pathogen. West J Med 1989;151:518.
197. Spriegel JR, Saag KG, Tsang T-K. Infectious diarrhea secondary to *Enteromonas hominis.* Am J Gastroenterol 1989;84:1313.
198. Saulsbury FT, Winkelstein JA, Yolken RH. Chronic rotavirus infection in immunodeficiency. J Pediatr 1980;97:61.
199. Willoughby RE, Wee SB, Yolken RH. Non-group A rotavirus infection associated with severe gastroenteritis in a bone marrow transplant patient. Pediatr Infect Dis J 1988;7:133.
200. Wood DJ, David TJ, Chrystie IL, Totterdell B. Chronic enteric virus infection in two T-cell immunodeficient children. J Med Virol 1988;24:435.
201. Yolken RH, Bishop CA, Townsend TR, et al. Infectious gastroenteritis in bone-marrow transplant patients. N Engl J Med 1982;306:1009.
202. Townshend TR, Bolyard EA, Yolken RH, et al. Outbreak of Coxsackie A1 gastroenteritis: A complication of bone-marrow transplantation. Lancet 1982;1:820.
203. Zahradnik JM, Spencer MJ, Porter DD. Adenovirus infection in the immunocompromised patient. Am J Med 1980;68:725.
204. Chandler FW, White EH, Callaway CS, et al. Unidentified virus-like particles in the intestine of patients with the acquired immunodeficiency syndrome. Ann Intern Med 1984;100:851.
205. Chachoua A, Dieterich D, Krasinski K, Greene J, Laubenstein L, Wernz J, Buhles W, Koretz S. 9-(1,3-dihydroxy-2-propoxymethyl) guanine (ganciclovir) in the treatment of cytomegalovirus gastrointestinal disease with the acquired immunodeficiency syndrome. Ann Intern Med 1987;107:133.
206. Weber JN, Thom S, Barrison I, et al. Cytomegalovirus colitis and oesophageal ulceration in the context of AIDS: Clinical manifestations and preliminary report of treatment with Foscarnet (phosphonoformate). Gut 1987;28:482.
207. Surawicz CM, Myerson D. Self-limited cytomegalovirus colitis in immunocompetent individuals. Gastroenterology 1988;94:194.
208. Underwood JCE, Corbett CL. Persistent diarrhoea and hypoalbuminaemia associated with cytomegalovirus enteritis. Br Med J 1978;1:1029.
209. Tajima T. An autopsy case of primary cytomegalic inclusion enteritis with remarkable hypoproteinemia. Acta Pathol Jpn 1974;i24:151.
210. Tytgat GN, Huibregtse K, Schellekens PT, Feltkamp-Vroom TH. Clinical and immunologic observations in a patient with late onset immunodeficiency. Gastroenterology 1979;76:1458.
211. Goodman ZD, Boitnott JK, Yardley JH. Perforation of the colon associated with cytomegalovirus infection. Dig Dis Sci 1979;24:376.
212. Gleaves CA, Lee CF, Kirsch L, et al. Evaluation of a direct fluorescein-conjugated monoclonal antibody for detection of cytomegalovirus in centrifugation culture. J Clin Microbiol 1987;25:1548.
213. Seidman EG, Walker WA. Gastroenterologic and liver disorders. In: Stiehm ER, ed. Immunologic disorders in infants and children, ed 3. Philadelphia: WB Saunders, 1989:503.
214. Sonsino E, Mouy R, Foucaud P, et al. Intestinal pseudoobstruction related to cytomegalovirus infection of myenteric plexus. N Engl J Med 1984;311:196.
215. McGregor RS, Zitelli BJ, Urbach AH, Malatack JJ, Gartner JC. Varicella in pediatric orthotopic liver transplant recipients. Pediatrics 1989;83:256.
216. Drew HL, Buhles W, Erlich KS. Herpesvirus infections (cytomegalovirus, herpes simplex virus, varicella-zoster virus). How to use ganciclovir (DHPG) and acyclovir. Infect Dis Clin North Am 1988;2:495.
217. Miller AI, Smith B, Rogers AI. Phlegmonous gastritis. Gastroenterology 1975;68:231.
218. Mittleman RE, Suarez RV. Phlegmonous gastritis associated with the acquired immunodeficiency syndrome/pre-acquired immunodeficiency syndrome. Arch Pathol Lab Med 1985;109:765.
219. Seligman BR, Rosner F, Ritz ND. Major surgery in patients with acute leukemia. Am J Surg 1972;124:629.
220. Skibber JM, Matter GJ, Pizzo PA, et al. Right lower quadrant pain in young patients with leukemia. Ann Surg 1987;206:711.
221. Schaller RT, Schaller JF. The acute abdomen in the immunologically compromised child. J Pediatr Surg 1983;18:937.
222. Stellato TA, Shenk RR. Gastrointestinal emergencies in the oncology patient. Semin Oncol 1989;16:521.
223. Varki AP, Armitage JO, Feagler JR. Typhlitis in acute leukemia. Cancer 1979;43:695.
224. Teefey SA, Montana MA, Goldfogel GA, Shuman WP. Sonographic diagnosis of neutropenic typhlitis. Am J Roentgenol 1987;149:731.
225. Fricke MP, Maile CW, Crass JR, et al. Computed tomography of neutropenic colitis. Am J Roentgenol 1984;143:763.
226. Carroll PR, Cattolica EW, Turzan CV, McAninch JW. Necrotizing soft-tissue infections of the perineum and genitalia. Etiology and early reconstruction. West J Med 1986;144:174.
227. Glenn J, Cotton D, Wesley R, Pizzo P. Anorectal infections in patients with malignant disease. Rev Infect Dis 1988;16:42.
228. Yousem DM, Fishman EK, Jones B. Crohn disease: Perirectal and perianal findings at CT. Radiology 1988;167:331.
229. Barnes SG, Sattler FR, Ballard JO. Perirectal infections in acute leukemia. Ann Intern Med 1984;10:515.
230. Hiatt JR, Kuchenbecker SL, Winston DJ. Perineal gangrene in the patient with granulocytopenia: The importance of early diverting colostomy. Surgery 1986;100:912.
231. Shaked AA, Shinar E, Freund H. Managing the granulocytopenic patient with acute perianal inflammatory disease. Am J Surg 1986;152:510.
232. Kalb RE, Grossman ME. Chronic perianal herpes simplex in immunocompromised hosts. Am J Med 1986;80:486.
233. Seigal FP, Lopez C, Hammer GS, et al. Severe acquired immunodeficiency in male homosexuals manifested by chronic perianal ulcerative herpes simplex lesions. N Engl J Med 1981;305:1439.
234. Stroud GM. Recurrent herpes simplex and prednisone dosage in a patient with nephrotic syndrome due to primary systemic amyloidosis. Arch Dermatol 1961;84:396.
235. Straus SE, Smith HA, Brickman C. Acyclovir for chronic mucocutaneous herpes simplex virus infection in immunosuppressed patients. Ann Intern Med 1982;96:270.
236. Hutto JO, Bryan CS, Greene FL, et al. Cryptococcosis of the colon resembling Crohn's disease in a patient with the hyperimmunoglobulinemia E-recurrent infection (Job's) syndrome. Gastroenterology 1988;94:808.
237. Quinn TC. Clinical approach to intestinal infections in homosexual men. Med Clin North Am 1986;70:611.
238. Laughon BE, Druckman DA, Vernon A, et al. Prevalence of enteric pathogens in homosexual men with and without acquired immunodeficiency syndrome. Gastroenterology 1988;94:984.

239. Lax JD, Haroutiounian G, Attia A, et al. Tuberculosis of the rectum in a patient with acquired immune deficiency syndrome. Report of the case. Dis Colon Rectum 1988;31:394.

240. Lee MH, Waxman M, Gillooley JF. Primary malignant lymphoma of the anorectum in homosexual men. Dis Colon Rectum 1986;29: 413.

241. Ioachim HL, Weinstein MA, Robbins RD, Sohn N, Lugo PN. Primary anorectal lymphoma. A new manifestation of the acquired immune deficiency syndrome. Cancer 1987;60:1449.

242. Frazer IH, Medley G, Crapper RM, et al. Association between anorectal dysplasia, human papillomavirus, and human immunodeficiency virus infection in homosexual men. Lancet 1986;2:657.

243. Peterson PK, Balfour HH, Marker SC, et al. Cytomegalovirus disease in renal allograft recipients: A prospective study of the clinical features, risk factors, and impact on renal transplantation. Medicine 1980;59:283.

244. Sutherland DER, Chan FY, Foucar E, et al. The bleeding cecal ulcer in transplant patients. Surgery 1979;86:386.

245. Foucar E, Mukai K, Foucar K, et al. Colon ulceration in lethal cytomegalovirus infection. Am J Clin Pathol 1981;76:788.

246. Cho RT, Tisnado J, Liu CI, et al. Bleeding cytomegalovirus ulcers of the colon: Barium enema and angiography. Am J Roentgenol 1981;136:1213.

247. West JC, Armitage SO, Mitros FA, et al. Cytomegalovirus cecal erosion causing massive hemorrhage in a bone marrow transplant recipient. World J Surg 1982;6:251.

248. Welsh RA, McClinton LT. Aspergillosis of lungs and duodenum with fatal intestinal hemorrhage. Arch Pathol 1954;57:379.

249. Fitzpatrick TJ, Neiman BH. *Histoplasma capsulatum* infection associated with gastric ulcer and fatal hemorrhage. Arch Intern Med 1953;91:49.

250. Anuras S, Summers R. Fulminant herpes simplex hepatitis in an adult: Report of a case in a renal transplant recipient. Gastroenterology 1976;70:425.

251. Marrie TJ, McDonald ATJ, Conen PE, et al. Herpes simplex hepatitis—Use of immunoperoxidase to demonstrate the viral antigen in hepatocytes. Gastroenterology 1982;82:71.

252. Goodman ZD, Ishak KG, Sesterhenn IA. Herpes simplex hepatitis in apparently immuno-competent adults. Am J Clin Pathol 1986;85: 694.

253. Shulman HM, McDonald GB. Liver disease after marrow transplantation. In: Sale GE, Shulman HM, eds. The pathology of bone marrow transplantation. New York: Masson, 1984:104.

254. Faden H, Jockin H, Talty MR, et al. Fatal disseminated adenovirus infection featuring liver necrosis and prolonged viremia in an immunosuppressed child with malignant histiocytosis. Am J Pediatr Hematol Oncol 1985;7:15.

255. Biggs DD, Toorkey BC, Carrigan DR, et al. Disseminated Echovirus infection complicating bone marrow transplantation. Am J Med 1990;88:421.

256. Galbraith RM, Eddleston AL, Williams R, Zuckerman AJ. Fulminant hepatic failure in leukaemia and choriocarcinoma related to withdrawal of cytotoxic drug therapy. Lancet 1975;2:528.

257. Hoofnagle JH, Dusheiko GM, Schafer DF, et al. Reactivation of chronic hepatitis B virus infection by cancer chemotherapy. Ann Intern Med 1982;96:447.

258. Hansen CA, Sutherland DE, Snover DC. Fulminant hepatic failure in an HBsAg carrier renal transplant patient following cessation of immunosuppressive therapy. Transplantation 1985;39:311.

259. Flowers MA, Heathcote J, Wanless IR, et al. Fulminant hepatitis as a consequence of reactivation of hepatitis B virus infection after discontinuation of low-dose methotrexate therapy. Ann Intern Med 1990;112:381.

260. Vergani D, Locasciulli A, Masera G, et al. Histological evidence of hepatitis B virus infection with negative serology in children with acute leukemia who develop chronic liver disease. Lancet 1982;1: 361.

261. Locasciulli A, Santamaria M, Masera G, et al. Hepatitis B virus markers in children with acute leukemia: The effect of chemotherapy. J Med Virol 1985;15:29.

262. Pao CC, Yang WL, Wu SY, et al. Presence of hepatitis B virus

DNA in serum of surface antigen seronegative immunocompromised patients. J Clin Microbiol 1987;25:449.

263. Dienstag JL. Viral hepatitis in the compromised host. In: Rubin RJ, Young LS, eds. Clinical approach to infection in the compromised host, ed 2. New York: Plenum Publishing, 1988:325.

264. Sengar DP, Rashid A, McLeish WA, et al. Hepatitis B surface antigen (HBsAg) infection in a hemodialysis unit. II. Factors affecting host immune response to HBsAg. Can Med Assoc J 1975;113:945.

265. Blumberg BS, Sutnick AI, London WT. Australia antigen as a hepatitis virus: Variation in host response. Am J Med 1970;48:1.

266. Degott C, Degos F, Jungers P, Naret C, et al. Relationship between liver histopathological changes and HBsAg in 111 patients treated by longterm hemodialysis. Liver 1983;3:377.

267. Jungers P, Naret C, et al. Histological and immunological survey of chronic active hepatitis in 650 hemodialyzed patients. In: Touraine JL, Traeger J, eds. Transplantation and clinical immunology. Amsterdam Excerpta Medica, 1979:38.

268. Bronsther O, Makowka L, et al. Occurrence of cytomegalovirus hepatitis in liver transplant patients. J Med Virol 1988;24:423.

269. Snover DC, Hutton S, Balfour HH, et al. Cytomegalovirus infection of the liver in transplant recipients. J Clin Gastroenterol 1987;9: 659.

270. Lewis JH, Patel HR, Zimmerman HJ. The spectrum of hepatic candidiasis. Hepatology 1982;2:479.

271. Moseley RH, Kris MG, Einzig A, et al. Respiratory alkalosis and abdominal pain heralding Candida hepatitis: Occurrence in patients with acute leukemia in remission. Arch Intern Med 1982;142:1495.

272. Tashjian LS, Abramson JS, Peacock JE. Focal hepatic candidiasis: A distinct clinical variant of candidiasis in immunocompromised patients. Rev Infect Dis 1984;6:689.

273. Fitzgerald EJ, Coblentz C. Fungal microabscesses in immunosuppressed patients—CT appearances. J Can Assoc Radiol 1988;39:10.

274. Gordon SC, Watts JC, Veneri RJ, Chandler FW. Focal hepatic candidiasis with perihepatic adhesions: Laparoscopic and immunohistologic diagnosis. Gastroenterology 1990;98:214.

275. Korinek JK, Guarda LA, Bolivar R, Strochlein JR. *Trichosporon* hepatitis. Gastroenterology 1983;85:732.

276. Young RC. The Budd–Chiari syndrome caused by Aspergillus. Two patients with vascular invasion of the hepatic veins. Arch Intern Med 1969;124:754.

277. Patel SA, Borges MC, Batt MD, Rosenblatz HJ. *Trichosporon cholangitis* associated with hyperbilirubinemia and findings suggesting primary sclerosing cholangitis on endoscopic retrograde cholangiopancreatography. Am J Gastroenterol 1990;85:84.

278. Vallaeys JH, Praet MM, Roels HJ, et al. The Budd–Chiari syndrome caused by a zygomycete. A new pathogenesis of hepatic vein thrombosis. Arch Pathol Lab Med 1989;113:1171.

279. Brems JJ, Hiatt JR, Klein AS, et al. Disseminated aspergillosis complicating orthotopic liver transplantation for fulminant hepatic failure refractory to corticosteroid therapy. Transplantation 1988;46:479.

280. Hagopian WA, Huseby JS. *Pneumocystis hepatitis* and choroiditis despite successful aerosolized pentamidine pulmonary prophylaxis. Chest 1989;96:949.

281. Fishman EK, Magid D, Kuhlman JE. *Pneumocystis carinii* involvement of the liver and spleen: CT demonstration. J Comput Assist Tomogr 1990;14:146.

282. Beschorner WE, Pino J, Boitnott JK, et al. Pathology of the liver with bone marrow transplantation. Effects of busulfan, carmustine, acute graft-versus-host disease, and cytomegalovirus infection. Am J Pathol 1980;99:369.

283. Davis JJ, Heyman MB, et al. Sclerosing cholangitis associated with chronic cryptosporidiosis in a child with a congenital immunodeficiency disorder. Am J Gastroenterol 1987;82:1196.

284. Lefkowitz JH. Bile ductular cholestasis: An ominous histopathologic sign related to sepsis and "cholangitis lenta." Hum Pathol 1982;13: 19.

285. Zimmerman HJ, Fang M, Utili R, et al. Jaundice due to bacterial infection. Gastroenterology 1979;77:362.

286. Fang MH, Ginsberg AL, Dobbins WO. Marked elevation in serum alkaline phosphatase activity as a manifestation of systemic infection. Gastroenterology 1980;78:592.

287. Navari RM, Sullivan KM, Springmeyer SC, et al. Mycobacterial

infections in marrow transplant patients. Transplantation 1983;36: 509.

288. Baker AL, Rosenberg IH. Hepatic complications of total parenteral nutrition. Am J Med 1987;82:489.

289. Mitchell RB, Wagner JE, Karp JE, et al. Syndrome of idiopathic hyperammonemia after high-dose chemotherapy: Review of nine cases. Am J Med 1988;85:662.

290. Krause W, Matheis H, Wulf K. Fungaemia and funguria after oral administration of *Candida albicans*. Lancet 1969;1:598.

291. McDonald GB, Vracko R. Systemic absorption of oral cholestyramine. Gastroenterology 1984;87:213.

292. Myerowitz RL. The pathology of opportunistic infections, with pathogenetic, diagnostic, and clinical correlations. New York: Raven Press, 1983:23.

293. Cohen ML, Murphy MT, Counts GW, et al. Prediction by surveillance cultures of bacteremia among neutropenic patients treated in a protective environment. J Infect Dis 1983;147:789.

294. Beschorner WE, Yardley JH, Tutschka P, Santos G. Deficiency of intestinal immunity with graft-vs-host disease in humans. J Infect Dis 1981;144:38.

295. Peterson WL, Mackowiak PA, Barnett CC, et al. The human gastric bactericidal barrier: Mechanisms of action, relative antibacterial activity and dietary influences. J Infect Dis 1989;159:979.

296. Remington JS, Schimpff SC. Please don't eat the salads. N Engl J Med 1981;304:433.

297. Pinegar JA, Cooke EM. *Escherichia coli* in retail processed food. J Hyg 1985;95:39.

298. Moe G. Low microbial diets for patients with granulocytopenia. In: Bloch AS, ed. Nutrition management of the cancer patient. Rockville, MD: Aspen Publishing, 1990:125.

299. Cleaning and disinfection of equipment for gastrointestinal flexible endoscopy: Interim recommendations of a working party of the British Society of Gastroenterology. Gut 1988;29:1134.

300. Shovron PJ, Eykyn SJ, Cotton PB. Gastrointestinal instrumentation, bacteremia and endocarditis. Gut 1983;24:1078.

301. Botoman VA, Surawicz CM. Bacteremia with gastrointestinal endoscopic procedures. Gastrointest Endosc 1986;32:342.

302. Bianco JA, Pepe MS, Higano C, et al. Prevalence of clinically relevant bacteremia following upper gastrointestinal endoscopy in bone marrow transplant recipients. Am J Med 1990;89:134.

303. Wade JC. Unpublished observations.

304. Berdonck LF, de Graan-Hentzen YCE, Dekker AW, et al. Cytomegalovirus seronegative platelets and leukocyte-poor red blood cells from random donors can prevent primary cytomegalovirus infection after bone marrow transplantation. Bone Marrow Transplant 1987;2: 73.

305. Wade JC, Schimpff SC. Epidemiology and prevention of infection in the compromised host. In: Rubin RH, Young LS, eds. Clinical approach to infection in the compromised host, ed 2. New York: Plenum Publishing, 1988:5.

306. Buckner CD, Clift RA, Sanders JE, et al. Protective environment for marrow transplant recipients. A prospective study. Ann Intern Med 1978;89:893.

307. Schimpff SC, Greene WH, Young VM, et al. Infection prevention in acute nonlymphocytic leukemia. Laminar air flow room reverse isolation with oral, nonabsorbable antibiotic prophylaxis. Ann Intern Med 1975;82:351.

308. Schimpff SC. Surveillance cultures. J Infect Dis 1981;144:81.

309. Gurwith MJ, Brunton JL, Lank BA, et al. A prospective controlled investigation of prophylactic trimethoprim-sulfamethoxazole in hospitalized granulocytopenic patients. Am J Med 1979;66:248.

310. Dekker AW, Rozenberg-Arska M, Sixma JJ, et al. Prevention of infection by trimethoprim-sulfamethoxazole plus amphotericin-B in patients with acute nonlymphocytic leukaemia. Ann Intern Med 1981;95:555.

311. Schmeiser T, Kurrie E, Arnold R, et al. Norfloxacin for prevention of bacterial infections during severe granulocytopenia after bone marrow transplantation. Scand J Infect Dis 1988;20:625.

312. Rozenberg-Arska M, Dekker AW, Verhoef J. Prevention of infections in granulocytopenic patients by fluorinated quinolones. Rev Infect Dis 1989;11(Suppl 5):S1231.

313. Peterson FB, Buckner CD, Clift RA, et al. Laminar air flow isolation and decontamination: A prospective randomized study of the effects

of prophylactic systemic antibiotics in bone marrow transplant patients. Infection 1986;14:115.

314. Peterson FB, Thornquist M, Buckner CD, et al. The effects of infection prevention regimens on early infectious complications in marrow transplant patients: A four arm randomized study. Infection 1988;16:199.

315. De Gregoria MW, Lee WMF, Ries CA. Candida infections in patients with acute leukemia: Ineffectiveness of nystatin prophylaxis and relationship between oropharyngeal and systemic candidiasis. Cancer 1982;50:2780.

316. Hahn DM, Schimpff SC, Fornter CL, et al. Infection in acute leukemia patients receiving oral nonabsorbable antibiotics. Antimicrob Agents Chemother 1978;13:958.

317. Levine AS, Siegel SE, Schreiber AD, et al. Protected environments and prophylactic antibiotics. A prospective controlled study of their utility in the therapy of acute leukemia. N Engl J Med 1973;288: 477.

318. Hofstra W, deVries-Hospers HG, Van der Waaij D. Concentrations of nystatin in faeces after oral administration of various doses. Infection 1979;4:166.

319. Hofstra W, deVries-Hospers G, Van der Waaij D. Concentration of amphotericin B in faeces and blood of healthy volunteers after the oral administration of various doses. Infection 1982;10:223.

320. Brincker H. Prophylactic treatment with miconazole in patients highly predisposed to fungal infection. Acta Med Scand 1978;204:123.

321. Hann IM, Corringham R, Keaney M, et al. Ketoconazole versus nystatin plus amphotericin-B for fungal prophylaxis in severely immunocompromised patients. Lancet 1982;1:826.

322. Brammer KW. Management of fungal infection in neutropenic patients with fluconazole. Hamatol Bluttransfus 1990;33:546.

323. Powderly WG, Kobayashi GS, Herzig GP, et al. Amphotericin B resistant yeast infection in severely immunocompromised patients. Am J Med 1988;84:826.

324. Tricot G, Joosten E, Boogaerts MA, et al. Ketoconazole vs. itraconazole for antifungal prophylaxis in patients with severe granulocytopenia: Preliminary results of two nonrandomized studies. Rev Infect Dis 1987;9(Suppl 1):S94.

325. Pizzo PA, Robichaud KJ, Gill KA, et al. Empiric antibiotic and antifungal therapy for cancer patients with prolonged fever and granulocytopenia. Am J Med 1987;72:101.

326. Winston DJ, Ho WG, Gale RP, Champlin RE. Prophylaxis of infection in bone marrow transplants. Eur J Cancer Clin Oncol 1988;24(Suppl 1):S15.

327. Stein R, Kayser J, Klenher J. Clinical value of empirical amphotericin B in patients with acute myelogenous leukemia. Cancer 1982;50: 2247.

328. EORTC International Antimicrobial Therapy Cooperative Group. Empiric antifungal therapy in febrile granulocytopenic patients. Am J Med 1989;86:668.

329. Wade JC, Newton B, Flournoy N, Meyers JD. Oral acyclovir for prevention of herpes simplex virus reactivation after marrow transplantation. Ann Intern Med 1984;100:823.

330. Nyerges G, Meszner Z, Gyarmati E, Kerpel-Fronius S. Acyclovir prevents dissemination of varicella in immunocompromised children. J Infect Dis 1988;157:309.

331. Chow AW. Infections of the oral cavity, neck and head. In: Mandell GL, Douglas RG, Bennett JE, eds. Principles and practice of infectious diseases, ed 3. New York: Churchill Livingstone, 1990:516.

332. Pollack M. *Pseudomonas aeruginosa*. In: Mandell GL, Douglas RG, Bennett JE, eds. Principles and practice of infectious diseases. New York: Churchill Livingstone, 1990:1673.

333. Rampling A, Warren RE, Bevan PC, et al. *Clostridium difficile* in haematological malignancy. J Clin Pathol 1985;38:445.

334. Cudmore MA, Silva J, Fekety R, et al. *Clostridium difficile* colitis associated with cancer chemotherapy. Arch Intern Med 1982;142: 333.

335. Miller SD, Koornhof HJ. *Clostridium difficile* colitis associated with the use of antineoplastic agents. Eur J Clin Microbiol 1984;3:10.

336. Delmer M, Vandercam B, Aresani V, Michaus JL. Epidemiology and prevention of *Clostridium difficile* infections in a leukemia unit. Eur J Clin Microbiol 1987;6:623.

337. Heard SR, O'Farrell S, Holland D, et al. The epidemiology of *Clostridium difficile* with use of a typing scheme: Nosocomial acquisition

and cross-infection among immunocompromised patients. J Infect Dis 1986;153:159.

338. Shaked A, Shinar E, Freund H. Neutropenic typhlitis: A plea for conservatism. Dis Colon Rectum 1983;26:351.

339. Jacobson MA, Hahn SM, Gerberding JL, et al. Ciprofloxacin for *Salmonella bacteremia* in the acquired immunodeficiency syndrome (AIDS). Ann Intern Med 1989;110:1027.

340. Laine L, Conteas C, DeBruin M, et al. A prospective randomized trial of fluconazole vs. ketoconazole for *Candida* esophagitis. Gastroenterology 1990;98:A458.

341. Gold JWM. Opportunistic fungal infections in patients with neoplastic diseases. Am J Med 1984;76:458.

342. Lopez-Berenstein G, Bodey GP, Fainstein V, et al. Treatment of systemic fungal infections with liposomal amphotericin B. Arch Intern Med 1989;149:2544.

343. Denning DW, Tucker RM, Hansen LH, Stevens DA. Treatment of invasive aspergillosis with itraconazole. Am J Med 1989;86:791.

344. Conti DJ, Tolkoff-Rubin NE, Baker GP, et al. Successful treatment of invasive fungal infection with fluconazole in organ transplant recipients. Transplantation 1989;48:692.

345. Tucker RM, Williams PL, Arathoon EG, Stevens DA. Treatment of mycoses with itraconazole. Ann NY Acad Sci 1988;544:451.

346. Meyers JD, Wade JC, Mitchell CD, Saral R, Lietman PS, Durack DT, Levin MJ, Segreti AC, Balfour HH. Multicenter collaborative trial of intravenous acyclovir for the treatment of mucocutaneous herpes simplex virus infection in the immunocompromised host. Am J Med 1982;73(Suppl 1A):229.

347. Shepp DH, Newton BA, Dandliker PS, Flournoy N, Meyers JD. Oral acyclovir therapy for mucocutaneous herpes simplex virus infections in immunocompromised marrow transplant recipients. Ann Intern Med 1985;102:783.

348. Sacks SL, Wanklin RJ, Reece DE, et al. Progressive esophagitis from acyclovir-resistant herpes simplex. Clinical roles for DNA polymerase mutants and viral heterogeneity? Ann Intern Med 1989;111:893.

349. England JA, Zimmerman ME, Swierkosz EM, et al. Herpes simplex virus resistant to acyclovir. A study in a tertiary care center. Ann Intern Med 1990;112:416.

350. Erlich KS, Jacobson MA, Koehler JE, et al. Foscarnet therapy for severe acyclovir-resistant herpes simplex virus type-2 infections in patients with the acquired immunodeficiency syndrome (AIDS). An uncontrolled trial. Ann Intern Med 1989;110:710.

351. Fletcher CV, Englund JA, Bean B, et al. Continuous infusion high-dose acyclovir for serious herpesvirus infections. Antimicrob Agents Chemother 1989;133:1375.

352. Sawyer MH, Ichauspe G, Biran KK, Waters DJ. Molecular analysis of the pyrimidine deoxyribonucleoside kinase gene of wild-type and acyclovir-resistant strains of varicella-zoster virus. J Gen Virol 1988;69:2585.

353. Rindgen O, Lonnqvist B, Paulin T, Ahlmen J, Klintmalm G, Wahren B, Lernestedt JO. Pharmacokinetics, safety, and preliminary clinical experiences using foscarnet in the treatment of cytomegalovirus infections in bone marrow and renal transplant recipients. J Antimicrob Chemother 1986;17:373.

354. Davidson GP, Whyte PB, Daniels E, Franklin K. Passive immunization of children with bovine colostrum containing antibodies to human rotavirus. Lancet 1989;2:709.

355. Janoff EN, Smith PD, Blaser MJ. Acute antibody responses to *Giardia lamblia* are depressed in patients with AIDS. J Infect Dis 1988;157:798.

356. Ament ME, Rubin CE. Relation of giardiasis to abnormal intestinal structure and function in gastrointestinal immunodeficiency syndromes. Gastroenterology 1972;62:216.

357. Smith PD, Gillin FD, Spria WW, Nash TE. Chronic giardiasis: Studies on drug sensitivity, toxin production and host immune response. Gastroenterology 1982;83:797.

358. Tomkins AM, Wright SG, Draser BS, James WPT. Bacterial colonization of jejunal mucosa in giardiasis. Trans R Soc Trop Med Hyg 1978;72:33.

359. Portnoy D, Whiteside ME, Buckley E, MacLeod CL. Treatment of intestinal cryptosporidiosis with spiramycin. Ann Intern Med 1984;101:202.

360. Connolly GM, Dryden MS, Shanson DC, Gazzard BG. Cryptosporidial diarrhoea in AIDS and its treatment. Gut 1988;29:593.

361. Meisel JL, Perera DR, Meligro C, Rubin CE. Overwhelming watery diarrhea associated with *Cryptosporidium* in an immunosuppressed patient. Gastroenterology 1976;70:1156.

362. Lewis IJ, Hart CA, Baxby D. Diarrhoea due to *Cryptosporidium* in acute lymphoblastic leukaemia. Arch Dis Child 1985;60:60.

363. Miller RA, Holmberg RE, Clausen CR. Life-threatening diarrhea caused by *Cryptosporidium* in a child undergoing therapy for acute lymphocytic leukemia. J Pediatr 1983;103:256.

364. Katz MD, Erstad BL, Rose C. Treatment of severe *Cryptosporidium*-related diarrhea with octreotide in a patient with AIDS. Drug Intell Clin Pharm 1988;22:134.

365. Saxon A, Weinstein W. Oral administration of bovine colostrum anti-cryptosporidia antibody fails to alter the course of human cryptosporidiosis. J Parasitol 1987;73:413.

366. Tzipori S, Roberton D, Cooper DA, White L. Chronic cryptosporidial diarrhoea and hyperimmune cow colostrum. Lancet 1987;2:344.

367. Ungar BLP, Ward DJ, Fayer R, Quinn CA. Cessation of *Cryptosporidium*-associated diarrhea in an acquired immunodeficiency syndrome patient after treatment with hyperimmune bovine colostrum. Gastroenterology 1990;98:486.

368. Petri WA, Ravdin JI. *Entamoeba histolytica*. In: Walzer PD, Genta RM, eds. Parasitic infections in the compromised host. New York: Marcel Dekker, 1989:385.

369. Norris SM, Ravdin JI. The pharmacology of antiamebic drugs. In: Ravdin JI, ed. Amebiasis: Human infection with Entamoeba histolytica. New York: John Wiley & Sons, 1988:734.

370. Douce RW, Brown AE, Khambooruang C, Walzer PD, Genta RM. Seroepidemiology of strongyloidiasis in a Thai village. Int J Parasitol 1987;17:1343.

371. Pelletier LL. Chronic strongyloidiasis in World War II Far East ex-prisoners of war. Am J Trop Med Hyg 1984;33:55.

372. Luft BJ. *Toxoplasma gondii*. In: Walzer PD, Genta RM, eds. Parasitic infections in the compromised host. New York: Marcel Dekker, 1989:179.

373. Sheehan DJ, Raucher BG, McKitrick JC. Association of *Blastocystis hominis* with signs and symptoms of human disease. J Clin Microbiol, 1986;24:548.

374. Markell EK, Udkow MP. *Blastocystis hominis*: Pathogen or fellow traveler? Am J Trop Med Hyg 1986;35:1023.

375. Westerman C, Christensen RP. Chronic *Isospora belli* infection treated with co-trimoxazole. Ann Intern Med 1979;91:413.

376. Gordon FM, Simon GL, Wofsy CB, Mills J. Adverse reactions to trimethoprim-sulfamethoxazole in patients with the acquired immunodeficiency syndrome. Arch Intern Med 1984;100:495.

377. Weiss LM, Perlman DC, Sherman J, Tanowitz H, Wittner M. *Isospora belli* infection: Treatment with pyrimethamine. Ann Intern Med 1988;109:474.

47

Approach to Gastrointestinal Problems Associated with Common Clinical Conditions

JAMES W. FRESTON
JAMES R. MOORE

Gastrointestinal (GI) diseases are often encountered in the form of disorders superimposed on such common conditions as pregnancy, cardiorespiratory disease, diabetes mellitus, rheumatoid arthritis, renal failure, and nervous system disorders. Moreover, the conditions may increase the frequency of certain digestive disorders, alter the expression of some, and influence the outcome of others. The GI diseases may, in turn, influence the underlying primary conditions. This chapter addresses the GI manifestations of several common clinical conditions.

DIABETES MELLITUS

General Considerations

The relationship between diabetes mellitus and the GI tract is complex. Weight loss, vomiting, or acute gastric distention may be prominent symptoms of diabetic ketoacidosis, but their presence does not necessarily mean that the GI tract has been damaged by diabetes. On the other hand, diabetic vomiting and diarrhea are entities usually seen in longstanding diabetics and may be presumed to be due to end-organ damage caused by the disease. Diabetes may result from gastroenterologic disorders, particularly pancreatic disease and cirrhosis. Finally, conditions such as autoimmune gastritis and celiac disease are neither the consequence nor the cause of diabetes, but appear with more frequency in diabetics than in the general population.

Gastroenterologic Complications

The prevalence of gastroenterologic symptoms in diabetics is unknown but probably is considerable.[1] Feldman found that only 28% of 136 diabetics had no gastroenterologic symptoms (see Table 47-1). Most of the symptoms described were attributable to abnormal esophageal or GI motility. Problems with disturbed GI motility may be more common than patient complaints would suggest. In many patients, disturbed motility is manifest not by overt gastroenterologic symptoms, but by unexplained worsening of diabetic control.[2]

The reasons for the longstanding motility disturbances encountered in diabetics are not entirely clear. Motility of the gastroenterologic tract, including the esophagus and biliary tree, is controlled in large part by the enteric nervous system. Many enteric neurotransmitters are amines or peptides that can act as hormones or paracrine agents (see ch 1, 2, 7–11). Central nervous system influences on motility are mediated by the autonomic nervous system (see ch 3). In principle, motor dysfunction of the GI tract might occur if the nerves of the autonomic nervous system were affected by the patchy demyelination that occurs in the somatic peripheral nerves of longstanding diabetics. Motor dysfunction might also occur if the enteric nervous system were disrupted by the same process, if neuropeptide regulation were abnormal, or if the effector muscles were damaged in some way by the diabetes.

Acute motility disturbances in diabetics occur during periods of ketoacidosis when many metabolic disturbances are present. Hyperglycemia itself may delay gastric emptying,[3] as may hypokalemia. However, other metabolic abnormalities are probably important also because the clinical manifestations of disordered motility are relatively unusual in nonketotic patients with hyperglycemia.

Diabetic Autonomic Neuropathy in the Gastrointestinal Tract

Much evidence supports the concept that autonomic neuropathy is a prerequisite for the development of clinically significant disorders of GI motility in diabetics. Most patients have longstanding

TABLE 47–1
Gastrointestinal Symptoms in 136 Diabetic Outpatients

SYMPTOM	OUTPATIENTS, *n* (%)
Constipation	82 (60)
Abdominal pain	46 (34)
Nausea and vomiting	39 (29)
Dysphagia	37 (27)
Diarrhea	30 (22)
Fecal incontinence	27 (20)
No gastrointestinal symptoms	32 (24)

Data from Feldman M, Schiller LR. Disorders of gastrointestinal motility associated with diabetes mellitus. Ann Intern Med 1983;98:378.

diabetes with symptoms of autonomic neuropathy, such as postural or exertional hypotension, impotence, or sweat gland instability.[1] Many have evidence of somatic peripheral neuropathy, as well as eye and renal complications of diabetes.[1]

Direct evidence of autonomic neuropathy involving the GI tract in humans comes from functional studies and a limited number of morphologic investigations. Sham feeding was ineffectual in eliciting an acid secretory response in diabetics, while the response to intragastric stimuli was maintained.[4] Similarly, the normal spike response to a meal was absent in the colon of longstanding diabetics with constipation.[5] These subjects responded normally to pentagastrin and bethanechol, respectively, showing that the problem was not one of end-organ damage and implying that a defect in the efferent arm of the autonomic nervous system was present. Morphologic studies of the autonomic nervous system have been less clear-cut. Disruption of nerve fibers in the thoracic vagi of diabetics occurs,[6] but no morphologic abnormalities were found in the abdominal vagi of patients with diabetic gastroparesis.[7]

Diabetes and the Enteric Nervous System

Morphologic studies have shown axonal degeneration and thickening of the basement membrane of Schwann's cells in Meissner's plexus of humans with diabetic autonomic neuropathy.[8] Similar findings have been found in Auerbach's plexus in rats with streptozotocin-induced diabetes.[9] These animals also had degeneration of the adrenergic and serotonergic innervation of the ileum[9] but no obvious change in the proximal colon.[10] Substance P-like immunoreactivity in the ileum and colon was unchanged from control. However, in the proximal gut substance P was decreased while VIP was increased.[11]

Whether or not similar anatomic or functional changes occur in humans with longstanding diabetes, and whether such changes are related to gastroenterologic symptoms seen in diabetics, is unknown. Also unknown is whether these changes are secondary to extraintestinal neuronal loss or a direct result of the diabetes itself.

Gut Endocrine Abnormalities

Many symptoms of disordered GI motility in diabetes are strikingly paroxysmal, suggesting the possibility that hormonal factors are involved. In diabetics with gastroparesis, glucagon levels are not suppressed by hyperglycemia, and hypoglycemia does not induce increased plasma glucagon levels.[12] Motilin levels show normal cyclic variations in diabetics with gastric motility disturbances but at increased levels.[13]

Features of Disordered Gastrointestinal Motility

ESOPHAGEAL DYSFUNCTION

Motor function of the esophagus is relatively simple to study by contrast radiology, manometry, or scintigraphy (see ch 7, 54, 114, 121, and 128). A plethora of studies have shown that abnormalities of motor function can be found in up to 80% of patients with diabetic peripheral neuropathy.[14,15] Barium studies have demonstrated esophageal dilatation, delayed emptying, and spontaneous aperistaltic contractions.[13,16] Manometric studies most commonly show decreased peristalsis, peristalsis with multipeaked pressure waves, or decreased esophageal velocities.[17] Lower esophageal sphincter pressures usually are reduced.[18] A smaller number of diabetics have increased peristalsis in the esophagus.[16] Abnormal manometric findings may be found more frequently in patients with psychiatric symptoms.[19] Radionuclide scintigraphy demonstrates diminished esophageal clearance in the overwhelming majority of patients with diabetes and peripheral neuropathy.[18]

The clinical manifestations of esophageal dysmotility are much less frequent than the laboratory abnormalities. The most typical complaint is heartburn, presumably caused by either increased gastroesophageal reflux or decreased clearance. Delayed gastric emptying is common in these patients and might also contribute to reflux.[18]

Dysphagia may be a consequence of the motor abnormalities, but its occurrence should not be ascribed to a diabetes-related motor disorder without further investigation. Diabetics are just as likely to develop carcinoma of the esophagus as other people.

Candida esophagitis is relatively common in diabetics and can cause severe odynophagia. Its presence can be inferred if the patient has thrush, but confirmation is best made by mucosal brushings obtained at endoscopy.

GASTRIC DYSFUNCTION

In 1958, Kassander[20] introduced the euphonious term "gastroparesis diabeticorum" to describe the atony and delayed gastric emptying observed in some diabetic patients. In these patients, the upper GI series showed gastric dilatation, diminished or absent peristalsis, prolonged retention of barium, and duodenal bulb atony.

Various techniques have been used to quantify gastric emptying in diabetics with autonomic neuropathy or gastroenterologic symptoms (see ch 8, 60, 114, 121, and 128). Radiolabeled test meals in which different isotopes have been used for solid and liquid phases of the meal have given results that are not entirely consistent. Delayed emptying of both solid and liquid meal components has been found.[21] Others have found no difference between diabetics and controls, and delay of the solid phase but not the liquid phase has been demonstrated.[22] Another approach to quantifying gastric dysfunction in diabetics has been the use of ingested radiopaque markers. In these studies, radiopaque solids are passed into the small intestine significantly more slowly in diabetics than controls.[23] Nuclear scanning or radiologic techniques do not discriminate well between diabetics with and without symptoms.[21] Many, perhaps the majority, of diabetics who have demonstrable abnormalities of gastric emptying by any given technique have no symptoms. Manometric studies have shown diabetics with nausea and vomiting to have abnormal antral,[24] pyloric,[25] and small intestinal motility.[26] The duration and frequency of antral contractions are reduced in the majority of patients. In some patients, low-amplitude antral contractions occur.[25] The pylorus is reported to show prolonged tonic contractions.[26] Unlike normal subjects, diabetic patients do not demonstrate the initiation of phase III migrating motor complex activity with each peak of motilin concentration.[13]

The typical patient with symptoms from diabetic gastroparesis has usually had diabetes for several years and is insulin-dependent with a history of poor control. Ketosis develops despite relative euglycemia. Diabetic complications such as retinopathy, renal failure, or peripheral neuropathy are usually present. Chronic satiety and nausea are common complaints, often with nonspecific epigastric discomfort or pain. Vomiting usually is paroxysmal, and it may precipitate metabolic disarray. Weight loss may be appreciable but is rarely progressive, perhaps because there are interludes of relative freedom from symptoms during which lost weight may be regained. Bezoars may develop, presumably as a consequence of disordered gastric emptying. This may cause exacerbation of symptoms as well as halitosis.[27]

Management should include active efforts to achieve perfect diabetic control, at least in the short term. Blood glucose estimations may not be adequate as an index of control of these patients' diabetes. Correction of the metabolic abnormalities may require intravenous electrolytes, water glucose, and insulin. Once achieved, remission of symptoms of gastroparesis may be prolonged. In some patients, nausea, epigastric discomfort, and satiety recur despite good metabolic control. These patients may be helped by a low-fat diet. Symptoms may be improved by antiemetic agents, such as prochlorperazine. Metoclopramide is widely used for this purpose. It has central antiemetic properties, as well as being a gastric prokinetic agent in normal subjects. In symptomatic diabetics with gastroparesis, the subjective improvement with metoclopramide therapy does not correspond with objective improvement in gastric emptying.[21] The drug's central effects may provide most relief. Unfortunately, metoclopramide may lose its effectiveness with prolonged use, and its side effects, including drowsiness, hyperprolactinemia, and extrapyramidal reactions, may prove troublesome. For these reasons, it is probably best used for periods up to 2 or 3 weeks.[28] Other prokinetic agents, which are less well-studied but may prove useful in this condition, include domperidone[29] and cisapride.[30] Erythromycin has motilin agonist properties and shows some promise as an agent for promoting normal gastric activity in these patients.[31,32]

In the routine management of these patients, objective measurements of gastric emptying, such as labeled test meals, are not particularly helpful because they do not discriminate well between symptomatic and asymptomatic patients, and they do not predict the response to treatment.[21]

Constipation

Constipation is by far the most common GI symptom in patients with longstanding diabetes and is much more common in diabetics than controls.[1] Constipation is more likely in patients with complaints suggesting diabetic neuropathy.

The onset of constipation is insidious. Patients may seek help when more common remedies such as bulk and osmotic laxatives no longer work. Investigations needed depend on the patient's age and whether or not other problems are present, such as GI bleeding. Diabetics, too, can develop colon cancer. In most patients, digital examination with guaiac testing of the stool, sigmoidoscopy, and barium enema are all that is required. Some patients may respond to increased fiber supplementation. Others may also need suppositories or enemas. A different approach is the use of prokinetic agents, such as metoclopramide, for this purpose.[1] Metoclopramide appears to have little effect on normal colon but appears to be effective in the short-term treatment of diabetic constipation.[33] Defective extrinsic innervation of the large bowel may, in some way, render the colon more sensitive to this agent.

Diarrhea

The incidence of diarrhea in longstanding diabetics is usually reported to be 10% to 20%.[1] These patients may have a wide variety of complaints. Classic diabetic diarrhea usually is found in younger males with longstanding diabetes who have symptoms of autonomic neuropathy and a history of poor control of their diabetes. They describe intermittent diarrhea, which may be nocturnal and precipitate. Incontinence of stool during these episodes is not unusual.[1] Some patients do not have diarrhea by the usual definition of daily stool weight greater than 200 g/day. Their complaint is of fecal incontinence involving liquid stools. Other patients may complain of typical symptoms of steatorrhea, with bulky, foul-smelling stools, and a voracious appetite.

Steatorrhea in diabetics has several causes. The most obvious is combined endocrine and exocrine insufficiency of the pancreas, usually resulting from chronic pancreatitis. Emulsification of triglyceride depends on shearing forces generated by normal gastric contractions, which may be absent in diabetics. Bile salts may be depleted either by deconjugation caused by bacterial overgrowth[34] or by failure of absorption.[35] Bacterial overgrowth is presumed to occur because of failure of propagation of the normal interdigestive migrating motor complex. Small intestinal bile salt malabsorption may be a consequence of disruption of the normal integrated secretory and contractile responses in the biliary tract. Finally, celiac disease coexists more frequently with diabetes than would be expected by chance.[36]

Evaluation of disabling diarrhea in a diabetic should begin with ascertaining that fecal weight is over 200 g/day. If so, a standard

3-day stool collection for fat should be instituted because many of the causes of steatorrhea are potentially correctable. Bacterial overgrowth of the small intestine may be detected by the glycocholate breath test or by part II of the Schilling test. A practical alternative is a 2-week course of tetracycline therapy. Pancreatic insufficiency may respond to a trial of pancreatic enzyme supplementation. Small intestinal biopsy detects coexisting celiac disease. This should be considered, particularly in patients who have developed steatorrhea before or shortly after their diabetes.

Patients with no other demonstrable cause for diarrhea are said to have idiopathic diabetic diarrhea. The cause remains an enigma. There is general presumption that it is a consequence of autonomic or enteric neuropathy,[37] but clear evidence for this is lacking. A specific defect in the absorption of fluid and electrolytes by the intestine of streptozotocin-treated rats was associated with loss of noradrenergic innervation of enterocytes.[38] In some patients the α_2-agonist clonidine may improve the diarrhea.[38] Another potential mechanism for diarrhea in these patients is spillage of bile salts into the large intestine, which can have a marked cathartic effect.[35]

In the absence of specific therapy, soluble fiber supplements, such as psyllium, may be helpful. Fiber adds bulk to liquid stools and may decrease their liquidity by adsorbing bile salts. Fiber may also even out the cyclic swings between incapacitating diarrhea and intractable constipation, which is the lot of many of these patients. Unfortunately, satiety from coexistent gastroparesis may make soluble fiber supplements difficult to tolerate. When diarrhea is present and persistent, loperamide or diphenoxylate may provide some symptomatic relief. Clonidine may be useful, and anecdotal reports suggest that somatostatin analogue may help incapacitating diarrhea.[39]

In practice, all of these measures may work for a short time. Then the symptom recurs, and some new therapeutic maneuver must be used. The patient becomes querulous, and the physician becomes dispirited. Much time is needed for patient counseling, advice, and encouragement.

Fecal Incontinence

Diabetic diarrhea results in incontinence much more frequently than other forms of chronic diarrhea, such as inflammatory bowel disease. In one study, 28 out of 30 patients with diabetic diarrhea also had episodes of incontinence.[1] The majority had at least one episode during sleep. Patients describe how they are aware of the need to defecate but can do nothing to prevent it. Their stool is liquid, but diarrhea by the usual definition of daily stool weight greater than 200 g/day may not be present.[1]

Incontinence occurs in diabetic patients with autonomic neuropathy. Resting anal sphincter tone is low.[40] Other possible contributing factors, such as loss of rectal sensation[41] or compliance, have been suggested but not demonstrated rigorously.

Treatment is based on the premise that incontinence is only a problem in patients with liquid feces. Some patients may benefit from soluble fiber, which makes liquid stools more viscous. Others may benefit from antidiarrheal agents. These may be taken when patients are going to sleep or leaving their homes. In these patients, the goal of treatment is not elimination of the diarrhea but avoidance of the severe embarrassment of fecal soiling. Biofeedback

conditioning can do no harm but may be disappointing in patients with neuropathy and sphincter disturbance.[42]

Gallstones

Gallstones are probably more common in patients with diabetes mellitus, particularly of the adult onset variety.[43] It is not clear that diabetes per se causes gallstones because obesity may be a factor common to both. One reason why diabetics with autonomic neuropathy might be more prone to develop gallstones is poor gallbladder emptying.[44,45] Management of gallstones in diabetics remains controversial. There is general agreement that symptomatic gallstones require treatment. Cholecystectomy is the standard therapy, but bile salt dissolution with or without shock wave lithotripsy is an option for patients with cholesterol gallstones who are poor surgical risks. The proper management of diabetic patients with asymptomatic gallstones is unclear. Symptoms of acute cholecystitis might be masked by autonomic neuropathy, and emergency surgery for gallstones in diabetics carries a high mortality. Elective surgery carries increased risk with diabetics compared to nondiabetics but is much safer than emergency surgery. More recent analyses suggest that diabetes itself does not increase the risks of elective surgery; rather, the frequent coexistence of ischemic heart disease or nephropathy may complicate postsurgical management and enhance the risk. Careful assessment of possible operative risk factors is needed in each individual patient. Elective cholecystectomy in diabetics with silent gallstones has been advocated,[46,47] however, decision analysis studies incorporating a wide range of assumptions about mortality from elective and emergency surgery for gallstone-related diseases suggest that silent gallstones in diabetics should be treated the same way as in the nondiabetic population. Surgery should be reserved for patients who develop evidence of biliary colic, acute cholecystitis, or other manifestations of biliary disease.[48]

RHEUMATOID ARTHRITIS

General Considerations

Arthritis in rheumatoid disease may be only the most prominent symptom of a multisystem disorder. Other organs, including those of the GI tract, may be affected (Table 47-2). Intraabdominal catastrophies may occur because of vasculitis, or more insidious dysfunction may occur because of amyloidosis (ch 106). And even if the gastroenterologic tract is unscathed by these processes, it is very likely to be affected by the drugs used in treating the arthritis.

Gastroenterologic Involvement

In chronic rheumatoid arthritis, temporomandibular joint involvement is common, frequently leads to difficulties chewing food,

TABLE 47–2

Gastrointestinal Manifestations of Rheumatoid Arthritis

Abnormal mastication
Dysphagia
Gastritis
Ischemic colitis
Bowel infarction
Pancreatitis
Cholecystitis
Protein-losing enteropathy
Gold-induced colitis

and may easily be overlooked.[49] Mastication and bolus formation may also be impaired by limited saliva production in those patients who have Sjögren's syndrome. Poorly chewed food may be difficult to swallow, leading to complaints of dysphagia. Dysphagia in patients with rheumatoid arthritis may also be a result of impaired esophageal motility. Manometric evidence of impaired esophageal motility is said to occur in about 25% of patients with longstanding rheumatoid arthritis,[49] although complaints of dysphagia or heartburn are much less common. A careful history usually differentiates between those patients with rheumatoid arthritis who have impaired mastication and those with symptomatic motor disorder of the esophagus. Reduced lower esophageal sphincter pressure and reduced peristalsis are more common in patients with "overlap" syndromes, which include features of systemic sclerosis.

Patients with rheumatoid arthritis are frequently found to have gastritis when subjected to mucosal biopsy.[50] The significance of such findings is unclear because gastritis occurs with increasing frequency as age advances and because almost all patients with rheumatoid arthritis have received prolonged courses of nonsteroidal antiinflammatory drugs. Atrophic gastritis is probably not significantly more common in patients with rheumatoid arthritis than controls, and achlorhydria occurs with about the same frequency in both groups.[51] For unexplained reasons, minor increases in gastrin levels are common in patients with rheumatoid arthritis.[52]

Vasculitis is a well-known complication of rheumatoid arthritis but is rare, occurring in a small minority of patients with severe arthritis, fever, subcutaneous nodules, and cutaneous ulceration.[53] These patients have high titers of rheumatoid factor. About 10% of patients with rheumatoid vasculitis have GI involvement in the form of ischemic colitis,[54] bowel infarction, pancreatitis, acute cholecystitis, or protein-losing enteropathy.[53,54,55]

The effects of nonsteroidal antiinflammatory drugs on the gastroduodenal mucosa are discussed in Chapters 6, 30, 31, and 61. Patients with rheumatoid arthritis who take these medications for prolonged periods are at increased risk of developing either of the two life-threatening complications of ulcers: hemorrhage or perforation. Gold salts used in the treatment of rheumatoid arthritis have the peculiar side effect of causing a colitis of uncertain pathophysiology.[56] Treatment should include withdrawal of therapy and general supportive measures. Sulfasalazine, cromolyn, and bowel rest have been used. Early reports suggested high mortality from this condition. However, more recent experience indicates a much more benign course, probably reflecting earlier recognition and treatment of this side effect of gold therapy.

PREGNANCY

The anatomic displacement of the gravid uterus and effects of increased circulating levels of sex hormones induce various changes in GI function and may alter the expression of some diseases (Table 47-3). This section addresses the gastroenterologic problems in pregnancy that are not discussed in detail elsewhere. It does not discuss the hepatic abnormalities or diseases associated with pregnancies, diseases that can be more frequent and serious than those discussed here.

Nausea and Vomiting

Nausea and vomiting occur in up to 90% and 55% of pregnant patients, respectively.[57–59] These symptoms may be classified as "nausea and vomiting of pregnancy" or "hyperemesis gravidarum" according to whether they cause disturbances in fluid and electrolyte balance or nutrition.

NAUSEA AND VOMITING OF PREGNANCY

The onset usually is shortly after the first missed menstrual period, and the condition is more common in primigravidas, obese women, young women, nonsmokers, women with less than 10 years of education, and women who had nausea and vomiting in a previous pregnancy.[58] Nausea and vomiting while taking oral contraceptive medication also increases the risk. Sleep disturbances and fatigue often accompany nausea and vomiting.

The etiology is unknown. Organic diseases such as gastritis, cholecystitis, and peptic ulcer disease rarely are responsible. Elevated serum levels of human chorionic gonadotropin (HCG),[60] progesterone, and androgens[61] have been reported inconsistently. Patients are more likely to have unwanted pregnancies and negative relationships with their mothers[59]; the significance of these findings is unknown.

Symptoms usually disappear before the 4th month of gestation. There is no evidence of increased fetal mortality. Treatment is supportive and consists largely of reassurance regarding the temporary nature of the symptoms and the favorable maternal and fetal outcome that can be anticipated.

TABLE 47–3

Gastrointestinal Manifestations of Pregnancy

Nausea and vomiting
Pancreatitis
Appendicitis
Gastroesophageal reflux
Cholelithiasis
Constipation
Ruptured splenic aneurysm
Ruptured spleen
Mallory-Weiss lesions
Acute granulomatous peritonitis

HYPEREMESIS GRAVIDARUM

Sometimes called pernicious vomiting, this condition is characterized by intractable vomiting, weight loss, dehydration, and electrolyte disorders. The condition likely represents a severe form of the spectrum of nausea and vomiting in pregnancy rather than a separate disorder. Like milder cases, the onset of symptoms follows the first menstrual period and usually resolves before the 4th month of gestation. In one study, however, 60% of cases persisted for more than half the duration of the pregnancy.[62] The incidence is increased with twin pregnancies, hydatidiform mole, younger age, and high body weight[63,64] but is not associated with differences in color, race, or desire for abortion.[63] Nulliparity may increase the risk,[64] but this is disputed.[63]

Various hormonal abnormalities have been described in afflicted patients. Abnormal thyroid function tests[65–68] and elevated HCG levels have been reported.[69] Elevated mean levels of total estradiol, unbound estradiol, and sex hormone binding-globulin binding capacity were reported to be elevated in afflicted women compared to pregnant patients matched for age and parity,[64] consistent with a hypothesis that elevated estrogen levels are responsible for excessive vomiting.[64] Most studies regarding pathogenesis, however, have focused on psychologic factors. Patients usually have vomited during previous emotional disturbances and have a high incidence of emotional immaturity, sexual maladjustment, and strong maternal attachment.[70] In a postpartum study, 15% of afflicted patients had evidence of hysteria compared to 2% in control subjects.[62] These observations, successful treatment by hypnosis in some instances, and a lower incidence during wartime support a psychosomatic basis or contribution to hyperemesis gravidarum.[70–73]

Treatment usually entails hospitalization for correction of fluid and electrolyte disturbances. Liquid meals may be given through a pediatric nasogastric tube; total parenteral hyperalimentation may be useful in some cases.[74,75] Some patients benefit from behavioral modification.[76]

Increased fetal mortality was not found in recent large series,[64] although low birth weights and congenital malformations are slightly more common. Women who have lost more than 5% of their prepregnancy weight are particularly prone to deliver infants with low birth weight and possibly more malformations.[77]

Pancreatitis

Most episodes of this rare condition in pregnancy occur in the third trimester and are associated with cholelithiasis.[78] Some cases may be caused by the effects of increased estrogen level on an underlying lipoprotein disorder.[79] As in nonpregnant patients, it may be a postoperative complication.[79] Acute pancreatitis in pregnancy generally carries a high risk of maternal and fetal mortality,[80] although management of "gallstone pancreatitis" by cholecystectomy and common duct exploration in the second trimester has been reported not to increase fetal or maternal mortality.[81] Most cases subside with medical management, allowing surgery to be delayed until the second trimester.

Appendicitis

Approximately 1 in 2000 pregnant women develop appendicitis[82–84]; it is the most common GI condition requiring surgery during pregnancy. It occurs in all trimesters but probably is most frequent in the second trimester and least frequent in the third.

The diagnosis is made with approximately equal difficulty as in nonpregnant patients. The symptoms usually are the same, but the location of abdominal tenderness is different. Because the enlarging uterus displaces the cecum cephalad, tenderness in the 5th month of pregnancy is more likely to be above the umbilicus. In the third trimester, tenderness may be just beneath the right costal margin. The effects of the large uterus also may contribute to maternal and fetal mortality because of the relationship of the enlarged uterus to the inflamed appendix. If the condition progresses to local perforation, peritonitis may not be immediately evident because the uterus forms a medial wall that contains the abscess. The abscess stimulates uterine contractions and premature delivery; as the uterus diminishes in size, the previously walled-off abscess rapidly causes generalized peritonitis.

Early surgery is indicated because maternal and fetal mortality increases with the development of peritonitis. Laparotomy with a normal appendix does not increase mortality, although delivery may ensue.[84] The normal appendix should not be removed because this increases fetal loss.

Gastroesophageal Reflux

Pregnant patients commonly experience heartburn and have reversible gastroesophageal reflux disease. This is attributed largely to high plasma levels of progesterone, which decrease lower esophageal sphincter tone, increase the percentage of nonperistaltic contractions, and increase gastric pressure.[85–87]

Treatment is based on the same nonpharmacologic foundation as in nonpregnant patients (see ch 55). Reduction of meal volume, especially fluids; cessation of smoking; avoidance of coffee, alcohol, citrus, mint, fatty foods, and chocolate; raising the head of the bed; and avoiding meals within 2 hours of lying down should be attempted before employing drug therapy. Agents that increase salivary secretion, such as lozenges and gum, should be encouraged. Drugs that are poorly absorbed, such as antacids and alginic acid preparations, can be added if necessary. Antacids containing low salt concentrations are preferred, and magnesium-containing antacids may serve an additional useful purpose in constipated patients. Sucralfate may be effective in some cases and is safe in pregnancy. Because the safety of H_2-receptor antagonists, omeprazole, and prokinetic agents in pregnancy is uncertain, management should be attempted without them, if possible, particularly in the first trimester. If symptoms remain uncontrolled, the H_2-receptor antagonists cimetidine or ranitidine, or the prokinetic agent metoclopramide, should be employed first because there is considerably more experience with their use in pregnancy than with the newer H_2-receptor antagonists, prokinetic agents, or omeprazole.

Gallstones

Gallstones are common in pregnancy because gallbladder emptying is impaired by high circulating levels of progesterone, and bile salt secretion is decreased by high plasma estrogen levels.[88] It is not known, however, if the complications of gallstones increase during a given pregnancy. Like others, pregnant patients with gallstones may be asymptomatic, have mild symptoms, or develop severe life-threatening cholecystitis (ch 94).

The presence of asymptomatic gallstones may be detected fortuitously during ultrasound examination of the uterus. The clinical expression and diagnosis of symptomatic cholecystitis are identical to those in nonpregnant patients except that deep palpation of the right upper quadrant may be difficult or even impossible, and oral cholecystography and isotope scans are to be avoided. Ultrasound of the gallbladder may be more difficult in late gestation due to gallbladder displacement, but this remains the preferred method for detecting gallstones and estimating gallbladder volume and wall thickness.

Most patients with cholecystitis experience resolution of symptoms with medical management with analgesics, intravenous fluids, and antibiotics. If the disease progresses, cholecystectomy can be done without increased risk to the mother or fetus.

Constipation

Gastrointestinal transit time to the cecum is prolonged in the second and third trimesters of pregnancy, an effect possibly due to the combination of bowel displacement and progesterone-induced smooth muscle inhibition.[79] The incidence of constipation in pregnancy varies, being low in Israel[89] and as high as 38% in the United Kingdom.[90]. Dietary fiber intake is not different between matched groups of constipated and nonconstipated women in the third trimester,[91] although the ingestion of 10 g of supplemental fiber daily improves constipation.[92] Constipation and the hemorrhoids that often accompany it respond to the daily ingestion of supplemental fiber and to exercise, nonabsorbable stool softeners, and glycerin suppositories.

Other Conditions

Ruptured splenic artery aneurysm is uncommon but carries a high maternal and fetal mortality rate.[93,94] Sudden unexplained signs of intravascular volume depletion with or without abdominal pain should raise suspicion of this diagnosis. Angiography confirms the diagnosis; surgery is indicated. Surgery also has been advocated for asymptomatic aneurysms because the natural course seems to be progression to rupture.[94] Nearly 100 cases of *splenic rupture* have been reported in pregnancy. Sudden left upper quadrant pain associated with signs of intravascular volume depletion suggests this diagnosis. Most ruptures occur in the third trimester, making assessment of abdominal distention an unreliable indicator of intraabdominal fluid accumulation. Emergency surgery is indicated.[95–97] *Mallory-Weiss lesions* occur[98]; conservative management usually suffices. *Acute granulomatous peritonitis* has been described

in women with abdominal pain in pregnancy and after cesarean section.[99,100] The mechanism appears to be due to premature rupture of fetal membranes or meconium spillage during cesarean section.

RENAL DISEASE

Uremia has numerous GI manifestations (Table 47-4). Hiccups, nausea, vomiting, anorexia, heartburn, epigastric pain, xerostomia, metallic taste, and GI bleeding occur commonly. With the exception of hemorrhage, the common GI symptoms usually are not associated with lesions detectable by endoscopy.[101] Nearly all symptoms are relieved by dialysis.

Gastrointestinal Hemorrhage

The most frequent life-threatening GI problem in both acute and chronic renal failure is hemorrhage (ch 30, 31, 61, and 108). Most patients experience bleeding, often due to gastric and duodenal ulcers[102]; multiple ulcers may be present. Stress-related mucosal damage ("stress ulcers") also may cause bleeding, particularly in patients with multiorgan failure. In patients with chronic renal failure, gastric angiodysplasia is responsible for bleeding more often than ulcers.[103]

The cause of gastroduodenal ulceration in renal failure is poorly understood. Serum gastrin levels are elevated in about half of patients with acute renal failure[104] and in most patients with chronic failure, presumably due to impaired renal inactivation of gastrin. Despite gastrin elevations, basal and stimulated gastric acid secretion may be low, normal, or high.[104–106] Furthermore, gastric acid secretion does not correlate with the lesions or symptoms.[104] The gastrin levels usually return to normal after successful transplantation.[106–108] However, gastrin levels may remain elevated in about one fourth of patients despite decreased acid secretion, suggesting the presence of an abnormality in the control of acid secretion.

The risk of upper GI hemorrhage is not eliminated by renal transplantation; bleeding from peptic ulcers and erosions is common.[109–111] The cause is obscure. Steroid usage has been implicated but correlates poorly with hemorrhage.[111,112] Cytomegalovirus in-

TABLE 47–4
Gastrointestinal Manifestations of Renal Disease

Angiodysplasia
Peptic ulcer
Pancreatitis
Duodenal polyposis
Bowel obstruction
Bowel perforation
Diarrhea
Uremic enterocolitis
Cecal and rectal ulcers
Stercoral ulcers
"Wasting syndrome"

festation of the gastric and duodenal mucosa is common[113,114] and may contribute to the development of multiple erosions, which can bleed.[113]

Vagotomy and drainage procedures before transplantation are no longer advocated. Similarly, screening of patients by gastric analysis or endoscopy is not helpful because there is no correlation between pretransplantation gastric analysis or ulcer disease and posttransplantation hemorrhage. The prophylactic use of H₂-receptor antagonists in the first month after transplantation has been found to be effective.[115]

Upper GI hemorrhage in patients with renal failure or in the posttransplantation period is difficult to manage. Treatment with H₂-receptor antagonists and antacids is standard but is not known to stop bleeding. Attempts to arrest hemorrhage and stop bleeding by endoscopic methods may be attempted, although there are no controlled trials in this patient population. Bleeding from angiodysplasia may be prevented by the use of oral chronic estrogen-progesterone preparations.[116]

Pancreatic Disease

Pancreatitis may occur more frequently in patients with renal failure.[117] The etiology is unknown. The diagnosis may be missed during life,[117] possibly because of difficulties in diagnosing the condition (see ch 88 and 89). Both salivary and pancreatic amylases may be elevated without pancreatitis, and the ratio of amylase clearance to creatinine clearance is misleading because it is elevated in chronic renal failure with or without pancreatitis.[118] Exocrine pancreatic insufficiency responsive to enzyme replacement has been documented.[119]

Other Conditions

A variety of disorders of the small and large intestine have been reported in patients with chronic renal failure. *Duodenal polyposis* due to *Brunner's gland hypertrophy*,[120] *ileus,* and *intestinal obstruction* with or without perforation have been reported.[121-124] *Diarrhea* may occur in some patients due to bacterial overgrowth,[125] abnormal bile acid metabolism with changes in intraluminal bile acid concentrations and the presence of unusual bile acids,[126] and so-called *uremic enterocolitis,* which is attributed to poor mucosal perfusion.[127] Colonic abnormalities in chronic renal failure may be expressed as hemorrhage, perforation, and obstruction. Profuse bleeding has been reported from *cecal* and *rectal ulcers.*[128,129] The incidence of perforation is increased due to *ruptured diverticula, cecal ulcers,* and *stercoromas.*[129] Obstruction due to *colonic intussusception* has been described.[130]

A *"wasting syndrome"* has been attributed to a combination of factors including increased catabolism due to infection, uremia itself, and frequent dialysis.[119] Malabsorption of calcium, magnesium, and phosphate has been reported[131-133]; the phosphate malabsorption may be due to low 1,25-dehydroxyvitamin D levels and the use of aluminum antacids.[133]

Renal Transplantation

The GI complications are not eliminated by renal transplantation. Nearly 20% of patients experience complications within a few months,[134] but complications are rare after 10 years. *Gastrointestinal hemorrhage* from erosions and ulcers is the most frequent serious complication, as described above in the context of renal failure. Suppression of immunity causes *esophageal candidiasis,* which may be fatal in diabetics,[135] *Kaposi's sarcoma,*[136] hyperinfestation with *Strongyloides stercoralis,*[137] and *abscesses.*[138] *Perforations* from diverticulitis continue after transplantation.[138] Lethal *necrotizing pancreatitis* occurred in patients taking azathioprine and prednisone in a large series of transplanted patients.[139]

NERVOUS SYSTEM DISEASE

Several common nervous system disorders have important GI manifestations (Table 47-5). The manifestations may change with the evolution of the diseases, particularly in patients with stroke and spinal cord injuries. In general, the GI disturbances result from abnormalities in motor function of the gut.

Cerebral Vascular Accidents (CVA)

Difficult swallowing is the most common GI consequence of an acute CVA, occurring in nearly half of patients.[140] Most cases are associated with a lesion in one cerebral hemisphere; those who survive usually regain their ability to swallow within 2 weeks.[140,141] Dysphagia is associated with an increased incidence of aspiration,[142,143] chest infections,[140] and mortality.[140,141]

A video fluorographic study disclosed that dysphagia is due to a combination of physiologic disturbances in swallowing rather than isolated disorders.[142] A delayed swallowing reflex was the most common abnormality, followed in order by reduced pharyngeal peristalsis and reduced tongue control. Cricopharyngeal dysfunction occurred in only 2 of 38 patients. Few differences in the nature of swallowing disorders were seen according to location of the CNS lesion. Most aspiration occurred because of delayed triggering of the swallowing reflex.

Bedside diagnosis of dysphagia usually is simple. Patients often have associated speech impairment (comprehension and expression) and facial weakness. They have difficulty in swallowing even a mouthful of water. Dysphonia is the most common clinical characteristic of aspirating patients.[143] Localizing the physiologic defect responsible for dysphagia and detecting aspiration, however, are more accurately accomplished by videofluorography than by experienced clinicians.[144]

Management of dysphagia and avoidance of aspiration after a CVA entails intravenous feeding acutely, followed by compensatory oral feeding programs.[145] While often useful, percutaneous placement of a gastrostomy tube for enteral feeding of a patient with chronic neurologic impairment has been reported to result in aspiration at high nutrient infusion rates.[145]

TABLE 47–5
Gastrointestinal Manifestations of Nervous System Disease

Cerebral Vascular Accidents	**Multiple Sclerosis**
Dysphagia	Oropharyngeal dysphagia
Esophagopulmonary aspiration	Gastric stasis
	Constipation
	Fecal incontinence
Spinal Cord Injury	
	Parkinson's Disease
Gastric stress	
Peptic ulcer	Dysphagia
Gastritis	Gastric stasis
Gastroesophageal reflux	Constipation
Cholelithiasis	
Premature Diverticulosis	**Peripheral Nervous System Disorders**
Solitary colonic ulcer	
Constipation	Dysphagia
Fecal impaction	Gastric stasis
Autonomic dysreflexia	Megacolon
	Diarrhea
	Steatorrhea

Spinal Cord Injury

Approximately 12,000 people in the United States are rendered paraplegic or quadriplegic by spinal cord injury each year. An array of GI problems attend those who survive; some of the problems differ according to the time elapsed after the cord injury.

Patients with acute spinal cord injury often have gastric stasis and ileus[146] and an increased incidence of upper GI bleeding and perforation. Of 439 patients, 6.1% hemorrhaged, 7 more than once.[147] Most episodes occurred within 4 weeks of injury; the mean was 22.5 days. The incidence was higher in patients with cervical injury. The most commonly diagnosed lesions were duodenal ulcers, followed by gastric ulcers and gastritis. A recent study found a 4.7% incidence of peptic ulceration with hemorrhage or perforation.[148] These patients generally were treated prophylactically with antacids with or without H_2-receptor antagonists. The complication rate of acid peptic lesions was 7.5% in spinal cord injury patients given nutrition in a haphazard manner in the first few days after injury and 2% in patients treated according to an organized nutrition protocol that resulted in providing total energy requirements within 48 hours.[148] There is controversy as to whether the use of steroids increases the risk of acid peptic lesions in spinal injury patients. Although no correlation has been found in some studies,[147] a study of patients with spinal cord *compression* showed an increased incidence of upper GI bleeding and perforation that appeared to be influenced by steroid administration.[149] Bleeding developed in 1.9% and perforation in 2.8% of patients with cord compression treated with 16 mg/day of dexamethasone. Of 226 patients being tapered from 100 mg/day of dexamethasone, GI hemorrhage occurred in 3.5% and perforation occurred in 2.7%. Ninety-one percent of perforations occurred within 30 days of starting steroids and were associated with more free peritoneal involvement but fewer signs and symptoms of peritonitis than in patients not treated with steroids.

The management of GI complications after acute cord injury entails the use of nasogastric suction for gastric stasis and ileus.

The prokinetic agents metoclopramide[150] and cisapride[151] have been effective in some patients because the enteric nervous system is intact. Medical management of upper GI bleeding is discussed in Chapter 30. In patients with spinal cord injury, ulcer surgery should not include vagotomy because of the risk of severe gastric retention.[152]

Patients surviving acute trauma but left with residual cord damage have an increased frequency of gastroesophageal reflux[146] and a threefold increase incidence of cholelithiasis.[153] The cause of the later is unknown; speculation has included impaired gallbladder motility with resultant stasis, altered GI transit leading to abnormal enterohepatic circulation, and metabolic alterations leading to abnormal lipid secretion.[153] Diverticulosis occurs prematurely with chronic spinal injury,[146] and bleeding from a solitary colonic ulcer has been reported.[154] Impaired gastric emptying can result in decreased bioavailability of some drugs, including theophylline.[155]

Severe constipation often follows spinal cord injury. The pathophysiology depends on the level of injury. Transection of the cord above the first lumbar vertebra abolishes the colonic response to a meal[156] and causes reduced colonic motility, compliance, and tolerance to luminal distention.[157] On the other hand, lower transection and injury to the cauda equina result in marked enhancement of compliance and gross colonic distention during fluid filling without a corresponding increase in intracolonic pressure. Both situations foster constipation and fecal impaction.

Management of constipation is discussed in detail in Chapter 39. Self-digital distention of the rectum on a regular basis is used to initiate defecation. Many patients use stool softeners, and some require stimulatory laxatives. Cisapride has relieved intractable constipation in some cases.[158]

Spinal section above the fifth thoracic route may result in autonomic dysreflexia. This abnormal autonomic reflex, triggered by fecal impaction or bladder distention, causes hypertension and tachycardia[159,160] and may cause subarachnoid hemorrhage, CVA, and seizures. Autonomic dysreflexia is prevented by avoidance of constipation and bladder catheterization on a regular basis.[159,160]

Multiple Sclerosis

Multiple sclerosis (MS) is one of the most common diseases capable of causing severe disabilities in young adults. Only trauma and rheumatic disease exceed MS in this respect. The number of MS patients in the United States is estimated at 250,000 to 500,000.[161] The GI manifestations include oropharyngeal dysphagia, gastroparesis, and abnormal bowel habit.[162-165] In a survey of 280 patients with MS, 68% had constipation, fecal incontinence, or both.[165] The nature of the bowel dysfunction has been difficult to characterize because constipation and fecal incontinence commonly coexist. Moreover, the disease fluctuates, resulting in acute chronic or intermittent bowel symptoms. The common occurrence of more than one neurologic lesion in a given patient adds to the complexity. Various bowel abnormalities have been described in afflicted patients. Seven patients evaluated with colometrograms, somatosensory evoked potentials, and myoelectric activity studies exhibited "hyperreflexic" rectums, low baseline colonic motor activity, and postprandial increase in colonic motility.[157] Transit time through the colon is delayed in different segments of the colon, although transit often is increased in patients with simultaneous urinary bladder dysfunction.[164] Some patients have hypertonicity of the anal canal, variable canal pressures, or decreased amplitude of the rectoanal inhibitory reflex. These manometric abnormalities constitute rectal outlet obstruction. This, coupled with impairment of activity of pelvic floor musculature, leaves some MS patients with impaired colonic propulsion and defecation.[165]

In MS patients, treatment is complicated by the fact that a fine line often exists between constipation and incontinence.[164] Some patients prefer constipation to soiling episodes. Management of fecal incontinence entails establishing a daily time for defecation and a routine schedule of enemas or suppositories to keep the rectum empty. Loperamide or diphenoxylate may reduce stool frequency and improve stool consistency.

Parkinson's Disease

This common movement disorder may cause swallowing abnormalities,[166] disturbed esophageal motility,[167] erratic gastric emptying,[168] and constipation. The distressing belching during "off" periods may be related to the disturbed esophageal motility, an effect abolished by the dopamine receptor antagonist apomorphine.[167] The erratic gastric emptying may contribute to the "random" fluctuations in parkinsonian mobility because stabilization of mobility occurs if levodopa is delivered intraduodenally rather than orally.[169]

Peripheral Nervous System Disorders

Among the common conditions affecting the peripheral nervous system are alcoholic neuropathy, which can impair esophageal peristalsis,[170] and diabetic neuropathy, which causes a host of problems including impaired esophageal peristalsis, gastroparesis,

gallbladder dysfunction, megacolon, diarrhea, and steatorrhea, as discussed in detail earlier in this chapter.

MUSCLE DISEASE

Muscle diseases are uncommon but one, myotonic dystrophy, is remarkable for its array of GI symptoms (Table 47-6). These include dysphagia, vomiting, heartburn, diarrhea, constipation, pseudo-obstruction, and steatorrhea.[171-174] Unlike most primary muscle diseases, myotonic dystrophy involves both striated and smooth muscles. This accounts for variable swallowing and esophageal function.[173,175] Striated muscle involvement accounts for impaired swallowing, secondary to myotonia of the tongue and oral musculature, as well as for oropharyngeal dysphagia and decreased amplitude of pharyngeal and upper esophageal sphincter contractions. The peristaltic sequence is normal. Smooth muscle involvement of the esophagus causes slow emptying of the body of the esophagus. Lower esophageal sphincter function is normal. Disorders distal to the esophagus, including impaired gastric emptying,[176] bezoar formation,[177] abnormal small bowel motility,[178] and collagenous sprue, have been reported.[172] Pseudo-obstruction[174] and various colonic abnormalities have been documented, including megacolon, volvulus, and segmental sigmoid narrowing.[176,179]

PULMONARY DISEASE

Chronic Pulmonary Disease

Chronic obstructive pulmonary disease is closely associated with duodenal ulcers. In patients with ulcers, the frequency of chronic lung disease is increased two- to threefold, and up to 30% of patients with chronic pulmonary disease have ulcers.[180-182] The expected death rate in peptic ulcer patients is increased fivefold in the presence of chronic lung disease.[181]

The mechanisms for the association of ulcers and chronic pulmonary disease are obscure. The association persists after adjusting for cigarette smoking.[182] Moreover, peptic ulcers do not appear to be a consequence of identified physiologic sequelae, because ulcers do not correlate with degree of CO_2 retention, clinical severity of pulmonary disease, or its treatment.[183] A genetic basis for this association has been suggested.[183]

Cystic fibrosis and α_1-antitrypsin deficiency are specific entities in which chronic pulmonary disease and peptic ulcers are asso-

TABLE 47–6
Gastrointestinal Manifestations of Myotonic Dystrophy

Dysphagia	Gastric stasis	Megacolon
Vomiting	Collagenous sprue	Volvulus
Heartburn	Pseudo-obstruction	

ciated. The relative risk for ulcers in cystic fibrosis is not yet established; risk appears to be increased by 50% to 300% in patients with α_1-antitrypsin deficiency.[183] The mechanisms are speculative. Patients with cystic fibrosis have decreased pancreatic bicarbonate secretion, which could impair buffering of acid in the duodenum. Studies of bicarbonate secretion in gastroduodenal epithelium have not been reported. In the case of α_1-antitrypsin deficiency, one can speculate that the unopposed proteolytic activity that presumably destroys lung tissue also in some way undermines gastroduodenal defense.

Asthma

The relationship between gastroesophageal reflux and pulmonary symptoms, including wheezing, is established (ch 55). Nocturnal asthma may be precipitated by reflux.[184–186] In these instances, the pulmonary problems are largely, if not entirely, a consequence of reflux. On the other hand, asthma may *cause* reflux, as suggested by the improvement of symptoms of reflux that result from medical management of asthma.[187] The pathophysiology is unknown.

HEART DISEASE

Cardiac Failure

Right-sided cardiac failure, whether caused by pulmonary hypertension, cardiac lesions, or constrictive pericarditis, is associated with protein-losing enteropathy.[188] Most of these patients have ascites because of the effects of high systemic venous pressures on the liver.

"Forward" failure of the left heart, or circulatory insufficiency secondary to shock, results in reduced splanchnic perfusion (ch 109). Stress ulceration results from a combination of mucosal hypoxemia and the presence of acid and pepsin. Low blood flow to abdominal viscera may result in ischemic colitis.[189,190] Ischemic colitis in patients may be precipitated by the use of vasoconstrictors, such as vasopressin[189] or digitalis.[190]

Aortic Stenosis and Angiodysplasia

Angiodysplasia, also known as vascular ectasias, is well-described as the cause of acute GI bleeding (ch 108). An association with aortic stenosis has been postulated but remains unproven.[191]

Cardiac Transplantation

The GI complications of heart transplantation have been elucidated in recent large series.[192,193] Of 86 patients treated with cyclosporine

A and prednisone for immunosuppression, 30 had complications resulting in general surgical consultation.[193] The pancreas and biliary system were most commonly affected. Pancreatitis occurred in 16 patients; 5 required surgery, resulting in a 40% mortality. Nine patients developed cholecystitis; cholecystectomy was performed in 5 with no mortality. Other GI complications included gastric outlet obstruction, ileus, perforation, and bleeding. In a series of 122 heart, 19 heart–lung and two heart–liver transplantations, "general surgery" complication developed in 40 patients (28%).[192] In addition to the complications mentioned previously, these authors reported instances of cecal ulceration with sepsis, perianal abscess, lymphocele of the groin, inguinal or ventral herniae, and false aneurysm of the femoral artery. Cytomegalovirus GI infection has been described,[194] including a case of fatal hemorrhage from cylomegalovirus-infected duodenitis and duodenal ulcer.[195] Pancreatitis appears to occur frequently after any transplantation surgery but is rarely symptomatic.[196]

The reader is directed to Chapter 6, Epithelia: Biologic Principles of Organization; Chapter 8, The Physiology of Gastric Motility and Gastric Emptying; Chapter 28, Approach to the Patient with Dysphagia; Chapter 30, Approach to the Patient with Gross Gastrointestinal Bleeding; Chapter 31, Approach to the Patient with Occult Gastrointestinal Bleeding; Chapter 38, Approach to the Patient with Diarrhea; Chapter 39, Approach to the Patient with Constipation; Chapter 55, Reflux Esophagitis; Chapter 60, Disorders of Gastric Emptying; Chapter 61, Acid-Peptic Disorders; Chapter 94, Gallstones; Chapter 108, Vascular Ectasias, Tumors, and Malformations; Chapter 109, Vascular Insufficiency; Chapter 114, Contrast Radiology; Chapter 121, Gastrointestinal Radionuclide Imaging Procedures; and Chapter 128, Evaluation of Gastrointestinal Motility: Methodological Considerations.

REFERENCES

1. Feldman M, Schiller LR. Disorders of gastrointestinal motility associated with diabetes mellitus. Ann Intern Med 1983;98:378.
2. Gupta KK, Hedge KP, Lai R. Diabetic gastric neuropathy with acute hypoglycaemic attacks. J Indian Med Assoc 1971;57:258.
3. MacGregor IL, Gueller R, Watts HD, et al. The effect of acute hyperglycemia on gastric emptying in man. Gastroenterology 1976;70:190.
4. Feldman M, Corbett DE, Ramsey EJ, et al. Abnormal gastric function in longstanding insulin dependent diabetic patients. Gastroenterology 1979;77:12.
5. Battle WM, Snape WJ, Alavi A, et al. Colonic dysfunction in diabetes mellitus. Gastroenterology 1980;79:1217.
6. Smith B. Neuropathology of the oesophagus in diabetes mellitus. J Neurol Neurosurg Psychiatry 1974;37:1151.
7. Yoshida MM, Schuffler MD, Sumi SM. There are no morphological abnormalities of the gastric wall or abdominal vagus in patients with diabetic gastroparesis. Gastroenterology 1988;94:907.
8. Schmidt H, Reiman JF, Schmid A, et al. Ultrastructure of diabetic autonomic neuropathy of the gastrointestinal tract. Klin Wochenschr 1984;62:399.
9. Monckton G, Pekovitch E. Autonomic neuropathy in streptozotocin-induced diabetes in rats. Can J Neurol Sci 1980;7:135.

10. Lincoln J, Bokor JT, Crowe R, et al. Myenteric plexus in strepto-zotocin treated rats. Neurochemical and biochemical evidence for diabetic neuropathy in the gut. Gastroenterology 1984;86:654.

11. Belai A, Lincoln J, Milner P, et al. Enteric nerves in diabetic rats; Increase in vasoactive intestinal polypeptide but not substance P. Gastroenterology 1985;89:967.

12. Reynold C, Molnar GD, Horwitz DL, et al. Abnormalities of en-dogenous glucagon and insulin in unstable diabetes. Diabetes 1977;26:36.

13. Achem-Karem S, Funakoshi A, Vinik A, et al. Plasma motilin con-centration and interdigestive migrating motor complex in diabetic gastroparesis; Effective of metroclopramide. Gastroenterology 1985;88:492.

14. Mandelstam P, Lieber A. Esophageal dysfunction in diabetic neu-ropathy gastroenteropathy. JAMA 1967;201:88.

15. Hollis JB, Castell DO, Braddom RL. Esophageal function in diabetes mellitus and its relationship to peripheral neuropathy. Gastroenter-ology 1977;73:1098.

16. Vix VA. Esophageal motility in diabetes mellitus. Radiology 1969;92:363.

17. Loo FD, Dodds WJ, Soergel KH, et al. Multipeaked esophageal peristaltic waves in patients with diabetic neuropathy. Gastroenter-ology 1985;88:485.

18. Russell COH, Gannon FR, Coatsworth J. Relationship among esophageal dysfunction, diabetic gastroenteropathy and peripheral neuropathy. Dig Dis Sci 1983;28:289.

19. Clouse RE, Lustman PJ, Reidel WL. Correlation of esophageal mo-tility abnormalities with neuropsychiatric status in diabetics. Gas-troenterology 1986;90:1146.

20. Kassander P. Asymptomatic gastric retention in diabetics (gastro-paresis diabeticorum). Ann Intern Med 1958;48:797.

21. Loo FD, Palmer DW, Soergel KH, et al. Gastric emptying in patients with diabetes mellitus. Gastroenterology 1984;86:485.

22. Wright RA, Clemente R, Wathen R. Diabetic gastroparesis: An ab-normality of gastric emptying of solids. Am J Med Sci 1985;289:240.

23. Feldman M, Smith HJ, Simon TR. Gastric emptying of solid ra-dioopaque markers: Studies in healthy subjects and diabetic patients. Gastroenterology 1984;87:895.

24. Malagelada JR, Reese WD, Mazzola LJ, et al. Gastric motor ab-normalities in diabetic and postvagotomy gastroparesis: Effect of metoclopamide and bethanechol. Gastroenterology 1980;78:286.

25. Mearin F, Camilleri M, Malagelada JR. Pyloric dysfunction in di-abetics with recurrent nausea and vomiting. Gastroenterology 1986;90:1919.

26. Camilleri M, Malagelada JR. Abnormal intestinal motility in diabetics with the gastroparesis syndrome. Eur J Clin Invest 1984;14:420.

27. Silver BJ, Rhodes JB, Schimke RN, et al. Gastric bezoars: a com-plication of diabetic gastroparesis. J Kansas Med Soc 1983;84:249.8.

28. Schade RR, Dugos MC, Lhotsky DM, et al. Effect of metoclopamide on gastric liquid emptying in patients with diabetic gastroparesis. Dig Dis Sci 1985;30:10.

29. Horowitz M, Harding PE, Chalterton BE, et al. Acute and chronic effects of domperidone on gastric emptying in diabetic autonomic neuropathy. Dig Dis Sci 1985;30:1.

30. Feldman M, Smith HJ. Effective cisapride on gastric emptying of undigestable solids in patients with gastroparesis diabeticorum. Gastroenterology 1987;92:171.

31. Vantrappen G, Janssens J, Tack J, et al. Erythromycin is a potent gastrokinetic in diabetic gastroparesis. Gastroenterology 1989;96:A525.

32. Janssens J, Vantrappen G, Urbain JL, et al. The motilin antagonist erythromycin normalizes impaired gastric emptying in diabetic gas-troparesis. Gastroenterology 1986;96:A237.

33. Snape WJ, Battle WM, Schwartz SS, et al. Metoclopramide to treat gastroparesis due to diabetes mellitus: A double blind controlled trial. Ann Intern Med 1982;96:444.

34. Scarpello JHB, Hague RV, Cullen DR, et al. The ^{14}C-glycocholate tests in diabetic diarrhoea. Br Med J 1976;2:673.

35. Molloy AM, Tomkin GH. Altered bile in diabetic diarrhoea. Br Med J 1978;2:1462.

36. Kotetzko S, Burgin-Wolff A, Koletzko B, et al. Prevalence of coeliac disease in diabetic children and adolescents. Eur J Pediatr 1988;148:113.

37. Taub S, Mariani A, Barkin JS. Gastrointestinal manifestations of diabetes mellitus. Diabetes Care 1979;2:437.

38. Fedorak RN, Field M, Chang EB. Treatment of diabetic diarrhea with clonidine. Ann Intern Med 1985;102:197.

39. Tsai ST, Vinik AI. Diabetic diarrhea and somatostatin. Ann Intern Med 1986;104:894.

40. Schiller LR, Santa Ana CA, Schmulen AC, et al. Pathogenesis of fecal incontinence in diabetes mellitus evidence for internal anal sphincter dysfunction. N Engl J Med 1982;307:1666.

41. Katz LA, Kaufman HJ, Spiro HM. Anal sphincter characteristics. Gastroenterology 1967;52:513.

42. Cerulli MA, Nikoomanes HP, Schuster MM. Progress in biofeedback conditioning for fecal documentation. Gastroenterology 1979;76:742.

43. Ponz de Leon MP, Ferenderes R, Coruli N. Bile lipid composition and bile acid pool size in diabetics. Am J Dig Dis 1978;23:710.

44. Gitelson S, Oppenheim D, Swartz A. Size of the gallbladder in pa-tients with diabetes mellitus. Diabetes 1969;18:493.

45. Hickman MS, Schwesinger WH, Page CP. Acute cholecystitis in the diabetic: A case control study of outcome. Arch Surg 1988;123:409.

46. Turrill FL, McCarron M, Mikkelsen WP. Gallstones and diabetes: An ominous association. Am J Surg 1961;102:184.

47. Mundth ED. Cholecystitis and diabetes mellitus. N Engl J Med 1962;267:642.

48. Friedman LS, Roberts MS, Brett AS, et al. Management of asymp-tomatic gallstones in the diabetic patient. A decision analysis. Ann Intern Med 1988;109:913.

49. Sun DCH, Roth SH, Mitchell CS, et al. Upper gastrointestinal disease in rheumatoid arthritis. Dig Dis 1974;19:405.

50. Dawes PT, Haslock I, Cooke WM. The importance of endoscopy in rheumatology. Results of a comparative study between a group of arthritic patients and controls. Br J Clin Pract 1987;41:738.

51. Grossman MI, Kirsner JB, Gillespie IE. Basal and histalog stimulate gastric secretion in control subjects and in patients with peptic ulcer or gastric ulcer. Gastroenterology 1963;45:14.

52. Yorke AJ, Davis P, Salims M. Hypergastrinemia in rheumatoid ar-thritis. Clin Exp Rheumatol 1986;4:49.

53. Dyer NJ, Kendell MJ, Hawkins CJ. Malabsorption in rheumatoid disease. Ann Rheum Dis 1979;30:151.

54. Scott DGI, Bacon PA, Tribe CR. Systemic rheumatoid vasculitis; A clinical and laboratory study of 50 cases. Medicine 1981;60:288.

55. Burt RW, Berensen MM, Samuelsen CO, et al. Rheumatoid vasculitis on the corner of presenting as pancolitis. Dig Dis Sci 1983;28:183.

56. Langer HE, Hartman MN, Heineman N. Gold colitis induced by auranofin treatment of rheumatoid arthritis: Case report and review of the literature. Ann Rheum Dis 1987;46:787.

57. Jarnfelt-Samsioe A, Samsioe G, Velinder GM. Nausea and vomiting in pregnancy—a contribution to its epidemiology. Gynecol Obstet Invest 1983;16:221.

58. Klebanoff MA, Koslowe PA, Kaslow R, et al. Epidemiology of vom-iting in early pregnancy. Obstet Gynecol 1985;66:612.

59. FitzGerald CM. Nausea and vomiting in early pregnancy. Br J Med Psychol 1985;57:159.

60. Masson GM, Anthony F, Chau E. Serum chorionic gonadotropin (HCG), schwangerschaftsprotein 1 (SP1), progesterone and oes-tradiol levels in patients with nausea and vomiting in early pregnancy. Br J Obstet Gynaecol 1985;92:211.

61. Jarnfelt-Samsioe A, Bremme K, Eneroth P. Steroid hormones in emetic and non-emetic pregnancy. Eur J Obstet Gynecol Reprod Biol 1986;21:87.

62. Guze SB, DeLong WB, Majerus PW, et al. Association of clinical psychiatric disease with hyperemesis gravidarum. A three-and-a-half year follow-up study of 48 patients and 45 controls. N Engl J Med 1959;261:1363.

63. Fitzgerald JPB. Epidemiology of hyperemesis gravidarum. Lancet 1956;1:660.

64. Depue RH, Bernstein L, Ross RK, et al. Hyperemesis gravidarum in relation to estradiol levels, pregnancy outcome, and other maternal factors: A seroepidemiologic study. Am J Obstet Gynecol 1987;156(5):1137.

65. Bruun TH, Kristoffersen K. Thyroid function during pregnancy with special reference to hydatidiform mole and hyperemesis. Acta Endocrinol 1978;88:383.
66. Bouillon R, Naesens M, Van Assche FA, et al. Thyroid function in patients with hyperemesis gravidarum. Am J Obstet Gynecol 1982;143:922.
67. Juras N, Banovac K, Sekso M. Increased serum reverse triiodothyronine in patients with hyperemesis gravidarum. Acta Endocrinol 1983;102:284.
68. Dozeman R, Kaiser FE, Cass O, et al. Hyperthyroidism appearing as hyperemesis gravidarum. Arch Intern Med 1983;143:2202.
69. Kauppila A, Huhtaniemi I, Ylikorkala O. Raised serum human chorionic gonadotrophin concentrations in hyperemesis gravidarum. Br Med J 1979;1:1670.
70. Harvey WA, Sherfey MJ. Vomiting in pregnanacy. A psychiatric study. Psychosom Med 1954;16:1.
71. Coppen AJ. Vomiting of early pregnancy. Psychological factors and body build. Lancet 1959;1:172.
72. Semmens JP. Female sexuality and life situations. An etiologic psychosocio-sexual profile of weight gain and nausea and vomiting in pregnancy. Obstet Gynecol 1971;38:555.
73. Wolkind S, Zajicek E. Psycho-social correlates of nausea and vomiting in pregnancy. J Psychosom Res 1978;22:1.
74. Levine MG, Esser D. Total parenteral nutrition for the treatment of severe hyperemesis gravidarum: Maternal nutritional effects and fetal outcome. Obstet Gynecol 1988;72(1):102.
75. Stellato TA, Danziger LH, Burkons D. Fetal salvage with maternal total parenteral nutrition: The pregnant mother as her own control. J Parenteral Enteral Nutr 1988;12(4):412.
76. Long MAD, Simone SS, Tucher JJ. Outpatient treatment of hyperemesis gravidarum with stimulus control and imagery procedures. J Behav Ther Exp Psychiatry 1986;17:105.
77. Gross S, Librach C, Cecutti A. Maternal weight loss associated with hyperemesis gravidarum: A predictor of fetal outcome. Am J Obstet Gynecol 1989;160(4):906.
78. McKay AJ, O'Neill J, Imrie CW. Pancreatitis, pregnancy and gallstones. Br J Obstet Gynecol 1980;87(1):47.
79. Bynum TE. Hepatic and gastrointestinal disorders in pregnancy. Med Clin North Am 1977;61:129.
80. Jouppila P, Mokka R, Larmi TKI. Acute pancreatitis in pregnancy. Surg Gynecol Obstet 1974;313:879.
81. Block P, Kelly TR. Management of gallstone pancreatitis during pregnancy and the postpartum period. Surg Gynecol Obstet 1989;168(5):426.
82. Anonymous Appendicitis in pregnancy. Lancet 1986;1:195.
83. Aranson M. Appendicitis during pregnancy. Ten year review at Maine Medical Center. J Maine Med Assn 1979;70:341.
84. Punnonen R, Aho AJ, Gronroos M, et al. Appendectomy during pregnancy. Acta Chir Scand 1979;145:555.
85. Van Thiel DH, Gavaler JS, Joshi SN, et al. Heartburn of pregnancy. Gastroenterology 1977;72:666.
86. Brock-Utne JG, Dow TG, Dimopoulos GE, et al. Gastric and lower oesophageal sphincter pressures in early pregnancy. Br J Anaesth 1981;53:381.
87. Dodds WJ, Dent J, Hogan WJ. Pregnancy and the lower esophageal sphincter. Gastroenterology 1978;74:1334.
88. Shaffer EA, Taylor PJ, Logan K, et al. The effect of progestin on gallbladder function in young women. Am J Obstet Gynecol 1984;148:504.
89. Levy N, Lemberg E, Sharf M. Bowel habit in pregnancy. Digestion 1971;4:216.
90. Anderson AS. Constipation during pregnancy. Incidence and methods used in its treatment in a group of Cambridgeshire women. J Health Visitor 1984;57:363.
91. Anderson AS. Dietary factors in the aetiology and treatment of constipation during pregnancy. Br J Obstet Gynaecol 1985;3:245.
92. Anderson AS, Whichelow MJ. Constipation during pregnancy: Dietary fibre intake and the effect of fibre supplementation. Hum Nutr Appl Nutr 1985;39A:202.
93. Lowry SM, O'Dea TP, Gallagher DI, et al. Splenic artery aneurysm rupture: The seventh instance of maternal and fetal survival. Obstet Gynecol 1986;67(2):291.
94. Jorgenson BA. Visceral artery aneurysms. A review. Dan Med Bull 1985;32(4):237.
95. de Graff J, Pijpers PM. Spontaneous rupture of the spleen in third trimester of pregnancy. Report of a case and review of the literature. Eur J Obstet Gynecol Reprod Biol 1987;25(3):243.
96. Trastek VF, Pariolero PC, Joyce JW, et al. Splenic artery aneurysms. Surgery 1982;91(6):694.
97. Denehy T, McGrath EW, Breen JL. Splenic torsion and rupture in pregnancy (Review). Obstet Gynecol Surv 1988;43(3):123.
98. Aviles E. Surgical emergencies during pregnancy. Rev Med Panama 1987;12(2):126.
99. Bokhari SI, Desser KB, Mouer JR, et al. Maternal meconium granulomatous peritonitis. Arch Intern Med 1981;141:658.
100. Schwartz IS, Bellow GV, Feigin G, et al. Maternal vernix caseosa peritonitis following premature rupture of fetal membranes. JAMA 1985;254:948.
101. Musola R, Franzin G, Mora R, et al. Prevalence of gastroduodenal lesions in uremic patients undergoing dialysis and after renal transplantation. Gastrointest Endosc 1984;30:343.
102. Ishikawa E, Nishi T, Matsuo M, et al. Clinical studies on the prognosis of 150 cases of acute renal failure. Hinyokika Kiyo 1983;29:169.
103. Zuckerman GR, Cornette, GL, Clouse RE, et al. Upper gastrointestinal bleeding in patients with chronic renal failure. Ann Intern Med 1985;102:588.
104. Wesdorp RI, Falcao HA, Banks PB, et al. Gastrin and gastric acid secretion in renal failure. Am J Surg 1981;141:334.
105. Gold CH, Morely JE, Vijoen M, et al. Gastric acid secretion and serum gastrin levels in patients with chronic renal failure on regular hemodialysis. Nephron 1980;25:92.
106. Paimela H, Harkonen M, Karonen SL, et al. Relation between serum group II pepsinogen concentration and the degree of Brunner's gland hyperplasia in patients with chronic renal failure. Gut 1985;26:198.
107. Paimela H, Harkonen M., Karonen SL, et al. The effect of renal transplantation on gastric acid secretion and on the serum levels of gastrin and group I pepsinogens. Ann Clin Res 1985;17:105.
108. Hansky J. Effect of renal failure on gastrointestinal hormones. World J Surg 1979;3:463.
109. Hadjiyannakis EJ, Evans DB, Smellie WAB, et al. Gastrointestinal complications after renal transplantation. Lancet 1971;2:781.
110. Lerut J, Lerut T, Grumez JA, et al. Surgical gastrointestinal complications in 277 renal transplantations. Acta Chir Belg 1980;79:383.
111. Schweizer RT, Bartus SA. Gastroduodenal ulceration in renal transplant patients. Conn Med 1978;42:85.
112. Conn HO, Blitzer BL. Nonassociation of adrenocorticoid therapy and peptic ulcer. N Engl J Med 1976;294:473.
113. Pranzin G, Muolo A, Griminelli T. Cytomegalovirus inclusions in the gastroduodenal muscosa of patients after renal transplantation. Gut 1981;22:698.
114. Kodama T, Fukuda S, Takino T, et al. Gastroduodenal cytomegalovirus infection after renal transplantation. Fiberscopic observations. Endoscopy 1985;17:157.
115. Walter S, Thorup-Anderson J, Christensen U, et al. Effect of cimetidine on upper gastrointestinal bleeding after renal transplantation: A prospective study. Br Med J [Clin Res] 1984;289:1175.
116. Bronner MH, Pate MB, Cunningham JT, et al. Estrogen-progesterone therapy for bleeding gastrointestinal telangiectasias in chronic renal failure. Ann Intern Med 1986;105:371.
117. Avvam MM. High prevalence of pancreatic disease in chronic renal failure. Nephron 1977;18:68.
118. Keogh B, McGeeney KF, Drury MI, et al. Renal clearance of pancreatic and salivary amylase relative to creatinine in patients with chronic renal insufficiency. Gut 1978;19:1125.
119. Sachs EF, Hurwitz FJ, Bloch HM, et al. Pancreatic exocrine hypofunction in the wasting syndrome of end-stage renal disease. Am J Gastroenterol 1983;78:170.
120. Paimela H, Tallgren LG, Stenman S, et al. Multiple duodenal polyps in uraemia: A little known clinical entity. Gut 1984;25:259.
121. Zizic TM, Shulman LE, Stevens MB. Colonic perforations in systemic lupus erythematosus. Medicine 1975;54:411.
122. Brandt LJ, Davidoff A, Berstein LH, et al. Small intestinal involve-

ment in Waldenstrom's macro-globulinaemia. Dig Dis Sci 1981;26:174.

123. Cooney DR. Small bowel obstruction and ileal perforation: Complication of uremia. J Indiana State Med Assoc 1976;69:781.

124. Rubenstein RB. Uremic ileus. Uremia presenting as colonic obstruction. NY State J Med 1979;79:248.

125. Mitch WE. Nitrogen metabolism in patients with chronic renal failure. Am J Clin Nutr 1978;31:1594.

126. Gordon SJ, Miller LJ, Haeffner LJ, et al. Abnormal intestinal bile acid distribution of azotaemic man: A possible role in the pathogenesis of uremic diarrhoea. Gut 1976;17:58.

127. Aubia J, Lloveras J, Munne A, et al. Ischemic colitis in chronic uremia. Nephron 1981;29:146.

128. Goldberg M, Hoffman GC, Wombolt DG. Massive hemorrhage from rectal ulcers in chronic renal failure. Ann Intern Med 1984;100:397.

129. Bischel MD, Reese T, Engel J. Spontaneous perforation of the colon in a hemodialysis patient. Am J Gastroenterol 1980;74:182.

130. Young R, Bryk D. Colonic intussusception in uremia. Am J Gastroenterol 1979;71:229.

131. Cryer PE, Kissane JM. Gastrointestinal symptoms and shock in a patient with chronic renal failure: Clinicopathologic conference. Am J Med 1980;69:595.

132. Mountokalakis TD, Virvidakis CE, Singhellakis PN, et al. Magnesium absorption in chronic renal failure. Gastroenterology 1981;80:632.

133. Davis GR, Zerwekh JE, Parker TF, et al. Absorption of phosphate in the jejunum of patients with chronic renal fialure before and after correction of vitamin D deficiency. Gastroenterology 1983;85:908.

134. Lerut J, Lerut T, Grumez JA, et al. Surgical gastrointestinal complications in 277 renal transplantations. Acta Chir Belg 1980;79:383.

135. Jones JM, Glass NR, Belzer FO. Fatal *Candida* esophagitis in two diabetics after renal transplantation. Arch Surg 1982;117:499.

136. Harwood AB, Osoba D, Hofstader SL, et al. Kaposi's sarcoma in recipients of renal transplants. Am J Med 1979;67:759.

137. Meyers WC, Harris N, Steel S, et al. Alimentary tract complications after renal transplantation. Ann Surg 1979;190:535.

138. Guice K, Rattazzi LD, Marchioro TL. Colon perforation in renal transplant patients. Am J Surg 1979;138:43.

139. Burnstein M, Salter D, Cardella C, et al. Necrotizing pancreatitis in renal transplant patients. Can J Surg 1982;25:547.

140. Gordon C, Hewer RL, Wade DT. Dysphagia in acute stroke. Br Med J [Clin Res] 1987;295:411.

141. Barer DH. The natural history and functional consequences of dysphagia after hemispheric stroke. J Neurol Neurosurg Psychiatry 1989;52(2):236.

142. Veis SL, Logemann JA. Swallowing disorders in persons with cerebrovascular accident. Arch Phys Med Rehabil 1985;66(6):372.

143. Horner J, Massey EW, Riski JE, et al. Aspiration following stroke: Clinical correlates and outcome. Neurology 1988;38(9):1359.

144. Splaingard ML, Hutchins B, Sulton LD, et al. Aspiration in rehabilitation patients: Videofluoroscopy vs bedside clinical assessment. Arch Phys Med Rehabil 1988;69(8):637.

145. Cole MJ, Smith JT, Molnar C, et al. Aspiration after percutaneous gastrostomy. Assessment by Tc-99m labeling of the enteral feed. J Clin Gastroenterol 1987;9(1):90.

146. Gore RM, Mintzer RA, Calenoff L. Gastrointestinal complications of spinal cord injury. Spine 1981;6:538.

147. Soderstrom CA, Ducker TB. Increased susceptibility of patients with cervical cord lesions to peptic gastrointestinal complications. J Trauma 1985;Nov 25(11):1030.

148. Kuric J, Lucas CE, Ledgerwood AM, et al. Nutritional support: A prophylaxis against stress bleeding after spinal cord injury. Paraplegia 1989;27;140.

149. Fadul CE, Lemann W, Thaler HT, et al. Perforation of the gastrointestinal tract in patients receiving steroids for neurologic disease. Neurology 1988;38(3):348.

150. Miller F, Fenzl TC. Prolonged ileus with acute spinal cord injury responding to metaclopramide. Paraplegia 1981;19:43.

151. Etienne M, Verlinden M, Brassinne A. Treatment with cisapride of the gastrointestinal and urological sequelae of spinal cord transection: Case report. Paraplegia 1988;26:162.

152. Osteen RT, Barsamian EM. Delayed gastric emptying after vagotomy and drainage in the spinal cord injury patient. Paraplegia 1981;19:46.

153. Apstein MD, Dalecki-Chipperfield K. Spinal cord injury is a risk factor for gallstone disease. Gastroenterology 1987;92:966.

154. Bernstein L, Joseph R, Staas WE, Jr. Solitary colonic ulcer in a spinal cord injured patient. Arch Phys Med Rehabil 1986;67:194.

155. Segal JL, Brunnemann SR, Gordon SK, et al. The absolute bioavailability of oral theophylline in patients with spinal cord injury. Pharmacotherapy 1986;6:26.

156. Aaronson MJ, Freed MM, Burakoff RB. Colonic myoelectric activity in persons with spinal cord injury. Dig Dis Sci 1985;30:295.

157. Glick ME, Meshkinpour H, Haldeman S, et al. Colonic dysfunction in patients with thoracic spinal cord injury. Gastroenterology 1984;86:287.

158. de Groot GH, de Pagter GF. Effects of cisapride on constipation due to a neurological lesion. Paraplegia 1988;26(3):159.

159. McGuire TJ, Kumar VN. Autonomic dysreflexia in the spinal cord injured. What the physician should know about this medical emergency. Postgrad Med 1986;80:81.

160. Bell J, Hannon K. Pathophysiology involved in autonomic dysreflexia. J Neurosci Nurs 1986;18:86.

161. Scheinberg L, Smith CR. Rehabilitation of patients with multiple sclerosis (Review). Neurol Clin 1987;5(4):585.

162. Kilman WJ. Disorders of pharyngeal and upper esophageal sphincter motor function. Arch Intern Med 1976;136:592.

163. Gupta YK. Gastroparesis with multiple sclerosis. JAMA 1984;252:42.

164. Sullivan SN, Ebers GC. Gastrointestinal dysfunction in multiple sclerosis. Gastroenterology 1984;84:1640.

165. Hinds JP, Wald A, Eidelman BH. Bowel dysfunction in a multiple sclerosis population. Gastroenterology 1988;94:187.

166. Robbins JA, Logemann JA, Kirshner HS. Swallowing and speech production in Parkinson's disease. Ann Neurol 1986;19:283.

167. Kempster PA, Lees AJ, Crichton P, et al. Off-period belching due to a reversible disturbance of oesophageal motility in Parkinson's disease and its treatment with apomorphine. Movement Disorders 1989;4(1):47.

168. Kurlan R, Rothfield KP, Woodward WR, et al. Erratic gastric emptying of levodopa may cause "random" fluctuations of parkinsonian mobility. Neurology 1988;38(3):419.

169. Kurlan R, Nutt JG, Woodward WR, et al. Duodenal and gastric delivery of levodopa in parkinsonism. Ann Neurol 1988;23(6):589.

170. Winship DH, Caflisch CR, Zboralski FF, et al. Deterioration of esophageal peristalsis in patients with alcoholic neuropathy. Gastroenterology 1968;55:173.

171. Dabaghi RE, Scott LD. Intestinal pseudo-obstruction in a patient with myotonic dystrophy. Tex Med 1986;82:42.

172. Woods CA, Foutch PG, Kerr DM, et al. Collagenous sprue as a cause for malabsorption in a patient with myotonic dystrophy: A new association. Am J Gastroenterol 1988;83(7):765.

173. Swick HM, Werlin SL, Dodds WJ, et al. Pharyngoesophageal motor function in patients with myotonic dystrophy. Ann Neurol 1981;10:454.

174. Dabaghi RE, Scott LD. Intestinal pseudo-obstruction in a patient with myotonic dystrophy. Tex Med 1986;84:42.

175. Eckardt VF, Nix W, Kraus W, et al. Esophageal motor function in patients with muscular dystrophy. Gastroenterology 1986;90:628.

176. Simpson AJ, Khilnani MT. Gastrointestinal manifestations of the muscular dystrophies. Am J Roentgenol 1975;125:948.

177. Kuiper DH. Gastric bezoar in a patient with myotonic dystrophy. Am J Dig Dis 1971;16:529.

178. Nowak TV, Anuras S, Brown BP, et al. Small intestinal motility in myotonic dystrophy patients. Gastroenterology 1984;86:808.

179. Weinter MJ. Myotonic megacolon in myotonic dystrophy. Am J Roentgenol 1978;130:177.

180. Langman MJS, Cooke AR. Gastric and duodenal ulcer and their associated diseases. Lancet 1976;1:680.

181. Bonnevie O. Causes of death in duodenal and gastric ulcer. Gastroenterology 1977;73:1000.

182. Monson RR. Duodenal ulcer as a second disease. Gastroenterology 1970;59:712.

183. Rotter JI. Peptic ulcer. In: Emery AEH, Rimoin DL, eds. The principles and practice of medical genetics. New York: Academic Press, 1980:31.

184. Barish CF, Wu WC, Castell DO. Respiratory complication of gastroesophageal reflux. Arch Intern Med 1985;145:1882.

185. Bernstein A, Temple JG. Gastro-oesophageal reflux and bronchial asthma relationship? In: Baron JH, ed. Cimetidine in the 80's. Edinburgh: Churchill Livingstone 1981;167.

186. Larrain A, Carrasco J, Gallequillos J, Pope CE. Reflux treatment improves lung function in patients with intrinsic asthma. Gastroenterology 1981;80:1204.

187. Singh V, Jain N. Asthma as a cause for, rather than a result of, gastroesophageal reflux. J Asthma 1983;20:241.

188. Davidson JD, Waldman TR, Goodman DS, et al. Protein losing enteropathy in congestive heart failure. Lancet 1961.894.

189. Lambert M, dePeyer R, Mauer AF. Reversible ischemic colitis after intravenous vasopressin use. JAMA 1982;247:666.

190. Gazes PC, Holmes CR, Mosely V. Acute hemorrhage and necrosis of the intestines associated with digitalization. Circulation 1961;23:358.

191. Greenstein RJ, McElhonny AJ, Ruben D, et al. Colonic vascular ectasias and aortic stenosis: Coincidence or causal relationship? Am J Surg 1986;151:347.

192. Steed DL, Brown B, Reilly J, et al. General surgical complication in heart and heart lung transplantation. Surgery 1987;98:739.

193. Colon R, Frazier OH, Kahan BD, et al. Complications in cardiac transplant patients requiring general surgery. Surgery 1988;103:32.

194. Sinnott JT IV, Cullison JP, Rogers K. Treatment of cytomegalovirus gastrointestinal ulceration in a heart transplant patient. J Heart Transplant 1987;6(3):186.

195. Bramwell NH, Davies RA, Koshal A, et al. Fatal gastrointestinal hemorrhage caused by cytomegalovirus duodenitis and ulceration after heart transplantation. J Heart Transplant 1987;6(5):303.

196. Fernandez JA, Rosenberg JC. Post transplantation pancreatitis. Surg Gynecol Obstet 1976;143:695.

48

Approach to the Patient Requiring Nutritional Supplementation

WILLIAM D. HEIZER
BEVERLY HOLCOMBE

NUTRIENT REQUIREMENTS AND RECOMMENDATION

For every healthy person there is a range of daily oral intake for each essential nutrient that is adequate and safe. At intakes below and above that range, evidence of deficiency and toxicity, respectively, will appear. The lower end of the range can be defined as the dietary requirement. An intravenous requirement could be defined similarly and would not necessarily be identical to the dietary requirement.

Approximately every 5 years the National Research Council of the National Academy of Sciences acting on a report from its Food and Nutrition Board publishes *Recommended Dietary Allowances* (RDAs). To allow for individual variability in requirements, these recommended allowances are set two standard deviations above the estimated mean dietary requirements for normal persons. In addition, the RDAs take into account other factors such as the effect of the dietary form in which nutrients are ingested and variations in absorption. Different RDAs are given for different ages, for males and females, and for conditions such as pregnancy and lactation. In 1989, to accompany the 10th and latest edition, two auxiliary tables were published, "Estimated Safe and Adequate Daily Dietary Intakes for Selected Vitamins and Minerals," dealing with certain vitamins and trace elements for which no RDAs have been established and "Estimated Minimum Requirements" for sodium, potassium, and chloride.[1] It should be noted that RDAs are amounts intended to be safe and adequate when consumed as part of a normal diet. They are neither minimal nor necessarily optimal levels of intake.

The RDAs are used in nutritional planning and in Food and Drug Administration labeling standards. For simplicity in food labeling, the multiple recommended *dietary* allowances were used to define a single set of recommendations called the U.S. Recommended *Daily* Allowance or "USRDA." The USRDAs are based on the 7th edition of the RDAs published in 1968 and are the highest RDA set for nonpregnant, nonlactating persons older than 4 years of age with a few exceptions. For most nutrients, the USRDA coincides with the RDA for adult males. A higher USRDA for iron is a notable exception. Throughout this chapter, the recommended values given will be the USRDA.

ETIOLOGIES OF NUTRIENT DEFICIENCIES

In this chapter we will discuss the practical aspects of detecting and managing mineral, vitamin, and protein–calorie deficiencies in which supplementation is indicated for immediate improvement in function, safety, or well-being. It is beyond the scope of this chapter to consider the evidence that ingestion of some nutrients in excess of the amounts currently eaten by many persons in developed countries or in excess of officially recommended amounts may decrease the incidence or severity of certain chronic diseases.[2]

Deficiency of a nutrient may result from a decrease in its intake or absorption or an increase in its loss or utilization. The gastrointestinal tract plays a critical role in these processes. Deficiencies may occur when disease alters any of the normal gastrointestinal functions, including ingestion, digestion, absorption, or secretion. Intestinal dysfunction can affect not only the assimilation of ingested nutrients but also the reabsorption of nutrients that are normally secreted and reabsorbed.

As a deficiency of any nutrient is developing, metabolic and physiologic derangements precede readily observable signs and symptoms. Therefore, it is important to anticipate potential deficiencies by appreciating the mechanisms that cause them and the disease states in which they frequently occur.

Inadequate Intake

Inadequate intake is probably the most frequent reason for nutrient deficiencies even in developed countries. More than 30% of the U.S. population ingest less than 70% of the RDAs for calcium, iron, magnesium, vitamin A, and vitamin B$_6$.[3] Therefore, deficiencies of these nutrients as well as others, including protein and calories, should be anticipated when disease causes a prolonged period of decreased food intake. Frequent causes of decreased intake include anorexia, nausea, dysphagia, depression, intoxica-

tion, pain or diarrhea induced by eating, therapeutic diets, and self-imposed diets. Decreased food intake contributes to most nutrient deficiencies, including those in which other mechanisms are primary.

Decreased Absorption

Among the malabsorption syndromes, nutrient deficiencies are most frequent and severe in those caused by a decrease in effective mucosal absorptive surface, such as short bowel syndrome, celiac sprue, and Whipple's disease. When mucosal absorption is diminished, not only is the absorption of ingested nutrients reduced but also a portion of the minerals, vitamins, and protein in gastric, pancreatic, biliary, and small bowel secretions may escape normal reabsorption. Divalent cations, most notably calcium, magnesium, and zinc, are especially vulnerable to malabsorption because they are less than 60% absorbed normally. Malabsorption further reduces uptake not only due to loss of absorptive surface but also because these ions combine with unabsorbed fatty acids in the lumen to form poorly absorbed soaps. Furthermore, since there is substantial secretion of calcium and zinc into the intestinal lumen, excessive loss of these ions from the gastrointestinal tract can occur even when there is little or no oral intake.[4,5] Under normal circumstances, absorption of water, sodium, potassium, and chloride is much more complete than absorption of the divalent cations. Nevertheless, deficiencies of the monovalent ions and water should be anticipated when malabsorption is severe, especially when the absorptive capacity of the colon is diminished or absent as, for example, in patients with a short intestine terminating in a jejunostomy.

Malabsorption of some nutrients should be anticipated during treatment with certain drugs.[6,7] Cholestyramine can induce a mild generalized malabsorption of fat and fat-soluble vitamins by binding bile salts. It further reduces vitamin D absorption by binding the vitamin. Neomycin may induce malabsorption by precipitating bile salts in the intestinal lumen. Sulfasalazine competitively inhibits folate absorption, colchicine inhibits the release of fat-soluble vitamins from enterocytes, and antacids in the form of hydroxides of magnesium or aluminum decrease absorption of phosphorus.

The biologic availability and absorption of some nutrients is influenced by other components in the diet.[7] Dietary phytate diminishes absorption of calcium, iron, phosphorus, and zinc. Excessive dietary phosphorus can decrease absorption of calcium and iron. Absorption of fat-soluble vitamins is diminished when there is very little fat in the diet. Raw egg white diminishes the absorption of biotin.

Increased Losses

Increased nutrient losses from the gastrointestinal tract may occur in the absence of malabsorption. Examples include depletion of water and various electrolytes, including sodium, potassium, chloride, hydrogen, bicarbonate, zinc, magnesium, calcium, and phosphate, which can occur as a result of diarrhea, high-output fistulae, vomiting, or nasogastric suction. Iron deficiency results from chronic loss of iron as blood, most often from the gastrointestinal tract or female genital tract.

Excessive loss in the urine is a frequent cause of nutrient deficiencies. Deficits of water, sodium, chloride, potassium, and phosphate should be anticipated in the face of osmotic diuresis. Renal wasting of potassium occurs during alkalosis. Some drugs, especially amphotericin and cisplatin, cause renal tubular defects resulting in excessive losses of potassium and magnesium, which can be profound and can last for months after the drug is stopped. Many diuretics increase urinary losses of potassium and magnesium. Urinary excretion of micronutrients, especially zinc and some vitamins, is increased during catabolic illnesses. This appears to result from direct effects of the neurohumoral mediators of the catabolic response as well as renal clearance of nutrients released from catabolized lean tissue.

Excessive sweating can deplete sodium, potassium, chloride, and water as well as trace minerals and nitrogen.

Increased Utilization

In pregnancy and lactation, the utilization of many nutrients is increased, including fat, carbohydrate, protein, calcium, and vitamins. The mother will experience a net loss if her nutrient intake does not meet the additional demands.

Nutrient utilization is also increased when there is net accretion of lean body tissue. If the full complement of nutrients required for synthesis of lean tissue is not provided, growth is slowed, and eventually other evidence of specific nutrient deficiency will develop. The need to supply adequate nutrients for growth in childhood is obvious. However, the need to provide extra vitamins and minerals for the person who is rapidly regaining lean body mass following recovery from a catabolic illness or malabsorption is more likely to be overlooked. The person who is body-building by means of exercise and weight lifting unequivocally requires additional nutrients for synthesis of new muscle tissue, but it appears unlikely that these demands are great enough to require supplementation over and above a well-balanced diet.

Increased utilization of nutrients, especially fat, carbohydrate, and proteins, is most frequently encountered by patients during catabolic conditions such as sepsis, trauma, and burns. Nutrients are required to support the increased synthesis of phagocytes, white blood cells, fibroblasts, immunoglobulins, collagen, and other proteins associated with the stress response and wound healing. The responses to stress, which are systemic and local and humoral and neural, are only beginning to be understood. The effects of these powerful responses is to release nutrients from endogenous sources and make them available to meet the increased demands. Fatty acids and glycerol are released from adipose stores and serve as fuels. As lean tissue is catabolized, amino acids and other nutrients are made available for synthesis of the cells and proteins associated with the stress response. Some of the amino acids are also oxidized for energy. Glutamine is used as fuel by intestinal epithelial cells, alanine is converted to glucose by the liver (gluconeogenesis), and other amino acids liberated by muscle catabolism, especially the branched-chain amino acids leucine, isoleucine, and valine, are used locally as fuel for the muscle. When amino acids are oxidized for energy their amino groups are converted to urea and excreted. This accounts for almost all of the increase in urinary nitrogen

that occurs during the stress response. The resulting erosion in lean body mass can be decreased but seldom eliminated entirely by nutrition support. Current research is approaching this problem by searching for more appropriate substrate mixtures to meet the increased demands of stress as well as for beneficial ways to avoid, block, or modify the neurocytohumoral responses that mediate the increase in lean body mass degradation.

CONDITIONS IN WHICH NUTRITIONAL SUPPLEMENTATION IS FREQUENTLY REQUIRED

In light of the foregoing discussion, it is apparent that a person's need for nutrient supplementation is determined by the balance between intake and absorption of the nutrient on one hand compared with loss and utilization on the other. Some conditions are especially likely to result in deficiencies.

Alcohol Abuse

Persons who abuse alcohol have a high incidence of nutrient deficiencies, which are often multiple. The reasons are many. Excessive alcohol intake can depress appetite for food, both directly in some persons and indirectly by causing nausea, vomiting, gastritis, diarrhea, and pancreatitis. Alcohol is toxic to the epithelial cells of the small intestine, causing decreased transport of nutrients including glucose, amino acids, folate, and thiamine.[8] Absorption is further compromised by alcohol-induced malnutrition, especially protein–calorie malnutrition, by folate and zinc deficiency, and by bile acid deficiency when cirrhosis is present. Increased urinary losses of folate, zinc, magnesium, and phosphate occur, and tissue utilization of folate is altered by alcohol abuse.[8]

Once cirrhosis develops, the likelihood of deficiencies is further increased by alterations in nutrient metabolism. Pyridoxal phosphate, the active product of vitamin B_6, is metabolized more rapidly by persons with cirrhosis than by normal subjects. Thiamine storage and conversion to its active metabolite, thiamine pyrophosphate, is diminished. Conversion of vitamin D to 25-hydroxy vitamin D is also decreased in the cirrhotic liver.

Inflammatory Bowel Disease (see ch 77)

Multiple nutritional deficiencies have been documented in patients with inflammatory bowel disease, especially Crohn's disease (Table 48-1).[9] Protein–calorie malnutrition is caused by decreased intake resulting from anorexia, nausea, and dietary restrictions as well as by increased utilization and loss resulting from inflammation and corticosteroid administration. In addition, nutrient absorption may be decreased by loss of functioning mucosa or by bile salt deficiency resulting from damage or resection of the distal ileum. Severe damage or resection of the terminal ileum results in vitamin B_{12} malabsorption. Iron deficiency from chronic intestinal bleeding and deficiencies of zinc and potassium resulting from chronic diarrhea can be anticipated. Urinary loss of zinc is increased by episodes of acute inflammation and corticosteroid administration. It is now well established that the growth failure that occurs in

TABLE 48-1
Frequency of Nutritional Deficiencies Reported in Inflammatory Bowel Disease

	CROHN'S DISEASE (%)	ULCERATIVE COLITIS (%)
Weight loss	65–75	18–62
Hypoalbuminemia	25–80	25–50
Intestinal protein loss	75	+
Negative nitrogen balance	69	+
Anemia	60–80	66
Iron deficiency	39	81
Vitamin B$_{12}$ deficiency	48	5
Folic acid deficiency	54	36
Calcium deficiency	13	+
Magnesium deficiency	14–33	+
Potassium deficiency	6–20	+
Vitamin A deficiency	11	NR
Vitamin C deficiency	+	NR
Vitamin D deficiency	75	+
Vitamin K deficiency	+	NR
Zinc deficiency	+	+
Copper deficiency	+	NR
Metabolic bone disease	+	+

+, Reported but incidence not described.
NR, Not reported.
Driscoll RH, Rosenberg IH. Total parenteral nutrition in inflammatory bowel disease. Med Clin North Am 1978;62:185.

up to 30% of children with Crohn's disease can usually be reversed by adequate intake of nutrients.[10,11]

Short Bowel Syndrome (see ch 74)

In short bowel syndrome, eating may be decreased as a result of food-induced diarrhea but intake is often two to three times greater than normal. Nutrient deficiencies are primarily the result of malabsorption of ingested and endogenous nutrients. Protein and calorie malnutrition and deficiencies of magnesium, zinc, calcium, potassium, B vitamins, and fat-soluble vitamins are especially likely.

RECOGNIZING AND TREATING NUTRITIONAL DEFICIENCIES

The following sections of this chapter are designed to be a practical guide summarizing when and how to supplement patients with individual nutrients. Usually, deficiencies can be anticipated or recognized at an early stage and corrected before the occurrence of classic deficiency syndromes. Nevertheless, it is important to recognize the classic signs and symptoms of deficiency (Table 48-2).

Deficiencies of Major Minerals

Major minerals are defined as those that are needed in quantities greater than 100 mg/d. Deficiencies of sodium, potassium, calcium, phosphorus, and magnesium will be discussed.

SODIUM[12–15]

Sodium, the principal cation in extracellular fluid, is necessary for the maintenance of intravascular fluid volume and membrane potentials. No RDA has been established, but the estimated minimum daily requirement for adults is 500 mg (22 mEq). Western societies consume more than adequate amounts. Sodium is abundant in both animal and plant sources, but in the United States the primary dietary source is table salt. Almost all ingested sodium is absorbed, and homeostasis is accomplished by renal excretion. Normally, only small amounts are lost in stool and through the skin as perspiration.

Deficiency as a consequence solely of inadequate intake is virtually unknown. Increased loss is usually from the gastrointestinal tract, as a result of vomiting, diarrhea, or drainage, from the kidneys as a result of diuresis, salt-wasting renal disease, or adrenal insufficiency, or from the skin as a result of excessive perspiration. Approximate mean concentrations of sodium in various fluids in milliequivalents per liter are as follows: bile, 145; pancreatic juice, 130; jejunal fluid, 115; ileal fluid, 100; sweat, 75; gastric fluid, 70; mature ileostomy output, 45; saliva, 10; and normal stool, 5.

Sodium depletion usually presents as symptoms of dehydration because of concomitant water loss. Severe depletion presents as nausea, vomiting, exhaustion, cramps, seizures, and ultimately cardiorespiratory collapse. To assess sodium deficiency, it is important to determine intravascular volume status as well as urine sodium concentration and osmolality. When sodium deficiency is the result of increased gastrointestinal or cutaneous losses, urine osmolality is increased and urine sodium concentration is less than 10 mEq/L. When sodium deficiency results from ongoing diuretic administration, urine osmolality is decreased and urine sodium concentration is greater than 10 mEq/L.

Serum sodium concentration primarily reflects water, not sodium, balance. Therefore, in sodium depletion the serum concentration may be low, normal, or high depending on the relative deficits of sodium and water. When the serum concentration is low, "pseudohyponatremia" due to a high blood lipid level must be ruled out. A real, but osmotically appropriate lowering of the serum sodium level occurs when excessive amounts of other osmotically active molecules such as glucose or urea are present. Serum osmolality estimated by the following formula should fall within the normal range (275–295 mOsm/kg) if sodium concentration is appropriately reduced:

Estimated serum osmolality

$$= 2[Na^+](mEq/L) + \frac{Glucose(mg/dL)}{18} + \frac{BUN(mg/dL)}{2.8}$$

Among hospitalized patients hyponatremia is most frequently the result of dilution by excess free water, not sodium depletion. The free water excess is usually caused by heart, liver, or renal

TABLE 48–2
Some Physical Signs of Nutritional Deficiency

	FINDING	DEFICIENCY
Hair	Thin, sparse	Protein, zinc, biotin
	Flag sign (transverse depigmentation)	Protein, copper
	Easy pluckability	Protein
Nails	Spoon-shaped (koilonychia)	Iron
	No luster, transverse ridging	Protein-energy
Skin	Dry, scaling (xerosis)	Vitamin A, zinc
	Seborrheic dermatitis	Essential fatty acids (EFA), zinc, pyridoxine, biotin
	Flaky paint dermatosis	Protein
	Follicular hyperkeratosis	Vitamin A, vitamin C, EFA
	Nasolabial seborrhea	Niacin (B_1), pyridoxine (B_6), riboflavin (B_2)
	Petechiae, purpura	Vitamin C, vitamin K, vitamin A
	Pigmentation, desquamation	Niacin (pellagra)
	Pallor	Folate, iron, cobalamin, copper, biotin
Eyes	Angular palpebritis	Riboflavin
	Blepharitis	B vitamins
	Corneal vascularization	Riboflavin
	Dull, dry conjunctiva	Vitamin A
	Bitot's spot	Vitamin A
	Keratomalacia	Vitamin A
	Fundal capillary microaneurysms	Vitamin C
	Ophthalmoplegia	Thiamine (Wernicke's encephalopathy)
Mouth	Angular stomatitis	B vitamins, iron, protein
	Cheilosis	Riboflavin, niacin, pyridoxine, protein
	Atrophic lingual papillae	Niacin, iron, riboflavin, folate, cobalamin
	Glossitis (scarlet, raw)	Niacin, pyridoxine, riboflavin, folate, cobalamin
	Decreased sense of taste and smell	Vitamin A, ?zinc
	Swollen, bleeding gums	Vitamin C
Glands	Parotid enlargement	Protein
	"Sicca" syndrome	Ascorbic acid
	Thyroid enlargement	Iodine
Heart	Enlargement, tachycardia, high output failure	Thiamine (wet beriberi)
	Small heart, decreased output	Protein-energy
	Cardiomyopathy	Selenium
	Cardiac arrhythmias	Magnesium, potassium
Extremities	Edema	Protein, thiamine
	Muscle weakness	Protein-energy, selenium
	Bone and joint tenderness (child)	Vitamin C, vitamin A
	Osteopenia, bone pain	Vitamin D, calcium, phosphorus, vitamin C
Neurologic	Confabulation, disorientation	Thiamine (Korsakoff's psychosis)
	Decreased position and vibratory senses, ataxia	Cobalamin, thiamine
	Decreased tendon reflexes	Thiamine
	Weakness, paresthesias	Cobalamin, pyridoxine, thiamine
	Mental disorders	Cobalamin, niacin, thiamine, magnesium
Other	Delayed wound healing	Vitamin C, protein, ?zinc, ?EFA
	Hypogonadism, delayed puberty	Zinc
	Glucose intolerance	Chromium

insufficiency, by overenthusiastic fluid administration, and less often by the syndrome of inappropriate secretion of antidiuretic hormone. Fluid excess can usually be documented by the presence of edema, weight gain, intake greater than output, and decreasing hematocrit. Appropriate treatment for dilutional hyponatremia is water restriction, not sodium supplementation.

Hyponatremia caused by true sodium depletion (sodium deficit exceeds water deficit) is treated by administering sodium chloride orally, enterally, or intravenously. The sodium deficit can be estimated as follows:

$$Na^+ \text{ deficit (mEq)} = (\text{desired } [Na^+] - \text{observed } [Na^+]) \text{ mEq/L}$$
$$\times 0.55 \times \text{body weight in kg.}$$

Symptomatic hyponatremia (seizures or marked lethargy) is treated with intravenous 0.9% sodium chloride or, rarely, 3% sodium chloride. One half of the estimated deficit is administered over the first 24 hours, and serum sodium concentration is monitored every 2 to 4 hours. Rapid correction of hyponatremia has been associated with permanent neurologic deficits from central pontine myelinolysis, although the actual etiology of the condition is debated.

Treatment of sodium depletion associated with hypernatremia (water deficit exceeds sodium deficit) includes the repletion of both sodium and water. Symptomatic volume depletion should be treated with 0.9% sodium chloride to achieve the maximum increase in intravascular volume. Asymptomatic depletional hypernatremia can be treated with 0.45% sodium chloride. The serum concentration of sodium should be decreased slowly to prevent cerebral edema and seizures. Treatment of sodium depletion associated with a normal serum sodium level (water deficit equals sodium deficit) is accomplished by balanced repletion of both sodium and water usually in the form of 0.9% sodium chloride.

Chronic excessive sodium losses in diarrhea or in patients who have an ileostomy should be treated by increasing the daily oral intake of sodium and water, in the form of oral rehydration solution if necessary. Commercial products designed to replace sweat loss are widely available and are usually satisfactory for adult patients with normal renal function. Efforts to diminish stool and ostomy losses of sodium and water should be encouraged, including the avoidance of caffeine and any other food substances observed to increase intestinal output. Antidiarrheal and anticholinergic agents are often helpful. Octreotide (synthetic somatostatin), 50 to 200 μg, subcutaneously one to three times daily shows promise for diminishing fluid and electrolyte losses in some patients with chronic excessive ostomy output or diarrhea.

Sodium toxicity and severe hypernatremia can result from excessive administration of oral sodium chloride or intravenous sodium chloride solutions more concentrated than 0.9%. Symptoms of toxicity include vomiting, diarrhea, peripheral vascular collapse, respiratory depression, and death.

POTASSIUM[12-15]

Potassium is the primary cation of intracellular fluid (140–160 mEq/L), where it helps maintain osmotic pressure and acid–base balance within the cell. The 2% of total body potassium present in the extracellular fluid plays an essential role in influencing rest-ing membrane function, especially in cardiac muscle. No RDA has been established, but the estimated minimum daily requirement for adults is 2000 mg (51 mEq) and most adults consume 2000 to 6000 mg daily. It is abundant in many foods, particularly meats, milk, fruits, and some vegetables (Table 48-3).

Potassium is absorbed in the upper gastrointestinal tract and eliminated primarily by the kidneys, which regulate potassium homeostasis. Only a small amount normally is lost in stool and perspiration. Renal excretion is influenced by plasma potassium concentration, systemic pH, renal tubular flow rate, aldosterone, glucocorticoids, and the presence of nonabsorbable anions in tubular fluid. In chronic renal failure, elimination by the kidney decreases and gastrointestinal tract elimination increases, but not enough to compensate adequately.

Hypokalemia is defined as a serum potassium concentration less than 3.5 mEq/L. Symptoms may appear when the level falls below 3 mEq/L. Decreased intake is a rare cause of hypokalemia because potassium is present in most foods and the kidneys normally can decrease excretion to between 3 and 5 mEq/d. Hypokalemia commonly occurs as the result of shifts from the extracellular to the intracellular compartment, but total-body potassium may remain essentially normal. This intercompartmental shift can result from alkalosis, administration of glucose or insulin, treatment with β_2-adrenergic agonists, untreated leukemia, treatment of megaloblastic anemia, and periodic paralysis. When hypokalemia is the result of alkalosis, potassium supplementation should be given only if symptoms of hypokalemia are present or if hypokalemia persists after correction of the alkalosis.

True total-body potassium depletion is usually the result of increased urinary or gastrointestinal losses. Excessive urinary loss is caused by diuretics, alkalosis, corticosteroid excess (primary aldosteronism, Cushing's syndrome, corticosteroid therapy), some antibiotics (aminoglycoside, amphotericin, penicillin, rifampin), cisplatin, and, rarely, renal tubular acidosis. Depletion may also result from excessive gastrointestinal losses due to vomiting, gastric

TABLE 48-3
Selected Foods Rich in Potassium

FOOD	AMOUNT
Excellent Sources (500–800 mg)	
Canteloupe	1/2
Potato, white, baked	1 medium
Dates	1/2 cup
Raisins	1/2 cup
Figs, dried	4 medium
Avocado	1/2
Prune juice	1 cup
Very Good Sources (400–500 mg)	
Skim milk	8 ounces
Banana	1 medium
Orange juice	8 ounces
Grapefruit	1 cup
Nectarine	1 large
Watermelon	2 cups

suctioning, enterocutaneous fistulae, diarrhea, laxative abuse, excessive enemas, and villous adenomas of the large bowel. The hypokalemia associated with vomiting and gastric suctioning is largely due to renal potassium loss stimulated by hypovolemia and alkalosis. Rarely, potassium loss by severe sweating is sufficient to produce hypokalemia. Hypokalemia may occur in patients with hypercalcemia, but the mechanism is uncertain. Rarely, hypokalemia is caused by hypomagnesemia, and potassium repletion may be difficult or impossible until the magnesium level is corrected.

Manifestations of potassium depletion include confusion, drowsiness, decreased mental status, muscle weakness and cramps, myalgias, and, occasionally, glucose intolerance. Gastrointestinal manifestations include nausea, vomiting, diarrhea, ileus, and gastric atony. The kidney responds by excreting an acid urine, and intracellular potassium is exchanged for hydrogen ion, resulting in alkalosis. Continued hypokalemia damages the kidney's tubular concentrating mechanism, causing polyuria, nocturia, and polydipsia.

Total-body potassium depletion resulting from losses in excess of intake should be treated with supplemental administration of potassium. The total-body deficit cannot be estimated accurately. As an approximate guide, when the serum potassium concentration is greater than 3.0 mEq/L, a 1-mEq/L decrease in serum concentration indicates a 100- to 200-mEq deficit. Below 3.0 mEq/L, a 1-mEq/L decrease in serum concentration suggests a deficit of 200 to 400 mEq. Intravenous potassium supplementation is usually indicated for patients with serum potassium concentrations less than 2.5 mEq/L as well as for those with less severe hypokalemia who are symptomatic, have severe liver disease, or are receiving digitalis. Potassium infusion usually should not exceed 10 mEq/h in the absence of electrocardiographic monitoring or 40 mEq/h with monitoring. Administration rates faster than this are painful and irritating to peripheral veins and may induce symptoms of hyperkalemia. When the serum potassium concentration is between 2.5 and 3.5 mEq/L and no symptoms of hypokalemia are present, oral or enteral supplementation with 20 to 40 mEq of potassium, one to four times daily, should be started. For mild deficiencies, foods rich in potassium may be sufficient (see Table 48-3).

For intravenous therapy, the chloride salt is usually best but potassium phosphate is often appropriate for patients receiving total parenteral nutrition (TPN) and for treating the hypophosphatemia of diabetic ketoacidosis. In the presence of acidosis, potassium acetate is usually most appropriate. For oral administration, a variety of potassium salts, including gluconate, citrate, acetate, bicarbonate, and chloride, are available. The chloride salt is preferred except when hypokalemia is secondary to diarrhea or renal tubular acidosis, in which case one of the alkalinizing salts should be used. Oral potassium supplementation products are available in slow-release, matrix, or microencapsulated formulations, which are better tolerated than the liquid preparations (Table 48-4).[16] The current slow-release forms have greatly reduced the likelihood

TABLE 48-4
Oral Potassium Products Comparison Chart

DOSAGE FORMS	POTASSIUM SALT	BRAND NAMES	POTASSIUM CONTENT	COMMENTS
Liquid	Potassium chloride	Various	Soln 10, 20, 30 40 mEq/15 mL	Rapid absorption; low frequency of gastrointestinal ulceration; unpleasant taste
	Potassium acetate/bicarbonate/citrate	Trikates, Tri-K	Soln 45 mEq/15 mL	Preferred forms in patients with delayed gastrointestinal transit time; avoid nonchloride salts in metabolic alkalosis
	Potassium gluconate	Kaon	Soln 20 mEq/15 mL	
Powder	Potassium chloride	Various	Packet 15, 20, 25 mEq	
	Potassium	K-Lyte	Packet 25 mEq	
	Bicarbonate/citrate	K-Lyte DS	Packet 50 mEq	Must be dissolved in water before use; avoid nonchloride salts in metabolic alkalosis
Effervescent tablets	Potassium chloride	Kaochlor-Eff	Tab 20 mEq	
		Klorvess	Tab 20 mEq	
		K-Lyte/Cl	Tab 25 mEq	
		K-Lyte/Cl 50	Tab 50 mEq	
Sustained-release capsules, tablets	Potassium chloride	Kaon-Cl	Tab 6.7 mEq	Wax matrix or polymer-coated crystals in gelatin capsule; bioequivalent to liquid forms; avoid in patients with delayed gastrointestinal transit time
		Micro-K, Slow-K	Cap 8 mEq	
		Kaon Cl 10, K-Tab, Klotrix	Tab 10 mEq	
		K-Dur	Tab 20 mEq	
Salt substitutes	Potassium chloride	Adolph's, Morton's, NuSalt, No Salt, Various	Pwdr 50–70 mEq/tsp	Inexpensive dietary source; prescribe specific amount to avoid hyperkalemia; contraindicated in oliguria, severe renal disease

Adapted in part from Knoben JE, Anderson PO. Handbook of clinical drug data. 6th ed. Hamilton, IL: Drug Intelligence Publications, 1988:607.
Adapted in part from Stanaszek WF, Romankiewicz JA. Current approaches to management of potassium deficiency. Drug Int Clin Pharm 1985;19:176.

of small bowel ulcers and strictures that resulted from previous formulations.

Adequate potassium supplementation will correct the serum potassium level within hours unless ongoing renal or gastrointestinal wasting is severe. However, in chronically depleted patients supplementation for weeks is required to restore total-body potassium levels to normal. Excessive supplementation will produce hyperkalemia especially in patients with renal insufficiency. Serum potassium levels greater than 6.5 mEq/L are associated with moderate risk and those above 8.0 mEq/L with severe risk. Cardiac effects of potassium excess include peaked T waves on the electrocardiogram, bradycardia, asystole, and ventricular fibrillation. Other signs include skeletal muscle weakness, fasciculations, areflexia or hyperreflexia, paralysis, fatigue, and lassitude.

Spurious hyperkalemia or spurious normalization of hypokalemia can result from red blood cell hemolysis during or after phlebotomy. Extreme leukocytosis may produce the same effect without signs of hemolysis, owing to release of potassium by the white cells. Thrombocytosis can also produce pseudohyperkalemia because the platelets release potassium during the clotting process. This can be avoided by using plasma instead of serum for potassium determination in patients with very high platelet counts.

CALCIUM

Calcium is the most abundant mineral in the body. Ninety-nine percent, about 1.2 kg, is in bone. The remaining 1% is crucial for nerve transmission, muscle contractility, coagulation, and enzyme regulation.[13]

The USRDA is 1200 mg/d. Typical American diets provide a mean of approximately 750 mg daily.[17] Milk and dairy products are rich sources of calcium as are leafy green vegetables (except spinach) and fish with edible bones such as sardines and salmon. Approximately 150 to 200 mg is secreted daily into the gastrointestinal tract.[18] Only about 30% of ingested calcium is absorbed. It is actively transported in the duodenum but most is absorbed more distally in the small bowel. The ion is filtered by the glomerulus, and 97% to 99% is reabsorbed by the tubular epithelial cells. Some calcium is eliminated in sweat.

Forty percent of serum calcium is bound to proteins, 15% is complexed with anions, and 45% is in the ionized, physiologically active form.[18] A change in serum albumin concentration will result in a change in the total serum calcium concentration and no significant change in the ionized calcium concentration. As a general rule, for each 1g/dL decrease in serum albumin, total serum calcium concentration deceases by 0.8 mg/dL.[19]

The conditions that can cause hypocalcemia requiring calcium supplementation include vitamin D deficiency, hypoparathyroidism, pseudohypoparathyroidism, hypomagnesemia, acute pancreatitis, neoplasms with osteoblastic metastases, malabsorption syndromes, and medications including aminoglycosides, cisplatin, mithramycin, citrated blood, phosphates, and anticonvulsants.[15] Signs and symptoms of hypocalcemia include latent tetany (positive Chvostek's or Trousseau's sign), frank tetany, hyperreflexia, paresthesias, seizures, mental status changes, increased intracranial pressure, and choreoathetotic movements. The electrocardiogram shows prolonged QT intervals with normal QRS complexes.[15,20]

Chronic calcium deficiency causes rickets in children and osteomalacia in adults. While osteomalacia results from inadequate intake, absorption, or metabolism of calcium, vitamin D, or phosphate, the etiology of osteoporosis is more controversial and probably involves additional factors, including estrogen and progesterone status, lifelong physical activity, and intake of other nutrients. Of the four clinical methods in current use to quantitate bone density, dual-energy radiographic absorptiometry (DRA) appears to be more precise and accurate than single-photon absorptiometry (SPA), dual-photon absorptiometry (DPA), or quantitative computed tomography (QCT).[21] Histologic examination of bone in conjunction with Tetracycline labeling is required for accurate distinction between osteomalacia and osteoporosis.

The treatment of asymptomatic hypocalcemia must be based on knowledge of the cause. For example, treatment with supplemental calcium may be inappropriate in chronic renal failure and hypoalbuminemia or only adjunctive in vitamin deficiency, hypoparathyroidism, and hypomagnesemia. Acute symptomatic hypocalcemia should be treated immediately to prevent life-threatening laryngospasm, seizures, and cardiac arrhythmias. Ten to 20 ml of 10% calcium gluconate solution (100 to 200 mg elemental calcium) is given over 5 minutes. This should be followed with an infusion of calcium gluconate in 5% dextrose at 1 to 2 mg/kg/h of elemental calcium.[20] Serum calcium level should normalize in 6 to 12 hours. Blood pressure, electrocardiogram, and serum calcium level should be monitored at 6- to 8-hour intervals until symptoms are controlled.

Patients who have chronic hypocalcemia or osteopenia on the basis of poor intake or decreased absorption should be treated orally with 500 to 2500 mg of elemental calcium daily administered in two to four doses. A number of oral calcium salts varying in elemental calcium content are available (Table 48–5). Calcium supplements may cause constipation, especially in the elderly. However, because it is poorly absorbed, oral calcium can occasionally cause diarrhea and dehydration in patients with short bowel syndrome. When calcium supplementation alone does not maintain adequate serum levels, vitamin D should be added to increase intestinal absorption of the ion. The dose varies greatly from patient to patient. The usual dose range is 25,000 to 150,000 units orally per day of ergocalciferol (vitamin D_2). To avoid hypercalciuria, renal damage and soft tissue calcifications, therapy should begin at a low dose and be titrated up at 3- to 4-week intervals based on 24-hour urine calcium and serum calcium values. A urine calcium level greater than 300 mg per 24 hours is an indication to reduce the vitamin D dose. Hypercalcemia is a late manifestation

TABLE 48–5
Selected Oral Calcium Supplements

SALT	% ELEMENTAL CALCIUM	TABLET SIZE (MG) (MG CALCIUM/TAB)
Calcium carbonate	40	
Caltrate		1500 (600)
Os-Cal 500		1250 (500)
Tums		500 (200)
Calcium lactate	13	
Generic		650 (85)
Calcium phosphate	38	
Posture		800 (300)
Calcium citrate	21	
Citracal		950 (200)

of vitamin D toxicity, which requires several weeks to resolve in patients receiving vitamin D_2. Other vitamin D preparations are described in the section on vitamin D.

Excessive calcium intake may predispose some persons to kidney stones but is rarely the cause of hypercalcemia except at doses exceeding 3 g/d or unless supplemental vitamin D is also being given. Symptoms and signs include anorexia, nausea, vomiting, constipation, polyuria, fatigue, weakness, decreased deep tendon reflexes, confusion, lethargy, shortened QT interval, prolonged PR interval, prolonged QRS interval, and cardiac arrest.[19]

PHOSPHORUS

Phosphorus is the predominant intracellular anion.[22,23] It is essential for the structural integrity of cells, regulation of enzyme systems, and generation and storage of energy. It effects delivery of oxygen to tissue by regulating the concentration of 2,3-diphosphoglycerate in red blood cells. However, 85% of the body's phosphorus is in bone.

The requirements for phosphorus parallel those of calcium. The USRDA is 1200 mg, and typical daily intake is 800 to 1500 mg. It is abundant in most foods, especially dairy products and in soft drinks. Fifty to 80% of ingested phosphorus along with some of that which is secreted by the gastrointestinal tract is absorbed, virtually all in the small intestine. Absorption is promoted by 1,25-dihydroxy vitamin D. The kidney regulates phosphorus homeostasis through glomerular filtration and tubular reabsorption. Eighty to 90% of the filtered phosphorus is normally reabsorbed, but this can increase to 99.8% when dietary intake of phosphorus is low.[22] Parathyroid hormone inhibits the tubular reabsorption of phosphorus.

Normal serum phosphorus concentration is 2.5 to 4.5 mg/dL in adults and substantially higher in children. A serum concentration between 1.0 and 2.5 mg/dL in an adult is considered moderate hypophosphatemia. Levels less than 1.0 mg/dL constitute severe hypophosphatemia and are usually symptomatic.[22,23] Hypophosphatemia is virtually nonexistent in healthy humans because of the abundance of phosphorus in foods and the efficient renal conservation mechanism.

Hypophosphatemia occurs among hospitalized patients more frequently than is generally appreciated since levels are often not measured. Causes include decreased intestinal absorption, increased urinary losses, and shifts of serum phosphorus into the intracellular compartment. Reduced absorption results from therapy with phosphate-binding antacids, malabsorption, vitamin D deficiency, and parathyroid hormone deficiency. Increased renal excretion occurs in diseases of the proximal tubule, diuretic therapy, osmotic diuresis, hyperparathyroidism, severe thermal burns, and chronic corticosteroid therapy.[22,23] Hypophosphatemia and phosphate depletion commonly occur as a result of insufficient administration of supplemental phosphorus when phosphate-rich lean tissue is being restored.[22] Carbohydrate infusion, enterally or parenterally, also lowers the serum phosphorus concentration by shifting it from the plasma to the intracellular compartment. The causes of hypophosphatemia are often multifactorial, especially in alcoholism, alcoholic withdrawal, and recovery from diabetic ketoacidosis.[22,23]

Signs and symptoms of severe hypophosphatemia include hemolytic anemia, impaired white blood cell function, metabolic encephalopathy, seizures, paresthesias, muscle weakness, rhabdomyolysis, and decreased glucose utilization. Hypophosphatemia promotes tissue hypoxia because it lowers red blood cell levels of 2,3-diphosphoglycerate. This shifts the hemoglobin-oxygen dissociation curve to the left, which means that less oxygen is released in the tissues where it is needed.

When hypophosphatemia is the result of antacid therapy, stopping the antacid is usually sufficient. Phosphate supplementation is indicated for hypophosphatemia of other etiologies, as prophylaxis during nutrition support, and, debatably, during the treatment of diabetic ketoacidosis. When oral or enteral intake is possible, phosphorus supplementation can be provided with milk or other oral preparations (Table 48-6).[22-25] Intravenous supplementation should be used for persons who are unable to take oral preparations or those with symptomatic or severe hypophosphatemia (serum level less than 1 mg/dL). One of two dosing regimens for adults is commonly used:

1. Infuse 0.08 mmol/kg for recent and uncomplicated hypophosphatemia and 0.16 mmol/kg for prolonged hypophosphatemia. Increase the dose 25% to 50% for symptomatic hypophosphatemia and decrease it 25% to 50% if hypercalcemia is present. The initial dose is infused over 6 hours and should not exceed 15 mmol.[26]
2. Infuse 0.32 mmol/kg over 12 hours if renal function is normal and there is no hypercalcemia.[27]

Serial serum concentrations should be monitored and additional supplementation given as necessary to maintain a serum phosphorus concentration greater than 2.0 mg/dL.[26,27]

Excessive oral administration of phosphate will cause diarrhea. Chronic excessive ingestion can cause hypocalcemia, osteopenia, and possibly renal stones. Too rapid or excessive intravenous infusion can precipitously lower the serum calcium level and cause damaging precipitation of calcium phosphate in the renal tubules and other tissues.

Doses and concentrations of phosphorus should be recorded in millimoles or milligrams of elemental phosphorus and not milliequivalents. This is because the number of milliequivalents varies with pH since the phosphate ion exists in physiologic solutions as a mixture of HPO_4^{--} and $H_2PO_4^-$ and the relative amounts are determined by pH.

MAGNESIUM

Magnesium is found intracellularly both in bone (60%) and soft tissue (40%). Only 1% is in the extracellular compartment. It is critical for many enzymatic functions, normal growth, wound healing, neuromuscular activity, myocardial contractility, membrane stability, and coagulation.[28]

The USRDA is 350 mg (29 mEq), and the typical adult diet provides 20 to 40 mEq of magnesium daily. Cocoa, nuts, cereals, seafood, meats, legumes, and green vegetables are rich food sources.[28,29] Only 30% to 60% of ingested magnesium is normally absorbed in the small intestine. Elimination occurs primarily in the kidney where it is filtered by the glomerulus and reabsorbed in the tubule so that normally only 2% to 3% of the filtered load is excreted.[28,29]

When renal and intestinal functions are normal, magnesium homeostasis is maintained over a wide range of dietary magnesium intake. The kidneys can excrete as much as 1000 mEq/d, but on very low intake, total renal and fecal losses decrease to less than

TABLE 48–6
Phosphate Products Comparison Chart

PRODUCT	PHOSPHORUS		SODIUM		POTASSIUM
	Mg	mmol	mg	mEq	mEq
Oral					
Fleets Phospho Soda (per mL)	128	4.1	111	4.8	0
K-Phos Modified Formula (per tablet)	125	4	67	2.9	1.4
K-Phos Neutral (per tablet)	250	8.1	301	13.1	1.4
Neutra-Phos Plain (per cap or 75 mL)	250	8.1	164	7.1	7.1
Neutra-Phos K (per cap or 75 mL)	250	8.1	0	0	14.3
Skim Milk (per quart)	1000	32	552	24	40
Intravenous					
Potassium Phosphate Abbott (per mL) Various	94	3	0	0	4.4
Sodium Phosphate Abbott (per mL)	94	3	93	4	0

From Knoben JE, Anderson PO. Handbook of clinical drug data. 6th ed. Hamilton, IL: Drug Intelligence Publications, 1988: 604.
Benberez K. Hypophosphatemia and potassium supplementation. Hosp Pharm 1980;15:611.

1 mEq/d. Because magnesium is primarily an intracellular cation, deficiency may exist in the presence of normal, increased, or decreased serum concentrations. Thus, subclinical deficiency secondary to decreased intake may occur in protein–calorie malnutrition, starvation, and alcoholism.[28]

Symptomatic magnesium deficiency is usually the result of decreased absorption of increased losses in urine or via the gastrointestinal tract. Intestinal absorption is decreased in malabsorption syndromes, especially in patients with extensive small bowel resection.[30] Excessive urinary loss, usually due to decreased tubular reabsorption, occurs in a variety of circumstances. Numerous medications promote renal loss of magnesium including diuretics, antibiotics (amphotericin B, gentamicin, ticarcillin, carbenicillin), antineoplastic agents (cisplatin), osmotic agents (mannitol), and cardiac glycosides.[28-30] Increased renal losses also occur in hypercalcemia, renal tubular dysfunction, acute and chronic alcoholism, diabetes mellitus, hyperparathyroidism, hyperaldosteronism, and hypophosphatemia. Prolonged losses of gastrointestinal fluids accompanied by infusion of magnesium-free parenteral fluids can also cause magnesium deficiency.[28,29] Hypomagnesemia due to a shift of magnesium from the extracellular to the intracellular compartment occurs with refeeding, with treatment of diabetic ketoacidosis, after parathyroidectomy, in acute pancreatitis, and with correction of acidosis in renal failure.[28] Hypomagnesemia is often associated with and can be a cause of hypocalcemia, hypokalemia, and hypophosphatemia.[28]

Hypomagnesemia affects neuromuscular and cardiac functions and mental status.[13] It may present as tremor of the extremities and tongue, myoclonic jerks, ataxia, tetany, coma, ventricular dysrhythmias, tachycardia, hypotension, or cardiac arrest. Psychiatric disturbances, which may be subtle, include apathy, depression, delirium, hallucinations, and psychosis.[28,30]

Serum magnesium concentrations do not correlate well with total-body stores, but it is reasonable to assume that there is magnesium depletion when the serum concentration is less than 1.0 mg/dL.[28] Patients with serum levels between 1.0 and 1.5 mg/dL may be significantly depleted and usually have detectable symptoms, although they may be subtle. A load test can be used to assess total-body deficiency. Twenty-four-hour urine magnesium concentration is measured on 3 consecutive days. On the second day, 40 mEq of magnesium is given intravenously over 5 to 8 hours and urine output of magnesium is compared with that of the day before and the day after. Normal patients retain 20% or less of the dose, while depleted patients retain more than 20%. The validity and reliability of the test still need to be assessed in a variety of conditions.

Patients with mild deficiency or ongoing magnesium losses should receive foods rich in magnesium and an oral magnesium supplement if required.[28] A variety of magnesium salts, including oxide, hydroxide, carbonate, chloride, and sulfate, are available (Table 48-7). Persons with normal renal function may be given 8 to 24 mEq (97 to 292 mg) of magnesium orally four times daily.[31] If renal function is even mildly decreased, the dose must be lowered and serum levels monitored closely since toxic serum levels can develop quickly.

The magnesium ion is poorly absorbed, accounting for its effectiveness as a saline cathartic. Therefore, it is best to give small doses frequently. Nevertheless, patients with magnesium deficiency due to malabsorption often cannot be repleted by oral supplementation. Magnesium gluconate is quite soluble but contains only up to 2.4 mEq of magnesium per tablet. An enteric-coated magnesium chloride formulation (Slo-Mag) and a sustained-release magnesium lactate preparation (Mag-Tab SR) have been released and may be better absorbed. Potassium-sparing diuretics such as spironolactone decrease urinary magnesium losses and may be useful especially for patients who are also hypokalemic.[29]

Parenteral magnesium should be given to hypomagnesemic patients who are unresponsive to oral therapy. Outpatients can be treated intramuscularly with 2.0 mL of 50% magnesium sulfate solution (8 mEq) in each buttock, every 1 to 7 days. Few patients will tolerate this for very long, and intermittent infusions of magnesium usually along with other electrolytes via an indwelling central venous catheter are sometimes required. Guidelines for acute parenteral magnesium replacement of symptomatic or severe hypomagnesemia are as follows:

1. To replace by the intravenous route, load with magnesium sulfate 6 g (49 mEq) intravenously over 5 hours. Follow with 10 g (83 mEq) during the next 24 hours and 6 g daily for the following 3 days.[32] Life-threatening symptoms including seizures and dysrhythmias can be treated initially with 4 g magnesium sulfate (40 mL of 10% solution, 33 mEq magnesium) intravenously over 4 minutes.[30]
2. To replace intramuscularly, load with 2 g magnesium sulfate (16 mEq) intramuscularly every 2 hours for four doses, then 2 g every 4 hours for four doses. On the second day give 1 g magnesium sulfate (8 mEq) intramuscularly every 4 hours for six doses.[30]

Serum levels usually increase to normal in a few days, but total-body repletion requires several weeks. The doses recommended should be reduced by 25% to 50% for patients with renal impairment. If hypocalcemia or hypokalemia co-exists with hypomagnesemia, magnesium should be administered first. The serum potassium level usually increases rapidly to normal, and the serum calcium level will usually return to normal within 4 days of magnesium replacement.[28]

Rapid administration of magnesium may cause transient hypotension, flushing, and sweating. Replacement therapy should include monitoring of clinical response, monitoring of respirations, assessment of deep tendon reflexes, and determination of serial serum magnesium concentrations.[28,30] Hypermagnesemia should be avoided. At serum concentrations of 3 to 9 mEq/L toxicity can include cutaneous vasodilation, nausea, vomiting, drowsiness, lethargy, hypotension, bradycardia, prolonged PR interval, and depressed deep tendon reflexes. Above concentrations of 10 mEq/L, muscle paralysis, respiratory depression, narcosis, widened QRS complexes, and occasionally fatal dysrhythmias can occur. Above concentrations of 14 mEq/L, asystole and cardiac arrest are likely.

Deficiencies of Trace Minerals

At present, approximately 15 trace minerals are known to be important in mammalian physiology. Deficiency states in humans have been reported for iron, iodine, zinc, copper, chromium, selenium, and possibly manganese and molybdenum. These minerals along with fluoride and cobalt are generally accepted as essential in humans.

Except for iron deficiency, trace mineral deficiencies are rarely diagnosed. This may be because they are rare or, more likely, because it is difficult to recognize and diagnose deficiencies until

TABLE 48–7
Magnesium Products Comparison Chart

PRODUCT	DOSAGE FORMS*	MAGNESIUM CONTENT† (mEq/g)	COMMENTS
Magnesium carbonate	Tab 500 mg	23.7	Poorly soluble; low absorption
Magnesium chloride	Soln 200 mg/mL	9.8	Used IV or orally as a 5% solution; alternative to parenteral $MgSO_4$
	Enteric coated tab 535 mg		Slo-Mag
Magnesium citrate	Soln 297 mg/5 mL	4.4	Oral use only
Magnesium gluconate	Tab 300, 500 mg	4.8	Very soluble; well absorbed; produces no diarrhea
Magnesium hydroxide	Susp 200–400 mg/5 mL	34.0	Readily available in combination antacid formulations. Start with 5-mL susp or 1 tab; increase as tolerated to qid. May require gastric acid to be absorbed; inexpensive
	Tab 300, 600 mg		
Magnesium lactate	Sustained release Tab 700 mg	9.8	Mag-Tab SR
Magnesium oxide	Cap 140 mg	49.6	Poorly soluble; net absorption low especially in malabsorptive states
	Tab 250, 400, 420, 500 mg		
Magnesium sulfate	Soln 10%, 12.5%, 50%	8.1	Use IV, IM, or PO

Magnesium products exhibit variable absorption; dose patient incrementally until no further rise in serum magnesium occurs or until diarrhea ensures. Oral magnesium alleviates diarrhea in some patients with malabsorption.
† *1 mEq = 12 mg = 0.5 mmol Mg.*
Adapted from Knoben JE, Anderson PO. Handbook of clinical drug data. 6th ed. Hamilton, IL: Drug Intelligence Publications, 1988:602.
Flink EB. Magnesium deficiency: Etiology and clinical spectrum. Acta Med Scand Supplement 1981;647:125.

they are far advanced. Much that has been learned in recent years about trace mineral deficiencies in humans has come from observations of patients on long-term TPN. TPN fluids are now generally supplemented with up to six trace minerals—zinc, copper, chromium, manganese, selenium, and molybdenum. Parenteral iron and iodine are also available.

IRON

The USRDA for iron is 18 mg. However, the intake recommended for menstruating females in the most recent edition of the RDA is 15 mg/d, a decrease from the previous RDA of 18 mg/d. The recommended amount during pregnancy is 30 mg/d. Rich dietary sources include red meat, fish, oysters, brewer's yeast, egg yolks, figs, dates, molasses, and dried beans.[33]

Iron is absorbed primarily in the duodenum and upper jejunum. Approximately 10% of ingested iron is normally absorbed, but this can increase to 30% in deficiency states. Absorption is also enhanced by gastric acid, by ascorbic acid and other organic acids, and during pregnancy, growth, and development.[33-35] Absorption is decreased when iron forms an insoluble complex as with phytates, phosphates, or antacids.[35-36] Once absorbed, iron is stored as ferritin in the liver, spleen, and bone marrow. Very little iron is excreted. Approximately 1 mg is lost daily via the gastrointestinal tract, and menstrual losses are approximately 15 mg per month.[35]

Iron deficiency may result from loss of blood, increased utilization, inadequate diet, or malabsorption. Common causes of iron deficiency include chronic gastrointestinal bleeding, excessive menstruation, and multiple pregnancies. Deficiency that is due in part to malabsorption occurs in celiac sprue, achlorhydria, and postgastrectomy states.[35,36]

Iron deficiency results in anemia characterized by microcytic and hypochromic red blood cells. There are decreased values for mean red blood cell volume, serum iron, and serum ferritin and elevated values for red blood cell distribution width, iron-binding capacity, transferrin, and free protoporphyrin. Percent saturation of transferrin is decreased. The absence of stainable iron in bone marrow aspirate provides the definitive diagnosis. None of the less invasive blood tests are specific for iron deficiency, but low serum ferritin followed by low percent transferrin saturation are most specific for adult patients of all ages.[37] Clinical signs and symptoms of iron deficiency reflect anemia and the resulting mismatch in the demands for oxygen and the diminished oxygen delivery to tissues. They include weakness, dizziness, decreased exercise tolerance, and increased heart rate. There is some evidence that symptoms due to iron deficiency may occur before red blood cell changes are apparent.

Therapy for iron deficiency anemia includes the identification and control of the underlying cause as well as correction of the anemia with supplemental iron. The goal of iron supplementation is to replete stores and correct the anemia. Hemoglobin concentration, mean red blood cell volume, and red blood cell distribution width are useful indicators of response. Therapy should be continued for at least 3 months after these measurements have stabilized. Based on the maximum rates of hemoglobin regeneration and iron absorption, the maximum adult oral dose of elemental iron need not exceed 200 mg/d.[34] Iron is better absorbed in the ferrous than ferric state and much better absorbed in organic forms such as heme. Inorganic iron is available as the sulfate, gluconate,

and fumarate salts. These are absorbed equally well but differ in the elemental iron content and therefore the number of tablets required to provide 200 mg of elemental iron. The usual adult dose is one tablet of ferrous sulfate USP 325 mg (65 mg iron) or equivalent administered three times a day between meals.[34] To optimize absorption, iron supplements should be taken in divided doses and on an empty stomach. However, this is more likely to cause abdominal pain, cramps, and nausea compared with taking the dose with meals. Iron repletion can be accomplished with less risk of gastrointestinal side effects by giving one or two tablets daily. Sustained-release and enteric-coated iron formulations are available. They are more expensive, there is no evidence that they decrease gastrointestinal side effects, and they may not be well absorbed if dissolution occurs distal to the primary absorption sites in the duodenum and upper jejunum.[34] Many iron supplements also contain ascorbic acid to enhance absorption or stool softeners to decrease constipation, but generally the dose of both is inadequate to produce the desired response.[34] Tetracycline and antacids impair absorption of iron, which should not be taken within 2 hours of these medications.

Parenteral iron therapy is used if oral therapy is not possible, if there is no response to oral therapy, or if iron loss from intractable bleeding exceeds absorption by the oral route. Iron dextran (Imferon) is available for intramuscular or intravenous use. The total dose required to replete stores can be calculated based on the patient's weight and observed hemoglobin using the equations or tables printed in the package insert. A test dose of 25 mg (0.5 mL Imferon) should be given initially, and thereafter the daily dose should not exceed 100 mg (2 ml Imferon). Intramuscular administration should be by deep injection using the Z-track technique to decrease the risk of permanent skin discoloration.[34] Because of this risk and pain at the injection site, the intravenous route is preferred.

The dose may be given intravenously over 2 to 3 hours diluted in normal saline. It can also be added to TPN mixtures that do not contain fat. Parenteral iron, especially intravenous therapy, has been associated with adverse reactions of anaphylaxis, urticaria, rashes, sweating, dizziness, fever, headache, nausea, and vomiting. The likelihood of adverse reactions appears to be directly related to the rate of administration.[34]

Iron overload as a result of excessive iron in the diet is rare in the United States but can occur as a result of excessive intake of iron supplements or frequent blood transfusions. The estimated minimum toxic oral dose for healthy adults is 100 mg/d,[38] but this amount may cause iron overload damage to a significant number of persons. Excess iron is stored in the liver, kidneys, heart, and other organs and results in hemosiderosis. Acute iron toxicity can occur after ingesting large amounts (> 20 mg/kg), and a lethal oral dose is between 200 and 250 mg/kg.

ZINC

Zinc is a cofactor for many enzymes that participate in the metabolism of carbohydrate, fat, and protein.[39] It is necessary for cell growth and proliferation, sexual maturation, reproduction, dark adaptation, and night vision and may play a role in taste acuity, wound healing, immune defenses, and hemostasis.[40]

The USRDA is 15 mg/d. Net absorption, primarily in the small intestine, is 20% or less. Consequently, the amount of zinc excreted in the stool each day is only a little less than the amount ingested and also the recommended amount of zinc intravenously is 3 mg/d. Homeostasis is maintained by losses in urine, about 2 mg/d, and a little is lost in sweat.[39] Food sources rich in zinc are meat, eggs, milk, and seafood, especially oysters.

Zinc deficiency is probably much more prevalent than is generally appreciated. Overt deficiency in otherwise healthy persons is not reported in the United States, but growth of children in certain areas of the country appears to be limited by inadequate dietary zinc.[41] Persons with gastrointestinal diseases, including Crohn's disease, ulcerative colitis, short bowel syndrome, jejunoileal bypass, cystic fibrosis, pancreatic insufficiency, and chronic diarrhea of other causes, are at increased risk of zinc deficiency because of increased gastrointestinal losses and decreased intake. Diarrheal stool contains approximately 17 mg/kg of zinc, while small bowel fluid averages about 12 mg/kg of zinc.[42] Other conditions predisposing to zinc deficiency are cirrhosis, alcoholism, anorexia nervosa, nephrotic syndrome, sickle cell anemia, pregnancy, pica, and the administration of penicillamine.[39,40,43]

Clinical manifestations of zinc deficiency are growth retardation, scaly skin lesions, alopecia, diarrhea, apathy, night blindness, poor wound healing, and dysgeusia.[40] Acute zinc deficiency manifested as a rash especially around the nose, mouth, and groin can develop within weeks in patients receiving TPN containing no zinc. Laboratory documentation of zinc status is difficult and unreliable. Serum or plasma concentrations are commonly used. They correlate poorly with total body zinc status, but plasma levels are usually low in patients who are severely deficient. Other measurements such as zinc content of white blood cells, platelets, saliva, and hair have been used but with little documented improvement in diagnostic accuracy.[40]

Zinc supplementation should be given to patients at risk of developing zinc deficiency and those with clinical signs and symptoms of deficiency.[40,44,45] Many oral multivitamin and mineral formulations contain zinc, usually 10 to 20 mg per dose. Zinc sulfate, 220 mg (50 mg zinc), given one to three times a day is more effective but may cause symptoms of gastric irritation, especially at the higher doses. For patients requiring parenteral therapy, zinc is available in several multiple trace element products and as a single entity for intravenous use. Parenteral zinc therapy should meet the normal daily parenteral needs (2.5–4.0 mg) and replace any deficits or increased losses.[44,46] It is not unusual for adult home TPN patients to receive 10 to 25 mg zinc daily in the TPN fluid.

Zinc is considered one of the least toxic heavy metals. The estimated minimum toxic oral dose for normal adults is 500 mg/d,[38] although long-term ingestion of lower doses may induce copper deficiency. Acute ingestion of 12 g of zinc sulfate produced only drowsiness and an increase in serum lipase and amylase concentrations.[39] Intravenous doses of 40 to 80 mg over a few hours have been administered to critically ill patients with no adverse effects.[39]

COPPER

Copper is an essential component of several metalloenzymes, including ceruloplasmin and superoxide dismutase.[47] It is critical for normal skeletal development, normal development of the central nervous system, taste sensation, iron absorption, and pigmen-

tation.[40,47,48] The recommended safe and adequate dietary intake for adults is 1.5 to 3 mg/d. Parenteral copper requirements are 0.3 mg/d[49] if losses are not abnormal. Requirements are increased if there is increased loss of gastrointestinal fluids.[49] Liver and legumes are good sources, and approximately 40% is absorbed, primarily in the stomach and small intestine. Most of the absorbed copper is excreted in bile and undergoes an enterohepatic circulation. Elimination is primarily in the stool. Less than 5% is eliminated renally, and dermal losses are insignificant.[47] It is present in plasma tightly bound to ceruloplasmin, a 160,000-dalton molecular weight protein made in the liver.

Copper deficiency in adults is exceedingly rare. It can occur in patients who are receiving TPN without copper and patients getting chelating agents such as D-penicillamine or large doses of zinc.[5] Deficiency has occurred in premature infants and in infants and children with generalized malnutrition, prolonged diarrhea, malabsorption syndromes, and Menkes' syndrome (a genetic defect in copper absorption) and during prolonged TPN without copper supplementation.[40,49] The laboratory assessment of copper status is difficult because serum concentrations do not correlate well with tissue levels. Copper concentrations in urine, hair, and red blood cells as well as serum ceruloplasmin concentrations have been used to assess copper status[40] but are not convincingly better than serum copper concentrations. Clinical manifestations of deficiency are microcytic and hypochromic anemia, leukopenia, neutropenia, and scurvy-like skeletal abnormalities.[40,48,49] In the appropriate setting these findings, especially neutropenia or anemia unresponsive to iron therapy, and a low serum copper value are sufficient to make the diagnosis.

Copper supplementation is indicated when deficiency is diagnosed and should also be considered when there are increased gastrointestinal fluid losses from diarrhea or fistulae, especially biliary tract fistulae.[49] Oral supplementation can be provided as multivitamin and mineral preparations. They usually contain copper sulfate, which provides 0.4 mg of elemental copper per milligram of the anhydrous salt. For adults, a daily oral dose of 2 to 3 mg elemental copper is adequate to treat deficiency states. For infants and children, the dose is 0.05 to 0.1 mg/kg/d. The estimated minimum toxic oral dose for normal adults is 100 mg/d.[38] Copper is a component of several intravenous trace mineral formulations and is available as a single entity for intravenous use. The amount recommended for TPN in adults is 0.3 to 0.5 mg/d of elemental copper, which should be reduced to 0.15 mg/d for patients with cholestasis.[50,51] The amount for TPN in children is 0.02 mg/kg/d. The intravenous doses that have been given for treatment of deficiency are 2 to 7 mg/d for adults and 0.05 mg/kg/d for infants.[52,53]

SELENIUM

Selenium is an essential part of the enzyme glutathione peroxidase. This enzyme protects against tissue damage from peroxides that occur during tissue oxidation. The antioxidant function of selenium is similar to that of vitamin E. There is no USRDA for selenium. Recommended dietary allowances, established for the first time in 1989, are 0.055 mg/d for women and 0.07 mg/d for men. Dietary sources are meat, poultry, fish, and cereal grains. Selenium is absorbed in the small intestine and excreted in urine and stool.[54,55]

Absorption of selenite solutions and selenomethionine is greater than 90%, but absorption from food is less certain.[56]

Selenium status can be assessed by measurement of plasma, serum, whole blood, or tissue concentrations of the element or by determination of glutathione peroxidase activity in red blood cells, white blood cells, or platelets.[40,55] Human deficiency secondary to inadequate dietary intake occurs in areas of China where the soil is low in selenium and presents as a dilated cardiomyopathy (Keshan disease). Below-normal blood selenium levels have been reported in patients with inflammatory bowel disease, celiac sprue, enterocutaneous fistulae, cirrhosis, and cancer as well as in patients receiving TPN and tube feeding. In addition, functional changes consistent with selenium deficiency have been reported in patients receiving long-term parenteral nutrition therapy. The changes, which included myositis, weakness, and cardiomyopathy, resolved with selenium supplementation,[57] but fatal cardiomyopathy was reported in an untreated patient.[58] For oral use the highest recommended adult intake is 0.2 mg/d and the estimated minimum toxic dose is 1.0 mg/d.[38] The optimal daily intravenous dose of selenium for long-term TPN patients is not established but 0.02 to 0.08 mg/d appears to be adequate.[50,51] It is usually given as sodium selenite, but sodium selenate or L-selenomethionine would also be suitable. To treat deficiency states, an intravenous dose of 0.1 to 0.2 mg/d has been used.[57]

CHROMIUM

Chromium potentiates the action of insulin at the cell receptor level. It exists in foods as a complex known as the "glucose tolerance factor." Chromium also may play a role in lipoprotein metabolism.[40,59] The estimated safe and adequate dietary intake for adults is 0.05 to 0.2 mg/d.[1] Rich sources of chromium are brewer's yeast, spices, vegetable oils, liver and kidney. Only 2% of dietary chromium is absorbed, so most is excreted in the stool. The small amount excreted in urine is increased by glucose loading and high insulin levels. The recommended amount in TPN is 0.015 to 0.025 mg/d.

Chromium deficiency has been reported in patients receiving long-term parenteral nutrition therapy after massive intestinal resections.[60–62] Clinical manifestations included hyperglycemia, relative insensitivity to exogenous insulin, peripheral neuropathy, and weight loss. Intravenous chromium supplementation resulted in normalization of serum glucose concentrations, weight gain, and resolution of the neuropathy. Assessment of chromium status is difficult since concentrations correlate poorly with body stores and reported normal serum levels have varied widely. Patients with normal chromium status will have an increase in urine and serum concentrations after a glucose load. Absence of such an increase may be an indication of deficiency. The test may be repeated after chromium supplementation as further verification.[40] Chromium deficiency should be considered in persons receiving long-term parenteral nutrition therapy who develop glucose intolerance in the absence of infection. Treatment consists of intravenous chromium chloride, 0.15 to 0.2 mg/d, for 2 weeks. Disappearance of glucose intolerance and neuropathy after treatment is currently the best diagnostic test for deficiency.

MOLYBDENUM

Molybdenum, a component of several oxidases, is important for the metabolism of purines and sulfur-containing compounds.[40] The estimated safe and adequate adult dietary intake is 0.075 to 0.25 mg/d.[1] Good sources are beef kidney, some cereals, and some legumes. Most diets provide 0.045 to 0.5 mg/d.[63] The use of body fluid and tissue concentrations of molybdenum to assess status is difficult and unreliable. Measurement of xanthine oxidase and sulfite oxidase enzyme activity may provide a better indication of deficiency. Dietary molybdenum deficiency has been implicated in a few cases of growth retardation. There is one report of probable molybdenum deficiency associated with long-term parenteral nutrition. After 6 months of TPN the patient developed tachycardia, tachypnea, headache, night blindness, nausea and vomiting, lethargy, and, ultimately, coma. High plasma concentrations of methionine and almost undetectable levels of uric acid were noted. Supplementation with ammonium molybdate in doses of 0.3 mg/d reversed the clinical and biochemical abnormalities.[64] Based on animal studies molybdenum is relatively nontoxic.[64]

MANGANESE

Manganese is a cofactor for several enzyme systems, including pyruvate carboxylase and superoxide dismutase. The estimated safe and adequate adult dietary intake is 2 to 5 mg/d. Foods rich in manganese include cereals, grains, and green leafy vegetables. It is poorly absorbed from the gastrointestinal tract and secreted in bile.[40,65] The major route of excretion is via the stool. Although manganese deficiency has been demonstrated in animals, no definitive case of deficiency in humans has been reported. One case report of suspected manganese deficiency presented as vitamin K deficiency accompanied by nausea, dermatitis, hypocholesterolemia, and changes in the growth rate and color of hair and beard.[66] Manganese is available as a component of many oral vitamin and mineral combination products or alone as the chloride or sulfate salts. It was recommended for inclusion in TPN solutions in 1977 and is usually added in amounts of 0.3 to 0.5 mg/day, although its essentiality in TPN has not been established.

IODINE

Iodine is an integral part of the thyroid hormones triiodothyronine and tetraiodothyronine (thyroxine) and is necessary for normal thyroid function.[33,67] The USRDA is 0.15 mg. Seafoods are rich in iodine, but iodized table salt is the most abundant source in the United States. About 30% of the amount absorbed is extracted by the thyroid gland.[33] The major route of excretion is the kidneys, but some is also excreted via the skin, lungs, and the gastrointestinal tract.[68]

Iodine deficiency is now rare in the United States. When it occurs it is most commonly the result of inadequate intake and causes hypothyroidism together with hyperplasia and hypertrophy of the thyroid gland. Naturally occurring goitrogens in food markedly effect the likelihood of goiter formation at any particular level of iodine intake. Iodine is not added to TPN mixtures for short-term or long-term therapy, and there have been no reports of deficiency in these patients. Presumably, sufficient iodine is present as a contaminant or is absorbed from the skin. Iodine status can be assessed by measuring triiodothyronine, thyroxine resin uptake, and thyroid-stimulating hormone. Deficiency should be treated by increasing the intake of iodide in the diet.[69]

FLUORIDE

Fluoride is necessary for normal growth, reproduction, and intestinal absorption of iron, and it activates some enzyme systems. An estimated safe and adequate dietary intake for adults is 1.5 to 4 mg/d.[1] Fluoride is found in small amounts in almost all foods. Tea and sardines are excellent sources, but the major source is drinking water. It is almost completely absorbed from the gastrointestinal tract, and it is avidly retained by bone. The major route of elimination is urine. Fluoride deficiency has not been described in humans, including those on home TPN to which fluoride is never added. A low intake is associated with an increased incidence of dental caries and possibly an increased susceptibility to osteoporosis. In areas where daily intake is inadequate to protect against dental caries, fluoride is usually added to drinking water to bring the concentration up to 1 mg/L.[70]

OTHER TRACE MINERALS

Vanadium, nickel, cobalt, tin, and silicon are considered essential in mammals since deficiencies have been produced experimentally, but human deficiencies have not been reported. Other elements, including cadmium, lead, boron, aluminum, arsenic, mercury, strontium, and lithium, may eventually prove to be essential. Most of these trace elements are probably present in sufficient quantities as contaminants in TPN, but that may not be true of boron.[71]

Deficiencies of Vitamins

Vitamin deficiencies can result from decreased intake, decreased absorption, increased utilization, or increased loss. The time of onset of deficiency is dependent on many factors. For example, deficiencies of fat-soluble vitamins (A,D,E, and K) and vitamin B_{12} take months to years to develop because relatively large stores are present in adipose tissue or in the liver. In addition, vitamin D is made endogenously in sun-exposed skin. Water-soluble vitamins other than vitamin B_{12} generally have smaller body stores, and, consequently, deficiencies can occur in weeks to months. Pyridoxine and biotin (as well as vitamin K) are exceptions since they are produced by enteric bacteria, and some amounts are absorbed from this source. Vitamins (or metabolized forms) that undergo enterohepatic circulation, which include vitamins A and D, folic acid, and cobalamin, are especially vulnerable to increased fecal loss when the patient has malabsorption. Blood levels of the water-soluble vitamins generally reflect body stores and begin to fall early in the course of deficiency, well before clinical manifestations occur. Therefore, blood levels are useful indices of water-soluble vitamin deficiencies. For the fat-soluble vitamins, interpretation of blood levels is less straightforward. Vitamins A and D are carried by specific binding proteins, the level of which can

affect the plasma vitamin levels. Liver or kidney disease may result in decreased blood levels of active hydroxylated vitamin D when total body stores of the vitamin are adequate.

VITAMIN A

Vitamin A is the collective term for vitamin A alcohol (retinol) and related biologically active forms. It is essential for growth and development, maintenance of epithelial cells, stability of cell membranes, reproduction, and vision in dim light.[72-75] Advances in organic chemistry have led to synthesis of more than 1000 new retinoids. These compounds have already had an impact on therapy for skin disease and hold promise for other fields, including cancer therapy. The β-carotenes are precursors of vitamin A but appear to have additional beneficial functions, probably as antioxidants.

The USRDA for vitamin A is 5000 IU or approximately 1500 μg retinol equivalents (RE). However, the most recent RDAs for adults are 1000 μg RE for males and 800 μg RE for females.[1] Animal products are rich sources and include liver, kidney, dairy products, and eggs. Carotenoid pigments, especially β-carotene, are found in green and yellow vegetables. Conversion of food carotenoids to vitamin A is dependent on many factors, but a conversion ratio of 6 μg β-carotene or 12 μg of mixed carotenoids to 1 μg retinol has been suggested.[74]

Vitamin A, which is present in animal products in the form of long-chain retinyl esters, is hydrolyzed to retinol by lipases and esterases in bile and pancreatic secretions. In contrast, carotene precursors of vitamin A are absorbed along with dietary lipids and enzymatically converted to retinol in gastrointestinal mucosal cells. About 90% of dietary vitamin A is absorbed, incorporated into chylomicrons, transported in the lymphatic circulation, and stored in the liver, which controls its release.[72] Retinoic acid is the form excreted in bile. Absorption of β-carotenes is less efficient, only 40% to 60%.[74] When vitamin A is released from the liver, it is transported in the plasma as a trimolecular complex with retinol-binding protein and transthyretin. If stores of the vitamin are adequate, any excess vitamin A is excreted in bile. A very small amount is excreted in urine along with metabolites.[76,77]

Vitamin A deficiency is usually the result of decreased intake or fat malabsorption. Contributing factors may include impaired conversion of carotenoids to vitamin A (mucosal disease), inability to store the vitamin (liver disease), deficiency of transport proteins (liver disease, protein malnutrition), and increased urinary losses (tuberculosis, cancer, pneumonia, urinary tract infections).[72] Inadequate intake is rare in the United States, but the number of new cases of corneal disease due to vitamin A deficiency worldwide may approach 1 million each year.[78] Several cases of vitamin A deficiency in home TPN patients resulted from loss of the vitamin from TPN mixtures during storage.[79] As a result, multivitamins are generally added to home TPN mixtures just before they are infused. Before deficiency occurs, liver stores of vitamin A must become depleted, which normally takes approximately 2 years. Symptoms of deficiency are night blindness, xerophthalmia, follicular hyperkeratosis, altered taste and smell, increased cerebrospinal fluid pressure, and increased infections, especially of the skin.[72,74,77] Plasma vitamin A concentration can be measured as an aid in diagnosis. The normal value is controversial, but 20 to 80 μg/dL is a reasonable normal range. Measurement of serum carotene is easier and correlates with vitamin A absorption,[77] but because carotene is not stored in humans it does not assess vitamin A deficiency.

Severe deficiency can be treated orally with vitamin A, 30,000 μg RE (100,000 IU) daily for 3 days followed by 15,000 μg RE (50,000 IU) daily for 2 weeks then 3000 to 6000 μg RE (10,000–20,000 IU) daily for 2 months. The same doses may be given intramuscularly.[76]

Doses of vitamin A greater than the RDA are contraindicated in pregnant women because of the potential for teratogenicity. The minimum toxic oral dose for normal adults is between 7500 and 15,000 μg RE (25,000 and 50,000 IU) daily.[38] Acute toxicity including dizziness, headache, drowsiness, and nausea may occur within hours of ingesting 600,000 RE. Symptoms of chronic toxicity include dry skin and mucous membranes, increased intracranial pressure, skeletal pain, alopecia, anorexia, irritability, psychiatric symptoms, hepatic dysfunction, exophthalmos, and hypercalcemia often associated with elevations of levels of serum cholesterol and triglycerides. Patients with advanced renal failure are at increased risk of toxicity.[80] Most symptoms disappear within weeks to months after the vitamin is discontinued. Carotene is not converted to vitamin A fast enough for even massive doses to be toxic, but large doses will impart a yellow-orange tint to the skin.

VITAMIN D

Vitamin D is the designation for a group of sterols and their metabolites that have antirachitic activity. Cholecalciferol (D_3) and ergocalciferol (D_2) are the most important. In the small intestinal mucosa, vitamin D in conjunction with parathyroid hormone and calcitonin promotes the absorption of calcium and phosphorus. The vitamin is necessary for normal bone formation and regulates calcium and phosphorus metabolism in bone and kidney.[76,81]

The USRDA is 0.01 mg of cholecalciferol (400 IU). Vitamin D occurs naturally in foods of animal origin such as fish-liver oils, eggs, liver, and dairy products. "Fortified" milk is also an important source. Dietary cholecalciferol is absorbed by the small intestine and transported in lymph in association with chylomicrons and lipoproteins. Cholecalciferol is also biosynthesized when 7-dehydrocholesterol, found in skin lipids, is exposed to ultraviolet light. The vitamin is stored in the liver, adipose tissue, and muscle and is slowly released. It is hydroxylated in the liver to 25-hydroxy vitamin D, which is further hydroxylated in the kidney to 1,25-dihydroxy vitamin D. Vitamin D compounds and metabolites are excreted in bile, but few of these compounds have antirachitic activity. Small amounts are excreted in the urine.[81,82]

Vitamin D deficiency secondary to inadequate intake is thought to be rare in the United States in part because milk products are fortified with the vitamin. Even persons who do not consume diary products usually get adequate sunlight exposure to prevent vitamin D deficiency. However, among those elderly persons who have little exposure to sunlight, deficiency may be rather prevalent and may contribute to the high incidence of bone fractures in this group.[83,84] Deficiency should be considered in any patient with steatorrhea or severe liver or kidney disease. Vitamin D deficiency causes hypocalcemia and hypophosphatemia, which in turn stimulates parathyroid hormone secretion to mobilize calcium from bone. In time this produces osteomalacia in adults. Patients at risk should be followed with periodic measurement of levels of serum 25-hydroxy vitamin D, calcium, phosphorus, and bone alkaline phosphatase, as well as of bone density (see section on calcium). Serum vitamin D_2 and D_3 concentrations can be measured; however, measurement of the hydroxylated metabolites, 25-hydroxy vitamin D and 1,25-dihydroxy vitamin D provides more information on vitamin D status, including the functions of hydroxylase systems in the liver and kidney. The level of 25-hydroxy vitamin D is a useful indicator of body stores.[85]

Adults with osteomalacia secondary to a nutritional deficiency of vitamin D should receive 0.1 to 0.2 mg (4000–8000 IU) of cholecalciferol daily by mouth. Much larger oral doses, up to 50,000 IU daily, may be required for patients with malabsorption. Serum 25-hydroxy vitamin D should be measured every 3 to 4 weeks and the dose adjusted to bring the serum level into the normal range. If necessary in severe malabsorption, intramuscular vitamin D should be used. Excessive vitamin D will cause hypercalcemia and renal damage and the effect persists long after administration is stopped. Therefore, if serum levels are not followed, the dose of vitamin D used to treat osteomalacia should be reduced as soon as bone symptoms are relieved and before the alkaline phosphatase level returns to normal or bone healing is complete.[82] Vitamin D deficiency secondary to liver or kidney disease may require treatment with 25-hydroxy vitamin D or 1,25-dihydroxy vitamin D, respectively.

Oral vitamin D supplements are available in various forms, including vitamin D_3 (cholecalciferol), vitamin D_2 (ergocalciferol), 25-hydroxy vitamin D, 1,25-dihydroxy vitamin D, and dihydrotachysterol, a synthetic product similar to 25-hydroxy vitamin D. Vitamin D_2 in sesame oil, 500,000 IU/mL, is available for intramuscular injection. Multivitamin products for intravenous use in TPN provide 200 IU of vitamin D_2 daily.

Signs of toxicity are hypercalcemia and hypercalciuria, which can result in irreversible renal failure. The estimated minimum toxic oral dose for healthy adults is 1.25 mg (50,000 IU) daily.[38] Unless renal damage is severe, vitamin D toxicity is usually reversible once administration is discontinued.

VITAMIN E

Vitamin E refers to two groups of lipid-soluble compounds, tocopherols and tocotrienes, found in plants. The most active and abundant is α-tocopherol. The most important function of vitamin E is as an antioxidant and free-radical scavenger. The current recommended dietary allowance for adult males is 10 mg α-tocopherol equivalents (TE). The richest source is vegetable oils, and adequate amounts are ingested in the usual diet. As the intake of polyunsaturated fatty acids increases, the need for vitamin E increases. Fortunately, foods high in polyunsaturated fatty acids are also good sources of vitamin E.[72,86] Absorption of the ingested vitamin, which ranges from 20% to 80% in various studies, occurs in the small intestine and requires bile salts and pancreatic enzymes. From the intestine, tocopherols enter the lymph, circulate attached to lipoproteins, and are stored in adipose tissue, muscle, and liver.

Vitamin E deficiency is well documented in animals but is very rare in humans. Newborns and premature infants are particularly at risk because of poor vitamin E absorption.[86,87] Deficiency occurs in abetalipoproteinemia, cystic fibrosis and other malabsorption syndromes, cirrhosis, and biliary obstruction and as a result of excessive mineral oil ingestion.[87] Abnormalities associated with vitamin E deficiency include a progressive neurologic syndrome of areflexia, gait disturbance, decreased vibratory and proprioceptive sensation and paresis of gaze, histologic changes in the spinal cord and medulla, and red blood cell hemolysis. Deficiency can be documented by low serum α-tocopherol concentration, best measured by high-performance liquid chromatography. Increased fragility of red blood cells on exposure to 2% hydrogen peroxide is another helpful test, although it is not entirely specific. The plasma concentration of α-tocopherol is influenced by plasma lipid content because the vitamin is carried exclusively by lipoproteins. Therefore, the ratio of α-tocopherol to total lipid, or to the sum of triglyceride and cholesterol, is more accurate than the vitamin level alone.[87]

For treatment of deficiency states oral or intramuscular doses up to 300 mg of d-α-tocopherol have been used. Pharmacologic doses up to 100 mg/kg in infants and up to a total dose of 600 mg/d in adults have been given in various conditions believed by some to benefit from the antioxidant properties of vitamin E.[82,88] Long-term use of vitamin E in doses of 300 to 600 mg/d has been reported to cause nausea, muscular weakness, fatigue, headache, elevation of blood pressure, thrombophlebitis, breast tenderness, and blurred vision. Symptoms resolve when excessive doses are discontinued.

VITAMIN K

The term *vitamin K* designates naphthoquinone compounds with antihemorrhagic activity. These compounds are critical for the production of plasma clotting factors II (prothrombin), VII, IX, and X. The recommended dietary allowance of vitamin K for adult males is 0.08 mg/d. The vitamin is abundant in most diets. It is also synthesized by intestinal bacteria, and approximately half the daily need is probably derived from this source. Vitamin K_1, or phylloquinone, is available in plants, especially green vegetables. Vitamin K_2, or menaquinone, is found in bacteria and animals. Menadione (vitamin K_3) and phytonadione are synthetic compounds. All vitamin K compounds are fat soluble and are absorbed in the small intestine. The vitamin is concentrated in the liver and excreted in bile, stool, and urine.[86,89,90]

Nutritional deficiency is uncommon in adults because of the large amount in foods and because bacteria synthesize the vitamin in the intestine. Deficiency is most often the result of fat malabsorption often compounded by poor intake and diminished liver function or diminished bile secretion, for example, in chronic alcoholics with cirrhosis. Inhibition of intestinal bacterial biosynthesis by antibiotic administration at times also appears to play a role.[86,90]

The only clinically applicable test for vitamin K deficiency is the one-stage prothrombin time. It is not a sensitive test since it becomes abnormal only after the deficiency is advanced. A prolonged prothrombin time is also not specific for vitamin K deficiency since it occurs in patients with liver disease, with consumptive coagulopathy, and with other clotting abnormalities in the absence of deficiency. However, restoration of normal prothrombin time by parenteral administration of 5 to 10 mg of vitamin K confirms a deficiency.

In adults the vitamin is nontoxic even in doses up to 40 mg/d.[76] Rarely, intravenous phytonadione has produced a severe anaphylactic-type reaction even when diluted and given slowly.

THIAMINE (VITAMIN B_1)

Thiamine is essential for the function of numerous enzyme systems and plays a major role in energy production. Requirements vary with the intake of energy, especially carbohydrate. The USRDA is 1.5 mg/d.

Thiamine deficiency, primarily in the form of beriberi, occurs in areas of the world where polished rice is the staple cereal in the diet. Adult beriberi presents as easy fatigability, weakness, paresthesias, and high-output congestive heart failure. In the United States where food is abundant in thiamine, deficiency most often occurs in alcoholics and occasionally in patients with malabsorption, prolonged febrile illnesses, and chronic renal failure on dialysis.[91] Other vitamin deficiencies and alcohol toxicity probably contribute to the abnormalities attributed to thiamine deficiency, which include peripheral neuropathy manifested by burning and weakness in the feet and legs, cerebellar dysfunction, subacute necrotizing encephalomyelopathy, and Wernicke's encephalopathy. Wernicke's encephalopathy is manifested by apathy, confusion, weakness, ataxic gait, and a number of eye signs, including photophobia, nystagmus, and paralysis of the extraocular muscles especially for upward gaze. Thiamine deficiency may also play a role in Korsakoff's syndrome.

When thiamine intake is inadequate, there is a fall in urinary thiamine levels, expressed per gram of urinary creatinine. A deficit in body stores is best estimated by the degree of enhancement of red blood cell transketolase activity by thiamine pyrophosphate added in vitro.[92,93]

Thiamine hydrochloride is available as a single entity in oral form (5 to 250 mg per dose) and parenteral form (5, 100, and 200 mg/mL) and in virtually all multivitamin preparations. Adults with mild deficiency should receive 10 to 20 mg intramuscularly or 25 to 50 mg orally twice daily for 1 week followed by an oral maintenance dose of 2 to 5 mg daily. Critically ill patients, especially those with central nervous system manifestations of thiamine deficiency should receive 50 to 100 mg intravenously, followed by a similar intramuscular dose daily for 3 days followed by oral supplementation of 5 to 30 mg daily until a normal diet is resumed. Signs of thiamine deficiency may be acutely precipitated or made worse by administration of carbohydrate, including 5% dextrose intravenous infusion. Therefore, patients at risk of deficiency should receive 50 mg of thiamine parenterally before carbohydrate is administered. Since thiamine deficiency is frequently associated with deficiencies of other B vitamins, multiple vitamins should be given.

Excess thiamine is excreted in the urine. The estimated minimum toxic oral dose for normal adults is 300 mg/d.[38] Sensitivity to parenteral thiamine therapy has been reported to cause feelings of warmth, tingling, pruritus, nausea, sweating, and occasionally an anaphylactic reaction.[82,76]

RIBOFLAVIN (VITAMIN B_2)

Riboflavin is a major component of two essential coenzymes, flavin adenine dinucleotide and flavin mononucleotide. The USRDA is 1.7 mg/d. The vitamin is abundant in milk, eggs, and leafy green vegetables. Absorption occurs by a site-specific, saturable system in the small intestine. The primary route of excretion is via the kidney as unmetabolized riboflavin.

Riboflavin deficiency is usually seen in conjunction with other B vitamin deficiencies especially in alcoholism and malabsorption syndromes. Deficiency is characterized by angular stomatitis (maceration and fissuring of the mucocutaneous junction at the angles of the mouth), cheilosis (inflammation of the lips), glossitis, seborrheic-like dermatitis, pruritus, photophobia, and visual impairment. Laboratory assessment of riboflavin status is accomplished by observing the change in activity of glutathione reductase, a flavin adenine dinucleotide–dependent enzyme, in lysed red blood cells following in vivo addition of flavin adenine dinucleotide.[94] However, there is seldom a clinical need for the determination.

Riboflavin is available in tablets of 3 to 100 mg and in a parenteral solution of 35 mg/mL. It is a component of virtually all oral and parenteral multivitamins. Deficiency states should be treated with 5 mg orally twice a day, usually along with other vitamins.[76] A response is generally seen in several days to weeks. Prophylaxis with 3 mg/d is appropriate in malabsorption syndromes.

No toxicity or adverse effects have been reported with oral or parenteral administration of riboflavin. The minimum oral toxic dose for normal adults is estimated to be 1000 mg/d, although no more than approximately 25 mg is absorbed from a single oral dose.[38]

NIACIN (VITAMIN B₃)

The term *niacin* encompasses nicotinic acid as well as its amide form, nicotinamide (niacinamide). It is a component of the coenzymes nicotinamide adenine dinucleotide and nicotinamide adenine dinucleotide phosphate, which participate in more than 50 metabolic reactions. Humans also can synthesize approximately 1 mg of niacin from 60 mg of the amino acid tryptophan, and deficiency does not occur unless both niacin and tryptophan availability are limited.[91,95] The USRDA for niacin is 20 mg. Animal proteins, beans, nuts, whole grains, and enriched bread and cereal are good dietary sources.

In contrast to years past, niacin deficiency (pellagra) is now rare in the United States and is most often a complication of alcoholism. It may very rarely be encountered in patients with malabsorption syndrome. Deficiency can occur in patients with carcinoid syndrome because a large amount of tryptophan is used by the tumor for serotonin production. Patients with Hartnup disease are also at risk because of a defect in tryptophan absorption.[95]

Clinical signs of pellagra are the "3 Ds": dermatitis, diarrhea, and dementia. The dermatitis is scaly, hyperpigmented, and localized to the sun-exposed areas such as the neck, face, dorsa of the hands and forearms, and anterior surfaces of the feet and legs. The tongue and mucous membranes of the mouth are also often painful and swollen. Diarrhea is probably due to the direct effect of niacin deficiency on epithelial cell function. Central nervous system dysfunction includes irritability, headache, insomnia and anxiety progressing to psychosis, hallucinations, and seizures.

There is no clinically relevant test for body stores of niacin.[95,96] The level of a niacin metabolite, N-methylnicotinamide, in urine reflects intake and absorption of the vitamin.

The vitamin is available in 20- to 500-mg tablets of nicotinic acid or nicotinamide and parenterally as nicotinamide. Pellagra should be treated with 100 mg of nicotinic acid or nicotinamide three times daily until signs and symptoms resolve. If necessary, nicotinamide, 100 mg, may be given intramuscularly.[76] The redness and swelling of the tongue disappear in 2 to 3 days. Mental and gastrointestinal symptoms also clear rapidly. The skin lesions may require several weeks to months to resolve. Pellagra is usually accompanied by other B vitamin deficiencies so multiple vitamins should be given.[76,82]

Small doses of niacin or niacinamide are nontoxic. The large doses used to treat pellagra and the even larger doses, up to 3 g/d of nicotinic acid, used to treat hypercholesterolemia often result in flushing, pruritus, sensation of burning, nausea, vomiting, heartburn, diarrhea, dizziness, and tachycardia. These symptoms usually disappear within 2 weeks if therapy is continued. Hyperglycemia and hepatic injury manifested by elevated transaminase and bilirubin levels may occur at doses as low as 750 mg/d.[97,98]

PYRIDOXINE (VITAMIN B₆)

Vitamin B₆ refers to three interconvertible compounds: pyridoxine, pyridoxal, and pyridoxamine. This vitamin is essential for the function of many transaminases and amino acid decarboxylases and is involved not only in the metabolism of all amino acids but also in the synthesis of acetylcholine, porphyrin, arachidonic acid, and bile acids. The USRDA is 2 mg daily. Animal protein and whole grain cereals are good dietary sources. The vitamin is produced by intestinal microorganisms and some may be absorbed from this source. Dietary vitamin B₆ is rapidly absorbed in the small intestine. It is excreted in the urine unchanged and as a metabolic by-product, 4-pyridoxic acid. Pyridoxine deficiency is rare in humans and has most often been reported as a result of treatment with pyridoxine antagonists, especially isoniazid, hydralazine, and penicillamine. Rarely, deficiency occurs in chronic alcoholism and malabsorption, usually in association with deficiencies of other B vitamins.[99]

Clinical manifestations of deficiency are peripheral neuropathy, seborrheic dermatitis around the eyes and nasolabial folds, and oral lesions, including glossitis, angular stomatitis, and cheilosis similar to that seen in niacin and riboflavin deficiencies. Seizures and anemia may also occur.[99] Biochemical assessment of deficiency is not necessary for clinical management. Urinary excretion of free pyridoxine or 4-pyridoxic acid primarily reflect recent intake. Deficiency can be assessed by measurement of serum pyridoxine concentration (normal > 50 ng/mL). Body stores are probably best determined by measuring the effect of pyridoxal phosphate on red blood cell transaminase activity in vitro.[99,100]

Pyridoxine hydrochloride is available in oral form, 5- to 100-mg tablets, and for parenteral use, 50 or 100 mg/mL. Suspected deficiency should be treated with improvement in dietary intake and the oral administration of 50 to 150 mg daily. A multiple vitamin should be continued for several weeks after clinical manifestations are corrected to provide an additional 2 to 5 mg/d along with other B vitamins. A prophylactic oral dose of 50 mg/d should be given to patients receiving isoniazid therapy.

It was previously concluded that pyridoxine was nontoxic. However, recent reports indicate that persons consuming 2 to 6 g/d of the vitamin can experience symptoms including paresthesias, loss of vibratory sense, difficulty walking, and decreased proprioception. The toxic dose may be less than 2 g/d.[38,91]

FOLATE (FOLACIN, FOLIC ACID)

The folate molecule consists of three components: a pteridine ring, paminobenzoate, and glutamate. It exists in many forms depending on the degree of reduction of the double bonds in the ring (e.g., tetrahydrofolate), the presence of 1-carbon groups (e.g., N5-methyl tetrahydrofolate) and the number of glutamyl residues in the peptide chain (e.g., folate pentaglutamate). Functioning as a carrier of 1-carbon groups from donor to recipient molecules, the vitamin is necessary for synthesis of nucleic acids, initiation of protein synthesis, synthesis of acetylcholine, and metabolism of several amino acids. Three other vitamins—cobalamin, ascorbic acid, and niacin—are involved in the conversion of folate to active coenzyme forms.[76,101]

The USRDA for folate is 0.4 mg, but the most recent RDA for adult males is 0.2 mg.[91] The vitamin is abundant in vegetables, legumes, kidney, liver, and nuts. It is absorbed in the small intestine and excreted in bile and urine. The chemical forms of folate present in food determine its stability, availability, absorption, and retention. The polyglutamate form, which is usually present in food, must be hydrolyzed to monoglutamate by a conjugase in the intestinal mucosa during absorption.

Folate deficiency is seen in areas of poor socioeconomic and dietary conditions. In developed countries, it is most commonly the result of poor intake due to chronic alcoholism or to decreased absorption resulting from malabsorption syndromes, sulfasalazine therapy, anticonvulsant therapy, or the effect of alcohol on small bowel mucosa. Deficiency also results from increased utilization in pregnancy and in conditions of rapid cell turnover such as hemolytic anemia, leukemia, and chronic myelofibrosis. Inhibition of dihydrofolate reductase, an enzyme that converts folate to the active coenzyme, can also cause folate deficiency. Drugs that inhibit the enzyme include methotrexate, trimethoprim, pyrimethamine, and triampterene.[101,102]

The primary manifestation of folate deficiency is macrocytic anemia often accompanied by thrombocytopenia and leukopenia. Other features may include glossitis, diarrhea, fatigue, and possibly neurologic signs. As folate deficiency progresses, decreased serum folate is the first abnormality to develop, followed in order by decreased red blood cell folate, multilobed polymorphonuclear white blood cells, and finally macrocytic anemia.[101] Because the serum level is so responsive to folate ingestion and absorption, it is not a good measure of body stores, which are better assessed by red blood cell folate levels. Most folate in the serum is bound to albumin; consequently, low total serum folate can be a result of hypoalbuminemia.

Oral folate supplements in the form of unreduced pteroylglutamic acid are available in tablets up to 1 mg. Body stores of folate can be repleted with 1 mg orally per day given for 2 to 3 weeks. The parenteral route is used only if oral therapy is impossible or malabsorption is severe. A reticulocyte response is seen within 3 to 5 days, and peak response occurs in 5 to 10 days. The hematocrit will begin to rise after about 2 weeks of therapy. Maintenance folate therapy may be necessary for persons with malabsorption or chronic alcoholism. Generally, a maintenance dose of 0.2 to 0.4 mg/d in a multivitamin preparation is adequate. A dose of 1 mg/d is recommended for patients receiving more than 1 g of sulfasalazine daily, although clinical folate deficiency is uncommon.

No folate toxicity has been reported, and the estimated minimum oral toxic dose for normal adults is 400 mg/d.[38] However, there are circumstances in which the vitamin can be harmful. Giving folate to a patient with cobalamin deficiency is likely to correct the anemia and thus mask the cobalamin deficiency until neurologic damage has occurred, which may be irreversible. Also, very large doses of folate given to treat the megaloblastic anemia caused by antiepileptic drugs may aggravate the seizure disorder.[91]

COBALAMIN (VITAMIN B₁₂)

A single cobalt atom in the cobalamin molecule is the site of attachment of key functional groups. As a result, naturally occurring active forms include hydroxo-, nitro-, and methylcobalamin while cyanocobalamin, the most frequently used therapeutic form, contains a cyanide group attached to the cobalt. The coenzyme forms, methyl- and 5′-deoxyadenosylcobalamin, function as a carrier for methyl groups and hydrogen. Cobalamin participates in the synthesis of nucleic acids, porphyrin, methionine, and some fatty acids.[101] The USRDA for cobalamin is 6 μg/d, but the current RDA for adults is 2 μg.[91] The vitamin is found only in animal products, including meat, liver, fish, eggs and milk. It is synthesized by colonic flora, but it is not absorbed from that source.

Absorption of cobalamin is complex. In food the vitamin is bound to enzymes and must be released by gastric proteases. It is then tightly bound by haptocorrin (R protein) present in the gastric fluid. In the upper small intestine, pancreatic proteases hydrolyze haptocorrin, releasing cobalamin, which can then bind to intrinsic factor, a glycoprotein that is secreted by gastric parietal cells and that is not hydrolyzed by pancreatic proteases. The intrinsic factor-cobalamin complex attaches to specific receptor sites in the terminal ileum where it is absorbed and free cobalamin is released. The free vitamin is then bound by several transport proteins, but only transcobalamin II delivers it to tissues. There is a large enterohepatic circulation of cobalamin that helps account for the fact that malabsorption causes a deficiency more frequently and rapidly than does dietary inadequacy. The liver can store 2 to 3 mg of cobalamin, and since daily losses normally do not exceed 3 μg, deficiency ordinarily does not become evident for 2 to 5 years after intake or absorption is stopped.[101]

Dietary deficiency of cobalamin occurs only in lacto-ovovegetarians who do not consume any foods of animal origin. The three common causes of cobalamin deficiency are (1) gastric lesions, especially pernicious anemia and gastrectomy; (2) lesions of the terminal ileum including resection and destruction of the mucosa; and (3) bacterial overgrowth in which bacteria in the small intestine bind dietary cobalamin and carry it away in the stool. Deficiency also results from a rare congenital deficiency of the carrier protein transcobalamin II, and, very rarely, in severe pancreatic insufficiency.

Cobalamin deficiency usually presents as a macrocytic anemia associated with a megaloblastic bone marrow and multilobed nuclei in the polymorphonuclear white blood cells. Fatigue, weakness, and dyspnea may accompany the anemia. Multiple nonspecific symptoms have been described, including anorexia, loss of taste, glossitis, diarrhea, dyspepsia, hair loss, and impotence. Neurologic symptoms generally begin with numbness and tingling, first noted in the feet and subsequently in the hands. If untreated, this will progress to loss of vibratory sense, loss of coordination, muscle weakness and atrophy, and, finally, irritability and memory disturbances. An occasional patient, usually elderly, will present with a psychiatric illness, most often depression, as the first manifestation of deficiency.

The diagnosis is usually suspected on the basis of hematologic findings. The level of serum cobalamin is generally a good indicator of body stores. However, normal serum levels in the face of inadequate body stores can occur when there is a deficiency of the carrier protein transcobalamin II, and when cobalamin analogues that interfere with the radioisotopic binding assay are present in the serum. Conversely, low serum cobalamin levels in the presence of normal body stores may occur in folate deficiency and in hypoproteinemia, although low serum levels must suggest cobalamin deficiency until proven otherwise. Absorption of free cobalamin is best assessed by the Schilling test; however, some postgastrectomy patients may absorb food cobalamin poorly but free cobalamin normally.[103]

When cobalamin deficiency is secondary to a strict vegetarian diet, it may be treated with 3 to 6 µg/d of oral cobalamin. Deficiency due to pernicious anemia or other absorptive defects is treated intramuscularly with 100 µg/d for 3 days and then 100 µg monthly or 1000 µg every 2 to 3 months. Increased well-being is usually noted within 24 hours, and reticulocytosis begins in 5 to 7 days. Neurologic findings may take 6 months or longer to improve. Cyanocobalamin is available for oral and parenteral use, and hydroxocobalamin can be used parenterally.[101,104]

No toxicity has been reported from oral or parenteral cobalamin. An exceedingly rare anaphylactic-like reaction has been reported with intramuscular administration, possibly due to impurities in the particular preparation.[104] Hypokalemia, which can be severe, may occur during the first few days of therapy for severe pernicious anemia.

ASCORBIC ACID (VITAMIN C)

Ascorbic acid functions as an essential cofactor for several hydroxylation reactions and plays a key role in the synthesis of collagen. The USRDA is 60 mg. Fruits, especially citrus fruits, and vegetables are rich in ascorbic acid, which is readily absorbed in the small intestine.[91,105]

Scurvy develops after 2 to 3 months of a diet very deficient in ascorbic acid. It is rare in the United States, where it is usually the result of alcoholism, food faddism, malabsorption, or Crohn's disease. Early symptoms are weakness, lassitude, irritability, aching joints and muscles, and weight loss. Later, perifollicular hyperkeratotic papules appear on the buttocks, thighs, and legs, followed by petechiae on the lower legs. In advanced deficiency, the gums become swollen, red, and spongy, and hemorrhaging occurs especially from the gums and in the skin and muscles. Serum and white blood cell ascorbic acid concentrations are used to document deficiency. Serum concentration decreases before there are clinical signs of deficiency. Among chronically ill patients there is a high prevalence of subclinical ascorbic acid deficiency indicated by low blood levels.[105] Deficiency in adults is treated with 250 mg ascorbic acid four times a day orally, which will replete stores within 1 week. Thereafter, 100 to 200 mg/d should be continued until skin lesions heal. The diet should be changed to include foods rich in ascorbic acid.

Ascorbic acid is relatively nontoxic, although large doses may cause gastrointestinal irritation and osmotic diarrhea. The estimated minimum toxic oral dose for normal adults is between 1000 and 5000 mg/d.[38]

BIOTIN

Biotin is one of the B vitamins and is a coenzyme for several carboxylases. No RDA has been established, but a safe and adequate dietary intake for adults is 0.03 to 0.1 mg/d. It is abundant in food, and a large amount is also synthesized by intestinal flora.[106] Dietary deficiency of biotin is exceedingly rare but can be produced by excessive consumption of raw egg white, which contains a biotin-binding glycoprotein, avidin. Deficiency occurred in a number of children and adults on TPN before biotin was included in commercial multivitamin preparations for TPN.[106] The effects of deficiency include anorexia, nausea, dermatitis, alopecia, mental depression, and organic aciduria. Symptoms disappear with biotin supplementation in doses of 0.15 to 0.3 mg parenterally or 0.2 to 10 mg orally per day for a few days. No adverse effects have been reported with either parenteral or oral biotin administration. The estimated oral minimum toxic dose for normal adults is 50 mg/d.[38]

PANTOTHENIC ACID

Pantothenic acid is a precursor of coenzyme A, which is essential for the metabolism of fats, carbohydrates, and proteins and for the synthesis of steroids and porphyrins.[107] No RDA has been established, but the estimated safe and adequate dietary intake for adults is 4 to 7 mg/d.[91] It is widely distributed in foods, absorbed in the small intestine, and excreted in the urine. Clinical deficiency has not been observed in humans, probably because it is so abundant in foods. It is available as a single entity for oral administration and is included in both oral and parenteral multiple vitamin products. Toxicity has not been reported in humans. Daily intake of 10 to 20 mg may occasionally cause diarrhea.[91] The estimated minimum oral toxic dose is 1000 mg/d.[38]

Essential Fatty Acid Deficiency

Essential fatty acids are long-chain fatty acids that cannot be synthesized by mammals. In humans they consist of three polyunsaturated fatty acids—linoleic, linolenic, and arachidonic acid. Of these, only linoleic acid and, to a much lesser degree, linolenic acid are required in the diet. Humans can synthesize arachidonic acid from linoleic acid. Essential fatty acids are required for a variety of functions, including membrane structure, platelet function, prostaglandin synthesis, wound healing, immunocompetence, and integrity of skin, hair, and nerve fibers.

The requirement for linoleic acid is 1% to 2% of the total calorie intake in adults. Vegetable oils including safflower, sunflower seed, corn, soybean, cottonseed, and peanut oils are rich dietary sources. Essential fatty acids are also produced by lipolysis of adipose tissue, which is approximately 10% linoleic acid. Absorption and metabolism of essential fatty acids in the diet is like that of other long-chain fatty acids. Intravenous lipid emulsions currently used for TPN consist of soybean and safflower oil and provide very large, perhaps excessive, amounts of linoleic acid.

Essential fatty acid deficiency was very rarely recognized before the use of TPN, which provided no fat prior to development of intravenous fat emulsions. Within 1 to 3 weeks after initiating fat-free parenteral nutrition, biochemical evidence of essential fatty acid deficiency can be documented by an increase in the triene (5,8,11-eicosatrienoic acid) to tetraene (arachidonic acid) ratio in the plasma. A ratio of greater than 0.4 is consistent with deficiency. Clinical manifestations of essential fatty acid deficiency can begin 3 to 6 weeks after fat-free TPN is begun. They include a scaly dermatitis on the lower extremities, groin, and axillae indistinguishable from the rash of zinc deficiency. Other signs include alopecia, coarsening of the hair, hepatomegaly, fatty liver, thrombocytopenia, mild diarrhea, and growth retardation in infants. Essential fatty acid deficiency has virtually disappeared among TPN patients because of the routine administration of intravenous fat emulsions. An increased plasma triene to tetraene ratio consistent with essential fatty acid deficiency has been demonstrated in patients with peripheral vascular disease, short bowel syndrome, burns, and polytrauma.[108]

Essential fatty acid deficiency associated with parenteral nutrition therapy can be prevented or treated if it occurs by providing 1% to 2% of total calories as intravenous fat emulsion. The emulsions are available as 10% (1.1 kcal/mL) and 20% (2.0 kcal/mL) products. Administration of oral essential fats will also correct the deficiency if they are absorbed. There are reports that cutaneous application of safflower oil or sunflower seed oil will prevent and correct essential fatty acid deficiency. This therapy appears to be effective only in infants and children in whom it reverses the triene-tetraene ratio after 7 to 10 days, but clinical manifestations may continue for 2 to 3 weeks.

PROTEIN–CALORIE DEFICIENCY REQUIRING NUTRITION SUPPORT

Surveys have documented that 20% to 60% of patients admitted to American hospitals are undernourished and that the average patient's nutritional status is worse at discharge than on admission.[109,110] What impact does undernutrition have on patient morbidity and mortality? This important question is proving to be very difficult to answer quantitatively because the effects of malnutrition are not easy to distinguish from those of the underlying disease. Consequently, there are no specific and sensitive methods for quantitating protein–calorie malnutrition that are suitable for clinical use.

Any discussion of protein–calorie supplementation must acknowledge the detrimental effects of protein–calorie excess. Obesity contributes substantially to the morbidity and mortality of hospitalized patients. Even more relevant are data indicating that mild to moderate undernutrition is protective. Several large longitudinal studies have demonstrated that among initially healthy U.S. populations, a weight approximately 10% below the average is associated with the lowest long-term mortality. Caged rats maintained on life-long, semi-starvation diets live dramatically longer than ad libitum fed controls. Finally, undernutrition may provide some protection against certain viruses and other intracellular pathogens.[111]

Nevertheless, it is obvious that malnutrition alone can cause morbidity and mortality. Healthy adults will die of starvation after 60 to 90 days of no protein or calorie intake. When the hypermetabolism of illness is added to starvation, lean body mass will decrease to a fatally low level in a shorter time, perhaps as little as 14 days.[112] Animal and human studies have documented clinically important effects of lesser degrees of malnutrition, including weakness, decreased immune responses, skin breakdown, infection (especially pneumonia), impaired wound healing, and emotional changes of apathy and irritability.[113] Physical performance begins to deteriorate when more than 10% of body cell mass is lost during starvation.[114] Furthermore, recovery from the detrimental effects of malnutrition is slow. Human volunteers who suffered 24% loss of body weight and 72% loss of exercise capacity during semi-starvation had not returned to baseline exercise capacity after 4 months of refeeding.[113] If malnutrition is severe, full recovery of cardiac and skeletal muscle function may be impossible due to irreversible damage.[115] These results emphasize the importance of attention to nutrition early in the course of illness.

Deciding to Institute Nutrition Support— Theoretical Considerations

The ultimate goals of nutrition support are to decrease morbidity and mortality related to deficits of energy, protein, and other nutrients. Intensive research efforts have been aimed at developing assessment methods that will identify patients most likely to benefit from nutrition support. Initially, these efforts concentrated on quantifying the degree of malnutrition.[116,117] The effectiveness of this approach has been hampered and called into question by the realization that measurements such as serum protein concentrations, delayed hypersensitivity, and even weight are neither sensitive nor specific for malnutrition, especially in critically ill patients.[112,118–120] In addition, as methods of nutrition support became safer, it became more difficult for many physicians to justify withholding nutrients from critically ill patients until they were clinically malnourished.[112] It can be argued that nutrition support of patients is appropriate even in the absence of documented efficacy because, unlike drug treatment, nutrient intake is the norm and, therefore, it is the prolonged withholding of nutrients from patients that must be justified. However, the expense and risks of tube feeding and TPN refute this argument and require that better methods be developed to identify patients who will truly benefit from these therapies. Recent work has focused on measurements and indices that predict outcome and are modifiable by nutrition support.[121] Measurements of function such as immune response and muscle function, which, when decreased, may directly cause a poor outcome and which can be maintained or improved by nutrition support, seem especially appealing.[122–124]

Randomized, controlled clinical trials of the efficacy of nutrition support have been somewhat disappointing but help define the proper role of this therapy. They indicate that perioperative TPN is probably helpful for severely malnourished patients undergoing major surgery and for well-nourished patients who are likely to be without adequate nutrition for prolonged periods (at least 10 to 14 days) as a result of surgery or complications.[125] A limited number of patients with hepatic encephalopathy may benefit from TPN with branched-chain amino acids.[126] Supplementary tube feeding improves clinical outcome in thin elderly women with fracture of the neck of the femur.[127] There is adequate evidence that nutrition support is beneficial for selected patients with short bowel syndrome and other forms of intestinal failure, Crohn's disease, enterocutaneous fistulae, burns, and cancer.[128] The impact of nutrition support on the outcome of patients with critical illness remains unsettled.[129] Finally, based on a meta-analysis that is not yet published, the American College of Physicians concluded that the routine use of TPN for patients undergoing cancer chemotherapy is likely to cause more harm than good,[130] but few would have argued that routine use was appropriate.

Deciding to Institute Nutrition Support— Practical Aspects

Nutrition support may be defined as the process of providing total nutrition by any means other than ordinary foods. It includes oral supplements, tube feeding (enteral nutrition), and intravenous feeding (peripheral and central TPN). Deciding when to begin nutrition support is a matter of informed clinical judgment—an endeavor that is currently as dependent on art and belief as it is on science. The goal is to provide nutrition support only to those patients in whom the benefits will exceed the risks.

Five Steps to Optimal Nutrition Support

The following are the five steps to optimal nutrition support. They form the framework for the remainder of this chapter:

1. Prevent malnutrition.
2. Establish energy and protein goals.
3. Select, establish, and maintain an access for feeding. Consider oral feeding first, then tube feeding, and finally the intravenous route.
4. Choose or design an optimal formula for the individual patient considering each component.
5. Monitor the patient to ensure that nutrition support is as effective and safe as possible.

Two memory aids—KCALS and FACE MTV—are useful for remembering each of the important steps for optimal nutrition support:

K—Keep the patient nourished. Is everything feasible being done to encourage intake of ordinary foods? Does the patient need nutrition support?

C—Calculate energy and protein goals.

A—Access. Can the patient's needs be met best by oral supplements, tube feeding, or intravenous feeding? Once selected, can the access route (feeding tube, peripheral intravenous line, or central catheter) be established and maintained?

L—List (or at least think about) components of the formula

and choose amounts best suited for the specific patient as follows:

F—Fluids: should fluids be restricted?

A—Amino acids/protein: are special formulas indicated?

C—Calories: what is the most appropriate mix of carbohydrate and fat calories?

E—Electrolytes: how much sodium, potassium, chloride, acetate, phosphate, calcium, magnesium?

M—Miscellaneous: should heparin, insulin, etc., be included?

T—Trace elements: are the standard amounts adequate, especially zinc?

V—Vitamins: are the standard amounts adequate?

S—Special monitoring to ensure safe and effective nutrition support.

Keeping the Patient Nourished

Hospital-acquired malnutrition may be diminished or prevented by encouraging intake of ordinary food where appropriate and by avoiding missed meals and unpalatable or restricted diets unless they are clearly required. Too often patients miss meals unnecessarily when diet orders are not written and NPO orders are not discontinued promptly. The usefulness of many restricted diets is not supported scientifically. Even when the diet is useful as, for example, a renal failure diet, the hospitalized patient may find it so unpalatable that very little is eaten. In that situation, patients should be given what they want to eat and the intake monitored.

Many undernourished hospitalized patients will eat more if they are given assistance at meal time. Family members and hospital volunteers should be encouraged to help the nursing staff provide feeding assistance. Patients can often be encouraged to eat more by providing ethnic foods and allowing supplementary food to be supplied by relatives and friends. Nutritionally complete liquids and puddings for oral use are commercially available, and the patient should be allowed to select among several of the brands and flavors available in the hospital formulary.

When it is obvious that oral intake will not suffice or is not appropriate, the risks of more aggressive nutrition support must be weighed against the benefits. Institutional as well as patient factors should be considered.

WEIGHING THE RISKS AND BENEFITS OF NUTRITION SUPPORT: INSTITUTIONAL FACTORS

The risks of enteral and parenteral nutrition support are minimized when those caring for the patient are experienced in the techniques, when written protocols are followed, and when a team of experienced professionals is available for consultation or management.

WEIGHING THE RISKS AND BENEFITS OF NUTRITION SUPPORT: PATIENT FACTORS

Three factors affecting protein–calorie nutrition status often overlap in the same patient (Fig 48-1). Each of the three should be explored by answering the following questions:

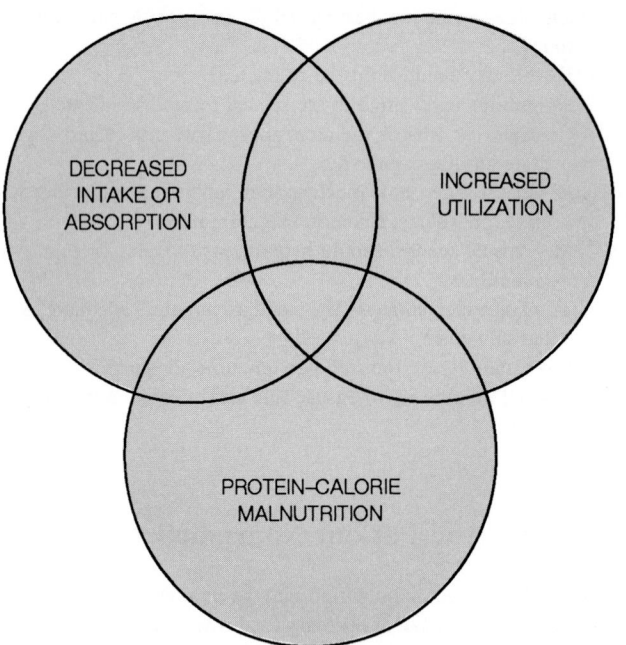

FIGURE 48–1. Indications for nutrition support. All three factors shown must be considered in judging the need for nutrition support. The decision to begin nutrition support is based on the number of factors present and the intensity of each factor.

1. Is the patient's protein and calorie intake inadequate? If so, how long is it likely to remain inadequate?
2. Is the patient using or likely to use protein and calories at a rate that is accelerated due to fever, infection, trauma, burns, corticosteroid therapy, or other catabolic condition?
3. Does the patient already have decreased protein–calorie stores?

The number of these factors present and the intensity of each determines the time when nutrition support should begin. Put simply, the questions to be answered are: How fast is fuel going in? How fast is it being used? How much is in the tank?

Assessment of Nutrient Intake. Nutrient intake is often zero and therefore easy to determine. If not, it can be estimated as a percentage of usual intake or, preferably, a calorie count can be done by the dietary staff. Allowance must be made for fecal wastage of oral calories and protein in the patient with malabsorption. However, inadequate intake is much more important than decreased absorption in almost all patients.

Assessment of Nutrient Utilization. As a general approximation, the rate of resting energy utilization (resting energy expenditure [REE]) for a healthy person is 20 kcal/kg. It is increased up to a maximum of approximately twofold by large burns and to a lesser extent by other severe catabolic conditions such as sepsis and trauma. Under the same circumstances, protein requirements may increase from 0.8 g/kg/d to a maximum of approximately 2.0 g/kg/d. Methods for quantifying calorie and protein utilization are discussed in more detail in a later section entitled "Calculating Calorie and Protein Goals."

Assessment of Protein and Energy Malnutrition. Many measurements, individual and grouped, have been proposed for quantifying protein–calorie malnutrition (Table 48-8).[109,117,118,120–124,131–169] They serve a useful purpose of drawing the attention of the health-care team to patient nutritional needs. However, enthusiasm for nutritional assessment must be tempered by the fact that there is no "gold standard" for quantifying malnutrition in hospitalized patients. Also, none of the measurements proposed for quantifying malnutrition in individual patients is sensitive and specific enough to be of much practical use, especially in critically ill patients. An approach taken by recent investigators has been to determine the relative value of various "nutritional markers" in predicting hospital morbidity and mortality ("nutrition-associated complications"). Buzby and colleagues[163] found that four of ten such variables measured preoperatively correlated with postoperative mortality and complications. They developed a linear predictive model relating the four factors to the percentage of risk of postoperative morbidity, mortality, or both as follows:

Prognostic nutritional index percent

$$= 158 - 16.6 \text{ (Alb)} - 0.78 \text{ (TSF)} - 0.2 \text{ (TFN)} - 5.8 \text{ (DH)}$$

where Alb = serum albumin (g/dL)
TSF = triceps skinfold thickness (mm)
TFN = serum (transferrin (mg/dL)
DH = delayed hypersensitivity to any one of three skin test antigens (mumps, streptokinase-streptodornase, *Candida*) graded as follows: 0, nonreactive; 1, <5 mm induration; 2, >5 mm induration.

The model functioned well in a prospective study of 100 patients undergoing gastrointestinal surgery.[163] In another, nonrandomized study, 7 days of preoperative nutritional support reduced postoperative morbidity and mortality below that predicted for the high-risk group, which comprised those with a prognostic nutritional index greater than 50%.[170] Some of the statistical assumptions underlying the prognostic nutritional index have been criticized.[117,121,134]

Serum albumin concentration is the predominant factor in the prognostic nutritional index. That is consistent with a number of other reports dating to the 1930s showing that serum albumin concentration is a good predictor of morbidity and mortality.[121,146] Its specificity and sensitivity in this regard and, of course, its predictive accuracy depend on the population studied.[121] The reduction in serum albumin levels encountered in hospitalized patients is often a result of the metabolic response to injury and infection and does not specifically reflect protein–calorie malnutrition.[120] However, by identifying the population at greatest risk, hypoalbuminemia may also identify those most likely to benefit from nutrition support.[171]

A subjective global assessment of nutrition status has been developed based entirely on the medical history and physical examination.[134,135,145] On the basis of specific factors in the history and physical examination patients are subjectively rated as (A) well nourished, (B) moderately malnourished, or (C) severely malnourished (Fig 48-2). The rating is most influenced by the patient's loss of subcutaneous tissue, muscle wasting, and percent weight loss, and the subjective global assessment correlates well with "objective" measures of nutritional status. It is as good as

TABLE 48–8
Partial Compilation of Methods Proposed for Assessing
Protein–Calorie Nutritional Status

History[109,117,118,131–135]

Physical Examination[109,117,131,134,135]

Body Measurements—Anthropometrics[117,131,136–142]

Method loss[143]
Weight/height
Weight as percent of usual
Skinfold thicknesses
Mid arm muscle circumference

Serum Protein Concentrations[120,144]

Total protein[122]
Albumin[134,145–149]
Transferrin[122,134,150]
Retinol binding protein[151]
Transthyretin (prealbumin)[151,152]
Fibronectin[153–155]

Enzyme Activities[122,156]

Immunologic Tests[157–159]

Delayed cutaneous hypersensitivity
Total lymphocyte count
Lymphocyte blastogenesis
Neutrophil chemotaxis
Complement levels

Creatinine-Height Index[134,142,160]

Skeletal Muscle Function

Hand grip dynamometry[123]
Stimulated contraction[124,161,162]

Prognostic indices[121,122,134,163–165]

Subjective Assessment[134,135,145,166,167]

Research Techniques[142,168,169]

Multiple isotope dilution
Total-body potassium
Computed tomography
Magnetic resonance imaging
Infrared interactance
Soft tissue radiography
Ultrasonography
Neutron activation analysis
Bioelectrical impedance
Total-body electrical conductivity (TOBEC)
Muscle biopsy analysis
Densitometry
Single- and dual-photon absorptiometry

serum albumin concentration in predicting major nutrition-associated complications, including death, wound healing problems, deep infections, and sepsis.[145] Combinations of serum albumin and subjective global assessment are somewhat better than either alone.[145] For predicting infection, the sensitivity (0.82) and specificity (0.72) of the subjective global assessment is better than the prognostic nutritional index. It is also superior to creatinine-height index, albumin value, transferrin value, skin testing, or skinfold thickness measurements.[134] Factors affecting the accuracy of nutritional assessment methods for predicting nutrition-related complications have been thoroughly reviewed.[121,134]

For clinical purposes, we recommend that the patient's nutritional status be assessed from the history, physical examination, and serum albumin concentration. Any of the following is an indication of malnutrition:

—Weight loss greater than 10% in 6 months and continuing
—Minimal subcutaneous fat in nonathletes (measure or estimate by pinching)
—Muscle wasting in the absence of a neurologic cause (estimate visually and by palpation)
—Serum albumin level less than 3 g/dL not resulting from overhydration, liver disease, or chronic excessive loss from the intestinal tract or kidneys.

TIME LIMITS FOR BEGINNING NUTRITION SUPPORT

Appropriate times for beginning nutrition support are summarized in Table 48-9. Within the ranges given, starting time should be based on the intensity of hypercatabolism and malnutrition. Therapy can begin earlier if it is clear the patient will not resume oral intake within the time limits indicated. The times listed will be considered inappropriately long by some and too short by others. No one should be dogmatic, especially about the critically ill, hypercatabolic patient in an intensive care unit, since there are no controlled data to indicate whether nutrition support given at any time is beneficial to these patients. For suitable patients, tube feeding can begin earlier than TPN because it is theoretically a safer, less expensive, and more effective therapy. Recent results of animal and human studies indicate that tube feeding begun immediately after resuscitation from burns and trauma (i.e., within the first 24 hours) may be particularly beneficial. Early enteral feeding appears to decrease the translocation of bacteria across the intestinal wall, decrease hypercatabolism, and reduce the incidence of sepsis and multiple organ failure.[172–176] If these results are confirmed in further human studies, early enteral feeding of patients with burns and trauma may become the standard of practice.

Calculating Calorie and Protein Goals*

The nonprotein calorie goals for the great majority of patients will fall between 25 and 35 kcal/kg/d and the protein goals usually fall between 1 and 2 g/kg/d. The basis for these practical recommendations should be understood.[177–186]

Throughout this chapter the term protein *will be used when referring to* amino acids, peptides, or whole proteins.

Select appropriate category with a checkmark or enter numerical value where indicated by "#"

A. History

1. Weight change

   Overall loss in past six months: amount = # _____ kg; % loss = # _____

   Change in past 2 weeks: _____ increase

   _____ no change

   _____ decrease

2. Dietary intake change (relative to normal)

   _____ No change

   _____ Change: duration = # _____ weeks

   type: _____ suboptimal solid diet _____ full liquid diet

   _____ hypocaloric liquids _____ starvation

3. Gastrointestinal symptoms (that persisted >2 weeks)

   _____ none _____ nausea _____ vomiting _____ diarrhea _____ anorexia

4. Functional capacity

   _____ No dysfunction (e.g., full capacity)

   _____ Dysfunction: duration = # _____ weeks

   type: _____ working suboptimally

   _____ ambulatory

   _____ bedridden

5. Disease and its relation to nutritional requirements

   Primary diagnosis (specify) _____

   Metabolic demand (stress): _____ no stress _____ low stress

   _____ moderate stress _____ high stress

B. Physical (for each trait specify: 0 = normal, 1+ = mild, 2+ = moderate, 3+ = severe)

   # _____ loss of subcutaneous fat (triceps, chest)

   # _____ muscle wasting (quadriceps, deltoids)

   # _____ ankle edema

   # _____ sacral edema

   # _____ ascites

C. SGA rating (select one)

   _____ A = Well nourished

   _____ B = Moderately (or suspected of being) malnourished

   _____ C = Severely malnourished

(From Detsky AS, McLaughlin JR, Baker JP, et al. What is subjective global assessment of nutritional status? JPEN 1987; 11:8)

FIGURE 48–2. Subjective global assessment of nutritional status.

The aim is to achieve nitrogen equilibrium or positive nitrogen balance without giving a harmful excess of calories or protein. Excessive calorie administration increases the likelihood of complications from hyperglycemia, fatty infiltration of the liver, excessive carbon dioxide production, and hypermetabolism. When the rate of intravenous glucose infusion is increased, glucose oxidation increases and reaches a plateau when the infusion rate reaches about 5 mg/kg/min (7 g/kg/d). Insulin administration does not increase the rate of glucose oxidation beyond this plateau rate.[187-189] Unoxidized glucose is diverted to synthesis of glycogen and fat, which consumes calories without any obvious functional benefit to the patient.

Taken together, the available studies indicate that optimum nitrogen balance and, therefore, presumably optimum benefit from nutrition support, will be achieved when the patient is administered calories equal to between 100% and 120% of his or her actual total daily energy expenditure. Total daily energy expenditure can be estimated knowing that it comprises the following seven components:

1. *Basal Energy Expenditure (BEE)* is the energy used for normal body functions when well, awake, in a thermoneutral environment, and in a basal fasting state after overnight bed rest. It cannot be measured in patients since they are not

TABLE 48-9
Appropriate Times for Beginning Nutrition Support
of Patients Who Are Not Eating*

	BEGIN TUBE FEEDING IF POSSIBLE	BEGIN TPN
Patient neither hypercatabolic nor malnourished	7 days	14 days
Patient either hypercatabolic or malnourished	1–5 days	6–10 days
Patient both hypercatabolic and malnourished	1–3 days	1–7 days

* Times can be doubled for patients ingesting as much as half their energy and protein requirements. Nutrition support should begin sooner than the times indicated when it is clear that the patient will not begin eating until well beyond the times shown.

well. BEE can be estimated as 20 kcal/kg/d or more accurately by means of the Harris-Benedict equations[190]:

$$\text{Women (kcal/d)} = 655 + (9.6 \times \text{Wt})$$
$$+ (1.7 \times \text{Ht}) - (4.7 \times \text{A})$$
$$\text{Men (kcal/d)} = 66 + (13.7 \times \text{Wt})$$
$$+ (5 \times \text{Ht}) - (6.8 \times \text{A})$$

where   Wt = actual weight in kg

Ht = height in cm

A = age in years

It should be noted that energy expenditure will be less than the basal rate during prolonged fasting (starvation), sleep, and hypotension.

These formulas will overestimate energy expenditure for obese patients. The estimate can be improved by using the mean of actual weight and desirable weight instead of actual weight. Desirable weight can be obtained from readily available tables or can be estimated based on height as: 100 pounds plus 5 pounds for each inch over 5 feet for women and 106 pounds plus 6 pounds for each inch over 5 feet for men.

2. *Stress hypermetabolism* is the additional energy expenditure caused by the patient's illness. It varies among patients with the same illness and during the course of illness and cannot be estimated with great accuracy for individual patients.[191] Average stress hypermetabolism expressed as a multiplier of calculated BEE ranges from 1.1 × BEE (i.e., 10% above calculated BEE) for the few days following uncomplicated abdominal surgery to 2 × BEE (i.e., 100% above BEE) for massive burns prior to skin grafting. Average stress factors estimated or measured for various conditions are shown in Table 48-10.[192]

3. *Nonshivering thermogenesis* is the energy required to maintain body temperature above ambient temperature. It is minimal for patients with intact skin in temperature-controlled environments and can be ignored.

4. *Diet-induced thermogenesis* is the energy required to digest, absorb, transport, metabolize, and store nutrients. It is de-

pendent on the type and amount of energy administered and minimally dependent on the route of administration. It probably does not exceed 10% to 15% of energy administered for most patients receiving nutrition support.

5. *Abnormal energy losses in urine, stool, and drainage from fistulae and wounds* are seldom significant and are ignored. They are most important as sources of nitrogen loss.

6. *Energy expenditure of activity* ranges from 10% to 30% of BEE for most hospitalized patients.

7. *Energy expenditure for weight gain.* The energy equivalent of 1 pound of weight gain is approximately 3500 kcal. Therefore, when weight gain is desired, 500 kcal/d can be added to the energy goal and should result in a gain of approximately 1 pound per week. Alternatively, the energy for weight gain can be set at 20% of BEE. Weight gain generally is not possible and should not be attempted in patients with stress factors above 1.2.

The sum of the first three of these components, BEE, stress hypermetabolism, and nonshivering thermogenesis, is resting energy expenditure (REE). It can be measured accurately at the bedside by indirect calorimetry, which makes use of the known relationship between energy expenditure and the volume of oxygen consumed and carbon dioxide produced. If the patient is receiving nutrients at the time of the indirect calorimetry then the fourth factor above, diet-induced thermogenesis, is also included in the measured REE. To determine total energy expenditure, the components not measured by indirect calorimetry must be estimated and added to the measured REE. The nutritional support group at the hospital of the University of Pennsylvania, which has extensive experience with indirect calorimetry for this purpose, recommends a nonprotein calorie intake of 130% REE for patients who do not require weight gain (fat repletion) and 150% REE for patients who need weight gain.[191] They compared the energy intake determined in this way for 100 patients with the intake that would have been prescribed for the same patients using 190 published

TABLE 48-10
Stress Factors*

CONDITION	STRESS FACTOR
Well-nourished, unstressed	1.0
Postabdominal surgery, uncomplicated	1.0–1.1
Multiple trauma (acute phase)	
Normotensive	1.1–1.5
Hypotensive	0.8–1.0
Multiple trauma (recovery)	1.0–1.2
Sepsis (acute phase)	
Normotensive	1.2–1.7
Hypotensive	0.5
Sepsis (recovery)	1.0
Burn, 20%–40% body surface, prior to skin graft	1.5–2.0
Burn, after successful grafting	1.0–1.3

* Multiply the estimated basal energy expenditure by the stress factor to yield an estimate of resting energy expenditure.
Adapted from Schlichtig R, Ayres SM. Nutritional support of the critically ill. Chicago: Year Book Medical Publishers, 1988:111.

guidelines for estimating calorie requirements of hospitalized patients.[191] They found little correlation between energy goals based on their measurements and those based on the guidelines. The guidelines estimated needs substantially above and below their measurement-derived goals for individual patients. On average, use of the published formulas would have resulted in administration of substantially more calories per day. Although these results argue for use of indirect calorimetry in estimating energy goals for hospitalized patients who are to receive nutrition support, it is not clear that any expense or risk of administering too little or too much energy to some patients justifies the expense of performing several indirect calorimetric measurements for each patient receiving nutrition support.

In practice, if a method for doing accurate indirect calorimetry is available, it should be used to measure REE especially for selected patients who would be least tolerant of overfeeding or underfeeding or for whom it would be most difficult to estimate energy requirements accurately. These include patients who are very malnourished, patients in respiratory or heart failure, and those with diabetes, morbid obesity, closed-head trauma, or paralysis. Nonprotein energy goals should be set at 130% REE for patients who do not require weight gain and 150% REE for those who do. When indirect calorimetry is not available or not needed, the energy goal may be calculated as shown in Table 48-11.

As stated at the beginning of this section, for practical purposes the majority of hospitalized patients requiring nutrition support may be given between 25 and 35 kcal/kg/d from nonprotein sources based on their current dry weight. Less stressed and older patients usually fall into the lower end of this range, while more stressed and younger patients fall into the upper range. For weight gain, amounts up to 40 or 45 kcal/kg/d may be appropriate.

Should the protein administered to a patient be counted as an energy source that contributes to meeting energy goals? Opinion is divided. Since the reason for giving protein is to provide nitrogen, not energy, many do not count protein calories toward the calorie goal. However, few patients achieve a sustained positive nitrogen balance of more than 2 to 3 g/d. Therefore, the great majority of protein given is actually oxidized as an energy source and, therefore, counting it as such is reasonable. We prefer not to count protein as a calorie source. The excess calories given when protein calories are not counted help make up for the fact that the amount of nutrient actually given to most patients is less than the amount ordered. For TPN the amount given averages approximately 90% of the amount ordered, and for tube feeding it is approximately 83%.[193]

Protein Goals

At any energy intake, nitrogen balance is directly dependent on protein intake.[194] However, there are methodologic problems in

TABLE 48-11
Calculating Energy Goals in the Absence
of Calorimetry Measurement

1. Estimate BEE (Harris-Benedict formula or 20 kcal/kg/d)
2. Multiply BEE by stress factor (see Table 48-10)
3. Add for activity: 10% to 30% of BEE
4. Add for weight gain if indicated: 500 to 1000 kcal/d

TABLE 48-12
Guidelines for Protein Administration

CONDITION	PROTEIN (g/kg/d)*
Renal failure, not on dialysis	0.8
Renal failure on hemodialysis	1.0
Renal failure on peritoneal dialysis	1.2
Malnourished, not metabolically stressed	1.0–2.0
Postoperative, no organ failure	1.2–1.5
Severely catabolic, no renal or liver failure	1.5–2.0

* Based on current dry weight unless patient is > 140% of desirable body weight, in which case use the mean of actual and desirable weight.

the measurement of both nitrogen balance and protein synthesis that have prevented the precise determination of optimal protein intake for patients.[192] Furthermore, while healthy persons can tolerate large amounts of protein without ill effects, patients often cannot. Excessive protein administration to patients may result in azotemia, osmotic diuresis, hyperammonemia, hepatic encephalopathy, or respiratory muscle fatigue owing to increased ventilatory sensitivity to carbon dioxide.[195] When energy intake is adequate, optimum protein intake for hospitalized patients ranges from 0.8 to 2.0 g/kg/d based on current dry body weight. Within this range, the appropriate intake depends on the level of metabolic stress, renal function, liver function, and the amount of any excessive nitrogen losses in urine, stool, drainage, and dialysis fluid. Guidelines are shown in Table 48-12. Occasionally, patients who are resorbing large hematomas will require even less than 0.8 g/kg/d of protein.

Nitrogen equilibrium is generally not obtainable at any energy or protein intake in patients who are severely septic[196] or traumatized.[197,198] These patients have elevated rates of whole-body protein catabolism and synthesis. Nutritional support reduces negative nitrogen balance primarily by further increasing whole-body protein synthesis and not by decreasing protein catabolism.[198] Intensive efforts are being made to find safe ways to block or blunt the neurocytohumoral mechanisms responsible for accelerated protein catabolism in stressed patients,[199] including most recently administration of recombinant human growth hormone. Immobilization accompanying illness and injury contributes to the muscle wasting and nitrogen loss.[200] Nitrogen balance may improve to the extent that mobilization of the patient can be achieved.

Access for Nutrition Support

Once the decision is made to initiate nutrition support and the goals for energy and protein are determined, the next step is selection of an access route. First, the oral route should be considered to be sure nothing has been overlooked that would allow the goals to be reached. Next the enteral route is considered. If that is not feasible or not successful, then the intravenous route, either peripheral or central, must be used.

The final two steps to optimum nutrition support, namely, listing (or at least thinking about) the individual components in the nutrition formula and special monitoring will be discussed separately for parenteral and enteral nutrition.

PARENTERAL (INTRAVENOUS) NUTRITION

Indications

TPN is indicated for those patients who cannot meet their nutritional needs for a prolonged period of time via the gastrointestinal tract. Guidelines for the use of TPN in the hospitalized adult patient have been published by the American Society for Parenteral and Enteral Nutrition.[201]

Peripheral TPN

The advent of safe intravenous lipid emulsions made peripheral TPN practical because the emulsions are calorically dense (up to 2 kcal/mL) and yet they are isotonic. Peripheral TPN fluid consists of a mixture with final concentrations of 5% to 10% glucose, 2% to 5% amino acid, and electrolytes. This crystalloid solution is mixed with 10% or 20% intravenous fat emulsion as an all-in-one mixture, or the lipid emulsion is infused piggyback simultaneously with the crystalloid solution. Delivery of nutrients into a peripheral vein is limited by the relatively low rate of blood flow in these veins (10 to 50 mL/min). As a result, peripheral TPN fluid, which is usually 600 to 900 mOsm/kg and is given at 2 to 3 L/d, raises osmolality in the vein substantially and causes phlebitis. The risk of phlebitis can be reduced by giving less TPN or by diluting it, but frequently neither approach is satisfactory.

Some groups have been successful in providing nutrition support to a substantial number of patients with peripheral TPN. In practice, we find that there are relatively few patients who need nutrition support for whom the peripheral route provides optimum nutrition. To use this technique patients should have good peripheral veins, be able to tolerate relatively large volumes of fluid, and have relatively low energy and protein needs. Generally, patients who meet these criteria can be fed orally or enterally or can tolerate several days without nutrient intake. Frequently, patients who are begun on peripheral TPN receive inadequate nutrition at a substantial cost for only a few days before being switched to the oral, enteral, or central TPN route. Occasionally, peripheral TPN can be used effectively to supplement suboptimal oral or enteral intake.

Central TPN

In central TPN, the problem of hypertonic fluid causing damage to the vein is avoided by delivering the nutrient mixture into a vein with a high volume flow, usually the superior vena cava. The rapid flow, 1.5 to 2.0 L/min, dilutes the hypertonic mixture, up to 3000 mOsm/kg, so quickly that there is little risk of hypertonic damage to the vein. It should be noted that any other vascular system with a high flow rate, such as the type of arteriovenous fistulae used for dialysis, can be used for "central TPN" with little risk of damage to the fistula, although use of the fistulae is usually restricted to dialysis.

Ideally, the hypertonic central TPN fluid should be administered into the middle to lower part of the superior vena cava via a central venous catheter inserted by way of the right subclavian vein. The left subclavian vein is the next best choice. The internal jugular veins may be used if subclavian access is not feasible due to coagulopathy, severe pulmonary disease, or local skin conditions. However, adequate dressing and site care for jugular catheters is difficult. Although the complication rate for insertion of jugular catheters is less than for subclavian catheters, the infection rate in the weeks after insertion is considerably higher for jugular catheters. For this reason, the subclavian vein is the preferred access route for central TPN. Use of the inferior vena cava via the femoral vein is discouraged except as a last resort because of the high risk of infection and thrombosis.

Insertion of Central Venous Catheters for TPN

Insertion of the central venous catheter should be performed or directly supervised by a physician thoroughly familiar with placement of catheters for central TPN. The Seldinger method is the standard and safest technique. The vein is entered with a small-gauge needle through which a wire is passed. The tapered catheter is passed over the wire, which is then withdrawn. Ideally, each hospital, certainly each teaching hospital, should provide a detailed printed protocol for central venous catheter insertion. A chest radiograph must be obtained as soon as possible after insertion, and only isotonic fluid should be infused until proper position of the catheter tip is verified. A procedure note in the patient's chart should document the date and time of the procedure, site of insertion, type and length of catheter, radiographic results, and any apparent complications.

The substantial risks of central venous catheter insertion include pneumothorax, arterial bleeding, brachial plexus injury, air embolism, guidewire embolism, hemothorax, cardiac tamponade, and death.[202,203] The risks are lower when the procedure is done by someone who has inserted more than 50 catheters and when less experienced operators are well supervised.[204] Pneumothorax and perforation of the superior vena cava or heart by the catheter tip may be delayed for several days after insertion.[202,203] Delayed perforation of the vein or heart can be caused by malposition of the catheter tip and movement of the tip relative to vascular structures during normal body movement and breathing.

Silastic catheters with a long skin tunnel and anchored by a Dacron cuff are usually used for patients receiving TPN and hydration at home. Some physicians favor using these catheters for inpatients who are deemed likely to require TPN for several weeks. This practice is based on the assumption, as yet unproven, that these catheters are less likely to become infected, less prone to accidental removal, and less likely to cause vascular injury and thrombosis, compared with temporary, nontunneled catheters. Randomized controlled trials are needed. We do not favor these catheters for adult inpatient use because physicians are too reluctant to remove them when catheter infection is in the differential diagnosis.

Maintenance of the Catheter

Successful central TPN requires that central venous access be maintained. Infection, accidental removal, and clogging are the most frequent reasons for loss of the catheter. Central catheters are suspected of causing infection about ten times more frequently than they actually are the cause.[205,206] The distinction is important because removing the catheter when it is not necessary increases risk and expense. However, there are no uniformly used criteria for identifying true catheter-related sepsis. Suggested criteria are listed below, but they include some that are more useful epidemiologically than clinically since they require removal of the catheter.[207]

1. Two or more positive blood cultures from the catheter and peripheral sites with the same organism isolated from the catheter tip on removal.
2. Persistently positive blood cultures from the catheter and negative cultures from peripheral sites associated with clinical signs of sepsis.
3. Quantitative blood cultures simultaneously collected from the catheter and peripheral sites that show a concentration of organisms five to ten times as great in the catheter sample compared with the peripheral sample.
4. Infection of the exit wound site or tunnel by the same organism isolated from blood culture.

Simultaneous, quantitative blood cultures from the catheter and periphery using the lysis centrifugation (Isolator) method helps to distinguish catheter-related sepsis from that which is not caused by the catheter.[206,207] Replacement of catheters over a guidewire appears to be a safe and convenient way to establish whether sepsis is catheter-related. If there is no change in the signs of infection after the exchange, then the catheter is not likely to have been at fault. However, when catheter-related sepsis is present the new catheter may become infected with the same organism.[205]

Catheter infections can occur in the fibrin sheath surrounding the intravascular portion of the catheter, in the tunnel between the skin entry site and the vein, and in the hub and lumen of the catheter. Infection in the fibrin sheath coating the intravascular portion of the catheter is most likely to be from a distant source. Little can be done to prevent it other than the usual precautions against hospital-acquired infections. There are conflicting data as to whether small amounts of heparin in the TPN fluid (1 to 2 units/mL) by decreasing fibrin sheath formation will decrease the rate of catheter infection. Whether some current catheter materials are better than others in this regard is also controversial.

Infections in the catheter tunnel can be minimized by proper attention to cleansing and dressing of the skin entry site.[208] Every hospital should have a written protocol for this procedure. One or a small group of persons should be charged with either doing the dressing changes for all patients or providing quality assurance if others are doing the procedure. Good results have been reported with traditional occlusive dressings changed every 2 or 3 days and with transparent dressings changed every 7 to 14 days. However, a recent meta-analysis concludes that transparent dressings are associated with a significantly higher rate of infection.[209] A silver nitrate–impregnated cuff surrounding the catheter and pushed into the subcutaneous portion of the skin tunnel may significantly reduce the incidence of catheter infection.[210]

The frequency of infections in the hub and lumen of the catheter is reduced by minimizing the number of times the administration system is entered and by applying povidone iodine to any junction in the central fluid administration system before it is opened. TPN fluids are almost never the source of infection. Injections should not be made into the TPN line, and no additions should be made to the TPN mixture except in the institution's pharmacy. Compared with single-lumen catheters, triple-lumen catheters are about three times more likely to become infected.[211,212] In-line filters do not reduce the incidence of infections associated with central catheters or TPN. Where they are still used the justification for filters is that they trap particulates and air.

To prevent accidental removal of the catheter, they are usually sutured to the skin near the entry site. This practice is forbidden by some experts because of concern that it increases the risk of tunnel infection. Whichever method is used, adequate taping of 1 or 2 loops of tubing to the dressing or to the patient's chest is essential. To prevent clogging of the catheter, a pump should be used to maintain flow through it at all times.

The protocol in some institutions is to change TPN catheters over a wire or to insert a new catheter on the opposite side at regular intervals such as every 3 to 7 days. This is a reasonable practice for patients who are repeatedly bacteremic, including burn patients, and for patients with recurrent or persistent fever or leukocytosis. However, changing central catheters on a routine basis in patients who show no signs of infection is of unproven benefit, expensive, and probably causes more harm than good.

TPN Via Multiple-Lumen Catheters

Whenever possible, TPN should be administered through single-lumen catheters and any parenteral medications that cannot be put into the TPN fluid in the institution's pharmacy should be administered via a peripheral vein. The single-lumen TPN catheter can be exchanged for a multiple-lumen catheter over a wire if additional central access is required subsequently. The superior vena cava port on hemodynamic monitoring catheters (Swan-Ganz) is suitable for short-term TPN. When using multiple-lumen catheters for TPN, one lumen should be designated for TPN administration and should not be used for any other purpose. All lumens should be managed by the same protocol used for TPN catheters.

Designing a TPN Formula

In addition to the energy and protein content of a TPN formula, seven other features must be considered. A mnemonic—FACE MTV—helps recall each component in an appropriate order. They are as follows:

Fluid. Should fluid be restricted? If the patient cannot tolerate more than 1000 to 1500 mL of additional fluid, calorie and protein goals may not be achievable. In this event, every effort should be made to reduce any other fluids the patient is receiving in order to make room for nutritional fluids. Peripheral TPN (dilute fluids) obviously cannot be used for nutrition support when volume must be restricted. The most concentrated intravenous nutrients commercially available are 70% dextrose in water (2.38 kcal/mL), 20% fat emulsion (2.0 kcal/mL) and 15% amino acid solution.

Amino Acids. Crystalline amino acids are currently the only source of nitrogen for parenteral nutrition therapy. Mixtures for general use are designed to be of high biologic value similar to egg albumin or casein. A typical standard amino acid mixture contains approximately 15 amino acids and, on a weight per weight basis, approximately 45% of the amino acids are essential, 20% branched chain (leucine, isoleucine, valine) and 12% methionine plus aromatic amino acids (phenylalanine, tyrosine, tryptophan). Amino acid solutions with different amino acid compositions may be more beneficial than the standard mixture for certain conditions.[213] The commercially available special mixtures for use in adult patients differ from standard amino acid mixtures as follows:

Renal failure mixtures with a much higher proportion of essential amino acids
Liver failure mixtures with more branched-chain amino acids and less methionine and aromatic amino acids
Stress mixtures with more branched-chain amino acids

These products are severalfold more expensive than the standard mixtures, and data regarding their benefit are conflicting and incomplete. We conclude that the renal failure mixtures offer little, if any, advantage because virtually all patients with chronic renal failure on TPN are being dialyzed and for them the standard amino acid mixtures are entirely adequate. A liver failure mixture may be useful in rare patients with liver disease who become encephalopathic on administration of standard amino acids at a rate less than the goal rate. A stress amino acid mixture may be more effective than the standard amino acid product in retarding erosion of body protein mass in patients with severe trauma or sepsis. However, these patients often require a fluid-restricted TPN formula and none of the stress amino acid mixtures are as concentrated as the most concentrated standard mixture currently available, which is 15%.

Calories. What proportion of the nonprotein calories should be given as fat versus carbohydrate? For most humans, fat makes up 10% to 45% of the nonprotein calories eaten. TPN formulas in which fat provides anywhere from 10% to 70% of the calories seem to be well tolerated. TPN formulas with 20% to 30% of the nonprotein calories as fat are associated with fewer complications and probably greater efficacy than formulas with less fat and more glucose.[214,215] A higher percentage of fat calories in TPN, up to 50% of nonprotein calories, is appropriate for patients with diabetes. A similar high-fat formula is also appropriate for patients with pulmonary failure resulting in carbon dioxide retention, because, calorie-for-calorie, fat oxidation produces less carbon dioxide than carbohydrate oxidation. When carbon dioxide retention is a problem it is also important to avoid feeding more calories than the patient needs since excess calorie administration further increases carbon dioxide production, hypermetabolism, and oxygen demand with no beneficial results except an increase in the patient's adipose tissue.

The relative nitrogen-sparing effects of glucose and lipid and the rate of lipid utilization in septic and injured patients is controversial.[198,216,217] The current intravenous lipid emulsions are polyunsaturated long-chain triglycerides from soybeans and/or safflower oils. Their use, especially in septic and injured patients, should be tempered by evidence that these emulsions can diminish clearance of bacteria from the bloodstream, impair macrophage function, blockade the reticuloendothelial system, impair pulmonary function, and alter immunocompetence.[192,218] Consequently, septic and injured patients probably should not receive more than 1 g/kg/d of the current emulsions and some recommend no more than 30 g/d.[219] Other intravenous fats, including medium-chain tryglycerides, fish oils, and structured lipids, are being studied and appear promising both as nutrients and as pharmacologic agents.[219-221]

Electrolytes. In choosing or designing a TPN mixture, the content of several electrolytes must be considered. In order of decreasing frequency with which serum abnormalities occur in patients on TPN, they are phosphorus, potassium, sodium, magnesium, calcium, and chloride/acetate (acid–base balance). Standard electrolyte mixtures are suitable for 50% to 80% of patients receiving TPN. A standard mixture will seldom be suitable for patients who already have an abnormal serum level of one of the electrolytes or for patients with congestive heart failure, renal failure, liver failure, or multiple organ failure.

Phosphorus. Generally 15 mmol of phosphorus should be provided per 800 glucose calories. Large quantities of phosphorus shift from the extracellular to the intracellular compartments under the influence of glucose and during tissue synthesis. If the TPN solution contains insufficient phosphorus, the serum concentration will decline slowly to reach a nadir, which usually occurs 2 to 4 days after beginning TPN. For this reason, severe hypophosphatemia (< 1.0 mg/dL) should be corrected before beginning central TPN. Antacids in the gastrointestinal tract will lower the serum phosphorus value even in the absence of oral or enteral feeding. When adding phosphorus to TPN mixtures, one must be aware of the amount of calcium also being administered in order to prevent the precipitation of calcium phosphate. Precipitation is unlikely to occur if twice the phosphorus concentration (mmol/L) plus the calcium concentration (mEq/L) does not exceed 45.

Potassium. Requirements for potassium are generally 30 to 40 mEq per 800 glucose calories. Potassium shifts rapidly from the extracellular to the intracellular compartments under the influence of glucose and during tissue synthesis. If the solution contains insufficient potassium, a significant fall in serum concentration may be observed as early as 6 to 12 hours after beginning TPN.

Sodium. Most patients receiving TPN are given 30 to 50 mEq of sodium per liter of formula. Mixtures containing less sodium, including sodium-free fluids, may be given to patients with fluid retention. Low serum sodium concentrations in patients receiving TPN are most often dilutional due to overhydration or to the syndrome of inappropriate secretion of antidiuretic hormone. Dilutional hyponatremia should be corrected by decreasing fluid intake, for example, by increasing the concentration of the TPN mixture. Occasional patients with large fluid losses from ileostomies, fistulae, or diarrhea or with renal wasting of sodium may have hyponatremia due to true depletion, and they will require higher concentrations of sodium in the TPN mixture. Hyperna-tremia due to free water deficit as a result of hyperventilation or excessive losses from drainage, diarrhea, or diuresis is managed by increasing the free water intake in the TPN or other fluids.

Magnesium. Most patients do well with a magnesium in-take of 5 to 10 mEq/L of TPN. Hypomagnesemia during TPN is most often encountered in patients receiving drugs that cause renal wasting of magnesium such as diuretics, cisplatin, or am-photericin.

Calcium. The quantity of calcium needed by resting adult patients receiving TPN has not been established. Typically TPN provides 5 to 10 mEq/L.

Chloride/Acetate. A small amount of chloride and a larger amount of acetate are provided by the manufacturer in virtually all amino acid mixtures to prevent acidosis resulting from metabolism of lysine and arginine. Standard electrolyte mixtures include additional acetate over and above that present in the amino acid mixture. To decrease the risk of metabolic alkalosis, the amount of additional acetate should be limited for patients with large gastric fluid losses who are not receiving a histamine receptor antagonist. The addition of more acetate to the mixture may be appropriate for patients who have metabolic acidosis that is cor-rectable by acetate.

Miscellaneous Additives. To avoid problems of in-compatibility, it is important to limit miscellaneous additives to TPN mixtures to those known to be compatible with a wide range of formulas. Additions may include heparin, insulin, and hista-mine—H_2 receptor antagonists. Heparin, 1 unit/mL, frequently is added to central TPN mixtures. It may minimize clotting in the catheter and decrease fibrin sheath formation on the surface of the catheter. Studies indicate that two to five times this amount is required to reduce the incidence, possibly as high as 30%, of silent subclavian vein thrombosis. This is seldom done because of the risk of bleeding. Heparin should be removed from the TPN when heparin-induced thrombocytopenia is suspected. Insulin should not be added routinely but only to manage documented hyperglycemia. If hyperglycemia occurs, the initial insulin dose usually should not exceed 10 units per 800 glucose calories. Ad-ditional insulin is given subcutaneously or intravenously on a slid-ing scale, and a similar amount is subsequently added to the TPN. Increasing the amount of insulin in the TPN mixture above 100 to 150 units per day is unlikely to be helpful. Instead, the amount of glucose administered should be reduced and the calories replaced by intravenous fat emulsion, if possible. Both cimetidine and ra-nitidine are compatible with TPN mixtures and effective when administered in this way.

Albumin is compatible with crystalloid TPN solutions but not with the "all-in-one" mixtures that contain intravenous lipid emulsion. The appropriateness of administering intravenous al-bumin is controversial. Available data support giving albumin to patients with serum levels below 2.5 g/dL who are receiving ad-equate TPN.[222] Any cost-effectiveness of intravenous albumin will be diminished if there are rapid losses of albumin from the plasma via capillary leak (severe sepsis or trauma), proteinuria, or protein-losing enteropathy. The dose of albumin required can be calculated based on a volume of distribution equal to 30% of body weight

or based on a regression equation.[223] It is usually best to give the total amount over 2 or 3 days to avoid intravascular volume over-load. Administration should be stopped once the serum concen-tration reaches 3.0 g/dL.

Trace Elements. Trace elements should be administered according to the guidelines of the expert panel for the Nutritional Advisory Group of the American Medical Association.[224] An extra 2 mg of zinc is often given to hypercatabolic patients. A typical trace element cocktail provides the following per day: zinc, 5.0 mg; copper, 1.0 mg; manganese, 500 μg; chromium, 10 μg; and selenium, 60 μg.

As noted in the first part of this chapter, there is no practical way to assess trace element status clinically. Serum levels are difficult to measure accurately and do not correlate adequately with other measures of deficiency. Our practice is to include ap-proximately the amounts indicated above in the daily TPN mixture for everyone receiving TPN, even those with renal failure and other organ failure. Zinc is the only trace element likely to be required in larger amounts than indicated above.[51] Zinc loss in upper small bowel fluid is approximately 17 mg/L of output, while losses in diarrhea or ileostomy output are approximately 12 mg/L.[42] Therefore, patients with diarrheal diseases or other large fluid losses from the intestine may require additional zinc, up to 25 mg/d.

Iron is not routinely put in TPN. If significant iron deficiency is documented, iron dextran, 1 to 2 mL/d, may be added to the crystalloid TPN solutions, but not to all-in-one mixtures.

Vitamins. Multivitamin cocktails for intravenous use should be added routinely to the TPN fluid each day unless there is a contraindication. The amount of each vitamin in the available standard cocktails is in accordance with the recommendations of the Nutrition Advisory Group of the American Medical Associ-ation.[225] Typical vitamin amounts administered daily in TPN are shown in Table 48-13.

Vitamin K is not present in the commercially available mul-tivitamin products. Phytonadione should be added daily, 1 mg, or

TABLE 48–13
Typical Vitamin Amounts Administered Daily in TPN

VITAMIN	AMOUNT
Vitamin A	3300 IU
Vitamin D	200 IU
Ascorbic acid (vitamin C)	100 mg
Folic acid	400 μg
Niacin	40 mg
Riboflavin (vitamin B_2)	3.6 mg
Thiamine (vitamin B_1)	3 mg
Pyridoxine (vitamin B_6)	4 mg
Cyanocobalamin (vitamin B_{12})	5 μg
Pantothenic acid	15 mg
Biotin	60 μg
Vitamin E	10 IU
Vitamin K	1 mg

weekly, 10 mg to the TPN mixture. Anaphylactic-like adverse reactions have not been documented with vitamin K in these doses administered via TPN mixtures. If the vitamin is not added routinely, prothrombin time should be determined at least weekly; however, it is an insensitive measure of vitamin K status. A patient with a normal prothrombin time and a marginal vitamin K status may develop prolonged prothrombin time and bleeding within hours if vitamin K availability is decreased such as by starting broad-spectrum antibiotics or if utilization of clotting factors is increased, as would occur during surgery. Vitamin K should be omitted for the rare patient on TPN who is being anticoagulated with warfarin.

The optimal amounts of parenteral vitamins for patients with various catabolic conditions is controversial. It is reasonable to double the amounts listed above for patients on TPN who are pregnant and those undergoing rapid repletion of lean body mass. Patients with trauma, sepsis, or burns may benefit from larger amounts of some vitamins, especially vitamins C and A.

24-Hour and All-in-One Systems

Traditionally, TPN has been prepared in 1-L containers. Most patients receive between 1.5 and 3.0 L of crystalloid solution. Lipid emulsion is given by piggyback or through a separate line daily or two to three times a week. Recent availability of large volume bags has made it possible to put a 24-hour supply of crystalloid solution in a single bag. This has a number of advantages, including decreasing the amount of time required by the nursing staff to administer TPN and decreasing the number of times each day that the TPN administration line is entered. There are few, if any, disadvantages. In this system, intravenous lipid emulsions are still given separately, usually using a second pump.

The all-in-one or total nutrient admixture system in which all of the TPN fluids for 24 hours including the lipid emulsion are placed in a single bag is becoming increasingly popular. The advantages are the same as those mentioned above, plus this system eliminates the nursing time, infection risk, and extra pump required to administer the lipid emulsion separately. Disadvantages of this method include inability to see particulates, inability to use amino acid solutions that have a low pH, and some limitations on the amounts of divalent cations and other additions that can be made to the mixture without risking a break in the lipid emulsion.

Special Monitoring for Patients Receiving Parenteral Nutrition

When patients are placed on TPN they should be monitored to assess the adequacy of nutrition support and also to anticipate and reduce risks of complications.

MONITORING TO ASSESS ADEQUACY OF NUTRITION SUPPORT

The TPN formula is designed to meet the patient's estimated energy and protein goals. Ideally, the patient should then be ob-served to determine that the amounts being given are optimal. For the reasons already discussed, there is no rigorous and practical way to make this determination. Weight changes over weeks are useful, but over shorter periods of time weight changes reflect fluid balance more than energy balance. There has been some enthusiasm for using serum concentrations of proteins with short half-lives such as transferrin, retinol-binding protein, and especially transthyretin (prealbumin) to follow changes in nutrition status. None is specific or sensitive enough as an indicator of nutritional repletion to be of much practical value. This is especially true for critically ill patients, because serum protein concentrations are influenced by changes in intravascular volume, capillary leak, and acute-phase response as well as by changes in nutrition status. Indirect calorimetry can be used to determine how the amount of energy being used per minute compares with the amount being given. It should be noted that calorimetry measures energy expenditure during a short period when the patient is resting. Energy use per minute will increase substantially when the patient is turned, suctioned, debrided, and disturbed in other ways, but these activities usually add only a few percent to the total daily energy expenditure.

When it is technically feasible, nitrogen balance is the most practical and effective way to estimate the adequacy of nitrogen and energy administration. The test requires a 24-hour urine collection for either urinary urea nitrogen, which can be measured by the same method as blood urea nitrogen, or total urinary nitrogen, usually determined by a chemiluminescence method. Most data indicate that total urinary nitrogen can be accurately approximated from urinary urea nitrogen by either of the following formulas:

$$TUN = UUN/0.8 \quad \text{or} \quad TUN = UNN + 2.$$

However, recent data indicate that urinary urea nitrogen cannot be used to reliably determine total urinary nitrogen in all patients receiving nutrition support.[226] For greatest accuracy in determining nitrogen balance, the patient should be on a constant calorie and nitrogen intake for at least 48 hours prior to starting the collection. Nitrogen balance measurements provide minimal information for the patient with large fluid losses from wounds and fistulae because a significant amount of nitrogen may be lost, resulting in a falsely high nitrogen balance. The calculation for nitrogen balance is as follows:

$$N_{Balance} = N_{in} - N_{out}$$

$$N_{in} = \text{g amino acids administered} \div 6.25^*$$

$$N_{out} = TUN \, (g)\dagger + 1 \, g\ddagger$$

---

* On average, there is 1 g nitrogen per 6.25 g of dietary protein. If known, the correct figure for the specific amino acids mixture received by the patient should be used in the calculation. This figure ranges from 6 to 7 g amino acid per 1 g nitrogen for various amino acid preparations.

† If UNN is measured, estimate TUN: TUN = UUN + 2.

‡ In the absence of oral or enteral feeding the loss of nitrogen from the skin and intestinal tract is estimated to be 1 g. For enteral feeding, the estimate is usually 2 g.

MONITORING TO ANTICIPATE AND REDUCE RISKS OF COMPLICATIONS

The potential complications of central TPN are numerous and life threatening. The frequency and type of metabolic monitoring must be tailored to the individual patient to avoid either inadequate or excessive monitoring. The important complications can be grouped into three categories: mechanical, septic, and metabolic. Mechanical complications are generally associated with insertion and care of the central venous catheter and are minimized by adherence to a written procedure and by adequate supervision.

Sepsis due to central TPN has been greatly reduced by the current methods of preparing the fluids and by strictly adhering to protocols for aseptic catheter insertion and care. When a patient receiving central TPN develops a fever or leukocytosis, it is seldom necessary to remove the catheter immediately. The following course of action is recommended:

1. Inspect the catheter entry site and change the dressing.
2. Evaluate the patient thoroughly for other possible sources of infection and obtain Isolator blood cultures peripherally and through the catheter.
3. If a source of fever or leukocytosis is found, treat it appropriately and continue TPN via the catheter. If quantitative cultures indicate a catheter-related infection, the catheter should be removed. Long-term Silastic catheters may be treated with antibiotics through the catheter. We also recommend a 1-hour treatment of the catheter lumen with urokinase.
4. If, after 24 hours, no source of fever has been identified and evidence of infection continues, remove and culture the catheter by rolling the intravascular portion and the tunnel portion of the catheter on separate culture plates. Evidence of septic shock from an unknown source is an indication for immediate catheter removal.
5. If the catheter is removed for suspected infection, close observation and repeat cultures are indicated. Generally, catheter-related infections will resolve within 24 hours after removal.
6. If the initial blood cultures are negative and fever subsides, reinsert the catheter in a new site after 24 hours and restart TPN.
7. If the initial blood cultures are positive, initiate appropriate antibiotic therapy. The catheter can be reinserted once blood cultures are negative.
8. Patients with bacteremia from a source other than the catheter may be treated with appropriate antibiotics while the catheter is left in place. Recurrent or persistent bacteremia is an indication for catheter removal.
9. When it appears to be in the patient's best interest, an infected catheter may be left in place during antibiotic treatment or the catheter may be exchanged for a new one over a guidewire, thus avoiding the potential complications of a new insertion. The percentage of cases in which these procedures are successful in eradicating catheter-related infections is not known.

Metabolic abnormalities occur frequently in patients on central TPN. Dangerously high and low serum concentrations of virtually every component present in TPN have been reported. The most frequent problems are hyperglycemia, hypophosphatemia, and hypokalemia.[227] All three are less likely to occur if 20% to 30% of the nonprotein calories are provided as fat. Appropriate monitoring of blood and urine will allow early detection of changes and avoidance of preventable complications.

Hyperglycemia, serum glucose greater than 200 mg/dL, occurs in a significant percentage of patients receiving central TPN. If not followed closely and treated appropriately, hyperosmolar dehydration, coma, and death may occur. The incidence of hyperglycemia may be decreased by 1) initiating central TPN with no more than 250 g of dextrose on the first day of therapy; 2) monitoring urine glucose concentrations; and 3) monitoring serum glucose concentrations if there is glucose in the urine or the patient has renal failure. If hyperglycemia occurs, regular insulin should be given on a sliding scale. The administration rate of the TPN should be reduced temporarily if the serum glucose concentration exceeds 350 mg/dL, and hyperglycemia should be controlled at less than 200 mg/dL before advancing the TPN rate again. Hyperglycemia in a previously stable patient usually indicates a new metabolic stress, most often infection, and the hyperglycemia may occur several hours before other signs of infection.

Hypophosphatemia occurs as a result of new tissue synthesis and a shift from the extracellular to the intracellular compartments caused by glucose. Patients who are chronic alcoholics, severely malnourished, or taking antacids are at increased risk. Severe hypophosphatemia (< 1.0 mg/dL) can result in hemolysis and serious effects on the cardiorespiratory system and white blood cell function. The TPN solution usually provides 15 to 45 mmole/d. Patients at risk of hypophosphatemia should receive an additional 10 to 20 mmol/d as should patients who develop mild to moderate hypophosphatemia (1.0 to 2.0 mg/dL) after beginning TPN. Severe hypophosphatemia (< 1 mg/dL) should be corrected with supplemental intravenous phosphorus via a separate intravenous line.

Hypokalemia also occurs as a result of new tissue synthesis and shifts into the intracellular compartments caused by glucose. This may require addition of extra potassium to the TPN solution, occasionally up to as much as 150 to 200 mEq/d. In the presence of alkalosis or hypomagnesemia, it may be difficult or impossible to correct the hypokalemia because of renal potassium wasting.

Hypomagnesemia is most likely to occur in patients who are chronic alcoholics, severely malnourished, or receiving diuretics or other drugs that cause renal magnesium wasting.[228] Severe hypomagnesemia (< 1.0 mEq/L) should be treated with up to 100 mEq of magnesium sulfate administered over 24 hours via a separate intravenous line.

Hyponatremia is most often dilutional and should be treated by reducing fluid intake.

Fluid overload/dehydration should be monitored by measurement of intake and output, checking of daily weights, and measurement of urine specific gravity. If fluid overload occurs, more concentrated substrates ($D_{70}W$, 15% amino acids, 20% fat emulsion) can be used to decrease fluid intake. Often, the total fluid intake can also be restricted by decreasing the volume used for administration of intravenous antibiotics and other drugs. If the patient is dehydrated, additional fluid can be given peripherally or additional water can be added to the TPN fluid.

Fat intolerance occurs in patients who do not clear intravenous fat emulsions normally. When emulsions are administered daily, it is appropriate to determine serum triglycerides two or three times a week initially and once or twice a week thereafter. If serum triglyceride levels obtained while the fat emulsion is infusing exceed 300 mg/dL, the amount of fat being administered should be decreased. To better assess clearance, serum triglyceride values can be determined 4 to 6 hours after intravenous fat emulsion has been stopped. If the concentration exceeds 200 mg/dL, the amount infused should be decreased. Infusion of intravenous fat emulsion at a rate faster than recommended by the manufacturer may cause chest, back, or arm pain. In spite of concern regarding their use in patients with acute or chronc pancreatitis, most human and animal studies have reported no ill effects of intravenous fat in these conditions. Intravenous fat emulsions may be harmful in septic patients as a result of blockade of the reticuloendothelial system and possibly other adverse effects on immune and inflammatory responses. The harmful effects can be minimized by limiting the dose of intravenous fats to 1.0 g/kg/d and administering the fats continuously over 24 hours.

Hypoglycemia occasionally occurs when central TPN infusion is stopped abruptly. The risk is increased if there is insulin in the TPN or the TPN infusion rate is unusually high. To minimize this risk, dextrose 10% in water, should be infused at the same rate the TPN was infusing for 4 hours after TPN is stopped or the TPN infusion rate should be tapered before stopping.

Hypercalcemia of unclear etiology occurring during TPN has been reported.[229,230]

Liver test abnormalities occur frequently in patients on TPN. The etiology is unclear and probably multifactorial, including factors unrelated to TPN, calculous and acalculous cholecystitis, and fatty liver.[231] The ratio of fat to dextrose in the TPN formula is not an important determinant.[232]

ENTERAL NUTRITION (TUBE FEEDING)

The delivery of nutrients into the gastrointestinal tract using a tube is the preferred method of feeding patients who cannot ingest adequate nutrients by mouth but have a functioning digestive tract. There is mounting evidence that, in addition to being less expensive, enteral nutrition provides important nutrients not present in TPN, including glutamine and short-chain fatty acids.[233,234] Benefits of enteral feeding compared with TPN include better preservation of both immune function and intestinal function and less hypercatabolism.[172,175,176,235,236] Therefore, only if the gastrointestinal tract cannot be used safely and effectively should TPN be considered. Guidelines for the use of enteral nutrition in adult patients were published by the American Society for Parenteral and Enteral Nutrition Board of Directors in 1987.[237]

Access for Tube Feeding

Patient acceptance, efficiency, and overall success of tube feeding are greatly enhanced by selection of the appropriate equipment.

Modern small-bore, flexible feeding tubes have eliminated many of the adverse effects and much of the discomfort of large-bore polyvinyl chloride tubes for feeding. The small size and flexible material extend the length of time the tube can be left in place without the complications of tissue irritation or pressure necrosis encountered with the larger tubes. Many patients are able to eat with the tube in place, which permits tube feeding to supplement oral intake.

Nasogastric feeding is usually the most appropriate route for cooperative patients. Removal of the tube by uncooperative or disoriented patients is a disadvantage. Delayed gastric emptying and regurgitation leading to aspiration is the major risk. Therefore, aspiration precautions are essential. The orogastric route can be used when there is head or nasal injury or gross nasal deformity. Nasoduodenal feeding has the theoretical advantage of bypassing the reservoir action of the stomach and using both the pyloric and gastroesophageal sphincters to help prevent reflux and aspiration. For this reason, it is especially useful in the intensive care setting and for patients with diminished gag reflex. However, fluid can reflux from the duodenum into the stomach, leading to regurgitation and aspiration. Consequently, nasoduodenal feeding may provide less protection than is generally assumed[238] and nasojejunal feeding may be preferrable. Nasojejunal feedings are also used to infuse nutrients distal to a duodenocutaneous fistula. Disadvantages to either location include the delay in feeding and the expense associated with getting the tube into position and verifying its location radiographically. A feeding tube with a pH probe at its tip permits more rapid and inexpensive duodenal placement. With the appropriate technique and practice, some individuals can learn to intubate the duodenum without fluoroscopy or pH probe guidance. An additional theoretical disadvantage of duodenal and jejunal feeding is that it bypasses the bactericidal action of gastric acid so that administration of a contaminated feeding product is more likely to result in diarrhea or sepsis.

A gastrostomy tube is indicated when transnasal passage of a tube is impossible because of obstruction or when long-term feeding is anticipated. The recent development of safe methods for placing gastrostomy tubes via endoscopic or radiographic guidance which require only sedation and local anesthesia has been a significant advance. Surgical or radiographic placement of the gastrostomy tube is necessary if the patient is not a candidate for endoscopy. Complications of gastrostomy placement and feeding include skin irritation, aspiration, and infection of the tract, including severe fasciitis. The latter complication appears to be most likely in obese diabetics.

A feeding catheter may be placed directly into the jejunum at the time of abdominal surgery. The small intestine is often less affected than the stomach and colon by postoperative ileus. Therefore, jejunostomy feedings can often be initiated soon after surgery. In the event that adequate oral intake is delayed, use of this enteral feeding route may avoid the need for TPN. Enthusiasm for placement of needle catheter jejunostomies at the time of abdominal surgery has waned somewhat owing to a relatively high complication rate. A large-bore feeding jejunostomy tube is usually preferable. It can be used for short-term postoperative feeding or for long-term tube feeding of patients in whom gastrostomy is inappropriate. Jejunal feeding tubes can be placed endoscopically or radiographically by inserting a smaller tube through the pylorus into the jejunum via an established gastrostomy.

Selecting the Tube

For most adults, a 10F tube strikes an appropriate balance between comfort on the one hand and the risk of clogging on the other. It is suitable for all enteral products, liquid medications, diluted antacids, and occasional well-crushed tablets. More viscous mixtures such as psyllium hydrophilic mucilloid and undiluted antacids require 12F or 14F tubes.

Modern small-bore feeding tubes, although much more expensive than simple small-bore polyethylene tubes, are usually worth the additional cost because of added features. These include radio-opacity, water-activated lubricant on the surfaces (to aid insertion of the tube and removal of the accompanying stylet and to decrease clogging), and designs that diminish the risk that the stylet will exit the tube and penetrate the bowel wall. The latter feature permits the stylet to be safely reinserted without removing the tube from the patient, if performed without excess force. Small-bore feeding tubes must be inserted with great care and under experienced supervision. The tip of the tube can easily enter the trachea and penetrate the lung or pleura, as indicated by a rapidly growing number of reports. A cuffed endotracheal tube offers no protection against this complication and, in fact, appears to predispose the patient to it. Comatose, obtunded, or uncommunicative patients are especially at risk.[239] Perforation of the esophagus or stomach and even penetration of the brain with these small-bore tubes has been reported. An abdominal radiograph to verify placement before feeding is begun is essential for comatose, obtunded, or uncooperative patients.

Selecting the Method of Administration

In most cases, continuous infusion of the enteral product using a pump is recommended since this method is generally better tolerated by hospitalized patients. Continuous infusion is usually essential when feeding directly into the duodenum or jejunum to decrease the risk of dumping syndrome. Continuous feeding should be initiated with full strength product at 20 to 25 mL/h. The rate may be increased every 6 to 8 hours in increments of 20 to 25 mL as tolerated by the patient until the goal rate is reached. Unless the patient needs additional free water, dilution of the formula should be avoided since it is time consuming and increases the risk of contaminating the product while offering no advantage over administering full strength formula at a slower rate.

At times, it is advantageous to give the daily amount of tube feeding product over 10 to 12 hours (cyclic infusion). Cyclic daytime feeding may be used for the patient at increased risk of nocturnal aspiration. Cyclic night-time feeding permits some patients to eat more food during the day.

Infusions may also be given intermittently, for example, 500 mL over 30 minutes three or four times daily. This has the advantage of freeing the patient from continuous attachment to a feeding device and is well tolerated by selected patients. This method is often preferrable for patients who are ambulatory, scheduled for regular treatments, or unable to be positioned with the head of the bed elevated continuously. Intermittent infusions are usually given by gravity drip, especially for home tube feeding. Patients may tolerate intermittent nasogastric feedings of 250 to 750 mL given at rates of up to 60 mL/min.

Maintaining the Patency and Position of the Feeding Tube

Each institution should have written policies for maintaining the patency and position of small-bore feeding tubes. Mechanical problems with the tube are a major reason why many patients on tube feeding do not receive adequate nutritional support.[193] Frequent flushing and avoiding pill fragments are most important for maintaining patency. Multiple techniques for unclogging tubes have been published and include the use of small quantities of carbonated beverage, pancreatic enzymes, and 95% ethyl alcohol gently infused into the tube. Excessive force, which could rupture the tube in the pharynx, must be avoided.

Maintaining a feeding tube in the appropriate position is often difficult. Adequate taping is essential. The length of tube extending from the nose should be noted at least every 8 hours. Disoriented patients usually require placement of mitts or restraints on the hands. Rarely, a "bridle" may be indicated, which is a small plastic tube passed posterior to the nasal septum and secured to the feeding tube.

Selecting a Tube Feeding Product

The number of tube feeding products commercially available is large and increasing rapidly. Description of specific products are readily available.[240,241] Many institutions have a formal method for selecting a limited number of tube feeding products and for informing the staff of the content and characteristics of the products selected. The many products available can be assigned to approximately 15 categories on the basis of medically important characteristics. It is efficient to select one product for each category and to review those selections once a year.

In selecting or creating a tube feeding mixture for a particular patient, the same seven features described for designing a TPN formula should be considered. The memory aid FACE MTV prompts one to consider the seven components (fluid, amino acids, calories, electrolytes, miscellaneous, trace elements, and vitamins) as follows:

Fluid Restrictions/Requirements. Most products have a caloric density of approximately 1 kcal/mL. They provide approximately 900 mL of free water per liter of formula, and this plus the amount of water used to flush the tube is adequate for patients who do not have excessive fluid losses. If fluid restriction is required, a product with a density of 1.5 to 2.0 kcal/mL should be used to provide the same nutrients in less volume. The nutrient density of tube feeding products can also be increased by adding individual (modular) preparations of protein, carbohydrate, or fat. Fluid intake can be further reduced by decreasing the volume of water used to flush the feeding tube to a minimum of 60 mL/d.

Formulas more concentrated than 1 kcal/mL are generally not suitable for long-term use in any patient who is unable to drink water in response to thirst or who is likely to have a blunted thirst response such as the elderly since hypernatremia, dehydration, and death may result.

Amino Acid/Protein. In choosing or designing a tube feeding formula, one should consider not only the total protein content, which ranges from 20 to 75 g/L in commercial products, but also the chemical form of the amino acids (free, peptide, whole protein) and the relative amounts of individual amino acids most suitable for various disease states. Products containing whole protein (polymeric formulas) are suitable for most patients. These provide the least expensive and most physiologic form of nitrogen for enteral use. The possible advantages of peptide formulas over whole protein for improving nitrogen absorption in patients with intestinal disease, decreasing the incidence of diarrhea, and stimulating protein synthesis remain to be confirmed. Formulas in which the nitrogen is predominantly in the form of essential amino acids may delay the need for dialysis in patients with renal failure. Formulas with a greater proportion of branched-chain amino acids and lower proportion of aromatic amino acids and methionine than the polymeric formulas may be useful in a very limited number of patients with liver failure. These products do not offer any substantive benefit over traditional treatments as primary therapy of hepatic encephalopathy.

Calories: Carbohydrate Versus Fat. Fat comprises 25% to 40% of nonprotein calories in most commercial products for tube feeding. For patients with glucose intolerance or carbon dioxide retention due to pulmonary disease, it is usually appropriate to select a product in which 50% or more of the calories are provided by fat, at least for short-term use.[242] Formulas with very little fat, primarily the "elemental diets," are appropriate for patients who are unable to absorb fat adequately, those recovering from pancreatitis, and those with slow gastric emptying.

Electrolytes. Enteral products vary considerably in electrolyte content, but product selection is seldom made primarily on this basis. A product low in sodium or low in all electrolytes is often appropriate for patients with renal, liver, or heart failure. It should be noted that some products designed for use in renal failure and hepatic failure contain no electrolytes. Electrolytes can be added to tube feeding products to supplement patients with deficiencies of potassium, phosphate, magnesium, or sodium. Mixing the electrolyte supplement with 500 to 1000 mL of formula is preferable to bolusing it into the feeding tube. Dilutional hyponatremia calls for a more concentrated formula, not sodium supplementation.

Miscellaneous Additives. Additives other than electrolytes may include antidiarrheal agents such as loperamide or deodorized tincture of opium.

Trace Elements. The volume of enteral product infused daily should be sufficient to provide at least 100% of the USRDA of zinc (15 mg). Most enteral products for adults contain known amounts of zinc, iron, copper, iodine, and manganese, and some contain known amounts of selenium, molybdenum, and chromium. Some products designed for use in patients with hepatic and renal disease are not supplemented with trace elements and should not be used for more than a few weeks unless the patient is given trace elements.

Vitamins. The volume of most enteral products required to provide 100% of the USRDA of vitamins is 1000 to 2000 mL/d. Some products for patients with hepatic failure and renal failure contain no vitamins or an incomplete vitamin profile. If the amount of enteral product given does not provide 100% of the RDA, supplemental vitamins should be given. Although the amount of vitamin K in several enteral products has been decreased in recent years, the amount is still sufficient to decrease prothrombin time in some patients on warfarin therapy. When a patient on warfarin is begun on an enteral product, prothrombin time should be monitored frequently for 7 to 10 days.

Special Monitoring for Patients Receiving Tube Feeding

Tube-fed patients should be monitored to access the adequacy of nutrition support and to anticipate and reduce the risks of complications.

MONITORING TO ASSESS ADEQUACY OF NUTRITION SUPPORT

The volume of formula actually administered each day should be recorded and compared with the goal amount. Unless a concerted effort is make, the amount given is likely to be 15% to 20% below the amount ordered.[193] Stable or increasing body weight is a useful indication of adequate nutrition over a period of weeks to months. Over shorter periods of time, a normal or increasing serum transthyretin (prealbumin) concentration and positive nitrogen balance are the best indicators, as discussed in the preceding section on TPN.

COMPLICATIONS OF TUBE FEEDING

In addition to the previously discussed bronchopulmonary and other mechanical complications of inserting feeding tubes, the major complications of tube feeding are aspiration, gastrointestinal problems including diarrhea, and metabolic abnormalities.

The risk of regurgitation and aspiration can probably be decreased by feeding into the duodenum and can be eliminated by jejunal feeding. During gastric feeding and for at least 1 hour afterward, the patient's upper body should be elevated at least 30 degrees above horizontal. Gastric residual volumes should be checked before each intermittent feeding or every 8 to 12 hours during continuous feeding. A residual volume exceeding 100 to 150 mL usually indicates delayed gastric emptying and an increased risk of regurgitation and aspiration. Failure to obtain a significant residual volume via a small bore feeding tube does not reliably rule out a large gastric residual volume. Strategies for reducing gastric residual volume include intravenous metoclopramide, continuous rather than intermittent feeding, and a feeding product with less fat.

Both the incidence and the etiology of diarrhea among tube-fed patients are uncertain. The incidence reported is between 6% and 60%, but the possibility that most of the "diarrrhea" is no more than incontinence remains to be disproven. The current products are probably not diarrheagenic in healthy persons.[243] When a tube-fed patient develops diarrhea, the following potential causes should be considered:

1. Diarrhea unrelated to the tube feeding, for example, drug-induced, especially antibiotics, antacids, sorbitol-containing elixirs.[244]
2. Too rapid rate of administration. Change to continuous infusion by pump.
3. Too little fiber so that inadequate short chain fatty acids (e.g., acetate, proprionate, butyrate) are made in the colon. Change to a formula with fiber or add psyllium.[245]
4. Formula with too high osmolality. This is an unlikely cause but try an isotonic formula.
5. Formula with improper composition for patient's digestive/absorptive capabilities. Patients with bile or pancreatic insufficiency or short bowel may require a low-fat formula.
6. Protein–calorie malnutrition. Malnutrition reduces digestive and absorptive capacity. It may be necessary to reduce the enteral feeding rate and use supplemental parenteral nutrition to allow time for nutritional recovery of the stomach and small intestine.
7. Deficiency of other nutrients. Diarrhea or absorptive defects can result from deficiencies of niacin, zinc, vitamin A, vitamin B_{12}, and folic acid.
8. Bacterial or fungal contamination of the tube feeding formula. This should not occur if appropriate protocols are followed for filling the reservoir and changing the reservoir and administration sets.
9. Low serum albumin concentration. If the serum albumin concentration is less than 2.5 g/dL and no other cause for diarrhea is found it is appropriate to give intravenous albumin to raise the level to 3.0 g/dL.

Other methods for decreasing diarrhea in tube-fed patients await further documentation, including low-fat formulas together with large amounts of vitamin A, peptide formulas, short-chain fatty acids, and glutamine.

When the cause of diarrhea cannot be found or eliminated, antidiarrheal agents can be used, including lopermide (Imodium), diphenoxalate and atropine (Lomotil), or deodorized tincture of opium.

The metabolic complications of tube feeding are essentially the same as those discussed for central TPN. Hyperkalemia is more frequent in tube feeding because the amount of potassium in most products is adequate for rapid restoration of lean body mass and is excessive for some patients, especially those with impaired renal function.

Specific Gastrointestinal Disease Indications for Nutrition Support

INTESTINAL FAILURE

The most unequivocal indication for nutrition support, usually long-term TPN, is intestinal failure, that is, any disease that renders the intestinal tract incapable of digesting or absorbing enough orally ingested nutrients to sustain life. Causes of intestinal failure

include massive small bowel resection, radiation enteritis, motility disorders (scleroderma and pseudoobstruction), chronic adhesive peritonitis, and mucosal diseases unresponsive to therapy, such as collagenous sprue. Diseases of the central nervous system, oropharynx, and esophagus that render the patient unable to ingest sufficient nutrients to sustain life are a frequent indication for tube feeding. Animal data as well as clinical experience indicate that after massive small bowel resection, adequate nutrition support with TPN beginning within the first few days after surgery as well as the stimulation from oral or enteral feeding are both important for optimal adaptation of the remaining small intestine.[246]

ENTEROCUTANEOUS FISTULAE

Improved management of enterocutaneous fistulae over the past 40 years has led to a dramatic decrease in mortality and an increase in the rate of spontaneous, nonsurgical closure.[246] The improvements are attributable to better management of problems such as sepsis and electrolyte imbalance as well as improved nutrition support. Sheldon and associates estimated that TPN is the primary therapeutic modality leading to closure in 30% to 50% of patients with enterocutaneous fistulae while it is a supportive tool that makes possible safe and definitive operative management in the other 50% to 70%.[247] The likelihood of closure without surgery is decreased if there is complete loss of bowel continuity, unresolved obstruction distal to the fistula, local infection or foreign body, a large output from the fistula, multiple complex fistulae, underlying inflammatory bowel disease, radiation damage, or cancer. If spontaneous closure does not occur after 30 to 60 days of TPN and conservative treatment, it is unlikely to occur with continuation of this therapy. However, very complex fistulae associated with extensive intra-abdominal infection occasionally benefit from more prolonged TPN prior to surgery. Tube feeding of an elemental or other very low residue diet may be tried when appropriate for patients with fistulae of the distal ileum or colon.

ULCERATIVE COLITIS

The role of nutrition support in management of patients with ulcerative colitis is essentially no different from the principles already enumerated. Neither bowel rest and TPN nor enteral nutrition with an elemental diet are useful as primary therapy for the disease. They do not decrease the need for surgery or for other traditional means of therapy. The same appears to be true for Crohn's colitis.

CROHN'S ENTERITIS

Nutrition support has a more important role in the modern management of Crohn's disease involving the small bowel. This may be due entirely to the fact that malnutrition is very prevalent among these patients, including not only protein–calorie malnutrition but also deficiencies of vitamins, especially vitamins A and D, and the trace element zinc (see Table 48-1). These deficiencies play a significant role in the morbidity of Crohn's disease. Thus, for example, growth failure among children with Crohn's disease responds to aggressive nutrition support whether given intravenously, enterally, or orally.[10,11]

A number of studies have investigated the effect of nutrition support with or without bowel rest in patients with Crohn's disease of the small bowel who were sick enough to require hospital admission. Taken together, these studies suggest that 40% to 80% of the patients treated with aggressive nutrition therapy for 2 to 3 weeks will respond symptomatically enough to be declared in remission and that oral or enteral administration of an elemental diet is as effective as TPN.[248] Relapse rates range from 25% to 85% after 1 year.[246] A controlled trial demonstrated that bowel rest was not a significant factor in achieving remission.[249] The mechanism by which nutritional repletion decreases symptoms experienced by patients with Crohn's disease remains unclear. Possibilities include improved immune function and improvement in the metabolism and differentiation of epithelial tissue, which enhances mucosal repair. An important result of these studies should be more emphasis by the medical community on preventing protein–calorie malnutrition and other nutrient deficiencies in patients with Crohn's disease. This should include avoiding restrictive diets except when it is clear that the restriction will decrease symptoms and enhance total nutrient intake. Supplements of vitamins (especially folate and vitamins B_{12}, A, and D), minerals, and trace elements (especially zinc) should be given whenever appropriate and somewhat more liberally than is currently the practice. Based on the data available to date, elemental diets or TPN should not be used as "primary therapy" for patients with Crohn's disease who would otherwise undergo surgery. Exceptions are patients with such extensive small bowel disease or a small bowel already so reduced in length by previous resections that surgery is likely to leave the patient with intestinal failure.

ACUTE PANCREATITIS

Severe acute pancreatitis induces a catabolic response similar to sepsis and burns. The victims are frequently already nutritionally depleted, and intestinal function may not return for weeks. Therefore, it is usually appropriate to begin nutrition therapy within the first week of the attack unless rapid recovery appears likely. In most cases, TPN is the therapy of choice in order to minimize pancreatic stimulation. Glucose intolerance should be anticipated. For unclear reasons, there is a higher incidence of catheter sepsis in patients with pancreatitis than in other patients receiving TPN.[246] Intravenous lipid emulsion is not contraindicated in patients with acute pancreatitis.[246] In less severe pancreatitis or in the recovery phase, nasoduodenal tube feeding with an elemental diet is appropriate.

LIVER DISEASE

There is some evidence that aggressive nutrition support decreases morbidity or mortality in acute or chronic liver disease.[246,250] Hepatic encephalopathy is associated with an abnormal plasma amino acid profile. Nutritional products, both enteral and parenteral, designed to correct the abnormal plasma amino acid profile are available.[213] These products have higher concentrations of branched-chain amino acids (leucine, valine, and isoleucine) and lower concentrations of methionine and aromatic amino acids (tyrosine, tryptophan, and phenylalanine) than ordinary diets. They are most appropriately used for patients who develop encephalopathy at an intake of ordinary protein below their requirements in spite of the usual treatment for hepatic encephalopathy. There is evidence that these products may be as effective as lactulose or neomycin as primary therapy for hepatic encephalopathy, but from a nutritional point of view there is nothing to recommend this treatment over standard therapy plus an ordinary diet.

HOME ENTERAL AND PARENTERAL NUTRITION

Patients who require tube feeding but are otherwise stable enough to leave the hospital should be evaluated for nutrition support at home or in a nonacute care facility. Enteral feeding outside of the hospital is most often used for patients with trouble swallowing due to neuromuscular disorders or head and neck cancers. Feeding is most often via a gastrostomy or jejunostomy. A fiber-containing feeding product is preferable.[251]

Home TPN is most appropriate for patients with uncorrectable intestinal failure. This therapy is increasingly being used for patients with malignancy, but it remains to be determined how often this is in the patient's best interest. In the absence of data to indicate that survival or quality of life of patients with malignancies is improved by home TPN, this expensive and burdensome technology should have a limited role in management of patients with malignancy. If oral hydration is inadequate and the enteral route cannot be used, the cancer patient who is not receiving intensive chemotherapy may be better served by home intravenous fluid and electrolytes since this therapy has fewer potential metabolic complications and requires less in-hospital learning time than home TPN. The American Society for Parenteral and Enteral Nutrition has published standards for home nutrition support and guidelines for use of home TPN. It should be emphasized that the availability of home therapy must not cause the premature discharge of patients prior to adequate stabilization of the medical condition or adequate preparation for safe home care. On the other hand, when life-long hospitalization is the only alternative to home TPN, it is usually in the patient's best interest to go home on TPN after every effort has been made to maximize safety and efficacy of the endeavor, even if they remain suboptimal.[252]

The reader is directed to Chapter 17, Carbohydrate Assimilation; Chapter 18, Intestinal Lipid Absorption; Chapter 19, Protein Digestion and Assimilation; Chapter 20, Vitamins and Minerals; Chapter 21, General Nutritional Principles; and Chapter 74, Short Bowel Syndrome.

REFERENCES

1. Food and Nutrition Board Subcommittee on the Tenth Edition of the RDA's. In: Recommended dietary allowance. Washington, DC: National Academy Press, 1989.

2. Committee on Diet and Health, Food and Nutrition Board, Commission on Life Sciences, National Research Council. Diet and health: implications for reducing chronic disease risks. Washington, DC: National Academy Press, 1989.

3. Pao EM, Mickle SJ. Problem nutrients in the United States. In: Prescott SC, Proctor BE, eds. Food technology. New York: McGraw-Hill Inc, 1981;35:69.

4. Avioli LV. Calcium and phosphorus. In: Shils ME, Young VR, eds. Modern nutrition in health and disease. 7th ed. Philadelphia: Lea & Febiger, 1988:142.

5. Solomons NW. Zinc and copper. In: Shils ME, Young VR, eds. Modern nutrition in health and disease. 7th ed. Philadelphia: Lea & Febiger, 1988:238.

6. Rosenberg IH, Alpers DH. Nutritional deficiency in gastrointestinal disease. In: Sleisenger MH, Fordtran JS, eds. Gastrointestinal disease. 4th ed. Philadelphia: WB Saunders, 1988:1983.

7. Altman PL, Dittmer DS. Metabolism. Bethesda, MD: Federation of American Societies for Experimental Biology, 1968.

8. Shaw S, Lieber CS. Nutrition and diet in alcoholism. In: Shils ME, Young VER, eds. Modern nutrition in health and disease. 7th ed. Philadelphia: Lea & Febiger, 1988:1423.

9. Drisoll RH, Rosenberg IH. Total parenteral nutrition in inflammatory bowel disease. Med Clin North Am 1978;62:185.

10. Kelts DG, Grand RJ, Shen G, et al. Nutritional basis of growth failure in children and adolescents with Crohn's disease. Gastroenterology 1979;76:720.

11. Kirschner BS, Klich JR, Kalman SS, et al. Reversal of growth retardation in Crohn's disease with therapy emphasizing oral nutritional restitution. Gastroenterology 1981;80:10.

12. Randall HT. Water, electrolytes, and acid–base balance. In: Shils ME, Young VR, eds. Modern nutrition in health and disease. 7th ed. Philadelphia: Lea & Febiger, 1988:108.

13. Cuddy PG. Fluid and electrolyte disorders. In: Young LY, Koda-Kimble MA, eds. Applied therapeutics: the clinical use of drugs. 4th ed. Vancouver, WA: Applied Therapeutics, 1988:635.

14. Mudge G. Agents affecting volume and composition of body fluids. In: Goodman LS, Gilman A, eds. The pharmacological basis of therapeutics. 7th ed. New York: Macmillan, 1985:846.

15. Just PM. Fluid and electrolyte therapy. In: Herfindal ET, Hirschman JL, eds. Clinical pharmacy and therapeutics. 3rd ed. Baltimore: Williams & Wilkins, 1984:605.

16. Knoben JE, Anderson PO. Handbook of clinical drug data. 6th ed. Section 40:00 Electrolytes, caloric and water balance. Hamilton, IL: Drug Intelligence Publications, 1988:607.

17. The NIH Consensus Conference: osteoporosis. JAMA 1984;252:799.

18. Popovtzer MM, Knochel JP. Disorders of calcium, phosphorus, vitamin D, and parathyroid hormone activity. In: Schrier RW, ed. Renal and electrolyte disorders. 3rd ed. Boston: Little, Brown & Co, 1986:251.

19. Burns Schaiff RA, Hall TG, Bar RS. Medical treatment of hypercalcemia. Clin Pharm 1989;8:108.

20. Zaloga GP, Chernow B. Hypocalcemia in critical illness. JAMA 1986;256:1924.

21. Sartoris DJ, Resnick D. Dual-energy radiographic absorptiometry for bone densitometry: current status and prospective. AJR 1989;152:241.

22. Juan D. The causes and consequences of hypophosphatemia. Surg Gynecol Obstet 1981;153:589.

23. Knochel JP. Hypophosphatemia. West J Med 1981;134:15.

24. Ensminger AH, Ensminger ME, Konlande JE, Robson JRK. Foods and nutrition encyclopedia. Clovis, CA: Pegus Press, 1983:1749.

25. Conner CS. Hypophosphatemia. Drug Intell Clin Pharm 1984;18:594.

26. Lentz RD, Brown DM, Kjellstrand CM. Treatment of severe hypophosphatemia. Ann Intern Med 1978;89:941.

27. Vanatta JB, Aldress DL, Whang R, et al. High-dose intravenous phosphorus therapy for severe complicated hypophosphatemia. South Med J 1983;76:1424.

28. Juan D. Clinical review: the clinical importance of hypomagnesemia. Surgery 1982;91:510.

29. Gums JG. Clinical significance of magnesium: a review. Drug Intell Clin Pharm 1987;21:240.

30. Graber TW, Yee AS, Baker FJ. Magnesium: physiology, clinical disorders, and therapy. Ann Emerg Med 1981;10:49.

31. Montgomery P. Treatment of magnesium deficiency. Clin Pharm 1987;6:834.

32. Flink EB. Nutritional aspects of magnesium metabolism. West J Med 1980;133:304.

33. Anderson CE. Minerals. In: Schneider HA, Anderson CE, Coursin DB, eds. Nutritional support of medical practice. 2nd ed. Philadelphia: Harper & Row, 1983:54.

34. Bolinger AM, Korman NR. Anemias. In: Young LL, Koda-Kimble MA, eds. Applied therapeutics: the clinical use of drugs. 4th ed. Vancouver, WA: Applied Therapeutics, 1983:1051.

35. Ross G. Iron metabolism: perspectives. Nutr Supp Serv 1982;2:28.

36. Herbert V. Hematology and the anemias. In: Schneider HA, Anderson CE, Coursin DB, eds. Nutritional support of medical practice. 2nd ed. Philadelphia: Harper & Row, 1983:386.

37. Guyatt GH, Patterson C, Ali M, et al. Diagnosis of iron-deficiency anemia in the elderly. Am J Med 1990;88:205.

38. Committee on Diet and Health, Food and Nutrition Board, National Research Council. Dietary supplements. In: Diet and health: implications for reducing chronic disease risk. Washington, DC: National Academy Press, 1989:509.

39. Flodin NW. Pharmacology of micronutrients. In: Albanese AA, Kritchevsky D, eds. Current topics in nutrition and disease. New York: Alan R. Liss, 1988:285.

40. Solomon NW. Trace minerals. In: Rombeau JL, Caldwell MD, eds. Parenteral nutrition. Philadelphia: WB Saunders, 1986:169.

41. Hambidge KM, Hambidge C, Jacobs M, Baum JD. Low levels of zinc in hair, anorexia, poor growth, and hypogeusia in children. Pediatr Res 1972;6:868.

42. Wolman SL, Anderson GH, Marliss EB, et al. Zinc in total parenteral nutrition: requirements and metabolic effects. Gastroenterology 1979;76:458.

43. Sandstead HH, Evans GW. Zinc. In: Present knowledge in nutrition. 5th ed. Washington: The Nutrition Foundation, 1984:479.

44. Jeejeebhoy KN. Zinc and chromium in parenteral nutrition. Bull NY Acad Med 1984;60:118.

45. Prasad AS. Trace elements in the elderly. In: Bales CV, ed. Mineral homeostasis in the elderly. New York: Alan R. Liss, 1989:69.

46. AMA Department of Foods and Nutrition. Guidelines for essential trace elements preparations for parenteral use. JAMA 1979;241:2051.

47. Flodin NW. Pharmacology of micronutrients. In: Albanese AA, Kritchevsky D, eds. Current topics in nutrition and disease. New York: Alan R. Liss, 1988:255.

48. Shike M. Copper in parenteral nutrition. Bull NY Acad Med 1984;60:132.

49. Shike M, Roulet M, Kurian R, et al. Copper metabolism and requirements in total parenteral nutrition. Gastroenterology 1981;81:290.

50. Fleming CR. Trace element metabolism in adult patients requiring total parenteral nutrition. Am J Clin Nutr 1989;49:573.

51. Szwanek M, Khalidi N, Wesley JR. Trace elements and parenteral nutrition. Nutr Supp Serv 1987;7:8.

52. Fujita M, Itakura J, Takagi Y, Okada A. Copper deficiency during total parenteral nutrition: clinical analysis of three cases. J Parenter Enter Nutr 1989;13:421.

53. Tokuda Y, et al. Copper deficiency in an infant on prolonged total parenteral nutrition. J Parenter Enter Nutr 1986;10:242.

54. Levander OA. The importance of selenium in total parenteral nutrition. Bull NY Acad Med 1984;60:144.

55. Flodin NW. Pharmacology of micronutrients. In: Albanese AA, Kritchevsky D, eds. Current topics in nutrition and disease. New York: Alan R. Liss, 1988:269.

56. Burk R. Selenium. In: Present knowledge in nutrition. 5th ed. Washington, DC: The Nutrition Foundation, 1984:519.

57. Brown MR, et al. Proximal muscle weakness and selenium deficiency associated with long-term parenteral nutrition. Am J Clin Nutr 1986;43:549.

58. Quercia RA, Korn S, O'Neill D, et al. Selenium deficiency and fatal cardiomyopathy in a patient receiving long-term home parenteral nutrition. Clin Pharm 1984;3:531.

59. Flodin NW. Pharmacology of micronutrients. In: Albanese AA,

Kritchevsky D, eds. Current topics in nutrition and disease. New York: Alan R. Liss, 1988:247.

60. Jeejeebhoy KN, Chu RC, Marliss EB, et al. Chromium deficiency, glucose intolerance, and neuropathy reversed by chromium supplementation, and a patient receiving long-term total parenteral nutrition. Am J Clin Nutr 1977;30:531.

61. Freund H, Atamian S, Fischer JE. Chromium deficiency during total parenteral nutrition. JAMA 1979;241:496.

62. Brown RO, Forloines-Lynn S, Cross, R, Heizer WD. Chromium deficiency after long-term parenteral nutrition. Dig Dis Sci 1986;31:661.

63. Nichoalds GE. Molybdenum. In: Baumgartner TG, ed. Clinical guide to parenteral micronutrition. Melrose Park, IL: Educational Publications, 1984:165.

64. Abumrad NN. Molybdenum—is it an essential trace metal? Bull NY Acad Med 1984;60:163.

65. Leach RM. Manganese in enteral and parenteral nutrition. Bull NY Acad Med 1984;60:172.

66. Doisy EA. Micronutrient controls on biosynthesis of clotting proteins and cholesterol. In: Hemphill DD, ed. Trace substances in environmental health. Columbia, MO: University of Missouri Press, 1972:6:193.

67. Molitch ME, Dahms WT. Endocrinology. In: Schneider HA, Anderson CE, Coursin DB, eds. Nutritional support of medical practice. 2nd ed. Philadelphia: Harper & Row, 1983:328.

68. Nichoalds GE. Iodide. In: Baumgartner TG, ed. Clinical guide to parenteral micronutrition. Melrose Park, IL: Educational Publications, 1984:157.

69. Jong BJ. Thyroid disorders. In: Young LL, Koda-Kimble MA, eds. Applied therapeutics: the clinical use of drugs. 4th ed. Vancouver, WA: Applied Therapeutics, 1988:1625.

70. Sweeney EA, Shaw JH. Nutrition in relation to dental medicine. In: Shils ME, Young VR, eds. Modern nutrition in health and disease. 7th ed. Philadelphia: Lea & Febiger, 1988:1069.

71. Berner YN, Shuller TR, Nielsen FH, et al. Selected ultratrace elements in total parenteral nutrition solutions. Am J Clin Nutr 1989;50:1079.

72. Anderson CE. Vitamins. In: Schneider HA, Anderson CE, Coursin DB, eds. Nutrition support of medical practice. 2nd ed. Philadelphia: Harper & Row, 1983:23.

73. Olson JA. Vitamin A, retinoids, and carotenoids. In: Shils ME, Young VR, eds. Modern nutrition in health and disease. 7th ed. Philadelphia: Lea & Febiger, 1988:292.

74. McLarery DS. Vitamin A deficiency and toxicity. In: Present knowledge in nutrition. 5th ed. Washington, DC: The Nutrition Foundation, 1984:192.

75. Commnittee on Diet and Health, Food and Nutrition Board, National Research Council. Fat-soluble vitamins. In: Diet and health: implications for reducing chronic disease risk. Washington, DC: National Academy Press, 1989:311.

76. Goldsmith GA. Curative nutrition—vitamins. In: Schneider HA, Anderson CE, Coursin DB, eds. Nutrition support of medical practice. 2nd ed. Philadelphia: Harper & Row, 1983:160.

77. Sitren HS. Vitamin A. In: Baumgartner TG, ed. Clinical guide to parenteral micro nutrition. Melrose Park, IL: Educational Publications, 1984:183.

78. Goodman DS. Vitamin A and retinoids in health and disease. N Engl J Med 1984;310:1023.

79. Riggle MA, Brandt RB. Decrease of available vitamin A in parenteral nutrition solutions. J Parenter Enter Nutr 1986;10:388.

80. Gleghorn EE, Eisenberg LD, Hack S, et al. Observations of vitamin A toxicity in three patients with renal failure receiving parenteral ailmentation. Am J Clin Nutr 1986;44:107.

81. DeLuca HF. Vitamin D and its metabolites. In: Shils ME, Young VR, eds. Modern nutrition in health and disease. 7th ed. Philadelphia: Lea & Febiger, 1988:313.

82. AMA Division of Drugs. Vitamins and minerals. In: AMA Drug Evaluations. 5th ed. Philadelphia: WB Saunders, 1983:1121.

83. Lips P, van Ginkel FC, Jongren MJM, et al. Determinants of vitamin D status in patients with hip fracture and in elderly control patients. Am J Clin Nutr 1987;46:1005.

84. Delvin EE, Imbach A, Copti M. Vitamin D nutritional status and related biochemical indices in an autonomous elderly population. Am J Clin Nutr 1988;48:373.

85. Fraser DR. Vitamin D. In: Present knowledge in nutrition. 5th ed. Washington, DC: The Nutrition Foundation, 1984:209.

86. Subcommittee on the Tenth Edition of the RDA. Fat-soluble vitamins. In: Recommended dietary allowances. 10th ed. Washington, DC: National Academy Press, 1989:78.

87. Farrell PM. Vitamin E. In: Shils ME, Young VR, eds. Modern nutrition in health and disease. 7th ed. Philadelphia: Lea & Febiger 1988:340.

88. Roberts HJ. Perspective on vitamin E as therapy. JAMA 1981;246:129

89. Flodin NW. Pharmacology of micronutrients. In: Albanese AA, Kritchevsky D, eds. Current topics in nutrition and disease. New York: Alan R. Liss, 1988:59.

90. Olson RE. Vitamin K. In: Shils ME, Young VR, eds. Modern nutrition in health and disease. 7th ed. Philadelphia: Lea & Febiger 1988:328.

91. Subcommittee on the Tenth Edition of the RDAs. Water-soluble vitamins. In: Recommended dietary allowances. 10th ed. Washington, DC: National Academy Press, 1989:115.

92. Tanphalichtr V, Wood B. Thiamin. In: Present knowledge in nutrition. 5th ed. Washington, DC: The Nutrition Foundation, 1984:273.

93. McCormic DB. Thiamin. In: Shils ME, Young VR, eds. Modern nutrition in health and disease. 7th ed. Philadelphia: Lea & Febiger, 1988:355.

94. McCormick DB. Riboflavin. In: Shils ME, Young VR, eds. Modern nutrition in health and disease. Philadelphia: Lea & Febiger, 1988:362.

95. McCormick DB. Niacin. In: Shils ME, Young VE, eds. Modern nutrition in health and disease. 7th ed. Philadelphia: Lea & Febiger, 1988:370.

96. Rao BSN, Gopalan C. Niacin. In: Present knowledge in nutrition. 5th ed. Washington, DC: The Nutrition Foundation, 1984:318.

97. McEvoy GK, ed. AHFS (American Hospital Formulary Service) drug information 90. Bethesda, MD: American Society of Hospital Pharmacists, 1990:2113.

98. Flodin NW. Pharmacology of micronutrients. In: Albanese AA, Kritchevsky D, eds. Current topics in nutrition and disese. New York: Alan R. Liss, 1988:129.

99. McCormick DB. Vitamin B$_6$. In: Shils ME, Young VR, eds. Modern nutrition in health and disease. 7th ed. Philadelphia: Lea & Febiger, 1988:376.

100. Henderson CM. Vitamin B$_6$. In: Present knowledge in nutrition. 5th ed. Washington, DC: The Nutrition Foundation, 1984:303.

101. Herbert VD, Colman N. Folic acid and vitamin B$_{12}$. In: Shils ME, Young VR, eds. Modern nutrition in health and disease. 7th ed. Philadelphia: Lea & Febiger, 1988:388.

102. Flodin NW. Pharmacology of micronutrients. In: Albanese AA, Kritchevsky D, eds. Current topics in nutrition and disease. New York: Alan R. Liss, 1988:161.

103. Carmel R, Sinow RM, Siegel ME, Samloff M. Food cobalamin malabsorption occurs frequently in patients with unexplained low serum cobalamin levels. Arch Intern Med 1988;148:1715.

104. Flodin NW. Pharmacology of micronutrients. In: Albanese AA, Kritchevsky D, eds. Current topics in nutrition and disease. New York: Alan R. Liss, 1988:179.

105. Hornig DH, Moser V, Glatthaar BE. Ascorbic acid. In: Shils ME, Young VE, eds. Modern nutrition in health and disease. 7th ed. Philadelphia: Lea & Febiger, 1988:417.

106. McCormick DB. Biotin. In: Shils ME, Young VR, eds. Modern nutrition in health and disease. 7th ed. Philadelphia: Lea & Febiger, 1988:436.

107. McCormick DB. Pantothenic acid. In: Shils ME, Young VR, eds. Modern nutrition in health and disease. 7th ed. Philadelphia: Lea & Febiger, 1988:383.

108. Linscheer WG, Vergroesen AJ. Lipids. In: Shils ME, Young VR, eds. Modern nutrition in health and disease. 7th ed. Philadelphia. Lea & Febiger, 1988:72.

109. Roubenoff R, Roubenoff RA, Preto J, Balke CW. Malnutrition among hospitalized patients: a problem of physician awareness. Arch Intern Med 1987;147:1462.

110. Weinsier RL, Hunker EM, Krumdieck CL, Butterworth CE. A prospective evaluation of general medical patients during the course of hospitalization. Am J Clin Nutr 1979;32:418.

111. Alexander JW. Nutritional management of the infected patient. In: Kinney JM, Jeejeebhoy KN, Hill JL, Owen OE, eds. Metabolism in patient care. Philadelphia: WB Saunders, 1988:625.

112. Negro F, Cerra FB. Nutritional monitoring in the ICU: rational and practical application. Crit Care Clin 1988;4:34.

113. Keys A, Brozek J, Henschel A, et al. The biology of human starvation. Minneapolis: University of Minnesota Press, 1950.

114. Daws TA, Consolazio CF, Hilty SL, et al. Evaluation of cardiopulmonary function of work performance in man during caloric restriction. J Appl Physiol 1972;33:211.

115. Schocken DD, Holloway D, Powers PS. Weight loss and the heart: effects of anorexia nervosa and starvation. Arch Intern Med 1989;149:877.

116. Butterworth CE, Blackburn GL. Hospital malnutrition and how to assess nutritional status of a patient. Nutr Today 1976:March/April.

117. Baker JP, Detsky AS, Wesson DE, et al. Nutritional assessment: a comparison of clinical judgement and objective measurements. N Engl J Med 1982;306:969.

118. McLaren DS, Meguid MM. Nutritional assessment at the crossroads. J Parenter Enter Nutr 1983;7:575.

119. Bozzetti F. Nutritional assessment from the prospective of a clinician. J Parenter Enter Nutr 1987;11:115S.

120. Fleck A. Acute phase response: implication for nutrition and recovery. Nutrition 1988;4:109.

121. Dempsey DT, Mullen JL. Prognostic value of nutritional indices. J Parenter Enter Nutr 1987;11:109S.

122. Bozzetti F, Migliavacca S, Gallus G, et al. "Nutritional" markers as prognostic indicators of postoperative sepsis in cancer patients. J Parenter Enter Nutr 1985;9:464.

123. Klidjian Am, Archer TJ, Foster KJ, Karran SJ. Detection of dangerous malnutrition. J Parenter Enter Nutr 1982;6:119.

124. Jeejeebhoy KN. Bulk or bounce—the object of nutritional support. J Parenter Enter Nutr 1988;12:539.

125. Detsky AS, Baker JP, O'Rourke K, Goel V. Perioperative parenteral nutrition: a meta-analysis. Ann Intern Med 1987;107:195.

126. Naylor CD, O'Rourke K, Detsky AS, Baker JP. Parenteral nutrition with branched-chain amino acids in hepatic encephalopathy: a meta-analysis. Gastroenterology 1989;97:1033.

127. Bastow MD, Rawlings J, Allison SP. Benefits of supplementary tube feeding after fractured neck of femur: a randomized controlled trial. Br Med J 1973;287:1589.

128. Silberman H. Nutrition therapy: clinical applications. In: Parenteral and enteral nutrition. 2nd ed. Norwalk, CT: Appleton & Lange, 1989:365.

129. Schlichtig R, Ayres SM. Nutritional status, nutritional therapy, and survival of critical illness. In: Nutritional support of the critically ill. Chicago: Year Book Medical Publishers, 1988:1.

130. McGeer AJ, Detsky AS, O'Rourke K. Parenteral nutrition in patients receiving cancer chemotherapy. Ann Intern Med 1989;110:734.

131. Grant JP, Custer PB, Thurlow J. Current techniques of nutritional assessment. Surg Clin North Am 1981;61:437.

132. Howard L, Meguid MM. Nutritional assessment in total parenteral nutrition. Clin Lab Med 1981;1:611.

133. Kudsk KA. Sheldon GF. Nutritional assessment. In: Fischer JE, ed. Surgical nutrition. Boston: Little, Brown, & Co, 1983:407.

134. Detsky AS, Baker JP, Mendelson RA, et al. Evaluating the accuracy of nutritional assessment techniques applied to hospitalized patients: methodology and comparisons. J Parenter Enter Nutr 1984;8:153.

135. Detsky AS, McLaughlin JR, Baker JP, et al. What is subjective global assessment of nutritional status? J Parenter Enter Nutr 1987;11:8.

136. Forse RA, Shizgal HM. The assessment of malnutrition. Surgery 1980;88:17.

137. Gray GE, Gray LK. Validity of anthropometric norms used in the assessment of hospitalized patients. J Parenter Enter Nutr 1979;3:366.

138. Bishop CW. Reference values for arm muscle area, arm fat area, subscapular skinfold thickness, and some of skinfold thicknesses for American adults. J Parenter Enter Nutr 1984;8:515.

139. Heymsfield SB, Casper K. Anthropometric assessment of the adult hospitalized patient. J Parenter Enter Nutr 1987;11:36S.

140. Forbes GB, Brown MR, Griffiths HJL. Arm muscle plus bone area: anthropometry and CAT scan compared. Am J Clin Nutr 1988;47:929.

141. Frisancho AR. New norms of upper limb fat and muscle areas for assessment of nutritional status. Am J Clin Nutr 1981;34:2540.

142. Lukaski HC. Methods for the assessment of human body composition: traditional and new. Am J Clin Nutr 1987;46:537.

143. Studley HO. Percentage of weight loss: a basic indicator of surgical risk in patients with chronic peptic ulcer. JAMA 1936;106:458.

144. Golden MHN. Transport proteins as indices of protein status. Am J Clin Nutr 1982;35:11590.

145. Detsky AS, Baker JP, O'Rourke K, et al. Predicting nutrition-associated complications for patients undergoing gastrointestinal surgery. J Parenter Enter Nutr 1987;11:440.

146. Rainey-McDonald CG, Holliday RL, Wells GA, Donner AP. Validity of a two-variable nutritional index for use in selecting candidates for nutritional support. J Parenter Enter Nutr 1983;7:15.

147. Hickman DM, Miller RA, Rombeau JL, et al. Serum albumin and body weight as predictors of postoperative course in colorectal cancer. J Parenter Enter Nutr 1980;4:314.

148. Rudman D, Feller AG, Nagraj SH, et al. Relation of serum albumin concentration to death rate in nursing home men. J Parenter Enter Nutr 1987;11:360.

149. Reinhardt GF, Myscofski JW, Wilkens DB, et al. Incidence and mortality of hypoalbuminemic patients in hospitalized veterans. J Parenter Enter Nutr 1980;4:357.

150. Roza AM, Tuitt D, Shizgal HM. Transferrin—a poor measure of nutritional status. J Parenter Enter Nutr1984;8:523.

151. Church JM, Hill GL. Assessing the efficacy of intravenous nutrition in general surgical patients: dynamic nutritional assessment with plasma proteins. J Parenter Enter Nutr 1987;11:235.

152. Tuten MB, Wogt S, Dasse F, et al. Utilization of prealbumin as a nutritional parameter. J Parenter Enter Nutr 1985;9:709.

153. Howard L, Dillon B, Saba TM, et al. Decreased plasma fibronectin during starvation in man. J Parenter Enter Nutr 1984;8:237.

154. Saba TM, Dillon BC, Lanser ME. Fibronectin and phagocytic host defense: relationship to nutritional support. J Parenter Enter Nutr 1983;7:62.

155. Sandstedt S, Cederblad G, Larsson J, et al. Influence of total parenteral nutrition on plasma fibronectin in malnourished patients with or without inflammatory response. J Parenter Enter Nutr 1984;8:493.

156. Waterlow JC, Stephen JML. Enzymes and the assessment of protein nutrition. Proc Nutr Soc 1969;28:234.

157. Dominioni L, Dionigi R. Immunological function at nutritional assessment. J Parenter Enter Nutr 1987;11:7OS.

158. Twomey P, Ziegler D, Rombeau J. Utility of skin testing in nutritional assessment: a critical review. J Parenter Enter Nutr 1982;6:50.

159. Miller CM. Immunological assays as measurements of nutritional status: a review. J Parenter Enter Nutr 1978;2:554.

160. Walser M. Creatinine excretion as a measure of protein nutrition in adults of varying age. J Parenter Enter Nutr 1987;11:73S.

161. Shizgal HM, Vasilevsky CA, Gardiner PF, et al. Nutritional assessment and skeletal muscle function. Am J Clin Nutr 1986;44:761.

162. Jeejeebhoy KN. The functional basis of assessment. In: Kinney JM, Jeejeebhoy KN, Hill JL, Owen OE, eds. Metabolism in patient care. Philadelphia: WB Saunders, 1988:739.

163. Buzby GB, Mullen JL, Matthews DC, et al. Prognostic nutritional index in gastrointestinal surgery. Am J Surg 1980;139:160.

164. Starker PM, Gump FE, Askanazi J, et al. Serum albumin levels as an index of nutritional support. Surgery 1982;91:194.

165. Pettigrew RA, Hill GL. Indicators of surgical risk and clinical judgement. Br J Surg 1986;73:47.

166. Pettigrew RA, Charlesworth PM, Farmilo RW, Hill GL. Assessment of nutritional depletion and immune competence: a comparison of clinical examination and objective measurements. J Parenter Enter Nutr 1984;8:21.

167. Jeejeebhoy KN, Baker JP, Wolman SL, et al. Critical evaluation of the role of clinical assessment and body composition studies in pa-

tients with malnutrition and after total parenteral nutrition. Am J Clin Nutr 1982;35:1117.

168. Heymsfield SB, Rolandelli R, Casper K, et al. Application of electromagnetic and sound waves in nutritional assessment. J Parenter Enter Nutr 1987;11:64S.

169. Beddoe AH, Hill GL. Clinical measurement of body composition using in vivo neutron activation analysis. J Parenter Enter Nutr 1985;9:504.

170. Mullen JL, Buzby GP, Matthews DC, et al. Reduction of operative morbidity and mortality by combined preoperative and postoperative nutritional support. Ann Surg 1980;192:604.

171. Bistrian BR. Value of serum albumin level in acute care. Nutrition 1988;4:175.

172. Moore FA, Moore EE, Jones TN, et al. TEN versus TPN following major abdominal trauma—reduced septic morbidity. J Trauma 1989;29:916.

173. Cerra FB, Shronts EP, Konstantinides NN, et al. Enteral feeding in sepsis: a prospective randomized, double-blind trial. Surgery 1985;98:632.

174. Moore EE, Jones TN. Benefits of immediate jejunostomy feeding after major abdominal trauma: a prospective, randomized study. J Trauma 1986;26:874.

175. Mochizuki H, Trocki O, Dominioni L, et al. Mechanism of prevention of post-burn hypermetabolism and catabolism by early enteral feeding. Ann Surg 1984;200:297.

176. Alexander JW, Gottschlich MM. Nutritional immunomodulation in burn patients. Crit Care Med 1990;18:5149.

177. Elwyn DH, Gump FE, Munro HN, et al. Changes in nitrogen balance of depleted patients with increasing infusions of glucose. Am J Clin Nutr 1979;32:1597.

178. Dreig P, Elwyn D, Askanazi J, Kinney J. Parenteral nutrition in septic patients: effect of increasing nitrogen intake. Am J Clin Nutr 1987;46:1040.

179. Greenberg GR, Marliss EB, Anderson GH, et al. Protein-sparing therapy in postoperative patients: effects of added hypocaloric glucose or lipid. N Engl J Med 1976;294:1411.

180. Iapichino G, Radrizzani D, Solca M, et al. The main determinants of nitrogen balance during parenteral nutrition in critically ill injured patients. Intensive Care Med 1984;10:251.

181. Jeejeebhoy KN, Anderson GH, Nakhooda AF, et al. Metabolic studies in total parenteral nutrition with lipid in man. J Clin Invest 1976;57:125.

182. Munro HN. Energy intake and nitrogen metabolism. In: Kinney JM, Lense E, eds. Assessment of energy metabolism in health and disease. Columbus, OH: Ross Laboratories, 1978:105.

183. Peters C, Fischer JE. Studies on calorie to nitrogen ratio for total parenteral nutrition. Surg Gynecol Obstet 1980;151:1.

184. Rutten, Blackburn GL, Flatt JP, et al. Determination of optimal hyperalimentation infusion rate. J Surg Res 1975;18:477.

185. Spanier AH, Shizgal HM. Calorie requirements of the critically ill patient receiving intravenous hyperalimentation. Am J Surg 1977;133:99.

186. Wilmore DW. Energy requirements for maximum nitrogen retention. In: Greene HL, Holliday MA, Munro HN, eds. Clinical nutrition update. Chicago: American Medical Association, 1977:47.

187. Wolfe RR, Allsop JR, Burke JF. Glucose metabolism in man: responses to intravenous glucose infusion. Metabolism 1979;28:210.

188. Burke JF, Wolfe RR, Mullany CJ, et al. Glucose requirements following burn injury: parameters of optimal glucose infusion and possible hepatic and respiratory abnormalities following excessive glucose intake. Ann Surg 1979;190:274.

189. Wolfe RR, O'Donnell TF, Stone MD, et al. Investigation of factors determining the optimal glucose infusion rate in total parenteral nutrition. Metabolism 1980;29:892.

190. Harris J, Benedict F. A biometric study of basal metabolism in man. Washington, DC: Carnegie Institute, 1919:40.

191. Foster GD, Knox LS, Dempsey DT, Mullen JL. Caloric requirements in total parenteral nutrition. J Am Coll Nutr 1987;6:231.

192. Schlichtig R, Ayres SM. Nutritional support of the critically ill. Chicago: Yearbook Medical Publishers, 1988:97.

193. Abernathy GB, Heizer WD, Holcombe BJ, et al. Efficacy of tube feeding in supplying energy requirements of hospitalized patients. J Parenter Enter Nutr 1989;13:387.

194. Chikenji T, Elwyn DH, Gil K, et al. The effects of increasing glucose intake on nitrogen balance and energy expenditure in malnourished adult patients receiving parenteral nutrition. Clin Sci 1987;72:489.

195. Askanazi J, Weissman C, LaSala PA, et al. The effect of protein intake on ventilatory drive. Anesthesiology 1984;60:106.

196. Shaw JHF, Wildbore M, Wolfe RR. Whole body protein kinetics in severely septic patients. Ann Surg 1987;205:66.

197. Streat SJ, Hill GL. Nutritional support in the management of critically ill surgical intensive care patients. World J Surg 1987;11:194.

198. Shaw JHF, Wolfe RR. An integrated analysis of glucose, fat, and protein metabolism in severely traumatized patients. Ann Surg 1989;209:63.

199. Nelson KM, Long CL. Physiological basis for nutrition in sepsis. Nutr Clin Prac 1989;4:6.

200. Shangraw RE, Stuart CA, Prince MJ, Wolfe RR. The effect of bed rest on leucine metabolic response to insulin in normal man. Fed Proc 1987;46:1087.

201. ASPEN Board of Directors. Guidelines for use of total parenteral nutrition in the hospitalized adult patient. J Parenter Enter Nutr 1986;10:441.

202. Seneff MG. Central venous catheterization: a comprehensive review: I. J Intensive Care Med 1987;2:163.

203. Seneff MG. Central venous catheterization: a comprehensive review: II. J Intensive Care Med 1987;2:218.

204. Bernard RW, Stahl WM. Subclavian vein catheterization: a prospective study: I. Non-infectious complications. Ann Surg 1971;173:184.

205. Pettigrew RA, Lang SDR, Hydock DA, et al. Catheter-related sepsis in patients on intravenous nutrition: a prospective study of quantitative catheter cultures and guidewire changes for suspected sepsis. Br J Surg 1985;72:52.

206. Mosca R, Curtas S, Forbes B, Meguid MM. The benefits of isolator cultures in the management of suspected catheter sepsis. Surgery 1987;102:718.

207. Merritt RJ, Mason W. Catheter-associated infections—1988. Nutrition 1988;4:247.

208. Schlichtig R, Ayres SM. Modes of delivery: rationale, implementation, and mechanical complications. In: Nutritional support of the critically ill. Chicago: Year Book Medical Publishers, 1988:143.

209. Hoffman KK, Weber DJ, Samsa GP, Rutala WA. A meta-analysis of transparent polyurethane for use as a central venous catheter dressing. Proceedings of the 3rd International Conference on Nosocomial Infections. Atlanta, GA, August 1990 (submitted for publication).

210. Maki DG, Cobb L, Garman JK, et al. An attachable silver-impregnated cuff for prevention of infection with central venous catheters: a prospective randomized multi-center trial. Am J Med 1988;85:307.

211. Hilton E, Haslett TM, Borenstein MP, et al. Central catheter infections: single- versus triple-lumen catheters: influence of guidewires on infection rates when used for replacement of catheter. Am J Med 1988;84:667.

212. Yeung C, May J, Hughes R. Infection rate for single-lumen versus triple-lumen subclavian catheters. Infect Control Hosp Epidemiol 1988;9:154.

213. Heyman MB. General and specialized parenteral amino acid formulations for nutrition support. J Am Diet Assoc 1990;90:401.

214. Meguid MM, Schimmel E, Johnson WC, et. al. Reduced metabolic complications in total parenteral nutrition: pilot study using fat to replace one-third of glucose calories. J Parenter Enter Nutr 1982;6:304.

215. Baker JP, Detsky AS, Stewart S, et al. Randomized trial of total parenteral nutrition in critical ill patients: metabolic effects of varying glucose-lipid ratios as the energy source. Gastroenterology 1984;87:53.

216. Long CL. Fuel preferences in the septic patient: glucose or lipid? J Parenter Enter Nutr 1987;11:333.

217. Frayn KN. Fuel preferences in the septic patient: glucose or lipid? J Parenter Enter Nutr 1988;12:319.

218. Wan JM-F, Teo TC, Babayan VK, Blackburn GL. Invited comment:

lipids and the development of immune dysfunction and infection. J Parenter Enter Nutr 1988;12:43s.

219. Blackburn GL. In search of the "preferred fuel." Nutr Clin Prac 1989;4:3.

220. Heird WC, Grundy SM, Hubbard VS. Structured lipids and their use in clinical nutrition. Am J Clin Nutr 1986;43:320.

221. Mascioli EA, Babayan VK, Bistrian BR, Blackburn GL. Novel triglycerides for special medical purposes. J Parenter Enter Nutr 1988;12:127s.

222. Brown RO, Bradley JE, Bekemeyer WB, Luther RW. Effect of albumin supplementation during parenteral nutrition on hospital morbidity. Crit Care Med 1988;16:1177.

223. Brown RO, Bradley JE, Luther RW. Response of serum albumin concentrations to albumin supplementation during central total parenteral nutrition. Clin Pharm 1987;6:222.

224. Expert panel for nutrition advisory group, AMA Department of Foods and Nutrition. Guidelines for central trace element preparations for parenteral use. JAMA 1979;241:2051.

225. The nutrition advisorty group of the Department of Foods and Nutrition, American Medical Association. Multivitamin preparations for parenteral use. A statement by the Nutrition Advisory Group. J Parenter Enter Nutr 1979;3:258.

226. Grimble GK, West MF, Acuti ABC, et al. Assessment of an automated chemiluminescence nitrogen analyzer for routine use in clinical nutrition. J Parenter Enter Nutr 1988;12:100.

227. Weinsier RL, Bacon J, Butterworth CE. Central venous alimentation: a prospective study of the frequency of metabolic abnormalities among medical and surgical patients. J Parenter Enter Nutr 1982;6:421.

228. Dickerson RN, Brown RO. Hypomagnesemia in hospitalized patients receiving nutritional support. Heart Lung 1985;14:561.

229. Izsak EM, Shike M, Roulet M, Jeejeebhoy KN. Pancreatitis in association with hypercalcemia in patients receiving total parenteral nutrition. Gastroenterology 1980;79:555.

230. Gilligan JE, Hagley S, Worthley LIG, et al. Hypercalcemia associated with parenteral amino acid and dextrose infusion. Am J Clin Nutr 1982;35:993.

231. Schlichtig R, Ayres SM. Monitoring and management of the metabolic sequelae of hyperalimentation. In: Nutritional support of the critically ill. Chicago: Yearbook Medical Publishers, 1988:169.

232. Tayek TA, Bistrian B, Sheard NF, et al. Abnormal liver function in malnourished patients receiving total parenteral nutrition: a prospective study. J Am Coll Nutr 1990;9:76.

233. O'Dwyer ST, Smith RJ, Hwang TL, Wilmore DW. Maintenance of small bowel mucosa with glutamine-enriched parenteral nutrition. J Parenter Enter Nutr 1989;13:579.

234. Koruda MJ, Rolandelli RH, Bliss DZ, et al. Parenteral nutrition supplemented with short-chain fatty acids: effect on the small-bowel mucosa in normal rats. Am J Clin Nutr 1990;51:685.

235. Herndon DN, Barrow RE, Stein M, et al. Increased mortality with intravenous supplemental feeding in severely burned patients. J Burn Care Rehabil 1989;10:309.

236. Fong Y, Marano MA, Barber A, et al. Total parenteral nutrition and bowel rest modify the metabolic response to endotoxin in humans. Ann Surg 1989;210:449.

237. ASPEN Board of Directors. Guidelines for the use of enteral nutrition in the adult patient. J Parenter Enter Nutr 1987;11:435.

238. Gustke RF, Varma RR, Soergel KH. Gastric reflux during perfusion of the proximal small bowel. Gastroenterology 1970;59:890.

239. Roubenoff R, Ravish WJ. Pneumothorax due to nasogastric feeding tubes: report of four cases, review of the literature, and recommendations for prevention. Arch Intern Med 1989;149:184.

240. MacBurney MM, Young LS. Formulas. In: Rombeau JL, Caldwell MD, eds. Enteral and tube feeding. Philadelphia: WB Saunders, 1984:171.

241. Heymsfield SB, Erbland M, Casper K, et al. Enteral nutritional support: metabolic, cardiovascular, and pulmonary interactions. Clin Chest Med 1986;7:41.

242. Al-Saady NM, Blackmore CM, Bennett ED. High fat, low carbohydrate, enteral feeding lowers P_{CO_2} and reduces the period of ventilation in artificially ventilated patients. Intensive Care Med 1989;15:290.

243. Pesola GE, Hogg JE, Yonnios T, et al. Isotonic nasogastric tube feedings: do they cause diarrhea? Crit Care Med 1989;17:1151.

244. Edes TE, Walk BE, Austin JL. Diarrhea in tube-fed patients: feeding formula not necessarily the cause. Am J Med 1990;88:91.

245. Scheppach W, Burghardt W, Bartram P, Kasper H. Addition of dietary fiber to liquid formula diets: the pros and cons. J Parenter Enter Nutr 1990;14:204.

246. Silberman H. Parenteral and enteral nutrition. In: Nutrition therapy: clinical applications. 2nd ed. Norwalk, CT: Appleton & Lange, 1989:365.

247. Sheldon GF, Gardner BN, Way LW, Dunphy JE. Management of gastrointestinal fistulas. Surg Gynecol Obstet 1971;133:385.

248. Payne-James JJ, Silk DBA. Total parenteral nutrition as primary treatment in Crohn's disease—RIP? Gut 1988;29:1304.

249. Greenberg GR, Fleming CR, Jeejeebhoy KN, et al. Controlled trial of bowel rest and nutritional support in the management of Crohn's disease. Gut 1988;29:1309.

250. Cabre E, Gonzalez-Huix F, Abad-Lacruz A, et al. Effect of total enteral nutrition on the short-term outcome of severely malnourished cirrhosis. Gastroenterology 1990;98:715.

251. Bastian CH, Driscoll RH. Enteral tube feeding at home. In: Rombeau JL, Caldwell MD, eds. Enteral and tube feeding. Philadelphia: WB Saunders, 1984:494.

252. Silberman H. Nutrition therapy: home care. In: Parenteral and enteral nutrition. 2nd ed. Norwalk, CT: Appleton & Lange, 1989:345.

49

Genetic Counseling for Gastrointestinal Patients

JEROME I. ROTTER
LINDA M. RANDOLPH

PART A: GENERAL PRINCIPLES

Genetics is the study of biologic variation. Medical genetics is the study of the genetic basis for variability in susceptibility to disease. Not everyone is equally susceptible to most gastrointestinal (GI) diseases. To a small or large degree, depending on the disorder, the differences in susceptibility are based on differences in the genetic constitution of individuals. These genetic differences are important for defining the etiology and classification of GI diseases, for diagnosing and managing patients with GI diseases, and for knowing when and how to evaluate family members. Therefore, every clinician must have an understanding of genetic principles and their application to GI diseases.

This chapter reviews the evidence that there are genetic components to specific GI diseases; how the genetic components are inherited; and how the information is used in the care and counseling of patients and their families.

CONTRIBUTION OF GENETICS TO GI DISORDERS

Diseases affecting the GI tract can be arranged on a continuum from those having strictly a genetic basis (e.g., familial polyposis coli) to those having strictly an environmental basis (e.g., *Salmonella* gastroenteritis). Most disorders fall somewhere between and result from the interaction of genetic and environmental factors (e.g., milk-induced diarrhea in patients with lactase deficiency).[1]

The genetic etiology of familial polyposis coli (an autosomal dominant disorder having a high degree of penetrance) can be appreciated from the study of a single pedigree. However, for many GI disorders, it is considerably more difficult to establish the presence of a genetic component. There are several reasons.[1]

One is that the disorder may not be inherited in a simple mendelian pattern. A second is that it is genetically heterogeneous (i.e., its clinical manifestations result from several disorders, each having a different etiology). (Patterns of mendelian inheritance and genetic heterogeneity are discussed on page 988.) A third reason is that the age of onset of clinical disease may be late or variable. This complicates the study of families of patients with the disorder because younger family members may have the ab-

normal gene or genes responsible for the disease but have not yet manifested clinical disease. A fourth reason is that environmental factors play a role in many disorders. Thus, to be clinically affected, a person must have the necessary genetic factor(s) and must be exposed to the necessary environmental agent(s). A good example is lactose intolerance, a disorder characterized by bloating, diarrhea, and malabsorption brought on by ingesting milk and other lactose-containing products. The underlying defect is an absence of intestinal lactase. Lactase deficiency is inherited in an autosomal recessive mendelian pattern, but disease (i.e., symptoms) occurs only after exposure to the necessary environmental factor, in this case, a large load of dietary lactose.

The first order of business is to review the methods that can establish whether a disease has a genetic component (Table 49-1).[1]

A genetic component to a disease may be suspected from the finding of (1) *familial aggregation* (a higher frequency of the disease in first-degree relatives of patients with the disease than in the general population) or (2) marked variation in its frequency among different ethnic groups. For example, duodenal ulcer, which is known to have a genetic component, shows both familial aggregation and marked variation in frequency in different ethnic groups.[2] The frequency of duodenal ulcer is two- to threefold greater in relatives of duodenal ulcer patients than in controls and is much higher in the Scottish population than in Southwest American Indians. Similarly, inflammatory bowel disease (IBD) has a frequency 30-fold or more greater in relatives and is found in increased frequency in Jewish populations compared to the non-Jewish populations in which they reside.[3-5] Familial aggregation has been observed for all the disorders listed in Table 49-2.

However, neither familial aggregation nor differences in disease frequency among ethnic groups proves a genetic component to a disease. The reason is that families and larger related population units (ethnic groups) share both common genes and common environmental factors (e.g., diet, geography, exposure to infectious agents). Thus, to prove a genetic component to a disease, it is necessary to separate common genetic from common environmental factors.

Animal models can provide indirect evidence for a genetic component (see Table 49-1). If a spontaneously occurring disease

TABLE 49–1
Evidence for Genetic Factors in GI Diseases

SUGGESTIVE EVIDENCE	EXAMPLE
Familial aggregation	Colon cancer increased among relatives of colon cancer patients; inflammatory bowel disease (IBD) increased among relatives of IBD patients
Ethnic differences	Marked ethnic differences in the frequency of peptic ulcer and of IBD
Genetic syndromes	Multiple endocrine neoplasia syndrome type I, with gastrinoma leading to peptic ulcer; familial polyposis coli leading to colon cancer; Hermansky-Pudlak syndrome associated with granulomatous colitis
Animal models	Spontaneous animal models of gallstones

DEFINITIVE EVIDENCE	EXAMPLE
Environmental Controls	
Twins	Increased concordance for peptic ulcer in monozygotic (MZ) compared to dizygotic (DZ) twin pairs; increased concordance of IBD in MZ versus DZ twins
Spouses	Colon cancer increased in relatives but not spouses of colon cancer patients; IBD increased in relatives but not in spouses of IBD cases; gallstones increased in siblings but not in spouses of gallstone patients
Genetic Markers	
Association	Blood group O associated with duodenal ulcer
	HLA DR3 associated with celiac disease
Linkage	Alleles of the *met* oncogene linked to cystic fibrosis

in animals is analogous to a disease in humans, the role of genetic factors in that species can be shown by defining differences among strains and by designing appropriate matings. However, even if a genetic contribution is unequivocally demonstrated for the disease in animals, it is reasoning by analogy to make the same conclusion for the disease in humans.

The existence of a genetic syndrome featuring the disease of interest is evidence that genetic factors can cause the disease in a subset of cases. For example, cancer of the colon in persons with familial polyposis coli clearly is genetic in origin. However, this finding suggests, but by itself does not prove a genetic component to common colon cancer.

Definitive evidence for a genetic component can be obtained by twin, spouse, and adoption studies, and by association and linkage studies using gene markers[1] (see Table 49-1).

The classic method to decide whether familial aggregation is due to common genetic versus common environmental factors is to study twin pairs. In this method, rates of concordance (i.e.,

whether one or both members of a twin pair are affected with the disease) are determined in monozygotic (MZ) and in dizygotic (DZ) twin pairs. (MZ twin pairs are genetically identical; DZ twin pairs are no more genetically alike than any pair of siblings). A higher concordance rate in MZ than in DZ twin pairs indicates that familial aggregation is due to a significant genetic component, while equal rates of concordance indicate that familial aggregation is determined largely by environmental factors. Peptic ulcer, celiac disease, and IBD are examples of disorders in which concordance rates are higher in MZ than in DZ twin pairs.

For some disorders, especially disorders with a late age of onset, an adequate sample of twin pairs may not be available. In this instance, spouses can be used as environmental controls. Studies of colon cancer, gallstones, and IBD have shown that, in contrast to genetically related persons, spouses sharing the same household environment do not have an increased risk for these diseases.

Another approach to separate genetic from environmental effects is to compare the frequency of a disease in adopted versus biologically related relatives. This type of investigation has been used mostly to study genetic contributions to behavioral and psychiatric disorders such as depression and alcoholism, but has also been applied to obesity. These studies have consistently shown a greater similarity of persons to their biologic as opposed to their adopted relatives.

The final category of evidence that proves a genetic component is the finding that the disease is associated with a well-delineated genetic marker (e.g., blood group, HLA antigen, serum enzyme polymorphism, or, more recently, molecular genetic markers). The topic of genetic markers is discussed further in the section entitled "The Gene Map, Linkage, and Association" (page 995).

Before turning to the question of how the genetic component is inherited, the nature of the genetic material is briefly reviewed.

ORGANIZATION OF GENETIC MATERIAL AND MOLECULAR GENETICS

The central biologic dogma is indicated in Figure 49-1.[6,7] Genetic material in all cells consists of deoxyribonucleic acid (DNA), which is organized into long double helices.

DNA consists of pentose sugars, phosphates, and four bases, two pyrimidines—cytosine (C) and thymidine (T), and two purines—adenine (A) and guanine (G). The backbone of each helix consists of pentose sugars and phosphates, while genetic information resides in the varying sequence of the four bases. The combination of pentose sugar, phosphate, and base is called a *nucleotide*. The nucleotide bases are arranged in a complementary fashion in that adenine in one chain always pairs with thymine in

TABLE 49–2
Common GI Disorders With a Genetic Component

Atrophic gastritis	Gastric cancer
Peptic ulcer	Lactase deficiency
Celiac disease	Inflammatory bowel disease
Colon cancer	Gallstones

THE GENETIC MATERIAL

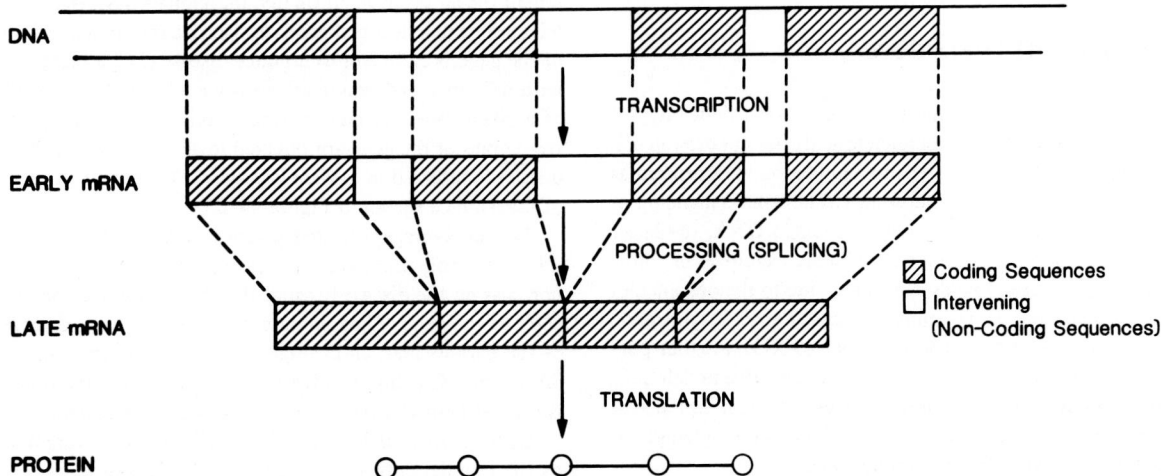

FIGURE 49–1. DNA is the primary genetic material, the genes. To convert genetic information in DNA into actual function, the DNA is transcribed into messenger RNA (mRNA) by a multistep process. The mRNA is then translated by the cell's protein synthesis mechanism, the ribosomes, into a sequence of amino acids that specifies a particular protein. The proteins are the functioning units of the cell. Each amino acid is coded for by a nucleotide triplet of the mRNA, which, in turn, was coded for by a corresponding triplet in the DNA. (Rotter Jl. In: Gitnick G, et al, eds. Principles and Practice of Gastroenterology and Hepatology. New York: Elsevier, 1988: 1501.)

the other chain, and cytosine always pairs with guanine. The complementary structure of the two chains provides a mechanism for its replication; each strand serves as the template for a new strand. The complementarity of the DNA strands also allows the identification of specific DNA sequences in a complex mixture, if one has available a radiolabeled probe consisting of the complementary sequences (also known as a DNA probe). This technique, nucleic acid hybridization, is critical for the success of molecular genetic techniques (see section entitled "Recombinant DNA and Restriction Fragment Length Polymorphisms" on page 996).

The entirety of human genetic material (genome) consists of approximately 3 billion nucleotide pairs and is organized into 23 pairs of chromosomes. Of the 23 pairs, 22 pairs are morphologically identical (homologous) in both sexes and are called *autosomes.* The remaining pair, the sex chromosome, consists of two X chromosomes in females and an X and a Y chromosomes in males.

DNA can either replicate itself (necessary for cell division and the formation of gametes [sperm and oval]) or can be transcribed into messenger ribonucleic acid (mRNA) for eventual translocation into proteins. The proteins, in turn, function either as structural units or as chemical catalysts (enzymes).

Genetic information in DNA is determined by the sequence of nucleotide bases. Different sequences of three bases, known as the genetic code, code for specific amino acids. Besides those sequences (sometimes more than one) coding for each individual amino acid, other sequences code for punctuation signals (e.g., the end of the gene). If the average protein consists of a few hundred amino acids, the average gene would consist of approximately 1000 base pairs, resulting in enough DNA for 3 million genes. However, much of the DNA in the genome is not coded into protein. The current estimate is that there are about 100,000 functional human genes. Because only some 4000 genes have been

recognized by either molecular, biochemical, or clinical techniques, biologists still have their work cut out for them. The genetic information encoded in DNA is transcribed by DNA-dependent RNA-polymerase into mRNA. This is a single-stranded ribonucleic acid that differs in composition from DNA in that uracil replaces cytosine and ribose replaces deoxyribose. The information encoded in mRNA is, in turn, translated by polyribosomes in the cytoplasm into proteins.

At one time, it was thought that genes were coded in their entirety into mRNA, which, in turn, was translated into the specific amino acid sequence making up a particular protein. We now know that most genes consist of coding sequences (exons), which are translated into specific amino acid sequences, and untranslated sequences (introns), which do not appear in the mRNA that is used by the cell's protein-synthesizing machines, the ribosomes (see Fig 49-1). It also is clear that DNA sequences on either side of the gene have important roles in regulating gene expression (promoters, enhancers). Thus, the functional genetic unit is considerably more complex than was considered a decade ago.

TYPES OF GENETIC DISEASES AND MODES OF INHERITANCE

Regardless of their complexity at the molecular level, genes still follow the laws of inheritance elucidated by Mendel in the 19th century. Now that we have reviewed the nature of the genetic material, it is appropriate to consider how these laws apply to genetic diseases and their modes of inheritance.

The three major categories of genetic disease are: (1) chromosomal disorders, (2) mendelian disorders, and (3) nonmendelian (multifactorial) disorders.[6,8–10]

Chromosomal Disorders

Chromosomal disorders are due to an excess or a deficiency of total genetic material. Deoxyribonucleic acid does not exist in cell nuclei as naked DNA, but rather in combination with protein as chromatin. Each of the 46 chromosomes of humans is made up of this chromatin, with a core of double-stranded DNA, the latter likely a single continuous molecule. Classic examples of chromosomal disorders are Down's syndrome, due to the presence of an extra chromosome 21 (trisomy 21) and Turner's syndrome, due the lack of a second sex chromosome (45 XO). Smaller portions of chromosomes can be missing or in excess, due to deletions or duplications of portions of chromosomes, or as consequence of their rearrangement in chromosomal translocations (exchanges of material between two different chromosomes).

An imbalance of total genetic material results in a variety of defects (e.g., multiple malformations and mental retardation). Although the underlying mechanism is poorly understood, the severity of the defects depends on the amount and the specificity of chromosomal material involved. Most chromosomal disorders are sporadic (i.e., arise from errors in forming gametes or early zygotes), but inherited forms (translocations) also occur.

While chromosomal disorders do include malformations of the GI tract (e.g., duodenal atresia in trisomy 21 and abdominal wall defects [omphalocele] in trisomy 13), constitutional (congenital) chromosomal disorders do not contribute greatly to the total burden of GI disease.

An important distinction should be made between constitutional and acquired chromosome abnormalities. *Constitutional* chromosomal disorders are congenital, represent germ-line changes, and are usually present in all tissues of an affected person. In contrast, *acquired* or somatic chromosomal aberrations are present only in specific tissues such as tumors. Most cancers are characterized by acquired chromosome abnormalities.[11] The observation of specific or recurring chromosome abnormalities in certain tumors has led to identification of the specific genes involved in oncogenesis in certain human tumors.[12] Examples have included point mutations in oncogenes (genes involved in cell growth that, when unregulated, can lead to cancer), gene amplification, gene rearrangements as a consequence of chromosomal translocations, and gene deletions leading to the loss of tumor suppressor genes (also known as anti-oncogenes). An excellent example of the latter is that of colon cancer, with such genes being identified on the short arm of chromosome 17 and the long arm of chromosome 18.[13–15]

Mendelian (Single Gene) Disorders

Mendelian disorders are due to abnormalities in single genes. They are so named because they follow the well-delineated patterns of inheritance first described by Mendel in the 19th century.[6,10,16,17] Examples of mendelian disorders affecting the GI tract are listed in Table 49-3. (A more extensive listing is given in Tables 49-12 through 49-17.)

AUTOSOMAL DOMINANT INHERITANCE

Autosomal dominant disorders are due to single genes located on one of the autosomes. Normally, individuals have two copies (alleles) of each autosomal gene. A disorder is dominant if one copy of the gene is sufficient to produce disease (i.e., a person affected with an autosomal dominant disorder has one "abnormal" copy of a given gene and one "normal" copy of the same gene). The two copies of the gene are referred to as the *genotype;* the clinical disease is referred to as the *phenotype.* This results in the pattern of inheritance shown in Figure 49-2.

On the average, affected persons pass the disease to 50% of their offspring. Unaffected offspring neither develop the disease nor pass on the disease because they have received the "normal" copy of the gene. Thus, in an autosomal dominant disorder, one of the parents and, on average, 50% of the parent's siblings and 50% of the offspring are affected. This pattern of inheritance often is termed *vertical transmission* or *vertical aggregation.*

Some additional features of mendelian disorders are illustrated by the familial polyposis syndromes (Table 49-4).

Example—The Familial Polyposes. The familial polyposis syndromes are characterized by multiple polyps in the GI tract (see ch 79). These may range from dozens to literally thousands. The two best known and most important of the familial polyposes syndromes are familial polyposis coli (FPC) and Gardner's syndrome. Both are characterized by a large number of adenomatous polyps, which are located primarily in the colon and rectum. In FPC, polyps are the only manifestation, but in Gardner's syndrome there are a variety of extraintestinal manifestations (osteomas of the jaw and sebaceous cysts are the most common).[18] These disorders are important both because of their frequency (approximately 1 in 10,000) and their inordinately high risk for colon cancer. (The risk for colon cancer in affected persons who survive into old age is close to 100%). As is discussed in the section entitled "The Gene Map, Linkage, and Association" (page 995), there is evidence that these two disorders are related genetically because both have been localized to the long arm of chromosome 5.

One concept illustrated by the polyposis syndromes is *delayed age of onset.* Because a disorder is genetic does not mean it is clinically evident at birth. Colonic polyps in FPC usually do not appear until affected persons are in their second or third decade of life. (If colon cancer is the basis for bringing a person to attention, the apparent age of onset is even later.)

A second concept is *pleiotropism,* which is a short way of saying multiple effects of a single gene. The multiple clinical manifestations of Gardner's syndrome—colonic polyps, osteomas of the jaw, and sebaceous cysts—represent the effect of a single gene on different organs. The same is true for Peutz-Jeghers syndrome (the hamartomatous polyps and buccal and palmar melanin spots represent the multiple effects of a single mutant gene).

A third concept is *variable expressivity.* This means that the quantitative and qualitative manifestations of a genetic disease may vary considerably among affected persons. For example, one patient with the gene for Gardner's syndrome may have multiple osteomas and sebaceous cysts, whereas another may exhibit only one or two sebaceous cysts.

A fourth concept, *penetrance,* is related to that of variable expressivity. Persons known to carry the gene (proved by trans-

TABLE 49–3
Examples of Mendelian Disorders That Affect the Gastrointestinal Tract

AUTOSOMAL DOMINANT DISORDERS	GI PRESENTATION
Tylosis (diffuse hyperkeratosis of the palms and soles) with esophageal cancer	Esophageal cancer
Multiple endocrine neoplasia syndrome, type I (tumors of pituitary, parathyroid, and of endocrine pancreas; pancreatic tumors include gastrinomas resulting in severe ulcer disease)	Duodenal ulcer
Hereditary hollow visceral myopathy	Intestinal pseudo-obstruction
Familial polyposis coli (multiple colonic adenomatous polyps with colonic cancer)	Colon cancer, GI bleeding
Gardner's syndrome (multiple colonic adenomatous polyps, sebaceous cysts, and osteomas of the jaw)	Colon cancer, GI bleeding
Peutz-Jeghers syndrome (hamartomatous polyps of the entire GI tract, melanin pigmentation of lips, oral mucosa, palms, and soles)	GI bleeding, intussusception
Hereditary pancreatitis	Pancreatitis
Hereditary hemorrhagic telangiectasia of Osler-Weber-Rendu syndrome	GI bleeding
Cancer family syndrome (colon, breast, and endometrial cancer)	Colon cancer, GI bleeding
Ehlers-Danlos type IV (thin translucent skin with arterial, bowel, and uterine rupture)	Diverticula, gut perforation

AUTOSOMAL RECESSIVE DISORDERS	GI PRESENTATION
Cystic fibrosis (pulmonary disease and exocrine pancreatic failure)	Malabsorption
Schwachman syndrome (pancreatic insufficiency and pancytopenia)	Malabsorption
Turcot syndrome (multiple colonic adenomatous polyps and cancer, malignant tumors of the central nervous system)	Colon cancer, GI bleeding
Familial Mediterranean fever (recurrent polyserositis)	Abdominal pain
Lactase deficiency	Malabsorption, diarrhea
Hermansky-Pudlak syndrome (oculocutaneous albinism, platelet dysfunction, pulmonary fibrosis, and inflammatory bowel disease)	Inflammatory bowel disease

mitting it to their offspring) yet who have no recognizable clinical manifestations of the disease (the far end of the spectrum of variable expressivity) are considered to be nonpenetrant.

Penetrance may be a function of the intensity of examination of at-risk persons. For example, in FPC, if colonoscopy is not performed, many affected persons would not be identified and would be considered nonpenetrant.

Penetrance also can be a function of the age of the patient. As noted previously, polyps in FPC and in Gardner's syndrome often do not appear until the second or third decade of life. Therefore, affected persons may be nonpenetrant while young. Conversely, in Peutz-Jeghers syndrome, melanin pigmentation of the palms and soles may diminish with age. Thus, older affected persons, examined for the first time, may be considered nonpenetrant.

The polyposis syndromes also illustrate dramatically the concept of *genetic heterogeneity for single gene disorders*. Genetic heterogeneity means that the clinical manifestations of a disease may have different etiologies; more formally that different mutations can cause an identical or similar phenotype. A further distinction is allelic heterogeneity, which refers to mutations at the same locus (same chromosomal location [i.e., same gene]), versus locus heterogeneity, which refers to mutations at different loci (i.e., different genes). Genetic heterogeneity within the polyposes syndromes has been established by histologic examination of polyps revealing adenomas in FPC and hamartomas in Peutz-Jeghers syndrome, by more complete clinical delineation of the syndrome (e.g., the presence in Gardner's syndrome of osteomas and sebaceous cysts and in Peutz-Jeghers syndrome of melanin pigmentation of the

AUTOSOMAL DOMINANT

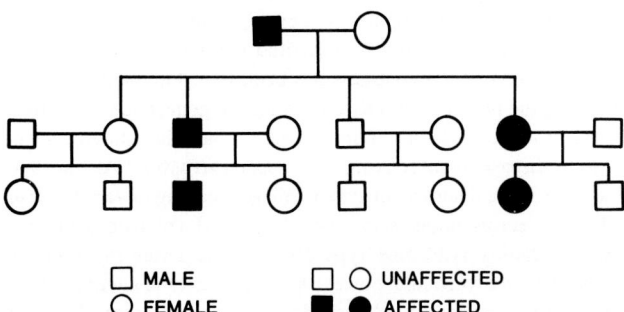

FIGURE 49–2. Idealized autosomal dominant pedigree demonstrating vertical transmission.

TABLE 49–4
Familial Polyposis Syndromes as Examples of Autosomal Dominant Disorders

DISORDER	HISTOLOGY OF POLYPS	LOCATION OF POLYPS	CANCER RISK	OTHER FEATURES	MODE OF INHERITANCE*
Familial polyposis coli	Adenoma	Colon	High (colon)	None	AD
Gardner's syndrome	Adenoma	Colon	High (colon), occasionally other sites	Sebaceous cysts, osteomas of jaw and skull, super-numerary teeth, fibromatosis	AD
Peutz-Jeghers syndrome	Hamartoma	Entire GI tract	Moderate (occasional small intestinal, ovarian; but moderate for non-GI malignancies)	Melanin spots of lips, buccal mucosa, palms, and soles	AD
Turcot syndrome	Adenoma	Colon	High (colon)	Medulloblastoma	AR
Juvenile polyposis coli	Juvenile	Predominantly colon, but also rest of GI tract	High (colon and gastric)	None	AD
Juvenile polyposis coli and A-V malformations	Juvenile	Predominantly colon	High (colon and gastric)	Arteriovenous malformations	AD
Cronkhite-Canada syndrome	Juvenile	Entire GI tract	Low	Alopecia, dystrophic nails, diffuse pigmentation, enteropathy	Sporadic

* *AD = autosomal dominant; AR = autosomal recessive.*

lips and buccal mucosa), and by delineation of different patterns of inheritance (autosomal dominant for FPC versus autosomal recessive for Turcot syndrome).

The clinical importance of separating the multiple colonic polyposis phenotype into distinct etiologic entities is that the disorders differ in their natural history and management. For example, the need for surveillance of index patients and their relatives is minimal for the polyposis syndromes that carry little or no risk for colonic cancer. But for others (e.g., FPC), identification of an affected person indicates a markedly high risk for colon cancer and a need for prophylactic total colectomy, and necessitates the intensive screening of at-risk relatives.

AUTOSOMAL RECESSIVE INHERITANCE

A disorder is inherited in an autosomal recessive fashion if two copies of an abnormal gene are needed for expression of the disease. Examples of autosomal recessive disorders affecting the GI tract are listed in Tables 49-3 and 49-5. (A more extensive listing is given in Tables 49-12 through 49-17.)

Because affected persons receive two copies of the abnormal gene, one from each parent, the pattern of inheritance usually is that the parents are not affected, but one fourth of the siblings of the nuclear family are affected. This pattern of inheritance is sometimes referred to as *horizontal aggregation* (Fig 49-3). Because most families in the developed world are small (two or three children), most cases are the only case in a family and appear to be sporadic (nongenetic). It is important that the possible genetic cause of an isolated disease in a family not be ignored simply because of the lack of a positive family history for that individual

case. As in autosomal dominant disorders, both sexes are affected with the same frequency.

Affected persons are known as *homozygotes* (or more formally as homozygous for the disease gene). Both parents and one half of all siblings carry one copy of the abnormal gene and are termed *heterozygotes*. The heterozygotes are clinically normal. The final one quarter of siblings are homozygous normal.

Autosomal recessive disorders include many of the classic inborn errors of metabolism (see Table 49-5).[19,20] While in a real sense all mendelian disorders are inborn errors, the term usually is reserved for disorders affecting enzymatic processing of a variety of substances. As shown in Table 49-5, sugars, fats, amino acids, vitamins, metals, and even ions can be involved.

Classically, recessive disorders have been hypothesized to code for enzyme proteins and dominant disorders for structural proteins. The reasoning is that because most enzymes are coded for in such large amounts, even 50% of normal enzyme concentration (coded for by one normal gene) is more than adequate for metabolic needs. Only with the complete absence of an enzyme (i.e., two abnormal genes) would disease develop. Indeed, the majority of recognized inborn errors are inherited in a recessive fashion.

In contrast, the hypothesis has been that dominant disorders, needing the presence of only one abnormal gene, code for a structural protein, which if abnormal even in half the amount, would lead to disease by interfering with normal structure. An excellent example is the disorders of type I collagen leading to various forms of osteogenesis imperfecta, and of type III collagen leading to Ehlers-Danlos syndrome type IV.[21,22] The latter disorder can present with diverticula, bowel rupture, or arterial aneurysms.[21,23] While this mechanism is undoubtedly true for many dominant disorders, others are due to enzyme deficiencies in tightly regulated metabolic systems (e.g., porphyrin synthetic enzymes in the por-

TABLE 49–5

Inborn Errors of Metabolism as Examples of Autosomal Recessive Disorders Involving the Gastrointestinal Tract

DISORDER	INHERITANCE*	ENZYME DEFICIENCY	METABOLITE(S)
Acrodermatitis enteropathica	AR	? Zinc-binding protein	Zinc
Sucrose-isomaltase deficiency	AR	Sucrase-isomaltase	Sucrose, maltose, isomaltose
Lactase deficiency, common adult type	AR	Lactase	Lactose (adolescence or adulthood)
Glucose-galactose malabsorption	AR	Na/glucose transporter	Glucose, galactose
Hartnup disease	AR	Transport protein for neutral amino acids	Neutral amino acids (e.g., tryptophan)
Cystinuria	AR	Transport proteins for dibasic amino acids	Cystine, ornithine, arginine, lysine
Pancreatic lipase deficiency	AR	Pancreatic lipase	Triglycerides
Congenital pernicious anemia	AR	Intrinsic factor	Cobalamin (vitamin B_{12})
Imerslund-Grasbeck	AR	? Postreceptor transport of intrinsic factor-B_{12} complex by ileum	Cobalamin (vitamin B_{12})
Congenital chloride diarrhea	AR	? Chloride-bicarbonate exchanger	Chloride

AR = autosomal recessive.

phyrias where only 50% of normal enzyme activity can lead to disordered metabolism and disease).

The disorders listed in Tables 49-3 and 49-5 illustrate several other principles of recessive disorders. Just like dominant disorders, recessive disorders can manifest anytime in life—from the newborn period (e.g., meconium ileus due to cystic fibrosis [CF]) to middle age (e.g., first appearance of lactose intolerance). Because recessive disorders require two abnormal genes, they are more likely to occur if the parents are related (i.e., consanguineous). The rarer the disorder (and hence the rarer the gene), the higher the frequency of increased consanguinity among the parents of affected persons.

The likelihood of a recessive disorder is increased if the frequency of the abnormal gene is high within an ethnic group. This is the reason for the higher frequency of a number of autosomal recessive disorders in certain ethnic groups (e.g., cystic fibrosis in U.S. and European white populations [see ch 92], familial Mediterranean fever (FMF) in Sephardic Jews and Armenians, and lactase deficiency in Oriental populations [see page 1015).

All the offspring of a person homozygous for a recessive disorder are obligatory heterozygotes and, therefore, usually clinically unaffected. At times, however, a recessive disorder may be so common that parent-to-offspring transmission (pseudodominant transmission) is observed. This is due to the mating of an affected homozygote and a heterozygote. In such a case, half the time the offspring are also homozygous for the mutant gene, and therefore affected. In the non-Ashkenazi Jewish population and in Armenians, the frequency of the recessive gene leading to FMF is extremely high, and, as a consequence, such vertical transmission is observed.[24,25] In fact, it has been estimated that one in seven Armenians is a carrier (heterozygote) for this disorder. For the same reason, vertical transmission is seen with lactase deficiency in high-incident populations.

AUTOSOMAL RECESSIVE

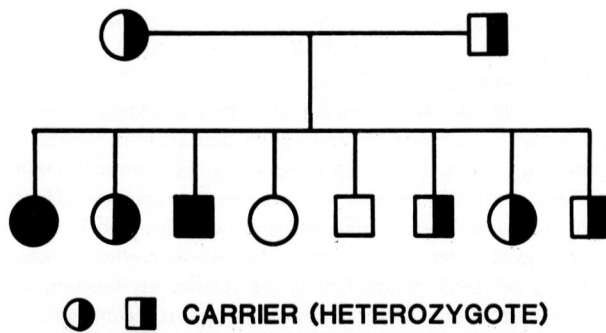

CARRIER (HETEROZYGOTE)
AFFECTED (HOMOZYGOTE)
HOMOZYGOUS NORMAL

FIGURE 49–3. Idealized autosomal recessive pedigree demonstrating horizontal aggregation.

X-LINKED INHERITANCE

What distinguishes men from women is one chromosome. Men have an X and a Y chromosome; women have two copies of the X chromosome. The Y chromosome is small and appears to carry mainly male-determining genes. Thus, in females, an abnormal gene located on an X chromosome may behave in a dominant or recessive fashion, but in males, who have only one X chromosome, the behavior is different.

A male affected with an X-linked condition is said to be hemizygous. The pattern of inheritance of an X-linked disorder (diagonal aggregation) is shown in Figure 49-4. The difference from an autosomal pattern of inheritance is that a male affected with an X-linked recessive disorder can pass the gene to none of his sons but to all of his daughters. Carrier (heterozygous) females yield four types of offspring, each accounting for 25% of the total—carrier females, normal females, normal males, and affected males.

Few recognized X-linked disorders involve the GI tract. One group of X-linked disorders that can present as a GI disorder is the hemophilias (A and B), but GI bleeding is not the usual presentation of these hemorrhagic diatheses.

MITOCHONDRIAL INHERITANCE

In eukaryotes, not all the DNA is located in the nucleus. Thus, in humans, besides the major DNA coding for genes in the nucleus, there is also DNA located in the mitochondria of the cell. This mitochondrial DNA encodes a number of subunits of the mitochondrial respiratory chain.[26,27] Mitochondria are located in the cytoplasm. When a zygote is formed, all the mitochondria are derived from the ovum, and none from the sperm. This leads to a distinctive pattern of inheritance for mutations in mitochondrial DNA. They are transmitted exclusively in the maternal line, from a mother to all her children. Males never transmit such a disorder. This applies not only to the affected males' children, but to all their descendants. This distinguishes this pattern of inheritance from X-linked disorders. Because mitochondria are located exclusively in cytoplasm, this has also been termed *cytoplasmic inheritance*.[28] An increasing number of disorders are being identified

TABLE 49-6
Nonmendelian Genetic Disorders

Characteristics

Demonstrate increased familial aggregation
Aggregation shown to be genetic
Aggregation doesn't fit mendelian ratios or patterns

Explanations

Many additive genes each of small effect—polygenic
Genes and environmental factors—multifactorial
Major gene and environmental factors—genetic susceptibility
Two (or more) major genes, both necessary—two locus (multilocus)
Different disorders, different genetics—genetic heterogeneity
All of the above

Examples

Rare—pyloric stenosis, Hirschsprung's (megacolon)
Common—peptic ulcer, inflammatory bowel disease, colon cancer (and most of Table 49-2)

as having this distinctive pattern of inheritance, such as Leber's hereditary optic neuropathy.[28,29]

Nonmendelian (Common or Multifactorial) Disorders

Most of the common GI disorders (including malformations) show familial aggregation (see Table 49-2), and, by the criteria listed in Table 49-1, the aggregation is due to a genetic component. However, for the majority of these disorders, the pattern of familial aggregation is not consistent with any simple mendelian mode of inheritance.

Several models have been proposed to resolve this seeming paradox (Table 49-6). One is the polygenic threshold model.[1,8] The concept of this model is that the genetic component is due to the aggregate effect of many genes (polygenes), each with a small effect. Thus, in this model, the disease would occur only if a person had a sufficient number of the disease-promoting genes, beyond a certain threshold. If environmental factors also play a role, the model is referred to as *multifactorial*.

The polygenic model can explain how a disorder can be both genetic and nonmendelian. Indeed, on first analysis, familial aggregation of several disorders—especially such common malformations as pyloric stenosis and congenital megacolon (Hirschsprung's disease)—appeared consistent with this model.

However, there are both practical and theoretical problems with the polygenic model. One is that it gives no direction as to how to identify the disease-promoting genes. A second is the underlying assumption that the disorder under study has the same etiology in all patients.

It is apparent that the genetic contribution to many common diseases is better explained by genetic heterogeneity.[1,30] The concept of *genetic heterogeneity for common diseases* is that what may appear to be one disease with one cause often consists of several

X-LINKED RECESSIVE

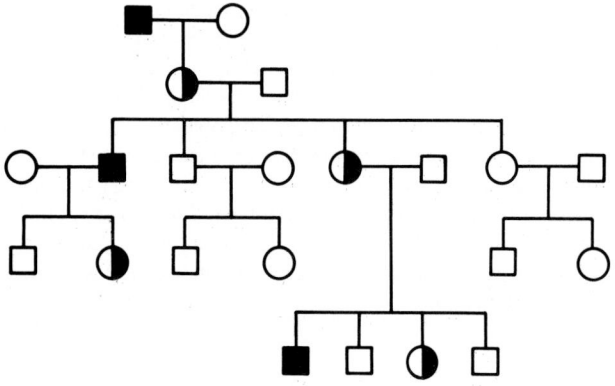

■ AFFECTED MALE (HEMIZYGOTE)
□ NORMAL MALE
◑ CARRIER FEMALE (HETEROZYGOTE)
○ NORMAL, NON–CARRIER FEMALE

FIGURE 49–4. Idealized pedigree of an X-linked recessive disorder. Note that affected males are related to one another through carrier females.

diseases, each with a different etiology. Because the etiologies may be genetic, environmental, or genetic–environmental, some forms of the disease may be inherited in a mendelian fashion, whereas others may exhibit a nonmendelian or multifactorial pattern. However, if heterogeneity of the disease is not recognized at the outset, the overall familial aggregation may resemble the pattern expected in multifactorial inheritance.

Examples—Peptic Ulcer and Inflammatory Bowel Disease.

The methods for demonstrating heterogeneity in common diseases such as peptic ulcer or inflammatory bowel disease are listed in Table 49-7 (see also ch 61 and 78). A comparison of Table 49-7 with Table 49-1 indicates that several of the findings that suggest a genetic component to a disease also provide evidence that the disease is genetically heterogeneous.[1,30] Thus, the fact that there are several rare genetic syndromes that feature peptic ulcer as one of their manifestations is immediate proof that at least some forms of ulcer are genetically heterogeneous, because these syndromes are due to mutations at different

loci in the human genome.[30,31] These syndromes also provide direct proof of pathogenetic heterogeneity (e.g., gastric acid hypersecretion due to increased gastrin secondary to gastrinoma in multiple endocrine neoplasia syndrome type I [MEN I] versus increased histamine in systemic mastocyosis). The same logic, although less well developed, applies to disorders with an increased frequency of IBD such as the Hermansky-Pudlak syndrome accompanied by granulomatous colitis.[5,32]

The finding of ethnic differences in a disease, particularly if these include differences in the clinical features, also suggests genetic heterogeneity. In the case of peptic ulcer, both the frequency of ulcer and the type of ulcer differ dramatically between Scottish whites and Southwest American Indians—duodenal ulcer is more common in whites; gastric ulcer is more common in American Indians.[2] Within duodenal ulcer, the type of complication differs dramatically from one continent to another. In Europe, hemorrhage is the most common complication; in Africa, duodenal stenosis is more common.

The finding of clinical differences within the same population also suggests heterogeneity of a disease. For example, gastric ulcer

TABLE 49-7
Criteria for Demonstrating Heterogeneity in Common Diseases (Peptic Ulcer and Inflammatory Bowel Disease as Examples)

CRITERION	EXAMPLE—PEPTIC ULCER	EXAMPLE—IBD
Rare genetic syndromes that feature the disease as part of the phenotype	Multiple endocrine neoplasia syndrome type I, and gastrinomas Systemic mastocytosis Tremor–nystagmus–ulcer syndrome Amyloidosis, type IV Pachydermoperiostosis Leukonychia–duodenal ulcer–gallstones	Turner's syndrome (XO) Hermansky-Pudlak syndrome Various immunodeficiency disorders
Ethnic variability in incidence and in clinical features	Duodenal ulcer more frequent in Europe, gastric ulcer more frequent in Japan Stenosis more common in Africa, hemorrhage more common in Europe	
Clinical evidence	*Gastric versus duodenal ulcer:* different age distributions *Within duodenal ulcer:* early and late age of onset associated with different clinical features and complications Association of ulcer with other diseases—chronic lung disease, renal stones (without hyperparathyroidism)	Ulcerative colitis versus Crohn's disease: different clinical features and complications Ulcerative colitis associated with sclerosing cholangitis
Clinical genetic evidence	*Gastric versus duodenal ulcer:* increased risk is families in site specific Concordant twins concordant for ulcer site	Concordance rates for monozygotic twins higher for Crohn's disease than for ulcerative colitis
Physiologic differences	*Gastric versus duodenal ulcer:* gastric acid secretion and serum pepsinogen I higher in duodenal than gastric ulcer *Within duodenal ulcer:* abnormalities (acid hypersecretion, hyperpepsinogenemia I, increased gastrin response to a meal, increased rate of gastric emptying, acid stimulatory antibodies) present in some but not all patients	Intestinal permeability abnormalities perhaps in Crohn's, not in ulcerative colitis Antineutrophil cytoplasmic antibodies in ulcerative colitis, in only a few Crohn's *Within Crohn's:* C3 functional abnormality present in some patients
Family studies using physiologic abnormalities as subclinical markers	*Within duodenal ulcer:* hyperpepsinogenemic I families versus normopepsinogenemic I duodenal ulcer families; familial rapid gastric emptying; familial antral G-cell hyperfunction; familial duodenogastritis	*Within Crohn's:* C3 functional abnormality in some families and not others
Heterogeneity of association with polymorphic genetic markers	*Gastric vs. duodenal ulcer:* blood group O associated with duodenal ulcer *Within duodenal ulcer:* blood group O and HLA antigens associated with older age of onset and normal acid secretion	Crohn's associated with C3 polymorphism Ulcerative colitis associated with HLA DR2

and duodenal ulcer differ in average age of onset and in their rates of complications. Also, patients who develop duodenal ulcer at an early age have a higher risk of bleeding and stronger family history of duodenal ulcer than patients who first develop the disease after age 30.[33] Conversely, the latter patients have a higher risk of other complications (e.g., perforations). Of course, the clinical differences in Crohn's disease and ulcerative colitis have long been part of evidence arguing for the separation of these disorders.

Heterogeneity of peptic ulcer is also suggested by its association with other diseases.[2] In the case of chronic lung disease, because the ulcer often precedes the onset of lung disease, it is possible that the ulcer and the lung disease are the common manifestation of an underlying abnormality. In other words, the association may well be another example of pleiotropism (i.e., multiple effects of a single gene). A similar concept may apply to the association of both forms of IBD with ankylosing spondylitis, and the association of the ulcerative colitis form of IBD with sclerosing cholangitis.[5]

Clinical genetic studies, which combine clinical evaluation within the context of family studies, can provide strong evidence for genetic heterogeneity of a disease. Such studies have shown that the increased risk for peptic ulcer in a family is specific for the type of ulcer observed in the index case.[2,34] Thus, relatives of gastric ulcer patients are at increased risk for gastric ulcer, but not for duodenal ulcer. Similarly, relatives of duodenal ulcer patients are at increased risk for duodenal ulcer, but not for gastric ulcer. This specificity (i.e., that the ulcer type "runs true" in families) is formally termed *independent segregation*. This, in turn, is good evidence that gastric ulcer and duodenal ulcer are genetically distinct disorders. Similar studies in IBD yielded a very different result, in that whether one began with either ulcerative colitis or Crohn's, both forms are increased in family members.[3,35] However, evidence in this regard for heterogeneity of IBD includes the much higher concordance rate in MZ twins with Crohn's disease than in those with ulcerative colitis, and the failure to observe mixed MZ twin pairs (i.e., one with Crohn's and one with ulcerative colitis).[5,36]

Another method to determine heterogeneity of a common disease is to search for major genes (i.e., genes that have a major effect on risk for the disease). Persons in the population or within families who possess such genes are at a significant risk for the disorder in question.

The search for major genes can be conducted from the *phenotype* down or from the *genotype* up.

As an example of the terms *phenotype* and *genotype,* let us consider a person who possesses the gene for multiple endocrine neoplasia syndrome type I (MEN I; see also ch 91). MEN I is an autosomal dominant disorder characterized by tumors of the pituitary, parathyroids, and pancreas.[37] These tumors often produce excessive amounts of their respective hormones (e.g., growth hormone and prolactin by pituitary tumors; parathyroid hormone [PTH] by parathyroid tumors; gastrin and insulin by pancreatic tumors). The genotype of this individual is determined by the presence of the MEN I gene. However, his or her phenotype (i.e., the clinical manifestations of the genotype) can be extremely variable. For example, the affected individual may present with symptoms of hypercalcemia such as renal stones due to excess PTH, peptic ulcer due to excess gastrin, or acromegaly due to excess growth hormone. Each of these may occur alone or in any combination, or the individual may be entirely free of symptoms.

In analyzing a common disease from the phenotype down, the first step is to understand the pathophysiology underlying the clinical abnormality. In the case of peptic ulcer, we started with the clinical phenotype of abdominal pain, with or without a complication such as upper GI bleeding. We proceeded to define the phenotype better by clinical, radiographic, and histologic examinations. In this way, an ulcer in the stomach or duodenum is detected by radiography or endoscopy. Histologic examination demonstrated that the ulcer is chronic and nonmalignant. By studying the physiology of the processes that could conceivably lead to a chronic ulcer, we learned that duodenal ulcer patients secrete more acid (on the average) than normal subjects or patients with gastric ulcer, and that some duodenal ulcer patients have high levels of serum pepsinogen I (a precursor of the stomach's digestive enzyme pepsin).[2,38] In explaining the phenotype, we have found physiologic heterogeneity within peptic ulcer (i.e., duodenal ulcer patients produce more acid and pepsin than gastric ulcer patients). Even within duodenal ulcer, patients can be further subdivided as to whether they are acid hypersecretors or normosecretors, hyperpepsinogenemic I or normopepsinogenemic I, produce an increased amount of gastrin in response to a meal, or empty their stomach contents more rapidly into the duodenum.[2,38] There is evidence for physiologic heterogeneity within the duodenal ulcer population.

Family studies are extremely useful in demonstrating that physiologic heterogeneity is fundamental to disease pathogenesis (i.e., that it precedes rather than follows the appearance of clinical disease).[1] One can study in families not just the aggregation of clinical disease, such as peptic ulcer, or clinical characteristics, such as ulcer site (gastric versus duodenal), but also the physiologic characteristics that are hypothesized to lead to the ulcer. If these physiologic abnormalities are also found in some clinically unaffected relatives, it can be concluded that the abnormalities likely precede rather than follow the disease. In the process of this type of study, the pattern of inheritance of the subclinical physiologic abnormality can be elucidated. The abnormality can serve as a subclinical marker of genetic predisposition to the disease. This process has demonstrated that the subclinical physiologic abnormality is a marker of a major gene, which, in many cases, is inherited in a mendelian fashion (i.e., the physiologic abnormality is genetically determined and those with the abnormal trait are at increased risk for disease).

The study of subclinical markers also can clarify the pattern of inheritance of genetic components to a disease. For example, the aggregation of duodenal ulcer in families of duodenal ulcer patients is not consistent with a simple mendelian mode of inheritance. In a number of these families, both the ulcer patients and a number of their clinically unaffected relatives have an elevated serum pepsinogen I level. Quite often, the aggregation of an elevated serum pepsinogen I in these families is consistent with autosomal dominant inheritance.[39,40] Approximately 40% of such relatives have recognized clinical duodenal ulcer. The genetic or environmental factors that convert this common genetic susceptibility into clinical disease are not known. In other families, all members, including those with the duodenal ulcer, have normal serum pepsinogen I levels.[41] The use of this subclinical genetic marker, an elevated serum pepsinogen I level, has (1) demonstrated genetic heterogeneity of duodenal ulcer, in that serum pepsinogen I levels (high or normal) are consistent within families; and (2) the genetic component of duodenal ulcer in hyperpepsinogenemic I patients and their families. Other subclinical genetic markers (e.g., the gastrin response to a protein meal and the rate of gastric emptying) have identified additional subtypes of duodenal ulcer.[2,31]

The approach of identifying major genetic susceptibilities by using subclinical genetic markers has been applied to a number of common GI disorders. For example, there are well-defined physiologic concomitants of severe atrophic gastritis, which is the underlying cause of pernicious anemia. The physiologic abnormalities include a low serum pepsinogen I level, a high serum gastrin, and, most specific, a low serum pepsinogen I to pepsinogen II ratio.[42] The use of these physiologic abnormalities as subclinical markers of atrophic gastritis has demonstrated that the aggregation of atrophic gastritis in family members of patients with pernicious anemia is consistent with dominant inheritance, with a late age of onset.

As another example, the presence of a few or single adenomatous polyps often accompanies common nonsyndromic colon cancer. Family studies using flexible sigmoidoscopy have revealed a significant excess of solitary polyps in relatives of ordinary colon cancer patients; with an aggregation consistent with dominant inheritance.[43,44] So, again, a major gene has been identified that predisposes to common colon cancer. In this instance, the subclinical manifestation is, at most, a few colonic polyps. Similar approaches in IBD have included the study of intestinal permeability or of complement function in the relatives of Crohn's patients; the latter study has provided evidence for genetic heterogeneity within Crohn's by observing that low levels of C3 activity appear to be a familial trait, but only in a subset of families.[45,46]

Finally, the last method to detect major genes and to demonstrate genetic heterogeneity of a disease consists of "working from the genotype up." This method is discussed in detail in the section entitled "The Gene Map, Linkage, and Association." Briefly, the approach is to determine whether a gene, with a known mode of inheritance (e.g., ABO blood groups or HLA antigens or DNA restriction fragment length polymorphisms [RFLPs]), is associated with a disease in the population or in families. An example of how this type of study can contribute to our knowledge of genetic heterogeneity is the association of blood group antigens with peptic ulcer.[2] The association of blood group O with duodenal ulcer, but not with gastric ulcer, demonstrates that duodenal ulcer and gastric ulcer are genetically distinct disorders.

The importance of delineating etiologic and genetic heterogeneity is that the several diseases that constitute a clinical phenotype (e.g., duodenal ulcer or IBD) may have different relationships to potential environmental risk factors such as nonsteroidal antiinflammatory agents or to potential infectious agents such as *Helicobacter pylori*, different natural histories, or different optimal therapies[47,48] (Table 49-8).

THE GENE MAP, LINKAGE, AND ASSOCIATION

The organization in humans of the estimated 100,000 genes on the 23 pairs of chromosomes is termed the *gene map*.[49] The location of each gene on its chromosome is termed the gene *locus*. The specific form of each gene is called an *allele*. Because the chromosomes are paired (homologous), each person has two copies (i.e., two alleles) of each gene, except for X-linked genes in the male. (It should be noted that whereas persons are limited to two

TABLE 49–8
Genetic and Etiologic Heterogeneity of Peptic Ulcer

Peptic ulcer associated with rare genetic syndromes
  Multiple endocrine neoplasia, type I
  Systemic mastocytosis
  Tremor–nystagmus–ulcer syndrome
  Amyloidosis, type IV
  Pachydermoperiostosis
  Leukonychia–duodenal ulcer–gallstones
Gastric ulcer
Combined gastric and duodenal ulcer
Hyperpepsinogenemic I duodenal ulcer (also usually acid hypersecretors)
Antral G-cell hyperfunction
Normopepsinogenemic I duodenal ulcer
Rapid gastric emptying
Childhood duodenal ulcer*
  Normal acid secretion
  Elevated acid secretion
Immunologic forms of duodenal ulcer*
  Subgroup with acid-stimulatory antibodies
Peptic ulcer associated with chronic diseases*
  Peptic ulcer and chronic lung disease
  Duodenal ulcer and renal stones (without hyperparathyroidism)
  Duodenal ulcer and coronary artery disease

Tentative subdivisions.

alleles of each gene, there may be hundreds of alleles of each gene in the population.)

Linkage

Because there are about 100,000 genes and only 23 pairs of chromosomes, any two pairs of different genes are most likely to have their loci on different pairs of chromosomes. When this is the case, each gene (more precisely the allele at each genetic locus) is transmitted to offspring randomly (segregates independently). The two pairs of genes are said to be *unlinked*.

Less often, two pairs of different genes have their loci on the same chromosome. When the two loci are sufficiently close together, the alleles at adjacent loci often are transmitted together (i.e., cosegregate). When this is observed, the two gene loci are said to be *linked*.

The *recombination fraction* is a measure of how often alleles at the two loci separate during meiosis (the formation of gametes) and are transmitted randomly. A recombination fraction of 10% means that 10% of the time the alleles at the two loci separate at meiosis (i.e., recombine with alleles on the homologous chromosome). The converse is that 90% of the time the alleles at the two loci do not recombine and are transmitted together. The recombination fraction can range from zero (completely linked) to 50% (unlinked). If the recombination fraction is a few percent or less, the two loci are very close (tightly linked) and the transmission of an allele at one locus can be used to predict the transmission of the other.

The clinical importance of linkage is that a disease gene that cannot be detected directly can still be traced in a family if it is closely linked to a *polymorphic marker gene*. The criteria for a polymorphic marker gene are that (1) the gene is polymorphic (i.e., occurs in different forms known as alleles, with the less frequent alleles having a frequency of 1% or more), (2) the alleles have a well-characterized mendelian mode of inheritance, and (3) the products of the alleles can be detected reliably (and usually easily). Examples of polymorphic marker genes include blood group antigens, enzyme electrophoretic polymorphisms, HLA antigens, and inherited variation at the DNA level itself.[50,51] If a polymorphic gene is closely linked to a disease gene, we can take advantage of inherited variation among individuals to follow the marker alleles and, therefore, the disease gene through a family.

In each family, the particular marker allele is defined by the affected member. Therefore, linkage studies can be done only in families that already have at least one affected member. It also should be noted that the marker allele is not the same in all families because, in general terms, the linkage relationship is between the loci of the disease gene and the marker gene and any allele can occupy the marker locus. This finding is in contrast to the concept of association in which a particular marker allele (or alleles) is involved in all families (see "Association," page 997).

Recombinant DNA and Restriction Fragment Length Polymorphisms

Although linkage is potentially an extremely powerful tool to screen for and prevent inherited disease, until the last few years it had been applied to very few GI (or other) disorders. The reason is that, until recently, only a relatively small number of polymorphic gene markers were available (approximately 30 to 40). These consisted of enzyme polymorphisms (usually defined by electrophoresis) and antigenic differences on red blood cells (e.g., blood groups) and white blood cells (HLA antigens).

The number of polymorphic markers has increased dramatically during the last few years. Modern molecular biologic methods (often referred to as recombinant DNA technology) have given us the ability to develop an essentially unlimited number of polymorphic gene markers.[50,51]

This ability is based on two advances. One advance is the ability to select specific pieces of DNA from the entire human genome, recombine them with viral or bacterial plasmid genes, and insert the *recombinant DNA* into a virus or bacteria, which can multiply rapidly and produce multiple copies of this recombinant DNA.[6,7,51] The human DNA that is being multiplied may be derived from a known gene (by knowing its protein sequence or by producing a complementary DNA from protein coding mRNA using an enzyme known as reverse transcriptase) or an unknown segment of DNA. The multiplied recombinant DNA is a chemically pure reagent that can be used as a *DNA probe*. That is, DNA–DNA interactions are so exact and specific, that this multiplied DNA probe representing a specific gene, when put in solution with many different DNA pieces derived from a sample of the entire human genome (or even with DNA from different species), combines (hybridizes) only with the specific human DNA from which it was derived

(that it is complementary to). This is what underlies the technique known as Southern blotting.

The second advance was the discovery of enzymes in bacteria that cut DNA at specific sites. These enzymes are termed *restriction endonucleases*. We can take any source of cellular DNA, such as white cells, cut it up into small fragments with restriction endonucleases, and pick out the few specific pieces of DNA that compose a specific gene of interest by hybridizing the digested DNA with a preselected DNA probe.

All previous linkage markers depended on inherited variation at the protein level, detected by immunologic or biochemical techniques. However, there is much more variation at the DNA level itself, because the DNA code is redundant (i.e., more than one DNA triplet can code for the same amino acid) and because a large amount (actually the majority) of DNA is not translated into protein. Furthermore, even if a protein is only expressed in one tissue such as liver, because all nucleated cells share all genes, we can study the genetics of a disorder at the molecular level using any source of DNA, such as white cells or skin fibroblasts.

These two advances allow us to measure inherited variation at the DNA level itself.[50] Using a restriction enzyme to digest a source of DNA obtained from a patient, a pattern of DNA fragments is seen by the technique of Southern blotting that consists of those pieces of DNA that hybridize with the specific synthetic DNA probe, which has been labeled radioactively so it gives a visible pattern on film. Such DNA fragment patterns often vary from one person to another. This inherited variation is termed *restriction fragment length polymorphism* (RFLP). Hundreds of polymorphic linkage markers have been identified by this method, and many thousands are possible.

Example—Cystic Fibrosis. Cystic fibrosis (CF; see also ch 92) is the most common genetic disorder of the pancreas.[52,53] It is also the most common lethal autosomal recessive disorder in white populations (estimated frequency, 1 in 2000 births). The disorder is characterized by viscous secretions and dysfunction of multiple exocrine glands, leading to pancreatic insufficiency and malabsorption, chronic pulmonary infection with emphysema, and high chloride concentration in sweat. While mild cases do survive into adulthood, the majority of affected persons die in childhood or young adulthood from chronic lung disease. The GI manifestations are discussed in more detail in "Cystic Fibrosis," page 1013. Here we focus on genetic linkage and genetic counseling considerations.

As contrasted to a disorder such as FPC where preclinical detection can lead to disease prevention, preclinical detection of affected persons with CF, such as is possible by determining the concentration of chloride in sweat, cannot prevent pancreatic and lung disease because there is no effective preventive treatment.

Genetic counseling is recommended for all patients and families with CF. Linkage studies using recombinant DNA methodology have demonstrated that the CF gene is located on the long arm of chromosome 7 and have identified a number of polymorphic DNA linkage markers.[54] Two closely linked markers are polymorphisms of the *met* oncogene and an anonymous DNA probe, termed PJ3.11. This molecular technology became available for prenatal diagnosis of CF and is offered routinely to those with a previously affected child and to other relatives of childbearing age. For this purpose, cells are obtained from either chorionic villi (at 8 to 10 weeks of gestation) or from amniotic fluid (at 14 to

20 weeks of gestation). These cells have the same genotype as the fetus; hence, they have the same DNA. Thus, if the fetus is found to have the same linkage markers as an affected child in the family, the fetus is predicted to be affected (Fig 49-5). An adjunctive test used in some situations is the measurement of alkaline phosphatase (low in CF) in the amniotic fluid of fetus at risk. The two tests together provide close to 99% accuracy for prenatal diagnosis. However, this has been improved with the identification of the actual gene for CF and delineation of mutations at the DNA level.[55] Because a significant proportion of the mutations are not yet identified, carrier screening for the general population is not yet recommended.[56]

Although prenatal diagnosis makes it possible to identify an affected fetus, because there is no effective preventive therapy for CF, the primary option for the parents is termination of pregnancy. Because CF is an autosomal recessive disorder, this option is faced only one quarter of the time. It is important to emphasize that, in the past, most parents who had an affected child with CF elected to stop having children altogether. This technology allows families the freedom to have children unaffected with this lethal disease.

Example—Familial Polyposis Coli.

Molecular linkage investigations have also identified the genetic region, although not yet the gene, for FPC and Gardner's syndrome (see also ch 79). The location was first suggested to be on the long arm of chromosome 5 by a case report of a mentally retarded person with polyposis who had an interstitial deletion of a portion of that chromosomal arm.[57] This was followed by studies of familial polyposis families using molecular DNA probes from chromosome 5 and, specifically, its long arm. These succeeded in establishing linkage of FPC to that gene region.[58,59] (This process was considerably faster than that for CF, because in CF all chromosomes were being examined before sufficient data were developed that established the location on chromosome 7.) An important result of these studies was that both FPC and the more complex Gardner's syndrome with its bone and soft tissue tumors, map to the same region of the long arm of chromosome 5.[60] This is evidence that they may be allelic disorders. This chromosomal region is being intensively studied, and cloning of the actual gene is expected to be forthcoming. Even now, however, with the available markers, preclinical or prenatal diagnosis based on DNA analysis of cells obtained from peripheral blood or prenatally (chronic villi or amniocentesis) is available from certain centers.

Association

The methodology of association studies differs from that of linkage studies[1,8] (Table 49-9). Whereas in linkage studies, families are

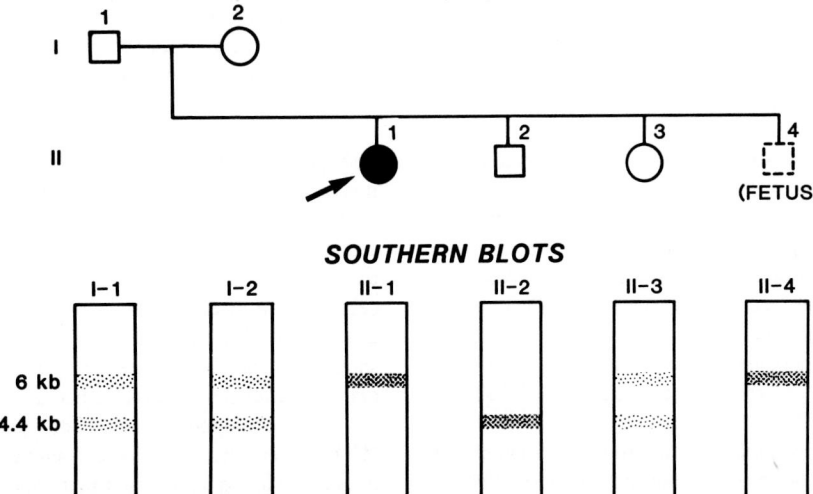

SOUTHERN BLOTS

FIGURE 49-5. Pedigree of cystic fibrosis (CF) illustrates linkage to a DNA probe and prenatal diagnosis. Having an affected child, the parents are obligate heterozygotes. The first child is affected (II-1). There are two unaffected siblings (II-2, II-3), and prenatal diagnosis has been performed on a male fetus at 25% mendelian risk (II-4). DNA has been obtained on all persons (from peripheral blood samples, except for the fetus where it was obtained from chorionic villi or amniotic fluid cells). The DNA samples have been digested by the restriction enzyme Taq 1, electrophoresed, and transferred to a filter. A DNA probe of the closely linked *met* oncogene has been applied. As can be seen, there is variation at the *met* oncogene locus. The heterozygous parents (I-1, I-2) each have a 6.0-kb and 4.4-kb (kb = kilobase) fragment. Their affected daughter (II-1) received the 6.0-kb fragment from each parent. Therefore, the CF gene can be presumed to be linked in both parents to the 6.0-kb fragment. This is confirmed by the siblings II-2 and II-3, who are clinically unaffected and can be inferred to be homozygous normal and heterozygous (like the parents), respectively. The fetus (II-4) has unfortunately received the same two alleles as the affected sister (II-1; i.e., he has received the 6.0-kb fragment from each parent). Barring the slight chance of recombination, he is predicted to have received a CF gene from each parent and therefore to be affected. (Rotter JI. In: Gitmick G, et al. eds. Principles and Practice of Gastroenterology and Hepatology. New York: Elsevier, 1988:1501.)

TABLE 49–9
Comparison of Linkage and Association

CHARACTERISTIC	LINKAGE	ASSOCIATION
Uses polymorphic gene markers	Yes	Yes
How discovered	Family studies	Population studies (cases and controls)
Relationship	Between two genetic loci (any allele can occupy the marker locus)	Between a specific allele and a disease (or between two alleles)
Explanation	Loci close together on the same chromosome (no interaction inferred)	Causal relation to disease, or linkage disequilibrium

tested to determine whether alleles at two different loci travel together; in association studies, the frequency of a marker allele is determined in persons with a specific disease (cases) and in disease-free persons from the same population (controls). If there is a significant difference in the frequency of the marker allele between cases and controls, the allele is regarded to have a role in the etiology of the disease. The *relative risk* (or odds ratio) for a disease for a specific marker can be calculated from the magnitude of the frequency difference in the marker allele. The magnitude of the relative risk is a measure of the strength of the biologic association of the marker with the disease.

The first disease association reported (in the 1950s) was that of blood group A with gastric cancer. Soon thereafter, blood group O was reported to be associated with peptic ulcer. In both cases, the relative risk was small (less than 1.5) and the reason for the associations remains obscure even today.

However, even these weak associations helped delineate genetic heterogeneity of peptic ulcer.[2] The blood group O association with peptic ulcer was shown to be specific for duodenal ulcer and pre-pyloric ulcer (but not with ulcer of the body of the stomach). Thus, even though of a low order of magnitude, the association helped separate duodenal ulcer from gastric ulcer. There is evidence that it may further separate duodenal ulcer, because some studies have indicated the blood group O association may be confined to older onset patients who tend to have gastric acid outputs within the normal range.[33,38]

In the 1970s, interest was rekindled by the observation of considerably stronger associations of certain diseases with alleles of the HLA system.[61,62] The HLA system is the major histocompatibility complex (MHC) of humans (i.e., the genetic region that determines, in large part, the success of transplantation of certain organs). In animals, autoimmune disease and susceptibility to certain tumors were found to be linked to the MHC. This led to a search for disease associations in humans.

Initial associations were described with alleles of the HLA class I loci (i.e., alleles at the HLA A and HLA B loci). The HLA A and B loci are closely linked. These alleles code for antigens that are found on all nucleated cells. The antigens are detected by antisera obtained from multiparous women or multiple-transfused persons.

The most spectacular initial finding was the discovery of the association of HLA B27 with ankylosing spondylitis, with a relative risk approaching 100. Somewhat less spectacular, but highly sig-

nificant HLA associations with GI diseases also were found. For example, the frequencies of antigen A3 at the HLA A locus and antigens B7 and B14 at the HLA B locus were found to be increased severalfold in patients with idiopathic hemochromatosis. (These associations led to the linkage studies that clarified the mode of inheritance of hemochromatosis.) Another prominent association is HLA B8 with gluten-sensitive enteropathy (GSE, also known as celiac disease), again with a severalfold relative risk.

One possible explanation for these associations is that the HLA alleles have a direct role in disease pathogenesis. This does not seem to be the case for either the HLA A3-hemochromatosis association or the HLA B8-GSE association. The primary reason for this conclusion is that the majority of people in the population who have HLA A3 or HLA B8 do not have hemochromatosis or GSE.

The generally accepted explanation for these associations is *linkage disequilibrium* (also known as allelic association). That is, it is believed that many of the recognized disease-associated HLA alleles are not involved directly in the pathogenesis of their associated disease, but rather are innocent bystanders located next to actual disease genes that directly determine the increased susceptibility to disease. This relationship is clear for the HLA A3 association with hemochromatosis; the disease is inherited as a simple autosomal recessive disorder, but most persons who have two A3 alleles do not have hemochromatosis.

This phenomenon of linkage disequilibrium also applies to the HLA antigens themselves. For example, certain alleles at the HLA A locus are found with greater than expected frequency with certain alleles at the HLA B locus (e.g., HLA A1 at the A locus and HLA B8 at the B locus). Therefore, A1 and B8 are associated. But A1 and B8 are entirely separate genes and gene products. However, the HLA A and B loci are linked, in fact tightly linked. What appears to have happened is that the alleles are at loci that are so closely linked that there has not been adequate time to separate them evolutionarily (i.e., to come to linkage equilibrium). The result is linkage disequilibrium. This may have occurred simply due to lack of time for sufficient recombinations to have occurred. Or, it may be because since the HLA gene region has a major role in the body's immune response, selection has kept together certain advantageous combinations of alleles.

In any case, because the HLA alleles themselves are in linkage disequilibrium, the favored hypothesis to explain HLA-disease associations is that they are secondary to linkage disequilibrium between the associated alleles and the actual disease genes. An implication of this hypothesis is stronger associations may exist with other genes in the HLA region. When it became possible to measure the products of the HLA class II region genes, also known as the HLA D region, stronger associations were found between gluten-sensitive enteropathy and antigen DR3 of the HLA DR locus, stronger than the B8 association.[63] There have been other advances (e.g., the detailed molecular structure of the HLA class II region is being delineated).[64] It is clear that even the DR3–GSE association is not specific enough, and molecular methods are being used to identify the actual susceptibility gene or genes.[65]

In the case of the HLA-disease associations, as contrasted to ABO blood group-disease associations, major genes determining disease susceptibility have been identified. Thus, using either the method of linkage or association, one can work from the genotype up to identify major genetic susceptibilities.

The HLA-disease association studies also indicate that, even if major genes are involved, susceptibility to a disease is not always inherited in a simple mendelian fashion. For example, in GSE, DR3 appears to identify a major HLA susceptibility gene, but one or more non-HLA, nonchromosome 6 genes appear required for disease susceptibility.[63] Thus, GSE may be thought of as a two-locus disorder (or multilocus, if more than two loci are involved).

Gluten-sensitive enteropathy (see also part B of this chapter and ch 71) is termed a two-locus or multilocus disease, rather than a polygenic disease, because susceptibility can be ascribed to two or more major genes.[66] The clinical significance is that, by determining the segregation of polymorphic marker genes within families, family members at significantly increased risk for these diseases can be identified. For example, siblings of a GSE patient who share the same DR3 allele or HLA haplotypes have a significantly increased risk for GSE.[67] In such siblings, small bowel biopsy can be done to detect subclinical GSE, which, if detected, can be treated by a gluten-free diet.

CLINICAL GENETICS

Clinical genetics and genetic counseling are the application of the principles of medical genetics to the care of patients and families with genetic disease.[10] As should be apparent, this applies not only to mendelian disorders but also to the several common GI disorders with a major genetic component discussed in this chapter.[1,68]

The clinical geneticist, like any clinician, is concerned about three things: what is it? (diagnosis), what's going to happen? (prognosis), and what can be done about it? (therapy and prevention). The difference is that the clinical geneticist asks these questions not just about the patient, but also about the patient's family, and the patient's and family's potential offspring.

Genetic Diagnosis

There are several lessons from genetics for clinical diagnosis. One is to use the family as an additional investigative tool. This is done most effectively by examining relatives who are potentially at risk. A relative cannot be said to be unaffected unless he or she

has been evaluated by a physician who is searching for the specific disorder segregating in the family.

A second lesson relates to the nature of the history, physical, and subsequent examinations. In evaluating patients, directed questions should be asked about and patients should be examined for findings that may indicate a syndromic form of what otherwise is a common disease. For example, in evaluating a patient with duodenal ulcer, one should always inquire about the personal and family history of renal stones and pituitary tumors. In evaluating a patient for colonic cancer, the patient should be examined for sebaceous cysts and osteomas of the jaw that would suggest Gardner's syndrome, and should be asked about a history in relatives, not only of colon cancer, but also of breast and endometrial cancer because their presence may suggest the dominantly inherited cancer family syndrome.

Genetic Prognosis and Counseling

Genetic prognosis deals both with the prognosis for the individual affected with a specific GI disorder, and also with delineating disease risks for various relatives. *Genetic counseling* is the process by which such risks for a disease and the potential options for dealing with those risks are communicated to the individual and family at risk. Thus, as in genetic diagnosis, not just the individual, but often the whole family is properly considered the patient.

Communicating the risk for a disease has two components. One is the numerical risk; the other is the burden or severity of the disorder. For example, both lactose intolerance and CF are inherited as autosomal recessives. When a child is found to be affected for either disorder, the risk to other children of the same parents is 25%. However, the burden for the individual and family is very different. Lactose intolerance usually causes only modest symptoms and, in any case, is readily treated by limitation of the amount of lactose-containing foods in the diet. In contrast, CF is a disorder that requires enormous medical attention and cost, and still almost invariably leads to death by young adulthood. Thus, even though the numeric risk is the same for the two disorders, the consequences are very different in terms of individual and family suffering and economic costs, and it is important that this information be conveyed to the family.

Nevertheless, it is important to delineate the quantitative risk for disease to family members as accurately as possible so they can make well-informed reproductive and health-care decisions. Our ability to quantify a given relative's disease risk varies tremendously (Table 49-10). When a given GI disorder can be reliably diagnosed as a specific mendelian disorder, accurate counseling can be given based on well-known mendelian rules (e.g., the risk to siblings of an affected individual is 25% for an autosomal recessive disorder such as FMF, or 50% for an autosomal dominant disorder such as heredity hemorrhagic telangiectasia).

For the many nonmendelian (multifactorial) disorders, however, well-defined mathematical rules predicting risk are not available. In these cases, we rely on empiric recurrence risks (i.e., the frequency of relatives actually observed to be affected in a large series of families). While such empiric risk counseling is considerably less precise than counseling based on mendelian risks, it is often reassuring in that the risks are often low, often 5% or

TABLE 49–10
Categories of Genetic Prediction and Counseling

BASIS FOR PREDICTION	EXAMPLE*
Empiric	Pyloric stenosis
	Megacolon (Hirschprung's disease)
	Inflammatory bowel disease
Mendelian	Cancer family syndrome (AD)
	Hereditary hemorrhagic telangiectasia (AD)
	Familial Mediterranean fever (AR)
Empiric or mendelian and subclinical marker	Lactase deficiency (AR) (marker: lactose intolerance)
	Atrophic gastritis (marker: serum pepsinogen I:pepsinogen II ratio)
Mendelian and linkage	Huntington's disease (AD) (linkage: chromosome 4)
Mendelian, subclinical marker, and linkage	Familial polyposis coli (AD) (marker: colonic polyposis) (linkage: chromosome 5)
	Multiple endocrine neoplasia, type I (AD) (marker: elevated gastrin, PTH, pituitary hormones) (linkage: chromosome 11)
Mendelian, subclinical marker, linkage, and the gene defect	Cystic fibrosis (AR) (marker: sweat chloride) (linkage: chromosome 7) (gene defect: defined at molecular level in 70–80% of mutations)

* *(AD) = autosomal dominant; (AR) = autosomal recessive.*

less. For example, the disease risk to siblings of an IBD patient is 5% to 8%, depending on the population studied.[3] The offspring risk may be similar but is less well defined.

For many GI disorders, the best information we may be able to obtain is either the mendelian or empiric risks. Clearly, the patients, their families, and their physicians would like to do better. Instead of counseling a relative for FPC, a dominant disorder, as having a 50% risk, we would like to divide this risk group into those who actually have the disorder (100% risk) and those who do not (0% risk). A number of methods allow us to further refine a family member's disease risk, and these can be applied to FPC (see Table 49–10). These are discussed in "Genetic Screening, Therapy, and Parenthood," page 1001.

Finally, an important component of genetic counseling is conveying to the patient and the family the various options of dealing with the disorder and its risk of recurrence. For some disorders, especially those that are treatable (e.g., lactose intolerance or vitamin B_{12} deficiency of atrophic gastritis), preclinical screening is recommended to diagnose the disorder at a stage when intervention can ameliorate or even prevent clinical disease. For others (e.g., CF) that are virtually incompatible with a healthy existence, the option of prenatal diagnosis, if available for that specific disorder, should be discussed. This must be done with appropriate sensitivity and respect for the widely varying attitudes and ethical concerns that different couples bring to this discussion and the subsequent decision-making process.

Genetic Screening, Therapy, and Prevention

For many GI disorders, not only can we provide counseling for genetic risks, but we can refine those risks by additional studies performed in the patient and at-risk family members, the process of family-based *genetic screening* (see Table 49–10).

For example, a relative at risk for dominantly inherited FPC (FPC) should be screened by periodic colonoscopy to detect the presence of multiple adenomatous polyps. The multiple polyps are a subclinical marker of the predisposition to colonic cancer. Those found to be affected (i.e., those who have multiple polyps) should undergo prophylactic colectomy. Conversely, those found to lack polyps do not need such surgery. This screening can even be further refined with the genetic linkage markers on the long arm of chromosome 5 discussed earlier. Those who inherit the same chromosome 5 as the affected persons in the family should undergo even more intensive screening, and those who do not share that chromosome with the affected persons are at a reduced risk. (This latter risk is still not zero, given the possibility of recombination between the FPC gene and the linked marker genes.) Similarly, relatives of multiple endocrine neoplasia I patients should be screened for subclinical hyperparathyroidism and subclinical pituitary tumors. This disorder has been localized to chromosome 11, and linkage can be used here as well to focus further screening efforts.[69]

Even if the mode of inheritance of a disorder is not fully clarified, or if it is clearly a nonmendelian disorder, subclinical markers may be available to identify those at higher risk who need to undergo more frequency screening. Thus, the serum pepsinogen I: pepsinogen II ratio, which is a sensitive and specific marker for gastritis, should be used to screen relatives of pernicious anemia and gastric cancer patients. Those relatives with abnormal screening tests can be followed aggressively with serum B_{12} levels (for vitamin B_{12} deficiency) or with endoscopy or double-contrast radiography (for early gastric cancer). Similarly, relatives of patients with common (nonsyndromic) colon cancer should be screened for isolated colonic adenomatous polyps. When polyps are found, they should be removed, and such persons need to undergo repeated similar investigations.

As the human gene map is filled in, genetic linkage markers increasingly will be used for family screening and risk assessment.[10,16,49] This is possible for a significant number of disorders, including many involving the GI tract. Examples of the latter include CF, FPC, and multiple endocrine neoplasia type I. Once a diagnosis is made, family members can be screened with the linked genetic markers for the specific chromosome (e.g., chromosomes 7, 5, and 11, respectively, for the above disorders). Following these linked markers through a family can identify who has the disease gene and is at risk for developing clinical disease. Depending on the circumstances, such information can be applied preclinically or prenatally.

The basic purpose of genetic family screening is to identify those persons at sufficiently high risk that an intervention can be recommended. In the case of disorders for which therapeutic intervention is possible (the majority of disorders listed in Table 49–11), such as vitamin B_{12} deficiency consequent to atrophic gastritis (treatment—vitamin B_{12} replacement), the single ade-

TABLE 49–11

Diseases for Which Genetic Screening of Relatives and/or Referral for Genetic Counseling are Indicated

	RELATIVES SHOULD BE SCREENED	FAMILY SHOULD BE REFERRED FOR GENETIC COUNSELING
Atrophic gastritis (pernicious anemia)	X	
Gastric cancer	X	
Multiple endocrine neoplasia I	X	X
Celiac disease	X	
The familial polyposes	X	X
Cancer family syndrome	X	X
Colon cancer (nonsyndromic)	X	
Cystic fibrosis	X	X
The majority of disorders listed in Tables 49–3, 49–4, and 49–5	X	X

referral for formal genetic consultation is indicated for the purposes of genetic evaluation, counseling, and design of an individualized screening program (see Table 49-11).

It is important to emphasize that just because a disorder is genetic, or has a genetic component, does not mean that it is untreatable. In fact, as should be apparent from the entire range of GI disorders that have been discussed in this chapter, the exact opposite is true. Not only are the many GI diseases with a genetic component treatable, but many are preventable. The existence of a genetic susceptibility to the majority of GI disorders means that not everybody in the population is at equal risk, but that there are persons at specific high risk to whom screening can be most effectively applied. As those at specifically high risk are identified by the methods discussed in this chapter, the physician will use this information not only for improved therapy, but for disease prevention as well. Thus, the clinical genetic approach, emphasizing human variation and individuality, will be used increasingly to diagnose, treat, and prevent disease in persons susceptible to the many disorders that involve the GI tract.

nomatous polyp predisposing to colon cancer (treatment—polypectomy), or the multiple polyposis of FPC (treatment—colectomy), the goal should be *preclinical diagnosis* and therapy that prevents or minimizes clinical disease. If a disorder is not treatable and is incompatible with a normal existence, the option of *prenatal diagnosis* should be discussed with the family. This is available for an increasing number of GI malformations, inborn errors, and other GI disorders discussed in this chapter.

To recommend screening, two basic guidelines should be followed. First, there must be accurate methods for assessing and refining a given relative's risk for disease. Second, there should be an acceptable intervention, either for clinical disease prevention or reproductive decision making. For several disorders, the principles of screening are straightforward and should be applied by any physician. In others, there are a number of complexities, and

SUMMARY

This part of the chapter has reviewed genetic principles as they are applied to the care of patients and their families with GI disease. Numerous lines of evidence indicate that the majority of both rare and common GI disorders have a genetic component. The categories of genetic disease—chromosomal, mendelian, and nonmendelian (multifactorial)—and the genetic classification of numerous GI disorders have been reviewed. An increasing number of the genes responsible for these GI disorders are being specifically localized to defined chromosomal locations in the human gene map by linkage analysis and recombinant DNA techniques. Methods for genetic risk assessment, preclinical diagnosis, and prenatal diagnosis have been discussed. The clinician can increasingly identify those family members at risk for specific GI disorders, and this enables not only improved therapy but, in many cases, a dramatic ability to prevent or minimize clinical disease by intervening before its onset.

PART B: SPECIFIC GENETIC DISORDERS

IMMUNOGENETIC DISORDERS

Pernicious Anemia—Atrophic Gastritis

Pernicious anemia is characterized by megaloblastic anemia secondary to vitamin B_{12} deficiency. Vitamin B_{12} is a compound required for normal hematopoiesis and functioning of the central

nervous system. To be absorbed, it must attach to a specific carrier protein called intrinsic factor (IF), which comes from the gastric parietal cells. The IF-B_{12} complex is taken up by receptors in the ileum. There, the vitamin B_{12} attaches to another carrier protein called transcobalamin II (TCII), which enters the bloodstream.[70-72]

The importance of vitamin B_{12} derives from its being a cofactor in two reactions, the synthesis of methionine from homocysteine and the conversion of methylmalonic acid to succinic acid. An inadequate supply of methionine leads to inadequate formate formation, which is necessary for the methylation of deoxyuridine to form thymidine.

Almost all causes of vitamin B_{12} deficiency have a genetic basis. They include impaired vitamin B_{12} absorption due to a lack of normal IF; impaired absorption in the ileum; or impaired transport mechanisms for the ileum to the bloodstream.[70-72] The resulting lack of vitamin B_{12} produces a failure of the marrow cells to respond properly to folic acid, and immature and abnormal red cells are produced, resulting in a characteristic morphologic pattern termed *megaloblastic anemia.*

The most common cause of pernicious anemia is a particular, familial type of atrophic gastritis of the fundic gland mucosa of the stomach.[70,73] This type of atrophic gastritis, type A, is distinguished by primary involvement of the fundic gland mucosa with essential sparing of the gastric antrum. It is commonly accompanied by evidence of immunologic derangements such as the presence of parietal cells and IF autoantibodies.[70,74] The destruction of parietal cells by the inflammatory process results in a lack of acid secretion and impaired IF production. The autoantibodies can also directly interfere with IF production or binding. Therefore, there is less binding of IF with dietary vitamin B_{12} in the stomach. As a consequence, less IF-B_{12} complex presents to the specific receptors in the terminal ileum, absorption is impaired, and vitamin B_{12} deficiency results.

Type A gastritis has an estimated prevalence of about 5%.[70] It is most common in persons of Northern European descent. Relatives of patients with pernicious anemia may have a 20-fold increased risk of developing pernicious anemia as compared with the general population. Besides the increased family aggregation of clinical pernicious anemia, further evidence for a genetic component to the severe atrophic gastritis is the association of pernicious anemia with blood group A and certain HLA antigens, and the increased frequency in relatives of subclinical abnormalities such as parietal cell antibodies, atrophic gastritis on biopsy, low or absent gastric acid secretion, an elevated serum gastrin level, a low serum pepsinogen I level, and a low serum pepsinogen I: pepsinogen II ratio.[42,75] The familial aggregation of such subclinical abnormalities is most consistent with dominant inheritance with a very late age at onset.

The clinical implications of the genetic nature of pernicious anemia/atrophic gastritis are twofold. First, the affected person is at risk for other autoimmune disorders, most commonly autoimmune thyroid disease.[70,73,74] Second, first-degree relatives are at risk both for autoimmune thyroid disease and atrophic gastritis. Relatives can be screened by endoscopic biopsy, assessment of gastric acid secretion, or measurement of serum gastrin, pepsinogen I, and pepsinogen II.[42] Because the type A gastritis of pernicious anemia affects primarily the oxyntic gland mucosa of the gastric fundus and spares the antrum, the serum pepsinogen I level (which reflects the chief cell mass) is usually greatly reduced. However, because the antrum is spared, the serum pepsinogen II level (which originates from cells in both the fundus and antrum) is maintained. In addition, lack of acid results in lack of inhibitory feedback to the G cells of the antrum and, hence, a rise in serum gastrin levels. The serum pepsinogen I:pepsinogen II ratio has been shown to have the greatest screening efficiency for atrophic gastritis, but the serum gastrin and pepsinogen I levels may be used as well.[42] Thus, these tests may be used to determine which family members have atrophic gastritis, and these persons should have their serum

vitamin B_{12} levels measured to detect the earliest deficiencies and to determine when they should be treated.

Other genetically determined causes of vitamin B_{12} deficiency occur much earlier in life. A lack of vitamin B_{12} absorption is noted in congenital IF deficiency due to absence of IF or presence of a biologically inert IF and in congenital selective vitamin B_{12} malabsorption (Imerslund-Grasbeck syndrome), which appears to be due to a defect in the ileal receptor for IF-B_{12} complex. These syndromes are autosomal recessive in their inheritance, and none is accompanied by atrophic gastritis.

In congenital IF deficiency, children develop normally for a year and then show clinical stigmata of megaloblastic anemia, with irritability, constipation or diarrhea, pallor, anorexia, organomegaly, and diminished deep tendon reflexes.[72,76] Vitamin B_{12} levels are very low. Clinical signs return to normal with the administration of IF orally or vitamin B_{12} parenterally. Congenital IF deficiency due to production of biologically inert IF is clinically similar to congenital IF deficiency.

Patients with Imerslund-Grasbeck syndrome present at any time between ages 2 and 15 with pallor, weakness, irritability, vomiting, pyrexia, glossitis, and constipation.[71,77,78] Megaloblastic anemia is found, along with leukopenia and thrombocytopenia. Serum vitamin B_{12} levels are very low, and folic acid levels are usually normal. Investigation reveals impaired intestinal absorption of vitamin B_{12} that is not corrected by the addition of more IF.[72] More than 90% of patients also have proteinuria that is not correctable by the administration of parenteral vitamin B_{12}. The treatment consists of monthly intramuscular doses of 250 μg hydroxycobalamin or intramuscular doses every 2 to 3 months of 1000 μg hydroxycobalamin. Mental retardation may ensue from delay or lack of treatment, so siblings of an affected person should be screened.

Gluten-Sensitive Enteropathy

The clinical manifestations of gluten-sensitive enteropathy, also known as nontropical or celiac sprue, are described in Chapter 71. The disorder appears to be a genetically determined immunologic reaction to gluten (a principal protein of wheat), in which the small intestinal mucosa is severely damaged and malabsorption results.[79] Persons who are most at risk for the development of gluten-sensitive enteropathy are those of Northern European and especially Irish descent. The incidence is 1 in 1000 to 2000 in Great Britain, 1 in 1000 in Sweden and Norway, and as much as 1 in 600 in Western Ireland.[80] The mode of inheritance is not fully understood, but it is thought that there is more than one disease susceptibility gene.[63,66] One gene has been linked to the HLA region of chromosome 6, where it has been associated with the HLA-B8, HLA-DR3, and HLA-DR7 alleles. There are also clinical associations with other HLA-DR3-associated diseases such as insulin-dependent diabetes.

The disorder is another example in which family-based screening is recommended. All first-degree relatives of patients with gluten-sensitive enteropathy should be evaluated for subclinical malabsorption. Because these tests are not reliable (e.g., the only manifestations of gluten-sensitive enteropathy may be growth deficiency in a child or spontaneous abortions in a woman of reproductive age), the presence of disease can be determined reliably only by small bowel biopsies. Such a test is indicated in the evaluation of all siblings and should strongly be considered for other first-degree relatives, such as parents and offspring who have a 5% risk for disease. HLA typing and antigliadin antibodies can aid in the assessment of risk in more distant relatives.[67]

Inflammatory Bowel Disease

There is substantial evidence that genetic factors play a role in the predisposition to the inflammatory bowel diseases (IBD).[5] In fact, the most established risk factor for IBD is a positive family history. The lines of evidence indicating that genetic factors are important include ethnic differences and familial aggregation, genetic syndromes associated with IBD, genetic marker studies, and physiologic studies within families.

Epidemiologic data on IBD demonstrate dramatic differences in disease frequency between geographic areas and ethnic groups (see also ch 78). IBD is more common among whites than among American blacks, Latin Americans, and Japanese. The highest rates are reported for the Jewish populations in the United States and Europe, while a lower rate is reported for the Jewish population in Israel.[81]

The familial aggregation of IBD is well documented.[3,5] The proportion of IBD patients with a positive family history varies among different studies and is in the range of 10% to 20%. Crohn's disease (CD) patients have a positive family history more often than ulcerative colitis (UC) patients, suggesting that genetic factors may either be relatively more important or more penetrant in the pathogenesis of Crohn's disease.[82] The empiric risks (i.e., the reported actual risks to first-degree relatives of IBD patients) are 2% to 5% for siblings and 1% to 4% for parents and offspring, depending on the specific study.[3,5] However, these risks are likely an underestimate, and when the lifetime risk for these various classes of relatives is determined, estimates are as high as 8% to 9% in Ashkenazi Jews.[3] These risks are as much as 30- to 60-fold greater than in the general population. They do not seem to be attributable to a common familial environment. This is so because there is no increased risk to spouses, the disease appears widely separated in time and place in many families, and the twin data demonstrate an increased concordance rate in MZ twins, whereas DZ twins are affected at the sibling rate. In addition, the monozygotic concordance rate is considerably higher for CD than for UC.[36]

Interestingly, there is a crossover within families between types of IBD. A patient with IBD who has a relative with ulcerative colitis has a 15% to 20% chance of having Crohn's disease and a corresponding 80% to 85% chance of having ulcerative colitis. In contrast, a patient with a relative who has Crohn's disease is almost as likely to have ulcerative colitis as Crohn's disease. These data suggest that a number of cases of Crohn's disease and ulcerative colitis share a common, but as yet unidentified, underlying genetic susceptibility.

Important evidence that IBD has genetic determinants comes from the observations of marked increased frequency in certain genetic disorders. Both UC and CD occur more often in Turner syndrome patients than in the general population.[83] Another genetic syndrome associated with IBD is the Hermansky-Pudlak syndrome, which is an autosomal recessive disorder featuring oculocutaneous

albinism, a defect in platelet aggregation, accumulation of a ceroidlike pigment, and, commonly, interstitial pulmonary fibrosis. A significant proportion of patients develop a granulomatous colitis that histologically resembles the findings in CD with non-necrotizing granulomas, yet with brown granular pigment.[32] In addition, IBD has also been reported in families with various inherited immunodeficiencies, including agammaglobulinemia, inherited deficiency of the second component of the complement, as well as in hereditary angioedema.[5]

Because of the evident immunologic dysfunction present in these diseases, attempts to find a genetic basis for IBD have focused on the HLA region as well as other genetic markers of the immune system.[5,46,84–87] The available data are not yet definitive, but suggest the involvement of the HLA region and certain complement genes in a subset of IBD patients.

The biologic mechanisms by which the genetic susceptibility to IBD leads to disease are not known. Given the importance of genetic predisposition, emerging clues are likely to come from family studies. These have revealed certain abnormalities of complement function, abnormalities of intestinal permeability, and various autoantibodies in clinically normal relatives.[45,46,88] The available data are most consistent with the concept of genetic heterogeneity for IBD—that different genes results in distinct and different pathophysiologic abnormalities that result in etiologically different forms of IBD.

GENETIC DISORDERS OF NUTRIENT ASSIMILATION (MALABSORPTION)

Disorders of Carbohydrate Absorption

Several familial disorders of carbohydrate malabsorption are recognized (Table 49-12). These include familial lactose intolerance, lactase deficiency, sucrase-isomaltase deficiency, and glucose-galactose malabsorption. Of these, only late-onset lactase deficiency, or adult type hypolactasia, is common.

LACTASE DEFICIENCY (HYPOLACTASIA)

In almost all mammals, lactase activity peaks in the newborn period. Shortly thereafter, it can diminish to about 10% of maximal activity, which is the usual activity found in adults with lactase deficiency. This is particularly true of non-white adults, of whom three fourths or more are lactase deficient. In whites, the prevalence of lactase deficiency ranges from 5% to 30% in adults, depending on the specific ethnic group[89,90] (see also ch 72).

Persons who are members of ethnic groups with greater than 50% prevalence of late-onset lactase deficiency, or hypolactasia, present between the ages of 1 and 5 years with diarrhea and crampy abdominal pain after the administration of lactose-containing foods. In whites destined to have hypolactasia, symptoms usually do not appear until later, at approximately age 13.

There are three primary ways to confirm the diagnosis of lactase deficiency.[89–91] A peroral intestinal biopsy of at least 3 mg tissue

(text continues on page 1006)

TABLE 49–12
Genetic Disorders of Nutrient Assimilation

CONDITION	INHERITANCE*	FEATURES
Defects in Carbohydrate Absorption		
Late-onset lactase deficiency (hypolactasia)	AR	Abdominal pain, bloating, diarrhea after lactose ingestion, present in >75% of nonwhites and in about 20% of whites
Familial lactose intolerance	?AD	Lactase normal, lactose has toxic effect on small intestine, and an excess of lactose is absorbed
Sucrase-isomaltase deficiency	AR	Symptoms similar to lactase deficiency except evoked by table sugar not milk
Glucose-galactose malabsorption	AR	Symptoms of bloating, abdominal pain, and diarrhea occur with ingestion of most carbohydrates. Treatment: substitute fructose for other carbohydrates
Defects in Amino Acid Absorption		
Iminoglycinuria	AR	Membrane transport defect causing excretion of excess proline, hydroxyproline, and glycine; no clinical consequences
Hartnup disease	AR	Intermittent red, scaly rash after sun exposure; cerebellar ataxia and psychiatric changes in about 15% of those affected; massive aminoaciduria of neutral amino acids
Cystinuria	AR	Renal tubule and intestinal epithelium transport abnormalities of all dibasic amino acids; nephrolithiasis due to insolubility of cystine in urine; three subtypes; symptoms in second or third decade
Lysinuric protein intolerance (dibasic aminoaciduria I and II)	AR	Two similar disorders involve abnormal transport of dibasic amino acids (arginine, lysine, ornithine) across basolateral membranes of intestinal and renal tubular cells. Onset is in infancy after cow's milk formula introduced. Vomiting, diarrhea, failure to thrive, organomegaly, mental retardation, lens opacities, stretchy skin, and sparse hair occur. Hyperammonemia is due to deficient hepatic uptake of amino acids. Treatment is protein restriction and citrulline supplementation.
Blue diaper syndrome	?AR	Hypercalcemia, nephrocalcinosis, and indicanuria due to intestinal tryptophan transport defect; presents in infancy
Oasthouse syndrome (methionine malabsorption)	AR	Patients may have odor of oasthouse (a kiln for drying hops); mental retardation, diarrhea, convulsions; onset in infancy
Lowe oculocerebrorenal syndrome	XLR	Impaired intestinal and renal absorption of lysine and arginine, leading to cataracts, mental retardation, vitamin D-resistant rickets, glaucoma, and generalized aminoaciduria and organic aciduria
Lysine intolerance	AR	Episodic vomiting, rigidity, and coma in infancy relieved by low-protein diet; hyperammonemia and high lysine and arginine levels, apparently due to defective L-lysine: NAD-oxidoreductase activity in liver
Lysine malabsorption syndrome	?AR	Physical and mental retardation in association with impaired intestinal absorption of lysine; also hyperlysinuria and hypolysinemia; probably due to lysine transport defect
Glutamate-aspartate transport defect	?AR	Defective intestinal and renal transport of glutamic and aspartic acids, leading to moderate hyperprolinemia and hypoglycemia
Defects in Vitamin and Mineral Absorption		
Pernicious anemia (vitamin B_{12} deficiency, atrophic gastritis)	?AD	Due to severe atrophic gastritis of the gastric fundus, leading to absence of intrinsic factor
Pernicious anemia as part of polyglandular autoimmune syndromes	AR, ?AD	Two autoimmune polyendocrine syndromes can include atrophic gastritis. One features candidiasis, hypoparathyroidism, and Addison disease. The other features autoimmune thyroid disease, insulin-dependent diabetes, and Addison disease
Congenital pernicious anemia due to defect of intrinsic factor	AR	Presents with megaloblastic anemia in childhood, although diagnosis has been made in adults; due to functional absence or abnormal intrinsic factor, no gastritis

(continued)

TABLE 49–12 (Continued)

CONDITION	INHERITANCE*	FEATURES
Defects in Vitamin and Mineral Absorption		
Pernicious anemia due to selective intestinal malabsorption of vitamin B_{12} (Imerslund-Grasbeck syndrome)	AR	Megaloblastic anemia due to malabsorption of vitamin B_{12} not corrected with exogenous intrinsic factor; disorder is in ileal receptor; associated proteinuria
Folic acid transport defect	AR	Defective intestinal absorption of folic acid and defect in transport of folic acid into cerebrospinal fluid, causing megaloblastic anemia, mental retardation, convulsions, and movement disorder; parenteral administration of folic acid corrects anemia
Pseudo-vitamin D deficiency (rickets)	AR	Defective intestinal absorption of calcium leads to rickets and short stature, myopathy, hypocalcemia, and hypophosphatemia, distinct from X-linked vitamin D-resistant rickets; several subtypes; responds to large doses of vitamin D
Acrodermatitis enteropathica	AR	Zinc malabsorption produces intermittent diarrhea, bullous dermatitis; failure to thrive; alopecia of scalp, eyebrows, and eyelashes; and thymic hypoplasia. Manifestations resolve with oral zinc supplementation
Hypomagnesemia	AR	Primary intestinal malabsorption of magnesium leads to hypomagnesemia and hypocalcemia; presents as convulsions in newborn period
Defects in Electrolyte Absorption		
Congenital chloride diarrhea	AR	May present in utero with polyhydramnios, presumably due to diarrhea. Newborn may present with distended abdomen. Voluminous, watery stools containing large amounts of chloride, leading to hypochloremia, hypokalemia, and metabolic alkalosis
Congenital sodium diarrhea	AR	Clinically similar to congenital chloridorrhea, except sodium and bicarbonate are excreted
Congenital adrenal hypoplasia	AR	Deficiency in any one of several enzymes in cortisol synthesis pathway, which may lead to virilization, especially in females; renal and intestinal salt losing and/or hypertension
18-Oxidation defects of aldosterone	AR	18-Hydroxylase and 18-hydroxysteroid dehydrogenase deficiencies present in infancy with dehydration, occasional vomiting, hypernatremia, and hypokalemia
Disorders That Can Lead to Defects in Intestinal Protein and Fat Absorption		
Pancreatic disorders		For malabsorption due to pancreatic exocrine abnormalities, see Table 49–16
Deafness with mesenteric diverticula of small intestine	?AR	Progressive sensory neuropathy including nerve deafness with onset in first three decades. Vagal nerve abnormality leads to diminished gastric motility. Also seen are multiple diverticula with jejunoileal ulceration, malabsorption of fat, and intestinal loss of protein
Protein-losing enteropathy	AR	Hepatic vein stenosis causes Budd-Chiari syndrome in childhood, leading to edema, growth retardation, diarrhea, abdominal pain, clubbing, iron-deficiency anemia, and hypoproteinemia
Intestinal lymphagiectasia	AD	Leg edema, ulcers in males, dysproteinemia, variety of congenital malformations, and high incidence of stillbirth; intestinal loss of protein due to lymphangiectasia; dilated lymphatic spaces in small bowel and partial vilous atrophy; results in lymphopenia, hypogammaglobulinemia, and skin anergy; can present as neonatal edema
Hereditary lymphedema	AD	Birth onset of edema that is particularly severe below the waist; paucity of lymph nodes above inguinal ligaments; loss of albumin via the intestines; thought to be distinct from hereditary lymphedema type II, which has onset at puberty

* AR = autosomal recessive; AD = autosomal dominant; XLR = X-linked recessive.
Modified from Randolph LM, Rotter JI. In: Kelley WN, ed. Textbook of internal medicine. Philadelphia: JB Lippincott, 1989:630.

to assay for oligosaccharidase is possibly the most definitive method, but oral lactose tolerance tests or breath tests are adequate for clinical purposes and are not invasive. The oral lactose tolerance test involves administering 1 g/kg lactose (50 g maximum) and drawing blood at 0, 15, 30, 60, 90, and 120 minutes to measure plasma glucose. Normally, the plasma glucose should rise by 20 mg/dl. A tentative diagnosis of lactase deficiency can be made if abdominal cramping pain and diarrhea are seen along with failure of the plasma glucose rise. The best and most clinically available breath test for establishing a diagnosis of lactase deficiency is the hydrogen breath test. The subject is given sugar (1 g/kg) to ingest, and his or her breath is collected for a specified period and analyzed by gas chromatography. Hydrogen, along with carbon dioxide, is produced by colonic bacteria's action on the carbohydrate. If lactase is normal, much less carbohydrate reaches the large bowel, and less than 3 ppm hydrogen is produced by the lungs. Persons with disaccharidase deficiencies, including lactase deficiency, have greater than 50 ppm hydrogen in exhaled air 90 minutes after ingestion of the sugar.

The treatment for lactase deficiency is restriction of dietary lactose. Usually patients can tolerate one or two 8-oz. glasses of milk (12–24 g lactose) per day without symptoms, so there usually is no need for absolute elimination of lactose. The physician should caution the patient that there are many foods (including prepackaged and ready-to-eat) that contain lactose of which they may not be aware. Calcium supplements should also be considered to prevent osteoporosis in susceptible persons.

Crossed immunoelectrophoresis of small-intestinal biopsies of Scandinavian persons with hypolactasia, as well as other studies, have shown that the molecular defect in adults with hypolactasia is a decreased amount of active brush-border lactase protein.[90,91] Further studies designed to explain the differences in adult lactase activities in different ethnic groups have shown that human lactase activity is independent of lactose intake; therefore, it appears clear that the differences are on a genetic basis.

It is well documented that the inheritance of hypolactasia is autosomal recessive.[92] One would first expect that only siblings would be affected in families, but it is commonly observed that parents and offspring are affected as well. As was discussed earlier under recessive inheritance, this is due to the inordinate high frequency of the gene for hypolactasia. This results in a homozygote affected often marrying a heterozygote carrier; on average, half the offspring are affected in such matings.

The reason why lactase deficiency is the rule among human populations (and lactase persistence the exception) has yielded interesting speculation.[89,90] There is little evidence that suggests large segments of the population of the world depended on milk for nutrition. However, milk contains a sizable amount of calcium, and lactose appears to increase intestinal calcium absorption; therefore, populations receiving low ultraviolet radiation or insufficient dietary vitamin D may have been protected against rickets by maintenance of intestinal lactase.

FAMILIAL LACTOSE INTOLERANCE

In contrast, intestinal lactase is present in normal amounts in this disorder. It is a much more severe disorder and can be fatal unless diagnosed promptly.[91,93] It is characterized by vomiting, diarrhea, failure to thrive, severe dehydration, and cachexia. Lactose appears to have a direct toxic effect on the intestine. Aminoaciduria and disacchariduria are present in early infancy. There is normal lactose tolerance or only a transient lactase deficiency (due to damage to the intestinal lining). When lactose is withdrawn, symptoms resolve. It is thought to be due to excess absorption of lactose. The disorder spontaneously resolves between 12 and 18 months of age. The inheritance is thought to be autosomal dominant.

SUCRASE-ISOMALTASE (S-I) DEFICIENCY

Also known as sucrase-alpha-dextrinase deficiency (see also ch 72), this disorder presents with a wide variety of symptoms, from severe diarrhea in infancy to occasional "stomach upsets" in adults.[91,93] The disorder affects 0.2% of North Americans and 10% of Greenland Eskimos. Symptoms are similar to those of lactase deficiency except that they are evoked by table sugar and not by milk. Starch is well tolerated. Symptoms begin with the ingestion of sweetened foods and fruits. The diagnosis is made using the same techniques as in lactase deficiency. Tolerance to the offending sugars increases with age. It has been found that ingesting live yeast (preferably on a full stomach) can ameliorate symptoms after sucrose ingestion. Fresh bakers' yeast has sucrase activity.

Attempts to elucidate the nature of the defect have shown that the isomaltase part of the S-I complex is labile in the absence of sucrase, suggesting the primary defect is in the sucrase, with secondary effects on isomaltase. Other studies, using polyacrylamide gel electrophoresis of membrane fractions, have shown that in some cases the normal S-I band is replaced by an abnormal protein band; in other cases, not only was no normal S-I band found, but no abnormal band was detected either. This suggests that the enzyme may be either structurally modified or entirely absent, which may explain at least part of the clinical variability seen in this disorder. These findings illustrate well the biochemical heterogeneity present even within a relatively uncommon, single-gene disorder. The inheritance is autosomal recessive.

GLUCOSE-GALACTOSE MALABSORPTION

Intestinal monosaccharidase deficiency presents in a clinically indistinguishable way from intestinal disaccharidase deficiency.[91] In glucose-galactose malabsorption, diarrhea and dehydration are seen after ingestion of almost any carbohydrate, because virtually all contain at least one of these sugars. The diagnosis is suggested by examination of the stools, which are acidic and contain glucose and galactose. It can be distinguished from disaccharidase deficiency by virtue of the fact that there is no significant rise in plasma glucose in the course of a glucose-galactose oral tolerance test. Patients who have been carefully evaluated have also been found to have a mild defect in renal tubular reabsorption of glucose; they excrete 250 to 1000 mg/dl glucose in the urine. Treatment is to substitute fructose for other carbohydrates in the diet.

The underlying abnormality is in the transport mechanism in the small intestine; the mucosa is unable to take up glucose and galactose. As with sucrase-isomaltase deficiency, tolerance to the offending sugars improves with age. The inheritance is autosomal recessive.

Disorders of Peptide Absorption

Proteins are normally absorbed by two major mechanisms. One involves transport of liberated free amino acids by group-specific sodium-dependent amino acid transport systems, and the other involves uptake of unhydrolyzed peptides by means independent of the specific entry mechanisms. There are at least three major group-specific active transport systems: monoamino monocarboxylic (neutral) amino acids; dibasic amino acids and cystine; and dicarboxylic (acidic) amino acids. The genetic disorders of protein absorption involve deficiencies in one or more of these transport mechanisms.[94]

IMINOGLYCINURIA

Iminoglycinuria consists of five subtypes. All are benign inborn errors of imino acid (proline and hydroxyproline) and glycine absorption in the kidneys, and two of the subtypes also involve the intestine.[95] In most cases, iminoglycinuria has been discovered during investigations carried out for other purposes. The diversity of clinical abnormalities in probands with familial iminoglycinuria suggests that there is probably no direct relationship between the inherited disorder and the accompanying illness, and no treatment is necessary.

When any of the three amino acids is given orally, excretion of the other two increases, indicating a group-specific membrane transport defect. Heterogeneity in the disorder is suggested by several lines of evidence, including the fact that some homozygotes show no proline transport defect. Obligate heterozygotes may be hyperglycinuric or not. At least four alleles for the disorder are known, but it is not known whether they are all at the same locus. The condition is inherited in an autosomal recessive pattern and occurs most often in Ashkenazi Jews. The frequency of affected persons among whites is about 1 in 15,000, giving a heterozygote frequency of about 2%.

The existence of an autosomal dominant form of glycinuria with oxalate urolithiasis has been postulated. This type also occurs more often in Ashkenazi Jews. It probably is actually a particular heterozygote form of iminoglycinuria that predisposes some persons to urolithiasis.[95]

HARTNUP DISEASE

Hartnup disease is a rare disorder with an incidence of 5 per 100,000, as observed in a Massachusetts urine screening program. The disorder produces virtually no symptoms or signs in more than 90% of patients. In those with symptoms, onset is in childhood, with the presentation of an intermittent, red, scaly, pellagralike rash after exposure to sunlight, attacks of cerebellar ataxia, and occasional psychiatric disorders. Some persons are of low normal or subnormal intelligence. The single constant feature and the only diagnostic test is massive aminoaciduria involving a group of neutral and aromatic monoamino monocarboxylic amino acids that share a common renal (proximal tubule) reabsorption mechanism.[96] These patients also have a diminished capacity for jejunal absorption of these amino acids because of a transport defect at the brush border. This results in the retention of the amino acids

in the intestine for abnormally long periods, allowing intestinal bacteria to convert them into dipeptide decomposition products, some of which are absorbed. A subgroup of patients with Hartnup's disease has been identified in which intestinal absorption is normal and the patients are clinically normal. There is inadequate nicotinamide synthesis because of diminished tryptophan absorption, thus causing pellagra. The formation of decomposition products that are toxic to the central nervous system, coupled to pellagra, leads to the cerebellar and psychiatric manifestations. In addition, general nutritional deficiency results from the diminished availability of essential amino acids. Patients are treated by administration of nicotinamide.

Although the disorder is autosomal recessive, the fact that only a small group of patients have the typical manifestations has led to the theory that other genes may affect the clinical outcome.[97]

CYSTINURIA

Cystinuria is an autosomal recessive disorder characterized by cystine, lysine, ornithine, and arginine transport abnormalities in both the renal tubule and in the intestinal epithelium.[98] The clinical manifestations are confined to nephrolithiasis resulting from the insolubility of cystine in urine.

Three types of cystinuria have been recognized. Urinary stones form in all three types, and investigation of the stones leads to the diagnosis. The stones are radiopaque and are present as hexagonal cystine crystals in the urine. Treatment is directed at reducing the concentration of cystine in urine by increasing urine volume, increasing solubility by alkalinization, and, as a last alternative, reducing free cystine excretion by administration of D-penicillamine.

Classification of the three types of cystinuria has been accomplished by evaluating the excretion rates of amino acids in obligate heterozygotes. In type I, heterozygotes excrete no excess amino acids. Excretion of up to twice the normal amount characterizes type III heterozygotes, and type II is assigned to those heterozygotes who excrete 9 to 15 times the normal amount but still less than that necessary for the formation of stones.

Although cystinuria is a relatively rare disease in most populations, it is thought to have an incidence of 1 in 2500 in Israeli Jews of Libyan origin. The incidence in the United States, based on screening of newborns, is 1 in 15,000. The second and third decades of life are the peak times for expression of the disorder. It affects males more severely than it does females, although the disorder occurs equally in both sexes.

LYSINURIC PROTEIN INTOLERANCE

Lysinuric protein intolerance is characterized by abnormal transport of dibasic amino acids across the basolateral membranes of intestinal and renal tubular cells.[99] Its onset is in infancy when cow's milk or cow's-milk formula is introduced. It is associated with vomiting, diarrhea, failure to thrive, severe growth retardation, hepatosplenomegaly, and often mental retardation. Lens opacities are common, the skin may be stretchy, and the joints may be hyperextensible. Often the hair is sparse and brittle. Affected infants show a markedly diminished rise in plasma levels of arginine, lysine, and ornithine after an oral load, indicating malabsorption of these amino acids. In addition, the kidney has reduced tubular reabsorption of these same amino acids. Analysis of plasma amino acids indicates subnormal levels of arginine, lysine, ornithine, leucine, and tyrosine. Serine and citrulline levels are normal, and glutamine and alanine levels may be markedly increased. Lysinuria is present. The diagnosis is based on the finding of dibasic aminoaciduria without cystinuria, impaired intestinal absorption of basic amino acids, and protein intolerance. Hyperammonemia occurs due to deficient hepatic uptake of the amino acids, which gives rise to a deficiency of some intermediate products of the urea cycle.

Treatment consists of protein restriction with citrulline and lysine supplements. Some of the abnormalities resolve on this therapy. The disorder is autosomal recessive, and consanguinity is common. Some heterozygotes manifest partial intestinal malabsorption after an oral load.

BLUE DIAPER SYNDROME

Blue diaper syndrome is a rare, probably autosomal recessive disorder of tryptophan malabsorption.[94] Unlike the previously described abnormalities, the kidney is apparently not affected. The unabsorbed tryptophan is converted to indoles in the intestine by bacteria. The indoles are absorbed and converted in the liver to indican, which, when oxidized, becomes indigo blue in the urine. Infants present with failure to thrive, recurrent fever, infections, irritability, and constipation, besides the bluish discoloration of the diapers. Hypercalcemia and nephrocalcinosis also occur because of increased absorption of calcium.

OASTHOUSE SYNDROME

Oasthouse syndrome is a disorder of methionine absorption so named because affected patients excrete urine containing alpha-hydroxybutyric acid, a product of bacterial metabolism of methionine that has the odor of an oast house, a kiln for drying hops.[94] A methionine-free diet improves the findings of mental retardation, diarrhea, and convulsions.

LOWE'S OCULOCEREBRORENAL SYNDROME

Lowe's oculocerebrorenal syndrome is an X-linked recessive disorder characterized by cataracts, mental retardation, vitamin D-resistant rickets, glaucoma, generalized aminoaciduria, and organic aciduria, leading to death before adolescence from renal failure.[94] Intestinal and renal absorption of lysine and arginine is impaired. The responsible gene has been localized to a particular band of the long arm of the X-chromosome, and flanking DNA markers may be used for carrier detection.[100]

Disorders of Electrolyte Absorption

There are three major genetic causes of electrolyte/water malabsorption in the intestine. These include congenital chloride diarrhea, congenital sodium diarrhea, and disorders of aldosterone metabolism causing significant salt wasting.[101]

CONGENITAL CHLORIDE DIARRHEA

Congenital chloride diarrhea is a disorder that may present in utero with polyhydramnios, presumably due to diarrhea. The infant may be born prematurely with a distended abdomen. Voluminous, watery stools containing large amounts of chloride are produced, leading to hypochloremia, hypokalemia, and metabolic alkalosis. With later presentation or with inadequate replacement therapy, weight and height gains are affected. The diagnosis is made by measuring the chloride content of the stools, as well as the characteristic serum electrolyte changes. Treatment consists of administering prostaglandin inhibitors (primarily indomethacin) and potassium chloride. The secretory diarrhea in this condition results from deficiency in intestinal brush border chloride–bicarbonate exchange. The inheritance is autosomal recessive (see also ch 72).

CONGENITAL SODIUM DIARRHEA

Congenital sodium diarrhea presents similarly to congenital chloride diarrhea with polyhydramnios, premature birth, and voluminous, watery stools in the first days of life. Diagnosis is based on stool electrolyte measurement, which reveals excess sodium and bicarbonate. Treatment consists of replacement therapy with sodium and bicarbonate. Perfusion studies show that the jejunum is in a net secretory state with intact hexose transport but with abnormal intestinal sodium–hydrogen exchange activity. The inheritance is probably autosomal recessive.

PSEUDO-OBSTRUCTION

Intestinal pseudo-obstruction is suggested clinically by recurrent signs and symptoms of intestinal obstruction in the absence of mechanical obstruction, as proven by appropriate radiologic, endoscopic, or surgical investigations. There are several causes of pseudo-obstruction, many of which are listed in Table 49-13. These include pseudo-obstruction due to visceral myopathy and visceral neuropathy.[102]

In the adult, a longstanding history of symptoms suggestive of GI dysmotility, such as dysphagia, early satiety, and constipation or diarrhea, may precede the onset of acute symptoms. These usually occur in the second to fourth decades of life, although some of the rarer, sporadic cases occur in the neonatal period. The acute symptoms, regardless of the underlying cause, are usually abdominal pain and distention, early satiety, and diarrhea. In contrast, infants with the disorder usually present with severe abdominal distention and obstruction after feeding. The presence and severity of complications depend on the age of the patient (whether infant or adult), primary site of involvement, and degree of functional impairment. Malnutrition is common and results either from decreased food intake, impaired digestion, or malabsorption. In infants, reflux esophagitis and aspiration pneumonia occur due to impaired gastroesophageal motility.

TABLE 49–13
Genetic Disorders Associated With Gastrointestinal Pseudo-Obstruction

CONDITION	INHERITANCE*	FEATURES
Visceral myopathy with megaduodenum and/or megacystis	AD	Megaduodenum is associated with thinning and fibrosis of the longitudinal muscle; absence of contractions in smooth muscle of esophagus. Megacystis occurs without obstruction but with vesicoureteral reflux. Severity varies; diagnosis often made in adults. Family study can prevent unnecessary surgery for pseudo-obstruction.
Visceral myopathy with external ophthalmoplegia	?AR	Ptosis, ophthalmoplegia, progressive intestinal pseudo-obstruction leading to malnutrition and death before 30 years of age
Visceral neuropathy type a	?AR	Megaduodenum, generalized dilation of small intestine, redundant colon; mental retardation and calcification of basal ganglia; onset of hypomotility in childhood
Visceral neuropathy type b	?AR	Dilation and nonperistaltic hyperactivity of esophagus, stomach, small intestine; extensive colonic diverticulosis; gait ataxia, autonomic dysfunction, absent deep tendon reflexes, sensory neuropathy; onset of hypomotility in childhood
Visceral neuropathy type c	?AD	Delayed gastric emptying; generalized dilatation of small intestine. Diarrhea and obstructive symptoms have onset in adolescence.
Visceral neuropathy type d	?AD	Abnormal gastric emptying, segmental dilation of jejunum and ileum; onset in adolescence or middle age with early satiety, painful abdominal distention, and diarrhea. Vomiting is uncommon.
Deficiency of argyrophil myenteric plexus	AR	Failure of development of argyrophil myenteric plexus leading to short small intestine, malrotation, functional intestinal obstruction, and pyloric hypertrophy. Bowel wall thickening is noted at laparotomy. Onset is in infancy, but diagnosis is often made in adulthood.
Hirschsprung's disease (aganglionic megacolon)	Probably multifactorial	Absence of innervation of short or long segment of colon; a heterogeneous disorder with empiric recurrence risks of 7% for siblings of affected females and 2.6% for siblings of affected males; also seen in 5% of patients with Down's syndrome.
Aganglionosis, total intestine	?AR	Distinct from Hirschsprung's disease in that entire intestine is involved.
Hirschsprung's disease with ulnar polydactyly, polysyndactyly of big toes, and ventricular septal defect	?AR	An apparently rare disorder described in two brothers
Microcolon	?AR	Microcolon occurs with aganglionosis of entire colon and part of small intestine. Obstruction of small intestine; can be due to another disorder such as cystic fibrosis with meconium ileus
Waardenberg syndrome	AD	Hirschsprung's disease is reported with increased frequency in this disorder, which features widely set eyes, heterochromia iridis, frontal white blaze of hair, white eyelashes, piebaldism, and cochlear deafness.
Oculopharyngeal muscular dystrophy	AD, and rarely AR	Onset late in life; characterized by dysphagia, ptosis, and weakness and wasting of facial, neck, and distal limb muscles. Mitochondrial abnormalities are seen on electron microscopy.

* AR = autosomal recessive; AD = autosomal dominant.
From Randolph LM, Rotter JI. In: Kelley WN, ed. Textbook of internal medicine. Philadephia: JB Lippincott, 1989:630.

When mechanical obstruction has been ruled out by appropriate means, diagnostic studies to evaluate pseudo-obstruction include esophageal and intestinal manometry, gastric emptying studies, and full-thickness biopsy with silver stains. Esophageal manometry shows aperistalsis and incomplete relaxation of the lower esophageal sphincter. Intestinal manometry usually shows a hypomotile pattern. Gastric emptying studies show a delay for solids and a variable pattern for liquids. Silver stains delineate neuropathic from myopathic forms.

Clinical GI manifestations of the visceral myopathic and neuropathic forms are similar. In the myopathic form, however, other evidence of myopathy such as megacystis, vesico-ureteral reflux, ophthalmoplegia, ptosis, and small intestine diverticulosis can be present. The pathogenesis of the GI manifestations appears to be degenerative changes and thinning of intestinal smooth muscle, especially of the longitudinal layers. Neurons are normal.

In the neuropathic forms, autonomic neurologic abnormalities such as ataxia, abnormal pupillary reflexes, and abnormal tendon reflexes are present. One type is also associated with basal ganglia calcification and mental retardation. Histologic sections of tissues stained with a silver stain reveal degenerative changes of myenteric plexus neurons.

Males and females are equally likely to be affected with the pseudo-obstruction disorders, some of which are autosomal dominant, some autosomal recessive, and others possibly multifactorial or sporadic.

The treatment in mild cases is the administration of small, frequent feedings and the use of metoclopramide or cisapride. In more severe cases, gastrostomy tube placement or resections of the involved portion of the GI tract may be useful. Long-term parenteral nutrition is indicated in the remainder of cases.

The prognosis depends on the age of onset, the extent of involvement, and the response to treatment. Patients with onset in infancy and with diffuse involvement are likely to require the administration of long-term parenteral nutrition. In the forms with known autosomal recessive or dominant inheritance, detection of subclinically affected persons can often be accomplished through the use of gastric emptying studies and manometry.[102]

HEREDITARY DISORDERS CAUSING GASTROINTESTINAL BLEEDING

In the evaluation of GI hemorrhage, a variety of genetic disorders, each one individually rare, should be considered. These include disorders of the hematologic system (platelets and clotting factors) and abnormalities of vessel walls or supporting structures such as occur in some of the connective tissue disorders. There are many genetic defects in platelets and clotting factors, some of which predispose to GI bleeding.

Several other disorders predispose to GI bleeding through nonhematologic mechanisms (Table 49-14). These include the polyposis syndromes (described in ch 79 and in part A of this chapter). These syndromes, particularly Peutz-Jeghers syndrome, can result in acute GI hemorrhage from the individual polyp but can more likely present with mild persistent or recurrent bleeding resulting in chronic iron deficiency anemia. Rarely, hematemesis may occur as a result of polyps in the stomach, duodenum, or jejunum.[103]

TABLE 49–14
Genetic Nonhematologic Disorders Predisposing to Gastrointestinal Bleeding

CONDITION	INHERITANCE*	FEATURES
Polyposis syndromes		See ch. 79
Neurofibromatosis (NF-1 type)	AD	Neurofibromas in the bowel can ulcerate into the lumen.
Elhers-Danlos syndrome type IV	AD, AR	Rupture of viscera and great vessels due to faulty collagen synthesis
Pseudoxanthoma elasticum	AD, AR	Angioid streaks on fundoscopic examination; thickened, grooved skin in neck, axillae, other flexural areas; hematemesis more common than melena; at least four subtypes described
Osler-Rendu-Weber syndrome (hereditary hemorrhagic telangiectasia)	AD	Telangiectasias of the tip of the tongue and mucosal surfaces of the lips and also in conjunctivae and gastrointestinal mucosa; cirrhosis of liver a complication; prolonged, frequent epistaxis and severe intestinal bleeding
Blue rubber bleb nevus syndrome	AD	Skin lesions look like bluish nipples that compress easily and refill; associated with intestinal hemangiomas
Cavernous hemangiomas of the small intestine	AD	Intestinal hemangiomas without other manifestations
Enterocolitis	?AR	Apparently rare disorder in which abdominal distention and bloody diarrhea cause death in the first month of life. Autopsies have shown ulcerative colitis or pseudomembranous enterocolitis.
Hermansky-Pudlak syndrome	AR	Storage disorder characterized by oculocutaneous albinism, inflammatory bowel disease, and platelet dysfunction, as well as by restrictive lung disease; high frequency in Puerto Ricans

* AD = autosomal dominant; AR = autosomal recessive.
Modified from Randolph LM, Rotter JI. In: Kelley WN, ed. Textbook of internal medicine. Philadelphia: JB Lippincott, 1989: 630.

Neurofibromatosis

Von Recklinghausen neurofibromatosis (known as NF-1 to differentiate it from the neurofibromatosis associated with bilateral acoustic neuromas) is a fairly common disorder present in about 1 in 4000 live births in the United States. It is a neurocutaneous disorder in which café au lait spots of the skin and neurofibromas of the skin and viscera are prominent.[104] Such neurofibromas can occur in the ileum and can ulcerate into the lumen of the bowel, resulting in severe bleeding. The diagnosis of NF-1 is established by the presence of six or more café au lait spots of 1.5 cm or larger in postpubertal patients. It is inherited as an autosomal dominant trait. The responsible gene is located on chromosome 17, and the actual gene has been identified.[105]

Ehlers-Danlos Syndrome

Connective tissue disorders in which the strength of structural tissues is impaired may predispose to GI bleeding. One such disorder is Ehlers-Danlos syndrome type IV. There are at least ten subtypes of Ehlers-Danlos syndrome; the classic form, known as type I, involves stretchy skin and joints, easy bruising, and atrophic scarring.[21,22] In type IV, however, patients have extremely thin, fragile skin and tissues, and they are subject to rupture of large vessels and of the bowel wall.[23] They are also subject to colonic diverticula, which can rupture and bleed. A variety of genetic defects (with different modes of inheritance) leading to the defective synthesis of type III collagen cause Ehlers-Danlos syndrome type IV. The other types of Ehlers-Danlos syndrome are due to other collagen defects and are not associated with the life-threatening bleeding that typifies type IV.

Pseudoxanthoma Elasticum

Pseudoxanthoma elasticum primarily affects the skin of the neck, axillae, and other flexural areas; the Bruch's membrane of the eye, resulting in angioid streaks on funduscopic examination; and the arteries producing GI and urinary tract hemorrhage, precocious calcification, and occlusive vascular changes.[106] Recurrent severe hematemesis was the presenting feature of one of the first reported cases.

Hematemesis is much more common than melena; superficial hemorrhages and erosions may be seen in the stomach. Bleeding tends to occur as early as the first decade of life, before the skin and eye changes are evident. Pregnant women are more susceptible to bleeding.

The diagnosis is made on the basis of clinical examination. At least four subtypes are thought to exist: two autosomal dominant and two autosomal recessive types.[106] The dominant type I is characterized by peau d'orange skin, severe vascular complications, and severe choroiditis. The dominant type II is more common than type I and is characterized by macular or focal changes in the skin, which is very stretchy, and by myopia, high-arched palate, blue sclerae, and loose jointedness. The recessive type I is similar to the dominant type I and is much more common than the recessive type II, which is characterized by generalized skin changes with no ocular or vascular abnormalities.

Osler-Rendu-Weber Syndrome

Another genetic disorder that predisposes to GI bleeding is the Osler-Rendu-Weber syndrome, or hereditary hemorrhage telangiectasia.[107,108] Telangiectasias of the tip of the tongue and mucosal surfaces of the lips are typical; they also occur on the conjunctiva, ears, fingers, face, and mucosa of the GI tract, bladder, and nasopharynx. In some cases, pulmonary arteriovenous fistulas may occur, leading to clubbing. Frequent, prolonged epistaxis is common, and GI bleeding can be life-threatening. The disorder is autosomal dominant.

Blue Rubber Bleb Nevus Syndrome

A prominent feature of blue rubber bleb nevus syndrome is the presence of skin lesions that feel like rubber nipples. They are easily compressible and refill quickly after compression. The most common sites are the trunk and upper arms, but the mucosa of the nasopharynx and GI tract, particularly the small bowel, can also be affected by hemangiomatous formation, leading to bleeding. Treatment is supportive. The inheritance is autosomal dominant.[109]

Hermansky-Pudlak Syndrome

Hermansky-Pudlak syndrome occurs most frequently in Puerto Rico, where the prevalence is 1 in 2000 population.[110,111] It is a storage disorder of a ceroidlike substance that leads to its characteristic features of partial albinism, restrictive lung disease, and a platelet abnormality. Although the platelet count in patients with this syndrome is normal, part of this pigment storage disorder includes a deficiency of the granule storage pool in platelets. As a result, and also because many patients with Hermansky-Pudlak syndrome have IBD as a component, GI bleeding can occur as a further complication.[32] The inheritance is autosomal recessive.

MALFORMATIONS OF THE GI TRACT

Most GI malformations have much more bearing on the pediatric population than they do on adults (Table 49-15).[16,112] Some of these malformations, however, may present in adulthood. One such disorder is gut malrotation, which can present in adults with symptoms and signs of intestinal obstruction. Malrotation can exist alone (the usual case in otherwise healthy adults) or as part of a syndrome. Another exception is duodenal stenosis, which may occur in adults with annular pancreas. Some evidence suggests that

TABLE 49–15
Malformations of the Gastrointestinal Tract

CONDITION	INDIVIDUAL*	FEATURES
VATER association	Sporadic	Vertebral defects, anal atresia, tracheoesophageal fistula with esophageal atresia, and radial and renal abnormalities. Nearly all cases have been sporadic.
Achalasia-microcephaly syndrome	?AR	Apparently rare syndrome with microcephaly, mental deficiency, and onset in early childhood of symptoms of achalasia
Familial esophageal achalasia	AR	Onset in childhood of achalasia. Some patients with Sjögren's syndrome or glucocorticoid deficiency plus achalasia in childhood have been described. Consideration of adrenal insufficiency should be made in any child with achalasia.
Congenital deafness with vitiligo and achalasia	AR	Deafness with achalasia, short stature, and vitiligo. Achalasia and leukoderma alone have also been described in at least two families with the same inheritance pattern.
Hiatal hernia; congenital short esophagus	?AD	Several families have been described in which members in two or more generations have been affected.
Microcephaly, hiatal hernia and nephrotic syndrome (Galloway syndrome)	AR	Albuminuria and vomiting of feedings begin at birth; ears are large, and kidneys show microcystic dysplasia and focal glomerulosclerosis. Death usually occurs by age three
Tracheoesophageal fistula with or without esophageal atresia	Probably multifactorial	Many familial cases have been reported; this seems to be distinct from the VATER association (see above).
Cutis laxa	AR	One of two recessive types of cutis laxa; disorder is a deficiency of elastic fibers producing diaphragmatic and other hernias, diverticula of the gastrointestinal and urinary tract, infantile emphysema, and death in the first year of life. The other recessive type and a dominant type do not affect the gastrointestinal tract.
Pyloric atresia	AR	Congential pyloric atresia due to the reduction of the pylorus to a fibrous band or being obstructed by the diaphragm.
Pyloric stenosis	Multifactorial, AD	Present at about 1 month of age with vomiting, no diarrhea, excellent appetite; due to hypertrophy of pyloric muscle. After one affected child, recurrence risk as about 10% for male relatives and 2% for females. Striking male preponderance and some dominant pedigrees have been described.
Smith-Lemli-Opitz syndrome	AR	Syndrome of multiple dysmorphic features, plus pyloric stenosis in some. Other features are microcephaly, mental retardation, hypotonia, incomplete development of the male genitalia, hypospadias, a high forehead, and syndactyly of the second and third toes.
Duodenal atresia	AR and feature of some syndromes	Presents in infancy as isolated finding; may also be part of a syndrome (e.g., Down's syndrome and multiple intestinal atresia)
Situs inversus viscerum	?AR	Abnormal situs of viscera may be due to abnormal gene(s) that normally control locations of body organs; may be a subset of Kartagener syndrome.
Kartagener syndrome (immotile cilia syndrome)	AR	Situs inversus viscerum plus dextrocardia, bronchiectasis, and sterility in males; may be associated with intestinal obstruction and/or duodenal atresia. Probably all manifestations are due to structural abnormalities in cilia; cilia play an important role in locating viscera normally during early embryonic development.
Jejunal atresia	AR	Agenesis of the mesentery leading to distal small bowel coming straight off cecum and twisting around the marginal artery. This creates the apple-peel appearance seen at surgery. Primary abnormality may be obliteration of the superior mesenteric artery.
Volvulus of midgut	?AD	Midgut malrotation presents at infancy or childhood. One patient had multiple congenital abnormalities; in the rest, it is an isolated finding
Diverticulosis of bowel, femoral or inguinal hernia, and retinal detachment	?AR	Recurrent femoral and/or inguinal hernias with diverticula of large or small bowel and/or urinary bladder with marfanoid habitus, severe myopia, internal strabismus, and retinal detachment; presents in childhood
Multiple intestinal atresia	AR	Involves stomach to anus; intraluminal calcifications seen on roentgenograms; may lead to early death or can cause less severe involvement
Cornelia de Lange syndrome	Unknown (2%–5% recurrence risk)	Characteristic facial features include hirsutism, synophrys, broad nasal root, micrognathia, and malformed ears. Abnormal hands, congenital heart disease, and severe mental retardation occur. Minority of patients also have intestinal atresia.
Anal-sacral anomalies	?AR	Apparently rare disorder featuring anterior sacral meningocele, anal canal duplication cyst, and covered anus

(continued)

TABLE 49–15 (Continued)

CONDITION	INDIVIDUAL*	FEATURES
Imperforate anus	?AR and ?XLR	Usually sporadic; occasionally more than one sibling affected
Other anorectal anomalies	?AD	Anal stenosis with rectovaginal fistula has been seen in mother and two daughters. Anal stenosis may occur fairly commonly as a dominant disorder with incomplete penetrance.
Imperforate anus with hand, foot, and ear anomalies (Rear or Townes Brochs syndrome)	AD	Imperforate anus, triphalangeal thumbs or other radial abnormalities, sensorineural deafness, deformed external ears, and renal anomalies (mainly hypoplastic kidneys)
Cat's eye syndrome (with imperforate anus)	Chromosomal	Imperforate anus, vertical pupil due to iris coloboma; preauricular tags or fistulas; heart and urinary tract malformations; and mild to moderate mental retardation. Due to extra, small acrocentric chromosome, a deletion of either No 14 or No 22
Polydactyly, imperforate anus, and vertebral anomalies	?AD	These three findings were present in 8 of 186 cases of polydactyly; none was familial. Other cases have also been reported
Reiger syndrome	AD	Anal stenosis, iris coloboma, broad nasal root, umbilical malformation, glaucoma, similar features seen in a number of chromosomal abnormalities
Schinzel syndrome	?AD	Anal atresia, abnormalities of the fourth and fifth fingers, hypoplastic ulnas, small penis, delayed puberty, obesity, and pyloric stenosis

* AR = autosomal recessive; AD = autosomal dominant; XLR = X-linked recessive.
From Randolph LM, Rotter JI. In: Kelley WN, ed. Textbook of internal medicine. Philadelphia: JB Lippincott, 1989:630.

annular pancreas can be inherited as an autosomal dominant condition.

GALLSTONES

Cholelithiasis is an excellent example of a genetically heterogeneous disorder. Although many gallstones are composed of bile supersaturated with cholesterol, some are caused by excess cholesterol and others by undersecretion of bile acids. One of the important lines suggesting the importance of genetic factors in gallstone disease has been the large variation in frequency among ethnic groups, being especially high in Mexican-Americans and American Indians.[113,114]

One difficulty in assessing the role of genetic factors in such a common disease as cholelithiasis is that there is a fairly high likelihood that the relative of a patient could be affected by chance alone and not because of a genetic factor. However, well-controlled studies comparing siblings and spouses of affected patients have shown that there is, indeed, familial clustering due to genetic factors (i.e., siblings are affected much more commonly than the spouses of the same sex). Further supportive evidence for genetic factors is a Danish study of twin pairs surviving to the age of 40, which showed concordance in 14 of 25 MZ pairs, whereas, in the like-sexed DZ twins, concordance was seen in only 6 of 40 pairs.[115] Formal studies of the genetics of gallstone disease have encountered the problem of silent disease. Postmortem studies have shown that about half of the cases of cholelithiasis are unrecognized during life. Thus, clinical studies alone underestimate the degree of family studies. Studies using oral cholecystography have shown that silent gallstones are increased in family members as well.[116] Studies of biliary lipid composition in siblings and twins further indicate that the contributing factors to gallstone formation—molar percentage of biliary cholesterol, bile acid composition, cholesterol synthesis, and bile cholesterol saturation—are under significant genetic control.[117,118]

DISORDERS OF THE PANCREAS
(Table 49–16)

Cystic Fibrosis

As was discussed in part A, the most common genetic disorder of the pancreas is cystic fibrosis (Table 49-16; see also ch 92). Indeed, it is the most common lethal autosomal recessive disorder in the white population, occurring with a frequency of one in 2000 births. The disorder is characterized by viscous secretions and dysfunction of multiple exocrine glands, leading to pancreatic insufficiency and malabsorption, chronic pulmonary infection with emphysema, and high chloride concentration in sweat.

The GI manifestations of CF are emphasized here (also see ch 92). Because of the life-threatening nature of the pulmonary complications of CF, less emphasis is paid to the GI complications. However, their importance is underscored by the fact that CF is the leading cause of malabsorption in children. Moreover, more than one third of patients with CF survive to adulthood and develop many of the GI complications with time.[52,53,119,120]

Close to 90% of patients with CF have pancreatic insufficiency leading to achylia. Most are born with insufficiency and require replacement therapy by the first birthday. Pancreatic secretions are abnormal, and the pancreatic ducts also become plugged by the viscous substance, leading to destruction of distal ducts. Proximal to the ducts, autodigestion and inflammation lead to fibrosis

TABLE 49–16
Genetic Disorders of the Pancreas

CONDITION	INHERITANCE*	FEATURE
Cystic fibrosis	AR	Exocrine disease that presents with respiratory infection and steatorrhea in infancy or childhood; occurs in 1 in 2000 whites
Hyperlipoproteinemia type I (familial hyperchylomicronemia, idiopathic hyperlipemia of Berger-Grutz type, essential familial hyperlipemia)	AR	Abdominal pain, hepatosplenomegaly, xanthomas in childhood or adulthood; due to deficient lipoprotein lipase; responds dramatically to fat-free diet; apparently does not cause precocious atherosclerosis
Lipase or colipase (or combined), congenital absence of, pancreatic	AR	Chronic diarrhea in childhood responds to exogenous administration of lipase or colipase
Pancreas, annular	?AD	Rare condition presenting in childhood with signs of high intestinal obstruction; secondary duodenal atresia; surgical repair necessary
Pancreatic insufficiency and bone marrow dysfunction (Shwachman-Bodian syndrome)	AR	Exocrine cells in pancreas are replaced with fat, sparing the endocrine pancreas. Skeletal changes (metaphyseal dysostosis) lead to moderate dwarfism, some with pancytopenia. Patient is predisposed to hematologic malignancies.
Johanson-Blizzard	AR	Developmental and dental abnormalities, short stature
Trypsinogen deficiency	AR	Failure to thrive, edema, and hypoproteinemia with normal sweat electrolytes; onset in infancy; responds to oral protein hydrolysate
Enterokinase deficiency	AR	Clinically similar to trypsinogen deficiency
Pancreatitis, hereditary	AD	Clinically similar to nonfamilial chronic pancreatitis except age at onset averages 13 years. Five to 10% also have diabetes mellitus and pancreatic pseudocysts
Pancreatitis, sclerosing cholangitis, and sicca complex	AR	Leukocyte migration inhibited in presence of bile antigen, suggesting immune mechanism
Congenital pancreatic hypoplasia	AR	Exocrine and endocrine abnormalities including early onset type I diabetes

* AR = autosomal recessive; AD = autosomal dominant.
From Randolph LM, Rotter JI. In Kelley WN, ed. Textbook of internal medicine. Philadelphia: JB Lippincott, 1989:630.

and exocrine insufficiency. With the identification of the actual CF gene and the most common mutation, there is evidence that specific mutations have a higher risk for pancreatic insufficiency than others (i.e., that the occurrence of pancreatic disease within CF is under significant genetic control), and much of that is due to different mutations at the CF locus.[121,122]

Malabsorption, primarily of fats, leads to malnutrition, hemorrhage due to lack of vitamin K absorption, and tetany due to hypocalcemia from losses in the stool. Vitamins D and A are relatively unaffected by the pancreatic deficiency. The lack of vitamin E leads to neurologic disease in some patients, which manifests as abnormal eye movements, diminished reflexes, ataxia, and weakness. Untreated persons may absorb an excess of iron and develop hemosiderosis of the liver. They may also develop vitamin B_{12} deficiency. The islets of Langerhans are secondarily affected by fibrosis of the pancreas, leading to glucose intolerance in about one half of patients with CF. This usually resembles the pattern of non-insulin-dependent, or type II, diabetes mellitus.

More than 12 pancreatic replacement products on the market; two of the most effective are Pancrease, a capsule containing porcine pancreatic enzyme concentrate, and Cotazym, which comes in capsules or as a powder, which is useful for administration in an infant's food or formula. These products should be given with all meals and snacks. Besides pancreatic replacement, patients need to maintain adequate caloric intake and should be counseled by a nutritionist.

Hepatic changes from CF occur in about one third of affected children, but symptomatic hepatic disease occurs in only 2% to 5% of patients. The thick secretions plug bile ducts, resulting in secondary inflammation and fibrosis. An elevated serum alkaline phosphatase or gamma-glutamyl transpeptidase (GGTP) level signal focal biliary changes. Gallstones are a fairly common manifestation of CF but are usually clinically insignificant.

The best known intestinal manifestation of CF is meconium ileus, which presents as obstruction in 1% to 20% of affected children. If Gastrografin enema and oral N-acetylcysteine do not resolve it, surgery is necessary. After the newborn period, an equivalent of meconium ileus is occasionally encountered, presenting as colicky pain and constipation. On physical examination, a fecal impaction can sometimes by palpated. If volvulus or intussusception is present, surgery is required; otherwise, medical treatment with Gastrografin enema, mineral oil, increased pancreatic enzymes, and acetylcysteine can be attempted. Rectal prolapse occurs in up to one fourth of patients before age 2, but it usually does not occur in patients given pancreatic replacement therapy. The mechanism for the prolapse is not known.[119]

Genetic linkage assessment by molecular techniques for the purpose of prenatal diagnosis is widely available and was discussed earlier under "Linkage" in part B of this chapter (page 995).

Pancreatic Insufficiency

The Shwachman-Bodian syndrome of pancreatic insufficiency and bone marrow dysfunction involves replacement of the exocrine pancreas with fat, sparing the endocrine pancreas.[123] Skeletal changes of the metaphyseal dysostosis type, leading to moderate dwarfism, are also present. Some patients have pancytopenia with susceptibility to infection. They are predisposed to hematologic malignancies such as those noted in Fanconi's anemia. Respiratory difficulties are not a feature. The diagnosis is established by documentation of the exocrine deficiency in association with characteristic metaphyseal changes on roentgenograms and CT scan findings in the pancreas. The inheritance is autosomal recessive.

Much rarer is the Johanson-Blizzard syndrome, which includes many developmental abnormalities as well as exocrine pancreatic insufficiency.[124] Short stature is probably part of this syndrome but is also contributed to by the accompanying hypothyroidism, urinary tract infections, and repair of anal abnormalities, often imperforate anus. Although the original reports included these abnormalities, as well as deafness, unusual hair growth patterns, and hypoplastic alae nasi, many of the subsequent cases (22 in all) have not had the exact same phenotype.

Hereditary Pancreatitis

Hereditary pancreatitis is a genetic disorder that is similar clinically to nonfamilial chronic pancreatitis. It is characterized by steatorrhea and recurrent attacks of severe abdominal pain, fever, and marked elevation of serum amylase levels. This last finding differentiates the disorder from FMF. Mean age at onset is 13 years. Five to 10% of affected persons have pancreatic insufficiency, diabetes mellitus, and pseudocysts. As in chronic pancreatitis, attacks can be precipitated by emotional stress, alcohol, or a diet rich in fat. The disorder is autosomal dominant with 80% penetrance.[125]

FAMILIAL MEDITERRANEAN FEVER

Familial Mediterranean fever (FMF) is an autosomal recessive disorder with protean manifestations and an obscure etiology.[24,126] The clinical disorder of FMF has a frequency of approximately 1 in 2400 in Israel, a country in which it has been studied intensively.[24] Half the patients are of Sephardic Jewish descent, about 20% are Armenian, 20% are Turkish or Arabic, and the rest are Italian, Greek, or Ashkenazi Jews. The disease occurs rarely in northern Europeans. Its pattern of inheritance is an autosomal

recessive disorder. As discussed above, nearly half the patients do not have a positive family history.

The manifestations usually appear during childhood or adolescence and are characterized by brief episodic febrile attacks, recurring in varying intervals and associated with painful inflammation in a variety of serosal surfaces, including the abdomen, chest, joints, and skin, hence the alternative name of recurrent familial polyserositis. Attacks last typically for 1 to 2 days and occur once or twice a month. The natural history of the attacks can be quite variable, even in an individual patient. Clinical features include fever, abdominal pain, and signs of peritonitis in nearly all the patients. Common but less constant features include pleuritic pain, mild arthritis of the large joints, and a transient erysipelaslike skin lesion on the lower extremities. In 1% of patients, meningitis also occurs. When arthritis occurs, it is an episodic monarthritis or oligoarthritis of the large joints, mimicking oligoarthritic forms of juvenile rheumatoid arthritis. The attacks usually last days to weeks but may last for months and are associated with radiographic changes of periarticular osteopenia but without erosions. The peritonitis is indistinguishable from other causes of that disorder, so that other acute febrile conditions must be considered, such as appendicitis, cholecystitis, pancreatitis, and intestinal obstruction.

Laboratory tests are nonspecific during the attacks of pain and fever. The white blood cell count averages 16,000 cells per microliter but may go as high as 40,000 cells per microliter. The erythrocyte sedimentation rate increases, as do other acute phase reactants (fibrinogen, C-reactive protein). Albuminuria and microscopic hematuria also occur. The obstructive series may show bowel edema and air–fluid levels in the small bowel, causing confusion with mechanical obstruction. The diagnosis is made in patients, often with the appropriate ethnic background, who have typical, self-limited, and recurrent attacks of fever and abdominal pain.

The most severe feature of the disease is the progressive accumulation of a specific protein known as amyloid fibrillar protein AA in the kidney, which manifests clinically as a nephropathy. There is considerable ethnic variation in the incidence of amyloidosis in FMF, which does not mirror the apparent prevalence of the underlying gene. Amyloidosis occurs least frequently in Armenians with the disorder, even though FMF occurs most commonly in Armenians (1 in 400). The disease occurs next most commonly in non-Ashkenazi Jews (1 in 2400), whereas the incidence of amyloidosis in FMF is most common in Moroccan Jews in Israel (up to 30%). In some patients, the amyloidosis develops before any other clinical sign. The genetic or environmental factors that account for these differences in the incidence of amyloidosis are not clear.[127] The amyloidosis appears to be a secondary phenomenon due to the periodic inflammation, because its occurrence is reduced by therapy.

The etiology of FMF is unknown.[128] The best possibility seems to be that it involves a genetically determined defect in the regulation of inflammatory responses. Research into the etiology of FMF has included studies of suppressor T cells, leukocyte chemotaxis, lysosome release from neutrophils, and immune globulins, all without a definite identification of the pathophysiologic defect.[128] The most recent finding is that complement component C5a was found to be decreased to a level less than 10% of controls in the peritoneal fluid of five patients with FMF.[129] The proposed hypothesis is that a deficiency in the inhibitory activity of C5a in the inflammatory response in synovial and other fluids may play

TABLE 49–17
Hereditary Neoplasias of the Gastrointestinal Tract (Excluding Polyposis Syndromes and Colon Cancer)

CONDITION	INHERITANCE*	FEATURES
Keratosis palmaris et plantaris with esophageal cancer (congenital sliding hiatal hernia, lower esophagus lined by gastric mucosa)	AD	Distinct from keratosis palmaris et plantaris familiaris in that this entity is associated with esophageal cancer and also with the later onset of tylosis. Palms and soles are diffusely hyperkeratotic (onset in first year of life). Low serum vitamin A level is evident in some cases.
Multiple endocrine neoplasia type III (IIb), mucosal neuroma syndrome	?AD	Multiple true neuromas, pheochromocytoma, hypertrophy of lips, medullary thyroid cancer, megacolon with plexus hyperplasia, and colonic diverticula. Neuromas often involve face and tongue. Prophylactic thyroidectomy is indicated. No parathyroid disease is present.
Multiple endocrine adenomatosis type I	AD	Triad of islet cell adenomas includes insulinomas, which cause hypoglycemia; gastrinomas, which cause peptic ulcers; and parathyroid adenomas, which cause hyperparathyroidism. Pituitary tumors are also a feature.
Intestinal carcinoid	?AD	Familial incidences of appendiceal and ileum carcinoid have been reported. Duodenal carcinoid is also seen in multiple endocrine neoplasia types I–III
Pancreatic carcinoma	?AR	Presents at age 66–75 with pancreatic acinar carcinoma; no tumors at other sites
Carney's syndrome (myxoma, spotty pigmentation and endocrine overactivity; includes NAME and LAMB syndromes)	?AD	Café au lait spots and subcutaneous myxoid neurofibromas, atrial myxoma and bilateral adrenocortical nodular dysplasia; about half of males have bilateral large-cell calcifying Sertoli cell tumors. Occasionally there is freckling around lips and in mouth, but much less common than in Peutz-Jeghers syndrome. Gastric leiomyosarcoma and palatal myxomas are associated.
Basal cell nevus syndrome (Gorlin-Goltz syndrome)	AD	Many basal cell nevi appear, usually at the time of puberty and rarely at birth. Associated tumors are hamartomas of the stomach, medulloblastoma, astrocytoma, and ovarian fibromas. Patients are exquisitely sensitive to the effects of therapeutic amounts of ionizing radiation and may develop many more basal cell nevi at the sites of radiation. Cleft lip and/or palate and mental retardation occur in about 5% of those affected. Probable gene location is chromosome 1.
DiGeorge syndrome	?AD	Abnormalities in the development of derivatives of the third and fourth pharyngeal pouches, absence of the parathyroids (leading to hypocalcemia) and thymus. Cellular immunity is impaired, often leading to death due to infection; transplantation of fetal thymus provides effective immune reconstitution. Associated abnormalities include tumors of the oropharynx, as well as deformities of the ear, nose, mouth, and aortic arch. Small deletions of chromosome 22 and spontaneous mutations have been implicated, in addition to the autosomal dominant pattern of inheritance seen in some families.
Dyskeratosis congenita (Zinsser-Cole-Engman syndrome)	XLR usually; AD in one family	Cutaneous pigmentation; continuous lacrimation due to atresia of the lacrimal ducts; leukoplakia of the oral mucosa and sometimes the anal mucosa; nail dystrophy; testicular atrophy; and thrombocytopenia and anemia are features. Opportunistic infections are also associated.
Epidermolysis bullosa dystrophica	AD, AR	There are at least 18 varieties of epidermolysis bullosa, of which six are of the dystrophica type. Others include the junctionalis, lethalis, pretibial, and simplex types. A feature common to all types is blistering, which can be lethal in the newborn period (in the letalis types), or it can present as localized traumatic blistering in childhood or adolescence.

(continued)

TABLE 49–17 (Continued)

CONDITION	INHERITANCE*	FEATURES
Epidermolysis bullosa dystrophica	AD, AR	Because the blisters in the dystrophica type are subepidermal (as opposed to epidermal in the simplex types), healing leads to scarring and sometimes to malignancy; most are commonly in the oropharynx and esophagus.
Neurofibromatosis (NF)	AD	Neurofibromas of the colon are a recognized feature of type I neurofibromatosis, but there are also two subtypes of NF specifically separated from other NF cases by the presence of gastrointesinal tumors. One is familial intestinal neurofibromatosis, or type III NF, in which multiple neurofibromas of the intestine without cutaneous manifestations have been observed in several generations within families. The other is neurofibromatosis–pheochromocytoma–duodenal carcinoid syndrome, which has been observed in several patients and for which it has been suggested that it be reclassified a multiple endocrine neoplasia type IIIa. One of the cases was familial, and all had characteristic cutaneous manifestations of classic NF. Patients may present with jaundice (due to obstruction by the duodenal carcinoid) or with manifestations of the pheochromocytoma (flushing, tachycardia, sweating).

* *AD = autosomal dominant; AR = autosomal recessive; XLR = X-linked recessive.*
Modified from Randolph LM, Rotter JI. In: Kelley WN, ed. Textbook of internal medicine. Philadelphia: JB Lippincott, 1989: 630.

an important role in the pathogenesis of the characteristic recurrent attacks in FMF.

Colchicine, 0.6 mg orally two to three times per day, is an effective treatment in the prevention of the acute febrile attacks of the disease. A very low fat diet (20 g) can also prevent attacks.[130] Colchicine also favorably influences the course of renal amyloidosis. Colchicine does not allay symptoms when taken during attacks. Some patients use it intermittently to forestall attacks when they recognize that one is imminent.

The responsible gene has not been identified.[127] Genetic counseling is that for an autosomal recessive disorder, with the added complexity of the high gene frequency in certain ethnic groups. Knowledge of the disorder in a family helps clarify the diagnosis in relatives.

GASTROINTESTINAL CANCER

One of the most exciting contributions of genetics to oncology and gastroenterology has been the realization that there is a strong heritable component to many GI malignancies. The importance of this finding is the possibility of early treatment and even prevention of malignancy in at-risk relatives of affected persons. The clinical features of GI malignancies are covered elsewhere in this volume (ch 57, 62, 63, 70, 78, 84, 90, 91, and 96). The several genetic syndromes that feature an increased risk for noncolonic GI tract cancer are listed in Table 49–17. The familial polyposes have been considered earlier in part A and in Chapter 79.

SUMMARY

This chapter has reviewed genetic principles as they are applied to the care of patients and their families with GI disease. Numerous lines of evidence indicate that the majority of both rare and common GI disorders have a genetic component. Two categories of genetic disease—mendelian and nonmendelian—and the genetic classification of numerous GI disorders have been reviewed. An increasing number of genes responsible for these GI disorders are being specifically localized to defined chromosomal locations in the human gene map by linkage analysis and recombinant DNA techniques. Methods for genetic risk assessment, preclinical diagnosis, and prenatal diagnosis are increasingly available. The consequence for the clinician is that we can increasingly identify those family members at risk for specific GI disorders, and this enables not only improved therapy but, in many cases, a dramatic ability to prevent or minimize clinical disease by intervening before its onset.

The reader is directed to Chapter 72, Specific Mucosal Protein Deficiency States; Chapter 79, Polyposis Syndromes; and Chapter 92, Congenital and Hereditary Disease of the Pancreas.

REFERENCES

1. King RA, Rotter JI, Motulsky AG, eds. The genetic basis of common diseases. New York: Oxford University Press, 1991, in press.

2. Rotter JI. The genetics of peptic ulcer disease—more than one gene, more than one disease. Prog Med Genet 1980;4:1.

3. Roth M-P, Petersen GM, McElree C, Vadheim CM, Panish JF, Rotter JI. Familial recurrence risk estimates of inflammatory bowel disease in Ashkenazi Jews. Gastroenterology 1989;96:1016.

4. Roth M-P, Petersen GM, McElree C, Feldman E, Rotter JI. Geographic origins of Jewish patients with inflammatory bowel disease. Gastroenterology 1989;97:900.

5. Shohat T, Vadheim CM, Rotter JI. The genetics of inflammatory bowel diseases. In: Gitnick G, ed. Inflammatory bowel diseases: A physician's guide. New York: Igaku-Shoin, 1991, in press.

6. Gelehrter TD, Collins FJ. Principles of medical genetics. Baltimore: Williams & Wilkins, 1989.

7. Lewin B. Genes IV. Oxford: Oxford University Press, 1990.

8. Vogel F, Motulsky AG. Human genetics. Problems and approaches, ed 2. Berlin: Springer-Verlag, 1986.

9. Thompson MW. Genetics in medicine, ed 4. Philadelphia: WB Saunders, 1986.

10. Harper PS. Practical genetic counselling, ed 3. London: Wright, 1988.

11. Le Beau MM, Rowley JD. Chromosomal abnormalities in leukemia and lymphoma: Clinical and biological significance. Adv Hum Genet 1986;15:1.

12. Bishop JM. The molecular genetics of cancer. Science 1987;235:305.

13. Vogelstein B, Fearon ER, Hamilton SR, et al. Genetic alterations during colorectal-tumor development. N Engl J Med 1988;319:525.

14. Baker SJ, Fearon ER, Nigro JM, et al. Chromosome 17 deletions and p53 gene mutations in colorectal carcinomas. Science 1988;244:217.

15. Fearon ER, Cho KR, Nigro JM, et al. Identification of a chromosome 18q gene that is altered in colorectal cancers. Science 1990;247:49.

16. McKusick VA. Mendelian inheritance in man—Catalogs of autosomal dominant, autosomal recessive, and X-linked phenotypes, ed 9. Baltimore: Johns Hopkins University Press, 1990.

17. Emery AEH, Rimoin DL, eds. Principles and practice of medical genetics, ed 2. Edinburgh: Churchill Livingstone, 1991, in press.

18. Gardner EJ. Genetic and clinical study of intestinal polyposis, a predisposing factor for carcinoma of colon and rectum. Am J Hum Genet 1951;3:167.

19. Scriver CR, Beaudet AL, Sly WS, Valle D, eds. The metabolic basis of inherited disease, ed 6. New York: McGraw-Hill, 1989.

20. Harries JT, ed. Familial inherited abnormalities. Clin Gastroenterol 1982;11(1).

21. Byers PH. Disorders of collagen biosynthesis and structure. In: Scriver CR, Beaudet AL, Sly WS, Valle D, eds. The metabolic basis of inherited disease. New York: McGraw-Hill, 1989:2805.

22. Cohn DH, Byers PH. Clinical screening for collagen defects in connective tissue diseases. Clin Perinatol 1990;17:793.

23. Kahn T, Reiser M, Gmeinwieser J, Heuck A. The Ehlers-Danlos syndrome, type IV, with an unusual combination of organ malformations. Cardiovasc Intervent Radiol 1988;11:288.

24. Eliakim M, Levy M, Ehrenfeld M. Recurrent polyserositis. Amsterdam: Elsevier, 1981.

25. Rogers DA, Shohat M, Petersen GM, et al. Familial Mediterranean fever in Armenians: Autosomal recessive inheritance with high gene frequency. Am J Med Genet 1989;34:168.

26. Hatefi Y. The mitochondrial electron transport and oxidative phosphorylation system. Annu Rev Biochem 1985;54:1015.

27. Chomyn A, Cleeter MWJ, Ragan CI, Riley M, Doolittle RF, Attardi G. URF6, last unidentified reading frame of human mtDNA code for an NADH dehydrogenase subunit. Science 1986;234:614.

28. Shoffner JM, Wallace DC. Oxidative phyosphorylation diseases—Disorders of two genomes. Adv Hum Genet 1990;19:267.

29. Wallace DC, Singh G, Lott MT, et al. Mitochondrial DNA mutation associated with Leber's hereditary optic neuropathy. Science 1988;242:1427.

30. Rotter JI, Samloff IM, Rimoin DL. Genetics and heterogeneity of common gastrointestinal disorders. New York: Academic Press, 1980.

31. Rotter JI, Shohat T. Peptic ulcer. In: Emery AEH, Rimoin DL, eds. Principles and practice of medical genetics, ed 2. Edinburgh: Churchill Livingstone, 1991;1097.

32. Schinella RA, Greco A, Cober BL, Denmark LW, Cox RP. Hermansky-Pudlak syndrome with granulomatous colitis. Ann Intern Med 1980;92:20.

33. Lam SK, Ong GB. Duodenal ulcers, early and late onset. Gut 1976;17:169.

34. Doll R, Kellock TD. The separate inheritance of gastric and duodenal ulcer. Annals of Eugenics 1951;16:231.

35. Kirsner JB. Genetic aspects of inflammatory bowel disease. Clin Gastroenterol 1973;2:557.

36. Tysk C, Lindberg E, Jarnerot G, Floderus-Myrhed B. Ulcerative colitis and Crohn's disease in an unselected population of monozygotic and dizygotic twins. A study of heritability and the influence of smoking. Gut 1988;29:990.

37. Schimke RN. Multiple endocrine adenomatosis syndromes. Adv Intern Med 1976;21:249.

38. Lam SK. Pathogenesis and pathophysiology of duodenal ulcer. Clin Gastroenterol 1984;13:447.

39. Rotter JI, Sones JQ, Samloff IM, et al. Duodenal ulcer disease associated with elevated serum pepsinogen I: An inherited autosomal dominant disorder. N Engl J Med 1979;300:63.

40. Sumii K, Uemura N, Inbe A, et al. Familial aggregation of duodenal ulcer and an autosomal dominant inheritance of hyperpepsionogenimia I. Hiroshima J Med Sci 1986;35:171.

41. Rotter JI, Petersen GM, Samloff IM, et al. Genetic heterogeneity of hyperpepsinogenemic I and normopepsinogenemic I duodenal ulcer disease. Ann Intern Med 1979;91:372.

42. Samloff IM, Varis K, Ihamaki T, Siurala M, Rotter JI. Relationships among serum pepsinogen I, serum pepsinogen II, and gastric mucosal histology. A study in relatives of patients with pernicious anemia. Gastroenterology 1982;83:204.

43. Burt RW, Bishop DT, Cannon LA, Dowdle MA, Lee RG, Skolnick MH. Dominant inheritance of adenomatous colonic polyps and colorectal cancer. N Engl J Med 1985;312:1540.

44. Cannon-Albright LA, Skolnick MH, Bishop DT, Lee RG, Burt RW. Common inheritance of susceptibility to colonic adenomatous polyps and associated colorectal cancers. N Engl J Med 1988;319:533.

45. Hollander D, Vadheim CM, Brettholz E, Petersen GM, Delahunty T, Rotter JI. Increased intestinal permeability in Crohn's patients and their relatives: An etiological factor? Ann Intern Med 1986;105:883.

46. Elmgreen J, Both H, Binder V. Familial occurrence of complement dysfunction in Crohn's disease: Correlation with intestinal symptoms and hypercatabolism of complement. Gut 1985;26:151.

47. Roth SH. Nonsteroidal anti-inflammatory drugs: Gastropathy, deaths, and medical practice. Ann Intern Med 1988;109:353.

48. Bartlett JG. *Campylobacter pylori*: Fact or fancy? Gastroenterology 1988;94:229.

49. Kidd KK, Klinger HP, Ruddle FH, eds. Human gene mapping 10. Cytogenet Cell genet 1989;51(1).

50. White RL. Diagnosis when the gene locus is unknown. Hosp Pract 1985;20:103.

51. Weatherall DJ. The new genetics and clinical practice, ed 2. Oxford: Oxford University Press, 1985.

52. Lloyd-Still JD. Textbook of cystic fibrosis. Boston: John Wright. 1983.

53. Taussig LM. Cystic fibrosis. New York: Thieme-Stratton, 1984.

54. Beaudet A, Bowcock A, Buchwald M, et al. Linkage of cystic fibrosis to two tightly linked DNA markers: Joint report from a collaborative study. Am J Hum Genet 1986;39:681.

55. Rommens JM, Iannuzzi MC, Kerem B, et al. Identification of the cystic fibrosis gene: Chromosome walking and jumping. Science 1989;245:1059.

56. Lemna WK, Feldman GL, Kerem B, et al. Mutation analysis for heterozygote detection and the prenatal diagnosis of cystic fibrosis. N Engl J Med 1990;322:291.

57. Herrera L, Kakati S, Gibas L, Pietrazak E, Sandberg AA. Gardner syndrome in a man with an interstitial deletion of 5q. Am J Med Genet 1986;25:473.

58. Bodmer W, Bailey CJ, Bodmer J, et al. Localization of the gene for familial adenomatous polyposis on chromosome 5. Nature 1987;328:614.

59. Leppert M, Dobbs M, Scambler P, et al. The gene for familial polyposis coli maps to the long arm of chromosome 5. Science 1987;238:1411.

60. Nakamura Y, Lathrop M, Leppert M, et al. Localization of the genetic defect in familial adenomatous polyposis within a small region of chromosome 5. Am J Hum Genet 1988;43:638.

61. Simons MJ, Tait BD. Detection of immune-associated genetic markers of human disease. Edinburgh: Churchill Livingstone, 1984.

62. Tiwari JL, Terasaki PI. HLA and disease associations. New York: Springer-Verlag, 1985.

63. Pena AS, Mann DL, Hague NE, et al. Genetic basis of gluten-sensitive enteropathy. Gastroenterology 1978;75:230.

64. Bell JI, Todd JA, McDevitt HO. The molecular basis of HLA-disease association. Adv Hum Genet 1989;18:1.

65. Bugawan TL, Angelini G, Larrick J, Auricchio, Ferrara GB, Erlich HA. A combination of a particular HLA-DP beta allele and an HLA-DQ heterodimer confers susceptibility to coeliac disease. Nature 1989;339:470.

66. Greenberg DA, Rotter JI. Two locus models for gluten sensitive enteropathy: Population genetic considerations. Am J Med Genet 1981;8:205.

67. Lin HJ, Rotter JI, Conte WJ. Use of HLA marker associations and HLA haplotype linkage to estimate disease risks in families with gluten sensitive enteropathy. Clin Genet 1985;28:185.

68. Lubin MB, Lin HJ, Vadheim CM, Rotter JI. Genetics of common diseases of adulthood, implications for prenatal counseling and diagnosis. Clin Perinatol 1990;17:889.

69. Larsson C, Skogseid B, Boerg K, Nakamura Y, Nordtgold M. Multiple endocrine neoplasia type I maps to chromosome 11 and is lost in insulinoma. Nature 1988;332:85.

70. Chanarin I. The megaloblastic anaemias, ed 2. Oxford: Blackwell, 1979.

71. Chanarin I. Disorders of vitamin absorption. Clin Gastroenterol 1982;11:73.

72. Fenton WA, Rosenberg LE. Inherited disorders of cobalamin transport and metabolism. In: Scriver CR, Beaudet AL, Sly WS, Valle D, eds. The metabolic basis of inherited disease, ed 6. New York: McGraw-Hill, 1989:2065.

73. Kass L. Pernicious anemia. Philadelphia: WB Saunders, 1976.

74. Irvine WJ. Autoimmune atrophic gastritis. In: Rotter JI, Samloff IM, Rimoin DL, eds. Genetics and heterogeneity of common gastrointestinal disorders. New York: Academic Press, 1980:149.

75. Varis K, Samloff IM, Tiilikainen A, et al. Gastritis in first-degree relatives of pernicious anemia, gastric cancer patients, and controls. In: Rotter JI, Samloff IM, Rimoin DL. Genetics and heterogeneity of common gastrointestinal disorders. New York: Academic Press, 1980:177.

76. Carmel R. Gastric juice in congenital pernicious anemia contains no immunoreactive intrinsic factor molecule: Study of three kindreds with variable ages at presentation, including a patient first diagnosed in adulthood. Am J Hum Genet 1983;35:67.

77. Imerslund O. Idiopathic chronic megaloblastic anemia in children. Acta Pediatrica Scand 1960;49(Suppl 119):1.

78. Grasbeck R, Gordin R, Kantero I, Kuhlback B. Selective vitamin B_{12} malabsorption and proteinuria in young people. A syndrome. Acta Med Scand 1960;167:289.

79. Strober W. Genetic factors in gluten-sensitive enteropathy. In: Rotter JI, Samloff IM, Rimoin DL, eds. Genetics and heterogeneity of common gastrointestinal disorders. New York: Academic Press, 1980;243.

80. McConnell RB, ed. The genetics of coeliac disease. Lancaster: MTP Press, 1981.

81. Gilat T, Grossman A, Fireman Z, Rozen P. Inflammatory bowel disease in Jews. In: McConnell R, Rozen P, Langman M, Gilat T, eds. The genetics and epidemiology of inflammatory bowel disease. Basel: Karger, 1986:135.

82. Farmer RG, Michener WM, Mortimer EA. Studies of family history among patients with inflammatory bowel disease. Clin Gastroenterol 1980;9:221.

83. Weinrieb IJ, Fineman RM, Spiro HM. Turner syndrome and inflammatory bowel disease. N Engl J Med 1976;294:1221.

84. Asakura H, Tsuchiya M, Aiso S, et al. Association of human lymphocyte-DR2 antigen with Japanese ulcerative colitis. Gastroenterology 1982;82:413.

85. Fujita K, Naito S, Okabe N, Yao T. Immunologic studies in Crohn's disease. I. Association with HLA systems in the Japanese. J Clin Lab Immunol 1984;14:99.

86. Cottone M, Bunce M, Taylor CJ, Ting A, Jewell DP. Ulcerative colitis and HLA phenotype. Gut 1985;26:952.

87. Elmgreen J, Sorensen H, Berkowicz A. Polymorphism of complement C3 in chronic inflammatory bowel disease. Predominance of the C3F gene in Crohn's disease. Acta Med Scand 1984;215:375.

88. Fiocchi C, Roche JK, Michener WM. High prevalence of antibodies to intestinal epithelial antigens in patients with inflammatory bowel disease and their relatives. Ann Intern Med 1989;110:786.

89. Paige DM, Bayless TM, eds. Lactose digestion. Clinical and nutritional implications. Baltimore: Johns Hopkins University Press, 1981.

90. Flatz G. The genetic polymorphism of lactase activity in adult humans. In: Scriver CR, Beaudet AL, Sly WS, Valle D, eds. The metabolic basis of inherited disease, ed 6. New York: McGraw-Hill, 1989:2999.

91. Harries JT. Disorders of carbohydrate absorption. Clin Gastroenterol 1982;11:17.

92. Sahi T. Genetics and epidemiology of hypolactasia. In: Rotter JI, Samloff IM, Rimoin DL, eds. Genetics and heterogeneity of common gastrointestinal disorders. New York: Academic Press, 1980:215.

93. Semenza G, Auricchio S. Small-intestinal disaccharidases. In: Scriver CR, Beaudet AL, Sly WS, Valle D. The metabolic basis of inherited disease, ed 6. New York: McGraw-Hill, 1989:2975.

94. Silk DBA. Disorders of nitrogen absorption. Clin Gastroenterol 1982;11:47.

95. Scriver CR. Familial renal iminoglycinuria. In: Scriver CR, Beaudet AL, Sly WS, Valle D. The metabolic basis of inherited disease, ed 6. New York: McGraw-Hill, 1989:2529.

96. Levy HL. Hartnup disorder. In: Scriver CR, Beaudet AL, Sly WS, Valle D. The metabolic basis of inherited disease, ed 6. New York: McGraw-Hill, 1989:2515.

97. Scriver CR, Mahon B, Levy HL, et al. The Hartnup phenotype: Mendelian transport disorder, multifactorial disease. Am J Hum Genet 1987;40:401.

98. Segal S, Thier SO. Cystinurias. In: Scriver CR, Beaudet AL, Sly WS, Valle D. The metabolic basis of inherited disease, ed 6. New York: McGraw-Hill, 1989:2479.

99. Simell O. Lysinuric protein intolerance and other cationic aminoacidurias. In: Scriver CR, Beaudet AL, Sly WS, Valle D. The metabolic basis of inherited disease, ed 6. New York: McGraw-Hill, 1989:2497.

100. Wadelius C, Fagerholm P, Pettersson U, Anneren G. Lowe oculocerebrorenal syndrome: DNA-based linkage of the gene to Xq24-q26, using tightly linked flanking markers and the correlation to lens examination in carrier diagnosis. Am J Hum Genet 1989;44:241.

101. Milla PJ. Disorders of electrolyte absorption. Clin Gastroenterol 1982;11:31.

102. Mayer EA, Schuffler MD, Rotter JI, Hanna P, Mogard M. A familial visceral neuropathy with autosomal dominant transmission. Gastroenterology 1986;91:1528.

103. Utsunomiya J, Iwama T, Taimura M, Hirayama R. Clinical and population genetics of the hereditary gastrointestinal polyposes. In: Rotter JI, Samloff IM, Rimoin DL. Genetics and heterogeneity of common gastrointestinal disorders. New York: Academic Press, 1980:391.

104. Riccardi VM, Eichner JE. Neurofibromatosis. Phenotype, natural history, and pathogenesis. Baltimore: Johns Hopkins University Press, 1986.

105. Wallace MR, Marchuk DA, Andersen LB, et al. Type 1 neurofibromatosis gene: Identification of a large transcript disrupted in three NF1 patients. Science 1990;249:181.

106. Goodman RM. Pseudoxanthoma elasticum and related disorders. In: Emery AE, Rimoin DL, eds. Principles and practice of medical genetics, ed 2. New York: Churchill Livingstone, 1991;1083.

107. Zentler-Munro PL, Howard ER, Karani J, Williams R. Variceal hemorrhage in hereditary hemorrhage telangiectasia. Gut 1989;30:1293.

108. Peery WH. Clinical spectrum of hereditary hemorrhagic telangiectasia (Osler-Weber-Rendu disease). Am J Med 1987;82:989.

109. Walshe MM, Evans CD, Warin RP. Blue rubber bleb naevus. Br Med J 1966;2:931.

110. Witkop Jr CJ, Quevedo Jr WC, Fitzpatrick TB, King RA. Albinism. In: Scriver CR, Beaudet AL, Sly WS, Valle D. The metabolic basis of inherited disease, ed 6. New York: McGraw-Hill, 1989:2905.

111. Shanahan F, Randolph L, King R, et al. Hermansky-Pudlak syndrome: An immunologic assessment of 15 cases. Am J Med 1988;85:823.

112. Jones, KL. Smith's recognizable patterns of human malformation, ed 4. Philadelphia: WB Saunders, 1988.

113. Bennion LJ, Knowler WC. Epidemiology of gallstones. In: Rotter JI, Samloff IM, Rimoin DL. Genetics and heterogeneity of common gastrointestinal disorders. New York: Academic Press, 1980:297.

114. Diehl AK, Haffner SM, Knapp JA, Hazuda HP, Stern MP. Dietary intake and the prevalence of gallbladder disease in Mexican Americans. Gastroenterology 1989;97:1527.

115. van der Linder W. Genetics of cholelithiasis. In: Rotter JI, Samloff IM, Rimoin DL, eds. Genetics and heterogeneity of common gastrointestinal disorders. New York: Academic Press, 1980:313.

116. Gilat T, Feldman C, Halpern Z, Dan M, Bar-Meir S. An increased familial frequency of gallstones. Gastroenterology 1983;84:242.

117. Danzinger RG, Gordon H, Schoenfield LJ, Thistle JL. Lithogenic bile in siblings of young women with cholelithiasis. Mayo Clin Proc 1972;47:762.

118. Kesaniemi YA, Koskenvuo M, Vuoristo M, Miettinen TA. Biliary lipid composition in monozygotic and dizygotic pairs of twins. Gut 1989;30:1750.

119. Zentler-Munro PL. Cystic fibrosis—A gastroenterological cornucopia. Gut 1987;28:1531.

120. Shepherd RW, Cleghorn GJ. Cystic fibrosis: Nutritional and intestinal disorders. Boca Raton: CRC Press, 1989.

121. Kerem B, Buchanan JA, Durie P, et al. DNA marker haplotype association with pancreatic sufficiency in cystic fibrosis. Am J Hum Genet 1989;44:827.

122. Kerem B, Rommens JM, Buchanan JA, et al. Identification of the cystic fibrosis gene: Genetic analysis. Science 1989;245:1073.

123. Shwachman H, Diamond LK, Oski FA, Khaw KT. The syndrome of pancreatic insufficiency and bone marrow dysfunction. J Pediatr 1964;65:645.

124. Hurst VA, Saraitser M. Johanson-Blizzard syndrome, J Med Genet 1989;26:45.

125. Sibert JR. Hereditary pancreatitis in England and Wales. J Med Genet 1978;15:189.

126. Schwabe AD, Peters RS. Familial Mediterranean fever in Armenians. Analysis of 100 cases. Medicine 1974;53:453.

127. Shohat M, Shohat T, Rotter JI, et al. Serum amyloid A and P protein genes in familial Mediterranean fever. Genomics 1990;8:83.

128. Shohat M, Korenberg JI, Schwabe AD, Rotter JI. Hypothesis: Familial Mediterranean fever—A genetic disorder of the lipocortin family? Am J Med Genet 1989;34:163.

129. Matzner Y, Brzezinski A. C5a-inhibitor deficiency in peritoneal fluids from patients with familial Mediterranean fever. N Engl J Med 1984;311:283.

130. Mellinkoff SM, Schwabe AD, Lawrence JS. A dietary treatment for familial Mediterranean fever. Arch Intern Med 1961;108:80.

50

Approach to the Patient with Drug or Alcohol Dependency

DAVID W. CRABB

INTRODUCTION

A large number of Americans abuse drugs or alcohol; for instance, approximately 18 million Americans abuse alcohol,[1] and 700,000 are addicted to heroin. The magnitude of drug use is nearly always underestimated, because denial by patients of loss of control over drug and alcohol use makes the diagnosis of substance abuse difficult. In addition, the use of the drugs may have effects that simulate other pathologic conditions, and hospitalized individuals may undergo withdrawal syndromes and still not report the use of drugs to the physician. Finally, many patients with chronic abdominal pain become addicted to prescribed pain medications. For these reasons, it is important for the practitioner to be alert to the presence of occult alcohol and drug abuse, to understand the biology of drug dependence, to recognize personality disorders in patients susceptible to drug addiction (see ch 130), and to know how drug abuse can mimic and complicate other illnesses. This chapter will cover the traditional drugs of abuse (such as narcotics, alcohol, sedative-hypnotics, amphetamines, cannabis, tobacco, and cocaine) as well as hallucinogens, laxatives, diuretics, and anabolic steroids. Many terms are used to describe aberrant drug-seeking behavior, and the definitions are continuously modified. Physical dependence has been defined[2] as "an adaptive state that manifests itself by intense physical disturbances when the administration of the drug is suspended." Psychic dependence[2] is "a condition in which a drug produces a feeling of satisfaction and a psychic drive that requires periodic or continuous administration of the drug to produce pleasure or to avoid discomfort." There may not be a valid neurobiologic basis for this division. The prototypical physical withdrawal syndromes are the violent ones related to opiate, barbiturate, and alcohol addiction. However, psychologic withdrawal symptoms may be quite severe, and the avoidance of these symptoms undoubtedly is important in perpetuating drug-seeking behavior. Cocaine is an example of a drug of this class; it produces intense craving for the euphoric effect of the drug and a prolonged period of anhedonia (i.e., an inability to obtain enjoyment from life) after stopping the drug. The current DSM-III-R criteria for psychoactive substance dependence and abuse are given in Tables 50-1 and 50-2.[3] This general definition applies to all psychoactive substances, including alcohol. These definitions emphasize the behaviors leading to increased consumption of drugs or alcohol, rather than withdrawal and tolerance. However, most drugs of abuse produce tolerance with continued use. This requires the abuser to increase the dose used to achieve the desired psychic effect. Tolerance may be due to increased rates of drug metabolism (e.g., of alcohol or barbiturates). This pharmacokinetic tolerance results from induction of drug-metabolizing enzymes in the liver (especially cytochrome P450–linked systems). Pharmacodynamic tolerance denotes decreased activity of the drug in the central nervous system (CNS) and may result from decreased receptor number or action. An additional form of tolerance is learned or conditioned tolerance. This term refers to the ability of an individual to perform better in an environment in which he has pre-

TABLE 50-1

DSM-III-R Diagnostic Criteria for Psychoactive Substance Dependence

A. At least three of the following:
  1. Substance often taken in larger amounts or over a longer period than the person intended
  2. Persistent desire or one or more unsuccessful efforts to cut down or control substance use
  3. A great deal of time spent in activities necessary for obtaining the substance, taking the substance, or recovering from its effect
  4. Frequent intoxication or withdrawal symptoms when expected to fulfill major role obligations at work, school, or home, or when substance use is physically hazardous
  5. Important social, occupational, or recreational activities given up or reduced because of substance abuse
  6. Continued substance use despite knowledge of having a persistent or recurrent social, psychologic, or physical problem that is caused by or exacerbated by the use of the substance
  7. Marked tolerance: the need for markedly increased amounts of the substance (i.e., at least a 50% increase) in order to achieve intoxication or desired effect, or markedly diminished effect with continued use of the same amount
  8. Characteristic withdrawal symptoms
  9. Substance often taken to relieve or avoid withdrawal symptoms
B. Some symptoms of the disturbance have persisted for at least 1 month or have recurred repeatedly over a longer period of time

Reprinted with permission from Diagnostic and Statistical Manual of Mental Disorders. 3rd ed, revised. Copyright, 1987: American Psychiatric Association.

1021

TABLE 50-2
DSM-III-R Criteria for Psychoactive Substance Abuse

A. A maladaptive pattern of substance use indicated by at least one of the following:
1. Continued use despite knowledge of having a persistent social, occupational, psychologic, or physical problem that is caused by or exacerbated by the use of the psychoactive substance
2. Recurrent use in situations when use is physically hazardous

B. Some of the symptoms of the disturbance have persisted for at least 1 month, or have recurred repeatedly over a longer period of time

C. Never met the criteria for psychoactive substance dependence for this substance

Reprinted with permission from Diagnostic and Statistical Manual of Mental Disorders. 3rd ed, revised. Copyright, 1987: American Psychiatric Association.

viously used the drug. Conditioning also plays an important role in drug craving.

Several medical complications of intravenous drug use can be seen with any injected drug and will be summarized here.[4] They include skin infections, tetanus, septicemia, infectious endocarditis (most commonly staphylococcal), venous thrombosis and pulmonary embolism, pulmonary granulomas, and acquisition of hepatitis B, non-A non-B hepatitis, δ hepatitis, and HIV infection. The threat of transmission of malaria may be the reason why heroin is commonly cut with quinine.[4] The injected drug may have been cut with other compounds with additional toxicity or may

not be the substance anticipated. Thus, even the history of use of a certain drug must be viewed skeptically. Other complications of drug abuse are listed in Table 50-3.

INDIVIDUAL PSYCHOACTIVE DRUGS OF ABUSE

Ethanol

PHARMACOLOGY

Despite the large amount of research performed on the effects of ethanol on the CNS, it is not yet clear exactly how ethanol affects the brain. Ethanol certainly interacts with cell membranes, although the concentrations required to change laboratory measures of molecular order ("fluidity") of the membranes are quite high. It is hypothesized that ethanol interacts with certain microdomains within the membrane.[1] One microdomain may be that in the vicinity of the benzodiazepine–barbiturate–$GABA_A$ receptor–chloride channel. Ethanol at low concentrations (20–100 mM) stimulates chloride uptake by isolated brain vesicles.[5] This effect is blocked by Ro15-4513, a benzodiazepine receptor inverse agonist. In turn, this effect of Ro15-4513 can be reversed by a benzodiazepine antagonist, Ro15-1788. The effect of Ro15-4315 is probably not solely related to its weak inverse agonist effects, because

TABLE 50-3
Medical Complications of Drug Abuse

Nervous System

Intracranial bleeding

Seizures

Organic psychosis

Wernicke's encephalopathy

Hyperpyrexia

Blindness (methanol)

Polyneuropathy

Suicide

Respiratory

Pulmonary granulomata

Nasal septal perforation

Paraquat poisoning (contaminated marijuana)

Pulmonary edema

Aspiration pneumonia

Lung abscess

Cardiovascular

Infective endocarditis

Cardiac arrhythmia

Angina/infarction (secondary to hypertension or tachycardia)

Vasculitis

Alcoholic cardiomyopathy

Gastrointestinal

Hepatitis virus transmission

Cocaine hepatotoxicity

Narcotic bowel syndrome

Precipitation of hepatic encephalopathy

Renal

Glomerulonephritis (heroin)

Musculoskeletal

Subcutaneous abscess

Tetanus

Cellulitis

Septic arthritis

Osteomyelitis

Metabolic

Precipitation of porphyria

Metabolic acidosis (ethylene glycol)

more potent inverse agonists do not antagonize ethanol effects.[6] Thus, ethanol may selectively change the microenvironment of the channel in a way that enhances GABAergic transmission. This would account for the antianxiety effects of ethanol and the cross-tolerance between ethanol, barbiturates, and benzodiazepines. The neuroanatomic location of this effect is unknown. Other neurotransmitter systems are probably also involved in the reinforcing effects of ethanol, because the anxiolytic effects are not the only reward experienced. More recently, ethanol has been shown to be a potent inhibitor of the glutamate NMDA receptor.

A predisposition to drink ethanol and the CNS responses to it are in part genetically determined. Studies with selected lines of rodents have shown differences in alcohol preference, innate sensitivity to ethanol, and the rate of development of tolerance.[1] Work with rats bred for their preference for alcohol has implicated both serotonergic and enkephalinergic pathways in the reward system for alcohol consumption and has suggested that serotonin uptake inhibitors may reduce alcohol craving.[7]

MECHANISMS OF DEVELOPMENT OF TOLERANCE

Neuroadaptive tolerance to ethanol may involve changes in the membrane near the chloride channel. The homeoviscous adaptation hypothesis suggests that the membrane becomes more ordered after chronic ethanol use to oppose the fluidizing effect of ethanol. This allows individuals to remain conscious at blood levels of alcohol (over 200–300 mg/dl) that would deeply intoxicate inexperienced drinkers. Higher doses of ethanol produce intoxication symptoms in rats that cannot be reversed with Ro15-4315, indicating other effects of ethanol not directly involving the GABA$_A$ receptor–chloride channel.[5] Tolerance to these very high levels is only partial, and alcoholics can certainly die of respiratory depression from very high doses of alcohol.

Prolonged ethanol use also induces pharmacokinetic tolerance, in part by induction of the ethanol-metabolizing cytochrome P450 isoenzyme, p450j or p450IIE1.[8] This enzyme system also metabolizes a number of drugs, which may increase their clearance or hepatotoxicity (Table 50-4). Alcohol-tolerant individuals may metabolize alcohol as much as 30% faster than nondrinkers, although this is difficult to study given the large interindividual variation in alcohol metabolic rates. Lastly, it is becoming clear that expectancy (i.e., the anticipation of drinking ethanol) alters the biologic response of ethanol. Drinkers develop conditioned tolerance to drinking in familiar environments.

MECHANISMS OF DEPENDENCE AND WITHDRAWAL

Alcohol withdrawal is thought to be a consequence of the adaptation of neuronal membranes. During ethanol withdrawal, the increased rigidity of the membrane may interfere with GABAergic transmission. This alteration in inhibitory neural systems results in CNS and sympathetic nervous system overactivity. The results are stereotyped: in the first day or two, tremor, sweating, flushing, and tachycardia occur. Ten to twenty percent of individuals experience hallucinations during withdrawal. Seizures occur in the first 24 to 48 hours and are followed by delirium tremens in a minority of patients. This delirium is characterized by hallucinations and evidence of severe sympathetic overactivity. The proposed interaction between ethanol and the GABA receptor is consistent with the efficacy of barbiturates or benzodiazepines in preventing alcohol withdrawal. These drugs both augment GABAergic transmission and facilitate inhibition of the nervous system. They prevent delirium but do not ameliorate it after it is fully developed.

CLINICAL FEATURES AND DIAGNOSIS

The risk of experiencing alcohol-related problems is quite high in western cultures. (See ch 61, 88, and 89 for discussions of the effects of alcohol on stomach and pancreas.) The lifetime risk is 19% to 25% for men and 4% to 6% for women. Although about 20% to 45% of skid-row, homeless individuals are alcoholic, they account for only 7% of all alcoholics.[1] The risk of alcoholism

---

TABLE 50-4
Drug–Alcohol Interactions

Increased Clearance	Increased Hepatotoxicity
Meprobamate	Vitamin A
Pentobarbital	Isoniazide
Tolbutamide	Acetaminophen
Propranolol	Nitrosamines
Rifampin	Carbon tetrachloride
Warfarin	Cocaine
Phenytoin	
Isoniazide	**Synergistic Effects**
	Barbiturates
Antabuselike Reactions	Benzodiazepines
Metronidazole	Narcotics (includes diphenoxylate)
Chloramphenicol	
Griseofulvin	
Sulfonylureas	

involves a genetic component. Cloninger has delineated two groups of alcoholics based on adoption studies of children of alcoholics.[9] Type I alcoholics are men or women with a predisposition to alcoholism that requires environmental factors to precipitate drinking problems. Type II alcoholism is limited to men who also have antisocial personality characteristics. Sons of type II alcoholics have a ninefold increase in risk of becoming alcoholics compared with the general population. They also have abnormalities in electroencephalographic event-related potential measurements that antedate alcohol use. Because there are over 28 million children of alcoholics in the U.S.,[1] there is great impetus for research into biologic markers for risk of alcoholism.

The features of the alcohol dependence syndrome are given in Table 50-5.[10] The most important diagnostic tool is simply asking the patient and members of the family carefully about alcohol use and any difficulties related to it. The CAGE test is a simple, non-threatening question list[11]: the patient is asked if he has felt the need to *Cut* down on drinking, if he is *Annoyed* by questions about his drinking behavior, if he feels *Guilty* about his drinking and its effects, and if he needs an *Eye-opener* (an early morning drink) to feel better. Positive answers to two or more questions is highly suggestive of occult alcohol abuse, with a 93% sensitivity and 76% specificity. In addition, increased values of blood tests such as the mean corpuscular volume, uric acid, triglycerides, or γ-glutamyl transpeptidase should alert the physician to the possibility of alcohol abuse.[12] Unfortunately, there is no widely available biochemical test to quantify drinking behavior. Two promising markers are acetaldehyde-protein adducts and carbohydrate-deficient transferrin. The adducts form in liver[13] and blood from the condensation of acetaldehyde with proteins. Carbohydrate-deficient transferrin is formed in the liver of heavy drinkers and can be detected immunologically or electrophoretically. The test seems to be highly specific for alcohol consumption in excess of 60 g per day and has a sensitivity of about 90%.[14]

TABLE 50-5
Alcohol Dependence Syndrome

1. Narrowing of the drinking repertoire
   With increased severity of dependence, there is little variability of drinking pattern between drinking days and occasions.
2. Salience of drinking behavior
   Negative social, family, and/or health consequences will not deter drinking behavior. Highest priority is given to securing alcohol.
3. Subjective awareness of a compulsion to drink
   Severely dependent alcoholics are aware of an impaired capacity for moderate drinking. In the past, this characteristic was called "loss of control" drinking; in some cultures, it is characterized by an inability to abstain.
4. Tolerance
   With increased severity of dependence, and prior to the development of severe liver damage, alcoholics are less sensitive to the effects of alcohol.
5. Physical dependence
6. Relief avoidance drinking
   With increased severity of dependence, drinking occurs earlier in the day (e.g., upon awakening) in order to avoid the discomfort of "morning-after" symptoms.
7. Rapid reinstatement of the syndrome with recurrent drinking

From Meyer RE, Kranzler HR. Alcoholism: Clinical implications of recent research. J Clin Psychiatry 1988;49(suppl):8.

TREATMENT

The treatment of alcoholism includes detoxification and long-term help in maintaining sobriety. Detoxification may be performed outside the hospital for patients who do not have major medical illnesses or severe withdrawal symptoms (i.e., delirium tremens or seizures).[15] A current practice for the rehabilitation phase is inpatient hospitalization with intensive counseling, behavior modification, and involvement with Alcoholics Anonymous and other support groups. However, the outcome for therapy seems to be better predicted by characteristics of the patient rather than the specific type of therapy. Individuals with intact support (married, stable job, no antecedent psychopathology, middle- to upper-class) have abstinence rates of up to 60% at 12 to 18 months after treatment, while unemployed individuals in the lower economic class have only a 30% abstinence rate. Even without any therapy, about 20% of individuals will achieve abstinence. There is great interest in developing tests to monitor alcohol consumption during treatment. Acetaldehyde-protein adducts or carbohydrate-deficient transferrin may be useful in the future.

Much attention has been directed toward discovering pharmacologic agents that will reduce the craving for alcohol.[16] Certainly in those alcoholics with coexistent psychiatric diagnoses, such as schizophrenia, affective disorders, or anxiety disorders, therapy for the psychiatric disorder is indicated. Lithium, benzodiazepines, bromocriptine, and even opiates have been shown to reduce alcohol consumption in animals, and lithium and benzodiazepines have been used in humans, albeit without dramatic success. Serotonin uptake inhibitors, such as fluoxetine and zimelidine, reduce alcohol drinking in rodent models and have been somewhat effective in the small number of human subjects tested. Alcohol-sensitizing drugs (disulfiram [Antabuse] and cyanamide) have been used for many years to modify drinking behavior. These drugs, as well as some used for other reasons (Table 50-4), inhibit aldehyde dehydrogenase. The consumption of ethanol while using these drugs results in the accumulation of acetaldehyde and a dysphoric reaction consisting of nausea, tachycardia, facial flushing, and hypotension. The theoretic basis for this form of therapy is firm: Japanese with the alcohol-flush reaction have a genetic deficiency in aldehyde dehydrogenase and have a very low risk of becoming alcoholic.[17] However, in the largest controlled trial, with over 200 patients in each group,[18] disulfiram, placebo disulfiram (1-mg tablets), and control groups had nearly identical 1-year abstinence rates (approximately 20%).

Sedative-Hypnotics

This class of drugs is represented by the barbiturates and benzodiazepines. Although initially used for sedation, they are now more commonly used for anxiety. As many as 15% of the American population uses benzodiazepines in a given year. Both classes of drugs interact with the benzodiazepine–barbiturate–GABA$_A$ receptor–chloride channel, and they facilitate the inhibitory action of GABA. This explains the dangerous interaction between alcohol and these sedatives (Table 50-4). Behavioral effects of these drugs include emotional lability, loquacity, slurred speech, and ataxia. Occasionally the drugs induce a delirium with incoherence, disorientation, and disturbances of perception.[4] As is the case for alcohol, an initial phase of stimulation may occur as a result of disinhibition; this may lead to violent or unexpected behavior. It is of interest that users of benzodiazepines develop tolerance to the sedative effects of the drugs but not to the anxiolytic effects. It is well known that barbiturates induce hepatic microsomal enzymes that metabolize these drugs. The benzodiazepines are much less potent inducers of the microsomal enzymes. Pharmacodynamic tolerance to the effects of the drugs is partial. Dependence upon barbiturates can occur in about a month of use of high doses; benzodiazepine dependence requires substantially longer use, probably on the order of 20 weeks. Withdrawal from these drugs causes tremor, hyperreflexia, anxiety, and, in severe cases, seizures. Barbiturate withdrawal in particular can be as dangerous as delirium tremens and shares the intense sympathetic overactivity. Withdrawal is accomplished by reducing the dose of the barbiturate or benzodiazepine by about 10% per day.

Opiates

PHARMACOLOGY

Opiate abuse is probably as old as alcohol abuse. *Opion* is the Greek word for juice of the opium poppy, from which morphine is derived. Repeated efforts have been made to modify the opiate structure to eliminate its abuse potential; notable failures include heroin and methadone. The action of opiates and the mechanism of withdrawal from them are rather well understood.[19] Opiates act through CNS receptors that normally interact with endogenous peptides called enkephalins and endorphins. At least five classes of opioid receptors have been distinguished: μ, κ, σ, δ, and ϵ. μ

receptors have high affinity for morphine, other alkaloid opiates, and β-endorphin and mediate the euphoric and addictive effects of opiates. These compounds inhibit neural activity by increasing K^+ conductance, resulting in relaxation and euphoria (Table 50-6). The reported effects of intravenous opiates are an initial intense euphoria followed by a dreamlike, tranquil state. Heroin is the drug of abuse in over 90% of narcotic addicts; however, codeine and oxycodone are commonly prescribed by internists and are widely abused. Underground chemists have modified the anesthetic fentanyl, producing 3-methyl-fentanyl, an opiate with over a thousand-fold greater potency than morphine and a high risk of overdose. Fentanyl is not detected on usual toxicology screening tests. A modification of meperidine produced methylphenyl-tetrahydropyridine (MTPT), which destroys dopaminergic neurons in the substantia nigra and caused an outbreak of toxic parkinsonism on the West Coast.[20]

MECHANISMS OF TOLERANCE AND WITHDRAWAL

Tolerance to the effects of opiates varies with the effect considered: no tolerance is observed for the production of miosis or constipation. Thus, requests of patients treated with codeine for diarrhea do not indicate tolerance to the drug but either worsening of the underlying disease or abuse of the drug. Forty-five milligrams of codeine, 5 mg of diphenoxylate, and 2 mg of loperamide are approximately equal in their constipating effects. Chronic use of opiates does not reduce the number of opiate receptors on neurons; tolerance appears to be due to uncoupling of the receptor from the K^+ conductance. The noradrenergic neurons of the locus cae-

TABLE 50-6
Pharmacologic Actions of Drugs of Abuse

DRUG	ACTION
Depressants	
Ethanol	Fluidize membranes (ethanol), induce P450 (ethanol and barbiturates)
Barbiturates	Facilitate Cl^- conductance by effects on $GABA_A$–barbiturate–benzodiazepine
Benzodiazepines	receptor–Cl^- channel
Opiates	Interact with opioid receptors; μ receptors increase K^+ conductance
Cannabis	Unknown
Stimulants	
Cocaine	Blocks uptake of dopamine and norepinephrine
Amphetamines	Release norepinephrine, inhibit monoamine uptake, activate serotonergic and dopaminergic receptors
Phencyclidine	Blocks dopamine uptake, increases dopamine release, anticholinergic, interacts with σ opioid receptors
Hallucinogens	Sympathomimetic, inhibit serotonergic neurons
Nicotine	Activates ganglionic nicotinic receptors
Anabolic Steroids	Activate muscle and CNS (?) androgen receptors, increase growth hormone (?)
Laxatives	Stimulate intestinal movement and secretion
	Mechanisms not clearly established
Diuretics	Inhibit electrolyte reabsorption in renal tubules

ruleus become tolerant to opiates, and within 10 hours of stopping a short-acting drug like heroin, these neurons become hyperactive.[19] Fully developed withdrawal symptoms include lacrimation, rhinorrhea, dilated pupils, piloerection (hence the term "cold turkey"), sweating, yawning, hypertension, tachycardia, and fever. The appearance of hallucinations, tremor, or delirium is not typical and suggests that the patient is also withdrawing from another drug.

TREATMENT

It is documented that making patients experience severe withdrawal symptoms does not enhance their ability to remain abstinent in the future. Withdrawal can be blocked by the use of the central adrenergic agonist clonidine, given in 0.1- to 0.3-mg doses four times a day. This drug acts on presynaptic receptors and inhibits neural activity in the locus caeruleus.[21] Subsequent opiate use can be blocked by chronic use of the orally active opiate antagonist naltrexone. Unfortunately, these patients, or those maintained on methadone, often abuse other drugs whose actions are not blocked by naltrexone or methadone, especially alcohol and cocaine. It is of interest that naloxone has been reported to increase fecal output in a few patients with idiopathic constipation and intestinal pseudo-obstruction. Of the opiates used for the treatment of diarrhea, loperamide has the advantage of a very low incidence of CNS effects, due in part to its concentration in the gastrointestinal tract. Very high doses of loperamide have been used in an uncontrolled fashion for severe diarrhea; responses to these doses may not be mediated by the opioid receptors. Diphenoxylate at doses only five times the usual dose can induce opiate dependence, and overdose causes the usual features of a narcotic overdose. For this reason, atropine was added to diphenoxylate (Lomotil) to reduce the likelihood of abuse.

Cocaine and Other Stimulants

The abuse of cocaine has accelerated in the last several years, predominantly because of the increased use of free-base cocaine (crack), which is smoked. Crack is available at quite low prices relative to other illicit drugs of abuse. Cocaine offers a good example of the dissociation of addictive potential from the induction of physical dependence. Cocaine does induce tolerance, but the withdrawal syndrome is relatively mild. Nonetheless, smoking of crack seems capable of dominating an individual's life and interests within a rather short period of time, certainly less time than for alcohol abuse. Thus, it may have the highest abuse potential of any drug in current use. The effects of amphetamines are generally similar to those of cocaine.

PHARMACOLOGY

Cocaine can be absorbed from the lungs, gastrointestinal tract, and nasal mucosa. The first-pass metabolism of cocaine to benzoylegconine and methoxyegconine by the liver renders the oral route impractical and is responsible for the short half-life of cocaine taken by more direct routes (20–40 minutes after a dose). Cocaine hydrochloride is used nasally (snorting) or intravenously. Cocaine

free-base is now cheaply made from the salt by treatment with sodium bicarbonate and is vaporized by heating in a pipe. It is absorbed from the pulmonary circulation and reaches the brain even faster than after injection. Amphetamines are taken orally or intravenously. Cocaine and amphetamines produce intense feelings of euphoria and well-being.

The neuronal effects of cocaine are biphasic. It initially blocks the reuptake of norepinephrine and especially dopamine, increasing the concentrations of these transmitters in the synaptic cleft. The euphoric effect of cocaine appears to require an intact dopaminergic pathway between the ventral tegmental area and the nucleus accumbens.[19] Presynaptic feedback subsequently reduces the release of these transmitters and leads to increases in postsynaptic receptor numbers after chronic use. It is postulated that this late decrease in neurotransmitter concentration induces postcocaine dysphoria (crash) and may facilitate craving for and dependence on the drug. Amphetamines release norepinephrine in the CNS, inhibit monoamine uptake, and possibly activate serotonergic and dopaminergic receptors (Table 50-6). Users of amphetamines and cocaine increase their doses to achieve euphoric effects, indicating the development of tolerance. The sympathetic effects are predictable: pupillary dilation, tachycardia, and hypertension. To reduce these side effects, stimulant users commonly use other drugs with relaxing properties, such as alcohol, marijuana, barbiturates, or benzodiazepines. Amphetamines can produce hallucinations and a delirium that persists beyond the duration of intoxication. Several other amphetamine derivatives are used on the street. These include methylenedioxyamphetamine (MDA), methylenedioxymethamphetamine (MDMA), paramethoxyamphetamine (PMA), methylenedioxyethylamphetamine (MDEA), and methyldimethoxyamphetamine (DOM). Typically, intoxication with these compounds leads to sympathetic stimulation and hallucinations. Stimulant users are at risk for cardiac arrhythmia, acute hypertensive crises, and seizures, which may account for an occasional sudden death. A rare form of necrotizing angiitis is associated with intravenous amphetamine use.

Withdrawal from these drugs produces a mild physical abstinence syndrome characterized by depression, fatigue, disturbed sleep with increased dreaming, and intense craving. Craving can also be elicited by conditioned cues (i.e., environmental stimuli that the abuser associates with psychic effects of the drug). Responses to conditioned cues appear to persist much longer than the physical abstinence syndrome.

THERAPY

Stimulant abusers are often treated as outpatients because of the relatively mild withdrawal syndrome. Complete abstinence is deemed essential and is documented by mandatory urine testing. The craving for cocaine is treated by intensive counseling and may be helped by pharmacologic therapy. The use of tricyclic antidepressants has been best studied.[21–23] By blocking reuptake of amine transmitters, tricyclics may reduce the mood effects of withdrawal. Other drugs, including bromocriptine, methylphenidate, and lithium, have been tried, but controlled clinical trials have not yet been reported. Another form of treatment is extinction therapy. It consists of allowing the patient to watch videotapes depicting the use of cocaine or to handle drug paraphernalia without the reward of cocaine. It is hoped that this treatment will extinguish conditioned cues.

Cannabis

The active constituent of marijuana is Δ9-tetrahydrocannabinol, THC. THC causes euphoria, relaxation, subjective intensification of perception, alteration of the sense of time, and impaired psychomotor function. THC also causes vasodilation (which is responsible for tachycardia and conjunctival injection) and stimulation of appetite. Cannabis dependence is recognized by DSM-III-R,[3] and withdrawal symptoms of restlessness, insomnia, and nausea have been observed. Patients with prior histories of schizophrenia have increased risk of precipitating psychosis if they use cannabis. Attacks of anxiety or paranoia occur in about 5% of episodes of cannabis use. Prolonged use of cannabis is reported to result in an "amotivational syndrome" characterized by preoccupation with drug use, passivity, and decreased drive and memory.

Phencyclidine

This compound (PCP) was originally used as an anesthetic but was discontinued because of delirium that occurred in about 10% of patients awakening from the drug. It can be taken by any route but is commonly smoked. The pharmacologic actions of phencyclidine include (Table 50-6): inhibition of dopamine reuptake (similar to the action of cocaine), stimulation of dopamine release, blockade of cholinergic receptors, and possibly interaction with sigma opioid receptors (which may account for its analgesic action). Inhibition of proprioceptive afferents may explain the sensation of weightlessness reported by users. Animal studies document that phencyclidine can produce tolerance and a withdrawal syndrome that includes auditory-induced seizures. It produces euphoria at low doses and stimulation of the sympathetic nervous system, hyperactivity, and hallucinations at higher doses. The hallucinations are frequently auditory, and the behavior of the abuser can closely resemble that of schizophrenics. It can cause paranoia and violent behavior. Intoxication is notable for vertical and horizontal nystagmus, evidence of sympathetic overactivity, numbness and increased pain threshold, ataxia, and dysarthria. Phencyclidine is sometimes sold as LSD or psilocybin on the street. It can be synthesized rather easily; a related compound PHP is synthesized from pyrrolidine instead of pyridine and cannot be detected in urine screening assays.

Hallucinogens

Hallucinogens may be decreasing in popularity. Currently available drugs include lysergic acid diethylamide (LSD), PCP, and amphetamine derivatives. All hallucinogens are sympathomimetic, producing hypertension, pupillary dilation, tachycardia, and hyperreflexia, as well as disturbances of perception. They carry the risk of loss of control, flashbacks (transient re-experiencing of previous drug-induced perceptions), and terrifying hallucinations ("bad trips"). Hallucinogens offer an interesting example of dissociation of tolerance and dependence; tolerance appears to develop rapidly (after three to four doses) by unknown mechanisms, but there appears to be little physical or psychic dependence or craving. It is of interest that LSD suppresses serotonergic neurons in the raphe nuclei, which are also suppressed during REM sleep. Perhaps hallucinogens act upon the normal neuroanatomic substrates of dreams (Table 50-6).

Laboratory Detection of Substance Abuse

Recent alcohol use can be detected by analysis of breath, blood, or urine. Alcohol is eliminated at about 100 mg/kg/h, but this rate varies by two- to threefold between individuals. The need for a test for chronic alcohol abuse was discussed earlier in this chapter. Detection of the other drugs can be divided into two phases—screening and confirmation.[24,25] Routine toxicologic screening tests (usually using thin-layer chromatography), which are used for patients suspected of taking a drug overdose, are less sensitive than the immunologic tests. More sensitive tests include immunologic tests (radioimmunoassay or enzyme-multiplied immunoassay technique [EMIT]) and gas chromatographic methods. The EMIT tests are the most widely available and are inexpensive. Confirmation is generally by GC-mass spectrometry, which is nearly absolutely specific and extremely sensitive. The detection of drug abuse also entails careful collection of the urine sample (to prevent substitution or adulteration of the specimen) and attention to the "chain of custody" required to prove that a given patient was in fact using the drug detected. It must be recalled that urine testing requires informed consent of individuals over 18 years of age except in medical emergencies.

Δ9-THC and PCP are lipophilic and can be detected in the urine for several days after a single use. Cocaine metabolites can be detected for up to 48 hours after use; freezing of the urine is recommended if the analysis cannot be performed rapidly. Urinary LSD can be detected by radioimmunoassay. The detection of amphetamines and PCP is complicated by cross-reactions with over-the-counter medications. Occasional false-positives have been observed for PCP tests when the patient uses the decongestant combinations Rondec or Dimetapp. Several sympathomimetics can give positive results on amphetamine screening: ephedrine, pseudoephedrine, phenylpropanolamine, phentermine hydrochloride, fenfluramine hydrochloride, and others.[25] Tests for opiates may give positive results if the patient has consumed poppy seeds. Dextromethorphan (in Robitussin DM) does not give a false-positive result at usual doses.[25] Surreptitious use of diuretics can be detected by measuring blood furosemide or urinary thiazide concentrations.

Management of Acute Drug Overdose or Toxicity

The information summarized in Table 50-7 illustrates the effects of several classes of drugs of abuse. Obviously, it is important to ensure that the apparently intoxicated individual does not have an additional medical problem, such as alcoholic hypoglycemia, head injury, meningitis, Wernicke's encephalopathy, seizures, intracranial bleeding, or hepatic coma. Generally, patients in coma need circulatory and respiratory support, and care to avoid pressure complications. A specific diagnosis needs to be made if possible. Any suspicion of opiate overdose warrants a trial of naloxone, 0.4 mg intravenously. Specific antagonists are not otherwise available. Multiple drug use and attempted suicide or homocide should be

TABLE 50-7
Recognition of Drug Intoxication and Overdose

DRUG	SYMPTOMS OF INTOXICATION	SPECIAL CONSIDERATIONS
Depressants	Somnolence, dysarthria, ataxia, nystagmus	Alcoholic hypoglycemia
Alcohol		Multidrug use
Sedatives		Ethylene glycol or methanol poisoning
Opiates	Miosis, shallow coma, depressed respirations	Reverse with naloxone
		Normal pupils with propoxyphene, dilated with meperidine
		Pulmonary edema
Cannabis	Conjunctival injection, tachycardia	Panic attacks
		Toxic psychosis
Stimulants	Hypertension, tachycardia, agitation, paranoia, hallucinations, seizures, mydriasis, hyperthermia	
Cocaine		
Amphetamines		Adsorb with charcoal
Phencyclidine (PCP)		Vertical nystagmus
		Coma with open eyes
		Mimics mania, schizophrenia
		Excretion increased in acid urine
Hallucinogens		Street ''LSD'' may be PCP

kept in mind. Seizures, agitation, or delirium from cocaine, stimulants, and PCP may be managed with diazepam or haloperidol and by reducing sensory stimulation.

ABUSE OF OTHER COMPOUNDS AND EATING DISORDERS

Tobacco

Tobacco use is extremely common; perhaps 30% of adult Americans smoke or use other forms of tobacco. It has major implications for health. For the gastroenterologist, tobacco use predisposes to cancer of the upper gastrointestinal tract and is a major reason for failure of peptic ulcer healing. The major pharmacologic compound in tobacco is nicotine.[26] This alkaloid is absorbed from the oral mucosa (in the cases of cigar and pipe smoking and the use of chewing tobacco or snuff) or lungs. Smokers have the remarkable ability to unconsciously regulate the amount of nicotine they absorb by altering how they smoke. As a result, nicotine intake is not reduced very much by the use of low-nicotine cigarettes or by reduction in the number of cigarettes smoked per day.[26] The major actions of nicotine are an increase in sympathetic outflow, resulting in an acceleration of heart rate, and a general mental arousal. Stimulation of Renshaw cells may result in muscle relaxation because of inhibition of anterior horn cells. Tolerance to the effects of nicotine on the brain, although partial, occurs very rapidly (within several hours), and a withdrawal syndrome is well recognized. The symptoms include restlessness, irritability, anxiety, impatience, and inability to concentrate. It is of interest that these symptoms can be ameliorated by clonidine.[27] This finding suggests the involvement of noradrenergic systems in the craving of tobacco as well as opiates. Another way to reduce the withdrawal syndrome is to substitute nicotine chewing gum for cigarettes. Controlled trials of the gum, used in combination with other behavior modification counseling, have shown an improvement in quitting smoking (27%) compared with placebo (18%). Of interest, many individuals appear to become dependent upon the gum and are unable to quit chewing. There is no information to indicate whether use of nicotine gum influences healing rates in peptic disease. Another effect of smoking, probably not mediated by nicotine, is the induction of hepatic drug–metabolizing enzymes. Smokers have increased rates of metabolism of imipramine, desmethyldiazepam, lidocaine, oxazepam, pentazocine, propranolol, and theophylline. It is important to recognize that this altered metabolic rate will decline toward normal within a week or two of abstinence, which may require a change in drug dosing during a hospitalization.

Anabolic Steroids

Perhaps a million athletes, mostly males, use anabolic steroids to augment their training, particularly in power sports such as weight lifting and football.[28] Very recently, steroid use has emerged among teenaged boys who simply wish to improve their appearance. A number of commonly used steroids are listed in Table 50-8; some are veterinary preparations. It has not been easy to document the efficacy of these drugs; nonetheless, the use of high doses of anabolic steroids in combination with intensive physical conditioning probably increases lean muscle mass and strength. It is not clear how the drugs work: they may induce an anabolic state by interaction with skeletal muscle androgen receptors, block the catabolic effects of corticosteroids by antagonizing the glucocorticoid receptors, or increase aggressiveness and therefore make training more effective. There is also evidence that growth hormone secretion is increased in some individuals using the drugs.

Typically, these drugs are used in cycles of 4 to 12 weeks during heavy training. Several drugs are used together ("stacking"). Oral androgens, alkylated at the C-17 position to prevent first-pass metabolism by the liver, are taken daily, and injectable steroids are taken daily to weekly. The doses used are often orders of magnitude greater than doses used for other clinical conditions. There may be substantial differences in the side effects of the drugs given continuously (for medical indications) or intermittently (for athletic training), and in fact many of the side effects described below have mainly been observed in patients receiving long-term androgen therapy.

The liver may be affected by any of the C-17 alkyl androgens.[29] Typical problems include abnormalities of dye excretion and, much more rarely, jaundice. Surprisingly, this occurs with low levels of alkaline phosphatase and mild increases in transaminases. It appears to be reversible in all cases. Of greater concern is the development of liver cell hyperplasia, liver cell adenoma, hepatocellular carcinoma, and angiosarcoma of the liver. There have been instances of liver malignancies that have regressed with discontinuation of the steroid, which strongly implicates them in the pathogenesis of the tumor. A very unusual disorder is peliosis hepatis, in which blood-filled cysts appear in communication with the sinusoids. It can cause death by rupture of the cysts and bleeding. The cardiovascular system may be affected by the use of the steroids. LDL (low-density lipoproteins) cholesterol increases, while HDL (high-density lipoproteins) cholesterol decreases. This usually reverts to normal within months of stopping the drugs. The long-term effects are as yet unknown, but there have been case reports of myocardial infarction and stroke in athletes using steroids. Endocrine effects of the steroids are many. Gonadotropins are greatly diminished by the use of the androgens, a fact used to prove that

TABLE 50-8
Anabolic Steroids Used by Athletes

Bolasterone	Methyltestosterone†
Boldenone*‡	Nandrolone‡
Clostebol	Norethandrolone
Dehydrochlormethyltestosterone	Oxandrolone†
Fluoxymesterone	Oxymesterone
Mesterolone	Oxymetholone†
Methandienone†	Stanozolol†‡
Methenolone‡	Testosterone‡
Methandrostenolone†‡	Trienbolone*‡

* *Veterinary preparation*
† *Orally active*
‡ *Used parenterally*

TABLE 50-9
DSM-III-R Diagnostic Criteria for Bulimia Nervosa

A. Recurrent episodes of binge eating (rapid consumption of a large amount of food in a discrete period of time)
B. Feeling of a lack of control over eating behavior during the eating binges
C. The person regularly engages in either self-induced vomiting, use of laxatives or diuretics, strict dieting or fasting, or vigorous exercise in order to prevent weight gain
D. A minimum average of two binge-eating episodes a week for at least 3 months
E. Persistent overconcern with body shape and weight

American Psychiatric Association: Diagnostic and Statistical Manual of Mental Disorders. Third Edition, Revised. Washington, DC, American Psychiatric Association, 1987.

the presence of steroid metabolites in the urine of an athlete is the result of chronic usage. As a result, testicular atrophy and decreased spermatogenesis are common, although probably reversible. Plasma sex hormone–binding globulin and thyroxine binding–globulin are substantially decreased, estradiol is increased (probably from aromatization of some of the androgens), and circulating thyroxine and triiodothyronine levels are low. This probably does not reflect tissue thyroid hormone deficiency, because TSH (thyroid-stimulating hormone) levels are also decreased. Cortisol levels are normal. Marked increases in growth hormone levels have been observed in individuals taking these drugs. The adverse effects of these drugs are most pronounced in adolescent boys who may undergo premature closure of the epiphyses, and in women who may have irreversible deepening of the voice, clitoromegaly, hirsutism, and male-pattern baldness.

Lastly, the use of androgenic steroids probably induces neuropsychiatric disturbances. Several surveys have uncovered significant mood changes and some evidence of psychotic episodes during steroid use. Aggressive behavior appears to be common. There is even a suggestion that the steroids have an addictive potential, due to dysphoria and depression that can follow the cycle of steroid use or occur after discontinuation of the drugs.

Steroid abuse is easy to suspect because of the muscular development of the patient. It should be considered in young athletes with hypercholesterolemia, abnormal liver tests or hepatomegaly, and psychiatric disturbances. Needle marks are often visible on the thighs or buttocks of these patients. The use of the drugs can be further documented by detection of the steroid or metabolites in the urine by GC-mass spectrometry and measurement of serum gonadotropins.

Bulimia and Laxative and Diuretic Abuse

In the last decade, several disorders of eating behavior have been recognized and are rather prevalent.[30] These include anorexia nervosa and several variants of binge eating variously called bulimia ("ox hunger"), bulimia nervosa, or bulimarexia (Table 50-9). Anorexia nervosa usually is not difficult to diagnose because the patients have substantial weight loss (>15% of premorbid body weight). This disorder is discussed further in Chapter 32. On the other hand, bulimia patients are usually near ideal body weight, although they consider themselves to be overweight. Strictly defined, bulimia is binge eating; the term bulimarexia is applied to patients who seek to control the results of the binge by self-induced vomiting, or laxative or diuretic abuse. The term bulimia will be used here to include those individuals who binge and purge; they are susceptible to drug as well as food overuse.

The prevalence of bulimia may be quite high. Estimates have ranged as high as 40% of college-age women and 10% of college-age men; lower prevalences of perhaps 3% have been reported from a family planning clinic in Britain. It is largely a disorder of young white women. The eating and purging practices are almost always secretive; hence the true prevalence is unknown. The average patient is about 25 years old and has been binging for 7 years. Around 88% of bulimic patients induce vomiting, 61% abuse laxatives, 50% use over-the-counter diet pills (typically sympathomimetics), 33% use diuretics for weight loss, and 64% report chewing food and spitting it out.[31] Over one third self-report problems with alcohol or drug abuse. Presenting complaints are nonspecific and include weakness, abdominal pain and bloating, sore throat, and puffy cheeks. It is certainly worth suspecting an eating disorder in young women with the following signs or laboratory abnormalities[32]: enlarged salivary glands, erosion of the dental enamel on the lingual side of the teeth (from exposure to hydrochloric acid), conjunctival hemorrhage or ecchymosis of the neck and face (from vomiting), and Russell's sign (scarring of the first metacarpophalangeal joint of the dominant hand from inducing vomiting); hypokalemia, metabolic alkalosis, and chronic diarrhea (Table 50-10). Abnormal electrolytes are found in about half of the patients, most commonly the bicarbonate level. Hypokalemia and dehydration may rarely result in chronic renal impairment. Diuretic abuse can be suspected from hypokalemia and confirmed by blood or urine testing for furosemide and thiazides. Gastrointestinal complications of bulimia and purging include esophagitis, Mallory–Weiss tears, Boerhaave's syndrome (esophageal rupture), gastric dilation or rupture, dilation of the duodenum or proximal jejunum, elevated serum amylase in as many as 28% (either from the salivary glands or the pancreas), melanosis coli, and cathartic colon. Rarely, these patients use other medications such as thyroid hormone preparations in an attempt to lose weight. The use of syrup of ipecac (emetine) to induce vomiting has been linked to the development of skeletal and cardiac myopathy. Both anorectic and bulimic patients seem to have a higher than average risk of suicide. The therapy of these patients is based upon psychologic counseling and antidepressants. They are probably best managed by referral to a psychiatrist or to a primary care physician working with a psychologist. Several placebo-controlled, double-blinded studies have demonstrated the effectiveness of tricyclic antidepressants for bulimia.[33,34]

Laxative abusers are also predominantly female. No systematic studies have been undertaken to determine the frequency of bulimia among laxative abusers, but the detection of laxative abuse should strongly suggest bulimia.[31] The laxatives may be taken to reduce distention following a binge, or because of the perception that dehydration following their use speeds weight loss. Careful studies of the effectiveness of cathartics in weight control show at most about a 10% reduction in energy absorption, and reviews of dietary intake and body weight of vomiters and purgers demonstrate that the purgers ate significantly less and weighed more than the vomiters.[35] It is puzzling that patients abuse laxatives and yet consult physicians for diarrhea. The typical case is a woman with several complaints, commonly weakness, nausea or vomiting, diarrhea or constipation, and abdominal pain. Cutaneous signs such as clubbing, skin eruptions (from phenolphthalein use), and hyperpigmentation have also been observed.[36] These patients have often been examined repeatedly by many physicians, without a diagnosis having been made. In fact, laxative abuse is one of the more common causes of chronic unexplained diarrhea referred to a university medical center.[37] The diagnosis rests upon detection of the laxative in the stool (alkalinization to detect phenolphthalein) or urine (bisacodyl, danthron, rhein, and phenolphthalein); methods are available for the determination of the latter by thin-layer chromatography.[38] In some cases, a room search may be necessary. Although it is important to make this diagnosis to prevent unnecessary testing, long-term improvement in these patients is not often seen.

The reader is directed to Chapter 27, Psychosocial Factors in the Care of Patients with Gastrointestinal Disease; and Chapter 130, Psychiatric Evaluation and Management in Gastrointestinal Illness.

TABLE 50-10
Medical Complications of Bulimia

Gastrointestinal

Enamel erosion, parotid gland enlargement, increased amylase, esophagitis, esophageal rupture, gastric dilation, pancreatitis, cathartic colon, melanosis coli

Chest

Aspiration, pneumomediastinum

Cardiac

Dehydration, arrhythmia (secondary to hypokalemia), ipecac toxicity

Metabolic

Dehydration, metabolic alkalosis, hypochloremia, hypokalemia, hyponatremia

Skin

Calluses (fingers, hands), eruptions due to laxatives or diuretics

REFERENCES

1. Sixth Special Report to the U.S. Congress on Alcohol and Health, January 1987. U.S. Department of Health and Human Services, Public Health Service; Alcohol, Drug Abuse and Mental Health Administration, National Institute on Alcohol Abuse and Alcoholism.
2. Eddy NB, Halbach H, Isbell H, Seevers MH. Drug dependence: Its significance and characteristics. Bull World Health Organ 1965;32: 721.
3. Diagnostic and statistical manual of mental disorders. 3rd ed, revised. Washington, DC, American Psychiatric Association, 1987.
4. Senay EC. Substance abuse disorders in clinical practice. Boston: John Wright PSG, 1983.
5. Suzdak PD, Glowa JR, Crawley JN, Schwartz RD, Skolnick P, Paul SM. A selective imidazobenzodiazepine antagonist of ethanol in the rat. Science 1986;234:1243.
6. Lister RG, Nutt DJ. Is Ro15-4513 a specific alcohol antagonist? Trends in Neurosci 1987;10:223.

7. McBride WJ, Murphy JM, Lumeng L, Li T-K. Effects of Ro15-4513, fluoxetine, and desipramine on the intake of ethanol, water and food by the alcohol-preferring (P) and –non-preferring (NP) lines of rats. Pharmacol Biochem Behav 1988;30:1045.

8. Lieber CS, DeCarli LM. Ethanol oxidation by hepatic microsomes: Adaptive increases after ethanol feeding. Science 1968;162:917.

9. Cloninger CR. Neurogenetic adaptive mechanisms in alcoholism. Science 1987;236:410.

10. Meyer RE, Kranzler HR. Alcoholism: Clinical implications of recent research. J Clin Psychiatry 1988;49(suppl):8.

11. Mayfield D, McLeod G, Hull P. The CAGE questionnaire: Validation of a new alcoholism screening instrument. Am J Psychiatry 1974;131:1121.

12. Skinner HA, Holt S, Schuller R, Roy J, Israel Y. Identification of alcohol abuse using laboratory tests and a history of trauma. Ann Intern Med 1984;101:847.

13. Lin RC, Smith RS, Lumeng L. Detection of a protein-acetaldehyde adduct in the liver of rats fed alcohol chronically. J Clin Invest 1988;81:615.

14. Stibler H, Borg S. The role of carbohydrate-deficient transferrin as a marker of high alcohol consumption. In: Kuriyama K, Takada A, Ishii H, eds. Biomedical and social aspects of alcohol and alcoholism. Amsterdam: Elsevier, 1988:503.

15. Hayashida M, Alterman AI, McLellan AT, et al. Comparative effectiveness and costs of inpatient and outpatient detoxification of patients with mild-to-moderate alcohol withdrawal syndrome. N Engl J Med 1989;320:358.

16. Sinclair JD. The feasibility of effective psychopharmacological treatments for alcoholism. Br J Addict 1987;82:1213.

17. Harada S, Agarwal DP, Goedde HW, Tagaki S, Ishikawa B. Possible protective role against alcoholism for aldehyde dehydrogenase isozyme deficiency in Japan. Lancet 1982;ii:827.

18. Fuller RK, Branchey L, Brightwell DR, et al. Disulfiram treatment of alcoholism: A Veterans Administration Cooperative Study. JAMA 1986;256:1449.

19. Koob GF, Bloom FE. Cellular and molecular mechanisms of drug dependence. Science 1988;242:715.

20. Langston JW, Ballard P, Tetrud JW, Irwin I. Chronic parkinsonism in humans due to a product of meperidine analog synthesis. Science 1983;219:979.

21. Gold MS, Dackis CA. New insights and treatments: Opiate withdrawal and cocaine addiction. Clin Ther 1984;7:6.

22. Gawin FH. Chronic neuropharmacology of cocaine: Progress in pharmacotherapy. J Clin Psychiatry 1988;49(suppl):11.

23. Horberg LK, Schnoll SN. Treatment of cocaine abuse. In: Masserman JH, ed. Current Psychiatric Therapy. Vol 22. New York: Grune & Stratton, 1983:177.

24. Gold MS, Dackis CA. Role of the laboratory in the evaluation of suspected drug abuse. J Clin Psychiatry 1988;47(suppl):17.

25. Schwartz RH. Urine testing in the detection of drugs of abuse. Arch Intern Med 1988;148:2407.

26. Benowitz NL. Pharmacologic aspects of cigarette smoking and nicotine addiction. N Engl J Med 1988;319:1318.

27. Glasman AH, Jackson WK, Walsh BT, Roose SP, Rosenfeld B. Cigarette craving, smoking withdrawal, and clonidine. Science 1984;226:864.

28. Windsor RE, Dumitru D. Anabolic steroid use by athletes. How serious are the health hazards. Postgrad Med 1988;84:37.

29. Ishak KG, Zimmerman HJ. Hepatotoxic effects of the anabolic/androgenic steroids. Semin Liver Dis 1987;7:230.

30. Caspar RC. The pathophysiology of anorexia nervosa and bulimia nervosa. Annu Rev Nutr 1986;6:299.

31. Mitchell JE, Hatsukami D, Eckert ED, Pyle RL. Characteristics of 275 patients with bulimia. Am J Psychiatry 1985;142:482.

32. Mitchell JE, Seim HC, Colon E, Pomeroy C. Medical complications and medical management of bulimia. Ann Intern Med 1987;107:71.

33. Bond WS, Crabbe S, Sanders MC. Pharmacotherapy of eating disorders: A critical review. Drug Intell Clin Pharm 1986;20:659.

34. Pope HG, Hudson JI. Antidepressant drug therapy for bulimia: Current status. J Clin Psychiatry 1986;47:339.

35. Lacey JN, Gibson E. Does laxative abuse control body weight? A comparative study of purging and vomiting bulimics. Hum Nutr Appl Nutr 1985;39A:36.

36. Slugg PH, Carey WD. Clinical features and follow-up of surreptitious laxative users. Cleve Clin Q 1984;51:167.

37. Read NW, Krejs GJ, Read JG, Santa Ana CA, Morawski SG, Fordtran JS. Chronic diarrhea of unknown origin. Gastroenterology 1980;78:264.

38. de Wolff FA, de Haas EJM, Verweij M. A screening method for establishing laxative abuse. Clin Chem 1981;27:914.

51

Advice to Travelers

EDGAR C. BOEDEKER
PATRICK W. KELLEY

GENERAL CONSIDERATIONS

An estimated 8 million Americans will travel from the industrialized world to the developing world each year. The risk of health problems and infectious diseases is greatly increased in travel to developing nations as compared to industrialized nations. Steffen and colleagues[1] determined a 15% incidence of significant health problems in Swiss travelers visiting developing countries. Diarrheal illness, particularly the self-limited syndrome known as traveler's diarrhea, is the syndrome most commonly experienced by travelers to developing nations. In addition, returning travelers may experience persistent diarrhea; thus, gastroenterologists may frequently be consulted concerning health problems related to travel.

Pretravel History

This should include considerations of destinations, a detailed itinerary, and plans or duties overseas in order to determine the relative risk of exposure to specific infectious agents or other hazardous conditions. This should be coupled with a medical history focused on determining those chronic illnesses or health conditions which might increase susceptibility to travel-related disease or render treatment or prophylaxis more difficult.

1. The itinerary should include a chronologic list of specific locales to be visited and the length of anticipated stay. Disease risk for infectious diseases varies greatly not only by country[2] but also within different regions (rural versus urban) of a country (e.g., malaria in Thailand). Thus, this type of detailed information may determine the need for prophylaxis. Travel from countries where diseases such as cholera or yellow fever are endemic may generate a governmental (administrative) demand for evidence of vaccination prior to entering certain other countries, even though the traveler may not have visited endemic areas, and even though this practice (in the case of cholera vaccination) does not conform to World Health Organization (WHO) guidelines. A list of current requirements, by country, can be found in the annual Public Health Service Publication "Health Information for International Travel."[3]

The dates and duration of travel are important considerations. Some diseases, such as traveler's diarrhea, have their peak incidence soon after arrival in an appropriate locale,[4] whereas others have a cumulative risk that increases with length of stay. Other diseases may be seasonal in incidence. Scheduling of multiple immunizations may be limited by the time available before departure. Ideally, a traveler should seek consultation at least 6 weeks prior to travel.

The types of activities to be undertaken during travel influence the risk of illness. Increased risk is associated, for example, with "adventure vacations" taken off the usual tourist routes as compared with guided tours. Self-conducted tours have an intermediate risk. Risk may also be related to the type of accommodation planned and will differ for stays in hotels (depending on standard of quality), private homes (primitive versus modern), or camps. Professional activities may expose the traveler to additional environmental risks. The extent of possible animal exposure should be evaluated along with the availability of quality medical care for prompt postexposure prophylaxis of rabies.

2. Important aspects of the medical history include the traveler's sex (considering the possibility of pregnancy, or need for breastfeeding), age (with particular attention to risks associated with extremes of age), allergies (with emphasis on drugs that might be used for prophylaxis or treatment, including vaccine constituents), immune status (including factors that might compromise systemic or mucosal defenses, such as gastrointestinal [GI] surgery, antacids or H2 blockers, asplenism, and immunosuppressing drugs or diseases), and chronic medical problems (including chronic obstructive pulmonary disease [COPD], diabetes, malabsorptive states, and G-6PD deficiency). These illnesses may be complicated during travel. They may also render individuals more susceptible to, or may complicate therapy of, travel-related illness.

The opinions expressed herein are those of the authors and not necessarily those of the United States Army or the Department of Defense.

General Advice

DEALING WITH MODES OF TRAVEL

Air Travel. This is the almost universal means of long-distance travel, and it is associated with the disruption of cycles of sleep and wakefulness known as "jet lag." It is useful to attempt to gradually shift the sleep cycle to that of the new time zone prior to departure, realizing that about 1 day of adjustment in the new environment is required for each time zone change. The short-duration benzodiazepine triazolam (Halcion) has also been recommended to adjust the sleep cycle. However, retrograde amnesia has been reported with previously recommended doses of 0.5 mg taken with alcohol on short flights.[5] This drug should be used after arrival in the time zone, or at low dose to induce sleep during flights of at least 6 hours, and alcohol should not be taken concurrently. Diets have been devised, such as the Argonne Anti–Jet Lag Diet, to readjust the cycle of food intake to correspond to breakfast time at the destination on the day of arrival.

Reduced pressures in aircraft cabins contribute to dehydration, an effect that is enhanced by alcohol. Adequate hydration should be maintained with nonalcoholic beverages. Forced inactivity on flights, together with dehydration, leads to venous stasis and increased risk of thromboembolic disease.[6] Travelers should be aware of this risk and should undertake frequent leg and body exercises and frequent walks in the aisles. In subjects at high risk, low-dose aspirin therapy should be considered. Persons with COPD may experience dyspnea at reduced oxygen tensions present in airline cabins.

Sea Travel. This form of travel may induce motion sickness. The sustained-release, dermal patch preparation of scopolamine (Transdermscop)[7] may be preferable to over-the-counter preparations such as diphenhydramine. In severe cases, promethazine HCl (Phenergan) or prochlorperazine (Compazine) may be useful in suppository form.

DRINKING WATER

Unpurified water can be the source of a variety of bacterial, viral, and parasitic pathogens. Carbonated beverages are usually safe, but bottled water cannot be relied upon. Several methods are available for disinfecting water. Water boiled for 15 minutes is safe. Water obtained from the "hot" tap if maintained at 140° to 160°F may provide some protection, but this is clearly unreliable. Instead, tap water should be disinfected by halogen treatment or filtration if boiling is not possible. Available filter kits do not reliably remove enteric viruses; however, filtration to remove particulate matter improves the efficiency of halogen treatment. Halogen treatment is also less effective in cold water. Methods for halogen treatment include the addition of:

1 tablet of iodine (tetraglycine hydroperiodide) to one quart of warm, clear water (or two tablets to cool or cloudy water) to achieve levels of 7 (or 14) ppm, or sufficient chlorine tablets (cal-

cium hypochlorite) to achieve levels between 5 and 10 ppm, as determined by a portable colorimetric kit.

MEDICAL CARE OVERSEAS

Travelers should consult with their medical insurance company prior to departure to determine the extent of their coverage during travel and to determine the need for supplemental coverage. It is advisable to contact the U.S. embassy or consulate in the country being visited to obtain recommendations for physicians, hospitals, or emergency medical services.

Travelers should take adequate supplies of their own medications as well as medications for prophylaxis and treatment of travel-associated diseases. Medications obtained overseas may differ (in name and strength) from those in the U.S. Potentially dangerous drugs may be included in over-the-counter preparations available overseas.

IMMUNOPROPHYLAXIS—DISEASES FOR WHICH IMMUNIZATION IS AVAILABLE

Some vaccines may be required by law, others are medically recommended in appropriate circumstances, and other vaccines, which are generally recommended regardless of travel, may be particularly important to the traveler. In the following sections we will discuss relevant risk factors providing indications for immunization with each of the available vaccines. Once the required and recommended vaccinations for an individual traveler are determined, a schedule of vaccination should be developed.

The vaccination schedule should take into consideration the interactions of live vaccines with each other, the interaction of live and inactivated vaccines (i.e., yellow fever and cholera vaccines), and interactions of immune serum globulin (ISG) with live vaccinations. The physician may also have to deal with the prospect of immunization with less than the recommended time before travel. When possible, live-virus vaccinations should be separated by 30 days or should be given simultaneously at separate sites. Yellow fever and cholera vaccines should be separated by a 3-week interval if possible. If both are required, the yellow fever vaccine should have priority of administration (but both should be administered in order to avoid quarantine, denial of entry, or requirement for vaccination overseas in less than optimal circumstances). To maximize the immunologic response to a live virus vaccine, avoid live virus vaccination for at least 6 weeks (and preferably 3 months) after giving ISG. Conversely, do not give ISG for 14 days after a live viral vaccine to avoid impairing the immune response. If ISG use following live viral vaccination has an overriding priority, the antiviral titer should be checked and the possibility of reimmunization at 3 months should be considered. The live virus smallpox vaccine is no longer recommended because smallpox has been eradicated.

Other factors influencing recommendations for vaccination are hypersensitivity and altered immunocompetence. Live virus vaccines (yellow fever, measles, mumps, flu) may contain egg protein. Some states of altered immunocompetence, or loss of host defense mechanisms, may increase the need for vaccination. Patients with an altered gastric barrier may have increased risk of enteric infections. However, in individuals with immune deficiency syndromes, live viral vaccines are usually contraindicated. The risk[8] to immunologically impaired close contacts of vaccinees should also be considered (e.g., with oral polio vaccine). Malaria chemoprophylaxis with chloroquine may induce some degree of immune system depression that could interfere with active immunization (e.g., against rabies).

Vaccines That May Be Required for Travel

CHOLERA

The risk of cholera in travelers is extremely low, even when visiting endemic areas. Morger and colleagues estimated an incidence of 1/500,000 for travelers to Asia or Africa.[8] Given the availability of treatment (rehydration and tetracycline), the low incidence of cholera among travelers, the relatively high reactogenicity to vaccination, and the relatively limited efficacy of the present vaccine, cholera vaccination will seldom be medically recommended for the usual tourist.[9] It may be considered for travelers who will be living and working under unsanitary conditions in highly endemic areas of the world.

Some countries (but not the U.S.) require cholera vaccination for travelers from places reporting current cholera infection in the biweekly "Summary of Health Information for International Travel" or "blue sheet" published by the Centers for Disease Control (CDC). This requirement usually does not apply to all visitors arriving from a country reporting infection but only to those travelers who have visited regions of that country where infection is reported. To satisfy this legal requirement, cholera vaccination should have been given 6 days to 6 months prior to entering the country. A single dose of vaccine will usually meet this requirement. A list of countries with this requirement is provided in the CDC publication "Health Information for International Travel."[3] Failure to satisfy these requirements may result in quarantine for up to 6 days, denial of entry, or a demand for vaccination overseas. Consult "Health Information for International Travel" for current requirements.[3]

The currently available cholera vaccine is a killed whole-cell bacterial vaccine given parenterally that causes significant local reactogenicity in 1% to 2% of recipients. It has a demonstrated efficacy of 50% with a duration of 3 to 6 months, but with greatest effect in the first 2 months. Therefore, boosting every 6 months is required for continued efficacy. However, efficacy is best demonstrated for inhabitants of, or long-term visitors to, endemic areas in whom it most likely serves to boost naturally acquired immunity. Better cholera vaccines are under development, including an oral combination of killed whole cholera cells supplemented with the B (or binding) subunit of cholera toxin, which has demonstrated efficacy, but no side effects, in populations in endemic areas.

YELLOW FEVER

This disease is limited to tropical Africa (15°N to 10°S) and northern South America, including Panama (10°N to 15°S). The Orient and the Indian subcontinent have been spared, although they have competent insect vectors. In endemic areas, the risk of disease is greatest in forested areas, and measures to avoid mosquitoes are important. Fatality rates can be as high as 40%; thus, vaccination is important. The requirement for yellow fever vaccine is greatest for travelers who will leave urban areas, although urban outbreaks can occur, especially in Africa.

The vaccine[10] is a highly efficacious (95+%) live viral vaccine that is well tolerated, although it should not be given to the immunocompromised. The vaccinee may be considered to be protected 10 days after vaccination. Boosting is recommended at 10-year intervals. The vaccine can be given only at designated yellow fever vaccine centers because it is expensive and degrades rapidly upon reconstitution. Use is not recommended in infants less than 6 months of age or in pregnant women.

Many Asian countries appropriately require yellow fever vaccine for travelers from infected areas because of the strong concern about importing infection. Six-day quarantines may be required for nonvaccinated travelers from these regions. Consult "Health Information for International Travel" for current requirements.[3]

Active and Passive Immunizations Recommended for Other Infections

VIRAL HEPATITIS

Hepatitis A. Hepatitis A virus (HAV) is prevalent in many countries of Africa, Asia, and Central and South America, where it is usually a mild childhood disease. Risk is greatest in rural or unsanitary urban areas, but cases occur along usual tourist routes. Transmission is by way of contaminated food, beverages, or ice, or by way of person-to-person contact. Risk is cumulative with increasing duration of exposure. Thus, duration of travel may be a major determinant of a decision for prophylaxis with immune serum globulin (ISG). The dose of ISG is 0.02 ml/kg for trips less than 3 months and 0.06 ml/kg for longer trips up to 5 months.[11] Passive immunization is indicated for those residing in developing countries, especially if they travel to rural areas or to other areas with poor sanitation, or if they have close contact with the local populace, especially young children. Because 20% to 35% of U.S. adults may be immune to HAV, determination of HAV antibody titers may obviate the need for ISG prophylaxis. The preparation of ISG by cold ethanol fractionation removes the risk of transmission of blood-borne viruses, including human immunodeficiency virus (HIV) and hepatitis B virus (HBV).[12]

Hepatitis B. Hepatitis B virus (HBV) risk is elevated in the developing world, especially Asia, the South Pacific, and sub-Saharan Africa, where HB surface antigen carrier rates range from 5% to 20%. Risk factors are related to parenteral blood exposure by way of contaminated needles, sexual activity, transfusions, and medical exposures, but casual transmission may also occur in highly endemic areas. Both plasma-derived and yeast-recombinant HBV vaccines are available in the U.S.. Neither product carries risk of HIV infection. The immunization schedule requires three doses over 6 months (days 0, 30, and 180); however, one or two doses may give some protection. If a compressed schedule is used, antibody titers should be checked subsequently and an additional dose considered. HBV immunization is recommended for healthcare workers, long-term (>6 months) residents, those sexually active with the local populace, and those who may receive local medical care.[13]

TYPHOID FEVER

Typhoid is prevalent in many countries of Africa, Asia, and South and Central America.[14] Vaccination against *Salmonella typhi* is not required but is recommended for travelers to areas at risk. Vaccination is particularly indicated for travelers with prolonged exposure to potentially contaminated food and water in smaller cities, villages, or rural areas off the usual tourist route. Risk increases with increasing duration of exposure; therefore, vaccination is especially recommended for those remaining at risk for more than 2 weeks. For a 1-week stay, relative risks of typhoid are 14 to $19/10^6$ in the western hemisphere as compared with 93 to 140 in the Indian subcontinent, 13 to 21 in Africa, and only 1.9 in the Far East.

The current vaccine consists of parenterally administered acetone- or phenol-killed *S. typhi*.[15] Two doses at 4-week intervals are recommended but can be replaced by three doses at weekly intervals if time is short. Booster doses are recommended at 3-year intervals. The protection rate is high (70%–90% efficacy), but caution in sanitary practices is still required by the vaccinated traveler, because large inocula of *S. typhi* can overwhelm the protective effect of vaccination. Marked local reactions at the injection site with fever and malaise are the major disadvantages of the current vaccine. Parenteral typhoid vaccination is not recommended in pregnancy. Two additional vaccines, with negligible side effects, have been developed. These are the purified Vi capsular polysaccharide of *S. typhi*[16] and the live oral attenuated *S. typhi* strain Ty21a.[17] The Vi capsular polysaccharide is not available in the United States. The live *S. typhi* strain Ty21a is now available as Vivotif Berna enteric coated capsules containing 2 to 6×10^9 colony forming units. Four doses are required to be administered on alternate days (1, 3, 5, 7) for 1 week. This vaccine is indicated for adults and children older than 6 years. It should not be administered to individuals who are immunosuppressed or during febrile or gastrointestinal illness. Efficacy of Ty21a is comparable to the acetone and phenol-killed vaccine. The optimum booster dose has not been described and there is no experience with Vivotif Berna vaccine as a booster for those previously immunized with parenteral typhoid vaccine. A tentative booster schedule of four vaccine capsules on alternate days every 5 years is suggested.

RABIES

Canine rabies is widespread in Asia, Africa, and parts of Latin America. Less common vectors include mongooses in the Carib-bean and vampire bats in Latin America. The risk is present in many urban and rural areas. Children are at greatest risk because of their relative lack of caution in dealing with potentially rabid animals. Bite avoidance and prompt cleansing of bites with soap and water are of great importance. Pre-exposure prophylaxis with the human diploid cell rabies vaccine (HDCV),[18] or the rabies vaccine absorbed (RVA),[19] is recommended for those visiting threat areas for 30 days or more, and particularly for those with delayed access to medical care. For primary immunization, three doses of HDCV are given over 21 to 28 days, either intradermally (0.1 ml) or intramuscularly (1 ml). The need for booster doses after 2 years may be determined by checking titers. HDCV prophylaxis does not eliminate the need for postexposure immunization should a bite occur, although it reduces the postexposure HDCV dose series from five to two injections and eliminates the need for rabies immune globulin (which may be unavailable locally). The administration of chloroquine phosphate for malaria prophylaxis concurrent with rabies vaccination can significantly interfere with the immune response to intradermal, but not intramuscular, vaccine.

MENINGOCOCCAL DISEASE

There is a low, but definite, risk for travelers to the savanna regions of sub-Saharan Africa, particularly those with close contact with the local populace. Epidemics are common in this area during the dry season (December to June). Other risk areas include New Delhi, Nepal, and Saudi Arabia.[20] The available vaccine is a tetravalent (serogroups A, C, Y, W-135) capsular polysaccharide parenteral vaccine that has minimal reactogenicity. The vaccine is 75% to 100% efficacious for serogroups A and C, but it is less effective in infants and young children.

PLAGUE

Plague is endemic among rodent populations in many rural mountainous or upland areas of the world, including the western United States, South America, Africa, the Middle East, and central and southeast Asia.[21] This occasionally leads to outbreaks among rodents in small rural villages and towns, which increases the risk of human disease. Risk is very small for urban travelers staying in modern hotels. The available vaccine is a parenteral formalin-killed preparation of the plague bacillus that is administered in a primary series of three injections at 4-week intervals, with booster doses at 6 months to 2 years.[22] Local reactogenicity is moderately high. The vaccine should be considered in individuals who will be living in plague-endemic rural areas where it is difficult to avoid rodents and fleas.

VIRAL ENCEPHALITIS

Vaccines for Japanese B encephalitis and tick-borne encephalitis are unlicensed in the United States.

1. Japanese B encephalitis is a mosquito-borne disease that is endemic in tropical zones of central and southeast Asia and

may be epidemic in the more northern regions of these countries.[23] Risk is greatest in rural areas where rice culture and pig farming are common, and in the rainy season (June to September). An inactivated vaccine produced by Biken (Japan) was formerly available at regional vaccination centers in the U.S. through the CDC. This vaccine is now available only to military populations in the U.S.; thus, if needed by civilians who will be spending more than 2 weeks in endemic rural areas in season, it will have to be obtained overseas. Risk for most travelers to the Orient is low.[24]

2. Tick-borne encephalitis occurs in the U.S.S.R. and Central and Eastern Europe, where risks are increased in forested areas. Transmission also occurs by way of unpasteurized dairy products from infected animals. Vaccination with the vaccine produced in Austria is effective but is not indicated for most travelers.[25] Protective measures against ticks and avoidance of unpasteurized dairy products are advised.

Vaccines Recommended for All, Even Nontravelers

POLIO

Polio is prevalent in the developing world. Whether traveling or not, persons should be immunized against polio consistent with CDC Immunization Practices Advisory Committee (ACIP) recommendations.[26] All travelers to countries with endemic or epidemic polio should be fully immunized. Persons previously immunized may need an additional vaccine dose prior to travel.

Oral live polio vaccine (OPV or Sabin vaccine) is easy to administer and provides for the possibility of immunization of contacts by way of fecal shedding. It is recommended for primary vaccination of infants, children, and adolescents. The primary series consists of three doses. Doses 1 and 2 are given 6 to 8 weeks apart, and the third dose is given at least 6 weeks later but is usually given 8 to 12 months later. If time is not available for the complete primary series, a single dose is recommended. The vaccine carries a small risk of paralytic polio (1/500,000 for the first dose), which is greatest in adults. Therefore, it should not be used to primarily immunize adults, although it is recommended for adolescents to age 18.[27] Risk drops to 1/12 million, however, for subsequent doses. Adult travelers should be given one additional dose if they have already received only the primary series. A need for subsequent booster doses has not been established. Immunocompromised individuals should not receive this vaccine.

Enhanced inactivated polio vaccine (eIPV) requires parenteral injection but has a lower likelihood of serious side effects. It is recommended for the primary immunization of adults or the immunocompromised. Three primary doses are required. Doses 1 and 2 are given 4 to 8 weeks apart, and dose 3 is given 6 to 12 months later. If time is not adequate for at least two eIPV doses (less than 4 weeks), then a single eIPV (or OPV for normal adults) dose is recommended. Following primary immunization, a single booster dose should be administered to travelers. The need for more than a single booster dose has not been established.

MEASLES, MUMPS, AND RUBELLA

These diseases are common in the developing world. Indications are the same as for nontravelers, except that the need for compliance is greater. For those born after 1956, a dose of measles vaccine is recommended prior to travel regardless of immunization history.[28]

TETANUS AND DIPHTHERIA

Tetanus and diphtheria boosters are routinely indicated at 10-year intervals, but a 5-year schedule may be useful for travelers with the significant possibility of dirty wounds, particularly if they are traveling to countries where practice of immunization hygiene is questionable.

DISEASES FOR WHICH CHEMOPROPHYLAXIS IS RECOMMENDED

Malaria

Although there are four species of the human malaria parasite (*Plasmodium falciparum*, *P. malariae*, *P. ovale*, and *P. vivax*), most severe disease (and almost all fatalities) is caused by *P. falciparum*. Although infection with some strains of *P. falciparum* can be prevented by chemoprophylaxis with chloroquine, malaria has become an increasingly serious problem for travelers because of the emergence of chloroquine-resistant, and multiple drug–resistant, strains.[29] This problem is compounded by the occurrence of adverse reactions to alternative drugs.[30] Thus, the traveler should be advised that no antimalarial is 100% effective and that a multistage approach to the problem is required, including measures to prevent exposure, chemoprophylaxis, and rapid treatment if resistant malaria occurs despite chemoprophylaxis.[31]

The insect vector, the female *Anopheles* mosquito, actively feeds from dusk to dawn; thus, particular preventive care is required during this time period. Bites should be minimized by the use of long-sleeved clothing with repellents such as those containing 30% DEET or pyrethrum, and mosquito netting during sleep.[32]

Choice of prophylaxis and therapy will depend on information on drug resistance supplied from "Health Information for International Travel"[3] or from the CDC (404-639-1610). *Plasmodium falciparum* remains chloroquine-sensitive in some areas, but resistance is expanding in Africa, Southeast Asia, the Indian subcontinent, South America, and Oceania. Multiple drug–resistant strains are present in Southeast Asia, East Africa, and parts of South America.

Chloroquine phosphate is the drug of choice for sensitive malaria. For prophylaxis it is administered weekly (300 mg chloroquine base) starting 2 weeks before travel and continuing for at least 4 weeks after return from the endemic area. This dose is well tolerated, although retinopathy has been reported after prolonged use.

Mefloquine has recently been licensed in the U.S. for the prevention of chloroquine-resistant malaria. In most malarious areas of the world (excluding the Dominican Republic, Haiti, Central America west of the Panama Canal, the Middle East, and Egypt), mefloquine is now the drug of choice for the prevention of malaria. The adult dosage is 250 mg weekly for 4 weeks, then every other week. Prophylaxis should extend for 4 weeks after departing from the malarious area. It is recommended that mefloquine be started 1 or 2 weeks before entry into the malarious area. Rarely, serious adverse reactions have been noted at prophylactic doses (e.g., hallucinations, convulsions). Minor side effects observed with prophylactic doses, such as gastrointestinal disturbance and dizziness, tend to be transient and self-limited. Mefloquine should not be used in persons with a known hypersensitivity to the drug, in children less than 15 kg, in pregnant women, in travelers using beta blockers or other drugs that may prolong or alter cardiac conduction, in travelers involved in tasks requiring fine coordination and spatial discrimination, and in travelers with a history of epilepsy or psychiatric disorder. Experience with the long-term (more than 6 months) use of mefloquine is limited; additional adverse reactions may yet be reported.

Alternatives to mefloquine for use in persons potentially exposed to chloroquine-resistant malaria include taking doxycycline daily or taking weekly chloroquine while carrying a treatment dose of Fansidar for use when malaria symptoms arise and qualified medical care is not readily available. Doxycycline, when used for malaria prophylaxis, is administered at 100 mg per day for adults starting 1 to 2 days before exposure and continuing for 4 weeks after malaria exposure ends.[33] Doxycycline may cause photosensitivity, usually manifested by an exaggerated sunburn reaction. Avoiding prolonged exposure to the sun, taking the drug in the evening, and using a sunscreen that absorbs long-wave (UVA) radiation are advised. Doxycycline also increases the risk of monilial vaginitis and is associated with nausea and vomiting, particularly when taken on an empty stomach. Doxycycline should not be given to pregnant women or to children under 8 years of age. To reduce the risk of some adverse gastrointestinal consequences (e.g., invasive infections), it is desirable not to take doxycycline for longer than a month or two.

For travelers to chloroquine-resistant areas who cannot take either mefloquine or doxycycline, taking weekly chloroquine plus carrying a treatment dose of Fansidar (three tablets) is another alternative. The weekly use of Fansidar, which was once a common alternative, is now discouraged because of the risk of serious skin reactions to Fansidar, including Stevens–Johnson syndrome, with fatal reactions occurring in as many as 1/20,000 users.[30] The treatment dose of Fansidar should be taken promptly if a febrile illness occurs and professional medical care is not readily available. This is only a temporary measure and should be promptly followed up by a competent medical evaluation. Fansidar-resistant malaria is widespread in parts of Southeast Asia and in the Amazon Basin area of South America. Resistance has also been reported in sub-Saharan Africa.

Primaquine is indicated for terminal prophylaxis, to eradicate the asymptomatic extra-erythrocytic (tissue) stage of *P. vivax* and *P. ovale* after risk of malaria exposure ends (i.e., after the traveler leaves endemic areas). Terminal prophylaxis can be omitted in most travelers with short, low-intensity mosquito exposures. Primaquine for terminal prophylaxis is given as 45 mg orally each week for 8 weeks or, alternatively, 15 mg daily for 14 days. Testing for glucose-6-phosphate dehydrogenase (G-6PD) deficiency prior to treatment is indicated to avoid hemolytic reactions.

Leptospirosis

Leptospirosis can be acquired through wading or swimming in water contaminated by the urine of infected animals. This is a recognized public health problem in Central America and the Caribbean, particularly in field workers. Although this is not likely to be a usual problem for tourists, studies in U.S. troops deployed in jungle operations in Panama have demonstrated the prophylactic efficacy of a weekly dose of 200 mg of doxycycline.[34]

DISEASES REQUIRING INITIATION OF TREATMENT DURING TRAVEL

Traveler's Diarrhea (TD)

Traveler's diarrhea is a common, and all-too-familiar, syndrome characterized by the abrupt onset of loose or watery stools occurring with increased frequency. Associated symptoms include mild fever, abdominal cramps, nausea, bloating, and malaise. The syndrome is caused by the ingestion of defined bacterial pathogens in food or water by immunologically naive travelers from developed countries in countries where sanitation is poor and the pathogens are endemic. In high-risk areas (including many developing countries in Latin America, Africa, the Middle East, and Asia), attack rates in travelers range from 30% to 70%. Onset commonly occurs within 2 to 3 days of arrival and is greatest in the first week.[4] Because different pathogens may cause similar symptoms, more than one episode may occur, although these episodes decrease markedly after a 5- to 6-week stay in a region. Duration of diarrhea is usually 3 to 4 days and rarely longer than 1 week. Although the illness is not life-threatening, it may prove markedly disruptive and unpleasant for the traveler.

The most frequent organisms responsible for the TD syndrome remain the enterotoxigenic *Escherichia coli* (ETEC),[35] but other less frequently isolated bacterial species include shigellae, salmonellae, *Campylobacter jejuni*, and *Yersinia enterocolitica*. These are the same organisms that are responsible for endemic bacterial diarrhea in infants and children in developing countries. Viruses do not appear to be important causes of TD in adults. The parasites *Giardia lamblia*, *Entamoeba histolytica*, and even cryptosporidiae are occasionally found and may be more important in specific locales (e.g., giardiasis in Leningrad).

No vaccines are currently available for any of the bacterial species responsible for traveler's diarrhea, although vaccine development is being actively pursued. Passive protection against ETEC disease has been achieved in volunteer challenge studies by the ingestion of immunoglobulins derived from the milk of hyperimmunized cows,[36] but such products are not currently available, nor have they been tested in field studies. Thus, travelers must deal with this syndrome through a combination of preventive measures and self-treatment once the characteristic symptoms occur.

PREVENTIVE MEASURES

Preventive measures for TD include the use of dietary discretion and prophylactic drugs with antimicrobial activity. The practice of dietary discretion to avoid contaminated foods and beverages is highly recommended, whereas antimicrobial prophylaxis can only be suggested with great reservation in travelers who fully understand, and are willing to accept, the risk of adverse reactions to these agents.

Dietary Discretion. Untreated tap water, drinks with ice, fresh vegetables, and salads have been shown to be unsafe and should be avoided. Methods for disinfecting water have been mentioned above. Unpasteurized dairy products and raw seafood are unsafe. Foods from street vendors, which may have been prepared in advance, allowed to stand, and then reheated, are also hazardous. Safe foods include carbonated beverages, bottled beer and wine, and well-cooked foods served hot. The oft-quoted advice "If you can't boil it, cook it, or peel it, forget it" is generally sound. Nevertheless, as a practical matter, it is extremely difficult for travelers to prevent TD by dietary restriction.

Prophylactic Agents. Several agents have been shown to provide effective prophylaxis against TD in clinical trials; however, their routine use was not recommended at the most recent National Institutes of Health Consensus Development Conference[37,38] on TD because of concern over the strong probability of inducing some severe, or even fatal, side effects in an attempt to prevent a nonfatal disease. Because many travelers are aware of studies demonstrating the effectiveness of prophylactic agents, they may request them from their physician or obtain them in the countries to which they travel. Travelers who seek to obtain the benefit of prophylactic agents should be clearly advised of the potential for severe adverse reactions and be willing to accept this risk/benefit ratio.

Bismuth subsalicylate (BSS, as Pepto-Bismol) taken four times daily in liquid (60 ml q.i.d.) or solid (two 300-mg tablets) formulations decreases the incidence of TD by about 50%, but the actual minimal effective dose is not known.[39] Salicylate intoxication, in those with renal failure or those taking other forms of salicylate, is the major concern. Permanent neurologic side effects from bismuth intoxication are a potential risk but are unlikely with short-term administration. In addition, the preparation turns tongue and stools black, and the liquid preparation is bulky. Despite these concerns, the use of BSS can be an acceptable prophylactic measure.

Several antibiotic agents, including doxycycline, trimethoprim/sulfamethoxazole, trimethoprim alone, and norfloxacin, have been reported to decrease the incidence of TD by up to 90%.[40–42] Their routine use by travelers is discouraged because of the possibility of such serious side effects as Stevens–Johnson syndrome, aplastic anemia, or antibiotic-induced colitis. In addition, the effectiveness of some of these agents may be decreasing because of the documented emergence of antibiotic-resistant enteric strains in Third World countries where nonprescription use of antibiotics is wide-

spread. The possibility of actually increasing susceptibility to serious infections with antibiotic-resistant strains of *Salmonella* or *Campylobacter* has also been suggested.

TREATMENT

The recommended approach to TD[36,37] is to provide the traveler with effective treatment measures that can be initiated as soon as the syndrome is recognized. These measures include maintenance of adequate hydration and administration of antidiarrheal drugs alone or in combination with a short course of antibiotic therapy. This approach requires patient education of the traveler by the physician. Laboratory identification of the particular bacterial species causing the illness is neither practical nor necessary; however, the patient must be taught to distinguish between the TD syndrome and dysentery (characterized by bloody stools and/or high fever) in order to avoid opiates and seek medical care if dysentery occurs.

1. Maintenance of adequate hydration is the only essential treatment for most diarrheal illnesses, yet many individuals still have an unfortunate tendency to stop oral intake when diarrhea occurs. Travelers should begin fluid replacement when diarrhea is recognized, and oral intake should exceed stool losses. In most cases of TD, fluid replacement can be achieved with available safe liquids, preferably containing glucose sources, and a palatable source of salt. Alternatively, "homemade" solutions can be formulated by adding a pinch of salt, a pinch of bicarbonate, and a tablespoon of sugar to 1 L of water. Packets of oral rehydration salts containing glucose, NaCl, KCl, and sodium citrate have been developed by the World Health Organization and are marketed by several commercial companies. These salts can be mixed with water to provide effective fluid replacement, even in cases of severe purging. Such packets may be obtained before travel, but they are often more readily available in Third World countries where they are effectively used as an alternative to intravenous therapy for cases of severe diarrheal disease.[43]

2. Synthetic opiates rapidly control diarrheal symptoms and cramping in mild to moderate cases of TD. They can be safely used for up to 3 days in cases of watery diarrhea. Because of concern that they can decrease clearance of invasive pathogens, such as shigellae, synthetic opiates *should not* be used in the presence of bloody diarrhea or high fever (temperature greater than 101°F). The available synthetic opiates include diphenoxylate plus atropine (Lomotil) given initially (in adults) as 2 tablets q.i.d., then tapered over the next 2 days, and loperamide (Imodium) given (in adults) as 4 mg (two 2-mg capsules) initially, then 2 mg after each loose stool to a total of 16 mg/day.[44] A liquid "over-the-counter" formulation of loperamide is now available. These preparations should not be given to children under the age of 2 years.

3. Bismuth subsalicylate (BSS) given as 30 ml of the liquid Pepto-Bismol preparation every half hour for eight doses also shortens the course of TD[45]; however, it has less rapid onset of action than the antidiarrheal drug loperamide.[46]

4. Prompt initiation of a 3-day course of empiric b.i.d. antibiotic therapy is recommended to shorten the duration of

more severe cases of TD. Several regimens have been effective in field studies in shortening the duration of illness from 3 to 5 days to 1.5 days or less. These include:

Trimethoprim/sulfamethoxazole (160 mg/800 mg) b.i.d. × 3 days.[47]
Trimethoprim alone (200 mg) b.i.d. × 3 days.[46]
Doxycycline (100 mg) b.i.d. × 3 days.
Ciprofloxacin (500 mg) b.i.d. × 3 days.[48]

Choice of antibiotic therapy will depend on both the characteristics of the individual traveler and the patterns of developing drug resistance in different areas of the world. The trimethoprim/sulfamethoxazole combination remains the therapy of choice in most areas. Doxycycline may be recommended for travelers sensitive to sulfonamides, but resistance to this drug is increasing in Southeast Asia and Central America. Photosensitivity reactions and fungal overgrowth are concerns with doxycycline, and it should not be used in children because of permanent staining of teeth. Ciprofloxacin (or the older quinolone norfloxacin at 400 mg b.i.d.) may emerge as the treatment of choice in the near future. Clinical trials are currently testing the efficacy of single, larger-dose antibiotic therapy as an alternative to the 3-day courses currently recommended.

5. Combination therapy. A recent study indicated a synergistic therapeutic effect of combining a 3-day course of antibiotics with an antidiarrheal agent. In travelers to Mexico, 3 days of trimethoprim/sulfamethoxazole (160 mg/800 mg b.i.d.) together with loperamide (4-mg loading dose followed by 2 mg after each loose stool) was superior to either component alone in decreasing the duration of TD.[49] Combinations of loperamide with the fluoroquinolone antibiotics are currently being tested in field studies. Such combinations appear to be emerging as nearly ideal therapy for TD, and their effectiveness should further discourage the use of prophylactic regimens.

Altitude Sickness

Rapid ascent to altitudes above 8000 feet leads to insomnia, headache, nausea, and vomiting (acute mountain sickness), as well as more severe altitude sickness associated with pulmonary and/or cerebral edema.[50,51] Susceptibility of individuals to these symptoms is variable, but incidence is related to the degree of exertion and to the altitude attained. Sleeping at high altitude increases the likelihood of symptoms. The symptoms are the result of decreased vascular integrity associated with hypoxia. Prevention is best achieved by acclimatization by staying 2 to 4 days at intermediate altitudes (4000–6000 feet) and making the final ascent gradually (1000 ft/day). Such advice is often difficult to accommodate on tourists' schedules. Acetazolamide (a carbonic anhydrase inhibitor) improves acclimatization by inducing a degree of hyperchloremic metabolic acidosis, which induces a compensatory respiratory alkalosis. Dosage is 250 mg b.i.d. or t.i.d. begun 24 hours before ascent. This regimen can decrease the frequency of acute mountain sickness by 30% to 50%. Dexamethasone, 4 mg q6–8h, has also been shown to decrease the incidence of altitude sickness. Combined use of acetazolamide and dexamethasone is more effective than either drug alone. Mild cases of acute mountain sickness may not require descent but may be treated with rest, alcohol avoidance, and acetaminophen for headache. Hypnotics for sleep disturbance should be avoided. If high-altitude pulmonary or cerebral edema occurs, oxygen should be administered at 6 to 12 L/min if available, but immediate descent is mandatory. Treatment with dexamethasone[52] and acetazolamide, or with nifedipine (10 mg sublingually ×1 or ×2 plus 20 mg slow release q6h),[53] may be effective in relieving symptoms but should not be used to delay descent. In no case should drug treatment be used to permit individuals with acute mountain sickness to attempt to ascend to a higher altitude.

Typhus

The risk to travelers is low. Treatment with tetracycline or chloramphenicol is curative. A vaccine is no longer available in the U.S.

DISEASES WITHOUT SPECIFIC TREATMENT OR IMMUNOPROPHYLAXIS

Human Immunodeficiency Virus (HIV)

RISKS TO THE UNINFECTED TRAVELER

There is a high HIV infection rate in some areas, particularly in Africa. Because there is no effective vaccine or proven postexposure prophylaxis, and current treatment modalities are of limited effectiveness, the traveler must depend on preventive measures, most reliably abstinence, to avoid infection. Travelers at risk include those who use contaminated syringes or needles for illicit drug use or for medical procedures and those who have sexual intercourse with: infected persons, homosexuals, prostitutes or other persons with multiple sexual partners, or those whose infection status is unknown. Infected blood products and components are a source of disease. In some countries, blood and biologic products (particularly clotting factor concentrates) may not be screened for HIV antibody.

RISKS FOR PERSONS WITH HIV INFECTION

There is some theoretic concern that multiple vaccinations may accelerate the course of HIV infection because of possible stimulation to proliferation of infected T cells. Inactivated vaccines have not produced documented adverse reactions and are recommended although immune responses may be suboptimal. Live viral vaccines *should not* be administered because of concern for disseminated infection.

Although many countries do not restrict travel by HIV-infected persons, over 50 countries do have restrictions for at least certain categories of travelers.[54,55] Some countries also require HIV antibody tests for particular groups of travelers, usually as a function of length and purpose of stay.[55]

DISEASES IN THE RETURNING TRAVELER

Asymptomatic

Persons who experienced significant febrile or diarrheal illness during travel, or who resided for long periods in developing countries, may deserve some medical follow-up evaluation even if they are currently asymptomatic. Tests to be considered include complete blood count (CBC) (with attention to the presence of eosinophilia), liver function tests, examination of three fresh stool samples for ova and parasites, tuberculin testing, and serology for diseases known to be prevalent in the area of residence. Stool culture to detect a *Salmonella* carrier state might be considered, although this is likely to be of low yield given the frequency of self-limited traveler's diarrhea and the relative infrequency of *Salmonella* as a cause.

Symptomatic

Symptomatic patients deserve a more comprehensive and directed investigation, remembering that symptoms developing even months to years after return may be related to travel exposure.[56] It is useful to consider the symptoms of persistent diarrhea and persistent fever as separate groups.

DIARRHEA

Patients with persistent diarrhea should be evaluated for the presence of *Giardia*, amebiasis, recurrent *Salmonella* or *Shigella,* and helminth infection, particularly if eosinophilia is present. Schistosomiasis may cause persistent diarrhea. Recently, *Isospora belli* has been recognized as a cause of chronic traveler's diarrhea in a normal host.[57] An increasing risk of *Cryptosporidium* infection in travelers has been recognized in serologic studies,[58] although these organisms are unlikely to cause chronic disease in individuals with normal immune status. The possibility of tropical sprue should also be considered (see ch 69).

FEVER

In returned travelers who present with predominantly febrile illness, diseases to be considered include: malaria, amebic liver abscess, enteric fever (*Salmonella typhi*), hepatitis, and tuberculosis.

EOSINOPHILIA

The presence of eosinophilia should suggest the possibility of filariasis or liver flukes as well as helminthic infections.

> The reader is directed to Chapter 68, Small Intestine: Infections with Common Bacterial and Viral Pathogens; Chapter 69, Chronic Infections of the Small Intestine; Chapter 104, Parasitic Diseases: Protozoa; and Chapter 105, Parasitic Diseases: Helminths.

REFERENCES

1. Steffen R, Rickenbach M, Wilhelm U, et al. Health problems after travel to developing countries. J Infect Dis 1987;156:84.
2. Strickland GT, Weske JT. Geographic distribution of infectious diseases. In: Hunter's tropical medicine. Philadelphia: W. B. Saunders, 1984:965.
3. US Public Health Service. Health information for international travel. HHS Publication No. (CDC) 88-8280, May 1988.
4. Steffen R, Linde F, Gyr K, Schar M. Epidemiology of diarrhea in travelers. JAMA 1983;249:1176.
5. Morris HH, Estes ML. Traveler's amnesia—Transient global amnesia secondary to triazolam. JAMA 1987;258:945.
6. Cruickshank JM, Gorlin R, Jennet B. Air travel and thrombotic episodes: The economy class syndrome. Lancet 1988;2:497.
7. Anonymous. Transdermal scopolamine for motion sickness. Med Lett 1981;23:89.
8. Morger H, Steffen R, Schar M. Epidemiology of cholera in travellers, and conclusions for vaccination recommendations. Br Med J 1983;286:8.
9. CDC. Recommendations of the Immunization Practices Advisory Committee. Cholera vaccine. MMWR 1988;37:617,623.
10. CDC. Yellow fever vaccine. Recommendations of the Immunization Practices Advisory Committee. Ann Intern Med 1984;100:540.
11. CDC. Recommendations for protection against viral hepatitis. Recommendations of the Immunization Practices Advisory Committee. Ann Intern Med 1985;103:391.
12. CDC. Lack of transmission of human immunodeficiency virus through Rh$_o$(D) immune globulin (human). MMWR 1987;36:728.
13. Fagan EA, Williams R. Hepatitis B vaccination and the traveller. Travel Medicine International 1986;4:2,59.
14. Ryan CA, Hargrett-Bean NT, Blake PA. *Salmonella typhi* infections in the United States, 1975–1984: Increasing role of foreign travel. Rev Infect Dis 1989;11:1.
15. Warren JW, Hornick RB. Immunization against typhoid fever. Annu Rev Med 1979;30:457.
16. Acharya IL, Lowe CU, Thapa R, Gurubacharya VL, Shrestha MB, Cadoz M, Schulz D, Armand J, Bryla DA, Trollfors B, Cramton T, Schneerson R, Robbins JD. Prevention of typhoid fever in Nepal with the Vi capsular polysaccharide of *Salmonella typhi*. N Engl J Med 1987;317:1101.
17. Levine MM, Ferreccio C, Black RE, Germanier R, Chilean Typhoid Committee. Large scale field trial of Ty21 a live oral typhoid vaccine in enteric-coated capsule formulation. Lancet 1987;1049.
18. CDC. Rabies prevention—United States, 1984. Recommendations of the Immunization Practices Advisory Committee. MMWR 1984;33;393.
19. CDC. Rabies vaccine adsorbed: A new rabies vaccine for use in humans. MMWR 1988;37:217,223.
20. Moore PS, Harrison LH, Telzak EE, Ajello GW, Broome CV. Group A meningococcal carriage in travelers returning from Saudi Arabia. JAMA 1988;260:2686.

21. Anonymous, Plague infected areas. Weekly Epidemiological Record 1988;40:306.

22. CDC. Plague vaccine. Recommendations of the Immunization Practices Advisory Committee. Weekly Epidemiological Record 1982;43:332.

23. Monath TP. Japanese encephalitis—A plague of the Orient. N Engl J Med 1988;319:641.

24. CDC. Japanese encephalitis with special reference to the low risk for travelers to the 1988 Olympics to be held in Korea. Advisory Memorandum #93, January 7, 1988.

25. McNeil JG, Lednar WM, Stansfield SK, Prier RE, Miller RN. Central European tick-borne encephalitis: Assessment of risk for persons in the armed services and vacationers. J Infect Dis 1985;152:650.

26. CDC. Recommendations of the Immunization Practices Advisory Committee (ACIP). Poliomyelitis prevention. MMWR 1982;31:22.

27. Nkowane BM, Wassilak GF, Orenstein WA, Bart KJ, Schonberger LB, Hinman AR, Kew OM. Vaccine-associated paralytic poliomyelitis, United States: 1973 through 1984. JAMA 1987;257:1335.

28. Anonymous. Measles revaccination. Med Lett 1989;31:69.

29. Moran JS, Bernard KW. The spread of chloroquine-resistant malaria in Africa—Implications for travelers. JAMA 1989;262:245.

30. Miller KD, Lobel HQ, Satriale RF, Kuritsky JN, Stern R, Campbell CC. Severe cutaneous reactions among American travelers using pyrimethamine-sulfadoxine (Fansidar) for malaria prophylaxis. Am J Trop Med Hyg 1986;35:451.

31. CDC. Recommendations for the prevention of malaria in travelers. MMWR 1988;37:277.

32. Peto TEA, Gilks CF. Strategies for prevention of malaria in travelers: Comparison of drug regimens by means of risk-benefit analysis. Lancet 1986.1256.

33. Pang L, Limsomwong N, Singharaj P. Prophylactic treatment of vivax and falciparum malaria with low-dose doxycycline. J Infect Dis 1988;158:1124.

34. Takafuji ET, Kirkpatrick JW, Miller RN, Karwacki JJ, Kelley PW, Gray MR, McNeill KM, Timboe HL, Kane RE, Sanchez JL. An efficacy trial of doxycycline chemoprophylaxis against leptospirosis. N Engl J Med 1984;310:497.

35. Gorbach SL, Kean BH, Evans DG, Evans DJ, Bessudo D. Travelers' diarrhea and toxigenic *Escherichia coli*. N Engl J Med 1975;292,933.

36. Tackett CO, Losonsky G, Link H, Hoang Y, Guesry P, Hilpert H, Levine MM. Protection by milk immunoglobulin concentrate against oral challenge with enterotoxigenic *Escherichia coli*. N Engl J Med 1988;318:1240.

37. NIH Consensus Conference. Traveler's diarrhea. JAMA 1985;253:2700.

38. Gorbach SL, Edelman R, eds. Traveler's diarrhea. NIH Consensus Development Conference. Rev Infect Dis 1986;8:S109.

39. Steffen R, DuPont HL, Heusser R, Helminger A, Witassek F, Manhart MD, Schar M. Prevention of traveler's diarrhea by the tablet form of bismuth subsalicylate. Antimicrob Agents Chemother 1986;29:625.

40. Sack DA, Kaminsky DC, Sack RB, Itotia JN, Arthur RR, Kapikain AZ, Orskov F, Orskov I. Prophylactic doxycycline for travelers' diarrhea. Results of a prospective double blind study of Peace Corps volunteers in Kenya. N Engl J Med 1978;298:758.

41. DuPont HL, Galindo E, Cabada FJ, Sullivan P, Evans DJ. Prevention of traveler's diarrhea with trimethoprim-sulfamethoxazole and trimethoprim alone. Gastroenterology 1983;84:75.

42. Johnson PC, Ericsson CD, Morgan DR, DuPont HL, Cabada FJ. Lack of emergence of resistant fecal flora during successful prophylaxis of traveler's diarrhea with norfloxacin. Antimicrob Agents Chemother 1986;30:671.

43. Santosham M, Daum RS, Dillman L, Rodriquez JL, Luque S, Russell R, Kourany M, Ryder RW, Bartlett AW, Rosenberg A, Benenson AS, Sack RB. Oral rehydration therapy of infantile diarrhea. N Engl J Med 1982;306:1070.

44. Steffen R, Heusser R, Tschopp A, DuPont HL. Efficacy and side-effects of six agents in the self-treatment of traveller's diarrhoea. Travel Medicine International 1988;1:153.

45. DuPont HL, Sullivan P, Pickering LK, Ackerman MS. Symptomatic treatment of diarrhea with bismuth subsalicylate among students attending a Mexican university. Gastroenterology 1977;73:715.

46. Johnson PC, Ericsson CD, DuPont HL, Morgan DR, Bitsura JAM, Wood LV. Comparison of loperamide with bismuth subsalicylate for the treatment of acute travelers' diarrhea. JAMA 1986;255:757.

47. DuPont HL, Reves RR, Galindo E, Sullivan PS, Wood LV, Mendiola JG. Treatment of travelers' diarrhea with trimethoprim/sulfamethoxazole and with trimethoprim alone. N Engl J Med 1982;307:841.

48. Ericsson CD, Johnson PC, DuPont HL, Morgan DR, Bitsura AM, Cabada FJ. Ciprofloxacin or trimethoprim-sulfamethoxazole as initial therapy for traveler's diarrhea. Ann Intern Med 1987;106:216.

49. Erricsson CD, DuPont HL Mathewson JJ, West S, Johnson PC, Bitsura JAM. Treatment of traveler's diarrhea with sulfamethoxazole and trimethoprim and loperamide. JAMA 1990;263:2578.

50. Anonymous. High altitude sickness. Med Lett 1988;30:89.

51. Johnson TS, Rock PB. Current concepts. Acute mountain sickness. N Engl J Med 1988;319:841.

52. Levine BD, Yoshimura K, Kobayashi T, Fukushima M, Shimbato T, Ueda G. Dexamethasone in the treatment of acute mountain sickness. N Engl J Med 1989;321:1707.

53. Oelz O, Maggiorini M, Ritter M, Waber U, Jenni R, Vock P, Bartsch P. Nifedipine for high altitude pulmonary oedema. Lancet 1989;II:1241.

54. Gilmore N, Orkin AJ, Duckett M, Grover SA. International travel and AIDS. AIDS 1989;3(Suppl 1):S225.

55. Duckett M, Orkin AJ. AIDS-related migration and travel policies and restrictions: A global survey. AIDS 1989;3(Suppl 1):S231.

56. Wolfe MS. Management of the returnee from exotic places. J Occup Med 1979;21:691.

57. Shafer N, Moore L. Chronic traveler's diarrhea in a normal host due to *Isospora belli*. J Infect Dis 1989;159:596.

58. Ungar BLP, Mulligan M, Nutman TB. Serologic evidence of *Cryptosporidium* infection in US volunteers before and during Peace Corps service in Africa. Arch Intern Med 1989;149:894.

52

Public Health for Medical Staff

DAVID J. WEBER
WILLIAM A. RUTALA
ELLEN LI

Nosocomial infections are a cause of substantial morbidity and mortality for patients. The most representative data have been provided by the Centers for Disease Control (CDC) by way of its National Nosocomial Infection Surveillance System (NNIS). The 1984 data revealed that 2.2% to 4.1% of hospitalized patients developed a nosocomial infection.[1] The importance of nosocomial infections can be highlighted by noting that they extended hospitalization an average of 4 days per infection, and approximately 1% of nosocomial infections caused death while 3% contributed to death. The financial impact of nosocomial infections has been estimated by Haley, who used data obtained from the Study on the Efficacy of Nosocomial Infection Control (SENIC).[2] In 1985 dollars, each nosocomial infection resulted in average excess patient charges of $1,833, with an overall cost of approximately $4,000,000,000. Preventing the transmission of infectious agents between patients and between patients and staff is a duty of all health care providers. This chapter will provide an overview of hospital infection control, discuss the means of interrupting the transmission of infectious agents, and cover issues of infection control of special relevance to specialists in gastroenterology. For a more comprehensive overview of hospital epidemiology, the reader is referred to several excellent monographs.[3–5]

OVERVIEW OF HOSPITAL EPIDEMIOLOGY

Acquisition of Nosocomial Pathogens

The acquisition of nosocomial pathogens depends on a complex interplay of the host, pathogen, and environment. Host factors important in the development of nosocomial infection are underlying medical disorders, impairment of nonspecific host defenses, impairment of T- and B-cell–mediated immune function, extremes of age, and genetic factors. Microbial factors include minimum inoculating dose sufficient to cause infection, virulence (i.e., ability to produce disease), infectiousness (i.e., frequency of transmission), and ability to produce a latent infection. The environment may serve as a reservoir and/or source of an infectious agent. A reservoir is defined as the place where a microorganism maintains its presence, metabolizes, and replicates. The source is the location

from which the infectious agent passes to the host. Control of nosocomial infections requires an understanding of the hospital as a complex ecosystem.

Nosocomial infections may result from either endogenous flora (i.e., microbes that are normal commensals of skin, respiratory tract, gastrointestinal tract, or genitourinary tract), exogenous flora (i.e., microbes with an environmental reservoir), or reactivation of latent infectious agents (e.g., *Mycobacterium tuberculosis*, herpes viruses).

Iatrogenic breaches of body integrity are the major risk factor predisposing to infection by endogenous flora. Immunosuppression is the major risk factor for reactivation of latent infectious agents. Transmission of exogenous pathogens from an environmental reservoir or source to the patient may occur by one or more of four different routes: airborne, common vehicle, contact, or vector-borne. Airborne transmission describes organisms that have a true airborne phase as part of their pattern of dissemination. In common vehicle spread, a contaminated inanimate vehicle serves as the means of transmission of the infectious agent to multiple persons. Common vehicles may include the following: ingested food or water and infused products such as medications or intravenous fluids. In contact spread, the patient has had contact with the source that is either direct, indirect, or droplet. Hospital staff frequently serve as the source for direct contact spread of nosocomial pathogens. Indirect contact spread requires an intermediate object, which is usually inanimate (e.g., endoscopes, thermometers), in the transmission of the pathogen from the source to the patient. Droplet spread refers to the brief passage of the pathogen through the air when the source and the patient are within a few feet of each other. Exogenous pathogens may directly infect or colonize the patient. Vector-borne nosocomial infections have not been reported in the United States.

Infection Control in the Hospital

All hospitals should have an infection control program whose goal is to minimize the risks of transmission of infectious agents between patients and between patients and staff. Key aspects of this program should include an active employee health program[6,7]; a system of surveillance[8–10]; training in and implementation of isolation guidelines, including universal precautions[11–15]; investigation of potential epidemics[16,17]; audits of antibiotic use[18]; and a vigorous program of staff education. The employee health program should include pre-employment screening of personnel, including obtaining a history of immunizations, periodic reevaluation of employees' health status, evaluation of ill employees who might transmit infectious agents with a policy of work restriction or exclusion when appropriate,[6,7] provision for postexposure prophylaxis following exposure to infectious agents (i.e., parenteral exposure to hepatitis B; mucosal exposure to gonococci; cutaneous exposure to syphilis; close contact without mask precautions to patients with invasive meningococcal infections, pertussis, tuberculosis, or active varicella/zoster infection), and counseling of pregnant women regarding potential health hazards.[19]

Unless medically contraindicated, all health care personnel should meet current guidelines regarding immunization against mumps, measles, rubella, and diphtheria-tetanus.[20-22] Health care workers with significant exposure to blood or body fluids should be immunized against hepatitis B (HBV). Yearly influenza immunization is recommended. Health care workers in close contact with patients who might be excreting polio virus should be immune to poliomyelitis.

Clinicians should be aware that state law may require that public health authorities be notified when a patient is diagnosed with certain diseases of public health significance.[23]

NOSOCOMIAL TRANSMISSION OF BLOOD-BORNE PATHOGENS

Acquisition of blood-borne pathogens, such as human immunodeficiency virus (HIV-1) and HBV, is of ongoing concern to gastrointestinal (GI) endoscopy personnel because of their frequent contact with blood and secretions that are potentially infectious. Transmission of blood-borne pathogens occurs most commonly by percutaneous injury with a contaminated needle, but mucous membrane and nonintact skin contamination are other possible routes.

More than 20 diseases have been transmitted in hospital settings by needle sticks, including HIV-1, hepatitis B, hepatitis C, syphilis, and malaria.[24] Prevention of nosocomial transmission of these agents requires strict adherence to universal blood and body fluid precautions (Table 52-1),[15,25-27] use of proper techniques of blood drawing and appropriate disposal of needles and other sharps, screening of blood and organ donors (i.e., HIV-1, hepatitis B, human T lymphotropic virus-1 [HTLV-1]), and immunization of hospital personnel with significant exposure to blood or body fluids with hepatitis B vaccine.

It is recommended that all endoscopy personnel wear gloves, gowns, protective eyewear, and masks for all procedures. Care should be taken with handling sharp instruments, such as spiked biopsy forceps and sclerotherapy needles. All endoscopy personnel should be immunized against HBV.

Human Immunodeficiency Virus

Since its recognition in 1981, the acquired immunodeficiency syndrome (AIDS) has become the dominant public health problem. It is estimated that 1 to 1.5 million Americans are currently infected with the human immunodeficiency virus (HIV-1), the causative agent of AIDS (see ch 103). As of January 1, 1989, over 100,000 cases of AIDS had been reported to the CDC. Predicted numbers of AIDS cases are as follows: 60,000 in 1990, 71,000 in 1991, and 80,000 in 1992.

Although the seroprevalence of HIV-1 infection in the general population is unknown, the seroprevalence of HIV-1 has been determined for selected subpopulations[28]: civilian applicants for military service, 0.14% (1985–1988); Job Corps entrants, 0.41%; first-time blood donors, 0.042% (1985–1988); sentinel hospital patients, 0.12% to 0.80% (median, 0.24%); and newborn blood, 0% to 3.6%. Given the current endemic rate of HIV-1 infection, it is not surprising that health care workers may be exposed to HIV-1–infected patients or contaminated blood despite the labeling of known infected patients with blood and body fluid precautions. Among 506 patient specimens submitted to a hospital laboratory at an urban teaching hospital in Seattle, hepatitis B surface antigen was present in 6.3%, anti–HIV-1 in 3.0%, and either one of these in 8.7%.[29] Among unlabeled specimens, HIV-1 antibody or hepatitis B surface antigen, or both, were present in 5.7%. Studies in 1986 and 1987 in an inner-city hospital in Baltimore revealed that 3.0% and 4.0%, respectively, of patients presenting to the emergency room without a history of HIV-1 infection were in fact seropositive.[30,31] These studies emphasize the need for handling all blood specimens and patients as if contaminated with transmissible agents such a HIV-1 and HBV (Table 52-2).[32,33]

HIV-1 has three major modes of transmission: sexual contact with an infected person, exposure to infected blood or blood products (mainly through needle-sharing among intravenous drug users), and perinatal transmission from an infected woman to her fetus or infant.[34] Studies of household contacts of HIV-1–infected patients have consistently failed to demonstrate that "casual" contact can lead to HIV-1 transmission. As opposed to prevalence studies of hepatitis B, prevalence studies of HIV-1 infection have failed to reveal rates of infection in hospital personnel higher than those in the general population. Thus, it appears that care of HIV-1–infected patients involving only casual contact would not place hospital personnel at risk for HIV-1 acquisition.

There is little information on the risk to endoscopy personnel. In one study, all nine endoscopy unit health care workers remained seronegative after 1 year of performing procedures on AIDS patients.[35] Because the data concerning endoscopy personnel are limited, the risk must be extrapolated from data on health care workers in general.

Over 20 health care providers have been reported who may have acquired HIV-1 infection through occupational exposure. Most workers experienced needle-stick injuries, but mucous membrane or nonintact skin contamination was also noted. The magnitude of risk of acquiring HIV-1 infection following direct exposure to contaminated body fluids can be estimated by combining the results of ongoing prospective studies.[36] In these studies, 6 of 1404 health care workers seroconverted following parenteral injury by way of a needle-stick or sharp object, for a risk of 0.40% per exposure (95% confidence interval, 0.15%–0.84%) or 0.43% per person (95% confidence interval, 0.14%–0.79%). None of 746 exposures involving contamination of a mucous membrane or nonintact skin resulted in seroconversion, yielding a risk of <0.13% per exposure (95% confidence interval, 0%–0.38%). The actual infection rate following these exposures is likely to be much smaller than the upper bounds of the confidence interval.

TABLE 52–1

Universal Blood and Body Fluid Precautions to Prevent Occupational HIV-1 and HBV Transmission

1. In the hospital and other health care settings, "universal precautions" should be followed when workers are exposed to blood, certain other body fluids (amniotic fluid, pericardial fluid, peritoneal fluid, pleural fluid, synovial fluid, cerebrospinal fluid, semen, and vaginal secretions), or any body fluid visibly contaminated with blood.
2. "Universal precautions" should be employed for *all* patients.
3. Hands should be washed before and after patient contact and immediately if hands are contaminated with blood or other bloody body fluids; hands should also be washed after removing gloves.
4. Gloves should be worn for touching blood or body fluids, mucous membranes, or nonintact skin, for handling items or surfaces soiled with blood or body fluids, and for performing venipuncture and other vascular access procedures. Gloves should be changed after contact with each patient.
5. Masks are generally not needed; however, masks should be worn during procedures that are likely to generate blood or other body fluids. A mask alone does not offer adequate protection; masks should be worn in combination with protective eyewear.
6. Protective eyewear is not usually needed; however, protective eyewear should be worn during procedures that are likely to generate blood or other body fluids. Normal eyeglasses are not adequate; wraparound eyewear or facial shields should be used. Eyewear should always be worn in combination with a mask.
7. Gowns are not routinely needed; however, gowns should be worn if soiling of exposed skin or clothing is likely.
8. Sharp objects represent a major hazard. Contaminated needles should not be recapped, purposely bent or broken, removed from disposable syringes, or otherwise manipulated by hand. After they are used, disposable syringes and needles, scalpel blades, and other sharp instruments should be placed in puncture-resistant containers for disposal; the puncture-resistant containers should be located as close as practical to the use area.
9. Although saliva has not been implicated in HIV-1 transmission, to minimize the risks for exchange of body fluids during resuscitation procedures, pocket masks or mechanical ventilation devices should be readily available in areas in which resuscitation procedures are likely to be needed.
10. Health care workers who have exudative lesions or weeping dermatitis should refrain from direct patient care and from handling patient-care equipment until the condition resolves.
11. A private room is usually not needed; however, a patient requires a private room if his or her hygienic practices are poor or if the room environment is likely to be soiled with blood or body fluids.
12. Patients may receive regular food service on reusable dishes; no special precautions are indicated for meal service.
13. Contaminated equipment that is reusable should be cleaned of visible organic material, placed in an impervious container, and returned to central sterile supply for decontamination and reprocessing.
14. Spills of blood or blood-containing body fluids on noncritical environment surfaces should be cleaned up by use of the following procedure: first, put on gloves (and other barriers if indicated); and second, disinfect contaminated surfaces with a dilute solution (1:100 for smooth surfaces, 1:10 for porous surfaces) of household bleach (sodium hypochlorite) and water or an EPA-registered disinfectant/detergent. Diluted bleach stored for 30 days loses about 50% of the original concentration (e.g., 1000 ppm at day 0 to about 500 ppm at day 30). In certain situations, the use of a tuberculocidal agent may be appropriate, for example, significant blood contamination of a noncritical item such as a stethoscope or a substantial blood spill on a work surface. Spills containing broken glass or sharp objects should first be covered with disposable towels, then, saturated with 1:10 bleach solution and allowed to stand for at least 10 minutes, and finally, cleaned up.
15. Compliance with these precautions is the responsibility of the health care employee. Employers must provide orientation, training, continuing education of all health care workers, and provision of adequate supplies.

(Adapted from references 15, 25–27.)

The later stages of HIV-1 infection are characterized by an increased prevalence of a variety of infections, many of which are incorporated into the Centers for Disease Control Case Definition of AIDS.[37] Most infectious agents associated with HIV-1 infection, such as *Toxoplasmosis gondii, Mycobacterium avium* complex, *Cryptococcus neoformans,* and *Pneumocystis carinii,* are not believed to represent a nosocomial hazard. However, a variety of infectious agents associated with HIV-1 infection may pose a nosocomial hazard to other patients or staff (Table 52–3). Special vigilance is required to ensure that proper precautions are employed, because persons with cutaneous infections due to herpes zoster, herpes simplex, and *Treponema pallidum* may present with

unusual manifestations, including an atypical clinical appearance or prolonged duration. Of special note is the high incidence of tuberculosis, 5% to 10%, among HIV-1–infected persons. In a majority of cases, clinical tuberculosis precedes the development of AIDS by a median of 8 to 10 months. Delays in diagnosis and institution of respiratory precautions may occur because the presentation of tuberculosis in these patients is characterized by a higher likelihood of anergy, negative smears and cultures with the use of expectorated sputum, and an atypical chest radiographic appearance.

As knowledge has increased regarding transmission routes of HIV-1, the Centers for Disease Control and American Medical

TABLE 52–2
Comparison of HIV-1 and Hepatitis B

	HIV-1	HEPATITIS B
No. of Carriers in U.S.	1–1.5 million	1 million
Subpopulations at High Risk of Infection	Homosexual men, I.V. drug users, prostitutes, recipients of blood products 1978–85, sexual partners of above, children of HIV+ mothers, emigrants/refugees from areas of high HIV-1 endemicity	Homosexual men, I.V. drug users, clients in institutions for the mentally retarded, patients in hemodialysis units, emigrants/refugees from areas of high HBV endemicity
Percent of Hospital Patients Infectious	0.3% nonendemic areas 3–4% in ER, endemic areas	1–1.5%
Percent of Patients Without Risk Factors by History	3%	30%
Risk of Transmission Following Needlestick	0.4%	10–30%
No. Cases/Yr. U.S. Health Care Workers	Total 20–30 cases worldwide	12,000/yr, 200–300 deaths/yr

(Adapted from Becherer P, Weber DW. The needle and the damage done?: Responding to a needle stick. NC Med J 1989; 50:281.)

TABLE 52–3
HIV-1–Associated Infections That Represent a Nosocomial Hazard

INFECTION	ADDITIONAL ISOLATION PRECAUTIONS (BEYOND UNIVERSAL PRECAUTIONS)
Pulmonary	
Mycobacterium tuberculosis	Respiratory
Cutaneous	
Herpes zoster	Respiratory/contact
Herpes simplex	Contact
Staphylococcus aureus	Contact (significant disease)
Treponema pallidum (syphilis)	Contact
Gastrointestinal	
Cryptosporidium sp.	Enteric
Salmonella sp.	Enteric
Shigella sp.	Enteric
Systemic	
Cytomegalovirus	None
Epstein–Barr virus	None
Hepatitis B	None

(Adapted from Weber DJ, Rutala WA. Management of HIV-1 infection in the hospital setting. Infect Control Hosp Epidemiol 1989;10:3.)

Association have continued to develop and publish guidelines to minimize the risk of nosocomial acquisition.[15,25,26,38,39]

Perception of the potential risk of transmitting HIV to endoscopic personnel has had an impact on endoscopic practice.[35] Of note in one questionnaire survey, 20% of responding institutions stated that AIDS was considered a relative contraindication to performing endoscopy.[35] In certain settings, such as the problem of dysphagia in AIDS patients, it may be appropriate to recommend empiric therapy for candidiasis prior to investigating further with endoscopy. There is much interest in developing alternative procedures for diagnosis.[40] Advances in instrumentation, such as the use of video equipment, may reduce exposure of the endoscopist to splashes with contaminated material. A device that reduces the volume of fluid escaping from the biopsy valve has recently been described.[41]

In the event that a health care worker has a parenteral or mucous membrane exposure to blood or another potentially infectious secretion, the CDC recommends that the HIV antibody status of the source patient be determined if consent for testing can be obtained.[42] If the source patient is HIV antibody–positive or refuses testing, the health care worker should undergo HIV testing immediately and at 6 weeks, 12 weeks, and 6 months postexposure if initial tests are negative. The exposed health care worker should seek medical attention for any febrile illness during the first 12 weeks after exposure.

Postexposure prophylaxis with zidovudine (AZT) following parenteral exposure to HIV-1–infected blood has been suggested.[43] However, a definitive recommendation cannot be made at this time because the efficacy and safety of this treatment modality have not been determined.[42]

Hepatitis B (HBV)

In 1987, the CDC estimated the total number of HBV infections in the United States to be 300,000 per year, with 75,000 infected persons developing acute hepatitis. The CDC has estimated that the United States contains a pool of 500,000 to 1,000,000 virus carriers, with a high prevalence (5%–15%) of hepatitis B surface antigen (HB_sAg) being found in "high-risk" subpopulations (Table 52-2).[44,45]

TRANSMISSION OF HEPATITIS B IN THE HOSPITAL

The CDC has estimated that 12,000 American health care workers whose jobs entail exposure to blood become infected with HBV each year, that 500–600 will require hospitalization as a result of that infection, and that 250 will die (12–15 from fulminant hepatitis, 170–200 from cirrhosis, and 40–50 from liver cancer).[15] HB_sAg has been detected in a variety of body fluids, including blood and blood products, cord blood, tears, saliva, semen, breast milk, feces, urine, vaginal secretions, cerebrospinal fluid, and synovial fluid.[46] Like HIV-1, HBV is spread through exposure to body fluids by the parenteral route (transfusion of blood or blood products, sharing of contaminated needles or syringes, tattooing, and hemodialysis), sexual contact, or vertical transmission from infected mother to her infant. Percutaneous exposure to blood by way of needle stick has been reported to lead to HBV infection, despite the use of immune globulin preparations, in approximately 10% of health care workers if the source was HB_sAg-positive and 19% to 27% of recipients if the source was hepatitis B e antigen-positive.[47,48]

HBV is relatively stable in the environment, as demonstrated by its survival after drying and storage at 25°C and 42% relative humidity for 1 week.[49] Hence, it is not surprising that indirect transmission has been reported between persons as a result of blood-contaminated instruments or other objects. Infection has been associated with a blood–contaminated jet gun injector,[50] endoscopes,[51,52] and a multidose heparin vial.[53] Environmental surfaces in clinical laboratories are frequently (34%) positive for HB_sAg,[54] and contaminated file cards have been reported to lead to transmission among laboratory technicians.[55]

Compared to the general population (blood donors), health care workers are four times more likely to have detectable markers of HBV infection. The prevalence ranges from approximately a 2-fold to 10-fold increase depending on the degree of blood exposure in the work environment.[56] One study states that the prevalence of HBV markers among gastroenterologists is equivalent to that of "low-risk" physicians and does not correlate with the length of endoscopy exposure.[57]

Health care personnel with acute HBV infection or who are asymptomatically HB_sAg-positive appear to be at low risk for transmitting hepatitis B to their patients.[58] However, occasionally HB_sAg-positive physicians,[59,60] dentists,[61,62] oral surgeons,[63,64] obstetricians,[65] and nurses[66] have been implicated in the transmission of HBV to multiple patients.

PREVENTION OF NOSOCOMIAL ACQUISITION OF HEPATITIS B

Prevention of hepatitis B requires adherence to universal precautions, use of the hepatitis B vaccine, and appropriate postexposure prophylaxis (Table 52-4).[44,45]

Two hepatitis B vaccines, both made with recombinant technology, are available: Recombivax-HB (Merck, Sharp & Dohme) and Engerix-B (Smith Kline & French Laboratories).[46] HBV vaccines are administered by intramuscular injection into the deltoid as a three-dose series, with the second and third doses administered

TABLE 52–4

Recommendations for Hepatitis B Prophylaxis Following Percutaneous or Mucosal Exposure

EXPOSED PERSON	TREATMENT WHEN SOURCE IS FOUND TO BE:		
	HB_sAg-Positive	HB_sAg-Negative	Source Not Tested or Unknown
Unvaccinated	HBIG × 1* and initiate HB vaccine†	Initiate HB vaccine†	Initiate HB vaccine†
Previous vaccinated known responder	Test exposed for anti-HB_s 1. If adequate‡, no treatment 2. If inadequate, HB vaccine booster dose	No treatment	No treatment
Known nonresponder	HBIG × 2 or HBIG × 1 plus 1 dose HB vaccine	No treatment	If known high-risk source, may treat as if source were HB_sAg-positive
Response unknown	Test exposed for anti-HB_s 1. If inadequate‡, HBIG × 1 plus HB vaccine booster dose 2. If adequate, no treatment	No treatment	Test exposed for anti-HB_s 1. If inadequate‡, HB vaccine booster dose 2. If adequate, no treatment

* HBIG (Hepatitis B immunoglobulin) dose 0.06 ml/kg I.M. given immediately after exposure.
† HB vaccine dose. First dose within 1 wk, second dose 1 month later, third dose 6 months after first dose.
‡ Adequate anti-HB_s is >10 SRU by RIA or positive by EIA.
(Adapted from Centers for Disease Control. Protection against viral hepatitis: Recommendations of the Immunization Practices Advisory Committee [ACIP]. MMWR 1990;39:[No. RR-2])

1 and 6 months after the first dose. Currently recommended doses are as follows (check current package insert): Recombivax-HB (10 μg/ml)—10 μg for adults, 5 μg for children 11 to 19 years, 2.5 μg for children (HB$_s$Ag-negative mothers) from birth through 10 years, and 5 μg for neonates born to HB$_s$Ag-positive mothers; Recombivax-HB (40 μg/ml)—40 μg for predialysis and hemodialysis patients; and Engerix-B (20 μg/ml)—40 μg for adult dialysis patients, 20 μg for adults, and 10 μg for children. Whether the increased dose of antigen present in Engerix-B versus Recombivax-HB leads to higher antibody levels requires additional study.

Both the plasma-derived vaccine, Heptavax-B, and the currently available recombinant vaccines have resulted in the development of protective antibody levels in more than 95% of immunologically normal recipients.[46] Older age, heavy smoking, higher body mass indices, injection into the buttock, and genetic factors have been associated with lower rates of seroconversion. Hemodialysis, chronic renal failure, and HIV-1–infected patients exhibit both lower seroconversion rates and lower geometric mean titers among responders than do normal hosts. The administration of immune globulin preparations simultaneously with hepatitis B vaccine does not affect the development of antibody to HB$_s$Ag (anti-HB$_s$).

Long-term follow-up studies demonstrated that HBV vaccines were efficacious in preventing HBV infection[67–70] and antibody levels greater than 10 sample ratio units (SRU) provided protection.[68,71] Despite marked reduction of antibody levels with time, vaccine responders have generally not developed clinical illness.[70]

Side effects with all currently licensed vaccines are similar. Fifteen to twenty percent of recipients will experience soreness at the injection site, and approximately 15% experience one or more mild systemic symptoms (fever, headache, nausea, and fatigue). Postlicensure surveillance of the plasma-derived vaccine conducted between 1982 and 1985 revealed a borderline significant risk for Guillain–Barré syndrome; however, the risk for this event was insignificant compared with the morbidity and mortality associated with HBV infection.[72] Other serious side effects have not been reported. Concerns that HIV-1 may be transmitted by the plasma-derived vaccine have proved to be unfounded. Adverse reactions to the yeast-derived proteins in the recombinant vaccines have been exceedingly rare. There is no evidence that hepatitis B vaccine is not efficacious or safe in pregnancy. Fetal toxicity has not been reported. However, toxicity studies in pregnant animals or humans have not been performed.

Controversies in vaccine management include: the need for booster doses, screening and reimmunization of vaccine nonresponders, and the use of intradermal immunization. Antibody levels decline with time; therefore, although booster doses at set intervals are not currently recommended, it is likely that routine boosters will be required at an interval yet to be determined to maintain protective immunity. Given the high efficacy of hepatitis B vaccine and the poor response of initial nonresponders to reimmunization, it is unlikely to be cost-effective to screen for and reimmunize vaccine failures. The use of intradermal administration of hepatitis B vaccine should be postponed until large-scale studies demonstrate efficacy comparable to intramuscular administration.

In the event that an unvaccinated worker has a parenteral or mucous membrane exposure to blood, that health care worker should begin vaccination against HBV immediately (Table 52-4). If the source is known to be HB$_s$Ag-positive or is at high risk for being positive, hepatitis B immune globulin (HBIG) should also be given. It is not necessary to routinely screen the exposed health care worker for previous exposure to HBV prior to vaccination. If the exposed health care worker has been previously vaccinated against HBV, anti-HB$_s$ levels should be tested. If the antibody level is inadequate (<10 SRU), the health care worker should be treated as an unvaccinated patient.

Cytomegalovirus (CMV)

CMV, a member of the herpes virus family, rarely causes symptomatic disease in immunologically normal persons. However, it contributes significantly to the morbidity and mortality of immunocompromised persons, such as HIV-1–infected patients, transplant recipients, and other immunosuppressed patients, and is also the most common congenital viral pathogen in the United States.[73,74] The most important sources of horizontal transmission in the hospital are blood transfusion and organ transplantation.[75,76] Horizontal transmission between hospitalized patients is uncommon but has been demonstrated.[77]

The issue of transmission of CMV between patients and health care workers is a matter of controversy because of the adverse effects of fetal infection in pregnant health care workers and of infection of immunocompromised hosts. However, the high risk of *nonoccupational* exposure due to the high prevalence of infection in the community (30%–40% in middle-class communities and nearly 100% in lower socioeconomic urban groups) makes it difficult to measure an increased risk of nosocomial infection.[73] More recently, studies using DNA restriction analysis to type the CMV strain have failed to demonstrate nosocomial transmission between patients and staff.[73]

It appears that good hand washing is sufficient to prevent transmission of CMV between patients and staff. For seronegative patients at high risk for complications associated with CMV infection, measures to provide CMV-negative blood and/or organs should be used.[78,79] The role of passive immunization, antiviral therapy, and vaccine in preventing CMV disease in these patients is currently under investigation.[73]

Non-A, Non-B Hepatitis

The term *non-A, non-B hepatitis* (NANBH) has been used to refer to acute hepatitis occurring in patients when serologic tests and epidemiologic evidence exclude other hepatotropic viruses, including hepatitis A, hepatitis B, hepatitis D (delta virus), cytomegalovirus, and Epstein–Barr virus.[80–83] NANBH accounts for 70% to 100% of post-transfusion hepatitis.[84] Approximately 5% to 10% of the 3 million individuals transfused each year develop NANBH.[80–85] The incidence of NANBH is higher in recipients of blood derived from paid donors compared with volunteers, and the risk increases with the number of units transfused and the degree of elevation of alanine aminotransferase (ALT) in the donor blood.[80] Studies employing intensive surveillance methods have revealed that 20% to 40% of acute hepatitis may be due to NANBH. Intravenous drug use is the major risk factor for acquisition of NANBH.[85] Sexual transmission has also been reported.[86]

At least two distinct agents have been associated with parenterally transmitted NANBH. The first agent (hepatitis C) contains a positive-stranded RNA molecule, is 30 to 80 nm in size, and appears to be related to the flaviviruses or togaviruses. The virus has recently been cloned and a serologic test has been developed.[87-89] A majority of cases of transfusion-related NANBH appear to be due to hepatitis C.[90-93] Many but not all donors capable of transmitting hepatitis C will have evidence of elevated ALT. Anti-hepatitis C antibodies have been found in 0.7% to 1.4% of blood donors from New York,[94] the United Kingdom,[95] France,[96] Italy,[97] and Germany.[98] Intrafamilial spread of hepatitis C has also been demonstrated.[99] The magnitude of the risk of developing hepatitis C following a contaminated needle stick has not yet been assessed. In addition, the efficacy of immune serum globulin in preventing hepatitis C when used as postexposure prophylaxis is unknown. The second agent causing parenteral NANBH is poorly characterized, but it is 25 to 30 nm in size and is not chloroform-sensitive.

Prevention of transfusion-related NANBH currently relies on the careful selection of blood donors and the use of surrogate markers for infection (i.e., elevated ALT or presence of anti-HB_c). Recent studies suggest that neither surrogate will eliminate donor blood containing NANBH.[88] Current studies are under way evaluating the utility of anti–hepatitis C detection assays as a means of reducing post-transfusion NANBH. By the time this chapter is published, it is likely that all blood products will be routinely screened for hepatitis C antibodies.

Epidemic water-borne NANBH (ENANBH or hepatitis E) has been recognized on the Indian subcontinent for years.[81,100,101] Nosocomial transmission has not been described.

NOSOCOMIAL GASTROENTERITIS

Diarrhea frequently develops in hospitalized patients and may lead to evaluation by a gastroenterologist.[102] Etiologies include nasogastric feedings, antibiotic administration, underlying disease, administration of drugs (e.g., antacids, cathartics), surgically altered anatomy, and infectious gastroenteritis. The subject of nosocomial gastroenteritis has been comprehensively reviewed.[103-106]

Definition

According to the CDC criteria,[8] nosocomial gastroenteritis must meet one of the two following criteria: (1) Acute onset of diarrhea (liquid stools for >12 hours) with or without vomiting or fever (>38°C) and no likely noninfectious cause (e.g., diagnostic tests, therapeutic regimen, acute exacerbation of a chronic condition, pyschologic stress). (2) Two of the following with no recognizable cause: nausea, vomiting, abdominal pain, or headache, and any of the following: (a) enteric pathogen isolated from stool culture or rectal swab, (b) enteric pathogen detected by routine or electron microscopy, (c) enteric pathogen detected by antigen or antibody assay on feces or blood, (d) evidence of enteric pathogen detected by cytopathic changes in tissue culture (toxin assay), or (e) diagnostic single antibody titer (IgM) or fourfold increase in paired serum samples (IgG) for pathogen.

Incidence and Significance

Data gathered by the CDC by way of the National Nosocomial Infections Study (NNIS) from 1980 to 1984 revealed that the nosocomial gastroenteritis infection rate was 1.3/10,000 discharges. Rates (per 10,000 discharges) varied by service (pediatrics, 4.2; newborn, 3.3; medicine, 1.1; surgery, 1.0; gynecology, 0.5; obstetrics, 0.2) and hospital category (0.5 for small, non–medical school affiliated to 1.8 for large, medical school–affiliated). Most cases of gastroenteritis occurred among children and the elderly (1–12 months, 41%; 1–19 years, 10.4%; 20–59 years, 21.5%; and ≥60 years, 27.1%). Overall, nosocomial gastroenteritis accounted for less than 1% of endemic nosocomial infections reported by hospitals participating in the NNIS.

Modes of Transmission

Hospitalized patients may develop nosocomial gastroenteritis as a result of overgrowth of a potential pathogen present at the time of admission, transmission from a colonized or infected patient or staff member, ingestion of contaminated food or water, or use of a contaminated instrument (e.g., endoscopes) (Table 52-5). Patient-to-patient transmission by way of the hands of hospital personnel, generally after contact with a child with diarrhea, is probably the most common mode of transmission.[107] Epidemics have most commonly involved nurseries[107-109] and psychiatric/psychogeriatric units[110-115] because of the enhanced possibility of transmission.

Hospitals represent a major site of risk for food-borne epidemics. According to data reported by the CDC, during 1979 to 1981, outbreaks in hospitals and nursing homes accounted for 3.3% of all reported outbreaks, 6.3% of all reported cases, and 39.4% of all reported deaths.[116] Food-borne epidemics related to hospital food services have involved patients,[117,118] hospital personnel,[119-122] and visitors.[123-125] The contaminated food may have been prepared elsewhere but served in the hospital.[119,121,126]

In order for a food-borne outbreak to occur, the food must become contaminated with pathogenic organisms or toxins, the food must be mishandled so that the organism can proliferate, and, finally, the food must be ingested by susceptible persons.[116] Secondary transmission may also occur in the hospital when patients or staff become infected and expose other patients or personnel as a result of poor hygiene or faulty patient-care techniques.[127,128]

Etiologic Agents

Clusters of infections have been reported with the following pathogens: hepatitis A,[123] rotavirus,[129,130] Norwalk-like agents,[114,115,131,132] *Bacillus cereus* food poisoning,[119,133,134] *Clostridium difficile*,[135-138] *C. perfringens* food poisoning,[117,118] *Escherichia coli*,[108] *Salmonella* sp.,[110,113,120,121,126-128,139-142] *Shigella* sp.,[107,111,112,122,124] *Yersinia enterocolitica*,[143] and *Cryptosporidium* sp.[144] Nosocomial acquisition of cryptosporidia by hospital personnel has also been reported.[145,146] There are only limited data regarding the relative frequency with which various etiologic agents cause nosocomial gastroenteritis, and much of the data are biased

TABLE 52–5
Relative Importance of Different Routes of Transmission and Fomites in the Spread
of Selected Agents Causing Epidemic Nosocomial Gastroenteritis

| | CONTACT | | | | COMMON |
AGENT	Direct	Indirect	DROPLET	FOMITES	VEHICLE
Adenovirus	+	?	?	?	?
Rotavirus	++	?	±	±	−
Norwalk agent	++	?	?	?	±
C. difficile	+	?	−	±	−
E. coli	++	?	−	−	−
Salmonella	++	+	±	±	++
Shigella	++	−	−	−	−
Y. enterocolitica	++	?	−	−	−
Cryptosporidia	+	?	−	−	+

++, common; +, occasional; ±, rare; −, little or no evidence; ?, unknown.
(Adapted from Hughes JM, Jarvis WR. Nosocomial gastrointestinal infections. In: Wenzel RP, ed. Prevention and control of nosocomial infections. Baltimore: Williams & Wilkins, 1987:405.)

because of selective patient populations and inadequate methodology to detect all potential pathogens. An etiologic agent was identified in 57% of cases of nosocomial gastroenteritis as part of the NNIS.[104] Bacterial agents, most commonly *C. difficile*, accounted for 78% of the reported agents. *Salmonella* sp. ranked second. However, many hospitals lacked diagnostic virology laboratories, and the relative importance of viruses was certainly underestimated. Most food-borne outbreaks occurring in the hospital were due to *Salmonella* sp., *Staphylococcus aureus*, or *C. perfringens*.[116,147]

Several prospective studies have evaluated the etiologic agents responsible for nosocomial diarrhea in adult patients by performing bacterial cultures, *C. difficile* assays, and examination for ova plus parasites.[148,149] Two of 1449 stool cultures (0.14%) were positive, none of 582 examinations for ova and parasites was positive (0%), but approximately 20% of stool samples tested positive for *C. difficile* cytotoxin. A similar study in children revealed a bacterial pathogen in less than 1%, rotavirus in 45%, and *C. difficile* cytotoxin in 17%.[150] Enteric adenovirus was occasionally discovered.[150] The high frequency of rotavirus as an etiology in pediatric nosocomial diarrhea is consistent with other reports.[151]

Based on these data, bacterial cultures and examination of the stool for ova and parasites should not be routinely performed as part of the evaluation of nosocomial diarrhea.[148,149,152] Because endoscopy provides a rapid means of making the diagnosis of pseudomembranous colitis (assays for *C. difficile* toxin take 2–3 days), this procedure may be useful in the evaluation of nosocomial diarrhea. Bacterial cultures should be considered when evaluating common-source epidemics, especially those related to food preparation.

Clostridium difficile

Current studies suggest that *C. difficile* (see ch 83) is the causative agent in 15% to 25% of antibiotic-associated diarrhea and 70% to 95% of antibiotic-associated colitis. The most common antibiotics

precipitating infection are clindamycin, ampicillin, and the cephalosporins. The least common are the aminoglycosides and vancomycin. The incidence of *C. difficile* disease is not related to the dose or duration of antibiotic therapy. Neoplastic agents may also lead to *C. difficile* colitis.

Several studies have linked *C. difficile* with outbreaks of diarrhea and colitis in hospitalized adults receiving antimicrobial therapy.[135,136,153–156] Gerding has summarized the basic hypotheses regarding the origin of *C. difficile* diarrhea. The first is endogenous activation (through antimicrobial or antineoplastic drug use) of asymptomatically carried pathogens, the second is exogenous acquisition of organisms (from the environment or human contacts) with resultant diarrhea in hosts predisposed by antimicrobial treatment.[157] This latter hypothesis is supported by recent studies using molecular analysis of *C. difficile* strains that indicate that unique organisms are responsible for multiple cases of epidemic and endemic nosocomial *C. difficile* disease and carriage.[135–137,155,156]

The means by which hospitalized patients acquire *C. difficile* is still unclear. Carriage on the hands of personnel has been documented.[137,158] In addition, environmental contamination by *C. difficile* spores is well described and may be found on objects in close proximity to infected patients, including sinks, toilets, commodes, and bedding.[137,138,158–160]

Efforts to reduce *C. difficile* infections by way of environmental control have not produced convincing results.[161] Cohorting carriers and cohorting infected patients have been shown to reduce *C. difficile* infection rates.[156] However, hand washing and the use of disposable gloves when handling body substances have also been effective and are more practical.[162,163]

Enteric Viruses

Nosocomial gastroenteritis has been reported to be caused by a variety of enteric viruses (see ch 68), including rotavirus,[129,130,164–174] Norwalk or Norwalk-like viruses,[131,132,175–178] enteric adenovirus,[179–181] astrovirus,[166] and calicivirus.[182,183] Infants[130,164,165,167-171,174] and elderly patients[132,177] appear to be the most vulnerable.

Rotavirus, the most common enteric pathogen in children, is isolated from a quarter to half of all children admitted to the hospital with gastroenteritis.[184,185] The majority of patients with rotavirus infection are between 6 and 24 months of age. Although infection may lead to copious diarrhea and significant vomiting, asymptomatic infection is common and may serve as a source for nosocomial transmission.

Both epidemic and endemic nosocomial infections due to rotavirus have been reported, most commonly involving neonatal nurseries. The modes of introduction of infection into the hospital setting and transmission within the hospital have been incompletely characterized. Sources of infection are most likely asymptomatically infected patients or staff.[186] Transmission is most likely person-to-person by way of the contaminated hands of hospital personnel.[187,188] Rotaviruses may persist for prolonged periods on environmental surfaces; thus, fomites may play a role in nosocomial transmission.[189] In addition, evidence also exists for aerosol droplet transmission.[190]

The rapid identification of patients infected with rotavirus has been shown to be ineffective in the prevention of nosocomial acquisition.[191] Prevention efforts should stress routine hand washing with virucidal disinfectants and proper institution of enteric precautions.

Salmonella Species

Information provided by hospitals to the CDC as part of the NNIS from 1980 to 1984 indicated that *Salmonella* sp. (see ch 68) ranked second, behind *C. difficile*, as a cause of nosocomial gastroenteritis.[104] Although nosocomial gastroenteritis due to viruses was undoubtedly underestimated, *Salmonella* continues to be an important cause of both sporadic and epidemic infections in the hospital.[104,106,116,142,192-195]

Most epidemics of *Salmonella* have resulted from common-vehicle transmission or cross-transmission between patients. The source in common-vehicle transmission is usually contaminated food, although epidemics due to contaminated pharmaceuticals (such as carmine dye, pancreatin, pepsin, bile salts, gelatin, and vitamins; extracts of thyroid, adrenal cortex, pancreas, pituitary, liver, and stomach; and human platelets for transfusion) have been reported.[192] Cross-transmission between patients may occur as a result of direct patient interaction, by way of the hands of hospital personnel, by way of contamination of medical instruments that have been inadequately disinfected (see page 1056), or by way of fomites such as dust, delivery-room resuscitators, bedside tables and cribs, thermometers, or water baths used to warm baby food.[192] Epidemics due to cross-transmission have been noted to occur more commonly than those due to common-vehicle transmission, but the latter mode of transmission involves more patients per outbreak and more patients in total.[106,142,195] Cross-infection occurred most commonly in nurseries and pediatric wards.[142] In contrast, common-vehicle transmission involved only patients on general hospital wards or in nursing homes. Mortality was highest for neonates, followed by hospitalized patients, and lowest for nursing home patients.

Foods incriminated in outbreaks due to *Salmonella* have included poultry, red meat, milk, dried coconut, and yeast.[192] However, the most frequent source of common-vehicle transmission has been eggs or egg products.[127,128,140,142] Intact eggs are now a frequently reported source of *Salmonella* epidemics.[196] Kitchen equipment may also become contaminated by either raw food or food handlers, leading to contamination of prepared foods.

Prevention of food-borne outbreaks due to *Salmonella* and other enteric pathogens depends on rigorous attention to local sanitary codes in hospital kitchens. Patients should never receive raw eggs or unpasteurized milk. In general, it would be wise for hospitals to use routinely only pasteurized egg products. Hospital employees with diarrheal diseases should be evaluated by employee health personnel. Hand washing, proper food hygiene, and proper cleaning plus disinfection of equipment are important elements in preventing common-vehicle transmission and cross-transmission of *Salmonella*.

Shigella Species

Outbreaks of nosocomial shigellosis (see ch 83) have been reported much less commonly than *Salmonella* outbreaks. Direct person-to-person transmission has been the primary mode of spread,[107,111,112] although common-source outbreaks due to contaminated food have occurred.[122,124] The low inoculum, 10^{1-2} organisms, capable of producing disease is of particular concern in hospital settings such as pediatric playrooms and the newborn nurseries, where frequent exposure to stool is common. Control of *Shigella* outbreak requires active case-finding, institution of enteric precautions, evaluation of ill employees, and attention to hand washing.[197]

NOSOCOMIAL INFECTIONS ASSOCIATED WITH GASTROINTESTINAL PROCEDURES

Endoscopes are routinely contaminated during clinical use. With increasing numbers of procedures being scheduled per day, there is increasing pressure on the staff to minimize the time spent in disinfecting equipment between patients. Despite the lack of uniformity in endoscopic cleaning techniques, documented endoscope-related infections are rare.[198,199] Nonetheless, serious infections related to GI procedures have occurred and have led to fatalities in a number of instances.[200] The recent emergence of the AIDS epidemic has raised concerns regarding patient-to-patient and patient-to-staff transfer of HIV infection. Because gastrointestinal symptoms are frequent in these patients, endoscopic procedures are performed frequently on these immunocompromised patients. Introduction of organisms, that in a normal host would lead to an asymptomatic or self-limiting illness, could lead to serious and potentially fatal infections in these patients. Finally, cross-infections due to contaminated endoscopes could lead to the spread of antibiotic-resistant organisms throughout the hospital.

Infectious complications affecting the patients involve the following settings[201]:

1. Transfer of pathogens related to contaminated equipment. Endoscopes may serve as a vector for transmitting GI pathogens, such as *Salmonella*, between patients. Improperly stored equipment, water bottles, or tubing may serve as a reservoir for opportunistic gram-negative bacilli, such as *Pseudomonas*.

2. Bacteremia. Gastrointestinal endoscopy and associated procedures (e.g., biopsy, sclerotherapy, laser treatment) can result in transient bacteremia, which could seed potentially susceptible tissues or prostheses.

3. Aspiration pneumonia. Regurgitation and inhalation of stomach contents may result in pneumonia and lung abscess. The incidence is estimated to be 0.1/1000.[198] It is most likely to occur during endoscopy of the bleeding patient.[198]

4. Perforation. The incidence of perforation has been estimated to be 0.3/1000 with routine upper endoscopy and 2/1000 with colonoscopy.[199] Therapeutic procedures such as esophageal dilatation (4–12/1000 depending on the instrument used[198]), sclerotherapy, coagulation, and laser therapy are associated with an increased risk of perforation.

The immune status of the patients is important in determining the risk of infections. Patients with severe neutropenia, those receiving immunosuppressive chemotherapy, or those with immunodeficiency syndromes, most notably AIDS, are at increased risk from infectious complications. Other host factors may include debility and achlorhydria.

Finally, the staff of endoscopy units are at risk for developing infections, most notably HBV and HIV, from contact with blood or bloody sputum or GI secretions of infected patients. This section will focus on infections related to cross-infection and bacteremia.

Analysis of documented instances of cross-infections transmitted by endoscopy, such as a recent outbreak of *S. newport*, suggests that the incidence of cross-infections is probably underestimated.[202] A number of the patients cultured during this outbreak were found to have asymptomatic infections. Because there may be prolonged incubation periods prior to the development of symptomatic infections and because patients involved in the same outbreak may be under the care of different physicians, an episode of cross-infection may not be recognized.[202] Transmission may be discovered because cultures are fortuitously obtained in a series of patients so that a cluster of infection may be detected.[202]

In cases where no cross-infection related to endoscopic procedures has been documented (as is the case for transmission of HIV), the risk must be estimated by extrapolating from currently available data based on existing data on other populations (discussed previously). Microbiologic surveillance of equipment has been used to assess the effectiveness of various decontamination procedures.

Infections Related to Contaminated Equipment

Infections that have been reported to be associated with contaminated equipment have been reported with the following procedures:

ESOPHAGOGASTRODUODENOSCOPY

The 1974 American Society for Gastrointestinal Endoscopy Survey[198] reported 17 infections during 211,410 procedures. The major pathogen reported was *Salmonella*.[200] Other organisms reported include *Helicobacter pylori*,[203–205] *Pseudomonas*,[200] hepatitis B,[200] and *Strongyloides*.[200]

Salmonella

Infections with *S. oslo, S. oranienburg, S. agona, S. typhi, S. typhimurium,* and *S. kedougou* associated with contaminated endoscopes and involving a total of 81 patients have been documented[200] (see ch 68). Although there were no fatalities, five of these patients developed septicemia.[200] These episodes were associated with the use of disinfectants such as hexachlorophene, cetrimide, and chlorhexidine, which are known to have relatively poor germicidal activity against gram-negative bacteria.[200] After the disinfectant was changed to povidone-iodine or 2% glutaraldehyde, endoscope cultures became negative and no new cases of *Salmonella* were reported.

Helicobacter Pylori

Three cases of symptomatic infections associated with upper endoscopy with biopsy have been reported.[203,204] The risk for iatrogenic infection with this organism associated with gastroscopy with biopsy has been estimated in one series to be 1.1%.[205]

Pseudomonas

Fourteen cases of *Pseudomonas* infections (with five fatalities) have been reported.[200] Two of the patients with fatal septicemia had leukemia and were severely neutropenic.[206] In several cases, the endoscopes had been inadequately disinfected by soaking in solutions in which *Pseudomonas* species readily survive (e.g., benzalkonium chloride, chlorhexidinecetrimide). Of note, ancillary equipment, especially water bottles and connecting tubes, may be colonized by *Pseudomonas* species.

Hepatitis B

Two cases of hepatitis B virus infections acquired at endoscopy have been reported. Existing data suggest that the risk of transmission of hepatitis B virus infection is small. In nine prospective studies, none of 230 patients inadvertently examined with an endoscope previously used on HBsAg-positive patients developed overt hepatitis, and one became HBsAg-positive.[200] In the case where a patient developed overt hepatitis, the air/water channel had been rinsed with water but not with activated glutaraldehyde.[51]

Strongyloides

In an outbreak of *Strongyloides* esophagitis involving four patients, evidence strongly suggested cross-infection from a single endoscope.[200]

ENDOSCOPIC RETROGRADE CHOLANGIOPANCREATOGRAPHY (ERCP)

Cholangitis is the second most common complication of ERCP (following pancreatitis), with a reported incidence of 0.8% to 6%.[200] It is the most common cause of death following ERCP.[200] Biliary stasis is clearly an important factor, because 90% of reported instances of cholangitis following ERCP and all fatal cases have occurred in patients with obstructed bile ducts. Most cases associated with contaminated equipment grew *Pseudomonas aeruginosa.*[200] Transmission of this organism stopped when decontamination procedures were changed to removal of residual moisture by suctioning alcohol through all channels followed by forced air drying.[207] In other cases where organisms belonging to Enterobacteriaceae, such as *E. coli,* have been isolated, there is evidence suggesting that instrumentation facilitated dissemination of gut organisms already contaminating the bile.[200] A recent retrospective study suggested that prophylactic antibiotics directed against aerobic bowel organisms will reduce the episodes of septicemia, particularly in patients with biliary obstruction.[208]

Pancreatic sepsis and abscess are rare, but serious complications of ERCP[200] are probably due to introduction of contaminated material into a stagnant duct system. Prophylactic broad-spectrum antibiotics, minimizing the amount of contrast agent injected into the duct, and early decompressive surgery have been recommended when a poorly draining pseudocyst or an obstructed pancreatic duct is present.

COLONOSCOPY

Compared with upper endoscopy, there are very few reported cases of transmission of infection at colonoscopy.[200] Recently, an outbreak of *Salmonella newport* was transmitted by colonoscopy during a 2-week period following colonoscopy and biopsy of a patient with acute *S. newport* gastroenteritis, causing two symptomatic infections and two asymptomatic infections.[202] The organism was subsequently cultured from a colonic biopsy forceps. The outbreak was stopped after all forceps were sterilized with ethylene oxide and the staff was reinstructed with respect to decontamination procedures (discussed in more detail above).

OTHER ORGANISMS

Although there are no reports of transmission of *Mycobacterium tuberculosis* by GI procedures, cross-infection with this organism has occurred after bronchoscopy with a fiberoptic bronchoscope disinfected for 10 minutes before use with povidone-iodine.[200] Cryptosporidia oocysts are resistant to many disinfectants.[209] This is of concern because infection of immunocompromised hosts, such as AIDS patients, could lead to severe diarrheal illnesses and because there may be a high prevalence of asymptomatic cryptosporidiosis in patients undergoing endoscopy.[210] Contamination of an endoscope with a fungal organism, *Trichosporon beigelii,* but without any incidence of invasive disease has been recently reported.[211]

Bacteremia and Endocarditis Associated With Gastrointestinal Procedures

Documented cases of endocarditis related to GI procedures are rare.[212-214] Although the incidence of endocarditis is not known, the paucity of reported cases indicates that it is an uncommon event. The evidence implicating upper endoscopy is poorly doc-

umented.[213] Two patients were reported to have developed endocarditis associated with esophageal dilation.[215,216] There have been several reported cases of endocarditis developing after sigmoidoscopy.[213] Most patients who developed endocarditis related to GI procedures had pre-existing valvular disease.

Prospective studies of endoscopy bacteremia show a wide variance in the incidence reported with any given procedure (Table 52-6), but overall procedures such as esophagogastroduodenoscopy, endoscopic retrograde cholangiopancreatography, colonoscopy, and sigmoidoscopy are associated with a low mean frequency (3%-6%) of bacteremia.[214] In fact, the greatest bacteremia associated with lower endoscopy may take place prior to the procedure with the "bowel prep," for which antibiotic prophylaxis is not routinely recommended.[217] Whether biopsy increases the incidence of bacteremia is debated.[218] Invasive therapeutic procedures, esophageal dilatation, sclerotherapy, and laser treatment of malignancy are associated with a higher mean frequency (18%-45%) of bacteremia.[214] Of note, the estimated incidence of bacteremia with tooth brushing is 40%.[219] Disinfection of the dilators just prior to use decreased the incidence of bacteremia with esophageal dilatation in several studies.[220] Decreasing the length of the needle and sterilizing the water used in sclerotherapy have also been associated with a decreased incidence of bacteremia in this procedure.[218]

The types of organisms involved are important. *E. coli* and *Bacteroides* species (found in the colon) rarely cause endocarditis. *Streptococcus viridans* and enterococcus, which have a relatively high affinity for heart valves, are more likely to cause endocarditis than are other bacteria.[214,217] Therefore, the incidence of bacteremia for specific organisms, such as enterococci, is more relevant than the total incidence of bacteremia. In one series, 25% of patients undergoing sclerotherapy had enterococcal bacteremia.[221] This same series also reported positive blood cultures for *Staphylococcus aureus,* an organism that is not covered by standard antibiotic prophylaxis in GI procedures. The incidence of enterococcal bacteremia associated with dilatation has been estimated to be 5%.[220]

Although there have been reported cases of endocarditis fol-

TABLE 52-6
Bacteremia with Gastrointestinal Procedures*

PROCEDURE	MEAN INCIDENCE	COMMENTS
EGD	4% (0–11%)	Endocarditis reported[212,213]
ERCP	6% (0–14%)	
Colonoscopy	3% (0–27%)	
Sigmoidoscopy	3% (0–9%)	Endocarditis reported[212,213]
Sclerotherapy	18% (5–52%)	Brain abscess reported[222]
		S. aureus bacteremia reported[221]
Laser	29% (0–40%)	
Esophageal dilatation	45% (0–54%)	Endocarditis reported[215,216]

* EGD, esophagogastroduodenoscopy; ERCP, endoscopic retrograde cholangiopancreatography.
(Adapted from Fleisher D. Recommendations for antibiotic prophylaxis before endoscopy. Am J Gastroenterol 1989;84:1489. Infection control during gastrointestinal endoscopy. Gastrointest Endosc 1988;34(Suppl 3): 37S.)

lowing GI procedures, it is difficult to determine, based on the available data, whether the risk of this complication following GI endoscopy is significantly higher than the risk incurred during daily activities, such as chewing food and cleaning teeth, which are also associated with transient bacteremias. Furthermore, there are no data available on whether antibiotic prophylaxis actually prevents endocarditis.

Complications other than endocarditis, also presumably due to bacteremias associated with GI procedures, have been reported. These include a brain abscess following sclerotherapy[222] and a *Listeria monocytogenes* septicemia following colonoscopy in a patient with ulcerative colitis receiving adrenocorticotropic hormone (ACTH).[223]

NOSOCOMIAL INFECTIONS RELATED TO NUTRITIONAL SUPPORT

Enteral Feeds

Enteral alimentation is a widely used modality for providing nutrition in critically ill patients. Infectious hazards associated with placement and maintenance of a nasogastric tube include nosocomial pneumonia,[224,225] inadvertent tube placement into a bronchus or the pleural space with resultant pneumonia or empyema,[226] and occlusion of sinus drainage into the nasal fossa with resultant sinusitis. Because enteral feeds can support the rapid proliferation of microorganisms, they represent an additional potential hazard to the hospitalized patient. Contaminated enteral feeds may lead to colonization by pathogenic bacteria, infection by opportunistic or recognized enteric pathogens, or food poisoning due to bacterial enterotoxins.[227]

Commercial and hospital-prepared enteral feeds are capable of supporting luxuriant growth of microorganisms (i.e., 10^6–10^8 organisms/ml). Microorganisms isolated from enteral feeds have included the following: *Enterobacter, E. coli, Klebsiella, Proteus, Salmonella enteritidis, Pseudomonas aeruginosa, Moraxella, Citrobacter, Bacillus, S. aureus*, coagulase-negative staphylococci, streptococci, and fungi.[227–232] Intrinsic contamination of tube feedings has also been reported,[233,234] including an episode in which four infants developed nosocomial infections secondary to infant formulas being intrinsically contaminated with *Enterobacter sakazakii*.[235] Contamination is likely in locally prepared (i.e., in the dietary department) or manipulated formulas.[236] Studies have revealed that 30% to 60% of manipulated or locally prepared feeds may become contaminated within 24 hours.[231,237–239] Reservoirs of pathogens demonstrated in the kitchen have included mixers, homogenizers, dish cloths, work surfaces, metal sieves, polypropylene jugs, and a detergent dispenser.[237,240,241] Strains similar to those contaminating enteral feeds have been isolated from the hands of hospital personnel, suggesting that manipulation of the system may have led to contamination.[231] Experimental work has verified that manipulation, unless done with strictly sterile techniques, may lead to contamination.[242]

Despite reports detailing frequent high-level contamination of enteral feeds, few reports have investigated the link between contamination and actual infection. Ingestion of 10^4 to 10^6 organisms

(*E. coli, Klebsiella,* or *Pseudomonas*) by healthy volunteers may produce detectable fecal counts of the ingested strains. Ingestion by hospitalized patients of 10^3 to 10^4 organisms of *P. aeruginosa* or *E. coli* has led to the acquisition of the same strains, as evidenced by finding the bacteria in the feces.[241,243] Recently, a prospective study that used plasmid analysis to identify bacterial strains demonstrated that contaminated enteral feeds may lead to gastrointestinal colonization.[244] Thus, enteral feeds may be a source for gastrointestinal colonization by gram-negative organisms. Gastroenteritis has been reported to result from the use of contaminated feeds.[230,236,245] In addition, septicemia resulting from contaminated enteral feeds is an increasingly recognized cause of nosocomial bloodstream infections.[239,246–249] Animal studies support the conclusion that bacterial contamination of enteral nutrient solutions may lead to sepsis.[250]

Because enteral feeds easily become contaminated and such contamination may lead to colonization of patients with potential pathogens, gastroenteritis and sepsis, it is imperative to follow guidelines designed to ensure that enteral feeding is indicated and provided in a safe manner.[251,252] These guidelines include the use of sterile commercial enteral feeds or feeds prepared by use of rigid aseptic conditions in the hospital, using a closed administration set, avoiding manipulation of the enteral set, and stressing careful hand washing by personnel. If individual patients require specially formulated feeds, all ingredients and equipment used for mixing them should be clean, and preparation should be carried out under aseptic conditions. Furthermore, delays between preparation and administration should be minimized, and the feeds should be refrigerated in a clean refrigerator if not immediately used. Preservatives such as 0.03% potassium sorbate have been shown to decrease microbial growth.[253,254] The feasibility of including bacteriostatic/bacteriocidal agents in enteral feeds is being explored.[229]

Total Parenteral Nutrition (TPN) (see also ch 48)

Infusion therapy is employed in over one half of the 40 million patients hospitalized in the United States each year in order to provide fluid and electrolytes, blood or blood products, or parenteral nutrition, or for hemodynamic monitoring.[255] Approximately one third of all outbreaks of nosocomial bacteremia, one third of all endemic nosocomial bacteremias, and over half of candidemias are infusion-related and derive mainly from vascular catheters.[255] Hospital-related risk factors associated with an increased risk of bacteremia include the following: type of catheter (plastic > steel), location of catheter (central > peripheral; femoral > jugular/subclavian), type of placement (cutdown > percutaneous), duration of placement (at least 72 hours > shorter than 72 hours), skill of venipuncturist (others > I.V. team), and need for catheter (emergency > elective).[256] Patient risk factors associated with device-related bacteremia include extremes of age (<1 or >60 years old), granulocytopenia, immunosuppressive chemotherapy, loss of skin integrity, severity of underlying illness, and presence of distant infection.[256] The risk factors associated with nosocomial bacteremia, the pathogens associated with infection, and the clinical management of intravascular device-related infections have been comprehensively reviewed.[255–258]

Hyperalimentation has emerged as a major risk factor for nosocomial bacteremia and fungemia for several reasons[256]: First, the composition of commercial hyperalimentation fluids, especially lipid emulsions, supports the growth of bacteria and fungi, especially *Candida*.[259,260] Although bacteria may multiply more readily, *Candida* sp. (*C. albicans* and *C. tropicalis*) are able to reach levels of 10^3 to 10^5 colony-forming units (CFU)/ml by 24 hours.[254–261] Furthermore, even very low inocula (2 CFU/ml), such as would be consistent with touch contamination during preparation or administration, resulted in increases in concentrations of 1 to 3 logs by 24 hours.[262] Second, TPN catheters often remain in place for extended periods of time. Third, the hypertonicity of the solution tends to cause thrombosis, which may result in an increased risk of infection. Septic thrombophlebitis by *Candida* sp. is a serious problem that most commonly occurs in the setting of TPN and involves the central veins.[263–265] Fourth, patients who require TPN often are critically ill with other risk factors that predispose to bacteremia (i.e., neutropenia, extensive burns, multiple trauma, and so forth).

Overall, the risk of septicemia in central venous catheters used for hyperalimentation is approximately 3 to 5 infections per 100 devices.[266–269] Tunneled catheters (i.e., Broviac, Hickman, and so forth) have a risk of approximately 0.5 to 1 episodes of sepsis per year. Risks may significantly vary among centers depending on patient mix. Major pathogens include *Candida* sp., coagulase-negative staphylococci, *S. aureus*, and gram-negative bacilli. Factors associated with an increased risk of infection include disruption of the integrity of the delivery system,[269,270] manipulation of the catheter (for blood drawing, intermittent medication administration, or flushing), multiple-lumen compared with single-lumen catheters,[258] and use of a transparent dressing (Hoffman K. Personal communication). Factors not proved to be effective in decreasing the incidence of sepsis associated with central venous catheterization for TPN include addition of heparin to the infusate, use of antiseptic ointments, routine changing of the dressing, and tunneling the catheter under the skin to increase the distance between the anatomic insertion site and the site at which the catheter enters the vessel.[256]

Candida sp. have been reported to be the most common pathogens associated with TPN. Investigators in the 1970s reported candidal retinal lesions and/or sepsis in up to 23% of patients receiving TPN.[271–273] Implementation of infection control guidelines developed by the Centers for Disease Control[274] and the use of "hyperalimentation teams"[275] have reportedly decreased the incidence of candidemia to between 1.4 and 2.5%.[275,276] However, some reports in the 1980s have noted a high incidence of retinal lesions (9.9%) and candidemia (6.9%) in patients receiving TPN.[277] Although most candidal infections associated with TPN are presumed to arise as a result of yeast contamination of the administration set or entrance at the skin--intravenous line interface, intrinsic contamination of infusates has led to epidemics.[278,279]

Malassezia furfur is a unipolar budding yeast that lacks the ability to synthesize medium- and long-chain fatty acids and, therefore, requires an exogenous supply of these lipids for growth. *M. furfur*, which is part of the normal skin flora in adolescents and adults, has been associated with a variety of clinical diseases, including pityriasis versicolor, folliculitis, seborrheic dermatitis, and dandruff.[280] In recent years, *M. furfur* has been noted to be a cause of fungemia and systemic infections, most notably in

TABLE 52–7

Guidelines to Minimize Central Venous Catheter (TPN)–Related Infections

1. TPN should be administered under the supervision of a team of health care personnel consisting of a physician, nurse, pharmacist, and dietitian.
2. Insertion and maintenance of central venous catheters should be detailed in rigidly-adhered-to protocols.
3. TPN solutions should be prepared with strict aseptic techniques (preferably in a laminar flow hood). Once prepared, the solution should be used immediately or stored at 4°C in a refrigerator dedicated to maintaining medications.
4. Persons inserting central venous catheters should be thoroughly familiar with the anatomy and technique. Insertion of the catheter should be performed with use of sterile technique. The patient's skin should be prepped with one of three antiseptic preparations (providone-iodine, alcohol, chlorhexidine) and allowed to dry. The antiseptic should not be removed with alcohol. All persons in the room, including the patient, should wear a mask. The operator and assistant should scrub and wear sterile gloves and gown. A large sterile field should be draped, and equipment should be manipulated (i.e., guide wire) so as not to touch anything outside the field.
5. A single-lumen catheter should be used whenever possible.
6. The preferred site for "temporary" central lines for TPN is as follows (in order of decreasing preference): right subclavian, left subclavian, right internal jugular, left internal jugular, right external jugular, left external jugular, right femoral, and left femoral. The order may not be best for patients with certain conditions such as severe coagulopathy, severe lung disease, or infected skin over an entry site.
7. For adults, tunneled central catheters (e.g., Hickman or Broviac catheters) should not be inserted *solely* for in-hospital use. Tunneled catheters may be appropriate for patients requiring long-term central venous access who will experience multiple admissions and discharges.
8. Once inserted, the catheter should be anchored to avoid movement. An occlusive dressing should be used.
9. Dressing should be changed whenever wet, soiled, or nonocclusive. It is reasonable to change the dressings at set intervals (e.g., three times per week).
10. A closed administration set should be used. The number of entries into the catheter should be held to the absolute minimum. Blood should always be drawn from a peripheral vein if one is available. For adults, the discomfort of a venipuncture is *not* a reason to risk infection by drawing from a central catheter. For neonates and infants, slightly more liberal use of central lines may be appropriate to avoid multiple venipunctures. If the catheter *must* be used for blood drawing, every possible effort should be made to draw blood no more than once per day.
11. A protocol should be available detailing the method of drawing blood from a central venous catheter. Key aspects include the following: use of sterile material; careful hand washing prior to blood drawing; the hub, cap, and threads must be saturated with povidone-iodine and allowed to dry before the catheter is opened; and stopcocks should not be used.
12. The TPN solutions should be changed every 24 hours. Tubing should be changed every 48 hours.
13. Central venous catheters should be changed only for the following reasons: (a) evidence of catheter infection, (b) a chronic or recurrent fever, (c) a chronic or recurrent white count elevation, or (d) large areas of burned or denuded skin. There is no evidence that the practice of changing catheter routines every 3 to 7 days is beneficial.
14. Central venous catheters should be removed promptly when they are no longer indicated.

(Adapted from Heizer W. UNC Hospitals Central Catheter Policy.)

low-birthweight infants provided with high-lipid-content infusions.[281–285] Infections in adults have also been reported.[286,287] Most but not all patients have been cured by removal of the infected catheter.[285] Of importance, the isolation of *M. furfur* from blood requires special techniques.[288]

A strict protocol for the management of TPN should be used (Table 52-7). The management of suspected line-related sepsis has been reviewed.[256,257]

PREVENTION OF NOSOCOMIAL INFECTIONS RELATED TO GASTROINTESTINAL PROCEDURES

Disinfection and Sterilization of Equipment

The need for appropriate sterilization or disinfection of patient-care items has been emphasized by published reports documenting infection after improper decontamination practices. Because it is neither necessary nor possible to sterilize all patient-care items, hospital policies must identify whether cleaning, disinfection, or sterilization is indicated, based primarily on an item's use.[289,290]

Definitions

Sterilization is defined as the complete elimination or destruction of all forms of microbial life. It is accomplished in the hospital by either steam under pressure, dry heat, ethylene oxide gas, or liquid chemicals. Disinfection describes a process that eliminates all pathogenic microorganisms on inanimate objects but not ordinarily bacterial spores; generally, disinfection is achieved by chemicals or pasteurization. Factors that have been shown to affect disinfection efficacy are the prior cleaning of the object, the organic load on the object, the type and level of microbial contamination, the concentration of and exposure time to the germicide, the physical configuration of the object, and the temperature and pH of the disinfection process. More extensive consideration of these and other factors that affect both disinfection and sterilization may be found in several reviews.[291–295]

Cleaning is the physical removal of soil and organic material from objects and is usually done with water and detergents. Cleaning must precede disinfection and sterilization procedures. Decontamination is a procedure that removes or inactivates pathogenic microorganisms on objects so that they are safe to handle.

Rational Approach to Disinfection and Sterilization

Recent guidelines[289] rely on the approach developed by E.H. Spaulding almost 25 years ago,[293] which divides all patient-care items into three categories: critical, semicritical, and noncritical (Table 52-8). Critical items are so named because of the high risk of infection if such an item is contaminated with any microorganism, including bacterial spores (e.g., surgical instruments, car-

TABLE 52–8
Classification of Devices According to Disinfection Processes

DEVICE CLASSIFICATION	SPAULDING PROCESS CLASSIFICATION	EPA PRODUCT CLASSIFICATION
Critical (Enters Sterile Tissue or Vascular System) Implants, scalpels, needles, surgical instruments, and so forth	Sterilization (sporicidal chemical—prolonged contact)	Sterilant/disinfectant
Semicritical (Touches Mucous Membranes or Nonintact Skin) Flexible endoscopes, laryngoscopes, endotracheal tubes, or other similar instruments	High-level disinfection (sporocidal chemical—short contact)	Sterilant/disinfectant
Noncritical (Touches Intact Skin) Stethoscopes, table tops, floors	Intermediate-level disinfection	Hospital disinfectant with label claim for tuberculocidal activity
	Low-level disinfection	Hospital disinfectant without label claim for tuberculocidal activity

(Modified from Favero MS, Bond WW. Chemical disinfection of medical and surgical material. In: Block SS, ed. Disinfection, Sterilization and Preservation, ed 4. Philadelphia: Lea & Febiger, 1991.)
(Reprinted from Rutala WA. APIC guidelines for selection and use of disinfectants. Am J Infect Control 1990; 18:99.)

diac catheters, implanted devices, and so forth). Critical items must be sterile. Endoscopes fall into the category of semicritical items—those which come into contact with mucous membranes or skin that is not intact. Semicritical items require at least high-level disinfection with the use of wet pasteurization or chemical disinfectants (Table 52-9). Noncritical items may touch only intact skin (e.g., blood-pressure cuffs, crutches, bed rails, and so forth). Manufacturers' recommendations should always be reviewed for any particular piece of equipment.

Cleaning and Disinfection/Sterilization of Endoscopes and Accessory Equipment

ENDOSCOPES

Mechanical cleaning of all parts of the endoscope is imperative because subsequent disinfection or sterilization procedures will be ineffective if debris is not removed.[296-298] Specifically, (a) the insertion tube should be washed with a sponge or cloth, (b) the endoscope tip should be washed using a soft toothbrush, (c) the biopsy and air/water ports should be cleaned with a cotton-tip applicator (d) all endoscopic channels should be brushed to remove particulate matter, (d) cleaning solution should be suctioned through all channels, (e) immersible equipment should be rinsed with water, and (f) the nonimmersible parts (e.g., control head) should be wiped with 70% isopropanol and towel-dried. A recent study suggested that the control head could also potentially transmit infection and recommended wiping with detergent and 70% ethanol.[299]

High-level disinfection is currently recommended for routine disinfection of endoscopes and their channels.[289,296-298] In choosing a disinfectant, it is important that it be compatible with the instrument used. The exact time for disinfecting semicritical items is somewhat illusive because of conflicting label claims and lack of agreement in the literature, especially concerning the mycobactericidal activity of glutaraldehydes. The longer the exposure of an item to a disinfectant, the more likely that all contaminating microorganisms will be inactivated. Unfortunately, extended exposure to a disinfectant can damage delicate and intricate instru-

TABLE 52-9
Disinfection of Equipment Between Cases*

EQUIPMENT	RECOMMENDATIONS	COMMENTS
Esophageal dilators	1. Mechanical cleaning 2. Soak in high-level disinfectant (e.g., 2% glutaraldehyde) for at least 20 min	Reduce bacteremia
Endoscopes	High-level disinfection: 1. Mechanical cleaning—brush all channels, clean all valves, wipe surfaces including handle and head	Disinfection may not be effective if organic material is not removed
	2. High level disinfection A. Nonimmersible—soak instrument and fill all channels with high-level disinfectant (e.g., 2% glutaraldehyde) for at least 20 min	All surfaces (i.e., all channels) must be in contact with disinfectant for microbial inactivation
	B. Immersible—automatic washing machine or immersion in high-level disinfectant for at least 20 min	
	3. Rinse disinfected endoscope with sterile water; if not feasible, follow tap water rinse with alcohol rinse and forced air drying	Tap water contains microorganisms (e.g., *P. aeruginosa*) that may recontaminate the endoscope
	Sterilization: 1. Mechanical cleaning—brush all channels, clean all valves, wipe surfaces including handle and head	
	2. Ethylene oxide sterilization	Requires 24 h processing time
Accessory equipment Semicritical—cytology brushes, cannula, balloons	1. Mechanical cleaning as above 2. High-level disinfection as above	

Critical—biopsy forceps or other cutting instruments, heater probes	1. Mechanical cleaning as above
	2. Sterilization
	  A. Heat resistant—autoclave
	  B. Heat sensitive—ethylene oxide
		Cross-transmission from biopsy forceps often cited

* *Based on references 296-298.*

ments such as endoscopes. Ten-minute exposure/immersion times using 2% glutaraldehyde preparations are currently used in many endoscopy units. These conditions should be sufficient to inactivate HBV and HIV-1.[291,297] However, under these conditions inactivation of mycobacteria is not complete.[289] For this reason, the infection control guideline recently prepared under the auspices of the Association for Practitioners in Infection Control recommends that the minimum time of exposure be 20 minutes at room temperature.[289]

In a preliminary communication, Casemore and associates[209] report that 30 minutes in 2% glutaraldehyde does not effectively disinfect oocytes of *Cryptosporidium*. Other disinfectants that are effective in inactivating cryptosporidia are not compatible with the equipment. Infections with this organism in immunocompetent individuals result in transient diarrhea, but in immunocompromised patients, they cause severe illness. At present, thorough mechanical cleaning may be the major means of preventing cross-infection with this organism. Although no cases of endoscopic transmission have been reported, further investigation of cryptosporidia susceptibility to disinfectants is warranted. Disinfection guidelines may need to be altered based on these studies.

Iodophors, alcohols, quaternary ammonium compounds, hexachlorophene, and chlorhexidine-cetrimide do not reliably kill all microorganisms (with the exception of bacterial spores) and should not be used to disinfect endoscopes. Routine high level disinfection is sufficient to inactivate HIV-1, HBV, and TB. Because many patients infected with these pathogens may be asymptomatic at the time of the procedure, the use of a two-tier system of disinfection/sterilization or the use of designated instruments is not recommended.

Sterilization of the endoscopes can be achieved by longer immersion times (e.g., 6–10 hours) with certain disinfectants/sterilants or by treatment with ethylene oxide. The latter procedure usually requires 24 hours before the instrument can be reused and is therefore not practical for routine use.

Precautions must be instituted to prevent toxicity from exposure to glutaraldehyde.[289,298] To limit exposure to the endoscopy staff, hospitals are moving toward the automatic endoscope washers or immersion baths with covers. For nonimmersible instruments, the insertion tube of the endoscope should be immersed in disinfectant, and disinfectant should be suctioned or pumped into all channels and clamped for at least 20 minutes.

Adequate rinsing must follow disinfection to remove any residual disinfectant. The use of sterile water is ideal; however, if this is not feasible, a tap water rinse should be followed with an alcohol rinse and forced air drying. Water bottles also should be sterilized or disinfected on a daily basis to prevent colonization with *Pseudomonas* and other gram-negative bacteria.

CLEANING AND STERILIZATION OF ACCESSORY EQUIPMENT

Instruments that break the mucosal surface, such as biopsy forceps, should undergo sterilization. In many instances, disposable instruments and accessories, such as cannulas, sphincterotomes, balloons, sclerotherapy needles, and cytology brushes, are being used. Nondisposable instruments should undergo thorough mechanical cleaning. Episodes of cross-infection have often been attributed to contaminated biopsy forceps. It is recommended that

biopsy forceps undergo ultrasonic cleaning to remove debris that hand cleaning cannot remove. Sterilization can be achieved by autoclaving (for heat-resistant equipment) or by treatment with ethylene oxide (for heat-sensitive equipment). Endoscopic instruments that come in contact with mucous membranes should be high level disinfected.[289]

Antibiotic Prophylaxis

Because of the lack of scientific data regarding the risk of endocarditis associated with GI procedures, the indications for antibiotic prophylaxis before endoscopy are controversial.[214,217,218] The recommendations from the American Heart Association[301] differ from those put forth by the American Society for Gastrointestinal Endoscopy[297] in terms of who should receive prophylaxis (Table 52-10). The AHA recommends prophylactic antibiotics for patients with prosthetic valves, most congenital heart malformations (not including isolated secundum atrial septal defect and ligated patent ductus arteriosus), surgically constructed systemic pulmonary shunts, rheumatic and other acquired valvular dysfunction, idiopathic hypertrophic subaortic stenosis, a previous history of bacterial endocarditis, and mitral valve prolapse with insufficiency.[301,302] The ASGE recommends prophylaxis only in patients with prosthetic valves, surgically constructed systemic pulmonary shunts, or a previous history of bacterial endocarditis.[297] The AHA recommends prophylaxis for gallbladder surgery, colonic surgery, esophageal dilatation, and sclerotherapy of esophageal varices.[302]

TABLE 52–10

Indications for Prophylaxis for Bacterial Endocarditis

	AHA	ASGE
Cardiac Lesions		
Prosthetic valve	+	+
Surgically constructed pulmonary shunts	+	+
Previous history of bacterial endocarditis	+	+
Most congenital heart malformations	+	
Not isolated secundum atrial septal defect		
Not ligated patent ductus arteriosus		
Rheumatic and other valvular dysfunction	+	
Idiopathic hypertrophic subaortic stenosis (IHSS)	+	
Mitral valve disease with insufficiency	+	
Procedure		
Esophageal dilation	+	
Sclerotherapy	+	
Endoscopy with or without biopsy*	−	
Barium enema	−	
Percutaneous liver biopsy	−	

* In patients with prosthetic valve, pulmonary shunts, and previous history of bacterial endocarditis, physicians may choose to administer prophylactic antibiotics.
AHA, American Heart Association (see refs. 301, 302).
ASGE, American Society of Gastrointestinal Endoscopy (see ref. 297).

TABLE 52–11
Antibiotics for Prophylaxis

PROCEDURE		AGENT
Upper GI instrumentation 　Esophageal dilatation 　Sclerotherapy 　Upper endoscopy**	Oral regimen for minor or repetitive procedures in low-risk patients	Amoxicillin* 3.0 g P.O. 1 h before procedure, 1.5 g 6 h after first dose
	Standard regimen	Ampicillin 2.0 g I.M. or I.V. ½ to 1 h before procedure, follow-up dose may be given 8 h after initial dose
Lower endoscopy**	Standard regimen	Ampicillin 2.0 g I.M. or I.V., plus gentamicin 1.5 mg/kg I.M. or I.V. ½ to 1 h before procedure; follow-up dose may be given 8 h after initial dose
	Penicillin-allergic patients	Vancomycin† 1.0 g I.V., slowly, over 1 h instead of ampicillin

* For children, 50 mg/kg of ampicillin.
† For children less than 60 lb, 20 mg/kg.
** For indications as outlined in Table 52–10.
(Adapted from Fleisher D. Recommendations for antibiotic prophylaxis before endoscopy. Am J Gastroenterol 1989;84: 1489; Neu HC. Recommendations for antibiotic prophylaxis before endoscopy. Am J Gastroenterol 1989;84:1488; Dajani AS et al. Prevention of bacterial endocarditis: Recommendations by The American Heart Association. JAMA 1990;264: 2919.)

The AHA does not recommend prophylaxis for GI endoscopy with or without biopsy, barium enema, or percutaneous liver biopsy.[301,302] However, physicians may still choose to administer prophylactic antibiotics to patients with prosthetic valves, surgically reconstructed pulmonary shunts, or a previous history of bacterial endocarditis for low risk procedures such as endoscopy. Procedures such as ERCP and lithotripsy are not specifically addressed by either society. Patients will frequently receive antibiotic prophylaxis to prevent septicemia related to ERCP. The ASGE did not make recommendations regarding selective use of prophylaxis for some GI procedures except to point out that the incidence of bacteremia may be higher with certain procedures such as injection sclerotherapy.[297]

Both societies subscribe to basically the same antibiotic regimens. Recommendations for antibiotic regimens for various procedures are summarized in Table 52-11. For instrumentation of the upper GI tract, oral amoxicillin or intravenous ampicillin is recommended. For instrumentation of the lower GI tract, ampicillin in combination with gentamicin is recommended (for coverage of enterococci). Vancomycin is recommended for penicillin-allergic patients. The indications for using parenteral as opposed to oral antibiotics are not clear. The bias of one expert is to give parenteral antibiotics particularly if an intravenous line is in place for the procedure.[217]

There is little evidence to support the use of antibiotics for patients with prosthetic devices other than prosthetic valves.[214,297] Antibiotic prophylaxis is recommended for ERCP in the setting of bile duct obstruction.[209] The antibiotics chosen should cover aerobic bowel organisms, such as ampicillin in combination with gentamicin.[209] Prophylaxis may be considered in patients with severe neutropenia or those who are immunocompromised.[214]

The reader is directed to Chapter 26, The Gastrointestinal Microflora.

REFERENCES

1. Horan TC, White JW, Jarvis WR, Emori TC, Culver DH, Munn VP, Thornsberry C, Olson DR, Hughes JM. Nosocomial infection surveillance, 1984. MMWR 1985;35:17SS.
2. Haley RW. Incidence and nature of endemic and epidemic nosocomial infections. In: Bennett JV, Brachman PS, eds. Hospital infections, ed 2. Boston: Little, Brown, 1986:359.
3. Bennett JV, Brachman PS, eds. Hospital infections, ed 2. Boston: Little, Brown, 1986.
4. Wenzel RP, ed. Prevention and control of nosocomial infections. Baltimore: Williams & Wilkins, 1987.
5. Weber DJ, Rutala WA. Nosocomial infections: New issues and strategies for prevention. Infect Dis Clin North Am 1989;3:1.
6. Williams WW. Guidelines for infection control in hospital personnel. Infect Control 1983;4(Suppl):326.
7. Patterson WB, Craven DE, Schwartz DA, Nardell EA, Kasmer J, Noble J. Occupational hazards to hospital personnel. Ann Intern Med 1985;102:658.
8. Garner JS, Jarvis WR, Emori TG, Horan TC, Hughes JM. CDC definitions for nosocomial infection, 1988. Am J Infect Control 1988;16:128.
9. Landry SL, Donowitz LG, Wenzel RP. Hospital-wide surveillance: Perspective for the practitioner. Am J Infect Control 1982;10:66.
10. Haley RW. Surveillance by objective: A new priority-directed approach to the control of nosocomial infection. Am J Infect Control 1985;13:78.
11. Garner JS, Simmons BP. Guidelines for isolation precautions in hospitals. Infect Control 1983;4(Suppl):245.
12. Larson E. Bringing the new isolation guidelines into focus. Am J Infect Control 1984;12:312.
13. Underwood MA. Cost-effective application of the Centers for Disease Control guidelines for isolation precautions in hospitals. Am J Infect Control 1985;13:269.
14. Lynch P, Jackson MM, Cummings MJ, Stamm WE. Rethinking the role of isolation practices in the prevention of nosocomial infections. Ann Intern Med 1987;107:243.
15. Centers for Disease Control. Guidelines for prevention of transmission of human immunodeficiency virus and hepatitis B virus to health-care and public-safety workers. MMWR 1989;38:1.
16. Dixon RE. Investigation of endemic and epidemic nosocomial infections. In: Bennett JV, Brachman PS, eds. Hospital infections, ed 2. Boston: Little, Brown, 1986:73.

17. Wenzel RP. Epidemics—Identification and management. In: Wenzel RP, ed. Prevention and control of nosocomial infection. Baltimore: Williams & Wilkins, 1987:94.

18. Bryan CS. Strategies to improve antibiotic use. Infect Dis Clin North Am 1989;3:723.

19. Votra EM, Rutala WA, Sarubbi FA. Recommendations for pregnant employee interaction with patients having communicable infectious diseases. Am J Infect Control 1983;11:10.

20. ACP Task Force on Adult Immunization, Infectious Diseases Society of America. Guide for adult immunization, ed 2. Philadelphia: American College of Physicians, 1990.

21. Immunization Practices Advisory Committee. Adult immunization: Recommendations of the immunization practices advisory committee. CDC, Public Health Service, U.S. Department of Health and Human Services, Atlanta, 1989.

22. Williams WW, Preblud SR, Reichelderfer PS, Hadler SC. Vaccines of importance in the hospital setting. Infect Dis Clin North Am 1989;3:701.

23. Chorba TL, Berklman RL, Safford SK, Gibbs NP, Hull HF. Mandatory reporting of infectious diseases by clinicians. JAMA 1989;262:3018.

24. Jagger J, Hunt EH, Brand-Elnaggar J, Pearson RD. Rates of needle-stick injury caused by various devices in a university hospital. N Engl J Med 1988;319:284.

25. Centers for Disease Control. Recommendations for prevention of HIV transmission in health-care settings. MMWR 1987;36(Suppl 2S):2S.

26. Centers for Disease Control. Update: Universal precautions for prevention of transmission of human immunodeficiency virus, hepatitis B virus and other bloodborne pathogens in health-care settings. MMWR 1988;37:377.

27. Henderson DK. AIDS and the health-care worker: Management of human immunodeficiency virus infection in the health-care setting. AIDS Updates 1988;1:1.

28. Centers for Disease Control. AIDS and human immunodeficiency virus infection in the United States: 1988 update. MMWR 1989;38:2.

29. Handsfield HH, Cummings MJ, Swenson PD. Prevalence of antibody to human immunodeficiency virus and hepatitis B surface antigen in blood samples submitted to a hospital laboratory: Implications for handling specimens. JAMA 1987;258:3395.

30. Baker JL, Kelen GD, Sivertson KT, Quinn TC. Unsuspected human immunodeficiency virus in critically ill emergency patients. JAMA 1987;257:2609.

31. Kelen GD, Fritz S, Qaqish B, et al. Unrecognized human immunodeficiency virus infection in emergency department patients. N Engl J Med 1988;318:1645.

32. Becherer P, Weber DW. The needle and the damage done?: Responding to a needle stick. N C Med J 1989;50:281.

33. Centers for Disease Control. Recommendations for protection against viral hepatitis. MMWR 1985;34:313.

34. Friedland GH, Klein RS. Transmission of the human immunodeficiency virus. N Engl J Med 1987;317:1125.

35. Raufman J, Straus EW. Endoscopic procedures in the AIDS patient, risks, precautions, indications and obligations. Gastroenterol Clin North Am 1988;17:495.

36. Weber DJ, Rutala WA. Management of HIV-1 infection in the hospital setting. Infect Control Hosp Epidemiol 1989;10:3.

37. Centers for Disease Control. Revision of the CDC surveillance case definition for acquired immunodeficiency syndrome. MMWR 1987;26:3S.

38. American Medical Association Board of Trustees. Prevention and control of acquired immunodeficiency syndrome. JAMA 1987;258:2097.

39. Centers for Disease Control. Semen banking, organ and tissue transplantation, and HIV antibody testing. MMWR 1988;37:57.

40. Rosario MT, Raso CL, Comer GM, Clain DJ. Transnasal brush cytology for the diagnosis of Candida esophagitis in the acquired immunodeficiency syndrome. Gastrointest Endosc 1988;35:102.

41. Laine L. A prospective trial of an anti-splatter device for the protection of endoscopic personnel from potentially AIDS-infective fluids. Gastrointest Endosc 1987;34:470.

42. Centers for Disease Control. Public health service statement on management of occupational exposure to human immunodeficiency virus, including considerations regarding zidovudine post-exposure use. MMWR 1990;29:1.

43. Henderson DK, Beekmann SE, Gerberding J. Post-exposure antiviral chemoprophylaxis following occupational exposure to the human immunodeficiency virus. AIDS Updates 1990;3:1.

44. Guidelines for prevention of transmission of human immunodeficiency virus and hepatitis B virus to health-care and public-safety workers. U.S. Department of Health and Human Services, 1989.

45. Centers for Disease Control. Protection against viral hepatitis: Recommendations of the Immunization Practices Advisory Committee (ACIP). MMWR 1990;39:1.

46. Weber DJ, Rutala WA. Hepatitis B immunization update. Infect Control Hosp Epidemiol 1989;10:541.

47. Seeff LB, Wright EC, Zimmerman HJ, et al. Type B hepatitis after needle-stick exposure: Prevention with hepatitis B immune globulin. Ann Intern Med 1978;88:285.

48. Werner BG, Grady GF. Accidental hepatitis-B-surface-antigen-positive inoculations: Use of "e" antigen to estimate infectivity. Ann Intern Med 1982;97:367.

49. Bond WW, Favero MS, Petersen NJ, Gravelle CR, Ebert JW, Maynard JE. Survival of hepatitis B virus after drying and storage for one week. Lancet 1981;1:550.

50. Centers for Disease Control. Hepatitis B associated with jet gun injection—California. MMWR 1986;35:373.

51. Birnie GG, Quigley EM, Clements GB, Follet EAC, Watkinson G. Endoscopic transmission of hepatitis B virus. Gut 1983;24:171.

52. Morris IM, Cattle DS, Smits BJ. Endoscopy and transmission of hepatitis B. Lancet 1975;2:1152.

53. Oren I, Hershow RC, Ben-Porath E, et al. A common-source outbreak of fulminant hepatitis B in a hospital. Ann Intern Med 1989;110:691.

54. Lauer JL, VanDrunen NA, Washburn JW, Balfour HH. Transmission of hepatitis B virus in clinical laboratory areas. J Infect Dis 1979;140:513.

55. Pattison CP, Boyer KM, Maynard JE, Kelly PC. Epidemic hepatitis in a clinical laboratory: Possible association with computer card handling. JAMA 1974;230:854.

56. West D. The risk of hepatitis B infection among health care professionals in the United States: A review. Am J Med Sci 1984;287:26.

57. Koretz R, Chin K, Gitnick G. The endoscopist's risks from endoscopic transmission of hepatitis. Gastroenterology 1985;88:1454A.

58. Alter HJ, Chalmers TC, Freeman BM, Lunceford JL, Lewis TL, Holland PV, Pizzo PA, Plotz PH, Meyer WJ. Health-care workers positive for hepatitis B surface antigen: Are their contacts at risk? N Engl J Med 1975;292:454.

59. Grob PJ, Bischof B, Naeff F. Cluster of hepatitis B transmitted by a physician. Lancet 1981;1:1218.

60. Grob PJ, Moeschlin P. Risk to contacts of a medical practitioner carrying HBsAG. N Engl J Med 1975;293:197.

61. Levin ML, Maddrey WC, Wands JR, Mendeloff AI. Hepatitis B transmission by dentists. JAMA 1974;228:1139.

62. Hadler SC, Sorley DL, Acree KH, et al. An outbreak of hepatitis B in a dental practice. Ann Intern Med 1981;95:133.

63. Centers for Disease Control. Outbreak of hepatitis B associated with an oral surgeon—New Hampshire. MMWR 1987;36:132.

64. Rimland D, Parkin WE, Miller GY, Schrack WD. Hepatitis B outbreak traced to an oral surgeon. N Engl J Med 1977;296:953.

65. Lettau LA, Smith JD, Williams D, Lundquist WD, Cruz F, Sikes RK, Hadler SC. Transmission of hepatitis B with resultant restriction of surgical practice. JAMA 1986;255:934.

66. Garibaldi RA, Rasmussen CM, Holmes AW, Gregg MB. Hospital-acquired serum hepatitis: Report of an outbreak. JAMA 1972;219:1577.

67. Francis DP, Hadler SC, Thompson SE, et al. The prevention of hepatitis B with vaccine: Report of the Centers for Disease Control multi-center efficacy trial among homosexual men. Ann Intern Med 1982;97:362.

68. Dienstag JL, Werner BG, Polk BF, Snydman DR, Craven DE, Platt R, Crumpacker CS, Quellet-Hellstrom R, Grady GF. Hepatitis B vaccine in health care personnel: Safety, immunogenicity, and indications of efficacy. Ann Intern Med 1984;101:34.

69. Mannucci PM, Zanetti AR, Gringeri A, et al. Long-term immu-

nogenicity of a plasma-derived hepatitis B vaccine in HIV seropositive and HIV seronegative hemophiliacs. Arch Intern Med 1989;149: 1333.

70. Hadler SC, Francis DP, Maynard JE, et al. Long-term immunogenicity and efficacy of hepatitis B vaccine in homosexual men. N Engl J Med 1986;315:209.

71. Krugman S, Davidson M. Hepatitis B vaccine: Prospects for duration of immunity. Yale J Biol Med 1987;60:333.

72. Shaw FE, Graham DJ, Guess HA, et al. Postmarketing surveillance for neurologic adverse events reported after hepatitis B vaccination. Am J Epidemiol 1988;127:337.

73. Gerberding JL. Risks to health care workers from occupational exposure to hepatitis B virus, human immunodeficiency virus, and cytomegalovirus. Infect Dis Clin North Am 1989;3:735.

74. Pomery C, Englund JA. Cytomegalovirus: Epidemiology and infection control. Am J Infect Control 1987;15:107.

75. Tolpin MD, Stewart JA, Warren D, et al. Transfusion transmission of cytomegalovirus confirmed by restriction endonuclease analysis. J Pediatr 1985;107:953.

76. Fiala M, Payne JE, Berne TV, et al. Epidemiology of cytomegalovirus infection after transplantation and immunosuppression. J Infect Dis 1975;132:421.

77. Spector SA. Transmission of cytomegalovirus among infants in hospital documented by restriction-endonuclease-digestion analyses. Lancet 1983;1:378.

78. Bowden RA, Sayers M, Flournoy N, et al. Cytomegalovirus immune globulin and seronegative blood products to prevent primary cytomegalovirus infection after marrow transplantation. N Engl J Med 1986;314:1006.

79. Gilbert GL, Hayes K, Hudson IL, James J, The Neonatal Cytomegalovirus Infection Study Group. Prevention of transfusion-acquired cytomegalovirus infection in infants by blood filtration to remove leucocytes. Lancet 1989;1:1228.

80. Dienstag JL. Non-A, non-B hepatitis: I. Recognition, epidemiology, and clinical features. II. Experimental transmission, putative virus agents and markers and prevention. Gastroenterology 1983;85: 439,743.

81. Lever AML. Non A/non B hepatitis. J Hosp Infect 1988;11:150.

82. Polesky HF, Hanson MR. Transfusion-associated hepatitis C virus (non-A, non-B) infection. Arch Pathol Lab Med 1989;113:232.

83. Sherlock S. Virus hepatitis B, A, non-A, non-B. J Hepatol 1989;8: 254.

84. Thomas HC. Non-A, non-B hepatitis. Q J Med 1987;65;793.

85. Centers for Disease Control. Hepatitis surveillance report No. 52, 1989.

86. Alter MJ, Coleman PJ, Alexander WJ, et al. Importance of heterosexual activity in the transmission of hepatitis B and non-A, non-B hepatitis. JAMA 1989;262:1201.

87. Choo Q-L, Kuo G, Weiner AJ, Overby LR, Bradley DW, Houghton M. Isolation of a cDNA clone derived from a blood-borne non-A, non-B viral hepatitis genome. Science 1989;244:359.

88. Kuo G, Choo Q-L, Alter HJ, et al. An assay for circulating antibodies to a major etiologic virus of human non-A, non-B hepatitis. Science 1989;244:362.

89. Miyamura T, Saito I, Katayama T, et al. Detection of antibody against antigen expressed by molecularly cloned hepatitis C virus cDNA: Application to diagnosis and blood screening for posttransfusion hepatitis. Proc Natl Acad Sci USA 1990;87:983.

90. Alter HJ, Purcell RH, Shih JW, et al. Detection of antibody to hepatitis C virus in prospectively followed transfusion recipients with acute and chronic non-A, non-B hepatitis. N Engl J Med 1989;321: 1494.

91. Esterban JI, Viladomiu L, Gonzalez A, et al. Hepatitis C virus antibodies among risk groups in Spain. Lancet 1989;2:294.

92. van der Poel CL, Reesink HW, Lelie PN, et al. Anti-hepatitis C antibodies and non-A, non-B post-transfusion hepatitis in The Netherlands. Lancet 1989;2:297.

93. Sansonno D, Dammacco F. Antibodies to hepatitis C virus in non-A, non-B post-transfusion and cryptogenetic chronic liver disease. Lancet 1989;2:798.

94. Stevens CD, Taylor PE, Pindyck J, et al. Epidemiology of hepatitis C virus. JAMA 1990;263:49.

95. Cash JD, McClelland DBL, Urbaniak SJ, Contreris M, Barbara JAJ. Screening for hepatitis C virus antibody. Lancet 1989;2:505.

96. Janot C, Courouce AM, Maniez M. Antibodies to hepatitis C virus in French blood donors. Lancet 1989;2:796.

97. Sirchia G, Bellobuono A, Giovanetti A, Marconi M. Antibodies to hepatitis C virus in Italian blood donors. Lancet 1989;2:797.

98. Kuhnl P, Seidl S, Stangel W, Beyer J, Sibrowski W, Flik J. Antibody to hepatitis C virus in German blood donors. Lancet 1989;2:324.

99. Ideo G, Bellati G, Pedraglio E, Bottelli R, Donzelli T, Putignano G. Intrafamilial transmission of hepatitis C virus. Lancet 1990;335: 353.

100. Cock DM, Bradley DW, Sandford NL, et al. Epidemic non-A, non-B hepatitis in patients from Pakistan. Ann Intern Med 1987;106: 227.

101. Ramalingaswami V, Purcell RH. Waterborne non-A, non-B hepatitis. Lancet 1988;1:571.

102. Kelly TW, Patrick MR, Hillman KM. Study of diarrhea in critically ill patients. Crit Care Med 1983;11:7.

103. DuPont HL, Ribner BS. Infectious gastroenteritis. In: Bennett JV, Brachman PS, eds. Hospital infections, ed 2. Boston: Little, Brown, 1986:495.

104. Hughes JM, Jarvis WR. Nosocomial gastrointestinal infections. In: Wenzel RP, ed. Prevention and control of nosocomial infections. Baltimore: Williams & Wilkins, 1987:405.

105. Pickering LK, Reves RR. Diarrhea. In: Donowitz LG, ed. Hospital-acquired infection in the pediatric patient. Baltimore: Williams & Wilkins, 1988:56.

106. Palmer SR, Rowe B. Investigation of outbreaks of Salmonella in hospitals. Br Med J 1983;287:891.

107. Beers LM, Burke TL, Martine DB. Shigellosis occurring in newborn nursery staff. Infect Control Hosp Epidemiol 1989;10:147.

108. Gerards LJ, Hennekam RCM, Dijk WCy, Roord JJ, Fleer A. An outbreak of gastroenteritis due to *Escherichia coli* 0142 H6 in a neonatal department. J Hosp Infect 1984;5:283.

109. Lam BCC, Tam J, Ng MH, Yeung CY. Nosocomial gastroenteritis in paediatric patients. J Hosp Infect 1989;14:351.

110. Galloway A, Roberts C, Hunt EJ. An outbreak of *Salmonella typhimurium* gastroenteritis in a psychiatric hospital. J Hosp Infect 1987;10:248.

111. Hunter PR, Hutchings PG. Outbreak of *Shigella sonnei* dysentery on a long stay psychogeriatric ward. J Hosp Infect 1987;10:73.

112. Horan MA, Gulati RS, Fox RA, Glew E, Ganguli L, Kaeney M. Outbreak of *Shigella sonnei* dysentery on a geriatric assessment ward. J Hosp Infect 1984;5:210.

113. Meara J, Mayon-White R, Johnston H. Salmonellosis in a psychogeriatric ward: Problems of infection control. J Hosp Infect 1988;11: 86.

114. Mitchell E, O'Mahony M, McKeith I, Sprott MS, Codd AA, Wright AG. An outbreak of viral gastroenteritis in a psychiatric hospital. J Hosp Infect 1989;14:1.

115. Sanyal D. Outbreaks of viral gastroenteritis caused by small round structure virus in psycho-geriatric patients. J Hosp Infect 1987;9: 302.

116. Hughes JM, Gangarosa EJ. Hospital food services: Role in prevention of nosocomial foodborne disease. In: Bennett JV, Brachman PS, eds. Hospital infections, ed 2. Boston: Little, Brown, 1986:257.

117. Thomas M, Noah ND, Male GE, et al. Hospital outbreak of *Clostridium perfringens* food-poisoning. Lancet 1977;1:1046.

118. Yamagishi T, Sakamoto K, Sakurai S, et al. A nosocomial outbreak of food poisoning caused by enterotoxigenic *Clostridium perfringens*. Microbiol Immunol 1983;27:291.

119. Baddour LM, Gaia SM, Griffin R, Hudson R. A hospital cafeterial-related food-borne outbreak due to *Bacillus cereus:* Unique features. Infect Control 1986;7:462.

120. Opal SM, Mayer KH, Roland F, Brondum J, Heelan J, Lyhte L. Investigation of a food-borne outbreak of salmonellosis among hospital employees. Am J Infect Control 1989;17:141.

121. Spitalny KC, Okowitz EN, Vogt RL. Salmonellosis outbreak at a Vermont hospital. South Med J 1984;77:168.

122. Centers for Disease Control. Shigellosis in a children's hospital—Pennsylvania. MMWR 1979;28:498.

123. Meyers JD, Romm FJ, Tihen WS, Bryan JA. Food-borne hepatitis A in a general hospital. JAMA 1975;231:1049.

124. Centers for Disease Control. Hospital-associated outbreak of *Shigella dysenteriae* type 2—Maryland. MMWR 1983;32:250.

125. Gellert GA, Tormey M, Rodriguez G, Brougher G, Dassey D, Pate C. Food-borne disease in hospitals: Prevention in a changing food service environment. Am J Infect Control 1989;19:136.

126. Centers for Disease Control. Multistate outbreak of salmonellosis caused by precooked roast beef. MMWR 1981;30:391.

127. Steere AC, Craven PJ, Hall WJ, et al. Person-to-person spread of *Salmonella typhimurium* after a hospital common-source outbreak. Lancet 1975;1:319.

128. Sanders E, Sweeney FJ, Friedman EA, Boring JR, Randall EL, Polk LD. An outbreak of hospital-associated infections due to *Salmonella derby*. JAMA 1963;186:984.

129. Noone C, Banatvala JE. Hospital acquired rotaviral gastroenteritis in a general paediatric unit. J Hosp Infect 1983;4:297.

130. Rodriguez WJ, Kim HW, Brandt CD, Fletcher AB, Parrott RH. Rotavirus: A cause of nosocomial infection in the nursery. J Pediatr 1982;101:274.

131. Gustafson TL, Kobylik B, Hutcheson RH, Schaffner W. Protective effect of anticholinergic drugs and psyllium in a nosocomial outbreak of Norwalk gastroenteritis. J Hosp Infect 1983;4:367.

132. Pether JVS, Caul EO. An outbreak of food-borne gastroenteritis in two hospitals associated with a Norwalk-like virus. J Hyg Camb 1983;91:343.

133. Giannella RA, Brasile L. A hospital food-borne outbreak of diarrhea caused by *Bacillus cereus:* Clinical, epidemiologic, and microbiologic studies. J Infect Dis 1979;139:366.

134. Jephcott AE, Barton BW, Gilbert RJ, Shearer CW. An unusual outbreak of food-poisoning associated with Meals-on-Wheels. Lancet 1977;2:129.

135. Clabots CR, Peterson LR, Gerding DN. Characterization of a nosocomial *Clostridium difficile* outbreak by using plasmid profile typing and clindamycin susceptibility testing. J Infect Dis 1988;158:731.

136. Degl'Innocenti R, Santis MD, Berdondini I, Dei R. Outbreak of *Clostridium difficile* diarrhoea in an orthopaedic unit: Evidence by phage-typing for cross-infection. J Hosp Infect 1989;13:309.

137. McFarland LV, Mulligan ME, Kwok RYY, Stamm WE. Nosocomial acquisition of *Clostridium difficile* infection. N Engl J Med 1989;320:204.

138. Testore GP, Pantosti A, Cerquetti M, Babudieri S, Panichi G, Gianfrilli PM. Evidence for cross-infection in an outbreak of *Clostridium difficile*-associated diarrhoea in a surgical unit. J Med Microbiol 1988;26:125.

139. Kumarasinghe G, Hamilton WJ, Gould JDM, Palmer SR, Dudgeon JA, Marshall WC. An outbreak of *Salmonella muenchen* infection in a specialist paediatric hospital. J Hosp Infect 1982;3:341.

140. Morse LJ, Rubenstein AD. A food-borne institutional outbreak of enteritis due to *Salmonella blockley*. JAMA 1967;202:115.

141. Robins-Browne RM, Rowe B, Ramsaroop R, et al. A hospital outbreak of multiresistant *Salmonella typhimurium* belonging to phage type 193. J Infect Dis 1983;147:210.

142. Schroeder SA, Aserkoff B, Brachman PS. Epidemic salmonellosis in hospital and institutions. N Engl J Med 1968;279:674.

143. Ratnam S, Mercer E, Picco B, Parsons S, Butler R. A nosocomial outbreak of diarrheal disease due to *Yersinia enterocolitica* serotype 0:5, biotype 1. J Infect Dis 1982;145:242.

144. Martino P, Gentile G, Caprioli A, et al. Hospital-acquired cryptosporidiosis in a bone marrow transplantation unit. J Infect Dis 1988;158:647.

145. Baxby D, Hart CA, Taylor C. Human cryptosporidiosis: A possible case of hospital cross infection. Br Med J 1983:287:1760.

146. Dryjanski J, Gold JWM, Ritchie MT, Kurtz RC, Lim SL, Armstrong D. Cryptosporidiosis: Case report in a health team worker. Am J Med 1986;80:751.

147. Sharp JCM, Collier PW, Gilbert RJ. Food poisoning in hospitals in Scotland. J Hyg Camb 1979;83:231.

148. Siegel DL, Edelstein PH, Nachamkin I. Inappropriate testing for diarrheal diseases in the hospital. JAMA 1990;263:979.

149. Yannelli B, Gurevich I, Schoch PE, Cunha BA. Yield of stool cultures, ova and parasite tests, and *clostridium difficile* determinations in nosocomial diarrheas. Am J Infect Control 1988;16:246.

150. Brady MT, Pacini DL, Budde CT, Connell MJ. Diagnostic studies of nosocomial diarrhea in children: Assessing their use and value. Am J Infect Control 1989;17:77.

151. Welliver RC, McLaughlin S. Unique epidemiology of nosocomial infection in a children's hospital. Am J Dis Child 1984;138:131.

152. Gilligan PH. Diarrheal disease in the hospitalized patient. Infect Control 1986;7:607.

153. Brunetto AL, Pearson ADJ, Craft AW, Pedler SJ. *Clostridium difficile* in an oncology unit. Arch Dis Child 1988;63:979.

154. Foulke GE, Silva J. *Clostridium difficile* in the intensive care unit: Management problems and prevention issues. Crit Care Med 1989;17:822.

155. Heard SR, O'Farrell S, Holland D, Crook S, Barnett MJ, Tabaqchali S. The epidemiology of *Clostridium difficile* with use of a typing scheme: Nosocomial acquisition and cross-infection among immunocompromised patients. J Infect Dis 1986;153:159.

156. Wust J, Sullivan NM, Hardegger U, Wilkins TD. Investigation of an outbreak of antibiotic-associated colitis by various typing methods. J Clin Microbiol 1982;16:1096.

157. Gerding DN. Disease associated with *Clostridium difficile* infection. Ann Intern Med 1989;110:255.

158. Fekety R, Kim K-H, Brown D, Battis DH, Cudmore M, Silva J. Epidemiology of antibiotic-associated colitis: Isolation of *Clostridium difficile* from the hospital environment. Am J Med 1981;70:906.

159. Mulligan ME, George WL, Rolfe RD, Finegold SM. Epidemiological aspects of *Clostridium difficile*-induced diarrhea and colitis. Am J Clin Nutr 1980;33:2533.

160. Silva J, Iezzi C. *Clostridium difficile* as a nosocomial pathogen. J Hosp Infect 1988;11:378.

161. Mulligan ME. Epidemiology of *Clostridium difficile*-induced intestinal disease. Rev Infect Dis 1984;6:S222.

162. Gerding DN, Johnson S, Olson M, Weiler M, Hughes R, Clabots C. Prospective controlled study of vinyl glove use to interrupt *Clostridium difficile* nosocomial transmission. Abstracts of the Eighty-Eighth Annual Meeting of the American Society for Microbiology, May 8–13, 1988, Miami Beach, Florida. Washington, DC: American Society for Microbiology, Abstract No. L-32, 1988:416.

163. Johnson S, Gerding DN, Olson MM, et al. Prospective, controlled study of vinyl glove use to interrupt *Clostridium difficile* nosocomial transmission. Am J Med 1990;88:137.

164. Cone R, Mohan K, Thouless M, Corey L. Nosocomial transmission of rotavirus infection. Pediatr Infect Dis J 1988;7:103.

165. Di Matteo A, Sarasini A, Scotta MS, Parea M, Licardi G, Gerna G. Nosocomial outbreak of infant rotavirus diarrhea due to the appearance of a new serotype 4 strain. J Med Virol 1989;27:100.

166. Lewis DC, Lightfoot NF, Cubitt WD, Wilson SA. Outbreaks of astrovirus type 1 and rotavirus gastroenteritis in a geriatric in-patient population. J Hosp Infect 1989;14:9.

167. Pacini DL, Brady MT, Budde CT, Connell MJ, Hamparian VV, Hughes JH. Nosocomial rotaviral diarrhea: Pattern of spread on wards in a children's hospital. J Med Virol 1987;23:359.

168. Vial PA, Kotloff KL, Losonsky GA. Molecular epidemiology of rotavirus infection in a room for convalescing newborns. J Infect Dis 1988;157:668.

169. Dearlove J, Latham P, Dearlove B, Pearl K, Thomson A, Lewis IG. Clinical range of neonatal rotavirus gastroenteritis. Br Med J 1983:286:1473.

170. Hjelt K, Krasilnikoff PA, Grauballe PC, Rasmussen SW. Nosocomial acute gastroenteritis in a paediatric department with special reference to rotavirus infections. Acta Paediatr Scand 1985;74:89.

171. Chan RCK, Tam JS, Fok TF, French GL. RNA-electrophoresis as a type of method for nosocomial rotavirus infection in a special-care baby unit. J Hosp Infect 1989;13:367.

172. Dennehy PH, Peter G. Risk factors associated with nosocomial rotavirus infection. Am J Dis Child 1985;139:935.

173. Holzel H, Cubitt DW, McSwiggan DA, Sanderson PJ, Church J. An outbreak of rotavirus infection among adults in a cardiology ward. J Infect 1980;2:33.

174. Rudd PT, Carrington D. A prospective study of chlamydial, mycoplasmal, and viral infections in a neonatal intensive care unit. Arch Dis Child 1984;59:120.

175. Greenberg HB, Valdesuso J, Yolken RH, Gangarosa E, Gary W, Wyatt RG, Konno T, Suzuki H, Chanock RM, Kapikian AZ. Role

of Norwalk virus in outbreaks of nonbacterial gastroenteritis. J Infect Dis 1979;139:564.

176. Halvorsrud J, Orstavik I. An epidemic of rotavirus-associated gastroenteritis in a nursing home for the elderly. Scand J Infect Dis 1980;12:161.

177. Sawyer LA, Murphy JJ, Kaplan JE, et al. 25- to 30-NM virus particle associated with a hospital outbreak of acute gastroenteritis with evidence for airborne transmission. Am J Epidemiol 1988;127:1261.

178. Leers W-D, Kasupski G, Fralick R, Wartman S, Garcia J, Gary W. Norwalk-like gastroenteritis epidemic in a Toronto hospital. Am J Public Health 1987;77:291.

179. Kotloff KL, Losonsky GA, Morris JG, Wasserman SS, Singh-Naz N, Levine MM. Enteric adenovirus infection and childhood diarrhea: An epidemiologic study in three clinical settings. Pediatrics 1989;84:219.

180. Yolken RH, Lawrence F, Leister F, Takiff HE, Strauss SE. Gastroenteritis associated with enteric type adenovirus in hospitalized infants. J Pediatr 1982;101:21.

181. Yolken RH, Franklin CC. Gastrointestinal adenovirus: An important cause of morbidity in patients with necrotizing enterocolitis and gastrointestinal surgery. Pediatr Infect Dis 1985;4:42.

182. Humphrey TJ, Cruickshank JG, Cubitt WD. An outbreak of calicivirus associated gastroenteritis in an elderly person's home: A possible zoonosis? J Hyg 1984;92:293.

183. Spratt HC, Marcks MI, Gomersall M, Gill P, Pai CH. Nosocomial infantile gastroenteritis associated with minirotavirus and calicivirus. J Pediatr 1978;93:922.

184. Champsaur H, Questiaux E, Prevot J, Henry-Amar M, Goldszmidt D, Bourjouane M, Bach C. Rotavirus carriage, asymptomatic infection, and disease in the first two years of life. I. Virus shedding. J Infect Dis 1984;149:667.

185. Vesikari T, Maki M, Sarkkinen HK, Arstila PP, Halonen PE. Rotavirus, adenovirus, and non-viral enteropathogens in diarrhoea. Arch Dis Child 1981;56:264.

186. Eiden JJ, Verleur DG, Vonderfecht SL, Yolken RH. Duration and pattern of asymptomatic rotavirus shedding by hospitalized children. Pediatr Infect Dis J 1988;7:564.

187. Samadi AR, Huq MI, Ahmed QS. Detection of rotavirus in handwashings of attendants of children with diarrhoea. Br Med J 1983;286:188.

188. Ansari SA, Sattar SA, Springthorpe VS, Wells GA, Tostowaryk W. Rotavirus survival on human hands and transfer of infectious virus to animate and nonporous inanimate surfaces. J Clin Microbiol 1988;26:1513.

189. Sattar SA, Lloyd-Evans N, Springthorpe VS, Nair RC. Institutional outbreaks of rotavirus diarrhoea: Potential role of fomites and environmental surfaces as vehicles for virus transmission. J Hyg 1986;96:277.

190. Prince DS, Astry C, Vonderfecht S, Jakab G, Shen F-M, Yolken RH. Aerosol transmission of experimental rotavirus infection. Pediatr Infect Dis 1986;5:218.

191. Dennehy PH, Tente WE, Fisher DJ, Veloudis BA, Peter G. Lack of impact of rapid identification of rotavirus-infected patients on nosocomial rotavirus infections. Pediatr Infect Dis J 1989;8:290.

192. Centers for Disease Control. Institutional salmonellosis. J Infect Dis 1973;128:357.

193. Cruickshank JG, on behalf of the Public Health Laboratory Service. Salmonella Subcommittee. The investigation of Salmonella outbreaks in hospitals. J Hosp Infect 1984;5:241.

194. Weikel CS, Guerrant RL. Nosocomial salmonellosis. Infect Control 1985;6:218.

195. Joseph CA, Palmer SR. Outbreaks of Salmonella infection in hospitals in England and Wales 1978–87. Br Med J 1998;298:1161.

196. Centers for Disease Control. Update: *Salmonella enteritidis* infections and grade A shell eggs—United States, 1989. MMWR 1990;38:877.

197. Gold R. Shigellosis in the nursery. Infect Control Hosp Epidemiol 1989;10:145.

198. Vennes JA. Infectious complications of gastrointestinal endoscopy. Dig Dis Sci 1981;26:60s.

199. Silvis SE, Nebel O, Rogers G, et al. Endoscopic complications: Results of the 1974 American Society for Gastrointestinal Endoscopy Survey. JAMA 1976;235:928.

200. O'Connor HJ, Axon ATR. Gastrointestinal endoscopy: Infection and disinfection. Gut 1983;24:1067.

201. Axon ATR, Cotton PB. Endoscopy and infection. Gut 1983;24:1064.

202. Dwyer DM, Klein EG, Istre GR et al. *Salmonella newport* infections transmitted by fiberoptic colonoscopy. Gastrointest Endosc 1987;33:84.

203. Graham D, Alpert L, Smith J, et al. Iatrogenic *Campylobacter pylori* infection is a cause of epidemic achlorhydria. Am J Gastroenterol 1988;83:1168.

204. Otten MH, de Jong J, Visser J, et al. *Campylobacter pylori* infection transmitted by gastroscopy. Neth J Med (In press)

205. Langenberg W, Rauws EAJ, Oudbier JH, Tytgat GNJ. Patient to patient transmission of *Campylobacter pylori* infection by fiberoptic gastroduodenoscopy and biopsy. J Infect Dis 1990;161:507.

206. Greene WH, Moody M, Hartley R, et al. Esophagoscopy as a source of *Pseudomonas aeruginosa* sepsis in patients with acute leukemia: The need for sterilization of endoscopes. Gastroenterology 1974;67:912.

207. Allen JI, Allen MO, Olsen MM, et al. *Pseudomonas* infection of the biliary system resulting from use of a contaminated endoscope. Gastroenterology 1987;92:759.

208. Siegman-Ingra Y, Spinrad S, Rutter J. Septic complications following endoscopic retrograde cholangiopancreatography: The experience in Tel Aviv Medical Center. J Hosp Infect 1988;12:7.

209. Casemore DP, Blewett DA, Wright SE. Letter: Cleaning and disinfection of equipment for gastrointestinal flexible endoscopy: Interim recommendations of a working party of the British Society of Gastroenterology. Gut 1989;30:1156.

210. Roberts WG, Green PHR, Ma J, et al. Prevalence of cryptosporidiosis in patients undergoing endoscopy: Evidence for an asymptomatic carrier state. Am J Med 1989;87:537.

211. Singh S, Singh N, Kochhar R, et al. Contamination of an endoscope due to *Trichosporon beigelii*. J Hosp Infect 1989;14:49.

212. Sharvon PJ, Eykyn SJ, Cotton PB. Gastrointestinal instrumentation bacteraemia and endocarditis. Gut 1983;24:1078.

213. Botoman VA, Surawicz CM. Bacteremia with gastrointestinal endoscopic procedures. Gastrointest Endosc 1986;32:342.

214. Fleisher D. Recommendations for antibiotic prophylaxis before endoscopy. Am J Gastroenterol 1989;84:1489.

215. Yin TP, Dellipiani AW. Bacterial endocarditis after Hurst bougienage in a patient with a benign esophageal stricture. Endoscopy 1983;15:27.

216. Niv Y, Bat L, Motro M. Bacterial endocarditis after Hurst bougienage in a patient with a benign stricture and mitral valve prolapse. Gastrointest Endosc 1985;31:265.

217. Neu HC. Recommendations for antibiotic prophylaxis before endoscopy. Am J Gastroenterol 1989;84:1488.

218. Meyer GW. Endocarditis prophylaxis and gastrointestinal procedures. Am J Gastroenterol 1989;84:1492.

219. Durack DT. Prophylaxis of infective endocarditis. In: Mandell FL, Douglas RG, Bennett JE, eds. Principles and practices of infectious diseases, ed 3. New York: Churchill Livingstone, 1989:716.

220. Meyer GW. Endocarditis prophylaxis and esophageal dilatation. Gastrointest Endosc 1989;35:129.

221. Cohen LB, Korsten MA, Scherl EJ, et al. Bacteremia after endoscopic injection sclerosis. Gastrointest Endosc 1983;29:198.

222. Cohen FL, Koerner RS, Taub SJ. Solitary brain abscess following endoscopic injection sclerosis of esophageal varices. Gastrointest Endosc 1985;31:331.

223. Shemesh O, Bornstein IB, Weissberg N, et al. Listeria septicemia after colonoscopy in an ulcerative colitis patient receiving ACTH. Am J Gastroenterol 1990;85:216.

224. Ciocon JO, Silverstone FA, Graver LM, Foley CJ. Tube feedings in elderly patients. Arch Intern Med 1988;148:429.

225. Pingleton SK. Enteral nutrition as a risk factor for nosocomial pneumonia. Eur J Clin Microbiol Infect Dis 1989;8:51.

226. McWey RE, Curry NS, Schabel SI, Reines HD. Complications of nasoenteric feeding tubes. Am J Surg 1988;155:253.

227. Anderton A. Microbiological aspects of the preparation and administration of naso-gastric and naso-enteric tube feeds in hospitals—A review. Hum Nutr Appl Nutr 1983;37A:426.

228. Bastow MD, Greaves P, Allison SP. Microbial contamination of enteral feeds. Hum Nutr Appl Nutr 1982;36A:213.

229. Department of Health and Human Services. Bacterial contamination of enteral formula products. FDA Drug Bulletin 1988;18:34.

230. Gill KJ, Gill P. Contaminated enteral feeds. Br Med J 1981;282: 1971.

231. Schreiner RL, Eitzen H, Gfell MA, Kress S, Gresham EL, French M, Moye L. Environmental contamination of continuous drip feedings. Pediatrics 1979;63:232.

232. White WT, Acuff TE, Sykes TR, Dobbie RP. Bacterial contamination of enteral nutrient solution: A preliminary report. J Parenter Enteral Nutr 1979;3:459.

233. Anderton A. Microbiological quality of products used in enteral feeds. J Hosp Infect 1986;7:68.

234. Bologna L, Marcina A, Daraio M, Gleich S. Infant feeding formula contaminated by Enterobacter cloacae. Infect Control 1984;5:115.

235. Simmons BP, Gelfand MS, Haas M, Metts L, Ferguson J. Enterobacter sakazakii infections in neonates associated with intrinsic contamination of a powdered infant formula. Infect Control Hosp Epidemiol 1989;10:398.

236. Anderson KR, Norris DJ, Godfrey LB, Avent CK, Butterworth CE. Bacterial contamination of tube-feeding formulas. J Parenter Enteral Nutr 1984;8:673.

237. Casewell M, Phillips I. Food as a source of Klebsiella species for colonisation and infection of intensive care patients. J Clin Pathol 1978;31:845.

238. Crocker KS, Krey SH, Markovic M, Steffee WP. Microbial growth in clinically used enteral delivery systems. Am J Infect Control 1986;14:250.

239. Schroeder P, Fisher D, Volz M, Paloucek J. Microbial contamination of enteral feeding solutions in a community hospital. J Parenter Enteral Nutr 1983;7:364.

240. Casewell MW. Bacteriological hazards of contaminated enteral feeds. J Hosp Infect 1982;3:329.

241. Cooke EM, Shooter RA, Komar PJ, et al. Hospital food as a possible source of Escherichia coli in patients. Lancet 1970;1:436.

242. Anderton A, Aidoo KE. The effect of handling procedures on microbial contamination of enteral feeds. J Hosp Infect 1988;11:364.

243. Shooter RA, Cooke EM, Gaya H, et al. Food and medicaments as possible sources of hospital strains of Pseudomonas aeruginosa. Lancet 1969;1:1227.

244. Thurn J, Crossley K, Gerdts A, Maki M, Johnson J. Enteral hyperalimentation as a cause of nosocomial infection. J Hosp Infect 1990;15:203.

245. Fagerman KE. Bacteriostatic enteral feeding solutions needed. Nutr Supp Serv 1986;6:32.

246. Levy J. Enteral nutrition: An increasingly recognized cause of nosocomial bloodstream infection. Infect Control Hosp Epidemiol 1989;10:395.

247. Levy J, Laethem YV, Verhaegen G, Perpete C, Butzler J-P, Wenzel RP. Contaminated enteral nutrition solutions as a cause of nosocomial bloodstream infection: A study using plasmid fingerprinting. J Parenter Enteral Nutr 1989;13:228.

248. Bladwin BA, Zagoren AJ, Rose N. Bacterial contamination of continuously infused enteral alimentation with needle catheter jejunostomy—Clinical implications. J Parenter Enteral Nutr 1984;8:30.

249. Casewell MW. Enteral feeds contaminated with Enterobacter cloacae as a cause of septicemia. Br Med J 1981;182:973.

250. Van Enk RA, Furtado D. Bacterial contamination of enteral nutrient solutions: Intestinal colonization and sepsis in mice after ingestion. J Parenter Enteral Nutr 1986;10:503.

251. Anderton A, Howard JP, Scott DW. Microbiological control in enteral feeding. Hum Nutr Appl Nutr 1986;40A:163.

252. American Society for Parenteral and Enteral Nutrition Board of Directors. Guidelines for the use of enteral nutrition in the adult patient. J Parenter Enteral Nutr 1987;11:435.

253. Fagerman KE, Paauw JD, Dean RE. Bacterial contamination of enteral solutions. J Parenter Enteral Nutr 1985;9:378.

254. Fagerman KE, Paauw JD, McCamish MA, Dean RE. Effects of time, temperature, and preservative on bacterial growth in enteral nutrient solutions. Am J Hosp Pharm 1984;41:1122.

255. Maki DG. Infections due to infusion therapy. In: Bennett JV, Brachman PS, eds. Hospital infections, ed 2. Boston: Little, Brown, 1986:561.

256. Henderson DK. Bacteremia due to percutaneous intravascular de-

vices. In: Mandell GL, Douglas RG, Bennett JE, eds. Principles and practices of infectious diseases, ed 3. New York: Churchill Livingstone, 1989:2189.

257. Hamory BH. Nosocomial bloodstream and intravascular device-related infections. In: Wenzel RP, ed. Prevention and control of nosocomial infections. Baltimore: Williams & Wilkins, 1987:283.

258. Perkins CM, Dascomb HE. Intravascular device-related infections. Prob Crit Care 1990;4:21.

259. Crocker KS, Noga R, Filibeck DJ, Krey SH, Markovick M, Steffee WP. Microbial growth comparisons of five commercial parenteral lipid emulsions. J Parenter Enteral Nutr 1984;8:391.

260. Kim CH, Lewis DE, Kumar A. Bacterial and fungal growth in intravenous fat emulsions. Am J Hosp Pharm 1983;40:2159.

261. Goldmann DA, Martin WT, Worthington JW. Growth of bacteria and fungi in total parenteral nutrition solutions. Am J Surg 1973;126: 314.

262. Keammerer D, Mayhall CG, Hall GO, Pesko LJ, Thomas RB. Microbial growth patterns in intravenous fat emulsions. Am J Hosp Pharm 1983;40:1650.

263. Bernard RW, Stahl WM, Chase RM. Subclavian vein catheterizations: A prospective study. II. Infectious complications. Ann Surg 1971;173: 191.

264. Jarrett F, Maki DG, Chan C-K. Management of septic thrombosis of the inferior vena cava caused by Candida. Arch Surg 1978;113: 637.

265. Strinden WD, Helgerson RB, Maki DG. Candida septic thrombosis of the great central veins associated with central catheters. Ann Surg 1985;202:653.

266. Dillon JD, Schaffner W, Van Way CW, Meng HC. Septicemia and total parenteral nutrition: Distinguishing catheter-related from other septic episodes. JAMA 1973;223:1341.

267. Sitzmann JV, Townsend TR, Siler MC, Bartlett JG. Septic and technical complications of central venous catheterization: A prospective study of 200 consecutive patients. Ann Surg 1985;202:766.

268. Young GP, Alexeyeff M, Russell DMcR, Thomas RJS. Catheter sepsis during parenteral nutrition: The safety of long-term opsite dressings. J Parenter Enteral Nutr 1988;12:365.

269. Snydman DR, Murray SA, Kornfeld SJ, Majka JA, Ellis CA. Total parenteral nutrition–related infections: Prospective epidemiologic study using semiquantitative methods. Am J Med 1982;73:695.

270. Ryan JA, Abel RM, Abbott WM, Hopkins CC, Chesney TMcC, Colley R, Phillips K, Fischer JE. Catheter complications in total parenteral nutrition: A prospective study of 200 consecutive patients. N Engl J Med 1974;290:757.

271. Ashcraft KW, Leape LL. Candida sepsis complicating parenteral feeding. JAMA 1970;212:454.

272. Curry CR, Quie PG. Fungal septicemia in patients receiving parenteral hyperalimentation. N Engl J Med 1971;285:1221.

273. Montgomerie JZ, Edwards JE. Association of infection due to Candida albicans with intravenous hyperalimentation. J Infect Dis 1978;137: 197.

274. Maki DG, Goldmann DA, Rhame FS. Infection control in intravenous therapy. Ann Intern Med 1973;79:867.

275. Nehme AE. Nutritional support of the hospitalized patient. JAMA 1980;243:1906.

276. Reinhardt GF, Gelbart SM, Greenlee HB. Catheter infection factors affecting total parenteral nutrition. Am Surg 1978;44:401.

277. Henderson DK, Edwards JE, Montgomerie JZ. Hematogenous Candida endophthalmitis in patients receiving parenteral hyperalimentation fluids. J Infect Dis 1981;143:655.

278. Plouffe JF, Brown DG, Silva J Jr, Eck T, Stricof RL, Fekety FR Jr. Nosocomial outbreak of Candida parapsilosis fungemia related to intravenous infusions. Arch Intern Med 1977;137:1686.

279. Solomon SL, Khabbaz RF, Parker RH, Anderson RL, Geraghty MA, Furman RM, Martone WJ. An outbreak of Candida parapsilosis bloodstream infections in patients receiving parenteral nutrition. J Infect Dis 1984;149:98.

280. Marcon MJ, Powell DA. Epidemiology, diagnosis, and management of Malassezia furfur systemic infection. Diagn Microbiol Infect Dis 1987;7:161.

281. Azimi PH, Levernier K, Lefrak LM, et al. Malassezia furfur: A cause of occlusion of percutaneous central venous catheters in infants in the intensive care nursery. Pediatr Infect Dis J 1988;7:100.

282. Long JG, Keyserling HL. Catheter-related infection in infants due to an unusual lipophilic yeast—*Malassezia furfur*. Pediatrics 1985;76:896.

283. Powell DA, Marcon MJ. Failure to eradicate *Malassezia furfur* Broviac catheter infection with antifungal therapy. Pediatr Infect Dis J 1987;6:579.

284. Powell DA, Aungst J, Snedden S, et al. Broviac catheter-related *Malassezia furfur* sepsis in five infants receiving intravenous fat emulsions. J Pediatr 1984;105:987.

285. Redline RW, Dahms BB. Malassezia pulmonary vasculitis in an infant on long-term intralipid therapy. N Engl J Med 1981;305:1395.

286. Garcia CR, Johnston BL, Corvi G, Walker LJ, George WL. Intravenous catheter-associated *Malassezia furfur* fungemia. Am J Med 1987;83:790.

287. Brooks R, Brown L. Systemic infection with *Malassezia furfur* in an adult receiving long-term hyperalimentation therapy. J Infect Dis 1987;156:410.

288. Marcon MJ, Powell DA, Durrell DE. Methods for optimal recovery of *Malassezia furfur* from blood culture. J Clin Microbiol 1986;24:696.

289. Rutala WA. APIC guidelines for selection and use of disinfectants. Am J Infect Control 1990;18:99.

290. Weber DJ, Rutala WA. Environmental issues and nosocomial infections. In: Farber BF, ed. Infection control in intensive care. New York: Churchill Livingstone, 1987:131.

291. Rutala WA. Disinfection, sterilization, and waste disposal. In: Wenzel RP, ed. Prevention and control of nosocomial infections. Baltimore: Williams & Wilkins, 1987:257.

292. Favero MS. Chemical disinfection of medical and surgical materials. In: Block SS, ed. Disinfection, sterilization and preservation, ed 3. Philadelphia: Lea & Febiger, 1983:469.

293. Spaulding EH. Chemical disinfection of medical and surgical material. In: Lawrence CA, Block SS, eds. Disinfection, sterilization and preservation, ed 1. Philadelphia: Lea & Febiger, 1968:517.

294. Bean HS. Types and characteristics of disinfectants. J Appl Bacteriol 1967;30:6.

295. Russell AD, Hugo WB, Ayliffe GAJ, eds. Principles and practice of disinfection, preservation and sterilization. Oxford: Blackwell Scientific Publications, 1982.

296. Society of Gastrointestinal Assistants. Recommended guidelines for infection control in gastrointestinal endoscopy settings. Rochester, NY: Society of Gastrointestinal Assistants, Inc, 1988.

297. American Society for Gastrointestinal Endoscopy Infection control during gastrointestinal endoscopy. Gastrointest Endosc 1988;34(Suppl 3):37S.

298. Cleaning and disinfection of equipment for gastrointestinal flexible endoscopy: Interim recommendations of a working party of the British Society of Gastroenterology. Gut 1988;29:1134.

299. Sobala GM, Lincoln C, Axon ATR. Does the endoscope control head need to be disinfected between examinations. Endoscopy 1989;21:19.

300. Hanson PJV, Gor D, Chadwick MV. Endoscopy and AIDS: An evaluation of the risk of cross-infection. Gut 1989;30:A742.

301. Shulman ST, Amien DP, Biano AL, et al. Prevention of bacterial endocarditis: A statement for health professionals by the Committee on Rheumatic Fever and Infective Endocarditis of the Council on Cardiovascular Disease in the Young. Circulation 1984;70:1123A.

302. Dajani AS, Bisno AL, Chung KJ, et al. Prevention of bacterial endocarditis: Recommendations by the American Heart Association. JAMA 1990;264:2919.

III

Gastrointestinal Diseases

A. Esophagus

53

Esophagus: Anatomy and Structural Anomalies

GREGORY A. BOYCE
H. WORTH BOYCE, JR.

Clinicians who assume responsibility for diagnosis and treatment of esophageal disorders must have a knowledge base of the details of esophageal anatomy. Recognition of pathologic alterations in their earliest stages can be accomplished only if one is aware of the normal anatomy and its variants. Optimum interpretation of every test of esophageal function and morphology is dependent upon such knowledge of the peculiarities of esophageal anatomy. As one's understanding of the manifestations of esophageal disease advances, knowledge of its anatomy will be increasingly recognized as being essential to clinical success.

EMBRYOLOGY

During the fourth week of embryologic development, a small diverticulum forms on the ventral surface of the foregut adjacent to the pharyngeal gut. This diverticulum (tracheobronchial) separates gradually from the dorsal foregut through the esophagotracheal septum with eventual separation into the trachea and esophagus.[1] With cranial growth of the embryonic body, the esophagus elongates rapidly. During the sixth week of gestation, the circular muscle coat and ganglion cells of the myenteric plexus form. During the seventh week, blood vessels enter the submucosa.

The esophageal epithelium rapidly proliferates and almost completely fills the lumen in the seventh and eighth week, leaving residual channels within the nearly occluded lumen.[2] A single esophageal lumen returns in the tenth week, leaving a superficial layer of ciliated epithelial cells.

In the fourth month, ciliated epithelial cells are replaced by stratified squamous epithelium, a process that continues until birth. Residual islands of ciliated epithelium at the proximal and distal ends of the esophagus remain and give rise to esophageal glands.[3]

ADULT ANATOMY

Gross Anatomy

The adult esophagus is a flattened muscular tube that arises proximally at the pharyngoesophageal junction (C5-C6 vertebral interspace) and courses through the posterior mediastinum to end at the gastroesophageal junction (T11 vertebral level). The esophageal lumen can distend to approximately 2 cm in anteroposterior diameter and up to 3 cm in lateral diameter. The length of the adult esophagus is variable but ranges in length from 18 to 26 cm.[4] The cervical esophagus extends from the pharyngoesophageal junction to the suprasternal notch (about 4 to 5 cm long). At this level the esophagus is surrounded by the trachea anteriorly, vertebral column posteriorly, and the carotid sheaths and thyroid laterally.

The thoracic esophagus passes just posterior to the tracheal wall and courses right posterior to the aortic arch (T4 vertebral level) and posterior to the tracheal bifurcation and left mainstem bronchus. At the T8 vertebral level, the esophagus turns left and crosses anterior to the aorta at the level of the diaphragmatic hiatus. At the T10 vertebral level the esophagus passes through an elliptical opening in the muscular diaphragm and enters into the cardiac portion of the stomach at an oblique angle.

The abdominal portion of the esophagus (so-called submerged segment) is short, varying in length from 0.5 to 2.5 cm.[5] At this level the left lobe of the liver lies anteriorly, the caudate lobe of the liver lies to the right, the fundus of the stomach is to the left, and the right crura of the diaphragm and aorta lie posterior. The borders of the esophageal hiatus are formed by the diaphragmatic crura and median arcuate ligament (when present). The crura arise from the first four lumbar vertebrae, intervertebral discs, and anterior longitudinal ligament. The fibers of the left and right crura pass upward and anteriorly to form the muscle borders of the hiatal ring and then insert in the transverse ligament of the central tendon of the diaphragm.[6] The crural origin of the muscle margins of the esophageal hiatus is quite variable.[7-9]

At the level of the diaphragm the esophagus is surrounded by collagen and elastic fibers of the phrenoesophageal membrane. This membrane extends from the hiatal margin to insert into the circumference of the esophagus both above and below the diaphragm.[10,11] It is most pronounced in infants. With age, the esophagus is less firmly fixed to the hiatus, and fat appears between the fibers.[12] This membrane does not exist in patients with long-standing hiatal hernia.[13]

The esophageal mucosal surface is rather homogeneous in color and topography throughout. The color is a pinkish gray from cricopharyngeus to squamocolumnar junction. Small, linearly oriented mucosal vessels may be seen on close inspection with good illumination. These and many other vessels are apparent when the esophagus is distended, as in achalasia. As a matter of fact, in achalasia the vascular pattern of the esophagus is difficult to differentiate from that of the rectum. The squamocolumnar mucosal junction is detected easily in normals by the abrupt disappearance of this vascular pattern and the dramatic color change to the reddish orange, slightly granular mucosa of the gastric cardia. This mucosal junction normally is located at or below the level of the diaphragmatic hiatus.

Blood Supply

The arterial blood supply to the esophagus is largely segmental with little vascular overlap (Fig 53-1). The cervical esophagus is supplied mainly by branches of the inferior thyroid artery. Branches of other arteries such as the common carotid, subclavian, vertebral, and ascending pharyngeal may provide additional blood supply. The thoracic esophagus is supplied by branches of the aorta, right intercostal, and bronchial arteries. The abdominal esophagus is supplied by branches of the left gastric, short gastric, and left inferior phrenic artery. Devascularization and ischemia of the esophagus is a concern during resectional operations because of the segmental nature of the blood supply.

The venous anatomy of the esophagus has been well defined (Fig 53-2). Fine intraepithelial channels drain into a subepithelial superficial venous plexus. This plexus drains into deep intrinsic veins in the submucosa. At the level of the gastroesophageal junction, the superficial venous plexus and deep intrinsic veins communicate with their gastric counterparts.[14]

Perforating veins connect the deep intrinsic veins to adventitial veins. At the level of the cervical esophagus, the adventitial veins drain into the inferior thyroid vein, deep cervical vein, vertebral vein, and peritracheal venous plexus.

At the thoracic level, adventitial veins drain into the azygous vein on the right, the hemiazygous vein on the left, and the intercostal veins when the hemiazygous is absent. At the gastro-

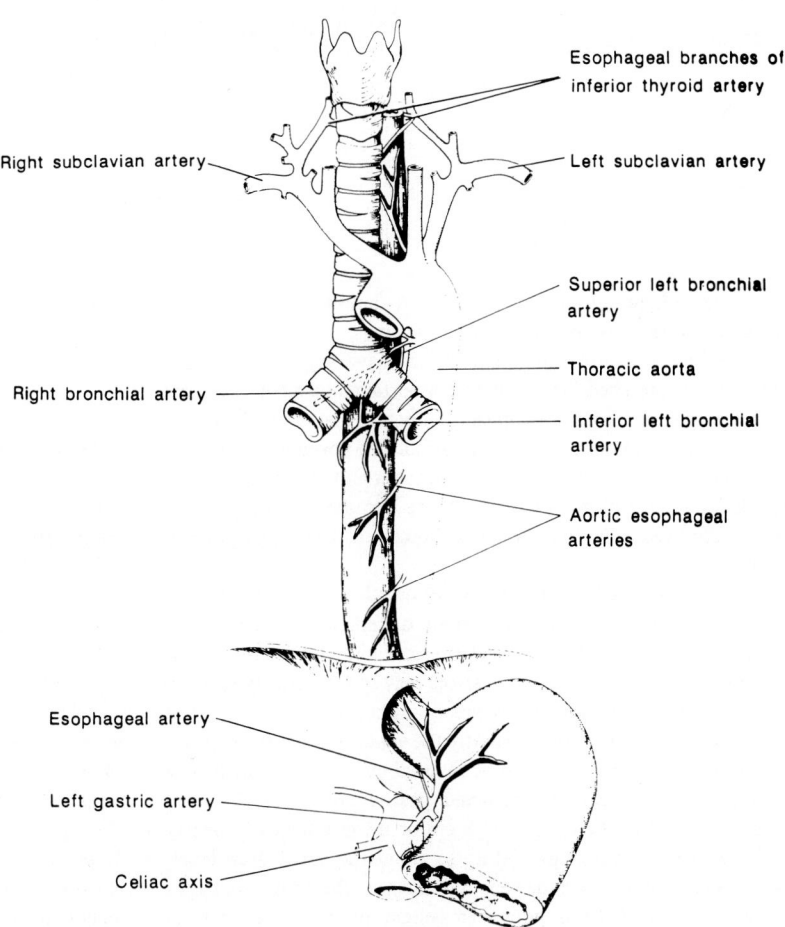

Right subclavian artery

Right bronchial artery

Esophageal branches of inferior thyroid artery

Left subclavian artery

Superior left bronchial artery

Thoracic aorta

Inferior left bronchial artery

Aortic esophageal arteries

Esophageal artery

Left gastric artery

Celiac axis

FIGURE 53–1. Arterial system of the esophagus.

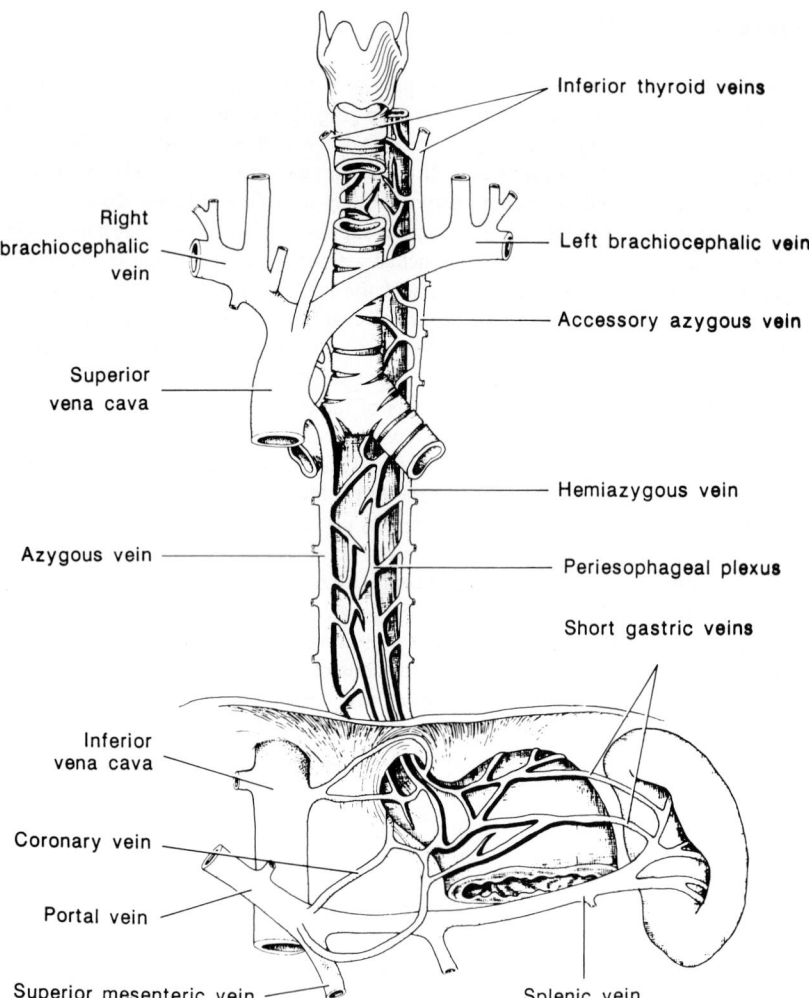

FIGURE 53–2. Venous drainage of the esophagus.

esophageal junction, portal systemic circulation involves venous drainage of the esophagus, stomach, pancreas, spleen, diaphragm, and retroperitoneum. Anatomic studies have suggested a high-pressure "watershed" region between portal and azygous systems at the region of the gastroesophageal junction that would be prone to venous dilation in portal hypertension.[15] In portal hypertension, the deep intrinsic veins in the submucosa and subepithelial superficial venous plexus dilate, protrude into the lumen, and may markedly stretch and thin the epithelial surface, forming esophageal varices.[14]

In patients with portal hypertension, these vessels serve as collateral channels to provide a route of return for portal blood to the systemic circulation. When pressure and flow become great enough, these dilated veins or varices may spontaneously rupture and lead to severe bleeding. The precise pathophysiology of variceal rupture is not known, but currently the explosion theory (rupture from high pressure) seems to be favored over the erosion theory (mucosal destruction by refluxed gastric contents). Variceal bleeding is from the distal 6 to 8 cm of the esophagus in nearly all cases. Varices may extend up to about the aortic arch level, the upper limit of where the venous drainage of the lower esophagus drains by way of the azygous vein system into the superior vena cava. Varices found cephalad to this level have been termed

"downhill varices." These result from either anomalies of the cervical venous system or superior vena cava obstruction.

Innervation

The vagus nerve supplies only parasympathetic innervation to the esophagus, although caudal to the neck the vagus nerve carries a mixture of parasympathetic and sympathetic nerve fibers (Fig 53-3). The cervical esophagus is innervated by the recurrent laryngeal nerves that arise from the vagus. Branches of the vagal nerves and left recurrent laryngeal nerve innervate the upper thoracic esophagus. The left and right vagus intertwine with sympathetic fibers to form the esophageal plexus.[16] Out of the esophageal plexus the anterior and posterior vagal trunks form at a variable distance above the diaphragm.[17] Below the diaphragm the anterior (left) vagal trunk splits into anterior gastric branches and hepatic branch. The posterior (right) vagal trunk splits into posterior gastric branches and a branch to the celiac plexus. Sympathetic innervation is supplied by the superior cervical ganglion, sympathetic chain, major splanchnic nerve, thoracic aortic plexus, and celiac ganglion.

A dense network of lymph vessels is found in the mucosa and

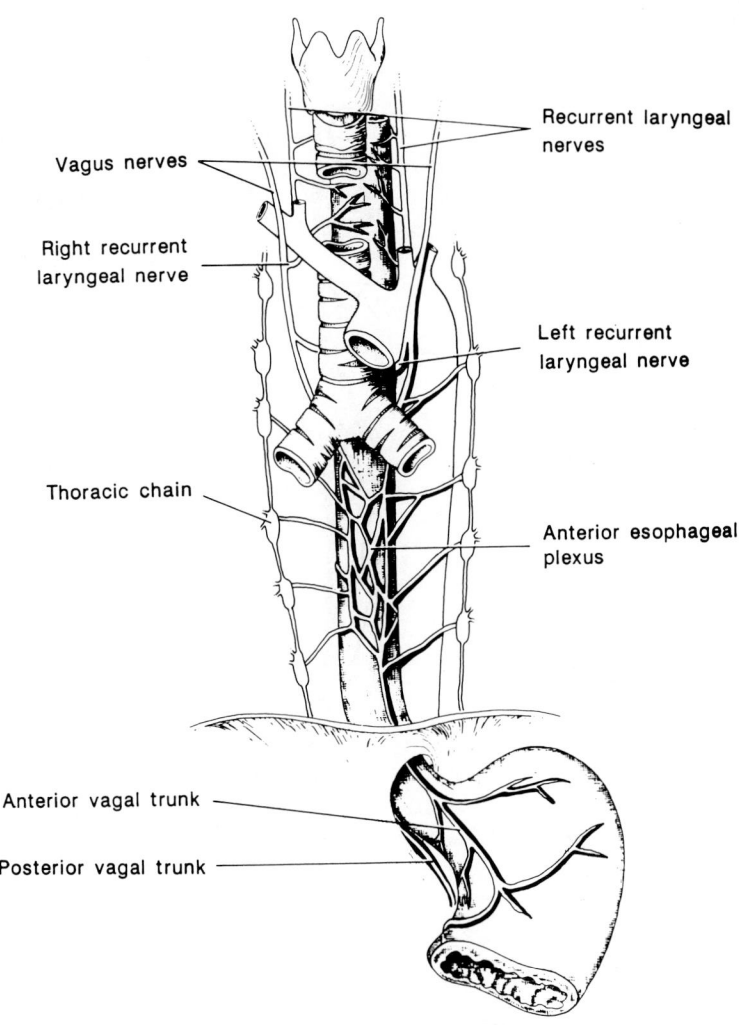

FIGURE 53–3. Innervation of the esophagus.

submucosa of the esophageal wall (Fig 53-4). These vessels travel a variable distance longitudinally before penetrating the muscular wall and draining into adventitial lymph nodes. The deep cervical lymph nodes drain the proximal esophagus. At more distal levels, the lymph vessels drain into the adjacent lymph node chain. Internal jugular, tracheal, tracheobronchial, posterior mediastinal, and pericardial nodes drain adjacent esophageal segments. Unlike the arterial supply, the lymphatic drainage of the esophagus is not segmental. Multiple interconnections exist between nodal chains. This arrangement accounts for the unfortunate frequency of the wide intramural and mediastinal lymphatic spread of esophageal carcinoma.

HISTOLOGY

Light Microscopy

The esophageal wall is composed of four layers: the mucous membrane (tunica mucosa), submucosa (tunica submucosa), muscularis externa (tunica muscularis), and the adventitia (tunica adventitia)

(Figs 53-5*A* and 53-5*B*). The absence of a serosal layer allows esophageal malignancies to spread more readily and makes esophageal anastomosis and surgical repair more difficult.

The innermost layer, the mucous membrane, is composed of nonkeratinized squamous epithelium, supporting connective tissue (lamina propria) and a thin layer of smooth muscle (muscularis mucosae). The squamous epithelium is composed of a basal cell layer (stratum basale), a prickle cell layer (stratum intermedium), and the superficial layer (stratum superficiale). The inner border of the epithelium is irregular because of protrusions of the lamina propria (dermal papillae or rete pegs).[18] The basal cell layer is composed of basophilic, cylindrical cells that have the capacity to divide and replenish the superficial layers.[19]

The esophagus contains cells that are a part of the gut-associated lymphoid tissue. Cytotoxic T cells (intraepithelial lymphocytes) and Langerhans cells (macrophages) are found in the squamous epithelium. Helper T cells and B lymphocytes are seen primarily in the lamina propria.[20] Intraepithelial melanocytes and argyrophil cells can be found in the basal cell layer.[21]

The muscularis mucosae is composed of smooth muscle cells that separate the lamina propria from the submucosa (Figs 53-5*A* and 53-5*B*). The submucosa consists primarily of loose connective tissue. A vascular network (Heller's plexus), nerve plexus, mucin-

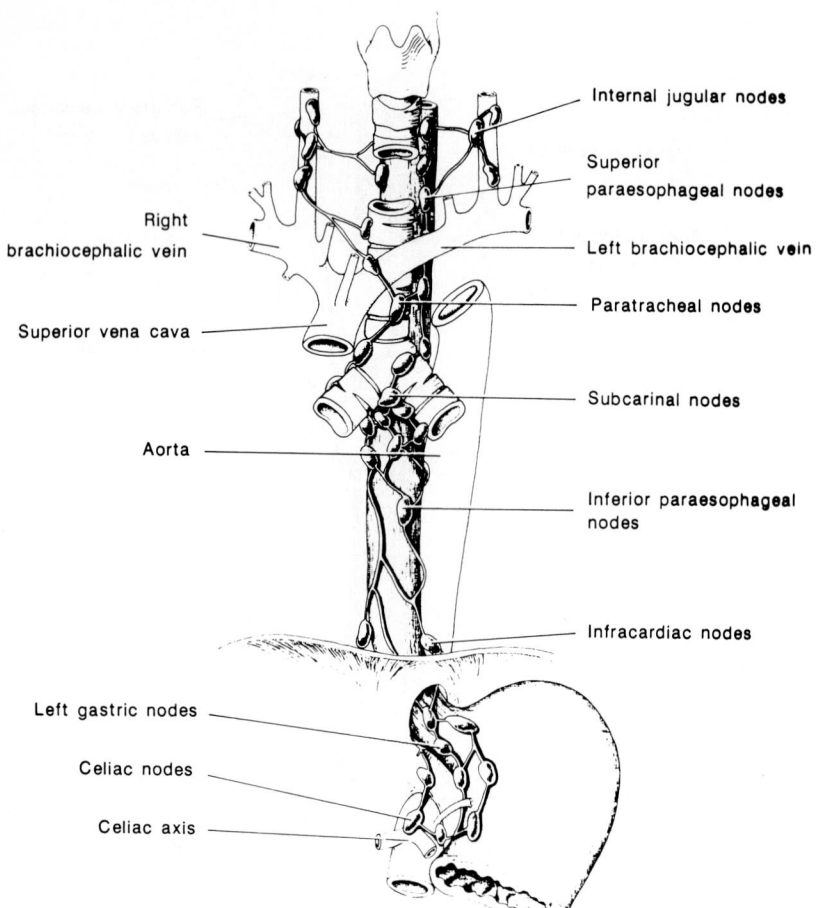

Right brachiocephalic vein

Superior vena cava

Aorta

Internal jugular nodes

Superior paraesophageal nodes

Left brachiocephalic vein

Paratracheal nodes

Subcarinal nodes

Inferior paraesophageal nodes

Infracardiac nodes

Left gastric nodes

Celiac nodes

Celiac axis

FIGURE 53–4. Lymphatic system of the esophagus.

secreting glands, lymph follicles, and lymphocytes are located at the level of the submucosa.

Striated muscle fibers of the inferior pharyngeal constrictor and cricopharyngeus muscles overlap with striated circular muscle fibers of the cervical esophagus at the level of the C5–C6 vertebral interspace. This corresponds to the level of the physiologic upper esophageal sphincter segment, of which the cricopharyngeus appears to be the major component.[22–25]

The muscular wall of the esophagus is composed of both an inner circular and outer longitudinal layer, the inner circular layer being the thicker of the two layers (Figs 53-5*A* and 53-5*B*). The first centimeter of the proximal esophagus is striated muscle alone, the next 6 to 8 cm are mixed (striated/smooth), and the remaining length is all smooth muscle.[9] In situ, longitudinal muscle fibers run in an elongated spiral. Circular muscle fibers run in an elliptical course with some fibers leaving their bundle to join higher or lower bundles.[26]

An area below the diaphragm and proximal to the angle of His (abdominal or submerged segment) has been described in fixed gastroesophageal specimens where the inner circular muscle layer thickens and the fibers become semicircular and interlaced. Oblique fibers of gastric type from the greater curve are also found. It has been suggested that this area corresponds to the physiologic lower esophageal sphincter, but by most observations the sphincter lies proximal to this level just cephalad to the diaphragmatic hiatus.[27]

The myenteric plexus (Auerbach's) is found between the inner circular and outer longitudinal muscle coat. The adventitial layer consists of connective tissue with networks of nerve plexus, vascular structures, and elastic fibers. Other specialized elements can be seen in the esophageal wall. Islands of gastric mucosa, sebaceous glands, taste buds, and foci of hyperplastic epithelial cells with intranuclear glycogen (glycogenic acanthosis) have been described.[28–31] The latter condition is commonly seen during fiberoptic esophagoscopy as focal white elevations several millimeters in diameter scattered randomly at any or all levels of the esophagus.

Electron Microscopy

With electron microscopy, basal cells appear as oblong or cuboidal structures with central nuclei. The cytoplasm contains mitochondria, small golgi apparatuses, free ribosomes, lysosomes, and little endoplasmic reticulum. No glycogen is seen in these cells. As these cells mature and leave the basal layer, they become larger and more flattened with cellular constituent similar to that of basal cells. They constitute the prickle cell layer or stratum intermedium. Glycogen is present in these cells, and membrane-coating granules believed to play a role in cell cohesion are seen

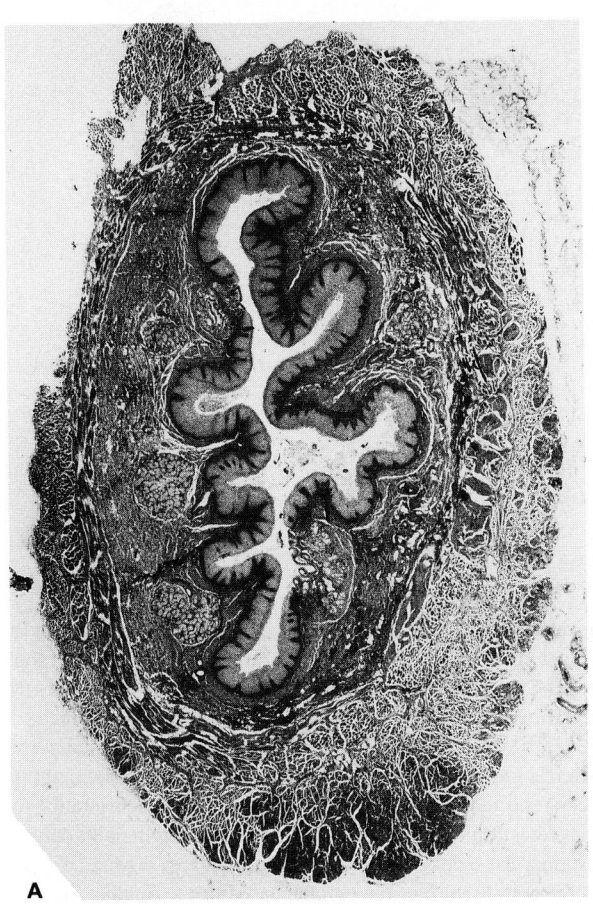

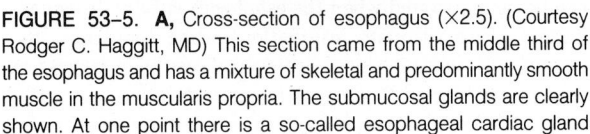

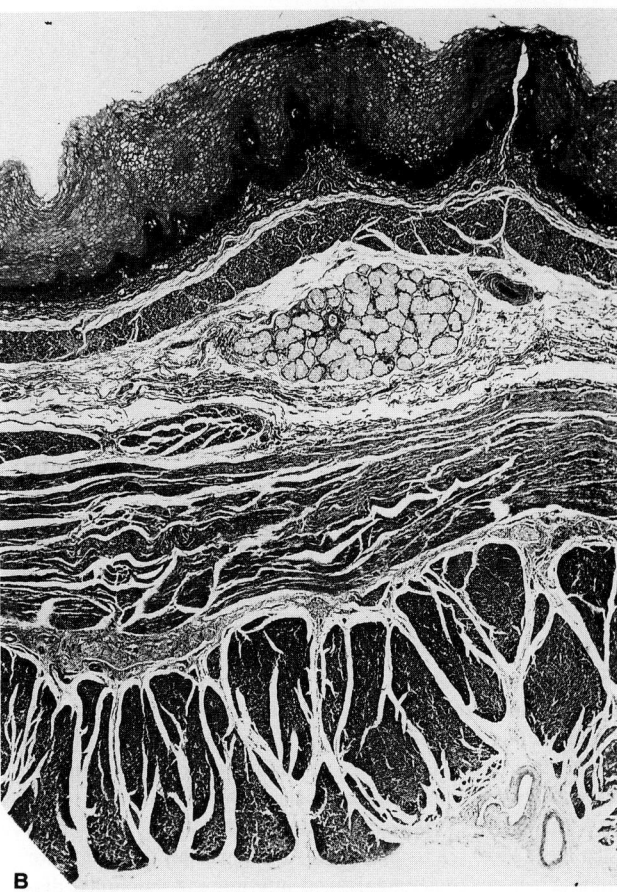

FIGURE 53-5. A, Cross-section of esophagus (×2.5). (Courtesy Rodger C. Haggitt, MD) This section came from the middle third of the esophagus and has a mixture of skeletal and predominantly smooth muscle in the muscularis propria. The submucosal glands are clearly shown. At one point there is a so-called esophageal cardiac gland where a small focus of glandular epithelium interrupts the squamous mucosa. This is a normal finding seen in at least 1% of all esophagi. **B,** Longitudinal section of esophageal wall (×10). (Courtesy Rodger C. Haggitt, MD)

in the superficial prickle cell layer.[32,33] The presence of glycogen in the superficial mucosal cells accounts for their brownish black staining by Lugol's iodine solution as applied for chromoendoscopy.

In the superficial layer, the squamous epithelial cells are more flattened and oriented parallel to the surface. The cell membrane becomes more prominent and the cell edges may overlap. Membrane-coating granules are present. Acid and neutral mucosubstances are found on all layers of epithelial cells. Acid mucosubstances are present in larger amounts on superficial cells and may play a protective role.[34,35] Microplicae seen on surface cells by scanning electron microscopy may function in holding the mucus in place.[36]

With electron microscopy, the submucosal nerve plexus is seen as an irregular network near the inner coat of the muscularis externa. The myenteric plexus (Auerbach's) is a more extensive network of nerve bundles. The density of ganglia in the myenteric plexus increases distally.[37] In the lower esophageal sphincter region, nerve endings are seen as multiple varicosities with close contact to differentiated smooth muscle cells (Cajal's cells) that play a role in initiation and coordination of contraction.[38]

DEVELOPMENTAL ANOMALIES

Tracheoesophageal Fistula and Atresia

During embryogenesis, disruption of the process of elongation and separation of the trachea and esophagus can occur. If fusion of the tracheoesophageal septum is incomplete, a *tracheoesophageal fistula* (TEF) will result. If elongation outstrips foregut cell proliferation, both ventral and dorsal cells may form tracheal tissue, and *esophageal atresia,*[1] with or without associated tracheoesophageal fistula, will develop. Five basic types of TEF and atresia have been described with the use of varying classification schemes (Fig 53-6). Esophageal atresia with lower-pouch fistula is by far the most common.[39–44] Hydramnios and prematurity are common in infants with atresia and/or TEF.[44–46] Up to 50% of infants may have other associated congenital anomalies.[47] Associated gastrointestinal anomalies include imperforate anus, midgut malrotation, duodenal atresia, and annular pancreas.[48]

Symptoms vary depending upon the type of tracheoesophageal

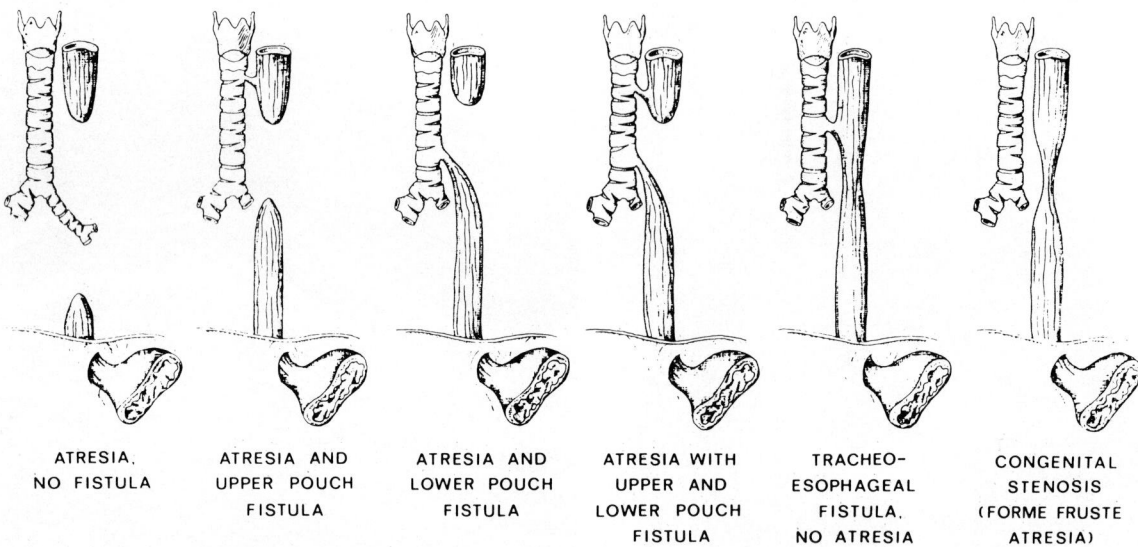

| ATRESIA, NO FISTULA | ATRESIA AND UPPER POUCH FISTULA | ATRESIA AND LOWER POUCH FISTULA | ATRESIA WITH UPPER AND LOWER POUCH FISTULA | TRACHEO-ESOPHAGEAL FISTULA, NO ATRESIA | CONGENITAL STENOSIS (FORME FRUSTE ATRESIA) |

FIGURE 53-6. The spectrum of esophageal atresia, tracheoesophageal fistula, and congenital stenosis.

anomaly. In infants with atresia alone, diagnosis is often made after birth. Unswallowed saliva fills the mouth and nostrils, and formula is regurgitated. In infants with atresia and distal fistula, excessive salivation and regurgitation occur along with cyanosis and pneumonia secondary to reflux of gastric contents. Infants with proximal fistula experience respiratory distress and cyanosis with feedings. In the case of proximal and distal fistula, the proximal fistula usually is the cause of most symptoms.

Isolated TEF (H-fistula) leads to cough and choking with feedings, recurrent pneumonia, and intermittent abdominal distention. This anomaly rarely has been initially diagnosed in adulthood. Adult patients present with a history of recurrent pneumonia and bronchiectasis.[49–51]

The diagnosis of TEF is often suspected on the basis of clinical findings. The presence of atresia can be documented by the inability to pass an esophageal catheter. Chest films may demonstrate a gasless abdomen or distention based upon the type of fistula present. Insufflation of air into the esophagus by way of catheter may be adequate to demonstrate the TEF radiographically. Radiographic contrast cautiously introduced by way of catheter is often used to delineate the atretic segment and fistula location. In patients with H-type TEF, repeated contrast examinations may be necessary before the fistulous tract is demonstrated.[52]

The surgical trend has been toward early primary repair, with staged repair reserved for infants with respiratory distress or severe associated congenital anomalies. If the esophageal segments cannot be approximated initially, repeated bougienage may be used to lengthen the atretic segments, allowing subsequent primary anastomosis.[53,54] Delayed colon interposition is used when primary anastomosis is impossible. Surgical mortality has declined dramatically in the last 30 years. Currently, the primary determinants of survival are coexistent congenital anomalies and severity of associated pulmonary disease.[55,56]

Congenital Esophageal Stenosis

Congenital esophageal stenosis is the least common congenital tracheoesophageal anomaly (Fig 53-6). It is estimated to occur

once per 25,000 live births. This anomaly is felt to result from failure of normal embryonic separation of trachea and esophagus.[57] Stenosis due to cartilage, residual respiratory epithelium, and muscular wall maldevelopment has been described (Fig 53-7).[58–62] As opposed to atresia and TEF, congenital stenosis often is not diagnosed until later in childhood. Several cases have been reported in adults.[63,64] Symptoms include regurgitation, prolonged eating time, and dysphagia with recurrent solid bolus impaction. An esophagram usually demonstrates segmental stenosis in the middle third of the esophagus. Multiple ringlike folds often can be demonstrated when the esophagus is fully distended with barium. With adequate insufflation during endoscopy, the appearance of multiple rings with normal overlying mucosa can be seen in most cases. Segmental resection has been advocated for these patients; however, bougienage has been reported to be safe in children and adults.[58,65]

Congenital Esophageal Duplications

Congenital esophageal duplications can be tubular or cystic. They are believed to arise as the result of failure of vacuoles to coalesce properly, preventing recanalization of the esophageal lumen. As a result, there is formation of a cyst or parallel tubular channel within the esophageal wall.[66]

Tubular duplications are rare. They may be asymptomatic or may present with dysphagia. Tubular duplications may communicate at both ends with the esophageal lumen or may be closed at one end.[67–70] Cystic duplications are less rare; they constitute 0.5% to 2.5% of esophageal tumors. However, they are the second most common benign esophageal tumor, leiomyoma being most common.[71,72] They occur within the wall of the esophagus and are surrounded by two layers of smooth muscle. These cysts are lined with squamous columnar, cuboid, pseudostratified, or ciliated epithelium.[73,74] Sixty percent of duplications arise in the distal third of the esophagus, 17% in the middle third, and 23% in the upper third.[75] These cysts are reported to be more common on the right side of the esophagus.[76]

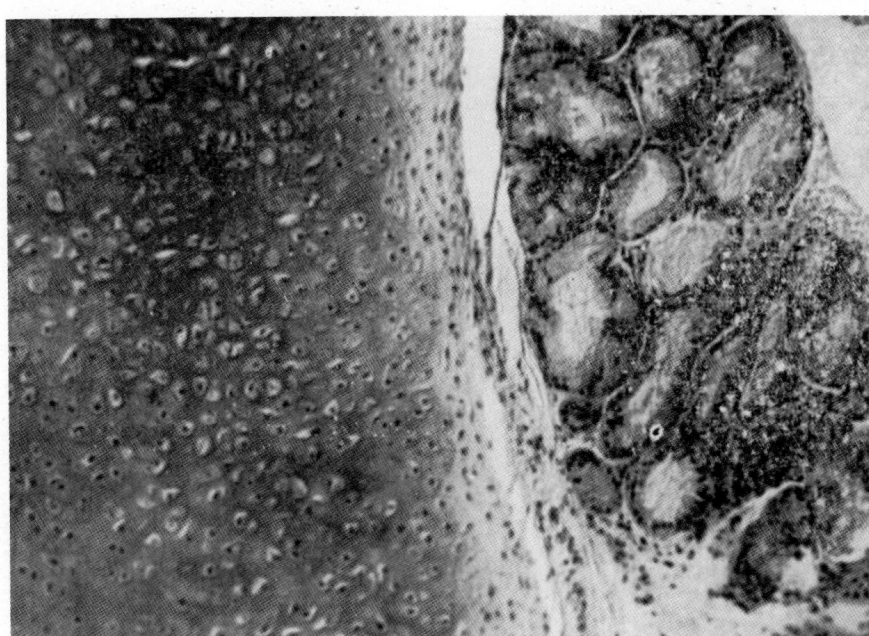

FIGURE 53–7. Histologic section from esophageal wall of resected segment of congenital stenosis. Note cartilage on the left and tracheal glands on the right. (Courtesy Ishida M, Tsuchida Y, Saito S, et al. Congenital esophageal stenosis due to tracheobronchial remnants. J Pediatr Surg 1969;4(3):340.)

Duplications of the proximal third of the esophagus are typically diagnosed in infancy because of symptoms of tracheobronchial compression. Such cysts in the distal two thirds of the esophagus may result in symptoms of dysphagia, epigastric discomfort, retrosternal pain, cough, dyspnea, or regurgitation, although many are diagnosed while asymptomatic.[77] Cysts located posterior to the heart have been associated with cardiac arrhythmias.[78]

Gastric cysts containing actively secreting ectopic gastric mucosa, *inclusion cysts* containing squamous or respiratory epithelium but without smooth muscle wall, *bronchogenic cysts* containing cartilage, and *neuroenteric cysts* also can be found in the esophageal wall but are less common. These cysts can present with symptoms similar to those of true duplication cysts.[75]

Congenital Duplication Cysts

Congenital duplication cysts can be seen on chest radiographs as posterior or middle mediastinal masses. On barium esophagram, a smooth, curved displacement of the esophagus is seen without the sharp, steplike proximal and distal margin seen with leiomyomas. Ultrasound has been used as an adjunct to distinguish cystic from solid masses.[79] Technetium 99m–sodium pertechnetate nuclear medicine scan has been used to diagnose a neuroenteric cyst in a child.[80]

Computed tomography (CT) can be helpful in determining location, size, and anatomic relationship to other organs. However, CT may not distinguish duplications from other submucosal esophageal lesions, and CT densitometry may be misleading in differentiating esophageal duplication cysts from other mediastinal masses.[81,82] At endoscopy, a soft compressible bulge into the esophageal lumen without overlying mucosal abnormality can be seen.[83] Endoscopic ultrasound should prove useful in further delineating the structure of duplication cysts as well as other intramural and paraesophageal lesions in adults.[84]

Surgical resection is recommended for definitive treatment and pathologic diagnosis. Complete excision of duplication cysts can be performed without disruption of the esophageal mucosa, and the morbidity of surgical excision is low.[85,86] Marsupialization has been used for treatment of large cysts, and needle aspiration has been used to relieve tracheal compression from a duplication cyst.[87,88] Although rare, development of malignancy within tubular or cystic duplication has been reported.[89–91]

Bronchopulmonary Foregut Malformations

Bronchopulmonary foregut malformations are pulmonary sequestrations with patent congenital communication to the upper gastrointestinal tract.[92] Bronchopulmonary foregut malformations develop when cell rests with respiratory potential arise from the esophagus caudal to the lung bud or when a portion of the lung bud arises from the dorsal esophagus rather than the ventral trachea.[93] The tract between the sequestered pulmonary lobe typically involutes because of outgrowth of its blood supply; incomplete involution of the tract leads to a gastrointestinal tract communication.[94] Bronchopulmonary foregut malformations are most commonly seen in the lower lobes. Arterial supply and venous drainage are variable.[95,96] Up to 40% of children with communicating bronchopulmonary foregut malformations have associated congenital anomalies.[97] Clinical presentation in infants is respiratory distress, exacerbated with feedings. Congestive heart failure also may occur. In adults and older children, recurrent pneumonia, bronchiectasis, hemoptysis, gastrointestinal bleeding, and dysphagia may develop.[95] Contrast esophagram, bronchography, and angiography are used for diagnosis and surgical planning.

Aortic Arch Vessel Abnormalities

It has been estimated that 3% of the population have a congenital abnormality of the aortic arch vessels, but only rarely does this

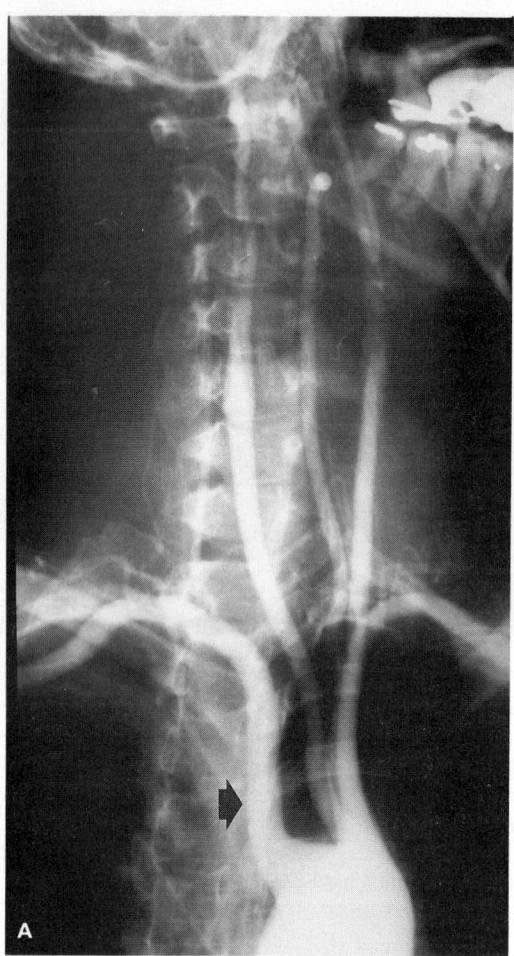
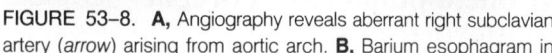
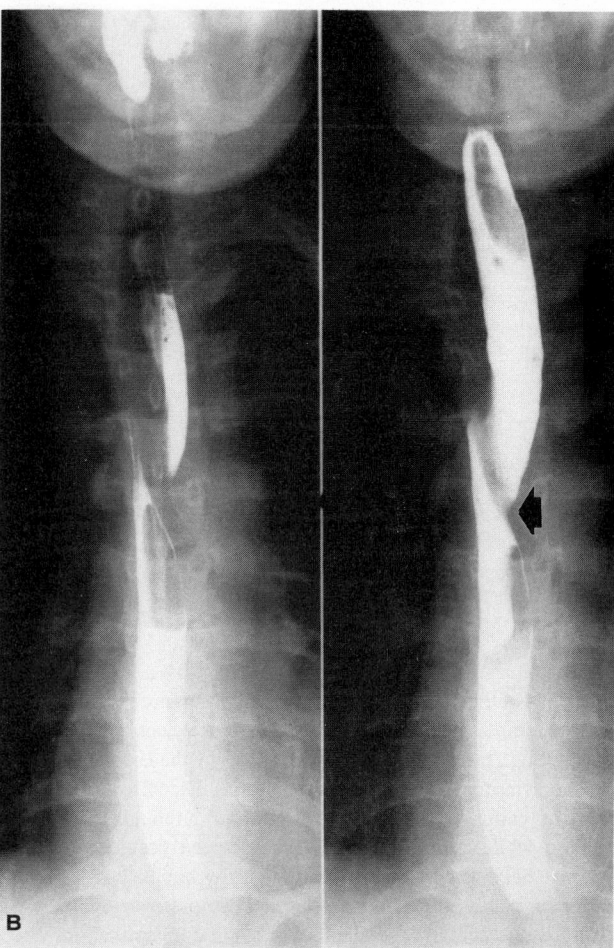

FIGURE 53–8. **A,** Angiography reveals aberrant right subclavian artery (*arrow*) arising from aortic arch. **B,** Barium esophagram in same patient reveals oblique esophageal compression (*arrow*) by the aberrant right subclavian artery posterior to the esophagus.

result in symptomatic compression of the esophagus.[98] In the embryo, the foregut is surrounded by vascular structures of the branchial arches. Normally, portions of the branchial arches obliterate to form the great vessels and aortic arch. Abnormalities in developmental obliteration of the branchial arches may lead to vascular compression of the trachea and esophagus.[99] The majority of symptomatic congenital vascular compressions become clinically apparent in infancy; however, certain types of vascular anomalies may present in adulthood. In infants, respiratory symptoms predominate; dysphagia is the primary complaint in adults.

Dysphagia lusoria (literally translated, lusoria means "a trick of nature") is the term used to describe symptomatic esophageal compression from an aberrant right subclavian artery. Symptoms of this anomaly may occur at the onset of semisolid feedings, later in childhood, or in adult life.

With this anomaly, the right subclavian artery arises from the left side of the aortic arch and courses obliquely upward and posterior, compressing the esophagus (Fig 53-8*A*). It is estimated that aberrant right subclavian artery occurs in 0.5% to 1% of the population, with only 10% of these having symptoms related to compression.[100] This is the vascular anomaly that most typically causes symptoms later in life.[101]

Barium esophagram demonstrates an oblique filling defect just above the level of the aortic arch (Fig 53-8*B*). Endoscopy may demonstrate a pulsatile compression of the lumen. The right radial pulse may be weakened or obliterated by endoscopic compression or during bougienage.[102,103] Correction is performed in children by division and ligation of the aberrant artery. In adults, reanastomosis to the ascending aorta is performed to avoid development of subclavian steal syndrome.[104,105] However, surgery is not always needed because many adult patients can easily tolerate minor degrees of dysphagia by simply modifying their diet.

Esophageal compression by *anomalous vertebral artery* and *right aortic arch* with constricting left ligamentum arteriosum have been reported in adults and can be successfully repaired surgically.[106,107]

Double aortic arch, right aortic arch with patent ductus arteriosus, cervical aortic arch, and *aberrant left pulmonary artery* are causes of tracheoesophageal compression in infants. Early surgical intervention is recommended for these anomalies.[108,109]

Heterotopic Gastric Mucosa

Heterotopic gastric mucosa can be seen occasionally in the esophagus during careful endoscopic inspection. In a series of 1000 autopsies in infants and children, Rector and Connerley found ectopic gastric mucosa in 7.8%. The majority of these were in the proximal one third of the esophagus.[110] Heterotopic gastric mucosa has been seen in 2.8% to 3.5% of consecutive endoscopies.[111,112] At endoscopy, these areas of gastric mucosa typically are small, distinct patches of reddish orange mucosa in the proximal esophagus. This heterotopic mucosa is referred to as the "inlet patch" when found in the cervical esophagus.[111] However, they can occur throughout the esophagus and have a linear appearance.[113] The slight reddish orange coloration usually contrasts nicely with the surrounding pinkish gray esophageal mucosa but can be dramatically demonstrated after staining the squamous mucosa around its margin with topical dilute iodine solution (Lugol's) injected by way of an endoscope cannula. On biopsy, corpus-fundic or antral-type mucosa is seen, sometimes containing parietal cells capable of acid secretion. The majority of cases of heterotopic gastric mucosa are felt to be clinically insignificant. Complications of tracheoesophageal fistula and adenocarcinoma arising from heterotopic gastric mucosa have been reported.[114–116]

MUCOSAL RINGS AND WEBS

Mucosal Rings

The lower esophageal mucosal ring (B ring) was initially described by Templeton in 1944.[117] Subsequently, in 1953 both Ingelfinger and Kramer, along with Schatzki and Gary, independently described the association of lower esophageal mucosal rings with dysphagia.[118,119]

Lower esophageal mucosal rings are located at the level of the squamocolumnar mucosal junction. These rings consist of mucosa and submucosa and are covered by squamous mucosa on the proximal side and either columnar mucosa or several millimeters of squamous mucosa on the distal (gastric) side.[120,121] The true ring is circumferential, symmetrical from all angles of radiographic view, and less than 3 mm in thickness. The majority of lower esophageal mucosal rings are asymptomatic; however, they may be a cause of intermittent dysphagia and typically present in patients over the age of 40 years.[122,123]

The degree of symptoms is dependent upon the diameter of the ring. Rings over 20 mm in diameter usually are asymptomatic; rings 13 to 20 mm cause variable degrees of dysphagia, depending upon type and size of bolus; and rings less than 13 mm regularly cause solid food dysphagia.[124,125] Studies have suggested that formation and progression of the lower esophageal mucosal ring are related to gastroesophageal reflux; however, such true rings usually are not associated with inflammation.[126,127] There has been much misunderstanding in the literature and in practice by confusing true rings with ringlike strictures due to acid reflux. Studies examining serial esophagrams have demonstrated development and progressive narrowing of true lower esophageal mucosal rings.[128]

On esophagram, lower esophageal mucosal rings appear as a thin transverse circumferential ridge above the hiatus of the diaphragm. To visualize the ring, the region of the esophagogastric junction must be adequately distended (Fig 53-9). By definition, a hiatal hernia is *always* present. Valsalva maneuver during the esophagram is helpful in demonstrating a ring.[129] Symptomatic mucosal rings are reproducible and do not disappear during radiographic examination. Barium esophagram using prone full-column technique is more sensitive than double-contrast radiography or endoscopy for detection of many lower esophageal mucosal rings.[130] Use of a barium tablet or marshmallow bolus may further improve the sensitivity of the barium esophagram to correlate dysphagia with the ring.

Asymptomatic mucosal rings often are demonstrable during barium esophagram or during endoscopy. When the lumen is adequately distended in a patient with a hiatal hernia, with either barium or air, a ring protrusion develops along the squamocolumnar

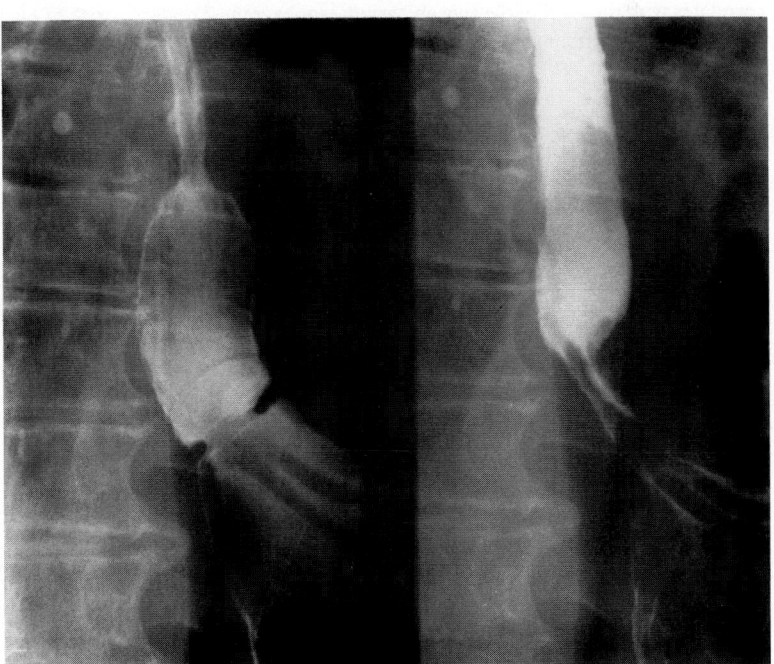

FIGURE 53–9. Barium esophagram on the left demonstrates a lower esophageal ring at the upper end of a hiatal hernia pouch. The esophagram on the right after the lumen collapses fails to reveal the ring.

mucosal junction and remains visible under fluoroscopy or endoscopy only while the lumen is adequately distended. Because of the failure to adequately distend the esophagus during the radiographic examination, mucosal rings with mild degrees of narrowing are commonly missed. This dynamic ring, just like the static, symptomatic Schatzki ring, is a relatively precise marker for the squamocolumnar mucosal junction and thereby for a hiatal hernia as well. Either type of ring can be demonstrated only when a hiatal hernia is present. Symptomatic lower esophageal rings should be treated (see ch 131). The vast majority of patients can be effectively treated with passage of a large (50–60 French) Maloney dilator.[131] Many clinicians use the standard gradual peroral sequential dilation technique rather than passage of a single large-diameter bougie. Treatment by pneumatic dilation or transendoscopic electrosurgical incision has been reported. These latter techniques are not necessary and should not be used because of their higher risk.

Muscular Rings

The lower esophageal muscular ring (A ring) occurs several centimeters proximal to the squamocolumnar junction at a level that corresponds to the upper portion of the lower esophageal sphincter segment. These rings consist of an annular ring of hypertrophied and/or hypertonic muscle covered with normal squamous epithelium.[132] Muscular rings are seen most often in patients with esophageal motor disorders, gastroesophageal reflux, and hiatal hernia. The most common symptom associated with muscular rings is intermittent dysphagia, although typically these rings are asymptomatic and are incidental findings during radiography. On barium esophagram, muscular rings are smooth symmetrical narrowings that are broader (4–5 mm) than mucosal rings. These rings may vary in caliber during radiographic examination and may disappear with full distention.[129] In some cases, esophageal manometry reveals a hypertensive lower esophageal sphincter that correlates with the level of the ring on barium esophagram. Treatment of symptomatic muscular rings is performed by passage of a large-caliber (50–60 French) Maloney dilator.

Webs

Esophageal webs are thin transverse membranes of squamous epithelium. They usually occur in the upper and midesophagus. Upper esophageal webs are typically found in the postcricoid area. In large series of patients evaluated by cineradiography for complaints of dysphagia, esophageal webs were found in up to 7%.[133] Webs usually involve the anterior wall of the cervical esophagus, occasionally extending laterally and less commonly involving the entire circumference, and occasionally they are multiple. The frequency of esophageal webs increases with age.

The association of postcricoid webs with iron deficiency anemia (Plummer–Vinson or Paterson–Kelly syndrome) is rare.[134–137] However, this group of patients may be at increased risk for development of pharyngeal and cervical esophageal carcinoma.[138,139] The majority of webs are asymptomatic. Intermittent solid food dysphagia is the usual complaint in symptomatic patients.

Midesophageal webs are rare. They may be single or multiple and are believed to be of congenital origin.[140–144] Midesophageal webs typically present with symptoms of dysphagia. When symptomatic, these webs are best treated with bougienage. Treatment with transendoscopic incision or surgical resection has been reported but is rarely necessary.[140,145]

ESOPHAGEAL DIVERTICULA

Zenker's Diverticula

Pharyngoesophageal diverticulum was first described by Ludlow in 1769.[146] Zenker and Ziemssen subsequently reviewed the world literature in 1877—thus the subsequent association of Zenker's name with this condition.[147] Pharyngoesophageal (Zenker's) diverticula form by protrusion of posterior hypopharyngeal mucosa between the oblique fibers of the inferior pharyngeal constrictor and the transverse fibers of the cricopharyngeus (triangle of Killian) proximal to the esophagus. Debate has long existed as to the mechanisms for formation of pharyngoesophageal diverticula.[148]

Recent evidence suggests that during swallowing, high hypopharyngeal pressures occur in some people because of poor compliance of the upper esophageal sphincter, and this may be important in the development of pharyngoesophageal (Zenker's) diverticulum.[149]

Patients typically present after age 50 with duration of symptoms ranging from weeks to years. Symptoms include solid and liquid dysphagia, regurgitation of undigested food, cough, and halitosis. When large diverticula are present, gurgling in the neck or a bulge in the left neck can be seen during eating. Aspiration pneumonia or significant weight loss can occur. Diagnosis is obtained by barium swallow with lateral views of the pharyngoesophageal junction (Figs 53-10*A* and 53-10*B*). Caution must be used during endoscopy or passage of nasogastric tubes because of risk of inadvertent perforation of the diverticulum. Passage of the endoscope over a fluoroscopically placed guidewire may be necessary in some instances in order to safely intubate the esophagus.

The usual approach to symptomatic pharyngoesophageal diverticulum is surgery. There is no consensus as to the best surgical approach.[150,151] Diverticulectomy, diverticulectomy with cricopharyngeal myotomy, diverticular inversion with myotomy, and myotomy alone all have been used. Endoscopic division of the septum between the esophageal lumen and the diverticulum under general anesthesia with diathermy knife or CO_2 laser has been used with low reported morbidity and good symptomatic response rates.[152,153] Surgical morbidity and recurrence rates vary widely in reported surgical series.

Postoperatively, radiographic recurrence appears to be more common than symptomatic recurrence.[154] Squamous cell carcinoma can complicate a long-standing pharyngoesophageal diverticulum. In a series of 1249 patients seen over a 53-year period, squamous cell carcinoma was found in 0.4%.[155] With barium swallow, carcinoma may appear as a persistent filling defect in an otherwise smooth-walled diverticulum.[156] Endoscopy is important in adequately evaluating the diverticulum either preoperatively or during definitive surgery. Spindle cell carcinoma and benign tumors also have been reported to arise in pharyngoesophageal diverticula.[156,157]

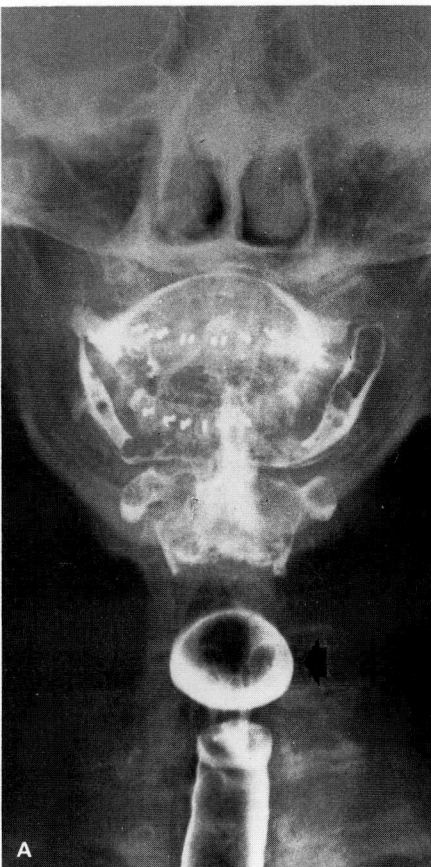
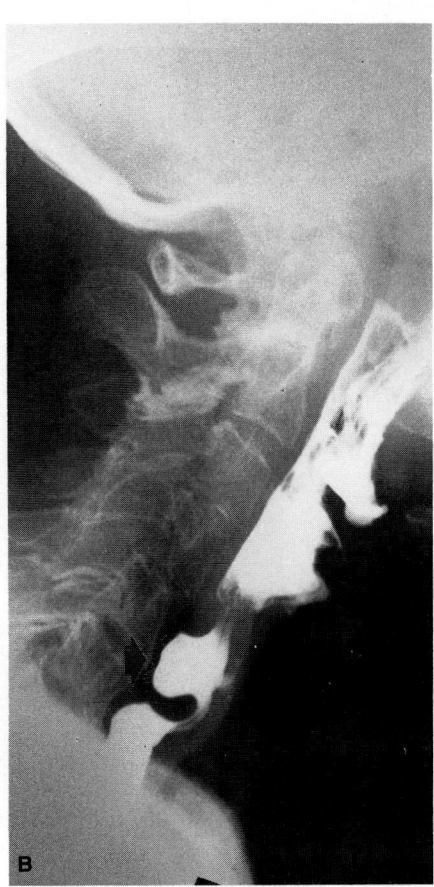

FIGURE 53–10. **A,** Anterior view of barium-filled Zenker's diverticulum (*arrow*). The narrowed segment just distal is the lumen of the cricopharyngeus. **B,** Lateral view of Zenker's diverticulum (*arrow*) in the same patient. The prominent closure of the cricopharyngeus muscle (upper esophageal sphincter) is shown just distal to this diverticulum.

Simple diverticulectomy has been recommended for localized tumor, with pharyngolaryngectomy reserved for more extensive disease. Five-year survival for reported cases is 14%.[158]

Midesophageal and Epiphrenic Diverticula

Diverticula also may occur in the mid or distal esophagus. In the past, *midesophageal diverticula* were believed to develop secondary to traction from contiguous mediastinal inflammation and adenopathy (fungal, tuberculosis). Current evidence indicates that these diverticula likely develop secondary to motility disorders.[159] Midesophageal diverticula can be large and wide-mouthed, small, or multiple. Diagnosis is typically made by barium swallow (Fig 53-11).

Distal esophageal diverticula (epiphrenic) also are thought to develop secondary to motility disorders but also may be seen in patients with long-standing distal esophageal stricture and achalasia. Symptoms such as dysphagia and chest pain likely are due to the underlying motility disorder or esophageal stricture.[160] An epiphrenic diverticulum is seen on barium swallow as a smooth lateral pouch just proximal to the region of the lower esophageal sphincter (Fig 53-11).

Endoscopy can be safely performed in patients with esophageal diverticula. Endoscopically, they appear as a smooth pouch off the axis of the esophageal lumen. Fluoroscopy and guidewire should be used when dilation is performed in patients with diverticula to avoid inadvertent diverticular perforation.

Diverticula are rarely symptomatic; thus, diverticulectomy is usually not necessary. Treatment is directed to the underlying motility disorder or stricture if present.

Esophageal Intramural Pseudodiverticulosis

Esophageal intramural pseudodiverticulosis is a rare condition, first described by Mendl and colleagues in 1960, in which multiple small pseudodiverticula form in the wall of the esophagus.[161] These pseudodiverticula are formed by dilatation of the excretory ducts of the submucosal esophageal glands.[162] The pathogenesis of esophageal intramural pseudodiverticulosis is unclear; however, it appears that stasis and inflammation may be two factors in its development. It has been proposed that blockage of intramural ducts by inflammatory debris leads to their dilatation.

The majority of patients present with chronic dysphagia. Esophageal strictures are seen in 70% to 90% of patients, and esophageal manometric abnormalities have been found in two thirds of those studied. Esophageal candidiasis has been described in up to 50% of reported cases; however, its role in the development of esophageal intramural pseudodiverticulosis is unknown.

Treatment of esophageal intramural pseudodiverticulosis is directed toward underlying conditions. Dilation of strictures, an-

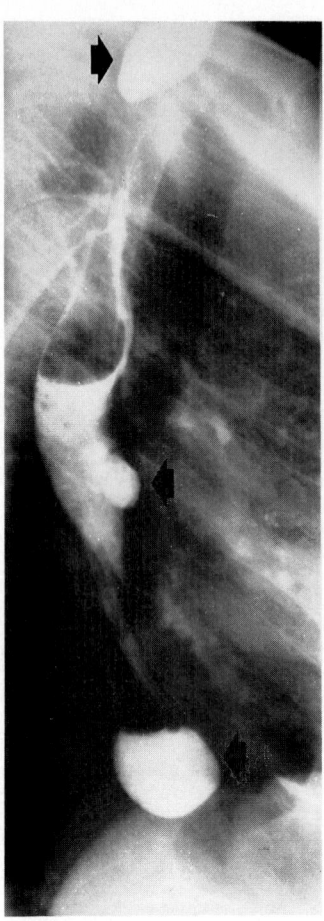

FIGURE 53–11. Barium radiograph demonstrating three diverticula: Zenker's (*upper arrow*), midesophageal (*middle arrow*), and barium-filled epiphrenic diverticulum (*lower arrow*). This occurrence of three types of diverticula in the same patient is distinctly rare!

tireflux therapy, and calcium channel blocking agents have been reported to relieve symptoms of this disorder.[163]

ESOPHAGEAL HIATAL HERNIA

Although a few instances are congenital, the vast majority of hiatal hernias appear later in life and are considered to be of acquired type. Concepts of causation include: (1) esophageal contraction secondary to reflux-induced injury with a pulling-up of the stomach, (2) increased intra-abdominal pressure pushing the stomach above the diaphragm, (3) atrophy or weakening of the hiatal region and phrenoesophageal membrane, and (4) combinations of the above.

The anatomic junction of esophagus with stomach normally lies at, or several centimeters caudad to, the esophageal hiatus of the diaphragm. Its location relative to the hiatus varies within a 2- or 3-cm range, depending upon body position, phase of respiration, intra-abdominal pressure, and the integrity of the surrounding structures that either confine or attach to the esophageal junction region. The phrenoesophageal membrane or fascia of Laimer arises from the crura of the diaphragm and inserts into the esophagus about 2 to 3 cm above the hiatus. This membrane

serves to anchor the esophagogastric junction region sufficiently to allow the necessary mobility with respiration but taut enough to prevent proximal movement of the upper margin of the stomach more than 1 to 2 cm above the diaphragmatic hiatus. Such cephalad movement also is limited by the hiatal diameter and configuration of the diaphragmatic crura that surround most of the hiatal circumference. The phrenoesophageal membrane fixes this region to the diaphragm and closes the potential space between the esophagus and diaphragm. Wolf concluded that the most basic feature of an acquired esophageal hiatal hernia is stretching of the fascial attachments of the esophagogastric junction region of the diaphragm.[164]

In order to understand the anatomy of an esophageal hiatal hernia, one must know the relative positions of the hiatal margins, the domes of the diaphragm, the true or muscular esophagogastric junction, the angle of His, and the gastric fundus. For clinicians, this need dictates that they must understand gross anatomy in addition to radiographic anatomy by way of barium contrast studies, and endoscopic anatomy with both direct and retroversion views. The anatomy of this region studied in the cadaver differs so much from that observed radiographically, endoscopically, and at operation that it offers little to enhance this review.

The level of the diaphragmatic hiatus is the zero point relative to which we measure movement and position of the proximal stomach. A direct or sliding esophageal hiatal hernia is best defined as being present when the stomach wall at its junction with the esophagus is displaced cephalad above the diaphragm into the thorax by a distance of 2 or more cm.

Radiographically, the position of the esophageal hiatus lies below the dome of the diaphragm in both the anteroposterior and lateral projections. This point is worthy of great emphasis, and the failure to recognize this anatomic fact has been confusing the diagnosis of hiatal hernia for decades—and it still does. Many gastric herniations are missed because the mucosal features of the stomach are considered significant only if they project cephalad above the radiographic dome of the diaphragm rather than simply cephalad to the hiatus.[164]

The radiographic anatomy and physiology of the diaphragm, distal esophagus and its abdominal segment, relative to the definition of hiatal hernia have been carefully and elegantly studied.[164–169] Modern radiologic techniques are very accurate for diagnosis of hiatal hernia when the criteria of Wolf are applied.[164] His criteria are easily understood and correlate closely with endoscopic observations. Wolf emphasized that widening of the hiatus alone is a valid sign of hiatal hernia and is the most significant sign of a potentially symptomatic hiatal hernia. Longitudinal mucosal folds regularly are seen in the hernia pouch. The upper or cephalad margins of these folds represent the level of the dislocated esophagogastric junction. As discussed previously, the presence of a lower esophageal or Schatzki ring on barium radiography also is indicative of a hiatal hernia (Fig 53-9).

The endoscopic signs of hiatal hernia include dislocation of the normally located squamocolumnar mucosal junction 2 cm or more above the diaphragmatic hiatus during quiet respiration without additional air inflation (Fig 53-12; Color Fig 17).[170–172] Another reliable sign is the finding of a patulous hiatus (1) when the proximal stomach can be viewed by way of the hiatus from the distal esophagus (antegrade view) (see Fig 53-12; Color Fig 17) or (2) when, at gastroscopy, retroflexion of the endoscope reveals a patulous hiatus around the shaft of the endoscope (ret-

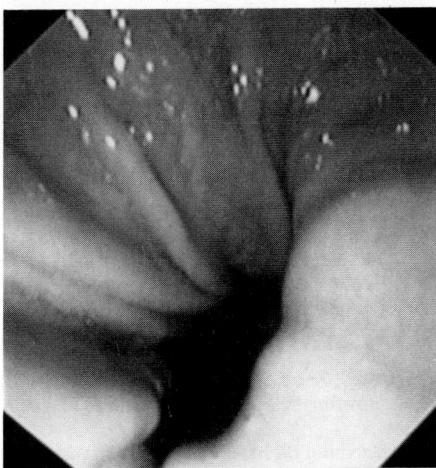

FIGURE 53–12. (See Color Fig 17) Antegrade endoscopic view into a hiatal hernia proximal to a patulous diaphragmatic hiatus. Note the gastric mucosal folds in the hernia pouch extending over the hiatal margin. The upper ends of the gastric mucosal folds are located about 1 cm distal to the squamocolumnar junction and coincide with the level of the true esophagogastric or muscular junction.

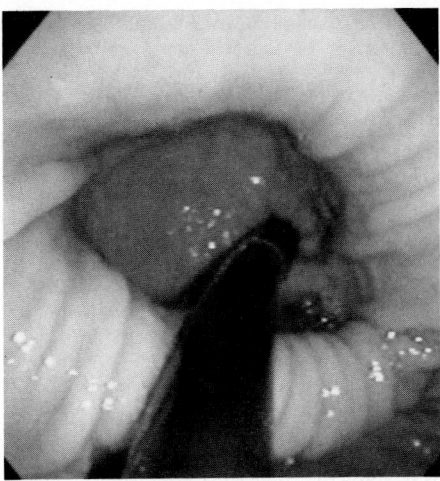

FIGURE 53–13. (See Color Fig 18) Retrograde view from the stomach into the hernia pouch through the patulous hiatus. Note the gastric folds coursing over the margin of the hiatal circumference.

rograde view) (Fig 53-13; Color Fig 18).[173] One or both of these findings, proximal dislocation of stomach and patulous cardia, are always present when there is reflux esophagitis, a reflux-related distal esophageal stricture, or a columnar-lined (Barrett) esophagus.

The study of Johnson and colleagues, who used clearly defined endoscopic criteria, showed that when either hiatal hernia and esophagitis or hiatal hernia with normal mucosa and patulous hiatus coexisted there was a 91% correlation with abnormal 24-hour *p*H monitoring.[173] Dodds has summarized the available evidence in his statement: "Although many patients with hiatal hernia do not exhibit reflux esophagitis, most patients with reflux esophagitis have an axial hiatal hernia."[169] The precise relationship between hiatal hernia, lower esophageal sphincter function and dysfunction, and gastroesophageal reflux disease has not yet been determined. However, one thing seems certain, that is, the pathogenesis of gastroesophageal reflux sequelae is related in some way to both the anatomic defect (hiatal hernia) and physiologic dysfunction in the esophageal body and hypotension in the lower esophageal sphincter.

Although the hiatal hernia per se rarely causes symptoms directly (incarceration with pain and/or bleeding), it is the anatomic companion of all the major complications of gastroesophageal reflux. Fortunately, proper medical therapy controls reflux-related problems sufficiently well that surgical intervention is needed in less than 5% of patients.[174]

Hiatal hernia is one of the most prevalent defects in the gastrointestinal tract in the western world.[175] Although there are variations in indications and techniques for barium radiography in different countries, there does appear to be a decreased incidence of hiatal hernia in Africa, India, and Korea.[176] There is evidence that hiatal hernias are more common in women and in both sexes with increasing age. Burkitt and James have proposed that frequent increases in intra-abdominal pressure caused by straining at stool may be a major factor.[175] Low-fiber diet is proposed as a likely cause for this problem. Burkitt supports this theory by emphasizing

the high prevalence of hiatal hernia in radiologic surveys from western countries (12%–69% depending on age) compared with very low prevalence in countries in Africa and Asia (between 1% and 5%). Hiatal hernia has been found to be more common in persons with peptic ulcer disease, scleroderma, kyphosis, and ankylosing spondylitis.[176] It is considered rare in association with achalasia in several reports, being in the range of 1.5% to 2.3%.[177,178] On the other hand, Palmer found the two entities associated in 12.5% of cases.[179] Variations in diagnostic criteria may have accounted for some of this difference in incidence.

The reader is directed to Chapter 7, Esophageal Motor Function; Chapter 28, Approach to the Patient with Dysphagia; Chapter 29, Approach to the Patient with Chest Pain; Chapter 54, Motility Disorders of the Esophagus; Chapter 55, Reflux Esophagitis; Chapter 58, Miscellaneous Diseases of the Esophagus; Chapter 59, Stomach: Anatomy and Structural Anomalies; Chapter 111, Upper Gastrointestinal Endoscopy; Chapter 114, Contrast Radiology; Chapter 118, Applications of Computed Tomography to the Gastrointestinal Tract; Chapter 122, Angiography; Chapter 128, Evaluation of Gastrointestinal Motility: Methodological Considerations; and Chapter 131, Gastrointestinal Dilation.

REFERENCES

1. Sadler TW. Digestive system. In: Langman's medical embryology, ed 5. Baltimore: Williams & Wilkins, 1985:224.
2. Schridde H. Uber die Epithelproliferationen in der embryonalen menschlichen Speiserohre. Virchows Arch 1908;191:179.
3. Gray SW, Skandalakis JE. The esophagus. In: Embryology for surgeons. Philadelphia: WB Saunders, 1972:63.
4. Meyer GW, Austin RM, Brady CE, et al. Muscle anatomy of the human esophagus. J Clin Gastroenterol 1986;8(2):131.
5. Harrington SW. Esophageal hiatal diaphragmatic hernia. Surg Gynecol Obstet 1955;100:277.
6. Hayward J. The lower end of the oesophagus. Thorax 1961;16:36.

7. Listerud MB, Harkins HN. Anatomy of the esophageal hiatus. Anatomic studies on two hundred four fresh cadavers. Arch Surg 1958;76:835.

8. Collis JL, Kelly TD, Wiley AM. Anatomy of the crura of the diaphragm and the surgery of hiatus hernia. Thorax 1954;9:175.

9. Low A. A note on the crura of the diaphragm and the muscle of Treitz. J Anat Physiol 1954;42:93.

10. Peters PM. Closure mechanisms at the cardia with special reference to diaphragmatic oesophageal elastic ligament. Thorax 1955;10:27.

11. Bombeck CT, Dillard DH, Nyhus LM. Muscular anatomy of the gastroesophageal junction and role of phrenoesophageal ligament. Autopsy study of sphincter mechanism. Ann Surg 1966;164:643.

12. Gray SW, Rowe JS Jr, Skandalakis JE. Surgical anatomy of the gastroesophageal junction. Ann Surg 1979;45:575.

13. Androulakis JA, Skandalakis JE, Gray SW. Contributions to the pathological anatomy of hiatal hernia. JAMA 1966;55:295.

14. Kitano S, Terblanche J, Kahn D, et al. Venous anatomy of the lower oesophagus in portal hypertension: Practical implications. Br J Surg 1986;73:525.

15. Vianna A, Hayes PC, Moscosa G, et al. Normal venous circulation of the gastroesophageal junction. Gastroenterology 1987;93(4):876.

16. Peden JK, Schneider CF, Bickel RD. Anatomic relations of the vagus nerves to the esophagus. Am J Surg 1950;80:32.

17. Chamberlin JA, Winship T. Anatomic variations of the vagus nerves. Their significance in vagus neurectomy. Surgery 1947;22:1.

18. Goetsch E. The structure of the mammalian oesophagus. Am J Anat 1910;10:1.

19. Geboes K, Desmet V. Histology of the esophagus. Front Gastrointest Res 1978;3:1.

20. Geboes K, De Wolf-Peeters C, Rutgeerts P, et al. Lymphocytes and Langerhans cells in the human oesophageal epithelium. Virchows Arch [A] 1983;401:45.

21. Tateishi R, Taniguchi H, Wada A, et al. Argyrophil cells and melanocytes in esophageal mucosa. Arch Pathol 1974;98:87.

22. Donner MW, Bosma JF, Robertson DL. Anatomy and physiology of the pharynx. Gastrointest Radiol 1985;10:196.

23. Ekberg O, Lindstrom C. The upper esophageal sphincter area. Acta Radiol 1987;28(2):173.

24. Kahrilas PJ, Dodds WJ, Dent J, et al. Upper esophageal sphincter function during deglutition. Gastroenterology 1988;95:95.

25. Welch RW. Manometry of the normal upper esophageal sphincter and its alterations in laryngectomy. J Clin Invest 1979;63:1036.

26. Kaugmann P. Die mushelandordsung in der speiserohre. Ergebn Anat Entwickl Gesch 1968;40:3.

27. Lieberman-Meffert D, Algower M, Schmid P, et al. Muscular equivalent of the lower esophageal sphincter. Gastroenterology 1979;76(1):31.

28. Rector LE, Connerley ML. Aberrant mucosa in the esophagus in infants and in children. Arch Pathol 1941;31:285.

29. Auld RM, Lukash WM, Bordin GM. Heterotopic sebaceous glands in the esophagus. Gastrointest Endosc 1987;33:332.

30. Desmet VJ, Tytgat GN. Histology and electron microscopy of the esophagus. In: von Trappen G, Hellemans J, eds. Diseases of the esophagus. Berlin, Heidelberg, New York: Springer-Verlag, 1974:24.

31. Rywlin AM, Ortega R. Glycogenic acanthosis of the esophagus. Arch Pathol 1970;90:439.

32. Al Yassin TM, Tones PG. Fine structure of squamous epithelium and submucosal glands of human esophagus. J Anat 1977;123:705.

33. Hopwood D, Logan KR, Bouchier IAD. The electron microscopy of normal human oesophageal epithelium. Virchows Arch [B] 1978;26:345.

34. Logan KR, Hopwood D, Milne G. Ultrastructural demonstration of cell coat on the cell surfaces of normal esophageal epithelium. Histochem J 1977;9:495.

35. Hopwood D, Logan KR, Milne G. Mucosubstances in the normal human oesophageal epithelium. Histochemistry 1977;54:67.

36. Hopwood D, Logan KR, Coghill G, et al. Histochemical studies of mucosubstances and lipids in normal human oesophageal epithelium. Histochem J 1977;9:153.

37. Geboes K, Mebis J, Desmet V. The esophagus: Normal ultrastructure and pathologic patterns. In: Motta PM, Fjuita H, Correr S, eds.

Ultrastructure of the digestive tract. Boston, Dordrect, Lancaster: Martinus Nijhoff, 1988:17.

38. Faussone-Pellegrini MS, Cortesini C, Romagnoli P. Ultrastructural features and localization of the interstitial cells of Cajal in the smooth muscle coat of the human esophagus. J Submicrosc Cytol 1985;17:187.

39. Vogt EC. Congenital esophageal atresia. Am J Roentgenol 1929;22:463.

40. Ladd WE. The surgical treatment of esophageal atresia and tracheoesophageal fistula. N Engl J Med 1944;230:625.

41. Gross RE. The surgery of infancy and childhood. Philadelphia: WB Saunders, 1953.

42. Swenson O, Lipman R, Fisher JH, et al. Repair and complications of esophageal atresia and tracheoesophageal fistula. N Engl J Med 1962;267:960.

43. Stephens CA, Mustard WT, Simpson JS Jr. Congenital atresia of the esophagus with tracheo-esophageal fistula. Surg Clin North Am 1956;36:1465.

44. Koop CE, Hamilton JP. Atresia of the esophagus: Factors effecting survival in 249 cases. Z Kinderchir 1968;5:319.

45. Waterston DJ, Bonham-Carter RE, Aberdeen E. Congenital tracheo-oesophageal fistula in association with oesophageal atresia. Lancet 1963;55.

46. Slim MS, Bickers WM. Esophageal atresia with tracheo-esophageal fistula. Arch Surg 1970;100:577.

47. Holder TM, Cloud DT, Lewis JE, et al. Esophageal atresia and tracheoesophageal fistula. A survey of its members by the Surgical Section of the American Academy of Pediatrics. Pediatrics 1964;34:542.

48. Andrassy RJ, Mahour GH. Gastrointestinal anomalies associated with esophageal atresia or tracheoesophageal fistula. Arch Surg 1979;114:1125.

49. Moorhead JM, Reid RA, Vontz FU. Congenital tracheoesophageal fistula in an adult. South Med J 1982;75:1030.

50. Enoksen A, Lovaas J, Haavik PE. Congenital tracheoesophageal fistula in the adult. Scand J Thorac Cardiovasc Surg 1979;13:173.

51. Holman WL, Vaezy A, Postlethwait RW, et al. Surgical treatment of H-type tracheoesophageal fistula diagnosed in an adult. Ann Thorac Surg 1986;41:453.

52. Beasley SW, Myers NA. The diagnosis of congenital tracheoesophageal fistula. J Pediatr Surg 1988;23(5):415.

53. Hendren WH, Hale JR. Electromagnetic bougienage to lengthen esophageal segments in congenital esophageal atresia. N Engl J Med 1975;293(9)8.

54. Howard R, Meyers NA. Esophageal atresia: A technique for elongating the upper pouch. Surgery 1965;58:725.

55. Louhimo I, Lindahl H. Esophageal atresia: Primary results of 500 consecutively treated patients. J Pediatr Surg 1983;18(3):217.

56. Pohlson EC, Schaller RT, Tapper D. Improved survival with primary anastomosis in the low birth weight neonate with esophageal atresia and tracheoesophageal fistula. J Pediatr Surg 1988;23(5):418.

57. Bluestone CD, Kerry R, Sieber WK. Congenital esophageal stenosis. Laryngoscope 1969;79:1095.

58. Ishida M, Tsuchida Y, Saito S, et al. Congenital esophageal stenosis due to tracheobronchial remnants. J Pediatr Surg 1969;4(3):339.

59. Sneed WF, LaGarde DC, Kogutt MS, et al. Esophageal stenosis due to cartilaginous tracheobronchial remnants. J Pediatr Surg 1979;14(6):786.

60. Anderson LS, Shackelford GD, Mancilla-Jimenez R, et al. Cartilaginous esophageal ring: A cause of esophageal stenosis in infants and children. Radiology 1973;108:665.

61. Ibrahim NBN, Sandry RJ. Congenital oesophageal stenosis caused by tracheobronchial structures in the oesophageal wall. Thorax 1981;36:465.

62. Groote AD, Laurini RN, Polman HA. A case of congenital esophageal stenosis. Hum Pathol 1985;16(11):1170.

63. Castleman B, Towne VW. Case 42411. Case records of Massachusetts General Hospital. N Engl J Med 1956;255(15):707.

64. Bergmann M, Charnas RM. Tracheobronchial rests in the esophagus. Their relation to some benign strictures and certain types of cancer of the esophagus. J Thorac Surg 1958;35(1):97.

65. Boyce GA, Boyce HW Jr. Congenital esophageal stenosis: Adult

presentation (abstr). International Society of Diseases of the Esophagus 1989.

66. Bremer JL. Congenital anomalies of the viscera. Cambridge: Harvard University Press, 1957.

67. Ciechanowski S, Glinski LK. Fistulae oesophageo-oesophageales congeniate. Virchows Arch [A] 1910;199:420.

68. Maier HC. Intramural duplication of the esophagus. Ann Surg 1957;145:395.

69. Ansell G, Edwards FR. Double esophagus. J Fac Radiol 1958;9:154.

70. Kelley ML Jr, Murtagh J, McCarty WC Jr. Reduplication of the esophagus. Presenting as midesophageal web and diverticulum. JAMA 1968;204(1):73.

71. Schmidt HW, Clagett OT, Harrison EG Jr. Benign tumors and cysts of the esophagus. J Thorac Cardiovasc Surg 1961;41:716.

72. Boyd DP, Hill LD III. Benign tumors and cysts of the esophagus. Am J Surg 1957;93:252.

73. Salyer DC, Salyer WR, Eggleston JC. Benign developmental cysts of the mediastinum. Arch Pathol Lab Med 1977;101:136.

74. Ildstad ST, Tollerud DJ, Weiss RG, et al. Duplications of the alimentary tract. Ann Surg 1988;208(2):184.

75. Arbona JL, Figueroa Fazzi JG, Mayoral J. Congenital esophageal cysts: Case report and review of the literature. Am J Gastroenterol 1984;79(3):177.

76. Sabiston DC Jr, Scott HW Jr. Primary neoplasms and cysts of the mediastinum. Ann Surg 1952;136(5):777.

77. Barlow D. Enterogenous cyst of oesophagus. Br J Surg 1957;45:100.

78. Creech O, DeBakey ME. Ciliated epithelial cysts of the esophagus associated with cardiac abnormalities. J Thorac Cardiovasc Surg 1954;28:64.

79. Hocking M, Young DG. Duplications of the alimentary tract. Br J Surg 1981;68:92.

80. Ferguson CC, Young LN, Sutherland JB, et al. Intrathoracic gastrogenic cyst—Preoperative diagnosis by technetium pertechnetate scan. J Pediatr Surg 1973;8(5):827.

81. Weiss LM, Fagelman D, Warhit JM. CT demonstration of an esophageal duplication cyst. Case report. J Comput Assist Tomogr 1983;7:716.

82. Marvasti MA, Micthell GE, Burke WA, et al. Misleading density of mediastinal cysts on computerized tomography. Ann Thorac Surg 1981;31(2):167.

83. McHardy G, Bruni H, Lilly J. Bronchogenic cyst of the esophagus, report of a case and review of the literature. Gastrointest Endosc 1971;18:31.

84. Yasuda K, Nakajima M, Yoshida S, et al. The diagnosis of submucosal tumors of the stomach by endoscopic ultrasonography. Gastrointest Endosc 1989;35(1):10.

85. Nehme AE, Rabiah F. Ciliated epithelial esophageal cyst: Case report and review of the literature. Am Surg 1977;43:114.

86. Salo JA, Ala-Kulju KV. Congenital esophageal cysts in adults. Ann Thorac Surg 1987;44:135.

87. Bishop HC, Koop CE. Surgical management of duplications of the alimentary tract. Am J Surg 1964;107:434.

88. Tarnay TJ, Chang CH(J), Nugent RG, et al. Esophageal duplication (foregut cyst) with spinal malformation. J Thorac Cardiovasc Surg 1970;59(2):293.

89. McGregor DH, Mills G, Boudet RA. Intramural squamous cell carcinoma of the esophagus. Cancer 1976;37(3):1556.

90. Boivin Y, Cholette JP, Lefebvre R. Accessory esophagus complicated by an adenocarcinoma. Can Med Assoc J 1964;90:1414.

91. Tapia RH, White VA. Squamous cell carcinoma arising in a duplication cyst of the esophagus. Am J Gastroenterol 1985;80(5):325.

92. Gerle RD, Jaretzki A III, Ashley CA, et al. Congenital bronchopulmonary foregut malformation. Pulmonary sequestration communicating with the gastrointestinal tract. N Engl J Med 1968;278(26):1413.

93. Leithhiser RE, Capitanio MA, Macpherson RI, et al. "Communicating" bronchopulmonary foregut malformations. AJR 1986;146:227.

94. Fowler CL, Pokorny WJ, Wagner ML, et al. Review of bronchopulmonary foregut malformations. J Pediatr Surg 1988;23(9):3.

95. Heithoff KB, Sane SM, Williams HJ, et al. Bronchopulmonary foregut malformations: A unifying etiological concept. Am J Roentgenol 1976;126(1):46.

96. Crawford DB, Cole S, Danielson KS, et al. Malformation of bronchopulmonary foregut with systemic and pulmonary arterial blood supply. Chest 1978;73(3):421.

97. Bowen AD III, Parry WH. Bronchopulmonary foregut malformation in the Goldenhar anomalad. AJR 1980;134:186.

98. Holder TM, Leape LL, Ashcroft KW. Congenital malformations of the trachea, bronchi and esophagus, In: Shumrick DA, Paparella MM, eds. Otolaryngology, ed 2. Philadelphia: WB Saunders, 1980:2561.

99. Edwards FR. Vascular compression of the trachea and oesophagus. Thorax 1959;14:187.

100. Lasher EP. Types of tracheal and esophageal constriction due to arterial anomalies of the aortic arch, with suggestions as to treatment. Am J Surg 1958;96:228.

101. Palmer ED. Dysphagia lusoria: Clinical aspects in the adult. Ann Intern Med 1955;42(6):1173.

102. Mustard WT, Trimble AW, Trusler GA. Mediastinal vascular anomalies causing tracheal and esophageal compression and obstruction in childhood. Can Med Assoc J 1962;87:1301.

103. Facquet J, Welti JJ, Alhomme P. Dysphagie lusoria mortelle par anomalie de la sous-clavierie droite. Nouveau Procede Diagnostique Arch Mal Coeur 1955;48:582.

104. Hallman GL, Cooley DA. Congenital aortic vascular ring. Arch Surg 1964;88:666.

105. Karlson KJ, Heiss FW, Ellis FH Jr. Adult dysphagia lusoria. Treatment by arterial division and reestablishment of vascular continuity. Chest 1985;87(5):684.

106. Vasquez MT, Garcia MAM, Wollrich FS, et al. Cervical dysphagia lusoria from vertebral arterial compression. Arch Surg 1983;118:125.

107. Adkins RB Jr, Maples MD, Graham BS, et al. Dysphagia associated with an aortic arch anomaly in adults. Am Surg 1986;52(5):238.

108. Lincoln JCR, Deverall PB, Stark J, et al. Vascular anomalies compressing the oesophagus and trachea. Thorax 1969;24:295.

109. Massumi R, Wiener L, Charif P. The syndrome of cervical aorta. Report of a case and review of the previous cases. Am J Cardiol 1963;11:678.

110. Rector LE, Connerley ML. Aberrant mucosa in the esophagus in infants and in children. Arch Pathol 1941;31(3):285.

111. Jabbari M, Goresky CA, Lough J, et al. The inlet patch: Heterotopic gastric mucosa in the upper esophagus. Gastroenterology 1985;89(2):352.

112. Feller SC, Weaver GA. Heterotopic gastric mucosa in the upper esophagus. Gastroenterology 1986;90(1):257.

113. Tytgat GNJ. Endoscopy of the oesophagus. In: Cotton PB, Tytgat GNJ, Williams CB, eds. Annual of gastrointestinal endoscopy. London: Gower Academic Journals, 1988:3.

114. Kohler B, Kohler G, Riemann JF. Spontaneous esophagotracheal fistula resulting from ulcer in heterotopic gastric mucosa. Gastroenterology 1988;95(3):828.

115. Schmidt H, Riddell H, Walter B, et al. Adenokarzinome in heterotoper magenschleimhaut des proximalen oesophagus. Leber Magen Darm 1985;15:144.

116. Yoshida M, Ide H, Yamada A, et al. Early detection of adenocarcinoma of the esophagus. Endoscopy 1986;18(Suppl 3):44.

117. Templeton FE. X-ray examination of the stomach. In: A description of roentgenologic anatomy, physiology and pathology of the esophagus, stomach and duodenum. Chicago: The University of Chicago Press, 1944:104.

118. Schatzki R, Gary JE. Dysphagia due to a diaphragm-like localized narrowing in the lower esophagus ("lower esophageal ring"). Am J Roentgenol 1953;70(6):911.

119. Ingelfinger FJ, Kramer P. Dysphagia produced by a contractile ring in the lower esophagus. Gastroenterology 1953;23(3):419.

120. Postlethwait RW, Musser AW. Pathology of lower esophageal web. Surg Gynecol Obstet 1965;120:571.

121. MacMahon HE, Schatzki R, Gary JE. Pathology of a lower esophageal ring. Report of a case, with autopsy, observed for nine years. N Engl J Med 1958;259(1):1.

122. Bartlett MK, Jones CM. Surgical experience with the lower esophageal ring. Ann Surg 1959;149:491.

123. Keyting WS, Baker GM, McCarver RR, et al. The lower esophagus. Am J Roentgenol 1960;84(6):1070.

124. Schatzki R. The lower esophageal ring: Long term follow up of symptomatic and asymptomatic rings. Am J Roentgenol 1963;90(4):805.

125. Eckardt V, Dagradi AE, Stempien SJ. The esophagogastric (Schatzki) rings and reflux esophagitis. Am J Gastroenterol 1972;58:525.

126. Paulson DL. Benign stricture of the esophagus secondary to gastroesophageal reflux. Ann Surg 1967;165(5):765.

127. Rinaldo JA Jr, Gahagan T. The narrow lower esophageal ring: Pathogenesis and physiology. Am J Dig Dis 1966;11:257.

128. Chen YM, Gelfand DW, Ott DJ, et al. Natural progression of the lower esophageal mucosal ring. Gastrointest Radiol 1987;12(2):93.

129. Ott DJ, Gelfand DW, Wu WC, et al. Esophagogastric region and its rings. AJR 1984;142:281.

130. Ott DJ, Chen YM, Wu WC, et al. Radiographic and endoscopic sensitivity in detecting lower esophageal mucosal ring. AJR 1986;147:261.

131. Webb WA. Esophageal dilation: Personal experience with current instruments and techniques. Am J Gastroenterol 1988;83(5):471.

132. Goyal RK, Bauer JL, Spiro HM. The nature and location of lower esophageal ring. N Engl J Med 1971;284(21):1175.

133. Ekberg O, Malmquist J, Lindren S. Pharyngo-oesophageal webs in dysphagical patients. Fortschr Rontgenstr 1986;145:75.

134. Kelly AB. Spasm at the entrance of the esophagus. J Laryngol Rhinol Otol 1919;24:285.

135. Paterson DR. A clinical type of dysphagia. J Laryngol Rhinol Otol 1919:34:289.

136. Vinson PP. Hysterical dysphagia. Minn Med 1922;5:107.

137. Waldenstrom J. Iron and epithelium. Some clinical observations. Part I. Regeneration of the epithelium. Acta Med Scand 1938;(Suppl 90):380.

138. McNab Jones RF. The Paterson-Brown-Kelly syndrome. Its relationship to iron deficiency and post-cricoid carcinoma. J Laryngol Otol 1961;75:529.

139. Chisholm M. The association between webs, iron and post-cricoid carcinoma. Postgrad Med J 1974;50:215.

140. Ikard RW, Rosen HE. Midesophageal web in adults. Ann Thorac Surg 1977;24(4):355.

141. Kelley ML, Frazer JP. Symptomatic mid-esophageal webs. JAMA 1966;197:(2):183.

142. Longstreth GF, Wolochow DA, Tu RT. Double congenital mid-esophageal webs in adults. Dig Dis Sci 1979;24(2):162.

143. Shiflett DW, Gilliam JH, Wu WC, et al. Multiple esophageal webs. Gastroenterology 1979;77:556.

144. Carlisle WR. A case of multiple esophageal webs and rings. Gastrointest Endosc 1984;30(3):184.

145. Mares AJ, Bar-Ziv J, Lieberman A, et al. Congenital esophageal stenosis. Transendoscopic web incision. J Clin Gastroenterol 1986;8(5):555.

146. Ludlow A. A case of obstructed deglutition, from a preternatural dilation of, and bag formed in, the pharynx. Medical Observations and Inquiries by a Society of Physician in London, ed 2. 1769;3:85.

147. Zenker FA, Ziemssen H. Krankheiten des oesophagus in handbuch des speciellen pathologie und therapie. Leipzig: FC Vogel, 1877;(Suppl 50):7.

148. Knuff TE, Benjamin SB, Castell DO. Pharyngoesophageal (Zenker's) diverticulum: A reappraisal. Gastroenterology 1982;82:734.

149. Cook IJ, Gabb M, Panagopoulos V, et al. Zenker's diverticulum: A defect in upper esophageal sphincter compliance? (abstr) Gastroenterology 1989;96(5, Part 2):A98.

150. Butcher RB II, Larrabee WF Jr. Surgical treatment of hypopharyngeal (Zenker's) diverticulum. Arch Otolaryngol 1979;105:254.

151. Bowdler DA, Stell PM. Surgical management of posterior pharyngeal pulsion diverticula: Inversion versus one-stage excision. Br J Surg 1987;74(11):988.

152. Van Overbeek JJM, Hoeksema PE. Endoscopic treatment of the hypopharyngeal diverticulum: 211 cases. Laryngoscope 1982;92:88.

153. Welch AR, Stafford F. Comparison of endoscopic diathermy and resection in the surgical treatment of pharyngeal diverticula. J Laryngol Otol 1985;99:179.

154. Bertelsen S, Aasted A. Results of operative treatment of hypopharyngeal diverticulum. Thorax 1976;31:544.

155. Huang B, Unni KK, Payne WS. Long-term survival following diverticulectomy for cancer in pharyngoesophageal (Zenker's) diverticulum. Ann Thorac Surg 1984;38(3):207.

156. Turner MJ, Chir B. Carcinoma as a complication of pharyngeal pouch. Br J Radiol 1963;36:206.

157. Hansen JB, Jagt T, Gundtoft JP, et al. Pharyngo-oesophageal diverticula. A clinical and cineradiographic follow-up study of 23 cases treated by diverticulectomy. Scand J Thorac Cardiovasc Surg 1973;7:81.

158. Bowdler DA, Stell PM. Carcinoma arising in posterior pharyngeal pulsion diverticulum (Zenker's diverticulum). Br J Surg 1987;74(7):561.

159. Evander A, Little AG, Ferguson MK, et al. Diverticula of the mid- and lower esophagus: Pathogenesis and surgical management. World J Surg 1986;10:820.

160. Debas HT, Payne WS, Cameron AJ, et al. Physiopathology of lower esophageal diverticulum and its implications for treatment. Surg Gynecol Obstet 1980;151:593.

161. Mendl K, McKay JM, Tanner CH. Intramural diverticulosis of the oesophagus and Rokitansky–Aschoff sinuses in the gall-bladder. Br J Radiol 1960;33:496.

162. Castillo S, Aburashed A, Kimmelman J, et al. Diffuse intramural esophageal pseudodiverticulosis. New cases and review. Gastroenterology 1977;72(3):541.

163. Umlas J, Sakhuja R. The pathology of esophageal intramural pseudodiverticulosis. Am J Clin Pathol 1976;65:314.

164. Wolf BS. Sliding hiatal hernia: The need for redefinition. Am J Roentgenol 1973;117(2):231.

165. Rinaldo JA Jr. Some observations concerning the physiology of the distal esophagus with comments on hiatal hernia. Henry Ford Hosp Med Bull 1966;14:77.

166. Heitmann P, Wolf BS, Sokol EM, et al. Simultaneous cineradiographic-manometry study of the distal esophagus: Small hiatal hernias and rings. Gastroenterology 1966;50:737.

167. Clark MD, Rinaldo JA Jr, Eyler WR. Correlation of manometric and radiologic data from the esophagogastric area. Radiology 1970;94:261.

168. Wolf BS, Cohen BR. Radiologic localization of the esophageal hiatus as determined by intraluminal pressure measurements. Radiology 1961;76:903.

169. Dodds WJ. Current concepts of esophageal motor function: Clinical implications of radiology. Am J Roentgenol 1977;128:549.

170. Dagradi AE, Stempien SJ. Symptomatic esophageal hiatus sliding hernia. Clinical, radiologic, and endoscopic study of 100 cases. Am J Dig Dis 1962;7(7):613.

171. Trujillo NP, Slaughter RL, Boyce HW Jr. Endoscopic diagnosis of sliding-type diaphragmatic hiatal hernias. Am J Dig Dis 1968;13(10):855.

172. Trujillo NP, Boyce HW Jr. Gastroscopy: An aid to the detection of small sliding-type hiatal hernias. South Med J 1968;61(1):1.

173. Johnson LF, DeMeester TR, Haggitt RC. Endoscopic signs for gastroesophageal reflux objectively evaluated. Gastrointest Endosc 1976;22(3):151.

174. Palmer ED. The hiatus hernia–esophagitis–esophageal stricture complex. Am J Med 1968;44:566.

175. Burkitt DP, James PA. Low-residue diets and hiatus hernia. Lancet 2 (July 21), 1973:128.

176. Earlam R. Hiatus hernia. In: Clinical tests of oesophageal function. New York: Grune & Stratton, 1975:127.

177. Binder HJ, Clemett AR, Thayer WR, et al. Rarity of hiatus hernia in achalasia. N Engl J Med 1965;272:680.

178. Taub W, Achkar E. Hiatal hernia in patients with achalasia. Am J Gastroenterol 1987;82(12):1256.

179. Palmer ED. Achalasia: Anatomy of cardia as it relates to regional pathophysiology. Radiology 1956;67:79.

54

Motility Disorders
of the Esophagus

JOEL E. RICHTER

INTRODUCTION

During the past 2 decades, there has been a remarkable resurgence of interest in studies of esophageal motility disorders. Improvements in methodology for accurate measurements of intraluminal pressures began this reawakening with greater sophistication in studies of the lower esophageal sphincter, and continued through more recent refinements in the measurement of esophageal peristaltic pressures and, finally, upper esophageal sphincter and pharyngeal function. In addition, advances in radiologic techniques, particularly cineradiography and radionuclide scintigraphy, permit accurate correlation of liquid and solid bolus movement with changes in esophageal pressures. These clinical and research tools have expanded our understanding of esophageal motility disorders and their relationship to symptoms, especially in patients with noncardiac chest pain and persons complaining of oropharyngeal dysphagia. Unfortunately, research in this area has been hampered by the inability to gather pathologic specimens of muscles and nerves in diseases that are not life-threatening. Likewise, technology has limited human studies of esophageal nerve conduction, membrane potential, and muscle function in vitro. This perspective may help to explain our understanding and effective therapies for achalasia. In contrast, our knowledge is quite incomplete about the spastic disorders of the esophagus and the complex interactions associated with swallowing. Nevertheless, multiple tools are available for evaluating esophageal function, which should help us with the diagnosis and treatment of patients with esophageal motility disorders.

DISORDERS OF THE HYPOPHARYNX, UPPER ESOPHAGEAL SPHINCTER, AND CERVICAL ESOPHAGUS

A large number of conditions can cause dysphagia in the region of the hypopharynx, upper esophageal sphincter, and cervical esophagus. In this area, swallowing is brought about by striated muscle as opposed to the smooth muscle in the distal esophagus and the rest of the gastrointestinal tract. As such, the lesions that cause difficulty are different from those encountered in the esophageal body and lower esophageal sphincter. Anything that might affect the brain stem swallowing center or the afferent or efferent nerves that modulate the process—cranial nerves V, VII, IX, X, and XII—may cause dysfunction of this portion of the esophagus with resulting oropharyngeal dysphagia. In addition, disorders of the striated muscles of this region, such as myasthenia gravis and polymyositis, can cause similar complaints. Oropharyngeal dysphagia is a common problem in the elderly population and is frequently associated with a poor prognosis. Studies of nursing home patients show that 30% to 40% of patients have eating and swallowing abnormalities.[1] The importance of abnormal swallowing mechanisms in the elderly is reflected by the high incidence of aspiration pneumonia in autopsy studies.[2] However, oropharyngeal dysphagia may be seen in younger patients, and these conditions may be more amenable to medical therapy. Table 54-1 lists conditions that may cause oropharyngeal dysphagia.

Clinical Disorders Associated With Oropharyngeal Dysphagia

UPPER ESOPHAGEAL SPHINCTER DISORDERS

Dysfunction of the upper esophageal sphincter can be broadly divided into alterations in resting tone and changes in sphincter relaxation.[3] Unfortunately, much of the data by which these disorders have been classified are based on older radiographic or manometric studies. Many of these diseases need to be restudied with modern cineradiographic techniques and high fidelity manometric systems with computerized analysis.

Cricopharyngeal Hypertension. This term has been used in the past to describe higher than normal upper esophageal sphincter pressure contributing to dysphagia in some patients with Plummer-Vinson syndrome, gastroesophageal reflux disease, or globus hystericus, and in postlaryngectomy patients.[4-7] In many cases, gastroesophageal reflux may be the common denominator. Initial studies suggested that acid perfusion of the distal esophagus caused an increase in upper esophageal sphincter tone.[8] However, more recent studies indicate that intraluminal distention is the

TABLE 54–1
Clinical Disorders Associated With Oropharyngeal Dysphagia

Motility Disorders of the Upper Esophageal Sphincter (UES)

Hypertensive UES

Hypotensive UES

Abnormal UES relaxation

    Incomplete relaxation (cricopharyngeal achalasia)

    Premature closure (Zenker's diverticulum?)

    Delayed relaxation (familial dysautonomia)

Neuromuscular Disorders

Neurologic diseases

    Cerebrovascular accidents

    Poliomyelitis

    Amyotrophic lateral sclerosis

    Parkinson's disease

    Multiple sclerosis

    Central nervous system diseases

    Wilson's disease

    Sydenham's and Huntington's chorea

    Tabes dorsalis

    Brain stem tumors

    Cranial nerve injuries

    Peripheral neuropathies (diptheria, botulism, rabies, diabetes mellitus)

Skeletal muscle diseases

    Inflammatory myopathies

        Polymyositis

        Dermatomyositis

    Muscular dystrophies

        Myotonic dystrophy

        Oculopharyngeal dystrophy

    Myasthenia gravis

    Metabolic myopathy (thyrotoxicosis, myxedema, steroid myopathy)

    Sarcoidosis

    Systemic lupus erythematosis

    Stiff man syndrome

Local Structural Lesions

Inflammatory (pharyngitis, tonsillar abscess, tuberculosis)

Neoplastic

Congenital webs

Plummer-Vinson syndrome

Extrinsic compression (thyromegaly, cervical spur, lymphadenopathy)

Surgical resection of the oropharynx

Postsurgical changes from other operations in this region

---

primary stimulus responsible for reflex upper esophageal sphincter contractions.[9,10] This was demonstrated by showing similar changes in sphincter tone with equal volumes of saline or acid solutions as well as intraluminal balloon distention. This may also be the reason some patients with distal esophageal abnormalities occasionally experience proximal dysphagia. Some patients with globus hystericus have been shown to have gastroesophageal reflux.[11] However, these patients also have a high prevalence of psychologic abnormalities, which may alter their pain perception and increase upper esophageal sphincter pressures.[12] The latter mechanism is supported by a recent study showing that acute emotional stress from a dichotic listening task significantly increased mean upper esophageal sphincter pressures in normal persons.[13]

Cricopharyngeal Hypotonia. Abnormally low pressures in the upper esophageal sphincter have been described in a variety of neuromuscular disorders including amyotrophic lateral sclerosis, myasthenia gravis, and myotonic dystrophy.[14] However, it is rarely an isolated disorder; most patients also have weakness of the pharyngeal musculature.[3] Welch found lowered resting upper esophageal sphincter pressures, increased sphincter length, and loss of upper esophageal sphincter asymmetry in postlaryngectomy patients.[15] Patients with esophagopharyngeal regurgitation also have been reported to have decreased resting upper esophageal sphincter pressures compared to healthy subjects and patients with heartburn but without regurgitation.[16]

Abnormalities of Upper Esophageal Sphincter Relaxation. Three types of abnormalities have been described in association with abnormal upper esophageal sphincter relaxation: incomplete relaxation, delayed relaxation, and premature closure. *Cricopharyngeal achalasia* is a term formerly used to describe incomplete upper sphincter relaxation occurring after the majority of swallows as the result of uncoordination with the pharyngeal phase of deglutition. It has been described as an isolated phenomenon in children and newborns; it usually resolves spontaneously within 2 weeks of birth.[17–19] However, in adults it is usually secondary to an underlying neuromuscular disorder or previous neck surgery including pharyngectomy, laryngectomy, and tracheostomy placement.[20–22] An increased amount of fibrous tissue has been detected in sections of the cricopharyngeal muscle obtained during myotomy in some patients with cricopharyngeal achalasia.[23] Other myopathic features also have been detected.[24] Radiographically, this entity may be suggested by the presence of a cricopharyngeal bar at the C6–7 level, occasionally with a functional delay in barium passage. However, correlation of this finding with manometric studies is poor. Patients with a prominent cricopharyngeal bar are usually found to have pressure values within the normal range with good relaxation.[25]

Delayed upper esophageal sphincter relaxation is a characteristic finding in familial dysautonomia or the Riley-Day syndrome.[26,27] This autosomal recessive disease, occurring in Jewish families of eastern European ancestry, is characterized by derangements in autonomic function including sucking and swallowing usually present from birth. Radiologic studies have shown delayed opening of the cricopharyngeus with normal pharyngeal motor activity and disordered distal esophageal motility.[26] No manometric confirmation for these findings has been reported.

It has been suggested that premature closure of the upper esophageal sphincter is important in the pathogenesis of a pharyngoesophageal (Zenker's) diverticulum, a protrusion of hypopharyngeal mucosa between oblique fibers of the inferior pharyngeal constrictor and transverse fibers of the cricopharyngeal muscle.[28,29] However, Kopicek and Creamer found no manometric abnormalities in eight patients with a Zenker's diverticulum.[30] Knuff et al found significantly lower upper esophageal sphincter pressures with complete relaxation and normal pharyngeal coordination in eight Zenker's patients compared to age-matched controls studied with an infused oval catheter system.[31] In another study of ten patients with Zenker's diverticulum treated with cricopharyngeal myotomy and diverticulum suspension, upper esophageal sphincter and pharyngeal coordination was abnormal in all swallows in two patients, normal in six patients, and normal in 60% to 80% of swallows in the remaining two patients.[32] In only one patient were over half the swallows associated with incomplete relaxation. Therefore, it appears that patients with Zenker's diverticulum constitute a heterogeneous group with a still ill-defined pathogenesis.

NEUROLOGIC DISORDERS

Cerebrovascular Accidents. By far the largest single group of neurologic conditions producing oropharyngeal dysphagia are cerebrovascular accidents. Symptoms are usually abrupt and associated with other evidence of neurologic damage particularly in the distribution of the cranial nerves. Occasionally, oropharyngeal dysphagia is the prominent complaint, and corroborating evidence of brain stem deficits is lacking. In these situations, computed tomography (CT) or magnetic resonance imaging (MRI) of the brain stem region usually reveals multiple infarctions. In a videofluorographic study of 38 patients studied within 4 months of their stroke, 82% had delayed triggering of the swallowing reflex, 58% had reduced pharyngeal peristalsis, 50% had reduced lingual control, and 32% had aspiration of barium.[33] Over three quarters of the patients exhibited more than one derangement, with right-sided stroke patients having a greater propensity for one component swallowing problems. In a recent prospective study, Gordon et al evaluated 91 consecutive stroke patients for dysphagia within 4 days of the event.[34] Forty-one patients (45%) presented with dysphagia, and older patients were significantly more likely to have dysphagia after their stroke. Forty-three percent of the dysphagia patients had a stroke confined to one cerebral hemisphere. The mechanism producing dysphagia with hemispheric strokes is unclear, but brain stem distortion secondary to cerebral edema is a likely possibility. Reduction of brain edema may explain the resolution of dysphagia within 2 weeks in the majority of the patients (86%) studied by Gordon and colleagues. In the same study, a significantly higher percentage of patients with cerebrovascular accidents and dysphagia have pulmonary infections and dehydration due to aspiration. This emphasizes the need to protect the patient's airway and provide for adequate fluids and nutrition until swallowing recovers. While hemispheric cerebrovascular accidents with dysphagia are often due to ischemic events in the distribution of the middle cerebral artery, others have found dysphagia in lesions involving the vertebrobasilar arteries or the posterior inferior cerebellar arteries.[35] Severe bulbar involvement with evidence of bilateral disease is most likely to be associated with measurable motor abnormalities.[36] Rarely, unilateral involvement has also been documented to produce upper esophageal sphincter dysfunction and symptoms.[37]

Motor Neuron Diseases. In chronic progressive bulbar palsy (upper motor neuron disease) or pseudobulbar palsy (lower motor neuron disease), degenerative neuronal changes lead to paralysis of the tongue and pharynx producing abnormalities in the oral and pharyngeal phases of swallowing.[3] Difficulty with swallowing is often the earliest symptom, and some patients may im-

prove with cricopharyngeal myotomy.[38,39] Bulbar poliomyelitis may cause oropharyngeal dysphagia usually due to pharyngeal abnormalities because of its predilection to involve the nucleus ambiguus.[40,41] Others have reported cricopharyngeal dysfunction in this disorder.[35] Amyotrophic lateral sclerosis is another progressive neurologic condition affecting lower motor neurons. In most patients, there is progressive weakness of the tongue and pharyngeal musculature.[42] Motor abnormalities may manifest as spontaneous and repetitive fasciculations ultimately leading to complete loss of voluntary deglutition.[43]

Parkinson's Disease. This degenerative lesion can affect the swallowing center. Patients may have difficulty in forming and manipulating the food bolus in the mouth. Hypopharyngeal stasis, aspiration, and upper esophageal sphincter dysfunction are other prevalent findings in untreated patients.[35,44] Once the bolus is pushed into the esophagus, normal deglutition usually follows. Despite the prevalence of these abnormalities, many patients remain relatively asymptomatic. Recognition of the disorder is important because selected, but not all, patients improve their dysphagia when treated with L-dopa.[45] Therefore, oropharyngeal dysphagia in Parkinson's disease has a better prognosis than many other untreatable neurologic causes.

Multiple Sclerosis. Oropharyngeal dysphagia is reported in up to 55% of patients with this demylinating disease of the central nervous system.[46] A variety of swallowing abnormalities occur including difficulties initiating a swallow, cricopharyngeal abnormalities, and uncoordinated swallowing and respiration leading to aspiration.

Other Neurologic Causes. Less common neurologic conditions producing oropharyngeal dysphagia include tumors of the brain stem and syringobulbia, both producing dysphagia similar to the motor neuron diseases.[3] Peripheral nerve diseases such as tetanus, botulism, lead poisoning, alcoholic neuropathy, and nerve injuries resulting from carcinoma, surgery, or radiation therapy may result in transfer dysphagia. In addition, extrapyramidal lesions such as Sydenham's and Huntington's chorea can lead to panpharyngeal hyperactivity and cricopharyngeal dysfunction.[35]

PRIMARY MUSCLE DISORDERS

Inflammatory Myopathies. Polymyositis and its cousin, dermatomyositis (associated with skin eruption), are characterized by diffuse inflammation of striated muscle manifested by weakness and atrophy of the proximal muscle groups.[47] The esophagus is involved manometrically or radiographically in 60% to 70%, with over half of patients experiencing dysphagia.[48] Corresponding pathologic changes in the striated portion of the esophagus include degeneration and necrosis of muscle fibers along with a chronic inflammatory infiltrate. Typical radiographic features include poor contraction of the pharyngeal constrictors, pooling and retention of barium in the valleculae, pharyngonasal reflux, and disorganized pharyngeal emptying. Manometrically, there is decreased upper esophageal sphincter tone, decreased contractions in the pharynx, and contraction waves in the proximal esophageal body are of low amplitude.[49] It has recently been noted that motor abnormalities in the distal esophagus are also common in this disorder.[50] Treatment with corticosteroids or other immunosuppressive agents often improves the dysphagia as well as the other general symptoms.

Muscular Dystrophies. Two forms of muscular dystrophy are associated with oropharyngeal dysphagia: myotonic dystrophy and oculopharyngeal dystrophy. Other forms of muscular dystrophy do not appear to be associated with upper esophageal motility disturbances.[51] A constellation of features characterizes patients with myotonic dystrophy including myopathic facies, swan neck, myotonia, muscle wasting, frontal baldness, testicular atrophy, and cataracts. Approximately one half of patients complain of oropharyngeal dysphagia, which usually presents several years after the development of other disease manifestations. Radiographic studies have shown impairment of pharyngeal emptying as well as abnormal peristalsis throughout the esophageal body.[52,53] A recent study using modern manometric and scintigraphic technology demonstrated markedly reduced upper esophageal sphincter pressures with decreases in peristaltic amplitude in both the striated and smooth muscle esophagus in patients with muscular dystrophy. No abnormalities in upper esophageal sphincter relaxation were found, and coordination with pharyngeal events remains normal. Although radionuclide esophageal transit was delayed, there was no clear relationship between the general severity of disease and the degree of esophageal dysfunction.[51] Successful treatment of the pharyngeal dysfunction has been reported with both quinine and procainamide.[54,55]

Oculopharyngeal dystrophy is a rare, autosomal dominant disorder, usually occurring after age 60. It is characterized by progressive bilateral ptosis, followed by the development of dysphagia.[56,57] This dysphagia is usually mild and is secondary to pharyngeal weakness. Upper esophageal sphincter tone, relaxation, and coordination have been reported to be normal.[58] Radiographic abnormalities are minimal, showing slow but unhindered passage of barium through the pharynx. Unlike patients with myotonic dystrophy, these patients do not exhibit abnormalities of other portions of the esophagus or gastrointestinal tract.

Myasthenia Gravis. This disorder of the motor endplate affects striated esophageal musculature, and approximately two thirds of patients experience oropharyngeal dysphagia.[3] As is typical for other skeletal muscles in this disorder, patients can usually swallow normally at the beginning of the meal but have progressive difficulty as they continue to eat. Radiographic studies demonstrate a decreased ability to form and move a food bolus, pooling of barium in the pharyngeal recesses, and ballooning of the pharynx with repeated swallowing, which may lead to aspiration or pharyngonasal regurgitation.[3,59] A manometric study of 25 patients with myasthenia gravis found evidence of decreased upper esophageal sphincter tone, but, otherwise, sphincter relaxation and pharyngeal coordination were normal.[60] Resting to allow reaccumulation of acetylcholine in nerve endings or administration of an anticholinesterase drug improves symptoms and pharyngoesophageal functions simultaneously.

Other Muscle Diseases. Oropharyngeal dysphagia occurs with other diseases that can affect striated muscle. Both hyperthyroidism and hypothyroidism have been incriminated.[61] One study reported incomplete relaxation of the sphincter in a patient with myxedema. Return of normal sphincteric function followed correction of the hypothyroidism.[62] Sarcoidosis and systemic lupus erythematosus also have been reported to produce swallowing disorders.[63] A rare cause of oropharyngeal dysphagia is the stiff man syndrome.[64] This disease, which affects all the striated muscles in the body, is thought to result from lack of inhibitory control of the anterior horn cells in the spinal cord. It responds to therapeutic doses of diazepam.

Clinical Manifestations

Neuromuscular diseases affecting the hypopharynx and upper esophagus produce a distinctive type of dysphagia. The patient is often unable to initiate swallowing and repeatedly has to attempt to swallow. The food bolus cannot be propelled successfully from the hypopharyngeal region, through the upper esophageal sphincter, and into the esophageal body. The resulting symptom is "oropharyngeal" or "transfer" dysphagia. The patient is aware that the bolus has not left the oropharynx and specifically locates the site of symptoms to the region of the cervical esophagus. The delay between the initiation of the swallow and the development of dysphagia can also accurately locate the site of dysfunction. Dysphagia within 1 second of swallowing is suggestive of an oropharyngeal abnormality.[65] Once started on its way, a liquid bolus may enter into the trachea or nose rather than the esophagus. Some patients describe recurrent bolus impactions that require manual dislodgement. In severe cases, saliva cannot be swallowed, and drooling occurs. Coughing episodes during a meal are indicative of a concomitant tracheobronchial aspiration. Pain is infrequent because dysphagia predominates.

Other symptoms are less frequent and may be progressive, constant, or intermittent. Swallowing associated with a gurgling noise may suggest the presence of a Zenker's diverticulum. Recurrent bouts of pulmonary infections may reflect spill-over of food into the trachea from inadequate laryngeal protection. Hoarseness may result from recurrent laryngeal nerve dysfunction or intrinsic muscular disease resulting in ineffective vocal cord movement. When weakness develops in the soft palate or pharyngeal constrictors, dysarthria and nasal speech as well as pharyngonasal regurgitation result. Finally, unexplained weight loss may be the only clue to a swallowing disorder because patients avoid eating due to the difficulties encountered.

Physical examination of patients with oropharyngeal dysphagia usually reflects a neurologic or neuromuscular condition contributing to this symptom. Hemiparesis reflective of a previous cerebrovascular accident; palpebral ptosis and end-of-the-day weakness indicative of myasthenia gravis; or a fenestrating gait and paucity of movement, characteristics of Parkinson's disease, can lead to a precise diagnosis. Specific cranial nerve deficits that are involved in deglutition may also aid in the diagnostic evaluation.

It has been stated that dysphagia always indicates the presence of esophageal dysfunction.[66] It is important, therefore, that one not confuse dysphagia with "globus hystericus." This sensation of cervical fullness or a "lump in the throat" is not necessarily accompanied by dysphagia. It is a more constant symptom that usually does not interfere with swallowing and, in fact, may be relieved during deglutition. As the name implies, globus hystericus has long been considered a symptom of the hysteric personality. However, this term may be a misnomer. A recent study revealed that, although almost all patients with globus hystericus had obsessive personalities and many were depressed, few had hysteric traits.[12] Despite this high prevalence of psychologic abnormalities, some patients may have their symptoms secondary to increased upper esophageal sphincter tone as the result of gastroesophageal reflux or emotional distress.[11,13]

Diagnostic Studies

The most commonly used studies in evaluating patients with oropharyngeal dysphagia are cineradiography and esophageal manometry. However, the literature is confusing about the usefulness of these studies for several reasons. All tests may be normal if the patient has only intermittent symptoms. Many of these patients are quite elderly, and a good database is not available about normal oropharyngeal and upper esophageal sphincter function in elderly persons. The diagnostic modalities of cineradiography and esophageal manometry measure different aspects of esophageal function, which frequently do not overlap. Esophageal manometry measures the presence of sphincter tone, the presence and characteristics of pressure waves, and the coordinated activity between these two physiologic processes. On the other hand, cineradiography defines pharyngeal and esophageal anatomy while simultaneously assessing bolus movement of fluids. Future investigation may show that more clinical information can be obtained by performing these studies simultaneously in patients with oropharyngeal dysphagia. Finally, these patients are usually studied with water or barium solutions, which may miss abnormalities only associated with semisolid or solid foods. Much improvement is needed in our diagnostic armamentarium in patients with oropharyngeal dysphagia. This is a particularly exciting new frontier for the esophagologist.

CINERADIOGRAPHY

Crucial to evaluating the patient with oropharyngeal dysphagia is cineradiography or videotape recordings of the mouth, pharynx, and upper esophagus during the barium swallow. Its superiority over the single film technique arises from the fact that it permits frame-by-frame analysis (30–100 frames/s) of individual swallows needed to delineate the complex and rapid sequence of events occurring in this region. In addition, a much more direct physiologic assessment of swallowing can be made. Therapeutic decisions can also be made by giving patients various consistencies of barium to swallow and determining the consistency that results in the least functional derangement.

A preliminary soft tissue lateral view of the neck should be taken to rule out structural problems as well as obtain information about the cervical spine, tongue position, relationship of the hyoid bone to the mandible, and contours of the pharynx and larynx. Dynamic recordings of the barium swallow should include both lateral and PA views. Serial cineradiographic images of the pharynx during normal swallowing are shown in Figure 54-1.[67]

Cineradiographic abnormalities during swallowing can be grouped into four major categories: (1) motility disturbances, (2) retention in the pharyngeal recesses, (3) pharyngeal stasis, and (4) misdirected swallowing (aspiration, laryngeal penetration).

Motility disturbances may manifest as delayed initiation of swallowing with a prolonged duration or a disturbance in the sequence of muscular activity. Repeated attempts at swallowing may be seen with the tongue moving backward several times before a swallow is initiated. Sluggish or completely disorganized motor activity may be present, often accompanied by stasis and aspiration. Retention of barium in the pharyngeal recesses may be due to altered mucosal sensitivity, decreased muscular tone, alterations in the shape and size of the recesses as may occur with atrophy of supporting elements, and neuromuscular disturbances. Pharyngeal stasis in the absence of distal mechanical obstruction is another reliable sign of disturbed pharyngeal motility.[68] Misdirected swallowing resulting in laryngeal penetration and aspiration is one of the most striking abnormalities often indicative of oropharyngeal dysphagia. Potentiating the problem may be the presence of retained pharyngeal contents in the pharyngeal recesses or delayed opening of the cricopharyngeus, an abnormality found in familial dysautonomia.[26]

Several studies have evaluated patients referred for acute and chronic oropharyngeal dysphagia with modern cineradiographic techniques. In a study of 250 patients, Ekberg and Nylander[69] found that 80% demonstrated functional swallowing abnormalities including epiglottic dysfunction in 33%, misdirected swallowing and laryngeal penetration in 41%, cricopharyngeal dysfunction in 22%, webs in 5%, and five patients demonstrated a Zenker's diverticulum. In this study, 37% of patients exhibited an isolated abnormality while 43% had two or more functional abnormalities, particularly in association with epiglottic dysfunction. In a smaller study of patients referred for evaluation of acute oropharyngeal dysphagia (less than 2 weeks), 34 of 45 patients exhibited a functional or anatomic abnormality similar to the above study.[70] Once again, almost half (21 patients) had two or more abnormalities.

Upper esophageal sphincter dysfunction, manifested by the presence of a visible cricopharyngeal muscle (bar), remains an area of controversy relevant to its contribution to symptomatic dysphagia. It has been speculated that the cricopharyngeal bar represents either pharyngoesophageal uncoordination or actual musculature hypertrophy.[70,71] In a retrospective study of 618 unselected patients who underwent upper gastrointestinal evaluation, Curtis et al found evidence of cricopharyngeal abnormalities in 77 (10.8%) patients.[72] However, dysphagia was found in less than 15% of these patients and did not correlate with radiographic findings. Most visible cricopharyngeal abnormalities were seen for only short intervals and were inconsistent in appearance from swallow to swallow. In another study of 16 asymptomatic normal persons, six demonstrated a visible cricopharyngeus, again emphasizing that its presence radiographically does not necessarily contribute to symptoms.[73] Furthermore, most patients with the radiographic diagnosis of cricopharyngeal bar have normal upper esophageal sphincter pressures with complete relaxation when studied manometrically.[25]

PHARYNGEAL AND UPPER ESOPHAGEAL MANOMETRY

To date, esophageal manometry has been less helpful in the evaluation of patients with presumed oropharyngeal dysphagia. Several technical problems may contribute to the overall low diagnostic yield of manometry. Pressure events within the oropharynx may

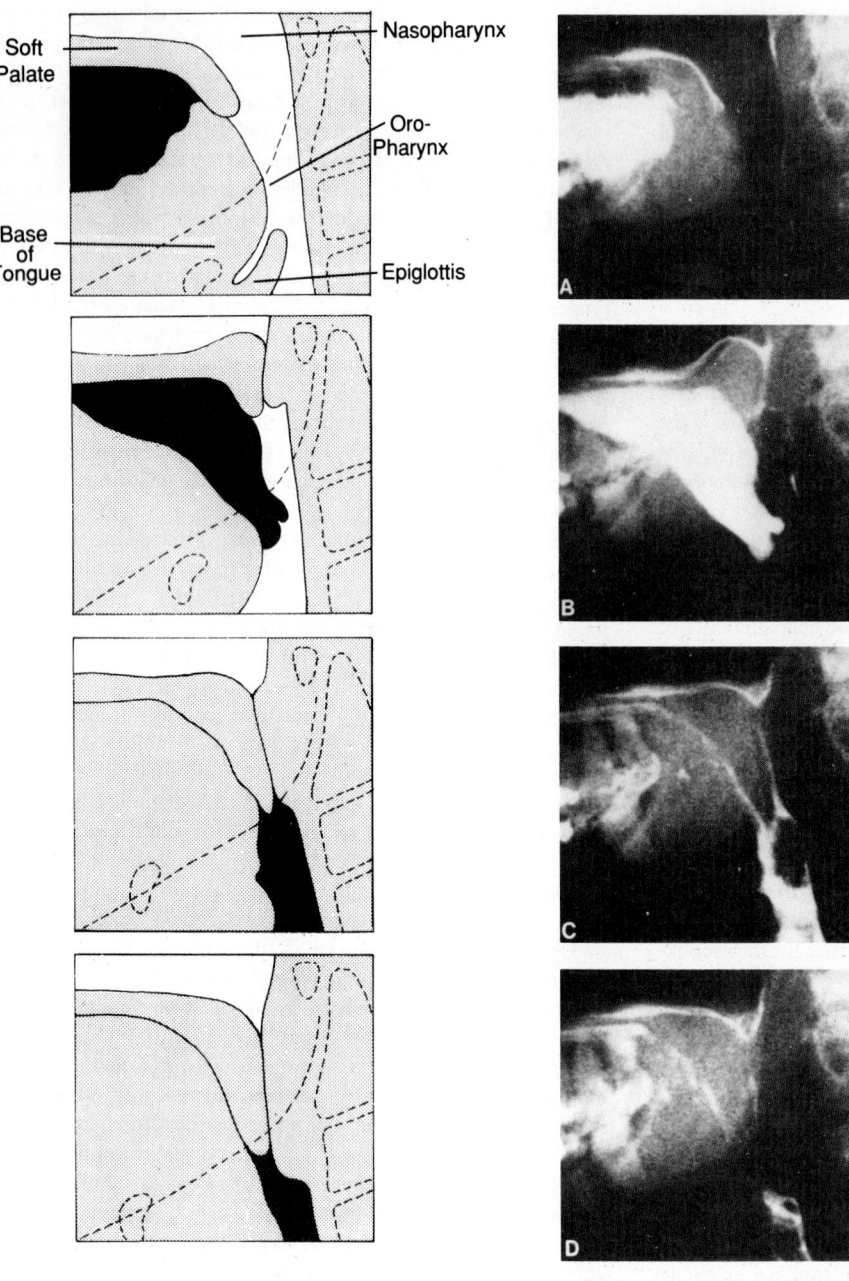

FIGURE 54–1. Cineradiographic imaging of the pharynx during normal swallow. **A,** Small amount of contrast has been introduced through the nose and is seen coating the posterior nasopharyngeal wall. Bolus (black on drawing, white in cineradiographs) is retained in the mouth by apposition of the posterior aspect of the superior portion of the tongue and the depressed soft palate. **B,** Bolus is then propelled into the oropharynx along with elevation of the soft palate apposing and perpendicular to the converging posterior pharyngeal wall. **C,** Contact between the soft palate and pharynx is further accentuated until the bolus has cleared the oropharynx. At this point, one begins to see the proximal stripping wave. **D,** Stripping wave then becomes more pronounced and proceeds distally.

(continued)

exceed 500 mm Hg/s and often are of short duration (less than 0.5 seconds). The fidelity of low compliance infusion catheter systems capable of recording pressure changes up to 400 mm Hg/s, while useful in studying motility in the distal esophagus, may be inadequate for pharyngeal and upper esophageal evaluation.[74] Additional limitations of fluid-filled catheter systems include a flat frequency response of only 5 Hz while pharyngeal wave forms occur with a frequency response of 50 Hz, and the undesirable effects of water infusion into the hypopharynx.[75] The radial asymmetry and variable resting pressures of the upper esophageal sphincter also can contribute to technical problems. Some investigators have suggested that an oval catheter, which more closely resembles the natural shape of the upper esophageal sphincter, might better measure pressure dynamics.[8] However, our laboratory found no significant differences in minimum or maximum upper esophageal sphincter pressure recorded with either a round or oval

catheter among 20 normal volunteers, ages 19 to 65 years.[76] More importantly, several studies have shown that the rapid pull-through technique produces 25% to 35% higher upper esophageal sphincter pressure measurements than the slow station pull-through technique, due either to direct stimulation or water perfusion stimulating the sphincter to contract.[76–78] Therefore, to avoid measuring a falsely high upper esophageal sphincter pressure, the station pull-through technique is required.

Several research laboratories have been measuring pressure events in the pharyngoesophageal region with a 6-cm, sleeve sensor or self-contained intraluminal transducer system (Fig 54-2). The major advantage of the sleeve sensor is its ability to remain within the sphincter throughout the swallow, thereby accurately recording sphincter pressure.[78] However, a recent study showed that a side-hole recording site, positioned 1.5 cm proximal to the peak of the high pressure zone, not only accurately records postswallow

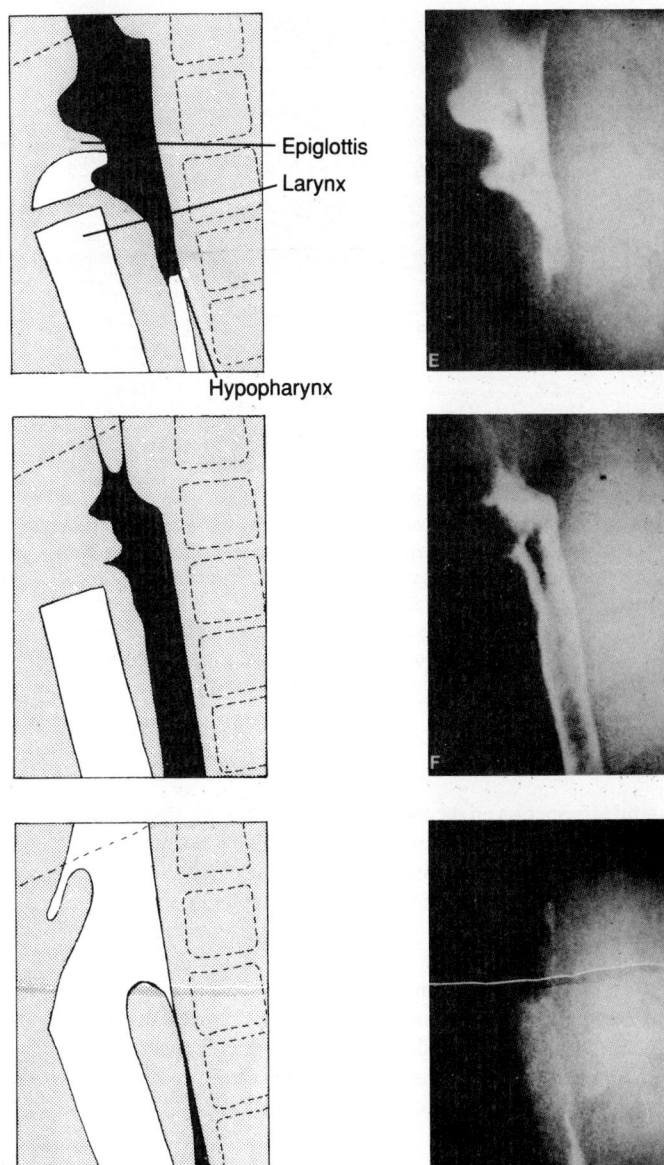

Epiglottis
Larynx
Hypopharynx

FIGURE 54–1. *(continued)* **E,** Next, the epiglottis completely inverts, and the laryngeal vestibule closes as the bolus begins to pass through the hypopharynx. **F,** With the epiglottis completely inverted and the larynx closed and elevated, the appearance of the conus is produced. The cricopharyngeal muscle is open, allowing passage of the bolus. Note the proximal pharyngeal stripping wave superiorly. **G,** Once the bolus has passed into the cervical esophagus, the larynx reopens, and the epiglottis assumes its resting upright position. Note absence of barium in hypopharynx after completed swallow. (From Jones B, Kramer SS, Donner MW: Dynamic imaging of the pharynx. Gastrointest Radiol 1985;10:213.)

sphincter contraction, but also a relaxation interval that closely corresponded to the fluoroscopically determined interval of sphincteric opening.[79] Our laboratory has demonstrated no difference in the upper esophageal sphincter relaxation profile using either the sleeve sensor or a single orifice infused catheter.[80] In addition, the sleeve sensor does not accurately record the offset of upper esophageal sphincter relaxation and cannot accurately measure pharyngeal contractions. The intraluminal transducer system consists of two portions—one or two proximal microtransducers for recording pharyngeal pressures and a distal transducer consisting of a glycerin-filled Silastic circumferential annulus surrounding a single miniature strain gauge used to assess upper esophageal sphincter pressure. The major advantage of this recording apparatus is a flat frequency response of up to 2000 Hz reducing distortion of the high-frequency signals generated in the pharyngoesophagus.[81] Although these are still primarily research tools, the widespread use of this new technology may identify many previously undescribed manometric abnormalities in patients with oropharyngeal dysphagia.

The techniques used to measure pressures in the pharynx and esophageal sphincter have been described elsewhere (ch 126). The primary measurements include resting upper esophageal sphincter pressure using a station pull-through technique, an approximation of the onset and offset of pharyngeal peristaltic waves, and the degree of relaxation and coordination between the upper esophageal sphincter and pharyngeal contractions (Fig 54-3). Due to the rapid nature of these pressure events, on-line computer analysis may afford a more accurate assessment of upper esophageal sphincter and pharyngeal dynamics.[82]

OTHER MODALITIES

Esophagoscopy may be important in the evaluation of patients with oropharyngeal dysphagia. It assists in excluding the presence of endoluminal lesions at the pharyngeal level, along with evaluating the distal esophageal body, which may be the source of proximally referred symptoms. Direct laryngoscopy also provides

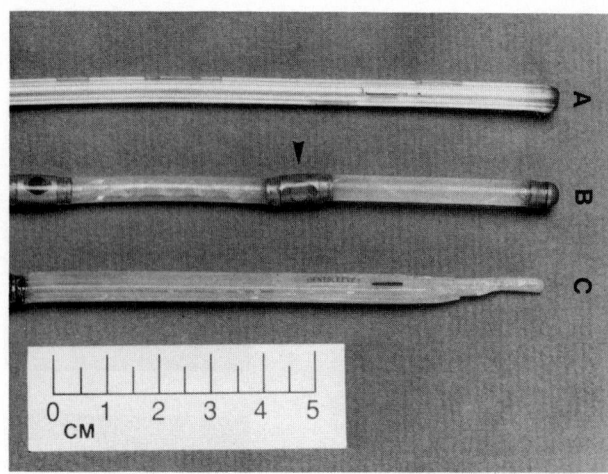

FIGURE 54–2. Manometry catheters used to assess upper esophageal sphincter. **A,** Standard round water-perfused catheter with external diameter of 4.8 mm. **B,** Intraluminal Konigsberg microtransducer system—proximal probe for recording pharyngeal pressures and a distal transducer (*arrow*) consisting of a glycerin-filled Silastic circumferential annulus surrounding a single miniature strain gauge used to assess upper esophageal sphincter pressure. **C,** Six-centimeter sleeve catheter can straddle the upper esophageal sphincter permitting constant pressure measurements.

useful information on the status of the hypopharynx, upper esophageal sphincter, and proximal esophagus. Radionuclide studies, using solid and liquid boluses labeled with technetium sulfur colloid, offer a potential technique for quantitating hypopharyngeal stasis, regurgitation, and tracheal aspiration before and after therapy.[40]

CT or MRI of the brain may be helpful in diagnosing some of the neurologic disorders associated with oropharyngeal dysphagia. The anticholinesterase, edrophonium chloride (Tensilon), may also be a useful diagnostic study in patients with suspected myasthenia gravis as the cause of their dysphagia.

Treatment

The treatment of oropharyngeal dysphagia consists of first recognizing and correcting potentially reversible causes including Parkinson's disease, myasthenia gravis, hyper- or hypothyroidism, and polymyositis. A trial of bougienage dilatation has been advocated for myogenic forms of dysphagia; however, sustained improvement is unlikely.[42] Dilatation may be effective in patients with cicatricial scarring from previous neck surgery. Blind bougienage dilatation is contraindicated in patients with a Zenker's diverticulum.[83]

The majority of patients with stroke-induced dysphagia generally improve over time.[34] Those with residual deficits may benefit from maneuvers directed at retraining swallowing function. The application of thermal stimulation to trigger the swallowing reflex has been used in neurologically impaired patients. This technique involves placing a cold stimulus (usually a laryngeal mirror) to the base of the anterior faucial arches. In theory, the sensitivity of this area is heightened such that subsequent voluntary swallows are more apt to trigger normal deglutition. In one study of 25

neurologically impaired patients, total transit time improved in 82% of patients for liquid swallows and 100% with paste swallows.[84] The effects of thermal stimulation tend to be immediate, but the long-term benefits are yet to be determined. Consultation with a speech pathologist should be considered both for evaluation and treatment for this group of patients.

Patients with oropharyngeal dysphagia frequently are considered for cricopharyngeal myotomy. This surgical procedure is designed to weaken or abolish the upper esophageal sphincter high-pressure zone by sectioning the cricopharyngeal muscle and the proximal 3 to 4 cm of striated muscle of the cervical esophagus. The results for myotomy vary according to the underlying cause of dysphagia and extent of pharyngeal dysfunction. The best results are obtained if oropharyngeal sensation is intact along with voluntary tongue and pharyngeal movements. Mills found that if the tongue could be protruded as far as the lower lip, there was enough propulsion to initiate deglutition.[39] Overall, patients with oropharyngeal dysphagia of neurologic origin have a good to excellent result in more than 50% of myotomies with a surgical mortality of 10%.[42] Patients with myogenic forms of oropharyngeal dysphagia also frequently have favorable responses to myotomy. For example, in patients with oculopharyngeal muscular dystrophy, excellent results have been reported in 75% of patients with sustained improvement for 2 to 4 years.[85] Although an uncommon entity, myotomy for patients with idiopathic dysfunction of the upper esophageal sphincter produces generally excellent results.[3] Myotomy alone for the treatment of Zenker's diverticula remains controversial. Some reports indicate the disappearance of diverticulum after cricopharyngeal myotomy alone while other studies suggest a possible reduction in diverticular recurrence if a myotomy is performed with the diverticulectomy.[86,87] However, recent experience indicates cricopharyngeal myotomy permanently controls symptoms in only 78% of patients with small diverticuli.[88] Contraindication for myotomy includes significant gastroesophageal reflux with regurgitation because most deaths are associated with aspiration.[83]

Obviously, it is essential that patients with oropharyngeal dysphagia have their nutritional status optimized. Enteral feedings, using either a Dobhoff or percutaneous endoscopic gastrostomy tube (PEG), may be necessary on either a temporary or permanent basis.

ACHALASIA

Achalasia, or cardiospasm, was the first motor disorder of the esophagus to be recognized clinically. In this disease, there is a double defect in esophageal function. The lower esophageal sphincter does not appropriately relax, offering resistance to the flow of liquids and solid materials from the esophagus into the stomach. In addition, there is a loss of peristalsis in the lower two thirds of the smooth muscle portion of the esophagus. Therefore, both the outflow tract and pumping mechanism of the esophagus are abnormal in achalasia.

The first case of achalasia was described in 1672 by Sir Thomas Willis, who, in his description of a patient with achalasia, stated "the mouth of the stomach (cardia) being always closed either by a tumor or palsied, nothing could be admitted into the ventricle (stomach) unless it was violently opened." For fifteen years, he treated his patient with a dilator made of whalebone with a sponge

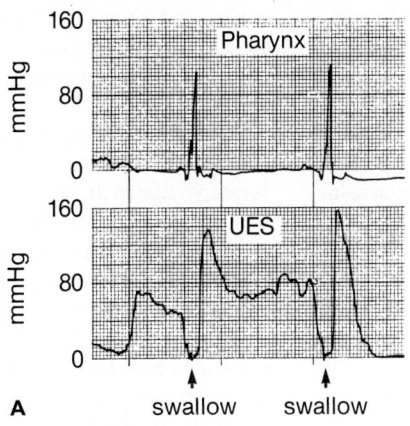

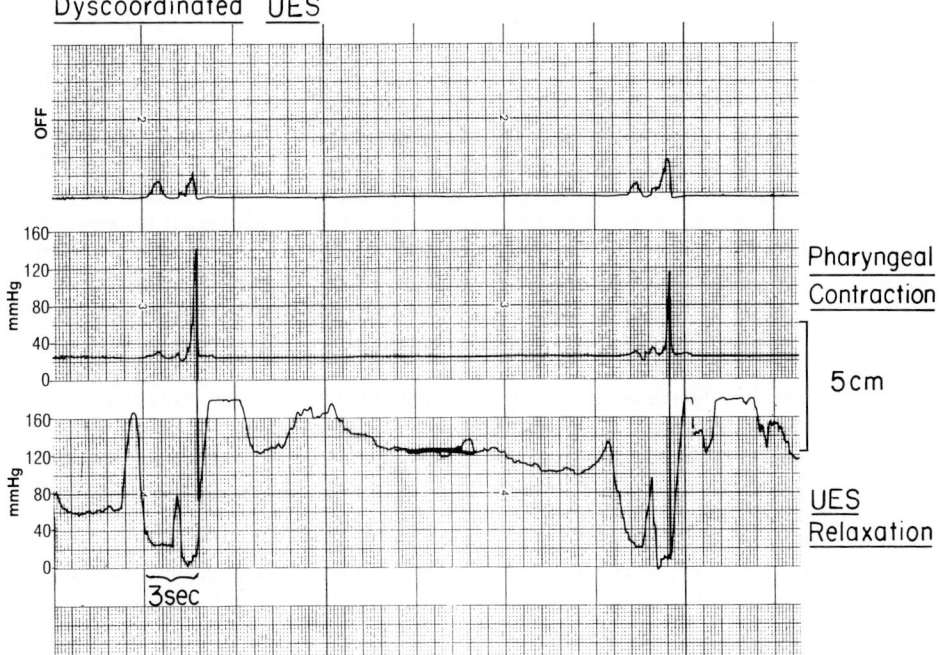

FIGURE 54–3. **A,** Pharyngeal and upper esophageal sphincter (UES) pressure measurements in a healthy subject. The peak of the pharyngeal contraction generally occurs at the nadir of UES relaxation during swallowing. **B,** Similar study in a stroke patient with oropharyngeal dysphagia and dyscoordinated UES. Intermittently (first swallow), the pharyngeal contraction occurs after UES pressure has begun to return to baseline. Symptoms improved after a cricopharyngeal myotomy.

at the end with which the patient forced his food into the stomach after eating.[89] Sporadic cases were reported in the next two centuries with all patients having esophageal dilatation and no obvious evidence of organic esophageal obstruction. This led Von Mikuliczi in 1881 to suggest that spasm of the cardia was present, hence the term *cardiospasm*.[90] Hurst and Rake in 1929, aware of the ease with which bougies could be passed into the stomach in patients with achalasia, questioned the spasm concept and coined the term *achalasia,* believing that the sphincter was unable to relax normally.[91] This term has survived historically because subsequent investigative techniques have confirmed failure of lower esophageal sphincter relaxation.

Epidemiology

Achalasia usually presents in persons between the ages of 25 to 60 years, but onset in childhood is well documented.[92,93] Achalasia

in early childhood should raise suspicion of a systemic syndrome associated with achalasia or a congenital syndrome, while achalasia in older age should raise the suspicion of malignancy (pseudoachalasia). Most studies find that men and women are affected equally. The disease most frequently occurs in whites. Achalasia has been reported in monozygotic twins,[94] in siblings,[95] and in parents and children.[96] However, the role of genetic factors in primary achalasia is still uncertain. The occurrence of achalasia in only one of a pair of monozygotic twins speaks against a strong genetic predisposition.[97] Furthermore, a recent study of 159 patients with achalasia found no proven cases of achalasia in 1012 first-degree relatives surveyed.[98] Therefore, coexistence of achalasia in these settings could be coincidental, caused by some genetic predisposing factor, or a result of common exposure to an environmental factor (eg, a virus).

Achalasia is uncommon but not rare. A study from the British Isles estimated a prevalence of achalasia of 10 cases/100,000 population. However, the frequency was different in various parts of the British Isles ranging from 13.4 cases/100,000 population in

Ireland to 7.1 cases/100,000 population in Wales.[99] Because achalasia is a chronic disease, its prevalence exceeds the number of newly diagnosed cases per year (incidence) by a considerable amount. The annual incidence of achalasia in the United States and Europe is estimated at 0.4 to 0.6 cases/100,000 while the incidence in black Africa appears to be much lower.[99-102] One study from England suggested that the incidence of achalasia increases in older age.[103] These regional and age-related differences seem to favor an environmental cause for achalasia.

Pathophysiology

NEUROPATHOLOGY

Abnormalities in both muscle and nerve components can be detected in achalasia, although the neural lesion is thought to be of primary importance. Three major neuroanatomic changes have been described: (1) loss of ganglion cells within the myenteric (Auerbach's) plexus, (2) degeneration of the vagus nerve, and (3) qualitative as well as quantitative changes in the dorsal motor nucleus of the vagus. Of these three findings, the loss of ganglion cells is best substantiated. Most observers agree that there are fewer ganglion cells in the body of the esophagus, and that the ganglion cells present are surrounded by mononuclear inflammatory cells.[91,104] Some have attributed the decreased ganglion cells to the mechanical separation of the plexus by esophageal dilatation. An actual decrease in ganglion cells, however, has been substantiated by the observation that neuronal bodies are less prevalent in the distal esophagus of patients with early, nondilated disease.[104] In addition, the degree of loss appears related to the duration of disease; ganglion cells are nearly absent in patients with symptoms of 10 years' duration or longer.[104] In the lower esophageal sphincter, the number of ganglion cells has been reported as normal, reduced, or absent. Histologic analysis of the manometrically defined lower esophageal sphincter segment in 17 patients with achalasia showed a complete disappearance of ganglion cells in 94% of the cases and a decrease in the number of neurons with marked chronic inflammatory cells in one case (6%). These authors could find no relationship between the histologic changes and resting lower esophageal sphincter pressure or the duration of symptoms.[105] Damaged ganglion cells may contain intracytoplasmic hyaline, spherical eosinophilic inclusions (Lewy bodies). Lewy bodies also are seen in the brain in Parkinson's disease and in degenerating ganglion cells of the esophagus in some parkinsonian patients with dysphagia.[106]

Along with the destruction of ganglion cells, there is a reduction in nerve fibers within the wall of the esophagus in achalasia. It has been postulated that postganglionic neurons that mediate lower esophageal sphincter relaxation are selectively damaged in achalasia. Recently, immunohistochemical studies have demonstrated a marked reduction of vasoactive intestinal peptide (VIP) staining neurons as well as the concentration of VIP in the lower esophagus of achalasia patients compared to the tumor-free portion of the lower esophagus of patients with esophageal or gastric carcinoma.[107] In view of the potent smooth muscle-relaxing effects of VIP, this could account for the incomplete relaxation and increased resting tone of the lower esophageal sphincter characteristic of achalasia. Because peristalsis in the smooth muscle portion of the esophagus

is triggered by an initial phase of inhibition by noncholinergic, nonadrenergic postganglionic neurons, selective destruction of these inhibitory neurons in achalasia conceivably could explain aperistalsis as well.

By light microscopy, vagal branches to the esophagus appear normal in achalasia patients. However, electron microscopic studies reveal Wallerian degeneration of the vagus nerve with disintegration of the axoplasm, changes in Schwann's cells, and degeneration of the myelin sheaths, findings that are characteristic of experimental nerve transection.[108] However, tests of vagal function in achalasia patients have revealed inconsistent results.[109-111]

Finally, qualitative and quantitative reports of changes in the brain stem have been described in patients with achalasia. Degenerative changes, including fragmentation and dissolution of nuclear material, have been reported in ganglia of the vagal dorsal motor nucleus.[112] Other investigators have reported a reduction in the number of ganglion cells in these nuclei.[104] These extraesophageal neuropathic changes have been demonstrated in only small numbers of achalasia patients. Nevertheless, lesions of the vagus nerve or its motor nuclei are plausible in this disease, because bilateral lesions in the cat dorsal motor nuclei can produce dysfunction resembling achalasia.[113]

The circular muscle of the lower esophagus in patients with achalasia is thickened. However, the smooth muscle cells are described as normal by light microscopy. Electron microscopic studies show detachment of myofilaments from the surface membranes and cellular atrophy.[114] It is not clear whether these changes are important in the pathogenesis of the disease or merely represent muscular adaptation to a primary neural disorder.

Not only is the site of primary neuropathology in achalasia uncertain, but also the nature of the pathologic process. Two theories exist: (1) achalasia is primarily a degenerative disease of neurons whose cell bodies are either in the medulla or the myenteric plexus; or (2) achalasia is primarily an infection of neurons by a virus or some other infectious agent. It has been suggested that achalasia may be caused by herpes zoster[115] or measles virus.[116] Another argument in favor of an infectious etiology is that the protozoan, *Trypanosoma cruzi*, produces ganglion damage and an achalasialike syndrome with megaesophagus.

NEUROPHYSIOLOGIC STUDIES

Physiologic studies have confirmed the presence of denervation of the smooth muscle segment of the esophagus in patients with achalasia. The major neuropathic process seems to involve the postganglionic noncholinergic, nonadrenergic inhibitory neurons. Muscle strips from the circular layer of the esophageal body in achalasia contract when directly stimulated by acetylcholine but not in response to ganglionic stimulation by nicotine.[117] Similarly, strips from the lower esophageal sphincter do not relax in response to ganglionic stimulation in achalasia patients, but they do in normal controls.[117] Further evidence of denervation is shown by the response to a synthetic acetylcholine, Mecholyl. Both the esophageal body[118] and the lower esophageal sphincter[119] respond with strong contractions when Mecholyl is injected. This heightened response has been interpreted as evidence of denervation hypersensitivity. Finally, cholecystokinin octapeptide (CCK-OP) generally reduces lower esophageal sphincter pressure in normal persons yet causes a paradoxical increase in many patients with achalasia.[120] This effect may represent loss of inhibitory neurons in the lower esophageal sphincter region, because these neurons normally produce a predominant relaxation response to CCK-OP stimulation. In conjunction with histologic evidence that ganglion cell loss may be partial, studies have suggested that postganglionic cholinergic stimulatory fibers to the lower esophageal sphincter may be spared in achalasia. Thus, the lower esophageal sphincter pressure in achalasia increases after administration of the ace-tycholinesterase inhibitor edrophonium and decreases after administration of the muscarinic antagonist atropine.[121]

Confirming histologic studies, physiologic observations reveal evidence of vagal dysfunction in patients with achalasia. An abnormal gastric secretory response to insulin-induced hypoglycemia has been demonstrated in nearly one third of achalasia patients.[109] All with inappropriate gastric responses were found to have normal gastric acid secretion in response to a histamine analogue. Furthermore, sham feeding techniques have documented decreased acid secretion and release of pancreatic polypeptide in some patients with achalasia.[110] Others have reported intact vagal function in patients with untreated achalasia.[111] However, a subnormal response was found in eight of ten patients who had previously undergone pneumatic dilatation and in three of four patients who had a myotomy. These abnormalities were thought to reflect the effect of treatment in disrupting the sphincter rather than impairment of its innervation.[111]

In summary, the etiology of primary achalasia is unknown. The disease is either a degenerative or infectious disease of nerve cells located in the dorsal motor nucleus of the vagus nerve, the myenteric plexus, or both sites. Axonal degeneration and smooth muscle changes probably are secondary to neuronal damage. The noncholinergic, nonadrenergic inhibitory nerves to the lower esophageal sphincter and perhaps to the esophageal body are selectively impaired while the cholinergic stimulatory nerves largely are spared. These changes result in increased basal lower esophageal sphincter pressure and poor relaxation. Degeneration of ganglion cells in the esophageal body itself eventually leads to permanent aperistalsis and allows esophageal dilatation.

Clinical Features

DYSPHAGIA

Symptoms, rather than physical findings, are the hallmarks of achalasia. All patients have solid food dysphagia, with the majority of patients also having variable degrees of liquid dysphagia.[92,122] The onset of dysphagia is usually gradual, beginning with solids but including liquids intermittently. The duration of symptoms at presentation averages 2 years, although a wide variation in duration is seen.[122] As might be expected, those with the mildest symptoms may have the longest histories because these patients are not bothered sufficiently to seek medical attention. Patients commonly describe the sensation of fullness or gurgling in the chest, and, as the meal progresses, the food seems to fill up and overflow. Many patients believe that emotional stress and eating rapidly worsens their dysphagia. The severity of dysphagia fluctuates but usually reaches a plateau and does not worsen with time. In others, however, it progresses to the point of severe dis-

comfort, and weight loss is pronounced. Patients may report the use of specific maneuvers to improve esophageal emptying. Certain postural maneuvers, such as throwing the shoulders back, lifting the neck, and performing a rapid Valsalva's maneuver, help the material to pass into the stomach. Slow, deliberate swallowing during a meal seems to alleviate retrosternal fullness in some patients. It has been suggested that this maneuver takes advantage of the 10- to 20-mm Hg increment in intraesophageal pressure produced by swallowing a food or liquid bolus, an increment that could encourage esophageal emptying.[122] Carbonated beverages also may improve dysphagia probably by increased intraesophageal pressure. An occasional patient states that alcohol is beneficial in helping the food to pass into the stomach. Whether this works directly on the sphincter or indirectly by relaxing the patient is not known.

REGURGITATION

Regurgitation of undigested food in the esophagus is a common complaint occurring in 60% to 90% of patients with achalasia.[122,123] The material brought up is often recognized as food that has been eaten many hours previously. It tends to be nonbilious and not to have an acid taste. Unprovoked regurgitation often occurs during or shortly after a meal. It is not unusual for some patients to induce vomiting manually to relieve chest discomfort. Typically, patients note food or saliva backing up in the mouth while asleep. Nocturnal regurgitation can be annoying or very severe. Regurgitated food and saliva may end up on the pillowcase or sometimes in the trachea producing severe bouts of coughing and choking. Occasionally in young women, these symptoms may be confused with those of eating disorders, especially anorexia nervosa or bulimia.[124]

CHEST PAIN

Chest pain is reported by one third to one half of patients with achalasia and tends to improve with the course of the disease.[92,122] Patients usually describe a squeezing pressurelike sensation retrosternally, and a minority have radiation to the neck, arms, jaw, and back. Chest pain is often precipitated by eating, can awake the patient at night, and may be so severe as to cause decreased food intake and weight loss. If chest pain persists and is a predominant complaint, this should indicate the likely presence of an atypical form of achalasia, such as vigorous achalasia.[125]

HEARTBURN

Some authorities have suggested that heartburn is absent in achalasia because of the increased basal lower esophageal sphincter pressure preventing gastroesophageal reflux.[126] However, more recent reports suggest that 25% to 45% of patients with achalasia may complain of symptoms compatible with heartburn.[92,122] Characteristically, the pyrosis is not immediately postprandial, frequently awakes the patient at night, and does not predictably improve with antacids or H_2 antagonists. Recent studies using 24-hour esophageal pH monitoring have shown that the pyrosis is not caused by acid reflux but rather results from the production of lactic acid by bacterial fermentation of retained food in the esophagus.[127]

OTHER SYMPTOMS

Weight loss is very common and usually increases with the duration of the disease. Weight loss may be the best historic parameter for assessing the severity of achalasia and usually correlates with the degree of esophageal emptying before and after treatment.[122] Approximately 10% of achalasia patients may have significant bronchopulmonary complications as the result of regurgitation of material from the esophagus.[128] Patients with esophageal symptoms of long duration may actually come to medical attention because of pulmonary complications. Organisms involved most commonly are aerobic and anaerobic oropharyngeal flora, which are aspirated, leading to bronchitis, bronchial pneumonia, or lung abscess. There also is an apparent increased incidence of pulmonary infection with mycobacteria in achalasia.[129] Rarely, the dilated, fluid-filled esophagus can lead to acute obstruction of the airway, usually the trachea.[130,131] Such patients may be difficult to intubate endotracheally, requiring decompression of the esophagus by a nasoesophageal tube[130] or rarely by pharyngotomy.[131] Bleeding is very rare in achalasia, although there has been one report of massive bleeding from an esophagopericardial fistula.[132]

Diagnosis

Achalasia is suspected from a compatible clinical history, and the diagnosis usually is not difficult. Early cases may be misdiagnosed because screening radiographs fail to reveal esophageal dilatation and marked distortion at the esophagogastric junction. However, the diagnosis is made correctly in virtually all cases if a systematic approach is taken for patients with symptoms suggestive of this motor disorder.

RADIOGRAPHIC STUDIES

Radiographic studies are the primary screening test in patients with achalasia. A plain chest film can occasionally show mediastinal widening and an outline of the esophageal wall as the result of megaesophagus (Fig 54-4). Another clue on an upright chest x-ray is the absence of a gastric air bubble. Lower esophageal sphincter hypertension may prevent air that is swallowed from entering the stomach in approximately 50% of cases.[133] Chronic aspiration as evidenced by pulmonary infiltrates may be seen in longstanding untreated achalasia.

Although plain films of the chest provide important clues, a barium swallow with fluoroscopy is the most appropriate first study in patients with suspected achalasia. The barium bolus enters the esophagus, and a peristaltic contraction may travel a short distance from the upper sphincter region through the skeletal muscle portion of the esophagus. In the supine position, peristalsis fails to clear the bolus from the esophagus. Contrast material may simply lay in the atonic organ or be moved up and down the esophageal body by repetitive, nonperistaltic contractions. The lower esophageal sphincter opens partially and intermittently, allowing small

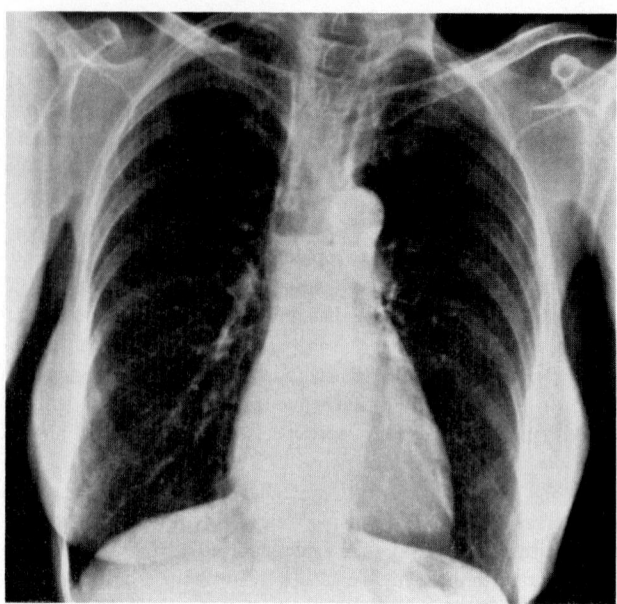

FIGURE 54–4. Chest x-ray showing features that may be seen in achalasia including a widened mediastinum and an air–fluid level in the midesophagus.

amounts of contrast material to squirt into the stomach. Relaxation does not appear to be associated temporarily with swallowing.

Once enough barium is swallowed to fill the esophagus, other typical features are seen (Fig 54-5A). The esophageal body is usually dilated, and dilatation is greatest in the distal esophagus. The column of barium terminates in a tapered point, the location of the nonrelaxing sphincter. This smooth, symmetric tapering is commonly called a "bird's beak." In patients with severe longstanding disease, the esophageal dilatation may be so severe to distort the esophagus, resembling a sigmoid colon. In cases with relatively short history of symptoms, the esophageal body may be only slightly or not at all dilated. In fact, it may take several years for esophageal dilatation to appear. In these cases, the radiographic diagnosis may be missed unless careful fluoroscopy is performed. An air–fluid level may be seen on the chest x-ray (see Fig 54-4) or barium swallow in addition to retained particulate matter in the esophagus. Mucosal irregularities should not be noted in achalasia, and, if present, malignancy should be considered. Spot films of the gastric cardia should always be performed to help rule out adenocarcinoma of the stomach. Occasionally, an epiphrenic diverticulum is observed in the patient with achalasia. This occurs immediately above the lower esophageal sphincter and usually extends to the right of the esophagus. Diverticuli can be massive, interfering significantly with other diagnostic tests and therapeutic maneuvers.

ENDOSCOPY

Endoscopic examination is always required to exclude neoplastic processes at the location of the gastroesophageal junction and evaluate the esophageal mucosa before therapeutic manipulations. In some patients with longstanding disease, it may be necessary to lavage the esophagus before endoscopy or even place them on clear liquids for several days to visualize the esophageal mucosa. Typical endoscopic findings include dilatation and atony of the esophageal body with normal mucosa. However, as the esophagus dilates, erythema, friability, or superficial ulcerations consistent with esophagitis may result from stasis of food and the effects of lactic acid production by bacterial fermentation. In some patients, these changes also can result from pill-induced injury producing esophagitis and even strictures, making the differentiation from cancer very difficult. Whitish plaque covering the epithelial surface may be seen as the result of *Candida* infection. If a mucosal biopsy reveals candidiasis, topical antifungal therapy before pneumatic dilatation is recommended as prophylaxis against mediastinal contamination should perforation occur.[134] The lower esophageal sphincter usually has a puckered appearance that does not open with air insufflation. However, the instrument should easily pass through the sphincter into the stomach with gentle pressure. Inability to pass the endoscope beyond the gastroesophageal junction or the necessity for undue force in entering the stomach should immediately raise the suspicion of malignancy or benign stricture. Careful examination for hiatal hernia is important. Although rare (4%) in patients with achalasia,[135] its presence may influence the method of treatment because esophageal perforation during pneumatic dilation is more common in these patients.[136] Once the endoscope is in the stomach, careful inspection of the gastroesophageal junction should be noted on retroflex view. Questionable mucosal abnormalities in this area should always be biopsied, especially in patients older than 50 years.

ESOPHAGEAL MANOMETRY

The diagnosis of achalasia should always be established by esophageal manometry. This is particularly important when radiographs are normal or inconclusive. Four manometric features are characteristic of achalasia (Table 54-2): (1) absence of peristalsis in the distal smooth muscle segment of the esophageal body, (2) incomplete or abnormal lower esophageal sphincter relaxation, (3) elevated lower esophageal sphincter pressure and, (4) elevated intraesophageal pressures relative to the gastric baseline.

Absent peristalsis is an absolute requirement for the diagnosis of achalasia and may be the only manometric finding if the manometry catheter cannot be passed blindly or under fluoroscopic guidance into the stomach. Dry or wet swallows induce no sequential propagated waves in the smooth muscle portion of the esophagus. Contraction waves that are measured are generally of low amplitude (10–40 mm Hg) and are simultaneous in onset. Pressure tracings from different parts of the esophagus show remarkable similarity (mirror image) indicating that the recording ports on the catheter are detecting pressure changes in a closed chamber (see Fig 54-5B). Contraction wave amplitudes diminish with increasing esophageal distention. When the esophagus is extremely dilated, no contractions are measured and the minor pressure changes simply result from the swallowed bolus entering the esophagus. Some patients may exhibit higher amplitude (greater than 60 mm Hg) simultaneous repetitive contractions in response to swallows. This manometric pattern is called vigorous achalasia and is usually seen in patients with a greater incidence of severe chest pain and less esophageal dilatation on x-ray (Fig 54-6)125. In the past, administration of methacholine (Mecholyl) has been

used to aid in the diagnosis of achalasia. A positive response after methacholine injection is indicated by a sustained increase in intraluminal pressure to greater than 25 mm Hg usually associated with an increase in the amplitude and repetitive characteristics of simultaneous contractions. Failure to respond to methacholine is strong evidence against the diagnosis of achalasia, but a positive test can be observed in patients with diffuse esophageal spasm. The pain and unpleasant cholinergic side effects do not justify its routine use considering the little additional information gained.

If the catheter can be passed into the stomach, it is preferable to perform the station pull-through technique of lower esophageal sphincter measurement. The station pull-through allows assessment of both sphincter pressure and relaxation, which cannot be done with the rapid pull-through technique. Lower esophageal sphincter relaxation should be assessed with wet water swallows (5 ml) because dry swallows may underestimate relaxation, giving the false impression of incomplete relaxation in normal persons.[137]

Lower esophageal sphincter resting pressures are usually elevated (above 35 mm Hg) in approximately 60% of patients, sometimes to three times normal.[138] The length of the high pressure zone is also longer than that seen in normal subjects. Low sphincter pressures are not seen in untreated patients with achalasia and should suggest another diagnosis, particularly scleroderma. In achalasia patients, intraesophageal resting pressures frequently are higher than intragastric pressure, an opposite relation to that seen in normal subjects. This intraesophageal pressure increment appears to be attributable to retained food and secretions within the esophagus. It is not always found and, if present, can be eliminated with esophageal evacuation.

More important to the diagnosis of achalasia than resting lower esophageal sphincter characteristics is the demonstration of impaired sphincter relaxation after a swallow (see Fig 54-5C). Over 80% of patients with achalasia have obvious incomplete relaxation (± 30% mean relaxation), with measurements of the actual percentage being relatively unimportant.[139] This is a marked contrast to normals in which the sphincter relaxes greater than 90% in response to wet swallows. This residual (nadir) lower esophageal sphincter pressure resulting from incomplete relaxation is responsible for obstructing passage of material from the esophagus into the stomach and helps to explain why these patients can support a column of barium in the esophagus when standing upright. Although underemphasized, approximately 20% to 30% of achalasia patients may have evidence of apparent complete lower esophageal relaxation intermittently or even after all swallows.[140,141] These patients usually have less weight loss, a shorter duration of dysphagia, and less esophageal dilatation than patients with classic achalasia.[141] Esophageal manometry demonstrates relaxation of the lower esophageal sphincter to the gastric baseline but a significantly shorter duration of relaxation than normals. This "complete" relaxation is probably artifactual. The normal lower esophageal sphincter should relax sufficiently to produce a luminal opening of greater than 20 mm diameter. Because the standard motility catheter has a diameter less than 4.8 mm, it is likely that a partial relaxation will allow the esophageal wall to move away from the catheter, producing manometric relaxation, yet still not provide the normal completely relaxed luminal opening.[141] This group of patients represents an early stage of achalasia, which frequently progresses to the more classic form with incomplete lower esophageal sphincter relaxation over a period of several years.

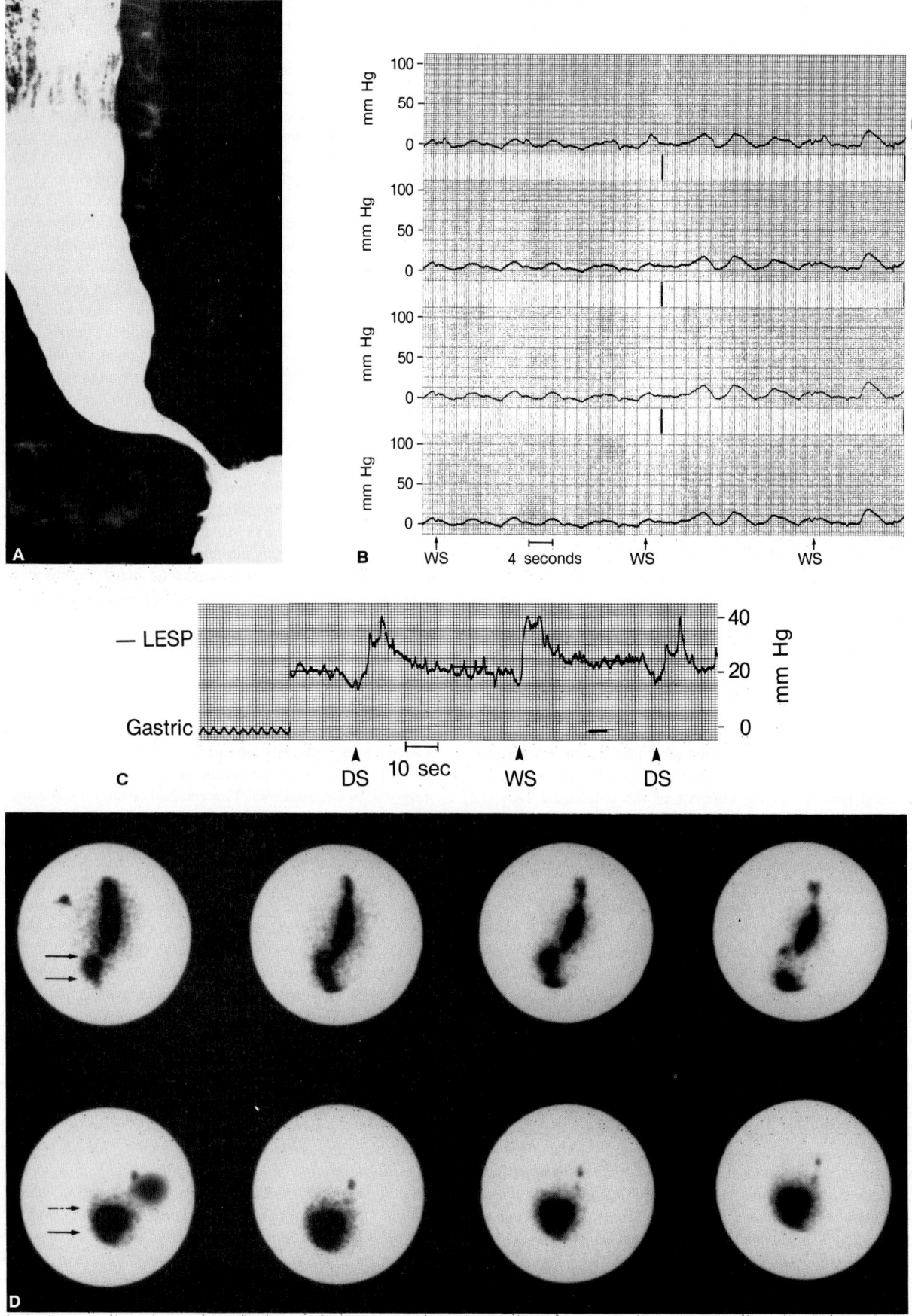

TABLE 54–2
Manometric Findings in Achalasia

1. Absent peristalsis in esophageal body (required for diagnosis).
2. Incomplete lower esophageal sphincter relaxation (usually present, not required). Complete relaxation of short duration may be seen in early achalasia.
3. Elevated resting lower esophageal sphincter pressure (common, not required).
4. Elevated intraesophageal pressure relative to gastric pressures (common, not required).

RADIONUCLIDE STUDIES

Radionuclide studies measure the rate at which radiolabeled liquid or solid test meals empty from the esophagus into the stomach. Liquid studies are usually performed in the supine position and show an adynamic pattern because the material lays in the atonic esophagus (Fig 54-7).[142] Unfortunately, emptying also is abnormally slow in other disorders of esophageal peristalsis or anatomic obstruction of the esophagus. Therefore, the tests lack the specificity of manometry and have not been widely used. On the other hand, esophageal emptying of a semisolid meal (usually egg salad sandwich or beef stew) in the upright position may be a useful diagnostic and therapeutic test.[141,143] This study reveals prolonged retention of the meal when compared with normals, and retention is also abnormal in patients with early achalasia and apparent complete lower esophageal sphincter relaxation.[141] Furthermore, it can be repeated post-treatment to assess the degree of improvement, which generally correlates with the changes in lower esophageal sphincter pressure (see Fig 54-5D). False-positive results have occasionally been seen in patients with isolated hypertensive lower esophageal sphincter, and, rarely, untreated achalasia patients may have a normal test.

Differential Diagnosis

A group of disorders that mimic idiopathic achalasia must be considered when making a diagnosis. These diseases may resemble achalasia so closely that conventional diagnostic tests are misleading.

MALIGNANCIES (PSEUDOACHALASIA)

The most alarming mimickers are the malignant neoplasms. Most commonly, these tumors are adenocarcinomas of the gastroesophageal junction, but reports exist of pancreatic, oat cell, squamous cell of the esophagus, prostate, and lymphomas invading the region of the lower esophageal sphincter.[92] These tumors usually produce achalasia as the result of one of two mechanisms: (1) the tumor mass encircles or compresses the distal esophagus producing a constricting segment, or (2) malignant cells infiltrate the esophageal Auerbach's plexus. However, there are other reports of apparently non-neurogenic involvement by tumors such as Hodgkin's disease, poorly differentiated bronchogenic carcinoma, and hepatoma that cause achalasia from a distance, leading to suspicion of a paraneoplastic syndrome.[92] Pseudoachalasia occurs mainly in the elderly and may represent about 10% of patients over 60 years of age with suspected achalasia.[92] At one time, it was thought that certain clinical features could help distinguish pseudoachalasia caused by cancer from primary achalasia, including duration of dysphagia for less than 1 year, age of more than 50 years, and weight loss of more than 15 lb.[144] However, these criteria have been shown to have poor predictive value and are not especially helpful when facing an individual patient.[145]

Esophageal manometry cannot distinguish patients with these neoplasms from patients with idiopathic achalasia.[92] On the other hand, endoscopy with biopsies usually results in a diagnosis of pseudoachalasia in the majority of patients reported in the literature. Ominous endoscopic findings include mucosal ulcerations or nodularity, reduced compliance of the esophagogastric junction, or the inability to pass the endoscope into the stomach. However, as many as 25% of patients with pseudoachalasia may have normal endoscopic examinations because of submucosal involvement by the malignancy.[92] Amyl nitrate administration during the barium study may improve the accuracy of this radiologic technique for differentiating achalasia from malignancy. In patients with idiopathic achalasia, amyl nitrate usually causes a measurable increase in maximal lower esophageal sphincter diameter of 3 mm or more while having no effect on lower esophageal sphincter diameter in patients with pseudoachalasia.[146] CT is also of value in detecting distal tumors. In idiopathic achalasia, the esophageal wall may appear somewhat thickened on CT scan, but any thickening in the lower sphincter region should be concentric and symmetric.[147] If the underlying tumor can be treated successfully, the clinical, radiographic, and manometric abnormalities sometimes, but not always, disappear, and esophageal peristalsis may even return.

CHAGAS' DISEASE

Chagas' disease is caused by a protozoan, *Trypanosoma cruzi*, and is transmitted by the bite from reduviid (kissing) bugs. It is endemic in areas of central Brazil, Venezuela, and northern Argentina, although cases in south Texas have been reported. After the bug

FIGURE 54–5: Classic radiographic, manometric, and scintigraphic findings in achalasia. **A,** Typical barium esophagogram showing a dilated esophagus with smooth tapering at the distal segment—"bird beaking." Typical manometric findings in the esophageal body, **B,** and lower esophageal sphincter, **C,** in achalasia. In the body, recording sites from proximal to distal portion of the esophagus (top to bottom of figure) with spacings at 5-cm intervals reveal a total absence of peristaltic activity during a series of wet swallows (WS). When the esophagus is extremely dilated, no contractions will be measured, and the minor pressure changes simply result from the water bolus entering the esophagus. Lower esophageal sphincter tracing reveals normal basal pressures (20 mm Hg) with incomplete relaxation to gastric baseline after both dry (DS) and wet (WS) swallows. (From Castell DO, Richter JE, Dalton CB, eds. Esophageal motility testing. Amsterdam: Elsevier, 1987.) **D,** Radionuclide emptying studies before (*top*) and after (*bottom*) pneumatic dilatation. Selective images at 1, 5, 10, and 15 minutes after ingestion of radiolabeled meal. Note marked retention in esophagus before treatment and normal emptying following dilatation (*arrows* represent gastric activity). (From Ott DJ, Richter JE, Chen YM, et al. Radiographic and manometric correlation in achalasia with apparent relaxation of the lower esophageal sphincter. Gastrointestinal Radiology 1989;14:1.)

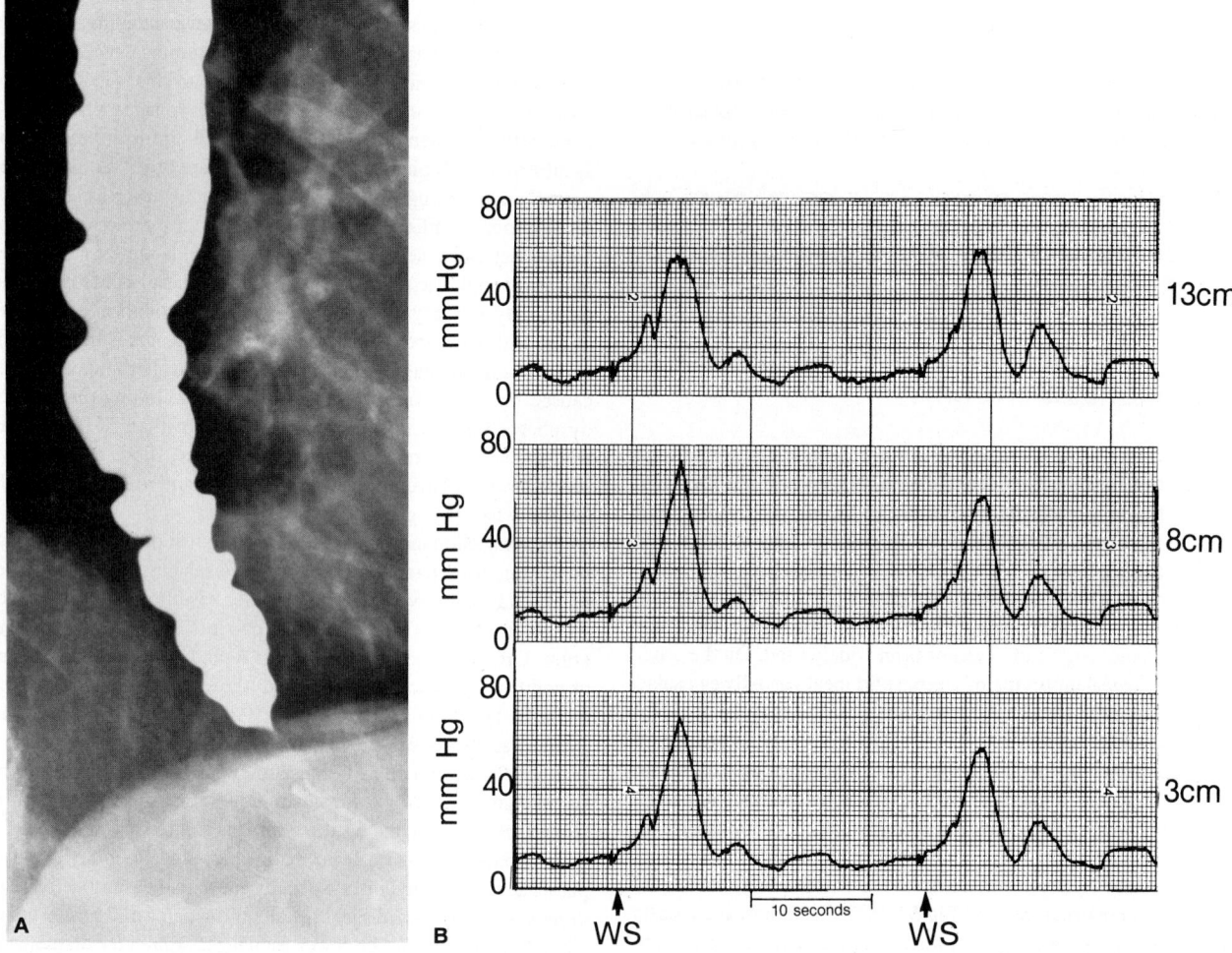

FIGURE 54–6. Radiographic and manometric features of vigorous achalasia. **A,** Barium esophagogram reveals a mildly dilated esophagus with tertiary contractions and smooth tapering of distal esophagus. **B,** Manometric tracing of esophageal body with recording sites 3, 8, and 13 cm above lower esophageal sphincter. All wet swallows (WS) were followed by simultaneous repetitive contractions of higher amplitude (50–70 mm Hg) than usually seen in classic achalasia.

bite, an acute septicemic phase of the illness develops that can be severe (even fatal) or so mild as to go unnoticed. A chronic phase of this disease develops many years later with the destruction of ganglion cells throughout the body, including the heart and the gastrointestinal, urinary, and respiratory tracts. Chronic cardiomyopathy with conduction system disturbances and arrhythmias is most frequent and the most common cause of death in these patients. In the digestive tract, the organs most frequently affected are the esophagus and the colon. The severity of esophageal motor dysfunction is directly related to the loss of intramural ganglion cells.[148] It is believed that abnormality of motility is found when 50% of these cells are destroyed and dilatation only when destruction affects 90%. Interestingly, during the initial stages of esophageal involvement, the motor disorder is confined to the body of the esophagus and involvement of the lower esophageal sphincter occurs only later in the course of the disease.[148] Evidence of other tubular organ involvement (megaureter, megaduodenum, megacolon, megarectum) is most useful in establishing the diagnosis in likely candidates. Otherwise, these patients have all the clinical, radiographic, and manometric features of idiopathic achalasia. If

suspected, the chronic form of the disease can be identified by complement fixation serologic tests. Treatment is similar to idiopathic achalasia because there is no specific therapy for Chagas' disease.

MISCELLANEOUS CAUSES OF SECONDARY ACHALASIA

Achalasialike syndrome secondary to esophageal infiltration by amyloid,[149] sphingolipids,[150] eosinophils,[151] and sarcoidosis[152] has been reported. Successful palliation of esophageal symptoms from amyloidosis has been observed using conventional pneumatic dilatation.[149] Patients with diabetes mellitus and autonomic neuropathy[153] as well as chronic idiopathic intestinal pseudo-obstruction[154] have been reported to have esophageal motor disorders resembling achalasia. In contrast to idiopathic form, these patients usually have minimal esophageal symptoms. Unusual diseases associated with secondary achalasia include pancreatic pseudocysts,[155] Recklinghausen's disease,[156] multiple endocrine neo-

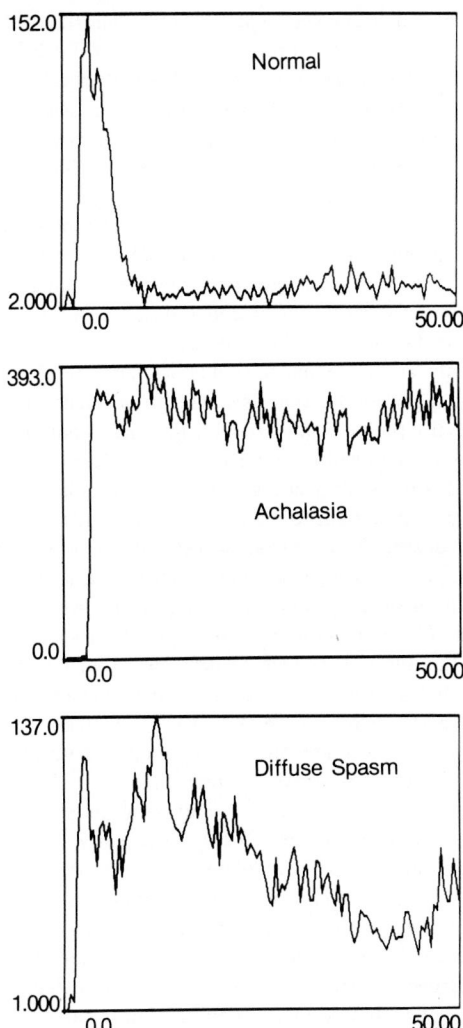

FIGURE 54–7. Esophageal radionuclide liquid transit studies in normal subject (*top*) and patients with achalasia (*middle*) and diffuse esophageal spasm (*bottom*). Radioactivity counts are on the vertical axis and time in minutes on horizontal axis. Achalasia has an adynamic pattern with delayed emptying time. In contrast, diffuse esophageal spasm demonstrates a chaotic, to-and-fro pattern with delayed transit time.

plasia, type IIB,[157] juvenile Sjögren's syndrome,[158] and familial adrenal insufficiency with alacrima.[159] The latter disease has its onset in childhood with an autosomal recessive inheritance. Autonomic nervous system dysfunction produces achalasia, the inability to tear (alacrima), sinoatrial dysfunction, abnormal pupillary responses to light, and delayed gastric emptying. The etiology of the adrenal dysfunction is unknown.

Treatment

The degenerative neural lesion of achalasia cannot be corrected. Therefore, treatment is directed at palliation of symptoms and prevention of complications. This is mainly accomplished by reducing lower esophageal sphincter pressure because peristalsis rarely, if ever, returns with therapy. Lower esophageal sphincter

pressure can be reduced by three modalities: drug therapy, forceful dilatation, and surgical myotomy. These therapies hope to overcome the obstructing lower esophageal sphincter by improving gravitational esophageal emptying through reduction of sphincter tone, while maintaining an adequate barrier against gastroesophageal reflux. Abnormal lower esophageal sphincter relaxation is not improved by any form of therapy.

PHARMACOTHERAPY

A number of drugs act on the lower esophageal sphincter smooth muscle directly or indirectly to reduce resting sphincter pressure in normal persons and in patients with achalasia. Anticholinergics,[160] amyl nitrate,[146] sublingual nitroglycerin,[161] theophylline,[161] and beta$_2$-agonist[161,162] have been tried with inconsistent results in achalasia patients. The most experience has been reported with isosorbide dinitrate and the calcium channel blockers, particularly nifedipine.

The sublingual use of isosorbide dinitrate (Isordil), 5 to 10 mg before meals, has been shown to decrease mean resting lower esophageal sphincter pressures by 66% with relaxation usually lasting at least 90 minutes.[163] Long-term therapy for up to 19 months may result in marked or complete relief of dysphagia.[163] A large drop in lower esophageal sphincter pressure in response to the drug predicts a good clinical response to chronic therapy. Side effects (headaches) are common but can be reduced when the route of administration is changed to oral administration (10 mg). Another study[164] found sublingual isosorbide dinitrate (5 mg) superior to sublingual nifedipine therapy (20 mg). Placebo-controlled trials, however, are not available.

Calcium channel blockers (diltiazem, nifedipine, verapamil) interfere with calcium uptake by smooth muscle cells producing relaxation of the lower esophageal sphincter as well as reducing the amplitude of peristaltic contractions in the body of the esophagus. Diltiazem[165] and verapamil[166] have been studied in achalasia patients and found to result in some reduction in lower esophageal sphincter pressure. The most experience has been with nifedipine, with one study finding it to be more effective than either diltiazem or verapamil.[167] After 20 mg nifedipine sublingually, lower esophageal sphincter pressure is reduced by 30% to 40%.[164,168] In a placebo-controlled clinical study of long-term drug therapy, nifedipine (30–40 mg/day) gave 70% excellent or good results in a group of 20 patients who were followed for 6 to 18 months.[169] Nifedipine can be administered in a dose of 10 to 30 mg sublingually (capsules are broken in the mouth) approximately 30 to 45 minutes before meals. The timing is important because plasma concentrations peak at 1 hour in achalasia patients rather than 30 to 40 minutes as in normals.[170] Increasing doses can lead to a higher incidence of side effects including flushing, dizziness, headaches, peripheral edema, and faintness. It probably is important to add a nocturnal dose of nifedipine to promote esophageal emptying overnight and to minimize regurgitation.

The role of pharmacologic agents in the long-term management of achalasia remains unclear. It is not known whether continued use prevents dilatation or complications. Available drugs have short peak durations of action, tachyphylaxis often results, and the meal frequency is limited to the interval of drug administration. Nevertheless, pharmacotherapy may have a primary role in the following settings: (1) elderly patients or those with significant medical problems making them poor candidates for pneumatic dilatation or myotomy; (2) patients who refuse invasive forms of treatment; (3) patients whose mental states preclude adequate acceptance or cooperation for dilatation or surgery; and (4) as a temporizing measure in otherwise healthy patients with mild or intermittent symptoms. However, in my experience, the latter group requires more definitive therapy over the next several years.

DILATATION

In the original case report of achalasia, Willis used bougienage therapy with a whalebone attached to a sponge to relieve his patient's symptoms.[89] Despite occasional reports to the contrary,[171] benefit from maximum dilatation, even with a 50 to 58 Fr dilator, is quite transient, and self-bougienage is required for long-term therapy. Not surprisingly, a recent study in patients with achalasia secondary to Chagas' disease found that lower esophageal sphincter pressure decreased by 65% 1 year after pneumatic dilatation but only by 15% 1 year after bougienage.[172] Therefore, pneumatic dilatation has replaced bougienage as the most effective nonsurgical method to treat achalasia.

Forceful dilatation to a diameter of approximately 3 cm is necessary to tear the circular muscle and effect lasting reduction of lower esophageal sphincter pressure in achalasia patients. Various types of dilators have been developed for this purpose (Fig 54-8). The Starck dilator is a mechanical device with expanding metal arms where the dilating diameter is determined by manual force.[173] It was the first commercially available dilator but generally has been replaced by pneumatic balloon dilators. Hydrostatic balloon dilators are distended with water under various pressures.[174,175] They were popular at one time, particularly in Europe. The most commonly used devices to treat achalasia are pneumatic balloon dilators, which are distended with air under various pressures. The maximum dilatation of these bags is fixed by a silk, nylon, or plastic cover. The first pneumatic dilator was the Mosher bag[176] followed by the Sippy dilators,[177] which were a series of bags from 3 to 5 cm in diameter that could be placed sequentially on a metal

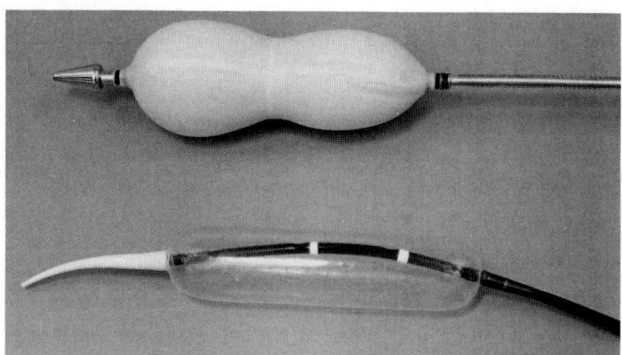

FIGURE 54–8. Two types of currently available pneumatic dilators for the treatment of achalasia. *Top,* Rider-Moeller balloon is dumb-bell shaped and attached to a semirigid metal post. A flanged tip on the dilator can be passed over a guidewire. Three balloon sizes are available: 2.9, 3.8, and 4.8 cm at maximum distention. *Bottom,* Rigidflex dilator has a cylindrical balloon and a double-lumen catheter that allows placement of the entire dilator over a guidewire. Balloons are available in three sizes: 3.0, 3.5, and 4.0 cm at maximum distention.

bougie. These dilators were replaced with cylindrical radiopaque balloons on mercury-filled rubber tubes (Hurst-Tucker, Brown-McHardy) or hourglass-shaped bags (Rider-Moeller) attached to a semirigid metal post.[178–180] Most recently, the Rigiflex dilator has been developed with a double lumen catheter that allows placement of the entire dilator over a guidewire.[181] This cylindrical balloon is similar in design to the Grunzig angioplasty catheter, being made of nonradiopaque polyethylene. Balloons are available in three diameters: 3.0, 3.5, and 4.0 cm. The last type of dilator (Witzel) is a nonradiopaque polyethylene pneumatic dilator mounted on a forward-viewing endoscope, making it possible to position the dilator under directed vision.[182]

Not only are there multiple dilators, but the technique of pneumatic dilatation for achalasia is far from standardized. Most authorities use premedication to allay the anxiety and pain. However, some recommend no premedication for fear it may unduly relax the lower esophageal sphincter.[183] Initial dilator diameter sizes range from 2.9 cm to 4.0 cm. A recent study suggests that larger size dilators have a higher success rate but also more complications, particularly perforation.[122] Therefore, it is reasonable to start with a smaller diameter and repeat the procedure if unsuccessful. The maximum pressure required for successful dilatation or the duration of balloon inflation is not known. In the literature, balloon dilatation pressures have ranged from 7 lb/in^2 (300 mm Hg) to 15 lb/in^2 (774 mm Hg).[184,185] Duration of inflation has ranged from several seconds to 5 minutes with several authors repeating the procedure two to three times.[186,187] Furthermore, until recently, there have been no comparison studies between the available pneumatic dilators. We have recently compared the Brown-McHardy and Rigiflex dilators in 20 randomized achalasia patients.[188] Successful end-points were defined as improvement of symptoms, weight gain, and improved emptying during an upright solid esophageal emptying study. All ten patients improved with the Brown-McHardy dilator, while seven of ten improved with the Rigiflex dilator. One patient not improved with the Rigiflex dilator had a myotomy, while the other two were successfully treated by the Brown-McHardy dilator. No complications occurred with either dilator.

The pneumatic esophageal dilatation technique described below has been used by the author for the last 12 years using the Brown-McHardy, Rider-Moeller, and, most recently, the Rigiflex balloon dilator. This procedure is usually done in an outpatient or day hospital setting. The patient is placed on a liquid diet the night before dilatation, and, if necessary, the esophagus is emptied with an Ewald tube before passage of the instrument. Before all pneumatic dilatations, the inflatable bag should be inspected for leaks, symmetry, and measurement of the maximum inflated circumference. Premedications include cetacaine spray, meperidine (Demerol, 50–100 mg IV), and diazepam (Valium, 2–10 mg IV) as needed to produce mild sedation. In adults, the author generally begins with a 3.5-cm-diameter dilator, increasing the size if the dilatation is unsuccessful. A smaller diameter dilator (3.0 cm) should be used in children. With the patient sitting, the dilator is passed through the mouth until it is about 40 to 50 cm from the teeth. The patient lies in the right anterior oblique position on the x-ray table. Under fluoroscopic guidance, the bag is positioned until it straddles the diaphragm. It is important to maintain the waist in the center of the bag (Fig 54-9A). As the diameter of the bag increases, the waist tends to ride up the bag, which can be prevented by upper traction on the dilator. After the bag is con-

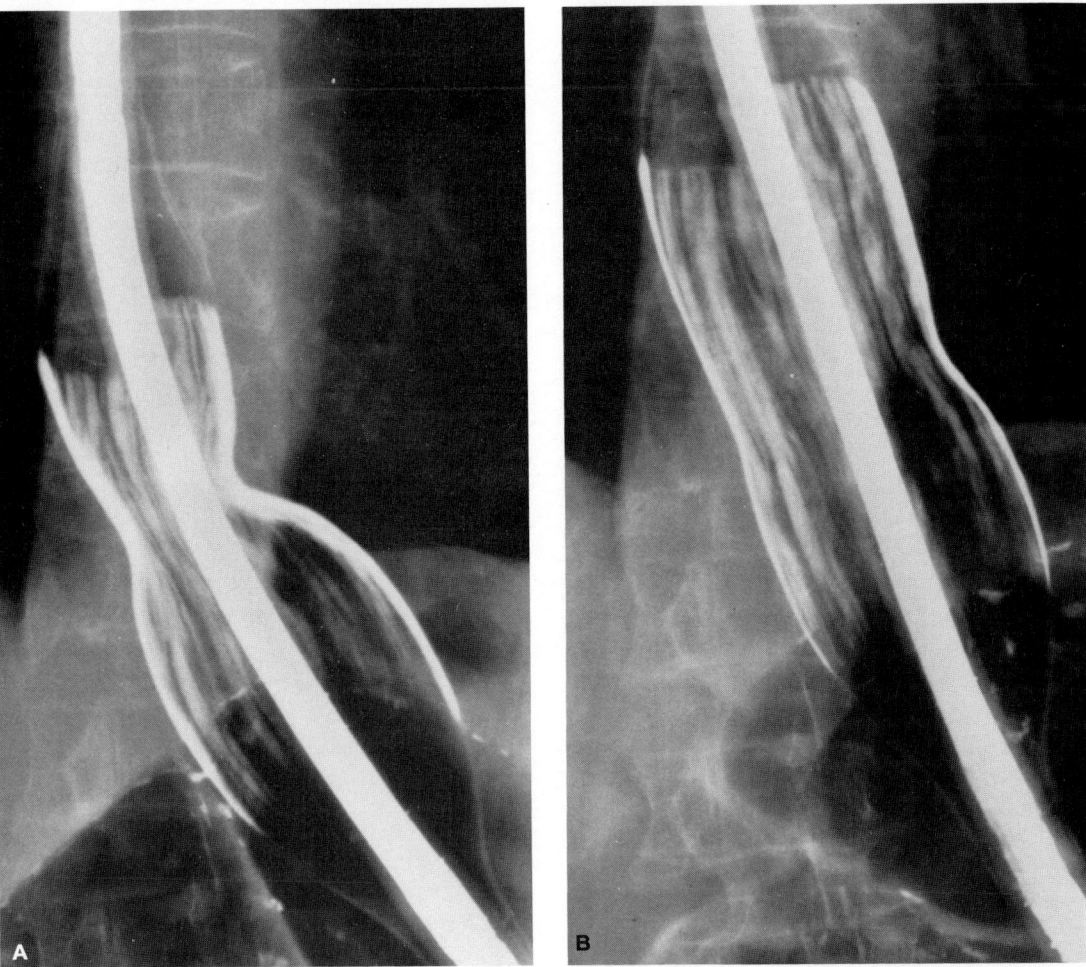

FIGURE 54–9. Pneumatic dilatation with the Brown-McHardy dilator. **A,** Dilator is shown straddling the esophagogastric junction with "waist" created by lower esophageal sphincter impinging on the bag, which is partially inflated with a pressure of 3 psi. **B,** Dilator is fully expanded to a pressure of 15 psi with nearly complete loss of waist.

firmed to be in proper position fluoroscopically, further rapid inflation increases the pressure until the waist is entirely obliterated (see Fig 54-9B). Usually the pressure required to dilate the adult esophagus is between 9 and 15 lb/in^2. At this point, patients usually experience moderate to severe discomfort across the lower chest. The high pressure is maintained for 60 seconds and released. The bag is next reinflated to determine the pressure required to obliterate the waist. If the dilatation has been effective, less pressure (3–6 lb/in^2) is required. If no change is noted, a second dilatation should be performed following the same procedure. No more than two dilatations are performed at a single session. A few streaks of blood are frequently seen on the balloon when it is withdrawn. However, the lack of blood does not indicate an unsuccessful dilatation.

After dilatation, the patient is placed in a semierect position, and the esophagus is examined radiographically first with water-soluble contrast material injected through a tube placed into the esophagus. If no obvious perforation is seen, this material is aspirated and the examination is repeated with barium sulfate suspension. Multiple films of the esophagogastric region are obtained and compared to the predilatation esophagogram when available. The purpose of the test is to examine for distal esophageal leaks

near the region of the esophagogastric junction and not to determine the adequacy of dilatation.[189] If no leak is seen, the patient is observed carefully over the next 6 to 12 hours, and the diet is gradually resumed. The patient with a small "confined" perforation or intramural hematoma is usually asymptomatic and can be managed conservatively. Antibiotics should be initiated, as should close observation for signs of worsening pain and fever suggesting extension of the perforation (Fig 54-10). If barium is observed to flow freely into the mediastinum and left chest, immediate thoracotomy and repair are indicated. If the tear is small, the repair and the myotomy can be performed in the same operation.

Studies indicate that 32% to 98% of patients had no further dysphagia after pneumatic dilatation[174,184,190–193] (Table 54-3). The response rate varies with patient's age (younger patients do less well than older patients)[193] and duration of symptoms (those with a shorter history respond less well), but it does not seem to be related to the degree of esophageal dilatation or tortuosity.[190] Efficacy of this procedure is reduced by half for each subsequent dilatation.[191] Thus, patients having a poor initial result or rapid recurrence of symptoms have less likelihood of responding to additional dilatations. In my experience, approximately 10% to 20% of patients may require further dilatation several to many years

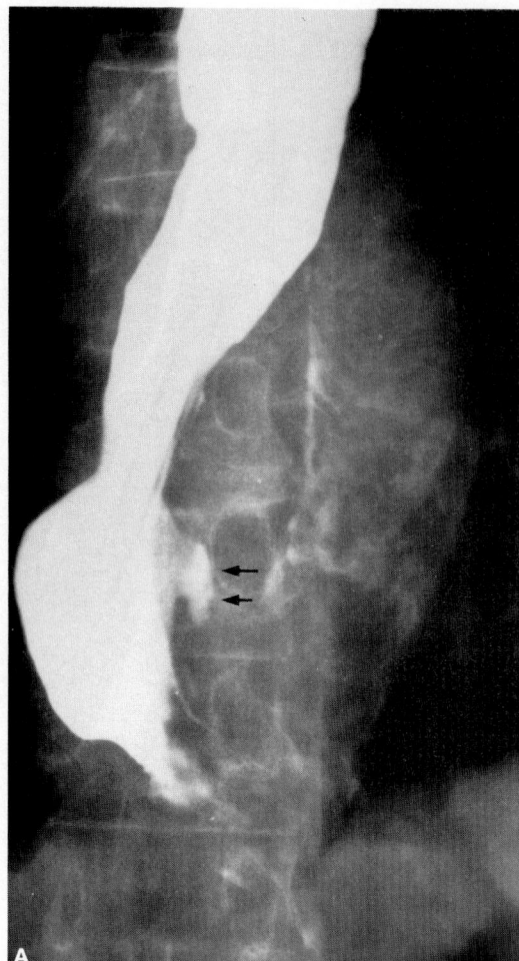 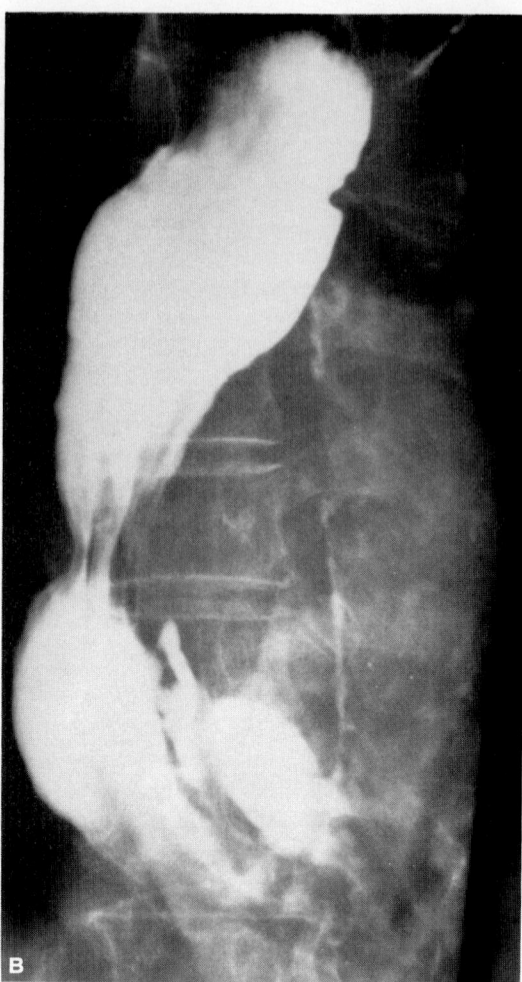

FIGURE 54–10. A, Small, confined contrast collection (*arrows*) immediately after pneumatic dilatation. Patient was free of symptoms at this time. **B,** Five hours later, patient developed severe chest pain and fever. Free perforation into the mediastinum is now present. Patient underwent emergency thoracotomy with repair of 5-cm laceration. One year later, he is free of dysphagia. (From Ott DJ, Richter JE, Wu WC, et al. Radiographic evaluation of esophagus immediately after pneumatic dilatation for achalasia. Dig Dis Sci 1987;32:962.)

after the initial procedure. These patients generally do very well with repeat dilatation, although occasionally they may require surgery. Response to myotomy is not influenced by previous dilatation.[192]

Significant decreases in lower esophageal sphincter pressure occur immediately after pneumatic dilatation but tend to increase slightly over a period of time. Relaxation of lower esophageal sphincter on swallowing does not return after dilatation. The traditional impression has been that esophageal peristalsis does not return after pneumatic dilatation or myotomy. This has been questioned by several case reports[194–196] and the experience reported by the Cleveland Clinic.[197] The latter group demonstrated the return of intermittent distal progressive peristaltic contraction in 7 of 34 (20%) patients with achalasia successfully treated by pneumatic dilatation. However, closer examination of these studies rarely finds evidence of normal bolus transit by fluoroscopy.

The incidence of immediate complications from pneumatic dilatation ranges from 1% to 16%.[184,192] The most feared complication is esophageal perforation ranging from 1% to 13% with the majority

of these cases being small, localized perforations. Despite widely held opinions to the contrary, the small perforations can be managed conservatively with antibiotics and hyperalimentation.[198,199] because pneumatic dilatation leaves some residual lower esophageal sphincter pressure (usually 10–15 mm Hg), gastroesophageal reflux is rare, occurring and persisting in fewer than 2% of patients. In my experience, patients may have variable degrees of chest discomfort and heartburn after returning home, which lasts for less than 4 weeks and can be temporarily relieved with antacids or H_2 antagonists. Mortality from pneumatic dilatation has only been rarely reported.[190,192]

SURGERY

The goal of surgical therapy is to reduce lower esophageal sphincter resting pressure without compromising the barrier so much as to promote gastroesophageal reflux. Most modern forms of surgical therapy for achalasia are variations on an esophageal myotomy,

TABLE 54–3
Series of Over 100 Patients Treated With Balloon Dilatation or Surgical Myotomy in Achalasia

AUTHOR	YEAR	NUMBER OF PATIENTS	RESPONSE GOOD–EXCELLENT (%)	MORTALITY (%)	COMPLICATIONS PERFORATION* (%)
Balloon Dilatation					
Olsen et al[190]	1951	452	60	0.4	2.2
Sanderson et al[191]	1970	408	81	0	3.5
Vantrappen et al[192]	1980	403	77	0.2	2.6
Surgical Myotomy					
Okike et al[202]	1979	456	85	0.2	——
Jara et al[203]	1979	121	80	0	——
Ellis et al[204]	1984	113	78	0	——
Black et al[205]	1976	108	65	0	——
Menzies-Gow et al[206]	1978	102	86	0	——
Csendes et al[207]	1988	100	92	0	——

* —— = not discussed or not relevant.

first performed by Heller in 1913.[200] In the original operation, an anterior and posterior myotomy was performed, either through an abdominal or thoracic approach. Most surgeons only perform an anterior myotomy through a transthoracic approach. In patients with classic achalasia, the myotomy extends less than 1 cm onto the stomach and to several centimeters above the palpated region of the lower sphincter. Patients with vigorous achalasia may have a longer region of muscle thickening and may require more extensive myotomy. In an attempt to prevent gastroesophageal reflux after myotomy, some authorities recommend that it be combined with various types of antireflux procedures and possibly a proximal gastric vagotomy.[201] However, these latter operations should be done very carefully because an improperly performed fundoplication may lead to severe and prolonged dysphagia.

Good to excellent results from myotomy occur in 65% to 92% of patients (see Table 54-3).[202,207] Myotomy reduces lower esophageal sphincter pressure more dependably than does pneumatic dilatation, and this appears to be responsible for its greater efficacy.[186] The most significant complication of myotomy is gastroesophageal reflux. Overall, the incidence of symptomatic reflux is usually less than 10%.[199] However, studies with longer follow-up have reported rates as high as 52%.[203] Reflux disease may be complicated by esophagitis, strictures, and Barrett's esophagus with or without adenocarcinoma.[208] Postmyotomy gastroesophageal reflux is especially damaging in patients with achalasia because esophageal clearance by primary or secondary peristalsis is absent. Postoperative reflux usually can be handled by the same methods used in the treatment of ordinary gastroesophageal reflux disease. Persistent severe dysphagia occurs in less than 10% of patients treated surgically.[186] The dysphagia appears soon after surgery if the initial myotomy has been inadequate or the fibers cut by the myotomy have regrown. Dysphagia may be a late postoperative complication if the myotomy has been too thorough, leading to reflux and a peptic stricture. Manometry and esophagoscopy are helpful in deciding which possibility is present. Additionally, the fundoplication sometimes done in addition to the myotomy may be too tight, resulting in severe dysphagia, a complication requiring additional surgical intervention. The mortality associated with a surgical myotomy is low (less than 2%).

CHOICE OF THERAPY

Today there are relatively few contraindications to balloon dilatation. Uncooperative patients and patients in whom a secondary carcinoma cannot be excluded should undergo myotomy. Children and infants, patients with previous myotomies, and patients with variant forms of achalasia can be treated successfully with pneumatic dilatation. Patients with marked esophageal dilatation and tortuosity also can be treated successfully with pneumatic dilators placed across the esophagogastric junction with the aid of endoscopically placed guidewire. Epiphrenic diverticuli and large hiatal hernias are still considered by most experts to be relative contraindications to pneumatic dilatation because of the high incidence of associated perforations.

It is difficult to compare pneumatic dilatation and surgical myotomy from literature reports because few comparative studies have been carried out. Csendes et al recently reported the final results of the only randomized controlled trial comparing these two modalities in 81 patients with achalasia.[186] After a 5-year follow-up, 95% of the operated patients were asymptomatic and two had mild heartburn, while 65% of the dilated patients were asymptomatic after one or more dilatations and none had heartburn. Positive acid reflux tests were noted in 28% of the postoperative versus 8% of the postdilatation group. In both groups, pretreatment lower esophageal sphincter pressures were similar and decreased significantly after treatment; the surgical group had a consistently lower mean sphincter pressure (8.4 mm Hg) than the postdilatation group (15.2 mm Hg). These results suggest that surgery may be more efficacious than pneumatic dilatation in treating achalasia. However, this study may have been biased against the dilated patients because of their more pronounced dysphagia. In addition, the technique of pneumatic dilatation may have been insufficient. The Mosher bag was rapidly inflated to 5.4 lb/in² for 5 to 20 seconds, this being less inflation pressure for a shorter duration than usually reported. In the era of DRGs, the cost, length of hospitalization, and recovery time also are important issues. Pneumatic dilatation has the advantage of requiring only an overnight hospitalization, compared to 7 to 10 days in the hospital for myotomy. The recovery period after pneumatic dilatation is usually less than 1 week in contrast to 4 to 6 weeks after myotomy. The cost of the two procedures varies greatly but generally ranges between $500 to $1000 for pneumatic dilatation and $2,000 to $5,000 for surgical myotomy.

My opinion is that the choice of therapy should be made after evaluating the risk status of the patient and the capabilities of the medical center (i.e., presence of an experienced gastroenterologist in performing pneumatic dilatation versus a surgeon accomplished in myotomy. As diagrammed in Figure 54-11, I favor pneumatic dilatation as the treatment of choice in low-risk patients. If a satisfactory result is not obtained, one repeat dilatation may be performed before turning to surgery. High-risk patients (elderly persons or patients with multiple medical problems) initially should be treated with pharmacotherapy or possibly static bougienage. If this is unsuccessful, patients showing further deterioration should undergo "gentle" pneumatic dilatation.

Complications of Achalasia

The complications of achalasia are related to retention and stasis in the esophagus. The majority of these complications already have been discussed including esophagitis, bronchopulmonary problems, acute airway obstruction, lower esophageal diverticulum, and, rarely, bleeding. The most feared complication of achalasia is the development of squamous cell carcinoma of the esophagus. This malignancy has been reported in association with achalasia with rates as high as 20%, but such series were contaminated by patients with primary tumors mimicking achalasia.[209–211] Nev-

ertheless, it appears that the prevalence of carcinoma is higher in achalasia patients, with rates ranging from 2% to 7% being found in the larger recent series. The tumors develop many years after the diagnosis of achalasia, usually in patients with unsatisfactory or no treatment. As the tumors often arise in a greatly dilated esophagus, symptoms can be quite delayed and the neoplasms frequently are large and advanced at the time of detection. The pathogenesis of the carcinoma is obscure, but stasis and mucosal irritation may be precipitating factors. The actual incidence of cancer after identifying patients with achalasia is not known, and this affects the yield from any endoscopic surveillance program.[211] My opinion is that patients with achalasia are at an increased risk for squamous cell carcinoma, but the relative risk is not known. Because marked esophageal dilatation and stasis may be important contributing factors, the diagnosis of achalasia must be systematically identified and aggressively treated. Although supporting data are not available, the author only performs surveillance endoscopy (every 1 to 2 years) in patients with marked residual esophageal dilatation and stasis.

SPASTIC MOTILITY DISORDERS OF THE DISTAL ESOPHAGUS

The development of precise infusion systems that permit accurate pressure recordings have brought studies of esophageal motility into the modern age. This new technology has allowed us to establish criteria from normals based on large numbers of healthy adults.[212,213] At the same time, a variety of new esophageal motility "disorders" have been recognized, particularly in patients with noncardiac chest pain syndromes. These manometric patterns are different from achalasia, being characterized by normal peristalsis intermittently interrupted by simultaneous contractions, high-amplitude or long-duration waves, or dysfunction of the lower esophageal sphincter. There has been great confusion in the literature whether these manometric abnormalities represent separate distinct entities or variations of diffuse esophageal spasm. This has resulted in manometric classifications with colorful terminology and segregation based on either a "lumper" or "splitter" approach. The lumpers prefer to talk about normal motility, achalasia, and diffuse esophageal spasm.[214] My group[215,216] and others[217,218] have been instrumental in splitting the latter group into diffuse esophageal spasm, nutcracker esophagus, hypertensive lower esophageal sphincter, and a group of nonspecific esophageal motility disorders. Others have further broken down these groups based on the presence or absence of simultaneous contractions, high-amplitude contractions, long-duration contractions, repetitive activity, and lower esophageal sphincter relaxation.[140,212] The splitters originally hoped that further definition would lead to a better understanding of pathophysiology and possibly different therapeutic approaches. However, this does not seem to be the case. It appears that these groups of patients have similar clinical presentations, a pathologic base has been determined for none, management approaches are similar for all, and a specific outcome for any one subset is not recognized. Therefore, it probably is appropriate to "group" these manometric disorders under the general term of *spastic motility disorders of the distal esophagus*. It has even be questioned whether these newer abnormal motility patterns represent important disturbances of esophageal function or simply "curious" manometric

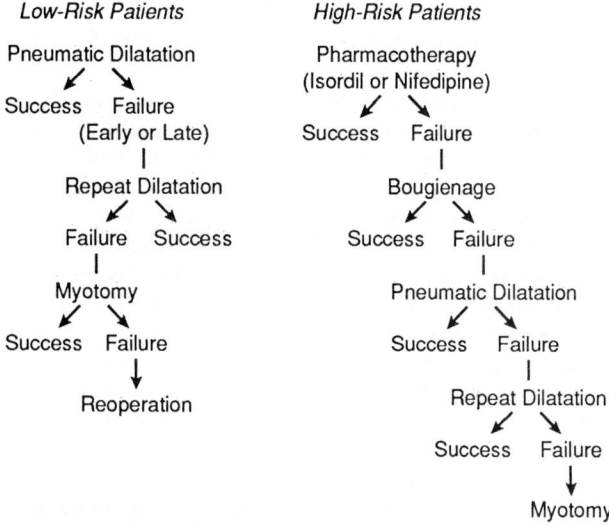

FIGURE 54–11. Flowchart for the suggested treatment of low- and high-risk patients with achalasia.

findings. One authority[219] recently suggested the following criteria to define a manometric finding as an important esophageal disease: (1) the motility event must be a major "alteration" of esophageal physiology, (2) motility changes must be associated temporally with symptoms of esophageal disease, (3) the abnormality of esophageal function must be demonstrated by other independent measures, and (4) the symptoms or signs of esophageal abnormality must be improved as the esophageal disorder is corrected. These may be worthwhile criteria, but, on closer scrutiny, they would permit only achalasia to be defined as a true clinical esophageal motility disorder. Many more studies are required to understand the clinical significance and complex pathophysiology of these spastic esophageal motility disorders.

Pathophysiology

Patients with spastic disorders of the esophagus rarely require surgery, and the diseases are not fatal. The esophageal muscles and neural plexus are not readily accessible for routine biopsy. Thus, very little material is available for pathologic examination and study. The most striking change reported grossly in the esophagus is diffuse muscular thickening, mainly of the lower two thirds of the esophagus. Thickening up to 2 cm has been reported in patients with clinical and manometric evidence consistent with diffuse esophageal spasm.[220,221] However, there are well-documented cases of these motility disorders in which thickening was not found at thoracotomy.[222] All patients with esophageal muscular thickening do not suffer from pain or dysphagia. In one report, five of six cases of muscular hypertrophy found at autopsy were asymptomatic in life.[223] Otherwise, the esophageal muscle has been shown to be essentially normal by light microscopy.[220]

Little specific evidence of neuropathology has been reported. Unlike achalasia, loss of ganglion cells in the intramural plexus has not been demonstrated. However, some of the patients with diffuse esophageal spasm have exhibited changes in the vagus nerve that were much more diffuse than those reported for patients with achalasia.[220] These findings include fragmentation of neural filaments, increase in endoneural collagen, and fragmentation of mitochondria. Because these changes were seen diffusely in the vagus nerve, the authors concluded that they probably represented afferent fibers because this type of fiber is predominant in the human vagus. However, sophisticated histochemical studies were not done to ascertain whether they actually were afferent or efferent nerves. Central nervous system abnormalities have not been reported in patients with spastic motility disorders.

Despite little evidence of neuropathology, physiologic studies suggest there may be some neural dysfunction. In these disorders, the esophagus is particularly sensitive to cholinergic stimulation, which produces an exaggeration of abnormal manometric findings in many patients.[224–226] Edrophonium chloride, a cholinesterase inhibitor, and ergonovine maleate, an α-adrenergic drug, also produce similar results.[227–229] However, these responses are not sensitive or specific for the spastic motility disorders. Similar manometric changes have been reported in achalasia and in normals, particularly when age-matched controls were used.[227] Furthermore, not all subjects with spastic motility disorders show a worsening of their manometric findings after these agents. Recent electromyographic studies in patients with diffuse esophageal spasm have demonstrated spike independent contractions of the esophageal body and increased excitability of spontaneous spike activity.[230] These findings may represent impaired noncholinergic, nonadrenergic inhibitory neural mechanisms. An imbalance between excitatory and inhibitory innervation could conceivably lead to the motility changes seen in the spastic disorders. However, some of these abnormalities are seen in healthy subjects in response to normal physiologic stimuli. For example, approximately 15% of dry swallows are followed by simultaneous contractions[213] and ingestion of very cold liquids may be associated with low-amplitude contractions and even aperistalsis.[231,232]

Increasing evidence indicates that central nervous system processing could participate and produce some of these spastic manometric abnormalities. Psychologically stressful interviews may produce simultaneous and repetitive contractions in normal subjects that resemble the described contraction abnormalities.[233] Loud noises or difficult mental tasks performed during manometry have been shown to increase contraction amplitude and produce simultaneous contractions in the distal esophagus.[234,235] In one study, these findings were observed in healthy control subjects, but the response was exaggerated in those with motility disorders, particularly nutcracker esophagus.[235] Other clinical observations complement the results of laboratory studies. Patients undergoing the stress of alcohol withdrawal have been observed to have very high-amplitude contractions in the distal esophagus and elevated lower esophageal sphincter pressures, which returned to normal after 1 month of abstinence.[236] During 24-hour ambulatory esophageal pressure monitoring, abnormal motility patterns can be seen as frequently after rather than preceding the onset of pain, suggesting a secondary phenomenon.[237] These findings may have a relationship to the observation that psychiatric disorders are unusually prevalent in symptomatic patients with spastic disorders compared to those with other manometric abnormalities (achalasia) or normal esophageal motility. Using the Diagnostic Interview Schedule, one group found that nearly 80% of symptomatic patients had psychiatric diagnoses, particularly anxiety disorders, panic attacks, depression, or somatization disorders.[238] Others who have administered self-report inventories to patients with nutcracker esophagus and hypertensive lower esophageal sphincter found response patterns suggesting that these patients have excessive concerns about somatic functions and have more frequent and severe gastrointestinal symptoms under stress.[239]

A proposed model for the interactions observed among the spastic motility disorders has recently been suggested.[134] As shown in Figure 54-12, the location of pathology (disease locus) is not known but appears to include both a motor (effector) and sensory component. These two limbs may not be involved equally in all cases and can be stimulated independently by various maneuvers. This is consistent with observations that cholinergic stimulation frequently precipitates motility changes with or without pain but can provoke pain without significantly altering esophageal contractions.[227] Likewise, acid instillation may stimulate sensitized neuroreceptors, producing pain independent of motility changes.[240,241] Balloon distention studies also have reproduced esophageal pain at low distending volumes without noticeable motor changes in these patients.[242] This evidence for lower visceral pain thresholds suggests a sensory disorder may play an important role in some patients. The high prevalence of psychiatric disorders found in these patients may alter sensory perception, a concept supported by other chronic pain disorders. It should be noted in

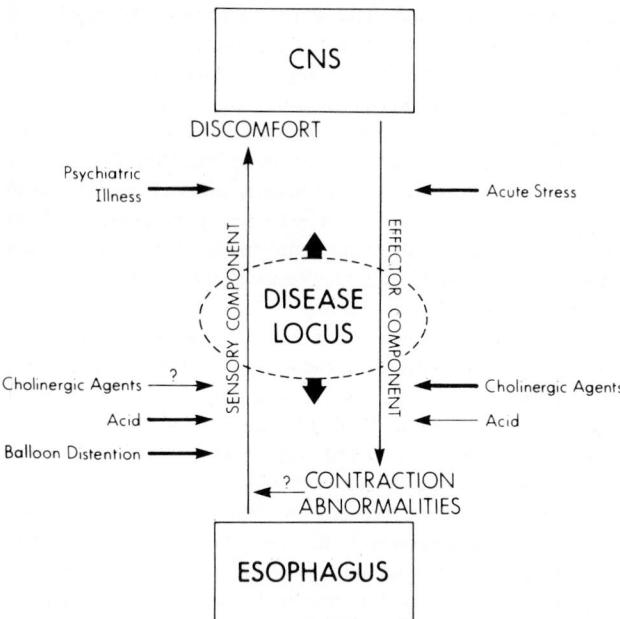

FIGURE 54–12. Model proposed by Clouse for the complex interactions in the spastic motility disorders. The location of the pathology in these disorders (disease locus) is not known but appears to include both a motor (effector) component and a sensory component. These two limbs may not be involved equally in all cases and can be stimulated independently by various stimuli (drugs, acid, distention). Emotional states may acutely affect the motor component, while chronic psychiatric illness may alter the sensory component. Contraction abnormalities measured in the esophagus are secondary markers for the disease and do not predictably provoke the sensory limb. (From Clouse RE. Motor disorders. In: Sleinsenger MH, Fordtran JS, eds. Gastrointestinal disease: Pathophysiology, diagnosis, management, ed 4. Philadelphia: WB Saunders, 1989:559.)

this model that the esophageal contraction abnormalities may be only markers or epiphenomena for the disease and only occasionally provoke the sensory limb. If so, spastic motility disorders associated with chest pain would resemble other stress-related chronic pain syndromes (i.e., tension headaches) in which increases in the physiologic markers for the syndromes (i.e., electromyographic activity) are not consistently related to episodes of pain.[243] This hypothetical model also has many similarities to the proposed interactions in patients with the irritable bowel syndrome. In fact, we and others[244] believe these two conditions actually may represent a spectrum of disease, the "irritable gut."

Manometric Features

The manometric features of the spastic motility disorders are restricted to the smooth muscle portion of the esophagus, particularly the 10-cm segment proximal to the lower esophageal sphincter. The motility findings of these disorders are discussed as if they were separate entities so as to emphasize specific manometric features and their prevalence. However, this segregation may be artificial because the spastic motility disorders are quite variable, changing patterns from day to day and even from hour to hour.

DIFFUSE ESOPHAGEAL SPASM

The clinical syndrome of diffuse esophageal spasm was first described by Hamilton Osgood in 1889.[245] The earliest manometric studies by Creamer and associates[246] and Roth and Flesher[247] identified the manometric feature common to patients with diffuse spasm: the simultaneous onset of pressure contractions recorded by two adjacent recording orifices in the esophagus. Simultaneous waves, usually in the distal esophagus, were mixed with normal peristaltic sequences, showing that the esophagus had not completely lost its ability to produce propagating contractions, thereby suggesting a partial or intermittent effect (Fig 54-13). Simultaneous onset of the contractions rather than simultaneous peaks is the important characteristic because radiologic studies have shown that the former changes are associated with disruption of bolus transit.[248,249]

The frequency of simultaneous contractions characterizing diffuse esophageal spasm has been a point of some controversy. Based on healthy controls, we found simultaneous contractions were distinctly uncommon after wet swallows.[213] Therefore, diffuse esophageal spasm was defined by the presence of greater than 10% simultaneous contractions.[215] In a review of 40 patients with symptomatic diffuse esophageal spasm, we observed simultaneous contractions after approximately 40% of wet swallows (range 20%–90%). A minimum of 30% simultaneous contractions has been proposed for the diagnostic criterion of diffuse esophageal spasm when using dry swallows.[225,250] However, dry swallows may result in overdiagnosing this disorder because simultaneous contractions may be seen after 80% and even 100% of dry swallows in healthy adults.[213] Simultaneous contractions are not specific for diffuse esophageal spasm and may be seen in other spastic motility disorders as well as patients with gastroesophageal reflux and neuropathies secondary to diabetes, collagen vascular disease, alcoholism, and pseudo-obstruction.

Other manometric abnormalities reported in diffuse esophageal spasm include repetitive contractions, high-amplitude contractions, contractions of prolonged duration, and abnormalities of the lower esophageal sphincter. These latter findings are usually not seen as isolated events but occur as variations of the basic abnormal response (i.e., intermittent simultaneous contractions). Repetitive contractions defined by three or more pressure peaks may be swallow-induced or spontaneous (not related to a swallow). Giant contraction waves of high amplitude and long duration have long been recognized as occurring with diffuse esophageal spasm.[246] Before the development of newer manometric equipment, a contraction pressure of more than 40 to 50 mm Hg was considered one of high amplitude. More recent experiences suggest that the amplitude of esophageal contraction in diffuse esophageal spasm is usually not increased, and prolonged duration waves are generally associated with repetitive contractions.[215] Frequent spontaneous contractions have been observed in these patients,[220] but this has not been a consistent observation.[215] Spontaneous esophageal activity may be seen in healthy adults and, therefore, must be interpreted cautiously in the diagnosis of diffuse esophageal spasm.[213] Finally, lower esophageal sphincter abnormalities may be seen in diffuse esophageal spasm. One group reported that sphincter relaxation was incomplete in 10 patients and hypertensive sphincters were found in 9 of 27 patients with diffuse esophageal spasm.[250] Incomplete sphincter relaxation occurred even more frequently (8 of 12 patients) in another series of patients with diffuse esophageal spasm.[251]

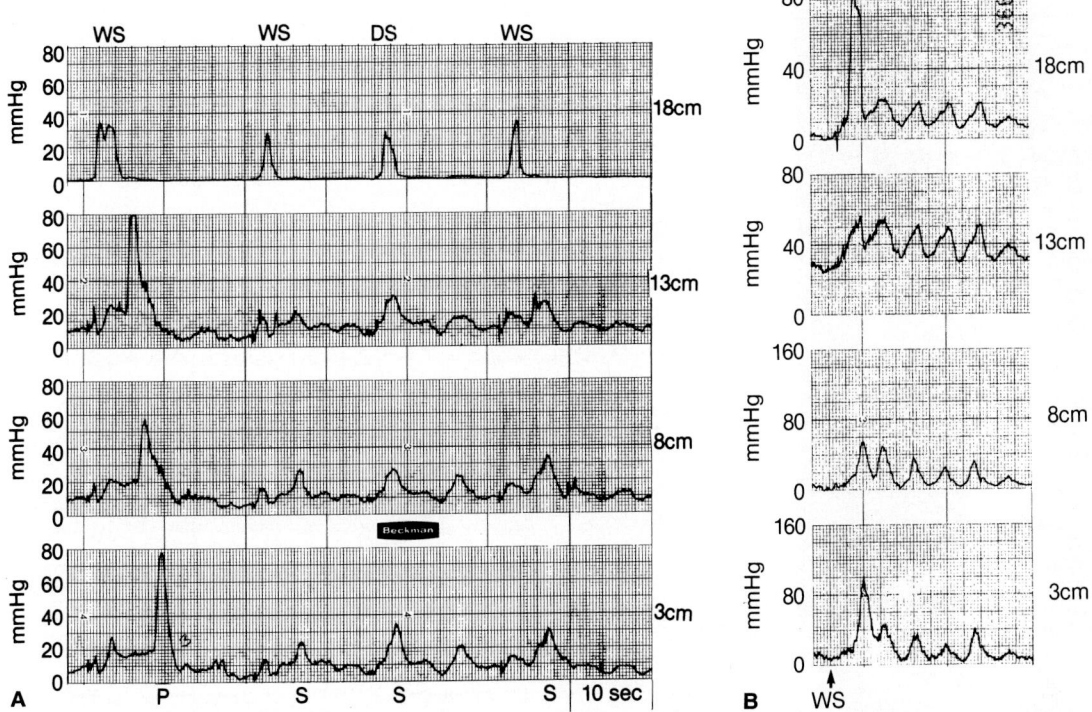

FIGURE 54–13. Manometric findings in patients with diffuse esophageal spasm. **A,** This study is characterized by simultaneous contractions (S) in the distal esophagus with the intermittent presence of normal peristaltic (P) activity (swallow on left). The tracing shows recording sites located 18, 13, 8, and 3 cm above the lower esophageal sphincter and the response to both wet swallows (WS) and dry swallows (DS). **B,** Classic example of repetitive contractions following a wet swallow (WS). Note that high-amplitude contractions are not seen in these examples and are uncommon findings in patients with diffuse esophageal spasm studied in our laboratory. (From Castell DO, Richter JE, Dalton CB, eds. Esophageal motility testing. Amsterdam: Elsevier, 1987.)

NUTCRACKER ESOPHAGUS

In 1977, Brand et al reported that 41% of noncardiac chest pain patients with abnormal esophageal manometry showed a pattern of high-amplitude peristaltic contractions.[217] Two years later, Benjamin and colleagues confirmed these observations and coined the term *nutcracker esophagus*.[252] Other terms that have been used to describe this motility disorder include *supersqueeze esophagus, symptomatic esophageal peristalsis, hypertensive peristalsis,* and *high-amplitude peristaltic contractions.* Regardless of the colorful terminology, this manometric diagnosis has been found in 27% to 48% of patients with noncardiac chest pain having abnormal esophageal motility reported from many laboratories throughout the world.[216–218,252,253]

Nutcracker esophagus is a descriptive term for the manometric findings in a patient with chest pain or dysphagia characterized by average distal esophageal peristaltic pressures greater than two standard deviations above a well-documented normal range. Initial reports identified nutcracker esophagus when average distal amplitudes were greater than 120 mm Hg based on normal studies in young healthy control subjects.[252] However, these values have been revised upward with our better understanding of the range of normal pressures, particularly in older healthy subjects.[212,213] In our laboratory, nutcracker esophagus is defined by average peristaltic pressures (mean of ten wet swallows) exceeding 180 mm Hg; other laboratories use average pressures from 150 to 200 mm Hg (Fig 54-14A). We have seen some patients with average unstimulated pressure in excess of 400 mm Hg. These extremely strong peristaltic waves can be shown to respond appropriately to

pharmacologic agents that attenuate esophageal contractions, such as atropine. Nutcracker esophagus is an extremely labile motility disorder. During a 3- to 5-year follow-up of 23 such patients, esophageal pressures were usually highest on the initial manometric study, and only 54% of subsequent studies showed high-amplitude contractions.[254] Up to one third of patients with nutcracker esophagus also have contractions of prolonged duration (greater than 6 seconds).[255]

The barium esophagogram[256] and radionuclide transit studies[248] are usually normal in patients with nutcracker esophagus as the result of orderly peristalsis propelling the bolus along the esophagus (see Fig 54-14B). Occasionally, a defect in esophageal transit is seen, but this likely results from intermittent simultaneous contractions.[257] Although high-amplitude esophageal contractions may be found more frequently in patients with noncardiac chest pain, these persons are usually asymptomatic when the diagnosis is made. Furthermore, chest pain improvement does not predictably correlate with amplitude reduction by pharmacotherapy[258] or surgical myotomy.[259] Therefore, the relationship of chest pain and high-amplitude peristaltic contractions does not appear to be causal.

HYPERTENSIVE LOWER ESOPHAGEAL SPHINCTER

The presence of an excessively high resting lower esophageal sphincter was first described in 1960 by Code et al at the Mayo Clinic.[260] Although many of these patients had other esophageal motility abnormalities (particularly diffuse esophageal spasm),

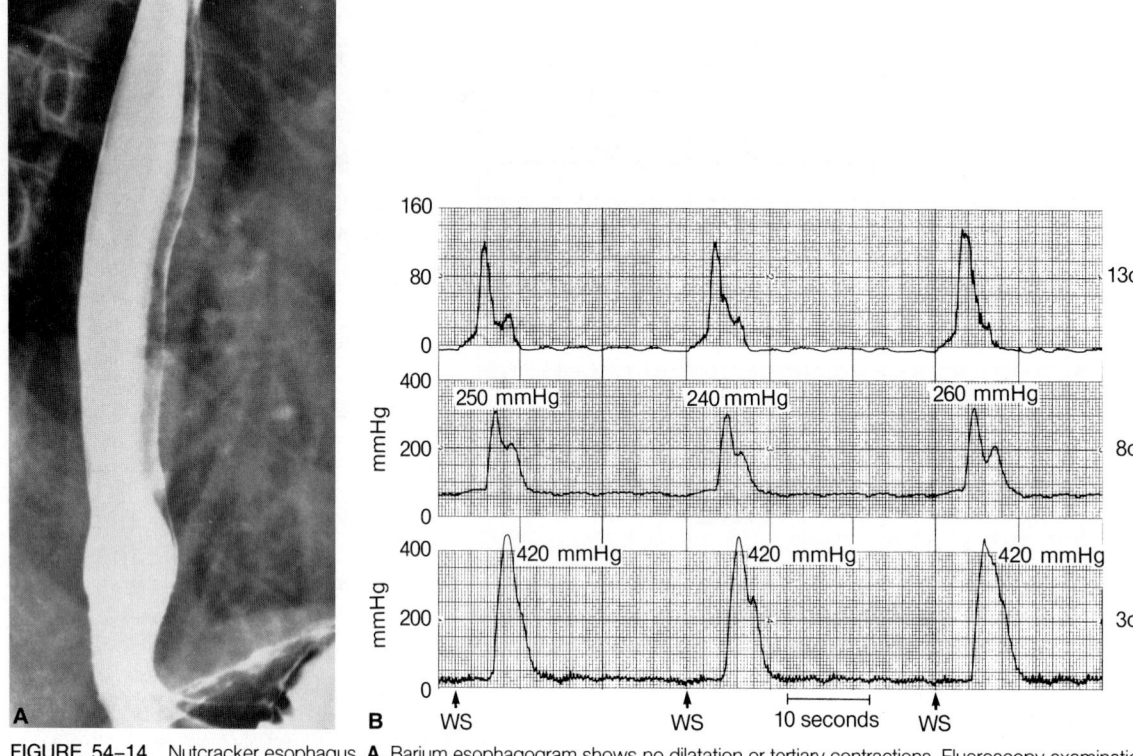

FIGURE 54–14. Nutcracker esophagus. **A,** Barium esophagogram shows no dilatation or tertiary contractions. Fluoroscopy examination of swallowing revealed normal peristaltic stripping waves. **B,** Esophageal manometry shows contractions in response to wet swallows (WS) that are clearly peristaltic in nature but characterized by excessively high-pressure amplitudes (240–420 mm Hg) in the distal esophagus 8 and 3 cm above the lower esophageal sphincter. The patient experienced no symptoms during the manometry study despite these high-amplitude contractions. (Manometric illustration from Castell DO, Richter JE, Dalton CB, eds. Esophageal motility testing. Amsterdam: Elsevier, 1987.)

approximately 50% showed only isolated abnormalities of the lower esophageal sphincter characterized by increased resting lower esophageal sphincter pressures associated with normal sphincter relaxation and normal peristalsis. A subsequent report also found excessively large and prolonged contractions of the sphincter after relaxation, a phenomenon called "hypercontracting or hyperreacting sphincter."[261] In our laboratory, the hypertensive lower esophageal sphincter is defined by sphincter pressures exceeding two standard deviations above the normal range (> 45 mm Hg). Recently, a computer-analyzed study of lower esophageal sphincter parameters in these patients suggested that there may be some impairment in sphincter relaxation when compared to healthy controls.[262] These manometric abnormalities could account for these patients' report of symptoms, however, radiographic and scintigraphic studies usually have found normal esophageal function without bolus retardation at the level of the lower sphincter.[262] Although by definition all patients with hypertensive lower esophageal sphincter have normal peristalsis, approximately 50% may have high-amplitude contractions consistent with nutcracker esophagus.

NONSPECIFIC ESOPHAGEAL MOTILITY DISORDERS

When evaluating large numbers of patients for potential esophageal motility disorders, one frequently finds esophageal contraction patterns that are outside the range of normal findings but that do not readily fit into the previously described categories. These miscellaneous manometric abnormalities include frequent nontransmitted contractions (greater than 20% of wet swallows), retrograde contractions, low-amplitude contractions (<30 mm Hg), prolonged duration peristaltic waves (>6 seconds), and isolated incomplete lower esophageal sphincter relaxation. We have classified these miscellaneous abnormalities into the general category of nonspecific esophageal motility disorders. These patterns represent a broad spectrum of abnormalities, and their clinical significance is unknown.

Clinical Features

Spastic disorders of the esophagus appear at any age; the mean age of presentation is approximately 40 years. In contrast to achalasia, a female predominance seems to be present in most studies.[216,263] The cardinal symptoms of spastic esophageal motility disorders are dysphagia and chest pain. Patients frequently present with a combination of both symptoms. The prevalence of chest pain is constant across the various spastic disorders, but the prevalence and severity of dysphagia increase as patients have more manometric features consistent with classic diffuse esophageal spasm.[263]

DYSPHAGIA

Dysphagia for liquids and solids is present in 30% to 60% of patients with spastic motility disorders.[216,263] The symptom is intermittent in nature, varying on a daily basis from mild to very severe, and there may be periods of relatively normal swallowing. The dysphagia does not necessarily accompany chest pain and may be related to swallowing specific substances such as large boluses of food, medications, or liquids of extreme temperatures. Regurgitation of food or liquids into the mouth or nasopharynx may accompany dysphagia, but this is infrequent compared to achalasia. Dysphagia is usually not progressive or severe enough to interfere markedly with eating and to produce weight loss. The symptoms of dysphagia are believed to be related to the previously described motility disturbances, particularly simultaneous contractions, nonconducted swallows, or low-amplitude waves that do not seal the esophageal lumen, thereby interfering with normal bolus transit. However, these nonpropulsive contractions do not consistently produce this symptom, suggesting that other factors (luminal distention, bolus size) may contribute to dysphagia.

CHEST PAIN

Intermittent anterior chest discomfort is reported by 80% to 90% of patients with spastic motility disorders.[216,263] Chest pain is usually described as squeezing, is substernal in location, and may radiate into the back, neck, jaw, or arms, making it sometimes indistinguishable from angina. Pain episodes may last from minutes to hours, and swallowing is generally not impaired during these episodes. The pain can be quite severe, causing the patient to become ashen and to perspire. Relief of symptoms may require narcotics or nitroglycerin, further confusing the distinction between esophageal and cardiac pain. Features suggesting esophageal rather than cardiac pain include pain that is nonexertional and continues for hours; pain that interrupts sleep or is meal-related; pain that is relieved with antacids; or the presence of associated esophageal symptoms including heartburn, dysphagia, or regurgitation.[264] Unfortunately, none of these features apply exclusively to esophageal pain.

The mechanism producing pain in these spastic motility disorders is poorly understood. Some patients may be experiencing occult acid reflux unrelated to their motility disorder.[265] A popular hypothesis has been that esophageal motility disorders produce chest pain as a result of high intramural esophageal tension inhibiting blood flow for a critical time period (i.e., myoischemia).[225] However, the arterial blood supply to the esophagus is extensive,[266] and, hence, it is unlikely that esophageal blood flow could be critically compromised by local contractions that are even two to three times greater than systolic blood pressure or that are sustained for up to 30 seconds. Furthermore, these patients are usually asymptomatic when these esophageal motility disorders are defined, and chest pain improvement does not predictably correlate with amplitude reduction produced by either pharmacotherapy[258] or surgical myotomy.[259] Other potential causes of esophageal chest pain include excitation of temperature receptors or acute luminal distention.[231,267] It is possible that chest pain experienced by patients with esophageal motility disorders is due to proximal distention of the esophageal body by an abnormal distal contraction or by the lack of coordination between lower esophageal sphincter

relaxation and the esophageal contraction advancing toward it.[251] However, the absolute degree of esophageal distention may not be the only factor because esophageal balloon distention studies suggest these patients also have lower visceral pain thresholds.[242]

OTHER SYMPTOMS

Heartburn is present in as many as 20% of patients with spastic motility disorders.[263] This symptom may reflect abnormal esophageal sensation rather than pathologic reflux, because it often is not reproduced by acid instillation and is poorly responsive to antireflux therapy. Symptoms compatible with the irritable bowel syndrome are common and may be seen in over 50% of these patients.[268,269] Female patients also often have symptoms of urinary and sexual dysfunction. Emotional disturbances, particularly anxiety and depression, are very common and should be identified and appropriately treated.

The general prevalence of spastic motility disorders is unknown. Studies from our laboratory suggest that the patient's chief complaint of either chest pain or dysphagia may be important factors in the prevalence and type of spastic motility disorder identified.[216] In a recent 3-year experience with 1161 patients referred for esophageal manometry, esophageal motility disorders were significantly more prevalent in patients evaluated for dysphagia (132 of 251, 53%) than in patients evaluated for noncardiac chest pain (255 of 910, 25%). As noted in Figure 54-15, nutcracker esophagus was the most common motility disorder seen in patients with noncardiac chest pain but was infrequent in patients with dysphagia. In contrast, achalasia was common in patients with dysphagia but rare in patients with noncardiac chest pain. In our experience, diffuse esophageal spasm, as previously defined, is an uncommon motility disorder associated with either chest pain or dysphagia.

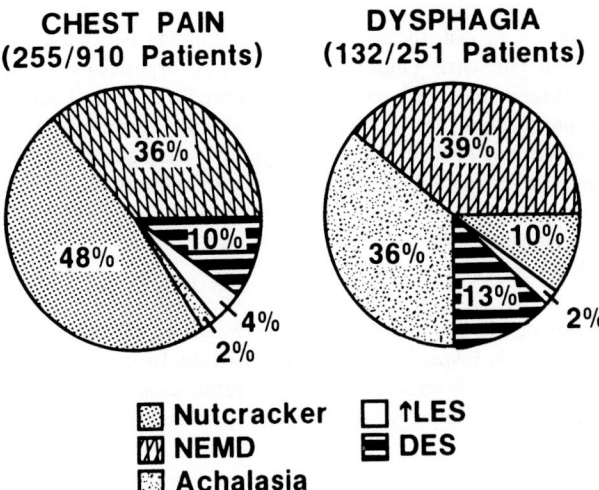

FIGURE 54–15. Pie diagram comparing incidence of esophageal motility disorders in patients with noncardiac chest pain (*left*) and dysphagia (*right*) studied over 3 years at the Bowman Gray School of Medicine. NEMD = nonspecific esophageal motility disorder; LES = hypertensive lower esophageal sphincter; DES = diffuse esophageal spasm. (From Katz PO, Dalton CB, Richter JE, et al. Esophageal testing in patients with non-cardiac chest pain and/or dysphagia. Ann Intern Med 1987;106:593.)

Diagnosis

Although spastic motility disorders are defined by esophageal manometry, the intermittent nature of these abnormalities frequently requires the use of other esophageal tests. In these patients, I often use several studies to better understand the cause of the patient's symptoms and functional abnormalities before beginning any therapeutic treatment. Furthermore, the pain of spastic motility disorders can mimic coronary artery disease sufficiently that extensive cardiac evaluation including coronary angiography is commonly required.

RADIOLOGIC STUDIES

A plain film of the chest reveals no characteristic findings in patients with spastic motility disorders. A barium esophagogram with fluoroscopy is the initial test in any patient with dysphagia and should also be considered in subjects with chest pain potentially of esophageal origin. In patients with severe motility disorders, particularly classic diffuse esophageal spasm, the peristaltic wave is observed to travel as far as the aortic arch before it is disrupted by isolated and uncoordinated movement of the lower two thirds of the esophagus. These indentions are produced by dysfunctional circular muscle contractions. The severe lumen obliterating "tertiary contractions" produce entrapment of barium, delay the bolus transit, and may produce to-and-fro bolus movement. This distorted radiographic appearance has solicited such descriptive terms as *corkscrew esophagus, rosary bead esophagus, pseudodiverticula,* and *curling* (Fig 54-16). Interestingly, these striking radiologic abnormalities are frequently not associated with symptoms of chest pain or dysphagia. It should be noted that not all tertiary contractions are associated with esophageal motility disorders. Mild, partial lumen indenting tertiary contractions can be seen in healthy controls and not be associated with disordered bolus movement. In all cases, whether mild or severe, the uncoordinated postswallow contractions are intermixed with swallows that have normal appearance. In fact, the spastic motility disorders associated with normal peristalsis (nutcracker esophagus, hypertensive lower esophageal sphincter) are usually associated with normal barium esophagograms. Patients with spastic motility disorders do not have beaking of their lower esophagus, but sliding hiatal hernias appear to be more frequent than in healthy subjects.[270]

ENDOSCOPY

Endoscopy is frequently done in the evaluation of patients with dysphagia or suspected esophageal chest pain. Its major role is to identify possible structural lesions or reflux esophagitis because the spastic motility disorders have no typical endoscopic features.

RADIONUCLIDE STUDIES

Radionuclide scintigraphy can measure esophageal transit time and define the pattern of bolus movement. Abnormal peristalsis and delayed emptying are readily detected. Russell et al found liquid radionuclide transit studies performed in the supine position to be 100% sensitive in 15 patients with identified motility dis-orders. In addition, 9 of 15 patients with dysphagia and normal esophageal manometry were found to have transit abnormalities.[142] Patients with classic diffuse esophageal spasm usually have a chaotic, to-and-fro pattern with delayed esophageal emptying (see Fig 54-7). False-negative studies occur from intermittent esophageal dysmotility or spastic motility disorders associated with orderly peristalsis such as nutcracker esophagus and hypertensive lower esophageal sphincter.[248,262] For these reasons, the radionuclide transit study never fulfilled its initial promise as a simple screening test for suspected motility disorders.

PROVOCATIVE TESTS

The majority of patients with spastic motility disorders are asymptomatic at the time of diagnosis. Therefore, one cannot be certain that the esophagus is the source of their pain. Hence, a number of physical and pharmacologic means have been tried to induce chest pain and abnormal motility. Intravenous ergonovine produces increased esophageal contractions and reproduces chest pain, but the risk of undesirable cardiac side effects has limited its routine use in the esophageal laboratory.[214,228,229,271] Intravenous edrophonium chloride (Tensilon) has emerged as the most popular and potentially most helpful pharmacologic test for esophageal chest pain. Recent experience with edrophonium has indicated a positivity rate (defined as reproduction of the patient's chest pain) of 24% in one large series using a dose of 80 μg/kg[227] and a positivity rate of 40% in another study using a dose of 10 mg.[272] Unfortunately, the changes in esophageal contractile activity after edrophonium have not predictably distinguished patients with chest pain from healthy subjects.[227,272,273] Furthermore, a positive Tensilon response can occur in patients with reflux esophagitis.[274] A recent report indicated that an exceptionally high positive response can be obtained using repeated large doses of bethanechol. In a study of 87 patients with noncardiac chest pain, 77% were found to have reproduction of their atypical chest pain after two subcutaneous injections of bethanechol (50 μg/kg) separated by 15 minutes. However, over half of these patients experienced troubling side effects during the testing procedure.[226]

Other innovative provocative tests have included inflation of a balloon in the esophagus and measurements of motility during food ingestion. We found that balloon distention produced chest pain in 18 of 30 (60%) noncardiac chest pain patients, but in only 6 of 30 (20%) healthy volunteers.[242] Balloon pressures and esophageal contractions did not distinguish chest pain patients from control subjects. Allen et al observed that food ingestion frequently brought out dysphagia and esophageal motility disorders missed by standard manometry. In a study of 77 patients, dysphagia occurred during food ingestion alone in 36 patients versus 6 patients with water swallows alone. In addition, all but six of the patients with food-provoked dysphagia had motility abnormalities seen within 10 seconds of reporting their symptoms.[275] Unfortunately, food ingestion has not helped in the evaluation of suspected esophageal chest pain.

24-HOUR AMBULATORY PH/MOTILITY TESTING

Patients with spastic motility disorders may concurrently have gastroesophageal reflux disease or acid reflux can be the primary

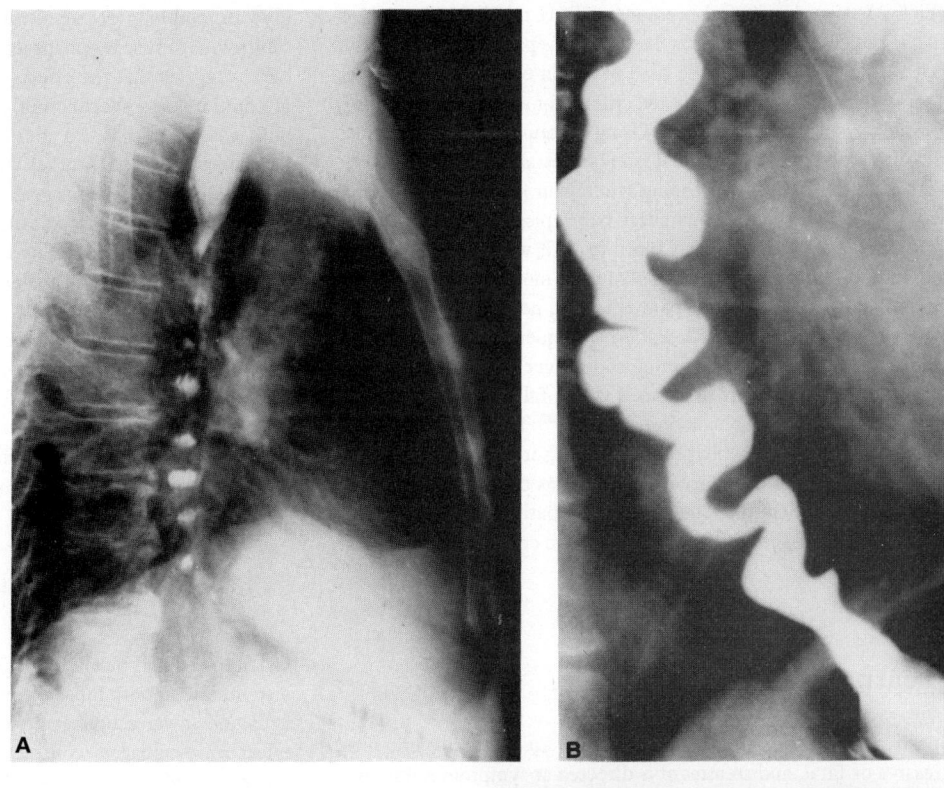

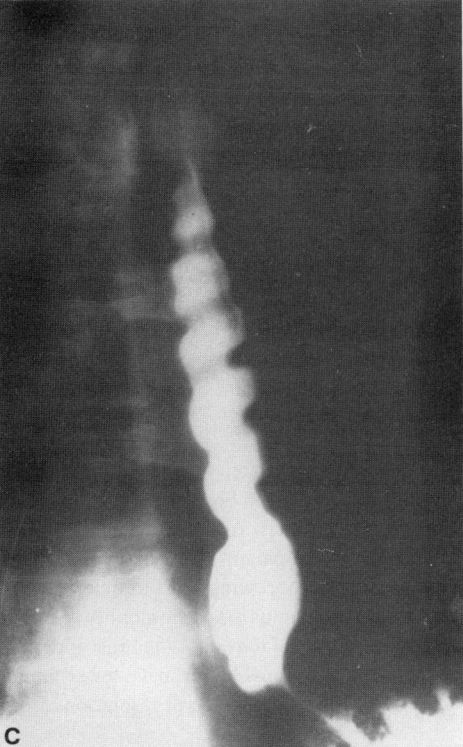

FIGURE 54–16. Barium esophagograms in patients with diffuse esophageal spasm revealing, **A,** segmentation of the barium column illustrating the "rosary bead esophagus," **B,** marked tortuosity forming "pseudo-diverticula," and, **C,** the extreme abnormalities producing the "corkscrew" esophagus. (Courtesy DO Castell, MD.)

cause of their motility disorders.[265] Because these patients usually have normal endoscopic examinations, 24-hour esophageal pH monitoring is the best diagnostic test to identify confidently abnormal acid reflux and its relationship to symptoms.

The critical test for evaluating patients with recurrent chest pain should be the identification of abnormal motility at the time of spontaneous pain events. The technology for ambulatory intraesophageal pressure monitoring has lagged behind pH monitoring but is emerging as a research tool. Janssens et al originally reported a group of 60 patients with noncardiac chest pain in which 24-hour esophageal pressure and pH monitoring revealed that 21 patients had an abnormal esophageal episode (38% motility, 19% reflux, 43% both) at the time of a pain event.[276] This report is somewhat confusing because the criteria for an abnormal motility episode were not clearly defined. Using a requirement for abnormal pressure based on an individual standard established for each patient from the 24-hour recording while pain free, we have found that 12% of 92 spontaneous chest pain episodes in 24 patients were associated with abnormal motility, 20% with reflux episodes, and an additional 4% with both abnormal motility and reflux. In the remaining 64% of chest pain episodes, no esophageal abnormalities could be identified. Patients frequently were found to experience multiple chest pain episodes over the 24-hour study, only some of which were associated with a fall in intraesophageal pH or an abnormal contraction pattern.[237] These early reports suggest that spastic esophageal motility disorders may not be as common a cause of esophageal chest pain as previously reported. Furthermore, the complex nature of these patients chest pain may account for their generally poor response to conventional medical therapies.

Treatment

Spastic disorders of the distal esophagus are generally not progressive or fatal, and treatment is directed at symptom reduction. Satisfactory therapy has been difficult for several reasons, including frequent uncertainties about the specific diagnosis, the availability of numerous therapies that have important side effects, the intermittent nature of the symptoms, and the evolving concept that many patients improve over time without the need for aggressive therapy.

Information gathered by ambulatory pH monitoring shows that gastroesophageal reflux is an important consideration in these patients. A trial of good antireflux therapy should be used for 1 to 2 months if evidence suggests this diagnosis. This is particularly important because many therapies aimed at decreasing esophageal contraction pressures may exacerbate reflux.

REASSURANCE

The most important step in patients with chest pain and spastic motility disorders is to be as certain as possible of its distinction from angina pectoris. A simple explanation of the phenomenon often relieves the patient who has been sure that the doctor has been missing or concealing heart trouble. In turn, relief of anxiety cuts down the stimulus to spastic motility disorders, which is closely related to emotional tension. When this approach is used, patients accept their symptoms better, have fewer limitations in lifestyle, and often have a diminution or resolution of their chest pain.[277]

NITRATES, ANTICHOLINERGICS, AND HYDRALAZINE

The rationale for using these drugs in treating spastic esophageal motility disorders relates to their ability to relax smooth muscle. Symptomatic improvement and a manometric response to nitro-

glycerin and long-acting nitrate agents have been reported in patients with diffuse esophageal spasm.[278] A more recent study, however, suggests that the effects of nitrates on esophageal pressures are minimal and short acting.[279] No controlled studies of patients with spastic esophageal motility disorders treated with nitrates have been reported. Studies with oral anticholinergic agents have shown decreased esophageal pressure in healthy adults,[280] but studies of patients with painful esophageal motility disorders have not been done. Although hydralazine does not affect the resting contraction pressures in the esophageal body, one study reported decreased pressure responses to cholinergic stimulation with bethanechol. In a limited uncontrolled experience in three patients with spastic motility disorders, regular administration of hydralazine (75–200 mg/day) was felt to produce a meaningful degree of symptom improvement.[281] Although clinical experience with these drugs is often disappointing, the individual patient should be given a trial of one of these agents because it might be effective.

CALCIUM CHANNEL BLOCKING AGENTS

Calcium channel blocking drugs (diltiazem, nifedipine, verapamil) also inhibit smooth muscle contractions in the body of the esophagus and lower esophageal sphincter. A dramatic dose–response effect on esophageal contraction pressure in patients with nutcracker esophagus has been shown with nifedipine therapy (10–30 mg orally).[282] Diltiazem therapy also decreases the amplitude and duration of peristaltic contraction in these patients, but changes were observed only with the highest tested dose (150 mg orally).[283] Recent double-blind, placebo-controlled studies with calcium blockers have been disappointing. Despite its more dramatic effect on esophageal pressures, nifedipine (10–30 mg, tid) was not superior to placebo in improving the overall pain response in 20 patients with nutcracker esophagus.[258] Similar results were found in eight patients with diffuse esophageal spasm.[283] The findings of preliminary studies with diltiazem therapy have been conflicting.[284,285] These studies indicate that decreases in esophageal pressures may not correlate with pain relief. Calcium channel blocking agents may be useful in treating patients with these disorders but need to be combined with other therapies or used to treat patients with pain episodes that clearly occur simultaneously with abnormal esophageal contractions.

PSYCHOTROPIC DRUGS AND BEHAVIOR THERAPY

Anecdotal reports have suggested that anxiolytic or antidepressant agents may effectively treat patients with symptomatic esophageal motility disorders clearly produced by stress. A recent double-blind, placebo-controlled study supports these observations.[286] Low doses of the antidepressant trazodone hydrochloride (Desyrel 100–150 mg/day) produced global improvement and reduced distress from esophageal symptoms. The overall improvement was not dependent on any change in manometric pattern during the course of the study. Successful management of symptoms associated with spastic motility disorders also have been reported using behavioral modification programs and biofeedback.[287,288]

ESOPHAGEAL DILATATION

Clinical experience has suggested that passing a large mercury-filled dilator may promote transient relief from dysphagia or chest pain in selected patients with spastic motility disorders. We found such bougie dilatation produces some relief of symptoms, but similar responses can be produced with either a large dilator (54 Fr) or a much smaller placebo dilator (24 Fr).[289]

Pneumatic dilatation has been used in severely symptomatic patients with diffuse esophageal spasm, especially when dysphagia is the predominant symptom.[199,290] In this situation, one may be treating an early transition phase of diffuse esophageal spasm into achalasia. In one large series, only 45% of the patients noted relief, in contrast to response rates of 80% in achalasia.[199] Patients with hypertensive lower esophageal sphincter pressure also have rarely been treated with pneumatic dilatation.[290] I reserve this therapy for patients with intractable symptoms in whom a delay in distal esophageal emptying can be documented.

ESOPHAGOMYOTOMY

When dysphagia becomes so severe that weight loss is noted or when pain becomes unbearable, surgical relief should be considered. This consists of a Heller myotomy across the lower esophageal sphincter with proximal extension of the incision to include the involved area of spasm. Success rates exceeding 50% have been reported, although results are better for patients with severe dysphagia than chest pain.[259] The author has not personally referred a patient for long myotomy. However, I have seen several patients who have undergone myotomy without relief of their symptoms. Charles Pope has suggested that myotomy for spastic esophageal motility disorders be reserved for patients in whom manometry has documented abnormal motor activity during an attack of pain.[66] Although a difficult requirement to fulfill, I believe this cautious approach is warranted. As DeMeester emphasizes, "the creation of a defect to correct a defect can never restore the function of a organ to normal."[291]

Spastic Motility Disorders— Part of a Spectrum of Diseases?

In 1967, a single case report indicated that an occasional patient showing the syndrome of diffuse esophageal spasm might eventually make a transition to classic achalasia.[292] A subsequent report by Vantrappen and colleagues indicated this was not an isolated phenomenon because 6 of 156 patients were observed to undergo this transition over a period of a few months or years.[140] Subsequently, isolated cases of patients with nutcracker esophagus evolving to diffuse esophageal spasm and even achalasia have been reported.[254,293] These patients present initially with a combination of chest pain and dysphagia. This transition to achalasia is heralded clinically by the loss of the chest pain component while the dysphagia may worsen. At that stage, the patient has definite achalasia, and the treatment should proceed as indicated. This phenomenon is probably not becoming more common but is being increasingly recognized as the result of easier availability of esophageal motility laboratories and the greater opportunity for follow-up of patients

with spastic motility disorders. Whether these observations represent a chance occurrence or a true spectrum of motility dysfunction cannot be established yet.

ESOPHAGEAL MOTILITY DISORDERS ASSOCIATED WITH SYSTEMIC DISEASES

Collagen Vascular Diseases

SCLERODERMA

Of all the generalized diseases producing esophageal motility abnormalities, scleroderma is the best characterized. Scleroderma is a diffuse disease involving fibrosis and degenerative changes in the skin, synovium, and parenchyma of certain organs, notably the heart, kidneys, lungs, intestines, and esophagus. Two forms of the generalized disease exist: progressive systemic sclerosis with diffuse scleroderma (a more fulminant form with early appearance of disease in various internal organs) and the CREST (calcinosis, Raynaud's phenomenon, esophageal dysfunction, sclerodactyly, telangiectasia) syndrome. Regardless of the form, the esophagus is involved in approximately 75% to 85% of all patients with scleroderma, by either manometric or radiographic criteria.[294,295] The patients tend to be middle-aged, 30 to 50 years old, and are more often women and white, which is a general reflection of the prevalence of scleroderma.

The basic pathologic process of scleroderma is primarily atrophy of the smooth muscle with subsequent replacement and fibrosis of the submucosa and muscularis. In the esophagus, pathologic changes are confined to the lower two thirds (the smooth muscle portion) of the esophagus, giving rise to diminished to absent muscle contractions in the distal esophagus and incompetency of the lower esophageal sphincter.[296] In some scleroderma patients, the esophageal muscle may still be responsive to cholinergic stimulation, suggesting that neural dysfunction has preceded muscle atrophy and fibrosis.[296] However, a distinct neuropathologic lesion has not been described in the esophagus or other parts of the gut. Perhaps more refined histochemical and electron microscopic studies may resolve these inconsistent findings.

The clinical manifestations of scleroderma are those of dysphagia and heartburn. Symptomatic patients usually have Raynaud's phenomenon, but the severity of the esophageal disease does not coincide with skin changes or other systemic manifestations of scleroderma.[297] Although the degree of motility dysfunction often is profound, the symptoms of heartburn or dysphagia may be found in less than 50% of patients, suggesting some impairment in sensory function.[298] Gastroesophageal reflux disease may be severe because of the loss of lower esophageal sphincter competency in conjunction with poor esophageal clearance. The prevalence of erosive esophagitis may be as high as 60%, with some patients developing Barrett's esophagus and subsequent adenocarcinoma.[299,300] Invariably, patients with esophagitis are those with underlying esophageal motility disorders from their scleroderma.[299] Dysphagia may result from the motor disturbance itself

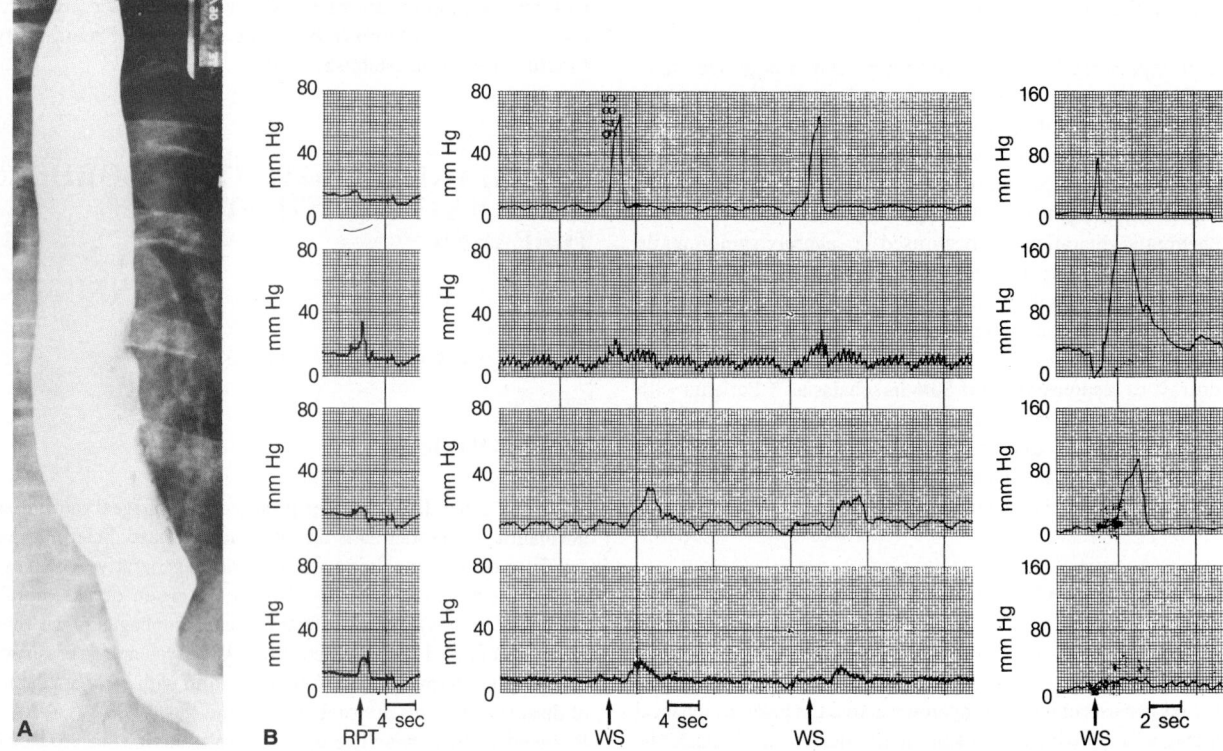

FIGURE 54–17. Scleroderma esophagus. **A,** Barium esophagogram reveals a dilated esophagus with aperistalsis of the distal smooth muscle portion. The esophagogastric junction is patulous with free gastroesophageal reflux. **B,** Esophageal manometry of the same patient. On the left, a rapid pull-through (RPT) across the lower esophageal sphincter reveals low sphincter pressure. In the center, the four recording sites are located at 5-cm intervals from proximal to distal (top to bottom of figure) in the body of the esophagus. Weak peristaltic contractions are seen with each of two wet swallows (WS) in the smooth muscle portion of the esophagus with a much stronger contraction in the single recording site located in the proximal (striated muscle) esophagus. On the right, normal contraction pressures are seen in the pharynx, upper esophageal sphincter, and upper esophagus (top three recording sites) with the low contraction pressure seen in the distal recording site located in the smooth muscle portion of the esophagus.

or from a stricture complicating reflux. Some patients may have dysphagia and odynophagia from *Candida* esophagitis.[299]

Radiographic examination of the esophagus characteristically shows a dilated esophagus with aperistalsis involving the distal smooth muscle portion. As long as the patient is standing, esophageal emptying is normal, but when the patient lies down, barium remains for hours in the esophagus. A hiatal hernia may be seen, and the lower esophageal sphincter is patulous with free gastroesophageal reflux (Fig 54-17A). This common cavity phenomenon may result in the esophagus containing air in the resting state. Radiologic changes or erosive esophagitis is common, and nearly one third of patients may have peptic strictures.[299] Wide mouth diverticula of the esophagus, similar to those described in the colon of scleroderma patients, also has been seen.[301]

Esophageal manometric abnormalities are present in approximately 75% of patients with scleroderma.[294,295] The characteristic features include low to absent lower esophageal sphincter pressure, weak to absent distal esophageal peristalsis, and normal upper esophageal peristalsis and sphincter pressure (see Fig 54-17B). Usually, dysfunction in the esophageal body becomes evident before the loss of lower sphincter tone,[302] and reduction in contraction strength precedes aperistalsis that is seen with advanced involvement.[303] However, any and all combinations of dysfunction in the distal body and sphincter have been reported in patients with scleroderma. Although characteristic of scleroderma, these manometric abnormalities are not specific because less than 40% of patients identified in a motility laboratory with these findings have any evidence of connective tissue diseases.[304] Manometry appears to be more sensitive than radiography for detecting early esophageal involvement by scleroderma.[295] Radionuclide transit studies correlate well with manometry in scleroderma, and these tests may be useful in staging the disease.[305]

There is no effective treatment for the patient whose esophagus is involved by scleroderma. Gastroesophageal reflux should be identified and aggressively treated with acid-suppressing drugs, particularly the H_2 antagonists.[306] Dysphagia without stricture may improve with treatment of reflux esophagitis. Stricture formation seems to be more insidious in scleroderma patients and may require frequent bougie dilatation therapy. In particularly severe cases of intractable esophagitis, antireflux surgery may be required. Although a fundoplication may be done, it should be "loose" or of the 270-degree variety so as to minimize problems with postoperative dysphagia.

MIXED CONNECTIVE TISSUE DISEASE

This disorder represents a mixture of clinical features found in scleroderma, polymyositis, and systemic lupus erythematosus, and is noted by the presence of high titers of a circulating antibody for a nuclear ribonucleoprotein antigen. More than 60% of patients have esophageal involvement defined by cineradiography.[307] Manometric abnormalities may be even more common, having been reported in up to 82% of mixed connective tissue disease patients.[308] Abnormalities of both smooth and skeletal muscle are common. In the largest report to date,[308] 5 of 17 patients had motility patterns consistent with scleroderma while 10 patients had diffuse aperistalsis of the esophageal body and low pressures in both the upper and lower sphincters. Although this latter motility abnormality has rarely been reported in other connective tissue disorders, its presence strongly suggests the diagnosis of mixed connective tissue disease. Some have reported improvement of the motility abnormalities with steroid therapy,[307] but these therapeutic changes have been disputed by others.[308]

OTHER COLLAGEN VASCULAR DISEASES

Esophageal symptoms are not common in systemic lupus erythematosus, although 25% to 35% of unselected patients have manometric abnormalities.[303,308,309] These findings appear to be a combination of the abnormalities seen in scleroderma and polymyositis with decreased upper and lower esophageal peristalsis and lower esophageal sphincter pressure. Findings consistent with diffuse esophageal spasm have also been described in one report.[310] Rheumatoid arthritis does not usually produce major esophageal symptoms. Manometric abnormalities that have been reported are rather mild, with only a decrease in esophageal peristaltic amplitude being noted in 30% of patients in one study.[311] Over 50% of patients with primary Sjögren's syndrome may complain of dysphagia. One study using dry swallows described decreased upper esophageal peristalsis in nine of ten patients.[312] However, another study using wet swallows found esophageal dysfunction in only 36% of 22 patients.[313] Because this disease is characterized by diminished lacrimal and salivary gland secretions, these patients' complaints of dysphagia are more likely secondary to a lack of saliva, making solid bolus passage difficult, rather than minor motility abnormalities.

Endocrine and Metabolic Disorders

DIABETES MELLITUS

Abnormalities in esophageal motility are frequently detected in patients with diabetes mellitus when they are studied by either radiography or manometry. More than 60% of diabetic patients with evidence of peripheral or autonomic neuropathy may have disordered esophageal motility,[314] but recent studies suggest that male diabetics without neuropathic changes may also have dysmotility.[315] The clinical significance of these abnormalities is uncertain because most of these patients are asymptomatic.[314] Histologic and pharmacologic studies suggest that the esophageal abnormalities are secondary to the degenerative effects of diabetes mellitus on the autonomic nervous system, rather than smooth muscle dysfunction. However, in one study, contraction abnormalities correlated with the presence of psychiatric disturbances but not with neuropathy,[316] a finding similar to observations in nondiabetic subjects with esophageal spasm symptoms.

The manometric abnormalities in diabetic patients include combinations of any of the following: decrease in the amplitude of peristalsis, decreased number of nontransmitted peristaltic waves, decreased lower esophageal sphincter pressure with impaired relaxation after swallowing, simultaneous contractions, and repetitive contractions.[314,317,318] When severe, these abnormalities can be identical to those of diffuse esophageal spasm. More recently, increased frequency of peristaltic double-peaked contractions has been reported in diabetics with peripheral neuropathy.[319] Pharmacologic responses to edrophonium and atropine suggest a possible increased cholinergic tone as the basis of these double-peaked contractions. The significance of this finding remains to be determined, because double-peaked waves do occur in normals,[213] and the high incidence of these contractions (greater than 95% of all peristaltic swallows) noted in this group of diabetics has not been confirmed by other manometric studies.[314,317,318]

THYROID DISEASES

Thyroid hormones may play a physiologic role in the control of esophageal motor function. An increase in the velocity of esophageal peristalsis has been described in 15 patients with Graves' disease, which reverted to normal with treatment.[320] All the patients were free of symptoms. Diffuse esophageal spasm has also been described in one patient with thyrotoxic myopathy.[321] With myxedema, on the other hand, dysphagia may be a common complaint, and, in fact, a decrease in the amplitude and velocity of peristaltic contractions and primary peristalsis have been noted in one group of patients studied.[322] Other case reports have noted a decrease in lower esophageal sphincter pressure and incomplete relaxation of the upper esophageal sphincter.[62] All these abnormalities revert to normal with thyroid replenishment.

AMYLOIDOSIS

Manometric abnormalities associated with amyloidosis include a decrease in lower esophageal sphincter pressure, a decrease in both upper and lower esophageal peristaltic amplitude, simultaneous contractions, and even an achalasialike picture.[323,324] In the largest series reported, greater than 60% of patients with systemic amyloidosis had esophageal manometric abnormalities.[324] These derangements have been attributed to random deposition of amyloid in muscle and possibly the nerves of the esophagus.[324,325] Similar manometric findings have also been noted in familial amyloid polyneuropathy.[326]

Alcohol and the Esophagus

Acutely, the oral ingestion of small quantities of alcohol sufficient to raise blood alcohol level to 110 mg/dl is associated with a minimal fall in the amplitude of peristaltic waves and no change in resting lower esophageal sphincter pressures.[327] The acute administration of intoxicating amounts of ethanol by the oral or intravenous route cause a decrease in the amplitude of peristaltic contractions and lower esophageal sphincter pressure, decreased primary peristalsis, and frequent simultaneous contractions.[328] These changes vanish within 8 to 24 hours of alcohol cessation.

In chronic alcoholics with peripheral neuropathy, a diminution of primary peristalsis with corresponding increase in nonperistaltic contractions has been reported in the distal esophagus.[329] Secondary peristalsis (the response to balloon distention) is also lost in these patients.[329] Studies in long-term alcoholics without neuropathy do not reveal these defects. Patients undergoing acute alcohol withdrawal may have marked elevation of lower esophageal sphincter pressures as well as amplitude of peristaltic contractions in the distal esophagus.[236] These hypertensive changes return to normal within 30 days of alcohol abstinence. The motility disorders associated with chronic alcoholism usually do not produce symptoms.

Gastroesophageal Reflux Disease

Acid reflux may produce esophageal motility disorders independent of the presence of esophagitis or strictures. In one report using long-term esophageal pH and pressure monitoring, one third of patients with chest pain and normal endoscopy had reflux-associated abnormal motility.[276] Patients with esophagitis may have manometric changes resembling diffuse esophageal spasm. These patients' symptoms worsen with nitrates and improve with antireflux therapy.[265] In a recent study of 177 patients with gastroesophageal reflux disease, a subset had abnormal esophageal peristalsis with decreased incidence of complete peristaltic sequences after swallowing, hypotensive peristaltic waves, or impaired responses to esophageal distention.[330] The prevalence of impaired peristaltic function increased with the more severe forms of esophagitis. For example, 3% of patients with normal endoscopic examination, 11% with mild esophagitis, and 30% with severe esophagitis had intermittent failure of the normal peristaltic sequence. Amplitude of peristaltic contractions and lower esophageal sphincter pressure also was inversely related to the severity of gastroesophageal reflux disease. Likewise, esophageal motility abnormalities may be present in up to 50% of patients with peptic strictures[331] and 40% of patients with Barrett's esophagus.[332] Whether these motility abnormalities predate the esophagitis or are secondary to acid injury is controversial. Animal studies suggest that acid-induced esophagitis may produce decreased lower esophageal sphincter pressures and contraction abnormalities of the distal esophagus.[333] These motility abnormalities resolve with healing of the esophagitis. However, these are acute studies and may not reflect the chronic effects of acid reflux seen in humans. In support of this fact, patients studied with erosive esophagitis show no improvement in esophageal motor function after healing of esophagitis.[334]

The Esophagus and Aging

Based on radiographic and manometric studies performed in the early 1960s, it was initially felt that the aging process produced certain patterns of esophageal dysfunction. These studies in patients over the age of 90 years demonstrated decreased primary peristalsis, decreased lower esophageal sphincter relaxation, and an increase in spontaneous contractions.[335,336] The presence and severity of symptoms correlated poorly with these motility abnormalities. However, patients with systemic diseases such as diabetes mellitus or other neurologic disorders were not usually excluded from these early studies.

More recently, a study of patients over the age of 70 years, carefully screened to rule out diabetes or nervous system abnormalities, has revealed quite different results.[337] In these otherwise healthy elderly subjects ranging in age from 71 to 87 years, the incidence of abnormal esophageal motility was no greater than that found in a control group of healthy young subjects. The only abnormality found was a significant decrease in the amplitude of esophageal peristalsis in the elderly group, particularly in those over 80 years of age. Using similar patients, other groups have reported that motility disturbances, consisting primarily of decreased peristaltic amplitude and a slight decrease in the frequency of primary peristalsis, were uncommon.[338,339] Taken as a whole, it would appear that the main effect of age on esophageal function is a mild decrease in the amplitude or force of the esophageal contractions. Severe motility abnormalities when encountered in the elderly are more often due to systemic diseases rather than to the aging process. Therefore, the term *presbyesophagus* should not be considered as a diagnostic entity.

> The reader is directed to Chapter 7, Esophageal Motor Function; Chapter 28, Approach to the Patient with Dysphagia; Chapter 29, Approach to the Patient with Chest Pain; Chapter 53, Esophagus: Anatomy and Structural Anomalies; Chapter 55, Reflux Esophagitis; Chapter 57, Esophageal Tumors; Chapter 111, Upper Gastrointestinal Endoscopy; Chapter 114, Contrast Radiology; and Chapter 128, Evaluation of Gastrointestinal Motility: Methodological Considerations.

REFERENCES

1. Sieben H, Trupe E, Siebens A, et al. Correlates and consequences of eating dependency in institutionalized elderly. J Am Geriatr Soc 1986;34:192.
2. Siebens AA. The cricopharyngeus. accessory muscle of respiration? John Hopkins Symposium, Baltimore, MD. February 28, 1986.
3. Kilman WJ, Goyal RK. Disorders of pharyngeal and upper esophageal sphincter motor function. Arch Intern Med 1976;136:592.
4. Brunner H. Cricopharyngeal muscle under normal and pathologic conditions. Arch Otolaryngol 1952;56:616.
5. Hunt PS, Connell AM, Smiley TB. The cricopharyngeal sphincter in gastric reflux. Gut 1970;11:303.
6. Watson WC, Sullivan SN. Hypertonicity of cricopharyngeal sphincter: Cause of globus sensation. Lancet 1984;2:1417.
7. Schobinger R. Spasm of the cricopharyngeal muscle as cause of dysphagia after total laryngectomy. Arch Otolaryngol 1958;67:271.
8. Gerhardt DC, Shuck TJ, Bordeaux RA, et al. Human upper esophageal sphincter: Response to volume, osmotic and acid stimuli. Gastroenterology 1978;75:268.
9. Thompson DG, Andreollo NA, McIntyre AS, et al. Studies of the oesophageal clearance responses to intraluminal acid. Gut 1988;29:881.
10. Andreollo NA, Thompson DG, Kendall GPN, et al. Functional relationships between cricopharyngeal sphincter and oesophageal body in response to graded intraluminal distension. Gut 1988;29:161.
11. Hollewell JD, Cole TB. Isolated head and neck symptoms due to hiatus hernia. Arch Otolaryngol 1970;92:499.
12. Lektinen V, Puhakka H. A psychosomatic approach to the globus hystericus syndrome. Acta Psychiatr Scand 1976;53:21.

13. Cook IJ, Dent J, Shannon S, et al. Measurement of upper esophageal sphincter pressure. Effect of acute emotional stress. Gastroenterology 1987;93:526.

14. Vantrappen G, Hellmans J. Diseases of the esophagus. New York: Springer-Verlag, 1974:399.

15. Welch RW, Luckman K, Ricks PM, et al. Manometry of the normal upper esophageal sphincter and its alterations in laryngectomy. J Clin Invest 1979;63:1036.

16. Gerhardt DC, Castell DO, Winship DH, et al. Esophageal dysfunction in esophagopharyngeal regurgitation. Gastroenterology 1980;78:893.

17. Benson PF. Transient dysphagia due to muscular incoordination. Proc R Soc Med 1962;55:237.

18. Macauley JC. Neuromuscular incoordination of swallowing in the newborn. Lancet 1951;1:1208.

19. Reichert TJ, Bluestone CD, Stool SE, et al. Congenital cricopharyngeal achalasia. Ann Otol Rhinol Laryngol 1977;86:603.

20. Bonanno PC. Swallowing dysfunction after tracheostomy. Ann Surg 1971;174:29.

21. Duranceau A, Jameson G, Hurwitz AL, et al. Alteration in esophageal motility after laryngectomy. Am J Surg 1976;131:30.

22. Litton WB, Leonard JR. Aspiration after partial laryngectomy. Cineradiographic studies. Laryngoscope 1969;79:877.

23. Cruse JP, Edwards DA, Smith JF, Wyllic JH. The pathology of cricopharyngeal dysphagia. Histopathology 1979;3:223.

24. Hanna W, Henderson RD. Nemaline rods in cricopharyngeal dysphagia. Am J Clin Pathol 1980;74:186.

25. Hurwitz AL, Nelson JA, Haddad JK. Oropharyngeal dysphagia: Manometric and cine esophagraphic findings. Am J Dig Dis 1975;20:313.

26. Marguiles SI, Brunt PW, Donner MW, et al. Familial dysautonomia: A cineradiographic study of the swallowing mechanism. Radiology 1968;90:107.

27. Riley CM. Familial dysautonomia. Adv Pediatr 1957;9:157.

28. Ardran GM, Kemp FA, Lund WS: The etiology of the posterior pharyngeal diverticulum: A cineradiographic study. J Laryngol Otol 1964;78:333.

29. Ellis FH Jr, Schlegel JF, Lynch VP, et al. Cricopharyngeal myotomy for pharyngoesophageal diverticulum. Ann Surg 1969;170:340.

30. Kopicek J, Creamer B. A study of pharyngeal pouches. J Laryngol Otol 1961;75:406.4

31. Knuff TE, Benjamin SB, Castell DO. Pharyngoesophageal (Zenker's) diverticulum: A reappraisal. Gastroenterology 1982;82:734.

32. Duranceau A, Rheault MJ, Jamieson GG. Physiologic response to cricopharyngeal myotomy and diverticulum suspension. Surgery 1983;94:655.

33. Veis SL, Logemann JA. Swallowing disorders in persons with cerebrovascular accident. Arch Phys Med Rehabil 1985;66:372.

34. Gordon C, Hewer RL, Wade DT. Dysphagia in acute stroke. Br Med J 1987;295:411.

35. Silbiger ML, Pikielney R, Donner MW. Neuromuscular disorders affecting the pharynx: Cineradiographic analysis. Invest Radiol 1967;2:442.

36. Fischer RA, Ellison GW, Thayer WR, Spiro HM, Galser GH. Esophageal motility in neuromuscular disorders. Ann Intern Med 1965;63:229.

37. Serebro HA, Mieny CJ, Webster A, Jackson H. Oesophageal manometric studies of dysphagia in Vernet's syndrome. Br J Surg 1971;58:461.

38. Christie AC. The roentgen findings in chronic progressive bulbar palsy. Am J Roentgen 1932;27:71.

39. Mills CP. Dysphagia in pharyngeal paralysis treated by cricopharyngeal sphincterotomy. Lancet 1973;1:455.

40. Bosma JF. Residual disability of pharyngeal area resulting from poliomyelitis: Clinical management of patients. JAMA 1957;165:216.

41. Faber HK, Silverberg RJ. A neuropathological study of acute human poliomyelitis with special reference to the initial lesion and to various portals of entry. J Exp Med 1966;83:329.

42. Duranceau A, Lafontaine ER, Taillefer R, et al. Oropharyngeal dysphagia and operations on the upper esophageal sphincter. Surg Annu 1987;19:317.

43. Carpenter RJ, McDonald TJ, Howard FM. The otolaryngologic presentation of amyotrophic lateral sclerosis. Otolaryngology 1978;86:479.

44. Calne DB, Shaw DG, Spiers ASD, et al. Swallowing in parkinsonism. Br J Radiol 1970;43:456.

45. Cotzias GC, Papavasiliou PS, Gellene E. Modification of parkinonism—Chronic treatment with L-dopa. N Engl J Med 1969;280:337.

46. Daly DD, Code CF, Anderson HA. Disturbances of swallowing and esophageal motility in patients with multiple sclerosis. Neurology 1962;12:250.

47. Bradley WG. Inflammatory diseases of muscle. In: Kelley WM, Harris ED Jr, eds. Textbook of rheumatology. Philadelphia: WB Saunders, 1985:1225

48. Jacob H, Berkowitz D, McDonald E, et al. The esophageal motility disorder of polymyositis. A prospective study. Arch Intern Med 1983;143:2262.

49. Scobey MW. Secondary motility disorders. In: Castell DO, Richter JE, Dalton CB, eds. Esophageal motility testing. Amsterdam: Elsevier, 1987:163.

50. Horowitz M, McNeil JD, Maddern GJ, Collins PJ, Shearman DJ. Abnormalities of gastric and esophageal emptying in polymyositis and dermatomyositis. Gastroenterology 1986;90:434.

51. Eckardt VF, Nix W, Kraus W, et al. Esophageal motor function in patients with muscular dystrophy. Gastroenterology 1986;90:628.

52. Garrett JM, Dubose TD, Jackson JE, et al. Esophageal and pulmonary disturbances in myotonia dystrophica. Arch Intern Med 1969;123:26.

53. Siegel CI, Hendrix TR, Harvey JC. The swallowing disorder in myotonia dystrophica. Gastroenterology 1966;50:541.

54. Casey EB. Dystrophica myotonica presenting with dysphagia. Br Med J 1971;2:443.

55. Leach W. Generalized muscular weakness presenting as pharyngeal dysphagia. J Laryngol Otol 1962;76:237.

56. Murphy SF, Drachman DB. The oculopharyngeal syndrome. JAMA 1968;203:1003.

57. Szobor A. Data on the oculopharyngeal syndrome. A clinico-pathological study. Eur Neurol 1973;9:242.

58. Bender MD. Esophageal manometry in oculopharyngeal dystrophy. Am J Gastroenterol 1972;62:215.

59. Kramer P, Atkinson M, Wyman SM, et al. The dynamics of swallowing: II. Neuromuscular dysphagia of pharynx. J Clin Invest 1957;36:589.

60. Huang M-H, King K-L, Chien K-Y. Esophageal manometric studies in patients with myasthenia gravis. J Thorac Cardiovasc Surg 1988;95:281.

61. Ellis FH. Upper esophageal sphincter in health and disease. Surg Clin North Am 1971;51:553.

62. Wright RA, Penner DB. Myxedema and upper esophageal dysmotility. Dig Dis Sci 1981;26:376.

63. Ramirez-Mata M, Reyes PA, Alarcon-Segovia D, et al. Esophageal motility in systemic lupus erythematosus. Am J Dig Dis 1974;19:132.

64. Sulway MJ, Baume PE, David E. Stiff-man syndrome presenting with complete esophageal obstruction. Am J Dig Dis 1970;15:79.

65. Edwards DAW. Discriminatory value of symptoms in the differential diagnosis of dysphagia. Clin Gastroenterol 1976;5:49.

66. Pope CE II. Symptoms of esophageal disease. In: Sleisenger MH, Fordtran JS, eds. Gastrointestinal disease, ed 2. Philadelphia: WB Saunders, 1978:196.

67. Jones B, Kramer SS, Donnner MW. Dynamic imaging of the pharynx. Gastrointest Radiol 1985;10:213.

68. Donner MW. Swallowing mechanisms and neuromuscular disorders. Semin Roentgen 1974;9:273.

69. Ekberg O, Nylander G. Cineradiography of the pharyngeal stage of deglutition in 250 patients with dysphagia. Br J Radiol 1982;55:258.

70. Ekberg O, Nylander G. Cineradiography in 45 patients with acute dysphagia. Gastrointest Radiol 1983;8:295.

71. Torres WE, Clements JL, Austin GE, et al. Cricopharyngeal muscle hypertrophy: Radiologic anatomic correlation. Am J Roentgen 1984;141:927.

72. Curtis DJ, Cruess DF, Berg T. The cricopharyngeal muscles: A video-recording review. Am J Roentgen 1984;142:497.

73. Curtis DJ, Creuss DF, Dachman AH. Normal erect swallowing. Normal function and incidence of variations. Invest Radiol 1985;20:717.

74. Arndorfer RC, Stef JJ, Dodds WJ, et al. Improved infusion system

for intraluminal esophageal manometry. Gastroenterology 1977;73:23.

75. Orlowski J, Dodds WJ, Linehan JH, et al. Requirements for accurate manometric recording of pharyngeal and esophageal peristaltic pressure waves. Invest Radiol 1982;17:567.

76. Green WER, Castell JA, Castell DO. Upper esophageal sphincter pressure recording: Is an oval manometry catheter necessary? Dysphagia 1988;2:162.

77. Hellmans J, Agg HO, Pelemans W, et al. Pharyngoesophageal swallowing disorders and the pharyngoesophageal sphincter. Med Clin North Am 1981;65:1149.

78. Kahrilas PJ, Dent J, Dodds WJ, et al. A method for continuous monitoring of upper esophageal sphincter pressure. Dig Dis Sci 1987;32:121.

79. Kahrilas PJ, Dodds WJ, Dent J, et al. Upper esophageal sphincter function during deglutition. Gastroenterology 1988;95:52.

80. Castell JA, Dalton CB, Castell DO. Pharyngeal and upper esophageal sphincter manometry in humans. Am J Physiol 1991;258:G173.

81. Dodds WJ, Kahrilas PJ, Dent J, et al. Considerations about pharyngeal manometry. Dysphagia 1986;1;209.

82. Castell JA. The computer in the motility laboratory. In: Castell DO, Richter JE, Dalton CB, eds. Esophageal motility testing. Amsterdam: Elsevier, 1987;91.

83. Hutwitz AL, Duranceau A. Upper esophageal sphincter dysfunction—Pathogenesis and treatment. Dig Dis Sci 1978;23:275.

84. Lazzara G, Lazarus C, Logemann JA. Impact of thermal stimulation on the triggering of the swallowing reflex. Dysphagia 1986;1:73.

85. Duranceau A, Forand MD, Fateux JP. Surgery in oculopharyngeal muscular dystrophy. Am J Surg 1980;139:33.

86. Blakeley WR, Garety EJ, Smith DE. Section of the cricopharyngeus muscle for dysphagia. Arch Surg 1968;96:745.

87. Welsh GF, Payne WS. The present status of one-stage pharyngoesophageal diverticulectomy. Surg Clin North Am 1973;53:953.

88. Payne WS, King RM. Pharyngoesophageal (Zenker's) diverticulum. Surg Clin North Am 1983;63:815.

89. Willis T. Pharmaceutice rationalis sive diatribe de medicamentorum operationibus in human corpore. London, Hagae-Comitis: A Leers, 1974

90. Von Mikuliczi R. J Zur Pathologie and Therupic des Cardiospasms. Dtsch Med Wochenschr 1904;30:17.

91. Lendrum FC. Anatomic features of the cardiac orifice of the stomach with special reference to cardiospasm. Arch Intern Med 1937;59:474.

92. Kahrilas PJ, Kishle SM, Helm JF, et al. Comparison of pseudoachalasia and achalasia. Am J Med 1987;82:439.

93. Berquist WE, Byrne WJ, Ament ME, et al. Achalasia: Diagnosis, management, and clinical course in 16 children. Pediatrics 1983;71:798.

94. Stein DT, Knauer CM. Achalasia in monozygotic twins. Dig Dis Sci 1982;27:636.

95. Bosher LP, Shaw A. Achalasia in siblings. Clinical and genetic aspects. Am J Dis Child 1981;135:709.

96. Freiling T, Berges W, Borchard F, et al. Family occurrence of achalasia and diffuse spasm of the oesophagus. Gut 1988;29:1595.

97. Eckrich JD, Winans CS. Discordance for achalasia in identical twins. Dig Dis Sci 1979;24:221.

98. Mayberry JF, Atkinson M. A study of swallowing difficulties in first degree relatives of patients with achalasia. Thorax 1985;40:391.

99. Mayberry JF, Atkinson M. Variations in the prevalence of achalasia in Great Britain and Ireland: An epidemiological study based on hospital admissions. Q J Med 1987;237:67.

100. Earlnam RJ, Ellis FH, Nobrega FT. Achalasia of the esophagus in a small urban community. Mayo Clin Proc 1969;44:478.

101. Golen EA, Switz DM, Zfass AM. Achalasia: Incidence and treatment in Virginia. Va Med 1982;109:183.

102. Stein CM, Gelfand M, Taylor HG. Achalasia in Zimbabwean blacks. S Afr Med J 1985;67:261.

103. Mayberry JF, Atkinson M. A studies of incidence and prevalence of achalasia in the Nottingham area. Q J Med 1985;56:451.

104. Cassella RR, Brown AL Jr, Sayre GP, Ellis F Jr. Achalasia of the esophagus: Pathologic and etiologic considerations. Ann Surg 1964;160:474.

105. Csendes A, Smok G, Braghetto I, et al. Gastroesophageal sphincter pressure and histologic changes in the distal esophagus in patients with achalasia of the esophagus. Dig Dis Sci 1985;30:941.

106. Qualman SJ, Haupt AM, Yang P, Hamilton SR. Esophageal Lewy bodies associated with ganglion cell loss in achalasia. Similarity to Parkinson's disease. Gastroenterology 1984;87:848.

107. Aggestrup S, Uddman R, Sundler F, et al. Lack of vasoactive intestinal peptide nerves in esophageal achalasia. Gastroenterology 1983;84:924.

108. Cassella RR, Ellis FH Jr, Brown AL Jr. Fine-structure changes in achalasia of the esophagus. I. Vagus nerves. Am J Pathol 1965;46:279.

109. Wollam GL, Maker FT, Ellis FH Jr. Vagal nerve function in achalasia of the esophagus. Surg Forum 1967;18:362.

110. Dooley CP, Taylor IL, Valenzuela JE. Impaired acid secretion and pancreatic polypeptide release in some patients with achalasia. Gastroenterology 1983;84:809.

111. Atkinson M, Ogilvie AL, Robertson CS, Smart HL. Vagal function in achalasia of the cardia. Q J Med 1987;240:297.

112. Kimura K. The nature of idiopathic esophagus dilatation. Jpn J Gastroenterol 1929;1:199.

113. Higgs B, Kerr FWL, Ellis FH Jr. The experimental production of esophageal achalasia by electrolytic lesions in the medulla. J Thorac Cardiovasc Surg 1965;50:613.

114. Koberle F. Chagas' disease and Chagas' syndrome. The pathology of American trypanosomiasis. Adv Parasitol 1968;6:63.

115. Smith B. The neurological lesion in achalasia of the cardia. Gut 1970;11:388.

116. Jones DB, Mayberry JF, Rhoades J, Munro J. Preliminary report of an association between measles virus and achalasia. J Clin Pathol 1983;36:655.

117. Misiewicz JJ, Walles SL, Anthony PP, Gummer JW. Achalasia of the cardia: Pharmacology and histopathology of isolated cardiac sphincteric muscle from patients with and without achalasia. Q J Med 1969;38:17.

118. Kramer P, Ingelfinger FJ. Esophageal sensitivity to Mecholyl in cardiospasm. Gastroenterology 1951;19:242.

119. Heitmann P, Espinoza J, Csendes A. Physiology of the distal esophagus in achalasia. Scand J Gastroenterol 1969;4:1.

120. Dodds WJ, Dent J, Hogan WJ, et al. Paradoxical lower esophageal sphincter contraction induced by cholecystokinin octapeptide in patients with achalasia. Gastroenterology 1981;80:327.

121. Holloway RH, Dodds WJ, Helms JF, et al. Integrity of cholinergic innervation of the lower esophageal sphincter in achalasia. Gastroenterology 1986;90:924.

122. Wong RKH, Johnson LF. Achalasia. In: Castell DO, Johnson LF, eds. Esophageal function in health and disease. New York: Elsevier Biomedical, 1983;99.

123. Olsen AM, Holman CB, Anderson HA. Diagnosis of cardiospasm. Dis Chest 1953;23:477.

124. Stacher G, Kiss A, Wiesnagrotzki S, et al. Oesophageal and gastric motility disorders in patients categorized as having primary anorexia nervosa. Gut 1986;27:1120.

125. Bondi JL, Godwin DH, Garrett JM. Vigorous achalasia. It's clinical interpretation of significance. Am J Gastroenterol 1972;58:145.

126. Pope CE II. Motor disorders. In: Sleisenger MH, Fordtran JS, eds. Gastrointestinal disease, ed 2. Philadelphia: WB Saunders, 1978:424.

127. Smart HL, Foster PN, Evans DF, et al. Twenty-four hour oesophageal acidity in achalasia before and after pneumatic dilatation. Gut 1987;28:883.

128. Vantrappen G, Hellmans J, Deloof W, et al. Treatment of achalasia with pneumatic dilatation. Gut 1971;12:268.

129. Aronchick JM, Miller WT, Epstein DM, Geflex WB. Association of achalasia and pulmonary *Mycobacterium fortuitum* infection. Radiology 1986;160:85.

130. Dominguez F, Hernandez-Ranz F, Boiveda D, Valdazo P. Acute upper-airway obstruction in achalasia of the esophagus. Am J Gastroenterol 1987;82:362.

131. Collins MP, Rabie S. Sudden airway obstruction in achalasia. J Laryngol Otol 1984;98:207.

132. Breatnach E, Han SY. Pneumopericardium occurring as a complication of achalasia. Chest 1986;90:292.

133. Orlando RC, Call DL, Bream CA. Achalasia and absent gastric air bubble. Ann Intern Med 1978;88:60.

134. Clouse RE. Motor disorders. In: Sleinsenger MH, Fordtran JS, eds. Gastrointestinal disease, ed 4. Philadelphia: WB Saunders, 1989: 559.

135. Taub W, Achkar E. Hiatal hernia in patients with achalasia. Am J Gastroenterol 1987;82:1256.

136. Vantrappen G, Hellemans J. Diseases of the esophagus. New York: Springer-Verlag, 1974:341.

137. Chobanian SJ, Benjamin SB, Spurling TJ, et al. Characterization of lower esophageal sphincter relaxation in normal (Abstract). Clin Res 1982;30:723.

138. Castell DO. Achalasia and diffuse esophageal spasm. Arch Intern Med 1976;136:571.

139. Cohen S, Lipschultz W. Lower esophageal sphincter dysfunction in achalasia. Gastroenterology 1971;61:814.

140. Vantrappen G, Janssen J, Hollemans J, Coremans G. Achalasia, diffuse esophageal spasm and related motility disorders. Gastroenterology 1979;76:450.

141. Katz PO, Richter JE, Cowan R, Castell DO. Apparent complete lower esophageal sphincter relaxation in achalasia. Gastroenterology 1986;90:978.

142. Russell COH, Hill LD, Holmes ER III, et al. Radionuclide transit: A sensitive screening test for esophageal dysfunction. Gastroenterology 1981;80:887.

143. Holloway RH, Krosin G, Lange RC, et al. Radionuclide esophageal emptying of a solid meal to quantitate results of therapy in achalasia. Gastroenterology 1987;84:771.

144. Tucker HJ, Snape WJ, Cohen S. Achalasia secondary to carcinoma: Manometric and clinical features. Ann Intern Med 1978;89:315.

145. Sandler RS, Bozymski EM, Orlando RC. Failure of clinical criteria to distinguish between primary achalasia and achalasia secondary to tumor. Dig Dis Sci 1982;27:209.

146. Dodds WJ, Stewart ET, Kishk SM, et al. Radiological amyl nitrate test for discriminating pseudoachalasia from idiopathic achalasia. AJR 1986;1:21.

147. Tischler JM, Shin MS, Stanley RJ, Koehler RE. CT of the thorax in patients with achalasia. Dig Dis Sci 1983;28:697.

148. Bettarello A, Pinotti HW. Oesophageal involvement in Chagas' disease. Clin Gastroenterol 1976;5:103.

149. Costigan DJ, Clouse RE. Achalasia-like esophagus from amyloidosis. Successful treatment with pneumatic bag dilatation. Dig Dis Sci 1983;28:763.

150. Roberts DH, Gilmore IT. Achalasia in Anerson-Fabry's disease. J R Soc Med 1984;77:430.

151. Landers RT, Kuster GGR, Strum WB. Eosinophilic esophagitis in a patient with vigorous pulmonary sarcoidosis. Surgery 1983;94:32.

152. Dulfresne CR, Jeyasingham K, Baker RR. Achalasia of the cardia associated with pulmonary sarcoidosis. Surgery 1983;94:32.

153. Hollis JB, Castell DO, Braddom RL. Esophageal function in diabetes and its relation to peripheral neuropathy. Gastroenterology 1977;73:1098.

154. Schuffler MD. Chronic intestinal pseudo-obstruction syndrome. Med Clin North Am 1981;65:1331.

155. Woods CA, Foutch PG, Waring JP, Sanowski RA. Pancreatic pseudocyst as a cause of secondary achalasia. Gastroenterology 1989;96:235.

156. Foster PN, Stewart M, Lowe JS, Atkinson M. Achalasia like disorder of the oesophagus in von Recklinghausen's neurofibromatosis. Gut 1987;28:1522.

157. Cuthbert JA, Gallaghen ND, Turtle JR. Colonic and oesophageal disturbance in a patient with multiple endocrine neoplasia. Type 2b. Aust NZ J Med 1978;8:518.

158. Simila S, Kokkonen J, Kaski M. Achalasia sicca—Juvenile Sjogren's syndrome with achalasia and gastric hyposecretion. Eur J Pediatr 1978;129:175.

159. Stuckey BG, Mastaglia FL, Reed WD, Pullan P. Glucocorticoid insufficiency, achalasia, alacriona with autonomic and motor neuropathy. Ann Intern Med 1987;106:62.

160. Lobis IF, Fisher R. Anticholinergics therapy for achalasia. A controlled trial (Abstract). Gastroenterology 1976;70:976.

161. Wong RK, Maydonovitch C, Garcia JE, et al. The effect of terbutaline sulfate, nitroglycerin, and aminophylline on lower esophageal sphincter pressure and radionuclide esophageal emptying in patients with achalasia. J Clin Gastroenterol 1987;9:386.

162. DiMarino AJ, Cohen S. Effect of an oral beta-2-adrenergic agonist on lower esophageal sphincter pressure in normal subjects and in patients with achalasia. Dig Dis Sci 1982;27:1063.

163. Gelfand M, Rozen P, Keren S, Gilat T. Effect of nitrates on LOS pressure in achalasia: A potential therapeutic aid. Gut 1981;22:312.

164. Gelfand M, Rozen P, Gilat T. Isosorbide dinitrate and nifedipine treatment of achalasia: A clinical, manometric and radionuclide evaluation. Gastroenterology 1982;83:963.

165. Silverstein BD, Kramer CA, Pope CE II. Treatment of esophageal motor disorders with a calcium channel-blocker, diltiazem (Abstract). Gastroenterology 1982;81:1181.

166. Becker BS, Burakoff R. The effect of verapamil on the lower esophageal sphincter pressure in normal subjects and in achalasia. Am J Gastroenterol 1983;78:773.

167. Orr WC, Allen ML, Mellow M, et al. Differential effects of calcium channel blocking and anticholinergic agents on esophageal function (Abstract). Gastroenterology 1984;86:1202.

168. Traube M, Hongo M, Magyar L, McCallum RW. Effects of nifedipine in achalasia and in patients with high-amplitude peristaltic esophageal contractions. JAMA 1984;252:1733.

169. Bortolotti M, Labo G. Clinical and manometric effects of nifedipine in patients with esophageal achalasia. Gastroenterology 1981;80:39.

170. Hongo M, Traube M, McAllister RG, McCallum RW. Effect of nifedipine on esophageal motor function in humans: Correlation with plasma nifedipine concentration. Gastroenterology 1984;86:8.

171. Mandelstam P, Block C, Newell L, Dillon M. The role of bougienage in the management of achalasia—The need for reappraisal. Gastrointest Endosc 1982;28:169.

172. Raizman RE, De Rezende JM, Neva FA. A clinical trial with pre- and post-treatment manometry comparing pneumatic dilatation with bougienage for treatment of achalasia. Am J Gastroenterol 1980;74:405.

173. Stark H. Die Behandlung der spasmogenen Speiserohrenerweiterung. Munch Med Wochenschr 1924;71:334.

174. Thomas S, Negus VE, Bateman GH. Disease of the nose and throat. In: A textbook for students and practitioners, ed 6. London: Cassal and Company, Ltd, 1955:776.

175. Plummer HS. Cardiospasm with a report of forty cases. JAMA 1908;51:549.

176. Mosher HP. Cardiospasm. Postgraduate Medical Journal 1923;26:240.

177. Van Goidsenhaven GE, Vantrappen G, Verbeke S. Treatment of achalasia of the cardia with pneumatic dilatation. Gastroenterology 1963;45:326.

178. Tucker G. Cardiospasm: A pneumatic-mercury dilator. Annals of Otolaryngology 1939;48:808.

179. Browne DC, McHardy G. A new instrument for use in esophagospasm. JAMA 1939;113:1963.

180. Rider JA, Moeller HC, Parletti EJ, Desai DC. Diagnosis and treatment of diffuse oesophageal spasm. Arch Surg 1969;99:435.

181. Cox J, Buckton GK, Bennett JR. Balloon dilatation in achalasia: A new dilator. Gut 1986;27:986.

182. Witzel L. Treatment of achalasia with a pneumatic dilator attached to a gastroscope. Endoscopy 1981;13:176.

183. Boyce HW, Palmer ED, eds. Techniques of clinical gastroenterology. Springfield: Charles C Thomas, 1975;241.

184. Kurlander DJ, Raskin HF, Kirsner JB, Palmer WL. Therapeutic value of the pneumatic dilator in achalasia of the esophagus: Long-term results in sixty-two living patients. Gastroenterology 1963;45:604.

185. Bennett JR, Hendrix TR. Treatment of achalasia with pneumatic dilatation. Mod Treat 1970;7:1207.

186. Csendes A, Braghetto I, Henriquez A, Cortes C. Late results of prospective randomized study comparing forceful dilatation and esophagomyotomy in patients with achalasia of the esophagus. Gut 1989;30:299.

187. Heimlich JJ, O'Connor TW, Flores DC. Case for pneumatic dilatation in achalasia. Annals of Otolaryngology 1978;87:519.

188. Stark GA, Castell DO, Richter JE, Wu WC. Prospective randomized comparison of Brown-McHardy and microinvasive balloon dilators in treatment of acholasia. Am J Gastroenterol 1990;15:1322.

189. Ott DJ, Richter JE, Wu WC, et al. Radiographic evaluation of esophagus immediately after pneumatic dilatation for achalasia. Dig Dis Sci 1987;32:962.

190. Olsen AM, Harrington SW, Moersch HJ, Anderson HA. The treatment of cardiospasm: Analysis of a twelve year experience. J Thorac Cardiovasc Surg 1951;22:164.

191. Sanderson DR, Ellis FH Jr, Olsen AM. Achalasia of the esophagus. Results of therapy by dilatation, 1950–1967. Chest 1970;58:116.

192. Vantrappen C, Janssens J. To dilate or to operate? That is the question. Gut 1983;24:1013.

193. Fellow IW, Ogilive AL, Atkinson M. Pneumatic dilatation in achalasia. Gut 1983;24:1020.

194. Mellow MH. Return of esophageal peristalsis in idiopathic achalasia. Gastroenterology 1976;70:1148.

195. Bianco A, Cagossi M, Scrimieri D, Greco AV. Appearance of esophageal peristalsis in treated idiopathic achalasia. Dig Dis Sci 1986;31:40.

196. Ponce J, Miralbes M, Garrigues V, Berenguer J. Return of esophageal peristalsis after Heller's myotomy for idiopathic achalasia. Dig Dis Sci 1986;31:545.

197. Lamet M, Fleshler B, Achkar E. Return of peristalsis in achalasia after pneumatic dilatation. Am J Gastroenterol 1985;80:602.

198. Cameron JL, Kieffer RF, Hendrix TR, et al. Selective non-operative management of contained intrathoracic disruptions. Ann Thorac Surg 1978;27:404.

199. Vantrappen G, Hellemans J. Treatment of achalasia and related motor disorders. Gastroenterology 1980;79:144.

200. Heller E. Extramukose Cardiaplastik beim chronischen Cardiospasmus mit Dilatation des Oesophagus. MiH. a.d. Grenzgeb d. Med. u Chin (Jena) 1913;27:141.

201. Belsey R. Functional disease of the esophagus. J Thorac Cardiovasc Surg 1966;52:164.

202. Okike N, Payne WS, Neufeld NT, et al. Esophagomyotomy versus forceful dilatation for achalasia of the esophagus. Results in 899 patients. Ann Thorac Surg 1979;28:119.

203. Jara FM, Toledo-Pereya LH, Lewis JH, Mulligan DJ. Long-term results of esophagomyotomy for achalasia of the esophagus. Arch Surg 1979;114:935.

204. Ellis FH Jr, Drozier RE, Watkins E. The operation for esophageal achalasia: Results of esophagomyotomy without an antireflux operation. J Thorac Cardiovasc Surg 1984;88:344.

205. Black J, Vorbach AN, Collis JL. Results of Heller's operation for achalasia of the esophagus: The importance of hiatal repair. Br J Surg 1976;63:949.

206. Menzies-Gow AR, Gummer JW, Edwards DA. Results of Heller's operation for achalasia of the cardia. Br J Surg 1978;65:483.

207. Csendes A, Braghetto I, Mascaro J, Henriquez A. Late subjective and objective evaluation of the results of esophagomytomy in 100 patients with achalasia of the esophagus. Surgery 1988;104:469.

208. Aghar FP, Keren DF. Barrett's esophagus complicating achalasia after esophagomyotomy. J Clin Gastroenterol 1987;9:232.

209. Wychalis AR, Woolan GL, Anderson HA, Ellis FH Jr. Achalasia and carcinoma of the esophagus. JAMA 1971;215:1638.

210. Hankins JR, McLaughlin JS. The association of carcinoma of the esophagus with achalasia. J Thorac Cardiovasc Surg 1975;69:355.

211. Chuong JJH, DuBovik S, McCallum RW. Achalasia as a risk for esophageal carcinoma. A reappraisal. Dig Dis Sci 1984;29:1105.

212. Clouse RE, Staiano A. Contraction abnormalities of the esophageal body in patients referred for manometry. Dig Dis Sci 1983;28:784.

213. Richter JE, Wu WC, Johns DN, et al. Esophageal manometry in 95 healthy adult volunteers. Dig Dis Sci 1987;32:583.

214. London RC, Ouyang A, Snape WJ, Cohen S. Provocation of esophageal pain by ergonovine or edrophonium. Gastroenterology 1981;81:10.

215. Richter JE, Castell DO. Diffuse esophageal spasm: A reappraisal. Ann Intern Med 1984;100:242.

216. Katz PO, Dalton CB, Richter JE, et al. Esophageal testing in patients with non-cardiac chest pain and/or dysphagia. Ann Intern Med 1987;106:593.

217. Brand DL, Martin D, Pope CE. Esophageal manometrics in patients with angina-like chest pain. Am J Dig Dis 1977;22:300.

218. Traube M, Abibi R, McCallum RW. High amplitude peristaltic esophageal contractions associated with chest pain. JAMA 1983;250:2655.

219. Cohen S. Esophageal motility disorders and their response to calcium channel antagonists. The sphinx revisited. Gastroenterology 1987;93:201.

220. Gillies M, Nicks R, Skyring A. Clinical, manometric and pathologic studies in diffuse esophageal spasm. Br Med J 1967;2:527.

221. Ferguson TB, Woodbury JD, Roper CL, Burford TH. Giant muscular hypertrophy of the esophagus. Ann Thorac Surg 1969;8:209.

222. Ellis FH, Olsen AM, Schlegel JF, Code CF. Surgical treatment of esophageal hypermotility disturbances. JAMA 1964;188:862.

223. Demian SDE, Vargas-Cortes F. Idiopathic muscular hypertrophy of the esophagus. Chest 1978;73:28.

224. Kramer P, Fleshler B, McNally E, Harris LD. Oesophageal sensitivity to Mecholyl in symptomatic diffuse spasm. Gut 1967;8:120.

225. Mellow M. Symptomatic diffuse esophageal spasm. Manometric follow-up and response to cholinergic stimulation and cholinesterase inhibition. Gastroenterology 1977;73:237.

226. Nostrant TT, Saves J, Haber T. Bethanechol increases the diagnostic yield in patients with esophageal chest pain. Gastroenterology 1986;91:1141.

227. Richter JE, Hackshaw BT, Wu WC, Castell DO. Edrophonium: A useful provocative test for esophageal chest pain. Ann Intern Med 1985;103:14.

228. Alban-Davies H, Kaye MD, Rhodes J. Diagnosis of oesophageal spasm by ergometrine provocation. Gut 1982;23:89

229. Eastwood GL, Weiner BH, Dickerson J. Use of ergonovine to identify esophageal spasm in patients with chest pain. Ann Intern Med 1981;94:768.

230. Ouyang A, Reynolds JC, Cohen S. Spike-associated and spike-independent esophageal contractions in patients with symptomatic diffuse spasm. Gastroenterology 1983;84:907.

231. Meyer GW, Castell DO. Human esophageal response during chest pain induced by swallowing cold liquids. JAMA 1981;246:2057.

232. Kaye MD, Kilby AE, Harper PC. Changes in distal esophageal function in response to cooling. Dig Dis Sci 1987;32:22

233. Rubin J, Nagler R, Spiro HM, Pilot ML. Measuring the effect of emotions on esophageal motility. Psychosom Med 1962;24:170.

234. Stacher G, Schmeierer C, Landgraf M. Tertiary esophageal contractions evoked by acoustic stimuli. Gastroenterology 1979;44:49.

235. Anderson KO, Dalton CB, Bradley LA, Richter JE. Stress: A modulator of esophageal pressures in healthy volunteers and non-cardiac chest pain patients. Dig Dis Sci 1989;34:83.

236. Keshavarzian A, Iber FL, Ferguson Y. Esophageal manometry and radionuclide emptying in chronic alcoholics. Gastroenterology 1987;92:751.

237. Peters LJ, Maas LC, Petty D, et al. Spontaneous non-cardiac chest pain: Evaluation by 24 hour ambulatory esophageal motility and pH monitoring. Gastroenterology 1988;94:878.

238. Clouse RE, Lustman PJ. Psychiatric illness and contraction abnormalities of the esophagus. N Engl J Med 1983;309:1337.

239. Richter JE, Obrecht WF, Bradley LA, et al. Psychological comparison of patients with nutcracker esophagus and irritable bowel syndrome. Dig Dis Sci 1986;31:131.

240. Richter JE, Johns DN, Wu WC, Castell DO. Are esophageal motility abnormalities produced during the intraesophageal acid perfusion test? JAMA 1985;253:1914.

241. Burns TW, Venturatos SG. Esophageal motor function and response to acid perfusion in patients with symptomatic reflux esophagitis. Dig Dis Sci 1985;30:529.

242. Richter JE, Barish CF, Castell DO. Abnormal sensory perception in patients with esophageal chest pain. Gastroenterology 1986;91:845.

243. Burish TG. EMG biofeedback in the treatment of stress-related disorders. In: Prokop CK, Bradley LA, eds. Medical psychology: Contributions to behavioral medicine. New York: Academic Press, 1981:395.

244. Schuster M. Esophageal spasm and psychiatric disorder. N Engl J Med 1983;309:1382.

245. Osgood H. A peculiar form of oesophagismus. Boston Medical and Surgical Journal 1989;120:401.

246. Creamer B, Donoghue FE, Code CF. Pattern of esophageal motility in diffuse spasm. Gastroenterology 1958;34:782.

247. Roth HP, Fleshler B. Diffuse esophageal spasm. Ann Intern Med 1964;61:914.

248. Richter JE, Blackwell JN, Wu WC, et al. Relationship of radionuclide

liquid bolus transport and esophageal manometry. J Lab Clin Med 1987;109:217.

249. Kahrilas PJ, Dodds WJ, Hogan WJ. Effect of peristaltic dysfunction on esophageal volume clearance. Gastroenterology 1988;94:73.

250. DiMarino AJ, Cohen S. Characteristics of lower esophageal sphincter function in symptomatic diffuse esophageal spasm. Gastroenterology 1974;66:1.

251. Kaye MD. Anomalies of peristalsis in idiopathic diffuse oesophageal spasm. Gut 1981;22:217.

252. Benjamin SB, Gerhardt DC, Castell DO. High amplitude, peristaltic esophageal contractions associated with chest pain and/or dysphagia. Gastroenterology 1979;77:478.

253. Orr WC, Robinson MG. Hypertensive peristalsis in the pathogenesis of chest pain. Am J Gastroenterol 1982;77:604.

254. Dalton CB, Castell DO, Richter JE. The changing face of the nutcracker esophagus. Am J Gastroenterol 1988;83:358.

255. Herrington JP, Burns TW, Balart LA. Chest pain anddysphagia in patients with prolonged peristaltic contractile duration of the esophagus. Dig Dis Sci 1984;29:134.

256. Ott DJ, Richter JE, Wu WC, et al. Radiologic and manometric correlation in "nutcracker esophagus." AJR 1986;692:1986.

257. Benjamin SB, O'Donnell JK, Hancock J, et al. Prolonged radionuclide transit in "nutcracker esophagus." Dig Dis Sci 1983;28:775.

258. Richter JE, Dalton CB, Bradley LA, Castell DO. Oral nifedipine in the treatment of non-cardiac chest pain in patients with the nutcracker esophagus. Gastroenterology 1987;93:21.

259. Ellis FH, Crozier RE, Shea JA. Long esophagomyotomy for diffuse esophageal spasm and related disorders. In: Siewart JR, Holscher AH, eds. Diseases of the esophagus: Pathophysiology, diagnosis, conservative and surgical treatment. New York: Springer-Verlag, 1988:913.

260. Code CF, Schlegel JF, Kelly ML. Hypertensive gastroesophageal sphincter. Proc Mayo Clinic 1960;35:391.

261. Garrett JM, Godwin DH. Gastroesophageal hypercontracting sphincter. JAMA 1969;208:992.

262. Waterman DC, Dalton CB, Ott DJ, et al. Hypertensive lower esophageal sphincter: What does it mean? J Clin Gastroenterol 1989;11:139.

263. Reidel WL, Clouse RE. Variations in clinical presentations of patients with contraction abnormalities. Dig Dis Sci 1985;30:1065.

264. Alban-Davies H, Johns DB, Rhodes J, Newcombe RJ. Angina-like esophageal pain: Differentiation from cardiac pain by history. J Clin Gastroenterol 1985;7:477.

265. Swamy N. Esophageal spasm: Clinical and manometric response to nitroglycerin and long-acting nitrates. Gastroenterology 1977;72:23.

266. Lieberman-Meffert DM, Luescher U, Neff U, et al. Esophagectomy without thoracotomy: Is there a risk of intramediastinal bleeding. Ann Surg 1987;206:184.

267. Kahrilas PJ, Dodds WJ, Hogan WJ. Dysfunction of the belch reflex. Gastroenterology 1987;93:818.

268. McMahan TP, Richter JE. Non-cardiac chest pain (NCCP) and irritable bowel syndrome (IBS). Part of a continuum? Gastroenterology 1986;90:1546A.

269. Clouse RE, Eckert TC. Gastrointestinal symptoms of patients with esophageal contraction abnormalities. Dig Dis Sci 1986;31:236.

270. Clouse RE, Eckert TC, Staiano A. Hiatus hernia and esophageal contraction abnormalities. Am J Med 1986;81:447.

271. Koch KL, Curry C, Feldman RL. Ergonovine-induced esophageal spasm in patients with chest pain resembling angina pectoris. Dig Dis Sci 1982;27:1073.

272. Lee CA, Reynolds JC, Ouyang A, Cohen S. Esophageal chest pain: Value of high-dose provocative testing with edrophonium chloride in patients with normal esophageal manometries. Dig Dis Sci 1987;32:682.

273. Castell DO, Richter JE. Edrophonium testing for esophageal pain. Concurrence and discord. Dig Dis Sci 1987;32:897.

274. Nasrallah SM, Hendrix EA. Comparison of hypertonic glucose to other provocative tests in patients with non-cardiac chest pain. Am J Gastroenterol 1987;82:406.

275. Allen ML, Orr WC, Mellow MH, Robinson MG. Water swallows versus food ingestion as manometric tests for esophageal dysfunction. 1988;95:831.

276. Janssens J, Vantrappen G, Ghillebert G. 24 hour recording of esophageal pressure and pH in patients with non-cardiac chest pain. Gastroenterology 1986;90:1978.

277. Ward BW, Wu WC, Richter JE, et al. Long-term follow-up of symptomatic status of patients with non-cardiac chest pain: Is diagnosis of esophageal etiology helpful? Am J Gastroenterol 1987;82:215.

278. Orlando RC, Bozymski EM. Clinical and manometric effects of nitroglycerin in diffuse esophageal spasm. N Engl J Med 1973;289:23.

279. Kikendall JW, Mellow MH. Effect of sublingual nitroglycerin and long-acting nitrate preparations on esophageal motility. Gastroenterology 1980;79:703.

280. Hongo M, Traube M, McCallum RW. Comparison of effects of nifedipine, propantheline bromide, and the combination of esophageal function in normal volunteers. Dig Dis Sci 1984;29:300.

281. Mellow MH. Effect of isosorbide and hydralazine in painful primary esophageal motility disorders. Gastroenterology 1982;83:364.

282. Richter JE, Spurling TJ, Cordova CM, Castell DO. Effects of oral calcium blocker, diltiazem, on esophageal contractions. Dig Dis Sci 1984;29:649.

283. Alban-Davies H, Lewis MJ, Rhodes J, Henderson AH. Trial of nifedipine for prevention of oesophageal spasm. Digestion 1987;36:81.

284. Frachtman RL, Botoman VA, Pope CE. A double-blind crossover trial of diltiazem shows no benefit in patients with dysphagia and/or chest pain of esophageal origin. Gastroenterology 1986;90:1420A.

285. Spurling TJ, Cattau EL, Hirszel R, et al. A double blind crossover study of the efficacy of diltiazem on patients with esophageal motility dysfunction. Gastroenterology 1985;88:1596A.

286. Clouse RE, Lustman PJ, Eckert TC, et al. Low-dose trazodone for symptomatic patients with esophageal contraction abnormalities: A double-blind, placebo-controlled trial. Gastroenterology 1987;92:1027.

287. Jacobson E. Spastic esophagus and mucus colitis: Etiology and treatment by progressive relaxation. Arch Intern Med 1927;39:433.

288. Latimer PR. Biofeedback and self-regulation in the treatment of diffuse esophageal spasm: A single-case study. Biofeedback Self Regul 1981;6:181.

289. Winters C, Artnak EJ, Benjamin SB, et al. Esophageal bougienage in symptomatic patients with the nutcracker esophagus. JAMA 1984;252:3630.

290. Ebert EC, Ouyang A, Wright SH, Cohen S. Pneumatic dilatation in patients with symptomatic diffuse esophageal spasm and lower esophageal sphincter dysfunction. Dig Dis Sci 1983;28:481.

291. DeMeester TR. Surgery for esophageal motor disorders. Ann Thorac Surg 1982;34:225.

292. Kramer P, Harris LD, Donaldson DM. Transition from symptomatic diffuse spasm to cardiospasm. Gut 1967;8:115.

293. Narducci F, Bassotti G, Graburri M, Morelli A. Transition from nutcracker esophagus to diffuse esophageal spasm. Am J Gastroenterol 1985;80:242.

294. Turner R, Lipshutz W, Miller W, et al. Esophageal dysfunction in collagen disease. Am J Med Sci 1973;265:191.

295. Clements PJ, Kadell B, Ippoliti A, et al. Esophageal motility in progressive systemic sclerosis (PSS). Comparison of cine-radiographic and manometric evaluation. Dig Dis Sci 1979;24:639.

296. Cohen S, Fisher R, Lipshutz W, Turner R, et al. The pathogenesis of esophageal dysfunction in scleroderma and Raynaud's disease. J Clin Invest 1972;51:2663.

297. Kaufman JH, Braverman IM, Spiro HM. Esophageal manometry in scleroderma. Scand J Gastroenterol 1968;62:1243.

298. Garrett JM, Winkelmann RK, Schlegel JF, Code CF. Esophageal deterioration in scleroderma. Mayo Clin Proc 1971;46:92.

299. Zamost BJ, Hirschberg J, Ippoliti AF, et al. Esophagitis in scleroderma. Prevalence and risk factors. Gastroenterology 1987;92:421.

300. Katzka DA, Reynolds JC, Saul SH, et al. Barrett's metaplasia and adenocarcinoma of the esophagus in scleroderma. Am J Med 1987;82:46.

301. Clements JL, Abernathy J, Weens HS. Atypical esophageal diverticula associated with progressive systemic sclerosis. Gastrointest Radiol 1978;3:383.

302. Treacy WL, Baggenstoss AH, Slocumb CH, Code CF. Scleroderma of the esophagus. A correlation of histologic and physiologic findings. Ann Intern Med 1963;59:351.

303. Stevens MB, Hookman P, Siegel CI, et al. Aperistalsis of the esophagus in patients with connective tissue disorders and Raynaud's phenomenon. N Engl J Med 1964;270:1218.

304. Schneider HA, Yonker RA, Longely S, et al. Scleroderma esophagus: A nonspecific entity. Ann Intern Med 1984;100:848.

305. Drane WE, Karvelis K, Johnson DA, et al. Progressive systemic sclerosis: Radionuclide esophageal scintigraphy and manometry. Radiology 1986;160:73.

306. Petrokubi RJ, Jeffries GH. Cimetidine versus antacid in scleroderma with reflux esophagitis. Gastroenterology 1979;77:691.

307. Winn D, Gerhardt D, Winship D, et al. Esophageal function in steroid-treated patients with mixed connective tissue disease. Clin Res 1976;24:545A.

308. Gutierrez F, Valenzuela JE, Ehresmann GR, et al. Esophageal dysfunction in patients with mixed connective tissue diseases and systemic lupus erythematosus. Dig Dis Sci 1982;27:592.

309. Ramirez-Mata M, Reyes PA, Alacron-Segovia D, et al. Esophageal motility in systemic lupus erythematosus. Am J Dig Dis 1974;19:132.

310. Peppercorn MA, Docken WP, Rosenberg S. Esophageal motor dysfunction in systemic lupus erythematosus. Two cases with unusual features. JAMA 1979;242:1895.

311. Sun DCH, Roth SH, Mitchell CS, et al. Upper gastrointestinal disease in rheumatoid arthritis. Am J Dig Dis 1974;19:405.

312. Ramirez-Mata M, Pena-Ancira FF, Alacron-Segovia D. Abnormal esophageal motility in primary Sjogren's syndrome. J Rheumatol 1976;3:63.

313. Tsianos EB, Chiras CD, Drosos AA, et al. Oesophageal dysfunction in patients with primary Sjogren's syndrome. Ann Rheum Dis 1985;44:610.

314. Hollis JB, Castell DO, Braddom RL. Esophageal function in diabetes mellitus and its relation to peripheral neuropathy. Gastroenterology 1977;73:1098.

315. Keshavarzian A, Iber FL, Nasrallah S. Radionuclide esophageal emptying and manometric studies in diabetes mellitus. Am J Gastroenterol 1987;82:625.

316. Clouse RE, Lustman PJ, Reidel WL. Correlation of esophageal motility abnormalities with neuropsychiatric status in diabetes. Gastroenterology 1986;90:1146.

317. Mandelstram P, Siegel CI, Lieber A, et al. The swallowing disorder in patients with diabetic neuropathy-gastroenteropathy. Gastroenterology 1969;56:1

318. Stewart IM, Hosking DJ, Preston BJ, et al. Oesophageal motor changes in diabetes mellitus. Thorax 1976;31:278

319. Loo FD, Dodds WJ, Soergel KH, et al. Multipeaked esophageal peristaltic pressure waves in patients with diabetic meuropathy. Gastroenterology 1985;88:485.

320. Meshkinpour H, Afrasiabi MA, Valenta LJ. Esophageal motor function in Grave's disease. Dig Dis Sci 1979;24:159.

321. Fischer RA, Ellison GW, Thayer WR, et al. Esophageal motility in neuromuscular disorders. Ann Intern Med 1965;63:229.

322. Eastwood GL, Braverman LE, White EM, et al. Reversal of lower esophageal sphincter hypotension and esophageal aperistalsis after treatment for hypothyroidism. J Clin Gastroenterol 1982;4:307.

323. Gilat T, Spiro HM. Amyloidosis and the gut. Am J Dig Dis 1968;13:619.

324. Rubinow A, Burakoff R, Cohen AS, et al. Esophageal manometry in systemic amyloidosis. A study of 30 patients. Am J Med 1983;75:951.

325. Liske E, Chou S, Thompson HG. Peripheral and automatic neuropathy in amyloidosis. JAMA 1963;186:432.

326. Burakoff R, Rubinow A, Cohen AS. Esophageal manometry in familial amyloid polyneuropathy. Am J Med 1985;79:85.

327. Mayer EM, Grabowski CJ, Fisher RS. Effects of graded doses of alcohol on esophageal motor function. Gastroenterology 1978;75:1133.

328. Hogan WJ, Viegas de Andrade SR, Winship DH. Ethanol-induced acute esophageal motor dysfunction. J Appl Physiol 1972;32:755.

329. Winship DH, Caflish CR, Zboralske FF, et al. Deterioration of esophageal peristalsis on patients with alcoholic neuropathy. Gastroenterology 1968;55:173.

330. Kahrilas PJ, Dodds WJ, Hogan WJ, et al. Esophageal peristaltic dysfunction in peptic esophagitis. Gastroenterology 1986;91:897.

331. Ahtaridis G, Snape WJ, Cohen S. Clinical and manometric findings in benign peptic strictures of the esophagus. Dig Dis Sci 1979;24:858.

332. Herlihy KJ, Orlando RC, Bryson JC, et al. Barrett's esophagus: Clinical, endoscopic, histologic, manometric and electrical potential difference characteristics. Gastroenterology 1984;86:436.

333. Higgs RH, Castell DO, Eastwood GL. Studies on the mechanism of esophagitis induced lower esophageal sphincter hypotension in cats. Gastroenterology 1976;71:51.

334. Eckardt VF. Does healing of esophagitis improve esophageal function? Dig Dis Sci 1988;33:161.

335. Zboralske FF, Amberg JR, Soergel KH. Presbyesophagus: Cineradiographic manifestations. Radiology 1964;82:463.

336. Soergel KH, Zboralske FF, Amberg JR. Presbyesophagus: Esophageal motility in nonagerians. J Clin Invest 1964;43:144.

337. Hollis JB, Castell DO. Esophageal function in elderly men. A new look at "presbyesophagus." Ann Intern Med 1974;80:371.

338. Khan TA, Shragge BW, Crispin JS, et al. Esophageal motility in the elderly. Am J Dig Dis 1977;22:1049.

339. Csendes A, Guiraldes E, Bancalari A, et al. Relation of gastroesophageal sphincter pressures and esophageal contractile waves to age in man. Scand J Gastroenterol 1978;13:443.

55

Reflux Esophagitis

ROY C. ORLANDO

Gastroesophageal reflux (GER) represents the effortless movement of gastric contents from stomach to esophagus. Because this phenomenon occurs in virtually everyone multiple times every day and in the majority without clinical consequences, GER, per se, is not a disease but a normal physiologic process. GER, however, can be pathologic, producing symptoms and signs of damage to esophagus, oropharynx, larynx, and respiratory tissue. The term "gastroesophageal reflux disease (GERD)" has been coined to reflect this broad range of damage.

The most common form of GERD is reflux esophagitis. Reflux esophagitis can be recognized clinically either by the presence of recurrent symptoms (heartburn) or by changes in epithelial morphology, the latter visualized radiologically, endoscopically, or histologically. Some investigators use the term "reflux esophagitis" more restrictively, limiting it, as the suffix -itis suggests, to subjects with mucosal damage accompanied by inflammation. In this context, subjects with symptoms but without inflammation are said to have either "reflux disease" or "symptomatic reflux." However, subjects with reflux disease or symptomatic reflux also have acid-damaged esophagi, although damage may only be demonstrable with techniques more powerful than light microscopy.[1,2] Therefore, the term reflux esophagitis is used in this chapter in the broader context to include both groups. This, however, does not imply that the distinction between groups is not important, and this becomes evident in the discussion of complications and therapy.

EPIDEMIOLOGY

Reflux esophagitis is an important disorder for a number of reasons. First, it is extremely common. Reports indicate that up to 36% of otherwise healthy Americans experience heartburn at least once a month, and 7% of Americans have heartburn as often as once a day.[3] In addition, up to 25% of pregnant women are reported to have reflux symptoms on a daily basis.[3] Second, it has serious clinical consequences. Reflux esophagitis can lead to obstruction through stricture formation, to bleeding and perforation through ulceration, and to cancer through the development of a columnar lining known as Barrett's esophagus. Third, it has considerable economic impact. As one of the major acid-peptic diseases, reflux esophagitis is in part responsible for the expenditure worldwide of 2 to 3 billion dollars per year for anti-ulcer prescription and nonprescription drugs.

ETIOLOGY

It is generally accepted that reflux esophagitis is a multifactorial disease whose initiating event is the reflux of gastric contents into the esophageal lumen. Esophagitis develops in susceptible persons when there is prolonged contact of esophageal epithelium with noxious substances in the refluxate. Fortunately for the majority of us, because we all reflux and are therefore at risk,[4,5] it is uncommon for this sequence to be carried to completion. This is due to the existence of a three-tiered defense system for esophageal protection against noxious gastric contents.[6] The three components of this defense system are (1) antireflux barriers, (2) luminal clearance mechanisms, and (3) tissue resistance (Fig 55-1).

Potency of the Refluxate

The substances found in stomach that can contribute to the noxious quality of the refluxate include: hydrochloric acid (HCl), pepsin, bile salts (conjugated and deconjugated), and pancreatic enzymes (trypsin, lipase). Each of these has been shown experimentally to produce esophageal injury, but not all under the same conditions.[7-13] One condition that predetermines which substances are noxious is gastric pH. Thus, in subjects in whom gastric pH is neutral or alkaline, as, for example, postgastrectomy patients or persons who have atrophic gastritis or pernicious anemia, the major injurious agents in the refluxate are deconjugated bile salts and pancreatic enzymes. These same agents, however, play essentially no role in esophageal damage when gastric pH is acidic. This is because, at acid pH, deconjugated bile salts are insoluble and pancreatic enzymes are inactive.

The overwhelming majority of subjects with reflux esophagitis secrete acid and have acidic refluxates. At acid pH, hydrogen ions (H^+) are the major injurious agents in the refluxate, and their capacity for injury to the esophageal epithelium is concentration-(pH) and time-dependent. Further, the rate and degree of mucosal damage are markedly accelerated if luminal pH is less than 2 or if pepsin or conjugated bile salts are present in the refluxate.[1,7-10,14] The relative importance of pepsin, bile salts, and rate of acid secretion to the development of reflux esophagitis is unclear. Subjects with reflux esophagitis have been reported to secrete gastric acid at rates equal to or greater than healthy subjects.[15,16] In either case, the pH of the refluxate can be less than 1, a value

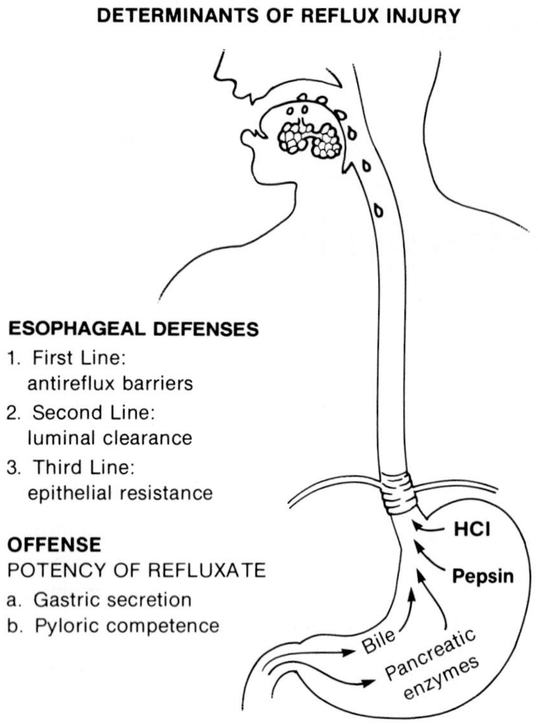

DETERMINANTS OF REFLUX INJURY

ESOPHAGEAL DEFENSES

1. First Line:
   antireflux barriers
2. Second Line:
   luminal clearance
3. Third Line:
   epithelial resistance

OFFENSE
POTENCY OF REFLUXATE
a. Gastric secretion
b. Pyloric competence

HCl

Pepsin

Bile

Pancreatic enzymes

FIGURE 55-1. Diagrammatic representation of the three-tiered system by which the esophagus defends itself from damaging agents contained in the gastric refluxate. The anti-reflux barriers act to minimize the frequency of reflux, the clearance mechanisms minimize the duration of contact with the refluxate, and factors comprising tissue resistance minimize the damage done during epithelial contact with the refluxate. (Orlando RC. Oesophageal defenses. In: Bennett JR, ed. Oesophagitis. London: Current Medical Literature, Ltd, in press, 1991.)

readily able to produce esophageal damage. Also, while acidified bile salts accelerate the rate of damage to esophageal epithelium experimentally, they appear to play little or no role in clinical (acid) reflux disease. This is supported by (1) the failure to detect bile salts using high performance liquid chromatography in the refluxate of subjects with esophagitis;[17] (2) the absence of two distinctive features of experimental bile salt injury—membrane microvesiculation and intracellular deposition of bile salts[18,19]—in human biopsies;[2] and (3) the ability of omeprazole, an agent that abolishes acid secretion, to achieve healing rates of well over 90% in subjects with reflux esophagitis.[20] Pepsin, as a normal component of gastric juice, likely contributes to esophageal damage in reflux disease. However, pepsin's effect, as distinct from acid, remains unclear because pepsin at neutral pH is innocuous and agents that heal esophagitis possibly through pepsin inactivation concomitantly raise pH or inhibit the action of H^+ on the epithelium.[20-23]

Esophageal Defense

ANTIREFLUX BARRIERS

The first tier of the three-tiered esophageal defense against acid damage is the antireflux barriers. These barriers that protect the

esophagus by *limiting the frequency* of reflux include: the lower esophageal sphincter (LES), intraabdominal segment of esophagus, diaphragm, phrenoesophageal ligament, mucosal rosette, and acute angle of His.

Lower Esophageal Sphincter. The major antireflux barrier is the LES, an area of specialized circular smooth muscle located at the most distal end of the esophagus.[24,25] In the resting state, the LES is contracted, creating a barrier (high pressure zone) to the transfer of acid-pepsin from stomach to esophagus. However, because reflux occurs in everyone, the LES is, by nature, an imperfect barrier (Fig 55-2). In healthy subjects, this imperfection is due to phenomena known as transient LES relaxations (TLESRs).[5,26,27] TLESRs are spontaneous, nonswallow-initiated events that permit reflux by obliterating the high pressure zone. TLESRs can be induced by gastric or subthreshold (for swallowing) pharyngeal stimulation, and these stimuli initiate a vagally mediated, noncholinergic inhibitory reflex to the LES.[27-29] Gastric distention, by increasing the frequency of TLESRs, accounts for the observed increase in reflux frequency that occurs normally after meals.

Subjects with reflux esophagitis, in general, reflux more frequently than healthy subjects (see Fig 55-2). This suggests that impaired barrier function is one factor important for the development of esophagitis. Dodds and colleagues[26] have identified in subjects with esophagitis three circumstances under which reflux can occur (Fig 55-3). The first and most frequent circumstance is spontaneous reflux accompanying TLESRs. This explains the apparent paradox of reflux disease developing in subjects with normal LES pressure. The second circumstance is stress reflux associated with a weak (low pressure) LES. In this case, an increase

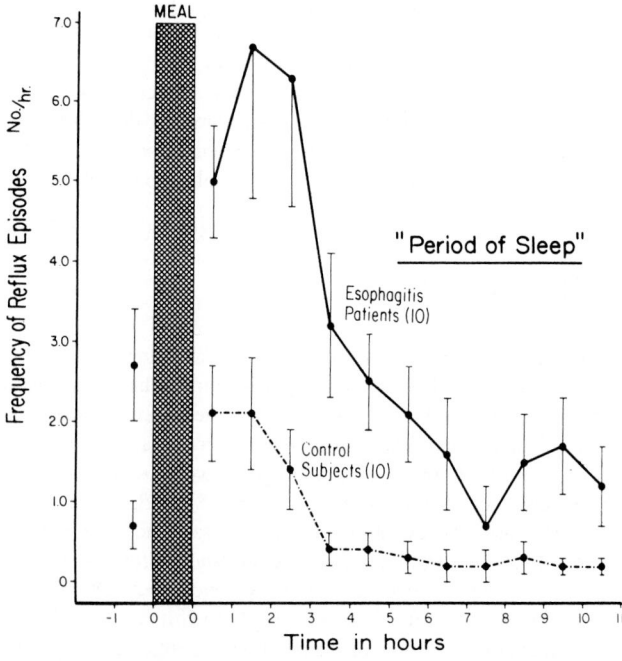

FIGURE 55-2. Gastroesophageal reflux during 12 hours of monitoring in control subjects and patients with reflux esophagitis. (From Dodds WJ, Dent J, Hogan WJ, et al. Mechanisms of gastroesophageal reflux in patients with reflux esophagitis. N Engl J Med 1982;307:1547.)

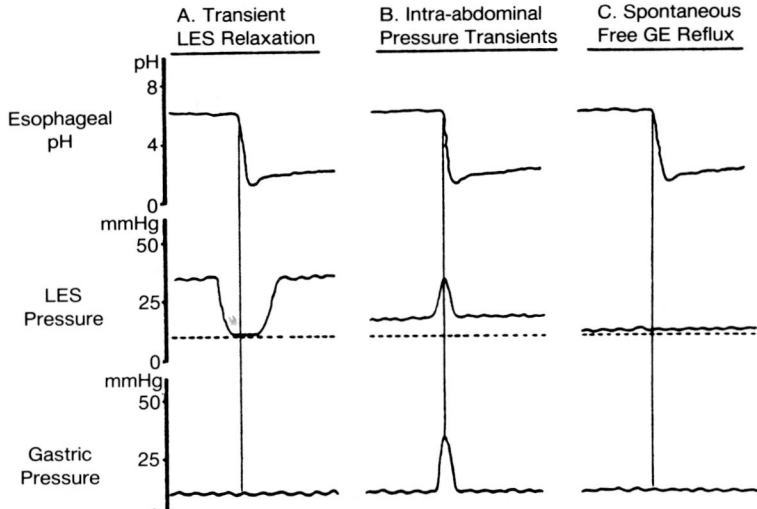

A. Transient LES Relaxation   B. Intra-abdominal Pressure Transients   C. Spontaneous Free GE Reflux

FIGURE 55–3. Schematic representation of three different mechanisms of gastroesophageal (GE) reflux. GE reflux events (*vertical lines*) may **A**, accompany a transient lower esophageal sphincter (LES) relaxation; **B**, develop as stress reflux during a transient increase in intra-abdominal pressure that overcomes LES resistance; or **C**, occur as spontaneous free reflux across an atonic sphincter. (From Dodds WJ, Dent J, Hogan WJ, et al. Mechanisms of gastroesophageal reflux in patients with reflux esophagitis. N Engl J Med 1982;307: 1547.)

in intraabdominal pressure precipitates reflux by creating enough force to overcome the weak squeeze of the LES. The third circumstance is free reflux; this can occur anytime across an essentially nonexistent (incompetent) LES.

In subjects with reflux esophagitis and a hypotensive LES, the mechanisms responsible for impaired LES contractility have not been established. One hypothesis suggests that LES incompetence is a primary neuromuscular defect.[30,31] An alternative proposal is that LES incompetence is a secondary defect, the result and not the cause of reflux esophagitis. In support of the latter hypothesis, acid perfusion of the cat esophagus resulted not only in esophagitis but a significant reduction in LES pressure, and cessation of perfusion was followed by gradual healing of lesions and return of the LES toward baseline.[32] A similar sequence has been sought in humans, but significant recovery in LES function has not been demonstrated after healing of esophagitis.[33–35] Although this failure of LES recovery, which is cited as one reason for the propensity of reflux esophagitis to relapse, supports the hypothesis that LES incompetence precedes not follows the development of esophagitis, one can argue that it just reflects less reversible damage due to the chronicity of disease.

The mechanisms responsible for TLESRs in subjects with esophagitis appear to be no different from those in healthy subjects.[26,36] However, because there are more of them, an abnormality could exist in sensory input from pharynx or stomach. Delayed gastric emptying by increasing both gastric volume and degree of distention could increase TLESR frequency, and this phenomenon has been observed in a subset of subjects with reflux esophagitis.[28,37,38]

Hiatus Hernia. The relationship between a sliding hiatus hernia and reflux esophagitis remains controversial. Once considered synonymous, they clearly are not. Most subjects with hernias do not have reflux esophagitis.[39–41] The functional state of the LES and not the existence of a hernia determines the development of reflux disease.[42] However, although most subjects with hernias do not have esophagitis, most subjects with esophagitis, particularly when severe, do have hernias.[43–45] It has been shown that the existence of a hernia in subjects with esophagitis can contribute to impaired barrier function.[46] From an anatomic perspective, the

reason for this is clear: there is reduced support of LES function from external structures such as the diaphragm.[47–49] Nonetheless, when the barrier function of the LES remains intact, clearly a hernia alone is inadequate to produce disease. The question that remains to be answered is whether a hiatus hernia can, with time, lead to the impairment of LES function.

LUMINAL ACID CLEARANCE

The second tier in the esophageal defense against reflux damage is luminal clearance. This mechanism comes into play after an episode of reflux to *limit the duration of epithelial contact* with acidic gastric contents. The factors contributing to luminal clearance include: gravity, peristalsis, salivary secretion, and possibly secretion from esophageal submucosal/mucosal glands.[6]

Gravity may increase the rate of bolus clearance when reflux occurs in the upright position[50] but does not operate when the subject is supine. Therefore, subjects with reflux are advised to sleep with the head of their beds elevated. Perhaps even more important than gravity is the contribution of peristalsis and salivary secretion to luminal acid clearance.[51,52] These factors are illustrated in Figure 55-4. After reflux occurs, the majority of the bolus volume is swept from esophagus to stomach by one or two swallow-induced peristaltic contractions. Despite bolus removal, the pH of the esophageal lumen remains acidic unless the swallows contain saliva. Saliva dilutes and, by its bicarbonate content, neutralizes the residual acid remaining within the lumen. Although not established in humans, the possibility exists that luminal acid may also be cleared by alkaline secretions from esophageal mucosal/submucosal glands. Such a mechanism may explain the occurrence of acid clearance from the esophageal lumen in recumbent subjects in the absence of swallowing.[5] Luminal acid clearance by the secretion of bicarbonate from submucosal glands has been observed in the opossum esophagus.[53] Like opossum esophagus, the human esophagus also contains such glands (although not as extensive a network).[54–56]

Duration, and not frequency, of epithelial contact with acid generally correlates with the severity of esophagitis.[57–59] This suggests that abnormal clearance is as important for the development

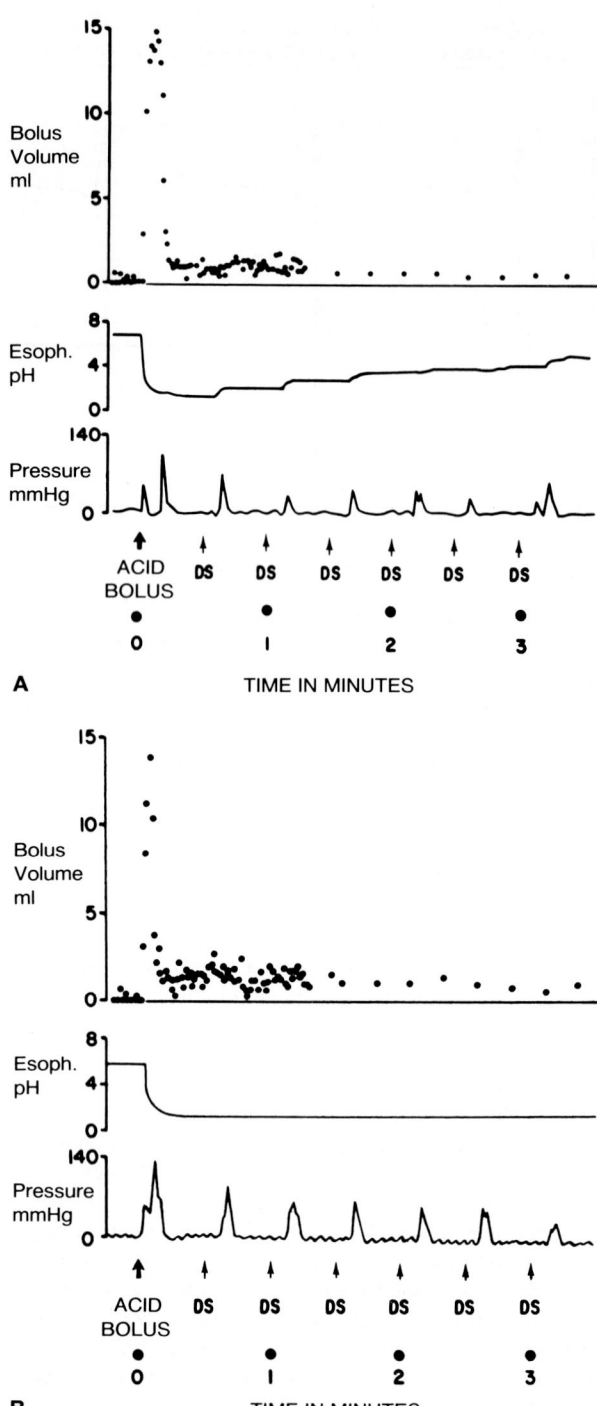

A

TIME IN MINUTES

B

TIME IN MINUTES

FIGURE 55–4. **A**, Relationship between esophageal acid clearance, motor activity, and emptying of fluid volume. Despite clearance of the injected bolus volume to less than 1 ml by the secondary peristaltic sequence, esophageal pH did not begin to rise until the first dry swallow (DS) 30 seconds after bolus injection and did not approach pH 7 until the sixth swallow. **B**, Effect of oral aspiration of saliva on esophageal acid clearance and emptying of fluid volume. Only peristaltic pressure complexes from the distal esophagus are shown. Despite nearly complete emptying of the bolus volume by the initial secondary peristaltic sequence, saliva aspiration effectively prevented esophageal acid clearance. (From Helm JF, Dodds WJ, Pelc LR, et al. Effect of esophageal emptying and saliva on clearance of acid from the esophagus. N Engl J Med 1984;310: 284.)

of esophagitis as the reflux event itself. However, most patients with reflux disease have normal salivary secretion,[60] and, although abnormalities in peristaltic function have been identified (e.g., increased numbers of low amplitude, aperistaltic and spontaneous contractions, and increased numbers of failed swallows),[50,57,61,62] these abnormalities generally delay luminal clearance only briefly. Nonetheless, a circumstance exists in all subjects when luminal clearance is delayed for prolonged periods of time, and this circumstance is sleep.[63–65] During sleep, there is neither swallowing nor salivation, and clearance by gravity is also negated.[66–68] Thus, sleeping is a high-risk (in)activity for prolonged acid exposure and, consequently, for the development of esophagitis. This is borne out by the common association between nocturnal (supine) reflux and esophagitis[4,58,59,69] and by the positive correlation between nocturnal reflux and severity of reflux disease (Fig 55-5).

Esophageal acidification in sleeping healthy subjects is usually followed by an arousal.[63,64] Because arousal from sleep restores swallowing and salivation, such a response improves the rate of luminal clearance. Notably, subjects with esophagitis are more rapidly aroused from sleep during esophageal acidification than healthy subjects; this is presumably due to increased permeability of their epithelium to the H^+ stimulus. Although these findings fail to document delayed arousal as a cause for disease in this study population, such a scenario might contribute to the development of esophagitis in those with a depressed sensorium (e.g., after ingestion of alcohol or hypnotics at bedtime).[70]

TISSUE RESISTANCE

Although clearance mechanisms are generally effective in reducing contact between acid and epithelium, the cumulative contact time even in healthy subjects remains considerable, 1 to 2 hours/day.[59] Furthermore, reflux occurring during sleep in healthy subjects (see Fig 55-2) can result in epithelial contact with acid that is continuous. The failure to develop esophagitis under these conditions suggests the existence of a third defense mechanism— "tissue resistance." Tissue resistance is not a single factor but a group of esophageal structure/functions that interact to prevent or minimize epithelial damage from noxious luminal contents.[6] For discussion purposes, they are subdivided into preepithelial, epithelial, and postepithelial defenses (Table 55-1).

In the stomach and duodenum, an important preepithelial defense mechanism is the mucus–unstirred water layer–bicarbonate complex.[71–73] The gel-like property of mucus prevents pepsin from gaining access to surface cells, while secreted bicarbonate protects by creating an alkaline microenvironment that buffers back-diffusing H^+. This mechanism, however, appears to be of minor importance for protection of the esophagus because the esophagus does not have a well-defined surface mucous layer and it does not maintain a significant lumen-to-surface pH gradient during acid exposure (Fig 55-6).

The esophageal epithelial defense consists of both structural and functional components (Fig 55-7). Structural components include the cell membranes and intercellular junctional complex; these protect against acid injury by limiting the rate of H^+ diffusion into the epithelium. The nature of the intercellular barrier has not been established for human esophageal epithelium. In mouse esophagus, the junctional barrier is created by a lamellar lipid material contained within the intercellular space, and, in rabbit

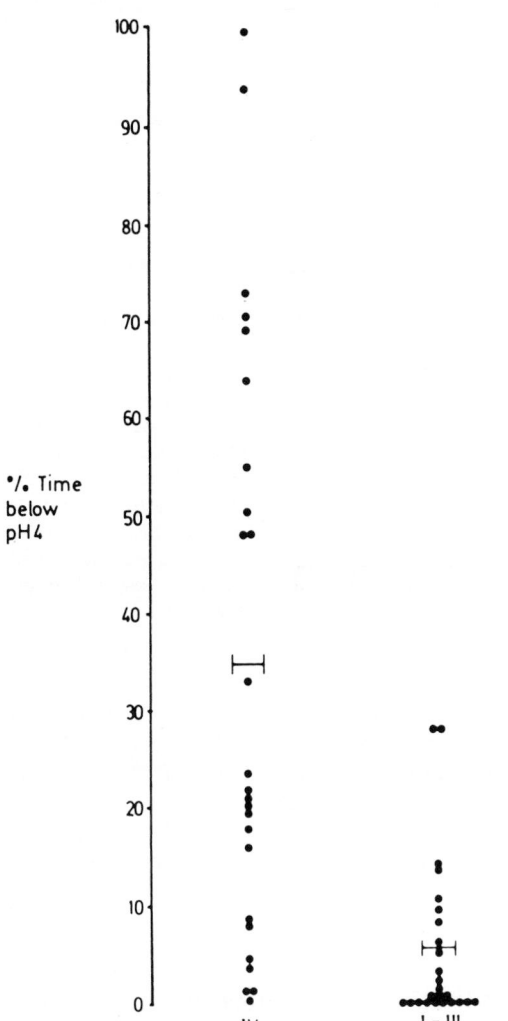

TABLE 55-1

Potential Components of "Tissue Resistance" Against Acid Injury in Esophagus

Preepithelial defenses
    1. Mucous layer
    2. Unstirred water layer
    3. Surface bicarbonate ion concentration
Epithelial Defenses
    Physical Barriers
    4. Cell membranes
    5. Intercellular junctional complex
        a. Tight junctions
        b. Intercellular lipid or mucin
    Functional Components
    6. Cellular defense against acidification
        a. Epithelial transport (e.g., Na^+/H^+ exchange)
        b. Intracellular buffering
            Basic proteins
            Bicarbonate ions
    7. Epithelial repair
        a. Epithelial restitution
        b. Cell replication
Postepithelial Defense
    8. Blood flow
        a. Delivery of protective agents
            Oxygen
            Metabolic substrates (nutrients)
            Bicarbonate ions (extracellular buffering)
        b. Removal of noxious agents
            CO_2
            H^+
            Metabolic byproducts
            Cellular debris

Modified from Orlando RC. Esophageal epithelial resistance. In: Castell DO, Wu WC, Ott DJ, eds. Gastroesophageal reflux disease: Pathogenesis, diagnosis, therapy. Mount Kisco, NY: Futura, 1985.

FIGURE 55-5. Nocturnal (midnight to 8:00 AM) pH data showing significantly greater nocturnal acid exposure in 25 patients with complications of oesophagitis (IV) compared to those with less severe (I–III) disease. Grade IV complications included strictures in 12, Barrett's esophagus in 7, and esophageal ulcers in 6 patients. (From Robertson D, Aldersley M, Shepherd H, Smith CL. Patterns of acid reflux in complicated oesophagitis. Gut 1987;28:1484.)

esophagus, the barrier appears to consist of tight junctions combined with a mucopolysaccharide cement within the intercellular space.[74,75] Similar mucopolysaccharides have been located within the intercellular space in the human esophagus.[76]

The functional components of the epithelial defense against acid injury have not been fully characterized in esophagus. Nonetheless, esophageal cells, like other vertebrate cells, have the ability to buffer and extrude H^+. The capacity of esophageal cells to handle H^+ depends on the buffering capacity of intracellular proteins, the ability to generate intracellular base (bicarbonate), and the ability of membrane pumps and channels to transport H^+. In most cells, intracellular bicarbonate is generated by carbonic anhydrase. This enzyme has not been sought in esophagus, although it is present in other stratified squamous epithelia (e.g., frog skin, ox rumen).[77] Esophageal cells do contain a Na-H antiport within

the membrane.[78] After cell acidification (e.g., after an episode of reflux), the esophageal cell can potentially raise intracellular pH by exchanging H^+ for extracellular Na^+ (see Fig 55-7).

The postepithelial defense of the esophagus against acid is accomplished principally by its blood supply. Blood flow delivers oxygen, nutrients, and bicarbonate and removes H^+ and CO_2, functions that maintain tissue acid–base balance in dynamic fashion. Perfusion of the esophagus with acid leads to an increase in esophageal blood flow;[79,80] and this could prevent interstitial and intracellular acidosis by increasing bicarbonate delivery to the mucosa. The importance of preventing interstitial acidosis has been demonstrated in an animal model of acid damage to the esophagus.[81] In this model, luminal acid damages the esophageal epithelium by traversing the paracellular route and acidifying the basolateral membrane. However, when basolateral membrane acidification is prevented by provision of an adequate supply of serosal buffer (i.e., bicarbonate), epithelial necrosis could be prevented (Fig 55-8).

When esophageal epithelium has sustained damage, containment of the injury depends in large part on rates of repair. In stomach and duodenum, rapid repair occurs for limited damage by a process known as epithelial "restitution."[82–85] Restitution oc-

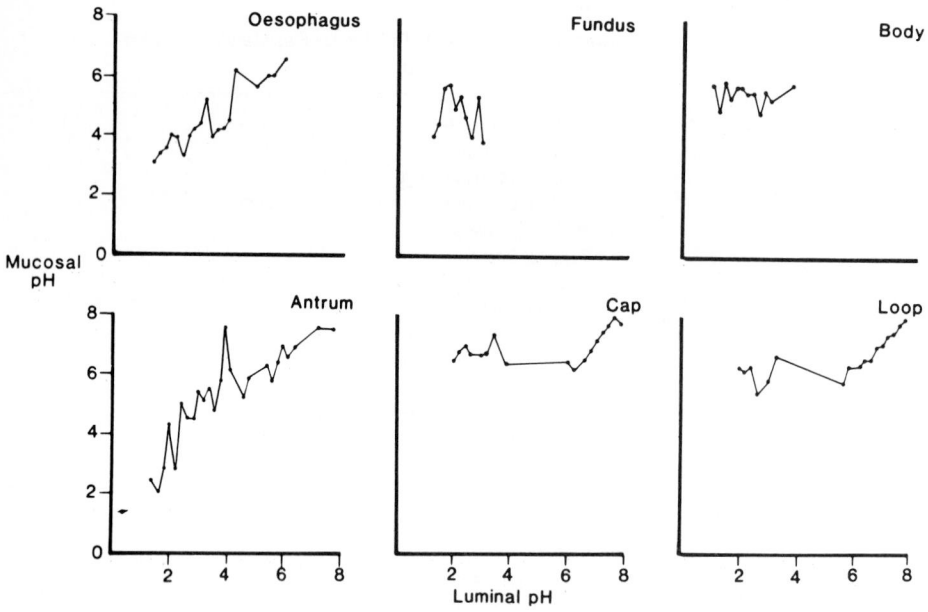

FIGURE 55–6. The relationship between juxtamucosal and luminal pH at each anatomic site in healthy subjects over a range of luminal pH values. Note the stability of juxtamucosal pH in fundus, body, duodenal cap, and duodenal loop in contrast to that observed in esophagus and gastric antrum. Mean values are shown. (From Quigley EMM, Turnberg LA. pH of the microclimate lining the human gastric and duodenal mucosa in vivo—studies in control subjects and duodenal ulcer patients. Gastroenterology 1987;92: 1876.)

curs rapidly (< 1 hour) because it does not require cell replication. Instead, viable epithelial cells repair the defect by migrating in amoebalike fashion over the regions of bare basement membrane. With more extensive injuries, such as when the basement membrane is damaged, considerably more time is required to repair the epithelium through the formation of granulation tissue and epithelial cell replication. Not surprisingly, an increase in cell replication has been observed in biopsy specimens of esophageal epithelium from subjects with reflux esophagitis.[86] The process of restitution has not been observed in esophageal epithelia despite being sought for up to 2¼ hours after acid damage.[81]

Data are not available to confirm the possibility that defects in "tissue resistance," either inherited or acquired, are a cause or a contributing factor in reflux esophagitis in humans. Nonetheless, esophageal exposure to cigarette smoke and alcohol has been linked to the development of esophageal damage, and each has been shown experimentally to have deleterious effects on epithelial function. For example, exposure of rabbit esophageal epithelium to either

nicotine or an aqueous extract of cigarette smoke inhibits active Na transport,[87] while exposure of dog esophageal epithelium to alcohol increases its permeability to H+.[88,89] However, smoking and alcohol also have negative effects on LES barrier function and luminal acid clearance,[50,57] and for this reason the contribution of these epithelial effects to the development of esophagitis are uncertain.

Conditions Associated with Reflux

A number of conditions are associated with the development of reflux esophagitis. All have in common the ability to either increase the noxious quality of the refluxate or decrease one or more of the three esophageal defenses. Examples of these conditions include the Zollinger-Ellison syndrome,[90] pregnancy,[91] scleroderma,[92] diabetes mellitus,[93] and prolonged nasogastric intubation. With the

EPITHELIAL DEFENSES
(Uppermost Living Cell Layer)

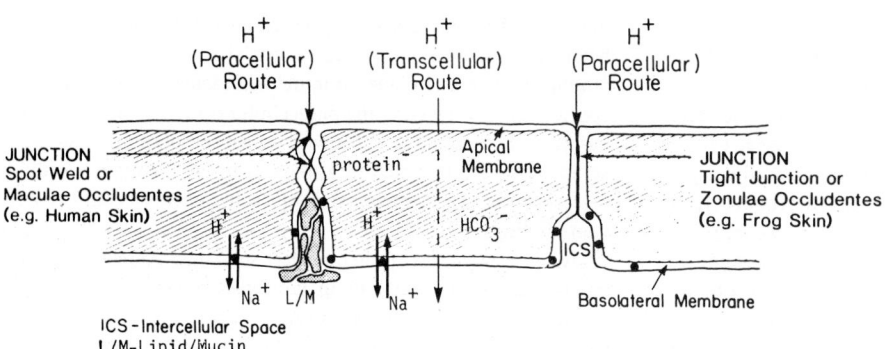

FIGURE 55–7. Tissue resistance. Some of the recognized epithelial defenses against acid injury are illustrated. Structural barriers to H+ diffusion include the cell membrane and intercellular junctional complex. Functional components include intracellular buffering by negatively charged proteins and HCO_3^- and H+ extrusion processes (e.g., Na^+/H^+ exchange) for regulation of intracellular pH. (Modified from Orlando RC. Esophageal epithelial resistance. In: Castell DO, Wu WC, Ott DJ, eds. Gastroesophageal reflux disease: Pathogenesis, diagnosis, therapy. Mount Kisco, NY: Futura, 1985.)

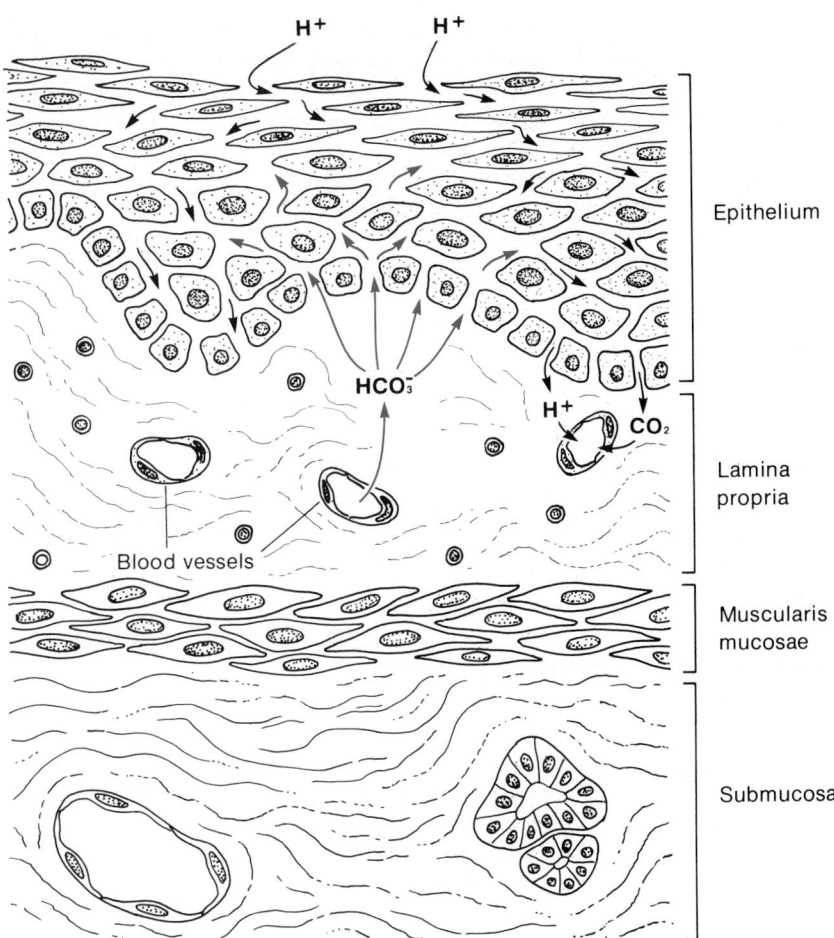

FIGURE 55–8. Tissue resistance. The major postepithelial defense against acid injury is an adequate blood supply. In addition to providing essential nutrients and oxygen for cell metabolism, the blood supply maintains tissue acid–base balance through the delivery of HCO_3^- and removal of H^+ and CO_2. The HCO_3^- contained in the interstitial fluid is important for neutralization of H^+ diffusing through the intercellular space. (From Orlando RC. Oesophageal defenses. In: Bennett JR, ed. Oesophagitis. London: Current Medical Literature Ltd., in press, 1991.)

Zollinger-Ellison syndrome, gastric acid hypersecretion undoubtedly contributes to the development of esophagitis by increasing the noxious quality of the refluxate. However, it is also likely that Zollinger-Ellison syndrome impairs defense by way of the ability of large gastric volumes to increase reflux through stimulation of TLESRs. Impaired defense in pregnancy, scleroderma, diabetes mellitus, and with prolonged nasogastric intubation also increases the risk for esophagitis. In pregnancy, the major inducement to reflux appears to be the relaxant effects of circulating estrogens and progesterones on the LES. The smooth muscle atrophy in scleroderma and the neuromuscular dysfunction in diabetes can result in dysfunction of both the LES, increasing reflux frequency, and esophageal peristalsis, delaying acid clearance. When such dysfunction is carried to extremes as it is in scleroderma, a severe form of esophagitis develops.[94] It is also likely that prolonged nasogastric intubation results in esophagitis by mechanically impairing both LES function and peristalsis.

CLINICAL MANIFESTATIONS

SYMPTOMS

The most common manifestation of pathologic reflux is heartburn. Heartburn is perceived as a substernal burning sensation that moves from the subxiphoid region up toward the manubrium. It most often occurs after meals and upon reclining at bedtime. Heartburn typically is relieved by antacids, baking soda, milk, or other buffering substances. When present on a recurrent basis, characteristic symptoms permit the diagnosis of reflux esophagitis to be confidently established by history alone. Although an aid to diagnosis, neither the frequency nor severity of heartburn is of value in predicting the degree of tissue damage. Indeed, severe damage can be asymptomatic.

Subjects with reflux esophagitis may also complain of atypical chest pain with a few or none of the characteristics of heartburn. At times, the chest pain more closely resembles that associated with cardiac disease. It may be sharp or dull and may radiate widely, including into the neck or arms. Because of overlapping neural pathways, the similarity in pain patterns for diseases of heart and esophagus is not surprising, and tests are needed to help distinguish the organ of origin (see section entitled Tests to Assess the Relationship of Atypical Chest Pain to [Acid] Reflux).

Pathologic reflux may also produce other symptoms including water brash, regurgitation, dysphagia, and odynophagia; and these may occur with or without accompanying heartburn. Regurgitation is the perception within the oral cavity of refluxed gastric contents (e.g., a bitter or acid taste). A history of bilious stains on the pillowcase in the morning may signal regurgitation occurring during sleep. Water brash is the spontaneous appearance of fluid in the mouth due to stimulated salivary secretion. Unlike regurgitated material, the fluid has a bland or slightly salty taste. Esophageal acid is believed to initiate this secretion through a vagally mediated esophago-salivary reflex. Dysphagia is an esophageal symptom that indicates the impairment in the movement of swallowed material from pharynx to stomach. It is usually described in terms of food "hanging up," "slowing down," or "getting stuck" substernally. In subjects with reflux esophagitis, the onset of dysphagia raises the concern that a stricture or carcinoma in a Barrett's esophagus has developed. Less frequently, dysphagia in esophagitis is a manifestation of abnormal peristalsis. If dysphagia is due to a stricture or cancer, the complaint is usually for solid food alone, while motor abnormalities are more likely to produce symptoms with ingestion of both solids and liquids. Odynophagia is defined as a sharp pain on swallowing and is usually localized under the sternum. It is far more common in esophagitis caused by infectious agents (*Candida*, herpes, cytomegalovirus) or by medications (tetracycline, KCl, quinine). When present, odynophagia usually reflects severe erosive/ulcerative disease and may be so uncomfortable that the subject is unable or afraid to eat.

Nonesophageal Signs/Symptoms of GERD

GER may damage regions other than esophagus, most notably the oropharynx, larynx, and respiratory tract. Damage to the oropharynx may give rise to sore throat, earache, gingivitis, poor dentition, and globus hystericus; reflux damage to the larynx and respiratory tract may cause hoarseness, wheezing, bronchitis, asthma, and aspiration pneumonia. In the pediatric age group, GER has been reported to cause apnea and the sudden infant death syndrome (SIDS).[95] Apnea and SIDS are presumably due to aspiration of refluxed gastric contents into the trachea or reflex bronchospasm with subsequent respiratory compromise or arrest.

Although aspiration of refluxed gastric contents into the upper airways and lungs can occur, the magnitude of this problem remains unclear. In a given patient, it is difficult to establish a cause-and-effect relationship between GER and pulmonary disease. Instead of cause and effect, the association of reflux and pulmonary disease may be through sharing of a common risk factor (e.g., smoking). Alternatively, the presence of one disease (e.g., pulmonary disease) may either directly or indirectly contribute to the other. The development of asthma or emphysema could enhance reflux by altering diaphragmatic location and function and by requiring medications, such as theophylline, that lower LES pressure. More importantly, a cause-and-effect relationship is difficult to establish because the available tests lack sufficient sensitivity and specificity to diagnosis reflux-related pulmonary disease. For example, one test devised to establish cause and effect involves ingestion of technetium 99 (^{99}Tc)-pertechnetate at bedtime to label gastric contents and gamma counter scanning of the subject in the morning for the presence of radiolabeled material within the lungs.[96-98] However, for the test to be positive, indicating reflux-induced aspiration, a scan also needs to be performed immediately after ingestion; this is done to exclude aspiration upon swallowing rather than through reflux. Even when the scan is positive, a judgment must be made as to whether the identified amount aspirated is of sufficient quantity to produce disease. Alternatively, when the scan is negative, and most are, the result is equally inconclusive. This

is because the label may have been emptied from the stomach and is made unavailable for reflux or because reflux-induced aspiration may not have occurred on the study night.

The relationship between reflux and asthma is even more complex when it is recognized that the refluxate need not enter the trachea for the production of pulmonary symptoms; bronchospasm can be elicited by acidification of the esophagus alone.[99-101] Bronchospasm appears mediated through cholinergic fibers in the vagus nerve because the response can be blocked by vagotomy or administration of atropine. Despite these observations, in clinical practice, the response to antireflux therapy in asthmatics is extremely variable,[102-105] being dependent upon the accuracy of diagnosis and the effectiveness of the antireflux regimen employed.

DIFFERENTIAL DIAGNOSIS AND DIAGNOSTIC STUDIES

Diagnostic Studies

A large number of tests have been devised for investigating subjects suspected of having reflux esophagitis (Table 55-2). In clinical practice, most are unnecessary to establish the diagnosis and initiate treatment. A history of recurrent heartburn alone is adequate to diagnosis reflux esophagitis and initiate therapy. This point bears emphasis because most "objective" tests for diagnosing reflux use this symptom as the gold standard for a positive test. Although a majority of subjects with heartburn are well served by an empiric trial of medical therapy without additional testing (see section entitled Therapy), it must be emphasized that the severity of heartburn correlates poorly with the severity of tissue injury. For this reason, it may be difficult to decide which subjects deserve

TABLE 55-2

Tests for Assessing the Presence of Gastroesophageal Reflux, Its Mechanisms, and Its Consequences

A. Tests for reflux
1. Upper gastrointestinal series
2. Tuttle (standard acid reflux) test
3. Continuous intraesophageal pH monitoring
4. Radionuclide (^{99}Tc) scintiscanning

B. Tests to assess symptoms
1. Bernstein (acid perfusion) test
2. Continuous intraesophageal pH monitoring

C. Tests to assess esophageal damage
1. Barium esophagram or upper gastrointestinal series
2. Upper endoscopy
3. Esophageal biopsy
4. Esophageal potential difference measurement*

D. Tests to assess pathogenesis of esophagitis
1. Acid clearance test*
2. Radionuclide (^{99}Tc) scintiscanning*
3. Esophageal manometry
4. Gastric analysis

* *Principally investigational procedures.*

radiologic or endoscopic investigation. Based on the goals of treatment being relief of symptoms and prevention of complications, investigations should be performed in those subjects with either persistent heartburn or symptoms and signs indicative of significant tissue injury (e.g., dysphagia, odynophagia, guaiac positive stool, anemia). Early investigation is also indicated for any subject in whom the diagnosis is uncertain.

TESTS TO ASSESS REFLUX

Barium Studies. The most readily available test for identifying pathologic reflux is the upper gastrointestinal series.[40] The unimpeded movement of barium from the filled stomach to esophagus in the head-down subject is considered positive for reflux. Although highly specific, this maneuver has very low sensitivity, missing up to 80% of subjects with reflux esophagitis.[40,106,107] To increase the sensitivity of the barium study, the water-siphon test was developed.[108] In this maneuver, reflux of barium was sought in the head-down subject sipping water through a straw. This test has been abandoned because of low specificity— the high false-positive rate for reflux being due to physiologic relaxation of the LES with swallows.[40,109]

Tuttle (Standard Acid Reflux) Test. This test, introduced by Tuttle and Grossman in 1958,[110] was the first to use an intraesophageal pH electrode for detection of pathologic reflux. After passing a pH electrode into the stomach of a supine, fasting subject to document the presence of gastric acid,[111] the probe is repositioned 5 cm above the manometrically defined LES to monitor for the presence of spontaneous free reflux (pH drops to less than 4).[111] If free reflux is not observed in the basal state, reflux is sought during straight leg raising, Valsalva and Müller maneuvers, and during manual abdominal compression. A positive test is recorded if pH falls to less than 4 during or shortly after two maneuvers. If the test is negative, the same maneuvers are repeated after adding 300 ml 0.1N HCl to the stomach. The sensitivity of this test ranges from 54% to 100% (average 80%), and the specificity ranges from 70% to 95% (average 83%).[112]

Continuous Intraesophageal pH Monitoring. Continuous intraesophageal pH monitoring is an excellent method for the diagnosis of pathologic reflux.[113-115] Continuous monitoring is performed with the nasally inserted pH probe affixed 5 cm above the LES. A reference electrode is taped to the skin, and both electrodes are connected to a battery-powered computer for continuous recording. An integral part of the computer is an event marker, which can be activated by the subject for correlation of reflux events with symptoms, activity, or body position. Monitoring is generally carried out for 24 hours, although shorter times have been suggested as providing equally discriminatory information. A reflux episode is counted when intraesophageal pH falls below 4. For this reason, subjects must avoid ingesting acidic foods (false-positive results) and must refrain from taking medications such as antacids, anticholinergics, or H_2-receptor antagonists (false-negative results). Using a computer program, the following parameters are usually assessed: total number of reflux episodes, total number of reflux episodes lasting longer than 5 minutes, and total duration that esophageal pH is less than 4. In most centers,

these same values are subdivided according to their occurrence in the upright (daytime) or supine (nocturnal) position.

The sensitivity and specificity of prolonged pH monitoring in identifying pathologic reflux are good to excellent. The sensitivity ranges from 48% to 100% (average 85%), and the specificity approaches 100%.[112] This level of specificity, however, has not been achieved by all. It is proposed that maximal sensitivity and specificity can best be achieved by considering the percentage of time esophageal pH is less than 4. By this criterion, a sensitivity of 93.3% and specificity of 92.9% were obtained using, as threshold, values of 10.5% in the upright position and 6% in the supine position.[116] Subjects were classified as "normal" if values for both upright and supine positions were below threshold, and "pathologic" if either was above threshold.

Radionuclide (^{99}Tc) Scintiscanning. Radiolabeled ^{99}Tc-sulfur colloid may be used as a semiquantitative test for detection of GER.[117] After instilling 300 ml of ^{99}Tc-sulfur colloid-laced saline into the stomach through a nasogastric tube, gamma counter counts over stomach and esophagus are obtained in supine subjects before and during abdominal compression, the latter standardized by means of an abdominal binder. Reflux is determined by a scoring system based on the number of counts over esophagus relative to the number of counts over stomach. Although the specificity of this method for detecting reflux averages 90%, the sensitivity varies from 14% to 90%.[118-120]

TESTS TO ASSESS THE RELATIONSHIP OF ATYPICAL CHEST PAIN TO (ACID) REFLUX

Bernstein Test. The Bernstein test is useful for determining if atypical chest pain is related to esophageal acidification.[121] The test is performed in a seated subject by positioning a nasogastric tube in midesophagus and initially infusing normal saline at 100 to 120 drops/min for 5 to 15 minutes, followed by infusion with 0.1N HCl. If symptoms develop within 30 minutes of acid infusion, saline is reinfused to assess relief. If symptoms resolve, HCl is reinfused. The subject should not be aware of what solution is being infused. The appearance of symptoms during acid infusion, but not saline, constitutes a positive test. Complete relief of symptoms by saline is not essential. In some centers, the Bernstein test is not considered positive unless a gastric origin for symptoms is excluded by failure to reproduce symptoms by acid-perfusion of the stomach.[122] The proper interpretation of a "positive" Bernstein test in assessing the origin of chest pain requires knowledge of the type of symptoms elicited during acid perfusion. If acidification reproduces the subject's spontaneous pain, an esophageal origin is supported. In contrast, if acid perfusion produces heartburn or a new type of pain, the esophagus is acid-sensitive but its relevance to the clinical complaint is indeterminate.

The sensitivity of the Bernstein test ranges from 32% to 100% (average 78%) for reflux disease, and its specificity ranges from 40% to 100% (average 84%).[112] When performed in subjects with atypical chest pain, however, its sensitivity in establishing the cause for symptoms is much lower, range 7% to 27%,[123,124] but its specificity is believed to be high.[125] Nonetheless, care must be taken in interpreting all positive Bernstein tests (i.e., reproducing the subject's spontaneous pain) as indicative of esophageal disease because it is known that esophageal acid perfusion can precipitate myocardial ischemia[126] and evidence is accumulating that normal coronary angiography does not completely exclude a possible cardiac cause for pain.[127,128]

Continuous Intraesophageal pH Monitoring.

The ability to correlate symptoms with an (acid) reflux event is an important role of continuous pH monitoring. The correlation of atypical symptoms with reflux events on pH monitoring in 12 of 50 subjects resulted in subsequent relief for all 12 by an antireflux program that included surgery in 8 and medical therapy in 4.[129] Despite these favorable results, such correlations can prove difficult. For example, it is unclear how confident the diagnosis of a reflux-related symptom is when multiple episodes occur during monitoring, only one of which is associated with a reflux event. Alternatively, it is unclear how confident the diagnosis of a reflux-related event is when multiple episodes of reflux occur without symptoms and symptoms occur during another such episode that is otherwise indistinguishable. Because our understanding of the origin and mechanisms of esophageal pain remains rudimentary, the possibility that such observations may prove coincidental rather than causal must be kept in mind.

TESTS TO ASSESS THE TYPE OR EXTENT OF ESOPHAGEAL INJURY

Esophageal mucosal damage can be identified macroscopically by radiologic or endoscopic study or microscopically by evaluation of esophageal biopsies. The pathologic findings in the esophagus resulting from reflux are presented in Table 55-3.

TABLE 55-3
Esophageal Pathology in Gastroesophageal Reflux

Noninflammatory changes
  1. Basal cell hyperplasia
  2. Increased papillary height
Inflammatory changes
  1. Acute
     a. Vascular congestion/stasis
     b. Mucosal edema
     c. Polymorphonuclear leukocytic infiltration (neutrophils/ eosinophils)
  2. Chronic
     a. Mononuclear leukocyte infiltration (macrophages)
     b. Increased macrophage activity
     c. Proliferation of fibroblasts
     d. Ingrowth of vascular endothelium
Epithelial necrosis
  1. Erosion
  2. Ulceration
Epithelial repair
  1. Granulation tissue
  2. Fibrosis (stricture formation)
  3. Epithelial regeneration
     a. Squamous replication
     b. Columnar metaplasia (Barrett's esophagus)

Orlando R. Pathology of reflux oesophagitis and its complications. In: Jamieson GG, ed. Surgery of the oesophagus. New York: Churchill Livingstone, 1988.

Barium Studies. A barium esophagram or upper gastrointestinal series is usually the initial procedure performed in subjects with reflux. Although less sensitive or specific than endoscopy, a single contrast study can readily identify strictures, ulcers, and a hiatus hernia.[40] If a double-contrast technique is employed, erosions and a reticulated mucosal pattern suggestive of Barrett's epithelium may also be identified.[130] The radiologic identification of a nonmalignant midesophageal stricture or ulcer usually indicates that the esophagus below is lined by columnar (Barrett's) epithelium.[131]

Endoscopy and Biopsy. Upper endoscopy with biopsy is the gold standard for documenting the type and extent of tissue injury from reflux. It should, however, be used judiciously because of the cost and the small, but real, potential for complications. Endoscopic findings in patients with reflux esophagitis include normal-appearing mucosa, erythema, edema, friability, exudate, erosions, ulcers, strictures, and Barrett's epithelium.[58,132,133] Some of these findings are subtle and subject to considerable interobserver variability,[132] and none are etiologically specific for reflux disease; they are also noted in subjects with esophageal injury from other causes. Esophageal biopsies should be routinely performed at the time of endoscopy to: (1) document the histology of gross abnormalities, (2) detect microscopic abnormalities in normal-appearing mucosa, and (3) aid in excluding infectious and neoplastic causes of esophageal injury.

Histology. Many subjects with recurrent heartburn have an endoscopically normal appearing mucosa. In this circumstance, random biopsies of the lower esophagus can provide histologic evidence of disease. The most sensitive hallmarks of reflux damage to esophageal mucosa were initially described on esophageal specimens obtained by Rubin-Quinton suction biopsy;[134] but these same changes are also evident on well-oriented specimens obtained with endoscopic jumbo biopsy forceps.[133] They are: (1) increased height of the esophageal papillae, papillae extending greater than or equal to two thirds of the way to the luminal surface, and (2) basal cell hyperplasia, basal layer thickness greater than or equal to one sixth of the epithelium (Fig 55-9). The increase in papillary height results from desquamation of acid-damaged surface cells; basal cell hyperplasia reflects an increased rate of cell replication, the reparative response. The basal layer thickens because these are the only cells within the epithelium capable of mitosis.[135,136] Heartburn is believed to be triggered by acid contact with sensory nerve endings within the lamina propria. The close proximity of papilla to lumen explains the frequent symptoms in subjects with these histologic changes. Although increased papillary height and basal cell hyperplasia are sensitive indicators of reflux damage, they lack specificity.[137-139] These abnormalities are noted on esophageal biopsies from the lower 2.5 cm of esophagus in 20% of healthy subjects.[137]

Acute inflammation is a specific hallmark of esophageal damage.[140-143] It is characterized by damage to the tissue's vascular bed, edema, and infiltration by polymorphonuclear leukocytes, which release the vasoactive substances that contribute to these changes. Prostaglandins may be one of the substances that mediate inflammation in the esophagus. This may be the reason that indomethacin, a cyclooxygenase inhibitor, appears to prevent the histologic appearance of esophagitis after acid or radiation exposure.[144,145] Vasoactive substances produce vasodilation and in-

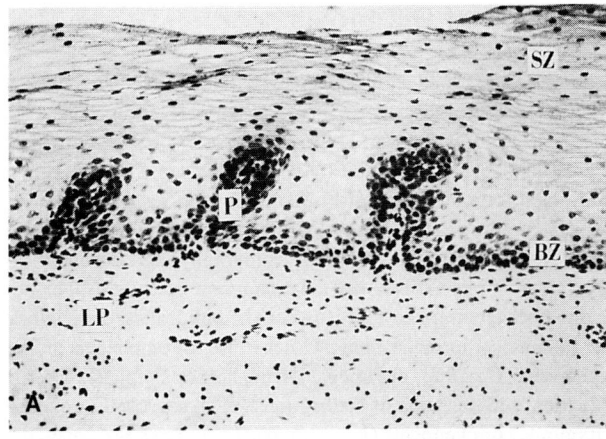

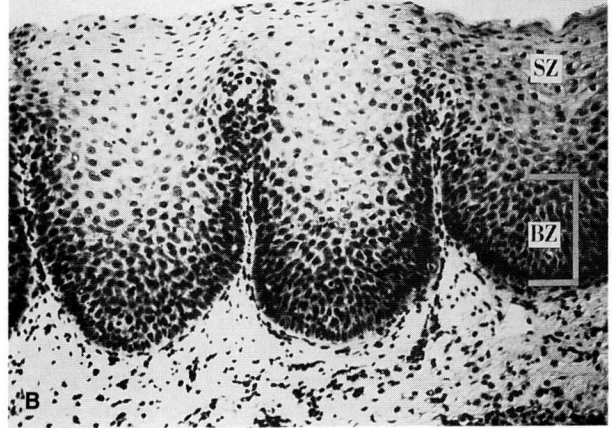

FIGURE 55–9. **A**, Normal esophageal suction biopsy from a healthy subject without reflux. Basal zone thickness is approximately 10% of total epithelial thickness; papillae extend approximately one half of the distance to the epithelial surface. **B**, Abnormal suction biopsy from a subject with symptomatic reflux. Basal zone thickness is approximately 35% of total epithelial thickness; papillae extend over two thirds of the distance to the epithelial surface. *BZ* = basal zone; *SZ* = stratified zone; *P* = papillae; *LP* = lamina propria. Hematoxylin-eosin, ×170. (Ismail-Beigi F, Horton PF, Pope CE. Histological consequences of gastroesophageal reflux in man. Gastroenterology 1970;58:163.)

creased vascular permeability leading to edema and stasis. The elaboration of chemotactic substances causes migration of neutrophils and eosinophils into the area.[146] The identification of neutrophils on esophageal biopsy is specific for acute esophageal damage; however, it is also an insensitive marker, being found in only 15% to 30% of subjects with reflux symptoms.[138,140,142,143] Eosinophils are found more often than neutrophils in those with reflux (19%–63% of subjects), but their presence is less specific, being found on biopsy in 10% to 33% of healthy adults.[138,142,143]

Acute inflammation is often intermixed with chronic inflammation in esophageal biopsies because reflux esophagitis is a chronic disease with superimposed episodes of acute injury. Chronic inflammation is characterized by the presence of macrophages (Langerhans' cells) and granulation tissue, the latter consisting of new vessel growth and fibroblast activity.[146] The macrophages are derived from blood monocytes and are important for scavenging cellular debris. These same macrophages are also responsible for stimulating fibroblast proliferation and new vessel growth of

granulation tissue. The fibroblasts, in turn, synthesize and deposit collagen for wound healing. In cases of severe injury, fibroblasts may deposit enough collagen to form a lumen-encroaching scar known as a stricture (see section entitled "Complications"). In addition to a stricture, severe injury may also lead to aberrant repair of the epithelial lining. In the latter case, the lower esophagus becomes lined by columnar epithelium, a condition known as Barrett's esophagus (see section entitled "Complications").

Esophageal PD Measurement. The spontaneous electrical potential difference (PD) across the esophageal epithelium is created by the combination of active Na transport from lumen to blood and the resistance of cell membranes and intercellular junctional structures to the passive diffusion of ions. Consequently, the presence of a normal PD is indicative of a structurally and functionally sound epithelium.[147–149] When esophageal tissues are exposed to acid, the damage that develops is heralded principally by a decline in PD.[1,147,150–152] This decline is initially the result of increased permeability through the intercellular junctions and later by inhibited Na transport. When PD is abolished by acid exposure, necrosis is evident histologically. However, with less severe injury the PD may be either low or normal. In cases where acid-damaged tissues have retained a normal PD, damage can be unmasked by monitoring PD during acid perfusion. The esophageal PD of patients with a positive Bernstein test declines to pathologically low levels during acid perfusion, while subjects with a negative test exhibit no fall in PD with similar exposure.[148]

The PD of healthy squamous epithelium differs from that of columnar epithelium such that the transition in values can be used to identify the squamocolumnar junction.[151,153,154] Because the PD of columnar epithelium in Barrett's esophagus is also typically high, the combination of PD and pressure measurements using a Ringer-perfused manometric catheter as a probe have been successful in detecting Barrett's esophagus.[153] Nonetheless, while PD measurements have utility both for identifying damaged tissue and screening for Barrett's esophagus, it is principally a research technique and does not abrogate the need for endoscopy and biopsy for histologic confirmation.

TESTS TO ASSESS THE MECHANISMS RESPONSIBLE FOR THE DEVELOPMENT OF ESOPHAGITIS

Acid Clearance Test. This test is based on the concept that delayed luminal clearance of acid contributes to the development of esophagitis. It is performed by injecting 15 ml of 0.1N HCl into midesophagus while monitoring esophageal pH 5 cm above the LES. After esophageal acidification, subjects are instructed to dry swallow, and the number of dry swallows needed to raise pH back to neutral is recorded. Initial studies showed that almost all healthy subjects cleared acid with 10 swallows and those with esophagitis required much more (15–40 swallows).[155] However, such discriminatory results have not been confirmed by others, and, consequently, this test is not used clinically because it is an insensitive indicator of reflux disease. However, in a given subject, the demonstration of delayed acid clearance may provide important information that a defect in peristalsis or salivary secretion may contribute to reflux disease.

Radionuclide (⁹⁹Tc) Scintiscanning. Scintiscanning, like the acid clearance test, has been used to monitor esophageal clearance.[52,156] This is done by monitoring with a gamma counter the disappearance from the esophageal lumen of a swallowed bolus labeled with ⁹⁹Tc-sulfur colloid. The same limitations apply to this method as to that for the acid clearance test described above.

Esophageal Manometry. Manometry by perfused-catheter technique is widely used for evaluating the contractility of the esophageal musculature.[157] A multilumen (usually triple) catheter assembly is passed through the nose into the esophagus and fixed in place such that the most distal orifice is located within the LES and the two or more upper orifices, spaced 5 cm apart, are in position to monitor peristalsis. By perfusing the catheters with water by way of a pneumohydraulic capillary infusion system, the pressures generated by esophageal contractions can be sensed, amplified, and recorded for study.

Mean LES pressure is one parameter that can be obtained from the tracing. Initially, it was thought that this parameter could discriminate between subjects with and without reflux esophagitis.[158,159] However, considerable overlap exists.[160] In fact, 30% to 50% of reflux subjects have normal LES pressure (10–30 mmHg), while low LES pressure (less than 10 mmHg) can be found in 10% of healthy subjects. Despite disillusionment with measurements of LES pressure for diagnosis, it has value for assessing prognosis. A low LES pressure in subjects with reflux is associated with a high failure rate on medical therapy[35] and a low LES pressure may predict which reflux subjects will subsequently relapse after medical treatment.[161] This would suggest that knowledge of LES pressure may help determine which subjects are more likely to benefit from antireflux surgery.[162]

In subjects with reflux, a variety of abnormalities of peristaltic function may be noted. While providing information relevant to an understanding of pathophysiology, in most cases these findings do not affect therapy. It may, however, serve to establish a correct diagnosis (e.g., achalasia in a subject referred for refractory esophagitis believed on the basis of reflux or as the first clue to the diagnosis of scleroderma). Manometric evaluation of peristaltic function also is important preoperatively because documentation of disordered peristalsis may influence the type of antireflux repair chosen (see section entitled Surgical Treatment).

Gastric Analysis. Gastric analysis is rarely used for assessing subjects with reflux esophagitis because of the general sense that most patients with symptomatic reflux have normal rates of acid secretion.[15] This approach, however, may change given the difficulty of standard doses of H₂-blockers to heal esophagitis[161,163,164] and the dramatic success of the more potent acid-reducing agent, omeprazole.[20] If it were shown that increasing gastric pH by using higher doses of H₂-blockers would also improve the healing rates in esophagitis, perhaps, as in the therapy of Zollinger-Ellison syndrome,[165] gastric analysis could be used to determine the proper dose of H₂-blocker in persons with refractory disease. Further, reflux esophagitis is common in subjects with the Zollinger-Ellison syndrome,[90] and a gastric analysis may be useful for raising this diagnostic possibility.

Differential Diagnosis

Symptoms associated with GER may be mimicked by other diseases such as cholelithiasis, peptic ulcer, gastritis, angina pectoris, and esophageal motor disease. However, these disorders can usually be distinguished from reflux by performing some of the same or additional tests including ultrasonography, upper gastrointestinal series, cine-esophagogram, endoscopy with gastric biopsy, esophageal manometry, stress electrocardiography, and coronary angiography. While GER is the most common cause of esophagitis, it must be remembered that it is not the only cause, especially in the immunocompromised host. Other causes of esophagitis include infections (*Candida*, cytomegalovirus, herpes simplex), chest irradiation, and ingestion of medications (KCl, tetracycline, quinine, vitamin C) or chemicals (lye, bleach). These areas are covered in greater detail in Chapters 56 and 58.

CLINICAL COURSE AND COMPLICATIONS

Clinical Course of Reflux Esophagitis

The clinical course of pathologic reflux is extremely variable. Subjects may have brief periods of heartburn that spontaneously resolve or readily respond to simple dietary measures or antacids, or they may have persistent symptoms whose severity and frequency are disruptive to their daily lives. Interestingly, whether intermittent or persistent, responsive or not to diet and antacids, symptoms do not predict or parallel the degree of esophageal mucosal damage from reflux. Subjects may complain of severe, persistent symptoms for months to years, yet on objective study, they are found to have little or no mucosal abnormalities. Alternatively, damage to esophageal mucosa may progress, with or without accompanying symptoms, from inflammation to ulceration and from ulceration to healing by stricture formation or the development of Barrett's esophagus. It is somewhat ironic to note that two of the more serious lesions in reflux esophagitis, strictures and Barrett's esophagus, arise directly from attempts at repair.

Complications

STRICTURES

Strictures are bands of submucosal fibrous tissue that encroach upon the esophageal lumen, and in so doing impede the passage of ingested material from mouth to stomach. Strictures are recognized clinically by the development of dysphagia, which usually progresses slowly over months to years. With dysphagia there is often a reduction in heartburn, reflecting the ability of strictures to act as a barrier to reflux.

Radiologically, peptic strictures are usually smooth-walled, tapered circumferential narrowings in the lower esophagus averaging 1 to 4 cm in length (Fig 55-10). At times, however, they may be

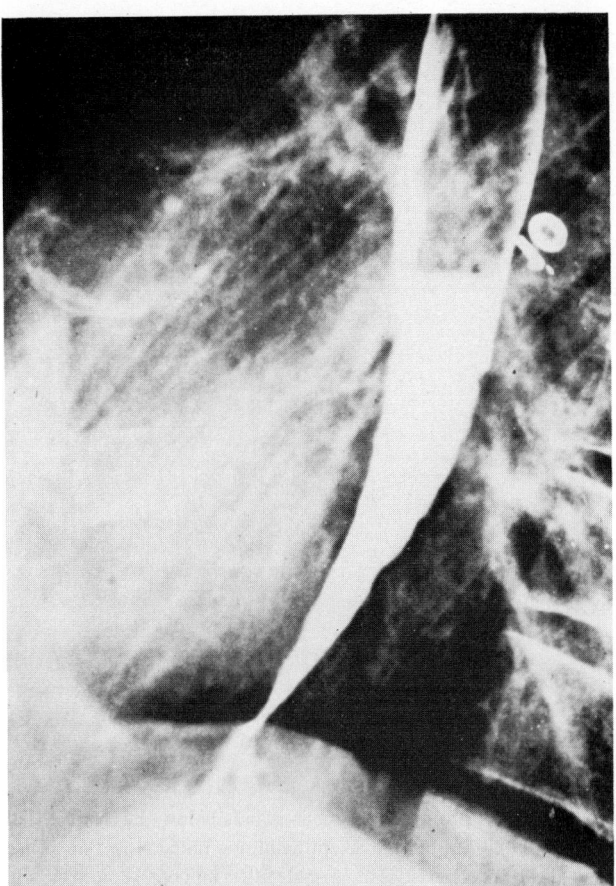

FIGURE 55–10. Barium esophagram showing a benign peptic stricture in the distal esophagus as a complication of longstanding reflux esophagitis.

much longer, irregular or eccentric in appearance, and located in mid or upper esophagus.[40] In all cases, the benign nature of the peptic stricture needs to be confirmed by endoscopy and biopsy. Endoscopy and biopsy are also valuable for documenting the occurrence of Barrett's epithelium below mid- and upper esophageal peptic strictures.[131]

BARRETT'S ESOPHAGUS

Barrett's esophagus denotes the presence of a simple columnar epithelium lining the lower esophagus rather than the normal stratified squamous epithelium.[166] Although in some cases a congenital origin seems possible, it is generally believed to be an acquired lesion that develops predominantly from reflux damage to the lining of the lower esophagus.[166–168] In Barrett's esophagus, the columnar epithelium is located in the distal esophagus and usually occurs in association with other features of reflux esophagitis. These features distinguish it from the inlet or herald patch, which is an island of columnar epithelium located in the upper esophagus.[169] The inlet patch appears to be of congenital origin and is usually asymptomatic. Occasionally, however, patients with inlet patches capable of acid secretion may develop dysphagia or other esophageal symptoms.[170] Replacement of stratified squamous

epithelium by columnar epithelium has been documented by serial endoscopies and biopsies in subjects with esophagitis[171–173] and can be produced experimentally in animal models of reflux esophagitis.[174,175] Because the columnar epithelium is more acid-resistant than stratified squamous epitheium,[176] the development of a Barrett's esophagus appears initially to be an effective protective manuever. This view is reinforced by the observation that subjects with Barrett's esophagus experience less pain during esophageal acid perfusion than do subjects with esophagitis in squamous linings.[177] However, the price for this protection comes high because Barrett's esophagus is a premalignant condition, leading to the development of adenocarcinoma of the esophagus in approximately 10% of subjects.[178–181] Although the prevalence of adenocarcinoma is estimated at 10%, the incidence of developing cancer from a nonmalignant Barrett's epithelium remains a controversial issue, with reports of developing cancer ranging from 1 in 442 patient-years to 1 in 52 patient-years[182–185] (see ch 57).

Barrett's esophagus was once considered an uncommon condition, but with the advent of endoscopy it has been observed in approximately 10% to 15% of subjects with esophagitis and up to 40% of subjects with peptic strictures.[153,186] Barrett's esophagus occurs more often in males than females (3:1 male predominance) and in all age groups, with the average age at the time of diagnosis being 55 years. It is common in whites and rare in blacks.[166,187] Barrett's esophagus itself produces no symptoms, but because it arises as a complication of reflux, the majority present with either heartburn or dysphagia. When dysphagia is the presenting complaint, it usually reflects the presence of a stricture or heralds the development of adenocarcinoma.

The diagnosis of Barrett's esophagus requires the demonstration of columnar epithelium within the lower esophagus (Fig 55-11). Its presence may be suggested by the finding of a midesophageal stricture or ulcer on upper gastrointestinal series. Alternatively, it may be demonstrated by ^{99}Tc pertechnetate scintiscanning, which shows uptake of radiolabel above the diaphragm, or by esophageal PD measurement, which demonstrates values greater than -25 mV.[40,131,153,188,189] However, Barrett's esophagus is usually diagnosed on endoscopy, the lesion being suspected by orad displacement of the squamocolumnar junction into the tubular lumen of the esophagus. The squamocolumnar junction can be visually appreciated by the juxtaposition of deep-red columnar mucosa with a lighter orange-pink squamous mucosa (Fig 55-12; Color Fig 19). Barrett's esophagus may also be recognized by the presence of red columnar islands within squamous mucosa or by the presence of lighter squamous islands within a circumferential columnar mucosa.[181] When distinction by color is not clear-cut, differential staining by instillation of Lugol's solution may be helpful.[186] Lugol's solution stains the glycogen-rich squamous epithelium blue-black, leaving unstained the glycogen-poor columnar epithelium. While color and staining characteristics are useful for localization of suspicious areas, the diagnosis of Barrett's esophagus ultimately requires biopsy for histologic confirmation. Endoscopic biopsies are adequate for the diagnosis when the columnar lining extends more than 3 cm into the tubular lumen. However, when a short segment of Barrett's esophagus is present, manometrically guided suction biopsies may be required for clear documentation that biopsies containing columnar mucosa were obtained above the LES.[190] The exception to this approach occurs when specialized columnar epithelium is obtained on endoscopic biopsy. This his-

BARRETT'S ESOPHAGUS: A DIAGNOSTIC APPROACH

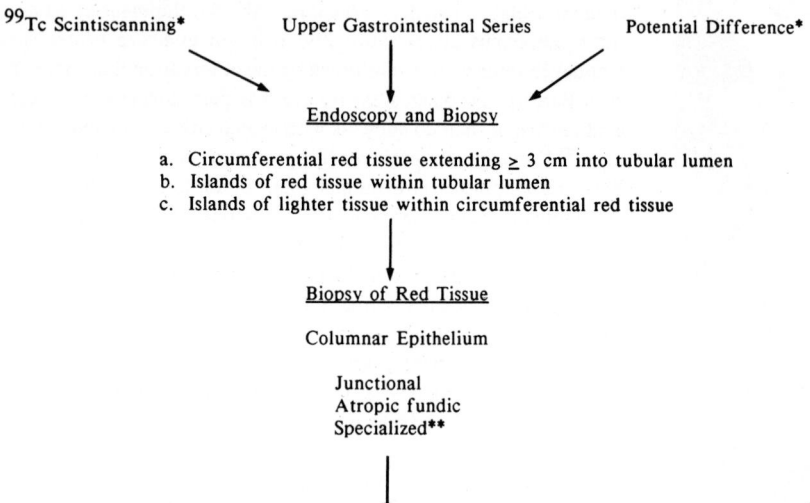

ANATOMIC LOCALIZATION OF COLUMNAR EPITHELIUM

^{99}Tc Scintiscanning*   Upper Gastrointestinal Series   Potential Difference*

Endoscopy and Biopsy

a. Circumferential red tissue extending ≥ 3 cm into tubular lumen
b. Islands of red tissue within tubular lumen
c. Islands of lighter tissue within circumferential red tissue

Biopsy of Red Tissue

Columnar Epithelium

Junctional
Atropic fundic
Specialized**

Manometrically-Guided Suction Biopsy

For all circumferential lesions < 3 cm unless
specialized columnar found on biopsy above

FIGURE 55–11. Diagnostic scheme for the diagnosis of Barrett's (columnar-lined lower) esophagus. *, Experimental techniques; **, Pathognomonic for Barrett's esophagus.

tology confirms Barrett's esophagus because, unlike junctional and atrophic fundic mucosa, it is not found in upper stomach.[140,166]

Barrett's epithelium is comprised of three different histologic types: atrophic gastric fundic, junctional, and specialized columnar epithelium (Fig 55-13). The atrophic gastric-fundic epithelium contains functioning parietal and chief cells and, consequently, is similar to tissue derived from the normal gastric fundus. Junctional epithelium is similar to tissue derived from the normal gastric

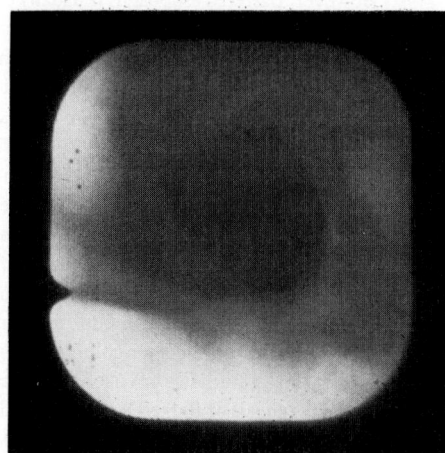

FIGURE 55–12. (See Color Fig 19) Endoscopic appearance of the distal esophagus in a patient with circumferential-type Barrett's esophagus. Note that the red columnar epithelium completely lines the lower esophagus but merges proximally with the lighter stratified squamous epithelium of the mid-esophagus. (From Herlihy KJ, Orlando RC, Bryson JC, et al. Barrett's esophagus: Clinical, endoscopic, histologic, manometric and electrical potential difference characteristics. Gastroenterology 1984;86: 436.)

cardia with its prominent mucous glands below the surface cell lining. Specialized columnar epithelium is unusual in that it has none of the characteristics of normal gastric mucosa. It more closely resembles the small intestinal epithelium with villi, microvilli, goblet and Paneth's cells.[190,191] While subjects with Barrett's esophagus may have only one epithelial type, they more often have a mosaic pattern comprising two or all three types. Given the variety of epithelia found, no clear agreement has been reached on their origin. One hypothesis is that Barrett's esophagus arises from orad migration of columnar cells from the stomach.[174] This is attractive because of the similarity between two of the types and normal gastric epithelia. Others suggest that the same columnar cells are derived, not from gastric epithelium, but from columnar cells lining the esophageal mucosal and submucosal glands.[192] However, because neither of these explanations accounts for the appearance of specialized columnar epithelium, a third hypothesis is that the columnar cells arise from a pluripotential cell type within squamous epithelium.[193]

HEMORRHAGE

While most subjects with reflux esophagitis have little or no evidence of gastrointestinal bleeding, those with esophageal erosions and ulcers may develop chronic bleeding and iron deficiency anemia. Also, although uncommon, life-threatening hemorrhage can develop, usually in the setting of deep ulcers.

PERFORATION

Esophageal perforation is a rare complication of reflux esophagitis. Like major hemorrhage, it usually develops as a consequence of

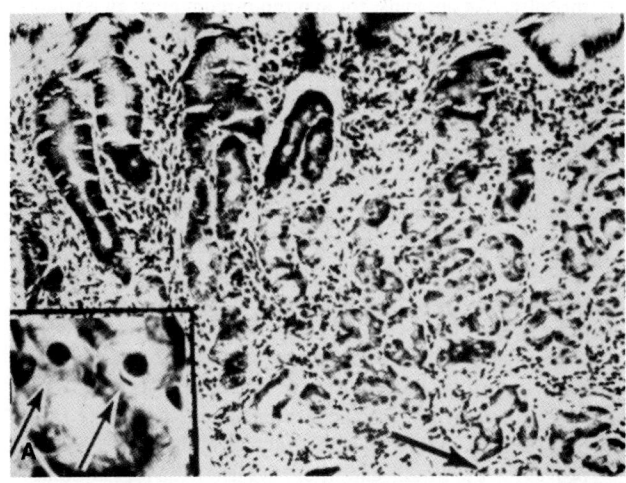

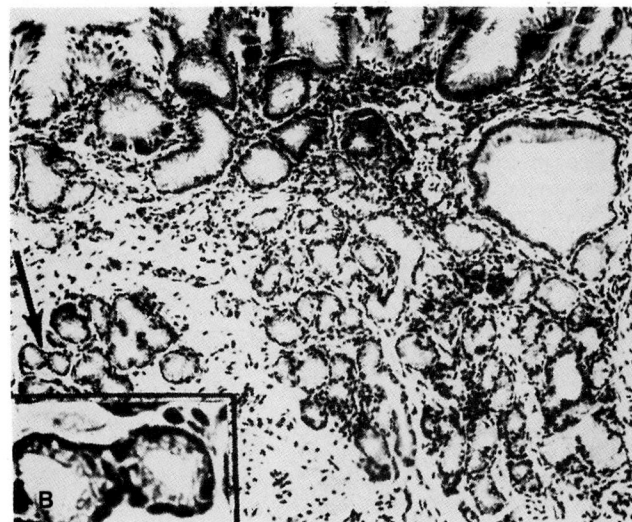

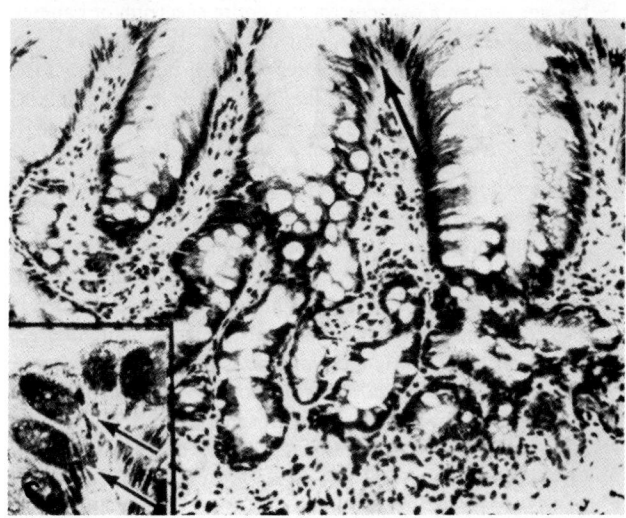

FIGURE 55–13. Light micrographs of epithelial types in Barrett's esophagus. **A,** Gastric-fundic type epithelium with mild inflammation and moderate glandular atrophy. The *large arrow* identifies inset (×100). The inset demonstrates parietal cells (*arrows*) in glandular layers (×500). **B,** Junctional type epithelium with mild inflammation (×100). The *large arrow* identifies inset, which shows mucous glands with no parietal cells (×425). **C,** Specialized columnar epithelium with villiform surface pattern and intestinal type goblet cells that appear empty in this hematoxylin-and-eosin-stained section (×175). The *large arrow* shows an area comparable to that of inset, which shows Alcian blue staining of intestinal-type goblet cells (*arrows*) on surface epithelium (×350). (From Paull A, Trier JS, Dalton MD, et al. The histologic spectrum of Barrett's esophagus. N Engl J Med 1976;295:476.)

an esophageal ulcer. Perforation and the resulting mediastinitis can be life-threatening unless rapidly recognized and treated.

THERAPY

Medical Management

Reflux esophagitis is a disease that, even untreated, usually progresses slowly and only rarely produces acute life-threatening events. For this reason, the vast majority of subjects should initially be managed medically. Medical management can be separated into two categories: (1) lifestyle modification and (2) drug therapy. Both therapies work to either reduce the noxious potency of the refluxate or increase the effectiveness of esophageal defenses (i.e., antireflux barriers, clearance mechanisms, epithelial resistance).[194]

LIFESTYLE MODIFICATION

Lifestyle modification should be part of the initial management in all subjects (Table 55-4). These measures may be effective in reducing symptoms and preventing recurrence and the price is right—costing almost nothing. Furthermore, the benefits accrued from lifestyle modification are not limited to improvement in reflux esophagitis because a low-fat diet, cessation of smoking, and reduction of alcohol intake also reduce the risk of serious hepatic, colonic, and cardiopulmonary disease.

The rationale for the lifestyle modifications recommended in Table 55-4 are as follows: elevation of the head of the bed or, for patients in whom this is intolerable, sleeping on a 10-inch wedge allows gravity to enhance the rate of acid clearance during sleep.[195,196] Cessation of smoking and alcohol is valuable because both agents lower LES pressure, reduce acid clearance, and directly alter epithelial cell function. Reducing the size of the meal and the intake of fat, carminatives and chocolate, may also reduce the frequency of reflux by avoiding foods that lower LES pressure and by reducing gastric distention (and TLESRs). Coffee (caffeinated and decaffeinated), tea, and cola beverages should be

TABLE 55-4
Lifestyle Modifications for Reflux Esophagitis

1. Elevate the head of the bed 6 inches.
2. Stop smoking.
3. Stop excessive alcohol consumption.
4. Reduce dietary fat.
5. Reduce meal size.
6. Avoid bedtime snacks.
7. Reduce weight (if overweight).
8. Avoid these foods:
   Chocolate
   Carminatives (spearmint, peppermint)
   Coffee (caffeinated and decaffeinated)
   Tea
   Cola beverages
   Tomato juice
   Citrus fruit juices
9. Avoid, when possible, these drugs:
   Anticholinergics
   Theophylline
   Diazepam
   Narcotics
   Calcium channel blockers
   β-adrenergic agonists (isoproterenol)
   Progesterone (some contraceptives)
   α-adrenergic antagonists (phentolamine)

Orlando RC. Gastroesophageal reflux: Medical treatment. In: Bayless TM, ed. Current therapy in gastroenterology and liver disease, ed 3. Philadelphia: BC Decker, 1990, p 7.

avoided because they stimulate acid secretion, and tomato juice, orange juice, and other citrus products may produce symptoms both because of their acidity[197] and because of their hyperosmolality.[198] Finally, reflux frequency may be reduced by avoiding, when possible, those drugs listed in Table 55-4 that are known to lower LES pressure.

CONVENTIONAL DRUGS

Drug therapy is important in the management of reflux esophagitis. Table 55-5 lists those in use and under active investigation and gives the important mechanisms by which each of these agents are thought to act to relieve symptoms and heal lesions.

1. Liquid antacids, on a prn basis, are the mainstay for rapid, safe, effective relief of symptoms. Antacids may also be effective in healing esophageal lesions, but, even in well-motivated patients, compliance with a regimen rigorous enough to accomplish this is limited.[108] Problems with compliance arise because of poor palatability and major bowel-habit altering side-effects (magnesium-containing agents producing diarrhea and aluminum-containing agents producing constipation). The potential for magnesium and aluminum toxicity further limits their use in patients with significant renal disease. Low-sodium antacids (e.g., Riopan) are preferable for those on salt-restricted diets.

2. Gaviscon, an antacid–alginate combination, can be used empirically, like antacids, for symptom relief or as an adjunct to therapy in those with more severe disease.[199] Although Gaviscon is safe, it contains aluminum, magnesium, and sodium, therefore the same precautions listed for antacids apply.

3. H$_2$-receptor antagonists. Just as antacids are the mainstay for immediate symptom relief, the H$_2$-antagonists are the mainstay for continuous treatment of GERD.[164] They are, in general, both safe and effective. Their capacity for inhibiting acid secretion renders the refluxate less noxious to the epithelium, providing both protection against the development of symptoms during reflux and increasing the chances for lesions to heal. Although doses and frequency of administration vary, all H$_2$-antagonists can reduce acid secretion and may be effective in chronic treatment of GERD.[200,201] However, to date, ranitidine is the only agent having FDA approval for use in this condition. While effective, ranitidine has not proven a panacea for the entire spectrum of patients with GERD. In particular, patients with gross (erosive) esophagitis do moderately better with full-dose therapy (150 mg, bid) than those on placebo, but relapse is similar to placebo when dosage is reduced for maintenance (150 mg at bedtime).[21]

4. Bethanechol is a cholinergic agonist that has been shown to be effective in reducing symptoms and healing lesions in some, but not all, trials.[35,202] Its usefulness is limited because of troublesome side-effects including flushing, blurry vision, headaches, abdominal cramps, and urinary frequency. It is also contraindicated in a number of common conditions, such as asthma, peptic ulcer disease, ischemic heart disease, and obstructive disease of the intestine or urinary tract. Many experts prefer to use bethanechol as an adjunct to H$_2$-antagonist therapy at bedtime (i.e., when the risk from reflux is greatest and side-effects are less bothersome).[203]

5. Metoclopramide is a dopamine antagonist that has limited efficacy in reducing symptoms.[204] It does not appear to heal esophageal lesions except when used in combination with H$_2$-antagonists.[161] Metoclopramide crosses the blood–brain barrier, and central nervous system (CNS) side-effects such as drowsiness, insomnia, agitation, tremor, and dyskinesias are common. Side-effects are frequently severe enough to require cessation of treatment.[34]

6. Sucralfate, the basic salt of aluminum hydroxide and sucrose octasulfate, may be useful in the treatment of reflux esophagitis. In one European trial, it has been reported to be more effective than placebo in reducing symptoms and healing lesions in GERD.[205] An American trial, however, has shown only marginal benefits with sucralfate, although interestingly, patients with the more severe (erosive) disease appeared to benefit most.[206] This inconsistency may reflect the greater retention of sucralfate within the esophagus of patients with larger epithelial defects (erosions, ulcers).[207] Sucralfate acts topically, and, because it has limited systemic absorption, it appears to be safe. The most common side-effect reported is constipation, a reflection of its aluminum content. However, because its aluminum content can be absorbed, it should be used cautiously and at reduced dosage in patients with renal disease.[208]

TABLE 55-5
Drug Therapy for Reflux Esophagitis

CONVENTIONAL DRUGS	DOSE	MECHANISM(S) OF ACTION*
Antacid:Liquid	15 ml/qid	Buffer HCl
(e.g., Mylanta II/Maalox TC) (HCl Neut. capacity 25 mEq/5 ml)†	1 h pc & qhs	↑ LESP
Gaviscon		
(Al hydroxide, Mg trisilicate, NaHCO₃, Alginic acid)	2–4 tabs qid	↓ Reflux by viscous mechanical barrier
	pc & qhs	Buffer HCl in esophagus
H₂-Receptor antagonists		
Cimetidine (Tagamet)	300 mg qid	↓ HCl secretion ⎫ by inhibiting
	pc & qhs	↓ Gastric volume ⎭ H₂-receptor
Ranitidine (Zantac)	150 mg bid	
	pc & qhs	
Famotidine (Pepcid)	40 mg qhs	same as cimetidine
Nizatidine (Axid)	300 mg qhs	
Bethanechol (Urecholine)	25 mg qid	↑ LESP
	½ h ac & qhs	↑ Esophageal acid clearance
Metoclopramide (Reglan)	10 mg qid	↑ LESP
	½ h ac & qhs	↑ Gastric emptying
Sucralfate (Carafate)	1 g qid	↑ Tissue resistance
	1 h pc & qhs	Buffer HCl in esophagus
		Bind pepsin/bile salts
Inhibitors of H⁺–K⁺-ATPase		
Omeprazole (Prilosec)	20 mg/da	↓ HCl secretion
		↓ Gastric volume
Agents under Investigation		
Cisapride	10 mg tid–qid	↑ LESP, ↑ gastric emptying
Domperidone	10–20 mg tid–qid	↑ LESP, ↑ gastric emptying

* *LESP = lower esophageal sphincter pressure; ↑ = increase; ↓ = decrease.*
† *Note: Patients with reflux are generally not known to be hypersecretors of gastric acid. Therefore therapeutic doses of antacids are based on capacity to buffer basal HCl secretion of ~ 1–7 mEq/hr (mean 2 mEq/hr) and peak meal-stimulated HCl secretion of ~ 10–60 mEq/hr (mean 30 mEq/hr).*
Orlando RC. Gastroesophageal reflux: Medical treatment. In: Bayless TM, ed. Current therapy in gastroenterology and liver disease, ed 3. Philadelphia: BC Decker, 1990, p 7.

7. Omeprazole, a substituted benzimidazole, has just been released in the United States for the short-term (4–8 weeks) treatment of endoscopically documented erosive esophagitis and symptomatic GERD refractory to customary medical therapy. Omeprazole, a potent inhibitor of acid secretion, produces complete achlorhydria with once-a-day dosing. This is due to the irreversible blockade of the parietal cell H⁺-K⁺-ATPase, the final common pathway for acid secretion. It is superior to H₂-antagonists in inhibiting acid secretion, and this appears to be responsible for the dramatic improvement in symptoms and rapid rate of lesion healing in GERD.[20,209,210] The effectiveness of omeprazole in the short-term treatment of GERD has not been challenged; however, because cessation of therapy is followed by high rates of recurrence (erosive esophagitis recurred in 50% of patients within 2 months and in 82% of patients within 6 months of stopping therapy[20]), its safety for long-term use has. Omeprazole is not approved for use as maintenance therapy in GERD because abolition of acid secretion, by enhancing gastrin release, has been shown to produce enterochromaffin tumors (carcinoids) in experimental animals.[211] In addition, complete acid suppression, by removing the acid barrier to ingested organisms, may also increase the potential for gastrointestinal and systemic infections or gastric carcinoma due to bacterial conversion of nitrogenous food components into carcinogenic nitrosamines.

INVESTIGATIONAL DRUGS

Clinical testing is underway for the following agents:

1. Domperidone, a dopamine antagonist, has fewer side-effects than metoclopramide because it crosses the blood–brain barrier less readily. However, domperidone has had little documented success in reducing symptoms and healing lesions in

GERD,[212] perhaps because of its limited ability to increase LES pressure when given orally.

2. Cisapride is a prokinetic agent that has been shown to be superior to placebo in reducing symptoms and healing lesions in GERD.[213] Cisapride increases gastric emptying and LES pressure through an action that releases acetylcholine from the myenteric plexus. Side-effects have been minimal, but a wider experience with this agent is needed.

TREATMENT STRATEGY

In the majority of patients presenting with recurrent heartburn, empiric treatment with lifestyle modification plus antacids or a short course of an H_2-receptor antagonist is reasonable for a finite period of time (e.g., 3–4 weeks). Those failing empiric therapy should have upper endoscopy with biopsy to rule out other diagnoses, to assess the type and extent of esophageal damage, and to guide further treatment.

Endoscopy helps guide treatment by subdividing reflux subjects into those with and without erosive (macroscopic) esophagitis.[194] Those without erosive esophagitis, regardless of symptom severity, are at *low risk* for the major complications, while those with erosive esophagitis are at *high risk* because major complications are likely to develop only in the context of extensive inflammation and epithelial necrosis. In the absence of erosive esophagitis (low risk for complications), the primary goal of therapy should be control of symptoms. Routine endoscopy for follow-up is not usually necessary. The primary goal of therapy for patients with erosive esophagitis (high risk) is the healing of lesions to prevent complications. Periodic follow-up endoscopy is required in these patients because of the poor correlation between symptom relief and lesion healing.

Whether in the high- or low-risk group, medical therapy is based on lifestyle modification (see Table 55-4) and the selective use of drugs (see Table 55-5). The first-line agents in treating reflux esophagitis are the H_2-receptor antagonists and antacids. In contrast to the use of H_2-antagonists in peptic ulcer disease, they should be given more than once per day, and one of the doses should be at bedtime. The bedtime dose is especially important because sleep carries with it the greatest risk of prolonged contact of acid with epithelium. Antacids may be used on a prn basis for symptom relief. In subjects for whom the goal is symptom relief, the effectiveness of the regimen can be assessed and modified if necessary within a few weeks. When the goal is lesion healing, therapeutic efficacy is better assessed endoscopically at 2- to 3-month intervals.

If this regimen is unsuccessful, higher and more frequent doses of the H_2-antagonist should be used, or other agents such as bethanechol, sucralfate, and metoclopramide should be added to the regimen. Bethanechol can be given orally up to four times a day, but a single 25-mg bedtime dose is better tolerated and may be effective. Sucralfate, 1 g, four times a day, can also be helpful but is best administered as a suspension or slurry prepared by mixing the tablets with 30 ml of water or glycerol. The recommended dosage for metoclopramide is 10 mg four times a day, but reduction in dosage or cessation of therapy may be required in many subjects because of CNS side-effects. The effectiveness of the modified regimen is reassessed in a few weeks for symptom relief and in a few months for lesion healing.

If the above modifications fail, a maximum medical regimen would include lifestyle modifications plus drugs that favorably alter each of the four major pathogenetic pathways leading to development of reflux esophagitis (see Fig 55-1). Such a regimen includes an H_2-antagonist to reduce the potency of the refluxate, bethanechol at bedtime to strengthen the antireflux barrier and increase luminal clearance, and sucralfate to increase tissue resistance. Alternatively, omeprazole, a new agent that completely abolishes acid secretion, can be prescribed alone in doses of 20 mg per day. These regimens, even if successful, may be difficult to maintain for prolonged periods either because of high cost, inconvenience, or, in the case of omeprazole, concern about long-term safety. High-risk subjects either failing to heal or relapsing on tolerable, safe maintenance regimens should be considered for surgery. (Note that the benefits of continuous full-dose omeprazole likely outweigh the risks in poor operative candidates.) Low-risk subjects failing these regimens should have repeat endoscopy to both reconfirm the diagnosis and reassess the severity of disease. If reflux esophagitis is confirmed and has clearly progressed under treatment, surgery is indicated. However, subjects with intractable symptoms but little (microscopic) or no esophagitis are better served by an updated history to assess life stresses that may impact on their capacity to cope with symptoms and by performing a Bernstein test and 24-hour pH monitoring. These latter tests are useful for providing some objective documentation of a relationship between esophageal acidification and the patient's complaints.

MEDICAL TREATMENT OF COMPLICATIONS

Strictures. Medical therapy is an option for the initial management of reflux esophagitis complicated by an esophageal stricture or Barrett's esophagus. For those with benign strictures narrow enough to produce dysphagia (lumen diameter generally less than or equal to 13 mm), esophageal dilation is performed. This can be accomplished using a variety of instruments and techniques (see ch 131). The simplest technique involves peroral passage of rubber Hurst (round ends) or Maloney (tapered ends) mercury-filled dilators of increasing size to stretch and ultimately disrupt the fibrous bands responsible for the narrowing.[214] Hurst and Maloney dilators come in diameters of 16 to 60 French (Fr) (3 Fr = 1 mm). An alternative method of bougienage that is more involved but generally safer and more effective in dilating the long or very narrow stricture uses the hollow-centered Savary plastic-covered polyvinyl dilator passed over a steel guide wire that has been previously inserted fluoroscopically beyond the stricture and into stomach.[215] The Savary dilator has largely supplanted the wire-guided Eder-Puestow dilator, which employed a metal push-rod with limited flexibility and metal olives. Wire-guided balloon (Gruntzig) dilators have been effectively employed for the dilation of esophageal strictures.[216,217] Unlike the mercury, plastic, or metal dilators, the balloon systems have the advantage of directing their entire dilating force outward at the stricture rather than having part translated into undesirable shear forces exerted downward through the lumen and tangential to the stricture.

Dilation is generally performed using only topical pharyngeal anesthetics supplemented, if necessary, by small amounts of Demerol or midazolam (Versed). Dilation is generally limited to three dilators of increasing size per session, and sessions are spaced at 1- to 2-week intervals. After satisfactory dilation, medical therapy combined with passage of the largest-sized dilator at gradually longer intervals can usually prevent return of symptoms.[218-220] Either failure to dilate a stricture successfully or failure to prevent its recurrence at least at an interval tolerable to the patient is a clear indication for surgery. Surgery in these cases has been successfully employed both for stricture dilation and for prevention of recurrence by performance of an antireflux procedure.[221,222]

Barrett's Esophagus. Like strictures, Barrett's esophagus can be managed medically.[223] Despite reports to the contrary, no therapy to date, either medical or surgical, has been convincingly shown to produce regression or prevent malignant degeneration. The therapeutic goals for subjects with Barrett's esophagus are the same as for uncomplicated reflux esophagitis—to reduce symptoms and heal esophageal lesions. However, because of the additional risk of malignant degeneration, endoscopic surveillance for dysplasia and carcinoma is recommended on a periodic basis (see ch 57). The only alternative to endoscopic surveillance for protection against esophageal cancer is to have an esophagectomy, a procedure associated with significant morbidity and mortality, which cannot be recommended routinely for prophylaxis.

Surgical Treatment

The general indications for antireflux surgery in subjects with GERD are: (1) the failure of medical therapy to heal and prevent the relapse of erosive (ulcerative) esophagitis, (2) the inability of medical therapy to prevent recurrence of a stricture, and (3) the development of aspiration pneumonia or airway compromise.

The Belsey and Nissen fundoplication and the Hill posterior gastropexy are the three procedures used most widely to control reflux (Figs 55-14 through 55-16). Each claims success in relieving symptoms and healing lesions in about 85% of cases.[112] Successful surgery, however, does not guarantee a permanent cure. Long-term follow-up indicates that symptoms recur in about 10% of cases.[112,224] Antireflux surgery in general carries morbidity rates of 2% to 8% with the most common complication being dysphagia and the gas-bloat syndrome (i.e., inability to belch or vomit). The mortality rate for these procedures is approximately 1%. Although the Nissen fundoplication, which is a complete (360-degree) wrap, has somewhat more complications than the incomplete Belsey repair, the former procedure is preferred by most surgeons because it can be performed through either an abdominal or thoracic incision and because it has a lower recurrence rate. The Belsey fundoplication, however, is usually preferred in subjects with impaired peristalsis because the incomplete wrap reduces the risk of severe postoperative dysphagia. The mechanism whereby fundoplication prevents reflux is incompletely understood. Among the factors contributing to its success may be: (1) the reduction of a hiatus hernia restoring the normal relationship between LES and external supports such as diaphragm, (2) the enhancement of LES contractility by improving length–tension relationships, and (3) the buttressing effect on LES contractility from an external wrap of gastric smooth muscle.

The Hill procedure is not a fundoplication but a gastropexy in which the gastroesophageal junction is anchored to the median arcuate ligament.[112] Although technically more difficult and requiring intraoperative manometry for calibrating the cardia, the

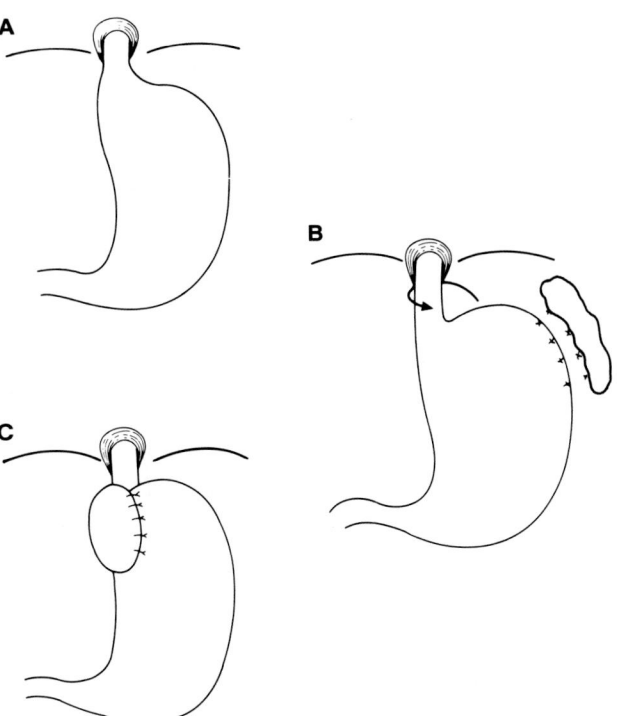

FIGURE 55–14. Nissen fundoplication. **A,** Before mobilization. **B,** Fundus and upper greater curvature mobilized and taken around the mobilized esophagus in the direction of the arrow. **C,** Completed fundoplication around the lower esophagus. (From Jamieson GG, Duranceau AC. The development of surgery for gastro-oesophageal reflux disease. In: Jamieson GG, ed. Surgery of the oesophagus. Edinburgh: Churchill Livingstone, 1988:233.)

Hill repair can be used to control reflux in subjects with prior gastric resection when little or no stomach is left to form a wrap.

The Angelchik prosthesis is a Silastic ring that served as an antireflux device by affixing it like a collar around the intraabdominal segment of esophagus (Fig 55-17). The beauty of the ring was in the ease of application.[225,226] However, the benefits of the device are offset by the risk of serious complications.[112] Dysphagia severe enough to require reoperation for removal of the prosthesis occurred in up to 30%, and ring migration, erosion, and slippage has been reported to produce pain, bleeding, or gastric outlet obstruction.

GASTROESOPHAGEAL REFLUX IN CHILDREN

Pathologic reflux in children, just as in the adult, is common and can produce a wide array of symptoms and tissue injury. Regurgitation, for example, is readily recognized, but reflux may present with other symptoms that could be considered the equivalents of "heartburn" in the adult. These are irritability, difficulty feeding, fussiness, rumination, and failure to thrive. In addition, reflux is considered a potential cause for a number of serious airway diseases in children including apnea, near SIDS, asthma, and aspiration pneumonia.[99,227]

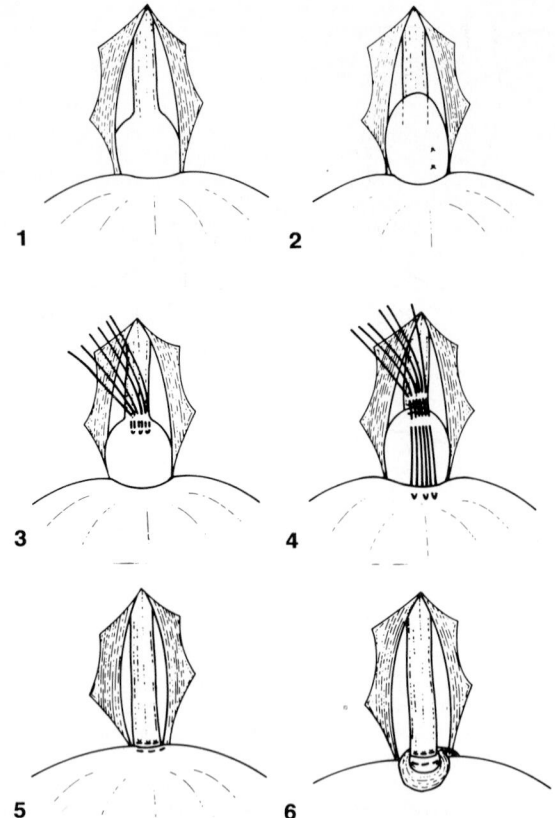

FIGURE 55–15. Belsey Mark IV repair. (1) mediastinal pleura opened showing sliding hernia; (2) stomach mobilized into chest; (3) first row of imbricating sutures; (4) second row of imbricating sutures showing them placed through diaphragm; (5) second row tied, taking repair below the diaphragm; (6) completed repair with the hiatus narrowed by posterior crural sutures. (From Jamieson GG, Duranceau AC. The development of surgery for gastro-oesophageal reflux disease. In: Jamieson GG, ed. Surgery of the oesophagus. Edinburgh: Churchill Livingstone, 1988:233.)

The pathogenesis of reflux esophagitis in children mirrors in many respects that in adults.[228] A notable difference, however, is that many children may "outgrow" their disease. This may, in part, be due to delayed maturation of the LES. In those who fail to improve, the damage to esophagus can run the full gamut of that seen in the adult from inflammation to ulceration with healing by stricture formation or Barrett's esophagus.[229,230] Two interesting observations in children that differ from adults are that intraepithelial eosinophils on esophageal biopsy appear relatively specific for esophagitis[231] and that the color of Barrett's columnar epithelium may not be visually distinct from that of normal squamous mucosa.[232] This latter finding makes suspecting the diagnosis more difficult in children and emphasizes the need for endoscopic esophageal biopsies in cases suspected of reflux.

Treatment of reflux esophagitis in infants includes the use of small thickened feedings and maintenance of the upright or prone position.[229,230] Otherwise, the same medications available for treatment as in the adult are used, but with appropriate reductions in dosage. Medical management in children is of particular value when it is believed that the disease will abate with further growth and development. However, when the disease has proved difficult

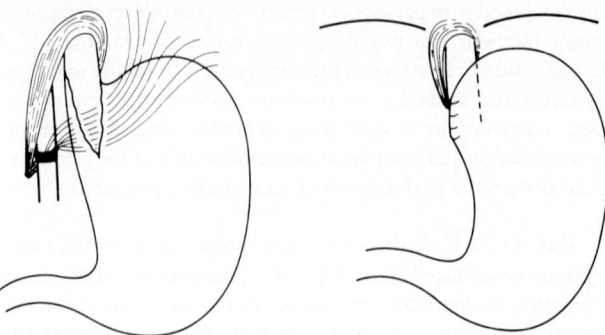

FIGURE 55–16. Hill repair (posterior gastropexy). *Left,* After mobilization of the gastroesophageal junction, imbricating sutures are used to anchor the junction to the median arcuate ligament. *Right,* when the sutures are tied they create a partial anterior fundic wrap of the oesophagus and also anchor the gastroesophageal junction posteriorly. (From Jamieson GG, Duranceau AC. The development of surgery for gastroesophageal reflux disease. In: Jamieson GG, ed. Surgery of the oesophagus. Edinburgh: Churchill Livingstone, 1988:233.)

to management in the very young or there is evidence to indicate that reflux is responsible for severe airway disease, surgery (Nissen fundoplication) should be performed.[95,231]

ALKALINE REFLUX ESOPHAGITIS

Alkaline reflux esophagitis is an uncommon clinical entity in which esophagitis develops from repeated and prolonged contact of esophageal epithelium with *nonacidic* gastric or intestinal con-

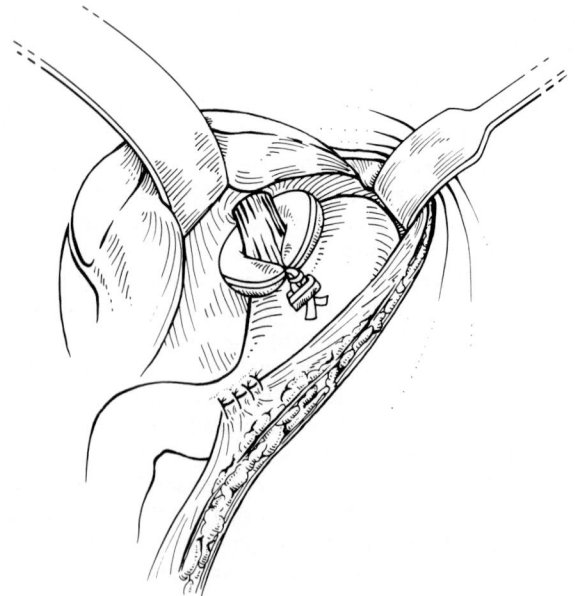

FIGURE 55–17. Diagrammatic representation of an Angelchik prosthesis tied in place and accompanied by a gastropexy. (Angelchik JP. The implantable oesophageal collar (Angelchik antireflux prosthesis). Chap. 29. In: Jamieson GG, ed. Surgery of the oesophagus. Edinburgh: Churchill Livingstone, 1988:283.)

tents.[233] This usually occurs in subjects who have had either total gastrectomy with esophagojejunostomy or vagotomy and antrectomy with a Billroth II gastroenterostomy. Even more rarely, unoperated subjects with achlorhydria have developed alkaline esophagitis.[234,235]

Alkaline esophagitis unlike acid-reflux esophagitis is not caused by the pH of the refluxate, which is usually in the range of 7 to 8. Thus, factors other than pH are responsible for damage, and the likely candidates are deconjugated bile salts and pancreatic enzymes.[11-13,233] These substances enter the gastrointestinal lumen distal to the pylorus, which may be the barrier that prevents the development of alkaline esophagitis. It is evident that the achlorhydric subject must have dysfunction of both pylorus and LES to enable lower intestinal contents to gain access repeatedly to the esophageal epithelium. Such a sequence has previously been documented in a subject with pernicious anemia and heartburn.[235] In this patient, symptoms could be elicited by esophageal perfusion with bile salts, and heartburn could be relieved by treatment with cholestyramine, an agent that binds bile salts.

The treatment of alkaline esophagitis is based on reducing contact between contents of the alkaline refluxate and esophageal epithelium. The frequent administration of bile salt-binding agents (cholestyramine, colestipol, and sucralfate) and agents with mucosal coating effects (antacids, colloidal bismuth) may be effective. Alternatively, when medical management fails, surgical creation of a Roux-en-Y to divert the intestinal contents away from the anastomotic site is useful in subjects with prior gastrectomy. Alternatively, a standard fundoplication may suffice for subjects with an intact stomach or adequate gastric remnant.

The reader is directed to Chapter 7, Esophageal Motor Function; Chapter 28, Approach to the Patient with Dysphagia; Chapter 29, Approach to the Patient with Chest Pain; Chapter 53, Esophagus: Anatomy and Structural Anomalies; Chapter 54, Motility Disorders of the Esophagus; Chapter 56, Esophageal Infections; Chapter 57, Esophageal Tumors; Chapter 58, Miscellaneous Diseases of the Esophagus; Chapter 111, Upper Gastrointestinal Endoscopy; Chapter 114, Contrast Radiology; Chapter 126, Endoscopic Mucosal Biopsy; Chapter 128, Evaluation of Gastrointestinal Motility: Methodological Considerations; and Chapter 131, Gastrointestinal Dilation.

REFERENCES

1. Orlando RC, Powell DW, Carney CN. Pathophysiology of acute acid injury in rabbit esophageal epithelium. J Clin Invest 1981;68:286.
2. Hopwood D, Milne G, Logan KR. Electron microscopic changes in human oesophageal epithelium in oesophagitis. J Pathol 1979;129:161.
3. Nebel OT, Fornes MF, Castell DO: Symptomatic gastroesophageal reflux: Incidence and precipitating factors. Am J Dig Dis 1976;21:953.
4. DeMeester TR, Johnson LF, Joseph GJ, Toscano MS, Hall AW, Skinner DB. Patterns of gastroesophageal reflux in health and disease. Ann Surg 1976;184:459.
5. Dent J, Dodds WJ, Friedman RH, et al. Mechanism of gastroesophageal reflux in recumbent asymptomatic human subjects. J Clin Invest 1980;65:256.
6. Orlando RC. Oesophageal defenses. In: Bennett JR, ed. Oesophagitis. London: Current Medical Literature, in press, 1991.
7. Chung RSK, Magri J, DenBesten L. Hydrogen ion transport in the rabbit esophagus. Am J Physiol 1975;229:496.
8. Harmon JW, Johnson LF, Maydonovitch CL. Effects of acid and bile salts on the rabbit esophageal mucosa. Dig Dis Sci 1981;67:91.
9. Goldberg HI, Dodds WJ, Gee S, Montgomery C, Zboralske FF. Role of acid and pepsin in acute experimental esophagitis. Gastroenterology 1969;56:223.
10. Salo J, Kivilaakso E. Role of luminal H^+ in the pathogenesis of experimental esophagitis. Surgery 1982;92:61.
11. Salo JA, Lehto V, Karonen S, Kivilaakso E. Role of lipase in the pathogenesis of experimental esophagitis in the rabbit. Arch Surg 1987;122:1160.
12. Lillemoe KD, Johnson LF, Harmon JW. Alkaline esophagitis: A comparison of the ability of components of gastroduodenal contents to injure the rabbit esophagus. Gastroenterology 1983;85:621.
13. Safaie-Shirazi S, DenBesten L, Zike WL: Effect of bile salts on the ionic permeability of the esophageal mucosa and their role in the production of esophagitis. Gastroenterology 1975;68:728.
14. Smith JL, Opekun AR, Larkai E, Graham DY. Sensitivity of the esophageal mucosa to pH in gastroesophageal reflux disease. Gastroenterology 1989;96:683.
15. Dubois A. Role of gastric factors in the pathogenesis of gastroesophageal reflux. In: Castell DO, Wu WC, Ott DJ, eds. Gastroesophageal reflux disease: Pathogenesis, diagnosis, therapy. Mount Kisco, NY: Futura, 1985:81.
16. Coleman S, Hirschowitz BI: Studies of gastric secretion as a risk factor for esophagitis. Gastroenterology 1984;86:1051A.
17. Mittal RK, Reuben A, Whitney JO, McCallum RW. Do bile acids reflux into the esophagus? Gastroenterology 1987;92:371.
18. Bateson MC, Hopwood D, Milne G, Bouchier IAD. Oesophageal epithelial ultrastructure after incubation with gastrointestinal fluids and their components. J Pathol 1981;133:33.
19. Schweitzer EJ, Bass B, Batzri S, Harmon J. Bile acid accumulation by rabbit esophageal mucosa. Dig Dis Sci 1986;31:1105.
20. Hetzel DJ, Dent J, Reed WD, et al. Healing and relapse of severe peptic esophagitis after treatment with omeprazole. Gastroenterology 1988;95:903.
21. Koelz HR, Birchler R, Bretholz A, et al. Healing and relapse of reflux esophagitis during treatment with ranitidine. Gastroenterology 1986;91:1198.
22. Schweitzer EJ, Bass BL, Johnson LF, Harmon JW. Sucralfate prevents experimental peptic esophagitis in rabbits. Gastroenterology 1985;88:611.
23. Orlando RC, Powell DW. Effect of sucralfate on esophageal epithelial resistance to acid in the rabbit. Gastroenterology 1984;86:1201.
24. Haddad JK. Relation of gastroesophageal reflux to yield sphincter pressures. Gastroenterology 1970;58:175.
25. Castell DO. The lower esophageal sphincter: Physiologic and clinical aspects. Ann Intern Med 1975;83:390.
26. Dodds WJ, Dent J, Hogan WJ, et al. Mechanisms of gastroesophageal reflux in patients with reflux esophagitis. N Engl J Med 1982;307:1547.
27. Mittal RK, McCallum RW. Characteristics of transient lower esophageal sphincter relaxation in humans. Am J Physiol 1987;252:G636.
28. Holloway RH, Hongo M, Berger K, McCallum RW. Gastric distention: A mechanism for postprandial gastroesophageal reflux. Gastroenterology 1985;89:779.
29. Martin CJ, Patrikios J, Dent J. Abolition of gas reflux and transient lower esophageal sphincter relaxation by vagal blockade in the dog. Gastroenterology 1986;91:890.
30. Higgs RH, Castell DO, Eastwood GL. Studies on the mechanism of esophagitis-induced lower esophageal sphincter hypotension in cats. Gastroenterology 1976;71:51.
31. Biancani P, Barwick K, Selling J, McCallum R. Effects of acute experimental esophagitis on mechanical properties of the lower esophageal sphincter. Gastroenterology 1984;87:8.
32. Eastwood GL, Castell DO, Higgs RH. Experimental esophagitis in cats impairs lower esophageal sphincter pressure. Gastroenterology 1975;69:146.
33. Wesdorp E, Bartelsman J, Pape K, et al. Oral cimetidine in reflux esophagitis: A double blind controlled trial. Gastroenterology 1978;74:821.

34. Bright-Asare P, El-Bassousi M. Cimetidine, metoclopramide or placebo in the treatment of symptomatic gastroesophageal reflux. J Clin Gastroenterol 1980;2:149.

35. Saco LS, Orlando RC, Levinson SL, Bozymski EM, Jones JD, Frakes JT. Double-blind controlled trial of bethanechol and antacid versus placebo and antacid in the treatment of erosive esophagitis. Gastroenterology 1982;82:1369.

36. Mittal RK, McCallum RW. Characteristics and frequency of transient relaxations of the lower esophageal sphincter in patients with reflux esophagitis. Gastroenterology 1988;95:593.

37. Maddern GJ, Chatterton BE, Collins PJ, Horowitz M, Shearman DJC, Jamieson GG. Solid and liquid emptying in patients with gastro-oesophageal reflux. Br J Surg 1985;72:344.

38. Velasco N, Hill LD, Gannan RM, Pope CE II. Gastric emptying and gastroesophageal reflux. Effects of surgery and correlation with esophageal motor function. Am J Surg 1982;144:58.

39. Ellis FH Jr. Current concepts. Esophageal hiatal hernia. N Engl J Med 1972;287:646.

40. Ott DJ. Barium esophagram. In: Castell DO, Wu WC, Ott DJ, eds. Gastroesophageal reflux disease: Pathogenesis, diagnosis, therapy. Mount Kisco, NY: Futura, 1985:109.

41. Johnson LF, DeMeester TR, Haggitt RC. Endoscopic signs for gastroesophageal reflux objectively evaluated. Gastrointest Endosc 1976;22:151.

42. Cohen S, Harris LD. Does hiatus hernia affect competence of the gastroesophageal sphincter? N Engl J Med 1971;284:1053.

43. Kramer P. Does a sliding hiatus hernia constitute a distinct clinical entity? Gastroenterology 1969;57:442.

44. Wright RA, Hurwitz AL. Relationship of hiatal hernia to endoscopically proved reflux esophagitis. Dig Dis Sci 1979;24:311.

45. Ott DJ, Wu WC, Gelfand DW. Reflux esophagitis revisited: Prospective analysis of radiologic accuracy. Gastrointest Radiol 1981;6:1.

46. Mittal RK, Lange RC, McCallum RW. Identification and mechanism of delayed esophageal acid clearance in subjects with hiatus hernia. Gastroenterology 1987;92:130.

47. Boyle JT, Altschuler SM, Nixon TE, Tuckman DN, Pack AI, Cohen S. Role of the diaphragm in the genesis of lower esophageal sphincter pressure in the cat. Gastroenterology 1985;88:723.

48. Welch RW, Gray JE. Influence of respiration on recording of LES pressure in humans. Gastroenterology 1982;83:590.

49. Mittal RK, Rochester DF, McCallum RW. Electrical and mechanical activity in the human lower esophageal sphincter during diaphragmatic contraction. J Clin Invest 1988;81:1182.

50. Kjellin G, Tibbling L. Influence of body position, dry and water swallows, smoking and alcohol on esophageal acid clearance. Scand J Gastroenterol 1978;13:283.

51. Helm JF, Dodds WJ, Hogan WJ. Salivary response to esophageal acid in normal subjects and patients with reflux esophagitis. Gastroenterology 1987;93:1393.

52. Helm JF, Dodds WJ, Pelc LR, Palmer DW, Hogan WJ, Teeter BC. Effect of esophageal emptying and saliva on clearance of acid from the esophagus. N Engl J Med 1984;310:284.

53. Hamilton BH, Orlando RC. In vivo alkaline secretion by mammalian esophagus. Gastroenterology 1989;97:640.

54. Al Yassin TM, Toner PG. Fine structure of squamous epithelium and submucosal glands of human esophagus. J Anat 1977;123:705.

55. Goetsch E. The structure of the mammalian oesophagus. Am J Anat 1910;10:1.

56. Johns BAE. Developmental changes in the oesophageal epithelium in man. Anatomy 1952;86:431.

57. Stanciu C, Bennett JR. Oesophageal acid clearing: One factor in the production of reflux oesophagitis. Gut 1974;15:852.

58. Johnson LF, DeMeester TR, Haggitt RC: Endoscopic signs for gastroesophageal reflux objectively evaluated. Gastrointest Endosc 1976;22:151.

59. Schindlbeck NE, Heinrich C, Konig A, Dendorfer A, Pace F, Muller-Lissner SA. Optimal thresholds, sensitivity, and specficity of long-term pH metry for the detection of gastroesophageal reflux disease. Gastroenterology 1987;93:85.

60. Sonnenberg A, Steinkamp U, Weise A, et al. Salivary secretion in reflux esophagitis. Gastroenterology 1982;83:889.

61. Heddle R, Dent J, Toouli J, Lewis I. Esophageal peristaltic dysfunction in peptic esophagitis (Abstract). Gastroenterology 1984;85:1109.

62. Kahrilas PJ, Dodds WJ, Hogan WJ, Kern M, Arndorfer RC, Reece A. Esophageal peristaltic dysfunction in peptic esophagitis. Gastroenterology 1986;91:897.

63. Orr WC, Johnson LF, Robinson MG. Effect of sleep on swallowing, esophageal peristalsis, and acid clearance. Gastroenterology 1984;86:814.

64. Orr WC, Robinson MG, Johnson LF. Acid clearance during sleep in the pathogenesis of reflux esophagitis. Dig Dis Sci 1981;26:423.

65. Sondheimer JM. Gastroesophageal reflux: Update on pathogenesis and diagnosis. Pediatr Clin North Am 1988;35:103.

66. Lear CSC, Flanagan JB Jr, Moorrees CFA. The frequency of deglutition in man. Arch Oral Biol 1965;10:83.

67. Lichter I, Muir RC. The pattern of swallowing during sleep. Electroencephalogr Clin Neurophysiol 1975;38:427.

68. Schneyer LH, Pigman W, Hanahan L, Gilmore RW. Rate of flow of human parotid, sublingual, and submaxillary secretions during sleep. J Dent Res 1956;35:109.

69. Robertson D, Aldersley M, Shepherd H, Smith CL. Patterns of acid reflux in complicated oesophagitis. Gut 1987;28:1484.

70. Vitale GC, Cheadle WG, Patel B, Sadek SA, Michel ME, Cuschieri A. The effect of alcohol on nocturnal gastroesophageal reflux. JAMA 1987;258:2077.

71. Flemstrom G, Garner A. Gastroduodenal HCO$_3^-$ transport: Characteristics and proposed role in acidity regulation and mucosal protection. Am J Physiol 1982;242:G183.

72. Allen A, Garner A. Gastric mucus and bicarbonate secretion and their possible role in mucosal protection. Gut 1980;21:249.

73. Williams SE, Turnberg LA. Studies of the "protective" properties of gastric mucus: Evidence for mucus bicarbonate barrier. Gut 1979;20:A922.

74. Lacy ER, Tobey NA, Cowart K, Orlando RC. The esophageal mucosal barrier: Structural correlates. Gastroenterology 1989;96:A281.

75. Elias PM, McNutt NS, Friend DS. Membrane alterations during cornification of mammalian squamous epithelia: A freeze-fracture, tracer and thin-section study. Anat Rec 1977;189:577.

76. Hopwood D, Logan KR, Coghill G, Bouchier IAD. Histochemical studies of mucosubstances and lipids in normal human oesophageal epithelium. Histochem J 1977;9:153.

77. Carter MJ: Carbonic anhydrase: Isoenzymes, properties, distribution, and functional significance. Biol Rev 1972;47:465.

78. Agnone LM, Schmidt LN, Goldstein JL, Layden TJ. Mechanisms of regulation of intracellular pH in isolated rabbit esophageal cells. Clin Res 1989;37:365A.

79. Bass BL, Schweitzer EJ, Harmon JW, Kraimer J. H$^+$ back diffusion interferes with intrinsic reactive regulation of esophageal mucosal blood flow. Surgery 1984;96:404.

80. Hollwarth ME, Smith M, Kvietys PR, Granger DN. Esophageal blood flow in the cat. Gastroenterology 1986;90:622.

81. Tobey NA, Powell DW, Schreiner VJ, Orlando RC. Serosal bicarbonate protects against acid injury to rabbit esophagus. Gastroenterology 1989;96:1466.

82. Silen W. Gastric mucosal defense and repair. In: Johnson LR, Christensen J, Jacobson ED, Jackson MJ, Walsh JH, eds. Physiology of the gastrointestinal tract, vol 2, ed 2. New York: Raven Press, 1987:1055.

83. Svanes K, Ito S, Takeuchi K, Silen W. Restitution of the surface epithelium of the in vitro frog gastric mucosa after damage with hyperosmolar sodium chloride. Gastroenterology 1982;82:1409.

84. Lacy ER, Ito S. Rapid epithelial restitution of the rat gastric mucosa after ethanol injury. Lab Invest 1984;51:573.

85. Feil W, Wenzl E, Vattay P, Starlinger M, Sogukoglut T, Schiessel R. Repair of rabbit duodenal mucosa after acid injury in vivo and in vitro. Gastroenterology 1987;92:1973.

86. Livstone EM, Sheahan DG, Behar J. Studies of esophageal epithelial cell proliferation in patients with reflux esophagitis. Gastroenterology 1977;73:1315.

87. Orlando RC, Bryson JC, Powell DW. Effect of cigarette smoke on esophageal epithelium of the rabbit. Gastroenterology 1986;91:1536.

88. Chung RSK, Johnson GM, DenBesten L. Effect of sodium tauro-

cholate and ethanol on hydrogen ion absorption in rabbit esophagus. Am J Dig Dis 1977;22:582.

89. Shirazi SS, Platz CD. Effect of alcohol on canine esophageal mucosa. J Surg Res 1978;25:373.

90. Richter JE, Pandol SJ, Castell DO, McCarthy DM. Gastroesophageal reflux disease in the Zollinger-Ellison syndrome. Ann Intern Med 1981;95:37.

91. Dodds WJ, Dent J, Hogan WF. Pregnancy and the lower esophageal sphincter. Gastroenterology 1978;74:1334.

92. Zamost BJ, Hirschberg J, Ippoliti AF, Furst DE, Clements PJ, Weinstein WM. Esophagitis in scleroderma. Gastroenterology 1987;92:421.

93. Parkman HP, Schwartz SS. Esophagitis and gastroduodenal disorders associated with diabetic gastroparesis. Arch Intern Med 1987;147:1147.

94. Recht MP, Levin MS, Katzka DA, Reynolds JC, Saul SH. Barrett's esophagus in scleroderma: Increased prevalence and radiographic findings. Gastrointest Radiol 1988;13:1.

95. Foglia RP, Fonkalsrud EW, Ament ME, et al. Gastroesophageal fundoplication for the management of chronic pulmonary disease in children. Am J Surg 1980;140:72.

96. Chernow B, Johnson LF, Janowitz WR, Castell DO. Pulmonary aspiration as a consequence of gastroesophageal reflux—a diagnostic approach. Dig Dis Sci 1979;24:839.

97. Ghaed N, Stein MR. Assessment of a technique for scintigraphic monitoring of pulmonary aspiration of gastric contents in asthmatics with gastroesophageal reflux. Ann Allergy 1979;42:306.

98. Reich SB, Earley WC, Ravin TH, Goodman M, Spector S, Stein MR. Evaluation of gastropulmonary aspiration by a radioactive technique: Concise communication. J Nucl Med 1977;18:1079.

99. Mansfield LE, Stein MR. Gastroesophageal reflux and asthma: A possible reflex mechanism. Ann Allergy 1978;41:224.

100. Mansfield LE, Hameister HH, Spaulding HS, Smith NJ, Glab N. The role of the vagus nerve in airway narrowing caused by intra-esophageal hydrochloric acid provocation and esophageal distention. Ann Allergy 1981;47:431.

101. Kjellin G, Tibbling L, Wranne B. Bronchial obstruction after esophageal acid perfusion in asthmatics. Clin Physiol 1981;1:285.

102. Goodall R, Earis J, Cooper DN, Berstein A, Temple JG. Relationship between asthma and gastro-oesophageal reflux. Thorax 1981;36:116.

103. Larrain A, Carrasco J, Gallesguillos J, Pope CE. Reflux treatment improves lung function in patients with intrinsic asthma. Gastroenterology 1981;80:A1204.

104. Ekstrom T, Lindgren BR, Tibbling L. Effects of ranitidine treatment on patients with asthma and a history of gastro-oesophageal reflux: A double blind crossover study. Thorax 1989;44:19.

105. Harper PC, Bergner A, Kaye MD. Antireflux treatment for asthma. Improvement in patients with associated gastroesophageal reflux. Arch Intern Med 1987;147:56.

106. Battle WS, Nyhus LM, Bombeck CT: Gastro-esophageal reflux: Diagnosis and treatment. Ann Surg 1973;177:560.

107. Ott DJ, Gelfand DW, Wu WC. Reflux esophagitis: Radiographic and endoscopic correlation. Radiology 1979;130:158.

108. Crummy AB. The water test in the evaluation of gastroesophageal reflux. Radiology 1966;78:501.

109. Linsman JF. Gastroesophageal reflux elicited while drinking water (water siphonage test). AJR 1965;94:325.

110. Tuttle SG, Grossman MI. Detection of gastro-oesophageal reflux by simultaneous measurement of intraluminal pressure and pH. Proc Soc Exp Biol Med 1958;98:2257.

111. Orlando RC. pH probe for reflux (Tuttle test). In: Drossman DA, ed. Manual of gastroenterologic procedures, ed 2. New York:Raven Press, 1987:51.

112. Jamieson GG, Duranceau AC. The development of surgery for gastro-oesophageal reflux disease. In: Jamieson GG, ed. Surgery of the oesophagus. Edinburgh: Churchill Livingstone, 1988:233.

113. Pattrick FG. Investigation of gastroesophageal reflux in various positions with a two lumen pH electrode. Gut 1970;11:659.

114. Spencer J. Prolonged pH recording in the study of gastro-esophageal reflux. Br J Surg 1969;54:912.

115. Johnson LF, DeMeester TR. Twenty-four hour pH monitoring of the distal esophagus. Am J Gastroenterol 1974;62:325.

116. Schindlbeck NE, Heinrich C, Dendorfer A, Pace F, Muller-Lissner S. Influence of smoking and esophageal intubation on esophageal pH-metry. Gastroenterology 1987;92:1994.

117. Fisher RS, Malmud LS, Roberts GS, Lobis IF. Gastroesophageal (GE) scintiscanning to detect and quantitate GE reflux. Gastroenterology 1976;70:301.

118. Hoffman GC, Vansant JH. The gastroesophageal scintiscan: Comparison of methods to demonstrate gastroesophageal reflux. Arch Surg 1979;114:727.

119. Menin RA, Malmud LS, Petersen RP, Maier WP, Fisher RS. Gastroesophageal scintigraphy to assess the severity of gastroesophageal reflux disease. Ann Surg 1980;191:66.

120. Velasco N, Pope CE, Gannan RM, Roberts P, Hill LD. Measurement of esophageal reflux by scintigraphy. Dig Dis Sci 1984;29:977.

121. Bernstein LM, Baker LA. A clinical test for esophagitis. Gastroenterology 1958;34:760.

122. Moraes-Filho JP, Bettarello A. Lack of specificity of the acid perfusion test in duodenal ulcer patients. Dig Dis Sci 1974;19:785.

123. Katz PO, Dalton CB, Richter JE, Wu WC, Castell DO. Esophageal testing in patients with noncardiac chest pain or dysphagia: Results of three years' experience with 1161 patients. Ann Intern Med 1987;106:593.

124. Janssens J, Vantrappen G, Ghillebert G. 24-hour recording of esophageal pressure and pH in patients with noncardiac chest pain. Gastroenterology 1986;90:1978.

125. Richter JE, Bradley LA, Castell DO. Esophageal chest pain: Current controversies in pathogenesis, diagnosis and therapy. Ann Intern Med 1989;110:66.

126. Mellow MH, Simpson AG, Watt L, Haye O, Schoolmeester L, Haye OL. Esophageal acid perfusion in coronary artery disease: Induction of myocardial ischemia. Gastroenterology 1983;83:306.

127. Ducrotte PH, Berland J, Denis PH, et al. Coronary sinus lactate estimation and esophageal motor abnormalities in angina with normal coronary angiogram. Dig Dis Sci 1984;29:305.

128. Brush JE Jr, Cannon RO III, Schenke WH, et al. Angina due to coronary microvascular disease in hypertensive patients without left ventricular hypertrophy. N Engl J Med 1988;319:1302.

129. DeMeester TR, Cimochowski GE, O'Drobinak J. Esophageal function in patients with angina-type chest pain and normal coronary angiograms. Ann Surg 1982;196:488.

130. Levine MS, Kressel HY, Caroline DF, Laufer I, Herlinger H, Thompson JJ. Barrett esophagus: Reticular pattern of the mucosa. Radiology 1983;147:663.

131. Trier JS. Morphology of the epithelium of the distal esophagus in patients with midesophageal peptic strictures. Gastroenterology 1970;58:444.

132. Geisinger KR, Wu WC. Endoscopy and biopsy. In: Castell DO, Wu WC, Ott DJ, eds. Gastroesophageal reflux disease: Pathogenesis, diagnosis, therapy. Mount Kisco, NY: Futura, 1985:149.

133. Kobayashi S, Kasugai T. Endoscopic and biopsy criteria for the diagnosis of esophagitis with a fiberoptic esophagoscope. Dig Dis Sci 1974;19:345.

134. Ismail-Beigi F, Horton PF, Pope CE. Histological consequences of gastroesophageal reflux in man. Gastroenterology 1970;58:163.

135. Eastwood GL. Gastrointestinal epithelial renewal. Gastroenterology 1977;72:962.

136. Messier B, Leblond CP. Cell proliferation and migration as revealed by radioautography after injection of thymidine-H³ into rats and mice. Am J Anat 1960;106:247.

137. Weinstein WM, Goboch ER, Bowes KL. The normal human esophageal mucosa: A histologic reappraisal. Gastroenterology 1975;68:40.

138. Seefeld U, Krejs GJ, Siebenmann RE, Blum AL. Esophageal histology of gastroesophageal reflux. Morphometric findings in suction biopsies. Am J Dig Dis 1977;22:956.

139. Goldman H, Antonioli DA. Mucosal biopsy of the esophagus, stomach, and proximal duodenum. Hum Pathol 1982;13:423.

140. Orlando R. Pathology of reflux oesophagitis and its complications. In: Jamieson GG, ed. Surgery of the oesophagus. Edinburgh: Churchill Livingstone, 1988:189.

141. Geboes K, Desmet V, Vantrappen G, Mebis J. Vascular changes in

the esophageal mucosa: An early histologic sign of esophagitis. Gastrointest Endosc 1980;26:29.

142. Mitros FA. Inflammatory and neoplastic diseases of the esophagus. In: Appelman HD, ed. Pathology of the oesophagus, stomach and duodenum. London: Churchill Livingstone, 1984:1.

143. Behar J, Sheahan GG, Biancani P. Medical and surgical management of reflux esophagitis. N Engl J Med 1975;293:263.

144. Eastwood GL, Beck BD, Castell DO, Brown FC, Fletcher JR. Beneficial effect of indomethacin on acid-induced esophagitis in cats. Dig Dis Sci 1981;20:601.

145. Northway MG, Bennett A, Carroll M, et al. Comparative effects of anti-inflammatory agents and radiotherapy on normal esophagus and tumors in animals. Gastroenterology 1980;78:1229.

146. Robbins SL, Cotran RS. Inflammation and repair. In: Robbins SL, Cotran RS, eds. Pathologic basis of disease, ed 2. Philadelphia: WB Saunders 1979:55.

147. Orlando RC, Powell DW, Bryson JC, et al. Esophageal potential difference measurements in esophageal disease. Gastroenterology 1982;83:1026.

148. Orlando RC, Powell DW. Studies of esophageal epithelial electrolyte transport and potential difference in man. In: Allen A, Flemstrom G, Garner A, Silen W, Turnberg LA, eds. Mechanisms of mucosal protection in the upper gastrointestinal tract. New York: Raven Press, 1984:75.

149. Orlando RC. Esophageal epithelial resistance. In: Castell DO, Wu WC, Ott DJ, eds. Gastroesophageal reflux disease: Pathogenesis, diagnosis, therapy. Mount Kisco, NY: Futura, l985:55.

150. Khamis B, Kennedy C, Finucane J, et al. Transmural potential difference: Diagnostic value in gastro-oesophageal reflux. Gut 1978;19:396.

151. Vidins EI, Fox JEF, Beck IT. Transmural potential difference (PD) in the body of the esophagus in patients with esophagitis, Barrett's epithelium and carcinoma of the esophagus. Am J Dig Dis 1971;16:991.

152. Eckardt VF, Adami B. Esophageal transmural potential difference in patients with symptomatic gastroesophageal reflux. Klin Wochenschr 1980;58:293.

153. Herlihy KJ, Orlando RC, Bryson JC, Bozymski EM, Carney CN, Powell DW. Barrett's esophagus: Clinical, endoscopic, histologic, manometric and electrical potential difference characteristics. Gastroenterology 1984;86:436.

154. Turner KS, Powell DW, Carney CN, et al. Transmural electrical potential difference in the mammalian esophagus in vivo. Gastroenterology 1978;75:286.

155. Booth DJ, Kemmerer WT, Skinner DB. Acid clearing from the distal esophagus. Arch Surg 1968;96:731.

156. Tolin RD, Malmud LS, Reilley J, Fisher RS. Esophageal scintigraphy to quantitate esophageal transit (quantitation of esophageal transit). Gastroenterology 1979;76:1402.

157. Orlando RC. Esophageal manometry. In: Drossman DA, ed. Manual of gastroenterologic procedures, ed 2. New York: Raven Press, 1987:30.

158. Winans CS, Harris LD. Quantitation of lower esophageal sphincter competence. Gastroenterology 1967;52:773.

159. Pope CE. A dynamic test of sphincter strength: Its application to the lower esophageal sphincter. Gastroenterology 1967;52:779.

160. Richter JE, Castell DO. Gastroesophageal reflux: Pathogenesis, diagnosis and therapy. Ann Intern Med 1982;97:93.

161. Lieberman DA. Medical therapy for chronic reflux esophagitis. Arch Intern Med 1987;147:1717.

162. DeMeester TR. Surgical management of gastroesophageal reflux. In: Castell DO, Wu WC, Ott DJ, eds. Gastroesophageal reflux disease: Pathogenesis, diagnosis, therapy. Mount Kisco, NY: Futura, 1985:243.

163. Castell DO. Medical therapy for reflux esophagitis: 1986 and beyond. Ann Intern Med. 1986;104:112.

164. Richter JE. A critical review of current medical therapy for gastroesophageal reflux disease. J Clin Gastroenterol 1986;8:72.

165. Raufman J-P, Collins SM, Pandol SJ, et al. Reliability of symptoms in assessing control of gastric acid secretion in patients with Zollinger-Ellison syndrome. Gastroenterology 1983;84:108.

166. Bozymski EM, Herlihy KJ, Orlando RC. Barrett's esophagus. Ann Intern Med 1982;97:103.

167. Mangla JC. Barrett's esophagus: An old entity rediscovered. J Clin Gastroenterol 1981;3:347.

168. Sjogren RW, Johnson LF. Barrett's esophagus: A review. Am J Med 1983;74:313.

169. Jabbari M, Goresky CA, Lough J, et al. The inlet patch: Heterotopic gastric mucosa in the upper esophagus. Gastroenterology 1985;89:352.

170. Steadman C, Kerlin P, Teague C, Stephenson P. High esophageal stricture: A complication of "inlet patch" mucosa. Gastroenterology 1988;94:521.

171. Mossberg SM. The columnar-lined esophagus (Barrett syndrome): An acquired condition? Gastroenterology 1966;50:671.

172. Goldman MC, Beckman RC. Barrett syndrome. Case report with discussion about concept of pathogenesis. Gastroenterology 1960;39:104.

173. Endo M, Kobayashi S, Kozu T, et al. A case of Barrett's epithelialization followed up for five years. Endoscopy 1974;6:48.

174. Bremner CG, Lynch VP, Ellis FH. Barrett's esophagus: Congenital or acquired. An experimental study of esophageal mucosal regeneration in the dog. Surgery 1970;68:209.

175. Wong J, Finckh ES. Heterotopia and ectopia of gastric epithelium produced by mucosal wounding in the rat. Gastroenterology 1971;60:279.

176. Kiriluk LB, Merendino KA. Comparative sensitivity of mucosa of different segments of alimentary tract in dog to acid peptic action. Surgery 1954;35:547.

177. Johnson DA, Winters C, Spurling TJ, Chobanian SJ, Cattau EL Jr. Esophageal acid sensitivity in Barrett's esophagus. J Clin Gastroenterol 1987;9:23.

178. Naef AP, Savary M, Ozzello L. Columnar-lined esophagus: An acquired lesion with malignant predisposition. Report on 140 cases of Barrett's esophagus with 12 adenocarcinomas. J Thorac Cardiovasc Surg 1975;70:826.

179. Hawe A, Payne WS, Weiland LH, Fronatana RS. Adenocarcinoma in the columnar epithelial lined lower (Barrett) esophagus. Thorax 1973;28:511.

180. Haggitt RC, Tryzelaar J, Ellis HF, Colcher H. Adenocarcinoma complicating columnar epithelium-lined (Barrett's) esophagus. Am J Clin Pathol 1978;70:1.

181. Thompson JJ, Zinsser KR, Enterline HT. Barrett's metaplasia and adenocarcinoma of the esophagus and gastroesophageal junction. Hum Pathol 1983;14:42.

182. Cameron AJ, Ott BJ, Payne WS. The incidence of adenocarcinoma in columnar-lined (Barrett's) esophagus. N Engl J Med 1985;313:857.

183. Spechler SJ, Robbins AH, Rubins HB, et al. Adenocarcinoma and Barrett's esophagus. An overrated risk? Gastroenterology 1984;87:927.

184. Robertson CS, Mayberry JF, Nicholson DA, et al. Value of endoscopic surveillance in the detection of neoplastic change in Barrett's esophagus. Br J Surg 1988;75:760.

185. Hameeteman W, Tytgat GNJ, Houthoff HJ, Van Den Tweel JG. Barrett's esophagus: Development of dysplasia and adenocarcinoma. Gastroenterology 1989;96:1249.

186. Burbige EJ, Radigan JJ. Characteristics of the columnar-cell lined (Barrett's) esophagus. Gastrointest Endosc 1979;25:133.

187. Eastwood GL, Bonnice CA. Barrett's esophagus—a special problem. In: Castell DO, Wu WC, Ott DJ, eds. Gastroesophageal reflux disease: Pathogenesis, diagnosis, therapy. Mount Kisco, NY: Futura, 1985:301.

188. Orlando RC. Transmural electrical potential difference measurements in Barrett's esophagus. In: Spechler SJ, Goyal RK, eds. Barrett's esophagus: Pathophysiology, diagnosis, and management. New York: Elsevier Science, 1985:121.

189. Berquist TH, Nolan NG, Carlson HC, et al. Diagnosis of Barrett esophagus by pertechnetate scintigraphy. Mayo Clin Proc 1973;48:276.

190. Paull A, Trier JS, Dalton MD, et al. The histologic spectrum of Barrett's esophagus. N Engl J Med 1976;295:476.

191. Schreiber DS, Apstein M, Hewrmos JA. Paneth cells in Barrett's esophagus. Gastroenterology 1978;74:1302.

192. Adler RH. The esophagus with columnar epithelium. Its clinical significance. Geriatrics 1965;20:109.

193. Dayal Y, Wolfe HJ. Gastrin-producing cells in ectopic gastric mucosa of developmental and metaplastic origins. Gastroenterology 1978;75:655.

194. Orlando RC. Gastroesophageal reflux: Medical treatment. In: Bayless TM, ed. Current therapy in gastroenterology and liver disease, ed 3. Philadelphia: BC Decker, 1990, p 7.

195. Johnson LF, DeMeester TR. Evaluation of elevation of the head of the bed, bethanechol, and antacid foam tablets on gastroesophageal reflux. Dig Dis Sci 1981;26:673.

196. Hamilton JW, Boisen RJ, Yamamoto DT, Wagner JL, Reichelderfer M. Sleeping on a wedge diminishes exposure of the esophagus to refluxed acid. Dig Dis Sci 1988;33:518.

197. Price SF, Smithson KW, Castell DO. Food sensitivity in reflux esophagitis. Gastroenterology 1978;75:240.

198. Lloyd DA, Borda IT. Food-induced heartburn: Effect of osmolality. Gastroenterology 1981;80:740.

199. Bernardo DE, Lancaster-Smith M, Strickland ID, Wright JT. A double-blind controlled trial of "Gaviscon" in patients with symptomatic gastroesophageal reflux. Curr Med Res Opin 1975;3:388.

200. Hine KR, Holmes GKT, Melikian V, Lucey M, Fairclough PD. Ranitidine in reflux oesophagitis. Digestion 1984;29:119.

201. Sherbanuik R, Wensel R, Bailey R, et al. Ranitidine in the treatment of symptomatic gastroesophageal reflux disease. J Clin Gastroenterol 1984;6:9.

202. Thanik KD, Chey WY, Shah AN, Grutierrez JH. Reflux esophagitis: Effect of oral bethanechol on symptoms and endoscopic findings. Ann Intern Med 1980;93:805.

203. Johnson LF, Peura D. Gastroesophageal reflux: Medical treatment. In: Bayless TM, ed. Current therapy in gastroenterology and liver disease, ed 1. Philadelphia: BC Decker, 1986:189.

204. McCallum RW, Fink SM, Winnam GR, Avella J, Callachari C. Metoclopramide in gastroesophageal reflux disease: Rationale for its use and results of a double-blind trial. Am J Gastroenterol 1984;79:165.

205. Weiss W, Brunne H, Buttner GR, et al. Treatment of reflux esophagitis with sucralfate [in German]. Dtsch Med Wochenschr 1983;108:1706.

206. Williams RM, Orlando RC, Bozymski EM, et al. Multicenter trial of sucralfate suspension for the treatment of reflux esophagitis. Am J Med 1987;83:61.

207. Goff JS, Adcock KA, Schmelter R. Detection of esophageal ulcerations with technetium-99m albumin sucralfate. J Nucl Med 1986;27:1143.

208. Robertson JA, Salusky IB, Goodman WG, Norris KC, Coburn JW. Sucralfate, intestinal aluminum absorption and aluminum toxicity in a patient on dialysis. Ann Intern Med 1989;111:179.

209. Dammonn HG, Blum AL, Lux G, Krankenhaus B. Differences in healing tendency of reflux oesophagitis with omeprazole and ranitidine. Results of an Austrian-German-Swiss multi-center trial. Dtsch Med Wochenschr 1986;111:123.

210. Havelund T, Laursen LS, Skoubo-Kristensen E, et al. Omeprazole and ranitidine in treatment of reflux oesophagitis: Double blind comparative trial. Br Med J 1988;296:89.

211. Hakanson R, Sundler F, Carlsson E, Mattsson H, Larsson H. Proliferation of enterochromaffin-like (ECL) cells in the rat stomach following omeprazole treatment. Hepatogastroenterology 1985;32:48.

212. Blackwell JN, Heading RC, Fetter MR. Effect of domperidone on lower esophageal sphincter pressure and gastroesophageal reflux in patients with peptic oesophagitis. Progress with domperidone. Roy Soc Med (Int Cong Symp Series) 1981;36:57.

213. Baldi F, Biachi Porro G, Dobrilla G, et al. Cisapride compared to placebo in healing reflux oesophagitis. A multicenter double-blind trial. J Clin Gastroenterol 1988;10:641.

214. Bozymski EM. Dilatation of the esophagus: Wire-guided bougies (Eder-Puestow and Savary Gilliard bougies). In: Drossman DA, ed. Manual of gastroenterologic procedures, ed 2. New York: Raven Press, 1987:169.

215. Dumon J, Meric B, Sivak MV, Fleisher D. A new method of esophageal dilatation using Savary-Gilliard bougies. Gastrointest Endosc 1985;31:379.

216. Kozarek R. Endoscopic Gruntzig balloon dilatation of gastrointestinal stenosis. J Clin Gastroenterol 1984;30:359.

217. Lindor KD, Ott BJ, Hughes RW Jr. Balloon dilatation of upper digestive tract strictures. Gastroenterology 1985;89:545.

218. Patterson DJ, Graham DY, Smith JL, et al. Natural history of benign esophageal stricture treated by dilatation. Gastroenterology 1983;85:346.

219. Lanza FL, Graham DY. Bougienage is effective therapy for most benign esophageal strictures. JAMA 1978;240:844.

220. Wesdorp E, Bartelsman J, Hartog Jager F, Huibregtse K, Tytgat G. Results of conservative treatment of benign esophageal strictures: A follow-up study in 100 patients. Gastroenterology 1982;82:487.

221. Mercer CD, Hill LD. Surgical management of peptic esophageal stricture: Twenty-year experience. J Thorac Cardiovasc Surg 1986;91:371.

222. Hill LD, Gelfand M, Bauermeister D. Simplified management of reflux esophagitis with stricture. Ann Surg 1979;1972:638.

223. Orlando RC. Barrett's esophagus. In: Bayless TM, ed. Current therapy in gastroenterology and liver disease, ed 2. Philadelphia: BC Decker, 1986:189.

224. Orringer MB, Skinner DB, Belsey RHR. Long term results of the Mark IV operation for hiatal hernia and analyses of recurrences and their treatment. J Thorac Cardiovasc Surg 1972;53:25.

225. Angelchik JP, Cohen R. A new surgical procedure for the treatment of gastro-esophageal reflux and hiatal hernia. Surg Gynecol Obstet 1979;148:246.

226. Starling JR, Reichelderfer MO, Pellett JR, Belzer FO. Treatment of symptomatic gastro-esophageal using the Angelchik prosthesis. Ann Surg 1982;195:686.

227. Herbst JJ, Minton SD, Books LS. Gastroesophageal reflux causing respiratory distress and apnea in newborn infants. J Pediatr 1979;95:763.

228. Sondheimer JM. Spontaneous swallowing, esophageal peristalsis and acid clearance in awake and sleeping infants. Clin Res 1988;36:206A.

229. Groben PA, Siegal GP, Shub MD, Ulshen MH, Askin FB. Gastroesophageal reflux and esophagitis in infants and children. Perspect Pediatr Pathol 1987;11:124.

230. Herbst JJ. Gastroesophageal reflux. J Pediatr 1981;98:859.

231. Winter HS, Madara JL, Stafford RJ, Grand RJM, Quinlah J-E, Goldman H. Intraepithelial eosinophils: A new diagnostic criterion for reflux esophagitis. Gastroenterology 1982;83:818.

232. Dahms BB, Rothstein FC. Barrett's esophagus in children: A consequence of chronic gastroesophageal reflux. Gastroenterology 1984;86:318.

233. Nath BJ, Warshaw AL. Alkaline reflux gastritis and esophagitis. Annu Rev Med 1984;35:383.

234. Palmer ED. Subacute erosive ("peptic") esophagitis associated with achlorhydria. N Engl J Med 1960;262:927.

235. Orlando RC, Bozymski EM. Heartburn in pernicious anemia—a consequence of bile reflux. N Engl J Med 1973;289:522.

56

Esophageal Infections

JEAN-PIERRE RAUFMAN

Only 5 years ago, it was stated that, with few exceptions, esophageal infections had become a rarity.[1] Today, as a consequence of the factors discussed below, we are witnessing an epidemic of esophageal infections. Patients with these infections may be asymptomatic, but more commonly they complain of odynophagia or dysphagia. Rarely, with severe mucosal involvement, complications such as hemorrhage, fistulas, or strictures may develop. Identification of the infecting organism and institution of therapy are important because, in contrast to the underlying diseases that predispose patients to their occurrence, esophageal infections commonly respond to appropriate treatment.

The most important factor associated with the increasing incidence of esophageal infection is the acquired immunodeficiency syndrome (AIDS) epidemic. Despite the protean manifestations of AIDS, one common feature is esophageal involvement with pathogens, most usually *Candida* species. These infections cause odynophagia and dysphagia and, thereby, contribute to the poor nutritional status of afflicted patients.[2] Because the number of patients with AIDS will continue to increase during this decade, the management of esophageal infection in this clinical setting merits special consideration.

Another factor in the upsurge of esophageal infections is the increase in organ transplantation and the attendant use of immunosuppressive therapy to prevent rejection. Colonization and infection of the esophagus with a variety of organisms in transplantation patients contribute significantly to postoperative morbidity and mortality.[3–5]

In this chapter, esophageal infections are classified by etiology: fungi, viruses, or bacteria (Table 56-1). The organisms in each category are reviewed in terms of clinical presentation, pathology, diagnosis, and therapy. This section concludes with a consideration of the approach to diagnosing and managing esophageal infection in AIDS.

EPIDEMIOLOGY

Epidemiologic data regarding infections of the esophagus are scarce and unreliable. Because these infections are not reported to governmental agencies, one can only estimate the incidence and prevalence of these disorders from medical literature, most of which deals with case reports or, at best, small series of patients. In the past, the most reliable estimates of the prevalence of these infections were derived from necropsy data. However, the decreasing autopsy rate in the United States has restricted this source of information. Nevertheless, a clear pattern emerges with respect to the groups of patients at risk for esophageal infection.

Primary esophageal infection is rare in an otherwise normal patient in whom no permissive factor, such as antibiotic use, impaired peristalsis, or esophageal trauma can be identified. The most common pathogen in this situation is herpes simplex virus,[6–10] although candidiasis may also be observed in elderly patients with no other predisposing factors.[11]

In general, immunocompetent patients who develop esophageal infection have conditions that weaken the normal esophageal defenses such as peristalsis and the normal oroesophageal flora that protect against colonization and subsequent infection of the esophagus with pathogenic organisms. Esophageal peristalsis may be impaired in diseases such as diabetes, scleroderma, or achalasia, thereby resulting in stasis of esophageal contents and providing a culture medium for pathogens. The normal flora of the oroesophageal region may be altered by the use of antimicrobial agents, also allowing overgrowth of a pathogen. In these situations, patients with an intact immune system may develop an esophageal infection, most frequently candidiasis. In other instances, infection in an adjacent organ may spread into and involve the esophagus. For example, mediastinal tuberculous lymphadenitis may result in fistula formation and drainage into the esophagus.

More commonly, some form of humoral or cellular immunodeficiency, such as that associated with cancer, cancer chemotherapy, posttransplantation immunosuppression, or AIDS, underlies esophageal infection. Corticosteroid use for a variety of conditions may also cause sufficient immunosuppression to permit

TABLE 56–1

Organisms Associated With Infectious Esophagitis

Fungi	Bacteria
Candida species (esp. *albicans*)	*Mycobacterium tuberculosis*
Aspergillus species	*Actinomyces israelii*
Histoplasma capsulatum	*Streptococcus viridans*
Blastomyces dermatitides	*Lactobacillus acidophilus*
Viruses	*Treponema pallidum*
Herpes simplex virus (type 1)	
Cytomegalovirus	
Varicella-zoster virus	

esophageal infection. The reported prevalence of esophageal infection, predominantly candidiasis, in patients with cancer ranges from 2.8% to 13%.[12-15] Patients with myeloproliferative disorders are at greater risk of esophageal candidiasis than those with solid tumors.[12-15] The reported prevalence of esophageal infection in posttransplantation patients is 11% for liver recipients,[5] and ranges from 4%[16] to 46%[4] in bone marrow recipients, and from 2%[17] to 24%[5] in kidney recipients. Whereas esophageal candidiasis predominates in kidney transplantation patients,[5,17] viral infection (cytomegalovirus [CMV] and herpes simplex) predominates in bone marrow and liver transplantation patients.[4,5] Although the frequency of esophageal candidiasis in AIDS is unknown, a survey of university training programs in digestive diseases[18] revealed that odynophagia and dysphagia were the most frequent indications for upper gastrointestinal endoscopy in AIDS patients and that esophageal candidiasis was the most common finding. At Kings County Hospital, a large municipal institution in New York City, we estimated that 75% of patients with AIDS have symptoms attributable to esophageal infection sometime during the course of their disease.[2] There is no difference in the predilection for esophageal infection between the major risk groups for AIDS. That is, the prevalence and clinical characteristics of these infections are the same among homosexuals, intravenous drug abusers, and heterosexual partners of patients infected with the human immunodeficiency virus (HIV).

SPECIFIC INFECTIONS

Fungal Infections

CANDIDA SPECIES

Epidemiology. The most common fungal infection of the esophagus is caused by *Candida* species, predominantly *Candida albicans*. Related organisms that may cause esophageal infection include *Candida tropicalis, Candida parapsilosis*, and *Torulopsis glabrata*.[19] These organisms are a normal component of the oral flora, and their growth is kept in check by bacterial commensals. Infection can be a consequence of increased fungal growth or impaired cell-mediated immunity. This may result from antibiotic (tetracycline, sulfonamides, and others) or immunosuppressive (corticosteroids, cyclosporine, and others) therapy, or the development of hematologic malignancies or AIDS.

Pathology. The gross pathologic appearance of esophageal candidiasis can range from a few white plaques on the mucosa to a dense white-gray pseudomembrane overlying friability and ulceration that covers the entire mucosal surface of the esophagus (Fig 56-1). These pseudomembranes are composed of fungal organisms, sloughed mucosal cells, and fibrin. Within these extremes of esophageal involvement is a spectrum of disease with varying degrees of edema, exudate, hyperemia, and ulceration. Fungal invasion may be associated with luminal narrowing and obstruction, and, depending on the depth of penetration, with the formation of fistulas or pseudodiverticuli. It is not clear whether *Candida*

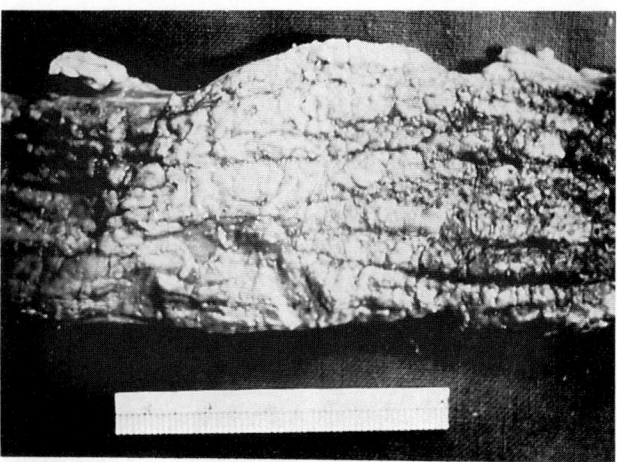

FIGURE 56-1. Diffuse ulcerative esophageal candidiasis in a post mortem specimen from a patient with AIDS. (Courtesy of Dr. S. Iyer, Kings County Hospital, New York.)

organisms are the cause of fistulas and diverticuli or whether they simply colonize previous anatomic defects.

Clinical Manifestations and Complications. The usual clinical presentation of esophageal candidiasis is dysphagia or odynophagia in a patient with one of the risk factors described above. These symptoms range from mild difficulty swallowing to pain on swallowing so intense that the patient avoids ingesting any food at all. Generally, as in other causes of dysphagia, symptoms are worse after ingestion of solids compared to liquids. Rarely, retrosternal pain or burning may occur independent of swallowing. Occasionally, esophageal candidiasis is detected fortuitously in an asymptomatic patient.

Physical examination may be helpful if oral candidiasis (thrush) or manifestations of mucocutaneous candidiasis are present. Oral candidiasis is commonly associated with esophageal candidiasis in AIDS,[20] but many patients have fungal infection limited to the esophagus. Patients with chronic mucocutaneous candidiasis may have fungal involvement of various mucous membranes, hair, nails, and skin with a history of adrenal or parathyroid dysfunction.

Complications of esophageal candidiasis, in order of decreasing frequency, include esophageal hemorrhage secondary to ulceration, luminal obstruction secondary to a mycetoma or fibrosis and stricture, fistulization into the bronchial tree, and sloughing of the entire esophageal mucosa with replacement by a pseudomembrane. Bleeding from esophageal candidiasis is usually mild and does not require transfusion; however, life-threatening hemorrhage has been reported.

Diagnosis. The clinical diagnosis of esophageal candidiasis should be suspected when a patient at high risk complains of odynophagia or dysphagia. The presence of oral candidiasis lends further support to this diagnosis, but the absence of oral involvement does not exclude esophageal disease. Radiographic or endoscopic examination of the esophagus are commonly used to confirm the diagnosis.

Classic barium swallow findings in esophageal candidiasis are mucosal inflammation and ulceration resulting in a "shaggy" appearance (Fig 56-2).[21] However, plaques, pseudomembranes,

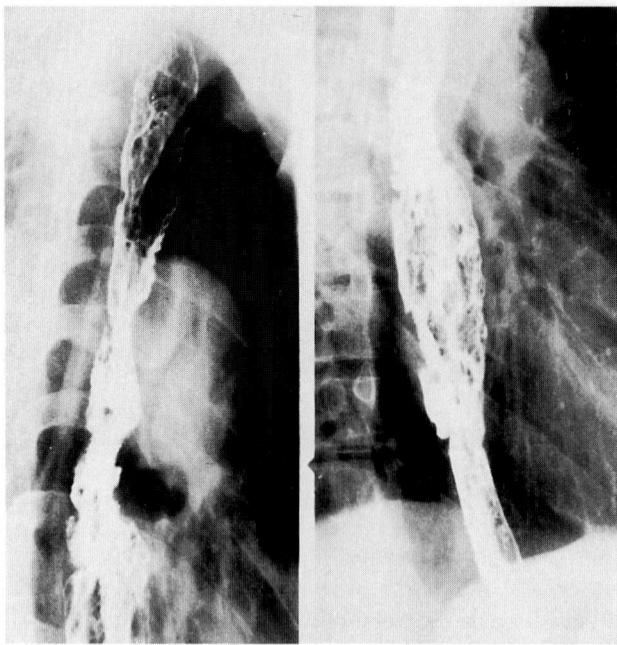

FIGURE 56–2. Barium esophagram showing typical "shaggy" appearance of diffuse ulcerative esophageal candidiasis. (Courtesy of Dr. R. de Silva, Kings County Hospital, New York.)

cobblestones, polypoid nodules, fungus balls, strictures, esophagopulmonary fistulas, and mucosal bridges have been reported.[22–33] Recently, we and others have reported focal esophageal lesions in patients with AIDS and esophageal candidiasis.[34,35] In some cases, large esophageal ulcers and masses were considered neoplastic by the radiologist before endoscopy revealed the correct diagnosis. These various x-ray appearances can occur in the same patient at different times in the course of the disease. Moreover, a normal barium esophagram does not exclude the presence of esophageal candidiasis. Using single column technique, a false-negative rate of 25% has been reported.[14] Although double contrast technique may decrease the false-negative rate to 10%,[36] it has been our experience that severe pain limits its use in some patients.[34]

Endoscopic examination of the esophagus is the most sensitive and specific way of diagnosing esophageal candidiasis. The gross endoscopic appearance of *Candida* esophagitis may be graded according to published criteria[11]: Grade 1—a few raised white plaques up to 2 mm in diameter, without ulceration; grade 2—multiple raised white plaques greater than 2 mm in diameter, without ulceration; grade 3—confluent, linear, and nodular elevated plaques with superficial ulceration; grade 4—findings of grade 3 plus narrowing of the esophageal lumen.

During endoscopy, mucosal lesions can be brushed for cytologic diagnosis. A sleeve can be used over the brush to prevent contamination by fungal organisms in the biopsy channel of the endoscope or in the mouth. At least three microscope slides should be smeared with the material obtained from brushings. One of these can be examined immediately after adding 10% potassium hydroxide, while the others are fixed in 95% ethanol before staining with the modified Papanicolaou or periodic acid–Schiff (PAS) methods (Fig 56-3). Similarly, lesions can be biopsied for histologic diagnosis

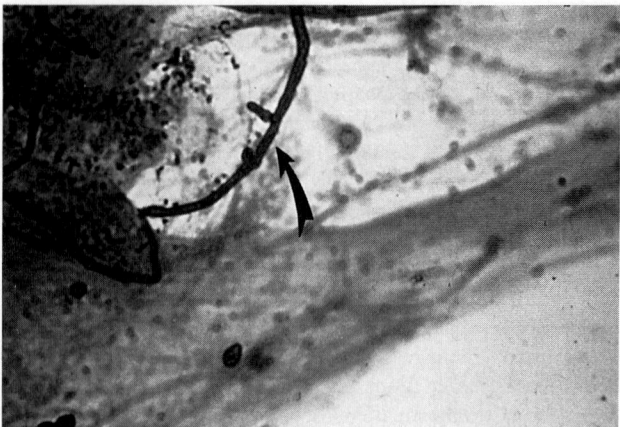

FIGURE 56–3. Periodic acid–Schiff stain of smear prepared from endoscopic brushings of esophageal candidiasis. *Arrow* indicates pseudohyphae.

(Fig 56-4). Biopsy specimens should be fixed rapidly in 10% formalin and subsequently embedded in paraffin before staining with hematoxylin-eosin, PAS, or Gomori's methenamine silver stains. Cytologic examination of esophageal brushings is more sensitive than histologic examination of biopsy specimens because organisms may be washed off tissue surfaces during processing of biopsy specimens from superficial (grades 1–2) candidiasis.[11] Rarely, positive cytology but negative histology indicates colonization rather than infection with *Candida*. If necessary, culture of brushings or biopsy material on appropriate fungal media allows for speciation of the *Candida* organisms and determination of the sensitivity of the fungus to various therapeutic agents.

Skin testing or serologic tests for candidiasis is generally not helpful in the diagnosis of *Candida* esophagitis. Immunodeficient patients with esophageal candidiasis are frequently anergic, and positive skin or serologic tests may reflect infection in another organ or superinfection of herpetic or CMV esophagitis. Moreover, in one study,[11] up to 17% of control subjects had positive serologic tests for candidiasis.

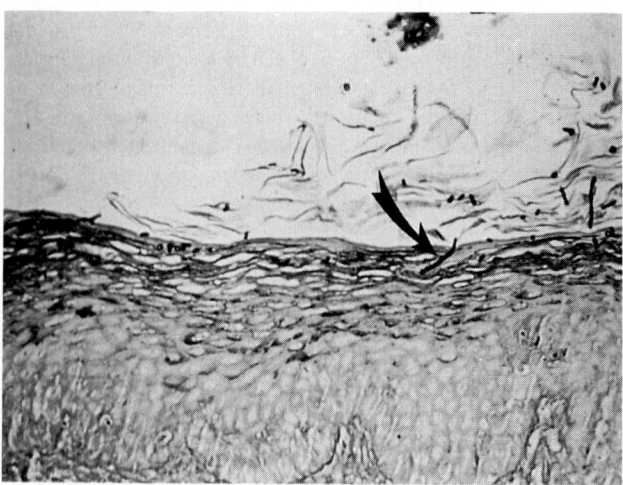

FIGURE 56–4. Endoscopic biopsy specimen from patient with esophageal candidiasis. *Arrow* shows mucosal invasion by fungal organisms.

Treatment. Esophageal candidiasis generally responds promptly to initiation of oral antifungal therapy. If possible, predisposing factors, such as antibiotic or corticosteroid use, should be discontinued. However, in many situations, such as AIDS, effective therapy for the underlying immunodeficiency is unavailable. Bougienage or other nonpharmacologic treatment for stricture or other complications of esophageal candidiasis is rarely needed.

Although many antifungal agents have been used to treat esophageal candidiasis, few studies have compared the efficacy of various regimens. Consequently, recommendations for therapy are based on uncontrolled clinical trials. In general, a stepwise progression of therapy from oral agents to more toxic parenteral agents is used.

Oral therapy with ketoconazole (Nizoral) has become the treatment of choice for esophageal candidiasis. Ketoconazole, like other imidazole derivatives, alters fungal cell membrane permeability by interference with the biosynthesis of sterols, particularly ergosterol. Abnormal ion fluxes resulting from altered membrane permeability cause fungal cell injury and death. Although other imidazoles, like clotrimazole and miconazole, may be effective for oral candidiasis and for prophylaxis against esophageal involvement, these agents are generally considered less effective as primary therapy for esophageal candidiasis.

Ketoconazole therapy (200 mg/day) has been reported to cause resolution of esophageal candidiasis within 8 days in patients without AIDS.[37] In nonresponders, the dose may be increased as needed to a maximum of 800 mg/day, although side-effects, especially nausea, may limit the dose used. Patients with AIDS generally require higher doses of ketoconazole, and a starting dose of 400 mg/day is recommended.[38] Optimal absorption of ketoconazole requires an acid milieu and may be decreased in situations of gastric hypoacidity such as pernicious anemia or those induced iatrogenically by the use of antacids or histamine$_2$-receptor antagonists. Studies demonstrating that many patients with AIDS have decreased gastric acid secretion[39] and consequent decreased bioavailabilty of ketoconazole[40] may explain why these patients require higher doses of this antifungal agent. Whether gastric reacidification in AIDS will improve the therapeutic response to ketoconazole remains to be determined.

Adverse effects of ketoconazole include dose-dependent nausea, hepatotoxicity, and inhibition of steroid production and cyclosporine metabolism. Mild hepatotoxicity, reflected by small increases in serum transaminases, is not unusual and does not necessarily require discontinuation of ketoconazole therapy. However, the development of symptomatic liver disease with jaundice reflects more serious damage that can lead to fatal hepatic necrosis if the drug is not withdrawn.[41] Inhibition of gonadal and adrenal steroid synthesis by ketoconazole has therapeutic potential for a variety of endocrine conditions.[42] Nevertheless, adrenal insufficiency may result from prolonged use of ketoconazole, especially if there are potentiating factors such as adrenal involvement with CMV or mycobacteria in AIDS. In males treated with ketoconazole, decreased testosterone levels may cause gynecomastia, oligospermia, loss of libido, and impotence. Finally, ketoconazole inhibits the metabolism of cyclosporine and may increase cyclosporine blood levels in transplantation recipients. Therefore, patients taking both drugs require frequent measurement of cyclosporine blood levels and a possible decrease of cyclosporine doses to avoid severe nephrotoxicity.

Despite the popularity of ketoconazole for the treatment of esophageal candidiasis, good results have been reported with older imidazoles such as clotrimazole (10 mg, four times daily) and miconazole (50 mg, four times daily).[43,44] Miconazole is also available for intravenous administration (200–600 mg every 8 hours), but use of this formulation has been associated with nausea, vomiting, pruritis, anemia, thrombocytopenia, hyponatremia, hyperlipidemia, and phlebitis at the infusion site. Rare instances of anaphylactic reactions, cardiorespiratory arrest, acute psychosis, and other central nervous system (CNS) toxicity with the use of intravenous miconazole require that a test dose (200 mg) be given with a physician in attendance. This drug can also increase blood levels of oral hypoglycemic agents and anticoagulants if taken concurrently. Clotrimazole may cause elevation in serum transaminases, nausea, vomiting, and neurotoxicity. The role of newer imidazole derivatives such as fluconazole and itraconazole remains to be determined. Although preliminary animal and human tests suggest that these agents have a greater volume of distribution, longer elimination half-life, and less toxicity than ketoconazole, further testing is required to determine their relative efficacy for treating fungal infections of the esophagus. Nevertheless, fluconazole (Diflucan) (100–200 mg daily), an imidazole derivative that does not require an acid environment for absorption, has been approved for the treatment of esophageal candidiasis. Like ketoconazole, this agent may increase blood levels of drugs like cyclosporine, phenytoin, and warfarin, but it does not appear to alter testicular or adrenal function.

The other major family of antifungal agents is the polyene antibiotics represented by amphotericin, nystatin, and others. These agents act by irreversibly binding to sterols in fungal cell membranes, thereby destroying the permeability characteristics of the membrane and causing cell death. Because the antifungal activity of amphotericin depends on binding to fungal membrane sterols and imidazoles inhibit sterol synthesis, it has been suggested that prior therapy with an agent like ketoconazole may promote the emergence of amphotericin-resistant isolates.[45] The clinical relevance of this theoretical risk is unclear.

Nystatin (Mycostatin) is most commonly used to treat oral candidiasis as a "swish and swallow" of 400,000 units suspended in 4 ml of water every 2 to 4 hours while the patient is awake. This dose has been increased sixfold in some patients with severe esophageal candidiasis.[46] Although nystatin is effective for treating thrush, imidazole derivatives, such as ketoconazole and fluconazole, are generally preferred for the treatment of esophageal candidiasis.

Although amphotericin B (Fungizone) is the most effective treatment for systemic mycoses, its severe side effects have relegated it to "last resort" status for the treatment of esophageal candidiasis. Patients with esophageal candidiasis resistant to treatment with ketoconazole, or other less toxic agents, can be treated with "low-dose" amphotericin B (10 mg daily). An initial test dose of 1 mg, dissolved in 50 to 150 ml of 5% dextrose in water, and infused over 20 to 30 minutes should be given. This test dose commonly causes a febrile reaction that begins 2 to 3 hours after the infusion and lasts about an hour. Rarely, this reaction may be severe and accompanied by delirium, hypo- or hypertension, wheezing, and hypoxemia. This reaction may be prevented or ameliorated by prior administration of antipyretics, antihistamines, meperidine, or hydrocortisone (25–50 mg). Higher doses of amphotericin B are rarely needed for the management of esophageal candidiasis in the absence of other organ involvement. If deemed necessary, after the test dose, the daily dose can be increased gradually in 5- to 10-mg increments to a maximum of 0.6 mg/kg/day. Renal toxicity is the most serious side effect of continued use of amphotericin B. Early, reversible renal toxicity is a function of the daily dose; however, late, potentially irreversible kidney damage is related to the total dose of amphotericin given. Cessation of therapy, or at least a decrease in dose, is recommended if serum creatinine exceeds 3 mg/dl. Other adverse effects of amphotericin include nausea, vomiting, headache, anorexia, hypokalemia, hypomagnesemia, bone marrow suppression, and thrombophlebitis. In general, these side effects are less common with the lower doses necessary to eradicate successfully esophageal candidiasis.

Flucytosine (Ancobon) is a fluorinated pyrimidine with a narrow spectrum of antifungal activity that acts by interfering with fungal translation of RNA. This oral agent (50–150 mg/kg/day taken every 6 hours) can be used in combination with amphotericin B but should not be used alone because fungi rapidly develop resistance to it. This agent can cause rash, hepatitis, severe diarrhea, and fatal bone marrow suppression. Flucytosine is excreted by the kidneys, therefore the dose should be lowered if it is used at all in the presence of renal failure. The advantage of using amphotericin in combination with flucytosine is that the synergistic antifungal action of these agents allows for the use of lower, less hazardous doses of each drug.

Because the patient's underlying propensity for developing candidiasis frequently persists despite successful treatment of the esophageal infection, consideration has been given to maintenance or prophylactic antifungal therapy. The prophylactic use of ketoconazole or nystatin for the prevention of esophageal candidiasis in cancer patients has yielded mixed results.[47–49] The benefits, risks, and costs of prophylactic antifungal therapy in immunosuppressed patients require further investigation.

ASPERGILLOSIS, HISTOPLASMOSIS, AND BLASTOMYCOSIS

Epidemiology. Esophageal involvement with these fungi is rare. Although uncommon, *Aspergillus* species may be second to *Candida* species as a cause of infectious esophagitis in cancer patients.[50] Mixed *Aspergillus-Candida* infection with tracheoesophageal fistula has been reported.[50] Most instances of histoplasmosis and blastomycosis esophagitis represent secondary esophageal involvement originating in paraesophageal lymph nodes and not a primary esophageal infection.[51–53] Although no particular geographic distribution within the United States has been reported for aspergillosis or blastomycosis,[50,54] histoplasmosis is endemic in the midwestern states, particularly Ohio, Indiana, Kentucky, Tennessee, Iowa, Missouri, and Kansas.

Clinical Manifestations, Pathology, and Complications. The symptoms of esophageal aspergillosis are similar to those of candidiasis, but more patients may present with severe odynophagia.[55] In contrast, in patients with esophageal histoplasmosis or blastomycosis, the predominant symptom is dysphagia for solids. Odynophagia occurs less frequently. The clinical manifestations of these infections are a consequence of the different pathologic effects of the fungi involved.

Esophageal infection with *Aspergillus* species causes an esoph-

agitis that is characterized by large deep ulcers, but may be grossly and microscopically indistinguishable from candidiasis.[55] In contrast, histoplasmosis and blastomycosis are more likely to cause focal lesions or abscesses of the esophagus as a consequence of extension from mediastinal lymph nodes. These focal lesions cause narrowing of the esophageal lumen, thereby mechanically obstructing the passage of food. Histoplasmosis may cause severe odynophagia if the muscle layers of the esophagus are involved in an inflammatory abscess. All three fungal infections can progress to the formation of fistulas from the esophagus to the bronchial passages or mediastinum.

Diagnosis. Although esophageal aspergillosis is uncommon, it should be considered in cases of apparent *Candida* esophagitis that are resistant to appropriate therapy. Endoscopy with brushings and biopsies for cytologic and histologic examination, respectively, may establish the diagnosis if the cytologist or pathologist is able to distinguish the septate hyphae of *Aspergillus* species from the pseudohyphae of *Candida* species. Culture of biopsy material using fungal media can be helpful, but these organisms may take a long time to grow.

Histoplasmosis should be considered in endemic areas (see above) and if extraesophageal manifestations such as hilar adenopathy, calcification, or atelectasis of adjacent pulmonary tissue, or splenic calcification are present. Barium esophagography or endoscopy may show a focal area of extrinsic compression of the esophagus, usually in the region of the carina. Because *Histoplasma capsulatum* does not generally invade the esophageal mucosa, endoscopic brushings or biopsies are not helpful. If a definitive diagnosis is required, this can usually be obtained by bronchoscopy, mediastinoscopy, or surgery. Serologic tests are not useful because of the high prevalence of positive results in endemic areas.

Esophageal blastomycosis, the least common of the three fungal infections described here, should be considered in patients with skin involvement and dysphagia. The diagnosis can be made on examination of direct smears or by fungal culture of infected material.

Therapy. Histoplasmosis frequently resolves without antifungal therapy. If therapy is necessary, ketoconazole and amphotericin B are effective against histoplasmosis and blastomycosis. Because of the toxicity associated with amphotericin (see section entitled "*Candida* Species: Treatment"), this agent should probably be reserved for severe infections or failures of ketoconazole therapy. Systemic aspergillosis should be treated with high-dose amphotericin B. Surgery may be required for drainage of abscesses or excision of fistulas.

Viral Infections

HERPES SIMPLEX VIRUS (TYPE 1)

Epidemiology. Herpes simplex virus (type 1) (HSV-1) is one of three herpes viruses that affect the esophagus, the others being CMV and varicella-zoster virus (see sections entitled Cytomegalovirus and Varicella-zoster Virus). After *Candida* species, HSV-1 is the next most frequent agent that causes infectious esophagitis. Although esophageal infection with HSV-1 has been reported most frequently in patients with immunosuppression or other predisposing factors, in contrast to esophageal candidiasis, it can also occur in otherwise healthy people without these risk factors.[8-10] As with candidiasis, precise figures for the incidence or prevalence of HSV-1 esophagitis are difficult to obtain. First described as an autopsy finding in 1943,[56] subsequent estimates of the prevalence of this esophageal infection at necropsy have ranged from 1.4% to 25%.[57,58]

Pathology. HSV-1 esophageal infection starts as a cluster of discrete vesicles affecting the lower third of the esophagus. As these vesicles enlarge and ulcerate, they may combine to form larger lesions (Fig 56-5). Microscopic examination of the squamous epithelial cells at the edge of the ulcers reveals multinucleation, ground-glass nuclei, and eosinophilic Cowdry type A inclusion bodies that may take up half of the nuclear volume. These inclusion bodies may be surrounded by a "halo." With time, the inclusion bodies may become more basophilic, filling, enlarging, and deforming the nucleus. Electron microscopic examination of these cells may reveal enveloped virions. Generally, the intervening mucosa between these lesions is normal. In immunocompetent patients, the host response to HSV-1 infection arrests and promotes healing of these lesions, but, in immunodeficient patients, there may be progression to a diffuse ulcerative, hemorrhagic esophagitis. The necrotic ulcers are prone to superinfection with *Candida* species.[59,60]

Clinical Manifestations and Complications. HSV-1 esophageal infection commonly presents with the sudden onset of severe odynophagia. The odynophagia may be so severe that there is an inability to swallow solids or liquids. Herpes labialis ("cold sores"), or skin infection, may antedate or occur during the esophageal infection. In untreated immunocompetent persons, resolution of HSV-1 esophageal infection occurs 1 to 2 weeks after the onset of symptoms. In immunodeficient patients, HSV-1 esophageal infection can result in severe hemorrhage[61,62] or perforation with tracheoesophageal fistula,[63] or may serve as a focus for dissemination.[57]

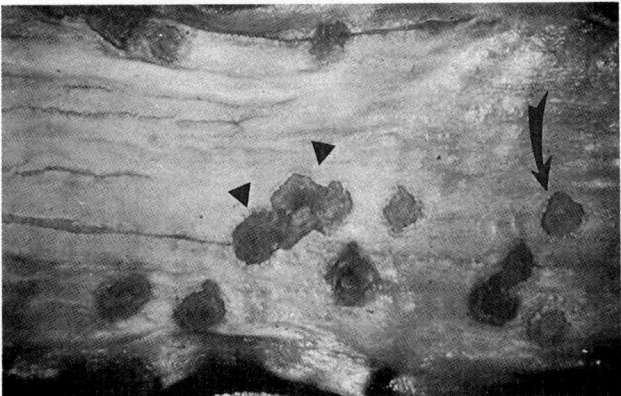

FIGURE 56-5. Multiple discrete ulcers of the esophagus caused by herpes simplex virus in an autopsy specimen from a patient with AIDS. *Arrow* indicates typical "punched-out" ulcer. *Arrowheads* indicate coalescence of ulcers. (From Raufman J-P. Odynophagia/dysphagia in AIDS. Gastroenterol Clin North Am 1988;17:599.)

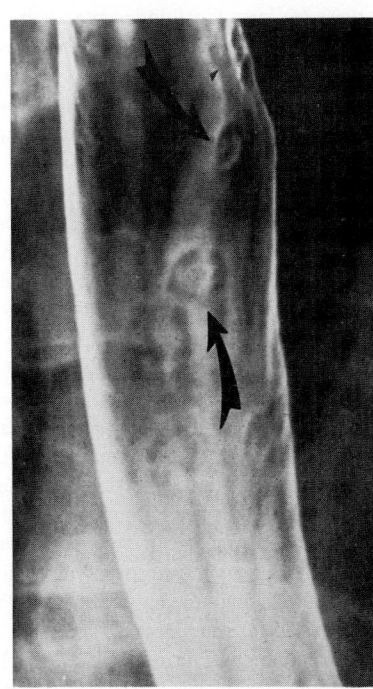

FIGURE 56-6. Double-contrast esophagram revealing discrete superficial ulcers with radiolucent halos (*arrows*) on a background of normal mucosa in a patient with herpes esophagitis. (From Levine MS, Woldenberg R, Herlinger H, Lanfer I. Opportunistic esophagitis in AIDS: Radiographic diagnosis. Radiology 1987;165:815.)

Diagnosis. The initial diagnostic test ordered by primary care physicians for patients with severe odynophagia is frequently a barium esophagram. Infection with HSV-1 generally appears as focal ulceration on a background of normal mucosa in the distal third of the esophagus (Fig 56-6). These ulcers have been described as "stellate" with less propensity to form the longitudinal or linear lesions that are seen in CMV infection.[64] Severe, diffuse herpetic esophagitis may result in a cobblestone or shaggy mucosal appearance similar to that observed with *Candida* esophagitis.[65]

Confirming the diagnosis of herpetic esophagitis requires endoscopy to obtain tissue for microscopic examination and culture. The gross endoscopic appearance of herpetic esophagitis reflects the pathologic changes and appears as discrete "punched-out" ulcers (0.3–2.0 cm in diameter). These ulcers may have raised yellow rims and have been given the eponym "volcano ulcer."[64] Bullous formation or coalescence of ulcers may give the mucosa an erosive, hemorrhagic appearance with exudates that may mimic esophageal candidiasis. Cytologic or histologic examination of brushings or biopsies taken from the edge of an ulcer may reveal multinucleate squamous cells with Cowdry type A intranuclear inclusion bodies. The diagnostic yield from brushings may be higher than from biopsies because more of the esophageal mucosa is sampled by the former technique.

These characteristic radiologic, endoscopic, and histologic findings in a patient with appropriate symptoms are usually sufficient to establish the diagnosis of herpetic esophagitis so that therapy can be started. If a definitive diagnosis is needed, biopsy material should be taken for viral culture. As with other causes of infectious esophagitis, serologic tests are of little help in establishing the diagnosis of HSV-1 esophagitis because a positive test without a clear rise (at least fourfold) in titers during the course of the infection indicates only that the patient has been exposed to the virus but does not prove the etiology of the esophagitis. Immunohistochemistry on biopsy samples using specific monoclonal antibodies to HSV is a research technique that is not readily available for clinical diagnostic purposes.[66]

Therapy. Analgesia with 2% viscous lidocaine suspension may be the only treatment needed for HSV-1 esophagitis in immunocompetent persons. Although a liquid diet can usually be tolerated during the symptomatic phase of the illness, parenteral alimentation is required for the occasional patient who is unable to take anything by mouth. Acyclovir [9-(2-hydroxyethoxymethyl)guanine] (Zovirax), a nucleoside analogue, has been found to shorten periods of viral shedding, lessen pain, and hasten healing in placebo-controlled trials in immunocompromised patients with HSV-1 and HSV-2 oral and genital infections. Although this agent has not been studied in a controlled fashion for HSV-1 esophagitis, intravenous acyclovir (250 mg/m^2 of body surface area every 8 hours for 7–10 days) appears to improve symptoms in this disorder.[67] Side-effects of acyclovir therapy appear limited to irritation of peripheral veins used for drug infusion and a low incidence of rash. Because of its apparent safety and efficacy, acyclovir therapy is commonly instituted in all patients with HSV-1 esophagitis regardless of their immune status.

CYTOMEGALOVIRUS

Epidemiology. Although clinical cases of CMV esophagitis were not reported before 1985,[1] the AIDS epidemic has changed this. Before AIDS, CMV infection of the esophagus was an infrequent autopsy finding. Although *Candida* and HSV-1 infection of the esophagus are more common in AIDS, CMV infection has become a well-recognized clinical complication of AIDS with involvement of the esophagus being less common than infection of other organs.[68,69]

Pathology. The most prominent feature of CMV esophagitis is mucosal ulceration. In some cases, the ulcers are numerous, round or serpiginous, and deep, often reaching the muscularis. In other cases, a solitary large ulcer is observed, perhaps representing a late-stage coalescence of smaller ulcers. Inclusion bodies may be seen in the cytoplasm of infected squamous cells. CMV infection of endothelial cells may cause vasculitis with ischemic injury to the mucosa that causes or contributes to ulceration.

Clinical Manifestations and Complications. In contrast to HSV-1 esophagitis, CMV esophagitis does not occur in immunocompetent persons. Therefore, the usual clinical presentation of CMV esophageal infection is the onset of dysphagia or odynophagia in a patient with AIDS or another immunodeficiency state. Patients may already have CMV infection diagnosed in another organ (e.g., CMV retinitis or colitis). As with HSV-1 esophageal infection, sitophobia resulting from the odynophagia associated with CMV esophagitis may require the institution of parenteral hyperalimentation.

Diagnosis. As with HSV-1, the radiologic appearance of CMV esophagitis is that of focal ulceration of otherwise normal esophageal mucosa occurring in the distal third of the esophagus. Barium esophagography in patients with CMV infection may reveal vertical, linear ulcers with central umbilication and occasionally, in severe, extensive disease, diffuse thickening of mucosal folds (Fig 56-7).[68–71] These ulcers have been classified as "giant ulcers" because they may exceed 2 to 3 cm in length.[72]

The gross endoscopic appearance of CMV is generally that of small (0.3–0.5 cm diameter) ulcers, but occasionally longitudinal or "giant" (1–3.5 cm) ulcers may be seen in the distal third of the esophagus. Sometimes CMV infection of the esophagus is associated with small polypoid masses.[68] Cytologic or histologic examination of esophageal brushings or biopsies, respectively, reveals epithelial or endothelial cytoplasmic inclusions. CMV can be grown in culture if tissue samples are placed in appropriate viral transport media and incubated in the proper cell line. Storing samples in a freezer before inoculation into cell culture decreases the yield.

Culture of CMV from blood or urine, or serologic tests for CMV are not helpful in diagnosing CMV esophagitis. A positive result with any of these tests does not localize the infection to the esophagus, and, as noted above, patients may have multiorgan infection with CMV.

Therapy. A new acyclovir derivative, 9-(1,3-dihydroxy-2-propoxymethyl)guanine (ganciclovir) appears to be effective for treating CMV esophagitis. A recent uncontrolled clinical trial reported symptomatic improvement with ganciclovir (Cytovene) (5 mg/kg intravenously every 12 hours for 14 days) in four of five

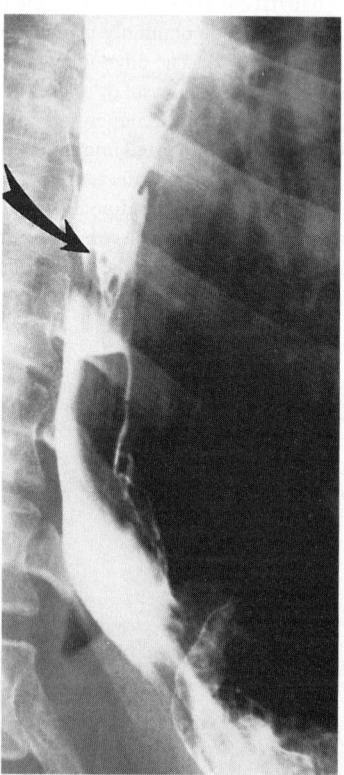

FIGURE 56–7. Barium esophagram showing large, longitudinal ulcer (*arrow*) typical of cytomegalovirus infection. Endoscopic biopsies revealed intracytoplasmic inclusions. (Courtesy of Dr. J. K. Amorosa, University of Medicine and Dentistry of New Jersey and Dr. R. de Silva, Kings County Hospital, New York.)

patients with AIDS and CMV esophagitis.[73] However, repeat endoscopy after therapy was not performed to determine the effect of therapy on the mucosal lesion. Toxicity with this agent includes neutropenia and rash. Although further testing is required to confirm the efficacy of this drug for CMV esophagitis, the rarity of spontaneous remission, uncontrolled reports suggesting improvement with therapy,[74,75] and the absence of an effective alternative supports use of ganciclovir for this indication.

Foscarnet (trisodium phophonoformate hexahydrate) is a pyrophosphate analogue that inhibits viral DNA polymerase and reverse transcriptase. Although this agent appears to have efficacy similar to that of ganciclovir for treating CMV retinitis, its utility for other CMV infections remains to be determined. Foscarnet may cause reversible renal failure and anemia.

VARICELLA-ZOSTER VIRUS

The frequency of esophageal involvement during the course of chickenpox or herpes zoster infections is unknown. Certainly, clinical esophagitis caused by varicella-zoster virus is very rare.[76,77] Presumptive varicella-zoster virus esophagitis has been reported in association with herpes zoster involving thoracic dermatomes.[76] In these cases, the esophageal lesions mimicked HSV-1 esophagitis with vesicles and ulcers involving the distal esophagus. Resolution of esophageal disease paralleled resolution of cutaneous lesions. Residual esophageal stricture is a reported complication of varicella-zoster virus esophagitis.[77] Although this virus is susceptible to acyclovir, experience with drug therapy for esophageal involvement is lacking.

Mycobacterial, Bacterial, and Treponemal Infections

MYCOBACTERIUM TUBERCULOSIS

Epidemiology. Previously, tuberculous involvement of the esophagus has been considered a rare autopsy finding that occurred in only 0.14 to 0.15% of necropsies.[78,79] However, the combination of the AIDS epidemic and the recent upsurge in reported cases of systemic tuberculosis may increase the incidence of esophageal infection.

Pathology. Most commonly, tuberculosis affects the middle third of the esophagus around the level of the carina. This is usually caused by spread of infection from tuberculous mediastinal lymph nodes by way of a draining fistula or by obstructed lymphatics. Ulceration of the esophageal mucosa may occur at the point of contact with infected fistulas or lymphatics. Less commonly, tuberculosis can involve the upper third of the esophagus by direct extension from tuberculous pharyngitis or laryngitis. Lesions of the esophagus, such as cancer or a benign stricture, may serve as a nidus for growth of swallowed mycobacteria. Hematogenous spread of tuberculosis to the esophagus is rare but can lead to a granular form of esophageal tuberculosis with multiple mucosal miliary granulomata. Primary esophageal tuberculosis in the absence of extraesophageal disease is exceedingly rare.[80] The fibrotic response of esophageal or mediastinal tissues to mycobacterial infection can result in esophageal obstruction.

Clinical Manifestations and Complications. The symptoms of esophageal tuberculosis depend on the degree and type of involvement. Patients with ulceration may complain of odynophagia, whereas a fibrotic stricture may result in dysphagia. Sitophobia as a consequence of odynophagia may contribute to emaciation caused by systemic tuberculosis.

The most common serious complication of esophageal tuberculosis is the formation of a fistula between the esophagus and the trachea, bronchi, or pleural space. This should be suspected clinically in a patient with known respiratory or esophageal tuberculosis who starts coughing after swallowing, especially if food is expectorated.[81] Unfortunately, some patients with this complication may be asymptomatic. As discussed above, fibrous reaction can result in the formation of long strictures or traction diverticula. Severe upper gastrointestinal hemorrhage from tuberculous esophageal ulcers[82] and tuberculous arterioesophageal fistulas[83,84] have been reported.

Diagnosis. Esophageal tuberculosis should be suspected in a patient with pulmonary or systemic tuberculosis who develops dysphagia or odynophagia. X-ray findings are nonspecific and include ulceration and stricture. An ulcerated tuberculous granulomatous mass may appear like an esophageal cancer on barium esophagography (Fig 56-8).[85-87] A sinus tract or fistulous connection to the bronchial tree or mediastinum is suggestive of tuberculosis but can also be seen with malignancy, syphilis, actinomycosis, or blastomycosis (Fig 56-9). Esophagoscopy may be very helpful in establishing the diagnosis. Although the gross appearance of ulcers or strictures is not diagnostic of tuberculosis, endoscopic biopsies around the edge of the lesions may reveal granulomas or acid-fast bacilli. Biopsy material may be cultured for further confirmation of the diagnosis and determination of sensitivities to antimycobacterial agents.

Therapy. Multidrug therapy for systemic tuberculosis usually heals esophageal tuberculosis and closes fistulas. If fistulas do not close with medical therapy, surgical intervention is necessary. Surgical options include colon interposition.[88] In addition to antimycobacterial agents, tuberculous esophageal strictures may require bougienage for relief of dysphagia. Hemorrhage from an arterioesophageal fistula requires emergency surgery.

BACTERIA

Epidemiology. Recent reports[4,89] indicate that bacterial esophagitis may be more common in immunocompromised patients than previously thought. Bacterial infection was found in 12% to 16% of autopsies and 11% of endoscopies in patients with infectious esophagitis. For the most part, the infecting pathogens are representative oral flora, particularly gram-positive organisms, including *Streptococcus viridans*, staphylococci, and *Bacillus* species. It may, therefore, be difficult to distinguish infection from colonization of damaged esophageal mucosa. Infection with *Actinomyces israelii*, *Corynebacterium diphtheria*, and *Lactobacillus acidophilus* have been reported rarely.[90–92]

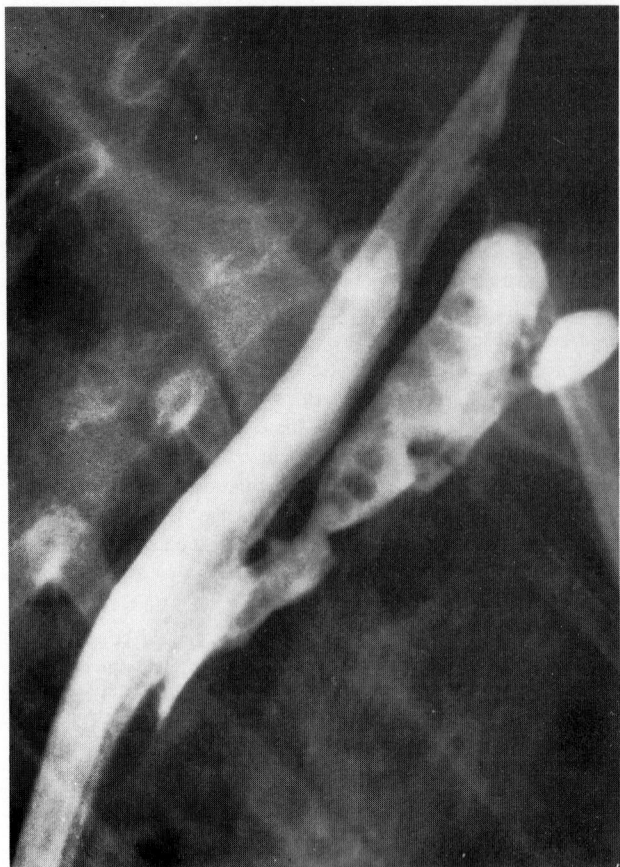

FIGURE 56–8. Barium esophagram showing perforation of a tuberculous esophageal ulcer. (Courtesy of Dr. J. Farman, Columbia-Presbyterian Medical Center, New York.)

Pathology. Bacterial esophagitis is probably a secondary event that follows esophageal injury from nasogastric tubes, cytotoxic chemotherapy, radiation therapy, or reflux esophagitis. The gross pathologic appearance of the esophagus in bacterial infection ranges from normal mucosa to ulcers associated with erythema, plaques, pseudomembranes, or hemorrhage.[89] Microscopic examination reveals pseudomembranes and bacterial invasion, which may extend only through the squamous epithelium or be transmural with infiltration of blood vessels (phlegmonous esophagitis).[89] Neutropenic patients have larger numbers of esophageal organisms with less inflammatory response.[89] Actinomycosis is characterized by granulomatous esophagitis and drainage of so-called sulfur granules from sinuses leading from abscess cavities.

Clinical Manifestations and Complications. Commonly, bacterial esophagitis is diagnosed in a neutropenic patient undergoing chemotherapy for a hematogenous malignancy who complains of dysphagia or odynophagia. The patient is usually febrile, but infection can occur without fever. Esophageal infection may serve as a focus for bacteremia and seeding of other organs.[93]

Diagnosis. The diagnosis of bacterial esophagitis should be considered in the clinical setting described above. Endoscopic examination of the esophagus with biopsy and culture is required to establish this diagnosis. Radiographic findings of mucosal inflammation and ulceration are nonspecific.

Therapy. If diagnosed promptly, bacterial esophagitis, caused by organisms such as streptococcus or actinomycosis respond to high doses of parenteral penicillin or another appropriate antimicrobial agent. If possible, therapy should be tailored to the drug sensitivities of cultured organisms. Mortality is related to the condition causing the underlying immunodeficiency rather than to bacterial esophagitis per se.

TREPONEMA PALLIDUM

Epidemiology. A computer-assisted search of the literature reveals no reports of syphilitic involvement of the esophagus after 1961. This esophageal infection is very rare.

Pathology. Tertiary syphilis of the esophagus may present as a submucosal gumma or diffuse inflammatory reaction with fibrosis most commonly affecting the upper third of the esophagus. As with other esophageal infections, mucosal ulcers are common. The classic microscopic appearance is that of syphilitic periarteritis.[94]

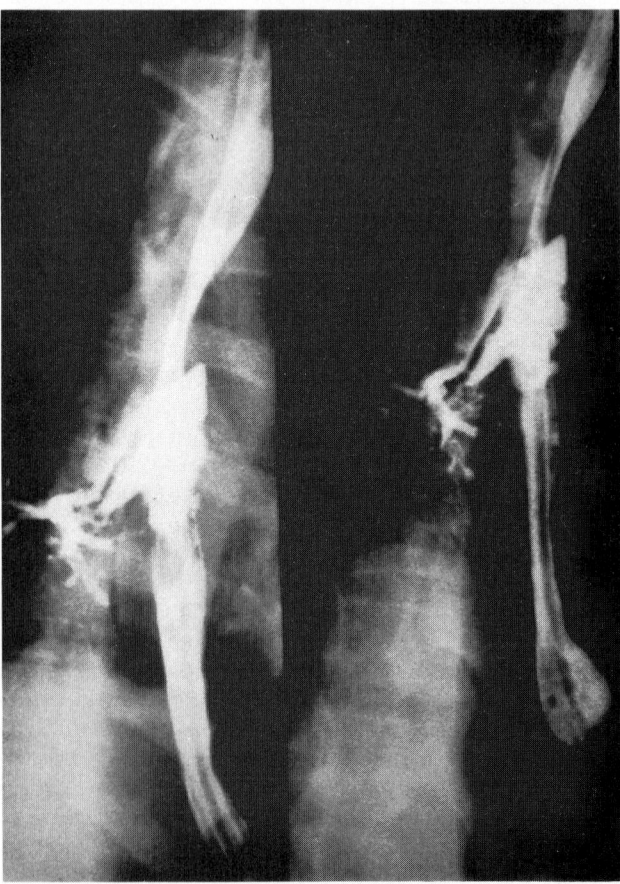

FIGURE 56–9. Two views of barium esophagram showing esophago-bronchial fistula in a patient with esophageal tuberculosis. (Courtesy of Dr. S. Iyer, Kings County Hospital, New York.)

Clinical Manifestations and Complications.
Dysphagia in a patient with syphilitic involvement of another organ or positive serologic tests for syphilis should suggest the diagnosis of esophageal syphilis. Nevertheless, the rarity of esophageal syphilis and comparative frequency of syphilis suggests that in most patients with infectious esophagitis and positive serologic test for syphilis, another pathogen is the cause of the esophagitis. Odynophagia appears to be less common in syphilitic esophagitis than in other infections.[94,95] The most common complications of luetic esophagitis are strictures and fistulas.

Diagnosis. Barium esophagography may show a long stenotic, ulcerated segment in the upper third of the esophagus. Endoscopy may reveal diffuse ulceration in the same region with a stiff esophageal wall. Biopsies may not be helpful in confirming the diagnosis, and the clinician may have to rely on the results of a therapeutic trial of antisyphilitic drugs.

Therapy. Penicillin therapy is generally sufficient to cure esophageal disease, including fistulas. Stenotic esophageal segments may require bougienage or surgical resection.

ESOPHAGEAL INFECTION IN AIDS

The AIDS epidemic has altered the clinical approach to the diagnosis and management of esophageal infection in several ways.

In AIDS, as in other immunodeficiency states, candidiasis is the most common esophageal infection. Nevertheless, several distinguishing features govern the physician's clinical strategy in this rapidly growing subset of patients with esophageal infections.

First, in AIDS patients with oral candidiasis, the presence of odynophagia or dysphagia almost always indicates *Candida* esophagitis.[2,20] As a consequence, these patients can be started on antifungal therapy without further diagnostic evaluation. Endoscopy may be reserved for patients who do not respond to therapy within a week, or who have clinical or laboratory findings suggestive of an esophageal disorder other than candidiasis. This diagnostic approach should obviate the need for many costly, time-consuming, potentially hazardous and uncomfortable endoscopies without jeopardizing care.

Second, in AIDS, the incidence of uncommon esophageal pathogens such as CMV is increasing.[70,71] Esophagitis with previously unknown esophageal pathogens such as cryptosporidiosis has been reported.[96] In addition, an ulcerating esophagitis of unknown cause has been reported coincident with HIV seroconversion.[97] Endoscopic biopsies revealed unidentified viruslike particles (100–140 nm in diameter) in electron microscopic sections from eight such patients. The esophagitis resolved after 2 to 4 weeks, but six patients subsequently developed esophageal candidiasis. The etiology of this apparently new esophageal disorder remains to be determined. These reports make it apparent that gastroenterologists evaluating esophagitis in AIDS patients must be prepared at the time of endoscopy to obtain multiple specimens for a variety of bacteriologic, parasitic, and viral studies.

Third, esophageal candidiasis is more resistant to therapy and more likely to recur in AIDS than in other clinical situations.[38] Adequate therapy may require higher doses of antifungal agents[38] or measures such as gastric acidification to increase the bioavailability of drugs like ketoconazole.[40] Moreover, the high likelihood of recurrence suggests that patients with AIDS would benefit from prophylactic antifungal drug regimens.[2]

Finally, the emergence of acyclovir- and ganciclovir-resistant strains of herpes simplex virus and CMV, respectively, has been reported recently in patients with AIDS.[98,99] Although these viruses may respond to other agents, like foscarnet,[100] an increase in the prevalence of resistant organisms in AIDS patients and the emergence of similar strains in non-AIDS viral esophagitis are issues of great concern.

The reader is directed to Chapter 28, Approach to the Patient with Dysphagia; Chapter 29, Approach to the Patient with Chest Pain; Chapter 46, Approach to Gastrointestinal Problems in the Immunocompromised Patient; Chapter 55, Reflux Esophagitis; Chapter 103, Gastrointestinal Complications of the Acquired Immunodeficiency Syndrome; Chapter 107, Gastrointestinal Manifestations of Immunologic Disorders; Chapter 126, Endoscopic Mucosal Biopsy; and Chapter 127, Microbiologic Studies.

REFERENCES

1. Kramer P, Burakoff R. Infections of the esophagus. In: Berk JE, ed. Bockus: Gastroenterology, ed 4. Philadelphia: WB Saunders, 1985: 787.
2. Raufman JP. Odynophagia/dysphagia in AIDS. In: Friedman SL, ed. Gastrointestinal manifestations of AIDS. Philadelphia: WB Saunders, 1988:599.
3. Jones JM, Glass NR, Belzer FO. Fatal *Candida* esophagitis in two diabetics after renal transplantation. Arch Surg 1982;117:499.
4. McDonald GB, Sharma P, Hackman RC, et al. Esophageal infections in immunosuppressed patients after marrow transplantation. Gastroenterology 1985;88:1111.
5. Alexander JA, Brouillette DE, Chien MC, et al. Infectious esophagitis following liver and renal transplantation. Dig Dis Sci 1988;33:1121.
6. Owensby JC, Stammer JL. Esophagitis associated with herpes simplex infection in an immunocompetent host. Gastroenterology 1978;74: 1305.
7. Springer DJ, DaCosta LR, Beck IT. A syndrome of acute self limiting ulcerative esophagitis in young adults probably due to herpes simplex virus. Dig Dis Sci 1979;24:535.
8. Depew WT, Prentice RSA, Beck IT, Blakeman JM. Herpes simplex ulcerative esophagitis in a healthy subject. Am J Gastroenterol 1977;68:381.
9. DeGaeta L, Levine MS, Guglielmi GE, Raffensperger EC, Laufer I. Herpes esophagitis in an otherwise healthy patient. AJR 1985;144: 1295.
10. Deshmukh M, Shah R, McCallum RW. Experience with herpes esophagitis in otherwise healthy patients. Am J Gastroenterol 1984;79: 173.
11. Kodsi BE, Wickremesinghe PC, Kozinn PJ, Iswara K, Goldberg PK. *Candida* esophagitis. A prospective study of 27 cases. Gastroenterology 1976;71:715.
12. Eras P, Goldstein MJ, Sherlock P. *Candida* infection of the gastrointestinal tract. Medicine 1972;51:367.
13. Prolla JC, Kirsner JB. The gastrointestinal lesions and complications of the leukemias. Ann Intern Med 1964;61:1084.
14. Jensen KB, Stenderup A, Thomsen JB, Bichel J. Oesophageal moni-

liasis in malignant neoplastic disease. Acta Med Scand 1964;175:455.

15. Ehrlich AN, Stadler G, Geller W, Sherlock P. Gastrointestinal manifestations of malignant lymphoma. Gastroenterology 1968;54:1115.
16. Winston DJ, Gale RP, Meyer DV, Young LS. Infectious complications of human bone marrow transplantation. Medicine 1979;58:1.
17. Frick T, Fryd DS, Goodale RL, Simmons RL, Sutherland DER, Najarian JS. Incidence and treatment of *Candida* esophagitis in patients undergoing renal transplantation. Am J Surg 1988;155:313.
18. Raufman JP, Straus EW. Gastrointestinal endoscopy in patients with acquired immune deficiency syndrome: An evaluation of current practices. Gastrointest Endosc 1987;33:76.
19. Tom W, Aaron JS. Esophageal ulcers caused by *Torulopsis glabrata* in a patient with acquired immune deficiency syndrome. Am J Gastroenterol 1987;82:766.
20. Tavitian A, Raufman JP, Rosenthal LE. Oral candidiasis as a marker for esophageal candidiasis in the acquired immunodeficiency syndrome. Ann Intern Med 1986;104:54.
21. Andren L, Theander G. Roentgenographic appearances of esophageal moniliasis. Acta Radiol 1956;46:571.
22. Goldberg HI, Dodds WJ. Cobblestone esophagus due to monilial infection. Am J Roentgenol 1968;104:608.
23. Guyer PB, Brunton FJ, Rooke HWP. Candidiasis of the esophagus. Br J Radiol 1971;44:131.
24. Holt JM. *Candida* infection of the oesophagus. Gut 1968;9:227.
25. Jones JM. Necrotizing *Candida* esophagitis. JAMA 1980;244:2190.
26. Lewicki AM, Moore JP. Esophageal moniliasis. Am J Radiol 1975;125:218.
27. Rohrman CA, Kidd R. Chronic mucocutaneous candidiasis: Radiologic abnormalities in the esophagus. AJR 1978;130:474.
28. Sheft DJ, Shrago G. Esophageal moniliasis: The spectrum of the disease. JAMA 1970;213:1859.
29. Ho CS, Cullen JB, Gray RR. An unusual manifestation of esophageal moniliasis. Radiology 1977;123:287.
30. Rattan J, Hallak A, Rozen P, et al. Esophageal moniloma and mucosal bridge. Gastrointest Endosc 1982;28:114.
31. Orringer MB, Sloan H. Monilial esophagitis: An increasingly frequent cause of esophageal stenosis? Ann Thorac Surg 1978;26:364.
32. Ott DJ, Gelfand DW. Esophageal stricture secondary to candidiasis. Gastrointest Radiol 1978;2:323.
33. Kowal LE, Goodman LR, Teplick SK, et al. Multiple infectious esophageal fistulae. Am J Gastroenterol 1983;78:309.
34. Farman J, Tavitian A, Rosenthal LE, et al. Focal esophageal candidiasis in acquired immunodeficiency syndrome (AIDS). Gastrointest Radiol 1986;11:213.
35. Bier SJ, Keller RJ, Krivisky BA, et al. Esophageal moniliasis: A new radiographic presentation. Am J Gastroenterol 1985;80:734.
36. Levine MS, Woldenberg R, Herlinger H, Laufer I. Opportunistic esophagitis in AIDS: Radiographic diagnosis. Radiology 1987;165:815.
37. Fazio RA, Wickremesinghe PC, Arsura EL. Ketoconazole treatment of *Candida* esophagitis—A prospective study of 12 cases. Am J Gastroenterol 1983;78:261.
38. Tavitian A, Raufman JP, Rosenthal LE, et al. Ketoconazole-resistant *Candida* esophagitis in patients with acquired immunodeficiency syndrome. Gastroenterology 1986;90:443.
39. Lake-Bakaar G, Quadros E, Beidas S, et al. Gastric secretory failure in patients with the acquired immunodeficiency syndrome (AIDS). Ann Intern Med 1988;109:502.
40. Lake-Bakaar G, Tom W, Lake-Bakaar D, et al. Gastropathy and ketoconazole malabsorption in the acquired immunodeficiency syndrome (AIDS). Ann Intern Med 1988;109:471.
41. Lewis JH, Zimmerman HJ, Benson GD, Ishak, KG. Hepatic injury associated with ketoconazole therapy. Gastroenterology 1984;86:503.
42. Sonino N. The use of ketoconazole as an inhibitor of steroid production. N Engl J Med 1987;317:812.
43. Ginsburg CH, Braden GL, Tauber AI, Trier JS. Oral clotrimazole in the treatment of esophageal candidiasis. Am J Med 1981;71:891.
44. Deschamps MH, Pape JW, Verdier RI, et al. Treatment of *Candida* esophagitis in AIDS patients. Am J Gastroenterol 1988;83:20.
45. Cosgrove RF, Beezer AE, Miles RJ. In vitro studies of amphotericin

B in combination with the imidazole antifungal compounds clotrimazole and miconazole. J Infect Dis 1978;138:681.
46. Sanders E, Levinthal C, Donner MW. Monilial esophagitis in a patient with hemoglobin SC disease. Ann Intern Med 1962;57:650.
47. Hann I, Prentice H, Corringham R, et al. Ketoconazole versus nystatin plus amphotericin B for fungal prophylaxis in severely immunocompromised patients. Lancet 1982;1:826.
48. Shepp DH, Klosterman A, Siegel MS. Comparative trial of ketoconazole and nystatin for prevention of fungal infection in neutropenic patients treated in a protective environment. J Infect Dis 1985;152:1257.
49. Hansen RM, Reinerio N, Sohnle PG, et al. Ketoconazole in the prevention of candidiasis in patients with cancer. Arch Intern Med 1987;147:710.
50. Obrecht WF, Richter JE, Olympio GA, Gelfand DW. Tracheoesophageal fistula: A serious complication of infectious esophagitis. Gastroenterology 1984;87:1174.
51. Fifer WR, Woellner RC, Gordon SS. Mediastinal histoplasmosis. Dis Chest 1965;47:518.
52. Jenkins DW, Fisk DE, Byrd RB. Mediastinal histoplasmosis with esophageal abscess. Gastroenterology 1976;70:109.
53. Wheat LJ, Slama TG, Eitzen HE, et al. A large urban outbreak of histoplasmosis: Clinical features. Ann Intern Med 1981;94:331.
54. Cherniss EI, Waisbren BA. North American blastomycosis: A clinical study of 40 cases. Ann Intern Med 1956;44:105.
55. Young RC, Bennett JE, Vogel CL, et al. Aspergillosis: The spectrum of the disease in 98 patients. Medicine 1970;49:147.
56. Pearce J, Dagradi A. Acute ulceration of the esophagus with associated intranuclear inclusion bodies. Arch Pathol 1943;35:889.
57. Buss DH, Scharyj M. Herpes virus infection of the esophagus and other visceral organs in adults: Incidence and clinical significance. Am J Med 1979;66:457.
58. Nash G, Ross JS. Herpetic esophagitis: A common cause of esophageal ulceration. Hum Pathol 1974;5:339.
59. Brayko DM, Kozarek RA, Sanowski RA, et al. Type I herpes simplex esophagitis with concomitant esophageal moniliasis. J Clin Gastroenterol 1982;4:351.
60. Mirra SS, Bryan JA, Butz WC, Miles ML. Concomitant herpesmonilial esophagitis: Case report with ultrastructural study. Hum Pathol 1982;13:760.
61. Fishbein PG, Tuthill R, Kressel H, et al. Herpes simplex esophagitis: A cause of upper gastrointestinal bleeding. Dig Dis Sci 1979;24:540.
62. Rattner HM, Cooper DJ, Zaman MB. Severe bleeding from herpes esophagitis. Am J Gastroenterol 1985;80:523.
63. Obrecht WF Jr, Richtert JE, Olympio GA, et al. Tracheoesophageal fistula: A serious complication of infectious esophagitis. Gastroenterology 1984;83:1174.
64. Agha FP, Horchang HL, Nostrant TT. Herpetic esophagitis: A diagnostic challenge in immunocompromised patients. Am J Gastroenterol 1986;81:246.
65. Levine MS, Loevner LA, Scott SH, et al. Herpes esophagitis: Sensitivity of double-contrast esophagography. AJR 1988;151:57.
66. Goldstein LC, McDougall JK, Nowinski RC. Monoclonal antibodies to herpes simplex viruses: Use in antigenic typing and rapid diagnosis. J Infect Dis 1983;147:829.
67. Kadakia SC, Oliver GA, Peura DA. Acyclovir in endoscopically presumed viral esophagitis. Gastrointest Endosc 1987;33:33.
68. Balthazar EJ, Megibow AJ, Hulnick DH. Cytomegalovirus esophagitis and gastritis in AIDS. Am J Radiol 1985;144:1201.
69. Frager DH, Frager JD, Brandt LJ, et al. Gastrointestinal complications of AIDS: Radiologic features. Radiology 1986;158:597.
70. Balthazar EJ, Megibow AJ, Hulnick D, et al. Cytomegalovirus esophagitis in AIDS: Radiographic features in 16 patients. AJR 1987;149:919.
71. Teixidor HS, Honig CL, Norsoph E, et al. Cytomegalovirus infection of the alimentary canal: Radiologic findings with pathologic correlation. Radiology 1987;163:317.
72. St. Onge G, Bezahler G. Giant esophageal ulcer associated with cytomegalovirus. Gastroenterology 1982;83:127.
73. Chachoua A, Dieterich D, Krasninsk K, et al. 9-(1,3- dihydroxy-2-propoxymethyl)guanine (ganciclovir) in the treatment of cytomeg-

alovirus gastrointestinal disease with the acquired immunodeficiency syndrome. Ann Intern Med 1987;107:133.

74. Stein DS, Verano AS, Levandowski RA. Successful treatment with ganciclovir of disseminated cytomegalovirus infection after liver transplantation. Am J Gastoenterol 1988;83:684.

75. Harbison MA, Girolami PC, Jenkins RL, Hammer SM. Ganciclovir therapy of severe cytomegalovirus infections in solid-organ transplant recipients. Transplantation 1988;46:82.

76. Gill RA, Gebhard RL, Dozeman RL, et al. Shingles esophagitis: Endoscopic diagnosis in two patients. Gastrointest Endosc 1984;30: 26.

77. Kroneke MK, Cuadrado MR. Esophageal stricture following esophagitis in a patient with herpes zoster: Case report. Milit Med 1984;149:479.

78. Carr DT, Spain DM. Tuberculosis in a carcinoma of the oesophagus. Am Rev Tuberculosis 1942;46:346.

79. Lockard LB. Oesophageal tuberculosis. A critical review. Laryngoscope 1913;23:561.

80. Seivewright N, Feehally J, Wicks ACB. Primary tuberculosis of the esophagus. Am J Gastoenterol 1984;79:842.

81. Wigley FM, Murray HW, Mann RB, et al. Unusual manifestation of tuberculosis: TE fistula. 1976;60:310.

82. Lewis RJ, Sisler GE. Reversible total esophageal exclusion. Ann Thorac Surg 1985;37:476.

83. Chase RA, Haber MH, Pottage JC Jr, et al. Tuberculous esophagitis with erosion into aortic aneurysm. Arch Pathol Lab Med 1986;110: 965.

84. O'Leary M, Nollet DJ, Blomberg DJ. Rupture of a tuberculous pseudoaneurysm of the innominate artery into the trachea and esophagus: Report of a case and review of the literature. Hum Pathol 1977;8:458.

85. de Mas R, Lombeck G, Riemann JF. Tuberculosis of the oesophagus masquerading as ulcerated tumour. Endoscopy 1986;18:153.

86. Ito Y, Kobayashi S, Kasugai T. Tuberculosis of the esophagus. Am J Gastroenterol 1976;65:454.

87. Laajam MA. Primary tuberculosis of the esophagus: Pseudotumoral presentation. Am J Gastroenterol 1984;79:839.

88. Montes I, Larsen E, Haiderer O, Kennedy JH. Tuberculous stricture of the esophagus: Report of a patient successfully treated by colon interposition. Chest 1971;60:194.

89. Walsh TJ, Belitsos NJ, Hamilton SR. Bacterial esophagitis in immunocompromised patients. Arch Intern Med 1986;146:1345.

90. Vinson P, Sutherland CG. Esophagobronchial fistula resulting from actinomycosis: Report of a case. Radiology 1926;6:63.

91. Kiviranta UK. Are any strictures of the esophagus due to diphtheria? Ann Otol 1949;58:429.

92. McManus JPA, Webb JN. A yeast-like infection of the esophagus caused by *Lactobacillus acidophilus*. Gastroenterology 1975;68:583.

93. Gilver RL. Esophageal lesions in leukemia and lymphoma. Dig Dis Sci 1970;15:31.

94. Hudson TR, Head JR. Syphilis of the esophagus. J Thorac Surg 1950;20:216.

95. Stone J, Friedberg SA. Obstructive syphilitic esophagitis. JAMA 1961;177:711.

96. Kazlow PG, Shah K, Bendov KJ, et al. Esophageal cryptosporidiosis in a child with acquired immune deficiency syndrome. Gastroenterology 1986;91:1301.

97. Rabeneck L, Boyko WJ, McLean DM, et al. Unusual esophageal ulcers containing enveloped viruslike particles in homosexual men. Gastroenterology 1986;90:1882.

98. Erlich KS, Mills J, Chatis P, et al. Acyclovir-resistant herpes simplex virus infections in patients with the acquired immunodeficiency syndrome. N Engl J Med 1989;320:293.

99. Erice A, Chou S, Biron KK, et al. Progressive disease due to ganciclovir-resistant cytomegalovirus in immunocompromised patients. N Engl J Med 1989;320:289.

100. Chatis PA, Miller CH, Schrager LE, Crumpacker CS. Successful treatment with foscarnet of an acyclovir-resistant mucocutaneous infection with herpes simplex virus in a patient with acquired immunodeficiency syndrome. N Engl J Med 1989;320:297.

57

Esophageal Tumors

BRIAN J. REID

SQUAMOUS CELL CARCINOMA

Squamous cell carcinoma is the most common neoplasm of the esophagus. Although it may be found at an early stage in areas of the world where its high incidence makes mass surveillance feasible, in the Western World esophageal carcinoma is usually detected only when it has become incurable. Of the estimated 10,600 patients diagnosed with esophageal cancer in the United States in 1988, fewer than 800 will survive 5 years.[1]

Epidemiology

Esophageal squamous cell carcinoma has one of the highest geographic variations in incidence of any malignant neoplasm with a 500-fold difference between areas of high and low risk (Table 57-1). Very high annual incidences are reported in the Caspian region of Iran, Northern China, and some regions of the Soviet Union. Large variations in incidence occur within small geographic confines. For example, rates in different regions of Iran vary from 7

TABLE 57–1
Epidemiology of Squamous Cell Carcinoma of the Esophagus

Sex: Male > Female

Race: Black > White

Geography (high risk):

Iran (Caspian region)

Northern China

Soviet Union (Turkmenistan and Uzbekistan)

South Africa

Social class: Higher risk in lower socioeconomic groups

Environmental factors:

Tobacco (smoking and chewing)

Alcohol

Betel nut chewing

Hereditofamilial factors:

Tylosis (70% to 95% incidence by age 65)

Concomitant/preexisting conditions:

Achalasia

Lye strictures

Head and neck squamous carcinoma

Plummer-Vinson syndrome

?Ionizing radiation

?Celiac sprue

?Esophageal diverticula

---

to 171 per 100,000, and in China there is a 70-fold difference between areas of high and low incidence.[2]

In the United States, blacks have a fourfold to fivefold increased risk relative to whites. Black men have an incidence of 15.1 per 100,000; the risk for black women is 4.1 per 100,000. The corresponding figures for white men and women are 2.9 and 1.1 per 100,000, respectively.[3,4] Between 1973 and 1982, the incidence of squamous cell carcinoma of the esophagus among blacks increased 30%.[4]

Etiology

Environmental factors appear to be responsible for the vast majority of esophageal squamous cell carcinomas. With the exception of the rare condition tylosis, there is little evidence of genetic predisposition to this disease. For example, one large study involving 877 relatives of 101 esophageal cancer patients and 2572 relatives of control patients failed to document any genetic influence, but found an association with alcohol abuse.[5]

It has been estimated that at least 90% of the risk for esophageal cancer in North America and Western Europe can be attributed to alcohol and tobacco.[2] Excessive use of alcohol has been documented to be a risk factor for esophageal cancer in numerous studies,[6–11] and the risk increases in a dose-response manner.[2,7,8,12] The type of alcohol may also influence the risk.[7]

Tobacco, smoked or chewed, is associated with an increased risk of esophageal cancer.[2,6,7,12–15] In cigarette smokers, the risk increases with increasing consumption, although it may level off at high doses.[2,16,17] Studies have shown an increased incidence of esophageal cancer in consumers of both alcohol and tobacco.[2,12,15] For example, in Brittany, the relative risk of esophageal cancer for men consuming more than 121 g of alcohol per day was 49.6, and the relative risk for smokers of more than 30 g of tobacco was 7.8. When the two risk factors were combined, the relative risk was 155.6.[18]

Although tobacco and alcohol are major determinants of the risk of esophageal squamous cell carcinoma in the Western World, other risk factors appear to be operating in some areas of the globe. For example, in northern Iran, alcohol and tobacco consumption contribute little to the overall risk.[2] In some areas, regional habits such as betel chewing or swallowing the residue of pipe tobacco or opium pipes may contribute to an increased risk.[2,19] The importance of environmental factors in esophageal carcinoma is accentuated by the finding that chickens in Northern China have a high incidence of spontaneously occurring esophageal cancer, which corresponds to the incidence of human cancer in the region.[20,21]

Esophageal cancer is a disease of lower socioeconomic groups,[2] and nutritional factors have been postulated to play a role in its pathogenesis.[7,8] In general, lack of a varied diet appears to have the most convincing association with the development of esophageal carcinoma, and diets deficient in fruits, vegetables, eggs, dairy products, and protein have been implicated.[7,19] Although deficiencies of some vitamins, minerals, and other micronutrients have been suggested to be involved in esophageal carcinogenesis,[19,22–24] the evidence for their role is inconclusive. Some populations with a high risk of esophageal carcinoma have diets containing high levels of nitrosamines or other potential carcinogens.[19,24–26]

A number of conditions have been postulated to predispose to esophageal carcinoma. Unfortunately, the contribution of each of these conditions to the overall risk of esophageal cancer is small,[27] and, in most cases, the magnitude of the risk cannot be estimated, making surveillance for early detection difficult.

Tylosis, a condition characterized by hyperkeratosis of the palms and soles, oral leukoplakia, and esophageal squamous cell carcinoma, is an autosomal dominant condition.[28–30] It was originally described in two Liverpool families, and the risk of affected members developing esophageal cancer by age 63 was estimated to be 95% if they did not die from some other cause.[28,29] Esophageal cancer has subsequently been confirmed in a small number of additional families with tylosis and in a few sporadic cases.[31–33] Given the predisposition of affected family members to develop esophageal carcinoma, endoscopic surveillance seems warranted.

Achalasia is frequently mentioned as a precancerous condition of the esophagus. A review of the literature to 1983 documented 281 patients who had both achalasia and esophageal carcinoma, although, in many cases, definitive evidence of achalasia was lacking.[34] The prevalence of esophageal carcinoma in patients with longstanding achalasia is approximately 5%.[35–40] Further evidence that achalasia is a premalignant condition comes from the earlier onset of esophageal cancer in achalasia patients than in the general population.[41] The mean duration from the onset of symptoms of achalasia to the development of carcinoma has been estimated to be 17 to 20 years.[40,41]

The magnitude of the risk to the individual patient with achalasia is controversial and difficult to establish. A recent study of 91 manometrically diagnosed patients with achalasia who did not initially have carcinoma showed that none developed cancer during 589 patient-years of follow-up.[35] At present, there appears to be insufficient evidence to support routine surveillance endoscopy in patients with achalasia.[34]

Lye stricture has also been postulated to be a premalignant condition,[42] although it is difficult to estimate the magnitude of the risk without prospective studies. Lye strictures are responsible for only a small fraction of esophageal carcinomas, and most agree that the duration from caustic exposure to development of cancer is approximately 40 years.[42,43]

Head and neck squamous carcinoma has been shown to have an association with esophageal squamous cell carcinoma (Fig. 57-1), probably reflecting the influence of alcohol and tobacco as causative agents for both cancers.[44,45] For patients with a primary

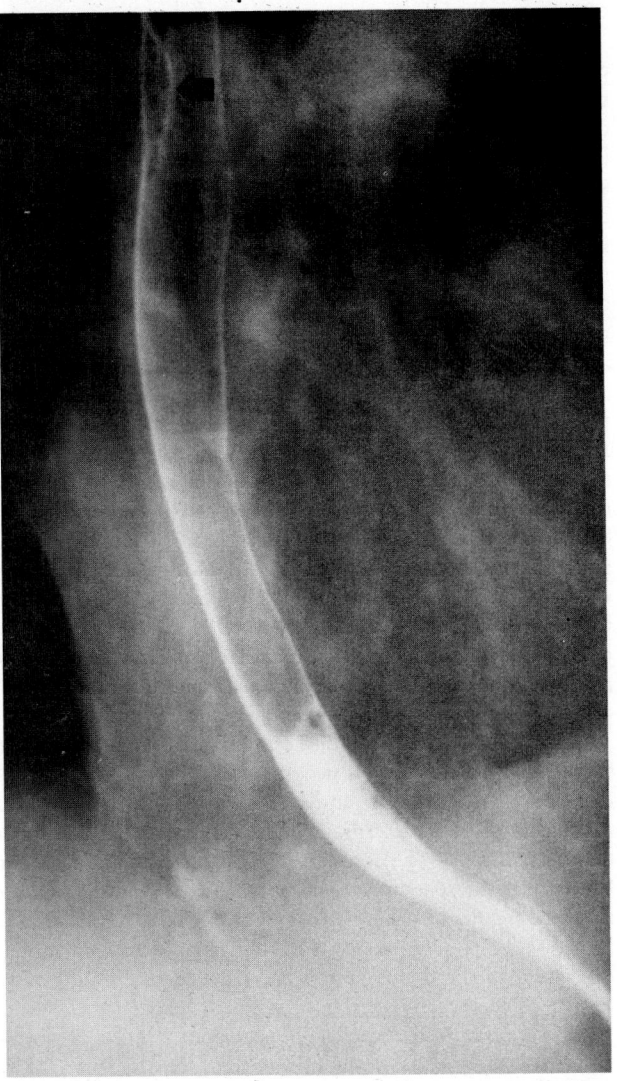

FIGURE 57–1. An early esophageal squamous cell carcinoma that was detected as a second malignancy during evaluation of a patient who had a head and neck primary squamous cell carcinoma. (Radiograph courtesy of Dr. Charles Rohrmann.)

head and neck tumor, the risk of a second, coexisting esophageal primary appears to be approximately 0.7% to 6.0%.[46–49] Endoscopic evaluation of the esophagus of all patients with head and neck cancers has been advocated.[46,47,49]

Exposure to ionizing radiation,[50,51] celiac sprue,[52] Plummer-Vinson syndrome,[53] and esophageal diverticula[54] have been implicated in the pathogenesis of some esophageal cancers.

Clinical Manifestations

In its early stages, esophageal carcinoma may be totally asymptomatic or may be manifested only by mild, nonspecific symptoms for which the patient may not seek medical attention.[55,56] Even early carcinomas may be associated with mild complaints related to eating such as retrosternal discomfort, mild or intermittent dysphagia, a foreign body sensation, or odynophagia.[57–59]

As the tumor grows, symptoms of advanced esophageal carcinoma appear. Progressive dysphagia is the most common presenting complaint, occurring in over 90% of patients.[60–62] Dysphagia usually signifies that more than 50% of the esophageal lumen is occluded. It typically begins with solids and can progress to the point at which liquids or even saliva cannot be swallowed. Dysphagia in a patient over 45 years of age should be considered to be due to esophageal carcinoma until proven otherwise.[61]

Anorexia and weight loss occur in approximately 75% of patients with advanced esophageal carcinoma.[62,63] Weight loss may be the result of inadequate intake secondary to dysphagia or a nonspecific effect of the cancer and predisposes to hypoalbuminemia and other nutritional deficits. Odynophagia occurs in 50% of patients. A gnawing pain felt retrosternally or in the back suggests mediastinal extension. Bleeding from esophageal carcinoma is most frequently occult and can lead to iron-deficiency anemia. Brisk bleeding is an uncommon presentation.

Cough may result from aspiration pneumonia or tracheoesophageal fistula. Local invasion of the cancer can produce pleural effusions and empyema. Hoarseness suggests involvement of the recurrent laryngeal nerve. Bone pain suggests skeletal metastases. Occasionally, the cancer may erode into the aorta with resulting exsanguination.

Physical findings are not a prominent part of the clinical presentation of esophageal carcinoma. Fixed supraclavicular lymphadenopathy or axillary lymph node metastases are a sign of advanced disease. Hepatomegaly secondary to metastatic disease is a sign of a poor prognosis.

Differential Diagnosis and Diagnostic Studies

In the patient with new-onset dysphagia, the main elements in the differential diagnosis are benign peptic stricture, corrosive stricture, esophageal motor disorders including achalasia, esophageal adenocarcinoma, and adenocarcinoma of the gastric cardia with distal esophageal involvement. Although less common, the other tumors described in this chapter may produce similar symptoms.

The patient with a benign peptic stricture may give a long history of heartburn or other regurgitant symptoms; unfortunately, patients with esophageal adenocarcinoma complicating Barrett's esophagus do so as well. The patient with a corrosive stricture usually gives a history of caustic ingestion. The patient with achalasia may present with a history of intermittent dysphagia and a characteristically dilated proximal esophagus and distal tapered "bird's beak" configuration on barium esophagogram. Nevertheless, the symptom of dysphagia, especially in a patient over 45 years of age, mandates a complete evaluation to rule out esophageal carcinoma.

The diagnostic evaluation of the patient with suspected esophageal carcinoma can be divided into two steps. The first step is to confirm the diagnosis of carcinoma through use of the barium esophagogram and upper gastrointestinal endoscopy with biopsy and cytology. The second step is to determine the spread of disease, or its stage, so that appropriate treatment can be instituted.

STAGING

Several staging systems have been proposed for esophageal cancer.[61] In general, surgical-pathologic staging is more accurate than pretreatment clinical staging for predicting survival. In a retrospective study of the surgical specimens of 3987 patients with esophageal carcinoma in Japan, the most important determinants of survival were depth of invasion, the presence or absence of lymph node metastases, and the presence or absence of distant metastases.[64] Survival decreases with increasing depth of tumor invasion. Submucosal invasion has a 5-year survival of 46.1%, which falls progressively with invasion of the muscularis propria (29.5%), the adventitia (21.7%), and extension to contiguous structures (7%).[64] Survival also decreases with involvement of lymph nodes that are increasingly distant from the primary tumor. Metastasis to distant organs reduces 5-year survival to 3.0%.[64] These results are consistent with those of other studies.[65]

DIAGNOSTIC STUDIES

The goal of the pretreatment evaluation is to determine the diagnosis, depth of tumor invasion, degree of nodal involvement, and the presence or absence of distant metastases. Clinical staging is still imprecise in achieving this goal. Barium esophagogram and endoscopy are useful in evaluating the primary tumor, whereas the clinical examination, biochemical profiles, and computed tomography (CT) scanning are useful, although imperfect, tools in assessing lymph node and distant organ involvement.[61] Radionuclide bone scans, ultrasonography, bronchoscopy, and biopsy of suspicious lesions are useful studies in some patients.[61]

Endoscopy.   Flexible fiberoptic endoscopy with direct vision biopsy and cytology represents the single most important test in the diagnosis of esophageal carcinoma and, unless contraindicated, should be performed in any patient in whom the diagnosis is suspected.[66-71] The overall low incidence of esophageal squamous cell carcinoma in the United States has made surveillance programs such as have been instituted in China for the early detection of esophageal cancer impractical. In the absence of identifiable high-risk groups, detection of early esophageal carcinoma depends on careful inspection of the esophageal mucosa in all patients undergoing endoscopy. Because early carcinomas have the highest cure rate, it is important for endoscopists to be aware of their appearance.

The endoscopic appearance of early esophageal carcinoma has been described in several studies.[72-76] In China, four types of endoscopic abnormality were reported: (1) The most common was the superficial erosive cancer with a slightly depressed lesion with gray erosions occurring in a reddish mucosa. The cancer was friable, and bleeding occurred when it was touched by the endoscope; (2) a slightly elevated plaque with granular or coarse mucosal surfaces; (3) a "congestive" cancer, characterized by red spots on the esophageal mucosa; and (4) a small polypoid lesion.[72]

Early esophageal carcinomas have been also described as white elevated plaques, red depressed areas, or both[74] or, alternatively, erosions consistent with gastroesophageal reflux disease.[75] Some investigators have used dyes such as toluidine blue and iodine (Lugol's solution) instilled by way of a thin catheter that is passed through the biopsy channel of the endoscope to aid in visualization of early esophageal squamous carcinomas.[74,76]

In the United States, the endoscopist is more commonly called on to evaluate a patient with progressive dysphagia in whom the barium esophagogram already suggests carcinoma. Such advanced carcinomas may appear as circumferential "apple core" lesions, exophytic masses, an infiltrating lesion that may mimic a benign stricture, or an ulcer.[77] Submucosal spread of the cancer can produce nodules that are covered with normal mucosa. If the endoscope can be passed beyond the malignant narrowing, the proximal and distal extent of the tumor, its circumferential extent, and any associated abnormalities should be recorded.[77] If possible, a retroflexed view of the gastric cardia should be obtained.

Biopsy and Cytology.   Direct vision biopsies and cytologies are complementary, and both should be obtained.[66-68,70] Ideally, multiple biopsies should be obtained using a large-channel endoscope and spiked, oval-cupped biopsy forceps. If the degree of obstruction precludes use of a large-channel endoscope, a pediatric endoscope may permit visualization of the entire lesion, although biopsies obtained through the smaller endoscope may not be as satisfactory. In some cases, the biopsy forceps and cytology brush may be passed gently beyond the narrowing to obtain additional samples for analysis. If necessary, the stenosis may be gently dilated for endoscopic evaluation, biopsies, and cytologies.[78,79]

Several factors influence the accuracy of endoscopic biopsy in the diagnosis of esophageal neoplasms. In general, accuracy increases with increasing numbers of biopsies.[66-69,77] When six to ten endoscopic biopsies are obtained, the diagnostic accuracy is 80% to 95%.[66,67,70] The accuracy of endoscopic biopsies can also be affected by the pattern of tumor growth; biopsies from exophytic tumors were more frequently positive than biopsies from stenotic lesions.[68,77] This may be due to the difficulty in passing the endoscope beyond a stenotic lesion and the tendency of infiltrative cancers to be partially covered by normal mucosa.

The accuracy of endoscopic brush cytology in upper gastrointestinal malignancies is most commonly reported as 70% to 90%.[66-68,70,80] In some cases, cytology may provide the only evidence of carcinoma.[81] By combining cytology with multiple endoscopic biopsies, accuracies of 90% to 100% can be attained.[66,68,70] Rarely, both biopsy and cytology fail to diagnose a cancer in cases with endoscopic or radiographic evidence of carcinoma. In these cases, repeat endoscopic biopsies and cytologies are indicated at the first possible opportunity.

In Northern China where there is a high incidence of esophageal carcinoma, mass screening programs have been instituted using cytologies obtained by a balloon covered with nylon mesh.[82,83] The detection rate for carcinoma using this technique is approximately 90%. Between 70% and 90% of the cancers were early with estimated 5- and 10-year survivals of 86% and 56% after surgical treatment.[82,84] Balloon cytology may be more accurate in the diagnosis of early carcinomas than barium esophagogram or fiberoptic endoscopy.[58,82]

Attempts to use such "blind" esophageal cytology in the United States have been less successful with sensitivities for detection of advanced esophageal cancer ranging from 72.4% to 93%.[85–87] The low yield of screening asymptomatic patients in the United States was illustrated by the absence of carcinoma among 99 asymptomatic alcoholics who were evaluated by balloon cytology.[88]

Radiology. Because patients with early esophageal carcinoma may have mild complaints relative to eating for which a barium esophagram may be ordered, it is important that the radiologist and gastroenterologist maintain a high degree of suspicion in evaluating any patient whose complaints are clearly related to the act of deglutition.[89] Although radiology is not as sensitive as endoscopy in detecting early esophageal cancer,[58] several studies indicate that a double-contrast barium esophagram can detect many early esophageal carcinomas.[89–93] The accuracy in diagnosing such early carcinomas was 73% with a 27% false-negative and a 37% false-positive rate.[91] It may be necessary to accept a high false-positive rate to ensure the highest degree of radiologic detection of small, early cancers.

The radiologic appearance of early esophageal carcinoma is subtle. Early, erosive carcinoma is characterized by disruption or loss of the normal smooth mucosal pattern and a granular mucosal appearance. Single or multiple tiny ulcerations or niches may be observed, and the wall may be irregular or stiff.[90,92] Plaquelike early carcinomas are seen as small filling defects. Polypoid lesions are characterized by small intraluminal filling defects that usually involve one wall of the esophagus and may contain central ulcerations (Fig. 57-2).[92] Radiologic detection of early elevated carcinomas is easier than detection of depressed lesions.[90]

The findings on barium esophagram in advanced esophageal carcinoma can be divided into three major categories: Polypoid, infiltrative, and ulcerative with some overlap between categories.[94] The most common presentation of advanced esophageal carcinoma is that of a polypoid intraluminal mass (see Fig. 57-2). The initial presentation may be a round, smooth-margined lesion that mimics a benign tumor. An exophytic cancer may produce a localized or extensive polypoid defect. The mass may have the characteristic appearance of an "apple core" lesion with circumferential involvement by the cancer leaving only a narrowed, irregular lumen (see Fig. 57-2).

Infiltrating carcinomas may produce regional loss of esophageal distensibility with or without narrowing of the esophageal lumen. The narrowing may be symmetric or asymmetric and can mimic a benign esophageal stricture. Although ulceration may occur in all types of esophageal carcinoma, the primary ulcerative type appears to be the rarest. Such cancers are characterized by a well-marginated meniscoid ulcer surrounded by a thin rim of lucency representing a collar of neoplastic tissue.[95]

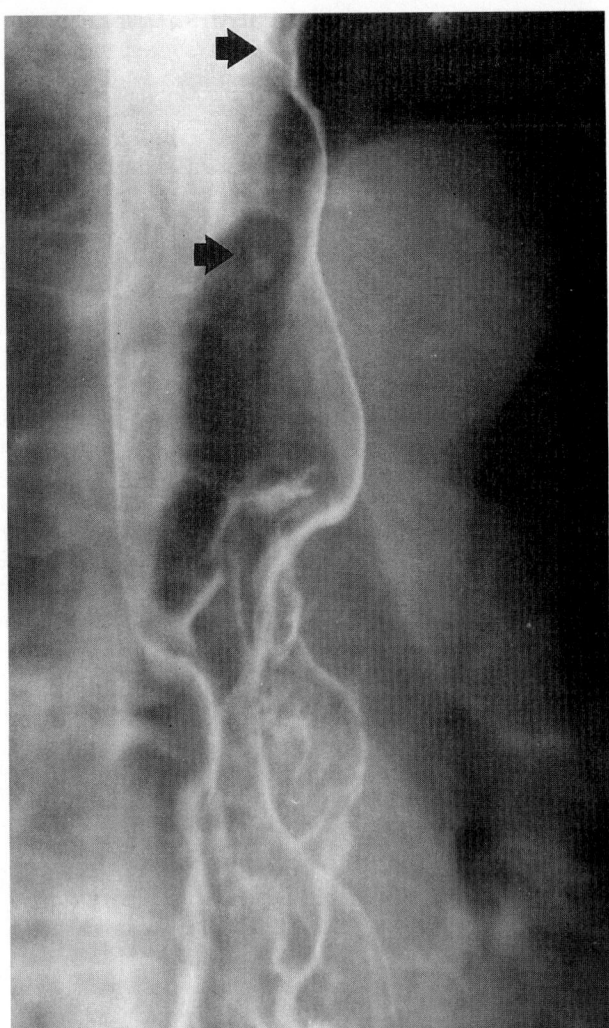

FIGURE 57-2. One large annular ulcerating squamous cell carcinoma and two small polypoid squamous cell carcinomas (*arrows*). (Radiograph courtesy of Dr. Charles Rohrmann.)

Imaging Studies. CT scanning has been used in the preoperative staging of patients with esophageal carcinoma.[96–102] The relatively small numbers of patients in most series, different imaging equipment, and some differences in the criteria for tumor involvement make comparison of different studies difficult. However, numerous series indicate that CT can be a useful, but not infallible, tool in the pretreatment evaluation of the patient with esophageal cancer. Overall accuracy of CT staging has been variously estimated at 39% to 100%.[97,98,101,103] For example, CT criteria for aortic invasion, which would preclude curative resection, have been reported to have a sensitivity of 80% to 100% and a specificity of 50% to 100%.[97,98,101] Similarly, CT can be useful in the preoperative assessment of tracheobronchial involvement by the tumor.[97–99,101]

When CT staging is compared with the final surgical-pathologic stage, it is clear that there are significant overstaging and understaging errors.[98,101,103] The major sources of error are in detection of lymph node involvement or early spread beyond the esophageal wall and both false-positive and false-negative assessments occur.[97,98,100,103]

Clinical Course and Complications

In the Western World, esophageal carcinoma usually presents in an advanced stage and follows a rapidly fatal course. Approximately 75% of untreated patients die within a year.[104] This course has led to the concept that esophageal carcinoma is a rapidly growing tumor. However, studies from regions that practice surveillance for early detection indicate that there may be a long interval during which dysplasia or early carcinoma may be diagnosed.[24,105,106] In both China and Iran, it has been estimated that the early stages of neoplastic progression in the esophagus might persist for 20 or more years.[107,108]

In China, balloon cytologies have been used to follow progression and regression of mucosal dysplasia. Of patients with severe dysplasia, 26.6% (21 of 79) developed cancer and 40.5% regressed to normal or mild dysplasia. Of patients with mild dysplasia, 15.2% (16 of 105) progressed to severe dysplasia and 44.8% (47 of 105) regressed to normal.[59] These studies suggest that both mild and severe dysplasia, at least as assessed cytologically, may be reversible intermediates in the progression to carcinoma and that 5 years may be required for severe dysplasia to progress to carcinoma.[24] Several more years may be required for early esophageal cancer to progress to advanced carcinoma. In China, 58% of 90 untreated early esophageal squamous carcinomas remained superficial when prospectively followed for 19 to 78 months.[106] The estimated median survival time for untreated early esophageal carcinoma was 75 months with an estimated 5-year survival of 62.5%. Whether the temporal progression and prognosis of these early lesions is similar in the Western World is unknown.

Based on the Oriental experience, it appears that cancer detected and treated at its early stages may carry a better prognosis, although this has not been conclusively established in Western populations.[55] For example, in China, resected early cancers have 5-year survivals of approximately 90%,[58] but, in other populations, the benefit of early diagnosis, while substantial, may not be as great. In a study of 51 European patients who had cancer limited to the mucosa and submucosa, only 49% were known to be alive and disease-free after a mean follow-up of 30 months.[55] In part, this may be due to differences in postoperative mortality (13.7% in the European study) and follow-up (6% of the European patients were lost to follow-up).

The average survival of untreated patients with advanced, symptomatic cancer is approximately 9.5 months.[104,108] It is at this stage of disease that many of the most devastating complications of esophageal carcinoma develop including progressive cachexia and weight loss, aspiration pneumonia, tracheoesophageal fistulae, recurrent laryngeal nerve paralysis, and superior vena cava obstruction.

Therapy

Unfortunately, in the Western World, most patients with esophageal carcinoma present with advanced disease that is incurable by existing therapeutic modalities. Only a few, fortunate patients who have their disease detected at an early stage will be cured by surgical resection. For most, the diagnosis of esophageal carcinoma signals the beginning of a life-long, but brief, battle for local tumor control in which palliation, not cure, is the goal. Overall 1- and 5-year survivals are approximately 18% and 5%, respectively.[109]

SURGERY

In 1980, Earlam and Cunha-Melo critically reviewed the outcome of surgery in 83,783 patients with esophageal carcinoma reported in 122 papers published between 1960 and 1979.[109] Their data suggested that "of 100 patients with the condition, 58 will be explored and 39 have the tumor resected, of whom 13 will die in the hospital. Of the 26 patients leaving the hospital with the tumor excised, 18 will survive for 1 year, 9 for 2 years and 4 for 5 years. Esophageal resection for squamous cell carcinoma has the highest operative mortality of any routinely performed surgical procedure today."

Recently, however, some surgeons who specialize in resection of esophageal carcinoma have reported series with much lower operative mortalities including several series with operative mortalities of less than 10%.[110–114] These improvements in surgical survival undoubtedly reflect improved patient selection as well as operative technique and perioperative care. Unfortunately, such improved survival statistics appear to be limited to a few centers, and many series continue to be published with hospital mortalities greater than 20%.

Esophagogastrectomy with primary esophagogastrostomy is the surgical procedure of choice for most patients.[111] When performed on appropriately selected patients by an experienced surgeon who has a low operative mortality rate, it may provide excellent palliation.[115] However, in spite of improvements in surgical mortality, esophagectomy has a disappointingly low cure rate, (e.g., a 5-year survival of 6%).[114] Even those patients who are resected for cure typically have 5-year survival rates of less than 25%.[115]

Although some uncontrolled studies have suggested benefit from pre- or postoperative radiation therapy for esophageal squamous carcinoma, this has not been confirmed by controlled studies. Three prospective, randomized trials of preoperative radiation therapy have not demonstrated a statistically significant improvement in 5-year survival by combined therapy.[116–118] The European Organization for Research and Treatment of Cancer concluded that ". . . there is no argument to recommend preoperative radiation as a routine procedure."[117]

RADIATION THERAPY

There have been no randomized trials of surgery versus radiation therapy for esophageal squamous cell carcinoma. Most centers use surgery rather than radiation therapy as the primary treatment modality for potentially resectable disease. Patients are usually referred for radiation therapy because they are not surgical candidates, either because preoperative assessment showed unresectable tumor or because of their general medical condition. Nevertheless, patients treated with radiation therapy have a 1-year survival of 18% and a 5-year survival of 6%, values that are comparable to surgery.[119]

Many patients receive significant and long-lasting palliation of dysphagia with radiation therapy, although in some patients dysphagia may temporarily worsen during the course of therapy.[119] The duration of palliation after radiotherapy can be quite variable.

Approximately 50% of patients obtain palliation of dysphagia for at least 2 months, but less than 15% have relief for more than 12 months.[120-123] Recently, intracavitary radiation has been reported to result in relief of dysphagia in 70% of patients with squamous cell carcinoma for 8 to 50 weeks (median 15 weeks).[124] Thus, radiation therapy can give relief of dysphagia, but, in many cases, the dysphagia recurs and may require additional therapy.[121,123]

The low mortality from radiation therapy, less than 1%,[121] probably reflects the tendency to stop if the patient becomes too ill during therapy.[119] The most common complication is radiation esophagitis, which can include stricture formation.[121,125] Other more serious complications such as skin burns, pulmonary fibrosis, and radiation myelitis are rare in modern radiation therapy units. The lack of significant therapy-related morbidity and mortality is an advantage for radiation therapy over surgery especially in the patient with advanced disease whose life expectancy is limited and who may, therefore, never develop recurrent local disease and dysphagia.

COMBINED MODALITY THERAPY

Because many patients in the United States have evidence of disseminated disease when their tumor is initially diagnosed, one recent approach to therapy has been to combine preoperative chemotherapy, with or without radiation, and surgery.[120,126-129] The chemotherapeutic regimens most commonly use a cisplatin-containing combination.[126,127,130-132]

In one study, 21 patients with "untreated and nonmetastatic" squamous cell carcinoma of the esophagus received preoperative 5-fluorouracil, cisplatin, and radiation.[130] Fifteen patients were resected for cure; seven had no residual carcinoma in the esophageal specimen although two had microscopic nodal disease. Of the 19 patients taken to surgery in this study, 5 (27%) died without leaving the hospital. All five patients who were free of disease at surgery remained disease-free during follow-ups of up to 39 months.

In a larger series of patients treated with 5-fluorouracil, cisplatin, and radiation, 71 of 113 eligible patients were operable (63%), and overall resectability was 49%.[133] Eighteen (17%) of 106 evaluable patients had a complete response as defined by no evidence of tumor in the resected specimen. Surgical mortality was 11%. Four patients with complete responses subsequently died of recurrent tumor.

In several series, response to chemotherapy has identified a subset of patients who have increased survival.[127,128,130,132-134] However, the role of chemotherapy in the management of squamous cell carcinoma of the esophagus depends on further investigation because there have been, as yet, no large-scale, randomized, controlled trials reported and because there have been adverse effects of the chemotherapy.[126,131,132]

PERORAL DILATATION

In the patient in whom dysphagia limits oral intake, peroral dilatation can be started soon after the diagnosis of esophageal squamous cell carcinoma to reestablish a lumen for fluid and caloric intake.[135] Dilatation using Maloney, Savary, or Eder-Peustow dilators is successful in establishing a lumen that permits soft or regular diet in over 90% of patients.[135,136] Complications are un-common and include perforation and bleeding.[135-137] Death due to dilatation is also rare.[135-138] Some patients may not have an adequate lumen maintained by dilatation and require other therapies.[135,136]

Several endoscopic methods of palliation are available, including esophageal prosthesis placement,[139-147] laser therapy,[148-157] and BICAP electrocoagulation therapy.[158] These are reviewed in detail in Chapter 135.

ESOPHAGEAL ADENOCARCINOMA

The vast majority of esophageal adenocarcinomas develop as a complication of Barrett's esophagus[159,160]; esophageal adenocarcinomas arising in esophageal glands[160,161] or heterotopic gastric mucosa[162] are rare. Although many studies have estimated that adenocarcinomas account for approximately 8% of all esophageal cancers,[160,163-165] several recent studies have reported substantially higher percentages.[166-168] Furthermore, many gastroesophageal junctional cancers arise in short segments of Barrett's esophagus,[169-171] further increasing the potential contribution of Barrett's metaplasia to upper gastrointestinal malignancy.

Epidemiology

Esophageal adenocarcinoma is a disease that predominantly affects whites.[163,170,172-174] Although cases have been reported in patients in their twenties, the incidence usually begins to increase after the age of 40 and rises with each succeeding decade.[4] It is a disease of men with a male:female predominance of 3 to 5.5:1.[159,173] During the decade between 1973 and 1982, the incidence of esophageal adenocarcinoma among white men in the United States rose 74%.[4] Some series,[172,173] but not all,[163] suggest that smoking may be a risk factor for carcinoma.

Etiology

Barrett's esophagus develops as a complication of chronic gastroesophageal reflux in which the normal squamous epithelium of the esophagus is replaced by a metaplastic columnar epithelium.[175-182] The exact magnitude of the risk of carcinoma developing in Barrett's esophagus has been difficult to ascertain. The prevalence of adenocarcinoma at the time of initial diagnosis of Barrett's esophagus is approximately 8%.[163,174,182-187] However, many factors may contribute to over- or underestimation of the prevalence of cancer in Barrett's esophagus. Because available evidence indicates that the specialized metaplasia represents the major risk for malignancy in Barrett's esophagus, some studies may have underestimated the prevalence of cancer by classifying patients who had only fundic or cardiac gland mucosa as "Barrett's esophagus." The prevalence of esophageal adenocarcinoma has probably also been underestimated because some cancers occurring in the distal esophagus were dismissed as gastric in origin.[188] The prevalence of adenocarcinoma could be overestimated because patients with cancer are more likely to have endoscopy.

The incidence of adenocarcinoma arising in Barrett's esophagus has been variously estimated at one cancer in 52 to 441 patient years of follow-up,[174,187,189–192] or approximately 500 cases per 100,000.[193] This incidence is higher than the reported incidence of esophageal squamous cell carcinoma in Northern China where mass surveillance has been practiced for almost 30 years.[193] Thus, Barrett's esophagus is a condition in which endoscopic surveillance for the early detection of carcinoma is warranted.[193,194] It has been demonstrated that endoscopic surveillance biopsies can detect adenocarcinomas in Barrett's esophagus at an early stage in which they are potentially curable.[195]

Clinical Manifestations

In its early stages, esophageal adenocarcinoma is silent. The only clinical manifestations may be those of gastroesophageal reflux and its complications, including heartburn, regurgitation, benign strictures with dysphagia, and bleeding from ulcerations.[195] If systematic endoscopic biopsies are not taken at this stage, dysplasia or early carcinoma may be missed.[195–198] The severity of gastroesophageal reflux symptoms cannot be used to identify the patient at risk for cancer because some patients may be minimally symptomatic before developing an advanced Barrett's adenocarcinoma.[159]

New symptoms may appear as the neoplasm grows. In general, these symptoms are similar to those of advanced squamous cell carcinoma and include progressive dysphagia, weight loss, odynophagia, chest pain, fatigue, vomiting, cough, and gastrointestinal bleeding, which is most commonly occult but may be brisk. Hemoccult-positive stools and iron-deficiency anemia may develop as a result of occult blood loss.

Differential Diagnosis and Diagnostic Studies

The differential diagnosis depends on the stage of the disease. In the patient whose only symptoms are those of chronic gastroesophageal reflux, there are three main elements in the differential diagnosis:

1. Gastroesophageal reflux disease without Barrett's esophagus,
2. Barrett's esophagus without high-grade dysplasia, or
3. Barrett's esophagus complicated by high-grade dysplasia or early adenocarcinoma.

In the patient who presents with dysphagia in the absence of symptoms of gastroesophageal reflux, the differential diagnosis is identical to that for squamous cell carcinoma.

ENDOSCOPY

When the diagnosis of Barrett's esophagus or esophageal adenocarcinoma is entertained, the single most important diagnostic study is upper gastrointestinal endoscopy with biopsy. At endoscopy, the position of three endoscopic landmarks, the squamocolumnar junction, the region of the lower esophageal sphincter, and the diaphragmatic pinchcock, should be noted and recorded.

The squamocolumnar junction (ora serrata) normally occurs as a wavy interface between the white stratified squamous epithelium of the esophagus and the salmon-pink epithelium of the stomach in the region of the lower esophageal sphincter.[199–201] In Barrett's esophagus, the squamocolumnar junction is displaced proximally and represents the junction between squamous epithelium and specialized metaplasia.[200–204]

In evaluating patients with suspected Barrett's esophagus, it is important to recognize hiatal hernias so that biopsies from them are not mistakenly classified as "Barrett's esophagus." A hiatal hernia pouch has gastric folds that run from the stomach through the diaphragmatic hiatus and disappear just distal to the lower esophageal sphincter region.[199,200] The diaphragmatic hiatus can be recognized as a concentric narrowing that varies with respiration. The normal lower esophageal sphincter region can usually be recognized at the distal end of the tubular esophagus by the presence of a circumferential rosette that can be opened by gentle insufflation with air. In Barrett's esophagus, the lower esophageal sphincter region is usually more patulous, but is still recognizable.

Early Barrett's adenocarcinomas can be detected in mucosa that is endoscopically remarkable only for a proximally relocated ora serrata.[195] In such cases a systematic protocol of endoscopic biopsy can establish the diagnosis.[195] Some early cancers may be associated with superficial erosions, plaquelike elevations, or areas of nodularity. As the cancer becomes more advanced, it may appear as an intraluminal polypoid mass (Fig. 57-3), a stricture (which may be asymmetric), or a deep ulceration.

ENDOSCOPIC BIOPSY AND CYTOLOGY

In the patient with Barrett's esophagus, the goal of the endoscopic evaluation is to detect by biopsy high-grade dysplasia or early adenocarcinoma that may not be apparent to gross visualization. A systematic protocol of four-quadrant endoscopic biopsies at 2-cm intervals in the Barrett's lining can detect such early neoplasia.[195] Multiple biopsies should also be taken of any abnormality, such as erosions, nodules, ulcers, or strictures, no matter how insignificant they appear.[195] Endoscopic surveillance should be performed with a large-channel endoscope and spiked, oval-cupped biopsy forceps.

Endoscopic brush cytology may detect early esophageal adenocarcinoma.[205] However, its value in surveillance has not been documented, and the use of cytology alone may not detect occult malignancy in Barrett's esophagus. A 24% false-negative rate for cytology has been reported for invasive esophageal adenocarcinoma in one study,[206] although a 90% to 100% detection rate has been reported by another group in a smaller number of patients.[207] Therefore, only a systematic protocol of endoscopic biopsy has been shown to consistently detect high-grade dysplasia or early adenocarcinoma arising in Barrett's esophagus. Prudence would suggest that cytology may be complementary in endoscopic surveillance, but it requires the interest and expertise of the cytopathologist and does not replace the need for endoscopic biopsies.

Flow cytometric detection of aneuploidy or increased G2/tetraploid fractions may provide additional information concerning

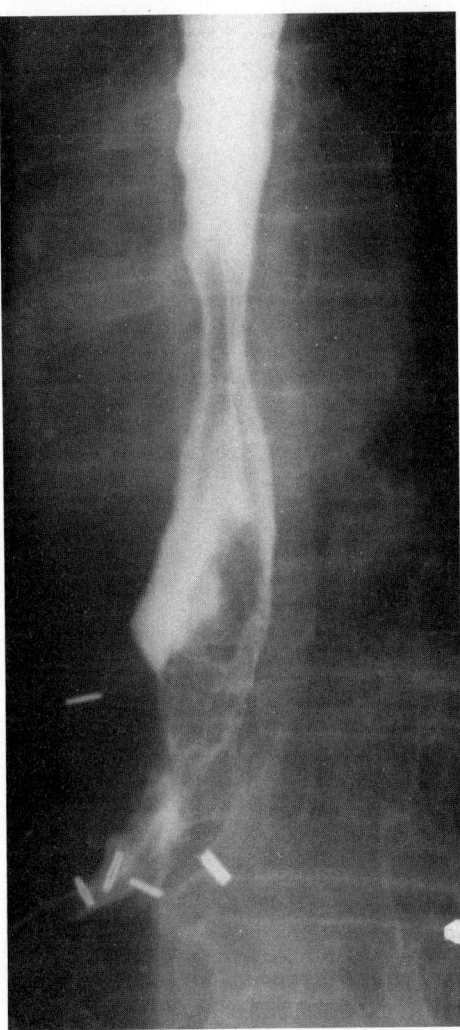

FIGURE 57–3. Polypoid Barrett's adenocarcinoma occurring in the distal esophagus above evidence of a prior antireflux surgery. (Radiograph courtesy of Dr. Charles Rohrmann.)

shown to be reproducible.[215] In coded review, interobserver agreement on high-grade dysplasia and intramucosal carcinoma was 86%, but agreement on indefinite for dysplasia and low-grade dysplasia was substantially lower.[215] Second, because high-grade dysplasia in Barrett's esophagus is relatively rare in unselected patients, most pathologists do not have the opportunity to review many cases. For this reason, the general pathologist would be wise to seek a second opinion before surgical resection is considered. Third, if a biopsy showing high-grade dysplasia was taken from an endoscopically visualized abnormality such as a mass, an ulcer, an area of nodularity, or a malignant-appearing stricture, repeat endoscopic biopsies at the first opportunity are indicated. Fourth, some adenocarcinomas are so well-differentiated that they can be distinguished from high-grade dysplasia only by demonstrating invasion below the muscularis mucosae. This may be difficult because endoscopic biopsies usually do not obtain sufficient amounts of submucosal tissue and because the recurring ulceration associated with Barrett's esophagus may obliterate the muscularis mucosae.

RADIOLOGY

Although certain findings on radiologic study may suggest Barrett's esophagus, such as a mid- or high esophageal stricture or ulcer, barium studies are insensitive in detecting uncomplicated Barrett's esophagus.[216-220] With the development of advanced adenocarcinoma, a barium esophagogram may show any of the abnormalities described for squamous cell carcinoma, although esophageal adenocarcinomas are usually located comparatively more distally. CT scans have been used preoperatively to help stage esophageal and gastroesophageal junction adenocarcinomas and have advantages and disadvantages similar to those described for squamous cell carcinoma.[221]

CLINICAL COURSE AND COMPLICATIONS

Esophageal adenocarcinoma develops by a multistep process. In response to chronic gastroesophageal reflux, the normal stratified squamous epithelium of the esophagus is replaced by a metaplastic columnar epithelium that may migrate proximally with continued reflux.[178-181] Although three different patterns of epithelium have been described in Barrett's esophagus,[222] only the specialized metaplastic epithelium has been seen in proximal biopsies in three careful endoscopic studies.[202-204] This specialized metaplastic epithelium has been found surrounding the majority of Barrett's adenocarcinomas and is probably the precursor of high-grade dysplasia and adenocarcinoma in Barrett's esophagus.[195,202,204,223]

Knowledge of the events in neoplastic progression in Barrett's esophagus has largely been inferred by studying the mucosa surrounding esophageal adenocarcinomas. The majority of Barrett's adenocarcinomas have high-grade dysplasia in the surrounding epithelium,[173,195,223-225] and several authors have proposed a model of neoplastic progression in which gastroesophageal reflux leads to metaplasia, which, in some patients, progresses to dysplasia

patients at risk for esophageal adenocarcinoma[208-210] (Fig. 57-4). Furthermore, aneuploidy or increased G2/tetraploid fractions can sometimes be detected months to years before the development of adenocarcinoma, suggesting that they may be intermediates in neoplastic progression in some cases.[211] Therefore, if the capability for flow cytometry exists, one biopsy at each level of the columnar-lined tubular esophagus should be evaluated for DNA content. Flow cytometry should be performed using a single-step detergent method on fresh or frozen biopsies because this minimizes clumping of cells or nuclei that may otherwise cause an artifactually high G2/tetraploid fraction.[208,212,213] Delays in processing or autolysis may lead to a false-positive near-diploid aneuploidy.[214]

In the patient who presents with dysphagia and at endoscopy is found to have a mass, ulcer, an area of nodularity, or a stricture, multiple biopsies should be taken and direct vision brush cytology should be performed. If biopsies and cytologies are not diagnostic, the biopsies and cytologies should be repeated.

Caution must be exercised in interpreting the histologic diagnosis of dysplasia in Barrett's esophagus. First, only the diagnoses of high-grade dysplasia and intramucosal carcinoma have been

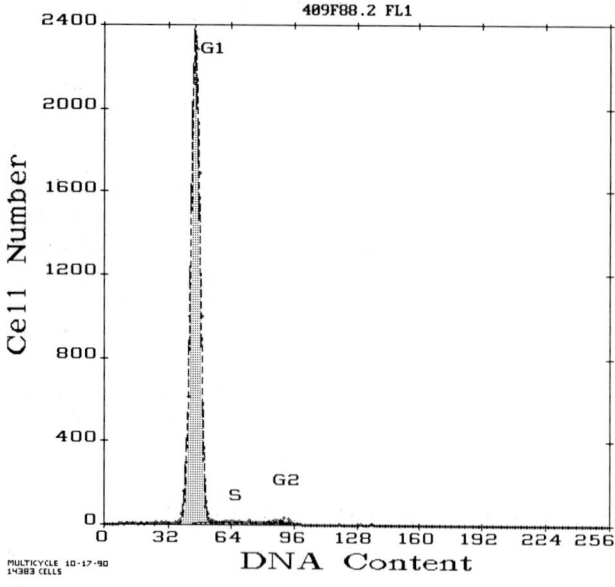

A

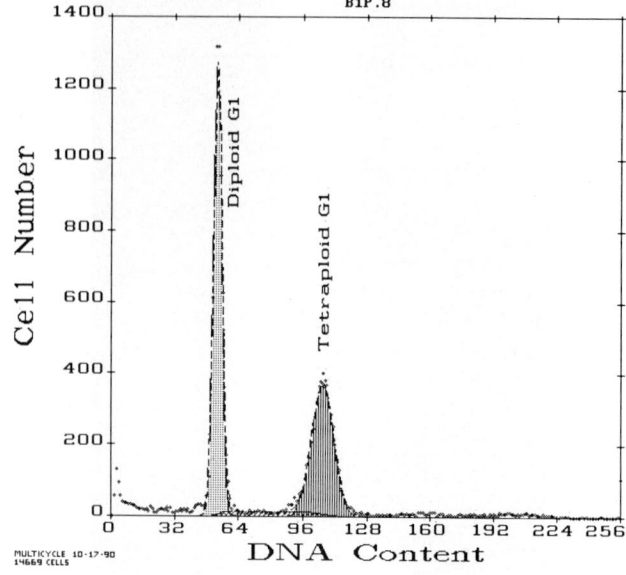

B

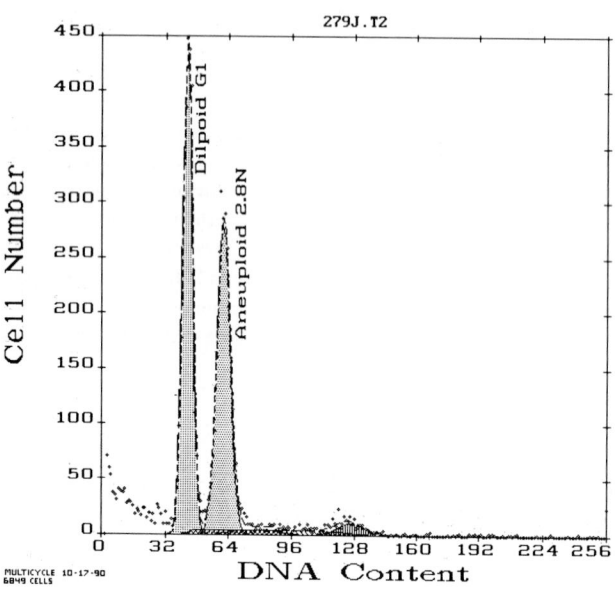

C

FIGURE 57–4. (A) A normal flow cytometry histogram of a biopsy taken from fundic gland mucosa. More than 95% of the cells are in the G1 peak with only small fractions of cells in S phase or the G2 interval of the cell cycle. (B) Flow cytometry histogram from an area of high-grade dysplasia in Barrett's esophagus. There is an abnormal population of cells with a DNA content of 4N (diploid G2 or tetraploid G1) comprising 42% of the cells. (C) Flow cytometry histogram taken from a Barrett's adenocarcinoma. There is an aneuploid population with a DNA content of 2.8N comprising 49% of the total cells.

and, ultimately, to adenocarcinoma.[203,223,224] Factors that promote the development of dysplasia and adenocarcinoma in Barrett's esophagus are poorly understood. Although it has been proposed that continued gastroesophageal reflux may be a factor,[226] several patients have been reported who developed esophageal adenocarcinoma after antireflux surgery.[172,182,187,227] There is no convincing evidence that eliminating reflux in the patient with Barrett's esophagus reduces the risk of malignancy.

In some patients, dysplasia appears to spread and involve large areas of esophageal mucosa before invasion occurs, while, in others, small areas of dysplasia already contain an invasive carcinoma.[195] The time required to progress from specialized metaplasia to dysplasia and, ultimately, to carcinoma is unknown and may be variable from patient to patient.[187,195,211,226] The natural history of high-grade dysplasia is poorly understood; it may regress, persist for

prolonged periods without progressing, or progress to adenocarcinoma.[187,195,197,228,229]

If cancer goes undetected in its early stages, it may spread to involve the muscularis propria, the adventitia, and adjacent organs. Metastatic spread may occur to regional lymph nodes in the thorax and abdomen, the liver, brain, bone, peritoneum, lung, and other sites.[230] Once cancer develops in Barrett's esophagus, there is a well-recognized propensity to develop multiple tumors.[231,232] In two series, multicentric cancers were found in 13% and 37% of Barrett's adenocarcinomas.[206,233]

The nature of the events controlling tumor progression from metaplasia through dysplasia to early and, ultimately, to advanced adenocarcinoma are unknown. Cancers appear to arise in Barrett's esophagus in association with a process of genomic instability that produces abnormal clones of cells that have abnormal DNA contents and proliferative abnormalities.[208,213,234] As many as 13 different aneuploid populations can be detected in the dysplasia and metaplasia surrounding some early Barrett's adenocarcinomas.[234] Ultimately, one of these clones acquires the capacity for invasion and becomes an early carcinoma.[235]

ENDOSCOPIC SURVEILLANCE INTERVALS

Several long-term prospective studies are in progress to determine how frequently patients with Barrett's esophagus should undergo endoscopic surveillance biopsy and cytology. The data generated thus far are insufficient to make conclusive recommendations. Based on present knowledge, if biopsies taken according to the above systematic protocol are negative for dysplasia, if they show no evidence of aneuploidy or abnormalities of proliferation by flow cytometry, and if the brush cytology is benign, repeat endoscopic evaluation at 2-year intervals is reasonable.[200] If the capacity for flow cytometry does not exist, annual endoscopic surveillance should be performed. For patients whose biopsies are judged only indefinite for dysplasia and have no associated endoscopic or flow cytometric abnormality, follow-up at 12-month intervals is appropriate. Shorter intervals should be used in patients in whom there is an increased clinical concern because of the nature of the histologic, flow cytometric, or endoscopic abnormalities.

If high-grade dysplasia is detected in a biopsy taken from mucosa that showed no gross endoscopic abnormalities, early reendoscopy with multiple biopsies should be undertaken to determine the extent of the high-grade dysplasia and to search for a coexisting adenocarcinoma. No general recommendation for management can be made if, at reendoscopy, only high-grade dysplasia is found. For each patient, the known risks of surgical therapy must be weighed against the unknown risk of coexisting or future carcinoma. Each patient with high-grade dysplasia must be evaluated individually, weighing the usual surgical risk factors including age, general medical, cardiac, and pulmonary status. The patient's wishes and ability to comply with endoscopic surveillance should also be considered.

For patients with high-grade dysplasia who are not deemed surgical candidates, but who would be if adenocarcinoma were documented, multiple endoscopic biopsies should be repeated 3 months after the initial two endoscopies and at 3- to 6-month intervals thereafter. Large areas of dysplasia are more difficult to survey than smaller ones.

Unsuspected adenocarcinomas have been discovered in surgical specimens of some patients who underwent esophagectomy because endoscopic biopsies showed high-grade dysplasia.[173,197] This has led some to advocate esophagectomy for all patients whose biopsies show high-grade dysplasia.[236] Unfortunately, most of these studies did not report the sites and numbers of endoscopic biopsies.[173,197] Furthermore, in some cases, endoscopic or radiologic abnormalities were noted that, in the presence of high-grade dysplasia, should have raised concern about the possibility of cancer.[197] The systematic biopsy protocol described above correctly predicted the presence or absence of adenocarcinoma in eight surgical specimens, suggesting that it could decrease the possibility of a missed, unsuspected carcinoma, especially in the patient who is a poor surgical candidate.[195]

Therapy

The prognosis for patients with esophageal adenocarcinoma has been dismal with a 5-year survival in the United States of only 7%. However, the identification of patients with Barrett's esophagus permits endoscopic surveillance for early detection of adenocarcinoma, and this could improve long-term survival. Surgery or palliative measures remain the primary modes of therapy. Once intramucosal adenocarcinoma is documented in Barrett's esophagus, the treatment is surgical resection if the patient is considered an acceptable surgical candidate and if preoperative clinical staging does not reveal definitive evidence of unresectable metastatic spread.[110,237,238] Because Barrett's adenocarcinomas are frequently multicentric or associated with extensive high-grade dysplasia and because specialized metaplasia can become dysplasia and adenocarcinoma, the entire columnar-lined segment should be removed.

Although reports of patients who had esophageal or gastroesophageal junction adenocarcinoma treated with radiation or chemotherapy have appeared,[239-242] the role of radiation or chemotherapy in the management of Barrett's adenocarcinoma is unclear.[243] Palliation with peroral dilatation, esophageal prostheses, and laser therapy is similar to that described for squamous cell carcinoma.

OTHER EPITHELIAL TUMORS

Benign Epithelial Tumors

Squamous cell papillomas of the esophagus are benign lesions usually discovered as incidental findings at endoscopy. They are typically small, white or pink sessile polypoid lesions.[244-246] Histologically, they are characterized by a papillated appearance with normal or hyperplastic squamous epithelium covering a core of connective tissue.[244] They can be readily removed by forceps biopsy[244] and do not usually recur.[245]

Malignant Epithelial Tumors

Squamous cell carcinoma with spindle cell component has been called by a number of different terms including carcinosarcoma and pseudosarcoma.[246,247] It is an unusual variant that contains both epithelial and prominent spindle cell elements suggestive of sarcoma.[246,247] Originally, carcinosarcoma was considered to be a tumor in which both the carcinomatous and spindle cell elements were malignant, while pseudosarcoma was considered to be a tumor in which the spindle cell elements were non-neoplastic reactive cells without the ability to metastasize. However, metastasis of spindle cells has been reported in some cases of pseudosarcoma.[247-250]

Spindle cell carcinomas are typically large, polypoid tumors.[246-250] They are usually single but can be multiple.[246,251] Histologically, they represent a spectrum of tumors characterized by varying mixtures of carcinomatous cells, usually squamous, and prominent spindle cells. The epithelial cells may only be dysplastic, or they can be represented by an invasive squamous cell carcinoma from which the spindle cells seem to arise.[246-249,251] Occasionally, the spindle cell elements are associated with evidence of mesenchymal differentiation such as the formation of cartilage or bone.[252]

Much of the debate about these tumors centers on the histogenesis of the spindle cell elements. Several theories have been proposed including the possibilities that they represent "collision carcinomas" that contain both a carcinoma and a sarcoma, that the spindle cells represent mesenchymal metaplasia of the squamous cells,[246,248] and that, in some cases, the spindle cells are reactive non-neoplastic mesenchymal cells.[253] Ultrastructural and immunohistochemical studies have not clarified the issue.[248,251,252] Some, but not all authors have reported that the spindle cells contain epithelial markers such as desmosomes, tonofilaments, and cytokeratins.[248,250-252] Whether these differences represent true biologic distinctions between tumors or sampling error is unclear.[248] Many pathologists believe that spindle cell carcinomas arise from squamous cell cancers that produce a spindle cell component.[246,248,252]

Verrucous squamous cell carcinoma of the esophagus is a slow growing malignant tumor that shows relentless local invasion but rarely metastasizes.[254] One case persisted for 7 years without developing metastases.[255] The slow growth rate and absence of metastases might result in a better prognosis, but many cases invade adjacent organs including the bronchial tree before diagnosis.[254,255]

Adenosquamous carcinomas are tumors that contain elements of both adenocarcinoma and squamous carcinoma.[256,257]

Adenoid cystic carcinoma of the esophagus is a rare tumor with only 23 cases reported in the world literature before 1986.[258] The average age of the patients was 65 years, and there was a male:female ratio of 15:8.[258] The tumors are typically multilobulated or ulcerated, and most cases have been discovered in an advanced stage.[259-261] In general, the prognosis is poor, although disease-free survival postresection has been reported for two patients whose tumors were confined to the submucosa.[258,260,262] Although some believe that these cancers arise from submucosal glands, other origins have been postulated.[258,262,263]

Melanoma is a rare esophageal cancer that can either be primary or metastatic. In one series of 1918 esophageal cancers, only two cases of primary malignant melanoma were reported.[264] Patients are usually in the sixth, seventh, or eighth decades of life with a mean age of approximately 60 years.[265-268] Dysphagia and weight loss are the most common symptoms, and the tumor is typically bulky and polypoid.[265,266] The extent of lateral spread of tumor is frequently underestimated at surgery as reflected by the prevalence of positive surgical margins.[266] The presence of esophageal melanocytes and junctional activity has been used to distinguish between primary and metastatic melanoma of the esophagus.[268,269]

Although metastatic melanoma frequently involves the gastrointestinal tract, the esophagus is an uncommon site for metastasis relative to the stomach, small bowel, and colon.[270] In one large series of patients with metastatic melanoma, 4% had esophageal metastases.[271]

Small-cell carcinoma of the esophagus is an uncommon tumor that may include both a small-cell variant of squamous carcinoma and oat cell carcinoma.[272-274] Oat cell carcinoma of the esophagus can be primary or secondary to spread from other sites. Primary oat cell carcinoma of the esophagus is a disease of the elderly with an average age at diagnosis of 64.5 years.[272] Dysphagia is the most common presenting symptom.[272] Ectopic endocrine syndromes

involving inappropriate antidiuretic hormone secretion or hypercalcemia have been reported in two cases.[275,276] The prognosis of primary oat cell carcinoma of the esophagus has been dismal with an average survival of 4.7 months.[272]

Macroscopically, esophageal oat cell carcinomas have been described as polypoid (47.5%), fungating (15%), ulcerating (15%), or stenotic (22.5%). Microscopically, oat cell carcinoma of the esophagus is an anaplastic small-cell carcinoma resembling small-cell carcinoma of the lung and which sometimes shows evidence of squamous differentiation.[272]

Carcinoid tumors of the esophagus are rare.[277,278] They often occur at the gastroesophageal junction and, in many cases, may represent gastric carcinoids that have secondarily involved the esophagus.[279-281] Carcinoid syndrome has not been reported.

Choriocarcinoma of the esophagus is an exceedingly rare tumor whose histogenesis is uncertain.[282] They may occur in association with esophageal adenocarcinoma.[283] Secretion of human chorionic gonadotropin has been reported.[282]

NONEPITHELIAL TUMORS

Benign Nonepithelial Tumors

Leiomyomas are the most common benign tumors of the esophagus.[284-287] Men are more frequently affected than women with a ratio of 2:1.[288] These tumors are typically single, and 56% occur in the lower third of the esophagus.[288] At least half of patients with esophageal leiomyomas are asymptomatic, and the lesion is discovered as an incidental finding at x-ray or at autopsy.[287,288] Among patients who have symptoms, dysphagia and retrosternal discomfort are the most common presenting complaints.[287,288] Hemorrhage is rare but has been reported.[289]

The diagnosis is usually made by barium esophagogram, which shows a smooth, round defect with sharp margins and no irregularity of the overlying or surrounding mucosa (Fig. 57-5). At endoscopy, the leiomyoma is a rounded mass with normal overlying mucosa. Biopsy is contraindicated because of potential secondary infection, bleeding, or perforation and because postbiopsy changes may make surgical enucleation difficult.[287,290] When biopsies have been attempted, they are usually nondiagnostic.[287] If symptoms require therapy, surgical enucleation of the leiomyoma is the procedure of choice.[287,288]

Granular cell tumor of the esophagus is an uncommon tumor that is being reported with increasing frequency as fiberoptic endoscopic examinations of the esophagus increase. It is usually benign and is believed to be derived from neural or Schwann's cell elements. Endoscopically, it is characterized as a smooth, sessile polyp with overlying normal mucosa.[291] Eighty percent of tumors occur in the distal esophagus, and they are usually single, although multiple tumors have been reported in 14% of cases.[291]

In 60% of patients, the lesions were asymptomatic and were incidental findings at endoscopy.[291,292] Patients who presented with dysphagia and substernal pain typically had larger tumors.[291,292] The tumors usually remain stable during serial endoscopic follow-up,[291-293] and only two cases of malignancy have been reported.[291] In neither of these cases could a multicentric benign tumor be

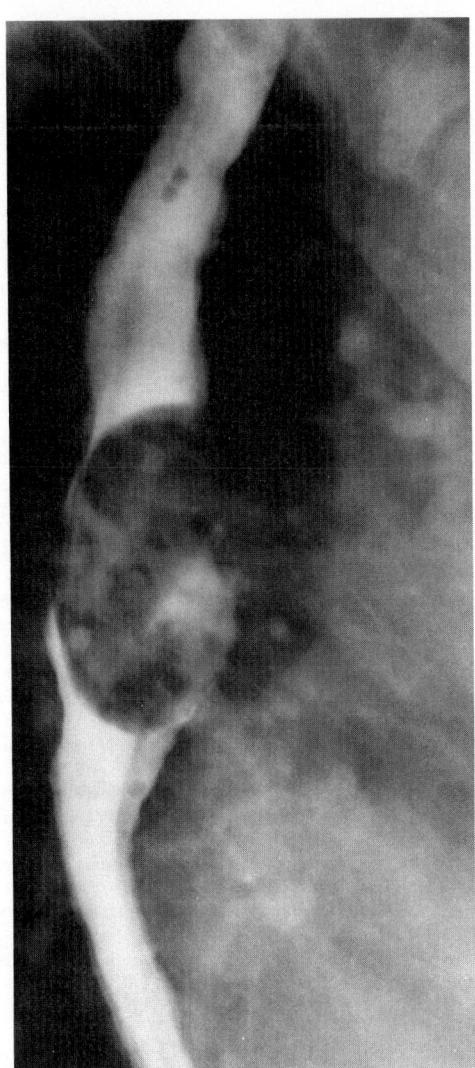

FIGURE 57-5. Large leiomyoma of the esophagus. (Radiograph courtesy of Dr. Charles Rohrmann.)

excluded, and one patient survived 22 years after an incomplete resection.[291]

Intraluminal fibrovascular polyps are rare lesions of the esophagus that may grow to large sizes and may present dramatically with prolapse into the larynx with resulting asphyxiation and death.[287,294] Other symptoms include dysphagia, regurgitation, vomiting, and, occasionally, hematemesis or melena secondary to mucosal ulceration. The polyps are covered by a smooth mucosa and are composed of fibrous and vascular tissue. When prominent adipose tissue is present, the lesion has been called a fibrolipoma or pedunculated lipoma.[287] In some cases, these benign lesions are covered in part by reactive squamous epithelium, which may be misinterpreted as carcinoma by the pathologist. In others, the granulation tissue in the polyp contains atypical mesenchymal cells that can be mistaken for carcinoma or sarcoma. If there is a discrepancy in the clinical impression and the histologic diagnosis, repeat biopsies are indicated to resolve the disparity.

Hemangiomas are infrequent tumors of the esophagus. They may present with dysphagia or bleeding, which can sometimes be massive.[295] Many hemangiomas are small, asymptomatic lesions that are found incidentally at autopsy.[295]

Lymphangiomas are very rare esophageal tumors. Endoscopically, they are seen as a translucent, easily compressed mass.[296] Histologically, they are characterized by dilated endothelial-lined spaces.[287]

Sessile submucosal nodules that are composed of adipose or fibrous tissue are called *lipomas* and *fibromas*, respectively.[294] They are rare, representing less than 5% of benign esophageal tumors.[294] A variety of congenital cysts lined by epithelia resembling that of the esophagus, bronchus, or stomach have been reported.[294] The patients are usually asymptomatic but may present with dysphagia or other symptoms.

Malignant Nonepithelial Tumors

Leiomyosarcoma is an uncommon tumor of the esophagus with only 45 cases reported in the world literature.[297–299] The tumors have been classified as either polypoid or infiltrative and can occur in all segments of the esophagus (Fig. 57-6). Sixteen of the 45 patients have survived for more than 1 year after treatment.[297]

Secondary Tumors of the Esophagus

Metastatic carcinoma to the esophagus is unusual. In one series of 1000 consecutive autopsies of patients who had malignant epithelial neoplasms, only 31 had esophageal metastases.[300] Excluding malignant melanoma, breast cancer is the most common tumor metastatic to the esophagus.[301] Other cancers that have been reported to metastasize to the esophagus include gastric, renal, liver, prostate, testicular, bone, and skin.[300] Carcinomas of the lung and head and neck have also been reported to be metastatic to the esophagus.[301]

When symptomatic, metastatic carcinomas involving the esophagus usually cause dysphagia by extrinsic compression.[302] The endoscopic appearance is that of an extrinsic stricture with normal mucosa or an intraluminal mass.[301,302] In one series of breast carcinomas metastatic to esophagus, dilatation was associated with a high frequency of perforation.[302]

LEUKEMIA

Microscopic infiltration of the esophagus with leukemic cells is relatively frequent in autopsy series of acute and chronic leukemia.[303] Rarely, the infiltration may be sufficient to become grossly evident and to produce dysphagia.[304]

LYMPHOMA

Primary esophageal lymphoma is a rare disease. Both primary esophageal Hodgkin's[305] and non-Hodgkin's lymphomas[306] may present with dysphagia or odynophagia. Recognition is important to guide therapy, and endoscopic biopsies have sometimes been insufficient to establish the diagnosis.[305] Patients with AIDS develop esophageal lymphomas presenting as dysphagia or hematemesis.[307]

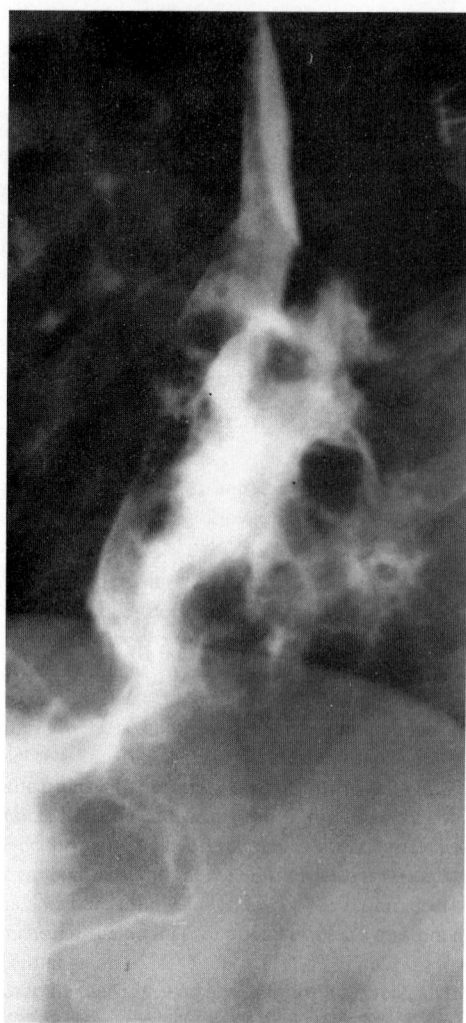

FIGURE 57–6. Ulcerated and perforating sarcoma of the esophagus. (Radiograph courtesy of Dr. Charles Rohrmann.)

Lymphomatous involvement of the esophagus is more often associated with widespread disease or infiltration from adjacent lymph nodes.[304] Although microscopic disease of the esophagus may be noted in careful autopsy studies in both Hodgkin's and non-Hodgkin's lymphomas, clinically evident disease is rare.[304]

The reader is directed to Chapters 24, Neoplasia of the Gastrointestinal Tract; Chapter 28, Approach to the Patient with Dysphagia; Chapter 29, Approach to the Patient with Chest Pain; Chapter 53, Esophagus: Anatomy and Structural Anomalies; Chapter 55, Reflux Esophagitis; Chapter 111, Upper Gastrointestinal Endoscopy; Chapter 114, Contrast Radiology; Chapter 117, Endoscopic Ultrasound; Chapter 118, Applications of Computed Tomography to the Gastrointestinal Tract; Chapter 126, Endoscopic Mucosal Biopsy; Chapter 131, Gastrointestinal Dilation; Chapter 134, Endoscopic Control of Nonvariceal Upper Gastrointestinal Hemorrhage; and Chapter 135, Endoscopic Therapy of Sessile Tumors.

REFERENCES

1. Silverberg E, Boring CC, Squires TS. Cancer statistics. CA 1990; 40:9.
2. Day NE, Muñoz N. Esophagus. In: Schotterfeld D, Fraumeni JF, eds. Cancer epidemiology and prevention. Philadelphia: WB Saunders, 1982:596.
3. Schoenberg BS, Bailar JC, Fraumeni JF. Certain mortality patterns of esophageal cancer in the United States, 1930–67. J Natl Cancer Inst 1971;46:63.
4. Ynag PC, Davis S. Incidence of cancer of the esophagus in the US by histologic type. Cancer 1988;61:612.
5. Mozbech J, Videbach A. On the etiology of esophageal carcinoma. J Natl Cancer Inst 1955;15:1665.
6. Burch PRJ. Esophageal cancer in relation to cigarette and alcohol consumption. J Chronic Dis 1984;37:793.
7. Yu MC, Garabrant DH, Peters JM, Mack TM. Tobacco, alcohol, diet, occupation, and carcinoma of the esophagus. Cancer Res 1988;48:3843.
8. Ziegler RG. Alcohol–nutrient interactions in cancer etiology. Cancer 1986;58:1942.
9. Monson RR, Lyon JL. Proportional mortality among alcoholics. Cancer 1975;36:1077.
10. Pottern LM, Morris LE, Blot WJ, et al. Esophageal cancer among black men in Washington, D.C. I. Alcohol, tobacco, and other risk factors. J Natl Cancer Inst 1981;67:777.
11. Hakulinen, T, Lehtimäki L, Lehtonen M, Teppo L. Cancer morbidity among two male cohorts with increased consumption in Finland. J Natl Cancer Inst 1974;52:1711.
12. Wynder EL, Mabuchi K. Etiological and environmental factors. JAMA 1973;266:1546.
13. Kahn HL. The Forn study of smoking and mortality among U.S. veterans: Report on eight and one-half years of observation. Natl Cancer Inst Monogr 1966;19:1.
14. Keller AZ. The epidemiology of esophageal cancer in the west. Prev Med 1980;9:607.
15. Wynder EL, Bross IJ. A study of etiological factors in cancer of the esophagus. Cancer 1961;14:389.
16. Doll R, Peto R. Mortality in relation to smoking: 20 years' observations on male British doctors. Br Med J 1976;2:1525.
17. Weir JM, Dunn JE. Smoking and mortality: A prospective study. Cancer 1970;25:105.
18. Tuyns AJ, Péquignot G, Jensen OM. Le cancer de l'oesophaage en Ille-et-Vilaine en fonction des niveaux de consommation d'alcool et de tabac. Des risques qui se multiplient. Bull Cancer 1977;64:45.
19. Duranceau A. Epidemiologic trends and etiologic factors of esophageal carcinoma. In: Delarue NC, Wilkins EW Jr, Wong J. International trends in general thoracic surgery. Vol 4: Esophageal cancer. St Louis: CV Mosby, 1988:3.
20. Priester WA. Esophageal cancer in North China: High rates in human and poultry populations in the same areas. Avian Dis 1975;19:213.
21. The Coordinating Group for Research on Etiology of Esophageal Cancer in North China. The epidemiology and etiology of esophageal cancer in North China. A preliminary report. Chin Med J 1975;1(3): 167.
22. Mellow MH, Layne EA, Lipman TO, et al. Plasma zinc and vitamin A in human squamous carcinoma of the esophagus. Cancer 1983;51;1615.
23. Thurnham DI, Zheng S-F, Munoz N, et al. Comparison of riboflavin, vitamin A, and zinc status of Chinese populations at high and low risk for esophageal cancer. Nutr Cancer 1985;7:131.
24. Yang CS. Research on esophageal cancer in China: A review. Cancer Res 1980;40:2633.
25. Lu S-H, Ohsima H, Fu H-M, et al. Urinary excretion of N-nitrosamino acids and nitrate by inhabitants of high- and low-risk areas for esophageal cancer in northern China: Endogenous formation of nitrosoproline and its inhibition by vitamin C^1. Cancer Res 1986;46: 1485.
26. Cheng SJ, Jiang YZ, Li MH, Lo HZ. A mutagenic metabolite produced by *Fusarium monoliforme* isolated from Linxian County, China. Carcinogenesis 1985;6:903.

27. Bennetts RW. Esophageal cancer in the United States: Diagnostic modalities and surveillance of high-risk groups. In: Stroehlein JR, Romsdahl MM, eds. Gastrointestinal cancer. New York: Raven Press, 1981:137.

28. Howel-Evans W, McConnell RB, Clarke CA, Sheppard PM. Carcinoma of the oesophagus with keratosis palmaris plantaris (tylosis). Q J Med 1958;27:413.

29. Harper PS, Harper RMJ, Howel-Evans AW. Carcinoma of the oesophagus with tylosis. Q J Med 1970;39:317.

30. Tyldesley WR, Hughes ROI. Tylosis, leukoplakia, and oesophageal carcinoma. Br Med J 1973;4:427.

31. Clarke CA, Evans WH, McConnell RB, Sheppard PM. Carcinoma of oesophagus in association with tylosis. Br Med J 1959;2:1100.

32. Parnell DD, Johnson SAM. Tylosis palmaris et plantaris. Arch Dermatol 1969;100:7.

33. Shine I, Allison PR. Carcinoma of the oesophagus with tylosis (keratosis palmaris et plantaris). Lancet 1966;1:951.

34. Matthews HR, Pattison CW. Esophageal carcinoma as a complication of achalasia: The screening controversy. In: Delarue NC, Wilkins EW Jr, Wong J, eds. International trends in general thoracic surgery. Vol 4: Esophageal cancer. St Louis: CV Mosby, 1988:11.

35. Chuong JJH, Dubovik S, McCallum RW. Achalasia as a risk factor for esophageal carcinoma. A reappraisal. Dig Dis Sci 1984;29:1105.

36. Carter R, Brewer LA III. Achalasia and esophageal carcinoma. Studies in early diagnosis for improved surgical management. Am J Surg 1975;130:114.

37. Norton GA, Postelthwait RW, Thompson WM. Esophageal carcinoma: A survey of populations at risk. South Med J 1980;73:25.

38. Barrett NR. Achalasia of the cardia: Reflections upon a clinical study of over 100 cases. Br Med J 1964;1:1135.

39. Belsey R. Functional disease of the esophagus. J Thorac Cardiovasc Surg 1966;52:164.

40. Ellis FG. The natural history of achalasia of the cardia [abridged]. Proc R Soc Med 1960;53:663.

41. Just-Viera JO, Haight C. Achalasia and carcinoma of the esophagus. Surg Gynecol Obstet 1969;128:1081.

42. Hopkins RA, Pustlethwait RW. Burns and carcinoma. Ann Surg 1981;194:146.

43. Appleqvist P, Salmo M. Lye corrosion carcinoma of the esophagus. A review of 63 cases. Cancer 1980;45:2655.

44. Wynder EL, Mushinski MH, Spivak JC. Tobacco and alcohol comsumption in relation to the development of multiple primary cancers. Cancer 1977;40:1872.

45. Goldstein HM, Zornoza J. Association of squamous cell carcinoma of the head and neck with cancer of the esophagus. Am J Roentgenol 1978;131:791.

46. Abemayer E, Moore DM, Hanson DG, Identification of synchronous esophageal tumors in patients with head and neck cancer. J Surg Oncol 1988;38:94.

47. Atkins JP, Keane WM, Young KA, Rowe LD. Value of panendoscopy in determination of secondary primary cancer. A study of 451 cases of head and neck cancer. Arch Otolaryngol 1984;110:533.

48. Maisel RH, Vermeersch H. Panendoscopy for second primaries in head and neck cancer. Ann Otol 1981;90:460.

49. Shapshay SM, Hong WK, Fried MP, et al. Simultaneous carcinomas of the esophagus and upper aerodigestive tract. Otolaryngol Head Heck Surg 1980;88:373.

50. Beebe GW, Kato H, Land CE. Studies of the mortality of A-bomb survivors. 6: Mortality and radiation dose, 1950–1974. Search 1978;75:138.

51. Goffman TE, McKeen EA, Curtis RE, Schein PS. Esophageal carcinoma following irradiation for breast cancer. Cancer 193;52:1808.

52. Selby WS, Gallagher ND. Malignancy in a 19-year experience of adult celiac disease. Dig Dis Sci 1979;24:687.

53. Larsson L-G, Sandström A, Westling P. Relationship of Plummer-Vinson disease to cancer of the upper alimentary tract in Sweden. Cancer Res 1975;35:3308.

54. Huang B-S, Unni KK, Payne WS. Long-term survival following diverticulectomy for cancer in pharyngoesophageal (Zenker's) diverticulum. Ann Thorac Surg 1984;38:207.

55. Froelicher P, Miller G. The European experience with esophageal cancer limited to the mucosa and submucosa. Gastrointest Endosc 1986;32:88.

56. Barge J, Molas G, Maillard JN, et al. Superficial oesophageal carcinoma: An oesophageal counterpart of early gastric cancer. Histopathology 1981;5:499.

57. Huang GU, K'ai WY. Clinical diagnosis. In: Huang GJ, K'ai WY, eds. Carcinoma of the esophagus and gastric cardia. Berlin, Heidelberg, New York, Tokyo: Springer-Verlag, 1984:238.

58. Huang GJ. Recognition and treatment of the early lesion. In: Delarue NC, Wilkins EW Jr, Wong J, eds. International trends in general thoracic surgery. Vol 4: Esophageal cancer. St Louis: CV Mosby, 1988:149.

59. The Coordinating Groups for the Research of Esophageal Carcinoma, Honan Province and Chinese Academy of Medical Sciences. Studies on relationship between epithelial dysplasia and carcinoma of the esophagus. Chin Med J 1975;1(2):110.

60. McKeown KC. Clinical presentation of carcinoma of the oesophagus. J R Coll Surg Edinb 1986;31:199.

61. DeMeester TR, Barlow AP. Surgery and current management for cancer of the esophagus and cardia: Part I. Curr Probl Surg 1988;25:477. Part II. Curr Probl Surg 1988;25:537.

62. Keagy BA, Murray GF, Starek PJK, et al. Esophagogastrectomy as palliative treatment for esophageal carcinoma: Results obtained in the setting of a thoracic surgery residency program. Ann Thorac Surg 1984;38:611.

63. Parker EF, Gregorie HB, Arrants JE, Ravenel JM. Carcinoma of the esophagus. Ann Surg 1970;171:746.

64. Mountain CF. Rationale in staging of cancer of the esophagus. In: Delarue NC, Wilkins EW Jr, Wong J, eds. International trends in general thoracic surgery. Vol 4: Esophageal cancer. St Louis: CV Mosby, 1988:73.

65. Watson A. Pathologic changes affecting survival in esophageal cancer. In: Delarue NC, Wilkins EW Jr, Wong J, eds. International trends in general thoracic surgery. Vol 4: Esophageal cancer. St Louis: CV Mosby, 1988:90.

66. Bruni HC, Nelson RS. Carcinoma of the esophagus and cardia. Diagnostic evaluation in 113 cases. J Thorac Cardiovasc Surg 1975;70:367.

67. Prolla JC, Reilly RW, Kirsner JB, Cockerham L. Direct-vision endoscopic cytology and biopsy in the diagnosis of esophageal and gastric tumors: Current experience. Acta Cytol 1977;21:339.

68. Winawer SJ, Sherlock P, Belladonna JA. Endoscopic brush cytology in esophageal cancer. JAMA 1975;232:1358.

69. Yoshii Y, Kuno N, Yagi M, Kasugai T. Endoscopic biopsy and cytology in esophageal and gastric carcinoma with the fiberesophagoscope. Gastrointest Endosc 1971;17:150.

70. Witzel L, Halter F, Grétillat PA, et al. Evaluation of specific value of endoscopic biopsies and brush cytology for malignancies of the oesophagus and stomach. Gut 1976;17:375.

71. Young JA, Hughes HE, Lee FD. Evaluation of endoscopic brush and biopsy touch smear cytology and biopsy in the diagnosis of carcinoma of the lower oesophagus and cardia. J Clin Pathol 1980;33:811.

72. Guanrei Y, He H, Sungliang Q, Yuming C. Endoscopic diagnosis of 115 cases of early esophageal carcinoma. Endoscopy 1982;14:157.

73. Endo M, Kobayashi S, Suzuki H, et al. Diagnosis of early esophageal cancer. Endoscopy 1971;2:61.

74. Monnier P, Savary M, Pasche R, Anani P. Intraepithelial carcinoma of the oesophagus: Endoscopic morphology. Endoscopy 1981;13:185.

75. Burke EL, Sturm J, Williamson D. The diagnosis of microscopic carcinoma of the esophagus. Dig Dis 1978;23:148.

76. Mandard AM, Tourneux J, Gignoux M, et al. In situ carcinoma of the esophagus. Macroscopic study with particular reference to the Lugol test. Endoscopy 1980;12:51.

77. Vinayek R, Levin B. Endoscopic diagnosis. In: DeMeester TR, Levin B, eds. Cancer of the esophagus. Orlando, San Diego, New York, London, Toronto, Montreal, Sydney, Tokyo: Grune & Stratton (Harcourt Brace Jovanovitch), 1985:43.

78. Barkin JS, Taub S, Rogers AI. The safety of combined endoscopy, biopsy and dilation in esophageal strictures. Am J Gastroenterol 1981;76:23.

79. Wong J, Branicki FJ. Esophagoscopy and bronchoscopy. In: Delarue NC, Wilkins EW Jr, Wong J, eds. International trends in general thoracic surgery. Vol 4: Esophageal cancer. St Louis: CV Mosby, 1988:36.

80. Hanson JT, Thoreson C, Morrissey JF. Brush cytology in the diagnosis of upper gastrointestinal malignancy. Gastrointest Endosc 1980;26:33.

81. Leiman G, Tim LO, Segal I. Diagnosis of upper gastro-intestinal lesions by endoscopy, cytology and biopsy. S Afr Med J 1979;55:619.

82. Shu Y-J. Cytopathology of the esophagus. An overview of esophageal cytopatholy in China. Acta Cytol 1983;27:7.

83. Coordinating Group for Research on Esophageal Cancer, Linhsien County, Honan. Early diagnosis and surgical treatment of esophageal cancer under rural conditions. Chin Med J 1976;2(2):113.

84. Guojun H, Lingfang S, Dawei Z, et al. Diagnosis and surgical treatment of early esophageal carcinoma. Chin Med J 1981;94(4):229.

85. Aste H, Saccomanno S, Munizzi F. Blind pan-esophageal brush cytology. Diagnostic accuracy. Endoscopy 1984;16:165.

86. Tim LO, Leiman G, Segal I, et al. A suction-abrasive cytology tube for the diagnosis of esophageal carcinoma. Cancer 1982;50:782.

87. Tsang T-K, Hidvegi D, Horth K, Ostrow JD. Reliability of balloon-mesh cytology in detecting esophageal carcinoma in a population of US veterans. Cancer 1987;59:556.

88. Korsten MA, Worner TM, Feinman L, et al. Balloon cytology in screening of asymptomatic alcoholics for esophageal cancer, Part I. Dig Dis Sci 1985;30:845.

89. Shirakabe H, Yamaki G, Maruyama T, Nishizawa M. Radiologic patterns of early esophageal carcinoma. In: Delarue NC, Wilkins EW Jr, Wong J, eds. International trends in general thoracic surgery. Vol 4: Esophageal cancer. St Louis: CV Mosby, 1988:19.

90. Itai Y, Kogure T, Okuyama Y, Akiyama H. Superficial esophageal carcinoma. Radiological findings in double-contrast studies. Radiology 1978;126:597.

91. Moss AA, Koehler RE, Margulis AR. Initial accuracy of esophagograms in detection of small esophageal carcinoma. Am J Roentgenol 1976;127:909.

92. Koehler RE, Moss AA, Margulis AR. Early radiographic manifestations of carcinoma of the esophagus. Radiology 1976;119:1.

93. Yamada A. Radiologic assessment of resectability and prognosis in esophageal carcinoma. Gastrointest Radiol 1979;4:213.

94. Wiot JW, Felson B. Radiographic differential diagnosis. JAMA 1973;226:1548.

95. Gloyna RE, Zornoaz J, Goldstein HM. Primary ulcerative carcinoma of the esophagus. Am J Roentgenol 1977;129:599.

96. Moss AA, Schynder P, Thoeni RF, Margulis AR. Esophageal carcinoma: Pretherapy staging by computed tomography. AJR 1981;136:1051.

97. Thompson WM, Halvorsen RA, Foster WL Jr, et al. Computed tomography for staging esophageal and gastroesophageal cancer: Reevaluation. AJR 1983;141:951.

98. Quint LE, Glaser GM, Orringer MR, Gross HH. Esophageal carcinoma: CT findings. Radiology 1985;155:171.

99. Quint LE, Glazer GM, Orringer MB. Esophageal imaging by MR and CT: Study of normal anatomy and neoplasms. Radiology 1985;156:727.

100. Picus D, Balfe DM, Koehler RE, et al. Computed tomography in the staging of esophageal carcinoma. Radiology 1983;146:433.

101. Becker CD, Barbier P, Porcellini B. CT evaluation of patients undergoing transhiatal esophagectomy for cancer. J Comput Tomogr 1986;10:607.

102. Inculet RI, Keller SM, Dwyer A, Roth JA. Evaluation of noninvasvie tests for the preoperative staging of carcinoma of the esophagus: A prospective study. Ann Thorac Surg 1985;40:561.

103. Lea JW, Prager RL, Bender HW Jr. The questionable role of computed tomography in preoperative staging of esophageal cancer. Ann Thorac Surg 1984;38:479.

104. Parker EF, Hanna CB, Postlethwait RW. Carcinoma of the esophagus. Ann Surg 1952;135:697.

105. Yanjin M. Gunangyi L, Xianzhi G, Wenheng C. Detection and natural progression of early oesophageal carcinoma: Preliminary communication. J Roy Soc Med 1981;74:884.

106. Guanrei Y, Songliang Q, He H, Guizen F. Natural history of early esophageal squamous carcinoma and early adenocarcinoma of the gastric cardia in the People's Republic of China. Endoscopy 1988;20:95.

107. Crespi M, Grassi A, Amiri G, et al. Oesophageal lesions in Northern Iran: A premalignant condition? Lancet 1979;2:217.

108. Huang GJ. Natural progression of esophageal carcinoma. In: Delarue NC, Wilkins EW Jr, Wong J, eds. International trends in general thoracic surgery. Vol 4: Esophageal cancer. St Louis: CV Mosby, 1988:87.

109. Earlam R, Cunha-Melo JR. Oesophageal squamous cell carcinoma: I. A critical review of surgery. Br J Surg 1980;67:381.

110. Ellis FH Jr. Cancer of the esophagus and cardia. Role of surgery in palliation. Postgrad Med 1984;75:139.

111. Ellis FH Jr, Gibb SP, Watkins E Jr. Esophagogastrectomy. A safe, widely applicable, and expeditious form of palliation for patients with carcinoma of the esophagus and cardia. Ann Surg 1983;198:531.

112. Akiyama H, Tsurumaru M. Kawamura T, Ono Y. Principles of surgical treatment for carcinoma of the esophagus. Analysis of lymph node involvement. Ann Surg 1981;194:438.

113. Orringer MB. Transhiatal esophagectomy without thoracotomy for carcinoma of the thoracic esophagus. Ann Surg 1984;200:282.

114. Galandiuk S, Hermann RE, Cosgrove DM, Gassman JJ. Cancer of the esophagus. The Cleveland Clinic experience. Ann Surg 1986;203:101.

115. Ellis FH Jr. Surgical palliation: Esophageal resection—A surgeon's opinion. In: Delarue NC, Wilkins EW Jr, Wong J, eds. International trends in general thoracic surgery. Vol 4: Esophageal cancer. St Louis: CV Mosby, 1988:375.

116. Launois B, Delarue D, Campion JP, Kerbaol M. Preoperative radiotherapy for cancer of the esophagus. Surg Gynecol Obstet 1981;153:690.

117. Gignoux M, Roussel A, Paillot B, et al. The value of preoperative radiotherapy in esophageal cancer: Results of a study of the E.O.R.T.C. World J Surg 1987;11:426.

118. Huang GJ, Gu X-Z, Wang LJ, et al. Combined preoperative irradiation and surgery for esophageal carcinoma. In: Delarue NC, Wilkins EW Jr, Wong J, eds. International trends in general thoracic surgery. Vol 4: Esophageal cancer. St Louis: CV Mosby, 1988:315.

119. Earlam R, Cunha-Melo JR. Oesophageal squamous cell carcinoma: II. A critical review of radiotherapy. Br J Surg 1980;67:457.

120. Kelsen D. Current concepts in the treatment of esophageal cancer. In: DeCosse JJ, Sherlock P, eds. Clinical management of gastrointestinal cancer. Boston: Martinus Nijhoff, 1984:123.

121. Pearson JG. Radiotherapy for esophageal carcinoma. World J Surg 1981;5:489.

122. Hancock SL, Glatstein E. Radiation therapy of esophageal cancer. Semin Oncol 1984;11:144.

123. Wara WM, Mauch PM, Thomas AN, Phillips TL. Palliation for carcinoma of the esophagus. Radiology 1976;121:717.

124. Rowland CG, Pagliero KM. Intracavitary irradiation in palliation of carcinoma of oesophagus and cardia. Lancet 1985;2:981.

125. Newwaishy GA, Read GA, Duncan W, Kerr GR. Results of radical radiotherapy of squamous cell carcinoma of the oesophagus. Clin Radiol 1982;33:347.

126. Kelsen DP. Preoperative chemotherapy in esophageal carcinoma. World J Surg 1987;11:433.

127. Leichman L, Steiger Z, Seydel HG, Vaitkevicius VK. Combined preoperative chemotherapy and radiation therapy for cancer of the esophagus: The Wayne State University, Southwest Oncology Group and Radiation Therapy Oncology Group Experience. Semin Oncol 1984;11:178.

128. Carey RW, Hilgenberg AD, Wilkins EW, et al. Preoperative chemotherapy followed by surgery with possible postoperative radiotherapy in squamous cell carcinoma of the esophagus: Evaluation of the chemotherapy component. J Clin Oncol 1986;4:697.

129. Wolfe WG, Burton GB, Seigler HF, et al. Early results with combined modality therapy for carcinoma of the esophagus. Ann Surg 1987;205:563.

130. Leichman L. Steiger Z, Seydel HG, et al. Preoperative chemotherapy and radiation therapy for patients with cancer of the esophagus: A potentially curative approach. J Clin Oncol 1984;2:75.

131. Kies MS, Rosen ST, Tsang T-K, et al. Cisplatin and 5-fluorouracil in the primary management of squamous esophageal cancer. Cancer 1987;60:2156.

132. Hilgenberg AD, Carey RW, Wilkins EW Jr, et al. Preoperative chemotherapy, surgical resection, and selective postoperative therapy for squamous cell carcimoma of the esophagus. Ann Thorac Surg 1988;45:357.

133. Poplin E, Fleming T, Leichman L, et al. Combined therapies for squamous-cell carcinoma of the esophagus, a Southwest Oncology Group Study (SWOG-8037). J Clin Oncol 1987;5:622.

134. Roth JA, Pass HI, Flanagan MM, et al. Randomized clinical trial of preoperative and postoperative adjuvant chemotherapy with cisplatin, vindesine, and bleomycin for carcinoma of the esophagus. J Thorac Cardiovasc Surg 1988;96:242.

135. Heit HA, Johnson LF, Siegel SR, et al. Palliative dilation for dysphagia in esophageal carcinoma. Ann Intern Med 1978;89:629.

136. Moses FM, Peura DA, Wong RKH, et al. Palliative dilation of esophageal carcinoma. Gastrointest Endosc 1985;31:61.

137. Cassidy DE, Nord HJ, Boyce HW. Management of malignant esophageal strictures—Role of esophageal dilation and peroral prothesis. Am J Gastroenterol 1981;76:173.

138. Tulman AB, Boyce HW Jr. Complications of esophageal dilation and guidelines for their prevention. Gastrointest Endosc 1981;27:229.

139. Buset M, Marez B, Baize M, et al. Palliative endoscopic management of obstructive esophagogastric cancer: Laser or prosthesis? Gastrointest Endosc 1987;33:357.

140. Jager DH, Bartelsman JFWM, Tytgat GNJ. Palliative treatment of obstructing esophagogastric malignancy by endoscopic positioning of a plastic prosthesis. Gastroenterology 1979;77:1008.

141. Diamantes T, Mannell A. Oesophageal intubation for advanced oesophageal cancer: The Baragwanath experience 1977–1981. Br J Surg 1983;70:555.

142. Earlam R, Cunha-Menlo JR. Malignant oesophageal strictures: A review of techniques for palliative intubation. Br J Surg 1982;69:61.

143. Gasparri G, Casalegno PA, Camandona M, et al. Endoscopic insertion of 248 prostheses in inoperable carcinoma of the esophagus and cardia: Short-term and long-term results. Gastrointest Endosc 1987;33:354.

144. Hine KR, Atkinson A. The diagnosis and management of perforations of esophagus and pharynx sustained during intubation of neoplastic esophageal strictures. Dig Dis Sci 1986;31:571.

145. Lux G, Groitl H, Ell C. Tumor stenoses of the upper gastrointestinal tract—Therapeutic alternatives to laser therapy. Endoscopy 1986;18:37.

146. Ogilvie AL, Dronfield MW, Ferguson R, Atkinson M. Palliative intubation of oesophagogastric neoplasms fibreoptic endoscopy. Gut 1982;23:1060.

147. Unruh HW, Pagliero KM. Pulsion intubation versus traction intubation for obstructing carcinomas of the esophagus. Ann Thorac Surg 1985;40:337.

148. Fleischer D, Kessler F. Endoscopic Nd:YAG laser therapy for carcinoma of the esophagus: A new form of palliative treatment. Gastroenterology 1983;85:600.

149. Fleischer D, Sivak MV. Endoscopic Nd:YAG laser therapy as palliative treatment for advanced adenocarcinoma of the gastric cardia. Gastroenterology 1984;87:815.

150. Fleischer D, Divak MV Jr. Endoscopic Nd:YAD laser therapy as palliation for esophagogastric cancer. Parameters affecting initial outcome. Gastroenterology 1985;89:827.

151. Felischer D. The Washington symposium on endoscopic laser therapy, April 18 and 19, 1985. Gastrointest Endosc 1985;31:397.

152. Krasner N, Barr H, Skidmore C, Morris AI. Palliative laser therapy for malignant dysphagia. 1987;28:792.

153. Mellow MH, Pinkas H. Endoscopic laser therapy for malignancies affecting the esophagus and gastroesophageal junction. Analysis of technical and functional efficacy. Arch Intern Med 1985;145:1443.

154. Lightdale CJ, Zimbalist E, Winawar SJ. Outpatient management of esophageal cancer with endoscopic Nd:YAG laser. Am J Gastroenterol 1987;82:46.

155. Bown SG, Hawes R. Matthewson K, et al. Endoscopic laser palliation for advanced malignant dysphagia. Gut 1987;28:799.

156. Bader M, Dittler HJ, Ultsch B, et al. Palliative treatment of malignant stenoses of the upper gastrointestinal tract using a combination of laser and afterloading therapy. Endoscopy 1986;18(Suppl 1):27.

157. Ell C, Riemann JF, Lux G, Demling L. Palliative laser treatment of malignant stenoses in the upper gastrointestinal tract. Endoscopy 1986;18(Suppl 1):21.

158. Johnson JH, Fleischer D, Petrini J, Nord HJ. Palliative bipolar electrocogulation therapy of obstructing esophageal cancer. Gastrointest Endosc 1987;33:349.

159. Sjogren RW, Johnson LF. Barrett's esophagus: A review. Am J Med 1983;74:313.

160. Smith JL. Pathology of adenocarcinoma of the esophagus and gastroesophageal region, and "Barrett's esophagus" as a predisposing condition. In: Stroehleim JR, Rombsdahl MM, eds. Gastrointestinal cancer. New York: Raven Press, 1981:125.

161. Bell-Thomson J, Haggitt RC, Ellis FH. Mucoepidermoid and adenoid cystic carcinomas of the esophagus. J Thorac Cardiovasc Surg 1980;79:438.

162. Schmidt H, Riddell RH, Walther B, et al. Adenocarcinoma in the upper third of the esophagus occurring in heterotopic gastric mucosa. Gastroenterology 1985;88:1574.

163. Haggitt RC, Dean PJ. Adenocarcinoma in Barrett's epithelium. In: Spechler J, Goyal R, eds. Barrett's esophagus: Pathophysiology, diagnosis and management. New York: Elsevier, 1985:153.

164. Cutler SJ, Young JL, eds. Third national cancer survey: Incidence data. Natl Cancer Inst Monogr 1975;41:402.

165. Bosch A, Frias Z, Caldwell WL, Adenocarcinoma of the oesophagus. Cancer 1979;43:1557.

166. Levine MS, Caroline D, Thompson JJ, et al. Adenocarcinoma of the esophagus: Relationship to Barrett mucosa. Radiology 1984;150:305.

167. Wang HH, Antonioli DA, Goldman H. Comparative features of esophageal and gastric adenocarcinomas: Recent changes in type and frequency. Hum Pathol 1986;17:482.

168. Dees M, Blankenstein M, Frenkel M. Adenocarcinoma in Barrett's esophagus: A report of 13 cases. Gastroenterology 1978;74:1119.

169. MacDonald WC, MacDonald JB. Adenocarcinoma of the esophagus and/or gastric cardia. Cancer 1987;60:1094.

170. Hamilton SR, Smith RRL, Cameron JL. Prevalence and characteristics of Barrett esophagus in patients with adenocarcinoma of the esophagus or esophagogastric junction. Hum Pathol 1988;19:942.

171. Schnell T, Sontag S, Chejfec G. Occurrence of adenocarcinoma in short segments or tongue of Barrett's esophagus. Gastroenterology 1989;96:A452.

172. Sanfey H, Hamilton SR, Smith RRL, Cameron JL. Carcinoma arising in Barrett's esophagus. Surg Gynecol Obstet 1985;161:570.

173. Skinner DB, Walther BC, Riddell RH, et al. Barrett's esophagus. Comparison of benign and malignant cases. Ann Surg 1983;198:554.

174. Spechler SJ, Robbins AH, Rubins HG, et al. Adenocarcinoma and Barrett's esophagus. An overrated risk? Gastroenterology 1984;87:927.

175. Barrett NR. Chronic peptic ulcer of the oesophagus and 'oesophagitis.' Br J Surg 1950;38:175.

176. Allison PR, Johnstone AS. The oesophagus lined with gastric mucous membrane. Thorax 1953;8:87.

177. Barrett NR. The lower esophagus lined by columnar epithelium. Surgery 1957;41:881.

178. Hamilton SR. Pathogenesis of columnar cell-lined (Barrett's) esophagus. In: Spechler SJ, Goyal R, eds. Barrett's esophagus: Pathophysiology, diagnosis and management. New York: Elsevier, 1985:29.

179. Mossberg SM. The columnar-lined esophagus (Barrett syndrome)—An acquired condition? Gastroenterology 1966;50:671.

180. Endo M, Kobayashi S, Kozu T, et al. A case of Barrett epithelization followed up for five years. Endoscopy 1974;6:48.

181. Halvorsen JF, Smith BKH. The "Barrett syndrome" (the columnar-lined lower oesophagus): An acquired condition secondary to reflux

oesophagitis. A case report with discussion of pathogenesis. Acta Chir Scand 1975;141:683.

182. Naef AP, Savary M, Ozzello L. Columnar-lined lower esophagus: An acquired lesion with malignant predisposition. Report on 140 cases of Barrett's esophagus with 12 adenocarcinomas. J Thorac Cardiovasc Surg 1975;70:826.

183. Menguy R. On the malignant potential of acquired short esophagus. Arch Surg 1979;114:260.

184. Hawe A, Payne WS, Weiland LH, Fontana RS. Adenocarcinoma in the columnar epithelial lined lower (Barrett) oesophagus. Thorax 1973;28:511.

185. Messian RA, Hermos JA, Robbins AH, et al. Barrett's esophagus. Clinical review of 26 cases. Am J Gastroenterol 1978;69:458.

186. Borrie J, Goldwater L. Columnar cell-lined esophagus: Assessment of etiology and treatment. A 22 year experience. J Thorac Cardiovasc Surg 1976;71:825.

187. Cameron AJ, Ott BJ, Payne WS. The incidence of adenocarcinoma in columnar-lined (Barrett's) esophagus. N Engl J Med 1985;313: 857.

188. American Joint Committee for Cancer Staging and End Results Reporting. Clinical staging system for carcinoma of the esophagus. CA 1975;25:50.

189. Veen AH, Dees J. Blankenstein JD, Blankenstein M. Adenocarcinoma in Barrett's oesophagus: An overrated risk. Gut 1989;30:14.

190. Sprung DJ, Ellis FH, Gibb SP. Incidence of adenocarcinoma in Barrett's esophagus. Am J Gastroenterol 1984;79:817.

191. Robertson CS, Mayberry JF, Nicholson DA, et al. Value of endoscopic surveillance in the detection of neoplastic change in Barrett's oesophagus. Br J Surg 1988;75:760.

192. Hameeteman W, Tytgat GNJ, Houthoff HJ, Tweel JG. Barrett's esophagus: Development of dysplasia and adenocarcinoma. Gastroenterology 1989;96:1249.

193. Spechler SJ. Endoscopic surveillance for patients with Barrett esophagus: Does the cancer risk justify the practice? Ann Intern Med 1987;106:902.

194. American Society for Gastrointestinal Endoscopy. Policy and procedure manual for gastrointestinal endoscopy: Guidelines for training and practice 1990, March.

195. Reid BJ, Weinstein WM, Lewin KJ, et al. Endoscopic biopsy can detect high-grade dysplasia or early adenocarcinoma in Barrett's esophagus without grossly recognizable neoplastic lesions. Gastroenterology 1988;94:81.

196. Spechler SJ, Goyal RK. Barrett's esophagus. N Engl J Med 1987;315: 362.

197. Lee RG, Dysplasia in Barrett's esophagus. A clinicopathologic study of six patients. Am J Surg Pathol 1985;9:845.

198. Berenson MM, Riddle RH, Skinner DB, Freston JW. Malignant transformation of esophageal columnar eipithelium. Cancer 1978;41: 554.

199. Boyce WH. The esophagogastric junction: 25 years looking and learning. ASGE Distinguished Lectureship, May 1984.

200. Reid BJ, Haggitt RC, Rubin CE. Barrett's esophagus: Medical and surgical management. Philadelphia: WB Saunders, 1988:157.

201. Reid BJ, Weinstein WM. Barrett's esophagus and adenocarcinoma. Annu Rev Med 1987;38:477.

202. Weinstein W, Van Deventer G, Ippoliti A. A histologic evaluation of Barrett's esophagus using a standardized endoscopic biopsy protocol. Gastroenterology 1984;86:1296.

203. Reid BJ, Rubin CE. When is the columnar-lined esophagus premalignant? Gastroenterology 1985;88:1552.

204. Gottfried MR, McClave SA, Boyce HW. Incomplete intestinal metaplasia in the diagnosis of columnar lined esophagus (Barrett's esophagus). Am J Clin Pathol 1989;92:741.

205. Belladonna JA, Hajdu SI, Bains MS, Winawer SJ. Adenocarcinoma in situ of Barrett's esophagus diagnosed by endoscopic cytology. N Engl J Med 1974;291:895.

206. Payne WS, McAfee MK, Trastek VF, et al. Adenocarcinoma of the columnar eipthelial-lined lower esophagus of Barrett. In: Delarue NG, Wilkins EW Jr, Wong J, eds. International trends in general thoracic surgery. Vol 4: Esophageal cancer. St Louis: CV Mosby, 1988:256.

207. Robey SS, Hamilton SR, Gupta PK, Erozan YS. Diagnostic value of cytopathology in Barrett esophagus and associated carcinoma. Am J Clin Pathol 1988;89:493.

208. Reid BJ, Haggitt RC, Rubin CE, Rabinovitch PS. Barrett's esophagus: Correlation between flow cytometry and histology in detection of patients at risk for adenocarcinoma. Gastroenterology 1987;93:1.

209. McKinley MJ, Budman DR, Grueneberg D, et al. DNA content in Barrett's esophagus and esophageal malignancy. Am J Gastroenterol 1987;82:1012.

210. Fennerty MB, Sampliner RE, Way D, et al. Discordance between flow cytometric abnormalities and dysplasia in Barrett's esophagus. Gastroenterology 1989;97:815.

211. Reid BJ, Blount PL, Rubin CE, et al. Predictors of progression to malignancy in Barrett's esophagus: Endoscopic, histologic and flow cytometric followup of a cohort. Gastroenterology 1990;98:A305.

212. Haggitt RC, Reid BJ, Rabinovitch PS, Rubin CE. Barrett's esophagus. Correlation between mucin histochemistry, flow cytometry, and histologic diagnosis for predicting increased cancer risk. Am J Pathol 1988;131:53.

213. Blount PL, Rabinovitch PS, Reid BJ. DNA content cytometry and neoplastic progression in the gastrointestinal tract. In: Eastwood G, ed. Premalignant conditions of the gastrointestinal tract: Pathogenesis, diagnosis, and management. New York: Elsevier, 1990 (in press).

214. Alanen KA, Joensu H, Klemi PJ. Autolysis is a potential source of false aneuploid peaks in flow cytometric DNA histograms. Cytometry 1989;10:417.

215. Reid BJ, Haggitt RC, Rubin CE, et al. Observer variation in the diagnosis of dysplasia in Barrett's esophagus. Hum Pathol 1988;19: 166.

216. Levine MS, Kressel HY, Caroline DF, et al. Barrett esophagus: Recticular pattern of the mucosa. Radiology 1983;147:663.

217. Agha FP. Radiologic diagnosis of Barrett's esophagus: Critical analysis of 65 cases. Gastrointest Radiol 1986;11:123.

218. Chen YM, Gelfand DW, Ott DJ, Wu WC. Barrett esophagus as an extension of severe esophagitis: Analysis of radiologic signs in 29 cases. AJR 1985;145:275.

219. Chernin MM, Amberg JR, Kogan FJ, et al. Efficacy of radiologic studies in the detection of Barrett's esophagus. AJR 1986;147:257.

220. Vincent ME, Robbins AH, Spechler SJ, et al. The reticular pattern as a radiographic sign of the Barrett esophagus: An assessment. Radiology 1984;153:333.

221. Freeny PC, Marks WM. Adenocarcinoma of the gastroesophageal junction: Barium and CT examination. AJR 1982;138:1077.

222. Paull A, Trier J, Dalton M, et al. The histologic spectrum of Barrett's esophagus. N Engl J Med 1976;295:476.

223. Thompson JJ, Zinsser KR, Enterline HT. Barrett's metaplasia and adenocarcinoma of the esophagus and gastroesophageal junction. Hum Pathol 1983;14:42.

224. Haggitt RC, Tryzelaar J, Ellis FH, Colcher H. Adenocarcinoma complicating columnar epithelium-lined (Barrett's) esophagus. Am J Clin Pathol 1978;70:1.

225. Smith RRL, Hamilton SR, Bointnott JK, Rogers EL. The spectrum of carcinoma arising in Barrett's esophagus: A clinicopathologic study of 26 patients. Am J Surg Pathol 1984;8:563.

226. Skinner DB, Walther BC, Little AG. Surgical treatment of Barrett's esophagus. In: Spechler SJ, Goyal R, eds. Barrett's esophagus: Pathophysiology, diagnosis and management. New York: Elsevier, 1985:211.

227. Hamilton SR, Hutcheson DF, Ravich WJ, et al. Adenocarcinoma in Barrett's esophagus after elimination of gastroesophageal reflux. Gastroenterology 1984;86:356.

228. Schnell T, Sontag S, Chejfec G, et al. High grade dysplasia in Barrett's esophagus: A report of experience with 43 patients. Gastroenterology 1989;96:A452.

229. Hamilton S. Discussion. In: Barrett's esophagus. Pathophysiology, diagnosis, and management. New York: Elsevier, 1985:240.

230. Dragutsky MS, Dean PJ. Recurrence and metastasis of resected adenocarcinoma arising in Barrett's esophagus. Gastroenterology 1987;92:1374.

231. McDonald GB, Brand DL, Thorning DR. Multiple adenomatous neoplasms arising in columnar-lined (Barrett's) esophagus. Gastroenterology 1977;72:1317.

232. Meuwissen SGM, Visser J, Leguit P, Wesdrop E. Quadruple cancer

in a columnar-lined (Barrett) esophagus. J Clin Gastroenterol 1983;5:71.

233. Witt TR, Bains MS, Zaman MB, Martini N. Adenocarcinoma in Barrett's esophagus. J Thorac Cardiovasc Surg 1983;85:337.

234. Rabinovitch PS, Reid BJ, Haggitt RC, et al. Progression to cancer in Barrett's esophagus is associated with genomic instability. Lab Invest 1988;60:65.

235. Blount PL, Rabinovitch PS, Haggitt RC, et al. Early Barrett's adenocarcinoma arises within a single aneuploid population. Gastroenterology 1990;98:A273.

236. Hamilton SR, Smith RRL. The relationship between columnar epithelial dysplasia and invasive adenocarcinoma arising in Barrett's esophagus. Am J Clin Pathol 1987;87:301.

237. Payne WS, Trastek VF, Piehler JM, et al. Current techniques for the surgical management of malignant lesions of the thoracic esophagus and cardia. Mayo Clin Proc 1986;61:564.

238. Harle IA, Finley RJ, Belsheim M, et al. Management of adenocarcinoma in a columnar-lined esophagus. Ann Thorac Surg 1985;40:330.

239. Weiden PL, Hill LD, Kozarek RA, et al. Neoadjuvant chemoradiotherapy for resectable gastroesophageal junction adenocarcinoma. Adjuvant Therapy of Cancer 1987;5:497.

240. Coia Lr, Engstrom PF, Paul A. Nonsurgical management of esophageal cancer: Report of a study of combined radiotherapy and chemotherapy. J Clin Oncol 1987;5:1783.

241. Wilson SE, Hiatt JR, Stabile BE, Williams RA. Cancer of the distal esophagus and cardia: Preoperative irradiation prolong survival. Am J Surg 1985;150:114.

242. Zhang DW. Surgical management of adenocarcinoma at the gastroesophageal junction. International trends in general thoracic surgery. Vol 4: Esophageal cancer. St Louis: CV Mosby, 1988:155.

243. Rein R, Kelsen DP, Geller N, et al. Adenocarcinoma of the esophagus and gastroesophageal junction. Cancer 1985;56:2512.

244. Sablich R. Benedetti G, Bignucolo S, Serraino D. Squamous cell papilloma of the esophagus: Report on 35 endoscopic cases. Endoscopy 1988;20:5.

245. Fernandez-Radriquez CM, Badia-Figuerola N, Ruiz del Arbol L, et al. Squamous papilloma of the esophagus: Report of six cases with long-term follow-up in four patients. Am J Gastroenterol 1986;81:1059.

246. Mastsusaka T, Watanabe H, Enjoji M. Pseudosarcoma and carcinosarcoma of the esophagus. Cancer 1976;37:1546.

247. Hughes JH, Cruickshank AH. Pseudosarcoma of the oesophagus. Br J Surg 1969;56:72.

248. Battifora H. Spindle cell carcinoma. Ultrastructural evidence of squamous origin and collagen production by tumor cells. Cancer 1976;37:2275.

249. Martin MR, Kahn LB. So-called pseudosarcoma of the esophagus. Nodal metastases of the spindle cell element. Arch Pathol Lab Med 1977;101:604.

250. Osamura RY, Shimamura K, Hata JI, Taoaoki N. Polypoid carcinoma of the esophagus. A unifying term for "carcinosarcoma" and "pseudosarcoma." Am J Surg Pathol 1978;2:201.

251. Gal AA, Martin SE, Kernen JA, Patterson MJ. Esophageal carcinoma with prominent spindle cells. Cancer 1987;60:2244.

252. Hanada M, Nakano K, Li Y, Yamashita H. Carcinosarcoma of the esophagus with osseous and cartilagenous production. Acta Pathol Jpn 1984;34(3):669.

253. Lane N. Pseudosarcoma (polypoid sarcoma-like masses) associated with squamous-cell carcinoma of the mouth, fauces, and larynx: Report of ten cases. Cancer 1957;10:19.

254. Minielly JA, Harrison EG Jr, Fontana RS, Payne WS. Verrucous squamous cell carcinoma of the esophagus. Cancer 1967;20:2078.

255. Meyerowitz BR, Shea LT. The natural history of squamous verrucosed carcinoma of the esophagus. J Thorac Cardiovasc Surg 1971;61:646.

256. Kuwano H, Nagamatsu M, Ohno S, et al. Coexistence of intraepithelial carcinoma and glandular differentiation in esophageal squamous cell carcinoma. Cancer 1988;62:1568.

257. Kuwano, H, Ueo H, Sugimachi K, et al. Glandular or mucus-secreting components in squamous cell carcinoma of the esophagus. Cancer 1985;56:514.

258. Akamatsu T, Honda T, Nakayma J, et al. Primary adenoid cystic carcinoma of the esophagus. Report of a case and its histochemical characterization. Acta Pathol Jpn 1986;36:1707.

259. Azzopardi JG, Menzies T. Primary esophageal adenocarcinoma. Confirmation of its existence by the finding of mucous gland tumors. Br J Surg 1962;59:497.

260. Jacobsohn WZ, Libson Y, Dollberg L. Adenoid cystic carcinoma of the esophagus. Gastrointest Endosc 1980;26:102.

261. Zardawi IM, Talbot IC, Primary adenoid cystic carcinoma of the oesophagus. Diagnostic Histopathology 1983;6:39.

262. Kabuto T, Taniguchi K, Iwanaga T, et al. Primary adenoid cystic carcinoma of the esophagus. A report of a case. Cancer 1979;43:2452.

263. Sweeney EC, Cooney T. Adenoid cystic carcinoma of the esophagus. A light and electron microscopic study. Cancer 1980;45:1516.

264. Turnbull AD, Rosen P, Goodner Jt, Beattie EJ. Primary malignant tumors of the esophagus other than typical epidermoid carcinoma. Ann Thorac Surg 1973;15:463.

265. DeCostanzo DP, Urmacher C. Primary malignant melanoma of the esophagus. Am J Surg Pathol 1987;11(1):46.

266. Ludwig ME, Shaw R, De Suto-Nagy G. Primary malignant melanoma of the esophagus. Cancer 1981;48:2528.

267. Lautz U-U, Schmidt FW, Cullen P. Primary malignant melanoma of the esophagus. Endoscopy 1986;18:240.

268. Milman PJ. Primary malignant melanoma of the esophagus. Gastrointest Endosc 1987;33:36.

269. Raven RW, Dawson I. Malignant melanoma of the oesophagus. Br J Surg 1964;51:551.

270. Patel JK. Didoikar MS, Pickren JW, Moore RH. Metastatic pattern of malignant melanoma. A study of 216 autopsy cases. Am J Surg 1978;135:807.

271. Gupta TD, Brasfield R. Metastatic melanoma. A clinicopathological study. Cancer 1964;17:1323.

272. Sabanatham S, Graham GP, Salama FD. Primary oat cell carcinoma of the oesophagus. Thorax 1986;41:318.

273. Rosen Y, Moon S, Kim B. Small cell epidermoid carcinoma of the esophagus. An oat-cell-like carcinoma. Cancer 1975;36:1042.

274. Briggs JC, Ibrahim NBN. Oat cell carcinoma of the oesophagus: a clinicopathological study of 23 cases. Histopathology 1983;7:261.

275. Reyes CV, Jao W, Gould VE. Neuroendocrine carcinomas of the esophagus. Ultrastruct Pathol 1980;1:367.

276. Doherty MA, McIntyre M, Arnott SJ. Oat cell carcinoma of esophagus: A report of six British patients with a review of the literature. Int J Radiat Oncol Biol Phys 1984;10:147.

277. Einspanier GR, Caleel RT, Milford AF. Carcinoid tumors of the esophagus. Report of a case. J Am Osteopath Assoc 1987;87:500.

278. Siegel A, Swartz A. Malignant carcinoid of oesophagus. Histopathology 1986;10:761.

279. Brenner S, Heimlich H, Widman M. Carcinoid of esophagus. NY State J Med 1969;69:1337.

280. Brodman HR, Pai BN. Malignancy carcinoid of the stomach and distal esophagus. Review of the literature and a case report. Am J Dig Dis 1968;13:677.

281. Oz MC, Ashley PF, Oz M. Atypical gastroesophageal carcinoid: A case report and review of the literature. Del Med J 1987;59:785.

282. Kikucki Y, Tsuneta Y, Kawai T, Aizawa M. Choriocarcinoma of the esophagus producing chorionic gonadotropin. Acta Pathol Jpn 1988;68(4):489.

283. McKechnie JC, Fechner RE. Choriocarcinoma and adenocarcinoma of the esophagus with gonadotropin secretion. Cancer 1971;27:694.

284. Postlethwait RW, Musser AW. Changes in the esophagus in 1,000 autopsy specimens. J Thorac Cardiovasc Surg 1974;68:953.

285. Plachta A. Benign tumors of the esophagus. Am J Gastroenterol 1962;38:639.

286. Schmidt HW, Clagett OT, Harrison EG Jr. Benign tumors and cysts of the esophagus. J Thorac Cardiovasc Surg 1961;41:719.

287. Watson RR, O'Connor TM, Weisel W. Solid benign tumors of the esophagus. Ann Thorac Surg 1967;4:80.

288. Seremetis MG, Lyons WS, DeGuzman VC, Peabody JW Jr. Leiomyomata of the esophagus. Cancer 1976;38:2166.

289. Stadler J, Orda R, Baratz M, Wiznitzer T. Giant leiomyoma of the

esophagus as a cause for gastrointestinal bleeding. J Clin Gastroenterol 1987;9:613.

290. Postlethwait RW. Benign tumors and cysts of the esophagus. Surg Clin North Am 1983;63:925.

291. Subramanyam K, Shannon CR, Patterson M, et al. Granular cell myoblastoma of the esophagus. J Clin Gastroenterol 1984;6:113.

292. Brady PG, Milligan FD. Lymphangioma of the esophagus—Diagnosis by endoscopic biopsy. Dig Dis 1973;18:423.

293. Miwa K, Hattori T, Hosokawa Y, Nakamura Y, et al. Granular cell tumor of the esophagus. Gastroenterol Jpn 1986;21:508.

294. Ming S-C. Tumors of the esophagus and stomach. In: Atlas of tumor pathology. Washington: Armed Forces Institute of Pathology, 1973: 17.

295. Gentry RW, Dockerty MB, Clagett OT. Vascular malformations and vascular tumors of the gastrointestinal tract. International Abstracts of Surgery 1949;88:281.

296. Brady PG, Nord HJ, Connar RG. Granular cell tumor of the esophagus: Natural history, diagnosis and therapy. Dig Dis Sci 1988;33: 1329.

297. Choh JH, Khazei AH, Ihm HJ. Leiomyosarcoma of the esophagus: Report of a case and review of the literature. J Surg Oncol 1986;32: 223.

298. Gaede JT, Postlethwait RW, Shelburne JD, et al. Leiomyosarcoma of the esophagus. Report of two cases, one associated with squamous cell carcinoma. Thorac Cardiovasc Surg 1978;75:740.

299. Rainer WG, Brus R. Leiomyosarcoma of the esophagus; Review of the literature and report of 3 cases. Surgery 1965;58:343.

300. Abrams HL, Spiro R, Goldstein N. Metastases in carcinoma. Analysis of 1000 autopsied cases. Cancer 1950;3:74.

301. Nussbaum M, Grossman M. Metastases to the esophagus causing gastrointestinal bleeding. Am J Gastroenterol 1976;66:467.

302. Atkins JP. Metastatic carcinoma to the esophagus. Ann Otol Rhinol Larygol 1966;75:356.

303. Prolla JC, Kirsner JB. The gastrointestinal lesions and complications of the leukemias. Ann Intern Med 1964;61:1084.

304. Givler RL. Esophageal lesions in leukemia and lymphomas. Am J Dig Dis 1970;15:31.

305. Stein HA, Murray D, Warner HA. Primary Hodgkin's disease of the esophagus. Dig Dis Sci 1981;26:457.

306. Matsuura H, Saito R, Nakajima S, et al. Non-Hodgkin's lymphomas of the esophagus. Am J Gastroenterol 1985;80:941.

307. Bernal A, del Junco GW. Endoscopic and pathologic features of esophageal lymphoma: A report of four cases in patients with acquired immune deficiency syndrome. Gastrointest Endosc 1986;32:96.

58

Miscellaneous Diseases of the Esophagus

EUGENE M. BOZYMSKI
JERRY F. LONDON

One of the main functions of the esophagus is the bolus transport of nutrients from the mouth to the stomach. Unfortunately, the esophagus may be exposed to a variety of substances, including medications, that may damage the squamous epithelial lining, leading to problematic clinical situations. Additionally, the esophagus may be inadvertently damaged as a consequence of treatment for various neoplasms. Finally, a wide range of ingested foreign bodies may traumatize or obstruct the esophagus.

Certain systemic illnesses such as sarcoidosis and Crohn's disease may involve the esophagus to varying degrees. The fact that the esophagus is lined by squamous epithelium places it at unique risk for involvement with dermatologic diseases. The esophagus may also be damaged by mechanical force developed either internally as in retching or externally as a result of trauma. In this section, we will address these various topics.

CAUSTIC INJURY TO THE ESOPHAGUS

Introduction and Epidemiology

A wide variety of biologically harmful products ranging from arsenic (ant killers) to sodium hydroxide and other caustics (drain cleaners) are available in every home and workplace. Children are at highest risk, and accidental ingestion occurs in approximately 5000 youngsters yearly.[1] Severe damage to the upper gastrointestinal tract may occur within seconds, and the extreme morbidity and occasional mortality that ensue are sufficient reasons to place a premium on prevention. Hazardous products should be kept out of the reach of children. Public education and the use of child-resistant containers have been of some benefit.[2] The practice of transferring poisons or caustic substances from their original container to a drink container may result in a catastrophe, such as in the case of nine youths mistaking liquid lye for wine.[3]

Ingestion of caustic agents with suicidal intent constitutes the second most common occurrence.[4] Additionally, the mentally retarded may ingest a variety of injurious materials. Lastly, caustic ingestion may occur as an unrecognized form of child abuse.[5] Ingested caustic substances can generally be classified as acid or alkali. The distinction is clinically important because the mechanism of tissue damage is quite different.

ALKALI

Liquid or granular lye (sodium hydroxide or potassium hydroxide) is widely available in household toilet bowl cleaners, drain cleaners, oven cleaners, and myriad others.[6] Because of ingestions, the maximum allowable concentration of alkali in these products has been reduced to 10%.[6] However, it is well documented that damage to the esophagus occurs with exposure to concentrations well below this level.[7] Farm and industrial caustics of higher alkali concentrations are available without poison-prevention safeguards.[8]

Clinitest tablets containing copper sulfate, sodium hydroxide, citric acid, and sodium carbonate are occasionally ingested accidentally or with suicidal intent.[9] If they get stuck in the esophagus, the presence of fluid initiates a vigorous chemical reaction with the production of excessive heat with damage that is additive to the caustic injury.

Small disc batteries of various sizes are tempting objects for children to swallow. If they lodge in the esophagus, severe injury will occur as the result of the leakage of potassium or sodium hydroxide.[10]

ACID

Acids account for approximately 15% of caustic ingestions.[6,11,12] Common sources include toilet bowl cleaners, swimming pool additives, antirust compounds, and soldering fluxes.[13] Household agents (Vanish, Sani-Flush, Lysol, and Mister Plumber) often contain sulfuric, hydrochloric, or phosphoric acid. The esophagus has some resistance to acid injury, and esophageal burns occur in only 6% to 20% of acid ingestions.[14] Generally, acids cause more severe damage to the stomach than to the esophagus.[15]

MISCELLANEOUS AGENTS

Products containing ammonia are occasionally ingested but usually do not result in severe esophageal damage, perhaps because the severe odor limits the amount ingested.[11] Bleaching agents containing sodium hypochlorite have a higher pH than other acids and are not as damaging to the esophagus.[11,16]

Etiology

Caustic injury to the gastrointestinal tract is categorized in a manner similar to that of skin burns.[12,17] First-degree burns are superficial, leading to mucosa hyperemia and edema; the mucosa may slough, but there is no scar formation (Fig 58-1). A second-degree burn extends through the submucosa into the muscular layers and is associated with exudate, mucosal loss, and deep ulcerations. Over a period of weeks to months, luminal stenosis may occur.[12] A third-degree burn is transmural, with erosion into the mediastinum, pleural cavity, or peritoneal cavity and with fistula formation and possibly death.

The actual physical form of the caustic agent plays an important role in determining the extent and location of mucosal damage. Crystalline caustics attach to oral mucosa, are more difficult to swallow, and may be spit out, leading to oropharyngeal burns often without much esophageal damage. On occasion, during suicide attempts, patients will ingest crystalline lye capsules. This may spare the pharynx and esophagus from injury, but severe gastric injury occurs.[18] Conversely, once a liquid caustic enters the posterior pharynx, the patient invariably swallows and will have burns in the esophagus.[11,19]

Upper gastrointestinal disease may compound this problem by delaying transit, leading to further damage. Regurgitation may allow a to-and-fro movement across the esophagogastric junction that repeatedly brings the caustic into contact with the esophagus.[13,20]

ALKALI

Alkalis lead to liquefaction necrosis.[21] The extent of mucosal damage is dependent upon the concentration and duration of mucosal contact.[22] Weak concentrations damage the mucosa and submucosa, whereas concentrations of 22.5% may cause severe inflammation and saponification of all esophageal layers.[22,23] Thrombosis of blood vessels further aggravates the situation. Microscopically, edema, cell necrosis, and infiltration with polymorphonuclear leukocytes are present and are followed by bacterial colonization. As little as 1 ml of a 30% solution (Liquid-Plumber) of sodium hydroxide will destroy a cat's esophagus.[1] Information such as this led to changes in the composition of such agents, and "new improved Liquid-Plumber" contains 5% potassium hydroxide rather than 30% sodium hydroxide.[24]

ACID

Acids produce coagulative necrosis. The more concentrated the acid, the more severe the injury.[11] A mucosal coagulum that may help limit the penetration of the acid into the esophageal wall develops immediately.[6,25] In patients with delayed esophageal

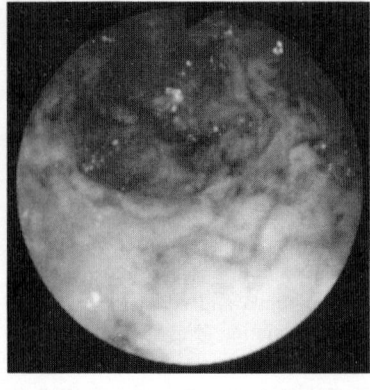
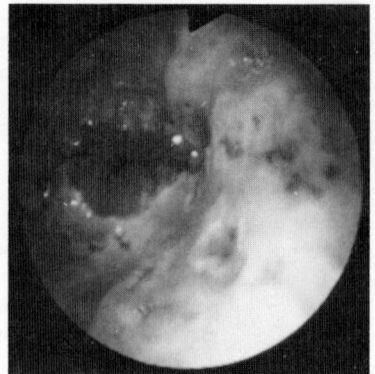
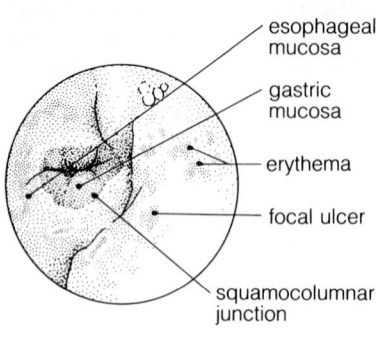
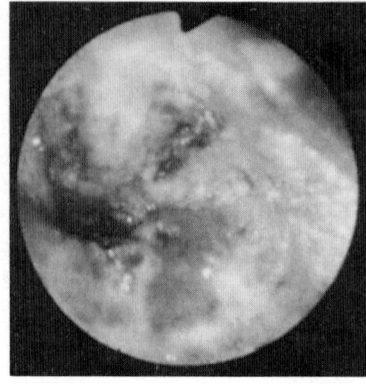

esophageal
mucosa

gastric
mucosa

erythema

focal ulcer

squamocolumnar
junction

FIGURE 58–1. **A,** Esophageal injury after caustic ingestion. The patient presented with retrosternal pain and was found to have mild to moderate esophageal damage with erythema. **B,** Focal ulceration noted proximal to the esophagogastric junction indicates more severe injury. **C,** The mucosa was extensively burned by caustic ingestion and is edematous. The lumen is narrowed. (Silverstein FE, Tytgat GNJ. Atlas of gastrointestinal endoscopy. Philadelphia: WB Saunders, 1987.)

emptying, more damage will occur. Generally, the stomach bears the brunt of injury in cases of concentrated acid ingestion.[11] If the stomach is empty, damage will occur along dependent areas, the greater curvature, and the antrum, with a tendency to spare the fundus.[26]

Clinical Manifestations

HISTORY

The ingestion of a caustic substance by adult patients is usually a suicide attempt and only rarely an accident. Children ingesting caustics generally do so accidentally, and the parent will usually know which agent was involved.[27] If there is a question as to what was ingested, the material should be brought in for inspection.

The extent or the severity of the burn cannot be reliably assessed by history.[6,28–30] Symptoms may include burning of the lips, tongue, and/or pharynx, dysphagia, odynophagia, drooling, vomiting, and dyspnea (Table 58-1). Hematemesis and abdominal pain may be indicative of gastric injury. Fifty percent of the patients with at least two of three symptoms (drooling, vomiting, stridor) will have serious esophageal injury as compared with no esophageal injury in those with only one symptom. Symptoms of third-degree burns include shock, mediastinitis, and peritonitis. Late or chronic manifestations of caustic ingestion include dysphagia secondary to esophageal stricture and vomiting due to antral scarring and gastric outlet obstruction.[18,31]

PHYSICAL FINDINGS

The presence of oropharyngeal burns does not help in identifying patients with esophageal damage.[6,29–31] Oral ulcers with white membranes and edema may be prominent. These lesions are quite painful and may bleed.[33] Excessive salivation is frequently noted.[32] Hoarseness, wheezing, and stridor are suspicious for airway involvement and deserve careful evaluation.[34] In severe cases, the patient may not be able to swallow oral secretions and will be sitting forward drooling over a basin. If perforation has occurred, the patient may present with signs of shock, mediastinitis, or peritonitis requiring acute surgical intervention.[35]

TABLE 58–1
Symptoms of Caustic Ingestion

Burning of the lips, tongue, or pharynx
Odynophagia
Dysphagia
Drooling
Vomiting
Dyspnea/stridor
Hematemesis
Abdominal pain

Differential Diagnosis and Diagnostic Studies

Unless the patient is unconscious when first seen, the diagnosis may be established by history. A parent or friend may actually bring the caustic container. The patient, family, or friends should be questioned regarding any previous history of esophageal or gastric problems potentially confounding management.

If the airway is intact and vital signs are stable, evaluation of the extent of injury can be undertaken. Chest x-rays and abdominal flat and upright views should be evaluated for signs of pneumonitis, pleural effusion, or possibly free air in the mediastinal or peritoneal cavity. In the case of battery ingestion, the chest films are extremely important in confirming and localizing the problem.[36] Radiographic findings will differentiate a battery from the more common esophageal foreign body (a coin) by a double-density appearance on frontal projection.

Poor correlation between symptoms plus the physical examination with the degree of mucosal damage make early endoscopy important in the evaluation of these patients.[3,4,11,15,24,28,30-32,35,37] With the use of smaller flexible endoscopes, patients can be examined carefully with intravenous conscious sedation. Endotracheal intubation is warranted if respiratory distress is present. Endoscopic examination should be gentle to protect against iatrogenic perforation[16,24,38,39] but has generally been safe.[30,33] If viability of the tissue is a concern, the endoscopic examination should be terminated. If perforation has occurred, intraoperative endoscopy may be of benefit to define the extent of luminal damage.

If one sees no esophageal or gastric damage in spite of a history of caustic ingestion or the presence of oropharyngeal burns, systemic antibiotics and corticosteroids can be avoided.[11] First-degree burns usually are indicated by scattered erythema or mucosal hemorrhage. Exudate and blisters are suggestive of more extensive injury, and ulcers with circumferential necrosis and black coagulum indicative of severe injury are harbingers of stricture formation.[11,35,40,41]

Barium studies of the upper gastrointestinal tract are not warranted in the acute setting of caustic ingestion. Furthermore, barium precludes adequate visualization during endoscopy. If done, esophagrams typically show atony, dilatation, ulceration, and sloughing of mucosa.[42] The presence of intramural air or contrast material within the wall of the esophagus is indicative of extensive injury.[43] On follow-up examinations, multiple strictures are often present. The radiologic abnormalities are similar regardless of whether the caustic ingested was alkali or acid. Antral or pyloric channel ulcers or gastric outlet obstruction may be seen following ingestion of a strong acid.[18,44,45]

Computed tomography of the chest and abdomen may play a role in assessing the extent of damage or determining if an abscess has developed.

Clinical Course and Complications

The clinical outcome of patients who have ingested caustics is directly related to the severity of the damage. Patients who suffer only first-degree burns usually do well. Those who develop second-degree burns, particularly with circumferential involvement of the esophagus, have a much poorer outcome and a greater risk of stricture formation.[6,11,19,21,30,31,35] Third-degree burns with erosion into the mediastinum or peritoneal cavity usually require surgical intervention and are associated with significant morbidity and mortality.[3,11,18,19,30,31,35]

Acute airway obstruction can occur as a consequence of aspirating the caustic. Infectious complications and tracheoesophageal fistula can be extremely problematic.[46] In the case of a third-degree burn, adjacent organs may be involved. Aortic rupture, usually occurring within the first 2 weeks, has been reported.[47] Disseminated intravascular coagulation has also been reported in association with acid ingestion, leading to a fatal outcome.[48]

ESOPHAGEAL STRICTURE

Predicting the risk of esophageal stricture formation in patients after caustic ingestion is difficult. Dysphagia that occurs immediately following a caustic injury is due to esophageal spasm and to acute edema.[24] Esophageal stenosis may occur as early as 2 weeks following a caustic burn.[49] It is clear that full-thickness circumferential burns predictably predispose to stricture development.[6,31] Strictures may be insidious, and careful follow-up is important.[24]

CARCINOMA OF THE ESOPHAGUS

Following lye ingestion, the risk of squamous cell carcinoma of the esophagus increases approximately 1000-fold beyond that of the general population (Fig 58-2).[50-52] Of 502 patients with esophageal cancer, 36 (7.2%) gave a prior history of lye ingestion.[51] The mean latent time between lye ingestion and esophageal cancer was 41 years.[50] The mean age of these patients is lower than that of patients with usual esophageal cancer, lending further support to the association.[50] The majority of lye-associated esophageal scar carcinomas are found in the area of the tracheal bifurcation.[50,53] Periodic surveillance endoscopy may be warranted.

GASTRIC DAMAGE

Gastric outlet obstruction, usually antral stenosis, generally occurs 2 to 6 weeks following the ingestion and may be confused with gastric carcinoma.[54-57] Squamous metaplasia and gastric carcinoma have also been reported after acid damage to the stomach, although it is not clear that an increased risk of gastric cancer exists.[58,59]

Therapy

Immediately after a caustic ingestion, questions of neutralization invariably arise. Dilution with water or milk has been suggested.[9,19,60] Mild acids or alkalis should not be used to neutralize ingested caustics because the exothermic reaction might add to the injury.[6,19]

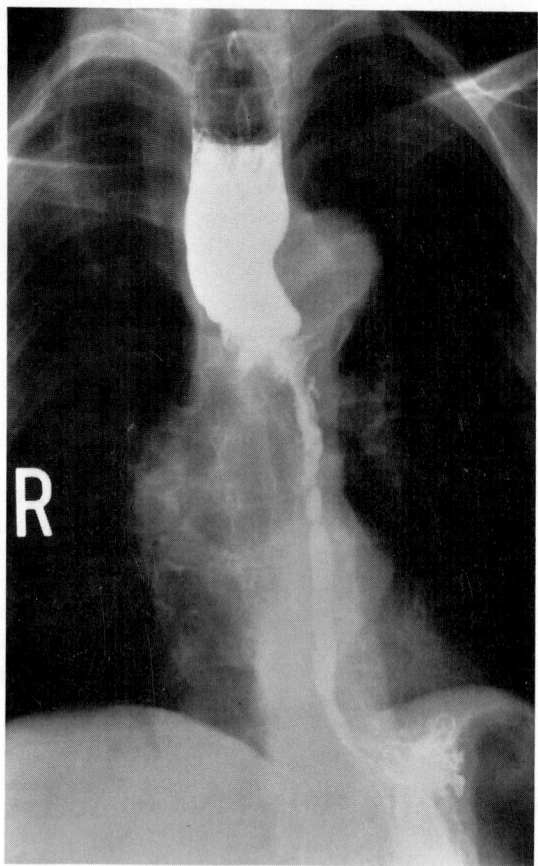

FIGURE 58–2. Multiple esophageal strictures and the development of squamous cell carcinoma 40 years after the ingestion of lye.

Once the patient arrives in the emergency room, the status of the airway should be evaluated and stabilized.[61] Induced emesis is contraindicated because vomiting has the potential of re-exposing the esophagus to the damaging agent and may cause tears or perforations in the damaged esophagus.[19] Intravenous fluids are administered as necessary, and oral intake is prohibited. These patients should be followed closely for symptoms and signs of mediastinitis or peritonitis. If clinical or radiographic findings suggest perforation, surgical intervention is indicated.[3] Early endoscopy aids not only in acute management but also in long-term planning.

ANTIBIOTICS

The use of antibiotics in the management of patients with caustic burns remains unsettled. Many authors suggest broad-spectrum antibiotics in this setting, aware that gram-positive organisms are frequently involved.[4,16,22,24,25,34,41] The use of antibiotics seems reasonable and appropriate in patients with second- and third-degree burns. If corticosteroids are used, antibiotics should be used concomitantly because of the increased risk of infection.[6,30]

CORTICOSTEROIDS

The use of corticosteroids remains largely empiric. Studies are controversial regarding the efficacy in decreasing stricture formation and fibrosis.[11–16,18,20–22,24–26,30,37,39,49,62,63] Many physicians recommend prednisone (60 mg in adults and 1–2 mg/kg in children) or its equivalent.[12,13,37] The duration of therapy recommended is variable; 3 weeks seems to be the minimum for extensive burns.[11,19,24] There is a valid concern that corticosteroids may mask or even potentiate the development of mediastinitis or peritonitis.[1,4,25,35,41,61]

Opinions vary, but corticosteroids should be reserved for those patients with circumferential esophageal burns with increased likelihood of stricture development. It may very well be that with a deep burn, stricture is unavoidable regardless of management.[24,31]

OTHER AGENTS

Experimental animal studies suggest that inhibitors of collagen formation, including penicillamine, B-aminopropionitrile, and N-acetylcysteine, might be useful, but no human data are available.[64–66] Sucralfate has been found to be of benefit in an uncontrolled report.[67]

ESOPHAGEAL DILATATION

Esophageal bougienage should be avoided during the acute phase of injury because instrumentation may increase the risk of perforation.[39] "Early" dilatation has been supported in an uncontrolled trial.[37] However, we and others recommend delaying dilatation for 2 to 4 weeks[4,35,39] and then proceeding very gently. Mild esophageal scarring will usually respond to dilatation, but patients with very tight, long strictures or multiple strictures are felt to be at increased risk from instrumental perforation during dilatation and usually require surgery.[24,31,35,39]

ESOPHAGEAL STENTS

Studies in cats have demonstrated that, following lye burns of the esophagus, intraluminal stenting with silicone rubber catheters can prevent stricture formation.[49] However, other experimental data indicate that the presence of a tube in the esophagus is detrimental.[22] Data are insufficient to allow one to judge the usefulness of this modality.[21,68]

SURGERY

Clearly, the patient with perforation or "impending perforation" requires surgery. Patients with multiple, very tight strictures may require surgery as well.[31,35,39] Colonic interposition has been found to be very useful in this situation.[39] In the case of gastric scarring, hydrostatic balloon dilatation has occasionally been successfully used, but treatment usually requires antrectomy.[69]

DISC BATTERIES

Fortunately, most disc batteries will pass through the gastrointestinal tract without causing damage. If a battery lodges in the esophagus, immediate removal is indicated.[2] Endoscopic techniques are preferred to directly assess the burn area and to prevent perforation during the extraction.[2,6,19,36]

MEDICATION-INDUCED ESOPHAGEAL INJURY

A host of medications may cause mucosal damage when delayed in their transit (Table 58-2).[12,70-74] The size and shape of the medication is an important determinant of esophageal transit time; round tablets take longer to pass than oval ones.[75] Gelatinous-coated tablets and capsules pass more readily when ingested with sufficient water.[76] Taking medication while lying down may cause it to be delayed above the lower esophageal sphincter; tablets swallowed in the upright position are more likely be delayed in the upper esophagus.[75] In young people, antibiotics are frequently the offending agent. In older patients, potassium chloride, nonsteroidal anti-inflammatory drugs, and Vitamin C may cause problems.

Although patients with pre-existing esophageal stenosis or disordered motility are at increased risk, most cases of esophageal injury occur in patients without prior esophageal problems. There is predilection for mucosal damage in areas where the esophagus is subject to external compression, such as the level of the aortic arch.[75] Medications such as aspirin, ascorbic acid, and tetracycline cause damage by specific tissue interactions. Doxycycline has a *p*H of 2.5 when dissolved and produces an acid injury.[12] Potassium chloride, particularly the slow-release tablets, are markedly hypertonic and may lead to venous thrombosis.[12]

Clinically, odynophagia and dysphagia usually occur abruptly several hours after the medication is ingested, but symptoms may

TABLE 58-2
Medications Reported to Cause Esophageal Damage

Aspirin	NSAIDs*
Chloral hydrate	Quinine
Clindamycin	Potassium chloride†
Cromolyn sodium	Quinidine
Emepronium	Tetracycline
Ferrous sulfate	Vitamin C

* Nonsteroidal anti-inflammatory drugs.
† Certain preparations.

be delayed for days or weeks.[72] Persistent retrosternal pain may develop, yet hematemesis occurs infrequently.[77]

The history is of major importance in suggesting the diagnosis. Upper endoscopy will frequently show a discrete ulcer in the mid-esophagus with varying degrees of exudate. Occasionally, remnants of the medication may be found. The lesion may be a single large ulcer or a cluster of shallow ones. The differential diagnosis includes gastroesophageal reflux and Barrett's esophagus, among others. Biopsies show inflammation with regenerative hyperplasia and are helpful in differentiating these ulcers from virus-associated ulcers[77,78] or neoplasm.[79] Esophagrams may show an ulcer or stricture (Fig 58-3). Subtle mucosal changes are best seen with double-contrast esophagrams.

If the situation is recognized and the offending medication discontinued, symptoms usually subside in several weeks; however, severe stricture formation may occur. If a deep ulcer has developed and the medication is inadvertently continued, perforation is a risk.[72]

Treatment centers upon diagnosing the problem and discontinuing the offending drug. Viscous lidocaine may provide temporary relief augmenting antacids and analgesics. The role, if any, for sucralfate or misoprostol awaits controlled trials. Medication

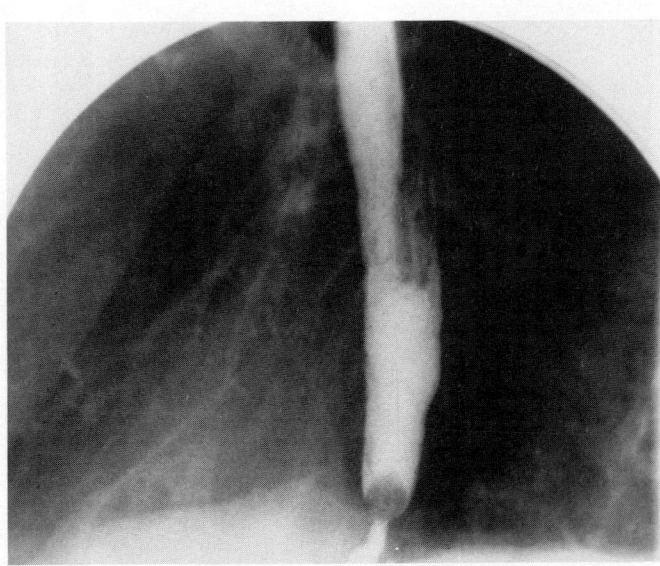

FIGURE 58-3. Radiolucent tablet (analgesic) lodged in the distal esophagus just above a pre-existing stricture.

should be changed to liquid or microencapsulated formulations. All patients, particularly those with esophageal abnormalities, should be advised to take medications in the upright position with sufficient water. Patients who are bedridden and whose medication cannot be changed from tablet form require sufficient quantities of fluid to ensure passage of the medication into the stomach.[75]

RADIATION ESOPHAGITIS

Radiation therapy is a useful adjunct in the treatment of many neoplasms. The development of esophagitis may be the major dose-limiting toxicity in the treatment of thoracic tumors.[80–82] The incidence and severity of esophageal damage are proportional to the radiation dose and the area of esophagus irradiated. Retrosternal burning and esophagitis are frequent with doses greater than 30 Gy; severe esophagitis occurs after 50 Gy; strictures and fistulas may occur after 60 Gy. Esophageal damage is increased by combining chemotherapy with radiotherapy.[80,83,84] Efforts to reduce these complications have included the use of specialized ports, shields, dose hyperfragmentation, and alternate-day schedules for chemotherapy and radiation treatments.[80,85,86]

Radiation doses needed to treat thoracic neoplasms frequently exceed esophageal tolerance. Acutely, radiation damages cells and inhibits mitosis in the germinal layer of the squamous epithelium, predisposing to ulceration and sloughing. The endothelium of esophageal submucosal arterioles is particularly radiosensitive, and damage leads to capillary dilation, edema, and leukocyte infiltration that potentiates the ulceration and sloughing of the epithelium. Over time, fibrosis of the submucosa and lamina propria damages both the smooth muscle fibers and the neuronal elements.

Clinically, acute esophagitis often begins during the third to fifth week of radiation therapy.[87] Patients frequently complain of retrosternal burning, odynophagia, and dysphagia.[88,89] Occasionally, the substernal chest pain may be so severe that myocardial ischemia is considered. The symptoms may be produced by the radiation injury alone or by opportunistic infection of the damaged esophagus. The radiographic or endoscopic appearance of the infected esophagus may be indistinguishable from changes induced by radiation alone.

If the patient has received less than 30 Gy, the symptoms of esophagitis usually subside within a week following therapy. As the total dose is increased, there may be progression to fibrosis and scarring. Typically, a smooth, elongated stricture forms with a thickened wall and loss of neuronal elements. Peristaltic waves terminate at the proximal end of the stricture, and tertiary contractions are evident distally and the lower esophageal sphincter fails to relax.[88] A chronic inflammatory state may develop leading to ulceration, psuedopolyp formation, and mucosal bridges.[90] Fistulas from the esophagus to the trachea, mediastinum, and even the aorta have occurred.[91]

The concomitant use of chemotherapeutic agents and radiotherapy potentiates injurious effects (Fig 58-4).[83,84] A "recall phenomenon" or "amnestic response" is recognized in which a patient who has undergone radiotherapy is subjected to chemotherapy and suffers a relapse of esophagitis.

Treatment includes a soft or liquid diet and local anesthetics

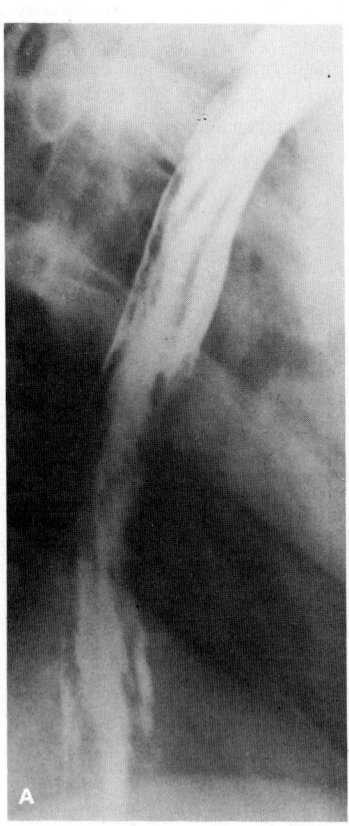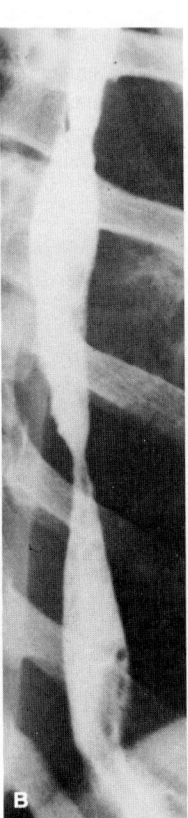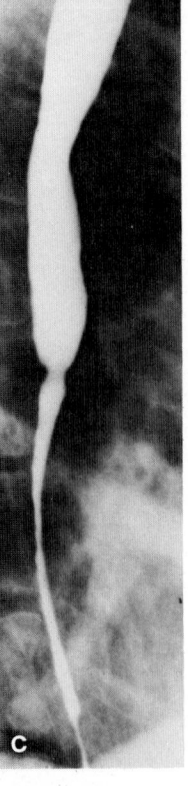

FIGURE 58–4. Esophagitis induced by combined radiation and chemotherapy (doxorubicin). **A,** Barium esophagram performed 10 days after the onset of symptoms demonstrates a dilated esophagus with thickened folds. Peristaltic activity was diminished at fluoroscopy. **B,** Esophagram 16 days after the onset of symptoms demonstrates a narrowed esophagus with markedly irregular mucosa and formation of a stricture in the distal half. No peristalsis was evident at fluoroscopy. **C,** High-grade stenosis involving about 9 cm of the distal esophagus with significant obstruction was found on follow-up examination 2 months after the onset of symptoms. The lumen of the stricture is irregular. The transition from the proximal esophagus, although abrupt, appears benign and is characterized by concentric narrowing. (Eisenberg RL. Gastrointestinal radiology: A pattern approach, ed 2. Philadelphia: JB Lippincott, 1990.)

such as viscous Xylocaine or antacids. Severe acute radiation esophagitis may require narcotic analgesics and brief interruption of radiotherapy or at least a 10% reduction in dosage.[88] Metoclopramide may assist impaired esophageal motility. Several patients improved when treated with nifedipine.[92] Opportunistic infections should be sought and treated accordingly, but persistent symptoms of dysphagia must be suspect for treatment failure and primary tumor growth. The late complications of esophageal stricture and dysmotility require a different approach; repetitive esophageal dilations may be necessary. Hydrocortisone injections into the strictured area to decrease the local inflammation have been useful,[93] as have drugs inhibiting the arachidonic acid cascade.[94]

FOREIGN BODIES IN THE ESOPHAGUS

The esophagus is the most common site of foreign-body impaction in the gastrointestinal tract.[95] Coins are the most frequent objects ingested by children; chicken or fish bones by adults.[96] Populations at increased risk for swallowing foreign bodies include adults who wear dentures, patients with psychiatric illnesses, and prisoners in whom ingesting a foreign body may result in the secondary gain of exchanging a prison cell for a hospital bed. Typically, these items tend to become lodged at an area of esophageal narrowing: the cervical esophagus, the level of the aortic arch, the distal esophagus just above the esophagogastric junction, or any area of structural abnormality. Food impactions usually occur in the setting of underlying esophageal disease, such as a Schatzki's ring or stricture (Fig 58-5; Color Fig 20).[97-99]

Patients may complain of sharp, sticking pain in the neck or chest area and occasionally are able to localize the site of the foreign object accurately. Dysphagia is the most common symptom, followed by odynophagia, choking, and drooling.[97,100,101] Coughing, dyspnea, and wheezing occur in 5% to 15% of patients and may

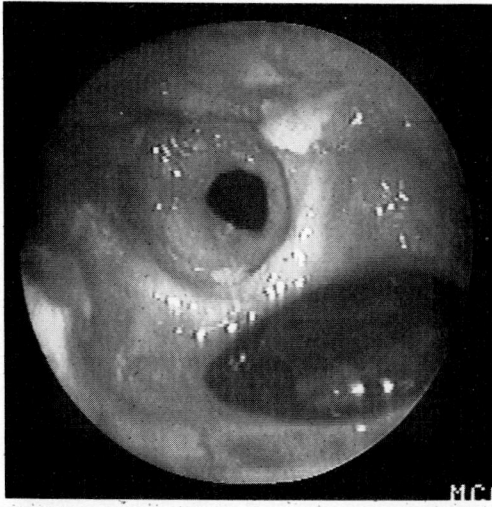

FIGURE 58-5. (See Color Fig 20) "Watermelon esophagus." A watermelon seed lodged in a pseudodiverticulum above a very narrow esophageal stricture.

be indistinguishable from symptoms caused by tracheal foreign bodies. In one case, a 20-month-old child presented with an 11-month history of stridor. Ultimately, a small plastic disc was found in an esophageal wall abscess.[102]

Frequently, a history of ingestion of a foreign body is offered, or, in the case of an infant, the ingestion has been witnessed. A history of prior ingestions or food impactions is common. The physical examination is usually unremarkable. Radiographs of the neck and chest will often detect radiopaque foreign bodies.[100,103,104] In the case of a radiolucent object, subcutaneous air or soft-tissue swelling may be a clue to the correct diagnosis. An esophagram, perhaps using barium-soaked cotton, may be helpful,[95,105] but aspiration precautions are needed. In the presence of a neck mass, computed tomography may delineate the foreign body[105] or the location of an abscess.[102] Flexible upper endoscopy will usually provide the diagnosis and an opportunity to remove the object.

Most ingested foreign bodies pass through the gastrointestinal tract uneventfully. Once an object becomes impacted in the esophagus, the size, shape, presence of sharp points, and location determine the clinical presentation. Esophageal obstruction, ulceration, and perforation may lead to cervical or mediastinal abscess formation.[95] Wheezing or dyspnea may result from tracheal compression or aspiration of esophageal contents. Long-standing foreign bodies of the esophagus may induce cricoid perichondritis, periesophagitis, esophageal diverticula, or esophageal stenosis.[102] Fistulous tracts to the trachea or bronchus and the aorta or innominate artery have been reported.[95,106,107]

Treatment of esophageal foreign bodies depends on the object's physical characteristics, its location, and the length of time it has been in place. In all cases, the risk of pulmonary aspiration and laryngeal obstruction must be guarded against and minimized. Removal of blunt, radiopaque esophageal foreign bodies has been accomplished by use of a Foley catheter under fluoroscopic guidance.[104,108] In a review of 2500 cases, the technique had a 95% success rate with only one serious, but reversible, complication.[104] There is some controversy regarding the safety of this technique and the reporting of serious complications.[109-111] Flexible endoscopy does not require general anesthesia, and when it is used in conjunction with an overtube or foreign body retrieval hood, it offers protection from tracheal aspiration of the foreign body.[112,113] There should always be a physician present who can manage the patient's airway in case of an emergency. If the object has been present for a long time, the patient may require surgery to not only remove the foreign body but also drain an abscess or repair a perforation. It is useful to perform an "in vitro" trial with a similar foreign body to determine which endoscopic accessory will be most useful in the actual removal.

Food impaction represents a special case. Usually food impacts in the distal esophagus and is almost always associated with underlying esophageal disease.[97] Sublingual nitroglycerin may produce smooth muscle relaxation and occasionally allows the food to pass.[114] Glucagon decreases the lower esophageal sphincter pressure, and when it is administered in 0.5-mg intravenous boluses up to 2.0 mg it has effectively relieved esophageal food impactions.[98]

Flexible upper endoscopy is generally successful in removing the impaction. Blindly pushing the bolus with the endoscope should be avoided because there is usually a stricture or other structural abnormality such as a tumor obstructing the lumen. With the use of endoscopy with an overtube and basket or snare techniques, the obstructing matter can usually be safely removed or advanced into the stomach. Once the esophagus has been cleared, the patient should be treated with acid-reducing therapy and a liquid diet. The underlying esophageal stricture should not be dilated at this time.

Occasionally the use of a large-bore orogastric tube advanced under fluoroscopic guidance will be successful in removing the food bolus by suction. Rarely, surgery will be necessary to clear an esophageal food impaction. Surgery is the treatment of choice if there is evidence of esophageal perforation or the material is imbedded in the esophageal wall.

SYSTEMIC DISEASES AFFECTING ESOPHAGUS (Table 58-3)

Sarcoidosis

Gastrointestinal involvement in patients with sarcoidosis has been exceedingly rare, occurring in only 2 of 1254 cases.[115] In biopsy materials, granulomas were found in the gastrointestinal tract of 10% of patients with known sarcoidosis, but the patients had rarely complained of gastrointestinal symptoms.[116] Granulomatous esophagitis usually presents in conjunction with generalized sarcoidosis.

Patients who have generalized sarcoidosis may develop dysphagia, more commonly due to gastroesophageal reflux or infection than to sarcoidosis. Dysphagia may be due to esophageal compression by enlarged lymph nodes[120] or achalasialike symptoms.[121] Granulomatous infiltration of the esophageal wall may produce symptoms by the formation of long strictures.[117-119]

Therapy is aimed at the systemic disease, but tight esophageal strictures may require dilatation. In selected cases, esophagojejunal interposition has been useful.[117]

Crohn's Disease

Crohn's disease involving the upper gastrointestinal tract is uncommon, occurring in 3% to 13% of patients with ileocolonic Crohn's disease.[122,123] Involvement of the esophagus is even more unusual, with only 1 case of Crohn's esophagitis noted among 383 patients with Crohn's disease.[124] Similarly, in another report, 9 cases of esophageal involvement were documented in a group of 500 patients with Crohn's disease.[125] The presence and degree of inflammation in the esophagus usually parallel the activity of the disease in other parts of the gastrointestinal tract.[126] However, dysphagia has occasionally been the presenting symptom leading to the diagnosis of Crohn's disease, and rarely esophageal involvement has been found in patients with no other manifestations of the disease.[127,128]

Patients with Crohn's esophagitis may complain of odynophagia, dysphagia, pyrosis, or substernal chest pain.[119,125,127-133] As the disease progresses, symptoms due to fistulous tracts to the bronchi, mediastinum, or stomach may predominate.[122,126,127] The diagnosis of esophageal involvement in Crohn's disease is difficult to establish.[134] The esophageal aphthous ulcerations may be due to acid-peptic disease, herpetic and mycotic infections, or Behçet's disease, or they may be drug-induced.[126] Later in the course, radiographs may show a cobblestone appearance or "crocodile skin" (Fig 58-6)[130] produced by linear ulcerations; decreased motility and decreased distensibility may also be present. Ultimately, esophageal strictures may form, and deep inflammatory fissures may be evident as sinus tracts or fistulas to adjacent structures.[119,122,126,127]

Endoscopy with biopsies is more helpful in eliminating other causes than in establishing the diagnosis of Crohn's esophagitis. Endoscopic biopsies are inadequate to demonstrate the transmural nature of the inflammation in Crohn's disease.[126,127] Unlike colonic biopsies, tissue from the esophagus very infrequently contains granuloma.[119,126-128,130,132]

The clinical course is highly variable. In patients with acute Crohn's esophagitis, excellent results have been achieved with systemic corticosteroids.[125] Sulfasalazine has been less successful.[129] Progressive stricture formation, the "garden hose deformity,"[130] has been reported. Surgical resection and esophagogastrostomy may be necessary in cases in which medical therapy and bougienage of strictures have not been adequate.[127,130] Recurrence at the anastomosis and complications of esophagocutaneous fistula have been noted.[119] Some patients have done well after bougienage and medical management for as long as 21 years.[130]

Behçet Disease

In 1937, Behçet described a syndrome characterized by a clinical triad of oral aphthous ulcers, genital ulcers, and ocular inflam-

TABLE 58-3
Systemic Diseases Affecting the Esophagus

DISEASE	ETIOLOGY	ESOPHAGEAL FINDINGS
Sarcoidosis	Granulomatous infiltration	Long strictures
Crohn's disease	Transmural inflammation	Aphthous ulcers, linear ulcers, decreased motility, strictures, sinus tracts
Behçet's disease	Immune complex disease	Superficial ulcers, diffuse esophagitis, perforated ulcers, severe stenosis
Graft-versus-host disease	Donor lymphocytes active against host antigens	Desquamative esophageal mucosa, webs, strictures, gastroesophageal reflux

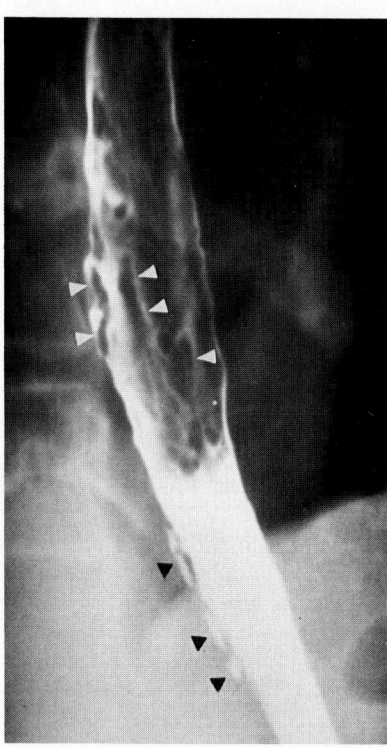

FIGURE 58–6. Crohn's esophagitis. Filiform polyps (*white arrowheads*) are associated with mucosal nodularity, deep ulcers, and intramural sinus tracts (*black arrowheads*). (Eisenberg RL. Gastrointestinal radiology: A pattern approach, ed 2. Philadelphia: JB Lippincott, 1990.)

mation; involvement of the skin, gastrointestinal tract, vascular system, nervous system, and articular cartilage is now recognized.[135,136] Typically presenting in young adults, this systemic inflammatory illness is most common in the Middle East and Japan.

Manifestations of Behçet's disease usually include oral and genital aphthous-type ulcerations.[137] Esophageal involvement was first reported in 1973, and more than 25 cases have now been reported.[136,138] Patients have presented with odynophagia, dysphagia, chest pain, epigastric pain, and hematemesis due to various lesions such as superficial erosions, diffuse esophagitis, perforated ulcers with mediastinal abscess, and severe esophageal stenosis. Most of the lesions have been found in the middle and distal esophagus. All of these patients had other manifestations of Behçet's disease concomitant with esophageal involvement.

Esophagrams may show mucosal lesions, ulceration, perforation, or esophageal stricture. Patients in whom the esophagram is normal may have esophageal ulceration detected at endoscopy.[139] Biopsies show ulceration with nonspecific inflammation and neutrophilic infiltration.[136]

The clinical course is that of the multisystem disease. The unpredictable exacerbations and remissions of the underlying disease have made evaluation of therapeutic agents difficult. Dysphagia due to esophageal ulcers may resolve spontaneously in a time course similar to that of the disappearance of oral ulcerations.[139] In other cases, the ulceration may persist and progress to perforation or esophageal stricture.[136,138,140] Large trials are lacking, but some success in treating Behçet's disease has been reported with whole-blood and plasma transfusions,[141,142] transfer factor,[143]

and immunosuppressive agents.[144,145] Corticosteroids have produced marked improvement of symptoms, but it has been suggested that they may mask ongoing inflammation and may contribute to the failure of ulcer healing.[140]

Graft-versus-host Disease

Allogeneic bone marrow transplants are increasingly successful for the treatment of aplastic anemia and leukemia. However, 25% to 40% of the long-term survivors develop chronic graft-versus-host disease (GVHD). This syndrome is characterized by sclerodermalike skin lesions, sicca syndrome, oral mucositis, diarrhea, chronic liver disease, infections, and disordered immune functions. Esophageal involvement is relatively uncommon and has been reported only in patients who have multisystem involvement with GVHD.

GVHD esophagitis may present as severe odynophagia, dysphagia, pyrosis, and severe retrosternal chest pain with radiation to the back. In one series, 8 of 63 patients with chronic GVHD developed esophageal symptoms.[146] All patients had evidence of other organ involvement.

Patients with GVHD are typically being treated with immunosuppressive agents; therefore, esophageal symptoms may be due to opportunistic infections. The differential diagnosis includes not only infectious etiologies but also autoimmune diseases such as progressive systemic sclerosis, systemic lupus erythematosus, lichen planus, and Sjögren's syndrome. Endoscopy is necessary to establish the diagnosis. In a majority of cases, the esophageal mucosa has appeared erythematous, friable, and peeling, appropriately termed desquamative esophagitis.[146] The presence of strictures and upper esophageal webs has also been noted. Esophagrams are useful to detect the mucosal lesions, strictures, and webs, but biopsy material is needed to rule out infectious etiologies. Manometric studies have demonstrated a high incidence of aperistalsis in symptomatic patients with GVHD. Gastroesophageal reflux with peptic esophagitis has also been found to be a significant factor in some patients.[147]

Some patients have improved on increased regimens of immunosuppressive therapy, while others have improved on antireflux therapy alone. Occasionally the symptoms are so debilitating that they require parenteral nutrition or gastrostomy. Esophageal strictures have been treated with repeated bougienage, but esophageal perforation has occurred in at least two cases. For most patients, a combined approach with immunosuppressives and antireflux therapy has been efficacious.

DERMATOLOGIC DISEASES AFFECTING ESOPHAGUS

Pemphigus Vulgaris

The squamous epithelium of the esophagus renders it susceptible to certain dermatologic diseases (Table 58-4). Pemphigus vulgaris (PV) is a chronic, blistering disease occasionally involving the esophagus. This disease usually presents in the fourth to the sixth decade of life with flaccid bullae of the skin and oral mucous

TABLE 58–4

Dermatologic Diseases with Esophageal Manifestations

DISEASE	ETIOLOGY	ESOPHAGEAL FINDINGS
Pemphigus vulgaris	IgG against ground substance, separation of superficial epithelium from basal layer	Erythema, hemorrhagic bullae, sheets of desquamating mucosa
Bullous pemphigoid	IgG against basement membrane	Intraepidermal bullae, esophagitis dissecans superficialis
Benign mucous membrane pemphigoid	Unknown, probably immune complex mediated	Bullae, webs, long strictures
Epidermolysis bullosa dystrophica	Genetic, separation of basal layer from dermis	Bullae, blebs, ulceration with deep scarring, long strictures, spontaneous dissection

membranes.[148,149] PV is slightly more prevalent in women than men and occurs with a greater frequency among people of Jewish and Mediterranean descent.

PV is an autoimmune disease characterized by the presence of IgG specific for ground substance of squamous epithelium.[148] The dissolution of intercellular bridges leads to rounding of the suprabasal cells, referred to as acantholysis.[148-151] Thus, the superficial epithelium is susceptible to separation from the basal layer after only minimal trauma.

Fifty percent of patients with PV may have esophageal involvement without clinical symptoms.[149] Complaints include dysphagia, odynophagia, epigastric pain, and pyrosis.

Endoscopy with biopsy is required to establish the diagnosis. Endoscopically, scattered erythema, whitish plaques, flaccid hemorrhagic bullae, erosions with adherent clots, and sheets of mucosa peeling from the esophageal wall have been described.[148,149,151] Biopsies typically show acantholysis with inflammation of the submucosal tissues.[150] Positive direct immunofluorescent staining of intraepithelial cells is considered diagnostic for PV esophagitis. However, the same findings have been reported as a drug effect in patients treated with penicillamine or thiopronine.[149,150] Frequently, PV patients are on corticosteroid therapy, predisposing them to opportunistic infections. Biopsies differentiating monilial or herpetic infections significantly alter the therapeutic approach. Rarely, patients have presented with hematemesis due to esophageal involvement.[148]

PV was a relatively fatal affliction until the advent of corticosteroid therapy. Esophageal PV may require high-dose intravenous corticosteroids, but the response is rapid and survival greatly enhanced.[150,152]

Bullous Pemphigoid

Bullous pemphigoid (BP) is a benign vesicobullous disease occurring primarily in older patients. The disease has a predilection for the flexor surfaces, and involvement of the oropharynx occurs in 20% of the patients.[153] The actual incidence of esophageal involvement in BP may be underestimated because symptoms are infrequent, even in the presence of active disease.[153]

The formation of bullae is the result of IgG autoantibodies directed against the basement membrane of squamous epithelium. The bullae form above the basement membrane because of the deposition of IgG and C3 activating the complement pathway and the membrane attack complex.[154] Intraepidermal bullae are characteristically found.

Esophageal involvement with BP is usually asymptomatic. Breakdown and healing of the bullae rarely lead to cicatrix formation. Rarely, patients have developed odynophagia and dysphagia. These symptoms may precede emesis of a cast of the esophagus containing the squamous mucosa, termed "esophagitis dissecans superficialis."[155] Even in this case, healing is very rapid and free of scarring. Massive upper gastrointestinal hemorrhage may rarely occur.[156]

The differential diagnosis of esophageal bullous lesions includes benign mucous membrane pemphigoid, junctional bullous epidermatosis (Herlitz's disease), familial benign chronic pemphigus (Hailey–Hailey disease), pemphigus vulgaris, and epidermolysis bullosa dystrophica (EBD).[153,157] Esophagrams, although safe, are of little diagnostic use in BP. The presence of anti–basement membrane antibody in serum is considered diagnostic, but only 70% of patients test positive. Immunohistochemical stains of biopsy material from active sites in BP show linear deposition of IgG and C3 along the basement membrane in virtually all cases.

The course of esophageal involvement in BP is generally chronic and uncomplicated. Hemorrhage and mucosal sloughing are rare. Sulfapyridine has occasionally been useful, but high-dose prednisone or combinations of prednisone and cyclophosphamide are more frequently efficacious.[158,159]

Benign Mucous Membrane Pemphigoid

Benign mucous membrane pemphigoid (BMMP) is a chronic blistering disease of the conjunctiva and oral mucosa. Involvement of the external genitalia and the pharyngeal and nasal mucosa is also seen. Of patients with documented BMMP, 2.3% to 13% develop esophageal involvement. One patient presented with esophageal BMMP and no other manifestations of the disease.[160] BMMP usually begins in the fourth decade of life or later[161] and is slightly more prevalent in women than men. Although immune complex deposition is present in the affected tissues, the etiology of BMMP remains unknown.

Esophageal involvement with BMMP may be seen initially or up to 10 years later in the course of the disease. Patients complain of dysphagia, odynophagia, and chronic cough due to aspiration.[161-163] Rarely, patients have been found to have active esophageal disease without evident symptoms.[161,164] Aspiration is manifest by chronic cough, and occasionally the development of aspiration pneumonia has led to death.[165]

Establishing the diagnosis of BMMP esophageal disease can be difficult because there are no truly pathognomonic findings. Esophagrams may show bullae as seen in bullous pemphigoid (BP) and epidermolysis bullosa dystrophica (EBD). Small esophageal webs in the upper esophagus are frequently present in BMMP, BP, EBD, pemphigus vulgaris, and Plummer–Vinson syndrome.[161] Esophageal strictures are typically located in the upper esophagus and are long and smoothly tapering (Fig 58-7).[161] Bullae are rarely seen endoscopically.[161] Biopsy samples show chronic inflammation of the subepithelial connective tissue.[162] There may be subepithelial bullae and a lack of acanthosis.[161] Immunofluorescent stains demonstrate intracellular and basement membrane deposition of IgG and C3.[162]

Long esophageal strictures may develop and respond only temporarily to dilatation, yet endoscopy may be hazardous in these patients. One patient had normal-appearing mucosa on passage of the endoscope, but on withdrawal, multiple 3- to 6-cm hemorrhagic bullae had formed. This has been equated with a Nikolsky's sign of the skin.[164] Systemic corticosteroids or dapsone has been of some benefit.[161,162] Colonic interposition has been suggested for refractory esophageal strictures.

Epidermolysis Bullosa Dystrophica

Epidermolysis bullosa dystrophica is a rare, genetic, vesiculobullous or mechanobullous disease[137,166,167] primarily affecting squamous epithelium. The various forms of epidermolysis bullosa are separated into dystrophic, scarring, and nondystrophic categories. Esophageal involvement is clinically important in only the autosomal-recessive, dystrophic form, epidermolysis bullosa dystrophica-recessive (EBD-R), and rarely in the autosomal-dominant, dystrophic forms.

The precise genetic defect leading to EBD-R has not been delineated. Histopathologically, there is a separation of the basal lamina from the underlying dermis due to a marked reduction or absence of anchoring fibrils between the lamina densa and the dermis.[168,169] In addition, skin from the bullae show a sixfold increase in collagenase activity compared to normal.[166] The end result is that the squamous epithelium forms bullae in response to minor trauma and heals by cicatrix formation, which may shorten the esophagus and lead to a traction hiatal hernia.

Cutaneous bullae are evident early in life. Over time, the loss of hair and nails, the formation of flexion contractures, and the formation of syndactyly by the scarring/healing process have been referred to as mummification (Fig 58-8). The same process also occurs in the mouth, oropharynx, and esophagus as a result of the trauma of mastication and swallowing. Esophageal sites most frequently involved include the area of the upper esophageal sphincter, the level of the carina, and the distal esophagus.[170] Esophageal bullae and blebs ulcerate and often bleed, then heal with scar formation. The resultant strictures are of variable length; 50% are in the upper one third of the esophagus and 25% are multiple (Fig 58-9).[170] Although the strictures are permanent, the patient may report waxing and waning dysphagia due to new bullae forming in the stricture and surrounding edema. Esophageal peristalsis proximal to the stricture is diminished and lost entirely in the strictured area. Upper esophageal webs form by postinflammatory healing and may contribute to dysphagia.[171] Younger patients may

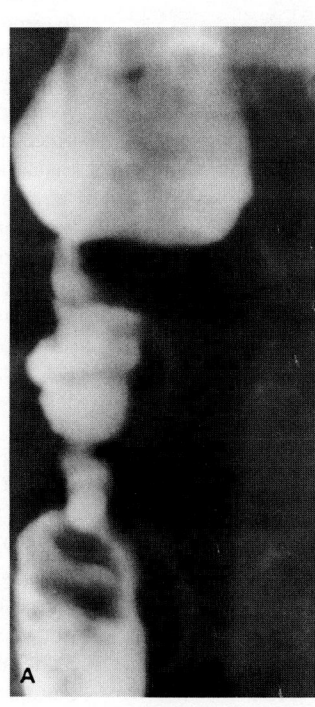
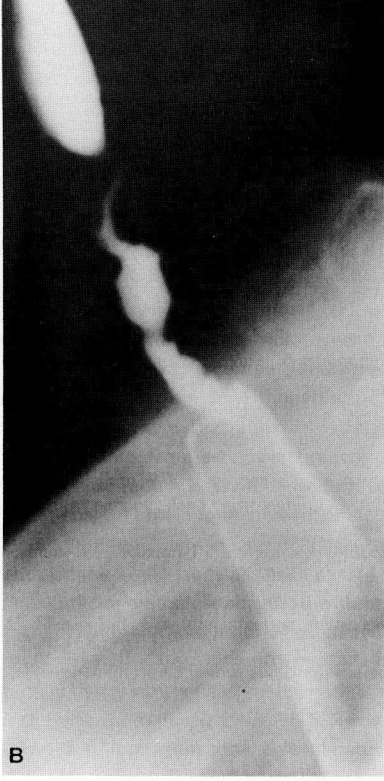

FIGURE 58–7. Benign mucous membrane pemphigoid. Postinflammatory scarring causes a long, irregular area of narrowing suggestive of a malignant process. (Eisenberg RL. Gastrointestinal radiology: A pattern approach, ed 2. Philadelphia: JB Lippincott, 1990.)

A

B

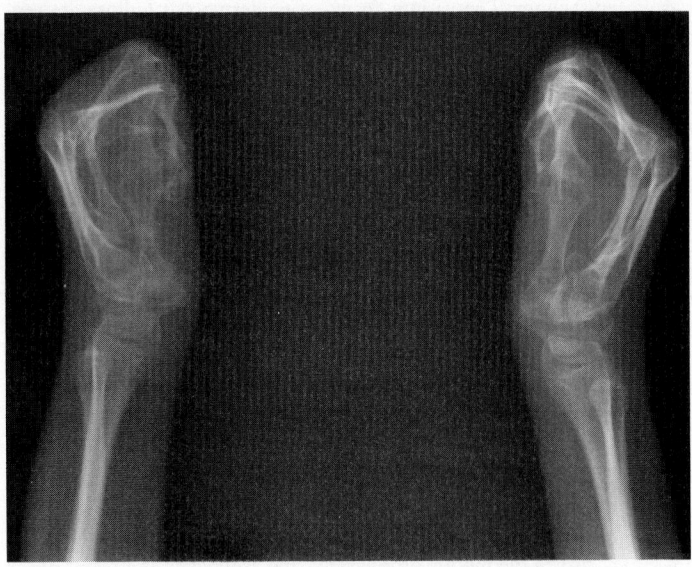

FIGURE 58–8. Radiograph showing severe contraction deformities of the hands referred to as mummification.

associate eating with pain and become severely malnourished. Esophageal occlusion occurs by food impacting in the strictured area or bullae forming in the stricture.[166]

Spontaneous dissection of the esophageal wall creating a "double-barrel" deformity on esophagram has been reported.[168] Esophageal rupture has occurred in patients who have tried to forcefully swallow solid food[168] and during bougienage.[170] Gastroesophageal reflux does not appear to be a major factor in the etiology of the lower esophageal strictures.[172]

The esophagram is the diagnostic test of choice for evaluating EBD-R patients with dysphagia because this produces almost no trauma to the mucosa. However, the radiographic picture may be similar to that of peptic esophagitis, esophageal cancer, candidal or herpetic infections, chemical- or irradiation-induced esophagitis, and scleroderma.[170] Endoscopy has no primary role in the diagnostic evaluation of these patients because trauma may induce further bulla formation. Careful endoscopy has been used to remove impacted food, to rupture lumen-occluding bulla, and to perform esophageal dilatations.[170]

The prognosis of esophageal involvement in EBD-R is poor.[166] Patients should be advised to avoid coarse foods and hot foods. In many cases, a pureed diet or nutritionally complete liquid diet may be necessary to avoid malnutrition. During periods of complete esophageal occlusion, total parenteral nutrition has been used. Dysphagia may be relieved by corticosteroid therapy, but failure to respond is also reported.[166,170,171] Dilantin has also been reported to be of some benefit in treating skin lesions, but an effect on esophageal lesions is not well documented.[173] Esophageal strictures, once formed, are permanent. Endoscopy with bougienage has been successful in a number of cases, but the potential for esophageal trauma and perforation is high.[166] In patients with severe esophageal stenosis and malnutrition or perforation, esophagectomy with colonic interposition has been performed.[166,170,171] Patients with interpositions have relief of dysphagia and improved nutrition in a 10-year follow-up period.[174] Nearly complete esophagectomy is advocated at the time of surgery because there is an increased risk of cancer formation in the esophageal mucosa of patients with EBD-R.[175]

Mallory–Weiss Laceration

In 1929, Mallory and Weiss described alcoholic patients who had retching and emesis followed by massive hematemesis due to linear mucosal tears of the gastric mucosa near the esophagogastric junction.[176] Subsequent reports have shown that the incidence of such tears among patients who present with upper gastrointestinal bleeding varies from 1% to 13%, with 5% being the most commonly

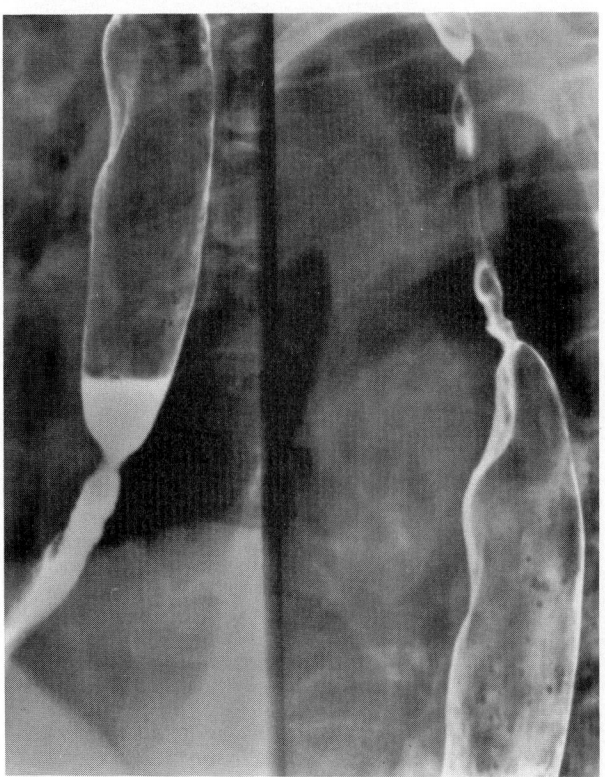

FIGURE 58–9. Patient with EBD-R demonstrating strictures of the proximal and distal esophagus.

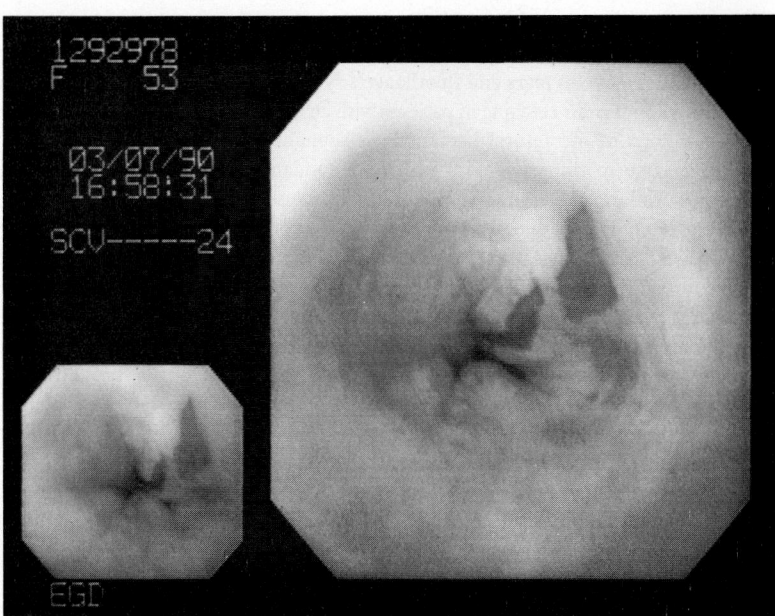

FIGURE 58–10. (See Color Fig 21) Nonpenetrating mucosal laceration following retching in a 53-year-old woman.

reported incidence.[177–183] Multiple mucosal lacerations have been found in up to 27% of the cases. Tears tend to occur more commonly in men than women, with a 4:1 ratio.[178,179,183] The patients are typically in the third to fifth decade of life, but patients as young as 3 weeks of age have been reported.[183,184] The widespread use of fiberoptic endoscopy has greatly increased our awareness of these tears and our understanding of their clinical significance.

Mallory–Weiss tears are characterized by the presence of nonpenetrating mucosal lacerations in either the distal esophagus or the proximal stomach (Fig 58-10; Color Fig 21). Although the etiology is not fully understood, these mucosal lacerations have been noted to be present after events that suddenly raise intra-abdominal pressure, such as retching, emesis, coughing, seizures, hiccups under anesthesia, closed-chest massage, straining with lifting or stooling, and blunt abdominal trauma.[177–179,184] During emesis, the esophageal transmural pressure rapidly changes as much as 100 mm Hg.[179] Emesis due to alcoholism has been the most frequently reported event associated with Mallory–Weiss tears, but emesis due to any cause, chemotherapy for example, may be responsible.[176–180,183,185] Hiatal hernias are found in 42% to 80% of these patients and may be a risk factor.[179,183] The intraluminal pressure in the herniated portion of the stomach is the same as in the subdiaphragmatic area despite its intrathoracic location. This may increase the change in transmural pressures during emesis and increase the potential for mucosal laceration. Some authors postulate that transient hiatal hernias may form in patients who develop such tears and do not have evidence of hiatal hernias.[178]

Patients will most often give a history of retching or nonbloody emesis prior to the onset of hematemesis.[177] Rarely, patients with actively bleeding tears have presented with hematochezia or no history of a forceful abdominal event.[170] The bleeding may vary from a self-limited episode of hematemesis to massive hemorrhage with melena and shock occasionally requiring intensive care and transfusions.

In patients with upper gastrointestinal bleeding, gastric ulcers, duodenal ulcers, and gastritis have been more common than Mallory–Weiss tears as the source of blood loss.[180,181,186] Conversely, in as many as 77% of patients who have bleeding tears, other pathologic lesions are present.[178,179] Patients with known esophageal varices are especially difficult to evaluate. Mallory–Weiss tears were the source of bleeding in 4.8% of these patients in one series.[182] However, whether variceal bleeding and emesis precipitated the tear or the tear precipitated massive variceal bleeding is unclear.

Early endoscopy is the most sensitive diagnostic modality to document the presence of a bleeding tear and offers the opportunity for therapeutic intervention.[178,179,184] Other tests such as Tc-99m sulfur colloid scan, esophagrams, and angiography have occasionally been positive but are not as reliable as endoscopy.[187]

A vast majority of patients with Mallory–Weiss tears will stop bleeding spontaneously and require no intervention other than hemodynamic support.[183] Endoscopic hemostatic therapy by injection of anhydrous ethanol (98%)[180] or multipolar electrocoagulation[186,188] has gained widespread acceptance as the first-line treatment of actively bleeding tears. Occasional failures have been due to poor visualization caused by torrential bleeding. Injection of epinephrine 1:10,000 in the area surrounding the lesion usually provides adequate temporary hemostasis to allow electrocoagulation. Surgery was once the only effective intervention[184,189] and may still be necessary if the bleeding cannot be controlled. Intravenous infusion of vasopressin has rarely been reported to control the hemorrhage.[179,184,190] Esophageal balloon tamponade is particularly hazardous because the tear may be extended or the frequently present hiatal hernia may be ruptured.[178,179,186] Angiographic arterial embolization has also been occasionally reported, but endoscopic diagnosis and therapy is the treatment of choice.

ESOPHAGEAL INTRAMURAL HEMATOMAS

In rare circumstances, intramural hematomas of the esophagus will develop spontaneously by dissection of the mucosa from the muscular layers. The hematoma may completely obstruct the esophagus, occasionally forming a second lumen, the "double-barrel" esophagus.[191] Intramural hematomas have occurred without gender predominance in patients ranging in age from 21 to 81 years.[192,193] These hematomas usually occur in settings similar to those of Mallory–Weiss tears and Boerhaave's syndrome but may also occur without prior retching in patients with coagulopathies.[194]

The etiology of intramural hematoma is thought to be mechanical damage to the esophageal wall by a sudden change in transmural wall pressures due to a variety of causes, such as coughing, retching, or sneezing.[192] In several reported cases of esophageal hematomas there has been suspicion of medication- or foreign body–induced esophageal damage preceding the event.[195–197] Also, an esophageal hematoma has been reported to occur after variceal sclerotherapy.[196] Patients with a coagulopathy, congenital or secondary to anticoagulant therapy, may develop spontaneous intramural hematomas with little or no history of esophageal barotrauma.[192,194]

Patients with hematomas often present with sharp substernal chest pain and dysphagia preceding hematemesis.[191,193–195,197] Many of these patients report retching or aborted sneezes prior to the onset of pain and hematemesis.[194] The amount of bleeding varies from lightly blood-tinged emesis to massive bleeding requiring up to 6 units of blood transfusion. In some cases, esophageal obstruction can be pronounced.

Patients presenting with severe substernal chest pain and hematemesis require early endoscopy as the evaluation of choice. Typically, a mass with bluish discoloration is seen protruding into the esophageal lumen. The appearance has been confused with carcinoma on occasion.[194] Esophagrams show a filling defect in the esophagus, and the true and false lumens may be separated by a thin "mucosal stripe" or give the "double-barrel" esophagus image.[191,198] Leiomyoma, carcinoma, and metastatic disease can have similar radiographic appearances, but the esophagrams are generally diagnostic.[194] Computed tomography with contrast is also very useful in the evaluation of esophageal hematomas. Typically, a nonenhancing esophageal mass that has the CT density of blood is evident.[193,195,197]

Although the acute presentation of an esophageal hematoma is dramatic, with dysphagia, esophageal occlusion, and often hematemesis, the clinical course and long-term consequences are relatively mild. Symptoms generally resolve in 2 to 10 days with conservative therapy.[191,194–197] Nutritional support and aspiration precautions are necessary, and underlying coagulopathy should be corrected. Blood transfusion is occasionally required. Rarely, the patient may develop fever and a pleural effusion due to an esophageal perforation that was not detected earlier.[198]

ESOPHAGEAL INJURY AND RUPTURE

Esophageal rupture is a life-threatening injury that is difficult to diagnose yet frequently requires early surgical intervention. It may be iatrogenic following instrumentation of the esophagus, may be secondary to external abdominal or thoracic trauma, or may occur spontaneously, as in Boerhaave's syndrome. Patients aged 1 to more than 80 years have presented with esophageal rupture, with a mean age ranging from 28 to 43 years, without a gender or race predominance.[199,200] Successful management of patients with rupture depends on early diagnosis and intervention.

The esophagus may rupture by intraluminal trauma from either foreign bodies or medical devices or by extracorporeal trauma to the abdomen or chest. In one series of 69 patients, 48% of the ruptures were iatrogenic, 33% were due to external trauma, and only 8% were spontaneous.[199] Iatrogenic esophageal rupture is a well-recognized risk of rigid or flexible endoscopy, bougienage or balloon dilation of esophageal strictures, and dilation of the lower esophageal sphincter for achalasia.[199,201–205] However, rupture has also been reported in conjunction with placement of nasogastric tubes, erroneous inflation of a gastric balloon in the esophagus, sclerotherapy, and balloon tamponade for bleeding esophageal varices.[199,206,207]

Trauma that involves penetration of the neck, thorax, or upper abdomen should always raise the suspicion of a penetrating esophageal injury.[208] Rarely, blunt thoracoabdominal trauma causes esophageal rupture by rapid changes of the esophageal transmural pressure[200,209] similar to the pathophysiology of Mallory–Weiss lacerations. However, the majority of these ruptures are found to be in the cervical and upper thoracic esophagus rather than distally.[200] The Heimlich maneuver is effective by rapidly raising intrathoracic pressure to dislodge a tracheal obstruction and occasionally has been reported to cause esophageal rupture with severe complications despite having saved the patient from asphyxia.[210,211] Motor vehicle accidents are frequently accompanied by blunt trauma to the chest by the steering wheel. The esophagus may also suffer contusion with interruption of the vascular supply, leading to necrosis and perforation some days later.[200,209]

Spontaneous esophageal rupture was first described in 1724 by Boerhaave. His patient, Baron von Wassenaer, died suddenly after severe retching and emesis and was found at autopsy to have an esophageal rupture and food contaminating the thorax.[212] Although spontaneous esophageal rupture (Boerhaave's syndrome) was initially thought quite rare, the number of reported cases has been increasing, probably because of heightened awareness and accurate diagnosis.[213,214] Any maneuver that transiently elevates the intra-abdominal pressure, such as lifting or straining, may result in spontaneous esophageal rupture. The majority of spontaneous ruptures occur in the distal esophagus.[199] Lack of a serosal membrane has been thought to contribute to the ease of esophageal rupture,[209] but careful histologic examination of surgically resected specimens from two patients demonstrated an absence of the muscularis mucosa in the esophageal wall surrounding the rupture site.[215] Thus, some patients may be predisposed to spontaneous rupture.

The clinical manifestations of esophageal rupture are diverse and dependent on the extent and acuity of the rupture. As many as 50% of patients with iatrogenic perforations may be asymptomatic for the first 8 hours.[199] Similarly, trauma victims may have esophageal injury overlooked in the urgency to treat more obvious injuries.[200] Cervical and upper esophageal ruptures may be accompanied by neck and chest pain, subcutaneous emphysema, dysphagia, odynophagia, nausea, vomiting, hematemesis, hoarseness, or aphonia.[199,200,204,216] More distal perforations present with similar findings, but in addition there may be abdominal pain, pneumothorax, or pneumomediastinum (Fig 58-11). Occasionally, the examiner may hear a "Hamman's crunch," a rasping crackle in cadence with the cardiac sounds, on auscultation of the chest. The symptoms of vomiting, chest pain, and subcutaneous emphysema referred to as Mackler's triad are nonspecific and only reported in a third of patient's with Boerhaave's syndrome.[199] Intense thirst for small sips of cold water has been reported in two patients with early spontaneous esophageal rupture.[217] Sudden massive esophageal rupture may be dramatic, presenting with tension pneumothorax, hypotension, and shock. The clinical outcome of such patients is dependent on early diagnosis and management.

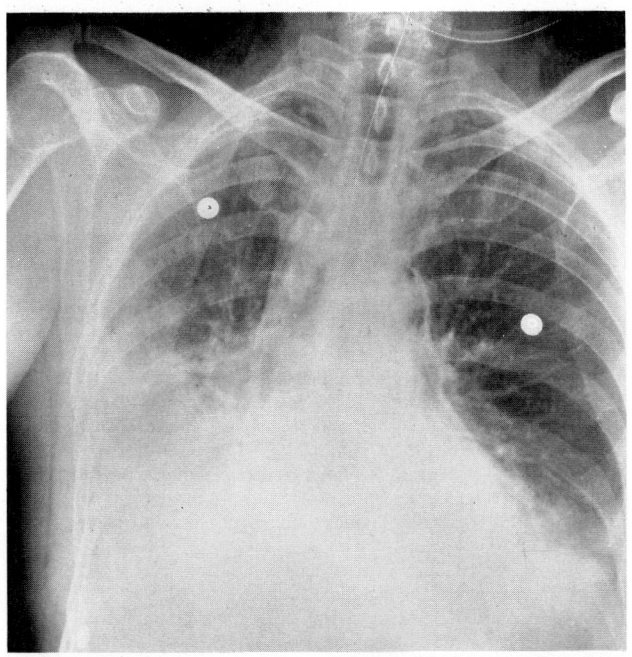

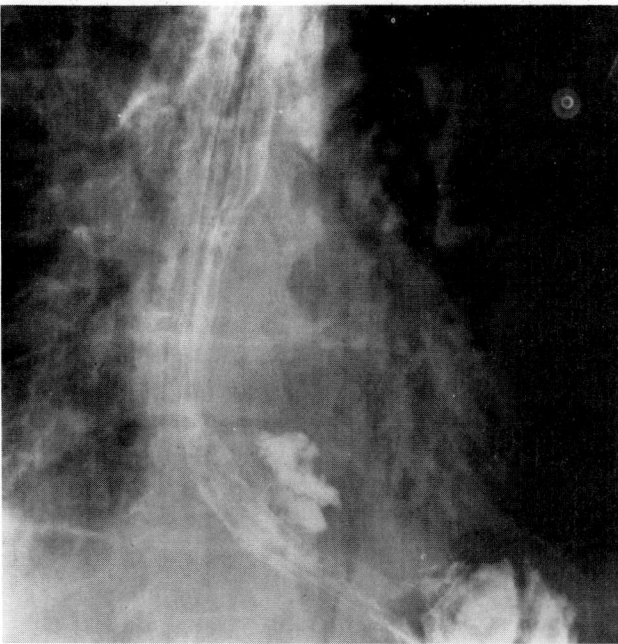

FIGURE 58–11. Boerhaave's syndrome in a 57-year-old who presented with chest pain following an episode of retching and vomiting. Chest radiograph (**A**) showing effusion and infiltrate in right lower lobe and subcutaneous air in soft tissues. Esophagram (**B**) demonstrates extravasation of barium from the site of perforation.

Evaluation of patients for the presence of an esophageal rupture requires a high index of suspicion. The presenting symptoms are vague and may be similar to those of patients with pulmonary embolus, myocardial infarction, aortic dissection, Mallory–Weiss laceration, spontaneous pneumothorax, pancreatitis, strangulated diaphragmatic hernia, or perforated peptic ulcer.[213] The physical examination may detect presence of crepitance. Chest and abdominal radiographs are helpful to detect subcutaneous emphysema, pneumothorax, pneumomediastinum, pleural effusion, and free

air in the peritoneal cavity[204,213] but may be normal in up to 33% of cases initially.[199] Esophagrams employing water-soluble contrast such as Gastrografin with multidirectional views are diagnostic in most cases.[199,200,213,215,216] If these are negative, barium esophagrams, which provide better definition, should be obtained. Upper endoscopy may be useful to establish the diagnosis but may miss small ruptures and increases the risk of extending the esophageal perforation. Cervical penetrating injuries are a special case. The cervical esophagus is difficult to fully evaluate at surgery, and pre- or intraoperative endoscopy is warranted.[208]

The diagnosis may be delayed for several days until the patient develops fever, mediastinitis, pleural effusion, or sepsis. Examination of the pleural fluid reveals an exudate with a pH as low as 6.0 due to a combination of gastric acid refluxed through the esophageal defect and the metabolism of leukocytes.[218,219] Elevated amylase in the pleural fluid is of salivary origin. Bacterial infection of the pleural fluid, empyema, is common, and thoracic myonecrosis rarely occurs.[220]

Therapy depends upon the site and size of the defect, the time elapsed between rupture and diagnosis, and the overall health status of the patient. Clearly, cardiorespiratory support and antibiotics are the initial concern. If the rupture is small and confined or in the cervical esophagus, medical management may be appropriate. The majority of patients who sustain an esophageal rupture and are diagnosed early will require surgical intervention.[199,200,204,213,216,221] Primary closure is the treatment of choice if there is no underlying esophageal disease.[199] Partial esophagectomy has occasionally been necessary. If the esophageal rupture is diagnosed later, the management goals are drainage of the infected area and prevention of further leakage. Multiple chest tubes and esophageal diversion may be appropriate.[221] The patient will have a prolonged hospital course requiring nutritional support and often multiple procedures.

The reader is directed to Chapter 7, Esophageal Motor Function; Chapter 28, Approach to the Patient with Dysphagia; Chapter 29, Approach to the Patient with Chest Pain; Chapter 44, Skin Lesions Associated with Gastrointestinal Diseases; Chapter 45, Approach to Gastrointestinal Problems in the Elderly; Chapter 46, Approach to Gastrointestinal Problems in the Immunocompromised Patient; Chapter 47, Approach to Gastrointestinal Problems Associated with Common Clinical Conditions; Chapter 53, Esophagus: Anatomy and Structural Anomalies; Chapter 54, Motility Disorders of the Esophagus; Chapter 55, Reflux Esophagitis; Chapter 56, Esophageal Infections; Chapter 57, Esophageal Tumors; Chapter 106, Gastrointestinal Manifestations of Systemic Diseases; Chapter 107, Gastrointestinal Manifestations of Immunologic Disorders; Chapter 111, Upper Gastrointestinal Endoscopy; Chapter 114, Contrast Radiology; Chapter 126, Endoscopic Mucosal Biopsy; Chapter 131, Gastrointestinal Dilation; and Chapter 139, Procedure-Related Complications.

REFERENCES

1. Leape LL, Ashcraft KW, Scarpelli DG, et al. Hazard to health—Liquid lye. N Engl J Med 1971;287:578.
2. Maves MD, Carithers JS, Birck HG. Esophageal burns secondary to disc battery ingestion. Ann Otol Rhinol Laryngol 1984;93:364.

3. Meredith JW, Kon ND, Thompson JN. Management of injuries from liquid lye ingestion. J Trauma 1988;8:1173.

4. Sellars SL, Spence RAJ. Chemical burns of the oesophagus. J Laryngol Otol 1987;101:1211.

5. Friedman EM. Caustic ingestions and foreign body aspirations: An overlooked form of child abuse. Ann Otol Rhinol Laryngol 1987;96:709,987.

6. Moore WR. Caustic ingestions: Pathophysiology, diagnosis, and treatment. Clin Pediatr 1986;25:192.

7. Vancura EM, Clinton JE, Ruiz E, et al. Toxicity of alkaline solutions. Ann Emerg Med 1980;9:118.

8. Edmonson MB. Caustic alkali ingestions by farm children. Pediatrics 1987;79:413.

9. Lacouture PG, Gaudreault P, Lovejoy FH. Clinitest tablet ingestion: An in vitro investigation concerned with initial emergency management. Ann Emerg Med 1986;15:143.

10. Rivera EA, Maves MD. Effects of neutralizing agents on esophageal burns caused by disc batteries. Ann Otol Rhinol Laryngol 1987;96:362.

11. Hawkins DB, Demeter MJ, Barnett TE. Caustic ingestion: Controversies in management. Laryngoscope 1980;90:98.

12. Hill L, Kozarek R, McCallum R, Mercer CD. The esophagus: Medical and surgical management. Philadelphia: WB Saunders, 1988:220.

13. Sleisenger MH, Fordtran JS. Gastrointestinal disease, vol 1, ed 4. Philadelphia: WB Saunders, 1989:203.

14. Maull KI, Scher LA, Greenfield LJ. Surgical implications of acid ingestion. Surg Gynecol Obstet 1979;148:895.

15. Isolauri J, Markkula H, Auvinen O. Copper sulfate corrosion and necrosis of the esophagus and stomach. Acta Chir Scand 1986;15:701.

16. Tucker JA, Yarington CT Jr. The treatment of caustic ingestion. Otolaryngol Clin North Am 1979;12:343.

17. Hollinger PH. Management of esophageal lesions caused by chemical burns. Ann Otol Rhinol Laryngol 1968;77:819.

18. Allen RE, Thoshinsky MJ, Stallone RJ, et al. Corrosive injuries of the stomach. Arch Surg 1970;100:409.

19. Wason S. The emergency management of caustic ingestions. J Emerg Med 1987;79:413.

20. Ritter F, Newman MH, Newman DE. A clinical and experimental study of corrosive burns of the stomach. Ann Otol Rhinol Laryngol 1968;77:830.

21. Coln D, Chang JHT. Experience with esophageal stenting for caustic burns in children. J Pediatr Surg 1986;21:588.

22. Krey H. On the treatment of corrosive lesions in the esophagus. Acta Otolaryngol (Stockh) 1952;102(Suppl):1.

23. Ritter FN. Lye burns of the esophagus and their treatments. Adv Otorhinolaryngol 1978;23:104.

24. Haller JA Jr, Andrews HG, White JJ, et al. Pathophysiology and management of acute corrosive burns of the esophagus: Results of treatment in 285 children. J Pediatr Surg 1971;6:578.

25. Ashcraft KW, Padula R. The effect of dilute corrosives on the esophagus. Pediatrics 1974;53:226.

26. Penner GE. Acid ingestion: Toxicology and treatment. Ann Emerg Med 1980;9:374.

27. Rothstein FC. Caustic injuries to the esophagus in children. Pediatr Clin North Am 1986;33:665.

28. Gaudreault P, Parent M, McGuigan MA, Chicoine L, Lovejoy FH Jr. Predictability of esophageal injury from signs and symptoms: A study of caustic ingestion in 378 children. Pediatrics 1983;71:767.

29. Sarfati E, Gossot D, Assens P, Celerier M. Management of caustic ingestion in adults. Br J Surg 1987;74:146.

30. Cello JP, Fogel RP, Boland CR. Liquid caustic ingestion: Spectrum of injury. Arch Intern Med 1980;140:501.

31. Moazam F, Talbert JL, Miller D, Mollitt DL. Caustic ingestion and its sequelae in children. South Med J 1987;80:187.

32. Crain EF, Gershel JC, Mezey AP. Caustic ingestions: Symptoms as predictors of esophageal injury. Am J Dis Childhood 1984;138:863.

33. Postlethwait RW. Chemical burns of the esophagus. Surg Clin North Am 1983;63:915.

34. Di Costanzo J, Noirclerc M, Jouglard J, et al. New therapeutic approach to corrosive burns of the upper gastrointestinal tract. Gut 1982;21:370.

35. Ferguson MK, Migliore M, Staszak VM, Little AG. Early evaluation and therapy for caustic esophageal injury. Am J Surg 1989;157:116.

36. Maves MD, Lloyd TV, Carithers JS. Radiographic identification of ingested disc batteries. Pediatr Radiol 1986;16:154.

37. Adam JS, Birck HG. Pediatric caustic ingestion. Ann Otol Rhinol Laryngol 1982;91:656.

38. Howell JM. Alkaline ingestions. Ann Emerg Med 1986;15:820.

39. Campbell GS, Burnett HF, Ransom JM, Williams GD. Treatment of corrosive burns of the esophagus. Arch Surg 1977;112:495.

40. Symbas PN, Vlasis SE, Hatcher CR. Esophagitis secondary to ingestion of caustic material. Ann Thorac Surg 1983;36:73.

41. Middlekamp JN, Ferguson TB, Roper CL, Hoffman FD. The management and problem of caustic burns in children. J Thorac Cardiovasc Surg 1969;57:341.

42. Muhletaler CA, Gerlock AJ, de Soto L, Halter SA. Acid corrosive esophagitis: Radiographic findings. AJR 1980;134:1137.

43. Kozarek FA, Sanowski RA. Caustic cicatrization of the pharynx associated with dysphagia and premalignant mucosal changes. Am J Gastroenterol 1982;77:5.

44. Chodak GW, Passaro E. Acid ingestion: Need for gastric resection. JAMA 1978;239:225.

45. Love L, Berkow AE. Trauma to the esophagus. Gastrointest Radiol 1978;2:305.

46. Burrington JD. Surgical management of the tracheoesophageal fistula complicating caustic ingestion. Surgery 1978;84:329.

47. Ottosson A. Late aortic rupture after lye ingestion. Arch Toxicol 1981;47:59.

48. Greif F, Kaplan O. Acid ingestion: Another cause of disseminated intravascular coagulopathy. Crit Care Med 1986;14:990.

49. Reyes HM, Lin CY, Schlunk FF, Replogle RL. Experimental treatment of corrosive esophageal burns. J Pediatr Surg 1974;9:317.

50. Appelqvist P, Salmo M. Lye corrosion carcinoma of the esophagus. Cancer 1980;45:2655.

51. Csikos M, Horvath O, Petri A, Petri I, Imre J. Late malignant transformation of chronic corrosive oesophageal strictures. Langenbecks Arch Chir 1985;365:231.

52. Kiviranta JK. Corrosion carcinoma of the esophagus: Cases of corrosion and nine cases of corrosion carcinoma. Acta Otolaryngol (Stockh) 1952;42:89.

53. Hopkins RA, Postlethwait RW. Caustic burns and carcinoma of the esophagus. Ann Surg 1981;194:146.

54. Appelqvist P, Mattila S, Jyrala A, Tala P. Surgical treatment of carcinoma of the oesophagus and cardia. Scand J Thorac Cardiovasc Surg 1977;11:278.

55. Bovill EG, Bulawa FA, Olivetti RG. Severe corrosive gastritis with antral stenosis following ingestion of Sani-Flush. Gastroenterology 1951;17:436.

56. Karon AB. The delayed gastric syndrome with pyloric stenosis and achlorhydria following the ingestion of acid—A definite clinical entity. Am J Dig Dis 1962;7:1041.

57. Steigmann F, Dolehide RA. Corrosive (acid) gastritis: Management of early and late cases. N Engl J Med 1956;254:981.

58. Eaton H, Tennekoon GE. Squamous carcinoma of the stomach following corrosive acid burns. Br J Surg 1972;59:382.

59. Maull KI. Surgical implications of acid ingestion. Surg Gynecol Obstet 1979;148:895.

60. Rumack BH, Burrington JD. Caustic ingestion: A rational look at diluents. Clin Toxicol 1977;11:27.

61. Kirsh MM, Ritter F. Caustic ingestion and subsequent damage to the oropharyngeal and digestive passages. Ann Thorac Surg 1976;21:74.

62. Weisskopf A. Effects of cortisone on experimental lye burns and strictures of the esophagus. J Thorac Surg 1954;24:483.

63. Oakes DD, Sherck JP, Mark JBD. Lye ingestion: Clinical patterns and therapeutic implications. J Thorac Cardiovasc Surg 1982;83:194.

64. Gehanno P, Guidon C. Prohibition of experimental esophageal lye strictures by penicillamine. Arch Otorhinolaryngol 1981;107:145.

65. Butler C, Madden JW, Davis WM, et al. Morphologic aspects of experimental esophageal stricture, II: Effect of steroid hormones, bougienage, and lathyrisms on acute lye burns. Surgery 1977;81:431.

66. Liu AJ, Richardson MA. Effects of N-acetylcysteine on experimen-

tally induced esophageal lye injury. Ann Otol Rhinol Laryngol 1985;94:477.

67. Reddy AN, Budhraja M. Sucralfate therapy for lye-induced esophagitis. Am J Gastroenterol 1987;83:71.

68. Reyes HM, Hill JL. Modification of the experimental stent technique for esophageal burns. J Surg Res 1976;20:65.

69. Hogan RB, Polter DE. Nonsurgical management of lye-induced antral stricture with hydrostatic balloon dilation. Gastrointest Endosc 1986;32:228.

70. Wienbeck M, Berges W, Lübke HJ. Drug-induced oesophageal lesions. Baillieres Clin Gastroenterol 1988;2:263.

71. Mason SJ, O'Meara TF. Drug-induced esophagitis. J Clin Gastroenterol 1981;3:115.

72. Kikendall JW, Friedman AC, Oyewole MA, Fleischer D, Johnson LF. Pill-induced esophageal injury: Case reports and review of the medical literature. Dig Dis Sci 1983;28:174.

73. Lambert JR, Newman A. Ulceration and stricture of the esophagus due to the oral potassium chloride (slow release tablet) therapy. Am J Gastroenterol 1980;73:508.

74. Delpre G, Kadish U, Stahl B. Induction of esophageal injuries by doxycycline and other pills: A frequent but preventable occurrence. Dig Dis Sci 1989;34:797.

75. Channer KS, Virjee JP. The effect of size and shape of tablets on their esophageal transit. J Clin Pharmacol 1986;26:141.

76. Marvola M, Rajaniemi M, Marttila E, Vahervuo K, Sothman A. Effect of dosage form and formulation factors on the adherence of drugs to the esophagus. J Pharm Sci 1983;72:1034.

77. McDonald GB. Esophageal diseases caused by infection, systemic illness and trauma. In: Sleisenger MH, Fordtran JS. Gastrointestinal disease, vol 1, ed 4. Philadelphia: WB Saunders, 1988:640.

78. Agha FP, Wilson JAP, Nostrand TT. Medication-induced esophagitis. Gastrointest Radiol 1986;11:7.

79. Ravich WJ, Kashima M, Donner MW. Drug-induced esophagitis simulating esophageal carcinoma. Dysphagia 1986;1:13.

80. Bunn PA, Lichter AS, Makuch RW, et al. Chemotherapy alone or chemotherapy with chest radiation therapy in limited stage small cell lung cancer. A prospective, randomized trial. Ann Intern Med 1987;106:655.

81. Coia LR, Engstrom PR, Paul A. Nonsurgical management of esophageal cancer: Report of a study of combined radiotherapy and chemotherapy. J Clin Oncol 1987;5:1783.

82. Stillwagon GB, Order SE, Guse C, et al. 194 hepatocellular cancers treated by radiation and chemotherapy combinations: Toxicity and response: A Radiation Oncology Group study. Int J Radiat Oncol Biol Phys 1989;17:1223.

83. Umsawsdi T, Valdivieso M, Barkley HT, et al. Esophageal complications from combined chemoradiotherapy (cyclophosphamide + Adriamycin + cisplatin + XRT) in the treatment of non–small cell lung cancer. Int J Radiat Oncol Biol Phys 1985;11:511.

84. D'Angio GJ, Farber S, Maddock CL. Potentiation of x-ray effects by actinomycin D. Radiology 1959;73:175.

85. Arcangeli G, Righini R, Nervi C, et al. Pilot study of multiple-fraction daily radiotherapy alternating with chemotherapy in patients with stage IV non–oat cell lung cancer. Cancer Treat Rev 1985;69:25.

86. Seydel HG, Diener-West M, Urtasun R, et al. Hyperfractionation in the radiation therapy of unresectable non–oat cell carcinoma of the lung: Preliminary report of a RTOG pilot study. Int J Radiat Oncol Biol Phys 1985;11:1841.

87. Northway MG, Eastwood GL, Libshitz HI, et al. Antiinflammatory agents protect opossum esophagus during radiotherapy. Dig Dis Sci 1982;27:923.

88. Chowhan NM. Injurious effects of radiation on the esophagus. Am J Gastroenterol 1990;85:115.

89. Rothstein RD, Ouyang A. Chest pain of esophageal origin. Gastroenterol Clin North Am 1989;18:257.

90. Papazian A, Capron JP, Ducroix JP, et al. Mucosal bridges of the upper esophagus after radiotherapy of Hodgkin's disease. Gastroenterology 1983;84:1028.

91. Fajardo LF, Lee A. Rupture of major vessels after radiation. Cancer 1975;36:904.

92. Finkelstein E. Letter: Nifedipine for radiation oesophagitis. Lancet 1986;1:1205.

93. Nelson RS, Hernandez AJ, Goldstein HM, Saca A. Treatment of irradiation esophagitis: value of hydrocortisone injection. Am J Gastroenterol 1979;71:17.

94. Nicolopoulos N, Mantidis A, Stathopoulos E, et al. Prophylactic administration of indomethacin for irradiation esophagitis. Radiother Oncol 1985;3:23.

95. Bloom J, Rapaport Y, Zikk D. Dairy product containers as a source of unusual esophageal foreign bodies. J Otolaryngol 1988;17:404.

96. Jackson C, Jackson CL. Bronchoesophagology. Philadelphia: WB Saunders, 1950:13.

97. Chaikouni A, Kratz JM, Crawford FA. Foreign bodies of the esophagus. Am J Surg 1985;51:173.

98. Trenkner SW, Maglinte DDT, Lehman GA, Chernish SM, Miller RE, Johnson CW. Esophageal food impaction: Treatment with glucagon. Radiology 1983;149:401.

99. Shaffer HA, Alford BA, deLange EE, et al. Basket extraction of esophageal foreign bodies. AJR 1986;147:1010.

100. Beg MH, Reyazuddin, Hasan A. Esophageal foreign bodies. Indian J Pediatr 1988;55:323.

101. Kramer TA, Riding KH, Salkeld LJ. Tracheobronchial and esophageal foreign bodies in the pediatric population. J Otolaryngol 1986;15:155.

102. Fernandes ET, Hollabaugh RS, Boulden T. Mediastinal mass and radiolucent esophageal foreign body. J Pediatr Surg 1989;24:1135.

103. Bendig DW. Removal of blunt esophageal foreign bodies by flexible endoscopy without general anesthesia. Am J Dis Child 1986;140:789.

104. Campbell JB, Condon VR. Catheter removal of blunt esophageal foreign bodies in children: Survey of the Society for Pediatric Radiology. Pediatr Radiol 1989;19:361.

105. Kobayashi T. Esophageal foreign bodies in children. Int J Pediatr Otorhinolaryngol 1984;7:193.

106. Lui RC, Johnson FE, Horovitz JH, Cunningham JN. Aortoesophageal fistula: Case report and literature review. J Vasc Surg 1987;6:379.

107. Schumacher KJ, Weaver DL, Knight MR, Presberg HJ. Aortic pseudoaneurysm due to ingested foreign body. South Med J 1986;79:146.

108. Alexander AA, Hayden CK, Swischuk LE. Catheter removal of esophageal foreign bodies: Push or pull? AJR 1988;151:835.

109. Healy GB. Removal of esophageal foreign bodies with a Foley catheter under fluoroscopic control [letter]. Can Med Assoc J 1988;138:490.

110. Crysdale WS. Removal of esophageal foreign bodies with a Foley catheter under fluoroscopic control [letter]. Can Med Assoc J 1987;137:988.

111. Crysdale WS. Removal of esophageal foreign bodies with a Foley catheter under fluoroscopic control [letter]. Can Med Assoc J 1988;138:490.

112. Mee AS, Wright JP. Endoscopic removal of sharp foreign objects using an oversleeve. S Afr Med J 1981;7:743.

113. Witzel L, Scheurer U, Muhlemann A, Halter F. Removal of razor blades from the stomach with fiberoptic endoscope. Br Med J 1974;8:539.

114. Spiro HM. Clinical gastroenterology, ed 3. New York: Macmillan Publishing Co. 1983;99:120.

115. Maycock RL, Bertrand P, Morrison CE, et al. Manifestations of sarcoidosis: Analysis of 145 patients, with a review of nine series selected from the literature. Medicine 1963;35:67.

116. Palmer ED. Note on silent sarcoidosis of the gastric mucosa. J Lab Clin Med 1958;52:231.

117. Wiesner PJ, Kleinman MS, Condemi JJ, Resnicoff SA, Schwartz SI. Sarcoidosis of the esophagus. Dig Dis 1971;16:943.

118. Oakley JR, Lawrence DAS, Fiddian RV. Sarcoidosis associated with Crohn's disease of ileum, mouth and oesophagus. J R Soc Med 1983;76:1068.

119. Maffei VJ, Zaatari GS, McGarity WC, Mansour KA. Crohn's disease of the esophagus. J Thorac Cardiovasc Surg 1987;94:302.

120. Cook DM, Dines DE, Dycus DE. Sarcoidosis: Report of a case presenting as dysphagia. Chest 1970;75:84.

121. Dufresne CR, Jeyasingham K, Baker RR. Achalasia of the cardia associated with pulmonary sarcoidosis. Surgery 1983;94:32.

122. Levine MS. Crohn's disease of the upper gastrointestinal tract. 1987;25:79.

123. Kurtz B, Steinhardt HJ, Malchow H. The radiological and endoscopic appearances of Crohn's disease of the upper gastro-intestinal tract. Fortschr Rontgenstr 1982;136:124.

124. Legee DA, Carlson HC, Judd ES. Roentgenologic features of regional enteritis of the upper gastrointestinal tract. AJR 1970;110:355.

125. Geboes K, Janssens J, Rutgeerts P, Vantrappen G. Crohn's disease of the esophagus. J Clin Gastroenterol 1986;8:31.

126. Gore RM, Ghahremani GG. Crohn's disease of the upper gastrointestinal tract. Crit Rev Diagn Imaging 1986;25:305.

127. Ghahremani GG, Gore RM, Breuer RI, Larson RH. Esophageal manifestations of Crohn's disease. Gastrointest Radiol 1982;7:199.

128. Freson M, Kottler RE, Wright JP. Crohn's disease of the oesophagus. A case report. S Afr Med J 1984;66:417.

129. Klein GL, Ament ME, Sparkes RS. Monozygotic twins with Crohn's disease: A case report. Gastroenterology 1980;79:931.

130. Madden JL, Ravid JM, Haddad JR. Regional esophagitis: A specific entity simulating Crohn's disease. Ann Surg 1969;170:351.

131. Huchzermeyer H, Paul F, Seifert E, Fröhlich H, Rasmussen CW. Endoscopic results in five patients with Crohn's disease of the esophagus. Endoscopy 1977;8:75.

132. Gelfand MD, Krone CL. Dysphagia and esophageal ulceration in Crohn's disease. Gastroenterology 1968;55:510.

133. LiVolsi VA, Jaretzki A. Granulomatous esophagitis. A case of Crohn's disease limited to the esophagus. Gastroenterology 1973;64:313.

134. Fröhlich H, Huchzermeyer H, St. Stender H. The radiological findings in oesophagitis due to Crohn's disease. Fortschr Rontgenstr 1976;125:497.

135. Behcet H. Uber rezidivierende apthose, durch ein Virus verursachte Geschwure am Munde, am Auge und an den Gentalien. Dermatol Wochenschr 1937;105:1152.

136. Mori S, Yoshihira A, Kawamura H, et al. Esophageal involvement in Behcet's disease. Am J Gastroenterol 1983;78:548.

137. Loeffel ED, Koya D. Cutaneous manifestations of gastrointestinal disease. Cutis 1978;21:852.

138. Brodie TE, Ochsner JL. Behcet's syndrome with ulcerative esophagitis: Report of the first case. Thorax 1973;28:637.

139. Shapiro LS, Notis WM, Romanoff NR. Letter: Self-limited esophageal ulcerations in Behcet's syndrome. Arthritis Rheum 1983;26:690.

140. Lebwohl O, Forde KA, Berdon WE, et al. Ulcerative esophagitis and colitis in a pediatric patient with Behcet's syndrome. Response to steroid therapy. Am J Gastroenterol 1977;68:550.

141. Haim S, Sherf K. Behcet's disease: Presentation of 11 cases and evaluation of treatment. Isr J Med Sci 1966;2:69.

142. O'Duffy JD, Carney JA, Deodhar S. Behcet's disease. Report of 10 cases, 3 with new manifestations. Ann Intern Med 1971;75:561.

143. Berhard GC, Hein LR. Transfer factor treatment in Behcet's syndrome. J Rheumatol 1974;(Suppl)1:34.

144. Buckley CE, Gills JP, Durham NC. Cyclophosphamide therapy of Behcet's disease. J Allergy 1969;43:273.

145. Foster GR. Behcet's colitis with oesophageal ulceration treated with sulphasalazine and cyclosporin. J R Soc Med 1988;81:545.

146. McDonald GB, Sullivan KM, Schuffler MD, Shulman HM, Thomas ED. Esophageal abnormalities in chronic graft-versus-host disease in humans. Gastroenterology 1981;80:814.

147. Ralph DD, Springmeyer SC, Sullivan KM, Hackman RC, Strob R, Thomas ED. Rapidly progressive air-flow obstruction in marrow transplant recipients. Am Rev Respir Dis 1984;129:641.

148. Wood DR, Patterson JB, Orlando RC. Pemphigus vulgaris of the esophagus. Ann Intern Med 1982;96:189.

149. Eliakim R, Goldin E, Livshin R, Okon E. Esophageal involvement in pemphigus vulgaris. Am J Gastroenterol 1988;83:155.

150. Yamamoto H, Kozawa Y, Otake S, Shimokawa R. Pemphigus vulgaris involving the mouth and esophagus. Int J Oral Surg 1983;12:194.

151. Barnes LM, Clark ML, Estes SA, Bongiovanni GL. Pemphigus vulgaris involving the esophagus: A case report and review of the literature. Dig Dis Sci 1987;32:655.

152. Goldin E, Lijovetzky G. Esophageal involvement by pemphigus vulgaris. Am J Gastroenterol 1985;80:828.

153. Sharon P, Greene ML, Rachmilewitz D. Esophageal involvement in bullous pemphigoid. Gastrointest Endosc 1978;24:122.

154. Dahl MV, Falk RJ, Carpenter R, Michael AF. Deposition of the membrane attack complex of complement in bullous pemphigoid. J Invest Dermatol 1984;82:132.

155. Stevens AE, Dove GAW. Oesophageal cast: Oesophageal dissecans superficialis. Lancet 1960;2:1279.

156. Eng TY, Hogan WJ, Jordon RE. Oesophageal involvement in bullous pemphigoid. A possible cause of gastrointestinal haemorrhage. Br J Dermatol 1978;99:207.

157. Kaplan RP, Touloukian J, Ahmed AR, Newcomer VD. Esophagitis dissecans superficialis associated with pemphigus vulgaris. J Am Acad Dermatol 1981;4:682.

158. Person JR, Rogers RS. Bullous pemphigoid responding to sulfapyridine and the sulfones. Arch Dermatol 1977;113:610.

159. Maciejowska E, Jablonska S, Chorzelski T. Is pemphigus herpetiformis an entity? Int J Dermatol 1987;26:571.

160. Benedict EB, Lever WF. Stenosis of the oesophagus in benign mucous membrane pemphigoid. Ann Otol Rhinol Laryngol 1952;61:1120.

161. Al-Kutoubi MA, Eliot C. Oesophageal involvement in benign mucous membrane pemphigoid. Clin Radiol 1984;35:131.

162. Isolauri J, Airo I. Benign mucous membrane pemphigoid involving the esophagus: A report of two cases treated with dilation. Gastrointest Endosc 1989;35:569.

163. Karasick S, Mapp E, Karasick D. Esophageal involvement in benign mucous membrane pemphigoid. J Can Assoc Radiol 1981;32:247.

164. Witte JT, Icken JN, Lloyd ML. Induction of esophageal bullae by endoscopy in benign mucous membrane pemphigoid. Gastrointest Endosc 1989;35:566.

165. Lever WF. Pemphigus and pemphigoid. Springfield, IL: Charles C Thomas, 1965.

166. Agha FP, Francis IR, Ellis CN. Esophageal involvement in epidermolysis bullosa dystrophica: Clinical and roentgenographic manifestations. Gastrointest Radiol 1983;8:111.

167. Holbrook KA. Extracutaneous epithelial involvement in inherited epidermolysis bullosa. Arch Dermatol 1988;124:726.

168. Warren RB, Warner TF, Gilbert EF, Pellet JR. Acquired double-barrel oesophagus in epidermolysis bullosa dystrophica. Thorax 1980;35:472.

169. Briggman RA, Wheeler C. Epidermolysis bullosa dystrophica recessive. A possible role of anchoring fibrils in pathogenesis. J Invest Dermatol 1975;65:203.

170. Tishler JM, Han SY, Helman CA. Esophageal involvement in epidermolysis bullosa dystrophica. Am J Roentgenol 1983;141:1283.

171. Hillemeier C, Touloukian R, McCallum R, Gryboski J. Esophageal web: A previously unrecognized complication of epidermolysis bullosa. Pediatrics 1981;67:678.

172. Bauer EA, Cooper TW. Therapeutic considerations in recessive dystrophic epidermolysis bullosa. Arch Dermatol 1981;117:529.

173. Orlando RC, Bozymski EM, Briggman RA, Bream CA. Epidermolysis bullosa: Gastrointestinal manifestations. Ann Intern Med 1974;81:203.

174. Bauer EA, Cooper TW. Therapeutic considerations in recessive epidermolysis bullosa. Arch Dermatol 1981;117:529.

175. Weschler HL, Krugh FJ, Domonkos AN, et al. Polydysplastic epidermolysis bullosa and the development of epidermal neoplasms. Arch Dermatol 1970;102:374.

176. Mallory GK, Weiss S. Hemorrhages from lacerations of the cardiac orifice of the stomach due to vomiting. Am J Med Sci 1929;178:506.

177. Fishman ML, Thirwell MP, Daly DS. Mallory-Weiss tear: A complication of cancer chemotherapy. Cancer 1983;52:2031.

178. Weaver DH, Maxwell JG, Castleton KB. Mallory-Weiss syndrome. Am J Surg 1969;118:887.

179. Michel L, Serrano A, Malt RA. Mallory-Weiss syndrome: Evolution of diagnostic and therapeutic patterns over two decades. Ann Surg 1980;192:716.

180. Sugawa C, Fujita Y, Ikeda T, Walt AJ. Endoscopic hemostasis of bleeding of the upper gastrointestinal tract by local injection of ninety-eight per cent dehydrated ethanol. Surg Gynecol Obstet 1986;162:159.

181. Walters K, Silver JR. Gastrointestinal bleeding in patients with acute spinal injuries. Int Reh Med 1986;8:44.

182. Tabibian N, Graham DY. Source of upper gastrointestinal bleeding in patients with esophageal varices seen at endoscopy. J Clin Gastroenterol 1987;9:279.

183. Watts HD, Admirand WH. Mallory–Weiss syndrome: A reappraisal. JAMA 1974;230:1674.

184. Cannon RA, Lee G, Cox KL. Gastrointestinal hemorrhage due to Mallory–Weiss syndrome in an infant. J Pediatr Gastroenterol Nutr 1985;4:323.

185. Griffiths JD. Mallory–Weiss tear and cytotoxic-induced emesis. Med J Aust 1986;144:110.

186. Laine L. Multipolar electrocoagulation in the treatment of active upper gastrointestinal tract hemorrhage. N Engl J Med 1987;316:1613.

187. Swayne LC, Samach M. Serendipitous detection of a Mallory–Weiss tear on hepatic imaging. Clin Nucl Med 1986;11:597.

188. Papp JP. Electrocoagulation of actively bleeding Mallory–Weiss tears. Gastrointest Endosc 1980;26:128.

189. Whiting EG, Barron G. Massive hemorrhage from laceration, apparently caused by vomiting in the cardiac region of the stomach with recovery. Calif Med 1955;82:188.

190. Dill JE, Wells RF. Use of vasopressin in the Mallory–Weiss syndrome. N Engl J Med 1971;284:852.

191. Natsuda Y, Kuwano H, Ezaki T, Sugimachi K, Inokuchi K. Spontaneous submucosal dissection of the esophagus: A case report. Jap J Surg 1983;13:354.

192. Atefi D, Horney JT, Eaton SB, Shulman M, Whaley W, Galambos JT. Spontaneous intramural hematoma of the esophagus. Gastrointest Endosc 1978;24:172.

193. Piccione PR, Winkler WP, Baer JW, Kotler DP. Pill-induced intramural esophageal hematoma. JAMA 1987;257:929.

194. Shay SS, Berendson KA, Johnson LF. Esophageal hematoma: Four new cases, a review, and proposed etiology. Dig Dis Sci 1981;26:1019.

195. Schweiger F, Depew WT. Spontaneous intramural esophageal hematoma. J Clin Gastroenterol 1987;9:546.

196. Low DE, Patterson DJ. Complete esophageal obstruction secondary to dissecting intramural hematoma after endoscopic variceal sclerotherapy. Am J Gastroenterol 1988;83:435.

197. Demos TC, Okrent DH, Studlo JD, Flisak ME. Spontaneous esophageal hematoma diagnosed by computed tomography. J Comput Assist Tomogr 1986;10:133.

198. Dallemand S, Amorosa JK, Morris DW, Iyers S. Intramural hematomas of the esophagus. Gastrointest Radiol 1983;8:7.

199. Flynn AE, Verrier ED, Way LW, Thomas AN, Pellegrini CA. Esophageal perforation. Arch Surg 1989;124:1211.

200. Beal SL, Pottmeyer EW, Spisso JM. Esophageal perforation following blunt trauma. J Trauma 1988;28:1425.

201. Nobrega J. Esophageal balloon dilatation: A follow-up study of 74 patients. Cardiovasc Intervent Radiol 1989;12:255.

202. LaBerge JM, Kerlan RK, Pogany AC, Ring EJ. Esophageal rupture: Complication of balloon dilatation. Radiology 1985;157:56.

203. LeBolt SA, Cho S-R. Dilatation of a stenotic esophageal segment containing a diverticulum. South Med J 1987;80:252.

204. Graeber GM, Niezgoda JA, Albus RA, et al. A comparison of patients with endoscopic perforations and patients with Boerhaave's syndrome. Chest 1987;92:995.

205. Gertler JP, Brophy C, Elefteriades J. Esophageal rupture after routine Maloney dilatation. J Clin Gastroenterol 1986;8:175.

206. Turner WW. Esophageal rupture: Fatal complication of balloon tamponade for acute variceal hemorrhage. Tex Med 1983;79:57.

207. Rubio PA. Esophageal rupture secondary to passage of a gastric bubble for weight control. Arch Surg 1988;123:394.

208. Wood J, Fabian TC, Mangiante EC. Penetrating neck injuries: Recommendations for selective management. J Trauma 1989;29:602.

209. Andrews J. Difficult diagnoses in blunt thoracoabdominal trauma. J Emerg Nurs 1989;15:399.

210. Haynes DE, Haynes BE, Yong YV. Esophageal rupture complicating Heimlich maneuver. Am J Emerg Med 1984;2:507.

211. Sams JS. Dangers of the Heimlich maneuver for esophageal obstruction. N Engl J Med 1989;321:980.

212. Derbes VJ, Mitchel RE. Herman Boerhaave's "Atroci nec descripti prius, morbi historia": First translation (from original Latin, 1724) of the classic case report of rupture of esophagus, with annotations. Bull Med Libr Assoc 1955;43:217.

213. Uehara DT, Dymowski JJ, Schwartz J, Turnbull TL. Chest pain, shock and pneumomediastinum in a previously healthy 56-year-old man. Ann Emerg Med 1987;16:359.

214. Abbott OA, Mansour KA, Logan WD, et al. Atraumatic so-called "spontaneous" rupture of the esophagus. J Thorac Cardiovasc Surg 1970;59:67.

215. Kuwano H, Matsumata T, Adachi E, et al. Lack of muscularis mucosa and the occurrence of Boerhaave's syndrome. Am J Surg 1989;158:420.

216. Curci MR, Dibbins AW, Grimes CK. Compressed air injury to the esophagus: Case report. J Trauma 1989;29:1713.

217. Ward WG. Cold water polydipsia: Unheralded marker of spontaneous esophageal rupture. South Med J 1986;79:1161.

218. Good JT, Antony VB, Reller LB, Maulitz RM, Sahn SA. The pathogenesis of the low pleural fluid pH in esophageal rupture. Am Rev Respir Dis 1983;127:702.

219. Houston MC. Pleural fluid pH: Diagnostic, therapeutic, and prognostic value. Am J Surg 1987;154:333.

220. LoCicero J, Vanecko RM. Clostridial myonecrosis of the chest wall complicating spontaneous esophageal rupture. Ann Thorac Surg 1985;40:396.

221. Lucas CE, Splittgerber F, Ledgerwood AM. Conservative therapy for missed esophageal perforation after blunt trauma. Am J Emerg Med 1986;4:520.

B. STOMACH

59

Stomach: Anatomy and Structural Anomalies

GREGORY L. EASTWOOD

GROSS ANATOMY OF THE STOMACH AND DUODENUM

The study of anatomy is prerequisite to the understanding of function. Indeed, the gross and microanatomy of the stomach and duodenum are intimately related to their physiologic behavior.

Because the stomach and the duodenum are closely related in function as well as in the pathogenesis and manifestations of disease, the anatomy of the two organs are considered here together.

Anatomic Relationships and Divisions

The stomach is located in the upper abdomen just beneath the diaphragm (Fig 59-1). It receives the distal end of the esophagus immediately after the esophagus penetrates the diaphragmatic hiatus, and empties into the beginning of the small intestine, the duodenum. Because it is distensible and on a free mesentery, the size, shape, and position of the stomach vary greatly with posture and contents. Empty, it is roughly the size of an open hand. Distended with food, it can fill much of the upper abdomen and may descend into the lower abdomen or pelvis when a person stands.

The stomach is somewhat arbitrarily separated into the cardia, fundus, body, antrum, and pylorus (Fig 59-2; Color Fig 22). The *cardia* is a 1- to 2-cm segment just distal to the esophagogastric junction. The *fundus* is the superior portion of the stomach that lies above an imaginary horizontal plane that passes through the esophagogastric junction. The *body* is the large main portion of the stomach between the fundus and the antrum. The *antrum* is the smaller distal one fourth to one third of the stomach, and the *pylorus* is the narrow 1- to 2-cm channel that connects the stomach with the duodenum. The medial, shorter border of the stomach is called the *lesser curve;* the opposite broad, lateral and inferior surface is the *greater curve.* Along the lesser curve at about the junction of the body and antrum is a bend that is accentuated during peristalsis called the *angularis.*

The duodenum extends from the pylorus to the ligament of Treitz in a sharp curve that almost completes a circle. It is so named because it is about equal in length to the breadth of 12 fingers, or 25 cm. It has no mesentery, is largely retroperitoneal, and its position is relatively fixed.

The duodenum is divided into four portions (Fig 59-3; Color Fig 23). The first part, or *superior portion,* is about 5 cm long and begins at the pylorus, passes backward, upward, and to the right, beneath the liver to the neck of the gallbladder. The first 2 to 3 cm of the superior portion is naturally dilated and is called the duodenal bulb. The duodenum takes a sharp curve and descends along the right margin of the head of the pancreas for 7 to 10 cm as the second part, or *descending portion.* The common bile duct and the pancreatic duct, together or separately, enter the medial aspect of the descending duodenum. The duodenum turns medially, becoming the third part, or *horizontal portion,* and passes from right to left across the spine, inclining upward for a length of about 5 to 8 cm. Finally, the fourth part, or *ascending portion,* begins at the left of the vertebral column, ascends to the left of the aorta for 2 to 3 cm, and ends at the ligament of Treitz, where the intestine angles abruptly forward and downward to become the jejunum.

Circulation

The stomach and duodenum derive their blood supply from the celiac axis and the superior mesenteric artery. The celiac axis arises from the aorta at about the twelfth thoracic vertebra and gives off the splenic, left gastric, and hepatic arteries (see ch 109). Branches from these vessels form a dense anastomotic network that encircles the stomach, providing a rich blood supply. The hepatic artery gives rise to the right gastric artery and the gastroduodenal artery, and the latter continues as the right gastroepiploic artery. The short gastric arteries and the left gastroepiploic artery are branches of the splenic artery.

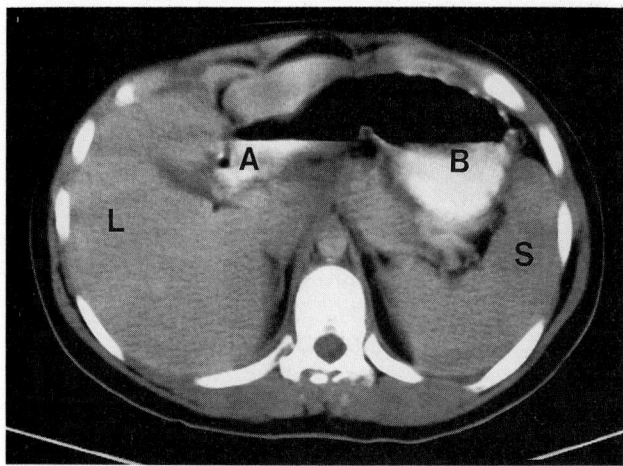

FIGURE 59-1. Computerized tomogram of the abdomen shows the relation of the stomach to adjacent structures. The stomach contains air (black) and barium contrast material (white). *A* = gastric antrum; *B* = gastric body; *L* = liver; *S* = spleen. (Courtesy of Dr. Sathyanarayana.)

The superior mesenteric artery comes off the aorta 3 to 4 cm below the celiac axis, just behind the pancreas between the first and second lumbar vertebrae (see ch 109). The inferior pancreaticoduodenal branch of the superior mesenteric artery not only sends branches to the distal stomach, but also supplies the duodenum. Other arteries supplying the duodenum are the right gastric and the superior pancreaticoduodenal, both arising from the hepatic artery.

The venous drainage of the stomach and duodenum generally accompanies the arterial supply. The right and left gastric veins drain the lesser curve of the stomach, and the right and left gastroepiploic and short gastric veins drain the greater curve. The veins from the stomach and duodenum lead either to the splenic or superior mesenteric veins, or directly into the portal vein.

Lymphatics

The lymph drainage of the stomach and duodenum mainly follows the blood vessels. The lymphatics of the stomach are continuous at the esophagogastric junction with those of the esophagus, and at the pylorus with those of the duodenum. Plexuses of lymphatics in the submucosa, muscular coat, and serosa anastomose and drain to four main groups from the stomach and two groups from the duodenum.

In the stomach, the first group of lymphatics accompanies the branches of the left gastric artery, receives tributaries from the surfaces of the upper portion of the stomach, and terminates in the *superior gastric nodes*. The second group of lymphatics drains the fundus and proximal body of the stomach, accompanying the short gastric and left gastroepiploic arteries, ending in the *pancreaticolienal* and *splenic nodes*. The third group drains the distal greater curve into the *inferior gastric nodes* with subsequent connections to the *subpyloric nodes*. The last group of gastric lymphatics drains the pyloric region and passes to the *superior gastric* and *hepatic nodes* as well as to the *subpyloric nodes*.

Extensive communications link the four groups of lymphatics. This means that neoplasms arising in one region of the stomach can spread easily elsewhere in the stomach and beyond. Furthermore, the regional groups of lymphatics drain to nodes that lie near the celiac axis, which also receives lymphatic drainage from the liver. The extensive lymphatic communications that serve the stomach and the propensity of metastases to spread beyond the stomach limit the surgical treatment of gastric carcinoma and contribute to its poor prognosis.

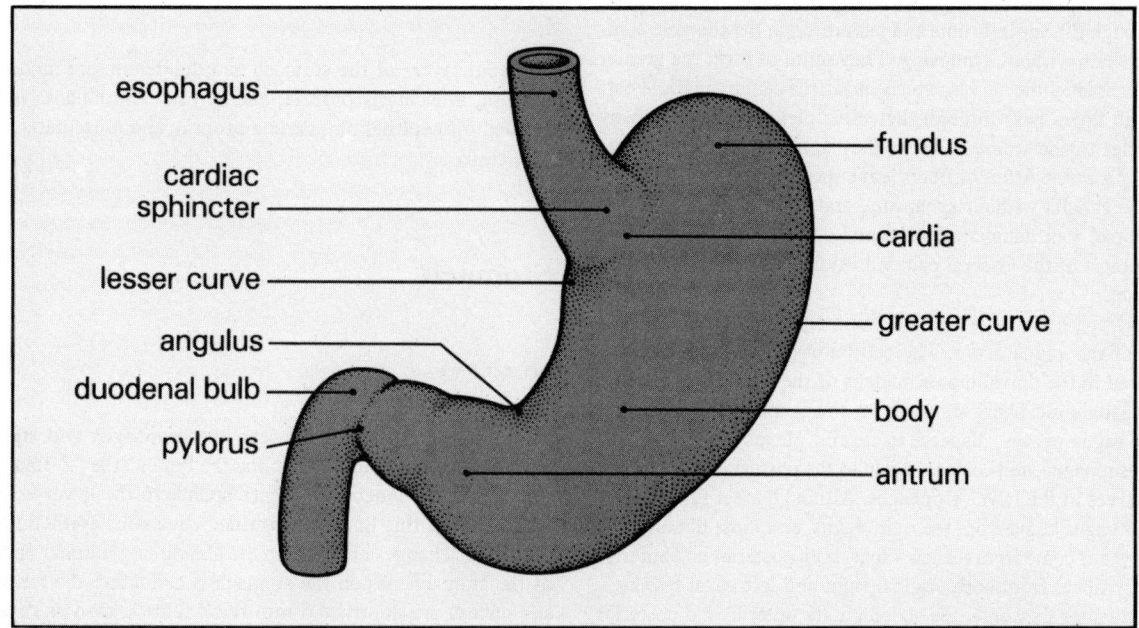

FIGURE 59-2. (See Color Fig 22) Diagram of the lower esophagus, stomach, and proximal duodenum. (Misiewicz JJ, Bartram CI, Cotton PB, Mee AS, Price AB, Thompson RPH. Atlas of clinical gastroenterology. London: Gower Medical Publishing, 1987.)

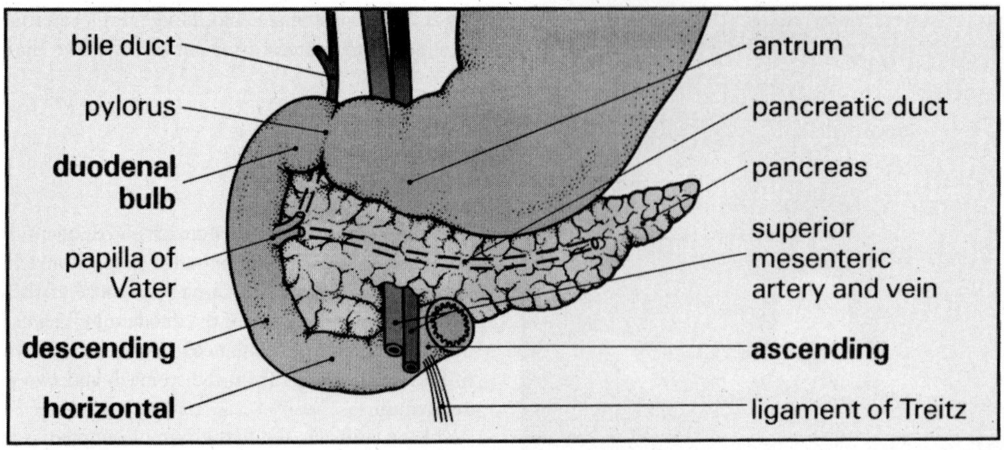

FIGURE 59–3. (See Color Fig 23) Diagram showing the anatomic relationships of the duodenum. (Misiewicz JJ, Bartram CI, Cotton PB, Mee AS, Price AB, Thompson RPH. Atlas of clinical gastroenterology. London: Gower Medical Publishing, 1987.)

The duodenal lymphatic vessels are composed of an anterior and a posterior set that converge into a series of small *pancreaticoduodenal nodes* on the anterior and posterior aspects of the junction between the pancreas and duodenum. Efferents from these nodes pass superiorly to the *hepatic nodes* and inferiorly to the *preaortic nodes* around the origin of the superior mesenteric artery.

Innervation

The stomach and duodenum receive both sympathetic and parasympathetic innervation. Of course, much of the innervation of the gut is under control of the enteric nervous system, which is not grossly visible (see ch 1).

The cell bodies of the sympathetic nerves reside in the gray matter of the anterior columns of the spinal cord from the fifth through twelfth thoracic segments. Their axons leave the spinal cord through the ventral roots and pass through the thoracic sympathetic chain without synapsing. They unite to form the greater and lesser splanchnic nerves, which end in the celiac ganglia. Postganglionic fibers pass through the celiac plexus and accompany the arteries to the stomach where they enter the intramural autonomic plexuses. Afferent fibers leave the stomach, pass through the celiac ganglia without synapsing, and reach their cell bodies in the dorsal root ganglia of the spinal cord. The afferent fibers conduct most of the visceral pain sensation from the stomach and duodenum.

Parasympathetic innervation of the stomach and duodenum is by way of the vagus nerve. The cell bodies of the vagus nerves are located in the dorsal motor nucleus of the medulla oblongata. The preganglionic fibers travel down the esophagus as the right and left vagus nerves, disperse to form a plexus that surrounds the midesophagus, and coalesce again as the posterior and anterior vagus nerves in the lower esophagus. Although most fibers in the posterior vagus come from the right vagus, and most fibers in the anterior vagus come from the left vagus, both posterior and anterior vagi carry fibers from both original right and left vagal trunks.

Shortly after they enter the abdomen, the anterior and posterior vagi branch (Fig 59-4; Color Fig 24). The anterior vagus divides into the hepatic and anterior gastric branches; the posterior vagus divides into the celiac and posterior gastric branches. The hepatic branch goes on to innervate the liver, gallbladder, pylorus, and proximal duodenum. The celiac branch innervates other abdominal viscera. The anterior and posterior gastric branches continue along the lesser curve of the stomach, giving off numerous branches to the fundus and body, and terminating in a "crow's foot" distribution to the antrum. Preganglionic vagal fibers synapse with neurons in the intrinsic plexuses of the gastric wall, Auerbach's plexus within the muscularis propria, and Meissner's plexus in the submucosa. Postganglionic fibers from the plexuses innervate the secretory cells and muscle. The vagal innervation to the body and fundus primarily stimulates acid secretion, whereas vagal innervation to the antrum primarily stimulates motility. Little is known about the function of the afferent fibers of the vagus nerve.

MICROSCOPIC ANATOMY

The four layers of the stomach and duodenum are mucosa, submucosa, muscularis propria, and serosa. The mucosa is further divided into epithelium, lamina propria, and muscularis mucosae (see ch 6).

Stomach

MUCOSA

The mucosal boundary between the esophagus and stomach is visible as a zig-zag line encircling the lumen (the "Z-line") at the location in the mucosa that corresponds to the lower esophageal sphincter. At this line, the stratified squamous epithelium of the esophagus changes abruptly to the glandular columnar epithelium of the stomach. When the stomach is collapsed, the mucosa and submucosa are contracted into thick folds known as rugae. The rugae generally appear as a honeycomb pattern except along the lesser curve and in the antrum, where they are arranged longi-

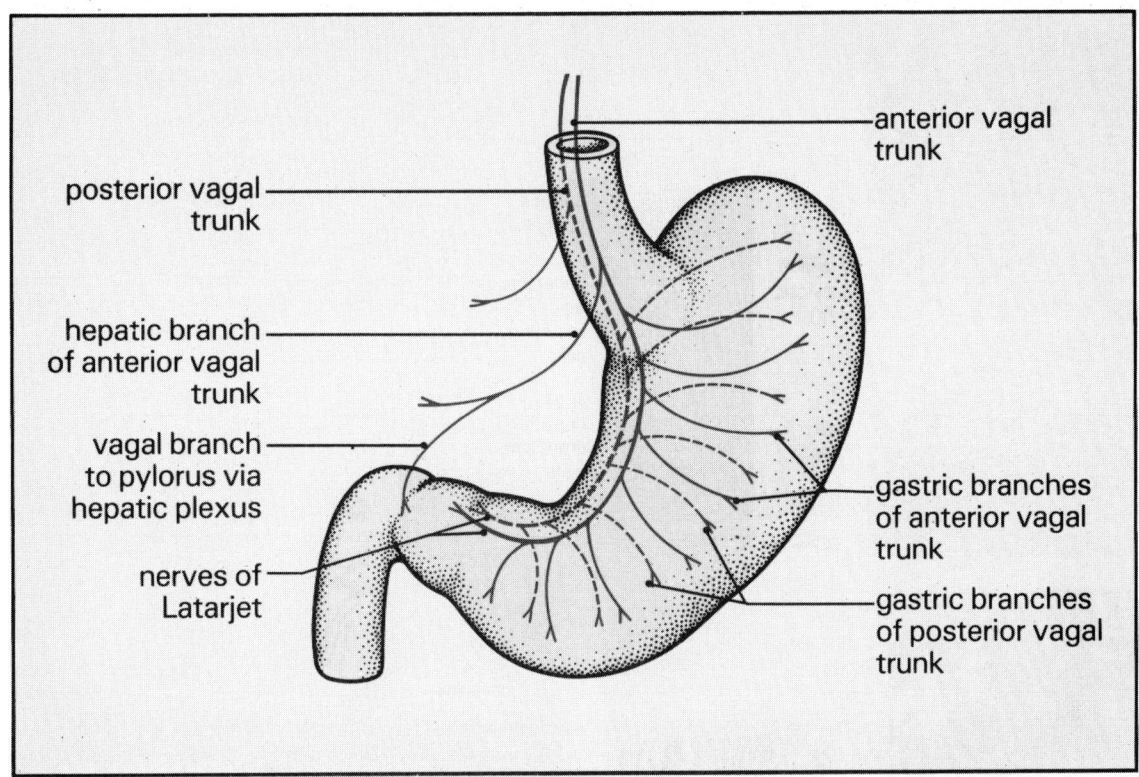

FIGURE 59–4. (See Color Fig 24) Diagram showing the anatomic arrangement of the vagus nerves. (Misiewicz JJ, Bartram CI, Cotton PB, Mee AS, Price AB, Thompson RPH. Atlas of clinical gastroenterology. London: Gower Medical Publishing, 1987.)

tudinally. Rugae flatten and disappear upon distention of the stomach.

The general architecture of the gastric mucosa consists of pits, or foveolae, that invaginate from the surface of the mucosa. Beneath the pits and emptying into them are glands. A single-cell-thick *epithelium* covers the surface and lines the pits and glands. The *lamina propria* of the stomach is less well developed than in the intestine. It is more abundant between the pits under the surface epithelium, but also includes the narrow space between the densely packed glands. The lamina propria consists of loose connective tissue containing bundles of collagen fibers, thin strands of smooth muscle, fibroblasts, macrophages, lymphatics, blood vessels, and nerves. A continuous sheet of smooth muscle, the *muscularis mucosae*, forms the inferior margin of the mucosa and separates it from the submucosa.

The mucosa of the stomach is divided into two major types, fundic and antral, which differ in structure and function (Fig 59-5*A,B*; Color Fig 25*A,B*). A third type, junctional or cardiac mucosa, is limited to the 1 to 2 cm in the cardia of the stomach just distal to the esophagogastric junction (see Fig 59-5*C*; Color Fig 25*C*).

Fundic type mucosa lines the body and fundus of the stomach (see Fig 59-5*A*; Color Fig 25*A*). Mucus-secreting cells are found on the surface, extending down into the pits (Fig 59-6). In fundic mucosa, the pits are shallow and the glands beneath them are long and convoluted. The glands are lined by parietal cells (Fig 59-7), which secrete hydrochloric acid and intrinsic factor, and by chief cells, which secrete pepsinogens. Although parietal and chief cells comingle, the density of parietal cells is greater in the upper and midportions of the glands, whereas chief cells are more numerous in the deeper portion of the glands.

Antral type mucosa is found in the antrum and pyloric channel (see Fig 59-5*B*). Here also mucus-secreting cells line the elongated pits, but the glands are virtually devoid of parietal and chief cells. Rather, the glandular cells elaborate an alkaline mucus that contains pepsinogens. Both antral and fundic mucosae contain endocrine cells that secrete a variety of hormones. In particular, gastrin is secreted from specific G cells located in the glands of the antrum.

Junctional mucosa occurs in a 1- to 2-cm narrow band at the cardia just distal to the Z-line between the esophagus and stomach (see Fig 59-5*C*). Junctional mucosa is architecturally similar to fundic mucosa in that it also is comprised of shallow pits and long tortuous glands, but the glands are devoid of parietal and chief cells.

EPITHELIAL CELL TYPES

Several epithelial cell types, some of which have been mentioned above, are found in the gastric mucosa. These include surface mucous cells, mucous neck cells, chief (zymogenic) cells, parietal (oxyntic) cells, and endocrine cells.[1-3]

Surface mucous cells line the mucosal surface and the gastric pits (see Fig 59-6). The cells are broad at the top and may narrow toward the base, allowing for a variable amount of intercellular space. As is typical of all columnar epithelial cells, surface mucous cells are attached to one another near their apical margins by a junctional complex, comprised of a tight junction and an intermediate junction (see ch 6). In addition to the junctional complexes, disklike desmosomes are scattered throughout the lateral plasma membranes to provide additional intercellular attachments.

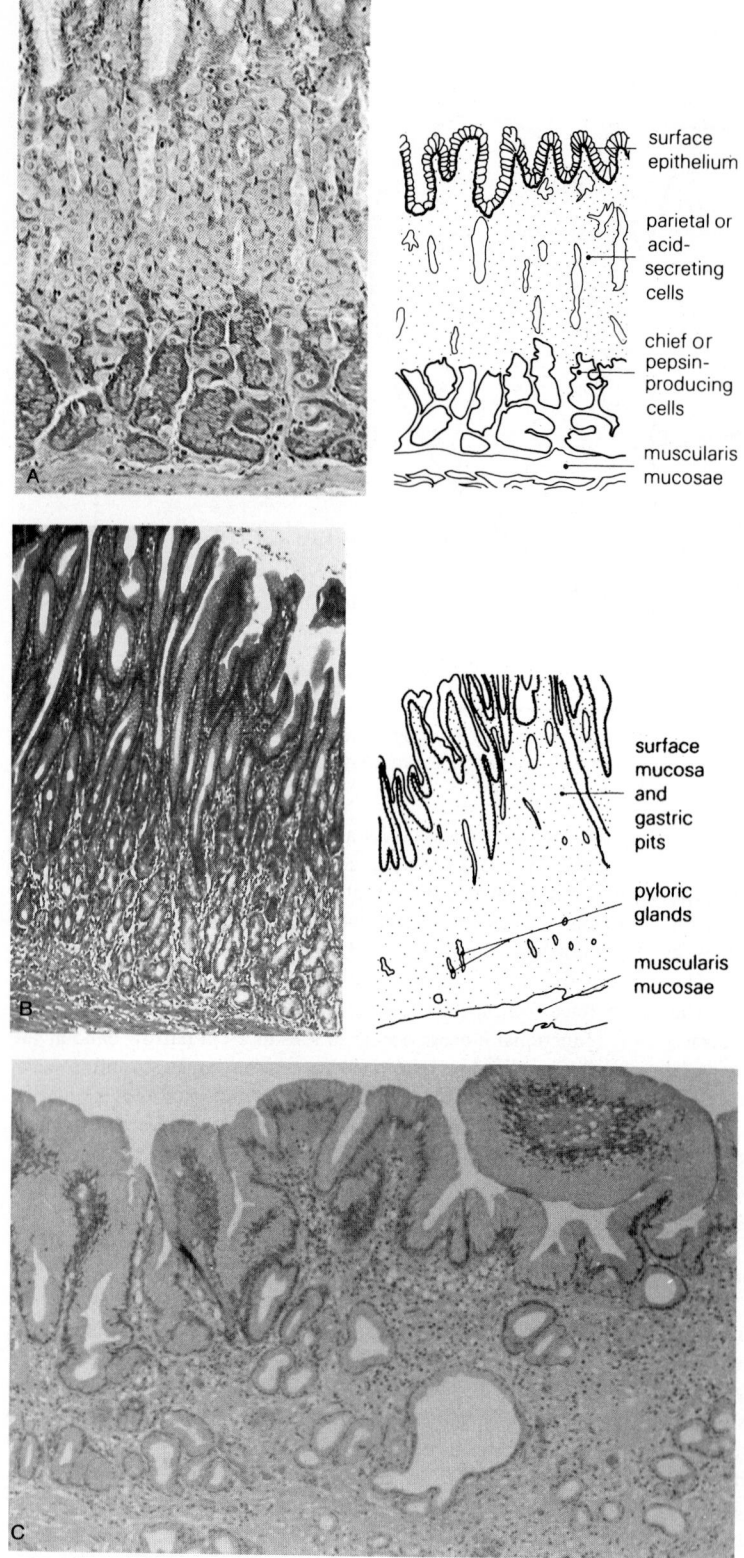

surface
epithelium

parietal or
acid-
secreting
cells

chief or
pepsin-
producing
cells

muscularis
mucosae

surface
mucosa
and
gastric
pits

pyloric
glands

muscularis
mucosae

FIGURE 59–5. A, (See Color Fig. 25A,B,C) Light photomicrograph of fundic-type gastric mucosa. Columnar mucus-secreting cells line the surface and pits, acid-secreting parietal cells (light staining cuboidal cells) predominate in the midportion of the mucosa, and pepsinogen-secreting chief cells (darker staining) are located deeper in the mucosa. Hematoxylin and eosin. (Courtesy of Dr. P. Wheater.) **B,** Light photomicrograph of antral-type gastric mucosa. The gastric pits are deeper than in fundic mucosa. Mucus-secreting glands are deep in the mucosa and empty into the pits. Hematoxylin and eosin. **C,** Light photomicrograph of junctional gastric mucosa. Although the architecture is similar to fundic mucosa, the mucosa is thinner and the loosely arranged glands are devoid of parietal and chief cells. Hematoxylin and eosin. (**A** and **B** from Misiewicz JJ, Bartram CI, Cotton PB, Mee AS, Price AB, Thompson RPH. Atlas of clinical gastroenterology. London: Gower Medical Publishing, 1987. **C** from Mitros FA. Atlas of gastrointestinal pathology. London: Gower Medical Publishing, 1988.)

The apical portion of surface mucous cells is occupied by closely packed, mucous granules, each bounded by a trilaminar membrane. Stubby, sparse microvilli protrude from the apical cell membrane, and there is a filamentous glycocalyx on the surface. The nucleus is located in the lower part of the cell. Between the nucleus and the mucous granules lies the Golgi complex. Free ribosomes are

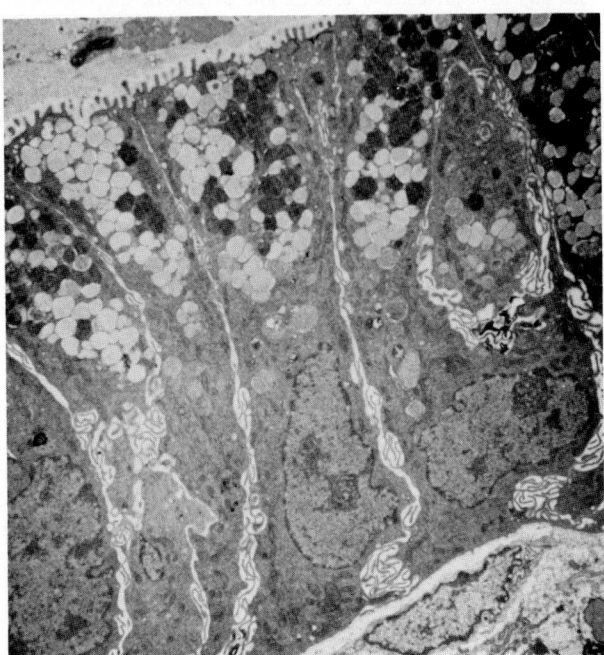

FIGURE 59-6. Transmission electron micrograph of surface, mucus-secreting cells of the stomach. Stubby microvilli protrude from the apical surface, closely packed mucous granules occupy the apical cytoplasm, and the nucleus lies near the base of the cell (×3200). (Misiewicz JJ, Bartram CI, Cotton PB, Mee AS, Price AB, Thompson RPH. Atlas of clinical gastroenterology. London: Gower Medical Publishing, 1987.)

abundant, but granular endoplasmic reticulum and mitochondria are sparse.

Mucous neck cells line the neck of the glands and also occur singly deeper within the glands. These cells are virtually identical to the cells that line the glands of junctional and antral mucosae. Mucous neck cells have a narrow apex and a broad base. The apical mucous droplets are bounded by a trilaminar membrane and appear less electron dense than those of surface mucous cells.

Parietal, or oxyntic, cells are concentrated in the mid and upper portions of the glands of fundic type mucosa (see Fig 59-7). They are responsible for secreting hydrochloric acid and intrinsic factor. Parietal cells are pyramidal in shape with centrally placed nuclei.[4] One or several canaliculi run through the cytoplasm, lined by numerous microvilli, and communicating with the gastric gland. Numerous tubovesicles fill much of the cell, particularly in the vicinity of the canaliculi. Considerable evidence indicates that the membranes lining the canaliculi and surrounding the tubovesicles are the same and interchange with each other. In fact, during resting, nonsecretory conditions, the tubovesicles are greatly increased at the expense of the canaliculi, whereas during the acid secretory state, tubovesicles diminish and the canaliculi become more elaborate.[5,6] The so-called proton pump, or H^+–K^+–ATPase, is located in the membrane of the canalicular microvilli. Hydrochloric acid is believed to be secreted across the microvillar membrane into the canaliculus. It then passes out of the cell into the gastric gland and, finally, is extruded into the gastric lumen (see ch 13). In keeping with the high metabolic demands of the parietal cell, mitochondria are abundant.

Chief, or zymogenic, cells predominate in the body and deeper portion of the glands (see Fig 59-5A) but comingle with the parietal cells up to the neck region. These cells secrete pepsinogens that are converted to pepsin in the gastric lumen. Granular endoplasmic reticulum and free ribosomes are abundant, and the Golgi complex is prominent. Closely packed pepsinogen-containing granules fill much of the cytoplasm, each surrounded by a trilaminar membrane. The pepsinogen is released into the lumen of the gland after the limiting membrane of the granule fuses with the luminal cell membrane.

Endocrine cells of various staining and morphologic characteristics are scattered throughout the mucosa of the stomach.[7] The endocrine cell that has been studied most extensively and that appears to have the most clinical relevance is the gastrin, or G, cell.[7,8] G cells are located in the midportions of the glands of the antrum and in the crypts of the duodenum. They are characterized by a broad base, which rests against the basement membrane that runs beneath the epithelium, and a narrow apex, which extends to the lumen of the gland. Microvilli protrude out into the gland lumen and may be involved in reception of stimuli that release gastrin. Gastrin-containing granules cluster toward the base of the cell. Stimulation of gastrin release occurs with eating. Specifically, distention of the antrum, contact of antral mucosa with peptides and amino acids, and vagal excitation all stimulate gastrin secretion from antral G cells. Although the basally oriented gastrin granules would seem to be an ideal location for secretion into the surrounding mucosa and submucosa, to be taken up by the circulation,

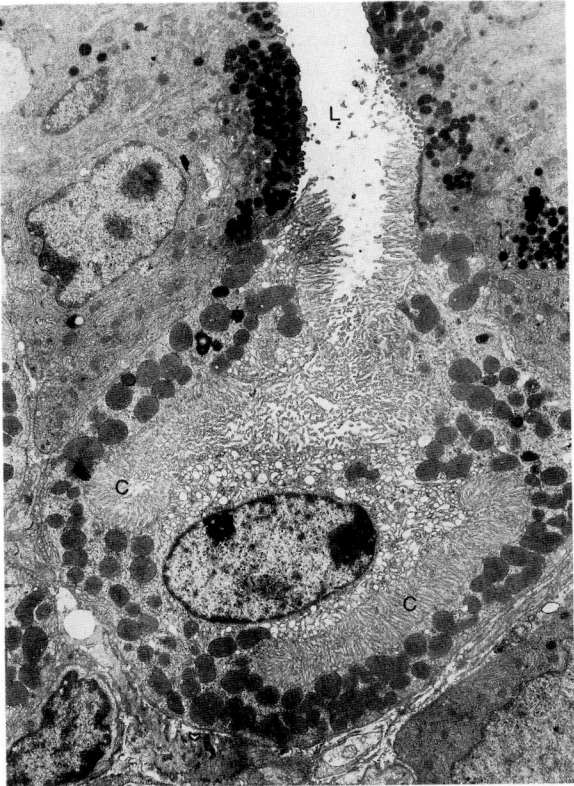

FIGURE 59-7. Transmission electron micrograph of a parietal cell. Around the central nucleus are clusters of tubovesicles. A canaliculus (C), lined by numerous microvilli, runs through the cell and empties into the lumen of the gland (L). Dark staining mitochondria are located at the periphery (×4000). (Eastwood GL. Acid-peptic disease. In: Eastwood GL, ed. Core textbook of gastroenterology. Philadelphia: JB Lippincott, 1984: 32.)

much of the gastrin actually is secreted into the lumen of the stomach.[9] Little is known about the function and fate of intraluminal gastrin, and most information about gastrin refers to its action as a bloodborne hormonal agent (see ch 2 and 13).

Several other types of endocrine cells also have been identified in the gastric mucosa. Some cells contain granules that reduce silver without pretreatment with a reducing substance; these are called argentaffin cells. Other endocrine cells must be exposed to a reducing substance before they react with silver; they are called argyrophilic cells. Some cells exhibit both argentaffin and chromaffin reactions and are called enterochromaffin cells. The function of all endocrine cells has not been determined, but some contain serotonin and others contain somatostatin.

SUBMUCOSA

The submucosa is a layer of connective tissue that lies immediately beneath the mucosa. It provides a loose framework for the passage of arteries, veins, lymphatics, and nerves.

MUSCULARIS PROPRIA

The major muscle layer of the stomach has a circular layer of smooth muscle which is surrounded by an outer longitudinal layer that is characteristic of the muscularis propria of the entire gastrointestinal tract. In addition, the stomach has a layer of oblique fibers. The circular layer is rather uniform throughout the stomach. The outer longitudinal layer is variable, becoming thicker along the greater and lesser curves. The oblique fibers are internal to the circular layer and are most prominent at the upper stomach, spreading over the anterior and posterior surfaces as they pass distally.

SEROSA

This outermost layer of the stomach consists of areolar tissue covered by a single layer of squamous mesothelial cells.

Duodenum

MUCOSA

The architecture of the mucosa changes abruptly within the pyloric channel from the pits and glands that are typical of antral type gastric mucosa to the mucosa of the small intestine. The latter is characterized by fingerlike projections, called villi, and intervening invaginations, called crypts, at the bases of the villi (see ch 66).

Mucosal biopsies from the distal duodenum are typical of the architecture of the proximal jejunum. Villi are tall and straight, and the villus:crypt ratio is about 4 to 5:1. In the proximal duodenum, villi normally are distorted, appearing shorter, broader, and sometimes leaflike. This lack of uniform appearance in the proximal duodenum is attributed to the effects of gastric acid and

other digestive juices. For this reason, diagnostic biopsies of the proximal small bowel should be taken from the third or fourth portion of the duodenum to ensure accuracy of interpretation[10,11] (see ch 126).

A continuous single cell layer of *epithelium* covers the villi and lines the crypts. The *lamina propria* occupies the cores of the villi and the contiguous space between the crypts. As in the stomach, it is composed of loose connective tissue and contains lymphatics (lacteals), blood vessels, nerves, and smooth muscle fibers. Furthermore, plasma cells and lymphocytes are found within the lamina propria in varying numbers. Beneath the crypts and perpendicular to them lies the *muscularis mucosae*.

EPITHELIAL CELL TYPES

Four major cell types are found within the epithelium of the duodenum, namely, absorptive cells, mucous cells, Paneth cells, and enteroendocrine cells.[12,13] These cells are described in detail in Chapter 66.

SUBMUCOSA

The submucosa of the duodenum serves a similar function as in the stomach in providing a connective tissue framework for the passage of blood vessels, lymphatics, and nerves. Furthermore, in the duodenum, the glands of Brunner, which secrete an alkaline mucus, are found in the submucosa. These glands extend through the muscularis mucosae to occupy a portion of the mucosa and empty into the crypts (Fig 59-8; Color Fig 26).

MUSCULARIS PROPRIA AND SEROSA

As elsewhere in the gastrointestinal tract, this is the major muscle coat of the duodenum. A layer of inner circular fibers is surrounded by a layer of fibers arranged longitudinally. The myenteric plexus of nerve fibers is situated between the two layers.

The serosa of the duodenum is similar to that of the stomach.

EPITHELIAL RENEWAL

General Comments

The epithelium of the stomach and duodenum undergoes constant rapid renewal[14,15] (see ch 6). The overall process of epithelial renewal includes the proliferation, migration, differentiation, senescence, and loss of epithelial cells.

The proliferative zone in gastric mucosa is located in the base of the pits and the contiguous upper portion of the glands. New cells migrate upward along the sides of the pits and onto the mucosal surface to replenish the surface mucous cells. The renewal of this population probably varies from one area of the stomach to another, but in humans is on the order of 2 to 6 days.[16]

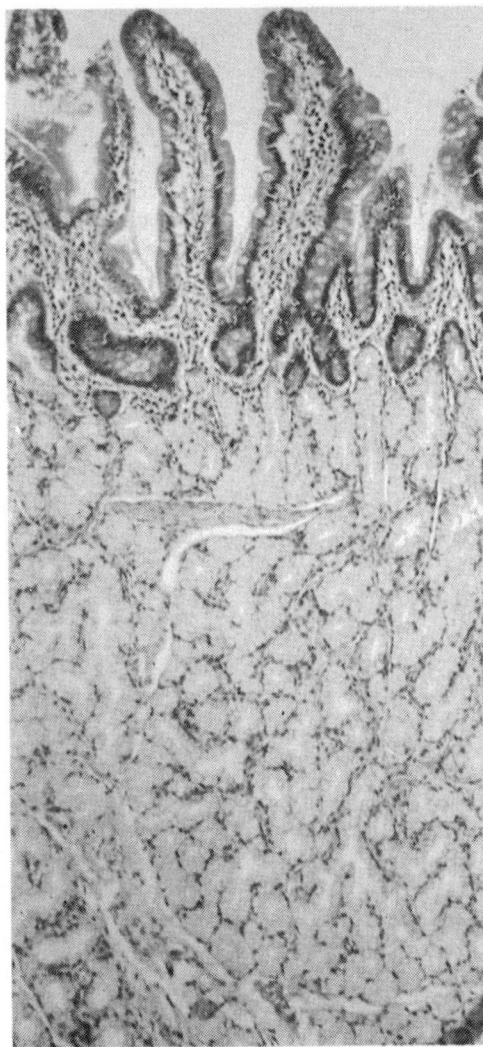

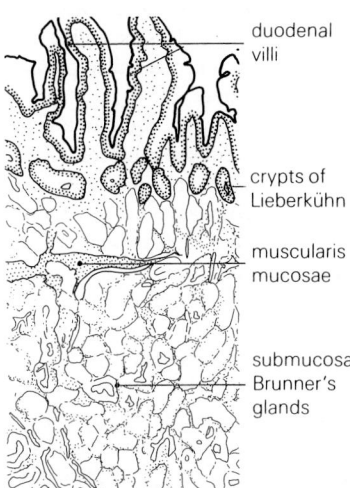

duodenal villi

crypts of Lieberkühn

muscularis mucosae

submucosal Brunner's glands

FIGURE 59–8. (See Color Fig 26) Light photomicrograph of duodenal mucosa. Villi protrude from the mucosal surface. Columnar absorptive cells and goblet (mucous) cells cover the villi and line the crypts at the base of the villi. Clusters of clear-staining cells that secrete an alkaline mucus, called Brunner's glands, are found above and below the muscularis mucosae and empty into the base of the crypts. Hematoxylin and eosin. (Misiewicz JJ, Bartram CI, Cotton PB, Mee AS, Price AB, Thompson RPH. Atlas of clinical gastroenterology. London: Gower Medical Publishing, 1987.)

The renewal of the glandular populations in the stomach is much slower than that of the surface epithelium. The progenitor cells of the parietal and chief cells originate in the proliferative zone and migrate slowly downward. Studies in animals indicate that the renewal of these populations is on the order of weeks to months.[17]

In the duodenum, epithelial proliferation occurs in the crypts. Cells migrate up the villi and eventually are extruded into the gut lumen at the villous tips. The entire process of cell generation, migration, and loss requires about 6 days in humans.[16] The crypts are surrounded by a sheath of fibroblasts within the lamina propria which undergoes proliferation and migration in synchrony with the epithelium.[18] In the villi, the fibroblasts continue to migrate toward the villous tips, although perhaps at an accelerated rate compared to epithelial migration. Whether the fibroblasts ultimately are sloughed into the lumen of the bowel, or whether they are "recycled" to deeper layers of the lamina propria, is unknown. The relationship between epithelial renewal and the fibroblast sheath in the stomach has not been studied well, but it is likely that fibroblast proliferation and migration accompany epithelial renewal in gastric mucosa as well.

Alterations of Epithelial Renewal in Gastroduodenal Disorders

Aspirin, indomethacin, and ethanol all have been shown to stimulate epithelial proliferation in the experimental setting.[19–22] The stimulatory effects of these agents may be a compensatory reaction to mild injury. On the other hand, corticosteroids appear to depress epithelial proliferation.[23] It is possible that the inhibition of epithelial proliferation by corticosteroids could render the mucosa susceptible to the effects of other ulcerogens as well as retard the healing of existing mucosal lesions.

Physiologic stress, in the form of water immersion restraint, also depresses fundic epithelial proliferation.[22] Although it is reasonable to expect circulating levels of corticosteroids to be elevated during stress, numerous other factors may affect epithelial proliferation and other mechanisms of mucosal protection. For example, stress in rats has been shown to reduce gastric mucosal prostaglandin generation.[24,25] Nevertheless, it is tempting to speculate that stress-induced depression of epithelial proliferation may contribute to the formation of mucosal lesions in humans, such as occurs in very ill patients in intensive care units.

Epithelial proliferation appears to be increased in all forms of chronic gastritis, ranging from chronic superficial gastritis to the gastric atrophy associated with pernicious anemia.[26,27] The zone of proliferating cells is expanded in these disorders, a finding that is common to other so-called premalignant conditions of the gastrointestinal tract.[26–29]

Gastric epithelial proliferation also has been shown to be accelerated in Zollinger-Ellison (Z-E) syndrome.[30] Serum gastrin levels, of course, are markedly elevated in the Z-E syndrome. Similarly, serum gastrin levels may be elevated in chronic gastritis as a consequence of parietal cell dropout and hyposecretion of acid. Thus, the stimulation of epithelial proliferation in both Z-E syndrome and chronic gastritis, which differ dramatically in clinical manifestations, is in keeping with the known trophic effects of gastrin on gastric mucosa.[31]

Information about epithelial proliferation in duodenal ulcer disease is limited. Autoradiographic studies of biopsies from mucosa adjacent to active duodenal ulcers as well as from nonulcerated duodenitis show that proliferation is increased when compared to normal-appearing mucosa from sites that are distant from the active ulceration or inflammation or from normal subjects.[32] The observed increase in epithelial proliferation may be due to the effects of inflammation, and it is not known whether ulcer patients have a defect in epithelial proliferation that precedes ulceration.

Because considerable interest has centered on the beneficial effects of prostaglandins on the gastroduodenal mucosa in recent years, it is reasonable to inquire whether prostaglandins affect epithelial proliferation. The weight of evidence indicates that prostaglandins do not have a primary effect on epithelial proliferation but rather retard senescence and loss of epithelial cells.[33–35] Thus, the result is thickening of the mucosa, which may contribute to the protective effects of prostaglandins.

EMBRYOLOGY OF THE STOMACH AND DUODENUM

The stomach and proximal duodenum are derived from the primitive foregut.[36,37] The duodenum beyond the origin of the liver bud (the future entry of the common bile duct) is formed from the cephalic end of the midgut.

In the fourth week of development, the stomach appears as a fusiform dilatation of the foregut. Over the next several weeks, the stomach rotates 90 degrees clockwise around its longitudinal axis, ending with its left side facing anteriorly and its right side posteriorly. This accounts for the left vagus nerve supplying the anterior wall of the stomach and the right vagus nerve supplying the posterior wall (see section titled "Innervation"). The original posterior wall of the stomach, now the left wall, grows faster than the anterior (right) wall, to become the greater and lesser curves, respectively. The rotation pulls the dorsal mesentery of the stomach, which attaches the stomach to the posterior body wall, to the left, forming the omental bursa, or lesser sac of the peritoneum. The ventral mesentery attaches the stomach and duodenum to the liver and antral body wall.

During the growth and rotation of the stomach, the cephalic end moves to the left and slightly downward and becomes the fundic and cardiac portions. Conversely, the caudal end moves upward and to the right to become the antrum and pylorus. Thus, the long axis of the stomach in its final position runs from above left to below right.

As the stomach rotates and enlarges, the duodenum also grows rapidly, forming a loop that projects ventrally, rotates to the right, and finally lies retroperitoneally. During the fifth and sixth weeks, because of the rapid proliferation of the epithelium, the lumen of the duodenum is temporarily obliterated. Subsequent vacuolization of the lumen and degeneration of some of the cells results in recanalization over the next several weeks.

The embryonic endoderm forms the epithelium of the digestive tract and is responsible for the epithelium and glands of the stomach and duodenum. The connective tissue, muscle, and serosa are derived from the mesoderm.

CONGENITAL ABNORMALITIES OF THE STOMACH

Atresia

In gastric atresia, the stomach ends blindly in the antrum or pyloric canal. The atretic portion may consist only of mucosa and submucosa with normal muscle and serosa surrounding, or the entire gastroduodenal wall may be atretic. The etiology is not clear. Failure of recanalization of the antrum and pylorus that is transiently occluded by epithelium during embryogenesis has been postulated. The condition may be familial.[38]

The diagnosis of gastric atresia is suggested when a newborn has nonbilious vomiting and there was a large volume of amniotic fluid at birth. Abdominal flat x-ray films typically show a stomach distended with air but no air in the bowel.

Treatment is surgical. If the atretic segment is short and involves only the mucosa, excision of the membrane plus a pyloroplasty may suffice. More extensive atresia requires excision and gastroduodenostomy or gastrojejunostomy.

Mucosal Membranes

Mucosal membranes may occur in the antrum or pylorus and encircle but typically do not occlude the lumen.[39,40] The membrane may contain either squamous or columnar epithelium. The etiology is probably related to the same factors that cause pyloric atresia. Acquired membranes have been attributed to peptic ulcer disease. Although vomiting may occur in infancy, symptoms usually do not develop until late childhood or adulthood, and are related to the narrowness of the aperture.

The diagnosis should be suspected when there is unexplained vomiting. Plain abdominal films usually are normal, but the barium contrast upper gastrointestinal series shows a sharply defined, bandlike defect in the prepyloric antrum. Gastric emptying may be delayed, and the portion of the antrum between the mucosal membrane and the pylorus may simulate a second duodenal bulb.

Treatment is simple surgical excision of the membrane with or without pyloroplasty.

Duplication of the Stomach

Gastric duplications contain mucosa, submucosa, and the three layers of muscle and are separate from the main portion of the stomach.[41,42] Rarely, they communicate with the stomach or the pancreas, but typically occur as a noncommunicating, extragastric mass. Gastric duplications may coexist with other duplications of the digestive tract.

Patients may present at any age with an abdominal mass, pain, or symptoms of gastric obstruction, but most become symptomatic in infancy. Occult bleeding may occur, accounting for unexplained anemia, or patients may present with hematemesis or melena if peptic ulceration develops at the site of communication. Rarely, the cyst perforates into the abdomen resulting in peritonitis. The diagnosis is suspected on upper gastrointestinal series by the appearance of a mass that protrudes into the lumen, extrinsic compression of the stomach, or filling of the cyst with barium. Treatment is surgical excision.

Microgastria

Microgastria is a failure of the stomach to develop from the foregut.[43] Thus, it does not enlarge, rotate, or differentiate into fundus, body, and antrum. The esophagus dilates and may provide some storage of ingested food, but patients with microgastria generally present with vomiting, malnutrition, and anemia shortly after birth. The condition usually is associated with developmental cardiac abnormalities. Most patients die within weeks to months. Treatment initially consists of frequent small feedings and intravenous alimentation. If the patient survives, surgical formation of a jejunal reservoir pouch can be considered.[44]

Gastric Teratoma

Teratomas are unusual congenital tumors that contain all three primary embryonic germ layers.[45] They may occur virtually anywhere in the body and are rare in the stomach. Gastric teratomas may present with upper gastrointestinal bleeding, signs of obstruction, or simply an upper abdominal mass. They are found almost exclusively in males. Although gastric teratomas usually are diagnosed in children, they may not be discovered until adulthood.[46]

Plain abdominal films may show calcification, which usually is either teeth or bone within the tumor, and barium contrast studies confirm a gastric mass.

Treatment is surgical resection of the tumor. Because of the large size of these tumors, total gastric resection with formation of a jejunal pouch may be necessary.[45] Gastric teratomas usually are not associated with other congenital abnormalities, and prognosis is good.

HYPERTROPHIC PYLORIC STENOSIS

Neonatal

Neonatal hypertrophic pyloric stenosis is due to hypertrophy and edema of the pyloric muscle, causing gastric outlet obstruction. It is common, occurring once in every 150 births in males, and once in every 750 births in females. It is the most common indication for surgery during the first 6 months of life.[47] The etiology is unknown. Cases tend to cluster in families.

Infants with hypertrophic pyloric stenosis typically remain asymptomatic until the third or fourth week after birth, when they develop regurgitation, then projectile vomiting. Vomiting may occur immediately after ingestion of food or may be delayed until the stomach is full. The vomitus is free of bile but may contain blood after repeated vomiting. Despite the vomiting, the infant continues to feed until malnutrition and weakness supervene, and interest in feeding wanes. Because so little of what is ingested reaches the intestine, constipation and oliguria are frequent complications, and the infant fails to gain weight.

On physical examination, the baby appears thin and dehydrated. The hypertrophied pyloric muscle characteristically is felt as a mass somewhere in the upper abdomen. The stomach is dilated, and gastric peristalsis may be visible. The palpable pyloric mass is most likely to be detected immediately after the infant has vomited, whereas the dilated stomach and visible peristalsis are more evident during or after feeding.

An upright plain film of the abdomen typically shows a large gastric air bubble but little or no air beyond the stomach in the intestine. Upper gastrointestinal x-ray series shows a long, narrow pyloric canal, typically giving the appearance of a "double channel" (Fig 59-9). The prepyloric antrum and the duodenal bulb may be indented by the mass. To minimize pulmonary aspiration and to enhance diagnostic visibility, the stomach should be evacuated before instilling barium. The characteristic hypertrophied muscle mass can be identified by ultrasound examination, which may obviate the need for barium contrast studies.[48]

The initial treatment of infants with hypertrophic pyloric stenosis is to replace fluid and electrolytes and correct the alkalosis that usually results from protracted vomiting. Definitive therapy is surgical division of the pyloric muscle from the serosa to the submucosa. After surgery, the infant may have some mild vomiting, but symptoms usually disappear in several days. Subsequent growth and development are normal, and long-term results are excellent.

Adult

Rarely, an adult may develop signs and symptoms of pyloric obstruction due to congenital hypertrophic pyloric stenosis.[49] However, most cases of adult hypertrophic pyloric stenosis are thought to develop secondary to chronic pyloric ulcer disease, severe gastritis, or cancer, which leads to hypertrophy of the pyloric muscle. In some patients, because of a familial occurrence, genetic predisposition is suspected.

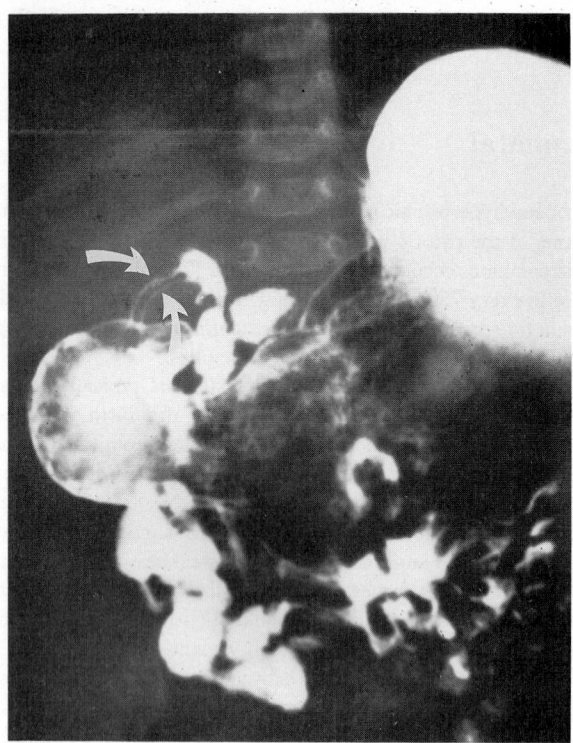

FIGURE 59–9. Barium contrast upper gastrointestinal series shows the long, narrow, "double-channel" of the pylorus (*arrows*) in a patient with hypertrophic pyloric stenosis.

Nausea, vomiting, early satiety, and epigastric pain, aggravated by eating, are typical complaints. Because these symptoms are similar to those of the associated disease, the diagnosis of hypertrophic pyloric stenosis may be delayed. The pyloric mass is relatively small and is not felt on physical examination.

The barium contrast study shows a long, narrow pyloric channel, delay in gastric emptying, and sometimes dilatation of the stomach. Upper gastrointestinal endoscopy is indicated to rule out carcinoma or confirm the diagnosis of peptic disease.

Surgical resection of the pyloric region, with a gastroduode-

nostomy, is the therapeutic procedure of choice to rule out a small focus of carcinoma within the hypertrophied muscle.

CONGENITAL DUODENAL OBSTRUCTIONS

Atresias and Membranes

These congenital obstructions are similar in etiology to those that occur in the stomach (see section titled "Congenital Abnormalities of the Stomach"). During early embryologic development, the duodenal lumen is filled completely with epithelium. Failure of subsequent recanalization results in stenosis of the duodenum. The obstruction may be a simple mucosal membrane or more extensive, involving all layers of the duodenum for a variable length. Duodenal atresias frequently are associated with other congenital anomalies, including Down's syndrome, malrotation of the gut, cardiac anomalies, tracheoesophageal fistula, renal anomalies, anorectal malformations, and annular pancreas.[50]

Infants with duodenal membrane or atresia develop vomiting shortly after birth. If the obstruction is proximal to the ampulla of Vater, the vomitus is devoid of bile; if it is distal to the ampulla, the vomitus is bile-stained. Rarely, duodenal membranes persist into adulthood or develop in adults for unknown reasons. These patients complain of epigastric fullness, vomiting, and loss of weight.

If the obstruction is distal to the duodenal bulb, plain abdominal films show the typical "double-bubble" appearance of a distended duodenal bulb and a distended stomach (Fig 59-10). Absence of gas distal to the duodenum suggests complete obstruction. Upper gastrointestinal contrast x-ray studies may not be necessary but can confirm the site of obstruction.

Treatment begins with nasogastric suction and correction of fluid and electrolyte abnormalities. Surgical treatment consists of gastrojejunostomy for proximal duodenal obstructions and duodenojejunostomy for mid and distal duodenal obstructions. Prog-

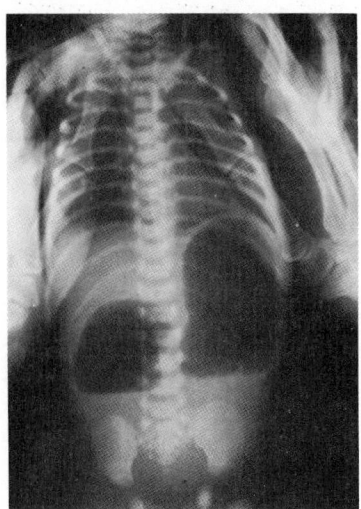

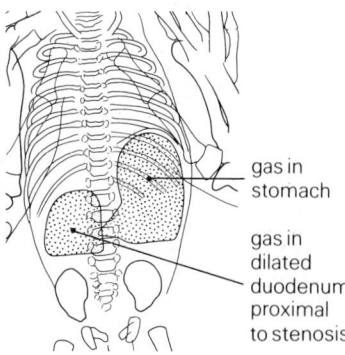

gas in stomach

gas in dilated duodenum proximal to stenosis

FIGURE 59–10. Plain abdominal radiograph in an infant with duodenal atresia shows the "double-bubble" sign. Both the stomach and the proximal duodenum are distended with air. (Misiewicz JJ, Bartram Cl, Cotton PB, Mee AS, Price AB, Thompson RPH. Atlas of clinical gastroenterology. London: Gower Medical Publishing, 1987.)

nosis depends on the severity of associated anomalies. Recently, endoscopic treatment of duodenal membranes in adults using laser or electrocautery has been reported.[51,52]

Annular Pancreas

Patients with annular pancreas may have complete or partial duodenal obstruction. They may present as neonates with intractable vomiting or as children or young adults with less dramatic vomiting and abdominal pain. The etiology of the condition is not clear but probably results from failure of complete migration of the ventral pancreatic bud during embryogenesis, resulting in either a remnant of pancreatic tissue within the duodenal wall or a portion of the pancreas that partially encircles the duodenum. Annular pancreas frequently is associated with other anomalies, such as malrotation, facial cleft, imperforate anus, cardiac malformations, tracheo-esophageal malformations, and Down's syndrome.[53]

The clinical presentation and plain abdominal x-ray films are consistent with duodenal obstruction, such as described above with duodenal atresia. Upper gastrointestinal x-ray series confirms the site of duodenal obstruction but cannot differentiate among the various causes of duodenal obstruction (Fig 59-11). In the adult, endoscopic retrograde cholangiopancreatography (ERCP) may make the diagnosis of annular pancreas when the duct supplying the annular pancreas is connected with the main pancreatic duct.[54]

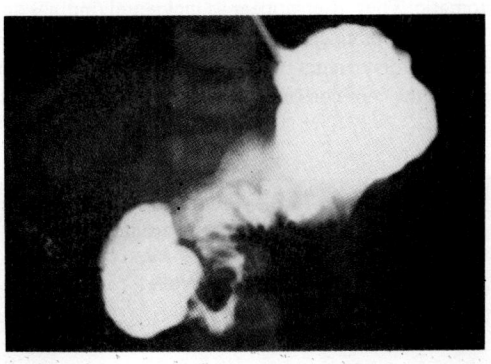

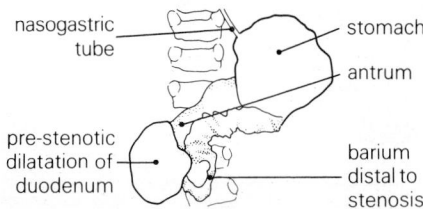

FIGURE 59–11. Barium contrast upper gastrointestinal series shows partial occlusion of the second part of the duodenum, consistent with annular pancreas, duodenal atresia, or other causes of duodenal obstruction. (Courtesy of Dr. K. J. Shah.) (Misiewicz JJ, Bartram Cl, Cotton PB, Mee AS, Price AB, Thompson RPH. Atlas of clinical gastroenterology. London: Gower Medical Publishing, 1987.)

Annular pancreas may also be associated with acute[54] and chronic[55] pancreatitis.

Management consists of nasogastric intubation for decompression of the stomach and correction of fluid and electrolyte abnormalities. Definitive treatment is either a duodenoduodenostomy or duodenojejunostomy.[53] Resection or division of the narrowed segment should not be attempted because of the risk of developing pancreatitis or a pancreatic fistula. As with duodenal membranes and atresias, the results of surgery in relieving the duodenal obstruction are good, and the prognosis depends on the outcome of associated anomalies.

Duplication

Duplications of the duodenum contain all the layers of the normal duodenum and, as in the stomach, may or may not communicate with the main duodenal lumen. They cause obstruction because of their mass effect, which compresses the duodenum. The clinical presentation and diagnosis are similar to other congenital duodenal obstructions. Rarely, duodenal duplications may perforate into the head of the pancreas and cause pancreatitis. The treatment is surgical and is dictated by the relationship of the cyst to the biliary and pancreatic ducts and the blood vessels.[56] If total resection is not possible, the cyst may be drained into adjacent bowel.

Incomplete Rotation of the Intestines

Incomplete or abnormal rotation of the large or small intestine is the most common cause of duodenal obstruction in childhood.[57,58] Mesenteric bands may compress the second or third parts of the duodenum either when the cecum fails to rotate completely into the right lower abdomen or when the hepatic flexure lies medial to the duodenum. Also, if the duodenum fails to complete its rotation (see section entitled "Embryology of the Stomach and Duodenum"), the ligament of Treitz may come to lie to the right of the midline, rather than to the left, resulting in kinking of the duodenum or obstruction by mesenteric bands. Over 50% of patients with malrotation have another developmental anomaly, such as duodenal atresia, annular pancreas, or Hirschsprung's disease.

Patients typically present within the first few weeks of life with bilious vomiting and abdominal distention. Peristalsis may be visible. Sometimes, volvulus of the intestine or cecum occurs because of the loose mesentery, which causes intestinal ischemia and bleeding. These patients have bloody stool and may develop perforation, peritonitis, and sepsis. Some patients with malrotation are asymptomatic as neonates but experience intermittent postprandial vomiting and distention later in childhood or as an adult. Still others remain asymptomatic throughout life.

As with other causes of duodenal obstruction, plain abdominal x-ray films typically show a large gastric air bubble and a distended duodenum proximal to the obstruction. An upper gastrointestinal x-ray series can confirm the site of obstruction and, if barium is able to pass to the distal bowel, may identify the type and extent of malrotation.

Treatment consists of surgical division of obstructing bands, fixation of the cecum to prevent further episodes of volvulus, and resection of infarcted segments of bowel. If the latter is extensive, the infants develop malabsorption and may require intravenous alimentation.

Superior Mesenteric Artery Syndrome

The superior mesenteric artery (SMA) passes over the third portion of the duodenum. Rarely, the SMA appears to obstruct the duodenum at this point, compressing the duodenum against the fixed retroperitoneal structures. This condition has been attributed to an acute angle of the SMA with the aorta, thereby trapping the duodenum, but the exact etiology is unknown.[59]

The clinical importance of the SMA syndrome has been questioned because of the nonspecific nature of the symptoms attributed to it and the difficulty in documenting SMA compression of the duodenum as the cause of the symptoms.[60] The typical patient with SMA syndrome complains of episodic epigastric distress, often associated with vomiting. Symptoms may be acute or chronic, sometimes dating back to early childhood. Compression of the duodenum by the SMA has been associated with rapid growth in children, marked weight loss in adults, immobilization in a body cast (which increases lordosis and accentuates the angle of the SMA with the aorta), previous abdominal surgery, and inflammatory conditions of the abdomen.

Plain abdominal films in adults usually are unremarkable, but in children a "double-bubble" sign may be evident (see section entitled "Atresias and Membranes" and Fig 59-10). Upper gastrointestinal barium contrast studies show a typical abrupt cutoff of the barium in the third portion of the duodenum with proximal dilatation.[61] Lateral views during abdominal aortography may show a narrowed angle of the SMA with the aorta. Because of the controversy about the clinical importance of the SMA syndrome, it is necessary to exclude other causes of abdominal pain before making the diagnosis of SMA syndrome.

Initial treatment includes small feedings or a liquid diet. The patient may benefit from lying prone or on the left side after eating. Recovery of lost weight or removal of a body cast typically improves symptoms. Surgical treatment of refractory cases is usually duodenojejunostomy.

Preduodenal Portal Vein

A preduodenal portal vein, sometimes in association with a preduodenal common bile duct, also can cause obstruction of the duodenum.[61–63] The condition is rare; only about 50 cases have been reported. The association of preduodenal vein with other congenital malformations, such as duodenal stenosis or atresia, annular pancreas, intestinal malrotation, and biliary tract abnormalities, is important for the surgeon to remember to avoid serious surgical accident at the time of correction of the other malformation. During early embryonic life, both retro- and preduodenal

veins drain the primitive gut.[61] Usually the preduodenal branch atrophies, leaving a normal retroduodenal portal vein. However, if the retroduodenal branch atrophies, the preduodenal vein remains patent and may compress the duodenum.

GASTRIC AND DUODENAL DIVERTICULA

Gastric and duodenal diverticula may be congenital or acquired.[64,65] Over 75% of gastric diverticula occur on the posterior wall within 2 cm of the esophagogastric junction and are thought to be congenital (Fig 59-12). The remaining gastric diverticula usually are found in the prepyloric antrum and develop as a result of the scarring and dilatation that may accompany peptic or neoplastic disease or because of surgery for those conditions. They usually cause no symptoms independent of the underlying cause and require no specific treatment.

Congenital gastric diverticula usually are discovered as incidental findings on barium contrast studies. The large majority are asymptomatic. Symptoms of pain, pressure, or dyspepsia, when they do occur, probably are related to other causes. However, bleeding and perforation have been reported and are treated surgically. Otherwise, no treatment is indicated.

Congenital duodenal diverticula predominate within 2 cm of the ampulla of Vater (Fig 59-13). In fact, the ampulla may empty into a diverticulum. Congenital duodenal diverticula usually are asymptomatic. They often appear as incidental findings on barium contrast studies and may interfere with attempts at ERCP. However, duodenal diverticula in the vicinity of the ampulla of Vater may obstruct the common bile duct, either by external compression

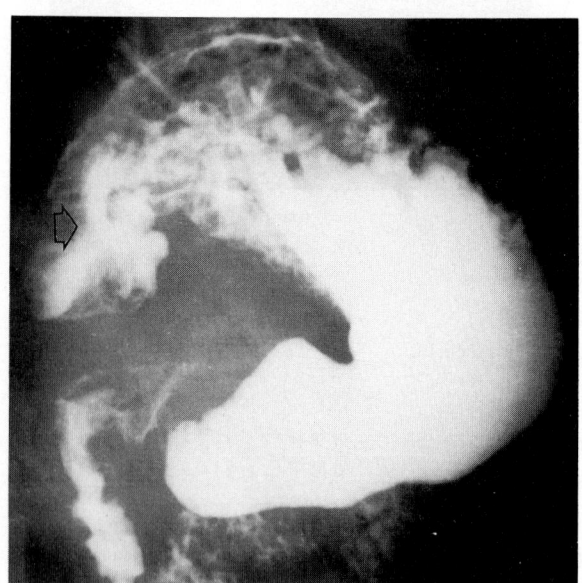

FIGURE 59–12. Barium contrast upper gastrointestinal series shows a large diverticulum originating on the lesser curve near the esophagogastric junction (*arrowhead*).

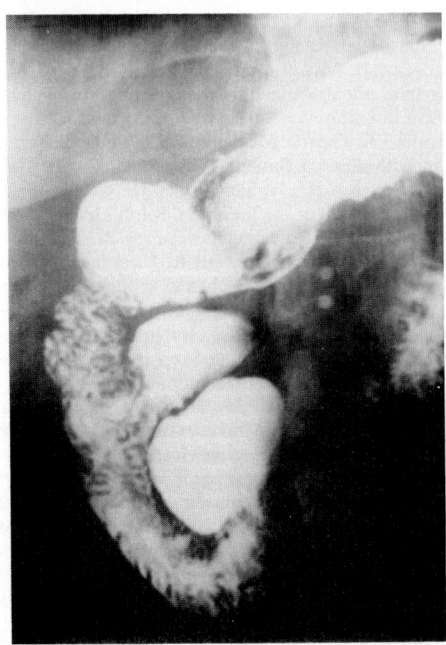

FIGURE 59–13. View of the duodenal loop during a barium contrast upper gastrointestinal series showing two large diverticula arising from the medial border of the descending duodenum. (Misiewicz JJ, Bartram CI, Cotton PB, Mee AS, Price AB, Thompson RPH. Atlas of clinical gastroenterology. London: Gower Medical Publishing, 1987.)

on the duct or by distorting the entry into the duodenum. Nevertheless, most cases of extrahepatic biliary obstruction in association with a duodenal diverticulum are due to some other cause, such as an obstructing common bile duct stone or a neoplasm.

If a duodenal diverticulum is proven to obstruct the common bile duct, the appropriate surgical treatment is either choledochoduodenostomy or Roux-en-Y choledochojejunostomy, and not excision of the diverticulum.

Acquired duodenal diverticula are found almost always in the duodenal bulb, which is the most common site of peptic ulcer disease. As with acquired antral diverticula, acquired duodenal diverticula usually do not require treatment.

ECTOPIC GASTRIC MUCOSA

Gastric mucosa has been identified in the esophagus,[66] small intestine,[67] and large intestine.[68] In the esophagus, a congenital mucosal rest may be present in as many as 5% of the normal population.[66] This usually occurs in the upper esophagus, ranging from a few millimeters to complete encirclement. Rarely, the patch may ulcerate and cause dysphagia or bleeding. Ectopic gastric mucosa of the small intestine may develop polypoid lesions that obstruct or bleed.[67] Of course, Meckel's diverticula that contain gastric mucosa may cause ulceration and bleeding.[69] Gastric mucosa in the colon and rectum has been described alone or in association with mucosal polypoid lesions and typically is manifested by rectal bleeding.[68]

The reader is directed to Chapter 1, The Enteric Nervous System and its Extrinsic Connections; Chapter 2, Gastrointestinal Hormones; Chapter 6, Epithelia: Biologic Principles of Organization; Chapter 8, The Physiology of Gastric Motility and Gastric Emptying; Chapter 13, Gastric Secretion; Chapter 53, Esophagus: Anatomy and Structural Anomalies; Chapter 60, Disorders of Gastric Emptying; Chapter 61, Acid-Peptic Disorders; Chapter 62, Zollinger-Ellison Syndrome; Chapter 63, Tumors of the Stomach; Chapter 64, Surgery for Peptic Ulcer Disease; Chapter 65, Miscellaneous Diseases of the Stomach; Chapter 66, Small Intestine: Anatomy and Structural Anomalies; Chapter 76, Colon: Anatomy and Structural Anomalies; Chapter 87, Pancreas: Anatomy and Structural Anomalies; Chapter 109, Vascular Insufficiency; Chapter 111, Upper Gastrointestinal Endoscopy; Chapter 114, Contrast Radiology; Chapter 122, Angiography; and Chapter 126, Endoscopic Mucosal Biopsy.

REFERENCES

1. Ito S. Anatomic structure of the gastric mucosa. In: Code CF, Heidel W, eds. Handbook of physiology, alimentary canal, secretion. Washington, DC: American Physiological Society, 1967;Section 6, 2:705.
2. Lillibridge CB. The fine structure of normal human gastric mucosa. Gastroenterology 1964;47:269.
3. Rubin W, Ross LL, Sleisenger MH, Jeffries GH. The normal human gastric epithelia. A fine structural study. Lab Invest 1968;19:598.
4. Rohrer GV, Scott JR, Joel W, Wolf S. The fine structure of human gastric parietal cells. Am J Dig Dis 1965;10:13.
5. Rosa F. Ultrastructure of the human gastric mucosa in the resting state and after stimulation with Histalog. Gastroenterology 1963;45:354.
6. Sedar AW. Fine structure of the stimulated oxyntic cell. Fed Proc 1965;24:1360.
7. Rubin W. Endocrine cells in the normal human stomach. A fine structural study. Gastroenterology 1972;63:784.
8. Greider MH, Steinberg V, McGuigan JE. Electron microscopic identification of the gastrin cell of the human antral mucosa by means of immunocytochemistry. Gastroenterology 1972;63:572.
9. Hengels KJ, Muller JE, Scholten T, Fritsch WP. Evidence for the secretion of gastrin into human gastric juice. Gut 1980;21:760.
10. Achkar E, Carey WD, Petras R, et al. Comparison of suction capsule and endoscopic biopsy of small bowel mucosa. Gastrointest Endosc 1986;32:278.
11. Trier JS. Diagnostic value of peroral biopsy of the small intestine. N Engl J Med 1971;285:1470.
12. Cheng H, Leblond CP. Origin, differentiation and renewal of the four main epithelial cell types in the mouse small intestine. V. Unitarian theory of the origin of the four main epithelial cell types. Am J Anat 1974;141:537.
13. Trier JS, Rubin CE. Electron microscopy of the small intestine: A review. Gastroenterology 1965;49:574.
14. Eastwood GL. Gastrointestinal epithelial renewal. Gastroenterology 1977;72:962.
15. Lipkin M. Growth and development of gastrointestinal cells. Annu Rev Physiol 1985;47:175.
16. MacDonald WC, Trier JS, Everett NB. Cell proliferation and migration in the stomach, duodenum, and rectum of man: Radioautographic studies. Gastroenterology 1964;46:405.
17. Ragins H, Wincz F, Liu SM, et al. The origin and survival of gastric parietal cells in the mouse. Anat Rec 1968;162:99.
18. Parker FG, Barnes EN, Kaye GI. The pericryptal fibroblast sheath. IV. Replication, migration, and differentiation of the subepithelial

fibroblasts of the crypt and villus of the rabbit jejunum. Gastroenterology 1974;67:607.

19. Yeomans ND, St John DJB, deBoer WGRM. Regeneration of gastric mucosa after aspirin-induced injury in the rat. Am J Dig Dis 1973;18:773.

20. Willems G, Vansteenkiste Y, Smets PH. Effects of ethanol on the cell proliferation kinetics in the fundic mucosa of dogs. Am J Dig Dis 1971;16:1057.

21. Eastwood GL, Quimby GF. Effect of chronic aspirin ingestion on epithelial proliferation in rat fundus, antrum, and duodenum. Gastroenterology 1982;82:852.

22. Kuwayama H, Eastwood GL. Effects of water immersion restraint stress and chronic indomethacin ingestion on gastric antral and fundic epithelial proliferation. Gastroenterology 1985;88:362.

23. Eastwood GL, Quimby GF, Laferriere JR. Effects of chronic steroid ingestion on gastroduodenal epithelial renewal in the rat. Cell Tissue Kinet 1981;14:405.

24. Basso N, Materia A, Forlini A, et al. Prostaglandin generation in the gastric mucosa of rats with stress ulcer. Surgery 1983;94:104.

25. Avunduk C, Eastwood GL, Polakowski NJ, Quimby GF, et al. Effects of stress on gastric mucosal prostaglandin generation in intact, adrenalectomized, and sham operated rats. J Clin Gastroenterol, 1990;12(Suppl 1):S48–S51.

26. Castrup HJ, Fuchs K. Cell renewal in inflammatory changes of the gastric mucosa. Dtsch Med Wochenschr 1974;99:892.

27. Bell B, Almy TP, Lipkin M. Cell proliferation kinetics in the gastrointestinal tract of man. III. Cell renewal in esophagus, stomach, and jejunum of a patient with treated pernicious anemia. J Natl Cancer Inst 1967;38:615.

28. Pellish LJ, Hermos JA, Eastwood GL. Cell proliferation in three types of Barrett's epithelium. Gut 1980;21:26.

29. Eastwood GL, Trier JS. Epithelial cell renewal in cultured rectal biopsies in ulcerative colitis. Gastroenterology 1973;64:383.

30. Castrup HJ, Fuchs K, Pieper HJ. Cell renewal of gastric mucosa in Zollinger-Ellison syndrome. Acta Hepatogastroenterol 1975;22:40.

31. Miller LR, Jacobson ED, Johnson LR. Effect of pentagastrin on gastric mucosal cells grown in tissue culture. Gastroenterology 1973;64:254.

32. Bransom CJ, Boxer ME, Clark JC, et al. Epithelial cell proliferation in duodenal ulcer. Scand J Gastroenterol 1984;19:515.

33. Uribe A, Rubio C, Johansson C. Cell kinetics of rat gastrointestinal mucosa. Autoradiographic study after treatment with 15(R)15-methyl-prostaglandin E$_2$. Scand J Gastroenterol 1986;21:246.

34. Uribe A, Johansson C, Rubio C. Cell proliferation of the rat gastrointestinal mucosa after treatment with E$_2$ prostaglandins and indomethacin. Digestion 1987;36:238.

35. Svendsen LB, Jorgensen FS, Hansen OH, et al. Influence of the prostaglandin E$_1$ analogue rioprostil on the human gastric mucosa. Digestion 1987;37:29.

36. Sadler TW. Langman's medical embryology, 5th ed. Baltimore: Williams & Wilkins, 1985:224.

37. Moore KL. Before we are born. Basic embryology and birth defects, 3rd ed. Philadelphia: WB Saunders, 1989:166.

38. Olsen L, Grotte G. Congenital pyloric atresia: Report of a familial occurrence. J Pediatr Surg 1976;11:181.

39. Haddad V, Macon WL IV, Islami MH. Mucosal diaphragms of the gastric antrum in adults. Surg Gynecol Obstet 1981;152:227.

40. Feliciano DV, Van Heerden JA. Pyloric antral mucosal webs. Mayo Clin Proc 1977;52:650.

41. Wieczorek RL, Seidman I, Ranson JHC, et al. Congenital duplication of the stomach: Case report and review of the English literature. Am J Gastroenterol 1984;79:597.

42. Parker BC, Guthrie J, France NE, Atwell JD. Gastric duplications in infancy. J Pediatr Surg 1972;7:294.

43. Gorman B, Shaw DG. Congenital microgastria. Br J Radiol 1984;57:260.

44. Shackelford GD, McAllister WH, Brodeur AF, et al. Management of congenital microgastria with a jejunal reservoir pouch. J Pediatr Surg 1980;15:882.

45. De Angelis VR. Gastric teratoma in a newborn infant: Total gastrectomy with survival. Surgery 1969;66:794.

46. Gray SW, Johnson HC Jr, Skandalakis JE. Gastric teratoma in an adult: With a review of the literature. South Med J 1964;57:1346.

47. Benson DC. Infantile pyloric stenosis. Prog Pediatr Surg 1970;1:63.

48. Ball TI, Atkinson GO Jr, Gay BB Jr. Ultrasound diagnosis of hypertrophic pyloric stenosis: Real-time application and the demonstration of a new sonographic sign. Radiology 1983;147:499.

49. Wellman KF, Kagan A, Fang H. Hypertrophic pyloric stenosis in adults. Survey of the literature and report of a case of the localized form (torus hyperplasia). Gastroenterology 1964;46:601.

50. Fonkalsrud EW, deLorimier AA, Hays DM. Congenital atresia and stenosis of the duodenum: A review compiled from the members of the surgical section of the American Academy of Pediatrics. Pediatrics 1969;43:79.

51. Gertsch P, Mosimann R. Endoscopic laser treatment of a congenital duodenal diaphragm in an adult. Gastrointest Endosc 1984;30:253.

52. Jex RK, Hughes RW Jr. Endoscopic management of a duodenal diaphragm in the adult. Gastrointest Endosc 1986;32:416.

53. Merrill JR, Raffensperger JG. Pediatric annular pancreas: Twenty years' experience. J Pediatr Surg 1976;11:921.

54. Chevillotte G, Sahel J, Raillat A, et al. Annular pancreas. Report of one case associated with acute pancreatitis and diagnosed by endoscopic retrograde pancreatography. Dig Dis Sci 1984;29:75.

55. Gilinsky NH, Lewis JW, Flueck JA, et al. Annular pancreas associated with diffuse chronic pancreatitis. Am J Gastroenterol 1987;82:681.

56. Soper RT, Selke AC. Duplication cyst of the duodenum: Case report and discussion. Surgery 1970;68:562.

57. Kiesewetter WB, Smith JW. Malrotation of the midgut in infancy and childhood. Arch Surg 1958;77:483.

58. Filston HC, Kirks DR. Malrotation: The ubiquitous anomaly. J Pediatr Surg 1981;16:614.

59. Akin JT Jr, Skandalakis JE, Gray SW. The anatomic basis of vascular compression of the duodenum. Surg Clin North Am 1974;54:1361.

60. Shandling B. The so-called superior mesenteric artery sundrome. Am J Dis Child 1976;130:1371.

61. Marchant EA, Alvear DT, Fagelman KM. True clinical entity of vascular compression of the duodenum in adolescence. Surg Gynecol Obstet 1989;168:381.

62. Braun P, Collin PP, Ducharme JC. Preduodenal portal vein: A significant entity? Report of two cases and review of the literature. Can J Surg 1974;17:316.

63. Makey DA, Bowen JC. Preduodenal portal vein: Its surgical significance. Surgery 1978;84:689.

64. Eras P, Beranbaum SZ. Gastric diverticula: Congenital and acquired. Am J Gastroenterol 1972;57:120.

65. Osnes M, Lotveit T, Larsen S, Aune S. Duodenal diverticula and their relationship to age, sex, and biliary calculi. Scand J Gastroenterol 1981;16:103.

66. Jabbari M, Goresky C, Lough J, et al. The inlet patch: Heterotopic gastric mucosa in the upper esophagus. Gastroenterology 1985;89:352.

67. Lee SM, Mosenthal WT, Weisman RE. Tumorous heterotopic gastric mucosa in the small intestine. Arch Surg 1970;100:619.

68. Wolff M. Heterotopic gastric epithelium in the rectum. Am J Clin Pathol 1971;55:604.

69. Weinstein EC, Cain JC, ReMine WH. Meckel's diverticulum: 55 years of clinical and surgical experience. JAMA 1962;182:251.

60

Disorders of Gastric Emptying

HENRY C. LIN
JAMES H. MEYER

A gastroenterologist is frequently faced with patients whose symptoms of early satiety, bloating, nausea, vomiting, or abdominal pain remain unexplained after the usual diagnostic studies of endoscopies, ultrasounds and computed tomography (CT) scans. Many of these patients complain of intermittent epigastric symptoms that are closely tied to meals. For these postprandial complaints, patients often either go through a cholecystectomy or become chronic users of antiulcer medications. Many, however, remain largely unrelieved despite these therapeutic attempts and continue to search for a cure. Depending on their medical histories, these patients often carry a variety of previous diagnoses, such as gastritis, spastic stomach, food intolerances, postgastrectomy or postcholecystectomy syndromes, irritable gut, functional bowel syndrome, and nonulcer dyspepsia. As a result of the availability of quantitative gastric emptying studies, delayed gastric emptying of food from the stomach has been found in many of these chronic sufferers. This finding has prompted the use of the more specific terms of gastric stasis and gastroparesis. In this chapter we will discuss different methods to assess gastric motility and various disorders of altered gastric emptying.

METHODS TO ASSESS GASTRIC MOTILITY

Quantification of Gastric Emptying

The development of reliable methods to quantify gastric emptying underlies much of recent progress in understanding normal and disordered gastric motility. Of the 14 methods available (Table 60-1), gamma scintigraphy has become the standard because of its precision and simplicity. It is noninvasive and exposes the patient to much less radiation than methods that use x-rays, yet it provides accurate measurements of gastric emptying.[1-3]

A newer method, applied potential tomography,[4,5] has the advantages of portability of equipment and freedom from radiation. These advantages, however, are offset by the method's limitation to liquid meals and requirement for pharmacologic inhibition of gastric secretions (which interfere with the measurement of gastric impedence). Real-time ultrasonography[6-8] is also noninvasive, but

equipment is currently limited to major centers, and it is difficult to use with solid meals or in obese subjects.

Gamma cameras can be used to track gastric emptying of liquids, solid foods, or indigestible solids, singly or in combinations. Solid foods are easily labeled with ^{99m}technetium sulfur colloid, which tightly binds to protein. Reliable methods include injecting the sulfur colloid into the matrix of meat[9,10] before cooking or intermixing the colloid in eggs or pancakes before solidifying the mixture during cooking.[11,12] Indigestible solids can be labeled by overcoating them with materials with which nuclides have been mixed.[13] Liquids are labeled with chelates of technetium or indium, which prevent the nuclides from binding to solid foods or gastric mucosa.[9,11]

Which of these should be used to measure gastric emptying? We now know that liquids (even those which contain nutrients), solid foods, and indigestible solids empty from the stomach in different temporal patterns that reflect differing motor phenomena (ch 8). Indigestible solids larger than 3 to 5 mm are emptied mostly by migrating motor complexes during periods of interdigestive motility. Digestible solid foods, when swallowed in the usual size of about 8 to 12 mm, commonly exhibit an initial lag (i.e., no or little emptying) during which the food is reduced by a combination of gastric motility and digestion to tiny particles (<1 mm) before it empties. These smaller particles are then carried from the stomach by liquids. Once emptying begins, solids continue to empty at a steady rate until less than 20% of the meal remains, after which their emptying slows. Thus, the overall shape of the time-course is typically sigmoid (Fig 60-1). On the other hand, liquids most often exhibit an initially rapid phase of emptying followed by a slower emptying phase, typically giving a biphasic time-course that resembles that of exponential decay (Fig 60-2). The rapid phase is most likely initiated by a combination of gravity and intragastric pressure generated by tone of the gastric wall pressing against the volume of the meal. The slower, second phase follows a reduction in gastric pressure and other reflex muscular adjustments to limit the rate of outflow.

The differing temporal patterns complicate assessments of emptying. A convenient measure of gastric emptying is the time taken to empty 50% of the tracked substances (T50%), and this simple measure has been used most often to discern disordered emptying. The rate of emptying during the steady emptying phase (with liquids or solids) is, however, not the only determinant of this measure. The duration and nature of the early emptying phase

TABLE 60–1
Principles of Methods Measuring Gastric Emptying

METHOD	MARKER	COMMENT
Radiographic		
Upper GI series	BaSO$_4$ suspension	Insensitive; not quantitative
Barium burger	Ba-impregnated food	More sensitive; not quantitative
Radiopaque tubes	Ba-filled plastic	Sensitive; quantitative
Intubation		
Saline load	Saline	Semiquantitative; insensitive
Serial test meal	Liquid nutrients	Quantitative; somewhat sensitive; impractical
Double sampling dye dilution	Liquid nutrients	Quantitative; somewhat sensitive
Intestinal dye dilution	Liquid or mixed meals	Quantitative; sensitive; cumbersome
Scintigraphic		
Scanner or single crystal	Liquid or mixed meals	Semiquantitative; sensitive
Gamma camera	Liquid or mixed meals; nondigestibles	Quantitative; sensitive; most versatile; now standard technique
Real-time ultrasound		
To measure gastric volume	Liquid meals	Quantitative; erect posture only; nonobese only
To measure gastric emptying time (antral cross-section)	Liquid or mixed meals	Semiquantitative; erect posture only; nonobese only
Gastric impedance		
Nontomographic; limited electrodes	Nonionic liquid or homogenized mixed meals	Quantitative; needs H$_2$ blockers
Tomographic	Nonionic liquid or homogenized mixed meals	Quantitative; needs H$_2$ blockers
Ferromagnetic	Iron suspension	Little experience

are also important. For solids, this is the length of time before emptying begins, and for liquids, this is the initially rapid emptying phase. With solid foods, the duration of the initial lag may vary quite a bit among normal subjects. As a result, the variation in T50% among normal subjects is wide. If the normal shape of the emptying time-course is distorted by disease, the T50% becomes even less accurate as a measure of emptying. For example, distal gastrectomy drastically alters the shape of the time-course. There often is an initially rapid emptying phase followed by an almost no emptying phase. In these circumstances, the T50% almost entirely reflects the magnitude of the initially rapid phase rather than the later rate of emptying. More sophisticated analyses have therefore tried to assess the shape of the curve as well as the T50%[14,15] or to measure the duration of the early phase.[16–18] These descriptive efforts to categorize the different shapes of emptying curves encountered in clinical practice hardly compensate for our ignorance of fundamental relationships between the shape of the emptying time-course and gastric motor events. Without such knowledge, it is almost impossible to use a simple test of gastric

emptying as a descriptor of diseased gastric motility other than as a screening test for disease. Even as screening tests, these techniques are less sensitive than they could be if we had a better understanding of the variables involved in normal gastric emptying. For example, the interpretation of gastric emptying results is hampered by our ignorance of those variables which underlie the marked day-to-day variation in the length of the initial lag phase among normal subjects.

Clinical data suggest that measuring gastric emptying of solids is more sensitive to the detection of disease than is measuring the emptying of liquids. A number of patients who were thought to have delayed gastric emptying on the basis of clinical symptoms have been studied with gamma cameras that tracked gastric emptying of solid food and liquid contents (most often water). Only 61% of the total were judged to have delayed gastric emptying (Table 60-2) by these tests. Of these, the majority (55%) had delayed gastric emptying of both liquids and solid food, but 45% exhibited normal gastric emptying of liquids, with delayed emptying of solid foods. Even before the advent of gamma cameras,

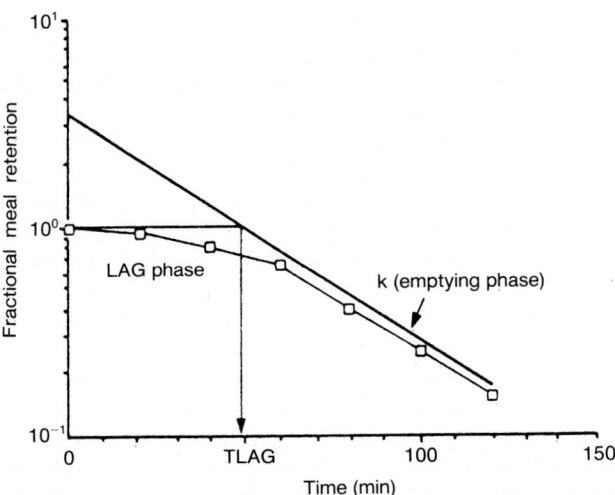

FIGURE 60–1. Solid emptying. (Siegel JA, Urbain JL, Adler LP, et al. Biphasic nature of gastric emptying. Gut 1988;29:85.)

gastroenterologists recognized that a barium burger test (i.e., solid food impregnated with barium sulfate) was more sensitive to disease than standard upper GI radiologic exams, which use aqueous suspensions of barium sulfate.[19,20] The lower sensitivity of liquid emptying to disorders of gastric motility may reflect the fact that solids require vigorous phasic contractions of the antrum for grinding and propulsion, whereas liquids can trickle from the stomach by gravity or can be propelled by the pressure of tonic contractions of the fundus (ch 8).

Gastric emptying of indigestible solids may also be measured. By impregnating them with barium sulfate, the number remaining in the stomach with time can be quantitated by serial radiographs. Feldman[21] has reported that 2 × 6-mm plastic cylinders are more sensitive in detecting delayed gastric emptying in diabetics than is radiolabeled food. It is as yet unknown whether these cylinders are retained by the food-filled stomach until the stomach is empty so that they are then expelled with the next migrating motor com-

LIQUID EMPTYING

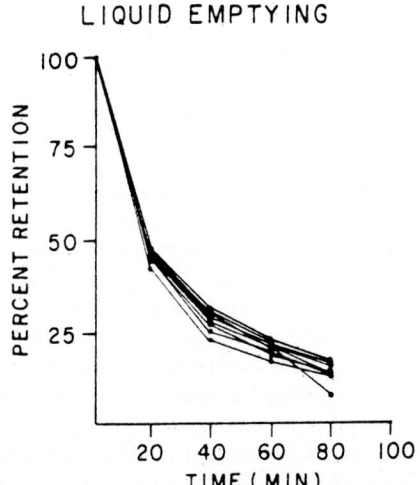

FIGURE 60–2. Liquid emptying. (Moore JF, Christian PE, Brown JA, et al. Influence of meal weight and caloric content on gastric emptying of liquids in man. Dig Dis Sci 1984;29:513.)

TABLE 60–2
Slow (s) Liquid (L) Versus Slow (s) Solid (S) Emptying*

	nL/nS	nL/sS	sL/ns	sL/sS
Diabetes mellitus				
Heading, 1977	9	0	1	2
Loo, 1984	10	4	0	5
Wright, 1985	0	10	0	0
Horowitz, 1985	4	1	0	7
Horowitz, 1986	19	5	10	11
Horowitz, 1987	2	0	5	13
Keshavarzian, 1987	22	4	0	4
Postgastrectomy†				
MacGregor, 1977	0	5	0	0
Gulsrud, 1979	6	1	0	0
Mayer, 1984	10	5	0	0
Dermatomyositis				
Horowitz, 1986	5	0	0	8
Scleroderma				
Horowitz, 1987	0	3	0	5
Gastric dysmotility				
Camilleri, 1986	0	0	0	13
Unspecified				
Siegel, 1987‡	14	10	0	13
Nonulcer dyspepsia				
Jian, 1989	18	2	2	6
Totals	119	50	18	87

n = normal, s = slow emptying, L = liquid, S = solid
* Almost all of the studied patients had clinical symptoms of gastric stasis. The number of patients in each category was not always stated but could be inferred from the texts of the papers. While this tabulation indicates a correlation between slowed liquid and solid emptying in the majority of abnormal subjects, about one third had slow solid emptying with normal liquid emptying. Many patients had no detectable emptying abnormality despite symptoms.
† All patients with vagotomy had abnormally rapid liquid (L) emptying, the normal outcome of this surgery and thus indicated as n.
‡ Abnormal by 50%-emptying criterion.

plex (MMC) or whether emptying of these cylinders is uniquely sensitive to diabetic gastropathy.

Most often, gamma scintigraphic methods have been used simply to measure gastric emptying as a transit phenomenon. Abnormalities of transit detected have not been easily related to abnormalities in gastric motility. Recently, however, the use of gamma cameras with better resolution and meals with high radioactivities have allowed observers to detect and interrelate antral contractions with gastric emptying.[22] Moreover, real-time ultrasonography can also provide information on gastric diameters,[7] antral contractions, and cyclical flows.[6] In view of the difficulties of studying gastric motility with manometry (discussed below), it is likely that these newer techniques, now in their infancy, will be further developed to study the relationship of gastric motility and transit. For example, the use of fast-frame nuclear magnetic resonance[23] may allow simultaneous tracking of gastric emptying of resonance markers in a test meal and patterns of contraction waves in three dimensions.

Whatever technique is used to study gastric emptying, clinicians should realize that a variety of factors other than disease may influence the observed rates. They are: (1) marker choice (digestible versus indigestible versus liquids),[24] (2) size and nutrient meal composition,[25] (3) meal temperature,[26] (4) time of day,[27] (5) subject posture (erect versus supine),[28] (6) patient's gender and/or female progesterone level,[29-33] (7) patient's age,[29,31,34-36] (8) drug intake (Table 60-3), (9) alcohol intake,[38] and (10) smoking.[36,37] Thus, it is imperative that test conditions be standardized and that each diagnostic unit establish individual standards of normal emptying to interpret test results. This procedure may appropriately include age and sex matching of control subjects. Even with these measures, day-to-day variations within normal subjects may be as high as 30%.[40] With such variation, tests of gastric emptying are probably insensitive to milder abnormalities of gastric motility, a possibility that may account for their inability to detect abnormality in up to a third of patients who complain of chronic nausea and vomiting (see Table 60-2).

Intraluminal Manometry

Most manometric studies have used either perfused, multilumen tubes with side holes connected to extracorporeal transducers or multiple, intraluminal solid-state transducers, devices similar to those used to study esophageal motility. Usually, a string of sensors is placed across the terminal antrum and pylorus so that the most distal probes are located in the duodenum, while more proximal probes record motility in the pylorus and distal antrum. This technique allows the investigator to record phasic contractions and determine which contractions were propagated along the antrum and/or across the pylorus. However, there are recording problems that are unique to the stomach. Unlike the esophagus or small intestine, the stomach is a cavernous, conical, rather than tubular, organ with its apex at the pylorus. Thus, manometric sensors positioned more proximally from the pylorus are farther away from the surrounding gastric wall. From animal studies in which records from serosal strain gauges were compared with intraluminal sensors,[41] it has been shown that the more proximal sensors may fail to record contractions. In the presence of food, and in some disorders of gastric emptying, most of the stomach, including the antrum,[7] dilates, a situation that can decrease the sensitivity of antral probes.

Another problem with manometry is that the recording may fail to accurately record pyloric contractions. Probes may slip in and out of the pyloric channel with gastric or even respiratory movements. One method of overcoming this difficulty is to decrease the spacing intervals between probes that lie across the pylorus so that there is a higher probability that one or another probe will always lie in the pylorus even with relative movement of the sensing assembly. An alternative is the use of a Dent manometric sleeve 6 cm in length. Because this apparatus is capable of detecting a contraction that impinges on any portion of its length, positioning the sleeve across the pylorus assures recording of sphincteric activity despite small dislocations.

Manometric sensors are best suited to record phasic contractions rather than alterations in gastric tone. Therefore, the tonic relaxation of the proximal stomach that allows the organ to store food and the postprandial increase in tone over time may be detected poorly (ch 8 and 128). Only recently has Azpiroz[42] developed an electronic barostat that is capable of sensing fundic tone. It remains to be seen whether such an apparatus will help clarify clinical disorders of gastric emptying. Manometric methods and their clinical application are discussed more thoroughly in Chapter 128.

TABLE 60-3
Effects of Medications on Gastric Emptying

Delays gastric emptying

Opiates

Atropine

Desmethylimipramine (tricyclic antidepressant)

Propantheline bromide

Aluminum hydroxide antacids

Sucralfate

Progesterone

Diphenhydramine (anticholinergic)

Beta agonist

L-dopa

Alcohol (high concentration)

Tobacco

Calcium channel blockers

Tetrahydrocannabinol

Glucagon

Accelerates gastric emptying

Histamine H_2 antagonist

Naloxone

Beta blockers

Metoclopramide

Domperidone

Cisapride

Electrogastrography

Normally, pacesetter potentials sweep the human antrum in an aboral direction at a frequency of three cycles per minute (ch 8). These slow waves can be detected in human subjects by surgical implantation of serosal electrodes[43] or by endoscopic siting of mucosal suction electrodes.[44] Such techniques have been used to demonstrate that some disorders that are manifested by abnormally slow gastric emptying are associated with abnormal pacesetter or slow wave activity: either the frequency of pacesetter cycles is slow (bradygastria) or an abnormally high-frequency, irritable focus of electrical activity in the distal antrum dominates electrical rhythms, driving the pacesetter activity in an abnormal, oral direction (tachygastria). Because phasic contractions of the antrum are triggered by the pacesetter, abnormalities in frequency or direction of pacesetter potentials may lead to abnormalities in frequency or direction of phasic contractions and as a result may alter gastric emptying. Because of the distinct frequency and strong directional orientation of the pacesetter, the potential may be detected through electrically filtered cutaneous recordings over and around the stomach region.[45,46] While electrogastrography is clinically useful in detecting pacesetter dysrhythmias, this test is not available in most medical centers. A more detailed discussion of this method can be found in Chapter 128.

PROKINETIC AGENTS

Because most disorders of gastric motility manifest as delayed emptying, therapy has focused on medications that increase gastric contraction. Prokinetic agents are drugs with facilitating action on gastrointestinal motility. Included in this group are metoclopramide and two newer agents, domperidone and cisapride, which are discussed in the following section (Table 60-4). Many other drugs are undergoing evaluation for their potential prokinetic effects. These are described in the section entitled Experimental Agents With Novel Modes of Action.

Established Agents

BETHANECHOL CHLORIDE

Bethanechol is a synthetic ester with cholinergic action primarily through stimulation of muscarinic receptors. When it is given orally or subcutaneously, the effects of the drug are limited to increasing contractile activities of the gastrointestinal and urinary tract.

The duration of action is 1 to 2 hours following an oral dose, peaking in 30 to 90 minutes. The elimination pathway of bethanechol is unknown. The usual oral dose is 25 mg four times a day.

Bethanechol has been used in a number of gastrointestinal motility disorders with variable efficacy. In the setting of gastroesophageal reflux disease, decreased lower esophageal pressure and delayed gastric emptying are commonly found in untreated patients. In this group, symptomatic improvement can be achieved with the use of this drug. The effects on esophageal and gastric motility, however, are mixed. Taken orally at a dose of 25 mg

four times per day, bethanechol increased lower esophageal sphincter pressure[47] but failed to have an accelerating effect on delayed gastric emptying.[48] Symptomatic response was easier to demonstrate. On 24-hour ambulatory pH monitoring, nocturnal reflux was reduced with this agent.[49] Furthermore, in a double-blind study, significant improvement in heartburn symptoms was also noted.[50]

In patients with severe diabetes mellitus, diminished esophageal peristalsis, decreased gastric motor activities, and absent interdigestive motor complex are all common abnormalities. In this setting, bethanechol increased esophageal peristalsis slightly,[51] markedly increased fundic and antral contractions, but did not trigger phase III activity.[52,53] However, no well controlled studies are available on the effects of bethanechol on gastric emptying and the upper gastrointestinal symptoms of diabetics. Because this drug lacks the central antiemetic advantage of the new prokinetic agents, its usefulness in diabetes is limited.

Adverse effects are rare when bethanechol is given orally. After an abnormally large dose, possible effects include abdominal cramps, skin flushing, sweating, lacrimation, salivation, nausea and vomiting, bronchoconstriction, urinary urgency, and miosis. Cardiovascular effects are infrequent with oral administration but may include a fall in blood pressure if the patient is hypertensive. Atrial fibrillation may occur in the hyperthyroid patient. The drug should not be given after recent gastrointestinal surgery or when a mechanical obstruction is suspected.[54]

METOCLOPRAMIDE

Metoclopramide (methoxychloroprocainamide) is a substituted benzamide with both dopamine-antagonistic and cholinergic-enhancing effects. In the gastrointestinal tract, dopamine is an inhibitor with the primary action of decreasing contractile activities in the esophagus and stomach.[55] The activities of metoclopramide are, however, principally the result of its potent cholinergic-enhancing effects. Dopamine antagonism also plays a role in the prokinetic effect of metoclopramide.[56] Atropine, but not vagotomy, decreases these cholinergic effects, indicating that the activity of the drug is at the level of the enteric cholinergic nerve. Unlike cholinergic drugs, the action of metoclopramide requires some endogenous cholinergic activity to be present. This requirement suggests that the cholinergic effect is the result of facilitation of acetylcholine release from cholinergic neurons. Moreover, a direct

TABLE 60-4
Prokinetic Agents

AGENT	ACTIVITY	MECHANISM(S)	DOSE
Metoclopramide	Proximal gut only	Central dopamine antagonism Cholinomimetic effect Sensitization of smooth muscle Muscarinic receptors	10 mg
Domperidone	Proximal gut only	Peripheral dopamine antagonism	20 mg q.i.d.
Cisapride	Esophagus to colon	Facilitation of acetylcholine Release from myenteric plexus Serotonin antagonism	10 mg q.i.d.

action on the smooth muscles of the gut by way of sensitization of muscarinic receptors is also likely to be important.[57]

The prokinetic properties of metoclopramide are mainly limited to the proximal gut. Only limited effect on the colon has been reported. Metoclopramide enhances transit of food from the esophagus to the ileocecal valve by increasing esophageal contraction, gastric emptying, and small intestinal motor activity.[58] Gastroduodenal coordination is facilitated by the drug's effect of simultaneously increasing antral contractions and relaxing the pylorus and duodenal bulb.[59] The dopamine-antagonistic action of metoclopramide inhibits fundic receptive relaxation, which further promotes gastric emptying.[60] Patients with delayed gastric emptying as a consequence of weakened antral contraction or incoordinated gastroduodenal activity may benefit from the actions of metoclopramide.

The peak plasma drug level is reached approximately 60 to 120 minutes after administration of an oral dose. This is delayed with impaired gastric emptying. The therapeutic plasma level ranges from 40 to 80 ng/ml. The onset of the prokinetic effect on the gastrointestinal tract occurs within 3 minutes of administration of an intravenous injection and within 60 minutes of administration of an oral dose. The plasma half-life is about 4 hours. With 80% of the drug excreted in the urine unchanged, reduced renal function delays drug elimination.[61]

In patients presenting with significant impaired gastric emptying, intravenous use of the drug may be required until sufficient symptomatic response permits oral drug administration. The usual adult oral dose is 10 mg four times per day, taken 30 minutes before meals and at bedtime. Initially, the therapy is for 2 to 8 weeks.[61] With symptomatic relief, an attempt should be made to discontinue the drug. Unfortunately, many clinical disorders of gastroparesis have a chronic relapsing course necessitating indefinite therapy.

Central nervous system (CNS) actions are important for both the beneficial and adverse effects of metoclopramide. The antiemetic activity of the agent is illustrated by its blocking action on apomorphine. Centrally, the emetic effects of apomorphine on the chemoreceptor trigger zone are blocked by the dopamine antagonism of metoclopramide, and peripherally, the retrograde vomiting reflex involving the proximal gut is inhibited.[62] Drowsiness, dystonic reactions, and nervousness are the most common side effects limiting the use of metoclopramide. Dystonic reactions are more common in patients younger than 30 years of age (25%) than in older adults (1.8%).[61] In spite of the frequency of these unwanted CNS symptoms, cases of overdose of metoclopramide involving 80 to 100 times the amount regularly used in therapy are not lethal.[56] Irreversible chronic tardive dyskinesia, especially in the elderly, has been reported as a catastrophic consequence of long-term therapy (2–4 years).[61] Concurrent use of other agents with sedative effects (barbiturates, alcohol) should be avoided. Inhibition of dopamine receptors may also lead to hyperprolactinemia, which leads to impotence, galactorrhea, or amenorrhea. These effects usually reverse when the medication is stopped.

The uses of metoclopramide in gastrointestinal motility disorders are in the management of gastroesophageal reflux disease and gastroparesis. In most clinical settings of gastroparesis where symptomatic response with metoclopramide is achieved, improvement in gastric emptying actually correlates poorly with symptomatic relief. Thus, the antiemetic effect of this drug may be as important to the beneficial action of metoclopramide as its prokinetic activity.

DOMPERIDONE

Domperidone, a benzimidazole derivative, is a peripheral dopamine antagonist with clinical beneficial effects similar to those of metoclopramide. The main advantage of domperidone is that this prokinetic agent does not cross the blood–brain barrier. The central nervous system side effects of metoclopramide that limit its usefulness are minimal with this drug. Because the chemoreceptor trigger zone is outside the blood–brain barrier, domperidone is also similar to metoclopramide in having a potent central antiemetic effect. In contrast to metoclopramide, however, atropine does not block the gastrointestinal motor-stimulating effects of domperidone.[63]

As with metoclopramide, the effects of domperidone are observed mainly in the proximal gastrointestinal tract. Primarily, this prokinetic agent increases lower esophageal pressure and accelerates gastric emptying, particularly by way of inhibition of receptive fundic relaxation and enhancement of gastroduodenal coordination.[64]

Like metoclopramide, domperidone is used mainly in the treatment of gastroesophageal reflux disease and gastroparesis. However, in placebo-controlled clinical studies, while symptomatic responses were seen, the beneficial effect of domperidone on gastric emptying could not be demonstrated.[65,66] Further limiting the potential use of this agent is the observation that the prokinetic effect of domperidone disappears with chronic administration.[67]

Peak plasma level is achieved within 30 to 120 minutes of oral ingestion. Domperidone is subject to extensive hepatic biotransformation. After an oral dose, 31% is eliminated in the urine and 60% in feces. The elimination half-life is 7.5 hours and is prolonged with severe renal dysfunction.[63] The usual oral dose is 20 to 40 mg given four times a day. There is only limited experience in the long-term use of this drug. The intravenous form of domperidone was withdrawn by the manufacturer after possible cardiac toxicity was identified with this route of administration.[68]

The side effects of domperidone are less than those reported with metoclopramide. Hyperprolactinemia is a significant side effect with resultant galactorrhea, amenorrhea, or impotence. Dystonic reactions are exceedingly rare. While the absence of serious neurologic side effects has stimulated a great deal of interest in domperidone, the role of this agent in the treatment of disorders of gastric emptying has yet to be established.

CISAPRIDE

Cisapride, a benzamide derivative, is a newer gastrointestinal prokinetic agent without dopamine-antagonistic or cholinomimetic effects. The drug exerts its action through facilitation of acetylcholine release from the myenteric plexus. Serotonin antagonism, established in the in vitro setting, may also account for the stimulating activity of the drug.[69] In contrast to metoclopramide, which is active only in the proximal gut, cisapride has effects along the entire gastrointestinal tract.[70–76] Cisapride increases lower esophageal sphincter pressure without altering esophageal peristalsis.[71]

Antral motility is stimulated and duodenogastric reflux is reduced with intravenous administration.[77] Liquid and solid emptying are accelerated with acute administration of cisapride.[73] In fasting humans, cisapride induced propulsive motility patterns in the jejunum.[75] Furthermore, prokinetic effects are also seen in the colon.[76]

Peak plasma level is achieved within 2 hours of a 10-mg oral dose. Half-life after an intravenous dose of 10 mg is 19.4 hours. Colonic activity has been observed with a dose of 5 mg.[76] The usual starting oral dose is 10 mg three times a day. Side effects are rare. In contrast to metoclopramide or domperidone, hyperprolactinemia is not seen with this drug.

The proper use of cisapride is not established. Considering its activity throughout the gut and the absence of significant adverse effects, cisapride may be the agent long sought after to treat motility disorders where the whole gut is involved, such as in diabetes mellitus. Colonic hypomotility disorders may also benefit from this drug. However, studies of long-term use and controlled clinical trials are still needed before any conclusions can be made on the usefulness of cisapride.

Experimental Agents With Novel Modes of Action

5-HYDROXYTRYPTAMINE (5 HT3) RECEPTOR ANTAGONIST

The effects of metoclopramide and cisapride may involve serotonin-antagonistic activity.[69,78] GR38032F is a highly selective 5-hydroxytryptamine (5 HT3) receptor antagonist that increases gastric emptying in the guinea pig. With its lack of action on dopamine receptors, a 5 HT3 receptor antagonist may offer an advantage over metoclopramide.[79] A similar agent, ICS 205-930, was found to accelerate solid emptying in normals when given as 10- or 20-mg intravenous doses. No adverse effects were noted.[80]

CCK ANTAGONISTS

At physiologic doses, CCK and gastrin inhibit gastric emptying. Proglumide, an antagonist of CCK with weak antagonistic action on gastrin, has been found to accelerate liquid emptying in rats when injected intraperitoneally.[81] A newer and more potent CCK antagonist has just been shown to accelerate gastric emptying in humans.[82] Presumably, these antagonists inhibit feedback regulation mediated by CCK. Because feedback inhibition is most likely diminished during abnormally slow gastric emptying of nutrients into the duodenum, it is moot whether these agents will be therapeutically effective.

NALOXONE

Morphine inhibits gastric emptying by way of mu opiate receptors. The opiate receptor antagonist naloxone given at 5-mg intravenous bolus did not significantly accelerate solid and liquid emptying in normal humans.[83] In the setting of small intestinal pseudo-obstruction, when given in a daily dose of 1.6 mg subcutaneously, naloxone accelerated solid emptying.[84] Recently, new information suggests that the interaction of opiate receptors and gastric emptying may be more complicated than previously realized. Both mu and kappa opiate receptors may be important in the regulation of emptying, and naloxone may actually be involved with both receptors. U-50488, a kappa opiate agonist, has been shown to accelerate solid emptying, but it delayed liquid emptying. Naloxone abolished both effects. Morphine, on the other hand, delayed only solid emptying.[85] Because enkephalins have been demonstrated in the neurons of the myenteric plexus,[86] a mu opiate antagonist or even a kappa agonist may well be useful in accelerating solid emptying. With no adverse effects, naloxone may offer a therapeutic advantage.

ERYTHROMYCIN

Abdominal discomfort is often a complaint after the use of erythromycin. Recently, these symptoms have been observed to be associated with enhanced gastric motor activity. After an intravenous administration of erythromycin, moderate to severe pains correlated with antral contraction of large amplitude and long duration in both the fasted and fed state. There was no change in plasma motilin.[87] This association has raised the possibility of a new therapeutic use for this drug. The use of erythromycin as a prokinetic agent was investigated in eight patients with severe diabetic gastroparesis. With use of a 40-mg intravenous dose, phase III of the MMC was induced in the antrum and the upper intestine in both patients and controls. The activity suggests that erythromycin may be a motilin agonist and binds to motilin receptors on gastrointestinal smooth muscles.[88,89] Strong antral contractions were also noted with a dose of 200 mg in both groups.[90] In a double-blind, placebo-controlled study involving 10 patients with diabetic gastroparesis, the intravenous administration of 200 mg of erythromycin shortened the gastric emptying times of both solids and liquids.[91] The accelerating effect on solids and liquids was similar. This finding was postulated to be related to the powerful antral contractions induced by this antibiotic. Even with these promising reports, the quest for an ideal prokinetic agent may not yet be over. In dogs fitted with duodenal fistulas, erythromycin was found to accelerate solid emptying by impairing the gastric sieving.[92] After erythromycin administration, the ability of the stomach to sieve was severely impaired. Compared with controls, the percentage of food particles ≥ 0.5 mm increased from 7.7% to 63.2%. This effect of erythromycin on gastric sieving can be described as "pharmacologic antrectomy." In patients with a distal gastric resection, maldigestion, early satiety, and weight loss are all well-recognized adverse consequences of impaired sieving; therefore, in the long run, the gastrokinetic potential of this antibiotic may be less promising. Very little is now known about the long-term effect of erythromycin. Janssens reported that improved gastric emptying in his group of 10 patients was still observed, although less dramatically, after 4 weeks of oral erythromycin.[91] More information is needed before the therapeutic role for this agent in the management of gastrointestinal motility disorders can be established.

DISORDERS WITH ALTERED GASTRIC EMPTYING

Even with the recent surge in the study of disorders of gastric emptying, our understanding of the nature of these disorders is very primitive indeed. With the availability of gamma scintigraphy, abnormal gastric emptying has been found in many disease states. In certain disease conditions, the association with the abnormal pattern of emptying is well studied and clinically significant. These disorders are grouped as disorders of gastric emptying in the section entitled Established Associations. With many other diseases, the association appears important, but the available information is too limited for a clear conclusion. These disorders of gastric emptying are grouped in the section Associations Likely to Be Important. In a number of diseases, there is still a substantial disagreement on whether the association even exists. In any case, the clinical significance of the gastric motor abnormality is uncertain. These disorders of gastric emptying are grouped in the section entitled Associations of Uncertain Significance. Conditions associated with accelerated gastric emptying will be described first, followed by disorders associated with delayed gastric emptying.

Accelerated Gastric Emptying

ESTABLISHED ASSOCIATIONS

Postulcer Surgery

Emptying of Liquids. All operations on the stomach for peptic ulcer disease result in rapid gastric emptying of liquid nutrients. Pyloric myotomy (i.e., pyloroplasty) or pylorectomy has a modest effect on the gastric emptying of liquids. In dogs, gastric emptying of liquid meals is accelerated in the first few minutes postprandially,[93] but this effect is small unless the meal is large in volume or a (truncal) vagotomy is added to the pyloric ablation.[94] Both conditions (large meal volume, truncal vagotomy) increase intragastric pressure and the gastroduodenal pressure gradient, thus promoting emptying of liquids from the stomach. Normally, gastric emptying is mainly regulated by feedback inhibition, which reduces gastric tone, pressure, and antral motility

(see ch 8), so pyloric contraction and resistance to outflow plays a secondary role. When intragastric tone or pressure is abnormally increased by large meal volumes or truncal vagotomy, however, the importance of pyloric control of outflow is increased. Similarly, when gastroduodenal pressure gradients are barostatically controlled in experimental animals (a situation in which control of gastric propulsion by fundic tone and antral contractions is replaced by barostatic control of pressures), the regulatory role of the pylorus in limiting outflow becomes evident.[95]

Vagal denervation of the stomach eliminates gastric accommodation and receptive relaxation reflexes, so intragastric pressure rises rapidly to abnormal levels as the volume of the meal entering the stomach increases. This defect results in precipitous emptying of liquids early after the meal. It is seen with truncal, selective gastric, or proximal gastric vagotomies.[96] As indicated in the previous paragraph, adding the pyloroplasty compounds the effect of the vagal denervation to greatly accelerate early postprandial emptying of liquids (Table 60-5). Proximal gastric vagotomy selectively denervates only the acid-secreting, proximal stomach, while leaving the vagal motor supply to the antrum intact. However, the loss of gastric accommodation reflexes after proximal gastric vagotomy is reflected by a small increase in acceleration of liquid emptying. If, for some reason, pyloroplasty is added to this operation, then liquids empty precipitously, about as fast as after truncal vagotomy with pyloroplasty.[97-100]

Subtotal gastrectomy (i.e., 75%–80% distal gastric resection) removes the antrum and pylorus and a significant portion of the body of the stomach. The resection has two major effects on the gastric emptying of liquids: (1) The loss of considerable capacity with the resection impairs the ability of the stomach to accommodate meal volume without an above-normal rise in intragastric pressure.[101] (2) The removal of the active resistance of the pyloric sphincter further accelerates the emptying of liquids (see Table 60-5).

Gastric emptying after any operation with truncal vagotomy seems to be even faster than after subtotal gastrectomy alone (see Table 60-5).[102] Perhaps this increased effect of truncal vagotomy is the result of both disruption of accommodation reflexes and the partial loss of additional reflexes from the intestine that feed back to inhibit gastric emptying in response to nutrients or to duodenal distention (ch 8).

The rapid emptying of liquid meals after truncal vagotomy or subtotal gastrectomy does not entirely result from loss of gastric accommodation to meal volume and consequentially high intragastric pressures. The effect of gravity is unmasked, as well, by

TABLE 60-5
Postulcer Surgery Gastric Emptying Patterns

TYPE	ANATOMIC CONSIDERATION	LIQUIDS	SOLIDS
Subtotal gastrectomy	75% resection	Accelerated	Variable, rapid
Truncal vagotomy plus antrectomy	50% resection	Accelerated	Rapid initially, followed by slowed
Truncal vagotomy plus pyloroplasty	Antrum intact, pyloric control disrupted	Accelerated	Rapid initially, followed by slowed
Proximal gastric vagotomy	Selective denervation of proximal stomach	Mild initial acceleration	Normal

the vagal denervation and/or antrectomy or pyloroplasty. Thus, gastric emptying of liquids in the erect versus recumbent posture is nearly double.[103,104] By contrast, in normal subjects, gravity is so checked by feedback reflexes that its effects are difficult to demonstrate. Not all control is lost, however, after vagal and/or pyloric disruption. Feeding fat before a meal slows liquid emptying.[105] Whether extravagal neural feedback and/or hormones control these responses is unknown.

Many believe that rapid gastric emptying of liquids results in a postprandial symptom complex called the "dumping syndrome."[106] This is characterized by the presence of early satiety, nausea, vomiting, abdominal pain, palpatations, sweating, dizziness, light-headedness, syncope, diarrhea, and flushing. Indeed, it is likely that unusual responses are triggered by nutrients that rapidly enter the small intestine. Normally, most nutrients are digested and absorbed as they traverse the proximal half of the small intestine.[107] After ulcer surgery, however, liquid meals empty so rapidly that digestive and absorptive mechanisms are overwhelmed. As a result, a considerable load of nutrients reaches the distal intestine.[108,109] The intensity of feedback control from the intestine depends on both how much is exposed to nutrients and whether it is mediated by nervous reflexes or hormones.[110,111] The abnormal exposure of the whole intestinal length to nutrients after these operations probably accounts for the excessive postcibal release of gut hormones that is commonly observed in these patients.[112]

While these ideas on the genesis of postcibal symptoms are quite plausible, several observations indicate that they are oversimplifications. Almost all patients who have had an ulcer operation and have been studied postoperatively exhibited rapid gastric emptying of liquids but no symptoms.[102] Furthermore, Gulsrud found that slowing the rate of nutrient entry into the small intestines of symptomatic patients did not ameliorate their "dumping syndrome."[104] Likewise, patients most commonly experience postprandial symptoms after meals of solid foods that do not empty so precipitously.

Despite these arguments, much therapy for postprandial symptoms is directed at slowing gastric emptying. Treatments include: the elimination of liquids with meals, the inclusion of viscous guar or pectin[112-115] in meals (to slow gastric emptying by increasing intragastric viscosity), surgical interposition of an antiperistaltic loop of jejunum between stomach and duodenum,[116,117] and the placement of serosal electrodes on the duodenum to allow reverse pacing of duodenal contractions in an effort to slow gastric emptying.[118] Each treatment has enjoyed some enthusiastic application, but none has entirely relieved symptoms, probably because the idea that symptoms arise only from rapid emptying of meal contents is not entirely correct.

Clinical evidence does suggest a more consistent relationship between rapid gastric emptying and postprandial diarrhea. First, diarrhea is more common in patients who have had truncal vagotomy (with pyloroplasty or gastroenterostomy) than in those who have had a subtotal gastrectomy.[119] Gastric emptying of liquids is faster after the former. Second, emptying of liquids is faster in the 10% or so of patients with vagotomy plus pyloroplasty who develop diarrhea than in those without diarrhea.[101] Third, patients with diarrhea have more rapid and extensive transit of nutrients to the terminal ileum than do those without diarrhea.[109,120] These patients with diarrhea also have a significantly greater postprandial flow of volume through the terminal ileum into the colon after a liquid meal.[121]

Emptying of Solids. The rate of gastric emptying of solid foods depends on both how fast the stomach is able to propel the food and how rapidly it can convert large pieces of swallowed food by digestion and grinding into small particles. Ulcer operations affect both processes. Distal gastric resection affects gastric sieving so that there is less resistance to the outflow of larger pieces of food, a situation that would speed emptying. Vagal denervation of the stomach markedly alters gastric motility, especially reducing antral contractility and emptying of solid foods. Antrectomy removes much or all of the peristaltic region of the stomach, which probably slows gastric emptying of solids. In addition, all ulcer operations reduce the gastric secretion of acid and gastric enzymes, so that the speed of chemical digestion or reduction of solid food to small particles is further reduced.[122] Thus, these operations give rise to a mixture of alterations that, on one hand, may speed gastric emptying of solid foods and, on the other hand, may slow expulsion. Correspondingly, the observed effects in these patients are quite variable. Unlike other ulcer operations, proximal gastric vagotomy or highly selective vagotomy does not alter the emptying rate of solid foods.[123-125] Other gastric operations frequently produce a rapid initial emptying phase followed by an abnormally slow phase of gastric emptying. Whether the overall emptying rate is decreased or increased depends on which of the two phases predominates. The following paragraphs will expand on this overview.

Normally, in dogs and humans, the stomach selectively retains radiolabeled solid foods of large size, allowing the passage of only smaller food particles less than 1 mm in diameter.[93,124,126,127] This selectivity was not lost when dogs underwent pyloroplasty or pylorectomy[93,127] but was altered by resection of the pylorus together with the distal 4 cm of antrum. Similarly, in humans with truncal vagotomy plus antrectomy (i.e., resection of antrum and pylorus), about 30% of ingested radiolabeled liver emptied from the stomach as particles larger than 1 mm, but patients with truncal vagotomy plus pyloroplasty emptied particles of radiolabeled liver of normal sizes.[124] Likewise, the human stomach after distal resection loses its ability to discriminate between large pieces of liver and smaller radiolabeled, indigestible solids.[128] After proximal gastric vagotomy (in which the distal stomach is neither surgically altered nor vagally denervated), the size of food particles emptied from the human stomach is normal.[124]

Vagal denervation of the stomach alters gastric motility in several ways. Truncal, complete gastric, or proximal gastric vagotomies reduce receptive relaxation and gastric accommodation to meal volume. While these alterations speed liquid emptying, it is not known how they might affect solid emptying. Vagal denervation of the antrum after truncal or complete gastric vagotomy reduces the force and frequency of antral contractions under fasting conditions or when antral contractions are reflexly stimulated by filling the stomach.[129-133] However, proximal gastric vagotomy preserves antral innervation and contractility. Because of the loss of antral contractility, a large percentage of patients who have had a truncal or complete gastric vagotomy will develop gastric obstruction unless a pyloroplasty or gastrojejunostomy is added to the vagotomy.[99,134] This so-called drainage procedure probably lowers resistance to outflow enough to prevent gastric stasis in the face of postvagotomy antral paresis. In contrast, gastric emptying of solid foods is normal[123] after a proximal gastric vagotomy without pyloroplasty. Vagal nerves also partially mediate feedback inhibition of gastric emptying by nutrients in the small intestine. These reflexes include those to the fundus (relaxation of tone induced by maltose in the intestine) and those to the antrum (decreased peristalsis in response to fat in the intestine) (ch 8). Truncal vagotomy also shortens the time of fed myoelectrical activity after a meal or may even abolish conversion of a fed to a fasting pattern.[135] It should be apparent from this brief discussion that the overall effects of vagal denervation of the stomach on emptying of solid foods cannot be predicted from available information. The reduction of antral motility under fasting conditions may be offset by the loss of inhibition of antral contractions when the intestine is filled with nutrients. Little is known about the effects of proximal gastric tone on redistribution of solid foods within the unresected stomach or the propulsion of solid foods from the proximal stomach after vagotomy plus antrectomy.

The majority of patients with truncal vagotomy plus antrectomy empty solid foods rapidly in the initial postprandial period. This phase of rapid emptying corresponds to the period in which abnormally large pieces of radiolabeled food empty from the stomach. While this loss of selective retention or resistance to outflow of large pieces of food may contribute to this rapid emptying, it does not appear to be the main reason for it. Rapid emptying in the early postprandial period was seen in patients who did not pass large pieces of radiolabeled food. Furthermore, some patients with vagotomy plus pyloroplasty who did not pass large particles of food still exhibited a rapid initial emptying similar to that seen in the patients with antrectomy. Patients with subtotal gastrectomy also frequently exhibit an early emptying phase similar to that seen in patients who have had truncal vagotomy with either pyloroplasty or antrectomy.[128,136,137] Presumably, some combination of reduced stomach capacity and loss of retention of larger pieces of food contributes to this rapid emptying phase.

Despite the initially rapid emptying that predominates in patients after these operations, overall emptying may vary because of a very slow, second emptying phase. Symptoms of the "dumping syndrome" do not correlate with these patterns. The loss of gastric sieving with the passage of larger-than-normal particles of solid food into the small intestine contributes to malabsorption, because larger pieces of food cannot be easily digested.[138-140]

Operative corrections have been tried on postulcer surgery patients suffering from intractable symptoms unrelieved by conservative therapies. These patients complain of severe postprandial distress and have been given diagnoses ranging from dumping syndrome to alkaline reflux gastritis. The procedures have included the placement of a Roux-en-Y diversion.[116,141-146] Available information on the effect of Roux-en-Y diversion on gastric emptying is confusing. In one report, previously accelerated emptying was slowed by the procedure. In this uncontrolled study of 22 patients undergoing Roux-en-Y gastrojejunostomy for dumping syndrome, pre- and postoperative solid emptying studies were performed on 7 patients. While 19 patients had symptomatic improvement with the diversion, the results of the emptying studies were far less encouraging.[141] Before diversion, only five of seven symptomatic patients had accelerated emptying. After Roux-en-Y, two of these patients developed delayed gastric emptying. The outcome, even in these patients, was not favorable. Near total gastrectomies were required later for severe gastric retention. No clear-cut effect of Roux-en-Y diversion on gastric emptying has been observed. In a prospective study of 15 patients with alkaline reflux gastritis,[145] solid emptying was found to be variable: rapid (45%), normal (25%), and delayed (30%). After diversion, nearly the same dis-

tribution was seen: rapid (40%), normal (30%), and delayed (30%). Further support against the association of Roux-en-Y diversion and impaired gastric emptying was provided by a report in which 117 consecutive patients were randomized to receive either Billroth I gastroduodenostomy or Roux-en-Y gastrojejunostomy following antrectomy and selective vagotomy for ulcer disease. There was no difference in postoperative results over an average follow-up period of 2 years. In both groups, postoperative gastric retention, symptoms, and delayed emptying of a semisolid meal occurred with similar frequency.[146] Because no consistent effect on gastric emptying has been identified with a Roux-en-Y diversion, little can be concluded about the etiology of stasis symptoms that may develop in a minority of these patients.

ASSOCIATIONS OF UNCERTAIN SIGNIFICANCE

Pancreatic Insufficiency. Because intestinal sensors, including those which inhibit gastric emptying, are triggered by digestive products rather than unhydrolyzed foods, one might predict that gastric emptying would be rapid in patients with severe pancreatic exocrine insufficiency. Indeed, gastric emptying of fatty liquid meals was noted by Long to be abnormally rapid in patients with marked steatorrhea from pancreatic insufficiency. The emptying rate was corrected with oral administration of pancreatic enzymes (Viokase).[147] In the only other reported study, however, patients with equally severe pancreatic insufficiency[148] had normal fractional rate of emptying of a mixed solid–liquid meal.

The opposite conclusions of these two studies leave open to question the effect of pancreatic insufficiency on gastric emptying. Of course, sampling errors inherent in studies with small numbers of patients could have accounted for the conflicting results, but another possibility is that the different natures of the test meals may account for the different outcomes. Because patients usually consume solid foods rather than liquid nutrients, Regan's study[148] is more clinically relevant than Long's.[147] Until further evidence to the contrary is forthcoming, it is fair to assume that gastric emptying of food in patients with pancreatic insufficiency is usually normal.

Peptic Ulcer Disease. Rapid entry of an acid load into the duodenum may exceed the buffering capacity of the proximal intestine. Accelerated gastric emptying has been considered as a possible factor for the development of duodenal ulcer because the rapid entry of acid might cause ulceration. A sizable number of studies seeking accelerated emptying in ulcer patients have been reported. The results have been conflicting.[149-159]

While there is uniform agreement that solid emptying is normal,[149,152] there is no consensus on liquid emptying. Some investigators have reported accelerated emptying,[151,153-155,157,159] while others have not.[149,150,152,157]

The discrepancies among studies of liquid emptying can be accounted for by differences in experimental design. In the positive studies, the acceleration of liquid emptying was minor and brief, seen only in the first few minutes after the meal. Studies of gastric emptying that measured at intervals longer than every 15 minutes missed these differences. A second, important design feature is the concentration of nutrients in the liquid test meal that inhibit gastric emptying. In the positive studies, differences between normals and patients with duodenal ulcer were discerned when the liquid meal contained concentrations of nutrients below maximum inhibiting doses. In the detailed study by Williams, most of these study design problems were eliminated. Acid, glucose, and fat liquid meals, each across a dose range, were tested in healed duodenal ulcer patients. The results were compared with normal controls. Ulcer patients emptied all three meals faster than controls, but the difference was observed only with the lower doses. With low-dose glucose and all concentrations of acids, the difference was present only in the first 5 minutes.[157] The duration of the initial, rapid emptying phase varies inversely with the concentration of inhibiting nutrient in the liquid meal.[158] At high concentrations, the initially rapid phase is very brief, and the duration may be so short that a defect in this early phase of regulation may be undetectable. Similar observations were made in a more recent study by Parr.[159]

The rapid initial emptying seen in these two studies is quite similar to the early rapid emptying noted in animals after pyloroplasty.[94] Thus, it is possible that peptic ulcer disease leads to pyloric distortion/scarring and subsequent pyloric dysfunction.

In the postprandial setting, it is unlikely that accelerated gastric emptying in duodenal ulcer disease has any clinical or even pathophysiologic relevance. In the fasting state, the impact on duodenal acid exposure may be greater. The various phases of the interdigestive migrating motor complex influence the rate of gastric emptying differently.[160] During phase I, when the rate of gastric emptying is the slowest, the small acceleration seen in duodenal ulcer patients may lead to higher entry of acid, causing ulceration.

Zollinger–Ellison Syndrome. Compared with normal controls, rapid gastric emptying of liquids[161] and solids[162] has been described in patients diagnosed as having Zollinger–Ellison syndrome. The emptying rate was probably not due to gastric hypersecretion because no change in the emptying rate was seen after an acid-suppressive dose of cimetidine. The abnormality may be related to dysfunction of the feedback mechanism. Fat, an inhibitor of gastric emptying, was found to be without any effect.[162]

Delayed Gastric Emptying

ESTABLISHED ASSOCIATIONS

Diabetes Mellitus. Gastrointestinal symptoms are common in patients with long-standing diabetes mellitus.[163,164] While esophageal manometric and scintigraphic abnormalities have been described as being quite common in diabetics, complaints of dysphagia and heartburn are surprisingly rare.[51,165–167] In contrast, along with constipation or diarrhea, upper gastrointestinal tract complaints of nausea, vomiting, and early satiety add considerably to the morbidity of the disease. These complaints are often, but not always, associated with abnormal gastric emptying.

While abnormal gastric emptying has been widely reported in patients with diabetes, clinical description is fragmentary. In the clinical literature, it is difficult to determine with certainty the relationships between abnormal gastric emptying and each of the following: (1) the duration of the diabetes, (2) the presence or absence of symptoms of nausea and vomiting, (3) the presence or absence of autonomic and/or peripheral neuropathy, (4) the presence or absence of nephropathy or retinopathy, (5) the presence of other gastrointestinal dysfunction (diarrhea, constipation), and even (6) the type of diabetes in patients with abnormal gastric emptying. Most authors, however, believe that abnormal gastric emptying complicates (usually type I) diabetes with neuropathy.[165,168,169]

Several factors have contributed to our present ignorance. In older reviews, in which testing was not systematic among all patients, the standard method of assessment was upper gastrointestinal radiography with aqueous suspensions of barium sulfate. It is now known that this technique is insensitive in detecting abnormalities of gastric transit. Thus, it is probable that only the most advanced cases of gastric dysfunction were tested and/or detected. This idea is supported by a reported prevalence rate of delayed gastric emptying of only 0.08% among 44,000 diabetics followed at the Joslin Clinic,[170] which was based on a radiographic survey of symptomatic diabetics. By contrast, abnormal gastric emptying is much more commonly recognized today on scintigraphic studies; for example, in one study, 27% of insulin-requiring diabetics (with the disease for more than 5 years) exhibited impaired gastric emptying of solid food.[171] But thus far, even the now widely used and more sensitive gamma scintigraphy has not greatly added to our information. Based on concepts from the older, radiologic studies,[170] modern investigators have often limited their scintigraphic studies to patients who most typically have symptoms of nausea and vomiting with long-standing, insulin-dependent diabetes complicated by neuropathy. While abnormal gastric emptying is indeed frequent in such patients, these studies provide little insight into the prevalence of this abnormality among subgroups of diabetics. More recent studies clearly demonstrated that asymptomatic diabetics may also exhibit abnormal gastric emptying[172] and, conversely, that some patients with symptoms may have normal scintigraphic tests of gastric emptying.[173] While systematic studies of large numbers of unselected diabetics to determine the true prevalence of abnormal emptying are still not available, information from a well-designed small study supports that it is a common finding even in the general diabetic population. Fifty-eight percent of a group of 45 randomly selected type I diabetics had delayed gastric emptying of either a liquid or solid meal.[165]

Several other factors also contribute to the confusion on the incidence of gastroparesis in diabetes mellitus. First, some studies have measured only liquid emptying, others only solid emptying; but few have measured both. Feldman[163] found that gastric emptying of indigestible objects was even more slowed in a few selected diabetics than gastric emptying of solid food. Thus, the detection of abnormality may depend on what marker is studied. Second, among several reports of abnormally slow emptying of solid food in diabetics, the nature of the slowing varied. Some authors reported mainly a slowing from a prolongation of the initial lag phase,[172] while others reported a slowed rate of emptying after a normal lag phase,[165,174] and still other authors reported both defects in the same subjects.[175] Third, hyperglycemia affects gastric emptying[165,166,177,178] and/or gastric motility.[176]

Most studies of gastric emptying have either not controlled the concentration of blood glucose at test or failed to mention this variable. In his report on type I diabetics, Horowitz did address the effects of hyperglycemia. He noted that there was a strong correlation with delayed gastric emptying of liquids when blood glucose was ≥15 mmol/L (270 mg/dL).[165] A similar finding was noted in type II diabetics.[166] The effects of blood glucose on both solid and liquid gastric emptying were recently investigated in the setting of experimentally stabilized blood glucose levels. In this study, the blood glucose varied between euglycemic and hyperglycemic levels in 10 type I diabetics. During hyperglycemia, there was slowing of solid but not liquid emptying, compared with euglycemic studies. This is consistent with other studies in which emptying of both phases was measured, which also suggested that the emptying of solid foods was more often and/or more profoundly slowed in diabetes than was the emptying of liquids (see Table 60-2). Finally, diabetic gastropathy may be a heterogeneous disorder. Few have directly studied gastrointestinal motility in diabetics, but those investigators who have used manometry to study diabetics with nausea and vomiting have uncovered a variety of defects.

Reduced or absent peristaltic contractions in the antrum together with residual food and prolonged gastric retention of barium sulfate at gastrointestinal radiography has long been recognized by radiologists as the triad that typifies diabetic gastroparesis.[169,170,179] These abnormalities of antral motility detected in early radiographic studies have been confirmed by more modern manometric studies of antral contractility. Interdigestive motor activity in the fasted state was absent or diminished in the stomachs of symptomatic patients with diabetic gastroparesis.[180] This finding was not seen in diabetic controls. While the fundic tone was normal, fundic and antral motility indices were less in patients with diabetic gastroparesis (Fig 60-3).[52,53,181] The absence of gastric interdigestive motor activity in diabetic gastroparesis may well explain the frequent findings of gastric bezoars in these patients.[52] While most of these studies were performed on fasting patients, decreased antral motility after a meal has also been observed in diabetics with symptoms of gastroparesis.[181,182] Even in normal subjects, however, high concentrations of blood glucose disrupt antral contractions.[176] Thus, it is unknown to what degree high blood sugars per se during these experiments may have contributed to diminished antral motility. In addition, other patterns of antral motor abnormalities that may be responsible for impaired gastric emptying have been observed in diabetic patients. Tachygastria and bradygastria are found in patients with severe diabetic gastroparesis. These gastric dysrhythmias may result in poorly coordinated antral contractions.[182,183]

Aside from diminished propulsive motor activity, gastric emptying may also be delayed as the result of increased resistance to outflow. Both the pylorus and the small bowel participate in regulating gastric outflow resistance. Normally, the regulation of gastric emptying by intestinal nutrients depends partly on the stimulation of isolated pyloric contractions, which impedes transpyloric flow.[184-187] This regulatory mechanism is muscarinic in origin, because pyloric contractions induced by lipid or dextrose in the duodenal lumen can be blocked with atropine.[184-186] The disorganized gastric motor behavior of diabetes may also involve pyloric spasm. Improperly timed pyloric contractions of abnormal intensity and duration lead to "pylorospasm" and functional outlet obstruction (Fig 60-4). Pylorospasm was defined as prolonged (>3 minutes) and intense (>10 mm Hg) tonic contractions and was observed in 14 out of 24 patients studied. The observed pyloric dysmotility was noted in both the fasted and fed states. Along with these periods of "pylorospasm," diabetics also exhibited prolongation of normal pyloric contractile activities.[188]

In addition to weak or absent antral contractions, electrically disorganized antral peristalsis, and pylorospasm, some diabetics also exhibit abnormal jejunal contractions with postprandial bursts of powerful contractions.[181] These motor activities further increase the resistance to forward flow. Weak antral contractions, pylorospasm, and frequent clusters of duodenal–jejunal contractions (perhaps acting as a brake on gastric outflow) may combine to slow gastric emptying.

The pathogenesis of these findings is not understood. Claiming a similarity between diabetic gastroparesis and impaired gastric emptying after truncal vagotomy, Rundles[189] proposed in the 1940s that a neuropathy of the vagus nerves may be important in the genesis of diabetic gastropathy. However, it is now known that vagal denervation of the proximal or whole stomach leads to an acceleration of gastric emptying of liquids in the first several postprandial minutes,[177,190] whereas liquid emptying in afflicted diabetics is often slowed in the first postprandial hour.[175,191] Further evidence against the vagal neuropathy explanation was provided by Horowitz. In his report, accelerated early emptying was found only in the minority of his patients.[165] Postmortem histologic ex-

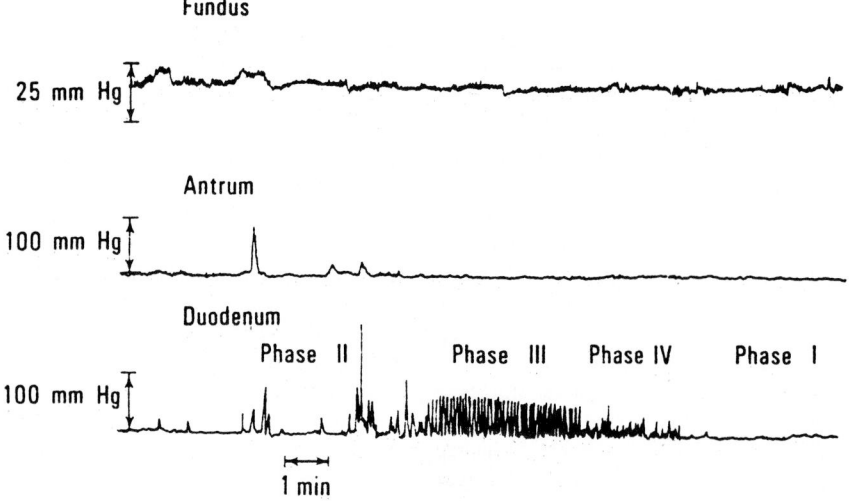

FIGURE 60–3. Absence of fundic and antral motor activities in diabetic gastroparesis. (Malagelada JR, Rees WDW, Mazzotta LJ, et al. Gastric motor abnormalities in diabetic and postvagotomy gastroparesis: Effect of metoclopramide and bethanecol. Gastroenterology 1980;78:286.)

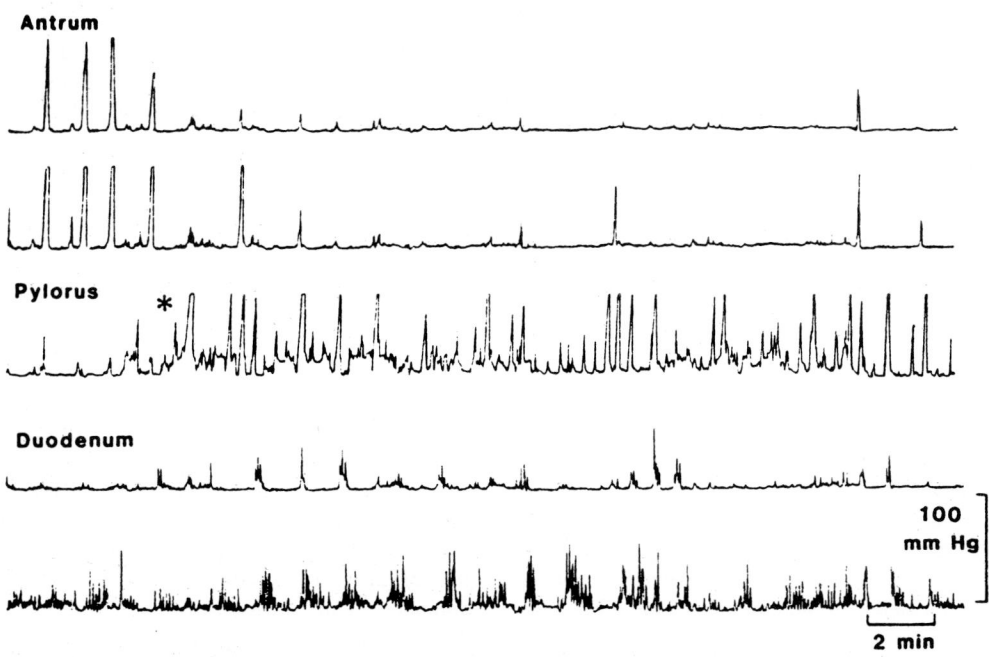

FIGURE 60–4. Pylorospasm in diabetic gastroparesis. (Mearin F, Camilleri M, Malagelada JR. Pyloric dysfunction in diabetics with recurrent nausea and vomiting. Gastroenterology 1986;90:1919.)

amination of the vagus nerves in afflicted diabetics has revealed degeneration of myelin in some patients[192] but not in others.[193] However, these conventional histologic studies do not detect abnormalities in the storage or release of neuropeptide transmitters in enteric nerves such as those described in diabetic animals.[194] The most convincing evidence for a functional derangement of the vagus nerves in diabetic patients was provided by Feldman,[195] who observed that these subjects had only one third the acid output of control subjects in response to sham feeding, although both groups secreted similar amounts of acid after exogenous pentagastrin. Many, but not all, patients with gastric stasis exhibit other evidence of autonomic dysfunction, such as the loss of vagotonic reflexes that slow the heart[171] and/or postural hypotension (sympathetic dysfunction). Because abnormal bursts of jejunal contractions in human diabetics were similar to those seen in jejuna of dogs after sympathectomy, Camilleri[181] has proposed that the loss of sympathetic nervous function plays an important role in diabetic gastropathy. Because the prokinetic agents (metoclopramide, domperidone, cisapride) improve gastric emptying in afflicted diabetics, at least temporarily, some[52,53,175] have argued that gastric muscle is normal (i.e., it is able to respond to exogenous stimuli), but such response to extra stimulation from exogenous drugs could equally well be interpreted as a loss of muscle responsiveness to normal levels of neural stimuli.

The clinical presentation of diabetic gastroparesis varies. On one end of the spectrum is the patient with diagnostic features of diabetic gastroparesis who may report no symptoms at all.[196] Poor diabetic control with frequent hypoglycemic episodes may be the only manifestation. Hypoglycemia is primarily the result of delayed emptying and absorption of food. Recurrent bezoar formation may be another presentation.[52] Much more commonly, nausea, vomiting of food eaten hours earlier, bloating, early satiety, and anorexia may be the presenting complaints.[197] Although symptom-free pe-

riods can be expected, the clinical course is likely to be chronic, with exacerbations lasting days to years.[179]

There are several ways of establishing the diagnosis of diabetic gastropathy. Retention of barium sulfate suspension during gastric radiography, together with gastric atony and the presence of residual food despite overnight fasting, is the classic radiographic triad of findings for diagnosis. Endoscopy should be used to exclude gastric mechanical obstruction in patients with abnormal radiography.[198] Because of its ease and low cost and apparently greater sensitivity than radiography, gamma scintigraphy is most commonly employed to establish delayed postprandial gastric emptying in diabetics who are thought to have gastropathy. A test showing delayed emptying is commonly accepted as diagnostic.

Nevertheless, there are problems with the use of gamma scintigraphy to establish the diagnosis. As already discussed, the sensitivity of the scintigraphic test depends on the type of marked substance that is tracked (see Table 60-2). Moreover, the interpretation of an abnormal study is complicated by the observation that symptoms often correlate poorly with either the solid or liquid emptying rate.[165,166,173,198] Patients with chronic nausea and vomiting suggestive of diabetic gastroparesis may have normal gastric emptying. In one report, six of seven diabetics with intermittent nausea and vomiting of unknown cause, suspected of having gastroparesis, were found to empty radiopaque markers normally.[199] On the other hand, entirely symptom-free patients may have abnormal emptying studies.[165,200,201] Even when a relatively insensitive means of detection was used, a surprisingly high prevalence of gastroparesis was found in symptom-free patients. A delayed emptying study is therefore meaningful clinically only if marked abnormality is found in the setting of symptoms of gastric stasis.

Prokinetic agents have been used in the treatment of diabetic gastroparesis. Metoclopramide enhanced gastric emptying acutely.[52,53,172,202,203] Chronically, however, the prokinetic effect has not been uniformly observed. In one study, a single oral dose of metoclopramide (10 mg) acutely improved emptying, but the effect was not maintained following 1 month of therapy.[203] This contrasted with another study in which sustained effect following 3 weeks of the same therapy was seen.[191] More than one mechanism is likely to be responsible for patients with diabetic gastroparesis, and responses to therapy are therefore unpredictable.[207] Symptoms of gastroparesis may be reduced even without correction of delayed gastric emptying.[172,191,203] The beneficial action of metoclopramide in gastroparesis is due to both enhanced emptying and central antiemetic activity. Antral and fundic motor activities are stimulated by this drug (Fig 60-5). Phase III interdigestive motor activity may be restored by metoclopramide with possible improvement of gastric clearing of indigestible solids, but the correlation of symptom reduction with this effect is unclear.[52,204,205] Five to twenty milligrams may be taken before meals and at bedtime. The dose should be titrated to the lowest possible level that will achieve the desired reduction of symptoms.

Bethanechol increases fundic and antral motility but does not trigger phase III activity.[52,53] Without the antiemetic action of metoclopramide and with the marked cholinergic side effects, this drug is less useful.

In a placebo-controlled study, cisapride accelerated the emptying of both liquid and solid meals and reduced symptoms.[199,206,207] In these limited studies, no side effect was noted. The beneficial effects were present even after 6 weeks.[206] In contrast to the study by Feldman, another placebo-controlled study reported no significant improvement of either symptoms or emptying with this drug.[173] Because the action of cisapride is thought to be entirely peripheral and limited to cholinergic enhancement of gastric motility, symptomatic improvement with cisapride may be useful only for the subgroup of patients with diabetic gastroparesis whose complaints are in fact due to delayed gastric emptying. The exact role of cisapride in the armamentarium of the gastroenterologist is not established. Because there are responders and nonresponders to metoclopramide, cisapride may be used as a second-line pro-

kinetic agent.[172] In contrast to metoclopramide, the continued use of this drug in a given patient should depend on the demonstration of enhanced emptying. The absence of side effects can be confirmed only with more extensive experience with this agent. Cisapride may be given as a 10-mg oral dose 30 minutes before meals.

Domperidone has also been tried in diabetic gastroparesis. In a placebo-controlled study, this agent accelerated both solid and liquid gastric emptying acutely. Symptomatic improvement was also achieved. However, after at least 1 month of therapy, the agent no longer had any effect on solid emptying. Liquid emptying was still increased. Like metoclopramide, there was no significant correlation between symptomatic improvement and any change in gastric emptying, raising the possibility for a still unidentified central effect.[175] With the use of cutaneous electrogastrography, the effect of long-term domperidone on the gastric myoelectrical activity of patients with diabetic gastroparesis was evaluated.[208] After 6 months of therapy, normal frequencies of three cycles per minute returned in all six patients. This was associated with symptomatic improvement in five out of six subjects, but a significant change in the gastric emptying rate was not demonstrated. Domperidone may be useful as the substitute prokinetic agent of choice in the acute setting when the clinician is confronted with the neurologic side effects of metoclopramide. Domperidone may be taken 30 minutes before meals as a 20-mg oral dose.

Most recently, erythromycin has been tried as a gastrokinetic agent in the treatment of diabetic gastroparesis. Acutely, with intravenous administration of 200 mg of erythromycin, both solid and liquid emptying were accelerated.[91] Little is known about the therapeutic efficacy of this antibiotic in the long-term treatment of diabetic gastroparesis. In 10 patients, after 4 weeks of erythromycin, Janssens reported that improvement of gastric emptying was still observed.[91] However, because the acceleration of solid emptying with this drug is at the expense of gastric sieving,[92] maldigestion is a potential complication of this therapy. The proper role of erythromycin is still unclear.

To date, few of the reported drug trials in diabetes have taken

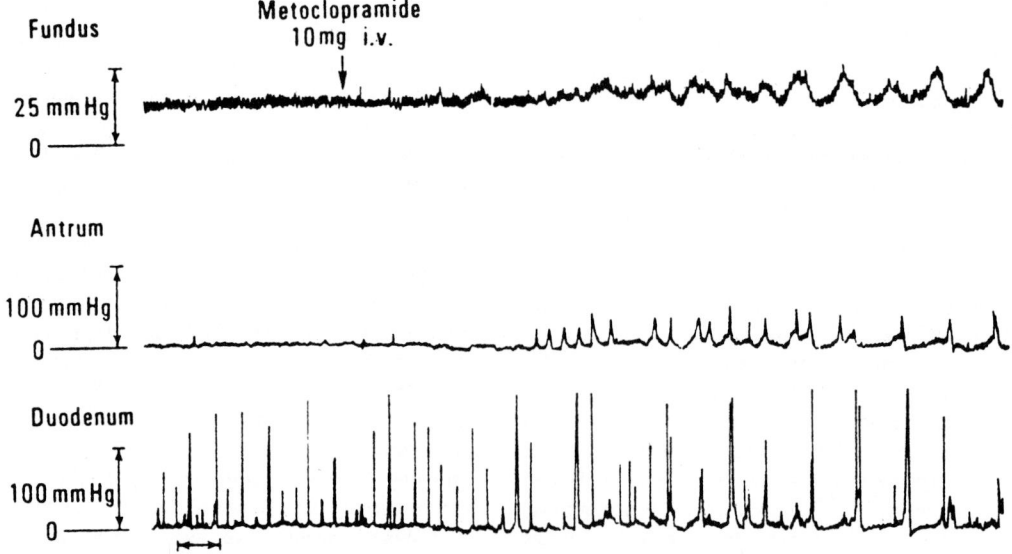

FIGURE 60-5. Metoclopramide stimulates fundic and antral motor activities. (Malagelada JR, Rees WDW, Mazzotta LJ, et al. Gastric motor abnormalities in diabetic and postvagotomy gastroparesis: Effect of metoclopramide and bethanecol. Gastroenterology 1980;78:286.)

into account the impact of blood glucose concentrations on gastric emptying. Thus, some of the reported benefits attributed to the drug may have actually resulted from lower blood glucoses at the time of the second test. Conversely, some of the apparent loss of benefit with sustained use may have actually resulted from chance elevations of blood glucose concentrations during follow-up examinations.

Diabetic patients with abnormal gastric emptying represent a heterogeneous group. We suspect that much of the high prevalence of abnormal emptying tests in as many as 58% of diabetics is an outcome of uncontrolled blood sugars during the tests of gastric emptying. A much smaller group of diabetics (perhaps as few as 0.08%) manifest delayed gastric emptying as the result of more permanent neuromuscular dysfunction. Furthermore, there are patients with severe gastrointestinal symptoms who have normal gastric emptying, and there are patients with markedly delayed gastric emptying who are asymptomatic. At the present time, management strategy is geared toward identifying the symptomatic patient with delayed gastric emptying. Response to therapy may then be followed by both symptom improvement and acceleration of gastric emptying.

Anorexia Nervosa. Anorexia nervosa is a neuropsychiatric disorder characterized by multiple gastrointestinal symptoms. Delayed gastric emptying, a common finding, often correlates with these symptoms and has been the target of therapy. Upper gastrointestinal symptoms such as postprandial bloating, nausea, heartburn, and epigastric pain are triggered by the ingestion of even small amounts of food. Relief is often possible only with self-induced vomiting. Early satiety, another symptom, results in low food intake and substantial weight loss. An abnormality in gastric motor function was suspected to be the etiology for these symptoms when acute dilatations of the stomach in anorectics were first reported. This complication, occasionally accompanied by perforations, was seen predominantly during refeeding attempts.[209–211]

Impaired gastric emptying of radiolabeled semisolid or solid foods has been found in almost all scintigraphic studies of patients with anorexia nervosa.[212–217] In contrast, liquid emptying was found to be either delayed[212–216] or normal.[217,218] Variables such as the severity of the gastric impairment, the degree of a patient's weight gain before the emptying study, the composition of the test meal, and the body position during imaging are probably responsible for much of the discrepancies with liquid emptying. In McCallum's study, the patients were age-matched with normal controls as well as weight-matched with controls with Crohn's disease.[219] Slowed solid but not liquid emptying was noted in 80% of anorectics when compared with either control group. There was no correlation with age, duration of symptoms, or percent of ideal body weight.

Electromechanical dysfunctions have been identified in patients with anorexia nervosa. Gastric dysrhythmias were found in all the study subjects, mainly occurring during both fasting and the postprandial period. Hypomotility was observed in the antral region. While antral contraction frequency was normal, low antral contraction amplitudes were frequently found.[220] These findings correlated with impaired emptying of solids. Because terminal antral contractions are probably crucial for the gastric emptying of solids, the observed motility abnormality may explain the nearly uniform observation of delayed emptying with solids but not liquids (ch 8). No significant change in the dysrhythmias or the emptying

rate was noted after completion of treatment. The exact nature of therapy, however, was not stated.[218] In this disorder with prominent psychiatric features, abnormal gastric motility may be the result of central nervous system effects. Cold stress inhibited antral contractions in humans.[221] Central nervous system stress, in the form of loud noises, induced altered gastric contractile activity in the dog.[222] Anorexia nervosa may be a clinical analogy to experimental stress-induced dysmotility.

Malnutrition alone can be associated with impaired gastric emptying.[223] The contribution of this factor was examined when gastric emptying was evaluated in 11 anorectics hospitalized for feeding under monitored conditions. Symptomatically, 81% of patients with delayed emptying had fullness, nausea, and/or vomiting. With completion of the program after weight gains of at least 3 kg, acceleration of both solid and liquid emptying was noted. While the psychiatric condition of the patients remained abnormal, the change in gastric emptying was still accompanied by symptomatic improvement. Because of the correction of emptying after weight gain, one might conclude that delayed gastric emptying is probably not a primary dysfunction of anorexia nervosa. The evidence is still insufficient for malnutrition to be the only culprit. Not only was there a lack of correlation between the amount of weight gained and the degree of improvement of emptying, but a few patients who gained weight have experienced a recurrence of delayed emptying.[224] Despite the uncertain relationship between gastric function and nutritional status, monitored feeding is the best therapeutic approach to correction of the patient's upper gastrointestinal symptoms. Simple weight gain, without the use of medication, may alone achieve the desired symptomatic response.

Several attempts at pharmacologic correction of the abnormal emptying have been reported. Bethanechol accelerated the emptying but failed to achieve complete restoration.[213] Although the studies were not placebo-controlled, metoclopramide successfully corrected delayed emptying.[219,225] Domperidone, in a double-blind randomized trial, accelerated the emptying rate in patients with severe delay.[226] In another well controlled trial, cisapride was also found to significantly improve emptying.[226] It is important to emphasize that a key question remains unanswered: whether modification of symptoms correlates with these pharmacologic accelerations of emptying.

Postoperative Gastric Atony After Surgery. Postoperative gastric atony is a diagnosis given to patients who do not have an anatomic obstruction but continue to experience nausea and vomiting. Their stomachs do not empty liquids or solids normally for 1 month or longer after ulcer surgery. Gastric atony is a rather uncommon condition, afflicting about 5% of patients who have had gastric surgery (vagotomy plus pyloroplasty, 1.25%; vagotomy plus antrectomy, 2.4%; subtotal gastrectomy, 3%; vagotomy plus subtotal gastrectomy, 9%).[227,228] A greater number of patients are able to empty liquid nutrients but very slowly expel solids. They may have the feeling of continuous bloating and fullness, and frequent vomiting if they try to eat normal meals. Other patients can usually tolerate small meals but may have episodes of vomiting or recurrent bezoars. Still other patients empty solid foods very slowly but have no symptoms. In short, there is a clinical spectrum of abnormally slow emptying of solid foods that may follow these operations.

The genesis of this problem is obscure. Authorities often cite the weakened antral peristalsis after truncal vagotomy plus pyloroplasty[93] as the cause. Diminished or absent antral MMCs are believed to contribute to the formation of bezoars. While asymptomatic postsurgical controls had normal phase III activity, eight out of nine patients with gastroparesis had no interdigestive motor cycles. Compared with postsurgical or healthy controls, little spontaneous fundic contractile activity was seen. However, the fundic tone was normal.[52] While these explanations fit well with currently held ideas that antral peristalsis grinds and propels solid foods from the stomach,[229] the spectrum of gastric emptying in patients who have had ulcer surgery points out our ignorance of relevant physiology. For example, patients who have had antrectomy (namely, with subtotal gastrectomy or with truncal vagotomy plus antrectomy) usually empty solid foods well, and most of the solid food emptied from their stomachs is ground to the normal size. How the aperistaltic proximal stomach accomplishes this feat is not understood. Many patients, however, present with gastric atony after antrectomy. In this setting, because the antrum has been resected, abnormal contractions of the (resected) antrum cannot be blamed.

Prokinetic drugs improve gastric emptying in some, but not all,[52] of the patients. It is not entirely clear how they produce an improvement. Agents like metoclopramide can enhance weak antral peristalsis in patients with vagotomy plus pyloroplasty, but because they also improve emptying in patients with gastric stasis after vagotomy plus antrectomy,[230] they must also have other actions, such as strengthening tone or motility in the proximal stomach. In a study of patients with vagotomy and partial gastrectomy, fundic and distal gastric motor activities were stimulated with metoclopramide. In five of nine patients, phase III activity was seen in the fundus after metoclopramide. Compared with placebo, the two patients on bethanechol exhibited a significant increase in fundic motility, but bethanechol did not induce phase III activity in the stomach.[52]

Some patients are so debilitated by their gastric atony symptoms that they consent to other surgical operations in the hope of obtaining relief. Reconstruction of the gastroenteric anastomosis (i.e., conversion of a Billroth I to a Billroth II or vice versa) is empirically the best available corrective method, but the chances are little better than 50% that these reoperations will produce an improvement.[231] While the majority had improvement in the vomiting symptom, only 5 of 15 such patients at the Mayo Clinic had complete relief with corrective surgery.[232]

It is important to emphasize that the pathogenesis of the symptoms experienced by patients who have undergone ulcer surgeries is still inadequately understood and is likely to involve explanations beyond just a change in gastric emptying pattern. Nausea and vomiting have been reported with exposure of the ileum to fatty acids.[233] Maldigestion is a complication of ulcer surgery.[229,234,235] Partially digested solids may reach the distal small intestine and be responsible for the reported postprandial symptoms and/or abnormal gastric emptying.[236] Clearly, much needs to be learned about this problem and its proper pharmacologic treatment.

ASSOCIATIONS LIKELY TO BE IMPORTANT

Gastric Dysrhythmias. Cyclical electrical activity of the stomach originates on the greater curvature at the junction between the proximal and distal parts of the organ. This region is called the gastric pacemaker. Analogous to the sino-atrial (SA) node of the heart, this pacemaker dominates the stomach by virtue of its fast firing rate. The rhythmic activity generated by the pacemaker is called the pacesetter potentials or basal electrical rhythm (BER). In man, the frequency is three cycles per minute, and in dog it is five to six cycles per minute. Pacesetter potentials partially depolarize muscle cells but do not result in muscle contraction. If the muscle cell is in an excitable state, the partial depolarization may be enough to trigger the occurrence of an action potential that causes the muscle cell to contract. Starting from the pacemaker site, pacesetter potentials spread circumferentially and toward the pylorus.[237] Because the occurrence of contractions is governed by these pacesetter potentials, contractile patterns in the antrum follow the spread of pacesetter potentials and are peristaltic (ch 8).

Similar to the heart, ectopic pacemakers in any other part of the stomach have the potential to be the controlling pacemaker. Two situations allow an ectopic pacemaker to take over: (1) if the normal one fails or (2) if a rival pacemaker develops an abnormally faster firing rate. In the first setting, a substituting, previously subservient pacemaker, with its slower firing rate, generates a "brady" rhythm. In the second setting, a rival pacemaker wins control by generating a "tachy" rhythm. An ectopic pacemaker is also likely to be less stable. The new rhythm is then highly irregular. An arrhythmia can also be generated by the normal pacemaker. Every now and then, even the normal pacemaker is susceptible to firing irregularly. This results in a wave of pacesetter potentials that has a rate falling within the normal range but has an irregular rhythm.

There are two ways by which an asynchronously firing ectopic gastric pacemaker disrupts the normal motor function of the stomach: (1) the abnormal pathway of spread may produce retrograde and poorly coordinated contraction[238] and (2) normal phasic contractions of the antrum are not generated by these abnormal pacesetter potentials.[239] That is, they do not produce as strong a contraction as normal pacesetter potentials.

Spontaneous Gastric Dysrhythmias. Gastric dysrhythmias have been found to occur spontaneously in normal dogs and healthy human volunteers.[182,218,238,240,241] In these groups, the dysrhythmic episodes were intermittent and very short-lived. In dogs, the spontaneous dysrhythmias were eliminated by eating.[242] Code and Marlett described several patterns of spontaneous gastric dysrhythmias in dog and man[238,243]: (1) *Bradygastria* is an abnormally slow but regular rhythm. (2) *Tachygastria* is an abnormally fast but regular rhythm. (3) *Tachyarrhythmia* is both abnormally fast in rate and irregular in rhythm. (4) *Gastric arrhythmia* is normal in rate but highly irregular in rhythm (Fig 60-6).

Drug-Induced Gastric Dysrhythmias. Aside from spontaneous occurrences, gastric dysrhythmias can also be induced by drugs. In dogs, the same gastric dysrhythmias observed to occur spontaneously were induced by glucagon, epinephrine, prostaglandin E2, and met-enkephalin.[239–241,244–246] Some promising clues on the origin of these electrical patterns were uncovered by use of these pharmacologic manipulations. Met-enkephalin- and epinephrine- but not glucagon-induced dysrhythmia were found to be blocked by indomethacin. This observation suggests that, in certain gastric dysrhythmias, a prostaglandin-mediated mechanism is important. Perhaps a prostaglandin synthesis inhibitor is useful to treat certain patients with gastric dysrhythmias.[247]

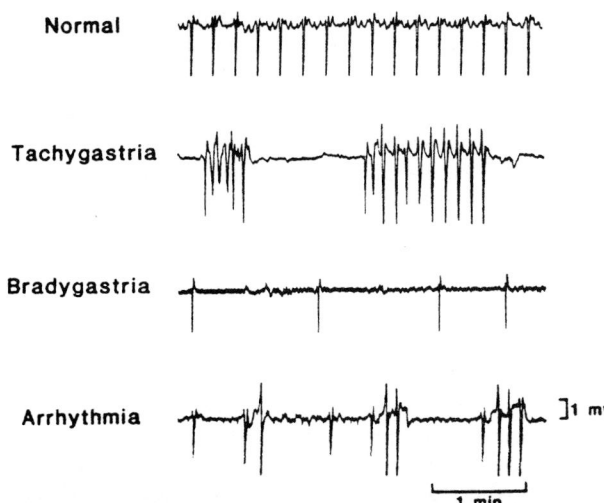

FIGURE 60–6. Types of gastric dysrhythmias. (Kim CH, Zinsmeister AR, Malagelada JR. Mechanisms of canine gastric dysrhythmia. Gastroenterology 1987;92:993.)

Sustained (Primary) Gastric Dysrhythmias. While spontaneous gastric dysrhythmias are found frequently in asymptomatic normals, these are characteristically very short-lived. If gastric dysrhythmias are sustained, motor function may be interrupted sufficiently to cause symptoms. In 1978, Telander reported a case of a 5-month-old infant who was persistently symptomatic from impaired gastric emptying. Because of severe vomiting, gastric distention, and failure to thrive, a transgastric feeding jejunostomy tube was placed. During this operation, an ectopic antral pacemaker generating a tachygastria pattern was identified by use of serosally implanted electrodes. Resection of the distal three fourths of the stomach resulted in resolution of vomiting and significant weight gain.[248] This report suggested that gastric dysrhythmia was the culprit for the symptoms.

Similar supportive evidence for the pathogenic role of sustained gastric dysrhythmias was provided by another case report in 1981. A 26-year-old female presented with an 18-month history of severe nausea, vomiting, pain, bloating, and early satiety. A weight loss of 89.3 kg was documented. Chronic serosal electrodes were implanted on her stomach and in her small intestine. Out of 944 minutes of total gastric recording time, she had 343 minutes of tachygastria and tachyarrhythmia. The dysrhythmias were associated with retrograde propagation of pacesetter potentials, reduced phase III of MMC, and asynchrony of duodenal and jejunal motility. After a hemigastrectomy and gastrojejunostomy, the symptoms decreased considerably.[243] Since this second case report, a sizable number of symptomatic patients with sustained gastric dysrhythmias have been reported. In this group of patients, normal antral contractions were absent with antral dysrhythmia.[245,246,249] The pathogenic effect of the dysrhythmias on gastric motor function is supported by the finding of delayed gastric emptying.

In dogs, spontaneous dysrhythmias were abolished with feeding.[242] It remains unknown whether sustained gastric dysrhythmia is related to a defect in the suppression of spontaneously occurring gastric ectopic pacemakers. The postprandial timing of the symptoms seen in these patients may well be due to the development of sustained gastric dysrhythmias when ectopic pacemakers are not suppressed properly by eating.

In contrast to the two extreme examples just described, a much larger population of patients presents to the gastroenterologist with symptom complexes that are far less debilitating but equally perplexing. Is there an association between these unexplained postprandial upper gastrointestinal symptoms and dysrhythmias? Recently, gastric dysrhythmias were actively pursued in this group of patients, and several studies reported that gastric dysrhythmias were found in many patients with unexplained upper gastrointestinal symptoms.[239,243–245,248–251] You and colleagues reported that gastric dysrhythmias were common in symptomatic patients. Out of 14 patients with unexplained nausea and vomiting, 9 were found to have tachygastria.[251] In a separate report of five patients, antral dysrhythmias along with retrograde propagated MMC were found in all the study patients with unexplained nausea, vomiting, and pain. Along with the dysrhythmias, impaired solid emptying was noted.[249]

In light of the frequent appearance of spontaneous gastric dysrhythmias in the asymptomatic normals, what do these dysrhythmias really mean? Is there any correlation with patient complaints? In a study in which motility findings were correlated with symptoms, this most important question was not answered to satisfaction. In a manometric study of 75 patients with functional upper gastrointestinal symptoms, 43 had gastric abnormalities and 32 had both gastric and small intestinal findings. The most common gastric abnormality was decreased antral phasic pressure activity. Symptoms, however, correlated poorly with the presence or absence of manometric abnormalities.[250] Electrical recordings were not made available, however.

In the future, actual electrical patterns of these patients can be obtained with the wider use of electrogastrography. Because of the strong directional orientation of the pacesetter, the potential may be detected through electrically filtered cutaneous recordings over and around the stomach region.[45,46] Recently, computerized analysis of electrogastrographic recordings has been greatly improved.[251a] This would simplify the procedure significantly and make electrogastrography a practical clinical tool to detect and investigate the clinical significance of gastric dysrhythmias.

Much work is needed before correct treatments can be developed for primary gastric dysrhythmias. There is only a limited experience with medical treatments using prokinetic agents. Metoclopramide provided some symptomatic relief but had no effect on the motility abnormalities.[249] In another report of a patient with antral tachygastria, initial treatment with domperidone or gastrojejunostomy alone was ineffective, but symptoms resolved after domperidone was reintroduced.[244]

Secondary Gastric Dysrhythmias. Gastric dysrhythmias are common in patients with anorexia nervosa. In fact, antral hypomotility is the most prevalent finding. Because terminal antral contractions are probably crucial for the gastric emptying of solids, the observed motility abnormality explains the nearly uniform observation of delayed emptying with solids but not liquids in this disease. Tachygastria with delayed gastric emptying is also observed during experimentally induced motion sickness. This finding offers a possible explanation for the nausea and vomiting associated with this syndrome.[252,253] It is well known that an anti-motion sickness medication, such as Dramamine, must be taken ahead of any anticipated trip to be effective. Could impaired gastric emptying secondary to motion sickness-induced tachygastria be the basis for this recommendation? A cutaneous delivery system, such as a scopolamine patch, offers a distinct advantage in light of the associated delay in gastric emptying.

Obesity/Bariatric Surgery.
The pathophysiology of obesity is not known. An inverse relationship between body size and the rate of gastric emptying was described in nonobese subjects. Slowing of gastric emptying occurred with an increase in weight. Abnormal weight gain may then result from an alteration of this homeostatic regulation. Solid but not liquid emptying was more rapid in 46 obese subjects when compared with normal controls, possibly suggesting the role of rapid emptying of food in the genesis of obesity. No correlation was found, however, between the rate of emptying and body surface area.[254] In contrast, other investigators reported that solid emptying was slowed compared with controls.[255-257] Gastric emptying rates did not correlate with weights of the patients.[258] These conflicting observations on gastric emptying in the overweight are consistent with the heterogeneous nature of obesity, as has been noted in studies focused on energy consumption.

Many gastric surgical procedures have been used for weight reduction in patients who fail conventional methods for weight control. Loss of appetite with weight reduction was observed in some of these attempts. Gastroplasty and gastric bypass are the two most commonly performed procedures. Gastroplasty (gastric partitioning) produces a 50-ml proximal pouch and a 10-mm gastrogastrostomy stoma. Gastric bypass divides the stomach in two, with the proximal compartment draining through a 12-mm gastroenterostomy. These procedures resulted in delayed gastric emptying and fundic distention, which may cause early satiety, loss of appetite, and weight reduction.

After gastric bypass, solid emptying was slower and liquid emptying was more rapid compared with controls. These findings may explain certain treatment failures in this group because rapid liquid emptying allows patients to tolerate larger volumes of high-calorie liquids.[259] Certain patients may experience a dumping syndrome similar to that of postulcer surgery patients. No correlation has been observed between the degree of weight loss, pouch or stomal size, and the rate of emptying.

In performing gastroplasty, surgeons have long focused on the optimal capacity of the proximal pouch along with the width and length of the gastrogastrostomy channel. This has been based on the assumption that a small pouch, by causing fundic distention, should induce early satiety, and a tighter channel will result in greater delay in pouch drainage. In a study in which the gastric pouch volume was measured preoperatively and postoperatively, the patient with the greatest weight loss had the largest increase in the pouch volume and the longest pouch drainage time. Both findings correlated with the tightest channel.[260] The rate of emptying from the whole stomach as well as from the proximal pouch has been evaluated to provide evidence for this assumption. With liquid emptying, no change was seen.[257,261-263] Solid or semisolid emptying from the whole stomach was reported to be varied: delayed,[263,264] normal,[261] or faster.[262] In addition, interpretations of these results are complicated by the absence of a predictable pattern of gastric emptying in the obese population. Furthermore, no correlation was seen between weight loss and any change in the the rate of emptying.[262]

The regulation of satiety is likely to be multifactorial, involving both intra- and extragastric mechanisms. Therefore, surgical interventions focused on altering the emptying of meals from the stomach can be expected to have only limited success.

Stress.
The activity of the brain is intimately linked to gut motility. Gastrointestinal responses to anxiety, fear, depression, and pain have been explored. While our understanding of the brain–gut axis is still incomplete, studies of experimental stress have clearly demonstrated the importance of the functional link between brain and gut (ch 8).[265]

Motion sickness, induced visually with a moving drum, was associated with the development of a rapidly firing ectopic antral pacesetter. A pattern of disorganized activity similar to tachygastria was observed.[266] Pain from submersion of a hand into 40°C water or labyrinthine stimulation markedly reduced postprandial antral phasic contraction. Norepinephrine and beta-endorphin levels were found to be elevated. Studies using receptor agonists and antagonists showed that naloxone[267] and adrenergic blockers[267,268] prevented stress-induced altered antral motility and gastric emptying. On the other hand, beta-adrenergic stimulation has been shown to delay gastric emptying.[269] These observations suggest that stress-induced gastric motility may be mediated by the opiate and sympathetic pathways.[269,270] It has been proposed that preoperative gastric stasis may be secondary to emotional stress and may increase the risk of aspiration of gastric contents. Paracetamol absorption, a technique for measuring gastric emptying without radioisotope exposure, was delayed in patients who developed high anxiety while awaiting minor surgery.[271,272]

Interdigestive gastric motility was altered by auditory stress in dogs. This effect was eliminated with bilateral vagotomy, indicating vagal mediation.[222] Cold stress alters gastric motility with a pattern similar to feedback inhibition of gastric motility by nutrients.[273] Antral motility was inhibited[267] and isolated pyloric pressure waves were increased, while duodenal pressure waves were reduced. This was accompanied by a delay in gastric emptying.

The relationship of stress to gastric motility and emptying is complex. Because different afferent and efferent pathways are involved in the response to pain, auditory stress,[274] anxiety, or other central stimuli, different patterns of altered gastroduodenal motility are observed. While the specific effects on motility and emptying are still debatable, considerable evidence is now available to support the importance of modulation of gastric motility by the central nervous system.

Neurologic Disorders.
Nausea and vomiting are commonly associated with a wide variety of neurologic disorders. These include illnesses with central lesions such as strokes, brain tumors, headaches, and seizures, and peripheral diseases such as Meniere's disease and labyrinthitis. Because gastric emptying can be altered by both the nucleus ambiguus and the dorsal motor nucleus of the vagus, it is not surprising that gastric motility is frequently affected by disorders involving the central nervous system. However, a cause-and-effect relationship is hard to establish from limited case reports.

An increase in intracranial pressure with direct effect on the vomiting center may explain the occurrence of nausea in patients with CNS lesion, although in certain cases altered gastric motility may also play a role.[275,276] Intermittent vomiting may represent simple partial seizure.[277] Stroke patients have been observed to have disturbed gastrointestinal motility,[278] and delayed gastric emptying was noted during migraine attacks.[279] Sympathetic outflow to the gastrointestinal tract is interrupted by a high cervical cord resection. Delayed postprandial gastric emptying in these patients has been reported.[280]

Diminished or absent antral activity along with abnormal migrating motor complexes originating in the stomach are commonly observed in patients with disorders of the enteric nervous system. While abnormal motility of the small bowel is the predominant feature, delayed gastric emptying is also seen in patients diagnosed as having idiopathic intestinal pseudo-obstruction.[281,282]

Thyroid Disorders.

Thyroid dysfunctions are often associated with gastrointestinal symptoms, with diarrhea and/or constipation being the most common complaints in hyperthyroidism and hypothyroidism, respectively. However, information on gastric motor activity in patients with hyperthyroidism and hypothyroidism is very limited. In the hyperthyroid state, studies using nutrient test meals noted normal postprandial gastric emptying.[283,284] In hypothyroid dogs, gastric and jejunal pacesetter potential activity as well as stimulated spike burst activities were all decreased,[285] but it is not known whether these disturbances are sufficient to alter gastric emptying.

Diseases Affecting the Gastric Wall.

Scleroderma is a multisystem vasculitis leading to deposition of collagen in involved organs. Gastrointestinal symptoms such as dysphagia, nausea, vomiting, and heartburn are common.[286] Abnormal motility of the esophagus has been extensively reported.[287–290] Reflux esophagitis with stricture formation, a significant complication of this disease, has been considered to be related to esophageal as well as gastric emptying dysfunctions. In a study of 12 patients, 7 had dysphagia and 8 had postprandial bloating. All the patients with dysphagia had abnormal esophageal emptying, and all the patients with bloating had delayed solid gastric emptying. The symptom severity, however, did not correlate with the magnitude of emptying abnormality.[291]

Fasting antral motor abnormalities have been observed.[292] Postprandial hypomotility of the antrum and small bowel were also noted in patients symptomatic for nausea, vomiting, or abdominal pain. In the majority, the amplitude of antral contractions was abnormally low, consistent with a myopathic process. In a minority, the findings were different. In this second group, while the contractile amplitudes were normal, incoordinated bursts of fasting activity were seen in the duodenum. These observations were suggestive of a neuropathic process. Antral motility was normal.[293] The different patterns of abnormalities were consistent with the two-staged progression of disease proposed for scleroderma: the neuropathic pattern associated with early scleroderma and the myopathic pattern with late disease.[294]

In a group of eight patients with gastrointestinal symptoms and abnormal esophageal and gastric emptying, cisapride in a placebo-controlled study improved solid and liquid emptying. Upper gastrointestinal symptoms were reduced after 1 month of oral cisapride 10 mg q.i.d. No effect, however, was seen on esophageal emptying.

A gastric emptying study should be performed as part of the evaluation of a scleroderma patient complaining of upper gastrointestinal symptoms. If delayed emptying is demonstrated, treatment with cisapride may be successful. Variable results can be expected and may be related to the stage of disease. Prokinetic therapy may be more effective in the earlier, neuropathic stage of scleroderma.

Isolated reports of delayed gastric emptying or gastric atony have also been observed in several other diseases: polymyositis and dermatomyositis,[295] dystrophia myotonica,[296,297] systemic lupus erythematosis,[298] and amyloidosis.[299]

Radiation.

Severe nausea, vomiting, and intolerance of both liquid and solid meals are common after irradiation, especially when the abdomen is in the treatment port. In a case report, gastroparesis was noted radiographically in association with absent antral motor activity.[300] In dogs experimentally treated with whole-body irradiation, gastric emptying of both liquids and solids was significantly delayed. While pretreatment with domperidone diminished the incidence of vomiting, there was no effect on the delayed gastric emptying.[301] The cause and effect of postradiation symptoms and delayed gastric emptying are therefore not established. Treatment should again be geared toward symptomatic improvement.

Abdominal Cancer.

In the setting of upper gastrointestinal cancer, nausea, vomiting, and early satiety are common. These symptoms may lead to poor food intake and inanition. Often, a correctable etiology is not found. Even without an obvious mechanical obstruction, severe symptoms of gastric stasis may be relieved by a palliative drainage procedure such as a gastrojejunostomy. A derangement of gastric motility may explain such symptoms. In a study involving 15 patients with nonobstructing pancreatic carcinoma, delayed gastric emptying was found in 60% of the subjects. The delayed emptying may even precede the onset of clinical stasis. The majority of patients with slowed emptying did not have symptoms.[302] While a direct disturbance of the neuromuscular controls of the stomach can be postulated to explain delayed gastric emptying in the setting of gastric carcinoma,[303,304] similar complications in the setting of gallbladder and pancreatic carcinomas are more difficult to explain.[305,306] Direct invasion into the surrounding nerves is often not found, and the size of the tumor is large enough to cause obstruction. This paraneoplastic syndrome-related impaired emptying was treated in an unrandomized trial with metoclopramide. Accelerated emptying correlated well with symptom improvement. Good response was reported as long as 3 months into therapy.[305] While well controlled studies are not available, abdominal cancer patients complaining of nausea, vomiting, or postprandial fullness with or without delayed emptying may benefit from metoclopramide. The presence of impaired motility of the stomach and/or duodenum leaves us with the challenging question of the usefulness of procedures designed to bypass a mechanical obstruction.[307]

Viral Gastroenteritis.

Upper gastrointestinal symptoms of anorexia, bloating, nausea, and vomiting are very common with acute viral gastroenteritis. Transient slowing of gastric emptying has been reported in this setting.[308] Further supporting this association, delayed gastric emptying has been observed in healthy subjects infected with parvoviruslike agents (Norwalk agent).[309] In a retrospective report of seven cases of postviral gastroparesis, four patients had antral hypomotility on manometry. Five of the seven patients recovered completely, with the remaining two still mildly symptomatic 29 to 37 months after the onset of symptoms.[310]

ASSOCIATIONS OF UNCERTAIN SIGNIFICANCE

Gastroesophageal Reflux Disease. The pathogenesis of gastroesophageal reflux disease has been considered to be multifactorial, including incompetent lower esophageal sphincter, decreased esophageal acid clearing, ineffective esophageal mucosal defense, and any factor that increases the reflux of gastric contents.[311] Reflux, in turn, depends partly on the intragastric volume. A significant delay in gastric emptying may increase the quantity of acid refluxed. Another effect of delayed emptying is reflex inhibition of lower esophageal sphincter tone. An increase in the gastric volume facilitates reflux by increasing the rate of transient lower esophageal sphincter relaxation.[312] Several studies have demonstrated that delayed gastric emptying of either liquids,[313-317] solids,[316,318,319] or mixed liquid/solid meals[48,314,320]) occurred in 41% to 57% of patients with gastroesophageal reflux disease. But these results are controversial, because absence of disturbances in gastric motility and emptying have also been reported. The precise role of delayed emptying in the pathogenesis of gastroesophageal reflux remains to be elucidated.[321-323]

Among the early studies, the degree of severity of the esophagitis in each studied patient was uncontrolled. This may be responsible for the inconsistent emptying results. Patients with Barrett's esophagus who have a more severe form of reflux disease may represent a more uniform study group. Because greater acid exposure has been identified in patients with Barrett's esophagus, delayed gastric emptying should be a more constant finding in these patients.[324] Contrary to expectations, however, delayed emptying was not found in this selected group of patients.[325,326]

In fact, delayed emptying, when present in patients with gastroesophageal reflux disease, failed to correlate with symptoms, lower esophageal sphincter pressure,[314,317] or 24-hour pH monitoring results.[321] The question is whether the delayed gastric emptying inconsistently associated with symptomatic reflux disease should even be the focus of a clinician's workup and management. The results of therapeutic trials with metoclopramide suggest that delayed gastric emptying is probably important only in a limited number of these patients. In these reports, metoclopramide enhanced gastric emptying in patients with gastroesophageal disease regardless of whether delayed emptying was initially present. Similarly, symptomatic improvement was achieved even with normal gastric emptying.[318] Metoclopramide may achieve good responses through its stimulatory effect on the lower esophageal sphincter pressure.[47] Bethanechol, an agent often used for treatment, did not improve gastric emptying.[48]

The majority of fundoplication patients complaining of recurring reflux symptoms had delayed emptying.[327] In this group there is a better correlation between the reflux symptom and delayed gastric emptying. Because patients with fundoplication are more likely to have symptoms refractory to acid-reduction measures, it is not surprising that an underlying motility disturbance is prevalent.

Nonulcer Dyspepsia of Various Types. Idiopathic dyspepsia is a common syndrome characterized by nonspecific postprandial symptoms in the setting of unremarkable upper gastrointestinal radiologic or endoscopic workup. These symptoms may include epigastric fullness, nausea, vomiting, excessive belching, and heartburn. Gastric stasis was considered to be a likely explanation for these complaints when the empiric use of domperidone, a prokinetic agent, was found to be effective in the symptomatic treatment of dyspepsia.[328-330] An early report described delayed gastric emptying of solids in a single patient with chronic dyspepsia. The slowed emptying was associated with weak antral activity.[331] In later studies, a significant fraction of patients with dyspepsia were found to have slowed emptying. The presence of delayed gastric emptying could not, however, be predicted based on the symptoms. In a group of 31 patients, all symptomatic with idiopathic dyspepsia, only 44% were found to have slowed solid and/or liquid emptying. In this group, the majority had only impaired liquid emptying.[332] In contrast, delayed emptying of solids[333,334] or solids and liquids was consistently observed by others.[335] Other prokinetic agents have been used to treat patients with dyspepsia and emptying. Cisapride accelerated the emptying of solids in double-blind randomized studies.[332,333] In an unrandomized study, intravenous cisapride was found to be more effective in correcting delayed solid emptying than were oral doses of 10 mg taken four times a day for 2 weeks.[335] Correlation of symptomatic improvement with enhancement of emptying was, however, absent. While cisapride alone accelerated emptying, both placebo and cisapride significantly improved dyspeptic symptoms. Even in this study, where patients were selected on the basis of having dyspeptic symptoms and delayed emptying, no association was established between clinical improvement and a change in emptying.[333] The majority of the motility studies were performed in the fasted state. The frequency of the interdigestive motility cycle was decreased in some patients with dyspepsia. Recently, long-term cisapride improved the infrequent antroduodenal interdigestive motility cycles seen in 20 dyspeptic patients.[336]

Nonulcer dyspepsia is likely to be found in a heterogeneous group of patients, with delayed gastric emptying present in only a subset of these patients. When therapy involves the use of an agent without central activity, such as cisapride, the dissociation between clinical response and change in emptying becomes apparent. The symptomatic improvement observed with domperidone is probably unrelated to any recognized motor abnormality.[337-339] Recently, a study designed to improve the understanding of patients with chronic idiopathic dyspepsia reported the following: (1) 16 out of 27 patients (59%) had delayed gastric emptying (8 with liquids only, 1 with solids only, and 7 with both); (2) no clinical feature clearly distinguished the subgroup with delayed gastric emptying from the other patients; (3) symptomatic improvement on cisapride was achieved mainly in the subgroup with objective evidence of gastric stasis; and (4) there was a trend over time toward improvement, even in the untreated group.[340] Currently, with our limited understanding, the diagnosis of nonulcer dyspepsia includes a whole host of unclassified disturbances. It is, therefore, not unexpected that only a fraction of patients exhibits delayed gastric emptying.

Delayed gastric emptying has been reported in gallbladder disease patients with dyspepsia. Similar delay was seen in postcholecystectomy patients with dyspepsia. The significance of this finding is unknown, because slowed gastric emptying was also observed in patients with gallbladder disease without dyspepsia.[341] Biliary disease may have an association with delayed gastric emptying. The dyspepsia of postcholecystectomy syndrome, however, is unlikely to be related to delayed gastric emptying.

Dyspeptic symptoms are common in patients with *Campylobacter pylori*-associated gastritis. An increased incidence of delayed gastric emptying was, however, not found when compared with either normal controls[342] or patients with *Campylobacter* culture-negative nonulcer dyspepsia.[343] Hence, the nonspecific symptoms of *Campylobacter pylori*-associated gastritis are not a result of gastric emptying disorders.

Bulimia. Patients with bulimia complain of symptoms of epigastric fullness, nausea, and vomiting suggestive of gastric retention. Liquid emptying was reported to be normal,[344-346] whereas semisolid or solid emptying was found to be either normal[345] or delayed.[344,346] Acceleration with cisapride was reported.[346] No information on clinical correlation is available.

Chronic Renal Failure. Nausea, vomiting, and anorexia are common complaints of patients with end-stage renal disease. These symptoms may continue even after the patient has been adequately dialyzed. In predialysis uremic patients, gastric emptying was noted to be either delayed with liquids[347] or normal.[348] In contrast, no delay in emptying was observed in patients receiving hemodialysis or chronic ambulatory peritoneal dialysis.[349-351] Even though correlation with symptoms was not reported, delayed gastric emptying is unlikely to be the explanation for the majority of renal failure patients complaining of nausea and vomiting.

Atrophic Gastritis. Gastric carcinoma is a known but uncommon complication of atrophic gastritis. Delayed gastric emptying, with prolonged contact time of carcinogens in the setting of a weakened mucosal barrier, may provide an explanation for this relationship. Delayed gastric emptying of solid but not liquid meals has been found in patients with atrophic gastritis.[352] This association with atrophic gastritis was observed with and without pernicious anemia.[353] The association of delayed emptying with atrophic gastritis may, however, simply be the result of poor intragastric processing of solid foods. Decreased gastric secretions in these patients may increase the time taken to fragment solid foods to tiny particles, a process that is in part dependent on peptic digestion.[354] Because a normal, functioning stomach will selectively retain larger pieces, emptying of these solids will be delayed, whereas liquids will be unaffected.

Total Parenteral Nutrition. In a study involving five patients on total parenteral nutrition, solid emptying was delayed.[355] Emptying rates off parenteral nutrition served as controls. The magnitude of the delay strongly correlated with the elevation of serum glucose. Because hyperglycemia is associated with reduced gastric motor activity and rate of emptying, the mechanism behind this observation may well be related to the effect of parenteral nutrition on serum glucose.[172,177] Because parenteral nutrition-induced hyperglycemia is now effectively managed with supplemental insulin, this association may be of limited importance. No information, however, is available on the gastric emptying rate when total parenteral nutrition is supplemented with insulin.

SUMMARY

The clinical descriptions of disordered gastric emptying and/or gastric motility discussed above are recent, which reflects the embryonic state of gastric motility as an area of clinical inquiry. As in any area of clinical description that has undergone recent and explosive growth, knowledge of these disorders is chaotic and difficult to comprehend. Part of the problem is in the clinical descriptions themselves. Some are too limited, with few cases (like those of CNS diseases), while others (like those in morbid obesity) are too conflicting to assure verity. These limitations do not apply to diabetic gastroparesis, postoperative dysfunction, or anorexia nervosa, where clinical descriptions of disordered gastric emptying abound, yet understanding of corresponding defects in motility lags.

One obvious problem is that classic techniques for measuring motility are too complex and invasive to be as widely applied as necessary to unravel pathophysiologic relations between disordered motility and abnormal transit. More important than technical limitation is the inadequacy of knowledge. We don't know enough about how the normal stomach works. Thus, we can't explain how the aperistaltic, proximal stomach fragments and empties food in asymptomatic patients who have had their antrums surgically removed. In this state of ignorance, we most certainly are at a loss to understand what ails those few postoperative patients who experience symptomatic gastric stasis. Like the electrocardiographers before the understanding of injury currents and vector analysis, we are reduced by our ignorance to a kind of pattern reading of emptying time-courses (albeit, with a diversity of methods for numerical analyses) without knowing what is important in these curves and thus where to concentrate our analysis.

Nevertheless, these descriptions provoke many questions that may be answered in the near future with investigative tools that are evolving rapidly. Given this promise, it is important for us to review what we have learned and what needs to be examined intensively.

Increasingly convincing is the idea that gastric emptying is controlled by the concerted action of different regions of the GI tract (proximal stomach, antrum, pylorus, small intestine). There is some redundancy among these controls: one region may compensate for the loss or dysfunction of other regions. Thus, to date we have seen no spontaneous disease of accelerated gastric emptying unless the surgeon disrupts more than one region. As an example, proximal gastric vagotomy alone speeds liquid emptying only moderately by altering fundic tone, intragastric pressure, and enterofundic reflexes, yet adding a pyloroplasty to proximal gastric vagotomy markedly accelerates emptying. This same idea rationalizes the observations of Camilleri and Malagelada in diabetic patients by showing that dysfunction at one or more of these sites in series may similarly lead to gastric stasis. Delayed gastric emptying in diabetic patients may be a result of (1) weakened antral peristalsis, (2) pylorospasm, or (3) altered duodenal motility.

Though still a hypothesis, this idea is important because we now are acquiring the tools to investigate regional interactions. These include the electronic barostat to measure fundic tone, the Dent sleeve to investigate pyloric pressures, real-time ultrasonography and improved gamma scintigraphy to visualize the magnitude and sequence of antral contractions, electrogastrography to characterize antral dysrhythmias, and a better overall concept of relations between intestinal contractions and intestinal receptive capacities. Furthermore, neuromuscular physiologists are providing us with an increasingly detailed (and complex) picture of regional differences in the neural circuits and their chemical messengers—for example, the prominent role of opioids in the control of the feline pylorus or the action of regulatory peptides on antral versus fundic muscle cells. It is most likely that in the future we will see the development of pharmacologic agents that have selective actions primarily on one region. If so, it is imperative that we understand what each region normally contributes and how disease may affect different regions of control.

While we have evident failure of gastric muscle (in starvation, polymyositis, scleroderma), which gives rise to gastric stasis, we are also beginning to understand the equal or greater importance of neural mechanisms in disordered gastric emptying. These include spinal nervous input as well as central nervous mechanisms (motion sickness, anorexia nervosa, and brain tumor). Here again, it is the prospect of selective pharmacologic intervention that should entice us to pursue most vigorously these early discoveries. After all, it is probably cheaper and more effective to treat motion sickness with the centrally acting agent Dramamine than to treat it with the prokinetic drug cisapride. In view of these bright prospects, the presently limited clinical descriptions should be regarded as seminal, not chaotic.

> The reader is directed to Chapter 3, The Brain–Gut Axis; Chapter 8, The Physiology of Gastric Motility and Gastric Emptying; Chapter 33, Approach to the Patient with Nausea and Vomiting; Chapter 64, Surgery for Peptic Ulcer Disease; Chapter 121, Gastrointestinal Radionuclide Imaging Procedures; and Chapter 128, Evaluation of Gastrointestinal Motility: Methodological Considerations.

REFERENCES

1. Delin NA, Axelsson B, Johansson C, Poppen B. Comparison of gamma camera and withdrawal methods for measurement of gastric emptying. Scand J Gastroenterol 1978;13:867.
2. VanDeventer G, Thomson J, Graham LS, Thomasson D, Meyer JH. Validation of correction for errors in collimation during measuring of gastric emptying of nuclide-labeled meals. J Nucl Med 1983;24:187.
3. Siegel JA, Wu RK, Knight LC, et al. Radiation dose estimates for oral agents used in upper gastrointestinal disease. J Nucl Med 1983;24:835.
4. Sutton JA, Thompson S, Sobnack R. Measurement of gastric emptying rates by radioactive isotope scanning and epigastric impedance. Lancet 1985;1:898.
5. Avill R, Mangnal YF, Bird NC, et al. Applied potential tomography. A new, noninvasive technique for measuring gastric emptying. Gastroenterology 1987;92:1019.
6. King PM, Adam RD, Pryde A, McDicken WN, Heading RC. Relationships of human antroduodenal motility and transpyloric fluid movement: Non-invasive observations with real-time ultrasound. Gut 1984;25:1384.
7. Bolondi L, Bortolotti M, Santi V, et al. Measurement of gastric emptying time by real time ultrasonography. Gastroenterology 1985;89:752.
8. Holt S, Cervantes J, Wilkinson A, Kirk Wallace JH. Measurement of gastric emptying rate in humans by real time ultrasonography. Gastroenterology 1986;90:918.
9. Wright RA, Thompson D, Syed I. Simultaneous markers for fluid and solid gastric emptying: New variations on an old theme. J Nucl Med 1981;83:1306.
10. Greenspan BS, Mayer FE, Meyer JH, Graham LS, Thomson JB. Comparison of in vitro and in vivo labeled chicken liver for evaluation of gastric emptying. J Nucl Med 1983;24:79.
11. Thomforde GM, Brown ML, Malagelada J-R. Practical solid and liquid phase markers for studying gastric emptying in man. J Nucl Med Tech 1985;13:11.
12. Knight LC, DeVegvar ML, Fisher RS, et al. Tc-99m-sulfur colloid vs. in vivo chicken liver in normal subjects. J Nucl Med 1982;23:21.
13. Meyer JH, Porter-Fink V, Elashoff J, Dressman J, Amidon GL. Human postcibal gastric emptying of 1–3 mm spheres. Gastroenterology 1988;94:1315.
14. Elashoff JD, Reedy TJ, Meyer JH. Analysis of gastric emptying data. Gastroenterology 1982;83:1306.
15. Siegel JA, Urbain J-L, Adler LP, et al. Biphasic nature of gastric emptying. Gut 1988;29:85.
16. Collins PJ, Horowitz M, Cook DJ, Harding PE, Shearman DJC. Gastric emptying in normal subjects—A reproducible technique using a single scintillation camera and a computer system. Gut 1983;24:1117.
17. Loo FD, Palmer DW, Soergel KH, Kalbfleisch JH, Wood CM. Gastric emptying in patients with diabetes mellitus. Gastroenterology 1984;86:485.
18. Camilleri A, Malagelada J-R, Brown ML, et al. Relation between antral motility and gastric emptying of solids and liquids in humans. Am J Physiol 1985;249:G580.
19. Raskin HF. Barium burger roentgen study for unrecognized clinically significant gastric retention. South Med J 1971;64:1227.
20. Pelot D, Dana ER, Berk JE, et al. Comparative assessment of gastric emptying by "barium burger" and saline load tests. Am J Gastroenterol 1972;58:411.
21. Feldman M, Smith HJ, Simon TR. Gastric emptying of solid, radiopaque markers: Studies in healthy subjects and diabetic patients. Gastroenterology 1984;87:895.
22. Abatzi Th-A, Bergmen S, Wiesnagrotzki G, et al. Gastric emptying and antral motor activity in 50 patients with anorexia nervosa (abstr). Gastroenterology 1988;94:A1.
23. Stripp D. Lab notes: Quicker pictures give look at organs in action. The Wall Street Journal 1989;B1, March 28.
24. Weiner K, Graham LS, Reedy T, et al. Simultaneous gastric emptying of two solids. Gastroenterology 1981;81:257.
25. Moore JG, Christian PE, Brown JA, et al. Influence of meal weight and caloric content on gastric emptying of meals in man. Dig Dis Sci 1984;29:513.
26. Sun WM, Houghton LA, Read NW, Grundy DG, Johnson AG. Effect of meal temperature on gastric emptying of liquids in man. Gut 1988;29:302.
27. Goo RH, Moore JG, Greenberg E, Alazraki NP. Circadian variation in gastric emptying of meals in humans. Gastroenterology 1987;93:515.
28. Chang CA, McKenna RD, Beck IT. Gastric emptying rate of water and fat phases of a mixed test meal. Gut 1968;9:420.
29. Hutson WR, Roehkasse RL, Wald A. Influence of gender and menopause on gastric emptying and motility. Gastroenterology 1989;96:11.
30. Datz FL, Christian PE, Moore J. Gender-related differences in gastric emptying. J Nucl Med 1987;28:1204.
31. Notivol R, Carrio I, Cano L, et al. Gastric emptying of solid and liquid meals in healthy young subjects. Scand J Gastroenterol 1984;19:1107.
32. McDonald I. Gastric activity during the menstrual cycle. Gastroenterology 1957;30:602.
33. Simpson KH, Stakes AF, Miller M. Pregnancy delays paracetamol absorption and gastric emptying in patients undergoing surgery. Br J Anaesth 1988;60:24.
34. Moore JG, Tweedy C, Christian PE, Datz FL. Effect of age on gastric emptying of liquid-solid meals in man. Dig Dis Sci 1983;28:340.
35. Evans M, Triggs E, Cheung M, et al. Gastric emptying rate in the elderly: Implications for drug therapy. J Am Geriatr Soc 1981;9:201.
36. Harrison A, Ippoliti A. Effect of smoking on gastric emptying (abstr). Gastroenterology 1979;76:1152.
37. McDonald WM, Owyang C. Smoking markedly inhibits gastric mo-

tility in smokers and nonsmokers (abstr). Gastroenterology 1989;96:A332.

38. Willson CA, Bushnell D, Keshavarzian A. The effect of acute and chronic ethanol administration on gastric emptying in cats. Dig Dis Sci 1990;35:444.

39. Moore JG, Datz FL, Christian PE. Exercise increases solid meal emptying rates in men. Dig Dis Sci 1990;35:428.

40. Brophy CM, Moore JG, Christian PE, et al. Variability of gastric emptying measurements in man employing standardized radiolabeled meals. Dig Dis Sci 1986;31:799.

41. You CH, Chey WY. Study of electromechanical activity of the stomach in humans and in dogs with particular attention to tachygastria. Gastroenterology 1984;86:1460.

42. Azpiroz F, Malagelada J-R. Intestinal control of gastric tone. Am J Physiol 1986;251:G727.

43. You CH, Lee KY, Chey WY, Menguy R. Electrogastrographic study of patients with unexplained nausea, bloating and vomiting. Gastroenterology 1980;79:311.

44. Stoddard CJ, Smallwood RH, Duthie HL. Electrical arrhythmias in the human stomach. Gut 1981;22:705.

45. Mirizzi N, Scafoglieri U. Optimal direction of the electrogastrographic signal in man. Med Biol Eng Comput 1983;21:385.

46. Abell TL, Malagelada J-R. Electrogastrography: Curent assessment and future perspectives. Dig Dis Sci 1988;33:982.

47. McCallum RW, Kline MM, Curry N, Sturdevant RAL. Comparative effects of metoclopramide and bethanechol on lower esophageal sphincter pressure in reflux patients. Gastroenterology 1974;68:1114.

48. McCallum RW, Fink SM, Lerner E, Berkowitz DM. Effects of metoclopramide and bethanechol on delayed gastric emptying present in gastroesophageal reflux patients. Gastroenterology 1983;84:1573.

49. Johnson LF, DeMeester TR. Evaluation of elevation of the head of the bed, bethanechol and antacid foam tablets on gastroesophageal reflux. Dig Dis Sci 1981;26:673.

50. Farrell RL, Roling GT, Castell DO. Cholinergic therapy of chronic heartburn. Ann Intern Med 1974;80:573.

51. Stewart IM, Hosking DJ, Preston BJ, Atkinson M. Oesophageal motor changes in diabetes mellitus. Thorax 1976;31:278.

52. Malagelada JR, Rees WD, Mazzotta LJ, Go VLW. Gastric motor abnormalities in diabetic and post vagotomy gastroparesis: Effect of metoclopramide and bethanechol. Gastroenterology 1980;78:286.

53. Fox S, Behar J. Pathogenesis of diabetic gastroparesis: A pharmacologic study. Gastroenterology 1980;78:757.

54. McEnvoy GK, ed. Bethanechol. American Hospital Service drug information. Bethesda, MD. American Society of Hospital Pharmacists, Bethanechol Chloride 1990:571.

55. Pinder RM, Brogden RN, Sawyer PR, et al. Metoclopramide: A review of its pharmacologic properties and clinical use. Drugs 1976;12:81.

56. Schultz-Dilrieu K. Metoclopramide. Gastroenterology 1979;77:768.

57. Eisner M. Gastrointestinal effects of metoclopramide in man: In vitro experiments with human smooth muscle preparations. Br J Med 1968;4:679.

58. Eisner M. Effect of metoclopramide on gastrointestinal motility in man: A manometric study. Am J Dig Dis 1971;16:409.

59. Johnson AG. Gastroduodenal motility and synchronization. Postgrad Med J 1973;4(Suppl):29.

60. Valenzuela JE. Dopamine as a possible neurotransmitter in gastric relaxation. Gastroenterology 1976;71:1019.

61. McEnvoy GK, ed. Metoclopramide. American Hospital Service drug information. Bethesda, MD. American Society of Hospital Pharmacists, 1988:1669.

62. Ramsbottom N, Hunt JN. Studies of the effect of metoclopramide and apomorphine on gastric emptying and secretion in man. Gut 1970;11:989.

63. Brogden RN, Carmine AA, Heel RC, et al. Domperidone: A review. Drugs 1982;24:360.

64. Friedman G. The GI drug column: Domperidone. Am J Gastroenterol 1983;78:679.

65. Davis RH, Clench MH, Mathias JR. Effects of domperidone in patients with chronic unexplained upper gastrointestinal symptoms: A double-blind, placebo-controlled study. Dig Dis Sci 1988;33:1505.

66. Nagler J, Miskovitz P. Clinical evaluation of domperidone in the treatment of chronic postprandial idiopathic upper gastrointestinal distress. Am J Gastroenterol 1981;76:495.

67. Horowitz M, Harding PE, Chatterton BE, et al. Acute and chronic effects of domperidone on gastric emptying in diabetic autonomic neuropathy. Dig Dis Sci 1985;30:1.

68. Champion MC. Domperidone, a new dopamine antagonist. Can Med Assoc J 1986;135:457.

69. Cooke HJ, Harvey HV. The effects of cisapride on serotonin-evoked mucosal response in guinea pig ileum. Eur J Pharmacol 1984;98:148.

70. Weinbeck M, Cinder-Wiesinger E, Bergges W. Cisapride acts as a motor stimulator in the human esophagus. Gastroenterology 1984;86:1298.

71. Wallin L, Kruse-Andersen S, Madsen T, Boesby S. Effect of cisapride on the gastro-oesophageal function in normal human subjects. Digestion 1987;37:160.

72. Muller-Lissner SA, Fraas C, Hartl A. Cisapride offsets dopamine-induced slowing of fasting gastric emptying. Dig Dis Sci 1986;31:807.

73. Jian R, Ducrot F, Piedeloup C, et al. Measurement of gastric emptying in dyspeptic patients: Effects of a new gastrokinetic agent (cisapride). Gut 1985;26:352.

74. Lazzaroni M, Sangaletti O, Bianchi Porro G. Effect of cisapride on gastric emptying and ileal transit time of balanced liquid meal in healthy subjects. Digestion 1987;37:110.

75. Coremans G, Janssens J, Vantrappen G, et al. Cisapride stimulates propulsive motility patterns in human jejunum. Dig Dis Sci 1988;33:1512.

76. Chey WY, Lee KY, You CH, et al. Effect of cisapride on colonic transit time in dogs and humans. Dig Dis Sci 1984;7:29.

77. Rezende J, Di Lorenzo C, Dooley CP, Valenzuela J. Cisapride stimulates antral motility and decreases duodenogastric reflux (DGR) (abstr). Gastroenterology 1988;94:A375.

78. Buchheit KH, Costall B, Engel G, et al. 5-Hydroxytryptamine receptor antagonism by metoclopramide and ICS 205-930 in the guinea-pig leads to enhancement of contractions of stomach muscle strips induced by electrical field stimulation and facilitation of gastric emptying in vivo. J Pharm Pharmacol 1985;37:664.

79. Costall B, Gunning SJ, Naylor RJ, Tyers MB. The effect of GR38032F, a novel 5-HT3-receptor antagonist, on gastric emptying in the guinea-pig. Br J Pharmacol 1987;91:263.

80. Akkermans LMA, Vos A, Hoekstra A, et al. Effect of ICS 205-930 (a specific 5-HT3 receptor antagonist) on gastric emptying of a solid meal (abstr). Gastroenterology 1988;94:A4.

81. Shillabeer G, Davison JS. Proglumide, a cholecystokinin antagonist, increases gastric emptying in rats. Am J Physiol 1987;252 (Regulatory Integrative Comp Physiol 21):R353.

82. Fried M, Lochner C, Eriacher U, et al. Role of CCK in the regulation of gastric emptying of pancreatic secretion in man. Gastroenterology 1989;96:A159.

83. Mittal RK, Frank EB, Lange RC, McCallum RW. Effects of morphine and naloxone on esophageal motility and gastric emptying in man. Dig Dis Sci 1986;31:936.

84. Schang JC, Devroede G, Perrault R. Naloxone therapy in small intestinal obstruction. Preliminary results about two cases. Am J Gastroenterol 1984;79:828.

85. Gue M, Honde C, Pascaud X, et al. Opposite effects of orally administered opiate agonists on gastric emptying of liquids and solids in dogs (abstr). Gastroenterology 1988;94:A159.

86. Edin R, Lundberg J, Terenius L, et al. Evidence for vagal enkephalinergic neural control of the feline pylorus and stomach. Gastroenterology 1980;79:294.

87. Sarna SK, Soergel KH, Koch TR, et al. Effects of erythromycin on human gastrointestinal motor activity in the fasted and fed states (abstr). Gastroenterology 1989;96:A440.

88. Depoortere I, Peeters TL, Matthijs G, Vantrappen G. Macrolide antibiotics are motilin receptor agonists (abstr). Hepatogastroenterology 1988;35:198.

89. Kondo Y, Torii K, Itoh Z, Omura S. Erythromycin and its derivatives with motilin-like biological activities inhibit the specific binding of 125I-motilin to duodenal muscle (abstr). Biochem Biophys Res Commun 1988;35:198.

90. Van Trappen G, Janssens J, Tack J, et al. Erythromycin is a potent

gastrokinetic in diabetic gastroparesis (abstr). Gastroenterology 1989;96:A525.

91. Janssens J, Peeters TL, Vantrappen G, Tack J, Urbain JL, De Roo M, Muls E, Bouillon R. Improvement of gastric emptying in diabetic gastroparesis by erythromycin. N Engl J Med 1990;322:1028.

92. Doty JE, Sanders SL, Gu YG, Lin HC. Erythromycin accelerates gastric emptying of solids at the expense of sieving (abstr). Gastroenterology 1990;98:A345.

93. Hinder RA, San-Garde BA. Individual and combined roles of the pylorus and antrum in the canine gastric emptying of a liquid and a digestible solid. Gastroenterology 1983;84:281.

94. Hinder RA, Bremner CG. Relative role of pyloroplasty size, truncal vagotomy and milk meal volume in canine gastric emptying. Am J Dig Dis 1978;23:210.

95. Miller J, Kauffman G, Elashoff J, Ohashi H, Carter D, Meye JH. Search for resistances controlling gastric emptying of liquid meals. Am J Physiol 1981;241:G403.

96. Wilbur BG, Kelly KA. Effect of proximal gastric, complete gastric, and truncal vagotomy on canine gastric electric activity, motility, and emptying. Ann Surg 1973;178:295.

97. Aeberhard P, Walther M. Results of a controlled randomized trial of proximal gastric vagotomy with and without pyloroplasty. Br J Surg 1978;65:634.

98. Binswager RO, Aeberhard P, Walther M, et al. Effect of pyloroplasty on gastric emptying: Long-term results obtained with a labeled test meal 14–43 months after operation. Br J Surg 1978;65:27.

99. Clarke RJ, Alexander-Williams J. The effect of preserving antral innervation and of a pyloroplasty on gastric emptying after vagotomy in man. Gut 1973;14:300.

100. Faxen A, Dotevall N, Kock G, et al. The influence of pyloroplasty on gastric emptying after parietal cell vagotomy (abstr). Scand J Gastroenterol 1973;(Suppl 20):14.

101. Williams NS, Miller J, Elashoff J, Meyer JH. Canine resistances to gastric emptying of liquids after ulcer surgery. Dig Dis Sci 1986;31:273.

102. MacGregor IL, Parent J, Meyer JH. Gastric emptying of liquid meals and pancreatic and biliary secretion after subtotal gastrectomy or truncal vagotomy and pyloroplasty in man. Gastroenterology 1977;72:195.

103. McKelvey STD. Gastric incontinence and postvagotomy diarrhea. Br J Surg 1970;57:741.

104. Gulsrud PO, Taylor IL, Watts HD, et al. How gastric emptying of carbohydrate affects glucose tolerance and symptoms after truncal vagotomy with pyloroplasty. Gastroenterology 1980;78:1463.

105. Kroop HS, Long WB, Alavi A, Hansell JR. Effect of water and fat on gastric emptying of solid meals. Gastroenterology 1979;77:997.

106. Ralphs DNL, Thomson JPS, Haynes S, et al. The relationship between the rate of gastric emptying and the dumping syndrome. Br J Surg 1978;65:637.

107. Borgstrom B, Dahlquist G, Lundh G, Sjovall J. Studies of intestinal digestion and absorption in the human. J Clin Invest 1957;36:1521.

108. Lundh G. Intestinal digestion and absorption after gastrectomy. Acta Chir Scand 1958;(Suppl 231):1.

109. Bond JH, Levitt MD. Use of breath hydrogen (H2) to quantitate small bowel transit time following partial gastrectomy. J Lab Clin Med 1977;90:30.

110. Lin HC, Doty JE, Reedy TJ, Meyer JH. Inhibition of gastric emptying by glucose depends on the length of the intestine exposed to the nutrient. Am J Physiol 1989;256:G404.

111. Fried M, Mayer EA, Jensen JBMJ, et al. Temporal relationships of cholecystokinin release, pancreatobiliary secretion and gastric emptying of a mixed meal. Gastroenterology 1988;95:1344.

112. Editorial. Dumping syndrome and gut peptides. Lancet 1980;2:1173.

113. Leeds AR, Ebeid F, Ralphs DNL, Metz G, Delawari JB. Pectin in the dumping syndrome. Lancet 1981;1:1075.

114. Meyer JH, Gu YG, Taylor IL. Intestinal action of guar on gastric emptying or hormone release. Gastroenterology 1986;90:1556.

115. Rydning A, Berstad A, Berstad T, et al. The effect of guar gum and fiber-enriched wheat bran on gastric emptying of a semisolid meal in healthy subjects. Scand J Gastroenterol 1985;20:230.

116. Sawyers JL, Herrington JL Jr. Superiority of antiperistaltic jejunal segments in management of severe dumping syndrome. Ann Surg 1973;178:311.

117. Mackie CR, Hall AW, Clark J, et al. The effect of isoperistaltic

118. Bjork S, Phillips SF, Kelly KA. Mechanisms of enhanced intestinal absorption with electrical pacing (abstr). Gastroenterology 1984;86:1029.

119. Goligher JC, Pulvertaft CN, deDombal FT, et al. Five to eight year results of Leeds-York controlled trial of elective surgery for duodenal ulcer. Br Med J 1968;2:781.

120. Madsen P, Peterson G. Postvagotomy diarrhea examined by means of a nutritional contrast medium. Scand J Gastroenterol 1968;3:545.

121. Ladas SD, Isaacs PET, Quereshi Y, et al. Role of the small intestine in postvagotomy diarrhea. Gastroenterology 1983;85:1088.

122. Ohashi H, Meyer JH. Effect of peptic digestion on gastric emptying of cooked liver in dogs. Gastroenterology 1980;79:305.

123. Lavigne ME, Wiley ZD, Martin P, Way LW, Sleisenger MH, MacGregor IL. Gastric, pancreatic, and biliary secretion, and the rate of gastric emptying after parietal cell vagotomy. Am J Surg 1979;138:644.

124. Mayer EA, Thomson JB, Jehn D, Reedy T, Elashoff J, Deveney C, Meyer JH. Gastric emptying and sieving of solid food and pancreatic and biliary secretions after solid meals in patients with nonresective ulcer surgery. Gastroenterology 1984;87:1264.

125. Mistiaen W, Van Hee R, Blockx P, Hubens A. Gastric emptying for solids in patients with duodenal ulcer before and after highly selective vagotomy. Dig Dis Sci 1990;35:310.

126. Meyer JH, Thomson JB, Cohen MB, et al. Sieving of food by the canine stomach and sieving after gastric surgery. Gastroenterology 1976;76:804.

127. Meyer JH, Thomson JB, Cohen MB, Schadchehr A, Mandiola SA. Sieving of solid food by the normal and ulcer-operated canine stomach. Gastroenterology 1979;76:804.

128. Holt S, Reid J, Taylor TV, Tothill P, Heading RC. Gastric emptying of solids in man. Gut 1982;23:292.

129. Aune S. Intragastric pressure after vagotomy in man. Scand J Gastroenterol 1969;4:447.

130. Staadas J, Aune S. Intragastric pressure/volume relationship before and after vagotomy. Acta Chir Scand 1970;136:611.

131. Staadas JO. Intragastric pressure/volume relationship before and after proximal gastric vagotomy. Scand J Gastroenterol 1975;10:129.

132. Kelly KA, Code CF. Effect of transthoracic vagotomy on canine gastric electrical activity. Gastroenterology 1969;57:51.

133. Malagelada J-R, Rees WDW, Mazzotta LJ, Go VLW. Gastric motor abnormalities in diabetic and postvagotomy gastroparesis: Effect of metoclopramide and bethanechol. Gastroenterology 1980;78:286.

134. Grimson KS, Taylor HM, Trent JC, et al. The effect of transthoracic vagotomy upon the function of the stomach and upon the early clinical course of patients with peptic ulcer. South Med J 1946;39:460.

135. Hall KE, El-Sharkawy TY, Diamant NE. Vagal control of migratory motor complex on the dog. Am J Physiol 1982;243:G276.

136. MacGregor IL, Martin P, Meyer JH. Gastric emptying of solid food in normal man and after subtotal gastrectomy and truncal vagotomy with pyloroplasty. Gastroenterology 1977;72:206.

137. Heading RC, Tothill P, McLoughlinn GP, et al. Gastric emptying rate measurement in man: A double isotope scanning technique for simultaneous study of liquid and solid components of a meal. Gastroenterology 1976;71:45.

138. Doty JE, Meyer JH. Vagotomy and antrectomy impairs intracellular but not extracellular fat absorption in the dog. Gastroenterology 1988;94:50.

139. Doty JE, Gu YG, Meyer JH. Vagotomy and antrectomy with gastrojejunostomy impairs fat absorption from liquid and solid food. Gastroenterology 1989;96:A128.

140. Meyer JH, Porter-Fink V, Crott R, Figeuroa W. Absorption of heme iron after truncal vagotomy with antrectomy. Gastroenterology 1987;92:1534.

141. Vogel SB, Hocking MP, Woodward ER. Clinical and radionuclide evaluation of Roux-en-Y diversion for postgastrectomy dumping. Am J Surg 1988;155:57.

142. Hocking MP, Vogel SB, Falasia CA, Woodward ER. Delayed gastric emptying of liquids and solids following Roux-en-Y biliary diversion. Ann Surg 1981;194:494.

143. Britten JP, Johnson D, Ward DL, et al. Gastric emptying and clinical outcome after Roux-en-Y diversion. Br J Surg 1987;74:900.

144. Vogel SB, Vair DB, Woodward ER. Alterations in gastrointestinal emptying of 99m technetium labelled solids following sequential antrectomy, truncal vagotomy and Roux-en-Y gastrojejunostomy. Ann Surg 1983;198:506.

145. Pellegrini CA, Patti MG, Lewin M, Waye LW. Alkaline reflux gastritis and the effect of biliary diversion on gastric emptying of solid food. Am J Surg 1985;150:166.

146. Haglund U, Janson R, Linhagen J, et al. Early postoperative results following antrectomy and selective vagotomy with gastroduodenostomy vs. Roux-en-Y gastrojejunostomy. Gastroenterology 1988;94:A164.

147. Long WB, Weiss JB. Rapid gastric emptying of fatty meals in pancreatic insufficiency. Gastroenterology 1974;67:920.

148. Regan PT, Malagelada J-R, DiMagno EP, Go VLW. Postprandial gastric function in pancreatic insufficiency. Gut 1979;20:249.

149. Malagelada JR, Longstreth GF, Deering TB, et al. Gastric secretion and emptying after ordinary meals in duodenal ulcer. Gastroenterology 1977;73:989.

150. Hunt JN. Influence of hydrochloric acid on gastric secretion and emptying in patients with duodenal ulcer. Br Med J 1957;1:681.

151. Griffith GH, Owen GM, Kirkman S, et al. Gastric emptying in health and in gastroduodenal disease. Gastroenterology 1968;54:1.

152. Holt S, Heading RC, Taylor TV, et al. Is gastric emptying abnormal in duodenal ulcer? Dig Dis Sci 1986;31:685.

153. Lam SK, Isenberg JI, Grossman MI, et al. Rapid gastric emptying in duodenal ulcer patients. Dig Dis Sci 1982;27:598.

154. Fordtran JS, Walsh JH. Gastric acid secretion rate and buffer content of the stomach after eating; results in normal subjects and in patients with duodenal ulcer. J Clin Invest 1973;52:645.

155. Stubbs DF, Hunt JN. A relation between the energy of food and gastric emptying in man with duodenal ulcer. Gut 1975;16:693.

156. Howlett PJ, Sheiner HJ, Barber DC, et al. Gastric emptying in control subjects and patients with duodenal ulcer before and after vagotomy. Gut 1976;17:542.

157. Williams NS, Elashoff J, Meyer JH. Gastric emptying of liquids in normal subjects and patients with healed duodenal ulcer disease. Dig Dis Sci 1986;31:943.

158. Brenner W, Hendrix TR, McHugh PR. Regulation of gastric emptying by glucose. Gastroenterology 1983;85:76.

159. Parr NJ, Grime S, Critchley M, et al. Abnormal pattern of gastric emptying of liquid in chronic duodenal ulcer. Digestion 1988;40:237.

160. Oberle RL, Chewn TS, Lloyd C, et al. The influence of the interdigestive migrating motor complex on gastric emptying of liquids. Gastroenterology 1988;94:A328.

161. Dubois A, Van Eerdewegh P, Gardner JD. Gastric emptying and secretion in Zollinger-Ellison syndrome. J Clin Invest 1977;59:255.

162. Harrison A, Ippoliti A, Cullison R. Rapid gastric emptying in Zollinger-Ellison syndrome (ZES) (abstr). Gastroenterology 1980;78:1180.

163. Feldman M, Schiller LR. Disorders of gastrointestinal motility associated with diabetes mellitus. Ann Intern Med 1983;98:378.

164. Atkinson M, Hosking DJ. Gastrointestinal complications of diabetes mellitus. Clin Gastroenterol 1983;12:633.

165. Horowitz M, Harding PE, Maddox A, et al. Gastric and esophageal emptying in insulin-dependent diabetes mellitus. J Gastroenterol Hepatol 1986;1:97.

166. Horowitz M, Harding PE, Maddox AF, et al. Gastric and esophageal emptying in patients with type II (non-insulin dependent) diabetes mellitus. Diabetologia 1989;32(3):151.

167. Hollis JB, Castell DO, Bradom RL. Oesophageal function in diabetes mellitus and its relation to peripheral neuropathy. Gastroenterology 1977;73:1098.

168. Ewing DJ, Clare BF. Diagnosis and management of diabetic autonomic neuropathy. Br Med J 1982;285:916.

169. Kassander P. Asymptomatic gastric retention in diabetes (gastroparesis diabeticum). Ann Intern Med 1958;48:797.

170. Zitomer BR, Gramm HF, Kozak GP. Gastric neuropathy in diabetes mellitus: Clinical and radiologic observations. Metabolism 1968;17:199.

171. Keshavarzian A, Iber FL, Vaeth J. Gastric emptying in patients with insulin-requiring diabetes mellitus. Am J Gastroenterol 1987;82:29.

172. Loo FD, Palmer DW, Soergel KH, et al. Gastric emptying in patients with diabetes mellitus. Gastroenterology 1983;86:485.

173. Havelund T, Oster-Jorgensen E, Larsen ML, Lauritsen K. Effects of cisapride on gastroparesis in patients with insulin-dependent diabetes mellitus. Acta Med Scand 1987;222:339.

174. Wright RA, Clemente R. Diabetic gastroparesis: An abnormality of gastric emptying of solids (abstr). Gastroenterology 1983;84:1355.

175. Horowitz M, Harding PE, Chatterton BE, et al. Acute and chronic effects of domperidone on gastric emptying in diabetic autonomic neuropathy. Dig Dis Sci 1985;30:1.

176. Barnett JL, Owyang C. Serum glucose concentration as a modulator of interdigestive gastric motility. Gastroenterology 1988;94:739.

177. MacGregor IL, Gueller R, Watts HD, Meyer JH. The effect of acute hyperglycemia on gastric emptying in man. Gastroenterology 1976;70:197.

178. Aylett P. Gastric emptying and change of blood glucose level as affected by glucagon and insulin. Clin Sci 1962;22:171.

179. Marshak RH, Marklansky D. Diabetic gastropathy. Am J Dig Dis 1964;9:366.

180. Achem-Karem SR, Funakoshi A, Vinik AI, et al. Plasma motilin concentration and interdigestive migratory motor complex in diabetic gastroparesis. Gastroenterology 1985;88:492.

181. Camilleri M, Malagelada J-R. Abnormal intestinal motility in diabetics with the gastroparesis syndrome. Eur J Clin Invest 1984;14:420.

182. Abell TL, Camilleri M, Malagelada J-R. High prevalence of gastric electrical dysrhythmias in diabetic gastroparesis (abstr). Gastroenterology 1985;88:1299.

183. Koch KL, Stern RM, Stewart WR, et al. Gastric emptying and gastric myoelectric activity in patients with diabetic gastroparesis: Effects of long-term domperidone treatment. Am J Gastroenterol 1989;84:1069.

184. Fraser R, Fone D, Horowitz M, et al. Pyloric motor response to intraduodenal lipid is sustained and atropine sensitive (abstr). Gastroenterology 1989;96:A157.

185. Hasler W, Bowling B, Owyang C. Intraduodenal lipids induce pyloric contractions. Role of cholecystokinin and the cholinergic and opiate pathways. Gastroenterology 1989;96:A200.

186. Fone D, Heddle R, Horowitz M, et al. Atropine blocks the pyloric motor response to intraduodenal dextrose in healthy volunteers. Gastroenterology 1988;95:A132.

187. Tougas G, Allescher HD, Li YY, et al. Effect of duodenal acidification on pyloroduodenal motor activity in humans. Gastroenterology 1988;94:A464.

188. Mearin F, Camilleri M, Malagelada J-R. Pyloric dysfunction in diabetics with recurrent nausea and vomiting. Gastroenterology 1986;90:1919.

189. Rundles RW. Diabetic neuropathy; general review with report of 125 cases. Medicine 1945;24:111.

190. Clarke RJ, Alexander-Williams J. Effect of preserving antral innervation and of a pyloroplasty on gastric emptying after vagotomy in man. Gut 1973;14:300.

191. Snape WJ Jr, Battle WM, Schwartz SS, et al. Metoclopramide to treat gastroparesis due to diabetes mellitus. A double-blind, controlled trial. Ann Intern Med 1982;96:444.

192. Kristensson K, Nordborg C, Olsson Y, et al. Changes in the vagus nerve in diabetes mellitus. Acta Pathol Microbiol Scand 1971;79:684.

193. Yoshida MM, Schuffler MD, Sumi SM. There are no morphologic abnormalities of the gastric wall or abdominal vagus in patients with diabetic gastroparesis. Gastroenterology 1988;94:907.

194. Gershon MD, Erde SM. The nervous system of the gut. Gastroenterology 1981;80:1571.

195. Feldman M, Corbett DB, Ramsey EJ, et al. Abnormal gastric function in longstanding insulin-dependent diabetic patients. Gastroenterology 1979;77:12.

196. Kassander P. Asymptomatic gastric retention in diabetes (gastroparesis diabeticum). Ann Intern Med 1958;48:797.

197. McCallum RW, Ricci DA, Rakatansky H, et al. A multicenter placebo-controlled clinical trial of oral metoclopramide in diabetic gastroparesis. Diabetes Care 1983;6:463.

198. Horowitz M, Maddox A, Harding PE, et al. Effect of cisapride on gastric and esophageal emptying in insulin-dependent diabetes mellitus. Gastroenterology 1987;92:1899.

199. Feldman M, Smith HJ. Effect of cisapride on gastric emptying of indigestible solids in patients with gastroparesis diabeticum: A comparison with metoclopramide and placebo. Gastroenterology 1987;92:171.

200. Atkinson M, Hosking DJ. Gastrointestinal complications of diabetes mellitus. Clin Gastroenterol 1983;12(3):633.

201. Yang R, Arem T, Chan L. Gastrointestinal tract complications of diabetes mellitus physiology and measurement. Arch Intern Med 1984;144:1251.

202. Longstreth GF, Malagelada J-R, Kelly KA. Metoclopramide stimulation of gastric motility and emptying in diabetic gastroparesis. Ann Intern Med 1977;86:195.

203. Schade RR, Duas MC, Lhotsky DM, et al. Effect of metoclopramide on gastric liquid emptying in patients with diabetic gastroparesis. Dig Dis Sci 1985;30:10.

204. Achem-Karem SR, Owyang C, Shapiro B, Vinik AI. Gastric motility and emptying studies predict clinical response to metoclopramide in diabetic gastroparesis (abstr). Gastroenterology 1983;84:1087.

205. Feldman M, Smith HJ, Simon TR. Gastric emptying of solid radio-opaque markers: Studies in healthy subjects and diabetic patients. Gastroenterology 1984;87:895.

206. McCallum RW, Petersen J, Dubovic S. Effect of cisapride on gastric emptying and symptoms associated with gastroparesis (abstr). Gastroenterology 1986;90:1541.

207. Petersen JM, Lange R, McCallum RW. Cisapride accelerates gastric emptying of solid and liquid meal component in patients with gastric stasis. Dig Dis Sci 1985;30:788.

208. Koch KL, Stern RM, Stewart WR, Vasey MW. Gastric emptying and gastric myoelectrical activity in patients with diabetic gastroparesis: Effect of long-term domperidone treatment. Am J Gastroenterol 1989;84:1069.

209. Russel GFM. Acute dilatation of the stomach in anorexia nervosa. Br J Psychiatry 1966;112:203.

210. Evans DS. Acute dilatation and spontaneous rupture of the stomach. Br J Surg 1968;55:940.

211. Jennings KP, Klidjian AM. Acute gastric dilatation in anorexia nervosa. Br Med J 1974;2:477.

212. Dubois A, Gross HA, Ebert MH, Castell DO. Altered gastric emptying and secretion in primary anorexia nervosa. Gastroenterology 1979;77:319.

213. Dubois A, Gross HA, Richter JE, Ebert MH. Effect of bethanechol on gastric functions in primary anorexia nervosa. Dig Dis Sci 1981;26:598.

214. Holt S, Ford MJ, Grant S, Heading RC. Abnormal gastric emptying in primary anorexia nervosa. Br J Psychiatry 1981;139:550.

215. Stacher G, Kiss A, Wiesnagrotzki S, Bergmann H, Hobart J, Schneider C. Oesophageal and gastric motility disorders in patients categorised as having primary anorexia nervosa. Gut 1986;27:1120.

216. Domstad PA, Shih W-J, Humphries L, Deland FH, Digenis GA. Radionuclide gastric emptying studies in patients with anorexia nervosa. J Nucl Med 1987;28:816.

217. McCallum RW, Grill BB, Lange R, Planky M, Glass EE, Greenfeld DG. Definition of a gastric emptying abnormality in patients with anorexia nervosa. Dig Dis Sci 1985;8:713.

218. Abell TL, Malagelada J-R, Lucas AR, et al. Gastric electromechanical and neurohormonal function in anorexia nervosa. Gastroenterology 1987;93:958.

219. McCallum RW, Grill BB, Lange R, et al. Definition of a gastric emptying abnormality in patients with anorexia nervosa. Dig Dis Sci 1985;30:713.

220. Abatzi Th-A, Bergmann H, Wiesnagrotzki S, et al. Gastric emptying and antral motor activity in 50 patients with anorexia nervosa (PAN) (abstr). Gastroenterology 1988;94:A1.

221. Stanghellini V, Malagelada J-R, Zinsmeister AR, et al. Effect of opiate and adrenergic blockers on the gut motor response to centrally acting stimuli. Gastroenterology 1984;87:1104.

222. Gue M, Fioramonti J, Frexino J, et al. Influence of acoustic stress by noise on gastrointestinal motility in dogs. Dig Dis Sci 1987;32:1411.

223. Keys A, Brozek J, Henschel A, et al. The biology of human starvation. Minneapolis: University of Minnesota Press, 1950:587.

224. Rigaud D, Bedig G, Merrouche M, Vulpillat M, Bonfils S, Apfelbaum M. Delayed gastric emptying in anorexia nervosa is improved by completion of a renutrition program. Dig Dis Sci 1988;8:919.

225. Saleh JW, Lebwohl P. Gastric emptying studies in patients with anorexia nervosa: Effect of metoclopramide (abstr). Gastroenterology 1979;76:1233.

226. Stacher G, Bergmann H, Wiesnagrotzki S, et al. Intravenous cisapride accelerates delayed gastric emptying and increases antral contraction amplitude in patients with primary anorexia nervosa. Gastroenterology 1987;92:1000.

227. Herman G, Johnson V. Management of prolonged gastric retention after vagotomy and drainage. Surg Gynecol Obstet 1970;130:1044.

228. Kraft RO, Fry WJ, DeWeese MS. Post-vagotomy gastric atony. Arch Surg 1964;88:865.

229. Meyer JH, Thomson JB, Cohen MB, et al. Sieving of food by the canine stomach and sieving after gastric surgery. Gastroenterology 1976;76:804.

230. Metzger WH, Cano R, Sturdevant RAL. Effect of metoclopramide in chronic gastric retention after ulcer surgery. Gastroenterology 1976;71:30.

231. Brooke-Cowden GL, Braasch J, Gibb SP, et al. Postgastrectomy syndromes. Am J Surg 1976;131:464.

232. Kelly KA, Becker JM, Van Heerden JA. Reconstructive gastric surgery. Br J Surg 1981;68:687.

233. Spiller RC, Trotman IF, Adrian TE, et al. Further characterisation of the 'ileal brake' reflex in man—Effect of ileal infusion of partial digests of fat, protein, and starch on jejunal motility and release of neurotensin, enteroglucagon, and peptide YY. Gut 1988;29:1042.

234. Mayer EA, Thomson JB, Jehn D, et al. Gastric emptying of solid food and pancreatic and biliary secretions after solid meal in patients with nonresective ulcer surgery. Gastroenterology 1987;87:1264.

235. Doty JE, Meyer JH. Vagotomy and antrectomy impairs intracellular but not extracellular fat absorption in the dog. Gastroenterology 1988;94:50.

236. Doty JE, Sanders SL, Gu YG, Meyer JH. Chyme from dogs with vagotomy, antrectomy and gastroenterostomy inhibits gastric emptying (abstr). Gastroenterology 1990;A346.

237. Kelly K, Code C. Canine gastric pacemaker. Am J Physiol 1971;220:112.

238. Code CF, Marlett JA. Canine tachygastria. Mayo Clin Proc 1974;49:325.

239. Abell TL, Malagelada J-R. Glucagon-evoked gastric dysrhythmias in humans shown by an improved electrogastrographic technique. Gastroenterology 1985;88:1932.

240. Kim CH, Azpiroz F, Malagelada J-R. Characteristics of spontaneous and drug-induced gastric dysrhythmias in a chronic canine model. Gastroenterology 1986;90:421.

241. Stoddard CJ, Smallwood RH, Duthie HL. Electrical arrhythmias in the human stomach. Gut 1981;22:705.

242. Sanders K, Menguy R, Chey W, et al. One explanation for human antral tachygastria (abstr). Gastroenterology 1979;76:1234.

243. You CH, Chey WY, Lee KY, et al. Gastric and small intestinal myoelectric dysrhythmia associated with chronic intractable nausea and vomiting. Ann Intern Med 1981;95:449.

244. Reynolds PPE, Bardakjianm BL, Diamant NE. A case of antral tachygastria: Symptomatic and myoelectric improvement with gastroenterostomy and domperidone therapy. Can Med Assoc J 1983;128:241.

245. You CH, Chey WY. Study of electromechanical activity of the stomach in humans and in dogs with particular attention to tachygastria. Gastroenterology 1984;86:1460.

246. Lee KY, Chey WY, Coy D. Experimental production of tachyarrhythmias in canine antrum (abstr). Gastroenterology 1979;76:1182.

247. Kim CH, Zinsmeister AR, Malagelada J-R. Mechanisms of canine gastric dysrhythmia. Gastroenterology 1987;92:993.

248. Telander RL, Morgan KG, Kreulen DL, et al. Human gastric atony with tachygastria and gastric retention. Gastroenterology 1978;75:497.

249. Cottrell CR, Sninsky CA, Martin JL, Mathias JR. Are alterations in gastroduodenal motility responsible for previously unexplained nausea, vomiting and abdominal pain? (abstr) Dig Dis Sci 1982;27:650.

250. Malagelada J-R, Stanghellini V. Manometric evaluation of functional upper gut symptoms. Gastroenterology 1985;88:1223.

251. You CH, Lee KY, Chey WJ, Menguy R. Electrogastrographic study of patients with unexplained nausea, bloating and vomiting. Gastroenterology 1980;79:311.

251a. Chen J, McCallum RW. Instantaneous determination of dysrhythmic events in gastric myoelectrical signals. Gastroenterology 1990;98: A336.

252. Stern RM, Koch KL, Stewart WR, Lindblad IM. Spectral analysis of tachygastria recorded during motion sickness. Gastroenterology 1987;92:92.

253. Wood MJ, Wood CD, Manno JE, et al. Nuclear medicine evaluation of motion sickness and medications on gastric emptying time. Aviat Space Environ Med 1987;58:1112.

254. Wright RA, Krindky S, Fleeman C, et al. Gastric emptying and obesity. Gastroenterology 1983;84:747.

255. Lavigne ME, Wiley ZD, Meyer JH, LacGregor IL. Gastric emptying as a function of body size. Gastroenterology 1978;74:1258.

256. Horowitz M, Collins PJ, Harding PE, Shearman DJC. Letter: Abnormalities in gastric emptying in obese patients. Gastroenterology 1983;85:983.

257. Christian PE, Datz FL, Moore JG. Gastric emptying studies in the morbidly obese before and after gastroplasty. J Nucl Med 1986;27: 1686.

258. Gannon MX, Pears DDJ, Chandler ST, et al. The effect of gastric partitioning on gastric emptying in morbidly obese patients. Br J Surg 1985;72:952.

259. Horowitz M, Cook DJ, Collins PJ, et al. Measurement of gastric emptying after gastric bypass surgery using radionuclides. Br J Surg 1982;69:655.

260. Backman L, Rosenborg M. The significance of gastric pouch size and emptying time for results of gastric surgery for massive obesity. Acta Chir Scand 1984;150:549.

261. Moore J, Moody F, Datz F, Christian P. Gastric emptying of liquids and solids following gastric partition in the morbidly obese (abstr). Gastroenterology 1981;80:1234.

262. Arnstein NB, Shapiro B, Eckhauser FE, et al. Morbid obesity treated by gastroplasty: Radionuclide gastric emptying studies. Radiology 1985;156:501.

263. Gannon MX, Pears DJ, Chandler ST, et al. The effect of gastric partitioning on gastric emptying in morbidly obese patients. Br J Surg 1985;72:952.

264. Villar HV, Patton DD, Norton LW, et al. Gastric emptying rate after gastric bypass and gastric partitioning (abstr). Dig Dis Sci 1980;25:716.

265. Gue M, Peeters T, Depoortere I, Vantrappen G, Bueno L. Stress-induced changes in gastric emptying, postprandial motility, and plasma gut hormone levels in dogs. Gastroenterology 1989;97:1101.

266. Stern RM, Kock KL, Stewart WR, et al. Spectral analysis of tachygastria recorded during motion sickness. Gastroenterology 1987;92: 92.

267. Stanghellini V, Malagelada J-R, Zinsmeister AR, et al. Effects of opiate and adrenergic blockers on the gut motor response to centrally acting stimuli. Gastroenterology 1984;87:1104.

268. Thompson DG, Richelson E, Malagelada J-R. Perturbation of upper gastrointestinal function by cold stress. Gut 1985;24:277.

269. Rees MR, Clark RA, Holdsworth CD, Barber DC, Howlett PJ. The effect of beta adrenergic agonist and antagonists on gastric emptying in man. Br J Pharmacol 1980;10:551.

270. O'Brien JD, Thompson DG, Day SJ, Burnham WR, Walker E. Perturbation of upper gastrointestinal transit and antroduodenal motility by experimentally applied stress: The role of beta-adrenoreceptor mediated pathways. Gut 1990;30:1530.

271. Heading RC, Nimmo J, Prescott LF, et al. The dependence of paracetamol absorption on the rate of gastric emptying. Br J Pharmacol 1973;47:415.

272. Simpson KH, Stakes AF. Effect of anxiety on gastric emptying in preoperative patients. Br J Anaesth 1987;59:540.

273. Fone DR, Horowitz M, Maddox A, Akkermans LM, Read NW, Dent J. Gastroduodenal motility during the delayed gastric emptying induced by cold stress. Gastroenterology 1990;98:1155.

274. Cann PA, Read NE, Cammack J, et al. Psychological stress and the passage of a standard meal through the stomach and small intestine in man. Gut 1983;24:236.

275. Livingston EH, Passaro EP, Garrick TR. Elevated intracranial pressure increases gastric contractility in the rat. Gastroenterology 1988;94:A255.

276. Wood JR, Camilleri M, Low PA, Malagelada J-R. Brainstem tumor presenting as an upper gut motility disorder. Gastroenterology 1985;89:1411.

277. Mitchell WG, Greenwood RS, Messenheimer JA. Abdominal epilepsy: Cyclic vomiting as the major symptom of simple partial seizures. Arch Neurol 1983;40:251.

278. Reynolds BJ, Eliasson SG. Colonic pseudoobstruction in patients with stroke. Ann Neurol 1977;1:305.

279. Volans GN. The effect of metoclopramide on the absorption of effervescent aspirin in migraine. Br J Clin Pharmacol 1975;2:57.

280. Fealey RD, Szurszewski JH, DiMagno EP. The effect of traumatic spinal cord transection on human upper gastrointestinal motility (abstr). Gastroenterology 1982;82:1053.

281. Mayer EA, Elashoff J, Hawkins R, et al. Gastric emptying of mixed solid–liquid meal in patients with intestinal pseudoobstruction. Dig Dis Sci 1988;33:10.

282. Schuffler MD. Chronic intestinal pseudoobstruction syndromes. Med Clin North Am 1981;65:1331.

283. Wiley ZD, Lavigne ME, Liu KM, MacGregor IL. The effect of hyperthyroidism on gastric emptying rates and pancreatic exocrine and biliary secretion in man. Am J Dig Dis 1978;23:1003.

284. Miller LJ, Owyang C, Malagelada J-R. Gastric, pancreatic and biliary responses to meals in hyperthyroidism. Gut 1980;21:695.

285. Kowalewski K, Kolodej A. Myoelectrical and mechanical activity of stomach and intestine in hypothyroid dogs. Am J Dig Dis 1977;22: 235.

286. Cohen S, Laufer I, Snape WJ Jr, et al. The gastrointestinal manifestations of scleroderma: Pathogenesis and management. Gastroenterology 1980;79:155.

287. Creamer B, Anderson HA, Code CF. Esophageal motility in patients with scleroderma and related diseases. Gastroenterology 1976;86: 763.

288. Kaufman HJ, Braverman IM, Spiro HM. Esophageal manometry in scleroderma. Scand J Gastroenterol 1968;3:246.

289. Clements PJ, Kadell B, Ippoliti A, Ross M. Esophageal motility in progressive systemic sclerosis. Dig Dis Sci 1979;24:639.

290. Orringer MB, Dabich L, Zarafonetis CJD, Sloan H. Gastroesophageal reflux in esophageal scleroderma: Diagnosis and implications. Ann Thorac Surg 1979;22:120.

291. Maddern GJ, Horowitz M, Jamieson GG, et al. Abnormalities of esophageal and gastric emptying in progressive systemic sclerosis. Gastroenterology 1984;87:922.

292. Rees WDW, Leigh RJ, Christofides ND, et al. Interdigestive motor activity in patients with systemic sclerosis. Gastroenterology 1982;83: 575.

293. Greydanus MP, Camilleri M. Abnormal postcibal antral and small bowel motility due to neuropathy or myopathy in systemic sclerosis. Gastroenterology 1989;96:110.

294. Cohen S, Fisher R, Lipshutz W, et al. The pathogenesis of esophageal function in scleroderma and Raynaud's disease. J Clin Invest 1972;51: 2663.

295. Horowitz M, McNeil JD, Madder GJ, et al. Abnormalities of gastric and esophageal emptying in polymyosis and dermatomyositis. Gastroenterology 1986;90:434.

296. Lewis TD, Daniel EE. Gastroduodenal motility in a case of dystrophia myotonica. Gastroenterology 1981;81:145.

297. Horowitz M, Maddox A, Maddern GJ, et al. Gastric and esophageal emptying in dystrophia myotonica: Effect of metoclopramide. Gastroenterology 1987;92:570.

298. Brown CH, Shirley EK, Haserick JR. Gastrointestinal manifestations of systemic lupus erythematosis. Gastroenterology 1956;31:649.

299. Gilat T, Spiro HM. Amyloidosis and the gut. Am J Dig Dis 1968;13: 619.

300. Layer P, Hotz J, Goebbell H. Gastroparesis after radiation: Successful treatment with carbachol. Dig Dis Sci 1986;31:1377.

301. Dubois A, Jacobus JP, Grissom MP, et al. Altered gastric emptying and prevention of radiation-induced vomiting in dogs. Gastroenterology 1984;86:444.

302. Barkin JS, Goldberg RI, Sfakianakis GN, Levi J. Pancreatic carcinoma is associated with delayed gastric emptying. Dig Dis Sci 1986;31:265.

303. Griffith GH, Gwen GM, Campbell H, Shields R. Gastric emptying in health, and in gastroduodenal disease. Gastroenterology 1968; 54:1.

304. Davies WT, Kilpatrick JR, Owen GM, Shields R. Gastric emptying

in atrophic gastritis and carcinoma of the stomach. Scand J Gastroenterol 1971;6:297.

305. Shivshanker K, Bennett RW Jr, Haynie TP. Tumor-associated gastroparesis: Correction with metoclopramide. Am J Surg 1983;145: 221.

306. Barkin JS, Goldberg RI, Sfakianakis GN, Levi J. Pancreatic carcinoma is associated with delayed gastric emptying. Dig Dis Sci 1986;31:265.

307. Sarr MG, Cameron JL. Surgical management of unresectable carcinoma of the pancreas. Surgery 1982;91:123.

308. Meerof JC, Schreiber DS, Trier JS, et al. Abnormal gastric motor function in viral gastroenteritis. Ann Intern Med 1980;92:370.

309. Ricci DA, McCallum RW. Diagnosis and treatment of delayed gastric emptying. Adv Intern Med 1988;33:357.

310. Oh JJ, Kim CH. Post-viral gastroparesis: Clinical features and prognosis (abstr). Gastroenterology 1989;96:A373.

311. Navad F, Texter C Jr. Gastroesophageal reflux: Pathophysiologic concepts. Arch Intern Med 1985;145:329.

312. Holloway RH, Hongo M, Berger K, McCallum RW. Gastric distention: A mechanism for postprandial gastroesophageal reflux. Gastroenterology 1985;89:779.

313. Ippoliti A, McCallum R, Sturdevant R. Gastric emptying in patients with gastroesophageal reflux. Clin Res 1976;24:535A.

314. McCallum RW, Berkowitz DM, Lerner E. Gastric emptying in patients with gastroesophageal reflux. Gastroenterology 1981;80:285.

315. Baldi F, Corinaldesi R, Ferrarini F, Stanghellini V, et al. Gastric secretion and emptying of liquids in reflux esophagitis. Dig Dis Sci 1981;26:886.

316. Velasco N, Hill LD, Gannon RM, Pope CE. Gastric emptying and gastroesophageal reflux. Am J Surg 1982;144:58.

317. Maddern GJ, Chatterton BE, Collins PJ, et al. Solid and liquid emptying in patients with gastroesophageal reflux disease. Br J Surg 1985;72:344.

318. Fink SM, Lange RC, McCallum RW. Effect of metoclopramide on normal and delayed gastric emptying in gastroesophageal reflux patients. Dig Dis Sci 1981;28:1057.

319. Little AG, DeMeester TR, Kirchner PT, et al. Pathogenesis of esophagitis in patients with gastroesophageal reflux. Surgery 1980;88: 101.

320. McCallum RW, Mensh R, Lange R. Definition of the gastric emptying abnormality in gastroesophageal reflux patients (abstr). Gastroenterology 1981;80:1226.

321. Shay SS, Eggli D, McDonald D, Johnson LF. Gastric emptying of solid food in patients with gastroesophageal reflux. Gastroenterology 1987;92:459.

322. Coleman SL, Rees WDW, Malagelada J-R. Normal gastric function in reflux esophagitis (abstr). Gastroenterology 1979;76:1115.

323. Csendes A, Henriquez A. Gastric emptying in patients with reflux esophagitis or benign strictures of the esophagus secondary to reflux compared to controls. Scand J Gastroenterol 1978;13:205.

324. Iascone C, DeMeester TR, Little AG, Skinner DB. Barrett's esophagus—Functional assessment, proposed pathogenesis and surgical therapy. Arch Surg 1983;118:543.

325. Kogan FJ, Kotler JA, Sampliner RE. Normal gastric emptying in Barrett's esophagus (abstr). Gastroenterology 1985;88:1451.

326. Johnson DA, Winters C, Drane WE, et al. Solid-phase gastric emptying in patients with Barrett's esophagus. Dig Dis Sci 1986;31: 1217.

327. Maddern GJ, Jamieson GG, Chatterton BE, Collina PJ. Is there an association between failed antireflux procedures and delayed gastric emptying. Ann Surg 1985;202:162.

328. Van De Mierop L, Rutgeerts J, Van Den Langenbergh B, Staessen A. Oral domperidone in chronic dyspepsia: A double-blind placebo controlled evaluation. Digestion 1979;19:244.

329. Englert W, Schlich D. A double-blind crossover trial of domperidone in chronic postprandial dyspepsia. Postgrad Med J 1979;55(Suppl 1):28.

330. Haarmann K, Lebkuchner F, Widmann A, et al. A double-blind study of domperidone in the symptomatic treatment of chronic postprandial upper gastrointestinal distress. Postgrad Med J 1979;55(Suppl 1):24.

331. Rees WDW, Miller LJ, Malagelada J-R. Dyspepsia, antral motor

dysfunction and gastric stasis of solids. Gastroenterology 1980;78: 360.

332. Jian R, Ducrot F, Piedeloup C, et al. Measurement of gastric emptying in dyspeptic patients: Effect of a new gastrokinetic agent (cisapride). Gut 1985;26:352.

333. Corinadesi R, Stanghellini V, Raiti C, et al. Effect of chronic administration of cisapride on gastric emptying of a solid meal and on dyspeptic symptoms in patients with idiopathic gastroparesis. Gut 1987;28:300.

334. Narducci F, Bassotti G, Granata MT, et al. Functional dyspepsia and chronic idiopathic gastric stasis; role of endogenous opiates. Arch Intern Med 1986;145:716.

335. Urbain J-L C, Spiegel JA, Debie NC, Pauwels SP. Effects of cisapride on gastric emptying in dyspeptic patients. Dig Dis Sci 1988;33:779.

336. Testoni PA, Bagnolo F, Fanti L, Passaretti S, Tittobello A. Longterm oral cisapride improves interdigestive antroduodenal motility in dyspeptic patients. Gut 1990;31:286.

337. Van De Mierop L, Rutgeerts J, Van Den Langenbergh B, Staessen A. Oral domperidone in chronic dyspepsia: A double-blind placebo controlled evaluation. Digestion 1979;19:244.

338. Englert W, Schlich D. A double-blind crossover trial of domperidone in chronic postprandial dyspepsia. Postgrad Med J 1979;55(Suppl 1):28.

339. Haarmann K, Lebkuchner F, Widmann A, et al. A double-blind study of domperidone in the symptomatic treatment of chronic postprandial upper gastrointestinal distress. Postgrad Med J 1979;55(Suppl 1):24.

340. Jian R, Ducrot F, Ruskoff A, et al. Symptomatic radionuclide and therapeutic assessment of chronic idiopathic dyspepsia. Dig Dis Sci 1989;34:657.

341. Watson RGP, Love AHG. Gastric emptying in patients with flatulent dyspepsia, with and without gallbladder disease. Scand J Gastroenterol 1987;22:47.

342. Prakach C, Marshal BJ, Planky MW, et al. Gastric emptying of solids in patients with Campylobacter pylori gastritis (abstr). Am J Gastroenterol 1987;82:935.

343. Wegener M, Borsch G, Schaffstein J, et al. Are dyspeptic symptoms in patients with Campylobacter pylori-associated type B gastritis linked to delayed gastric emptying. Am J Gastroenterol 1988;83: 737.

344. Grill BB, Greenfield D, Glass E, et al. Definition of the spectrum of gastric emptying in patients with bulimia. J Nucl Med 1983;24: 56.

345. Hutson W, Wald A, Mooney J, et al. Gastric emptying (GE) and antral motility (AM) in anorexia nervosa and bulimia (abstr). Gastroenterology 1988;94:A198.

346. Kiss A, Bergmann H, Abatzi Th-A, et al. Esophageal and gastric motor activity in bulimia (abstr). Gastroenterology 1988;94:A228.

347. McNamee PT, Moore GW, McGeown MG, et al. Gastric emptying in chronic renal failure. Br Med J 1985;291:310.

348. Freeman JG, Cobden I, Heaton A, Keir M. Letter: Gastric emptying in chronic renal failure. Br Med J 1985;291:1048.

349. Soffer EE, Geva B, Avni Y, Bar-Meir S. Gastric emptying in chronic renal failure patients on hemodialysis (abstr). Gastroenterology 1985;88:1592.

350. Wright RA, Clemente R, Wathen R. Gastric emptying in patients with chronic renal failure receiving hemodialysis. Arch Intern Med 1984;144:495.

351. Brown-Cartwright D, Smith HJ, Feldman M. Gastric emptying of an indigestible solid in patients with end-stage renal disease on continuous ambulatory peritoneal dialysis. Gastroenterology 1988;95: 49.

352. Davies WT, Kirkpatrick JR, Owen GM, Shields R. Gastric emptying in atrophic gastritis and carcinoma of the stomach. Scand J Gastroenterol 1971;6:297.

353. McCallum RW, Callahan C, Lange R. Abnormal gastric emptying of solid food in patients with or without pernicious anemia. (abstr) Dig Dis Sci 1980;25:717.

354. Ohashi H, Meyer JH. Effect of peptic digestion on gastric emptying of cooked liver in dogs. Gastroenterology 1980;79:305.

355. MacGregor IL, Wiley ZD, Lavigne ME, Way LW. Slowed rate of gastric emptying of solid food in man by high caloric parenteral nutrition. Am J Surg 1979;138:652.

61

Acid-Peptic Disorders

JON I. ISENBERG
KENNETH R. McQUAID
LOREN LAINE
WALTER RUBIN

The goal of this chapter is to emphasize recent advances in our understanding of the inflammatory diseases involving the stomach and duodenum: gastritis, duodenitis, and gastric and duodenal ulcer disease.

There has been a recent flurry of basic and clinical studies regarding the role of *Helicobacter pylori*, previously referred to as *Campylobacter pylori*, in the development of gastroduodenal inflammation and ulcer diseases. Although this presumed pathogen is found in most patients with ulcer, it is also commonly present in healthy control subjects, particularly those aged 60 years and older. Continued investigation will be required throughout the next decade to determine the precise role(s) of *H. pylori* in gastroduodenal mucosal injury. The status of *H. pylori* in the pathogenesis of gastritis, duodenitis, and ulcer disease is objectively reviewed here, as is the role of drugs directed at *H. pylori* in ulcer healing, prevention, and recurrence.

One of the most frequent presentations of ulcer disease is the sudden onset of upper gastrointestinal bleeding or the development of iron deficiency anemia in the enlarging geriatric population taking nonsteroidal anti-inflammatory drugs for arthritic symptoms. We review the magnitude of this important health care problem as well as the role of nonsteroidal anti-inflammatory drugs in prostaglandin formation, their effects on the gastroduodenal mucosa, and the treatment and potential preventative measures of this common form of mucosal injury.

Until recently, duodenal ulcer was considered to be largely secondary to increased gastric acid and pepsin secretion. This hypothesis served as the pharmacologic basis for the use of antacids, the development of the histamine H_2-receptor antagonists, and most recently the H^+/K^+ ATPase inhibitors. Of importance, however, is the enlarging body of data indicating that patients with duodenal ulcer have gastric acid secretory responses, both at rest and after a meal, that are very similar to those of normal subjects. Therefore, the pathogenesis of duodenal ulcer disease is not exclusively secondary to an increase in the so-called aggressive factors but is rather secondary to an imbalance between "aggressive" and "defensive" factors. Moreover, a host of additional elements (e.g., *Helicobacter pylori*, genetics, other diseases, psychologic stress, and so forth) of varying and as yet undetermined effects influence the development and natural history of duodenal ulcer diseases. This chapter will address these elements and attempt to establish a working hypothesis for ulcer pathogenesis.

The use and total costs of antiulcer drugs continue to expand in the United States. In contrast to the 1970s and early 1980s, ulcer therapy is not confined to drugs that either neutralize or suppress gastric acid secretion (and therefore also inhibit peptic activity). Drugs such as sucralfate and colloidal bismuth have been shown to expedite ulcer healing at rates similar to those of the histamine H_2-receptor antagonists without influencing acid/peptic secretion. Moreover, recent studies indicate that low doses of antacids are equally effective as other forms of ulcer treatment, but by mechanisms independent of their acid-neutralizing power. The evolution and pharmacologic aspects of antiulcer drugs are reviewed, and recommendations for acute and long-term therapy are developed.

Important aspects of gastroduodenitis and peptic ulcer disease not included in detail in this chapter include: gastric secretion (ch 13, 129), gastrointestinal hormones (ch 2), evaluation and treatment of upper gastrointestinal bleeding (ch 30, 31, 134), gastroduodenal biopsy (ch 126), gastrinoma—Zollinger–Ellison syndrome (ch 62), and gastric surgery (ch 64). The reader is referred to these chapters for more detailed discussions of these specific areas.

HELICOBACTER PYLORI

The description of *Helicobacter pylori* (HP) in 1983 has spawned an entirely new body of gastroenterologic literature. At the time of this writing, the exact role of HP in a variety of gastroduodenal pathologic processes remains uncertain, with opinions ranging from skepticism to zealotry. In this section we will attempt to provide an overview of available information, pointing out areas of controversy and providing summaries of our viewpoints in this rapidly developing field.

History

HP colonization of the stomach does not appear to be a new phenomenon. Descriptions of spirochetes in the gastric mucosa of animals date back to the 1890s, and similar organisms were reported in human stomachs at the beginning of the twentieth century.[1] In 1938, Doenges found spirochetes in 103 (43%) of 242 stomachs examined at autopsy.[2] In 1954, however, Palmer reported no evidence of spirochetes in 1180 gastric mucosal biopsies from 1000 patients; he suggested that organisms previously reported in normal stomachs represented an agonal or postmortem process and that the source of the bacteria was the oral cavity.[3] Although gram-negative bacteria were observed over the gastric mucosa in about 80% of patients with gastric ulcers (said to be *Pseudomonas aeruginosa*),[4] Warren[5] and Marshall,[6] in 1983, were the first to characterize *Helicobacter pylori* and to describe its close association with histologic gastritis.

Epidemiology

Gastritis has long been recognized to be a common finding in the normal population, and its histologic presence is closely paralleled by the presence of HP. The frequency of both gastritis and HP is related to age, geographic location, and ethnic background without evidence for a sexual predilection. Studies of asymptomatic subjects from the United States and Europe suggest that the prevalence of gastritis and HP increases with age.[7-11] Dooley and colleagues studied 113 asymptomatic volunteers in Los Angeles with endoscopy and biopsy and reported that the overall prevalence of HP increases from 10% in the 20s to 47% in the 60s (Fig 61-1).[10] Similar results were noted in a study of 73 healthy subjects from Dallas.[12] Indirect tests for HP (breath tests, serology) have also shown an age-related distribution of HP in asymptomatic subjects and blood donors from the United States,[13-15] the United Kingdom,[16] Australia,[17-19] and New Zealand.[20] In contrast, histologic gastritis and HP develop at an earlier age and with much greater frequency in parts of South and Central America, Asia, and Africa.[9,13,19,21-25]

Ethnic background also influences HP prevalence. Asymptomatic Hispanic subjects in the United States have approximately an 80% prevalence of HP (and associated histologic gastritis) with no variation at different age groups.[26] Asymptomatic blacks in the United States have an age-related rate of HP acquisition that parallels that of whites but is significantly (38%) higher, suggesting earlier infection in the black population.[15] This may be due to socioeconomic status: Klein and colleagues have reported that significantly more asymptomatic Peruvian children from low-income families than children from high-income families are HP-positive.[25] It is interesting, but of unclear significance, that of 274 Australian aborigines (in whom peptic ulcer is said to be almost unknown), only 2 subjects had serologic evidence of HP.[19]

In summary, the prevalence of HP and gastritis in the white United States and European population is very low in early adulthood and gradually increases to approximately 50% in persons over 50 or 60 years of age. Hispanics and blacks in the United States have a much higher prevalence. In contrast, HP is reported in a majority of people in many Third World countries, with a high prevalence often seen even in children and young adults.

Bacteriology and Transmission

Although originally classified as a *Campylobacter* species, HP has distinct structural, biochemical, and morphologic characteristics,[27-32] leading to its reclassification into the genus *Helicobacter*.[33] HP is a curved or S-shaped gram-negative rod approximately 0.5 X 3 μm in size, usually with four to six sheathed flagella at one pole.[34-37] Perhaps its most distinctive characteristic is the production of a highly active urease.[38] Culture of HP requires a supplemented medium (usually with blood or serum, as in chocolate agar or brain–heart infusion agar with serum); the addition of antibiotics to the culture medium also helps to decrease contamination by other bacteria.[39-42] HP grows within 3 to 5 days under microaerophilic conditions at 37°C.[40,43,44] Immediate culture of specimens is desirable, but storage at 4°C for up to 5 hours prior to culture should not interfere with recovery of the organism.[39] The natural habitat of HP, other than the human stomach, and its means of transmission are unclear. Reports of an increased prevalence in family members of patients with HP[45-47] and in institutionalized patients[17] (as well as the results of restriction endonuclease DNA analysis showing an identical HP strain in eight members of one family[48] and a separate identical strain in two patients in a chronic care facility[49]) suggest the possibility of person-to-person transmission or exposure to the same environmental source. Two outbreaks of presumed acute HP infection in volunteers participating in acid secretory studies[50-52] have been attributed to reinfusion of aspirated gastric juice contaminated by pH electrodes that were not thoroughly cleaned between uses.

Animal Models

HP species (identical to human HP by morphology, biochemistry, DNA–DNA hybridization, and monoclonal antibody) and associated chronic gastritis have been found in the stomachs of monkeys.[53-56] Because these animals were confined in research centers far removed from their native habitat, we cannot assume that HP is a normal pathogen in monkeys. In fact, none of 10 baboons caught in Africa and examined in the U.K. had HP identified.[53] Gastric HP infections

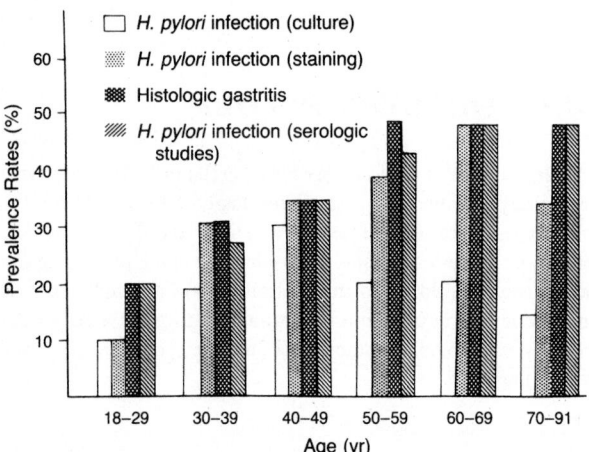

FIGURE 61–1. Prevalence of *Helicobacter pylori* (by culture, histology, and ELISA) and histologic gastritis in 113 asymptomatic volunteers. (Reproduced with permission from Dooley CP, Cohen H, Fitzgibbons PL, et al. Prevalence of Helicobacter pylori infection and histologic gastritis in asymptomatic persons. N Engl J Med 1989;321:1562.)

has been established in the gnotobiotic piglet[57,58] and germ-free rats[59] and may provide useful animal models for the study of HP. *"Campylobacter*-like" organisms have been identified in the stomachs of other animals, but these bacteria have characteristics that distinguish them from the human HP.[60-63]

Symptoms

Although HP is extremely common in humans, it is unclear whether it causes symptoms. Based on two self-inoculation studies[64,65] and two outbreaks in volunteers undergoing acid secretory studies,[50-52] HP does appear to cause a transient, acute clinical illness with upper abdominal pain, nausea, and vomiting that lasts for several days. Acute HP infection also causes hypochlorhydria that may last for months.[50,52,65] A role for chronic HP infection in gastrointestinal symptoms is much harder to document. Histologic gastritis has not been shown to be associated with abdominal symptoms, and there is either no significant difference in symptoms between HP-positive and HP-negative subjects[66-68] or only an increase in postprandial bloating or burping.[33,69,70] A study of 170 Finnish control subjects undergoing endoscopy revealed upper abdominal complaints in 15% of HP-positive volunteers and 12% of HP-negative subjects.[67] Prospective studies of 49 consecutive patients with nonulcer dyspepsia and 49 age-, sex-, and race-matched controls found no difference in the prevalence of HP or gastritis, although the HP prevalence in both groups of predominantly Hispanic patients was quite high (~80%).[71]

Methods of Diagnosis

Methods for the diagnosis of HP can be divided into two categories: invasive and noninvasive tests (Table 61-1).

HISTOLOGY

Because successful HP culture is dependent on proper microbiologic technique and requires several days, alternative methods of diagnosis are useful. Gram stain of a tissue smear of the biopsy specimen is a rapid test that has been used with good results by some investigators[35,72-75] but with unacceptably low sensitivities by others.[32,34,76,77] Histologic examination of the biopsy specimen provides an excellent means of diagnosis (Fig 61-2; Color Fig 27). HP can be identified by standard hematoxylin and eosin staining, but the Warthin–Starry silver stain (used by Marshall and Warren to first identify HP) and the preferred, easy-to-perform Giemsa stain (which may be modified by omitting the differentiation step) are probably the two best histologic methods for HP diagnosis.[34,35,72,74,75,78,79] Immunohistochemical methods of diagnosing HP have also been employed with good results.[80-82]

UREASE TESTS

In an effort to speed the diagnosis of HP, the urease activity of HP has been utilized. Endoscopic biopsy specimens are placed in

TABLE 61–1
Methods of Diagnosis—*Helicobacter Pylori*

I. Invasive (endoscopic biopsy required)
  A. Rapid diagnosis
    1. Gram stain of biopsy touch prep
    2. Urease test (broth, gel [CLOtest])
  B. Delayed diagnosis
    1. Histology (Giemsa, Warthin–Starry silver, hematoxylin & eosin, acridine orange, Gimenez, immunohistochemical)
    2. Bacterial culture
II. Noninvasive
  A. Urea breath test (^{13}C or ^{14}C)
  B. Serologic testing for antibodies to HP
    1. ELISA
      a. Vs. pooled whole extracts of HP
      b. Vs. high-molecular-weight cell–associated protein (urease)
    2. Others (immunoblot, complement fixation, passive hemagglutination)

a solution or gel containing urea and phenol red (a pH indicator). If urease is present from HP in the biopsy specimen, urea is hydrolyzed to release ammonia, and increasing pH in the solution or gel gives a pink color (Fig 61-3; Color Fig 28). These tests generally are read periodically over 2 to 3 hours after the biopsy and then again at 24 hours. The CLOtest, a commercially available test that has been most widely evaluated, has a sensitivity in the 80% to 90% range at 2 to 3 hours with few false positives; at least two thirds of patients develop a positive test in less than 30 minutes.[75,81,83-86] A small number of additional true positive specimens will be picked up by a 24-hour reading, but the incidence of false positives also may rise with some urease tests.[79,87]

UREA BREATH TESTS

A noninvasive method of detecting HP is desirable for large population studies and for routine diagnosis. ^{13}C- and ^{14}C-urea breath tests offer an excellent diagnostic yield without the need for endoscopic biopsy. Patients ingest a solution containing ^{13}C- or ^{14}C-labeled urea, and breath is sampled for isotope-labeled CO_2 released by HP urease activity. Sensitivities and specificities are in the 90% to 100% range,[88-93] and breath samples probably do not need to be collected beyond 20 minutes.[90,92,94] However, the breath tests require special material and equipment, are time-consuming, and, when ^{14}C is used, necessitate a small radiation exposure. In addition, very short courses of treatment may cause false-negative breath tests: 1 day of treatment with colloidal bismuth, sucralfate, or amoxicillin was shown to convert 9 of 29 patients (31%) from a positive to a negative test.[95] Thus, urea breath tests may be of limited use in patients receiving drug therapy.

SEROLOGY

Serologic testing should be the most acceptable method for detection of HP in both routine diagnosis and large epidemiologic studies. Enzyme-linked immunosorbent assays (ELISA) have been developed for detection of serum antibodies to HP,[14,16,96-100] as have complement fixation tests,[101] passive hemagglutination as-

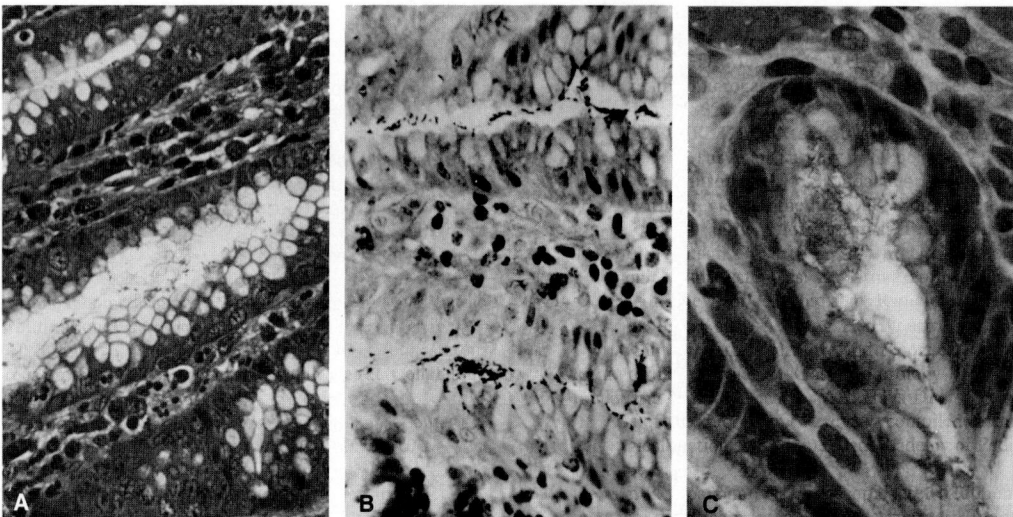

FIGURE 61–2. (See Color Fig 27) Gastric mucosal biopsy specimens positive for *Helicobacter pylori* with (**A**) Giemsa, (**B**) Warthin-Starry silver, and (**C**) hematoxylin and eosin stains. (Figures reproduced courtesy of Henry D. Appelman, University of Michigan Medical Center.)

says,[18] and immunoblot analysis.[102] In general, whole extracts of one or more sonicated HP strains have been pooled and used as antigens. Mean levels of IgG and IgA ELISA tests (but not IGM) are significantly higher in HP-positive subjects than in HP-negative subjects.[14,96,99,103] Comparison of immunologic tests from different centers is difficult, but sensitivities generally are 80% to 90%, while specificities vary widely, from 50% to over 90%.[14,18,91,97,98,101,102,104]

In an effort to improve the results obtained when whole HP extracts were used as antigens, Evans and co-workers developed an ELISA for an anti-HP antibody that detects IgG antibodies directed against high molecular weight cell–associated proteins of HP (this includes the enzyme urease).[94] The sensitivity and specificity in 300 subjects tested were 99% and 100%, respectively, using the urea breath test as the gold standard for HP infection and endoscopic biopsy to evaluate 4 individuals with nonconcor-

dant results. Serologic tests with this diagnostic yield seem ideal for the diagnosis of HP. Another simple, noninvasive test of potential usefulness is the measurement of HP-specific salivary IgG antibody levels.[103]

Little information is available regarding the long-term usefulness of serologic tests after HP eradication. Serum IgG antibodies against HP do appear to fall gradually over the 6 months after successful treatment, but they generally remain in the abnormal range.[105] Relapse of HP after eradication has also been associated with a rise in serum IgG antibodies against HP.[105]

SUMMARY

At present, the best diagnostic yield for HP in an institution without special interest and expertise (balancing diagnostic accuracy with cost and ease) would seem to be histologic examination of biopsy specimens, probably with a Giemsa stain. Should a rapid diagnosis be deemed necessary, use of a urease test or a Gram stain of a smear of an endoscopic gastric biopsy will provide reasonable results; a positive test will indicate HP infection, but a negative test will not rule out HP and a second test (e.g., histologic exam, culture) will still be necessary. If large-scale determination of HP status is required, noninvasive testing will be mandatory, and the development of accurate, standardized serologic tests should be the optimal method.

Gastroduodenal Disease and *Helicobacter Pylori*

ANTRAL GASTRITIS

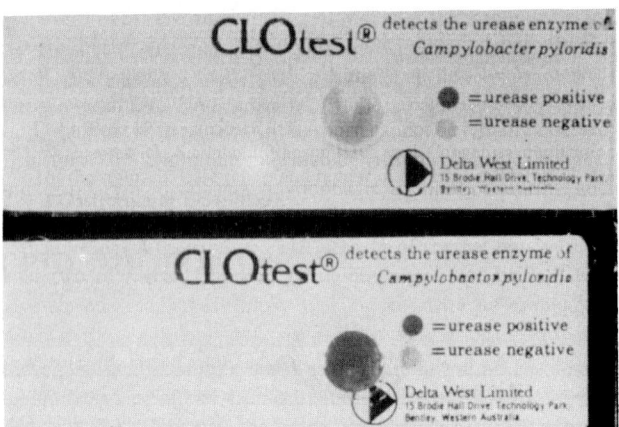

FIGURE 61–3. (See Color Fig 28) CLOtest: presence of *Helicobacter pylori* is indicated by pink color.

HP organisms reside in the gastric mucus layer adjacent to the epithelial cell surface (Fig 61-2).[76,106–110] The bacteria are more numerous in the region of epithelial cell junctions.[106,108,109] HP do penetrate into the junction between cells[76,108] and infrequently are seen inside epithelial cells.[37,111,112] Invasion beyond the epithelium virtually never occurs,[76,108,110] although bacteria have been reported within the parietal cell.[110] HP may be found in the gastrointestinal tract outside the stomach, but the organisms appear to colonize only areas of "gastric type" mucosa. HP may be identified on metaplastic glandular epithelium in Barrett's esophagus,[113–116] on areas of gastric metaplasia in the duodenum,[76,106,109,117] in gastric mucosa of Meckel's diverticulum,[118,119] and, in one case, on an island of gastric mucosa in the rectum.[120]

HP was first described in association with antral gastritis, and the antrum was considered to be its primary area of residence. However, HP is at least as common in the body and fundus of the stomach.[12,67,104,121,122] The concordance rate for HP in the antrum and body or fundus is over 80%,[10,12,67,85,122–124] and when HP is present in normal fundic gland mucosa, antral gastritis is usually present.[121,122,124,125] While HP in the antrum is almost always associated with inflammation, a number of patients with HP in biopsies from the proximal stomach will have normal fundic gland mucosa.[12,104,121,122] These findings have led to the speculation that HP may live merely as a commensal organism in the fundic gland mucosa.[104,122]

HP is present in the stomachs of 0% to 10% of individuals with histologically normally gastric mucosa.[32,33,43,75,76,101,107,117,125,126] In contrast, a majority of people with histologic gastritis have associated HP. In his original description of HP, Warren noted that bacilli were "*often* found in chronic gastritis" (an increase in mucosal round cell infiltration), while the "curved bacilli were almost *always* present in active chronic gastritis" (an increase in neutrophils as well as round cells).[5] Most (but not all) other investigators have confirmed that HP is more common in active gastritis than in inactive chronic gastritis. The prevalence of HP in subjects with active chronic gastritis ranges from approximately 70% to 95%, while HP prevalence in individuals with inactive chronic gastritis varies greatly from 15% to 90%.[14,32,33,67,75,76,107,123,125,127,128] Scores for both mononuclear cell infiltration and neutrophil infiltration are significantly higher in HP-positive gastric mucosal biopsies than in HP-negative specimens,[129–131] perhaps related to the fact that mucosal infiltration with neutrophils virtually always occurs in association with chronic gastritis.[127]

Although HP is clearly associated with mucosal inflammatory cell infiltration, epithelial changes are also considered a criterion for histologic gastritis. Warren's original report of HP in 1983 mentioned that "the surface epithelium was often irregular, with reduced mucinogenesis and a cobblestone surface."[5] Others have quantified a significantly greater incidence of epithelial abnormalities in HP-positive biopsy specimens.[129,131–133]

HP prevalence appears to be lower in atrophic gastritis than in superficial gastritis.[67,101,134] Siurala and colleagues[67] noted a decreasing prevalence of HP in the body of the stomach with increasing severity of gastritis (superficial gastritis: 91% prevalence; light, moderate, and severe atrophic gastritis: 60%, 22%, and 0% prevalence, respectively). Similar differences were not seen in antral biopsies, and others have failed to confirm this correlation.[43,107,125] At least some of this disparity may relate to a lower frequency of inflammatory cell infiltration (especially neutrophils) in patients with atrophic gastritis and the fact that HP prevalence may correlate more strongly with the presence of inflammatory

cells and active gastritis than it does with the severity of gastritis (superficial versus atrophic).[76,101]

Although a close association between histologic gastritis and HP is undeniable, the important question is whether HP is an etiologic agent for gastritis or whether it merely takes up residence in areas of mucosal inflammation caused by some other factor. Three lines of evidence suggest that HP is a cause, not a result, of histologic gastritis: (1) self-inoculation studies, (2) epidemic hypochlorhydria outbreaks, and (3) longitudinal treatment trials.

Two different physicians have voluntarily ingested an HP inoculum after documentation of a normal stomach by endoscopy, histology, culture, and, in one, pH testing.[64,65] On days 5 to 10, an acute inflammatory infiltrate was seen with abnormal epithelial cells noted in one case; HP was also identified. The acute inflammatory reaction resolved after 2 weeks and was replaced with a mononuclear cell infiltration. In one, a prolonged follow-up reported a mild increase in mononuclear cells still present in the lamina propria at 103 days in spite of treatment with doxycycline and bismuth subsalicylate. HP was not isolated.[65]

Two outbreaks of epidemic hypochlorhydria have been reported in participants in gastric secretory studies.[50,52] In both outbreaks, gastric juice was withdrawn, measured with a common, unsterilized pH electrode, and reinstilled for intragastric titration. Contamination of the electrode was presumed to be the source of the infection. In both instances these subjects developed prolonged hypochlorhydria with histologic gastritis, and over half of the volunteers also developed a transient clinical illness consisting of upper abdominal pain, nausea, and vomiting. "Severe fundal and antral gastritis" was seen in all hypochlorhydric subjects, and biopsies in four after recovery were "normal or showed minimal gastritis."[50] Retrospective analysis of stored acute and convalescent serum samples for IgG antibodies suggests that HP played a role in this outbreak.[51] Gastric biopsies from the four subjects in the second report showed superficial active gastritis ("most noticeable in the antrum") at 1 to 4 weeks after the onset of hypochlorhydria; at 8 months, 1 person had normal gastric mucosa and 3 had developed chronic gastritis with mononuclear cells replacing the neutrophils seen in earlier biopsy specimens.[52] No bacteria were reported in these patients, but HP has been suggested as the cause.

If HP is indeed a cause of histologic gastritis, then therapy that is specific for the bacteria should eradicate the organism and cause resolution of the gastritis. Evidence for this is discussed below under "Treatment of *Helicobacter pylori*."

PERNICIOUS ANEMIA

Patients with pernicious anemia have a specific gastritis (type A) characterized by chronic atrophic gastritis in the body of the stomach. The prevalence of HP in pernicious anemia is only 3% to 21% despite mean ages of 59 to 65 years.[135–138] In a prospective study of 20 patients compared to age- and race-matched controls, Fong and co-workers reported a significantly lower HP prevalence in the patients with pernicious anemia (15% versus 75%).[137]

POSTOPERATIVE STOMACH

Patients undergoing partial gastrectomies and gastroenterostomies for peptic ulcer disease would be expected to have a high prevalence of HP at the time of operation, and indeed these patients also develop a specific gastritis (see "Gastritis" section below). However, it has been suggested that reflux of duodenal contents, including bile acids, decreases HP infection.[139–142] Thirty-five patients with active duodenal ulcers and those treated with a highly selective vagotomy had HP prevalences of 97% and 94%, respectively, while 54 patients with previous Billroth-I or Billroth-II partial gastrectomies or truncal vagotomies with gastroenterostomy had significantly lower prevalences (22%, 47%, 50%, respectively).[139] Of eight patients who had a partial gastrectomy for peptic ulcers with Roux-en-Y anastomosis (preventing bile reflux into the stomach), all had continued HP infection, while HP was detected in only five of nine patients 6 months after undergoing a Billroth-II anastomosis.[142] In vitro, the growth of HP is reported to be reduced by 0.5% to 1% beef bile and inhibited by 5% beef bile, while other bacteria tested, including *Campylobacter jejuni*, grow well in 10% bile.[143]

ENDOSCOPIC GASTRITIS

A variety of endoscopic findings (erythema, friability, subepithelial hemorrhages, erosions) are frequently labeled as gastritis without histologic confirmation. However, no endoscopic finding other than a gastric or duodenal ulcer has been clearly documented to be associated with HP.[44,66,104,127,129,144]

NONSTEROIDAL ANTI-INFLAMMATORY DRUG (NSAID) GASTRITIS

Preliminary data suggest that gastric lesions induced by nonsteroidal anti-inflammatory drugs may be associated with a lower-than-expected prevalence of HP.[145]

SUMMARY OF HP ASSOCIATION WITH GASTRITIS

HP correlates closely with the histologic finding of gastritis, especially with that form accompanied by a neutrophilic infiltration. Mounting evidence does support the concept that HP is a cause of histologic gastritis rather than just an inhabitant of abnormal gastric mucosa. HP does not appear to be linked to, and the prevalence of HP may be lower in, atrophic gastritis associated with pernicious anemia or postgastrectomy gastritis. In addition, HP does not appear to be responsible for the endoscopic features frequently labeled as gastritis, such as erythema, subepithelial hemorrhages and erosions.

GASTRIC ADENOCARCINOMA

HP has been incriminated as a predisposing factor in the development of gastric adenocarcinoma.[1] Chronic gastritis is commonly associated with gastric adenocarcinoma and is more frequent in geographic locations and ethnic groups with a high incidence of gastric carcinoma.[9,22,26] The histologic gastritis in many of these patients may be associated with HP.[23,25,26] However, it is not certain whether the gastritis contributes to the development of gastric carcinoma, or both the gastritis and the cancer are products of the same genetic or environmental factors.

PEPTIC ULCER DISEASE

HP and histologic gastritis have a strong association with peptic ulcer disease. Approximately 85% to 100% of patients with duodenal ulcers and 70% to 90% of patients with gastric ulcers have gastric HP.[13,66,100,106,107,117,126,139,141,146–155] The lower prevalence of HP infection in patients with gastric ulcers may be due to some gastric lesions being caused by the ingestion of aspirin and NSAIDs,[156] and these drug-induced ulcers are reported to have a lower prevalence of associated histologic gastritis[157] and HP.[145] HP is significantly less frequent in patients with ulcers due to profound acid hypersecretion, as in Zollinger–Ellison syndrome.[158,159] Ulcers that occur in HP-negative patients taking NSAIDs or in Zollinger–Ellison syndrome prove that although HP may be a contributing factor in the pathogenesis of ulcer disease, it is not *the cause* of peptic ulcers.

In spite of the dramatic association between HP infection and peptic ulcer disease, a cause-and-effect relationship is not absolutely established at the present time. A clear-cut pathogenetic mechanism with experimental or clinical documentation is not available to explain how HP causes gastric and duodenal ulcers. The best evidence that HP is an important contributing cause in peptic ulcer disease is the mounting treatment data that suggest that drugs that eradicate HP also heal ulcers and prevent relapses as long as HP does not recur (Table 61-2).

DUODENITIS

The relationship of HP to duodenitis and gastric metaplasia of the duodenum is much less clear-cut than its relation to gastritis. Yet defining this relationship is necessary if HP is to be considered a contributing factor in the pathogenesis of duodenal ulcers. Duodenitis appears to be present in many healthy volunteers, although most have only a mild increase in mononuclear cells without neutrophilic infiltration.[11,160] In contrast, active duodenitis is found in a majority of patients with duodenal ulcers.[117,146,153] Wyatt and co-workers[117] and Johnston and co-workers[121] found duodenal HP in most cases of active duodenitis and state that HP never occurred in the absence of neutrophils. Other authors, however, find HP in a minority of duodenal biopsies and report no clear association

TABLE 61–2
Duodenal Relapse and *Helicobacter Pylori* Status

REFERENCE	FOLLOW-UP	DUODENAL ULCER RELAPSE		
		HP-Positive		HP-Negative
150	1 Yr	19/24 (79%)	*	4/15 (27%)
193	78 Wks	20/29 (69%)	*	0/7 (0%)
190, 216	? 62 Wks	30/41 (73%)	*	6/26 (23%)

* *P < 0.05 for duodenal relapse in HP-positive vs. HP-negative patients.*

with duodenal inflammation.[32,66,123,152,153,160,161] HP is commonly isolated on culture of duodenal biopsies without concomitant histologic identification of organisms.[123,153,160,161] This suggests that many positive duodenal cultures may represent contamination from the stomach.

Because HP is found only on gastric epithelia in the duodenum, the relation between gastric metaplasia of the duodenum and HP has been explored. Gastric metaplasia in the duodenum is a patchy, multifocal process present in 22% to 64% of healthy volunteers,[11,160] although it may be more common and/or more extensive in patients with active duodenitis or duodenal ulcers.[117,160] Wyatt and colleagues[117] found an association between gastric pH below 2.5 and the presence of gastric metaplasia and suggested that acid induces gastric metaplasia in the duodenum, allowing HP colonization and production of an acute inflammatory reaction. However, most patients with gastric metaplasia do not have associated duodenal HP,[117,123,160] and even patients with active duodenitis and gastric metaplasia have histologic evidence of duodenal HP in only 18% to 55% of cases.[117,123] Thus, available data do not allow us to accept this hypothesis of duodenal ulcer pathogenesis.

Pathogenesis of *Helicobacter Pylori*–Induced Injury

The mechanisms that might allow HP to damage the gastroduodenal mucosa have not been well defined. Production of ammonia by HP urease activity has been postulated as a cause of mucosal injury. In animals, ammonia deleteriously affects the gastric mucosal barrier.[163,164] In addition, exposure of a cultured human gastric cell line to HP caused morphologic changes as well as a significant decrease in cell viability, and these effects were prevented initially by concomitant treatment with a urease inhibitor.[165]

HP organisms elaborate a protease that degrades gastric mucus glycoproteins, increasing the permeability of mucus to hydrogen ions.[166,167] Lipase and phospholipase A activity have also been reported in filtrates of HP,[168] enzymes that theoretically could lead to an impairment in gastric mucosal defense.

Filtrates of HP have been shown to induce cytopathic effects in vitro in a variety of mammalian cell lines, and the toxic factor appears to be a protein.[169-171] Serologic recognition of a cytotoxic protein is present in almost 100% of HP-infected patients with peptic ulcers versus ~50% of asymptomatic patients with HP-positive gastritis,[171] suggesting that this protein may play a role in the pathogenesis of peptic ulcer disease. A cytotoxin is also reported to be significantly more common in HP strains from patients with peptic ulcers than in patients with chronic gastritis alone.[172]

HP-induced injury has also been postulated to occur by way of a gastrin-mediated mechanism. Two groups have reported elevated levels of gastrin in patients colonized with HP.[173,174] However, one group reported an associated elevation in peak acid output,[173] while the other found a lower 24-hour intragastric acidity in HP-positive patients.[174] In addition, treatment and eradication of HP did not result in a significant change in basal or maximal acid secretion in 10 patients.[175]

In summary, an etiologic role for HP appears to be best established in histologic gastritis. Based on the results of treatment studies (see "Treatment of *Helicobacter Pylori*"), HP also is likely to be a contributing factor in peptic ulcer disease. Evidence for a causative role of HP in gastric adenocarcinoma and duodenitis, however, is lacking at present. In addition, the mechanisms by which HP may cause gastroduodenal mucosal injury are poorly defined and require further investigation.

Treatment of *Helicobacter Pylori*

Although a large number of therapeutic regimens for HP have been evaluated in recent years, at the time of this writing *no definite indication for HP treatment exists*. The common finding of histologic gastritis does not require treatment, and any association of nonulcer dyspepsia and HP-positive gastritis is still tenuous. If HP is indeed an important factor in the pathogenesis of peptic ulcers, a potential use for HP therapy in the future will be to decrease ulcer recurrences by eradicating HP.

THERAPEUTIC AGENTS

A variety of antibiotics are effective against HP in vitro: penicillin, ampicillin, amoxicillin, erythromycin, gentamicin, cephalosporins, tetracyclines, ciprofloxacin, and imipenem; a majority of HP strains are also sensitive to metronidazole.[36,149,176-182] Bismuth compounds in the form of colloidal bismuth subcitrate (DeNol) and bismuth subsalicylate (Pepto-Bismol) are also effective in vitro against HP.[176,180,181,183-185] HP is not killed by other antiulcer drugs (histamine$_2$-receptor (H$_2$) antagonists, sucralfate, pirenzepine, misoprostol, and antacids).[180,181,186]

Although numerous antibiotics are active against HP in vitro, results of single-agent treatment in vivo are disappointing (Table 61-3). Clearance rates immediately after therapy range from 0% to 90%,[126,133,187-192] with amoxicillin providing perhaps the best initial clearance.[126,188] Colloidal bismuth subcitrate and bismuth subsalicylate generally have clearance rates higher than those of single-agent antibiotic therapy: ~50% or more with clearance rates ranging from 25% to 90% (Table 61-4).[70,75,126,133,190-197] However, initial clearance after therapy cannot be taken to represent eradication of HP because HP infection frequently is "rediscovered" in the days and weeks after treatment. Restriction endonuclease DNA analysis of HP strains before and after early relapse suggests that this "recurrence" represents persistent infection rather than eradication and reinfection.[198] Presumably, immediately after therapy HP density drops below detectable levels, but with time the number of bacteria gradually increases again. Examination at 1 month or more after cessation of therapy is considered necessary to verify HP eradication; most patients who are negative for HP at 1 month after therapy remain negative on prolonged follow-up.[126,199-201]

Single-agent antibiotic therapy rarely leads to long-term HP eradication,[133,188,190,192,199,202] and bismuth compounds alone also are unsuccessful in eradicating HP in a majority of patients.[190,192,195,203,204] Thus, combination therapies have been used in an attempt to increase rates of HP eradication (Table 61-5). The large array of combinations, dose schedules, and design flaws makes determination of the optimal treatment difficult. Triple therapy with bismuth, metronidazole, and either amoxicillin or tetracycline appears to be effective in initially clearing over 90%

TABLE 61–3

Treatment of Helicobacter Pylori: Single-Agent Antibiotic Therapy

MEDICATION	DAILY DOSE	DURATION	NO. SUBJECTS	HP CLEARANCE (0–2 WKS AFTER THERAPY)	HP ERADICATION (≥1 MO AFTER THERAPY)	REF. NO.
Amoxicillin	1 g b.i.d.	8 Days	22	0 Wk: 91%; 2 Wk: 0		188
	375 mg t.i.d.	?	22	68%	28%	126
Bacampicillin	800 mg b.i.d.	3 Wks	15		20%	191
Penicillin	600 mg t.i.d.	10 Days	6		0	191
Metronidazole	500 mg b.i.d.	3 Wks	5		20%	191
Tinidazole	500 mg b.i.d.	10 Days	29	3%	3%	190
Erythromycin	500 mg q.i.d.	2 Wks	15	7%		187
Ciprofloxacin	500 mg b.i.d.	2 Wks	13		0	191
Ofloxacin	200 mg b.i.d.	2 Wks	13		0	191
Furazolidone	100 mg q.i.d.	2 Wks	14	86%	40% (4/10)	133
	100 mg q.i.d.	4–8 Wks	15	27%	18%	202
Nitrofurantoin	100 mg q.i.d.	2 Wks	24	58%	0 (0/13)	133
	100 mg t.i.d.	10 Days	13	0		192
Rifampicin	600 mg q.d.	3 Wks	6		0	191
Doxycycline	200 mg—day 1, then 100 gm q.d.	9 Days	7	29%	0	182

and eradicating HP in at least 80% of cases.[200,201,203,205] Although bismuth is often given for 4 weeks and antibiotics have been given for 2 to 4 weeks, preliminary data suggest that combination treatment for only 1 week may provide similar eradication rates.[201] Therapy with bismuth and a single antibiotic gives eradication rates higher than those with single-agent treatment[190,199,203] and may approach the results with triple therapy.[203] In addition, therapy with two different antibiotics (amoxicillin and metronidazole or tinidazole)[105,201] may give a high rate of eradication.

TREATMENT OF GASTRITIS

Clearance and eradication of HP after medical therapy are associated with a significant decrease or resolution in histologic gastritis,

TABLE 61–4

Treatment of Helicobacter Pylori: Single-Agent Bismuth Therapy

MEDICATION	DAILY DOSE	DURATION	NO. SUBJECTS	HP CLEARANCE (0–2 WKS AFTER THERAPY)	HP ERADICATION (≥1 MO AFTER THERAPY)	REF. NO.
Colloidal bismuth subcitrate	120 mg q.i.d.	4 Wks	67	45%	15%	126
	120 mg q.i.d.	4 Wks	20	65%		195
	120 mg q.i.d.	4 Wks	23	43%		203
	120 mg q.i.d.	1 Mo	11	0		75
	108 mg q.i.d.	4 Wks	27	59%		197
	120 mg q.i.d.	8 Wks	20	70%	30%	192
	5 ml q.i.d.	6 Wks	?24–27	?48–54%		152
	180 mg q.i.d.	8 Wks	35	57%	34%	215
	240 mg b.i.d.	8 Wks	20	30%	15%	195
	240 mg b.i.d.	8 Wks	12	83%		70
	240 mg b.i.d.	1 Mo	16	50%		75
(Buffered)	240 mg b.i.d.	1 Mo	14	21%		75
(Chewable)	240 mg b.i.d.	1 Mo	22	23%		75
Bismuth subsalicylate	30 ml q.i.d.	3 Wks	18	78%		187
	300 mg t.i.d.	2 Wks	37	81%		193
	314 mg q.i.d.	3 Wks				
	900 mg t.i.d.	4 Wks	17	47%	?6–18%	192

especially the neutrophilic component.[75,133,152,187,188,197,200,206] This improvement is seen in patients with and without peptic ulcer disease, whereas the histologic gastritis associated with peptic ulcers does not improve and HP does not clear in patients treated with H_2-receptor antagonists or vagotomy, in spite of ulcer healing.[139,151-153,207] In contrast, both misoprostol and sucralfate cause no change in HP prevalence but caused statistically significant decreases in histologic gastritis in ulcer patients as compared with placebo.[208,209]

TREATMENT OF PEPTIC ULCERS

Colloidal bismuth subcitrate produces healing rates for peptic ulcers similar to those of cimetidine or ranitidine.[150,152,190,210-214] Bismuth compounds also may be more effective than continued H_2-receptor antagonists in healing ulcers refractory to cimetidine or ranitidine.[204,214] Of greater interest, significantly more patients treated with an H_2-receptor antagonist had recurrent ulcers in the year after treatment than did those treated with colloidal bismuth

TABLE 61–5
Treatment of Helicobacter Pylori: Multiple-Drug Therapy

MEDICATIONS	DAILY DOSE	DURATION	NO. SUBJECTS	HP CLEARANCE (0–2 WKS AFTER THERAPY)	HP ERADICATION (≥1 MO AFTER THERAPY)	REF. NO.
Amoxicillin + tinidazole	50 mg/kg	6 Wks	32		94%	105
	20 mg/kg	6 Wks				
Amoxicillin + metronidazole	500 mg t.i.d.	1 Wk	9		78%	201
	500 mg t.i.d.	1 Wk				
CBS + amoxicillin	120 mg q.i.d.	?	20	90%	40%	126
	375 mg t.i.d.	?				
CBS + amoxicillin	120 mg q.i.d.	4 Wks	18		50%	203
	500 mg t.i.d.	1 Wk				
CBS + metronidazole	120 mg q.i.d.	4 Wks	23		57%	203
	200 mg t.i.d.	1 Wk				
CBS + metronidazole	120 mg q.i.d.	4 Wks	20		85%	203
	400 mg t.i.d.	1 Wk				
CBS + tinidazole	120 mg q.i.d.	8 Wks	27	74%	70%	190
	500 mg b.i.d.	10 Days				
BSS + nitrofurantoin	900 mg t.i.d.	15 Days	6	0 Wk: 60% (3/5)		192
	100 mg t.i.d.	10 Days		2 Wk: 17%		
CBS + tetracycline + metronidazole	?120 mg t.i.d.	4 Wks	100	94%	94% (47 of 50) with initial HP clearance	200
	500 mg q.i.d.	4 Wks				
	200 mg q.i.d.	2 Wks				
CBS + amoxicillin + metronidazole	120 mg q.i.d.	4 Wks	20		85%	203
	500 mg t.i.d.	1 Wk				
	400 mg t.i.d.	1 Wk				
BSS + amoxicillin + metronidazole	600 mg t.i.d.	2 Wks	23	100%	90% (9 of 10)	205
	500 mg t.i.d.	2 Wks				
	500 mg t.i.d.	2 Wks				
BSS + amoxicillin + metronidazole	600 mg t.i.d.	2 Wks	26		81%	201
	500 mg t.i.d.	2 Wks				
	500 mg t.i.d.	2 Wks				
BSS + amoxicillin + metronidazole	600 mg t.i.d.	2 Wks	55		80%	201
	500 mg t.i.d.	1 Wk				
	500 mg t.i.d.	1 Wk				
BSS + amoxicillin + metronidazole	600 mg t.i.d.	1 Wk	15		80%	201
	500 mg t.i.d.	1 Wk				
	500 mg t.i.d.	1 Wk				

CBS, colloidal bismuth subcitrate; BSS, bismuth subsalicylate

subcitrate,[194,211,212] although other studies have failed to show a difference in relapse rates.[150,210] Colloidal bismuth subcitrate enhances mucosal defense in animal models,[208] and initially this was presumed to be its mechanism of action in healing ulcers. With the "discovery" of HP, however, the decrease in ulcer recurrence was thought to be due to eradication of HP. Certainly ulcers recur commonly in patients who continue to have evidence of HP infection; relapse is much less common in patients who are HP-negative (Table 61-2).[150,190,194,215,216]

The concept that eradication of HP by bismuth or other agents is solely responsible for decreasing ulcer recurrence must be viewed with reservation. Because colloidal bismuth subcitrate does not eradicate HP in a majority of patients, other factors (such as mucosal protection) may play a role in the excellent ulcer healing rates and lower relapse rates seen with bismuth treatment. Sucralfate treatment is accompanied by a recurrence rate lower than that found with cimetidine after ulcer healing,[209,213] yet sucralfate has no known effect on HP. In addition, both sucralfate and misoprostol, which enhance mucosal defense without clearing HP, decrease the histologic gastritis associated with peptic ulcers.[208,209] Furthermore, the antibiotic furazolidone is as effective as cimetidine in healing duodenal ulcers,[189,202,218] and in one small study the 6-month ulcer recurrence rate was significantly lower in furazolidone-treated patients than in cimetidine-treated patients.[202] However, less than a third of patients will have eradication of HP after therapy with furazolidone,[133,202] raising the possibility of another mechanism of action.

TREATMENT OF NONULCER DYSPEPSIA

In the absence of clear documentation that HP and/or histologic gastritis is associated with nonulcer dyspepsia, the role and treatment of HP in this syndrome are difficult to interpret. Three randomized, placebo-controlled studies of colloidal bismuth subcitrate provide data on treatment in HP-positive patients with nonulcer dyspepsia.[70,219,220] One study shows no significant improvement in symptoms despite a significant decrease in HP colonization and gastritis, a second shows a trend toward resolution of symptoms ($P = 0.055$), and the third reports significant improvement in symptoms but does not provide information on resolution of symptoms.[70] Two placebo-controlled studies using antibiotics (amoxicillin, nitrofurans) report no correlation of symptomatic improvement with active treatment or HP clearance.[133,188]

ADVERSE EFFECTS OF TREATMENT

Treatment of HP, especially with multiple drugs, may cause adverse effects. Nausea, vomiting, diarrhea, and thrush occur in patients receiving antibiotics as treatment for HP.[133,200] Few adverse effects have been identified with short-term ingestion of bismuth compounds, and these are discussed in detail under "Peptic Ulcer Disease: Pharmacology of Therapeutic Agents" for Acid-Peptic Diseases.

SUMMARY

At present, no definite indication for the treatment of HP exists. Evidence showing that eradication of HP may be associated with a significant decrease in peptic ulcer recurrence is accumulating. If confirmed, a single course of anti-HP treatment may become the treatment of choice in patients with ulcers. Eradication of HP requires treatment with at least two and perhaps three agents, including bismuth compounds (colloidal bismuth subcitrate or bismuth subsalicylate) and/or antibiotics such as amoxicillin, metronidazole, and tetracycline. Clear evidence that anti-HP therapy is beneficial in other disorders, such as nonulcer dyspepsia, is lacking.

PEPTIC ULCER DISEASES

The Problem

Peptic ulcer diseases (gastric and duodenal ulcer) represent serious medical problems largely because of their frequency: approximately 500,000 new cases and 4 million recurrences each year in the United States.[221] The mortality due to ulcer diseases is relatively low (i.e., less than 10,000 deaths per year in the United States) compared with diseases such as ischemic heart disease or cancer.[221] The high prevalence of ulcer diseases results in substantial pain and suffering as well as economic costs. However, the estimated annual direct costs for treatment of patients with ulcer disease (i.e., physician visits, diagnostic studies, medical treatment, and so forth) are approximately 3 to 4 billion dollars, and the indirect costs (i.e., cost related to time lost from work) are similar.[222] The total cost for antiulcer medications continues to increase, and it is now estimated to be at least 2 billion dollars per year in the United States.[223a]

In 1975 it was estimated that peptic ulcer contributed approximately 10% of the total $25 million in medical costs for digestive diseases.[223] It is likely that the expanding geriatric population in the United States, coupled with the enlarging use of NSAIDs that have inherent damaging effects to the gastroduodenal mucosa, has driven this cost substantially above 10% of total digestive disease expenditures.

Epidemiology

INCIDENCE AND PREVALENCE

It is not uncommon in everyday parlance for *incidence* to be incorrectly substituted for *prevalence*. *Incidence* represents a rate: the number of new cases of the disease in a specifically defined population at risk during a set time period (e.g., the number of new cases per population per year). *Prevalence*, however, refers to the number of patients with the specific disease under study in a specific population. Most commonly, prevalence refers to the "point prevalence" of a disease in a defined population at a specific point in time. However, prevalence may be expressed as "period prevalence" (i.e., the disease frequency in a population over a specified time period).[221]

In contrast to other diseases (e.g., colon cancer and acute myocardial infarction), a precise diagnosis of ulcer cannot be made easily. For example, a history of epigastric abdominal pain is an insensitive and nonspecific indicator of ulcer disease. Moreover, the most precise and readily available method of diagnosis, upper gastrointestinal endoscopy, is costly and not easily applied to a large random sample of the population. The lack of precision in the diagnosis of ulcer places many of the epidemiologic surveys in question quantitatively, but the reported qualitative time-trends are likely valid, particularly because similar observations have been reported by separate investigators in different population groups.[224–226] Ulcer complications, such as perforation and hemorrhage, usually require hospitalization and therefore can be assessed more accurately.

In spite of these limitations, Monson and MacMahon estimated in 1969 that in male physicians in the United States the lifetime prevalence of peptic ulcer was about 10% and the annual incidence was 0.3%. In those above the age of 45 years, 11% reported having duodenal ulcer (DU) and 1.2% reported having gastric ulcer (GU).[227] Therefore, at least in male physicians in the late 1960s, DU was about fivefold more common than GU and occurred in about 1 in 10 men.

The 1-year period prevalence of active combined gastric and duodenal ulcer in the United States in males and females is about 1.8%.[228] Therefore, with 250 million adults in the United States, 4.5 million will suffer annually from peptic ulcer diseases. In a recent large Japanese survey of male office workers above the age of 40, Kaneko and colleagues reported a 4.3% point prevalence of duodenal ulcer as determined by gastroduodenal photofluorography followed by endoscopic confirmation.[229] The explanation for the high prevalence of DU in Japanese males is unknown. No similar survey has been performed in the United States.

In the mid-1950s, the male:female ratio for deaths due to DU was about 5:1, but during the past decade this ratio has decreased to about 1.3:1.[230] This can be explained by the marked decrease in DU in males over the past 20 years, while there has been little change, and possibly a modest increase, in females.

Taken together, it can be estimated that there are between 200,000 and 400,000 new cases of duodenal ulcer in the United States annually, and because of the high recurrence rates for both DU and GU, about 4.5 million people suffer from peptic ulcer disease annually.

TIME AND GENDER TRENDS

Prior to the twentieth century, duodenal ulcer disease was distinctly unusual.[231] The major form of ulcer disease in the 1900s was gastric ulcer, particularly in women, and it was often associated with perforation. Duodenal ulcer disease increased progressively during the early 1900s, reaching a peak in about 1950.[232] Susser and Stein[233] attributed these changes to the urbanization of American society and proposed that factors introduced to the birth-cohort born between 1868 and 1908 predisposed this cohort to develop duodenal ulcer, while those born about 10 years earlier were more predisposed to develop gastric ulcer. Those born prior to and after these dates had a lower lifetime prevalence of ulcer disease. This finding suggests that some factor, possibly environmental, was introduced during the latter part of the nineteenth and early twentieth century that increased the incidence of ulcer. The temporal pattern suggests that the risk factors were introduced early in life, and these factors have decreased over the past 70 years. The birth-cohort phenomenon applies to data collected in the United States, Britain, Europe, and Japan.[234] (See recent review for more details.[234])

The elements that account for these time-related patterns are not known, and there are several postulates. The greater incidence of ulcer disease in those born around the turn of the century and immediately prior to the industrial revolution may be related to greater workloads and energy expenditure, decreased caloric intake, and so forth.[234] It may also be related to other factors, such as dietary constituents or cigarette smoking.[235,236] The recent decrease in ulcer disease may be related to the greater intake of polyunsaturated fats that serve as precursors of arachidonic acid and prostaglandins of the E and A class, agents that protect the gastroduodenal mucosa from damage and that expedite ulcer healing.[237] Furthermore, cigarette smoking, which also has decreased over the past 20 years, is causally associated with ulcer disease, an increased rate of ulcer complications, delayed ulcer healing, and higher recurrence rates.[238]

The incidence of ulcer disease (duodenal and gastric ulcer) decreased in the United States from 1970 through 1980 (Fig 61-4). For example, the 1965 hospitalization rate for ulcer disease, 252 per 100,000 population, decreased almost one half by 1981.[239] The major component of this decline was a decrease in hospitalizations for uncomplicated duodenal ulcers (Fig 61-5). Of note, there has been little change in the hospitalization rates for perforated duodenal ulcer and a modest decrease for gastrointestinal hemorrhage.

Furthermore, the mortality rates for duodenal and gastric ulcer have decreased. In 1962, the mortality rate for duodenal ulcer was 3.1 per 100,000, and for gastric ulcer it was 3.5 per 100,000; in 1979, each decreased to about 1 per 100,000.[240] GU has a greater mortality rate than DU, most likely because it occurs more commonly in older patients. Moreover, the number of physician office visits for duodenal ulcer decreased between 1958 and 1984.[241] These time-related variables have been observed in Europe as well as Asia.[242–244]

Recent surveys in Finland, Great Britain, and the United States report a substantial increase in the hospitalization of elderly patients with either ulcer hemorrhage or perforation.[245,246] Although the mortality from ulcer remained stable throughout the 1970s, it has risen significantly in patients over the age of 75. This has been attributed in large part to the intake of NSAIDs by an expanding geriatric population in whom the incidence of ulcer may increase independently.

It was anticipated that the availability of the H$_2$-receptor antagonists with their potent antisecretory and ulcer-healing effects might decrease the incidence of ulcer complications. However, in Denmark the incidence of ulcer complication has been unaltered since the introduction of the H$_2$-receptor antagonists.[247] This is believed to be true in Australia and the United States as well. Therefore, either treatment is ineffective in preventing ulcer complications or, more likely, patients become noncompliant over time.

In summary, duodenal ulcer reached a peak between 1950 and 1970 and decreased progressively until about 1980. During the past 30 years, the death rate, surgical rate, and physician visits

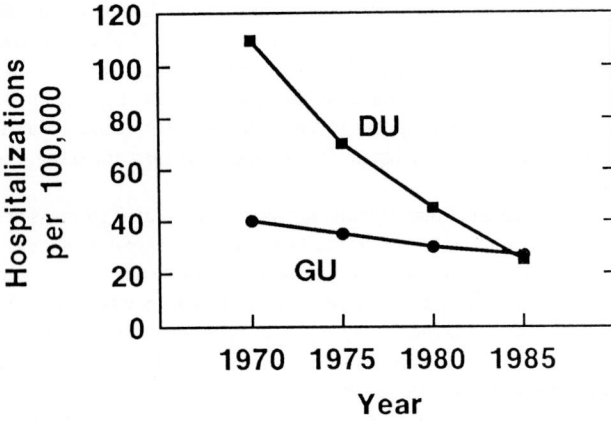

FIGURE 61-4. Hospitalization rates for duodenal ulcer (DU) and gastric ulcer (GU) from 1970 to 1985. There has been a marked decrease in DU, while GU has remained stable. In fact, with the increased use of nonsteroidal anti-inflammatory drugs (NSAIDs) there has been an increase in the incidence of gastric erosions and ulcers (see text). (Modified with permission from Kurata JH. Epidemiology of peptic ulcer disease. Clin Gastroenterol 1984;13:289.)

for ulcer decreased by more than 100%. This decrease has occurred predominantly in males.

GENETICS

Genetic factors play an important role in ulcer pathogenesis.[248] First, the concordance for peptic ulcer in identical (monozygotic) twins is approximately 50%.[249] Ulcer concordance is also increased in nonidentical twins, although not to the degree as in homozygous twins. Second, the lifetime prevalence of developing ulcer in first-degree relatives of ulcer patients is about threefold greater than that in the general population.[250] Interestingly, DU clusters in families, as does GU, but the prevalence of GU is not increased in DU families, or vice versa. Third, the inheritance of blood group O is associated with a modest (1.3-fold) increase in duodenal ulcer incidence.[251] While inheritance of a nonsecreting status of blood group antigens in body fluids (e.g., saliva, gastric secretion, and so forth) increases the risk by about 1.5-fold, the combined presence of both blood group O and nonsecretor status increases the risk of developing duodenal ulcer about 2.5-fold compared with the general population.[252] Furthermore, HLA subtypes (e.g., HLA-B5, -B12, and -Bw35) have been identified as genetic mark-

ers in DU. These findings are based on small pedigrees, and further study is needed. Fourth, the inheritance of the trait for elevated levels of serum pepsinogen I has served as a genetic marker in selected kindreds of duodenal ulcer families in whom ulcers occur significantly more commonly.[253] Finally, rare genetic syndromes associated with duodenal ulcer have been identified, for example, multiple endocrine neoplasia type I (MEN-I) (pancreatic islet cell gastrin-secreting adenoma, parathyroid adenoma, anterior pituitary adenoma, systemic mastocytosis, and other rare syndromes).[254]

Until quite recently, the prevailing hypothesis for the inheritance of peptic ulcer was the polygenic mode.[255] This implies that the constellation of genes, plus perhaps environmental factors, results in clinical disease.[256] Rotter and colleagues[257] have proposed that genetic heterogeneity is the preferred explanation for the familial aggregation of ulcer in the absence of simple Mendelian inheritance patterns. This implies that ulcer disease represents a group of distinct diseases of diverse etiologies, genetic and nongenetic, that produce identical clinical findings (other examples include the hyperlipemias, diabetes mellitus, and so forth). In support of genetic heterogeneity are pedigree studies in families with an increased incidence of ulcer that also have an inheritable marker for the development of ulcer (e.g., hyperpepsinogenemia I, increased gastric emptying, systemic mastocytosis, and so forth).[258] For example, only the minority of family members having hyperpepsinogenemia I develop ulcer disease.

In summary, as in many other diseases, one's genetic composition has an important impact on the subsequent development of disease. Considerable fundamental work is required to localize specifically these genetic markers.

MISCELLANEOUS FACTORS

The frequency, mortality, and complications of ulcer disease are somewhat more common in the winter months.[259] The explanation for the seasonal patterns in ulcer disease is unclear.

For unexplained reasons, although possibly related to genetic, environmental, or methodologic factors of data collection, regional differences in ulcer incidence exist. For example, the incidence of ulcer perforation is greater in Scotland than in England, and the incidence of duodenal ulcer is significantly less in northern India than in southern India.[260]

Although it was once considered that duodenal ulcer is an executive's disease, there is no evidence that distinct occupational factors influence ulcer incidence. In fact, peptic ulcer disease seems

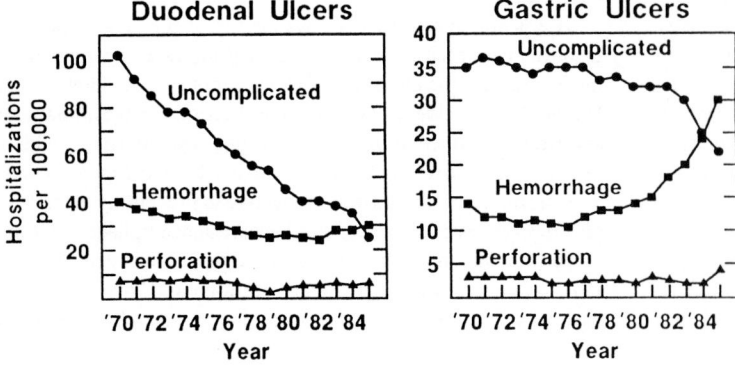

FIGURE 61-5. While the hospitalization rates for uncomplicated duodenal ulcers have decreased over the past decades, they are unchanged for hemorrhage and perforation. There has been a modest decrease in the hospitalization rate for uncomplicated gastric ulcer (note different scale on the gastric ulcer figure) and no significant change for perforation. However, there has been a marked increase in hospitalization rates for gastric ulcer hemorrhage likely due to increased use of nonsteroidal anti-inflammatory drugs. (Modified with permission from Kurata JH. Epidemiology of peptic ulcer disease. Clin Gastroenterol 1984;13:289.)

to be somewhat more common in those of lower economic strata.[261] The mortality due to ulcer disease is greater in nonwhites prior to the age of 65, and then it tends to equalize. These differences, however, are minor.

RISK FACTORS

Smoking. Most studies reveal a strong positive association between cigarette smoking and ulcer incidence, mortality, complications, recurrences, and delayed healing rates.[262–265] Such epidemiologic studies are open to question because of the retrospective collection of data and the lack of precise definitions of smoking, ulcer, and quantitation of smoking (i.e., is a person who smokes less than 10 cigarettes/day at comparable risk to one who smokes 2 or 3 packs/day?). It is therefore not surprising that there is lack of agreement between studies.[266–268]

In spite of these inherent methodologic limitations, a large, long-term follow-up of college students indicated that those who smoked in college had a modest (1.3-fold) increase in the subsequent risk of ulcer versus nonsmokers.[269] Furthermore, large retrospective studies reported that cigarette smokers were about twofold more likely to have ulcer disease than nonsmokers with a dose–response phenomenon: the number of cigarettes smoked per day and the number of pack-years were directly related to the incidence of ulcer.[270] Recently, in a 20-year study involving 5933 Hawaiian Japanese males, Stemmerman and co-workers reported that smoking was associated with an increased risk of both GU and DU.[271] However, the dose–response effect in pack-years was observed only for GU, and there was an association between poor pulmonary function and GU but not DU.

These findings suggest that decreased pulmonary function in ulcer patients is largely secondary to smoking and that smoking is related more to gastric than to duodenal ulcer. Chronic pulmonary disease is associated with an increased prevalence of ulcer disease, probably related to cigarette smoking. A recent endoscopic study in patients with rheumatoid arthritis taking NSAIDs revealed that 63% of those with gastric ulcer smoked, whereas in a similar, but ulcer-free, group 33% smoked.[272] This suggests that cigarette smoking further increases the risk of ulcer disease in patients receiving NSAIDs. It is possible that cigarette smoking and NSAID intake may be either independent or additive risk factors.

The mechanism(s) whereby cigarette smoking enhances ulcer pathogenesis is not understood. Cigarette smoking itself does not alter gastric acid secretion,[273] although DU patient smokers may have greater gastric acid secretion than nonsmokers[274] and a greater sensitivity to tetragastrin.[275] Cigarette smokers, with or without ulcers, have higher serum pepsinogen I (Pg-I) than their nonsmoking controls, and differences in serum Pg-I between smokers and nonsmokers were observed in DU but not GU patients.[276] The increase in serum Pg-I in nonulcer subjects was attributed to superficial fundic gastritis. Cigarette smoke has a number of effects in animals that may be operative in humans: decreased gastric and duodenal mucosal bicarbonate secretion, decreased mucosal blood flow, and increased duodenogastric reflux.

In summary, cigarette smokers are at an increased risk of developing ulcer disease and ulcer complications and have impaired healing rates. The precise pathophysiologic mechanisms that are operative require further investigation.

Nonsteroidal Anti-Inflammatory Drugs (NSAIDs). It is estimated that on any given day about 1 of 10 patients receiving NSAIDs has an active gastric ulcer.[277] NSAIDs represent one of the major causes of life-threatening complications such as upper gastrointestinal hemorrhage and perforation.[278,279] In the United States, NSAID gastropathy is reportedly the most frequent cause of severe untoward drug effects.[280]

The use of NSAIDs is extensive. About 3 million people, or 1.2% of the entire population, take NSAIDs daily in the United States. Furthermore, 50% of patients with arthritis are treated, or self-medicate, with NSAIDs on a daily basis.[281] It has been estimated that each year 2% to 4% of NSAID users suffer a serious GI drug-related complication.[282] In patients with rheumatoid arthritis who use NSAIDs on a regular basis, it is estimated that there are approximately 2,600 additional deaths/year and about 20,000 additional hospitalizations attributed to NSAID intake.[280] Because these estimates do not include patients with other arthritic conditions, such as osteoarthritis, the deaths and hospitalizations due to NSAIDs are undoubtedly even greater.

Overall, it has been estimated that there is a two- to threefold increased mortality due to gastrointestinal complications in chronic NSAID users.[283,284] Such complications occur largely in those above the age of 60 and in females, and, regrettably, they are usually not antedated by symptoms to forewarn the impending event. Furthermore, all classes of NSAIDs result in gastroduodenal damage. In fact, a prodrug, sulindac, which requires hepatic biotransformation to become biologically active and has no direct topical damaging effects (nor does the active compound), has at least the same relative risk for causing acute gastrointestinal bleeding as other NSAIDs.[285]

Although NSAIDs may produce serious life-threatening complications and are therefore a major health problem, the frequency of severe complications in the entire patient population receiving chronic NSAID treatment is low. Langman estimated that about 3 to 5 patients per 1000 who take NSAIDs on a daily basis are admitted for upper gastrointestinal hemorrhage, and only about 1 per 250,000 casual users are admitted.[286] Therefore, although NSAID-related complications are frequently observed by the gastroenterologist and general surgeon, they are far less commonly encountered by the family physician, internist, and even the rheumatologist. For example, when relative risk ratios are determined (i.e., the risk of a drug-induced complication in a specific disease population divided by an age- and sex-matched group with the same disease but not receiving the drug under study), the risk of GU and DU in Great Britain is about 3.2- and 2.7-fold greater, respectively.[287] McCarthy calculated the relative risk ratios for GU and DU in chronic NSAID users as about 45- and 8-fold greater, respectively.[288] Regardless of the precise relative risk ratios, the chances of developing either GU or DU are clearly increased in NSAID users relative to the general population, and gastric ulcer is about six times more common than duodenal ulcer. There is a direct dose–response relationship between NSAID dose and the likelihood of developing complications, particularly in those taking more than 22 aspirin tablets weekly.[289–291]

Unfortunately, the clinical markers that indicate who is predisposed to NSAID-induced complications are nonspecific and insensitive. The presence of a history of NSAID-related abdominal pain, concomitant intake of corticosteroids, history of antiulcer medications, prior ulcer disease, and smoking and/or alcohol intake have been identified as potential markers of NSAID-induced injury.[280,288] However, additional data are critically needed to identify those patients who are most likely to develop NSAID-induced ulcer complications so that they may be prevented.

In summary, in spite of their relatively low incidence of severe untoward side effects in the general population, NSAIDs represent a major health hazard throughout Western civilization primarily to the elderly, females, and those with prior ulcer disease. Moreover, the mortality in those who develop a major upper gastrointestinal complication secondary to NSAIDs is estimated at about 10%.[299,300] NSAIDs damage the gastric antrum predominantly, but also the duodenum, by both direct and indirect (inhibition of prostaglandin synthesis) mechanisms. It is not possible to determine which patients will have complications of NSAID therapy or, in a given patient, which NSAID will cause complications.

Adrenocorticosteroids. The role of corticosteroids in the development of peptic ulcer is controversial. Conn and Blitzer[301] reviewed 42 randomized trials and concluded that adrenocorticosteroids can be incriminated in ulcer pathogenesis in patients who receive daily corticosteroids for more than 1 month, in those who receive more than a total dose equivalent to 1 g of prednisone, and in those with prior ulcer disease. In a more recent survey, Messer and colleagues[302] failed to observe an association between corticosteroid intake and ulcer. For practical purposes, because the relationship between corticosteroids and ulcer disease is tenuous and, if present, of relatively low risk, there is no indication at present for the routine use of prophylactic antiulcer medications in patients placed on short-term corticosteroid therapy. However, in the patients with prior ulcer disease requiring prolonged adrenocorticosteroid treatment for a serious medical disease (e.g., a collagen vascular disease, after organ transplantation, severe chronic pulmonary disease, and so forth), the prophylactic use of antiulcer drugs is reasonable.[303]

Alcohol. Alcohol is an agent commonly used to induce gastric mucosal damage in animals.[304] However, in these models alcohol is often administered as absolute ethanol (i.e., pure ethanol or 200 proof!). Pure ethanol is lipid-soluble, traverses the gastric mucosa promptly, and results in frank acute mucosal damage.[305] Because most humans do not drink absolute ethanol, it is not likely that these experimental models have direct clinical counterpart. In fact, mucosal injury does not occur in humans at ethanol concentrations of less than 10% (20 proof).[306] At concentrations of 20% (40 proof) and greater, the transmucosal gastric potential difference decreases, and endoscopic evidence of acute injury is observed. Because of prompt mucosal restitution, it is unlikely that these acute and transient mucosal changes result in chronic mucosal damage. Furthermore, retrospective analysis of alcohol intake in patients with ulcer disease revealed that those who consumed modest amounts of alcohol had a decreased prevalence of ulcer disease compared with nondrinkers.[307] The only association between ethanol intake and ulcer disease exists in patients with portal cirrhosis.[308]

Although ethanol at low concentration (5%) may be a modest stimulant of gastric acid secretion, higher concentrations diminish acid secretion.[309] Wine and beer are each potent gastric acid secretagogues, and because of an unidentified constituent(s), red and white wine cause a marked increase in serum gastrin similar to that produced by a protein meal.[310,311] This is of physiologic interest but to date has no direct application to ulcerogenesis or therapy.

Diet. Although some types of foods and beverages are reported to cause dyspepsia, there are no convincing data that indicate that any specific diet causes ulcer. To the unseasoned palate, or gut, highly spiced foods (e.g., Mexican chile rellenos and Indian curries) are often reported to result in indigestion. However, the factors responsible for dyspepsia associated with ingestion of these types of foods are unknown. Of interest, duodenal ulcer is more common in the south of India (an area of low-fiber diet) than in the northern part (a wheat-eating area).[312] The explanation for this is not known, but it may be genetic or environmental or may be due to the effects of a high-residue diet on the release of epidermal growth factor (EGF) and/or prostaglandins. More recently, Berstad and colleagues reported that a diet containing high amounts of bran expedited duodenal ulcer healing and also prevented ulcer recurrences.[313] This interesting observation requires confirmation but suggests that fiber may play a therapeutic role in ulcer disease.

Both decaffeinated and caffeinated beverages (tea and coffee) are potent stimulants of gastric acid secretion (Fig 61-6).[310,314] Furthermore, cola-type beverages, beer, and milk are also potent secretagogues.[310] However, epidemiologic studies have failed to reveal an increased risk of ulcer disease in those who consume these beverages.

While bland meals and the frequent ingestion of milk were commonplace in the armamentarium of ulcer treatment in the early 1900s, they stimulate greater amounts of gastric acid secretion than three meals daily, and, more important, they do not expedite ulcer healing. Therefore, dietary alterations, other than instructions to avoid pain-causing foods, are unnecessary in ulcer patients.

ASSOCIATED DISEASES

There is epidemiologic evidence that duodenal ulcer occurs more commonly in patients with several other chronic medical diseases. Although the mechanisms (e.g., genetic and/or pathophysiologic) responsible for this relationship are known in some (e.g., gastrinoma—increased serum gastrin; systemic mastocytosis, basophilic leukemia—increased serum histamine), the precise mechanisms responsible for these relationships are for the most part unknown. Furthermore, in order to establish a definite association between two diseases, it is necessary to survey the disease prevalence in a large random sample of the population rather than in a referral population, as is present at all medical centers. The reason is that if patients with disease A, disease B, and a combination of diseases A and B are referred for treatment (and also undergo medical evaluation for other diseases), a falsely high prevalence of disease A accompanying disease B is often observed in a nonrepresentative sample of the population, as in medical centers. This is called "Berkson's fallacy" or referral bias.[315]

Table 61-6 lists those diseases associated with duodenal ulcer. There is a definite association between chronic pulmonary diseases and peptic ulcer.[316,317] The prevalence of ulcer disease in patients with chronic pulmonary diseases is about three- to fivefold greater, and deaths due to ulcer are about five times greater, than those of the general population.[317] Conversely, the frequency of chronic pulmonary diseases is reported to be about threefold greater in patients with ulcer disease. Interestingly, duodenal ulcer disease may antedate the recognition of pulmonary disease.[318] Although earlier studies tended to attribute the relationship to ulcers as being independent of cigarette smoking,[319] a large recent survey from Hawaii concluded that ulcer disease is in large part secondary

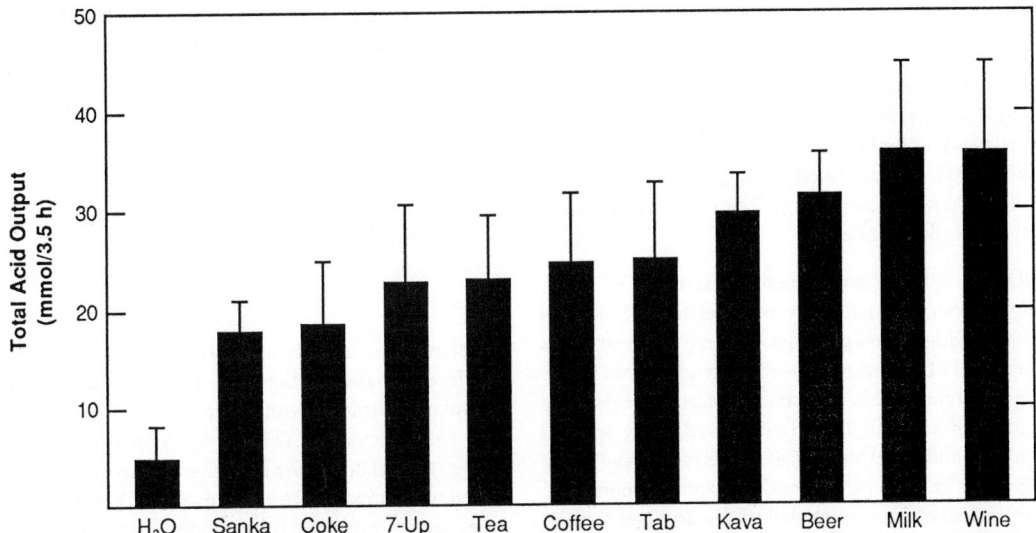

FIGURE 61-6. Mean total acid output over 3.5 hours after ingestion of 240 ml of wine or 360 ml of all other beverages in healthy subjects. Note that gastric acid secretion was unrelated to caffeine content (e.g., Coke contains 65 mg/360 ml, tea contains 92 mg/360 ml, and coffee and Kava coffee contain about 130 mg/360 ml); osmolalities varied from 0 with water to 928 mOsm/kg with beer; ionized calcium content was less than 2 mmol/L except for milk, 10.5 mmol/L. (Modified with permission from McArthur K, Hogan D, Isenberg JI. Relative stimulatory effects of commonly ingested beverages on gastric acid secretion in humans. Gastroenterology 1982;83:199, and Lenz HJ, Ferrari-Taylor J, Isenberg JI. Wine and 5 percent ethanol are potent stimulants of gastric acid secretion in humans. Gastroenterology 1983;85: 1082.)

to decreased pulmonary function (impaired FEV_1 [forced expiratory volume in 1 second]).[320] Because the vast majority of chronic pulmonary diseases in Western civilization are secondary to cigarette smoking, and because cigarette smoking is related to ulcer disease, it is difficult to extract the role of cigarette smoking as an independent variable in ulcerogenesis from chronic pulmonary disease. At present, the basic pathophysiologic mechanisms responsible for this association are not known. Moreover, patients with cystic fibrosis (possibly secondary to decreased pancreatic bicarbonate secretion) and alpha$_1$-antitrypsin deficiency (possibly due to lack of protease inhibitors) are also at increased risk of duodenal ulcer disease.[321]

Hepatic cirrhosis is also associated with an increased risk of duodenal ulcer (approximately a five- to eightfold increase compared with the general population).[322,323] The mechanisms are not understood, although it has been speculated that duodenal ulcer may be more frequent in cirrhotics because of impaired inactivation of gastrointestinal hormones (e.g., gastrin or other gastric secretagogues) that are normally inactivated within the liver.[324]

The other common medical disease associated with an increase in duodenal ulcer disease is chronic renal failure, sometimes associated with chronic hemodialysis and sometimes following renal transplantation.[325] Patients with uremia often develop angiodysplasia, associated with chronic gastrointestinal blood loss.[326] In addition, patients with chronic renal failure are reported to have an increased prevalence of endoscopic evidence of duodenal mucosal damage ("duodenitis").[327] The mechanisms responsible for ulcer disease and gastroduodenal mucosal damage under these circumstances are not known.

A decrease in the prevalence of duodenal ulcer occurs in patients with gastric atrophy (likely due to decreased acid/pepsin secretion) and patients with Addison's disease,[328] and possibly patients with diabetes mellitus.[329] Interestingly, a recent report described a pa-

tient with achlorhydria and a large postbulbar recurrent duodenal ulcer. The pathogenesis of this unusual ulcer is not known, but it suggests that the dictum "no acid—no ulcer" (Schwartz) may not apply to all duodenal ulcers.

TABLE 61-6

The Following Diseases Have Been Reported to be Associated With Duodenal Ulcer

Existing Evidence Strongly Supports An Association:

Zollinger–Ellison syndrome (gastrinoma)

Systemic mastocytosis

Multiple endocrine neoplasia type I

Chronic pulmonary diseases

Chronic renal failure

Hepatic cirrhosis

Kidney stones

Alpha antitrypsin deficiency

Evidence Is Only Suggestive Regarding Association With DU:

Crohn's disease

Hyperparathyroidism in the absence of multiple endocrine neoplasia type I

Coronary artery disease

Polycythemia vera

Chronic pancreatitis

Modified from Soll AF. Duodenal ulcer and drug therapy. In: Sleisenger JH, Fordtran JS, eds. Gastrointestinal diseases. Pathophysiology, diagnosis, management, ed 4. Philadelphia: WB Saunders, 1989: 832.

STRESS AND PSYCHOLOGIC FACTORS

The role of psychologic factors in the pathogenesis and natural history of peptic ulcer diseases has been the subject of numerous studies with conflicting conclusions. In light of the recent evidence describing the existence of brain peptides, the relationship between their release and gastrointestinal functions including secretion and motility,[330,331] it would not be surprising if central nervous system factors were to affect ulcer diseases.

Acute Stress. There are numerous examples of acute stress inducing gastric mucosal injury in experimental animals (e.g., cold-restraint, fatigue, and so forth).[332] These forms of stress are unphysiologic and often severe. The only circumstances where they may have any relationship to human disease is in patients subjected to acute and severe injuries or diseases who may develop acute gastric ulcers and/or erosions (also referred to as "acute hemorrhagic gastritis"). The pathogenesis of acute hemorrhagic gastritis is independent of conventional ulcer diseases (see section on "Gastritis" and ch 109).

Chronic Stress. The role of psychologic factors in the pathogenesis or natural history of gastric and duodenal ulcer disease is far from established. Early unblinded studies by Alexander[333] and Weiner and colleagues[334] described certain personality characteristics thought to be markers of ulcer-type personalities. These have included conflicts about dependency needs, hypochondriasis, low ego strength, and so forth.[335,336] However, these studies are open to criticism because of the lack of investigator blindness, retrospective nature, inadequate controls, inaccuracy of the diagnosis of ulcer (commonly made by X-ray), and imprecise tools to measure psychologic traits. Feldman and co-workers more recently observed that patients with ulcer had excessive dependency, lower ego strength, and hypochondriasis.[337] However, studies in patients in whom the diagnosis of duodenal ulcer disease was established endoscopically and with adequate control subjects (at least 50 subjects in each study arm) concluded that a number of emotional factors (e.g., anger, anxiety, unhappiness, emotional control, hostility) were not different between DU and normal subjects.[338,339]

In summary, there is no clearly established ulcer-type personality. Ulcer patients as a group tend to exhibit the same psychologic makeup as the general population. It is possible, but at present speculative, that the release of central nervous system (CNS) peptides may be influenced by certain psychologic factors; however, this requires study directly.

Pathology

PEPTIC ULCER

Benign peptic ulcers classically exhibit four layers or zones from surface to basal portion: (1) fibrinopurulent debris, (2) active cellular infiltration with neutrophils, (3) granulation tissue, and (4) collagenous scar (Fig 61-7; Color Fig 29).[340] By definition, ulcers extend below the muscularis mucosae; shallow lesions confined to the mucosa are called erosions. Ulcers that extend beyond the serosa are termed penetrating ulcer. The gastric or duodenal wall adjoining the ulcer crater is usually edematous and exhibits acute inflammation with neutrophilic infiltration. The superficial epithelium adjoining duodenal ulcers usually exhibits more gastric metaplasia (change of duodenal columnar epithelium to gastric-type surface mucous cells) than is observed in normal subjects. The muscularis mucosae and submucosa around ulcer craters are usually thickened. With healing, the edema and acute inflammation of the adjacent tissue improve, and epithelial cells migrate inward from the margins of the ulcer to cover the layer of granulation tissue. The basal fibrous zone contracts, diminishing the ulcer size but often resulting in a permanent scar.

GASTRITIS AND ULCER DISEASE

Most patients with duodenal ulcer disease have an associated, usually active, chronic antral gastritis (type B, see "Gastritis") but usually good preservation of the oxyntic (fundic) mucosa.[341-345] The pathogenesis of this antral gastritis has been unclear, although mounting evidence suggests that it is likely due to chronic *H. pylori* infection. It is interesting to note, however, that the

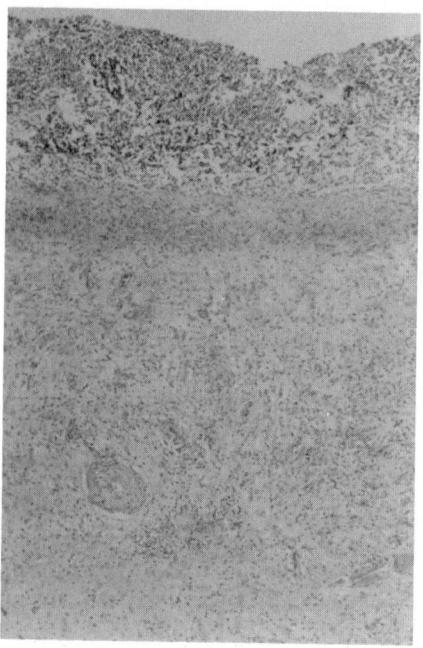

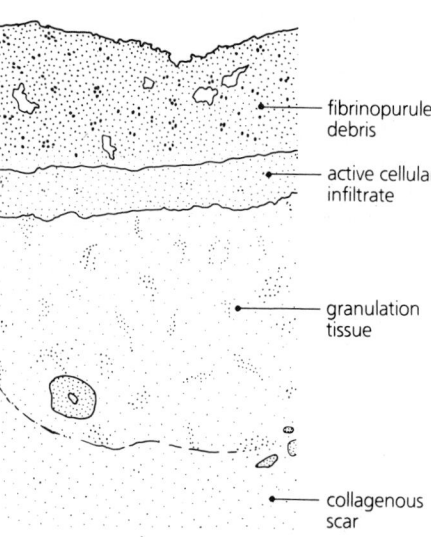

— fibrinopurulent debris

— active cellular infiltrate

— granulation tissue

— collagenous scar

FIGURE 61–7. (See Color Fig 29) The pathology of peptic ulcer. This ulcer crater shows the four classic zones of activity: fibrinopurulent debris, active cellular infiltrate with neutrophils, granulation tissue, and collagenous scar. Approximately 2.5×. (Mitros FA. Atlas of gastrointestinal pathology. Philadelphia: JB Lippincott, 1988: 3.15.)

gastritis has been reported to improve with healing of the ulcers, even when achieved with placebo therapy![344]

Gastric ulcers that are not associated with aspirin or other NSAID therapy almost always arise in the setting of type B chronic nonerosive atrophic gastritis.[346-354] Presumably the gastritis precedes the ulcer disease, predisposing the patient to ulcer development,[347,350,353,354] although this obligate sequence and implied causal relationship have not been clearly established. The gastric ulcers commonly develop near the junction of the antral gastritis and oxyntic mucosa, on the antral side, which is usually lined with pyloric or "pseudopyloric" type of epithelium. In about half the patients who develop gastric ulcers while chronically ingesting aspirin (and possibly other NSAIDs), the gastric mucosa appears normal and essentially free of gastritis.[355] This observation, reported in 1973, suggested even then that the pathogenesis of NSAID-associated gastric ulcers might be different from that of idiopathic ulcers.

DUODENITIS

Nonspecific or "peptic" duodenitis is characterized by acute and chronic inflammation of the duodenum, particularly the mucosa.[356-363] The lamina propria is infiltrated with increased numbers of plasma cells, lymphocytes, and occasionally eosinophils, and, in the case of acute or active duodenitis, with neutrophils as well. Neutrophils invade the superficial epithelium and occasionally even form crypt abscesses. The villous epithelium may exhibit degenerative changes and usually contains more gastric metaplasia (gastric surface mucous cells) than is normally observed. The villi may be shortened and edematous and their vessels may be congested, and the mucosal surface may be eroded and the crypts hyperplastic. Brunner's glands may be dilated and hyperplastic, and lymphoid hyperplasia—a prominence of lymph nodules in the submucosa and mucosa—may also be observed.

Duodenitis does not seem to be a common histologic finding in apparently healthy people.[364] Some increase in chronic inflammatory cells has been reported in about 12% of such people and neutrophilic infiltration in only about 4%.[364]

Acute duodenitis is observed adjacent to duodenal ulcers. Some patients, however, have more widespread duodenal inflammation.[365] With healing of the ulcers, this local inflammation often improves, but in many cases the active duodenitis persists.[365,366] Duodenitis, usually in association with antral gastritis, also occurs in patients without ulcers[343] and may precede the development of duodenal ulcers.[343,367,368] Is duodenitis in most patients secondary to the development of an ulcer or does duodenitis usually precede ulcer formation? Are duodenitis and ulcer two associated but independent pathologic processes? Today, the suspicion is that *H. pylori* infection may play an important role in the pathogenesis of both lesions, but even so, the sequences and interrelationships are uncertain.

Pathophysiology

DUODENAL ULCER

For 50 years, efforts have been made to understand the pathophysiologic abnormalities present in patients with duodenal ulcer diseases and, if possible, to apply these findings to the prevention or treatment. A simple formulation is that duodenal ulcer diseases result from an imbalance between aggressive and defensive factors. These factors, however, represent many separate constituents (e.g., genetic, environmental, infectious, or pathophysiologic), including some that are likely not yet identified.

Because DU disease is multifactorial, it is not surprising that no single pathophysiologic defect, or even a cluster of defects, is present in all DU patients. For example, at one extreme, about 10% of patients with gastrinoma and hypergastrinemia do not have ulcer disease (see ch 62), despite markedly increased gastric acid secretion.[369] Increased defensive factors likely prevent ulcer formation in this unique subset of Zollinger–Ellison patients, but the precise mechanism(s) involved is unknown.

The pathophysiology of DU diseases has been examined in selected, and usually relatively small, groups of ulcer and control subjects. In some studies, the criterion for DU was less strict than endoscopic documentation of ulcer, and in many studies potentially important factors such as age, smoking history, NSAID intake, ulcer duration and activity at the time of study, and so forth, were not controlled rigorously between ulcer and the control groups. It is not surprising, therefore, that discrepancies exist between studies because of the heterogeneity of DU disease itself as well as the heterogeneity of study populations.

In spite of these considerations, a series of pathophysiologic defects has been observed in DU patients (Fig 61-8).[370-372] There are a number of reasons to develop an understanding of the pathophysiology of DU. First, by understanding the pathophysiology, treatment modalities can be targeted to correct specific pathophysiologic defects. Second, definition of specific abnormalities and their prevalence could provide information that could identify subclinical DU disease. Third, specific pathophysiologic abnormalities may have an effect on the natural history or ulcer complication rate and therefore may serve to guide long-term therapy. The following section reviews the proposed defects in DU disease and attempts to place them in perspective.

Gastric Acid Secretion. Until recently, the focus of duodenal ulcer pathogenesis was directed largely at gastric acid and pepsin secretion. This was based on logical premises. About 40 years ago, it was observed that the gastric mucosa (i.e., the acid-secreting portion) was abnormally "thick" in about 20% of DU patients at surgery (clearly a selected population) and that the parietal cell number determined in autopsy tissue was greater in DU patients than in normal subjects.[373] However, there is about a two-thirds overlap between DU parietal cell number and that of the control group (Fig 61-9).[374] Why does DU develop in a patient when his/her total parietal cell mass is identical to the average of normal subjects, and, conversely, why does a control subject fail to develop ulcer disease when his/her parietal cell mass approaches the maximal observed in the DU group? The answer is likely because of the heterogeneity of DU diseases and the interplay between defensive, genetic, infectious, environmental, and other factors.

Parietal cell number/mass correlates with maximal stimulated gastric acid secretion.[375] Therefore, DU patients, as a group, secrete greater amounts of acid and pepsin at rest and in response to secretory stimulants including histamine, pentagastrin, and food.[370] As anticipated by the overlap in parietal cell number, there is also a large overlap in acid and pepsin secretion between DU and normal subjects, with only about one third of DU patients exceeding the upper limits of normal. However, there is a threshold in parietal cell number (about 1 billion cells/stomach) and maximal

Pathophysiologic Abnormalities in DU Vary in Frequency

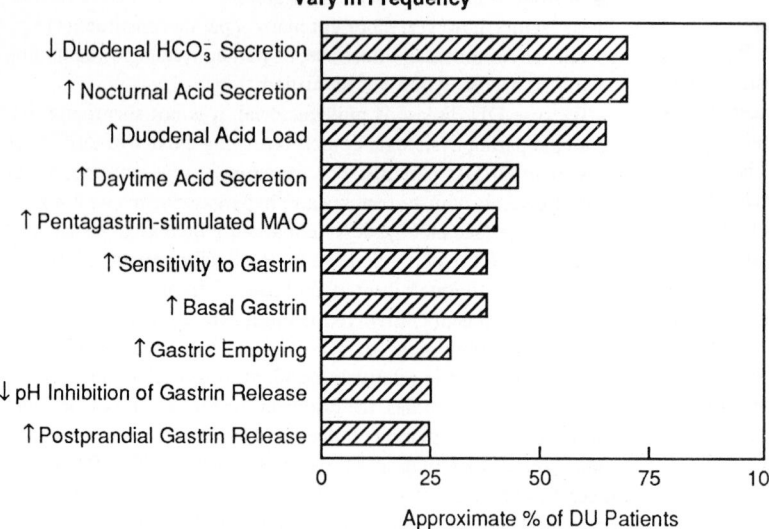

FIGURE 61–8. Pathophysiologic abnormalities in patients with duodenal ulcer vary in frequency. This figure depicts approximate percentages of duodenal ulcer patients with some of the abnormalities that have been described. It should be emphasized that these data come from many separate studies with different experimental conditions and patient populations. They are therefore meant to represent approximations of these abnormalities; for example, approximately 70% of duodenal ulcer patients have decreased proximal duodenal mucosal bicarbonate and/or increased nocturnal acid secretion.

histamine- or pentagastrin-stimulated acid output (about 10 mmol/h) below which duodenal ulcer does not occur.

The emphasis of DU pathogenesis was guided further toward acid/pepsin secretion by the fact that, until recently, the treatment of duodenal ulcer relied upon drugs and surgical procedures that decreased gastric acid and pepsin secretion. Only recently has it been recognized that 40% to 50% of patients with active DU heal in response to placebo treatment within 1 month, presumably in the absence of any changes in inherent acid/pepsin secretion. Elements other than secretory factors must be involved with ulcerogenesis and ulcer healing.

Basal Acid Output. Basal acid output (i.e., gastric acid secretion conventionally measured after an overnight fast for 1 hour in the absence of any stimulation [see ch 129]) tends to be related loosely to maximal secretory capacity. Because DU patients

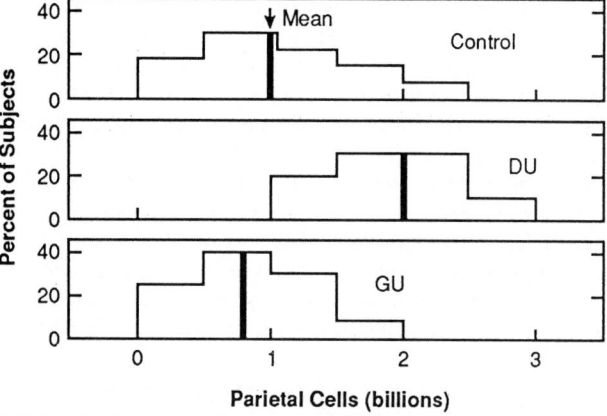

FIGURE 61–9. Mean parietal cell number in control (i.e., healthy) subjects, patients with duodenal ulcer (DU), and patients with gastric ulcer (GU). Note that while the mean (the broad vertical line) is about twofold greater in DU versus control, there is about a 66% overlap. Also, DU does not occur with less than about 1 billion parietal cells. GU patients are very similar to controls. (Modified with permission from Cox AJ. Stomach size and its relation to chronic peptic ulcer. Arch Pathol 1952;54:407.)

have an increased parietal cell mass, it is not surprising that DU patients as a group have an increased basal acid output (BAO) (Fig 61-10). In an analysis of seven separate studies, Lam observed that 10% to 40% of DU patients had an abnormal increase in BAO. When the BAO was normalized (BAO/MAO) for maximal acid output (MAO), 10% to 20% were beyond the normal range.[370] Therefore, basal acid output is increased in DU patients as a group, but, as with parietal cell number, there is a marked overlap with normal. The specific mechanism(s) responsible for increased basal acid output is not known.

An increase in interprandial or nocturnal acid secretion is probably more important than basal acid output.[376] Human gastric acid secretion follows a diurnal pattern, possibly related to circulating serum gastrin,[377] with the maximal secretion occurring in the late evening and early morning hours. It was recognized 40 years ago that nocturnal acid secretion was elevated in the majority of patients with DU[378–380]; this was attributed by Dragstedt to increased vagal "tone."[381] The finding of increased nocturnal acid secretion in DU has been the subject of recent interest because of its therapeutic implications.

With the refinement of small pH electrodes that can be positioned in the stomach without great inconvenience to the subject, recent studies have examined 24-hour gastric acidity (i.e., hydrogen ion concentration). Because secretory volumes are not collected, acid outputs are not measured by this technique. The integrated 24-hour acidity is greater in DU patients, but, as with other measures of gastric acid secretion, there is substantial overlap with normals.

Some, but not all, studies have observed an increased basal acid output/peak acid output (BAO/PAO) ratio.[382,383] An increase in the BAO/PAO ratio has been attributed to an increase in vagal "tone,"[384] although this explanation remains untested and speculative because vagal "tone" cannot be directly measured. Pancreatic polypeptide (PP) has been proposed as a measure of vagal-cholinergic activity, but no consistent abnormalities in PP secretion have been reported in DU patients.[385] Because (1) vagal-cholinergic stimulation is a potent stimulant of gastric acid secretion, (2) the release of some CNS peptides can alter gastric secretion by way of the vagus, and (3) vagotomy usually results in ulcer

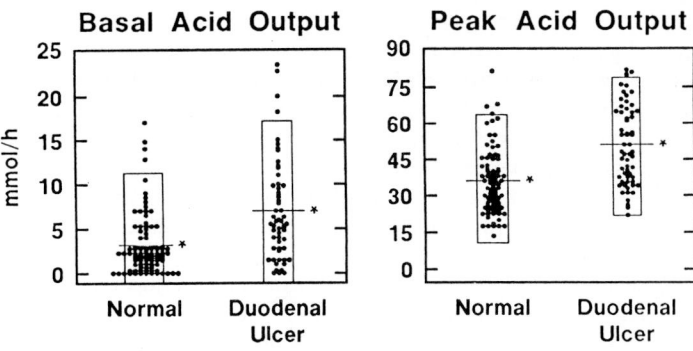

Boxes indicate ± 2 SDs, * Indicates means

FIGURE 61-10. Individual data points for basal and peak meal-stimulated gastric acid secretion in normal subjects and patients with duodenal ulcer. Although the mean (indicated by the horizontal line and the asterisk) is significantly greater in the duodenal ulcer patients, there is a marked overlap between populations. (Modified with permission from Blair AJ III, Feldman M, Barnett C, et al. Detailed comparison of basal and food-stimulated gastric acid secretion rates and serum gastrin concentrations in duodenal ulcer patients and normal subjects. J Clin Invest 1987;79:582.)

healing, it is attractive to incriminate vagal factors in DU pathogenesis. At this time, however, such a conclusion would be premature.

In summary, basal and nocturnal gastric acid secretion is, on average, increased in DU patients compared with normal subjects. The pathophysiologic explanation for this finding is not known. However, recent observations indicate that pharmacologic suppression of nocturnal acidity is more important than inhibition of acid secretion during the daytime in expediting ulcer healing (see Ulcer Treatment). Future studies on nocturnal acid secretion may provide information that will prove useful in a better understanding of the natural history of DU diseases.

Histamine and Pentagastrin Acid Secretion. In years past, histamine salts or synthetic analogues (e.g., betazole) were used to determine maximal acid output (MAO). Pentagastrin (Peptavlon), a synthetic analogue containing the C-terminal five amino acids of gastrin,[386] produces similar secretory responses without the untoward effects of histamine.[387] Because MAO is directly related to parietal cell mass, DU patients as a group have a greater MAO, but the overlap with normals is considerable. In a survey of 17 worldwide studies, Lam reported that the percentage of DU patients with an MAO or peak acid output (PAO) greater than the upper limits of normal ranged from 17% to 56%, with an average of 32%.[370] Therefore, as with parietal cell mass, only about one third of DU patients have an abnormally large secretory capacity.

Meal-Stimulated Acid Output. Meal-stimulated gastric acid secretion involves many interacting neural and humoral stimulatory and inhibitory events, and the response in DU patients is conflicting. Most studies report an increased meal-stimulated response in about 60% of DU patients.[370] Feldman and co-workers[388] recently failed to observe any substantial differences in peak meal-stimulated responses in a large group of DU subjects, although peak pentagastrin-stimulated acid output was significantly greater. Malagelada and colleagues observed that the duration of the secretory responses, rather than increased peak meal-stimulated acid secretory responses, tends to be prolonged (Fig 61-11).[389] This may explain the greater interprandial acid secretion observed in DU.

Sensitivity to Gastrin. A number of studies have examined whether the parietal cells in patients with DU are more sensitive to exogenous gastrin, its analogue pentagastrin, or to endogenous gastrin release.[390,391] It was postulated that although gastric acid secretion overlaps between DU and normal subjects,

the parietal cells of DU patients may exhibit an increased responsiveness, or sensitivity, to small doses of gastrin compared with normal subjects. This in turn would shift the dose-response curve to the left.

As in other areas involving pathophysiology of DU, the data are conflicting. Some reports indicate that 25% to 45% of DU patients demonstrate an increased sensitivity to exogenous pentagastrin, while others fail to observe any differences.[370] In a series of 200 DU patients in Hong Kong, Lam reported that hypersecretor patients who developed ulcer at an earlier age were more sensitive to pentagastrin than those hypersecretors who developed ulcer at later ages; among normosecretors, the late-onset DU patients were more sensitive.[392] Also, Lam and colleagues observed an increased sensitivity to endogenously released (meal-stimulated) gastrin.[393]

In summary, as with other pathophysiologic measures, the data are conflicting but suggest that some, but not all, DU patients have an increased responsiveness to circulating gastrin.

Gastrin. The increased gastric acid secretory drive and response to a protein meal could theoretically be explained by either a greater release of gastrin or the release of more potent or longer-acting molecular form (see ch 13). In humans, the 17- and 34-amino-acid-length gastrins predominate as the main circulating forms, G17 being in highest concentration in the gastric antrum and G34 being predominately in the duodenum.[394] The literature is conflicting regarding basal and postprandial gastrin concentra-

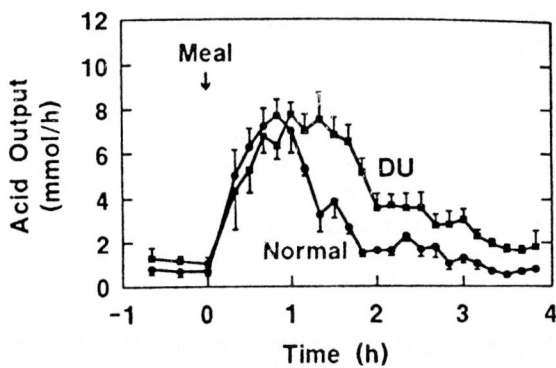

FIGURE 61-11. Although the acid secretory response in DU is similar to that in normal subjects in some studies, the duration of meal-stimulated gastric acid secretion is prolonged. (Reproduced with permission from Malagelada J, Longstreth GF, Deering TB, et al. Gastric secretion and emptying after ordinary meals in duodenal ulcers. Gastroenterology 1977;73:989.)

tions as well as antral gastrin content. Most have found resting plasma gastrins to be similar in DU and normal subjects.[395,396] Postprandial hypergastrinemia has been observed in some European studies, while most studies in the United States have not observed this finding.[394] Also, some have reported an increase in antral gastrin or a decrease in somatostatin stores, yet others have not.[397] At present, there is no established evidence for a primary change in either gastrin or somatostatin in patients with duodenal ulcer disease.

There is a rare syndrome of antral gastrin cell hyperfunction (also referred to as gastrin cell hyperplasia).[398] This may be familial and associated with DU, increased levels of fasting, and most particularly postprandial serum gastrin. It is rare, occurring in less than 0.1% of DU patients. It is diagnosed by the combination of fasting and marked postprandial hypergastrinemia, usually with gastric acid hypersecretion and a negative secretin provocative test (see ch 62).

Inhibitors of Gastric Secretion. Fat is a potent inhibitor of gastric acid secretion (see ch 13). Substitution of lipid for carbohydrate in a protein-containing meal resulted in a similar inhibitory effect on acid secretion in DU and normal subjects.[399,400]

Duodenal acidification releases secretin, a potent inhibitor of gastric acid secretion (see ch 2 and 13). An impaired duodenal acid feedback mechanism could result in diminished secretin release, decreased pancreatic bicarbonate secretion, and less inhibition of gastric acid secretion. Studies to examine the effects of duodenal acidification on these events in DU and normal subjects have not revealed any differences, indicating that duodenal acidification in DU releases secretin and stimulates the pancreas normally.[401] Furthermore, exogenous secretin reduced meal-stimulated gastric acid secretion similarly in DU and normal subjects.[402] In summary, fat- and acid-induced duodenal-to-gastric neurohumoral inhibitory events appear to be unaltered in DU.

Gastric Emptying. Increased entry of acid into the duodenum (duodenal acid load) could result from an increase in acid secretion, an increase in gastric emptying, or both. Early studies reported that liquid meals tended to empty more rapidly in DU patients.[403,404] More recent studies have revealed increased rates of gastric emptying in some, but not all, DU patients.[405] Lam and colleagues and Williams and colleagues reported that an acidified meal emptied more rapidly in DU patients compared with normal subjects.[406,407] Moreover, a few family pedigrees have been reported with the combination of increased rates of gastric emptying and DU.[408]

Again, and as with other reported pathophysiologic findings, it appears that some DU patients have increased rates of gastric emptying while many do not. In those with rapid emptying of gastric contents, duodenal acidification after a meal will be greater because the meal's buffering effect will leave the stomach rapidly, thereby permitting unbuffered acid to continue to enter the duodenum (Fig 61-12).[389,406]

Duodenal pH. Measurement of duodenal pH is fraught with methodologic problems. Although placement of a sensor (either an aspirator or pH probe) into the duodenal bulb is quite easy, it is not possible to assure that it will remain in place over prolonged periods of study. In addition, pH probes can come in contact with the duodenal mucosa, thereby recording juxtamucosal, rather than luminal, pH. Aspiration tubes can inadvertently result in collection of secretions from the more distal duodenum (i.e.,

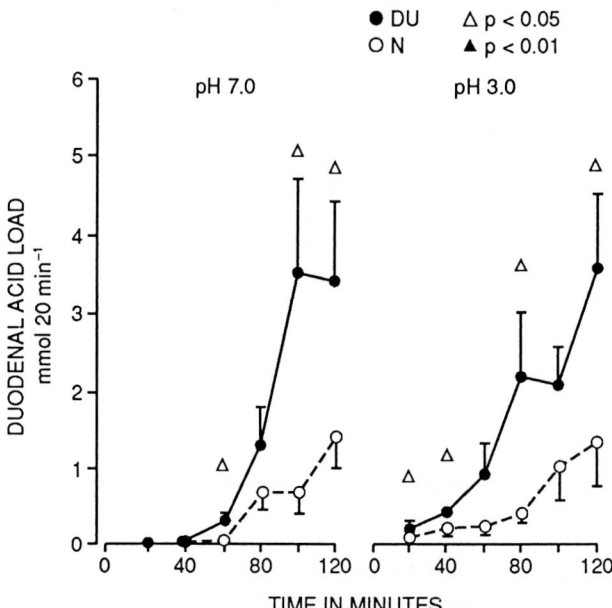

FIGURE 61–12. Duodenal acid load after intragastric instillation of protein meals at pHs 7 and 3 in patients with DU (solid lines and circles) and normals (N, open circles and dashed lines). Note the greater duodenal acid load at both pHs 7 and 3 in the DU group. As with other pathophysiologic abnormalities, there is a substantial overlap between groups. (Modified with permission from Lam SK, Isenberg JI, Grossman MI, et al. Rapid gastric emptying in duodenal ulcer patients. Dig Dis Sci 1982;27:598.)

near the entrance of the pancreatic ducts) or the stomach rather than the duodenal bulb.

Because of these methodologic difficulties, it is not surprising that the results of such studies are conflicting. Rune and co-workers attached multiple pH probes to include the stomach and duodenum and observed no significant differences in either bulbar or postbulbar duodenal pH between DU and control subjects.[409] Others, however, have reported that the duodenal bulb was more acidic in DU patients than in normals.[410,411] Of interest, when luminal and juxtamucosal pH is measured by passing a pH probe under direct vision through the biopsy channel of an endoscope, DU patients have a lower luminal and juxtamucosal pH both at rest and after luminal acidification.[412]

If gastric acid plays an important role in DU pathogenesis, one would anticipate that the pH in the duodenal bulb would be lower in DU patients. However, the pH, or acid/pepsin load, at which ulcerogenesis begins likely varies from patient to patient. This would explain why some gastrinoma patients, with massive acid hypersecretion and an acidic duodenum, can be ulcer-free and why some DU patients develop ulcer with perfectly normal rates of acid secretion and gastric emptying.

Duodenal Defense Factors. There are a number of elements that contribute to the capacity of the duodenum to withstand injury, as well as reparative processes that can result in prompt mucosal restitution.[413,414] Because the so-called aggressive factors are only modestly different between DU and normal subjects, attention recently has been focused on the proximal duodenum, the site of ulcer formation.

Mucus–Bicarbonate Layer. The gastrointestinal epithelium secretes a layer of water-insoluble mucus that overlies

FIGURE 61–13. There is a layer of mucus that overlies the gastroduodenal mucosa. This provides a barrier against the diffusion of acid (H+) from the lumen to the mucosa. The surface epithelial cells secrete bicarbonate into the base of this barrier. The right panel depicts the pH gradient as measured by a micro pH electrode passed from the stomach gradually into the mucus–bicarbonate barrier. Note that the lumenal pH is about 1.3 while the pH immediately adjacent to the surface cell is near 7.0. (Modified with permission from Flemstrom G, Kivilaakso E. Demonstration of a pH gradient at the luminal surface of rat duodenum in vivo and its dependence on mucosal alkaline secretion. Gastroenterology 1983;84:787.)

Mucus–Bicarbonate Barrier

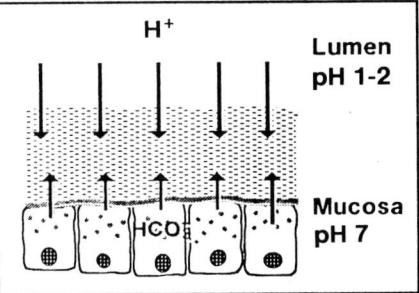

pH Gradient from Lumen to Epithelial Cell

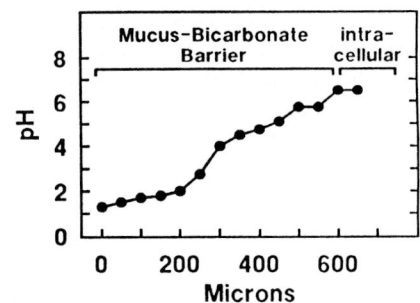

the mucosa.[415] Mucus contains about 95% water and 5% glycoproteins, which modestly impedes (about fourfold compared with water) the movement of hydrogen ion.[416] Mucus itself has little buffering capacity; it mainly serves as an unstirred water layer and the matrix into which surface epithelial bicarbonate is secreted (Fig 61-13). Surface mucus is dynamic, undergoing continuous renewal. Under normal circumstances, mucus is permeable to Vitamin B_{12} (MW=1350) but not to myoglobin (MW=17,500). Therefore, the permeation of pepsins with a molecular weight of approximately 35,000 is inhibited by mucus. However, pepsins are able to dissolve mucus by degrading the disulfide bridges in the regions of the protein core, and the resultant lower-molecular-weight subunits have a low viscosity and do not form a gel.[417] The thickness of gastric mucus as measured by a slit lamp is approximately 100 μm.[418] Preliminary data suggest that some patients with both gastric and duodenal ulcer have a mucus gel covering the mucosa that is somewhat structurally "weaker" than that of normal subjects.[419] The mechanism of this is unknown, but it has been postulated to be due to an increase in secretion of pepsin I, which digests mucus more readily than other forms of pepsin. There remain many unanswered questions regarding mucus secretion, its synthesis and degradation, and its role in ulcer diseases.

Mucosal Bicarbonate. The surface epithelial cells of the gastrointestinal mucosa are capable of transporting and/or synthesizing bicarbonate.[420] Bicarbonate, likely in association with sodium, enters immediately adjacent to the apical cell membrane and at the base of the mucus barrier. Therefore, in the stomach there is a pH gradient from the lumen to the apical cell membrane (Fig 61-13).[421] A few important observations regarding gastroduodenal mucosal bicarbonate secretion include: (1) proximal

duodenal mucosal bicarbonate secretion at rest is approximately twofold greater than bicarbonate secretion by the entire stomach, (2) there is a steep bicarbonate gradient from the proximal duodenum to the distal duodenum, (3) potent agonists of bicarbonate secretion include prostaglandins of the A and E class, luminal acidification, and some gastrointestinal hormones (e.g., vasoactive intestinal polypeptide [VIP]), and (4) epithelial bicarbonate secretion is inhibited by cyclooxygenase inhibitors (e.g., indomethacin), suggesting that endogenous prostaglandin production plays a role in maintaining basal bicarbonate production.[420]

In active duodenal ulcer disease, bicarbonate production by the duodenal bulb is markedly diminished compared with normal subjects both at rest and in response to luminal acidification (Fig 61-14).[421] However, resting and acid-stimulated bicarbonate production in the distal duodenum are comparable. In contrast to other pathophysiologic defects, there is less overlap (about one fourth) between ulcer and normal subjects. The mechanism of this defect, whether cause or effect, is currently under investigation. It is of interest, however, that PGE_2, a potent agonist of gastroduodenal bicarbonate production, produces significantly less bicarbonate production in inactive DU patients, suggesting a cellular or subcellular defect in bicarbonate secretion.[422] Moreover, histologic evaluation of the duodenum in inactive duodenal ulcer patients fails to reveal any striking morphologic differences from normal subjects to account for decreased mucus or bicarbonate secretion.[423]

Restitution. Under normal circumstances, the gastric mucosa, as well as the duodenal mucosa, undergoes prompt (within 15 to 30 minutes) restitution following injury.[413,414] Mucosal restitution, or reconstitution, involves the movement of surface ep-

FIGURE 61–14. Proximal and distal duodenal mucosal bicarbonate secretion in duodenal ulcer and normal subjects. Note that proximal duodenal mucosal bicarbonate secretion is significantly impaired in duodenal ulcer patients compared with normals, while distal duodenal mucosal bicarbonate production is similar in both. Also of note is the gradient from proximal to distal duodenum in the normal subjects. (Reproduced with permission from Isenberg Jl, et al. N Engl J Med 1987;316:374.)

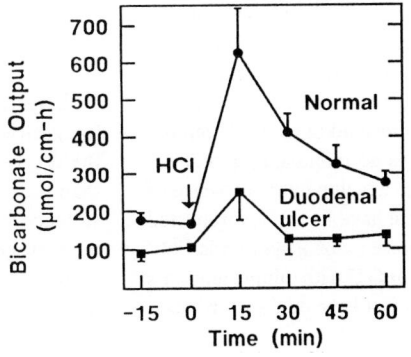

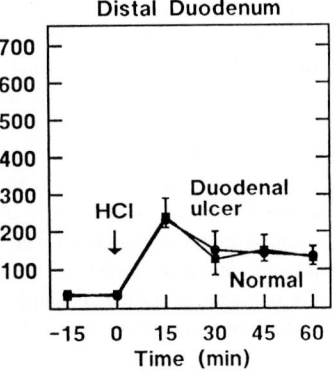

ithelial cells from the crypts upward along the basement membrane to cover the damaged epithelium. This process does not require cell division. Furthermore, recent evidence suggests that even individual cells are capable of undergoing cellular restitution.[424] That is, after damage, individual cells promptly restore wounded cell membranes. All the cellular and subcellular factors that regulate mucosal and cellular restitution are not yet established. However, this phenomenon likely explains the rapid repair that occurs in humans following superficial mucosal damage produced by drugs, ethanol, bile salts, and so forth.

GASTRIC ULCER

Although the pathophysiology of duodenal ulcer disease is far from being totally understood, the pathophysiology of the gastric ulcer disease not associated with NSAIDs is even less well understood. This section deals with idiopathic gastric ulcers, i.e., those which develop independent of an established exogenous cause such as NSAIDs. It is estimated that idiopathic gastric ulcers account for only about one fifth to one third of total gastric ulcer disease.[425]

Johnson has divided idiopathic gastric ulcers into three separate types: type I is represented by ulcers occurring in the body of the stomach and not associated with other gastroduodenal disease; type II ulcers are also located in the body of the stomach and are associated with a duodenal ulcer scar or active ulcer; and type III ulcers are located in the immediate prepyloric area and have pathophysiologic features similar to those of duodenal ulcer disease.[425]

Gastritis and Gastric Acid Secretion. Most gastric ulcers are localized to an area of about 2 cm in length on the antral side of the junction of the antral and oxyntic gland mucosas along the lesser curvature. There is usually widespread superficial gastritis involving the area around the ulcer as well as the gastric antrum (chronic superficial often atrophic antral gastritis).[426] Antral gastritis is prominent early in the history of gastric ulcer disease, and it progresses proximally to involve the oxyntic gland mucosa, sometimes proceeding on to gastric atrophy.[427] In fact, high lesser curvature ulcers, which would be expected to reside in oxyntic gland mucosa, are instead located in antral gland mucosa that has undergone metaplasia from oxyntic to antral gland mucosa.

The pathogenesis of the antral gastritis is not fully understood. It may be secondary to diminished pyloric tone, with reflux of noxious duodenal contents (e.g., bile acids, lysolecithin, and so forth) into the gastric antrum causing damage to the normal gastric mucosal barrier, leading to development of gastritis and in some cases ulcer.[428] However, with the recent documentation of *H. pylori*'s ability to produce chronic active gastritis, the role of this microorganism in gastric ulcer pathogenesis requires careful study.

Basal and stimulated gastric acid secretion in GU patients is, as a group, within normal limits. However, in contrast to DU patients, in whom there is an MAO threshold of about 10 mmol/h for ulcers to develop, in GU there is no minimal secretory response before ulceration occurs; ulcers develop in the presence of minimal amounts of acid. In fact, there have been a few reported patients with documented GU in the presence of achlorhydria.[429,430] The explanation for the development of GU with minute amounts of acid/pepsin is not known, but it is likely due to a marked impairment of gastric mucosal defensive factors. GU healing in some patients is unresponsive to standard doses of antiulcer drugs and may require larger doses with greater suppression of acid secretion. This suggests that the stomach, similar to the esophagus, in some GU patients is exquisitely sensitive to the presence of luminal acid.

Motility Abnormalities. Resting and acid- and fat-stimulated pyloric sphincter pressures may be diminished in small groups of patients with gastric ulcer.[431] It has been postulated that pyloric sphincteric dysfunction in GU permits a greater reflux of duodenal contents into the stomach, a phenomenon confirmed with barium studies.[432] Increased amounts of bile and lysolecithin have been reported in the stomachs of patients with GU.[433] Lysolecithin is particularly damaging to lipid membranes and may play a role in the altered mucosal permeability.

Gastric emptying and motility, particularly of solids, have also been reported to be abnormal in GU patients.[434,435] This is not surprising because the presence of an ulcer extending into the muscularis of the antrum would likely alter muscular function of the gastric antrum. Whether these effects are involved in pathogenesis or are secondary to the ulcer itself requires further study.

Duodenogastric Reflux. Bile acids (particularly deoxycholic acid), lysolecithin, and pancreatic peptidases are potential gastric mucosal damaging agents. With the use of various types of markers (e.g., barium, nonabsorbable markers, and ^{99m}Tc-EDTA), greater amounts of duodenogastric reflux have been observed in GU versus normal subjects both fasting and following a meal. It is difficult to know whether or not these findings represent cause or are secondary events. However, because they tend to persist after ulcer healing, they may serve as one of many factors in gastric ulcer pathogenesis.

These observations need to be balanced with the findings that patients with gastroenterostomies and copious amounts of duodenogastric reflux often have superficial gastritis (particularly surrounding the anastomosis) yet do not commonly develop gastric ulcers. Furthermore, gastric ulcer healing is not expedited with the bile salt–binding agent cholestyramine.[436]

Gastric Mucosal Barrier. The gastric mucosa, compared with the small intestine, is a "tight" epithelium resistant to the diffusion of hydrogen ion from the lumen.[437] The anatomic counterparts of this barrier are not fully defined but are likely due to cellular structures (i.e., the luminal cell membrane), tight junctions between surface cells, intracellular pH, and extracellular events (i.e., the pH/mucus barrier, mucosal blood flow, arterial pH, and so forth). In animals and humans, this barrier can be damaged by luminal agents (ethanol, NSAIDs, bile salts, and so forth).[438] Although *H. pylori* causes gastritis, it is not known if it also causes functional damage.

Mucosal Blood Flow. Gastric ulcers tend to occur near the gastric angulus, an area of prominent muscle bundles where the mucosa is directly supplied by the left gastric artery, rather than through a rich submucosal plexus like the remainder of the stomach.[454] Mucosal blood flow has been reported to be decreased in small groups of gastric ulcer patients.[455] It is possible that diminished blood flow may serve as a cofactor and may contribute to the ulceration.

NONSTEROIDAL ANTI-INFLAMMATORY DRUG–INDUCED MUCOSAL INJURY AND ULCERS

NSAID-induced mucosal injury can arbitrarily be divided into the effects of acute versus chronic ingestion. In a series of seminal experiments, Davenport and colleagues[439] reported that bathing the canine gastric mucosa with acidified aspirin resulted in a marked decrease in electrical potential difference (P.D.; a semi-quantitative measure of mucosal injury), back-diffusion of hydrogen ion from the gastric lumen into the mucosa, and the reciprocal entry of sodium into the gastric lumen. Prolonged or repeated exposure resulted in mucosal hemorrhage. These types of experiments have been reproduced with slight variations in a host of mammalian species, including humans.[440]

The observations in humans can be summarized as follows: The acute ingestion of aspirin (or other NSAIDs) in healthy volunteers, on a daily basis for 5 to 14 days, results in endoscopic evidence of mucosal injury (e.g., erythema, submucosal hemorrhage, superficial erosions, and rarely ulceration), a decrease in transmucosal P.D., and in many patients an increase in fecal blood loss.[440–442] Short-term (i.e., less than 2 weeks) aspirin intake results in acute gastric mucosal damage in 70% to 100% of subjects.[443] Some of the newer NSAIDs (e.g., ibuprofen) may cause less acute mucosal injury than aspirin, but all are capable of producing dose-dependent chronic mucosal injury,[444–446] including enteric-coated aspirin.

The major area of injury is the gastric antrum. Initially, NSAIDs were considered to limit their injury to the stomach.[447] However, recent endoscopic surveys in patients receiving NSAIDs both for short courses and chronically indicate that they also result in mucosal damage to the duodenum.[448,449] Unfortunately, there is no direct relationship between the acute endoscopic findings and the risk of developing potential life-threatening chronic lesions (e.g., ulcers, hemorrhage, perforation).[450] It is therefore not possible to extrapolate from short-term studies in healthy subjects which NSAIDs are most likely to cause severe upper gastrointestinal injury. For example, although some NSAIDs produce only minor injury relative to aspirin during acute studies, they often result in a greater degree of injury during chronic therapy.[451]

In a minority of patients (estimated at about 30%), continued NSAID intake after 1 to 2 weeks is followed by a decrease in mucosal injury.[452,453] The mechanism of this "adaptation" is not understood and tends to occur with modest doses, and it is not possible to determine prospectively in whom it will occur.

The mechanism responsible for NSAID-induced chronic mucosal injury is attributed in largest part to NSAID inhibition of cyclooxygenase, the key enzyme in the synthesis of prostaglandins.[292] Therefore, NSAIDs cause a significant decrease in mucosal prostaglandin content.[293] Prostaglandins of the E and A class protect the gastroduodenal mucosa, likely because of a number of effects (i.e., stimulation of mucus and bicarbonate secretion, increasing mucosal blood flow, and decreasing mucosal cell turnover).[294,295]

The late distinguished gastroenterologist–physiologist Morton I. Grossman said that aspirin has a one–two punch—a direct topical damaging effect as well as a systemic effect. Aspirin, in the presence of gastric acid, is un-ionized and lipid-soluble because of its pKa of 3.5. Therefore, at an acidic gastric pH, aspirin diffuses across the gastric mucosa and becomes ionized within mucosal cells and within the lamina propria where the pH is near 7.4. This results

in cell injury; vascular damage with extravasation of leukocytes; release of histamine, leukotrienes, and chemotactic factors; production of superoxides; and impaired mucosal proliferation.[296,297]

How do other NSAIDs cause mucosal damage? Their pKas range widely, from 3.5 for tolmetin sodium, to 4.5 for indomethacin, and to 6.3 for piroxicam.[298] Mucosal injury is not related directly to pKa alone but also to lipid solubility (i.e., the ability to diffuse across the gastroduodenal mucosal surface cell membrane) as well as their relative potency in inhibiting prostaglandin synthesis. This important area requires further fundamental investigation.

Clinical Manifestations

PAIN

Near the turn of the century, Lord Moynihan stated that 90% of cases with dyspepsia could be diagnosed based upon symptoms alone.[456] Spiro has referred to patients with symptoms of classic peptic ulcer as having "Moynihan's disease."[457] Prior to upper gastrointestinal endoscopy, the diagnosis of duodenal ulcer relied upon the patient's symptoms and was "confirmed" by radiographic findings of either a scarred, spastic duodenal bulb or an ulcer crater. Unfortunately, although most patients with peptic ulcer disease have abdominal pain, epigastric pain is more commonly not due to ulcer.[458] Therefore, both the sensitivity (symptoms positive/disease positive) and the specificity (symptoms negative/disease negative) of abdominal pain as a marker for ulcer disease are low. In a large survey of patients in a special dyspepsia clinic, Crean and Spiegelhalter reported that abdominal pain was present in 94% of patients with ulcer but was also present in 82% of patients without ulcer.[456] However, the criteria used to establish the diagnosis of ulcer (endoscopic versus radiographic) were not defined.

Abdominal pain in patients with ulcer disease is often localized to the epigastrium, nonradiating, and relieved by food. The most discriminating symptom, but still far from perfect, is the presence of pain that awakens the patient from sleep, usually between 12 and 3 A.M.[459] This symptom is present in approximately two thirds of patients with duodenal ulcer and one third of patients with gastric ulcer, but it is also present in about one third of patients with nonulcer dyspepsia.[460]

In a group of U.S. patients with dyspepsia, one fourth had ulcer disease at endoscopy.[461] However, of those with "classic ulcer dyspepsia," 40% had an ulcer crater while an additional 40% had gastroduodenitis without a crater. This study suggests that careful questioning improves diagnostic accuracy slightly.[462] Moreover, in Scandinavia, the clinical diagnosis of peptic ulcer based upon symptoms and determined by endoscopy portrayed a 60% to 70% sensitivity and specificity.[463] This is distinctly higher than others; for example, in Peru, the prevalence of endoscopic ulcer disease (either active or inactive) was only 12% in patients with abdominal pain.[464] Furthermore, approximately 10% of patients with peptic ulcer disease present with ulcer complications without an antecedent history. It is unknown why patients develop acute perforation or hemorrhage from ulcer disease without antecedent symptoms (see ch 64). It is possible that they are insensitive to pain; or, more likely, ulcer disease can indeed develop in the absence of pain.

A related and not yet fully understood issue is the relationship of gastroduodenitis to ulcer disease and to ulcer pain. Patients with ulcer disease may be pain-free, and, conversely, patients with healed ulcer disease may have pain.[465,466] Patients with classic ulcer symptoms may also have gastroduodenitis. In a group of 100 patients with ulcer symptoms evaluated clinically, radiographically, and with endoscopy, including biopsies of the stomach and duodenum, three fourths had no evidence of an ulcer crater, yet approximately 40% had either gastritis, duodenitis, or gastroduodenitis.[467] Only 10% of those with classic ulcer symptoms had no endoscopic or histologic abnormalities, and in the 49 patients with classic ulcer symptoms, 24 had ulcer craters while 25 had gastroduodenitis. This suggests that gastroduodenitis can cause the symptoms that are indistinguishable from those of classic ulcer disease.

Regrettably, there is lack of agreement both endoscopically and histologically as to what constitutes normal and abnormal gastroduodenal mucosa.[468] Some endoscopists will diagnose "gastritis" or "duodenitis" based entirely upon the appearance of the mucosa alone. This is inappropriate because there is poor agreement between gross visual assessment of the mucosa and the histologic assessment.[469] To make matters even more complicated, there are also differences between pathologists regarding the interpretation of biopsy tissue.[470]

Mechanism of Abdominal Pain. Although abdominal pain is commonly considered a prerequisite for peptic ulcer disease, its genesis remains undefined. In a blinded prospective study in which solutions of varying pH from 0.85 to 7.0 were infused into the stomachs of patients with endoscopically documented active DU, there was no consistent association between the pH of the infusate and the production of pain.[471] More recently, in an unblinded study, direct duodenal infusions of hydrochloric acid induced pain in patients with duodenitis[472] and duodenal ulcer.[473] Of interest, infusion of acid caused pain in 40% of patients with an active symptomatic DU, while saline infusion resulted in ulcer-type pain in 10%. Other factors, such as pepsin, bile acids, and motility events, likely also contribute to the pain.

Pain Relief. In all clinical trials of peptic ulcer treatment, abdominal pain resolves promptly in patients treated with either an active drug or placebo.[466,474] The data, although conflicting, suggest that active treatment is somewhat superior to placebo. Furthermore, there are many patients who have nonhealed ulcers and are asymptomatic as well as patients who have healed ulcers and yet are symptomatic.

Summary and Clinical Implications of Pain. Abdominal pain, a frequent clinical symptom of ulcer disease, is likely caused by a number of different entities, some with a pathologic counterpart and others without. Unfortunately, it is not possible to diagnose peptic ulcer disease with any great degree of accuracy based upon symptoms alone. There are, however, some clinical clues to suggest ulcer disease: prior documented ulcer, nocturnal pain, family history of ulcer, and antacid or antiulcer drug intake with pain relief.[456]

The dilemma that confronts the clinician is what course to pursue in the patient with ulcer symptoms, i.e., should the patient be placed on a trial of medical therapy, or should a diagnostic workup with its inherent costs be initiated? This is discussed under Diagnosis.

COMPLICATIONS

Complications of peptic ulcer include: hemorrhage, perforation or penetration, and obstruction (ch 64). Intractability, which previously was considered a complication of ulcer disease, is becoming progressively uncommon with the availability of more effective antiulcer drugs.

Hemorrhage is the most common complication, occurring in approximately 20% of patients.[475] Although ulcer hemorrhage occurs at all ages, it tends to be more common in patients in the sixth decade and beyond. This is related in large part to the increased use of NSAIDs, particularly in elderly women.[476,477] Approximately 10% to 20% of patients will bleed from either a gastric or duodenal ulcer without any antecedent symptoms. Furthermore, approximately one third of patients will have recurrent episodes of hemorrhage.[475] The diagnosis and the medical and surgical management of gastrointestinal hemorrhage are discussed elsewhere (see ch 30, 64, and 134).

Ulcer perforation is less common than hemorrhage yet more common than obstruction. Perforation occurs in approximately 7% of patients with peptic ulcer disease.[478] Duodenal ulcers tend to perforate anteriorly, while gastric ulcers perforate along the anterior wall of the lesser curvature of the stomach. Of note, with the increased use of NSAIDs, the incidence of perforation is increasing, particularly in women beyond the age of 60.

Penetration is similar pathologically to perforation except that the ulcer crater burrows through the entire wall of the intestine, and instead of leaking digestive contents into the peritoneal cavity, the crater bores into an adjacent viscus. Most commonly, gastric ulcers can penetrate into the left lobe of the liver, while duodenal ulcers penetrate into the adjacent pancreas. On rare occasions, gastric ulcers may penetrate into the colon, resulting in a gastrocolic fistula.

Gastric retention, commonly referred to as gastric outlet obstruction or "pyloric stenosis," can result from impaired antral motility due to the effects of acute inflammation and edema, or it can result from chronic fibrotic scarring near the gastroduodenal junction, a mechanical effect. The former tends to resolve with medical treatment, while the latter requires surgical or endoscopic (balloon dilatation) intervention. The prevalence of gastric retention is approximately 2% in patients with peptic ulcer disease. The symptoms of gastric retention tend to be insidious and can manifest themselves as gastroesophageal reflux, early satiety, weight loss, abdominal pain, and vomiting. As the degree of retention increases, the quantity of vomitus also increases, often containing food ingested 12 or more hours previously.

Diagnosis

ENDOSCOPY VERSUS RADIOGRAPHY

Prior to the 1960s, upper gastrointestinal endoscopy was performed with rigid and semirigid instruments.[479] Fiberoptic instruments were introduced in the late 1960s, followed by minute television chips in the 1980s (see ch 111). The instruments have become smaller and better tolerated by patients, and the optics have improved markedly. Upper gastrointestinal radiography has also been refined by the standard use of double-contrast techniques.[480]

The aim of any diagnostic test is to be both sensitive and specific, and therefore have a high diagnostic accuracy. Studies using double-contrast barium meals, for the most part, reveal equal accuracy between radiography and endoscopy in the diagnosis of ulcer (Table 61-7). Extrapolation of these studies to the conventional clinical practice is not warranted because both the radiography and endoscopy were performed by respective experts in each. Furthermore, such reports are biased in favor of endoscopy because this test is commonly used as the "gold standard." For example, lesions reported on x-ray, but not observed endoscopically, are assumed to be radiographic false positives, where indeed they may represent endoscopic false negatives (i.e., the ulcer was missed at endoscopy). With the current wide-angle instruments, visualization of the stomach and duodenum should be complete in almost all patients. However, in some series, up to 10% of duodenal ulcers have been missed by endoscopy.[481,482] Postbulbar duodenal ulcer disease can pose difficulty to the endoscopist if the lesion occurs in the distal part of the second portion of the duodenum or beyond. Lastly, the patient risk with endoscopy, although very small, is greater than that associated with radiography (see ch 111 and 114).

For the most part, although there is excellent agreement between endoscopy and double-contrast barium meal in the evaluation of patients with gastric ulcers,[479] radiography does not permit biopsies or cytologic brushings of the lesion in order to determine whether or not a gastric ulcer represents an ulcerating carcinoma.[483]

It was formerly thought that radiographic documentation of ulcer healing was an indication that the lesion was benign, although it is now clear that malignant ulcers may undergo partial as well as complete "healing."[484] Therefore, ulcer healing is not a reliable indicator of benignancy. Unfortunately, endoscopy with multiple biopsies of ulcerating lesions of the stomach is also imperfect in distinguishing gastric cancer from a benign ulcer. Approximately 4% of endoscopically and histologically benign ulcers are malignant on repeated examination.[485,486]

In summary, single-contrast radiographs of the stomach and duodenum are obsolete in the diagnosis of peptic ulcer disease. Double-contrast radiography performed by an experienced radiologist is comparable to upper GI endoscopy in diagnostic accuracy.[487] Endoscopy does permit simultaneous biopsy of gastric ulcers.

A DIAGNOSTIC APPROACH

A major tenet of the practice of medicine, that of establishing the precise diagnosis so that specific therapy can be prescribed, has been called into question when applied to patients with dyspepsia.[488,489] Most physicians prescribe highly effective antiulcer drugs without further investigation, and it is unusual in today's environment to encounter a patient with untreated dyspepsia. This approach has been endorsed in a recent policy statement by the American College of Physicians.[490] This policy of *treat first* is appropriate in the patient under the age of 40 with mild and intermittent epigastric symptoms but no other systemic symptoms, and without any evidence of ulcer complications. However, the therapeutic response should be evaluated to assure prompt symptomatic relief while on therapy as well as the absence of recurrence after therapy has been discontinued. In contrast, for the patient above the age of approximately 50 (those in whom symptoms have

TABLE 61-7
Diagnostic Accuracy of Upper Gastrointestinal Radiography Versus Upper Gastrointestinal Endoscopy

STUDY	TYPE OF MEAL	NUMBER OF PATIENTS IN STUDY	% AGREEMENT BETWEEN ENDOSCOPY AND RADIOLOGY	RADIOLOGIC FALSE NEGATIVES (%)
McColl, 1972	SCBM	330	66	11
Papp, 1973	SCBM	85	63	15
Barnes, et al, 1974	SCBM	50	60	10
Dellipiani, 1974	SCBM	248	60	21
Laufer, Mullens, and Hamilton, 1975	SCBM	175	78	11
	DCBM	65	94	3
Cumberland, 1975	SCBM	381	63	4
Moule, et al, 1975	SCBM	197	51	—
	DCBM	19	84	10
Salter, 1975	DCBM	414	80	4
Laufer, 1976	DCBM	225	93	5
Herlinger, Glanville, and Kreel, 1977	DCBM	50	82	6
Montagne, Moss, and Margulis, 1978	SC + DCBM	100	88–90	—
Knutson, et al, 1978	Not stated	453	77	3.5
Keto, et al, 1979	DCBM		90	7
Kiil and Anderson, 1980	SCBM	173	85	5
Miceli, et al, 1982	DCBM	214	98.5	1.5

SCBM, single-contrast barium meal; DCBM, double-contrast barium meal.
(Modified from Cotton PB, Shorvon PJ. Analysis of endoscopy and radiography in the diagnosis, follow-up and treatment of peptic ulcer disease. Clin Gastroenterol 1984;13:383.)

been of long duration, those with systemic symptoms [anorexia, weight loss, back pain, and so forth], or those in whom there is any suggestion of an occult malignancy or another disease process [e.g., pancreatic or biliary tract disease, and so forth]), the diagnosis should be established.

Which diagnostic procedure should be used? This depends, in large part, on the skill and experience of the personnel available. In a center in which there is superb GI radiography, this is a reasonable first course to pursue. However, because GI radiography is less emphasized than other imaging techniques (e.g., CT) among recent radiology trainees, the skills required to perform a thorough gastrointestinal study appear to be less than they were 10 to 20 years ago. In contrast, because the use of endoscopy has increased, the skills at performing thorough endoscopy have improved. In general, therefore, endoscopy is the preferred diagnostic test.

There is no justification for the *routine* use of one procedure followed by the other. There are instances, however, when a lesion (e.g., a gastric ulcer) that requires biopsy is observed on x-ray. Conversely, there can be endoscopic lesions (e.g., extrinsic displacement of the stomach or duodenum) that require radiographic studies. Therefore, the two procedures may, under certain circumstances, be complementary.

By tradition, endoscopy with biopsies has been considered the standard of practice in patients with gastric ulcer. However, with the increased intake of NSAIDs, the finding of a clearly benign-appearing gastric ulcer on x-ray in a 20-year-old patient with a history of recent NSAID intake doesn't necessarily warrant endoscopic examination with biopsies. However, all gastric ulcers should be observed until complete endoscopic healing because of the potential of an occult malignancy.[485,486]

Cost comparisons are complicated. Overall, the cost for upper GI endoscopy is approximately three to four times greater than the cost for upper GI radiography. However, some endoscopists are of the opinion that professional fees are excessive,[479] and this has led to the "screening endoscopy" at a cost similar to that of radiography. Additional cost:benefit studies are needed in patients with acid-peptic symptoms.

Pharmacology of Therapeutic Agents for Acid-Peptic Diseases

Prior to the 1970s, treatment of patients with acid-peptic diseases relied upon antacids, anticholinergics, and, in many centers, a bland diet and bed rest. Three important events that modified therapy occurred almost simultaneously: (1) the availability of fiberoptic endoscopy, (2) the recognition of the importance of randomized prospective double-blind controlled trials (RCTs) to determine the efficacy of treatment in medical diseases, and (3) the availability of the histamine H_2-receptor antagonist.

In the latter part of the 1970s, Peterson and co-workers reported that a large dose of a potent antacid (equivalent to a daily buffering capacity of 1000 mmol/d) resulted in approximately 80% of duodenal ulcers healing after 4 weeks of therapy compared with 45% of patients treated with an identical-appearing placebo.[491] Moreover, the first H_2-receptor antagonist, cimetidine, was introduced in the United States in 1977. The availability of a potent orally administered inhibitor of gastric acid secretion revolutionized the treatment of acid-peptic diseases. New and more potent H_2 blockers have been developed, and four are available for use in the United States at present: cimetidine, ranitidine, famotidine, and

nizatidine. Most recently, an H^+/K^+-ATPase inhibitor that blocks the final hydrogen ion transport process (omeprazole) has become available for gastrinoma patients and intractable esophagitis (see ch 55 and 62). Also, within the past 10 years, drugs that do not affect gastric acid secretion yet expedite ulcer healing with an efficacy comparable to antisecretory agents have become available. These include sucralfate and bismuth compounds (the latter not yet approved by the FDA). Finally, prostaglandin analogues of the E class, which have a moderate inhibitory effect on gastric acid secretion and also stimulate gastroduodenal mucus and bicarbonate secretion, are also available.

Both gastric and duodenal ulcer disease are chronic diseases with high recurrence rates. The recurrence rate of duodenal ulcer following complete healing and in the absence of maintenance therapy approaches 80% at 1 year, and the recurrence rate for gastric ulcer is equally high. Furthermore, gastric ulcers tend to recur sooner after healing.[888-890]

The goal of this section is not to review in detail the multitude of studies (well over 5000 clinical trials) that have been performed with these drugs. There are recent and comprehensive reviews that deal with these issues in great detail. Instead, this section will highlight important relevant information regarding the chemistry and pharmacokinetics, untoward effects, and therapeutic efficacy in the treatment of both acute gastric and duodenal ulcer. Prevention of ulcer recurrences and complications are also of primary importance and are reviewed here also.

The physiology of gastric acid secretion is reviewed elsewhere (ch 13). Briefly, the acid-secreting parietal cell contains receptors for histamine, gastrin, and acetylcholine on the basolateral membrane (Fig 61-15). Occupation of these receptors by an agonist results in the release of secondary messengers, cAMP or cytosolic calcium, that activate an array of intracellular protein kinases. These in turn activate the final common acid-secreting pump on the canalicular surface of the cell: the H^+/K^+-ATPase. The histamine receptor is of the H_2 class; hence, it is not blocked by conventional H_1-receptor antagonists but is blocked selectively and competitively by H_2-receptor antagonists.[492] Occupation of the H_2-receptor by histamine (released by adjacent histamine-containing cells) catalyzes by way of a G-protein, G_s, the production of cAMP by adenylate cyclase. Agonist occupation of the cholinergic (muscarinic, M1 subtype) or gastrin receptors stimulates acid secretion by a different mechanism: an increase in intracellular cytosolic ionized calcium, which, in turn, activates protein kinases. Of note, there appears to be a potentiating effect on acid secretion between agents activating the calcium pathway (acetylcholine and gastrin) and the cAMP pathway (histamine). Thus, receptor blockade of one pathway with an antagonist diminishes acid secretion in response to agents that are mediated through the alternative pathway.

H_2-RECEPTOR ANTAGONISTS

Structure. Of the thousands of compounds that have been developed and tested since the discovery of the first H_2-receptor antagonist, burimamide, in 1972,[493] four have been approved by the FDA for clinical use in the United States: cimetidine, ranitidine, famotidine, and nizatidine. A fifth, roxatidine,[494] is available elsewhere, and many others are in various stages of clinical and preclinical testing. These compounds share an aromatic ring system and a flexible side chain that is affixed to a polar, uncharged group (Fig 61-16). The precise structural requirements for H_2-receptor

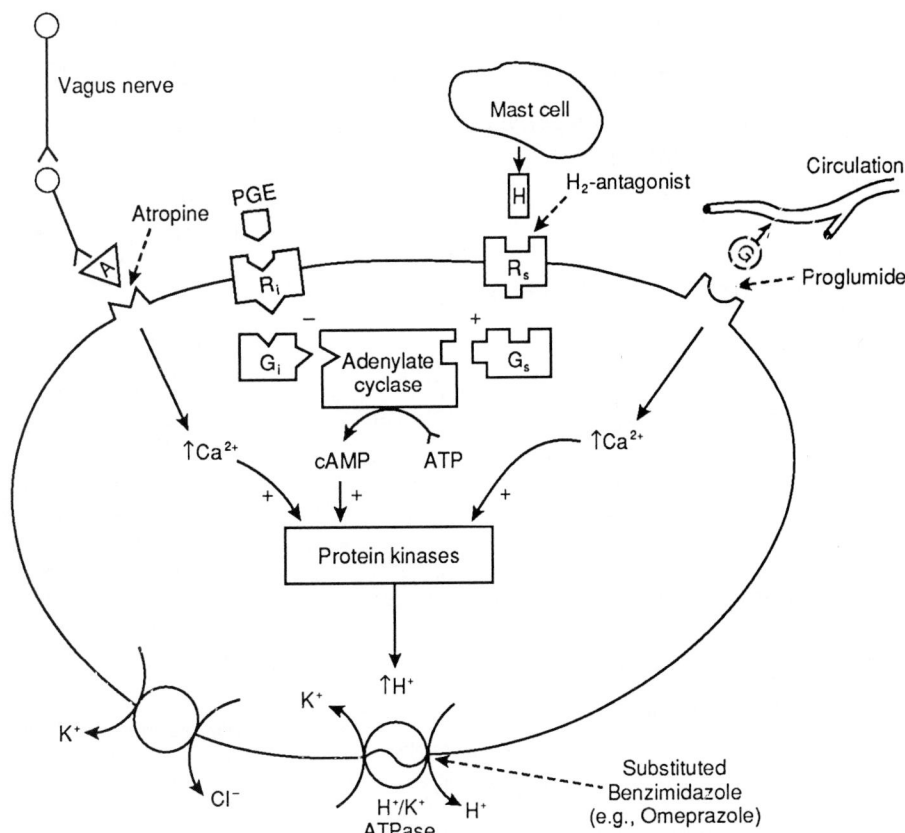

FIGURE 61–15. Schematic representation of a parietal cell, depicting pathways by which secretagogues stimulate acid secretion. Dashed arrows show sites of action of various inhibitors of acid secretion. *A,* acetylcholine; *H,* histamine; *PGE,* prostaglandins of E series; *G,* gastrin; G_i and G_r, inhibitory and stimulatory units of GTP-binding proteins (G proteins). (Wolfe MW, Soll AH. The physiology of gastric acid secretion. N Engl J Med 1988;319:1707.)

antagonism are not clear. Interestingly, several structural alterations have resulted in significant toxicity: oxmetidine (liver toxicity), metiamide (agranulocytosis), and tiotidine (gastric carcinoma).[495] If analogues with identical side chains are synthesized, the guanidino thiazole ring structure analogues (e.g., famotidine) have the highest receptor blocking activity, the aminomethyl furan ring structure analogues (e.g., ranitidine) have an intermediate activity, and the imidazole structure (cimetidine) has the lowest receptor blocking activity.[495]

Pharmacodynamics

Receptor Interactions. Currently available agents exhibit reversible competitive inhibition of histamine-stimulated acid secretion at the H_2-receptor in vivo.[495–501] That is, there is a dose-dependent shift to the right of histamine-stimulated acid secretion by H_2-antagonists without a suppression of the maximal acid secretory response. In vitro data from human gastric tissue indicate that famotidine has a slower onset of inhibition and dissociation from the receptor than cimetidine or ranitidine, suggesting some degree of noncompetitive inhibition; this may account for its longer half-life.[497,498] Very potent, extremely long-acting noncompetitive H_2-antagonists have been developed (loxtidine, lamitidine) but are not currently in clinical use.[495] None of the agents has any effects on the muscarinic, nicotinic, alpha, beta, gastrin, or H_1-receptors.[496,497]

Effects on Acid Secretion. In addition to their efficacy in inhibiting histamine-stimulated acid secretion, H_2-receptor antagonists also inhibit basal, sham-feed–, pentagastrin-, and meal-stimulated acid, volume, and pepsin secretion in a linear dose-dependent manner (Fig 61-17).[500–507] Up to 90% inhibition of

vagal- and gastrin-stimulated acid secretion occurs by histamine antagonists in a noncompetitive fashion and reflects the important role of histamine in potentiating the effects of cholinergic- and gastrin-stimulated secretion.[492] However, complete inhibition of pentagastrin- or meal-stimulated secretion has not been demonstrated with H_2-receptor antagonists.[503,505,508] On the basis of multiple pharmacologic studies, famotidine is 20 to 50 times more potent than cimetidine, and ranitidine is 4 to 8 times more potent than cimetidine on a molar basis. *Thus, equipotent oral doses are: famotidine 40 mg, ranitidine 300 mg, nizatidine 300 mg, and cimetidine 1200 to 1600 mg.*[496,497,498,509,510] However, increased potency does not necessarily confer a therapeutic advantage, providing that the drugs can be administered in equipotent doses without toxicity.

Perhaps more relevant are studies of oral dosing regimens of H_2-antagonists in which acid secretion and/or hydrogen ion [H^+] activity (pH) is measured over 24 hours in ambulatory subjects on a normal diet. A variety of formulations at various doses and dosing regimens have been tested.[503,511–520] Administration of cimetidine (300 mg q.i.d)[503] markedly raises the nocturnal pH in a sustained profile but has only a modest impact on the gastric daytime pH, with large peaks and troughs in the pH profile (Fig 61-18). More recently, single nocturnal dosing regimens have demonstrated efficacy equivalent to that of more frequent dosing regimens in the healing of duodenal and gastric ulcers (see below). These nocturnal regimens provide excellent nocturnal [H^+] suppression with almost no impact on the daytime pH profile.[511,516,521,522] If one compares the [H^+] activity profiles of twice-daily dosing regimens of H_2-receptor antagonists with equivalent single nocturnal doses, better suppression of gastric [H^+] activity is observed in the morning hours with the twice-daily regimens,

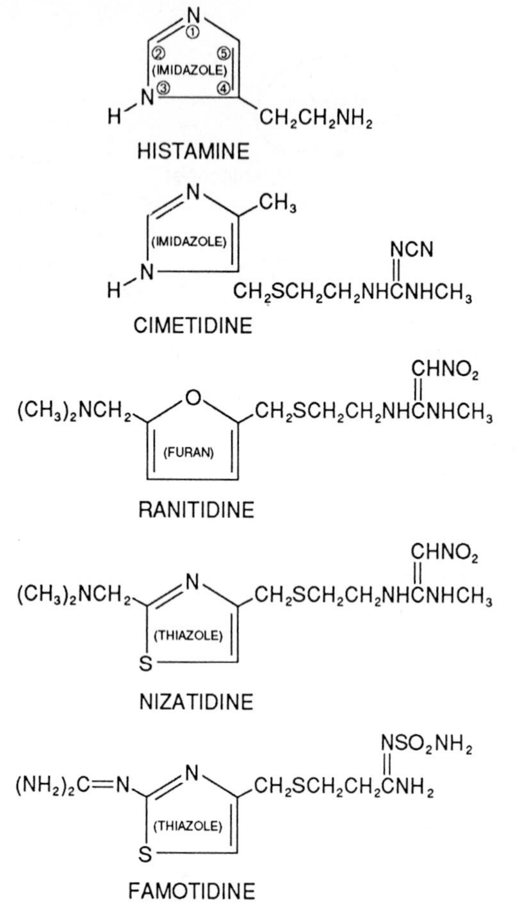

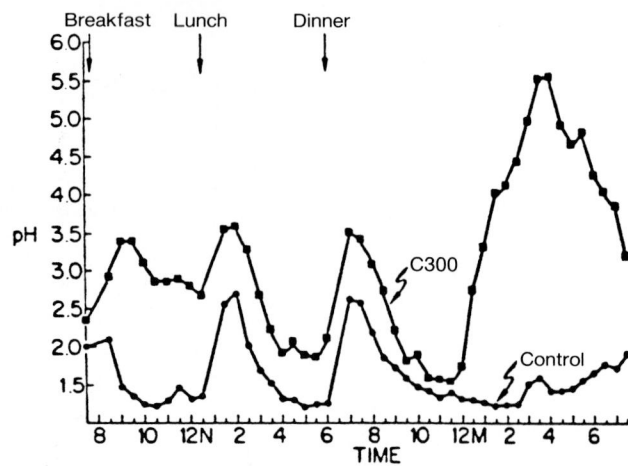

FIGURE 61–18. Mean gastric pH in duodenal ulcer patients during 24-hour control period (no medication) and with cimetidine 300 mg q.i.d. (taken with meals and at bedtime). Note the more modest impact of H$_2$ antagonists on the daytime pH versus the nocturnal pH profile. (Peterson WL, Barnett C, Feldman M, et al. Reduction of twenty-four-hour gastric acidity with combination drug therapy in patients with duodenal ulcer. Gastroenterology 1979;77:1015.)

near anacidity is obtained with both (Fig 61-19).[515] During a 24-hour period, the longest single period of unbuffered intragastric acidity includes the evening (after dinner) and the nocturnal periods. Administration of cimetidine 1600 mg, ranitidine 300 mg, or famotidine 40 mg in the early evening, after dinner, results in improved acid suppression in the evening hours with nocturnal suppression equivalent to that of the bedtime dosing regimens; hence, this may prove to be the optimal time of once-daily administrations (Fig 61-20).[509,517,525]

Summary. H$_2$-receptor antagonists suppress not only histamine-stimulated but basal, pentagastrin- and meal-stimulated acid secretion. Nevertheless, with twice-daily dosing regimens, the impact of these agents on daytime (meal-stimulated) activity is relatively modest compared with their pronounced suppression of nocturnal acidity. The degree of 24-hour, daytime, and nocturnal acid suppression with the various formulations and dosing regimens is included in Table 61-8.[521] When given in equipotent doses, the H$_2$-receptor antagonists are equivalent in their effects on acid suppression. A single nocturnal dose of an H$_2$-antagonist produces sustained acid suppression overnight. However, early evening ad-

FIGURE 61–16. Chemical structures of histamine and H$_2$-receptor antagonists. All four antagonists share an aromatic ring system with a flexible side chain attached to a polar uncharged group.

but the overall suppression of 24-hour acidity is nearly equivalent between b.i.d. and once-daily regimens (Fig 61-19).[518,520,521]

Interestingly, higher doses of ranitidine (200–300 mg b.i.d.) do not provide any additional degree of acid suppression.[513,519] The degree of nocturnal suppression of acidity is equivalent between the H$_2$-receptor antagonists when given at equipotent doses (i.e., cimetidine 800–1600 mg h.s., famotidine 20–40 mg h.s., and ranitidine 150–300 mg h.s.).[509,515,516,523,524] Although the higher doses result in overnight pH profiles that are significantly higher than the "half-dose" regimens, the [H$^+$] activity is so low that

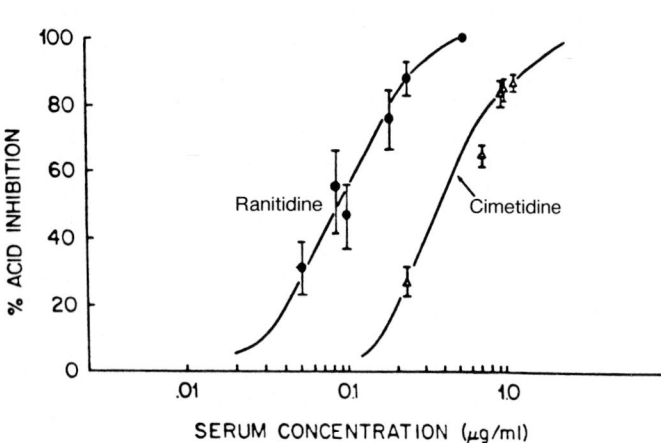

FIGURE 61–17. Dose–response curve of ranitidine and cimetidine for inhibition of meal-stimulated acid secretion. H$_2$ antagonists inhibit up to 90% of stimulated acid secretion in a linear dose-dependent manner. Ranitidine is approximately five times more potent than cimetidine. (Brater DC, Peters MN, Eshelman FN, Richardson CT. Clinical comparison of cimetidine and ranitidine. Clin Pharmacol Ther 1982;32:484.)

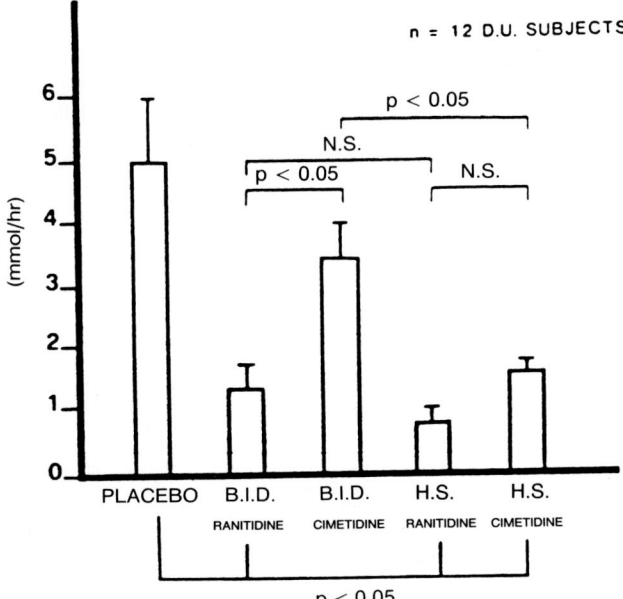

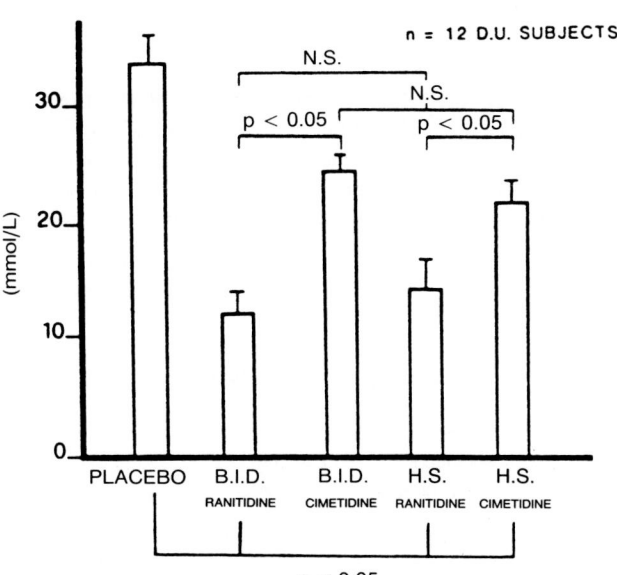

FIGURE 61–19. Upper graph: Mean hourly nocturnal acid secretion with administration of ranitidine 150 mg b.i.d., ranitidine 300 mg h.s., cimetidine 400 mg b.i.d., or cimetidine 800 mg h.s. Both ranitidine regimens and cimetidine 800 mg h.s. result in equivalent nocturnal acid inhibition. Lower graph: Mean 24-hour hydrogen ion activity with the four regimens listed above. Each agent provides comparable mean hydrogen ion activity whether administered once or twice daily. At these doses, ranitidine results in a mean hydrogen activity lower than that obtained with cimetidine. (Gledhill T, Howard OM, Buck M, Paul A, Hunt RH. Single nocturnal dose of an H₂ receptor antagonist for the treatment of duodenal ulcer. Gut 1983;24:904.)

ministration provides comparable nocturnal suppression with suppression of acid secretion in the evening hours as well and is probably preferable.

Pharmacokinetics

Absorption. (See Table 61-9) All H₂-antagonists are absorbed rapidly from the small intestine but not from the stomach.

Peak blood levels are obtained within 1 to 3 hours after oral administration.[496,497,510,526–529] The average bioavailability is 98% for nizatidine,[529] 70% to 75% for cimetidine,[528] 50% for ranitidine,[496] and 40% to 45% for famotidine.[497] Bioavailability is unaffected by concomitant food but may be decreased 30% to 40% by antacids[496,497,528–532]; thus, antacids should not be given within 2 hours of H₂-blocker doses. Sucralfate may also impair absorption.[496]

Distribution. All four agents are well distributed throughout the body with the exception of fat. The volume of distribution is approximately 1.2 L/kg because of a clinically insignificant (10%–20%) degree of binding by plasma protein.[496,497,528,529] H₂-antagonists cross the blood–brain barrier to a limited extent with all agents giving virtually identical CSF/serum ratios of 0.07 to 0.10.[533–535] Cimetidine and ranitidine are concentrated 10- to 20-fold in breast milk and excreted[496,528]; famotidine, although excreted, is not concentrated in breast milk.

Elimination. All four agents undergo elimination by a combination of renal excretion (glomerular filtration and tubular secretion) and hepatic metabolism. The principal mode of elimination varies depending on whether the drug is administered orally or intravenously. With intravenous dosing, approximately 60% to 80% of the drugs are cleared largely unchanged by the kidneys,[510,526,527] with the remainder excreted by the liver. After oral administration, these relative proportions are reversed for famotidine, ranitidine, and cimetidine,[496,497,526] but not for nizatidine, which is completely renally excreted.[527,529] Renal clearance of all four agents exceeds creatinine clearance because of extensive renal tubular secretion.[496,497,526,529] The serum half-lives of cimetidine, nizatidine, and ranitidine are similar at 1.5 to 3 hours.[496,503,526,529] However, because nizatidine and ranitidine are generally administered at doses twice the equipotent cimetidine dose, these agents provide acid suppression for a longer period of time. Famotidine has a significantly longer serum half-life of 3 to 3.5 hours[495,497,510,527];

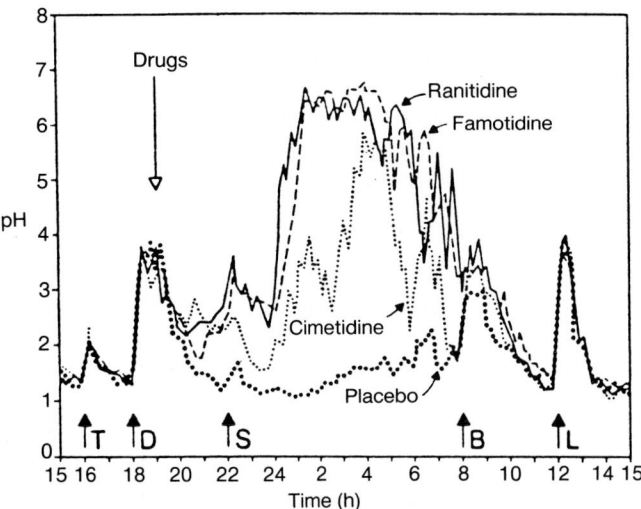

FIGURE 61–20. Twenty-four-hour pH profile in normal subjects administered cimetidine 800 mg, famotidine 40 mg, or ranitidine 300 mg after evening meal. Note sustained elevation of nocturnal pH as well as elevated pH profile in evening period. (Merki HS, Witzel L, Walt RP, et al. Double blind comparison of the effects of cimetidine, ranitidine, famotidine, and placebo on intragastric acidity in 30 normal volunteers. Gut 1988;29:81.)

TABLE 61–8
Duodenal Ulcer Healing Rates and Acid Suppression Achieved With Antisecretory Therapy

DRUG & DOSE	4-WEEK HEALING RATE (%)	% SUPPRESSION OF NOCTURNAL ACIDITY	% SUPPRESSION OF 24-HR ACIDITY	% SUPPRESSION OF DAYTIME ACIDITY
Omeprazole 40 mg q A.M.	98	99	98	97
Omeprazole 20 mg q A.M.	95	88	90	92
Ranitidine 300 mg q.h.s.	84	90	68	50
Famotidine 40 mg q.h.s.	82	95	64	39
Cimetidine 800 mg q.h.s.	80	79	48	23
Ranitidine 150 mg b.i.d.	79	70	68	66
Ranitidine 150 mg q.h.s.	75	76	45	20
Cimetidine 300 mg q.i.d.	74	68	65	63
Cimetidine 200 mg t.i.d. & 400 mg q.h.s.	74	72	56	43
Cimetidine 400 mg b.i.d.	72	54	37	23

Four-week healing rates and percentage suppression of 24-hour, daytime, and nocturnal acidity produced by various dose regimens of antisecretory drugs. Ordered by healing rate.
(Jones DB, Howden CW, Burget DW, Kerr GD, Hunt RH. Acid suppression in duodenal ulcer: A meta-analysis to define optimal dosing with antisecretory drugs. Gut 1987; 28:1120.)

in addition, it may have a slower rate of dissociation from the H_2-receptor. Thus, when equipotent doses are given, the duration of action of cimetidine, ranitidine, and nizatidine are similar, while the duration of action of famotidine is about 30% longer.[498,504]

Despite the importance of the liver in the elimination of H_2-receptor antagonists, plasma concentrations are affected to a much greater degree by renal insufficiency. The serum half-lives of cimetidine and ranitidine are increased two- to threefold, and the serum half-lives of nizatidine and famotidine are increased three- to sixfold, by renal insufficiency.[496,500,526] Recommendations for

TABLE 61–9
Comparisons of H_2-Receptor Antagonists

	CIMETIDINE	RANITIDINE	NIZATIDINE	FAMOTIDINE
Relative potency	1	4–8	4–8	20–50
Equivalent dose	1600 mg	300 mg	300 mg	40 mg
Bioavailability	60–80%	50–60%	90–100%	40–50%
Time to peak serum concentration (hrs)	1–2	1–3	1–3	1–3
Serum half-life (hrs)	1.5–2.5	2–3	1–2	2.5–4
Urinary excretion of oral dose	50%	30%	>90%	30%
Oral dosage forms available	200 mg 300 mg 400 mg 800 mg	150 mg 300 mg	150 mg 300 mg	20 mg 40 mg
Dose(s) for acute DU	300 mg q.i.d. 400 mg b.i.d. 800 mg h.s.	150 mg q.i.d. 300 mg h.s.	150 mg b.i.d. 300 mg h.s.	20 mg b.i.d. 40 mg h.s.
Dose(s) for acute GU	300 mg q.i.d. 400 mg b.i.d. 800 mg h.s.	150 mg b.i.d. 300 mg h.s.	Not approved	40 mg h.s.
Dose to prevent DU recurrence	400 mg h.s.	150 mg h.s.	150 mg h.s.	20 mg h.s.

DU, duodenal ulcer; GU, gastric ulcer.
From references 495–498, 510, 526, and 529.

dose reductions vary for each agent, but in general the doses are decreased by one half at a creatinine clearance of 15 to 30 ml/min for cimetidine, 50 ml/min for ranitidine and nizatidine, and 10 to 30 ml/min for famotidine.[496,497,526,529,536] Hemodialysis removes only 10% to 20% of the drug from the plasma; hence, replacement doses are not necessary after dialysis.[496,497,526,529,536] Peritoneal dialysis provides virtually no clearance of H_2-receptor antagonists.[496,497,536]

Hepatic dysfunction has minimal impact on H_2-antagonist pharmacokinetics, and therefore dose adjustment is not necessary in patients with compensated liver disease who maintain normal renal function.[496,497,526,534,537,538] However, in patients with decompensated cirrhosis, decreased hepatic clearance may be clinically important.[534,539-542] Furthermore, alterations in the blood–brain barrier in decompensated cirrhosis may increase the CSF:serum drug ratio, thereby increasing the likelihood of CNS toxicity.[533,542,543] For this reason, dose reductions of cimetidine, ranitidine, and famotidine should be instituted for patients with severe liver disease.[528]

The metabolism of H_2-blockers declines with age, and a dose reduction of up to 50% may be indicated in the geriatric population. Prolongation of drug clearance, principally due to an age-related decline in renal function,[496,497,526,529] results in increased plasma drug half-life, area under the curve and trough plasma levels. The relationship between serum drug levels, acid suppression, and ulcer healing have not been well established in the elderly.

Systemic Effects

Hemodynamic. Ventricular muscle histamine H_2-receptors mediate positive inotropic and chronotropic effects that are of little importance in normal physiology.[496,497,500,526,529] Hence, H_2-antagonists do not have any significant hemodynamic effects in most patients at the usual therapeutic doses.[496,497,500] Cimetidine and ranitidine have been reported to cause bradycardia and atrioventricular block and to inhibit the blood pressure and heart rate response to exercise,[496,500,544-546] while famotidine has been reported to decrease cardiac output about one fifth in healthy volunteers without affecting heart rate or blood pressure.[547] Thus, caution is warranted with the use of these agents in the hemodynamically unstable patient. Hypotension due to rapid intravenous infusion of cimetidine has been reported.[548-550] Therefore, it should be infused over 15 to 30 minutes. Infusion of intravenous ranitidine over 5 minutes appears to be without significant effects on systemic vascular resistance or blood pressure.[551,552]

Immunologic. Histamine has been shown in vitro to increase interleukin-2 production and to inhibit antigen- and mitogen-induced T-cell proliferation and production of other lymphokines by way of stimulation of an H_2-receptor on suppressor T cells.[496,553,554] Binding of lymphocyte H_2-receptor by cimetidine has been shown in vitro to enhance cell-mediated immunity[553] by inhibition of T-cell suppressor function. In vivo use of cimetidine to enhance immune function may be of theoretic benefit in certain immunodeficiencies such as common variable hypogammaglobulinemia, chronic mucocutaneous candidiasis, and herpes zoster, and certain tumors such as melanoma.[553-558] The effects of ranitidine on cell-mediated immunity are conflicting,[496,560,561] and effects of other H_2-antagonists have not been well studied.[562] Enhanced cellular immunity may be potentially deleterious in patients with renal allografts or chronic immunosuppression.[554,559,563-567]

Although the data are confusing, cimetidine should not be used in the transplant population.

Adverse Effects. The H_2-receptor antagonists have been shown to be well tolerated and to have a remarkably low frequency of side effects of less than 3%.[496,510,527,548,549,568-570] In fact, in a meta-analysis of randomized clinical trials, the overall rate of untoward side effects in those treated with H_2-antagonists was no different from that of placebo-treated patients.[570] Indeed, the voluminous literature that has accumulated regarding the adverse effects of these drugs is in vast disproportion to the low incidence of side effects. Cimetidine, as the first H_2-antagonist in clinical use, has undergone and continues to undergo the most extensive postmarketing surveillance.[569-575] The other H_2-antagonists have had much more limited surveillance of their side effects. Because cimetidine was the first and only H_2-antagonist available for several years, adverse effects attributed to cimetidine are less likely to be reported for newer agents of the same drug class. Furthermore, unusual side effects of the newer agents (famotidine and nizatidine) may not be apparent for several years after their release.[527,573] At present, there is no evidence that one H_2-antagonist has a distinctly superior profile. Indeed, in the only large study available, the adverse effects of cimetidine versus ranitidine were compared in over 37,000 patients in the Pennsylvania Medicaid population and were found to be virtually identical.[570]

Central Nervous System Toxicity. A variety of central nervous system reactions have been reported with all H_2-antagonists and include headache (0.2%–4.7%), lethargy (0.9%), dizziness (0.8%), confusion (0.2%), depression, memory impairment, and hallucinations.[527,535,568,571,573,576,577] The mechanism of action of CNS effects is not understood, but all H_2-antagonists appear to cross the blood–brain barrier with equivalent CFS:serum drug ratios. Histamine H_1- and H_2-receptors are present in the CNS; H_2-receptor stimulation may potentiate excitatory stimuli.[535] H_2-antagonists may interact with these receptors as well as with the GABA receptor complex.[535] At present, there is no evidence that one agent has any higher incidence of CNS side effects than another in the outpatient population.[549,569,570,574] The prevalence of CNS side effects attributable to intravenous H_2-antagonists is much more difficult to assess because the attributed clinical spectrum of CNS effects is not specific and may be caused by ICU psychosis, by other medications, or by the underlying medical illness. In the prospective Boston Collaborative Study of 1892 patients, a prevalence of 0.9% of CNS reactions was definitely attributable to intravenous cimetidine.[572] Similar large studies with other agents have not been published, but multiple case reports corroborate central nervous system toxicity with intravenous ranitidine and famotidine.[535,549,576-578] Surprisingly, toxicity is not related clearly to elevated serum drug levels[549,571]; however, elevated CSF drug levels may correlate better.[535,549] Impaired liver function may enhance CNS toxicity due to effects on the blood–brain barrier.[533,538,542,543,571] Age per se has not been found to be an independent risk factor of CNS toxicity.[549]

In summary, CNS side effects occur but are quite uncommon with all H_2-antagonists. In patients with underlying renal and liver disease, appropriate dose reductions should be employed.

Endocrine Abnormalities. Gynecomastia has been observed in approximately 0.2% of patients on long-term cimetidine at conventional doses[548,579] and rarely with ranitidine and famotidine.[496,549,570,579] In patients treated with high doses of cimetidine for hypersecretory states, it may be observed in up to 44%.[580] Impotence also appears to be dose-related, occurring frequently in patients treated with high doses of cimetidine.[580] These changes are readily reversed after discontinuing cimetidine or substituting another H$_2$-antagonist.[500,580,581] The pathophysiologic basis for these effects may be both displacement of dihydrotestosterone from peripheral antigen binding sites by cimetidine[500] and decreased hepatic cytochrome P-450 conversion of estradiol to the inactive 2-0H-estradiol, an effect not seen with other H$_2$-antagonists.[582] In addition, galactorrhea rarely has been reported with cimetidine. Intravenous cimetidine and ranitidine both increase prolactin secretion because of stimulation of H$_2$-receptors in the anterior pituitary.[575,579,583]

Drug Interactions. Clinically significant interactions of H$_2$-antagonists with other drugs may be due to an alteration in absorption, metabolism, or excretion of the drug. Drugs that require an acidic milieu for gastric absorption may have decreased uptake in the more alkaline milieu produced by H$_2$-antagonists.[584,585] With the exception of ketoconazole, the impact of H$_2$-antagonists on the absorption of other drugs has not been clinically significant.[585]

Cimetidine, and to a lesser extent ranitidine, binds to the hepatic cytochrome P-450 microsomal mixed-function oxidase enzyme system inhibiting phase I oxidation and dealkylation in a dose-dependent fashion[541,549,586]; phase II glucuronidation reactions and sulfation reactions are not inhibited.[549] Although cimetidine is reported to interact with multiple medications,[584,586–588] this inhibition is seldom of clinical significance. Problems arise most often with medications that are metabolized by the P-450 system and have a narrow therapeutic-to-toxic ratio: theophylline, phenytoin, lidocaine, and warfarin.[527,541,549,589,590] However, the metabolism of a variety of other P-450 metabolized medications is also impaired by cimetidine, and occasionally this is clinically significant. Altered metabolism has been demonstrated for beta-blockers, quinidine, calcium channel blockers, benzodiazepines, and tricyclic antidepressants.[541,584,587–590] Ranitidine, which binds 5 to 10 times less avidly to the P-450 enzyme system, has far less potential for significant adverse drug interactions.[532,541,589–592] Nizatidine and famotidine have negligible direct P-450 inhibition,[497,510,529] and there are few reports of significant drug interactions. Despite the infrequency with which serious adverse drug reactions occur with cimetidine, monitoring of theophylline, warfarin, and phenytoin levels is indicated if cimetidine is to be used in combination with these agents. It is more convenient and perhaps safer, however, to use another H$_2$-antagonist with less interactive potential.[541,549,585,590,592]

Cimetidine was recently reported to be a noncompetitive inhibitor of gastric alcohol dehydrogenase, an enzyme in the stomach that plays an important role in the first-past metabolism of oral ethanol. Increased peak blood levels and systemic bioavailability of oral ethanol have been demonstrated in patients taking cimetidine.[541,593,594] The systemic effects of alcohol may thereby be increased in patients receiving cimetidine. H$_2$-antagonists are secreted at the renal tubule, where they compete with the tubular secretion of creatinine and certain medications such as procainamide.[586] Clinically significant rises (10%–40%) in procaine levels may occur during H$_2$-antagonist therapy.[532,588] With normal renal function, clinically insignificant rises (15%) in serum creatinine

may occur because of impaired renal tubular creatinine secretion.[586,595] However, the glomerular filtration rate, as assessed by inulin clearance, is unaltered. Patients with renal transplants who are taking cyclosporin also have a small reversible rise in serum creatinine when taking H$_2$-antagonists without demonstrable nephrotoxicity or changes in renal function. H$_2$-antagonists do not affect serum cyclosporin levels and do not appear to potentiate cyclosporine nephrotoxicity.[595–597]

Other Adverse Effects. A variety of other severe idiosyncratic adverse effects have occurred with H$_2$-antagonists: reversible neutropenia, thrombocytopenia, agranulocytosis, and pancytopenia.[496,548,575,598–600] Rare cases of interstitial nephritis have been observed.[527,601] Asymptomatic elevations in hepatic transaminases as well as acute hepatitis have been observed with both cimetidine and ranitidine. These are extremely rare, generally mild, and reversible, and no deaths have been reported. The pattern is generally that of hepatocellular or a mixed injury.[541]

PROTON PUMP INHIBITORS—OMEPRAZOLE

Structure and Site of Action. Omeprazole is the first of a new class of antisecretory compounds: the hydrogen ion pump inhibitors. This agent inhibits the parietal cell H$^+$/K$^+$-ATPase, the acid secretory pump embedded within the canalicular membrane that is the final step in the acid secretory process.[602] This enzyme appears to be unique to the parietal cell. Omeprazole is a substituted benzimidazole derivative (Fig 61-21) that resembles H$_2$-receptor antagonists somewhat in structure but has a completely different mechanism of action.[603] As a weak base (pKa 3.97), it becomes protonated within an acidified compartment such as the parietal cell tubulovesicles and secretory canaliculus. Because charged molecules diffuse much more slowly through membranes than neutral compounds, the protonated omeprazole becomes concentrated within the tubulovesicles and the canaliculus.[602,604] Intact omeprazole is devoid of inhibitory activity and highly stable at neutral pH.[605] However, within acidified compartments, it rapidly undergoes transformation to its active derivative, a sulfonamide.[604] The sulfonamide compound has an extremely short half-life of 2 minutes, but it reacts rapidly with a mercapto group on the H$^+$/K$^+$-ATPase to form a covalent disulfide linkage. This leads to irreversible inhibition of the enzyme.[603,605,606] Thus, omeprazole is concentrated and converted to its active derivative close to its target of action, the gastric parietal H$^+$/K$^+$-ATPase.[604] Although other types of proton pumps are present in various mammalian cells, the H$^+$/K$^+$-ATPase is distinct structurally and mechanically from other H$^+$ transporting enzymes and appears to exist only in the parietal cell.[602]

Pharmacodynamics. The effects of omeprazole on basal and stimulated acid secretion by single dose and repeated doses have been studied.[607] Single oral omeprazole doses of 20 to 80 mg inhibit basal and pentagastrin-, betazole-, and meal-stimulated acid secretion in a dose-dependent fashion with near total acid suppression (98%) at the 80-mg dose.[606–609] Omeprazole effects on gastric secretory volume and pepsinogen secretion are less than its effects on gastric acid output.[603,606] With the enteric formulation presently used, maximal acid suppression occurs 3 to 6 hours after

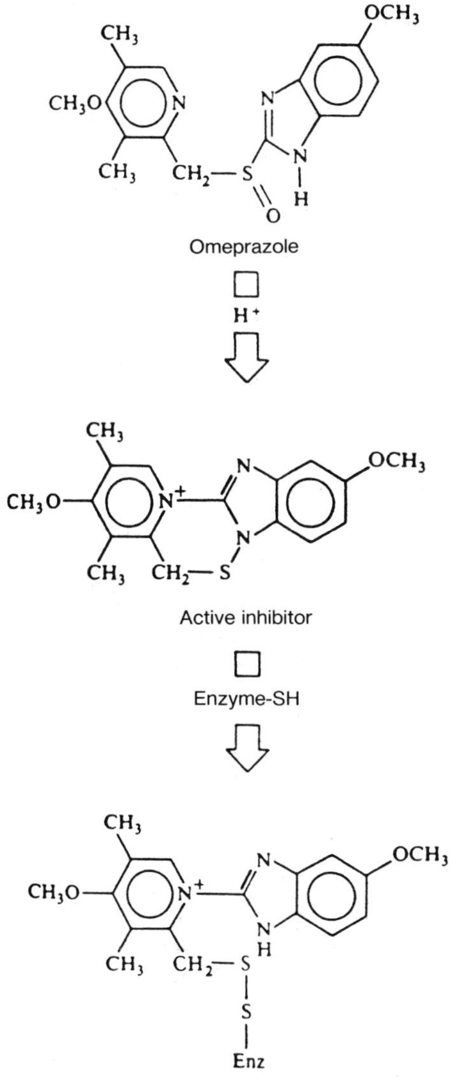

FIGURE 61–21. Omeprazole structure and activation. Within acidic secretory canaliculi of the parietal cell, omeprazole (a weak base) becomes protonated and subsequently transformed into a sulphenamide—the active inhibitor. The sulphenamide forms a disulfide complex with a cysteine group of the hydrogen ion pump, thereby inactivating it. (Modified from Wallmark B. Omeprazole: Mode of action and effect on acid secretion in animals. Scand J Gastroenterol 1988;24[suppl 166]:12.)

a single oral dose, and the degree of acid inhibition correlates well with the area under the plasma omeprazole concentration curve.[607]

With repeated daily doses of omeprazole, the degree of acid inhibition increases over the first few days, stabilizing within 3 to 5 days.[606,610] Thus, single daily dosing with 20 to 30 mg of omeprazole yields 70% inhibition of basal acid output and pentagastrin-stimulated secretion within 6 hours of the first dose, but more than 90% inhibition within 6 hours of the fifth to seventh daily doses.[606–608] After the last dose, 24-hour stimulated acid output remains inhibited by 60% to 70%. Although the serum half-life of omeprazole is less than 1.5 hours,[606] the irreversible inactivation of the proton pump provides long-lasting inhibition. In 24-hour studies of normal ambulatory subjects and duodenal ulcer patients

on a regular diet, omeprazole doses of 10, 20, and 30 mg per day for 1 week result in a 37%, 90%, and 97% decrease in 24-hour gastric acidity, respectively.[607,611] The optimal daily dosage of omeprazole for reduction of 24-hour acidity is 20 to 30 mg per day for most patients.[607] In a crossover study of omeprazole 20 mg per day compared with ranitidine 150 mg b.i.d., 24-hour intragastric acidity was suppressed 97% and 58%, respectively.[612] It is apparent from the 24-hour intragastric acidity profile (Fig 61-22) that omeprazole and ranitidine both provide potent suppression of nocturnal acid secretion. However, the impact of omeprazole on daytime (meal-stimulated) acid secretion is far greater than that provided by ranitidine. Because of the long duration of action of omeprazole, when 20 mg per day of it is given for just 3 consecutive days per week, it will take 4 treatment-free days before basal and peak acid output return to pretreatment values.[613]

Pharmacokinetics

Absorption. Omeprazole degrades very rapidly at an acidic pH. To prevent inactivation in the stomach, omeprazole was given initially as a suspension in a sodium bicarbonate solution.[603] More recently, an enteric-coated formulation has been developed to minimize intragastric degradation. The absorption of the enteric-coated granules may initially be erratic, with a peak serum concentration occurring 0.5 to 7 hours after administration.[603] Because omeprazole is acid-labile, its bioavailability increases over the first 3 to 5 days of administration because of the rise in gastric pH, which in turn results in less inactivation of the parent compound.[610] Absorption may be delayed by food[606]; hence, it should be administered on an empty stomach. Antacids, however, do not alter omeprazole's absorption. The systemic bioavailability of the enteric form is only 65%, compared with a buffered suspension.[603] Omeprazole undergoes extensive first-past hepatic metabolism, and the overall bioavailability of the enteric formulation is estimated at 30% to 40%.

Distribution. Omeprazole has a limited volume of distribution of 0.08 L/kg and initially is confined to extracellular water, where it is 95% protein-bound. Subsequently, it is concentrated within acidified compartments. By autoradiography, omeprazole has a rapid distribution and by 4 hours is limited to gastric mucosa, liver, and gallbladder. After 48 hours, radioactive omeprazole remains only in the gastric mucosa. Passage across the blood–brain barrier appears to be limited.[606]

Elimination. Omeprazole undergoes rapid elimination with a half-life of less than 1.5 hours.[606] Plasma levels are undetectable by 8 hours after oral administration. Omeprazole undergoes extensive hepatic metabolism to three metabolites, 80% of which are excreted in the urine and 20% in the bile.[603] Unchanged omeprazole is not recovered in the urine. The metabolites have no known acid-inhibitory activity. The pharmacokinetics of unchanged omeprazole are unaffected by renal insufficiency; however, the concentration of metabolites is increased. Omeprazole does not appear in dialysis fluid.[606] Therefore, it does not appear necessary to reduce the dosage of omeprazole for patients with chronic renal failure or those on dialysis. Insufficient information is available to date regarding the appropriate dosing for patients with hepatic failure. However, the extensive hepatic metabolism might suggest that an empiric dosage reduction will be appropriate,[603] but this requires direct study.

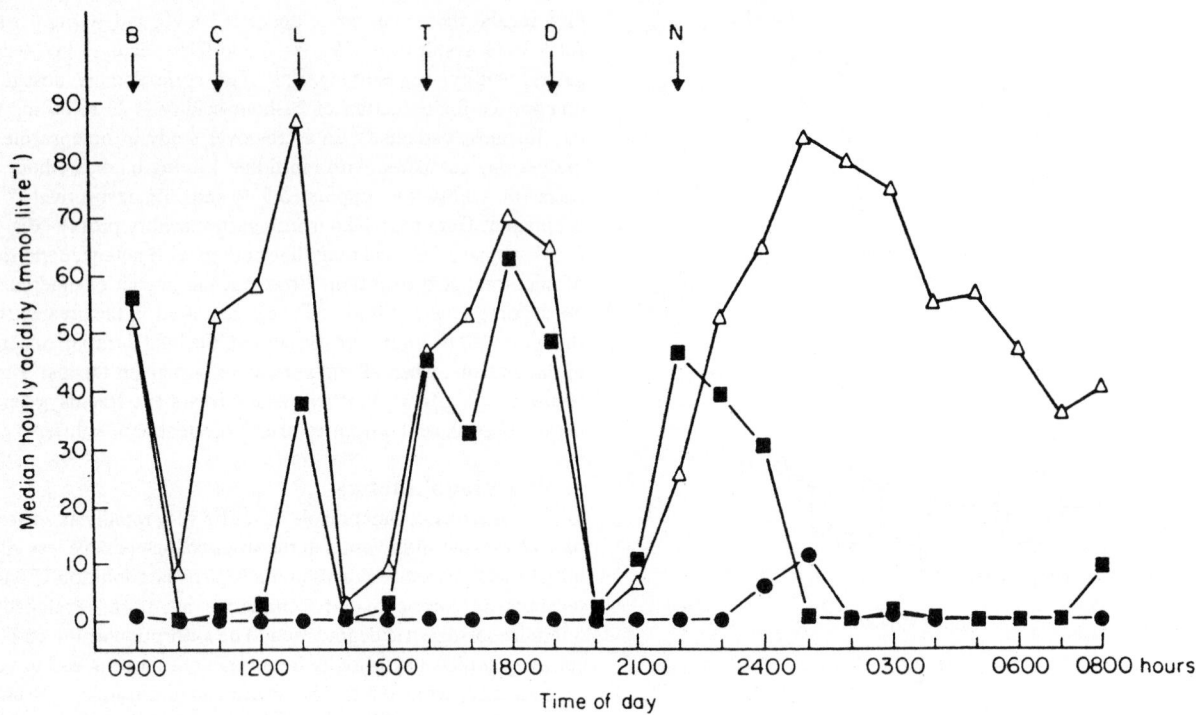

FIGURE 61–22. Median hourly intragastric acidity before (open triangles) and after treatment with ranitidine 150 mg b.i.d. (solid squares) or omeprazole 20 mg q.d. (solid circles). Note superior inhibition of meal-stimulated acid secretion provided by omeprazole.

(Lanzon-Miller S, Pounder R, Hamilton M, et al. Twenty-four-hour intragastric acidity and plasma gastrin concentration before and during treatment with either ranitidine or omeprazole. Aliment Pharmacol Ther 1987;1:239.)

Adverse Effects

General. Experience with omeprazole is limited. Therefore, one must be extremely cautious considering its safety profile. In multiple clinical trials using dosages of 20 to 60 mg per day for 4 to 8 weeks, the prevalence of reported adverse experiences has been similar to that of the placebo- or H_2-antagonist–treated population.[606,614,615] Omeprazole has been used for up to 4 years in dosages up to 360 mg per day in patients with Zollinger–Ellison syndrome with no serious adverse effects or irreversible laboratory abnormalities attributed to this drug.[616,617]

Drug Interactions. As with H_2-antagonists, drugs that require an acidic gastric milieu for absorption, such as ketoconazole and tetracycline, may have decreased absorption.[603] Both in vitro and in vivo, omeprazole has demonstrated a dose-related inhibition of hepatic cytochrome P-450 metabolism.[603,618–620] In healthy subjects, omeprazole prolongs the clearance of warfarin, phenytoin, and diazepam.[603,621,622] As with the H_2-receptor antagonists, caution is required when initiating omeprazole in patients taking these drugs. Interestingly, the metabolism of theophylline and propranolol may not be affected by omeprazole, suggesting that omeprazole may inhibit only a subset of the hepatic cytochrome P-450 enzyme system.[623,624]

Effects on Serum Gastrin. Single-dose studies of omeprazole in man have not demonstrated any significant effect on fasting or meal-stimulated gastrin levels.[603,606] Mild (less than two to three times basal) reversible elevations in serum gastrin have been noted in numerous clinical trials with omeprazole.[603,606,625,626] This typically occurs within 2 weeks of initiation

and normalizes within 1 to 4 weeks of discontinuation of therapy. In one duodenal ulcer trial of omeprazole 20 mg per day for 4 weeks, 12% of patients developed a rise in serum gastrin exceeding the upper limits of normal.[627] The elevation in serum gastrin is attributable to the suppression of gastric acidity, the principal inhibitor of antral gastrin release. As such, the rise in gastrin is not unique to omeprazole but is caused by other agents that suppress gastric acidity (e.g., ranitidine 150 mg b.i.d. raises fasting and 24-hour integrated gastrin levels in duodenal ulcer patients).[612,628] Indeed, there is a correlation between the degree of acid suppression induced by omeprazole or ranitidine and the median integrated 24-hour plasma gastrin concentration.[612] Of note, however, because of its more prolonged acid suppression, the rise in serum gastrin with omeprazole exceeds that with ranitidine (Fig 61-23).[612] Nevertheless, the elevation in gastrin likely has little clinical significance in short-term therapy.[626]

Gastric Carcinoid Tumors. In humans, prolonged hypergastrinemia associated with achlorhydria or Zollinger–Ellison syndrome has an increased risk of the development of gastric carcinoid tumors.[629,630] Therefore it is of some concern that lifelong (2-year) omeprazole treatment has led to gastric carcinoids in up to 40% of female rats.[631] Omeprazole has not been found to have any direct teratogenicity or mutagenicity in multiple genetic toxicology studies,[631] although this has been disputed recently.[632] It is hypothesized that sustained hypergastrinemia in the rat leads to hyperplasia of the oxyntic endocrine cells, of which the enterochromaffinlike (ECL) cell is the most abundant.[633] Gastric carcinoids may arise in the setting of ECL hyperplasia.[633] Hypergastrinemia, whether produced by proton pump inhibition, high-dose

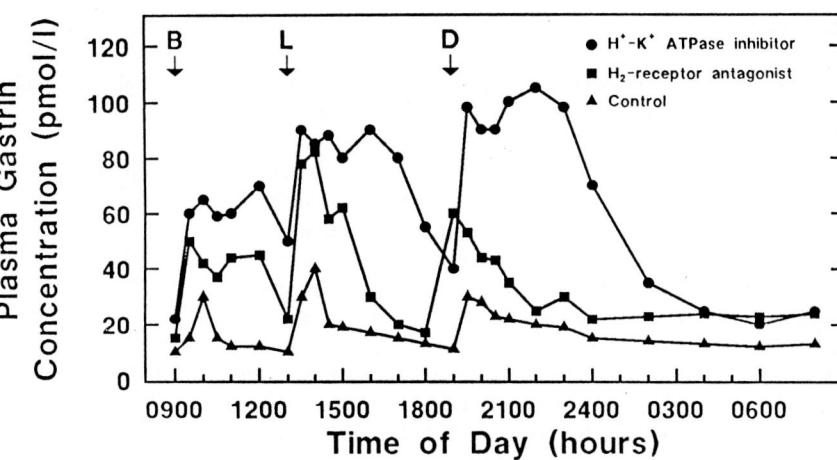

FIGURE 61-23. Median hourly plasma gastrin concentration before and after 28th day of treatment with either ranitidine 150 mg b.i.d. or omeprazole 20 mg q.am. A consistent rise in serum gastrin throughout the 24-hour period occurs with both regimens but is greater with omeprazole. (Lanzon-Miller S, Pounder R, Hamilton M, et al. Twenty-four-hour intragastric acidity and plasma gastrin concentration before and during treatment with either ranitidine or omeprazole. Aliment Pharmacol Ther 1987;1:239.)

H_2-receptor antagonists, infusions of gastrin, or partial fundectomy, results in gastric ECL cell hyperplasia in the rat and ultimately gastric carcinoids.[633–636] In these models, ECL cell hyperplasia and carcinoids are prevented by antrectomy (i.e., by prevention of secondary hypergastrinemia).[636] The time course for ECL growth appears to be rapid, with changes in cell density noted as early as 9 days after initiation of hypergastrinemia.[634] The degree of ECL cell hyperplasia is correlated with the plasma gastrin levels.[634,635] After 20 weeks of therapy with ranitidine or omeprazole in the rat, ECL cell changes are observed; these changes normalize within 10 weeks of discontinuation of antisecretory therapy.[636]

The risk of ECL cell hyperplasia in humans on long-term omeprazole is unclear. Studies of ECL cell changes in patients treated with long-term omeprazole for refractory esophagitis or ulcer disease are conflicting[637,638] but thus far do not support any substantial change in the ECL cell population.

In summary, the gastric ECL cell hyperplasia and carcinoids seen in rats are hypothesized to arise from persistent, profound hypergastrinemia secondary to acid suppression and are not due to specific carcinogenic properties of omeprazole. This hypothesis has been challenged vociferously by one authority.[639–641] In humans, the degree of gastrin elevation with omeprazole is far less than that seen in the rat and also far less than that seen in Zollinger–Ellison syndrome or pernicious anemia. Although further studies of the effect of long-term omeprazole on ECL hyperplasia in humans are critical, short-term therapy (up to 8 weeks) appears to be very safe. On the other hand, the safety of long-term use of this potent acid inhibitor is not established.[640,641]

SUCRALFATE

Structure. Sucralfate is a basic salt of sulfated sucrose in which the eight hydroxyl groups of sucrose have been replaced by sulfate and aluminum hydroxide (Fig 61-24).[642] It is insoluble in water and common organic solvents.[643] With the addition of dilute acid, as is found in the stomach, sucralfate powder becomes a viscous, tenacious paste and retains this property in the more alkaline duodenum.[644] Within an acidic milieu, there is a gradual dissociation of aluminum hydroxide into solution, leaving highly polar sulfate anions that may bind electrostatically to adjacent sucralfate molecules or to positively charged tissue proteins.[644] As a weak base, sucralfate has a theoretic buffering capacity of 13 mmol/g. However, sucralfate reacts with acid so slowly that 90% of the buffering capacity is retained. In vitro and in vivo, it has little or no acid-neutralizing activity.[642]

Pharmacodynamics. Sucralfate has efficacy as an acute cytoprotective agent against topical agents and stress ulceration and as a chronic therapeutic agent in peptic ulcer disease.[645,646] A variety of mechanisms of action are purported to account for its actions, but their relative importance is unknown. It is clear that sucralfate has minimal acid-neutralizing capacity and no effect on gastric acid secretion, so these mechanisms cannot account for its therapeutic properties.[646]

Sucralfate has a number of actions that are postulated to be important in ulcer therapy. One is the formation of a protective barrier over the base of ulcers and erosions.[644,647] As sucralfate dissociates, the sulfated sucrose compound binds to positively charged proteins in the ulcerated tissue, forming a potential barrier. This barrier may directly adsorb bile salts and pepsin and retard diffusion of pepsin, bile salts, and acid from the lumen to the ulcer. By binding to the exposed proteins, sucralfate limits access of pepsin to its protein substrate, decreasing further mucosal digestion.[642,647]

Sucralfate also has trophic effects that may be important in ulcer healing and epithelialization.[646] These include thickening of the surface, foveolar, and proliferative epithelial zones and an increase in the mucus content of surface cells.[645] Proliferation of cells at the ulcer margins may contribute to ulcer repair. Sucralfate also binds and concentrates epidermal growth factor (EGF) from saliva at the ulcer site,[648] perhaps stimulating epidermal growth

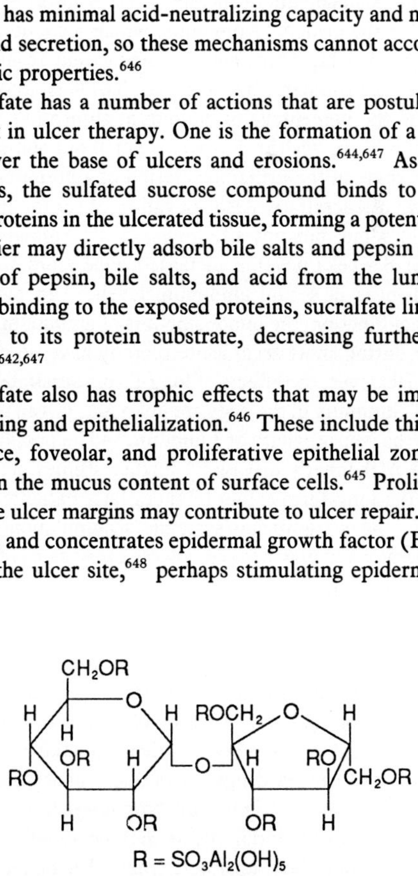

$$R = SO_3Al_2(OH)_5$$

FIGURE 61-24. Chemical structure of sucralfate.

and accelerating ulcer re-epithelialization. These actions warrant further study.

Sucralfate has a number of other actions that may be important for its acute cytoprotective actions but are of unclear importance in ulcer healing.[645,646] It stimulates gastric mucosal prostaglandin E_2 synthesis and luminal secretion,[645,649] although this is not seen in all studies.[650,651] Pretreatment with prostaglandin synthetase inhibitors (NSAIDs) decreases the cytoprotective activity of sucralfate against topical agents by more than 50%.[645] Sucralfate stimulates mucus and bicarbonate production in vitro and in vivo.[650–652] These important mucosal defensive factors may facilitate ulcer healing by protecting newly formed cells from peptic destruction. The aluminum salt that dissociates from sucralfate appears to be the active stimulant of gastroduodenal bicarbonate secretion.[652] Numerous other actions are attributed to sucralfate, including increased mucosal blood flow, protection of the microvasculature integrity, and increased macrophage activity, but these require more study.[645]

In summary, there is no shortage of potential explanations for the therapeutic effect of sucralfate. However, to date, the relative importance of each of its effects in ulcer healing and prevention of recurrence is unknown.

Pharmacokinetics.

Sucralfate is administered on an empty stomach two to four times daily.[642] After administration, binding to the ulcer site is demonstrated to last for up to 6 hours.[643] Sucralfate has minimal gastroduodenal absorption of only 3% to 5% of the parent compound; the remainder is excreted in the feces.[643] The small amount of sucralfate that is absorbed is excreted unchanged in the urine.[643] Aluminum, which accounts for 21% of sucralfate by weight, dissociates to some extent from sucralfate in an acidic environment, but less than 0.01% is absorbed. This is similar to the percentage of aluminum absorption that occurs with antacids.[653] In healthy subjects, a small but statistically significant increase in the urinary excretion of aluminum is evident after 2 days of sucralfate. Also, elevation of serum aluminum is observed in some, but not all, studies.[653–655] Animals given sucralfate for 8 weeks develop increased bone aluminum content without changes in serum aluminum levels.[655] In patients with normal renal function, the minor amounts of aluminum absorption that occur during short-term acute therapy have no clinical significance. However, the effects of long-term sucralfate in the disposition of aluminum in the body are unknown. Given the renewed interest in the neurotoxicity of aluminum and its possible involvement with Alzheimer's disease,[656] further studies are necessary regarding the long-term safety of sucralfate. Patients with renal insufficiency have significant systemic accumulation during sucralfate therapy and may occasionally manifest signs of acute aluminum toxicity.[655]

Adverse Effects.

Because of its minimal systemic absorption and its chemically inert structure, sucralfate is virtually devoid of systemic toxicity.[642,643] Side effects of constipation and nausea are reported in 2% to 3% of patients. Sucralfate may impair the absorption of certain drugs, particularly phenytoin and warfarin; however, clinically significant drug interactions are rare.[652] Nevertheless, these potential effects may be avoided by the administration of sucralfate separately from other medications. Sucralfate effectively binds phosphates in the gastrointestinal tract[657,658] and has been used in patients with chronic renal failure as a phosphate binder.

ANTACIDS

Structure and Formulations.

Antacids have been used for centuries in the treatment of patients with dyspepsia and acid-peptic diseases. Pliny reportedly used crushed coral (calcium carbonate) in the first century A.D. to treat patients with dyspepsia, and Paracelsus used the same to treat patients with heartburn.[659] They were the mainstay of antiulcer treatment until the availability of the H_2-receptor antagonists in the late 1970s.

Sodium Bicarbonate.

Sodium bicarbonate reacts promptly with hydrochloric acid to produce carbon dioxide, sodium chloride, and water. Because carbon dioxide is poorly soluble in water, it is largely in the form of gaseous CO_2. The stomach is quite impermeable to diffusion of carbon dioxide.[660] Therefore, in the event that a large quantity of CO_2 gas is generated in a patient who is unable to belch, acute gastric distention and even gastric rupture can result. In addition, because sodium does not form an insoluble product with other anions (e.g., the solubility of $NaHCO_3$ = 7 g/dl; Na_2CO_3 = 21 g/dl),[661] it is absorbed promptly from the small intestine, resulting in a base excess equal to the amount of sodium bicarbonate produced. In patients without renal or pulmonary disease, this base excess is promptly excreted principally by renal excretion.

Calcium Carbonate.

Calcium carbonate is quite similar to sodium bicarbonate, but it is less soluble in aqueous solutions (e.g., solubility of $CaCO_2$ = 0.0015 g/dl).[661] Therefore, it reacts less rapidly with gastric acid. In the presence of hydrochloric acid, calcium carbonate is converted to calcium chloride; the latter, being very soluble in water (solubility = 98 g/dl), can easily be absorbed from the small intestine. However, in the presence of carbonate, phosphate, or hydroxyl radicles in the duodenum, the calcium chelates produced again become quite insoluble (e.g., $Ca(H_2PO_4)_2$ = 1.8 g/dl). Because only a modest amount of calcium carbonate is absorbed, alkalosis is of much lesser magnitude than with sodium bicarbonate. In the presence of normal renal function, the absorbed calcium is excreted by the kidneys.

Magnesium Hydroxide.

Magnesium hydroxide is also a potent antacid that in many respects resembles calcium. When it interacts with hydrochloric acid, it results in magnesium chloride (solubility = 54 g/dl), but when it interacts with carbonate or phosphate in the small intestine, its solubility decreases to less than 0.4 g/dl. Magnesium antacids react with hydrochloric acid almost as rapidly as with sodium bicarbonate.[662] With both calcium and magnesium antacids, patients with renal insufficiency can develop hypercalcemia or hypermagnesemia because of poor renal excretion.

Aluminum Salts.

Aluminum salts, the hydroxide and oxide, is the fourth salt used as an antacid. It reacts slowly with hydrochloric acid and has limited buffering capacity. Aluminum chloride has a high water solubility (110 g/dl), while the phosphate salt is essentially insoluble. Plasma aluminum concentrations increase in patients receiving daily aluminum hydroxide antacids.[659] This aluminum can be deposited in tissues (e.g., the brain), and its role in the pathogenesis of Alzheimer's syndrome has been raised.[656] Furthermore, aluminum can bind with phosphate, resulting in insoluble aluminum phosphate, which in turn results in the loss of total body phosphate that can cause hypophosphatemia. Aluminum similarly binds with fluoride, impairing fluoride absorption.[663] Finally, aluminum hydroxide inhibits the absorption of some drugs (e.g., iron, tetracyclines, and so forth).[664]

The clinical pharmacology of antacids and their buffering effects have been reviewed extensively.[662] Of note, antacids have their greatest intragastric buffering effect when administered 1 hour following a meal.[665] It was previously thought that liquid antacids were substantially more potent than antacid tablets. However, recent studies indicate that antacid tablets are also effective buffers (see below).

Mechanisms of Action. Antacids were thought until recently to produce their therapeutic effect entirely because of their acid-neutralizing effects,[662] and on this basis the pharmaceutical industry synthesized more potent and concentrated antacid formulations. In fact, the use of large doses (1000 mmol/d) of antacid administered in divided doses in patients with DU was based upon the sound principle of wanting to effectively neutralize the bulk of the gastric acid secreted.[666,667] However, recent studies indicate that doses as low as 120 mmol/d of antacid tablets result in healing equivalent to that of the larger doses.[668] The buffering effect of this tiny antacid dose is modest at best. Therefore, the mechanism of action of low doses of antacids in expediting ulcer healing is currently the subject of study. Recent evidence suggests that some antacids release endogenous prostaglandins, but whether or not this contributes to their efficacy is not known. It is likely that the large doses (i.e., more than 500 mmol/d of buffer) act in large part by neutralization of gastric acid and secondarily by inactivation of pepsin, while doses of less than 200 mmol/d likely act by mechanisms independent of their acid-neutralizing effects.

Adverse Effects. The major adverse effects of antacids are the cathartic effect of the magnesium-containing antacids and the constipation of the aluminum- and calcium-containing antacids. These effects are dose-related and at high doses occur in up to two thirds of patients. Therefore, most antacid preparations available today contain a combination of magnesium and aluminum hydroxides. As mentioned, depending upon the solubility within the small intestine, a portion of the cations may be absorbed largely as chloride salts. This is of little concern in those with normal renal function. However, in patients with renal insufficiency, increases in serum calcium, magnesium, and aluminum (and tissue aluminum) concentrations may occur.[669] Furthermore, with sodium bicarbonate, which should not be used routinely as an antacid, systemic alkalosis and fluid overload can develop because of its intestinal absorption. Calcium antacids result in a transient increase in gastric acid secretion ("acid rebound") after their buffering effect has dissipated.[670] The mechanism of "acid rebound" is not fully understood but may be related to calcium's stimulatory effect on gastrin release and/or a direct effect on the parietal cell.

PROSTAGLANDINS

Structure. Prostaglandins were originally discovered in the prostate glands and human semen by Kurzrok,[671] Goldblatt,[672] and von Euler.[673] Prostaglandins are derivatives of 20-carbon-chain unsaturated fatty acids and therefore are also referred to as eicosanoids (eicosi = twenty). The major precursor for prostaglandins is arachidonic acid, which is present in the cell membranes and is released by activation of phospholipase A_2. Arachidonic acid may enter two metabolic pathways. It may be converted by cyclooxygenase to endoperoxides with the subsequent synthesis of prostacyclin, prostaglandins of the E or F class, or thromboxane. Alternatively, arachidonic acid can enter the lipoxygenase pathway, resulting in a number of leukotrienes that participate in the inflammatory response.[674] It is likely that under normal physiologic conditions, prostaglandins produce their effect by a paracrine action rather than functioning as classic hormones. Although they have a multitude of biologic effects, they tend to have a short biologic half-life. High doses of adrenocorticosteroids inhibit prostaglandin synthesis by inhibiting the activation of phospholipase A_2. Of clinical relevance is the observation by Vane that indomethacin, aspirin, and other NSAIDs are potent inhibitors of cyclooxygenase and thereby suppress prostaglandin formation.[675]

The human gastrointestinal mucosa contains and synthesizes prostaglandins. The primary prostaglandins synthesized are PGE_2 and $PGF_{2\alpha}$ in a ratio of about 2 to 1.[676] Only minor proportions of endoperoxides are converted to thromboxanes or 6-keto-$PGF_{1\alpha}$, the stable metabolite of prostacyclin.[677] Although luminal levels of prostaglandin can be measured, it is not known whether they accurately reflect localized biologic events.

A number of prostaglandins have undergone clinical trials in the United States. These include: misoprostol (a synthetic PGE_1 methyl analogue), arbaprostil (a dimethyl PGE_2 analogue), enprostil (a synthetic dehydro PGE_2 derivative), trimoprostil (a trimethyl PGE_2 analogue), and rioprostil (a 16-methyl 16-hydroxy analogue of PGE_1). To date, only misoprostol has been approved for use in humans by the Food and Drug Administration.

Pharmacodynamics/Mechanisms of Action. The precise mechanism of action of prostaglandin analogues in expediting the healing of peptic ulcer disease, as well as preventing drug-induced mucosal damage, is not fully understood. Prostaglandins have a multitude of plausible effects. Prostaglandin analogues stimulate mucus as well as bicarbonate secretion.[678] This, in turn, enhances the pH mucus barrier (Fig 61-13). The protective effect of prostaglandins is dissipated in the presence of mucolytic agents (such as N-acetyl cystine), drugs that inhibit bicarbonate secretion (such as acetazolamide),[679,680] and NSAIDs. The mucus-bicarbonate barrier alone cannot entirely account for the prostaglandin-induced mucosal protection because the pH gradient is dissipated at luminal pHs of less than approximately 1.8. Therefore, other factors must be involved. Prostaglandins of the E and I class enhance gastric mucosal blood flow. Recent evidence suggests that the maintenance of mucosal blood flow is of primary importance in preventing mucosal injury in animals. Mucosal blood flow is also of importance in ulcer healing. Furthermore, many of the prostaglandin analogues inhibit gastric acid secretion, although they are not as potent as the histamine H_2-receptor antagonists or the H^+/K^+-ATPase inhibitors. Some (e.g., enprostil) are quite potent. In addition, prostaglandins inhibit mucosal cell turnover,[681] which may also contribute to ulcer healing.

At this time, it appears likely that prostaglandin analogues expedite ulcer healing by more than one action. Inhibition of gastric acid secretion may be of major importance, but further investigation to dissect the relative roles of the prostaglandin effects in peptic ulcer disease is needed.

Pharmacokinetics. In order to be effective therapeutically, prostaglandins must come into direct topical contact with the gastroduodenal mucosa. They are, however, absorbed promptly from the small intestine and excreted principally by the kidneys. The half-life of misoprostol is approximately 1.5 hours, and 80% is recovered in the urine and feces within 24 hours.[682] The prostaglandins do not interact with the hepatic cytochrome P-450 drug-metabolizing enzyme system.

Natural PGE_2 has only a modest inhibitory effect on human gastric acid secretion[683] because of rapid intragastric inactivation by oxidation, which places a ketone group at the carbon-15 position. Some prostaglandin analogues (e.g., enprostil, 16,16 dimethyl PGE_2) are potent inhibitors of gastric acid secretion, likely because of inhibition of cyclic AMP generation by the parietal cells,[684] and some suppress meal-stimulated gastrin release (e.g., enprostil, 16,16 dimethyl PGE_2, arbaprostil) while others do not (e.g., misoprostol).[685] Others (e.g. arbaprostil, misoprostol) are only moderate inhibitors of gastric secretion and fail to substantially alter meal-stimulated gastric acid secretion. The explanation for why some inhibit gastrin release and why some are more potent inhibitors of gastric acid secretion is not understood.

Adverse Effects. The major untoward effects associated with prostaglandins are related to their pharmacologic actions on intestinal water and electrolyte transport and smooth muscle gastrointestinal and uterine motility. In humans, prostaglandins stimulate intestinal chloride, sodium, potassium, and water secretion in humans.[686] This effect is likely secondary to prostaglandin-induced stimulation of cyclic AMP in the enterocytes.[687] Diarrhea is reported in 10% to 30% of patients receiving prostaglandin analogues and is dose-related.[688] In comparative therapeutic ulcer studies, diarrhea occurs more commonly in those treated with prostaglandin analogues than in those in other therapeutic regimens (i.e., placebo, H_2-receptor antagonists, sucralfate, omeprazole, and so forth).

Furthermore, prostaglandins affect the smooth muscle of the uterus, increasing uterine pressure. Uterine bleeding has been reported in up to one third of females during the first trimester of pregnancy.[689] Therefore, the use of prostaglandin analogues in females who may potentially be pregnant is contraindicated. If used in this patient group, a pregnancy test is indicated prior to initiating therapy. Finally, prostaglandins can induce gastrointestinal mucosal hyperplasia in animals.[690] It is not known whether there is a clinical counterpart in humans.

COLLOIDAL BISMUTH SUBCITRATE

Structure and Formulations. As discussed in the *Helicobacter pylori* section, bismuth compounds in the form of colloidal bismuth subcitrate (CBS) and bismuth subsalicylate have been used alone and in combination with antibiotics for the treatment of *H. pylori*. In addition, colloidal bismuth subcitrate (also known as tripotassium dicitrato bismuthate) has been used extensively with good results as a single agent in the treatment of peptic ulcer disease. It is still under investigation in the United States but is approved for use in patients with ulcer disease in other countries. Colloidal bismuth subcitrate is available in solution and in chewable and coated tablets.

Mechanisms of Action. CBS is highly soluble in water but precipitates in an acid medium (pH less than 5) to form variously shaped crystals of bismuth oxychloride and bismuth citrate.[691] Colloidal bismuth has essentially no effect on gastric acid secretion and only minimal effects on peptic activity.[691] Besides its effect on *H. pylori*, colloidal bismuth subcitrate has several other actions that may account for its efficacy in the treatment of peptic ulcer disease. After CBS administration in the rat, bismuth preferentially coats ulcer craters as compared to surrounding normal mucosa.[692] CBS forms a glycoprotein–bismuth complex with mucus that creates a protective layer against acid-peptic digestion that also decreases the diffusion of hydrogen ion. CBS appears to be unique in forming a protective coating compared with other bismuth salts. Colloidal bismuth subcitrate also has mucosal defensive effects that appear, at least in part, to stimulate mucosal prostaglandin E_2 concentrations and thus bicarbonate secretion.[691,693,694] NSAIDs block the effect of CBS on PGE_2 and bicarbonate production. Nonetheless, CBS reduces the acute gastric mucosal damaging effects of NSAIDs, suggesting that it acts by both prostaglandin-mediated and prostaglandin-independent mechanisms.

The mucosal protective effects of CBS also may impart a therapeutic effect by stimulation of secretion of epidermal growth factor (EGF). CBS enhances the healing of gastric and duodenal ulcers induced in rats by acetic acid and augments the accumulation of epidermal growth factor in these experimental ulcers.[694] In addition, CBS inhibits peptic degradation of epidermal growth factor in vitro and prolongs epidermal growth factor availability in vivo.[695]

Pharmacokinetics. The majority of the ingested CBS is excreted in the feces as bismuth sulfide. However, minimal amounts of CBS are absorbed from the gastrointestinal tract, and small particles of bismuth precipitate have been observed in the duodenal epithelial cells after endocytosis.[696] Plasma bismuth concentrations rise in a dose-dependent manner during the first few weeks of therapy, plateau after about 4 weeks, and yet rarely exceed 50 μg/L.[691] Tissue accumulation occurs prinicpally in the kidneys, but small amounts occur also in other organs, such as the brain. Absorbed bismuth is eliminated in the urine, but this process is slow, and urinary concentrations remain high 2 weeks after cessation of CBS ingestion,[691] suggesting tissue accumulation and slow mobilization. Therefore, it should not be used, at least at present, in patients with renal insufficiency. Clearly, more work is needed to examine the pharmacokinetics of bismuth compounds in humans.

Adverse Effects. Few adverse effects occur with colloidal bismuth subcitrate. Blackening of the stools can be confused with melena. The solution form has an unpleasant ammoniacal smell. Chewable tablets cause staining of the tongue and mouth, although this is not seen with the coated tablets.[691] Diarrhea, headache, and mild dizziness have been reported occasionally.[691] The poor absorption of bismuth with colloidal subcitrate treatment makes it much less likely to cause encephalopathy, reported with other bismuth salts (e.g., bismuth subgallate, bismuth subnitrate), with short-term therapy.[691,697] However, a single case of paresthesias, fatigue, insomnia, and impaired concentration and memory after 20 months of CBS therapy has been reported.[697] The symptoms all improved over a period of 10 months after discontinuation of bismuth therapy. The toxicity of long-term bismuth therapy is unknown.

MISCELLANEOUS DRUGS

A number of other treatment modalities have been tested in patients with peptic ulcer diseases to relieve pain, expedite healing, and prevent recurrences. These range from dietary measures (to neutralize gastric acid; negative results) to recently testing acyclovir (to treat "latent" herpes infection; also negative results).[698] Anticholinergics, tricyclic antidepressants, and carbenoxolone have all been touted as active agents for the treatment of peptic ulcer disease and are reviewed briefly here. Of note, none of these agents is currently in the forefront of antiulcer therapy.

Anticholinergics.
The primary action of these drugs is to block the acetylcholine muscarinic receptor effect on the parietal cell and thereby decrease gastric acid secretion.[699] There are two subtypes of muscarinic receptors, M1 and M2.[700] The classic atropinelike anticholinergics act upon both the M1 and M2 receptors. The best known member of this class of drugs is atropine, and the class is often referred to as "atropinelike" drugs. The synthetic atropinelike agents have a quaternary ammonium structure (e.g., propantheline, L-hyoscyamine, butylscopolamine). As a group, they are poorly and unreliably absorbed.[701] In ordinary doses they do not cross the blood–brain barrier. Furthermore, their absorption is diminished when ingested with a meal.[702] Tertiary ammonium compounds (e.g., atropine) are better absorbed than the quaternary compounds. Pirenzepine, a tricyclic pyridobenzodiazepine derivative, has a low affinity for the M2 receptors (e.g., eye, urinary bladder) but a high affinity for the M1 receptors (e.g., the parietal cell).

The effect of the classic atropinelike anticholinergics on gastric acid secretion has been studied extensively.[702] They have only a modest inhibitory effect. At therapeutic doses (those which may cause untoward side effects—dry mouth, urinary retention, blurred vision), anticholinergics reduce basal acid secretion by about 50% and stimulated secretion (e.g., pentagastrin, meal) by only about 30%.[703] In individual patients, their inhibitory effects vary widely; for example, in one study, meal-stimulated gastric acid secretion was suppressed by 0% to 60%.[704]

The M1 antagonist pirenzepine also has a relatively modest effect on gastric acid secretion. An oral dose of 50 mg of pirenzepine decreases basal acid secretion by about 50% and pentagastrin-stimulated secretion by only about 40%.[705] As with the atropinelike anticholinergic agents, pirenzepine can cause dry mouth (about 15% of patients) and visual disturbances (about 2% of patients).[706] A newer M1 antagonist, telenzepine, is about 10 to 25 times more potent than the pirenzepine inhibitor of gastric acid secretion because of its greater bioavailability.[707]

In summary, it is apparent that the anticholinergic agents (either the combined M1/M2 inhibitors or the M1 antagonists) are in-

effective inhibitors of gastric acid secretion compared with the H_2-receptor antagonists and H^+/K^+-ATPase inhibitors. Furthermore, they are less effective in ulcer healing than current conventional treatment.

Tricyclic Antidepressants.
The tricyclic antidepressants have been used in patients with ulcer disease based on the hypothesis that many have "masked depression."[708] They have both a sedative and an anticholinergic effect. The prototype is imipramine, but there are numerous congeners (e.g., amitriptyline, desipramine, doxepin, nortriptyline, and so forth). However, they only slightly decrease acid and pepsin secretion,[709] they have CNS, cardiac, and other side effects, and they should not be used on a routine basis in patients with acid-peptic diseases.

Carbenoxolone.
Carbenoxolone is an extract of licorice that was used about 20 years ago primarily to treat gastric, and to a lesser extent duodenal, ulcers.[710] It has no significant effect on gastric acid secretion or motility.[711] Carbenoxolone inhibits peptic activity slightly, stimulates mucus secretion, and decreases mucosal cell loss.[711] Many of these actions are similar to those of prostaglandin E analogues, and carbenoxolone has been reported to decrease prostaglandin catabolism. It has an aldosteronelike effect and therefore results in fluid retention and hypokalemia and can precipitate congestive heart failure. These untoward effects can be obviated with the diuretic spirolactone. However, the administration of spirolactone impairs the modest therapeutic effect of carbenoxolone on ulcer healing. Importantly, the healing capacity of carbenoxolone contrasted with placebo is modest at best. It is not approved for use in the United States.

Acute Therapy of Duodenal Ulcers

H_2-RECEPTOR ANTAGONISTS

The histamine H_2-receptor antagonists have enjoyed a favored status for the acute treatment of duodenal ulcers for the past decade because of their efficacy, patient acceptance, and excellent safety profile. The various drug regimens of H_2-antagonists employed in DU therapy reflect an evolving understanding of ulcer pathogenesis.

Cimetidine was the first H_2-antagonist available for clinical use. It was initially administered in doses of 200 mg three times daily with meals and 400 mg h.s. (1 g/day) or 300 mg q.i.d., doses calculated to suppress basal and stimulated gastric acid secretion for as much of the 24-hour period as possible.[712,713] Multiple placebo-controlled trials in the late 1970s confirmed the efficacy of these regimens, with ulcer healing rates of 60% to 85% after 4 to 6 weeks of cimetidine therapy versus 20% to 70% in patients treated with placebo.[714] (For a complete compilation of H_2-antagonist trials from 1978 to 1982, see reference 714.)

The development of ranitidine precipitated a spate of further double-blind multicenter trials in the early 1980s in which either ranitidine 150 mg b.i.d. or cimetidine 400 mg b.i.d. was compared with cimetidine 1 g/day in a q.i.d. regimen (see reference 714 for a complete compilation). Both drugs administered twice daily produced healing rates of 60% to 75% after 4 weeks and 85% to

95% after 8 weeks of therapy, equivalent to the healing rates of the higher-dose q.i.d. cimetidine regimen.[714,715] It thus became apparent that twice-daily regimens were satisfactory alternatives for the treatment of acute duodenal ulcers.

The importance of nocturnal acid secretion in the pathogenesis of duodenal ulcer disease has been hypothesized for over 50 years.[712] With the success of initial trials of nocturnal doses of H_2-blockers in the early 1980s in the maintenance therapy of duodenal ulcers, the importance of nocturnal acid secretion in ulcer pathogenesis gained wider acceptance. A pharmacologic study by Hunt[520] demonstrated that single bedtime doses of cimetidine 800 mg or ranitidine 300 mg provided suppression of 24-hour gastric acid comparable to that of the equivalent total daily dosage administered b.i.d. and provided equal or superior suppression of nocturnal acidity (see above). A number of double-blind clinical trials comparing ranitidine 150 mg b.i.d. versus 300 mg h.s. or cimetidine 400 mg b.i.d. versus 800 mg h.s. in the acute healing of duodenal ulcers[496,716-722] demonstrated equivalent healing rates for twice-daily versus single bedtime regimens. Subsequently, famotidine and nizatidine have been released and tested with the same conclusions: twice-daily regimens have no therapeutic advantage to a single bedtime dosage.[497,529,723] In fact, all of the H_2-antagonists are approved and recommended for once-daily bedtime dosing in the treatment of uncomplicated duodenal ulcer disease. Hunt performed an extensive meta-analysis that compared the degree of gastric acid suppression derived from a number of pharmacologic studies of different H_2-antagonists with the ulcer healing rates from a number of controlled clinical trials.[521] The ulcer healing rates correlated better with the percentage suppression of nocturnal intragastric acidity than with the suppression of total or daytime acidity (Table 61-8; Fig 61-25).[724] Taken together, these data provide compelling evidence for the important role of nocturnal acid suppression in the healing of duodenal ulcers.

It must be acknowledged that the preeminent role of nocturnal acid suppression in ulcer therapy is not embraced by all investigators.[725-727] The sustained 24-hour acid suppression induced by the proton pump inhibitor omeprazole appears to result in more rapid healing of duodenal ulcers. In fact, a meta-analysis suggests that the ulcer healing rates with omeprazole correlate better with total 24-hour intragastric acid suppression than with nocturnal acid suppression.[521,712] Furthermore, a recent study reported comparable ulcer healing rates of morning versus bedtime doses of famotidine 40 mg.[727] Another study comparing three different cimetidine regimens (400 mg t.i.d. with meals, 1200 mg h.s., and 200 mg t.i.d. with meals plus 600 mg h.s.) found no difference in

the healing rates at 8 to 12 weeks but more rapid healing at 2 weeks with the mealtime regimen.[725] The relative importance of meal-stimulated acid secretion versus nocturnal acid secretion in the pathophysiology of duodenal ulcer disease merits further investigation. Notwithstanding these observations, H_2-antagonists are much more effective at inhibiting nocturnal acid secretion than meal-stimulated acid secretions, and the efficacy of nocturnal dosing regimens remains undisputed.

Regardless of the H_2-regimen employed, one can anticipate overall duodenal ulcer healing rates of approximately 75% at 4 weeks and 90% to 95% at 8 weeks with approved regimens. For uncomplicated duodenal ulcers, the nocturnal dosing regimen should be employed because of its ease of administration, improved patient compliance, and lower cost.

As noted above ("Pharmacology of Therapeutic Agents"), the administration of ranitidine or famotidine with dinner rather than at bedtime may provide equivalent nocturnal acid suppression and superior 24-hour acid suppression because of the improved acid suppression in the early evening hours. There are several studies comparing early evening and bedtime doses of ranitidine 300 mg in the healing of duodenal ulcers. Although the overall 4-week healing rates are no different between these regimens, either a statistically significant improvement or a trend toward improvement in the 2-week ulcer healing rates has been recorded with the early evening dosing.[517,728-730] It would appear that early evening dosing provides an effective alternative to the standard h.s. treatment regimens for ranitidine or famotidine.

H_2-Receptor Antagonists: Is There a Difference? If one accepts the primacy of nocturnal acid suppression in promoting ulcer healing, then minor differences in healing rates with different H_2-antagonist regimens are to be expected. Most comparative trials of different H_2-antagonists report no statistical differences; however, they generally have insufficient sample sizes to detect a difference in healing rates of less than 10% to 20%. Formal meta-analysis of 20 comparative trials of ranitidine with cimetidine has recently been performed.[715] There were 15 trials comparing ranitidine 150 mg b.i.d. with cimetidine 1 g/day (200 mg t.i.d. plus 400 mg h.s.) and five suitable trials comparing ranitidine 150 mg b.i.d. with cimetidine 400 mg b.i.d. Eighteen of these 20 trials had numerically higher healing rates after 4 weeks of ranitidine. In the two largest trials,[731,732] ranitidine was statistically superior to cimetidine; the sample size in most of the other studies was too small to detect a difference of less than 10%. The cumulative healing rates at 4 weeks were 77% for ranitidine (1114/

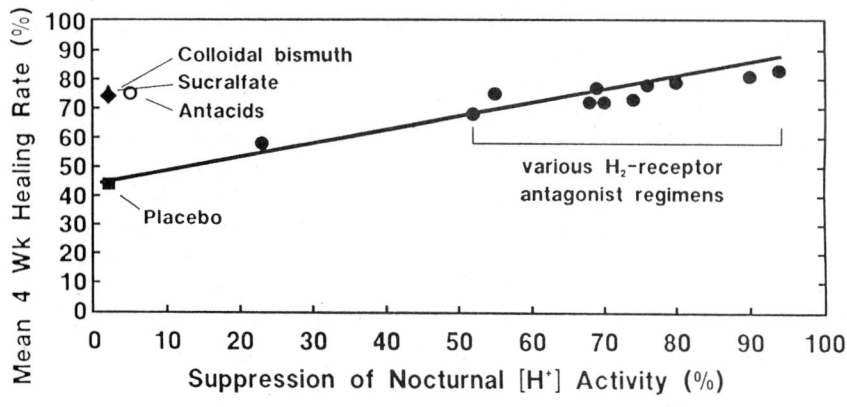

FIGURE 61-25. Correlation between suppression of nocturnal intragastric acidity and 4-week duodenal ulcer healing rates for different H_2-receptor antagonist regimens (listed in Table 61-8). (Modified from Hunt RH, Howden CW, Jones DB, Burget DW, Kerr GD. The correlation between acid suppression and peptic ulcer healing. Scand J Gastroenterol 1986;21(Suppl 125):22.)

1480 patients) and 70% for cimetidine (1013/1450 patients). By meta-analysis, ranitidine 150 mg b.i.d was statistically superior to both cimetidine regimens. From the Hunt analysis (Table 61-8; Fig 61-25), these two cimetidine regimens are less effective than ranitidine 150 mg b.i.d. in their nocturnal acid suppression, correlating with the inferior therapeutic results seen.

Far less data and no meta-analyses are available regarding the comparability of ulcer healing rates among nocturnal dosing regimens of the various H_2-receptor antagonists. Comparative studies of the currently recommended nocturnal dosing regimens (cimetidine 800 mg, ranitidine and nizatidine 300 mg, or famotidine 40 mg) report statistically similar 4-week healing rates, although limited study size may not permit detection of small differences.[496,497,529,733-737] All four regimens provide 90% to 100% of nocturnal acid suppression[515,516,522,524]; therefore, equivalent healing rates might be anticipated. In fact, nizatidine and ranitidine 150 mg and famotidine 20 mg, which are equipotent with cimetidine 800 mg, provide degrees of nocturnal acid inhibition that are similar to those of the corresponding standard full doses (300 mg and 40 mg, respectively).[515,516,523] Therefore, these lower dose regimens might be expected to yield healing rates comparable to those of the higher dose regimens and to cimetidine 800 mg h.s. This has been confirmed in one recent pilot study.[738]

In summary, standard doses of cimetidine, ranitidine, nizatidine, and famotidine administered as a once-daily bedtime dose appear to be comparable in the treatment of duodenal ulcer. Half-dose regimens of the other H_2-antagonists are comparable to cimetidine 800 mg in their suppression of nocturnal acidity and warrant further study in the therapy of duodenal ulcers. Early evening administration of a standard dose of ranitidine, nizatidine, or famotidine is an equally effective alternative to the bedtime dosing regimen.

OMEPRAZOLE

Omeprazole has proved efficacious in doses of 10 mg to 60 mg per day for acute duodenal ulcers in dose-comparative studies,[518,739-743] placebo-controlled studies,[627] and H_2-receptor antagonist controlled studies (Table 61-10).[615,744-748] On the basis of pharmacologic studies in DU patients, the optimal dose for maximal 24-hour intragastric acid suppression is 20 to 30 mg/d, doses that yield a mean of 90% and 97% acid suppression, respectively.[611,625] However, there is much more variability of individual patient response at 20 mg/d, with up to one third of patients exhibiting incomplete acid suppression.[625] In multiple dose-comparative trials, the 4-week cumulative healing rates are greater than 90% with omeprazole at 20 to 60 mg/d, with no distinct therapeutic advantage to doses above 20 mg/d. However, the healing rates at 2 weeks demonstrate an obvious linear dose dependency.[606,615] Therefore, doses greater than 20 mg/d heal DUs more rapidly, but there is a prompt "catch-up" thereafter.

A number of multicenter double-blind comparative trials of omeprazole versus H_2-receptor antagonists have been performed (Table 61-10),[615,628,744-749] although a meta-analysis has not been reported. Omeprazole doses of 20 to 40 mg/d yield 4-week healing rates of 82% to 100% versus 74% to 80% for cimetidine and 63% to 96% for ranitidine. Omeprazole was found to be statistically superior to cimetidine and ranitidine at 4 weeks in five out of six and five out of seven studies, respectively. Even if one considers only trials in which omeprazole 20 mg/d was compared with H_2-antagonists, omeprazole demonstrated statistically significant improvement in 4-week healing in six out of seven studies. Omeprazole 20 mg/d also demonstrated significantly higher 2-week healing rates compared with the H_2-antagonists in five out of eight

TABLE 61-10
Comparative Trials of Omeprazole Vs. H_2-Antagonists in Duodenal Ulcer Healing

STUDY	DESIGN	DRUG	DOSE	N	HEALING RATES (%) 2 Wks	4 Wks
Lauritsen[744]	R, DB	Omeprazole	30 mg/d	60†	73*	92*
	MC	Cimetidine	1 g/d	58†	46	74
Bardhan[748]	R, DB	Omeprazole	20 mg/d	33	83*	97*
	MC		40 mg/d	36	83*	100*
		Ranitidine	150 mg b.i.d.	33	53	82
McFarland[746]	R, DB	Omeprazole	200 mg/d	125	79*	91*
	MC	Ranitidine	300 mg h.s.	122	61	80
Classen[749]	R, DB	Omeprazole	20 mg/d	146†	72*	96
	MC	Ranitidine	150 mg b.i.d.	160†	59	92
Van Deventer[628]	R, DB	Omeprazole	20 mg/d	59	42	82*
	MC	Ranitidine	150 mg b.i.d.	65	34	63
Archambault[745]	R, DB	Omeprazole	20 mg/d	85	58	84
	MC	Cimetidine	600 mg b.i.d.	84	46	80
Mulder[747]	R, DB	Omeprazole	20 mg/d	91	60	87
	MC	Ranitidine	150 mg b.i.d.	90	64	91

* $P < 0.05$.
DB, double-blind; MC, multicenter; R, randomized.
† Protocol analysis.

studies, although the 2-week healing rates are less dramatic than with higher omeprazole doses.[615] It should be pointed out that the 2-week and 4-week healing rates with omeprazole 20 mg/d have been less impressive in the North American multicenter trials[627,628,745] than in studies done abroad. Notwithstanding, omeprazole 20 mg/d appears to offer a therapeutic gain over H_2-antagonists of approximately 15% after 2 and 4 weeks of therapy.[615]

Omeprazole also appears to provide more rapid ulcer pain relief than H_2-antagonists. Most studies demonstrate either a significant difference or a trend toward earlier pain relief at 1 to 2 weeks.[615,744-746,748]

In summary, omeprazole 20 to 40 mg/d has significantly higher DU healing rates at 2 weeks and, in most cases, also at 4 weeks than conventional doses of H_2-antagonists. This therapeutic advantage may translate into more rapid pain relief in some patients. The optimal dose for most patients is probably 20 mg/d. However, the dose-related variability of omeprazole on gastric acid suppression and the differences in 2- and 4-week healing rates suggest that 30 to 40 mg/d may yield more predictable responses. Although the duodenal ulcer healing rates for H_2-antagonists correlate better with the degree of nocturnal acid suppression, the healing rates for other antisecretory agents such as omeprazole correlate better with 24-hour gastric acid suppression.[521] It is not surprising that omeprazole, which inhibits 90% to 99% of gastric acid secretion in 24 hours, should yield significantly higher healing rates compared with conventional doses of H_2-antagonists, which inhibit 40% to 68% of 24-hour gastric acidity.[521] Recently, higher doses of ranitidine (300 mg b.i.d. to q.i.d.) have been compared with conventional doses (300 mg/d) in DU patients. These higher dose regimens suppress up to 79% of 24-hour gastric acidity and result in significantly higher 2- and 4-week ulcer healing rates than the conventional 300-mg bedtime ranitidine dose.[750-753] Direct comparisons between omeprazole and higher doses of H_2-receptor antagonists have not been performed.

SUCRALFATE

Sucralfate in a dose of 1 g q.i.d. is superior to placebo in several controlled treatment trials of duodenal ulcers.[754-757] A complete compilation of sucralfate therapeutic trials is provided in reference 758. The healing rates after 4 weeks of sucralfate treatment range from 50% to 80%, and the 4-week placebo healing rates varied markedly from about 25% to 65%. In most of these studies, superior symptomatic relief is reported in the sucralfate-treated group. Sucralfate 2 g b.i.d. has also been compared with the 1-g q.i.d. regimen, with approximately 75% 4-week healing rates observed with both regimens.[759-761]

There are several double-blind[762-765] and single-blind trials[766-770] comparing sucralfate with H_2-receptor antagonists in the treatment of acute DUs. In none of these studies is there a significant difference in healing rates between sucralfate 1 g q.i.d. and ranitidine 150 mg b.i.d. or cimetidine 0.8 to 1.2 g/d. Most of these studies are of inadequate size to detect a small therapeutic difference between these agents; therefore, a meta-analysis is needed. Cumulative ulcer healing rates of 70% to 80% and 85% to 95% are reported at 4 and 8 weeks with either sucralfate or H_2-receptor antagonists. It must be concluded that there is no discernible difference in acute ulcer healing rates at 4 or 8 weeks between sucralfate and H_2-antagonists.

There is controversy regarding the relative efficacy of various ulcer therapeutic agents on ulcer healing in nonsmokers versus smokers.[758] Most reports, and a recent meta-analysis, observed that ulcer healing is delayed in smokers versus nonsmokers.[771] Moreover, there appears to be a relationship between the number of cigarettes smoked and the risk of ulcers not healing.[771,772] These differences in ulcer healing rates are observed in multiple clinical therapeutic trials, regardless of whether the patient is treated with an active agent or placebo.[771-775] That is, placebo-treated smokers have much lower healing rates than nonsmokers. A recent single-blind trial claimed that ulcer healing with sucralfate was equally high in smokers and nonsmokers, in contrast to delayed healing rates in smokers treated with cimetidine.[770] This study has been criticized,[776] and this purported advantage of sucralfate in smokers has not been observed in other comparative trials.[763,764,768]

It is premature to conclude that sucralfate or other mucosal protective agents offer advantages for the smoking patient. Future therapeutic trials need to prestratify patients according to smoking status, number of cigarettes smoked, and ulcer size for this question to be properly answered.

ANTACIDS

In 1977, Peterson and colleagues[491] reported in a double-blind prospective trial that 1008 mmol/d of liquid antacid (30-ml doses 1 and 3 hours after meals and at bedtime) healed 78% of patients with DU over 4 weeks versus 45% with placebo, a significant difference. Numerous clinical trials have since examined the effect of high as well as low doses of antacids, including antacid tablets, in patients with acute DUs.[777] Daily doses of antacid as low as 120 to 200 mmol/d of buffering result in healing rates of approximately 70%, equivalent to those of higher doses of antacids (Fig 61-26).[778] This was confirmed by Lam and co-workers in Hong Kong with only a 175-mmol/d dose resulting in 77% healing.[779] Dose–response healing has been observed with liquid aluminum antacid with healing rates of 88% at the maximal dose of 414 mmol/d; placebo healing was 33%.[780]

When compared with cimetidine treatment, DU healing rates

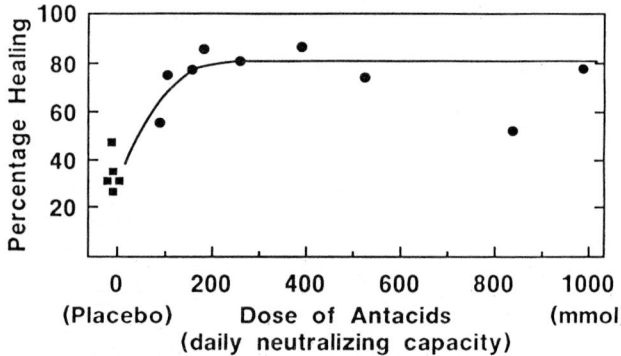

FIGURE 61–26. Healing rates of duodenal ulcer after one month's treatment with varying doses of antacid from 0 (placebo) to over 1000 mmol/d (equal to seven 30-ml doses of a potent liquid antacid). Of note, ulcer healing reaches a plateau with about 200 mmol/d. Each point represents results of a single clinical trial. (Reproduced with permission from Berstad A. Antacids in the treatment of gastrointestinal ulcer. Scand J Gastroenterol 1986;21:385.)

with antacids have been similar: healing after 4 and 6 weeks of therapy was 63% and 82% with either Mylanta-II (1008 mmol/ d) or cimetidine (1200 mg/d).[781] More recently, Weberg and colleagues[782] observed in a double-blind study that a low-dose antacid tablet, only 120 mmol/d of buffer, resulted in 71% DU healing after 1 month, similar to the 78% healing observed with 800 mg of cimetidine nightly; pain relief was also similar in the two groups. Variations on the theme exist[784,785] with the same results: small doses of antacid appear to be equal to ranitidine[784] or to the combination of liquid antacid plus cimetidine.[785] Therefore, combination therapy, at least as tested thus far, is of no greater efficacy than single-drug treatment.

The superiority of antacids in pain relief in patients with DU is controversial: some studies report that antacids and placebo produce equivalent pain relief,[491,786] while others report that antacids are superior to placebo.[787]

In summary, antacids are highly effective in expediting duodenal ulcer healing. They are therapeutic both as liquid and tablet formulations and at low (i.e., about 200 mmol/d) as well as higher doses. Antacids are, however, no longer the first-line therapy in spite of being less costly than other therapeutic agents. There are proponents, however, who state that "It seems . . . reasonable to recommend antacids as the first drug of choice when treating gastroduodenal ulcer."[788] If further studies indicate that low-dose antacid therapy is similar in efficacy to the more potent H_2-receptor antagonists and/or omeprazole and is less expensive and without toxicity, it is indeed reasonable for it to be reconsidered for primary therapy of DU.

PROSTAGLANDINS

Numerous prospective therapeutic studies with synthetic prostaglandin analogues for the treatment of acute duodenal ulcer are available,[789] although it is unlikely that the currently available prostaglandins will be used to any great extent in the treatment of acute DU because of the availability of more effective drugs with fewer untoward effects. Misoprostol (400 μg b.i.d.), arbaprostil (50 μg q.i.d.), enprostil (35 μg b.i.d.), and rioprostil (300 mg b.i.d.) have each been shown to be significantly more effective (60% to 80% healing) than placebo in expediting duodenal ulcer healing at 4 or 6 weeks.[791-796] Furthermore, a single nighttime dose of 100 μg of arbaprostil resulted in 86% of duodenal ulcers healing at 4 weeks.[790] Of note, non-antisecretory doses of prostaglandins (e.g., arbaprostil at doses of 25 μg q.i.d. or less) result in duodenal ulcer healing equivalent to that of placebo. Therefore, prostaglandin efficacy seems to be largely related to antisecretory effects.

A number of acute DU studies have compared synthetic prostaglandin analogues with the histamine H_2-receptor antagonists.[791-798] Overall, they indicate a distinct trend in favor of the H_2-receptor antagonists. Relief of ulcer pain in general is also somewhat greater with H_2-blockers than with the synthetic prostaglandin analogues.

In summary, prostaglandins account for only a modest amount of the existing antiulcer market. Although at antisecretory doses they are more effective than placebo, they are generally less effective than H_2-receptor antagonists. It is likely that they will be even less effective than omeprazole. Finally, current formulations result in dose-related diarrhea and abdominal cramps in a substantial proportion of patients.[792]

BISMUTH-CONTAINING COMPOUNDS

Colloidal bismuth subcitrate (CBS) has been compared with placebo and H_2-receptor antagonists in multiple controlled trials of duodenal ulcer therapy since 1974.[214,800] Initial trials were conducted with 120 mg q.i.d. of the liquid formulation of CBS, a formulation no longer generally available because of taste and smell (which also obviated true blinded trials). Nevertheless, CBS liquid has demonstrated clear superiority to placebo in multiple controlled trials, with 4-week healing rates of approximately 75%.[800] Similarly, multiple comparison trials of CBS liquid 120 mg q.i.d. with cimetidine 1 g q.i.d. failed to detect a significant difference in healing rates after 4 to 8 weeks.[214,800]

CBS chewable tablets, introduced in the early 1980s, had a significant improvement in taste and thereby improved patient acceptance. However, blackening of the teeth and tongue continued to make double-blind study design problematic. The chewable CBS tablets, 120 mg q.i.d., have demonstrated efficacy equivalent to that of the liquid CBS formulation in two duodenal ulcer trials,[800] and a large number of randomized double-blind comparison trials[214,800-802] have failed to detect a statistically significant difference in ulcer healing after 4 to 8 weeks between CBS tablets and cimetidine[214,800,803] or ranitidine.[801,802,804] There is a trend, however, toward earlier ulcer healing in CBS-treated patients at 4 weeks.[805]

Most recently, a coated CBS tablet improves patient acceptability even further.[806] A single-blind, randomized, multicenter trial comparing CBS chewable and coated tablets could demonstrate no significant difference in efficacy between these formulations.[806] Further comparison studies of CBS coated tablets with placebo and H_2-receptor antagonists are required.

In summary, CBS is an effective agent in the acute treatment of DU. In doses of 120 mg q.i.d., it is at least comparable in efficacy to H_2-receptor antagonists. Ulcer healing rates of 70% to 80% after 4 weeks and greater than 90% after 8 weeks of CBS therapy may be anticipated. CBS is not yet approved by the FDA for acute DU therapy.

Of greater importance than the efficacy of CBS in acute DU healing is its apparent impact on reducing subsequent ulcer recurrences. When compared with acute treatment with H_2-receptor antagonists, the duodenal ulcer recurrence rate 6 months after acute CBS therapy is approximately 17% lower.[805,807] The possible reasons for this reduction in ulcer recurrence are discussed in the section on *H. pylori* and ulcer recurrence.

MISCELLANEOUS DRUGS

Additional agents not in current use and not approved for the treatment of acute duodenal ulcer include: anticholinergics (combined M1 and M2 inhibitors), specific M1 anticholinergics, and the tricyclic antidepressants.[808,809]

Anticholinergics. The nonselective M1 and M2 anticholinergics, used commonly prior to the availability of the H_2-receptor antagonists, are only modest inhibitors of gastric acid and pepsin secretion. Furthermore, in the early clinical trials (many unblinded and without endoscopic assessment of healing), nonselective anticholinergics were at best only slightly better than placebo.[810] They were, therefore, appropriately discarded for antiulcer therapy. Prior to the availability of the H^+/K^+-ATPase inhibitor omeprazole, anticholinergic drugs were recommended in combination with H_2-receptor antagonists in patients with gastrinoma (see ch 62) because of their additive effect in suppressing gastric acid secretion.

Specific M1 Anticholinergics.

A few controlled and blinded trials with the specific M1 anticholinergic pirenzepine suggest that it is superior to placebo but less effective than H_2-receptor antagonists in expediting acute duodenal ulcer healing.[811] Although no meta-analysis has been reported to date, H_2-receptor antagonists are superior to pirenzepine in about three fourths of trials. Moreover, with doses of 150 mg of pirenzepine daily, about 15% of patients complain of dry mouth and 5% of visual disturbances.[812] Clearly, pirenzepine is inferior to the conventional drugs used to treat acute duodenal ulcer.

Tricyclic Antidepressants.

Limited trials with the tricyclic antidepressants,[809] performed on small numbers of patients, have shown healing rates with the tricyclic antidepressants that are superior to those of placebo but inferior to those observed with H_2-receptor antagonists.[811] Furthermore, the tricyclic antidepressants can cause somnolence and anticholinergiclike side effects. They should be used only as indicated in patients requiring antidepressant medication, and in the DU patient who is depressed, it is sensible to use standard antiulcer treatment as well.

RECOMMENDATIONS FOR ACUTE THERAPY

The goals of acute treatment of duodenal ulcer are to relieve pain, expedite healing, and prevent complications during ulcer healing. However, the steps involved in clinical decision making are complex.[813–815] The factors that direct physician choice of medications vary widely from anecdotal or last-case observation to the awareness of carefully performed and meticulously analyzed prospective randomized controlled trial (RCT) data. Furthermore, it is often assumed, albeit incorrectly, that the results obtained in RCTs will apply to the patient population that is being treated. Although RCTs have provided a wealth of valuable information regarding healing of peptic ulcer disease, the data from these studies may or may not apply to the individual patient. They are, however, the standards upon which clinical practice should be based. It should be noted that patients in RCTs tend to be closely monitored, undergo frequent endoscopic examinations, and are instructed repeatedly about proper medication intake. The standard of practice outside an RCT is often different, either more or less intense, depending upon the physician's style and standard of practice and the patient's response.

The choice of drugs for the treatment of acute duodenal ulcer, given the numerous drugs of established efficacy approved for use, rests upon factors such as: required dose frequency (which is related to patient compliance), patient acceptability, cost, likelihood of recurrences after healing, and untoward side effects. Drug selection, therefore, is in large part subjective.

The H_2-receptor antagonists are each highly effective in expediting acute duodenal ulcer healing. Furthermore, each can be given in a single evening or bedtime dose with prompt DU healing. The choice between specific H_2-receptor antagonists then rests with factors such as concomitant drug intake, which could interact unfavorably with the H_2-antagonist (e.g., cimetidine and warfarinlike drugs), cost, and patient acceptance. At this time, the use of either ranitidine 300 mg, nizatidine 300 mg, or famotidine 40 mg with supper or cimetidine 800 mg h.s. seems the most reasonable.

Sucralfate is an alternative to the H_2-receptor antagonists in the treatment of acute duodenal ulcer. However, it requires at least twice-daily dosing, and the current formulation is a rather large pill, which is difficult to swallow for some patients. In general, cost is quite similar to that of the H_2-receptor antagonists.

Antacids, likely because of the large volumes and frequent dosing (i.e., four times daily) used in the initial RCTs coupled with their effects on bowel habit, are not commonly used. However, in the event that there are additional clinical trials from North America and Europe confirming efficacy at modest doses, they are indeed worthy of use. They offer considerable cost savings.

Prostaglandin E analogues are not approved for use in the therapy of acute duodenal ulcer. They require multiple daily dosing and have an inferior healing profile when contrasted to H_2-receptor antagonists. At doses required to produce healing, there is frequently diarrhea and/or abdominal cramps. At present, they are not recommended for routine use in patients with acute duodenal ulcers.

In initial studies, omeprazole is as effective as the H_2-receptor antagonists, and in fact it reportedly promotes earlier duodenal ulcer healing (i.e., at 2 to 4 weeks) than the H_2-receptor antagonists. Omeprazole also requires only single-day dosing.

Colloidal bismuth subcitrate (CBS) is of clinical interest because of its therapeutic efficacy coupled with its reported low incidence of duodenal ulcer recurrences after healing (likely secondary to its effect on *H. pylori*). Current reports indicate that it has to be given at least twice daily. With both omeprazole and CBS, additional long-term toxicity data are needed.

In summary, at the time of this writing, the use of H_2-receptor antagonists as a single evening dose is recommended for the routine treatment of acute duodenal ulcers. In the near future, omeprazole may be approved for use. Colloidal bismuth suspension may become a choice for the acute treatment of duodenal ulcer disease if it is free of acute and chronic side effects, is documented to be associated with an ulcer recurrence rate after healing that is lower than that of competitive drugs, is well accepted by patients, and is of similar or lesser cost.

Acute Therapy of Gastric Ulcers

H_2-RECEPTOR ANTAGONISTS

H_2-antagonists are well established as effective therapeutic agents for acute gastric ulcers. Because the vast majority of gastric ulcer patients have normal or reduced levels of acid secretion, and there appears to be impairment of gastric mucosal defensive factors, it may seem paradoxical to treat such patients with acid inhibitory agents. However, it is clear that further reduction of gastric acidity with such agents promotes ulcer healing, even if the correlation between acid reduction and gastric ulcer healing is not as strong as with duodenal ulcers.[816]

The multiple placebo-controlled clinical drug trials of cimetidine, ranitidine, and famotidine in the treatment of acute GUs have been compiled in several recent reviews.[496,497,817-821] These studies reveal a great deal of variability in the rate of gastric ulcer healing with both active therapy and placebo. Although cumulative healing rates appear to be comparable to those of duodenal ulcers (i.e., 80% to 90% after 8–12 weeks of therapy),[816,822] the time for treatment-to-healing is delayed approximately 2 to 4 weeks.

An analysis of the factors influencing GU healing rates reveals some important differences from duodenal ulcers. With or without therapy, there is a strong correlation between GU healing and the duration of treatment or observation. Placebo healing rates increase progressively with time, approaching 50% to 60% at 8 weeks.[724] In contrast, DU healing rates with placebo do not increase significantly beyond 4 weeks.[712] Although GU healing rates with H₂-antagonists are related to the degree of suppression of intragastric acidity, the relationship is not nearly as strong as with duodenal ulcers.[816] Healing rates correlate better with the degree of 24-hour acid suppression than with nocturnal acid suppression. However, there is, in fact, very little difference in GU healing rates between the different antisecretory agents administered in a variety of regimens.[724,816] Direct comparative trials of ranitidine 150 mg b.i.d. with cimetidine 1 g/d (200 mg t.i.d. with 400 mg h.s.) reveal no differences in rate of healing or cumulative healing.[823-827] A limited number of comparative studies of nocturnal dosing versus a twice-daily regimen have been conducted with ranitidine, famotidine, and nizatidine, and these studies seem to confirm the equal efficacy of nocturnal dosing in the healing of GUs despite the apparently weaker correlation of GU healing with nocturnal acid suppression.[497,529,828-831] Although nocturnal dosing for GUs is approved for cimetidine, ranitidine, and famotidine, further studies are desirable before these regimens should be adopted as first-line therapy for all GU patients.[830]

OMEPRAZOLE

Omeprazole 20 to 40 mg/d has a demonstrated efficacy in the acute treatment of GUs and is equivalent or superior to H₂-antagonists.[832] The optimal dose is not established. Open noncomparative studies suggest that omeprazole 30 to 40 mg/d results in nearly 100% healing of GUs by 6 to 8 weeks, with faster healing evident at the higher dose.[832] In several comparative studies, omeprazole 20 to 30 mg/d results in significantly higher 4-week healing rates than ranitidine 150 mg b.i.d.,[833,834] cimetidine 400 mg b.i.d.,[835] or cimetidine 1 g/d.[836] The cumulative healing rate at 8 weeks is numerically, but not significantly, greater in omeprazole-treated patients (Table 61-11).[832]

Some studies,[832,833] but not all,[835] suggest that ulcers of the gastric corpus heal more slowly than ulcers in the antrum or prepyloric regions. In a recent multicenter comparative trial, omeprazole 40 mg/d had significantly higher healing rates than ranitidine 150 mg b.i.d. and a lower dose of omeprazole, 20 mg/d, at both 4 and 8 weeks.[834] In addition to fostering more rapid GU healing, omeprazole appears to provide more rapid pain relief than H₂-antagonists within the first 2 weeks of therapy. However, by 4 weeks these differences have disappeared.[832] The superiority of omeprazole 20 to 40 mg/d versus H₂-antagonists in providing earlier pain relief and gastric ulcer healing confirms the importance of gastric acid in the healing of gastric ulcers.[816] The results with

TABLE 61–11
Comparative Trials of Omeprazole Vs. H₂-Antagonists in Gastric Ulcer Healing

STUDY	DESIGN	DRUG	DOSE	N	HEALING RATES (%)		
					2 Wks	4 Wks	8 Wks
Classen[749]	R, DB	Omeprazole	20 mg/d	83	43	81	95
	MC	Ranitidine	150 mg b.i.d.	74	45	80	90
Barbara[833]	R, ? DB	Omeprazole	20 mg/d	80	35*	74*	96*
	MC	Ranitidine	150 mg b.i.d.	80	9	53	85
Lauritsen[1008]	R, DB	Omeprazole	30 mg/d	81	54*	81	86
	MC	Cimetidine	1 g/d	82	39	73	78
Bate[835]	R, DB	Omeprazole	20 mg/d	102		73*	84
	MC	Cimetidine	400 mg b.i.d.	87		58	75
Walan[834]	R, DB	Omeprazole	20 mg/d	172†		69*	89
	MC		40 mg/d	171†		80*	96*
		Ranitidine	150 mg b.i.d.	169†		59	85
Danish Omeprazole	R, DB	Omeprazole	30 mg/d	68†	41	77	88‡
Study Group[836]	MC	Cimetidine	1 g/d	65†	41	58	82‡

* *P < 0.05 compared with H₂-antagonist*
† *Data provided on per-protocol analysis*
‡ *6 weeks (not 8 weeks)*
R, randomized; DB, double-blind; MC, multicenter

omeprazole in GU are of interest because they suggest that the greater degree of acid suppression, the greater the GU healing rates—despite being a disease characterized by low amounts of gastric acid secretion.

SUCRALFATE

It is paradoxical that sucralfate, a drug proposed for its beneficial effects on mucosal defense mechanisms, has not been comprehensively studied for the treatment of gastric ulcers. Accordingly, it still lacks FDA approval for this indication. In a carefully conducted placebo-controlled, double-blind trial, a significantly higher healing rate was documented for sucralfate 1 g q.i.d. at 4 and 8 weeks.[837] In multicenter double-blind comparison trials of sucralfate 1 g q.i.d. versus ranitidine 150 mg b.i.d. and cimetidine 400 mg b.i.d., healing rates were numerically higher at 4 to 6 weeks in patients treated with an H_2-antagonist (approximately 70%) than they were in those treated with sucralfate (approximately 60%).[838,839] However, by 12 weeks, the cumulative healing rates were comparable at 85% to 95%. This trend toward lower 4-week healing rates in patients treated with sucralfate as compared with H_2-antagonists is also suggested in additional single-blind or unblinded studies.[767,840] More recently, sucralfate 2 g b.i.d. has been compared with cimetidine 400 mg b.i.d. in a single-center double-blind trial, with comparable healing rates observed at 4, 8, and 12 weeks.[841]

Overall, the various trials conducted to date[758] suggest that sucralfate has efficacy in the acute treatment of GUs, with healing rates of 50% to 60% and greater than 80% anticipated after 4 and 8 weeks of therapy, respectively. However, there is a dearth of well-conducted multicenter double-blind trials with sucralfate. Its comparability to H_2-antagonists, particularly in the first 4 to 6 weeks of therapy, requires further study.

ANTACIDS

As with duodenal ulcer, the use of antacids as the sole drug has become unfashionable in the treatment of gastric ulcer. Moderately large doses of antacid (560 mmol/d) and cimetidine (1200 mg/d) resulted in similar GU healing rates, about 60% at 6 weeks.[842] A modest dose of liquid antacid (320 mmol/d, 80 mmol q.i.d.) was reported to be arithmetically less effective than cimetidine (1200 mg/d) after 4 and 8 weeks of therapy, but after 12 weeks of therapy healing rates were 89% and 84%, respectively.[843] Pain relief was similar in all treatment groups. However, diarrhea occurred in one fifth of the antacid-treated group versus only 5% in the cimetidine or placebo groups. In Scandinavian studies, GU healing was 67% after 6 weeks of treatment with only 10 ml of antacid q.i.d. (120 mmol/d) compared with 25% healing with placebo,[844] whereas seven 10-ml doses of antacid (600 mmol/d) in a different study resulted in GU healing after 4 and 6 weeks similar to that with ranitidine 150 mg b.i.d., approximately 60% and 75%, respectively.[845] Pain relief was superior to that of placebo with this low-dose antacid program.

In summary, moderate to large doses of antacids are effective in expediting GU healing similar to that observed with H_2-receptor antagonists. The data on lower-dose antacid treatment of GU are conflicting and require additional studies. However, at present,

antacids are not used exclusively in the treatment of gastric ulcer. Therapeutic efficacy, patient acceptability, and the absence of altered bowel function make the H_2-receptor antagonists the preferred form of therapy.

PROSTAGLANDINS

Numerous trials have been performed contrasting the synthetic analogues of prostaglandin E with placebo and/or histamine H_2-receptor antagonists in the treatment of gastric ulcer. The findings are quite comparable to those observed in DU: at antisecretory doses, most, but not all, studies suggest that prostaglandins are more effective than placebo. For example, 8-week gastric ulcer healing of 62% was observed in patients treated with misoprostol 100 mg q.i.d. versus 45% with placebo,[846] and enprostil 35 μg daily compared with placebo showed 4-week healing rates of 59% and 33%, respectively.[847] As with duodenal ulcer, gastric ulcer healing rates tend to be less with the prostaglandin analogues compared with histamine H_2-receptor antagonists.[848,849] However, some report similar healing rates.[850] Of note, Euler and colleagues recently reported that a non-antisecretory dose of arbaprostil was no different from placebo in expediting gastric ulcer healing.[851] This would suggest that doses that do not reduce gastric acid secretion but theoretically should have a cytoprotective effect are ineffective.

In summary, the studies in gastric ulcer reveal that in general prostaglandin analogues tend to be less effective than H_2-receptor antagonists. They will no doubt be even less effective than omeprazole. At present, only misoprostol is approved for use in the United States, and it will likely be used only in specific patients, such as those with gastric ulcer disease requiring daily NSAID treatment. However, because gastric ulcers tend to heal, albeit slower, with H_2-receptor antagonists in patients with NSAID-induced ulcers, the precise role of misoprostol requires further study (see below).

BISMUTH-CONTAINING COMPOUNDS

In prospective, reportedly blinded studies (bismuth is difficult to blind because of its odor, taste, and buccal effects), gastric ulcer healing after 4 weeks of colloidal bismuth (120–240 mg q.i.d.) ranged from about 65% to 90% in contrast to approximately 35% with placebo. There have been a few studies with relatively small numbers of gastric ulcer patients contrasting CBS with H_2-receptor antagonists.[214,852-856] Tytgat and co-workers reported that the healing rates after 4 weeks of therapy with CBS 120 mg q.i.d., cimetidine 1 g/d, and placebo were 61%, 43%, and 18%, respectively.[855] CBS was significantly superior to placebo. When contrasted with ranitidine 150 mg b.i.d., CBS 120 mg q.i.d. resulted in equivalent healing after 4 (63% and 70%, respectively) and 8 weeks (79% and 88%, respectively) of treatment.[856]

In summary, there are quite limited data on gastric ulcer healing with colloidal bismuth subcitrate. The results, however, suggest that CBS is therapeutically effective and likely as effective as other established treatment modalities.[214] CBS has not been approved for use in the United States, and its long-term side effect profile is not established.

MISCELLANEOUS DRUGS

Although carbenoxolone has been shown to be more effective than placebo in expediting gastric ulcer healing,[857] it is less effective than other standard treatment programs. Furthermore, its aldosteronelike side effects limit its utility.

There are limited data on the effectiveness of tricyclic antidepressants in the treatment of gastric ulcer disease.[858] In a single study, the 1-month healing was 60% with trimipramine, 50 mg h.s., versus 20% with placebo.[859] However, there were more drug-related side effects (e.g., drowsiness) in the trimipramine-treated group. Because the efficacy of tricyclics is inferior to that of other standard forms of therapy and is associated with frequent side effects, they are not recommended for routine use. However, their use, preferably with other conventional antiulcer drugs, is appropriate in those patients with depression requiring drug treatment.

RECOMMENDATIONS FOR ACUTE TREATMENT OF GASTRIC ULCER

The healing rates of non–NSAID-related gastric ulcers are, in general, similar with all the H_2-receptor antagonists: cimetidine (300 mg q.i.d., 400 mg b.i.d., and 800 mg h.s.), ranitidine (150 mg b.i.d., 300 mg h.s.), and famotidine (40 mg q.h.s.); nizatidine is not approved by the FDA for treatment of GU at this time. The H^+/K^+-ATPase inhibitor omeprazole (20–40 mg/d), sucralfate (1 g q.i.d.), bismuth subcitrate (120 mg q.i.d.), and moderate- to high-dose antacids (500 to 1000 mmol/d) are also effective, but are not FDA approved, for gastric ulcer therapy. In addition, pain relief overall is similar between patients treated with these drugs.

How, then, should the physician decide between the various therapeutic choices? First, it is important to assure that the patient is not taking NSAIDs unless absolutely required, because their continued intake delays gastric ulcer healing. Second, smoking should be discontinued because in most studies it prolongs ulcer healing. The choice of the specific drug should be based upon efficacy, incidence and severity of untoward side effects, cost, and frequency of dosing (compliance is improved with less frequent dosing). All approved antiulcer drugs are for the most part very safe.

At present, the use of one of the H_2-receptor antagonists is most reasonable. They are approved for treating GUs, effective, safe, and can be taken as a single nocturnal dose. Sucralfate has not been extensively studied in GU patients and has not yet established efficacy equivalent to that of H_2-receptor antagonists. Although antacids are effective, they require multiple daily dosing, and they also may cause diarrhea. The prostaglandin E_1 analogue misoprostol, although effective in expediting GU healing, tends to be less potent than H_2-receptor antagonists, requires multiple daily dosing, and causes diarrhea and abdominal cramps in an appreciable percentage of patients. If further comparative studies demonstrate more rapid GU healing with omeprazole than with H_2-antagonists, it may become the preferable therapeutic agent. Similarly, if colloidal bismuth subcitrate demonstrates equivalent healing with lower ulcer recurrence rates than H_2-antagonists, it may become the agent of choice. Further therapeutic trials are needed.

Ulcer Recurrence

NATURAL HISTORY

There are limited data regarding the natural history of ulcer disease prior to the introduction of the H_2-receptor antagonists. Furthermore, because these early reports were retrospective and were performed before the ready availability of endoscopy, they are confounding because the initial diagnosis of ulcer was based on the clinical findings and radiography, both less than precise methods in establishing the diagnosis of ulcer. In spite of these limitations, a 13-year follow-up is available on 154 DU patients.[860] Of interest, 13 years after diagnosis, 57% of those interviewed reported no symptoms during the previous year; about three fourths of these denied any symptoms of ulcer during the prior 5 years, and one half had been symptom-free for more than 11 years. Only 12% reported moderate to severe symptoms. Five percent required emergency surgery for complications, and 17% had undergone elective surgery. In 1964, Fry, a general practitioner in Great Britain, reported that 10 years after diagnosis of duodenal ulcer, about 60% of his patients were symptom-free and less than 10% reported severe symptoms.[861] Over a 15-year period of follow-up, about 15% percent developed upper gastrointestinal hemorrhage and 10% developed a perforation.

Taken together, these studies suggest that the frequently quoted adage "once an ulcer, always an ulcer" is incorrect, at least as far as symptoms are concerned. They instead suggest that, at least in the pre-endoscopy and pre–H_2-receptor antagonist era, symptomatic duodenal ulcer disease tended to "burn out," and only one in five patients developed complications.

The waters have become murky. Numerous studies of H_2-receptor antagonists have reported that the 1-year incidence of duodenal ulcer recurrence in placebo-treated patients ranges from 50% to 90% (Fig 61-27).[862,863] This is in contrast to a 10% to 30% symptomatic recurrence rate over 1 year in patients maintained

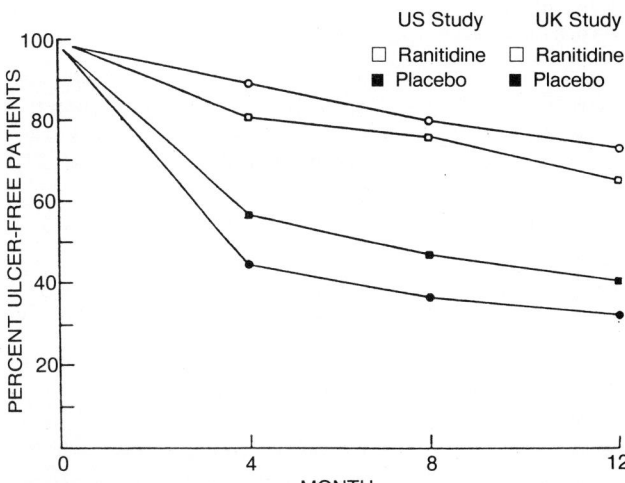

FIGURE 61–27. Duodenal ulcer recurrence rates during maintenance treatment. Results of two multicenter studies comparing placebo with ranitidine 150 mg h.s. in the maintenance treatment of patients with duodenal ulcers.[894,895] (Silvis SE. Results of the United States ranitidine maintenance trials. Am J Med 1984;77(Suppl 5B):33.)

on continuous, nocturnal H_2-receptor antagonist therapy.[864] In a study of duodenal ulcer recurrence rates in patients in whom the acute ulcer had healed with cimetidine and who were then placed on intermittent therapy as needed only for recurrences, over the year 26% reported no relapse, 83% reported two or fewer relapses, and 17% reported three or more relapses.[865] Similar results were observed by Frederiksen.[866] These findings suggest that in many patients ulcer disease tends to be responsive to initial treatment, and many patients have only a modest incidence of symptomatic recurrences. Furthermore, it is difficult to predict the course of the ulcer disease for any individual at the disease onset. Some patients may have relapses at regular intervals, while others have marked variations in intervals between relapses. There are, however, certain factors that tend to be associated with a greater ulcer recurrence rate (see below).

The above observations apply as well to non–NSAID-induced gastric ulcers. Early studies of the natural history of gastric ulcer reported recurrence rates of between 15% and 80% over the subsequent 2 to 5 years.[867-869] These results have been confirmed in more recent studies (Table 61-12). In addition, gastric ulcer recurrences were similar after acute healing with either placebo, antacids, or cimetidine, approximately 30% within 9 months of healing.[870] Of interest, as with duodenal ulcer, a substantial percentage of patients have asymptomatic recurrences (in some series up to one third), while some patients develop recurrent symptoms yet at endoscopy are ulcer-free (up to about 20%).[871]

In summary, there is limited prospective information on the natural history of both gastric and duodenal ulcer. Available data suggest that non–NSAID-associated gastric ulcers have a relatively high recurrence rate of about 40% to 60% over the subsequent 1 to 2 years after healing. The findings in duodenal ulcer are conflicting. Some studies suggest that the placebo or no-treatment 1-year endoscopic recurrence rate, after acute healing has occurred with H_2-receptor antagonists, approaches 80%,[872] while others[865] suggest that the symptomatic recurrence rate may be closer to 30%. Clearly, further study is indicated.

FACTORS ASSOCIATED WITH ULCER RECURRENCE

Because both gastric and duodenal ulcer disease (as well as combined GU plus DU) are associated with substantial recurrence rates, it would be important to be able to predict, and thereby discriminately treat, those who are destined for a recurrence. Unfortunately, thus far the studies that have examined factors that influence ulcer recurrence have been retrospective; that is, patients with healed ulcers were followed for various time periods, ulcer recurrences were determined, and attempts were made to relate various specific factors to recurrence rates.[864,873,874] In addition, studies have been conducted in defined populations, such as male veterans, and have been performed in relatively small groups of patients, which makes the extraction of single predictive elements difficult. This permits an increased risk of a type II error (i.e., concluding that no difference exists when one would be apparent with larger groups). The use of meta-analysis may permit a better understanding of this area.[875,876]

In spite of these limitations, some tentative conclusions can be made regarding factors that influence ulcer recurrences. Investigators at the Center for Ulcer Research and Education (CURE) have examined this important area.[864,877,878] In one study, DU patients whose ulcers healed promptly, who were younger, females, and nonsmokers, and who had a more recent onset of ulcer disease, fewer pain episodes at entry, and a low basal or peak acid output had fewer ulcer recurrences than those without these variables.[878] In a follow-up study of up to 6 years in 250 male veteran patients with DU and DU plus GU, Elashoff and colleagues observed that 11% of the total population developed ulcer complications.[877] The annual complication rate was twofold greater (5% and 2.7%, respectively) in those with a previous ulcer complication than in those who were complication-free. Also, recurrences were threefold greater comparing those with a prior ulcer complication plus hospitalization to those without these criteria, 27% versus 8%, re-

TABLE 61–12
Gastric Ulcer Recurrences After Healing

AUTHOR	INITIAL TREATMENT	FOLLOW-UP (YEARS)	RECURRENCES (%)	METHOD OF DIAGNOSIS
Sutton	Colloidal bismuth	3.5	13/29 (45)	Endoscopy
Jorde, et al.	Not specified	4–8	22/40 (55)	Endoscopy
Marks, et al.	Not specified	0.5	21/30 (70)	Endoscopy
Classen, et al.	Not specified	0.5	11/25 (44)	Endoscopy
Dawson, et al.	Not specified	0.5	10/24 (42)	Endoscopy
Hentschel, et al.	Cimetidine	1	23/42 (55)	Endoscopy
Machel, et al.	Cimetidine	1	12/14 (86)	Endoscopy
Battaglia, et al.	Multiple Rx	1	6/13 (46)	Endoscopy
Jorde, et al.	Ranitidine	1	19/22 (76)	Endoscopy
Wolosin, et al.	Cimetidine	0.75	9/22 (41)	Endoscopy
	Antacid		6/18 (33)	
	Placebo		5/18 (28)	

Modified with permission from Wolsin JD, Gertler SL, Peterson WL, et al. Gastric ulcer recurrence: Follow-up of a double-blind, placebo-controlled trial. J Clin Gastroenterol 1989;11:12.

spectively. However, and regrettably, no other variables or markers were identified to assist in predicting complication rates. In addition, patients with a longer ulcer history, less sleep (possibly because of night pain), greater milk intake (possibly to relieve pain), and greater emotional "upsets" and tranquilizer intake had a more severe course of DU. Of interest, age, age at onset of ulcer disease, and family history were unrelated to severity of disease. About two thirds of patients had a decrease in their pain over the follow-up period.

Recently, Van Deventer developed a "risk index" consisting of cigarette smoking, alcohol intake, early onset (before age 40) or repeated duodenal ulcers, and endoscopic evidence of duodenal scarring or erosions as additive factors in the prediction of DU recurrence (Fig 61-28).[864] Those with a risk index of less than 2 (each item given a value of 1) had about a 20% recurrence rate after 1 year compared to a 100% recurrence rate in those with a score of 4. These findings agree with the therapeutic recommendations by Bardhan that intermittent DU treatment is suitable for "low-risk" patients.[865]

Although gastric ulcer disease is also associated with a high recurrence rate, there are no data that permit precise identification of specific factors associated with high versus low ulcer recurrence rates. However, it is very likely that continued NSAID intake, smoking, and possibly continued ethanol intake may contribute to gastric ulcer recurrences.

DOES INITIAL THERAPY AFFECT ULCER RECURRENCE RATE?

The bulk of current evidence suggests that the duodenal ulcer recurrence rates following acute healing with antacids, H_2-receptor antagonists, H^+/K^+-ATPase inhibitors, sucralfate, or prostaglandin analogues are quite similar, approximately 70% to 80% within 1 year.[879–881] Chiverton and Hunt critically analyzed the effect of initial DU therapy on relapse rates.[882] They concluded that, in spite of the limitations due to methodologic issues, there is an increased relapse rate of DU after treatment with H_2-receptor antagonists compared with placebo or other classes of drugs. Furthermore, they calculated that the DU relapses 6 months after treatment with H_2-receptor antagonists were about 17% per month

greater than those with non–H_2-antagonists drugs; this is quite similar to the relapse rate reported by others.[883] Of interest, a number of trials have reported that duodenal ulcer recurrences were significantly less 1 year after healing with colloidal bismuth subcitrate (CBS) followed by no maintenance treatment.[884] In fact, in nonconcurrent treatment groups, the recurrence rates after acute treatment with CBS, without further maintenance therapy, have been reported to be similar to those observed with acute followed by prophylactic treatment with the H_2-receptor antagonists cimetidine and ranitidine.[884] These data, as well as other comparative trials, are open to question because recurrence rates were often obtained from separate, nonconcurrent trials.

More recently, Lane and Lee reported on a 4-year single-blind follow-up of 436 patients with endoscopically healed duodenal ulcer after a standard course of either cimetidine, ranitidine, pirenzepine, sucralfate, placebo, or tripotassium dicitrato-bismuthate (TDB).[880] Of note, DU recurrence 6 months after treatment with TDB was 19% compared with about 30% to 45% after the other drugs. This pattern persisted up to 1 year, when the recurrence rate in those healed with TDB was only 37% versus about 60% to 70% with the other agents. From 2 years to 4 years, recurrence rates approached 90% in all treatment groups, including those initially treated with TDB. This suggests that the beneficial effect of TDB treatment is self-limited—effective for the first 12 months after acute healing.

Because of the potential role of *H. pylori* in the rate of DU recurrences, colloidal bismuth preparations have been the subject of intense study. In a follow-up trial, patients with intractable DU (i.e., frequent relapses and/or recurrence while on maintenance H_2-receptor antagonist therapy) were randomized to CBS, or CBS plus amoxicillin and metronidazole ("triple" therapy).[885] One month after stopping treatment, about 80% had healed ulcers. *H. pylori* was eradicated in 15 of 17 treated with "triple" therapy, and none of these 15 patients developed recurrent DU over the 1-year follow-up. *H. pylori* was eradicated in only 2 of 21 treated with CBS alone, and 17 of these 21 *H. pylori*–positive patients developed a DU relapse. They concluded that because both groups received CBS, while only one group received antibiotics, the variable explaining relapses cannot be due to CBS but instead must be due to *H. pylori* infection. These highly provocative findings require confirmation.

Chronic Maintenance Therapy

For the majority of patients and for society as a whole, peptic ulcer disease is a chronic, recurrent, and expensive illness.[886,887] When treatment is discontinued after successful ulcer healing, the recurrence rate is 50% to 90% within 12 months for both duodenal ulcers[888,889] and gastric ulcers.[890] Numerous clinical trials confirm the efficacy of continuous maintenance drug therapy in reducing the number of ulcer recurrences.[888,889,891]

WHAT PHARMACOLOGIC AGENTS ARE EFFECTIVE?

A variety of pharmacologic agents and dosing regimens have been submitted to controlled clinical trials for maintenance treatment of peptic ulcers. The majority of these have been conducted with

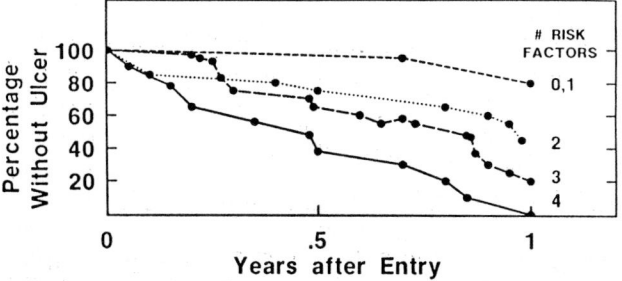

FIGURE 61-28. Duodenal ulcer recurrences over 1 year after complete healing. As the number of risk factors increases, so does the chance of having an ulcer recurrence. The risk factors include: alcohol use, cigarette smoking, ulcer disease onset prior to age 40, and evidence of duodenal scarring or an erosion at the time of entry into the study. (Reproduced with permission from Van Derventer G, Elashoff JD, Reedy T, et al. A randomized study of maintenance therapy with ranitidine to prevent the recurrence of duodenal ulcer. N Engl J Med 1989;320:1113.)

duodenal ulcers, and the response to treatment of gastric ulcers is less well established.[888] Currently, only H_2-receptor antagonists and sucralfate have FDA approval for maintenance therapy of duodenal ulcers; no agent has approval for maintenance therapy of gastric ulcers.

H_2-Receptor Antagonists

Duodenal Ulcers. Compilations of controlled trials of maintenance treatment with H_2-antagonists are available elsewhere.[497,509,529,888,889] Generally, these trials consist of placing patients with healed ulcers on a nightly dose of an H_2-receptor antagonist or placebo; endoscopy is performed at fixed intervals and also if ulcer symptoms recur. Comparison of different studies is hampered by important differences in the study design, including differences in entry and exclusion criteria, frequency of scheduled endoscopy, duration of follow-up, patient risk factors, definition of ulcer healing or recurrence, concurrent antacid use, patient drop-out rates, and the manner in which results are expressed: crude-rate analysis, life-table analysis, or ulcer point prevalence.[888,889,892,893] These limitations notwithstanding, it is clear that a nightly dose of cimetidine 400 mg, ranitidine or nizatidine 150 mg, or famotidine 20 mg reduces the ulcer recurrence rate to 20% to 50% at 1 year versus 50% to 90% in placebo-treated patients (see Fig 61-28; Color Fig 31).[889,891]

A recent meta-analysis of eight direct comparison trials of ranitidine 150 mg versus cimetidine 400 mg h.s. in duodenal ulcer maintenance demonstrated that the odds ratios favored ranitidine treatment in six out of eight studies.[891] Two of these were large multicenter studies that documented 1-year ulcer recurrence rates of approximately 20% for ranitidine-treated versus ~40% for cimetidine-treated patients.[894,895] Despite arguments to the contrary,[896] the superiority of ranitidine 150 mg to cimetidine 400 mg seems clear.[889]

This difference in ulcer relapse rates may be attributable to the differences in acid suppression: ranitidine 150 mg is more closely equipotent to 800 to 900 mg of cimetidine than to 400 mg.[509,515,523,524,889] When the utility of cimetidine 800 mg h.s. for 6 months followed by 400 mg h.s. or placebo for 6 months was studied, a significantly lower relapse rate occurred during the first 6 months when the higher cimetidine dose was administered. Famotidine 40 mg h.s. (which is equipotent to ranitidine 300 mg) has been compared with 20 mg h.s. in a large multicenter trial; no advantage was noted with the higher dose.[897]

Therefore, it would appear that the optimal H_2-antagonist regimen for maintenance therapy of duodenal ulcers is ranitidine or nizatidine 150 mg h.s. or famotidine 20 mg h.s.; cimetidine 400 mg h.s. appears to be somewhat inferior.

Gastric Ulcer.

Gastric ulcers unassociated with NSAIDs recur in 45% to 85% of patients within 1 year without maintenance.[890] H_2-receptor antagonists have been tested in a variety of dosing regimens for GU maintenance treatment[497,898–902]: ranitidine 150 mg h.s. or cimetidine 40 mg h.s., 400 mg b.i.d., or 1 g/day. All reduce 1-year gastric ulcer recurrence rates significantly compared with placebo, with 1-year ulcer recurrence rates on maintenance therapy ranging from 6% to 36%, similar to recurrence rates reported with duodenal ulcers. Bearing in mind the limitation of these small studies, nighttime doses of H_2-receptor antagonists appear to be effective in maintenance treatment of gastric ulcers.

Sucralfate

Duodenal Ulcers. Sucralfate has also demonstrated efficacy in the maintenance treatment of duodenal ulcers: three double-blind controlled trials confirm the superiority of sucralfate 1 g b.i.d. to placebo.[903–906] One-year ulcer recurrence rates range from 27% to 45% in sucralfate-treated patients versus 68% to 81% in placebo-treated patients. Sucralfate 1 g b.i.d. appears superior to 1 g h.s. in a single-blind study,[888] but further dosing studies are necessary.

Only one[907] of several comparison studies of sucralfate 1 g b.i.d. or 2 g q.h.s. with cimetidine 400 mg h.s. or ranitidine 150 mg h.s. has been conducted in a double-blind fashion.[905,907–910] These preliminary observations suggest comparable efficacy of sucralfate with H_2-receptor antagonists h.s. in the maintenance of duodenal ulcers. However, before sucralfate can be accepted as an alternative to H_2-receptor antagonists for duodenal ulcer maintenance treatment, more rigorous long-term, multicenter, double-blind comparative trials are necessary.

Gastric Ulcers. Limited studies have not consistently documented a significant advantage of sucralfate versus placebo in the maintenance treatment of gastric ulcers.[888,911–914] A recent blinded comparative study found sucralfate 1 g t.i.d. to be significantly inferior to ranitidine 150 mg b.i.d. in preventing GU recurrence over 1 year.[898] Further double-blind multicenter studies are necessary.

Even if sucralfate proves to be as effective as H_2-receptor antagonists in the maintenance treatment of peptic ulcers, questions relating to tissue aluminum accumulation with long-term sucralfate use must be resolved. The two studies measuring serum aluminum levels have not detected a significant rise at 1 year.[903,909] However, serum levels may not accurately reflect tissue aluminum accumulation.

Other Agents. A variety of other pharmacologic agents have undergone preliminary testing in maintenance treatment for ulcer disease, but their utility is unproved. Antacids 160 mmol b.i.d were superior to placebo and equivalent to cimetidine 400 mg h.s. in one double-blind multicenter maintenance trial.[915] Serum aluminum levels rose at 6 and 12 months in the antacid treatment groups, although this rise was not statistically significant. The principal advantage of antacid therapy in the maintenance treatment of ulcer disease is the lower cost relative to H_2-receptor antagonists. This advantage may be outweighed by the inconvenience of more frequent dosing, diarrhea, and the uncertainties of the long-term risks of aluminum ingestion.

Duodenal ulcer recurrence on maintenance treatment with colloidal bismuth subcitrate (CBS) 120 mg h.s. was 39% at 6 months, which was superior to placebo in a small single-blind study.[916] Serum bismuth levels rose significantly during the maintenance study. Long-term risks of bismuth are uncertain. Although bismuth compounds may play an increasingly important role in the acute treatment of peptic ulcers, a role in maintenance therapy appears unlikely.

The recurrence rates with rioprostil 600 mg h.s. (a prostaglandin E_1 analogue) were not statistically better than those with ranitidine in double-blind randomized maintenance trials, with 6-month recurrence rates of 15% versus 10%.[917] Further studies of prostaglandin analogues are warranted, although their questionable efficacy and high degree of side effects cast doubt on any utility in maintenance therapy.

The M_1-muscarinic anticholinergic antagonist pirenzepine 75 to 100 mg/d was superior to placebo and appeared to be comparable to cimetidine 400 mg h.s. in efficacy.[918,919] Dose-limiting side effects restrict the utility of anticholinergics in long-term ulcer maintenance therapy.

Omeprazole administered either as 10 mg daily or as 20 mg for 3 days consecutively out of 7 yielded recurrence rates of 26% to 29% at 6 months versus 83% for placebo-treated patients. Dose-ranging studies with omeprazole are necessary to determine the minimal optimal maintenance dose, and safety questions relating to long-term omeprazole must be addressed.[640]

DOES MAINTENANCE THERAPY DECREASE THE TOTAL NUMBER OF ULCER RECURRENCES OR MERELY THE NUMBER OF SYMPTOMATIC RECURRENCES?

Maintenance therapy with H_2-receptor antagonists changes the proportion of symptomatic to asymptomatic ulcer recurrences. Although the true incidence of asymptomatic ulcers in the general populace is unknown, 30% of endoscopically documented ulcer recurrences are asymptomatic in patients on placebo treatment.[889,920] In contrast, 50% to 70% of ulcer recurrences are asymptomatic in patients on maintenance therapy with H_2-receptor antagonists.[892,921,922]

The notion that the majority of asymptomatic ulcer recurrences do not undergo spontaneous healing in the absence of full-dose H_2-receptor antagonist treatment[920] was refuted by a recent study in which patients on maintenance treatment with ranitidine 150 mg h.s. underwent monthly endoscopy.[892] Ulcer recurrence rates were 48% within 1 year: 15% were symptomatic and 33% were asymptomatic. One third of asymptomatic ulcer recurrences healed within 1 month on continued maintenance therapy. This study suggests that maintenance trials in which scheduled endoscopies are performed at 6 to 12 months or for symptom recurrence underestimate the true frequency of ulcer recurrence in patients on active maintenance treatment (who are more likely to be asymptomatic) relative to patients on placebo (who are more likely to be symptomatic and therefore undergo endoscopic assessment). Thus, previous maintenance trials have underestimated the total number of ulcer recurrences in patients on maintenance treatment compared with placebo. It must be concluded that maintenance H_2-antagonists decrease total ulcer recurrences; however, they are most efficacious in decreasing symptomatic recurrences.[892,921]

DOES MAINTENANCE THERAPY REDUCE THE NUMBER OF ULCER COMPLICATIONS?

The risk of serious complications in patients with chronic peptic ulcer disease is 2% to 3% per year, with a lifetime risk that approaches 20%.[889,923]

Most maintenance studies have been limited to 12 months or less of observation and are of insignificant sample size to address whether long-term maintenance treatment reduces this significant complication rate. Reviews of placebo-controlled maintenance trials demonstrate a low rate of complications in both active treat-

ment and placebo treatment groups,[922,924] although complications are numerically higher in the latter.

The results of three long-term maintenance studies are available.[922,925,926] Only 6 complications were reported in 379 patients on active cimetidine treatment followed up to 6 years, representing only 1 ulcer complication per 178 years of patient follow-up.[926] Similarly, in over 1800 patients followed for up to 4 years while receiving cimetidine, there were 31 reported complications, or 1 per 113 patient years of treatment.[925]

Patients with prior ulcer complications have a twofold risk of subsequent complications. Retrospective assessment of chronic maintenance trials suggests that such patients have an extremely low complication rate on maintenance therapy.[922,924,926] In a prospective study of patients with a history of bleeding peptic ulcers, in 28 patients who were deemed compliant with their maintenance regimen, rebleeding occurred in 3.5%. In contrast, in 39 patients deemed noncompliant with the maintenance treatment, rebleeding occurred in 26%.[927]

Taken in aggregate, these data suggest that maintenance treatment may decrease the long-term ulcer complication rate. The low rate of complications observed in placebo treatment groups in maintenance studies suggests that close patient follow-up may also be important in decreasing ulcer complication rates. Clearly, more data from long-term placebo-controlled maintenance trials are necessary to answer this important clinical question.

There is no evidence that the increased proportion of asymptomatic ulcers to symptomatic ulcers occurring on maintenance treatment poses an increased risk of silent ulcer complications. Asymptomatic ulcer recurrences discovered incidentally in maintenance trials are observed to undergo a significant degree of spontaneous healing in the absence of any increase in H_2-antagonist therapy and may be of little clinical relevance.[892,920,921] Given the very low incidence of ulcer complications in patients on maintenance treatment, it is difficult to ascertain whether patients who developed complications are more likely to be asymptomatic.

IN WHAT SUBSET OF ULCER PATIENTS SHOULD MAINTENANCE THERAPY BE EMPLOYED?

The number of ulcer recurrences experienced over time is highly variable. Although 50% to 80% of patients will experience at least one ulcer relapse in 1 year in the absence of maintenance therapy, less than 20% experience three or more ulcer relapses in 1 year.[928] A number of factors may predict early and more frequent ulcer recurrences. These are reviewed under "Factors Associated With Ulcer Recurrence."

HOW LONG SHOULD MAINTENANCE THERAPY BE CONTINUED?

The safety and efficacy of H_2-receptor antagonists for at least 2 years in the maintenance therapy of peptic ulcers is well established. It is highly controversial whether maintenance H_2-receptor antagonists should be continued for even longer periods. The appropriate length of therapy is dependent on the natural history of ulcer disease, which is poorly defined. Although limited longitudinal observations suggest that peptic ulcer disease may "burn out" over 10 to 15 years in many patients, there are some in whom ulcer disease activity continues unabated for much longer periods with associated morbidity.[929] There is at present no way of identifying patients likely to have a more aggressive course. It may be reasonable to withdraw ulcer maintenance therapy and reassess the ulcer frequency after 1 to 2 years in most patients. Patients with continued recurrences occurring two to three times per year or high-risk patients (prior complications, multiple medical problems, continued NSAID therapy) may warrant indefinite maintenance treatment.

Ongoing, large, open clinical trials of maintenance cimetidine for up to 4 to 6 years for gastric and duodenal ulcers document its continued efficacy in reducing ulcer recurrence.[925,926] The rate of development of the first ulcer recurrence is highest in the first year and decreases in successive years.[922,925,926] The cumulative total ulcer recurrence rate at 5 years is 60% for duodenal ulcers and 45% for gastric ulcers. It appears that with sufficient time the majority of patients will experience at least one ulcer recurrence despite continued maintenance treatment.

The data from maintenance trials traditionally have been presented in a life-table analysis fashion as a cumulative first-ulcer relapse rate over time. Such an analysis provides little information about the disease activity in the population with time. In actual clinical practice and in longer clinical maintenance studies, patients who have an ulcer relapse while on maintenance treatment are usually treated with full-dose therapy for 4 to 8 weeks. Therefore, monthly ulcer prevalence rates (i.e., the proportion of all patients under observation with active ulceration in a given month) provide a more realistic means of assessing the efficacy of long-term maintenance therapy.[889,930]

Analyzed in this way, the monthly prevalence rates of symptomatic ulcers are 2% to 3% in patients on maintenance treatment.[925,926] The prevalence rates appear to decrease slightly with time, suggesting that ulcer disease may, in fact, "burn out" over time. The multiple inherent biases in long-term maintenance studies in which patients who are more symptomatic or less compliant tend to become lost to follow-up[893] render such a conclusion speculative at best.

In summary, with the limited number of long-term trials available, it can be concluded that H$_2$-antagonists continue to be effective for at least several years in the maintenance therapy of DUs.

WHAT ARE THE RISKS OF LONG-TERM MAINTENANCE TREATMENT?

Concerns have been raised regarding the potential effects of prolonged hypochlorhydria associated with H$_2$-antagonist maintenance therapy: bacterial overgrowth and hypergastrinemia.[931] Gastric acidity suppresses microorganism growth in the stomach and upper small intestine,[932] and patients with sustained hypochlorhydria due to atrophic gastritis, gastric surgery, or H$^+$/K$^+$-ATPase inhibitors[931-934] have an increased risk of cholera, salmonellosis, and parasitic infestation with *Giardia, Amoeba, Strongyloides,* and *Diphyllobothrium latum.* However, an increased risk of such infections has not been seen in patients receiving standard doses of H$_2$-receptor antagonists.[931] In Third World countries or in areas

with poorly prepared food, the impact of hypochlorhydria on the development of gastrointestinal infections is unknown.[931,934]

Bacterial overgrowth in the upper gastrointestinal tract may also convert nitrates to nitrites and to N-nitroso derivatives,[640,934] agents believed to be potential carcinogens. There is little evidence thus far that these carcinogens are increased in patients receiving H$_2$-receptor antagonists. Moreover, postmarketing surveillance studies do not support the relationship between H$_2$-receptor antagonists and gastric cancer.[640] It seems unlikely that nocturnal maintenance H$_2$-receptor antagonist therapy, which permits normal daytime pH, will promote bacterial overgrowth. However, serious concerns persist with the long-term acid suppression of omeprazole.[640]

Another side effect of some concern with long-term H$_2$-receptor antagonists is secondary hypergastrinemia. There is a reciprocal relationship between the degree of acid suppression produced with antisecretory drugs and serum gastrin levels. Treatment with short courses of therapeutic doses of omeprazole or H$_2$-receptor antagonists increases serum gastrin[612,807,935,936]; however, these increases resolve 1 to 2 weeks after discontinuation of acute therapy.[606,935] This transient hypergastrinemia has been postulated to be a factor in the increased rate of early ulcer recurrence in patients treated with antisecretory agents versus bismuth or sucralfate.[807]

Prolonged hypergastrinemia of any cause is implicated in the development of enterochromaffinlike (ECL) cell hyperplasia and carcinoid tumors (see Pharmacology: Omeprazole). While this is of significant concern with potent long-acting antisecretory agents, such as omeprazole,[633,634,636,640] there is no evidence to date that nightly maintenance therapy with H$_2$-receptor antagonists causes either significant hypergastrinemia or ECL cell hyperplasia. Surveillance studies do not suggest any serious sequelae in patients treated with H$_2$-receptor antagonists for up to 15 years.[889] Nevertheless, continued vigilance is warranted. The theoretic risks of hypochlorhydria from chronic H$_2$-receptor antagonist therapy may be weighed against the possible increased risk of gastric carcinoma that occurs after surgical therapy for peptic ulcer disease.[889,937]

WHAT ARE THE RELATIVE ADVANTAGES AND DISADVANTAGES OF VARIOUS TREATMENT STRATEGIES FOR PEPTIC ULCER DISEASE?

Peptic ulcer disease is a recurrent problem for the majority of patients. Options for managing these recurrent ulcers include: (1) Intermittent full-dose courses of ulcer therapy for 4 to 8 weeks when typical ulcer symptoms occur; after ulcer healing, the ulcer medication is discontinued until the next symptomatic relapse. (2) Continuous nighttime H$_2$-receptor antagonist maintenance therapy as above (to decrease the number of ulcer recurrences). Full-dose ulcer therapy is resumed for 4 to 8 weeks if symptomatic relapses occur despite maintenance treatment. (3) Ulcer surgery. Each of these options has its advantages and disadvantages, its proponents and critics.[928,929,938,939] In deciding among these treatment options, a number of factors must be considered.

Intermittent Full-Dose Therapy. After initial ulcer healing, 60% of patients will experience zero to one ulcer recurrences within 1 year without therapy, relatively mild disease that might not warrant continuous maintenance therapy. The ulcer recurrences pose a potential risk of complications, however, and result in associated suffering and time lost from work.[929,939] On the other hand, there is no compelling evidence that chronic maintenance therapy actually decreases the long-term risk of complications.[887] Moreover, maintenance therapy is costly, and the long-term risks of maintenance suppression are unknown.

Some have argued that all patients with a documented ulcer recurrence—even those with mild disease—should be placed on maintenance therapy indefinitely.[929] However, most argue that selected patients with mild disease do not require continuous maintenance therapy and instead should be treated with intermittent courses of full-dose therapy as necessary for symptomatic recurrences.[928,940]

Intermittent therapy is most appropriate for patients filling certain criteria: less than two ulcer recurrences per year that respond readily to medical therapy, age less than 60, no prior history of ulcer complications, no underlying serious medical illness, and no regular NSAID therapy (see below).[928] To put it simply, young, healthy patients with infrequent recurrences of symptomatic ulcers that respond readily to ulcer therapy are optimal candidates for intermittent therapy.

Continuous Maintenance Therapy. Many patients with recurrent ulcer disease will be better served by long-term H_2-receptor antagonist maintenance therapy. Approximately 30% to 50% of ulcer patients will experience two or more symptomatic ulcer recurrences per year.[928] Maintenance treatment is warranted in this subset with more aggressive disease to mitigate the associated suffering and morbidity.[889] The elderly and patients with serious underlying medical illness in whom a serious ulcer complication could prove fatal should also remain on continuous long-term maintenance treatment. Recognizing that absolute proof is lacking that maintenance therapy decreases the risk of ulcer complications in these patients,[887] it is felt nonetheless that the minimal risks of such treatment are far outweighed by the potential benefits. As discussed, patients with prior ulcer complications have at least a twofold increase of subsequent complications and therefore should be placed on continued maintenance therapy indefinitely.[923]

Gastric Surgery. The important role of surgery in peptic ulcer disease is covered in another chapter (see ch 64). Proximal gastric vagotomy, a safe, effective procedure with extremely low morbidity, is the surgical procedure of choice for uncomplicated recurrent duodenal ulcer disease.[941] More extensive surgery is generally reserved for recalcitrant duodenal ulcer disease or reoperations.

After proximal gastric vagotomy (PGV), the duodenal ulcer recurrence rate is approximately 3% per year, with a cumulative ulcer recurrence rate approaching 15% in 5 years.[889,940–942] These postsurgical recurrence rates are much lower than those reported with chronic maintenance medical therapy. Furthermore, ulcer recurrences after PGV generally are felt to be responsive to medical treatment.[889,943] Mortality for PGV is 0.1%,[889] and the incidence of postsurgical diarrhea, dumping, or gastric stasis is less than 3%.[941] Therefore, PGV is a safe, highly effective alternative to chronic maintenance therapy in patients with recurrent duodenal ulceration. Nonetheless, the role of PGV in the treatment of peptic ulcer disease is controversial.[929,938,944] For patients with frequent ulcer recurrences despite medical maintenance therapy, PGV may decrease lifelong morbidity and suffering.[889,941] Patients with com-

plications who are noncompliant with maintenance therapy, patients with complications despite continuous maintenance therapy, and patients with prior complications who live or work in settings in which surgical therapy is not immediately available should be considered for PGV.[889,940,941]

There is controversy whether gastric resective operations are associated with an increased risk of gastric carcinoma in the gastric remnant 15 to 20 years following surgery. The most recent and carefully performed studies suggest that if there is an increased risk of gastric cancer after ulcer surgery, it is only modestly greater than that of the general population.[937] To date, PGV does not appear to be associated with an increased carcinoma risk.

A cost–benefit analysis may be useful in deciding among the options of intermittent therapy, continuous therapy, or ulcer surgery in the treatment of chronic recurrent ulcer disease.[887,945] Such analyses attempt to take into account direct costs of ulcer treatment (hospital costs, physician charges, medication costs, laboratory charges, endoscopy charges) and indirect costs (absenteeism from work, death), as well as the amount of time spent free of ulcer symptoms. Such analyses, which involve many imprecise and calculated determinants, suggest that continuous maintenance therapy is equal in cost to intermittent therapy but provides more time free of ulcer symptoms. Maintenance therapy may be more cost-effective in the United States than PGV, but in Europe it surpasses the cost of PGV after 6 to 8 years.[887] While the financial costs of various treatment strategies are important from a public policy standpoint, they may not help in the decision making for individual patients. At this time it must be conceded that there is room for disagreement in the optimal management of patients with recurrent peptic ulcer disease. Bearing the advantages and limitations of each strategy in mind, one may select a different treatment program for different patients. In the absence of large, long-term, randomized treatment trials in chronic peptic ulcer disease, there is likely to be continued debate.

Recommendations for the Treatment of Recurrent Ulcer. The appropriate management of recurrent peptic ulcer disease depends upon the numerous factors outlined above. Only broad, tentative recommendations are given here. All ulcer patients should be admonished to give up smoking. Where possible, NSAIDs should be discontinued. In patients presenting with their first episode of documented, uncomplicated peptic ulcer, it is appropriate after the acute ulcer has healed to stop all antiulcer medications and observe for symptomatic ulcer recurrences. Approximately 20% of patients will not experience a recurrence and therefore would not benefit from maintenance treatment. Patients with recurrent ulcer symptoms should probably have an endoscopic or radiologic examination to confirm ulcer recurrence before embarking on either recurrent intermittent courses of antiulcer therapy or continuous maintenance therapy. This program, however, has not undergone cost-analysis.

At present, it is difficult to decide which patients with recurrent ulcers are best treated with intermittent acute therapy versus chronic maintenance therapy. For younger, healthy patients without prior ulcer complications having only one or two symptomatic recurrences per year, intermittent acute therapy is the most reasonable, least expensive, and most convenient. Patients who are elderly, who have prior ulcer complications, who smoke, who have a long history of ulcer disease, or who have multiple medical problems should be placed on continuous medical therapy for an indefinite period regardless of the frequency of their prior ulcer recurrence. Patients with frequent ulcer recurrences (greater than or equal to two per year) or early ulcer relapse (less than 3 months) after stopping acute ulcer therapy should, in most cases, also be placed on maintenance therapy for about 2 years. Fasting serum gastrin levels should be obtained in patients with frequent relapses to exclude Zollinger–Ellison syndrome.

In view of the gradual amelioration of ulcer symptomatology that occurs in some patients over time and the uncertainty of safety of long-term maintenance treatment, maintenance therapy may be electively discontinued in low-risk patients (those without prior ulcer complications or serious medical illnesses) after 1 to 2 years, and the patient should be observed for ulcer recurrence. High-risk patients or those patients who continue to have frequent recurrences off maintenance therapy should be left on maintenance treatment indefinitely. PGV or other ulcer surgery should be performed in the patient with recurrent ulcer complications that occur either despite continuous maintenance treatment or because of medical noncompliance. Likewise, otherwise healthy patients with frequent ulcer recurrences that require either high-dose H_2-antagonist or omeprazole for maintenance therapy should be considered for PGV. Finally, younger patients in whom long-term continuous maintenance therapy is being considered should also be offered proximal gastric vagotomy as a viable option. In the final analysis, the optimal treatment strategy will be determined jointly between the patient and the physician.

Refractory Ulcers

Although most duodenal and gastric ulcers heal within 4 to 8 weeks of standard antiulcer treatment, a subset of 5% to 10% of ulcers remain unhealed after 8 to 12 weeks of conventional therapy.[946] Such ulcers are labeled "resistant" or "refractory." The management of these ulcers constitutes a therapeutic challenge and is the subject of several excellent recent reviews.[947–949] The definition of refractory peptic ulcer is arbitrary and varies among different investigators.[949] Because most peptic ulcers are treated with H_2-receptor antagonists, the definition of refractoriness has commonly related to failure to heal an ulcer after a specified period of therapy with these agents.[947] For the purpose of this discussion, refractory peptic ulcers will refer to any endoscopically verified ulcer that fails to heal after 8 weeks (duodenal ulcer) or 12 weeks (gastric ulcer) of standard doses of H_2-antagonists.

RISK FACTORS FOR REFRACTORY ULCER

Little is known about the pathophysiologic mechanisms that underlie the development of refractory peptic ulcers. Several risk factors have been associated, including medical noncompliance, male gender, young age or old age, cigarette smoking, excessive alcohol intake, NSAID consumption, long history of ulcer disease, family history, and psychologic stress.[947–949] Smoking appears to be the most important predictor.[948]

Duodenal Ulcers. The relative importance of increased aggressive factors (acid-pepsin) versus altered mucosal defense mechanisms in the development of refractory ulcers is not estab-

lished. Acid hypersecretion, increased basal or nocturnal acid output, and increased maximal output have been reported by several investigators.[950,951] For example, of 75 DU patients prospectively treated with H_2-receptor antagonists for 8 weeks, the mean BAO was 20.0 mEq/hr in 20 patients in whom ulcers failed to heal, compared with 6.6 mEq/hr in the 55 healed ulcer patients.[950] In contradistinction to these studies, several other investigators do not find evidence of increased basal or maximal acid output in patients with refractory ulcers.[946,952–954]

It is likely that gastric acid hypersecretion plays a contributory role in a subset of patients with refractory ulcers. The overlap of gastric acid secretion between ulcer patients with and without refractory ulcers, however, is great, and the measurement of BAO or MAO is seldom useful in evaluating refractory DUs or guiding therapy. Acid hypersecretion due to Zollinger–Ellison syndrome is a rare cause of refractory DUs but should be excluded with a fasting serum gastrin level and/or secretin stimulation test.[949]

Increased vagal "tone" has been postulated by one investigator to be important in the pathogenesis of refractory DUs.[954] Nocturnal acid secretion was lower in refractory DU patients treated with a combination of H_2-receptor antagonists and atropine than in those treated with H_2-receptor antagonists alone.

Decreased responsiveness to the H_2-receptor antagonists could in theory contribute to the development of refractory ulcers. It has been noted by some, but not all, investigators that refractory DUs seldom occur with the first course of H_2-receptor antagonist therapy.[946,947] There is in vivo evidence that chronic H_2-receptor antagonists may lead to enhanced sensitivity or "up-regulation" of the H_2-receptor over time.[936,955,956] In theory, changes in receptor sensitivity could decrease responsiveness to H_2-receptor antagonists and retard ulcer healing. In support of this, a decreased gastric acid inhibition in response to cimetidine has been observed in patients with refractory DUs compared with patients with nonrefractory ulcers.[954] However, another study did not find such a difference.[946] This issue warrants further study.[882]

The importance of altered mucosal defense factors in the pathogenesis of refractory ulcers has not been studied. In particular, the role of *H. pylori* in refractory DUs requires investigation. Its presence in refractory ulcers has now been reported, and a trial of specific therapy to eradicate *H. pylori* has been reported for refractory ulcers.[977] (See Therapy of Refractory Ulcers—Mucosal Protective Agents.)

Gastric Ulcers and the Specter of Cancer. The pathophysiologic factors contributing to refractory GUs are even less well understood. Standard clinical practice up to now has been to recommend that refractory GUs undergo surgical resection to prevent complications and to exclude malignancy.[957,958] As a result, there has been an insufficient number of unresected patients to permit any meaningful evaluation of potential etiologic risk factors.

The possibility that underlying gastric malignancy may masquerade as a chronic nonhealing gastric ulcer is of major clinical importance. The more important clinical question, however, is what percentage of benign-appearing gastric ulcers are, in fact, malignant. The ability of the endoscopist to differentiate benign from malignant gastric ulcers by visual criteria alone is severely limited. In up to 50% of cases, the endoscopist is unable to categorize an ulcer as either benign or malignant with any degree of confidence.[959] One to eight percent of gastric ulcers labeled at endoscopy as benign are determined subsequently to be malignant.[937,958-962] In prospective clinical GU trials, 3% of patients initially enrolled with presumptive benign-appearing gastric ulcers were found subsequently to have gastric malignancy.[817,818]

Given the obvious limitations of the endoscopist to visually distinguish between benign and malignant ulcers, gastric biopsies are generally performed in patients with non–NSAID-associated gastric ulcers. But how reliable are endoscopic biopsies? A prospective study with biopsies of 202 consecutive patients, including 22 with gastric carcinoma, suggested that forceps biopsies yielded a correct diagnosis in more than 95% of gastric malignancies.[961] However, this accuracy pertains to biopsies of all gastric malignancies; the accuracy of endoscopic biopsy in patients with benign-appearing ulcers is less certain. One series reported 169 gastric adenocarcinomas in which 10 patients had benign-appearing gastric ulcers; in 6 of these 10 the initial endoscopic biopsies did not reveal cancer.[960] The correct diagnosis was subsequently detected 2 to 14 months later with repeated endoscopic biopsies. Another GU trial reported six patients in whom gastric ulcers were found to be malignant; two of the six had initial negative gastric biopsies.[959] Finally, Farini followed 113 patients with benign-appearing, biopsy-negative gastric ulcers; 7 of these patients were found on follow-up endoscopy over 2 to 12 months to have gastric carcinoma.[962] When a malignancy is suspected, multiple gastric biopsies as well as brushings of the lesion for cytologic examination are indicated.

There are several reports of malignant gastric ulcers that have undergone healing initially with H₂-receptor antagonists.[959,960] Although such events are rare, one cannot assume that partial, or even complete, healing is proof of the benignancy of an ulcer.[484,959]

Other causes of nonhealing gastric ulcers warrant mention. Gastric hypersecretion is a rare cause of gastric ulcers but should be excluded. Other unusual causes of chronic gastric ulcerations include Crohn's disease, amyloidosis, sarcoidosis, eosinophilic gastroenteritis, lymphoma, and infections such as tuberculosis, syphilis, and cytomegalovirus.

THERAPY OF REFRACTORY ULCERS

In managing the patient with a refractory peptic ulcer, it is important to verify patient compliance with the medication regimen. Noncompliance is the most common cause of a nonhealing ulcer and should be excluded. All patients should be counseled to discontinue smoking and NSAIDs where possible.[948,964] Fasting serum gastrin levels should be obtained to exclude Zollinger–Ellison syndrome.

Refractory Duodenal Ulcers

H₂-Receptor Antagonists. H₂-receptor antagonists may be continued at standard or increased doses.[946,947,965] If H₂-receptor antagonists are continued at standard doses (cimetidine 1 g/day or ranitidine 300 mg/day), approximately 50% to 60% of ulcers may heal with an additional 6 to 8 weeks of therapy.[947,949,965,966] At recommended standard doses for duodenal ulcers, cimetidine has less gastric acid inhibition than other H₂-receptor antagonists. Therefore, patients treated initially with cimetidine may derive some small therapeutic gain in being placed on an alternative agent. Of four comparative randomized trials testing this hypothesis, however, only one reported a significantly higher healing rate with ranitidine 300 mg than with continued cimetidine therapy, 1 g/day.[949,966]

Higher doses of H₂-receptor antagonists may be superior to conventional doses in refractory DUs.[946,947,950,951] Collen treated 20 refractory DU patients with 600 to 1200 mg per day of ranitidine in order to decrease basal acid output to <10 mEq/hr; complete ulcer healing was achieved in all patients.[950] Thus far, prospective, randomized, double-blind trials comparing standard and higher-dose H₂-receptor antagonists have not been performed.

Combination regimens of H₂-antagonists and anticholinergics have been postulated to offer superior control of acid secretion in patients with refractory ulcers.[951,954] However, a large multicenter double-blind trial could find no difference in healing of refractory ulcers treated with cimetidine 800 mg/day with or without pirenzepine 100 mg/day.[967] Other clinical trials of combination therapy have yielded conflicting results.[947,949] More recently, suppression of nocturnal acidity in patients with refractory DUs was found to be more effective with high-dose H₂-receptor antagonists than with H₂-receptor antagonists plus pirenzepine.[951] Therefore, the pathophysiologic importance of vagal stimulation in patients with refractory DUs appears to be minimal.

Omeprazole. Omeprazole appears to be an extraordinarily effective therapeutic agent for refractory DUs. Several open studies of omeprazole 40 mg/d in patients with DUs unhealed after at least 3 months of higher-dose ranitidine (450–600 mg/d) report 80% to 100% ulcer healing within 4 to 8 weeks.[947,968-972] Comparing omeprazole with continued H₂-receptor antagonist therapy, healing rates of refractory DUs at 4 weeks were not significantly different between omeprazole 20 mg/day and ranitidine 150 mg b.i.d. (80% and 75%, respectively).[973] In contrast, another European multicenter, double-blind trial confirmed significantly greater healing at both 4 and 8 weeks with omeprazole 40 mg/d compared with ranitidine 150 mg b.i.d.; healing rates at 8 weeks were 98% and 60%, respectively.[974] In summary, preliminary studies affirm the utility of omeprazole 40 mg/day in refractory DUs and suggest that it is at least equivalent and likely superior to continued therapy with H₂-receptor antagonists. Direct comparisons of higher-dose H₂-receptor antagonists with omeprazole in refractory DUs are necessary.

Mucosal Protective Agents. Two randomized studies of bismuth subcitrate (CBS) support the efficacy of this agent in refractory DUs. The 8-week healing rate of patients treated with CBS 120 mg q.i.d. (82%) was significantly greater than that with cimetidine 400 mg t.i.d. (39%).[975] In a separate randomized crossover trial, 85% of refractory DU patients healed during CBS therapy (120 mg q.i.d.) compared with 40% of patients during cimetidine therapy (400 mg q.i.d.).[976] A recent randomized study by Tytgat[977] demonstrated the superiority of combination therapy with CBS plus two antibiotics over CBS alone in the eradication of *H. pylori* in patients with aggressive ulcer disease manifested by frequent ulcer occurrences. Ulcer patients in whom *H. pylori* was eradicated had a significantly lower ulcer recurrence rate during follow-up than did those in whom *H. pylori* persisted (see "Ulcer Recurrence"). The efficacy of CBS, an agent with apparent activity against *H. pylori*, in healing refractory DUs is exciting. Further testing of CBS with and without antibiotics is needed in patients with refractory DUs to see not only whether healing can be expedited but whether ulcer recurrence rates can be diminished.

The role of sucralfate in refractory DUs has not been adequately studied. One study of DU patients unhealed after 8 weeks of sucralfate demonstrated 96% healing in patients who were switched to H_2-receptor antagonists versus 46% healing in those continued on sucralfate for 8 weeks.[978]

Surgery. The advent of potent H_2-receptor antagonists and H^+/K^+-ATPase inhibitors has decreased the number of refractory duodenal ulcers that require ulcer surgery. The role of elective ulcer surgery for the maintenance treatment of DUs is discussed above. A number of centers have reported higher ulcer recurrence rates after PGV in patients with refractory DUs than in patients with nonrefractory ulcers.[947,949,952] Furthermore, the responsiveness of these postsurgical ulcers to medical therapy may be poor.[947] Because PGV decreases BAO only 70% to 80%[941] and MAO only 50%, it theoretically should not offer any distinct therapeutic advantage over pharmacologic therapy with potent H_2-receptor antagonists or omeprazole.[949] The role of this procedure in refractory DUs compared with other surgical procedures, which carry higher attended morbidity and mortality, requires clarification.

Summary. In the era of potent H_2-receptor antagonists and proton pump inhibitors, the number of truly refractory duodenal ulcers is decreased. Regardless of the underlying pathophysiologic mechanism, it appears that a marked reduction in gastric acid secretion with these agents will result in healing in the majority of cases. Omeprazole is likely to be superior in this regard but requires further prospective double-blind comparison trials with higher doses of H_2-receptor antagonists. As discussed later (see "Maintenance Therapy of Refractory Ulcers," below), the bigger problem now in the treatment of refractory DUs is not the initial acute healing but the frequent, early ulcer recurrences that occur in these patients despite H_2-receptor antagonist maintenance therapy. The preliminary studies of bismuth regimens that proved efficacious not only in healing refractory ulcers but also in decreasing ulcer recurrence are extremely tantalizing and deserve study in refractory DUs.

Refractory Gastric Ulcers. There is a dearth of information regarding the efficacy of therapeutic regimens for refractory GUs because nonhealing GUs have generally been regarded as an indication for elective surgery.[957,958] Four open therapeutic trials of omeprazole 40 mg/d in refractory peptic ulcers have included a total of 61 patients with refractory GUs. More than 95% of these refractory GUs healed within 12 weeks of omeprazole treatment.[968,969,971,979] Prospective comparative studies of H_2-receptor antagonists versus omeprazole in refractory GUs are needed.[970] Studies are also necessary to clarify whether certain gastric ulcers (e.g., Types I, II, III, and so forth) are more or less amenable to medical treatment. Likewise, studies of bismuth and sucralfate in refractory GUs are lacking.

The decision to continue medical therapy or to recommend surgical treatment for refractory benign-appearing GUs is difficult and needs to be carefully considered. The surgical procedure performed for GU depends on the gastric ulcer type and location (see ch 64). In the past, surgical resection was recommended for nonhealing GUs in order to reduce morbidity (pain, bleeding, perforation) and to be certain an underlying malignancy had not been overlooked.[958] Preliminary studies with omeprazole suggest that this agent may be efficacious in the healing of many benign refractory GUs, thereby obviating the need for surgery. Whether this agent might transiently heal undiagnosed malignant ulcers, resulting in an unfortunate delay in diagnosis, is unknown. This risk must be weighed against the risk of gastric surgical procedures with their attendant morbidity and mortality. The prognosis of patients with benign-appearing ulcers that later prove malignant is quite good, with 5-year survival rates of greater than 50%.[960] Therefore, it behooves the patient to have such a malignancy detected in a timely fashion.

For the present, only tentative recommendations can be made. Patients with gastric ulcers not associated with continued NSAIDs that are unhealed after 2 to 3 months of therapy should be carefully assessed endoscopically and undergo four to seven biopsies.[961] Benign-appearing ulcers with negative biopsies may be followed on higher doses of H_2-receptor antagonists or on omeprazole. Repeated endoscopies with biopsies should be performed every 1 to 2 months until complete healing is documented. Ulcers that are not decreasing in size or that have dysplasia on biopsy should undergo surgical therapy.[980] Likewise, refractory GUs associated with complications are best managed surgically.

Maintenance Therapy of Refractory Ulcers. There are limited data regarding the utility of long-term maintenance treatment in patients with prior refractory ulcers. Maintenance therapy with conventional bedtime doses of cimetidine 400 mg appears to be ineffective in preventing ulcer recurrences.[949] In one controlled trial of patients with healed refractory ulcers, continuous medical treatment with cimetidine 800 mg h.s. or 400 mg h.s. yielded 1-year recurrence rates of 50% and 69%, respectively,[949] approximately double that of patients without refractory ulcers. Maintenance trials with more potent H_2-receptor antagonists are lacking. However, omeprazole 40 mg/day has recently been used as maintenance treatment in 59 patients with refractory gastric, duodenal, and esophageal ulcerations for 1 to 4 years with no documented ulcer recurrences,[979] a remarkable finding. In summary, refractory ulcers have an extremely high ulcer recurrence rate despite maintenance therapy with conventional doses of nighttime H_2-receptor antagonists. Higher doses of H_2-receptor antagonists or omeprazole likely offer some advantage but require further controlled testing.

NSAID-Associated Gastroduodenal Lesions

Nonsteroidal anti-inflammatory drugs (NSAIDs) are associated with a host of acute and chronic mucosal abnormalities in the stomach and the duodenum. (See "Peptic Ulcer Diseases, Epidemiology and Pathophysiology" and "Gastritis," as well as several recent reviews.[280,964,981-983])

ACUTE NSAID-INDUCED MUCOSAL LESIONS

Acute mucosal injury due to NSAIDs is seldom of clinical significance. Rapid healing occurs without therapy when the offending agent is discontinued. Because these lesions tend to be superficial, bleeding, when it occurs, is seldom severe and perforation does not occur.[964,981]

Prostaglandin analogues and to a lesser extent H_2-receptor antagonists have been shown to reduce the severity of NSAID-induced acute mucosal lesions[981] in a dose-dependent fashion.[964] Sucralfate, however, has shown rather limited efficacy in this regard.[981] Misoprostol, a prostaglandin E_2 analogue, results in a major reduction in acute NSAID-induced mucosal injury at doses of 100 to 200 μg q.i.d.[984-986] In an acute double-blind comparative study of volunteers given tolmetin for 6 days, misoprostol was significantly more effective than cimetidine in preventing acute mucosal lesions.[984]

In summary, acute mucosal lesions occur with a variety of NSAIDs primarily because of direct topical effects, but these lesions are generally of little clinical consequence. While it might seem likely that agents that cause acute mucosal damage would be more likely to cause dyspepsia, this is unproved. In fact, there is a poor correlation between the degree of acute mucosal injury and dyspepsia[983] (see below). Although effective, there is generally little need for prophylaxis with misoprostol or H_2-receptor antagonists in patients given an acute course of NSAID therapy.

CHRONIC NSAID-INDUCED MUCOSAL LESIONS

Clinical Aspects of Chronic NSAID-Associated Ulcers. Chronic NSAID ingestion is associated with the development of mucosal ulceration in 10% to 20% of patients.[981,987,988] Although ulcerations may occur after as early as 1 week of therapy, these deeper mucosal lesions typically emerge after 1 to 3 months.[964,981] In contrast to acute mucosal lesions, chronic ulcerations tend to be larger and deeper, extending through the lamina propria.[981] NSAIDs are most commonly associated with gastric antral ulcerations, where the prevalence in chronic NSAID users is almost 40-fold greater than that of the general population. Also, there is an estimated eightfold increase in the relative risk of duodenal ulcers.[981,987]

Unlike acute NSAID-induced mucosal injury, chronic NSAID injury is hypothesized to result from systemic effects of NSAIDs on mucosal defensive mechanisms, likely because of decreased mucosal prostaglandin production.[964,981,982,987] As such, all NSAIDs are capable of producing chronic NSAID mucosal injury, and at equal anti-inflammatory doses, no agent has established a superior safety profile.[983,987]

NSAID-associated ulcers are associated with severe ulcer complications. Although the precise risk is unknown, chronic NSAID users are at least four to seven times more likely to experience significant gastrointestinal hemorrhage or perforation than are age-matched controls.[280,989,990] It is estimated that 2% to 4% of chronic NSAID users per year will experience a gastroduodenal complication.[280] When one considers that 1.2% of the population uses NSAIDs daily, the number of patients at risk is sizable. Indeed, NSAID-associated mucosal lesions have been called the most severe drug side effect in the United States.[280]

The majority of patients on chronic NSAIDs, however, do not develop complications. The elderly, females, and patients with prior peptic ulcer disease appear to be at increased risk, as do those, to a lesser extent, who smoke, use alcohol chronically, have an underlying medical illness, or are on treatment with steroids or immunosuppressive agents.[280,964] In patients with multiple risk factors, the decision to use NSAIDs should be carefully considered, and close medical follow-up should be ensured.[280] Unfortunately, it is precisely the patient population that is at highest risk (i.e., the elderly with multiple medical problems) in whom NSAIDs are most likely to be needed.

The presence or absence of dyspeptic symptoms in patients on chronic NSAIDs has limited predictive value for determining which patients have serious mucosal lesions. Up to 50% of patients on chronic NSAIDs complain of some dyspepsia; frequent dyspepsia is reported in 25%.[981,991-993] However, 15% of patients treated with NSAID-placebo also complain of severe dyspepsia.[983] Of NSAID users with dyspepsia, at least 50% do not have important mucosal abnormalities.[981,994] More problematic is that up to one third of patients with significant mucosal ulcerations may be asymptomatic.[280,983,993] Of chronic NSAID users who develop complications, 60% have no heralding ulcer symptoms.[995] It is speculated that the analgesic properties of NSAIDs may diminish the patient's perception of ulcer pain.[964] Therefore, dyspepsia is of no discriminate utility in identifying that subset of chronic NSAID users most likely to have a mucosal ulceration or ulcer complication. Indeed, the presence of dyspeptic symptoms may prompt a diagnostic evaluation and/or therapy; in contrast, the clinically silent ulcer remains undiagnosed, untreated, and at risk of complications.[964]

Treatment of Chronic NSAID-Associated Ulcers. In patients with NSAID-associated gastroduodenal ulcers, it is self-evident that whenever possible the inciting agent should be discontinued. In many cases, NSAIDs are being used simply for analgesic purposes rather than for anti-inflammatory effects. Analgesia may be provided with alternative agents that do not affect mucosal PGE_2 synthesis, such as acetaminophen or nonacetylated salicylates.[988] If NSAIDs are discontinued, both gastric and duodenal ulcers respond rapidly to conventional therapy.[981,996] In some patients with severe inflammatory conditions, discontinuation of NSAIDs, even in the face of gastroduodenal ulceration, may be undesirable. A number of mostly unblinded, open, and nonrandomized small studies of such patients who continued NSAIDs have been reported,[981,996-1002] although it is difficult to draw firm conclusions from these limited data. It appears that H_2-receptor antagonists in conventional doses are capable of healing greater than 90% of small (less than 5 mm) gastric and duodenal ulcers within 8 weeks despite continuation of NSAIDs,[981,996] whereas the healing rate of larger (greater than 5–10 mm) ulcerations appears to be markedly retarded.[981,996,997,1001] With extended therapy over 3 to 6 months, the majority of these ulcerations heal gradually.[996,997] The effect of ulcer size on slower ulcer healing appears to be most prominent with gastric ulcers.[981] Because larger ulcerations are associated with a higher risk of complications and heal more slowly with H_2-receptor antagonists, it cannot be concluded that continued NSAID therapy in the presence of larger mucosal lesions is safe or advisable.[981,988] The risks, in fact, are unknown.

Omeprazole appears to be promising in the treatment of NSAID-associated ulcers. In a recent large multicenter, double-blind, randomized trial of omeprazole versus ranitidine, 39 patients with acute gastric ulcer therapy were allowed to continue NSAID therapy. Gastric ulcers healed within 8 weeks in 96% of patients treated with omeprazole versus 33% of the ranitidine-treated group.[834] Although the inciting pathogenetic defect in NSAID ulceration is presumed to be an alteration in mucosal defense, it would appear that significant acid inhibition with omeprazole nonetheless permits healing of NSAID-induced ulcers. Higher doses of H_2-receptor antagonists have not been tested extensively in the treatment of NSAID-induced ulcerations.

Mucosal protective agents have undergone limited assessment in the treatment of NSAID-induced lesions. A randomized double-blind trial of sucralfate 1 g q.i.d. versus placebo in patients who continued NSAIDs demonstrated a marginal improvement in an endoscopic lesion score that was not significantly different from that of placebo.[1002] Conversely, a randomized, double-blind, placebo-controlled study of misoprostol demonstrated 67% healing of gastric or duodenal ulcers at 8 weeks despite continued NSAIDs, compared with 26% in the placebo-treated group.[999]

Summary of Recommendations for Treatment of Chronic NSAID-Associated Ulcers.

Given the frequency of dyspeptic symptoms in patients on chronic NSAID therapy and the limited sensitivity and specificity of symptoms as a marker for mucosal abnormalities, it is neither feasible nor desirable to pursue a diagnostic evaluation of all patients on NSAIDs with gastrointestinal symptoms. Symptomatic high-risk patients and patients with iron deficiency anemia or hemoccult-positive stools warrant upper gastrointestinal endoscopic evaluation. In other patients, symptoms may be improved by changing to an alternative agent, reducing current therapy to the lowest effective dosage, and administering NSAIDs with meals.

Patients with persistent dyspepsia despite conservative measures should undergo endoscopic evaluation.[994] Up to one half of symptomatic patients will not have important mucosal abnormalities. Nevertheless, in a recent study, symptomatic therapy with H_2-receptor antagonists was moderately better than placebo in providing symptomatic relief in these ulcer-negative patients, 92% versus 72%.[1003] The merit of treating NSAID-associated symptoms in the absence of duodenal ulceration requires further study.

In patients with endoscopically documented duodenal or gastric ulceration, it is recommended that NSAIDs be discontinued, where possible, and conventional antiulcer therapy with H_2-receptor antagonists be initiated. If NSAID therapy must be continued, the optimal therapeutic approach is uncertain. Although smaller ulcerations will heal expeditiously on H_2-receptor antagonists alone, larger gastric or duodenal ulcerations may be better treated with omeprazole. Further endoscopic studies comparing omeprazole, H_2-receptor antagonists, and prostaglandin analogues in the healing of gastroduodenal ulcerations during NSAID therapy are needed.

Prevention of Chronic NSAID-Induced Lesions.

Antiulcer agents have been given chronically with NSAIDs in an attempt to prevent gastroduodenal lesions and concomitant complications. H_2-receptor antagonists (ranitidine 150 mg b.i.d.) have been tested in two prospective, randomized, placebo-controlled trials of arthritis patients on chronic NSAID therapy.[993,1004] The prevalence of duodenal lesions in both studies was significantly lower in the ranitidine-treated patients (less than 1.5%) than in the placebo group (6%–7%). However, there were no significant differences in gastric lesions between the ranitidine and placebo treatment groups. It would appear that H_2-receptor antagonists are effective prophylactic agents for NSAID-induced duodenal lesions but not gastric lesions.

The prostaglandin E_1 analogue misoprostol has demonstrated efficacy in the prevention of NSAID-associated gastric lesions in a double-blind, placebo-controlled trial. Misoprostol 200 μg q.i.d. dramatically reduced the cumulative incidence of gastric ulcers at 3 months from 22% to about 2% in patients with osteoarthritis treated with NSAIDs. The number of duodenal lesions in both treatment groups was too small to permit meaningful comparison.[1005] However, extrapolating from studies of the prophylaxis of acute NSAID-mucosal lesions that demonstrated excellent efficacy in the prevention of both acute duodenal and gastric lesions,[1006] misoprostol is likely to be effective in the prevention of chronic NSAID-associated gastric ulcerations. However, its benefit in duodenal ulcer prevention relative to H_2-receptor antagonists requires further study. Misoprostol is approved by the FDA for the prevention of chronic NSAID-associated gastric ulceration. Its patient acceptance is often limited because of untoward side effects, especially diarrhea.

It is unknown whether the reduction in the number of ulcerations seen in relatively short trials of prophylactic therapy will continue with long-term treatment. It is also unknown whether a reduction in the NSAID-associated ulcerations will result in a proportional decline in life-threatening complications. Long-term prospective clinical trials will be necessary to answer these important questions.[964] Given the large number of patients on chronic NSAID therapy and the relatively small number of ulcer complications, the costs and benefits of prophylactic therapy must be carefully considered.[1006,1007]

For the present, only the most tenuous of recommendations may be proffered. Patients at high risk for NSAID complications might be better served if NSAIDs are avoided entirely or given at the lowest effective dose. Therefore, NSAIDs must be used judiciously in the elderly, especially females, alcoholics, and smokers. Similarly, NSAIDs should be avoided in patients with multiple medical problems, prior peptic ulcer disease, prior ulcer complications, or current steroid therapy. If NSAIDs must be given in these high-risk patients, one should consider prophylactic therapy with misoprostol 200 μg q.i.d., recognizing that its utility in the prevention of duodenal lesions is uncertain. At this time, patients with prior duodenal ulceration on chronic NSAID therapy may be better treated with chronic H_2-receptor antagonists. At present, there are more questions than answers. The answers await prospective, comparative, randomized clinical trials.

GASTRITIS

Definitions and Classification

Gastritis is an acute, chronic, focal, or diffuse inflammatory disease of the stomach. It may present with a variety of symptoms, such as abdominal pain, nausea, vomiting, or upper GI bleeding, or it may be asymptomatic, only to present at some later time accompanied by anemia, gastric ulcer, or gastric cancer. Epigastric pain, nausea, and vomiting are commonly associated with gastritis; however, the vast majority of cases of acute and chronic gastritis probably do not produce symptoms unless accompanied by peptic ulceration or gastric outlet obstruction. Acute infectious diarrhea with abdominal pain, nausea, and vomiting is often called "acute gastroenteritis." If nausea and vomiting predominate, the term "acute gastritis" may be used. While it is now clear that acute infection with *H. pylori* can produce an acute gastritis with epigastric pain, nausea, and vomiting, there is little evidence that gastric inflammation is actually a feature of the common cases of acute infectious "gastroenteritis."[1009]

Previous classifications of the gastritides have been somewhat arbitrary and will continue to change with increasing knowledge of etiology and pathogenesis. Here, the classifications will be similar to those used by other authors (Table 61-13).[1010–1013]

Acute Erosive or Hemorrhagic Gastritis

Superficial ulcerations (erosions) of the stomach confined to the mucosal layer are produced by a variety of conditions, agents, and drugs, including pronounced physiologic stress ("stress erosions"), aspirin and other nonsteroidal anti-inflammatory drugs (NSAIDs), alcohol, direct local trauma, x-radiation, caustics, the reflux of bile into the stomach, uremia, mucosal ischemia, and a number of other drugs. The erosions vary in size and number, may be focal or diffuse, and may involve any portion of the stomach and sometimes the adjoining duodenum and esophagus. The erosions are associated with varying degrees of edema, subepithelial hemorrhage, and inflammation of adjoining mucosa, although in most instances inflammation tends to be minimal. Some of the lesions may be deeper, extending below the muscularis mucosae, and thus represent "ulcers"—either acute ulcers or, if associated with granulation tissue and fibrosis, chronic ulcers.

CLINICAL MANIFESTATIONS

Erosive gastritis is usually asymptomatic. A small number of patients experience epigastric discomfort, anorexia, nausea, and/or vomiting, but whether these symptoms are related to the superficial lesions or to the inciting cause is not always clear. Patients taking NSAIDs, for example, often have dyspeptic symptoms, but the presence or absence of symptoms does not correlate well with the presence or absence of gastric lesions.[1014] The most common manifestation of gastric erosions is upper GI bleeding, at which times the disease is called hemorrhagic gastritis. The bleeding may present overtly as hematemesis, melena, "coffee grounds," or blood in the aspirate of a patient on nasogastric suction, or with the symptoms of acute blood loss. Sometimes the bleeding is occult, detected by a guaiac test or presenting with symptoms of chronic iron deficiency anemia, especially in patients taking aspirin or other NSAIDs. On occasion, a deep ulcer accompanying erosive gastritis perforates. This is a rare complication of NSAID-induced erosive gastritis, but it is somewhat more common in "stress" erosive gastritis, especially with the Cushing's erosions or ulcers (see below).

DIAGNOSIS

Gastric erosions may be detected by a careful double-contrast barium study, but endoscopy is a more sensitive method of diagnosis. The endoscopist sees small, shallow, gray-based ulcerations, with or without associated hemorrhage. If the endoscopist thinks they have appreciable depth and extend below the mucosa, they are termed ulcers rather than erosions. The mucosa may also appear edematous, erythematous, and friable, as though truly inflamed. In addition, frequently there are small subepithelial hemorrhages (i.e., mucosal "petechiae" and red linear streaks). Because erosive gastritis is largely asymptomatic, most cases remain undiagnosed unless there is bleeding or the patient is endoscoped for some reason. It is estimated, for example, that perhaps half the arthritic patients chronically taking NSAIDs have undiagnosed gastric erosions.[1014]

PATHOGENESIS

The Gastric Mucosal Barrier. The pathogenesis of acute gastric mucosal injury is not well understood, although much new exciting knowledge has been gained in recent years. During the 1960s, a major cause of acute gastric mucosal injury was thought to be the disruption of the gastric mucosal barrier to acid back-diffusion.[1015–1018] The lining epithelium of the normal stomach is very impermeable, a property attributable to the "tightness" of the tight junctions ("zonulae occludens") between the apices of adjoining epithelial cells lining the surface and pits. As a result, the gastric surface is quite impermeable to most substances, including H^+ and other ions, so that the acid secreted into the lumen does not leak back into the mucosa, and the stomach can maintain an electric potential difference (PD) of approximately −40 mV across the epithelium. The mechanisms whereby agents such as NSAIDs "break" this barrier are described in detail under "Peptic Ulcer Diseases."

Prostaglandins and Cytoprotection. During the latter part of the 1970s and early 1980s, a protective role of mucosal prostaglandins was proposed and the concept of "cytoprotection" was developed.[1019–1025] Certain prostaglandins, produced in the gastric mucosa, were thought to play a significant role in maintaining the structural and functional integrity of the gastric mucosa (see NSAID sections of "Peptic Ulcer Diseases").

Subsequent studies by other investigators demonstrated that pretreatment of experimental animals with prostaglandins did not completely protect their stomachs from the injurious effects of alcohol; while the surface and pit epithelium was indeed damaged, the prostaglandins prevented deeper necrosis and hemorrhage of the gastric mucosa, permitting the mucosa to heal more rapidly after the injurious agent was removed.[1026] In fact, after destruction of superficial areas of the gastric epithelium, the surface was quickly re-epithelialized by the rapid migration of epithelial cells from the pits across an intact basal lamina over the denuded surface.[1026–1029] This rapid repair process is termed "restitution" and does not require cell replication.

The concept that the local production of certain prostaglandins in the gastric mucosa serves to maintain its integrity and protect it from erosion and ulceration provided a hypothesis for the pathogenesis of the erosive gastritis and ulcers produced by aspirin

TABLE 61–13
Classification of Gastritis

TYPE	DIAGNOSIS	HISTOLOGY	SYMPTOMS	CAUSES
1. Acute erosive or hemorrhagic gastritis	Endoscopy	Erosions with hemorrhage and inflammation	Bleeding	NSAIDs, alcohol, stress, ischemia, uremia, irradiation, caustics, gastroduodenal reflux (bile, alkaline, postoperative, or stomal gastritis)
2. Diffuse varioliform or chronic erosive gastritis	Endoscopy and biopsy	Aphthous-type ulcers with acute and chronic inflammation, often with intraepithelial lymphocytes	Dyspepsia, anorexia, occult bleeding	Unknown
3. Chronic nonerosive gastritis:				
Type A	Biopsy, Schilling test, acid secretion	Fundic mucosal atrophy	None (hypergastrinemia)	Autoimmune (pernicious anemia)
Type B	Biopsy	Antral inflammation	Dyspepsia	*H. pylori* infection
Postgastrectomy, nonerosive gastritis	Biopsy	Atrophy of remnant	None (?premalignant)	?Loss of trophic hormones
4. Granulomatous gastritis	Biopsy and culture	Acute and chronic inflammation with granuloma	Dyspepsia, bleeding, obstruction	Crohn's disease, sarcoidosis, idiopathic, tuberculosis, syphilis, fungi (histoplasmosis, Candidiasis, blastomycosis, actinomycosis)
5. Eosinophilic gastritis	Biopsy	Eosinophilic inflammation	Dyspepsia, obstruction, bleeding	?Allergy, chronic inflammation
6. Eosinophilic granuloma	Biopsy	Nodular fibrosis with eosinophilic infiltration	Dyspepsia, obstruction, bleeding	?Chronic inflammation
7. Other infectious gastritides:				
Phlegmonous or emphysematous gastritis	Surgical biopsy and culture	Purulent inflammation of submucosa, occasionally with gas	Peritonitis and shock	Gram-positive infection with alpha-hemolytic strep, *Clostridium septicum*, other pyogenic organisms
Viral gastritis	Biopsy and culture	Intranuclear inclusions	Dyspepsia, ?protein-losing	CMV and herpes
Parasitic gastritis	Biopsy and parasite exam	Presence of organisms	Dyspepsia	Anisakiasis, Cryptosporidiosis, Strongyloidasis, amebiasis, schistosomiasis
8. Hypertrophic gastropathy:				
Ménétrier's disease (hypertrophic gastritis)	Full-thickness mucosal biopsy	Hyperplasia of foveolar mucus cells forming elongated, tortuous, dilated glands	Dyspepsia and protein-losing (edema)	?Cause, sometimes due to allergy and possibly infection
Gastric pseudolymphoma	Full-thickness mucosal biopsy	Lymphoid hyperplasia with germinal centers	Dyspepsia	?Cause

and other nonsteroidals (see NSAID sections of "Peptic Ulcer Diseases," above).

Mucus, Bicarbonate, and Blood Flow. The role that surface mucus, HCO3⁻, and blood flow play in protecting the gastric mucosa from injury and in the pathogenesis of gastrodu-

odenal mucosal injury has been described in detail above in the section on "Peptic Ulcer Diseases."

Replication of Epithelial Cells. The epithelial cells lining the pits and surface of the gastric mucosa are replenished approximately every 3 to 5 days by the replication, differentiation, and migration of undifferentiated epithelial cells located in the upper glands (the neck region) and the base of the pits.[1030,1031] This process seems essential for maintaining populations of these cells and the structural integrity of the gastric surface. Interruption of this process by agents such as antimetabolites, other chemotherapeutic agents, and x-radiation may produce mucosal erosions and may interfere with the eventual repair of erosions produced by whatever means.[1030–1032] The rapid re-epithelialization of surface cells and erosions following necrosis by an agent such as aspirin or alcohol, however, would seem to be, as noted above, independent of this replication/differentiation/migration process. Replication is a more important process when the basal lamina has been destroyed (e.g., with true peptic ulcers).

Arachidonic Acid Metabolites, Mucosal Ischemia, and Free Radicals.

In contrast to "cytoprotective" prostaglandins, other arachidonic acid metabolites may play a causative role in the pathogenesis of some types of acute mucosal injury, some perhaps by affecting mucosal blood flow. Thromboxane A_2 is a potent gastric vasoconstrictor and can experimentally produce mucosal ulceration in animals.[1033–1035] Absolute alcohol, which produces mucosal ulceration in rats, also increases mucosal production of leukotriene C4, another vasoconstrictor.[1033,1036,1037] Pretreatment of rats with a 5-lipoxygenase inhibitor to inhibit the synthesis of leukotriene C4 protects the mucosa from damaging effects of ethanol.[1037] In fact, the earliest effects of ethanol seem to be directed against the gastric vasculature, resulting in mucosal capillary dilatation, stasis, and the leakage of red cells into the lamina propria in the superficial mucosa.[1038]

In addition, the local production of oxygen-derived free radicals in the gastric mucosa may lead to mucosal injury. Ischemia can cause mucosal ulceration in rats in the presence of gastric acid; the lesions can be prevented by inhibiting the formation of superoxide radicals with allopurinol or by "scavenging" them with superoxide dismutase.[1039] In other studies, the production of gastric mucosal damage by ethanol was shown to be accompanied by enhanced lipid peroxidation; prostaglandins could prevent both the injury and the increased peroxide formation.[1040]

TREATMENT

Obviously, avoidance or minimization of conditions and agents that cause acute erosive gastritis will minimize the chances of its occurrence. When it occurs, elimination of the causative conditions or agents will usually permit an eroded gastric mucosa to heal rapidly, often within a few days. Medical therapy of NSAID gastritis has been described in detail in the section on "Peptic Ulcer Diseases." The treatment of upper gastrointestinal bleeding secondary to gastritis is detailed in Chapter 30.

ETIOLOGIES

Stress Erosions.

Severe physiologic stress is a common, usually predictable, and rapid producer of "stress erosions" or erosive gastritis.[1041–1043] Common etiologies of stress erosions include significant trauma; extensive surgery; injury to the central nervous system produced by trauma or by surgery (Cushing's erosions or ulcers); burns (Curling's erosions or ulcers), especially when involving over one third of the body surface; sepsis; shock; respiratory failure; renal failure; and hepatic failure. Most patients placed in surgical or medical intensive care units can be expected to develop stress erosions. The more severe the physiologic stress or abnormality (i.e., the sicker the patient), the more extensive the erosions are apt to be and the more likely they are to hemorrhage.[1044] The likelihood of hemorrhage has been correlated with the intramural pH of the stomach wall, and bleeding is unusual above a pH of 7.24 and is more frequent in the presence of significant metabolic acidosis.[1045]

The erosions develop rapidly, usually within 24 hours of the "stressful" event. They tend to begin in the proximal stomach and may progress distally to involve the rest of the body and perhaps the antrum as well. The incidence of erosions and their complications varies with the severity of the stress and the etiology and has varied among reports. If no prophylactic therapy is given, it is thought that the vast majority of patients in medical and surgical intensive care units will develop erosions (see ch 109).[1041] Perhaps 10% to 30% of untreated patients at risk develop occult or modest overt GI bleeding, and approximately 1% to 3% develop overt hemorrhage requiring blood transfusions, although some studies have reported incidences even below and above these wide ranges.[1044,1046–1048] While most patients develop erosions within 24 hours of the stressful event, massive hemorrhage usually occurs 3 to 4 days later, although it may occur earlier or even 2 or 3 weeks later. Most cases with mild bleeding do well, at least in respect to their gastric erosions, but those with overt hemorrhage requiring transfusions have a high mortality, perhaps as much as 50%. Variations in frequency and mortality probably result from differences in definitions, accuracy of diagnosis, and severity of illness but may also result from the rapidity and effectiveness with which different institutions identify and treat the underlying stressful conditions such as sepsis, shock, and respiratory failure.

Curling's Ulcers.

Although stress erosions seem to be similar in their clinical behavior, there may be some qualitative and quantitative differences among the erosions associated with different types of stress. Erosions or ulcers associated with burns are called Curling's ulcers.[1049–1052] Burn patients may have more associated duodenal ulceration; about 15% of these patients have both duodenal and gastric ulceration.[1052] The duodenal ulcers are usually single and sharply demarcated, they may exhibit chronic inflammatory changes, and they may be deep. While the overall perforation rate of about 12% for Curling's ulcer patients[1051] is probably no different from that of most types of stress erosive gastritis,[1053] the duodenum is the more common site of perforation in the Curling's cases.

Cushing's Ulcers.

The erosions or ulcers associated with CNS trauma or surgery are called Cushing's ulcers.[1054] They tend to be deeper and perforate more often than other types of stress erosions/ulcers.[1055] They may also bleed more often than other types; perhaps as many as 40% to 80% of ulcers associated with head injuries bleed.[1056,1057] The Cushing's erosions are often associated with elevated serum gastrin levels[1055] and increased acid secretion,[1058–1060] which may account perhaps for their apparently more virulent behavior.

Pathogenesis.

The pathogenesis of stress erosions is not well understood. Although the presence of gastric acidity seems essential, only sepsis and CNS trauma/surgery seem to produce hypersecretion.[1058-1061] In fact, most patients in ICUs seem to be hyposecretors of acid. Some, but not all, predisposing conditions disrupt the mucosal barrier to acid back-diffusion, which may play a role in the pathogenesis in those instances.[1015] A major factor in the pathogenesis of stress gastritis is thought to be mucosal ischemia,[1062-1065] possibly, at least in part, by producing oxygen-derived free radicals (see ch 108).[1039] The role that local metabolites, such as prostaglandins, thromboxanes, leukotrienes, and so forth, may play has yet to be defined.[1033-1036]

Prophylaxis of Stress Erosions.

The most effective therapy for stress erosions is prophylaxis. The many known "stressful" conditions that produce the erosions, such as shock, sepsis, pulmonary failure, renal failure, and so forth, should be avoided if possible, rapidly identified if not avoided, and immediately and effectively treated. The general improvement in the care of acutely and severely ill patients and the advent of intensive care units have undoubtedly reduced the incidence of stress erosions and the mortality from their complications. Incidence and complications have also been markedly reduced by the development of effective prophylactic therapy in patients identified to be at risk. The "gold standard" has been the aspiration of gastric contents through a nasogastric tube every 1 to 2 hours to check the pH and the introduction through the tube of enough antacid (usually 30 or 60 ml of a potent antacid) to maintain the luminal pH above a selected level, usually between 3.5 and 5, but sometimes up to 7.[1066] The method is effective but costly, especially in terms of nursing requirements, and may produce side effects such as diarrhea, metabolic alkalosis, hypermagnesemia, and so forth. Antiulcer drugs are being used, although their use has not yet received FDA approval for this purpose. The H$_2$-blockers were attractive alternatives because they were easier to use and also suppressed gastric secretion, a feature with possible advantages. While H$_2$-blockers did not seem initially to be as effective as antacid titration, subsequent studies demonstrated their effectiveness when the gastric acidity was monitored and titrated with effective doses of H$_2$-blockers.[1044,1048,1057,1067-1071] Now a selected dose is usually administered to all patients, without pH monitoring. Individual patients may vary in their response to a given dose, and some groups of patients, such as hypersecretors with sepsis or CNS injury, may actually require higher doses to control gastric acidity. Longer-acting, more potent H$_2$-blockers may provide good persistent control of gastric acidity with bolus administrations, but shorter-acting, less potent ones (e.g., cimetidine) may provide more level, persistent control with continuous IV infusion.[1072]

Concern has been raised in recent years that the elevation of gastric pH in these acutely ill patients may increase the incidence of nosocomial pneumonias, particularly with gram-negative organisms.[1073,1074] These patients are frequently on antibiotics and have pharyngeal colonization with resistant gram-negative bacilli. When swallowed, the bacteria are usually killed by stomach acid. If gastric acidity is neutralized, however, the organisms may survive in the stomach and gain access to the lungs if gastric contents are aspirated. Indeed, some studies have suggested that nosocomial gram-negative pneumonias may be increased in intensive-care patients, especially those on ventilators, when gastric pH is raised by antacids or H$_2$-blockers to prevent stress erosions.[1073,1074] Clearly this important issue needs further study. At any rate, there are two drugs that have little effect on gastric pH that may prove effective in preventing stress erosions. Sucralfate 1 g suspended in saline (a commercial suspension may soon be available) and administered q4h or q6h appears promising,[1073-1077] as does misoprostol when 200 μg tablets are suspended in water and administered orally or by nasogastric tube q4h.[1078]

Drug- and Chemical-Induced Erosive Gastritis

Aspirin and Other NSAIDs. Aspirin and NSAIDs gastritis is discussed in detail under "Peptic Ulcer Diseases."

Ethanol. Ethanol is a well-recognized gastric mucosal toxin that disrupts the mucosal barrier to acid back-diffusion and is a common cause of erosive gastritis. The earliest toxic effect produced by ethanol, however, may be on the mucosal vasculature, leading to capillary stasis, dilation, endothelial damage, and subepithelial hemorrhage.[1038,1079] The results of studies of gastric mucosal damage in animals and humans are reviewed under "Peptic Ulcer Diseases: Epidemiology; Risk Factors; Alcohol."

Others. Additional drugs and chemicals have been implicated in the production of acute mucosal injury, including iron, potassium chloride, antitumor drugs, and caustics.[1080-1084] Caustics (strong acids and bases) can cause severe gastric damage (see ch 58).

Stomal (Postoperative, Bile, or Alkaline Reflux) Gastritis.

Patients who have undergone ulcer surgery commonly have reflux of duodenal contents into their stomachs or gastric remnants, and often gross abnormalities of the gastric mucosa are visible endoscopically.[1085-1089] The mucosa may appear erythematous and friable and may be eroded. The changes are most prominent near a gastroenterostomy; therefore, the lesion has been called "stomal gastritis." Because the mucosal changes have been thought to be due to the reflux of bile acids and/or other components of the duodenal contents, it has also been called "bile or alkaline reflux gastritis." This visible, often erosive gastritis is a separate entity from the chronic nonerosive gastritis observed in postgastrectomy gastric remnants.

On rare occasion, stomal gastritis is the source of acute GI hemorrhage, and occasionally it is suspected of being the cause of occult GI bleeding and iron deficiency anemia. Postgastrectomy symptoms, usually worse after eating and including epigastric pain or discomfort, nausea, and bilious vomiting, are frequently attributed to the stomal gastritis. However, because reflux and gastritis are so common in these postoperative patients, most of whom are asymptomatic, the cause of the symptoms remains uncertain. Oral cholestyramine therapy in such patients has generally been unsuccessful,[1090,1091] but operations designed to prevent the reflux, such as Roux-en-Y diversion, have been reported as helpful for some patients.[1086,1089,1092]

Trauma.

Acute mucosal injury is commonly produced by local trauma. Nasogastric suction is a frequent cause of focal mucosal erosions and subepithelial hemorrhages. Vomiting and retching are recognized causes of mucosal tears (Mallory–Weiss tears) just below or above the esophagogastric junction, but they may also be responsible for "petechiae" and erosions sometimes observed in the upper stomach, near the junction or in a bit of gastric mucosa prolapsed into the distal esophagus.[1093] Linear erosions observed in herniated gastric mucosa of patients with large hiatal hernias may also result from local traumatic mechanisms (ch 31 and 65).[1094] Physical techniques used in therapeutic endoscopy, such as a heater probe, electrocoagulation, and lasers, may also produce erosions around the region of therapy (ch 134).[1095]

Ischemia. Mucosal ischemia with the possible generation of oxygen-derived free radicals may be an important mechanism by which many conditions and agents produce acute mucosal injury. In fact, a major postulated mechanism by which mucosal prostaglandins provide cytoprotection is the promotion of mucosal blood flow through vasodilatation or by inhibiting vasoconstriction. In addition, primary vascular disease of the stomach, which results in ischemia such as vasculitis[1096] and embolization of cholesterol atheromata,[1097] may produce acute mucosal injury with erosions and/or ulcers.[1096–1099]

Other Etiologies. Erosive gastritis may be produced by other etiologies. *X-radiation* of the stomach was used in years past to treat severe refractory peptic ulcer disease or reflux esophagitis, especially in patients who were poor surgical candidates.[1100,1101] It caused a hemorrhagic necrosis of the gastric mucosa with destruction of the parietal cells and a consequent loss of acid secretion that promoted healing of acid-peptic related diseases. Parietal cells regenerated and acid secretion usually returned several months after the injury. Radiation gastritis with erosions or ulcers may still occasionally occur in patients receiving large-dose abdominal x-ray therapy.[1102] Gastric inflammation, fibrosis, and stricture formation may lead to outlet obstruction.

Uremia may disrupt the gastric mucosal barrier. Both chronic and acute renal failure may cause erosive gastritis. Cases associated with acute renal failure are often diagnosed as acute stress erosions.

Mucosal erosions and/or subepithelial hemorrhages are sometimes observed in patients without recognizable underlying causes and are termed *idiopathic erosive gastritis*. In reported studies of asymptomatic and dyspeptic patients, unexplained mucosal erosions and/or subepithelial hemorrhages were observed in 2.5% to 14% of subjects.[1103–1105]

Diffuse Varioliform Gastritis

Diffuse varioliform gastritis or chronic erosive gastritis is an uncommon disorder characterized by recurrent or persistent multiple gastric erosions unassociated with any known etiology.[1106–1114] Classically, the gastric folds (rugae) are irregularly thickened and studded with multiple small (usually less than 1 cm) nodules, many with central craters (aphthous nodules), located on the crests of the folds. Some patients have more classical erosions without the nodules. The disease may involve the whole stomach or predominately the body.[1112] If such injury is restricted to the antrum, it may possibly represent instead chronic type B gastritis with erosions (presumably *H. pylori* gastritis), bile reflux gastritis, or lymphocytic gastritis.[1108,1110,1112]

Patients may experience a variety of symptoms, often intermittent, including ulcerlike pain, atypical abdominal pain, nausea, vomiting, anorexia, weight loss, and occult or overt GI bleeding.[1106,1109,1113,1114] Patients may also be anemic or hypoalbuminemic.

A double-contrast barium study may suggest the diagnosis, but endoscopy and multiple biopsies are usually required, especially to exclude other diseases such as lymphoma, carcinoma, and other types of gastritis (see below). Biopsies near the lesions usually reveal an active gastritis, hyperplasia of foveolar mucous cells, and often a prominence of lymphocytes within the surface and foveolar epithelium.[1109,1110,1112] The prominence of intraepithelial lymphocytes has led to the description of a disease named *lymphocytic gastritis*,[1112,1115] which is probably the same entity as varioliform gastritis.[1112]

The etiology of varioliform gastritis remains unclear and the prognosis is uncertain. Patients may improve after several months, or symptoms may be intermittent or persistent for years. Effective therapy has not been established.[1109,1113,1114] Ulcer-type therapy should probably be tried before considering others, such as sodium cromoglycate or steroids.[1109,1113,1114]

Chronic Nonerosive Gastritis (Types A and B)

Chronic inflammation of the gastric mucosa, "chronic gastritis," without associated mucosal erosion or ulceration is a common histologic abnormality.[1010–1013,1116–1129] The lesion may be patchy, detected fortuitously in a gastric biopsy or surgical specimen, or it may be extensive, involving the entire gastric mucosa. The prevalence and extent of the abnormality vary among geographic areas and ethnic groups and increase with age such that the majority of people over the age of 50 have chronic gastritis.[1118–1134]

PATHOLOGY

The pathology is characterized by inflammation, epithelial abnormalities, and varying degrees of atrophy. This latter characteristic accounts for its commonly being called "atrophic gastritis" (Fig 61-29; Color Fig 30).[1010–1013,1116,1117] The lamina propria is infiltrated with increased numbers of chronic inflammatory cells (i.e., lymphocytes and plasma cells). When appreciable numbers of neutrophils are also present, the term "active gastritis" or "active chronic gastritis" has been commonly used (Fig 61-30). Inflammatory cells, particularly lymphocytes and neutrophils, when present, also frequently invade the epithelium (Fig 61-30) of the gastric pits (foveolae) and surface, and occasionally the glands as well.

The epithelium may appear normal, but often the surface cells show degenerative changes, and the pit and surface cells may contain little mucus. Increased numbers of undifferentiated or regenerative epithelial cells appear, especially in the bases of the pits and the glands. These are recognized as cuboidal or low-columnar basophilic cells with large hyperchromatic vesicular nuclei and prominent nucleoli. The epithelium may exhibit even more pronounced cytologic changes, such as atypia or even dysplasia and metaplasia.

Atrophy is a frequent feature of chronic nonerosive gastritis. In normal oxyntic mucosa of the body and fundus of the normal stomach, the gastric glands fill most of the mucosa below the level of the pits and are composed mainly of parietal (oxyntic) and chief cells with fewer undifferentiated neck, mucous gland, and endocrine cells.[1135,1136] Chronic gastritis commonly leads to loss of parietal and chief cells, a diminution of the gastric glands, an increase in the lamina propria or connective tissue between the

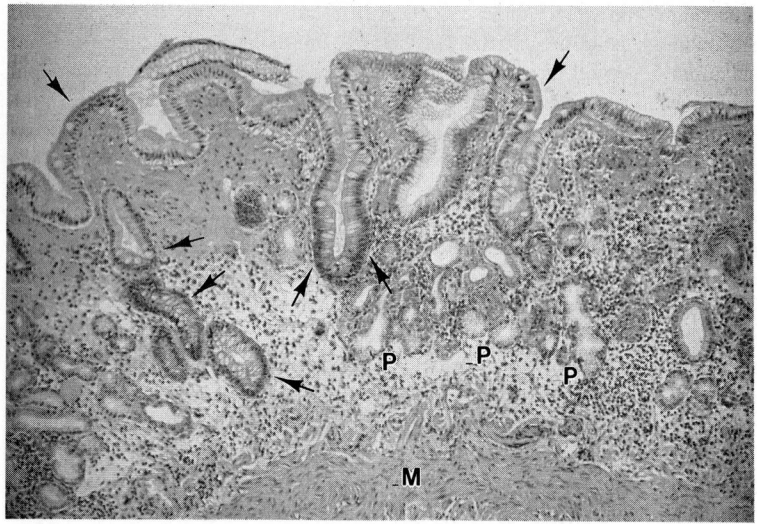

FIGURE 61–29. (See Color Fig 30) Pernicious anemia with severe atrophic gastritis (type A). A biopsy specimen from the body of the stomach shows that the area occupied by gastric glands is reduced, and the lamina propria is reciprocally expanded and infiltrated predominantly by chronic inflammatory cells. Parietal and chief cells—normal constituents of gastric glands—cannot be seen and are replaced by mucous cells normally observed in pyloric glands (pseudopyloric metaplasia) and by intestinal-type cells (intestinal metaplasia). *P* denotes glands with pseudopyloric metaplasia; the arrows denote some areas of intestinal metaplasia; and *M* denotes the muscularis mucosae. Approximately 100×.

glands, and thus atrophy or thinning of the mucosa (Fig 61-29; Color Fig 30). In addition, the parietal and chief cells are replaced with mucous cells that resemble those normally lining pyloric or cardiac glands ("pseudopyloric metaplasia") and/or with epithelial cells normally observed in the small intestine ("intestinal metaplasia") (Figs 61-31 and 61-32).[1137] Often there is also an increased number of endocrine cells.[1138]

In the antrum (pylorus or pyloric-antrum) of the normal stomach, the pyloric glands normally contain few or no parietal and chief cells and are surrounded by more connective tissue. Thus, in the absence of intestinal metaplasia, mild degrees of atro-

phy in antral specimens are more difficult to appreciate by conventional histologic techniques. In fact, if the location of a gastric specimen is not known, markedly atrophic mucosa from the body or fundus that contains few parietal and chief cells, but has extensive pseudopyloric metaplasia but no intestinal metaplasia,

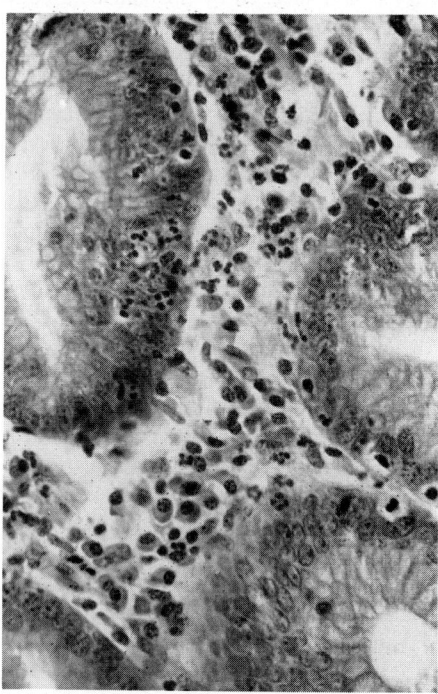

FIGURE 61–30. Active chronic gastritis. The lamina propria is infiltrated with neutrophils as well as plasma cells and other chronic inflammatory cells. The epithelium of the gastric pits and glands is also infiltrated with neutrophils and lymphocytes. Approximately 350×.

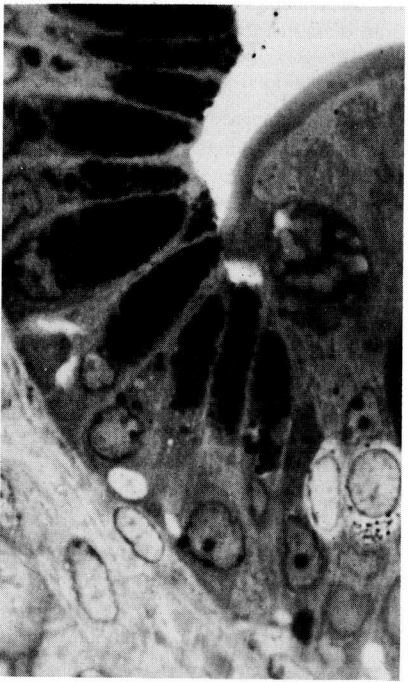

FIGURE 61–31. Atrophic gastritis and intestinal metaplasia. On the surface or in the gastric pits (shown here), mucous cells (on the left) may be seen in continuity with metaplastic intestinal cells (on the right) that resemble the differentiated villous epithelial cells of the normal intestine. Note the mucous granules in the gastric-type cells on the left and the prominent brush (striated) border on the intestinal-type cells on the right. This gastric biopsy specimen had been embedded in plastic (epon) and the semithin (1 μ) section stained with toluidine blue. Approximately 2200×. (Rubin W, Ross LL, Jeffries GH, Sleisenger MH. Intestinal heterotopia. A fine structural study. Lab Invest 1966;15:1024.)

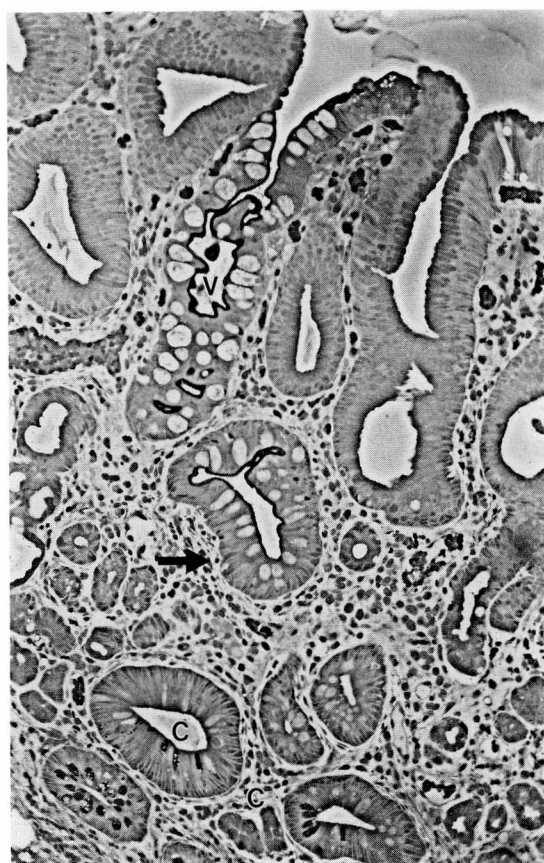

FIGURE 61–32. Pernicious anemia (type A gastritis) with intestinal metaplasia. Phase microscopy of a cytochemically reacted stomach demonstrates alkaline phosphatase activity by a black reaction product. The lateral areas of the section contain gastric-type epithelial cells, but the central area contains mainly intestinal-type cells (intestinal metaplasia). Most of the glands in the lower part of this central area, labeled "C," resemble crypts of the normal small intestine. They are lined largely by undifferentiated crypt cells, Paneth cells (with the dark granules), and goblet cells—the endocrine cells are not apparent. As the undifferentiated crypt cells in these metaplastic "crypts" migrate up the mucosa, they differentiate into mature villous cells, like the ones illustrated in Figure 61–31. At the level of the arrow, approximately in the middle of the mucosa, the maturing intestinal-type cells are developing into differentiated villous cells, which now have a visible brush border exhibiting alkaline phosphatase activity. This level of the mucosa corresponds to the junction of the crypts and villi in the normal small intestine—the region where the undifferentiated crypt cells undergo most morphologic, biochemical, and functional maturation into differentiated villous cells (enterocytes). (See the comparative region in the small intestine in Figure 66–5 in ch 66.) The metaplastic intestinal cells that extend above this area to the surface, along the pit or gland labeled "V," exhibit a prominent brush border with strong alkaline phosphatase activity. They correspond to the differentiated villous cells that line normal intestinal villi and have presumably acquired the biochemical maturation to function as enterocytes; they are able, for example, to absorb lipid, as illustrated in Figure 61–33. If serial sections were performed, the metaplastic intestinal cells would presumably be shown to be continuous: i.e., cells lining the crypts (C) would be continuous with ones lining the gland in the center (*arrow*), which in turn would be continuous with ones extending superiorly along the pit labeled "V" to the surface. Approximately 150×. (See Rubin W. Maturation of heterotopic intestinal epithelium. Clin Res 1969;17:310.)

might be interpreted as normal antrum or antrum with mild inflammation. Additional histologic features of chronic atrophic gastritis include the presence of dilated glands (cystic dilatation), a feature probably more common in the atrophic gastritis associated with the gastric remnant following partial gastrectomy, and prominent mucosal lymph follicles with germinal centers. There may be atrophy with little or no inflammation; such lesions, usually observed in type A gastritis (see below), have been termed "gastric atrophy" rather than atrophic gastritis.

The pathologic classification of chronic nonerosive gastritis has been somewhat arbitrary.[1010-1013] The presence of just superficial inflammation, confined largely to the lamina propria between the pits and perhaps the upper glands, has commonly been called "superficial gastritis." More severe lesions, with deeper inflammation and progressive degrees of atrophy, have been termed "mild," "moderate," and "severe" gastritis or "atrophic gastritis." Chronic nonerosive gastritis has been further classified into two major types, types A and B.[1013]

TYPE A CHRONIC GASTRITIS

Type A involves the body and fundus of the stomach (i.e., the so-called oxyntic or fundic mucosa) but largely spares the antrum. This variety of gastritis is the usual cause of pernicious anemia (PA): the loss of parietal cells leads eventually to inadequate secretion of intrinsic factor (as well as acid), malabsorption of Vitamin B_{12} (cyanocobalamin), and Vitamin B_{12} deficiency. The major etiology of this type A chronic atrophic gastritis is thought to be "autoimmune," and patients regularly exhibit a variety of positive immunologic tests.[1139,1140] For example, over 90% of patients have humoral antibodies directed against parietal cells (probably against their H^+,K^+-ATPase),[1141] and a majority of patients have antibodies against intrinsic factor. Patients with pernicious anemia often have other associated "autoimmune" diseases, such as Hashimoto's thyroiditis and Graves' disease.[1139,1140] Steroid therapy can actually produce some regeneration of parietal cells and some enhancement of Vitamin B_{12} absorption (Schilling test).[1142] The effect, however, is only modest at best, and patients should be treated with Vitamin B_{12} injections, not steroids.

Because the antrum is largely spared in type A gastritis, the population of endocrine cells that produce gastrin, the antral G cells, is maintained. With the loss of parietal cells and their acid secretion, the feedback inhibition of gastrin secretion by acid is also lost, and thus the G cells produce increased amounts of gastrin. Over 70% of patients with PA have elevated levels of serum gastrin, often in ranges commonly observed in Zollinger–Ellison (Z-E) patients.[1143] Patients with PA may also have an actual proliferation of antral G cells,[1144] so that elevated serum gastrin levels may be only partially reduced by the introduction of acid into the stomach.[1145]

TYPE B CHRONIC GASTRITIS

Type B gastritis, the more common variety of chronic nonerosive gastritis, involves mainly the antrum but may progress proximally, especially along the lesser curvature, to involve the oxyntic mucosa.[1010-1013,1146] Because the antrum, which contains the G cells, is involved, serum gastrin levels are usually not elevated, even though acid secretion may become appreciably reduced. Several possible etiologies have been suggested for type B gastritis, such as decreased pyloric tone with the reflux of bile and pancreatic secretions or the presence of a peptic ulcer. Increasing evidence suggests that infection with *H. pylori* may be the cause of most cases of type B chronic nonerosive gastritis.

EFFECTS OF GASTRITIS ON PARIETAL, CHIEF, AND OTHER EPITHELIAL CELLS

Most of the principal physiologic functions of the stomach and much of its metabolism are dependent upon its populations of differentiated epithelial cells.[1135,1136] Alterations in the numbers and types of epithelial cells in chronic nonerosive gastritis, especially when associated with appreciable atrophy, result in significant physiologic changes. The reduction in parietal cells leads to diminished secretion of acid and intrinsic factor, and a loss of chief cells results in reduced production of type I pepsinogens.[1147,1148] The development of pseudopyloric metaplasia probably results in increased production of mucus characteristic of pyloric glands, and, more dramatically, the development of intestinal metaplasia confers intestinal properties upon the stomach.

INTESTINAL METAPLASIA

Perhaps the most dramatic epithelial transformation is the development of intestinal metaplasia—the acquisition of epithelium that is normally observed only in the intestine.[1137] The most common type of intestinal metaplasia in stomachs is "complete metaplasia." This type resembles normal small intestinal epithelium with regard to the types of cells, ultrastructure, and histologic arrangement.[1137,1149-1152] Indeed, short villi may form on the surface of the stomach.[1137] Gastric glands, located in the lower portions of atrophic gastric mucosae and lined by intestinal-type cells, resemble crypts of the small intestine (Fig 61-32).[1137] They are lined by undifferentiated crypt cells, sometimes observed in mitosis, as well as Paneth cells, goblet cells, and intestinal types of endocrine cells.[1137] As the undifferentiated cells in these glands migrate upward toward the mucosal surface, they differentiate morphologically so as to resemble differentiated villous epithelial cells (enterocytes) with tall columnar cells that have prominent striated borders (microvilli) (Figs 61-31 and 61-32).[1137] They also differentiate biochemically and acquire enzymes characteristic of small intestinal enterocytes, such as alkaline phosphatase (Fig 61-32)[1149] and lactase.[1153]

In contrast to the small intestine, where morphologic and biochemical differentiation occur near the junction of the crypts and villi,[1152] the corresponding zone of differentiation of the aberrant intestinal epithelium in the atrophic stomach is near the middle of the mucosa (Fig 61-32).[1149] In the upper mucosa, goblet cells are interspersed among the differentiated "enterocytes," and both types of differentiated intestinal cells may be continuous with gastric-type mucous cells on the surface or in the pits (Fig 61-33; Color Fig 31).[1137]

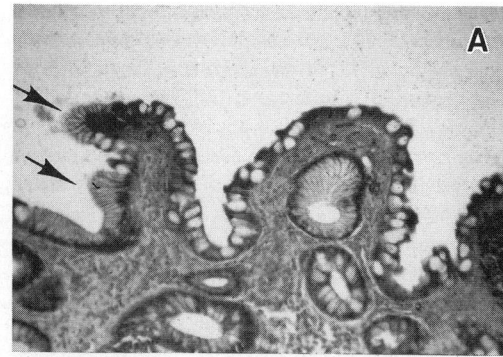

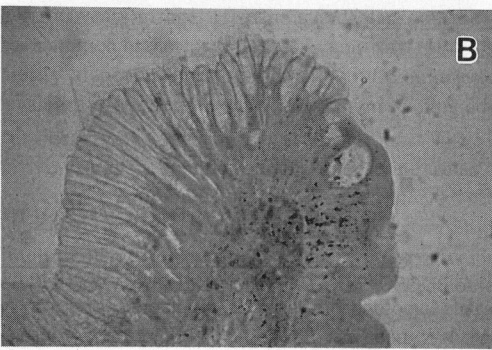

FIGURE 61–33. (See Color Fig 31) As intestinal-type cells in complete intestinal metaplasia differentiate morphologically and biochemically from undifferentiated "crypt" cells, as illustrated in Figure 61–32, they also develop the ability to function as differentiated intestinal villous cells (enterocytes). These two photomicrographs illustrate their ability to absorb lipid. Gastric specimens were frozen, and frozen sections were stained with oil red O to demonstrate lipid. The specimen in **A** was from a fasting patient with pernicious anemia. Lipid (in red) is observed in the lamina propria just below metaplastic surface intestinal cells, especially at or near the tips of short villi that have formed on the gastric surface. The arrows indicate small patches of gastric-type mucous cells; the remainder of the surface epithelial cells are intestinal-type. Little lipid is observed beneath the surface epithelium of the normal stomach or beneath gastric-type surface cells in atrophic stomachs. The specimen illustrated in **B** was obtained from the same patient 2 hours after a micellar solution of fatty acid and monoglyceride was infused into his stomach. The metaplastic intestinal cells on the right absorb the lipid; whereas the gastric-type surface mucous cells on the left do not. When serial biopsy specimens are studied by light and electron microscopy, the differentiated villous cells of complete intestinal metaplasia appear identical to normal small intestinal enterocytes as they absorb lipid.[1150] Thus, the presence of complete intestinal metaplasia seems to change the stomach from a primarily secretory organ to one that is more absorptive in nature.[1151] **A**, approximately 105×. **B**, approximately 500×. (Rubin W, Ross LL, Jeffries GH, Sleisenger MH. Some physiologic properties of heterotopic intestinal epithelium. Its role in transporting lipid into the gastric mucosa. Lab Invest 1967;16:813.)

Intestinal metaplasia has not only morphologic and biochemical properties of the small intestinal epithelium but also functional ones (Fig 61-33; Color Fig 31).[1150,1151,1153] The metaplastic stomach changes from a secretory organ to an "intestinal" organ capable of the "absorption" of certain substances, such as lipid, from the gastric lumen (Fig 61-33; Color Fig 31).[1150,1151] The mucus secreted by the goblet cells in "complete metaplasia" resembles that of the small intestine,[1154] and the endocrine cells not only morphologically resemble those of the small intestine[1137,1138,1155-1158] but produce at least some of the peptides usually secreted in the small intestine (e.g., secretin, CCK, glicentin, motilin, and gastric inhibitory polypeptide [GIP]).[1157-1160]

The so-called incomplete intestinal metaplasia is not as common and is seen more often in association with carcinoma of the stomach.[1161-1171] This epithelium usually does not exhibit well-developed striated borders, usually has morphologic and biochemical properties more suggestive of the large intestine rather than the small intestine, and often exhibits dysplastic changes. Stomachs may contain foci of both "complete" and "incomplete" intestinal metaplasia.

EFFECTS OF GASTRITIS ON ENDOCRINE CELL POPULATIONS AND THE DEVELOPMENT OF CARCINOIDS

The intestinal-type endocrine cells are often very abundant in foci of intestinal metaplasia, occasionally forming hyperplastic nodules or intestinal-type carcinoid tumors.[1158,1160,1172,1173] In addition, stomachs with severe atrophic gastritis and little or no acid secretion (e.g., type A gastritis associated with pseudopyloric metaplasia and pernicious anemia) often exhibit a proliferation of gastric-type endocrine cells in the nonintestinalized glands (Fig 61-34).[1138,1143,1155,1174,1175] The increased endocrine cells in the body and fundus of the stomach resemble those normally found in oxyntic mucosa.[1155] Enterochromaffinlike cells (ECL) predominate (Fig 61-34).[1136,1155] In the rat, ECL cells produce histamine.[1176-1178] This may be true of the ECL cells in the normal human stomach and of the numerous ones in atrophic stomachs, although histamine production by human ECL cells is less clearly established.[1179]

Patients with type A gastritis and pernicious anemia (PA) are at risk for developing gastric carcinoid tumors, presumably originating from the proliferated ECL cells.[1156,1159,1180-1186] These tumors tend to be small, micronodular, and often multiple, and they may form polypoid masses that may bleed. They are usually benign but may be of low-grade malignancy, exhibiting local invasion or occasionally even metastasis to the liver. Carcinoid tumors probably develop after many years of achlorhydria and are rarely, if ever, a cause of death. (The authors have heard of no documented cases of death from metastatic gastric carcinoids in PA patients as of December 1990). Anecdotal reports, yet to be verified, have described the regression of multiple gastric carcinoids in stomachs of PA patients following antrectomy with the subsequent reduction of serum gastrin levels.

A proliferation of gastric ECL cells also occurs in the Zollinger–Ellison (ZE) syndrome[1187,1188] and can be produced in rats by chronic (weeks) elevations of their serum gastrin levels created either by surgical procedures or by the profound chronic suppression of their acid secretion by means of omeprazole or a potent H_2-blocker.[1189-1195] ZE patients, like PA patients, also develop gastric carcinoids,[1188,1196-1198] and, if profound acid suppression and elevated gastrin levels are maintained for most of the life of the rats, a number of them, especially females, develop gastric carcinoid tumors, some malignant.[1189,1192-1195] These observations have led to the hypothesis that the chronic stimulation of the human or rat stomach by a yet-undetermined level of serum gastrin

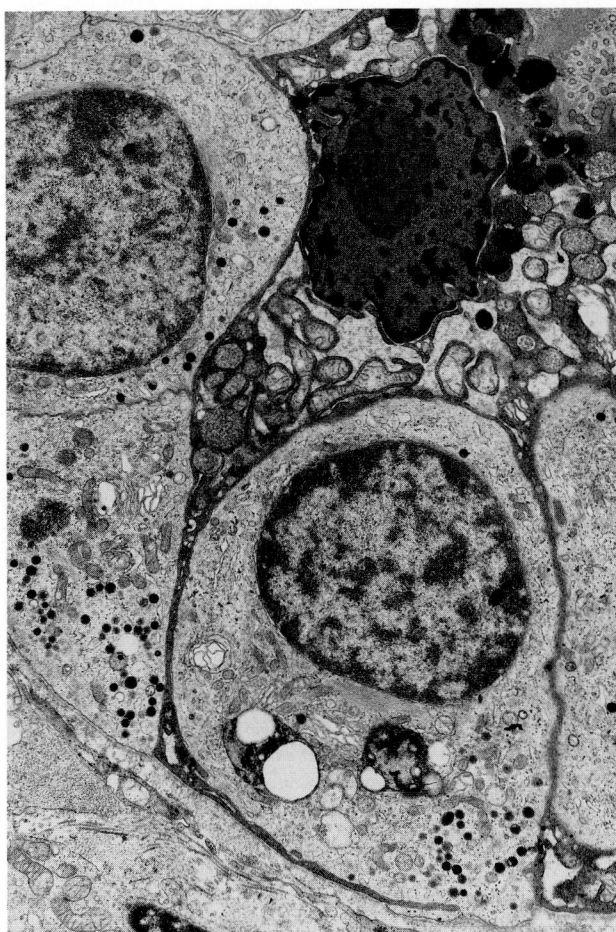

FIGURE 61–34. Electron micrograph of a "pseudopyloric" gland in the body of the stomach of a patient with pernicious anemia. This type A atrophic gastritis illustrates proliferated endocrine cells.[1138] The numerous endocrine cells in these glands ("crypts") with complete intestinal metaplasia resemble endocrine cells normally observed in the small intestine,[1137,1138] whereas the proliferated endocrine cells in the pseudopyloric glands in type A gastritis resemble endocrine cells observed in the normal oxyntic (gastric) glands.[1136,1155] Most of these endocrine cells are ECL cells, the predominant endocrine cell in normal oxyntic glands.[1136,1155] Note the small, dense, regular round granules that are characteristically observed in well-fixed human ECL cells.[1136] Approximately 12,000×. (Rubin W. A fine structural characterization of the proliferated endocrine cells in atrophic gastric mucosa. Am J Pathol 1973;70:109.)

leads to ECL cell proliferation and, eventually, in some subjects to carcinoid tumors.[1187,1189-1199] These considerations have led to some concern about the long-term use of very potent antisecretory agents such as omeprazole (see section on "Peptic Ulcer Diseases: Pharmacology of Therapeutic Agents").

RELATIONSHIP TO GASTRIC CARCINOMA AND ULCER

Chronic atrophic gastritis has been associated with carcinoma of the stomach[1131,1133,1200-1210] as well as carcinoids, polyps, and gastric ulcer.[1132,1134,1185,1211,1212] The risk of developing carcinoma in the stomach with type A gastritis has been thought, arguably,[1185,1210] to be increased by three to four times, probably after 15 to 30 years of achlorhydria.[1200,1201,1208,1209] The carcinomas in PA stomachs are often located in the fundus and cardia and are often multicentric and polypoid. Some of the previously diagnosed gastric carcinomas in PA patients may actually have been carcinoids ("carcinomalike"). The association of carcinoma of the stomach with chronic atrophic gastritis is further suggested by the fact that almost all stomachs resected for gastric carcinoma or polyps usually have an appreciable amount of atrophic gastritis with intestinal metaplasia, usually in the area of the carcinoma.[1132,1134,1213] Moreover, neoplastic cells in gastric carcinomas and polyps often have morphologic and histochemical features of intestinal epithelium.[1154,1214-1222] Either many of these neoplasms arise from intestinal metaplasia or, alternatively, intestinal metaplasia, dysplasia, and the intestinal type of carcinoma arise coincidentally without an obligate sequence.[1223] "Incomplete intestinal metaplasia," which is frequently abundant in stomachs with carcinoma, often exhibits features of colonic epithelium and tends to be more dysplastic than the "complete intestinal metaplasia." Some believe it may play a special role in the histogenesis of gastric cancer.[1161,1162,1166-1168]

Chronic atrophic gastritis, particularly of the type B variety, appears to be pathogenically associated with benign gastric ulcers (see "*Helicobacter Pylori:* Peptic Ulcer Disease" and "Peptic Ulcer Diseases: Gastric Ulcer"). Patients with PA or latent PA (type A gastritis), however, who have essentially no parietal cells and secrete no (or little) acid, rarely, if ever, develop benign ulcers.

CLINICAL CONSIDERATIONS

As discussed above, chronic nonerosive gastritis is asymptomatic in the vast majority of patients. Some patients with pernicious anemia (type A gastritis) have dyspeptic symptoms, but it is not clear whether such symptoms are more common in PA or are even related to the gastritis. Acute *H. pylori* infection (type B gastritis) can cause dyspeptic symptoms. However, it is not yet established whether chronic *H. pylori* infection and its associated gastritis produce chronic dyspeptic symptoms (see "*Helicobacter Pylori,*" above). Thus, chronic gastritis may be more important because of the diseases to which it may lead rather than the symptoms it may possibly produce. What effort, then, should be made to detect its presence in asymptomatic people, and when detected, either serendipitously or by intention, how should chronic gastritis be evaluated and managed?

Chronic nonerosive gastritis probably cannot be definitively diagnosed by endoscopy alone; biopsies are required. The erythema, subepithelial hemorrhage, or erosions observed in erosive gastritis are not seen in this form of gastritis; however, the endoscopist may appreciate a prominence of the submucosal vessels and/or a flattening of the gastric folds (rugae) if appreciable atrophy is present. In some cases with severe atrophy, the folds may actually be prominent or even nodular, an appearance that may suggest a hypertrophic gastropathy.

A variety of tests may suggest the presence of gastritis or reflect its severity. The maximal or peak acid output as determined by a gastric secretory study reflects the number of parietal cells; a low value usually suggests the presence of atrophic gastritis. Over 90% of patients with type A gastritis have serum antibodies to parietal cells, and 50% will have antibodies to intrinsic factor.[1139] A high serum gastrin in the presence of achlorhydria indicates type A

gastritis as seen in 70% of PA patients.[1143] A low serum pepsinogen I level or a low ratio of pepsinogen I to pepsinogen II suggests a loss of chief cells and atrophic gastritis.[1224] A variety of noninvasive, economical tests for the detection of *H. pylori* infection are being developed.

Type A Gastritis. Type A gastritis is usually diagnosed when patients present with the hematologic or neurologic manifestations of pernicious anemia. If a patient, however, is found in some way to have a severe atrophic gastritis compatible with a type A gastritis, he should probably have a pentagastrin-stimulated gastric analysis to determine if he has achlorhydria, or possibly he should have a Schilling test to assess Vitamin B_{12} absorption. If the patient is truly achlorhydric or is shown to have inadequate Vitamin B_{12} absorption, he should receive regular Vitamin B_{12} injections to prevent the development of pernicious anemia.

It is controversial whether the patient with PA should be placed under a surveillance program with regular gastroscopies, multiple gastric biopsies, and/or gastric cytologies. The gastric carcinoids that arise in these patients probably do not pose a great threat to life, while the danger of developing carcinoma has been controversial and may vary among populations (at most the risk is increased three- to fourfold after 15 to 20 years of achlorhydria).[1185,1200,1201,1208-1210] A reasonable program is for all PA patients to have gastroscopy and multiple gastric biopsies at the time of diagnosis. If the patient has no carcinoma, carcinoid, adenoma, or high-grade dysplasia, then regular surveillance endoscopy may not be warranted, especially if the patient does not have a personal or family history of cancer and does not live in an endemic area.[1185,1208] Any detected cancers and adenomas should be treated surgically if possible, and then the patient should be placed on a surveillance program for his remaining high-risk stomach. The proper management of high-grade dysplasia, which is believed to be a premalignant lesion, is also uncertain.[1225] Patients with dysplasia and carcinoids should at least be followed with endoscopies and biopsies if more aggressive therapy is not deemed advisable. Unverified anecdotal reports have noted the regression of carcinoids following antrectomy and supposedly the consequent reduction in circulating gastrin.

Type B Gastritis. The linkage of type B chronic gastritis with *H. pylori* infection in recent years may dramatically affect the approach to this disease and its treatment. If *H. pylori* infection is indeed proved to be the cause of type B gastritis and consequently of gastric carcinoma and ulcer, then the routine detection and elimination of the infection may become warranted. Before the adoption of such a radical practice, however, the feasibility and cost-effectiveness of such an approach should be demonstrated by careful clinical studies.

POSTGASTRECTOMY NONEROSIVE GASTRITIS

Following gastrectomy, especially after a Billroth II anastomosis, patients frequently develop an erosive gastritis near the stoma (stomal gastritis). Also, after partial gastrectomy, chronic atrophic gastritis commonly develops in the remaining stomach (the gastric stump or remnant), most rapidly during the 2 years following surgery.[1085,1087,1088,1226-1236] Because non-NSAID gastric ulcers and gastric carcinomas are regularly associated with atrophic gastritis, the presence of atrophic gastritis in the stump after surgery for these diseases is not surprising. Even in these patients, however, the gastrectomy is thought to promote the progression of whatever atrophic gastritis may have already existed at the time of surgery. While patients with duodenal ulcer disease commonly have associated antral gastritis, possibly due to *H. pylori* infection, their oxyntic glands are usually well preserved. Thus, the common development of atrophic gastritis in the stump of duodenal ulcer patients after partial gastrectomy is undoubtedly related to the surgery.

Certain pathologic features seem more common or more prominent in the chronic nonerosive gastritis observed in gastric stumps. These include: (1) hyperplasia of surface and pit (foveolar) cells,[1085] (2) the presence of gastric xanthelasma or mucosal islands of lipid-containing histiocytes, usually appearing as small yellowish white patches just below the surface epithelium,[1237,1238] and (3) the cystic dilatation of gastric glands in the superficial and/or deep mucosa, sometimes even in the submucosa, producing polypoid projections of the surface, especially near the stoma (gastritis cystica polyposa).[1085,1230,1233,1234,1239–1242]

Because *H. pylori* infection is much less common in the postgastrectomy stomach, the organism is not thought to be a likely cause of stump gastritis, especially in patients who had duodenal ulcer. The pathogenesis of the gastritis is more likely related to the antrectomy with the loss of antral G cells and the trophic hormone gastrin, and/or perhaps to the reflux of damaging intestinal juices that contain bile and pancreatic secretions.

Although gastrectomy patients frequently have a variety of GI symptoms, such as dumping, neither the stomal gastritis nor the nonerosive stump gastritis is a likely cause of dyspepsia. The risk of developing carcinoma in gastric stumps, however, has been reported, at least in some countries, to be increased some 15 or more years after gastrectomy.[1243–1246] An increased risk has not yet been established in the United States, where the incidence of gastric cancer in general is low. Whether repeated surveillance endoscopies and biopsies of stumps should be performed in patients 15 or more years after gastrectomy for ulcer disease remains controversial. Furthermore, it has not been established that early cancers or premalignant changes (dysplasia) can be detected and treated so as to effectively alter outcome.

Specific Gastritides

GRANULOMATOUS GASTRITIS

The gastric mucosa and deeper layers of the stomach may occasionally be involved with a chronic granulomatous inflammation caused by a variety of systemic diseases such as Crohn's disease, sarcoidosis, tuberculosis, syphilis, and fungal infections. Cases in which no etiology can be established are termed idiopathic granulomatous gastritis, and these are particularly difficult to differentiate from Crohn's disease or sarcoidosis of the stomach.[1247–1252] Small focal granulomas found fortuitously in gastric biopsy specimens may represent a reaction to some foreign material occasionally also visualized in the sections.

Granulomatous gastritis may affect any portion of the stomach, but most commonly the antrum. Inflammation, edema, and fibrosis may cause thickening of the mucosa and of the other layers as well, resulting in enlargement of gastric folds and narrowing of the lumen (Fig 61-35). The mucosal surface may become nodular, irregular, ulcerated, and/or eroded. The ulcers may hemorrhage or perforate, and, depending upon the etiology, the inflammation may occasionally form fistulas or sinus tracts.

Clinical Aspects. Patients may be asymptomatic or may experience a variety of symptoms related to associated gastric mucosal ulceration, to partial gastric outlet obstruction, or to extragastric involvement of the systemic diseases. Ulcerlike pain, postprandial epigastric discomfort, nausea, vomiting, and GI bleeding are common. Anemia may result from GI blood loss or to suppression of the bone marrow as seen in systemic disease.

Physical examination and routine laboratory tests, including a chest x-ray, may suggest the presence of an underlying systemic disease. However, it is usually a GI series (Fig 61-35) or endoscopy that detects the presence of a gastric abnormality that may be initially misinterpreted as gastric malignancy or peptic ulcer disease. The GI series may reveal narrowing of the antrum and pylorus (Fig 61-35); occasionally narrowing of the body, sometimes an "hourglass" deformity; and mucosal irregularity, nodularity, "cobblestoning," ulceration, and/or erosion; and it may even suggest tumor infiltration of the mucosa.

Deep gastric biopsies reveal the granulomatous gastritis (Fig 61-36), sometimes establishing a specific etiology and excluding other suspected diseases, such as gastric carcinoma or lymphoma. When the diagnosis of granulomatous gastritis is appreciated, additional sections of the biopsies should be processed with special stains in an effort to identify tubercle bacilli, fungi, spirochetes, and other organisms. If necessary, additional biopsies should be obtained for culture, and the proximal duodenum should be carefully visualized and biopsied so as to detect the presence of Crohn's disease. Additional tests (radiology or endoscopy) may have to be performed in an effort to establish a specific etiology by deter-

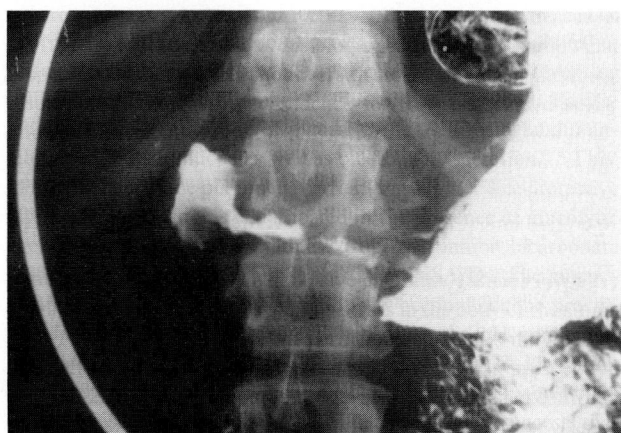

FIGURE 61-35. Granulomatous gastritis. GI series on a patient presenting with postprandial abdominal discomfort and nausea reveals antral narrowing and partial outlet obstruction. Suspected etiologies included a gastric malignancy, antral scarring from peptic ulcer disease, granulomatous gastritis, and eosinophilic gastritis. Endoscopy revealed mucosal irregularity, nodularity, and erosions. Biopsy specimens, illustrated in Figure 61-36, revealed granulomatous gastritis.

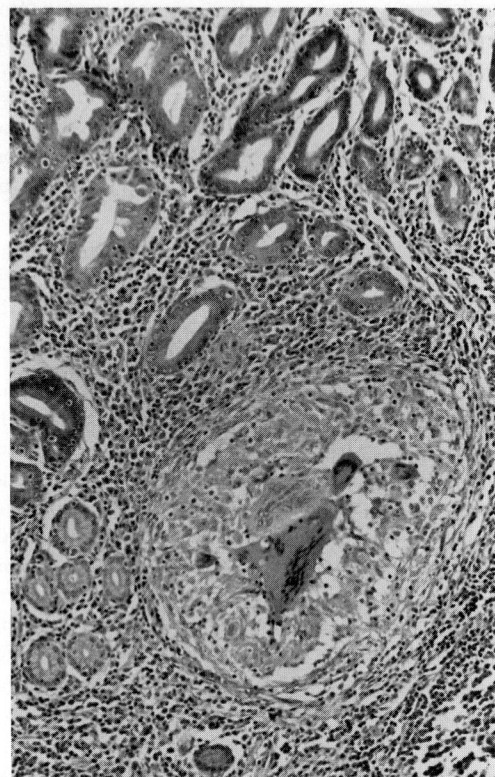

FIGURE 61-36. Antral biopsy specimens of granulomatous gastritis from the patient mentioned in Figure 61-35. Although the duodenum appeared normal by both the GI series and endoscopy, at surgery it too was found to be involved. The resected distal stomach and proximal duodenum both revealed granulomatous inflammation consistent with Crohn's disease. If the duodenum had been normal, the diagnosis would have been idiopathic granulomatous gastritis.

mining the presence of systemic disease (e.g., Crohn's disease in the more usual areas of the bowel or pulmonary sarcoidosis or tuberculosis).

Treatment. The treatment of granulomatous gastritis depends upon the specific etiology (see below). Symptoms due to gastric ulceration may improve with conventional ulcer therapy. Symptomatic gastritis due to Crohn's disease or sarcoidosis may improve with steroid therapy. Outlet obstruction or appreciable symptomatology unresponsive to medical therapy might require operative intervention.

Specific Etiologies

Crohn's Disease. Although Crohn's disease may affect the gastric mucosa, at least histologically, more frequently than previously appreciated, clinically apparent Crohn's gastritis is nevertheless uncommon and can be diagnosed with certainty only if extragastric disease is also present.[1253-1259] Gastric Crohn's disease involves the antrum and pylorus. Usually the proximal duodenum and other parts of the small or large intestine are involved as well. If Crohn's disease involves only the stomach, the gastritis will be diagnosed as idiopathic granulomatous gastritis. Rarely a case of granulomatous gastritis progresses to involve other areas of the intestine, and thus an "idiopathic" gastritis becomes a Crohn's gastritis. Crohn's gastritis may be asymptomatic and may be de-

tected fortuitously during contrast radiographs performed to study the small bowel of a patient with known or suspected Crohn's disease. On the other hand, the gastritis may be an important cause of symptoms, particularly those of gastric outlet obstruction or gastric ulceration.

Sarcoidosis. Sarcoidosis produces scattered silent granulomas in the GI tracts of a small number of patients, and even more rarely does it cause clinically evident gastrointestinal disease.[1249,1260-1262] It may, however, produce the same structural changes, symptoms, and radiographic and endoscopic findings as other types of granulomatous gastritis. If involvement of other organs or other manifestations of sarcoidosis cannot be demonstrated, then an isolated gastritis is appropriately diagnosed as idiopathic granulomatous gastritis.

Tuberculosis. Tuberculosis rarely involves the stomach,[1263-1267] although with the AIDS epidemic perhaps its incidence will increase.[1267] Tuberculous granulomatous gastritis is usually diagnosed from the gastric biopsies by demonstrating caseation necrosis in the sections or culturing the organisms from the tissue. The organism is usually not observed in the tissue sections, despite acid-fast staining. Detection of tuberculosis in other organs, such as the lungs, suggests tuberculosis as the cause of a granulomatous gastritis. As in Crohn's gastritis, the duodenum is also commonly involved. Antituberculous therapy should be effective, but gastric outlet obstruction may sometimes require surgery.

Syphilis. Late secondary and tertiary syphilis are very rare causes of granulomatous gastritis, sometimes producing "hourglass" deformities of the body of the stomach.[1268,1269] More commonly, early secondary lues causes a gastritis with thick folds, erosions, and mucosal infiltration with mononuclear cells but does not produce granulomas.[1270-1274] Diagnosis of syphilitic gastritis may be made by demonstrating *Treponema pallidum* in fixed biopsies by immunofluorescent or silver stains or by dark-field microscopy of a fresh biopsy specimen. Positive serologic tests for syphilis may be a helpful clue to the diagnosis. The nonspecific gastritis associated with early secondary syphilis should respond to penicillin or other appropriate antibiotics, but the response of the granulomatous gastritis of tertiary lues is less certain.

Fungal disease. A number of fungal infections are rare causes of granulomatous gastritis, including histoplasmosis,[1275-1277] candidiasis,[1278,1279] phycomycosis (mucormycosis),[1280,1281] and actinomycosis.[1282] Gastric histoplasmosis is usually a rare accompaniment of disseminated disease. Gastric candidiasis has been described in uncompromised patients.[1278,1279] However, when *Candida albicans* is found in gastric erosions and ulcers in immunocompromised patients,[1283-1286] it usually represents a colonization rather than a disease. Whether the *Candida* should be treated to minimize the risk of dissemination is not clear.[1283,1284] Mucormycosis may cause primary infections in debilitated or immunocompromised patients and may affect several organs, but gastric disease has also been reported in nondebilitated subjects.[1280,1281] Mucoraceae invade the gastric (and other) vessels, causing thrombosis, necrosis, ulceration, hemorrhage, and perforation. It is a virulent, lethal disease that is often unresponsive to amphotericin B and may require gastric surgery.

Idiopathic Granulomatous Gastritis.

If a specific etiology, such as Crohn's disease or sarcoidosis, cannot be identified, the granulomatous gastritis is said to be idiopathic.[1247,1249–1252] Effective medical therapy of the underlying disease is not established, and spontaneous resolution has rarely been reported.[1250] While it cannot be differentiated clinically from Crohn's or sarcoid gastritis, patients with idiopathic disease tend to be older.[1247]

EOSINOPHILIC GASTRITIS

Eosinophilic gastritis is a rare disorder of unknown etiology characterized by an eosinophilic infiltration of the stomach, particularly the antrum, and usually by peripheral eosinophilia.[1287–1289] The disease often involves the proximal small intestine as well, in which case the disease is called eosinophilic gastroenteritis. The eosinophilic infiltration may involve all layers of the wall or may predominate in the mucosa, the muscle layer, or the serosa. Mucosal involvement may produce mucosal ulceration, nodularity, and prominent folds; muscle involvement may lead to luminal narrowing; and serosal infiltration may lead to peritonitis and ascites. Possible symptoms include ulcerlike pain, the satiety, postprandial discomfort, nausea, and vomiting of gastric outlet obstruction, GI hemorrhage, and symptoms of anemia from chronic blood loss. GI series and endoscopy may reveal prominent antral folds, mucosal irregularity, nodularity, ulceration, and luminal narrowing. The x-ray and endoscopic findings may be confused with those of granulomatous gastritis or gastric malignancy. Endoscopic biopsies, peripheral eosinophilia, and the presence of proximal small bowel involvement usually provide the diagnosis, but in instances of mucosal sparing, the diagnosis may be more difficult. Symptoms usually respond to steroid therapy, but surgery may be necessary for persistent outlet obstruction or for diagnostic purposes.

EOSINOPHILIC GRANULOMA

This is an inflammatory polyp, usually arising from the submucosa in the antrum, composed largely of fibrous and vascular tissue, infiltrated with eosinophils, but not associated with peripheral eosinophilia.[1290–1294] They may be symptomatic, usually by obstructing the gastric outlet or by ulcerating and causing pain or bleeding. They must be differentiated from other polypoid lesions such as an adenoma, carcinoma, or leiomyoma. Diagnosis as well as therapy may require surgery.

BACTERIAL, VIRAL, AND PARASITIC GASTRITIS

On rare occasion the stomach may be infected by agents other than tuberculosis, syphilis, and fungi. The increasing number of patients immunocompromised as a result of AIDS, organ transplantation, and cancer chemotherapy may increase the incidence of these infectious gastritides due to bacteria, viruses, and parasites.

Phlegmonous Gastritis.

This is a rare, life-threatening, suppurative infection usually associated with alpha-hemolytic streptococci in the majority of cases but occasionally associated with other pyogenic bacteria such as pneumococci, staphylococci, *Escherichia coli, Proteus vulgaris,* anthrax, and *Clostridium perfringens.*[1295–1301] The purulent inflammation affects mainly the submucosa and may lead to sloughing of the mucosa, extension to the serosa, and often perforation and purulent peritonitis. The stomach is usually dilated and has thickened walls with a reddish or purplish color, and the submucosa and serosa may ooze pus. Small gastric vessels are commonly thrombosed. When the gas-forming organisms, such as *C. perfringens,* are present, a particularly dangerous form of phlegmonous gastritis called emphysematous gastritis may result.[1297,1301–1303] The striking abdominal x-ray reveals bubbles of gas within the stomach wall. A similar x-ray of gastric emphysema may also be seen in pneumatosis cystoides intestinalis or after trauma to the stomach as may be seen after a perforation with an endoscope or the rupture of a pulmonary bulla into the wall of the esophagus.[1304] The patient with emphysematous gastritis, however, is usually more acutely ill. The predisposing factors for the development of phlegmonous and emphysematous gastritis include debilitation, malnutrition, systemic infection, trauma, and even endoscopic polypectomy.[1298,1299,1302–1305] Emphysematous gastritis has been associated with gastric malignancy and previous ingestion of corrosives.

Patients with phlegmonous gastritis usually present with an acute abdomen characterized by the sudden onset of epigastric pain, nausea, and vomiting, accompanied by varying degrees of fever, chills, and prostration. The patient may have hematemesis and occasionally vomits frank pus or even a necrotic cast of the gastric wall. Abdominal examination frequently reveals findings of peritonitis. Plain films of the abdomen, ultrasonography, or a CT scan may show thickening of the stomach wall and, in the case of emphysematous gastritis, may reveal the presence of gas in the stomach wall.

Medical therapy alone usually fails, but rapid diagnosis and gastrectomy can usually reduce mortality to 20%. The patient should receive broad antibiotic coverage and have surgery as soon as possible. A local gastric resection may be adequate for focal involvement, but total gastrectomy may be required.

Cytomegalovirus.

This virus may involve the stomach, particularly in the immunocompromised patient with AIDS[1306,1307] or after marrow or organ transplantation,[1308–1311] but is occasionally found in noncompromised patients as well.[1312–1314] Because the virus is so prevalent in the immunocompromised host, its recovery from the stomach does not prove it is the cause of observed inflammation and erosions rather than an innocent bystander (colonizer). Identification in gastric biopsy specimens of classical cytomegalic cells with intranuclear inclusions along with positive cultures provides the diagnosis. CMV gastric infection in AIDS patients[1306,1307] and in children[1313,1314] may provide a Ménétrier-like disease with enlarged gastric folds and hypoproteinemia. The disease, at least in children, may be reversible.

Herpes Virus.

Rare gastric infections have been reported in immunocompromised patients with herpes simplex.[1311,1315]

Parasitic Gastritis.

Cryptosporidia,[1321] *Strongyloides,*[1297,1317,1318] and, rarely, *Entaemoba histolytica,*[1319] *Schistosoma species,*[1320] and *Necator americanus*[1321] are parasites that may colonize or infect the stomach.

Anisakiasis may cause an ulcerating eosinophilic granulomatous lesion of the gastric mucosa by the penetration of larvae of this nematode, which are 2 to 3.5 cm long and are acquired by eating raw or inadequately cooked fish.[1322-1325] The disease is seen mainly in Japan, but cases have also been reported in the United States. Severe abdominal pain results from the penetration of the parasites and may last a few days, supposedly until the larvae die. The worms may be seen by double-contrast barium x-rays or at endoscopy, and pain allegedly may subside within hours of removing the worms endoscopically. The worms may also be seen in sections of biopsy specimens. Local resection has been used for persistent lesions and symptoms.

HYPERTROPHIC GASTROPATHY

The term "hypertrophic gastropathy" refers to a group of disorders, most not well defined, that are characterized by enlarged gastric folds in the body and fundus of the stomach and hypertrophy of the gastric mucosa. Ménétrier's disease,[1326-1331] or hypertrophic gastritis, is the classic example, but the term is also applied to the stomachs of patients with Zollinger–Ellison syndrome and the so-called hypersecretory hypertrophic gastropathy, syndromes that are not truly gastrides.[1326,1332] The detection of enlarged gastric folds by endoscopy or a barium study in a symptomatic or even asymptomatic patient can pose a problem to the clinician. Are the folds really abnormal and therefore of clinical significance, and do they represent a hypertrophic gastropathy or even a more serious disease such as lymphoma or infiltrating carcinoma? How extensively, aggressively, and rapidly should the patient be studied? The history, physical examination, and initial ancillary laboratory studies are important aids in this decision.

Ménétrier's Disease (Hypertrophic Gastritis).

Ménétrier's disease is a rare disorder of unknown etiology characterized by a hypertrophic gastropathy that is produced mainly by a hyperplasia of gastric pit (foveolar) mucous cells. It is usually accompanied by protein-losing gastropathy (enteropathy) and often by atrophy of normal gastric glands and thus decreased gastric acid secretion.[1326-1331] While a few familial cases have been reported, heredity does not usually play a significant role in the pathogenesis.[1333] The disease may be focal or extensive. It is usually confined to the oxyntic (fundic) mucosa of the body and fundus but sometimes involves the antrum as well. The gastric folds are usually markedly enlarged, often tortuous, and may appear nodular or polypoid. The endoscopist may be unable to flatten them completely with air insufflation. Erosions, ulcers, and even hemorrhage may sometimes be observed on the folds.

In the past, a surgical specimen was often needed to establish a tissue diagnosis. The ability to obtain large, nearly full-thickness mucosal biopsy specimens by way of the endoscope now makes surgical diagnosis rarely necessary. The lesion is characterized by a thickened mucosa due to hyperplasia of the pit (foveolar) mucous cells forming elongated, tortuous, branched glands that are often markedly dilated (cystic dilatation). These mucous glands extend deep into the mucosa, even to the submucosa, replacing normal oxyntic (fundic) glands with their parietal and chief cells. The lamina propria may be infiltrated with mononuclear cells, especially in the superficial mucosa. Patches of normal oxyntic mucosa may survive within areas of abnormal mucosa.

The mechanism by which affected stomachs weep excessive amounts of plasma proteins into the gastric lumen is not entirely clear. Plasma proteins have been thought to move paracellularly between epithelial cells,[1330] and the possible presence of submucosal lymphangiectasia may promote such exudation.[1331]

Patients with Ménétrier's hypertrophic gastropathy may be asymptomatic or may present with gastrointestinal symptoms, anemia from GI blood loss, or, most characteristically, edema or a fortuitously detected low serum albumin and hypoproteinemia as a result of the protein-losing gastropathy. Gastrointestinal symptoms include epigastric pain, vomiting, and diarrhea. The detection of giant gastric folds by endoscopy or a GI series is usually the first diagnostic suggestion of this disorder, even if a low serum albumin is not present or appreciated. Successful full-thickness mucosal biopsies may provide histologic confirmation. The diagnosis may be supported by the demonstration of an abnormal gastroenteric loss of plasma proteins by a suitable test, such as measurement of the gastrointestinal clearance of alpha$_1$-antitrypsin,[1334] and by the demonstration of diminished secretion of gastric acid, a feature that is often, but not always, present.

The detection of apparently enlarged gastric folds presents a not uncommon diagnostic dilemma to the physician. A gastric lymphoma or carcinoma can usually be excluded by multiple deep mucosal biopsies and by cytology of brush specimens. In rare cases, a CT scan or perhaps the newer technique of endoscopic ultrasonography may be helpful. The hypertrophic gastropathy of Zollinger–Ellison syndrome should not pose a diagnostic problem because biopsy specimens should appear normal or reveal hyperplasia of the normal glandular cells and ulcers, gastric hypersecretion, and elevated serum gastrin levels usually are present. The rare, poorly defined, non-Zollinger–Ellison form of hypersecretory gastropathy is characterized by excessive gastric plasma protein loss, gastric hypersecretion of acid, and absence of the Zollinger–Ellison syndrome.[1326,1332]

While Ménétrier's hypertrophic gastropathy usually presents in middle-aged and older men, the disease—at least the presence of large gastric folds and hypoproteinemia—also occurs in children.[1313,1314,1335-1337] In childhood, however, the disease is usually reversible and is thought to be likely due to infection. CMV infection is one probable cause.[1313,1314] Acute, reversible cases are also seen in adults, possibly as a result of allergic reactions. It is not clear whether these acute, reversible cases actually represent functional changes of mucosal edema and abnormal vascular leakage of plasma proteins rather than a true Ménétrier's with histologic changes. The Ménétrier-like hypertrophic gastropathy with giant gastric folds has also been seen in AIDS patients and is also possibly related to CMV infection.

Treatment for Ménétrier's has not been established and should probably be judiciously individualized for each patient. Physicians should not be reluctant to employ minimal therapy, especially in patients with mild symptoms and little disability. Patients with dyspeptic symptoms, especially ones with ulcers, may benefit from conventional ulcer therapy. Antisecretory therapy with anticholinergics and histamine H$_2$-receptor blockers has been reported to improve symptoms and hypoalbuminemia in some cases.[1328] Partial gastric resections may be considered for patients with localized disease and unresponsive dyspeptic symptoms and hypoproteinemia. More extensive resections for diffuse disease should be considered only in severe, unremitting cases. It has been suggested that Ménétrier's disease is associated with or is a precursor of carcinoma, but this has not been established.[1328,1338] Edema should be treated by mechanical means, such as leg elevation and elastic stockings. Vascular, thromboembolic, and infectious complications may be significant and should be treated early and vigorously.[1329]

GASTRIC PSEUDOLYMPHOMA

Gastric "pseudolymphoma" is a rare condition of unknown etiology characterized by the marked focal hyperplasia of lymph follicles, usually with germinal centers, in the mucosa and submucosa and sometimes the deeper layers of the stomach.[1339–1342] As its name suggests, this lymphoid hyperplasia must be differentiated from a gastric lymphoma, and this differentiation can sometimes be difficult to make. In fact, an occasional patient with lymphoid hyperplasia has actually had an associated gastric lymphoma or has progressed to a lymphoma.[1340,1341] Patients may present with symptomatic gastric ulcers that, by endoscopy, either appear benign or, because of adjacent thick folds, appear to be infiltrating malignancies. Sometimes a GI series, obtained for whatever indication, suggests this disease because of localized, enlarged, irregular folds. Deep biopsies of the edge of the ulcer or of the suspicious folds reveal the lesion. The pathologists usually apply immunocytochemical staining techniques to help differentiate the benign lesion from an actual lymphoma and may request additional, deeper endoscopic biopsies to help them. Cases that remain questionable or suspicious should probably have a local surgical resection.

> The reader is directed to Chapter 2, Gastrointestinal Hormones; Chapter 30, Approach to the Patient with Gross Gastrointestinal Bleeding; Chapter 31, Approach to the Patient with Occult Gastrointestinal Bleeding; Chapter 49, Genetic Counseling for Gastrointestinal Patients; Chapter 58, Miscellaneous Diseases of the Esophagus; Chapter 62, Zollinger-Ellison Syndrome; Chapter 64, Surgery for Peptic Ulcer Disease; Chapter 106, Gastrointestinal Manifestations of Systemic Diseases; Chapter 109, Vascular Insufficiency; Chapter 111, Upper Gastrointestinal Endoscopy; Chapter 114, Contrast Radiology; Chapter 126, Endoscopic Mucosal Biopsy; Chapter 129, Tests of Gastric and Exocrine Pancreatic Function and Absorption; and Chapter 134, Endoscopic Control of Nonvariceal Upper Gastrointestinal Hemorrhage.

REFERENCES

1. Dooley CP, Cohen H. The clinical significance of Campylobacter pylori. Ann Intern Med 1988;108:70.
2. Doenges JL. Spirochaetes in the gastric glands of Macacus rhesus and humans without definite history of related disease. Proc Soc Exp Med Biol 1938;38:536.
3. Palmer ED. Investigation of the gastric mucosa spirochetes of the human. Gastroenterology 1954;27:218.
4. Steer HW, Colin-Jones DG. Mucosal changes in gastric ulceration and their response to carbenoxolone sodium. Gut 1975;16:590.
5. Warren JR. Letter: Unidentified curved bacilli on gastric epithelium in active chronic gastritis. Lancet 1983;1:1273.
6. Marshall B. Letter: Unidentified curved bacilli on gastric epithelium in active chronic gastritis. Lancet 1983;1:1273.
7. Siurala M, Isokoski M, Varis K, Kekki M. Prevalence of gastritis in a rural population: Bioptic study of subjects selected at random. Scand J Gastroenterol 1968;3:211.
8. Villako K, Tamm A, Savisaar E, Ruttas M. Prevalence of antral and fundic gastritis in a randomly selected group of an Estonian rural population. Scand J Gastroenterol 1976;11:817.
9. Imai T, Kubo T, Watanabe H. Chronic gastritis in Japanese with reference to high incidence of gastric carcinoma. J Natl Cancer Inst 1971;47:179.
10. Dooley CP, Cohen H, Fitzgibbons PL, et al. Prevalence of Helicobacter pylori infection and histologic gastritis in asymptomatic persons. N Engl J Med 1989;321:1562.
11. Kreuning J, Bosman FT, Kuiper G, Wal AM, Lindeman J. Gastric and duodenal mucosa in "healthy" individuals: An endoscopic and histopathological study of 50 volunteers. J Clin Pathol 1978;31:69.
12. Podolsky I, Lee E, Cohen R, Peterson WL. Prevalence of C. pylori in healthy subjects and patients with peptic diseases (abstr). Gastroenterology 1989;96:A394.
13. Graham DY, Klein PD, Opekun AR, Boutton TW. Effect of age on the frequency of active Campylobacter pylori infection diagnosed by the [13C] urea breath test in normal subjects and patients with peptic ulcer disease. J Infect Dis 1988;157:777.
14. Perez-Perez GI, Dworkin BM, Chodos JE, Blaser MJ. Campylobacter pylori antibodies in humans. Ann Intern Med 1988;109:11.
15. Graham DY, Adam E, Klein PD, et al. Comparison of the prevalence of asymptomatic C. pylori infection in the United States: Effect of age, gender and race (abstr). Gastroenterology 1989;96:A180.
16. Jones DM, Eldridge J, Fox AJ, Sethi P, Whorwell PJ. Antibody to the gastric Campylobacter-like organism ("Campylobacter pyloridis")—Clinical correlations and distributions in the normal population. J Med Microbiol 1986;22:57.
17. Berkowicz J, Lee A. Letter: Person-to-person transmission of Campylobacter pylori. Lancet 1987;2:680.
18. Marshall BJ, McGechie DB, Francis GJ, Utley PJ. Letter: Pyloric Campylobacter serology. Lancet 1984;2:281.
19. Dwyer B, Kaldor J, Tee W, Marakowski E, Raios K. Antibody response to Campylobacter pylori in diverse ethnic groups. Scand J Infect Dis 1988;20:349.
20. Morris A, Nicholson G, Lloyd G, Haines D, Rogers A, Taylor D. Seroepidemiology of Campylobacter pyloridis. N Z Med J 1986;99:657.
21. Russell PK, Aziz MA, Ahmad N, Kent TH, Gangarosa EJ. Enteritis and gastritis in young asymptomatic Pakistani men. Am J Dig Dis 1966;11:296.
22. Correa P, Cuello C, Duque E, et al. Gastric cancer in Colombia. III. Natural history of precursor lesions. J Natl Cancer Inst 1976;57:1027.
23. Gutierrez O, Sierra F, Gomez MC, Camargo H. Campylobacter pylori in chronic environmental gastritis and duodenal ulcer patients (abstr). Gastroenterology 1988;94:A163.
24. Megraud F, Brassens-Rabbe MP, Denis G, Touhami M, Hoa DQ. Campylobacter pylori infection—Evidence for a worldwide distribution and a high prevalence in developing countries (abstr). Gastroenterology 1989;96:A338.
25. Klein PD, Graham DY, Opekun AR, Sekeley S, Evans DG, Evans DJ Jr. High prevalence of Campylobacter pylori infection in poor and rich Peruvian children determined by 13C urea breath test (abstr). Gastroenterology 1989;96:A260.
26. Dehesa M, Dooley CP, Cohen H, Fitzgibbons P, Perez-Perez GI, Blaser MJ. High prevalence of Campylobacter pylori in an asymptomatic Hispanic population (abstr). Gastroenterology 1989;96:A115.
27. Romaniuk PJ, Zoltowska B, Trust TJ, et al. Campylobacter pylori, the spiral bacterium associated with human gastritis, is not a true Campylobacter sp. J Bacteriol 1987;169:2137.
28. Goodwin S, Blincow E, Armstrong J, McCulloch R. Campylobacter pyloridis is unique: GCLO-2 is an ordinary Campylobacter. Lancet 1985;2:38.
29. Goodwin CS, McCulloch RK, Armstrong JA, Wee SH. Unusual cellular fatty acids and distinctive ultrastructure in a new spiral bacterium (Campylobacter pyloridis) from the human gastric mucosa. J Med Microbiol 1985;19:257.
30. Lambert MA, Patton CM, Barrett TJ, Moss CW. Differentiation

of Campylobacter and Campylobacter-like organisms by cellular fatty acid composition. J Clin Microbiol 1987;25:706.

31. McNulty CAM, Dent JC. Rapid identification of Campylobacter pylori (C. pylori) by preformed enzymes. J Clin Microbiol 1987;25:1683.

32. Nedenskov-Sorensen P, Bjorneklett A, Fausa O, Bukholm G, Aase S, Jantzen E. Campylobacter pylori infection and its relation to chronic gastritis: An endoscopic, bacteriologic, and histomorphologic study. Scand J Gastroenterol 1988;23:867.

33. Goodwin CS, Armstrong JA, Chilvers T, et al. Transfer of Campylobacter pylori and Campylobacter mustelae to Helicobacter gennov as Helicobacter pylori comb-nov and Helicobacter mustelae comb-nov, respectively. Int J Syst Bacteriol 1989;39:397.

34. Marshall BJ, Warren JR. Unidentified curved bacilli in the stomach of patients with gastritis and peptic ulceration. Lancet 1984;1:1311.

35. Pinkard KJ, Harrison B, Capstick JA, Medley G, Lambert JR. Detection of Campylobacter pyloridis in gastric mucosa by phase contrast microscopy. J Clin Pathol 1986;39:112.

36. Taylor DE, Hargreaves JA, NG L, Sherbaniuk RW, Jewell LD. Isolation and characterization of Campylobacter pyloridis from gastric biopsies. Am J Clin Pathol 1987;87:49.

37. Bode G, Malfertheiner P, Ditschuneit H. Pathogenetic implications of ultrastructural findings in Campylobacter pylori related gastroduodenal disease. Scand J Gastroenterol 1988;23(Suppl 142):25.

38. Mobley HLT, Cortesia MJ, Rosenthal LE, Jones BD. Characterization of urease from Campylobacter pylori. J Clin Microbiol 1988;26:831.

39. Goodwin CS, Blincow ED, Warren JR, Waters TE, Sanderson CR, Easton L. Evaluation of cultural techniques for isolating Campylobacter pyloridis from endoscopic biopsies of gastric mucosa. J Clin Pathol 1985;38:1127.

40. Buck GE, Smith JS. Medium supplementation for growth of Campylobacter pyloridis. J Clin Microbiol 1987;25:597.

41. Megraud F, Bonnet F, Garnier M, Lamouliatte H. Characterization of "Campylobacter pyloridis" by culture, enzymatic profile, and protein content. J Clin Microbiol 1985;22:1007.

42. Buck GE, Gourley WK, Lee WK, Subramanyam K, Latimer JM, DiNuzzo AR. Relation of Campylobacter pyloridis to gastritis and peptic ulcer. J Infect Dis 1986;153:664.

43. Jones DM, Lessells AM, Eldridge J. Campylobacter like organisms on the gastric mucosa: Culture, histological, and serological studies. J Clin Pathol 1984;37:1002.

44. Langenberg M-L, Tytgat GNJ, Schipper MEI, Rietra PJGM, Zanen HC. Letter: Campylobacter-like organisms in the stomachs of patients and healthy individuals. Lancet 1984;1:1348.

45. Mitchell HM, Bohane TD, Berkowicz J, Hazell SL, Lee A. Letter: Antibody to Campylobacter pylori in families of index children with gastrointestinal illness due to C. pylori. Lancet 1987;2:681.

46. Cadranel S, Verhas M, Zeghlache S, De Prez C, Glupscinsky G. Campylobacter pylori in the families of children with primary ulcers and chronic gastritis (abstr). Gastroenterology. 1989;96:A69.

47. Drumm B, Perez-Perez GI, Blaser MJ, et al. Intrafamilial clustering of Helicobacter pylori infection. N Engl J Med 1990;322:359.

48. Rauws EAJ, Langenberg W, Oudbier J, Mulder CJJ, Tytgat GNJ. Familial clustering of peptic ulcer disease colonized with C. pylori of the same DNA composition (abstr). Gastroenterology 1989;96:A409.

49. Kim F, Mobley HLT, Burken M, Morris JG. Molecular epidemiology of Campylobacter pylori infection in a chronic care facility (abstr). Gastroenterology 1989;96:A256.

50. Ramsey EJ, Carey KV, Peterson WL, et al. Epidemic gastritis with hypochlorhydria. Gastroenterology 1979;76:1449.

51. Peterson W, Lee E, Skoglund M. The role of Campylobacter pyloridis in epidemic gastritis with hypochlorhydria (abstr). Gastroenterology 1987;92:1575.

52. Gledhill T, Leicester RJ, Addis B, et al. Epidemic hypochlorhydria. Br Med J 1985;290:1383.

53. Baskerville A, Newell DG. Naturally occurring chronic gastritis and C. pylori infection in the rhesus monkey: A potential model for gastritis in man. Gut 1988;29:465.

54. Dubois A, Tarnawski A, Fiala N, et al. Direct evidence for parietal cells invasion and injury by Campylobacter pylori–like organisms in rhesus monkeys. An animal model for gastritis? (abstr) Gastroenterology 1988;94:A105.

55. Bronsdon MA, Schoenknecht FD. Campylobacter pylori isolated from the stomach of the monkey, Macaca nemestrina. J Clin Microbiol 1988;26:1725.

56. Newell DG, Hudson MJ, Baskerville A. Isolation of a gastric Campylobacter-like organism from the stomach of four rhesus monkeys, and identification as Campylobacter pylori. J Med Microbiol 1988;27:41.

57. Lambert JR, Borromeo M, Pinkard KJ, Turner H, Chapman CB, Smith ML. Letter: Colonization of gnotobiotic piglets with Campylobacter pyloridis—An animal model? J Infect Dis 1987;155:1344.

58. Krakowka S, Morgan KR, Kraft WG, Leunk RD. Establishment of gastric Campylobacter pylori infection in the neonatal gnotobiotic piglet. Infect Immun 1987;55:2789.

59. Droy-Lefaix MT, Bonneville F, Moyen EN, Geraud G, Combrier E, Fauchere JL. Campylobacter pylori and gastritis: A new animal model in germ-free rats (abstr). Gastroenterology 1989;96:A130.

60. Fox JG, Cabot EB, Taylor NS, Laraway R. Gastric colonization by Campylobacter pylori subsp. mustelae in ferrets. Infect Immun 1988;56:2994.

61. Tompkins KS, Wyatt JI, Rathbone BJ, West AP. The characterization and pathological significance of gastric Campylobacter-like organisms in the ferret: A model for chronic gastritis? Epidemiol Infect 1988;101:269.

62. Yang P, Dahms B, Carr H, Czinn S. Naturally occurring ferret Campylobacter associated gastric disease: Characterization and response to non-steroidal anti-inflammatory agents (abstr). Gastroenterology 1989;96:A557.

63. Lee A, Hazell SL, O'Rourke J, Kourprach S. Isolation of a spiral-shaped bacterium from the cat stomach. Infect Immun 1988;56:2843.

64. Marshall BJ, Armstrong JA, McGechie DB, Glancy RJ. Attempt to fulfill Koch's postulates for pyloric Campylobacter. Med J Aust 1985;142:436.

65. Morris A, Nicholson G. Ingestion of Campylobacter pyloridis causes gastritis and raised fasting gastric pH. Am J Gastroenterol 1987;82:192.

66. Borsch G, Schmidt G, Wegener M, et al. Campylobacter pylori: Prospective analysis of clinical and histological factors associated with colonization of the upper gastrointestinal tract. Eur J Clin Invest 1988;18:133.

67. Siurala M, Sipponen P, Kekki M. Campylobacter pylori in a sample of Finnish population: Relations to morphology and functions of the gastric mucosa. Gut 1988;29:909.

68. Loffeld FJLF, Potters HVPJ, Arends JW, Stobberingh E, Flendrig JA, Van Spreeuwel JP. Campylobacter associated gastritis in patients with non-ulcer dyspepsia. J Clin Pathol 1988;41:85.

69. Rokkas T, Pursey C, Uzoechina E, et al. Campylobacter pylori and non-ulcer dyspepsia. Am J Gastroenterol 1987;82:1149.

70. Rokkas T, Pursey C, Uzoechina E, et al. Non-ulcer dyspepsia and short term De-Nol therapy: A placebo controlled trial with particular reference to the role of Campylobacter pylori. Gut 1988;29:1386.

71. George A, Dooley CP, Dehesa M, Cohen H, Arandia D. Evidence against a role for Campylobacter pylori in the pathogenesis of non-ulcer dyspepsia (abstr). Gastroenterology 1989;96:A170.

72. Montgomery EA, Martin DF, Peura DA. Rapid diagnosis of Campylobacter pylori. Am J Clin Pathol 1988;90:606.

73. Humphreys H, O'Morain C. Culture of the organisms and histochemical identification. Scand J Gastroenterol 1988;23(Suppl 142):16.

74. Madan E, Kemp J, Westblom U, Subik M, Sexton S, Cook J. Evaluation of staining methods for identifying Campylobacter pylori. Am J Clin Pathol 1988;90:450.

75. Morris A, Brown P, Ali MR, Lane M, Palmer R. Treatment of Campylobacter pylori gastritis: A pilot study using pirenzepine dihydrochloride (Gastrozepin) and three formulations of colloidal bismuth subcitrate (De-Nol). N Z Med J 1988;101:651.

76. Andersen LP, Holck S, Povlsen CO, Elsborg L, Justesen T. Campylobacter pyloridis in peptic ulcer disease. I. Gastric and duodenal infection caused by C. pyloridis: Histopathologic and microbiologic findings. Scand J Gastroenterol 1987;22:219.

77. Morris A, Arthur J, Nicholson G. Campylobacter pyloridis infection in Auckland patients with gastritis. N Z Med J 1986;99:353.

78. Aymard B, Labouyrie E, de Korwin JD, Ferry R, Duprez A. Histological staining methods for detection of gastric Campylobacter like organisms: A comparative study (abstr). Gastroenterology 1988;94:A16.

79. Westblom TU, Madan E, Kemp J, Subik MA. Evaluation of a rapid urease test to detect Campylobacter pylori infection. J Clin Microbiol 1988;26:1393.

80. Barbosa AJA, Queiroz DMM, Mendes EN, Rocha GA, Lima GF Jr, Oliveira CA. Immunocytochemical identification of Campylobacter pylori in gastritis and correlation with culture. Arch Pathol Lab Med 1988;112:523.

81. Negrini R, Lisato L, Cavazzini L, et al. Monoclonal antibodies for specific immunoperoxidase detection of Campylobacter pylori. Gastroenterology 1989;96:414.

82. Andersen LP, Holck S, Povlsen CO. Campylobacter pylori detected by indirect immunohistochemical technique. APMIS 1988;96:559.

83. Marshall BJ, Warren JR, Francis GJ, Langton SR, Goodwin CS, Blincow ED. Rapid urease test in the management of Campylobacter pyloridis–associated gastritis. Am J Gastroenterol 1987;82:200.

84. Morris A, McIntyre D, Rose T, Nicholson G. Letter: Rapid diagnosis of Campylobacter pyloridis infection. Lancet 1986;1:149.

85. Borsch G, Adamek R, Sandmann M, et al. Comparison of biopsy urease test and histologic examination for detection of Campylobacter pylori in duodenal, antral, and fundic biopsies. Hepatogastroenterology 1987;34:236.

86. Borromeo M, Lambert JR, Pinkard KJ. Evaluation of "CLO-test" to detect Campylobacter pyloridis in gastric mucosa. J Clin Pathol 1987;40:462.

87. Hazell SL, Borody TJ, Gal A, Lee A. Campylobacter pyloridis gastritis. I: Detection of urease as a marker of bacterial colonization and gastritis. Am J Gastroenterol 1987;82:292.

88. Graham DY, Klein PD, Evans DJ, et al. Campylobacter pylori detected noninvasively by the ^{13}C-urea breath test. Lancet 1987;1:1174.

89. Rauws EAJ, van Royen EA, Langenberg W, et al. C-14 urea breath test in C. pylori gastritis. Gut 1989;30:798.

90. Marshall BJ, Surveyor I. Carbon-14 urea breath test for the diagnosis of Campylobacter pylori associated gastritis. J Nucl Med 1988;29:11.

91. Jalali S, van Zanten SV, Goldie J, et al. ^{14}C-urea breath test, ELISA, and symptom score compared with histology and culture for detection of Campylobacter pylori (abstr). Gastroenterology 1989;96:A235.

92. Marshall BJ, Plankey MW, Hoffman S, McCallum RW. Simplifying the urea breath test for C. pylori (abstr). Gastroenterology 1989;96:A321.

93. Eggers RH, Tegeler R, Geletneky JV, Ludtke FE, Lepsien G, Bauer FE. ^{13}C-urea breath test—A new and noninvasive method for the diagnosis of Campylobacter pylori infections in health and disease (abstr). Gastroenterology 1989;96:A136.

94. Evans DJ Jr, Evans DG, Graham DY, Klein PD. A sensitive and specific serologic test for detection of Campylobacter pylori infection. Gastroenterology 1989;96:1004.

95. Vantrappen G, Hiele M, Rutgeerts P, Ghoos Y, Henneresse PE. A one-day treatment with colloidal bismuth, sucralfate or amoxicillin may already result in a false negative ^{13}C-urea breath test (abstr). Gastroenterology 1989;96:A525.

96. Booth L, Holdstock G, MacBride H, et al. Clinical importance of Campylobacter pyloridis and associated serum IgG and IgA antibody responses in patients undergoing upper gastrointestinal endoscopy. J Clin Pathol 1986;39:215.

97. Goodwin CS, Blincow E, Peterson G, et al. Enzyme-linked immunosorbent assay for Campylobacter pyloridis: Correlation with presence of C. pyloridis in the gastric mucosa. J Infect Dis 1987;155:488.

98. Faisal MA, Santogade PJ, Bokkenheuser V, Scholes JV, Holt PR, Kotler DP. Sensitivity and specificity of the serologic diagnosis of Campylobacter pylori infection (abstr). Gastroenterology 1988;94:A121.

99. Rathbone BJ, Wyatt JI, Worsley BW, et al. Systemic and local antibody responses to gastric Campylobacter pyloridis in non-ulcer dyspepsia. Gut 1986;27:642.

100. Gnarpe H, Unge P, Blomqvist C, Makitalo S. Campylobacter pylori in Swedish patients referred for gastroscopy. APMIS 1988;96:128.

101. Sethi P, Banerjee AK, Jones DM, Eldridge J, Hollanders D. Gastritis and gastric Campylobacter-like organisms in patients without peptic ulcer. Postgrad Med J 1987;63:543.

102. Von Wulffen H, Grote HJ, Gatermann S, Loning T, Berger B, Buhl C. Immunoblot analysis of immune response to Campylobacter pylori and its clinical associations. J Clin Pathol 1988;41:653.

103. Czinn S, Carr H, Yang P. Antibody response to Campylobacter pylori—A comparison of the systemic and mucosal immune system (abstr). Gastroenterology 1989;96:A106.

104. Peterson WL, Lee E, Feldman M. Relationship between Campylobacter pylori and gastritis in healthy humans after administration of placebo or indomethacin. Gastroenterology 1988;95:1185.

105. Oderda G, Vaira D, Holton J, Ainley C, Altare F, Ansaldi N. Amoxicillin plus tinidazole for Campylobacter pylori gastritis in children: Assessment by serum IgG antibody, pepsinogen I, and gastrin levels. Lancet 1989;1:690.

106. Steer HW. The gastro-duodenal epithelium in peptic ulceration. J Pathol 1985;146:355.

107. Price AB, Levi J, Dolby JM, et al. Campylobacter pyloridis in peptic ulcer disease: Microbiology, pathology, and scanning electron microscopy. Gut 1985;26:1183.

108. Hazell SL, Lee A, Brady L, Hennessy W. Campylobacter pyloridis and gastritis: Association with intercellular spaces and adaptation to an environment of mucus as important factors in colonization of the gastric epithelium. J Infect Dis 1986;153:658.

109. Steer HW. Surface morphology of the gastroduodenal mucosa in duodenal ulceration. Gut 1984;25:1204.

110. Rollason TP, Stone J, Rhodes JM. Spiral organisms in endoscopic biopsies of the human stomach. J Clin Pathol 1984;37:23.

111. Thomas JM, Poynter D, Gooding C, et al. Letter: Gastric spiral bacteria. Lancet 1984;2:100.

112. Lee WK, Gourley WK, Buck GE, Subramanyam K. A light and electron microscopic study of a Campylobacter-like bacteria inhabiting the human stomach (abstr). Gastroenterology 1985;88:1470.

113. Paull G, Yardley JH. Gastric and esophageal Campylobacter pylori in patients with Barrett's esophagus. Gastroenterology 1988;95:216.

114. Talley R, Weinstein WM, Marin-Sorensen M, Schneidman D, Reedy TJ, Van Deventer G. Campylobacter pylori colonization of Barrett's esophagus (abstr). Gastroenterology 1988;94:A454.

115. Hazell SL, Carrick J, Lee A. Campylobacter pylori can infect the oesophagus when gastric tissue is present (abstr). Gastroenterology 1988;94:A178.

116. Talley NJ, Cameron AJ, Shorter RG, Zinsmeister AR, Phillips SF. Campylobacter pylori and Barrett's esophagus. Mayo Clin Proc 1988;63:1176.

117. Wyatt JI, Rathbone BJ, Dixon MF, Heatley RV. Campylobacter pyloridis and acid induced gastric metaplasia in the pathogenesis of duodenitis. J Clin Pathol 1987;40:841.

118. de Cothi GA, Newbold KM, O'Connor HJ. Campylobacter-like organisms and heterotopic gastric mucosa in Meckel's diverticula. J Clin Pathol 1989;42:132.

119. Morris A, Nicholson G, Zwi J, Vanderwee M. Campylobacter pylori infection in Meckel's diverticula containing gastric mucosa. Gut 1989;30:1233.

120. Dye KR, Marshall BJ, Frierson HF, et al. Campylobacter pylori colonizing heterotopic gastric tissue in the rectum. Am J Clin Pathol 1990;93:144.

121. Johnston BJ, Reed PI, Ali MH. Prevalence of Campylobacter pylori in duodenal and gastric mucosa—Relationship to inflammation. Scand J Gastroenterol 1988;23(Suppl 142):69.

122. Cohen H, Gramisu M, Fitzgibbons P, Appleman M, Skoglund M, Valenzuela JE. Campylobacter pylori: Associations with antral and fundic mucosal histology and diagnosis by serology in patients with upper gastrointestinal symptoms. Am J Gastroenterol 1989;84:367.

123. Blomberg B, Jarnerot G, Kjellander J, Danielsson D, Kraaz W. Prevalence of Campylobacter pylori in an unselected Swedish pop-

ulation of patients referred for gastroscopy. Scand J Gastroenterol 1988;23:358.

124. Strauss RM, Wang TC, Kelsey PB, Ferraro MJ, Compton CC. The clinical importance of Campylobacter pyloris and the importance of fundal biopsies (abstr). Gastroenterology 1988;94:A447.

125. Wyatt JI, Rathbone BJ, Heatley RV. Local immune response to gastric Campylobacter in non-ulcer dyspepsia. J Clin Pathol 1986;39:863.

126. Rauws EAJ, Langenberg W, Houthoff HJ, Zanen HC, Tytgat GNJ. Campylobacter pyloridis-associated chronic active antral gastritis. A prospective study of its prevalence and the effects of antibacterial and antiulcer treatment. Gastroenterology 1988;94:33.

127. Berstad A, Alexander B, Weberg R, Serck-Hanssen A, Holland S, Hirschowitz BI. Antacids reduce Campylobacter pylori colonization without healing the gastritis in patients with nonulcer dyspepsia and erosive prepyloric changes. Gastroenterology 1988;95:619.

128. Pettross CW, Appleman MD, Cohen H, Valenzuela JE, Chandrasoma P, Laine L. Prevalence of Campylobacter pylori and association with antral mucosal histology in subjects with and without upper gastrointestinal symptoms. Dig Dis Sci 1988;33:649.

129. Laine L, Marin-Sorensen M, Weinstein WM. Campylobacter pylori in alcoholic hemorrhagic "gastritis." Dig Dis Sci 1989;34:677.

130. Chodos JE, Dworkin BM, Smith F, Van Horn K, Weiss L, Rosenthal WS. Campylobacter pylori and gastroduodenal disease: A prospective endoscopic study and comparison of diagnostic tests. Am J Gastroenterol 1988;83:1226.

131. Karttunen T, Niemela S, Lehtola J, Heikkila J, Maentausta O, Rasanen O. Campylobacter-like organisms and gastritis: Histopathology, bile reflux, and gastric fluid composition. Scand J Gastroenterol 1987;22:478.

132. The Gastrointestinal Physiology Working Group. Rapid identification of pyloric Campylobacter in Peruvians with gastritis. Dig Dis Sci 1986;31:1089.

133. Morgan D, Kraft W, Bender M, Pearson A. Nitrofurans in the treatment of gastritis associated with Campylobacter pylori. Gastroenterology 1988;95:1178.

134. Chen XG, Correa P, Offerhaus J, et al. Ultrastructure of the gastric mucosa harboring Campylobacter-like organisms. Am J Clin Pathol 1986;86:575.

135. O'Connor HJ, Axon ATR, Dixon MF. Letter: Campylobacter-like organisms unusual in type A (pernicious anemia) gastritis. Lancet 1984;2:1091.

136. Flejou JF, Bahame P, Smith AC, Stockbrugger RW, Rode J, Price AB. Pernicious anaemia and Campylobacter like organisms; is the gastric antrum resistant to colonization? Gut 1989;30:60.

137. Fong TL, Dehesa M, Dooley CP, et al. The prevalence of Campylobacter pylori in patients with pernicious anemia (abstr). Gastroenterology 1989;96:A154.

138. Charasz N, Roucayrol AM, Chaplain C, Cattan D, Dublanchet A. Prevalence of Campylobacter pylori in fundic atrophic gastritis with or without achlorhydria (abstr). Gastroenterology 1989;96:A83.

139. O'Connor HJ, Dixon MF, Wyatt JI, et al. Effect of duodenal ulcer surgery and enterogastric reflux on Campylobacter pyloridis. Lancet 1986;2:1178.

140. Offerhaus GJA, Rieu PNMA, Hansen JBMJ, Hoosten HJM, Lamers CBHW. Gastritis after gastric surgery; role of bile reflux and Campylobacter pylori (abstr). Gastroenterology 1988;94:A330.

141. O'Connor HJ, Dixon MF, Wyatt JI, Axon ATR, Dewar EP, Johnston D. Letter: Campylobacter pylori and peptic ulcer disease. Lancet 1987;2:633.

142. Offerhaus GJA, Rieu PNMA, Jansen JBMJ, et al. Prospective comparative study of the influence of postoperative bile reflux on gastric mucosal histology and Campylobacter pylori infection. Gut 1989;30:1552.

143. Tompkins DS, West AP. Letter: Campylobacter pylori, acid, and bile. J Clin Pathol 1987;40:1387.

144. Andersen LP, Elsborg L, Justesen T. Campylobacter pylori in peptic ulcer disease. II. Endoscopic findings and cultivation of C. pylori. Scand J Gastroenterol 1988;23:760.

145. Laine L, Marin-Sorensen M, Weinstein WM. Is Campylobacter pylori prevalence lower in gastric ulcers because of nonsteroidal antiinflammatory drug use? (abstr) Gastroenterology 1989;96:A282.

146. Blanco M, Pajares JM, Jimenez ML, Lopez-Brea M. Effect of acid inhibition on Campylobacter pylori. Scand J Gastroenterol 1988;23(Suppl 142):107.

147. Von Wulffen H, Heesemann J, Butzow GH, Loning T, Laufs R. Detection of Campylobacter pyloridis in patients with antrum gastritis and peptic ulcers by culture, complement fixation test, and immunoblot. J Clin Microbiol 1986;24:716.

148. McNulty CAM, Watson DM. Letter: Spiral bacteria of the gastric antrum. Lancet 1984;1:1068.

149. Marshall BJ, McGechie DB, Rogers PA, Glancy RJ. Pyloric Campylobacter infection and gastroduodenal disease. Med J Aust 1985;142:439.

150. Coghlan JG, Gilligan D, Humphries H, et al. Campylobacter pylori and recurrence of duodenal ulcers—A 12-month follow-up study. Lancet 1987;2:1109.

151. Hui WM, Ho H, Lam SK. Persistence of Campylobacter pylori during remission and subsequent relapse in duodenal ulcer (abstr). Gastroenterology 1988;94:A196.

152. Dooley CP, McKenna D, Humphreys H, et al. Histological gastritis in duodenal ulcer: Relationship to Campylobacter pylori and effect of ulcer therapy. Am J Gastroenterol 1988;83:278.

153. Hui WM, Lam SK, Chau PY, et al. Persistence of Campylobacter pyloridis despite healing of duodenal ulcer and improvement of accompanying duodenitis and gastritis. Dig Dis Sci 1987;32:1255.

154. Lambert JR, Hansky J, Eaves ER, Korman MG, Pinkard K, Medley G. Campylobacter like organisms in human stomach (abstr). Gastroenterology 1985;88:1463.

155. Graham DY, Jordan PH, Opekun AR, David IA, Klein PD. Campylobacter pylori is not the cause of duodenal ulcers (abstr). Gastroenterology 1988;94:A152.

156. Silvoso GR, Ivey KJ, Butt JH, et al. Incidence of gastric lesions in patients with rheumatic disease on chronic aspirin therapy. Ann Intern Med 1979;91:517.

157. MacDonald WC. Correlation of mucosal histology and aspirin intake in chronic gastric ulcer. Gastroenterology 1973;65:381.

158. Koop H, Stumpf M, Eissele R, Lamberts R, Creutzfeldt W, Arnold R. Antral Campylobacter pylori in different states of gastric acid secretion (abstr). Gastroenterology 1989;96:A267.

159. Saeed ZA, Evans DJ Jr, Evans DG, et al. Campylobacter pylori and the Zollinger Ellison Syndrome (ZES) (abstr). Gastroenterology 1989;96:A433.

160. Fitzgibbons PL, Dooley CP, Cohen H, Appleman MD. Prevalence of gastric metaplasia, inflammation, and Campylobacter pylori in the duodenum of members of a normal population. Am J Clin Pathol 1988;90:711.

161. Hazell SL, Hennessy WB, Borody TJ, et al. Campylobacter pyloridis gastritis. II: Distribution of bacteria and associated inflammation in the gastroduodenal environment. Am J Gastroenterol 1987;82:297.

162. Sipponen P, Varis K, Cederberg A, et al. Campylobacter pylori is associated with chronic gastritis but not active peptic ulcer disease. APMIS 1988;96:84.

163. Murakami M, Yoo J, Seiki M, Inada M, Mitake T. Destruction of the gastric mucosal barrier by ammonia in rats and dogs (abstr). Gastroenterology 1988;94:A317.

164. Saita H, Murakami M, Teramura S, Yoo JK, Kita T, Ishibashi A. Effect of exposure of Campylobacter pylori to gastric mucosa in rats on restitution of surface epithelial cells (abstr). Gastroenterology 1989;96:A435.

165. Smoot DT, Mobley HLT, Resau JH. Inhibition of Campylobacter pylori urease activity prevents gastric epithelial cell injury in vitro (abstr). Gastroenterology 1989;96:A480.

166. Sarosiek J, Slomiany A, Slomiany BL. Evidence for weakening of gastric mucus integrity by Campylobacter pylori. Scand J Gastroenterol 1988;23:585.

167. Slomiany BL, Bilski J, Sarosiek J, et al. Campylobacter pyloridis degrades mucin and undermines gastric mucosal integrity. Biochem Biophys Res Commun 1987;144:307.

168. Sarosiek J, Slomiany A, VanHorn K, Zalesna G, Slomiany BL. Lipolytic activity of Campylobacter pylori: Effect of sofalcone (abstr). Gastroenterology 1988;96:A399.

169. Leunk RD, Johnson PT, David BC, Kraft WG, Morgan DR. Cy-

totoxic activity in broth-culture filtrates of Campylobacter pylori. J Med Microbiol 1988;26:93.

170. Hubertz V, Czinn S. Demonstration of a cytotoxin from Campylobacter pylori. Eur J Clin Microbiol Infect Dis 1988;7:576.

171. Cover TL, Blaser MJ. Human serologic response to Campylobacter pylori cytotoxin-associated proteins (abstr). Gastroenterology 1989;96:A101.

172. Figura N, Guglielmetti P, Rossolini A, et al. Cytotoxin production by Campylobacter pylori strains isolated from patients with peptic ulcers and from patients with chronic gastritis only. J Clin Microbiol 1989;27:225.

173. Levi S, Beardshall K, Haddad G, et al. Campylobacter pylori and duodenal ulcers: The gastrin link. Lancet 1989;1:1167.

174. Smith JTL, Pounder RE, Evans DJ, et al. Inappropriate 24 hour hypergastrinemia in asymptomatic *C. pylori* infection (abstr). Gastroenterology 1989;96:A479.

175. Montbriand JR, Appelman HD, Cotner EK, et al. Treatment of Campylobacter pylori does not alter gastric acid secretion. Am J Gastroenterol 1989;84:1513.

176. McNulty CM, Dent J, Wise R. Susceptibility of clinical isolates of Campylobacter pyloridis to 11 antimicrobial agents. Antimicrob Agents Chemother 1985;28:837.

177. Lambert T, Megraud F, Gerbaud G, Courvalin P. Susceptibility of Campylobacter pyloridis to 20 antimicrobial agents. Antimicrob Agents Chemother 1986;30:510.

178. Shungu D, Nalin DR, Gilman RH, et al. Comparative susceptibilities of Campylobacter pylori to norfloxacin and other agents. Antimicrob Agents Chemother 1987;31:949.

179. Van Caekenberghe DL, Breyssens J. In vitro synergistic activity between bismuth subcitrate and various antimicrobial agents against Campylobacter pyloridis (C. pylori). Antimicrob Agents Chemother 1987;31:1429.

180. Lambert JR, Hansky J, Davidson A, Pinkard K, Stockman K. Campylobacter like organisms—In vivo and in vitro susceptibility to antimicrobial and antiulcer therapy (abstr). Gastroenterology 1985;88:1462.

181. Glupczynski Y, Delmee M, Burck C, Labbe M, Avesani V, Burette A. Susceptibility of clinical isolates of Campylobacter pylori to 24 antimicrobial and anti-ulcer agents. Eur J Epidemiol 1988;4:154.

182. Unge P, Gnarpe H. Pharmacokinetic, bacteriological and clinical aspects on the use of doxycycline in patients with active duodenal ulcer associated with Campylobacter pylori. Scand J Infect Dis 1988;Suppl 53:70.

183. Lambert JR, Way DJ, King RG, Eaves ER, Hansky J. Bismuth pharmacokinetics in the human gastric mucosa (abstr). Gastroenterology 1988;94:A248.

184. Skoglund ML, Watters K. Bismuth concentration at site of Campylobacter pylori colonization (abstr). Gastroenterology 1988;94:A430.

185. Lambert JR, Way DJ, King RG, Eaves ER, Lianeas K, Wan A. Denol vs Pepto-Bismol—Bismuth pharmacokinetics in the human gastric mucosa (abstr). Gastroenterology 1989;96:A284.

186. Graham DY, Klein PD, Opekun AR, et al. In vivo susceptibility of Campylobacter pylori. Am J Gastroenterol 1989;84:233.

187. McNulty CAM, Gearty JC, Crump B, et al. Campylobacter pyloridis and associated gastritis: Investigator blind, placebo controlled trial of bismuth salicylate and erythromycin ethylsuccinate. Br Med J 1986;293:645.

188. Glupczynski Y, Burette A, Labbe M, Deprez C, De Reuck M, Deltenre M. Campylobacter pylori–associated gastritis: A double-blind placebo-controlled trial with amoxicillin. Am J Gastroenterol 1988;83:365.

189. Huai-Yu Z, Guozhen L, Jundong G, et al. Letter: Furazolidone in peptic ulcer. Lancet 1985;2:276.

190. Marshall BJ, Goodwin CS, Warren JR, et al. Prospective double-blind trial of duodenal ulcer relapse after eradication of Campylobacter pylori. Lancet 1988;2:1437.

191. Hirschl AM, Hentschel E, Schutze K, et al. The efficacy of antimicrobial treatment in Campylobacter pylori–associated gastritis and duodenal ulcer. Scand J Gastroenterol 1988;23(Suppl 142):76.

192. Borsch G, Mai U, Muller KM. Monotherapy or polychemotherapy in the treatment of Campylobacter pylori-related gastroduodenal disease. Scand J Gastroenterol 1988;23(Suppl 142):101.

193. Malfertheiner P, Stanescu A, Bode G, Baczako K. Bismuth subsalicylate treatment in Campylobacter pylori related chronic erosive gastritis (abstr). Gastroenterology 1988:94:A279.

194. Smith AC, Price AB, Borriello P, Levi AJ. A comparison of ranitidine and tripotassium dicitrato-bismuth in relapse rates of duodenal ulcer. The role of Campylobacter pylori (abstr). Gastroenterology 1988;94:A431.

195. Lambert JR, Borromeo M, Eaves ER, Hansky J, Korman M. Efficacy of different dosage regimes of bismuth in eradicating Campylobacter pylori (abstr). Gastroenterology 1988;94:A248.

196. Lambert JR, Borromeo M, Korman MG, Hansky J. Role of Campylobacter pyloridis in non-ulcer dyspepsia—A randomized controlled trial (abstr). Gastroenterology 1987;92:1488.

197. Lambert JR, Borromeo M, Korman MG, Hansky J. Campylobacter pylori and nonulcer dyspepsia—Randomized controlled trial (abstr). Gastroenterology 1989;96:A284.

198. Langenberg W, Rauws EAJ, Widjojokusmo A, Tytgat GNJ, Zanen HC. Identification of Campylobacter pyloridis isolates by restriction endonuclease DNA analysis. J Clin Microbiol 1986;24:414.

199. Bayerdorffer E, Ottenjann R. The role of antibiotics in Campylobacter pylori associated peptic ulcer disease. Scand J Gastroenterol 1988;23(Suppl 142):93.

200. Borody T, Cole P, Noonan S, et al. Recurrence of duodenal ulcer and Campylobacter pylori infection after eradication. Med J Aust 1989;151:431.

201. Borsch G, Mai U, Opferkuch W. Short- and medium-term results of oral triple therapy to eradicate C. pylori (abstr). Gastroenterology 1989;96:A53.

202. Coelho LGV, Queiroz DMM, Barbosa AJA, et al. Furazolidone x cimetidine in duodenal ulcer C. pylori positive patients (abstr). Gastroenterology 1989;96:A91.

203. O'Riordan TO, Tobin A, Beattie S, O'Morain C, Sweeney E, Keane C. Adjuvant antibiotic treatment improves eradication of Campylobacter pylori in duodenal ulcer (abstr). Gastroenterology 1989;96:A378.

204. Wagner S, Freise J, Bar W, Schulz M, Schmidt FW. Bismuth subsalicylate in the treatment of refractory peptic ulcers in patients with Campylobacter pylori infection (abstr). Gastroenterology 1989;96:A532.

205. Borsch G, Mai U, Opferkuch W. Oral triple therapy may effectively eradicate Campylobacter pylori in man: A pilot study (abstr). Gastroenterology 1988;94:A44.

206. Drum B, Sherman P, Chiasson D, Karmali M, Cutz E. Treatment of Campylobacter pylori–associated antral gastritis in children with bismuth subsalicylate and ampicillin. J Pediatr 1988;113:908.

207. Meikle DD, Taylor KB, Truelove SC, Whitehead R. Gastritis, duodenitis, and circulating levels of gastrin in duodenal ulcer before and after vagotomy. Gut 1976;17:719.

208. Ho J, Lui I, Hui WM, Ng MMT, Lam SK. A study on the correlation of duodenal-ulcer healing with Campylobacter-like organisms. J Gastroenterol Hepatol 1986;1:69.

209. Lam SK, Hui WM, Lan WY, et al. Sucralfate overcomes adverse effect of smoking on duodenal ulcer healing and prolongs subsequent remission. Gastroenterology 1987;92:1193.

210. Kang JY, Piper DW. Cimetidine and colloidal bismuth in treatment of chronic duodenal ulcer. Comparison of initial healing and recurrence after healing. Digestion 1982;23:73.

211. Hamilton I, O'Connor HJ, Wook NC, Bradbury I, Axon ATR. Healing and recurrence of duodenal ulcer after treatment with tripotassium dicitrato bismuthate (TDB) tablets or cimetidine. Gut 1986;27:106.

212. Martin DF, Hollanders D, May SJ, Ravenscroft MM, Tweedle DEF, Miller JP. Difference in relapse rates of duodenal ulcer after healing with cimetidine or tripotassium dicitrato bismuthate. Lancet 1981;1:7.

213. Bianchi Porro G, Lazzaroni M, Petrillo M, De Nicola C. Letter: Relapse rates in duodenal ulcer patients formerly treated with bismuth subcitrate or maintained with cimetidine. Lancet 1984;2:698.

214. Wagstaff AJ, Benfield P, Monk JP. Colloidal bismuth subcitrate: A review of its pharmacodynamic and pharmacokinetic properties, and its therapeutic use in peptic ulcer disease. Drugs 1988;36:132.

215. Lambert JR, Borromeo M, Korman MG, Hansky J, Eaves ER. Effect of colloidal bismuth (De-Nol) on healing and relapse of duodenal ulcers—Role of Campylobacter pyloridis (abstr). Gastroenterology 1987;92:1489.

216. Goodwin CS, Marshall BJ, Blincow ED, et al. Prevention of mitroimidazole resistance in Campylobacter pylori by coadministration of colloidal bismuth subcitrate: Clinical and in vitro studies. J Clin Pathol 1988;41:207.

217. Tovey FI, Husband EM, Yiu YC, et al. Comparison of relapse rates and of mucosal abnormalities after healing of duodenal ulceration after one year's maintenance with cimetidine or sucralfate: A light and electron microscopy study. Gut 1989;30:586.

218. Zhi-Tian Z, Zheng-ying W, Ya-Xian C, et al. Letter: Double-blind short-term trial of furazolidone in peptic ulcer. Lancet 1985;1:1048.

219. Borody T, Hennessy W, Daskalopoulos G, Carrick J, Hazell S. Double blind trial of De-Nol in non-ulcer dyspepsia associated with Campylobacter pyloridis gastritis (abstr). Gastroenterology 1987;92:1324.

220. Loffeld RJLF, Potters VJP, Stobberingh E, et al. Campylobacter associated gastritis in patients with non-ulcer dyspepsia: A double blind placebo controlled trial with colloidal bismuth subcitrate. Gut 1989;30:1206.

221. Kurata JH. Ulcer epidemiology: An overview and proposed research framework. Gastroenterology 1989;96:569.

222. Von Haunalter G, Chandler VV. Cost of ulcer disease in the United States. Stanford, CA: Stanford Research Institute Project 5894, 1977.

223. Paringer L, Berk A. Costs of illnesses and disease fiscal year 1975. Report No. 2, Contract No. 1-0D-5-2121. Washington, DC: Public Services Laboratory, Georgetown University, 1977.

223a. Smith-Kline Beecham Internal Report, 1989:32.

224. Kurata JH, Honda GD, Frankl H. The incidence of duodenal and gastric ulcers in a large health maintenance organization. Am J Public Health 1985;75:625.

225. Langman MJS. Peptic ulcer. In: The epidemiology of chronic digestive disease. Chicago: Year Book Medical Publishers, 1979:9.

226. Sonnenberg A, Sengupta A, Bauerfeind P. Epidemiology of peptic ulcer disease. In: Rees WDW, ed. Advances in peptic ulcer pathogenesis. Lancaster, PA: MTP Press, 1988:1.

227. Monson RR, MacMahon B: Peptic ulcer in Massachusetts physicians. N Engl J Med 1969;281:11.

228. Kurata JH, Haile BM. Epidemiology of peptic ulcer disease. Clin Gastroenterol 1984;13:289.

229. Kaneko E, Ooi S, Ito G, Honda N. Natural history of duodenal ulcer detected by the gastric mass surveys in men over 40 years of age. Scand J Gastroenterol 1989;24:165.

230. Kurata JH. Ulcer epidemiology: An overview and proposed research framework. Gastroenterology 1989;96:569.

231. Jenning D. Perforated peptic ulcer. Changes in age-incidence and sex-distribution during the last 150 years (parts 1 and 2). Lancet 1940;i:395, 444.

232. Coggon D, Lambert P, Langman MJS. Twenty years of hospital admissions for peptic ulcer in England and Wales. Lancet 1981;1302.

233. Susser M. Period effects, generation effects and age effects in peptic ulcer mortality. J Chronic Dis 1982;35:29.

234. Sonnenberg A, Sengupta A, Bauerfeind P. Epidemiology of peptic ulcer disease. In: Rees WDW, ed. Advances in peptic ulcer pathogenesis. Lancaster, PA: MTP Press, 1988:1.

235. Friedman GD, Siegelaub AB, Seltzer CC. Cigarettes, alcohol, coffee and peptic ulcer. N Engl J Med 1974;290:469.

236. Tovey F. Duodenal ulcer in black populations in Africa south of the Sahara. Gut 1975;16:564.

237. Hollander D, Tarnawski A. Dietary essential fatty acids and the decline in peptic ulcer disease—A hypothesis. Gut 1986;27:239.

238. Harrison AB, Elashoff JD, Grossman MI. Peptic ulcer disease. In: Smoking and health, report of the Surgeon General. Washington, DC: US Public Health Service, Office on Smoking and Health, DHEW Publication No. 79-50066, 1979;9.

239. Kurata JH, Haile BM. Epidemiology of peptic ulcer disease. Clin Gastroenterol 1984;13:289.

240. Kurata JH, Elashoff JD, Haile BM, Honda GD. A reappraisal of time trends in ulcer disease and factors related to changes in ulcer hospitalization and mortality rates. Am J Public Health 1983;73:1066.

241. Sonnenberg A. Changes in physician visits for gastric and duodenal ulcer in the United States during 1958-1984 as shown by National Disease and Therapeutic Index (NDTI). Dig Dis Sci 1987;32:1.

242. Langman MJ. Trends in ulcer frequency. Postgrad Med J 1988;64(Suppl 1):37.

243. Tilvis RS, Vuoristo M, Varis K. Changed profile of peptic ulcer disease in hospital patients during 1969-1984 in Finland. Scand J Gastroenterol 1987;22:1238.

244. Sonnenberg A, Fritsch A. Changing mortality of peptic ulcer disease in Germany. Gastroenterology 1983;84:1553.

245. Walt R, Katchinski B, Logan R, et al. Occasional survey: Rising frequency of ulcer perforation in elderly people in the United Kingdom. Lancet 1986;1:489.

246. Jolobe OMP, Montgomery RD. Changing clinical pattern of gastric ulcer: Are anti-inflammatory drugs involved? Digestion 1984;29:164.

247. Christensen A, Bousfield R, Christiansen J. Incidence of perforated and bleeding peptic ulcers before and after the introduction of H_2-receptor antagonists. Ann Surg 1988;207:4.

248. Rimoin DL, Rotter JI. Genetic factors in peptic ulcer disease: An update. In: Peptic ulcer disease: An update. New York: BMI Information Publications, 1979:165.

249. McConnell RB. Peptic ulcer: Early genetic evidence—Families, twins, and markers. In: Rotter JI, Samloff IM, Rimoin DL, eds. The genetics and heterogeneity of common gastrointestinal disorders. New York: Academic Press, 1980:31.

250. Doll R, Kellock TD. The separate inheritance of gastric and duodenal ulcers. Ann Eugen 1951;16:231.

251. Aird I, Bewtall HH, Mehigan JA, Roberts JAP. The blood groups in relation to peptic ulceration and carcinoma of colon, rectum, breast and bronchus. Br Med J 1954;ii:315.

252. Clarke CA, Edwards JW, Haddock DRW, et al. A B O blood groups and secretor character in duodenal ulcer. Br Med J 1956;ii:725.

253. Rotter JI, Sones JQ, Samloff IM, Richardson CT, Gursky JM, et al. Duodenal ulcer disease associated with elevated serum pepsinogen I. An inherited autosomal dominant disorder. N Engl J Med 1979;300(63):63.

254. Rotter JI. Peptic ulcer. In: Emery AEH, Rimoin DL, eds. The principles and practice of medical genetics. New York: Churchill Livingstone, 1983:863.

255. Rimoin DL, Rotter JI. Genetic factors in peptic ulcer disease: An update. New York: BMI Publications, 1979:165.

256. Rotter JI, Rimoin DL. Peptic ulcer disease—A heterogeneous group of disorders? Gastroenterology 1977;73:604.

257. Rotter JI, Samloff IM, Rimoin DL. Genetics and heterogeneity of common gastrointestinal disorders. New York: Academic Press, 1980:111.

258. Ammann RW, Vetter D, Deyhle P, Tschen H, et al. Gastrointestinal involvement in systemic mastocytosis. Gut 1976;17:107.

259. Fich A, Goldin E, Zimmerman J, Rachmilewitz D. Calendary variations in the frequency of endoscopically diagnosed duodenal ulcer in Israel. J Clin Gastroenterol 1988;10:380.

260. Kurata JH, Haile BM. Epidemiology of peptic ulcer disease. Clin Gastroenterol 1984;13:289.

261. Pulvertaft CN. Peptic ulcer in town and country. Br J Prev Soc Med 1959;13:131.

262. Piper DW, Sasiry R, McIntosh J, et al. Smoking, alcohol, analgesics, and chronic duodenal ulcer. Scand J Gastroenterol 1984;19:1015.

263. Sonnenberg A, Muller-Lissner SA, Vogel E, et al. Predictors of duodenal ulcer healing and relapse. Gastroenterology 1981;81:1061.

264. Doll R, Jones FA, Pygott F. Effect of smoking on the production and maintenance of gastric and duodenal ulcers. Lancet 1958;657.

265. Rogot E, Murray JL. Smoking and causes of death among US veterans: 16 years of observation. Public Health Rep 1980;95:213.

266. Collen MJ, Stanczak VJ, Ciarleglio CA. Refractory duodenal ulcers (non-healing duodenal ulcers with standard doses of antisecretory medication). Dig Dis Sci 1989;34:233.

267. Reynolds JC. Famotidine therapy for active duodenal ulcers. A multivariate analysis of factors affecting early healing. Ann Intern Med 1989;111:7.

268. Rosch W. A comparison of roxatidine acetate 150 mg once daily

and 75 mg twice daily in ulcer healing. Drugs 1988;35(Suppl 3): 96.

269. Paffenbarger RS, Wing AL, Hyde RT. Chronic disease in former college students XIII. Early precursors of peptic ulcer. Am J Epidemiol 1974;100:307.

270. Chiverton SG, Hunt RH. Smoking and duodenal ulcer disease. J Clin Gastroenterol 1989;11(Suppl 1):529.

271. Stemmerman GN, Marcus EB, Buist AS, et al. Relative impact of smoking and reduced pulmonary function on peptic ulcer risk. Gastroenterology 1989;96:1419.

272. Farah D, Sturrock RD, Russell RI. Peptic ulcer in rheumatoid arthritis. Ann Rheum Dis 1988;47:478.

273. Bauerfeind P, Cilluffo T, Fimmel CJ, et al. Does smoking interfere with the effect of histamine H_2-receptor antagonists on intragastric acidity in man? Gut 1987;28:549.

274. Corinaldesi R, Stanghellini V, Paparo GF, et al. Gastric acid secretion and gastric emptying of liquids in 99 male duodenal ulcer patients. Dig Dis Sci 1989;34:251.

275. Akinori Y, Muto H. Increased parietal cell responsiveness to tetragastrin in patients with recurrent duodenal ulcer. Dig Dis Sci 1988;33:1459.

276. Malesci A, Basilico M, Bersani M, et al. Serum pepsinogen I elevation in cigarette smokers. Scand J Gastroenterol 1988;23:602.

277. Graham DY. Prevention of gastroduodenal injury induced by chronic nonsteroidal anti-inflammatory drug therapy. Gastroenterology 1989;96:675.

278. Hazleman BL. Incidence of gastropathy in destructive arthropathies. Scand J Rheumatol Suppl 1989;78:1.

279. Prichard PJ, Hawkey CJ. Aspirin and gastroduodenal injury. Dig Dis 1989;7:28.

280. Fries J, Miller S, Spitz P. Toward an epidemiology and gastropathy associated with nonsteroidal antiinflammatory drug use. Gastroenterology 1989;96:647.

281. Baum C, Kennedy DL, Forbes MD. Utilization of anti-inflammatory drugs. Arthritis Rheum 1984;28:686.

282. FDC reports. November 29, 1987:8.

283. Pincus T, Callahan LF. Taking mortality in rheumatoid arthritis seriously—Predictive markers, socioeconomic status and comorbidity. J Rheumatol 1986;14:841.

284. Armstrong CP, Blower AL. Nonsteroidal anti-inflammatory drugs and life threatening complications of peptic ulceration. Gut 1987;28:527.

285. Lanza FL, Nelson RS, Rack MF. A controlled endoscopic study comparing the toxic effects of sulindac, naproxen, aspirin, and placebo on the gastric mucosa of healthy volunteers. J Clin Pharmacol 1984;24:89.

286. Langman MJS. Drug-induced mucosal damage. In: Rees WDW, ed. Advances in peptic ulcer pathogenesis. Lancaster, PA: MTP Press, 1988:81.

287. Somerville KW, Faulkner G, Langman MJS. Nonsteroidal anti-inflammatory drugs and bleeding peptic ulcer. Lancet 1986;462.

288. McCarthy DM. Nonsteroidal anti-inflammatory drug-induced ulcers: Management by traditional therapies. Gastroenterology 1989;96:662.

289. Carson JL, Strom BL, Soper KA, et al. The association of nonsteroidal anti-inflammatory drugs with upper gastrointestinal tract bleeding. Arch Intern Med 1987;147:85.

290. Graham DY, Smith JL. Aspirin and the stomach. Ann Intern Med 1986;104:390.

291. Caruso I, Bianchi-Porro G. Gastroscopic evaluation of anti-inflammatory agents. Br Med J 1980;1:75.

292. Whittle BJR. Mechanisms underlying gastric mucosal damage induced by indomethacin and bile salts and the actions of prostaglandins. Br J Pharmacol 1977;60:455.

293. Konturek SJ, Obtulowicz W, Sito E, et al. Distribution of prostaglandins in gastric and duodenal mucosa of healthy subjects and duodenal ulcer patients: Effects of aspirin and paracetamol. Gut 1981;22:283.

294. Flemström G, Turnberg LA. Gastroduodenal defense mechanisms. Clin Gastroenterol 1984;13:327.

295. Hogan DL, Isenberg JI. Gastroduodenal bicarbonate production. Adv Intern Med 1988;33:385.

296. Rainsford KD. Mechanisms of gastrointestinal ulceration by non-steroidal anti-inflammatory/analgesic drugs. In: Rainsford KD, Velo GP, eds. Advances in inflammation research side effects of anti-inflammatory/analgesic drugs, Vol 6. New York: Raven Press, 1984.

297. Hawkey CJ, Rampton DS. Prostaglandins and gastrointestinal mucosa: Are they important in its function, disease or treatment? Gastroenterology 1985;89:1162.

298. Silen W, Ito S. Mechanisms for rapid re-epithelialization of the gastric mucosal surface. Annu Rev Physiol 1985;47:217.

299. Mitchell DM, Spitz PW, Young DY, et al. Survival, prognosis, and causes of death in rheumatoid arthritis. Arthritis Rheum 1986;29:706.

300. Vandenbroucke JP, Hazevoet HM, Cats A. Survival and cause of death in rheumatoid arthritis: A 25-yr prospective follow-up. J Rheumatol 1984;11:158.

301. Conn HO, Blitzer BL. Nonassociation of adrenocorticosteroid therapy and peptic ulcer. N Engl J Med 1976;294:433.

302. Messer J, Reitman D, Sacks H, Smith H Jr, et al. Association of adrenocorticosteroid therapy and peptic ulcer disease. N Engl J Med 1983;309:21.

303. Spiro H. Is the steroid ulcer a myth? N Engl J Med 1983;309:45.

304. Robert A. Cytoprotection by prostaglandins. Gastroenterology 1979;77:761.

305. Tarnawski A, Brzozowski T, Sarfeh IJ, et al. Prostaglandin protection of human isolated gastric glands against indomethacin and ethanol injury. Evidence for direct cellular action of prostaglandin. J Clin Invest 1988;81:1081.

306. Stern AI, Hogan DL, Isenberg JI. A new method for quantitation of ion fluxes across the *in-vivo* human gastric mucosa: Effect of aspirin, acetaminophen, ethanol and hyperosmolar solutions. Gastroenterology 1984;86:60.

307. Friedman GD, Siegelaub AB, Seltzer CC. Cigarettes, alcohol, coffee and peptic ulcer. N Engl J Med 1974;290:469.

308. Bonnevie O. Causes of death in duodenal and gastric ulcer. Gastroenterology 1977;73:1000.

309. Lenz HJ, Ferrari-Taylor J, Isenberg JI. Wine and five percent ethanol are potent stimulants of gastric acid secretion in man. Gastroenterology 1983;83:1082.

310. McArthur K, Hogan D, Isenberg JI. Relative stimulatory effects of commonly ingested beverages on gastric acid secretion in man. Gastroenterology 1982;83:199.

311. Peterson WL, Barnett C, Walsh JH. Effect of intragastric infusions of ethanol and wine on serum gastrin concentration and gastric acid secretion. Gastroenterology 1986;91:1390.

312. Malhotra SL. A comparison of unrefined wheat and rice diets in the management of duodenal ulcer. Postgrad Med J 1978;54:6.

313. Ryding A, Berstad A, Aadland E, et al. Prophylactic effect of dietary fibre in duodenal ulcer disease. Lancet 1982;2:736.

314. Cohen S, Booth GH Jr. Gastric acid secretion and lower-esophageal-sphincter pressure in response to coffee and caffeine. N Engl J Med 1975;293:897.

315. Donaldson RM Jr. Factors complicating observed associations between peptic ulcer and other diseases. Gastroenterology 1975;68:1608.

316. Langman MJS, Cooke AR. Gastric and duodenal ulcer and their associated diseases. Lancet 1976;680.

317. Bonnevie O. Causes of death in duodenal and gastric ulcer. Gastroenterology 1977;73:1000.

318. Stemmerman GN, Marcus EB, Buist AS, et al. Relative impact of smoking and reduced pulmonary function on peptic ulcer risk. Gastroenterology 1989;96:1419.

319. Kellow JE, Tao Z, Piper DW. Ventilatory function in patients with gastric and duodenal ulcer. Gastroenterology 1986;91:590.

320. Stemmerman GN, Marcus EB, Buist AS, et al. Relative impact of smoking and reduced pulmonary function on peptic ulcer risk. Gastroenterology 1989;96:1419.

321. Rotter JI. Peptic ulcer. In: Emery AEH, Rimoin DL, eds. The principles and practice of medical genetics. New York: Churchill Livingstone, 1983:863.

322. Kirk AP, Dooley JS, Hunt RH. Peptic ulceration in patients with chronic liver disease. Dig Dis Sci 1980;25:10.

323. Phillips MM, Ramsby GR, Conn HO. Portacaval anastomosis and peptic ulcer: A nonassociation. Gastroenterology 1975;68:121.

324. Lenz HJ, Hogan DL, Isenberg JI. The intestinal phase of gastric

acid secretion in humans with and without portacaval shunt. Gastroenterology 1985;89:791.

325. Jones RH, Rudge CJ, Bewick M, et al. Cimetidine: Prophylaxis against upper gastrointestinal hemorrhage after renal transplantation. Br Med J 1978;398.

326. Gilmore PR. Angiodysplasia of the upper gastrointestinal tract. Gastroenterology 1988;10(4):396.

327. Kang JY, Wu AYT, Sutherland IH, et al. Prevalence of peptic ulcer in patients undergoing maintenance hemodialysis. Dig Dis Sci 1988;33(7):774.

328. Eisenbarth GS, Lebovitz HE. Minireview. Immunogenetics of the polyglandular failure syndrome. Life Sci 1978;22:1675.

329. Langman MJS, Cooke AR. Gastric and duodenal ulcer and their associated diseases. Lancet 1976;680.

330. Tache Y. Central nervous system regulation of gastric acid secretion. In: Johnson LR, ed. Physiology of the gastrointestinal tract, ed 2. New York: Raven Press, 1987;911.

331. Tache Y, Brown M, Collu R. Central nervous system actions of bombesin-like peptides. In: Collu R, ed. Brain neurotransmitters and hormones. New York: Raven Press, 1982;183.

332. Silen W. Experimental models of gastric ulceration and injury. Am J Physiol 1988;255:395.

333. Alexander F. Psychosomatic medicine. New York: Norton, 1950.

334. Weiner H, Thaler M, Reiser MF, et al. A. Etiology of duodenal ulcer. I. Relation of specific psychological characteristics to rate of gastric secretion (serum pepsinogen). Psychosom Med 1957;19:1.

335. Feldman M, Walker P, Green JL, et al. Life events stress and psychosocial factors in men with peptic ulcer disease. A multidimensional case-controlled study. Gastroenterology 1986;91:1370.

336. Weisman AD. A study of the psychodynamics of duodenal ulcer exacerbations. With special reference to treatment and the problem of "specificity." Psychosom Med 1956;18:2.

337. Feldman M, Walker P, Green JL, et al. Life events stress and psychosocial factors in men with peptic ulcer disease. A multidimensional case-controlled study. Gastroenterology 1986;91:1370.

338. Talley NJ, Ellard K, Jones M, et al. Suppression of emotions in essential dyspepsia and chronic duodenal ulcer. A case-control study. Scand J Gastroenterol 1988;23:337.

339. Adami HO, Bergstrom R, Nyren O, et al. Is duodenal ulcer really a psychosomatic disease? A population-based case-control study. Scand J Gastroenterol 1987;22:889.

340. Magnus HA. The pathology of peptic ulceration. Postgrad Med J 1954;30:131.

341. Kekki M, Sipponen P, Siurala M. Progression of antral and body gastritis in active and healed duodenal ulcer and duodenitis. Scand J Gastroenterol 1984;19:382.

342. Meikle DD, Taylor KB, Truelove SC, Whitehead R. Gastritis, duodenitis, and circulating levels of gastrin in duodenal ulcer before and after vagotomy. Gut 1976;17:719.

343. Greenlaw R, Sheahan DG, DeLuca V, Miller D, Myerson D, Myerson P. Gastroduodenitis. A broader concept of peptic ulcer disease. Dig Dis Sci 1980;25:660.

344. Hui WM, Lam SK, Ho J, Ng MM, Lui I, Lai CL, Lok AS, Lau WY, Poon GP, Choi S, Choi TK. Chronic antral gastritis in duodenal ulcer. Natural history and treatment with prostaglandin E₂. Gastroenterology 1986;91:1095.

345. Cheli R, Giacosa A. Duodenal ulcer and chronic gastritis. Endoscopy 1986;18:125.

346. Oi M, Oshida K, Sugimura S. The location of gastric ulcer. Gastroenterology 1959;36:45.

347. Gear MWL, Truelove SC, Whitehead R. Gastric ulcer and gastritis. Gut 1971;12:639.

348. Aukee S. Gastritis and acid secretion in patients with gastric ulcers and duodenal ulcers. Scand J Gastroenterol 1972;7:567.

349. Zaterka S, Vieira FE, Neves DP, daSilva EP, Carneiro-Leao G, Bettarello A. Chronic gastritis and peptic ulcer. Acta Hepatogastroenterol 1977;24:381.

350. Maaroos HI, Salupere V, Uibo R, Kekki M, Sipponen P. Seven-year follow-up study of chronic gastritis in gastric ulcer patients. Scand J Gastroenterol 1985;20:198.

351. Marks IN, Shay H. Observations on the pathogenesis of gastric ulcer. Lancet 1959;1:1107.

352. Capper WM. Factors in the pathogenesis of gastric ulcer. Ann R Coll Surg Engl 1967;40:21.

353. Tatsuta M, Iishi H, Okunda S. Location of peptic ulcers in relation to antral and fundal gastritis by chromoendoscopic follow-up examinations. Dig Dis Sci 1986;31:7.

354. Moore SC, Malagelada JR, Shorter RG, Zinsmeister AR. Interrelationships among gastric mucosal morphology, secretion, and motility in peptic ulcer disease. Dig Dis Sci 1986;31:673.

355. MacDonald WC. Correlation of mucosal histology and aspirin intake in chronic gastric ulcer. Gastroenterology 1973;65:381.

356. Goldman H, Antonioli DA. Mucosal biopsy of the esophagus, stomach, and proximal duodenum. Hum Pathol 1982;13:423.

357. Schmitz-Moormann P, Pittner PM, Reichmann L, Massarat S. Quantitative histology study of duodenitis in biopsies. Pathol Res Pract 1984;178:499.

358. Schmitz-Moormann P, Schmidt-Slordahi R, Peter JH, Massarat S. Morphometric studies of normal and inflamed duodenal mucosa. Pathol Res Pract 1980;167:313.

359. Gelfand DW, Dale WJ, Ott DJ, et al. Duodenitis: Endoscopic-radiologic correlation in 272 patients. Radiology 1985;157:577.

360. Shousha S, Spiller RC, Parkins RA. The endoscopically abnormal duodenum in patients with dyspepsia. Biopsy findings in 60 cases. Histopathology 1983;7:23.

361. Hasan M, Sircus W, Ferguson A. Duodenal mucosal architecture in non-specific and ulcer associated duodenitis. Gut 1981;22:637.

362. Jaffe SN, Lee FD, Blumgart LH. Duodenitis. Clin Gastroenterol 1978;7:635.

363. Whitehead R, Roca M, Meikle DD, et al. The histological classification of duodenitis in fibreoptic biopsy specimens. Digestion 1975;13:129.

364. Kreuning J, Bosman FT, Kuiper G, Wal AM, Lindeman J. Gastric and duodenal mucosa in "healthy" individuals. J Clin Pathol 1978;31:69.

365. Paoluzi P, Pallone F, Zaccardelli E, Ripoli F, Marcheggiano A, Carratu R. Outcome of ulcer-associated duodenitis after short-term medical treatment. Dig Dis Sci 1985;30:624.

366. Fullman H, Van Deventer G, Schneidman D, Walsh J, Elashoff J, Weinstein W. "Healed" duodenal ulcers are histologically ill. Gastroenterology 1985;88:1390.

367. Cheli R. Duodenitis and duodenal ulcer. Digestion 1968;1:175.

368. Thomson WO, Robertson AG, Imrie CW, et al. Is duodenitis a dyspeptic myth? Lancet 1977;1:119.

369. Isenberg JI, Walsh JH, Grossman MI. Zollinger-Ellison syndrome. Gastroenterology 1973;65:140.

370. Lam SK. Pathogenesis and pathophysiology of duodenal ulcer. Clin Gastroenterol 1984;13:447.

371. Holt KM, Isenberg JI. Peptic ulcer disease: Physiology and pathophysiology. Hosp Pract 1985;20:89.

372. Soll AH. Duodenal ulcer and drug therapy. In: Sleisenger MH, Fordtran JS, eds. Gastrointestinal disease. Pathophysiology, diagnosis, management. Philadelphia: WB Saunders, 1989:814.

373. Hebbel R. Chronic gastritis; its relation to gastric and duodenal ulcer and to gastric carcinoma. Am J Pathol 1943;19:43.

374. Cox AJ. Stomach size and its relation to chronic peptic ulcer. Arch Pathol 1952;54:407.

375. Cheng FCY, Lam SK, Ong GB. Maximal acid output to graded doses of pentagastrin and its relation to parietal cell mass in Chinese patients with duodenal ulcer. Gut 1977;18:827.

376. Moore JG, Halberg F. Circadian rhythm of gastric acid secretion in men with active duodenal ulcer. Dig Dis Sci 1986;31:1185.

377. Moore JG, Wolfe M. Circadian plasma gastrin patterns in feeding and fasting man. Digestion 1974;11:226.

378. Winkelstein A. One hundred and sixty-nine studies in gastric secretion during the night. Am J Dig Dis 1935;778.

379. Levin E, Kirsner JB, Palmer WL, et al. A comparison of the nocturnal gastric secretion in patients with duodenal ulcer and in normal individuals. Gastroenterology 1948;10:952.

380. Levin E, Kirsner JB, Palmer WL. Twelve-hour nocturnal gastric secretion in uncomplicated duodenal ulcer patients: Before and after healing. Proceedings of the Society of Experimental Biology 1948;69:153.

381. Dragstedt LR. Editorial: Gastric secretion tests. Gastroenterology 1967;52:587.

382. Feldman M, Richardson CT, Fordtran JS. Effect of sham feeding on gastric acid secretion in healthy subjects and duodenal ulcer patients. Evidence for increased basal vagal tone in some ulcer patients. Gastroenterology 1980;79:796.

383. Kirkpatrick PM Jr, Hirschowitz BI. Duodenal ulcer with unexplained marked basal gastric acid hypersecretion. Gastroenterology 1980;79:4.

384. Feldman M, Richardson CT, Fordtran JS. Effect of sham feeding on gastric acid secretion in healthy subjects and duodenal ulcer patients: Evidence for increased basal vagal tone in some ulcer patients. Gastroenterology 1980;79:796.

385. Soll AH. Duodenal ulcer and drug therapy. In: Sleisenger MH, Fordtran JS, eds. Gastrointestinal disease. Pathophysiology, diagnosis, management. Philadelphia: WB Saunders, 1989:814.

386. Isenberg JI. Gastric secretory testing. In: Sleisenger MH, Fordtran JS, eds. Gastrointestinal disease, ed 2. Philadelphia: WB Saunders, 1978:714.

387. Brooks FP. The pathophysiology of peptic ulcer: An overview. In: Brooks FP, Cohen S, Soloway RD, eds. Peptic ulcer disease. New York: Churchill Livingstone, 1985:45.

388. Blair AJ III, Feldman M, Barnett C, et al. Detailed comparison of basal and food-stimulated gastric acid secretion rates and serum gastrin concentrations in duodenal ulcer patients and normal subjects. J Clin Invest 1987;79:582.

389. Malagelada JR, Longstreth GF, Deering TB, et al. Gastric secretion and emptying after ordinary meals in duodenal ulcer. Gastroenterology 1977;73:989.

390. Isenberg JI, Grossman MI, Maxwell V, et al. Increased sensitivity to stimulation of acid secretion by pentagastrin in duodenal ulcer. J Clin Invest 1975;55:330.

391. Lam SK, Isenberg JI, Grossman MI, et al. Gastric acid secretion is abnormally sensitive to endogenous gastrin released after peptone test meals in duodenal ulcer patients. J Clin Invest 1980;65:555.

392. Lam SK, Koo J, Sircus W. Early and late onset duodenal ulcers in Chinese and Scots. Scand J Gastroenterol 1983;18:651.

393. Lam SK, Isenberg JI, Grossman MI, et al. Gastric acid secretion is abnormally sensitive to endogenous gastrin released after peptone test meals in duodenal ulcer patients. J Clin Invest 1980;65:555.

394. Calam J, Dockray GJ, Walker R, et al. Molecular forms of gastrin in peptic ulcer: Comparison of serum and tissue concentrations of G17 and G34 forms in gastric and duodenal ulcer subjects. Eur J Clin Invest 1980;20:241.

395. Walsh JH. Gastrointestinal peptide hormones. In: Sleisenger MH, Fordtran JS, eds. Gastrointestinal disease, ed 4. Philadelphia: WB Saunders, 1989:78.

396. Taylor IL, Dockray GJ, Calam J, et al. Big and little gastrin responses to food in normal and ulcer subjects. Gut 1979;20:957.

397. Creutzfeldt AR, Ebert R, Becker HD, et al. Serum gastric inhibitory polypeptide (GIP) in duodenal ulcer disease: Relationship to glucose tolerance, insulin, and gastric release. Scand J Gastroenterol 1978;13:41.

398. Taylor IL, Calam J, Rotter JI, et al. Family studies of hypergastrinemic, hyperpepsinogenemic I duodenal ulcer. Ann Intern Med 1981;95:421.

399. Gross RA, Hogan D, Isenberg JI. The effect of fat on meal-stimulated duodenal acid load, duodenal pepsin load, and serum gastrin in duodenal ulcer and normal subjects. Gastroenterology 1978;75:357.

400. Kihl B, Olbe L. Fat inhibition of gastric acid secretion in duodenal ulcer patients before and after proximal gastric vagotomy. Gut 1980;21:1056.

401. Isenberg JI. Conventional therapy for duodenal ulcer in North America. In: Beck IT, ed. North American Symposium on Carbenoxolone, Montreal. Excerpta Medica 1975:123.

402. Dalton MD, Eisenstein AM, Walsh JH, et al. Effect of secretin on gastric function in normal subjects and in patients with duodenal ulcer. Gastroenterology 1976;71:24.

403. Hurst AF. New views on the pathology, diagnosis and treatment of gastric and duodenal ulcer. Br Med J 1920;1:559.

404. Shay H. The pathologic physiology of gastric and duodenal ulcer. Bull N Y Acad Med 1944;20:264.

405. Brömster D. Gastric emptying rate in gastric and duodenal ulceration. Scand J Gastroenterol 1969;4:193.

406. Lam SK, Isenberg JI, Grossman MI, et al. Rapid gastric emptying in duodenal ulcer patients. Dig Dis Sci 1982;27:598.

407. Williams NS, Elashoff J, Meyer JH. Gastric emptying of liquids in normal subjects and patients with healed duodenal ulcer disease. Dig Dis Sci 1986;31(9):943.

408. Rotter JI, Rubin R, Meyer JH, et al. Rapid gastric emptying—An inherited pathophysiologic defect in duodenal ulcer? (abstr) Gastroenterology 1979;76:1229.

409. Rune SJ. Diagnostic evaluation: Gastric acid secretion and pH. Scand J Gastroenterol 1988;23(Suppl 155):37.

410. Archambault AP, Rovelstad RA, Carlson HC. In situ pH of duodenal bulb contents in normal and duodenal subjects. Gastroenterology 1967;52:940.

411. Atkinson M, Henley KS. Levels of intragastric and intraduodenal acidity. Clin Sci 1955;14:1.

412. Quigley EMM, Turnberg LA. pH of the microclimate lining human gastric and duodenal mucosa in-vivo. Gastroenterology 1987;92:1876.

413. Silen W, Ito S. Mechanism for rapid re-epithelialization of the gastric mucosal surface. Annu Rev Physiol 1985;47:217.

414. Garner A. Enhancing mucosal defense and repair mechanisms. In: Rees WDS, ed. Advances in peptic ulcer pathogenesis. Lancaster, PA: MTP Press, 1988:225.

415. Allen A, Hutton DA, Leonard AJ, et al. The role of mucus in the protection of the gastroduodenal mucosa. Scand J Gastroenterol 1986;21(Suppl 125):71.

416. Snary D, Allen A, Pain RH. Structural studies on gastric mucoproteins. Lowering of molecular weight after reduction with 2-mercaptoethanol. Biochem Biophys Res Commun 1970;40:844.

417. Scawen M, Allen A. The action of proteolytic enzymes on the glycoprotein from pig gastric mucus. Biochem J 1977;163:363.

418. Sellers LA, Allen A. Mucus and gastroduodenal mucosal protection. In: Rees WDW, ed. Advances in peptic ulcer pathogenesis. Lancaster, PA: MTP Press, 1988:121.

419. Roberts SH, Heffermann C, Douglas AP. The sialic acid and carbohydrate content and the synthesis of glycoprotein from radioactive precursors by tissues of the normal and diseased upper intestinal tract. Clin Chim Acta 1975;63;121.

420. Flemström G. Gastric and duodenal mucosal bicarbonate secretion. In: Johnson LR, Christensen J, Jackson MJ, Jacobson ED, Walsh JH, eds. Physiology of the gastrointestinal tract, ed 2. New York: Raven Press, 1987:1011.

421. Kivilaakso E, Flemström G. Surface pH gradient in gastroduodenal mucosa. Scand J Gastroenterol 1984;19(Suppl 105):50.

422. Isenberg JI, Selling JA, Hogan DL, et al. Impaired proximal duodenal mucosal bicarbonate secretion in duodenal ulcer patients. N Engl J Med 1987;316:374.

423. Basuk PM, Hogan DL, Marin M, et al. Diminished duodenal mucosal bicarbonate secretion in duodenal ulcer is independent of mucosal histologic abnormalities: A prospective study. Gastroenterology 1989;95:A33.

424. Wallace JL. Gastric resistance to acid: Is the "mucus-bicarbonate barrier" functionally redundant? Am J Physiol (Gastrointest Liver Physiol) 1989;256:G31.

425. Johnson HD. Gastric ulcer: Classification, blood group characteristics, secretion pattern and pathogenesis. Ann Surg 1965;162:996.

426. Leading article. Gastric ulcer and gastritis. Lancet 1966;2:481.

427. Marks IN, Shay H. Observations on the pathogenesis of gastric ulcer. Lancet 1959;1:1107.

428. Richardson CT. Gastric ulcer. In: Gastrointestinal disease. Pathophysiology, diagnosis, management, ed 4, Vol 1. 879.

429. Richardson CT. Gastric Ulcer. In: Sleisenger MH, Fordtran JS, eds. Gastrointestinal disease. Philadelphia, Pa: WB Saunders, 1989:879.

430. Reid J, Taylor TV, Holt S, et al. Benign gastric ulceration in pernicious anemia. Dig Dis Sci 1980;25:148.

431. Fisher R, Cohen S. Physiological characteristics of the human pyloric sphincter. Gastroenterology 1973;64:67.

432. Flint FJ, Grech P. Pyloric regurgitation and gastric ulcer. Gut 1970;11:735.

433. Johnson AG, McDermott SJ. Lysolecithin: A factor in the pathogenesis of gastric ulceration. Gut 1974;15:710.

434. Miller LJ, Malagelada JR, Longstreth GF, et al. Dysfunctions of the stomach with gastric ulceration. Dig Dis Sci 1980;25:857.

435. Garrett JM, Summerskill WHJ, Code CF. Antral motility in patients with gastric ulcer. Am J Dig Dis 1966;11:780.

436. Niemela S, Heikkila J, Lehtola J. Duodenogastric bile reflux in patients with gastric ulcer. Scand J Gastroenterol 1984;19:896.

437. Macherey HJ, Petersen KU. Rapid decrease in electrical conductance of mammalian duodenal mucosa in-vitro. Gastroenterology 1989;97:1448.

438. Stern AI, Hogan DL, Isenberg JI. A new method for quantitation of ion fluxes across the *in-vivo* human gastric mucosa: Effect of aspirin, acetaminophen, ethanol and hyperosmolar solutions. Gastroenterology 1984;86:60.

439. Davenport HW, Warner HA, Code CF. Functional significance of gastric mucosal barrier to sodium. Gastroenterology 1964;47:147.

440. Stern AI, Hogan DL, Isenberg JI. A new method for quantitation of ion fluxes across the *in-vivo* human gastric mucosa: Effect of aspirin, acetaminophen, ethanol and hyperosmolar solutions. Gastroenterology 1984;86:60.

441. Graham DY, Smith JL. Aspirin and the stomach. Ann Intern Med 1986;104:390.

442. Belcon MC, Rooney PJ, Tugwell P. Aspirin and gastrointestinal hemorrhage: A methodologic assessment. J Chronic Dis 1985;38:101.

443. Llewelyn JG, Pritchard MH. Acute gastric hemorrhage and its relationship to the use of anti-inflammatory analgesics (NSAIDs). Ann Rheum Dis 1983;42:228.

444. Trondstad RI, Aadland E, Holler T, et al. Gastroscopic findings after treatment with enteric-coated and plain naproxen tablets in healthy subjects. Scand J Gastroenterol 1985;20:239.

445. Graham DY, Smith JL, Holmes GI, et al. Nonsteroidal anti-inflammatory effect of sulindac sulfoxide and sulfide on gastric mucosa. Clin Pharmacol Ther 1985;38:65.

446. Eliakim R, Ophir M, Rachmilewitz D. Duodenal mucosal injury with nosteroidal anti-inflammatory drugs. J Clin Gastroenterol 1987;9:395.

447. Levy M. Aspirin use in patients with major upper gastrointestinal bleeding and peptic ulcer disease. N Engl J Med 1974;290:1158.

448. Osnes M, Larsen S, Eidsaunet W, et al. Effect of diclofenac and naproxen on gastroduodenal mucosa. Clin Pharmacol Ther 1979;26:399.

449. Kurata JH. Epidemiology of peptic ulcer disease. Pract Gastroenterol 1983;7:13.

450. Langman MJS. Drug-induced mucosal damage. In: Rees WDW, ed. Advances in peptic ulcer pathogenesis. Lancaster, PA: MTP Press, 1988.

451. Larkai EN, Smith JL, Lidsky MD, et al. Gastroduodenal mucosa and dyspeptic symptoms in arthritis patients during chronic nonsteroidal anti-inflammatory drug use. Am J Gastroenterol 1987;82:1153.

452. Graham DY, Smith JL, Dobbs SM. Gastric adaptation occurs with aspirin administration in man. Dig Dis Sci 1983;28:1.

453. Graham DY, Smith JL, Spjut HJ, et al. Gastric adaptation: Studies in humans during continuous aspirin administration. Gastroenterology 1988;95:327.

454. Barlow TE, Bentley FH, Walden DN. Arteries, veins and arteriovenous anastomoses in the human stomach. Surg Gynecol Obstet 1951;93:657.

455. Kamada T, Kawano S, Nobuhiro S, et al. Gastric mucosal blood distribution and its changes in the healing process of gastric ulcer. Gastroenterology 1983;84:1541.

456. Crean GP, Spiegelhalter DJ. Symptoms of peptic ulcer. In: Brooks FP, Cohen S, Soloway RD, eds. Peptic ulcer disease. New York: Churchill Livingstone, 1985:1.

457. Spiro HM. Moynihan's disease? The diagnosis of duodenal ulcer. N Engl J Med 1974;291:567.

458. Ross P, Dutton AM. Computer analysis of symptom complexes in patients having upper gastrointestinal examinations. Am J Dig Dis 1977;17:248.

459. Horrocks JC, De Dombal FT. Clinical presentation of patients with "dyspepsia." Gut 1978;19:19.

460. Soll AH. Duodenal ulcer and drug therapy. In: Sleisenger MH, Fordtran JS, eds. Gastrointestinal disease—Pathophysiology, diagnosis, management. Philadelphia: WB Saunders, 1989:814.

461. DeLuca VA, Winnan GG, Sheahan DG, et al. Is gastroduodenitis part of the spectrum of peptic ulcer disease? J Clin Gastroenterol 1981;3(Suppl 2):17.

462. DeLuca VA, Winnan GG, Sheahan DG, et al. Is gastroduodenitis part of the spectrum of peptic ulcer disease? J Clin Gastroenterol 1981;3(Suppl 2):17.

463. Petersen H, Johannessen T, Kleveland P, Fjosne U, Dybdahl JH, Waldum HL. Do we need to listen to the patient? The predictive value of symptoms. Scand J Gastroenterol 1988;23(Suppl 155):30.

464. Leon-Barua R, Bonilla JJ, Rodriguez C, Gilman RH, Biber M, Watanabe J. Hunger pain: A poor indicator of peptic ulcer in a developing country. J Clin Gastroenterol 1989;11:621.

465. Gibinski K. Step by step towards the natural history of peptic ulcer disease. J Clin Gastroenterol 1983;5:299.

466. Isenberg JI, Peterson WL, Elashoff JD, et al. Healing of benign gastric ulcer with low-dose antacid or cimetidine. A double-blind randomized, placebo-controlled trial. N Engl J Med 1983;308:1319.

467. Greenlaw R, Sheahan DG, DeLuca V, et al. Gastroduodenitis: A broader concept of peptic ulcer disease. Dig Dis Sci 1980;25:660.

468. Cotton PB, Shorvon PJ. Analysis of endoscopy and radiography in the diagnosis, follow-up and treatment of peptic ulcer disease. Clin Gastroenterol 1984;13:383.

469. Black DD. Duodenitis. J Pediatr Gastroenterol 1988;7:353.

470. Whitehead R. Morphological aspects of duodenitis. Scand J Gastroenterol 1981;17(Suppl 79):80.

471. Harrison A, Isenberg JI, Schapira M, Hagie L. Most patients with active symptomatic duodenal ulcers fail to develop ulcer-type pain in response to gastroduodenal acidification. J Clin Gastroenterol 1982;4:105.

472. Joffee SN, Primrose J. Pain provocation test in peptic duodenitis. Gastrointest Endosc 1983;29:282.

473. Kang JY, Yap I, Guan R, Tay HH. Acid perfusion of duodenal ulcer craters and ulcer pain: A controlled double blind study. Gut 1986;27:942.

474. Peterson WL, Sturdevant RAL, Frankl HD, et al. Healing of duodenal ulcer with an antacid regimen. N Engl J Med 1977;297:341.

475. Graham DY. Complications of peptic ulcer disease and indications for surgery. In: Sleisenger MH, Fordtran JS, eds. Gastrointestinal disease—Pathophysiology, diagnosis, management. Philadelphia: WB Saunders, 1989:925.

476. Bartle WR, Gupta AK, Lazor J. Nonsteroidal anti-inflammatory drugs and gastrointestinal bleeding: A case-control study. Arch Intern Med 1986;146:2365.

477. Smart HL, Langman MJS. Late outcome of bleeding gastric ulcers. Gut 1986;27:926.

478. Richardson CT. Gastric ulcer. In: Sleisenger MH, Fordtran JS, eds. Gastrointestinal disease—Pathophysiology, diagnosis, management. Philadelphia: WB Saunders, 1989:879.

479. Cotton PB, Shorvon PJ. Analysis of endoscopy and radiography in the diagnosis, follow-up and treatment of peptic ulcer disease. Clin Gastroenterol 1984;13:383.

480. Laufer I. Assessment of the accuracy of double contrast gastroduodenal radiology. Gastroenterology 1976;71:874.

481. Fraser GM, Earnshaw PM. The double contrast barium meal: A correlation with endoscopy. Clin Radiol 1983;34:121.

482. Rogers IM, Sokhi GS, Moule B, et al. Endoscopy and routine double contrast barium meal in the diagnosis of gastric and duodenal disorders. Lancet 1976.901.

483. Thompson G, Somers S, Stevensons GW. Benign gastric ulcer—A reliable radiologic diagnosis? Am J Radiol 1983;141:331.

484. Sakita T, Oguro Y, Takasu S, et al. Observations on the healing of ulcerations in early gastric cancer. The life cycle of the malignant ulcer. Gastroenterology 1971;60:835.

485. Farini R, Farinati F, Cardin F, et al. Evidence of gastric carcinoma during follow up of apparently benign gastric ulcer. Gut 1983;24:A486.

486. Isenberg JI, Peterson WL, Elashoff JD, et al. Healing of benign gastric ulcer with low-dose antacid or cimetidine. A double-blind randomized, placebo-controlled trial. N Engl J Med 1983;308:1319.

487. Brown P, Salmon PR, Burwood RJ, Knox AJ, Clendinnen BG,

Read AE. The endoscopic, radiological, and surgical findings in chronic duodenal ulceration. Scand J Gastroenterol 1978;13:557.

488. Health and Public Policy Committee, American College of Physicians. Endoscopy in the evaluation of dyspepsia. Ann Intern Med 1985;102:266.

489. Kahn KL, Greenfield S. The efficacy of endoscopy in the evaluation of dyspepsia. J Clin Gastroenterol 1986;8(3):346.

490. Health and Public Policy Committee, American College of Physicians. Endoscopy in the evaluation of dyspepsia. Ann Intern Med 1985;102:266.

491. Peterson WL, Sturdevant RAL, Frankl HD, et al. Healing of duodenal ulcer with an antacid regimen. N Engl J Med 1977;297;341.

492. Wolfe MM, Soll AH. The physiology of gastric acid secretion. N Engl J Med 1988;319:1707.

493. Black JW, Duncan WAM, Durant GJ, Ganellin CR, Parsons ME. Definition and antagonism of histamine H2-receptors. Nature 1972;236:385.

494. Bender W, Brockmeier D. Pharmacokinetic characteristics of roxatidine. J Clin Gastroenterol 1989;11(Suppl 1):S6.

495. Schunack W. What are the differences between the H2-receptor antagonists? Aliment Pharmacol Ther 1987;1:493S.

496. Grant SM, Langtry HD, Brogden RN. Ranitidine—An updated review of its pharmacodynamic and pharmacokinetic properties and therapeutic use in peptic ulcer disease and other allied diseases. Drugs 1989;37:801.

497. Langtry HD, Grant SM, Goa KL. Famotidine—An updated review of its pharmacodynamic and pharmacokinetic properties, and therapeutic use in peptic ulcer disease and other allied diseases. Drugs 1989;38:551.

498. Howard JM, Chremos AN, Collen MJ, et al. Famotidine, a new, potent, long-acting histamine H2-receptor antagonist: Comparison with cimetidine and ranitidine in the treatment of Zollinger–Ellison syndrome. Gastroenterology 1985;88:1026.

499. Aadland E, Berstad A. Inhibition of histamine- and pentagastrin-stimulated gastric secretion by cimetidine in man. In: Cautzfeldt W. Proceedings of an international symposium on histamine H2-receptor antagonists, Gottingen, Germany, November 10–11, 1977. New York: Elsevier Science Publishing (Excerpta Medica), 1978: 47.

500. Richards DA. Comparative pharmacodynamics and pharmacokinetics of cimetidine and ranitidine. J Clin Gastroenterol 1983;5(Suppl 1):81.

501. Konturek SJ, Obtulowicz W, Kwiecien N, et al. Comparison of ranitidine and cimetidine in the inhibition of histamine, sham-feeding, and meal-induced gastric secretion in duodenal ulcer patients. Gut 1980;21:181.

502. Lebert PA, MacLeod SM, Mahon WA, Soldin SJ, Vandenberghe HM. Ranitidine kinetics and dynamics. Clin Pharmacol Ther 1981;30:539.

503. Brater DC, Peters MN, Eshelman FN, Richardson CT. Clinical comparison of cimetidine and ranitidine. Clin Pharmacol Ther 1982;32:484.

504. McCallum RW, Chremos AN, Kuljian B, Tupy-Visich MA, Huber PB. MK-208, a novel histamine H2-receptor inhibitor with prolonged antisecretory effect. Dig Dis Sci 1985;30:1139.

505. Brimblecombe RW. Evolution of the cimetidine dosing schedule. Postgraduate Medicine: Custom Communications, November 1985.

506. Aadland E, Berstad A, Semb LS. Inhibition of pentagastrin-stimulated gastric secretion by cimetidine in healthy subjects. In: Burland WL, Simkins MA, eds. Cimetidine—Proceedings of the Second International Symposium on Histamine H2-Receptor Antagonists. Amsterdam–Oxford: Excerpta Medica, 1977:87.

507. Sewing K-FR, Billian A, Malchow H. Comparative study with ranitidine and cimetidine on gastric secretion in normal volunteers. Gut 1980;21:750.

508. Merki HS, Witzel L, Kaufman D, et al. Continuous intravenous infusions of famotidine maintain high intragastric pH in duodenal ulcer. Gut 1988;29:453.

509. Deakin M, Glenny HP, Ramage JK, et al. Large single daily dose of histamine H2 receptor antagonist for duodenal ulcer. How much and when? A clinical pharmacological study. Gut 1987;28:566.

510. Berardi RR, Tankanow RM, Nostrant TT. Comparison of famotidine with cimetidine and ranitidine. Clin Pharm 1988;7:271.

511. Merki HS, Witzel L, Walt RP, et al. Double blind comparison of the effects of cimetidine, ranitidine, famotidine, and placebo on intragastric acidity in 30 normal volunteers. Gut 1988;29:81.

512. Pounder RE, Williams JG, Hunt RH, et al. The effects of oral cimetidine on food-stimulated gastric acid secretion and 24-hour intragastric acidity. In: Burland WL, Simkins MA, eds. Cimetidine—Proceedings of the Second International Symposium on Histamine H2-Receptor Antagonists. Amsterdam–Oxford: Excerpta Medica, 1977:189.

513. Walt RP, Male P-J, Rawlings J, et al. Comparison of the effects of ranitidine, cimetidine and placebo on the 24 hour intragastric acidity and nocturnal acid secretion in patients with duodenal ulcer. Gut 1981;22:49.

514. Orr WC, Finn AL, Allen M, Robinson MG, Wilson T. The timing of evening meal and ranitidine administration—Effects on patterns of 24 hour intragastric acidity. Aliment Pharmacol Ther 1988;2: 541.

515. Savarino V, Mela GS, Scalabrini P, et al. Overnight comparable anacidity by standard large and half-single bedtime doses of H2 antagonists in duodenal ulcer patients: A clinical pharmacological study. Am J Gastroenterol 1988;83:917.

516. De Gara CJ, Burget DW, Silletti C, Hunt RH. A double-blind randomized study comparing different dose regimens of H2-receptor antagonists on 24-hour gastric secretion in normal subjects and duodenal ulcer patients. Am J Gastroenterol 1987;82:36.

517. Merki HS, Wilder-Smith C, Halter F. Treatment with H2-receptor antagonists: When is the best time to dose? Scand J Gastroenterol 1988;23(Suppl 153):15.

518. De Gara CJ, Gledhill T, Hunt RH. Nocturnal gastric acid secretion: Its importance in the pathophysiology and rational therapy of duodenal ulcer. Scand J Gastroenterol 1986;21(Suppl 121):17.

519. Fimmel C, Etienne A, Cilluffo T, et al. Long-term ambulatory gastric pH monitoring: Validation of a new method and effect of H2-antagonists. Gastroenterology 1985;88:1842.

520. Gledhill T, Howard OM, Buck M, Paul A, Hunt RH. Single nocturnal dose of an H2 receptor antagonist for the treatment of duodenal ulcer. Gut 1983;24:904.

521. Jones DB, Howden CW, Burget DW, Kerr GD, Hunt RH. Acid suppression in duodenal ulcer: A meta-analysis to define optimal dosing with antisecretory drugs. Gut 1987;28:1120.

522. Celle G, Savarino V, Mela GS, et al. Once and twice daily doses of H2 antagonists revisited, using continuous intragastric pH monitoring. Scand J Gastroenterol 1988;23:385.

523. Savarino V, Mela GS, Zentilin P, et al. Low bedtime doses of H2-receptor antagonists for acute treatment of duodenal ulcer. Dig Dis Sci 1989;34:1043.

524. Chambers JB, Pryce D, Bland JM, Northfield TC. Effect of bedtime ranitidine on overnight gastric acid output and intragastric pH: Dose/response study and comparison with cimetidine. Gut 1987;28: 294.

525. Merki H, Witzel L, Harre K, et al. Single dose treatment with H2-receptor antagonists: Is bedtime administration too late? Gut 1987;28:451.

526. Brogden RN, Heel RC, Speight TM, Avery GS. Cimetidine: A review of its pharmacological properties and therapeutic efficacy in peptic ulcer disease. Drugs 1978;15:93.

527. Lipsy RJ, Fennerty B, Fagan TC. Clinical review of histamine 2 receptor antagonists. Arch Intern Med 1990;150:745.

528. Abate MA, Hyneck ML, Cohen IA, Berardi RR. Cimetidine pharmacokinetics. Clin Pharm 1982;1:225.

529. Price AH, Brogden RN. Nizatidine: A preliminary review of its pharmacodynamic and pharmacokinetic properties, and its therapeutic use in peptic ulcer disease. Drugs 1988;36:521.

530. Barzaghi N, Gatti G, Crema F, Perucca E. Impaired bioavailability of famotidine given concurrently with a potent antacid. J Clin Pharmacol 1989;29:670.

531. Steinberg WM, Lewis JH, Katz DM. Antacids inhibit absorption of cimetidine. N Engl J Med 1982;307:400.

532. Kirch W, Hoensch H, Janisch HD. Interactions and non-interactions with ranitidine. Clin Pharmacokinet 1984;9:493.

533. Schentag JJ, Calleri G, Rose JQ, et al. Pharmacokinetic and clinical studies in patients with cimetidine-associated mental confusion. Lancet 1979;1:177.

534. Cello JP, Oie S. Cimetidine disposition in patients with Laennec's cirrhosis during multiple dosing therapy. Eur J Clin Pharmacol 1983;25:223.

535. Berlin RG. Effects of H2-receptor antagonists on the central nervous system. Drug Dev Res 1989;17:97.

536. Bjoeldager PAL, Jensen JB, Nielsen LP, Larsen NE, Hvidberg EF. Pharmacokinetics of cimetidine in patients undergoing hemodialysis. Nephron 1983;34:159.

537. Smith IL, Ziemniak JA, Bernhard H, et al. Ranitidine disposition and systemic availability in hepatic cirrhosis. Clin Pharmacol Ther 981;35:487.

538. Schentag JJ, Cerra FB, Calleri GM, et al. Age, disease, and cimetidine disposition in healthy subjects and chronically ill patients. Clin Pharmacol Ther 1981;29:737.

539. Grahnen A, Jameson S, Loof L, Tyllstrom J, Lindstrom B. Pharmacokinetics of cimetidine in advanced cirrhosis. Eur J Clin Pharmacol 1984;26:347.

540. Gugler R, Muller-Liebenau B, Somogyi A. Altered disposition and availability of cimetidine in liver cirrhotic patients. Br J Clin Pharmacol 1982;14:421.

541. Lewis JH. Hepatic effects of drugs used in the treatment of peptic ulcer disease. Am J Gastroenterol 1987;82:987.

542. Ziemniak JA, Bernhard H, Schentag JJ. Hepatic encephalopathy and altered cimetidine kinetics. Clin Pharmacol Ther 1983;34:375.

543. Kimelblatt BJ, Cerra FB, Calleri G, et al. Dose and serum concentration relationships in cimetidine-associated mental confusion. Gastroenterology 1980;78:791.

544. Matthews SJ, Michelson PA, Cersosimo RJ. Cimetidine-induced sinus bradycardia. Clin Pharm 1982;1:556.

545. Hughes DG, Dowling EA, DeMeersman RE, Garnett WR, Karnes H. Cardiovascular effects of H2-receptor antagonists. J Clin Pharmacol 1989;29:472.

546. Tanner LA, Arrowsmith JB. Letter: Bradycardia and H2 antagonists. Ann Intern Med 1988;109:434.

547. Kirch W, Halabi A, Linde M, Santos SR, Ohnhaus EE. Negative effects of famotidine on cardiac performance assessed by noninvasive hemodynamic measurements. Gastroenterology 1989;96:1388.

548. Sax MJ. Clinically important adverse effects and drug interactions with H2-receptor antagonists: An update. Pharmacotherapy 1987;7:110S.

549. Freston JW. Safety perspectives on parenteral H2-receptor antagonists. Am J Med 1987;83(Suppl 6A):58.

550. Kiowski W, Frei A. Bolus injection of cimetidine and hypotension in patients in the intensive care unit. Arch Intern Med 1987;147:153.

551. Coursin DB, Farin-Rusk C, Springman SR, Goelzer SL. The hemodynamic effects of intravenous cimetidine versus ranitidine in intensive care unit patients: A double-blind, prospective, crossover study. Anesthesiology 1988;69:975.

552. Onofrey D, Kelly KM, Gentili DR, Benjamin E, Iberti TJ. The hemodynamic effects of intravenous ranitidine in intensive care unit patients: A double-blind prospective study. J Clin Pharmacol 1988;28:1098.

553. Mavligit GM. Immunologic effects of cimetidine: Potential uses. Pharmacotherapy 1987;7(6 Pt 2):120S.

554. Gifford RM, Tilberg AF. Cimetidine reduces cyclosporin inhibition of interleukin-2 production. J Surg Res 1988;45:276.

555. White WB, Ballow M. Modulation of suppressor-cell activity by cimetidine in patients with variable hypogammaglobulinemia. N Engl J Med 1985;312:198.

556. Van der Spuy S, Levy DW, Levin W. Cimetidine in the treatment of herpesvirus infections. S Afr Med J 1980;58:112.

557. Timm EG, Rozek SL. Cimetidine in malignant melanoma. DICP 1989;23:689.

558. Sandstrom E. Antiviral therapy in human immunodeficiency virus infection. Drugs 1989;38:417.

559. Masamori D, Anderson PO. Cimetidine and allograft rejection. Drug Intell Clin Pharm 1981;15:278.

560. Hellstrand K, Hermodsson S. Differential effects of histamine receptor antagonists on human natural killer cell activity. Int Arch Allergy Appl Immunol 1987;84:247.

561. Aweeka F, Lizak P, Garovoy M, et al. Interleukin-2 and immunoglobulin increases with H2-antagonists in humans. Transplant Proc 1989;21:1718.

562. Pierri I, Rogna S, Stagnaro R, et al. Comparison between famotidine and ranitidine immunomodulatory effects in man. Int J Immunother 1988;4:243.

563. Ahonen J, Paimela H, Kauste A, et al. Ranitidine and cimetidine in renal transplantation: A clinical trial. Int J Tissue React 1983;4:373.

564. Gifford RR, Schmidtke JR, Ferguson RM. Cimetidine modulation of lymphocytes from renal allograft recipients. Transplant Proc 981;13:663.

565. Jacob ER, Papa M. Cimetidine and allograft rejection. Isr J Med Sci 1983;19:161.

566. Burleson RL, Kronhaus RJ, Marbarger PD, Jones DM. Cimetidine, posttransplant peptic ulcer complications, and renal allograft survival. Arch Surg 1982;117:933.

567. Watson AJ, Dalbrow MH, Stachura I, et al. Immunologic studies in cimetidine-induced nephropathy and polymyositis. N Engl J Med 1983;308:142.

568. Saigenji K, Fukutomi H, Nakazawa S. Famotidine: Postmarketing clinical experience. Scand J Gastroenterol 1987;22(Suppl 134):34.

569. Richter JM, Colditz GA, Huse DM, Delea TE, Oster G. Cimetidine and adverse reactions: A meta-analysis of randomized clinical trials of short-term therapy. Am J Med 1989;87:278.

570. Das AF, Freston JW, Jacobs J, Fox NA, Morton RE. An evaluation of safety in 37,252 patients treated with cimetidine or ranitidine. Internal Medicine for the Specialist 1990;11:3.

571. Cerra FB, Schentag JJ, McMillen M, et al. Mental status, the intensive care unit, and cimetidine. Ann Surg 1982;196:565.

572. Porter JB, Beard K, Walker AM, et al. Intensive hospital monitoring study of intravenous cimetidine. Arch Intern Med 1986;146:2237.

573. Gifford LM, Aeugle ME, Myerson RM, Tannenbaum PJ. Cimetidine postmarket outpatient surveillance program. JAMA 1980;243:1532.

574. Humphries TJ, Myerson RM, Gifford LM, et al. A unique postmarket outpatient surveillance program of cimetidine: Report on phase II and final summary. Am J Gastroenterol 1984;79:593.

575. McGuigan JE. A consideration of the adverse effects of cimetidine. Gastroenterology 1981;80:181.

576. Henann NE, Carpenter DU, Janda SM. Famotidine-associated mental confusion in elderly patients. Drug Intell Clin Pharm 1988;22:976.

577. Haug MT, Slugg PH, Pippenger CE. Ranitidine pharmacokinetics and adverse CNS effects (abstr). Clin Pharmacol Ther 1989;45:PIIK.

578. Reid SR, Bayliff CD. The comparative efficacy of cimetidine and ranitidine in controlling gastric pH in critically ill patients. Can Anaesth Soc J 1986;33:287.

579. Ehrinnpreis MN, Dhar R, Narula A. Cimetidine-induced galactorrhea. Am J Gastroenterol 1989;84:563.

580. Jensen RT, Collen MJ, Pandol S, et al. Cimetidine-induced impotence and breast changes in patients with gastric hypersecretory states. N Engl J Med 1983;308:883.

581. Spence RW, Celestin LR. Gynaecomastia associated with cimetidine. Gut 1979;20:154.

582. Galbraith RA, Michnovicz JJ. The effects of cimetidine on the oxidative metabolism of estradiol. N Engl J Med 1989;321:269.

583. Delitala G, Devilla L, Pende A, Canessa A. Effects of the H2-receptor antagonist ranitidine on anterior pituitary hormone secretion in man. Eur J Clin Pharmacol 1982;22:207.

584. Sedman AJ. Cimetidine-drug interactions. Am J Med 1984;76:109.

585. Powell JR, Donn KH. Histamine H2-antagonist drug interactions in perspective: Mechanistic concepts and clinical implications. Am J Med 1984;77(Suppl 5B):57.

586. Nazario M. The hepatic and renal mechanisms of drug interactions with cimetidine. Drug Intell Clin Pharm 1986;20:342.

587. Gerber MC, Tejwani GA, Gerber N, Bianchine JR. Drug interactions with cimetidine: An update. Pharmacol Ther 1985;27:353.

588. Somogyi A, Gugler R. Drug interactions with cimetidine. Clin Pharmacokinet 1982;7:23.

589. Baciewicz AM, Baciewicz FA. Effect of cimetidine and ranitidine on cardiovascular drugs. Am Heart J 1989;118:144.

590. Hansten PD, Horn JH. H2-receptor antagonist interactions—Myths and misconceptions. Drug Interact News 1988;8:39.

591. Hussey EK, Dukes GE. Do all histamine2-antagonists cause a warfarin drug interaction? DICP 1989;23:675.

592. Smith SR, Kendall MJ. Ranitidine versus cimetidine. Clin Pharmacokinet 1988;15:44.

593. Caballeria J, Baraona E, Rodamilans M, Lieber C. Effects of cimetidine on gastric alcohol dehydrogenase activity and blood ethanol levels. Gastroenterology 1989;96:388.

594. Frezza M, Padova C, Pozzato G, et al. The role of decreased alcohol dehydrogenase activity and first-pass metabolism. N Engl J Med 1990;322:95.

595. Pachon J, Lorber MI, Bia M. Effects of H2-receptor antagonists on renal function in cyclosporine-treated renal transplant patients. Transplantation 1989;47:254.

596. Groen PC. Cyclosporine: A review and its specific use in liver transplantation. Mayo Clin Proc 1989;64:680.

597. Ptachcinski RJ, Venkataramanan R, Burckart GJ. Clinical pharmacokinetics of cyclosporin. Clin Pharmacokinet 1986;11:107.

598. Aymard JP, Aymard B, Netter P, et al. Haematological adverse effects of histamine H2-receptor antagonists. Med Toxicol 1988;3:430.

599. Agura ED, Vila E, Petersen FB, Shields AF, Thomas ED. The use of ranitidine in bone marrow transplantation. Transplantation 1988;46:53.

600. Gafter U, Zevin D, Komlos L, Livni E, Levi J. Thrombocytopenia associated with hypersensitivity to ranitidine: Possible cross-reactivity with cimetidine. Am J Gastroenterol 1989;84:560.

601. Freeman HJ. Ranitidine-associated interstitial nephritis in a patient with celiac sprue. Can J Gastroenterol 1988;2:35.

602. Sachs G, Wallmark B. The gastric H^+/K^+-ATPase: The site of action of omeprazole. Scand J Gastroenterol 1989;24(Suppl 166):3.

603. Adams M, Ostrosky J, Kirkwood C. Therapeutic evaluation of omeprazole. Clin Pharm 1988;7:725.

604. Wallmark B. Omeprazole: Mode of action and effect on acid secretion in animals. Scand J Gastroenterol 1989;24(Suppl 166):12.

605. Wallmark B, Lindberg. Mechanism of action of omeprazole. ISI Atlas of Sci: Pharmacology 1987:158.

606. Clissold S, Campoli-Richards D. Omeprazole. A preliminary review of its pharmacodynamic and pharmacokinetic properties, and therapeutic potential in peptic ulcer disease and Zollinger–Ellison syndrome. Drugs 1986;32:15.

607. Cederberg C, Ekenved G, Lind T, et al. Acid inhibitory characteristics of omeprazole in man. Scand J Gastroenterol 1985;20(Suppl 108):105.

608. Howden CW, Forrest JA, Reid JL. Effects of single and repeated doses of omeprazole on gastric acid and pepsin secretion in man. Gut 1984;25:707.

609. Lind T, Cederberg C, Ekenved G, et al. Effect of omeprazole—a gastric proton pump inhibitor—on pentagastrin stimulated acid secretion in man. Gut 1983;24:270.

610. Prichard P, Yeomans N, Mihaly G, et al. Omeprazole: A study of its inhibition of gastric pH after morning or evening dosage. Gastroenterology 1985;88:64.

611. Sharm B, Walt R, Pounder R, et al. Optimal dose of oral omeprazole for maximal 24 hours decrease of intragastric acidity. Gut 1984;25:957.

612. Lanzo-Miller S, Pounder R, Hamilton M, et al. Twenty-four-hour intragastric acidity and plasma gastrin concentration before and during treatment with either ranitidine or omeprazole. Aliment Pharmacol Ther 1987;1:239.

613. Hewson E, Yeomans, Angus P, et al. Effect of "weekend therapy" with omeprazole on basal and stimulated acid secretion and fasting plasma gastrin in duodenal ulcer patients. Gut 1988;29:1715.

614. Walan A. The clinical utility and safety of omeprazole. Scand J Gastroenterol 1989;24(Suppl 166):140.

615. Bianchi Porro G, Parente F. Omeprazole in the treatment of duodenal ulcer. Scand J Gastroenterol 1989;24(Suppl 166):48.

616. Maton P, Vinayek R, Frucht H, et al. Long-term efficacy and safety of omeprazole in patients with Zollinger–Ellison syndrome: A prospective study. Gastroenterology 1989;97:827.

617. Lloyd-Davies KA, Rutgersson K, Solvell L. Omeprazole in the treatment of Zollinger–Ellison syndrome: A 4-year international study. Aliment Pharmacol Ther 1988;2:13.

618. Jensen JC, Gugler R. Inhibition of human liver enzyme cytochrome P450 by omeprazole. Br J Clin Pharm 1986;21:328.

619. Henry DA, Gerkens JF, Brent P, et al. Inhibition of drug metabolism by omeprazole. Lancet 1984;2:46.

620. Gugler R, Jensen J. Omeprazole inhibits oxidative drug metabolism. Studies with diazepam and phenytoin in vivo and 7-ethoxycoumarin in vitro. Gastroenterology 1985;89:1235.

621. Prichard PJ, Walt RP, Kitchingman GK, et al. Oral phenytoin pharmacokinetics during omeprazole therapy. Br J Clin Pharmacol 1987;24:543.

622. Sutfin T, Balmer K, Bostrom H, et al. Stereoselective interaction of omeprazole with warfarin in healthy men. Ther Drug Monit 1989;11:176.

623. Gugler R, Jensen JC. Drugs other than H_2-receptor antagonists as clinically important inhibitors of drug metabolism *in vitro*. Pharmacol Ther 1987;33:133.

624. Henry D, Brent P, Whyte I, et al. Propranolol steady-state pharmacokinetics are unaltered by omeprazole. Eur J Clin Pharmacol 1987;33:369.

625. Naesdal J, Bankel M, Bodemar G, et al. The effect of 20 mg omeprazole daily on serum gastrin, 24-h intragastric acidity, and bile acid concentration in duodenal ulcer patients. Scand J Gastroenterol 1987;22:5.

626. Karvonen A, Keyrilainen O, Uusitalo A, et al. Effects of omeprazole in duodenal ulcer patients. Scand J Gastroenterol 1986;21:449.

627. Graham D, McCullough A, Sklar M, et al. Omeprazole versus placebo in duodenal ulcer healing—The United States experience. Dig Dis Sci 1990;35:66.

628. Van Deventer G, Cagiola A, Whipple J, et al. Duodenal ulcer healing with omeprazole: A multicenter, double-blind, ranitidine controlled study (abstr). Gastroenterology 1988;94:A476.

629. Solcia E, Capella C, Sessa F, et al. Gastric carcinoids and related endocrine growths. Digestion 1986;35(Suppl 1):3.

630. Borch K, Renvall H, Liedberg G, et al. Relations between circulating gastrin and endocrine cell proliferation in the atrophic gastric fundic mucosa. Scand J Gastroenterol 1986;21:357.

631. Ekman L, Hansson E, Havu N, et al. Toxicological studies on omeprazole. Scand J Gastroenterol 1985;20(Suppl 108):53.

632. Editorial: Omeprazole and genotoxicity. Lancet 1990;1:386.

633. Carlsson E. A review of the effects of long-term acid inhibition in animals. Scand J Gastroenterol 1989;24(Suppl 166):19.

634. Tielemans Y, Hakanson R, Sundler F, et al. Proliferation of enterochromaffinlike cells in omeprazole-treated hypergastrinemic rats. Gastroenterology 1989;96:723.

635. Larsson H, Carlsson E, Mattsson H, et al. Plasma gastrin and gastric enterochromaffinlike cell activation and proliferation: Studies with omeprazole and ranitidine in intact and antrectomized rats. Gastroenterology 1986;90:391.

636. Larsson H, Carlsson E, Hakanson R, et al. Time-course of development and reversal of gastric endocrine cell hyperplasia after inhibition of acid secretion. Studies with omeprazole and ranitidine in intact and antrectomized rats. Gastroenterology 1988;95:1477.

637. Solcia E, Rindi G, Havu N, et al. Qualitative studies of gastric endocrine cells in patients treated long-term with omeprazole. Scand J Gastroenterol 1989;24(Suppl 166):129.

638. Creutzfeldt W, Lamberts R, Stockman F, et al. Quantitative studies of gastric endocrine cells in patients receiving long-term treatment with omeprazole. Scand J Gastroenterol 1989;24(Suppl 166):122.

639. Penston J, Wormsley K. Achlorhydria: Hypergastrinaemia: Carcinoids—A flawed hypothesis? Gut 1987;28:488.

640. Wormsley K. Is chronic long-term inhibition of gastric secretion really dangerous? Scand J Gastroenterol 1988;23(Suppl 146):166.

641. Wormsley K. Risks of therapeutic achlorhydria. Scand J Gastroenterol 1988;23(Suppl 153):35.

642. Brogden RN, Heel RC, Speight TM, et al. Sucralfate. A review of its pharmacodynamic properties and therapeutic use in peptic ulcer disease. Drugs 1984;27:194.

643. Garnett W. Sucralfate—Alternative therapy for peptic-ulcer disease. Clin Pharm 1982;1:307.

644. Nagashima R. Development and characteristics of sucralfate. J Clin Gastroenterol 1981;3(Suppl 2):103.

645. Szabo S. Pathways of gastrointestinal protection and repair: Mechanisms of action of sucralfate. Am J Med 1989;86(Suppl 6A):23.

646. Tarnawski A, Hollander D, Gergely H. The mechanism of protective, therapeutic and prophylactic actions of sucralfate. Scand J Gastroenterol 1987;22(Suppl 140):7.

647. Nagashima R. Mechanisms of action of sucralfate. Mechanisms of action of sucralfate. J Clin Gastroenterol 1981;3(Suppl 2):117.

648. Konturek S, Brzozowski T, Bielanski W, et al. Epidermal growth factor in the gastroprotective and ulcer-healing actions of sucralfate in rats. Am J Med 1989;86(Suppl 6A):32.

649. Crampton JR, Gibbons LC, Rees WD. Effect of sucralfate on gastroduodenal bicarbonate secretion and mucosal prostaglandin E_2 metabolism. Scand J Gastroenterol 1987;22(Suppl 140):15.

650. Shorrock C, Rees W. Effect of sucralfate on human gastric bicarbonate secretion and local prostaglandin E_2 metabolism. Am J Med 1989;86(Suppl 6A):2.

651. Shea-Donohue T, Steel L, Montcalm E, et al. Gastric protection by sucralfate. Role of mucus and prostaglandins. Gastroenterology 1986;91:660.

652. Crampton JR, Gibbons LC, Rees WD. Stimulation of amphibian gastroduodenal bicarbonate secretion by sucralfate and aluminium: Role of local prostaglandin metabolism. Gut 1988;29:903.

653. Haram E, Weberg R, Berstad A. Urinary excretion of aluminium after ingestion of sucralfate and an aluminium-containing antacid in man. Scand J Gastroenterol 1987;22:615.

654. Sudhakar P, Pharm B, Melethil S, et al. Elevation of serum aluminum in humans on a two-day sucralfate regimen. J Clin Pharmacol 1987;27:213.

655. Robertson J, Salusky I, Goodman W, et al. Sucralfate, intestinal aluminum absorption, and aluminum toxicity in a patient on dialysis. Ann Intern Med 1989;111:179.

656. Birchall J, Chappel J. Aluminum, chemical physiology, and Alzheimer's disease. Lancet 1988;2:1008.

657. Roxe DM, Mistovich M, Barch DH. Phosphate-binding effects of sucralfate in patients with chronic renal failure. Am J Kidney Dis 1989;13:194.

658. Sherman R, Hwang E, Walker J, et al. Reduction in serum phosphorus due to sucralfate. Am J Gastroenterol 1983;78:210.

659. Walan A. Antacids and anticholinergics in the treatment of duodenal ulcer. Clin Gastroenterol 1984;13(2):473.

660. Stevens MH, Thirlby RC, Feldman M. Mechanism for high PCO_2 in gastric juice: Roles of bicarbonate secretion and CO_2 diffusion. Am J Physiol 1987;253:G527.

661. Carlson GL, Malagelada JR. Chemistry of the antacids: Its relevance to antacid therapy. In: Halter, ed. Antacids in the eighties. Munich: Urban and Schwarzenberg, 1982:7.

662. Peterson WL, Fordtran JS. Reduction of gastric acidity. In: Sleisenger MH, Fordtran JS, eds. Gastrointestinal disease, ed 2. Philadelphia: WB Saunders, 1978:891.

663. Dent CE, Winter CS. Osteomalacia due to phosphate depletion from excessive aluminium hydroxide ingestion. Br Med J 1974;551.

664. Ekenved G, Halvorsen L, Solvell L. Influence of a liquid antacid on the absorption of different iron salts. Scand J Haematol (Suppl) 1976;28:65.

665. Fordtran JS, Collyns JAH. Antacid pharmacology in duodenal ulcer. Effect of antacids on postcibal gastric acidity and peptic activity. N Engl J Med 1968;274:921.

666. Peterson WL, Sturdevant RAL, Frankl HD, et al. Healing of duodenal ulcer with an antacid regimen. N Engl J Med 1977;297:341.

667. Fordtran JS, Morawski SG, Richardson CT. In-vivo and in-vitro evaluation of liquid antacids. N Engl J Med 1973;288:923.

668. Berstad A, Weberg R. Antacids for peptic ulcer: Do we have anything better? Scand J Gastroenterol 1986;Suppl 125:32.

669. Kaehny WD, Hegg AP, Alfrey AC. Gastrointestinal absorption of aluminum from aluminum-containing antacids. N Engl J Med 1977;296:1389.

670. Fordtran JS. Acid rebound. N Engl J Med 1968;279:900.

671. Kurzrok R, Lieb CC. Biochemical studies of human semen II. The action of semen on the human uterus. Proc Soc Exp Biol Med 1930;28:268.

672. Goldblatt MW. A depressor substance in seminal fluid. J Soc Chem Ind (London) 1933;52:1056.

673. vonEuler US. Zur kenntnis der pharmakologischen wirkungen von nativsekreten und extrakten mannlicher accessorischer geschlechtsdrusen. Arch Pharmakol 1934;175:78.

674. Wallace JL. Lipid mediators of inflammation in gastric ulcer. Am J Physiol 1990;258;G1.

675. Vane JR. Inhibition of prostaglandin synthesis of a mechanism of action for aspirin-like drugs. Nature New Biol 1971;231:232.

676. Johansson C, Bergstrom S. Prostaglandins and protection of the gastroduodenal mucosa. Scand J Gastroenterol 1982;21(Suppl 77):21.

677. Aly A, Green K, Johansson C. Prostaglandin synthesis in gastric and duodenal mucosa in man. Scand J Gastroenterol 1981;16:1099.

678. Rees WDW, Turnberg LA. Editorial review mechanisms of gastric mucosal protection: A role for the mucus-bicarbonate barrier. Clin Sci 1982;62:343.

679. Kollberg B, Aly A, Johansson C. Acetazolamide interfered with the protective effect of prostaglandin E_2 in the rat gastric mucosa. Scand J Gastroenterol 1981;16:385.

680. Zlotoff RA, Lake AM, Hamilton SR, et al. N-acetylcysteine attenuates the cytoprotective effect of topical PGE_2 in rat stomach (abstr). Gastroenterology 1982;82:1218.

681. Tytgat GN, Henzen Longmans SC, Van Minnen AJ. Human gastric mucosal changes after oral 15(R)-15 methyl prostaglandin E_2 administration (abstr). Gastroenterology 1982;82:1200.

682. Schoenhard G, Oppermann J, Kohn FE. Metabolism and pharmacokinetic studies of misoprostol. Dig Dis Sci 1985;30:11.

683. Reele SB, Bohan D. Oral antisecretory activity of prostaglandin E_2 in man. Dig Dis Sci 1984;29:5.

684. Chen MC-Y, Amerian D, Toomey M, et al. Prostanoid inhibition of canine parietal cells: Mediation by the inhibitory GTP-binding protein of adenylate cyclase. Gastroenterology 1988;94:1121.

685. Thomas FJ, Koss MA, Hogan DL, et al. Enprostil, a synthetic prostaglandin E_2 analogue, inhibits meal-stimulated gastric acid secretion and gastrin release in patients with duodenal ulcer. Am J Med 1986;81(Suppl 2A):44.

686. Hawkey CJ, Rampton DS. Prostaglandins and the gastrointestinal mucosa: Are they important in its function, disease, or treatment? Gastroenterology 1985;89:1162.

687. Rampton DS. Prostaglandins and intestinal physiology. In: Curtis-Prior PB, ed. Prostaglandins and related fatty acid metabolites. Edinburgh: Churchill Livingstone (In press)

688. Misoprostol. Med Lett 1989;31:21.

689. Wengrower D, Fich A, Goldin E, et al. Cytoprotective doses of arbacet with minimal antisecretory properties are not effective in duodenal ulcer healing. Dig Dis Sci 1987;32:857.

690. Johansson C, Uribe A, Rubio C, et al. Effect of oral prostaglandin E_2 on DNA turnover in gastric and intestinal epithelia of the rat. Eur J Clin Invest 1986;16:509.

691. Wagstaff AJ, Benfield P, Monk JP. Colloidal bismuth subcitrate: A review of its pharmacodynamic and pharmacokinetic properties, and its therapeutic use in peptic ulcer disease. Drugs 1988;36:132.

692. Koo J, Ho J, Lam SK, et al. Selective coating of gastric ulcer by tripotassium dicitrato bismuthate in the rat. Gastroenterology 1982;82:864.

693. Konturek SJ, Kwiecien N, Obtulowicz W, et al. Effects of colloidal bismuth subcitrate on aspirin-induced gastric microbleeding, DNA loss and prostaglandin formation in humans. Scand J Gastroenterol 1988;23:861.

694. Konturek SJ, Dembinski A, Warzecha Z, et al. Epidermal growth factor (EGF) in the gastroprotective and ulcer healing actions of colloidal bismuth subcitrate (De-Nol) in rats. Gut 1988;29:894.

695. Slomiany BL, Bilski J, Sarosiek J, et al. Colloidal bismuth subcitrate (De-Nol) inhibits peptic degradation of epidermal growth factor (abstr). Gastroenterology 1988;94:A431.

696. Coghill SB, Meehan SE, Milne G, et al. Localization of De-Nol (tripotassium dicitratobismuthate) in gastric ulcers and normal upper gastrointestinal tract of man and rodents by light and electron microscopy. J Pathol 1983b;139:487.

697. Weller MPI. Neuropsychiatric symptoms following bismuth intoxication. Postgrad Med J 1988;64:308.

698. Rune SJ, Linde J, Bonnevie O, Draminsky Petersen H. Acyclovir in the prevention of duodenal ulcer recurrence. Gut 1990;31:151.

699. Ivey KJ. Anticholinergics: Do they work in peptic ulcer? Gastroenterology 1975;68:154.

700. Goyal RK, Rattan S. Neurohormonal, hormonal and drug receptors for the lower oesophageal sphincter. Gastroenterology 1978;74:598.

701. Beermann B, Hellstrom K, Rosen A. The gastrointestinal absorption of atropine in man. Clin Sci 1971;40:95.

702. Walen A. Antacids and anticholinergics in the treatment of duodenal ulcer. Clin Gastroenterol 1984;13:473.

703. Feldman M, Richardson CT, Peterson WL, et al. Effect of low dose Propantheline on food stimulated acid secretion. N Engl J Med 1977;297:1427.

704. Bieberdorf FA, Walsh JH, Fordtran JS. Effect of optimum therapeutic dose of poldine on acid secretion, gastric acidity, gastric emptying and serum gastrin concentration after a protein meal. Gastroenterology 1975;68:50.

705. Texter EC, Reilly PA. The efficacy and selectivity of pirenzipine. Review and commentary. Scand J Gastroenterol 1982;17(suppl 72):237.

706. Conciato G, Daniotti M, Ferrari S, et al. Efficacy and safety of pirenzepine in peptic ulcer and in non-ulcerous gastroduodenal diseases. A multicentre controlled clinical trial. Scand J Gastroenterol 1982;17(Suppl 81):1.

707. Londong W. Present status and future perspectives of muscarinic receptor antagonists. Scand J Gastroenterol 1986;Suppl 125:55.

708. Ries RK, Gilbert DA, Katon W. Tricyclic antidepressant therapy for peptic ulcer disease. Arch Intern Med 1984;144:566.

709. Tytgat GN, Hameeteman W, Van Olffen GH. Sucralfate, bismuth compounds, substituted benzimidazoles, trimipramine and pirenzepine in the short- and long-term treatment of duodenal ulcer. Clin Gastroenterol 1984;13:2.

710. Baron H, Sullivan FM, eds. Carbenoxolone sodium. London: Butterworths, 1970:103.

711. Koelz HR. Protective drugs in the treatment of gastroduodenal ulcer disease. Scand J Gastroenterol 1986;21(Suppl 125):156.

712. Chiverton SG, Hunt RH. Relationship between inhibition of acid secretion and healing of peptic ulcers. Scand J Gastroenterol 1989;24(Suppl 166):43.

713. Barbara L, Corinaldesi B, Stanghellini V, et al. The evolution of anti-ulcer therapy with cimetidine. Is a single large nocturnal dose of cimetidine the right therapy for duodenal ulcer? Scand J Gastroenterol 1986;21(Suppl 121):1.

714. Thomas JM, Misiewicz G. Histamine H2-receptor antagonists in the short- and long-term treatment of duodenal ulcer. Clin Gastroenterol 1984;13:501.

715. McIsaac R, McCanless I, Summers K, Wood J. Ranitidine and cimetidine in the healing of duodenal ulcer: Meta-analysis of comparative clinical trials. Aliment Pharmacol Ther 1987;1:369.

716. Kildebo S, Aronsen B, Bernersen R, et al. Cimetidine, 800 mg at night, in the treatment of duodenal ulcers. Scand J Gastroenterol 1985;20:1147.

717. Valenzuela JE, Dickson B, Dixon W, et al. Efficacy of a single nocturnal dose of cimetidine in active duodenal ulcer. Results of a United States multicenter trial. Postgraduate Medicine: Custom Communications, November 1985.

718. Capurso L, Dal Monte PR, Mazzeo F, et al. Comparison of cimetidine 800 mg once daily and 400 mg twice daily in acute duodenal ulceration. Br Med J 1984;289:1418.

719. Dickson B. Cimetidine, 800 mg once daily: Preliminary European clinical data evaluation. Scand J Gastroenterol 1986;21(Suppl 121):11.

720. Ireland A, Colin-Jones DG, Gear P, et al. Ranitidine 150 mg twice daily vs 300 mg nightly in treatment of duodenal ulcers. Lancet 1984;2:274.

721. Simon B, Bianchi Porro G, Cremer M, et al. A single nighttime dose of ranitidine 300 mg versus ranitidine 150 mg twice daily in the acute treatment of duodenal ulcer: A European multicenter trial. J Clin Gastroenterol 1986;8:367.

722. Lee FI, Reed PI, Crowe JP, McIsaac RL, Wood JR. Acute treatment of duodenal ulcer: A multicentre study to compare ranitidine 150 mg twice daily with ranitidine 300 mg once at night. Gut 1986;27:1091.

723. Gitlin N, McCullough AJ, Smith L, et al. A multicenter, double-blind randomized, placebo-controlled comparison of nocturnal and twice-a-day famotidine in the treatment of active duodenal ulcer disease. Gastroenterology 1987;92:48.

724. Hunt RH, Howden CW, Jones DB, Burget DW, Kerr GD. The correlation between acid suppression and peptic ulcer healing. Scand J Gastroenterol 1986;21(Suppl 125):22.

725. Lam SK, Hui WM, Matthew NG, et al. Reducing meal-stimulated acid secretion versus reducing nocturnal acid secretion for healing of duodenal ulcer. Dig Dis Sci 1989;34:1494.

726. Lam SK, Ching-Lung L, Matthew NG, Fok KH, Hui WM. Duodenal ulcer healing by separate reduction of postprandial and nocturnal acid secretions have different pathophysiology. Gut 1985;26:1038.

727. De Pretis G, Dobrilla G, Ferrari A, et al. Comparison between single morning and bedtime doses of 40 mg famotidine for the treatment of duodenal ulcer. Aliment Pharmacol Ther 1989;3:285.

728. Merki H, Witzel L, Huttemann W, et al. Early evening ranitidine administration promotes faster duodenal ulcer healing. Am J Gastroenterol 1988;83:362.

729. Castelli G, Squassante L, Uleri S, Zanferrari G. Do different ranitidine dosage regimens influence the rate of duodenal ulcer healing? (abstr) Gastroenterology 1990;98:A28.

730. Kogut DG, Agrawal N, Collen MJ, Johnson JA. 300 mg ranitidine administered at 6pm and at 10pm in the treatment of duodenal ulcer disease (abstr). Gastroenterology 1990;98:A233.

731. Laverdant C. A multicentre international comparative trial of ranitidine and cimetidine in the short term treatment of duodenal ulcer. Gastroenterol Clin Biol 1983;7:480.

732. Cortot A, Henry AM, Pappo M, Paris JC. A comparison of ranitidine (150 mg X 2) versus cimetidine (400 mg X 2) in the treatment of acute duodenal ulcer. Gastroenterol Clin Biol 1987;11:136.

733. Rodrigo L, Viver J, Conchillo F, et al. A multicenter, randomized, double-blind study comparing famotidine with cimetidine in the treatment of active duodenal ulcer disease. Digestion 1989;42:86.

734. Lee FI, Booth SN, Cochran KM, et al. Single night-time doses of 40 mg famotidine or 800 mg cimetidine in the treatment of duodenal ulcer. Aliment Pharmacol Ther 1989;3:505.

735. Cherner JA, Cloud ML, Offen WW, et al. Comparison of nizatidine and cimetidine as once-daily treatment of acute duodenal ulcer. Am J Gastroenterol 1989;84:769.

736. Alcala-Santaella R, Guardia J, Pajares J, et al. A multicenter, randomized, double-blind study comparing a daily bedtime administration of famotidine and ranitidine in short-term treatment of active duodenal ulcer. Digestion 1989;42:79.

737. Pace F, Colombo E, Ferrara A, et al. Nizatidine and ranitidine in the short-term treatment of duodenal ulcer: A cooperative double-blind study of once-daily bedtime administration. Am J Gastroenterol 1988;83:643.

738. Celle G, Savarino V, Picciotto A, et al. A single-blind pilot study comparing standard (300 mg) and half (150 mg) bedtime doses of ranitidine in the short-term healing of duodenal ulcer. J Clin Gastroenterol 1990;12:255.

739. Meyrick-Thomas J, Misiewicz J, Trotman I, et al. Omeprazole in duodenal ulceration: Acid inhibition, symptom relief, endoscopic healing, and recurrence. Br Med J 1984;289:525.

740. Prichard PJ, Rubinstein D, Jones DB, et al. Double blind comparative study of omeprazole 10 mg and 30 mg daily for healing duodenal ulcers. Br Med J 1985;290:601.

741. Gustavsson S, Adami H, Loof L, Nyberg A, Nyren O. Rapid healing of duodenal ulcers with omeprazole: Double-blind dose-comparative trial. Lancet 1983;2:124.

742. Belgian Multicentre Group. Rate of duodenal ulcer healing during treatment with omeprazole. A double-blind comparison of a daily dose of 30 mg versus 60 mg. Scand J Gastroenterol 1986;21(Suppl 118):175.

743. Naesdal J, Lind T, Bergsaker-Aspoy J, et al. The rate of healing of duodenal ulcers during omeprazole treatment. Scand J Gastroenterol 1985;20:691.

744. Lauritsen K, Rune SJ, Bytzer P, et al. Effect of omeprazole and cimetidine on duodenal ulcer. A double-blind comparative trial. N Engl J Med 1985;312:958.

745. Archambault A, Pare P, Bailey R, et al. Omeprazole (20 mg daily) versus cimetidine (1200 mg daily) in duodenal ulcer healing and pain relief. Gastroenterology 1988;94:1130.

746. McFarland RJ, Bateson MC, Green JRB, et al. Omeprazole provides quicker symptom relief and duodenal ulcer healing than ranitidine. Gastroenterology 1990;98:278.

747. Mulder CJJ, Tijtgat GNJ, Cluysenaer OJJ, et al. Omeprazole (20 mg o.m.) versus ranitidine (150 mg b.d.) in duodenal ulcer healing and pain relief. Aliment Pharmacol Ther 1989;3:445.

748. Bardhan KD, Bianchi Porro G, Bose K, et al. A comparison of two different doses of omeprazole versus ranitidine in treatment of duodenal ulcers. J Clin Gastroenterol 1986;8:408.

749. Classen M, Dammann H-G, Domschke W, et al. Omeprazole heals duodenal, but not gastric ulcers more rapidly than ranitidine. Hepatogastroenterology 1985;32:243.

750. McIsaac RL, Mills JG, Wood JR. Relationship between reduction in 24-hour intragastric acidity and duodenal ulcer healing for different ranitidine dosage regimens (abstr). Gastroenterology 1990;98:A87.

751. Mills JG, Lee FI, Johnson NJ, Wood JR. Effects of higher dose ranitidine therapy on duodenal ulcer healing (abstr). Gastroenterology 1990;98:A89.

752. Wood JR, Mills JG, Ebbutt AF. Higher dose ranitidine: Meta-analysis of duodenal ulcer trials (abstr). Gastroenterology 1990;98:A150.

753. Page MC, Lacey LA, Mills JG, Wood JR. Can higher doses of an H2-receptor antagonist accelerate duodenal ulcer healing? Aliment Pharmacol Ther 1989;3:425.

754. Sung JL, Yu JY, Wang TH, Wang CY, Chen DS. A placebo-controlled, double-blind study of sucralfate in the short-term treatment of duodenal ulcer. Scand J Gastroenterol 1983;18(Suppl 83):21.

755. Martin F. Sucralfate suspension 1 g four times per day in the short-term treatment of active duodenal ulcer. Am J Med 1989;86(Suppl 6A):104.

756. McHardy GG. A multicenter, double-blind trial of sucralfate and placebo in duodenal ulcer. J Clin Gastroenterol 1981;3(Suppl 2):147.

757. Moshal M, Spitaels J, Khan F. Sucralfate in the treatment of duodenal ulcers—A double-blind endoscopically controlled trial. S Afr Med J 1980;57:742.

758. Lam SK. Implications of sucralfate-induced ulcer healing and relapse. Am J Med 1989;86:122.

759. Brandstaetter G, Kratochvil P. Comparison of two sucralfate dosages (2 g twice a day versus 1 g four times a day) in duodenal ulcer healing. Am J Med 1985;79(Suppl 2C):36.

760. Marks I, Wright J, Gilinsky N, et al. A comparison of sucralfate dosage schedule in duodenal ulcer healing. J Clin Gastroenterol 1986;8:419.

761. Coste T, Rautureau J, Beaugrand M, et al. Comparison of two sucralfate dosages presented in tablet form in duodenal ulcer healing. Am J Med 1987;83(Suppl 3B):86.

762. Martin F, Farley A, Gagnon M, Bensemana D. Comparison of the healing capacities of sucralfate and cimetidine in the short-term treatment of duodenal ulcer: A double-blind randomized trial. Gastroenterology 1982;82:401.

763. Glise H, Carling L, Hallerback B, et al. Short-term treatment of duodenal ulcer. Scand J Gastroenterol 1986;21:313.

764. Van Deventer G, Schneidman D, Walsh J. Sucralfate and cimetidine as single agents and in combination for treatment of active duodenal ulcers. Am J Med 1985;79(Suppl 2C):39.

765. Koelz HR, Halter F. Sucralfate and ranitidine in the treatment of acute duodenal ulcer. Am J Med 1989;86(Suppl 6A):98.

766. Hentschel E, Schutze K, Dufek W. Controlled comparison of sucralfate and cimetidine in duodenal ulcer. Scand J Gastroenterol 1983;18(Suppl 83):31.

767. Pop P, Nikkels R, Thys O, Dorrestein G. Comparison of sucralfate and cimetidine in the treatment of duodenal and gastric ulcers. A multicenter study. Scand J Gastroenterol 1983;18(Suppl 83):43.

768. Rey JF, Legras B, Vicari F, Gorget C. Comparative study of su-

cralfate versus cimetidine in the treatment of acute gastroduodenal ulcer. Am J Med 1989;86(Suppl 6A):116.

769. Nielsen MCL, Nielsen OV, Moesgaard F. Ulcer healing after treatment with sucralfate emulsion or ranitidine. J Clin Gastroenterol 1988;10:377.

770. Lam SK, Hui WM, Lau WY, et al. Sucralfate overcomes adverse effect of cigarette smoking on duodenal ulcer healing and prolongs subsequent remission. Gastroenterology 1987;92:1193.

771. Chiverton S, Hunt R. Smoking and duodenal ulcer disease. J Clin Gastroenterol 1989;11(Suppl 1):S29.

772. Korman M, Hansky J, Eaves E, Schmidt G. Influence of cigarette smoking on healing and relapse rate in duodenal ulcer disease. Gastroenterology 1983;85:871.

773. Chiverton S, Burget D, Hunt R. Smoking does not impair the response to therapy in duodenal ulcer healing (abstr). Gastroenterology 1988;94:A69.

774. Kikendall J, Evaul J, Johnson L. Effect of cigarette smoking on gastrointestinal physiology and non-neoplastic digestive disease. J Clin Gastroenterol 1984;6:65.

775. McCarthy D. Editorial: Smoking and ulcers—Time to quit. N Engl J Med 1984;311:726.

776. Fordtran J, Schiller L, Shapowal S. Letter: Sucralfate, smoking and ulcer healing. Gastroenterology 1988;94:1107.

777. Walen A. Antacids and anticholinergics in the treatment of duodenal ulcer. Clin Gastroenterol 1984;13(2):473.

778. Berstad A, Weberg R. Antacids for peptic ulcer: Do we have anything better? Scand J Gastroenterol 1986;21(Suppl 125):32.

779. Lam SK, La KC, Lai CL. Treatment of duodenal ulcer with antacid and sulpiride. Gastroenterology 1979;76:315.

780. Kumar N, Vij JC, Karol A. Controlled therapeutic trial to determine the optimum dose of antacids in duodenal ulcer. Gut 1984;25:1199.

781. Ippoliti AF, Sturdevant R, Isenberg JI, et al. Cimetidine versus intensive antacid therapy for duodenal ulcer—A multicenter trial. Gastroenterology 1978;74:393.

782. Weberg R, Aubert E, Dahlberg O. Low-dose antacids or cimetidine for duodenal ulcer? Gastroenterology 1988;95:1465.

783. Jönsson KA, Bodemar G, Norrby K, et al. Are endoscopic and/or histologic findings in gastroduodenal mucosa a predictor of clinical outcome in peptic ulcer disease? Scand J Gastroenterol 1988;23:299.

784. Hunter JO, Crowe J, Gillies RR, et al. A double-blind randomized multicentre study comparing Maalox TC tablets and ranitidine in the healing of duodenal ulcer. Gut 1987;28:A1337.

785. Kunert H, Ottenjann R. Treatment with small doses of an antacid and combined with cimetidine. In: Halter F, ed. Antacids in the eighties. Munich: Urban & Schwarzenberg, 1982:87.

786. Sturdevant RAL, Isenberg JI, Secrist D. Antacid and placebo produced similar pain relief in duodenal ulcer patients. Gastroenterology 1977;72:1.

787. Rune SJ, Zachariasson A. Acute relief of epigastric pain by antacid in duodenal ulcer patients. Scand J Gastroenterol 1979;14(suppl 58):41.

788. Berstad A, Weberg R. Antacids for peptic ulcer: Do we have anything better? Scand J Gastroenterol 1986;21(Suppl 125):32.

789. Hawkey CJ, Walt RP. Prostaglandins for peptic ulcer: A promise unfulfilled. Lancet 1986;2:1084.

790. Euler AR, Krawiec J, Odes H. An evaluation of arbaprostil at multiple doses for the treatment of acute duodenal ulcer: A randomized double-blind placebo-controlled international trial. Am J Gastroenterol 1990;85:2.

791. Penston JG, Wormsley KG. Histamine H2-receptor antagonists versus prostaglandins in the treatment of peptic ulcer disease. Drugs 1989;37:391.

792. Lauritsen K, Rask-Madsen J. Prostaglandins and clinical experience in peptic ulcer disease. Scand J Gastroenterol 1986;21(Suppl 125):174.

793. Euler AR, Popiela T, Tytgat GN. A multiclinic trial evaluating arbaprostil [15R-15-methyl prostaglandin E2] as a therapeutic agent for gastric ulcer. Gastroenterology 1989;96:967.

794. Wengrower D, Fich A, Goldin E. Cytoprotective doses of arbacet with minimal antisecretory properties are not effective in duodenal ulcer healing. Dig Dis Sci 1987;32:857.

795. Bianchi-Porro PG, Parente F, Hentschel E. Rioprostil in the short-term treatment of duodenal ulcer: A multicentre double-blind trial vs cimetidine. Scand J Gastroenterol 1989;24(Suppl 164):219.

796. Dammann HG, Dreyer M, Muller P, et al. A single evening dose of rioprostil, 600 micrograms, in the treatment of acute duodenal ulcers. Scand J Gastroenterol 1989;24(Suppl 164):215.

797. Whorwell PJ. Rioprostil in the healing of duodenal ulceration: A short report. Scand J Gastroenterol 1989;24(Suppl 164):214.

798. Coremans G, Vantrappen G, Businger JA, et al. Efficacy and safety of rioprostil 300 micrograms b.d. in the treatment of duodenal ulcer: A double-blind controlled multicentre clinical study vs. ranitidine. Scand J Gastroenterol 1989;(Suppl 164):198.

799. Euler AR, Bailey RJ, Zinny MA, et al. Arbaprostil [15R-15-methyl prostaglandin E$_2$] in a single nighttime dose of either 50 or 100 micrograms in acute duodenal ulcer. Gastroenterology 1989;97:98.

800. Barbara L, Corinaldesi R, Rea E, Paternico A, Stanghellini V. The role of colloidal bismuth subcitrate in the short-term treatment of duodenal ulcer. Scand J Gastroenterol 1986;21(Suppl 122):30.

801. Lee FI, Samloff IM, Hardman M. Comparison of tri-potassium di-citrato bismuthate tablets with ranitidine in healing and relapse of duodenal ulcers. Lancet 1985;1:1299.

802. Bianchi Porro G, Lazzaroni M, Barbara L, et al. Tripotassium dicitrate bismuthate and ranitidine in duodenal ulcer—Healing and influence on recurrence. Scand J Gastroenterol 1988;23:1232.

803. Hamilton I, O'Connor H, Wood N, Bradbury I, Axon A. Healing and recurrence of duodenal ulcer after treatment with tripotassium dicitrato bismuthate (TDB) tablets or cimetidine. Gut 1986;27:106.

804. Ward M, Halliday C, Cowen A. A comparison of colloidal bismuth subcitrate tablets and ranitidine in the treatment of chronic duodenal ulcers. Digestion 1986;34:173.

805. Miller JP. Colloidal bismuth in the treatment of duodenal ulceration: The benefit for the patient. Scand J Gastroenterol 1989;24(Suppl 157):16.

806. Dekker W, Dal Monte P, Bianchi Porro G, et al. An international multi-clinic study comparing the therapeutic efficacy of colloidal bismuth subcitrate coated tablets with chewing tablets in the treatment of duodenal ulceration. Scand J Gastroenterol 1986;21(Suppl 122):46.

807. Chiverton SG, Hunt RH. Initial therapy and relapse of duodenal ulcer: Possible acid secretory mechanisms. Gastroenterology 1989;96:632.

808. Walan A. Antacids and anticholinergics in the treatment of duodenal ulcer. Clin Gastroenterol 1984;13:473.

809. Ries RK, Gilbert DA, Katon W. Tricyclic antidepressant therapy for peptic ulcer disease. Arch Intern Med 1984;144:566.

810. Ivey KJ. Anticholinergics: Do they work in peptic ulcer? Gastroenterology 1975;68:154.

811. Tytgat GNJ, Hameeteman W, Van Olffen GH. Sucralfate, bismuth compounds, substituted benzimidazoles, trimipramine and pirenzepine in the short- and long-term treatment of duodenal ulcer. Clin Gastroenterol 1984;13:543.

812. Texter EC, Reilly PA. The efficacy and selectivity of pirenzepine. Review and commentary. Scand J Gastroenterol 1982;72:237.

813. Wulff HR. Rational diagnosis and treatment. An introduction to clinical decision-making. Oxford: Blackwell Scientific Publications, 1981:209.

814. Chalmers TC. In: Blum A, Buyse M, Hewitt P, Koch M, eds. Data analysis for clinical medicine: The quantitative approach to patient care in gastroenterology. New York: International University Press, 1988.

815. Sturdevant RAL. How should results of controlled trials affect clinical practice? Gastroenterology 1977;73:1179.

816. Howden CW, Hunt RH. The relationship between suppression of acidity and gastric ulcer healing rates. Aliment Pharmacol Ther 1990;4:25.

817. Isenberg JI, Peterson WL, Elashoff JD, et al. Healing of benign gastric ulcer with low-dose antacid or cimetidine. A double-blind, randomized, placebo-controlled trial. N Engl J Med 1983;308:1319.

818. Graham D, Dyck W, Englert E, et al. Healing of gastric ulcer: Comparison of cimetidine and placebo in the United States. Ann Intern Med 1985;102:573.

819. Dyck W, Belsito A, Fleshler B, et al. Cimetidine and placebo in the treatment of gastric ulcer. Gastroenterology 1978;74:410.

820. Freston JW. Cimetidine in the treatment of gastric ulcer. Review and commentary. Gastroenterology 1978;74:426.

821. Hirschowitz B, DeLuca V, Graham D, et al. Treatment of benign chronic gastric ulcer with ranitidine. A randomized, double-blind, and placebo-controlled six week trial. J Clin Gastroenterol 1986;8:371.

822. Bauerfeind P, Koelz HR, Blum AL. Ulcer treatment—Regimens and duration of inhibition of acid secretion: How long to dose. Scand J Gastroenterol 1988;23(Suppl 153):23.

823. Dawson J, Jain S, Cockel R. Effect of ranitidine and cimetidine on gastric ulcer healing and recurrence. Scand J Gastroenterol 1984;19:665.

824. Baron H, Perrin V, et al. Gastric ulcer healing with ranitidine and cimetidine. A multicentre study. Scand J Gastroenterol 1983;18:973.

825. Belgian Peptic Ulcer Study Group. Single blind comparative study of ranitidine and cimetidine in patients with gastric ulcer. Gut 1984;25;999.

826. Kellow J, Barr G, Cowen A, et al. Comparison of ranitidine and cimetidine in the treatment of chronic gastric ulcer. A double-blind trial. Digestion 1983;27:105.

827. Wright J, Marks I, Mee A, et al. Ranitidine in the treatment of gastric ulceration. S Afr Med J 1982;61:155.

828. Ryan F, Jorde R, Ehsanullah R, Summers K, Wood J. A single night time dose of ranitidine in the acute treatment of gastric ulcer: A European multicentre trial. Gut 1986;27:784.

829. Jorde R, Burhol P. A single-centre study of gastric ulcer healing with 300 mg ranitidine at night versus 150 mg ranitidine twice daily. Scand J Gastroenterol 1986;21:833.

830. Brazer S, Tyor M, Pancotto F, et al. Randomized, double-blind comparison of famotidine with ranitidine in treatment of acute, benign gastric ulcer disease. Dig Dis Sci 1989;34:1047.

831. Cremer M, Keohane P, Mulder H, et al. Nizatidine versus ranitidine in gastric ulcer disease. A European multicentre trial. Scand J Gastroenterol 1987;22(Suppl 136):71.

832. Schepp W, Classen M. Omeprazole in the acute treatment of gastric ulcer. Scand J Gastroenterol 1989;24(Suppl 166):58.

833. Barbara L, Saggioro A, Olsson J, Cisternino M, Franceschi AM. Omeprazole 20 mg om and ranitidine 150 mg bd in the healing of benign gastric ulcers—An Italian multicentre study (abstr). Gut 1987;28:A1341.

834. Walan A, Bader J-P, Classen M, et al. Effect of omeprazole and ranitidine on ulcer healing and relapse rates in patients with benign gastric ulcer. N Engl J Med 1989;320:69.

835. Bate CM, Wilkinson SP, Bradby GVH, et al. Randomised, double blind comparison of omeprazole and cimetidine in the treatment of symptomatic gastric ulcer. Gut 1989;30:1323.

836. Danish Omeprazole Study Group. Omeprazole and cimetidine in the treatment of ulcers of the body of the stomach: A double blind comparative trial. Br Med J 1989;298:645.

837. Lam SK, Lau WY, Lai CL, et al. Efficacy of sucralfate in corpus, prepyloric and duodenal ulcer-associated gastric ulcers. Am J Med 1985;79(Suppl 2c):24.

838. Kagevi I, Anker-Hansen O, Carling L, et al. Swedish multicenter study on prepyloric and gastric ulcer. Scand J Gastroenterol 1987;22(Suppl 127):67.

839. Blum AL, Bethge H. Sucralfate in the treatment and prevention of gastric ulcer (abstr). Gastroenterology 1988;94:A39.

840. Marks IN, Wright JP, Denyer M, Garish JAM, Lucke W. Comparison of sucralfate with cimetidine in the short-term treatment of chronic peptic ulcers. S Afr Med J 1980;57:567.

841. Hjortrup A, Svendsen LB, Beck H, Hoffmann J, Schroeder M. Two daily doses of sucralfate or cimetidine in the healing of gastric ulcer. Am J Med 1989;86(Suppl 6A):113.

842. Englert E Jr, Freston JW, Graham DY, et al. Cimetidine, antacid and hospitalization in the treatment of benign gastric ulcer. Gastroenterology 1978;74:416.

843. Isenberg JI, Peterson WL, Elashoff JD, et al. Healing of benign gastric ulcer with low dose antacid or cimetidine: A double-blind, randomized, placebo-controlled trial. N Engl J Med 1983;308:1319.

844. Berstad A, Weberg R. Antacids for peptic ulcer: Do we have anything better? Scand J Gastroenterol 1986;21(Suppl 125):32.

845. Lauritsen K, Bytzer P, Hansen J, et al. Comparison of ranitidine and high-dose antacid in the treatment of prepyloric or duodenal ulcer. Scand J Gastroenterol 1985;10:123.

846. Agrawal NM, Saffouri B, Kruss DM. Healing of benign gastric ulcer. A placebo-controlled comparison of two dosage regimens of misoprostol, a synthetic analog of prostaglandin E_1. Dig Dis Sci 1985;30(suppl 11):1645.

847. Schubert TT, Frizzell JA, Meier PB, et al. A U.S. multicenter study of enprostil 35 micrograms twice daily for treatment of prepyloric, pyloric channel, and duodenal bulb ulcers. Dig Dis Sci 1989;34:1355.

848. Rachmilewitz D. Efficacy of prostanoids in the treatment of gastric ulcer. Clin Invest Med 1987;10:238.

849. Lauritsen K, Laursen LS, Havelund T, et al. Rioprostil and ranitidine in the treatment of prepyloric gastric ulcer. A double-blind comparative trial. Scand J Gastroenterol 1989;24:368.

850. Quinton A, Goldfain D, Weber F, et al. Treatment of benign gastric ulcer. A comparative clinical trial of rioprostil and ranitidine. Scand J Gastroenterol 1989;164:178.

851. Euler AR, Popiela T, Tytgat GN, et al. A multiclinic trial evaluating arbaprostil [15R-15-methyl prostaglandin E_2] as a therapeutic agent for gastric ulcer. Gastroenterology 1989;96(4):967.

852. Shou-Po C, Guo-Zong P. Short-term treatment with colloidal bismuth subcitrate (De-Nol) and cimetidine in Chinese patients with gastric ulcer. Clinical Trials Journal 1986;23:215.

853. Gibinski K, Nowak A, Marlicz K, et al. Dicytrynianobizmutan trojpotasowy w leczeniu wrzodu trawiennego i zapobieganiu nawrotowi wrzodu. Pol Tyg Lek 1984;39:1547.

854. Tanner AR, Cowlishaw JL, Cowen AE, Ward M. Efficacy of cimetidine and tri-potassium di-citrato bismuthate (De-Nol) in chronic gastric ulceration: A comparative study. Med J Aust 1979;1:1.

855. Tytgat GNJ, Van Bentem N, Van Olffen G, et al. Controlled trial comparing colloidal bismuth subcitrate tablets, cimetidine and placebo in the treatment of gastric ulceration. Scand J Gastroenterol 1982;17(80):31.

856. Parente F, Lazzaroni M, Petrillo M, Bianchi Porro G. Colloidal bismuth subcitrate and ranitidine in the short-term treatment of benign gastric ulcer: An endoscopically controlled trial. Scand J Gastroenterol 1986;21(122):42.

857. Langman MJS. Carbenoxolone in the treatment of ulcer disease. In: Holtermuller KH, Malagelada JR, eds. Advances in ulcer disease—Proceedings of a symposium on the pathogenesis and therapy of ulcer disease. Amsterdam: Excerpta Medica, 1980:406.

858. Ries RK, Gilbert DA, Katon W. Tricyclic antidepressant therapy for peptic ulcer disease. Arch Intern Med 1984;154:566.

859. Valnes K, Myren J, Qvigstad T. Trimipramine in the treatment of gastric ulcer. Scand J Gastroenterol 1978;13:497.

860. Greibe J, Bugge P, Gjorup T, et al. Long-term prognosis of duodenal ulcer: Follow-up study and survey of doctors' estimates. Br Med J 1977;2:1572.

861. Fry J. Peptic ulcer: A profile. Br Med J 1964;2:809.

862. Bardhan KD, Saul DM, Edwards JL, et al. Double-blind comparison of cimetidine and placebo in the maintenance of healing of chronic duodenal ulceration. Gut 1979;20:158.

863. Burland WL, Hawkins BW, Beresford J. Cimetidine treatment for the prevention of recurrence of duodenal ulcer: An international collaborative study. Postgrad Med J 1980;56:173.

864. Van Deventer GM, Elashoff JD, Reedy TJ, et al. A randomized study of maintenance therapy with ranitidine to prevent the recurrence of duodenal ulcer. N Engl J Med 1989;320:1113.

865. Bardhan KD. Intermittent treatment of duodenal ulcer for long-term medical management. Postgrad Med J 1988;64(Suppl 1):40.

866. Frederiksen HJ, Matzen P, Madsen P, et al. Spontaneous healing of duodenal ulcers. Scand J Gastroenterol 1984;19:417.

867. Hanscom DH, Buchman E. The follow-up period. Gastroenterology 1971;61:714.

868. Baume PE, Hunt JH, Piper DW. Glycopyronium bromide in the treatment of chronic gastric ulcer. Gastroenterology 1972;63:399.

869. Horwich L, Galloway R. Treatment of gastric ulceration with carbenoxolone sodium: Clinical radiologic evaluation. Br Med J 1965;2:1274.

870. Wolosin JD, Gertler SL, Peterson WL, et al. Gastric ulcer recurrence: Follow up of a double-blind, placebo-controlled trial. J Clin Gastroenterol 1989;11:12.

871. Thorat VK, Misra SP, Anand BS. Conventional versus on-demand therapy for duodenal ulcer: Results of a controlled therapeutic trial. Am J Gastroenterol 1990;85:243.

872. Freston JW. On-demand treatment for duodenal ulcers: Has its time come? Am J Gastroenterol 1990;85:241.

873. Elashoff JD, Van Deventer G, Reedy TJ, et al. Long-term follow-up of duodenal ulcer patients. J Clin Gastroenterol 1983;5:509.

874. Sonnenberg A, Muller-Lissner SA, Vogel E, et al. Predictors of duodenal ulcer healing and relapse. Gastroenterology 1981;81:1061.

875. Chalmers TC. In: Blum A, Buyse M, Hewitt MS, et al, eds. Data analysis for clinical medicine: The quantitative approach to patient care in gastroenterology. Rome: International University Press, 1988;217.

876. Elashoff JD. Combining results of clinical trials. Gastroenterology 1978;75:1170.

877. Elashoff JD, Van Deventer G, Reedy TJ, et al. Long-term follow-up of duodenal ulcer patients. J Clin Gastroenterol 1983;5:509.

878. Ippoliti A, Elashoff J, Valenzuela J. Recurrent ulcer after successful treatment with cimetidine or antacid. Gastroenterology 1983;85:875.

879. Miller JP, Faragher EB. Relapse of duodenal ulcer: Does it matter which drug is used in initial treatment? Br Med J 1986;293:1117.

880. Lane MR, Lee SP. Recurrence of duodenal ulcer after medical treatment. Lancet 1988;1:1147.

881. Gudmand-Hoyer E, Jensen KB, Drag E, et al. Prophylactic effect of cimetidine in duodenal ulcer disease. Br Med J 1978;1:1095.

882. Chiverton SG, Hunt RH. Initial therapy and relapse of duodenal ulcer: Possible acid secretory mechanisms. Gastroenterology 1989;96:632.

883. McLean AJ, Harrison PM, Ioannides-Demos L, et al. The choice of ulcer healing agent influences duodenal ulcer healing rate and long-term clinical outcome. Aust N Z J Med 1985;15:367.

884. Porro GB, Lazzaroni M, Parente F, et al. The influence of colloidal bismuth subcitrate on duodenal ulcer relapse. Scand J Gastroenterol 1986;21(Suppl 122):35.

885. Rauws EAJ, Tytgat GNJ. Eradication of Helicobacter pylori cures duodenal ulcer. Gastroenterology 1990;98:A111.

886. Strum WB. Prevention of duodenal ulcer recurrence. Ann Intern Med 1986;105:757.

887. Jensen DM. Economic and health aspects of peptic ulcer disease and H2-receptor antagonists. Am J Med 1986;81(Suppl 4B):42.

888. Berardi RR, Savitsky ME, Nostrant TT. Maintenance therapy for prevention of recurrent peptic ulcers. Drug Intell Clin Pharm 1987;21:493.

889. Sontag SJ, ACG Committee on FDA-related matters. Current status of maintenance therapy in peptic ulcer disease. Am J Gastroenterol 1988;83:607.

890. Wolosin J, Gertler S, Peterson W, Sandersfeld MA, Isenberg J. Gastric ulcer recurrence: Follow-up of a double-blind, placebo-controlled trial. J Clin Gastroenterol 1989;11:12.

891. Palmer RH, Frank WO, Karlstadt R. Maintenance therapy of duodenal ulcer with H2-receptor antagonists—A meta-analysis. Aliment Pharmacol Ther 1990;4:283.

892. Boyd EJS, Johnston DA, Penston JG, Wormsley KG. Does maintenance therapy keep duodenal ulcers healed? Lancet 1988;1:1324.

893. Underwood DD, Amos JC, Venables CW, et al. Three computer models for the calculation of prevalence of peptic ulcer disease during long-term treatment. Aliment Pharmacol Ther 1988;2:407.

894. Gough KR, Bardhan KD, Crowe JP, et al. Ranitidine and cimetidine in prevention of duodenal ulcer relapse. Lancet 1984;2:659.

895. Silvis SE. Results of the United States ranitidine maintenance trials. Am J Med 1984;77(Suppl 5B):33.

896. Freston JW. H2-receptor antagonists and duodenal ulcer recurrence: Analysis of efficacy and commentary on safety, costs, and patient selection. Am J Gastroenterol 1987;82:1242.

897. Texter EC, Navab F, Mantell G, Berman R. Maintenance therapy of duodenal ulcer with famotidine. Am J Med 1986;81(Suppl 4B):25.

898. Takemoto T, Namiki M, Ishikawa M, et al. Ranitidine and sucralfate

as maintenance therapy for gastric ulcer disease: Endoscopic control and assessment of scarring. Gut 1989;30:1692.

899. Hentschel E, Schutze K, Weiss W, et al. Effect of cimetidine treatment in the prevention of gastric ulcer relapse: A one year double blind multicentre study. Gut 1983;24:853.

900. Alstead E, Ryan F, Holdsworth C, Ashton M, Moore M. Ranitidine in the prevention of gastric and duodenal ulcer relapse. Gut 1983;24:418.

901. Barr G, Kang J, Canalese J, Piper D. A two-year prospective controlled study of maintenance cimetidine and gastric ulcer. Gastroenterology 1983;85:100.

902. Jorde R, Burhol P, Hansen T. Ranitidine 150 mg at night in the prevention of gastric ulcer relapse. Gut 1987;28:460.

903. Paakkonen M, Aukee S, Janatuinen E, et al. Sucralfate as maintenance treatment for the prevention of duodenal ulcer recurrence. Am J Med 1989;86(Suppl 6A):133.

904. Bolin TD, Davis AE, Duncombe VM, Billington B. Role of maintenance sucralfate in prevention of duodenal ulcer recurrence. Am J Med 1987;83(Suppl 3B):91.

905. Bolin TD. Sucralfate maintenance therapy in duodenal ulcer disease. Am J Med 1989;86(Suppl 6A):148.

906. Behar J, Roufail W, Thomas E, et al. Efficacy of sucralfate in the prevention of recurrence of duodenal ulcers. J Clin Gastroenterol 1987;9(Suppl 1):23.

907. Takemoto T, Kimura K, Okita K, et al. Efficacy of sucralfate in the prevention of recurrence of peptic ulcer—Doule blind multicenter study with cimetidine. Scand J Gastroenterol 1987;22(Suppl 140):49.

908. Tovey F, Husband E, Yiu Y, et al. Differences in mucosal appearances and in relapse rates in duodenal ulceration treated with sucralfate or cimetidine. Am J Med 1989;86(Suppl 6A):141.

909. Masoero G, Rocchia F, Rossanino A, et al. Comparison of ranitidine and sucralfate in the long-term treatment of duodenal ulcer. J Clin Gastroenterol 1986;8:624.

910. Rodrigo M, Berenguer J, Hinojosa J, Balanzo JM, Segu JL. Sucralfate and cimetidine as maintenance treatment in the prevention of duodenal ulcer recurrence. Am J Med 1987;83(Suppl 3B):99.

911. Classen M, Bethge H, Brunner G, et al. Effect of sucralfate on peptic ulcer recurrence: A controlled, double-blind multicenter study. Scand J Gastroenterol 1983;18(Suppl 83):61.

912. Miyake T, Ariyoshi J, Suzaki T, Oishi M, Sakai M, Ueda S. Endoscopic evaluation of the effect of sucralfate therapy and other drug parameters on the recurrence rate of gastric ulcers. Dig Dis Sci 1980;25:1.

913. Marks I, Wright J, Girdwood A, Gilinsky N, Lucke W. Maintenance therapy with sucralfate reduces rate of gastric ulcer recurrence. Am J Med 1985;79(Suppl 2C):32.

914. Marks I, Girdwood A, Wright J, et al. Nocturnal dosage regimen of sucralfate in maintenance of gastric ulcer. Am J Med 1987;83(Suppl 3B):95.

915. Bardhan KD, Hunter JO, Miller JP, et al. Antacid maintenance therapy in the prevention of duodenal ulcer relapse. Gut 1988;29:1748.

916. Bianchi Porro G, Lazzaroni M, Cortvriendt WRE. Maintenance therapy with colloidal bismuth subcitrate in duodenal ulcer disease. Digestion 1987;37(Suppl 2):47.

917. Businger JA, Fumagalli I, Michel H, Delas N, Stocker H. Rioprostil, a new prostaglandin E1 analogue, in the once-daily treatment for the prevention of duodenal ulcer recurrence: A comparison with ranitidine. Scand J Gastroenterol 1989;24(Suppl 164):152.

918. Moshal MG, Spitaels J-M, Khan F, Manion GL. Pirenzepine, cimetidine and placebo in the long-term treatment of duodenal ulceration. S Afr Med J 1982;62:12.

919. Marks IN, Wright JP, Bank L, et al. Comparison of pirenzepine with cimetidine in duodenal ulcer disease. S Afr Med J 1986;70:27.

920. Boyd EJS, Wilson JA, Wormsley KG. The fate of asymptomatic recurrences of duodenal ulcer. Scand J Gastroenterol 1984;19:808.

921. Pounder R. Silent peptic ulceration: Deadly silence or golden silence? Gastroenterology 1989;96:626.

922. Van Deventer GM, Elashoff JD, Reedy TJ, Schneidman D, Walsh JH. A randomized study of maintenance therapy with ranitidine to prevent the recurrence of duodenal ulcer. N Engl J Med 1989;320:1113.

923. Elashoff JD, Van Deventer G, Reedy TJ, et al. Long-term follow-up of duodenal ulcer patients. J Clin Gastroenterol 1983;5:509.

924. Boyd EJS, Wilson JA, Wormsley KG. Safety of ranitidine maintenance treatment of duodenal ulcer. Scand J Gastroenterol 1984;19:394.

925. Walan A, Bianchi-Porro G, Hentschel E, Bardhan KD, Delattre M. Maintenance treatment with cimetidine in peptic ulcer disease for up to 4 years. Scand J Gastroenterol 1987;22:397.

926. Bardhan KD. Six years of continuous cimetidine treatment in peptic ulcer disease: Efficacy and safety. Aliment Pharmacol Ther 1988;2:395.

927. Jensen D, Machicado G, Kovacs T, et al. Long-term recurrence rates of peptic ulceration and rebleeding with H2 maintenance therapy (abstr). Gastroenterology 1989;98:A239.

928. Bardhan KD. Intermittent treatment of duodenal ulcer for long term medical management. Postgrad Med J 1988;64(Suppl 1):40.

929. Wormsley KG. Long-term treatment of duodenal ulcer. Postgrad Med J 1988;64(Suppl 1):47.

930. Pounder RE. Model of medical treatment for duodenal ulcer. Lancet 1981;1:29.

931. Axon ATR. Potential hazards of hypochlorhydria in the treatment of peptic ulcer. Scand J Gastroenterol 1986;21(Suppl 122):17.

932. Hill M. Normal and pathological microbial flora of the upper gastrointestinal tract. Scand J Gastroenterol 1985;20(Suppl 111):1.

933. Cook GC. Infective gastroenteritis and its relationship to reduced gastric acidity. Scand J Gastroenterol 1985;20(Suppl 111):17.

934. Stockbrugger RW. Bacterial overgrowth as a consequence of reduced gastric acidity. Scand J Gastroenterol 1985;20(Suppl 111):7.

935. Forrest JAH, Fettes MR, McLoughlin GP, Heading RC. Effect of long-term cimetidine on gastric acid secretion, serum gastrin, and gastric emptying. Gut 1979;20:404.

936. Sewing KF, Hagie L, Ippoliti AF, et al. Effect of one-month treatment with cimetidine on gastric secretion and serum gastrin and pepsinogen levels. Gastroenterology 1978;74:376.

937. Lundegardh G, Adami H, Helmick C, Zack M, Meirik O. Stomach cancer after partial gastrectomy for benign ulcer disease. N Engl J Med 1988;319:195.

938. Andersen D. Prevention of ulcer recurrence—Medical vs surgical treatment. The surgeon's view. Scand J Gastroenterol 1985;20(Suppl 110):89.

939. Walan A, Strom M. Prevention of ulcer recurrence—Medical vs surgical treatment. The physician's view. Scand J Gastroenterol 1985;20(Suppl 110):83.

940. Van Deventer GM. Approaches to the long-term treatment of duodenal ulcer disease. Am J Med 1984;77(Suppl 5B):15.

941. Schirmer B. Current status of proximal gastric vagotomy. Ann Surg 1989;209:131.

942. Jensen H-E, Kjaergaard J, Meisner S. Ulcer recurrence two to twelve years after parietal cell vagotomy for duodenal ulcer. Surgery 1983;94:802.

943. Berstad A, Aadland E, Bjerke K. Cimetidine treatment of recurrent ulcer after proximal gastric vagotomy. Scand J Gastroenterol 1981;16:891.

944. Harling H, Balslev I, Bentzen E. Parietal cell vagotomy or cimetidine maintenance therapy for duodenal ulcer. Scand J Gastroenterol 1985;20:747.

945. Sonnenberg A. Costs of medical and surgical treatment of duodenal ulcer. Gastroenterology 1989;96:1445.

946. Bardhan KD. Refractory duodenal ulcer. Gut 1984;25:711.

947. Bardhan KD. Omeprazole in the management of refractory duodenal ulcer. Scand J Gastroenterol 1989;24(Suppl 166):63.

948. Walt RP, Daneshmend TK. Resistant duodenal ulcer: When, why and what to do? Postgrad Med J 1988;64:369.

949. Bianchi Porro G, Parente F. Duodenal ulcers resistant to H2 blockers: An emerging therapeutic problem. Scand J Gastroenterol 1988;23(Suppl 153):81.

950. Collen M, Stanczak V, Ciarleglio C. Refractory duodenal ulcers (nonhealing duodenal ulcers with standard doses of antisecretory medication). Dig Dis Sci 1989;34:233.

951. Deakin M, Colin-Jones DG, Williams JG. Pharmacological response to cimetidine and healing of duodenal ulceration: Effects of high-

dose cimetidine and combination of cimetidine with pirenzepine. Aliment Pharmacol Ther 1988;2:83.

952. Primrose JN, Axon ATR, Johnston D. Highly selective vagotomy and duodenal ulcers that fail to respond to H$_2$-receptor antagonists. Br Med J 1988;296:1031.

953. Strom M, Berstad A, Bodemar G, et al. Results of short and long-term cimetidine treatment in patients with juxtapyloric ulcers, with special reference to gastric acid and pepsin secretion. Scand J Gastroenterol 1986;21:521.

954. Gledhill L, Buck M, Hunt RH. Effect of no treatment, cimetidine 1 g/day, cimetidine 2 g/day and cimetidine combined with atropine on nocturnal gastric secretion in cimetidine non-responders. Gut 1984;25:1211.

955. Jones DB, Howden CW, Burget DW, Silletti C, Hunt RH. Alteration of H2 receptor sensitivity in duodenal ulcer patients after maintenance treatment with an H2 receptor antagonist. Gut 1988;29:890.

956. Prichard PJ, Jones DB, Yeomans ND, et al. The effectiveness of ranitidine in reducing gastric acid-secretion decreases with continued therapy. Br J Clin Pharmacol 1986;22:663.

957. Kelly K, Malagelada J. Medical and surgical treatment of chronic gastric ulcer. Clin Gastroenterol 1984;13:621.

958. Adkins R, Delozier J, Scott H, Sawyers J. The management of gastric ulcers. A current review. Ann Surg 1985;201:741.

959. Mountford RA, Brown P, Salmon PR, et al. Gastric cancer detection in gastric ulcer disease. Gut 1980;21:9.

960. Podolsky I, Storms P, Richardson C, et al. Gastric adenocarcinoma masquerading endoscopically as benign gastric ulcer. Dig Dis Sci 1988;33:1057.

961. Graham D, Schwartz J, Cain GD, et al. Prospective evaluation of biopsy number in the diagnosis of esophageal and gastric carcinoma. Gastroenterology 1982;82:228.

962. Farini R, Farinati F, Cardin F, et al. Evidence of gastric carcinoma during follow up of apparently benign gastric ulcer. Gut 1983;141:A486.

963. Ciclitira P, Machell R, Farthing M, Dick A, Hunter J. Double-blind controlled trial of cimetidine in the healing of gastric ulcer. Gut 1977;20:730.

964. Soll AH, Kurata J, McGuigan J. Ulcers, nonsteroidal antiinflammatory drugs, and related matters. Gastroenterology 1989;96:561.

965. Pounder RE. Duodenal ulcers that are difficult to heal. Reinvestigate and change the treatment. Br Med J 1988;297:1560.

966. Quatrini M, Basilisco G, Bianchi Porro E. Treatment of "cimetidine-resistant" chronic duodenal ulcers with ranitidine or cimetidine: A randomised multicentre study. Gut 1984;25:1113.

967. Bardhan KD, Thompson M, Bose K, et al. Combined anti-muscarinic and H$_2$-receptor blockade in the healing of refractory duodenal ulcer. A double blind study. Gut 1987;28:1505.

968. Tytgat G, Wormsley K. 100% healing with omeprazole of peptic ulcers resistant to histamine H$_2$-receptor antagonists. Gastroenterology 1985;88:A1620.

969. Sontag S, Hendrix T, Hirschowitz B, et al. Omeprazole for esophagitis and ulcer refractory to H$_2$-blockers. Gastroenterology 1988;94:A436.

970. Bardhan K, Naesdal J, Bianchi Porro E, et al. Omeprazole in the treatment of refractory peptic ulcer. Gastroenterology 1988;94:A22.

971. Pen JH, Michielsen PP, Pelckmans, PA et al. Omeprazole in the treatment of H$_2$-resistant gastroduodenal ulcers. Gastroenterology 1988;94:A348.

972. Guerreiro AS, Neves BC, Quina MG. Omeprazole in the treatment of peptic ulcers resistant to H$_2$-receptor antagonists. Aliment Pharmacol Ther 1990;4:309.

973. Delchier JC, Isal JP, Eriksson, et al. Double blind multicentre comparison of omeprazole 20 mg once daily versus ranitidine 150 mg twice daily in the treatment of cimetidine or ranitidine resistant duodenal ulcers. Gut 1989;30:1173.

974. Bardhan K, Naesdal J, Bianchi P, et al. Omeprazole in the treatment of refractory peptic ulcer (RPU). Gastroenterology 1988;94:A22.

975. Bianchi Porro G, Parente F, Lazzaroni M. Tripotassium dicitrato bismuthate (TDB) versus two different dosages of cimetidine in the treatment of resistant duodenal ulcers. Gut 1987;28:907.

976. Lam SK, Lee NW, Koo J, et al. Randomised crossover trial of tripotassium dicitrato bismuthate versus high dose cimetidine for duodenal ulcers resistant to standard dose of cimetidine. Gut 1984;25:703.

977. Tytgat GNJ, Rauws EAJ. Eradication of Helicobacter pylori cures duodenal ulcer. Lancet 1990;355:1233.

978. Chilovi F, Piazzi L, Dobrilla G. Sucralfate (S) v H$_2$-antagonists (H$_2$-A) in DU non-responders (non-R) to initial treatment with sucralfate. Gut 1988;29:A1442.

979. Brunner G, Greutzfelt W. Therapy with omeprazole in patients with peptic ulcerations resistant to extended high-dose ranitidine treatment. Digestion 1988;39:80.

980. Farinati F, Cardin F, Di Mario F, et al. Early and advanced gastric cancer during follow-up of apparently benign gastric ulcer: Significance of the presence of epithelial dysplasia. J Surg Oncol 1987;36:263.

981. McCarthy D. Nonsteroidal antiinflammatory drug–induced ulcers: Management by traditional therapies. Gastroenterology 1989;96:662.

982. Schoen R, Vender R. Mechanisms of nonsteroidal anti-inflammatory drug–induced gastric damage. Am J Med 1989;86:449.

983. Butt J, Barthel J, Moore R. Clinical spectrum of the upper gastrointestinal effects of nonsteroidal anti-inflammatory drugs. Am J Med 1988;84(Suppl 2A):5.

984. Lanza F, Aspinall R, Swabb E. Double-blind, placebo-controlled endoscopic comparison of the mucosal protective effects of misoprostol versus cimetidine on tolmetin-induced mucosal injury to the stomach and duodenum. Gastroenterology 1988;95:289.

985. Aadland E, Fausa O, Vatn M. Protection by misoprostol against naproxen-induced gastric mucosal damage. Am J Med 1987;83(Suppl 1A):37.

986. Jiranek GC, Kimmey MB, Saunders DR, et al. Misoprostol reduces gastroduodenal injury from one week of aspirin: An endoscopic study. Gastroenterology 1989;96:656.

987. Graham D. Prevention of gastroduodenal injury induced by chronic nonsteroidal antiinflammatory drug therapy. Gastroenterology 1989;96:675.

988. Roth S, Bennett R. Nonsteroidal anti-inflammatory drug gastropathy. Recognition and response. Arch Intern Med 1987;147:2093.

989. Griffin M, Ray W, Schaffner W. Nonsteroidal anti-inflammatory drug use and death from peptic ulcer in elderly persons. Ann Intern Med 1988;109:359.

990. Roth S. Nonsteroidal anti-inflammatory drugs: Gastropathy, deaths, and medical practice. Ann Intern Med 1988;109:353.

991. Larkai E, Lacey Smith J, Lidsky M, et al. Dyspepsia in NSAID users: The size of the problem. J Clin Gastroenterol 1989;11(2):158.

992. Larkai E, Lacey Smith J, Lidsky M, et al. Gastroduodenal mucosa and dyspeptic symptoms in arthritic patients during chronic nonsteroidal anti-inflammatory drug use. Am J Gastroenterol 1987;82:1153.

993. Ehsanullah RSB, Page MC, Tildesley G, et al. Prevention of gastroduodenal damage induced by non-steroidal anti-inflammatory drugs: Controlled trial of ranitidine. Br Med J 1988;297:1017.

994. Barrier C, Hirschowitz B. Controversies in the detection and management of nonsteroidal antiinflammatory drug–induced side effects of the upper gastrointestinal tract. Arthritis Rheum 1989;32:926.

995. Armstrong CP, Blower AL. Non-steroidal anti-inflammatory drugs and life threatening complications of peptic ulceration. Gut 1987;28:527.

996. Manniche C, Malchow-Moller A, Andersen JR, et al. Randomised study of the influence of non-steroidal anti-inflammatory drugs on the treatment of peptic ulcer in patients with rheumatic disease. Gut 1987;28:226.

997. O'Laughlin JC, Silvoso GR, Ivey KJ. Healing of aspirin associated peptic ulcer disease despite continued salicylate ingestion. Arch Intern Med 1981;141:781.

998. Bijlsma JWJ. Treatment of NSAID-induced gastrointestinal lesions with cimetidine—An international multicenter collaborative study. Aliment Pharmacol Ther 1988;2(Suppl 2):85.

999. Roth S, Agrawal N, Mahowald M, et al. Misoprostol heals gastroduodenal injury in patients with rheumatoid arthritis receiving aspirin. Arch Intern Med 1989;149:775.

1000. Jaszewski R, Calzada R, Dhar R. Persistence of gastric ulcers caused by plain aspirin or nonsteroidal antiinflammatory agents in patients treated with a combination of cimetidine, antacids, and enteric-coated aspirin. Dig Dis Sci 1989;34:1361.

1001. O'Laughlin J, Silvoso G, Ivey K. Resistance to medical therapy of gastric ulcers in rheumatic disease patients taking aspirin. Dig Dis Sci 1982;27:976.

1002. Caldwell J, Roth S, Wu W, Semble E. Sucralfate treatment of nonsteroidal anti-inflammatory drug-induced gastrointestinal symptoms and mucosal damage. Am J Med 1987;83(Suppl 3B):74.

1003. Bijlsma JWJ. Treatment of endoscopy negative NSAID-induced upper gastrointestinal symptoms with cimetidine—An international multicenter collaborative study. Aliment Pharmacol Ther 1988;2(Suppl 2):75.

1004. Lanza F, Robinson M, Bowers J, et al. A multi-center double-blind comparison of ranitidine vs. placebo in the prophylaxis of non-steroidal anti-inflammatory drug (NSAID) induced lesions in gastric and duodenal mucosae (abstr). Gastroenterology 1988;94:A250.

1005. Graham D, Agrawal N, Roth S. Prevention of NSAID-induced gastric ulcer with misoprostol: Multicentre, double-blind, placebo-controlled trial. Lancet 1988;2:1277.

1006. Hillman A, Bloom B. Economic effect of prophylactic use of misoprostol to prevent gastric ulcer patients taking nonsteroidal anti-inflammatory drugs. Arch Intern Med 1989;149:2061.

1007. Editorial. Misoprostol: Ulcer prophylaxis at what cost? Lancet 1988;2:1293.

1008. Lauritsen K, Rune SJ, Wulff HR, et al. Effect of omeprazole and cimetidine on prepyloric gastric ulcer: Double blind comparative trial. Gut 1988;29:249.

1009. Widerlite L, Trier JS, Blacklow NR, et al. Structure of the gastric mucosa in acute infectious nonbacterial gastroenteritis. Gastroenterology 1975;68:425.

1010. Whitehead R. Mucosal biopsy of the gastrointestinal tract, Vol 3. Philadelphia: WB Saunders, 1985.

1011. Weinstein WM. Gastritis. In: Sleisenger MH, Fordtran JS, eds. Gastrointestinal disease. Philadelphia: WB Saunders, 1989:792.

1012. Fenoglio-Preiser CM, Lantz PE, Listrom MB, Davis M, Rilke FO. Gastrointestinal pathology. An atlas and text. New York: Raven Press, 1989.

1013. Strickland RG, Mackay IR. A reappraisal of the nature and significance of chronic atrophic gastritis. Am J Dig Dis 1973;18:426.

1014. Larkai EN, Smith JL, Lidsky MD, Graham DY. Gastroduodenal mucosa and dyspeptic symptoms in arthritic patients during chronic nonsteroidal anti-inflammatory drug use. Am J Gastroenterol 1987;82:1153.

1015. Davenport HW, Warner HA, Code CF. Functional significance of gastric mucosal barrier to sodium. Gastroenterology 1964;47:142.

1016. Davenport HW. Salicylate damage to the gastric mucosal barrier. N Engl J Med 1967;276:1307.

1017. Kauffman G. Aspirin-induced mucosal injury: Lessons learned from animal models. Gastroenterology 1989;96:606.

1018. Stern AI, Hogan DL, Isenberg JI. A new method for quantitation of ion fluxes across in-vivo human gastric mucosa: Effect of aspirin, acetaminophen, ethanol and hyperosmolar solutions. Gastroenterology 1984;86:60.

1019. Robert A. Cytoprotection by prostaglandins. Gastroenterology 1979;77:761.

1020. Robert A. Prostaglandins and the gastrointestinal tract. In: Johnson LR, ed. Physiology of the gastrointestinal tract. New York: Raven Press, 1981:1407.

1021. Miller TA. Protective effects of prostaglandins against gastric mucosal damage: Current knowledge and proposed mechanisms. Am J Physiol 1983;245:G601.

1022. Olson GA, Leffler CW, Fletcher AM. Gastroduodenal ulceration in rabbits producing antibodies to prostaglandins. Prostaglandins 1985;29:475.

1023. Redfern JS, Blair AJ, Lee E, Feldman M. Gastrointestinal ulcer formation in rabbits immunized with prostaglandin E. Gastroenterology 1987;93:744.

1024. Robert A, Nezamis JE, Lancaster C, Davis JP, Field SO, Hanchar AJ. Mild irritants prevent gastric necrosis through "adaptive cytoprotection" mediated by prostaglandins. Am J Physiol 1983;245:G113.

1025. Konturek SJ, Brzozowski T, Piastucki I, Radecki T, Dembinski A, Dembinski-Kiec A. Role of locally generated prostaglandins in adaptive gastric cytoprotection. Dig Dis Sci 1982;27:967.

1026. Ito S, Lacy ER. Morphology of rat gastric mucosal damage, defense, and restitution in the presence of luminal ethanol. Gastroenterology 1985;88:250.

1027. Lacy ER, Ito S. Rapid epithelial restitution of the rat gastric mucosa after ethanol injury. Lab Invest 1984;51:573.

1028. Silen W, Ito S. Mechanisms for rapid re-epithelialization of the gastric mucosal surface. Annu Rev Physiol 1985;47:217.

1029. Silen W. Gastric mucosal defense and repair. In: Johnson LR, ed. Physiology of the gastrointestinal tract, ed 2. New York: Raven Press, 1987:1055.

1030. Neutra MR. The gastrointestinal tract. In: Weiss L, ed. Cell and tissue biology. Baltimore: Urban & Schwarzenberg, 1988:643.

1031. Lipkin M. Proliferation and differentiation of gastrointestinal cells in normal and disease states. In: Johnson LR, ed. Physiology of the gastrointestinal tract, ed 2. New York: Raven Press, 1987:255.

1032. Kim YS, Kerr R, Lipkin M. Cell proliferation during the development of stress erosions in mouse stomach. Nature 1967;215:1180.

1033. Whittle BJR, Oren-Wolman N, Guth PH. Gastric vasoconstrictor actions of leukotriene C_4, $PGF_{2\alpha}$, and thromboxane mimetic U-46619 on rat submucosal microcirculation in vivo. Am J Physiol 1985;248:G580.

1034. Whittle BJR, Kauffman GL, Moncada S. Vasoconstriction with thromboxane A_2 induces ulceration of the gastric mucosa. Nature 1981;292:472.

1035. Kauffman GL Jr, Whittle BJR. Gastric vascular actions of prostanoids and the dual effect of arachidonic acid. Am J Physiol 1982;242:G582.

1036. Gulati N, Philpot ME, Gulati OP, Mahnsten C, Huggel H. Effects of leukotriene C_4 and prostaglandin E_2 on the rat mesentery in vitro and in vivo. Prostaglandins Leukot Med 1983;10:257.

1037. Peskar BM, Lange K, Hoppe U, Peskar BA. Ethanol stimulates formation of leukotriene C_4 in rat gastric mucosa. Prostaglandins 1986;31:283.

1038. Trier JS, Szabo S, Allan CH. Ethanol-induced damage to mucosal capillaries of rat stomach. Gastroenterology 1987;92:13.

1039. Itoh M, Guth PH. Role of oxygen-derived free radicals in hemorrhagic shock-induced gastric lesions in the rat. Gastroenterology 1985;88:1162.

1040. Mizui T, Doteuchi M. Lipid peroxidation: A possible role in gastric damage induced by ethanol in rats. Life Sci 1986;38:2163.

1041. Lucas CE, Sugawa C, Riddle J, Rector F, Rosenburg B, Walt AJ. Natural history and surgical dilemma of "stress" gastric bleeding. Arch Surg 1971;102:266.

1042. Skillman JJ, Bushnell LS, Goldman H, Silen W. Respiratory failure, hypotension, sepsis and jaundice: A clinical syndrome associated with lethal hemorrhage from acute stress ulceration of the stomach. Am J Surg 1971;123:25.

1043. Marrone GC, Silen W. Pathogenesis, diagnosis and treatment of acute gastric mucosal lesions. Clin Gastroenterol 1984;13:635.

1044. Zinner MJ, Zuidema GD, Smith PL, Mignosa M. The prevention of upper gastrointestinal tract bleeding in patients in an intensive care unit. Surg Gynecol Obstet 1981;153:214.

1045. Fiddian-Green RG, McGough E, Pittenger G, Rothman E. Predictive value of intramural pH and other risk factors for massive bleeding from stress ulceration. Gastroenterology 1983;85:613.

1046. Stremple JF, Mori H, Lev R, Glass GBJ. The stress ulcer syndrome. Curr Probl Surg 1973;10(4):3.

1047. Schuster DP, Rowley H, Feinstein S, McGue MK, Zucherman GR. Prospective evaluation of the risk of upper gastrointestinal bleeding after admission to a medical intensive care unit. Am J Med 1984;76:623.

1048. Peura DA, Johnson LF. Cimetidine for prevention and treatment of gastroduodenal mucosal lesions in patients in an intensive care unit. Ann Intern Med 1985;103:173.

1049. Curling TB. On acute ulceration of the duodenum in cases of burns. Med Surg Trans (London) 1842;25:260.

1050. Czaja AJ, McAlhany JC, Pruitt BA. Acute gastroduodenal disease after thermal injury: An endoscopic evaluation of incidence and natural history. N Engl J Med 1974;291:925.

1051. Pruit BA, Goodwin CW. Stress ulcer disease in the burned patient. World J Surg 1981;5:209.

1052. Sevitt S. Duodenal and gastric ulceration after burning. Br J Surg 1967;54:32.

1053. David E, McIlrath DC, Higgins JA. Clinical experience with acute peptic gastrointestinal ulcers. Mayo Clin Proc 1971;46:15.

1054. Cushing H. Peptic ulcers and the interbrain. Surg Gynecol Obstet 1932;55:1.

1055. Bowen JC, Fleming WH, Thompson JC. Increased gastrin release following penetrating central nervous system injury. Surgery 1974;75:720.

1056. Kamada T, Fusamoto H, Kawano S, Hoguchi M, Hiramatsu K, Masazawa M, Abe H, Fuggi C, Sugimoto T. Gastrointestinal bleeding following head injury, a clinical study of 433 cases. J Trauma 1977;17:44.

1057. Haloran LG, Zfass AM, Gayle WE, Wheeler CB, Miller JD. Prevention of acute gastrointestinal complications after severe head injury: A controlled trial of cimetidine prophylaxis. Am J Surg 1980;139:44.

1058. Gordon MJ, Skillman JJ, Zervas WT, Silen W. Divergent nature of gastric mucosal permeability in gastric acid secretion in sick patients with general and neurosurgical disease. Ann Surg 1973;178:285.

1059. Watts C, Clark K. Gastric acidity in the comatose patient. J Neurosurg 1969;30:107.

1060. French JD, Porter RW, von Amerongen FK, Raney RB. Gastrointestinal hemorrhage and ulceration associated with intracranial lesions. Surgery 1952;32:395.

1061. Odonkor P, Mowat C, Himal HS. Prevention of sepsis-induced gastric lesions in dogs by cimetidine via inhibition of gastric secretion and by prostaglandin via cytoprotection. Gastroenterology 1981;80:375.

1062. Murakami M, Lam SK, Inada M, Miyake T. Pathophysiology and pathogenesis of acute gastric mucosal lesions after hypothermic restraint stress in rats. Gastroenterology 1985;88:660.

1063. Robert A, Leung FW, Guth PH. Ulcer potentiation by stress and aspirin: Role of acid, mucosal blood flow and prostaglandins. Gastroenterology 1989;97:1147.

1064. Payne JG, Bowen JC. Hypoxia of canine gastric mucosa caused by Escherichia coli sepsis and prevented with methylprednisolone therapy. Gastroenterology 1981;80:84.

1065. Garrick T, Leung FW, Buack S, Hirabayashi K, Guth PH. Gastric motility is stimulated but overall blood flow is unaffected during cold restraint in the rat. Gastroenterology 1986;91:141.

1066. McAlhany JC, Czaja AJ, Pruitt BA. Antacid control of complications from acute gastroduodenal disease after burns. J Trauma 1976;16:645.

1067. Jones RH, Rudge CJ, Bewick M, Parsons V, Weston MJ. Cimetidine: Prophylaxis against upper gastrointestinal haemorrhage after renal transplantation. Br Med J 1978;1:398.

1068. McElwee HP, Sirinek KR, Levine BA. Cimetidine affords protection of stress ulceration following thermal injury. Surgery 1979;86:620.

1069. Priebe HJ, Skillman JJ, Bushnell LS, Long PC, Silen W. Antacids versus cimetidine in preventing acute gastrointestinal bleeding: A randomized trial of 75 critically ill patients. N Engl J Med 1980;302:426.

1070. Groll A, Simon JB, Wigle RD, Tagichi K, Todd RJ, Depew WT. Cimetidine prophylaxis for gastrointestinal bleeding in an intensive care unit. Gut 1986;27:135.

1071. Poleski MH, Spanier AH. Cimetidine versus antacids in the prevention of stress erosions in critically ill patients. Am J Gastroenterol 1986;81:107.

1072. Ostro MJ, Russell JA, Soldin SJ, Mahon WA, Jeejeebhoy KN. Control of gastric pH with cimetidine: Boluses versus primed infusion. Gastroenterology 1985;89:532.

1073. Driks MR, Craven DE, Celli BR, Manning M, Burke RA, Garvin GM, Kunches LM, Farber HW, Wedel SA, McCabe WR. Nosocomial pneumonia in intubated patients given sucralfate as compared with antacids or histamine type 2 blockers: The role of gastric colonization. N Engl J Med 1987;317:1376.

1074. Tryba M. The risk of acute stress bleeding and nosocomial pneumonia in ventilated ICU patients: Sucralfate vs antacids. Am J Med 1987;83:117.

1075. Borrero E, Margolis IB, Bank S. A randomized trial of sucralfate vs antacid in preventing acute gastrointestinal bleeding in 100 critically ill patients. Am J Surg 1984;148:809.

1076. Borrero E, Ciervo J, Chang JB. Antacids vs sucralfate in preventing acute gastrointestinal tract bleeding in abdominal aortic surgery. Arch Surg 1986;121:810.

1077. Tryba M, Zevourow F, Torok M, Zeng M. Prevention of acute stress bleeding with sucralfate, antacids, or cimetidine: A controlled study with pirenzepine as a basic medication. Am J Med 1985;79(Suppl 2C):55.

1078. Zimmer MJ, Rypins EB, Martin LR, et al. Misoprostol versus antacid titration for preventing stress ulcers in postoperative surgical ICU patients. Ann Surg 1989;210:590.

1079. Guth PH. Gastric blood flow in ethanol injury and prostaglandin cytoprotection. Scand J Gastroenterol 1986;21(Suppl 125):86.

1080. Laine L, Bentley E, Chandrasoma P. The effect of oral iron therapy on the upper gastrointestinal tract: A prospective evaluation. Dig Dis Sci 1988;33:172.

1081. Moore JG, Alsop WR, Freston JW, Tolman KG. The effect of oral potassium chloride on upper gastrointestinal mucosa in healthy subjects: Healing of lesions despite continuing treatment. Gastrointest Endosc 1986;32:210.

1082. Lowe JE, Graham DY, Boisaubin EV, Lanza FL. Corrosive injury to the stomach: The natural history and role of fiberoptic endoscopy. Am J Surg 1979;137:803.

1083. Cello JP, Fogel RP, Boland R. Liquid caustic ingestion spectrum of injury. Arch Intern Med 1980;140:501.

1084. Di Costanzo J, Noirclerc M, Jouglard J, Escoffier JM, Cano N, Martin J, Gauthier A. New therapeutic approach to corrosive burns of the upper gastrointestinal tract. Gut 1982;21:370.

1085. Weinstein WM, Buch KL, Elashoff J, Reedy T, Tedesco FJ, Samloff IM, Ippoliti AF. The histology of the stomach in symptomatic patients after gastric surgery: A model to assess selective patterns of gastric mucosal injury. Scand J Gastroenterol 1985;20(Suppl 109):77.

1086. Meyer JH. Editorial: Reflections on reflux gastritis. Gastroenterology 1979;77:1143.

1087. Hoare AM, Jones EL, Alexander-Williams J, Hawkins CF. Symptomatic significance of gastric mucosal changes after surgery for peptic ulcer. Gut 1977;18:295.

1088. Saukkonen M, Sipponen P, Varis K, Siurala M. Morphologic and dynamic behavior of the gastric mucosa after partial gastrectomy with special reference to the gastroenterostomy area. Hepatogastroenterology 1980;27:48.

1089. Ritchie WP. Alkaline reflux gastritis: A critical reappraisal. Gut 1984;25:975.

1090. Meshkinpour H, Elashoff J, Steward H, Sturdevant RAL. Effect of cholestyramine on the symptoms of reflux gastritis. Gastroenterology 1977;73:441.

1091. Malagelada JR, Phillips SF, Higgins JA. A prospective evaluation of alkaline reflux gastritis. Bile acid binding agents and Roux-en-Y diversion. Gastroenterology 1979;76:1192.

1092. Warshaw AL. Intragastric alkali infusion. Simple, accurate provocative test for diagnosis of symptomatic alkaline reflux gastritis. Ann Surg 1983;194:297.

1093. Shepherd HA, Harvey J, Jackson A, Colin-Jones DG. Recurrent retching with gastric mucosal prolapse: A proposed prolapse gastropathy syndrome. Dig Dis Sci 1984;29:121.

1094. Cameron AJ, Higgins JA. Linear gastric erosion. A lesion associated with large diaphragmatic hernia and chronic blood loss anemia. Gastroenterology 1986;91:338.

1095. Bown SG, Swain CP, Storey DW, Collins C, Matthewson K, Salmon PR, Clark CG. Endoscopic laser treatment of vascular anomalies of the upper gastrointestinal tract. Gut 1985;26:1338.

1096. Shepherd HA, Patel C, Bamforth J, Isaacson P. Upper gastrointestinal endoscopy in systemic vasculitis presenting as an acute abdomen. Endoscopy 1983;15:307.

1097. Bourdages R, Prentice RSA, Beck IT, Dacosta LR, Paloschi GB. Atheromatous embolization to the stomach: An unusual cause of gastrointestinal bleeding. Am J Dig Dis 1976;21:889.

1098. Cherry RD, Jabbari M, Goresky CA, Herba M, Reich D, Blundell PE. Chronic mesenteric vascular insufficiency with gastric ulceration. Gastroenterology 1986;91:1548.

1099. Hojgaard L, Krag E. Chronic ischemic gastritis reversed after revascularization operation. Gastroenterology 1987;92:226.

1100. Clayman CB, Palmer WL, Kirsner JB. Gastric irradiation in the treatment of peptic ulcer. Gastroenterology 1968;55:403.

1101. Goldgraber MB, Rubin CE, Palmer WL, Dobson RL, Massey BW. The early gastric response to irradiation, a serial biopsy study. Gastroenterology 1954;27:1.

1102. Berthrong M, Fajardo LF. Radiation injury in surgical pathology. Part II. Alimentary tract. Am J Surg Pathol 1981;5:153.

1103. Akdamar K, Ertan A, Agrawal NM, McMahon FG, Ryan J. Upper gastrointestinal endoscopy in normal asymptomatic volunteers. Gastrointest Endosc 1986;32:78.

1104. Ihamaki T, Varis K, Siurala M. Morphological, functional and immunological state of the gastric mucosa in gastric carcinoma families: Comparison with a computer-matched family sample. Scand J Gastroenterol 1979;14:801.

1105. Nesland AA, Berstad A. Erosive prepyloric changes in persons with and without dyspepsia. Scand J Gastroenterol 1985;20:222.

1106. O'Brien TK, Saunders DR, Templeton FE. Chronic gastric erosions and oral aphthae. Am J Dig Dis 1972;17:447.

1107. Morgan G, McAdam WAF, Pyrah RD, Tinsley EGF. Multiple recurring gastric erosions (aphthous ulcers). Gut 1976;17:633.

1108. Lambert R, Andre C, Moulinier B, Bugnon B. Diffuse varioliform gastritis. Digestion 1978;17:159.

1109. Elta GH, Fawaz KA, Dayal Y, McLean AM, Phillips E, Bloom SM, Paul RE, Kaplan MM. Chronic erosive gastritis—A recently recognized disorder. Dig Dis Sci 1983;28:7.

1110. Franzin G, Manfrini C, Musola R, Rodella S, Fratton A. Chronic erosions of the stomach—A clinical, endoscopic and histological evaluation. Endoscopy 1984;16:1.

1111. Haot J, Berger F, Andre C, Moulinier B, Lambert R, Mainguet P. Lymphocytic gastritis versus varioliform gastritis. A historical series revisited. J Pathol 1989;158:19.

1112. Haot J, Jouret A, Willette M, et al. Lymphocytic gastritis—Prospective study of its relationship with varioliform gastritis. Gut 1990;31:282.

1113. Farthing MJG, Fairclough PD, Hegarty JE, Swarbrick ET, Dawson AM. Treatment of chronic erosive gastritis with prednisolone. Gut 1981;22:759.

1114. Andre C, Gillon J, Moulinier B, Martin A, Fargier MC. Randomised placebo-controlled double-blind trial of two doses of sodium cromoglycate in treatment of varioliform gastritis: Comparison with cimetidine. Gut 1982;23:348.

1115. Haot J, Hamichi L, Wallez L, Mainguet P. Lymphocytic gastritis: A newly described entity, a retrospective endoscopic and histological study. Gut 1988;29:1258.

1116. Wood IJ, Taft LI. Diffuse lesions of the stomach. London: Edward Arnold, 1958.

1117. MacDonald WC, Rubin CE. Gastric biopsy—A critical evaluation. Gastroenterology 1967;53:143.

1118. Haenszel W, Correa P, Cuello C, Guzman N, Burbano LC, Lores H, Munoz J. Gastric cancer in Colombia. II. Case-control epidemiologic study of precursor lesions. J Natl Cancer Inst 1976;57:1021.

1119. Kreuning J, Bosman FT, Kuiper G, Wall AM, Lindeman J. Gastric and duodenal mucosa in "healthy" individuals. J Clin Pathol 1978;31:69.

1120. Cheli R, Simon L, Aste H, Figus IA, Nicolo G, Bajtai A, Puntoni R. Atrophic gastritis and intestinal metaplasia in asymptomatic Hungarian and Italian populations. Endoscopy 1980;12:105.

1121. Siurala M, Varis K, Kekki M. New aspects of epidemiology, genetics, and dynamics of chronic gastritis. In: van der Reis L, ed. Frontiers of gastrointestinal research. The Stomach. Basel: S. Karger 1980;6:148.

1122. Pettross CW, Appleman MD, Cohen H, Valenzuela JE, Chandrasoma P, Laine LA. Prevalence of Campylobacter pylori and association with antral mucosal histology in subjects with and without upper gastrointestinal symptoms. Dig Dis Sci 1988;33:649.

1123. Rauws EA, Langenberg W, Houthoff HJ, Zanen HC, Tytgat GN. Campylobacter pyloridis–associated chronic active antral gastritis: A prospective study of its prevalence and the effects of antibacterial and antiulcer treatment. Gastroenterology 1988;94:33.

1124. Barthel JS, Westblom TU, Havey AD, Gonzalez F, Everett ED. Gastritis and Campylobacter pylori in healthy, asymptomatic volunteers. Arch Intern Med 1988;148:1149.

1125. Siurala M, Isokoski M, Varis K, Kekki M. Prevalence of gastritis in a rural population: Bioptic study of subjects selected at random. Scand J Gastroenterol 1968;3:211.

1126. Ihamaki T, Varis K, Siurala M. Morphological, functional and immunological state of the gastric mucosa in gastric carcinoma families: Comparison with a computer-matched sample. Scand J Gastroenterol 1979;14:801.

1127. Villako K, Tamm A, Savisaar E, Ruttas M. Prevalence of antral and fundic gastritis in a randomly selected group of an Estonian rural population. Scand J Gastroenterol 1976;11:817.

1128. Correa P, Cuello C, Duque E, et al. Gastric cancer in Colombia. III. Natural history of precursor lesions. J Natl Cancer Inst 1976;57:1027.

1129. Dooley CP, Cohen H, Fitzgibbons P, et al. Prevalence of Helicobacter pylori infection and histologic gastritis in asymptomatic persons. N Engl J Med 1989;321:1562.

1130. Krasinski SD, Russell RM, Samloff IM, Jacob RA, Dallal GE, McGandy RB, Hartz SC. Fundic atrophic gastritis in an elderly population. Effect on hemoglobin and several serum nutritional indicators. J Am Geriatr Soc 1986;34:800.

1131. Imai T, Kubo T, Watanabe H. Chronic gastritis in Japanese with reference to high incidence of gastric carcinoma. J Natl Cancer Inst 1971;47:179.

1132. Magnus HA. Observations on the presence of intestinal epithelium in the gastric mucosa. J Pathol Bacteriol 1937;44:389.

1133. Stout AP. Gastric mucosal atrophy and carcinoma of the stomach. N Y State J Med 1945;45:973.

1134. Morson BC. Intestinal metaplasia of the gastric mucosa. Br J Cancer 1955;9:365.

1135. Rubin W, Ross LL, Sleisenger MH, Jeffries GH. The normal human gastric epithelia. A fine structural study. Lab Invest 1968;19:598.

1136. Rubin W. Endocrine cells in the normal human stomach. A fine structural study. Gastroenterology 1972;63:784.

1137. Rubin W, Ross LL, Jeffries GH, Sleisenger MH. Intestinal heterotopia. A fine structural study. Lab Invest 1966;15:1024.

1138. Rubin W. Proliferation of endocrine-like (enterochromaffin) cells in atrophic gastric mucosa. Gastroenterology 1969;57:641.

1139. Field SP, Sachar DB. The immunology of pernicious anemia. In: Shorter RG, Kirsner JB, eds. Gastrointestinal immunity for the clinician. Orlando: Grune & Stratton, 1985:61.

1140. Leshin M. Southwestern internal medicine conference; Polyglandular autoimmune syndromes. Am J Med Sci 1985;290:77.

1141. Karisson FA, Burman P, Loof L, Mardh S. Major parietal cell antigen in autoimmune gastritis with pernicious anemia is the acid-producing H+, K+-adenosine triphosphatase of the stomach. J Clin Invest 1988;81:475.

1142. Jeffries GH, Todd JE, Sleisenger MH. The effect of prednisolone on gastric mucosal histology, gastric secretion, and vitamin B12 absorption in patients with pernicious anemia. J Clin Invest 1966;45:803.

1143. Borch K, Renvall H, Liedberg G, Andersen BN. Relations between circulating gastrin and endocrine cell proliferation in the atrophic gastric fundic mucosa. Scand J Gastroenterol 1986;21:357.

1144. Arnold R, Hulst MV, Neuhof CH, Schwarting H, Becker HD, Creutzfeldt W. Antral gastrin-producing G-cells and somatostatin-producing D cells in different states of gastric acid secretion. Gut 1982;23:285.

1145. Yalow RS, Berson SA. Further studies on the nature of immunoreactive gastrin in human plasma. Gastroenterology 1971;60:203.

1146. Kimura K. Chronological transition of the fundic–pyloric border determined by stepwise biopsy of the lesser and greater curvatures of the stomach. Gastroenterology 1972;63:584.

1147. Samloff IM. Cellular localization of group I pepsinogens in human gastric mucosa by immunofluorescence. Gastroenterology 1971;61:185.

1148. Cornaggia M, Capella C, Riva C, Finzi G, Solcia E. Electron immunocytochemical localization of pepsinogen I (PG I) in chief cells, mucous-neck cells and transitional mucous-neck/chief cells of the human fundic mucosa. Histochemistry 1986;85:5.

1149. Rubin W. Maturation of heterotopic intestinal epithelium. Clin Res 1969;17:310.

1150. Rubin W, Ross LL, Jeffries GH, Sleisenger MH. Some physiologic properties of heterotopic intestinal epithelium. Its role in transporting lipid into the gastric mucosa. Lab Invest 1967;16:813.

1151. Rubin W. Editorial: Intestine in the stomach. Transformation of the gastric mucosa into an absorptive tissue. Gastroenterology 1968;54:116.

1152. Rubin W. The epithelial "membrane" of the small intestine. Am J Clin Nutr 1971;24:45.

1153. Klein NC, Sleisenger MH, Weser E. Disaccharidases, leucine aminopeptidase, and glucose uptake in intestinalized gastric mucosa and in gastric carcinoma. Gastroenterology 1968;55:61.

1154. Lev R. The mucin histochemistry of normal and neoplastic gastric mucosa. Lab Invest 1965;14:2080.

1155. Rubin W. A fine structural characterization of the proliferated endocrine cells in atrophic gastric mucosa. Am J Pathol 1973;70:109.

1156. Bordi C, Gabrielli M, Missule G. Pathological changes of endocrine cells in chronic atrophic gastritis. Arch Pathol Lab Med 1978;102:129.

1157. Bordi C, Ravazzola M. Endocrine cells in the intestinal metaplasia of gastric mucosa. Am J Pathol 1979;96:391.

1158. Bordi C, Ravazzola M, DeVita O. Pathology of endocrine cells in gastric mucosa. Ann Pathol 1983;3:19.

1159. Borch K, Renvall H, Liedberg G. Gastric endocrine cell hyperplasia and carcinoid tumors in pernicious anemia. Gastroenterology 1985;88:638.

1160. Tsutsumi Y, Nagura H, Watanabe K, Yanaihara N. A novel subtyping of intestinal metaplasia of the stomach, with special reference to the histochemical characterizations of endocrine cells. Virchows Arch [A] 1983;401:73.

1161. Teglbjaerg PS, Nielsen HO. "Small intestinal type" and "colonic type" intestinal metaplasia of the human stomach. Acta Pathol Microbiol Scand 1978;86:351.

1162. Heilmann KL, Hopker WW. Loss of differentiation in intestinal metaplasia in cancerous stomachs. A comparative morphological study. Pathol Res Pract 1979;164:249.

1163. Jass J, Filipe MI. A variant of intestinal metaplasia associated with gastric carcinoma: A histochemical study. Histopathology 1979;3:191.

1164. Jass J, Filipe MI. The mucin profile of normal gastric epithelium, intestinal metaplasia and gastric carcinoma. Histochem J 1981;13:831.

1165. Segura DI, Montero C. Histochemical characterization of different types of intestinal metaplasia in gastric mucosa. Cancer 1983;52:408.

1166. Matsukura N, Suzuki K, Kawachi T, et al. Distribution of marker enzymes and mucin in intestinal metaplasia in human stomach and relation of complete and incomplete types of intestinal metaplasia to minute gastric carcinomas. J Natl Cancer Inst 1980;65:231.

1167. Sipponen P, Kekki M, Siurala M. Atrophic chronic gastritis and intestinal metaplasia in gastric carcinoma. A comparison with a representative population sample. Cancer 1983;52:1062.

1168. Filipe MI, Potet F, Bogomoletz WV, Dawson PA, Fabiani B, Chauveine P, Fenzy A, Gazzard B, Goldfain D, Zeegen R. Incomplete sulphomucin-secreting intestinal metaplasia for gastric cancer. Preliminary data from a prospective study from three centres. Gut 1985;26:1319.

1169. Sipponen P, Seppala K, Varis K, Hjelt L, Ihamaki M, Siurala M. Intestinal metaplasia with colonic-type sulphomucins in the gastric mucosa; its association with gastric carcinoma. Acta Pathol Microbiol Scand 1980;88:217.

1170. Matsukura N, Kawachi T, Sugimura T, Ohnuki T, Higo M, Itabashi M, Hirota T, Kitaoka H. Variety of phenotypical expression of intestinal marker enzymes and mucin in human stomach intestinal metaplasia. Acta Histochem Cytochem 1980;13:499.

1171. Nardelli J, Bara J, Rosa B, Burtin P. Intestinal metaplasia and carcinomas of the human stomach. J Histochem Cytochem 1983;31:366.

1172. Solcia E, Capella C, Buffa R, Usellini L, Frigerio B, Fontana P. Endocrine cells of the gastrointestinal tract and related tumors. Pathobiol Ann 1979;9:163.

1173. Solcia E, Capella C, Buffa R, Frigerio B, Sessa F, Tenti P. Histopathology and cytology of gastroenteropancreatic endocrine tumors. In: Friedman M, Ogawa M, Kisner D, eds. Diagnosis and treatment of upper gastrointestinal tumors. Amsterdam: Excerpta Medica, 1981:32.

1174. Rode J, Dhillon AP, Papadaki L, Stockbrugger R, Thompson RJ, Moss E, Cotton PB. Pernicious anaemia and mucosal endocrine cell proliferation of the non-antral stomach. Gut 1986;27:789.

1175. Bordi C, Ferrari C, D'Adda T, Pilato F, Carfagna G, Bertele A, Missale G. Ultrastructural characterization of fundic endocrine cell hyperplasia associated with atrophic gastritis and hypergastrinaemia. Virchows Arch [A] 1986;409:335.

1176. Rubin W, Schwartz B. Electron microscopic radioautographic identification of the ECL cell as the histamine-synthesizing endocrine cell in rat gastric oxyntic glands. Gastroenterology 1979;77:458.

1177. Rubin W, Schwartz B. An electron microscopic radioautographic identification of the "enterochromaffin-like" APUD cells in murine oxyntic glands. Demonstration of a metabolic difference between rat and mouse gastric A-like cells. Gastroenterology 1979;76:437.

1178. Rubin W, Schwartz B. Identification of the APUD endocrine cells of rat fundic mucosa by means of combined amine-fluorescence and electron microscopy. J Histochem Cytochem 1984;32:67.

1179. Lonroth H, Hakanson R, Lundell L, Sundler F. Histamine containing endocrine cells in the human stomach. Gut 1990;31:383.

1180. Creutzfeldt W, Arnold R, Creutzfeldt C, Feurle G, Ketterer H. Gastrin and G-cells in the antral mucosa of patients with pernicious anaemia, acromegaly, and hyperparathyroidism and in a Zollinger-Ellison tumour of the pancreas. Eur J Clin Invest 1971;1:461.

1181. Black WC, Haffner HE. Diffuse hyperplasia of gastric argyrophil cells and multiple carcinoid tumors. An historical and ultrastructural study. Cancer 1968;21:1080.

1182. Harris AI, Greenberg H. Pernicious anemia and the development of carcinoid tumors of the stomach. J Am Med Assoc 1978;239:1160.

1183. Carney JA, Go VLW, Fairbanks VF, Moore SB, Alport EC, Nora FE. The syndrome of gastric argyrophil carcinoid tumors and nonantral gastric atrophy. Ann Intern Med 1983;99:761.

1184. Rode J, Dhillon AP, Papadaki L, Stockbrugger R, Thompson RJ, Moss E, Cotton PB. Pernicious anaemia and mucosal endocrine cell proliferation of the non-antral stomach. Gut 1986;27:789.

1185. Stockbrugger RW, Menon GG, Beilby JOW, Mason RR, Cotton PB. Gastroscopic screening in 80 patients with pernicious anaemia. Gut 1983;24:1141.

1186. Moses RE, Frank BB, Leavitt M, Miller R. The syndrome of type A chronic atrophic gastritis, pernicious anemia, and multiple gastric carcinoids. J Clin Gastroenterol 1986;8:61.

1187. Bordi C, Cocconi G, Togni R, Vezzadini P, Missale G. Gastric endocrine cell proliferation. Association with Zollinger-Ellison syndrome. Arch Pathol 1974;98:274.

1188. Lehy T, Mignon M, Cadiot G, et al. Gastric endocrine cell behavior in Zollinger-Ellison patients upon long-term potent antisecretory treatment. Gastroenterology 1989;96:1029.

1189. Hakanson R, Bottcher G, Sundler F, Vallgren S. Activation and hyperplasia of gastrin and enterochromaffin-like cells in the stomach. Digestion 1986;35:23.

1190. Larsson H, Carlsson E, Mattson H, Lundell L, Sundler F, Sundell G, Wallmark B, Watanabe T, Hakanson R. Plasma gastrin and gastric enterochromaffin-like cell activation and proliferation. Studies with omeprazole and ranitidine in intact and antrectomized rats. Gastroenterology 1986;90:391.

1191. Sundler F, Carlsson E, Hakanson R, Larsson H, Mattsson H. Inhibition of gastric acid secretion by omeprazole and ranitidine. Effects on plasma gastrin and gastric histamine, histidine decarboxylase activity, and ECL cell density in normal and antrectomized rats. Scand J Gastroenterol 1986;21(Suppl 118):39.

1192. Eckman L, Hansson E, Havu N, Carlsson E, Lundberg C. Toxicological studies on omeprazole. Scand J Gastroenterol 1985;20(Suppl 108):53.

1193. Poynter D, Pick CR, Harcourt RA, Selway SA, Ainge G, Harman

IW, Spurling NW, Fluck PA, Cook JL. Association of long lasting unsurmountable histamine H2 blockade and gastric carcinoid tumors in the rat. Gut 1985;26:1284.

1194. Elder JB. Inhibition of acid and gastric carcinoids. Gut 1985;26:1279.

1195. Penston J, Wormsley KG. Achlorhydria: Hypergastrinaemia: Carcinoids—A flawed hypothesis? Gut 1987;28:488.

1196. Solcia E, Capella C, Sessa F, et al. Gastric carcinoid and related endocrine growths. Digestion 1986;35(Suppl 1):3.

1197. Mignon M, Lehy T, Bonnefond A, Ruszniewski PH, Labeille D, Bonfils S. Development of gastric argyrophil carcinoid tumors in a case of Zollinger–Ellison syndrome with primary hyperparathyroidism during long-term antisecretory treatment. Cancer 1986;59:1959.

1198. Bordi C, D'Adda T, Pilato FP, Ferrari C. Carcinoid (ECL cell) tumor of the oxyntic mucosa of the stomach: A hormone-dependent neoplasm? Prog Surg Pathol 1987;8:177.

1199. Bordi C, Costa A, Missale G. ECL cell proliferation and gastrin levels. Gastroenterology 1975;68:205.

1200. Rigler LG, Kaplan HS. Pernicious anemia and tumors of the stomach. J Natl Cancer Inst 1947;7:327.

1201. Mosbech J, Videbaek A. Mortality from and risk of gastric carcinoma among patients with pernicious anemia. Br Med J 1950;ii:390.

1202. Correa P, Cuello C, Duque E, et al. Gastric cancer in Colombia. III. Natural history of precursor lesions. J Natl Cancer Inst 1976;57:1027.

1203. Imai T, Kubo T, Watanabe H. Chronic gastritis in Japanese with reference to high incidence of gastric carcinoma. J Natl Cancer Inst 1971;47:179.

1204. Stemmermann G, Haenszel W, Locke F. Epidemiologic pathology of gastric ulcer and gastric carcinoma among Japanese in Hawaii. J Natl Cancer Inst 1977;58:13.

1205. Sipponen P, Kekki M, Haapakoski J, Ihamaki T, Siurala M. Gastric cancer risk in chronic atrophic gastritis: Statistical calculations of cross-sectional data. Int J Cancer 1985;35:173.

1206. Sipponen P, Kekki M, Siurala M. Atrophic chronic gastritis and intestinal metaplasia in gastric carcinoma. Comparison with a representative population sample. Cancer 1983;52:1062.

1207. Svendsen JH, Dahl C, Svendsen LB, Christiansen PM. Gastric cancer risk in achlorhydric patients. A long-term follow-up study. Scand J Gastroenterol 1986;21:16.

1208. Borch K. Epidemiologic, clinicopathologic, and economic aspects of gastroscopic screening of patients with pernicious anemia. Scand J Gastroenterol 1986;21:21.

1209. Joergensen J. The mortality among patients with pernicious anemia in Denmark and the incidence of gastric carcinoma among the same. Acta Med Scand 1951;139:472.

1210. Schafer LW, Larson DE, Melton LJ III, Higgins JA, Zinsmeister AR. Risk of development of gastric carcinoma in patients with pernicious anemia: A population-based study in Rochester, Minnesota. Mayo Clin Proc 1985;60:444.

1211. Oi M, Oshida K, Sugimura S. The location of gastric ulcer. Gastroenterology 1959;36:45.

1212. Gear MWL, Truelove SC, Whitehead R. Gastric ulcer and gastritis. Gut 1971;12:639.

1213. Teir H, Rasanen TA. A study of mitotic rate in renewal zones of non diseased portions of gastric mucosa in cases of peptic ulcer and gastric cancer with observations on differentiation and so-called intestinalization of gastric mucosa. J Natl Cancer Inst 1961;27:949.

1214. Jarvi O, Lauren P. On the role of heterotopias of the intestinal epithelium in the pathogenesis of gastric cancer. Acta Pathol Microbiol Scand 1951;29:26.

1215. Morson BC. Carcinomas arising from areas of intestinal metaplasia in the gastric mucosa. Br J Cancer 1955;9:377.

1216. Lauren P. The two histological main types of gastric carcinoma; diffuse and so-called intestinal type carcinoma. An attempt at a histo-clinical classification. Acta Pathol Microbiol Scand 1965;64:31.

1217. Ming SC, Goldman H, Freiman DG. Intestinal metaplasia and histogenesis of carcinoma in human stomach. Light and electron microscopic study. Cancer 1967;20:1418.

1218. Wattenberg LW. Histochemical study of aminopeptidase in metaplasia and carcinoma of the stomach. Arch Pathol 1959;67:281.

1219. Planteydt HT, Willighagen RGJ. Enzyme histochemistry of gastric carcinomas. J Pathol Bacteriol 1965;90:393.

1220. Stemmermann GN. Comparative study of histochemical patterns in non-neoplastic and neoplastic gastric epithelium. A study of Japanese in Hawaii. J Natl Cancer Inst 1967;39:375.

1221. Goldman H, Ming SC. Histochemical distribution of mucins in normal and neoplastic gastrointestinal epithelium. Arch Pathol 1968;85:580.

1222. Lev R, Siegel HI, Glass GBJ. The enzyme histochemistry of gastric carcinoma in man. Cancer 1969;23:1086.

1223. Hattori T. Development of adenocarcinomas in the stomach. Cancer 1986;57:1528.

1224. Samloff IM, Varis K, Ihamaki T, Siurala M, Rotter JI. Relationships among serum pepsinogen I, serum pepsinogen II and gastric mucosal histology. A study in relatives of patients with pernicious anemia. Gastroenterology 1982;83:204.

1225. Ming SC, Bajtai A, Correa P, Elster K, Jarvi OH, Munoz N, Negayo T, Stemmermann GN. Gastric dysplasia. Significance and pathologic criteria. Cancer 1984;54:1794.

1226. Park HK, Sinar DR, Sloss RR, et al. Histologic and endoscopic studies before and after gastric bypass surgery. Arch Pathol Lab Med 1986;110:1164.

1227. Correa P. The epidemiology and pathogenesis of chronic gastritis: Three etiologic entities. Front Gastrointest Res 1980;6:98.

1228. Pulimood BM, Knudsen A, Coghill NF. Gastric mucosa after partial gastrectomy. Gut 1976;17:463.

1229. Kekki M, Saukkonen M, Sipponen P, Varis K, Siurala M. Dynamics of chronic gastritis in the remnant after partial gastrectomy for duodenal ulcer. Scand J Gastroenterol 1980;15:509.

1230. Janunger KG, Domellof L, Eriksson S. The development of mucosal changes after gastric surgery for ulcer disease. Scand J Gastroenterol 1978;13:121.

1231. Schrumpf E, Serck-Hanssen A, Stadaaj J, Aune S, Myren O, Osnes H. Changes in the gastric stump 20-25 years after partial gastrectomy. Lancet 1977;2:467.

1232. Kleins G, Paquet KS, Lindstaedt H, Miedere S. Atrophic gastritis after Billroth I gastrectomy. Endoscopy 1979;2:127.

1233. Savage A, Jones S. Histological appearance of the gastric mucosa 15–27 years after partial gastrectomy. J Clin Pathol 1979;32:179.

1234. Gyeruldsen ST, Myren J, Frethem B. Alteration of gastric mucosa following a graded partial gastrectomy for duodenal ulcer. Scand J Gastroenterol 1968;3:465.

1235. Stempien SJ, Dagaradi AE, Tan DTD. Endoscopic aspects of the gastric mucosa ten years or more after vagotomy–pyloroplasty. Gastrointest Endosc 1971;18:21.

1236. Du Plessis DJ. Gastric mucosal changes after operation on the stomach. S Afr Med J 1962;36:471.

1237. Domellof L, Eriksson S, Helander HF, Janunger KG. Lipid islands in the gastric mucosa after resection for benign ulcer disease. Gastroenterology 1977;72:14.

1238. Terruzzi V, Minoli G, Butti GC, Rossini A. Gastric lipid islands in the gastric stump and in non-operated stomach. Endoscopy 1980;12:58.

1239. Franzin G, Musola R, Zamboni G, Manfrini C. Gastritis cystica polyposa: A possible precancerous lesion. Tumori 1985;71:13.

1240. Koga S, Watanabe H, Enjoji M. Stomal polypoid hypertrophic gastritis. A polypoid gastric lesion at gastroenterostomy site. Cancer 1979;43:647.

1241. Littler ER, Gleibermann E. Gastritis cystica polyposa. Cancer 1972;29:205.

1242. Griffel B, Engelgerg M, Reiss R. Multiple polypoid cystic gastritis in old gastroenteric stoma. Arch Pathol 1974;97:316.

1243. Schafer LW, Larson DE, Melton LJ, Higgins JA, Ilstrup DM. The risk of gastric carcinoma after surgical treatment for benign ulcer disease. A population-based study in Olmsted County, Minnesota. N Engl J Med 1983;309:1210.

1244. Offerhaus GJA, Huibregtse K, DeBoer J, Verhoeven T, Van Olffen GH, van de Stadt J, Tytgat GN. The operated stomach: A premalignant condition. A prospective endoscopic follow-up study. Scand J Gastroenterol 1984;19:521.

1245. Sonnenberg A. Endoscopic screening for gastric stump cancer—Would it be beneficial? A hypothetical cohort study. Gastroenterology 1984;87:489.

1246. Caygill CPJ, Hill MJ, Kirkham JS, Northfield TC. Mortality from gastric cancer following gastric surgery for peptic ulcer. Lancet 1986;1:929.

1247. Fahimi H, Deren J, Gottlieb L, Zamcheck N. Isolated granulomatous gastritis: Its relationship to disseminated sarcoidosis and regional enteritis. Gastroenterology 1963;45:161.

1248. Case records of the Massachusetts General Hospital (case 46—1974). N Engl J Med 1974;291:1127.

1249. Present D, Lindner A, Janowitz H. Granulomatous disease of the gastrointestinal tract. Annu Rev Med 1966;17:243.

1250. Weinstock JV. Idiopathic isolated granulomatous gastritis. Spontaneous resolution without surgical intervention. Dig Dis Sci 1980;25:233.

1251. Compton CC, Von Lichtenberg F. Necrotizing granulomatous gastritis and gastric perforation of unknown etiology: A first case report. J Clin Gastroenterol 1983;5:59.

1252. Hanada M, Takami M, Hirata K, Nakajima T. Hyalinoid giant cell gastritis. A unique gastric lesion associated with eosinophilic hyalinoid degeneration of smooth muscle. Acta Pathol Jpn 1985;35:749.

1253. Fielding JF, Toye DKM, Beton DC, Cooke WT. Crohn's disease of the stomach and duodenum. Gut 1970;11:1001.

1254. Rutgeerts P, Onette E, Vantrappen G, Geboes K, Broeckaert L, Talloen L. Crohn's disease of the stomach and duodenum: A clinical study with emphasis on the value of the endoscopy and endoscopic biopsies. Endoscopy 1980;12:288.

1255. Schmitz-Moormann P, Malchow H, Pittner PM. Endoscopic and bioptic study of the upper gastrointestinal tract in Crohn's disease patients. Pathol Res Pract 1985;179:377.

1256. Gore RM, Ghahremani GG. Crohn's disease of the upper gastrointestinal tract. CRC Crit Rev Diagn Imaging 1985;25:305.

1257. Tanaka M, Kimura K, Sakai H, Yoshida Y, Saito K. Long-term follow-up for minute gastroduodenal lesions in Crohn's disease. Gastrointest Endosc 1986;32:206.

1258. Jacobson IM, Schapiro RH, Warshaw AL. Gastric and duodenal fistulas in Crohn's disease. Gastroenterology 1985;89:1347.

1259. Priebe WM, Simon JB. Crohn's disease of the stomach with outlet obstruction: A case report and review of therapy. J Clin Gastroenterol 1983;5:441.

1260. Palmer ED. Note on silent sarcoidosis of the gastric mucosa. J Lab Clin Med 1958;52:231.

1261. Sprague R, Harper P, McClain S, Trainer T, Beeken W. Disseminated gastrointestinal sarcoidosis. Case report and review of the literature. Gastroenterology 1984;87:421.

1262. Chinitz MA, Brandt LJ, Frank MS, Frager D, Sablay L. Symptomatic sarcoidosis of the stomach. Dig Dis Sci 1985;30:682.

1263. Palmer E. Tuberculosis of stomach and stomach in tuberculosis: Review with particular reference to gross pathology and gastroscopic diagnosis. Am Rev Tuberc 1950;61:116.

1264. Chazan B, Aitchison J. Gastric tuberculosis. Br Med J 1960;2:1288.

1265. Talib S, Chawhan R, Zaheer A, Talib V. Primary tuberculosis of stomach. J Assoc Physicians India 1975;23:291.

1266. Palmer KR, Patil DH, Basran GS, Riordan JF, Silk DBA. Abdominal tuberculosis in urban Britain—A common disease. Gut 1985;26:1296.

1267. Brody JM, Deborah KM, Zeman RK, Klappenbach RS, Jaffe MH, Clark LR, Benjamin SB, Choyke PL. Gastric tuberculosis: A manifestation of acquired immunodeficiency syndrome. Radiology 1986;159:347.

1268. Knight W, Falk A. Tertiary gastric syphilis. Gastroenterology 1947;9:17.

1269. Cooley R, Childers J. Acquired syphilis of the stomach. Gastroenterology 1960;39:201.

1270. Reisman T, Leverett F, Hudson J, Kalser M. Syphilitic gastropathy. Am J Dig Dis 1975;20:588.

1271. Mitchell R, Bralow S. Acute erosive gastritis due to early syphilis. Ann Intern Med 1964;61:933.

1272. Sachar DB, Klein RS, Swerdlow F, Bottone E, Khilnani MT, Waye JD, Wisniewski M. Erosive syphilitic gastritis: Dark-field and im-munofluorescent diagnosis from biopsy specimen. Ann Intern Med 1974;80:512.

1273. Butz WC, Watts JC, Rosales-Quintana S, Hicklin MD. Erosive gastritis as a manifestation of secondary syphilis. Am J Clin Pathol 1975;63:895.

1274. Morin ME, Tan A. Diffuse enlargement of gastric folds as a manifestation of secondary syphilis. Am J Gastroenterol 1980;74:170.

1275. Fisher JR, Sanowski RA. Disseminated histoplasmosis producing hypertrophic gastric folds. Dig Dis Sci 1978;23:282.

1276. Orchard JL, Luparello F, Brunskill D. Malabsorption syndrome occurring in the course of disseminated histoplasmosis. Case report and review of gastrointestinal histoplasmosis. Am J Med 1979;66:331.

1277. Perez C, Sturim J, Kouchoukos N, Kamberg S. Some clinical and radiographic features of gastrointestinal histoplasmosis. Radiology 1966;86:482.

1278. Nelson R, Bruni M, Goldstein M. Primary gastric candidiasis in uncompromised subjects. Gastrointest Endosc 1975;22:92.

1279. Binder R, Nelson J. Candida albicans ulcer within hiatus hernia sac presenting as an ulcerated mass. Gastroenterology 1975;68:587.

1280. Lyon DT, Schubert TT, Mantia AG, Kaplan MH. Phycomycosis of the gastrointestinal tract. Am J Gastroenterol 1979;72:379.

1281. Lawson H, Schmaman A. Gastric phycomycosis. Br J Surg 1974;61:743.

1282. Van Olmen G, Larmuseau MF, Geboes K, Rutgeerts P, Penninckx F, Vantrappen G. Primary gastric actinomycosis: A case report and review of the literature. Am J Gastroenterol 1984;79:512.

1283. Eras P, Goldstein MJ, Sherlock P. Candida infection of the gastrointestinal tract. Medicine 1972;51:367.

1284. Peters M, Weiner J, Whelan G. Fungal infection associated with gastroduodenal ulceration: Endoscopic and pathologic appearances. Gastroenterology 1980;78:350.

1285. Gotlieb-Jensen K, Andersen J. Occurrence of Candida in gastric ulcers. Significance for the healing process. Gastroenterology 1983;85:535.

1286. DiFebo G, Miglioli M, Calo G, Biasco G, Luzza P, Gizzi G, Cipollini F, Rossi A, Barbara L. Candida albicans infection of gastric ulcer. Frequency and correlation with medical treatment. Results of a multicenter study. Dig Dis Sci 1985;30:178.

1287. Katz AJ, Goldman H, Grand RJ. Gastric mucosal biopsy in eosinophilic (allergic) gastroenteritis. Gastroenterology 1977;73:705.

1288. Klein NC, Hargrove RL, Sleisenger MH, Jeffries GH. Eosinophilic gastroenteritis. Medicine 1970;49:299.

1289. Cello JP. Eosinophilic gastroenteritis—A complex disease entity. Am J Med 1979;67:1097.

1290. O'Neill T. Eosinophilic granuloma of the gastrointestinal tract. Br J Surg 1970;57:704.

1291. Schwinger A. Eosinophilic granuloma of the upper GI tract. Am J Dig Dis 1965;10:58.

1292. Vazquez J, Ayestaran J. Eosinophilic granuloma of the stomach similar to that of bone. Virchows Arch [A] 1975;366:107.

1293. Johnstone JM, Morson BC. Inflammatory fibroid polyp of the gastrointestinal tract. Histopathology 1978;2:349.

1294. Ishikura H, Sato F, Naka A, Kodama T, Aizawa M. Inflammatory fibroid polyp of the stomach. Acta Pathol Jpn 1986;36:327.

1295. Nevin N, Eakins D, Clarke S, Carson D. Acute phlegmonous gastritis. Br J Surg 1969;56:268.

1296. Miller A, Smith B, Rogers A. Phlegmonous gastritis. Gastroenterology 1975;68:231.

1297. Williford ME, Foster WL, Halvorsen RA, Thompson WM. Emphysematous gastritis secondary to disseminated strongyloidiasis. Gastrointest Radiol 1982;7:123.

1298. Mittleman RE, Suarez RV. Phlegmonous gastritis associated with the acquired immunodeficiency syndrome/preacquired immunodeficiency syndrome. Arch Pathol Lab Med 1985;109:765.

1299. Blei ED, Abrahams C. Diffuse phlegmonous gastroenterocolitis in a patient with an infected peritoneojugular venous shunt. Gastroenterology 1983;84:636.

1300. Dutz W, Saidi F, Kohout E. Gastric anthrax with massive ascites. Gut 1970;11:352.

1301. Gonzalez LL, Schowengerdt C, Skinner HH, Lynch P. Emphysematous gastritis. Surg Gynecol Obstet 1963;116:79.

1302. Meyers H, Parker J. Emphysematous gastritis. Radiology 1967;89:426.

1303. Smith T. Emphysematous gastritis associated with adenocarcinoma of the stomach. Am J Dig Dis 1966;11:341.

1304. Kussin SZ, Henry C, Navarro C, Stenson W, Clain DJ. Gas within the wall of the stomach. Report of a case and review of the literature. Dig Dis Sci 1982;27:949.

1305. Lifton LJ, Schlossberg D. Phlegmonous gastritis after endoscopic polypectomy. Ann Intern Med 1982;97:373.

1306. Balthazar EJ, Megibow AJ, Hulnick DH. Cytomegalovirus esophagitis and gastritis in AIDS. Am J Roentgenol 1985;114:1201.

1307. Elta G, Turnage R, Eckhauser FE, Agha F, Ross S. A submucosal antral mass caused by cytomegalovirus infection in a patient with acquired immunodeficiency syndrome. Am J Gastroenterol 1986;81:714.

1308. Strayer DS, Phillips GB, Barker KH, Winokur T, DeSchryver-Kecskemeti K. Gastric cytomegalovirus infection in bone marrow transplant patients: An indication of generalized disease. Cancer 1981;48:1478.

1309. Franzin G, Musola R, Mencarelli R. Changes in the mucosa of the stomach and duodenum during immunosuppressive therapy after renal transplantation. Histopathology 1982;6:439.

1310. Komorowski RA, Cohen EB, Kauffman HM, Adams MB. Gastrointestinal complications in renal transplant recipients. Am J Clin Pathol 1986;86:161.

1311. McDonald GB, Shulman HM, Sullivan KM, Spencer GD. Intestinal and hepatic complications of human bone marrow transplantation. Part II. Gastroenterology 1986;90:770.

1312. Campbell DA, Piercy JRA, Shnitka TK, Goldsand G, Devine RDO, Weinstein WM. Cytomegalovirus-associated gastric ulcer. Gastroenterology 1977;72:533.

1313. Coad NAG, Shah KJ. Menetrier's disease in childhood associated with cytomegalovirus infection: A case report and review of the literature. Br J Radiol 1986;59:615.

1314. Marks MP, Lanza MV, Kahlstrom EJ, Mikity V, Marks SC, Kvalstad RP. Pediatric hypertrophic gastropathy. Am J Roentgenol 1986;147:1031.

1315. Howiler W, Goldberg HI. Gastroesophageal involvement in herpes simplex. Gastroenterology 1976;70:775.

1316. Garone MA, Winston BJ, Lewis JH. Cryptosporidiosis of the stomach. Am J Gastroenterol 1986;81:465.

1317. Scowden EB, Schaffner W, Stone WJ. Overwhelming strongyloidiasis. An unappreciated opportunistic infection. Medicine 1978;57:527.

1318. Ainley CC, Clark DG, Timothy AR, Thompson RPH. Strongyloides stercoralis hyperinfection associated with cimetidine in an immunosuppressed patient: Diagnosis by endoscopic biopsy. Gut 1986;27:337.

1319. Wongpaitoon V, Kanjanapanjapol S, Nithiyanant P, Nirapathpongporn S. Gastric ameboma, a complication of amebic liver abscess: A case report. J Med Assoc Thai 1985;68:378.

1320. Capdevielle P, Coignard A, LeGal E, Boudon A, Delprat J. Ulcere pre-pylorique et bilharziose gastrique. Gastroenterol Clin Biol 1979;3:153.

1321. Dumont A, Seferian V, Barbier P. Endoscopic discovery and capture of Necator americanus in the stomach. Endoscopy 1983;15:65.

1322. Asami K, Watanuki T, Sakai H, Imano H, Okamoto R. Two cases of stomach granuloma caused by Anisakis-like larval nematodes in Japan. Am J Trop Med Hyg 1965;14:119.

1323. Sugimachi K, Inokuchi K, Ooiwa T, Fujino T, Ishii Y. Acute gastric anisakiasis. Analysis of 178 cases. JAMA 1985;253:1012.

1324. Kliks MM. Anisakiasis in the western United States: Four new case reports from California. Am J Trop Med Hyg 1983;32:526.

1325. Kusuhara T, Watanabe K, Fukuda M. Radiographic study of acute gastric anisakiasis. Gastrointest Radiol 1984;9:305.

1326. Appelman HD. Localized and extensive expansions of the gastric mucosa: Mucosal polyps and giant folds. In: Appelman HD, ed. Pathology of the esophagus, stomach, and duodenum. Contemporary issues in surgical pathology, ed 4. New York: Churchill Livingstone, 1984:79.

1327. Berenson MM, Sannella J, Freston JW. Menetrier's disease. Serial morphological, secretory and serological observations. Gastroenterology 1976;70:257.

1328. Scharschmidt BF. The natural history of hypertrophic gastropathy (Menetrier's disease). Report of a case with 16 year follow-up and review of 120 cases from the literature. Am J Med 1977;63:644.

1329. Searcy RM, Malagelada JR. Menetrier's disease and idiopathic hypertrophic gastropathy. Ann Intern Med 1984;100:565.

1330. Kelly DG, Miller LJ, Malagelada JR, Huizenga KA, Markowitz H. Giant hypertrophic gastropathy (Menetrier's disease): Pharmacologic effects on protein leakage and mucosal ultrastructure. Gastroenterology 1982;83:581.

1331. Miura S, Asakura H, Tsuchiya M. Lymphatic abnormalities in protein-losing gastropathy, especially in Menetrier's disease. Angiology 1981;32:345.

1332. Overholt BF, Jeffries GH. Hypertrophic, hypersecretory protein-losing gastropathy. Gastroenterology 1970;58:80.

1333. Larsen B, Tarp U, Kristensen E. Familial giant hypertrophic gastritis. Gut 1987;28:1517.

1334. Hill RE, Herez A, Corey ML, Gilday DL. Fecal clearance of alpha-1-antitrypsin: A reliable measure of enteric protein loss in children. J Pediatr 1981;99:416.

1335. Knight JA, Matlak ME, Condon VR. Menetrier's disease in children: Report of a case and review of the pediatric literature. Pediatr Pathol 1983;1:179.

1336. Baker A, Volberg F, Sumner T, Moran R. Childhood Menetrier's disease: Four new cases and discussion of the literature. Gastrointest Radiol 1986;11:131.

1337. Kraut JR, Powell R, Hruby MA, Lloyd-Still JD. Menetrier's disease in childhood: Report of two cases and a review of the literature. J Pediatr Surg 1981;16:707.

1338. Wood GM, Bates C, Brown RC, Losowsky MS. Intramucosal carcinoma of the gastric antrum complicating Menetrier's disease. J Clin Pathol 1983;36:1071.

1339. Ranchod M, Lewin KJ, Dorfman RF. Lymphoid hyperplasia of the gastrointestinal tract. A study of 26 cases and review of the literature. Am J Surg Pathol 1978;2:383.

1340. Orr RK, Liniger JR, Lawrence W. Gastric pseudolymphoma. A challenging clinical problem. Ann Surg 1984;200:185.

1341. Brooks JJ, Enterline HT. Gastric pseudolymphoma. Its three subtypes and relation to lymphoma. Cancer 1983;51:476.

1342. Eimoto T, Futami K, Naito H, Takeshita M, Kikuchi M. Gastric pseudolymphoma with monotypic cytoplasmic immunoglobulin. Cancer 1985;55:788.

62

Zollinger-Ellison Syndrome

JOHN DEL VALLE
TADATAKA YAMADA

INTRODUCTION

"Fortunate indeed is the surgical service that does not have one or more problem cases of recurrent marginal ulceration despite the adequacy of the surgical attack" notes the opening sentence of Zollinger and Ellison's landmark description of the syndrome that today bears their names.[1] Benign ulceration of the upper jejunum associated with extremely high gastric acid secretion and the presence of a non-β cell adenoma of the pancreas was the triad of clinical findings described in two patients who eventually required total gastrectomy for relief of their severe ulcer disease. Although earlier reports[2,3] described a similar clinical scenario, it was Zollinger and Ellison who hypothesized that the components of this clinical triad were intimately related and produced by a humoral agent that induced gastric acid hypersecretion and its sequelae. This hypothesis was confirmed by Gregory and coworkers when they established that the tumor extract from a patient with Zollinger-Ellison syndrome contained a substance that was chemically and physiologically indistinguishable from the antral hormone gastrin.[4,5] Subsequent development of a sensitive and specific radioimmunoassay for gastrin[6,7] facilitated the measurement of this peptide in the sera of patients with Zollinger-Ellison syndrome, confirming that their circulating gastrin concentrations exceeded by severalfold the plasma levels found in a normal control population. This sensitive assay also permitted earlier tumor detection, a circumstance that has led to a steady increase in the reports of patients with gastrinoma. The past 3 decades have served witness to a dramatic change in the diagnostic strategy, treatment, and long-term survival of these patients. Potent inhibitors of gastric acid secretion and sophisticated preoperative and intraoperative diagnostic procedures have transformed Zollinger-Ellison syndrome from an illness in which total gastrectomy and tumor progression were the norm to a condition in which a cure is feasible in many of the afflicted patients.

EPIDEMIOLOGY

The true incidence and prevalence of the Zollinger-Ellison syndrome is unknown. The estimated incidence has ranged from 0.1% to 1% of patients who present with peptic ulcer disease in the United States.[8] Attempts to study the epidemiology of this syndrome have been limited by a number of factors. The heterogeneous clinical manifestations, the generalized use of histamine H_2 receptor antagonists for the treatment of acid peptic disease and its sequelae, and the high incidence of silent pancreatic endocrine neoplasms[9] have all contributed to an underestimation of the incidence and prevalence of Zollinger-Ellison syndrome. The age range of affected persons has varied from 7 to 90 years old, with the majority of patients being diagnosed between the ages of 30 and 50. Males with the disorder predominate over females by ratios varying from 2:1 to 3:2.[8,10,11]

Gastrinomas can be subdivided into tumors that are sporadic[12] and those that are genetically transmitted and associated with multiple endocrine neoplasia type I (MEN I).[13] Sporadic gastrinomas, the more common of the two, frequently behave as malignant tumors. Zollinger-Ellison tumors associated with MEN I occur at an earlier age than the sporadic tumors and are characterized by a more benign course. There are various distinguishing features between these two subtypes that will be discussed later in this chapter.

PATHOPHYSIOLOGY

Gastric acid hypersecretion and severe peptic ulcer diathesis secondary to unbridled release of gastrin from a non-β cell endocrine neoplasm are the essential elements leading to Zollinger-Ellison syndrome. The neoplastic pancreatic cells secreting gastrin are believed to arise from the ductular epithelium and not from cells of the islets of Langerhans, despite the appellation of gastrinomas as "islet cell tumors."[1] Normally the adult pancreas does not secrete gastrin but the fetal pancreas contains large quantities of this peptide.[14] After birth, the gastrin-secreting cells in the pancreas disappear and are not seen again except as benign or malignant neoplasms in Zollinger-Ellison syndrome. Although a detailed review of gastrin's biologic actions is beyond the scope of this chapter (see ch 2), two of its primary functions as a peptide hormone should be examined in order to comprehend the pathophysiology of the syndrome. Gastrin is found predominantly in the gastric antrum[15] and functions as the primary stimulant of postprandial gastric acid secretion.[16,17] Its stimulatory action occurs directly on the parietal cell[18] through specific cell surface receptors[19,20] that are linked to the phosphoinositide/protein kinase C second messenger system.[21] Gastrin also has a well-established trophic effect on gastrointestinal tissues.[22,23] In small doses the peptide has been shown to increase protein and DNA synthesis and total DNA content of gastric mucosa and other tissues. In Zollinger-Ellison syndrome, the hypergastrinemia that results from the release of peptide from an endocrine neoplasm free of the usual regulatory restraints has two synergistic effects: (1) overstimulation of gastric parietal cells to secrete acid and (2) increased mass of parietal cells susceptible to overstimulation. The potentiated gastric acid hypersecretion that results is presumably the cause of the clinical manifestations (i.e., acid peptic disease and diarrhea) of the gastrinoma syndrome.

Although it is well established that gastrinomas contain and secrete large concentrations of the biologically active fully processed molecular forms of gastrin, studies indicate that altered post-translational processing of progastrin may be a feature of the disorder as well. As reviewed in Chapter 2, gastrin is synthesized as a large precursor molecule that subsequently undergoes a series of post-translational processing steps involving proteolytic cleavage as well as carboxylterminal amidation. The end products are a variety of molecular forms of amidated gastrin including those of 17 (G17) and 34 (G34) amino acids in length[24] that are found not only in normal antral tissues but also in sera[25] and tumors of patients with gastrinoma.[4,26] Kariya and coworkers[27] examined the expression of the human gastrin gene by Southern blot analysis and observed that DNA from gastric antrum and gastrinoma were indistinguishable from each other without evidence of genomic rearrangements in the tumor tissues. By immunochemical analysis, however, Dockray and Walsh[28] observed an unusual component of gastrin in the sera of some patients with Zollinger-Ellison syndrome. Using region-specific antisera directed toward the amino terminus of G17 these investigators detected high circulating concentrations of what appeared to be the amino terminal tridecapeptide fragment of G17 (G17$_{1-13}$). This was the first evidence, albeit indirect, suggesting the presence of altered gastrin processing in gastrinoma tissues. On the basis of information obtained from the gastrin cDNA sequence[29-31] several investigators have developed region specific antisera toward progastrin and its processing intermediates and used them to examine the post-translational processing of the peptide in patients with gastrinomas.[32,33] These studies have confirmed that gastrin processing is altered in tumor tissue. The biologic significance of these observations is unclear, but one hypothesis is that the degree of altered processing may correlate with the state of de-differentiation of a tumor. This correlation was examined by Kothary and coworkers,[34,35] who suggested that a high ratio of amino terminal G17 to carboxyl-terminally amidated G17 immunoreactivity indicative of incomplete post-translational processing may signal the presence of tumor metastasis. These potentially important observations require further confirmation.

TUMOR DISTRIBUTION

Although initial studies observed that the majority of gastrinomas occur within the pancreas,[10] modern diagnostic studies coupled with aggressive surgical intervention have revealed that a large number are extrapancreatic and extraintestinal.[36,37] More than 80% of gastrinomas have been localized in the anatomic area known as the gastrinoma triangle.[38] The boundaries of this triangle include the confluence of the cystic and common bile ducts superiorly, the junction of the second and third portions of the duodenum inferiorly, and the junction of the neck and body of the pancreas medially. The most common extrapancreatic site is the duodenum,[39] wherein up to 15% of gastrinomas arise. Other less common extrapancreatic sites include the stomach, bones, ovaries, liver, and lymph nodes, which together account for less than 10% of gastrinomas. More than 50% of gastrinomas are considered to be malignant. Solitary pancreatic lesions were found in less than 30% of the earliest reported patients with gastrinomas.[10] With the more recent trend toward earlier measurement of serum gastrin and exploratory surgery,[40] the incidence of metastatic disease at the time of operation has decreased. Nevertheless, multiple tumors or metastatic lesions are still observed in 30% to 50% of patients at the time of diagnosis.

The morphology of the neoplastic cells in gastrinomas is heterogeneous.[41,42] The gastrin-producing cells are generally well differentiated and contain histologic markers that are characteristic of endocrine neoplasms in general; that is, they contain chromogranin, neuron-specific enolase, and tyrosine hydroxylase (see ch 91). Gastrinomas contain various types of secretory granules that can vary in ultrastructural appearance from those typically found in antral G-cells to those found in A-cells, D-cells, and abnormal islet D-cells and type IV cells. The degree of malignancy does not appear to correlate with a gastrinoma's histologic appearance, however, this observation must be tempered by the knowledge that tumor aggressiveness is usually determined retrospectively.

As is the case with other endocrine neoplasms (see ch 91), gastrinomas have been found to express a variety of neuroendocrine peptides besides gastrin, including somatostatin, pancreatic polypeptide (PP), adrenocorticotropic hormone (ACTH), and vasoactive intestinal peptide (VIP). Although the clinical manifestations are generally associated with overproduction of one hormone, case reports illustrating combined syndromes have been described.[43-47] Of these, Cushing's syndrome in association with gastrinoma is the mixed syndrome most frequently described.[48,49]

Clinical Manifestations

Symptoms and signs in patients with Zollinger-Ellison syndrome are primarily related to gastric acid hypersecretion and its consequences. More than 90% of patients with gastrinomas develop ulcers in the upper gastrointestinal tract at some point during their disease.[10-12] Presenting ulcer symptoms are indistinguishable from those associated with benign peptic ulcer disease (see ch 61), but frequently they will be less responsive to standard therapy. As in benign peptic ulcer disease, ulcers in patients with Zollinger-Ellison syndrome occur most frequently in the first portion of the duodenum (75%) and are usually solitary. However, ulcers in patients with gastrinomas also may occur in the second, third, and fourth portion of the duodenum (14%) and in the jejunum (11%).[11] The ulcers are usually less than 1 cm in diameter but can occasionally present as giant lesions. Peptic ulcer disease refractory to standard medical therapy, recurrent ulcers after prior gastric surgery, diarrhea in patients with ulcers, or peptic disease presenting with complications such as obstruction, perforation, or bleeding should lead to the suspicion of Zollinger-Ellison syndrome. Esophageal symptoms caused by acid reflux are seen in as many as two thirds of patients with Zollinger-Ellison syndrome.[50,51] The pathology found in the esophagus may range from mild to severe esophagitis complicated by stricture formation and Barrett's mucosa.

Aside from peptic ulcers, the other common feature of Zollinger-Ellison syndrome is diarrhea. Diarrhea can be present in over half of patients with gastrinoma and can occur in the absence of peptic ulcer symptoms.[10,12,52,53] Diarrhea may also precede the diagnosis of Zollinger-Ellison syndrome by many years. The pathogenesis of diarrhea is believed to be multifactorial, but its dependence on acid hypersecretion is demonstrated by amelioration of symptoms on continuous nasogastric suction or inhibition of acid secretion.[8,54] Thus, the severe volume load represented by the acid that can be secreted at the rate of several liters per day can account for some of the diarrhea. Added features of the diarrhea are steatorrhea and maldigestion,[55,56] which result from the inactivity of pancreatic enzymes at the low pH of the duodenum caused by the excessive acid load. The acidic pH of the small bowel may also lead to damage of the intestinal mucosa, resulting in a spruelike state with flattened intestinal villi and accompanying malabsorption.[57] Bile acids are poorly soluble in an acid milieu; thus Zollinger-Ellison syndrome may result in decreased micelle formation and subsequent malabsorption of vitamin B_{12} and other lipid-soluble nutrients and vitamins.[55] It is possible that in the presence of markedly high serum gastrin levels, gastrin itself may increase secretion of potassium and reduce absorption of sodium and water by the small intestine,[58,59] thus potentially leading to a secretory diarrhea. Secretory diarrhea may also occur in Zollinger-Ellison syndrome in association with the secretion of another hormone besides gastrin, such as VIP.

Twenty-five percent of patients with gastrinoma have MEN I syndrome.[13] As reviewed elsewhere in this textbook (see ch 91), the primary sites of organ involvement in this autosomal dominant genetic disorder include the parathyroid, pancreas, pituitary, and, less commonly, adrenal cortex and thyroid.

Hyperparathyroidism and its associated hypercalcemia have direct bearing on the gastric acid hypersecretory state found in patients with Zollinger-Ellison syndrome and MEN I. Intravenous infusion of calcium in healthy human volunteers induces gastric acid hypersecretion. In addition, calcium has been shown both in vivo[60] and in vitro[61] to stimulate gastrin release directly from gastrinomas. Indeed, previous reports[62,63] have demonstrated that

TABLE 62-1
When to Evaluate Serum Gastrin in Patients With Peptic Ulcer

Multiple ulcers
Ulcers in unusual locations
Ulcers associated with severe esophagitis
Ulcers resistant to therapy with frequent recurrences
Ulcer patients awaiting surgery
Extensive family history for peptic ulcer disease
Postoperative ulcer recurrence
Basal hyperchlorhydria
Unexplained diarrhea or steatorrhea
Hypercalcemia
Family history of pancreatic islet, pituitary, or parathyroid tumor
Prominent gastric or duodenal folds

TABLE 62-2
Hypergastrinemia: Differential Diagnosis

Hypochlorhydria or achlorhydria with or without pernicious anemia
Retained gastric antrum
G-cell hyperplasia
Renal insufficiency
Massive small bowel resection
Gastric outlet obstruction
Others: rheumatoid arthritis, vitiligo, diabetes, pheochromocytoma

resolution of hypercalcemia by parathyroidectomy reduces basal acid output and fasting serum gastrin concentrations in patients with gastrinoma with MEN I; thus resolution of hypercalcemia may play an important role in the therapy for this subgroup of patients with gastrinomas.

DIFFERENTIAL DIAGNOSIS AND DIAGNOSTIC STUDIES

The hallmark of Zollinger-Ellison syndrome is the presence of circulating hypergastrinemia.[6,7] The various clinical circumstances in which a serum gastrin value should be obtained because of a suspected gastrinoma are outlined in Table 62-1. Fasting serum gastrin levels in normal subjects and in patients with routine peptic ulcer disease are usually less than 150 pg/mL.[64] The degree of hypergastrinemia in patients with Zollinger-Ellison syndrome varies greatly. Although occasional reports of normal levels[65] and values that vary from day to day[66,67] have been described, virtually all patients with a gastrinoma have fasting levels greater than 150 pg/mL, with levels exceeding 100,000 pg/mL in some. A serum gastrin level of greater than 1000 pg/mL in the right clinical setting is virtually diagnostic of Zollinger-Ellison syndrome; however, many patients do not have this level of hypergastrinemia. Elevated serum gastrin levels are reported in a number of other clinical conditions as well (Table 62-2). The most common cause of hypergastrinemia is gastric atrophy.[68] Gastric acid is the primary inhibitor of gastrin release; therefore, its absence leads to uninhibited secretion of the hormone with concomitant hyperplasia of antral G-cells and hypergastrinemia as observed in pernicious anemia.[69-71] Up to 75% of patients with pernicious anemia have substantial hypergastrinemia. The gastrin levels in these patients can approximate those found in patients with gastrinomas, reaching values greater than 1000 pg/mL. Chronic atrophic gastritis and gastric carcinoma are two other conditions associated with hypochlorhydria, or achlorhydria and hypergastrinemia.[72] Hypergastrinemia occurs in association with normal or slightly increased gastric acid secretion in pheochromocytoma, rheumatoid arthritis, diabetes mellitus, vitiligo, gastroparesis, gastric outlet obstruction, renal insufficiency, retained antrum, and massive resection of the small bowel.[73,74] Rarer causes of fasting hypergastrinemia include G-cell hyperplasia and G-cell hyperfunction, which are also associated with gastric acid hypersecretion.[75,76]

To differentiate between the many causes of hypergastrinemia a variety of gastrin provocative tests[77-85] have been developed (Table 62-3). The secretin test has proved to be the easiest and

TABLE 62–3
Gastrin Provocative Testing

DISORDER	CALCIUM INFUSION	SECRETIN INJECTION	TEST MEAL
Gastrinoma	Increase in serum gastrin level by more than 400 pg/mL	Increase is usually greater than 200 pg/mL	Increase is less than 50%
Antral G cell hyperfunction	May or may not have increase in serum gastrin level greater than 400 pg/mL	Decrease, no change, or slight increase in serum gastrin level	Increase is greater than 200%
Common duodenal ulcer	Small increase in serum gastrin level	Increase is less than 200 pg/mL	Moderate increase in serum gastrin level

most reliable study to perform. Isenberg and associates, in seeking to determine whether the putative enterogastrone secretin (see ch 2) could inhibit acid secretion, made the serendipitous observation that, instead, the peptide induced a dramatic rise in plasma gastrin and acid secretion in patients with Zollinger-Ellison syndrome.[79] Since secretin did not have a stimulatory effect on gastrin release in normal subjects, the response noted in patients with a gastrinoma was a paradoxic one. There are some recent reports, however, that secretin can induce a significant early rise (albeit low) of serum gastrin levels in a few normal subjects and patients with common duodenal ulcer disease[84] and rarely in persons with achlorhydria.[85] The mechanism by which secretin stimulates release of gastrin from endocrine neoplasms is unclear. Studies using dispersed gastrinoma cells indicate that secretin directly stimulates gastrin release through a cyclic adenosine monophosphate (AMP)–dependent mechanism[61,86–88]; however, no such stimulation was observed when similar experiments were performed with cultured antral G-cells. The fundamental biologic difference between gastrin-releasing cells present in gastrinomas and G-cells found in normal gastrointestinal mucosa remains unknown. It is possible that the different ontogenic origins of these two cell populations account for their different behavior. As noted previously, gastrinoma cells are believed to arise in the pancreas from pluripotent ductular elements that may retain the functional characteristics of their normal counterparts that secrete bicarbonate in response to secretin.

In conducting the secretin provocative test it is important to ascertain the purity of the peptide to be injected. In the past a preparation of secretin (Boots) was commonly used and resulted in a host of false-positive test results because it contained numerous impurities, some of which cross-reacted with gastrin in radioimmunoassay. Today, the secretin used by virtually all laboratories is obtained from Kabi (GIH secretin) and is known to be pure. In the standard protocol, 2 μg of secretin per kilogram of body weight is infused by intravenous bolus, and serum for gastrin measurement is obtained 10 minutes and 1 minute before, and at 2, 5, 10, 15, 20, and 30 minutes after secretin injection. More than 90% of patients with a gastrinoma exhibit a rise in serum gastrin level within 15 minutes of secretin administration. Based on several studies comprising small numbers of patients, various criteria for establishing the positivity of a secretin provocative test have been proposed, including rises in serum gastrin levels of 100 pg/mL, 200 pg/mL, or 50% above basal levels. Although it has been suggested that an increment in serum gastrin value of greater than 200 pg/mL above basal levels has a sensitivity and specificity of more than 90% for the diagnosis of Zollinger-Ellison syndrome, it was not until recently that a large scale study examined this

carefully. Frucht and colleagues[89] prospectively evaluated the secretin provocative test and the calcium infusion study (see later) in 80 patients with gastrinoma. In accord with previous studies, the secretin test was found to be positive in 87% to 93% of all patients with Zollinger-Ellison syndrome and proved to be more advantageous than the calcium infusion study because of its greater sensitivity, shorter sampling time, ease of performance, and lack of side effects. Of all the three criteria for positivity the parameter recommended by the authors for establishing the diagnosis of Zollinger-Ellison syndrome was a rise in serum gastrin of 200 pg/mL or greater. The false-positive secretin tests reported in other studies[90,91] were not seen with these criteria.

The less commonly employed gastrin provocative test is the calcium infusion study. Calcium gluconate is administered at a concentration of 5 mg/kg/h for 3 hours, with simultaneous measurement of serum gastrin levels at 30-minute intervals. More than 80% of patients with a gastrinoma demonstrate an increase in gastrin levels of more than 400 pg/mL during the third hour of calcium infusion. This study is less sensitive and specific than secretin stimulation for identifying patients with Zollinger-Ellison syndrome. A rise is usually not seen in patients with common peptic ulcer disease or in normal subjects, but it may be observed in 50% of patients with hypergastrinemia of gastric origin. As outlined previously, lack of specificity, diminished sensitivity, and the potential adverse effects of administering intravenous calcium have made this provocative test less useful than the secretin test in diagnosing Zollinger-Ellison syndrome. It is usually reserved for patients with a negative secretin test in the presence of gastric acid hypersecretion and a strong clinical suspicion of gastrinoma.[89]

Standard meal gastrin provocative studies have been employed to distinguish hypergastrinemia of gastric origin (as in G-cell hyperplasia/hyperfunction) from that of pancreatic origin (gastrinoma). According to the prevailing dogma, patients with Zollinger-Ellison syndrome have less than a 50% rise in serum gastrin level in response to a meal, and a postprandial rise in serum gastrin of more than 100% is characteristic of G-cell hyperplasia/hyperfunction. However, data by Frucht and colleagues[92] suggest that 50% of patients with Zollinger-Ellison syndrome have a greater than 50% rise in serum gastrin postprandially. Thus, some caution should be maintained in applying the standard meal study for evaluation of patients with hypergastrinemia.

The net effect of hypergastrinemia is increased gastric acid secretion; thus it is not surprising that basal acid output (BAO) of 15 mEq/h or greater is found in as many as 90% of patients with a gastrinoma.[53,67,93–95] It is important to note, however, that 12% of patients with common duodenal ulcer disease can manifest similar levels of acid secretion. BAO greater than 5 mEq/h is found in 55% of patients with Zollinger-Ellison syndrome even after surgery.[93] To enhance the sensitivity of the gastric secretory studies, maximal acid output (MAO) values may also be measured. Since patients with gastrinomas are presumed to have near maximal secretion of gastric acid even under basal conditions, the acid secretory response to exogenously administered secretagogue (pentagastrin) is diminished. Accordingly, a BAO/MAO ratio of greater than 0.6 is highly suggestive of Zollinger-Ellison syndrome,[8] although a ratio of less than 0.6 does not exclude the diagnosis.[53,67,93] There has been controversy over the use of gastric analysis in view of the sensitivity and specificity of serum gastrin values with or without secretin stimulation. However, as discussed previously, the specificity of secretin stimulation is not 100%. Indeed, studies by Spindel and coworkers[78] have indicated that 59% of patients with elevated serum gastrin levels were either hypochlorhydric or achlorhydric, and thus the ability to diagnose Zollinger-Ellison syndrome was enhanced by performing gastric analysis prior to conducting secretin stimulation tests. Accordingly, under optimal circumstances, acid secretory studies should be part of the diagnostic evaluation in patients suspected of having gastrinomas. If the equipment needed for this test is not available, a simple basal gastric pH determination of more than 3.0 essentially rules out the diagnosis of Zollinger-Ellison syndrome.

In summary, no single diagnostic test has a sensitivity or specificity of 100% in evaluating patients for Zollinger-Ellison syndrome. One must juxtapose the information obtained from the various tests with the clinical presentation. A fasting gastrin value of more than 1000 pg/mL and a basal acid output more than 15 mEq/h in a patient with recalcitrant peptic ulcer is virtually diagnostic of Zollinger-Ellison syndrome. In the absence of this triad of findings, provocative testing may be required. Of these, the secretin stimulation test offers the greatest sensitivity and specificity.

TUMOR LOCALIZATION

Gastrinomas are notoriously difficult to localize. No tumor is found in approximately 50% of patients with Zollinger-Ellison syndrome who eventually undergo surgery, and more than 20% of patients are found to have metastatic disease at laparotomy.[96–98] The availability of potent antisecretory drugs has decreased the morbidity and mortality associated with uncontrollable acid hypersecretion significantly; thus emergency or urgent total gastrectomy is rarely, if ever, needed. However, studies indicate that the tumor itself, rather than the acid hypersecretion, is responsible for the bulk of the adverse sequelae associated with Zollinger-Ellison syndrome. Early intervention with resection of a localized tumor presents the only opportunity to cure this disease.[99,100] In addition, detection of metastatic disease will prevent unnecessary surgery. Accordingly, every effort should be made to localize the tumor preoperatively. A diagnostic plan for localizing gastrinomas in patients with Zollinger-Ellison syndrome is shown in Figure 62-1.

Many approaches have been used for the purpose of localizing gastrinomas. These include abdominal ultrasound,[101,102] computed axial tomography (CT scanning),[102–106] abdominal arteri-

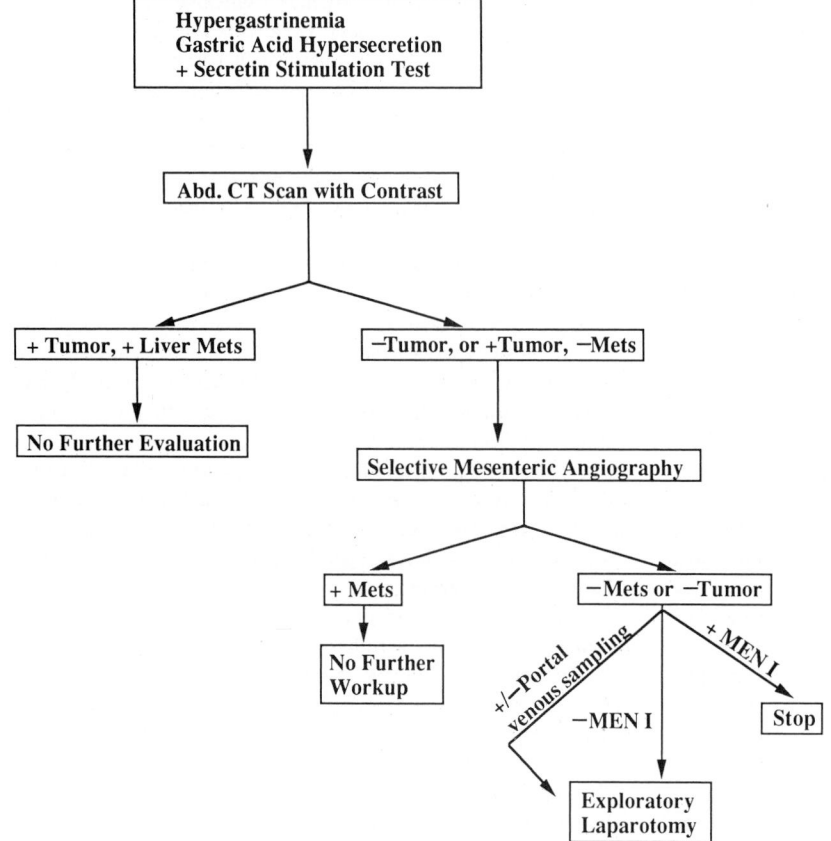

FIGURE 62–1. Diagnostic plan for localizing gastrinomas in patients with Zollinger-Ellison syndrome.

ography,[107-110] and selective portal venous sampling for gastrin[109,111-114] (Table 62-4).

In general, ultrasonography is considered useful for the diagnosis of gastrinomas only if a tumor can be detected. The sensitivity of this test is quite low, as suggested by a prospective study[115] in which ultrasonographically localizable tumors were found in only 20% of patients who were later shown by surgery to have gastrinomas. Nevertheless, the specificity of ultrasound as a diagnostic test was 90% to 100% in the patients who were diagnosed prospectively.

The diagnostic efficacy of CT scanning appears to be improving with the technology itself. A recent prospective study[106] examined the value of CT scanning in localizing tumors in 61 consecutive patients with gastrinomas. For extrahepatic gastrinoma, CT scanning with intravenous contrast media had a specificity of 95%, a sensitivity of 59%, a positive predictive value of 96%, and a negative predictive value of 54%. For gastrinomas metastatic to liver, CT scanning had a specificity of 98%, sensitivity of 72%, a positive predictive value of 93%, and a negative predictive value of 90%. Tumor size and location appear to be the key determinants in the successful diagnosis of gastrinoma by CT scanning. Approximately 80% of tumors in the pancreas and tumors greater than 3 cm in size are detected. Only 40% of extrapancreatic lesions and no tumors measuring less than 1 cm in diameter are detectable by CT scanning. The sensitivity and specificity of CT scanning does not appear to be enhanced by performing dynamic studies; therefore, routine scans with oral and intravenous contrast media will suffice.

Selective abdominal angiography has proven to be useful in some patients with Zollinger-Ellison syndrome.[108-110] Maton and coworkers[110] examined prospectively the role of selective angiography in the diagnosis of 20 consecutive patients who were subsequently diagnosed as having gastrinomas by surgery, autopsy, or percutaneous biopsy. In addition, they compared the results obtained via angiography with those obtained via CT scanning in 58 patients who underwent both tests. For hepatic gastrinoma, angiography had a specificity of 100% and a sensitivity of 86%, with a positive predictive value of 97% and a negative predictive value of 53%. In combination with CT scanning, 100% of the hepatic tumors were detected. Extrahepatic lesions were not as easily detected inasmuch as CT scanning detected only 57%, angiography 70%, and the combination 73%, with a false-positive rate of 7%. This study suggests that after a CT scan, selective abdominal angiography will detect an additional 28% of patients with liver lesions and an incremental 16% of patients with extra-

hepatic tumors. Unfortunately, 24% of the extrahepatic lesions will be missed even when both tests are used. Nevertheless, angiography is a useful adjunct to CT scanning in patients with Zollinger-Ellison syndrome who will undergo surgery.

Even under the best circumstances the combination of ultrasonography, CT scanning, and angiography fails to find tumors in anywhere from 20% to 50% of the patients with biochemical evidence of Zollinger-Ellison syndrome. Thus, percutaneous transhepatic selective portal venous sampling for gastrin has been explored as a means to improve the diagnostic yield.[109,111-114] In this technique a catheter is inserted into the portal vein and multiple samples from the vessels draining the pancreas are taken for measurement of gastrin immunoreactivity. Simultaneous blood samples are taken from either the peripheral venous circulation, hepatic artery, or hepatic vein. A gastrin gradient between the samples from the selectively cannulated vessels and the simultaneously obtained peripheral blood is determined. A step-up in the gastrin value suggests the presence of a gastrinoma. This technique is highly specialized and relies on expert angiographers as well as a sensitive radioimmunoassay for gastrin. There is general agreement with the relative sensitivity of this test in identifying the presence of gastrinomas (70%–90%), but there is considerable debate over its specificity, with values ranging from 33% to 90% depending on the series. The investigators at the National Institutes of Health reported on 27 consecutive patients with Zollinger-Ellison syndrome who were studied prospectively using this technique.[114] Their data suggest that the technique of selective venous gastrin sampling has no better sensitivity than imaging studies in localizing gastrinomas and, furthermore, that imaging studies have higher specificity and positive and negative predictive values. It is not surprising that the conclusion of these studies was to avoid selective venous sampling in evaluating patients with gastrinoma. Before accepting these conclusions, however, it is important to consider some nuances of the study. Even in the presence of a positive gastrin gradient, no patients in the study underwent excision of the head of the pancreas unless a palpable tumor was identified because of the high morbidity and mortality associated with the procedure and the relatively benign clinical course experienced by patients with negative laparotomies. Yet, 8 of the 12 patients who were considered to have false-positive results in the study were noted to have significant gastrin gradients in the region of the head of the pancreas. It is possible, therefore, that patients with microscopic lesions in that region were misdiagnosed. Others who have pursued a more aggressive approach toward excising the pancreatic head have observed a much higher specificity for

TABLE 62-4
Sensitivity and Specificity of Imaging Studies in Zollinger-Ellison Syndrome

STUDY	PRIMARY GASTRINOMA		METASTATIC GASTRINOMA	
	Sensitivity (%)	Specificity (%)	Sensitivity (%)	Specificity (%)
Ultrasound	21–28	92–93	14	100
CT scan	35–59	83–100	35–72	98–100
Selective angiography	35–68	84–94	33–86	96–100
Portal venous sampling	70–90	33–90		

selective portal venous gastrin sampling (90%) in patients with Zollinger-Ellison syndrome.[109] Furthermore, there is evidence to suggest that the technique is particularly useful in detecting extrapancreatic tumors, which are the most difficult to diagnose by other means. Despite the potential usefulness of the selective venous sampling technique, its complexity limits its availability to only a few specialized centers; thus it is not recommended for the evaluation of Zollinger-Ellison syndrome on a routine basis.

A new approach that appears to hold promise in the localization of small gastrinomas is intraoperative ultrasonography.[116–119] Initial studies suggest that tumors[119] not detected by the surgeon by manual inspection may be imaged through this technique. Other diagnostic approaches include magnetic resonance imaging,[120] venous sampling and radiographic imaging after selective arterial injection of secretin,[121] and receptor-targeted nuclear scanning following injection of a radioiodinated analogue of somatostatin.[122] These techniques have potential usefulness but are in the very early stages of development.

THERAPY

When considering therapy for Zollinger-Ellison syndrome it is important to consider two objectives: (1) control of gastric acid hypersecretion and (2) treatment of the malignant neoplasm. The emphasis placed on each of these objectives has shifted over the past 3 decades. Initially, total gastrectomy appeared to be the only alternative for effective treatment of the potentially lethal ulcer disease, and less attention was directed at tumor excision since many of the patients died of ulcer complications long before their tumors became problematic. With the advent of histamine, H₂ blockers, and effective ulcer therapy, long-term medical management became the favored approach, with tumor excision only a secondary consideration since the likelihood of finding and removing a gastrinoma seemed relatively remote.[123] Recently, the availability of highly effective antisecretory therapy through H^+,K^+-ATPase antagonists such as omeprazole has led to a significant reduction in mortality related to the complication of acid peptic disease. Under these circumstances it has become increasingly apparent that the major cause for morbidity and mortality in Zollinger-Ellison syndrome is widespread metastatic disease[124]; thus early tumor detection and excision has assumed primary importance.

Medical Therapy

The primary aim of medical therapy in Zollinger-Ellison syndrome is control of gastric acid hypersecretion. The development of histamine H₂-receptor antagonists was a major breakthrough toward this aim. Cimetidine, the first of these agents, proved to be very efficacious in controlling acid hypersecretion and prompted ulcer healing and symptom improvement in over 80% of patients with Zollinger-Ellison syndrome treated on a short-term basis.[125,126] However, over a longer term, these patients often required progressive increases in the frequency and dose of medication. To correct this problem, anticholinergic agents were used as adjunctive therapy but significant adverse effects were noted.[127,128] H₂-receptor

antagonists with greater potency and duration of action, such as ranitidine and famotidine, have since been developed and have proved to be efficacious in relieving symptoms and promoting ulcer healing in patients with gastrinomas.[129–133] Famotidine has a longer duration of action and is approximately eightfold and thirty-two-fold more potent than ranitidine and cimetidine respectively.[131] These features, coupled with its efficacy and safety, make famotidine the H₂-receptor antagonist of choice for the treatment of Zollinger-Ellison syndrome.

Despite excellent initial ulcer healing and symptom resolution with H₂-receptor antagonists, long-term studies indicate failure rates that may vary from 7% with famotidine to as high as 60% with cimetidine.[134,135] A major factor that may contribute to treatment failure is inadequate dosing of medication. This occurs all too frequently because of the relatively weak antisecretory action of even the most potent H₂ antagonists and because of the lack of correlation between ulcer symptoms and ulcer activity.[136,137] One approach to avoiding the high ulcer relapse rate is to individualize the treatment regimen so that dosing of medication is adjusted to maintain basal acid output (measured 1 hour prior to the next dose of medication) at less than 10 mEq/h[137] in nonoperated patients and less than 5 mEq/h in patients who have undergone a partial gastrectomy or in those having severe esophagitis.[51,138] Because the dose of medication required for suppression of gastric acid secretion may increase on a yearly basis, periodic gastric secretory studies should be performed. The reason for the increased requirement of H₂ blockers for adequate acid suppression is unknown but may be related to the trophic effects of gastrin on the oxyntic mucosa coupled with disease progression.[139,140]

The median H₂ antagonist dose ranges used in treatment of Zollinger-Ellison syndrome are shown in Table 62-5. Even though high doses of these agents have been used over prolonged periods of time their safety profile is encouraging. Despite the antiandrogenic side effects that have been reported in up to 50% of male patients on high-dose therapy with cimetidine,[141] few significant side effects have been observed in female patients. Treatment of gastrinoma with high doses of ranitidine and famotidine has proven to be safe, without dose-related hepatic, central nervous system, or hematologic side effects.

An important new class of drugs recently made available for the treatment of Zollinger-Ellison syndrome is the substituted benzimidazoles, of which omeprazole is the first.[142,143] These compounds are the most potent acid inhibitory agents available because they covalently bind to H^+,K^+-ATPase, the enzyme responsible for the generation of H^+ in the parietal cell (see ch 13). Their efficacy in inhibiting acid secretion, relieving dyspeptic symptoms, and promoting ulcer healing in patients with gastrinomas has been established.[144–146] Although omeprazole requirements for effective inhibition of acid secretion in patients with gastrinomas are higher than in patients with standard peptic ulcers (see Table 62-5), a single daily dose is capable of inhibiting gastric acid secretion completely in 80% of patients with Zollinger-Ellison syndrome, at least initially. The additional 20% of patients require twice-a-day dosing of medication. Tachyphylaxis may be observed less frequently with omeprazole than with H₂ blockers. Fewer than 10% of the patients being treated with omeprazole require yearly dosage adjustments. One concern with long-term omeprazole therapy has been its potential for inducing enterochromaffin cell hyperplasia. A recent prospective study following 40 patients with Zollinger-Ellison syndrome who were treated with omeprazole for

TABLE 62–5
Median Dose of Antisecretory Agents Used
in Patients With Gastrinoma

AGENT	MEDIAN DAILY DOSES (Range)
H$_2$ Blockers	3.6 g (1.2–12.6 g)
Cimetidine	
Ranitidine	1.2 g (0.45–6 g)
Famotidine	0.25 g (0.05–0.8 g)
H$^+$-K$^+$ ATPase inhibitor	60 mg
Omeprazole	

a mean of 29 months (6–51 months), found no evidence of hematologic, biochemical, or gastric toxicity.[147] Their marked potency, prolonged duration of action, and safety profile make substituted benzimidazoles the treatment of choice for peptic disease in patients with Zollinger-Ellison syndrome.

As discussed in Chapter 2, somatostatin is a known peptide inhibitor of gastric acid secretion[148] and gastrin release.[149] The recently developed biochemically stable analogue of somatostatin octreotide has been used with varying success in patients with gastrinomas.[150–153] One rationale for the use of somatostatin analogues is that they can inhibit the secretion of gastrin from the tumor as well as the action of gastrin on the oxyntic mucosa. At present, however, these compounds are available only in injectable form; thus they are rarely used as the first-line agent in the treatment of patients with Zollinger-Ellison syndrome.

Surgical Therapy

Prior to the advent of potent antisecretory agents, total gastrectomy was the operative procedure of choice in patients with gastrinomas. Although initial operative mortality was very high (15%–20%),[154] a total gastrectomy offered better long-term survival than more conservative approaches.[10] Increased experience and earlier diagnostic testing has reduced the operative mortality associated with total gastrectomy to less than 5%.[155] Nevertheless the new gastric antisecretory agents have obviated the need for total gastrectomy, and presently this procedure should be considered only in the rare patient with nonresectable gastrinoma in whom aggressive medical therapy has failed or in those persons who cannot take oral medications.

Another operation applied in the past as an adjunct to medical therapy in patients with Zollinger-Ellison syndrome is proximal gastric vagotomy. The rationale for this operation was the high failure rate with H$_2$ antagonists. Richardson and associates[156,157] reported on a series of 22 patients with gastrinomas who underwent surgery to remove any visible tumor and then were treated with parietal cell vagotomies. Selective vagotomy decreased basal acid output significantly in all of the patients, even if the tumor was incompletely resected or not localized at all. When compared with preoperative values, basal acid outputs were reduced by 41% to 69% in patients who had residual tumor and the dosage of H$_2$ antagonist required for therapy was reduced in 21 of 22 patients.

Despite these data, the availability of omeprazole has virtually eliminated the need for this operation in patients with Zollinger-Ellison syndrome.

As discussed earlier in this chapter, the hypercalcemia found in patients with MEN I may be associated with a gastric acid hypersecretory state that is refractory to medical therapy. A previous report[158] demonstrated that in addition to lowering both basal acid output and fasting hypergastrinemia in these patients, parathyroidectomy facilitates the management of peptic disease with H$_2$ antagonists. Although the availability of H$^+$-K$^+$ ATPase inhibitors may make this operation unnecessary, one should keep in mind that parathyroidectomy is a surgical option that may facilitate the medical management of patients with gastrinoma with MEN I and hyperparathyroidism who are refractory to medical management.

Clearly the appropriate surgical approach for therapy for Zollinger-Ellison syndrome today is curative resection of neoplasm. Although initial series reported less than 10% chance of total cure following tumor resection, present data indicate that this may be possible in as many as 30% of the cases. Improved diagnostic capabilities have led not only to a reduction in unnecessary surgery on patients with metastatic disease but also to the identification of extrapancreatic neoplasms with increasing frequency.[37,39,159–161] Recent studies have reported the incidence of extrapancreatic lesions to be as high as 66% and resection of these lesions to be associated with a high likelihood of long-term cure.[162]

Patients with gastrinoma with MEN I represent a particularly difficult problem to the surgeon. Because of the multicentric nature[163] of this disease curative resection is virtually impossible.[113,155,164,165] Thus, if the diagnostic evaluation does not reveal a resectable tumor, operative exploration should not be considered. If a single tumor is found during the preoperative evaluation, some would advocate an attempt at surgical resection[166] because a larger tumor may be associated with a higher likelihood of metastasis.

Operative management of Zollinger-Ellison syndrome should be undertaken by a surgeon with expertise in the treatment of islet cell tumors. Careful and detailed mobilization and exploration of the entire pancreas and surrounding areas should be performed. Duodenotomy[161] and meticulous evaluation of the duodenal mucosa is essential. Any tumors that are found in the region of the pancreatic head should be enucleated, and tumors located elsewhere should be resected with great care. In the event that a tumor is not found at surgery, distal pancreatectomy should be avoided because more then 80% of the gastrinomas are located within the gastrinoma triangle.[38] If a lesion is found in the head of the pancreas, a Whipple procedure should not be performed since the mortality of this surgical procedure outweighs its potential benefit.

Therapy for Metastatic Gastrinoma

Although major advances have been made in the diagnosis and medical and surgical therapy for Zollinger-Ellison syndrome, an effective approach to the management of patients with metastatic disease has yet to be developed. Metastatic disease occurs in 25% to 40% of patients with gastrinoma and at present is the most common source of morbidity and mortality in this disease. The dictum that the efficacy of the therapy is inversely proportional to the number of therapeutic modalities available certainly holds true in the case of metastatic Zollinger-Ellison syndrome. One major difficulty in evaluating the effectiveness of the various therapeutic regimens is that most clinical trials have examined very small numbers of patients.

Antineoplastic chemotherapy has been of limited usefulness in Zollinger-Ellison syndrome. Combined treatment with streptozotocin, 5-fluorouracil, and doxorubicin has provided the most promising results. In one series of 42 patients with metastatic islet tumors of various types[167] initial response rates of 63% and complete response rates of 33% were reported with this regimen. However, gastrinomas comprised a small percent of the cases studied and the response to chemotherapy may have varied according to the cell type of the tumor. In another study using a similar treatment regimen, Bonfils and coworkers[168] reported disappearance of the gastrinoma as assessed by imaging studies in 20% of their patients with Zollinger-Ellison syndrome with metastatic tumors.

A recent prospective study[169] by the investigators at the National Institutes of Health provided a more sobering perspective on treatment of metastatic gastrinoma with chemotherapy. Ten consecutive patients with the disorder were treated with a regimen of streptozotocin, 5-fluorouracil, and doxorubicin and, although a modest objective response was observed initially in 4 patients, the response lasted for less than 10 months. All of the patients were considered as treatment failures thereafter with no significant change in short-term survival, and many side effects of therapy including nausea and vomiting (100%), alopecia (80%), proteinuria (40%) and leukemia (20%) were noted. At 10 months after initiation of therapy all patients had evidence of tumor growth over the preceding 6 months. The question as to when to treat patients having metastatic gastrinoma with chemotherapy remains unanswered. Although an occasional patient with metastatic disease may survive up to 20 years, it appears that the majority will die within 5 years. Two approaches to this issue include beginning chemotherapy when the patient is symptomatic[167] from the metastasis, or reassess the patient 3 to 6 months after the initial presentation and use chemotherapy if the metastasis is increasing.[170] Both of these approaches are based on studies including relatively small numbers of patients; therefore future studies specifically addressing this question are needed before firm recommendations can be given.

Aggressive surgical resection has been offered as an alternative approach to treating metastatic gastrinoma and a longer survival has been claimed,[171] but controlled studies using such an approach are unavailable. Erickson and co-workers[172] have reported successful therapy for refractory metastatic endocrine neoplasms with human leukocyte interferon, but confirmatory studies are necessary. Hepatic artery embolization,[173] selective hepatic artery infusion of chemotherapeutic agents, and liver directed radiation therapy are treatment modalities under recent investigation, but the effectiveness of treating widespread disease in such fashion will probably be limited. Hormonal therapy with the stable somatostatin analogue octreotide has been attempted in metastatic gastrinoma,[174,175] and although this approach results in decreased gastric acid secretion and partial reduction of hormone release from tumors, it probably does not have predictable long-standing antitumoral effects as reported in other endocrine neoplasms.[166]

PROGNOSIS

Zollinger-Ellison syndrome can follow either a benign or a malignant course.[176] This classification is not based on tumor histopathology or level of hypergastrinemia but on a series of retrospectively determined clinical characteristics. Of these characteristics tumor extent is an important prognostic indicator. As reviewed by Maton and coworkers,[166] 5-year survival for all patients with a gastrinoma varies between 62% and 75% and 10-year survival varies between 47% and 53%. If one segregates the survival data according to extent of tumor present at the time of diagnosis, patients who have a negative laparotomy or have all of their tumor removed surgically have a 5- and 10-year survival rate of more than 90%. In contrast, patients with tumors that were incompletely resected have a 5- and 10-year survival of 43% and 25%, respectively. A summary of prognostic indicators is outlined in Table 62-6. Favorable outcome in Zollinger-Ellison syndrome is associated with primary duodenal tumors, isolated lymph node tumors, or tumors not detectable at the time of laparotomy.[177,178] Although the association of gastrinomas with MEN I has been considered a good prognostic indicator in the past,[177] recent studies[176,179] have cast doubt on this presumption.

Presence of hepatic metastasis clearly indicates a poor outcome in Zollinger-Ellison syndrome. In a review of 36 patients with gastrinoma[165] those found to have tumors in the liver at the time of initial evaluation had a mortality of more than 80% over a 5-year period. Absence of a detectable tumor or metastasis limited to lymph nodes was associated with a remarkably good outcome (see Table 62-6). More recently the presence of Cushing's syndrome in patients with sporadic gastrinoma has been reported as a poor prognostic indicator,[49] with a 0% survival at 3 years. We

TABLE 62-6
Prognostic Indicators

FAVORABLE OUTCOME	POOR OUTCOME
Primary duodenal wall tumor	Hepatic metastasis
Isolated lymph node tumor	Cushing's syndrome in sporadic Zollinger-Ellison syndrome
Tumor not found at laparotomy	Altered amino carboxyl terminal gastrin ratio (possible)
Presence of MEN type I (possible)	

have not found the combination of Cushing's syndrome and gastrinoma to have such drastic consequences. Altered amino to carboxyl terminal gastrin-17 ratios[34,35] and the presence of an aneuploidy state in the tumor[180] seem to suggest a poor prognosis, but confirmatory studies are needed.

The reader is directed to Chapter 2, Gastrointestinal Hormones; Chapter 13, Gastric Secretion; and Chapter 91, Endocrine Neoplasms of the Pancreas.

REFERENCES

1. Zollinger RM, Ellison EH. Primary peptic ulceration of the jejunum associated with islet cell tumors of the pancreas. Ann Surg 1955;142: 709.
2. Sailer S, Zinninger MM. Massive islet cell tumor of the pancreas without hypoglycemia. Surg Gynecol Obstet 1946;82:301.
3. Forty R, Barrett GM. Peptic ulcerations of third part of duodenum associated with islet cell tumors. Br J Surg 1952;40:60.
4. Gregory RA, Tracy HJ, French JM, Sircus W. Extraction of a gastrin-like substance from a pancreatic tumor in a case of Zollinger-Ellison syndrome. Lancet 1960;1:1045.
5. Gregory RA, Grossman MI, Tracy HJ, Bentley PH. Nature of gastric secretagogue in Zollinger-Ellison tumors. Lancet 1967;2:543.
6. McGuigan JE, Trudeau WL. Immunochemical measurements of elevated gastrin in the serum of patients with pancreatic tumors of the Zollinger-Ellison variety. N Engl J Med 1968;278:1308.
7. Yalow RS, Berson SA. Radioimmunoassay of gastrin. Gastroenterology 1970;58:1.
8. Isenberg JI, Walsh JH, Grossman MI. Zollinger-Ellison syndrome. Gastroenterology 1973;65:140.
9. Grimelius L, Hultquist GT, Stenkiuist B. Cytological differentiation of asymptomatic pancreatic islet cell tumors in autopsy material. Virchows Arch 1975;365:275.
10. Ellison EH, Wilson SD. The Zollinger-Ellison syndrome: reappraisal and evaluation of 260 registered cases. Ann Surg 1964;160:512.
11. Stage JG, Stadil F. The clinical diagnosis of the Zollinger-Ellison syndrome. Scand J Gastroenterol 1979;14(suppl 33):79.
12. Deveney CW, Deveney KE. Zollinger-Ellison syndrome (gastrinoma): current diagnosis and treatment. Surg Clin North Am 1987;67:411.
13. Ballard HS, Frame B, Havtsock RJ. Familial multiple endocrine adenoma–peptic ulcer complex. Medicine 1964;43:481.
14. Brand SJ, Andersen BN, Rehfeld JF. Complete tyrosine O-sulphation of gastrin in neonatal rat pancreas. Nature 1984;309:456.
15. Walsh JH. Gastrointestinal hormones. In: Johnson LR, ed. Physiology of the gastrointestinal tract. 2nd ed. New York: Raven Press, 1987: 182.
16. Richardson CT, Walsh JH, Hicks M, Fordtran JS. Studies on the mechanisms of food-stimulated gastric acid secretion in normal human subjects. J Clin Invest 1976;58:623.
17. Feldman M, Walsh JH, Wong HC, Richardson CT. Role of gastrin heptadecapeptide in the acid secretory response to amino acids in man. J Clin Invest 1978;61:308.
18. Soll AH, Amirian DA, Thomas LP, et al. Gastrin receptors on isolated parietal cells. J Clin Invest 1984;73:1434.
19. Soumarmon A, Cheret AM, Lewis JM. Localization of gastrin receptors in intact isolated and separated rat fundic cells. Gastroenterology 1977;73:900.
20. Matsumoto M, Park J, Yamada T. Gastrin receptor characterization: affinity crosslinking of the gastrin receptor on canine gastric parietal cells. Am J Physiol 1987;252:G143.
21. Chiba T, Fisher SK, Agranoff BW, Yamada T. Autoregulation of protein kinase C activity in gastric parietal cells via down-regulation of muscarinic and gastrin receptors. Am J Physiol 1989;256:G356.
22. Johnson LR. The trophic action of gastrointestinal hormones. Gastroenterology 1976;70:278.
23. Johnson LR. New aspects of the trophic action of gastrinitis hormones. Gastroenterology 1977;72:788.
24. Dockray GJ, Gregory RA. Gastrin. In: Schultz SG, Makhlouf GM, Raurer BB, eds. Handbook of physiology, section 6: The gastrointestinal system. Bethesda, MD: American Physiological Society, 1989: 311.
25. Rehfeld JF, Stadil F. Gel filtration studies on immunoreactive gastrin in serum from Zollinger-Ellison patients. Gut 1973;14:369.
26. Gregory RA, Tracy HJ, Agarwal KL, Grossman MI. Amino acid constitution of two gastrins isolated from Zollinger-Ellison tumour tissue. Gut 1969;10:603.
27. Kariya Y, Kato K, Yoshihide H, et al. Expression of human gastrin gene in normal and gastrinoma tissues. Gene 1986;50:345.
28. Dockray GJ, Walsh JH. Amino terminal gastrin fragment in serum of Zollinger-Ellison syndrome patients. Gastroenterology 1975;68: 222.
29. Noyes B, Mevarech M, Stein R, Agarwal K. Detection and partial sequence analysis of gastrin mRNA by using an oligonucleotide probe. Proc Natl Acad Sci USA 1979;76:1770.
30. Yoo O, Powell C, Agarwal K. Molecular cloning and nucleotide sequence of full length cDNA coding for porcine gastrin. Proc Natl Acad Sci USA 1982;79:1049.
31. Boel E, Vrust J, Norris F, et al. Molecular cloning of human gastrin cDNA: evidence for evolution of gastrin gene by duplication. Proc Natl Acad Sci USA 1983;80:2866.
32. Pauwels S, Desmond H, Dimaline R, Dockray GJ. Identification of progastrin in gastrinomas, antrum and duodenum by a novel radioimmunoassay. J Clin Invest 1986;77:376.
33. DelValle J, Sugano K, Yamada T. Progastrin and its glycine extended posttranslational processing intermediates in human gastrointestinal tissues. Gastroenterology 1987;92:1908.
34. Kothary PC, Fabri PJ, Gower W, et al. Evaluation of NH_2-terminus gastrins in gastrinoma syndrome. J Clin Endocrinol Metab 1986;62: 970.
35. Kothary PC, Mahoney WC, Vinik AI. Identification of gastrin molecular molecular variants in gastrinoma syndrome. Regul Pept 1987;17:71.
36. Wolfe MM, Alexander RW, McGuigan JE. Extrapancreatic, extraintestinal gastrinoma: effective treatment of surgery. N Engl J Med 1982;306:1533.
37. Bhagavan BS, Slavin RE, Goldberg J, Rao RN. Ectopic gastrinoma and Zollinger-Ellison syndrome. Hum Pathol 1986;17:584.
38. Stabile BE, Morrow DJ, Passaro E. The gastrinoma triangle: operative implications. Am J Surg 1984;147:25.
39. Hofman JW, Fox PS, Wilson SD. Duodenal wall tumors of the Zollinger-Ellison syndrome: surgical management. Arch Surg 1973;107:334.
40. Ellison EC, Carey LC, Sparks J, et al. Early surgical treatment of gastrinoma. Am J Med 1987;82(suppl 5B):17.
41. Creutzfeldt W, Arnold R, Creutzfeldt C, Track NS. Pathomorphologic, biochemical and diagnostic aspects of gastrinomas (Zollinger-Ellison syndrome). Hum Pathol 1975;6:47.
42. Grieder MH, Rosai J, McGuigan JE. The human pancreatic islet cells and their tumors: II. Ulcerogenic and diarrheogenic tumors. Cancer 1974;33:1423.
43. Dawson J, Bloom SR, Cockel R. A unique apudoma producing the glucagonoma and gastrinoma syndromes. Postgrad Med J 1983;59: 315.
44. Barragry TP, Wick MR, Delaney JP. Pancreatic islet cell carcinoma with gastrin and vasoactive intestinal polypeptide production. Arch Surg 1985;120:1178.
45. Ferrara JJ, Fucci JC, Benson JB. Metastatic pancreatic islet cell carcinoma causing manifestations of glucagon and gastrin hypersecretion. Conn Med 1985;49:777.

46. Wilson DM, Ceda GP, Bostwick DG, et al. Acromegaly and Zollinger-Ellison syndrome secondary to an islet cell tumor: characterization and quantification of plasma and tumor human growth hormone releasing factor. J Clin Endocrinol Metab 1984;59:1002.

47. Sardi A, Singer JA. Insulinoma and gastrinoma in Werner's disease (MEN I). Arch Surg 1987;122:835.

48. Lyons DF, Eisen BR, Clark MR, et al. Concurrent Cushing's and Zollinger-Ellison syndromes in a patient with islet cell carcinoma. Am J Med 1984;76:729.

49. Maton PN, Gardner JD, Jensen RT. Cushing's syndrome in patients with the Zollinger-Ellison syndrome. N Engl J Med 1986;315:1.

50. Richter JE, Pandol SJ, Castell DO, McCarthy DM. Gastroesophageal reflux disease in the Zollinger-Ellison syndrome. Ann Intern Med 1981;95:37.

51. Miller LS, Vinayek R, Frucht H, et al. Reflux esophagitis in patients with Zollinger-Ellison syndrome. Gastroenterology 1990;98:341.

52. Cameron AJ, Hoffman HN. Zollinger-Ellison syndrome: clinical features and long-term follow-up. Mayo Clin Proc 1974;49:44.

53. Regan PT, Malagelada JR. A reappraisal of clinical roentographic and endoscopic features of the Zollinger-Ellison syndrome. Mayo Clin Proc 1978;53:19.

54. King LE, Toskes PP. Nutrient malabsorption in the Zollinger-Ellison syndrome: normalization during long-term cimetidine therapy. Arch Intern Med 1983;143:349.

55. Shimoda SS, Saunders DR, Rubin LE. The Zollinger-Ellison syndrome with steatorrhea: II. The mechanism of fat and vitamin B_{12} malabsorption. Gastroenterology 1968;55:705.

56. Go VLW, Poley JR, Hofman AF, Summerskill WHJ. Disturbances in fat digestion induced by acidic jejunal pH due to gastric hypersecretion in man. Gastroenterology 1970;58:638.

57. Mansbach II CM, Wilkins RM, Dobbins WO, Tyor MP. Intestinal mucosal function and structure in the steatorrhea of Zollinger-Ellison syndrome. Arch Intern Med 1968;121:487.

58. Moshal MC, Broitman SA, Zamcheck N. Gastrin and absorption: a review. Am J Clin Nutr 1970;23:336.

59. Wright HK, Hersh T, Floch MH, Weinstein LD. Impaired intestinal absorption in the Zollinger-Ellison syndrome independent of gastric hypersecretion. Am J Surg 1970;119:250.

60. Deveney CW, Deveney KS, Jaffe BM, et al. Use of calcium and secretin in the diagnosis of gastrinoma. Ann Intern Med 1977;87:680.

61. Elouaer-Blanc L, Sobhani I, Ruszniewski P, et al. Gastrin secretin by gastrinoma cells in long-term culture. Am J Physiol 1988;255:G596.

62. McCarthy DM, Peiken SR, Lopatin RN, et al. Hyperparathyroidism—a reversible cause of cimetidine resistant gastric hypersecretion. Br Med J 1979;1:1765.

63. Norton JA, Cornelius MJ, Doppman JL, et al. Effect of parathyroidectomy in patients with hyperparathyroidism, Zollinger-Ellison syndrome, and multiple endocrine neoplasia type I: a prospective study. Surgery 1987;102:958.

64. Trudeau WL, McGuigan JE. Serum gastrin levels in patients with peptic ulcer disease. Gastroenterology 1970;59:6.

65. Wolfe MM, Jain DK, Edgerton JR. Zollinger-Ellison syndrome associated with persistently normal fasting serum gastrin concentrations. Ann Intern Med 1985;103:215.

66. Walsh JH, Grossman MI. Gastrin. N Engl J Med 1975;292:1324.

67. Thompson JC, Reeder DD, Villar HV, Roberts F. Natural history and experience with diagnosis and treatment of the Zollinger-Ellison syndrome. Surg Gynecol Obstet 1975;140:721.

68. Strickland RG, Bhathal PS, Korman MG, Hansky J. Serum gastrin and the antral mucosa in atrophic gastritis. Br Med J 1971;4:451.

69. McGuigan JE, Trudeau WL. Serum gastrin concentration in pernicious anemia. N Engl J Med 1970;282:358.

70. Korman MG, Strickland RG, Hansky J. Serum gastrin in chronic gastritis. Br Med J 1971;2:16.

71. Ganguli PC, Cullen DR, Irvine WJ. Radioimmunoassay of plasma gastrin in pernicious anemia, achlorhydria without pernicious anemia, hypochlorhydria and in controls. Lancet 1971;1:155.

72. McGuigan JE, Trudeau WL. Serum and tissue gastrin concentrations in patients with carcinoma of the stomach. Gastroenterology 1973;64:22.

73. Korman MG, Laver MC, Hansky J. Hypergastrinemia in chronic renal failure. Br Med J 1972;1:209.

74. Straus E, Gerson CD, Yalow RS. Hypersecretion of gastrin associated with the short bowel syndrome. Gastroenterology 1974;66:175.

75. Ganguli PC, Polak JM, Pearse AGE, et al. Antral-gastrin-cell hyperplasia in peptic ulcer disease. Lancet 1974;1:583.

76. Walsh JH, Nair PK, Kleibeuker J, et al. Pathological acid secretion not due to gastrinoma. Scand J Gastroenterol 1983;82(suppl):45.

77. Malagelada JR, Davis CS, O'Fallon WM, Go VLW. Laboratory diagnosis of gastrinoma: I. A prospective evaluation of gastric analysis and fasting serum gastrin levels. Mayo Clin Proc 1982;57:211.

78. Spindel E, Harty RF, Leibach JR, McGuigan JE. Decision analysis in evaluation of hypergastrinemia. Am J Med 1986;80:11.

79. Isenberg JI, Walsh JH, Passaro E Jr, et al. Unusual effect of secretin on serum gastrin, serum calcium and gastric acid secretion in a patient with suspected Zollinger-Ellison syndrome. Gastroenterology 1972;62:626.

80. Lamers CBH, Van Tongeren JHM. Comparative study of the value of calcium secretin and meal stimulated increase in serum gastrin in the diagnosis of the Zollinger-Ellison syndrome. Gut 1979;18:128.

81. McGuigan JE, Wolfe MM. Secretin injection test in the diagnosis of gastrinoma. Gastroenterology 1980;79:1324.

82. Basso N, LeZoche E, Materia A, et al. Studies with bombesin in the Zollinger-Ellison syndrome. Br J Surg 1981;68:97.

83. Romanus ME, Neal JA, Dilley WG. Comparison of four provocative tests for the diagnosis of gastrinoma. Ann Surg 1983;197:608.

84. Brady CE III, Utts SJ, Dev J. Secretin provocation in normal and duodenal ulcer subjects: is the gastrin rise in Zollinger-Ellison syndrome paradoxic or exaggeration? Dig Dis Sci 1987;32:232.

85. Feldman M, Schiller LR, Walsh JH, et al. Positive intravenous secretin test in patients with achlorhydria-related hypergastrinemia. Gastroenterology 1987;93:59.

86. Imamura M, Adachi H, Takahashi K, et al. Gastrin release from gastrinoma cells stimulated with secretin. Dig Dis Sci 1982;27:1130.

87. Gower WR Jr, Buzogany JA, Ellison EC, et al. Control of gastrin release in cultured gastrinoma derived G-cells. Surgery 1988;104:424.

88. Chiba T, Yamatani T, Yamaguchi A. Mechanism for increased gastrin release by secretin in Zollinger-Ellison syndrome. Gastroenterology 1989;96:1439.

89. Frucht H, Howard JM, Slaff JI, et al. Secretin and calcium provocative tests in the Zollinger-Ellison syndrome. Ann Intern Med 1989;111:713.

90. Mihas AA, Hirschowitz BI, Gibson RG. Calcium and secretin as provocative stimuli in the Zollinger-Ellison syndrome. Digestion 1978;17:1.

91. Primrose JN, Ratcliffe JG, Joffe SN. Assessment of the secretin provocation test in the diagnosis of gastrinoma. Br J Surg 1980;67:744.

92. Frucht H, Howard JM, Stark HA, et al. Prospective study of the standard meal provocative test in Zollinger-Ellison syndrome. Am J Med 1989;87:528.

93. Ayogi T, Summerskill WHJ. Gastric secretion with ulcerogenic islet cell tumor: importance of basal acid output. Arch Intern Med 1966;117:667.

94. Kaye MD, Rhodes J, Beck P. Gastric secretion in duodenal ulcer, with particular reference to the diagnosis of Zollinger-Ellison syndrome. Gastroenterology 1970;58:476.

95. McCarthy DM. Zollinger-Ellison syndrome. Ann Rev Med 1982;33:197.

96. Bonfils S, Landor JH, Mignon M, Hervoir P. Results of surgical management in 92 consecutive patients with Zollinger-Ellison syndrome. Ann Surg 1981;194:692.

97. Deveney CW, Deveney KE, Stark D, et al. Resection of gastrinomas. Ann Surg 1983;198:546.

98. Zollinger RM, Ellison EC, O'Dorisio TM, Sparks J. Thirty years' experience with gastrinoma. World J Surg 1984;8:427.

99. Ellison EC, Carey LC, Sparks J, et al. Early surgical treatment of gastrinoma. Am J Med 1987;82(suppl):17.

100. Harmon JW, Norton JA, Collin MJ, et al. Removal of gastrinomas for control of Zollinger-Ellison syndrome. Ann Surg 1984;200:396.

101. Hancke S. Localization of hormone producing gastrointestinal tumors by ultrasonic scanning. Scand J Gastroenterol 1979;14(suppl):115.

102. Gunther RW, Klose KJ, Ruckert K, et al. Islet cell tumors: detection of small tumors with computed tomography and ultrasound. Radiology 1983;148:485.

103. Dunnick NR, Doppman JL, Mills SR, McCarthy DM. Computed tomographic detection of non-beta pancreatic islet cell tumors. Radiology 1980;135:117.

104. Krudy AG, Doppman JL, Jensen RT. Localization of islet cell tumors by dynamic CT: comparison with plain CT, arteriography, sonography and venous sampling. Am J Radiol 1984;143:585.

105. Stark DD, Moss AA, Goldberg HI, Deveney CW. CT of pancreatic islet cell tumors. Radiology 1984;150:491.

106. Wank SA, Doppman JL, Miller DL, et al. Prospective study of the ability of computed axial tomography to localize gastrinomas in patients with Zollinger-Ellison syndrome. Gastroenterology 1987;92:905.

107. Boijsen E, Samuelsson L. Angiographic diagnosis of tumors arising from pancreatic islets. Acta Radiol [Diagn] (Stockh) 1970;10:161.

108. Mills S, Doppman JL, Dunnick NR, McCarthy DM. Evaluation of angiography in Zollinger-Ellison syndrome. Radiology 1979;131:317.

109. Roche A, Raisonnier A, Gillon-Savouret M-C. Pancreatic venous sampling and arteriography in localizing insulinomas and gastrinomas: procedure and results in 55 cases. Radiology 1982;145:621.

110. Maton PN, Miller DL, Doppman JL, et al. Role of selective angiography in the management of patients with Zollinger-Ellison syndrome. Gastroenterology 1987;92:913.

111. Ingemansson S, Larsson L-I, Lunderquist A, Stadil F. Pancreatic vein catheterization with gastrin assay in normal patients and in patients with the Zollinger-Ellison syndrome. Am J Surg 1977;134:558.

112. Burcharth F, Stage JG, Stadil F, et al. Localization of gastrinomas by transhepatic portal catheterization and gastrin assay. Gastroenterology 1979;77:444.

113. Glowniak JV, Shapiro B, Vinik AI, et al. Percutaneous venous sampling of gastrin value in sporadic and familial islet cell tumors and G-cell hyperfunction. N Engl J Med 1982;307:293.

114. Cherner JA, Doppman JL, Norton JA, et al. Selective venous sampling for gastrin to localize gastrinomas: a prospective assessment. Ann Intern Med 1986;105:841.

115. Norton JA, Doppman JL, Collen MJ, et al. Prospective study of gastrinoma localization and resection in patients with Zollinger-Ellison syndrome. Ann Surg 1986;204:468.

116. Rueckert KF, Klotter HJ, Kummerle F. Intraoperative ultrasonic localization of endocrine tumors of the pancreas. Surgery 1984;96:1045.

117. Sigel B, Machi J, Ramos JR, et al. The role of imaging ultrasound during pancreatic surgery. Ann Surg 1984;200:486.

118. Cromack DT, Norton JA, Sigel B, et al. The use of high-resolution intraoperative ultrasound to localize gastrinomas: An initial report of a prospective study. World J Surg 1987;11:648.

119. Norton JA, Cromack DT, Shawker TH, et al. Intraoperative ultrasonographic localization of islet cell tumors: a prospective comparison to palpation. Ann Surg 1988;207:160.

120. Tjon A, Tham RT, Falke TH, et al. CT and MR imaging of advanced Zollinger-Ellison syndrome. J Comput Assist Tomogr 1989;13:821.

121. Imamura M, Takahashi K, Adachi H, et al. Usefulness of selective arterial secretin injection test for localization of gastrinoma in the Zollinger-Ellison syndrome. Ann Surg 1987;205:230.

122. Krenning EP, Breeman WAP, Kooij PPM, et al. Localization of endocrine related tumors with radioiodinated analogue of somatostatin. Lancet 1989;1:242.

123. Fox PS, Hofman JW, Wilson SD, DeCosse JJ. Surgical management of the Zollinger-Ellison syndrome. SurgClin North Am 1974;54:395.

124. Richardson CT, Walsh JH. The value of histamine H₂ receptor antagonists in the management of patients with the Zollinger-Ellison syndrome. N Engl J Med 1976;294:133.

125. McCarthy DM. Report on the United States experience with cimetidine in Zollinger-Ellison syndrome and other hypersecretory states. Gastroenterology 1978;74:453.

126. Bonfils S, Mignon M, Gatton J. Cimetidine treatment of acute and chronic Zollinger-Ellison syndrome. World J Surg 1979;3:597.

127. Mignon M, Vallot T, Galmicher JP, et al. Interest of a combined antisecretory treatment, cimetidine and prirenzepin, in the management of severe forms of Zollinger-Ellison syndrome. Digestion 1980;20:56.

128. McCarthy DM, Hyman PE. Effects of opropanide on response to oral cimetidine in patients with Zollinger-Ellison syndrome. Dig Dis Sci 1982;27:353.

129. Collen MJ, Howard JM, McArthur KE, et al. Comparison of ranitidine and cimetidine in the treatment of gastric hypersecretion. Ann Int Med 1984;100:52.

130. Jensen RT, Collen MJ, McArthur KE, et al. Comparison of the effectiveness of ranitidine and cimetidine in inhibiting acid secretion in patients with gastric hypersecretory states. Am J Med 1984;77:90.

131. Howard JM, Cheremos AN, Collen MJ, et al. Famotidine, a new, potent, long-acting histamine H₂-receptor antagonist: comparison with cimetidine and ranitidine in the treatment of Zollinger-Ellison syndrome. Gastroenterology 1985;88:1026.

132. Vinayek R, Howard JM, Maton PN, et al. Famotidine in the therapy of gastric hypersecretory states. Am J Med 1986;81:49.

133. Howard JM, Vinayek R, Maton PN, et al. Famotidine: effective treatment of Zollinger-Ellison syndrome. J Clin Gastroenterol 1987;9:23.

134. Deveney CW, Stein S, Way LW. Cimetidine in the treatment of Zollinger-Ellison syndrome. Am J Surg 1983;146:116.

135. Stabile BE, Ippoliti AF, Walsh JH, Passaro E. Failure of histamine H₂-receptor antagonist therapy in Zollinger-Ellison syndrome. Am J Surg 1983;145:17.

136. Ippoliti AF, Stardevant RA, Isenberg JI, et al. Cimetidine versus intensive antacid therapy for duodenal ulcer. Gastroenterology 1978;74:393.

137. Raufman J-P, Collins SM, Pandol SJ, et al. Reliability of symptoms in assessing control of gastric acid secretion in patients with Zollinger-Ellison syndrome. Gastroenterology 1983;84:108.

138. Maton PN, Frucht H, Vinayek S, et al. Medical management of patients with Zollinger-Ellison syndrome who have had previous gastric surgery: a prospective study. Gastroenterology 1988;94:294.

139. Jensen RT. Basis for failure of cimetidine in patients with Zollinger-Ellison syndrome. Dig Dis Sci 1984;29:363.

140. Andersen BN, Lansen NE, Rune SJ, Woining H. Development of cimetidine resistance in the Zollinger-Ellison syndrome. Gut 1985;26:1263.

141. Jensen RT, Collen MJ, Pandol SJ, et al. Cimetidine induced impotence and breast changes in patients with gastric hypersecretory states. N Engl J Med 1983;308:883.

142. Larsson H, Carlsson E, Junggren U, et al. Inhibition of gastric acid secretion by omeprazole in the dog and rat. Gastroenterology 1983;85:900.

143. Lind T, Lederberg C, Ekenued G, et al. Effect of omerprazole—a gastric proton pump inhibitor—on pentagastrin stimulated acid secretion in man. Gut 1983;24:270.

144. Lamers CBHW, Lind T, Moberg S, et al. Omeprazole in Zollinger-Ellison syndrome. N Engl J Med 1984;310:758.

145. McArthur KE, Collen MJ, Maton PN, et al. Omeprazole: effective, convenient therapy for Zollinger-Ellison syndrome. Gastroenterology 1985;88:939.

146. McArthur KE, Jensen RT, Gardner JD. Treatment of acid peptic diseases by inhibition of gastric H⁺,K⁺-ATPase. Ann Rev Med 1986;37:97.

147. Maton PN, Vinayek R, Frucht H, et al. Long-term efficacy and safety of omeprazole in patients with Zollinger-Ellison syndrome: a prospective study. Gastroenterology 1989;97:827.

148. Park J, Chiba T, Yamada T. Mechanisms of direct inhibition of canine gastric parietal cells. J Biol Chem 1987;262:14190.

149. Sugano K, Park J, Soll AA, Yamada T. Stimulation of gastrin release by bombesin and canine gastrin releasing peptides: studies with isolated canine G-cells in primary culture. J Clin Invest 1987;79:935.

150. Ellison EL, O'Dorisio TM, Woltering EA, et al. Suppression of gastrin and gastric acid secretion in the Zollinger-Ellison syndrome

by long-acting somatostatin (SMS 201-995). Scand J Gastroenterol 1985;21(suppl 119):206.

151. Ellison EC, O'Dorisio TM, Sparks J, et al. Observations on the effects of a somatostatin analog in the Zollinger-Ellison syndrome: implications for the treatment of apudomas. Surgery 1986;100:437.

152. Campagnolo D, Gower WR, Fabri PJ, et al. Effect of somatostatin analogue (SMS 201-995) on molecular species of gastrin in gastrinoma. Surgery 1987;102:982.

153. Souquet J-C, Sassolas G, Forichon J, et al. Clinical and hormonal effects of a long-acting somatostatin analogue in pancreatic endocrine tumors and in carcinoid syndrome. Cancer 1987;59:1654.

154. Fox PS, Hofmann JW, Wilson SD, DeCosse JJ. Surgical management of the Zollinger-Ellison syndrome. Surg Clin North Am 1974;54:395.

155. Thompson JC, Lewis BG, Wiener I, Townsend CM Jr. The role of surgery in the Zollinger-Ellison syndrome. Ann Surg 1983;197:594.

156. Richardson CT, Feldman M, McClelland RN, et al. Effect of vagotomy in Zollinger-Ellison syndrome. Gastroenterology 1979;77:682.

157. Richardson CT, Peters MN, Feldman M, et al. Treatment of Zollinger-Ellison syndrome with exploratory laparotomy, proximal gastric vagotomy, and H_2 receptor antagonists: a prospective study. Gastroenterology 1985;89:357.

158. Norton JA, Cornelius MJ, Doppman JL, et al. Effect of parathyroidectomy in patients with hyperparathyroidism and Zollinger-Ellison syndrome and multiple endocrine neoplasia type I: a prospective study. Surgery 1987;102:958.

159. Thompson NW, Vinik AI, Eckhauser FE, Strodel WE. Extrapancreatic gastrinomas. Surgery 1985;98:1113.

160. Vogel SB, Wolfe MM, McGuigan JE, et al. Localization and resection of gastrinomas in Zollinger-Ellison syndrome. Ann Surg 1987;205:550.

161. Thompson NW, Vinik AI, Eckhauser FE. Microgastrinomas of the duodenum: a case of failed operations of the Zollinger-Ellison syndrome. Ann Surg 1989;209:396.

162. Norton JA, Collen MJ, Gardner JD, et al. Prospective study of gastrinoma localization and resection in patients with Zollinger-Ellison syndrome. Ann Surg 1986;204:468.

163. Thompson NW, Lloyd RV, Nishiyama RH, et al. MEN I pancreas: a histological and immunohistochemical study. World J Surg 1984;8:561.

164. Malagelada JR, Edis AJ, Adson MA, et al. Medical and surgical options in the management of patients with gastrinoma. Gastroenterology 1983;84:1524.

165. Mignon M, Ruszniewski P, Haffar S, et al. Current approach to the management of tumoral process in patients with gastrinoma. World J Surg 1986;10:703.

166. Maton PN, Gardner JD, Jensen RT. Diagnosis and management of Zollinger-Ellison syndrome. Endocrinol Metab Clin North Am 1989;18:519.

167. Moertel CG, Hanley JA, Johnson LA. Streptozocin alone compared with streptozocin plus fluorouracil in the treatment of advanced islet-cell carcinoma. N Engl J Med 1980;303:1189.

168. Bonfils S, Ruszniewski P, Haffar S, Laucournet H. Chemotherapy of hepatic metastases (HM) in Zollinger-Ellison syndrome (ZES): report of a multicentric analysis. Dig Dis Sci 1986;31(suppl):abstr WS52.

169. Von Schrenck T, Howard JM, Doppman JL, et al. Prospective study of chemotherapy in patients with metastatic gastrinoma. Gastroenterology 1988;94:1326.

170. Jensen RT, Gardner JD, Raufman J-P, et al. Zollinger-Ellison syndrome: current concepts and management. Ann Intern Med 1983;98:59.

171. Norton JA, Sugarbaker PH, Doppman JL, et al. Aggressive resection of metastatic disease in selected patients with malignant gastrinoma. Ann Surg 1986;203:352.

172. Eriksson B, Alm G, Lundquist G, et al. Treatment of malignant endocrine pancreatic tumours with human leukocyte interferon. Lancet 1986;2:1307.

173. Carrasco CH, Chuang VP, Wallace S. Apudoma metastatic to the liver: treatment by hepatic artery embolization. Radiology 1983;149:79.

174. Shepherd JJ, Senator GH. Regression of liver metastases in patients with gastrin secreting tumor treated with SMS 201-995. Lancet 1986;2:274.

175. Ruszniewski P, Laucournet H, Elouaer-Blanc L, et al. Long-acting somatostatin (SMS 201-995) in the management of Zollinger-Ellison syndrome: evidence for sustained efficacy. Pancreas 1988;3:145.

176. Stabile BE, Passaro E. Benign and malignant gastrinoma. Am J Surg 1985;149:144.

177. Zollinger RM. Gastrinoma: factors influencing prognosis. Surgery 1985;97:49.

178. Delcore R, Cheung LY, Friesen SR. Outcome of lymph node involvement in patients with the Zollinger-Ellison syndrome. Ann Surg 1988;208:291.

179. Wolfe MM, Jensen RT. Zollinger-Ellison syndrome: current concepts in diagnosis and management. N Engl J Med 1987;317:1200.

180. Stipa F, Arganini M, Bibbo M, et al. Nuclear DNA analysis of insulinomas and gastrinomas. Surgery 1987;102:988.

63

Tumors of the Stomach

C. RICHARD BOLAND
JAMES M. SCHEIMAN

INTRODUCTION

Carcinoma of the stomach is the most common cancer in the world. This comes as a surprise to many North Americans because the incidence of stomach cancer is conspicuously low in this region. However, in portions of the Eastern Hemisphere, stomach cancer accounts for one quarter to one half of all new cancers. Furthermore, a dramatic and surprising fall in the incidence of stomach cancer has occurred throughout the world over the past 50 years, for which there is no simple explanation (Fig 63-1). Thus, the study of stomach cancer is important because of its clinical impact worldwide; moreover, the falling incidence of this disease suggests that it is possible to modify environmental factors that produce gastrointestinal cancers. A detailed understanding of this phenomenon could result in a profound impact on our approach to controlling cancers of other organs. This chapter focuses on adenocarcinoma of the stomach, which accounts for the vast majority of cancers in the stomach; polyps, lymphomas, carcinoid tumors, and other sarcomas are dealt with at the end of the chapter.

EPIDEMIOLOGY

The estimated crude rates of cancer incidence indicate that gastric cancer accounts for approximately 10.5% of cancers worldwide (Table 63-1).[1] The distribution of this disease throughout the population is nonuniform. Stomach cancer has a predilection for men in virtually every population studied, occurring 1.4 to 1.7 times as frequently in men.

When evaluated by geographic region, there is great variation in the relative incidence of this disease (Table 63-2). For example, the incidence in Japan is more than 10 times higher than in certain parts of Africa and 6.5 times that observed in North America. The stomach is a major site of cancer incidence in portions of Europe (including Finland, Poland, and Iceland), the Soviet Union, Chile, and China. Gastric carcinoma accounts for more than 9% of the deaths in the tiny Republic of San Marino, and San Marinese continue to develop this disease after emigration to North America.[2] In the United States, the annual incidence of gastric cancer is approximately 9.6 cases per 100,000 population, making it only one fifth as prevalent as colon cancer. The disease is quite rare in parts of Africa (such as Uganda) and in India.[3]

Epidemiologists have attempted to discern the etiology of stomach cancer by studying its geographic distribution. In general, gastric carcinoma is a larger problem in developing nations than in industrialized nations. Incidence and mortality in lower socioeconomic status groups are up to three times as high as those in the upper socioeconomic groups (Table 63-3).[4] A north–south gradient of decreasing gastric cancer mortality has been noted in several countries, including the United States, Japan, and China.[4] Several migration studies have confirmed that first-generation emigrants tend to experience incidence rates similar to the country of origin, whereas subsequent generations develop the incidence rate of the host country.[5] When taken as a whole, the epidemiologic data strongly implicate the influence of incompletely identified environmental factors in the causation of stomach cancer.

Finally, a dramatic drop in the incidence of stomach cancer has been observed worldwide over the past 30 to 50 years[5] (Table 63-4). In the United States, a 67% decrease has been observed from 1950 to 1979. A similar decrease has been seen in high- and low-incidence countries but has been most prominent among the industrialized countries. However, one study performed in New Mexico indicated that stomach cancer mortality declined among Hispanic and non-Hispanic whites between 1958 and 1982, but did not fall among American Indians during this period, and actually increased twofold among American Indian women during the second half of this period.[6] Populations in discrete geographic regions with divergent changes in gastric cancer incidences may provide an opportunity to identify the most important environmental influences in this disease.

ETIOLOGY OF GASTRIC CARCINOMA

Dietary Factors

The striking variation in regional stomach cancer incidence has prompted investigators to scrutinize dietary practices in high- and low-risk areas. The situation appears to be very complex. No single factor accounts for all the differences in cancer incidence. The consumption of a carbohydrate-rich diet has been associated with an increased risk of gastric cancer; among the foods implicated are fava beans,[7] potatoes,[7,8] and "sour pancakes" (Shandong

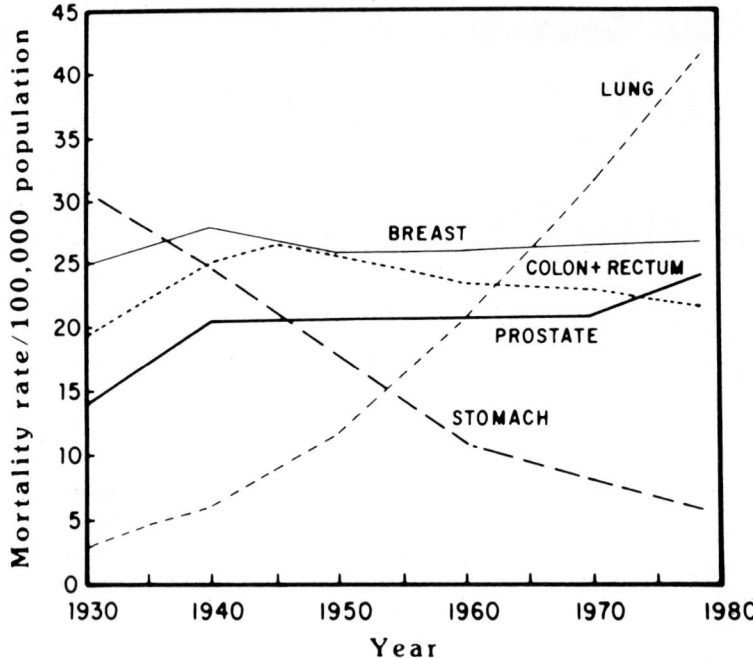

FIGURE 63–1. Time trends in the annual age-adjusted mortality rates for five prevalent cancers in the United States from 1930 to 1980. Rates for breast and prostate cancer are adjusted for sex. The marked rise in lung cancer draws a striking contrast to the falling mortality rates for stomach cancer, while rates for breast, colorectal, and prostate cancers show little age-adjusted change. (From Hill MJ. Environmental and genetic factors in gastrointestinal cancer. In: Sherlock P, Morson BC, Barbara L, Veronesi V, eds. Precancerous lesions of the gastrointestinal tract. New York: Raven Press, 1983:1.)

Province in China).[9] Unfortunately, the implicated foods cannot be consistently found in all of the high-risk regions. Moreover, carbohydrate-rich diets often overlap with high-salt intake,[7–9] contamination of grain supplies with mold,[9] and reduced intake of fresh fruits and vegetables.[7,9,10] The consumption of dried fish, soy sauce, and pickled foods correlates with stomach cancer risk in Japan,[5,11,12] but ingestion of dried fish and pickled foods overlaps with diets that are saltier and lower in fresh fruits and vegetables.

Moreover, preservation of foods by pickling or drying is seen where access to refrigeration is limited. It has been suggested that the widespread use of the home refrigerator and the growth of the frozen food industry has been a key factor in the reduction of gastric cancer incidence in North America and Western Europe. It is not yet clear whether improved refrigeration is actually responsible for reducing the incidence of gastric cancer; nor is it known whether this factor impacts on carcinogenesis by reducing

TABLE 63–1
The Most Frequent Cancers Worldwide (1980)*

MALES	Number†	%	FEMALES	Number	%	BOTH SEXES	Number	%
1. Lung	513.6	(15.8)	1. Breast	572.1	(18.4)	1. Stomach	669.4	(10.5)
2. Stomach	408.8	(12.6)	2. Cervix	465.6	(15.0)	2. Lung	660.5	(10.4)
3. Colon/rectum	286.2	(8.8)	3. Colon/rectum	285.9	(9.2)	3. Breast	572.1	(9.0)
4. Mouth/pharynx	257.3	(7.9)	4. Stomach	260.6	(8.4)	4. Colon/rectum	572.1	(9.0)
5. Prostate	235.8	(7.3)	5. Corpus uteri	148.8	(4.8)	5. Cervix	465.6	(7.3)
6. Esophagus	202.1	(6.2)	6. Lung	146.9	(4.7)	6. Mouth/pharynx	378.5	(6.0)
7. Liver	171.7	(5.3)	7. Ovary	137.6	(4.4)	7. Esophagus	310.4	(4.9)
8. Bladder	167.7	(5.2)	8. Mouth/pharynx	121.2	(3.9)	8. Liver	251.2	(4.0)
9. Lymphoma	139.9	(4.3)	9. Esophagus	108.2	(3.5)	9. Lymphoma	237.9	(3.7)
10. Leukemia	106.9	(3.3)	10. Lymphoma	98.0	(3.2)	10. Prostate	235.8	(3.7)
11. —	—	—	11. —	—	—	11. Bladder	219.4	(3.5)
12. —	—	—	12. —	—	—	12. Leukemia	188.2	(3.0)

* Taking all areas and both sexes together, the most frequent cancer in 1980 was stomach cancer, which comprised 10.5% of the total.
† Number refers to an estimate of thousands of new cases during 1980, worldwide.
Parkin DM, Laara E, Muir CS. Estimates of the worldwide frequency of sixteen major cancers in 1980. Int J Cancer 1988;41: 184.

TABLE 63-2

Stomach Cancer Incidence by Sex and Geographic Region: Crude Stomach Cancer Incidence Per 100,000 Population (1980)

REGION	MEN	WOMEN
North America	12.1	7.1
Japan	78.8	46.3
China	24.6	15.6
USSR	43.6	30.9
Western Europe	28.4	20.9
Eastern Europe	36.4	21.3
Northern Europe	28.2	18.2
Southern Europe	42.5	26.9
Central America	9.1	6.4
Tropical South America	21.2	11.8
Temperate South America	24.7	13.6

Modified from Parkin DM, Laara E, Muir CS. Estimates of the worldwide frequency of sixteen major cancers in 1980. Int J Cancer 1988; 41:184.

TABLE 63-4

The Decline in Gastric Cancer*

COUNTRY	1950–1952	1977–1979	% DECREASE
Finland	109	29	−73.4
Switzerland	56	16	−71.4
Norway	61	19	−68.9
United States	27	9	−66.7
Sweden	46	16	−65.2
Denmark	43	15	−65.1
Belgium	47	18	−61.7
Canada	35	14	−60.0
West Germany	66	27	−59.1
France	41	17	−58.5
Australia	32	14	−56.3
Ireland	60	27	−55.0
England and Wales	45	22	−55.1
Scotland	54	27	−50.0
Czechoslovakia	75	42	−44.0
Japan	130	73	−43.8
Italy	62	35	−43.5
Northern Ireland	54	32	−40.7

* Illustrated are the annual age-adjusted mortality rates for gastric cancer in 1950–1952 compared with rates obtained in 1977–1979. The rates have been age-adjusted to the 1951 population of England and Wales for ages 45–64 years, both sexes combined.
Modified from Hill MJ, Environmental and genetic factors in gastrointestinal cancer. In: Sherlock P, Morson BC, Barbara L, Veronesi V, eds. Precancerous lesions of the gastrointestinal tract. New York: Raven Press, 1983:1.

the intake of potential mutagens or alternatively by increasing the intake of anticarcinogens. Some foods may serve to counteract the effects of certain carcinogens. For example, it has been suggested that there are *protective* effects conferred to persons who consume increased amounts of allium vegetables, such as garlic, onions, scallions, and so forth.[13]

Gastric cancer is prevalent in Columbia and has been extensively studied in this South American country.[14–16] High- and low-risk regions have been identified within Colombia, and the population groups have been investigated for differences in dietary characteristics. High-risk groups tend to obtain their drinking water from wells with significantly higher nitrate concentrations than found in the low-risk regions, and excrete higher amounts of nitrate in the urine.[14] The high-risk groups have higher incidences of

TABLE 63-3

Relationship Between Social Class and Gastrointestinal Cancer*

	STOMACH CANCER	COLON CANCER
Standardized incidence, United Kingdom	1.00	1.00
Social Class		
I. (Professional/managerial)	0.49	1.20
II. ———	0.63	0.99
III. (Skilled workers)	1.01	1.05
IV. (Partly skilled)	1.14	0.92
V. (Unskilled workers)	1.13	1.09

* Note the stepwise increase in gastric cancer from class I to V among the population in the United Kingdom. Colonic cancer rates are not related to social class except for an apparent increase in class I, indicating that the relationship between social class and stomach cancer is simply not due to differences in ascertainment.
Hill MJ. Environmental and genetic factors in gastrointestinal cancer. In: Sherlock P, Morson BC, Barbara L, Veronesi V, eds. Precancerous lesions of the gastrointestinal tract. New York: Raven Press, 1983:1.

chronic atrophic gastritis and intestinal metaplasia.[15] In the highest-risk regions, three quarters of the population has developed chronic atrophic gastritis by age 45, whereas this change has occurred in less than half of the intermediate and lower-risk populations by that age.[15,16] This is discussed in more detail in the subsequent section entitled "Pathology of Gastric Cancer."

Increased use of tobacco and alcohol has been associated with an elevated risk of gastric cancer in the United States.[10] However, tobacco use is an unlikely candidate as a gastric carcinogen because the incidence of this disease has fallen dramatically during the first half of the 20th century, while tobacco use increased markedly and has been associated with an epidemic of lung cancer. Therefore, tobacco and alcohol use may be intermediate epidemiologic markers for some other agent, such as a diet deficient in retinoids or vitamin C, which may be common factors in all of the high-risk regions.[5,9–11] The cumulative effects of 20th century industrialization, including the introduction of plastics, solvents, and other novel substances into the food chain and general environment, have been associated with no increase in gastric cancer. Furthermore, the use of the outdoor charcoal grill, which has increased dramatically in the United States over the past 30 to 40 years has had no adverse impact on this disease. Likewise, alcohol use or abuse cannot be implicated in the hyperendemic regions of Eastern Asia.

The quality of drinking water has been scrutinized for a possible etiologic role in stomach cancer. Elevated nitrate levels in well water have been reported in several high-risk regions of South

America and Europe. Vegetables are the principal source of nitrates in some diets. Nitrates also enter the diet as preservatives of meat, fish, and vegetables. Dietary nitrates are potentially dangerous in the presence of nitrate-reducing bacteria in the mouth and stomach. These bacteria produce nitrate reductase that converts nitrates to nitrites, which are substrates for the formation of nitrosamides and nitrosamines. This is discussed in more detail in the next section. The role of numerous other contaminants of water have been suspected to play a role in stomach cancer, including aflatoxin, pepper, vitamin or mineral deficiencies, soft water, and so forth, however, a compelling case has emerged for none of them.[17] Also, contamination of the drinking water with asbestos does not increase the risk of stomach cancer, even in communities where sufficient asbestos is absorbed to result in a high incidence of pleural plaques.[18]

The epidemiology of gastric cancer suggests that the incidence rates are primarily determined by environmental, probably dietary, factors. This hypothesis has been strengthened by three arguments. First, experimental models have been developed whereby chemical carcinogens are administered to animals resulting in gastric cancer. These models have been used to determine how modifications in the diet influence the development of cancer. Second, dietary components have been identified that are chemically similar to compounds that are potent carcinogens in animals and are suspected to play a role in cancer risk for humans. Third, there is a well-documented pathologic sequence leading to stomach cancer in which the gastric epithelium is damaged by an unknown agent and becomes atrophic and achlorhydric; the bacterial flora in the stomach changes in response to the reduced secretion of acid and permits the generation of potential carcinogens; the gastric epithelium undergoes intestinal metaplasia; neoplasia ultimately develops within the metaplastic tissue. This progression of events is most commonly seen in those areas where gastric carcinoma has its greatest incidence. These three bodies of evidence provide a hypothetical framework in which to consider the etiology of cancer in the stomach.

Experimental Models of Gastric Carcinoma

Carcinoma of the stomach may be readily induced in rodents using the nitrosamine N-methyl-N′-nitro-N-nitrosoguanidine (MNNG). Much has been learned from this model, however, it is difficult to know how much of the insight gained is directly applicable to human disease. Nonetheless, several provocative observations have been made. For example, although the administration of MNNG is a paradigm of environmental carcinogenesis, species-dependent susceptibility to the carcinogen has been demonstrated among different species of rodents, ranging from 0 to 80% using identical doses of the compound.[19] At least one biochemical mechanism for species differences in gastric carcinogenesis is related to the ability of the gastric tissue to metabolize and inactivate MNNG by denitrosation.[20] The metabolism of carcinogens is complex, and denitrosation is only one of a variety of possible metabolic fates for nitrosamines. The ability of tissue to activate procarcinogens has been less well studied in this model. Of particular interest, in several species, males are substantially more susceptible than females.[19] Although it has not been explored,

this may be relevant to the observation in humans, in which males have consistently had higher rates of stomach cancer in virtually every population group.

After exposure to MNNG, the pyloric glands become larger, and the pool of proliferating epithelial cells expands. These early changes are significantly greater among the more susceptible species of rodents.[21] Within 16 weeks after exposure to MNNG, susceptible animals begin to develop intestinal metaplasia, which is part of the aging process that normally begins after 40 weeks in untreated control animals.[22] Adenomatous hyperplasia is a pathologic process that begins to appear at 32 to 40 weeks in the MNNG-treated animals (depending on dose), does not occur in control animals not treated with MNNG, and appears to be the pathologic focus from which cancer arises.[22] The important observation is that the chemical carcinogen may produce a variety of pathologic changes, some of which resemble other processes that frequently occur with aging in animals fed an "ordinary" laboratory diet.

The MNNG model permits the introduction of manipulations that may increase or decrease the likelihood of developing tumors. For example, gastrin is trophic to some cells in the stomach, and hypergastrinemia typically occurs in the setting of atrophic gastritis. Therefore, different models of hypergastrinemia have been developed in rodents to test its effect on carcinogenesis in the stomach. The prolonged administration of exogenous gastrin to MNNG-treated animals results in a significant increase in acid secretion but a decrease in the incidence of adenocarcinoma in the glandular stomach.[23,24] The effect of gastrin on epithelial proliferation in the stomach is complex; hypergastrinemia increases proliferation in the fundic mucosa but inhibits proliferation in the antral mucosa of the rat.[24] However, a model of hypergastrinemia and acid hypersecretion has been created by dividing the rodent stomach, performing a Billroth II gastrojejunostomy, and anastomosing the antral stump to the colon ("antral implant"). When compared to animals given antrectomy and Billroth II anastomosis, only the animals with the antral implant developed hypergastrinemia and acid hypersecretion. Significantly fewer MNNG-induced tumors developed in the gastric remnants of animals with the antral implants when compared with the antrectomized animals, but the alkalinized antral stumps continued to develop a high rate of tumors, leading the authors to suggest that acid secretion protected against gastric cancer.[25] This contention was supported by an experiment in which cysteamine was added to the MNNG model to stimulate gastrin release and acid secretion. Cysteamine-treated animals developed hypergastrinemia, increased secretion of acid, decreased indices of cellular proliferation in the fundus and antrum, and fewer MNNG-induced tumors.[26]

One can develop the model further by using multiple agents to manipulate the secretion of gastrin and acid. The concomitant administration of both cysteamine and propranolol further augments acid secretion but reduces the serum gastrin level. This maneuver produces a significant fall in gastric cancer incidence. Contrariwise, cysteamine plus cimetidine resulted in higher gastrin levels, inhibited acid secretion, increased proliferative indices in the antrum, and produced significantly more cancers than found in the cysteamine plus propranolol group.[27] The administration of exogenous histamine, another acid secretagogue, also decreased the number of MNNG-induced adenocarcinomas in the glandular stomach.[28] Contrariwise, a truncal vagotomy inhibits acid secretion and increases carcinogenesis.[29] Thus, although gastrin may exert a trophic effect on the gastric fundus, this hormone does not increase the development of adenocarcinoma in the carcinogen-treated rodent and can inhibit the development of cancer in the antrum. These experiments strongly suggest that acid secretion protects against carcinogen-induced gastric cancers. Of interest, the MNNG model also produces carcinoid tumors in the fundus of the rodent stomach, whereas the administration of exogenous gastrin has a minimal effect on the production of these tumors.[30]

This model has been used to study the influence of other putative cancer-modifying agents in the stomach. Transplantation of the bile duct to the stomach or administration of exogenous sodium taurocholate significantly increased the number of neoplastic lesions in the MNNG-treated rat.[31] The administration of aspirin twice a week in the MNNG model also markedly increased the number of tumors compared to animals treated with carcinogen alone.[32]

The animal model of gastric cancer has been used to study the effect of gastrojejunostomy and enterogastric reflux on the development of gastric tumors. Significantly more cancers develop in MNNG-treated animals after gastrectomy and jejunostomy compared with unoperated carcinogen-treated animals.[33] Of interest, a substantial number of animals develop gastric adenocarcinomas after gastrectomy and gastrojejunostomy even when not administered carcinogen, although spontaneous tumors in this region are very rare in control rats.[33-35] Furthermore, the number of tumors may be increased by administering a high-cholesterol diet to animals subjected to this operation, whether or not they had been treated with MNNG. This diet produces a significant increase in the secretion of bile into the stomach and increases fecal bile acid excretion.[35]

In summary, a nitrosamine induces gastric adenocarcinomas in rats. Acid-reducing maneuvers increase the number of tumors produced, whereas acid-stimulating agents are protective. Antrectomy and gastrojejunostomy, which is suspected to be a carcinogenic operation in humans, also enhances tumor development in rodents, as do other measures that increase the exposure of the stomach to bile.

Possible Carcinogens in the Human Diet: N-nitroso Compounds

N-nitroso compounds are strong carcinogens suspected to play a role in upper gastrointestinal carcinogenesis because of their spontaneous synthesis from dietary components and their ability to alkylate nucleic acids. Nitrosamides are a subset of the N-nitroso group formed in the stomach from nitrite and amides. Their spontaneous formation is favored by low pH, and no enzymes are required for their synthesis. They are unstable and likely to react near the site of their formation. Nitrosamines such as MNNG are more stable than most nitrosoureas or other nitrosamides, which makes them useful for animal studies of gastric carcinogenesis. However, the compounds actually involved in human carcinogenesis may be more ephemeral reaction products generated locally in the stomach, such as nitrosamides or compounds activated by mucosal enzymes from dietary procarcinogens.

The formation of nitrosamides in the stomach requires the presence of nitrites. Drinking water contains variable amounts of nitrate, which is readily absorbed from the gastrointestinal tract and actively secreted into saliva. Nitrate may be reduced to nitrite by the flora of the mouth or stomach. Human saliva typically contains 6 to 10 mg nitrite/L and 15 to 35 mg nitrate/L.[36] Nitrite levels of gastric juice are substantially lower but increase with rising gastric pH in the presence of nitrate-reducing bacteria, which may be seen in the setting of pernicious anemia or after acid-reducing surgery. As demonstrated in Table 63-5, salivary nitrate and nitrite levels rise to very high levels after a challenge dose of nitrate and are high in populations that have high rates of stomach cancer. Gastric nitrite has a number of possible metabolic fates;

TABLE 63-5
Nitrate and Nitrite Levels in Human Saliva and Gastric Juice*

MATERIAL ANALYZED	AVERAGE NITRATE (MG/L)	AVERAGE NITRITE (MG/L)
Saliva of Boston inhabitants		
Base value	5–35	6–10
After receiving a 100- to 500-mg dose of nitrate	≤500	≤100
Gastric contents		
Fasting: Normal subjects in England	———	0.12
Fasting: Pernicious anemia patients, contents pH > 5	———	0.55
Fasting: Colombian subjects with, e.g., gastritis, contents pH > 5	27 95	2.5 2.7
After high-nitrate-level meal; Normal subjects in France	55	5.0

* *Nitrate and nitrite levels in human saliva and gastric juice in Boston, Great Britain, Colombia, and France, demonstrating the elevated levels in fasting Colombian subjects (at greater risk of gastric cancer), and the marked response to oral nitrate challenge.*
Modified from Mirvish SS. Intragastric nitrosamide formation and other theories. JNCI 1983;71:629.

it may spontaneously decompose, bind to scavenger compounds, or react with amines to give rise to N-nitroso compounds.

The sources of gastric nitrites have been estimated based on current typical dietary practices in North America. The most prominent source of *dietary nitrate* is vegetables, which account for 85% of the intake. It is estimated that 25% of dietary nitrate participates in the "entero-salivary circulation." Approximately 20% of the salivary nitrate is reduced to nitrite by the oral flora, and this accounts for the majority (80%) of *gastric nitrite*.[37] The other 20% of gastric nitrite is derived directly from the diet. There is a high degree of correlation between nitrate intake and mortality from gastric cancer. This was noted previously in reference to studies within Colombia but has also been demonstrated by comparing nitrate intake in countries with differing risks for stomach cancer (Fig 63-2).[38] The ability of the host to reduce nitrate to nitrite may be equally important. In addition, the amine content of the diet is critical to the hypothesis that these compounds are active in gastric carcinogenesis. Nitrosamide precursor substances include a wide range of compounds, many of which are prominent in the diets of high-risk regions. Several compounds, such as vitamins C and E, have been found to inhibit the formation of nitrosamides from secondary amines and nitrites. The urinary secretion of nitrosamine degradation products may be dramatically inhibited in humans by the addition of only 1 g of ascorbic acid to the diet,[37,39] and a similar inhibition of nitrosamine excretion has been achieved using 400 mg of α-tocopherol.[39] The concentration of N-nitroso compounds has been measured in the gastric juice of patients with normal and diseased stomachs. An increase in the extractable N-nitrosamines occurred as the pH of the gastric

juice rose from 1 to 7 (Fig 63-3). The highest levels of these potentially carcinogenic compounds have been found in patients with gastric carcinoma, pernicious anemia, and partial gastrectomy (Fig 63-4). Elevated pH in the gastric juice correlated significantly with gastric nitrite levels and the numbers of nitrate-reductase producing bacteria. Of interest, men had significantly higher concentrations of N-nitrosamines than women.[40] Thus, the nitrosamide theory provides a potential explanation for some geographic regions at very high risk for gastric cancer. This concept is a complex one that requires a source of dietary nitrate, a mechanism for its reduction to nitrite, and a source of nitrosamide precursors. The situation is complicated by the ubiquitous presence of compounds that inhibit the metabolism of nitrate and the formation of nitrosamides.

Role of Chronic Atrophic Gastritis in Gastric Carcinogenesis

Atrophic gastritis occurs in 80% to 90% of patients with gastric carcinoma, and this close association has led to the assumption that it is etiologically related in this disease.[41] Atrophic gastritis is a curious entity in which mucosal atrophy and cellular hyperproliferation occur together.[42] This process begins with superficial inflammation limited to the upper half of the gastric gland, typically starts in the antrum, and, over time, progresses in severity and distribution throughout the stomach. Eventually, inflammation may involve the entire gland, and in the later stages of the disease, a

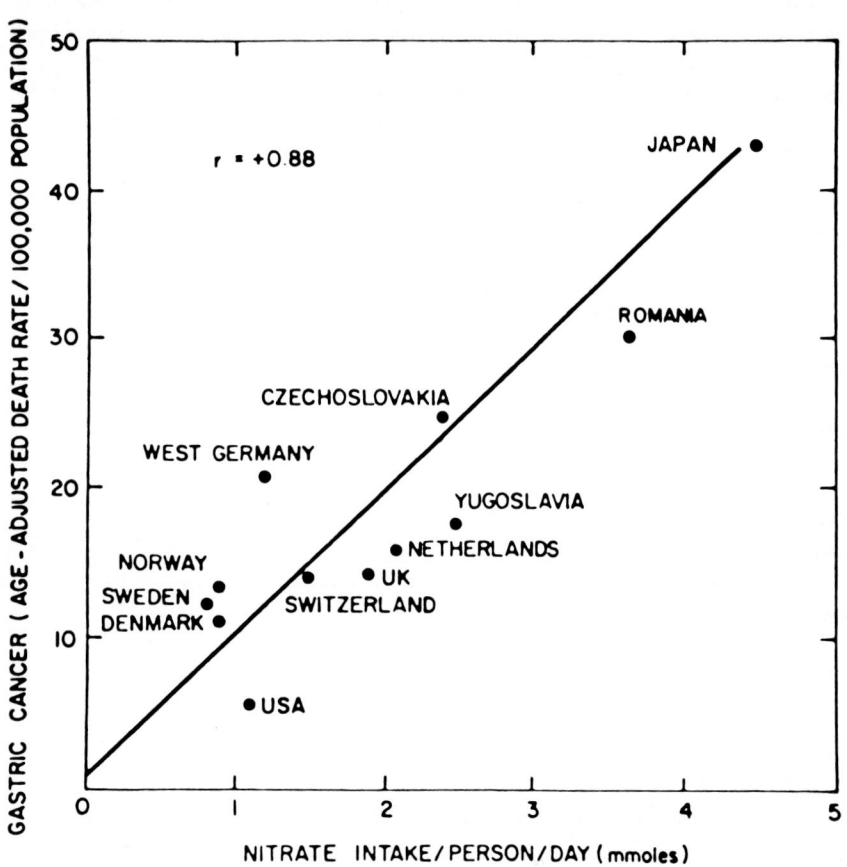

FIGURE 63-2. A high degree of correlation may be drawn between per capita intake of nitrates and age-adjusted mortality for gastric cancer. (From Mirvish SS. Intragastric nitrosamide formation and other theories. JNCI 1983;71:629.)

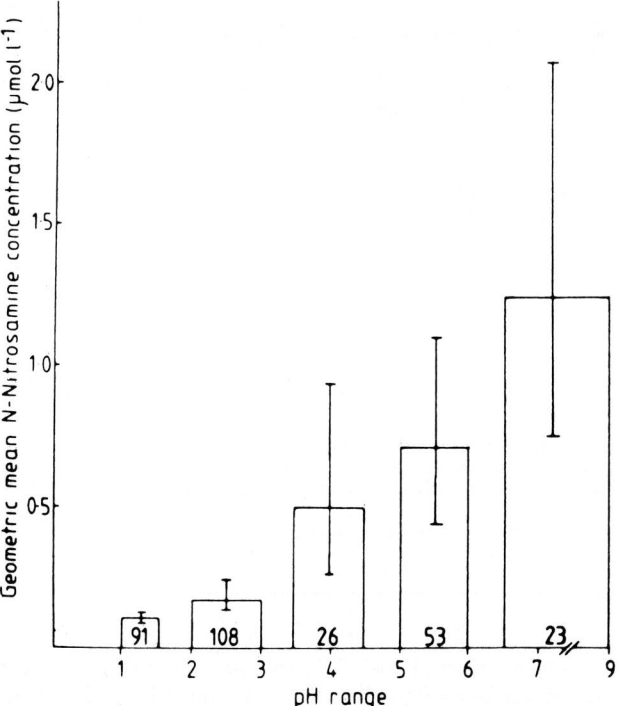

FIGURE 63–3. Relationship between gastric pH and extractable N-nitrosamines. (From Reed Pl, Smith PLR, Haines K, et al. Gastric juice N-nitrosamines in health and gastroduodenal disease. Lancet 1981;2:550.)

reduction in the inflammatory infiltrate and mucosal atrophy occur. The parietal cells do not disappear until late in the disease process, so most patients continue to secrete acid and have normal levels of gastrin. This contrasts with the less common variety of chronic gastritis that begins in the fundus, is associated with parietal cell antibodies and destruction of the gastric glands that contain parietal and chief cells, and produces pernicious anemia. The variety

of chronic atrophic gastritis that begins in the antrum is sometimes referred to as type B gastritis and is thought to be caused by a toxic or infectious environmental etiology. This is associated with a high incidence of antral ulcers and is very common in countries where carcinoma of the stomach is prevalent. Chronic atrophic gastritis that begins in the fundus, the type A variant, is a less common entity, is thought to have an autoimmune etiology, and is associated with gastric cancer in both high- and low-risk populations.

In its later stages, chronic atrophic gastritis may be complicated by the appearance of intestinal metaplasia. This entity also begins in the antrum and may spread to involve the entire stomach. Intestinal metaplasia is characterized by a series of morphologic changes, changes in histochemical staining,[43] and alterations in tissue glycoprotein expression.[44,45] "Intestinal type" gastric cancer (see section entitled "Pathology of Gastric Cancer") is highly associated with the presence of intestinal metaplasia and frequently arises within it.[46] A study of five geographically distinct Colombian population groups with different risks of stomach cancer has demonstrated a relationship between the annual incidence of gastric cancer and the prevalence of chronic atrophic gastritis and intestinal metaplasia, as illustrated in Table 63-6. In the highest risk regions of Colombia, 75% of the population had developed some type of gastritis by the age 45, whereas only 30% of the population had developed such changes in the lowest risk region.[16] For reasons that are not understood, these pathologic changes in the stomach begin to occur in adult life and increase in prevalence with age. Because it is not possible to know when this process begins in any individual patient, it is difficult to predict a timetable for neoplastic progression in the setting of chronic atrophic gastritis. However, several studies from Scandinavia, Italy, and Great Britain indicate that approximately 10% of patients with chronic atrophic gastritis develop gastric carcinoma approximately 15 years later (Table 63-7).[41,47–49] A control group consisting of subjects with normal gastric mucosa or superficial gastritis developed no gastric carcinomas during the 15-year follow-up.[49] Some insight into the

FIGURE 63–4. Gastric pH and N-nitrosamine concentrations in different patient groups. N = normal controls, DU = duodenal ulcer, Oes = esophagitis, V = vagotomy, Gas = chronic gastritis, GU = gastric ulcer, PG = partial gastrectomy. Carc = carcinoma of stomach, and PA = pernicious anemia. (From Reed Pl, Smith PLR, Haines K, et al. Gastric juice N-nitrosamines in health and gastroduodenal disease. Lancet 1981;2:550.)

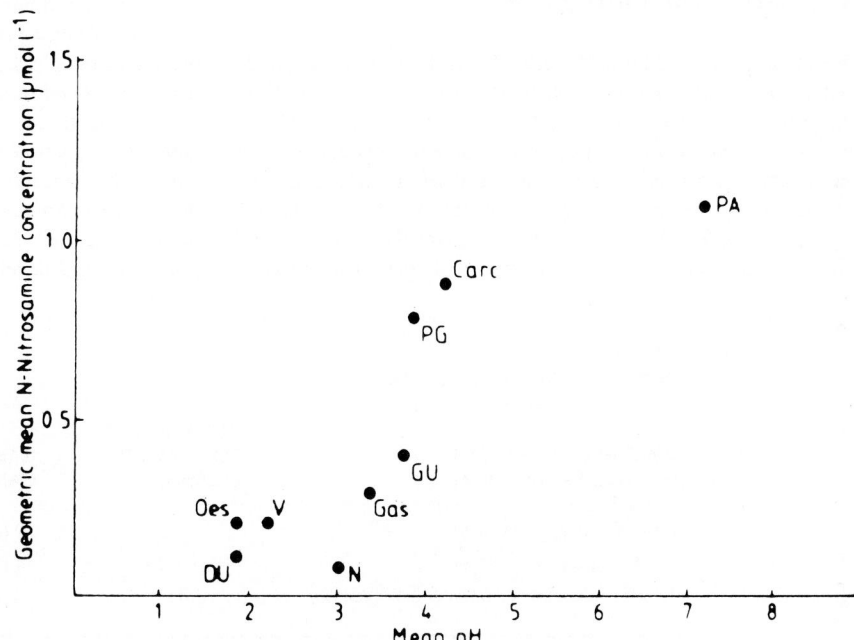

TABLE 63–6

Gastric Cancer and Precursor Lesions in Five Geographically Distinct Colombian Population Groups With Different Risks of Cancer*

| | ANNUAL INCIDENCE OF GASTRIC CANCER PER 100,000 | GASTRIC HISTOLOGY | | | |
GROUP	POPULATION	Normal (%)	Superficial Gastritis (%)	Chronic Gastritis (%)	Intestinal Metaplasia (%)
A (high-risk region)	150	25	19	56	22
B (emigres from A and C)	68	38	24	38	18
C (low risk)	40	29	28	34	11
D (Cali natives)	23	46	28	26	7
E (Cartagena natives)	6	70	17	13	6

* Groups A and C are high- and low-risk populations from a mountainous region of southwest Colombia; Group D represents the natives of a nearby city (Cali) with a low risk of stomach cancer, and Group B represents emigrants born in the mountainous regions (A and C) who moved to Cali. Population E is a northern Colombian city on the Atlantic coast with a low cancer risk (Cartagena).

Modified from Correa P, Cuello C, Duque, et al. Gastric cancer in Colombia. III. Natural history of precursor lesions. JNCI 1976;57:1027.

time required for the development of cancer was obtained from a study of 100 patients with atrophic gastritis in which no cases of gastric cancer developed within a 5-year follow-up.[50]

Therefore, in any given population of patients, chronic atrophic gastritis and intestinal metaplasia are indices of the risk of gastric carcinoma in that group and are markers within individuals of the high risk to develop gastric cancer. It is usually difficult to date the onset of the process, and a relatively long period of time appears to be required for the development of neoplasia. Moreover, only 10% of patients with this preneoplastic condition might be expected to develop cancer, even when followed for 10 to 20 years.

Role of Ulcer Surgery in Gastric Carcinogenesis

Operations performed for peptic ulcer disease have been associated with an increased risk for gastric cancer. The mechanism underlying carcinogenesis in this setting has been controversial. In 1980, Schlag et al[51] studied the appearance of potential carcinogens in the stomach after ulcer surgery. The gastric pH of single aspirated specimens was significantly elevated in the Billroth II patients (mean pH = 6.5 ± 0.5) compared to unoperated controls (mean pH = 2.1 ± 0.4) or patients who had undergone parietal cell

vagotomies (mean pH = 2.2 ± 0.6); patients with a Billroth I anastomosis had intermediate values (mean pH = 4.5 ± 1.0). Significant increases in gastric juice nitrite and N-nitroso compounds were found in the antrectomy patients compared with controls or those with vagotomy alone, and the increase was especially marked in the patients with Billroth II anastomoses. The levels of N-nitroso compounds correlated significantly with gastric pH. Measurements of gastric pH, nitrite, N-nitroso compounds, and nitrate-reducing bacteria obtained from patients with Billroth I or Billroth II gastrectomies have been reported to be similar to those seen in patients with carcinoma of the stomach.[52]

However, other investigators have challenged these findings. A small British study reported that patients who had undergone antrectomy and truncal vagotomy developed higher mean pH, increased counts of nitrate-reducing bacteria and nitrite concentrations, but no difference in concentrations of N-nitroso compounds.[53] Another study has reported a significant relationship between gastric pH and nitrite concentration, but no correlation between pH and total N-nitroso compound concentrations in the stomach. In that investigation, patients who had undergone vagotomy and gastrojejunostomy had significantly higher gastric pH and nitrite concentrations only if the gastric mucosa contained intestinal metaplasia or dysplasia.[54] This group of investigators has also reported that patients with vagotomy and gastrojejunostomy who had developed intestinal metaplasia or dysplasia had

TABLE 63–7

Chronic Atrophic Gastritis and Gastric Cancer

NUMBER OF SUBJECTS (GASTRIC PATHOLOGY)	DURATION OF FOLLOW-UP (YEARS)	GASTRIC CANCER	REFERENCE
N = 116 (atrophic gastritis)	15	9 (8%)	49
N = 40 (atrophic gastritis)	9–21	4 (10%)	47
N = 65 (atrophic or "preatrophic" gastritis)	11–18	9 (13%)	41, 48

significantly higher fasting intragastric bile acid concentrations compared to patients who had undergone the same operation but had merely gastritis, mucosal atrophy, or mild dysplasia.[55] These reports suggest that the relationship between operations for duodenal ulcer and N-nitroso compounds is, at the very least, complex and may involve the degree of anacidity and bile reflux. When assessing this literature, it should be kept in mind that the measurement of N-nitroso compounds is difficult, particularly in gastric juice. These compounds are intrinsically unstable, and there are no simple methods to measure all of the varieties and degradation products of these compounds. Furthermore, additional N-nitroso compounds may be generated in vitro after sample collection. Methods to measure nitrite are also complex, and in vitro degradation is more rapid at low pH. These complexities may explain some of the discrepancies that have been reported in this setting.[56]

CLINICAL MANIFESTATIONS OF GASTRIC CANCER

Symptoms of Gastric Cancer

The clinical features of stomach cancer are typically so vague and nonspecific that they rarely lead to an early diagnosis. Patients may complain of epigastric pain, early satiety, abdominal bloating, or meal-induced dyspepsia. Symptoms usually do not occur until the tumor is advanced. In Japan, where the disease is very common, screening programs have been developed to find tumors in asymptomatic subjects. Screening before the development of symptoms is the only way to find early stage tumors and improve the surgical outcome. Careful history and physical examination are unlikely to provide any benefit in the management of this disease; symptoms simply do not appear until the disease has become invasive and, in most instances, metastatic. In geographic locations where the incidence of gastric cancer is low, attention should be directed toward screening patients in high-risk groups, such as patients with chronic atrophic gastritis, pernicious anemia, gastric adenomatous polyps, and patients who have undergone prior surgery for peptic ulcer disease. There does not appear to be a relationship between chronic gastric ulcer and gastric carcinoma.[57] In general, benign ulcers do not undergo "malignant degeneration." However, a cancer may present as an ulcerated lesion, therefore all ulcers should be carefully examined for malignancy. Patients with late-onset hypogammaglobulinemia (also known as common variable immunodeficiency, not to be confused with AIDS) are at very high risk to develop pernicious anemia and gastric cancer.[58] In one study published in the pre-AIDS era, 3 of 39 (8%) patients with late onset immunoglobulin deficiency had a coincident carcinoma of the stomach.[59]

The incidence of stomach cancer varies as a geometric function of age, and the largest number of affected patients is found in the 50 to 70 year age group. A small percentage of patients develop gastric carcinoma before age 40, and, in North America, there is an excess of immigrants from high-risk countries and patients with positive family histories in this group. The detection of this disease in a young patient should raise the possibility that the patient comes from a cancer family syndrome or Lynch syndrome II kindred.[60] Gastric cancer in young patients is more likely to be of the diffuse type and associated with a poorer prognosis.[61-64]

The paucity of symptoms of early disease has prompted a search to identify markers that predict stomach cancer noninvasively. The use of "tubeless analysis" was initiated over 30 years ago but has never enjoyed widespread clinical use. The object of this test was to detect achlorhydria by administering a dye bound to a resin (Diagnex Blue) that would disassociate in the presence of gastric acid and be excreted in the urine. Serum pepsinogen levels are also abnormally low in patients with gastric atrophy and achlorhydria. A study of nearly 7000 patients from Japan has demonstrated a significant correlation between patients with low serum pepsinogens plus an abnormal Diagnex Blue test and the subsequent development of stomach cancer.[65] However, these tests have never been applied to populations at low risk for stomach cancer.

In summary, stomach cancer is difficult to diagnose until it reaches an advanced stage. A variety of noninvasive approaches have been evaluated to detect groups with gastric cancer or at high risk to develop the disease. In general, high-risk groups must be screened radiologically or endoscopically because no other approach is sufficiently sensitive or specific.

Pathology of Gastric Cancer

Adenocarcinoma accounts for approximately 95% of all gastric cancers, with the remainder consisting of lymphomas, carcinoids, and other sarcomas. The pathology of gastric adenocarcinoma may be classified in several ways.

First, neoplasms may occur in any of the anatomic regions of the stomach. Traditionally, it has been reported that approximately 50% of gastric cancers occur in the antrum, with the rest being distributed throughout the body, fundus, and gastroesophageal junction. However, several groups in the United States have reported a marked proximal shift in the distribution of stomach cancers in the past three decades; as many as 27% to 44% of adenocarcinomas now originate in the fundus, cardia, or gastroesophageal junction.[66,67]

Second, tumors may be classified by their gross morphologic configuration. Approximately 40% to 50% of gastric cancers are fungating or polypoid masses (Fig 63-5). A similar portion may be described as ulcerating lesions, which represent necrosis and excavation of an exophytic mass or infiltrating plaque. Two less common morphologic configurations with vastly different prognostic implications are linitis plastica and superficial spreading types of tumor, which account for 7% and 2% of stomach cancers, respectively. The linitis plastica lesion is an aggressively infiltrating tumor consisting of high-grade tumor cells accompanied by a marked desmoplastic reaction that produces the rigid, "leather-bottle" stomach. This tumor spreads through the submucosal plane to involve large portions of the stomach, produces metastases, and is accompanied by an especially poor prognosis. The superficial spreading carcinoma grows without invading the muscularis propria, is frequently amenable to successful resection, and is discussed in the context of early gastric cancer.

In the 1920s, Borrmann classified gastric cancers into four types; this classification applies principally to advanced gastric cancers (Fig 63-6). A Borrmann's type I tumor is a polypoid

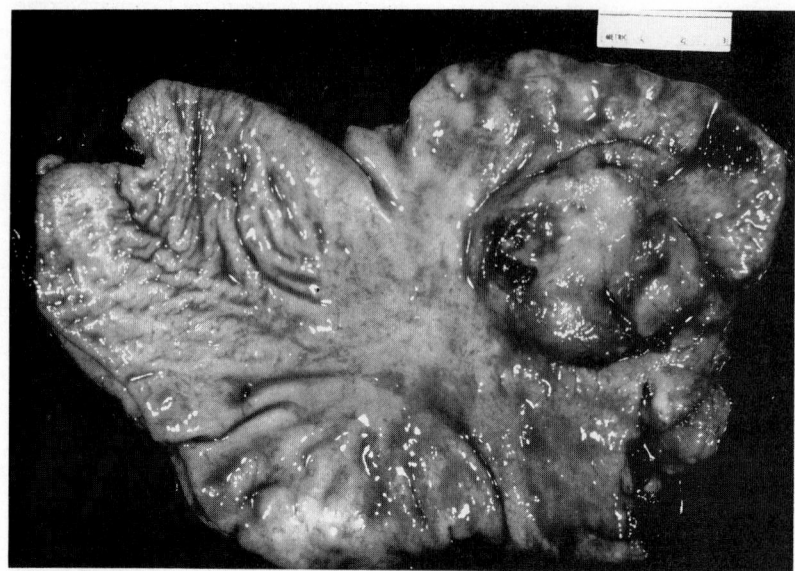

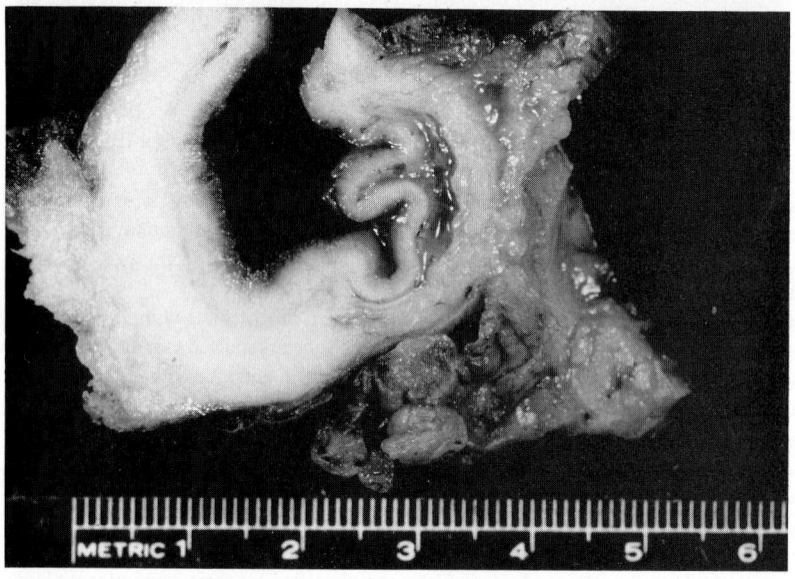

FIGURE 63–5. Gross pathology of stomach cancer. **A,** Fungating gastric carcinoma. This resected stomach contains a 4-cm fungating carcinoma in the setting of chronic atrophic gastritis. The cancer is on the right, and the rest of the epithelium is pale and atrophic. **B,** Infiltrating antral carcinoma. This cross section demonstrates the marked infiltration of the submucosa by this carcinoma, producing the linitis plastica or "leather bottle deformity" in the gastric antrum. Note that the infiltrating tumor (white tissue) is much thicker than the gastric mucosa itself.

lesion projecting into the gastric lumen without necrosis or ulceration. A Borrmann's type II lesion is described as "fungating" and may contain superficial ulcerations. Closely related to this is the Borrmann's type III cancer, in which there is a central ulcer within a large tumor mass. Finally, a Borrmann's type IV lesion is an infiltrative tumor, which would include the more extensive linitis plastica lesion as well. Although this classification is frequently referred to in the literature, there is a good deal of overlap among gastric cancers, and these morphologic variants provide relatively little insight into the biology of the tumor or the clinical outcome in any individual patient.

Early gastric cancer refers to a carcinoma that is limited to the mucosa or submucosa of the stomach without invading the submucosa. The definition is not limited by the diameter of the tumor nor the presence of a polypoid mass or ulceration. Early gastric cancer may be accompanied by regional lymph node metastases. This lesion is of particular importance because it is associated with a more favorable outcome after surgical resection; for prog-

nostic purposes, it should be considered separately from all other varieties of gastric carcinoma. These lesions are principally detected in high-risk populations that are subjected to screening, and are less frequently found in Western Europe and North America. Early gastric cancer may be divided into three subtypes (Fig 63-7). Type I is a protruded, polypoid lesion. Type II is a superficial lesion, which may be further divided into three subgroups, IIa, IIb, or IIc, depending on whether the lesion is elevated, flat, or depressed, respectively. A type III early gastric cancer is an excavated ulcer, but the tumor still does not penetrate the muscularis propria. The general classification of a tumor as an early gastric cancer is of greater prognostic significance than are any of the morphologic variants.

The microscopic pathology of stomach has also been subjected to different conceptual classification groups. The most widely used among these is the Lauren classification, which broadly allocates the tumors into two groups: intestinal type and diffuse type (Fig 63-8). The intestinal type of carcinoma is characterized by epi-

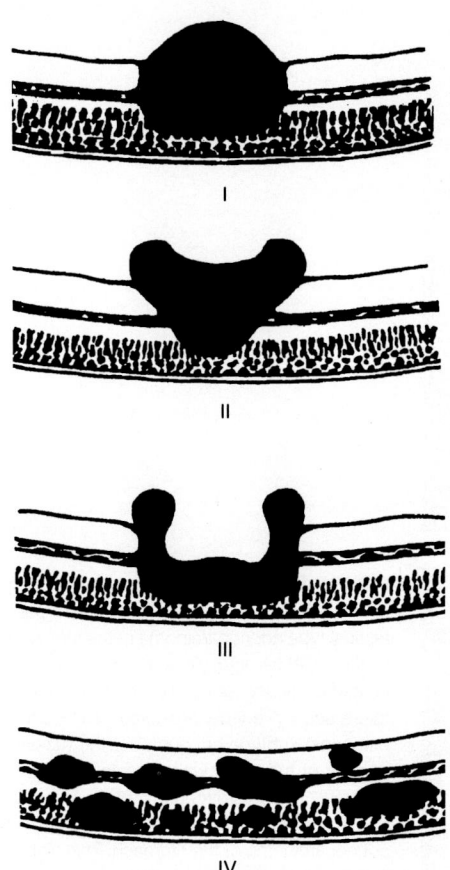

FIGURE 63–6. Borrmann's classification of advanced gastric cancer. Type I—polypoid; type II—fungating with surface ulceration and hemorrhage; type III—ulcerated without major luminal components; type IV—infiltrative (linitis plastica).

thelial cells that form discrete glands, either densely packed or surrounded by connective tissue. In fact, this lesion resembles a colonic carcinoma microscopically. The intestinal type of carcinoma is the most frequent variety in countries with high incidences of stomach cancer. They frequently arise within intestinal metaplasia and are more likely to present as a protruding, polypoid lesion. This pathologic variant generally has a better surgical outcome than the diffuse variety. Diffuse type carcinomas are characterized by sheets of epithelial cells or cells scattered in a stromal matrix without evidence of gland formation. Diffuse cancers tend to be cytologically less differentiated and may contain signet ring cells or secrete large amounts of extracellular mucin. These tumors, which make up a larger proportion of stomach cancers in the low-risk populations such as in North America, are less likely to be seen in a setting of intestinal metaplasia and are associated with a poorer prognosis.

All of the above classifications have been presented in an attempt to develop prognostic parameters for surgical therapy. However, the most important histologic factors are the depth of penetration of tumor into the muscularis propria and the distribution of lymph node metastases. The simple presence of regional lymph node metastases does not exclude resectability of a gastric cancer nor the possibility for long-term survival.

Rarely, variant histologies may be found that mimic adenocarcinoma of the stomach clinically or endoscopically. Carcinoid

tumors and lymphomas are discussed later in this chapter. The adenosquamous tumor variant contains both adenocarcinoma cells and squamous metaplasia in a single tumor. Adenosquamous carcinomas are subdivided into differentiated types and undifferentiated types depending on the adenocarcinomatous component, which determines the biologic behavior of the tumor. In general, the prognosis of adenosquamous carcinomas of the stomach is less favorable than typical adenocarcinomas because of more extensive tumor depth and the higher likelihood of metastasis.[68] Another rare variety is the parietal cell tumor, which may have a slightly better prognosis than other adenocarcinomas.[69]

More than 50 cases of primary choriocarcinoma of the stomach have been reported, most containing an admixture of adenocarcinoma of varying degrees of differentiation. This tumor is seen in both sexes; it is more common in men, and the mean age of onset is approximately 57 years. The origin of these tumors is

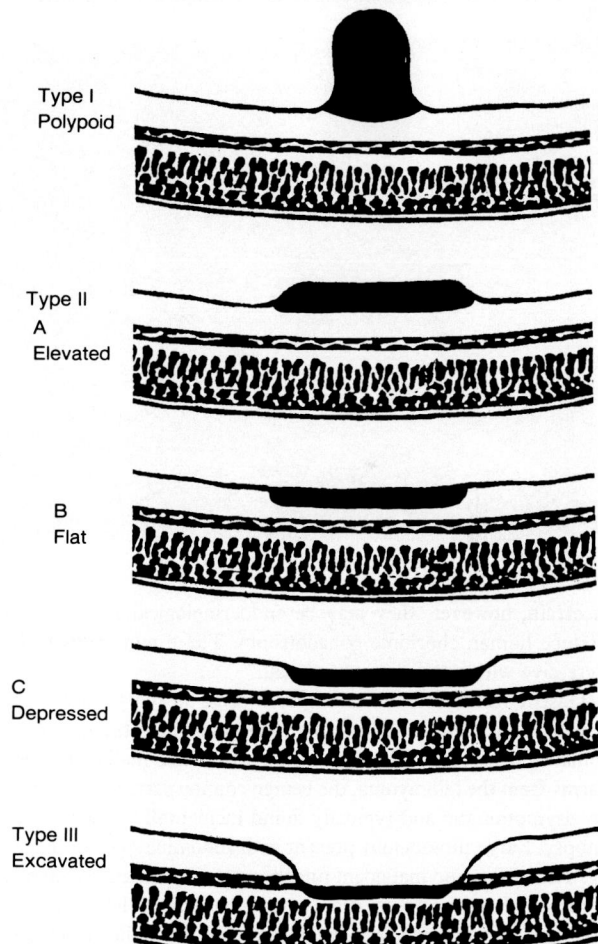

FIGURE 63–7. Macroscopic subtypes of early gastric cancer. Type I projects into the lumen and may be polypoid, nodular, or villous. Type II, or the superficial type, is characterized by an uneven surface and is further subdivided into three subtypes: IIa, elevated—well circumscribed, plaque-like and slightly raised; IIb, flat—may only be noticed by a subtle color change of the mucosa; IIc, depressed—does not exceed the thickness of the normal mucosa. Type III, or the excavated type, includes ulceration of the stomach involving more than mucosal thickness, and is usually seen in combination with other forms. Tumor growth is limited to the mucosa and submucosa in all types.

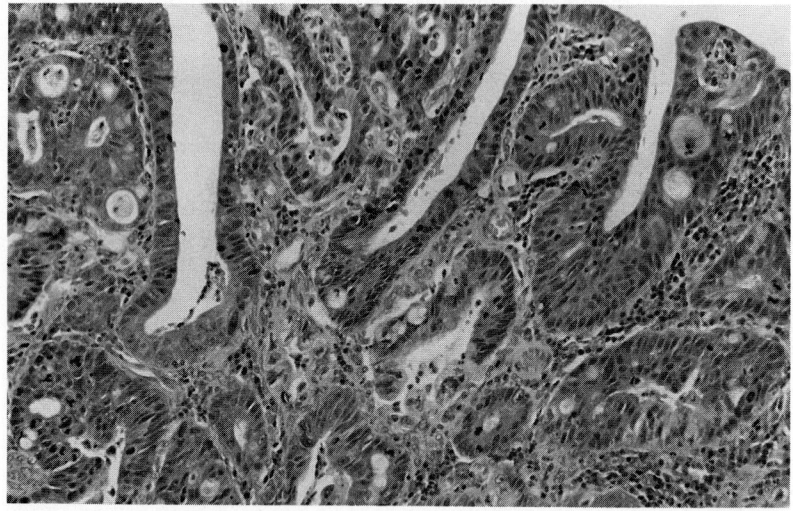

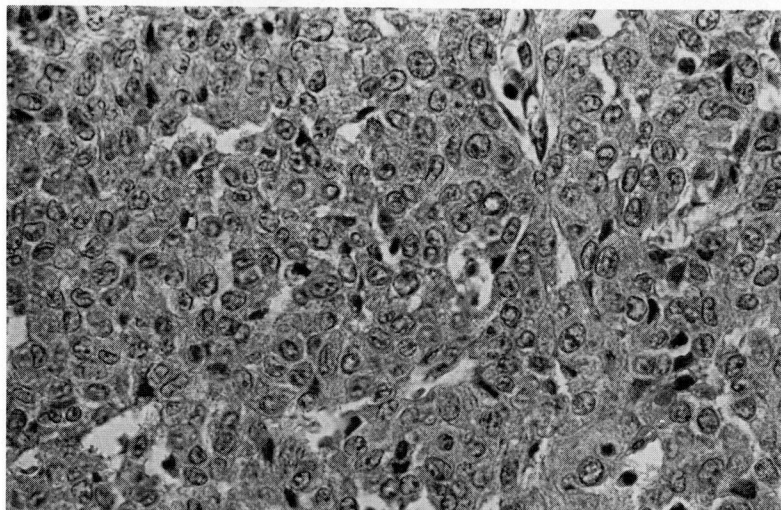

FIGURE 63–8. Microscopic pathology of gastric carcinoma. **A,** This low power photomicrograph of an intestinal-type adenocarcinoma of the stomach has been stained with hematoxylin and eosin. This type of tumor characteristically forms glandular structures similar to those seen in adenocarcinoma of the colon. This microscopic subtype accounts for the majority of cases in parts of the world where gastric carcinoma is more frequent. This microscopic subtype is frequently seen in the setting of chronic atrophic gastritis. **B,** Diffuse adenocarcinoma of the stomach. This high-power photomicrograph of a diffuse adenocarcinoma of the stomach demonstrates the large nuclei with poorly condensed chromatin, mitotic figures, and the general absence of glandular structures. This pathologic subtype is associated with a worse prognosis than that seen with intestinal types of cancer and makes up a greater proportion of the gastric cancers in parts of the world where gastric carcinoma is less frequently seen.

uncertain, however, they may be endocrinologically active and produce human chorionic gonadotropin. The tumor tends to be aggressive with a low rate of survival.[70]

Gastric leiomyosarcomas may also occur in the stomach, but they make up less than 1% of all primary malignant tumors of the stomach. It may be difficult to distinguish these malignant neoplasms from the leiomyoma, the benign counterpart, which is usually asymptomatic and typically found incidentally at surgery or autopsy. Large tumors may present with abdominal pain or bleeding. The benign and malignant tumors are distinguished principally by the number of mitoses; leiomyosarcomas have at least five mitoses per ten high-powered fields and have the ability to invade and metastasize. Unfortunately, aggressive metastasizing behavior may occur in some smooth muscle tumors that fail to meet the histologic criteria for malignancy. A variant tumor, the leiomyoblastoma, has been defined based on the characteristic pathologic features. These tumors have approximately the same clinical behavior as leiomyosarcomas, all of which have 5- and 10-year survival rates of approximately 56% and 43%, respectively.[71,72]

The ovary is an occasional site of metastasis from another primary tumor, frequently in the stomach, giving rise to the "Krukenberg's tumor." Krukenberg's tumors may be unilateral or bi-

lateral, and associated with spread throughout the peritoneum, mesentery, or other sites. In one series of 27 such tumors, 16 (59%) were derived from the stomach. These tumors are typically made up of mucinous, signet-ring carcinoma cells, surrounded by a cellular, non-neoplastic ovarian stroma. The ovarian tumor may become evident before the diagnosis of the gastrointestinal tumor. The presence of bulky, mucinous ovarian tumors should suggest the possibility of a gastric or colonic primary carcinoma.[73]

Pathology of Premalignant Gastric Lesions

Adenocarcinoma of the stomach frequently arises in the setting of chronic atrophic gastritis and intestinal metaplasia. It has been suggested that carcinomas arise in the proliferative cell zone in the neck region of intestinalized glands.[74] Intestinal metaplasia may be classified according to the histologic staining of the mucin. Intestinalized gastric tissue containing mature absorptive cells and goblet cells secreting sialomucins is termed complete, or type I, metaplasia. Incomplete intestinal metaplasia contains "intermediate cells" of various stages of differentiation and is further subdivided into types II and III depending on the cell dedifferentiation and presence of goblet cells secreting sulfomucins, both of which are more advanced in type III. Intestinal metaplasia occurs in association with greater than 70% of gastric carcinomas but may also be seen in non-neoplastic disease. Although type I intestinal metaplasia is the most commonly occurring variant, type III intestinal metaplasia is more highly associated with carcinoma.[75] In spite of this association, a prospective study of patients with chronic atrophic gastritis and sulfomucin-positive intestinal metaplasia has suggested that this marker may be of poor prognostic value for predicting gastric cancer.[76] In summary, incomplete intestinal metaplasia in the setting of chronic atrophic gastritis appears to be the site from which well-differentiated, intestinal type adenocarcinoma of the stomach arises. This relationship is not seen with the diffuse variant of gastric carcinoma. The long and unpredictable timeframe in which gastric cancer develops in this setting makes it difficult to determine screening schedules for patients with these pathologic variants.

Chronic Atrophic Gastritis and Gastric Cancer

The role of chronic atrophic gastritis in gastric carcinoma is discussed earlier in the section entitled "Etiology of Gastric Carcinoma." Populations at increased risk for gastric carcinoma have high rates of superficial gastritis at younger ages, which may evolve into gastric atrophy and intestinal metaplasia with advancing age.[14–16] In those populations, however, most patients with chronic atrophic gastritis do not develop cancer. The type A variant, which involves the fundus and is associated with achlorhydria, is the premalignant condition of greater concern. A prospective study of Finnish patients with type A gastritis revealed an 8% incidence of gastric cancer by 10 to 15 years, which was similar to a retrospective study of Italian patients with a cancer incidence of 14% by 11 to 18 years. This suggests that the incidence of gastric cancer in this setting is no greater than 1% per year.[41,48]

Pernicious anemia is a clinical entity that may occur as a sequela of type A chronic atrophic gastritis.[77] In Denmark, where the incidence of pernicious anemia is relatively high, 2.2% of all new cases of gastric cancer occur in patients with pernicious anemia.[78] However, the degree of risk associated with this disease is a matter of controversy, and recommendations for endoscopic surveillance must be made with an awareness of the rather low yield of adenocarcinoma if all such patients are screened on an annual basis. An endoscopic surveillance study of 80 British patients with pernicious anemia led to the diagnosis of 1 case of gastric cancer, 33 cases of dysplasia (24 mild, 6 moderate, 3 severe), and 18 patients with gastric polyps, most of which were non-neoplastic, but included one case of carcinoid tumor and one polyp containing mucosal dysplasia. The patients were drawn from a previously unscreened group for which the mean duration of pernicious anemia was 4.8 years.[79] A similar study from the Mayo Clinic detected only one gastric carcinoma among 152 patients observed for pernicious anemia for a total of 1550 patient-years, suggesting that the risk of this complication may be less in low-risk regions.[80]

Gastric Carcinoma in the Postantrectomy Stomach

It has been well established that the incidence of gastric carcinoma is increased in patients who have undergone a partial gastrectomy for peptic ulcer disease. This observation has been documented in several centers, but the magnitude of the increased risk has been debated repeatedly in the literature. Postgastrectomy patients incur a twofold or greater increase in risk of cancer, depending on the design and location of the study and duration of patient follow-up.[81–87] The risk appears to be greatest after a Billroth II procedure.[85] Retrospective autopsy studies that select all cases of gastric cancer have found the greatest degree of risk for postgastrectomy patients. Norwegian patients with gastric surgery at least 25 years before death had a sixfold increase in cancer.[81] Italian patients undergoing resections before age 45 had a 6.5% incidence of gastric cancer, and 8 of 39 (21%) patients ≥ 40 years postgastrectomy died with gastric stomach cancer.[83] British patients ≥ 20 years after operation had a four- to fivefold increase in deaths from gastric carcinoma.[85,86]

In spite of this apparent daunting risk, prospective surveillance studies of patients after partial gastrectomy have provided less alarming data that are useful for planning rational screening programs. In the first 15 years after surgery, no significant increase in cancer occurs, and no benefit may be expected from any surveillance program.[86,88] After 15 to 25 years of latency, however, a significant increase in carcinoma has been reported.[87] Nevertheless, at least one study found no increase in cancer after 33 years of follow-up.[89] Thus, the data are inconsistent and do not provide a strong case for annual screening in all patients who have undergone ulcer surgery.

It has been suggested that specific histologic abnormalities might permit the selection of high-risk patients among those who have undergone prior partial gastrectomy. The presence of severe mucosal dysplasia is the strongest marker of a heightened risk and warrants careful endoscopic follow-up with repeated biopsy.[90] The presence of chronic atrophic gastritis, intestinal metaplasia, or type III incomplete metaplasia does not appear to add substantial prognostic information to screening programs.[91,92] Of interest, patients who are more than 20 years postgastrectomy have a 3.3-fold excess number of cancers at all sites, including the biliary tree, pancreas, breast, and lung.[86] Although an increase in "stump cancers" appears to occur in patients operated on for peptic ulcer disease, this complication occurs late (i.e., over two decades after surgery), the risk is difficult to quantitate prospectively, and no pathologic abnormalities short of severe dysplasia identify subgroups at particularly increased risk.

DIAGNOSIS OF GASTRIC CANCER

The most important determinant of survival in patients with gastric cancer is the pathologic stage at the time of detection; therefore, it is essential that the physician maintain a high index of suspicion for the diagnosis. Most studies in nonscreened populations have found a low frequency of disease limited to the stomach at presentation and, consequently, a poor prognosis.[93] Because the symptoms produced by gastric cancer are nonspecific, the clinician must be aware of high-risk settings and be prepared to recognize an early gastric cancer when examining the stomach for unrelated complaints. Those patients with a history of chronic atrophic gastritis, especially when complicated by intestinal metaplasia, pernicious anemia, gastric polyps, prior gastric surgery, or immunodeficiency, in addition to elderly patients with new onset of dyspepsia, early satiety, or weight loss, should be groups targeted for early diagnostic investigation. Upper gastrointestinal tract radiology and endoscopy are the traditional diagnostic studies used in evaluation of these patients. Both techniques have intrinsic strengths and weaknesses.

Radiographic Diagnosis

The double-contrast technique of upper gastrointestinal radiography, developed in Japan as a screening test for early gastric carcinoma, employs an effervescent agent for gastric distention, a high-density barium suspension with good mucosa-coating properties, and radiographic maneuvers designed to ensure adequate views of the stomach and duodenum.[94] There is general agreement that this technique has offered a significant improvement in diagnostic accuracy over the single-contrast technique, with reports of diagnostic accuracy as high as 93% to 96%.[95,96] Findings typical of gastric carcinoma include mass lesions with or without luminal obstruction or ulceration, mucosal irregularity with a lack of distensibility, enlarged folds, and polypoid masses. In a large Japanese series that used endoscopy as the "gold standard," a correct diagnosis of advanced gastric cancer was made radiographically in 79% of cases, but, in 94% of cases, the radiologist identified the abnormality as an ulcer, cancer, or possible cancer. The technique was less sensitive for early gastric cancers, detecting 74% if all "vague mucosal abnormalities" are included. Anterior wall lesions were those most frequently missed.[96]

The ability to distinguish a benign from malignant gastric ulcer by radiography alone is controversial. When expert gastrointestinal radiologists used strict criteria for the appearance of benign ulcers, no malignant ulcers were missed.[97,98] Unequivocally benign gastric ulcers were characterized by a round or oval ulcer crater surrounded by a smooth mound of edema or regular, symmetric mucosal folds that radiated to the edge of the crater or the adjacent edematous mound. The mucosa surrounding benign ulcers had normal or enlarged areae gastricae (fine mucosal relief of the stomach) without evidence of nodularity, mass effect, or tumor infiltration. On tangential views, benign ulcers were characterized by projection of the crater outside the gastric lumen, often associated with a Hampton line or a smooth, symmetric ulcer mound or collar. Malignant ulcers were characterized en face by an asymmetric ulcer crater eccentrically located in an irregular mass with distortion or obliteration of the normal areae gastricae surrounding the ulcer. Nodularity, clubbing, fusion, or amputation of radiating folds also suggested malignancy. An indeterminate lesion was one with both benign and malignant characteristics, and endoscopy was recommended to ensure the diagnosis.[98]

This enthusiasm for the accuracy of radiographic diagnosis has included consideration of the differential cost of radiography in addition to concerns regarding the safety of upper gastrointestinal endoscopy. Some analyses have suggested that, instead of endoscopy, a more cost-effective approach may be to follow definitely

benign ulcers with radiography alone.[99] Because the observation has been made that malignant gastric ulcers may appear to heal[100] and other reports have suggested a lower rate of routine radiographic accuracy,[101] it seems prudent to follow up all patients who have gastric ulceration to complete healing by using gastroscopy and biopsy. The role of barium studies as the initial diagnostic test appears most appropriate in the low-risk patient who is able to cooperate with a radiologist highly skilled in the performance and interpretation of the double-contrast study. Any suspicious lesion requires immediate endoscopic evaluation.

Endoscopy

Panendoscopy of the upper gastrointestinal tract is a safe, accurate, and easily tolerated procedure. In skilled hands, the procedure has a mortality rate of 1:15,000 and a morbidity rate of 1:1000.[102] Patients appear to make little distinction in terms of comfort and acceptability between endoscopy and x-ray and may actually prefer endoscopy.[101] The endoscopic appearance of gastric carcinoma corresponds to Borrmann's pathologic classification (see Fig 63-6), which characterizes both the growth pattern of the lesion (exophytic or infiltrating) and the presence or absence of ulceration.[103]

A number of studies have evaluated the accuracy of endoscopy and biopsy in the diagnosis of gastric cancer. In a large prospective study from Osaka, Japan, Tatsuta et al found only 32 (3.7%) false-negative diagnoses of malignancy among 858 cases given benign diagnoses, and 3 (0.6%) false-positive diagnoses among 473 patients with a diagnosis of cancer.[104] Of those patients with false-negative biopsy diagnoses, 16 of 31 had a positive aspiration cytology using a tube introduced through the biopsy channel. In 5 of the 31 patients, atypia was noted on biopsy and a follow-up biopsy was positive, while in 7 patients, the endoscopic impression of cancer was strong enough to dictate surgery or repeat biopsy, both of which confirmed cancer. Three cases had all negative studies, and the delay in diagnosis averaged 21.3 months. The three false-positive cases were all associated with active ulceration, and malignancy was not found at the time of surgery. In this study, endoscopic biopsy had a sensitivity of 93.8% and a specificity of 99.6% with an overall accuracy of 97.4%. When one considers that the combination of endoscopic impression, biopsy, and aspiration cytology leads to appropriate detection and management without complication in 99.7% of those patients with gastric cancer, this study provides a strong argument for the use of endoscopy as the primary approach in the diagnosis of gastric cancer.

The high level of diagnostic accuracy with upper GI tract endoscopy with biopsy has been confirmed by other investigators. Dekker and Tytgat used at least 10 biopsy specimens of gastric ulcers and suspicious lesions and determined that the combination had an accuracy rate of 99.8%. They also confirmed that the endoscopic appearance alone was inadequate to ensure the proper diagnosis.[105]

The site of biopsy of potential malignant lesions is also important. Using freshly resected gastric carcinomas, Hatfield et al found that a high yield was obtained by biopsy of both the base and the rim of the malignant ulcer, and that the combination of the two sites yielded more than 95% accuracy.[106] The number of biopsy specimens necessary in the diagnosis of upper GI tract malignancies has been prospectively evaluated. Graham et al demonstrated that seven biopsies yielded the correct diagnosis in 98% of carcinomas, and the addition of salvage cytology (i.e., aspiration of material from the endoscopic biopsy channel) led to the correct diagnosis in all patients.[107] Although other studies have not been as successful in confirming the diagnostic value of biopsy (74%–86%) and brush cytology (77%–85%), the combination is clearly superior to either alone (88%–91%).[108,109] These results likely reflect differences in the nature of the lesions sampled (i.e., infiltrating lesions are more difficult to sample) and the experience of the cytologist. The use of a sheathed cytologic brush is a convenient method to prevent the loss of malignant cells on withdrawal from the endoscope. Brushing the lesion before biopsy has the added potential advantage of avoiding the dilution of malignant cells with blood and the difficulty of finding the lesion after biopsy-induced bleeding. The use of aspiration cytology has no apparent advantage over brush cytology, and gastric lavage cytology is largely of historic interest.

The endoscopic appearance of early gastric cancer, as classified by the Japanese Society for Gastroenterological Endoscopy, is divided into three main types (see Fig 63-7).[110] Early gastric cancer represents a challenge to the accuracy of endoscopic diagnosis because it can be much more difficult to recognize. The endoscopic diagnostic accuracy of early gastric cancer is in the range of 90%,[111,112] and repeated biopsy can raise this to 96%. The endoscopic diagnosis of lesions less than 5 mm is even more difficult.[113] Because particular difficulty is noted with flat, depressed, minute lesions, investigators in Japan have used the Congo red–methylene blue test to improve the diagnostic accuracy of endoscopy. In this test, acid-secreting areas appear blue or black due to color change of the Congo red, areas of intestinal metaplasia stain blue, but neoplasms bleach the dyes 2 to 5 minutes after the application. Using this technique, a significant improvement in identification of lesions was observed, allowing directed biopsy.[114]

Intramucosal and submucosal lesions are more difficult to biopsy due to the restricted accessibility of the abnormal tissue to the biopsy forceps. The combined use of a snare and biopsy forceps to lift and cut or the "well technique" of repeated deeper biopsies in a single location is occasionally helpful but may be hazardous and should be used with caution.[115]

Differential Diagnosis of Gastric Mass Lesions

The endoscopic appearance of gastric lymphoma may mimic that of adenocarcinoma. The presence of large, diffusely ulcerated folds that involve the entire body or the antrum may cause stenosis that may be indistinguishable from an infiltrative gastric cancer. The "classic" appearance of a volcanolike ulcer with a deep ulcer base within a prominent raised margin is observed less frequently. Multiple polypoid masses may also be observed. Biopsy and cytology are usually helpful in diagnosis.

Metastatic disease of the stomach may be confused with a primary tumor. The most common tumors that give rise to gastric metastases are from the lung, breast, and melanomas. These patients may not have widespread metastatic disease and may present with nonspecific gastrointestinal symptoms or bleeding. In patients with AIDS, Kaposi's sarcoma may involve the gastrointestinal tract, including the stomach, where discrete polypoid lesions with ulceration may be observed. Finally, the enlarged folds of Menetrier's disease may be confused with infiltrative adenocarcinoma. In those patients with large gastric folds and weight loss, a deep snare biopsy may be indicated to differentiate this lesion from cancer.[116]

Role of Tumor Markers

There are no tumor markers for gastric cancer with sufficient sensitivity or specificity to allow an early diagnosis of cancer. Carcinoembryonic antigen (CEA) has proven useful in the management of some patients with colorectal cancer and has been studied in patients with gastric cancer. Serum CEA has been noted to be elevated in 31% to 65%[117] of cases, but there is considerable overlap with benign gastric conditions and poor correlation with prognosis among patients with cancer. Gastric juice CEA is somewhat more promising than serum measurements. Several investigators have demonstrated a significant increase in gastric CEA in patients with gastric cancer, atrophic gastritis, and gastric ulcer.[118-120] Although these studies suggest that gastric CEA cannot help distinguish between benign and malignant lesions, it may be useful to target high-risk patients for additional investigation.

Gion et al have suggested that variation in the pH of gastric juice leads to difficulties with gastric tumor marker radioimmunoassay because low pH leads to decreased recovery and occasional irreversible loss of antigen. In addition to CEA, these investigators have studied other tumor markers including the monoclonal antibody-defined tumor-associated antigen CA19-9, tissue polypeptide antigen, and "neoplastic ferritin." These markers have been noted to be positive in 62% to 67%, 74% to 77%, and 42% to 60%, respectively, of gastric cancer patients' sera. These methodologic improvements may infuse some hope for the future in an area where there is little practical usefulness of tumor markers due to poor sensitivity and specificity.[121] Fetal sulfoglycoprotein antigen (FSA), another tumor-associated but not tumor-specific antigen, should also be mentioned. FSA is detectable in the gastric secretions of 96% of patients with gastric cancer, but there is no correlation with tumor stage, and the antigen is present in 14% of patients with benign disease.[122]

Noninvasive Markers of Chronic Atrophic Gastritis

Because intestinal metaplasia is associated with gastric cancer, investigators have endeavored to find other noninvasive markers of this association. In a cohort of patients that developed gastric cancer, a low serum pepsinogen I level was found in 31%, while matched controls had a significantly lower frequency (6.3%).[123] Similarly, serum gastrin levels were significantly elevated in patients with gastric cancer, which correlated with hypochlorhydria, consistent with earlier observations that achlorhydria is associated with carcinoma of the stomach.[124] Therefore, diminished acid secretion, low serum pepsinogen, and increased serum gastrin are all markers of the high-risk state but are insufficiently predictive to justify routine clinical use.

CLINICAL COURSE

Natural History

The prognosis in gastric cancer is affected by the intrinsic biologic properties of the tumor, its host, and the treatment. Five-year survival is used as a measure of treatment efficacy because survival beyond that point matches that of a control population.[125]

Staging

The extent of disease has been repeatedly demonstrated to be the most important factor determining whether a radical, potentially curative excision of the tumor is possible. The literature is somewhat difficult to interpret because there are three major TNM classifications of gastric cancer. Although all follow the tumor, node, metastasis (TNM) method of classification, the AJC (American Joint Committee for Cancer Staging and End Results Reporting), UICC (Union Internationale Contre de Cancer), and JRSGC (Japanese Research Society for Gastric Cancer) use different TNM classes within each stage. This has led to wide variations in survival among subgroups belonging to some stages. The size of the tumor, which has been included in some staging systems, has no significant prognostic role. Further, early gastric cancer, which may include the presence of local lymph node metastasis, requires recognition as a distinct stage with a favorable prognosis.

Maruyama has reviewed survival in 4734 patients who underwent resection and were treated at the National Cancer Center in Tokyo, Japan, from 1962 to 1984.[126] Those factors of prognostic importance were the presence of distant metastasis, the histologic depth of invasion, the pattern of lymph node metastasis, the macroscopic type of advanced cancer (i.e., Borrmann's classification), the location (upper third worse), and the degree of tumor differentiation (worse prognosis with less differentiation). Multivariate analysis indicated that the depth of invasion and lymph node metastasis were the most significant prognostic factors, and a new TNM classification was proposed and accepted in a joint meeting of the cancer societies in 1984. The new TNM categories are illustrated in Figure 63-9, and the clinical stages are described in Table 63-8. The value of this schema is outlined in the survival figures depicted in Figure 63-10. This staging classification represents the currently used staging system[127] and correlates best with survival.

The poor prognosis with cancer of the upper third of the stomach and among larger advanced gastric cancers has been confirmed in other reviews. In the case of Borrmann type I and II lesions, the mean 5-year survival rates were 34% and 38%, respectively. Type III and IV lesions have mean 5-year survival rates of 19% and 10%, respectively.[125] The histologic degree of differentiation is not independently predictive of prognosis, nor is the presence of stromal fibrosis;[125] there have been reports of both favorable[128] and unpredictable[126] prognostic value for desmoplastic reaction.

The effect of age and sex on prognosis is also variable.[125,129] While persons less than age 30 appear to have an aggressive disease, survival seems to improve with age until later in life, when postoperative mortality increases due to the presence of comorbid

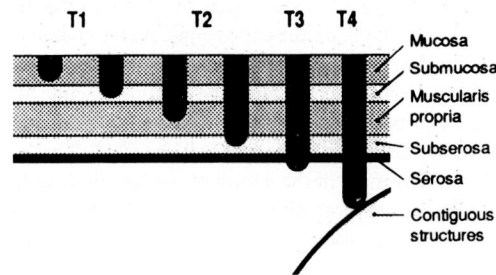

T-Classificattion of Gastric Cancer

T1 T2 T3 T4

Mucosa
Submucosa
Muscularis propria
Subserosa
Serosa
Contiguous structures

N-Classification of Gastric Cancer

C LG
CH S
PG>3cm
3 cm
N1   N2

perigastric (PG) < 3 cm

perigastric (PG) > 3 cm
left gastric (LG)
common hepatic (CH)
splenic (S)
celiac (C)

M-Classification of Metastasis

M_0 = No distant metastasis
M_1 = Distant Metastasis

FIGURE 63–9. TNM classification of gastric cancer. (Modified from Maruyama M. Treatment results of gastric cancer staged by the new TNM classification. In: Maruyama M, Kimura K, eds. Review of clinical research in gastroenterology. Tokyo: Igaku-Shoin, 1988:112.)

conditions. The survival difference between males and females is also of little prognostic importance. Another potentially important host determinant of survival may be HLA type; long-term survivals among patients with stage III disease and HLA-DR4 have been observed in one study.[130]

Another tumor characteristic correlated with poor prognosis is the presence of epidermal growth factor in the tumor. The authors postulated a functional role for this peptide in mediating invasiveness and desmoplasia.[131]

With the development of methods to analyze nuclear DNA content, flow cytometric studies of gastric carcinoma have demonstrated that early cancers have less aneuploid cells than do advanced tumors. The presence of cell populations with high ploidy within tumors has been correlated with age, decreased survival, increased incidence of vascular invasion, and metastasis.[132,133] Multiple subpopulations with DNA aneuploidy have been observed within tumors, which may represent potential foci from which resistance to cancer chemotherapy develops.[134]

Individuals with the best prognosis are those with disease discovered early, which tend to be less aggressive tumors, and disease resectable for cure. This has been repeatedly demonstrated by

TABLE 63–8
The New TNM Stage Grouping of Gastric Cancer*

STAGE	T	N	M
IA	T_1	N_0	M_0
IB	T_1	N_1	M_0
	T_2	N_0	M_0
II	T_1	N_2	M_0
	T_2	N_1	M_0
	T_3	N_0	M_0
IIIA	T_2	N_2	M_0
	T_3	N_1	M_0
	T_4	N_0	M_0
IIIB	T_3	N_2	M_0
	T_4	N_1	M_0
IV	T_4	N_2	M_0
	Any T	Any N	M_1

* Note the correlation between TNM stage and survival in Figure 63-10. Maruyama M. Treatment results of gastric cancer staged by the new TNM classification. In Maruyama M, Kimura K, eds. Review of clinical research in gastroenterology. Tokyo: Igaku-Shoin, 1988:112.

studies from Japan that use screening techniques that detect a large percentage (42%–46%) of early cancers and lead to an overall 5-year survival of 63% to 70%.[135,136] As the stage of disease at

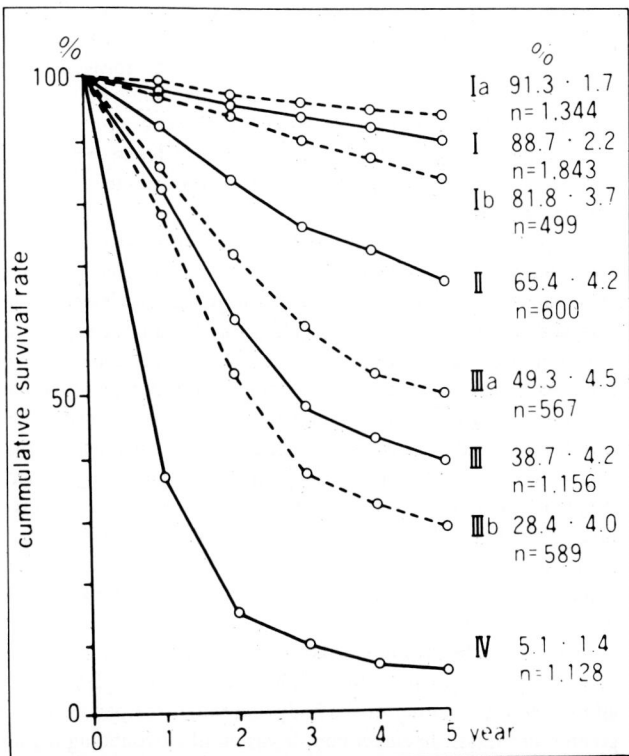

FIGURE 63–10. Survival rates of gastric cancer of patients using TNM stage grouping. (From Maruyama M. Treatment results of gastric cancer staged by the new TNM classification. In: Maruyama M, Kimura K, eds. Review of clinical research in gastroenterology. Tokyo: Igaku-Shoin, 1988: 112.)

detection increases, the presence of poor prognostic factors increases concomitant with poor surgical risk and a significantly decreased chance for curative resection.

ASSESSMENT OF DISEASE

The spread of gastric cancer occurs by four major routes (Table 63-9). The recognition of spread is necessary before surgery because the presence of disseminated metastasis indicates inability to perform a curative resection. Physical examination, with particular attention to the abdomen, rectum, vagina, and lymph nodes, remains the first step in the work-up for metastatic disease. As these patients are also at risk for second primary neoplasms, particularly in the lung, abnormal findings on routine examination should be carefully pursued.[137]

The role of computed tomography (CT) in the preoperative staging of gastric cancer remains a source of controversy between radiologists and surgeons. The initial enthusiasm for the accuracy of preoperative CT scanning reported by Moss et al[138] has been challenged. They reported a very close correlation between the CT and the operative findings, including a suggestion that it may replace laparotomy as a cost-effective alternative; however, this has been tempered by reports that CT evaluation is much less accurate. Cook et al reviewed 37 patients who underwent both CT and laparotomy and found that 51% had more extensive disease

TABLE 63–9
Gastric Cancer: Pattern of Spread

Direct Extension

Lesser and greater omentum
Liver
Pancreas
Spleen
Transverse colon

Lymphatic

Local-perigastric
Regional-celiac, common hepatic, left gastric, splenic
Distant
   Supraclavicular (Virchow's)
   Left axillary (Irish's)
   Umbilical (Sister Mary Joseph's)

Hematogenous

Hepatic
Pulmonary
Bone
CNS

Peritoneal

Disseminated
Pelvic
   Ovarian—Krukenberg's tumor
   Rectal shelf (Blumer's)

than predicted by CT.[139] Of greatest concern, six patients were predicted to have widespread disease by CT, but, at operation, three were found to have disease limited to the stomach or regional lymph nodes, allowing a potentially curative resection. While other radiologic studies such as angiography and radionuclide scans have little role in staging, CT still plays an important role preoperatively. Because CT scans are not 100% accurate, when widespread disease is suggested, percutaneous CT-directed biopsy seems appropriate to confirm a suspected metastatic lesion. If CT suggests that a surgical resection with a clear margin is at all possible, laparotomy and an attempt at resection are appropriate.

Endoscopy adds useful preoperative information, including an assessment of gastric distensibility, peristalsis, pyloric function (paralysis suggests vagal infiltration, particularly in lesions in the cardia), and the proximal and distal extent of tumor.[140] When available, endoscopic ultrasonography may offer additional information regarding the depth of invasion of gastric cancer. This instrument allows clear tomographic images of the gastric wall, and the accuracy of this technique in assessing the depth of invasion is approximately 85%.[141,142] Improvements in instrumentation and operator experience will, in all likelihood, improve the ability of endoscopic ultrasonography to help significantly in the differential diagnosis of gastric lesions and the staging of gastric cancer.

Because patients with carcinoma of the stomach are frequently chronically ill at the time of presentation, patients should be evaluated for the presence of significant malnutrition. The use of intravenous hyperalimentation for 10 to 14 days in addition to aggressive pulmonary toilet and an antibiotic bowel preparation to reduce gastric flora and prepare the colon in the event it is involved with disease, may improve operative success.[140]

TREATMENT OF GASTRIC CANCER

Surgery for Cure

Surgical resection remains the only therapy available that has curative potential. Every attempt should be made to identify those patients who will benefit from surgery through accurate clinical staging and optimal preoperative preparation.

While there is little debate that total removal of the area involved with tumor is the only curative therapy, the extent of the surgical procedure required has engendered some controversy. As noted earlier, preoperative studies may underdiagnose potential resectability, therefore, a suitable patient should always be considered for resection. Furthermore, the surgeon's intraoperative assessment of the extent of disease may not be reliable. Because lymphadenopathy may be due to either benign reactive changes or infiltration by neoplasm, and tumor invasion microscopically may be more extensive than is apparent macroscopically, the decision to proceed with a complete resection should be based on intraoperative frozen sections.[143]

Another debate centers around the value of routine total gastrectomy versus stage-dependent subtotal gastrectomy with lymph node dissection. The increased morbidity and mortality of extensive surgery must be weighed against a realization that surgical failures

after subtotal gastrectomy are usually due to tumor recurrence from extensive intramural invasion or regional lymph node metastases.[144] The surgical mortality in total gastrectomy series published before 1978 averaged 28%, however, other groups have subsequently reported 12.5%[145] and 15% surgical mortalities from experienced centers.[144] The major postoperative morbidity of total gastrectomy is related to the severity of alkaline esophageal reflux, which can be ameliorated by procedures designed to improve the reservoir function of the gastric reconstruction, such as Roux-en-Y esophagojejunostomy[144] or jejunal pouch with jejunoplication.[143] The only controlled randomized trial comparing subtotal gastrectomy with total gastrectomy for carcinoma of the antrum found no difference in operative mortality or 5-year survival.[146] The improved postoperative survival with radical or standard subtotal gastrectomy versus total gastrectomy may not reflect differences in the surgical procedure as much as it reflects differences in patient selection and the stage of disease operated on, because total gastrectomy is usually performed for more extensive disease.[147] Surgical margins of 5 to 10 cm beyond the cancer are recommended; total removal of the stomach may be necessary to achieve this goal. Small Borrmann I or II tumors of the antrum are exceptions, and subtotal resection is adequate for these lesions.[143,144] A report of an improved rate of perioperative mortality for the surgical management of gastric carcinoma as low as 4.6%[148] may reflect an improvement in surgical techniques and perioperative support in addition to patient selection. The operability rate in this series was 90.7%, and resectability rate was 78.1%, which is considerably greater than earlier series.

The decision to remove regional and perigastric lymph nodes is another source of debate within the surgical literature. Reports from Japan[149] suggest that extension of the resection to include regional lymphadenectomy leads to a significant improvement in survival, in contrast to earlier reports from the United States. This surgical approach appears to improve postoperative mortality and survival in general; however, the experience in Japan may reflect both earlier stage at diagnosis and increased operative experience with the disease.

Douglass and Nava[140] have suggested a surgical strategy for resection of gastric cancer. In the distal stomach, antrum, and lesser curve, resection should include the greater and lesser omentum and lymph node dissection along the hepatic artery to the liver hilum and along the left gastric artery to the celiac axis. A celiac axis lymph node dissection is added if nodes along the left gastric artery are involved, as are the superior pancreatic nodes and those along the splenic artery when these are enlarged. Routine splenectomy is not recommended, and the authors suggest that, if splenic hilar nodes are involved, systemic disease precluding resection is likely. For pyloric tumors, superior mesenteric artery nodes should be removed. Any tumor adherent to liver or duodenum mandates removal of the involved tissue with tumor-free margins of 5 cm or more.

Tumors of the greater curvature and posterior gastric wall require splenectomy, removal of lymph nodes along the splenic artery and the superior border of the body and tail of the pancreas, and greater and lesser omentectomy. Invasion of surrounding organs mandates their resection, as well as extending the lymph node resection beyond areas of involvement, and including tumors that involve the transverse colon and adherent mesocolon. Tumors of the fundus or esophagogastric junction are treated by proximal gastric resection or total gastrectomy if necessary. The left gastric artery is removed along with node dissection along the celiac axis to the aorta. The esophagus should be dissected, and tumor-free margins should be established; a combined abdominal and thoracic approach may be required for tumors in nonreducible hiatal hernias or those involving the distal esophagus. An abdominocervical approach has been used in patients with poor cardiopulmonary reserve.

The poor results of surgical treatment for gastric cancer in general reflect the inability to perform a curative resection at the time the lesion is diagnosed. Reports from countries outside of Japan reveal operability rates in the range of 62% to 82% with resection possible in 40% to 48% of patients.[93,146] Operative mortality is reported in the range of 13.7% to 26.5%.[147,150] Overall 5-year survival is quite poor, in the range 7.4% to 16.5%, and those resected for cure have a 20.5% to 42.8% 5-year survival.[93,147] Once again, it appears that the stage of disease at presentation is the most critical prognostic factor.

The Japanese results in the management of patients with gastric cancer reflect their extensive pioneering efforts in screening, surgery, and attempts at adjuvant therapy. In a recent review of the surgical treatment of 8000 cases of gastric cancer at the Cancer Institute Hospital in Tokyo from 1945 to 1986, the authors report dramatically improved results compared to surgical series from Europe and North America. The resectability rate in their series was 89.6%, with an operative mortality rate of 1.9%. Their overall 5-year survival was 37.4% for all patients, 59.4% for those who underwent curative surgery, and 5% for those with noncurative surgery.[151] These results are typical of the Japanese experience and highlight three major points: (1) the improvement in surgical results reflects early stage of disease at diagnosis; (2) increased surgical experience leads to improvements in operative mortality and long-term survival; and (3) patients with advanced gastric cancer in Japan have the same dismal outcome as elsewhere in the world.

Palliative Surgery

Because nonresectability is present in as many as 60% of patients operated on, the decision to perform a biopsy and a bypass procedure, or proceed with a palliative resection, is frequently encountered. No randomized controlled studies address this issue. Most surgical series suggest that resection is preferred to biopsy alone or bypass surgery.[152,153] Lawrence has suggested that palliative resection is preferred if it does not require total gastrectomy or anastomosis at the line of transected tumor and if the procedure does not add unacceptable operative risks.[154] Gastrojejunostomy is not recommended unless the patient is obstructed, because of the increased surgical morbidity and mortality.[152] These decisions must be placed in perspective with the overall prognosis of the patient, because extensive surgery may prolong the hospitalization of a patient who has a short time to live. Radiation therapy can often control bleeding associated with unresectable tumor,[154] and the endoscopic placement of stents or use of laser is available to treat obstructing lesions. Thus, palliative resection is most appropriate when preoperative staging has failed to predict unresectability and survival is expected beyond a few months.

RESECTION OF LOCAL RECURRENT DISEASE

Because the majority of patients who undergo resection suffer recurrent disease, the management of surgical treatment failures remains a major challenge facing the physician treating patients with gastric cancer. Although local or regional recurrence is the predominant pattern of relapse in one half[155] to two thirds[143] of patients, surgical resection appears to have little or no role in the management of these patients. With the exception of patients who develop an anastomotic recurrence after subtotal gastrectomy, surgical procedures for recurrent disease appear to be at high risk for complications and have little potential for long-term survival.[143] Patients who have undergone a tumor resection who then present with symptoms suggesting recurrence, such as dysphagia, should be evaluated with endoscopy. CT scans with directed biopsy may assist in determining if the cancer has recurred. As most patients have widespread disease not amenable to surgical resection, nonsurgical approaches are the principal considerations.

RESECTION OF METASTATIC DISEASE

During initial surgery for gastric cancer, every attempt should be made to remove the tumor en bloc, even if adjacent organs are involved. While some investigators have demonstrated that hepatic metastases are amenable to surgical resection at the time of gastrectomy, which appears to improve the efficacy of chemotherapy,[156] the value of this type of aggressive therapy has not been shown in controlled trials.[157] Isolated, potentially resectable distant metastatic disease appears quite rare in patients with gastric cancer.

Nonsurgical Therapy

CHEMOTHERAPY FOR METASTATIC DISEASE

Major difficulties exist in the assessment of the role of chemotherapy in patients with gastric cancer. Results from uncontrolled phase II studies, which are designed to test the antitumor activity of new pharmacologic agents, cannot be applied to clinical practice without confirmation in phase III randomized controlled studies, because the response of patients participating in phase II studies often reflects selection bias. The major problems in interpreting most trials are related to the use of response rate (i.e., 50% reduction in measurable tumor) as the measured outcome parameter and the lack of stratification of patients for prognostic factors. The role of chemotherapy in patients with unresectable disease continues to evolve. Trials suggest that combination chemotherapy is more active than single-agent therapy, however, treatment appears to produce only partial responses and has no significant effect on survival.[158]

Most drugs used as single agents have low partial response rates, and complete responses (i.e., no evidence of tumor) are extremely rare. The agents of greatest potential are 5-fluorouracil (5-FU), mitomycin-C, and doxorubicin (adriamycin), which have response rates of 25% to 30% in phase II studies; cisplatin and triazinate produce 14% to 22% response rates.[158] These agents have been combined in hopes of improved treatment responses.

The combination of 5-FU, doxorubicin, and mitomycin-C (FAM), the three most effective single agents, is the most commonly used regimen. The response rate reported in a large number of phase II trials is in the range of 35%.[158] A randomized trial comparing 5-FU versus 5-FU and doxorubicin versus FAM confirmed an increase in partial response with the combinations but failed to demonstrate improved survival.[159] Substituting methyl-CCNU for mitomycin-C in the FAM regimen (FAMe) to avoid the hematologic toxicity of the drug has been shown to be equivalent or less effective than FAM.[160]

Another combination with potential efficacy is 5-FU, doxorubicin, and cisplatin (FAP). Response rates in phase II trials as high as 50% and complete responses have been reported.[161] In an uncontrolled trial, this combination, in addition to the combination of 5-FU, doxorubicin, and triazinate, was reported to have improved 1-year survival.[162] If these results are confirmed in a phase III study currently in progress, this combination may offer the most effective chemotherapeutic regimen.[158]

Other combinations with potential for study based on early reports include mitomycin-C plus triazinate, and methotrexate plus 5-FU (FAMTx). Response rates of 35% to 59% have been reported for FAMTx in phase II trials, and complete responses in 12% provide some encouragement for the combination.[158]

Adjuvant Chemotherapy After Surgery "for Cure"

Because survival in those patients with gastric cancer resected "for cure" remains unacceptably low, attempts have been made to eradicate residual tumor postoperatively with adjuvant chemotherapy. Several randomized controlled trials of adjuvant chemotherapy have produced generally disappointing results. The first major study by the Gastrointestinal Tumor Study Group (GITSG) reported encouraging results for adjuvant 5-FU plus MeCCNU, including improved survival at 2 years after surgical resection.[163] Unfortunately, these results could not be reproduced in two similar cooperative trials.[164,165]

In a recent trial from Great Britain, 5-FU and mitomycin-C with or without induction therapy did not lead to improved survival.[166] Furthermore, the British trial noted a high incidence of deaths due to hemolytic-uremic syndrome, which has been attributed to mitomycin-C. Adjuvant therapy remains without any proven benefit and has potentially life-threatening toxicity. There appears to be no role for adjuvant chemotherapy outside of future controlled clinical trials.

Radiation Therapy

RADIOTHERAPY

Although the patterns of local or regional recurrence[155] suggest that adjuvant radiotherapy should improve survival when used alone, the dose and volume limitations necessary to spare adjacent organs preclude the delivery of adequate therapy. A few uncontrolled studies have suggested beneficial and possibly curative potential for radiation therapy, but others have failed to document this effect.[167] Whether better external radiation techniques will improve these limited results awaits further studies.[160] The Japanese experience with intraoperative adjuvant radiotherapy suggests that this treatment may have significant potential to improve survival.[168]

COMBINED RADIATION AND CHEMOTHERAPY

Early uncontrolled reports of the efficacy of combined radiation and chemotherapy (5-FU) prompted the GITSG to initiate a controlled trial of combined therapy versus chemotherapy alone for locally advanced gastric cancer.[169] The protocol included 5-FU plus methyl-CCNU with or without 5000 rad of radiation therapy. Early results favored chemotherapy alone because of the toxicity of the combined treatment, but the survival curves crossed during the third year of follow-up and remained in favor of combination therapy. Patients with gastric resection responded better than those whose cancers were never resected. Based on these encouraging results, other combined modality trials are in progress.[160]

Chemoimmunotherapy

The therapeutic administration of agents that stimulate immune function may be useful in patients with gastric cancer. Because tumor burden and chemotherapy lead to immunosupression, the use of immunostimulants has some theoretical rationale. Several studies from Japan have used bacterial cell wall extracts as adjuvant therapy in combination with chemotherapy and have suggested that certain subgroups of patients may have improved survival.[170,171] A trial from Italy, however, failed to show benefit of adjuvant chemoimmunotherapy when levamisole was combined with multiple agent chemotherapy.[172] An intriguing report from Denmark suggested that administration of cimetidine to patients with gastric cancer improved survival[173] and hypothesized this effect may be due to an immunomodulatory effect of the drug. The role of monoclonal antitumor antibodies and biologic response modifiers in the treament of gastric cancer remains an area for future investigation.[174] Results thus far fail to identify the usefulness of these therapies in patients with gastric cancer.

Treatment of Inoperable Disease

Because current chemotherapy protocols have not been demonstrated to improve survival, the use of chemotherapy for metastatic disease or as adjuvant therapy is not the standard of care, and new regimens should be studied in the setting of controlled clinical trials. Based on the earlier studies, combination chemotherapy using FAM or FAP remains most likely to attain partial remission and potential palliation. Its use must be balanced by concerns about the toxicity these agents produce. The future holds prospect for innovative chemotherapy regimens, including regional therapy with intraperitoneal cytotoxic agents.[158,175]

ENDOSCOPIC TREATMENT

For those patients who are not candidates for surgical resection because of widespread metastatic disease, laser photocoagulation is an effective palliative therapy. This treatment has been successful both in relieving obstruction and controlling bleeding without development of major complications.[176,177] Endoscopic laser treatment of polypoid early gastric cancers has been used with some success in Japan as a potential therapy when surgical resection is not possible.[178]

GASTRIC POLYPS

Gastric polyps are primarily of interest because of their potential relationship to gastric carcinoma. Gastric polyps are uncommon, occurring in less than 1% of autopsy or other surveys. They are almost always asymptomatic and are usually discovered as an incidental finding at endoscopic or radiologic examination. The majority of gastric polyps are benign and without malignant potential. The most frequent among these are hyperplastic polyps, which make up 74% to 79% of all gastric polyps.[179,180] The hyperplastic polyp consists of a proliferation of superficial epithelial elements without evidence of atypia. The histologic appearance led to the earlier name "regenerative polyps" for these lesions.[179] These usually remain small (<15 mm), are not premalignant lesions, and are not an adequate explanation for gastrointestinal blood loss.

The less common but pathologically more important lesion is the adenomatous polyp, which appears similar to the colonic adenoma and accounts for 10% to 20% of gastric polyps. These lesions may give rise to, or coexist with, gastric adenocarcinoma[179,180] and are not uncommon in pernicious anemia.[181] These lesions continue to grow larger and more progressively neoplastic and should always be removed. Patients with gastric adenomatous polyps require annual gastroscopic follow-up because of the risk of cancer.

Multiple gastric polyps are most often encountered in the fundus and frequently consist of dilated and distorted fundic glands. Fundic gland polyposis may occur in familial polyposis coli (or Gardner's syndrome), but two thirds of cases are not associated with syndromic gastrointestinal polyposis.[182,183] The polyps are usually small (<10 mm), occur in large numbers (from 10 to >100), but do not give rise to specific symptoms other than epigastric discomfort.[183] Fundic gland polyposis does not involve the antrum, and no clinical or pathologic differences are found between the familial and nonfamilial cases.[182,183]

Polyps present at the gastroenterostomy site are frequently due to displaced, hypertrophied gastric glands, called "gastritis cystica polyposa."[184] The principal significance of this lesion is its distinction from a carcinoma in the postoperative stomach.

Hypertrophic gastropathy is often interpreted radiologically or endoscopically as multiple gastric polyps. The epithelium is often made up of dilated gastric glands and hypertrophic pits. The classification of the forms of hypertrophic gastropathy (including Menetrier's disease) can be difficult because of the variable clinical features associated with this condition. The essential clinical point is that some proportion of these patients, perhaps 10%, develop carcinoma, and it may require considerable attention to subtle abnormalities in mucosal detail, and multiple biopsies, to identify the early appearance of neoplasia amidst a mass of hypertrophied folds.[185,186]

GASTRIC LYMPHOMA

Clinical Features

Lymphomas make up less than 5% of all gastric malignancies but make up the largest group after adenocarcinoma. Gastric lymphoma is most often indistinguishable grossly from adenocarcinoma, presenting as a polypoid lesion, ulcerated mass, or infiltrating submucosal lesion. Lymphomas do not have a predilection to occur in any particular region of the stomach but are more likely than other cancers to present with diffuse infiltration and enlarged rugal folds. The symptoms of gastric lymphoma are also nonspecific and include abdominal discomfort, nausea, vomiting, anorexia, weight loss, and hemorrhage.

The gastrointestinal tract is the most common extranodal site for the occurrence of lymphoma, and the majority of these occur in the stomach and small intestine. Most series indicate that 41% to 46% of primary gastrointestinal lymphomas originate in the stomach.[187,188] Diffuse histocytic lymphomas make up the largest pathologic group of gastric lymphoma, with the remainder scattered among a large number of other varieties.[187,189] Of interest, gastric lymphomas frequently arise in the setting of chronic gastritis (60%) and often within intestinal metaplasia (29%).[190]

Prognostic factors in this disease are, in part, similar to those for epithelial malignancies. Five-year survival is significantly worsened by serosal penetration and regional lymph node involvement.[190] Other adverse prognostic factors include involvement of the lesser curvature of the stomach, increasing stage of disease (see page 1374), and larger tumor size.

Diagnosis and Management of Gastric Lymphoma

Diagnosis and management of gastric lymphoma are overlapping issues because of the critical decision that must be made regarding the need for staging laparotomy and gastrectomy. Primary gastric lymphoma is most often first diagnosed by endoscopic biopsy. The use of CT has permitted an assessment of nodal involvement above and below the diaphragm, and, when this is combined with adequate pathologic samples obtained endoscopically (which may require snare biopsy of a polypoid mass or large rugal fold), abdominal exploration may not be needed to plan therapy. Total gastrectomy has been the traditional means of treating gastric lymphoma because it provided definitive tissue for pathologic exam, provided exploration of other abdominal structures, reduced tumor burden, and obviated concern that gastric hemorrhage or perforation would complicate medical eradication of the lymphoma. The accumulating experience on this subject suggests that not all patients require surgery.[191]

Although many staging systems have been proposed to classify non-Hodgkin's lymphomas, the Ann Arbor classification is suitable and widely used (Table 63-10).[192] The distribution in these categories varies largely as a function of patient selection. The 5-year survival for all patients with current treatment is about 50%, but outcome is strongly correlated with disease stage. For example, patients with stage I or II tumors less than 5 cm in diameter have greater than 80% 10-year survival, and at least one study has reported no 2-year survivors among those with stage III or IV disease.[193]

The therapeutic approach is highly controversial and must be individually determined. The first decision concerns the role of laparotomy and gastrectomy. When there is uncertainty regarding the histopathologic grade or tumor stage, or if there is bulky transmural lymphoma or the appearance of isolated I_E gastric lymphoma in a good surgical candidate, then laparotomy plays an important therapeutic role. However, if the diagnosis of grade II_E or worse disease has been established with biopsy and radiologic studies, then surgery is useful only in preventing treatment-induced perforation or hemorrhage—which may be expected in one quarter to one third of patients. In addition, total gastrectomy may be curative in the case of stage I_E disease. This must be weighed against an expected 10% surgical mortality and the considerable morbidity of a total gastrectomy. Many surgeons think that total gastrectomy is unnecessary and that a limited resection with adequate margins is appropriate. Although different surgical approaches have not been evaluated prospectively in this disease, a complete resection of all gross tumor with pathologic confirmation of negative resection margins is the current standard of management and is associated with an improvement in the operative mortality and postoperative morbidity.[194,195]

Once the decision regarding surgery has been addressed, the roles of radiation and chemotherapy must be determined. Postoperative radiation therapy may improve survival and is often added to the surgical plans, but a more aggressive approach including chemotherapy may further improve the outcome, even in stage I_E patients.[192] Combination chemotherapy consisting of cyclophosphamide, doxorubicin, vincristine, and prednisone (CHOP) is the standard approach for all advanced stages of the disease

TABLE 63-10
Ann Arbor Classification of Non-Hodgkin's Lymphoma as Applied to the Stomach

STAGE	EXTENT OF DISEASE	RELATIVE INCIDENCE (%)
I	Disease limited to the stomach	26–38
II	Extension to abdominal lymph nodes by biopsy or lymphangiography	43–49
III	Involvement of the stomach, abdominal lymph nodes, and nodular involvement above the diaphragm	13–31
IV	Disseminated lymphoma	

(i.e., stage III and IV). The role of radiation therapy is less clear. Radiation may be effective as primary treatment in controlling local disease, but lethal treatment failures occur outside of the irradiated field; the addition of radiation to gastrectomy does not seem to improve survival.[196]

In summary, exploratory laparotomy and gastrectomy are indicated when the clinical data for diagnosis are inadequate, or when stage I_E disease is suspected. When stage II_E, III_E, or IV_E are known, gastrectomy may obviate complications of treating the lymphoma, but chemotherapy is the primary therapeutic modality. Chemotherapy or radiation therapy may be added postoperatively in stage I_E disease. If a diagnosis of II_E or greater is made before surgery, and surgical resection is deemed unnecessary or inappropriate, combination chemotherapy is usually administered. Radiation therapy may be elected for the control of localized disease. Unfortunately, no regimen has been tested in controlled clinical trials because of the large number of different clinical stages and pathologic variants of the disease.

Other Considerations in Gastric Lymphoma

Three histologic variants of gastric pseudolymphoma have been identified and represent potential pitfalls that must be considered by the pathologist.[197] These lesions may present with clinical symptoms and endoscopic appearances that simulate adenocarcinoma or lymphoma. Pseudolymphoma is a mass of non-neoplastic lymphocytes that grossly simulates a malignant tumor. The cells that comprise these tumors are small lymphocytes without evidence of atypia. Multifocal hyperplastic lymphoid aggregates may occur in the stomach (or elsewhere in the gut) but are distinguishable by the presence of well-differentiated lymphocytes in characteristic follicles with germinal centers. Pseudolymphoma may account for 10% to 15% of all gastric lymphoid tumors and, therefore, is not a trivial consideration. A total gastric resection may be required in this circumstance to exclude the diagnosis of non-Hodgkin's lymphoma. One case has been reported in which a focal pseudolymphoma was diagnosed by partial gastrectomy and was followed by a true lymphoma 45 months later.[198]

Finally, patients who have received conservative, stomach-sparing therapy for gastric lymphoma may be at risk for the subsequent development of adenocarcinoma or gastric carcinoid.[199] It is not clear whether this reflects common causative agents in the genesis of all gastric cancers, or whether the second neoplasms occur as a consequence of radiation or chemotherapy.

GASTRIC CARCINOIDS

The term *carcinoid* was used initially to describe tumors with a characteristic pathologic appearance arising in the epithelial layer that had a less aggressive clinical course than typical adenocarcinomas. Carcinoid tumors can produce a panoply of functionally active substances including serotonin, histamine, gastrin, somatostatin, pituitary hormones, catecholamines, kinins, and prostaglandins, just to name a few. The different hormones produced by these tumors can give rise to a wide range of paraneoplastic syndromes, but most carcinoids secrete small amounts of product, which are quickly inactivated so they are clinically silent. The tumors do not form typical glands but grow in nests; they are not encapsulated, and the interface between the tumor and surrounding tissues may be distinct, show invasion, or be ambiguous, making the diagnosis of benign and malignant tumors difficult until metastases appear. Most gastric carcinoids occur in the body of the stomach, may be single or multiple (in approximately 14%), and may look like an ordinary ulcer, polyp, or tumor mass to the endoscopist.[200]

The stomach is the location of approximately 2% to 3% of all carcinoids, but gastric carcinoids represent only 0.3% of all gastric tumors.[201] Carcinoids of foregut origin characteristically synthesize 5-hydroxytryptamine (serotonin) and, therefore, are capable of producing the classic flushing of the carcinoid syndrome; actually, however, most gastric carcinoids do not produce symptoms related to vasoactive peptides and are frequently discovered incidentally.

Recently, interest has been directed toward the pathogenesis of carcinoid tumors. Carcinoids occur more frequently in patients with pernicious anemia and atrophic gastritis with achlorhydria.[202] They also appear to be more common in patients with Zollinger-Ellison syndrome. Furthermore, experimental models of carcinoid tumors may be created by inhibiting acid secretion using a potent H$_2$ receptor antagonist or omeprazole.[202,203] Each of these clinical situations is associated with hypergastrinemia. Any clinical condition in which serum levels of gastrin are elevated for a prolonged period should heighten one's awareness that gastric carcinoid tumors may develop.

The most common clinical decision encountered is the management of the incidentally discovered small gastric carcinoid tumor. The treatment of choice is always complete excision. Many of these tumors can be totally removed endoscopically, either using the "hot biopsy" forceps or snare cautery. Most carcinoids are slow-growing and have low invasive or metastatic potential, and, in these cases, endoscopic removal is adequate. An individualized decision rests on the completeness of local excision and an assessment of the malignant behavior of the tumor by the pathologist.

The carcinoid syndrome is rare in gastric carcinoids and most often reflects the presence of hepatic metastases. The treatment of metastatic carcinoid tumors involves two strategies. Cytotoxic therapy is often administered in an attempt to reduce the burden of tumor cells. Because of the indolent biologic behavior of these tumors, they tend not to respond particularly well to combination chemotherapy. Regimens that have been tried typically include 5-fluorouracil and streptozotocin plus one or more additional agents. Response rates (generally limited to objective reductions in tumor size) have been in the range of 30% and are not dramatic. As a result, most attention has been directed to the control of the paraneoplastic symptoms.

Patients with prominent secretion of serotonin from gastric carcinoid may respond to methyldopa, which inhibits the decarboxylation of 5-hydroxytryptophan to serotonin.[204] Control of other symptoms requires inhibition of the production or action of the specific hormone produced and can include a long list of drugs including indomethacin or other cyclooxygenase inhibitors, corticosteroids, H$_2$-antagonists, and various catecholamine antagonists. However, the advent of somatostatin for the control of a wide range of symptomatology is a promising innovation in the control of this syndrome. The somatostatin analogue octreotide acetate (Sandostatin, Sandoz Pharmaceuticals) administered sub-cutaneously in doses 50 μg to 500 μg, two to three times per day, can control flushing, diarrhea, and other symptoms in 79% of patients[205] and can inhibit the secretion of a wide range of tumor-produced autacoids. This approach, in most instances, is preferred to the administration of multiple drugs for individual symptom complexes in the patient with metastatic disease and is the treatment of choice in this situation.

The reader is directed to Chapter 24, Neoplasia of the Gastrointestinal Tract; Chapter 61, Acid-Peptic Disorders; Chapter 111, Upper Gastrointestinal Endoscopy; and Chapter 114, Contrast Radiology.

REFERENCES

1. Parkin DM, Laara E, Muir CS. Estimates of the worldwide frequency of sixteen major cancers in 1980. Int J Cancer 1988;41:184.
2. Jackson CE, Brownlee RW, Schuman BM, et al. Observations on gastric cancer in San Marino. Cancer 1980;45:599.
3. Boyd J, Langman M, Doll R. The epidemiology of gastrointestinal cancer with special reference to causation. Gut 1964;5:196.
4. Hill MJ. Environmental and genetic factors in gastrointestinal cancer. In: Sherlock P, Morson BC, Barbara L, Veronesi U, eds. Precancerous lesions of the gastrointestinal tract. New York: Raven Press, 1983:1.
5. Howson CP, Hiyama T, Wynder EL. The decline in gastric cancer; Epidemiology of an unplanned triumph. Epidemiol Rev 1986;8:1.
6. Wiggins CL, Becker TM, Key CR, et al. Stomach cancer among New Mexico's American Indians, Hispanic whites and non-Hispanic whites. Cancer Res 1989;49:1595.
7. Correa P, Cuello C, Fajardo LF, et al. Diet and gastric cancer: Nutrition survey in a high-risk area. JNCI 1983;70:673.
8. Hu J, Zhang S, Jia E, et al. Diet and cancer of the stomach: A case-control study in China. Int J Cancer 1988;41:331.
9. You W-C, Blot WJ, Chang Y-S, et al. Diet and high risk of stomach cancer in Shandong, China. Cancer Res 1988;48:3518.
10. Correa P, Fontham E, Pickle LW, et al. Dietary determinants of gastric cancer in South Louisiana inhabitants. JNCI 1985;75:645.
11. Nomura A, Yamakawa H, Ishidate T, et al. Intestinal metaplasia in Japan: Association with diet. JNCI 1982;68:401.
12. Hirayama T. Epidemiology of stomach cancer in Japan. Jpn J Clin Oncol 1984;14:159.
13. You W-C, Blot WJ, Chang Y-S, et al. Allium vegetables and reduced risk of stomach cancer. JNCI 1989;81:112.
14. Cuello C, Correa P, Haenzel W, et al. Gastric cancer in Colombia. I. Cancer risk and suspect environmental agents. JNCI 1976;57: 1015.
15. Haenzel W, Correa P, Cuello C, et al. Gastric cancer Colombia. II. Case-control epidemiologic study of precursor lesions. JNCI 1976;57: 1021.
16. Correa P, Cuello C, Duque E, et al. Gastric cancer in Colombia. III. Natural history of precursor lesions. JNCI 1976;57:1027.
17. Zemla B. Malignant neoplasms of the stomach and the quality of drinking water. Nutr Cancer 1988;11:1.
18. Neuberger M, Kundi M, Friedl HP. Environmental asbestos exposure and cancer mortality. Arch Environ Health 1984;39:261.
19. Ohgaki H, Kawachi T, Matsukura N, et al. Genetic control of susceptibility of rats to gastric carcinoma. Cancer Res 1983;43:3663.
20. Chen J, Barnes WS, Maiello J, et al. Biochemical mechanisms on species differences in gastric carcinogenesis. Cancer Res Clin Oncol 1984;108:135.
21. Ohgaki H, Tomihari M, Sato S, et al. Differential proliferative response of gastric mucosa during carcinogenesis induced by N-methyl-

N'-nitro-N-nitrosoguanidine in susceptible ACI rats, resistant Buffalo rats, and their hybrid F$_1$ cross. Cancer Res 1988;48:5275.

22. Tatematsu M, Furihata C, Katsuyama T, et al. Independent induction of intestinal metaplasia and gastric cancer in rats treated with N-methyl-N'-nitro-N-nitrosoguanidine. Cancer Res 1983;43:1335.

23. Tatsuta M, Yamamura H, Taniguchi H, et al. Gastrin protection against chemically induced gastric adenocarcinomas in Wistar rats: Histopathology of the glandular stomach and incidence of gastric adenocarcinoma. JNCI 1982;69:59.

24. Tatsuta M, Iishi H, Yamamura H, et al. Effect of cimetidine on inhibition by tetragastrin of carcinogenesis induced by N-methyl-N'-nitro-N-nitrosoguanidine in Wistar rats. Cancer Res 1988;48:1591.

25. Deveney CW, Freeman HJ, Way LW. Experimental gastric carcinogenesis in the rat. Am J Surg 1980;139:49.

26. Tatsuta M, Iishi H, Yamamura H, et al. Inhibitory effect of prolonged administration of cysteamine on experimental carcinogenesis in rat stomach induced by N-methyl-N'-nitro-N-nitrosoguanidine. Int J Cancer 1988;41:423.

27. Tatsuta M, Iishi H, Baba M, et al. Effects of propranolol and cimetidine on cysteamine inhibition of gastric carcinogenesis induced in Wistar rats by N-methyl-N'-nitro-N-nitrosoguanidine. Int J Cancer 1989;43:464.

28. Tatsuta M, Yamamura H, Ichii M, et al. Promotion by histamine of carcinogenesis in the forestomach and protection by histamine against carcinogenesis induced by N-Nitroso-N-methylinitroguanidine in the glandular stomach in W rats. JNCI 1983;71:361.

29. Tatsuta M, Yamamura H, Iishi H, et al. Promotion by vagotomy of gastric carcinogenesis induced by N-methyl-N'-nitro-N-nitrosoguanidine in Wistar rats. Cancer Res 1985;45:194.

30. Tahara E, Shimamoto F, Taniyama K, et al. Enhanced effect of gastrin on rat stomach carcinogenesis induced by N-methyl-N'-nitro-N-nitrosoguanidine. Cancer Res 1982;42:1781.

31. Kobori O, Shimizu T, Maeda M, et al. Enhancing effect of bile and bile acid on stomach tumorigenesis induced by N-methyl-N'-nitro-N-nitrosoguanidine in Wistar rats. JNCI 1984;73:853.

32. Chang F-H, Lee Y-C, Lee K-Y, et al. Cocarcinogenic action of aspirin on gastric tumors induced by N-nitroso-N-methyinitro-guanidine in rats. JNCI 1983;70:1067.

33. Kondo K, Suzuki H, Nagayo T. The influence of gastro-jejunal anastomosis on gastric carcinogenesis in rats. Gann 1984;75:362.

34. Nishidoi H, Koga S, Kaibara N. Possible role of duodenogastric reflux on the development of remnant gastric carcinoma induced by N-methyl-N'-nitro-N-nitrosoguanidine in rats. JNCI 1984;72:1431.

35. Makino M, Kaibara N, Koga S. Enhanced induction by high-cholesterol diet of remnant gastric carcinogenesis by N-methyl-N'-nitro-N-nitrosoguanidine in rats. JNCI 1989;81:130.

36. Tannenbaum SR, Sinskey AJ, Weisman M, et al. Nitrite in human saliva: Its possible relationship to nitrosamine formation. JNCI 1974;53:79.

37. Mirvish SS. Intragastric nitrosamide formation and other theories. JNCI 1983;71:629.

38. Hartman PE. Review: Putative mutagens and carcinogens in foods. I. Nitrate/nitrite ingestion and gastric cancer mortality. Environ Mutagen 1983;5:111.

39. Wagner DA, Shuker DEG, Bilmazes C, et al. Effect of vitamins C and E on endogenous synthesis of N-nitrosamino acids in humans: Precursor-product studies with [^{15}N]Nitrate. Cancer Res 1985;45:6519.

40. Reed PI, Smith PLR, Haines K, et al. Gastric juice N-nitrosamines in health and gastroduodenal disease. Lancet 1981;2:550.

41. Cheli R, Giacosa A. Atrophic gastritis. In: Sherlock P, Morson BC, Barbara L, Veronesi U, eds. Precancerous lesions of the gastrointestinal tract. New York: Raven Press, 1983:55.

42. Deschner EE, Winawer SJ, Lipkin M. Patterns of nucleic acid and protein synthesis in normal human gastric mucosa and atrophic gastritis. JNCI 1972;48:1567.

43. Jass JR, Strudley I, Faludy J. Histochemistry of epithelial metaplasia and dysplasia in human stomach and colorectum. Scand J Gastroenterol 1984;19(Suppl 104):109.

44. Bara J, Paul-Gardais A, Loisillier F, et al. Isolation of a sulfated glycopeptidic antigen from human gastric tumors: Its localization in normal and cancerous gastrointestinal tissues. Int J Cancer 1978;21:133.

45. Shimamoto C, Weinstein WM, Boland CR. Glycoconjugate expression in normal, metaplastic, and neoplastic human upper gastrointestinal mucosa. J Clin Invest 1987;80:167.

46. Sipponen P, Kekki M, Siurala M. Age-related trends of gastritis and intestinal metaplasia in gastric carcinoma patients and in controls representing the population at large. Br J Cancer 1984;49:521.

47. Walker IR, Strickland RG, Ungar B, et al. Simple atrophic gastritis and gastric cancer. Gut 1971;12:906.

48. Cheli R, Santi L, Ciancamerla G, et al. A clinical and statistical follow-up study of atrophic gastritis. Am J Dig Dis 1973;18:1061.

49. Siurala M, Isokoski M, Varis M, et al. Prevalence of gastritis in a rural population. Bioptic study of subjects selected at random. Scand J Gastroenterol 1968;3:211.

50. Findley JW, Kirsner JB, Palmer WL. Atrophic gastritis: A follow-up study of 100 patients. Gastroenterology 1950;16:347.

51. Schlag P, Ulrich H, Merkle P, et al. Are nitrite and N-nitroso compounds in gastric juice risk factors for carcinoma in the operated stomach? Lancet 1980;1:727.

52. Reed PI, Smith PLR, Summers K, et al. The influence of enterogastric reflux on gastric juice bacterial growth, nitrite, and N-nitroso compound concentrations following gastric surgery. Scand J Gastroenterol 1984;19(Suppl 92):232.

53. Keighley MRB, Youngs D, Poxon V, et al. Intragastric N-nitrosation is unlikely to be responsible for gastric cocarcinoma developing after operations for duodenal ulcer. Gut 1984;25:238.

54. Watt PCH, Sloan JM, Donaldson J, et al. Relation between gastric histology and gastric juice pH and nitrite and N-nitroso compound concentrations in the stomach after surgery for duodenal ulcer. J Clin Pathol 1984;37:511.

55. Watt PCH, Sloan JM, Kennedy TL. Relation between intragastric bile acid concentration and mucosal abnormality in the stomach after vagotomy and gastroenterostomy for duodenal ulcer. J Clin Pathol 1984;37:506.

56. Ruddell WSJ, Walters CL. Nitrite and N-nitroso compounds in gastric juice (letter). Lancet 1980;1:1187.

57. Hole DJ, Quigley EMM, Gillis CR, et al. Peptic ulcer and cancer: An examination of the relationship between chronic peptic ulcer and gastric carcinoma. Scand J Gastroenterol 1987;22:17.

58. Kinlen LJ, Webster ADB, Bird AG, et al. Prospective study of cancer in patients with hypogammaglobulinemia. Lancet 1985;1:263.

59. Hermans PE, Huizenga KA. Association of gastric carcinoma with idiopathic late-onset immunoglobulin deficiency. Ann Intern Med 1972;76:605.

60. Boland CR. Cancer family syndrome. A case report and literature review. Am J Dig Dis 1978;23:25s.

61. Bloss RS, Miller TA, Copeland EM. Carcinoma of the stomach in the young adult. Surg Gynecol Obstet 1980;150:883.

62. Holburt E, Freedman SI. Gastric carcinoma in patient younger than age 36 years. Cancer 1987;60:1395.

63. Mecklin JP, Nordling S, Saario I. Carcinoma of the stomach and its heredity in young patients. Scand J Gastroenterol 1988;23:307.

64. Grabiec J, Owen DA. Carcinoma of the stomach in young persons. Cancer 1985;56:388.

65. Pastore JO, Kato H, Belsky JL. Serum pepsin and tubeless gastric analysis as predictors of stomach cancer. N Engl J Med 1972;286:279.

66. Antonioli DA, Goldman H. Changes in the location and type of gastric adenocarcinoma. Cancer 1982;50:775.

67. Meyers WC, Damiano RJ, Postlethwait PW, et al. Adenocarcinoma of the stomach changing pattern over the last 4 decades. Ann Surg 1987;205:1.

68. Mori M, Iwashita A, Enjoji M. Adenosquamous carcinoma of the stomach: A clinocopathologic analysis of 28 cases. Cancer 1986;57:333.

69. Byrne D, Holley MP, Cuschieri A. Parietal cell carcinoma of the stomach: Association with long-term survival after curative resection. Br J Cancer 1988;58:85.

70. Fenoglio-Preiser C, Lantz PE, Listrom MB, et al. Neoplastic stomach. In: Fenoglio-Preish CM, Lantz PE, Listrom MB, et al, eds. Gastrointestinal pathology: An atlas and text. New York: Raven Press, 1989:215.

71. Shiu MH, Farr GH, Papachristou DN, et al. Myosarcomas of the stomach: Natural history, prognostic factors and management. Cancer 1982;49:177.

72. Knapp RH, Wick MR, Goellner JR. Leiomyoblastomas and their relationship to other smooth-muscle tumors of the gastrointestinal tract. Am J Surg Pathol 1984;8:449.

73. Holtz F, Hart WR. Krukenberg tumors of the ovary: A clinico-pathologic analysis of 27 cases. Cancer 1982;50:2438.

74. Hattori T. Development of adenocarcinomas in the stomach. Cancer 1986;57:1528.

75. Filipe MI, Potet F, Bogomoletz WV, et al. Incomplete sulphomucin-secreting intestinal metaplasia for gastric cancer. Preliminary data from a prospective study from three centres. Gut 1985;26:1319.

76. Ectors N, Dixon MF. The prognostic value of sulphomucin positive intestinal metaplasia in the development of gastric cancer. Histopathology 1986;10:1271.

77. Walker IR, Strickland RG, Ungar B, et al. Simple atrophic gastritis and gastric carcinoma. Gut 1971;12:906.

78. Elsborg L, Mosbech J. Pernicious anaemia as a risk factor in gastric cancer. Acta Med Scand 1979;206:315.

79. Stockbrugger RW, Menon GG, Beilby JOW, et al. Gastroscopic screening in 80 patients with pernicious anaemia. Gut 1983;24:1141.

80. Schafer LW, Larson DE, Melton LJ, et al. Risk of development of gastric carcinoma in patients with pernicious anemia: A population-based study in Rochester, Minnesota. Mayo Clin Proc 1985;60:444.

81. Stalsberg H, Taksdal S. Stomach cancer following gastric surgery for benign conditions. Lancet 1971;2:1175.

82. Stokkeland M, Schrumpf E, Hanssen AS, et al. Incidence of malignancies of the Billroth II operated stomach. Scand J Gastroenterol 1981;16(Suppl 67):169.

83. Giarelli L, Melato M, Stanta G, et al. Gastric resection—a cause of high frequency of gastric carcinoma. Cancer 1983;52:1113.

84. Offerhaus GJA, Huibregtse K, DeBoer J, et al. The operated stomach: A premalignant condition? Scand J Gastroenterol 1984;19:521.

85. Gaygill CPJ, Hill MJ, Kirkham JS, et al. Mortality from gastric cancer following gastric surgery for peptic ulcer. Lancet 1986;929.

86. Gaygill CPJ, Hill MJ, Hall CN, et al. Increased risk of cancer at multiple sites after gastric surgery for peptic ulcer. Gut 1987;28:924.

87. Offerhaus GJA, Tersmette AC, Huibregtse K, et al. Mortality caused by stomach cancer after remote partial gastrectomy for benign conditions: 40 years of follow up of an Amsterdam cohort of 2,633 postgastrectomy patients. Gut 1988;29:1588.

88. Schafter LW, Larson DE, Melton LJ, et al. The risk of gastric carcinoma after surgical treatment for benign ulcer disease. N Engl J Med 1983;309:1210.

89. Lundegardh G, Adami H-O, Helmick C, et al. Stomach cancer after partial gastrectomy for benign ulcer disease. N Engl J Med 1988;319:195.

90. Offerhaus GJA, Stadt J, Huibregtse K, et al. Endoscopic screening for malignancy in the gastric remnant: The clinical significance of dysplasia in gastric mucosa. J Clin Pathol 1984;37:748.

91. Domellof S, Eriksson S, Janunger K-G. Carcinoma and possible precancerous changes of the gastric stump after Billroth II resection. Gastroenterology 1977;73:462.

92. Bedossa P, Lemaigre G, Martin ED. Histochemical study of mucosubstances in carcinoma of the gastric remnant. Cancer 1987;60:2224.

93. Faivre J, Justrabo E, Hillon P, et al. Gastric carcinoma in Cote d'Or (France), a population based study. Gastroenterology 1985;88:1874.

94. Laufer I. Assessment of the accuracy of double contrast gastroduodenal radiology. Gastroenterology 1976;71:874.

95. Herlinger H, Glanville JN, Kreel L. An evaluation of the double contrast barium meal (DCBM) against endoscopy. Clin Radiol 1977;28:307.

96. Hamada T, Kaji F, Shirakabe H. Detectability of gastric cancer by radiology as compared to endoscopy. In: Maruyama M, Kimura K, eds. Review of clinical research in gastroenterology. Tokyo: Igaku-Shoin, 1988:36.

97. Thompson G, Somers S, Stevenson GW. Benign gastric ulcer: A reliable radiologic diagnosis? AJR 1983;141:331.

98. Levine MS, Creteur V, Kressel HY, et al. Benign gastric ulcers: Diagnosis and follow-up with double contrast radiography. Radiology 1987;164:9.

99. Armington WGN, Mann FA, Nelson JA. Cost-effective means of diagnosing and following benign and malignant gastric ulcers. Invest Radiol 1985;20:171.

100. Sakita T, Oguro Y, Takasu S, et al. Observations on the healing of ulcerations in early gastric cancer: The life cycle of the malignant ulcer. Gastroenterology 1971;60:835.

101. Dooley CP, Lavsor AW, Stace NH, et al. Double contrast barium meal and upper gastrointestinal endoscopy: A comparative study. Ann Intern Med 1984;101:538.

102. Shamir M, Schuman BM. Complications of fiberoptic endoscopy. Gastrointest Endosc 1980;26:86.

103. Fenoglio-Preiser C, Lantz PE, Listrom MB, et al. Neoplastic stomach. In: Fenoglio-Preish CM, Lantz PE, Listrom MB, et al, eds. Gastrointestinal pathology: An atlas and text. New York: Raven Press, 1989:200.

104. Tatsuta M, Iishi H, Okuda S, et al. Prospective evaluation of diagnostic accuracy of gastrofiberscopic biopsy in diagnosis of gastric cancer. Cancer 1989;63:1415.

105. Dekker W, Tytgat GN. Diagnostic accuracy of fiberendoscopy in the detection of upper intestinal malignancy: A follow-up analysis. Gastroenterology 1977;73:710.

106. Hatfield ARW, Slavin G, Segal AW, et al. Importance of the site of endoscopic gastric biopsy in ulcerating lesions of the stomach. Gut 1975;16:884.

107. Graham DY, Schwartz JT, Cain GD, et al. Prospective evaluation of biopsy number in the diagnosis of esophageal and gastric carcinoma. Gastroenterology 1982;82:228.

108. Shanghai Gastrointestinal Endoscopy Cooperative Group, People's Republic of China. Value of biopsy and brush cytology in the diagnosis of gastric cancer. Gut 1982;23:774.

109. Cook IJ, deCarle DJ, Haneman B, et al. The role of brushing cytology in the diagnosis of gastric malignancy. Acta Cytol 1988;32:461.

110. Bogomoletz WV. Early gastric cancer. Am J Surg Pathol 1984;8:381.

111. Itabashi M, Hirota T, Unakami M, et al. The role of the biopsy in diagnosis of early gastric cancer. Jpn J Clin Oncol 1984;142:253.

112. Green PHR, O'Toole KM, Slonim D, et al. Increasing incidence and excellent survival of patients with early gastric cancer: Experience in a United States Medical Center. Am J Med 1988;85:658.

113. Iishi H, Tatsuta M, Okuda S. Endoscopic diagnosis of minute gastric cancer less than 5 mm in diameter. Cancer 1985;56:655.

114. Tatsuta M, Iishi H, Okuda S, et al. Diagnosis of early gastric cancers in the upper part of the stomach by the endoscopic Congo-red-methylene blue test. Endoscopy 1984;16:131.

115. Winawer SJ. Tissue diagnosis in upper gastrointestinal malignancy. Gastroenterology 1982;82:379.

116. Blackstone MO. Endoscopic interpretation. New York: Raven Press, 1984:137.

117. Ellis DJ, Speirs C, Kingston RD, et al. Carcinoembryonic antigen levels in advanced gastric carcinoma. Cancer 1978;42:623.

118. Bunn PA, Cohen MI, Widerlite L, et al. Simultaneous gastric and plasma immunoreactive plasma carcinoembryonic antigen in 1,087 patients undergoing gastroscopy. Gastroenterology 1979;76:734.

119. Micali B, Flono MG, Artemisia A, et al. Usefulness of carcinoembryonic antigen measurement in gastric juice of patients with gastric disorders. J Clin Gastroenterol 1983;5:411.

120. Nitti D, Farini R, Grassi F, et al. Carcinoembryonic antigen in gastric juice collected during endoscopy: Value in detecting high-risk patients and gastric cancer. Cancer 1983;52:2334.

121. Gion M, Dittaci R, Munegato G, et al. Tumor marker radioimmunoassays in gastric juice: Methlogic drawbacks due to pH variations. Gastroenterology 1988;94:1271.

122. Heymer B, Quentmeir A. Biological markers for staging of gastric cancer, In: Herfarth CH, Schlag P, eds. Gastric cancer. Berlin: Springer-Verlag, 1979:157.

123. Nomura AHY, Stemmermann GN, Samloff IM. Serum pepsinogen I as a predictor of stomach cancer. Ann Intern Med 1980;93:537.

124. McGuigan JE, Trudeau WKL. Serum and tissue gastrin concentrations in patients with carcinoma of the stomach. Gastroenterology 1973;64:22.

125. Schmitz-Moormann P, Heider H-A, Thomas C. Cancer of the

stomach—prognosis, independent of therapy. In: Herfarth CH, Schlag P, eds. Gastric cancer. Berlin: Springer-Verlag, 1979:172.

126. Maruyama M. Treatment results of gastric cancer staged by the new TNM classification. In: Maruyama M, Kimura K, eds. Review of clinical research in gastroenterology. Tokyo: Igaku-Shoin, 1988: 112.

127. American Joint Committee on Cancer. Manual for staging of cancer, ed 3. Philadelphia: JB Lippincott, 1988:69.

128. Okada M, Kojimas S, Murakami M, et al. Human gastric carcinoma: Prognosis in relation to macroscopic and microscopic features of the primary tumor. JNCI 1983;71:275.

129. Armstrong CP, Dent DM. Factors influencing prognosis in carcinoma of the stomach. Surg Gynecol Obstet 1986;162:343.

130. Hayashi R, Ochiai T. HLA type and survival in gastric cancer. Cancer Res 1986;46:3701.

131. Tahara E, Sumiyoshi H, Hata J, et al. Human epidermal growth factor in gastric carcinoma as a biologic marker of high malignancy. Jpn J Cancer Res (Gann) 1986;77:145.

132. Baba H, Korenaga D, Okamura T. Prognostic significance of DNA content with special reference to age in gastric cancer. Cancer 1989;63:1768.

133. Aretxabala X, Yonemura Y, Sugiyma K, et al. DNA ploidy in early gastric cancer and its relationship to prognosis. Br J Surg 1988;75(8): 770.

134. Sasaki K, Hashimoto T, Kawachino CT, et al. Intratumoral regional differences in DNA ploidy of gastrointestinal carcinomas. Cancer 1988;62:2569.

135. Kaneko E, Nakamura T, Uneda N, et al. Outcome of gastric carcinoma detected by gastric mass survey in Japan. Gut 1977;18:626.

136. Yamakazi H, Oshima A, Murakami R, et al. A long term follow-up study of patients with gastric cancer detected by mass screening. Cancer 1989;63:613.

137. Olearchyk AS. Gastric carcinoma: A critical review of 243 cases. Am J Gastroenterol 1978;70:25.

138. Moss AA, Schnyder P, Marks W, et al. Gastric adenocarcinoma: A comparison of the accuracy and economics of staging by CT and surgery. Gastroenterol 1981;80:45.

139. Cook AO, Levine BA, Sirinek KR, et al. Evaluation of gastric adenocarcinoma: Abdominal CT does not replace celiotomy. Arch Surg 1986;121:603.

140. Douglass HO, Nava HR. Gastric adenocarcinoma—management of the primary disease. Semin Oncol 1985;12:32.

141. Yamanaka T, Kimura K. The use of ultrasonographic endoscopy in the assessment of depth of invasion of gastric cancer. In: Maruyama M, Kimura K, eds. Review of clinical research in gastroenterology. Tokyo: Igaku-Shoin, 1988:93.

142. Tio TL, Schouwink MH, Cikot RJLM, et al. Preoperative TNM classification of gastric carcinoma by endosonography in comparison with the pathological TNM system: A prospective study of 72 cases. Hepatogastroenterology 1989;36:51.

143. Schlag P. Considerations for surgical treatment of gastric carcinoma. Eur J Surg Oncol 1986;12:225.

144. Schrock TR, Way LW. Total gastrectomy. Am J Surg 1978;135: 348.

145. Pichlmayr R, Meyer HJ. Value of the gastrectomy "de Principe." In: Herfarth CH, Schlag P, eds. Gastric cancer. Berlin: Springer-Verlag, 1979:196.

146. Gouzi JL, Huguier M, Fagniez PL, et al. Total versus subtotal gastrectomy for adenocarcinoma of the gastric antrum. Ann Surg 1989;209:162.

147. Dupont JB, Lee JR, Burton GR, Cohn I. Adenocarcinoma of the stomach: Review of 1,497 Cases. Cancer 1978;41:941.

148. Yan C, Brroks JR. Surgical management of gastric adenocarcinoma. Am J Surg 1985;149:771.

149. Kodama Y, Sugimachi K, Soejima K, et al. Evaluation of extensive lymph node dissection for carcinoma of the stomach. World J Surg 1981;5:148.

150. Bizer LS. Adenocarcinoma of the stomach: Current results of treatment. Cancer 1983;51:743.

151. Nakajima T, Nishi M. Surgery and adjuvant chemotherapy for gastric cancer. Hepatogastroenterology 1989;36:79.

152. Boddie AW, McMurtrey MJ, Glacco GG, et al. Palliative total gastrectomy and esophagogastrectomy: A reevaluation. Cancer 1983;51: 1195.

153. Lawrence W Jr, McNeer G. The effectiveness of surgery for palliation of incurable gastric cancer. Cancer 1958;11:28.

154. Lawrence W, Jr. Gastric cancer. CA 1986;36:216.

155. Gunderson LL, Sosin H. Adenocarcinoma of the stomach: Areas of failure in a reoperation series (second or symptomatic look) clinicopathologic correlation and implications for adjuvant therapy. Int J Radiat Oncol Biol Phys 1982;8:1.

156. Okuyama K, Isono K, Juan I-K, et al. Evaluation of treatment for gastric cancer with liver metastasis. Cancer 1985;55:2498.

157. Clark PI, Slevin ML. Chemotherapy for stomach cancer. Br Med J 1987;295:870.

158. MacDonald JS, Gohmann JJ. Chemotherapy of advanced gastric cancer: Present status, future prospects. Semin Oncol 1988;15:42.

159. Cullinan SA, Moertel CG, Fleming TR, et al. A comparison of three chemotherapeutic regimens in the treatment of advanced pancreatic and gastric carcinoma. Fluororacil vs. fluororacil and doxorubicin vs. fluorouracil doxorubicin and mitomycin. JAMA 1985;253:2061.

160. LeChevalier T, Smith FP, Harter WK, et al. Chemotherapy and combined modality therapy for locally advanced and metastatic gastric carcinoma. Semin Oncol 1985;12:46.

161. Moertel C, Rubin J, O'Connel MJ, et al. A phase II study of combined 5-FU, doxorubicin and cisplatinum in the treatment of advanced upper gastrointestinal adenocarcinomas. J Clin Oncol 1986;4:1053.

162. Gastrointestinal Tumor Study Group. Triazinate and platinum efficacy in combination with 5-fluorouracil and doxorubicin: Results of a three-arm randomized trial in metastatic gastric cancer. JNCI 1988;80:1011.

163. Gastrointestinal Tumor Study Group. Controlled trial of adjuvant chemotherapy following curative resection for gastric cancer. Cancer 1982;49:1116.

164. Engstrom PF, Lavin PT, Douglass HO, et al. Postoperative adjuvant 5-FU plus methyl-CCNU therapy for gastric cancer patients. Cancer 1985;55:1868.

165. Higgins GA, Amadeo JH, Smith DE, et al. Efficacy of prolonged intermittent therapy with combined 5-FU and methyl CCNU following resection for gastric carcinoma: A Veterans Administration Surgical Oncology Group Report. Cancer 1983;52:1105.

166. Allum W, Hallissey MT, Kelley KA. Adjuvant chemotherapy in operable gastric cancer. 5 year follow-up of the first British Stomach Cancer Group Trial. Lancet 1989.571.

167. Weissberg JB. Role of radiation therapy in gastrointestinal cancer. Arch Surg 1983;118:96.

168. Abe M, Takahashi M. Intraoperative radiotherapy: The Japanese experience. Int J Radiat Oncol Biol Phys 1981;7:863.

169. Gastrointestinal Tumor Study Group. A comparison of combination chemotherapy and combined modality therapy for locally advanced gastric carcinoma. Cancer 1982;49:1771.

170. Ochiai T, Sato H, Sato H, et al. Randomly controlled study of chemotherapy versus chemoimmunotherapy in postoperative gastric cancer patients. Cancer Res 1983;43:3001.

171. Akiyosh T, Kawaguchi M, Arinaga S, et al. A trial of adjuvant combination chemoimmunotherapy for stage III carcinoma of stomach. J Surg Oncol 1984;26:86.

172. The Italian Gastrointestinal Tumor Study Group. Adjuvant treatments following curative resection for gastric cancer. Br J Surg 1988;75:1100.

173. Tonnesen H, Bulow S, Fischerman K, et al. Effect of cimetidine on survival after gastric cancer. Lancet 1988;ii:991.

174. Guillou PJ, Monson JRT. Immunological contributions to the management of gastric cancer. Hepatogastroenterology 1989;36:86.

175. Kaibara N, Hamazoe R, Iitouka Y, et al. Hyperthemic peritoneal perfusion combined with anticancer chemotherapy as prophylactic treatment of peritoneal recurrence of gastric cancer. Hepatogastroenterology 1989;36:75.

176. Mathus-Vliegen EMH, Tytgat GNJ. Laser photocoagulation in the palliative treatment of upper digestive tract tumors. Cancer 1986;57: 396.

177. Fleischer D, Sivak MV. Endoscopic Nd:YAG laser therapy as palliative treatment for advanced adenocarcinoma of the gastric cardia. Gastroenterology 1984;87:815.

178. Oguro Y, Hirashima T, Tajiri H, et al. Endoscopic treatment of early gastric cancer: Polypectomy and laser treatment. Am J Clin Oncol 1984;14(2):271.

179. Ming S-C, Goldman H. Gastric polyps, a histogenetic classification and its relation to carcinoma. Cancer 1985;18:721.

180. Tomasulo J. Gastric polyps, Histologic types and their relationship to gastric carcinoma. Cancer 1971;27:1346.

181. Laxen F. Gastric carcinoma and pernicious anaemia in long-term endoscopic follow-up of subjects with gastric polyps. Scand J Gastroenterol 1984;19:535.

182. Lee RG, Burt RW. The histopathology of fundic gland polyps of the stomach. Am J Clin Pathol 1986;86:498.

183. Iida M, Yao T, Watanabe H, et al. Fundic gland polyposis in patients without familial adenomatosis coli: Its incidence and clinical features. Gastroenterology 1984;86:1437.

184. Koga S, Watanabe H, Enjoju M. Stomal polypoid hypertrophic gastritis. Cancer 1979;43:647.

185. Scharschmidt BF. The natural history of hypertrophic gastropathy (Menetrier's disease). Report of a case with 16 year follow-up and review of 120 cases from the literature. Am J Med 1977;63:644.

186. Case Records of the Massachusetts General Hospital. N Engl J Med 1988;318:100.

187. Lewin KJ, Ranchod M, Dorfman RF. Lymphomas of the gastrointestinal tract. Cancer 1978;42:693.

188. Herrmann R, Panhon AM, Barcos MP, et al. Gastrointestinal involvement in non-Hodgkin's lymphoma. Cancer 1980;46:215.

189. Brooks JJ, Enterline HT. Primary gastric lymphomas, a clinicopathologic study of 58 cases with long-term follow-up and literature review. Cancer 1983;51:701.

190. Shimm DS, Dororetz DE, Anderson T, et al. Primary gastric lymphoma, an analysis with emphasis on prognostic factors and radiation therapy. Cancer 1983;52:2044.

191. Maor MH, Maddux B, Osborne BM, et al. Stages I_E and II_E non-Hodgkin's lymphomas of the stomach: Comparison of treatment modalities. Cancer 1984;54:2330.

192. Haber DA, Mayer RJ. Primary gastrointestinal lymphoma. Semin Oncol 1988;15:154.

193. Weingrad DN, Decosse JJ, Sherlock P, et al. Primary gastrointestinal lymphoma: A 30-year review. Cancer 1982;49:1258.

194. Shiu MH, Nisce LZ, Pinna A, et al. Recent results of multimodal therapy of gastric lymphoma. Cancer 1986;58:1389.

195. Rosen CB, van der Heerden JA, Martin JK, et al. Is an aggressive surgical approach with gastric lymphoma warranted? Ann Surg 1987;205:635.

196. Dworkin B, Lightdale CJ, Weingrad DN, et al. Primary gastric lymphoma: A review of 50 cases. Am J Dig Dis 1982;27:986.

197. Brooks JJ, Enterline HT. Gastric pseudolymphoma: Its three subtypes and relation to lymphoma. Cancer 1983;51:476.

198. Wolf JA, Spjut HJ. Focal lymphoid hyperplasia of the stomach preceding gastric lymphoma: Case report and review of the literature. Cancer 1981;48:2518.

199. Baron BW, Bitter MA, Baron JM, et al. Gastric adenocarcinoma after gastric lymphoma. Cancer 1987;60:1876.

200. Wilander E, El-Salhy M, Pitkanen P. Histopathology of gastric carcinoids: A survey of 42 cases. Histopathology 1984;8:183.

201. Godwin DJ. Carcinoid tumors: An analysis of 2,837 cases. Cancer 1975;36:560.

202. Creutzfeldt W. The achlorhydria-carcinoid sequence: Role of gastrin. Digestion 1988;39:61.

203. Poynter D, Pick CR, Harcourt RA, et al. Association of long lasting insurmountable H_2 blockade and gastric carcinoid tumors in the gut. Gut 1985;26:1284.

204. Moertel CG. Treatment of the carcinoid tumor and the malignant carcinoid syndrome. J Clin Oncol 1983;1:727.

205. Gorden P, Comi RJ, Maton PW, et al. Somatostatin and somatostatin analogue (SMS 201-995) in treatment of hormone-secreting tumors of the pituitary and gastrointestinal tract and non-neoplastic diseases of the gut. Ann Intern Med 1989;110:35.

64

Surgery for Peptic Ulcer Disease

HAILE T. DEBAS
SUSAN L. ORLOFF

The advent of powerful antiulcer drugs (H_2-receptor antagonists, omeprazole, and so forth) has made elective surgery for peptic ulcer a rare event. The advances in medical therapy have coincided with the advent of highly selective or proximal gastric vagotomy, an operation based on sound physiologic principles and one not associated with the severe undesirable side effects previously seen with gastric resection and truncal vagotomy. This operation has been accepted as the elective operation of choice for duodenal ulcer worldwide. Because of the rarity of elective operations for this disease, however, the experience and training of most North American surgeons in this operation have been limited. Despite the precipitous fall in elective ulcer surgery, neither the incidence of nor the need for surgery for the emergent complications of ulcer, perforation, and bleeding has changed significantly over the past 15 years.

SURGERY FOR DUODENAL ULCER DISEASE

Physiologic Basis of Ulcer Operations

Surgery for duodenal ulcer has evolved from simple gastroenterostomy, to subtotal gastrectomy, to truncal vagotomy and drainage, to more selective types of vagotomy (see Figs 64-1 through 64-4).

GASTROENTEROSTOMY

This was a popular operation in the early part of the century and was performed in order to divert gastric acid away from the duo-

denum to allow the ulcer to heal. Most ulcers healed but eventually recurred because the operation did nothing to reduce the acid-peptic factors considered etiologic in the disease.[1] The operation became obsolete 50 years ago.

SUBTOTAL GASTRECTOMY

The rationale for this operation was to reduce acid secretion by removing the entire antrum and variable amounts of the parietal cell mass.[2] Operations that removed 75% of the stomach were performed in the 1940s and 1950s. While those operations cured the peptic ulcer disease, they also produced many "gastric cripple" patients. In many patients, the sequelae proved worse than the primary ulcer disease, with severe weight loss, anemia, and the dumping syndrome. Less radical gastric resections of 60% to 65% were found to be just as effective and associated with fewer side effects. After gastric resection, the surgeon has two options for gastrointestinal (GI) reconstruction: a gastroduodenal anastomosis (Billroth I) or a gastrojejunal anastomosis (Billroth II) (Fig 64-1). The choice often depended on the state of the duodenum and on the amount of stomach resected.

GASTRIC RESECTIVE PROCEDURES

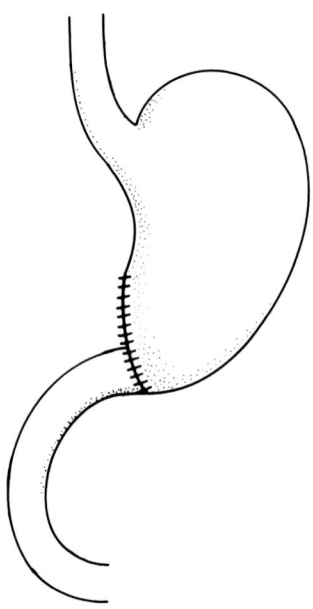
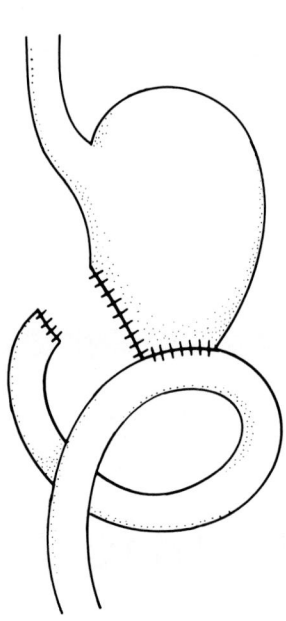
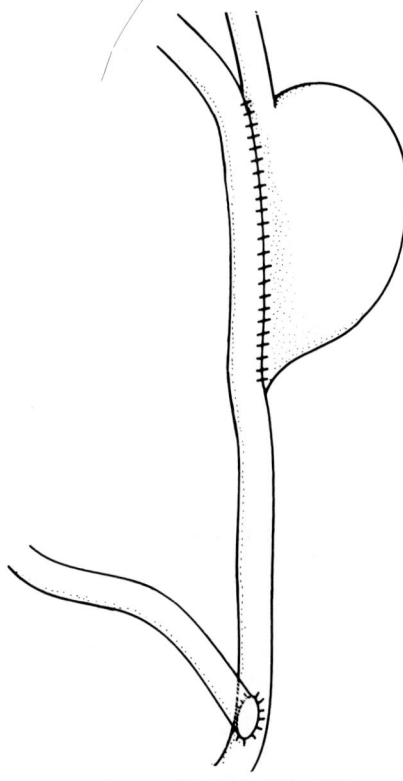

BILLROTH I ANASTOMOSIS
- Gastroduodenal hook-up
- Procedure of choice for gastric ulcer
- Used in combination with vagotomy for duodenal ulcer

BILLROTH II ANASTOMOSIS
- Gastrojejunal hook-up
- Used in duodenal ulcer surgery when subtotal gastrectomy was in vogue

CSENDES PROCEDURE
- Roux-en-Y esophago-gastro-jejunostomy
- Useful in high-lying gastric ulcers

FIGURE 64-1. Gastric Resective Procedures.

TRUNCAL VAGOTOMY AND DRAINAGE

The concept that section of the vagus nerves might cure ulcer disease was developed experimentally by the French surgeon Latarjet in 1921.[3] However, it was not popularized clinically until Dragstedt's landmark paper of 1943.[4] The physiologic effects of truncal vagotomy are described in Table 64-1. Truncal vagotomy reduces basal acid secretion by 85% and maximal acid output to gastrin or histamine by 50%.[5] Following vagotomy, the sensitivity of the parietal cell to gastrin is markedly reduced such that the dose–response curve is shifted to the right. Pepsin secretion by the chief cell is under vagal control, and following vagotomy marked reduction occurs in both basal and stimulated pepsin secretion. The efficacy of truncal and other types of vagotomy (Fig 64-2), therefore, lies not only in the reduction of acid secretion but also in the significant suppression of pepsin secretion. It should be remembered that H_2-receptor antagonists reduce acid secretion but do little to pepsin secretion. Following truncal or any other vagotomy, a state of basal and postprandial hypergastrinemia develops.[6] The mechanism of postvagotomy hypergastrinemia is not known but is thought to be due to both reduced acid secretion and the interruption of inhibitory vagal fibers.[7] Some have postulated, although proof is lacking, that the hypergastrinemia may have beneficial effects on mucosal growth and healing because gastrin has a trophic action on the oxyntic cell as well as the duodenal mucosa.

The efferent secretory fibers in the vagus account for only 2% to 3% of all the fibers in the vagal trunk.[8] Most of the remainder are either motor-efferent or -afferent fibers. The vagus is important in the regulation of motor function of the stomach, and following truncal vagotomy, receptive relaxation of the fundus is lost and pyloric sphincter relaxation is impaired. Unless a gastric drainage procedure is performed by either destroying the pyloric sphincter or bypassing it, severe impairment of gastric emptying of both solids and liquids results.[9] When a drainage procedure is added, however, emptying of liquids is accelerated, while the emptying of solids improves but remains slower than normal. Thus, after truncal vagotomy, all patients require a drainage procedure. Five drainage procedures are available (Fig 64-3). The Heineke–Mikulicz pyloroplasty is most commonly employed. In this procedure, a longitudinal incision is made at the pyloroduodenum, completely dividing the pylorus.[10] The incision then is closed transversely. The second most common drainage procedure is gastrojejunostomy, a procedure preferred by most surgeons when it is unsafe to perform pyloroplasty because of severe disease or inflammatory mass in the duodenum. Two additional procedures that are appropriate in selected situations are the Finney and the Jaboulay procedures.[11,12] In Finney pyloroplasty, a longitudinal incision over the antrum and duodenum much longer than that in Heineke–Mikulicz is used. The Jaboulay procedure is not a pyloroplasty but rather a gastroduodenostomy in which the pylorus is not divided. The last two procedures are believed to promote more satisfactory gastric emptying.

SELECTIVE GASTRIC VAGOTOMY

In this operation, the extragastric vagal branches (i.e., the hepatic and celiac) are spared but the entire stomach is vagally denervated (see Fig 64-2).[13,14] Because the antropyloric region is also denervated, a drainage procedure is required as with truncal vagotomy.

HIGHLY SELECTIVE OR PROXIMAL GASTRIC VAGOTOMY

In this operation, only the proximal stomach (the parietal cell mass) is vagally denervated (Fig 64-4).[15] The innervation of the antrum and pylorus is preserved by sparing the anterior and posterior antral nerves of Latarjet. Of course, the extragastric branches are also spared so that vagal innervation of the liver, biliary tree, pancreas, and small intestine is left intact. Unlike truncal or selective gastric vagotomy, highly selective vagotomy preserves the innervation of the antrum; hence, no drainage procedure is required. The reduction in acid and pepsin secretion after highly selective vagotomy is similar to that seen after truncal or selective gastric vagotomy.

INTRACTABLE DUODENAL ULCER

Ulcer intractability is one of the indications for surgery. Intractability is difficult to define because the definition must usually be based on subjective symptoms of the patient. Indeed, there is no agreed-upon definition. Failure of medical therapy is always implied, but there is no consensus on what this means. Often a patient is referred for surgery for intractability when both patient and treating physician agree that the patient's life-style and/or ability to maintain a job is threatened despite what is considered an ad-

---

TABLE 64-1
Physiologic Consequences of Truncal Vagotomy

Gastric

Secretory
85% reduction in basal acid secretion
50% reduction in maximal acid output
80% reduction in basal and stimulated pepsin secretion
Basal and postprandial hypergastrinemia (2–3 times normal)

Motor
Loss of fundic receptive relaxation
Loss of pyloric sphincter relaxation
Defective antral grinding function

Pancreas

Decreased basal enzyme secretion
Loss of cephalic and gastric phases of pancreatic secretion

Gallbladder

Defective gallbladder contraction
Loss of gastrocholecystic reflex

Small Intestine

Loss of regulated absorptive, secretory, and propulsive activity
Development of poorly understood "postvagotomy diarrhea"

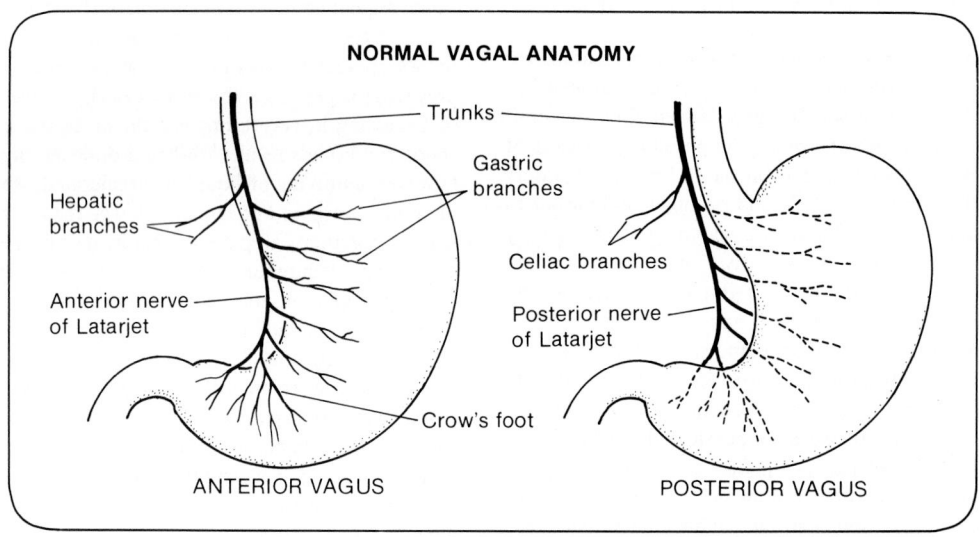

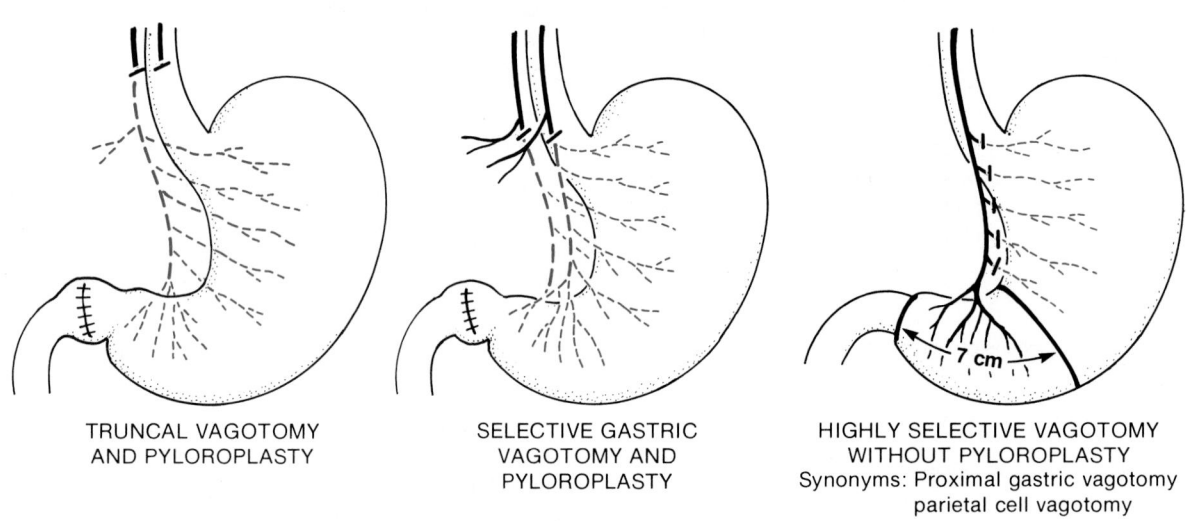

FIGURE 64–2. Types of vagotomy.

equate course of medical treatment. In the age of H$_2$-receptor antagonists, failure of medical therapy usually means recurrence of ulcer symptoms despite several courses of full-dose H$_2$-receptor antagonist therapy, including intervening maintenance therapy. Occasionally, however, intractability may be defined endoscopically by demonstrating failure of an ulcer to heal. The issue of such "cimetidine-resistant" ulcers becomes important particularly when there has been a history of prior complications (bleeding, perforation) or when the ulcer is a "giant" ulcer (>2 cm in diameter). It is probably advisable to perform gastric acid secretory studies in patients who fail H$_2$-receptor antagonist therapy while they are on drug therapy. Whether these patients could be successfully and safely treated with omeprazole, the potent proton-pump inhibitor, remains to be seen.

A more quantitative definition of ulcer severity has recently been provided by Elashoff and colleagues.[16] These investigators assigned a "pain score" from 0 to 180 by multiplying the number of days in the last 60 days the patient experienced pain by pain

intensity (0 = no pain; 1 = mild pain; 2 = moderate pain interfering with daily activities; and 3 = severe pain causing the patient to be bedridden). Patients with a "pain score" greater than 80 are considered to have severe ulcer disease.

Elective Operation for Intractability

Intractability is the main indication for elective operation. Occasionally, however, an elective operation may be indicated because of recurrent attacks of bleeding or chronic blood loss despite medical therapy. A number of elective operations are potentially applicable. These include various types of vagotomy (truncal, selective gastric, highly selective or proximal gastric) (Fig 64-2), gastric resection (Fig 64-1), or the combination of vagotomy and gastric resection. Numerous attempts have been made in the past to try to select the appropriate operation for a given patient based on his/her acid secretory capacity. Unfortunately, no convincing

GASTRIC DRAINAGE PROCEDURES

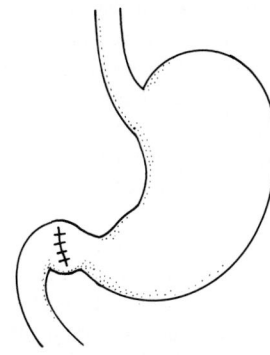

HEINKE-MICULICZ PYLOROPLASTY

Most commonly used drainage procedure in combination with truncal vagotomy and selective gastric vagotomy

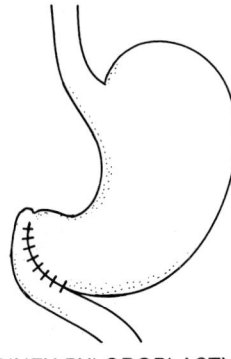

FINNEY PYLOROPLASTY

Longer pyloroplasty with incision of pyloric sphincter

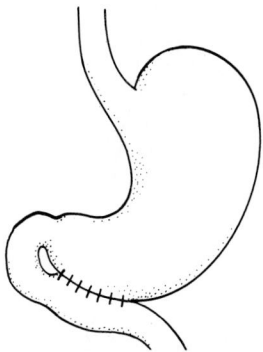

JABOULET PYLOROPLASTY

Gastroduodenal anastomosis without pyloric incision

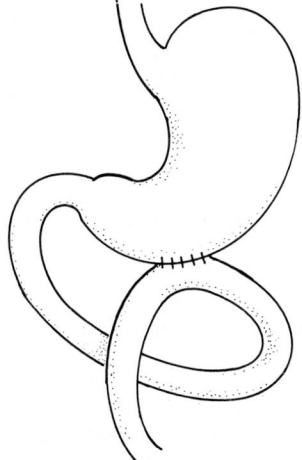

LOOP GASTRO-JEJUNOSTOMY

Used in combination with truncal or selective gastric vagotomy when pyloroplasty is unsafe because of severe inflammation or scaring

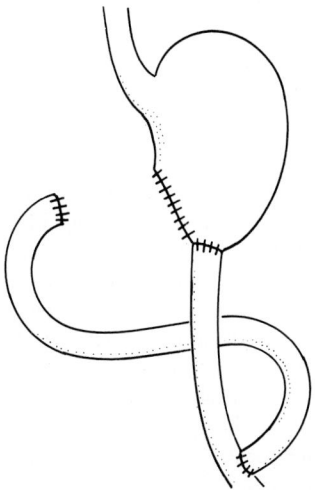

ROUX-EN-Y-GASTROJEJUNOSTOMY

Used to divert biliary-pancreatic secretion away from stomach

FIGURE 64–3. Gastric Drainage Procedures.

data have been provided that the selection of operation will be to the patient's advantage. The important considerations in the choice of an operation should, therefore, be: (1) freedom from severe side effects or undesirable sequelae, (2) low mortality rate, and (3) acceptable recurrence rate. The two operations that have emerged as the preferred procedures are proximal gastric vagotomy and truncal vagotomy and antrectomy. Proximal gastric vagotomy has few undesirable side effects and extremely low mortality but has a higher ulcer recurrence rate.[17-19] Vagotomy and antrectomy, on the other hand, has the lowest rate of ulcer recurrence (< 1%) but has a higher mortality rate and incidence of undesirable sequelae.[20,21] Truncal vagotomy and drainage has supporters, but it has little to recommend it as a routine elective operation.[22-24] Selective vagotomy and drainage has not shown significant advantages over truncal vagotomy and drainage.[25]

PROXIMAL GASTRIC VAGOTOMY

Of the operations mentioned above, our choice is proximal gastric vagotomy. The immediate advantages of this operation include the following: (1) vagal innervation of the antrum and pylorus are preserved; hence, no drainage procedure is required, (2) the gastrointestinal tract is not entered, thus minimizing the potential for infection, (3) no suture lines are left behind, eliminating any risk for suture-line dehiscence, (4) worldwide, the operative mortality has been shown to be less than 0.3% in a survey of nearly 5000 patients,[26] and (5) long-term undesirable side effects (dumping, diarrhea, anemia, weight loss, and so forth) are significantly less than with other ulcer operations. As can be seen in Table 64-2, dumping as a serious side effect is virtually eliminated. Such dumping symptoms as are reported in prospective studies

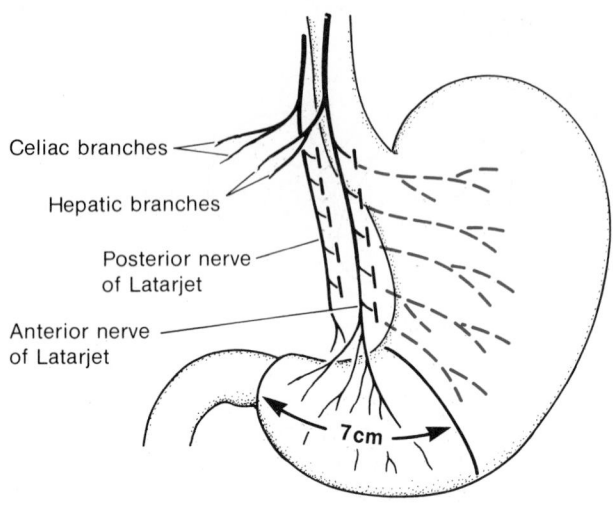

VAGOTOMY
- Selective proximal
- Highly selective
- Parietal cell
- Proximal gastric

Celiac branches
Hepatic branches
Posterior nerve of Latarjet
Anterior nerve of Latarjet

7 cm

is usually 7 cm from the pylorus, (2) denervation of the distal 6 to 8 cm of the esophagus, (3) division of the "criminal nerve" of Grassi, which courses behind the cardia toward the greater curvature, (4) sparing of the hepatic branches of the anterior vagus and the celiac branches of the posterior vagus, and (5) imbrication of the lesser curve of the stomach, a step in the operation not always carried out but useful in eliminating a leak if lesser curve necrosis does occur and also, theoretically, in preventing gastric reinnervation from nerve regeneration. To ensure completeness of vagotomy, two additional steps have been proposed.

First, intraoperative monitoring of completeness of gastric vagotomy may be accomplished in several ways. In Burge's test, the vagi are stimulated electrically with an electrode around the distal esophagus while intragastric pressures are monitored.[29] The Grassi test exploits the potentiating interaction of the vagus and gastrin.[30] The response to pentagastrin by an intragastric pH electrode and the completeness of vagotomy are indicated by failure of acid response when the electrode is brought in contact with the wall of the proximal stomach after pentagastrin administration. In another test, Congo red is sprayed on the gastric wall, and change in color brought about by acid secretion is monitored endoscopically.[31] The second recommendation to reduce ulcer recurrence is surgical and involves division of vagal fibers that may be distributed to the proximal stomach on the greater curvature along the right gastroepiploic vessels.[32] Thus, the greater curvature is cleared of vessels and nerves for a short distance at the point of anastomosis of the right and left gastroepiploic vessels. The entire operation usually takes 2 to 3 hours, and the immediate postoperative course is smooth and uncomplicated.

Vagotomy and Antrectomy

In the United States, vagotomy and antrectomy is perhaps the most commonly performed elective ulcer operation. The reason is twofold. First, the low recurrence rate and the ability to perform the operation with low (< 2%) mortality rate has led American surgeons to accept this operation as the most definitive.[33] Second, by the time proximal gastric vagotomy became popular, the incidence of elective ulcer surgery had already declined markedly, so most surgeons in this country have not learned the operation.

where patients are systematically interrogated are mild. Similarly, the incidence of diarrhea, maldigestion, anemia, weight loss, and other side effects is exceedingly small. The single most important shortcoming of proximal gastric vagotomy is the high incidence of ulcer recurrence. The high incidence of recurrence reported by some authors is undoubtedly related to poor surgical technique. Most of the technical failures are related to inadequate denervation of the distal 6 to 7 cm of the esophagus.[27] In an experimental study in dogs, it was shown that the vagal fibers over the distal esophagus are responsible for about 30% of acid secretion in response to central vagal stimulation by insulin hypoglycemia.[28] Incompleteness of proximal gastric vagotomy appears to relate much less to the distal extent of nerve section on the antrum. The operation is depicted in Fig 64-4. The essential elements of the operation include: (1) division of all gastric branches, but sparing the anterior and posterior antral nerves of Latarjet; the distal extent

TABLE 64–2
Chronic Side Effects Following Ulcer Surgery

COMPLICATION	RATE AFTER VARIOUS OPERATIONS			
	PGV (%)	TV + D (%)	V + A (%)	SG (%)
Dumping syndrome	5	10–15	10–20	10–20
Diarrhea	2–5	15–30	5–40	2–18
Anemia	0.5	3–15	7	10–40
Bone disease		?	20	30
Weight loss	2–10	5–20	10–30	20–40

PGV = proximal gastric vagotomy; TV + D = truncal vagotomy plus drainage; V + A = vagotomy plus antrectomy; SG = subtotal gastrectomy.

Hence, proximal gastric vagotomy, which is the elective operation of choice worldwide, is performed mostly in academic centers in the United States.

In vagotomy and antrectomy, a standard truncal vagotomy is performed by dividing the vagi over the abdominal esophagus cephalad to the origin of all extragastric and gastric branches. The gastric resection is limited to the antrum and usually resects about 30% to 40% of the stomach. A new lesser curve is constructed by closing the cut end of the stomach partially or completely, and gastrointestinal continuity is restored by gastroduodenal rather than gastrojejunal anastomosis, although the latter procedure is preferable when the first portion of the duodenum is badly scarred. When a gastrojejunostomy is elected, the anastomosis should be (1) performed at a point only a few inches distal to the ligament of Treitz, (2) retrocolic, and (3) infracolic. These details are designed to minimize problems of the afferent loop syndrome and torsion and jejunogastric intussusception that are occasionally seen when a long afferent limb or antecolic anastomosis is performed. The introduction of autosuture equipment has led to the performance of antecolic rather than retrocolic anastomosis, a practice that may have more long-term problems.

Truncal Vagotomy and Drainage

Although some surgeons continue to use vagotomy and drainage as their choice of elective operation, most reserve it for elderly or high-risk patients when expediency is desirable.[34] The choice of drainage procedure depends on the state of the proximal duodenum. In most patients, a Heineke–Mikulicz pyloroplasty is appropriate (Fig 64-3). In situations where the first portion of the duodenum is involved in severe scarring or in an inflammatory mass, a loop gastrojejunostomy is the procedure of choice. As mentioned above, the gastrojejunostomy should be retrocolic and infracolic and should have a short afferent limb. Although some surgeons have advocated a Roux-en-Y gastrojejunostomy in primary ulcer surgery, we think the procedure is generally ill-advised because of the potential for the "Roux syndrome" in which functional gastric outlet obstruction and inability to eat occur.[35]

COMPLICATIONS OF DUODENAL ULCER

Perforation

Perforation is present in about 7% of patients hospitalized for peptic ulcer disease and is the first manifestation of ulcer disease in about 2% of patients with duodenal ulcer.[36] After the diagnosis of duodenal ulcer, 0.3% of patients will perforate annually in the first 10 years. In the United States, perforation is about one fourth as common as hemorrhage as a complication of ulcer disease. The ulcers that perforate are in the anterior wall of the duodenum. The aphorism "anterior ulcers perforate, posterior ones bleed" is correct. However, perforation may be accompanied by bleeding in 10% of cases when a "kissing" ulcer is present in the posterior wall of the duodenum opposite the one that perforates anteriorly.[37]

CLINICAL PRESENTATION

Classically, the patient experiences sudden, severe epigastric pain. This is rapidly followed by generalized abdominal pain. Rarely the pain is referred to the shoulders. On examination, the patient is very ill, with signs of generalized peritonitis with a rigid, flat or scaphoid, silent abdomen exhibiting severe rebound tenderness.[38] The patient is almost never hypotensive early in the course of the disease but will have tachycardia and fever. Hypotension will develop late when bacterial peritonitis develops. If hypotension is seen early with the onset of pain, other diagnoses such as ruptured aortic aneurysm, acute pancreatitis, or mesenteric infarction should be suspected. Leukocytosis will be present, and occasionally mild elevation of serum amylase will be seen. Plain x-ray films of the abdomen (supine, upright, and right decubitus) should be obtained. Free air under the diaphragm on the upright film and/or under the lateral abdominal wall on decubitus views will be seen in about 75% of cases. When the diagnosis is in doubt, Hypaque or Gastrografin swallow should be obtained to demonstrate free perforation. Extravasation of dye will be seen except in the few patients who may have already sealed their perforation.

This classic presentation may be modified if certain conditions prevail. In the very old or the very young, signs and symptoms may be less severe. In the patient who is recovering from an abdominal operation for another disease, the pain and tenderness may be ascribed to routine postoperative events. In patients who are on steroids, the abdominal findings may be masked. Rarely, fluid may flow down the paracolic gutters, and the point of maximal pain and tenderness may be in the right lower quadrant, simulating acute appendicitis, or in the left lower quadrant, suggesting sigmoid diverticulitis.

Except in the rare situation when the patient presents late after perforation and the perforation is shown to be sealed, the treatment of choice is emergency surgery.

EMERGENCY OPERATION FOR PERFORATION

Emergency operation is required in duodenal ulcer disease when the complications of perforation and hemorrhage occur. The goals of surgery are twofold: (1) to close the perforation and (2) to perform definitive ulcer surgery when (a) proper indications exist and (b) certain conditions prevail to ensure safety.

Closure of Perforation

This is accomplished in one of two ways: (1) When the ulcer edges are edematous and friable, a tongue of vascularized omentum is laid over the perforation, and with the use of two or three interrupted sutures, the omentum is tied in place effectively, closing the perforation. The procedure is known as the "Graham Omental Patch."[39] (2) Sometimes the tissue at the ulcer edges is neither very edematous nor friable. In this case, the duodenal edges are approximated with two or three interrupted sutures, and a vascularized omental patch is placed over the closure to re-enforce it. The abdomen is then thoroughly washed and closed without a drain.

Definitive Ulcer Surgery

It was once said that about 40% of perforated duodenal ulcers are acute and that once the perforation is closed, no further ulcer symptoms would develop.[40] On the basis of this, definitive ulcer surgery was considered only in those patients with chronic peptic ulcer disease. The chronicity of ulcer disease is established by history or by findings of chronic duodenal scarring and foreshortening of the first portion of the duodenum at the time of operation. Recent studies suggest, however, that all patients with perforated duodenal ulcers should be considered for definitive surgery whether the ulcer is deemed acute or chronic.[41-43] The evidence for this conclusion is given in Table 64-3. It is clear from these reported studies that the addition of proximal gastric vagotomy significantly reduces postoperative recurrence of ulcer without increasing mortality or morbidity of the emergency operation.

A definitive ulcer operation in the face of perforated duodenal ulcer should be considered only if (1) the perforation is less than 24 hours long, (2) gross abdominal contamination with food and debris does not exist, and (3) the patient's general condition is good. The definitive ulcer operation of choice is proximal gastric vagotomy. Earlier fears that the esophageal dissection necessary for this operation may lead to spread of infection into the mediastinum have not been borne out by extensive clinical experience to date.

Whenever perforation is associated with either frank upper GI bleeding or the presence of blood in the nasogastric tube, it is necessary to extend the perforation by surgical incision of the duodenum in order to examine for a bleeding posterior ulcer, the so-called kissing ulcer.[37] Bleeding is then controlled by suture ligature of the ulcer bed. Under these conditions, the performance of a definitive ulcer operation, proximal gastric vagotomy, or truncal vagotomy and pyloroplasty is mandatory.

NONOPERATIVE MANAGEMENT OF PERFORATION

In our opinion, all patients with perforated duodenal ulcer should be treated operatively except for those who present late (24-36 hours after perforation) or those who are not surgical candidates because they are deemed not to tolerate anesthesia. Even when a patient presents with late perforation, nonoperative treatment is considered only if the patient is stable, no signs of generalized peritonitis are present, and Gastrografin swallow reveals no free leak into the peritoneal cavity. Once the decision is made for nonoperative management, nasogastric suction must be maintained and the patient treated with a full-dose antiulcer regimen with intravenous H_2-receptor antagonists or omeprazole. In addition, antibiotics should be given intravenously to cover gram-negative rods, gram-positive cocci, and anaerobes. Operative intervention should be considered anytime the patient's condition deteriorates.

Bleeding

INCIDENCE

About 20% of patients with duodenal ulcer will bleed (see ch 30).[44] On the average, bleeding occurs in the fifth and sixth decades of life. Thus, the mean age at which this complication is seen is about 20 years later than that at which perforation occurs. About 90% of patients admitted with a bleeding duodenal ulcer will stop bleeding within 8 hours of admission.

TABLE 64–3
Impact of Proximal Gastric Vagotomy in the Emergency Treatment of Perforated Duodenal Ulcer

	NUMBER OF PATIENTS	POSTOPERATIVE COMPLICATIONS	RECURRENT ULCERATION
Boey et al[128]			
Simple closure	41	7.3%	36.6%
Closure & PGV	37	10.8%	10.6%
Christiansen et al[129]			
Simple closure	25	8%	52%
Closure & PGV	25	20%	16%
Ceneviva et al[130]			
Simple closure	38	?	58%
Closure & PGV	38	?	5%
Combined Experience			
Simple closure	104	4.8%	48.1%
Closure & PGV	100	9.0%	10.0%

PGV = proximal gastric vagotomy.

PATTERNS OF BLEEDING

Most patients who have a significant episode of bleeding will present with hematemesis and/or melena without shock. Only 15% to 20% will present in hypovolemic shock with hematocrit levels less than 30%.[45] At least 33% of the patients will have had a previous episode of bleeding.[46] Bleeding may occur in the absence of ulcer pain, and sometimes any pre-existing ulcer pain may improve when the bleeding starts.

MANAGEMENT

The amount of blood loss is initially best assessed not by the hematocrit levels but clinically. Tachycardia over 100 per minute and/or a systolic blood rapid pressure of less than 100 mm Hg usually signifies blood loss of at least 1000 ml. Similarly, the presence of postural hypotension (fall in blood pressure of greater than 10 mm Hg on sitting up) is indicative of significant hemorrhage. Resuscitation should begin during initial evaluation. Two large-bore intravenous catheters (one preferably in a central vein) are inserted. Blood samples are obtained for laboratory values and for crossmatch of at least 4 units if the patient is hypotensive. Saline or Ringer's lactate solution is given intravenously. If the systolic blood pressure is unobtainable, either O-negative or group-specific Rh-negative blood may need to be administered. If plasma expanders such as dextran are used, their volume should be limited to less than 1000 ml.

A large-bore tube should be inserted into the stomach to remove blood. Gastric lavage with cold water or saline is begun. Intravenous administration of H_2-receptor antagonists is also started. As soon as the patient with a major bleed is stable, we prefer an urgent examination of the upper gastrointestinal tract by panendoscopy. From the surgical viewpoint, one of the most important values of such a study is to rule out the esophagus as the source of bleeding. A definitive diagnosis of the bleeding source is possible in over 90% of patients. In some patients, a visible vessel in the ulcer base may be encountered. Whether the visible vessel is bleeding or not, the likelihood of continuing or recurrent bleeding, and hence the need for early surgical intervention, increases.[47,48] Selective abdominal angiogram is rarely necessary. It becomes an attractive alternative when the bleeding is so severe that endoscopy cannot be done and especially in the high-risk patient when angiographic control of bleeding is sought.[49]

As mentioned above, some 90% of patients bleeding from a duodenal ulcer will stop bleeding within 8 hours. Once this occurs, the gastric *p*H should be kept continually above 6.0 with antacids. In selected patients, continuing bleeding may be controlled endoscopically by use of the heater-probe or laser. Attempts at endoscopic control when a "visible vessel" is present may aggravate the bleeding, and an operation may be more advisable.

EMERGENCY OPERATION FOR BLEEDING

Duodenal ulcer accounts for about 40% of cases of upper GI bleeding, and bleeding accounts for nearly 40% of deaths due to peptic ulcer disease.[50]

The indications for emergency operation to control bleeding vary with the patient's age and associated medical conditions. In general, however, the following indications are widely accepted: (1) massive exsanguinating bleeding where resuscitation to restore stable vital signs is impossible, (2) the need of 6 to 8 units of blood to maintain stable blood pressure in the first 24 hours, (3) slow but continuous bleeding for more than 48 hours, (4) recurrence of bleeding after it stopped while the patient was on medical treatment, a situation that most commonly suggests bleeding from the gastroduodenal artery, and (5) a visible, bleeding vessel on endoscopy, and perhaps even a "visible" vessel that may not be bleeding.

As mentioned above, the patient's age, the severity of the ulcer history, and the general condition may modify these indications. For example, a younger patient tolerates bleeding better than an older patient. However, when more than 8 to 10 units of blood are administered to a patient, a coagulopathy may develop. A number of patients who have received in excess of 15 units of blood may die of diffuse bleeding from coagulopathy despite successful surgical control of the bleeding ulcer. Finally, wherever feasible, endoscopic control of bleeding should be attempted. The temptation to perform repeated therapeutic endoscopic procedures while the amount of blood transfusion mounts must, however, be resisted.

The goals of emergency surgery in bleeding duodenal ulcer are twofold: (1) to control bleeding and (2) to perform definitive ulcer operation.

Control of Bleeding

The first step in the operation is to open the duodenum and control bleeding by suturing the bleeding vessels in the ulcer bed. Occasionally, despite the use of several appropriately placed sutures, oozing may persist from the ulcer bed. This may require additional sutures or ligation of the gastroduodenal artery outside the duodenum. Sometimes the first portion of the duodenum is severely scarred and foreshortened and the ulcer deeply penetrates the posterior wall. It is in circumstances like this that the sutures placed to control bleeding may inadvertently cause obstruction of the common bile duct. Whenever this danger is deemed to be present, the common bile duct is opened and a red rubber catheter is placed within it before the sutures are applied to the ulcer bed. After all the sutures are tied in the ulcer bed, the red rubber catheter is moved up and down in the bile duct. If it can be so moved, the common bile duct has not been incorporated in the suturing.

Definitive Ulcer Operation

The choices are vagotomy and pyloroplasty, vagotomy and antrectomy, and proximal gastric vagotomy. In this setting, truncal vagotomy and pyloroplasty has a 5% to 10% mortality and a bleeding rate in the immediate postoperative period of 15% to 25%.[51,52] Emergency vagotomy and antrectomy for bleeding has a mortality rate of up to 15% and a rebleeding rate of less than 5%.[53] These figures are, however, from the older literature, and the mortality rate now is likely much lower. Enthusiasm for proximal gastric vagotomy and control of bleeding by way of duodenostomy is increasing in Europe.[54] Mortality and rebleeding rates of 9% and 10%, respectively, have been reported by Hoffmann and colleagues. In the United States, it is generally accepted that vagotomy and pyloroplasty should be employed in the massively bleeding patient in whom expediency is considered a safety factor. Vagotomy and antrectomy is reserved for healthier, younger patients in whom the application of this more extensive operation is not considered to increase the mortality significantly. Proximal vagotomy has not received wide acceptance in the United States, but it is a procedure that can be performed safely and with a low mortality rate, when the addition of an extra hour to the operating time is deemed not to be unsafe. The authors' choice is vagotomy and pyloroplasty in the elderly or unstable patient and proximal vagotomy otherwise.

Obstruction

INCIDENCE

Chronic duodenal or channel ulcers are responsible for 80% of all cases of gastric outlet obstruction.[55] Gastric outlet obstruction occurs in 2% to 4% of patients with duodenal ulcer, and the incidence increases with duration of disease.[56] Succeeding ulcers in the duodenal bulb heal with scarring, causing a "clover leaf" deformity. Eventually a critical narrowing of the lumen occurs, causing symptoms. The type of duodenal ulcer that leads to obstruction often has a virulent course. Thus, 20% may have a history of previous bleeding, and a similar number previous perforation.[57] Occasionally, obstruction occurs as a result of inflammatory swelling from an active ulcer. However, when this occurs there is usually underlying severe scarring and anatomic narrowing that has not become critical, so that initial improvement on conservative therapy is often followed by organic narrowing, requiring more aggressive intervention.

CLINICAL FEATURES

The earliest symptom is early satiety in a patient who has had usually a decade or more of peptic ulcer disease. Early satiety will be shown to antedate vomiting by several months if a careful history is obtained.[58] Vomiting typically occurs after the evening meal as a result of the cumulative effect of the day's meals. As the disease progresses, however, vomiting may occur at any time. The vomitus is typically nonbilious and may contain undigested food, sometimes food eaten 12 or more hours earlier. Patients who have gastroesophageal incompetence will have aggravation of their reflux symptoms. A minority of patients will present with severe weight loss without too much vomiting. In such patients, the stomach dilates chronically and may come to occupy most of the left abdomen. Such patients present with a picture of malignant cachexia and are subsequently found to have benign gastric outlet obstruction. The advent of flexible endoscopy has made this type of presentation an extreme rarity. On the other extreme, patients may present with severe vomiting, dehydration, and metabolic disturbance. Typically, such patients develop contracted extracellular fluid volume, and a hypochloremic, hypokalemic metabolic alkalosis. The urine pH will be paradoxically acid, because in order to conserve volume, the kidney will exchange H^+ for Na^+ under the renin–aldosterone regulatory pathway.

The classic physical findings in patients with gastric outlet obstruction are weight loss and a succussion splash elicited by shaking the patient's abdomen. Nasogastric aspiration will result in the evacuation of a large amount of foul-smelling fluid sometimes containing vegetable debris. Upper GI examination will identify the site of obstruction and may suggest the nature of the underlying disease. However, the definitive diagnostic study is endoscopy, at which time biopsy specimens may be obtained to rule out malignancy. Typically, the endoscope cannot be passed into the duodenum, and an active ulcer may or may not be present or seen. In patients with subclinical obstruction, the Hunt saline load test may be used for diagnosis. By way of the mesogastric tube, 750 ml of saline is inserted into the stomach, and 30 minutes later the stomach contents are completely aspirated. A residual volume of more than 300 ml indicates gastric retention.[59]

MANAGEMENT

The initial management requires the insertion of a nasogastric tube and aspiration and lavage of the stomach. This should be done early to prevent aspiration. The status of extracellular fluid volume is assessed clinically and by urine output. Dehydrated patients will require a Foley catheter and a central vein pressure catheter to monitor fluid replacement. Metabolic alkalosis is usually readily corrected by the administration of saline and potassium chloride. When severe, however, an intravenous infusion of isotonic hydrochloric acid may be necessary. The use of ammonium chloride to correct metabolic alkalosis poses a danger, especially to patients with pre-existing liver disease, and is rarely indicated.

Peptic ulcer therapy with H_2-receptor antagonists is started, and an early decision is made regarding whether the patient requires total parenteral nutrition to correct any existing malnutrition.

SURGERY FOR OBSTRUCTION

The patient with gastric outlet obstruction may present a number of problems that must be attended to preoperatively. Some patients will be nutritionally depleted, and a course of preoperative total parenteral nutrition may be necessary. Occasionally, significant disturbances in electrolytes and in acid–base balance may be present. These disturbances require preoperative correction. In patients with long-standing obstruction and a grossly atonic stomach, a period of several days of nasogastric suction may help restore some gastric tone preoperatively and may minimize prolonged difficulties with gastric emptying postoperatively. Finally, the obstructed stomach is nearly always colonized by bacteria. It is judicious, therefore, to lavage the stomach, culture its contents, and place nonabsorbable antibiotics in its lumen preoperatively, and to treat the patient with broad-spectrum antibiotics in the preoperative period.

The choice of operation is between (1) truncal vagotomy and drainage and (2) vagotomy and antrectomy. Balloon dilatation of the obstruction and proximal gastric vagotomy was initially advocated by Johnston and colleagues.[60] The enthusiasm for the procedure has now waned because (1) in a number of cases balloon dilatation had caused perforation and (2) the rate of recurrent stenosis is unacceptably high.[61] Prior to the selection of operation, the surgeon must examine the pyloroduodenal region carefully. Sometimes a severe inflammatory process and scarring may exist. Should this be the case, the surgeon will wisely avoid tackling the region and may decide that neither pyloroplasty nor antrectomy can be performed safely. The safest procedure then becomes truncal vagotomy and loop gastrojejunostomy. In most situations, however, the pyloroduodenal area can be safely incised or excised. In the latter case, the choice is between truncal vagotomy and pyloroplasty and vagotomy and antrectomy. A prevalent thought among surgeons is that truncal vagotomy and pyloroplasty results in more prolonged problems in postoperative gastric emptying than vagotomy and antrectomy. No data exist to prove or disprove this contention, and either procedure is acceptable.

Whenever surgery is performed for gastric outlet obstruction, it is highly advisable to perform at the time of surgery a feeding jejunostomy. This procedure will obviate the need for expensive total parenteral nutrition should a protracted course of difficulty in gastric emptying follow the operation. In addition, in patients with a grossly dilated and atonic stomach, a tube gastrostomy may be constructed to avoid the prolonged use of nasogastric intubation.

Penetration

An ulcer located on the posterior wall of the duodenum may erode through the entire wall of the duodenum without causing free perforation. The process is slow and incites dense surrounding scarring, confining the penetration and preventing surrounding leakage. The posterior wall of the penetration is often the pancreas or the gastrohepatic membrane but is at times the prevertebral fascia. Extremely rarely, the penetration may involve the common bile duct and lead to duodenobiliary fistula. The incidence of penetration is unknown, but about 15% to 20% of intractable ulcers will be found at operation to have penetrated beyond the wall of the duodenum.[62]

CLINICAL PRESENTATION

The most important symptom that indicates penetration is radiation of the ulcer pain through to the middle back in the region of the first lumbar vertebra. The pain becomes gradually unresponsive to antacids or H_2-receptor antagonists. Penetration is a common cause of intractable ulcer disease. A small percentage of patients may have an elevated serum amylase without overt manifestation of acute pancreatitis. On rare occasion, a giant duodenal ulcer may result from destruction of the posterior wall of the duodenum over a large area. Typically, such giant ulcers may be missed on radiologic examination, and endoscopy is the best way to assess them. It is very important for the surgeon to be aware of such a lesion preoperatively in order to avoid mobilization of the duodenum, which can lead to a large defect that may be hard to close.

TREATMENT OF PENETRATION

Penetration usually indicates intractability, and if it has occurred despite adequate antiulcer therapy, operative intervention is required. The surgical options are those described above for intractable duodenal ulcer. Many surgeons consider this complication to represent high ulcer virulence and prefer to treat it with vagotomy and antrectomy rather than with proximal gastric vagotomy. However, no data exist to support this choice.

Fistula Formation

Rarely, a penetrating duodenal ulcer will bore into an adjacent hollow viscus that might have formed its base. The result is fistula formation. Such fistulas develop between the duodenum and the common bile duct or the gallbladder, but their incidence is exceedingly low.[63] A telltale sign of a fistula is the presence of gas within the biliary tree. Contrast studies document the presence of a duodenobiliary fistula. It must be remembered that a previous papillotomy or surgical choledocho-duodenostomy or erosion of a gallstone into the duodenum is more common as a cause of air in the biliary tree.

The treatment of duodenal ulcer complicated by fistulation into the biliary tree is treatment of the underlying peptic ulcer. Vagotomy and antrectomy with Billroth II anastomosis will both treat the ulcer and exclude the fistula. Before antrectomy is attempted, the surgeon must determine that the duodenal stump can be closed safely. If this is deemed not to be possible, nonresectional therapy with vagotomy should be considered while the fistula is left alone.

SURGERY FOR BENIGN GASTRIC ULCER

RATIONALE FOR SURGERY IN GASTRIC ULCER

Peptic ulcer disease is said to develop when there is an imbalance of acid-peptic aggressive factors and the defense mechanisms of the gastroduodenal mucosa. As discussed in Chapter 61, an increase in the aggressive factors is more important in the pathogenesis of duodenal ulcer—hence, the choice of procedures that reduce acid and pepsin secretion when treating duodenal ulcer. In gastric ulcer, a defect in the mucosa is considered the more important pathogenetic factor. Although the presence of acid is necessary for a gastric ulcer to develop, hypersecretion of acid is present only in a minority of patients. Indeed, about 25% to 30% of patients with gastric ulcer are hyposecretors of acid.[64] In addition, gastric ulcers almost always occur in non–acid-secreting mucosa, often near the junction with the acid-secreting mucosa. Patients with gastric ulcer show chronic atrophic gastritis involving the entire antrum. Even when an ulcer occurs high in the lesser curvature, it usually does so in mucosa that has undergone metaplasia from acid-secreting to non–acid-secreting mucosa. All these pieces of evidence collectively suggest that the non–acid-secreting mucosa of the stomach in patients with gastric ulcer has inherent susceptibility to acid-peptic damage, even when the acid and pepsin secretory capacity of the stomach is normal or subnormal.

The above line of reasoning would, therefore, suggest that gastric ulcer procedures that reduce acid secretion are less likely to be successful than those that resect the susceptible target tissue. Therefore, it is generally accepted that antrectomy is the procedure of choice in the surgical treatment of benign gastric ulcer.[65,66] We need to distinguish, however, between *four types of gastric ulcer.*[67] Type I gastric ulcers occur in the body of the stomach, most often at the lesser curvature. They account for 55% to 60% of all gastric ulcers. Hypersecretion of acid is rarely seen in this type of ulcer. Type II ulcers are gastric ulcers that occur in association with duodenal ulcers. They account for 20% to 25% of gastric ulcers and exhibit pathophysiologic alterations, including acid hypersecretion, similar to duodenal ulcers. Type III ulcers are those which occur in the prepyloric region and account for about 20% of all gastric ulcers. These ulcers are frequently associated with acid hypersecretion and exhibit a significant recurrence rate when treated with antrectomy only. In the United States, high-lying gastric ulcers at or near the gastroesophageal junction are seen rarely. In Chile, however, they are said to account for 27% of gastric ulcers. These ulcers have been recently named type IV ulcers.[68] Elective surgery for benign gastric ulcer, therefore, must take into account the differing characteristics of these ulcers in both their physiology and anatomy.

MALIGNANCY AND GASTRIC ULCER

The problem of an ulcerated cancer masquerading as a benign ulcer is more common than a benign gastric ulcer degenerating into a malignant one. Prior to the advent of routine flexible endoscopy, about 4% of patients diagnosed radiologically as having had a benign ulcer had an ulcerated cancer.[69] With the advent of endoscopy, the problem is much reduced but not eliminated. In the United States, carcinoma has been found in only 3% of resected gastric cancers.[70]

Selection of Operation for Gastric Ulcer

Because malignancy in a gastric ulcer cannot be totally excluded from biopsy alone, all elective operations should remove the ulcer in toto either as part of the resected distal stomach or by local excision when this is not feasible. Rarely, an ulcer lying high at the gastroesophageal junction may not be amenable to excision. In this case, a four-gradient biopsy of the ulcer margin is advocated. As mentioned above, the choice of elective operation depends on the type of gastric ulcer (Table 64-4).

TYPE I GASTRIC ULCER

The operation of choice is antrectomy with gastroduodenal anastomosis (Billroth I) without vagotomy. Usually 40% to 50% of the stomach including the ulcer is resected. The overall mortality of this procedure is 2%.[66] This low mortality rate is partly due to the fact that the duodenal bulb is normal in these patients. The ulcer recurrence rate is also about 2%. Although Pheils and colleagues[71] have reported a 6% recurrence rate with resection and gastroduodenal anastomosis and 3% with resection and gas-

TABLE 64-4
Surgical Options in Gastric Ulcer

INDICATION	FIRST CHOICE	SECOND CHOICE
Elective		
Type I	Antrectomy (B-I)	Highly selective vagotomy and ulcer excision
Type II	Vagotomy and antrectomy	Highly selective vagotomy and pyloroplasty
Type III	Vagotomy and antrectomy	Highly selective vagotomy and ulcer excision
Emergency		
Perforation	Antrectomy (B-I)	Excision and vagotomy
Obstruction	Antrectomy (B-I)	Vagotomy and pyloroplasty
Bleeding	Antrectomy (B-I)	Vagotomy and pyloroplasty, suture-control
High-lying Ulcer		
<2 cm from gastroesophageal junction	Csendes procedure	Kelling–Madlener
>2 cm from gastroesophageal junction	Pauchet or Schoemaker procedure	Csendes or Kelling–Madlener

From Cameron J, ed. Current surgical therapy. Toronto, Philadelphia: BC Decker, 1989:38.

trojejunostomy, most believe on empirical grounds that gastroduodenal anastomosis produces a more physiologic hookup. Both vagotomy and drainage and proximal gastric vagotomy have been used to treat gastric ulcer. The ulcer recurrence rate, however, is unacceptably high, with figures of 8% to 36%.[72,73]

TYPE II GASTRIC ULCER

Vagotomy and antrectomy is the treatment of choice because it treats the duodenal ulcer and removes the susceptible target, the antrum, and the ulcer. There is a place for truncal vagotomy and pyloroplasty, or even proximal vagotomy, in selected, high-risk patients. When either of the latter procedures is performed, the ulcer should be excised for histologic study. The recurrence rate is high when only vagotomy and ulcer excision is used.

TYPE III GASTRIC ULCER

Again, vagotomy and antrectomy encompasses best the goals of reducing acid secretion and removing both the antrum and the ulcer. Proximal gastric vagotomy has been shown to be associated with ulcer recurrence rates of 35% to 40% and hence is not recommended.[74] In selected patients, truncal vagotomy and pyloroplasty with ulcer excision may be employed, although the recurrence rate is high.

TYPE IV GASTRIC ULCER

This type of ulcer may be located at the gastroesophageal junction or at a point greater than 2 cm distally. Ulcers in the latter location can usually be removed with the antrum by extending the resection margin up the lesser curve (Pauchet procedure).[75] When the ulcer is more proximal, however, this maneuver is unlikely to be feasible. In that case, the surgeon has two choices. Antrectomy can be performed, leaving the ulcer behind (Kelling–Madlener procedure).[76] If this course of action is taken, it is essential to obtain four-quadrant biopsy of the ulcer. Ulcer recurrence after the Kelling–Madlener procedure is about 5%. A more satisfactory choice is to extend the resection line to include the ulcer and hence a portion of the distal esophagus. When this is done, gastrointestinal continuity can be restored with a Roux-en-Y esophagogastrojejunostomy (Csendes procedure).[77]

Emergency Operation for Gastric Ulcer

BLEEDING

Bleeding from a gastric ulcer is usually more serious than bleeding from a duodenal ulcer for two reasons. First, the bleeding is often more marked and is less likely to stop spontaneously. Second, bleeding gastric ulcers tend to occur more often in the elderly patient. The treatment of choice is distal gastric resection including the ulcer with gastroduodenal anastomosis. In the poor-risk patient, however, ulcer excision and either truncal vagotomy and pyloroplasty or proximal gastric vagotomy may be elected. When the ulcer cannot be removed safely, bleeding is controlled by suture followed by vagotomy. The mortality rate for emergency gastric resection in bleeding gastric ulcer has been reported to be as high as 10% to 40%, and the majority of deaths are in elderly patients.[50]

PERFORATION

Again, the operation of choice is antrectomy that includes the ulcer. In high-risk or unstable patients, the perforation may be treated by local excision or by closure with omental graft. Depending upon the patient's condition, vagotomy may be added.

OBSTRUCTION

This is a rare complication in gastric ulcer but may occur when the ulcer is pyloric or prepyloric. The treatment of choice is antrectomy with Billroth I anastomosis, an operation made simple by the fact that the proximal duodenum is normal.

RECURRENT ULCER AFTER SURGERY

Recurrence after surgery for peptic ulcer disease depends upon (1) the type of primary ulcer (i.e., duodenal or gastric) and (2) the type of surgical procedure employed to treat the primary ulcer. The data supporting this statement are given in Table 64-5.

TABLE 64-5
Recurrent Ulcer After Surgery

PRIMARY ULCER	INITIAL OPERATION	RECURRENCE RATE
Duodenal	Gastroenterostomy	40–50%
	Vagotomy and drainage	8–12%
	Selective vagotomy and drainage	8–12%
	Proximal gastric vagotomy	10–25%
	Vagotomy and antrectomy	1%
	Subtotal gastrectomy	2–6%
Gastric	Antrectomy	2%
	Vagotomy and drainage	10–25%
	Proximal gastric vagotomy	10–40%*

* *Highest recurrence rate after proximal gastric vagotomy has been recorded when the procedure has been used for pyloric and prepyloric ulcers.*

TABLE 64-6
Causes of Postoperative Recurrent Ulcer

Inadequate Operation

Incomplete vagotomy

Inadequate drainage

Inadequate resection

   Insufficient gastric resection

   Retained antrum

Long afferent limb in B-II resection

Poor Selection of Primary Operation

Gastroenterostomy alone

Vagotomy for gastric ulcer

Hypersecretory States

Zollinger–Ellison syndrome

Multiple endocrine neoplasia-I (MEN-I)

G-cell hyperplasia/hyperfunction

Retained antrum syndrome

Hypercalcemia

Other endocrinopathies (e.g., Cushing's syndrome, adrenal cortical tumor)

Ulcerogenic Drugs

Salicylates

Nonsteroidal anti-inflammatory drugs

Steroids

Reserpine

Pathophysiology of Ulcer Recurrence

The causes of postoperative recurrent ulcer are listed in Table 64-6. Gastroenterostomy does not reduce acid secretion and is therefore an inappropriate operation.

INADEQUATE OPERATION

The most common cause of recurrence after vagotomy is incomplete section of the vagi.[78] When truncal vagotomy has been the primary operation, the most common cause of incompleteness of vagotomy is a missed posterior vagal trunk. When proximal gastric vagotomy is done, the most common cause of incompleteness is inadequate clearance of all vagal fibers over the distal 6 to 8 cm of the esophagus. Additional causes of incompleteness of vagotomy in the latter operation might be failure to resect the criminal nerve of Grassi and perhaps also failure to divide vagal distribution at the greater curvature of the stomach. The experience of the individual surgeon in performing proximal gastric vagotomy is considered an important variable. Poor antral drainage after pyloroplasty or gastroenterostomy may also contribute to recurrent ulcer formation because gastric retention may stimulate acid secretion. The Finney and Jaboulay techniques of pyloroplasty are considered to provide better antral drainage than the Heineke–Mikulicz pyloroplasty, but the latter is simpler and is an adequate procedure for the great majority of patients. No convincing evidence has been produced about the superiority of gastroenterostomy over pyloroplasty, or vice versa. Gastric resection may be inadequate because either insufficient amount of stomach is resected or a portion of the antrum is left with the duodenal stem in the performance of a Billroth II resection. When gastric resection without vagotomy is employed as the primary procedure for duodenal ulcer, the recurrence rate is 36% after 30% to 50% gastric resection but only 12% after 50% to 70% gastric resection.[79]

POOR SELECTION OF PRIMARY OPERATION

Gastroenterostomy does not reduce acid secretion and hence is an inappropriate operation when employed without vagotomy. Recurrence rates of 40% to 50% led to its abandonment some 50 years ago. In general, the recurrence rate after any type of vagotomy for gastric ulcer is high when unaccompanied by resection. Particularly high rates of recurrence have been reported following proximal gastric vagotomy for pyloric and prepyloric ulcers.

HYPERSECRETORY STATES

The incidence of the Zollinger–Ellison syndrome (see ch 62) in patients with duodenal ulcer disease is only 1 in 1000. In patients with postoperative recurrent ulcer, the incidence rises to 1 in 50.[79] It is not cost-effective to investigate fully all patients with primary duodenal ulcer for the Zollinger–Ellison syndrome. We think it is useful, however, to determine fasting serum gastrin concentration preoperatively. The presence of the following clinical features in a patient with duodenal ulcer warrant full investigation for the Zollinger–Ellison syndrome (i.e., fasting serum gastrin, secretin test, and a meal test): (1) hypercalcemia or renal stones, (2) diarrhea, (3) multiple ulcers, (4) ulcer in the distal duodenum or jejunum, and (5) a family history of endocrinopathy, particularly of the MEN-I (multiple endocrine neoplasia) syndrome.

A second rare cause of hypergastrinemia is G-cell hyperplasia/hyperfunction (see ch 62), a congenital condition inherited as a mendelian dominant trait.[80] The disease is treated effectively by antrectomy and can thus be a cause of recurrent ulcer if only vagotomy without resection was the primary procedure. As mentioned above, if a piece of antrum is left with the duodenal bulb in Billroth II gastrectomy, the retained antrum is excluded from the acid stream and instead is continuously bathed by alkaline fluid.[81] G-cell hyperplasia and hypergastrinemia results, causing acid hypersecretion and recurrent ulcer. The incidence of this syndrome is extremely low. Hypercalcemia and other endocrinopathies are rare causes of hypersecretion and recurrent ulcer. A 10-fold increase in the prevalence of duodenal ulcer has been reported in patients with hyperparathyroidism.[82] Few cases of recurrent ulcer have been described that have been attributable to hyperparathyroidism or other endocrinopathies, such as Cushing's syndrome or functioning adrenal cortical syndrome.

ULCEROGENIC DRUGS

Good evidence exists that the use of nonsteroidal anti-inflammatory drugs is associated not only with the etiology of recurrent ulcer but also with acute developments of complications of recurrent ulcer.[83]

Management of Postoperative Recurrent Ulcer

DIAGNOSIS

Pain is the most important presenting symptom, being present in up to 95% of cases.[84] The pain is typical and is relieved by antacids. Hemorrhage and anemia due to occult bleeding may be presenting symptoms in 20% to 63% of patients.[85,86] Free perforation and obstruction are less frequent, occurring in 1% to 9% and 5% to 19%, respectively.[87,88] When diarrhea is associated with recurrent ulcer, especially when pyrosis and feculent vomiting are present, a gastrojejunocolic fistula must be suspected if the primary operation included a gastrojejunostomy.[89]

The most definitive diagnosis is made by endoscopy. While contrast study of the upper gastrointestinal tract may show an ulcer niche, the yield is far less than in endoscopy. At times, the two studies are complementary. A fasting serum gastrin should be obtained, and if elevated, or even when not elevated if one suspects a gastrinoma, a secretin test should be obtained. Fasting serum gastrin is frequently elevated after vagotomy. However, postvagotomy hypergastrinemia, unlike hypergastrinemia due to a gastrinoma, is not exacerbated by secretin. An elevation of serum pepsinogen I, according to Samloff, correlates well with acid secretory capacity and may indicate incomplete vagotomy.[90]

Acid secretory studies are not very helpful in diagnosis in primary ulcer disease. In postoperative recurrent ulcer, however, they are very useful. One-hour basal acid output is normally less than 5 mEq in patients who have undergone ulcer surgery. A basal acid output of greater that 5 mEq/hour is suggestive of incomplete vagotomy. The incidence of a recurrent ulcer in patients having greater than 10 mEq/hour of basal acid is 80%.[83] Completeness of vagotomy, however, is best assessed by measuring acid response to stimulation of central vagal centers. This can be done either by inducing hypoglycemia with insulin or by modified sham-feeding. The insulin test is both dangerous and nonspecific.[91] Modified sham-feeding, where the patient chews meat and spits it out, is the best and most physiologic test currently available to assess completeness of vagotomy.[92]

The retained antrum syndrome may be diagnosed by the occurrence of basal hypergastrinemia, a negative secretin test, the presence of bulbous dilatation at the duodenal stump on barium swallow, or by a positive technetium pertechnetate radioisotope scan. A gastrojejunocolic fistula is rarely diagnosed by the upper gastrointestinal series. It is best demonstrated by either upper gastrointestinal endoscopy or barium enema.

TREATMENT

In the precimetidine era, postoperative recurrent ulcer was considered a surgical disease always requiring operative treatment. This position has to be modified because H_2-receptor antagonists have been shown to be effective particularly in the treatment of recurrent ulcer after vagotomy. In the absence of a surgically treatable cause of the recurrence (retained antrum, gastrinoma, long afferent loop), medical treatment should be attempted and surgery considered if medical therapy fails.

The choice of the type of operative procedure to be employed depends on both the cause of the recurrence and the type of the primary ulcer operation. If the cause is identified as an ulcerogenic tumor, surgical therapy is directed to the tumor. If a gastrinoma is diagnosed and identified by localization studies, the tumor should be resected. If no tumor is identified by localization studies, including thorough surgical exploration of the pancreas, duodenum, and retroperitoneum, the choice is between H_2-receptor antagonist therapy and total gastrectomy. The decision has to be individualized and should take into consideration the presence and absence of complications, the response to medical therapy, and so forth. Ulcerogenic tumors of the parathyroid, adrenal, and other endocrine glands should be treated by appropriate excision or ablation of the tumor. In the MEN-I syndrome, where hyperparathyroidism may coexist with Zollinger–Ellison syndrome, the hyperparathyroidism should be treated first because regression of gastrointestinal symptoms will occur frequently. Similarly, if the cause of recurrence has been identified as retained antrum or a mechanical problem (long afferent limb), the operation is directed at resecting the retained antrum or correcting the mechanical problem.

In most patients, however, none of the above causes will be identified. If the recurrence has occurred after proximal gastric vagotomy, the best procedure is antrectomy.[93] If vagotomy and drainage was the primary treatment, antrectomy with re-vagotomy is indicated.[94] Sometimes, a missed posterior vagus is found intact, and completion of the vagotomy may suffice. Recurrence after vagotomy and antrectomy, a rare happening, is treated by re-vagotomy and re-resection.

Complications of recurrent ulcer require not only treatment of the complication but also a further acid-reducing procedure. Bleeding and perforated recurrent ulcers are best treated by resection and vagotomy or re-vagotomy. A gastrojejunocolic fistula is best treated with a preoperative course of broad-spectrum antibiotics and total parenteral nutrition, mechanical and bacteriologic bowel preparation, and a single-stage resection of the fistula, including a portion of the stomach, jejunum, and transverse colon. Reconstruction is then accomplished by gastrojejunostomy or gastroduodenostomy and colo-colic anastomosis. A truncal vagotomy should always be added or re-vagotomy performed if one had been done previously.

POSTGASTRECTOMY SYNDROMES

The term postgastrectomy syndromes is usually used to indicate chronic complications of any ulcer surgery whether or not a gastrectomy had been performed.

Pathophysiologic Consideration

The normal functions of the stomach include the secretion of acid, pepsin, and intrinsic factor as well as motility. The stomach has the capacity to accommodate when food is ingested so that the intraluminal pressure is not increased. This receptive relaxation requires intact vagal innervation.[95] The motility of the antrum is required to grind and triturate solids into small particles 1 mm or less in size.[96] The coordination of gastric motility and pyloric sphincter relaxation then results in the metered delivery of liquids and finely ground solids into the proximal duodenum. These motor activities are controlled by the gastric pacemaker and by a pacesetter potential. Ulcer operations disrupt, to a greater or lesser degree, both the secretory functions and the motility of the stomach, resulting in postgastrectomy syndromes. All forms of vagotomy disrupt the neural reflex that mediates receptive relaxation. Truncal and selective vagotomy disrupt, in addition, the motor function of the antropyloric complex. The pylorus tends to remain in a contracted state, and, unless it is destroyed by pyloroplasty or bypassed by gastrojejunostomy, gastric emptying is significantly slowed. Proximal gastric vagotomy preserves the vagal innervation of the antropyloric region and hence does not disrupt the motor function of the region. As a result, proximal gastric vagotomy affects little the emptying of solids and the size of food particles leaving the stomach.[97] By contrast, truncal vagotomy and drainage or antrectomy results in severe alterations in both the rate of emptying and the size of food particles leaving the stomach.

The effects of decreased gastric secretion are many. The hypochlorhydria that follows ulcer operations may result in increased bacterial colonization of the stomach and duodenum. Bacterial overgrowth may cause malabsorption and may generate nitrosamines, carcinogens that may contribute to the development of cancer. The hypochlorhydria may also lead to a chronic infection of the antral mucosa by *Helicobacter pylori*,[98] although a cause and effect cannot be precisely identified. Gastric acidification is also necessary for the solubilization of iron and calcium for optimal absorption. Following ulcer surgery, therefore, impaired absorption of calcium and particularly of iron may occur, leading to bone disease and iron-deficiency anemia, respectively.[99,100] Intrinsic factor is secreted by the parietal cells. Extensive gastric resection leads to loss of intrinsic factor, and Vitamin B_{12} deficiency is seen not infrequently after vagotomy and antrectomy.[101,102]

Specific Syndromes

DUMPING SYNDROME

When the antropyloric mechanism is either destroyed (resection, pyloroplasty) or bypassed (gastrojejunostomy), large quantities of hyperosmolar chyme can be "dumped" into the upper small intestine. The consequences are: (1) distention and activation of the distention reflex, leading to stimulation of motility, (2) osmotic shift of fluid from the intravascular compartment into the gut lumen, further aggravating the distention and leading to relative hypovolemia and hemoconcentration, and (3) release of vasoactive substances (substance P, neurotensin, vasoactive intestinal peptide, bradykinin, serotonin) that may cause peripheral vasodilatation and flushing. The mechanisms described above cause the *early dumping syndrome*, which has abdominal and systemic components.[103-106] The abdominal symptoms include pain, borborygmi, and diarrhea. Systemic manifestations include weakness, sweating, flushing (rarely), tachycardia, and palpitations. The abdominal

symptoms are thought to be induced by volume distention and the production of serotonin. The systemic effects are due to hypovolemia and peripheral vasodilatation caused by vasoactive substances. The early dumping syndrome occurs within 1 hour of eating.

With rapid entry of chyme into the intestine, rapid absorption of glucose results in hyperglycemia, provoking hyperinsulinemia. The hyperinsulinemia outlasts the hyperglycemia, resulting in secondary hypoglycemia in the second hour after eating. These hypoglycemic symptoms constitute the *late dumping syndrome*.[107] An exaggerated release of enteroglucagon is said to contribute to the development of these symptoms.[108]

Dumping can be prevented by preserving the innervated pylorus as in proximal gastric vagotomy. Dietary treatment is usually effective in controlling symptoms. A low-carbohydrate diet (which has a low osmolality), avoiding intake of liquids for 30 minutes (so that hyperosmolar materials are not washed out of the stomach) and lying down after eating for 20 to 30 minutes (so that gravity does not hasten emptying), is usually effective. Medical treatment with pectin and ephedrine is sometimes helpful. The long-acting somatostatin analogue octreotide has been shown recently to improve the symptoms of dumping.[109] The mechanisms of action are probably related to its ability to inhibit the release and action of vasoactive peptides from the intestine as well as its ability to inhibit the motor and secretory activities of the intestine. Somatostatin also inhibits the release of insulin and thereby prevents the late dumping symptoms of hypoglycemia. Intractable cases may require surgical treatment. Corrective operations are not always successful but may include conversion of Billroth I to Billroth II or vice versa, the construction of a Roux-en-Y gastrojejunostomy, or the insertion of a 10-in reversed jejunal segment between the pylorus and the duodenum.[110,111]

DIARRHEA

Chronic diarrhea may occur after both vagotomy and subtotal gastrectomy. Because it occurs more frequently after vagotomy, it is often referred to as *postvagotomy diarrhea* (see ch 38). The cause of postvagotomy diarrhea is unknown.[112,113] Several etiologic factors have been determined: (1) rapid gastric emptying, (2) rapid small intestinal transit, (3) increased ileal fluid delivery to the colon, (4) increased delivery of bile acids to the colon, (5) carbohydrate wastage with delivery to the colon, and (6) colonization of the upper gastrointestinal tract by bacteria and malabsorption.

The diarrhea typically occurs 1 to 2 hours after eating and is associated with urgency and the passage of excessive gas. The diarrhea also tends to be episodic. Although some 20% to 30% of patients develop looseness of bowel movements after truncal vagotomy, only about 5% have frank diarrhea and 1% intractable diarrhea.[114]

One of the measures described for the control of dumping is avoidance of certain food items (milk, bananas, sweetened juices, and soft drinks). The thought that bile acids in the colon may be etiologic has led to treatment with cholestyramine. The results are unimpressive.[115] Similarly, courses of broad-spectrum antibiotics have been recommended from time to time on the assumption that bacterial colonization of the gut may be pathogenetic. The results are equally poor. Attempts at surgical correction by interposing a 12-inch, retroperistaltic segment of jejunum some 50 cm beyond the duodenojejunal flexure are not uniformly successful.

ALKALINE REFLUX GASTRITIS

Following gastric resection or ablation or bypass of the pylorus, excessive reflux of bile, pancreatic, and intestinal secretion into the stomach may occur. In some patients, the reflux is thought to produce a distinctive postgastrectomy syndrome consisting of burning midepigastric pain unresponsive to antacids and aggravated by eating and recumbency. Bilious vomiting, anemia, and profound weight loss may also occur. Little or no acid is present in the stomach. Endoscopically, the gastric mucosa may be hyperemic, friable, and edematous. Biopsy shows poorly defined gastritis. Unfortunately, because alkaline reflux occurs in almost all patients undergoing the procedures listed above, and because few patients complain of this symptom complex, it is difficult to make a definitive diagnosis. The diagnosis is that of exclusion and is often uncertain. Surgical correction of alkaline reflux is effectively accomplished by construction of a 40 to 50–cm Roux-en-Y gastrojejunostomy. Unfortunately, poor results are seen in 40% to 70% of cases, stressing the difficulty in diagnosis.[116,117] Even the application of such diagnostic maneuvers as provocative testing with alkali, measurements of intragastric bile acid concentration, and scintigraphic determination of enterogastric reflux and gastric emptying improve little the results of surgical treatment. In some patients, the construction of a Roux-en-Y gastrojejunostomy results in the "Roux syndrome," a functional gastric outlet syndrome that often requires surgical reversal of the Roux-en-Y procedure.[118]

MALDIGESTION

Some degree of maldigestion probably occurs after all types of ulcer operation, except proximal gastric vagotomy. Possible reasons are several: (1) accelerated gastric emptying, (2) delivery of larger than normal food particles into the intestine, (3) more rapid transit through the small intestine, (4) impaired pancreatic enzyme response and gallbladder contractility to food following truncal vagotomy, (5) arrival of food in the intestine in procedures with gastrojejunostomy earlier than that of biliary-pancreatic secretions, and (6) bacterial colonization of the upper gastrointestinal tract.[119–121] Maldigestion per se is rarely a severe problem, but in patients who have other postgastrectomy problems it may become an aggravating factor.

ANEMIA

Chronic anemia is not an insignificant problem after major gastric resection. It develops largely because of deficiencies in iron, Vitamin B$_{12}$, and folate absorption.[122,123] Iron deficiency is the main cause, because with reduced postoperative acid secretion there is reduced ability to dissociate ferric iron from food and dissolve the mineral for absorption (see ch 31). Postgastrectomy patients handle ferrous iron much better, and ferrous iron supplements should be provided. Defective digestion of meals, the major source of dietary iron, is an important contributory cause of iron defi-

ciency. Generally, anemia occurs less frequently after vagotomy than after gastric resection. Megaloblastic anemia secondary to Vitamin B$_{12}$ deficiency is rare except in patients who have undergone radical subtotal or total gastrectomy. Monthly administration of parenteral Vitamin B$_{12}$ prevents and corrects the problem.

BONE DISEASE

Bone disease is more common after gastrectomy than after vagotomy and occurs more commonly in older patients.[124] It usually takes many years for the clinical picture to appear. Bone demineralization occurs because of defective calcium absorption and malabsorption of Vitamin D. A picture of osteomalacia is indicated by loss of radiodensity in bones, low serum calcium, avid retention of infused calcium, and sometimes elevated serum levels of immunoreactive parathyroid hormone.

WEIGHT LOSS

Weight loss is common after surgery, but severe weight loss is usually seen only with gastrectomy. Several explanations have been suggested: (1) reduced food intake, (2) malabsorption, and (3) maldigestion. Increased losses of fecal fat and nitrogen frequently accompany weight loss. In some patients, ulcer surgery unmasks gluten-sensitive enteropathy (sprue). In years past, severe weight loss (malnutrition) postgastrectomy was not infrequently due to reactivation of latent pulmonary tuberculosis.

GASTRIC CANCER

In European studies, the incidence of gastric cancer is three to four times greater in peptic ulcer patients treated surgically than in those treated medically.[125,126] The increased incidence begins 15 to 20 years after surgery and is greater after gastrectomy than after vagotomy. The incidence of cancer in the gastric remnant appears to be much less common in North America.[127]

The reader is directed to Chapter 1, The Enteric Nervous System and Its Extrinsic Connections; Chapter 2, Gastrointestinal Hormones; Chapter 3, The Brain–Gut Axis; Chapter 8, The Physiology of Gastric Motility and Gastric Emptying; Chapter 13, Gastric Secretion; Chapter 22, Gastrointestinal Blood Flow; Chapter 30, Approach to the Patient with Gross Gastrointestinal Bleeding; Chapter 31, Approach to the Patient with Occult Gastrointestinal Bleeding; Chapter 36, Approach to the Patient with Acute Abdomen and Fever of Abdominal Origin; Chapter 59, Stomach: Anatomy and Structural Anomalies; Chapter 60, Disorders of Gastric Emptying; Chapter 61, Acid-Peptic Disorders; Chapter 62, Zollinger–Ellison Syndrome; Chapter 63, Tumors of the Stomach; Chapter 65, Miscellaneous Diseases of the Stomach; Chapter 91, Endocrine Neoplasms of the Pancreas; Chapter 98, Abdominal Cavity: Anatomy and Structural Anomalies; Chapter 111, Upper Gastrointestinal Endoscopy; Chapter 114, Contrast Radiology; Chapter 128, Evaluation of Gastrointestinal Motility: Methodological Considerations; Chapter 129, Tests of Gastric and Exocrine Pancreatic Function and Absorption; Chapter 134, Endoscopic Control of Nonvariceal Upper Gastrointestinal Hemorrhage; Chapter 135, Endoscopic Therapy of Sessile Tumors; and Chapter 137, Exploratory Laparotomy.

REFERENCES

1. Thompson JE, Dailey TH. Recurrent ulceration after operation for peptic ulcer. Results after gastroenterostomy, gastrectomy, and vagotomy in 64 cases. Ann Surg 1966;163:704.
2. Goligher JC, Pulvertaft CN, deDombal ST, et al. Five to eight years results of Leeds/York controlled trial of elective surgery for duodenal ulcer. Br Med J 1968;2:781.
3. Latarjet A, Wertheimer P. Quelque results de l'inervation gastrique. Presse Med 1923;2:993.
4. Dragstedt LR, Owens FM Jr. Supradiaphragmatic section of the vagus nerves in treatment of duodenal ulcer. Proc Soc Exp Biol Med 1943;53:125.
5. Debas HT. Peripheral regulation of gastric acid secretion. In: Johnson LR, ed. Physiology of the gastrointestinal tract, ed 2. New York: Raven Press, 1987:931.
6. Debas HT, Hollinshead J, Seal A, Soon-Shiang P. Vagal control of gastrin release in the dog: Pathways for stimulation and inhibition. Surgery 1984;95:34.
7. Debas HT. Proximal gastric vagotomy interferes with a fundic inhibitory mechanism: A hypothesis for the high recurrence of peptic ulceration. Am J Surg 1983;146:51.
8. Grossman MI. Neural and hormonal stimulation of gastric secretion of acid. In: Handbook of physiology. Washington, DC: American Physiology Society, Section 6:835.
9. Yamagishi T, Debas HT. Control of gastric emptying: Interaction of the vagus and pyloric antrum. Ann Surg 1978;187:91.
10. Hayden WF, Read RC. A comparative study of Heineke-Mikulicz and Finney pyloroplasty. Am J Surg 1968;116:755.
11. Finney JMT. A new method for pyloroplasty. Bull Johns Hopkins Hosp 1902;13:155.
12. Jaboulay M. Le gastroenterostomie, le jejuno-duodenostome, la resection du pylore. Arch Prov Chir (Paris) 1892a;1:1.
13. Jackson RG. Anatomic study of the vagus nerves; with a technic of transabdominal selective gastric vagus resection. Arch Surg 1948;57:333.
14. Franksson C. Selective abdominal vagotomy. Acta Chir Scand 1948;96:409.
15. Johnston D, Wilkinson AR. Highly selective vagotomy without a drainage procedure in the treatment of duodenal ulcer. Br J Surg 1970;57:289.
16. Elashoff JD, Van Deventer G, Reedy TJ, Ippoliti A, Samloff IM, Durata J, Billings M, Isenberg M. Long-term follow-up of duodenal ulcer patients. J Clin Gastroenterol 1983;5:509.
17. Amdrup E, Jensen HE, Johnston D, Walder BE, Goligher JC. Clinical results of parietal cell vagotomy (highly selective vagotomy) two to four years after operation. Ann Surg 1974;180:279.
18. Jordan PH Jr. Indications for parietal cell vagotomy without drainage in gastrointestinal surgery. Ann Surg 1989;210:29.
19. Meisner S, Jorgensen LN, Jensen HE. The Kaplan and Meier and the Nelson estimate for the probability of ulcer recurrence 10 and 15 years after parietal cell vagotomy. Ann Surg 1988;207:1.
20. Herrington JL Jr. Truncal vagotomy with antrectomy—1976. Surg Clin North Am 1976;56:1335.
21. Thoroughman JC, Walker LG Jr, Raft D. A review of 504 patients with peptic ulcer treated by hemigastrectomy and vagotomy. Surg Gynecol Obstet 1964;119:257.
22. Jordan PH Jr, Condon RE. A prospective evaluation of vagotomy-pyloroplasty and vagotomy-antrectomy for treatment of duodenal ulcer. Ann Surg 1970;172:547.
23. Stempien SJ, Dagradi AE, Lee ER, Simonton JH. Status of duodenal ulcer patients ten years or more after vagotomy–pyloroplasty (V-P). Gastroenterology 1970;58:997.
24. Goligher JC, Pulvertaft CN, Irvin TT, Johnston D, Walker B, Hall RA, Wilson-Pepper J, Matheson TS. Five to eight year results of truncal vagotomy and pyloroplasty for duodenal ulcer. Br Med J 1972;1:7.
25. Kronborg O, Malmstrom J, Christiansen PM. A comparison between the results of truncal and selective vagotomy in patients with duodenal ulcer. Scand J Gastroenterol 1970;5:519.
26. Johnston D. Operative mortality and postoperative morbidity of highly selective vagotomy. Br J Surg 1975;62:160.
27. Taylor TV. Parietal cell vagotomy: Long-term follow-up studies. Br J Surg 1987;74:971.
28. Trout HH, Lewis CD, Harmon JV. The relative effects of lesser curvature vagotomy and esophageal vagotomy on the acid secretory effect of proximal gastric vagotomy. Ann Surg 1978;135:102.
29. Burge H, Vane JR. Method of testing for complete nerve section during vagotomy. Br Med J 1958;1:615.
30. Grassi G, Oreccechia C, Cantarelli I, Ibullz B. Intraoperative relation of gastric secretion acidity and complete vagotomy. Surg Gynecol Obstet 1972;134:35.
31. Donnahue PE, Bombeck CT, Yoshida Y, Nyhus LM. Endoscopic Congo red test during proximal gastric vagotomy. Ann Surg 1987;153:249.
32. Braghetto I, Csendes A, Lazo M, et al. A prospective randomized study comparing highly selective vagotomy and extended highly selective vagotomy in patients with duodenal ulcer. Ann Surg 1988;199:443.
33. Herrington JL Jr. Truncal vagotomy with antrectomy—1976. Surg Clin North Am 1976;56:1335.
34. Jordan PH Jr, Condon RE. A prospective evaluation of vagotomy-pyloroplasty and vagotomy-antrectomy for treatment of duodenal ulcer. Ann Surg 1970;172:547.
35. Gustavsson S, Illstrup DM, Morrison P, et al. Roux-Y stasis syndrome after gastrectomy. Ann Surg 1988;155:490.
36. Cohen MM. Treatment and mortality of perforated peptic ulcer: A survey of 852 cases. Can Med Assoc J 1971;105:263.
37. Stabile BE, Hardy HH, Passaro E Jr. "Kissing" duodenal ulcer. Arch Surg 1979;114:1153.
38. Kozoll DD, Meyer KA. Symptoms and signs in the prognosis of gastroduodenal ulcers: An analysis of 1,904 cases of acute perforated gastroduodenal ulcer. Arch Surg 1961;82:528.
39. Graham RR. The treatment of perforated duodenal ulcers. Surg Gynecol Obstet 1937;64:235.
40. Nemanich GJ, Nicoloff DM. Perforated duodenal ulcer; long-term followup. Surgery 1970;67:727.
41. Ceneviva R, de Castro E, Silva O Jr, et al. Simple suture with or without proximal gastric vagotomy for perforated gastroduodenal ulcer. Br J Surg 1986;73:427.
42. Choi S, Boey J, Alagaratnam TT, Poon A, Wong J. Proximal gastric vagotomy in emergency peptic ulcer perforation. Surg Gynecol Obstet 1986;163:531.
43. Jordan PH Jr. Proximal gastric vagotomy without drainage for treatment of perforated duodenal ulcer. Gastroenterology 1982;83:179.
44. Graham DY. Should emergency endoscopy be utilized in the management of upper gastrointestinal bleeding of unknown cause? Negative. In: Gitnick G, ed. Controversies in gastroenterology. New York: Churchill Livingstone, 1984:153.
45. Crook JN, Gray LW Jr, Nance FC, Cohn I Jr. Upper gastrointestinal bleeding. Ann Surg 1972;175:771.
46. Donaldson RM Jr, Handy J, Papper S. Five year follow-up study of patients with bleeding duodenal ulcer with and without surgery. N Engl J Med 1958;259:201.
47. Griffiths WJ, Neumann DA, Walsh JD. The visible vessel as an indicator of uncontrolled or recurrent gastrointestinal hemorrhage. N Engl J Med 1979;300:1411.
48. Storey DW, Bown SG, Swain CP, Salmon PR, Kirkham JS, Northfield TC. Endoscopic prediction of recurrent bleeding in peptic ulcers. N Engl J Med 1981;305:915.
49. Janicki P, Alfidi R. Selective visceral angiography in the diagnosis and treatment of gastroduodenal hemorrhage. Surg Clin North Am 1976;56:1365.
50. Grossman MI. Complications. In: Grossman MI, ed. Peptic ulcer: A guide for the practicing physician. Chicago, London: Year Book Medical Publishers, 1981, Vol 12, p 93.
51. Foster JH, Hall AD, Dunphy JE. Surgical management of bleeding ulcers. Surg Clin North Am 1966;46:387.
52. Kelley HG, Grant GN, Elliott DW. Massive gastroduodenal hemorrhage. Changing concepts of management. Arch Surg 1963;87:6.
53. Scott HW, Sawyers JL, Gobbel WG Jr, Herrington JL Jr. Definitive surgical treatment in duodenal ulcer disease. Curr Probl Surg 1968;10:3.

54. Hoffmann J, DeVantier A, Koelle T, Jensen HE. Parietal cell vagotomy as an emergency procedure for bleeding peptic ulcer. Ann Surg 1987;206:583.

55. Kozoll DD, Meyer KA. Obstructing gastroduodenal ulcers: General factors influencing incidence and mortality. Arch Surg 1964;88:793.

56. Rimer DG. Gastric retention without mechanical obstruction. A review. Arch Intern Med 1966;117:287.

57. Goldstein H, Janin M, Schapiro M, Boyle JD. Gastric retention associated with gastroduodenal disease: A study of 217 cases. Am J Dig Dis 1966;11:887.

58. Moody FG, Cornell GN, Beal JM. Pyloric obstruction complicating peptic ulcer. Arch Surg 1962;84:462.

59. Goldstein H, Boyle JD. The saline load test—A bedside evaluation of gastric retention. Gastroenterology 1965;49:375.

60. Johnston D, Lyndon PJ, Smith RB, Humphrey CS. Highly selective vagotomy without a drainage procedure in the treatment of hemorrhage, perforation, and pyloric stenosis due to peptic ulcer. Br J Surg 1973;60:790.

61. Rossi RC, Dial PF, Georgi B, et al. A five-ten year followup study of parietal cell vagotomy. Surgery 1986;162:301.

62. Jordan GL Jr, DeBakey ME, Duncan JM Jr. Surgical management of perforated peptic ulcer. Ann Surg 1974;179:628.

63. Feller ER, Warshaw AL, Schapiro RH. Observations on management of choledochoduodenal fistula due to penetrating peptic ulcer. Gastroenterology 1980;78:126.

64. Johnson HD, Love AHG, Rogers NC, Wyatt AP. Gastric ulcers, blood groups and acid secretion. Gut 1964;5:402.

65. Sun DCH, Stempien SJ. Site and size of the ulcer as determinants of outcome. The Veterans Administration cooperative study of gastric ulcer. Gastroenterology 1971;61:576.

66. Duthie HL, Moore KTH, Bardsley D, Clark RG. Surgical treatment of gastric ulcers. Controlled comparison of Billroth I gastrectomy and vagotomy and pyloroplasty. Br J Surg 1970;57:784.

67. Mulvihill SJ, Debas HT. Benign gastric ulcer. In: Cameron JL, ed. Current surgical therapy, ed 3. Toronto, Philadelphia: B.C. Decker 1989:38.

68. Csendes A, et al. Type IV gastric ulcer: A new hypothesis. Surgery 1987;101:361.

69. Gear MWL, Truelove SC, Williams DG, Massarella GR, Boddington MM. Gastric cancer simulating benign gastric ulcer. Br J Surg 1969;56:739.

70. Theenold S, Wetteland P. Ulcer-carcinoma of the stomach in a 10-year biopsy series: A follow-up study of 19 patients. Arch Pathol Microbiol Scand 1962;56:155.

71. Pheils MT, Mayday GB, Gillett DJ, Dunn RM. Surgery for benign gastric ulcer. Med J Aust 1970;1:56.

72. Stemmer EA, Zahn RL, Hom LW, Connolly JE. Vagotomy and drainage procedure for gastric ulcer. Arch Surg 1968;96:586.

73. Duthie HL, Bransom CJ. Highly selective vagotomy with excision of ulcer compared with gastrectomy for gastric ulcer in a randomized trial. Br J Surg 1979;66:43.

74. Anderson D, Amdrup E, Hostrup H, Sorensen FH. The Aarhus County vagotomy trial: Trends in the problem of recurrent ulcer after parietal cell and selective gastric vagotomy with drainage. World J Surg 1982;6:86.

75. Maingot R. The Billroth II operations. In: Maingot R, ed. Abdominal operations, ed 75. New York: Appleton-Century-Crofts, 1983, Vol.29, p.385.

76. Kelling G. Ueber die operative Behandlung des chronischen Ulcus ventriculi. Arch Klin Chir 1918;109:775.

77. Cseudes A, Braghetto I, Calvo F, et al. Surgical treatment of high gastric ulcer. Am J Surg 1985;149:765.

78. Fratkin LB. A review of surgical therapy for treatment of peptic ulcer disease 1942-1968. Am Surg 1973;39:470.

79. Stabile BE, Passaro E Jr. Recurrent peptic ulcer. Gastroenterology 1976;70:124.

80. Friesen SR, Tornita T. Pseudo Zollinger-Ellison syndrome: Hypergastrinemia, hyperchlorhydria without tumor. Ann Surg 1981;194:489.

81. Kiefer ED, Sedgewick CE. Marginal ulcer following partial or subtotal gastrectomy. Surg Clin North Am 1964;44:641.

82. Black BM. Primary hyperparathyroidism and peptic ulcer. Surg Clin North Am 1971;51:955.

83. Cleater RGM, Holubitsky JB, Harrison RC. Anastomotic ulceration. Ann Surg 1974;179:339.

84. Nieboer JF. Recurrent ulceration after surgical treatment of gastroduodenal peptic ulcer. Ann R Coll Surg Engl 1961;28:303.

85. Everson TC, Allen MJ. Gastrojejunal ulceration. Arch Surg 1954;69:140.

86. Balint JA, Cooper GW, Price ELC, et al. The management of anastomotic ulcer. Lancet 1957;2:551.

87. Thompson JE, Daily TH. Recurrent ulceration after operation for peptic ulcer: Results after gastroenterostomy, gastrectomy and vagotomy in 64 cases. Ann Surg 1966;163:704.

88. Stuart M, Hoerr SO. Recurrent peptic ulcer following primary operations with vagotomy for duodenal ulcer. Arch Surg 1971;103:129.

89. Condon JR, Tanner NC. Retrospective review of 208 proved cases of anastomotic ulcer. Gut 1968;91:438.

90. Samloff RM, Liebman WM, Secrest DE, et al. Effect of betazole on serum group I pepsinogen levels. Gastroenterology 1973;64:795.

91. Grossman MI. Some minor heresies about vagotomy. Gastroenterology 1974;67:1016.

92. Feldman M, Richardson CT, Fordtran JS. Experience with sham feeding as a test for vagotomy. Gastroenterology 1980;79:792.

93. Kennedy T, Green WER. Stomach and recurrent ulceration: Medical or surgical management? Am J Surg 1980;139:18.

94. Thirlby RC, Feldman M. Transthoracic vagotomy for postoperative peptic ulcer: Effects on basal, sham feeding and pentagastrin-stimulated acid secretion and on clinical outcome. Ann Surg 1985;201:648.

95. Meyer JH. Motility of the stomach and gastroduodenal junction. In: Johnson LR, ed. Physiology of the gastrointestinal tract, ed 2. New York: Raven Press, 1987.

96. Meyer JH, Thomson JB, Cohen MB, et al. Sieving of solid food by the normal and ulcer-operated canine stomach. Gastroenterology 1979;76:804.

97. Mayer EA, Thomson JB, Jehn D, Reedy T, Elashoff J, Deveney C, Meyer JH. Gastric emptying, sieving of solid food and pancreatic and biliary secretions after solid meals in patients with nonresective ulcer surgery. Gastroenterology 1984;87:1264.

98. Goodwin CS, Armstrong JA, Marshall BJ. *Campylobacter pyloridis*, gastric and peptic ulceration. J Clin Pathol 1986;39:353.

99. Blake J, Rechnitor PA. The hematological and nutritional effects of gastric operations. Q J Med 1953;22:419.

100. Deller DJ. Radiocalcium absorption after partial gastrectomy. Am J Dig Dis 1966;11:10.

101. Johnson HD, Kahn TA, Srivata R, et al. The late nutritional and hematological effects of vagal section. Br J Surg 1969;56:4.

102. Deller DH, Witts LJ. Changes in blood after partial gastrectomy with special reference to vitamin B_{12}. Q J Med 1952;31:71.

103. Roberts KE, Randall HT, Farr HW, et al. Cardiovascular and blood volume alterations resulting from intrajejunal administration of hypotonic glucose to gastrectomized patients: The relationship of these changes to the dumping syndrome. Ann Surg 1954;140:631.

104. LeQuesne LP, Hobsley M, Hand BH. The dumping syndrome—I. Factors responsible for symptoms. Br Med J 1960;1:141.

105. Editorial. Dumping syndrome and gut peptides. Lancet 1980;2:1173.

106. Sagar GR, Bryant MG, Ghatel MA, et al. Release of vasoactive intestinal peptide and the dumping syndrome. Br Med J 1981;282:507.

107. Weber BM, Bender MA, Moore GE. Dumping syndrome: An evaluation of some current etiological concepts. N Engl J Med 1957;265:285.

108. Sultz KT, Neelan FA, Nelson LB, et al. Mechanisms of postgastrectomy hypoglycemia. Arch Intern Med 1971;128:240.

109. Hopman WP, Wolberink RG, Lamers CB, Tongeren JH. Treatment of the dumping syndrome with the somatostatin analogue SMS 201-995. Ann Surg 1988;207(2):155.

110. Reber HA, Way LW. Surgical treatment of late postgastrectomy syndromes. Am J Surg 1975;129:71.

111. Brooke-Cowden GL, Braasch JW, Gibb SO, et al. Postgastrectomy syndromes. Am J Surg 1976;131:464.

112. Madsen P, Peterson G. Postvagotomy diarrhea examined by means of a nutritional contrast medium. Scand J Gastroenterol 1968;3:545.

113. McKelvey STD. Gastric incontinence and postvagotomy diarrhea. Br J Surg 1970;57:741.

114. Goligher JC, Pulvertaft CN, deDombal FT, et al. Five to eight year results of Leeds-York controlled trial of elective surgery for duodenal ulcer. Br Med J 1968;2:781.

115. Fromm H, Tunuguntla AK, Malavolti M, et al. Absence of significant role of bile acids in diarrhea of a heterogeneous group of postcholecystectomy patients. Dig Dis Sci 1987;32:33.

116. Vogel SB, Hocking MP, Woodward ER. Clinical and radionuclide evaluation of Roux-Y diversion for postgastrectomy dumping. Am J Surg 1988;155:56.

117. Ritchie WP Jr. Alkaline reflux gastritis: Late results on a controlled trial of diagnosis and treatment. Ann Surg 1986;203:537.

118. Ritchie WP Jr. Alkaline reflux gastritis: An objective assessment of its diagnosis and treatment. Ann Surg 1980;192:228.

119. MacGregor IL, Parent JA, Meyer JH. Gastric emptying of liquid meals and pancreatic and biliary secretion after subtotal gastrectomy or truncal vagotomy with pyloroplasty in man. Gastroenterology 1977;72:195.

120. Lundh G. Intestinal digestion and absorption after gastrectomy. Acta Chir Scand (Suppl)1958;231:1.

121. Tabaqchali S. The pathophysiological role of small intestinal flora. Scand J Gastroenterol 1970;5(Suppl 6):139.

122. Baird IM, Blackburn EK, Wilson GM. The pathogenesis of anemia after partial gastrectomy. Q J Med 1959;28:21.

123. Rygvold O. Hypovitaminosis B$_{12}$ following partial gastrectomy by Billroth II method. Scand J Gastroenterol (Suppl)1974;29:57.

124. Eddy RL. Metabolic bone disease after gastrectomy. Am J Med 1971;50:442.

125. Ellis J, Kingston RD, Brookes VS, Waterhouse JAH. Gastric carcinoma and previous peptic ulceration. Br J Surg 1979;66:117.

126. Pickford IR, Craven JL, Hall R, et al. Endoscopic examination of the gastric remnant 31-39 years after subtotal gastrectomy for peptic ulcer. Gut 1984;25:393.

127. Schuman BM, Walbaum JR, Hiltz SW. Carcinoma of the gastric remnant in a U.S. population. Gastrointest Endosc 1984;30:71.

128. Boey J, Branicki FJ, Alagaratnam TT, Fok PJ, Choi S, Poon A, Wong J. Proximal gastric vagotomy: The preferred operation for perforations in acute duodenal ulcer. Ann Surg 1988;208:169.

129. Christiansen J, Andersen OB, Bonnesen T, Baekgaard N. Perforated duodenal ulcer managed by simple closure versus closure and proximal gastric vagotomy. Br J Surg 1987;74:286.

130. Ceneviva R, de Castro e Silva O, Castelfranchi PL, Modena JLP, Santos RF. Simple suture with or without proximal gastric vagotomy for perforated duodenal ulcer. Br J Surg 1986;73:427.

65

Miscellaneous Diseases of the Stomach

ROBERT S. SANDLER

GASTRIC BEZOARS

Bezoars are persistent concretions of foreign matter found in the stomach. They may consist of a wide variety of substances, but the most common are composed of plant and vegetable fibers (phytobezoars), persimmons (disopyrobezoars), or hair (trichobezoars).

The term *bezoar* is believed to be a corruption of the Persian word *padzahr*,[1] which denotes counterpoison or antidote.[2] The original bezoars appear to have been calculi found in the belly of wild goats that inhabited the northeast corner of Persia.[1] Bezoars were originally believed to be antidotes for snakebite, poison, and the sting of venomous insects. Later, their curative effects were extended to include plague, epilepsy, dysentery, leprosy, smallpox, and certain fevers. They were endowed with marvelous medicinal properties, and were often worn as charms and amulets to protect against evil.[2] In England, bezoar stones were so highly regarded that Queen Elizabeth I carried one in a ring on her finger.[1] The medical literature on bezoars is fascinating and colorful. Bezoars are no longer regarded as antidotes and cures, however. Rather, they are currently considered a hazard to health and have been targets of ultrasound machines and lasers. Despite hundreds of reports in the literature, our understanding of the epidemiology and etiology is incomplete and therapy remains empiric.

Epidemiology

Although we do not know the precise incidence of bezoars, they are not common. Information about them comes mostly from case reports. Many bezoars are asymptomatic so that the reported cases seriously underestimate the prevalence in the population.

Bezoars were found in 0.4% of patients in two large endoscopic series.[3,4] While these figures tell us little about the incidence of bezoars, they suggest that bezoars are rare. They have been reported to occur in 10% to 25% of patients with antrectomies who underwent endoscopy to determine the cause of their symptoms.[5]

The distribution of bezoars in the population reflects predisposing factors. Trichobezoars, for example, are more common in women whose long hair enables them to put the strands in their mouths and swallow them. Men wearing long hair may also be at risk.[6] Because phytobezoars may complicate gastric surgery, they are found more commonly in middle-aged men, who are more likely to have undergone operations for peptic ulcer disease. The occurrence of certain bezoars may be seasonal. Persimmon bezoars are generally confined to periods when persimmons are available.[7]

Etiology

Bezoars develop when foreign material accumulates in the stomach. Simply stated, bezoars result when the material that enters the stomach is unable to exit because of large size, indigestibility, gastric outlet obstruction, or poor gastric motility. Inadequate chewing, missing or carious teeth, dentures, and rapid swallowing are often found in the history,[8,9] although they are not necessarily the only factors leading to bezoars in such cases.

Bezoars (usually phytobezoars) have occurred following various types of gastric surgery, including vagotomy and pyloroplasty, antrectomy, and partial gastrectomy (Table 65-1). Indeed, the vast majority of patients with phytobezoars have had previous surgery.[10] In these patients, the bezoars are a consequence of decreased secretion of acid and pepsin and reduced gastric propulsive activity. Stenosis at the site of an anastomosis may also predispose to bezoars.[10] The chronic gastritis that sometimes follows partial gastrectomy may lead to mucus secretion whose cementing effect may contribute to bezoar formation.[11] Bezoars may complicate gastric partitioning or gastric bypass procedures for massive obesity.

Gastric stasis from any cause can predispose to bezoars. Conditions that lead to delayed gastric emptying such as diabetic gastroparesis,[4,12] mixed connective tissue disease,[13] myotonic dystrophy,[14] and hypothyroidism[15] have been associated with bezoars.

In one report, the delayed gastric emptying reported in association with a bezoar resolved once the bezoar dissolved, suggesting that, in some instances, gastric stasis is secondary to the bezoar.[16]

A number of foods have been implicated, including grapes, oranges, prunes, raisins, figs, cherries, coconuts, peaches, apples, bran, oats, celery, pumpkins, sauerkraut, peanuts, cabbage, and potato peels.[8,17] Nonfood bezoars composed of hair, prune pits, plastic, paper, string, cotton,[17] Styrofoam (from eating Styrofoam cups[18]), toilet paper,[19] and string[8] have been found as well. A lactobezoar was reported in a child with cow's milk intolerance, although the mechanism is unclear.[20]

Persimmon bezoars are termed *disopyrobezoars* from the Greek *diospyron* (meaning "Jove's grain") which is the generic name for the wild persimmon.[2] The mechanism of persimmon bezoar formation has been well described. A soluble tannin termed *shibuol* forms a coagulum when astringent unripe fruit comes in contact with dilute hydrochloric acid in the stomach. The unripe fruit has an especially high concentration of tannin monomer that undergoes polymerization in the stomach, resulting in a tannin–cellulose–hemicellulose–protein complex.[21] This sticky precipitate is the basis of the bezoar mass.

Trichobezoars are composed of large quantities of hair of varying length firmly matted together, sometimes attaining enormous proportions. The surface is usually covered by a slimy mucoid substance. Undigested food and fat are often mixed with the hair.[2] Regardless of the color of the patient's hair, the trichobezoar is dark greenish brown or black. Trichophagia is generally considered more of a manifestation of a personality maladjustment (akin to nail biting) rather than a sign of psychosis or thought disorder.

Yeast bezoars, or *fungus balls*, have been reported as relatively late complications of gastric surgery. Postoperative gastric mycosis is generally a benign condition that does not require treatment unless symptoms are severe.[22] Gastric lavage and antimycotics have been used, but the majority of fungus balls disappear without any therapy.[23] Reconstruction of the gastric outlet has been effective in some patients.[22]

Concretions are hard masses of varying composition that are distinguished from softer bezoars by some authors. Concretions were first described in painters and furniture workers who drank furniture polish because of its high alcohol content.[2] Drinking water would then precipitate the resin into a mass weighing as much as 2000 g.[2] Cement ingestion is the paradigm for concretions

TABLE 65-1
Gastric Bezoars: Types, Constituents, and Predisposing Factors

TYPE	CONSTITUENTS	PREDISPOSING FACTORS
Phytobezoars	Vegetable matter (e.g., apples, bran, cabbage, celery, grapes, oranges, peaches)	Gastric surgery (decreased secretion of acid and pepsin, atony, stenosis, gastritis)
		Gastric stasis (diabetes, hypothyroidism, myotonic dystrophy)
Trichobezoars	Hair	Long hair
Disopyrobezoars	Persimmons	Eating unripe persimmons
Concretions	Foreign material (e.g., shellac, cement, aluminum hydroxide)	Ingestion of foreign matter
Fungus balls	Yeast	Gastric surgery

in the stomach.[24] Cement may be ingested accidentally by children or by adults who are mentally or emotionally deranged. Medication concretions may also occur but are rare (e.g., aluminum hydroxide antacid concretions in patients with renal failure).[25] Enteric-coated aspirin, which has a pH-sensitive surface layer of cellulose acetate phthalate, has accumulated in the stomach,[26] as has bismuth carbonate following ingestion for radiographic purposes.[27] Concretions have developed from highly compressed alkaline tablets of calcium and magnesium carbonate that are not readily dissolved in the achlorhydric stomach with pyloric obstruction.[27] The polymerized sucrose octasulfate molecule of sucralfate may form a concretion, even after standard doses.[28] Thus sucralfate is not recommended for the patient with gastric outlet obstruction. Oral administration of exchange resins for the treatment of hyperkalemia has led to concretions in low-birth-weight infants.[29]

Clinical Manifestations

The symptoms produced by gastric bezoars are vague and nonspecific. Indeed, bezoars may be asymptomatic,[30] a concept that is supported by recent experience with the gastric balloon for obesity, a form of iatrogenic bezoar. Among a group of patients with the balloon in place, 19% were unaware of the balloon and believed that they were in the sham balloon group.[31] Patients may have trichobezoars for 15 or 20 years before developing symptoms.[2]

The signs and symptoms depend, in large part, on the size, location, and degree of disturbance of gastric physiology.[27] Reported features include anorexia, bloating, early satiety, dyspepsia, malaise, weakness, weight loss, headaches, and a feeling of fullness or heaviness in the epigastrium.[2,8,27] Nausea, vomiting, and episodic epigastric abdominal pain may occur. The pain varies from slight epigastric discomfort to severe and violent colicky pain.[2] Foul breath has been mentioned in cases of trichobezoars.[27]

In some cases, symptoms have persisted after the bezoar resolved,[30] suggesting that symptoms were due to an underlying gastric motility disorder rather than the bezoar. Given the fact that bezoars may be asymptomatic, some of the symptoms reported to be a consequence of bezoars may be due to other independent conditions that are included in the differential diagnosis.

Differential Diagnosis and Diagnostic Studies

The differential diagnosis includes gastritis, peptic ulcer disease, gastric cancer, biliary tract disease, and other abdominal conditions.[10] These conditions may accompany bezoars and may, on occasion, produce symptoms that are attributed to the bezoar.

Inquiry about unusual eating habits or ingestion may provide important clues. In patients with trichobezoars, strands of hair may be found in the gastric contents or stool.[32] On occasion a large bezoar presents as an abdominal mass.

Plain films of the abdomen may reveal a gastric bezoar. A mass may be visible in the left upper quadrant. A different projection may reveal an air shadow or a mottled appearance that defines the bezoar mass (Fig 65-1).[33] Gastric emphysema may rarely be

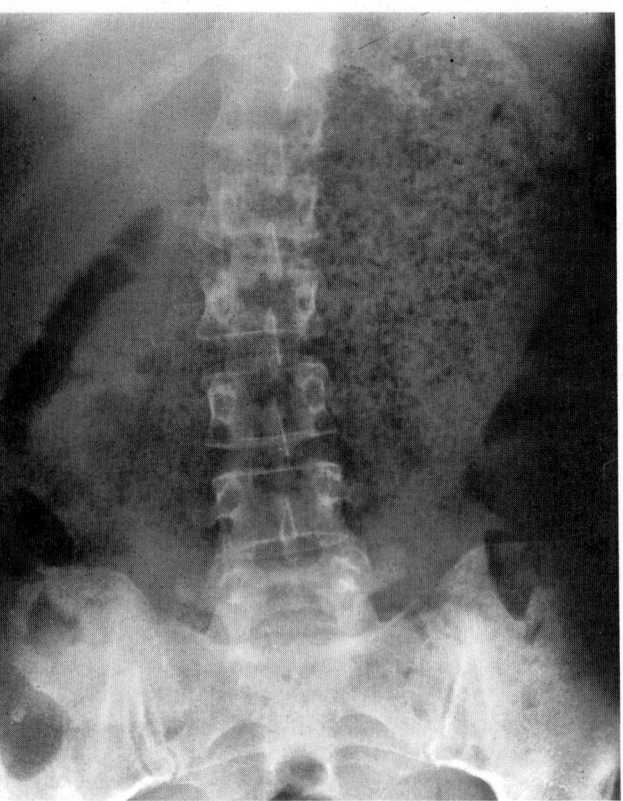

FIGURE 65–1. This radiograph from an upper gastrointestinal series of a patient following a partial gastrectomy (note surgical clips) demonstrates the mottled appearance of a bezoar. (Courtesy of C. Wilcox.)

seen on a plain film as well. A barium study of the stomach may demonstrate a spherical mass in the stomach around which the barium flows. This is movable and not attached.[8] Barium will often permeate the bezoar, demonstrating a characteristic mottled density. On delayed films the mass is unchanged.[33] Radiography is not completely reliable, however, and the bezoar may be missed as often as 55% to 76% of the time.[10,34]

Endoscopy is the most sensitive diagnostic test. In addition to detecting the bezoar and assessing mucosal integrity, endoscopy can help to define its composition and to confirm the absence of neoplasia.[34] On endoscopy, phytobezoars are masses varying in color from yellow to brown or green.[35] Persimmon bezoars are dark green or black.[21] Associated findings on endoscopy may be gastritis, ulcer, or carcinoma.[10]

Ultrasound is a noninvasive technique that may demonstrate a solid, complex bezoar mass.[33] It is unlikely that ultrasound will be an important diagnostic modality for gastric bezoars.

Clinical Course and Complications

Gastric outlet obstruction, anemia, hematemesis, and melena may occur as complications.[35] As the condition progresses, ulceration, perforation, and peritonitis may result. Bezoars that migrate from the stomach may lead to intestinal obstruction.

Therapy

MEDICAL THERAPY

Medical treatment for gastric bezoars can be divided into three categories: (1) enzymatic, including proteolytic, mucolytic, and cellulolytic; (2) mechanical, namely lavage and endoscopy; and (3) other modalities such as observation, metoclopramide therapy, or clear liquid diet (Table 65-2).[36] These various modalities have all been reported to be successful. Because unsuccessful attempts are not generally reported, and because the various techniques have not been compared in a randomized clinical trial, it is impossible to determine the most effective method. Moreover, because bezoars are heterogeneous in their makeup, no single therapy will be effective in all cases and treatment must be individualized.[37]

Enzymatic. A number of enzymatic agents have been tested based on their ability to dissolve cellulose, protein, and mucus. These have included dilute hydrochloric acid, Adolph's Meat Tenderizer (Adolph's Ltd, N. Hollywood, CA), papain, pancrelipase, and pancreatin (all known proteolytic agents); zinc chloride and cellulase, known cellulolytic reagents; and acetylcysteine, a mucolytic agent.[17,38]

Bezoars that are made up of fibers can be dissolved enzymatically. Success has been reported using papain, a proteolytic enzyme from the papaya, in the form of papase tablets, 10,000 U, one or two chewed with each meal, or Adolph's Meat Tenderizer, one teaspoon in a half glass of water before each meal.[17] Cellulase may be effective. Cellulase tablets may be crushed and given after meals or 1 L of cellulase solution (5 g in 300–500 mL of water) may be sipped over 24 hours for 2 days.[17,39] Both cellulase and papain can be obtained from biochemical supply companies. Because the phytobezoar mass is often cemented with mucus, a mucolytic agent may be helpful. Acetylcysteine has been used in amounts of 15 mL of acetylcysteine in 50 mL of saline instilled via a nasogastric tube three times a day for 2 days.[40] Mucolytic or cellulase preparations may work faster than proteolytic compounds.[36]

Enzyme treatments are generally safe but have been associated with complications. The high sodium concentration of Adolph's Meat Tenderizer has led to clinically significant hypernatremia.[36]

The presence of gastrointestinal ulceration along with the bezoar is believed to be a contraindication to use of enzymes by some authors[34] but not by others.[21] In the presence of ulceration, one might choose cellulolytic or mucolytic therapy rather than proteolytic enzymes.

Mechanical. Bezoars that are insoluble, such as prune pits, plastic, paper, hair, or cotton balls must be removed mechanically.[17] Endoscopic forceps, baskets, and snares have been used to remove these objects. An endoscopic overtube can be used to eliminate the potential of aspiration during endoscopic removal of foreign bodies.[5,41] Less dense objects may be fragmented into particles of small enough size to aspirate through the endoscope or to pass through the pylorus. These objects should be small enough so that they do not produce small bowel obstruction.

An interesting endoscopic approach involves using a Teledyne Water Pik (Teledyne Corp, Fort Collins, CO) oral hygiene instrument.[38] A long plastic tube is inserted through the scope and the proximal end attached to the water pik. A pulsating jet stream of water or enzyme solution can then be directed against the bezoar mass to fragment it.[17,38] Once the bezoar is fragmented it may be removed using large-bore orogastric tube lavage. Water pik therapy is believed to be especially useful when the gelatinous nature of the bezoar resists attacks with snares and forceps.[42]

A recent report documented the successful use of the neodymium:yttrium–aluminum–garnet (Nd:YAG) laser in two cases of patients with bezoars.[43] These bezoars had resisted dissolution attempts with cellulase. One patient required three laser sessions. The authors thought that a more powerful YAG laser might shorten treatment time and that when enzymatic dissolution or endoscopic destruction is unsuccessful, Nd:YAG laser therapy might avoid an unnecessary operation.

Treatment of bezoars that complicate gastroplasty for massive obesity may require dilating the surgical stoma with a Gruntzig balloon or Fogarty catheter.[44,45] Endoscopic diathermy incision using a papillotome has also been performed for this purpose.[46]

Authors who favor the mechanical method point to its speed and reliability and believe that it is the treatment of choice.[42] Others believe that endoscopic fragmentation and removal risks local injury and obstruction.[11] At times endoscopic treatment is impossible because the mass is too hard, too friable, or too mobile or is stuck to the wall.[11]

Other Medical Treatments. Metoclopramide given by drip infusion of 40 mg over 24 hours along with a clear liquid diet has been effective when used alone and as an adjunct to endoscopic treatment.[11] Long-term metoclopramide may prevent recurrence of bezoars,[47] and might be considered in patients with known gastric motility problems. A clear liquid diet may lead to dissolution of bezoars, but this may be a slow process. Nasogastric lavage with saline and nasogastric suction are other modalities that have been reported to be successful.[8] Some bezoars resolve spontaneously.[3]

Surgical Therapy

Surgical treatment is sometimes required. Surgery should generally be reserved for acute complications of bezoars such as perforation,

---

TABLE 65-2
Therapy for Gastric Bezoar

Medical Therapy

Enzymatic	Proteolytic	Papase tablets
		Adolph's meat tenderizer
	Cellulolytic	Cellulase tablets
	Mucolytic	Acetylcysteine
Mechanical	Removal	Endoscopic snares, baskets, and forceps
	Fragmentation	Water pik, endoscopic forceps
Other	Motility enhancers	Metoclopramide

Surgical Therapy

hemorrhage, or obstruction. Certain bezoars, such as large trichobezoars, are not amenable to medical treatment. Surgery may become necessary for bezoars that resist medical dissolution and cannot be removed or fragmented endoscopically. On the other hand, surgery sometimes fails because the basic defect causing the bezoar in the first place is not amenable to mechanical correction.[11]

Approach to Therapy

Bezoars may resolve spontaneously.[3] In the absence of gastric outlet obstruction, small bowel obstruction, or other serious problems due to bezoars, they may not need aggressive treatment.[3] If a bezoar is discovered incidentally on radiography or endoscopy in a patient without clear-cut symptoms from the bezoar, then either no therapy or a trial of enzymes or metoclopramide may be reasonable. If the patient is mildly symptomatic, therapy should begin with the cheapest and least invasive method that is likely to be successful. A trial of enzyme therapy for phytobezoars may be safer than endoscopic attempts at disruption. If symptoms are severe or if the bezoar persists, one of the endoscopic techniques should be undertaken. Endoscopy should be the primary modality for bezoars that are resistant to dissolution or are causing acute problems such as gastric outlet obstruction. Surgery should be reserved for failure of the above therapies or for complications.

In order to prevent bezoars, patients who have undergone gastric surgery should be instructed to chew slowly and to avoid raw fruits and stringy vegetables.[8] They should be warned of the risks of ingestion of persimmons.[7]

FOREIGN BODIES

A wide assortment of foreign bodies has been retrieved from the stomach. Foreign bodies may be swallowed either intentionally or accidentally. Small household items and toys are accidentally swallowed by children while playing (Fig 65-2). Objects normally placed in the mouth such as dental prostheses and toothbrushes may be swallowed accidentally by adults as a result of carelessness, rapid eating, poor eyesight, or alcohol intoxication.[48,49] Psychotic and demented patients are the major adult population at risk for intentional ingestion of foreign bodies.[50,51] Intentional ingestion of foreign bodies is also a problem for prisoners seeking the secondary gain associated with hospitalization.[48] There are 1500 to 1600 persons in the United States who die from ingestion of foreign bodies each year.[52]

Between 80% to 93% of the foreign bodies that reach the stomach will pass spontaneously.[48] Most traverse the stomach and exit uneventfully, producing few if any symptoms.[50] Symptoms are due to penetration or perforation of the bowel wall, causing localized or generalized peritonitis or obstruction. There may also be risk from the absorption of toxic substances contained in the foreign body.[50] The most common complications related to retained foreign bodies are pressure necrosis causing gastritis, mucosal tears or ulceration, perforation, abscess, hemorrhage, and fistulas.[48,49] Perforation is more common with sharp, pointed objects such as animal bones (fish and chicken primarily), metallic objects, and wood splinters.[48]

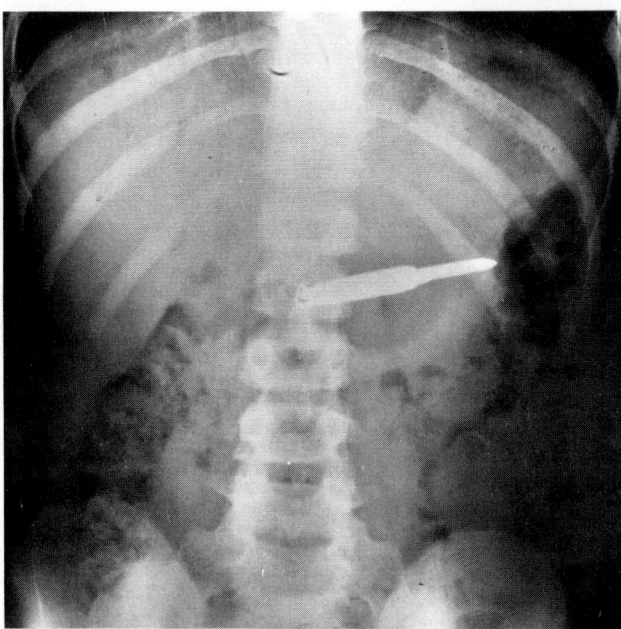

FIGURE 65-2. Radiograph of an open penknife swallowed by a child. Such an object could be removed using an endoscopic overtube. (Courtesy of F. Kelvin.)

Guidelines for the removal of gastric foreign bodies have not been established. One should consider removing objects that are greater than 2 cm in width or diameter or greater than 5 cm in length because they are unlikely to pass through the duodenum.[53] Sharp, pointed objects should probably be removed to eliminate the risk of perforation. Potentially toxic agents should also be removed. The most appropriate management of smooth objects that have remained in the stomach for weeks and that do not produce symptoms or evidence of mucosal damage is less certain.[50]

Many foreign bodies can be safely removed with an endoscope. The plan for extracting the object should be carefully thought out in advance. Most objects can be grasped with standard biopsy forceps and snares, although a variety of grasping gadgets specifically designed for foreign body removal are available.[53,54] Protective overtubes have been developed to reduce the dangers of aspiration, asphyxiation, and additional injury as sharp objects are removed.[41,55] The sharp object can be pulled into the overtube and then extracted. It is important to know when not to proceed with endoscopy.[53] Surgery may be advisable for large, jagged objects.

GASTRIC RUPTURE

Nontraumatic gastric rupture refers to a tear in the stomach wall in an area that is devoid of any pathology. The condition has been referred to as *spontaneous* gastric rupture, but this may be something of a misnomer because the rupture is rarely spontaneous. *Unexpected* gastric rupture may be a more descriptive term,[56] although gastric rupture is always unexpected.

The tear in the stomach ranges in size from a few to more than 15 cm. Edema, hemorrhage, and tearing of the muscle layers are seen, but an inflammatory reaction is absent.[57] The rupture begins as a mucosal tear followed by dissection in the deeper layers of the stomach with a longer tear in the serosa. Although the stomach has a generous blood supply, ischemia and infarction may result when intragastric pressure exceeds gastric venous pressure.[58] Sometimes the rupture occurs in such a necrotic area.

Epidemiology

There are no reliable estimates of its incidence, but the condition is extremely uncommon. Spontaneous gastric perforation has been found in 0.12% of 5160 unselected patients at autopsy.[59] Reviews of isolated case reports suggest a mean age of 43 with a female preponderance.[60] In the neonatal period, gastric rupture has been reported in 1 per 2900 live births among blacks in Washington, D.C.[61]

Etiology

The stomach is relatively resistant to rupture. It is a mobile and distensible organ situated deep within the abdomen protected by ribs and liver. Gastric rupture from blunt abdominal trauma is rare and occurs in less than 1.7% of cases of trauma.[62] The stomach muscles have an enormous capacity to relax with increasing intragastric volume, a phenomenon known as receptive relaxation.[63] It is not known how great a volume is necessary before gastric pressure begins to rise, but an early study by Revilliod suggested that the wall of the healthy stomach could be distended with 4000 mL of fluid before rupture occurred.[57]

In addition to flaccid walls that resist increases in pressure, the stomach can decompress through the pylorus and gastroesophageal junction. Gastric rupture may occur in an overdistended stomach when the pylorus and gastric cardia are obstructed. Cases have been reported in association with several conditions, including obstructing tumors of the esophagus, pancreas, pylorus, or duodenum[64]; Nissen fundoplication[65]; peptic ulcer disease; and congenital duodenal obstruction[65] that disturb the normal pressure release mechanism. The obstruction of the cardia and pylorus may be functional rather than fixed.[66] Positive pressure within the stomach tends to close the cardiac sphincter under normal conditions. An abnormally high pressure might accentuate this situation, leading to a functional obstruction.[65] Overdistention of the stomach might also occlude the cardioesophageal junction by angulating the esophagus against the right crus of the diaphragm.[60] A full dependent stomach might similarly cause angulation at the pylorus, thus blocking outflow.[67]

The site of the rupture is at the lesser curve near the cardia or at the fundus in about 60% of cases associated with gastric distention.[57] Under experimental conditions it has been observed that the distended stomach assumes a spherical shape with greatest stress imposed on the lesser curve.[60] Less frequently the rupture occurs on the greater curve, on the posterior or anterior wall, or near the pylorus.

The location of perforations that follow emesis are different from those resulting from distention. Whereas rupture following distention is generally located on the lesser curve, the greater curve and fundus predominate in cases associated with vomiting.[68] These lesions are located in the upper half of the stomach and lie near the esophageal hiatus. The rupture is believed to be a consequence of herniation of the stomach into the chest during forceful vomiting. In order for rupture to occur there must be a pressure gradient across the stomach. Because the forces brought to bear on the stomach during vomiting would be expected to compress rather than expand the stomach, a pressure gradient can only occur during gastric herniation into the chest.[68] This should be contrasted to the Boerhaave lesion, a transmural perforation of the esophagus, which may also occur with forceful vomiting. It has been proposed that the Boerhaave lesion occurs in the absence of a hiatus hernia so that the major forces are exerted across the wall of the esophagus leading to rupture[68] (see ch 58).

There are three major categories of conditions that have been reported to cause gastric rupture: *trauma*, *emesis*, and *distention*. These may occur alone or in combination. Examples of traumatic causes include coughing, grand mal seizure,[69] exertion involved in lifting heavy objects,[61] and the Heimlich maneuver.[70] Although the stomach is in a protected position, seat belt trauma may cause gastric rupture when an empty stomach is compressed against the vertebral column by a seat belt.[71] The stomach may be inadvertently ruptured during fiberoptic endoscopy. Therapeutic endoscopy with electrical instruments and lasers is more hazardous than simple diagnostic endoscopy, but current reliable incidence figures for rupture after diagnostic and therapeutic endoscopy are not available.

Vomiting may lead to gastric rupture. Examples include rupture following emesis during labor or the postpartum period,[72] retching with pyloric stenosis,[73] vomiting following ipecac administration,[74] and overeating in a patient with anorexia nervosa.[75]

Distention of the stomach from a number of causes has led to gastric rupture. Examples include administration of nasal oxygen, mouth-to-mouth resuscitation followed by external cardiac massage,[64] aerophagia, air sucking,[69] inadvertent inflation of the stomach during anesthesia,[58] gas producing fermentation of food in stomach,[65] and administration of oxygen by nasal catheter.[76] There have been several reports of upper gastrointestinal tract bleeding prior to gastric rupture. Presumably massive bleeding distends the stomach and thus predisposes to gastric rupture during vomiting.[67] In other cases a nonfunctioning Sengstaken tube probably occluded the cardioesophageal junction,[58,77] Gastric rupture has also occurred following diving accidents.[78,79] As the divers ascended, normal mechanisms to vent gas failed, gastric air expanded under lower pressure, and the stomach ruptured.

The stomach may not simply rupture, it may explode. Fermentation can occur in an obstructed stomach producing explosive mixtures similar to those known to occur in the colon. Failure to completely empty an obstructed stomach before cutting diathermy may lead to a gastric explosion.[80]

Sodium bicarbonate ingestion may lead to distention and rupture. Sodium bicarbonate is sometimes used as a remedy for the indigestion that results from overindulgence in food and drink. This practice may be hazardous because the carbon dioxide liberated in the stomach may be of sufficient volume to rupture an overdistended stomach.[64,81] For example, if a person ingested the recommended half teaspoon dose of baking soda containing about 1.8 g of sodium bicarbonate, its ingestion would produce 21.4 mmol of CO_2, assuming the stomach contained adequate hydrochloric acid to support the reaction.[63] If the gas remained in solution, the volume would not expand. If it entered the gas phase, the gastric volume would be increased by 475 mL. Fordtran and colleagues[63] have reported that even though bicarbonate reacts instantaneously with gastric hydrochloric acid, the resulting gas production is low because the carbon dioxide produced from the dehydration of carbonic acid dissolves in water and is only slowly released into the gas phase. A number of factors determine the rate of carbon dioxide release in vitro, including the volume of the solution, the quantity of reactants, the air volume over the reaction mixture, the partial pressure of carbon dioxide of the acid solution, and the stirring rate. The presence of food and alcohol has little effect. Although ingestion of the recommended dose of half a teaspoon of sodium bicarbonate results in only small amounts of sudden gas release, the larger doses selected by some persons could result in the rapid release of several hundred milliliters of gas. If taken when the stomach was already distended, bicarbonate could be an important factor in gastric rupture.[63]

Clinical Manifestations

The patient with gastric rupture may give a history of a recent large meal, ingestion of alkaline drugs, a preexisting gastric condition, and vomiting.[60] Some patients have correctly reported that their stomach burst.[64,75] The onset of symptoms is abrupt following rupture. There is rapid deterioration, severe pain, dyspnea, and abdominal distention.[65] Patients may present with the tetralogy of a *distended abdomen, shock, subcutaneous emphysema,* and physical findings consistent with *diffuse peritoneal irritation.*[60] Subcutaneous emphysema, an inconsistent finding, arises from free air in the abdominal cavity that passes through the retroperitoneal space and mediastinum to the neck.[66] Shock is a consequence of gross contamination of the peritoneum, blood loss, and tension pneumoperitoneum. The pneumoperitoneum compresses the inferior vena cava and compromises venous return to the heart, resulting in decreased cardiac output that is unlikely to respond to volume replacement alone.[67]

Differential Diagnosis and Diagnostic Studies

The differential diagnosis includes all forms of intra-abdominal catastrophe with peritonitis such as perforated peptic ulcer, appendicitis, pancreatitis, bowel infarction, rupture of the gallbladder or spleen, esophageal rupture (Boerhaave's), and carcinoma with perforation. Plain films of the abdomen show pneumoperitoneum that may also be apparent on the chest film. Because patients present in shock there is generally little time for diagnostic studies.

Clinical Course and Complications

Mortality without surgery is 100%.[58] Even with surgery, the mortality exceeds 60%. The slightly diminished mortality in recent years may be due to a greater understanding of the pathophysiology and management of shock.[61] Death following gastric rupture is

due to widespread peritonitis, air embolism, respiratory failure, bleeding, and sepsis.[67] Mediastinitis may result from the presence of gastric contents in the thoracic cavity.[61] The high mortality may be a function of the size of the rent in the stomach. Perforated ulcers are rarely larger than 1.5 cm, whereas most gastric ruptures are about 5 cm and some even larger.[81] The large size permits massive peritoneal soiling.

Therapy

The treatment for gastric rupture is surgery; there is no place for conservative therapy.[72] Shock must be managed aggressively. If abdominal pressure is dominant, a decompressing paracentesis may be beneficial.[58] Repair may require resection of necrotic areas of the stomach. If a predisposing obstructing lesion is discovered this may need to be attended to. Extensive peritoneal lavage is necessary at surgery in order to adequately clear debris. Broad-spectrum antibiotics should be given.

GASTRIC VOLVULUS

The term *volvulus* refers to an acquired twist of a viscus on itself and is derived from the Latin word *volvere* meaning "to twist around." Gastric volvulus is defined as an abnormal degree of rotation of one part of the stomach around another.[82] The rotation may occur around a line joining the pylorus to the esophagogastric junction (*organoaxial volvulus*) (Fig 65-3). In organoaxial volvulus the greater curvature usually swings anteriorly and upward so that the posterior surface of the stomach becomes the anterior. This rotation results in an upside-down stomach, with the greater curvature on the top and the lesser curvature on the bottom. In the less common *mesenteroaxial volvulus*, the axis of rotation is a horizontal line that runs from the center of the greater curvature to the porta hepatis (see Fig 65-3). The pyloroantral area rotates from right to left so that the posterior surface of the stomach becomes the anterior. In contrast to the organoaxial volvulus, the greater curvature remains on the bottom. Thus, in a mesenteroaxial volvulus the stomach is right-side up, but backward. In a review by Wastell and Ellis of over 200 cases, 59% were organoaxial, 29% mesenteroaxial, 2% combined, and the remaining 10% not classified.[83] The exact type of volvulus may be difficult to determine because mixed or intermediary forms occur. The distinction between types is rarely critical because the classification is of descriptive rather than prognostic importance.[85]

The volvulus may be partial or complete. Although the stomach has an extensive blood supply, complete volvulus may produce vascular compromise leading to ischemia. The tightness and the rapidity of the twist are more likely to predict gangrene than the type of volvulus.

Epidemiology

We know little of the epidemiology of gastric volvulus. Our only information comes from isolated case reports or case series. Vol-

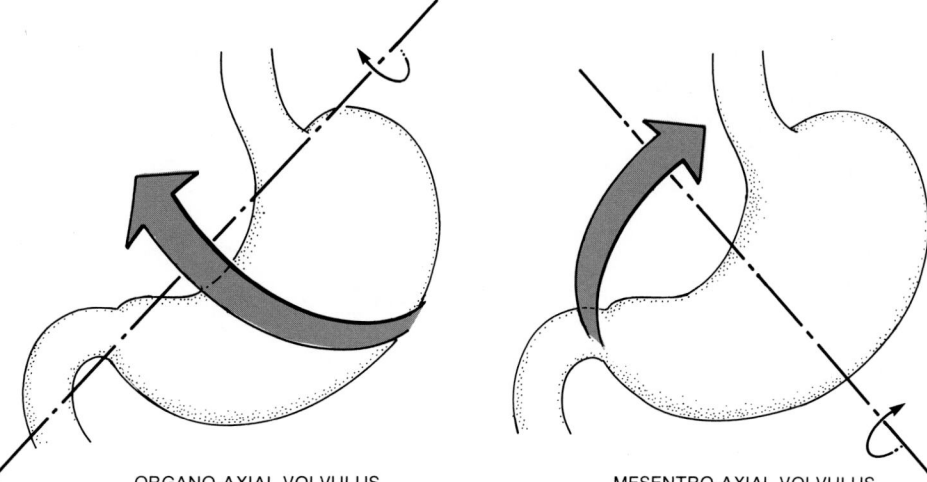

FIGURE 65-3. Schematic representation of the two types of gastric volvulus. **A,** Organoaxial volvulus. **B,** Mesenteroaxial volvulus. The line represents the axis of rotation.

ORGANO-AXIAL VOLVULUS

MESENTRO-AXIAL VOLVULUS

vulus has been described in the newborn and the elderly, with the peak incidence in the fifth decade.[83] The condition affects both sexes. Certain predisposing factors are seen in 50% of cases, including eventration of the diaphragm, hiatal hernia, phrenic nerve crush, history of trauma, or congenital abnormalities of mesenteric fixation.[85]

Etiology

The stomach is relatively fixed at the esophageal hiatus and the pylorus but has four ligamentous attachments—the gastrophrenic, gastrohepatic, gastrosplenic, and gastrocolic ligaments—that permit considerable changes in shape and position.[86] The most frequent cause of gastric volvulus is absence or abnormal laxity of one or more of these suspensory ligaments. The majority also involve diaphragmatic abnormalities such as eventration, hiatal hernia, or diaphragmatic paralysis.[84] In some cases adhesions may form an axis of rotation for the stomach.[87]

With large hiatus hernias, the entire fundus and proximal antrum may migrate into the posterior mediastinum. Because the lesser curve side is short, and because the duodenum and esophagogastric junctions are relatively fixed, the body and greater curve are free to rotate. The greater curve side ultimately occupies the highest position, resulting in an organoaxial volvulus (Fig 65-4). When the gastric suspensory ligaments are lax, the weight of a large fluid-filled stomach may result in the approximation of the pylorus and the cardia, thus predisposing to mesenteroaxial volvulus[87] (Fig 65-5).

Clinical Manifestations

The clinical signs and symptoms depend on the degree of rotation and the amount of obstruction. Gastric volvulus can present as either an acute abdominal emergency or as a chronic recurrent problem.

Acute gastric volvulus is a surgical emergency. Patients experience the sudden onset of severe left upper quadrant pain followed by retching and an inability to vomit. There is progressive distention of the upper abdomen, but the lower abdomen remains relatively soft and lax. There may be minimal abdominal signs when the stomach is in the chest.[85,88] Percussion reveals tympany, but tenderness is not initially marked. The triad consisting of (1)

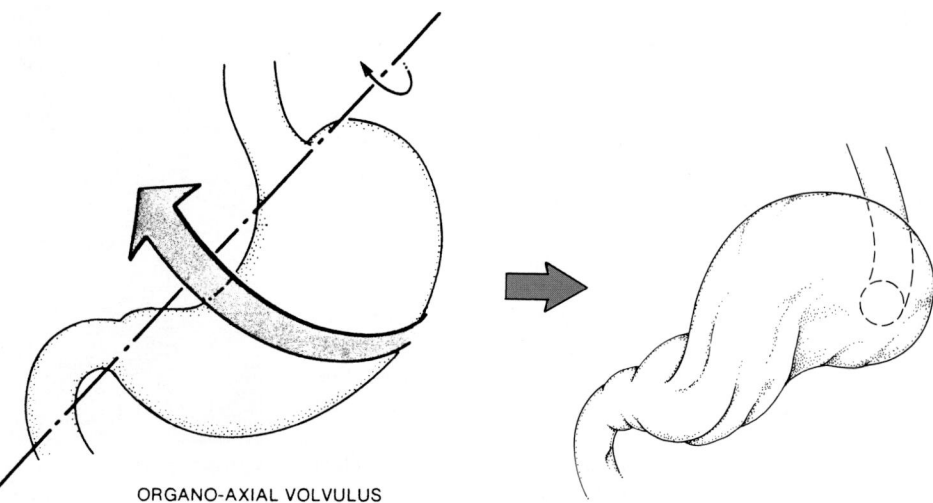

FIGURE 65-4. Diagrammatic representation of organoaxial volvulus.

ORGANO-AXIAL VOLVULUS

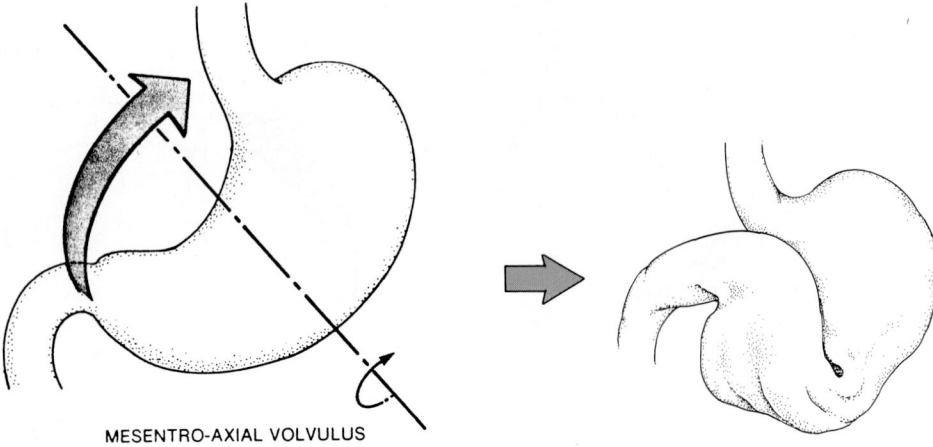

MESENTRO-AXIAL VOLVULUS

FIGURE 65–5. Diagrammatic representation of mesenteroaxial volvulus.

unproductive retching; (2) *acute localized epigastric distention*; and (3) *inability to pass a nasogastric tube* is believed to be diagnostic for acute gastric volvulus. Vascular occlusion, infarction, shock, perforation, and death may occur if surgery is not prompt. The mortality for acute gastric volvulus is 30% to 50%.[85]

Chronic gastric volvulus, reported more frequently than acute volvulus, has vague clinical features.[85] Chronic volvulus may present as an incidental radiologic finding on barium meal or chest film. When symptoms occur they are frequently those of mild, continuous or intermittent upper abdominal discomfort that may be impossible to differentiate from that due to peptic ulcer or cholecystitis.[88] Distortion of the esophagogastric junction may lead to dysphagia. The patient may complain of distress or bloating during or after meals, sometimes followed by retching or vomiting. There may be bouts of upper abdominal pain, eructation, and fullness, and a mass may even be noted.[85] Symptoms frequently come after a heavy meal and last variable periods of time after which they are completely relieved. If a good deal of air or fluid is swallowed, the distended and twisted stomach may prevent belching of the air or vomiting and the patient may simply bring up white frothy swallowed saliva.[88] The symptoms are sometimes relieved by self-induced vomiting or change in position.[85]

Differential Diagnosis and Diagnostic Studies

Acute gastric volvulus could be confused with myocardial infarction, acute pancreatitis, perforated peptic ulcer, or rupture of the gallbladder.[85] The symptoms of chronic gastric volvulus mimic those of gastric atony, acute gastric dilatation, pyloric obstruction,[84] peptic ulcer disease, or cholecystitis.[88]

The radiographic findings in gastric volvulus are characteristic. In mesenteroaxial volvulus the stomach is spherical on supine plain film and two fluid levels show on the erect film—one in the fundus (the lower) and one in the antrum (upper)[86] (Fig 65-6). These findings may also be seen on the chest radiograph. Frequently, diaphragmatic eventration and/or hiatal hernia are present.

Organoaxial volvulus is less easy to diagnose on plain films, especially if it is not associated with diaphragmatic defects, and it may be missed during barium study. The stomach lies rather

horizontally on plain film with a single air–fluid level.[86] Depending on the degree of torsion, a small amount of barium may pass into the stomach and reveal marked dilatation, the area of the twist, and poor passage of contrast medium past the site of the volvulus. There may be a paucity of gas in the remainder of the gastrointestinal tract.[84]

Therapy

In acute gastric volvulus immediate surgical intervention is necessary to avoid ischemic strangulation, perforation, shock, or death.[84] The volvulus is reduced surgically, and if necrosis has

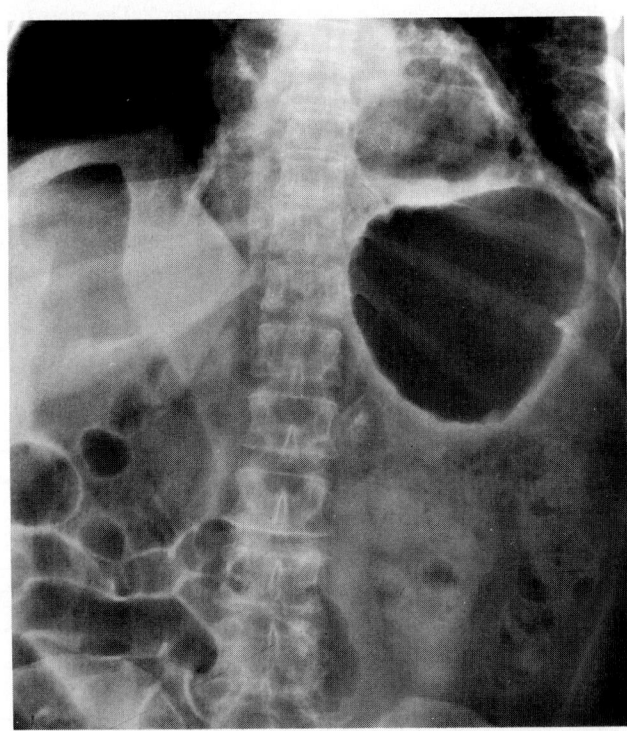

FIGURE 65–6. Plain film of abdomen in patient with gastric volvulus demonstrating two air–fluid levels. The upper represents the antrum and the lower the fundus. (Courtesy of F. Kelvin.)

taken place, local excision, subtotal gastrectomy, or even total gastrectomy may be required.[88] The objectives of surgery are to reduce the volvulus and prevent recurrence. The preferred surgical procedure to prevent recurrence is anterior gastropexy in which the greater curve of the stomach is fixed to the anterior abdominal wall.[89] Anatomic defects that predispose to volvulus such as large hiatus hernias should be repaired at the same time.

There have been several reports of endoscopic reduction of gastric volvulus.[90,91] Rotational maneuvers with the endoscope and air insufflation may successfully reduce the volvulus. Although this form of therapy might be contemplated in the poor-risk patient,[90] the underlying predisposition to volvulus remains and definitive therapy should be considered. A more permanent repair has been reported using dual percutaneous endoscopic gastrostomies, one in the antrum and one in the body.[92]

Although at least nine patients with acute or chronic volvulus have been "cured" with acupuncture,[93] more conventional therapy may be warranted. When the symptoms of chronic recurrent volvulus are disabling, operative repair may be indicated.[88] If patients have massive hernias, these should be repaired because gastric volvulus is an almost inevitable occurrence, and some patients will develop severe complications, including gangrene, perforation, and massive hemorrhage.[94] When the patient has mild chronic symptoms, or when the volvulus is discovered incidentally, the decision to perform surgery is more difficult. The proportion of patients who develop complications is not known. The success of volvulus reduction using endoscopy or acupuncture suggests that some patients with chronic volvulus may do well without therapy.

The reader is directed to Chapter 8, The Physiology of Gastric Motility and Gastric Emptying; Chapter 58, Miscellaneous Diseases of the Esophagus; Chapter 59, Stomach: Anatomy and Structural Anomalies; Chapter 60, Disorders of Gastric Emptying; Chapter 64, Surgery for Peptic Ulcer Disease; and Chapter 111, Upper Gastrointestinal Endoscopy.

REFERENCES

1. Elgood C. A treatise on the bezoar stone: by the late Mahmud bin Masud the Imad-ul-Din the physician of Ispahan. Ann Med Hist 1935;7:73.
2. DeBakey M, Ochsner A. Bezoars and concretions. Surgery 1938;4:934.
3. Kadian RS, Rose JF, Mann NS. Gastric bezoars: spontaneous resolution. Am J Gastroenterol 1978;70:79.
4. Ahn YH, Maturu P, Steinheber FU, Goldman JM. Association of diabetes mellitus with gastric bezoar formation. Arch Intern Med 1987;147:527.
5. Blackstone MO. Endoscopic interpretation. New York: Raven Press, 1984:186.
6. Singh A, Khanna RC, Jolly SS. Three unusual cases of trichobezoar. Gastroenterology 1961;40:441.
7. Moriel EZ, Ayalon A, Eid A, et al. An unusually high incidence of gastrointestinal obstruction by persimmon bezoars in Israeli patients after ulcer surgery. Gastroenterology 1983;84:752.
8. Allred-Crouch AL, Young EA. Bezoars—when the 'knot in the stomach' is real. Postgrad Med 1985;78:261.
9. Hayes PG, Rotstein OD. Gastrointestinal phytobezoars: presentation and management. Can J Surg 1986;29:419.
10. Diettrich NA, Gau FC. Postgastrectomy phytobezoars— endoscopic diagnosis and treatment. Arch Surg 1985;120:432.
11. Delpre G, Glanz I, Neeman A, et al. New therapeutic approach in postoperative phytobezoars. J Clin Gastroenterol 1984;6:231.
12. Brady PG, Richardson R. Gastric bezoar formation secondary to gastroparesis diabeticorum. Arch Intern Med 1977;137:1729.
13. Tsianos EB, Drosos AA. Gastroscopic removal of a phytobezoar formed in a patient with mixed connective tissue disease. Endoscopy 1988;20:122.
14. Kuiper DH. Gastric bezoar in a patient with myotonic dystrophy: a review of the gastrointestinal complications of myotonic dystrophy. Am J Dig Dis 1971;16:529.
15. Kaplan LR. Hypothyroidism presenting as a gastric phytobezoar. Am J Gastroenterol 1980;74:168.
16. Singh A, Barthel J. Delayed gastric emptying associated with gastric bezoar. Semin Nucl Med 1988;18:173.
17. Rider JA, Foresti-Lorente RF, Garrido J, et al. Gastric bezoars: treatment and prevention. Am J Gastroenterol 1984;79:357.
18. Finley CR Jr, Hellmuth EW, Schubert TT. Polystyrene bezoar in a patient with polystyrenomania. Am J Gastroenterol 1988;83:74.
19. Majeski JA. Paper bezoar in the stomach. South Med J 1985;78:1520.
20. Lemoh JN, Watt J. Lactobezoar and cow's milk protein intolerance. Arch Dis Child 1980;55:128.
21. Krausz MM, Moriel EZ, Ayalon A, et al. Surgical aspects of gastrointestinal persimmon phytobezoar treatment. Am J Surg 1986;152:526.
22. Konok G, Haddad H, Strom B. Postoperative gastric mycosis. Surg Gynecol Obstet 1980;150:337.
23. Perttala Y, Peltokallio P, Leviska T, Sipponen J. Yeast bezoar formation following gastric surgery. AJR 1975;125:365.
24. Visvanathan R. Cement bezoars of the stomach. Br J Surg 1986;73:381.
25. Moh P, Gold B. Gastric anatacid bezoar in a patient with chronic renal failure. NY State J Med 1987;87:235.
26. Bogacz K, Caldron P. Enteric-coated aspirin bezoar: elevation of serum salicylate level by barium study: case report and review of medical management. Am J Med 1987;83:783.
27. Siffert G. Foreign bodies in the stomach. In: Henry L. Bockus, ed. Gastroenterology, ed 3. Philadelphia, WB Saunders, 1974;1:1065.
28. Reddy AN. Sucralfate bezoar. Am J Gastroenterol 1986;81:149.
29. Ohlsson A, Hosking M. Complications following oral administration of exchange resins in extremely low-birth-weight infants. Eur J Pediatr 1987;146:571.
30. Zarling EJ, Thompson LE. Nonpersimmon gastric phytobezoar: a benign recurrent condition. Arch Intern Med 1984;144:959.
31. Benjamin SB, Maher KA, Cattau EL, et al. Double-blind controlled trial of the Garren-Edwards gastric bubble: an adjunctive treatment for exogenous obesity. Gastroenterology 1988;95:581.
32. DeBakey M, Ochsner A. Bezoars and concretions. Surgery 1939;5:132.
33. DeLuca SA, Sacknoff R. Gastric bezoars. Am Fam Physician 1986;33:123.
34. Stein DT, Ballin R, Stone BG. Endoscopic removal of gastric phytobezoars. J Clin Gastroenterol 1982;4:329.
35. Ishioka S, Sakai P, Regis OEC, et al. Obstructive syndrome due to bezoar in a B-II gastric stump: endoscopic treatment. Endoscopy 1983;15:44.
36. Zarling EJ, Moeller DD. Bezoar therapy: complications using Adolph's meat tenderizer and alternatives from literature review. Arch Intern Med 1981;141:1669.
37. Wortzel E, Ferrer JP, DeLuca RF. Medical treatment of postgastrectomy bezoar: report of four cases treated with a cellulase enzyme preparation and review. Am J Gastroenterol 1977;67:565.
38. Klamer TW, Max MH. Recurrent gastric bezoars: a new approach to treatment and prevention. Am J Surg 1983;145:417.
39. Smith BH, Mollot M, Berk JE. Use of cellulase for phytobezoar dissolution. Am J Gastroenterol 1980;73:257.
40. Schlang HA. Acetylcysteine in removal of bezoar. JAMA 1970;214:1329.
41. Gutierrez JG, Altman AR. A multipurpose overtube for diagnostic and therapeutic flexible fiberoptic endoscopy. Gastrointest Endosc 1986;32:274.
42. Lange V. Gastric phytobezoar: an endoscopic technique for removal. Endoscopy 1986;18:195.

43. Naveau S, Poynard T, Zourabichvili O, et al. Gastric phytobezoar destruction by Nd:YAG laser therapy. Gastrointest Endosc 1986;32: 430.

44. Strodel WE, Knol JA, Eckhauser FE. Endoscopy of the partitioned stomach. Ann Surg 1984;200:582.

45. Kretzschmar CS, Hamilton JW, Wissler DW, et al. Balloon dilation for the treatment of stomal stenosis complicating gastric surgery for morbid obesity. Surgery 1987;102:443.

46. Fryen J, Rosseland AR, Helsingen N. Endoscopic diathermy incision in the treatment of stoma obstruction. Endoscopy 1985;17:91.

47. Delpre G, Kadish U, Glanz I. Metoclopramide in the treatment of gastric bezoars. Am J Gastroenterol 1984;79:739.

48. Henderson CT, Engel J, Schlesinger P. Foreign body ingestion: review and suggested guidelines for management. Endoscopy 1987;19:68.

49. Kirk AD, Bowers BA, Moylan JA, Meyers W-C. Toothbrush swallowing. Arch Surg 1988;123:382.

50. Roark GD, Subramanyam K, Patterson M. Ingested foreign material in mentally disturbed patients. South Med J 1983;76:1125.

51. Proctor MH. Assault by battery. N Engl J Med 1987;316:554.

52. Bloom RR, Nakano PH, Gray SW, Skandalakis JE. Foreign bodies of the gastrointestinal tract. Am Surg 1986;52:618.

53. Soergel KH, Hogan WJ. Therapeutic endoscopy. Hosp Pract 1983;18(5):81.

54. Hennig AE, Seuberth K. Endoscopic removal of foreign bodies using a newly developed extractor. Endoscopy 1988;20:70.

55. Garrido J, Barkin JS. Endoscopic modification for safe foreign body removal. Am J Gastroenterol 1985;80:957.

56. Christoph RF, Pinkham EW. Unexpected rupture of the stomach in the postpartum period. Ann Surg 1961;154:100.

57. Baglio CM, Fattal GA. Spontaneous rupture of the stomach in the adult. Am J Dig Dis 1962;7:75.

58. Harling H. Spontaneous rupture of the stomach: a case report. Acta Chir Scand 1984;150:101.

59. McCormick WF. Rupture of the stomach in children; a review of the literature and report of seven cases. Arch Pathol 1959;67:416.

60. Albo R, Delorimier AA, Silen W. Spontaneous rupture of the stomach in the adult. Surgery 1963;53:797.

61. Demetriades D, Van der Veen BW, Hatzitheophilous C. Spontaneous rupture of the stomach in an adult. S Afr Med J 1982;61:23.

62. Brunsting LA, Morton JH. Gastric rupture from blunt abdominal trauma. J Trauma 1987;27:887.

63. Fordtran JS, Morawski G, Santa Ana CA, Rector FC Jr. Gas production after reaction of sodium bicarbonate and hydrochloric acid. Gastroenterology 1984;87:1014.

64. Brismar B, Strandberg A, Wiklund B. Stomach rupture following ingestion of sodium bicarbonate. Acta Chir Scand [Suppl] 1986;530: 97.

65. Kurgan A, Hoffmann J, Abramowitz HB. Spontaneous rupture of the stomach: a rare complication of Nissen's fundoplication. Int Surg 1984;69:357.

66. Ziv Y, Wolloch Y, Dintsman M. Spontaneous rupture of the stomach. Isr J Med Sci 1984;20:427.

67. O'Doherty DP, Baker AR, Barrie WW. Rupture of the stomach after hemorrhage from a gastric ulcer. Gastroenterology 1986;91:212.

68. Watts HD. Lesions brought on by vomiting: the effect of hiatus hernia on the site of injury. Gastroenterology 1976;71:683.

69. Chandrasekhara KL, Iyer SK, Sutton AL, Stanek AE. Spontaneous rupture of the stomach. Am J Med 1986;81:1062.

70. Croom DW. Rupture of the stomach after attempted Heimlich maneuver. JAMA 1983;250:2602.

71. Carragher AM, Cranley B. Seat-belt stomach transection in association with "Chance" vertebral fracture. Br J Surg 1987;74:397.

72. Graham WB. Spontaneous rupture of the stomach in the adult. J R Coll Surg Edinburgh 1982;27:368.

73. Jefferiss CD. Spontaneous rupture of the stomach in an adult. Br J Surg 1972;59:79.

74. Knight KM, Doucet JH. Gastric rupture and death caused by ipecac syrup. South Med J 1987;80:786.

75. Matikainen M. Spontaneous rupture of the stomach. Am J Surg 1979;138:451.

76. Van der Loos ThLJM, Lustermans FATh. Rupture of the normal stomach after therapeutic oxygen administration. Intens Care Med 1986;12:52.

77. Kristiansen B, Burcharth F. Rupture of the stomach complicating bleeding oesophageal varices. Acta Chir Scand 1982;148:203.

78. Halpern P, Sorkine P, Leykin Y, Geller E. Rupture of the stomach in a diving accident with attempted resuscitation: a case report. Br J Anaesth 1986;58:1059.

79. Cramer FS, Heimbach RD. Stomach rupture as a result of gastrointestinal barotrauma in a SCUBA diver. J Trauma 1982;22:238.

80. Earnshaw JJ, Keane TK. Gastric explosion: a cautionary tale. Br Med J 1989;298:93.

81. Lazebnik N, Iellin A, Michowitz M. Spontaneous rupture of the normal stomach after sodium bicarbonate ingestion. J Clin Gastroenterol 1986;8:454.

82. Tanner NC. Chronic and recurrent volvulus of the stomach. Am J Surg 1968;115:505.

83. Wastell C, Ellis H. Volvulus of the stomach, a review with a report of eight cases. Br J Surg 1971;58:557.

84. Gean AD, DeLuca S. Acute gastric volvulus. Am Fam Physician 1986;34:99.

85. Smith RJ. Volvulus of the stomach. J Natl Med Assoc 1983;75:393.

86. Cameron AE, Howard ER. Gastric volvulus in childhood. J Pediatr Surg 1987;22:944-947.

87. Carter R, Brewer LA, Hinshaw DB. Acute gastric volvulus: a study of 25 cases. Am J Surg 1980;140:99.

88. Ellis H. Diaphragmatic hernia—a diagnostic challenge. Postgrad Med J 1986;62:325.

89. Cybulsky I, Himal HS. Gastric volvulus within the foramen of Morgagni. Can Med Assoc J 1985;133:209.

90. Lowenthal MN, Odes HS, Fritsch E. Endoscopic reduction of acute gastric volvulus and volvulus of the sigmoid colon. J R Soc Med 1986;79:240.

91. Patel NM. Endoscopic correction of chronic gastric volvulus. Gastrointest Endosc 1983;29:63.

92. Eckhauser M, Ferron J. The use of dual percutaneous endoscopic gastrostomy (DPEG) in the management of chronic intermittent gastric volvulus. Gastrointest Endosc 1985;31:340.

93. Yaoguang W, Liyou Y. Volvulus of the stomach successfully treated with acupuncture: report of 9 cases. J Tradit Chin Med 1981;1:39.

94. Pearson FG, Cooper JD, Ilves R, et al. Massive hiatal hernia with incarceration: a report of 53 cases. Ann Thorac Surg 1983;35:45.

Index

Page numbers followed by t or f indicate tables and figures, respectively.
Page numbers in **boldface** indicate major discussions of the concept.

Enteric neuron(s), type II (*continued*)
 fast ESPs, 10, 10f
 resting membrane potentials, 11t
 slow ESPs, 13
Enteric neuropathy, 58, 1231
 constipation in, 781–782
Enteric vasodilator neurons, 9
Enteritis. *See also* Eosinophilic enteritis; Gastroenteritis; Radiation enteritis
 bacterial, 1749
  in acquired immunodeficiency syndrome,
   treatment, 2091t
 with chemotherapy, 1570
 erosive, drug-induced, 1565–1566
 infectious, diarrhea with, 1531
 ulcerative, 1488
Enteritis necroticans, 1571
Enteritis phlegmonosa, 1571
Enterobacter
 abscesses caused by, 2058
 infection, with enteral nutrition, 1053
 peritonitis, in CAPD, 2076
Enterobacter cloacae, in tropical sprue, 1473
Enterobacteria, in normal flora, 717
Enterobacteriaceae, 1457, 1749
 bacteremia, in granulocytopenic patient, 916
 infection
  in bone marrow transplant patient, 903
  in cardiac transplant patient, 902
  with corticosteroid therapy, 904
  in immunocompromised patient, 917
  in liver transplant patient, 902
 metabolic activities, 537
 in spontaneous bacterial peritonitis, 854t
Enterobacter sakazakii, contamination of infant formulas, 1053
Enterobiasis, in homosexual men, 2120
Enterobius vermicularis, 2119, **2120–2122**, 2123f.
   See also Pinworm
 clinical manifestations of, 2120–2122
 diagnosis of, 2122, 2528–2529
 drug treatment for, **2121t**
 epidemiology, 2120
 ova, 2124f
  size of, 2123f
 prevention, 2122
 pruritus ani caused by, 1828
 treatment, 2122
Enterocele(s), intermittent, 1832
Enteroceptors, **53–54**
Enterocholecystic reflex, 205
Enterochromaffin cells, 734, 1204, 1412–1413
Enterochromaffinlike cell(s), 1307
 hyperplasia, 1274–1275, 1292–1293
Enteroclysis, 1494
 for diagnosis of small-bowel sources of bleeding, 610, 610f
 for diagnosis of small bowel tumors, 1486
 indications for, 759, 1439
 with small bowel adenocarcinoma, 1498
Enterococcus
 abscess caused by, antibiotic therapy for, 2063
 in bile ducts, 1975
 endocarditis, with gastrointestinal procedures,
   1052
 peritonitis, in CAPD, 2076
 postoperative infection, 712
Enterocolitis, 1010t
 Clostridium difficile, **1756–1762**
 experimental, platelet-activating factor in, 469
 gold-induced, 2140
 neutropenic, 704
  in immunocompromised patient, 706t
 uremic, 935
Enterocyte(s), 1411f, 2163
 apical membrane, drug transport across, 521f,
   521–522
 basolateral membrane, drug transport across,
   521f, 521–522
 cytoskeleton of, 1414, 1417f
 damage/cell death
  direct, 742f
  immune system-mediated, 742f

 with inflammation, 741, 743t
  diarrheas characterized by, **740–741**
 mechanisms of, 741, 742f
 drug metabolism in, 523, 525–527
 fatty acid–binding proteins, 360–361
 isolated
  radionuclide uptake and efflux studies in,
   283
  for study of intestinal water and electrolyte
   transport, 281
 morphology, during lipid absorption, 365, 367f
 in starvation, 348
 triglyceride pools, 365, 368f
Enterocyte barrier, breakdown of, protein-losing
   enteropathy with, 1573
Enterocytozoon bieneusi, 2090
Enteroendocrine cell(s)
 formation, 486
 types, 487
Enteroenteric reflexes, 2. *See also* Sympathetic
   enteroenteric inhibitory reflexes
Enterofundic reflex, 142t
Enterogastric reflex(es), 20–21, 142t, 142–143,
   164
Enterogastric reflux, in animal model of gastric
   cancer, 1357
Enterogastrone, 234, 246
 definition of, 36, 40
 effects of, on gastric acid secretion, 243t
Enteroglucagon, **38**
 biologic action, 37t
 cell of origin, 37t
 effects of, on gastric acid secretion, 241, 242t
 endocrine function, 29t
 function, 30
 in ileal brake mechanism, 165
 in intestinal adaptation, 434
 promotion of small bowel tumors, in rat-AOM
   model, 1487
 release, 42, 45
 role in intestinal adaptation, 1544
 secretion, in gastric mucosa, 235
 serum level, effects on growth and development in gastrointestinal tract, 494
Enterohepatic circulation, 324–326, 325f
 dynamics, defects in, 327
 short-circuiting of, 327
Enterokinase, 296, 1533
 activity, 1862
  development of, 482
  after intestinal resection, 1543
 in bacterial overgrowth, 1535
 deficiency, **1525**
  congenital, 1948
   diagnosis of, 1948
   treatment of, 1948
  diarrhea caused by, 739t, 1525
Enteromonas hominis, infection, in immunocompromised patient, 910
 treatment, 919
Entero-oxyntin, 245
 effects of, on gastric acid secretion, 243t
Enteropancreatic reflex, 299, 305–306, 308–309
Enteropathic arthritis syndrome, 869
Enteropathogens, epidemiology of, 1447, 1448t
Enteropeptidase(s)
 action of, 1862
 activity, 385, 385f
 brush border, 386, 386t
Enteropyloric reflexes, 142–143, 164
Enterosalivary circulation, 510
Enteroscopy. *See also* Endoscopy; Push-entero-
   scopy; Total enteroscopy
 indications for, 610
 small bowel, in angiodysplasia, 2176
Enterotoxin(s), 97
 diarrhea caused by, 740t, 744, 1457–1458,
   1463
  signs and symptoms of, 745t
 effects of, on epithelium, 283–284
 of food-borne illness, 653, 1452t–1455t
 host defense against, 98
 as intestinal secretory stimuli, 276t, 734

Enterovirus
 infection
  in immunocompromised patient, prevention, 916
  proteases in, 390
  portal of entry, 97
  recovery of, from stool cultures, 2526
  in X-linked hypogammaglobulinemia, 2158
Entropy, 412
Enuresis, 779
Enzygnost, 1469
Enzyme(s). *See also* Digestive enzymes
 deficiencies, genetics of, 990–991, 991t
 and susceptibility to carcinogens, 505
Enzyme-linked immunoabsorbent assay, 2106,
   2165
 for *Helicobacter pylori* serum antibodies, 1243–
   1244
Enzyme-multiplied immunoassay technique, in
   detection of drug abuse, 1027
EOE-13, 2368
Eosinophilia
 peripheral, diseases associated with, 2166
 in returned traveler, 1040
Eosinophilic enteritis
 CT appearance of, 2364
 diarrhea caused by, 739t
 duodenal, 818
 histology, 757t
Eosinophilic gastroenteritis, **2166–2167**
 and biliary obstruction, 2011t
 chronic gastric ulcer in, 1295
 clinical manifestations of, 2166
 diarrhea caused by, 743t, **767**
 differential diagnosis, 1512, 2166–2167
 endoscopic mucosal biopsy in, 2506
 gastric involvement in, 2498
 iron deficiency caused by, 618
 occult bleeding with, 620
 pathophysiology of, 2166
 protein-losing enteropathy with, 767, 1573
 small bowel lesions in
  clinical features of, 2503t
  histologic description of, 2503t
 steatorrhea caused by, 751–752
 treatment, 2167
Eosinophilic granuloma, **1311**, 2166
 upper esophageal sphincter, 2348
Eosinophils
 esophageal infiltration by, 1098
 in esophagitis, 1133
 in host defense, 93
 in intestinal electrolyte transport, 278
 in intestinal mucosa, 268, 268f
 in perineurial space, with recent alcohol consumption, 1880
Ephedrine
 effect on laboratory detection of drug use,
   1027
 for postvagotomy dumping syndrome,
   1394
Epidemic collapse, 653
Epidemic nausea and vomiting, 653
Epidermal growth factor. *See also* Urogastrone/
   epidermal growth factor
 effect of sucralfate on, 1275–1276
 effects of
  on cell proliferation, 115, 503
  on gastric acid secretion, 243t
  on growth and development in gastrointestinal tract, 484–486, 491, 493–494
  on intrinsic factor secretion, 255
 in intestinal adaptation, 434
 and prognosis for gastric cancer, 1368
 receptors, 493–494
  internalization, 31
 role in intestinal adaptation, 1544
 in salivary ducts, 219
 salivary secretion of, 226t
 secretion, stimulation of, 1278
Epidermal inclusion cyst, presacral, 1819
Epidermoid carcinoma, of lip, 1436
Epidermolysis bullosa, **875**

ISBN 0-397-51227-9

90000